HARRISON'S
PRINCIPLES OF
INTERNAL
MEDICINE
TWELFTH EDITION

VOLUME 2

HARRISON'S

PRINCIPLES OF
INTERNAL
MEDICINE

TWELFTH EDITION

VOLUME 2

Editors

JEAN D. WILSON, M.D.
Professor of Internal Medicine, The University of Texas
Southwestern Medical Center, Dallas

EUGENE BRAUNWALD, A.B., M.D.,
M.A. (Hon.), M.D. (Hon.)
Hersey Professor of the Theory and Practice of Physic,
Harvard Medical School; Chairman, Department of Medicine,
Brigham and Women's Hospital, Boston

KURT J. ISSELBACHER, A.B., M.D.
Mallinckrodt Professor of Medicine, Harvard Medical School;
Director, Cancer Center, Massachusetts General Hospital,
Boston

ROBERT G. PETERSDORF, A.B., M.D.,
M.A. (Hon.), D.Sc. (Hon.), M.D. (Hon.),
L.H.D. (Hon.)
President, Association of American Medical Colleges,
Washington, D.C.

JOSEPH B. MARTIN, M.D., Ph.D.,
F.R.C.P.(C), M.A. (Hon.)
Professor of Neurology and Dean, School of Medicine,
University of California at San Francisco, San Francisco

ANTHONY S. FAUCI, M.D.
Director, National Institute of Allergy and Infectious Disease;
Chief, Laboratory of Immunoregulation; Director, Office of
AIDS Research, National Institutes of Health, Bethesda

RICHARD K. ROOT, M.D.
Professor of Medicine and Associate Dean for Clinical
Education, School of Medicine, University of California
at San Francisco, San Francisco

McGRAW-HILL, Inc.
Health Professions Division
New York   St. Louis   San Francisco   Colorado Springs
Auckland   Bogotá   Caracas   Hamburg   Lisbon   London
Madrid   Mexico   Milan   Montreal   New Delhi   Paris
San Juan   São Paulo   Singapore   Sydney   Tokyo   Toronto

HARRISON'S
PRINCIPLES OF INTERNAL MEDICINE
Twelfth Edition

1 2 3 4 5 6 7 8 9 0   DOW DOW   9 8 7 6 5 4 3 2 1 0

Foreign Editions
FRENCH (Eleventh Edition)—Flammarion, © 1988
GERMAN (Tenth Edition)—Schwabe and Company, Ltd., © 1986
GREEK (Eleventh Edition)—Parissianos, © 1990
ITALIAN (Twelfth Edition)—McGraw-Hill Libri Italia S.r.l. © 1992 (est.)
JAPANESE (Tenth Edition)—Hirokawa, © 1985
PORTUGUESE (Eleventh Edition)—Editora Guanabara Koogan, S.A., © 1988
SPANISH (Twelfth Edition)—McGraw-Hill/Interamericana de Espana, © 1991 (est.)

This book was set in Times Roman by Monotype Composition Company. The editors were J. Dereck Jeffers and Stuart D. Boynton. The indexer was Irving Tullar; the production supervisor was Robert Laffler; the designer was Marsha Cohen; R. R. Donnelley & Sons Company was printer and binder.

Library of Congress Cataloging-in-Publication Data

Harrison's principles of internal medicine—12th ed./editors, Jean D.
   Wilson . . . [et al.]
      p.   cm.
   Also issued in 2 v.
   Includes bibliographical references.
   ISBN 0-07-070890-8 (1-vol. ed.)—ISBN 0-07-079749-8 (2-vol. set),
   0-07-070891-6 (vol. 1), 0-07-070892-4 (vol. 2)
   1. Internal medicine.   I. Harrison, Tinsley Randolph, Date.
II. Wilson, Jean D., Date.   III. Title: Principles of internal medicine.
   [DNLM: 1. Internal Medicine.   WB 115 P957]
RC46.H333   1991
616—dc20
DLC
for Library of Congress   90-5814
                                                                    CIP

A salute to Raymond D. Adams by the editors of Harrison's

We dedicate this twelfth edition of *Harrison's Principles of Internal Medicine* to Raymond D. Adams. Dr. Adams joined the Harrison's editorial board for preparation of the second edition, which was published in 1954. Together with the other members of the editorial board at the time, Tinsley R. Harrison, William R. Resnik, Maxwell M. Wintrobe, George W. Thorn, and Paul B. Beeson, he established *Harrison's* as a serious competitor in the field.

Ray Adams left an indelible mark on the textbook with his first contributions. He advocated what was to become the chief feature of the book, namely, the use of the introductory chapters to discuss symptoms and signs—the "Cardinal Manifestations of Disease." He argued forcibly for including diseases of the nervous system as a major component. He developed over time a systematic syndromic approach to understanding diseases of the nervous system that came to be the foundation for teaching a substantial portion of the emerging community of academic neurologists in the United States. With the assistance of his able collaborator, Maurice Victor, and other members of the neurological staff at the Massachusetts General Hospital, the section on neurology became a major instrument for teaching several generations of medical students and house officers. Because of the way that he formulated neurology as an essential component of medicine, he has had an equally important impact on the training of internists. At times the arguments over how much neurology to include in a textbook of general medicine became thunderous, leading Tinsley Harrison on one occasion to suggest (only half-facetiously) that the title be changed to *The Principles of Internal Medicine and Details of Neurology*.

The syndromic approach to diseases that affect the nervous system arose from Ray Adams' enormous personal experience with patients, an experience that continues to the present day. A complete exposition of this approach has now appeared in four editions of *Principles of Neurology*, written with Maurice Victor.

Raymond Adams was graduated from Duke University Medical School. With support from a Rockefeller fellowship he trained with James Ayer and Charles Kubik in neurology at the Massachusetts General Hospital and with Eugen Kahn in psychiatry at Yale. He returned to Boston to Harvard's service at the City Hospital as head of the Neuropathology Laboratory in 1939 where, over the course of the next decade, he made major contributions in studies of neurosyphilis, meningitis, muscle disease, and the effects of alcohol on the nervous system. He became Bullard Professor of Neuropathology at Harvard Medical School and chief of the Neurology Service at the Massachusetts General Hospital in 1951 and continued in these positions until 1978. During those years he created the leading neurological service in the country and participated in the training of a generation of academic leaders who would populate many of the university chairs of neurology in the United States and elsewhere. During this time he contributed a series of landmark studies on clinicopathologic correlations of diseases affecting the nervous system. He produced some of the first evidence for autoimmune disease of the brain and made major contributions to the understanding of developmental diseases of the nervous system. He is an expert neuropathologist and a fine neuropsychiatrist. It is difficult to find a topic in neurology that has not been advanced by the scholarship of Ray Adams.

To those who have studied under Dr. Adams and to those who have worked with him in the development of *Harrison's*, he has always been a wise and congenial colleague who demanded excellence of himself and expected it of others. His generosity, wisdom, and creativity have meant much to us, and we affectionately dedicate this volume to him.

ABBREVIATED CONTENTS

CONTENTS

PART SEVEN
DISORDERS OF THE RESPIRATORY SYSTEM

PART EIGHT
DISORDERS OF THE KIDNEY AND URINARY TRACT

PART NINE
DISORDERS OF THE GASTROINTESTINAL SYSTEM

Section 1: Disorders of the alimentary tract

Section 2: Liver and biliary tract disease

Section 3: Disorders of the pancreas

PART TEN
DISORDERS OF THE IMMUNE SYSTEM,
CONNECTIVE TISSUE, AND JOINTS

Section 1: Disorders of the immune system

**PART ELEVEN
HEMATOLOGY AND ONCOLOGY**

PART THIRTEEN
NEUROLOGIC DISORDERS

Section 1: The central nervous system

Section 2: Disorders of nerve and muscle

PART FOURTEEN
PSYCHIATRY

Section 1: Psychiatric disorders

Section 2: Alcoholism and drug dependency

COLOR PLATES *After page 1218*

1 Atlas of common skin lesions encountered during the physical examination of the skin

A1-1 Dermatofibroma **A1-2** Acrochordon **A1-3** Angiokeratomas **A1-4** Café au lait macules **A1-5** Acne **A1-6** Dermatophytosis **A1-7** Eczematous dermatitis **A1-8** Localized lichenification **A1-9** Melasma (chloasma) **A1-10** Milia **A1-11** Psoriasis **A1-12** Perlèche **A1-13** Acrochordon **A1-14** Rosacea **A1-15** Seborrheic dermatitis **A1-16** Seborrheic keratosis **A1-17** Senile angioma ("cherry red spot") **A1-18** Senile lentigo **A1-18** Senile sebaceous adenoma **A1-19** Solar keratosis **A1-20** Spider nevus **A1-21** Tinea versicolor **A1-22** Verruca vulgaris **A1-23** Xanthelasma **A1-24** Systemic lupus erythematosus **A1-25** Necrotizing vasculitis syndrome **A1-26** Glucagonoma (*A*) and acquired zinc deficiency (*B*) **A1-27** Porphyria cutanea tarda **A1-28** Necrobiosis lipoidica **A1-29** Kaposi's sarcoma **A1-30** Carcinoid **A1-31** Malignant melanomas **A1-32** Dysplastic melanocytic nevi **A1-33** Malignant melanoma–dysplastic nevus syndrome

2 Atlas of infectious diseases

A2-1 Varicella **A2-2** Measles (rubeola) **A2-3** Rocky Mountain spotted fever **A2-4** Rocky Mountain spotted fever **A2-5** Meningococcemia **A2-6** Disseminated gonococcal infection **A2-7** Pseudomonas septicemia **A2-8** Facial erysipelas **A2-9** and **A2-10** Lyme disease: erythema chronicum migrans **A2-11** Secondary syphilis **A2-12** Papulosquamous lesions of secondary syphilis **A2-13** Macular syphilids **A2-14** Molluscum contagiosum **A2-15** Esthiomene **A2-16** Severe primary HSV infection **A2-17** Primary HSV pharyngitis **A2-18** Neonatal HSV infection **A2-19** Herpetic whitlow **A2-20** Keratodermia blenorrhagica **A2-21** Scabies excoriations **A2-22** Cervicofacial actinomycosis **A2-23** and **A2-24** Kaposi's sarcoma

3 Atlas of endoscopic findings

A3-1 Normal esophagus **A3-2** Peptic regurgitant esophagus **A3-3** Ulcerated squamous cell carcinoma **A3-4** Moniliasis of the esophagus **A3-5** Barrett's metaplasia of the esophagus with adenocarcinoma **A3-6** Normal body of the stomach with rugal folds **A3-7** Benign gastric ulcer of the lesser curve **A3-8** Gastric polyp **A3-9** Arteriovenous malformation of the gastric mucosa **A3-10** Normal pylorus **A3-11** Normal duodenal bulb **A3-12** Normal papilla of Vater **A3-13** Periampullary carcinoma **A3-14** Endoscopic papillotomy **A3-15** Normal colon **A3-16** Colonic adenomatous polyp **A3-17** Multiple small colonic adenomatous polyps **A3-18** Colon adenocarcinoma **A3-19** Crohn's colitis **A3-20** Severe ulcerative colitis **A3-21** Kaposi's sarcoma involving the colon

4 Atlas of fundoscopic examination

A4-1 Normal optic nerve and retina **A4-2** Central retinal artery occlusion **A4-3** Central retinal vein occlusion **A4-4** Early papilledema **A4-5** Drusen of the optic nerve head **A4-6** Anterior ischemic optic neuropathy **A4-7** Primary optic atrophy **A4-8** Angioid streaks **A4-9** Retinitis pigmentosa **A4-10** Band keratopathy **A4-11** Glaucomatous optic disk with secondary atrophy **A4-12** Diabetic retinopathy with microaneurysms **A4-13** Proliferative diabetic retinopathy **A4-14** Cytomegalovirus retinitis in AIDS **A4-15** Retinal arteriovenous malformation in the Wyburn-Mason syndrome

5 Atlas of hematology

A5-1 Normal blood smear **A5-2** Megaloblastic anemia **A5-3** Liver disease **A5-4** Iron-deficiency anemia **A5-5** β thalassemia intermedia **A5-6** Sickle cell anemia **A5-7** Traumatic hemolysis **A5-8** Spur cell anemia **A5-9** Uremia **A5-10** Hereditary spherocytosis **A5-11** Immunohemolytic anemia **A5-12** Myeloid metaplasia **A5-13** Normal granulocyte (*A*); normal monocyte and lymphocyte (*B*) **A5-14** Normal eosinophil (*A*); basophil (*B*) **A5-15** Normal granulocyte precursors in marrow **A5-16** Neutrophils with toxic granulation **A5-17** Band with Döhle body **A5-18** Hypersegmentation **A5-19** Chédiak-Higashi anomaly (*A*); Pelger-Huet anomaly (*B*) **A5-20** Reactive lymphocytes **A5-21** Chronic granulocytic leukemia **A5-22** Leukemic cell in acute promyelocytic leukemia **A5-23** Chronic lymphocytic leukemia **A5-24** Leukemic cells in acute lymphoblastic leukemia **A5-25** Hodgkin's disease **A5-26** Non-Hodgkin's nodular lymphoma **A5-27** Multiple myeloma

LIST OF CONTRIBUTORS

ITAMAR B. ABRASS, M.D.
Professor of Medicine and Head, Division of Gerontology and Geriatric Medicine, University of Washington School of Medicine, Seattle

ELIAS ABRUTYN, M.D.
Professor and Assistant Chairman, Department of Medicine, Medical College of Pennsylvania; Associate Chief, Medical Service, Veterans Administration Medical Center, Philadelphia

RAYMOND D. ADAMS, B.A., M.A., M.D., M.A. (Hon.), D.Sc. (Hon.), M.D. (Hon.)
Bullard Professor of Neuropathology, Emeritus, Harvard Medical School; Consultant Neurologist and formerly Chief of Neurology Service, Massachusetts General Hospital; Emeritus Director, Eunice K. Shriver Research Center, Boston; Médicin Adjoint, L'Hôpital Cantonale de Lausanne, Lausanne

JOHN ADAMSON, M.D.
President, The New York Blood Center, New York

SETH L. ALPER, M.D., Ph.D.
Instructor in Medicine, Harvard Medical School; Section of Molecular Medicine and Nephrology, Beth Israel Hospital, Boston

ROBERT J. ANDERSON, M.D.
Professor of Medicine, University of Colorado Health Sciences Center, Denver

JACK P. ANTEL, M.D.
Professor and Chairman, Department of Neurology and Neurosurgery, McGill University; Neurologist-in-Chief, Montreal Neurological Institute and Hospital, Montreal

BARRY G.W. ARNASON, M.D.
Raymond Professor and Chairman, Department of Neurology, and Director of Brain Research Institute, University of Chicago Pritzker School of Medicine, Chicago

ARTHUR K. ASBURY, M.D.
Ruth Wagner Van Meter and J. Ray Van Meter Professor of Neurology, University of Pennsylvania School of Medicine and Hospital of the University of Pennsylvania, Philadelphia

K. FRANK AUSTEN, M.D.
Theodore Bevier Bayles Professor of Medicine, Harvard Medical School; Chairman, Department of Rheumatology and Immunology, Brigham and Women's Hospital, Boston

ROBERT AUSTRIAN, M.D., D.Sc. (Hon.)
Professor Emeritus and Chairman, Department of Research Medicine, University of Pennsylvania School of Medicine, Philadelphia

BERNARD M. BABIOR, M.D., Ph.D.
Head, Division of Biochemistry, Department of Molecular and Experimental Medicine, and Member, Division of Hematology and Oncology, Department of Medicine, Scripps Clinic and Research Foundation, La Jolla

KAMAL F. BADR, M.D.
Assistant Professor of Medicine, Vanderbilt University School of Medicine, Nashville

DONALD S. BAIM, M.D.
Associate Professor of Medicine, Harvard Medical School; Director of Invasive Cardiology, Beth Israel Hospital, Boston

M. FLINT BEAL, M.D.
Associate Professor, Harvard Medical School; Assistant Neurologist, Massachusetts General Hospital, Boston

ARTHUR L. BEAUDET, M.D.
Investigator, Howard Hughes Medical Institute; Professor of Pediatrics and Cell Biology, Baylor College of Medicine, Boston

JOHN E. BENNETT, M.D.
Head, Clinical Mycology Section, National Institute of Allergy and Infectious Diseases, National Institutes of Health, Bethesda

MICHAEL S. BERNSTEIN, M.D.
Fellow, Department of Medicine, University of California, San Francisco

DAVID R. BICKERS, M.D.
Professor and Chairman, Department of Dermatology, Case Western Reserve University School of Medicine; Director, Department of Dermatology, University Hospitals of Cleveland, Cleveland

EDWIN L. BIERMAN, M.D.
Professor of Medicine and Head, Division of Metabolism, Endocrinology, and Nutrition, University of Washington School of Medicine, Seattle

ALAN L. BISNO, M.D.
Professor of Medicine, University of Miami School of Medicine; Chief, Medical Service, Veterans Administration Medical Center, Miami

JEAN BOLOGNIA, M.D.
Assistant Professor of Dermatology, Department of Dermatology, Yale University School of Medicine, New Haven

WALTER G. BRADLEY, M.D.
Chairman and Professor of Neurology, University of Vermont College of Medicine; Chairman, Department of Neurology, University Health Center, Burlington

DAVID L. BRAFF, M.D.
Professor of Psychiatry, University of California at San Diego; Director of Psychiatry, U.C.S.D. Medical Center, San Diego

KENNETH D. BRANDT, M.D.
Professor of Medicine and Head, Rheumatology Division, Indiana University School of Medicine; Director, Indiana University Specialized Center of Research in Osteoarthritis, Indianapolis

EUGENE BRAUNWALD, A.B., M.D., M.A. (Hon.), M.D. (Hon.)
Hersey Professor of the Theory and Practice of Physic, Harvard Medical School; Chairman, Department of Medicine, Brigham and Women's Hospital, Boston

IRWIN M. BRAVERMAN, M.D.
Professor of Dermatology, Department of Dermatology, Yale University School of Medicine, New Haven

BARRY M. BRENNER, B.S., M.D., M.A. (Hon.)
Samuel A. Levine Professor of Medicine, Harvard Medical School; Senior Physician and Director, Renal Division, Brigham and Women's Hospital, Boston

KENNETH R. BRIDGES, M.D.
Assistant Professor of Medicine, Harvard Medical School; Brigham and Women's Hospital, Boston

KAREN THATCHER BRITTON, M.D., Ph.D.
Associate Professor of Psychiatry, School of Medicine, University of California at San Diego, La Jolla

MARTIN M. BROWN, M.A., M.D., M.R.C.P.
Senior Lecturer in Neurology, St. Georges Hospital Medical School, London

MICHAEL S. BROWN, M.D.
Paul J. Thomas Professor, Department of Molecular Genetics, The University of Texas Southwestern Medical Center, Dallas

ROBERT H. BROWN, Jr., M.D., D.Phil.
Assistant Professor, Harvard Medical School; Associate Neurologist, Massachusetts General Hospital, Boston

H. FRANKLIN BUNN, M.D.
Professor of Medicine, Harvard Medical School; Senior Physician and Director, Hematology Research, Brigham and Women's Hospital, Boston

RONALD M. BURDE, M.D.
Professor and Chairman, Department of Ophthalmology, Ophthalmologist and Neuroophthalmologist, Albert Einstein College of Medicine, New York

JOHN BUTLER, M.D.
Professor of Medicine, University of Washington School of Medicine, Seattle

ROBERT N. BUTLER, M.D.
Chairman, Brookdale Professor of Geriatrics and Adult Development, Ritter Department of Geriatrics and Adult Development, The Mount Sinai Medical Center, New York

ALFRED E. BUXTON, M.D.
Associate Professor of Medicine, University of Pennsylvania School of Medicine; Director, Clinical Electrophysiology Laboratory, Hospital of the University of Pennsylvania, Philadelphia

EDWIN C. CADMAN, M.D.
Ensign Professor of Medicine and Chairman, Department of Medicine, Yale University Medical School, New Haven

CHARLES B. CARPENTER, M.D.
Professor of Medicine, Harvard Medical School; Director, Laboratory of Immunogenetics and Transplantation, Brigham and Women's Hospital, Boston

CHARLES C.J. CARPENTER, M.D.
Professor of Medicine, Brown University; Physician-in-Chief, The Miriam Hospital, Providence

BRUCE R. CARR, M.D.
Professor, Department of Obstetrics and Gynecology and Cecil and Ida Green Center for Reproductive Biology Sciences, The University of Texas Southwestern Medical Center, Dallas

EDWIN H. CASSEM, M.D.
Associate Professor of Psychiatry, Harvard Medical School; Acting Chief, Psychiatric Service, Massachusetts General Hospital, Boston

AGUSTIN CASTELLANOS, M.D.
Professor of Medicine, University of Miami School of Medicine; Director, Clinical Electrophysiology, Jackson Memorial Hospital, Miami

VERNE S. CAVINESS, Jr., M.D., Ph.D.
Joseph and Rose Kennedy Professor of Child Neurology and Mental Retardation, Harvard Medical School; Interim Chief, Neurology Service, and Chief, Child Neurology, Massachusetts General Hospital, Boston

RICHARD CHAMPLIN, M.D.
Associate Professor of Medicine and Director, Leukemia/Bone Marrow Transplant Service, School of Medicine, University of California at Los Angeles

KEITH H. CHIAPPA, M.D.
Associate Professor of Neurology, Harvard Medical School; Director, EEG and Evoked Potentials Unit of the Clinical Neurophysiology Laboratory and Department of Neurology, Massachusetts General Hospital, Boston

JOHN S. CHILD, M.D.
Professor of Medicine, School of Medicine, University of California at Los Angeles; Associate Chief, Division of Cardiology, and Director, Adult Cardiac Imaging and Hemodynamics Laboratories, UCLA Medical Center, Los Angeles

WALLACE A. CLYDE, Jr., M.D.
Professor of Pediatrics and Microbiology, University of North Carolina School of Medicine; Attending Physician, North Carolina Memorial Hospital, Chapel Hill

FREDRIC L. COE, M.D.
Professor of Medicine and Physiology and Chief, Nephrology Program, University of Chicago Pritzker School of Medicine, Chicago

ALAN S. COHEN, M.D.
Chief of Medicine and Director, Thorndike Memorial Laboratory; Conrad Wesselhoeft Professor of Medicine, Boston University School of Medicine, Boston

HARVEY R. COLTEN, M.D.
Professor and Chairman, Department of Pediatrics, Washington University School of Medicine; St. Louis Children's Hospital, St. Louis

WILSON S. COLUCCI, M.D.
Associate Professor of Medicine, Harvard Medical School; Associate Physician, Brigham and Women's Hospital, Boston

PATRICIA C. COME, M.D.
Associate Professor of Medicine, Harvard Medical School; Harvard Community Health Plan, West Roxbury

MAX D. COOPER, M.D.
Investigator, Howard Hughes Medical Institute; Professor of Medicine, Pediatrics, and Microbiology and Director, Division of Developmental and Clinical Immunology, University of Alabama at Birmingham, Birmingham

RICHARD A. COOPER, M.D.
Professor of Medicine, Executive Vice-President and Dean, Medical College of Wisconsin, Milwaukee

LAWRENCE COREY, M.D.
Professor of Laboratory Medicine and Microbiology and Head, Virology Division, University of Washington School of Medicine, Seattle

MARK A. CREAGER, M.D.
Assistant Professor of Medicine, Harvard Medical School; Director, Noninvasive Vascular Laboratory, Division of Vascular Medicine and Atherosclerosis, Brigham and Women's Hospital, Boston

RONALD G. CRYSTAL, M.D.
Chief, Pulmonary Branch, National Heart, Lung and Blood Institute, National Institutes of Health, Bethesda

JOHN J. CUSH, M.D.
Assistant Professor, Department of Internal Medicine, The University of Texas Southwestern Medical Center, Dallas

CHARLES A. CZEISLER, Ph.D., M.D.
Associate Professor of Medicine, Harvard Medical School; Associate Physician, Brigham and Women's Hospital; Director, Center for Circadian and Sleep Disorders, Boston

DAVID C. DALE, M.D.
Professor of Medicine, University of Washington School of Medicine, Seattle

THOMAS M. DANIEL, M.D.
Professor of Medicine, Case Western Reserve University, Cleveland

GILBERT H. DANIELS, M.D.
Associate Professor of Medicine, Harvard Medical School; Physician, Massachusetts General Hospital, Boston

ROBERT B. DAROFF, M.D.
Gilbert W. Humphrey Professor and Chairman, Case Western Reserve University School of Medicine; Director, Department of Neurology, University Hospitals of Cleveland; Neurology Service, Cleveland Veterans Administration Medical Center, Cleveland

JOHN R. DAVID, M.D.
John LaPorte Given Professor and Chairman, Department of Tropical Public Health, Harvard School of Public Health; Chief, Division of Tropical Medicine, Brigham and Women's Hospital, Boston

KENNETH DAVIS, M.D.
Professor of Radiology, Harvard Medical School; Director of Neuroradiology, Massachusetts General Hospital, Boston

MARC A. DICHTER, M.D., Ph.D.
Professor of Neurology, University of Pennsylvania School of Medicine, Philadelphia

JULES L. DIENSTAG, M.D.
Associate Professor of Medicine, Harvard Medical School; Associate Physician, Gastrointestinal Unit, Massachusetts General Hospital, Boston

ROBERT G. DLUHY, M.D.
Associate Professor of Medicine, Harvard Medical School; Associate Program Director of the Clinical Research Center, Brigham and Women's Hospital, Boston

RAPHAEL DOLIN, M.D.
Professor of Medicine, Microbiology and Immunology, and Head, Infectious Diseases Unit, University of Rochester School of Medicine and Dentistry, Rochester

DANIEL B. DRACHMAN, M.D.
Professor of Neurology and Neurosciences and Director, Neuromuscular Unit, The Johns Hopkins University School of Medicine, Baltimore

JEFFREY M. DRAZEN, M.D.
Professor of Medicine, Harvard Medical School; Chief, Pulmonary Division, Brigham and Women's and Beth Israel Hospitals, Boston

HENRY J. DURIVAGE, Pharm.D.
Associate Research Scientist and Director of Clinical Research, Section of Medical Oncology, Department of Internal Medicine, Yale University School of Medicine, New Haven

JOHANNA T. DWYER, D.Sc., R.D.
Professor of Medicine and Community Health, Tufts University School of Medicine; Senior Scientist, USDA Human Nutrition Research Center on Aging, Tufts University; Director, Frances Stern Nutrition Center, New England Medical Center Hospital, Boston

VICTOR J. DZAU, M.D.
William G. Irwin Professor and Chief, Division of Cardiovascular Medicine, Stanford University School of Medicine; Stanford University Hospital, Stanford

KENNETH H. FALCHUK, M.D.
Associate Professor of Medicine, Harvard Medical School; Physician, Brigham and Women's Hospital, Boston

ANTHONY S. FAUCI, M.D.
Director, National Institute of Allergy and Infectious Diseases, and Chief, Laboratory of Immunoregulation, and Director, Office of AIDS Research, National Institutes of Health, Bethesda

MURRAY J. FAVUS, M.D.
Professor of Medicine, University of Chicago Pritzker School of Medicine, Chicago

BERNARD N. FIELDS, M.D.
Adele Lehman Professor of Microbiology and Molecular Genetics, and Professor of Medicine and Chairman, Department of Microbiology and Molecular Genetics, Harvard Medical School, Boston

STUART C. FINCH, M.D.
Professor of Medicine, Robert Wood Johnson Medical School, University of Medicine and Dentistry of New Jersey, Camden

J. STEPHEN FINK, M.D.
Assistant Professor, Harvard Medical School; Assistant Neurologist, Massachusetts General Hospital, Boston

ADAM FINN, M.D.
Lecturer in Immunology, Institute of Child Health; Honorary Senior Registrar, The Hospital for Sick Children, London

DANIEL W. FOSTER, M.D.
Donald W. Seldin Distinguished Chair in Internal Medicine and Chairman, Department of Internal Medicine, The University of Texas Southwestern Medical Center, Dallas

MICHAEL M. FRANK, M.D.
Chief, Laboratory of Clinical Investigation, National Institute of Allergy and Infectious Diseases, National Institutes of Health, Bethesda

STANLEY D. FREEDMAN, M.D.
Head, Division of Infectious Diseases, Scripps Clinic and Research Foundation; Clinical Professor of Medicine, University of California at San Diego, La Jolla

BISHARA J. FREIJ, M.D.
Assistant Professor of Pediatrics, Division of Infectious Diseases, Department of Pediatrics, Georgetown University School of Medicine, Washington, D.C.

MICHAEL FREISSMUTH, M.D.
Instructor, Department of Pharmacology, University of Vienna

HARVEY M. FRIEDMAN, M.D.
Associate Professor, Department of Medicine, University of Pennsylvania School of Medicine, Philadelphia

LAWRENCE S. FRIEDMAN, M.D.
Associate Professor of Medicine and Vice Chairman of the Department of Medicine, Division of Gastroenterology and Hepatology, Thomas Jefferson University Hospital, Philadelphia

PAUL J. FRIEDMAN, M.D.
Professor of Radiology, University of California, San Diego

WILLIAM F. FRIEDMAN, M.D.
J.H. Nicholson Professor of Pediatric Cardiology and Executive Chairman, Department of Pediatrics, School of Medicine; UCLA Medical Center, Los Angeles

LAWRENCE A. FROHMAN, M.D.
Professor of Medicine, Director of Division of Endocrinology and Metabolism, University of Cincinnati College of Medicine, Cincinnati

JOHN I. GALLIN, M.D.
Director, Intramural Research Program, National Institute of Allergy and Infectious Diseases, National Institutes of Health, Bethesda

ROBERT C. GALLO, M.D.
Chief, Laboratory of Tumor Cell Biology, National Cancer Institute, National Institutes of Health, Bethesda

DONALD E. GANEM, M.D.
Associate Professor of Medicine and Microbiology, Division of Infectious Disease, Department of Medicine, University of California, San Francisco

PIERCE GARDNER, M.D.
Professor of Medicine and Associate Dean for Academic Affairs, School of Medicine, State University of New York at Stony Brook, Stony Brook

MARC B. GARNICK, M.D.
Associate Clinical Professor of Medicine, Dana-Farber Cancer Institute, Harvard Medical School; Vice President for Clinical Development, Genetics Institute, Cambridge

JAMES L. GERMAN III, M.D.
Professor (Genetics), Department of Pediatrics, Cornell University Medical College; Senior Investigator and Director, Laboratory of Human Genetics, The New York Blood Center, New York

ELOISE R. GIBLETT, M.D.
Executive Director Emeritus, Puget Sound Blood Center, Seattle

BRUCE C. GILLILAND, M.D.
Associate Dean for Clinical Affairs, University of Washington School of Medicine, Seattle

J. CHRISTIAN GILLIN, M.D.
Professor of Psychiatry, University of California at San Diego, and Director of U.C.S.D. Mental Health Research Center; Director of U.C.S.D. Fellowship in Psychopharmacology and Psychobiology, La Jolla

ALFRED G. GILMAN, M.D., Ph.D.
Raymond and Ellen Willie Professor of Molecular Neuropharmacology and Chairman, Department of Pharmacology, The University of Texas Southwestern Medical Center, Dallas

SID GILMAN, M.D.
Professor and Chairman, Department of Neurology, The University of Michigan Medical Center, Ann Arbor

RICHARD J. GLASSOCK, M.D.
Professor of Medicine, School of Medicine, University of California at Los Angeles; Chairman, Department of Medicine, Harbor-UCLA Medical Center, Torrance

ROBERT M. GLICKMAN, M.D.
Herrman L. Blumgart Professor of Medicine, Harvard Medical School; Physician-in-Chief, Beth Israel Hospital, Boston

DAVID W. GOLDE, M.D.
Professor of Medicine and Chief, Division of Hematology/Oncology, School of Medicine, University of California, Los Angeles

STEPHEN E. GOLDFINGER, M.D.
Associate Dean, Department of Continuing Education, and Associate Professor of Medicine, Harvard Medical School; Physician, Gastrointestinal Unit, Massachusetts General Hospital, Boston

PAUL GOLDHABER, D.D.S.
Dean and Professor of Periodontology, Harvard School of Dental Medicine, Boston

LEE GOLDMAN, M.D.
Professor of Medicine, Harvard Medical School; Vice-Chairman, Department of Medicine, Brigham and Women's Hospital; Chief, Division of Clinical Epidemiology, Brigham and Women's and Beth Israel Hospitals, Boston

JOSEPH L. GOLDSTEIN, M.D.
Paul J. Thomas Professor and Chairman, Department of Molecular Genetics, The University of Texas Southwestern Medical Center, Dallas

RAJ K. GOYAL, M.D.
Rabb Professor of Medicine, Harvard Medical School; Chief, Division of Gastroenterology, Beth Israel Hospital, Boston

JOHN W. GRAEF, M.D.
Associate Clinical Professor of Pediatrics, Harvard Medical School; Director, The Lead/Toxicology Clinic, The Children's Hospital, Boston

IGOR GRANT, M.D.
Professor and Acting Chairman, Department of Psychiatry, School of Medicine, University of California at San Diego, La Jolla

HARRY B. GREENBERG, M.D.
Professor of Medicine, Microbiology, and Immunology and Chief, Gastroenterology Division, Stanford University School of Medicine, Stanford

NORTON J. GREENBERGER, M.D.
Peter T. Bohan Professor and Chairman, Department of Medicine, University of Kansas School of Medicine, Kansas City

BRUCE M. GREENE, M.D.
Professor of Medicine, and Director, Division of Geographic Medicine, Department of Medicine, University of Alabama at Birmingham, Birmingham

JOHN S. GREENSPAN, Ph.D.
Professor and Chairman, Division of Oral Biology, University of California School of Dentistry, San Francisco Medical Center, San Francisco

JAMES E. GRIFFIN III, M.D.
Professor of Internal Medicine, The University of Texas Southwestern Medical Center, Dallas

J. McLEOD GRIFFISS, M.D.
Professor of Laboratory Medicine and Medicine, University of California San Francisco; Chief of Microbiology, Veterans Administration Medical Center, San Francisco

ROBERT C. GRIGGS, M.D.
Edward A. and Alma Vollertsen Rykenboer Professor of Neurophysiology, Professor of Neurology and Medicine, and Chairman, Department of Neurology, University of Rochester School of Medicine and Dentistry, University of Rochester Medical Center, Rochester

WILLIAM GROSSMAN, M.D.
Dana Professor of Medicine, Harvard Medical School; Chief, Cardiovascular Division, Beth Israel Hospital, Boston

JOHN H. GROWDON, M.D.
Associate Professor of Neurology, Harvard Medical School; Associate Neurologist and Director, Memory Disorders Unit, Massachusetts General Hospital, Boston

VLADIMIR C. HACHINSKI, M.D.
Richard and Beryl Ivey Professor and Chairman, Department of Clinical Neurological Sciences, University of Western Ontario, University Hospital, London, Ontario

BEVRA H. HAHN, M.D.
Chief of Rheumatology, University of California, Los Angeles

ROBERT I. HANDIN, M.D.
Associate Professor of Medicine, Harvard Medical School; Director, Hematology Division, Brigham and Women's Hospital, Boston

H. HUNTER HANDSFIELD, M.D.
Professor of Medicine, University of Washington School of Medicine; Director, Sexually Transmitted Disease Control Program, Seattle-King County Department of Public Health, Seattle

DONALD G. HARTER, M.D.
Senior Scientific Officer and Director, HHMI-NIH Research Scholars Program, Howard Hughes Medical Institute, Bethesda; Clinical Professor of Neurology, George Washington University School of Medicine and Health Sciences, Washington, D.C.

BARTON F. HAYNES, M.D.
Frederick M. Hanes Professor of Medicine and Chief, Division of Rheumatology and Immunology, Duke University School of Medicine, Durham

STEVEN C. HEBERT, M.D.
Associate Professor of Medicine, Harvard Medical School; Associate Physician, Brigham and Women's Hospital, Boston

CRAIG HENDERSON, M.D.
Associate Professor of Medicine, Harvard Medical School; Division of Medical Oncology, Dana-Farber Cancer Institute, Boston

FRED J. HENDLER, M.D., Ph.D.
Associate Professor of Medicine and Biochemistry, University of Louisville School of Medicine; James Graham Brown Cancer Center, Division of Hematology/Oncology, Louisville; Consulting Physician, Veterans Administration Medical Center, Dallas

FREDERICK P. HEINZEL, M.D.
Associate Professor of Medicine, Division of Infectious Disease, Department of Medicine, University of California, San Francisco

CHARLES B. HIGGINS, M.D.
Professor of Radiology and Chief, Magnetic Resonance Imaging, University of California School of Medicine, San Francisco

RAYMOND L. HINTZ, M.D.
Professor of Pediatrics and Head, Division of Pediatric Endocrinology, Stanford University School of Medicine, Stanford

MARTIN S. HIRSCH, M.D.
Associate Professor of Medicine, Harvard Medical School; Associate Physician, Infectious Diseases Unit, Massachusetts General Hospital, Boston

JAN V. HIRSCHMANN, M.D.
Associate Professor of Medicine, University of Washington School of Medicine; Assistant Chief, Medical Service, Seattle Veterans Administration Medical Center, Seattle

FRED HOCHBERG, M.D.
Associate Professor of Neurology, Harvard Medical School; Neurologist, Massachusetts General Hospital, Boston

PAUL D. HOEPRICH, M.D.
Professor of Medicine, Section of Medical Myocology, Division of Infectious and Immunologic Diseases, School of Medicine, University of California, Davis

GARY S. HOFFMAN, M.D.
Senior Investigator, Laboratory of Immunoregulation, National Institute of Allergy and Infectious Diseases, National Institutes of Health, Bethesda

JOHN H. HOLBROOK, M.D.
Professor of Internal Medicine, University of Utah School of Medicine, Salt Lake City

MICHAEL F. HOLICK, M.D., Ph.D.
Professor of Medicine, Chief of Endocrinology, and Director of the Clinical Research Center, Boston University School of Medicine, Boston

KING K. HOLMES, M.D., Ph.D.
Director, Center for AIDS and Sexually Transmitted Diseases; Professor of Medicine, University of Washington School of Medicine, Seattle

RANDALL K. HOLMES, M.D., Ph.D.
Professor and Chairman, Department of Microbiology, and Associate Dean for Academic Affairs, Uniformed Services University of the Health Sciences, Bethesda

THOMAS H. HOSTETTER, M.D.
Professor of Medicine, University of Minnesota School of Medicine; Director, Division of Renal Disease, University Hospital, Minneapolis

LYN J. HOWARD, B.M., D.Ch., F.R.C.P.
Professor of Medicine and Associate Professor of Pediatrics, and Head, Division of Clinical Nutrition, Albany Medical College, Albany

GARY W. HUNNINGHAKE, M.D.
Professor of Internal Medicine and Director, Pulmonary and Critical Care Medicine, University of Iowa College of Medicine, Iowa City

SIDNEY H. INGBAR, M.D., D.Sc. (Deceased)
Former William Bosworth Castle Professor of Medicine, Harvard Medical School; former Director, Thorndike Laboratory, Beth Israel Hospital, Boston

ROLAND H. INGRAM, Jr., M.D.
Professor and Vice-Chairman of Medicine, University of Minnesota Medical School; Chief of Medicine, Hennepin County Medical Center, Minneapolis

KURT J. ISSELBACHER, A.B., M.D.
Mallinckrodt Professor of Medicine, Harvard Medical School; Director, Cancer Center, Massachusetts General Hospital, Boston

RICHARD JACOBS, M.D., Ph.D.
Associate Clinical Professor of Medicine, Division of Infectious Disease, Department of Medicine, University of California, San Francisco

MARK E. JOSEPHSON, M.D.
Robinette Professor of Medicine (Cardiovascular Diseases), University of Pennsylvania School of Medicine; Chief, Cardiovascular Section, Hospital of the University of Pennsylvania, Philadelphia

LEWIS L. JUDD, M.D.
Director, National Institute of Mental Health, Rockville

LEE M. KAPLAN, M.D., Ph.D.
Assistant Professor of Medicine, Harvard Medical School; Assistant in Medicine, Gastrointestinal Unit, Massachusetts General Hospital, Boston

DENNIS L. KASPER, M.D.
William Ellery Channing Professor of Medicine, Harvard Medical School; Chief, Infectious Disease Division, Beth Israel Hospital, Boston

SATISH KATHPALIA, M.D.
Assistant Professor of Medicine, University of Chicago Pritzker School of Medicine; Attending Physician, Michael Reese Hospital and Medical Center, Chicago

DONALD KAYE, M.D.
Professor and Chairman, Department of Medicine, The Medical College of Pennsylvania, Philadelphia

WILLIAM N. KELLEY, M.D.
Professor of Medicine and Dean, School of Medicine, University of Pennsylvania, Philadelphia

GERALD T. KEUSCH, M.D.
Professor of Medicine, Tufts University School of Medicine; Chief, Division of Geographic Medicine and Infectious Diseases, New England Medical Center Hospital, Boston

MICHAEL B. KIMMEY, M.D.
Assistant Professor of Medicine and Director of Therapeutic Endoscopy, Division of Gastroenterology, University of Washington School of Medicine, Seattle

LOUIS V. KIRCHHOFF, M.D., M.P.H.
Assistant Professor of Medicine, Department of Internal Medicine, University of Iowa College of Medicine; Staff Physician, Veterans Administration Medical Center, Iowa City

J. PHILLIP KISTLER, M.D.
Associate Professor of Neurology, Harvard Medical School; Associate Neurologist, Massachusetts General Hospital, Boston

JOSEPH J. KLIMEK, M.D.
Associate Professor of Medicine, University of Connecticut Health Center; Acting Director, Department of Medicine, Hartford Hospital, Hartford

JAMES P. KNOCHEL, M.D.
Professor of Internal Medicine, The University of Texas Southwestern Medical Center; Chairman, Department of Medicine, Presbyterian Hospital, Dallas

HOWARD K. KOH, M.D.
Associate Professor of Dermatology, Medicine, and Public Health, Boston University Schools of Medicine and Public Health, Boston

WILLIAM J. KOVACS, M.D.
Assistant Professor of Medicine, Division of Endocrinology, Vanderbilt University School of Medicine, Nashville

KAREN KOVALOV-ST. JOHN, M.D.
Rheumatology Fellow, Indiana University School of Medicine, Indianapolis

STEPHEN M. KRANE, M.D.
Persis, Cyrus, and Marlow B. Harrison Professor of Medicine, Harvard Medical School; Physician and Chief, Arthritis Unit, Massachusetts General Hospital, Boston

J. THOMAS LaMONT, M.D.
Professor of Medicine, Boston University School of Medicine; Chief, Section of Gastroenterology, The University Hospital, Boston

LEWIS LANDSBERG, M.D.
Professor of Medicine, Harvard Medical School; Chief, Division of Endocrinology and Metabolism, Beth Israel Hospital, Boston

H. CLIFFORD LANE, M.D.
Deputy Clinical Director, National Institute of Allergy and Infectious Diseases, National Institutes of Health, Bethesda

PAUL N. LANKEN, M.D.
Associate Professor of Medicine, University of Pennsylvania School of Medicine; Medical Director, Medical Intensive Care Unit, Hospital of the University of Pennsylvania, Philadelphia

THOMAS J. LAWLEY, M.D.
Professor and Chairman, Department of Dermatology, Emory University School of Medicine, Atlanta

ALEXANDER R. LAWTON III, M.D.
Professor of Pediatrics and Microbiology, Division of Pediatrics, Immunology, and Rheumatology, Vanderbilt University School of Medicine, Nashville

J. MICHAEL LAZARUS, M.D.
Associate Professor of Medicine, Harvard Medical School; Physician, Brigham and Women's Hospital, Boston

ROBERT LEBOVICS, M.D.
Chief, Otolaryngology/Head, Neck Surgery, National Institute on Deafness and Other Communication Disorders, National Institutes of Health, Bethesda

NORMAN G. LEVINSKY, M.D.
Wade Professor and Chairman, Department of Medicine, Boston University School of Medicine; Physician-in-Chief and Director, Evans Memorial Department of Clinical Research, University Hospital, Boston

CHRISTOPHER H. LINDEN, M.D.
Assistant Professor of Medicine, University of Massachusetts Medical School; Director, Regional Poisoning Treatment Center, Worcester, Massachusetts

PETER E. LIPSKY, M.D.
Director, Harold C. Simmons Arthritis Research Center; Professor, Department of Internal Medicine, The University of Texas Southwestern Medical Center, Dallas

RICHARD M. LOCKSLEY, M.D.
Associate Professor of Medicine and Chief, Division of Infectious Disease, Department of Medicine, University of California, San Francisco

HARVEY F. LODISH, Ph.D.
Professor, Department of Biology, Massachusetts Institute of Technology; Member, Whitehead Institute for Biomedical Research, Cambridge

DAN L. LONGO, M.D.
Director, Biological Response Modifiers Program, Division of Cancer Treatment, National Cancer Institute-Frederick Cancer Research Facility, Frederick

FREDERICK H. LOVEJOY, JR., M.D.
Professor of Pediatrics, Harvard Medical School; Associate Physician-in-Chief, The Children's Hospital, Boston

SHEILA A. LUKEHART, Ph.D.
Research Associate Professor, Department of Medicine, Division of Infectious Diseases, University of Washington School of Medicine, Seattle

ROB ROY MacGREGOR, M.D.
Professor of Medicine and Chief of Infectious Diseases Division, Department of Medicine, University of Pennsylvania School of Medicine, Philadelphia

RAYMOND MACIEWICZ, M.D.
Associate Professor of Neurology, Harvard Medical School; Associate Neurologist, Massachusetts General Hospital, Boston

JON T. MADER, M.D.
Professor of Medicine, Division of Infectious Diseases, Department of Internal Medicine, The University of Texas Medical Branch, Galveston

HENRY J. MANKIN, M.D.
Edith M. Ashley Professor of Orthopedic Surgery, Harvard Medical School; Chief, Orthopedic Services, Massachusetts General Hospital, Boston

FRANCIS E. MARCHLINSKI, M.D.
Associate Professor of Medicine, University of Pennsylvania School of Medicine; Director, Arrhythmia Evaluation Center, Hospital of the University of Pennsylvania, Philadelphia

JOSEPH B. MARTIN, M.D., Ph.D., F.R.C.P.(C), M.A.(Hon.)
Professor of Neurology and Dean, School of Medicine, University of California, San Francisco

JOEL B. MASON, M.D.
Assistant Professor of Medicine, Tufts University School of Medicine; Scientist, USDA Human Nutrition Research Center on Aging, Tufts University, Boston

HENRY MASUR, M.D.
Deputy Chief, Critical Care Medicine, Clinical Center, National Institutes of Health, Bethesda

ROBERT J. MAYER, M.D.
Associate Professor of Medicine, Harvard Medical School; Division of Medical Oncology, Dana-Farber Cancer Institute, Boston

JOHN D. McCONNELL, M.D.
Assistant Professor of Urology, The University of Texas Southwestern Medical Center, Dallas

GEORGE H. McCRACKEN, JR., M.D.
Professor of Pediatrics and Chief, Division of Infectious Diseases, Department of Pediatrics, The University of Texas Southwestern Medical Center, Dallas

E. R. McFADDEN, JR., M.D.
Argyl J. Beams Professor of Medicine and Director, Airway Disease Center, Case Western Reserve University School of Medicine, Cleveland

JAMES E. McGUIGAN, M.D.
Professor of Medicine and Chairman, Department of Medicine, University of Florida College of Medicine, Gainesville

NANCY K. MELLO, Ph.D.
Professor of Psychology, Department of Psychiatry (Neuroscience), Harvard Medical School, Boston; Co-Director, Alcohol and Drug Abuse Research Center, McLean Hospital, Belmont

JERRY R. MENDELL, M.D.
Professor of Neurology, Ohio State University College of Medicine, Columbus

JOHN MENDELSOHN, M.D.
Winthrop Rockefeller Chair in Medical Oncology and Chairman, Department of Medicine, Memorial Sloan-Kettering Cancer Center, New York

JACK H. MENDELSON, M.D.
Professor of Psychiatry (Neuroscience), Harvard Medical School, Boston; Co-Director, Alcohol and Drug Abuse Research Center, McLean Hospital, Belmont

URS A. MEYER, M.D.
Professor of Pharmacology and Chairman, Department of Pharmacology, Biocenter of the University of Basel, Basel, Switzerland

EDGAR L. MILFORD, M.D.
Associate Professor of Medicine, Harvard Medical School; Associate Physician, Brigham and Women's Hospital, Boston

RICHARD A. MILLER, M.D.
Assistant Professor of Medicine, University of Washington School of Medicine; Chief, Infectious Disease Division, Seattle Veterans Administration Medical Center, Seattle

JOHN D. MINNA, M.D.
Chief, NCI-Navy Medical Oncology Branch, National Cancer Institute, National Institutes of Health; Professor of Medicine, Uniformed Services University for the Health Sciences, Naval Hospital, Bethesda

JAY P. MOHR, M.D.
Sciarra Professor of Clinical Neurology, College of Physicians and Surgeons of Columbia University Neurological Institute, New York

STEPHEN A. MORSE, MSPH, Ph.D.
Director, Division of Sexually Transmitted Diseases Laboratory Research, Centers for Disease Control, Atlanta

KENNETH M. MOSER, M.D.
Professor of Medicine, School of Medicine, University of California at San Diego; Director, Pulmonary and Critical Care Division, U.C.S.D. Medical Center, La Jolla

ARNOLD M. MOSES, M.D.
Professor of Medicine and Director, Clinical Research Center, State University of New York Health Science Center; Chief, Endocrinology Section, Veterans Administration Medical Center, Syracuse

HARALAMPOS M. MOUTSOPOULOS, M.D.
Professor and Head of Medicine, Department of Internal Medicine, University of Ioannina Medical School, Ioannina, Greece

HENRY W. MURRAY, M.D.
Professor of Medicine, Cornell University School of Medicine; Chief, Infectious Diseases, The New York Hospital-Cornell Medical Center, New York

ROBERT J. MYERBURG, M.D.
Professor of Medicine and Physiology and Director, Division of Cardiology, University of Miami School of Medicine, Miami

LEE M. NADLER, M.D.
Associate Professor of Medicine, Harvard Medical School; Division of Tumor Immunology, Dana-Farber Cancer Institute, Boston

THEODORE E. NASH, M.D.
Medical Officer, Laboratory of Parasitic Diseases, National Institute of Allergy and Infectious Diseases, National Institutes of Health, Bethesda

LAURENCE NEEDLEMAN, M.D.
Assistant Professor of Radiology, Jefferson Medical College, Philadelphia

PAUL NEIMAN, M.D.
Professor of Medicine and Adjunct Professor of Pathology, University of Washington School of Medicine; Fred Hutchinson Cancer Research Center, Seattle

HAROLD C. NEU, M.D.
Professor of Medicine and Pharmacology and Chief, Division of Infectious Diseases, College of Physicians and Surgeons, Columbia University, New York

JOHN A. OATES, M.D.
Professor and Chairman, Department of Medicine, Vanderbilt University School of Medicine; Physician-in-Chief, Vandberbilt University Hospital, Nashville

JERROLD M. OLEFSKY, M.D.
Professor of Medicine and Head, Division of Endocrinology and Metabolism, School of Medicine, University of California at San Diego, La Jolla

STUART H. ORKIN, M.D.
Leland Fikes Professor of Pediatric Medicine, Harvard Medical School; Children's Hospital, Boston

ROBERT A. O'ROURKE, M.D.
Charles Conrad Brown Distinguished Professor of Medicine, University of Texas Health Science Center at San Antonio; Chief of Cardiology, University of Texas Health Science Center Teaching Hospitals, San Antonio

THOMAS D. PALELLA, M.D.
Associate Professor of Internal Medicine and Chief, Division of Rheumatology, University of Michigan Medical School, Ann Arbor

DARWIN L. PALMER, M.D.
Professor of Medicine and Chief, Division of Infectious Disease, University of New Mexico School of Medicine, Albuquerque

JOSEPH E. PARRILLO, M.D.
James B. Herrick Professor of Medicine, Rush Medical College; Chief, Section of Cardiology, Chief, Section of Critical Care Medicine, Medical Director, Rush Heart Institute, Rush-Presbyterian-St. Luke's Medical Center, Chicago

RICHARD C. PASTERNAK, M.D.
Assistant Professor of Medicine, Harvard Medical School; Director, Coronary Care Unit, Beth Israel Hospital, Boston

PETER L. PERINE, M.D.
Professor and Director, Division of Tropical Public Health, Uniformed Services University of the Health Sciences, Bethesda

ROBERT G. PETERSDORF, M.D.
President, Association of American Medical Colleges; Clinical Professor of Medicine, Georgetown University School of Medicine, Washington, D.C.

ELIOT A. PHILLIPSON, M.D.
Professor of Medicine, University of Toronto; Physician-in-Chief, Mount Sinai Hospital, Toronto

DAVID J. PIERSON, M.D.
Professor of Medicine, University of Washington School of Medicine; Medical Director of Respiratory Care, Harborview Medical Center, Seattle

JAMES J. PLORDE, M.D.
Professor of Medicine, Departments of Laboratory Medicine and Microbiology, University of Washington School of Medicine; Chief, Microbiology Laboratory, Seattle Veterans Administration Hospital, Seattle

STANLEY A. PLOTKIN, M.D.
Professor of Pediatrics and Microbiology, University of Pennsylvania; Chair, Division of Infectious Diseases, The Children's Hospital of Philadelphia, Philadelphia

FRANCIS A. PLUMMER, M.D., F.R.C.P.(C)
Associate Professor, Department of Medical Microbiology, University of Manitoba, Winnipeg

DANIEL K. PODOLSKY, M.D.
Associate Professor of Medicine, Harvard Medical School; Chief, Gastrointestinal Unit, Massachusetts General Hospital, Boston

JOHN T. POTTS, Jr., M.D.
Jackson Professor of Clinical Medicine, Harvard Medical School; Chief of the General Medical Service, Massachusetts General Hospital, Boston

LAWRIE W. POWELL, M.D.
Professor of Medicine, University of Queensland; Physician, Royal Brisbane Hospital, Brisbane, Australia

DARWIN J. PROCKOP, M.D., Ph.D.
Professor and Chairman, Department of Biochemistry, Jefferson Medical College of Thomas Jefferson University; Director, Department of Biochemistry, Jefferson Institute of Molecular Medicine, Philadelphia

AMY PRUITT, M.D.
Assistant Professor of Neurology, Harvard Medical School; Associate Neurologist, Massachusetts General Hospital, Boston

PAUL G. RAMSEY, M.D.
Associate Professor and Associate Chairman, Department of Medicine, University of Washington School of Medicine, Seattle

JOEL M. RAPPEPORT, M.D.
Professor of Medicine, Yale University School of Medicine; Director, Bone Marrow Transplantation Program, Yale New Haven Hospital, New Haven

C. GEORGE RAY, M.D.
Professor, Departments of Pathology and Pediatrics, College of Medicine, The University of Arizona Health Sciences Center, Tucson

RICHARD C. REICHMAN, M.D.
Associate Professor of Medicine, Microbiology, and Immunology, The University of Rochester Medical Center, Rochester

HERBERT Y. REYNOLDS, M.D.
J. Lloyd Huck Professor of Medicine and Chairman, Department of Medicine, The Pennsylvania State University College of Medicine; University Hospital, The Milton S. Hershey Medical Center, Hershey

STUART RICH, M.D.
Associate Professor of Medicine and Chief, Section of Cardiology, University of Illinois College of Medicine, Chicago

EDWARD P. RICHARDSON Jr., M.D.
Bullard Professor of Neuropathology, Harvard Medical School; Senior Neurologist, Massachusetts General Hospital, Boston

GARY S. RICHARDSON, M.D.
Instructor in Medicine, Harvard Medical School; Associate Physician, Brigham and Women's Hospital, Boston

HAL B. RICHERSON, M.D.
Professor of Internal Medicine and Director, Allergy-Immunology Division, University of Iowa College of Medicine, Iowa City

JAMES M. RICHTER, M.D.
Assistant Professor of Medicine, Harvard Medical School; Chief, Gastrointestinal Clinic, Massachusetts General Hospital, Boston

S. CRAIG RISCH, M.D.
Professor of Psychiatry and Director of Clinical Research Programs, Emory University, Atlanta

R. PAUL ROBERTSON, M.D.
Professor of Medicine, Director of Clinical Research Center, and Director, Diabetes Center, University of Minnesota, Minneapolis

ALLAN R. RONALD, M.D.
H. E. Sellers Professor and Head, Department of Medicine, The University of Manitoba, Winnipeg

RICHARD K. ROOT, M.D.
Professor of Medicine, Department of Medicine, and Associate Dean for Clinical Education, School of Medicine, University of California, San Francisco

ALLAN H. ROPPER, M.D.
Associate Professor of Neurology, Harvard Medical School; Associate Neurologist and Director of Neurological/Neurosurgical Intensive Care Unit, Massachusetts General Hospital, Boston

IRWIN H. ROSENBERG, M.D.
Professor of Medicine, Nutrition, and Physiology, Tufts University School of Medicine; Director, USDA Human Nutrition Research Center on Aging, Tufts University, Boston

LEON E. ROSENBERG, M.D.
Dean and C.N.H. Long Professor of Human Genetics, Medicine, and Pediatrics, Yale University School of Medicine, New Haven

DANIEL ROTROSEN, M.D.
Bacterial Diseases Section, National Institute of Allergy and Infectious Diseases, National Institutes of Health, Bethesda

JODI ROY, M.S., R.D.
Frances Stern Nutrition Center, New England Medical Center Hospital, Boston

ARTHUR H. RUBENSTEIN, M.D.
Professor and Chairman, Department of Medicine, University of Chicago Pritzker School of Medicine, Chicago

JEREMY N. RUSKIN, M.D.
Associate Professor of Medicine, Harvard Medical School; Director of Cardiac Arrhythmia Service, Massachusetts General Hospital, Boston

ARTHUR I. SAGALOWSKY, M.D.
Professor of Urology and Director of Renal Transplantation, The University of Texas Southwestern Medical Center, Dallas

JAY P. SANFORD, M.D.
President and Dean, Uniformed Services University of the Health Sciences, Bethesda

DENNIS R. SCHABERG, M.D.
Professor of Internal Medicine, The University of Michigan Medical School, Ann Arbor

I. HERBERT SCHEINBERG, M.D.
Professor of Medicine and Head, Division of Genetic Medicine, Albert Einstein College of Medicine; Attending Physician, Hospital of the Albert Einstein College of Medicine, New York

ALAN L. SCHILLER, M.D.
Irene Heinz Given and John LaPorte Given Professor and Chairman of Pathology, The Mount Sinai School of Medicine, New York

R. NEIL SCHIMKE, M.D.
Professor of Pediatrics and Internal Medicine and Director, Division of Metabolism, Endocrinology, and Genetics, The University of Kansas College of Health Sciences, Kansas City

RUDI SCHMID, M.D., Ph.D.
Professor of Medicine and Associate Dean, University of California, San Francisco

ROBERT T. SCHOOLEY, M.D.
Associate Professor of Medicine, Harvard Medical School; Assistant Physician, Infectious Disease Unit, Department of Medicine, Massachusetts General Hospital, Boston

ROBERT W. SCHRIER, M.D.
Professor and Chairman, Department of Medicine, University of Colorado School of Medicine, Denver

JOHN S. SCHROEDER, M.D.
Professor of Medicine, Cardiology Division, Stanford University School of Medicine; Stanford University Medical Center, Stanford

MARC A. SCHUCKIT, M.D.
Professor of Psychiatry, School of Medicine, University of California at San Diego; Director, Alcohol Research Center, San Diego Veterans Administration Medical Center, La Jolla

PETER H. SCHUR, M.D.
Professor of Medicine, Department of Rheumatology, Brigham and Women's Hospital, Boston

DAVID S. SEGAL, Ph.D.
Professor of Psychiatry, School of Medicine, University of California at San Diego, La Jolla

JULIAN L. SEIFTER, M.D.
Assistant Professor of Medicine, Harvard Medical School; Associate Physician, Brigham and Women's Hospital, Boston

ANDREW P. SELWYN, M.D.
Associate Professor of Medicine, Harvard Medical School; Director of Cardiac Catheterization, Brigham and Women's Hospital, Boston

BHAGWAN T. SHAHANI, M.B., B.S.
Associate Professor of Neurology, Harvard Medical School; Associate Neurologist, Massachusetts General Hospital, Boston

GORDON C. SHARP, M.D.
Department of Medicine, Division of Immunology and Rheumatology, University of Missouri-Columbia School of Medicine, Columbia

ELIZABETH M. SHORT, M.D.
Director, Division of Biomedical Research and Faculty Development, American Association of Medical Colleges, Washington, D.C.

WILLIAM SILEN, M.D.
Johnson and Johnson Professor of Surgery, Harvard Medical School; Surgeon-in-Chief, Beth Israel Hospital, Boston

FRED E. SILVERSTEIN, M.D.
Professor of Medicine, Director, Gastrointestinal Endoscopy, Division of Gastroenterology, University of Washington School of Medicine, Seattle

THOMAS L. SLAMOWITZ, M.D.
Vice Chairman of Ophthalmology and Associate Professor of Ophthalmology and Neuroophthalmology, Albert Einstein College/ Montefiore Medical Center, New York

JAMES B. SNOW, Jr., M.D.
Director, National Institute on Deafness and Other Communication Disorders, National Institutes of Health, Bethesda

ARTHUR SOBER, M.D.
Associate Professor of Dermatology, Harvard Medical School; Associate Chief of Dermatology, Massachusetts General Hospital, Boston

FRANK E. SPEIZER, M.D.
Professor of Medicine, Harvard Medical School; Co-Director, Channing Laboratory, Brigham and Women's Hospital, Boston

WALTER E. STAMM, M.D.
Professor of Medicine, University of Washington School of Medicine; Head, Division of Infectious Diseases, Harborview Medical Center, Seattle

ALLEN C. STEERE, M.D.
Professor of Medicine and Chief, Division of Rheumatology, Department of Medicine, Tufts University School of Medicine, Boston, Massachusetts

ROBERT S. STERN, M.D.
Associate Professor of Dermatology, Harvard Medical School; Beth Israel Hospital, Boston

CHARLES F. STEVENS, M.D., Ph.D.
Professor of Molecular Neurobiology, Salk Institute, La Jolla

GENE H. STOLLERMAN, M.D.
Professor of Medicine, Boston University School of Medicine; Clinical Director, Bedford Division of The Geriatric Research, Educational, and Clinical Center, Veterans Administration Medical Center, Bedford

DAVID H.P. STREETEN, M.B., D. Phil, F.R.C.P.
Professor of Medicine and Head, Section of Endocrinology, State University of New York Upstate Health Science Center, Syracuse

NEIL A. SWANSON, M.D.
Professor of Dermatology, Otolaryngology, and Surgery (Plastic), Division of Plastic Surgery, Oregon Health Sciences University, Portland

ROBERT A. SWERLICK, M.D.
Department of Dermatology, Emory University School of Medicine, Atlanta

RUP TANDAN, M.D., M.R.C.P.
Assistant Professor, Department of Neurology, University of Vermont College of Medicine, Burlington

JOEL D. TAUROG, M.D.
Assistant Professor, The University of Texas Southwestern Medical Center; Southwestern Medical School, Dallas

E. DONNALL THOMAS, M.D.
Professor of Medicine, University of Washington School of Medicine; Member, Fred Hutchinson Cancer Research Center, Seattle

PHILLIP P. TOSKES, M.D.
Professor of Medicine and Chief, Division of Gastroenterology, University of Florida College of Medicine, Gainesville

MARVIN TURCK, M.D.
Professor of Medicine, University of Washington School of Medicine, Seattle

DAVID VALLE, M.D.
Professor of Pediatrics and Molecular Virology and Genetics, Johns Hopkins University School of Medicine; Investigator, Howard Hughes Medical Institute, Baltimore

MAURICE VICTOR, M.D.
Professor of Medicine (Neurology), Dartmouth Medical School, Hanover

DAVID C. WAAGNER, M.D.
Assistant Professor of Pediatrics, Department of Pediatrics, The University of Texas Health Sciences Center, Houston

JAMES F. WALLACE, M.D.
Professor of Medicine, University of Washington School of Medicine; Associate Physician-in-Chief, University Hospital, Seattle

PETER D. WALZER, M.D.
Associate Professor of Medicine, University of Cincinnati College of Medicine; Chief, Infectious Disease Service, Cincinnati Veterans Administration Medical Center, Cincinnati

JACK R. WANDS, M.D.
Associate Professor of Medicine, Harvard Medical School; Molecular Hepatology Laboratory, Cancer Center, Massachusetts General Hospital, Charlestown

LEONARD WARTOFSKY, M.D.
Professor of Medicine and Physiology, Uniformed Services University of the Health Sciences, Bethesda; Chief of Endocrinology and Metabolism, Walter Reed Army Medical Center, Washington, D.C.

STEVEN E. WEINBERGER, M.D.
Associate Professor of Medicine, Harvard Medical School; Clinical Director, Pulmonary Unit, Beth Israel Hospital, Boston

NICHOLAS J. WHITE, M.D., M.R.C.P.
Tropical Medicine Unit, Nuffield Department of Clinical Medicine, Oxford University, England; Faculty of Tropical Medicine, Mahidol University, Bangkok, Thailand

RICHARD J. WHITLEY, M.D.
Professor of Pediatrics, Microbiology, and Medicine, Department of Pediatrics, School of Medicine, The University of Alabama at Birmingham, Birmingham

GRANT R. WILKINSON, M.D.
Professor of Pharmacology, Vanderbilt University School of Medicine, Nashville

GORDON H. WILLIAMS, M.D.
Professor of Medicine, Harvard Medical School; Chief, Endocrine-Hypertension Division, Brigham and Women's Hospital, Boston

LEWIS T. WILLIAMS, Jr., M.D., Ph.D.
Associate Professor of Medicine, University of California at San Francisco School of Medicine; Cardiovascular Research Institute, Howard Hughes Medical Institute, San Francisco

JEAN D. WILSON, M.D.
Professor of Internal Medicine, The University of Texas Southwestern Medical Center, Dallas

BRUCE U. WINTROUB, M.D.
Professor and Chairman, Department of Dermatology, University of California, San Francisco

SHELDON M. WOLFF, M.D.
Endiocott Professor and Chairman, Department of Medicine, Tufts University School of Medicine; New England Medical Center, Boston

ALASTAIR J.J. WOOD, M.B., Ch.B., F.R.C.P. (Edin)
Professor of Medicine and Professor of Pharmacology, Vanderbilt University School of Medicine; Attending Physician, Vanderbilt University Hospital, Nashville

THEODORE E. WOODWARD, M.D.
Professor of Medicine Emeritus, University of Maryland School of Medicine, Baltimore

SHIRLEY H. WRAY, M.D., Ph.D., F.R.C.P.
Associate Professor of Neurology, Harvard Medical School; Director, Unit for Neurovisual Disorders, Department of Neurology, Massachusetts General Hospital, Boston

JOSHUA WYNNE, M.D.
Professor of Internal Medicine and Chief, Division of Cardiology, Wayne State University School of Medicine; Chief, Section of Cardiology, Harper Grace Hospitals, Detroit

KIM B. YANCEY, M.D.
Department of Dermatology, Uniformed Services University of the Health Sciences, Bethesda

JAMES B. YOUNG, M.D.
Associate Professor of Medicine, Harvard Medical School; Associate Physician, Beth Israel Hospital, Boston

PREFACE

In the twelfth edition of *Harrison's Principles of Internal Medicine* the editors have again attempted to incorporate the latest advances in the biology, pathophysiology, diagnosis, and treatment of disease and simultaneously to build appropriate bridges between the basic sciences and clinical medicine and emphasize the advances in medical science while retaining those facts which, while not new, remain clinically useful. Although in a preface we cannot describe all of the new and extensively updated parts of the eleventh edition, we would like to call the reader's attention to several of these:

"Introduction to Clinical Medicine" contains articles on the practice of medicine, clinical reasoning, cost awareness in medicine, and geriatric medicine.

"The Biological Basis of Disease," Part One, has been expanded and given added emphasis as the text's first major topic. It focuses on disorders affecting multiple organ systems, especially genetic diseases and disturbances of the immune system. The section provides more detailed coverage of cell growth and regulation with new chapters on normal cell growth and growth factors and on cell membranes and their receptors.

Now Part Two, "Cardinal Manifestations of Disease" remains a mainstay of this edition and serves as a comprehensive introduction to clinical medicine. Major patient symptoms, reviewed by organ system, are correlated with specific disease states—the basis of differential diagnosis. The twelfth edition contains new or rewritten chapters on chills and fever, visual disturbances, assessment of patients with disorders of cognition, disorders of sleep and circadian rhythm, prevention of cardiovascular collapse and death, and management of the resuscitated patient. The section on skin disease has been completely reorganized.

Part Three, "Clinical Pharmacology," and Part Four, "Nutrition," also have been reorganized. Chapters on clinical pharmacology review the fundamentals of clinical pharmacokinetics and individualized drug therapy. Up-to-date coverage of the physiology and pharmacology of the autonomic nervous system explores its key role in many disease states and the various ways in which drugs interact with this system. Included here as well is a new chapter on cyclic AMP and cellular messengers that work through G proteins.

Coverage of nutrition in clinical medicine encompasses nutritional requirements, the assessment of nutritional status, eating disorders such as anorexia nervosa, bulimia, and obesity, vitamin deficiency and excess, and disturbances in trace element metabolism. New discussions are featured on diet therapy and enteral and parenteral nutrition.

A primarily etiologically oriented review, Part Five, "Infectious Disease," details the latest approaches to the diagnosis, prevention, and treatment of bacterial, viral, and fungal infections and parasitic infestations. A new section focusing on commonly encountered clinical syndromes reviews septicemia and septic shock, infectious endocarditis, localized infections and abscesses, acute infectious diarrheal diseases, sexually transmitted diseases, pelvic inflammatory disease, acute urinary tract infections, infectious arthritis and osteomyelitis, and animal bite and scratch infections. Chapters on the treatment of bacterial, viral, mycotic, and parasitic infections have been grouped together and follow the section on the syndromic approach to infectious diseases.

In addition, a new chapter, "Infectious Diseases and the New Biology," accompanies major updates on host-microbe interactions, immunization, diphtheria, tetanus, botulism, meningococcal infections, salmonella infections, shigellosis, *Haemophilus* infections, cholera, Lyme disease, human retroviruses, Epstein-Barr virus, cytomegalovirus infection, leishmaniasis, trypanosomiasis, and filariasis.

"Disorders of the Organ Systems," the core of *Harrison's*, encompass Parts Six through Fourteen and include succinct accounts of the pathophysiology of major diseases—with emphasis on disease manifestations, diagnostic procedures, differential diagnosis, and treatment strategies. This comprehensive review of organ system disorders includes new chapters on therapeutic applications of cardiac catheterization, mechanical ventilatory support, endocrine tumors of the gastrointestinal tract and pancreas, cancer chemotherapy, breast cancer, benign and malignant skin lesions, gastrointestinal and pancreatic tumors, cognitive disorders, disorders of sleep and circadian rhythm, paraneoplastic diseases that affect the central nervous system, myasthenia gravis, and disorders of phosphorus and magnesium metabolism. Of particular note, the chapter on the acquired immunodeficiency syndrome has been expanded and revised to provide in-depth understanding of all aspects of this disease.

In the twelfth edition the comprehensive review of organ system disorders is complemented by a series of new chapters highlighting the impact of cellular and molecular biology on the understanding of cardiovascular, pulmonary, hematologic, renal, and neurologic disease. The impact of newer imaging techniques on diagnoses is described in chapters on the use of such techniques in diseases of the cardiovascular, pulmonary, hepatobiliary, and central nervous systems.

Finally Part Fifteen is an expanded and reorganized section on "Environmental and Occupational Hazards."

In organizing this edition of *Harrison's* the editors faced the special problem of the dual systems of laboratory nomenclature within the United States. Since July of 1988 virtually all medical journals throughout the world have utilized the International System (SI) of units for clinical laboratory values whereas most hospital laboratories in the United States use the conventional system of laboratory nomenclature. The net consequence is that the student of medicine uses one system in reading medical literature and another in dealing with patients. This dual system will probably be in operation for the indefinite future, and consequently we have decided to use both systems in the text, listing the SI units first and the conventional units in parentheses for all measurements except blood pressure, which is given only in millimeters of mercury, and for those measurements in which the numbers are the same for both systems (mmol/L or meq/L for sodium). In most instances the interconversion between SI and conventional units is straightforward. In other cases, however, the best way to convert from one system to the other is not always clearcut since there are different ways to express values in both. It is imperative that each reader consult his own laboratory for normal values. Perhaps the greatest potential danger inherent in the existence of the two systems is in the interpretation of plasma glucose and plasma calcium, but caution should be observed in the interpretation of all laboratory values.

In view of the requirements for continuing education for licensure and relicensure and of the emphasis on certification and recertification, a revision of the *PreTest Self-Assessment and Review* will appear with this edition. *PreTest Self-Assessment and Review* consists of several hundred questions based upon the textbook, along with answers and explanations for the answers. In addition, the *Companion Handbook* that was pioneered for the eleventh edition for use as a supplement to the text will be revised and updated.

One of the strengths of *Harrison's* is the close-knit relationships among the editors. Dr. Richard K. Root, Professor of Medicine and Associate Dean for Clinical Education at the University of California, San Francisco, worked together with Robert G. Petersdorf to edit the infectious disease coverage of the twelfth edition. We welcome Dr. Root as a valuable member of the editorial group.

We also wish to express our appreciation to our many associates and colleagues who as experts in their fields have helped us with constructive criticism and helpful suggestions: Raymond D. Adams, Carmen Allegra, Julian L. Ambrus, Jr., W. French Anderson, David

W. Bilheimer, Homer Boushey, George A. Bray, Barry M. Brenner, Neil A. Breslau, Michael S. Brown, William J. Burke, Harold A. Chapman, Allen W. Cheever, William W. Chin, Fred Cohen, Shaun Coughlin, George T. Curlin, Pat O. Daley, Richard T. Davey, Jr., Gregory J. Dehmer, Victor J. Dzau, Judith Falloon, Robert Fishman, Daniel W. Foster, Stephen Friend, Joseph L. Goldstein, Mark R. Green, James E. Griffin, Donald H. Harter, Jane E. Henney, Gary Hoffman, Allan Hunter, Steve Hyman, Roland H. Ingram, Jr., Seigo Izumo, Michael Jenike, Stephanie L. James, T. Scott Johnson, William S. Jordan, Jr., Lewis L. Judd, Robert E. Kalina, Robert Katzman, Joyce V. Kelly, Jeff Klein, Joseph A. Kovacs, Thomas J. Lawley, Robert S. Lebovics, John Leddy, Kenneth Luskey, James D. Marsh, Michael Matthay, Dale E. McFarlin, Steve McPhee, John Mendelsohn, John Mills, Eva J. Neer, Arthur W. Niehnuis, Frederick P. Ognibene, Steve Perkins, Dorothy Perloff, Stephen Petersdorf, Michael A. Polis, Herbert Y. Reynolds, William O. Robertson, Mark Rosenblum, Burton D. Rose, Daniel Rotrosen, Eugene H. Rubin, Walter Rubin, Kenneth Sack, Steven Schnittman, Christine E. Seidman, Julian Seifter, James H. Shelhamer, Gordon Strewler, Anthony F. Suffredini, Martin Tauber, Mark Taubman, Steven E. Weinberger, J. Woodrow Weiss, Scott Weiss, J.B. West, Peggy Wintroub, Daniel T. Wright, and Charles F. Zormuski.

This book could not have been edited without the dedicated help of our coworkers in the editorial offices of the individual editors. We are especially indebted to Patricia A. Clougherty, Hilda Gardner, Christy K. Gonzales, Brenda H. Hennis, Ann London, Joyce McKinney, Lucy A. Renzi, Kathryn A. Saxon, S. Horatio Slawson, Sandra Taylor, and Betsy Zickler.

Finally, we need to say a word of thanks to our colleagues at McGraw-Hill, J. Dereck Jeffers, Editor-in-Chief, and Stuart Boynton, Development Editor. They are an effective team who gave the editors constant encouragement and were of enormous help in the efforts involved in bringing this edition to fruition.

THE EDITORS

HARRISON'S
PRINCIPLES OF
INTERNAL
MEDICINE

TWELFTH EDITION

VOLUME 2

199 IMPACT OF CELL AND MOLECULAR BIOLOGY ON PULMONARY DISEASE

RONALD G. CRYSTAL

The major function of the lung is to exchange gases with the environment. As such, its essential role is mechanical—to bring the ambient air into close proximity to the output of the right heart, permitting efficient gas exchange at little energy cost. The traditional methods used to assess the lung in health and disease reflect this role, with chest x-rays used to evaluate lung anatomy and physiologic tests to assess lung function. These approaches define the type and extent of lung abnormalities associated with various categories of lung disease, but they give little insight into the underlying pathogenic processes.

These traditional methods have now been supplemented with the disciplines of cell and molecular biology. For this to become a reality, it was first necessary to have access to sufficient numbers of purified cellular and extracellular components of the lung so that they could be evaluated in vitro. Two developments made this possible: (1) techniques permitting the purification and in vitro culture of lung inflammatory and parenchymal cells; and (2) the use of the fiberoptic bronchoscope to sample the components of the epithelial surface of the lung by bronchoalveolar lavage.

The adaptation of tissue culture techniques to lung cells made it possible to study purified human lung alveolar macrophages and T lymphocytes, as well as lung parenchymal cells including bronchial and alveolar epithelial cells, endothelial cells, and mesenchymal cells.

Bronchoalveolar lavage (BAL) is a simple extension of fiberoptic bronchoscopy and typically yields 1 to 3 mL of epithelial lining fluid containing 10 to 30 $\times$ 10⁶ inflammatory cells from normal individuals and up to 200 $\times$ 10⁶ cells from subjects with chronic inflammatory diseases. Both the extracellular and cellular components can be assessed by the techniques of cellular and molecular biology.

Four disorders will be discussed to illustrate how these techniques have led to major advances in the understanding of human lung disease: idiopathic pulmonary fibrosis, chronic beryllium disease, alpha₁ antitrypsin deficiency, and cystic fibrosis.

IDIOPATHIC PULMONARY FIBROSIS (IPF) IPF is a chronic inflammatory fibrotic disorder localized to the lower respiratory tract and characterized by an alveolitis dominated by alveolar macrophages and neutrophils and, to a lesser extent, lymphocytes and eosinophils (see Chap. 211). The disease usually presents as dyspnea on exertion, the chest x-ray shows diffuse reticulonodular infiltrates, and analysis of lung function reveals restrictive abnormalities. Evaluation of the inflammatory cells recovered by BAL has lead to the concept that the cell responsible for directing the process of scar formation is the alveolar macrophage, a cell that normally defends the alveolar structures by phagocytosing infectious agents and particulates. In IPF, for reasons not completely understood but likely related to immune complexes formed in the local milieu, the alveolar macro-

phages express several genes that code for potent polypeptide mediators capable of recruiting fibroblasts and signaling them to proliferate. The consequence is that fibroblasts are abundant in the milieu of chronic damage. Since fibroblasts secrete a collagenous extracellular matrix, more collagen, i.e., a scar, forms.

Among the polypeptide mediators released by alveolar macrophages of IPF patients is fibronectin, a 220-kDa dimeric glycoprotein that interacts with the connective tissue matrix and with specific receptors on fibroblasts. Studies of fibronectin gene expression in alveolar macrophages demonstrate that fibronectin mRNA levels correlate with fibronectin release. Indeed, alveolar macrophages recovered from IPF patients contain more fibronectin mRNA than alveolar macrophages of normals (Fig. 199-1A and B).

Perhaps the most potent alveolar macrophage "growth factor" is platelet-derived growth factor (PDGF), a glycoprotein that in human alveolar macrophages is composed of dimers of A and B chains or homodimers of B chains. The genes for the A and B chains of PDGF are on different chromosomes and are modulated independently. Interestingly, the B chain is encoded by the c-sis gene, a cellular proto-oncogene on chromosome 22 with close homology to the v-sis gene, a transforming viral oncogene. Alveolar macrophages recovered from the lower respiratory tract of individuals with IPF express c-sis mRNA transcripts, and the PDGF protein product of the c-sis gene is released by these cells at a level fourfold greater than by normal macrophages (Fig. 199-1C). Thus, a gene homologous to a viral oncogene is expressed in an exaggerated fashion in one site and contributes to a localized proliferation of mesenchymal cells and eventual organ fibrosis. Furthermore, glucocorticoid therapy (the conventional treatment) does not affect PDGF release by the macrophages. Consequently, it is no surprise that most IPF patients continue to deteriorate even when treated in this fashion.

CHRONIC BERYLLIUM DISEASE Multiple exposures to airborne beryllium dusts, salts, or fumes can result, in susceptible individuals, in a chronic interstitial lung disorder characterized by the accumulation of lymphocytes and mononuclear phagocytes and the formation of noncaseating granulomas in the lower respiratory tract (see Chap. 206). The alveolitis is dominated by alveolar macrophages and T lymphocytes, in particular, activated CD4+ helper-inducer T cells, characteristic of the T cells in sites of chronic, delayed-type hypersensitivity reactions (Fig. 199-2A). Most noteworthy, the lung T cells proliferate in response to beryllium and do so to a greater extent than do blood T cells from the same individual, i.e., the antigen-specific T cells are compartmentalized to the site of the disease (Fig. 199-2B). Furthermore, the lung T cells proliferating in response to beryllium are confined to the helper-inducer subset. The proliferative response of these lung T cells is truly beryllium specific in that the cells do not proliferate in response to other metal salts or to typical recall antigens such as tetanus toxoid or streptokinase.

Together, these observations define chronic beryllium disease as a chronic hypersensitivity disease in which beryllium-primed lung CD4+ T cells play a central role in its pathogenesis. Beryllium presumably acts as an antigen by combining (as a hapten) with one or more proteins. However, since chronic beryllium disease develops in only a small proportion of those exposed to the agent, individual susceptibility must play a major role in determining who is at risk. The proliferative response of lung T cells to beryllium provides a

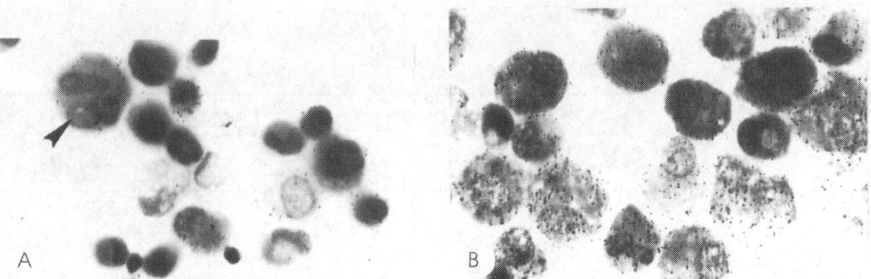

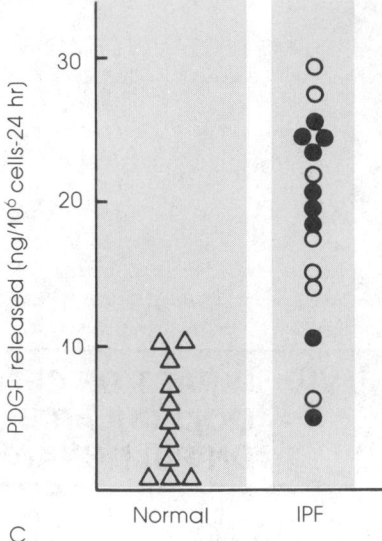

FIGURE 199-1 Exaggerated expression of alveolar macrophage genes coding for polypeptide mediators that modulate fibroblast accumulation in the alveolar walls of patients with idiopathic pulmonary fibrosis. *A.* Example of in situ hybridization analysis of fibronectin mRNA transcripts in alveolar macrophages of a normal individual. The mRNA transcripts in macrophages recovered by bronchoalveolar lavage were assessed with a ^{35}S-labeled fibronectin antisense cRNA probe and autoradiography. The grains above the macrophage (arrow) indicate fibronectin mRNA transcripts ($\times 500$). *B.* Similar to panel *A,* but with alveolar macrophages of a patient with IPF. On the average, there are twofold more fibronectin mRNA transcripts per macrophage than in normals ($\times 500$). *C.* Spontaneous exaggerated release of PDGF by alveolar macrophages recovered from the lower respiratory tract of individuals with IPF. Macrophages recovered by bronchoalveolar lavage were cultured for 24 h. Supernatants were evaluated for the presence of PDGF using a specific immunoassay. Each symbol represents one individual. For the IPF patients, closed circles represent untreated patients and open circles represent those receiving prednisone. Note that therapy has no effect on the release of this potent mediator.

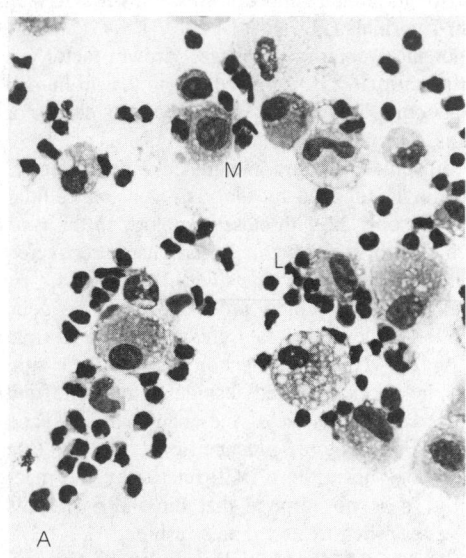

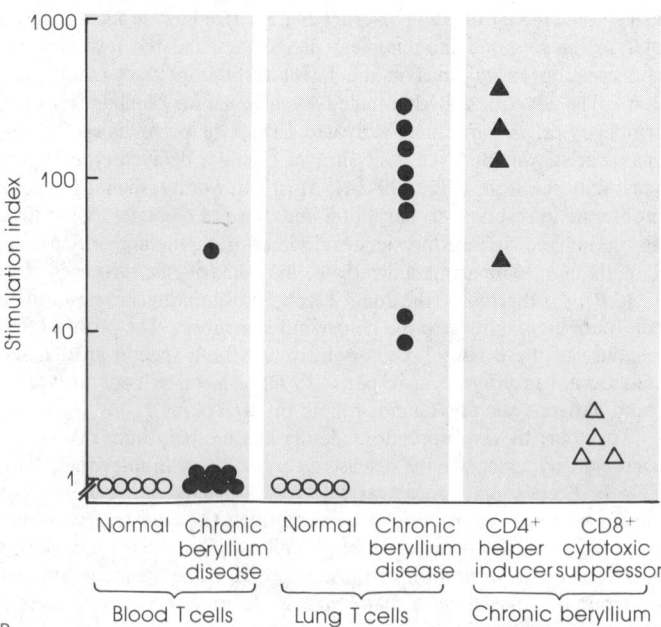

diagnostic tool to identify individuals with this disorder, thus obviating the need for chemical analysis of the lung parenchyma.

ALPHA₁ ANTITRYPSIN DEFICIENCY   Alpha$_1$ antitrypsin ($\alpha 1$AT) deficiency is a hereditary disorder characterized by reduced serum levels of $\alpha 1$AT, an antiprotease that provides the major defense for the lower respiratory tract against the ravages of neutrophil elastase, a powerful destructive protease. The loss of this protective screen of the fragile alveolar walls results in emphysema (Chap. 210).

The emphysema is the result of a variety of mutations in the $\alpha 1$AT gene on chromosome 14 (Fig. 199-3*A*). The two $\alpha 1$AT genes are codominantly expressed and together define the $\alpha 1$AT level in serum. The gene is pleomorphic with approximately 75 known alleles, of which at least 20 can cause a clinically relevant deficiency state. Most normal $\alpha 1$AT alleles are classified as M-type. Most $\alpha 1$AT is synthesized by liver hepatocytes; the enzyme is a typical secretory glycoprotein that is translated on the rough endoplasmic reticulum (RER), glycosylated in the cisternae of the RER, translocated to the Golgi, and then secreted (Fig. 199-3*B*). The two most common "deficiency" mutations are Z (exon V, Glu^{342} *GAG* → Lys *AAG*) and S (exon III, Glu^{264} *GAA* → Val G*T*A).

The Z mutation, carried by 1 in 50 Caucasians of European descent, causes hepatocytes of homozygotes to secrete only 10 to 15 percent of the normal amount of $\alpha 1$AT. Because the Glu^{342} → Lys substitution reverses the charge at this residue, the Z-type $\alpha 1$AT molecules aggregate in the RER, less $\alpha 1$AT is translocated to the Golgi, and hence $\alpha 1$AT deficiency results.

The S mutation, carried by up to 1 in 25 persons, causes a different derangement of $\alpha 1$AT processing. The hepatocytes degrade an

FIGURE 199-2 Beryllium-specific inflammatory processes in the lower respiratory tract of individuals with chronic beryllium disease. *A.* Inflammatory cells recovered by bronchoalveolar lavage of an individual with chronic beryllium disease. The alveolitis is dominated by lymphocytes (L) and alveolar macrophages (M) ($\times 500$). Flow cytometric analysis with appropriate monoclonal antibodies demonstrates that the lymphocytes are predominantly CD4$^+$ helper-inducer T lymphocytes. *B.* In vitro proliferation of blood and lung T lymphocytes of patients with chronic beryllium disease and normals in response to beryllium. The data are presented as a stimulation index (values >1 represent proliferation above control) and each symbol represents one individual. Normal blood and lung T cells rarely proliferate in response to beryllium. In contrast, lung, but not blood, T cells from individuals with chronic beryllium disease respond briskly to beryllium, with the CD4$^+$ helper-inducer T cells dominating the proliferative response.

increased proportion of the newly synthesized α1AT, resulting in less α1AT for secretion and hence the deficiency state. However, the relative "deficiency" associated with the S allele is less than that associated with Z. Consequently, S homozygotes are not at risk for emphysema, but SZ heterozygotes are at mild risk.

Z homozygotes have reduced α1AT in the lung and hence have a deficient screen against proteolytic attack by neutrophil elastase (Fig. 199-3C). While S homozygotes also have reduced α1AT levels, the amount is sufficient to afford protection, i.e., the "threshold" protective level is between that of S and Z homozygotes. Based on this concept, strategies to prevent the emphysema associated with α1AT deficiency have focused on augmenting the protective screen of the lower respiratory tract with α1AT. In this regard, intravenous administration of 60 mg/kg body weight of α1AT once a week results in α1AT serum levels sufficient to maintain lung levels above that necessary to provide sufficient antielastase protection to the alveoli, i.e., augmentation therapy reverses the biochemical abnormalities at the site of the target organ and thus is a rational approach to prevent the emphysema.

CYSTIC FIBROSIS (CF) CF is an autosomal recessive disorder of exocrine glands characterized in lung by accumulation of thick mucus, chronic bacterial infections, and chronic obstructive lung disease associated with severe bronchiectasis and parenchymal derangements (see Chap. 209). It is the most common lethal genetic disorder affecting Caucasian populations, with a heterozygote frequency of 1 in 20 to 25 individuals.

The technique of "chromosomal walking" was utilized to locate the cystic fibrosis gene to within approximately 300 kb in the q21-31 region of chromosome 7 (Fig. 199-4A). Family studies suggest that a single mutation of the CF gene is predominant. Even before the specific gene was identified, chromosomal markers were sufficiently close to permit accurate identification of CF homozygotes and of most heterozygotes and thus make possible genetic counseling.

Sequencing of the CF "gene" predicts that it codes for a protein of 168 kDa that spans the plasma membrane and contains a domain capable of binding adenosine triphosphate. Despite the fact that the function of the CF "protein" (called the *cystic fibrosis transmembrane conductance regulator*) is not known, it is possible to speculate about the pathogenesis of the disease (Fig. 199-4B). Measurement of potential differences across the tracheal epithelium of CF homozygotes has demonstrated a higher voltage than in normals, consistent with the known abnormality in electrolyte transport. In CF subjects who have received lung transplants the abnormal potential differences are no longer present. Cultured epithelial cells of CF patients exhibit abnormal potential differences similar to those observed in vivo. Importantly, the cultured epithelial cells are not capable of transporting Cl⁻ to the apical surfaces in a normal fashion. Together, these observations suggest that the abnormality of the CF gene is expressed in airway epithelial cells and implicate a dysfunction in the regulation of airway epithelial apical Cl⁻ channels as the fundamental abnor-

mality. It is hypothesized that the defect in Cl channel function causes CF lung disease by modifying the quantity and composition of the airway epithelial fluid. Presumably, such changes alter the

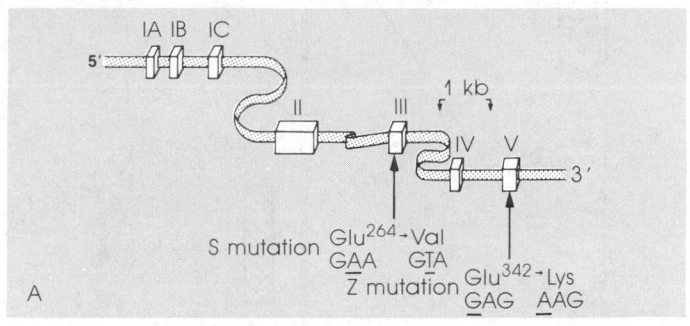

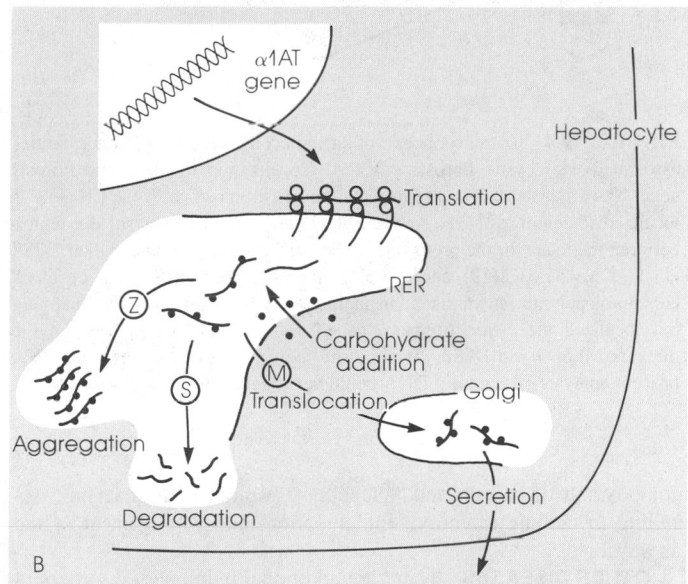

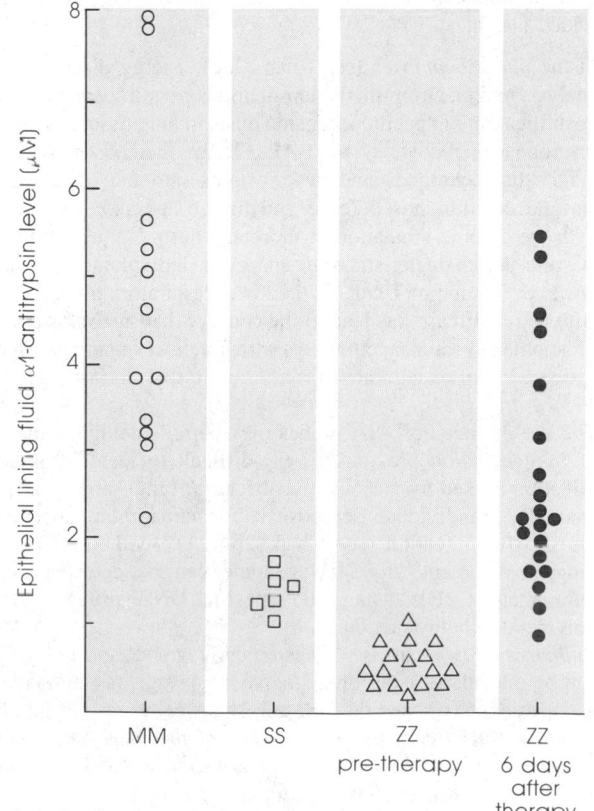

FIGURE 199-3 Pathogenesis and therapy of alpha₁ antitrypsin (α1AT) deficiency. *A.* Schematic of the 12.2-kb, 7-exon (I$_A$-I$_C$, II-V) α1AT gene. The two most common mutations of the normal M gene are S and Z. *B.* Synthesis and secretion of α1AT by hepatocytes. The normal M α1AT mRNA protein is translated on the rough endoplasmic reticulum (RER), carbohydrates are added, the molecule is translocated to the Golgi and secreted. The Z mutation results in aggregation of newly synthesized α1AT in the RER while the S mutation results in degradation. *C.* Consequences of mutations in the α1AT gene at the level of the alveoli. Shown are α1AT levels in alveolar epithelial lining fluid recovered by bronchoalveolar lavage. Each symbol represents a single individual. S and Z homozygotes have "deficient" amounts of α1AT in the lung, with the level for Z homozygotes below the threshold levels necessary to protect the lung. With once weekly intravenous augmentation therapy with purified human α1AT, the lung epithelial lining fluid α1AT level of Z homozygotes is restored above the protective threshold, thus protecting the lung from emphysema.

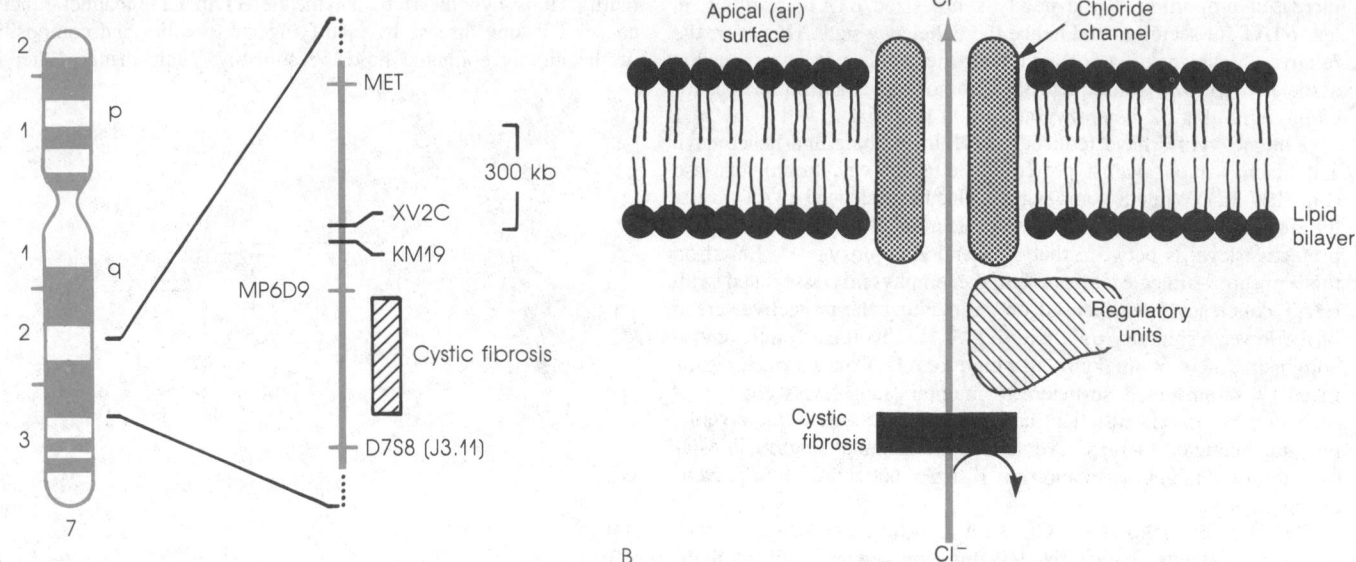

FIGURE 199-4 Current concepts of the molecular and biologic abnormalities associated with cystic fibrosis (CF). *A.* Localization of the cystic fibrosis gene. Shown at the left is a representation of chromosome 7; the CF gene is localized to region q21-31. At the right is an expanded view of the region between the locus for the proto-oncogene MET and the genomic marker D7S8 (J3.11); XV2C, KM19, and MP6D9 are other marker regions of DNA containing polymorphisms useful in haplotype analysis. Chromosomal mapping has localized the cystic fibrosis "gene" to a 250-kb region between the markers MP6D9 and D7S8. Even before the gene was identified with DNA probes, analysis of genomic DNA could accurately predict the inheritance of CF, permitting family planning. Now, specific probes have made accurate diagnosis rapid and simple. *B.* Schematic of the apical (air) membrane of an airway epithelial cell expressing the cystic fibrosis gene. In vivo measurements of electric potentials in the tracheal epithelium together with in vitro studies of cultured airway epithelial cells suggest the abnormality is related to the chloride channel on the apical surface of the epithelial cell, either directly involving a component of the channel or in regulatory units modulating its function. The control of Na^+, K^+, Cl^- through cotransporters and sodium-potassium pumps on the basolateral (serosal) surface of the epithelial cells appears normal, as does ion movement through tight junctions between cells.

composition of mucus and mucociliary clearance mechanisms, resulting in chronic infection, inflammation, and derangement of the airways.

OTHER DISEASES   There are additional pulmonary disorders in which the application of cell and molecular biology methods has provided insight.

1 In the *pneumoconioses* (see Chap. 206), energy dispersive x-ray analysis and electron diffraction methods permit identification and quantification of specific inorganic dusts in lung tissue and alveolar macrophages recovered by BAL. These methods provide new diagnostic techniques and new insights into the relationship of particle retention, host defense, and disease susceptibility associated with the chronic inhalation of inorganic dusts.

2 Despite the characteristic skin anergy in individuals with *sarcoidosis,* evaluation of T cells in the lower respiratory tract of patients with active disease has lead to the concept that sarcoid is a disease of heightened cellular immunity, with T cells responding to specific antigens in an exaggerated fashion at sites of disease (see Chap. 277).

3 The use of specific DNA probes now permits definitive diagnosis of *lung infection* previously very difficult to identify, including infection caused by various mycobacteria, fungi, and viruses. For example, in individuals seropositive for human immunodeficiency virus (HIV) infection (see Chap. 264), but without evidence of lung involvement, the HIV genome can be detected in lung inflammatory cells using HIV-specific DNA primers and the polymerase chain reaction.

4 *Pulmonary histiocytosis X* (eosinophilic granuloma of the lung) can be diagnosed using bronchoalveolar lavage and a monoclonal antibody (OKT6) specific for Langerhans cells (see Chap. 211).

5 In the *respiratory distress syndrome of the newborn,* immature alveolar type II cells do not produce sufficient surfactant to maintain alveolar stability, leading to lung collapse (see Chap. 201). The control of surfactant biosynthesis in alveolar type II cells has been delineated using cell culture techniques, strategies have been developed to accelerate the expression of the surfactant system using pharmacologic agents, and the biochemical nature of surfactant has been fully defined. This definition has led to cloning of the apoproteins of surfactant, allowing in vitro reconstitution of an artificial surfactant for use in therapy.

6 In *asthma,* cell biology methodologies have led to the identification of a broad armamentarium of naturally occurring mediators that likely play a role in the pathogenesis of reversible airway disease, and several genes related to these mediators have been cloned and characterized (see Chap. 204).

7 Finally, capitalizing on the identification, cloning, and in vitro production of a variety of potent "inflammatory" polypeptides, much attention has been given to the concept that mediators such as tumor necrosis factor play a role in modulating the parenchymal dysfunction characteristic of the respiratory failure of *adult respiratory distress syndrome.*

CONCLUSIONS   The application of modern cell and biology methods to investigate human disease depends on the capacity to obtain appropriate biologic materials relevant to the pathogenesis of the disease. For most diseases, the relevant biologic material must be obtained directly from the target organ, and this is a difficult task for internal organs. Utilizing cell culture techniques and the fiberoptic bronchoscope to gain access to the epithelial surface of the lung, many pulmonary disorders can now be investigated by the techniques of cell and molecular biology. As a consequence there has been a remarkable advance in the understanding of the pathogenesis of a variety of lung disorders and for several new insights into therapy.

REFERENCES

ADACHI K et al: Evaluation of fibronectin gene expression by *in situ* hybridization: Differential expression of the fibronectin gene among populations of human alveolar macrophages. Am J Pathol 138:193, 1988

BRANTLY M et al: Molecular basis of α1-antitrypsin deficiency. Am J Med 84:13, 1988

CRYSTAL RG et al: Interstitial lung disease of unknown cause: Disorders characterized by chronic inflammation of the lower respiratory tract. N Engl J Med 310:154, 235, 1984

——— ct al: Thc α1-antitrypsin gcnc and its mutations: Clinical conscqucnccs and strategies for therapy. Chest 95:196, 1989

MARTINET Y et al: Exaggerated spontaneous release of a platelet-derived growth factor by alveolar macrophages from patients with idiopathic pulmonary fibrosis. N Engl J Med 317(4):202, 1987

REYNOLDS HY: Bronchoalveolar lavage. Am Rev Respir Dis 135:250, 1987

RIORDAN JR et al: Identification of the cystic fibrosis gene: Cloning and characterization of complementary DNA. Science 245:1066, 1989

ROMMENS JM et al: Identification of the cystic fibrosis gene: Chromosome walking and jumping. Science 245:1059, 1989

SALTINI C et al: Chronic pulmonary berylliosis: Maintenance of the alveolitis by proliferation of beryllium-specific helper T-cells. N Engl J Med 230:1103, 1989

WELSH MJ, FICK RB: Cystic fibrosis. J Clin Invest 80:1523, 1987

WEWERS MD et al: Replacement therapy for alpha 1-antitrypsin deficiency associated with emphysema. N Engl J Med 316:1055, 1987

YAMAUCHI K et al: Modulation of fibronectin gene expression in human mononuclear phagocytes. J Clin Invest 80(6):1720, 1987

200 APPROACH TO THE PATIENT WITH DISEASE OF THE RESPIRATORY SYSTEM

EUGENE BRAUNWALD

As in other branches of medicine, a careful and detailed history and physical examination are the cornerstones for establishing an accurate diagnosis in patients with disorders of the respiratory system. In addition, the roentgenographic examination occupies a particularly important role in the evaluation of patients with lung disease. Since abnormalities of the respiratory system are frequently a manifestation of a systemic process, attention must be focused not only on the chest but also a comprehensive evaluation of the patient's entire health status is essential. For example, the presence of a pulmonary lesion on x-ray may be due to metastatic disease with the primary tumor elsewhere, and hemoptysis may be due to a disorder of hemostasis. Diffuse scleroderma may result in diffuse pulmonary infiltrative disease (Chap. 271), and multiple pulmonary cavities may be a manifestation of Wegener's granulomatosis (Chap. 276). All of the so-called collagen vascular diseases may have prominent pulmonary manifestations. Carcinoma of the lung (Chap. 215) may be accompanied by prominent extrathoracic manifestations, which may overshadow the pulmonary lesion. These include myopathy, peripheral neuropathy, hypertrophic pulmonary osteoarthropathy, and a variety of endocrine and metabolic manifestations, including Cushing's syndrome, the carcinoid syndrome, a hyperparathyroid-like picture, inappropriate secretion of antidiuretic hormone, gonadotropin (Chap. 309), and increased frequency of pulmonary infections.

HISTORY In eliciting the history of patients with pulmonary disease, it must be appreciated that an increasing fraction of the population is exposed to materials which are potentially toxic to the lung (Chap. 206). The history must therefore contain a detailed *occupational and personal history* with a description of exposure to hazards such as asbestos, coal, silica, beryllium, bagasse, iron oxide, tin oxide, cotton dust, titanium oxide, silver, nitrogen dioxide, animals, moldy hay, air conditioners, and furnace humidifiers. It is useful to construct a work history, which includes the patient's duties, duration of exposure, use of protective devices, and illness in fellow workers. The occupational history should include information on a job-by-job basis as well as the military service. Contact with both wild and domestic animals may result in pulmonary symptoms, such as bronchospasm in subjects allergic to pets, or, less commonly, acute pneumonitis in patients with psittacosis (Chap. 155), tularemia (Chap. 120), or Q fever. Because it is such an important risk factor for many forms of lung disease, history of tobacco consumption,

especially cigarette smoking, must be sought and should be quantified, generally in "pack-years." It is important to record the residence and travel histories; histoplasmosis and coccidioidomyosis (Chap. 151) are indigenous to certain regions. The habits of the patient with pulmonary disease must be gone into. Aspiration pneumonia and pneumococcal and *Klebsiella* pneumonia are often seen in alcoholics; lung abscess occurs in intravenous drug abusers.

Pneumocystis carinii pneumonia and other lung infections are frequent complications of the acquired immunodeficiency syndrome (Chap. 264), and a history of intravenous drug abuse or of sexual relations with individuals at high risk for this condition should be obtained, especially in patients with a pulmonary infiltrate and fever. A record of the patient's *previous residence* is of considerable importance in the diagnosis of histoplasmosis (the south and mid-western United States), coccidioidomycosis (the southwestern United States), tropical eosinophilia, and South American blastomycosis. For example, pulmonary mass lesions in patients in the Mediterranean Basin may be due to hydatid cysts, hemoptysis in patients from central China may be caused by paragonimiasis (Chap. 171), and cor pulmonale in Egypt frequently results from schistosomiasis (Chap. 170).

It is vitally important to elicit a history of *drug exposure* since essentially every class of drugs can produce pulmonary toxicity (Chap. 205), and all parts of the respiratory apparatus can be affected, including the alveoli, tracheobronchial tree, mediastinum, pleural cavities, pulmonary vessels, respiratory muscles, and the medullary respiratory center. Examples include the interstitial infiltrative diseases caused by bleomycin, cyclophosphamide, methotrexate, and nitrofurantoin; noncardiogenic pulmonary edema caused by aspirin; bronchospasm caused by beta-adrenergic blockers and nonsteroidal anti-inflammatory drugs; pulmonary vasculitis from intravenous drug abuse; pulmonary thromboembolism in women receiving oral contraceptives; (drug-induced) systemic lupus erythematosus with pleural involvement caused by hydralazine and procainamide; and weakness of the respiratory muscles caused by the aminoglycoside antibiotics.

The *family history* should consider pulmonary diseases which may be genetic, such as cystic disease of the lung, pulmonary emphysema due to alpha₁ antitrypsin deficiency (Chap. 210), cystic fibrosis (Chap. 209), asthma (Chap. 204), hereditary telangiectasia, Kartagener's syndrome, and alveolar microlithiasis, as well as infections due to the tubercle bacilli, fungi, and schistosoma where exposure to involved family members is important.

Dyspnea is a cardinal manifestation of diseases involving the respiratory and cardiovascular systems (Chap. 36). A detailed physical examination of both organ systems is therefore mandatory in every patient with this symptom. Dyspnea secondary to cardiac disease is often recognized by the presence of other evidence of heart failure, such as cardiac enlargement, gallop rhythms, and cardiac murmurs. It may be difficult to differentiate paroxysmal nocturnal dyspnea due to pulmonary edema of cardiac origin from nocturnal attacks of bronchial asthma and from chronic pulmonary disease with pooling of the secretions in the recumbent position, but a detailed description of the circumstances in which this symptom occurs is most useful. Dyspnea also is a common functional complaint, and an important clue in the identification of this form is the observation that shortness of breath often occurs at rest and is relieved during cxcrtion; thc opposite is the case in patients in whom this symptom is secondary to disease of the lungs or heart. Equally important in the differential diagnosis is a careful elucidation of the relationship of dyspnea to other symptoms such as cough or angina pectoris.

Patients with diseases involving the respiratory system may also present with *chest pain* which is frequently caused by inflammation of the pleura, occurring in pneumonia, pulmonary thromboembolism, tuberculosis, and malignancy (Chap. 16). Pleuritic pain is usually localized to one side of the chest and is related to respiration and to movements of the thorax. Lesions confined to the pulmonary parenchyma do not produce pain, while diseases involving the organs in the mediastinum (Chap. 216) may cause local discomfort with radiation characteristic of the specific organ. Pain may also originate in or be referred to the chest wall; it may be due to intercostal neuritis, as in herpes zoster, or to compression of the intercostal nerves as they leave the spinal cord. Such pain is often superficial in character and may be related to coughing and straining. Thoracic pain may also be due to myositis, costochondral disturbances, myocardial ischemia, pericarditis, esophageal disease, and aortic dissection and aneurysm (Chap. 16). The most common causes of pain related to respiration are disorders of the chest wall, pleurisy, intercostal neuritis, and costochondral disease. The latter condition characteristically causes chest pain intensified by palpation. A major task is to distinguish chest pain due to abnormalities of the bronchopulmonary system from that due to myocardial ischemia (see Chap. 16).

Cough and *expectoration* are also cardinal features of pulmonary disease (Chap. 35). Few patients can describe the severity of cough or quantity of expectoration reliably, and it is therefore desirable for the physician to inspect a 24-h collection of sputum. A cough productive of sputum is usually caused by an inflammatory process, while a nonproductive cough is caused by an irritative process. Cough is often precipitated by foreign materials irritating nerve endings in airways and is frequently caused by inflammation of the bronchi; the latter may be persistent (as in patients with a cigarette cough and chronic bronchitis) or acute (as in a variety of viral and bacterial infections). The time of occurrence of the cough and the character and quantity of expectorated material may point to the diagnosis. For example, bronchiectasis, lung abscess, and necrotizing pneumonia can produce purulent sputum which may have an offensive odor or be streaked with blood (Chaps. 207 and 208). In pulmonary edema, the sputum is pink, frothy, and watery (Chap. 36). Mucoid (translucent, viscid, shiny, white or gray) or mucopurulent (mucoid with flecks of yellow or green pus) sputum is characteristic of acute and chronic bronchitis. Sputum is bloody or rusty in pneumonia; it is thick, gelatinous, brick red, and laced with pus in *Klebsiella* pneumonia. Paroxysmal cough may also be the presenting feature in patients with bronchial asthma, in whom physical examination reveals wheezing respirations and squeaking musical sounds (Chap. 204), as well as in patients with left ventricular failure, in whom it generally occurs at night and in the recumbent position (Chap. 182). Pulmonary tuberculosis (Chap. 125), though less common than previously, remains a common cause of chronic cough, as does primary neoplasm of the lung (Chap. 215). A change in the character of a chronic cough, unaccompanied by an acute infection, should alert the physician to the need of carrying out a detailed examination.

Hemoptysis is often a frightening symptom (Chap. 35). Faint streaking of the sputum with blood may be observed in acute infections of the respiratory tract. However, many patients with bloody sputum have serious disease, such as pulmonary thromboembolism, tuberculosis, critical mitral stenosis, neoplasm of the lung, or bronchiec-

tasis. In all instances it is necessary to exclude sources of blood in the nasopharynx and bleeding of gastric or esophageal origin. The character of the bloody expectorate should be defined, since it may be helpful in identifying the underlying disease process. Sputum which is frankly bloody without mucus or pus may be due to pulmonary thromboembolism (Chap. 213). When pus is present, pneumonia, bronchiectasis, or lung abscess should be considered. Dilute, pink, frothy sputum is observed in acute pulmonary edema (Chap. 36).

PHYSICAL EXAMINATION   A careful examination of the thorax, including inspection, palpation, percussion, and auscultation, often provides the clue to the diagnosis of many common pulmonary disorders (Table 200-1). In addition, a meticulous *general physical examination* is mandatory in patients with disorders of the respiratory system. Enlarged lymph nodes in the cervical and supraclavicular regions should be sought. Disturbances of mentation or even coma occur in patients with acute carbon dioxide retention and hypoxemia. Telltale stains on the fingers point to heavy cigarette smoking; infected teeth and gums may occur in patients with aspiration pneumonitis and lung abscess; characteristic cutaneous lesions may point to sarcoidosis (Chap. 277), collagen vascular disease, Wegener's granulomatosis, and berylliosis, all of which may have prominent pulmonary manifestations. Clubbing of the fingers or, when advanced, osteoarthropathy (Chap. 284) may suggest carcinoma (Chap. 215) or suppurative disease (Chap. 207) of the lung; chronic hypoxemia, as occurs in patients with chronic bronchitis (Chap. 210); pulmonary arteriovenous fistula; or congenital heart disease with right-to-left shunt (Chap. 186). However, clubbing is also seen in some patients with biliary cirrhosis, regional enteritis, and ulcerative colitis. A careful search for infection in the teeth, gums, tonsils, or sinuses is recommended in patients suspected or known to have bronchiectasis or lung abscess. Neurologic findings including headache, drowsiness, papilledema, and other evidence of increased intracranial pressure may occur in patients with pulmonary disease who have hypoxemia and hypercapnia. Vascular collapse is a late complication of carbon dioxide intoxication and is characterized by hypotension, flushed skin, sweating, and tachycardia. A detailed examination of the cardiovascular system (Chap. 174) is mandatory in patients suspected of having respiratory disease and in patients with unexplained dyspnea, cough, or cyanosis because of the frequent difficulty of differentiating disorders of the respiratory and cardiovascular systems.

DIAGNOSTIC TESTS   The *roentgenographic examination* of the chest represents the cornerstone of the diagnostic workup of the patient with suspected pulmonary disease, and it is the integration of the information obtained from the clinical examination and the roentgenogram which often provides the key to diagnosis. Every effort must be made to obtain past chest x-rays. Unfortunately, physical examination of the chest has been deemphasized, largely because of the recognition of the enormous value of radiographic

---

TABLE 200-1   Physical findings in some common pulmonary disorders

Disorder	Inspection	Palpation	Percussion	Auscultation
Bronchial asthma (acute attack)	Hyperinflation; use of accessory muscles	Impaired expansion; decreased fremitus	Hyperresonant; low diaphragm	Prolonged expiration; inspiratory and expiratory wheezes
Pneumothorax (complete)	Lag on affected side	Absent fremitus	Hyperresonant or tympanitic	Absent breath sounds
Pleural effusion (large)	Lag on affected side	Decreased fremitus; trachea and heart shifted away from affected side	Dullness or flatness	Absent breath sounds
Atelectasis (lobar obstruction)	Lag on affected side	Decreased fremitus; trachea and heart shifted toward affected side	Dullness or flatness	Absent breath sounds
Consolidation (pneumonia)	Possible lag or splinting on affected side	Increased fremitus	Dullness	Bronchial breath sounds; bronchophony; pectoriloquy; crackles

SOURCE: JF Murray, in *Textbook of Respiratory Medicine*, JF Murray, JA Nadel (eds), p 449.

techniques. However, abnormalities such as small or moderate amounts of fluid in the alveoli or in the mediastinum, bronchospasm, and pleural effusions can often be detected more accurately by physical examination than by chest roentgenography. Tracheal deviation can be readily recognized on physical examination and may be observed in obstruction of a major bronchus and in atelectasis.

Chest roentgenograms obtained in the lateral decubitus position frequently reveal small pleural effusions not evident in the upright posture. A number of other abnormalities may be associated with normal roentgenograms. These include solitary lesions less than 6 mm in diameter, acute pulmonary thromboembolism without infarction, early interstitial pneumonia, diffuse granulomatous disease such as miliary tuberculosis, interstitial disease such as scleroderma and systemic lupus erythematosus, bronchiectasis, acute chronic bronchitis, mild to moderate emphysema, endobronchial masses only partially obstructing the airways, and the majority of instances of hypoventilation due to disorders of the central nervous system or neuromuscular disease. On the other hand, gross abnormalities of thoracic structure; pulmonary, mediastinal, and pleural masses; parenchymal consolidation, cysts, cavities, and abnormalities of the pulmonary vascular bed are all detected more reliably by roentgenographic than by physical examination.

An abnormal chest roentgenogram may be the presenting feature in an asymptomatic patient. In such circumstances the physician must make every effort to obtain earlier films in order to determine whether the lesion is new or old. Laminography, computed tomography, magnetic resonance imaging (Chap. 202), angiocardiography, and pulmonary scintigraphy are additional procedures which may be helpful in establishing a diagnosis in a patient with an abnormality on the plain chest roentgenogram.

A variety of other diagnostic procedures are helpful in the workup of the patient with known or suspected pulmonary disease. These are discussed in Chap. 203 and include skin tests for tuberculosis; scratch or intradermal tests to detect atopic reactions; appropriate serum complement fixation tests; and examination and culture of the sputum, pleural fluid, and bronchial washings. Bronchoscopy, bronchial brushings, and bronchoscopic biopsy have been greatly facilitated by the development of the fiberoptic bronchoscope. Mediastinoscopy, scalene node and mediastinal node biopsy, and pleural and lung biopsy may also be instrumental in establishing a diagnosis in an otherwise asymptomatic patient. Particularly important points which must be investigated in the history of the asymptomatic patient with an abnormality discovered on a routine chest roentgenogram include exposure to individuals with tuberculosis; previous tuberculin and fungal skin tests; residence in or visits to areas where fungal disease is endemic; a history of smoking and of exposure to dusts; and symptoms of systemic disease such as fever, sweat, fatigue, and weight loss. Physiologic (lung function) studies (Chap. 201) are of limited value in establishing an etiologic diagnosis in the patient with pulmonary diseases. They are, however, very helpful in assessing the physiologic consequences of disorders of the respiratory system and chest wall, as well as in following the effects of their progression or remission. Simple functional tests, such as observing the patient climbing one or two flights of stairs, are often valuable in determining whether or not the patient is grossly disabled.

In the approach to a patient with pulmonary disease, consideration must be given to the observation that substantial changes in the relative incidence of disease affecting the respiratory system have taken place in the United States during the past three decades. The prevalence of chronic infectious disorders such as tuberculosis, lung abscess, and bronchiectasis have decreased. On the other hand, patients with chronic bronchitis and with emphysema now survive longer and form an increasing fraction of patients with chronic respiratory disease, as do patients with environmental lung disease and with drug-induced disease. Modern intercontinental travel has increased the appearance in the western world of parasitic infestations of the lung. Also, the reduction of immunologic competence which occurs in patients with the acquired immunodeficiency syndrome

(Chap. 264) and in diabetics as well as in the treatment of patients with a variety of malignancies and those receiving immunosuppressive drugs has led to an increasing incidence of opportunistic infections of the lungs with a variety of microorganisms rarely pathogenic in the past.

REFERENCES

FISHMAN AP (ed): *Pulmonary Diseases and Disorders*, 2d ed. New York, McGraw-Hill, 1988

MURRAY JF: History and physical examination in *Textbook of Respiratory Medicine*, JF Murray, JA Nadel (eds). Philadelphia, WB Saunders, 1988, pp 431–451

BAUM GL, WOLINSKY E: *Textbook of Pulmonary Diseases*, 4th ed. Boston, Little, Brown, 1989

201 DISTURBANCES OF RESPIRATORY FUNCTION

STEVEN E. WEINBERGER / JEFFREY M. DRAZEN

The respiratory system includes the lungs, the central nervous system, the chest wall (with the diaphragm and intercostal muscles), and the pulmonary circulation. The CNS is the system controller, regulating the activity of the muscles of the chest wall, which serve as the respiratory system pump. As these components of the respiratory system act in concert to achieve gas exchange, malfunction of an individual component or alteration of the relationships among components can lead to disturbances in function. In this chapter, we consider three major aspects of disturbed respiratory function: (1) disturbances in ventilatory function, (2) disturbances in the pulmonary circulation, and (3) disturbances in gas exchange. Disorders relating to CNS control of ventilation are discussed in Chap. 217.

DISTURBANCES IN VENTILATORY FUNCTION

Ventilation is the process whereby the lungs provide fresh air to the alveoli. Measurements of ventilatory function in common diagnostic use consist of quantification of the air contained within the lungs under certain circumstances and the rate at which air can be expelled from the lungs. Two measurements of lung volume commonly used for respiratory diagnosis are total lung capacity (TLC) and residual volume (RV). The former is the volume of gas contained within the lungs after a maximal inspiration, while the latter is the volume of gas remaining within the lungs at the end of a maximal expiration. The volume of gas that is exhaled from the lungs in going from TLC to RV is called the vital capacity (VC) (Fig. 201-1).

Common clinical measurements of airflow are obtained from maneuvers in which the subject inspires to TLC and then forcibly exhales to RV. Three measurements are commonly made from a volume-time recording; i.e., a spirogram, obtained during such a forced expiratory maneuver: (1) the volume of gas exhaled during the first second of expiration (forced expiratory volume in 1 s or FEV_1); (2) the total volume exhaled (forced vital capacity of FVC); and (3) the average expiratory flow rate during the middle 50 percent of the vital capacity (maximal midexpiratory flow rate or MMFR; also called forced expiratory flow from 25 to 75 percent of the vital capacity, or $FEF_{25-75\%}$) (Fig. 201-2A).

PHYSIOLOGIC FEATURES The lungs are elastic structures, containing collagen and elastic fibers which resist expansion. In order for normal lungs to contain air, they must be distended by either a positive internal pressure, i.e., within the airways and alveolar spaces, or a negative external pressure, i.e., outside of the lung. The relationship between the volume of gas contained within the lungs

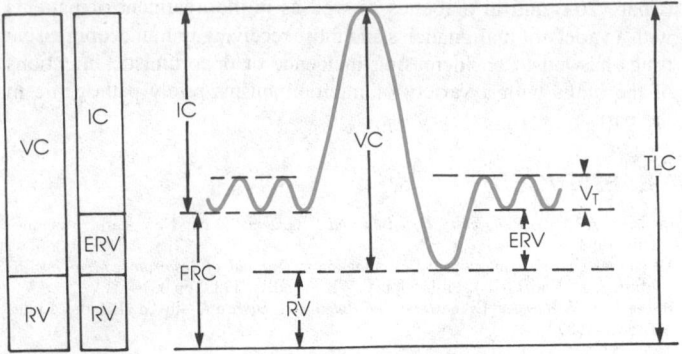

FIGURE 201-1 Lung volumes, shown by block diagrams (*left*) and by a spirographic tracing (*right*). TLC = total lung capacity; VC = vital capacity; RV = residual volume; IC = inspiratory capacity; ERV = expiratory reserve volume; FRC = functional residual capacity; V_T = tidal volume. (*From Weinberger*.)

and the distending pressure (transpulmonary pressure or P_{TP}, defined as internal pressure minus external pressure) is described by the pressure-volume curve of the lungs (Fig. 201-3*A*).

The chest wall is also an elastic structure, with properties similar to that of an expandable and compressible spring. The relationship between the volume enclosed by the chest wall and the distending pressure for the chest wall is described by the pressure-volume curve of the chest wall (Fig. 201-3*B*). For the chest wall to assume a volume different from its resting volume, the internal or external pressures acting on it must be altered. A positive distending pressure expands the chest wall, while a negative distending pressure compresses it.

Under normal circumstances, the lungs sit within the chest wall, so that the pressures and the forces acting on these structures are interrelated (Fig. 201-3*C*). At functional residual capacity (FRC), i.e., at the end of a normal exhalation, the lungs are partially inflated, so that their elastic recoil exerts a force tending to empty the lungs. At the same time, chest wall volume is such that its elastic recoil promotes outward expansion. Functional residual capacity occurs at the lung volume at which the tendency of the lungs to contract is

FIGURE 201-2 Spirographic tracings of forced expiration, comparing a normal tracing (*A*) and tracings in obstructive (*B*) and parenchymal restrictive (*C*) disease. Calculation of FVC, FEV_1, and MMFR is shown only for the normal tracing. Since there is no measure of absolute starting volume with spirometry, the curves are artificially positioned to show the relative starting lung volumes in the different conditions.

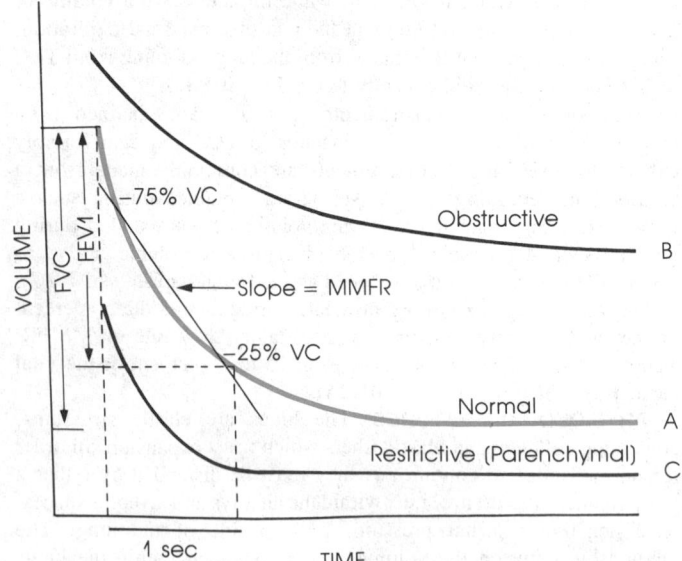

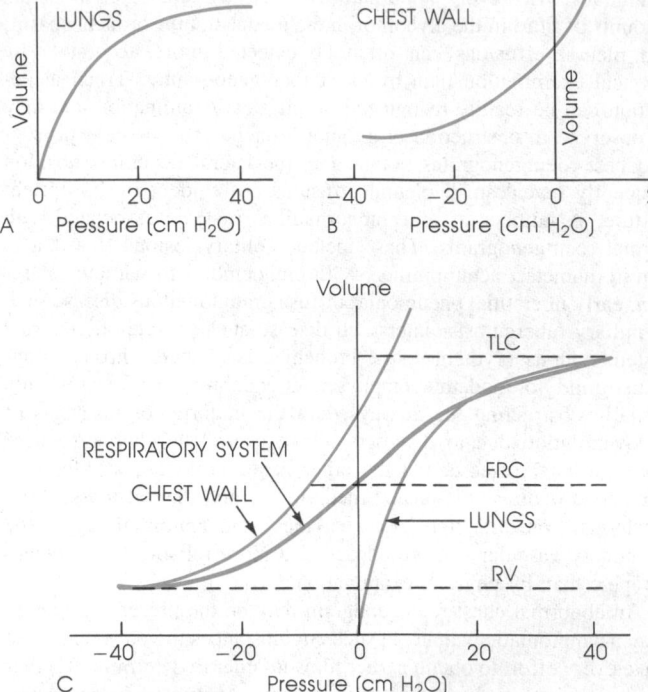

FIGURE 201-3 *A*. Pressure-volume curve of the lungs. *B*. Pressure-volume curve of the chest wall. *C*. Pressure-volume curve of the respiratory system, showing the superimposed component curves of the lungs and the chest wall. RV = residual volume; FRC = functional residual capacity; TLC = total lung capacity. (*From Weinberger*.)

opposed by the equal and opposite tendency of the chest wall to expand (Fig. 201-3*C*).

In order for the lungs and the chest wall to achieve a volume other than the resting volume or FRC, either the pressures acting upon them can be changed passively, e.g., with a mechanical ventilator delivering positive pressure to the airways and alveoli, or the respiratory muscles can actively oppose the tendency of the lungs and the chest wall to return to FRC. During inhalation to volumes above FRC, the inspiratory muscles must actively overcome the tendency of the respiratory system to decrease volume back to FRC. During active exhalation below FRC, expiratory muscle activity must overcome the tendency of the respiratory system to increase volume back to FRC. At TLC, the force applied by the inspiratory muscles to expand the lungs is balanced by the inward recoil of the lungs. As a consequence, the major determinants of TLC are the stiffness of the lungs and inspiratory muscle strength. If the lungs become stiffer, i.e., less compliant, TLC is decreased. If the lungs become less stiff, i.e., more compliant, TLC is increased. If the inspiratory muscles are significantly weakened, they are less able to overcome the inward elastic recoil of the lungs, and TLC is lowered.

At RV, the force exerted by the expiratory muscles to decrease lung volume further is balanced by the outward recoil of the chest wall, which becomes extremely stiff at low lung volumes. Two factors influence the volume of gas contained within the lungs at RV. The first is the ability of the subject to exert a prolonged expiratory effort, which is related to muscle strength and to the ability to overcome sensory stimuli from the chest wall. The second is the ability of the lungs to empty to a small volume. In normal lungs, as P_{TP} is lowered, lung volume decreases. In lungs with diseased airways, as P_{TP} is lowered, flow-limitation or airway closure can limit the amount of gas that is expired. Consequently, both weak chest wall muscles or intrinsic airways disease can result in an elevation in measured RV.

Dynamic measurements of ventilatory function are made by having the subject inhale to TLC and then perform a forced expiratory maneuver. If a subject performs a series of such expiratory maneuvers using increasing muscular intensity, expiratory flow rates will increase until a certain level of effort is reached. Beyond this level, additional effort will not result in an increment in forced expiratory flow rates; this phenomenon is known as the *effort independence* of forced expiratory flow. The physiologic mechanisms determining the flow rates during this effort-independent phase of forced expiratory flow have been shown to be the elastic recoil of the lung, the airflow resistance of the airways between the alveolar zone and the physical site of flow limitation, and the airway wall compliance at the site of flow limitation. Physical processes which decrease elastic recoil, increase airflow resistance, or increase airway wall compliance will decrease the flow rate that can be achieved at any given lung volume. Conversely, processes that increase elastic recoil, decrease resistance, or stiffen airway walls increase the flow rate that can be achieved at any given lung volume.

MEASUREMENT OF VENTILATORY FUNCTION Ventilatory function is measured under static conditions for determination of lung volumes and under dynamic conditions for determination of forced expiratory flow rates. VC, expiratory reserve volume (ERV), and inspiratory capacity (IC) (Fig. 201-1) are measured by having the patient breathe into and out of a spirometer, a device capable of measuring expired or inspired gas volume while plotting volume as a function of time. Other volumes, specifically RV, FRC, and TLC, cannot be measured in this way because they include the volume of gas present within the lungs even after a maximal expiration. One of two techniques is commonly used to measure these volumes: helium dilution or body plethysmography. In the helium dilution method, the subject repeatedly breathes in and out from a reservoir of a known volume of gas containing a trace amount of helium. The helium is diluted by the gas previously present in the lungs and is not absorbed into the pulmonary circulation. From knowledge of reservoir volume and initial and final helium concentrations, the volume of gas present within the lungs can be calculated. With the helium dilution method, the volume of gas present within the lungs may be underestimated if there are slowly communicating airspaces, such as bullae. In this situation, lung volumes can be more accurately measured with a body plethysmograph, a sealed box in which the patient sits while panting against a closed mouthpiece. Because there is no airflow into or out of the plethysmograph, pressure changes within the thorax during panting cause compression and rarefaction of the gas within the lungs and simultaneous rarefaction and compression of gas within the plethysmograph. By measuring pressure changes in the plethysmograph and at the mouthpiece, the volume of gas present within the thorax can be calculated by using Boyle's law.

Lung volumes and measurements made during forced expiration are interpreted by comparing the values measured with the values expected based on the age, height, sex, and race of the patient. Regression curves have been constructed based on data obtained from large numbers of normal, nonsmoking individuals without any evidence of lung disease. Predicted values for a given patient can then be obtained by using the patient's age and height in the appropriate regression equation. As there is variability among normal individuals, values between 80 and 120 percent of predicted are generally considered to be normal. The normal ratio FEV_1/FVC is approximately 0.75 to 0.80, though this value does fall somewhat with advancing age. The MMFR is often a more sensitive measurement of early airflow obstruction, particularly in small airways. However, the MMFR must be interpreted cautiously in the patient with abnormally small lungs (low TLC and VC). In this setting, less volume is exhaled during forced expiration, and the MMFR may appear abnormal when compared with the predicted value for the patient's age, height, and sex, even though it is normal relative to the size of the patient's lungs.

It is also a common practice to plot expiratory flow rates against lung volume (rather than against time); the resulting *flow-volume curve* is useful in that flow rates are closely linked to lung volumes (Fig. 201-4). In addition, the spirometric values mentioned above can be calculated from the flow-volume curve. Commonly, flow rates

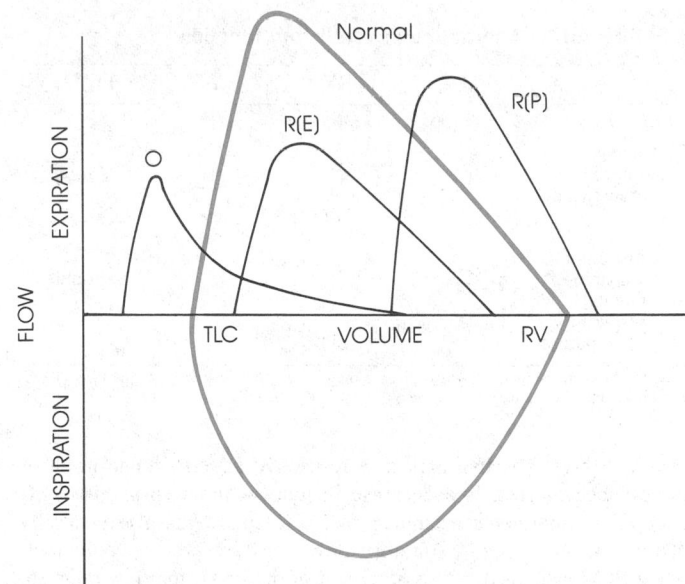

FIGURE 201-4 Flow-volume curves in different conditions: O = obstructive disease; R(P) = parenchymal restrictive disease; R(E) = extraparenchymal restrictive disease with limitation in inspiration and expiration. Forced expiration is plotted in all conditions; forced inspiration is shown only for the normal curve. TLC = total lung capacity; RV = residual volume.

during a maximal inspiratory effort performed as rapidly as possible are plotted as well, making the flow-volume curve into a *flow-volume loop*. At TLC, before expiratory flow starts, the flow rate is 0. During forced expiration, a high peak-flow rate is rapidly achieved. As expiration continues and lung volume approaches RV, the flow rate falls progressively, in a nearly linear fashion for a person with normal lung function. During maximal inspiration from RV to TLC, inspiratory flow is maximal at the midpoint of inspiration, so that the inspiratory portion of the loop is U-shaped or saddle-shaped. The flow rates achieved during maximal expiration can be analyzed quantitatively, by comparison of the flow rates at specified lung volumes with the predicted values, or qualitatively, by analysis of the shape of the descending limb of the expiratory curve.

PATTERNS OF ABNORMAL FUNCTION The two major patterns of abnormal ventilatory function, as measured by static lung volumes and spirometry, are restrictive and obstructive patterns. In the obstructive pattern, the hallmark is a decrease in expiratory flow rates. With fully established disease, the ratio FEV_1/FVC is decreased, as is the MMFR (Fig. 201-2, line *B*). The expiratory portion of the flow-volume loop demonstrates decreased flow rates for any given lung volume. Nonuniform emptying of airways is reflected by a coved (concave upward) configuration of the curve (Fig. 201-4). With early obstructive disease, which originates in the small airways, FEV_1/FVC may be normal; the only abnormalities noted on routine testing of pulmonary function may be a depression in MMFR and an abnormal configuration in the terminal portion of the forced expiratory flow-volume curve.

In *obstructive disease*, the TLC is normal or increased. When helium equilibration tests are used for measurement of lung volumes, the measured volume may be less than the actual volume, if helium was not well distributed to all airways and to all regions of the lung. Residual volume is elevated due to trapping of air during expiration, and the ratio RV/TLC is increased. Vital capacity is frequently decreased in obstructive disease, not because of low lung volumes, as is the case in restrictive disease, but because of the striking elevation in RV.

A *restrictive pattern* can be broadly subdivided into subgroups, depending on the location of the pathology—pulmonary parenchymal vs. extraparenchymal. For extraparenchymal disease, dysfunction can be predominantly in inspiration or in both inspiration plus expiration

TABLE 201-1   Alterations in ventilatory function

	TLC	RV	VC	FEV_1/FVC
Obstructive	N to ↑	↑	↓	↓*
Restrictive				
Pulmonary parenchymal	↓	↓	↓	N to ↑
Extraparenchymal— inspiratory	↓	N to ↓	↓	N
Extraparenchymal— inspiratory + expiratory	↓	↑	↓	variable

* Mild obstructive (small airways) disease may have ↓ MMFR with normal FEV_1/FVC. For abbreviations see text.

(Table 201-1). The hallmark of a restrictive pattern, found in all of these subcategories, is a decrease in lung volumes, primarily TLC and VC. In pulmonary parenchymal disease, RV is also generally decreased, and forced expiratory flow rates are preserved. In fact, when FEV_1 is considered as a percent of the FVC, the flow rates are often supranormal, i.e., disproportionately high relative to the size of the lungs (Fig. 201-2, line C). The flow-volume curve may graphically demonstrate this disproportionate relationship between flow rates and lung volumes, since the expiratory portion of the curve appears relatively tall (preserved flow rates) but narrow (decreased lung volumes), as shown in Fig. 201-4.

In the extraparenchymal pattern characterized by *inspiratory dysfunction,* due to either inspiratory muscle weakness or a stiff chest wall, adequate distending forces are prevented from being exerted on an otherwise normal lung. As a result, achieved TLC values are less than predicted, RV is often not significantly affected, and expiratory flows are preserved. In the extraparenchymal pattern characterized by inspiratory and expiratory dysfunction, the ability to expire to a normal RV is also limited, either because of expiratory muscle weakness or a deformed chest wall that is abnormally rigid at volumes below FRC. Consequently, RV is often elevated, unlike the pattern observed in the other restrictive subcategories. The ratio FEV_1/FVC is variable and depends upon expiratory muscle strength. If expiratory muscle strength is significantly decreased, then the ability to expire rapidly is impaired, and FEV_1/FVC may be decreased even though there is no airflow obstruction. If expiratory muscle strength is normal but the chest wall is abnormally stiff below FRC, then FEV_1/FVC may be increased.

In Table 201-1, the expected alterations in ventilatory function as indicated by pulmonary function testing are summarized. One reason to establish a ventilatory diagnosis is to categorize the functional disorder. This in turn can provide diagnostic information as outlined in Table 201-2. Note that lung disease can be present without abnormal ventilatory function, but the presence of specific diagnostic findings is an aid in differential diagnosis.

DISTURBANCES IN THE PULMONARY CIRCULATION

PHYSIOLOGIC FEATURES   The pulmonary vasculature normally must handle the entire output of the right ventricle, approximately 5 L/min in a normal adult at rest. The comparatively thin-walled vessels of the pulmonary arterial system provide relatively little resistance to flow, and are capable of handling this large volume of blood at low perfusion pressures compared with those of the systemic circulation. The normal mean pulmonary artery pressure of 15 mmHg is much less than the normal mean aortic pressure of approximately 95 mmHg. Regional pulmonary blood flow within the lung is dependent upon hydrostatic forces. In the upright person, pulmonary arterial pressure is lowest at the apex of the lung and highest at the lung bases. As a result, in the upright position, perfusion is least at the apex and greatest at the lung bases. When cardiac output increases, as occurs during exercise, the pulmonary vasculature is capable of recruiting previously unperfused vessels and distending underperfused vessels. As a result, the pulmonary vascular system is capable of handling the increase in flow with a decrease in pulmonary vascular resistance, so that the increment in mean pulmonary arterial pressure is small.

METHODS OF MEASUREMENT   Assessment of circulatory function within the pulmonary vasculature depends upon measuring pulmonary vascular pressures and cardiac output. Clinically, these measurements are commonly made in intensive care units capable of invasive monitoring and in cardiac catheterization laboratories. With a flow-directed pulmonary arterial (Swan-Ganz) catheter, pulmonary arterial and pulmonary capillary wedge pressures can be measured directly, and cardiac output can be obtained by the thermodilution method. Pulmonary vascular resistance can then be calculated according to the equation:

$$PVR = 80(PAP - PCW)/CO$$

where PVR = pulmonary vascular resistance
     PAP = mean pulmonary arterial pressure (mmHg)
    PCW = pulmonary capillary wedge pressure (mmHg)
     CO = cardiac output (L/min)

The normal value for pulmonary vascular resistance is approximately 50 to 150 $(dyn \cdot s)/cm^5$.

MECHANISMS OF ABNORMAL FUNCTION   (See Chap. 191) With disease, pulmonary vascular resistance may increase by a variety of mechanisms. Pulmonary arterial and arteriolar vasoconstriction is a prominent response to alveolar hypoxia. Pulmonary vascular resistance also increases if intraluminal thrombi or proliferation of smooth muscle within vessel walls diminishes the luminal cross-sectional area. If small pulmonary vessels are destroyed, either by scarring or by loss of alveolar walls, the total cross-sectional area of the pulmonary vascular bed diminishes, and pulmonary vascular resistance increases. When pulmonary vascular resistance is elevated, pulmonary arterial pressure rises to maintain normal cardiac output, or cardiac output falls if pulmonary arterial pressure does not increase.

CLINICAL CORRELATION   Disturbances in function of the pulmonary vasculature as a result of primary cardiac disease, either congenital heart disease or conditions which elevate left atrial pressure such as mitral stenosis, are beyond the scope of this chapter and are discussed in Chaps. 186 and 188, respectively. Instead, the focus will be on the pulmonary vasculature as its function is affected by diseases primarily involving the respiratory system, including the pulmonary vessels themselves.

TABLE 201-2   Common respiratory diseases by diagnostic categories

Obstructive
  Asthma
  Chronic obstructive lung disease (chronic bronchitis, emphysema)
  Bronchiectasis
  Cystic fibrosis
  Bronchiolitis
Restrictive—parenchymal
  Sarcoidosis
  Idiopathic pulmonary fibrosis
  Pneumoconiosis
  Drug- or radiation-induced interstitial lung disease
Restrictive—extraparenchymal
  Neuromuscular
    Diaphragmatic weakness/paralysis
    Myasthenia gravis*
    Guillain-Barré syndrome*
    Muscular dystrophies*
    Cervical spine injury*
  Chest wall
    Kyphoscoliosis
    Obesity
    Ankylosing spondylitis*

* Can have inspiratory and expiratory limitation (see text).

All diseases of the respiratory system causing hypoxemia are potentially capable of increasing pulmonary vascular resistance, since alveolar hypoxia is a very potent stimulus for pulmonary vasoconstriction. The more prolonged and intense the hypoxic stimulus, the more likely that a significant increase in pulmonary vascular resistance and pulmonary hypertension will result. In practice, patients with hypoxemia caused by chronic obstructive lung disease, interstitial lung disease, chest wall disease, and by the obesity hypoventilation–sleep apnea syndrome are particularly prone to developing pulmonary hypertension. If there are additional structural changes in the pulmonary vasculature secondary to the underlying process, these will increase the likelihood of developing pulmonary hypertension.

With diseases primarily affecting the pulmonary vessels, a decrease in the cross-sectional area of the pulmonary vascular bed is primarily responsible for increased pulmonary vascular resistance, while hypoxemia generally plays a lesser role. In the case of recurrent pulmonary emboli, parts of the pulmonary arterial system are occluded by intraluminal thrombi originating in the systemic venous system. With primary pulmonary hypertension (Chap. 212) or with pulmonary vascular disease secondary to scleroderma, the small pulmonary arteries and arterioles are affected by a generalized obliterative process that narrows and occludes these vessels. Pulmonary vascular resistance increases, and significant pulmonary hypertension often results.

DISTURBANCES IN GAS EXCHANGE

PHYSIOLOGIC FEATURES The primary functions of the respiratory system are to remove the appropriate amount of CO_2 from blood entering the pulmonary circulation and to provide adequate O_2 to blood leaving the pulmonary circulation. In order for these functions to be carried out properly, there must be adequate provision of fresh air to the alveoli for delivery of O_2 and removal of CO_2 (ventilation), adequate circulation of blood through the pulmonary vasculature (perfusion), adequate movement of gas between alveoli and pulmonary capillaries (diffusion), and appropriate contact between alveolar gas and pulmonary capillary blood (ventilation-perfusion matching).

A normal individual at rest inspires approximately 12 to 16 times per minute, each breath having a tidal volume of approximately 500 mL. A portion (approximately 30 percent) of each breath does not reach the alveoli, but remains in the conducting airways of the lung. This component of each breath, which is not generally available for gas exchange, is called the anatomic dead space component. The remaining 70 percent reaches and rapidly mixes with the gas resident in the alveolar zone and can participate in gas exchange. In this example, total ventilation each minute is approximately 7 L, composed of 2 L/min of dead space ventilation and 5 L/min of alveolar ventilation. In certain disease settings, some alveoli are ventilated but not perfused, so that additional ventilation is wasted beyond that portion related to the anatomic dead space. If total dead space ventilation is increased but total minute ventilation is unchanged, then alveolar ventilation must fall correspondingly.

GAS EXCHANGE This is dependent upon alveolar ventilation rather than total minute ventilation, as outlined below. The partial pressure of CO_2 in arterial blood (Pa_{CO_2}) is directly proportional to the amount of CO_2 produced per minute ($\dot{V}_{CO_2}$) and inversely proportional to alveolar ventilation ($\dot{V}_A$), according to the relationship:

$$Pa_{CO_2} = 0.863 \times \dot{V}_{CO_2}/\dot{V}_A$$

where $\dot{V}_{CO_2}$ is expressed in mL/min, $\dot{V}_A$ in L/min, and Pa_{CO_2} in mmHg. At fixed $\dot{V}_{CO_2}$, when alveolar ventilation increases, Pa_{CO_2} falls, and when alveolar ventilation decreases, Pa_{CO_2} rises. Maintaining a normal level of O_2 in the alveoli (and consequently in arterial blood) also depends upon provision of adequate alveolar ventilation to replenish alveolar O_2. This principle will become more apparent from the alveolar gas equation below.

Both O_2 and CO_2 diffuse readily down their respective concentration gradients through the alveolar wall and pulmonary capillary endothelium. Under normal circumstances this process is rapid, and equilibration of both gases is complete within one-third of the transit time of erythrocytes through the pulmonary capillary bed. Even in disease states where diffusion of gases is impaired, it is unlikely to be so severe that diffusion equilibration is not reached. Consequently, a diffusion abnormality rarely results in arterial hypoxemia at rest. If erythrocyte transit time in the pulmonary circulation is shortened, as occurs with exercise, and diffusion is impaired, then diffusion limitation may contribute to hypoxemia. Exercise testing can often demonstrate such physiologically significant abnormalities due to impaired diffusion. Even though diffusion limitation rarely makes a clinically significant contribution to resting hypoxemia, clinical measurements of what is known as *diffusing capacity* (see below) can be a useful measure of the integrity of the alveolar-capillary membrane.

Ventilation-perfusion matching In addition to the absolute level of ventilation and perfusion reaching the lung, gas exchange is critically dependent on the proper matching of ventilation and perfusion. The spectrum of possible ventilation-perfusion ($\dot{V}/\dot{Q}$) ratios within an alveolar-capillary unit ranges from zero, in which ventilation is totally absent and the unit behaves as a shunt, to infinity, in which perfusion is totally absent and the unit behaves as dead space. The P_{O_2} and P_{CO_2} of blood leaving each alveolar-capillary unit depend on the gas tension (blood and air) entering that unit and on the $\dot{V}/\dot{Q}$ ratio of that particular unit. At one extreme, when an alveolar-capillary unit has a $\dot{V}/\dot{Q}$ ratio = 0 and behaves as a shunt, blood leaving the unit has the composition of mixed venous blood entering the pulmonary capillaries. Under normal circumstances $P\bar{v}_{O_2} \sim 40$ mmHg and $P\bar{v}_{CO_2} \sim 46$ mmHg. At the other extreme, when an alveolar-capillary unit has a high $\dot{V}/\dot{Q}$ ratio and thus behaves almost like dead space, the small amount of blood leaving the unit has partial pressures of O_2 and CO_2 ($P_{O_2} \sim 150$ mmHg, $P_{CO_2} \sim 0$ mmHg while breathing room air) approaching the composition of inspired gas.

In the ideal situation, all alveolar-capillary units have equal matching of ventilation and perfusion, i.e., with a ratio of approximately 1 when each is expressed in L/min. But, even in the normal individual, some $\dot{V}/\dot{Q}$ mismatching is present, as there is normally a gradient of blood flow from the apices to the bases of the lungs. Moreover, there is a similar gradient of ventilation from the apices to the bases, but the gradient is less marked for ventilation than for perfusion. As a result, ventilation-perfusion ratios are higher at the lung apices than at the lung bases. Therefore, blood coming from the apices has a higher P_{O_2} and lower P_{CO_2} than blood coming from the bases. The net P_{O_2} and P_{CO_2} of the resulting mixture of blood coming from all areas of the lung is a weighted average of the individual components, which takes into account the relative amount of blood from each unit and the O_2 and CO_2 *content* of blood coming from each unit. Because of the sigmoid shape of the oxyhemoglobin dissociation curve, it is important to distinguish between the partial pressure and the content of O_2 in blood. Hemoglobin is almost fully saturated at a $P_{O_2} = 60$ mmHg, and little additional O_2 is carried by hemoglobin even with substantial elevations of P_{O_2} above 60 mmHg (see Fig. 290-4, p. 1517). On the other hand, significant O_2 desaturation of hemoglobin occurs once P_{O_2} falls below 60 mmHg onto the steep descending limb of the curve. As a result, blood coming from regions of the lung with a high $\dot{V}/\dot{Q}$ ratio, a high P_{O_2}, but only a small elevation in O_2 content, cannot compensate for blood coming from regions with a low $\dot{V}/\dot{Q}$ ratio, a low P_{O_2}, and a significant decrease in O_2 content. Although $\dot{V}/\dot{Q}$ mismatching can influence P_{CO_2}, this effect is less marked and often is overcome by an increase in overall minute ventilation.

MEASUREMENT OF GAS EXCHANGE Arterial blood gases The most commonly used measures of gas exchange are the partial pressures of O_2 and CO_2 in arterial blood, i.e., Pa_{O_2} and Pa_{CO_2}, respectively. These partial pressures do not measure directly the quantity of O_2 and CO_2 in blood, but rather the driving pressure for the gas to be carried in blood. The actual quantity or content of each of these gases in blood depends upon the solubility of the gas in plasma and the ability of any component of blood to react with or to bind the gas of interest. Since hemoglobin is capable of binding large amounts of O_2, oxygenated hemoglobin is the primary form in which O_2 is transported in blood. The actual content of O_2 in blood therefore depends both on the hemoglobin concentration and on the P_{O_2}. The P_{O_2} determines what percentage of hemoglobin is saturated with O_2, based upon the position on the oxyhemoglobin dissociation curve. Oxygen content in normal blood (at 37°C, pH 7.4) can be determined by adding the amount of O_2 dissolved in plasma to the amount bound to hemoglobin, according to the equation

$$O_2 \text{ content} = 1.34 \times (\text{hemoglobin}) \times \text{saturation} + 0.0031 \times P_{O_2}$$

since each gram of hemoglobin is capable of carrying 1.34 mL O_2 when fully saturated, and the amount of O_2 that can be dissolved in plasma is proportional to the P_{O_2}, with 0.0031 mL O_2 dissolved per deciliter of blood per mmHg P_{O_2}. In arterial blood, the amount of O_2 transported dissolved in plasma (approximately 0.3 mL O_2/dL blood) is trivial compared with the amount bound to hemoglobin (approximately 20 mL O_2/dL blood).

Most commonly, P_{O_2} is the measurement used to quantitate the adequacy of oxygenation of arterial blood. Arterial O_2 saturation can also be measured by oximetry and is particularly important in selected clinical conditions. For example, in patients with carbon monoxide exposure, carbon monoxide preferentially displaces O_2 from hemoglobin, essentially making a portion of hemoglobin unavailable for binding to O_2. In this circumstance, carbon monoxide saturation is high and O_2 saturation is low, even though the driving pressure for O_2 to bind to hemoglobin, reflected by P_{O_2}, is normal. Measurement of O_2 saturation, in order to determine O_2 content, is also important when mixed venous blood is sampled from a pulmonary arterial catheter to calculate cardiac output by the Fick technique. In mixed venous blood, the P_{O_2} is normally about 40 mmHg, but small changes in P_{O_2} may reflect relatively large changes in O_2 saturation.

A useful calculation in the assessment of oxygenation is the alveolar-arterial O_2 difference ($P_{A_{O_2}}$–$P_{a_{O_2}}$), commonly called the alveolar-arterial O_2 gradient (or A-a gradient). This calculation takes into account the fact that alveolar and, hence, arterial P_{O_2} can be expected to change depending on the level of alveolar ventilation, reflected by the arterial P_{CO_2}. When a patient hyperventilates and has a low P_{CO_2}, alveolar and arterial P_{O_2} will rise; conversely, hypoventilation and a high P_{CO_2} are accompanied by a decrease in alveolar and arterial P_{O_2}. These changes in arterial P_{O_2} are independent of abnormalities in O_2 transfer at the alveolar-capillary level, and reflect only the dependence of alveolar P_{O_2} on the level of alveolar ventilation.

In order to determine the alveolar-arterial O_2 difference, the alveolar P_{O_2} ($P_{A_{O_2}}$) must first be calculated. The equation most commonly used for this purpose, a simplified form of the alveolar gas equation, is

$$P_{A_{O_2}} = F_{I_{O_2}} \times (P_B - P_{H_2O}) - P_{a_{CO_2}}/R$$

where $F_{I_{O_2}}$ = fractional concentration of inspired O_2 (~0.21 when breathing room air)

P_B = barometric pressure (approximately 760 mmHg at sea level)

P_{H_2O} = water vapor pressure (47 mmHg when air is fully saturated at 37°C)

R = respiratory quotient (the ratio of CO_2 production to O_2 consumption, usually assumed to be 0.8)

If the above values are substituted into the equation for the patient breathing air at sea level, the equation becomes

$$P_{A_{O_2}} = 150 - 1.25 P_{a_{CO_2}}$$

The alveolar-arterial O_2 difference can then be calculated by subtracting measured $P_{a_{O_2}}$ from calculated $P_{A_{O_2}}$. In a healthy young person breathing air, the $P_{A_{O_2}}$–$P_{a_{O_2}}$ is normally less than 15 mmHg; this value increases with age and may be as high as 30 mmHg in elderly patients.

Adequacy of CO_2 elimination is measured by the partial pressure of CO_2 in arterial blood, i. e., $P_{a_{CO_2}}$. A more complete understanding of the mechanisms and chronicity of abnormal levels of P_{CO_2} also requires measurement of pH and/or bicarbonate (HCO_3^-), since P_{CO_2} and the patient's acid-base status are so closely intertwined (see Chap. 51).

Diffusing capacity The ability of gas to diffuse across the alveolar-capillary membrane is ordinarily assessed by the diffusing capacity of the lung for carbon monoxide ($D_{L_{CO}}$). In this test, a small concentration of carbon monoxide is inhaled, usually in a single breath that is held for approximately 10 s. The carbon monoxide is diluted by the gas already present in the alveoli, and is also taken up by hemoglobin as the erythrocytes course through the pulmonary capillary system. The concentration of carbon monoxide in exhaled gas is measured, and $D_{L_{CO}}$ is calculated as the quantity of carbon monoxide absorbed per min per mmHg pressure gradient from the alveoli to the pulmonary capillaries. The value obtained for $D_{L_{CO}}$ depends upon the alveolar-capillary surface area available for gas exchange and upon the pulmonary capillary blood volume. In addition, the thickness of the alveolar-capillary membrane, the degree of V/Q mismatching, and the patient's hemoglobin level will affect the measurement. The value for $D_{L_{CO}}$, ideally corrected for hemoglobin, can then be compared with a predicted value, based either on age, height, and sex or on the lung volume at which the value was obtained. Because of the effect of hemoglobin levels on $D_{L_{CO}}$, the measured $D_{L_{CO}}$ is frequently corrected to take the patient's hemoglobin level into account.

MECHANISMS OF ABNORMAL FUNCTION Arterial blood gases Hypoxemia is a common manifestation of a variety of diseases affecting the lungs or other parts of the respiratory system. The broad clinical problem of hypoxemia is often best characterized according to the underlying mechanism. The four basic mechanisms of hypoxemia are (1) decrease in inspired P_{O_2}, (2) hypoventilation, (3) shunt, and (4) V/Q mismatching. Diffusion block contributes to hypoxemia only under selected clinical circumstances and is not usually included among the general categories of hypoxemia. Determining the underlying mechanism for hypoxemia depends upon measurement of the $P_{a_{CO_2}}$, calculation of the $P_{A_{O_2}}$–$P_{a_{O_2}}$, and knowledge of the response to supplemental O_2. A flow chart summarizing the approach to the hypoxemic patient is found in Fig. 201-5.

Decrease in the inspired P_{O_2} and hypoventilation both cause hypoxemia by lowering $P_{A_{O_2}}$ and therefore $P_{a_{O_2}}$. In each case, gas exchange at the alveolar-capillary level is occurring normally, and $P_{A_{O_2}}$–$P_{a_{O_2}}$ is not elevated. Hypoxemia due to depression in inspired P_{O_2} can be diagnosed by knowledge of the clinical situation. Inspired P_{O_2} is lowered either because the patient is at a high altitude, where barometric pressure is low, or, much less commonly, because the patient is breathing a gas mixture containing less than 21 percent O_2. The hallmark of hypoventilation as a cause of hypoxemia is an elevation in $P_{a_{CO_2}}$. This is associated with an increase in $P_{A_{CO_2}}$ and a fall in $P_{A_{O_2}}$. When hypoxemia is due purely to a low inspired P_{O_2} or to alveolar hypoventilation, $P_{A_{O_2}}$–$P_{a_{O_2}}$ is normal. If $P_{A_{O_2}}$–$P_{a_{O_2}}$ and $P_{a_{CO_2}}$ are both elevated, then an additional mechanism, such as V/Q mismatching or shunt, is contributing to hypoxemia.

Shunting is a cause of hypoxemia when desaturated blood effectively bypasses oxygenation at the alveolar-capillary level. This occurs either because of a structural problem that allows desaturated blood to bypass the normal site of gas exchange, or because ventilation to perfused alveoli is absent. Shunting is associated with an elevation in the $P_{A_{O_2}}$–$P_{a_{O_2}}$. When shunting is an important contributing factor to hypoxemia, the lowered P_{O_2} is relatively refractory to improvement by supplemental O_2.

Finally, the largest clinical category of hypoxemia is V/Q mismatching. With V/Q mismatching, regions with low V/Q ratios contribute blood with a low P_{O_2} and a low O_2 content. Corresponding regions with high V/Q ratios contribute blood with a high P_{O_2}. However, because blood is already almost fully saturated with a normal P_{O_2}, elevation of the P_{O_2} to a high value does not significantly

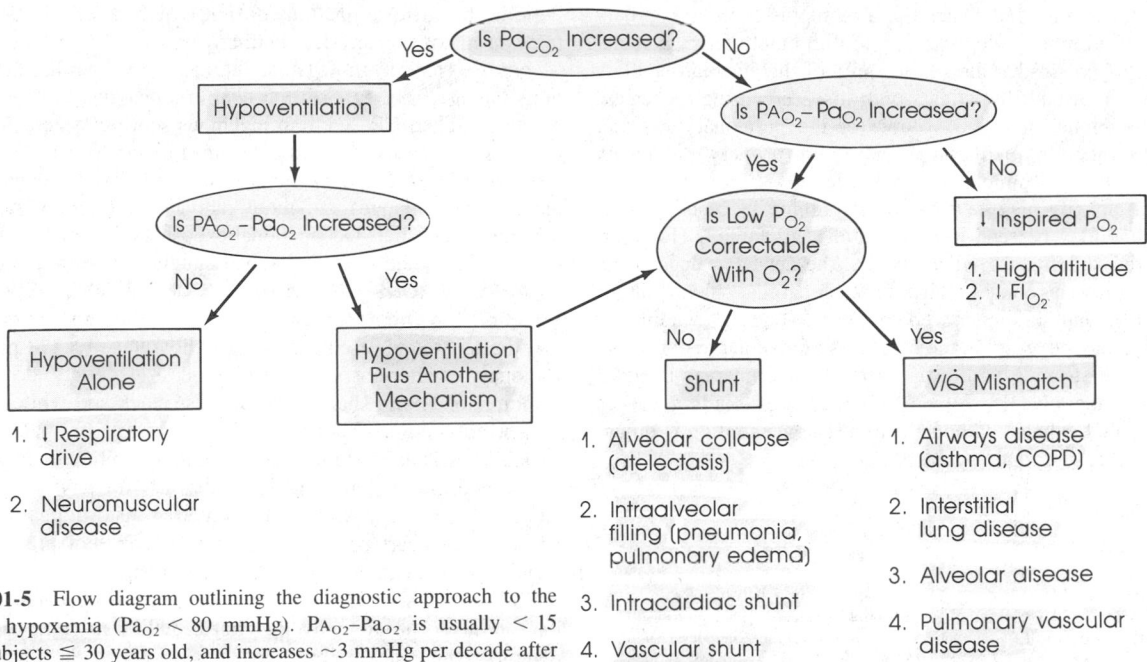

FIGURE 201-5 Flow diagram outlining the diagnostic approach to the patient with hypoxemia ($Pa_{O_2} < 80$ mmHg). $PA_{O_2}-Pa_{O_2}$ is usually < 15 mmHg for subjects ≤ 30 years old, and increases ~3 mmHg per decade after age 30.

increase O_2 saturation or content, and therefore cannot compensate for the reduction of O_2 saturation and content in blood coming from regions with a low V̇/Q̇ ratio. When V̇/Q̇ mismatch is the primary cause of hypoxemia, $PA_{O_2}-Pa_{O_2}$ is elevated, and P_{CO_2} is generally normal. Supplemental O_2 corrects the hypoxemia by raising the P_{O_2} in blood coming from regions with a low V̇/Q̇ ratio; this response distinguishes hypoxemia due to V̇/Q̇ mismatch from that due to true shunt.

The essential mechanism underlying all cases of hypercapnia is inadequate alveolar ventilation for the amount of CO_2 produced. It is conceptually useful to characterize CO_2 retention further, based on a more detailed examination of the potential contributing factors. These include: (1) increased CO_2 production; (2) decreased ventilatory drive ("won't breathe"); (3) malfunction of the respiratory pump or increased airways resistance, making it more difficult to sustain adequate ventilation ("can't breathe"); and (4) inefficiency of gas exchange (increased dead space or V̇/Q̇ mismatch) necessitating a compensatory increase in overall minute ventilation. In practice, more than one of these mechanisms is commonly responsible for hypercapnia, as increased minute ventilation is capable of compensating for increased CO_2 production and for inefficiencies of gas exchange.

Diffusing capacity Although the two main components affecting DL_{CO}, i.e., the membrane component and the pulmonary capillary blood volume, can be measured separately, this separation is made infrequently in clinical practice. Rather, the measurement is used in a more general way to assess the functional integrity of the alveolar-capillary membrane, which includes the pulmonary capillary bed. Diseases purely affecting the airways generally do not lower DL_{CO}, whereas diseases affecting alveolar walls or the pulmonary capillary bed will have an effect on DL_{CO}. Even though DL_{CO} is a useful marker to assess whether disease affecting the alveolar-capillary bed is present, an abnormal DL_{CO} does not necessarily imply that diffusion limitation is responsible for hypoxemia in a particular patient.

CLINICAL CORRELATIONS Arterial blood gases Useful clinical correlations can be made with the mechanisms underlying hypoxemia (Fig. 201-5). A lowered inspired P_{O_2} contributes to hypoxemia either at high altitude or if the concentration of inspired O_2 is less than 21 percent. The latter problem occurs if a patient receiving anesthesia or ventilatory support is inadvertently given a low-O_2 gas mixture to breathe, or if O_2 is consumed from ambient gas, as can occur during smoke inhalation from a fire. The primary

feature of hypoventilation as a cause of hypoxemia is an elevation in Pa_{CO_2}. The clinical correlates with hypoventilation are discussed in Chap. 217.

Shunt as a cause of hypoxemia can reflect transfer of blood from the right to the left side of the heart without it ever entering the pulmonary circulation, as occurs with an intracardiac shunt. This problem occurs most commonly in the setting of cyanotic congenital heart disease, when an interatrial or interventricular septal defect is associated with pulmonary hypertension, so that shunting is in the right-to-left rather than left-to-right direction. Shunting of blood through the pulmonary parenchyma is most frequently due to disease causing absence of ventilation to perfused alveoli. This can occur if the alveoli are atelectatic or if they are filled with fluid, as in pulmonary edema (both cardiogenic and noncardiogenic) or with extensive intraalveolar exudation of fluid due to pneumonia. Less commonly, vascular anomalies with arteriovenous shunting in the lung can cause hypoxemia. These anomalies can be hereditary, as found with hereditary hemorrhagic telangiectasia (Osler-Rendu-Weber syndrome), or acquired, as in pulmonary vascular malformations secondary to hepatic cirrhosis, which are similar to the commonly recognized cutaneous vascular malformations ("spider hemangiomas").

Ventilation-perfusion mismatch is the most common cause of hypoxemia clinically. Most of the processes affecting either the airways or the pulmonary parenchyma are distributed unevenly throughout the lungs and do not necessarily affect ventilation and perfusion equally. Some areas of lung may have good perfusion and poor ventilation, whereas others have poor perfusion and relatively good ventilation. Important examples of airways diseases in which V̇/Q̇ mismatch causes hypoxemia are asthma and chronic obstructive lung disease. Parenchymal lung diseases causing V̇/Q̇ mismatch and hypoxemia include interstitial lung disease and pneumonia.

Clinically important alterations in CO_2 elimination range from excessive ventilation and hypocapnia to inadequate CO_2 elimination and hypercapnia. These clinical problems are discussed in Chap. 217.

Diffusing capacity Measurement of DL_{CO} may be useful for assessing disease affecting the alveolar-capillary bed or the pulmonary vasculature. In practice, three main categories of disease are associated with lowered DL_{CO}—interstitial lung disease, emphysema, and pulmonary vascular disease. With interstitial lung disease, scarring of alveolar-capillary units diminishes the area of the alveolar-capillary bed as well as pulmonary blood volume. With emphysema, alveolar walls are destroyed, so that the surface area of the alveolar-capillary bed is again diminished. In patients with disease causing a decrease in the cross-sectional area and volume of the pulmonary vascular bed, such as recurrent pulmonary emboli or primary pulmonary hypertension, DL_{CO} is commonly diminished.

Diffusing capacity may be elevated if pulmonary blood volume is increased, as may be seen in congestive heart failure. However, once interstitial and alveolar edema ensue, the net DL_{CO} depends on the opposing influences of increased pulmonary capillary blood volume elevating DL_{CO} and pulmonary edema decreasing it. Finding an elevated DL_{CO} may be useful in the diagnosis of alveolar hemorrhage, such as in Goodpasture's syndrome. Hemoglobin contained in erythrocytes within the alveolar lumen is capable of binding carbon monoxide, so that exhaled carbon monoxide concentration is diminished and the measured DL_{CO} is increased.

REFERENCES

GOLD WM, BOUSHEY HA: Pulmonary function testing, in *Textbook of Respiratory Medicine*, JF Murray, JA Nadel (eds). Philadelphia, Saunders, 1988, pp 611–682

WEINBERGER SE: *Principles of Pulmonary Medicine*. Philadelphia, Saunders, 1986

WEST JB: *Pulmonary Pathophysiology—The Essentials*, 3d ed. Baltimore, Williams & Wilkins, 1987

WEST JB: *Respiratory Physiology—The Essentials*, 3d ed. Baltimore, Williams & Wilkins, 1985

---

202   IMAGING IN PULMONARY DISEASE

PAUL J. FRIEDMAN

Radiologic examination of the lungs and pleura has grown beyond the capability—great as it is—of the plain chest film or radiograph and includes the imaging modalities of computed tomography, nuclear magnetic resonance, ultrasound, and nuclear medicine. This chapter will focus on their applications, best understood in relation to the traditional chest film.

THE BASIC PRINCIPLES OF CLINICAL IMAGING

Defining the problem The first step in the imaging examination is to define the problem clearly enough to indicate what new information needs to be provided by an imaging study.

Consultation The next step is to decide if a plain chest radiograph (CR) will suffice, whether special radiographic views are necessary, or if the problem demands more expensive and time-consuming techniques. In this era of growing specialization, rapidly changing technology, and cost consciousness, it is increasingly useful to get radiologic consultation for this step.

Getting the results The value of a radiographic report often depends on whether the radiologist was aware of the question being asked. It has been shown that radiologic interpretation is far more accurate when an appropriate history is provided. Even with a history the false-negative error rate (the "misses") is 30 to 40 percent on average, when measured in controlled situations. It is therefore important to (1) provide a history; (2) read the report carefully but skeptically; (3) look at the films yourself; and (4) review them with a radiologist.

Screening The routine posteroanterior (PA) and lateral CR are an exception to problem-based imaging, but admission films are needed only if there is suspicion of cardiac or pulmonary disease.

Periodic health examinations do not require a CR unless there is a relevant history or physical finding.

OCCUPATIONAL HEALTH SCREENING Evaluating the extent of lung damage from exposure to coal or silica dust has been achieved by standardized CR, with an ingenious scoring system for pneumoconiosis. Health risks from exposure to asbestos dust are currently monitored by radiography, though with improved industrial hygiene the expected plaques are more rare and pulmonary fibrosis from asbestos is unusual. Occupational exposures to agents more likely to cause asthma than pneumoconiosis should not be monitored by CR.

APPLICATIONS OF IMAGING TECHNOLOGY, NEW AND OLD

Variations on chest radiography Chest radiologists uniformly agree that the technique of choice is high kilovoltage (>120 pkV), with a stationary scatter-absorbing grid, and a wide-latitude film-screen combination (more shades of gray, less black-and-white).

Portable films Though clearly necessary in many cases, the portable CR is deficient in detail resolution, latitude, penetration, and the normal gravitational gradient necessary for physiologic interpretation. It also has increased geometric distortion, more lung is obscured by heart or diaphragm, and it does not provide a lateral view. Lateral decubitus or prone positions may be useful in bedside radiography to show parts of the lung otherwise obscured by effusion; the lateral decubitus and other horizontal-beam films are good for demonstrating pneumothorax or fluid levels in the lung or pleural space. Portable radiographic examinations are also useful in assessing the positions of tubes and catheters commonly used in the intensive care unit.

Conventional tomography Essentially obsolete for most chest work, tomography is still used for studying the hilar regions, but far more information can be obtained about the hilar structures and the adjacent mediastinum from computed tomography (CT) or magnetic resonance (MR) imaging. Screening the lungs for metastases, formerly a major application of conventional tomography, is better done with CT. Conventional tomography should be used only in facilities where more advanced technology is not available.

COMPUTED TOMOGRAPHY

The x-ray absorption of each point (pixel) in a cross section of the body can be calculated by measuring the absorption of many fine x-ray beams at many angles within the plane of the cross section. The calculated numbers are displayed as radiographic densities with far more shades of gray than with CR (Fig. 202-1). In addition, CT eliminates the superimposition of structures that makes CR anatomy so difficult, and though the images are "noisy," there is less problem in detecting an abnormality because of obscuration by normal structures with CT than with CR. However, a set of images is needed to encompass the chest, since each represents only the information in a 1-cm thick transverse cross section. Each set of data is collected during suspended respiration, taking 1 to 4 s, and requires patient cooperation in taking and holding a comparable breath each time for good results.

MEDIASTINAL CT After less than a decade of use in the chest, CT is well established as the diagnostic procedure of choice for studying the mediastinum (Fig. 202-1B). The most common use is the assessment of lymph node size in the staging of lung cancer (Chap. 215). Detection of enlarged nodes may lead to biopsy, since enlargement of nodes by inflammation cannot be distinguished from that by tumor spread using only CT images. Most investigators find the false-negative error rate comparable to that of mediastinoscopy and somewhat better than cervical mediastinoscopy with left-sided lung cancers.

Lumps and bumps of the mediastinum, detected on CR, are readily analyzed using CT. Mediastinal cysts, tumors, fat, and calcification are readily distinguished because of the good density resolution. CT is also excellent for distinguishing vascular from nonvascular structures and for recognizing vascular anatomic variants or aneurysms.

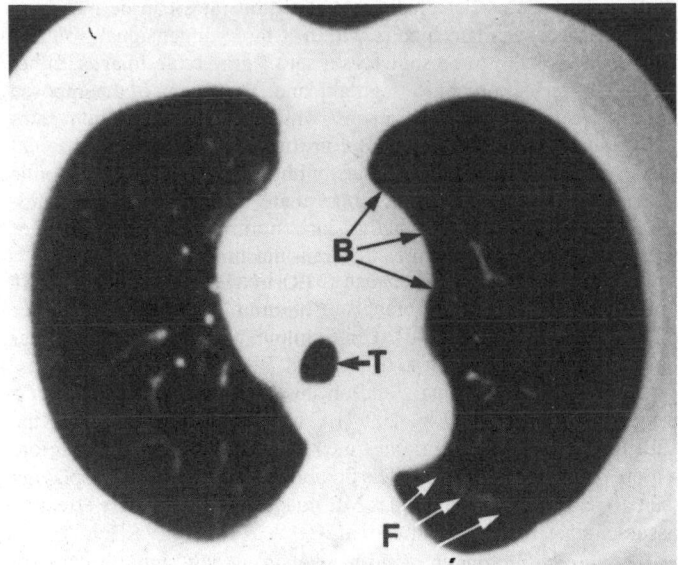

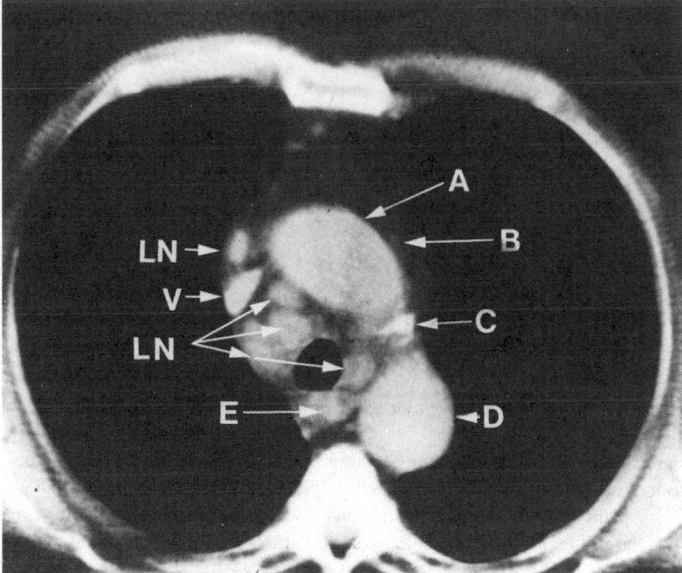

FIGURE 202-1 Normal CT of the chest, supine, standard 1 cm section, after intravenous contrast material. *A.* Typical "lung window" settings, with normal pulmonary vessels and the top of the oblique fissure (F) of the left lung visible. The dark circle within the mediastinum is the tracheal air column (T). Note bulge (B) along left mediastinum. *B.* Mediastinal settings show a clear delineation between the enlarged lymphomatous nodes (LN) and the surrounding fat. The soft tissue structure dorsal to the trachea is the esophagus (E). The major vessels visible are the superior vena cava (V) and ascending (A) and descending (D) aorta; small veins are also seen in the fat in front of the spine, behind the esophagus, and ventrally, behind the sternum, as well as in the generous layer of subcutaneous fat. The calcification (C) is a plaque in the aortic arch rather than a calcified lymph node. The mediastinal bulge (B) alongside the ascending aorta on the left is simply mediastinal fat, not an enlarged node.

CT is the best method for revealing fibrosing mediastinitis, since the important calcification is invisible with MR imaging.

CONTRAST MATERIAL There is no consensus about the indications for using intravenous contrast material in chest CT. Some institutions use contrast material universally and may even use the high dose–rapid infusion method known as *dynamic CT*. Others use contrast material regularly in studies of vessels or tumors but not for routine lung cancer staging. Injection of traditional hypertonic contrast media adds to the cost and risk of the study, since allergic and idiosyncratic reactions occur regularly. Serious reactions are uncommon, however, and death occurs no more than about once in every 40,000 intravenous injections. Newer agents are less toxic but are still several times as expensive.

CT OF THE PLEURA CT imaging resolves complex abnormalities which might involve the lung or pleura or both. For example, the diagnosis of bronchopleural fistula requires distinguishing pleural pockets from lung abscesses or cysts.

Tumors of the pleura are demonstrated in the transverse plane much more clearly than on CR, where they are hard to distinguish from inflammatory pleural thickening. The true extent of malignant mesothelioma or metastatic adenocarcinoma is therefore best shown on CT. The solid and fluid components of a pleural collection, which are the same density on CR, can be usefully distinguished on CT because of its greater density resolution (Fig. 202-2). Another asbestos-related application is the detection of pleural plaques and calcifications (Chap. 206). Though routine health screening of asbestos-exposed workers relies on the posteroanterior CR, sometimes it is necessary to use the much greater sensitivity of CT to detect pleural plaques or the characteristic small pleural calcifications.

CT OF THE LUNG AND AIRWAYS Since the CR has such excellent resolution and shows the air/tissue density differences so well, this application of CT has been the slowest to develop. The trachea and main bronchi are shown well in cross section (Fig. 202-2), and CT shows the mediastinal extent of endobronchial lesions, though longitudinal images of the trachea would be more useful clinically. Intrinsic tumors or deformity from other mediastinal primary or secondary neoplasms are demonstrable, but do not provide an indication for CT unless endoscopy is contraindicated. CT has much greater sensitivity for bronchial abnormality (thickening, dilatation, mucoid impaction) than CR. CT has practically replaced bronchography in screening for surgical bronchiectasis (Chap. 208), missing only minimal or localized cylindrical bronchiectasis.

Details of both alveolar and interstitial lung diseases can be

FIGURE 202-2 High-resolution CT, supine, 1.5 mm section, with edge-sharpening technique and standard "lung window." Patient with chronic thromboembolic pulmonary hypertension. Right pleural effusion (E). Airways are shown well, from the carina of the trachea (T) to segmental bronchi (arrowheads). Many visible peripheral pulmonary vessels are smaller than normal. Background vascularity is reduced in most regions, as contrasted to the subsegmental regions of more normal vascularity shown by the lighter density in the anterior segment of the right upper lobe (R) and, less clearly, in the axillary subsegment on the left (L). High-resolution CT can provide useful anatomic information about medium-sized vessels and bronchi. *(Courtesy of L. Olson.)*

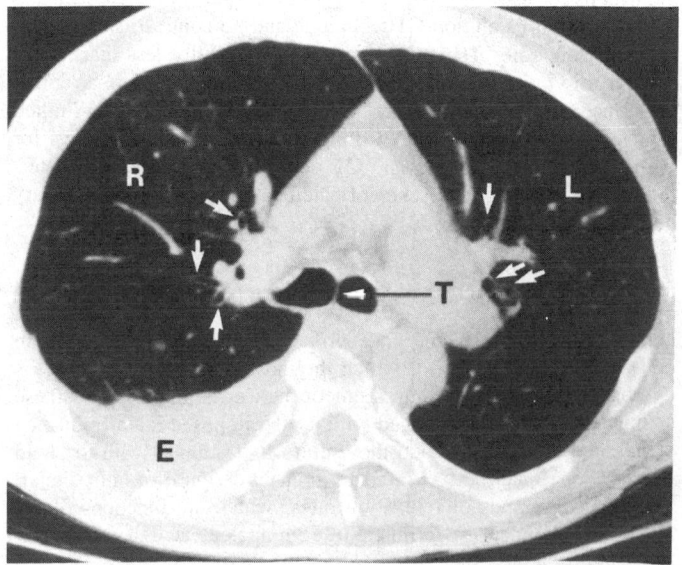

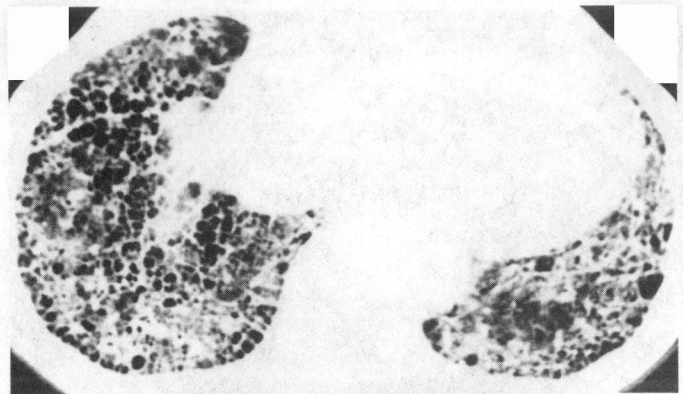

FIGURE 202-3 High-resolution CT, prone, 1.5 mm section, with edge-sharpening image processing, shown as a light ''lung window.'' Chronic interstitial fibrosis with severe honeycombing: a graphic portrayal, comparable to looking directly at a lung specimen. High-resolution CT can show detailed gross pathologic findings in many lung diseases, with great sensitivity for alveolar filling, for interstitial alterations of various kinds, and for emphysema. *(Courtesy of I. Feuerstein.)*

demonstrated on CT. The utility of studying parenchymal abnormalities is still unclear, since characteristic changes have been described in only a few diseases such as carcinomatosis, interstitial fibrosis (Fig. 202-3), and emphysema.

HIGH-RESOLUTION CT   The demonstration of parenchymal and bronchial abnormalities is enhanced by using high-resolution CT (Figs. 202-2 and 202-3). The geometric resolution of ordinary CT is nearly tenfold less than CR, but high-resolution brings it up to within a factor of two or three. The method uses a thin image plane, usually 1 to 2 mm instead of the conventional 10 mm, to reduce volume averaging of densities; often a smaller field of view to provide more pixels of computer resolution per unit area of lung; and a higher contrast or edge-enhancing image calculation. The result is comparable to a pathologist's naked-eye view of a slice of lung (Fig. 202-3). The trade-off is that the number of these thin slices that can be made is limited by radiation exposure, which precludes covering the entire lung; the method is used to sample the lung, like a noninvasive biopsy. Firm clinical indications have not developed yet, though this experimental technique should prove useful in the differential diagnosis of suspected interstitial lung diseases and is a preferred technique for excluding bronchiectasis.

LIMITED CT STUDIES   CT scans of the chest initially were complete, top to bottom, without and with contrast injection. With more confidence in the anatomy as displayed on the scan and widened indications for using CT, studies of a limited part of the chest, using regular or high-resolution CT technique and no contrast, should play an increasing role. Their cost can be substantially less than a full scan, hardly more than adding a couple of oblique views to a routine CR. Uncertain CR findings can often be solved rapidly using limited CT studies, in preference to waiting a few costly hospital days for the diagnosis to become clear. CT densitometry is useful in determining the presence or absence of calcification in solitary pulmonary nodules.

MAGNETIC RESONANCE IMAGING

Nuclear magnetic resonance is a property of atomic nuclei with an odd number of nucleons, of which the most abundant in the body is hydrogen. While in a strong magnetic field, the alignment of these spinning nuclei can be changed with a superimposed radio-frequency signal, and the rate at which they return to alignment with the field (''relaxation'') can be measured by their emission of a faint signal. There are two kinds of relaxation rates, which are functions of the atomic and chemical environment of each nucleus, and therefore they differ in different tissues.

By ingenious use of gradients, relaxation rates can be measured simultaneously at many points within a three-dimensional volume, which allows them to be shown as a set of gray scale images, either in the transverse, coronal, or sagittal plane. The timing of the imposed radio-frequency signal determines which of the relaxation rates predominates, and therefore the constructed images have different shades of gray for the same tissue, though the underlying anatomic structure is unchanged. At this time, there is only limited standardization of technique, especially since optimum differentiation of specific abnormalities requires different machine settings.

Transverse magnetic resonance (MR) images look much like CT images except for the different substitutions of light and dark for different tissues (Fig. 202-4). For example, fat is darker than water on CT, but is the brightest tissue on ''T_1-weighted'' MR images. Water (e.g., cerebrospinal fluid) becomes as bright as fat on T_2-weighted MR images (Fig. 202-4). The values, T_1 and T_2, are the half-times of the relaxation rates mentioned above, and are therefore a property of the tissue itself. The flexibility of eliciting and displaying the two relaxation rates provides MR images with even more effective tissue characterization contrast than CT.

Though the protons in blood have a strong MR signal because of the atomic environment of the iron and should therefore appear bright, flowing blood is seen as black, a signal void, on images. During the pause after the radio-frequency signal is triggered, while waiting to measure relaxation signals, the blood containing the altered protons has time to flow out of the plane of interest and is replaced by blood that is emitting no signal. Therefore, normal blood vessels as well as bronchi appear black on MR images (Fig. 202-4), but the distinction between nodes and vessels in the hilar regions is greatly facilitated compared to CT. There are artifactual signals from blood vessels, however, when blood flow is slow, notably on scans gated to diastole in the cardiac cycle (which are essential for studying the heart and hilar regions of the mediastinum) and on multisection simultaneous scans, when altered protons from one section will arrive at another level just in time for their signal to be detected. Finally, new methods of faster scanning result in images with flowing blood looking bright, as in an angiogram. The technology is evolving.

At present, MR scanning has important limitations compared with CT. A wide variety of artifacts complicate the interpretation of MR

FIGURE 202-4 Patient with ectopic ACTH syndrome caused by a bronchial carcinoid. Magnetic resonance image shows one bright region (high signal) in the posterior part of the left lower lobe (T). Normal pulmonary vessels are not visible because the MR signal of moving blood is emitted beyond the plane of the image. The carcinoid tumor was indistinguishable from vessels on the CT scan. This is a T_2-weighted image, as revealed by the bright appearance of the cerebrospinal fluid (C). The image is noisier than a CT image. The heart is blurred because of its motion (not a pulse-gated image), but the greater tissue resolution makes the tumor (T) visible compared to CT. There is absence of signal from the flowing blood in the descending aorta (d). *(Courtesy of I. Feuerstein and J. Doppman.)*

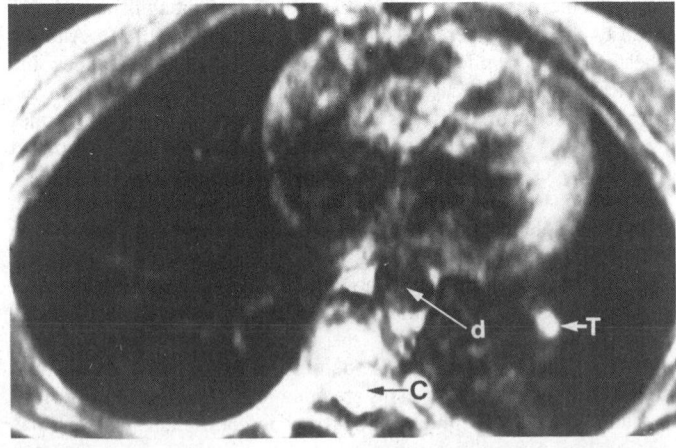

images and the images are also noisier and less uniform than those of CT. The geometric resolution of whole-body scans is inferior to CT, though superficial small regions can be shown with superb detail using special surface antennae to detect the faint relaxation signals. The advantage of being able to display data in any planar direction is weakened by the necessity (at present) of leaving a gap between the image slices. The collection of data (except with experimental fast-scan techniques) requires several minutes, which means that there are breathing artifacts in addition to those from cardiac motion. The narrow magnet tunnel into which the patient is inserted promotes claustrophobia, and the changes in the magnetic field cause a distressing noise. Ferromagnetic materials, including those in the patient, cannot be brought into the magnet room safely, for they will fly toward the center of the magnet. Other metal in the patient will merely ruin the image in its vicinity. Finally, the cost of MR scanning is substantial, approximately twice that of a contrast CT.

MR APPLICATIONS Gated cardiac studies are of great promise (Chap. 178), but are outside the scope of this discussion. The spine can be displayed with the perspective of an anatomic diagram, because of the availability of sagittal projections. This enables MR scanning to be particularly useful in questions of paraspinal, intraspinal, or intraosseous tumor. Tumors in the mediastinum can be analyzed by their T_1 and T_2 properties, but the hope for a way to distinguish inflammatory enlargement of nodes from that of tumor has not been realized yet. As noted, MR imaging is more sensitive than CT for distinguishing nonvascular tissue in the complex hilar regions and in the central portions of the lung (Fig. 202-4), but is probably less satisfactory in the mediastinum. Detection of intravascular pulmonary emboli or thrombi has been demonstrated experimentally, but clinical application is still remote.

Use of sagittal and coronal or oblique images in the mediastinum facilitates study of the arteries, so that MR scanning of the aorta is the preferred noninvasive way to detect aortic dissection or aneurysm (Chap. 197). These projections should be ideal for studying the trachea, but the trachea and bronchi are poorly displayed, with an artifactual narrowing of the lumen. The lungs and pleura do not usually benefit from MR study, in comparison with CT. The staging of lung cancer by mediastinal scanning has about the same effectiveness using MR as CT.

SPECTROSCOPY When chemists use MR to analyze mixtures and determine chemical structure, they study many nuclei in addition to hydrogen. Only hydrogen is sufficiently abundant in the body to provide enough signal to form images, but other substances can be quantitated in a volume that would be unsuitable for imaging. The most important is phosphorus, which has different resonant frequencies in its various molecular positions as part of ATP, AMP, creatine phosphate, inorganic phosphorus, etc. A limited number of relatively abundant cellular metabolites can also be measured by detecting protons with specific resonance values, if the very strong proton signal from water is suppressed. Metabolic processes can therefore be monitored by in vivo MR spectroscopy, a research technique of potential future clinical application.

NUCLEAR MEDICINE IMAGING

Injected or inhaled radioisotopes (radionuclides) incorporated into carefully chosen substances can provide anatomic, physiologic, and pathologic information from their distribution and disposition, as revealed on gamma camera images. Nuclear medicine remains the primary technique for the clinical problem of pulmonary thromboembolism (Chaps. 203 and 213) and the regional assessment of obstructive lung diseases.

ULTRASOUND IN THE CHEST

Imaging with ultrasound requires the computerized reconstruction of series of echoes of high-frequency sound emitted at various angles from a piezoelectric crystal transducer. The echoes arise as the radiating sound encounters surfaces of different acoustic impedance at right angles to its path. Ultrasound does not pass through air or bone, so the lungs themselves and the ribs are major limitations on its usefulness in the chest. A fluid collection such as a cyst or abscess will be echo-free, or *sonolucent*, unless it has debris in it, and will transmit sound and deeper echoes without attenuation. In solid tissues, the signal is attenuated as the sound is absorbed, so that the echoes become weaker as their depth in the tissue increases. Air-containing lung has no echo beyond the pleural interface at its surface, although consolidated lung may look like solid tissue.

APPLICATIONS The principal application of ultrasonography in the mediastinum is cardiac, discussed in detail in Chap. 177, including the detection of pericardial fluid and cysts. Bronchogenic cysts, in their most common subcarinal location, may also be confirmed to be fluid-containing by ultrasound. The most common pulmonary application is detection of fluid or pus in the pleural space. For diagnosis, ultrasound is convenient, since it can be performed with bedside apparatus, but it is not as accurate as CT (or MR) as it may confuse homogeneous pleural fibrosis or pulmonary consolidation with sonolucent pleural fluid. If the pleural fluid collection is loculated or small in amount, then localization by ultrasound enhances the safety and usefulness of thoracentesis.

INTERVENTIONAL RADIOLOGY

Advances in imaging with ultrasound and CT have brought with them a renaissance of percutaneous procedures for biopsy and drainage. Though fluoroscopically guided percutaneous needle biopsy of the lungs has been established for at least 20 years, CT has made it possible to pursue smaller targets and those close to vital structures. Under CT control, needle biopsy of enlarged nodes in the mediastinum can replace mediastinoscopic node biopsy, particularly when inoperability is being established by biopsy.

A more recent interventional innovation is drainage of pleural effusions, pneumothorax, and empyema in the thorax and abscesses in the abdomen by catheters inserted over guidewires that have been introduced through percutaneous needles, using techniques originally developed for angiography. The fluid or air pocket is localized and the needle position confirmed using ultrasound or CT, the specific technique depending on the ease with which the fluid can be delineated with ultrasound. Even lung abscesses can be drained percutaneously. Transcatheter embolization with particulate matter, coils, or detachable balloons has become widely used in the treatment of massive hemoptysis and arteriovenous malformations of the lung. Considerable savings are achieved in risk, pain, recovery time, and cost by avoiding major surgery with these methods.

REFERENCES

CARROLL FE JR: Lungs, in *Magnetic Resonance Imaging*, CL Partain et al (eds). Philadelphia, Saunders, 1988

FRASER RG et al: *Diagnosis of Diseases of the Chest*, 3d ed. Philadelphia, Saunders, 1988

FRIEDMAN PJ: Practical radiology of the hila and mediastinum. Postgrad Radiol 1:269, 1981

HAAGA JR, ALFIDI RJ (eds): *Computed Tomography of the Whole Body*, 2nd ed. St. Louis, Mosby, 1988

HIGGINS CB, HRICAK H: *Magnetic Resonance Imaging of the Body*. New York, Raven, 1987

PROTO AV: Mediastinal anatomy: Emphasis on conventional images with anatomic and computed tomographic correlations. J Thorac Imag 2:1, 1987

SAGEL SS, STANLEY RJ: *Computed Body Tomography with MRI correlation*, 2nd ed. New York, Raven, 1989

VAN SONNENBERG E et al: CT- and ultrasound-guided catheter drainage of empyemas after chest-tube failure. Radiology 151:349, 1984.

WEBB WR: Magnetic resonance imaging of the hila and mediastinum. Cardiovasc Intervent Radiol 8:306, 1986

———: *Mediastinum and hila*, in *Magnetic Resonance Imaging*, CL Partain et al (eds). Philadelphia, Saunders, 1988

203   DIAGNOSTIC PROCEDURES IN RESPIRATORY DISEASES

KENNETH M. MOSER

In seeking a definitive diagnosis in the patient with respiratory disease, a wide choice of diagnostic procedures is available. These procedures vary considerably, not only in diagnostic reliability and specificity, but also in terms of the discomfort and hazard to the patient. Hence, an orderly sequence of test selection is mandatory. This sequence should begin with procedures involving little risk and, only if necessary, move on to those which entail higher morbidity and potential mortality.

NONINVASIVE PROCEDURES

RADIOGRAPHIC PROCEDURES (See also Chap. 202)   The *chest roentgenogram* serves two major roles in the search for a diagnosis in the patient with respiratory disease: *detector* and *guide*. Occasionally, in its role as a detector, the routine chest roentgenogram initiates the diagnostic search by disclosing an abnormality in an asymptomatic individual. However, routine chest roentgenography (e.g., as an element of all hospital admissions) is neither necessary nor cost-effective. Therefore, more commonly, it detects pulmonary involvement in someone already ill. Rarely, detection may coincide with diagnosis; e.g., in spontaneous pneumothorax or when a radiopaque foreign body has been aspirated.

Far more frequently, however, the roentgenogram, having detected potential disease, provides a guide to the selection of subsequent diagnostic procedures. Many radiographic findings are quite characteristic of certain diseases. A number of radiographic patterns are sufficiently repetitive to warrant descriptive names, such as bilateral hilar adenopathy, solitary pulmonary nodule, diffuse interstitial infiltrate, alveolar filling pattern, multinodular lesion, and honeycomb lung. Thus, a particular radiographic finding, combined with other pertinent data, often permits establishment of a reasonable list of possible diagnoses. For example, the roentgenographic detection of bilateral hilar adenopathy in an asymptomatic, 26-year-old black male immediately places sarcoidosis at the top of the list. A chest roentgenogram disclosing upper lobe cavities in a febrile male whose brother recently was admitted to a tuberculosis sanitarium would make tuberculosis the most likely entity. Or a "diffuse interstitial" infiltrate—for which more than 100 causes exist—may yield a prompt diagnosis of varicella pneumonia when combined with the classic skin lesions. Multinodular lesions, with some cavitating, in a patient with sinusitis and red cell casts on urinalysis makes Wegener's granulomatosis a primary diagnostic possibility. However, no roentgenographic pattern is sufficiently specific to *establish* a diagnosis. Lung cancer (primary and metastatic) can present many roentgenographic patterns, as can both infectious and noninfectious lung disorders. For example, cardiogenic pulmonary edema may present as a perihilar or diffuse alveolar filling pattern, as an interstitial process and, rarely, as a lobar infiltrate or interlobar collection of fluid ("pseudotumor")—all with or without a pleural effusion.

In some instances, special radiographic techniques may provide valuable diagnostic insights.

Fluoroscopy allows visualization of the thoracic contents in a dynamic rather than static manner and also permits a wide range of special views. It also indicates whether a lesion is pulsatile, what its precise location in the thorax is, whether the hemidiaphragms move normally, i.e., whether they are fixed or move paradoxically, and how various zones of the lung behave during inspiration and expiration. Thus, fluoroscopy can define whether a roentgenographic density is actually in a rib or in the pleura rather than in the parenchyma; and may distinguish between a unilateral hyperlucent lung due to emphy-

sema (mediastinum shifts toward the normal lung on expiration) or to unilateral pulmonary arterial obstruction (no shift).

Thoracic *computed tomography* (*CT*) *scanning* has essentially replaced standard tomography (laminography, planigraphy). Both techniques provide a sequence of images, each representing a "slice of the lung" at a different depth. Ordinarily, "cuts" are made at 0.5- to 1.0-cm distances through the areas of interest. These procedures can identify a number of features which are not appreciated on the "routine" roentgenogram, including calcium in a solitary nodule (which if diffuse or in concentric rings signifies a benign etiology); a cavity within a mass lesion; and the presence of hilar, paratracheal, and subcarinal node enlargement. The CT scan is particularly useful in the definition of pleural disease (e.g., differentiating fluid from tumor; identifying calcium in asbestos-exposed individuals); with contrast injections, in differentiating tissue masses from vascular structures; and in identifying small parenchymal nodules. However, to some extent, the sensitivity of CT is a mixed blessing because it is still not known how many "normal" individuals have pleural or parenchymal abnormalities by CT and how these small, benign, hitherto undetected lesions can be distinguished from neoplastic lesions.

Magnetic resonance (MR) imaging remains, in terms of its value in pulmonary diseases, an investigational technique. It has potential value in achieving fine definition of mediastinal lesions and, perhaps, in defining embolic occlusion of major pulmonary arteries.

SKIN TESTS   Having arrived at a tentative list of diagnostic possibilities based on the history, physical examination, and radiographic appearance, the physician should move to other procedures. One of the simplest and most commonly overlooked is the application of *skin tests* with specific antigens. Antigens are now available to assist in the diagnosis of tuberculosis, histoplasmosis, coccidioidomycosis, blastomycosis, trichinosis, toxoplasmosis, and aspergillosis. These tests vary with respect to sensitivity and cross-reactivity, and attention to scrupulous technique in performance and interpretation is vital. Also, some antigens (e.g., histoplasmosis) may confound serologic tests performed subsequently. A positive skin test indicates only that the antigen has been encountered previously by the host; it does not, regardless of reaction intensity, imply active disease. Furthermore, drugs or diseases which depress cell-mediated immunity (e.g., prednisone, cyclophosphamide, lymphomas, sarcoidosis, disseminated tuberculosis, or coccidioidomycosis) may cause skin anergy. Indeed, a negative battery of skin tests, if it incorporates antigens such as mumps, streptokinase-streptodornase, *Trichophyton*, and *Candida*, suggests that a cause of skin anergy should be sought.

SEROLOGIC TESTS   These tests also may be useful in the diagnosis of histoplasmosis, blastomycosis, coccidioidomycosis, toxoplasmosis, *Mycoplasma* pneumonia, Legionnaires' disease, a variety of other infectious diseases involving the lungs, and certain immunologically mediated lung diseases (e.g., lupus erythematosus). Often, more extensive diagnostic procedures can be avoided if appropriate serologic tests are obtained. However, there is substantial interinstitutional variability with respect to the sensitivity, specificity, and types of serologic tests available. Therefore, their appropriate use requires close interaction with the responsible laboratory.

SPUTUM EXAMINATION   Another rapid, innocuous diagnostic procedure is *sputum examination*. It is important that the specimen contain sputum, not saliva, the latter being identified by the presence of squamous (mouth) rather than epithelial (bronchial) cells. The gross nature of the sputum—color, odor, and the presence of blood—may provide valuable clues; e.g., foul sputum suggesting anaerobic pulmonary infection, and blood, in any amount, indicating an abnormality that mandates further investigation. Carefully stained smears of the sputum should be examined next, for these may disclose the causative organism in many bacterial pneumonias, tuberculosis, *Pneumocystis* pneumonia, and in some fungus infections. Sputum eosinophilia can suggest the presence of reversible airway disease responsive to glucocorticoids; hemosiderin-laden macrophages suggest the possibility of Goodpasture's syndrome. Often valuable time is lost because the sputum smear is not examined and results of culture are awaited instead. Sputum samples can be obtained from patients who are not coughing by having them inhale a heated mixture of a mildly irritative solution that induces cough. Such induced samples have been particularly useful in the diagnosis of *P. carinii* pneumonia and in obtaining cytologic specimens for the diagnosis of carcinoma of the lung (Chap. 215). Careful handling of such specimens and interpretive expertise heavily determine the diagnostic yield.

Culture of expectorated sputum (spontaneous or induced) has fallen into disrepute because of uncertain yield and, particularly, because of frequent and unavoidable contamination by the oropharyngeal bacterial flora. Although such cultures are invaluable for identification of organisms responsible for tuberculous and fungus infections, their utility in detection of other bacterial agents responsible for pulmonary infection is often uncertain and can be misleading, particularly in patients who are immunocompromised, intubated, or receiving antimicrobial therapy. Five procedures, described below, are now gaining wide acceptance because they limit oropharyngeal contamination and/or can be used to obtain representative samples of lung secretions from the area of lung involvement: (1) catheter-brush sampling, (2) bronchoalveolar lavage, (3) transtracheal aspiration, (4) transbronchial lung biopsy, and (5) percutaneous needle aspiration of the lung.

PULMONARY FUNCTION TESTS (See also Chap. 201) Certain "patterns" of derangement in spirometric tests, arterial blood gases, diffusing capacity, and other functional parameters are particularly suggestive of certain pulmonary diseases. For example, diffuse interstitial fibrotic diseases of the lungs (Chap. 211) produce a "restrictive" spirometric defect, reduced pulmonary compliance, a reduced diffusing capacity, and an alveolar-arterial oxygen tension difference which is widened at rest and widens further with exercise. Emphysema (Chap. 210) characteristically causes expiratory obstruction, lung hyperinflation, decreased static elastic recoil (increased compliance), and a reduced diffusing capacity.

PULMONARY SCINTIPHOTOGRAPHY Scintiphotographs ("scans") of intrathoracic structures are obtained by a variety of "scanning" devices which record the pattern of intrathoracic radioactivity after intravenous injection or inhalation of gamma-emitting radionuclides. Direct photographic or computer-derived images, or digital data, reflecting radionuclide distribution are used for diagnostic purposes. The most commonly used images are those which reflect the distribution of pulmonary blood flow (perfusion) and ventilation. Such scans have multiple diagnostic applications. For example, a normal perfusion scan excludes the diagnosis of acute pulmonary embolism (Chap. 213). When perfusion scans showing defects are combined with ventilation scans, ventilation-perfusion patterns are provided which assist in the diagnosis of parenchymal lung diseases and vascular occlusive disorders, including pulmonary embolism.

Another type of scan involves intravenous injection of radionuclides which have an affinity for intrathoracic inflammatory and neoplastic tissues. Gallium 67 is the most useful of such radionuclides now available. Concentration of such agents, defined by scanning, may permit detection of neoplastic or inflammatory disease in the lungs or mediastinal lymph nodes. Uptake by the lungs may, in some patients, reflect the intensity of inflammatory activity associated with diffuse interstitial pneumonitis, sarcoidosis, and granulomatous infections. Inapparent extrapulmonary foci of granulomatous or neoplastic diseases also may be detected by body scanning.

New radionuclides continue to emerge which, when complexed with such materials as platelets, white blood cells (e.g., indium 111), fibrinogen, and albumin, may allow imaging of intrathoracic vessels, thrombi, inflammation, and neoplasms. Tomographic and other image-processing methods are emerging which may further extend the value of these techniques.

All the above procedures involve minimal risks and discomfort to the patient. Where applicable, these approaches should be considered before the more invasive techniques discussed below are considered, unless the condition of the patient demands immediate diagnosis.

INVASIVE PROCEDURES

BRONCHOSCOPY The primary objectives of bronchoscopy include direct visualization of the tracheobronchial tree, including abnormalities such as tumors or granulomatous lesions; biopsy of suggestive or obvious endobronchial lesions; and lavage, brushing, or biopsy of lung regions for cultural and cytologic examinations. Both the *diagnostic reach of* and *accessibility to* bronchoscopy have been expanded by the flexible fiberoptic bronchoscope (FOB). This can be understood best by comparing the FOB with the "standard" rigid bronchoscope.

The rigid bronchoscope is a wide-bore metal tube which incorporates a lighted mirror-lens system. The FOB is composed of fiberoptic bundles which provide both illumination and visualization pathways. A small channel with a diameter of 1 to 3 mm traverses the FOB, through which instruments can be passed, fluids delivered, and suction applied. The rigid bronchoscope comes in various external diameters limited only by the feasibility of introducing the rigid device orally and through the larynx. Biopsy and other procedures are carried out through the rather capacious interior of the rigid tube. The FOB also is available in various external diameters, but all are substantially smaller than rigid bronchoscopes (since no "wall" exists in the FOB). The distal tip of the FOB can be *flexed* easily to 90° and usually to 130° or more from the vertical.

Thus, the rigid bronchoscope permits visualization only of lobar bronchi and the orifices of some segmental bronchi. The flexible, smaller FOB extends the range of *view* to all segmental and subsegmental bronchi and the range for *biopsy and sampling* to the pulmonary parenchyma itself. A biopsy forceps, catheter, or brush passed through the FOB can be directed well beyond the tip of the bronchoscope itself, permitting *transbronchial lung biopsy, brushings,* or *aspiration of secretions* for culture and cytologic examination from the most distal regions of the lung. Indeed, both forceps and brush can reach and perforate the pleura, leading to pneumothorax. Therefore, when the lesion being approached is distal, fluoroscopic guidance is essential. Not only does this permit placement of the FOB, forceps, catheter, or brush directly into the area of interest, but also it ensures that the pleura will not be inadvertently reached and punctured. The FOB also allows *regional* lung lavage to obtain materials for cytologic examination and culture. The use of specially designed catheters (see below) placed through the FOB is quite useful in obtaining representative, noncontaminated secretions for culture, thus avoiding the problems mentioned previously with expectorated sputum.

Thus, the FOB has sharply increased the limited diagnostic reach previously available with rigid bronchoscopy. Equally important, the FOB has made bronchoscopy more available to the physician and more acceptable to the patient. The performance of rigid bronchoscopy requires the supine position for peroral insertion of the device; can be performed safely by a relatively few trained physicians; and is often carried out under general anesthesia in an operating room. Therefore, it has been a procedure requiring significant preparation and hence delay. Fiberoptic bronchoscopy can be performed in the sitting or supine position, since the FOB is easily inserted transnasally; can be performed by a large number of trained pulmonary specialists as well as surgeons; usually requires only local anesthesia; and can be performed safely on the wards, in diagnostic rooms equipped with a "dentist-type" chair, and in intensive care units. The FOB can be used easily in intubated patients on ventilators with simple "side-arm" adapters attached to the endotracheal tube. Therefore, when bronchoscopy is indicated, it is not surprising that fiberoptic bronchoscopy is now commonly the first choice. The roomier rigid bronchoscope is now usually reserved for situations in which the small biopsy-suction channel in the FOB may be inadequate (e.g., for removal of large foreign bodies, for laser surgery). The FOB also has a widening range of therapeutic applications including aspiration or lavage of secretions in patients with airway obstruction or atelectasis due to retained secretions; obstruction of bleeding areas of the lung, with a wedged FOB itself or with a balloon catheter passed via the

FOB, in patients who are poor surgical risks; removal of small foreign bodies; and placement of radionuclides in tumors. Transtracheal needle aspiration of paratracheal and subcarinal nodes also can be performed via the FOB, a procedure which is particularly useful in the staging of carcinoma of the lung.

The hazards of bronchoscopy are modest but should be recognized. In addition to the risk of general anesthesia which rigid bronchoscopy usually requires, they can include hypoxemia, laryngospasm, bronchospasm, pneumothorax, and, of course, bleeding following biopsy. Proper management before, during, and after bronchoscopy should prevent most of these complications. There is no absolute contraindication to FOB. Even in the presence of massive hemoptysis, FOB with appropriate precautions can yield useful information. Patients with bronchospasm (or a history of bronchospasm) are at particular risk of acute enhancement of spasm and should be approached after good preparation and with resources for intubation-ventilation at hand. The primary contraindication to both rigid and fiberoptic bronchoscopy is the same: performance by inexperienced personnel. Lack of experience sharply reduces diagnostic and therapeutic yield while increasing risks.

BRONCHOGRAPHY In this method, radiopaque material is instilled into the tracheobronchial tree via a catheter or bronchoscope. Positioning of the patient and catheter permits the material to coat all portions of the tracheobronchial tree for a sufficient period so that their outline can be recorded on chest roentgenograms. Bronchography is indicated for the diagnosis of bronchiectasis, for the identification of obstruction in distal bronchi, and for the detection of other types of congenital and acquired forms of tracheobronchial distortion or malformation. Like FOB, bronchography may induce bronchospasm; also, the irritative effects of the contrast medium may persist for some days. In many situations in which bronchography was used in the past (e.g., for the diagnosis of bronchiectasis), it is being replaced by chest CT.

TRANSTRACHEAL, CATHETER-BRUSH, AND PERCUTANEOUS NEEDLE ASPIRATION OF THE LUNG All three of these procedures are used to obtain material for culture and microscopic examination. In the case of culture, all three techniques bypass the oropharyngeal flora, though transtracheal aspiration is the least certain in this regard.

Transtracheal aspiration involves needle puncture of the cricothyroid membrane, insertion of a plastic cannula, and instillation of a saline solution, followed by suctioning of a sample. The procedure cannot be performed in intubated patients; contamination rates are high in previously intubated patients or those who have aspirated oropharyngeal contents. Because the procedure entails risks, although these are minimized by meticulous technique and experience, clear indications for its use should exist. These include apparent pulmonary infections in patients who are unable to cough, in whom cough is nonproductive, or in whom there has been a lack of response to therapy based on smears or cultures from expectorated sputum.

In these same contexts, *catheter-brush devices* specially designed with a distal plug to avoid oropharyngeal contamination can be used. These are manipulated (through an FOB or without it) under fluoroscopic guidance into the involved lung area. The distal absorbable plug is then ejected and the inner brush or catheter advanced for sampling. Finally, an alternative procedure is direct percutaneous aspiration, which can be performed using a small (23- or 25-gauge), thin-walled, *noncutting* needle. The needle, connected to a syringe, is introduced percutaneously into the area of the lung of interest; 2 to 3 mL saline is injected and then aspirated into the syringe and the needle withdrawn. Both the catheter-brush and needle approaches are high-yield, low-contamination procedures. In experienced hands, the risks are low, consisting chiefly of pneumothorax and bleeding. Patients should be carefully monitored for both.

The presence of a hemorrhagic diathesis is a relative contraindication to all three of the above procedures.

BRONCHOALVEOLAR LAVAGE (BAL) This procedure is usually performed by lightly wedging a fiberoptic bronchoscope in distal airways, gently irrigating the air spaces beyond with saline, and analyzing the cells obtained. A "liquid biopsy" of the contents of the distal air spaces is obtained. The procedure has value in the diagnosis of *P. carinii* pneumonia and other infections, in alveolar proteinosis, and in some patients with interstitial pneumonitis of uncertain cause. Maximum diagnostic yield requires careful techniques and expert sample processing.

THORACENTESIS AND PLEURAL BIOPSY Thoracentesis should be performed to obtain pleural fluid in all pleural effusions of uncertain etiology and may be indicated for relief of symptoms in some patients with effusion of known cause. In effusions of uncertain cause, closed (needle) pleural biopsy should be performed as part of the same procedure.

When pleural fluid is small in amount or when its presence or location is uncertain from routine or lateral decubitus roentgenograms, performance of the thoracentesis and biopsy under fluoroscopic, ultrasound, or CT scan guidance enhances both yield and safety. Pleural fluid obtained should be examined for specific gravity, white blood cell count and differential, protein and glucose concentrations, lactic acid dehydrogenase (LDH), pH, P_{CO_2} (sample collected anaerobically), and amylase. Gram stain, cultures, and exfoliative cytologic specimens should be obtained; and in some instances, rheumatoid factor and complement levels are measured. The gross appearance of the fluid, the quantity obtained, and the precise location of the thoracentesis should be recorded. A combination of a pleural fluid LDH above 200 IU, a pleural fluid/serum protein ratio greater than 0.5, and a pleural fluid/serum LDH ratio greater than 0.6 all indicate that an "exudative" rather than "transudative" process is present. A low pH (<7.20) often indicates that an empyema, probably requiring tube drainage, is present (Chap. 216). Specific diagnostic findings in pleural fluid may include the opalescent, pearly fluid characteristic of chylothorax; positive smears or cultures for tuberculosis or other infections; a marked elevation of amylase indicative of effusion secondary to pancreatitis or a ruptured esophagus; and the very low glucose values often seen in effusions associated with rheumatoid arthritis.

As already noted, closed (needle) pleural biopsy should follow thoracentesis whenever the diagnosis is uncertain. It is important to leave some fluid in the pleural space as this makes biopsy easier and safer. Bleeding, pneumothorax, and bronchopleural fistula induced by cutting through the visceral pleura are all more likely in the absence of fluid, and a satisfactory biopsy specimen is less likely to be obtained. Several special needles are available for biopsy of the parietal pleura. All have a cutting edge and some device for retaining the biopsy. The needle is inserted into the pleural effusion, then withdrawn until it is seated on the parietal pleura, from which a biopsy is obtained with the cutting edge. Usually, three biopsies are taken from different sites at the same session. Care should be exercised to place the needle in a position least likely to impinge on the intercostal vessels. All fluid to be used for diagnosis should be removed before biopsy since postbiopsy bleeding may obscure the true character of the fluid.

Pleuroscopy, using a modified FOB inserted through an intercostal trocar, also can be used for both direct inspection and biopsy of the pleura. In the absence of a pleural effusion, two other options exist for obtaining tissue from pleural-based lesions: aspiration needle biopsy and open biopsy. The technique for aspiration biopsy is the same as that described above, although some physicians use "cutting" needles (see "Lung Biopsy" below). Open pleural biopsy involves a limited thoracotomy, requiring anesthesia. A small intercostal incision is made, and the parietal pleura is biopsied under direct visualization. The incision is then closed, often without an intercostal tube. Open biopsy has several advantages because a larger specimen is obtained and the pleura and underlying lung can be seen and palpated. When pleural involvement is "spotty," open biopsy increases the possibility of establishing a diagnosis.

PULMONARY AND BRONCHIAL ANGIOGRAPHY Visualization of the pulmonary arteries by *pulmonary angiography* is achieved by direct, rapid injection of radiopaque materials into the main pulmonary artery or its branches, preferably via cardiac catheterization. Nonionic radiopaque materials, while more expensive, reduce the frequency and severity of unwanted respiratory and hemodynamic responses (e.g., cough, elevation in pulmonary arterial pressure). Multiple, large films can be obtained by an automatic filmchanger; or motion picture or video film (cineangiography) can be used. If visualization of smaller pulmonary vessels is required, magnification techniques can be used. Digital subtraction pulmonary angiography, providing computer-derived images of digital data, may allow imaging of the larger pulmonary arteries with contrast injected more proximally (into superior or inferior vena cava or peripheral vein) or at lower concentrations; however, motion artifacts limit its sensitivity and specificity. Angiography is frequently used to detect pulmonary emboli and a variety of congenital and acquired lesions of the pulmonary vessels. The procedure carries some risk, particularly in patients with pulmonary hypertension, and clear indication for it must exist as well as personnel experienced in its performance and interpretation.

Angioscopy, an experimental technique for direct visualization of the right cardiac chambers and pulmonary arterial system, can be accomplished by insertion of a fiberoptic device via a peripheral vein. The diagnostic role of this procedure in embolic and other disorders remains to be defined.

Bronchial arteriography is of value to identify and control (embolotherapy) otherwise obscure bleeding sites in the lungs. Transarterial placement of a catheter into the orifices or parent vessels of bronchial arteries can be accomplished by experienced operators. Radiopaque material is then injected so that these arteries can be visualized. If a bleeding site is identified, emboli can be injected via the catheter as a means for halting hemoptysis.

MEDIASTINOSCOPY AND MEDIASTINOTOMY Another favored site for biopsy is the lymph nodes in the mediastinum. Because they receive lymphatic drainage from the lungs, these nodes often disclose intrathoracic diseases such as carcinoma, granulomatous infections, and sarcoidosis. As noted above, transtracheal needle aspiration of mediastinal nodes via the FOB is one approach to such nodes. Another is mediastinoscopy, which involves insertion of a lighted mirror-lens system, much like a bronchoscope, through an incision at the base of the neck anteriorly. The instrument is advanced under visual control into the mediastinum, where inspection and biopsy can be carried out. Because of its higher yield of diagnostic lymph nodes, mediastinoscopy has virtually replaced biopsy of the *scalene fat pad* for nodes of interest on the right side of the mediastinum. However, for anatomic reasons, mediastinoscopy on the left is less satisfactory and more hazardous. Nodes in this location are usually approached through a limited left anterior thoracotomy (mediastinotomy) or, occasionally, by scalene fat pad biopsy. Needle aspiration, mediastinoscopy, and mediastinotomy are low-risk, high-yield procedures. They are invaluable in the "staging" of patients with known or suspected pulmonary malignancy.

LUNG BIOPSY Finally, if the diagnosis still remains unclear, biopsy of the lung may be required. Again, "closed" and "open" approaches are available. Closed biopsies are of three types: transbronchial, aspiration, and "cutting needle." Transbronchial biopsy, carried out through the fiberoptic bronchoscope, is a highly useful procedure, particularly since larger forceps have been introduced and the taking of multiple biopsies during one procedure has become routine.

However, when lesions are small and/or anatomically located beyond the reach of the FOB, direct aspiration needle biopsy is often more rewarding. *Aspiration* biopsy, mentioned previously, provides cytologic material but does not actually obtain a specimen of lung whose architecture can be examined, a feature which may be necessary to establish a diagnosis. Various "cutting" needles are available which do provide a "core" of the involved lung. However, this approach has waned in popularity because of the high incidence of pneumothorax and bleeding, occasional deaths due to air embolism, and the small size of the biopsy specimen, which may limit diagnostic

interpretation. Fluoroscopic guidance is essential in all these closed approaches, and they are contraindicated if pulmonary hypertension or a hemorrhagic diathesis is present.

Open-lung biopsy, requiring thoracotomy, is the final diagnostic resort. It is, however, a relatively safe procedure even in patients with respiratory failure, hemorrhagic diathesis, or pulmonary hypertension if meticulous surgical and anesthetic techniques are observed. Direct visualization allows selection of an optimum biopsy site, and of course, a specimen of adequate size is obtained. In selecting among these closed and open options, consideration of local expertise in their performance is a key factor.

All specimens obtained by biopsy should be both cultured and processed for pathologic examination.

REFERENCES

BORDELON JY JR et al: The telescoping plugged catheter in suspected anaerobic infections: A controlled series. Am Rev Respir Dis 128:465, 1983

BORDOW RA, MOSER KM: *Manual of Clinical Problems in Pulmonary Medicine.* Boston, Little, Brown, 1985

HASLAM PL: Bronchoalveolar lavage. Semin Respir Med 6:55, 1984

NAIDICH P et al (eds): *Computed Tomography of the Thorax.* New York, Raven Press, 1984

NICOD P et al: Pulmonary angiography in severe chronic pulmonary hypertension. Ann Intern Med 107:565, 1987

SHURE D (ed): *Diagnostic Technics: Clinics in Chest Medicine.* Philadelphia, Saunders, 1987

TURNER-WARWICK M, HASLAM PL: The value of serial bronchoalveolar lavage in assessing the clinical progress of patients with cryptogenic fibrosing alveolitis. Am Rev Respir Dis 135:26, 1987

WESSELIUS LJ et al: Computer-assisted versus usual lung gallium-67 index in normals and patients with interstitial lung disorders. Am Rev Respir Dis 128:1084, 1983

204 ASTHMA

E. R. McFADDEN, JR.

DEFINITION Asthma is a disease of airways that is characterized by increased responsiveness of the tracheobronchial tree to a multiplicity of stimuli. Asthma is manifested physiologically by a widespread narrowing of the air passages, which may be relieved spontaneously or as a result of therapy, and clinically by paroxysms of dyspnea, cough, and wheezing. It is an episodic disease, acute exacerbations being interspersed with symptom-free periods. Typically, most attacks are short-lived, lasting minutes to hours, and after them the patient seems to recover completely clinically. However, there can be a phase in which the patient experiences some degree of airway obstruction daily. This phase can be mild, with or without superimposed severe episodes, or much more serious, with severe obstruction persisting for days or weeks, a condition known as *status asthmaticus.*

PREVALENCE AND ETIOLOGY The prevalence and incidence of asthma is difficult to assess with certainty because of the lack of reliable population-based figures which have used uniform diagnostic criteria. However, it has been suggested that approximately 5 percent of adults and 7 to 10 percent of children in the United States and Australia have the disorder. Bronchial asthma occurs at all ages but predominantly in early life. About one-half of the cases develop before age 10 and another third occur before age 40. In childhood, there is a 2:1 male/female preponderance, which equalizes by age 30.

From an etiologic standpoint, asthma is a heterogeneous disease, and attempts to define it in etiologic or pathologic terms have proved difficult. It is useful for epidemiologic and clinical purposes to classify the forms of this disease by the principal stimuli that incite or are associated with acute episodes. However, it is important to emphasize that the distinction between various types of asthma may often be artificial, and the response of a given subclassification usually can be initiated by more than one type of stimulus. With this reservation in mind, one can describe two broad groups: allergic and idiosyncratic.

Allergic asthma is often associated with a personal and/or family history of allergic diseases such as rhinitis, urticaria, and eczema; positive wheal-and-flare skin reactions to intradermal injection of extracts of airborne antigens; increased levels of IgE in the serum; and/or positive response to provocation tests involving the inhalation of specific antigen.

A significant segment of the asthmatic population will present with negative family or personal histories of allergy, negative skin tests, and normal serum levels of IgE, and therefore cannot be classified on the basis of defined immunologic mechanisms. These we term *idiosyncratic*. Many of these will develop a typical symptom complex upon contracting an upper respiratory illness. The initial insult may be little more than a common cold, but after several days the patient begins to develop paroxysms of wheezing and dyspnea that can last for days to months. These individuals should not be confused with persons in whom the symptoms of bronchospasm are superimposed upon chronic bronchitis or bronchiectasis (see Chap. 210).

Unfortunately, many patients will not clearly fit into either of the above categories but will fall into a mixed group with features of each. In general, those patients whose onset of disease is in early life will tend to have a strong allergic component to their illness, while those who develop their asthma late tend to be nonallergic or to have mixed etiologies.

PATHOGENESIS OF ASTHMA The common denominator underlying the asthmatic diathesis is a nonspecific hyperirritability of the tracheobronchial tree. In asthmatics it correlates well with the clinical features of the illness. When airway reactivity is high, lung function becomes more unstable, symptoms are more severe and persistent, the acute response to bronchodilators is larger, and the amount of therapy required to control the patient's complaints increases. In addition, the magnitude of diurnal fluctuations in lung function becomes greater and the patient tends to awaken at night or in the early morning with breathlessness.

In both normal and asthmatic subjects, airway reactivity is known to rise following viral infections of the respiratory tract and exposure to oxidant air pollutants such as ozone and nitrogen dioxide. Viruses have more profound consequences, and following a seemingly trivial upper respiratory tract infection, airway responsivity may remain elevated for many weeks. In contrast, with exposure to ozone airway reactivity remains high for only a few days. Airway reactivity has also been shown to increase in normal individuals with the exogenous administration of platelet activating factor. Allergens can cause airway responsiveness to rise within minutes, and to remain elevated for weeks. If the dose of antigen is high enough, acute episodes of obstruction may occur daily for a prolonged period of time following a single exposure.

A number of causes have been postulated for the increased airway reactivity of asthma; however, the basic mechanism remains unknown. The most popular hypothesis at present is that of airway inflammation. Following exposure to an initiating stimulus, mast cells, basophils, and macrophages can be activated to release a variety of mediators which produce direct effects on airway smooth muscle and capillary permeability, thereby evoking an intense local reaction which can then be followed by a more chronic one. The latter may be brought about by the release of chemotactic factors which recruit cellular elements to the site of injury. In addition, it is thought that the acute and chronic effects of mediator release and cellular infiltration may result in epithelial damage with involvement of neural endings within the airways and the activation of an axon reflex. In this fashion, an essentially local phenomenon can be amplified to have widespread effects throughout the tracheobronchial tree.

The stimuli that increase airway responsiveness and incite acute episodes of asthma can be grouped into seven major categories:

allergenic, pharmacologic, environmental, occupational, infectious, exercise-related, and emotional.

Allergens Allergic asthma is dependent upon an IgE response controlled by T and B lymphocytes and activated by the interaction of antigen with mast cell–bound IgE molecules. Most of the allergens that provoke asthma are airborne, and in order to induce a state of sensitivity, they must be reasonably abundant for considerable periods of time. Once sensitization has occurred, however, the patient can then exhibit exquisite responsivity, so that minute amounts of the offending agent can produce significant exacerbations of the disease. Immunologic mechanisms appear to be causally related to the development of asthma in 25 to 35 percent of all cases, and contributory in perhaps another third. Allergic asthma is frequently seasonal, and it is most often observed in children and young adults. A nonseasonal form may result from allergy to feathers, animal danders, molds, and other antigens present continuously in the environment. Exposure to antigen typically produces an immediate response in which airway obstruction develops in minutes and then resolves. In 30 to 50 percent of patients a second wave of bronchoconstriction, the so-called late reaction, develops 6 to 10 h later. In a minority only a late reaction occurs. In some individuals following a single exposure marked cyclic changes in airway lability may recur daily for a variable period.

The mechanism by which an inhaled antigen can provoke an acute episode of asthma is unknown but seems to depend, in part, upon antigen-antibody interactions on the surface of pulmonary mast cells with the subsequent generation and release of the mediators of immediate hypersensitivity. Current postulates hold that very small antigenic particles penetrate the lung's defenses and come in contact with mast cells that are interdigitating with the epithelium at the luminal surface of the central airways. The subsequent elaboration of mediators then produces the sequence outlined above. The mediators released—histamine; bradykinin; the leukotrienes C, D, and E; platelet activating factor; prostaglandins PGG_2, $PGF_{2\alpha}$, and PGD_2, and thromboxane A_2—produce an intense inflammatory reaction with bronchoconstriction, vascular congestion, and edema formation. In addition to their ability to produce prolonged contraction of airway smooth muscle and mucosal edema, the leukotrienes also produce some of the other pathophysiologic features of asthma such as increased mucus production and impaired mucociliary transport mechanisms. The chemotactic factors that are elaborated, such as eosinophil and neutrophil chemotactic factors of anaphylaxis and leukotriene B_4, bring eosinophils, platelets, and polymorphonuclear leukocytes to the site of the reaction. One of the most important of these may be the eosinophil; when activated, these cells can produce leukotriene C_4 and platelet activating factor and thereby contribute directly to airway narrowing and edema. They also can cause mast cells to release histamine and chemotactic factors which could set up a self-sustaining cycle in which additional secondary effector cells including more eosinophils are brought to the site of the reaction. Equally important, degranulation of eosinophils can release major basic protein and eosinophil cationic protein into the airways, thus causing cilia to stop beating and a disruption of mucosal integrity with exfoliation of cells into the bronchial lumen in the form of Creola bodies.

Pharmacologic stimuli The drugs most commonly associated with the induction of acute episodes of asthma are aspirin, coloring agents such as tartrazine, beta-adrenergic antagonists, and sulfiting agents. The typical aspirin-sensitive respiratory syndrome primarily affects adults, although the condition may be seen in childhood. This problem usually begins with perennial vasomotor rhinitis that is followed by a hyperplastic rhinosinusitis with nasal polyps. Progressive asthma then appears. On exposure to even very small quantities of aspirin, affected individuals typically develop ocular and nasal congestion and acute, often severe, episodes of airway obstruction. The prevalence of aspirin sensitivity in asthmatic subjects varies from study to study, but many authorities feel that 10 percent is a reasonable figure. There is a great deal of cross reactivity between aspirin and other nonsteroidal anti-inflammatory compounds. Indomethacin, fenoprofen, naproxen, zomepirac sodium, ibuprofen, mefenamic acid, and phenylbutazone are particularly important in this regard. On the other hand, acetaminophen, sodium salicylate, choline salicylate, salicylamide, and propoxyphene are well tolerated. The exact frequency of cross reactivity to tartrazine and other dyes in aspirin-sensitive asthmatic subjects is also controversial, and again 10 percent is the commonly accepted figure. This peculiar complication of aspirin-sensitive asthma is particularly insidious, however, in that tartrazine and other potentially troublesome dyes are widely present in the environment and may be unknowingly ingested by sensitive patients.

Patients with aspirin sensitivity can be desensitized by daily administration of the drug. Following this form of therapy cross tolerance also develops to other nonsteroidal anti-inflammatory agents. The mechanism by which aspirin and other such drugs produce bronchospasm is unknown; however, immediate hypersensitivity does not seem to be involved.

Beta-adrenergic antagonists regularly produce airway obstruction in asthmatics as well as in others with heightened airway reactivity and should be avoided in such individuals. Even the selective beta$_1$ agents have this propensity, particularly at higher doses. In fact, even the local use of beta$_1$ blockers in the eye for the treatment of glaucoma has been associated with worsening asthma.

Sulfiting agents, such as potassium metabisulfite, potassium and sodium bisulfite, sodium sulfite, and sulfur dioxide, which are widely used in the food and pharmaceutical industry as sanitizing and preservative agents, can also produce acute airway obstruction in sensitive individuals. Exposure usually follows ingestion of food or beverages containing these compounds, e.g., salads, fresh fruit, potatoes, shellfish, and wine. Exacerbation of asthma has been reported following the use of sulfite-containing topical ophthalmic solutions, intravenous glucocorticoids, and some inhalational bronchodilator solutions. The incidence and mechanism of action of this phenomenon are unknown. When suspected, the diagnosis can be confirmed by either oral or inhalational provocations.

Environment and air pollution (See Chap. 206) Environmental causes of asthma are usually related to climatic conditions that promote the concentration of atmospheric pollutants and antigens. These conditions tend to develop in heavy industrial or densely populated urban areas and are frequently associated with thermal inversions or other situations associated with stagnant air masses. In these circumstances, although the general population can develop respiratory symptoms, patients with asthma and other respiratory diseases tend to be more severely affected. The air pollutants known to have this effect are ozone, nitrogen dioxide, and sulfur dioxide. The last needs to be present in high concentrations and produces its greatest effects during periods of high ventilation.

Occupational factors (See Chap. 206) Occupational-related asthma is a significant health problem, and acute and chronic airway obstruction has been reported to follow exposure to a large number of compounds used in many types of industrial processes: bronchoconstriction can result from working with, or exposure to, *metal salts* (platinum, chrome, and nickel); *wood and vegetable dusts* (oak, western red cedar, grain, flour, castor bean, green coffee bean, mako, gum acacia, karay gum, and tragacanth); *pharmaceutical agents* (antibiotics, piperazine, and cimetidine); *industrial chemicals and plastics* (toluene diisocyanate, phthalic acid anhydride, trimellitic anhydride, persulfates, ethylenediamine, paraphenylenediamine, and various dyes); *biologic enzymes* (laundry detergents and pancreatic enzymes); and *animal and insect dusts, serums, and secretions*. It is important to recognize that exposure to sensitizing chemicals, particularly those used in paints, solvents, and plastics, can also occur during leisure or non-work-related activities.

The underlying mechanisms for this airway obstruction appear to be three in number: (1) in some cases the offending agent results in the formation of a specific IgE, and the cause seems immunologic

(the immunologic reaction can be immediate, late, or dual); (2) materials being employed, in other cases, cause a direct liberation of bronchoconstrictor substances; and (3) work-related irritant substances, in still other cases, directly or reflexly stimulate the airways of either latent or frank asthmatics. With occupational exposures, other than those that give an immediate and dual immunologic reaction, the patients give a characteristic cyclic history. They are well when they arrive at work; symptoms develop toward the end of the shift, progress after leaving the work site, and then regress. Absence from work during weekends or vacation periods brings about a remission. Frequently, there are similar symptoms in fellow employees.

Infections Respiratory infections are the most common of the stimuli that evoke acute exacerbations of asthma. Well-controlled investigations have demonstrated that respiratory viruses and not bacteria or allergy are the major etiologic factors. In young children, the most important infectious agents are respiratory syncytial virus and parainfluenza virus. In older children and adults, rhinovirus and influenza virus predominate as pathogens. Simple colonization of the tracheobronchial tree is insufficient to evoke acute episodes of bronchospasm, and attacks of asthma occur only when symptoms of an ongoing respiratory tract infection are, or have been, present. The mechanism by which viruses induce asthma is unknown, but it is probable that the resulting inflammatory changes in the airway mucosa alter host defenses and make the tracheobronchial tree more susceptible to exogenous stimuli. Supporting evidence for this concept is derived from the fact that the airway responsiveness of even normal (non-asthmatic) subjects to nonspecific stimuli is transiently increased after a viral infection. Increased airway responsiveness can last from 2 to 8 weeks after the infection in both normals and asthmatics.

Exercise Asthma can also be induced or made worse by physical exertion. Provocation of bronchospasm by exercise is probably operative to some extent in every asthmatic patient, and in some it may be the only trigger mechanism that will produce symptoms. In the latter circumstance, when such patients are followed for sufficient periods of time, they often develop recurring episodes of airway obstruction independent of exercise: thus, the onset of this problem can frequently serve as the first manifestation of the full-blown asthmatic syndrome. The mechanism by which exercise produces acute exacerbations of asthma is related to the thermal changes that develop in the intrathoracic airways as heat and water are transferred from the mucosa to the inspired air to bring the latter to body conditions before it reaches the alveoli. The higher the ventilation and the colder, hence drier, the inspired air, the more the airway temperature falls, and so there is a significant interaction between the stress of the exercise task, the climatic environment in which it is performed, and the magnitude of the postexertional obstruction. Thus, for the same inspired air conditions, running will produce a more severe attack of asthma than will walking. Conversely, for a given task, the inhalation of cold air during its performance will markedly enhance the response, while warm, humid air will blunt or abolish it. Consequently, activities such as ice hockey, cross-country skiing, or ice skating are more provocative than is swimming in an indoor heated pool. The mechanism by which airway thermal changes evoke obstruction may be related to the hyperemia and engorgement of the microvasculature of the bronchial circulation brought about by rapid rewarming after the loss of heat described above.

Emotional stress Abundant objective data now exist which demonstrate that psychological factors can interact with the asthmatic diathesis to worsen or ameliorate the disease process. The pathways and nature of the interactions are complex but have been shown to be operational to some extent in almost half of the patients studied. Changes in airway caliber seem to be mediated through modification of vagal efferent activity. The most frequently studied variable has been that of suggestion, and the weight of current evidence is that it can be quite an important influence in selected asthmatics. When psychically responsive individuals are given the appropriate suggestion, they can actually decrease or increase the pharmacologic effects of adrenergic and cholinergic stimuli on their airways. The extent to which psychological factors participate in the induction and/or continuation of any given acute exacerbation is unknown but probably varies from patient to patient and in the same patient from episode to episode.

PATHOLOGY In a patient who has died of acute asthma, the most striking feature of the lungs at necropsy is their gross overdistention and failure to collapse when the pleural cavities are opened. When the lungs are cut, numerous gelatinous plugs of exudate are found in the majority of the bronchial branches down to the terminal bronchiole. Histologic examination shows hypertrophy of the bronchial smooth muscle, hyperplasia of mucosal and submucosal vessels, mucosal edema, denudation of the surface epithelium, pronounced thickening of the basement membrane, and eosinophilic infiltrates in the bronchial wall. In asthmatic patients who die from trauma and causes other than asthma itself, mucous casts, basement membrane thickening, and eosinophilic infiltrates are frequently observed. In both situations there is an absence of any of the well-recognized forms of destructive emphysema.

PATHOPHYSIOLOGY AND CLINICAL CORRELATES The pathophysiologic hallmark of asthma is a reduction in airway diameter brought about by contraction of smooth muscle, edema of the bronchial wall, and thick tenacious secretions. Although the relative contributions of each component to the patient's ventilatory impairment are unknown, the net result is an increase in airway resistance, decreased forced expiratory volumes and flow rates, hyperinflation of the lungs and thorax, increased work of breathing, alterations in respiratory muscle function, changes in elastic recoil, abnormal distribution of both ventilation and pulmonary blood flow, mismatched ratios, and altered arterial blood gases. Thus, although asthma is considered to be primarily a disease of airways, virtually all aspects of pulmonary function are compromised during an acute attack. In addition, in very symptomatic patients there frequently is electrocardiographic evidence of right ventricular hypertrophy, and pulmonary hypertension can be found. Quantification of the changes that develop during an acute episode of asthma demonstrate that when a patient presents for therapy, his or her forced vital capacity tends to be ≤50 percent of normal. The 1-s forced expiratory volume (FEV_1) averages 30 percent of predicted, while the maximum and minimum midexpiratory flow rates are reduced to 20 percent or less of expected. In keeping with the alterations in mechanics, the associated air-trapping is substantial. In acutely ill patients, residual volume (RV) frequently approaches 400 percent of normal, while functional residual capacity doubles. The patients tend to report that their attacks have ended clinically when their RV has fallen to 200 percent of its predicted value and when the FEV_1 rises to 50 percent.

Hypoxia is a universal finding during acute exacerbations, but frank ventilatory failure is relatively uncommon, being observed in 10 to 15 percent of patients presenting for therapy. Most asthmatics have hypocapnia and a respiratory alkalosis. Statistically, the finding of normal arterial carbon dioxide tension tends to be associated with quite severe levels of obstruction and consequently, when found in a symptomatic individual, should be viewed as impending respiratory failure and treated as such. Equally, the presence of metabolic acidosis in the setting of acute asthma heralds severe obstruction. Usually, there are no clinical counterparts to the derangements in blood gases. Cyanosis is a very late sign. Thus, a dangerous level of hypoxia can go undetected. Likewise the signs which are attributable to carbon dioxide retention such as sweating, tachycardia, and wide pulse pressure or to acidosis such as tachypnea do not tend to be of great value in predicting the presence of hypercapnia or hydrogen ion excess in individual patients, for they are too frequently seen in anxious patients with more moderate disease to be of much use. Consequently, trying to judge the state of an acutely ill patient's ventilatory status on clinical grounds alone can be extremely hazardous and should not be relied upon with any confidence. Arterial blood gas tensions, therefore, must be measured.

The symptoms of asthma consist of a triad of dyspnea, cough, and wheezing, the latter often being regarded as the *sine qua non*. In its most typical form asthma is an episodic disease, and all three symptoms coexist. Attacks often occur at night, for reasons which are not clear but may relate to fluctuations in airway receptor thresholds that may result from circadian variations in the circulating levels of endogenous catecholamines and histamine. Attacks may also abruptly follow exposure to a specific allergen, physical exertion, a viral respiratory infection, or emotional excitement. At the onset the patient experiences a sense of constriction in the chest, often with a nonproductive cough. Respiration becomes audibly harsh, and wheezing in both phases of respiration becomes prominent, expiration becomes prolonged, and patients frequently have tachypnea, tachycardia, and mild systolic hypertension. The lungs rapidly become overinflated, and the anterior-posterior diameter of the thorax increases. If the attack is severe or prolonged, the accessory muscles become visibly active and frequently a paradoxical pulse will develop. These two signs have been found to be extremely valuable in indicating the severity of the obstruction. In the presence of either, pulmonary function tends to be significantly more impaired than in its absence. It is important to note that the development of these signs depends upon the generation of large negative intrathoracic pressures. Thus, if the patient's breathing is shallow, these signs could be absent even though obstruction is quite severe. The other signs and symptoms of asthma imperfectly reflect the physiologic alterations that are present, so much so that if one relies upon the loss of subjective complaints, or even the sign of wheezing, as being the end point at which therapy for an acute attack should be terminated, an enormous reservoir of residual disease is missed.

Termination of the episode is frequently marked by a cough producing thick stringy mucus which often takes the form of casts of the distal airways (Curschmann's spirals), and when examined microscopically often shows eosinophils and Charcot-Leyden crystals. In extreme situations, wheezing may markedly lessen or even disappear completely, cough may become extremely ineffective, and the patient may begin a gasping type of respiratory pattern. These findings imply extensive mucous plugging and impending suffocation. Ventilatory assistance by mechanical means may be required. Atelectasis due to inspissated secretions may occasionally occur with asthmatic attacks. Other complications such as spontaneous pneumothorax and/or pneumomediastinum are rare.

Less typically, a patient with asthma may complain of intermittent episodes of nonproductive cough or dyspnea only on exertion. Unlike other asthmatics when examined during their symptomatic periods, these patients tend to have normal breath sounds but may wheeze after repeated forced exhalations and/or may show dynamic ventilatory impairments when tested in the laboratory. In the absence of both, a bronchoprovocation may be required to make the diagnosis.

The differentiation of asthma from other diseases associated with dyspnea and wheezing is usually not difficult, particularly if the patient is seen during an acute episode. The physical findings and symptoms listed above, and the history of periodic attacks, are quite characteristic. A personal or family history of allergic diseases such as eczema, rhinitis, or urticaria is valuable contributory evidence. *Upper airway obstruction by tumor* or *laryngeal edema* can occasionally be confused with asthma. Typically, such a patient will present with stridor, and the harsh respiratory sounds can be localized to the area of the trachea. Diffuse wheezing throughout both lung fields is usually absent. However, differentiation can sometimes be difficult, and indirect laryngoscopy or bronchoscopy may be required. Asthmalike symptoms in patients with glottic dysfunction have been described. These individuals close their glottis during inspiration and produce episodic attacks of severe airway obstruction, yet they do not respond to standard therapy. Frequently they produce enough obstruction to develop carbon dioxide retention. However, unlike asthma the arterial oxygen tension is well preserved, and the alveolar-arterial gradient for oxygen narrows during the episode and does not widen as is the case with lower airway obstruction. To establish the diagnosis of glottic dysfunction, the glottis should be examined when the patient is symptomatic. A normal examination at this time excludes the diagnosis; normal findings during asymptomatic periods do not.

Persistent wheezing localized to one area of the chest in association with paroxysms of cough indicates *endobronchial disease* such as foreign-body aspiration, neoplasms, or bronchial stenosis.

The signs and symptoms of *acute left ventricular failure* can occasionally mimic asthma, but the findings of moist basilar rales, gallop rhythms, blood-tinged sputum, and other signs of heart failure (Chap. 182) allow the appropriate diagnosis to be reached.

Recurrent episodes of bronchospasm can occur with *carcinoid tumors* (Chap. 262), *recurrent pulmonary emboli* (Chap. 213), and *chronic bronchitis* (Chap. 210). In the last there are no true symptom-free periods in that one can usually obtain a history of chronic cough and sputum production as a background upon which acute attacks of wheezing are superimposed. Recurrent emboli, particularly in young women on oral contraceptives, are occasionally very difficult to separate from asthma. Frequently, these patients will present with episodes of breathlessness, particularly on exertion, and they can sometimes wheeze. Pulmonary function studies may show evidence of peripheral airway obstruction (Chap. 201), and when these changes are present, lung scans may also be abnormal. The therapeutic response to bronchodilators, discontinuation of the contraceptives, and institution of anticoagulant therapy may be helpful, but pulmonary angiography may be necessary in order to establish the correct diagnosis.

Eosinophilic pneumonias (Chap. 205) are often associated with asthmatic symptoms as are various chemical pneumonias and exposures to insecticides and cholinergic drugs. Bronchospasm can occasionally be a manifestation of *systemic vasculitis* with pulmonary involvement.

LABORATORY FINDINGS It is difficult to establish the diagnosis of asthma in the laboratory, for no single test is conclusive. Positive wheal-and-flare reactions to skin tests can be demonstrated to various allergens, but that finding does not necessarily correlate with the intrapulmonary events. Sputum and blood eosinophilia and measurement of serum IgE levels are also helpful but are not specific for asthma. Chest roentgenograms showing hyperinflation are nondiagnostic, as are tests of pulmonary function. The latter, however, are quite useful in that one can measure the degree of obstruction present, document its reversible nature, and, when combined with provocational challenges, demonstrate the airway hyperirritability so characteristic of this disease. Furthermore, the performance of forced vital capacity maneuvers is very helpful in the evaluation of acute asthmatic attacks. A reduction in the FEV_1 to less than 25 percent of that predicted or to less than 0.75 liters with little or no response following the administration of a bronchodilator indicates that the patient should receive very careful surveillance in conjunction with intensive treatment.

THERAPY Elimination of the causative agent(s) from the environment of an allergic asthmatic is the most successful means available for treating this condition (for details on avoidance see Chap. 267). Desensitization or immunotherapy with extracts of the suspected allergens has enjoyed widespread favor, but controlled studies are limited and have not proved it to be highly effective.

Acute episodes of bronchial asthma represent one of the most common respiratory emergencies seen in the practice of medicine, and it is essential that the physician recognize which episodes of airway obstruction are life threatening and which patients demand what level of care. This can be readily accomplished by assessing selected clinical parameters in combination with measures of expiratory flow and gas exchange. The presence of a paradoxical pulse, use of accessory muscles, and marked hyperinflation of the thorax signify severe airway obstruction, and failure of these signs to remit within short order following aggressive therapy mandates objective monitoring of the patient using arterial blood gases and some index of pulmonary mechanics.

In general, there is a direct correlation between the severity of the obstruction with which the patient presents and the time that it takes to resolve it. Those individuals with the most impairment typically have multiple causes for their airway narrowing and require the most extensive therapy for resolution. In these circumstances, if the clinical signs of a paradoxical pulse and accessory muscle use are diminishing, and/or if peak expiratory flow rate is increasing, there is no need to change medications or doses. One need only to continue to follow the patient. If, however, peak flow is falling or if the magnitude of the pulsus paradoxicus is increasing, serial measures of arterial blood gases are required as well as a reconsideration of the therapeutic modalities being employed. If the patient has hypocarbia, one can afford to continue the current approaches a while longer. On the other hand, if the Pa_{CO_2} is within the normal range, or if it is elevated, the patient should be monitored in an intensive care setting and therapy should be intensified in order to reverse or arrest the patient's respiratory failure.

Drug treatment The drugs used in the treatment of asthma may be conveniently grouped into five major categories: beta-adrenergic agonists, methylxanthines, glucocorticoids, chromones, and anticholinergics. No one group is effective against all of the pathologic processes producing the disease, and since the degree of relief of airway obstruction is frequently incomplete with the use of a single agent, multiple drug regimens are commonplace.

ADRENERGIC STIMULANTS The drugs in this category consist of the catecholamines, resorcinols, and saligenins. These agents are analogues and produce airway dilatation through stimulation of beta receptors with the resultant formation of cyclic AMP. The catecholamines in widespread clinical use are epinephrine, isoproterenol, isoetharine, rimiterol, and hexoprenaline. The latter two are not available in the United States. As a group these compounds are short-acting and effective only by inhalational or parenteral routes. Epinephrine and isoproterenol are not beta$_2$-selective and have considerable chronotropic and inotropic cardiac effects. Epinephrine also has substantial alpha-stimulating effects. The usual dose is 0.3 to 0.5 mL of a 1:1000 solution administered subcutaneously. Isoproterenol is devoid of alpha activity and is the most potent agent of this group. It is usually administered in a 1:200 solution by inhalation. Controlled studies have shown that repetitive doses of epinephrine or isoproterenol are considerably more efficacious than the use of methylxanthines in the therapy of acute exacerbations of asthma. Isoetharine is the most beta$_2$-selective compound of this class, but is a relatively weak bronchodilator. It is employed as an aerosol and supplied as a 1% solution. The pharmacologies of hexoprenaline and rimiterol are similar to isoetharine.

The commonly used resorcinols are metaproterenol, terbutaline, and fenoterol, and the most widely known saligenin is albuterol, or salbutamol. With the exception of metaproterenol, these drugs are highly selective for the respiratory tract and virtually devoid of significant cardiac effects except in high doses. They are active by all routes of administration, and because their chemical structures allow them to bypass the metabolic processes used to degrade the catecholamines, their effects are long-lasting, exceeding 6 h in many studies.

Multiple studies now exist that demonstrate that the sympathomimetics are the drugs of choice in treating acute episodes of asthma. Based upon in vivo and in vitro data, there is little question that there is a range of potency among the currently available adrenergic agonists. However, the clinical importance of these observations is unclear, and in the main, differences in potency and duration between agents can be eliminated by adjusting doses and/or administration schedules. Non-beta$_2$ selective drugs tend to produce greater side effects such as tachycardia and nervousness, and most authorities recommend using long acting selective beta$_2$ agonists as initial therapy. The major side effect of the latter class is tremor.

The method by which beta agonists are administered is of great importance since it influences both the clinical response and the metabolic fate. Inhalation is the route of choice in that it increases the bronchial selectivity of these drugs and allows maximal bronchodilation to occur with fewer side effects than other routes of administration. This is true not just in maintenance therapy but also during the treatment of severe acute obstruction. In the past it was fashionable to treat episodes of severe asthma with intravenous sympathomimetics such as isoproterenol. This approach no longer appears justifiable. Isoproterenol infusions clearly can induce myocardial damage and even the beta$_2$ selective agents such as terbutaline and albuterol when given intravenously offer no advantages over the inhaled route.

METHYLXANTHINES   Theophylline, and its various salts, are medium potency bronchodilators. Like the beta agonists, they improve the movement of airway mucus and may decrease the release of mediators. Although efficacious, the drugs in this class are not as potent as the sympathomimetics, and they have a narrower therapeutic-toxic window. The mechanism responsible for the bronchodilator effect of the methylxanthines is unknown. It was formerly thought that these drugs increased cyclic AMP by the inhibition of phosphodiesterase. However, the available evidence does not support this concept. The therapeutic plasma concentrations of theophylline lie between 10 and 20 µg/mL. But the dose required to achieve this level varies widely from patient to patient due to differences in the metabolism of the drug. Theophylline clearance, and thus dosage requirements, is decreased substantially in neonates and the elderly and those with acute and chronic hepatic dysfunction, cardiac decompensation, and cor pulmonale. Clearance is also decreased during febrile illnesses. Clearance is increased in children. In addition a number of important drug interactions can alter theophylline metabolism. Clearance falls with the concurrent use of erythromycin and troleandomycin, allopurinol, cimetidine, and propranolol. It rises with cigarettes, marijuana, phenobarbital, and phenytoin or any other drug that has the capability of inducing hepatic microsomal enzymes.

For maintenance therapy long-acting theophylline compounds are available and are usually given twice per day or once daily. The dose is adjusted on the basis of the clinical response with the aid of serum theophylline levels. There is some evidence that single dose administration in the evening may reduce nocturnal symptoms. In contrast to the large number of oral compounds, aminophylline is the only compound available for intravenous use. The recommendations for intravenous therapy in children aged 9 to 16 and young adult smokers not currently receiving theophylline products are as follows: a loading dose of 6 mg/kg is given followed by an infusion of 1.0 mg/kg per hour for the next 12 h and then 0.8 mg/kg per hour thereafter. In nonsmoking adults, older patients, and those with cor pulmonale, congestive heart failure, and liver disease, the loading dose remains the same but the maintenance dose is reduced to between 0.1 and 0.5 mg/kg per hour. In those patients already receiving theophylline, the loading dose is frequently withheld or in extreme situations given in a reduced amount at 0.5 mg/kg.

The most common side effects of theophylline are nervousness, nausea, vomiting, anorexia, and headache. At plasma levels greater than 30 µg/mL there is a risk of seizures and cardiac arrhythmias.

GLUCOCORTICOIDS   Glucocorticoids have been used for many years in the treatment of asthma, but controversy still surrounds such basic issues as their specific indication and dose. Glucocorticoids are not bronchodilators, and their major use is in reducing airway inflammation. Although it is difficult to provide precise recommendations because objective data are lacking, there are several situations in the management of acute and chronic asthma in which all would agree that steroids should be employed. In acute illness, that is, when severe airway obstruction is not resolving, or is even worsening despite intense optimal bronchodilator therapy, and in chronic disease, steroids are most helpful when there has been failure of a previously optimal regimen with frequent recurrences of symptoms of progressive severity.

The dose that one should use is a matter of debate. Most would agree that sufficient quantities should be administered to achieve a plasma cortisol level of 100 µg/dL, but objective data supporting this figure do not yet exist. However, data are accumulating that indicate that very high doses do not offer advantage over more conventional amounts. For example, 6 mg/kg per day of hydrocortisone has been shown to produce the same effects as 80 mg/kg per day in status asthmaticus, and 15 to 20 mg of methylprednisolone every 6 h has the same consequences as doses eight to ten times greater. In most acute situations the intravenous administration of 4 mg/kg of hydrocortisone (or equivalent) as a loading dose, followed several hours later by an infusion regulated to deliver 3 mg/kg every 6 h will suffice. It should be emphasized that the effects of steroids in acute asthma are not immediate and may not be seen for 6 h or more after their initial administration. Consequently, it is mandatory to continue vigorous bronchodilator therapy during this interval. After 24 to 72 h, depending upon response, the patient can be switched to oral agents. A usual starting point is 40 to 60 mg prednisone as a single daily morning dose. The amount can then be reduced by half every third to fifth day. More rapid tapering frequently results in recurrent obstruction. In situations in which it appears that continued steroid therapy will be needed, an alternate-day schedule should be instituted to minimize side effects. This is particularly important in children, since continuous corticosteroid administration interrupts growth. Long-acting preparations such as dexamethasone should not be used in this approach for they defeat the purpose of alternate-day schedules by causing prolonged suppression of the pituitary-adrenal axis.

Several inhaled steroids of high topical potency are available and greatly facilitate the withdrawal of oral agents. They are also useful in reducing airway reactivity and as an alternative to oral glucocorticoids in situations where asthma symptoms are escalating. The former effect is quite important and data are accumulating that a reduction in airway reactivity can result in decreased morbidity. Hyperadrenal corticism and adrenal suppression are not major issues, and the most frequent side effect is symptomatic oropharyngeal candidiasis. This can be controlled by the use of a spacing device on the metered-dose inhaler.

CHROMONES   Cromolyn sodium is not a bronchodilator. Its major therapeutic effect is the inhibition of degranulation of mast cells, thereby preventing the release of the chemical mediators of anaphylaxis. The drug does not inhibit the combination of antigen with antibody, nor does it affect the fixation of IgE to mast cells. Cromolyn has been shown to be of use in atopic and nonatopic asthmatics, and it blunts exercise-induced asthma in both children and adults. Numerous trials have shown that about 75 percent of patients derive worthwhile benefits from the drug in terms of reduction of medications and improvement in symptoms. Cromolyn, like inhaled steroids, can lower airway reactivity, and both drugs together may produce additive effects. Therapy with cromolyn is best initiated between attacks or in periods of relative remission. If no response is noted by 4 to 6 weeks, the drug can be discontinued. A newer agent, nedocromil, with a greater spectrum of activity, is available in Europe.

ANTICHOLINERGICS   Anticholinergic drugs, such as atropine sulfate, are known to produce bronchodilatation in patients with asthma, but their use has been limited by systemic side effects. Nonabsorbable quaternary ammonium (atropine methylnitrate and ipratropium bromide) aerosol agents have undergone extensive trials and have been found to be both effective and remarkably free of untoward effects. They may be of particular benefit for patients with coexistent heart disease, in whom use of methylxanthines and beta stimulants may be dangerous. Furthermore, evidence is accumulating that addition of anticholinergics may enhance the bronchodilatation achieved by sympathomimetics. However, they are less potent and are slow to act (60 to 90 min may be required before peak bronchodilatation is achieved).

MISCELLANEOUS   Opiates, sedatives, and tranquilizers should be absolutely avoided in the acutely ill asthmatic because the risk of depressing alveolar ventilation is great and respiratory arrest has been reported to occur shortly after their use. Admittedly most individuals are anxious and frightened, but experience has shown that they can be calmed equally well by the physician's presence and reassurances. Beta-adrenergic blockers and parasympathetic agonists should be avoided, or used with great caution, for they can cause marked deterioration in lung function.

Expectorants and mucolytic agents have enjoyed great vogue in the past, but they do not add significantly to the treatment of the acute or chronic phases of this disease. Mucolytic agents such as acetylcysteine may actually produce bronchospasm when administered to susceptible asthmatics. This can be overcome by aerosolizing them in solution with a beta-adrenergic agent. The use of intravenous fluids in the treatment of acute asthma has also been advocated. There is little evidence to indicate that this adjunct hastens recovery.

SPECIAL INSTRUCTIONS   The treatment of patients with asthma who have coexisting conditions such as heart disease or pregnancy does not differ materially from that outlined above. Inhaled therapy with beta$_2$ selective agents is the mainstay, and the doses administered should be the lowest possible quantities required to produce the desired therapeutic effects. Such patients should routinely be given cromolyn and/or inhaled steroids to prevent acute episodes.

PROGNOSIS AND CLINICAL COURSE   Death from asthma is uncommon. Statistics for the United States indicate a death rate of approximately 0.3 per 100,000 persons. In the last several years, there has been concern that asthma death rates are increasing. The data, however, are not sufficiently compelling to result in uniform acceptance.

Information on the clinical course of asthma suggests a good prognosis for 50 to 80 percent of all patients, particularly those whose disease is mild and develops in childhood. The number of children still having asthma 7 to 10 years after the initial diagnosis varies from 26 to 78 percent with an average of 46 percent; however, the percentage who continue to have severe disease is relatively low (6 to 19 percent). The natural course of asthma in adult life has been little investigated. Some studies suggest that spontaneous remissions occur in approximately 20 percent of those who develop the disease as adults and 40 percent or so can be expected to improve with less frequent and severe attacks as they grow older.

REFERENCES

BURROWS B: The natural history of asthma. J Allergy Clin Immunol 80:373, 1987
FANTA CH, McFADDEN ER JR: Status Asthmaticus, in *Current Therapy in Internal Medicine*, TM Bayless et al (eds). Philadelphia, Decker, 1984, pp 6–10
KALINER MA, McFADDEN ER JR: Bronchial asthma, in *Immunological Diseases*, M Samter et al (eds). Boston, Little Brown, 1988, pp 1067–1118
McFADDEN ER JR: Asthma: Airway dynamics, cardiac function, and clinical correlates, in *Allergy: Principles and Practice*, E Middleton et al (eds). St Louis, CV Mosby, 1988, pp 1018–1036
SHELLER JR: Asthma: Emerging concepts and potential therapies. Am J Med Sci 293:298, 1987

205   HYPERSENSITIVITY PNEUMONITIS

GARY W. HUNNINGHAKE/HAL B. RICHERSON

DEFINITION   Hypersensitivity pneumonitis (HP), or extrinsic allergic alveolitis, is an immunologically induced inflammation of the lung parenchyma, involving alveolar walls and terminal airways, secondary to repeated inhalation of a variety of organic dusts and other agents by a susceptible host. In contrast to many of the other interstitial lung diseases, the etiology of this interstitial and alveolar filling disease is known. Although a number of etiologic agents have been identified, most are rare, and a few well-documented syndromes are associated with the vast majority of cases. The diagnosis of HP requires a constellation of clinical, radiographic, physiologic, pathologic, and immunologic criteria, each of which by itself is rarely pathognomonic, and the preferred treatment is avoidance of the causative antigen.

ETIOLOGY   Agents implicated as causes of HP include those listed in Table 205-1. Many cases of HP occurring in various occupations involve exposure to similar agents, particularly the thermophilic actinomycetes. Except for exotic occupational exposures, the usual sources of causative antigens are "moldy" hay, silage, or grain; pet birds; and heating, cooling, and humidification systems. Simple chemicals, such as isocyanates, may also cause hypersensitivity pneumonitis.

PATHOGENESIS   The finding that precipitating antibodies against extracts of moldy hay were demonstrable in most patients with farmer's lung led to the early conclusion that HP was an immune-complex-mediated reaction. Subsequent investigations of HP in human beings and animal models provided evidence for the importance of cell-mediated hypersensitivity. The very early (acute) reaction is characterized by an increase in polymorphonuclear leukocytes in the alveoli and small airways. This early lesion is followed by an influx of mononuclear cells into the lung and the formation of granulomas. The latter lesion appears to be a classic delayed hypersensitivity reaction to repeated inhalation of antigen and adjuvant-active materials.

Bronchoalveolar lavage in patients with HP consistently demonstrates an increase in T lymphocytes in lavage fluid (a finding which is also observed in patients with other granulomatous lung disorders). Patients with recent or continual exposure to antigen may also have an increase in polymorphonuclear leukocytes in lavage fluid. Increased numbers of mast cells have also been reported. In most patients examined during recovery from acute disease, the T lymphocytes in lavage fluid are predominantly the suppressor-cytotoxic T-cell subset, which expresses surface antigens (CD8) detected by OKT8 or Leu 2a monoclonal antibodies. In patients with very recent exposure to antigen, however, the numbers of CD4-bearing helper T cells (OKT4$^+$ or Leu 3a$^+$) may increase in lavage fluid. Similar findings may be present in similarly exposed, asymptomatic individuals. These observations suggest that there is an active modulation of granuloma formation in the lung by immunoregulatory T cells in this disorder.

CLINICAL PRESENTATION   The *clinical picture* varies from patient to patient and is related to the frequency and intensity of exposure to the causative antigen and perhaps other host factors. The presentation can be *acute, subacute,* or *chronic*. In the *acute form*, symptoms such as cough, fever, chills, malaise, and dyspnea may occur 6 to 8 h after exposure to the antigen and usually clear within a few days if there is no further exposure to antigen. The *subacute form* often appears insidiously over a period of weeks marked by cough and dyspnea and may progress to cyanosis and severe dyspnea requiring hospitalization. In some patients, a subacute form of the disease may persist after an acute presentation of the disorder, especially if there is continued exposure to antigen. In most patients with the acute or subacute form of HP, the symptoms, signs, and other manifestations of HP disappear within days, weeks, or months if the causative agent is no longer inhaled. Transformation to a chronic form of the disease may occur in patients with continued antigen exposure, but the frequency of such progression is uncertain. The *chronic form* may also present as a gradually progressive interstitial disease associated with cough and exertional dyspnea without a prior history consistent with acute or subacute manifestations. Such a gradual onset frequently occurs with low-dose exposure to the antigen.

DIAGNOSIS   Following acute exposure to antigen, neutrophilia and lymphopenia are frequently present. Eosinophilia is not a feature. All forms of the disease may be associated with elevations in erythrocyte sedimentation rate, C-reactive protein, rheumatoid factor, and serum immunoglobulins. Antinuclear antibodies are rarely present.

Examination for *serum precipitins* against suspected antigens, such as those listed in Table 205-1, is an important part of the diagnostic workup. If found, precipitins indicate sufficient exposure to the causative agent for generation of an immunologic response. The diagnosis of HP is not established solely by the presence of

TABLE 205-1 Selected examples of hypersensitivity pneumonitis (HP)

Disease	Antigen	Source of antigen
Bagassosis	Thermophilic actinomycetes	"Moldy" bagasse (sugar cane)
Bird fancier's, breeder's, or handler's lung	Parakeet, budgerigar, pigeon, chicken, turkey proteins	Avian droppings or feathers
Cephalosporium HP	Contaminated basement (sewage)	Cephalosporium
Cheese washer's lung	*Penicillium casei*	Moldy cheese
Chemical worker's lung	Isocyanates	Polyurethane foam, varnishes, lacquer, foundry casting
Coffee worker's lung	Coffee bean dust	Coffee beans
Compost lung	*Aspergillus*	Compost
Detergent worker's disease	*Bacillus subtilis* enzymes	Detergent
Familial HP	*Bacillus subtilis*	Contaminated wood dust in walls
Farmer's lung	Thermophilic actinomycetes*	"Moldy" hay, grain, silage
Fish meal worker's lung	Fish meal dust	Fish meal
Furrier's lung	Animal fur dust	Animal pelts
Hot tub lung	*Cladosporium* sp.	Mold on ceiling
Humidifier or air-conditioner lung (ventilation pneumonitis)	*Aureobasidium pullulans* or other microorganisms	Contaminated water in humidification and forced-air air-conditioning systems
Japanese summer house HP	*Trichosporon cutaneum*	House dust? Bird droppings
Laboratory worker's HP	Male rat urine	Laboratory rat
Lycoperdonosis	*Lycoperdon* puffballs	*Puffball* spores
Malt worker's lung	*Aspergillus fumigatus* or *A. clavatus*	Moldy barley
Maple bark disease	*Cryptostroma corticale*	Maple bark
Miller's lung	*Sitophilus granarius* (wheat weevil)	Infested wheat flour
Mushroom worker's lung	Thermophilic actinomycetes,* other	Mushroom compost
Paulis HP	Paulis reagent	Laboratory reagent
Pituitary snuff taker's lung	Animal proteins	Heterologous pituitary snuff
Potato riddler's lung	Thermophilic actinomycetes,* *Aspergillus*	"Moldy" hay around potatoes
Sauna taker's lung	*Auerobasidium* sp., other	Contaminated sauna water
Sequoiosis	*Aureobasidium*, *Graphium* sp.	Redwood sawdust
Streptomyces albus HP	*Streptomyces albus*	Contaminated fertilizer
Suberosis	Cork dust mold	Cork dust
Tap water lung	Unknown	Contaminated tap water
Thatched roof disease	*Sacchoromonospora viridis*	Dried grasses and leaves
Tobacco worker's disease	*Aspergillus* sp.	Mold on tobacco
Winegrower's lung	*Botrytis cinerea*	Mold on grapes
Wood trimmer's disease	*Rhizopus* sp., *Mucor* sp.	Contaminated wood trimmings
Woodman's disease	*Pencillium* sp.	Oak and maple trees
Woodworker's lung	Wood dust; *Alternaria*	Oak, cedar, and mahogany dusts; pine and spruce pulp

*Thermophilic actinomycetes species include *Micropolyspora faeni*, *Thermoactinomyces vulgaris*, *T. saccharrii*, *T. viridis*, and *T. candidus*.

precipitins, however, since precipitins merely indicate a significant exposure to an antigen source. Precipitins are found in sera of many individuals exposed to appropriate antigens who demonstrate no other evidence of HP. False-negative results may occur because of poor-quality antigens or an inappropriate choice of antigens. Extraction of antigens from the patient's environment may at times be helpful.

No specific or distinctive *chest roentgenogram* occurs in HP. It can be normal even in symptomatic patients. The acute or subacute phase may be associated with poorly defined, patchy, or diffuse infiltrates or with discrete, nodular infiltrates. In the chronic phase, the chest x-ray usually shows a diffuse reticulonodular infiltrate. Honeycombing may eventually develop as the condition progresses. Abnormalities rarely seen in hypersensitivity pneumonitis include pleural effusion or thickening, and hilar adenopathy.

Pulmonary function studies in all forms of HP may show a restrictive pattern with loss of lung volumes, impaired diffusion capacity, decreased compliance, and an exercise-induced hypoxemia. A resting hypoxemia may be found. Functional abnormalities may gradually increase in severity or may occur rapidly following acute or subacute exposure to antigen. As the chronic stage progresses, changes consistent with airway obstruction may also become increasingly prominent.

Bronchoalveolar lavage is used in some centers to aid in diagnostic evaluation, and the characteristic features of the lavage fluid are described above.

Lung biopsy may be indicated in patients without sufficient other criteria to make a definitive diagnosis. The initial biopsy procedure is usually a transbronchial biopsy. In some patients, an open-lung biopsy may be necessary, since this procedure will provide adequate material for pathologic studies whereas transbronchial biopsy may not. Although the histopathology is distinctive, it may not be

pathognomonic of HP. When the biopsy is taken during the active phase of disease, typical findings include an interstitial alveolar infiltrate consisting of plasma cells, lymphocytes, and occasional eosinophils and neutrophils, usually with accompanying granulomas. Interstitial fibrosis may be present but most often is mild in earlier stages of the disease. Some degree of bronchiolitis is found in about half the cases, whereas vasculitis is not a feature of the disorder.

The lack of standardized, nonirritating antigens and of proven controlled protocols makes *skin testing* and *inhalational challenge* useful only for experimental purposes. Similarly, *in vitro tests of cell-mediated (delayed) hypersensitivity* have not been shown to consistently correlate with clinical HP and cannot be recommended in the routine diagnostic workup.

In summary, the diagnosis in most cases is established by (1) consistent history, physical findings, pulmonary function tests, and chest x-ray, (2) exposure to a recognized antigen, and (3) finding an antibody to that antigen. In a few circumstances, bronchoalveolar lavage and/or lung biopsy may be needed. Provocation tests are research procedures and are not indicated.

Chronic HP may often be difficult to distinguish from a number of other interstitial lung disorders such as idiopathic pulmonary fibrosis, interstitial lung disease associated with a collagen vascular disorder, and drug-induced lung diseases. A negative history for use of appropriate drugs and no evidence of a systemic disorder usually exclude the presence of drug-induced lung disease or a collagen vascular disorder. In some patients, a lung biopsy may be required to differentiate chronic HP from idiopathic pulmonary fibrosis.

The lung disease associated with acute or subacute HP may clinically resemble other disorders which present with systemic symptoms and recurrent pulmonary infiltrates. These disorders include the collagen vascular disorders, drug-induced lung disease, allergic bronchopulmonary aspergillosis, and other eosinophilic pneumonias. Eosinophilic pneumonia is often associated with asthma and is typified by peripheral eosinophilia; neither of these is a feature of HP. Allergic bronchopulmonary aspergillosis is sometimes confused with HP because of the presence of precipitating antibodies to *Aspergillus fumigatus*. It is an obstructive rather than a restrictive lung disease, however, that is associated with allergic (atopic) asthma.

TREATMENT Because effective treatment depends largely on avoiding the antigen, identification of the causative agent and its source is essential. This is usually possible if the physician takes a careful environmental and occupational history or, if necessary, visits the patient's environment.

The simplest way to avoid the incriminated agent is to remove the patient from the environment or the source of the agent from the patient's environment. This recommendation cannot be taken lightly when it completely changes the life-style or livelihood of the patient. In many cases, however, the source of exposure (birds, humidifiers) can easily be removed. If occupational exposure is involved, an initial attempt can be made at antigen avoidance maneuvers least disruptive to the patient's livelihood, which usually means avoiding areas associated with heavy exposure and wearing an appropriate mask. This will not suffice for small-molecular-weight agents such as isocyanates, which require elaborate filtration devices. Pollen masks, personal dust respirators, airstream helmets, and ventilated helmets with a supply of fresh air are increasingly efficient means of purifying inhaled air. If symptoms recur or physiologic abnormalities progress in spite of these measures, then more effective measures to avoid antigen exposure must be pursued.

Compromises with environmental control pertain only to the acute, recurrent, transient clinical form of HP and must be accompanied by careful follow-up. Subacute forms are ordinarily the result of a heavy, sustained exposure. The chronic form typically results from low-grade exposure over many months to years, and the lung disease may already be partially irreversible. These patients should be advised to avoid completely all possible contact with the offending agent.

Patients with the *acute*, recurrent form of HP usually recover without need for glucocorticoids. *Subacute* HP may be associated with severe symptoms and marked physiologic impairment, and may continue to progress for several days despite hospitalization. Urgent establishment of the diagnosis and prompt institution of glucocorticoid treatment are indicated in such patients. Such therapy may also hasten recovery in patients with lesser involvement. Prednisone at a dosage of 1 mg/kg per day or its equivalent is continued for 7 to 14 days, and then tapered over the ensuing 2 to 6 weeks at a rate which depends on the patient's clinical status.

Patients with *chronic* extrinsic allergic alveolitis may gradually recover without therapy following environmental control. In many patients, however, a trial of prednisone may be useful to obtain maximal reversibility of the lung disease. Following initial prednisone therapy (1 mg/kg per day for 2 to 4 weeks), the drug is tapered to the lowest dosage that will maintain the functional status of the patient. Many patients will not require or benefit from long-term therapy if there is no further exposure to antigen.

THE EOSINOPHILIC PNEUMONIAS

The eosinophilic pneumonias are composed of distinct individual syndromes characterized by eosinophilic pulmonary infiltrates and, commonly, peripheral blood eosinophilia. Since Loeffler's initial description of a transient, benign syndrome of migratory pulmonary infiltrates and peripheral blood eosinophilia of unknown cause, this group of disorders has been enlarged to include diseases of known and unknown etiology (Table 205-2). These diseases may be considered as examples of hypersensitivity lung disease but are not to be confused with hypersensitivity pneumonitis (extrinsic allergic alveolitis) in which eosinophilia is not a feature.

When an eosinophilic pneumonia is associated with bronchial

TABLE 205-2 The eosinophilic pneumonias

1 Etiology known
  a Allergic bronchopulmonary aspergillosis
  b Parasitic infestations
  c Drug reactions
2 Idiopathic
  a Loeffler's syndrome
  b Chronic eosinophilic pneumonia
  c Allergic granulomatosis of Churg and Strauss
  d Hypereosinophilic syndrome

asthma, it is important to determine if the patient has extrinsic (allergic, atopic) asthma and has wheal-and-flare skin reactivity to *Aspergillus* allergens. If so, other criteria should be sought for diagnosis of *allergic bronchopulmonary aspergillosis* (ABPA) (Table 205-3). *A. fumigatus* is the most common etiologic agent, although other *Aspergillus* species have also been implicated. The chest roentgenogram in ABPA may show transient, recurrent infiltrates or may suggest the presence of proximal bronchiectasis. The bronchial asthma of ABPA likely involves an IgE-mediated hypersensitivity whereas the bronchiectasis associated with this disorder is thought to result from a deposition of immune complexes in proximal airways. Adequate treatment usually requires the long-term use of systemic glucocorticoids.

Tropical eosinophilia is usually caused by filarial infection; however, eosinophilic pneumonias also occur with other parasites such as *Ascaris, Ancyclostoma* species, *Toxocara* species, and *Strongyloides stercoralis*. Tropical eosinophilia due to *Wuchereria bancrofti* or *W. malayi* occurs most commonly in southern Asia, Africa, and South America, and is treated successfully with diethylcarbamazine.

Drug-induced eosinophilic pneumonias are typified by acute reactions to nitrofurantoin which may begin 2 h to 10 days after nitrofurantoin is started, with symptoms of dry cough, fever, chills, and dyspnea; an eosinophilic pleural effusion accompanying patchy or diffuse pulmonary infiltrates may also occur. Other drugs associated with eosinophilic pneumonias include sulfonamides, penicillin, chlorpropamide, thiazides, tricyclic antidepressants, hydralazine, mephenesin, mecamylamine, nickel carbonyl vapor, gold salts, isoniazid, para-aminosalicylic acid, and others. Treatment consists of withdrawal of the incriminated drugs and the use of glucocorticoids, if necessary.

The idiopathic eosinophilic pneumonias consist of a group of diseases of varying severity. *Loeffler's syndrome* is a benign, acute eosinophilic pneumonia characterized by migrating pulmonary infiltrates and minimal clinical manifestations. *Chronic eosinophilic pneumonia* presents with significant systemic symptoms including fever, chills, night sweats, cough, anorexia, and weight loss lasting several weeks to months. The chest x-ray frequently shows peripheral infiltrates which have been described as a photographic negative of pulmonary edema. Some patients also have bronchial asthma which

TABLE 205-3 Diagnostic features of allergic bronchopulmonary aspergillosis (ABPA)

MAIN DIAGNOSTIC CRITERIA

1 Bronchial asthma
2 Pulmonary infiltrates
3 Peripheral eosinophilia (> 1000 per cubic microliter)
4 Immediate wheal-and-flare response to *Aspergillus fumigatus*
5 Serum precipitins to *A. fumigatus*
6 Elevated serum IgE
7 Central bronchiectasis

OTHER DIAGNOSTIC FEATURES

1 History of brownish plugs in sputum
2 Culture of *A. fumigatus* from sputum
3 Elevated IgE (and IgG) class antibodies specific for *A. fumigatus*

is of the intrinsic or nonallergic type. Dramatic clearing of symptoms and chest x-rays is often noted within 48 h after initiation of glucocorticoid therapy.

Allergic angiitis and granulomatosis of Churg and Strauss is a multisystem vasculitic disorder that frequently involves the skin, kidney, and nervous system in addition to the lung (Chap. 276). The disorder may occur at any age and favors persons with a history of bronchial asthma. The asthma often is progressive until the onset of fever and exaggerated eosinophilia at which time the symptoms of asthma may ease. The illness may be fulminating and the prognosis grave unless treated aggressively with glucocorticoids and immunosuppressive therapy.

The hypereosinophilic syndrome is characterized by a peripheral blood eosinophilia over 1500 eosinophils per microliter for 6 months or longer; lack of evidence for parasitic, allergic, or other known causes of eosinophilia; and signs or symptoms of multisystem organ dysfunction. Consistent features are blood and bone marrow eosinophilia with tissue infiltration by relatively mature eosinophils. The organs affected typically include the heart, lungs, liver, spleen, skin, and nervous system. Therapy of the disorder consists of glucocorticoids and/or hydroxyurea plus therapy as needed for cardiac dysfunction, which is frequently responsible for much of the morbidity and mortality in this syndrome.

REFERENCES

Hypersensitivity pneumonitis

HASLAM PL et al: Mast cells, atypical lymphocytes, and neutrophils in bronchoalveolar lavage in extrinsic allergic alveolitis: Comparison with other interstitial lung disease. Am Rev Respir Dis 135:35, 1987

HUNNINGHAKE GW, BEDELL GN: Interstitial lung disease: Concepts of pathogenesis. Semin Respir Med 6:31, 1984

———— et al: Inflammatory and immune processes in the human lung in health and disease: Evaluation by bronchopulmonary lavage. Am J Pathol 97:149, 1979

LEATHERMAN JW et al: Lung T cells in hypersensitivity pneumonitis. Ann Intern Med 100:390, 1984

RICHERSON HB: Hypersensitivity pneumonitis (extrinsic allergic alveolitis), in *Pulmonary Diseases and Disorders*, 2d ed, AP Fishman (ed). New York, McGraw-Hill, 1988, p 667

————: Hypersensitivity pneumonitis—pathology and pathogenesis. Clin Rev Allergy 1:469, 1983

SALVAGGIO JE: Hypersensitivity pneumonitis. J Allergy Clin Immunol 79:558, 1987

SEMENZATO G et al: Different types of cytotoxic lymphocytes recovered from the lungs of patients with hypersensitivity pneumonitis. Am Rev Respir Dis 137:70, 1988

The eosinophilic pneumonias

GREENBERGER PA, PATTERSON R: Allergic bronchopulmonary aspergillosis: A model of bronchopulmonary disease with defined serologic, radiologic, pathologic and clinical findings from asthma to fatal destructive lung disease. Chest 91:165S, 1987

MALO JL et al: Studies in chronic allergic bronchopulmonary aspergillosis. 1. Clinical and physiological findings. 2. Radiological findings. 3. Immunological findings. 4. Comparison with a group of asthmatics. Thorax 32:254, 262, 269, 275, 1977

MAYCOCK RL, SALDANA MJ: Eosinophilic pneumonia, in *Pulmonary Diseases and Disorders*, 2d ed, AP Fishman (ed). New York, McGraw-Hill, 1988, p 683

SCHATZ M et al: The eosinophil and the lung. Arch Intern Med 142:1515, 1982

SCHOENBERGER CI, CRYSTAL RG: Drug-induced lung disease, in *Update IV: Harrison's Principles of Internal Medicine*, KJ Isselbacher et al (eds). New York, McGraw-Hill, 1983, p 49

SLAVIN RG: Allergic bronchopulmonary aspergillosis. Clin Rev Allergy 3:167, 1985

206 ENVIRONMENTAL LUNG DISEASES

FRANK E. SPEIZER

This chapter is designed to provide perspectives on ways to assess pulmonary diseases for which environmental causes are suspected. This assessment is important because removal of the patient from a harmful environment is often the only intervention that might prevent further significant deterioration or lead to improvement in a patient's condition. Furthermore, the identification of an environmentally associated disease in a single patient may lead to primary preventive strategies in other similarly exposed people who have not yet developed disease. Unless the physician specifically considers environmental exposures, these diseases and their causes will go undetected.

The exact magnitude of the problem is unknown, but there is no question that large numbers of people are at risk of developing serious respiratory disease as a result of occupational or environmental exposures. For example, even if only 5 percent (a conservative estimate) of workers currently exposed to asbestos, cotton dust, or silica are to suffer from respiratory disease as a result of their exposure, this represents more than 100,000 individuals in the United States.

Although industries are required to spend substantial amounts of capital in efforts to protect their workers, occupationally related respiratory diseases continue to occur. These diseases are often attributed to exposures in the distant past at a time when we were not aware of or at least did not consider worker protection to the degree that we do today. We have, as a society, elected to pay compensation to affected individuals, and the physician is often called upon to judge not only the physical condition of such a patient but also the degree to which the illness can be related to, or aggravated by, a particular occupational exposure.

HISTORY AND PHYSICAL EXAMINATION The patient history is of paramount importance in assessing any potential occupational or environmental exposure. Often one is dealing with potential exposures in industries or environmental settings in which the physician has little personal experience. The physician must, therefore, ask the patient to describe a suspected environmental exposure in detail.

Inquiry into specific work practices should include questions about specific contaminants involved, the availability and use of personal respiratory protection devices, the size and ventilation of workspaces, the numbers of other workers potentially at risk of exposure, and whether other coworkers have similar complaints. In addition, the patient must be questioned about alternative sources for potentially toxic exposures, including hobbies or other environmental exposures at home. Short-term exposures to potential toxic agents in the distant past also must be considered. This information can be best elicited by a detailed occupational history which inquires about every job (beginning even with part-time jobs during schooling), about the nature of the work, the materials handled, and the duration and chronologic years of employment.

Many people are aware of the potential hazards in their workplaces, and recent legislation has made it a requirement in many states that employees be informed about potentially hazardous exposures. These requirements include the provision of specific educational materials (including Material Safety Data Sheets), personal protective equipment and instructions in their use, and information on environmental control procedures. Reminders posted in the workplace may warn workers about hazardous substances. Protective clothing, lockers, and shower facilities may be considered necessary parts of the job. However, even in these ideal settings, the introduction of new processes, particularly when related to the use of new chemical compounds, may change exposure significantly, and often only the employee on the production line is aware of the change. For the physician who regularly sees patients from a particular industry, a visit to the work site can be very instructive.

The physical examination of patients with environmentally related lung diseases may help to determine the nature and severity of the pulmonary condition. Unfortunately, the pulmonary response to most injurious agents is the development of a limited number of nonspecific physical signs. These findings do not point to the specific causative agent, and other types of information must be used to arrive at an etiologic diagnosis.

PULMONARY FUNCTION TESTS AND CHEST RADIOGRAPH The use of pulmonary function tests and radiographic examinations of the chest can provide insight into the nature of the exposures which have led to the current condition of the patient and the level of impairment. Many mineral dusts produce characteristic alterations in the mechanics of breathing and lung volumes which clearly indicate a restrictive pattern (Chaps. 201 and 211). Exposures to a number of organic dusts or chemical agents capable of producing occupational asthma result in pronounced obstructive patterns of pulmonary dysfunction that may be reversible (Chap. 204). Standardized approaches for measuring the mechanics of breathing and diffusion across the alveolar membrane (Chap. 201) have been proposed for screening large industrial groups. Measurement of change in forced expiratory volume (FEV$_1$) before and after a working shift can be used to detect an acute bronchoconstrictive response. An acute decrement of FEV$_1$ over the Monday work shift is a characteristic feature of cotton textile workers with byssinosis.

For many years the chest radiograph has been used to detect and monitor the pulmonary response to mineral dusts. To provide a standardized method of recording judgments about the kind and severity of radiographic abnormalities, the International Labour Organization (ILO) International Classification of Radiographs of Pneumoconioses was developed. The ILO scheme involves classifying chest roentgenograms according to the nature and size of opacities seen and the extent of involvement of the parenchyma. However, judgments based only on chest radiographs may over- or underestimate the functional impact of pneumoconiosis. With dusts causing rounded, regular opacities, such as in coal worker's pneumoconiosis, the degree of involvement on the chest radiograph may be extensive, while pulmonary function may be only minimally impaired. In contrast, in pneumoconiosis causing linear, irregular opacities, as seen in asbestosis, the radiograph may lead to underestimation of the severity of the impairment. It is possible to have a history of exposure, moderately reduced forced vital capacity (FVC), and a reduced diffusion in asbestosis with a relatively normal chest radiograph. The radiographic findings of irregular or linear opacities are simply more difficult to separate from normal markings until relatively late in the disease. When shadows become large (radiographic lesions greater than 1 cm in diameter), the condition is termed *complicated pneumoconiosis,* sometimes called *progressive massive fibrosis* (PMF). Chest CT scanning can sometimes contribute additional useful information. However, the additional cost and radiation involved militate against using this technique except in cases where clinical and radiographic data are in conflict.

Other diagnostic procedures of use in identifying environmentally induced lung disease include evaluating heavy metal exposures (arsenic, cadmium in battery plant workers); bacteriologic studies (tuberculosis in medical care personnel, anthrax in wool sorters); fungal studies (coccidioidomycosis in southwestern farm workers, histoplasmosis in poultry or pigeon handlers); or serologic studies (psittacosis in pet shop workers or owners of sick birds, Q fever in tanners or slaughterhouse workers). Ultimately, a lung biopsy may be required both to make a morphologic diagnosis of the underlying pulmonary disease and to attempt to identify the specific etiologic agent.

MEASUREMENT OF EXPOSURE If reliable environmental sampling data are available, these sources of information should be used in assessing a patient's exposure. Since many of the chronic diseases result from exposure over many years, current environmental measurements should be combined with work histories to arrive at estimates of past exposure. However, the dose of any environmental agent is a complex interaction of chemical reaction, both at the emission source and in the ambient atmosphere, and physiologic factors, including ventilation rate and depth, which may affect transport and deposition of aerosols and gases in the lung. Even in acute conditions, when monitoring of exposure may be possible, little may be known about the actual dose received by the lung. Most of the research on health effects of air pollutants (discussed later in this chapter) has relied upon fixed-station monitoring of outdoor air, often at locations somewhat distant from the residences of the people being studied. In addition, most people spend less than 20 percent of their time outdoors. Efforts to determine the penetration rate of outdoor contaminants into the indoors suggest that these penetration rates are highly pollutant specific. Therefore, outdoor measurements can be used only in a relative sense, and they cannot be relied upon to estimate actual dose.

In situations where individual exposure to specific agents has been determined, either in a work setting or for ambient air pollutants, transport of these agents through the airways may be an important factor affecting dose. The upper airways are remarkably effective filters of both particles and gases. For example, virtually 100 percent of sulfur dioxide, a highly soluble gas, is absorbed in the upper airways during quiet breathing, and even during exercise sulfur dioxide is unlikely to penetrate beyond the large bronchi. On the other hand, nitrogen dioxide, which is less soluble, may reach the bronchioles and alveoli in sufficient quantities to result in an acute life-threatening disease in farmers exposed even briefly to the gas evolved from moldy hay in silos (silo filler's disease).

Particle size and chemistry of air contaminants also must be considered. Particles above 10 to 15 μm, because of their settling velocities in air, do not penetrate beyond the upper airways. These larger particles are often referred to as "fugitive dusts" and include pollens, other windblown dusts, and dusts resulting from mechanical industrial processes. They have little or no role in chronic respiratory disease except as possibly related to cancer (see below).

Particles below 10 μm in size are created by the burning of fossil fuel or high-temperature industrial processes resulting in condensation products from gases, fumes, or vapors. These particles are divided into two size fractions on the basis of their chemical characteristics. Particles approximately 2.5 to 10 μm (coarse-mode fraction) contain crustal elements, such as silica, aluminum, and iron. These particles mostly deposit relatively high in the tracheobronchial tree. Particles less than approximately 2.5 μm (fine-mode fraction or accumulation mode) contain sulfates, nitrates, and organic compounds. The deposition of the fine-mode particles is more often in the terminal bronchioles and alveoli. The smallest particles, those less than 0.1 μm in size, remain in the airstream and deposit in the lung only on a random basis as they come into contact with the alveolar walls through thermal forces and/or Brownian movement.

Besides the size characteristics of particles and the solubility of gases, the actual chemical composition, mechanical properties, and immunogenicity or infectivity of inhaled material determine in large part the nature of the diseases found among exposed persons.

OCCUPATIONAL EXPOSURES AND PULMONARY DISEASE

INORGANIC DUSTS   Asbestos exposure   Except in localized regions with single industrial exposures, such as coal-mining or granite-quarrying regions, the most frequent inorganic dust–related chronic pulmonary diseases are associated with industries using *asbestiform fibers.* Asbestos is a generic term for several different mineral silicates, including chrysolite, amosite, anthophyllite, and crocidolite. Approximately 9.1 million workers in the United States who had exposure to the various forms of asbestos fibers were estimated to be alive in 1980 and therefore subsequently at risk of asbestos-related diseases. Besides mining, milling, and manufacturing of asbestos products, the exceptional thermal and electric insulation properties of asbestos led to its widespread use in construction, leading to exposure of pipe fitters, boiler makers, and other workers in the building trades. In addition, asbestos is used in the manufacture of fire-smothering blankets and safety garments, as filler for plastic materials, in cement and floor tiles, and in friction materials, such as brake and clutch linings.

Exposure to asbestos is not limited to persons who directly handle the material. Cases of asbestos-related diseases have been encountered in individuals with only moderate exposure, such as the painter or electrician who works alongside the insulation worker in a shipyard, or the housewife who does no more than shake out and wash her husband's work clothes. Community exposure has probably resulted from the use of asbestos-containing material sprayed on steel girders in many large buildings as a safety feature to prevent buckling in case of fire. Clusters of cases of mesothelioma have been noted in the neighborhood of an asbestos plant in London and in the communities near asbestos mines in South Africa.

Asbestos was first used extensively in the 1940s. Starting in 1975 it has been mostly replaced with man-made mineral fibers, such as fiberglass or slag wool. However, asbestos is still used in the manufacture of brake linings, and remains as pipe and boiler insulation in hundreds of thousands of workplaces and homes. Despite current regulations mandating adequate training for any worker potentially exposed to asbestos, exposure probably continues among inexperienced demolition workers. The major health effects from exposure to asbestos are pulmonary fibrosis (asbestosis) and cancers of the respiratory tract and pleura and, rarely, peritoneum.

Asbestosis is a diffuse interstitial fibrosing disease of the lung which is directly related to the intensity and duration of exposure. Except for a history of exposure to asbestos (generally in a work setting), asbestosis resembles the other forms of diffuse interstitial fibrosis (Chap. 211). Usually at least 10 years of moderate to severe exposure has occurred before the disease becomes manifest.

Physiologic studies reveal a restrictive pattern with a decrease in lung volumes. Flow rates are commonly reduced less than would be predicted on the basis of the volume reduction. An early sign of severe disease may be a reduction in diffusing capacity.

Pulmonary fibrosis may occur following sufficient exposure to any of the asbestiform fiber types. The fibrotic lesions do not appear to relate to either shape or chemical composition of any fiber type. Recent studies indicate that during phagocytosis of the asbestos fiber, the membrane of the macrophage is damaged, which results in the release of lysosomes containing enzymes which may act to damage the lung parenchyma. The clinical manifestations are typical of those physical findings in any patient with pulmonary fibrosis (Chap. 211).

The chest radiograph can be used to determine a number of manifestations of asbestos exposure, as well as to identify specific lesions. Past exposure is specifically indicated by pleural plaques, which are characterized by either thickening or calcification along the parietal pleura, particularly along the lower lung fields, the diaphragm, and the cardiac border. Without additional manifestations, pleural plaques imply only exposure, not pulmonary impairment. Benign pleural effusions may occur, particularly in patients with abestosis, but are not necessarily restricted to those with overt disease. The fluid is sterile, but may be a serous or blood-stained exudate and may occur bilaterally. The effusion may be slowly progressive or may resolve spontaneously.

The radiographic diagnosis of asbestosis depends upon the presence of irregular or linear opacities, usually first noted in the lower lung fields and spreading into the middle and upper lung fields as the disease progresses. An indistinct heart border or a "ground glass" appearance in the lung fields is seen in some cases. As the fibrotic changes in the parenchyma begin to coalesce, the patient develops obliteration of entire acinar units with eventual formation of the classical honeycombed lung, which appears on chest radiographs as coarse infiltrates with small (about 7- to 10-μm) air spaces. No specific therapy is available in the management of patients with asbestosis. The supportive care is that of any patient with diffuse interstitial fibrosis from any cause.

In general, newly diagnosed cases will have resulted from exposure levels that were present many years before and, in spite of the patients' having left the industry, are attributable to that former exposure. Since the patient may be eligible for compensation within a specific time frame after the diagnosis of an asbestos-related disease is made, the physician making the diagnosis should be certain to inform the patient promptly. On occasion, the physician may have reason to suspect ongoing exposure from a patient's current job description or actual monitoring data. In such cases, federal or state

health authorities may need to be notified. Present-day occupational safety and health regulations, if followed properly, protect workers from exposure. Because the association of smoking and asbestosis increases the risk of developing lung cancer (see below), it is extremely important to advise such patients to stop smoking.

Lung cancer (Chap. 215), either squamous cell or adenocarcinoma, is the most frequent cancer associated with asbestos exposure. The excess frequency of lung cancer in asbestos workers is associated with a minimum lapse of 15 to 19 years between first exposure and development of the disease. Persons with more exposure are at greater risk of disease. In addition, there appears to be a significant multiplicative effect which leads to a far greater risk of lung cancer in persons who are cigarette smokers and have asbestos exposure than would be expected by taking the sum of both risks. Efforts to consider these high-risk individuals for special surveillance studies, including sputum cytologic examinations and repeated chest x-rays as frequently as every 4 to 6 months, suggest that cancers can be detected at an earlier stage and that the survival of these patients may be prolonged.

Mesotheliomas (Chap. 216), both pleural and peritoneal, are also associated with asbestos exposure. In contrast to lung cancer there does not appear to be any association with smoking. Relatively short-term exposures of 1 to 2 years or less occurring some 20 to 25 years in the past have been associated with the development of mesotheliomas (which stresses the point of obtaining a complete environmental exposure history). The risk for this type of tumor peaks 30 to 35 years after initial exposure. Although approximately 50 percent of mesotheliomas metastasize, the tumor generally is locally invasive, and death usually results from local extension. Most patients present with effusions that may obscure the underlying pleural tumor. In contrast to other causes of effusion, because of the restriction placed on the chest wall no shift of mediastinal structures toward the opposite chest will be seen. The major diagnostic problem is differentiation from peripherally spreading pulmonary adenocarcinoma or adeno-carcinoma metastatic to pleura from an extrathoracic primary site. Although a needle biopsy may be diagnostic, an open biopsy is often necessary and even when performed may not provide a definitive diagnosis of the origin of the tumor.

One concern in making a definitive diagnosis of a mesothelioma relates to potential compensation to the survivors of a patient with this usually fatal disease. Since epidemiologic studies have shown that more than 80 percent of mesotheliomas may be associated with asbestos exposure, documented mesothelioma in a worker with occupational exposure to asbestos may be compensable in many parts of the United States.

Other naturally occurring asbestiform material (e.g., erionite, a fibrous zeolite) induces mesotheliomas in test animals and has been associated with an excess incidence of lung cancer and mesotheliomas in a population in central Turkey exposed to it in volcanic rock. Man-made mineral fibers (MMMF) have similar physiochemical properties to naturally occurring asbestiform fibers. However, recent studies of exposure suggest that if excess risks of lung cancer do occur, they are less than with naturally occurring fibers. To date no cases of mesotheliomas from MMMF without exposure to asbestos have been reported. Part of the difficulty in assessing the effects of MMMF is that they have been used for relatively shorter periods and generally at lower exposure levels than for asbestos. Fortunately, recent concern has led to better worker protection.

Silicosis   In spite of the technical adequacy of existing protective equipment, *free silica* (SiO_2), or crystalline quartz, is still a major occupational hazard. In the United States estimates of potential numbers of exposed workers range between 1.2 to 3 million people. The major occupational exposures include mining, stone cutting, abrasive industries, foundry workers, packers of silica flour, and quarrying, particularly of granite. Most often the progressive pulmonary fibrosis (silicosis) occurs in a dose-response fashion after many years of exposure.

Workers exposed to sandblasting in confined spaces, tunneling through rock with high quartz content (15 to 25 percent), and engaged in the manufacture of abrasive soaps may develop acute silicosis with as little as 10 months' exposure. The disease may be rapidly fatal in less than 2 years in spite of the worker being removed from exposure. A radiographic picture of profuse miliary infiltration or consolidation is characteristic of acute silicosis.

In long-term, relatively less intense exposure, radiographic changes of rounded, small opacities in the upper lobes with retraction and hilar adenopathy classically appear after 15 to 20 years of exposure. Calcification of hilar nodes may occur in as many as 20 percent of cases and produces the characteristic "eggshell" pattern. These changes may be preceded by or be associated with a reticular pattern of irregular densities which are uniformly present throughout the upper lung zones.

The nodular fibrosis may be progressive in the absence of further exposure, with coalescence and formation of nonsegmental conglomerates of irregular masses in excess of 1 cm in diameter. These masses become quite large and are characteristic of progressive massive fibrosis (PMF). Significant functional impairment with both restrictive and obstructive components may be associated with this form of silicosis. In the late stages of the disease ventilatory failure may develop. Patients with silicosis are at greater risk of acquiring *Mycobacterium tuberculosis* infections (silicotuberculosis), although tuberculosis is not always involved in the progression of the disease to PMF. Because the frequency with which tuberculosis has been found at autopsy in patients with PMF exceeds considerably the frequency of premorbid diagnosis, treatment for tuberculosis is indicated in any patient with silicosis and a positive tuberculin test.

Other less hazardous silicates include fuller's earth, kaolin, mica, diatomaceous earths, silica gel, soapstone, carbonate dusts, and cement dusts. The production of fibrosis in workers exposed to these agents is believed to be related to either the free silica content of these dusts or, for substances which contain no free silica, to the potentially large dust loads to which these workers may be exposed.

Other silicates, including *talc dusts,* may be contaminated with asbestos and/or free silica. Accidental exposure to significant quantities of talc may result in an acute syndrome with cough, cyanosis, and labored breathing (acute talcosis). Severe progressive fibrosis with respiratory failure may ensue within a few years. Far more common is the fibrosis and/or pleural or lung cancer associated with chronic exposure in rubber workers who use commercial talc as a lubricant in tire molds. Pure talc does not produce fibrosis; thus, it is difficult to sort out whether the effects are due to the contamination of commercial talc by asbestos or by free silica.

Coal worker's pneumoconiosis (CWP) *Coal dust* is associated with CWP, which has enormous social, economic, and medical significance in every nation in which coal mining is an important industry. Simple radiographically identified CWP is seen in 12 percent of all miners and in as many as 50 percent of anthracite miners with more than 20 years' work on the coal face. The prevalence of disease is lower in workers in bituminous coal mines. Since much of the western United States coal is bituminous, CWP is less prevalent in that region.

Much of the symptomatology associated with simple CWP appears to be similar and additive to the effects of cigarette smoking on the development of chronic bronchitis and obstructive lung disease (Chap. 210). In the early stages of simple CWP, radiographic abnormalities consist of small, irregular opacities (reticular pattern). With prolonged exposure, one sees small, rounded, regular opacities, 1 to 5 mm in diameter (nodular pattern). Calcification is generally not seen, although approximately 10 percent of older anthracite miners have calcified nodules.

Complicated CWP is manifested by the appearance on the chest radiograph of nodules ranging from 1 cm in diameter to the size of an entire lobe, generally confined to the upper half of the lungs. This condition, considered a form of PMF, is accompanied by a significant reduction in diffusing capacity and with premature mortality. In contrast to patients with silicosis, only a relatively small percentage

of underground miners with simple CWP (5 to 15 percent, depending on the type of coal) develop PMF.

The mechanism whereby PMF occurs in CWP is not fully understood. Several hypotheses have been proposed, including (1) sufficient free silica is present in the dust; (2) normal clearance mechanisms are unable to clear the excessive dust loads; (3) an interplay occurs between an intrinsic immunologic mechanism and the dust and/or damaged lung tissue; and (4) atypical reactions to *Mycobacterium tuberculosis* occur. As previously described, PMF in silicosis is associated with prolonged duration and high intensity of exposure to free silica. Heavy exposure to carbon particles free of silica occurs in carbon black, graphite, and charcoal workers. The prolonged exposure of these workers may result in sufficient accumulation of carbon in the lung to produce PMF. The mechanism appears to relate to a breakdown of the clearance capacity of the airways.

Caplan's syndrome, which includes seropositive rheumatoid arthritis with characteristic PMF, is consistent with an immunopathologic mechanism. The syndrome was first described in coal miners but subsequently has been found in a number of pneumoconioses. Similarly, the high prevalence of antinuclear antibodies in sandblasting workers with silicosis and the elevation of gamma globulin levels in silicotic individuals suggest an immunologic mechanism. Although mycobacterial infections are found more often in coal miners than PMF is found in silicotic patients, tuberculosis does not appear to be associated with most of the cases of PMF in coal miners.

Berylliosis Beryllium may produce an acute pneumonitis or, far more commonly, a chronic interstitial pneumonitis. Unless one inquires specifically about occupational exposures to beryllium in the manufacture of alloys, ceramics, high-technology electronics, and, before the 1950s, in the production of fluorescent lights, one may miss entirely the etiologic relationship to an occupational exposure. Nonspecific pulmonary function tests may be normal or may indicate evidence of restrictive disease. Between 2 and 15 years of exposure, depending on its intensity, is required for the disease to become manifest. On open lung biopsy granulomatous formation similar to that seen in sarcoidosis (Chap. 277) may make differentiation impossible unless tissue levels of beryllium are measured.

Rarely, other hard metals, including aluminum powders, chromium, cobalt, titanium dioxide, and tungsten, may produce an interstitial pneumonitis.

Other inorganic dusts Other dusts are considered *nuisance dusts* because their major impact seems to be reduction in visibility and irritation of eyes, ears, nasal passages, and other mucous membranes. If they penetrate to the lower airways, they do not affect the architecture of the terminal bronchioles or acinar spaces or destroy collagen. Generally, clinical effects are reversible. Pulmonary function tests are usually normal unless another disease process coexists. If radiodense, macular collections of these dusts may produce striking radiographic pictures which are so characteristic that patients with a history of significant exposure are easily diagnosed as having the condition which bears the name reflecting the nature of the dust. Examples are iron and iron oxides from welding or silver finishing (*siderosis*); tin oxide used in metallurgy, color stabilization, printing, and the manufacture of porcelain, glass, and fabric (*stannosis*); and barium sulfate used as a catalyst for organic reactions, drilling mud components, and electroplating (*baritosis*). Other metal dusts producing similar radiodense pictures include *cerium dioxide* and *antimony salts.*

Most of the inorganic dusts discussed thus far are associated with the production of either dust macules or interstitial fibrotic changes in the lung. Another set of dusts (see Table 206-1), along with some of the dusts previously discussed, is associated with chronic mucous hypersecretion (chronic bronchitis), with or without reduction of expiratory flow rates. These conditions may be caused by cigarette smoking, and any effort to attribute some component of the disease to occupational and environmental exposures must take cigarette smoking into account. Most studies suggest an additive effect of dust

TABLE 206-1 Selected occupational dusts believed to be associated with mucous hypersecretion and/or obstructive airway disease and other respiratory diseases*

Agent (Exposure)	Mucous hyper-secretion	Ob-struc-tion	Other con-ditions†
INORGANIC DUST			
Antimony (Storage batteries, solder, ceramics, glass, plastics)	X		P
Arsenic (Manufacture of pesticides, pigments, glass, alloys)	X		C
Barium and compounds including BaO, BaSO₄, BaCO₃ (Catalyst, drilling mud, electroplating)	X		P
Cadmium dust (Electroplating, battery manufacture, welding, smelting, aluminum soldering)	X	X	P
Cement dust (Construction trades, manufacture of cement blocks)	X	X	
Chromium and CrO₃, CrF₂ (Corrosion inhibitor pigment, metallurgy, electroplating)	X		C
Coal dust (Mining)	X		P
Coke oven emissions (Retort house, coke ovens)	X	X	P, C
Graphite (Steelmaking, lubricants, pencils, paints, stove polish)	X	X	P
Iron dust (Steel and nonferrous foundry workers, welding)	X		P
Mica (Insulation, roofing shingles, oil refining, rubber manufacturing)	X		P
Phosphorus, elemental chlorides, sulfides (Manufacture of fireworks, agricultural chemicals, insecticides, pesticides)	X	X	
Rock dusts (Miners, tunnelers, quarry workers)	X		P
Vanadium pentoxide (Welding electrodes, additive to steel, by-product in ash from oil burning)	X	X	
ORGANIC DUST (see Chap. 205)			
Cotton dust, flax, hemp (Manufacture of yarns for linen, rope, cotton; ginning, cottonseed crushing; waste fiber processing)	X	X	
Grain dusts (Farmers, workers in grain elevators, barge and grain ship crewmembers)	X	X	
Moldy hay (Farmers, other animal attendants)	X		HP

* The table excludes agents associated with asthma as the primary disease (see Chap. 204).
† Other conditions include hypersensitivity pneumonitis (HP), pneumoconiosis (P), and cancers (C).
NOTE: X indicates that mucous hypersecretion or obstruction are associated with exposure.

exposure and smoking. The pattern of the effect is similar to that of cigarette smoking, suggesting that small airways may be the initial site of pathologic response to those cases associated with the development of obstructive lung disease. Cigarette smoke is usually the more noxious agent, and dust effects may be discernible only in nonsmokers.

ORGANIC DUSTS Some of the specific diseases associated with organic dusts are discussed in detail in the chapters on asthma (Chap. 204) and on hypersensitivity pneumonitis (Chap. 205). Many of these diseases are named for the specific setting in which the disease is found, e.g., farmer's lung, malt worker's disease, or mushroom worker's disease. Occupational and other environmental exposures must be sought when these conditions are suspected. Often the temporal relation of symptoms to exposure furnishes the best evidence for the diagnosis. Three occupational groups are singled out for discussion because they represent the largest proportion of people affected by the diseases resulting from organic dusts.

Cotton dust (byssinosis) Estimates of the number of exposed persons in the United States vary, but probably over 800,000 are exposed occupationally to cotton, flax, or hemp in the production of yarns for cotton, linen, and rope making. Although this discussion focuses on cotton, the same syndrome to a somewhat lesser degree has been reported in exposure to flax, hemp, and jute.

Although cotton dust–related disease was first described in the seventeenth century, it is only in the last 40 years that the disease has been recognized as a worldwide problem in the textile industry. Exposure occurs throughout the manufacturing process but is most pronounced in those portions of the factory involved with the treatment of the cotton prior to spinning—i.e., blowing, mixing, and carding (straightening of fibers). Cases reported from spinning rooms are believed to be due to secondary contamination from carding rooms. Recent attempts to control dust levels by use of exhaust hoods, general increase in ventilation, and wetting procedures in some settings have been highly successful. However, respiratory protective equipment appears to be required during certain operations to prevent workers from being exposed to levels of dust that exceed the current United States cotton dust standard.

Byssinosis is characterized clinically as occasional (early stage) and then regular (late stage) chest tightness toward the end of the first day of the workweek (Monday chest tightness). In epidemiologic studies, up to 80 percent of carding room employees may show a significant drop in their FEV_1 over the course of a Monday shift, depending on the level of exposure in the carding room air.

Initially the symptoms do not recur on subsequent days of the week. However, in 10 to 25 percent of workers, the disease may be progressive with chest tightness recurring or persisting throughout the workweek. After more than 10 years of exposure, workers with recurrent symptoms are more likely to have an obstructive pattern on pulmonary function testing. These higher grades of impairment are seen in workers exposed both to high levels of dust and for greater durations. There is an additive effect of cotton dust exposure plus cigarette smoking. The highest grades of impairment are generally seen in smokers.

Treatment in the early stages of the disease is directed toward reversing the bronchospasm with bronchodilators; however, the chest tightness appears at least in part to relate to histamine release, and antihistamines have been shown to lessen anticipated fall in FEV_1 the first day of the week. Clearly, reduction of dust exposure is of primary importance. All workers with persistent symptoms or significantly reduced levels of pulmonary function should be moved to areas of lower risk of exposure. Regular surveillance of pulmonary function in the industry has made it easier to identify affected persons. Persons with reduced pulmonary function, a personal history of respiratory allergy, and positive history of continued cigarette smoking should be considered at increased risk of developing byssinosis in association with working in the cotton industry.

Grain dust Although the exact number of workers at risk in the United States is not known, at least 500,000 people work in grain elevators, and over 2 million farmers are potentially at risk. The presentation of disease in grain elevator employees or workers in flour or feed mills is virtually identical to the characteristic finding in cigarette smokers, i.e., persistent cough, mucus hypersecretion, wheeze and dyspnea on exertion, and reduced FEV_1 and FEV_1/FVC ratio (Chap. 201).

Dust concentrations in grain elevators vary greatly but appear to be in excess of 10,000 μg/m³ with approximately one-third of the particles by weight being in the respirable range. The effect of grain dust exposure is additive to that of cigarette smoking with approximately 50 percent of workers who smoke having symptoms. Among nonsmoking grain elevator operators, approximately one-quarter have mucous hypersecretion, about five times the number that would be expected in unexposed nonsmokers. However, evidence of obstruction on pulmonary function studies is observed only in workers who smoke. It is not clear if this results from an enhancement of cigarette smoking effect in exposed workers or if smokers are more susceptible to the effects of grain dust.

Farmer's lung This condition results from exposure to moldy hay containing spores of thermophilic actinomycetes that produce a hypersensitivity pneumonitis (Chap. 205). There are few good population-based estimates of the frequency of occurrence of this condition in the United States. However, among farmers in Great Britain the rate of disease ranges from approximately 10 to 50 per 1000. The prevalence of disease varies in association with rainfall, which determines the amount of fungal growth, and with differences in agricultural practices related to turning and stacking hay.

The patient with acute farmer's lung presents 4 to 8 h after exposure with fever, chills, malaise, cough, and dyspnea without wheezing. The history of exposure is obviously essential to separate this disease from similar symptoms that might occur in influenza or pneumonia. In the chronic form of the disease, the history of repeated attacks after similar exposure is important to separate this syndrome from other causes of patchy fibrosis, e.g., sarcoidosis.

A wide variety of other organic dusts are associated with the occurrence of hypersensitivity pneumonitis (Chap. 205). For those patients who present with hypersensitivity pneumonitis, specific and careful inquiry about occupations, hobbies, or other home environmental exposures will, in most cases, reveal the source of the etiologic agent.

ASSESSMENT OF DISABILITY Significant reduction of dust levels in coal mines has resulted from federal legislation, enacted in the United States in 1969, which requires that respirable dust levels in underground mines be reduced to less than 2000 μg/m^3. This same legislation authorized payment to coal miners (or their survivors) totally disabled by CWP. The criteria for disability from CWP remain unclear and arbitrary. Much of the difficulty relates to the inability to determine in an individual with simple CWP what proportion of an observed respiratory impairment is related to coal dust and what proportion is due to cigarette smoking. The laws as currently interpreted suggest that to be eligible for payment of a claim, one need only show that an underlying condition (i.e., chronic bronchitis with obstruction, presumably due to cigarette smoking) is aggravated by CWP. Thus, it becomes critical that physicians involved in occupational lung disease claim cases be aware of detailed exposure histories of their patients, both in terms of occupational exposures and other environmental exposures (cigarette smoking). In addition, these physicians must understand that the extent to which the level of physiologic impairment incapacitates an individual may not be the sole criterion for determining disability. To assess disability properly may require input not only from physicians but also from experts in ergonomics and vocational rehabilitation, lawyers, and employer and employee representatives.

TOXIC CHEMICALS Exposure to toxic chemicals affecting the lung generally occurs in the form of gases and vapors. A common accident is one in which the victim is trapped in a confined space where the chemicals have accumulated to toxic levels. In addition to the specific toxic effects of the chemical, the victim will often sustain considerable anoxia, which can play a dominant role in determining whether the individual recovers.

Table 206-2 lists a variety of toxic agents which can produce acute and sometimes life-threatening reactions in the lung. All of these agents in sufficient concentrations have been demonstrated, at least in animal studies, to affect the lower airways and disrupt alveolar architecture, either acutely or as a result of chronic exposure. Some of these agents may be generated acutely in the environment. For example, when plastics burn, a number of compounds, including hydrogen cyanide and hydrochloric acid, may be formed and released. The effects and treatment of exposure to these toxic gases are discussed elsewhere (Chap. 374).

Fire fighters and fire victims are at risk of *smoke inhalation*, a numerically important cause of acute cardiorespiratory failure. Smoke inhalation kills more fire victims than does thermal injury. Carbon monoxide poisoning with resulting significant hypoxemia can be life-threatening (Chap. 374). Fire fighters may inappropriately use the "blackness" of the smoke to indicate the degree to which incomplete combustion and, thus, elevation of carbon monoxide levels are present. The increased use of synthetic materials (plastic, polyurethanes), which, when burned, may release a variety of other toxic agents, must be considered when evaluating smoke inhalation victims. Exposed victims may suffer some degree of lower respiratory tract inflammation, similar to that seen with exposure to other irritant gases, e.g., chlorine. Severe cases may develop pulmonary edema.

Fire fighters and victims also may be exposed to large quantities of particulate smoke. Significant long-term effects are not clearly associated with this particulate exposure except as related to the production of irritating effects on the upper airways. Studies attempting to demonstrate either an increased risk of cardiovascular events, presumably from recurrent exposure to carbon monoxide, or excess incidence of chronic respiratory disease from repeated smoke inhalation, are inconclusive, partly because of the difficulties in measuring exposure. Recent studies suggest increased airways responsiveness in firefighters with repeated episodes of smoke inhalation.

Some agents used in the manufacture of synthetic materials such as plastics, polyurethanes, and other polymers have resulted in some workers being sensitized to extremely low levels of *isocyanates, aromatic amines,* or *aldehydes*. Repeated exposure to these agents causes some workers to develop chronic cough and sputum production, asthma, or episodes of low-grade fever and malaise. Occasionally, as in byssinosis, these symptoms occur early in the workweek, but usually recur without workweek periodicity. In the case of exposure to diisocyanate in the production of polyurethane, chronic and persistent asthma in selected individuals appears to result from exposure to concentrations well below the recognized industrial standard. Methods to identify susceptible individuals are needed. At present, challenge testing is being used to determine if a given patient is sensitive. These challenges can be carried out in special environmental chambers where the physician can simulate the work exposure. Alternatively, nonspecific challenges with either pharmacologic agents, such as methacholine and histamine, or isocapneic cold air breathing are being used to identify patients with hyperreactive airways. The usefulness of this nonspecific approach as a method to screen potential sensitive workers has yet to be established.

An unusual route of exposure occurs in *polymer fume fever*. Polymers, notably fluorocarbons, which at normal temperatures produce no reaction, may be transmitted from a worker's hands to his or her cigarettes. Upon burning the cigarette, the polymer is volatilized, and the inhaled agent causes a characteristic syndrome of fever, chills, malaise, and occasionally mild wheezing. The same condition occurs in workers exposed to heated polymers without cigarette use. The syndrome is obviously controlled by proper attention to hygiene in the workplace. A similar self-limited, influenza-like syndrome—*metal fume fever*—results from acute exposure to fumes or smoke of zinc, copper, magnesium, and other volatilized metals. The syndrome may begin several hours after work and resolves within 24 h, only to return on repeated exposure. A proper occupational history should make the diagnosis evident.

ENVIRONMENTAL RESPIRATORY CARCINOGENS Historically, it has been the astute clinician who has recognized a higher incidence of malignant tumors associated with certain environmental exposures. When these observations are linked to an occupational setting, they must be pursued by epidemiologic studies of relatively large groups of both current and former workers. Often the concentration and/or exact nature of the substances contained in the putative exposures cannot be determined. Rarely, the possibility that a substance can play an etiologic role in cancer is supported by observing that a few cases of a very rare tumor in a particular group represent "an epidemic." Examples of this are nasal sinus and lung

TABLE 206-2   Selected common toxic chemical agents

Agents	Selected exposures	Acute effects from high or accidental exposure	Chronic effects from relatively low exposure
Acid fumes; H_2SO_4, HNO_3	Manufacture of fertilizers, chlorinated organic compounds, dyes, explosives, rubber products, metal etching, plastics	Mucous membrane irritation, followed by chemical pneumonitis 2–3 days	No data
Ammonia	Refrigeration, petroleum refining, manufacture of fertilizers, explosives, plastics, and other chemicals	Same as for acid fumes	Chronic bronchitis
Cyanides	Electroplating, extraction of gold or silver, manufacture of mirrors, fumigants, photo supplies	Increase in respiratory rate followed by respiratory arrest, lactic acidosis, pulmonary edema, death	No data
Diazomethane	Methylating agent for acid compounds; laboratory workers	Violent coughing, dyspnea, wheezing, pulmonary edema	No data
Formaldehyde	Manufacture of resins, leathers, rubber, metals, & woods; laboratory workers, embalmers; emission from urethane foam insulation	Same as for acid fumes	Cancers in one species of animals; no data on humans
Halides (Cl, Br, F)	Bleaching in pulp, paper, textile industry; manufacture of chemical compounds; synthetic rubber, plastics, disinfectant, rocket fuel, gasoline	Mucous membrane irritation, pulmonary edema; possible reduced FVC 1–2 yrs after exposure	Dryness of mucous membrane, epistaxis, dental fluorosis, tracheobronchitis
Hydrogen sulfide	By-product of many industrial processes, oil, other petroleum processes and storage	Low exposure: conjunctival irritation; higher: respiratory paralysis similar to cyanides	Chronic bronchitis, recurrent pneumonitis
Isocyanates (TDI, HDI, MDI)	Production of polyurethane foams, plastics, adhesives, surface coatings	Mucous membrane irritation, dyspnea, cough, wheeze, pulmonary edema	Upper respiratory tract irritation, cough, asthma, allergic alveolitis
Nitrogen dioxide	Silage, metal etching, explosives, rocket fuels, welding, by-product of burning fossil fuels	Cough, dyspnea, pulmonary edema may be delayed 4–12 h; possible result from acute exposure: bronchiolitis obliterans in 2–6 wks	Emphysema in animals, ? chronic bronchitis
Ozone	Arc welding, flour bleaching, deodorizing, emissions from copying equipment, photochemical air pollutant	Mucous membrane irritant, pulmonary hemorrhage and edema, reduced pulmonary function transiently in children exposed to summer haze	Chronic eye irritation
Phosgene	Organic compound, metallurgy, volatization of chlorine-containing compounds	Delayed onset of bronchiolitis and pulmonary edema	Chronic bronchitis
Phthalic anhydride	Manufacture of resin esters, polyester resins, thermoactivated adhesives	Nasal irritation, cough	Asthma, chronic bronchitis
Sulfur dioxide	Manufacture of sulfuric acid, bleaches, coating of nonferrous metals, food processing, refrigerant, burning of fossil fuels, wood pulp industry	Mucous membrane irritant, epistaxis	? Chronic bronchitis

cancer in nickel workers, angiosarcomas in vinyl chloride workers, and adenocarcinomas of the nose in woodworkers.

Only in those few cases in which animal studies have been carried out can one confirm that a given suspected agent is really a carcinogen. For example, bis(chloromethyl) ether (BCME) has been shown to produce tumors in animals and oat cell cancer of the lung in humans. In this particular case, BCME, used as a chemical intermediary in the manufacture of a number of organic compounds, was known to produce tumors in animals almost before the substance was introduced into industry. (This case is one of the prime examples of why federal legislation was enacted in the United States in the 1970s to control the release of toxic substances, particularly new chemicals.)

In addition to the asbestos trades, other occupational exposures associated with either proven or suspected respiratory carcinogens include acrylonitrile, arsenic compounds, beryllium (animal studies only), BCME, chromium, coke ovens (exposure to polycyclic hydrocarbons), iron oxide, isopropyl oil (nasal sinuses), mustard gas, the various ores used to produce pure nickel, talc (possible asbestos contamination in both mining and milling), vinyl chloride, welding, wood used in woodworking (nasal cancer only), and uranium. The occurrence of excess cancers in uranium miners raises the possibility

that there exists a large number of workers at risk by virtue of exposure to similar radiation hazards. This includes not only workers involved in processing uranium, up to and including its use in nuclear power plants and in military nuclear hardware, but also workers exposed in underground mining operations where radon daughters may be emitted from rock formations. In the latter case, the levels of exposure are generally considered to be relatively low; however, specific consideration must be given to the possibility of excess exposure for any hard rock miner.

GENERAL ENVIRONMENTAL EXPOSURES

AIR POLLUTION Dramatic and disastrous episodes of air pollution inversion have been documented in many industrialized centers in the world. Each of these episodes has been associated with excess acute mortality in the very old, the very young, and in those with chronic cardiopulmonary diseases. The most dramatic event was the London fog of 1952, in which approximately 4000 excess deaths occurred over a 2-week period following 5 days of severe cold and dense fog. Similar episodes in the United States, although less dramatic in terms of total deaths, occurred in Donora, Pennsylvania, in 1948, and in New York City in the 1960s. In these episodes, generally associated with cold temperature and air stagnation, patients with underlying cardiopulmonary disease were most severely affected.

In addition to significant excess mortality during these episodes, a large number of people required medical care for cardiorespiratory complaints. Subsequent follow-up studies failed to implicate these episodic disasters in the etiology of chronic respiratory disease in adults. On the other hand, many epidemiologic studies of both international and regional differences in the prevalences of chronic respiratory disease suggest that long-term exposures in polluted areas in the early to middle part of the twentieth century were associated with excess chronic respiratory disease.

In 1970, the U.S. federal government established air quality standards for several pollutants believed to be responsible for excess cardiorespiratory diseases. Primary standards regulated by the Environmental Protection Agency (EPA) designed to protect the public health with an adequate margin of safety exist for sulfur dioxide, total suspended particulates, nitrogen dioxide, ozone, lead, and carbon monoxide. These standards vary in their averaging times and levels, in part related to the differences in the known physiologic responses and epidemiologic evidence for each pollutant.

Pollutants are generated from both stationary sources (power plants and industrial complexes) and mobile sources (automobiles), and none of the pollutants occur in isolation. Thus, except for the change in carboxyhemoglobin from carbon monoxide exposure, it becomes extremely difficult to relate any specific health effect to any single pollutant. Furthermore, pollutants may be changed by chemical reactions after being emitted. For example, reducing agents, such as sulfur dioxide and particulate matter from a power plant stack, may react in air to produce acid sulfates and aerosols, the precursors of acid rain, which can be transported long distances in the atmosphere. Oxidizing substances, such as oxides of nitrogen and oxidants from automobile exhaust, may react with sunlight to produce ozone. Although originally a problem confined to the southwestern part of the United States, in recent years, at least during the summertime, elevated ozone and sulfate levels can occur throughout the United States. Both acute and chronic effects of these exposures are currently under investigation.

The symptoms and diseases associated with air pollution are the same as the nononcogenic conditions commonly associated with cigarette smoking. In addition, respiratory illness in early childhood has been associated with chronic exposure to only modestly elevated levels of SO_2 and total suspended particulates. It is not known whether persistent chronic exposure to a relatively constant level of pollutant(s) and recurrent short-term peak exposures which average to the same mean level have different effects. For a patient with significant cardiopulmonary impairment, one can only advise the individual to stay indoors during periods when pollution exceeds current standards.

INDOOR EXPOSURE Because of increased concern about energy costs, efforts to become energy efficient have led to reduced air exchange rates in indoor environments. The effects of these efforts have been to increase exposures to a variety of air contaminants heretofore not considered important. Two examples of potential health effects from exposure to indoor pollutants are discussed to indicate the magnitude of possible problems.

Until recently, little attention, beyond its nuisance effect, was given to the effects of *passive cigarette smoking*. The implication was that passive smoking exposures were too low to be of any consequence. Now studies have shown that the respirable particulate load in any household is directly proportional to the number of cigarette smokers living in the home. Increases in prevalence of respiratory illnesses and reduced levels of pulmonary function measured with simple spirometry have been found in children of smoking parents in a number of studies. The long-term consequences in terms of nononcogenic respiratory diseases are unknown. Two expert panels, however, have concluded that lung cancer risk is significantly higher in nonsmokers with long-standing residence in the households of smokers.

A novel source of indoor exposure to *formaldehyde* results from the curing process involved in the placement of urea-formaldehyde insulating foam or in several wood products used in modern furniture and the construction of mobile homes. Natural "degassing" of formaldehyde occurs during the first few months after the foam has been blown into the walls, with concentrations of formaldehyde as high as 5 ppm rapidly dropping off to less than 0.1 ppm. Chronic exposure to low levels of urea-formaldehyde (generally less than 1 ppm) may result if the foam is improperly installed. Patients apparently sensitive to concentrations of formaldehyde generally well below 1 ppm will complain of upper airway irritation with occasional epistaxis and sore throats. Lower respiratory complaints, such as chest pain and wheeze, however, are uncommon, and often the most disturbing complaints are mild memory and mood disorders. Formaldehyde is a proven animal carcinogen. Whether it causes cancer in humans is not established.

Radon gas is believed to be a risk factor for lung cancer. The main radon product (randon 222) is a gas that results from the decay series of uranium 238 with the immediate precursor being radium 226. The amount of radium in earth materials determines how much radon gas will be emitted. Outdoors the concentrations are trivial. Indoors levels are dependent on the ventilation rate and the size of space into which the gas is emitted. Levels associated with excess lung cancer risk may be present in as many as 10 percent of the houses in the United States. Where smoking exists in the household, the problem is potentially greater since the molecular size of radon particles readily attaches to smoke particles that are inhaled. Fortunately the technology is available for assessing and reducing the level of exposure.

PORTAL OF ENTRY The lung is a primary source of entry into the body for a number of toxic agents that affect other organ systems. For example, the lung is the route of entry for benzene (bone marrow), carbon disulfide (cardiovascular and nervous systems), cadmium (kidney), and mercury (kidney, central nervous system). Thus, in any disease state of obscure origin, it is important to consider possible inhaled environmental agents. Such consideration can sometimes furnish the clue needed to identify a specific external cause for a disorder that might otherwise be labeled "idiopathic."

REFERENCES

BECKLAKE MR et al: The relationship between acute and chronic airway responses to occupational exposures. Curr Pulmonol 9:25, 1988

COCHRANE AL, MOORE FA: A 20-year follow-up of men aged 55–64 including coal miners and foundry workers in Stavley. Br J Ind Med 37:226, 1980

CRAIGHEAD JE, MOSSMAN BT: The pathogenesis of asbestos-associated diseases. N Engl J Med 306:1446, 1982

Guidelines for the Use of International Labour Office Classification of Radiographs of Pneumoconiosis. Occupational Safety and Health Sciences 22 (Revised 1980). Geneva, ILO, 1980

KOSKINEN H: Symptoms and clinical findings in patients with silicosis. Scan J Work Environ Health 11:101, 1985

LARUNERYS RR: Occupational toxicology, in *Casarett and Doull's Toxicology, The Basic Science of Poison*, 3d ed, CD Kloassen, MD Amden, J Doull (eds). New York, MacMillan, 1986, chap 29

National Research Council: *Asbestiform Fibers, Nonoccupational Health Risks.* National Academy Press, Washington DC, 1984, chaps 2, 5, 6

PARKES WR: *Occupational Lung Disorders*, 2d ed. London, Butterworth, 1982

PETO R, SCHNEIDERMAN M (eds): *Quantification of Occupational Cancer*, Banbury Report, 9. Cold Spring Harbor, 1981

ROM WN (ed): *Environmental and Occupational Medicine*. Boston, Little, Brown, 1983, chaps 13, 20

SIMONATO L et al: The man-made mineral fiber European historical cohort study. Extension of the follow up. Scan J Work Environ Health 12:Suppl 1, 34, 1986

WEILL J: Occupational pulmonary diseases and acute and accidental exposures to irritant gases, in *Pulmonary Diseases and Disorders*, 2d ed, A P Fishman (ed). New York, McGraw-Hill, 1987, chap. 54

207 PNEUMONIA AND LUNG ABSCESS

HERBERT Y. REYNOLDS

PNEUMONIA

DEFINITION Pneumonia is inflammation affecting the parenchyma of the lung—that portion distal to the conducting airways and involving the respiratory bronchioles and the alveolar units. Histologically, pneumonitis or an inflammatory reaction causes alveolitis and accumulation of an exudate and is most often due to infection. With spread to the interstitium around alveoli, consolidation and a degree of impaired gas exchange occur in the involved lung tissue. With successful inactivation of the infecting agent, resolution occurs and normal lung structure is usually restored. Exceptions to complete healing occur with certain necrotizing pneumonias, as caused by staphylococci or gram-negative bacteria, after which scars or fibrosis may develop in the lung. Bronchopneumonia denotes patchy and diffuse areas of involvement and often implies that a less severe form of disease exists because signs and radiographic evidence of consolidation are absent. Pneumonia is a commonly encountered disease and, in one form or another, continues to be a leading cause of death in the United States.

PATHOGENESIS Microorganisms These reach lung tissue in several ways: (1) by direct inhalation of infectious particles from ambient air, (2) by aspiration of secretions from the mouth and nasopharynx, (3) by deposition in lung vasculature following hematogenous spread from another site, and rarely, (4) by penetration of lung tissue or spread from a contiguous site. Aspiration of microbes colonizing the naso-oropharynx provides the most frequent entry to the lung. The normal microbial flora of the upper respiratory tract is a complex mixture of aerobic bacteria such as *Streptococcus* sp., *Streptococcus pneumoniae*, *Branhamella catarrhalis*, *Corynebacteria*, *Neisseria* sp. (including *N. meningitidis*), *Staphylococcus* sp., and *Haemophilus* sp. Aerobic gram-negative bacilli, such as *Pseudomonas aeruginosa*, *Klebsiella pneumoniae*, or *Escherichia coli*, are harbored there rarely in healthy people. Anaerobic bacteria, localized in crevices of the gums and teeth, are very numerous and can reach 10^8 organisms per milliliter of saliva (see Chap. 108). Viruses are not usual flora.

Pulmonary infection may follow acquisition of a virulent new strain in the nasooropharynx or an unusually large inoculum of microbes in the lung. The normally symbiotic relationship between colonizing bacteria on the nasooropharyngeal mucosa can be affected by a number of host conditions that promote selection of different pathogenic organisms. Cigarette smoking and chronic bronchitis favor colonization with *S. pneumoniae*, *H. influenzae*, and, perhaps, *Legionella pneumophila*; alcoholism, poorly controlled diabetes mellitus, uremia, prior use of antibiotics, poor nutrition, and many critical illnesses favor acquisition of aerobic gram-negative bacilli. The stress of hospitalization, confinement to a high-level-care nursing facility or intensive care unit, surgery, and treatment with antineoplastic chemotherapy or immunosuppressive drugs all promote rapid colonization with potentially pathogenic organisms. Nosocomial pneumonia can occur in a sizeable percentage of such patients (5 to 25 percent), and its morbidity and mortality are appreciable.

Host defense mechanisms Although a common disease, pneumonia is a relatively rare occurrence in normal people. This attests to the effectiveness of the respiratory host defense system—a complex mixture of anatomic barriers and cleansing mechanisms present in the nasopharynx and upper airways and local cellular and humoral factors in the terminal air-exchange units (alveoli). Normal lungs are generally kept sterile below the first major bronchial divisions.

In the upper respiratory tract and large airways, *mechanical mechanisms* exclude particulate material. These mechanisms include: (1) anatomic barriers, such as the epiglottis and tight apical cellular junctions between epithelial lining cells of the mucosa; (2) reflex closure of the glottis; (3) frequent branching of the pulmonary tree, which leads to aerodynamic filtering of inspired air; (4) mucociliary clearance of particulates that impact on the mucosa; and (5) the cough response. When infectious agents, bacteria in particular, elude these defenses and are deposited in the alveoli, another group of host factors takes over. The terminal units (alveolar ducts and alveoli) do not contain ciliated epithelium and mucus-secreting cells (goblet cells and mucous glands) and coughing does not effectively clear material from the alveoli. Clearance is dependent on phagocytic cells and humoral factors. These mechanisms are shown in Fig. 207-1.

OPSONINS When bacteria or particles reach the alveolar surface, most are rapidly ingested by phagocytes. Although alveolar macrophages avidly phagocytose some inert particles, they usually ingest viable bacteria more slowly. Coating or opsonizing the organisms will enhance phagocytosis approximately tenfold. Nonimmune opsonins are found in the film of fluid on the alveolar surface (lipoprotein surfactant from type II pneumocytes and large fragments of the glycoprotein, fibronectin, produced locally by alveolar macrophages or delivered from intravascular sources). Immune opsonins include IgG antibody and a complement factor, C3b, that augment attachment to specific plasma membrane receptors (see Chap. 13). These opsonins are produced locally or are delivered as part of systemic humoral immunity.

IgG and its subclasses are present in bronchoalveolar lavage (BAL) fluid from normal subjects in approximately the same proportions as found in serum (see Chap. 13). The IgG2 subclass contains antibodies made to capsular polysaccharides of respiratory pathogens such as *S. pneumoniae* and *H. influenzae*, to teichoic acid present in *Staphylococcus aureus*, and to gram-negative lipopolysaccharides. Cytophilic or adherent IgG on alveolar macrophage plasma membranes is of the IgG1 and IgG4 subclasses. Macrophage Fc gamma receptors are most numerous for IgG3 and to a lesser amount, IgG1. IgG2 and IgG4 receptors are masked or buried.

In the airways the complement system can be activated along the alternative pathway. This can lead to lysis of a susceptible organism or to generation of opsonic C3b. Once phagocytosis has occurred, intracellular killing proceeds, but often at a slower rate than that measured in polymorphonuclear leukocytes (PMNs) and by less well-

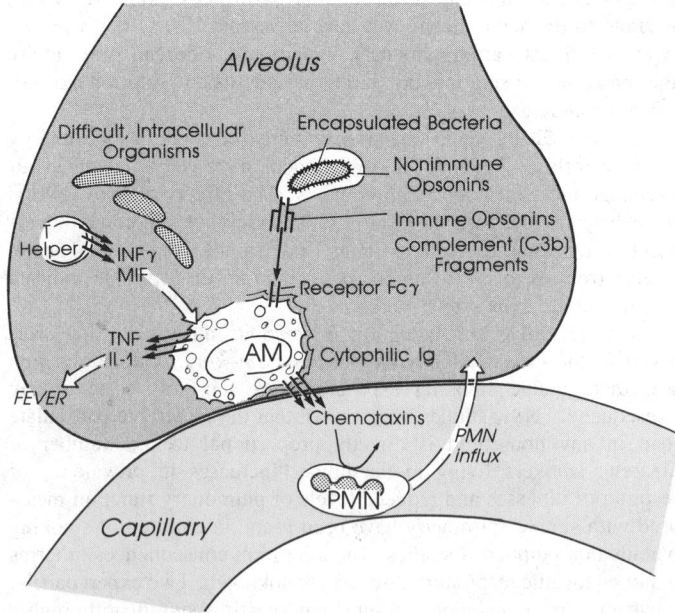

FIGURE 207-1 Alveolar host defense mechanisms (see text for details). Abbreviations: AM = alveolar macrophage; PMN = polymorphonuclear leukocytes; T-lym = T lymphocyte; INFγ = γ-interferon; MIF = migration inhibitory factor; TNF = tumor necrosis factor; IL-1 = interleukin 1.

defined mechanisms involving both oxygen-dependent and -independent pathways. In contrast to PMNs, macrophages usually lack myeloperoxidase; production of superoxide and H_2O_2 are enhanced by macrophage "activation" (see Chaps. 13 and 81).

MACROPHAGE-LYMPHOCYTE INTERACTIONS In addition to phagocytosis, subsequent containment and destruction of microbes hinge on the effectiveness of the macrophages to kill the organisms and the development of an inflammatory reaction. Alveolar macrophages are long-lived tissue cells that can survive months to years and presumably are capable of handling repeated microbial challenges. Because they are motile cells, they can migrate quickly to other alveoli through the pores of Kohn or move to more proximal areas of the respiratory tract. Macrophages are instrumental in degrading antigenic material and presenting it to appropriate alveolar lymphocytes that, in turn, may initiate specific immune responses (see Chap. 13). In addition, macrophages gain entry into lung lymphatics in respiratory bronchioles and are transported to regional lymph nodes that are sites of humoral and cellular immune responses for the lung. The many secretory products of macrophages are essential participants in the immune effector system and can contribute to chronic inflammation and to fibrogenesis or granuloma formation (see Chap. 81). Lymphocytes are important in regulation of lung macrophage functions related to cellular activation and inflammation. They are also directly involved in the formation and regulation of antibody responses and activation of dormant cytotoxic lymphocytes (see Chap. 13).

Lymphocytes retrieved from normal alveoli account for about 10 percent of airway cells. Seventy percent of these are T lymphocytes and proportions of the major subpopulations are similar to those in peripheral blood. Among the helper T cells is a small percentage of HLA-DR–positive lymphocytes (7 percent) that secrete the major amount of interleukin 2. Killer T cells may be dormant but can be activated by γ-interferon. Several important cytokines produced by T lymphocytes activate alveolar macrophages (Fig. 207-1) and include γ-interferon and macrophage-inhibitory factor. Acquired cell-mediated immunity (CMI) is necessary if the macrophage population is to contain or kill certain intracellular microbes. Examples include: *Mycobacterium tuberculosis* and other species, *L. pneumophila*, *Pneumocystis carinii*, *Listeria monocytogenes*, and cytomegalovirus. Because of suppression of CMI pneumonias caused by *P. carinii*, various fungi, *M. tuberculosis,* and cytomegalovirus are common in patients receiving high doses of glucocorticoids or with the acquired immunodeficiency syndrome (AIDS) (see Chap. 264).

INFLAMMATORY MECHANISMS PMNs are usually separated from alveolar spaces by three planes: tissue-capillary endothelium, interstitial space, and alveolar epithelium. PMN movement by chemotaxis into the alveoli is an orderly reaction initiated from the alveolar side. Several pathways can be involved. Macrophages help promote the acute inflammatory response, including chemotaxis. Production of chemotactic factors, particularly leukotriene B4, from macrophages can attract PMNs from pulmonary capillaries and venules and alter pulmonary capillary permeability. Other chemotactic and capillary permeability–altering factors include C3a and C5a and components of the kinin systems (see Chap. 81). The combined action of these agents promotes the accumulation of PMNs, fluid, and other humoral substances in alveoli. With the appearance of an inflammatory response, clinical illness usually occurs and a chest roentgenogram reveals an infiltrate. Production of interleukin 1 (IL-1) and tumor necrosis factor by alveolar macrophages can contribute to many of the systemic effects of pneumonia—such as chills and fever, malaise, and myalgias (see Chap. 20).

Ultimately the lung tissues may become consolidated. Release of proteolytic enzymes (e.g., PMN-derived elastase) can contribute to lung injury. Their neutralization by several inhibitor proteins, alpha$_1$ antiprotease, and possibly alpha$_2$ macroglobulin can minimize destruction of lung tissue. Pending successful containment of the infection, resolution and healing eventually occur. Little is known about the processes that halt the acute inflammatory reaction in pneumonia and initiate recovery.

CLINICAL MANIFESTATIONS The major symptoms of pneumonia are usually cough, fever, production of sputum, chest pain, and dyspnea. Pneumonia can develop acutely in a previously healthy person, or can be discovered almost incidentally from a chest radiograph of a chronically ill patient without major symptoms, but with another underlying disease. Coryza or mild upper respiratory symptoms and malaise often precede the onset of pneumonia. Typically, a pyogenic bacterial pneumonia, as caused by *S. pneumoniae,* follows a viral upper respiratory tract infection and has an abrupt onset with chills, a sustained fever, cough which will become productive of mucopurulent sputum, and chest aching or pleuritic pain. In contrast, a viral or mycoplasmal pneumonia also may have a prodromal upper respiratory tract phase, but malaise, headache, and cough linger for days; coughing and fever gradually increase, but pleuritic chest pain and respiratory distress are not usual. The symptoms produced by these major etiologic forms of pneumonia may overlap so that a suspected diagnosis cannot be made with confidence from the patient's initial presentation. Furthermore, the patient's overall condition and ability to cooperate and communicate can affect how the illness may present to the physician.

Young adults often have the classic acute symptoms that readily point to the lower respiratory tract. Occasionally, a lower lobe infection can irritate the diaphragmatic surface so that upper abdominal pain, referred pain to the shoulder, or eructation and hiccups are part of the symptom complex and can divert attention away from the lung to another diagnosis. Elderly or severely ill patients may have little cough, scant sputum production, little evidence of respiratory symptoms, and a deceptive absence of fever. In a hospitalized or immunocompromised patient, the major initial manifestations may be limited to fever, tachypnea, agitation, or altered mentation because of changes in oxygenation. Pneumonia may be apparent only after systematically excluding infection in other organ systems.

Important historical information includes knowledge of hemoptysis, chills, pleuritic chest pain, or use of antibiotics; risk factors or prior or underlying illnesses that increase susceptibility to a specific microbial infection (see Chap. 82); special epidemiologic or travel considerations, i.e., contact with ill family members, pets or other animals; recurrences of pneumonia.

PHYSICAL FINDINGS The breathing pattern and the position assumed in bed can indicate the patient's discomfort, reveal tachypnea, and demonstrate splinting of the chest to minimize pleuritic pain.

Percussion and auscultation of the chest may reveal signs of lung consolidation (dullness, inspiratory crackles, or bronchial breath sounds). However, the lung examination may be normal, particularly with interstitial pneumonias, even though radiographic changes can be seen. Appearance of the skin and mucous membranes can help assess fluid status, indicate jaundice or cyanosis, or reveal needle tracks in users of illicit drugs. The presence of clubbing may indicate underlying lung disease. The condition of the teeth and gingiva and adequacy of the gag reflex may provide a clue to aspiration. The cardiac examination may reveal murmurs consistent with associated endocarditis or pleuropericardial rubs. Upper abdominal tenderness may reflect diaphragmatic irritation resulting from inflamed pleural surfaces, rather than an intraabdominal process. Abdominal distention due to paralytic illness is common in bacterial pneumonia, particularly if it involves the lower lobes. An altered mental status may be due to high fever, hypoxemia, or a complicating meningitis.

DIAGNOSTIC STUDIES The *chest radiograph* is essential to confirm the presence of pneumonitis and its location, but its appearance will not accurately predict the etiology. A well-penetrated frontal film that allows good visualization of the retrocardiac area on the left and a lateral view film are desirable. Certain radiographic appearances are more typical of some organisms than others. Pneumonias tend to conform to one of three pathologic and radiographic patterns (Fig. 207-2): (1) alveolar or air space pneumonia, (2) interstitial pneumonia, or (3) bronchopneumonia. In air space pneumonia the organism causes an inflammatory exudate that involves many contiguous alveoli. Segmental boundaries are not preserved, and the bronchi, relatively

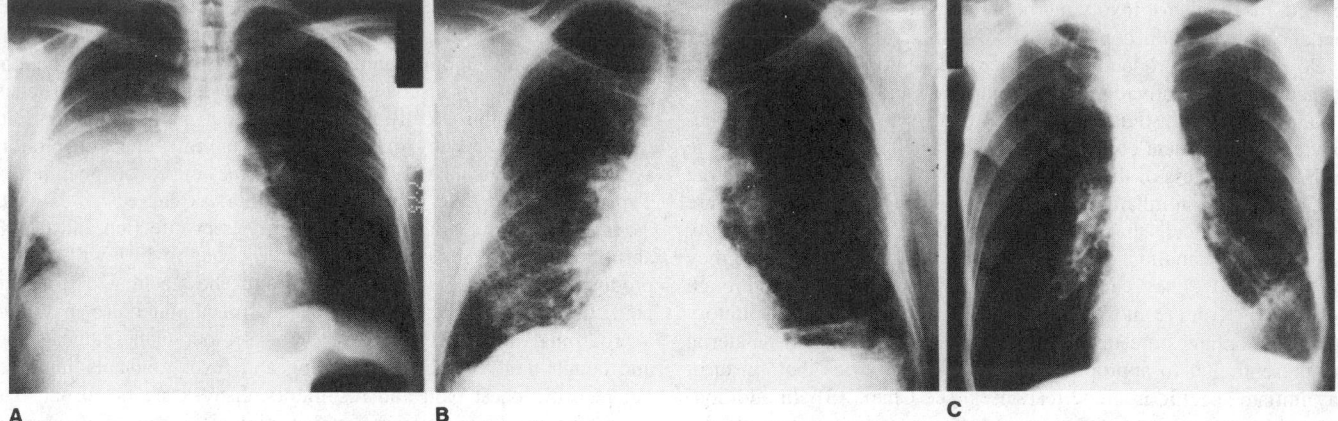

FIGURE 207-2   Roentgenographic appearances of pneumonia. *A.* Air space pneumonia. There is a dense, homogeneous, nonsegmental consolidation in the right lower lobe with a visible air bronchogram. *B.* Interstitial pneumonia. A linear or reticular pattern involves the lower lung fields bilaterally, more on the right. *C.* Bronchopneumonia. A segmental infiltrate without a visible air bronchogram appears in the left lower lung field.

uninvolved, remain patent. The radiologic result is nonsegmental consolidation with air bronchograms. A classic example is pneumococcal pneumonia. *Mycoplasma pneumoniae, P. carinii,* and viruses often cause an interstitial pneumonia, where inflammation is predominantly in the interalveolar septa, producing a reticular radiographic appearance. In bronchopneumonia, inflammation is restricted to the conducting airways, especially terminal and respiratory bronchioles, and the surrounding alveoli. Atelectasis may be present and air bronchograms are absent. *Staphylococcal pneumonia* is a typical example. The chest radiograph may also reveal diseases that can mimic pneumonia, such as pulmonary emboli with infarction (see Chap. 213), congestive heart failure (see Chap. 36), or neoplasms. Appropriate diagnostic studies should be carried out to exclude these possibilities, if indicated.

Bacterial pneumonias typically are associated with leukocytosis with a high percentage of PMNs and with a "left shift" (see Chap. 81), whereas changes in leukocyte counts may be minimal in viral and other pneumonias. The adequacy of the bone marrow reserves, use of glucocorticoid or cytotoxic therapy, and conditions such as alcoholism and renal or liver failure may have independent effects that make the white blood count a less predictable indicator of the nature of the inflammatory response. Arterial blood gases often reveal hypocarbia and respiratory alkalosis from hyperventilation and hypoxemia from perfusion of involved nonventilated alveoli. Respiratory and metabolic acidosis could be present from complicating severe bronchospasm, respiratory failure, or systemic sepsis.

Microscopic examination and *culture of respiratory secretions* are essential for the rational treatment of pneumonia; a vigorous attempt must be made to obtain adequate specimens. Several blood cultures should be obtained since they may reveal the etiologic agent and, if positive, can affect the prognosis and potential for metastatic infection.

A freshly obtained specimen of expectorated sputum should be prepared for a Gram's stain and culture (see Chap. 80). Examination of a wet-mounted specimen (purulent fleck of sputum emulsified with a few drops of saline on a microscopic slide, a coverslip placed over it, and viewed at $100\times$) can permit a decision about the adequacy of the sample from the cell types present. A sputum specimen representative of the lower respiratory tract will have PMNs and possibly alveolar macrophages visible and very few oral squamous epithelial cells (less than one or two per high-power field). Use of a mixture of anticapsular antibodies to cause capsular swelling or a quellung reaction for species of *S. pneumoniae* in a wet specimen can improve accuracy of sputum analysis.

If the patient is not producing sputum, an attempt to induce secretions by ultrasonic nebulization of water or saline particles is reasonable. Such particles (which may vary in size between 0.8 and 10 μm in diameter) serve as an irritant and stimulate most subjects to cough. As an example, *P. carinii* can be identified in the induced sputum of about 80 percent of patients with this pneumonia who have AIDS and in a smaller percentage of patients with non-HIV disease (see Chaps. 163 and 264). Attempts to obtain lung secretions by passing a small catheter through the nose or mouth rarely get beyond the vocal cords of an alert patient and may only obtain a sample of oropharyngeal fluids. This practice should be discouraged.

If it is impossible to induce an adequate respiratory sample, other, more invasive measures should be considered. The situation arises most often in the debilitated, chronically ill patient or the immunosuppressed host. Factors such as patient tolerance, hematologic parameters, probability of opportunistic infection, and expertise with a particular procedure all affect the choice of procedures; these might include transtracheal aspiration, fiberoptic bronchoscopy, percutaneous transthoracic needle aspiration, thoracentesis, or open-lung biopsy.

Percutaneous transtracheal aspiration is a direct approach that eliminates much of the contaminating oral microbial flora, but it carries a risk to the patient and is now rarely employed in most centers. A needle containing a polyethylene catheter is inserted through the cricothyroid membrane into the airway lumen, and material is aspirated after a small injection of saline solution which makes the patient cough. Although transtracheal specimens can become contaminated with mouth flora, both anaerobic and aerobic cultures should be done. Minor complications include air leak leading to subcutaneous or mediastinal emphysema, or blood-tinged sputum. Serious complications from subcutaneous emphysema and tracheal hemorrhage occur in less than 0.5 percent of procedures performed by experienced practitioners. This procedure should not be carried out by inexperienced operators or in uncooperative patients or those with thrombocytopenia or other coagulation disorders, since it may induce fatal hemorrhage or serious injury.

Fiberoptic bronchoscopy with BAL and a protected brush catheter provides another approach. The risk of bronchoscopy is small, even in patients with extensive pneumonia. Administration of supplemental oxygen during the procedure is necessary. Use of oximetry to monitor its effect is recommended. Platelet transfusions should be given to correct thrombocytopenia. A direct view of the affected lung anatomy, particularly if a loss of volume in the lung lobe accompanies the infection, may disclose an endobronchial obstruction. Removal of secretions or a mucus plug could make the procedure of therapeutic as well as diagnostic value. Usually, the lavage fluid or catheter brush culture will contain the offending pathogen; however, microbial cultures from the bronchoscopy specimens also contain contaminating flora from the nasopharynx, and interpretation can be confusing. Transbronchial biopsy can be added to the procedure to provide lung tissue for culture and histology. Multiple biopsies of pieces 2 to 3 mm in size are usually obtained from at least two segments of a lobe if a diffuse infiltrate is present.

Depending upon the pathogen, the combination of catheter brush and transbronchial biopsy cultures from immunocompromised hosts with lung infection will yield a specific etiologic diagnosis in 50 to 95 percent of cases.

Complications arising from bronchoscopy include hemorrhage and/or pneumothorax in about 5 percent of cases. Occasionally, a chest tube will be needed to treat the pneumothorax. About 25 percent of patients develop a postbronchoscopy fever about 4 to 8 h after the procedure. This usually lasts less than 24 h and is not a complicating pneumonia but a febrile reaction, due perhaps to cellular mediators produced in the lavaged lung segment (see Chap. 20). This episode can usually be managed with antipyretic therapy alone and without an additional antibiotic.

Percutaneous transthoracic needle aspiration is a diagnostic modality that is sometimes helpful in pneumonia, although needle aspiration guided by computed tomography (CT) is performed more frequently to diagnose discrete lung lesions. Spread of microorganisms along the needle track or soilage of pleural surfaces rarely occur, but pneumothorax is a complication.

With primary bacterial pneumonia a parapneumonic effusion may occur in 10 to 30 percent of cases; pleural effusions of small size can occur with *Mycoplasma* and *Legionella* infection as well, and pleural tuberculosis characteristically causes effusions (see Chap. 125). Decubitus chest radiographs or ultrasonography is used to confirm the presence of fluid in the pleural space. A diagnostic *thoracentesis* is indicated to determine whether the fluid contains organisms and/or has the characteristics of an empyema. Cellular analysis and certain chemical tests (pH, lactic dehydrogenase, glucose, and total protein) will identify pleural fluid to be a transudate or exudate (see Chap. 216). Empyema can develop with pneumonitis or lung abscess in adjacent lung tissue; the fluid is exudative and like pus. Microorganisms may be seen on stained smear and usually grow from cultures. If an empyema exists, repeated thoracentesis to drain the fluid or use of an indwelling chest tube to effect continuous drainage is usually necessary to hasten healing and to prevent or minimize future pleural adhesions.

If a parapneumonic effusion develops in the course of pneumonia, thoracentesis is indicated if: (1) fever has persisted for 72 h after beginning treatment with appropriate antibiotics; (2) a large effusion develops that is contributing to discomfort and impairing breathing or is increasing in size; and (3) there is evidence that once freely movable fluid has become loculated. In the absence of these findings, small effusions usually disappear, the patient continues to improve, and thoracentesis is usually not indicated.

Needle biopsy of the pleura should be included with a thoracentesis if malignancy or tuberculosis is suspected, or prior pleural fluid cellular analysis suggests an unsuspected primary pleural disease (see Chap. 216).

If bronchoscopy is unrevealing or contraindicated, diagnostic *open-lung biopsy* is often necessary in the immunocompromised patient with an advancing, pulmonary infiltrate (see Chap. 82). Problems with the procedure include delay until severe hypoxemia or other complications make the risk excessive; or handling of the tissue is poorly coordinated between the operator, the microbiologist, and the pathologist, and an optimal analysis is not performed. The radiologist or pathologist can often suggest the best area of lung to biopsy, and the microbiology laboratory can be prepared to ensure that the most appropriate cultures are processed quickly. A properly performed and handled open-lung biopsy will reveal a specific etiology for pulmonary infiltrates in over 90 percent of patients.

THERAPY The history, physical examination, chest radiograph, Gram stain of sputum, and other diagnostic measures will provide knowledge about predisposing factors of the illness, potential causes, and probable extent of pneumonia. These factors and the results of microbiologic studies will determine initial and subsequent therapy. The differential diagnosis will vary according to the status of certain host defenses and the epidemiologic setting. The more common microbiologically identifiable causes of a community-acquired pneu-

monia include *S. pneumoniae* (60 to 75 percent) (see Chap. 99), *Mycoplasma pneumoniae* (1 to 2 percent) (see Chap. 154), *Staph. aureus* (1 to 2 percent) (see Chap. 100), and *L. pneumophila* (2 to 15 percent) (see Chap. 124). No etiologic agent may be clearly defined in 20 to 40 percent of cases. *Haemophilus influenzae* (see Chap. 115) is an unusual cause of primary pneumonia and is more likely to be part of an infectious exacerbation of bronchitis in a person with chronic lung disease. With exposure to infected animals or birds rare causes of pneumonia, including *Coxiella burnetii* (Q fever) (see Chap. 153), *Chlamydia psittaci* (see Chap. 155), and *Francisella tularensis* (see Chap. 120), should be considered. Pneumonia can complicate a viral exanthem such as varicella (see Chap. 136) and, rarely, measles (see Chap. 141). Adenovirus (see Chap. 140) can be a cause of epidemic pneumonia in a young adult. In endemic areas, *Histoplasma capsulatum* and *Coccidioides immitis* (see Chap. 151) need to be considered as causes of acute illness. Respiratory infections, especially with *P. carinii*, are often the presentation of AIDS (see Chaps. 163 and 264).

A nosocomial pneumonia that develops during a patient's confinement to a specialized nursing home unit or hospital is likely to be caused by aerobic gram-negative enteric bacilli (see Chap. 111) or *Staph. aureus*. Similarly, hospitalized patients who have impaired host defenses or who are immunocompromised because of an underlying disease or therapy are at increased risk for pneumonias caused by organisms spread hematogenously from other body sites. Neutropenia and prolonged antibiotic use predispose to infection with fungi such as *Aspergillus fumigatus* (see Chap. 151).

Treatment entails appropriate support with fluids, antipyretic drugs, oxygen, airway suction or gravity (postural) drainage, and bronchodilator drugs if bronchospasm is present (see Chap. 204). Antibiotic therapy remains the cornerstone of medical management.

The initial antimicrobial therapy should be chosen on the basis of interpretation of clinical findings and in severely ill patients must be heavily weighed toward protecting the patient against the most dangerous of the conceivable infectious agents. Results of cultures and antibiotic susceptibilities for common bacterial pathogens take several days. Organisms that are not grown easily may require a diagnosis based on rising antibody titers in acute and convalescent serum (e.g., Q fever) or recognition by specific immunofluorescence (*Legionella* sp. in sputum). As a consequence, an element of uncertainty is often present, and initial antibiotic therapy is somewhat empiric. Three principles of antimicrobial therapy deserve emphasis: (1) all necessary specimens for appropriate bacteriologic cultures should be obtained before therapy is initiated so that there is a reasonable chance to recover the organism; (2) initial drug therapy should be as specific as the evidence pointing to the etiologic agent allows, yet sufficiently broad to cover the common microorganisms; and (3) a few days of broad-spectrum antimicrobial treatment usually will not cause superinfection or selection of drug-resistant bacteria; however, final antimicrobial treatment should be adjusted to use specific narrow-spectrum drugs, if possible, when the results of cultures and susceptibilities are available.

Certain categories of pneumonia suggest a choice of antibiotics for initial therapy. For a community-acquired pneumonia (CAP) in a previously healthy young or middle-aged adult, erythromycin (500 mg intravenously every 6 h) would be effective for most strains of *S. pneumoniae*, *L. pneumophila*, and *M. pneumoniae*, but not suitable for *Haemophilus* sp. and *Staph. aureus*. Cefotaxime (1 to 2 g intravenously every 8 h), or ceftizoxime (2 g intravenously every 12 h), or cefuroxime (750 mg intravenously every 8 h) would provide therapy for *S. pneumoniae*, *Haemophilus* sp., and *Staph. aureus*, but not for *Legionella*. In older adults with CAP, the probability increases that gram-negative bacteria are the cause, i.e., *K. pneumoniae*, *H. influenzae*, and *Enterobacter aerogenes*, favoring the use of the cephalosporins cited above. Reduced dosages will be required with renal failure (see Chap. 85).

Initial treatment for nosocomial pneumonia should consider aerobic gram-negative bacilli such as *K. pneumoniae*, *Pseudomonas aeru-*

ginosa, Serratia marcescens, or *Staph. aureus* as potential causes. In a nonimmunosuppressed adult with nosocomial pneumonia, initial therapy with a third-generation cephalosporin such as cefotaxime, ceftizoxime, ceftazidime (1 to 2 g intravenously every 8 to 12 h), or cefoperazone (1 to 2 g intravenously every 12 h) is acceptable. If the patient is neutropenic, it is preferable to use two antibiotics, an aminoglycoside such as gentamicin (1 to 1.5 mg/kg intravenously every 8 h), tobramycin (1 to 1.5 mg/kg intravenously every 8 h), or amikacin (5 mg/kg intravenously every 8 h) with ceftazidime or a semisynthetic broad-spectrum penicillin such as ticarcillin (40 mg/kg intravenously every 4 h) or piperacillin (40 mg/kg intravenously every 6 h); synergistic action will be provided against the most deadly bacterium in this patient setting, *Pseudomonas aeruginosa.* Reduced dosages are necessary in renal failure (see Chap. 85). If the neutropenic patient has already received extensive antimicrobial therapy, then infection with fungi is more likely and amphotericin B should be utilized (see Chaps. 82 and 151).

Aspiration pneumonia as part of a CAP is polymicrobial and will contain a variety of anaerobic flora such as *Bacteroides melaninogenicus, Fusobacterium nucleatum,* and anaerobic streptococci; several antibiotic regimens have been successfully employed (see Chap. 108). These include penicillin G, (1.0 million units intravenously every 4 to 6 h), or clindamycin (600 mg intravenously every 8 h). Amoxicillin or ampicillin (as 500 to 750 mg orally every 6 h) combined with metronidazole (as 500 mg orally every 6 h) is an effective oral regimen, especially if a lung abcess had developed that will require prolonged treatment. If aspiration occurs within the hospital, then treatment should be directed toward enteric gram-negative bacilli and *Staph. aureus* with a third-generation cephalosporin as outlined above.

Once the patient's therapy is underway, attention must be focused on possible complications. A resurgence of fever after an initial period of defervescence is a frequent clue to a complication. Poor coughing and an accumulation of secretions or a mucus plug can obstruct an airway, leading to partial collapse of a lobe or segment of lung. Chest percussion, gravity drainage, and/or endotracheal suction to remove secretions and help reexpand the atelectatic segment should be tried for 24 h before resorting to bronchoscopy. The development of loculated pleural fluid usually requires thoracentesis and possible chest tube drainage. Secondary bacterial infection following a viral pneumonia or superinfection occurring after broad-spectrum antimicrobial therapy may cause fever and worsening of the patient's condition; repeat culturing of the sputum and blood is necessary to confirm the diagnosis. Drug allergy may cause lingering fever, sometimes accompanied by mild eosinophilia and rash; improvement after discontinuation or substitution in the antibiotic regimen will aid in establishing this diagnosis. Finally, evidence of resolution of the pneumonic process must be observed radiographically. In uncomplicated cases repeat radiographs are indicated at 3 to 5 day intervals for the first week, with a follow-up chest x-ray 1 month after discharge or completion of treatment. In severely ill patients or those who do not respond promptly to treatment, radiography should be performed more frequently. Failure of the pneumonia to resolve may require sputum cytologies and bronchoscopy to rule out a partially obstructing airway lesion or an endobronchial tumor, or to establish more precisely the microbial etiology.

LUNG ABSCESS

DEFINITION AND PATHOGENESIS Lung abscesses form as a complication of a localized area of pneumonia or when a neoplasm becomes necrotic and contains purulent material that cannot drain easily from the area because of partial or complete bronchial obstruction. When the local pulmonary artery blood supply is occluded by emboli or by vasculitis (e.g., Wegener's granulomatosis) or is inadequate to support a rapidly growing neoplasm (primary bronchogenic carcinoma, usually squamous cell carcinoma), necrosis and

---

TABLE 207-1 Lung abscesses classified according to cause

I Necrotizing infections
  A Pyogenic bacteria (*Staphylococcus aureus, Klebsiella pneumoniae, Pseudomonas aeruginosa,* group A streptococcus, *Legionella* sp., *Bacteroides, Fusobacterium,* anaerobic and microaerophilic cocci and streptococci, other anaerobes including *Actinomyces* sp., *Nocardia* sp.)
  B Mycobacteria (*Mycobacterium tuberculosis, M. kansasii, M. avium-intracellulare*)
  C Fungi (*Histoplasma capsulatum, Coccidioides immitis, Aspergillus* sp.
  D Parasites (amebas, lung flukes)
II Cavitary infarction
  A Bland embolism
  B Septic embolism (*Staph. aureus,* various anaerobes, *Candida* sp.)
  C Vasculitis (Wegener's granulomatosis)
III Cavitary malignancy
  A Primary bronchogenic carcinoma
  B Metastatic malignancies (very uncommon)
IV Other
  A Infected cysts
  B Necrotic conglomerate lesions (silicosis, coal miner's pneumoconiosis)

---

cavity formation may occur. Existing bullae and cysts can become infected or develop secondary air-fluid levels when surrounding infection exists and resemble an abscess. When large areas of inflamed, fibrotic lung tissue coalesce, as found in advanced silicosis, vascular insufficiency may lead to cavity formation (see Table 207-1). Although the terms abscess and cavity tend to be used interchangeably, abscess is preferable because it implies the presence of necrosis, inflammation, or associated infection. A cavity is often a radiographic description that may be used to suggest a more static or quiescent process.

In the context of pneumonia, tissue necrosis may be due to properties of the infecting organisms. Infection with *Staph. aureus,* especially when bacteremic with septic lung emboli, can produce multiple abscesses that may evolve into pneumatoceles (see Chap. 100). Gram-negative bacilli, such as *Pseudomonas aeruginosa,* secrete exotoxins that can create vasculitis in addition to pneumonitis (see Chap. 111). Cavitation may develop as a complication of *Legionella* pneumonia (Chap. 124). In contrast, pneumococci, *H. influenzae, M. pneumoniae,* and viral infections almost never cause abscess formation. An abscess resulting from aspiration of nasopharyngeal secretions or gastroesophageal reflux is polymicrobial, with a prevalence of aerobic and facultatively anaerobic organisms (see Chap. 108). These mixed infections can be fulminant or indolent; airway obstruction by particulate material may facilitate abscess formation.

CLINICAL PRESENTATION A pulmonary abscess may evolve as part of a severe and rapidly progressing pneumonia. Its appearance is recognized radiographically and is accompanied by delayed resolution or worsening of the patient's anticipated clinical course, with persisting fever, copious expectoration of sputum, possibly hemoptysis, pleurisy, and even a pneumothorax. Sometimes, with an established pneumonia, it can be difficult to distinguish between a parenchymal abscess and/or a contiguous pleural effusion and empyema. Septic pulmonary emboli can cause multiple areas of infiltration on the radiograph and appear as patches of bronchopneumonia; later cavitation may occur. Staphylococcal endocarditis of the tricuspid or pulmonary valves, which is most often a complication of the use of illicit intravenous drugs, is the usual cause. Fever, chest pain, and occasionally hemoptysis are prominent manifestations. A cavity within the pneumonic area may be more evident with CT views of the lung.

A chronic lung abscess is often less dramatic in presentation: Cough, productive of foul-smelling and -tasting sputum; dyspnea; intermittent fever; weight loss; anorexia; and chest pain are the predominant features. Aspiration of oral or gastric secretions is the usual cause. Poor dentition with periodontal disease and conditions that promote aspiration are the common predisposing factors. Typical locations in the lung for aspiration-caused abscesses are the posterior segment of the upper lobe and superior segment of the right lower lobe. Endobronchial obstruction from a tumor must be considered as well, particularly if the right middle lobe is involved. The characteristic presentations of pulmonary tuberculosis, or necrotizing pulmonary infection caused by fungi, nocardia, or actinomyces species are discussed in Chaps. 151 and 152, respectively.

Physical examination may vary to include signs of consolidation with bronchial breath sounds, rales, and dullness or cavernous or amphoric breath sounds. Clubbing can occur and may develop in a few weeks. The chest radiograph often reveals a radiolucency in an opaque area of consolidation. An air-fluid level establishes that partial airway patency exists. Because the differentiation between a parenchymal abscess, an empyema, a bronchopleural fistula creating an empyema, an infected cyst, or a fluid level in an emphysematous bulla can be difficult, special radiographic views or CT scanning may be needed for clarification. Further laboratory evaluation including sputum analysis, cultures, and blood tests is similar to that described for pneumonia. Sputum cytologies should be obtained. The role of bronchoscopy in the initial evaluation of an abscess is controversial. Cultures obtained by bronchoalveolar lavage and protected catheters have limitations, but it may be useful to view the endobronchial anatomy to rule out obstruction. Bronchoscopy in the presence of a large fluid-filled cavity must be done cautiously because a sudden discharge of fluid into the airways is a hazard. Bronchoscopy is also indicated in an abscess that does not close in 4 to 6 weeks following appropriate treatment.

TREATMENT Antibiotic choice is predicated on identification of the organisms or the most likely ones present. The antibiotic choices suggested for aspiration pneumonia are appropriate for aspiration-caused abscess and are discussed in detail in Chap. 108. Other measures are similar to those described for treatment of pneumonia, with the additional goals of promoting good drainage of secretions and providing adequate nutrition. Pleural space drainage may be required for loculated fluid and empyema if these complicate the lung abscess. Surgical resection is rarely needed for a persistent abscess cavity; however, massive hemoptysis, localized malignancy, and possibly bronchiectasis may require this approach.

REFERENCES

Pneumonia

MANGI RJ et al: Cefoperazone *versus* combination antibiotic therapy of nosocomial pneumonia. Am J Med 84:68, 1988
PENNINGTON JE (ed): Hospital-acquired pneumonias. Semin Resp Infect 2:1, 1987
REYNOLDS HY: Bacterial adherence to respiratory tract mucosa—a dynamic interaction leading to colonization. Semin Resp Med 2.8, 1987
————: Lung inflammation: Normal host defense or a complication of some diseases. Ann Rev Med 38:295, 1987
————: Immunoglobulin G and its function in the human respiratory tract. Mayo Clin Proc 63:161, 1988
————: Pulmonary host defense. Chest 95S:223, 1989
VERGHESE A, BERK SL: Bacterial pneumonia in the elderly. Medicine 62:271, 1983

Lung abscess

JOHANSON WG et al: Aspiration pneumonia, anaerobic infections, and lung abscess. Med Clin North Am 64:385, 1980
MAHLER DA, D'ESOPO ND: Peri-emphysematous lung infection. Clin Chest Med 2:51, 1981
SCHACTER EN: Suppurative lung disease: Old problems revisited. Clin Chest Med 2:41, 1981

208 BRONCHIECTASIS AND BRONCHOLITHIASIS

HERBERT Y. REYNOLDS / RICHARD K. ROOT

BRONCHIECTASIS

DEFINITION Bronchiectasis is the permanent abnormal dilatation of one or more bronchi. Ectasia, or expansion and dilatation, can develop in any segment of the cartilage-containing tracheobronchial conducting airways when persisting inflammation in the lumen and adjacent wall causes destruction of the ciliated epithelium and submucosa and degeneration of elastic and muscular tissue. The diagnosis of bronchiectasis is suspected in patients with chronic cough with excessive expectoration of phlegm or purulent mucus or in those who have diffuse or localized recurrent bronchopulmonary infections, especially if associated with recurrent sinusitis and otitis media. The clinical picture may be difficult to distinguish from chronic bronchitis, however, and the two conditions may coexist. The diagnosis of bronchiectasis can be confirmed by bronchography, but tracheobronchitis, pneumonia, or atelectasis can produce bronchographic findings consistent with bronchiectasis which, unlike the findings in bronchiectasis, reverse with successful treatment. Traditionally, bronchiectasis has been classified on the basis of structural abnormalities seen on bronchography and is divided into localized and diffuse forms.

ETIOLOGY AND PATHOGENESIS Inflammation usually initiates the destructive process that results in bronchiectasis. Such injury can be caused by a primary microbial infection or by localized obstruction from either an intrinsic lesion in an airway, bronchial stenosis, or external compression. Stagnation of secretions in the presence of obstruction leads to secondary infection with inflammation and accumulation of leukocytes. The cumulative effects of proteolytic enzymes (collagenase and elastase) and toxic oxygen radical species released by neutrophils (see Chap. 81), as well as other products of inflammation, contribute to tissue necrosis. The effects of increased pressure due to retained inspissated secretions in the lumen may contribute to mucosal injury. Pathology often reveals exudative debris in and occluding the dilated bronchi.

The general size or segmental level of bronchi involved has provided descriptive terms for the pathologic findings of bronchiectasis. *Saccular* or *cystic* bronchiectasis affects major or proximal bronchi that end in large sacs by the fourth generation of branching. *Cylindrical* or *fusiform* dilatation is found in the sixth to eighth generation, produces an uneven involvement, and is probably a less severe form of disease. Clinically, the cylindrical type is a "dry" bronchiectasis with a less productive cough and fewer secretions. Varicose bronchiectasis is intermediate between saccular and cylindrical in form. If fibrosis has developed in the peribronchial area or extensively in the parenchyma thereby forming cysts, a telescoping or wrinkling effect in the subtending bronchi and bronchioles can be produced that is described as *traction* bronchiectasis. It is more often found with end-stage fibrocystic interstitial fibrosis; infection and excessive formation of secretions are unusual. The anatomic lesions of bronchiectasis may be visualized with bronchography or inferred from the appearance of bronchial structure in the chest radiograph or ultrathin (0.5-cm) sections of computed tomographic (CT) scans. Overlapping of all lesions can be found in any patient; thus, the anatomic pattern is not useful for etiologic diagnosis or correlation with clinical severity and has little therapeutic or prognostic significance.

With well-developed bronchiectasis, the bronchial artery circulation becomes more pronounced; vessels may be hypertrophied and more vulnerable to rupture. Whether the lack of supporting tissue for the vessels or increased exposure to irritation and pressure changes induced by coughing makes hemoptysis more likely is uncertain; certainly this problem is important clinically.

Localized bronchiectasis This entity is caused by a variety of bronchopulmonary infections or by the obstruction of bronchi. Measles and whooping cough were important causes before the development of effective immunization; currently, infection with adenovirus or respiratory syncytial virus leads to bronchiectasis in a small percentage of children with these conditions. Pulmonary tuberculosis was once a frequent cause but is now rare in the United States. More effective treatment of severe, necrotizing bacterial pneumonias with antibiotics has helped to minimize residual airway injury, reducing the frequency of resultant bronchiectasis. Childhood respiratory infection as the inciting cause of bronchiectasis remains prominent in developing countries or among the disadvantaged in places where immunization and health care are scarce. Localized bronchiectasis may result from obstruction by aspirated foreign bodies; these can usually be retrieved promptly with fiberoptic bronchoscopy, and irreversible injury is less likely now than before the availability of this modality. Local endobronchial obstruction from a primary tumor or metastases or external bronchial compression from enlarged hilar lymph nodes remains an important cause of postobstructive pneumonitis and/or atelectasis that can lead to bronchiectasis. Recurrent aspiration of orogastric secretions can be an important cause of localized bronchiectasis in patients with neurologic impairment. Rarely, a congenital abnormality in bronchial formation can create a cul-de-sac or bronchial malacia, thus causing localized bronchiectasis.

Diffuse bronchiectasis Bronchiectasis involving multiple lobes is usually the consequence of inherited or acquired defects in the defense mechanisms which normally protect the airways from infection or inflammation (see Chap. 207). The acquired conditions may include those which lead to repeated aspiration of orogastric contents (altered states of consciousness, neuromuscular impairment of swallowing or cough, gastroesophageal sphincter incompetence, and nasogastric intubation) or which cause chronic bronchitis (see Chap. 210) or, rarely, asthma (Chap. 204). The congenital conditions may involve alterations in the function of the mucociliary blanket or other aspects of pulmonary host defense. The congenital disorders are often associated with repeated respiratory tract infections including sinusitis, otitis media, and pneumonias or, in the case of immunoglobulin deficiencies, with systemic bacterial infections (see Chap. 263). Specific congenital disorders causing diffuse bronchiectasis include cystic fibrosis, the dyskinetic ciliary syndromes, Young's syndrome (sinopulmonary infections and obstructive azospermia), the hypogammaglobulinemias, or deficiencies of specific IgG subclasses. Less likely causes are congenital forms of tracheobronchomegaly; a cartilage disorder which leads to short stature, thoracic deformities, and bronchomalacia (Williams-Campbell syndrome); and α_1-antitrypsin deficiency.

DISORDERS OF MUCOCILIARY FUNCTION Intrinsic defects in the ultrastructure of cilia throughout the body can impair ciliary motion in several organ systems, particularly ciliated epithelium in the nasal and conducting airways and in the fallopian tubes; sperm are also immotile. Three basic defects have been identified in the doublet tubular structure of cilia—absent inner or outer dynein arms (causing Kartagener's syndrome), absent radial spokes, and absence of the central doublet of the axoneme of the cilium. As ciliary function is not entirely absent but lacks coordination, these are now described as *dyskinetic* (rather than *immotile*) ciliary syndromes. These congenital illnesses feature recurrent sinopulmonary infections, dextrocardia or situs inversus (in about half the cases of Kartagener's syndrome), and infertility. Recurrent bronchitis and pneumonias leading to diffuse bronchiectasis are a consequence of impaired removal of airway secretions normally aspirated during sleep.

The pathogenesis of cystic fibrosis and the mechanisms by which bronchiectasis might occur as a complication are discussed in Chap. 209.

IMMUNODEFICIENCY DISORDERS An absence of immunoglobulins, systemically and in the airway secretions, predisposes to sinopulmonary infections that ultimately lead to bronchiectasis. The absence of IgA and/or IgG neutralizing antibodies against viruses in tracheobronchial secretions or IgG opsonizing antibodies against encapsulated bacteria creates the conditions for recurrent infections. Secretory IgA is the principal immunoglobulin present in upper airway secretions and in those from the trachea and major bronchi (see Chaps. 13 and 207). Isolated absence of IgA may not have any infectious consequences unless associated with deficiencies of IgG2 and IgG4 (see Chap. 263). Common variable hypogammaglobulinemia, which involves all immunoglobulin classes, can develop acutely at any age (see Chap. 263). Selective deficiencies of IgG2 and/or IgG4 occur also and are associated with recurrent sinopulmonary infections which may result in diffuse bronchiectasis. While pneumonias are common in neutropenic subjects and those with neutrophil dysfunction (see Chap. 81), bronchiectasis does not appear to be as frequent or prominent as in the immunoglobulin disorders.

CLINICAL MANIFESTATIONS A raspy, frequent cough that produces purulent sputum in amounts that can total several hundred milliliters daily is a cardinal manifestation of bronchiectasis. Chronic low-grade respiratory infection can be interspersed with bouts of more severe bronchitis and bronchopneumonia accompanied by fever and chest pain. The sputum may vary in daily volume, appearance, and thickness; in some patients these characteristics may not correlate well with exacerbations or resolution of acute infection. Flecks of blood may be periodically admixed with the sputum, and frank hemoptysis can occur. Although hemoptysis is worrisome, it usually subsides quickly, and it does not necessarily portend a major hemorrhage.

Constitutional or systemic symptoms and signs are variable and include intermittent fever, lassitude, fatigue, and poor appetite. These are more pronounced with acute exacerbations of pulmonary infection. Dyspnea is variable and depends upon the extent of lung involvement as well as the presence or absence of acute infection. Wheezing due to associated asthma or bronchospasm may be a feature. Colonization of the bronchiectatic airways with *Aspergillus* species or, rarely, other fungi can precipitate acute asthmatic episodes due to an allergic IgE-mediated mechanism (see Chap. 51). This is accompanied by coughing up of gelatinous, rubbery mucous plugs containing many eosinophils; fungal hyphae may be seen.

Bronchiectasis that is associated with conditions leading to recurrent sinusitis and otitis media may have prominent symptomatic involvement of these organs. Postnasal secretions are increased, throat clearing is common, tinnitus, diminished hearing, frontal headache, and maxillary and dental pain may occur. All patients with bronchiectasis are prone to exacerbations of acute bacterial pneumonia (see Chap. 207). In fact, if pneumonia occurs repeatedly in an isolated or dependent lung segment, bronchiectasis should be suspected.

Physical findings will vary depending upon whether an underlying systemic disease is present and upon the extent of the pulmonary involvement. Many patients with limited localized bronchiectasis appear healthy and have minimal or no physical abnormalities. With more extensive disease chest auscultation will reveal coarse crackles over the affected areas, and wheezing may be present. With complicating pneumonia or atelectasis, diminished breath sounds and dullness to percussion may be found. With advanced disease, clubbing of fingers and toes is common and nailbed cyanosis may be evident. With end-stage disease, signs of secondary pulmonary hypertension and cor pulmonale usually develop (see Chap. 191).

LABORATORY STUDIES AND DIAGNOSTIC EVALUATION Results of laboratory and chest imaging studies vary with the underlying systemic disease and type of bronchiectasis. The total white blood cell count may be mildly elevated with a neutrophilic leukocytosis; this will be more pronounced and a left shift of neutrophils may be present with complicating pneumonia or sepsis. The erythrocyte sedimentation rate is often elevated. Anemia is rare. Arterial blood gas values may show a respiratory alkalosis or hypoxemia; they may be altered further by complicating pneumonia or bronchospasm (see Chap. 207). Initially, with diffuse bronchiectasis, pulmonary function tests may show obstruction, but with advanced disease and after many infections, a restrictive pattern evolves. Sputum cultures often disclose only mixed oral flora, and the intermittent presence of pathogens such as *Haemophilus influenzae*, *Streptococcus pneumoniae*, *Staphylococcus aureus*, or gram-negative enteric bacilli. A foul odor to the sputum suggests a predominance of anaerobes. Mucoid strains of *Pseudomonas auruginosa* are commonly and persistently isolated in patients with the later stages of cystic fibrosis (CF) (see Chap. 209).

In advanced cases, conventional radiographs may reveal 1- to 2-cm cystic-appearing lesions with or without fluid levels consistent with saccular bronchiectasis. Often the chest film shows linear streaks (tram tracks), on-end thickened bronchi, or signet-ring deformity, and groups of small curvilinear shadows, called grape clusters; these findings can be subtle. Lung CT scanning using ultrathin sections is a sensitive way to detect bronchiectasis, especially the saccular form, and to define its distribution. Bronchography is now rarely needed to document bronchiectasis, and when used should not be performed until several months have elapsed after an acute pneumonia to avoid misdiagnosis of reversible bronchiectasis.

Fiberoptic bronchoscopy is usually required to evaluate recurrent, segmental disease and atelectasis or collapsed areas to eliminate endobronchial obstruction. It is not the recommended way, however, to visualize bronchiectatic areas, particularly if these are distal to the third or fourth generation of bronchi and out of reach.

With diffuse bronchiectasis attention should be paid to defining the associated disorders. Impaired swallowing, cough, or gastroesophageal reflux should be evident from the history and physical examination. A family history of affected siblings, infant deaths, kindred with similar symptoms, or problems with infertility can reveal mucociliary or immune-deficiency disorders. Preliminary screening tests should include: analysis of electrolytes contained in a sample of sweat (see Chap. 209); quantitative serum immunoglobulins, including subclasses of IgG, and assessment of sperm motility.

Patients with asthma and suspected allergic bronchopulmonary aspergillosis should have the sputum cultured for *Aspergillus*, measurements of serum IgE values (usually in excess of 2500 ng/mL), and serologic studies for *Aspergillus* precipitins (positive in >90 percent). In referral centers additional studies might include measurement of secretory IgA in parotid fluid or nasal washings; assessment of ciliary clearance with an aerosolized, isotopic tracer; and biopsy of nasal mucosal for electron-microscopic cross-sectional views of cilia to define ultrastructure.

TREATMENT   Treatment is directed at controlling complicating infections and providing effective drainage of secretions.

With bacterial infection often responsible for initiating bronchiectasis as well as causing acute exacerbations with complicating pneumonitis, antibiotic treatment remains a mainstay in prevention and management. During exacerbations, microbial cultures will yield a mixture of bacteria, and it may be difficult to identify a discrete pathogen, with the exception of *P. aeruginosa* in patients with advanced CF. When no specific pathogen is identified and the patient is not so ill as to require hospitalization, use of an oral agent such as amoxicillin, ampicillin, tetracycline, trimethoprim-sulfamethoxazole, or the fixed combination of amoxicillin and clavulanic acid (Augmentin) are all reasonable initial choices (for dosages see Chap. 85). Parenteral antibiotics are usually reserved for more seriously ill patients with pneumonitis. Again the initial choice should be guided by results of Gram stain evaluation of the sputum and altered by culture results which reveal specific pathogens. When *S. aureus* is present or suspected, a penicillinase-resistant penicillin (nafcillin or oxacillin) or a cephalosporin (e.g., cefazolin) should be utilized. Infections with *P. aeruginosa*, as are common in patients with advanced CF, should be treated with a combination of an antipseudomonal penicillin or ceftazidime and an aminoglycoside such as tobramycin administered parenterally until a response occurs (see Chaps. 85 and 111). Favorable responses are usually defined by a decrease in and thinning of sputum and the resolution of systemic

symptoms. These effects generally occur over 5 to 7 days. Clearing of radiologic evidence of pneumonitis may take weeks. In some patients treatment may need to be prolonged for several weeks. Since the sputum culture is not likely to be sterilized by treatment, repeat culturing is indicated only in the event of suspected superinfection with resistant organisms. Antibiotic treatment is usually reserved for acute exacerbations since prolonged and prophylactic use of antibiotics has not been shown to prevent exacerbations and may lead to the development of resistant organisms. Nebulized antibiotics have not been shown to be effective in treating acute exacerbations or as prophylaxis.

Respiratory therapy, in the form of chest percussion and gravity drainage, can promote removal of thick secretions. If bronchospasm is a complicating factor, therapy with inhaled bronchodilators is indicated (see Chaps. 204 and 210). Oral theophylline has been employed as an adjunct to enhance respiratory muscle performance and perhaps ciliary activity; however, its benefits in this regard are unproven. Expectorants and mucolytic agents are usually not helpful. Bronchoscopy may be required to remove inspissated secretions. If allergic bronchopulmonary aspergillosis is suspected, a trial of moderate doses of oral glucocorticoids (20 mg prednisone daily) may be employed to help reduce airway inflammation. Larger doses of oral or parenteral glucocorticoids may be required if asthma unresponsive to bronchodilators supervenes (Chap. 204). Immunoglobulin deficiency should be treated with human immune serum globulin (see Chap. 263).

Smoking of cigarettes should be interdicted. There should be yearly vaccination against influenza as well as vaccination against pneumococcal infection. Episodes of sinusitis should be promptly treated and may require joint management with an otolaryngologist for sinus drainage procedures and relief of nasal obstruction. Nasal oxygen may be required on a chronic basis to maintain adequate oxygenation. A program of graded exercise, routine deep breathing, and maintenance of good nutrition should be part of general management.

If a localized area of bronchiectasis is found to be the site of recurring infections, hemorrhage, or other symptoms, surgical removal of the segment or lobe or an approach to correct a partial obstruction may be indicated. CT scanning and perhaps bronchography should be performed to exclude a more generalized process. Pulmonary function studies should be performed before surgery to determine the capacity of the patient to tolerate lung resection and to estimate pulmonary reserve after operation. With aggressive deployment of antibiotics and other respiratory therapy procedures, resection surgery is rarely necessary. Severe bronchial hemorrhage may be controlled by bronchial artery embolization rather than surgery. Conversely with very extensive pulmonary involvement and lung destruction, transplantation surgery may offer the only hope for survival.

PREVENTION   Prevention of bronchiectasis is promoted by prompt diagnosis and antimicrobial treatment of bronchopulmonary bacterial infections and by vaccination against measles and pertussis. Chronic bronchitis and asthma should be managed as outlined in Chaps. 204 and 210. Localized bronchiectasis due to obstruction can be prevented by prompt removal of foreign bodies, preferably by fiberoptic bronchoscopy; other causes of local obstruction should be surgically treated if feasible. For chronic aspiration of orogastric secretions, correction of the underlying cause should be carried out if possible. In some cases of swallowing disorders a feeding gastrostomy or even laryngeal closure with tracheostomy may be necessary. Immunoglobulin therapy should be administered to IgG-deficient patients as outlined in Chap. 263. Patients and their families with dyskinetic ciliary syndromes or CF should receive appropriate genetic counseling.

BRONCHOLITHIASIS

A broncholith represents a calcified fragment of tissue that is loose within the bronchial lumen. Broncholiths usually form from disorders that lead to calcification of pulmonary tissue or of lymph nodes which then impinge upon and erode into a bronchus. Most commonly, pulmonary calcification follows an infection that elicits a granulomatous response such as tuberculosis, histoplasmosis, or coccidioidomycosis. Tuberculosis is the leading cause of calcified pulmonary granulomas worldwide; however, in the United States histoplasmosis is probably more common. With bronchiectasis necrosis and calcification of bronchial cartilage may occur leading to fragmentation and the formation of broncholiths. Rarely, aspirated food or other tissues may be retained in the airway for a long time and become calcified.

Movements of the calcified particles into or within the airway cause the clinical manifestations of broncholithiasis: paroxysms of cough, symptomatic postobstructive bronchopulmonary infection, and episodic hemoptysis. The cough can be productive of a mixture of gritty, sandy particles or small stones admixed with purulent phlegm and blood.

Broncholithiasis should be considered in patients who have these symptoms, particularly if the chest x-ray discloses multiple calcifications in the lung and in hilar or mediastinal lymph nodes. Examination of the sputum may reveal calcified particles. CT scanning of the chest can be helpful in more precisely localizing areas of calcification. Some episodes of broncholithiasis are self-limited and require no further diagnostic evaluation or treatment. With persistence of symptoms, particularly if there is postobstructive infection, atelectasis, or significant hemoptysis, bronchoscopy is indicated to visualize the area of obstruction and, if possible, to extract the stone. Antibiotics as outlined for the treatment of bronchiectasis should be administered to treat associated infection. Rarely, thoracotomy and resection of involved pulmonary segments is required to manage persistent bronchial obstruction or massive hemoptysis.

REFERENCES

Bronchiectasis

BARKER AF, BARDANA EJ: Bronchiectasis: Update of an orphan disease. Am Rev Respir Dis 137:969, 1988

REYNOLDS HY: Host defense impairments that lead to respiratory infections. Clin Chest Med 8:339, 1987

SCHUYLER MR: Allergic bronchopulmonary aspergillosis. Clin Chest Med 4:15, 1983

STURGESS JM, TURNER JAP: Recurrent illness due to immotile cilia syndrome. J Respir Dis 3:48 1982

SWARTZ MN: Bronchiectasis, in *Pulmonary Disease and Disorders*, 2d ed, AP Fishman (ed). New York McGraw-Hill, 1988, pp 1553–1581

Broncholithiasis

COLE FH et al: Management of broncholithiasis: Is thoracotomy necessary? Ann Thoracic Surg 42:255, 1986

HAINES JD: Coughing up a stone. What to do about broncholithiasis. Postgrad Med 83:83, 1988

209 CYSTIC FIBROSIS

HARVEY R. COLTEN

Cystic fibrosis (CF) is an inherited multisystem disorder which is characterized by an abnormality in exocrine gland function. Nearly all patients develop chronic progressive disease of the respiratory system. Pulmonary disease is the most common cause of death and morbidity in patients with cystic fibrosis. Pancreatic dysfunction (exocrine or endocrine) occurs in 85 percent of patients; hepatobiliary and genitourinary disease are also frequent. Prior to the 1930s the syndrome was confused with several other disorders with signs and symptoms of intestinal malabsorption.

CF is common in populations of European origin. Estimates of the incidence of the disorder range from about 1/500 in Amish (Ohio)

to 1/90,000 in Hawaiian Orientals. For the white American population the disease occurs in 1/1600 to 1/2000 live births. The disease is recognized less frequently in black Africans. From the autosomal recessive mode of inheritance the gene frequency in white Americans is estimated at 1/20. A series of DNA probes that detect sequences close to the "CF gene" on the long arm of chromosome 7 have been used to detect restriction fragment length polymorphisms and to isolate the "cystic fibrosis gene," permitting antenatal diagnosis and carrier detection. The use of these genetic data, coupled with cell physiologic studies indicating a defect in regulation of a chloride channel in epithelia facilitated a better understanding of the molecular pathophysiology of cystic fibrosis. Based on studies of several hundred families, it is clear that a three-base-pair deletion resulting in loss of a phenylalanine at position 508 accounts for 30 to 75 percent of CF cases in different populations. Other mutations within this gene are responsible for most, if not all, of the remaining CF cases.

Currently, the median survival for patients with CF is about 20 years, and many patients survive to the third and fourth decades. A few have survived to age 50 and beyond. Even though survival of CF patients has improved, the mutation is semilethal. More than 98 percent of males with CF are infertile (see below), and fertility is reduced in women with the disease. This, together with the high incidence of the disease, suggests a selective advantage for the individual heterozygous for the CF gene, but this remains speculative in the absence of precise information about the gene defect.

CLINICAL MANIFESTATIONS General The majority of CF patients are diagnosed in infancy or childhood, but some escape detection until adulthood. Table 209-1 summarizes the multiple

---

TABLE 209-1 Principal clinical manifestations of cystic fibrosis

I Respiratory/cardiovascular
  A Bronchitis, bronchopneumonia, bronchiectasis, lung abscesses, aspergillosis (allergic)
  B Atelectasis
  C Sinusitis, nasal polyposis
  D Pulmonary hypertension
  E Cor pulmonale and congestive heart failure
  F Hemoptysis
  G Pneumothorax
  H Respiratory failure
II Gastrointestinal
  A Intestinal
    1 Meconium ileus
    2 Volvulus
    3 Ileal atresia
    4 Rectal prolapse
    5 Intussusception
    6 Fecal impaction
    7 Pneumatosis intestinalis
  B Pancreatic
    1 Nutritional deficit and growth failure due to pancreatic insufficiency
    2 Steatorrhea
    3 Diabetes mellitus
    4 Recurrent pancreatitis
  C Hepatobiliary
    1 Atrophic gallbladder, cholelithiasis
    2 Loss of bile salts
    3 Focal biliary cirrhosis
    4 Portal hypertension
      a Esophageal varices
      b Hypersplenism
      c Hemorrhoids
III Reproductive system
  A Males: sterility; absent or defective vas deferens, epididymis, and seminal vesicles in about 99 percent of males
  B Females: decreased fertility; increased viscosity of vaginal secretions
IV Skeletal
  A Retardation of bone age
  B Demineralization
  C Hypertrophic osteoarthropathy
V Other
  A Salt depletion
  B Heat stroke
  C Salivary gland hypertrophy
  D Retinal hemorrhage
  E Hypertrophy of apocrine glands

clinical features of this disease. Substantial pancreatic disease is more common in patients diagnosed early in life, because acute intestinal obstruction (meconium ileus at birth) or malnutrition and poor growth or development alerts the pediatrician and family. Patients with minimal or absent gastrointestinal complaints and atypical respiratory symptoms may be diagnosed for the first time when adult. The finding of microorganisms typically isolated from sputum of CF patients (a mucoid form of *Pseudomonas aeruginosa*) or male infertility in association with evidence of obstructive pulmonary disease suggests CF in a previously undiagnosed adult.

Respiratory All levels of the respiratory tract may be affected in CF. Nasal polyposis, sinusitis, and lower respiratory tract disease are common. Abnormalities in water and electrolyte transport across the respiratory epithelium are said to be uniquely abnormal in patients with CF. Primary qualitative or quantitative alterations in mucous secretion that are characteristic for CF have been suggested, but most if not all that have been experimentally determined appear similar to findings in patients with chronic bronchitis or bronchiectasis of diverse etiologies. Autopsy studies of infants dying of meconium ileus suggest that the lungs of newborns with CF are normal. The earliest pulmonary changes are hypertrophy of bronchial glands followed by mucous plugging and obstruction of small airways. Subsequent infection leads to a bronchiolitis, and centripetal progression of endobronchial disease results in chronic bronchitis, bronchiectasis, and peribronchial inflammation. The release of toxic oxygen species and proteolytic enzymes by bacterial and inflammatory cells probably contributes to the progression of airway disease. Specific and nonspecific systemic host defenses are normal or increased, though chronic inflammatory disease may lead to mechanical interference with local defense mechanisms.

Three major bacterial organisms chronically colonize or infect the airways of patients with CF. *Staphylococcus aureus* and *Haemophilus influenzae* are recovered from sputum in a minority, and *P. aeruginosa*, especially mucoid forms, are detected in more than 90 percent of CF patients. Once the *P. aeruginosa* is acquired, the organism is rarely if ever eliminated. Other bacteria (mucoid forms of *Escherichia coli*, *Legionella*, etc.) and other microorganisms, including viruses, mycoplasma, and fungi, may be present in the sputum of patients with CF. Colonization with *Pseudomonas cepacia* may herald a more unfavorable short-term prognosis. The mucoid *Pseudomonas* strains are detected almost exclusively in the CF population. Even family members of patients with CF are not colonized by this organism, so that recovery of a mucoid form of *P. aeruginosa* from patients with chronic pulmonary disease should prompt further diagnostic studies to rule out CF.

Acute and chronic pulmonary parenchymal involvement leads to loss of tissue, extensive fibrosis, and changes in lung and airway mechanics. The inflammatory and structural changes in airways and lung parenchyma lead to airway obstruction, hyperinflation, and ventilation-perfusion imbalance. The upper lobes are generally more involved than lower lobes. Pleural involvement is rare, and extrathoracic infection with respiratory pathogens is virtually absent. Secondary changes in pulmonary and bronchial vasculature in patients with advanced respiratory disease may lead to the substantial hemoptysis often observed in older patients. Pulmonary hypertension develops frequently in CF patients with severe airway obstruction and hypoxemia, resulting in progressive right ventricular failure (cor pulmonale). Clubbing is seen in nearly all patients.

TREATMENT Treatment of CF pulmonary disease is directed toward increasing mechanical drainage, as in patients with chronic bronchitis (Chap. 210), with the use of chest physiotherapy, exercise programs, etc. Control of bacterial infection or colonization is effected by antibiotic therapy specific for the common bacterial organisms isolated from CF sputum. Antibiotic-resistant strains of *P. aeruginosa* are frequently isolated from patients with advanced disease, but in general intravenously administered aminoglycosides in combination with modified penicillins or cephalosporins are employed for treatment of pulmonary exacerbations. Preliminary studies support the use of

aerosolized antibiotics (generally aminoglycosides) in the management of chronic pulmonary infection with *Pseudomonas aeruginosa*, but the success of this approach is highly dependent on technical details of the delivery system. Management of the bronchospastic component of the disease involves the use of systemic and aerosolized bronchodilators. Occasionally surgery (e.g., lobectomy) is required when infection or tissue destruction is localized. Prompt attention to and specific therapy of complications of pulmonary disease have been important factors in the improved survival of patients with CF. Small pneumothoraxes can generally be managed expectantly, while many will respond to tube thoracostomy alone. However, the best evidence suggests that this approach is associated with high recurrence rates. Therefore most episodes are treated with pleural sclerosis (with agents such as tetracycline or quinacrine), open pleurectomy, or pleurodesis. Massive hemoptysis is treated most safely and effectively by bronchial artery embolization via a percutaneous catheter. Congestive heart failure is managed as described elsewhere (Chaps. 182 and 191). Finally, for patients with advanced pulmonary disease, lung or heart-lung transplantation has been employed on an experimental basis at a limited number of institutions.

Gastrointestinal Pancreatic insufficiency leading to fat and protein malabsorption is a feature in the majority of cases (Chap. 261). Deficiencies of fat-soluble vitamins, caloric deprivation, failure to grow and develop, and other manifestations such as rectal prolapse occur in patients with untreated pancreatic insufficiency. About 5 percent of patients with CF are born with meconium ileus, i.e., intestinal obstruction secondary to inspissated meconium in the terminal ileum. Occasionally perforation and meconium peritonitis can occur. Treatment of pancreatic insufficiency with oral pancreatic enzymes corrects most of the deficits. For instance, it decreases the number and bulk of stools; the amount of flatulence, abdominal pain, and distention; and it largely corrects the malabsorption and hence corrects the nutritional deficiencies.

In patients with intact or partial pancreatic exocrine function, recurrent acute pancreatitis may occur. A minority of patients (2 to 5 percent) develop overt diabetes mellitus requiring exogenous insulin, but subclinical abnormalities in glucose metabolism can be detected in a much larger group of CF patients. The longer survival of patients with CF may allow the development of typical diabetic complications such as retinal and glomerular lesions. These should prompt more aggressive efforts to maintain optimal diabetic control.

Hepatobiliary disease is common in older patients. There is chronic cholestasis, inflammation, fibrosis, and even cirrhosis. All of the features of portal hypertension have been recognized. Extrahepatic disease of the biliary system is common.

Genitourinary Abnormalities of the genitourinary tract are present in 98 percent of males. These are due to an interruption in wolffian duct structures (atresia of the vas deferens) which results in azoospermia and decreased ejaculate volume (Chap. 321). Sexual development and potency are unaffected by the genitourinary abnormalities. Women have abnormal cervical mucus. Sexual development, the menstrual cycle, and fertility in women are less affected by direct effects of the mutation than by the effects of poor nutrition and/or chronic pulmonary disease. Women with CF can conceive and deliver healthy infants, but the maternal and fetal risks are functions of the extent of pulmonary disease and its complications. Close monitoring and prompt therapy in centers expert in high-risk obstetrical management are indicated.

Sweat glands The abnormality in the eccrine sweat gland function provides the most reliable diagnostic test for CF at present. Sodium, potassium, and chloride are elevated in sweat of patients with CF. The chloride concentration exceeds 70 mmol per liter, and the sodium concentration is greater than 60 mmol per liter in sweat of nearly all patients, though some individuals with "borderline values" may have many other manifestations of the disease. The corresponding values for chloride and sodium in normals rarely exceed 50 and 40 mmol per liter, respectively. Sweat electrolytes are measured most reliably by the pilocarpine iontophoresis method.

Even when qualitative screening methods are used, the diagnosis cannot be made without a quantitative sweat electrolyte measurement. The increased electrolyte content results from a failure of reabsorption in the sweat duct. Electrolyte losses may lead to significant salt depletion, especially in young children.

CONCLUSION Increasing survival of patients with typical findings of CF as well as patients undiagnosed until adult life requires an increased awareness of this disorder among physicians. The relatively high prevalence of this disorder and the enormous resources required to treat patients with CF has stimulated research activity to define the basic genetic defect responsible for the protean clinical manifestations of CF.

REFERENCES

BOAT TF et al: Cystic fibrosis, in CR Scriver et al (eds): *The Metabolic Basis of Inherited Disease,* 6th ed. New York, McGraw-Hill, 1989, pp 2649–2680

DAVIS PB: Cystic fibrosis. Semin Resp Med 6:243, 1985

DI SANT'AGNESE PA, DAVIS PB: Cystic fibrosis in adults: 75 cases and a review of 232 cases in the literature. Am J Med 66:121, 1979

FELLOWS KE et al: Bronchial artery embolization in cystic fibrosis: Technique and long-term results. J Pediatr 95:959, 1979

KEREM B et al: Identification of the cystic fibrosis gene: Genetic analysis. Science 245:1073, 1989

KNOWLES M et al: Increased bioelectrical potential difference across respiratory epithelia in cystic fibrosis. N Engl J Med 305:1489, 1981

PARK RW, GRAND RJ: Gastrointestinal manifestations of cystic fibrosis: A review. Gastroenterol 81:1143, 1981

RIORDAN JR et al: Identification of the cystic fibrosis gene: Cloning and characterization of complementary DNA. Science 245:1066, 1989

ROMMENS JM et al: Identification of the cystic fibrosis gene: Chromosome walking and jumping. Science 245:1059, 1989

SCANLIN TF: Cystic fibrosis (including assessment of pulmonary performance), in *Pulmonary Diseases and Disorders,* 2d ed, AP Fishman (ed). New York, McGraw-Hill, 1987, chap 76

SHWACHMAN H et al: The sweat test: Sodium and chloride values. J Pediatr 98:576, 1981

210 CHRONIC BRONCHITIS, EMPHYSEMA, AND AIRWAYS OBSTRUCTION

ROLAND H. INGRAM, JR.

Chronic bronchitis and emphysema are two distinct processes, often present in combination in patients with chronic airways obstruction. The diagnosis of chronic bronchitis is made by history, chronic airways obstruction is assessed physiologically, and emphysema can be diagnosed with certainty only by histologic examination of sections of whole lung fixed at inflation. Although the relationships between clinical characteristics, physiologic derangements, and morphologic changes have been diligently studied for many years, reasonably certain and uniform clinical criteria are still not available. Definitions and classifications have evolved, but these are not universally accepted. Nonetheless, the following definitions along with brief qualifications and descriptions are currently used by most persons involved in the diagnosis, treatment, and epidemiology of the chronic obstructive airways syndromes.

DEFINITIONS *Chronic bronchitis* is a condition associated with excessive tracheobronchial mucus production sufficient to cause cough with expectoration for at least 3 months of the year for more than 2 consecutive years. Several subclassifications have been proposed. *Simple chronic bronchitis* describes a condition characterized by mucoid sputum production. *Chronic mucopurulent bronchitis* is characterized by persistent or recurrent purulence of sputum in the absence of localized suppurative diseases such as bronchiectasis. Since there may or may not be obstruction as assessed by the use of the forced expiratory vital capacity maneuver, *chronic bronchitis with obstruction* deserves a separate classification. There is a further subset of patients with chronic bronchitis and obstruction who experience severe dyspnea and wheezing in association with inhaled irritants or during acute respiratory infections. Such patients are said to have *chronic infective asthma* or *chronic asthmatic bronchitis.* Since there is considerable but not complete reversibility of airflow obstruction with bronchodilator treatment and abatement of inflammation and since hyperresponsiveness of airways to nonspecific stimuli is seen in this group of patients, confusion is possible between patients with this condition and those with asthma who may also have *chronic airways obstruction* (Chap. 204). The differentiation is based mainly upon the history of the clinical illness. The patient with chronic asthmatic bronchitis has a long history of cough and sputum production with a later onset of wheezing, whereas the asthmatic with chronic obstruction gives a long history of wheezing with later onset of chronic productive cough.

Emphysema is defined as distention of the air spaces distal to the terminal bronchiole with destruction of alveolar septa. *Chronic obstructive lung disease* is defined as a condition in which there is chronic obstruction to airflow due to chronic bronchitis and/or emphysema (see below). Although the degree of obstruction may be less when the patient is free from respiratory infection and may improve somewhat with bronchodilator drugs, significant obstruction is always present.

PREVALENCE Approximately 20 percent of adult males have chronic bronchitis, yet only a minority of these are clinically disabled. According to all surveys males are more often affected than females. With increased cigarette smoking in women, however, the prevalence of bronchitis in them is increasing. Although cigarette smoking is the single most important etiologic factor, occupational and environmental exposures are now receiving more attention, mainly as contributors to the effects of cigarette smoking (Chap. 206).

Since no criteria have been agreed upon for making the diagnosis of emphysema during life, the incidence data are derived solely from postmortem surveys. It is rare to find adult lungs completely free of emphysema. There is a distinct increase in the extent of emphysema in the fifth decade with further increases through the seventh decade and little increase after that. Approximately two-thirds of adult males and one-fourth of females (most without recognized dysfunction) will have well-defined emphysema, which is often limited in extent. Therefore, the majority of those with emphysema will not have had disability or even symptoms associated with it. The situation is analogous to atherosclerosis in that the morphologic changes are far more frequent than the clinical manifestations attributable to the changes.

PATHOLOGY *Chronic bronchitis* is associated with hyperplasia and hypertrophy of the mucus-producing glands found in the submucosa of large cartilaginous airways. Quantitation of this anatomic change, known as the *Reid index,* is based upon the ratio of the thickness of the submucosal glands to that of the bronchial wall. In persons without a history of chronic bronchitis the mean ratio is 0.44 with a standard deviation ± 0.09, whereas in those with such a history the mean ratio is 0.52 ± 0.08. Although a low index is *rarely* associated with symptoms and a high index is commonly associated with symptoms during life, there is a great deal of overlap. Therefore many persons will have morphologic changes in large airways without having had chronic bronchitis.

Perhaps more important than the abnormalities in large airways are the changes often found in the small noncartilaginous airways. Goblet-cell hyperplasia, mucosal and submucosal inflammatory cells, and edema, peribronchial fibrosis, intraluminal mucus plugs, and increased smooth muscle are characteristic findings in small airways. The frequency of these latter findings in relation to premortem clinical and functional status has not been determined. However, in lungs from patients with chronic obstructive lung disease which have been studied at postmortem, the major site of airflow obstruction has been shown to be in the small airways.

Emphysema is classified according to the pattern of involvement of the gas-exchanging units (acini) of the lung distal to the terminal bronchiole. Although several morphologic patterns have been described, the two most important in the context of this discussion are those involving the respiratory bronchioles and alveolar ducts in the center of the acinus (centriacinar emphysema) and those involving the entire acinus (panacinar emphysema). Quite often both morphologic patterns are present in a single lung of a patient dying from chronic obstructive lung disease, although one type may predominate over the other.

With centriacinar emphysema the distention and destruction are mainly limited to the respiratory bronchiole and alveolar ducts, with relatively less change peripherally in the acinus. Because of the large functional reserve in the lung, many units must be involved in order for overall dysfunction to be detectable. The centrally destroyed regions of the acinus have a high ventilation/perfusion ratio because the capillaries are missing yet ventilation continues. This results in increased wasted ventilation (Vd/Vt), while the peripheral portions of the acinus have crowded and small alveoli with intact, perfused capillaries giving a low ventilation/perfusion ratio. This results in wasted blood flow to give a high alveolar-arterial P_{O_2} difference ($PA_{O_2} - Pa_{O_2}$) (Chap. 201). Mild degrees of centriacinar emphysema, often limited to the lung apices, are extremely common in lungs from persons above age 50 and are practically considered a normal finding.

Panacinar emphysema involves both the central and peripheral portions of the acinus which results, if the process is extensive, in a reduction of the alveolar-capillary gas exchange surface and loss of elastic recoil properties. When emphysema is severe, it may be difficult to distinguish between the two types which most often coexist in the same lung.

CONTRIBUTORY FACTORS Smoking Cigarette smoking is the most commonly identified correlate with both chronic bronchitis during life and extent of emphysema at postmortem. Experimental studies have shown that prolonged cigarette smoking impairs ciliary movement, inhibits function of alveolar macrophages, and leads to hypertrophy and hyperplasia of mucus-secreting glands; massive exposure in dogs can produce emphysematous changes. In addition to these chronic effects, it is probable that smoke inhibits antiproteases and causes polymorphonuclear leukocytes to release proteolytic enzymes acutely. Inhaled cigarette smoke can produce an acute increase in airways resistance due to vagally mediated smooth-muscle constriction, presumably by way of stimulating submucosal irritant receptors. The relationship of such recurrent episodes of acute bronchial constriction to the development and progression of chronic airways obstruction is uncertain. Recent studies, however, indicate that increased airways responsiveness is associated with more rapid progression in those with chronic airways obstruction.

It is now well established that some young asymptomatic smokers have considerable obstruction in small airways without there being either an increase of airway resistance or a diminution in the forced expiratory volume in 1 s. Since small airways, because of their large total cross-sectional areas, contribute very little to overall airflow resistance, more sensitive tests must be used to detect mild degrees of small-airways obstruction. Some tests, such as a decrease in compliance and resistance at rapid breathing rates, are based upon nonuniform behavior of the lung which is apparent only at increased frequencies. Obstruction of small airways also results in airways closure at higher lung volumes than in persons of the same age with unobstructed airways (Chap. 201). The measurements of closing volume and frequency dependence of resistance and compliance require special equipment not often available to clinicians. However, the simple spirogram is useful since flow rates at or below the mid-vital capacity range are often diminished in persons with mild small-airways obstruction. It has been shown that obstruction of small airways is the earliest demonstrable mechanical defect in young cigarette smokers and that the obstruction may disappear after cessation of smoking. It is possible, but has not been established with certainty, that those with small-airways obstruction are at greater risk of developing disabling chronic airways obstruction at some future time.

Not only is cigarette smoking the most common single factor leading to chronic airways obstruction, it also interacts with virtually every other contributory factor to be discussed below.

Air pollution The incidence and mortality rates of both chronic bronchitis and emphysema may be higher in heavily industrialized urban areas. Exacerbations of bronchitis are clearly related to periods of heavy pollution with sulfur dioxide (SO_2) and particulate matter. While nitrogen dioxide (NO_2) can produce small-airways obstruction (bronchiolitis) in experimental animals exposed to high concentrations, there are no data convincingly implicating NO_2, at even the highest pollutant levels, in the pathogenesis or worsening of airways obstruction in humans (Chap. 206).

Occupation Chronic bronchitis is more prevalent in workers who engage in occupations exposing them to either inorganic or organic dusts or to noxious gases. Epidemiologic surveys have succeeded in demonstrating an accelerated decline in lung function in many such workers—e.g., workers in plastics plants exposed to toluene diisocyanate and carding room workers in cotton mills (Chap. 206)—suggesting that their occupational exposure contributes to their future disability.

Infection Morbidity, mortality, and frequency of acute respiratory illnesses are higher in patients with chronic bronchitis. Many attempts have been made to relate these illnesses to infection with viruses, mycoplasmas, and bacteria. However, only the rhinovirus is found more often during exacerbations; that is to say, pathogenic bacteria, mycoplasmas, and viruses other than rhinovirus are found just as often between as during exacerbations. It is intuitively appealing to assign some role to respiratory infections in the pathogenesis and progression of chronic obstructive lung disease, and although this question is under study, there has been no conclusion to date. Recent epidemiologic studies, however, implicate acute respiratory illness as one of the major factors associated with the etiology as well as the progression of chronic airways obstruction. It has been shown that cigarette smokers may either transitorily develop or worsen small-airways obstruction in association with even mild viral respiratory infections. There is also some evidence that severe viral pneumonia early in life may lead to chronic obstruction, predominantly in small airways.

Familial and genetic factors Familial aggregation of chronic bronchitis has been well demonstrated in the past. Recent surveys have shown that children of smoking parents may experience more frequent and severe respiratory illnesses and have a higher prevalence of chronic respiratory symptoms. In addition, nonsmokers who remain in the presence of cigarette smokers (passive smokers) have increased blood levels of carbon monoxide which indicate that they are significantly exposed to smoke. Another well-documented form of indoor air pollution relates to the use of natural gas for cooking. The role of such pollution, however, remains controversial. Thus a part of the familial aggregation may be related to home air pollution. However, some studies of monozygotic twins have suggested some genetic predisposition to the development of chronic bronchitis independent of personal or familial smoking habits and other indoor air pollution. The exact genetic mode of transmission, if it exists at all, is uncertain.

The protease inhibitor alpha$_1$ antitrypsin is an acute-phase reactant, and normally the serum levels rise in association with many inflammatory reactions and with estrogen administration. Either deficient or absent serum levels of alpha$_1$ antitrypsin are found in some patients with the early onset of emphysema. By use of the techniques of acid starch gel and immunoelectrophoresis, genetic typing of the protease inhibitor (Pi) types has been possible. Most of the normal population have two M genes, designated as Pi type MM, and have serum alpha$_1$-antitrypsin levels in excess of 2.5 g/L. Several genes are associated with alterations in levels of serum alpha$_1$ antitrypsin, but the commonest ones associated with emphysema are the Z and S genes. Individuals who are homozygous ZZ or SS have serum levels often near 0 but always less than 0.5 g/L and develop severe panacinar emphysema in the third and fourth decades of life. The panacinar process predominates at the lung bases. Progressive dyspnea with minimal cough characterizes the clinical presentation, although chronic bronchitis is prominent in smokers. Given that alpha$_1$-protease inhibitors can be chemically synthesized or biologically produced in significant quantities and can be shown with intravenous infusion to restore the protease-antiprotease balance in liquid lavaged from the lungs of ZZ patients, it has been suggested that replacement therapy should be of value in preventing the development of emphysema; limited clinical trials are underway. The MZ and MS heterozygotes have intermediate levels of serum alpha$_1$ antitrypsin (i.e., between 0.5 and 2.5 g/L); hence the genetic expression is that of an autosomal codominant allele. It is a matter of some controversy whether the heterozygous state is associated with lung function abnormalities. Published studies are in direct conflict on this point, and further data are needed to be certain. The matter is of some importance, since the heterozygous state is common, with incidence estimates varying between 5 and 14 percent of the general population.

The precise way in which antitrypsin deficiency produces emphysema is unclear. In addition to inhibition of trypsin, alpha$_1$ antitrypsin is an effective inhibitor of elastase and several other proteolytic enzymes. There is experimental evidence that the structural integrity of lung elastin depends upon this antienzyme, which protects the lung from proteases released from leukocytes. It is tempting to speculate that recurrent inflammatory reactions related to infection and pollutants play some role in pathogenesis by calling forth leukocytes whose released proteases are uninhibited and are free to cause the damage.

The role of proteolytic enzymes in the induction of emphysema is not restricted to patients with alpha$_1$-antitrypsin deficiency. Evidence is accumulating that proteolytic enzymes derived from neutrophilic leukocytes and alveolar macrophages can produce emphysema even in subjects with normal circulating levels of antiproteases. It is possible that local concentrations of proteolytic enzymes may exceed the inhibitory capacity of antiproteases, that some proteases present are not susceptible to the available antiproteases, or that some of the proteolytic enzymes may be physically inaccessible to the antiprotease activity. The ultimate clinical utility of exogenously produced protease inhibitors currently under development will undoubtedly depend upon which of the protease-antiprotease interactions predominates in the production of emphysema.

PATHOPHYSIOLOGY   On the basis of the use of flow rates from forced expiratory vital capacity maneuvers and more sophisticated measures of airways resistance and elastic recoil properties of the lung, it has become clear that both chronic bronchitis and emphysema can exist without evidence of obstruction. However, by the time a patient begins to experience dyspnea as a result of these processes, obstruction is always demonstrable. Since chronic bronchitis and emphysema are usually combined, it might appear fruitless to determine the role of each in producing an individual patient's disability. However, one process may dominate over the other, and to the extent that inflammatory airways disease, secretions, and bronchospasm are present, there are therapeutic possibilities with some hope for improvement. Therefore it is of value to understand the mechanisms of airways obstruction in order to guide therapy and anticipate results.

Both chronic bronchitis and emphysema result in airways narrowing. In addition to the primary airways processes of chronic bronchitis, loss of elastic recoil of the lung in emphysema accounts for a decrease in airways caliber through loss of radial traction on airways. Narrowing of airways is often associated with both an increase in airways resistance and a diminution in maximal expiratory flow rates.

There are occasions in which a normal or only slightly elevated airways resistance is accompanied by low maximal expiratory flow rates. Under such circumstances an increase in the dynamic collapsibility of intrathoracic airways during forced exhalation is a possible explanation. Also in this context, the elastic recoil pressure of the lung must be considered in a slightly different way. In addition to providing radial support to airways during quiet breathing, the elastic recoil properties of the lung serve as a major determinant of maximal expiratory flow rates. The static recoil pressure of the lung is the difference between alveolar and intrapleural pressure. During forced exhalations, when alveolar and intrapleural pressures are high, there are points in the airway at which bronchial pressure equals pleural pressure. Flow does not increase with higher pleural pressure after these points become fixed so that the effective driving pressure between alveoli and such points is the elastic recoil pressure of the lung (Fig. 210-1). Hence maximal expiratory flow rates represent a complex and dynamic interplay between airways caliber, elastic recoil pressures, and collapsibility of airways. As a direct consequence of the altered pressure-airflow relationships, the work of breathing is increased in bronchitis and emphysema. Since flow-resistive work is flow rate–dependent, there is a disproportionate increase in the work of breathing with increased ventilation.

The designated subdivisions of the lung volume outlined in Chap. 201 are abnormal to varying degrees in both bronchitis and emphysema. The residual volume (RV) and functional residual capacity (FRC) are almost always higher than normal. Since the normal FRC is the volume at which the inward recoil of the lung is balanced by the outward recoil of the chest wall, loss of elastic recoil of the lung would clearly result in a higher static FRC. In addition, prolongation of expiration in association with obstruction would lead to a dynamic increase in FRC if inspiration is initiated before the respiratory system

FIGURE 210-1   *A.* A schematic diagram of the lung and intrathoracic airways with no airflow. The alveolar pressure (Palv) is greater than pleural pressure (Ppl) by an amount equal to the elastic recoil pressure of the lung (Pel)—i.e., Palv is the algebraic sum of Ppl + Pel. With no airflow Palv = P atmospheric, and for all of the intrathoracic airways, pressure outside is less than the pressure inside due to the Pel. *B.* The same schematic lung during forced exhalation when pleural pressure becomes quite positive. Palv is still greater than Ppl by an amount equal to Pel. However, there is a pressure drop along the airway associated with flow, and at some point Ppl equals local bronchial pressure (so-called equal pressure point, EPP). Mouthward from this point, Ppl exceeds local bronchial pressure and hence acts to compress the airways. *C.* Pressure within the airways from alveoli to the intrathoracic trachea is shown as a dashed line (---) and Ppl is shown as a constant (———). Therefore, the driving pressure from alveoli to EPP is equal to Pel, and a decrease in Pel (i.e., loss of elastic recoil) would mean a smaller driving pressure and smaller flow rates.

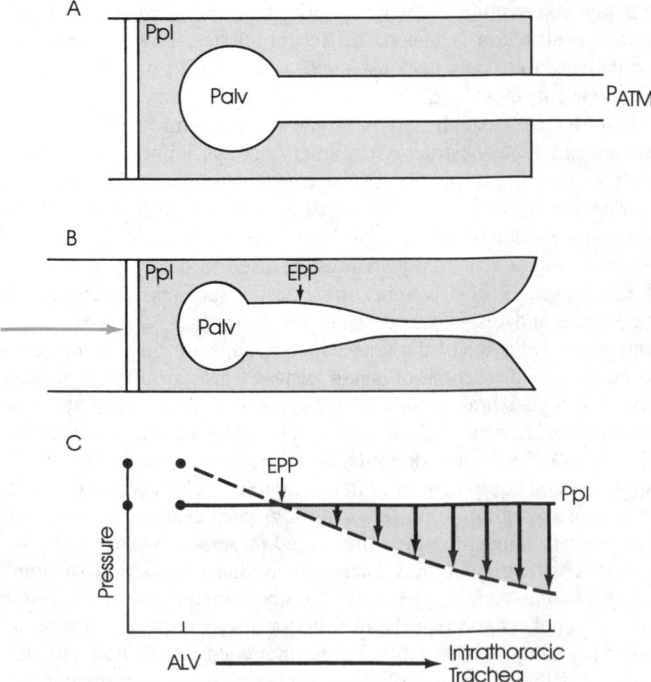

reaches its static balance point. Elevations of total lung capacity (TLC) are frequent. The exact cause is uncertain, but increases in TLC are often found in association with decreases in the elastic recoil of the lung. The vital capacity is frequently decreased, yet significant airways obstruction can be present with a normal to near-normal vital capacity.

The consequences of the airways and parenchymal processes are far more extensive than just the mechanical alterations discussed above. Maldistribution of inspired gas and blood flow is always present to some extent. When the mismatching is severe, impairment of gas exchange is reflected in abnormalities of arterial blood gases. There are regions of the lung with ventilation in excess of perfusion which increase the wasted ventilation ratio (that is, Vd/Vt; Chap. 201). At a normal resting CO_2 production, the net effective alveolar ventilation, as reflected by the arterial P_{CO_2}, may be excessive, normal, or insufficient depending upon the relationship of the overall minute volume to the wasted ventilation ratio. The net contribution of regions with perfusion in excess of ventilation can be assessed by either estimating or measuring the alveolar-arterial P_{O_2} difference (that is, $PA_{O_2} - Pa_{O_2}$; Chap. 201). Whatever the clinical syndrome associated with chronic bronchitis and emphysema, there are to some degree increases in both wasted ventilation and wasted blood flow.

The clinical manifestations depend, in large part, upon the ventilatory response to the disordered lung function. Some patients, at the cost of extremely high effort of breathing and chronic dyspnea, will maintain a strikingly increased minute volume, which results both in a normal to low arterial P_{CO_2}, despite the high Vd/Vt, and a relatively high arterial P_{O_2}, despite the high difference, $PA_{O_2} - Pa_{O_2}$. Other patients with only modest increases in effort of breathing and less dyspnea will maintain a normal to only moderately elevated minute volume at the cost of accepting a high arterial P_{CO_2} and a severely depressed arterial P_{O_2}.

Factors which account for clear differences in ventilatory responses between patients have been studied and debated for years. The bulk of available evidence suggests that those patients who maintain relatively normal or low arterial P_{CO_2} levels are those with an increased ventilatory drive relative to their blood gas values and those who chronically maintain high arterial P_{CO_2} and lower P_{O_2} levels have a diminished ventilatory drive in relation to their more severely deranged blood gas values. It is not at all certain whether individual differences are accounted for by variations in peripheral or central chemoreceptor sensitivity or through other afferent pathways. Perhaps of more immediate value is the fact that patients with predominant emphysema are either normally or excessively responsive both to hypercapnia and to exercise, whereas those with predominant bronchitis are less responsive to both, despite similar degrees of airways obstruction by spirometry.

The pulmonary circulation malfunctions not only in terms of regional distribution of blood flow but in terms of abnormal overall pressure-flow relationships. There is often mild to severe pulmonary hypertension at rest with further increases disproportionate to cardiac output elevations during exercise. A reduction in the total cross-sectional area of the pulmonary vascular bed can be attributed to anatomic changes and constriction of vascular smooth muscle in pulmonary arteries and arterioles as well as destruction of alveolar septa with loss of capillaries. Rarely does loss of capillaries alone lead to severe pulmonary hypertension with cor pulmonale, except as a near-terminal event. Of more importance is the constriction of pulmonary vessels in response to alveolar hypoxia. The constriction is reversible upon increase in alveolar P_{O_2} with therapy. There is a synergism between hypoxia and acidosis which assumes importance during episodes of acute or chronic respiratory insufficiency. Chronic hypoxia leads not only to pulmonary vascular constriction but also to secondary erythrocytosis. The latter, although not proved to be a significant contributor to pulmonary hypertension, could add an unfavorable rheologic load. As discussed in Chap. 191, the chronic afterload on the right ventricle leads to hypertrophy and, in association with disordered blood gases, ultimately to failure.

CLINICAL-FUNCTIONAL CORRELATIONS Dyspnea and impairment of physical work capacity are characteristic only of severe to moderately severe airways obstruction. There is considerable variation among patients, and those with predominant emphysema have greater dyspnea and restriction of physical activity with lesser degrees of obstruction than those in whom chronic bronchitis predominates. The majority of patients have functionally mixed disease, will usually experience exertional dyspnea when the forced expiratory volume in 1 s (FEV_1) falls below 50 percent of that predicted, and will have dyspnea at rest when the FEV_1 is less than 25 percent of that predicted. In addition to dyspnea at rest, carbon dioxide retention and cor pulmonale frequently occur when the FEV_1 falls to 25 percent of that predicted. However, those with predominant bronchitis often have carbon dioxide retention and cor pulmonale with FEV_1 values above 25 percent of normal, in contrast to patients with predominant emphysema whose FEV_1 usually falls well below that level before the onset of carbon dioxide retention and cor pulmonale. With a respiratory infection, small changes in the degree of obstruction can make a large difference in symptoms and gas exchange. Thus small therapeutic gains have rewarding results.

In general, the more severe the obstruction, the poorer the prognosis. Despite the general relationship, 20 to 30 percent of patients with severe obstruction and carbon dioxide retention will survive beyond 5 years.

CLINICAL SYNDROMES It is clear that the clinical presentation can vary in severity from simple chronic bronchitis without disability to the severely disabled state with chronic respiratory failure. From a practical standpoint, it is well to consider that any symptom or any measurable abnormality may foreshadow the development of severe disabling disease; hence cessation of smoking and avoidance of environmental irritants and toxins are to be advised. However, the advice to modify behavior and life patterns is rarely taken, and most physicians are called upon to categorize and treat patients with fully developed, chronic airways obstruction. Thus the approach taken here is to describe two polar opposite types of fully developed, chronic obstructive pulmonary disease with the realization that the majority of patients will have some features of both types. The salient features of each type are outlined in Table 210-1.

Predominant emphysema These patients often give a long history of exertional dyspnea with minimal cough which is productive of only small amounts of mucoid sputum. Mucopurulent exacerbations

TABLE 210-1 Chronic obstructive lung disease: Salient features of the two types

	Predominant emphysema	Predominant bronchitis
Age at time of diagnosis, y	60±	50±
Dyspnea	Severe	Mild
Cough	After dyspnea starts	Before dyspnea starts
Sputum	Scanty, mucoid	Copious, purulent
Bronchial infections	Less frequent	More frequent
Respiratory insufficiency episodes	Often terminal	Repeated
Chest film	"Hyperinflation" ± bullous changes, small heart	Increased bronchovascular markings at bases, large heart
Chronic Pa_{CO_2}, mmHg	35–40	50–60
Chronic Pa_{O_2}, mmHg	65–75	45–60
Hematocrit, %	35–45	50–55
Pulmonary hypertension:		
Rest	None to mild	Moderate to severe
Exercise	Moderate	Worsens
Cor pulmonale	Rare, except terminally	Common
Elastic recoil	Severely decreased	Normal
Resistance	Normal to slight increase	High
Diffusing capacity	Decreased	Normal to slight decrease

in association with infections are not frequent. The body build is asthenic with evidence of weight loss. The patient appears distressed with obvious use of accessory muscles of respiration which serve to lift the sternum in an anterosuperior direction with each inspiration. There is tachypnea with a relatively prolonged expiration through pursed lips, or expiration is begun with a grunting sound. While sitting, these patients often lean forward, extending the arms to brace themselves. The neck veins may be distended during expiration, yet they collapse briskly with inspiration. The lower intercostal spaces retract with each inspiration, and by palpation the lower lateral chest wall can be felt to move inward. The percussion note is hyperresonant, and by auscultation the breath sounds are diminished, with faint, high-pitched rhonchi heard toward the end of expiration. The cardiac impulse, if at all visible, is seen only in the xiphoid and subxiphoid regions, and cardiac dullness is either absent or severely reduced. By palpation there is frequently a sustained forward and downward right ventricular impulse in the subxiphoid region, and a presystolic gallop accentuated during inspiration is commonly heard.

The arterial P_{O_2} is often in the mid-70s (mmHg), and the P_{CO_2} is low to normal. Because of the maintained increase in minute volume and the maintenance of arterial P_{O_2} sufficient to nearly saturate hemoglobin, these patients have been referred to as "pink puffers." Their increased ventilatory drive probably accounts for their relatively preserved oxygenation and lack of hypercapnia; however, this increased drive with attendant increases in ventilation undoubtedly contributes to the severity of their dyspnea.

The TLC and RV are invariably increased, the vital capacity is low, and the maximal expiratory flow rates are diminished. The elastic recoil properties of the lung are severely impaired, and in direct proportion to this impairment, the capacity of the lung to transfer carbon monoxide is lowered.

On radiographic examination the diaphragms are low and flattened, the bronchovascular shadows do not extend to the periphery of the lung, and the cardiac silhouette is lengthened and narrowed. These findings in association with a large retrosternal translucency on lateral chest radiographs are interpreted as hyperinflation, which correlates well with increases in TLC and loss of elastic recoil. Peripheral attenuation of bronchovascular markings and increased retrosternal lucency correlate best with subsequent postmortem demonstration of extensive and severe emphysema which is predominantly of the panacinar type. Recently computed tomography (CT) has been shown to localize and quantitate emphysema. However, determining the localization of such regions most often is of little practical value and the overall quantitative assessments from elastic recoil properties and carbon monoxide transfer are just as good. Hence use of CT scans for this purpose is not ordinarily employed.

It is fortunate that the patient with predominant emphysema is less prone to mucopurulent relapses than is the patient with predominant bronchitis, since such relapses frequently lead to severe respiratory failure and death. That is to say, right-sided heart failure and hypercapnic respiratory failure are often terminal events in those patients with predominant emphysema. In the absence of such relapses, the clinical course is characterized by severe and progressive dyspnea for which little can be done. The physician's role is to seek out and treat any factor that is possibly reversible and strive to avoid pollutants and infections.

Predominant bronchitis   The patient with predominant bronchitis usually has an impressive history of cough and sputum production for many years with an immodest history of cigarette smoking. Initially the cough is present only in the winter months, and the patient is apt to seek medical attention, if at all, only during the more severe of the frequent mucopurulent relapses. Over the years the cough progresses from hibernal to perennial, and mucopurulent relapses increase in frequency, duration, and severity. After beginning to experience exertional dyspnea, the patient often seeks medical help and will be found to have a severe degree of obstruction. Occasionally such a patient will seek out a physician only after the onset of peripheral edema secondary to overt right ventricular failure.

More rarely the initial medical contact is made by family members who present the physician with a deeply cyanotic, edematous, and stuporous patient with acute respiratory insufficiency.

The patient with predominant bronchitis is often overweight and cyanotic. There is usually no apparent distress at rest, the respiratory rate is normal or only slightly increased, and there is no apparent usage of accessory muscles. The chest percussion note is normally resonant, and by auscultation, one can usually hear coarse rhonchi and wheezes which change in location and intensity after a deep and productive cough. There may be a sustained heave along the lower left sternal border which indicates right ventricular hypertrophy. In the presence of right ventricular failure there are often an early diastolic gallop and occasionally a holosystolic murmur, both of which are accentuated by inspiration. The latter finding is indicative of functional tricuspid regurgitation which is frequently accompanied by neck vein distention characterized by large v waves and brisk y descents. With right ventricular failure the cyanosis deepens and peripheral edema becomes prominent. Clubbing of the digits is unusual.

With or without right ventricular failure, the minute volume is only slightly increased due to an overall diminution in ventilatory drive which modulates the level of dyspnea. However, failure to increase minute volume greatly in the face of significant proportions of wasted ventilation and blood flow results in severely deranged arterial blood gases, with arterial P_{CO_2} values which are chronically increased to the range of the high 40s to low 50s (mmHg). The lowered P_{O_2} produces desaturation of hemoglobin, serves to stimulate erythropoiesis, and results in hypoxic pulmonary vasoconstriction. Desaturation and erythrocytosis combine to produce the cyanosis, and hypoxic pulmonary vasoconstriction accentuates the right-sided heart failure. Because of cyanosis and edema secondary to heart failure, such patients have been referred to as "blue bloaters." It has been proposed, with some supporting data, that one of the pathophysiologic events in the blue bloaters is the occurrence of repeated episodes of severe nocturnal oxygen desaturation in association with episodes of sleep apnea or periods of worsening hypoventilation. Such sleep-related ventilatory events worsen the degree of pulmonary hypertension and secondary erythrocytosis.

The TLC is often normal, and there is a moderate elevation of RV. The vital capacity is mildly diminished, and maximal expiratory flow rates are invariably low. The elastic recoil properties of the lung are normal or only slightly impaired, and the capacity of the lung to transfer carbon monoxide is either normal or minimally decreased.

On radiographic examination the diaphragms are well rounded, the bronchovascular markings are increased in the lower lung fields, and the cardiac silhouette is somewhat enlarged. In association with right ventricular failure the cardiac silhouette enlarges further, pulmonary arteries become more prominent, and an antigravity distribution of perfusion is apparent.

Despite well-planned management (see below) the patient with predominant bronchitis may experience many episodes of respiratory failure from which recovery is frequent with proper therapy (see p. 1080). The ability to recover from such repeated episodes in those patients is in striking contrast to the frequently fatal outcome of such events in those with predominant emphysema. Ultimately, the lungs at postmortem will be found to have severe bronchitic changes in both large and small airways and only moderate emphysema, predominantly of the centriacinar variety.

It should be reemphasized that the above syndromes are described as polar ends of a continuous spectrum of clinical features. Hence most patients will have some characteristics of each syndrome. The usefulness of recognizing and understanding the pathophysiologic bases for these lies in the planning of appropriate management strategies for each patient.

PRINCIPLES OF MANAGEMENT   Intelligent management must be based upon as complete knowledge as possible of the degree of obstruction, the extent of disability, and the relative reversibility of the patient's illness. To the extent that obstructive processes in the airways are contributory, there is a chance for treatment to be effective. Since emphysema is an irreversible process, prevention of progression and avoidance of acute insults constitute the main approach. History, physical examination, and chest radiographs should be supplemented by tests of lung function performed during a symptomatically stable period. Ideally, complete spirometry, plethysmographic lung volumes, transfer of carbon monoxide, arterial blood gases, and lung elastic recoil properties should be measured. Spirometry and lung volumes should be remeasured after the administration of bronchodilators in order to assess the degree of acutely reversible airways obstruction. Failure to see an acute change with bronchodilator drugs does not rule out the possibility of improvement with more prolonged administration of these agents. In instances in which the degree of exertional dyspnea appears to be disproportionately greater than the degree of obstruction, measurements of blood gases, minute volume, CO_2 production, and O_2 consumption during exercise are indicated in order to determine whether impaired lung function is sufficient to account for the symptoms. After the initial assessment the physician has some idea of the relative emphasis to be placed upon patient education, rehabilitative and preventive measures, and direct therapeutic interventions in management of the patient and the illness.

Cessation of smoking is the only certain means of influencing the progression of the chronic obstructive airways syndromes, and although such behavior modification is most effective at early stages of the disease processes, it is effective in slowing the rate of decline in lung function, even when such function is severely compromised. In the instances in which occupational or environmental exposures are thought to play a significant role, change of occupation or relocation of dwelling is advisable. The validity of such advice should be carefully considered since the impact on both the patient and the family is likely to be great. A simpler environmental change is that of eliminating aerosol sprays such as deodorants, hair sprays, and insecticides from the household. Hair sprays have been shown to produce acute airways responses even in normal subjects. Other preventive measures include yearly vaccination against the common or expected influenza virus strains. The patient should be given pneumococcal polysaccharide vaccine only once. Recognition of severe Arthus-type immunologic reactions following repeat pneumococcal vaccination has led to this "once-in-a-lifetime" recommendation.

Infections cannot be totally avoided, and the patient should be made aware that increasing purulence, viscosity, or volume of secretions signals the onset of an infection which should be treated early. The commonest pathogenic bacteria found are *Haemophilus influenzae* and *Streptococcus pneumoniae*. As mentioned above, however, the role of such bacteria is in question since they are just as often isolated during periods of relative clinical quiescence. Nonetheless, tetracycline or ampicillin should be given for a 7- to 10-day course. It is practical to have the patient keep a 7- to 10-day supply of antibiotics at home and to begin treatment at the onset of symptoms. In Great Britain it is common practice to give continuous antibiotic therapy during winter months in order to prevent mucopurulent relapses. Although there is evidence that viruses are frequent causes of mucopurulent relapses, clinical studies have shown that the standard antibiotic regimens decrease the duration and severity of infective episodes unrelated to culturable bacterial pathogens. Microscopic examination and culture of sputum are indicated if there are chills, fever, or chest pain or if purulence fails to respond to usually administered antibiotics.

It has been shown repeatedly that exercise programs, although not accompanied by measurable improvement in lung function, result in increased exercise tolerance and an improved sense of well-being. The improvement is usually task-specific, so that most physicians advise walking in preference to the use of special apparatus, such as stationary bicycles or wall gyms.

If malnutrition as assessed by body weight less than 85 percent of ideal is present, oral dietary supplements can result in improved

muscle strength, less fatigability, and lessening of breathlessness. A carefully taken dietary history and elimination of other serious causes for low body weight and weight loss should precede the start of any major nutritional supplement effort. As with exercise programs, there is not a direct and measurable effect on lung function from treating malnutrition; yet subjective relief and objective improvement in strength and exercise performance have been of great benefit in such patients.

Bronchodilator drugs are often quite helpful in alleviating symptoms, especially in those patients who respond to them acutely in the laboratory. These drugs form three categories: the methylxanthines, sympathomimetics with strong beta$_2$-adrenergic-stimulating properties, and anticholinergics. Theophylline, the most commonly used methylxanthine, can be given orally, rectally, or parenterally; in addition to bronchodilatation, it stimulates respiration and has cardiotonic and diuretic properties. Selective beta$_2$-stimulating drugs such as albuterol and metaproterenol can be given both orally and by aerosol with fewer cardiac side effects than are experienced with isoproterenol. Anticholinergic agents such as atropine have been avoided in the past because of their tendency to desiccate secretions; however, ipratroprium bromide, an anticholinergic agent in metered dose inhaler form, is an extremely effective bronchodilator in chronic bronchitic patients. It is considered by many to be the bronchodilator of choice for these patients.

The use of systemic glucocorticoids is, at our present state of knowledge, based upon very little scientific data from properly controlled clinical trials. Since these agents have time- and dose-related side effects that vary from deleterious to catastrophic, the almost invariable subjective benefit must be supported by objective measurements. There is little room for doubt in the minds of physicians that some patients respond well, even dramatically, to these agents in both objective and subjective terms. The real problem is how to select those patients most likely to benefit. Eosinophilia in the sputum, rather than in the blood, appears in some instances to identify that subgroup in advance. However, the best guidelines are, first, to try these agents only after maximal bronchodilator and bronchopulmonary drainage measures have been tried without success; second, to begin prednisone 30 mg once per day; third, to confirm the objective change in terms of spirometry and gas exchange, stopping these agents if no objective benefit is seen; and fourth, to decrease to the smallest dose that will maintain the improved level of function. The role, if any, of inhaled glucocorticoid agents for these patients, in contrast to asthmatic patients, has not been established in the syndromes with chronic obstruction.

Bronchopulmonary drainage should be maintained in patients with hypersecretion. If the coughing mechanism is ineffective or if paroxysms of coughing are exhausting, postural drainage is often a useful adjunct. Although liquefaction of secretions by means of orally administered expectorants or aerosol delivery of mucolytic agents is an appealing idea, it has never been shown by properly designed trials to be more effective than simple maintenance of total-body hydration.

Intermittent positive pressure breathing (IPPB) devices were formerly advocated for home management. The various rationales included diminution in the work of breathing, promotion of bronchopulmonary drainage, and more efficient delivery of bronchodilator drugs. The first of the rationales has been shown to have no basis in fact, and the goals of the last two have been shown to be as well accomplished by postural drainage and use of less elaborate aerosol generators. Hence the use of IPPB for home management cannot be justified.

When arterial hypoxia is persistent and severe (Pa_{O_2} of 55 to 60 mmHg) in association with cor pulmonale (see Chap. 191) and signs of right heart failure, continuous oxygen therapy is indicated. If the Pa_{O_2} is persistently <55 mmHg, with or without cor pulmonale, continuous oxygen supplementation should also be prescribed. The available data indicate that supplemental oxygen improves both exercise tolerance and neuropsychological function and alleviates pulmonary hypertension and right heart failure. In patients with severe hypoxemia the need for hospitalization occurs less frequently and life span is lengthened by the use of supplemental oxygen. In view of the expense of such therapy and the dangers of uncontrolled oxygen delivery (see below), it should be given only when it can be carefully monitored and its beneficial effects objectively verified.

Since most patients with chronic airways obstruction, especially those with features of predominant bronchitis, can be shown to decrease their Pa_{O_2} values significantly during sleep, most prominently during the REM phase, nocturnal oxygen administration has been suggested. While the rationale is clear and the results quite good, a recent cooperative clinical trial that compared nocturnal with continuous O_2 supplementation in severely hypoxic patients found that continuous O_2 administration was associated with a significantly lower mortality rate. Patients in both treatment groups experienced neuropsychological and hemodynamic benefits. Thus, supplemental nocturnal oxygen is better than none, but continuous oxygen is better than nocturnal in such severely ill patients.

Secondary erythrocytosis with the hematocrit in excess of 0.50 is most easily viewed as a mechanism allowing greater oxygen delivery to compensate for the chronically lowered arterial Pa_{O_2}; hence improvement in oxygenation through improved lung function or by oxygen administration is the most physiologic means to reverse erythrocytosis. Since erythrocytosis results in elevation of blood viscosity at all shear rates, the proposal has been made that pulmonary vascular hypertension is aggravated by its presence. Although no study has demonstrated an objective improvement in hemodynamics, lung mechanics, or gas exchange at rest following phlebotomy, ventilatory and cardiovascular function during exercise improve. Some patients who complain of headaches and a sense of head fullness show a favorable subjective response to periodic phlebotomy when the hematocrit is in excess of 0.55 percent. In support of this subjective improvement is the demonstration that, following phlebotomy, cerebral blood flow, previously diminished, returns toward normal.

ACUTE RESPIRATORY FAILURE

DIAGNOSIS Although it may be strongly suspected on clinical grounds, the firm diagnosis of acute respiratory failure in chronic airways obstruction is based upon measurements of arterial blood gas (Pa_{O_2}, Pa_{CO_2}) and pH values that must be interpreted in relation to the patient's chronic status. Since many patients will have chronically lowered Pa_{O_2} levels and increased Pa_{CO_2} values, the diagnosis is based upon the degree of change from the usual state of the individual patient. With regard to oxygenation, an acute decrease in Pa_{O_2} from a usual mid-70 range to the low 60s (mmHg) is just as indicative of acute respiratory failure as is an acute drop from a chronic mid-50 range to the mid-40s (mmHg). Thus a drop in Pa_{O_2} equal to or greater than 10 to 15 mmHg indicates acute failure.

Since renal compensation for chronic hypercapnia results in adjustment of arterial pH to near-normal values, the acuteness of the increase in Pa_{CO_2} can often be judged by the pH, unless there is a concomitant metabolic acidemia. As a practical guide, any level of hypercapnia associated with an arterial pH value less than 7.30 should be considered as acute respiratory failure.

PRECIPITATING FACTORS Increases in volume, viscosity, and/or purulence of secretions, presumably due to infection of the tracheobronchial tree, are the most common antecedents of acute respiratory failure in chronic obstructive lung disease. Increasing airways obstruction with airways inflammation and secretion, especially in association with a relatively blunted ventilatory drive, leads to worsening hypoxia and increasing CO_2 retention. Agitation, insomnia, and increasing dyspnea with impending respiratory failure are occasionally treated, mistakenly, with either sedatives or narcotics, and these, too, may precipitate frank respiratory failure. In fact such depressant drugs which impair ventilatory drive should be avoided

at all times in patients with severe chronic obstructive lung disease. Major episodes of air pollution can also lead to respiratory failure, and the physicians responsible for patients with severe bronchitis and emphysema should be alert to these environmental events.

Pneumonia, thromboembolism, left ventricular failure, and pneumothorax occasionally precipitate acute respiratory failure and are extremely difficult to detect unless considered and specifically sought. As a minimum, chest radiographs, electrocardiograms, and sputum examinations should be obtained in addition to arterial blood gas measurements in all patients with respiratory failure.

TREATMENT OF RESPIRATORY FAILURE The treatment of respiratory failure consists of two simultaneous processes: (1) maintaining acceptable levels of oxygenation and ventilation; and (2) treatment of infection, removal of secretions, and reversing any airway constriction present.

With regard to the first, these patients *need* oxygen when they are severely hypoxic, and while fears of respiratory depression due to the removal of the hypoxic respiratory stimulus are realistic, O_2 must be used, yet in the smallest concentration possible, to give a Pa_{O_2} in the mid-50-mmHg range while the patient's Pa_{CO_2}, pH, and clinical status are carefully monitored. It is best to begin with only modest increases in $F_{I_{O_2}}$ to approximately 0.24 (cf. air at 0.21), which can be accomplished using nasal prongs with O_2 flows at 1 to 2 liters per minute or, more precisely, with the use of a 0.24 Venturi mask. These latter masks, based upon Bernoulli's principle, deliver a fixed concentration of O_2 irrespective of the O_2 flow rate by entraining air in direct proportion to O_2 flow rate. They are high-flow masks (oxygen plus air entrained from the room), each designed for a specific $F_{I_{O_2}}$ (0.24, 0.28, 0.35, 0.40). Even small increases in Pa_{O_2} when starting from low levels result in significant increases in arterial oxygen content due to the shape of the oxygen-hemoglobin saturation curve over this range (Chap. 290). With improved oxygenation some patients will concomitantly increase their Pa_{CO_2} values. The standard explanation has been that this increase is due to the removal of the hypoxic drive to ventilation leading to further hypoventilation. While this is the most important mechanism, recent data indicate that worsening ventilation-perfusion relationships (Chap. 201) occur with O_2 treatment. This is attributed to reversal of hypoxic pulmonary arterial constriction in the more initially hypoxic, less well ventilated regions, which in turn leads to decreased perfusion of initially less hypoxic, better ventilated regions. The result is an increase in the wasted ventilation ratio (Vd/Vt, Chap. 201) leading to a smaller effective alveolar ventilation. In either case, the $F_{I_{O_2}}$ should be increased as little as possible to achieve a Pa_{O_2} in the mid-50-mmHg range. Some increase in Pa_{CO_2} can be expected and should not cause alarm if the patient is alert. The majority of patients can be managed in this conservative way with excellent results. However, occasionally large increases in Pa_{CO_2} occur and lead to stupor and coma. This can be explained by CO_2-induced cerebral vascular dilatation with increased intracranial pressure, including the development of papilledema, combined with the effect of hypercapnia and hypoxia on cerebral function. It must be emphasized that if stupor and coma supervene, stopping the administration of oxygen is the *worst possible* course of action. When CO_2 narcosis is present, respirations are sufficiently depressed from the CO_2 itself so that the patient will no longer respond to the rapidly worsening hypoxia, and fatal arrhythmias, generalized seizures, and death may ensue. The only alternative is to intubate the trachea and provide mechanical ventilatory support. Mechanical ventilators are described in Chap. 219.

Once mechanical ventilation has been instituted, the tidal volume and frequency should be set gradually to decrease the Pa_{CO_2} only down to the chronically elevated level rather than attempt to decrease it to or below a normal value. Since such patients have renal compensation for their chronic hypercapnia, Pa_{CO_2} values at or below the normal level result in significant alkalemia which in turn can lead to severe tachyarrhythmias and generalized seizures.

As mentioned above, maintaining oxygenation and ventilation serves to buy time while secretion removal, bronchial dilatation, and treatment of infection are instituted. Removal of secretions is accomplished by urging the patient to cough or by passing suction catheters into the trachea which, in addition to removing secretions that are present, stimulate cough that brings more secretions up to the region of the catheter tip. The advantage, if any, from the use of mucolytic agents in this process has yet to be demonstrated. However, beta$_2$-adrenergic bronchodilating agents have been shown to increase the rate of transport of particles by the mucociliary blanket, and, thus, in addition to bronchodilatation, such agents should improve the clearance of airway secretions. Postural drainage and chest percussion are other often-used adjuncts that have been shown, especially when secretions are voluminous, to improve tracheobronchial clearance, to increase sputum volume beyond that produced by cough, and to reduce airways obstruction.

Bronchodilatation with aminophylline given orally or by infusion and beta$_2$-adrenergic agonists by inhalation or subcutaneous injection has assumed a prominent role in treatment of acute respiratory failure in chronic airways obstruction. In addition to bronchodilatation these agents improve bronchopulmonary clearance and may help induce diuresis and hemodynamic improvement when there is cor pulmonale with failure (Chap. 191). Unless there is clearly an acute pneumonia, the use of antibiotics is more controversial in the setting of acute respiratory failure than in mucopurulent relapses without failure. Nonetheless, broad-spectrum antibiotics, if no single agent is suspected or isolated, or erythromycin, if legionellae or mycoplasmas are suspected, should be added to the regimen.

Complications arising in the course of treatment for acute respiratory failure are cardiac arrhythmias, most often multifocal supraventricular tachycardias, left ventricular failure, pulmonary emboli, and gastrointestinal hemorrhage from stress ulceration. Cardiac arrhythmias resulting from rapid decreases in oxygenation or increases in pH due to overventilation can be readily avoided. However, when giving multiple drugs having cardiotonic properties, the question always arises as to whether the arrhythmias are related to these. Keeping serum theophylline levels in the 10 to 20 mg per liter range and using relatively selective beta agonists, such as isoetharine by inhalation, can minimize these effects.

Left ventricular failure, usually attributable to coronary atherosclerosis with acute myocardial infarction, systemic hypertension, or aortic valvular disease, is difficult to detect in the presence of cor pulmonale. Fortunately, improving lung function and oxygenation most often reverse the pulmonary hypertension and right ventricular failure (Chap. 191) and induce a brisk diuresis. If signs of congestive failure persist or worsen after providing adequate oxygenation, consideration must be given to left ventricular failure; an assessment in such patients is best made through echocardiography or radioventriculography since the usual physical and radiographic findings are obscured in such patients. Only in the presence of adequate gas exchange and only with either the firm demonstration of, or strong clinical suspicion of, left ventricular failure should digitalis be used. Diuretic agents should also be reserved for left ventricular failure. They almost invariably produce hypokalemic, hypochloremic metabolic alkalemia that results in depression of ventilatory drive and interference with removal from mechanical ventilatory support.

Pulmonary emboli are suspected to be common in the setting of acute respiratory failure and are extremely difficult to detect since the lung scan is totally nonspecific and signs of cor pulmonale fluctuate in concert with the degree of lung dysfunction. Hence low-dose heparin prophylaxis should be used to prevent this complication. Gastrointestinal hemorrhage commonly complicates acute respiratory failure and is thought to be due to stress ulceration of the gastric mucosa. Awareness of this complication enhances the ability to detect it and act quickly. Antacids, coating agents such as sucralfate, nasogastric suction, and/or cimetidine have been used to diminish the frequency.

For those patients who have required mechanical ventilatory support, the process of removal from that support is largely empirical. In general, improving gas exchange and lung mechanics along with alertness and responsiveness of the patient signal that the support can be removed. Data such as maximal voluntary inspiratory mouth pressures greater than 20 cmH$_2$O, vital capacity greater than 10 mL per kilogram of body weight, and spontaneous tidal volume greater than 5 mL per kilogram of body weight are reassuring. However, many patients can be removed from such support with lesser values than these.

Failure to maintain gas exchange after removal of mechanical ventilatory support can usually be explained. *First* on the list is the continued administration or persistence of sedative and tranquilizing drugs that may have been prescribed earlier for agitation. These should be discontinued and time allowed for their metabolism. *Second* is the possibility that the endotracheal tube is of small bore and imposes a resistive load. If so, it should be replaced by a larger one. *Third* is worsening airways obstruction and accumulation of secretions; continued bronchial dilatation and airway suctioning avoid these. *Fourth* is a metabolic alkalemia, with or without diuretic therapy, that should be treated with potassium chloride. *Fifth* is having maintained a Pa$_{O_2}$ and Pa$_{CO_2}$ while being on mechanical ventilation that are too high and too low, respectively. This can be avoided by using an F$_{I_{O_2}}$ just sufficient to keep the Pa$_{O_2}$ around 60 mmHg and using the assist mode with small enough tidal volumes to keep the Pa$_{CO_2}$ at the expected chronic level (i.e., that associated with a normal or slightly low arterial pH) before discontinuing mechanical support. *Sixth* is poor nutrition, hypokalemia, or neuromuscular disease, making the patient too weak to maintain breathing or resulting in fatigue of the respiratory muscles. Nutrition, of course, is a longer range problem that should be anticipated, while hypokalemia is often handled along with the metabolic alkalemia. Muscle fatigue, especially diaphragmatic, has received a great deal of attention. From a practical standpoint, paradoxical (inward) movement of the upper abdomen with inspiration is the key clinical finding. Experimental evidence suggests that therapeutic levels of aminophylline or beta$_2$ agonists, such as fenoterol, reverse the manifestations of fatigue but the role of respiratory stimulants continues to be debated and the data to be inconclusive. In those patients with severely blunted ventilatory drive and improving lung function, stimulants may be tried cautiously. If there is severe metabolic alkalemia, acetazolamide can be tried as a stimulant while chloride replacement is being carried out. Medroxyprogesterone, a central stimulant, or almitrine, a peripheral chemoreceptor stimulant, appear to be safe and, in some instances, effective. Hypothyroidism is a metabolic condition with neuromuscular consequences and is difficult to detect in this clinical setting. Thus any prolonged and difficult weaning process should lead to the assessment of thyroid function.

PROGNOSIS On the average, data collected on large populations demonstrate a slow and relentless diminution in ventilatory function in patients with chronic airways obstruction. Although slow, the decrement in function with time far exceeds the rate of change seen with normal aging. In general, the likelihood of episodes of acute respiratory failure increases when the FEV$_1$ falls below 25 percent of predicted normal values. Although the in-hospital mortality rate averages 30 percent for a single episode and the 5-year survival rate after the initial episode of respiratory failure averages only 15 to 20 percent, the clinical syndrome is extremely important in determining both the short- and long-range prognosis. As noted above, those patients with predominant emphysema have a poorer prognosis after the onset of respiratory failure than do those with predominant bronchitis. In either case long-term oxygen treatment in those with severe hypoxemia results in prolongation of life and improvement in the quality of life.

BULLOUS EMPHYSEMA Confluent air spaces with diameters in excess of 1 cm are occasionally congenital but most often are found in association with generalized emphysema or progressive fibrotic processes. Gradual increases in size of such air spaces (or bullae) result from traction applied by regions with better elastic recoil properties, and such regions lose volume as the bullae become enlarged. If disability is severe, if the bulla is extremely large, and if either lobar gas sampling or ventilation and perfusion scans demonstrate that sufficient function remains in the nonbullous regions, surgical excision of the bulla may lead to functional improvement. Usually, however, improvement is relatively transitory because other emphysematous regions gradually enlarge into bullae after surgery.

VARIANTS OF EMPHYSEMA   In addition to the centriacinar and panacinar forms of emphysema described above, other structural patterns have been described but are functionally less important. Often there is overdistention and alveolar septal destruction in lung regions surrounding scar tissue (paracicatricial or scar emphysema) or along the borders of the acinus (paraseptal emphysema). The latter form, when it occurs at the visceral pleural surface, may predispose to episodes of spontaneous pneumothorax (Chap. 216). Infants rarely develop a check valve mechanism in a lobar bronchus which leads to rapid and life-threatening overdistention (congenital lobar emphysema). Unilateral emphysema may be an incidental radiographic finding (Macleod's or Swyer-James's syndromes). Since, in this condition, the airways are normal in number and structure but the alveoli are reduced in number, this form of unilateral emphysema has been attributed to disease occurring before the age of 8 years when alveoli are normally increasing in number. Overdistention and alveolar septal destruction are not present, and so this condition does not fit the definition of true emphysema. Most often the pulmonary artery on the affected side is hypoplastic. Although usually an incidental finding, the affected lung may become repeatedly infected so that surgical excision may be indicated.

MISCELLANEOUS DIFFUSE OBSTRUCTIVE SYNDROMES   *Bronchiolitis obliterans* is a term applied to widespread inflammatory and fibrotic obstruction of small airways. Initially this syndrome was thought to be restricted to those persons who had suffered severe viral infections in childhood, particularly those due to parainfluenza virus. However, recently this syndrome has also been described in adult patients with rheumatoid arthritis. The response to bronchodilator treatment is poor, as would be expected from the histopathologic findings, and fatal respiratory failure often ensues within 2 years. There have been reports suggesting a relationship between penicillamine therapy and the development of bronchiolitis obliterans in patients with rheumatoid arthritis; however, it is clear that this syndrome can develop in patients who have never received penicillamine.

A syndrome with similar histopathology has been described in recipients of autologous bone marrow transplants. Although most often interstitial pneumonitis and fibrosis are sequelae, it has been documented that some patients develop a bronchiolitis obliterans picture. It appears that the development of this process occurs most often in the setting of a chronic graft-versus-host syndrome; however, it is clear that diffuse airways obstruction has developed without evidence of this syndrome in bone marrow recipients.

Cystic fibrosis in the adult with chronic airways obstruction is discussed elsewhere (Chap. 209).

REFERENCES

ANTHONISEN NR: Home oxygen therapy, in *Update VI: Principles of Internal Medicine*, RG Petersdorf et al (eds). New York, McGraw-Hill, 1985, p 203

BLOCK ER: Oxygen therapy, in *Update: Pulmonary Diseases and Disorders*, AP Fishman (ed). New York, McGraw-Hill, 1982, p 349

CAMPBELL AH et al: Factors affecting the decline of ventilatory function in chronic bronchitis. Thorax 40:741, 1985

CATTERAL JR et al: Mechanism of transient nocturnal hypoxemia in hypoxic chronic bronchitis and emphysema. J Appl Physiol 59:1698, 1985

COHEN AB (ed): Proteases and antiproteases in the lung. Am Rev Resp Dis 127 (Suppl):S1, 1983

CHETTY KG et al: Improved exercise tolerance of the polycythemic lung patient following phlebotomy. Am J Med 74:415, 1983

EFTHIMOU J et al: The effect of supplementary oral nutrition in poorly nourished patients with chronic obstructive pulmonary disease. Am Rev Resp Dis 137:1075, 1988

FISHMAN AP: The spectrum of chronic obstructive disease of the airways, in *Pulmonary Diseases and Disorders*, 2d ed, AP Fishman (ed). New York, McGraw-Hill, 1987, Chap 68

LAROS CD et al: Bullectomy for giant bullae in emphysema. J Thorac Cardiovasc Surg 91:63, 1986

PUSA T, TCHERZEWSKI H: Analysis of proteolytic enzymes and their natural inhibitors in serum and bronchial lavage fluid in atopic bronchial asthma, chronic bronchitis and pneumonia. Allerg Immunol 31:169, 1985

THURLBECK WM: A pathologist's approach to clinical bronchitis and emphysema, in *Update: Pulmonary Diseases and Disorders*, AP Fishman (ed). New York, McGraw-Hill, 1982, p 137

---

211   INTERSTITIAL LUNG DISEASES

HERBERT Y. REYNOLDS

The interstitial lung diseases (ILDs) are a heterogeneous group of conditions that involve the alveolar walls and perialveolar tissue. The ILDs are nonmalignant and are not caused by any defined infectious agents. Although an acute phase of illness may occur, the onset is often insidious, and the disease is usually chronic in duration. The initial response of the host to the disease process is inflammation in the air spaces and alveolar walls, causing an acute phase of intraluminal and mural alveolitis. If the disease is chronic and smoldering, inflammation will spread to adjacent portions of the interstitium and vasculature and eventually produce interstitial fibrosis. The resultant scarring and distortion of lung tissue leads to significant derangement of gas exchange and ventilatory function. Inflammation can also involve the conducting airways, and bronchiolitis obliterans associated with an organizing pneumonia is probably part of the spectrum of an ILD.

This diverse group of diseases have many features in common, including similarity of symptoms, comparable appearance of chest radiographs, consistent alterations in pulmonary physiology, and typical histologic features. However, ILDs have been difficult to classify, because approximately 180 known individual diseases are characterized by interstitial lung involvement, either as primary disease or as a significant part of a multiorgan process, as occurs in the collagen vascular diseases. The chest radiograph is of limited aid in classification since it can have a similar appearance in many of the ILDs as well as in other unrelated lung diseases. One useful approach for classification is to separate ILDs into two groups, those with known causes and those with unknown causes; each of these groups can be divided into subgroups according to the presence or absence of histologic evidence of granulomas in interstitial or vascular areas (Table 211-1). For each ILD there may be an acute phase, and there is usually a chronic one as well.

Among the ILDs of known cause, the largest group comprises occupational and environmental inhalant exposures; these include diseases due to inhalation of inorganic dusts (Chap. 206), organic dusts, and various irritative or noxious gases (Chap. 205). The number of ILDs of unknown cause is also very large. The major ones within this category are idiopathic pulmonary fibrosis (IPF), sarcoidosis, and the ILD often associated with collagen vascular disorders. ILD secondary to inorganic dust exposure usually can be recognized if the occupational history is pursued. For the myriad (Table 211-1) of other diffuse ILDs, however, a precise diagnosis is obtained with difficulty, usually only after interpretation of an open-lung biopsy specimen; most of these diseases are relatively rare.

Although the initiating agent(s) or circumstances of the various ILDs may be diverse, and many are unknown, the immunopathogenic responses of lung tissue are limited, so that the initial mechanisms of injury, the development of alveolitis, and the attempts at repair sometimes leading to fibrosis will have common features. Idiopathic pulmonary fibrosis is discussed as the prototype ILD, as it is encountered relatively frequently and much of the recent research on mechanisms of lung fibrosis has focused on this disease.

TABLE 211-1 Major categories of alveolar and interstitial inflammatory lung diseases (ILDs)

Known cause	Unknown cause
LUNG RESPONSE: ALVEOLITIS, INTERSTITIAL INFLAMMATION, AND FIBROSIS	
Asbestos	Idiopathic pulmonary fibrosis
Fumes, gases	Collagen vascular diseases
Drugs (antibiotics) and chemotherapy drugs	Systemic lupus erythematosus, rheumatoid arthritis, ankylosing spondylitis,
Radiation	systemic sclerosis, Sjögren's syndrome,
Aspiration pneumonia	polymyositis-dermatomyositis
Residual of adult respiratory distress syndrome	Pulmonary hemorrhage syndromes
	Goodpasture's syndrome, idiopathic pulmonary hemosiderosis
	Pulmonary alveolar proteinosis
	Lymphocytic infiltrative disorders (lymphocytic interstitial pneumonitis)
	Eosinophilic pneumonias
	Lymphangioleiomyomatosis
	Amyloidosis
	Inherited diseases
	Tuberous sclerosis, neurofibromatosis, Niemann-Pick disease, Gaucher's disease, Hermansky-Pudlak syndrome
	Gastrointestinal or liver diseases (Crohn's disease, primary biliary cirrhosis, chronic active hepatitis, ulcerative colitis)
	Graft vs. host disease (bone marrow transplantation)
LUNG RESPONSE: AS ABOVE BUT WITH GRANULOMA	
Hypersensitivity pneumonitis (organic dusts)	Sarcoidosis
Inorganic dusts: beryllium silica	Langerhans cell granulomatosis (eosinophilic granuloma)
	Granulomatous vasculitides
	Wegener's granulomatosis, allergic granulomatosis of Churg-Strauss, lymphomatoid granulomatosis
	Bronchocentric granulomatosis

IDIOPATHIC PULMONARY FIBROSIS (IPF)

Many patients who present with nonproductive cough, progressive dyspnea, a chest radiograph showing lower lung zone reticular shadows, and pulmonary function tests showing a restrictive pattern (Chap. 201) will be said to have IPF after the diagnostic evaluation is completed. This condition is also known as *cryptogenic fibrosing alveolitis*. Although the terms *idiopathic* and *cryptogenic* mean that the etiologic agent is unknown, this is not a nebulous, wastebasket diagnosis or just a diagnosis of exclusion but rather a well-defined clinical entity.

IMMUNOPATHOGENESIS Several parts of the alveolar structure are affected in IPF, including the alveolar walls lined with type I and type II pneumocytes and the interstitial supporting structure composed of mesenchymal cells, especially fibroblasts and myofibroblasts, collagen, and various adhesive proteoglycans. The capillary endothelium may also be involved. The disease process does not affect the upper or conducting airways, but bronchiolitis of respiratory bronchioles may be present and alveolar units are always involved.

Normally, overlying or interspersed in the alveoli are a variety of immune cells including alveolar macrophages, dendritic macrophages, interstitial monocytes, lymphocytes, and inflammatory cells, such as polymorphonuclear leukocytes (PMNs) and eosinophils. The cellular content of normal bronchoalveolar lavage (BAL) fluid consists of approximately 80 percent alveolar macrophages, 10 percent lymphocytes (of which 70 percent are T lymphocytes), 1 to 5 percent B lymphocytes or plasma cells, 1 to 3 percent polymorphonuclear leukocytes, and 1 percent eosinophils.

In the earliest, reversible forms of alveolar injury, leakiness of the alveolar type I cells and the adjacent capillary endothelial cells

occurs, causing alveolar and interstitial edema and the formation of intraalveolar hyaline membranes. With persistence of the disease, increased alveolar-capillary permeability and desquamation of intraalveolar cells (alveolitis), mural inflammation, and interstitial fibrosis are present on biopsy. This process is also reflected in the composition of cells and enzymes recovered in BAL fluid (Table 211-2) and in cellular components present in lung biopsy tissue. The presence and severity of the disease process are spotty in distribution; a continuum of inflammatory and fibrotic changes can be found throughout the affected lung.

Figure 211-1 depicts schematically immunopathogenic mechanisms that interconnect the intraalveolar (luminal) and alveolar mural tissue with the interstitial space and capillary vascular areas. The inciting agent or stimulus is often unknown but is likely an antigen that can initiate an immunoglobulin response. This is reflected by an increased ratio of IgG subclasses IgG1 and G3, an increased number of IgG-releasing cells, and perhaps the formation of immune complexes. IgG may function as an opsonin or as part of an immune complex that interacts with the surface of the alveolar macrophage.

An increased number of macrophages, which are activated phagocytes capable of producing many cytokines that affect other lung cells, are a hallmark of the alveolitis. These macrophage cytokines or mediators could operate in two directions. First, through the production of chemotaxins, which may include leukotriene LTB_4, inflammatory cells such as PMNs and eosinophils are attracted into the alveoli. An increased percentage of PMNs (20 percent or more) and eosinophils (1 to 4 percent) in the profile of BAL cells is usual in IPF. Lymphocytes are not usually increased, unless the IPF is part of a collagen vascular disease. Enzymes or oxidant radicals from inflammatory cells and histamine may cause local injury or alter the permeability of type I cells. Second, macrophages are also capable of secreting substances that stimulate mesenchymal cells. For fibroblasts to replicate in the interstitium and in the alveolar walls, they must first be attracted and adhere to a connective tissue matrix and then be primed to enter the G_1 phase of a growth cycle to proliferate.

Several products from alveolar macrophages can participate in these steps. Platelet-derived growth factor (PDGF) (see p. 60) is a

TABLE 211-2 Cellular and immunologic changes in various IPF specimens

BLOOD

IgG (IgG1,3) elevated immune complexes, cryoglobulins
Serologic titers (low)
T lymphocytes (sensitized to type I collagen)

BRONCHOALVEOLAR FLUID

Alveolitis characterized by increased percentage of PMNs (20%) and eosinophils (2–4%), but lymphocytes can be increased also (20%)
Alveolar macrophages: activated macrophages and their secretory components are numerous:
   Chemotaxins to attract PMNs and muscle cells
   Plasminogen activator
   Macrophage-derived growth factor
   Fibronectin
   Platelet-derived growth factor (by c-*sis* oncogene)
Steroid receptors increased; mitotic index increased
Collagenase (PMN origin)
IgG increased (G3, G1 subclasses)
Immune complexes detectable
IgG-releasing cells present
Histamine elevated

LUNG TISSUE

Interstitial inflammation
Plasma cells, muscle cells, fibroblasts increased
Collagen synthesis increased
Fibrosis but no granuloma
Bronchiolitis obliterans can develop

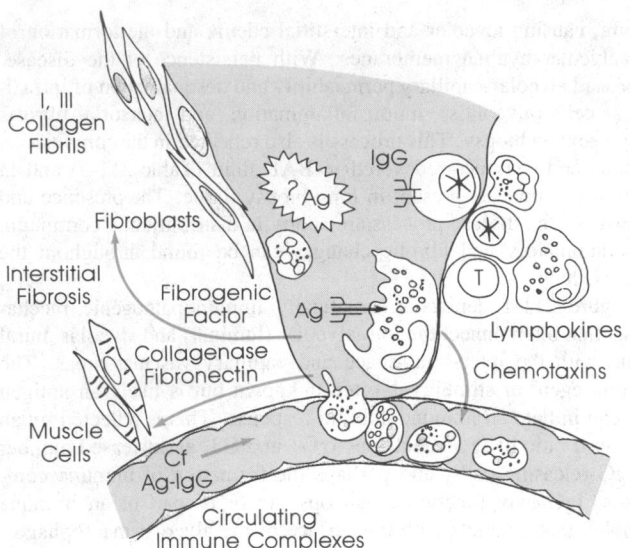

FIGURE 211-1 Immunologic mechanisms within the alveolar space, alveolar walls, and interstitium that can lead to inflammation and eventual fibrosis. The focus is on the alveolor macrophage, which is activated, possibly by an immune complex and an as yet unidentified antigen (Ag). Through mediators such as chemotaxins, the macrophage attracts PMNs and other cells from the circulation to the alveolar space, or it can initiate fibrogenesis with various mediators that can stimulate fibroblasts and muscle cells to proliferate. Interstitial fibrosis may result. *(From Reynolds, 1986.)*

chemoattractant for mesenchymal cells and a stimulus for fibroblasts to change from resting cells to cells entering G_1. Although PDGF is not produced by normal monocytes or macrophages, alveolar macrophages obtained from patients with IPF make it abundantly. This is correlated with c-*sis*, a proto-oncogene that codes for the beta chain of PDGF, which is increased in IPF-derived macrophages and which may drive the exaggerated release of PDGF. This mediator acts as a chemoattractant and a growth factor for fibroblasts. Later in the fibroblast replication cycle, alveolar macrophage-derived growth factor (AMDGF) can accelerate proliferation. Insulin and other cellular or metabolic substances are also needed in these growth-regulatory steps. Smooth-muscle cells can also proliferate. With continued activity of macrophages, fibrosis becomes more widespread and may involve the vasculature. Obliteration of functional alveolar structures occurs with scar tissue formation, and cystic areas develop from retraction of the terminal airways that once subtended the alveolar unit.

CLINICAL PRESENTATION   History On the average, patients are 50 years old, although the range spans infancy to old age. Several family clusters have been reported, and it is possible that genetic factors may determine susceptibility to the disease. The first clinical manifestations of ILD are dyspnea, effort intolerance, and a dry cough without other obvious cause. A detailed work history is essential. For example, casual exposure to asbestos many years previously may provide a crucial clue to the etiology. Work-related compensation may influence complaints for some individuals.

Approximately one-third of patients can pinpoint their awareness of dyspnea to the aftermath of a viral respiratory illness. Usually months or years elapse between the onset of exertional dyspnea and its progression perhaps to the point of breathlessness at rest. Dyspnea and frequent coughing are often accompanied by other constitutional symptoms such as fatigue, anorexia, weight loss, and arthralgias.

Physical findings Initially, the physical examination may not be revealing and auscultation of the chest may be normal. As the disease advances, dry rales, or coarse crackles on inspiration, are usually heard at the lung bases. There may be tachypnea at rest, cyanosis, and clubbing of the fingers and toes, usually without hypertrophic osteoarthropathy. In later stages, cor pulmonale (Chap.

191) is evident, with findings of pulmonary hypertension, such as an accentuated pulmonic second sound or a right-sided lift, and eventually signs of right heart failure. The right ventricular ejection fraction determined by radionuclide ventriculography is often depressed in the face of normal left ventricular performance.

LABORATORY AND DIAGNOSTIC TESTS   Imaging studies The chest radiograph usually reveals a pattern of diffuse reticular markings, prominent in the lower lung zones. Several radiographic patterns can be seen which correlate roughly with the duration of the disease. Early, a hazy "ground glass" appearance of the lower lung fields coincides with the stage of acute alveolitis. Later, curvilinear shadows predominate and may coalesce into nodular infiltrates. With end-stage disease, the linear opacities are seen in all lung fields, the lung fields appear contracted, and ring-shaped opacities resulting from cystic and bronchiectatic changes are obvious, creating the *honeycombed* or *swiss cheese* appearance of the lung. Biopsy-proven forms of diffuse IPF occasionally occur in patients with normal chest radiographs despite significant exercise intolerance, abnormal pulmonary function tests, including a reduced diffusing capacity, and dry rales.

Use of gallium 67 citrate scanning can be helpful in assessing inflammation of the lung parenchyma, as its uptake may correlate with the presence of PMNs in the airways and lung tissue. CT scanning, utilizing ultrathin cuts of 0.5 cm, is a sensitive means of documenting tissue infiltration and the presence of bronchiectasis or pleural changes.

Laboratory examination The erythrocyte sedimentation rate is usually elevated, circulating immune-complex titers and serum immunoglobulin levels may be increased, and cryoimmunoglobulins may be present. Serologic tests to screen for collagen vascular diseases are necessary to exclude these diagnoses. Although serum rheumatoid factor, antinuclear antibodies, depressed levels of complement, and other parameters of autoimmune diseases may be detected in approximately 10 percent of patients with IPF, the titers are generally quite low.

Lung function tests In patients with advanced disease, reductions in total lung capacity, vital capacity, and residual volume are found (Chap. 201). Usually evidence of airway obstruction is minimal and the FEV_1/FVC ratio is normal or increased. A restrictive respiratory functional pattern is usually present, reflecting the stiff, noncompliant lungs characteristic of IPF and its common aftermath, fibrosis. There is usually resting arterial hypoxemia, but the carbon dioxide tension is normal or decreased. Blood pH is normal. The alveolar-arterial oxygen gradient during exercise is elevated, and exercise tolerance is reduced. The carbon monoxide diffusing capacity is usually reduced by 30 to 50 percent. Changes in these variables are useful in monitoring the course of the illness and in assessing the effectiveness of treatment.

Bronchoscopy Direct investigation of the airways by fiberoptic bronchoscopy is part of the evaluation, and four to six transbronchial biopsies are taken to obtain lung tissue for diagnosis. These provide a sufficient quantity of tissue for a definitive pathologic diagnosis in approximately one-fourth of all cases of IPF. In some diffuse granulomatous interstitial diseases, such as sarcoidosis (Chap. 277), transbronchial biopsy will provide a tissue diagnosis in about 80 percent of cases. Bronchoscopy also permits bronchoalveolar lavage, which provides useful information about cells and proteins in the airways that generally correlates with histologic changes in the interstitial and alveolar tissues. An analysis of BAL fluid and cells can reveal a number of changes in IPF (Table 211-2).

Lung biopsy The importance of an adequate sample of lung tissue to permit a full histologic evaluation, good microbial cultures, immunofluorescence and electron-microscopic studies, and analysis of inorganic substances cannot be overemphasized. Therefore, if a transbronchial biopsy does not yield sufficient tissue for a confident diagnosis, open-lung biopsy should be considered. It is prudent to substantiate a tissue diagnosis before embarking on immunosuppressive therapy with its attendant complications.

DIAGNOSTIC APPROACH AND STAGING OF DISEASE ACTIV-ITY Following the clinical examination, chest radiograph, pulmonary function tests [lung volumes, FEV_1/FVC, and diffusing capacity (Chap. 201)], and arterial blood gas determination, the functional disability from the lung disease can be estimated. However, a histologic analysis of lung tissue should be made before the disease is diagnosed definitively. Fiberoptic bronchoscopy is usually the first invasive procedure and is important for ruling out infection, malignancy, and other specific diseases. Although transbronchial biopsy has a lower diagnostic yield in IPF than in sarcoidosis and other granulomatous diseases, it is nevertheless a useful, low-risk procedure with a 20 to 30 percent success rate for obtaining an adequate sample for a confident pathologic diagnosis. BAL for cellular and protein analysis may be useful in judging the nature of alveolar inflammation and immunologic activity (Table 211-2). However, the value of the periodic use of BAL analysis to monitor disease activity or its response to therapy has not been established. Use of gallium 67 lung scanning does not add diagnostic accuracy but may be an indication of general cellular activity in the lung.

If the diagnosis is still in doubt after the bronchoscopy and related procedures, an open-lung biopsy should be considered. The referring physician and the thoracic surgeon should cooperate in choosing the most representative area of the lung for biopsy, and the proper microbial cultures and immunologic studies can be obtained.

THERAPY Treatment is usually offered to patients with IPF, even to patients with advanced fibrotic disease. About 2 weeks after the open-lung biopsy, a trial of oral prednisone can be instituted in a dose of 1 mg/kg daily and continued for 8 to 12 weeks. If lung disease shows objective improvement, the dose is tapered to a maintenance level. Should the disease not respond or be progressive, the dosage of prednisone can be increased, but immunosuppression with cyclophosphamide should be considered. Cyclophosphamide is given at a dose of about 1.0 mg/kg daily (50 to 75 mg) with the patient continuing on a daily maintenance dose of oral prednisone (0.25 mg/kg). The dosages of cyclophosphamide may be increased as necessary by 50-mg increments at 7 to 10-day intervals. The objective is to reduce the white blood cell count to approximately half the normal baseline value, causing a distinct drop in the total blood lymphocyte count. However, a minimum count of 1000 polymorphonuclear leukocytes per microliter should be maintained.

Several other measures may help respiratory function. It is imperative that patients discontinue cigarette smoking. Since there is frequently a marked drop in Pa_{O_2} with exercise, supplemental oxygen therapy may be useful, sometimes using transtracheal catheter oxygen delivery. As the pulmonary vascular bed is destroyed by progressive fibrosis, pulmonary hypertension and cor pulmonale can develop; right-sided congestive heart failure can be difficult to control. Judicious use of diuretics is advised, and digitalis may be required, although adequate oxygenation is probably the best treatment for right heart failure (Chap. 191). Some patients may also develop obstruction to airflow and wheezing and coughing which may respond to bronchodilators. Infection may occur during immunosuppressive therapy and should be treated promptly and aggressively. Prophylactic use of pneumococcal and influenza vaccines is indicated. If refractory disease limited to the chest is present, the possibility of lung transplantation should be considered. Recent successes with single-lung transplantation for ILD make this therapy a reality for some patients.

INDIVIDUAL FORMS OF ILD

ILD ASSOCIATED WITH COLLAGEN VASCULAR DISORDERS In these diseases, various pulmonary structures can be affected, especially the pleura, so that ILD is but one manifestation of intrathoracic involvement and often a minor part of the multiorgan process. Analysis of BAL fluid and cells from patients with ILD associated with rheumatoid arthritis and systemic sclerosis is similar to that found in IPF (Table 211-2) and suggests similar pathogenetic mechanisms for fibrosis. A lymphocytic alveolitis may accompany some cases of ILD in rheumatoid disease and is a harbinger of a better response to immunosuppressive therapy.

Systemic lupus erythematosus (SLE) (See Chap. 269) About half of patients with SLE ultimately develop overt lung disease. Pleuritis, pleural effusion(s), or acute pneumonitis are the most frequent forms of lung disease, while a chronic, progressive ILD is uncommon. Although pleuropulmonary involvement may not be evident clinically, pulmonary function testing, particularly the diffusing capacity for carbon monoxide, reveals abnormalities in many patients.

Rheumatoid arthritis (See Chap. 270) A variety of pulmonary manifestations can occur, including pleural disease (pleural effusion and subpleural nodules), parenchymal nodular infiltrates associated with pneumoconiosis in miners (Caplan's syndrome), and diffuse interstitial fibrosis. The ILD can develop before joint disease becomes evident, particularly in men, and is accompanied by high titers of rheumatoid factor. Rarely, upper airway obstruction can occur from arthritis of the cricoarytenoid joint. Patients with rheumatoid arthritis who are receiving treatment with methotrexate or gold may develop ILD that represents a drug hypersensitivity, which must be differentiated from a preexisting or developing ILD associated with the underlying disease. Penicillamine therapy in patients with rheumatoid arthritis has been implicated in causing bronchiolitis obliterans (p. 1082).

Ankylosing spondylitis (See Chap. 274) Bilateral upper lobe fibrosis, which can be complicated by fibrocavitary disease, may develop late in the course.

Systemic sclerosis (See Chap. 271) Radiographic evidence of lung involvement develops in a majority of patients, but its severity or progression is variable. Because distal esophageal motor dysfunction is present in many patients, reflux with regurgitation and chronic aspiration is common. In addition, cutaneous scleroderma can involve the anterior chest wall and abdomen, causing restrictive lung function.

Sjögren's syndrome (See Chap. 273) General dryness and lack of airways secretions cause the major problems of hoarseness, cough, and bronchitis. Presence of an ILD in these patients may signify a lymphocytic infiltrate in lung tissue which can behave as a low-grade lymphoma.

Polymyositis and dermatomyositis (See Chap. 364) Although ILD is reported to occur in only 5 to 10 percent of patients, its presence is more common in the subgroup of patients with an anti-Jo-1 antibody that is directed to tRNA synthetase. Weakness of respiratory muscles contributing to aspiration pneumonitis is a common occurrence.

SYNDROMES OF ILD WITH PULMONARY HEMORRHAGE Recurrent hemoptysis, dyspnea, and hypoxemia in the presence of a chest radiographic pattern of diffuse alveolar opacities should raise the possibility of alveolar hemorrhage. An association between vasculitis involving the kidney (lung-renal syndromes) or other organ systems should be investigated. Alveolar hemorrhage occurs rarely in all collagen vascular disorders, but it is described most often with systemic lupus erythematosus. It can occur with systemic vasculitis and is described as an initial presentation of Wegener's granulomatosis; with Behçet's disease, in which aneurysm formation and rupture of small muscular arteries is a manifestation of necrotizing vasculitis; in allergic Churg-Strauss granulomatosis; in Henoch-Schönlein purpura syndrome; and in essential (mixed) cryoimmunoglobulinemia. Exposure to the toxic aerosol trimellitic anhydride may cause alveolar hemorrhage. Serologic tests for antinuclear antibody, anti-glomerular basement membrane antibody, and complement to document a vasculitis and immunologic disorder are the first steps, but renal biopsy and possibly lung biopsy may be required for a definitive diagnosis. Some specific syndromes in this category will be discussed next.

Goodpasture's syndrome (See Chap. 228) Pulmonary hemorrhage and glomerulonephritis are the features of this disease in which most patients have antibodies to renal glomerular and lung alveolar basement membranes.

Idiopathic pulmonary hemosiderosis   Diffuse alveolar hemorrhage can occur in the absence of other organ involvement or an obvious immunologic cause and is therefore a diagnosis of exclusion after considering the many causes of alveolar bleeding associated with collagen vascular and vasculitic diseases. A lung biopsy is usually necessary to document the lack of inflammatory injury in the lung tissues and to exclude other diseases with confidence. The clinical course can be variable, ranging from a recurrent and fulminant one with development of progressive interstitial fibrosis to minimal disease that may remit without sequelae. Children and young adults are usually affected. Glucocorticoid treatment is useful for control of bleeding acutely but is not a predictable long-term remedy for keeping the disease suppressed and preventing recurrence.

PULMONARY ALVEOLAR PROTEINOSIS   Similar clinical symptoms and the general appearance of the chest radiograph, showing diffuse alveolar consolidation and/or nodular shadows typically radiating from the hilar regions, place pulmonary alveolar proteinosis (PAP) in the ILD category. Histologically the alveoli are filled with granular material that stains with periodic acid Schiff reagent, but they exhibit no inflammation and have relatively normal septal structure. Strictly speaking, then, PAP is an intraalveolar process which resembles, but is not, an ILD. Because the proteinaceous response can be associated with inhaled dust exposure (silica and aluminum), malignancy, and chronic infection, termed *secondary PAP*, these disorders should be differentiated from primary PAP by lung biopsy. The intraalveolar material is a combination of surfactant phospholipid produced by type II pneumocytes and of other proteins and immunoglobulins found in alveolar lining fluid. The cytoplasm of alveolar macrophages appears engorged with inclusions. The "stuffed" macrophages with large phagolysosomes have diminished microbial killing capacity in vitro, but lung infections with unusual organisms are not frequent. Whole-lung lavage(s) will provide relief to many patients with dyspnea and progressive deterioration of arterial oxygenation and may also provide long-term benefit.

LYMPHOCYTIC INFILTRATIVE DISORDERS   This is a group of disorders that feature lymphocyte and plasma cell infiltration of the lung parenchyma and either are benign or can behave as low-grade lymphomas. Within the spectrum of chronic interstitial pneumonias, referred to as IPFs, a subset has been described with lung histology that shows diffuse interstitial infiltration with lymphocytes and plasma cells. In some of these patients an autoimmune disease or dysproteinemia exists. However, lymphocytic interstitial pneumonia (LIP) is probably not a distinct entity, belongs within the IPF group, and can be associated with Sjögren's syndrome. LIP has been reported in patients, particularly children, with AIDS.

Included among these disorders is immunoblastic lymphadenopathy, also termed *angioimmunoblastic lymphadenopathy*, which usually is a fulminant lymphoma-like disease that may have an element of ILD in some cases. *Lymphomatoid granulomatosis* can be included, but its granulomatous response also places it with the granulomatous ILDs (Table 211-1).

EOSINOPHILIC PNEUMONIAS (See Chap. 205)   These pneumonias encompass a spectrum of diseases in which lung hypersensitivity plays a role and in which a specific cause may or may not be identified. For example, with extrinsic asthma and exposure to fungal antigens, allergic bronchopulmonary mycosis can develop; filarial and other parasitic infections can cause tropical pulmonary eosinophilia; many common drugs can induce eosinophilic pneumonia. Chronic eosinophilic pneumonia has features that make it difficult to distinguish from IPF and other forms of progressive ILD. The disease, which more commonly affects older females, has several radiologic characteristics that are helpful in diagnosis: (1) a peripheral pattern of dense lung infiltrates that appear to cross anatomic lobar boundaries with sparing of the central lung regions; (2) regression but reappearance of infiltrates in the same lung locations; and (3) extreme sensitivity of the infiltrates (and disease symptoms) to modest doses of oral glucocorticoids. The diagnosis can be established by lung biopsy, which shows an eosinophilic inflammatory process.

LYMPHANGIOLEIOMYOMATOSIS   Immature smooth-muscle cells can proliferate in lung tissue around and throughout bronchial, vascular, and lymphatic structures, causing local obstruction or creating constricting lesions that develop into cysts. Lymphatics and lymph nodes in other organs are also usually affected. Because this disorder occurs predominantly in females of reproductive age, an association between estrogens and the disease is probable. Pulmonary symptoms consist of dyspnea, cough, and hemoptysis; a more overt presentation occurs with spontaneous pneumothorax, which can be recurrent, or with chylous effusion. In addition, the chest radiograph shows reticulonodular shadows and small cyst-like areas or honeycombing throughout the lung fields. In contrast to most forms of ILD, lung volumes are normal or increased, as is also the case with Langerhans cell granulomatosis (see below). Therapy for progressive lung disease has not been particularly effective. Pneumothoraxes and effusions may require chemical or surgical pleurodesis. Treatment with progesterone combined with ovariectomy has been used. Lung transplantation may be considered for some patients.

AMYLOIDOSIS (See Chap. 266)   Deposits of amyloid in the form of plaques or nodules can develop at all sites of the respiratory tract. Tracheal and endobronchial mucosal plaques or incidental parenchymal nodules can be difficult to diagnose clinically, but they usually coexist with extrapulmonary manifestations of primary or, less commonly, secondary amyloidosis. Lung biopsy is necessary for definitive diagnosis. As part of primary systemic amyloidosis or a plasma cell dyscrasia, an ILD may occur from amyloid deposits in alveolar septa and associated blood vessels, producing dyspnea, radiographic findings of diffuse reticulonodular shadows, and restrictive pulmonary function.

INHERITED DISORDERS ASSOCIATED WITH ILD   Pulmonary infiltrates and respiratory symptoms typical of mild ILD can develop in related family members and in several inherited diseases. These include the phacomatoses (Chap. 358) tuberous sclerosis and neurofibromatosis and the lysosomal storage diseases (Chap. 331), such as Niemann-Pick disease and Gaucher's disease. The *Hermansky-Pudlak syndrome* is an autosomal recessive disorder, in which granulomatous colitis and ILD may occur. It is characterized by oculocutaneous albinism, bleeding diathesis from platelet dysfunction, and the accumulation of a chromolipid, lipofuscin material in cells of the reticuloendothelial system. The pulmonary fibrosis is similar to IPF, but the alveolar macrophages may contain cytoplasmic ceroid-like inclusions.

GASTROINTESTINAL AND LIVER DISEASE   Rarely, inflammatory bowel disease and chronic hepatitis may be associated with a mild form of ILD. Crohn's disease, which has a number of similarities with sarcoidosis, may also be accompanied by asymptomatic lymphocytic alveolitis.

GRAFT VS. HOST DISEASE (GVHD) (See Chap. 299)   Some degree of GVHD occurs in all patients receiving bone marrow transplantation. However, in about 10 percent a chronic phase may ensue with the onset of dry cough, mucositis, dyspnea, and airflow obstruction in the small airways, as demonstrated by pulmonary function testing. Chest radiographs reveal peribronchiolar infiltrates, and lung biopsy shows focal areas of interstitial infiltration with a mixture of lymphocytes and PMNs. The lesions are consistent with bronchiolitis; no vasculitis is present. Some recipients of heart-lung transplants also develop bronchiolitis. Bronchiolitis in chronic GVHD may stabilize and disappear or may be progressive and fatal. Treatment includes increasing the doses of the immunosuppressive drugs together with bronchodilators and antibiotics. Infection, especially with viral agents, is a common complication.

ILD WITH A GRANULOMATOUS RESPONSE IN LUNG TISSUE OR VASCULAR STRUCTURES   Inhalation of organic dusts, which causes hypersensitivity pneumonitis, or of inorganic particles such as silica, which causes alveolitis and elicits a granulomatous inflammatory reaction leading to ILD, produces diseases of known etiology (Table 211-1) that are discussed in Chaps. 205 and 206. Sarcoidosis (Chap. 277) is prominent among granulomatous diseases of *unknown cause* in which ILD is an important feature.

Langerhans cell granulomatosis (eosinophilic granuloma or histiocytosis X) (See Chap. 63) This condition is being recognized with increasing frequency and may account for about 1 to 5 percent of ILD of unknown etiology. Previously, the proliferation of tissue macrophages (histiocytes) was thought to be characteristic of this disease that affects the lung, bones, and viscera. Now it is recognized that the precursor cell is the *dendritic cell*, which has potent stimulatory and accessory cell immune function, is normally found in the interstitium and alveolar septal areas, and is distinctly different from a tissue macrophage. The dendritic cell can evolve into the Langerhans cell, characterized by a specific CD1a surface antigen that reacts with a monoclonal antibody identified as T_6, and by intracytoplasmic organelles seen by electron microscopy that are called X bodies or Birbeck granules. Langerhans cells can be identified in skin and are present in bronchiolar epithelium of normal lung. Cigarette smoking or a similar irritant seems to be a stimulus for their proliferation. An increased number of these cells can be recovered in BAL from normal smokers, patients with bronchoalveolar carcinoma, and patients with IPF. However, in Langerhans cell granulomatosis of the lung, 3 percent or more of the BAL cells may be so identified, which greatly exceeds the percentage found in these other disorders. However, the Langerhans cells are not pathognomonic for this disease. The number of alveolar macrophages is also increased. Early in the disease a focus of Langerhans and surrounding inflammatory cells can be found adjacent to respiratory and terminal bronchioles, causing bronchiolitis. Later, alveolar structures are involved in progressive interstitial inflammation and fibrosis. In advanced disease, lung histology does *not* reveal the discrete typical granulomas that are found in sarcoidosis and hypersensitivity pneumonitis, nor are eosinophils greatly increased—two reasons that the prior appellation, "eosinophilic granuloma," was really a misnomer.

The pulmonary form of this disease occurs in young and middle-aged adults, usually males, and in those who use tobacco heavily; it may remain focal or involve one or several bony sites (long bones, spine, skull, or jaw). Occasionally, multifocal disease can affect the posterior pituitary gland, causing diabetes insipidus, a condition that is termed *Hand-Schüller-Christian disease*. In infants, *Letterer-Siwe disease* is a more fulminant visceral form of this disorder that mimics a malignant lymphoma. In adults, the presenting symptoms and signs do not distinguish this disease from other forms of ILD unless signs of a bone lesion exist. A spontaneous pneumothorax may herald the disease. Chest radiographs will show diffuse micronodular shadows and cystic spaces, sparing the costophrenic angles and preserving lung volume, as occurs in lymphangioleiomyomatosis. Pulmonary function tests may disclose a combination of obstructive and restrictive defects. As the disease progresses, greater airway obstruction may develop, and the chest radiograph can resemble that in advanced chronic obstructive lung disease. Treatment involves a mandatory cessation of tobacco use, which may cause the pulmonary disease to stabilize or regress. Glucocorticoids usually are not helpful. Penicillamine has been used in an attempt to prevent fibrosis with variable success. Local bone lesions may require radiation. For patients with increasing symptoms of airway obstruction, supportive therapy and bronchodilators may be tried, but their success has been modest.

Granulomatous vasculitis (See Chap. 276) Certain forms of vasculitis, accompanied by a granulomatous response, can involve the respiratory tract as part of a multiorgan process or can occasionally be localized to the respiratory tract, as occurs with a predominantly pulmonary form of Wegener's granulomatosis in which glomerulonephritis may not be prominent. It is very important to differentiate these conditions from lymphomatoid granulomatosis. Allergic angiitis and the granulomatosis of Churg and Strauss are forms of granulomatous vasculitis affecting many organs but especially the lungs; a history of asthma and the presence of eosinophilia are distinguishing features.

Lymphomatoid granulomatosis (See Chaps. 63 and 276) This involves primarily the lungs and less frequently the skin, central and peripheral nervous systems, and kidneys with an infiltration of lymphocytoid, plasmalike cells and macrophages creating a necrotic granulomatous inflammatory reaction, especially in or near blood vessels. The disease can progress as a lymphoproliferative disorder and evolve into malignant lymphoma in as many as 50 percent of patients. Treatment of lymphomatoid granulomatosis with glucocorticoids and cyclophosphamide may induce a remission, and if this occurs, subsequent relapse and development of lymphoma are not likely.

BRONCHOCENTRIC GRANULOMATOSIS In contrast to the necrotizing granulomatous reaction in lung vessels, i.e., angiocentric vasculitis, granulomatous destruction of bronchioles occurs in this condition. There is usually associated parenchymal inflammation causing ILD. Eosinophils can be present if asthma and hypersensitivity to fungal antigens within the bronchi have occurred. In other cases without these associated conditions, hypersensitivity to other microbial antigens is postulated. Bronchocentric granulomatosis must be differentiated from hypersensitivity pneumonitis caused by inhalation of organic dusts (see Chaps. 205 and 206).

REFERENCES

Idiopathic pulmonary fibrosis

CRYSTAL RG et al: Interstitial lung diseases of unknown cause: Disorders characterized by chronic inflammation of the lower respiratory tract. N Engl J Med 310:154, 235, 1984

EPLER GR et al: Bronchiolitis obliterans with organizing pneumonia. N Engl J Med 312:152, 1985

REYNOLDS HY: Idiopathic interstitial pulmonary fibrosis: Contribution of bronchoalveolar lavage analysis. Chest 89:139, 1986

————: Idiopathic pulmonary fibrosis, in *Current Therapy in Allergy, Immunology, and Rheumatology*, LM Lichtenstein, AS Fauci (eds). Toronto, Decker, 1988, vol 3, pp 214–220

TORONTO LUNG TRANSPLANT GROUP: Experience with single-lung transplantation for pulmonary fibrosis. JAMA 259:2258, 1988

Other interstitial lung diseases

ADAMSON D et al: Successful treatment of pulmonary lymphangiomyomatosis with oophorectomy and progesterone. Am Rev Respir Dis 132:916, 1985

ALLEN JN et al: Acute eosinophilic pneumonia as a reversible cause of noninfectious respiratory failure. N Engl J Med 321:569, 1989

BITTERMAN PB et al: Familial idiopathic pulmonary fibrosis. N Engl J Med 314:1343, 1986

CHAN CK et al: Small-airways disease in recipients of allogenic bone marrow transplants. Medicine 66:327, 1987

FAUCI AS et al: Lymphomatoid granulomatosis—prospective clinical and therapeutic experience over 10 years. N Engl J Med 306:68, 1982

HANCE AJ et al: Pulmonary and extrapulmonary manifestations of Langerhans cell granulomatosis (histiocytosis X). Semin Respir Med 9:349, 1988

KARIMAN K et al: Pulmonary alveolar proteinosis: Prospective clinical experience in 23 patients for 15 years. Lung 162:223, 1984

REYNOLDS HY: Bronchoalveolar lavage. Am Rev Respir Dis 135:250, 1987

ROSSI GA et al: Evidence for chronic inflammation as a component of interstitial lung disease associated with progressive systemic sclerosis. Am Rev Respir Dis 131:612, 1985

SEGGEN JS et al: Bronchiolitis obliterans. Chest 83:169, 1983

STRIMLAN CV et al: Lymphocytic interstitial pneumonitis. Ann Intern Med 88:616, 1978

212 PRIMARY PULMONARY HYPERTENSION

STUART RICH

Primary pulmonary hypertension is an uncommon disease characterized by increased pulmonary artery pressure and pulmonary vascular resistance without an obvious cause. The diagnosis can be made only after all etiologies for pulmonary hypertension have been excluded. There is a female-to-male preponderance (1.7:1), with patients most commonly presenting in the third and fourth decades, although the age range is from infancy to greater than 60 years. Because the predominant symptom of primary pulmonary hypertension is dyspnea, which can have an insidious onset in an otherwise healthy person, the disease is typically diagnosed late in its course. By that time the clinical and laboratory findings of severe pulmonary hypertension are usually present.

PATHOLOGY Three histologic patterns have been described in patients with primary pulmonary hypertension. *Plexogenic pulmonary arteriopathy* is the result of severe pulmonary hypertension from a variety of etiologies and is found in 30 to 60 percent of patients with primary pulmonary hypertension. It is more prevalent in younger women. The histology is characterized by changes in the pulmonary arteriolar bed including medial hypertrophy, concentric laminar intimal fibrosis, and plexiform lesions. Although the exact cause for the plexiform lesions remains unknown, they are only found when the pulmonary hypertension originates at the precapillary level. Plexogenic pulmonary arteriopathy also occurs in patients with pulmonary hypertension associated with congenital heart disease, with cirrhosis of the liver, and in pulmonary hypertension of collagen vascular disease. Some patients who present with primary pulmonary hypertension with high titers of antinuclear antibodies probably have a collagen vascular disease confined to the pulmonary vascular bed.

Thrombotic pulmonary arteriopathy accounts for approximately 40 to 50 percent of the cases of primary pulmonary hypertension and affects men and women equally. Histologically it is characterized by eccentric intimal fibrosis with medial hypertrophy, fibroelastic intimal pads in the arteries and arterioles, and scattered evidence of old recanalized thrombus appearing as fibrous webs. Although it has been proposed that recurrent microembolism is the cause for these lesions, no source for the emboli has been consistently found in these patients. Injury to the pulmonary vascular endothelium can create a procoagulant environment within the pulmonary arterial bed that might predispose to the development of thrombosis in situ, and abnormalities in fibrinolysis have recently been described in some patients. Whether the microthrombi represent a primary or secondary phenomenon is unknown, as microthrombi are also found in some patients with plexogenic pulmonary arteriopathy. Thrombotic pulmonary arteriopathy is also seen in patients with atrial septal defects and elevated pulmonary vascular resistance.

Pulmonary venoocclusive disease occurs in less than 10 percent of patients with primary pulmonary hypertension. Histologically it is manifest by widespread intimal proliferation and fibrosis of the intrapulmonary veins and venules, occasionally extending to the arteriolar bed. The pulmonary venous obstruction explains the increased pulmonary capillary wedge pressure observed in patients with advanced disease. These patients may develop orthopnea that can mimic left ventricular failure.

It is difficult to distinguish these three subsets of primary pulmonary hypertension on clinical grounds, as the symptoms are similar and the severity of the pulmonary hypertension is comparable in all three types. A chest radiograph and perfusion lung scan may be helpful, however. Patients with plexogenic pulmonary arteriopathy have normal perfusion lung scans, whereas those with thrombotic pulmonary arteriopathy and venoocclusive disease have an abnormal, patchy distribution of the radionuclide tracer. Patients with venoocclusive disease also have increased bronchovascular markings at the lung bases on chest radiograph.

ETIOLOGY The underlying cause for primary pulmonary hypertension is unknown. The high frequency of antinuclear antibodies suggests that some cases may be immunologically mediated, but specific etiologic agents for any of the three subtypes have not been identified. Insight into possible mechanisms was provided from the experience in Europe in the late 1960s in which the number of patients with unexplained pulmonary hypertension increased with the introduction of aminorex fumarate, an amphetamine-like drug used for appetite suppression. Use by susceptible individuals caused development of chronic pulmonary hypertension, the mechanism possibly pulmonary vasoconstriction from endothelial injury. Histologically, plexogenic pulmonary arteriopathy has been described in such cases.

The median survival of patients with pulmonary hypertension from aminorex was almost three times longer than that of patients with primary pulmonary hypertension. While some patients improved when the aminorex was discontinued, others had a progressive downhill course, even though the causative agent had been withdrawn.

Pregnancy and oral contraceptives had been proposed as etiologic factors, but this has not been substantiated by other studies. Their frequent association is more likely related to the prevalence of primary pulmonary hypertension in young women.

PATHOPHYSIOLOGY The underlying hemodynamic derangement in primary pulmonary hypertension is an increased resistance to pulmonary blood flow. Early in the disease there is a marked elevation in pulmonary artery pressure with relatively normal cardiac function. Over time the cardiac output becomes progressively reduced rather than the pulmonary artery pressure becoming progressively increased. Initially the pulmonary arteries may respond to vasodilators, but as the disease progresses, the elevated pulmonary vascular resistance becomes fixed. The pulmonary capillary wedge pressure remains normal until the late stages when it tends to rise in response to impaired diastolic filling of the left ventricle due to the altered configuration of the intraventricular septum. Eventually, as the right ventricle fails, the right atrial and right ventricular end-diastolic pressures rise in an attempt to compensate for the myocardial depression that has developed in response to chronic severe right ventricular pressure overload.

Pulmonary function is usually normal in primary pulmonary hypertension, although a mild restrictive pattern (see Chap. 201) is sometimes seen. Hypoxemia is common and is believed to be due to mismatching between pulmonary ventilation and perfusion, magnified by a low cardiac output. Occasional patients develop a patent foramen ovale which can also contribute to systemic arterial desaturation.

DIAGNOSIS A thorough diagnostic evaluation to look for all potential etiologies should be undertaken (see Fig. 212-1 and Table

FIGURE 212-1 An algorithm for the workup of a patient with unexplained pulmonary hypertension. (*Adapted with permission from S Rich.*)

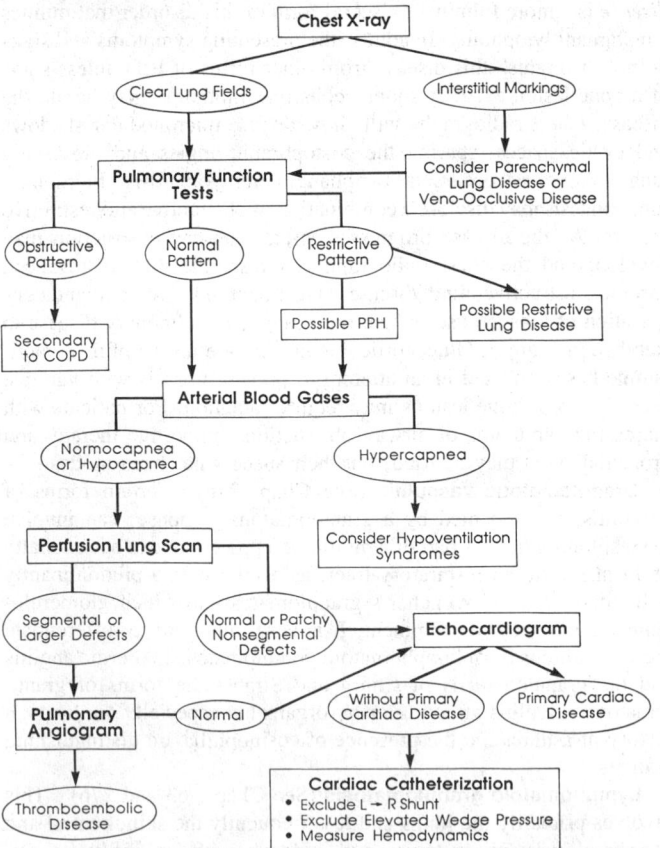

TABLE 212-1 Secondary causes of chronic pulmonary hypertension

Persistent fetal circulation
Congenital heart disease
Valvular heart disease
Primary myocardial disease
Pulmonary thromboembolic disease
Obstructive lung disease
Interstitial lung disease
Arterial hypoxemia with hypercapnea
Collagen vascular disease
Parasitic disease involving the lung
Sickle cell anemia
Intravenous drug abuse
Granulomatous lung disease
Chronic liver disease
Pulmonary artery stenosis
Pulmonary venous hypertension
Aminorex fumarate ingestion

SOURCE: From S Rich, Prog Cardiovasc Dis 31:205, 1988; used with permission.

212-1). The history usually reveals the gradual onset of shortness of breath with effort, progressing until the patient is dyspneic with minimal activity. The average duration from symptom onset until diagnosis is 2.5 years. Other common symptoms are fatigue, angina pectoris which likely represents right ventricular ischemia, syncope, near syncope, and peripheral edema. Approximately 7 percent of the cases are familial with the features of an autosomal dominant defect with variable expression.

The physical examination is characteristic. Increased jugular venous pressure, a reduced carotid pulse, and an easily palpable right ventricular lift are typical. Most patients have an increased pulmonic component of the second heart sound and right-sided third and fourth heart sounds. Tricuspid and pulmonic regurgitation and peripheral cyanosis and edema may be noted. Clubbing is not a feature.

The chest x-ray generally shows enlarged central pulmonary arteries and clear lung fields. The electrocardiogram usually reveals right axis deviation and right ventricular hypertrophy. The echocardiogram demonstrates right ventricular enlargement, a reduction in left ventricular cavity size, and abnormal septal configuration consistent with right ventricular pressure overload. Doppler studies have revealed a marked dependence upon atrial systole for ventricular filling. This would imply that atrial fibrillation could result in inadequate left ventricular filling and might be one cause for sudden death, as no patient with primary pulmonary hypertension and atrial fibrillation has been described. A mild restrictive pattern on pulmonary function tests is consistent with pulmonary hypertension and does not necessarily indicate restrictive lung disease. Hypoxemia, hypocapnia, and an abnormal diffusing capacity for carbon monoxide are almost invariable findings. Evidence of airways obstruction suggests a secondary etiology for the pulmonary hypertension. A perfusion lung scan may be normal or abnormal with multiple diffuse patchy filling defects of a nonsegmental nature and not suggestive of pulmonary thromboembolism. If the lung scan reveals perfusion defects of a segmental or subsegmental nature, a pulmonary angiogram must be done. Severe pulmonary hypertension in a patient with a high-probability lung scan should suggest a chronic process and not acute pulmonary embolism, as the nonconditioned right ventricle is unable to generate high systolic pressures acutely in the face of pulmonary thromboembolism. Chronic thromboembolic obstruction of the large pulmonary arteries can mimic primary pulmonary hypertension (see Chap. 213) but can be amenable to treatment with surgical thromboendarterectomy. Defining the precise location and extent of the clots is imperative for surgical removal.

There is risk in performing pulmonary angiography in patients with primary pulmonary hypertension, particularly in the presence of right ventricular failure with elevated right ventricular end-diastolic pressure. In these patients it is recommended that selective or subselective injections with smaller amounts of contrast be made to minimize the risks, and the use of low-osmolar, nonionic contrast

may also diminish risk. One mechanism for cardiac arrest in this setting is hypotension and bradycardia that may be vagally mediated; the pretreatment of selected patients with 1 mg atropine is also advocated.

Cardiac catheterization is mandatory to characterize the disease and exclude an underlying cardiac shunt as the etiology. The use of balloon-flotation catheters, especially those with removable guidewires, can facilitate right heart catheterization, which can be technically difficult. A right-to-left shunt might be attributable to a patent foramen ovale, but any left-to-right shunting implies the presence of a congenital defect. Though it may be difficult to obtain an accurate pulmonary capillary wedge pressure tracing in some patients, the wedge pressure is not falsely elevated. If recordings suggest that the wedge pressure is increased, left heart catheterization should also be performed to exclude mitral stenosis or increased left ventricular end-diastolic pressures as the cause. Although the diagnostic evaluation of these patients can be hazardous, experience from a national multicenter study revealed no mortality or serious morbidity in more than 300 patients whose evaluation included pulmonary angiography and cardiac catheterization. It is not necessary to perform an open lung biopsy in these patients to make an accurate diagnosis. If the diagnostic evaluation is undertaken as outlined, a correct diagnosis will almost always be made.

On occasion a patient may have marked elevations in pulmonary artery pressure and a relatively mild disease that is known to cause pulmonary hypertension. It would be a mistake to characterize these patients as having primary pulmonary hypertension on the belief that the pulmonary hypertension is out of proportion to the underlying associated condition. Since the pulmonary vascular bed has variable vasoreactivity, these cases probably reflect an exaggerated pulmonary vasoconstrictive response to the associated condition. Thus, severe pulmonary hypertension can coexist with mild chronic obstructive pulmonary disease, small intracardiac shunts, mild mitral stenosis, and even ischemic heart disease. The distinction, however, is important since the treatment of pulmonary hypertension should always be focused toward the underlying etiology.

NATURAL HISTORY The natural history of primary pulmonary hypertension is unknown because the initial disease is largely asymptomatic. Several series have reported a mean survival of 2 to 3 years for patients from the time of diagnosis. Occasional patients survive more than 10 years. Functional class is a strong predictor of survival, as patients who are functional class II and III have a mean survival of 3.5 years compared to those who are functional class IV in whom the mean survival is 6 months. The cause of death is usually right ventricular failure or sudden death; sudden death appears to be a late feature of the disease. Increased right atrial pressure above 15 mmHg and reduced cardiac index below 2 (L/min)/m² are hemodynamic predictors of a poor prognosis.

MANAGEMENT The treatment of primary pulmonary hypertension is unsatisfactory. Because the pulmonary vascular resistance increases dramatically with exercise, patients should be cautioned against participating in activities that demand increased physical stress. The use of digoxin remains controversial, as no studies have documented a benefit or detriment. Diuretic therapy may relieve dyspnea and peripheral edema and may be useful in reducing right ventricular volume overload in the presence of tricuspid regurgitation.

The main focus of therapy is vasodilator drugs. Virtually every class of vasodilator drug has been investigated, including beta-adrenergic agonists, alpha-adrenergic blockers, smooth-muscle vasodilators, nitrates, angiotensin converting enzyme inhibitors, and calcium channel antagonists. Most studies reporting favorable acute effects document a reduction in the pulmonary vascular resistance that is manifest by an increase in cardiac output, without a reduction in the mean pulmonary artery pressure. Although patients may feel better initially from increased oxygen transport to the systemic tissues, this results in increased stroke work of the right ventricle, which can result in worsening of right ventricular function and precipitate right ventricular failure over time. For vasodilators to have sustained beneficial effects, they must lower the pulmonary artery pressure substantially while preserving cardiac output and systemic blood pressure. To date no study has documented that vasodilators prolong life. However, the calcium channel antagonists are effective over the short term in some patients. When given in high doses that are titrated to the hemodynamic response, dramatic reductions in pulmonary artery pressure and pulmonary vascular resistance may be associated with improvement in symptoms and regression of right ventricular hypertrophy. However, less than half of the patients with primary pulmonary hypertension respond to this regimen. It is not known whether the response depends upon the histologic subtype, but the therapy is more successful in patients who are diagnosed early and have less advanced disease.

The administration of vasodilators can have serious acute and chronic adverse effects. Maintenance of adequate systemic blood pressure is crucial since right ventricular coronary blood flow is already compromised due to the loss of the normal systolic gradient for myocardial perfusion between the aorta and right ventricle. Vasodilator drugs can provoke acute right ventricular ischemia, and deaths have been reported. For these reasons the pharmacologic evaluation of primary pulmonary hypertension should always be undertaken with direct monitoring of systemic and pulmonary arterial pressures and cardiac output. Infusions of the pulmonary and systemic vasodilator prostacyclin have been utilized to test pulmonary vaso-reactivity of patients with primary pulmonary hypertension. Preliminary studies suggest that the response to prostacyclin may be predictive of the response to oral calcium blockers at higher doses.

Anticoagulant therapy has also been advocated based upon the evidence that thrombosis in situ is common. One retrospective study suggested that anticoagulants increase the survival of patients with primary pulmonary hypertension. Anticoagulants should not be expected to cause regression of the disease, however.

Patients who fail to respond to vasodilator drugs should be considered as possible candidates for heart-lung transplantation (see Chap. 183). The operation is best reserved for patients who are in the advanced stages of the disease in whom it may be predicted that survival is likely to be less than 1 year. A number of patients with primary pulmonary hypertension have undergone heart-lung transplantation, and to date recurrence of the disease has not been reported in a transplanted patient.

REFERENCES

Bjornsson J, Edwards WD: Primary pulmonary hypertension: A histopathologic study of 80 cases. Mayo Clin Proc 60:16, 1985

Fuster V et al: Primary pulmonary hypertension: Natural history and the importance of thrombosis. Circulation 70:580, 1984

Packer M: Vasodilator therapy for primary pulmonary hypertension. Ann Intern Med 103:258, 1985

Reitz BA: Heart-lung transplantation, in *Pulmonary Diseases and Disorders*, 2d ed, AP Fishman (ed). New York, McGraw-Hill, 1987, part 18

Rich S: Primary pulmonary hypertension. Prog Cardiovasc Dis 31:205, 1988

——— et al: High-dose calcium blocking therapy for primary pulmonary hypertension: Evidence for long-term reduction in pulmonary artery pressure and regression of right ventricular hypertrophy. Circulation 76:135, 1987

——— et al: Primary pulmonary hypertension: A national prospective study. Ann Intern Med 107:216, 1987

——— et al: Primary pulmonary hypertension: Radiographic and scintigraphic patterns of histologic subtypes. Ann Intern Med 105:499, 1986

——— et al: Pulmonary hypertension from chronic pulmonary thromboembolism. Ann Intern Med 108:425, 1988

Rubin LJ et al: Prostacyclin-induced pulmonary vasodilation in primary pulmonary hypertension. Circulation 66:334, 1982

213 PULMONARY THROMBOEMBOLISM

KENNETH M. MOSER

Pulmonary thromboembolism (PTE) is a leading cause of morbidity and mortality and can appear in many clinical contexts. Epidemiologic surveys indicate that PTE is responsible for more than 50,000 deaths in the United States annually. Many patients dying of PTE have serious underlying illnesses such as cancer and congestive heart failure. However, available data suggest that less than 10 percent of all pulmonary emboli result in death. Thus, the incidence of fatal plus nonfatal emboli probably exceeds 500,000 annually. This overall incidence seems verified by autopsy statistics. Evidence of recent or old embolism is detected in 25 to 30 percent of routine autopsies; with special techniques, this figure exceeds 60 percent. Even these data underestimate incidence, since many emboli resolve without trace and are not found at postmortem examination. The high incidence of PTE at autopsy contrasts sharply with the incidence of antemortem diagnosis. Available information suggests that an antemortem diagnosis has been made in only 10 to 30 percent of all cases in which old or recent embolism is demonstrated at autopsy.

VENOUS THROMBOSIS

PATHOGENESIS Available data indicate that more than 95 percent of pulmonary emboli arise from thrombi in the deep venous system of the lower extremities. Furthermore, it appears that the larger leg veins (popliteal vein and above) are by far the most common source of those pulmonary emboli which reach clinical attention. Thrombi occurring in the right cardiac chambers or in other veins account for the remainder. In situ pulmonary arterial thrombosis is rare. Thus, embolism should be viewed as a *complication* of deep venous thrombosis (DVT) in the lower extremity veins. Finally, some 90 percent of the deaths due to embolism occur within an hour or two—before a diagnostic-therapeutic plan can be implemented. These facts have several important implications with respect to PTE: (1) prevention of DVT is the most effective approach to prevention of, and death due to, embolism; (2) prompt treatment of DVT may limit the frequency of embolism; (3) techniques which identify the patient at high risk of DVT and allow prompt diagnosis are the key to reduction of embolic risk.

The three factors which promote DVT (and, therefore, embolic risk), as defined by Virchow in the nineteenth century, are stasis, abnormalities of the vessel wall, and alterations in the blood coagulation system. Coagulation alterations have been studied extensively, but as yet there is no reliable test for a state of "hypercoagulability," i.e., a test which will predict the risk of DVT. However, there is a growing list of conditions in which thrombotic risk is increased: deficiencies of antithrombin III, protein C, protein S, and components of the fibrinolytic system; presence of a lupus anticoagulant; and homocystinuria. But such discrete abnormalities are uncommon in the population that develops DVT and are usually discovered after the event. Therefore, the risk of DVT is best assessed by recognizing the presence of known "clinical" risk factors. Conditions associated with a high risk of venous thromboembolism include any surgical procedure requiring 30 min or more of general anesthesia, the postpartum period, left and right ventricular failure, fractures or other injuries of the lower extremities, chronic deep venous insufficiency of the legs, prolonged bed rest, carcinoma, obesity, and the use of estrogens.

NATURAL HISTORY In the contexts noted above, deep venous thrombi usually develop in the region of a venous valve. Platelets aggregate, forming a nidus (white thrombus), followed by development of a large fibrin (red) thrombus. The process is apparently a rapid one; large, extensive thrombi can develop within minutes. Growth occurs by continued fibrin and platelet accretion. Beyond formation, two processes may contribute to resolution: fibrinolysis and organization. Fibrinolysis may result in complete resolution within hours to several days. Any remaining thrombus undergoes organization, leaving behind a fibrotic zone that becomes reendothelialized. Valves are often rendered incompetent by this process, and modest or extensive luminal narrowing may occur. Once thrombus growth has halted, available data indicate that fibrinolysis/organization reaches a stable state in 7 to 10 days. It is during the first few days after formation, therefore, that embolic risk is highest.

DETECTION The clinical diagnosis of DVT is difficult. DVT is frequently present in the absence of clinical signs (e.g., pain, heat, swelling), and it is absent in 50 percent of patients in whom clinical signs or symptoms suggest its presence. Therefore a number of diagnostic tests have been developed. The gold standard is *ascending contrast venography;* but the application of this test is limited by technical and logistic considerations, and repetitive venography is impractical. Among available noninvasive techniques, two have been well-validated against venography: (1) impedance plethysmography (IPG), which detects venous outflow obstruction, is highly sensitive to acute above-knee thrombosis, but fails to detect many below-knee thrombi; and (2) the radiofibrinogen method, which is very sensitive to thrombus formation in calf veins and lower thigh veins, but not sensitive to thrombi which form in the upper thigh or above (also, 24 h is required for a definitive answer). The combination of IPG and radiofibrinogen leg scanning is equal in accuracy to contrast venography. Other available techniques await validation including Doppler ultrasound ("Duplex") studies, which are highly operator-dependent; radiovenography; and the use of other radiolabeled materials (^{111}In-platelets, antifibrin antibodies).

PROPHYLAXIS Application of these noninvasive approaches to the early diagnosis and follow-up of patients at high risk of DVT has led to significant changes in the approach to the prevention of DVT (and therefore of PTE). One validated prophylactic method is the use of small doses of subcutaneous heparin. Multiple studies, utilizing chiefly radiolabeled fibrinogen, have shown the high incidence of DVT in certain groups: patients over the age of 40 years with fractures of the pelvis and/or lower extremities; patients with myocardial infarction and/or severe congestive heart failure; patients undergoing major abdominal, thoracic, or gynecologic surgery. Furthermore, in the last group of patients, investigations have demonstrated a significant reduction in the incidence of DVT, PTE, and lethal PTE when heparin is given subcutaneously, in a dose of 5000 units every 12 h, beginning *before* operation (or on admission to the hospital) and continued until the patient is ambulatory. There is general agreement that this prophylactic approach, which has limited effect on coagulation tests and is associated with little risk of hemorrhage, should also be applied to *medical* patients at high risk of DVT and PTE. In the case of acute myocardial infarction, high risk would be imposed by the development of congestive failure, the presence of severe obesity, chronic venous insufficiency, or a prior history of DVT or PTE. Devices which compress the calf intermittently (usually once a minute) appear an effective alternative for prophylaxis in patients at risk of hemorrhage with low-dose heparin (neurosurgery, spinal cord trauma) or in whom low-dose heparin has proved ineffective (hip surgery, prostate surgery). Warfarin, started at the conclusion of lower extremity surgery, also is effective. Combinations (e.g., heparin plus venous compressive devices) are being explored in patients at particularly high risk. With these multiple options, some prophylaxis is available for almost every patient at risk of DVT.

NATURAL HISTORY OF PULMONARY EMBOLISM

THE ACUTE EVENTS The immediate result of thromboembolism is complete or partial obstruction of the pulmonary arterial blood flow to the distal lung. This obstruction leads to a series of pathophysiologic events which can be categorized as the "respiratory" and "hemodynamic" consequences of PTE.

Respiratory consequences Embolic obstruction produces a zone of the lung which is ventilated but not perfused—an intrapulmonary "dead space" (Chap. 201). Because it cannot participate in the process of gas exchange, ventilation of this nonperfused area is "wasted," in the functional sense. A potential consequence of embolic obstruction is constriction of the air spaces and airways in the affected lung zone. This pneumoconstriction, which might be viewed as a homeostatic mechanism to reduce wasted ventilation, appears to be due to the marked bronchoalveolar hypocapnia that results from cessation of pulmonary capillary blood flow, because it is abolished by inhalation of carbon dioxide–enriched air. While it occurs in animal experiments in which a double-lumen tube separates the ventilation from each lung, it probably occurs very rarely in patients who inhale dead space air (rich in carbon dioxide) into embolized lung zones.

Another disturbance caused by embolic obstruction—loss of alveolar surfactant—does not occur immediately. This surface-active lipoprotein is required to maintain alveolar stability. In its absence, alveolar collapse occurs. Cessation of pulmonary capillary blood flow leads to reduction in surfactant within 2 or 3 h, which becomes severe at 12 to 15 h. Frank atelectasis—the morphologic expression of alveolar instability—can be detected 24 to 48 h after interruption of blood flow.

Arterial hypoxemia is a common, though by no means universal, consequence of embolism. Several mechanisms can contribute to hypoxemia: ventilation-perfusion disturbances; cardiac failure with a lowered mixed venous P_{O_2} (widened arteriovenous difference); and obligatory perfusion through hypoventilated lung zones. Such obligatory perfusion develops because elevation of pulmonary arterial pressure due to embolic obstruction can overcome the vasoconstriction normally present in hypoventilated lung zones.

Hemodynamic consequences The primary hemodynamic consequence of thromboembolic obstruction is a reduction in the cross-sectional area of the pulmonary arterial bed. This loss of vascular capacity increases the resistance to pulmonary blood flow, which, if marked, leads to pulmonary hypertension and acute failure of the right ventricle. Tachycardia and often a decline in cardiac output also occur.

The factors that determine the severity of these hemodynamic changes have been the subject of continued debate. There is agreement that the *extent of embolic obstruction* is a key factor. However, the reserve capacity of the pulmonary arteriocapillary bed is so extensive that more than 50 percent of the vascular area must be obstructed before significant elevation in pulmonary arterial pressure results. Because pulmonary hypertension occurs in some patients with occlusion of lesser extent, investigators have searched for reflex or humoral vasoconstrictor mechanisms associated with embolism. Despite long and careful search for such mechanisms, their extent and frequency in human PTE remains unknown. Hence, some workers maintain that the degree of embolic obstruction itself is the only determinant of hemodynamic impairment. They suggest that instances of apparent disparity between the extent of embolism and clinical response reflect only clinical underestimation of the magnitude of the embolism. Other investigators, however, have presented compelling evidence to support the occurrence of pulmonary vasoconstriction with embolism. Some have demonstrated that constriction is associated with obstruction of the smaller, but not the larger, pulmonary arterial vessels. Another thesis holds that serotonin or thromboxane, known pulmonary vasoconstrictive-bronchoconstrictive substances, are released from platelets, which coat fresh emboli as they lodge in the pulmonary tree. This thesis introduces the attractive concept that an embolus might be regarded, in part, as a packet with pharmacologic, as well as obstructive, potential. A consensus view is that, while the extent of embolism is a key factor, humoral and/or reflex influences probably operate in certain patients and compromise the pulmonary circulation to a greater extent than might be expected on an anatomic basis alone.

The cardiopulmonary status of the patient prior to embolism is also critical in determining the clinical severity of embolism. A small embolus may have limited impact upon an otherwise healthy individual but may have serious consequences in someone with advanced cardiac or pulmonary disease.

Both experimental and clinical studies have established that infarction—death of lung tissue—rarely accompanies embolic occlusion. It is likely that less than 10 percent of emboli in humans lead to infarction. That infarction rarely follows embolism should occasion little surprise. The lung has three avenues for obtaining oxygen: the pulmonary arterial circulation, the bronchial arterial circulation, and the airways. Thus, infarction occurs infrequently, and its appearance usually is associated with compromise of bronchial arterial flow and/or airways to the involved area. Such compromise is promoted by the existence of other cardiac or pulmonary diseases, such as left ventricular failure, mitral stenosis, and chronic obstructive lung disease. Thus, infarction may occur in 30 percent or more of such patients, while it is quite rare in individuals who are free of cardiopulmonary disease.

BEYOND THE ACUTE STATE   The vast majority of pulmonary emboli resolve, and resolve rather quickly. Resolution of fresh emboli begins within the first few days and is well advanced in 10 to 14 days. As in DVT, two mechanisms promote restoration of vascular patency: the fibrinolytic system and the process of organization. However, the fibrinolytic system appears capable of more rapid dissolution of emboli than of venous thrombi.

The availability of these two efficient mechanisms raises the question as to why not all emboli resolve. There may be some impairment of the intrinsic fibrinolytic system. The emboli may have been well organized prior to their lodgment in the lung so that they are subject to neither fibrinolytic attack nor further organization. Alternatively, some emboli may be recurrent, so that their failure to resolve is more apparent than real.

Another important element of the natural history of thromboembolism is the development of bronchial arterial collateral circulation. If pulmonary arterial obstruction persists, bronchial arterial flow increases substantially over a period of several weeks, restoring flow to the capillary bed. With the return of flow, surfactant production is restored, so that alveolar stability is regained and atelectasis resolves.

DIAGNOSTIC FEATURES

While sequential studies of patients with venous thrombosis have demonstrated that embolism, often of substantial magnitude, can occur without causing symptoms, *sudden onset of unexplained dyspnea* is the most common, and often the only symptom of pulmonary embolism. *Pleuritic chest pain and hemoptysis are present only when infarction has occurred* and, because bland embolism rarely leads to infarction, are usually absent. With extensive embolism, severe substernal oppressive discomfort may be present, probably due to right ventricular ischemia. Patients also may present with syncope, suggesting a neurologic disorder. Other "occult" presentations in which embolism should be considered include repetitive bouts of otherwise unexplained supraventricular tachyarrhythmias; sudden onset or worsening of congestive heart failure (Chap. 182); sudden deterioration in the patient with chronic obstructive lung disease; and as an alternative to the diagnosis of "psychic" (anxiety-associated) hyperventilation. The most reliable symptom, however, is breathlessness. Severe, persistent dyspnea is an ominous sign, for it usually indicates extensive embolic occlusion.

PHYSICAL EXAMINATION   Findings on physical examination, like the history, may be deceptively normal. Examination of the lungs may disclose a few atelectatic rales; localized wheezes rarely are heard. A pleural friction rub or evidence of pleural effusion will not be present unless infarction has occurred.

On cardiac examination, the single consistent finding is tachycar-dia. Only in the rare cases of massive embolism will signs such as a right ventricular gallop, a palpable "lift" over the right ventricle (along the left sternal border), a loud pulmonary closure sound, or prominent *a* waves in the jugular venous pulse be found. A scratchy systolic ejection-type murmur may be heard in the pulmonic area. Also, a systolic or continuous murmur accentuated by inspiration may be audible over the lung fields. These murmurs appear to be generated by turbulence of flow in vessels partially obstructed by emboli since they disappear after resection or resolution of emboli. They should be carefully sought in any patient suspected of having PTE. Wide splitting of the second heart sound may be present. This indicates extensive embolic obstruction and implies both severe pulmonary hypertension and right ventricular failure. As embolic resolution occurs, this finding disappears. Absence of an accentuated pulmonic closure sound is not a reliable guide to the severity of PTE, since when embolism is sufficiently massive to reduce cardiac output, pulmonary arterial pressure falls, and the pulmonary closure sound may be normal or diminished.

The detection of *deep venous thrombosis* qualifies as an excellent clue to the diagnosis of embolism, but its absence does not exclude embolism, because the entire venous thrombus may embolize. Even when sought with diligence, *clinical* evidence of thrombophlebitis is found in less than half of patients with PTE. *Fever* in patients with pulmonary embolism is uncommon without complicating infection or infarction. With infarction, fever of 37.5 to 38.5°C (oral) is the rule; but temperature elevations to 39°C or above may occur, making the differentiation between pulmonary infarction and infection difficult.

On clinical grounds alone, then, a firm diagnosis of embolism cannot be made; the clinical *suspicion* of embolism requires confirmation by laboratory studies (Fig. 213-1).

LABORATORY STUDIES   Routine laboratory studies contribute little toward the diagnosis. Leukocytosis and elevation of the sedimentation rate are rarely present in the absence of infarction. A variety of other blood tests, such as assay for specific fibrinopeptides, fibrin degradation products, or enzymes, have been proposed; none has been shown to be diagnostically sensitive or specific.

Aside from tachycardia, the *electrocardiogram* is normal in most patients. With extensive embolization, there may be evidence of acute pulmonary hypertension (rightward shift of the QRS axis, a tall, peaked P wave), and ST-T changes indicative of right ventricular strain (Chap. 176). These changes are often transient, lasting minutes to hours, but when persistent, suggest severe pulmonary vascular obstruction.

The *chest roentgenogram* may show a parenchymal infiltrate and evidence of a pleural effusion if *infarction* has occurred. Characteristically, the infiltrates caused by infarction abut against the pleura. However, their shape varies, and they do not usually appear until 12 to 36 h after the embolism has occurred. The effusion, which often precedes the infiltrate, is characteristically small. Thoracentesis usually, but by no means invariably, yields hemorrhagic fluid, with the characteristics of an exudate.

The radiographic findings with embolism alone are more subtle. Elevation of the hemidiaphragm may occur. *Differences in diameter between vessels that should be of equivalent size* should raise the suspicion of embolism. For example, embolic obstruction of the right main pulmonary artery can lead to dilation of the left main pulmonary artery because that vessel must accept the entire pulmonary flow. There may be *abrupt "cutoff"* of a vessel; i.e., as the vessel is traced distally, it suddenly disappears. Clot has the same radiodensity as blood, accounting for the proximal shadow; the absence of flow beyond the clot explains the sudden radiographic "disappearance" of the vessel.

Organization of a clot within a pulmonary artery may lead to retraction of the vessel's walls and a so-called rattail configuration, in which the vessel is relatively normal proximally and suddenly tapers to a sharp point. Finally, there may be *abnormal radiolucency* in some lung zones due to absent or decreased flow. Such abnormally

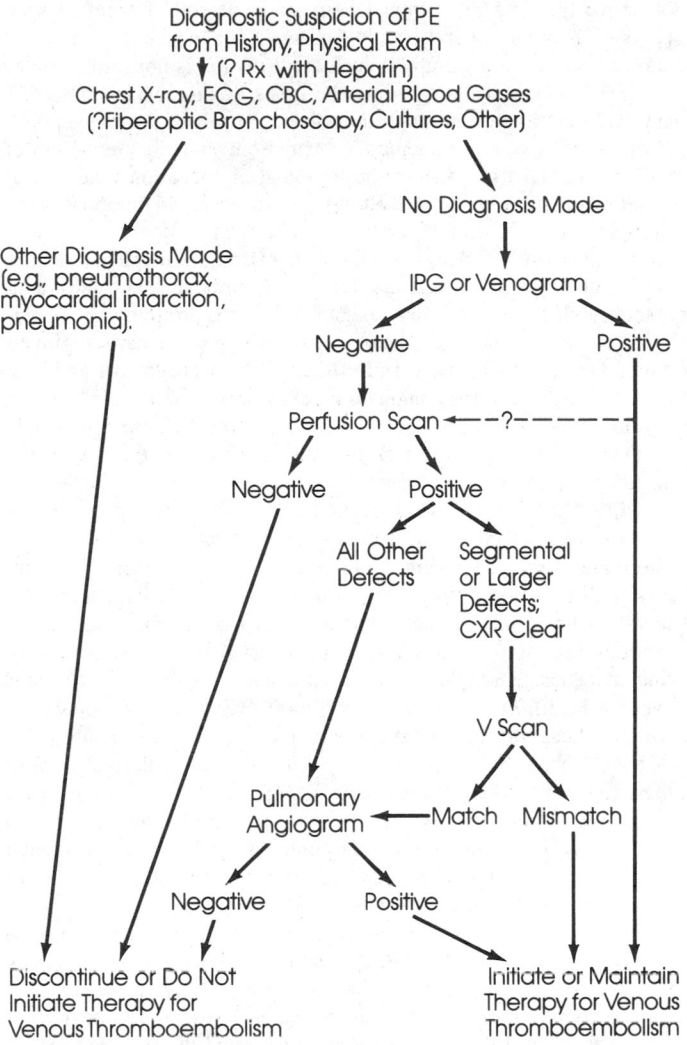

FIGURE 213-1 Flow chart used in diagnosis of pulmonary embolism (PE). IPG, impedance plethysmogram; V scan, ventilation scan.

lucent areas, indicative of proximal arterial obstruction, are best appreciated by examining comparable areas in the two lung fields.

Even in embolization without infarction, the roentgenogram may show small infiltrates, which appear in about 24 h and reflect atelectasis secondary to surfactant depletion. They are not associated with effusion, may fail to touch a pleural surface, and disappear without the linear scarring characteristic of infarction. It should be emphasized that a *normal chest roentgenogram does not exclude the diagnosis of PTE*. Indeed, a *normal* chest roentgenogram is the *most common* finding in embolic disease.

Analysis of arterial blood gases Massive embolism is commonly associated with arterial hypoxemia, hypocapnia, and respiratory alkalosis. In addition, the difference between alveolar P_{CO_2} and arterial P_{CO_2} ($PA_{CO_2} - Pa_{CO_2}$) may be widened owing to the increase in alveolar dead space (Chap. 201). However, a normal P_{O_2} does not exclude the diagnosis.

The laboratory tests discussed thus far are often negative in PTE and are relatively nonspecific. Therefore, it is usually necessary to proceed to two more definitive techniques: pulmonary perfusion and ventilation radiophotoscans and the pulmonary angiogram.

Pulmonary perfusion and ventilation scintiphotography Perfusion scintiphotographs (photoscans) are obtained by gamma camera imaging of the distribution of intravenously injected, gamma-emitting radionuclides. The most commonly used radionuclides are microspheres or macroaggregates of albumin (MAA), labeled with a gamma-emitting isotope such as technetium 99m. The radioactive particles, 50 to 100 μm in diameter, are trapped in the pulmonary

capillary bed because the pulmonary capillaries approximate 10 μm in diameter. Alternatively, xenon 133 gas, dissolved in saline solution, may be used, but patients must hold their breath. The distribution of labeled particles entrapped in capillaries, or of xenon 133 evolved from them, accurately depicts the distribution of pulmonary blood flow.

The camera-generated perfusion image can be recorded on radiographic film, on special photographic film, on a television screen, or on videotape. Normal scans exhibit homogeneous distribution of radioactivity, smooth margins, and a configuration which corresponds to the normal anatomy of the lungs. Any deviation from these characteristics requires explanation because it represents an abnormality in blood flow distribution.

The perfusion lung photoscan is quite valuable in the diagnosis of embolism. A properly performed perfusion scan which is *normal* excludes the diagnosis of clinically significant pulmonary embolism, as indicated by reports of the excellent outcomes of persons suspected of embolism, who had normal scans and who were not treated. On the other hand, a scan demonstrating zones of absent or sharply decreased radioactivity in the patient whose other findings are compatible with PTE keeps the diagnosis of embolism among the possibilities. Scanning is simple, safe, and rapid. It can be repeated to define the resolution, or recurrence, of obstructive vascular phenomena. Like any laboratory test, however, the photoscan must be applied and interpreted with care. It is important, for example, to obtain multiple scan views because lesions not apparent in one view may be easily detected in others. Furthermore, the lung photoscan demonstrates only abnormalities of the *distribution of blood flow*. It does not provide anatomic information. Many disorders other than PTE are associated with abnormalities in the distribution of pulmonary blood flow. Any disease process, such as pneumonia, atelectasis, or pneumothorax, which reduces the ventilation of a lung zone will decrease its perfusion. Parenchymal diseases, such as emphysema, sarcoidosis, bronchogenic carcinoma, and tuberculosis, can all produce scan defects. Therefore a perfusion defect lacks specificity. One approach to enhancing specificity is the performance of a ventilation scan, best achieved by having patients breathe a radioactive gas such as xenon 127 or xenon 133. To assist in deciding whether a ventilation scan may be useful and when pulmonary angiography is required, two factors should be considered: the size of the perfusion defect(s) and the chest roentgenographic findings. If all defects are subsegmental in size *or* if all defects (of any size) are limited to areas of roentgenographic infiltration, ventilation scanning will not be useful, and pulmonary angiography is required, if a definitive diagnosis is necessary. If defect(s) are segmental or larger in size, and one or more are in areas clear by x-ray, a ventilation scan should be done. If the radioactive gas enters ("washes in") and is cleared ("washes out") from the area(s) of perfusion defect(s), this "mismatch" of ventilation and perfusion is characteristic of vascular obstruction (Fig. 213-2). Pulmonary vascular obstruction is present in 90 percent or

FIGURE 213-2 Perfusion scan (left), posterior view, shows multiple segmental and larger perfusion defects in right upper and lower lobes, left lower lobe, and lingula. Ventilation scan (right) is normal at equilibrium. Xenon 133 washed in and out normally. Multiple emboli were confirmed angiographically.

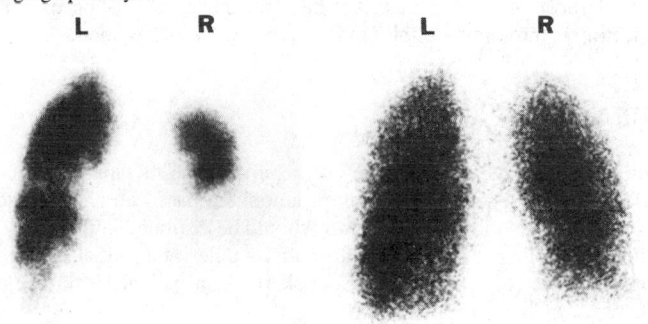

more of patients with this pattern. However, if ventilation is also abnormal (i.e., ventilation-perfusion "match" is present), no reliable diagnostic conclusion can be reached; pulmonary angiography is required. (It may not be required if DVT is present and already mandates therapy.) In some centers, ^{99m}Tc-DTPA particles are used for ventilation studies; this approach provides multiple views but does not allow "wash-out" evaluation.

Pulmonary angiography   This is the only established means for providing anatomic information about the pulmonary vasculature. Radiopaque material is injected, preferably through a cardiac catheter advanced into the pulmonary artery. Cardiac catheterization and angiography require specialized personnel, and a reasonable period for preparation and performance, and they entail more risk than the procedures discussed above. However, angiography provides a visual image of the pulmonary vessels, and catheterization can provide potentially important hemodynamic data (pulmonary artery and wedge pressures, cardiac output). Interpretive limitations of angiography are of three types: (1) *Injection artifacts* may occur which suggest absence of flow to a vessel. Injection should be repeated whenever the question of such artifacts exists. (2) The inability to evaluate the patency of small vessels is another limitation. Emboli in vessels below the resolving capability of the method cannot be detected with certainty, although magnification techniques can extend resolving capability. (3) Interpretive errors may also be a consequence of *not looking for the proper type of defect*. There are only two findings diagnostic of acute embolism. One is the *abrupt "cutoff"* of a vessel at the point of embolic impaction. However, complete embolic obstruction is uncommon. Therefore, *filling defects* are the most frequent finding; i.e., the embolus creates a "negative" shadow as the radiopaque material flows around it. The major contraindication to angiography is the absence of personnel who are experienced in both performing the procedure and interpreting the results. Serious diagnostic errors are commonplace if optimal techniques are not used or the complexities of interpretation are not appreciated. However, the risks of angiography are low in experienced hands. Injection of large boluses of contrast medium into the main pulmonary artery should be avoided in favor of small injections into vessels supplying lung regions identified as abnormal on the perfusion scan.

How far one should proceed down the diagnostic pathway outlined above depends on many factors, the major ones being the presence or absence of documented venous thrombosis, the severity of the patient's symptoms, and the hazards of contemplated therapy. In each condition, there is a need for precise diagnosis. If IPG or venography already has documented deep venous thrombosis of the popliteal vein or above, one is committed to anticoagulant therapy; thus, proceeding beyond perfusion scanning is rarely necessary. This means that evaluation for venous thrombosis is an essential part of the evaluation of the embolic suspect. Unfortunately, the absence of venous thrombosis cannot be used to exclude the diagnosis of pulmonary embolism. More than 20 percent of patients with embolism have no evidence of venous thrombosis, apparently because the entire venous thrombus has embolized. Therefore, in such patients, if symptoms are severe and/or the hazards of therapy are substantial, diagnostic precision is mandatory, and there should be no hesitancy in proceeding to angiography. Substantial hazards of therapy which mandate angiography include a high risk of bleeding on, or absolute contraindication to, anticoagulant therapy and consideration of embolectomy, thrombolytic therapy, or vena caval interruption.

TREATMENT

Initial intravenous administration of heparin is the therapy of choice for PTE. With a strong *suspicion* of embolism based on clinical and routine laboratory tests, such therapy should be instituted immediately, without awaiting diagnostic confirmation, unless the initial dose of heparin places the patient at clear risk (i.e., in patients with recent or active bleeding or a known hemostatic defect). Except in such patients, heparin therapy should not await diagnostic confirmation; one can always stop therapy if such confirmation is not forthcoming.

There is consensus regarding the goals of therapy in both DVT and PTE: (1) immediate inhibition of the growth of thromboemboli, (2) promotion of thromboembolic resolution, and (3) prevention of recurrence. Heparin achieves the first goal; it encourages the second by allowing fibrinolytic dissolution to be achieved unopposed by thrombus growth; and it assists in, although it does not ensure, prevention of recurrence. In addition, heparin inhibits platelet aggregation (and therefore potential release of thromboxane and serotonin) at the embolic site, and its anticoagulant action is promptly reversible.

There is *not* consensus, however, regarding (1) heparin regimens which best combine safety and efficacy; (2) the need for, and type of, tests for monitoring coagulation behavior during heparin therapy; (3) how long, and with what agents, antithrombotic therapy should be maintained; or (4) in which patients thrombolytic therapy should antedate antithrombotic therapy.

REGIMENS   In DVT, three methods of heparin administration have been advocated by various investigators: continuous intravenous, intermittent intravenous, intermittent subcutaneous. Continuous intravenous heparin is usually given in a dose of approximately 1000 units per hour. Intermittent intravenous heparin is commonly given in a dose of approximately 5000 units every 4 h or 7500 every 6 h. Subcutaneous heparin has been recommended at a dose of 5000 units every 4 h, 10,000 every 8 h, or 20,000 every 12 h. Studies exist which indicate that each of these regimens is more efficacious, safer, or both. Therefore, at this time, one can conclude only that *each* of these regimens (which approximate 30,000 units per 24 h) represents an acceptable treatment regimen. However, the continuous intravenous regimen, delivered by an infusion pump, is by far the most popular in the United States. *Intramuscular* injection of heparin is to be avoided because hematomas will develop.

It should also be recognized that there is a growing consensus that DVT that remains confined to the calf veins need *not* be treated with anticoagulant therapy. No increase in morbidity or mortality has been reported among patients in this category who are not treated. However, since 15 to 20 percent of calf-limited thrombi will extend to the popliteal veins and above during a 10- to 12-day period, such patients *must* be followed by serial IPG tests until this period has elapsed. If they cannot be followed in this manner, they should be treated.

In PTE, the same options for heparin therapy exist. The only additional question is whether an initial large intravenous bolus (10,000 to 20,000 units) should be given to inhibit the aggregation (and release reaction) of platelets adherent to the embolus. Most workers advocate such a dose, with one of the "standard" regimens being started 2 to 4 h later.

MONITORING   The value of clotting times (CT), partial thromboplastin times (PTT), or other coagulation tests to monitor the safety and efficacy of heparin remains a complex issue. With regard to safety, the risk of hemorrhage (the principal complication of heparin therapy) is not clearly related to coagulation test alterations; rather, it appears related to factors such as the coexistence of other diseases associated with bleeding risk (gastric or duodenal ulcer, coagulopathies, uremia) and advanced age. Likewise, achievement of the desired effect of heparin (cessation of thrombus growth in vivo) has not been related consistently to coagulation tests. Therefore, it is questionable whether monitoring with such tests is superior to empiric use of one of the regimens described above. While animal investigations have disclosed that maintaining the PTT above 1.5 times control does prevent growth of venous thrombi, limited data are not available documenting this in human patients. If done improperly or poorly timed, the CT or PTT tests are worthless and may be misleading. Furthermore, even with continuous intravenous therapy, the CT and PTT may vary substantially during a 24-h period. Despite these vagaries, a majority of experts currently recommend attempting to keep the CT or PTT, measured *just prior to the next* intermittent dose, at or above 1.5 times the baseline CT or PTT and at 1.5 to 2.0 times control with continuous infusion.

DURATION OF THERAPY In DVT, full anticoagulant protection is usually maintained for 7 to 10 days, the rationale being that this is the period required for dissolution and/or organization of the thrombus. In PTE, for the same reasons, a similar duration of therapy is advised. Bed rest is indicated until cardiopulmonary or leg symptoms subside. Carefully applied elastic support hose should be used (to encourage venous flow) as soon as leg pain, if present, subsides and the patient is ambulated.

During and beyond the acute phase there are several options for achieving proper anticoagulant protection. In deciding among these options, it should be recognized that the major question being addressed is: Does the patient need continued protection against the risk of *recurrent* DVT (and, therefore, PTE)? If the risk factor(s) that precipitated the acute episode of DVT-PTE is no longer present, the patient is asymptomatic, and the IPG is normal, it is acceptable to reduce heparin to a lower dose starting on day 7, ambulate the patient, and, if no symptoms develop, discontinue heparin on day 9 or 10. If these criteria are not met, as is the case in most patients, prolonged prophylactic therapy is warranted. Two options exist for such prophylaxis. The most common one is to initiate a prothrombinopenic agent (e.g., warfarin) as soon as the decision for long-term protection is made. Often, this can be done on day 2 or 3 of heparin therapy. Prothrombinopenic drugs are not suitable for initial therapy in thromboembolism, as their onset of action is too slow. Their only role is in maintaining anticoagulant protection for prolonged periods. If they are initiated early in the acute treatment course, the patient must be "in range," as defined by a prothrombin time of 1.5 to 1.8 times the control time for 3 to 5 days *before heparin is discontinued*. A second option for long-term protection is the use of self-injected subcutaneous heparin. Current data suggest that a dose of 7500 to 10,000 units every 12 h is adequate, is well-tolerated, and need not be monitored with coagulation tests.

There is no consensus regarding the period for which anticoagulant protection should be maintained beyond hospital discharge because firm data on this point are lacking. If *reversible* risk factors are present (e.g., immobilization after a leg fracture), therapy should be continued until the risk factors present have resolved. If the risk factors present are nonreversible (e.g., severe left and/or right ventricular failure), if the IPG remains positive, or if major lung scan defects persist at discharge, empiric decisions are made. At a minimum, 3 months of therapy seems wise, because recurrence is relatively common during this period. Beyond 3 months, however, continuation depends upon the balance among specific risk factors exhibited by the patient, IPG results, lung scan results, and the risks of continued therapy. In some instances, this balance may warrant lifetime maintenance on anticoagulant drugs.

Thrombolytic therapy The place of *thrombolytic (fibrinolytic)* agents (Chap. 189) in the management of acute venous thromboembolism remains to be defined. There is no question that available agents (streptokinase, urokinase), as well as the second-generation (tissue plasminogen activator, tPA) and potential third-generation agents, can hasten the resolution of venous thrombi and pulmonary emboli. They do not replace antithrombotic therapy. When used, thrombolytic agents must be followed by a standard course of antithrombotic therapy. Despite extensive study, it has not been established that such agents alter short-term or long-term morbidity, mortality, or recurrence rates among patients with DVT or PTE. These drugs, despite high fibrin specificity in the case of tPA, are associated with hemorrhagic risk in patients who have had, or require, any invasive procedure (e.g., vein puncture, arterial puncture, angiography, Swan-Ganz catheterization); and in patients with localized vascular lesions due to recent operation, trauma, or concomitant disease (e.g., peptic ulcer, stroke). If thrombolytic agents prove to have a therapeutic advantage, it would appear to be (1) in patients

with extensive, large-vein DVT (e.g., iliofemoral); and (2) in patients with massive embolism and persistent systemic hypotension in whom embolectomy would otherwise be contemplated.

Surgical therapy for DVT (thrombectomy) is now rarely considered because the results have not been encouraging. In PTE, surgical therapy should be reserved for those patients in whom heparin therapy is deemed inadequate or impractical. Anticoagulant therapy may be contraindicated by the presence of a bleeding diathesis, or the patient may be in such critical condition that it is felt unwise to await a response to medical therapy. In such instances *venous interruption* and *pulmonary embolectomy* must be considered.

The objective of venous interruption is to prevent immediate recurrence of embolism from lower extremity venous thrombi. While multiple ligation and clipping procedures have been used in the past, these have been largely supplanted by the use of filters placed in the inferior vena cava by a transvenous approach (jugular, femoral veins). Ligation of the inferior vena cava requires surgery, obstructs venous return acutely, and encourages collateral vein formation which bypasses the ligation. Clips require surgery for placement, may obstruct caval flow, and may thrombose. The filters, typified by the Greenfield filter, which has been the most widely used in recent years, are inserted transvenously, do not obstruct caval flow, protect against emboli greater than 2 mm in diameter, and are rarely subject to thrombosis.

There are two major indications for placement of a caval filter: (1) as a lifesaving procedure in patients with massive embolism who could not tolerate an embolic recurrence; and (2) to prevent embolism in patients with documented venous thrombosis in whom anticoagulant therapy is contraindicated.

There is one instance, however, in which prompt caval ligation is the therapy of choice: septic thrombophlebitis of pelvic origin with multiple septic pulmonary emboli. If these patients do not respond promptly to a heparin-antibiotic regimen, they may die unless caval (and left ovarian vein) ligation is carried out promptly.

Two criteria should be met before emergency pulmonary embolectomy is performed: (1) there must be evidence of severe hemodynamic compromise due to embolism, particularly sustained systemic hypotension, which is not responsive to supportive measures; and (2) the personnel and equipment required for embolectomy carried out with the aid of cardiopulmonary bypass must be available. Even with these criteria satisfied, it now appears likely that management of such patients by alternative approaches (placement of a caval filter plus heparin therapy; thrombolytic therapy) will be associated with lower mortality rates than is emergency embolectomy.

SPECIAL CONSIDERATIONS Total resolution of emboli does not always occur. Why some patients (perhaps 0.1 percent) fail to resolve their emboli is not yet known. However, if residual vascular obstruction is substantial, the patient may present, months or years after the actual embolic events, with dyspnea and pulmonary hypertension of uncertain cause, often with right ventricular failure. Such patients commonly are misdiagnosed, for months or years, as having "asthma," "chronic lung disease," "primary" pulmonary hypertension (Chap. 212), or cor pulmonale of unclear etiology (Chap. 191).

Such patients should be studied by appropriate techniques, since emboli in the main or lobar arteries can be surgically removed (thromboendarterectomy), allowing cure of this otherwise fatal form of pulmonary hypertensive disease. This entity, once an autopsy curiosity, is more common than previously appreciated: some 200 patients have been reported to have undergone thromboendarterectomy. Because surgical mortality is heavily conditioned by the severity of right ventricular dysfunction at the time of operation, early recognition is important.

PROGNOSIS IN PULMONARY EMBOLISM The prognosis of the patient with pulmonary embolism *in whom therapy is promptly instituted* is excellent. As stated at the outset of this chapter, less than 1 embolic event in 10 is lethal. The majority of these deaths occur suddenly and can be avoided only by prophylaxis (see above). The remainder appear to be due to embolic extension or recurrence, which therapy can moderate. Thus, for patients who survive long enough to reach medical attention and receive heparin, the outlook is quite good. Morbidity following embolism is uncommon since embolic resolution is the rule, and few patients develop the pulmonary hypertensive problem noted above.

Limited reliable data are available regarding recurrence rates in the months and years after a single embolic event (with or without prolonged postembolic anticoagulant therapy). In the absence of risk factors, or a positive IPG, recurrence appears to be uncommon, but more precise data are needed.

Whether the therapeutic approaches discussed here will be altered by new agents, such as low-molecular-weight heparin and newer thrombolytic agents, remains to be seen.

NONTHROMBOTIC EMBOLISM

Because the lung vasculature serves as a filter of the venous circulation, it is the recipient of diverse materials which can gain entry into venous blood, including bone marrow, foreign bodies, parasites, and tumor cells. The most frequently encountered form of nonthrombotic embolism is *fat embolism*. This dramatic and controversial entity follows the introduction of neutral fat into the venous circulation, most commonly after bone trauma or fracture (marrow fat), but occasionally after trauma to adipose tissue or liver infiltrated by fat. The clinical sequence is characteristic. After a latent period of 12 to 36 h or more, during which the patient is asymptomatic, sudden cardiopulmonary and neurologic deterioration appears. Mental aberrations, delirium, and coma develop. Dyspnea, tachypnea, and tachycardia occur, and the chest roentgenographic and physiologic components of the "adult respiratory distress syndrome" appear (see Chap. 218). Anemia and thrombocytopenia are common, as are petechiae on the upper thorax and arms. The pathogenesis of the syndrome is not clear, but it seems likely that two events occur: release of free fatty acids (by action of lipases on the neutral fat), which induces a toxic vasculitis, followed by platelet-fibrin thrombosis; and actual obstruction of small pulmonary arteries by macroaggregates of fat. Several forms of therapy have been proposed (corticosteroids, heparin, ethanol), but none has proved effective; treatment remains supportive and mortality rate high.

Another dramatic form of nonthrombotic embolism is *amniotic fluid embolism*. This occurs during both spontaneous delivery and cesarean section. Sudden and massive obstruction of the pulmonary microvasculature occurs, leading to shock and, often, death. With survival of the initial phase of the disease, the picture of disseminated intravascular coagulation appears. The syndrome is due to the entrance of a significant quantity of amniotic fluid into the venous circulation. This fluid is a potent thromboplastic agent which induces thrombosis in the pulmonary vasculature and elsewhere. The fluid also contains particulates which lodge in the lung. Treatment consists of supportive measures.

Nonembolic pulmonary arterial obstruction due to *vasculitis* has become a common problem among intravenous drug users. This vasculitis, caused by the drugs per se or materials (e.g., talc) mixed with the drugs, can induce thrombosis. This entity may be difficult to distinguish from PTE. Repetitive episodes may lead to irreversible and severe pulmonary hypertension.

REFERENCES

FEDULLO PF et al: ¹¹¹-Indium labelled platelets: Effect of heparin on uptake by venous thrombi and relationship to the activated partial thromboplastin time. Circulation 66:632, 1982

FISHMAN AP, KELLEY MA: Pulmonary thromboembolism (including prophylaxis, treatment, sickle cell disease and multiple pulmonary thrombi), in *Pulmonary Diseases and Disorders*, 2d ed, AP Fishman (ed). New York, McGraw-Hill, 1987, chap 66.

GOLDHABER SZ (ed): *Pulmonary Embolism and Deep Venous Thrombosis*. Philadelphia, Saunders, 1985

HUISMAN MV et al: Serial impedance plethysmography for suspected deep venous thrombosis in outpatients. N Engl J Med 314:823, 1986

HULL R et al: Pulmonary angiography, ventilation lung scanning and venography for clinically suspected pulmonary embolism in the abnormal perfusion scan. Ann Intern Med 98:891, 1983

—— et al: Adjusted subcutaneous heparin versus warfarin sodium in the long-term treatment of venous thrombosis. N Engl J Med 305:189, 1982

—— et al: Combined use of leg scanning and impedance plethysmography in suspected venous thrombosis. N Engl J Med 296:1497, 1977

KAKKAR VV et al: Prevention of post-operative embolism by low-dose heparin: An international multicenter trial. Lancet 2:45, 1975

KIPPER MS et al: Long-term follow-up of patients with suspected pulmonary embolism and a normal lung scan. Chest 82:411, 1982

MERCANDETTI A et al: Influence of perfusion and ventilation scans on therapeutic decision-making and outcome among embolic suspects. West J Med 142:208, 1985

MOSER KM et al: Thromboendarterectomy for chronic, major vessel thromboembolic pulmonary hypertension: Immediate and long-term results in 42 patients. Ann Intern Med 107:560, 1987

——, FEDULLO PF: Venous thromboembolism: Three simple decisions. Chest 83:117, 256, 1983

NIH Consensus Conference: Prevention of venous thrombosis and pulmonary embolism. JAMA 256:744, 1986

PHILBRICK JT, BECKER DM: Calf deep venous thrombosis: A wolf in sheep's clothing? Arch Intern Med 148:2131, 1988

SALZMAN EW et al: Intraoperative external pneumatic calf compression to afford long-term prophylaxis against deep vein thrombosis in urologic patients. Surgery 87:239, 1980

SASAHARA AA, DALEN JE: Controversy: Should fibrinolytic drugs be used to treat acute pulmonary embolism? J Cardiovasc Med 5:793, 1980

WESSLER S et al: *Dimensions of Warfarin Prophylaxis*. New York, Plenum, 1987

214   DISEASES OF THE UPPER RESPIRATORY TRACT

ROBERT LEBOVICS

The upper respiratory tract includes the nose and mouth, the paranasal sinuses, the ears and mastoids, the pharynx, and larynx. Its functions include the exchange and filtering of air, the intake of food and liquids and their separation from the air stream entering the tracheobronchial tree, the expression of speech, and the senses of taste, smell, and hearing. Respiratory ciliated epithelium lines those portions involved in air exchange and filtration; squamous cells line the oral cavity, tongue, and oropharynx. A complex neural network and collection of lymphoid tissues are involved in the operation of the senses and local immunity, respectively. This chapter will consider disorders involving specific regions of the upper respiratory tract. Disorders of taste, smell, and hearing and vestibular function are covered elsewhere (see Chaps. 24 and 26).

NOSE

EXTERNAL NASAL DISORDERS The nose is subject to the same skin diseases as those affecting the face. *Furunculosis* is common around the nasal vestibule in the region of the hair follicles. *Staphylococcus aureus* is the usual organism. Infection in that site can be dangerous because of the potential for spread to the cavernous sinus via draining veins. Treatment should be prompt and consists of local heat and antibiotics with antistaphylococcal activity (see Chap. 100). If there is marked local edema, fever, and signs of generalized sepsis, hospitalization and parenteral antibiotic therapy are necessary, with close evaluation for sinus or intracranial involvement. Incision and drainage of large lesions are usually required. Impetigo and erysipelas caused by group A *Streptococcus* can affect the outer nose; their recognition and management are discussed in Chap. 101.

Rhinophyma is a disease caused by chronic inflammation and hypertrophy of the skin, producing bulbous violaceous nasal tips, commonly in alcoholic men. Pathologically, sebaceous gland hypertrophy occurs with scarring and acanthosis. Treatment, when warranted, is surgical.

EPISTAXIS The nose receives major arterial vessels from both the internal and external carotid artery systems. Most nosebleeds come from Kiesselbach's plexus on the nasal septum. Disorders that produce a generalized bleeding diathesis such as the acute leukemias, thrombocytopenia, aplastic anemia or severe liver disease have general evidence of bruising, petechiae, or bleeding, but rarely can present as isolated epistaxis. Similarly, anticoagulant and antiplatelet drugs usually cause a more generalized bleeding diathesis, but epistaxis may be prominent. While hypertension does not cause epistaxis directly, it can perpetuate a nosebleed; prompt control of blood pressure is an essential part of treatment. A history of delayed nosebleeds after trauma often indicates bleeding from the anterior and posterior ethmoidal artery systems. Foreign body reactions, substance abuse (e.g., cocaine), and local infection may cause nosebleeds. Rare causes of repeated bouts of epistaxis include Osler-Weber-Rendu syndrome or von Willebrand's disease. A positive family history of epistaxis or gastrointestinal bleeding may suggest the diagnosis.

Treatment In many cases pressure or a small amount of packing will suffice to stop an anterior bleed. Additional medical management of acute but not life-threatening nosebleeds includes gentle suctioning of blood clots from the nose, locating the bleeding site, and electric or chemical cautery after anesthetizing the nose topically. Topical vasoconstrictors such as phenylephrine or oxymetazoline hydrochloride may facilitate control, as may local pressure. Underlying hematologic disorders should be identified and, if required, platelets and/or fresh frozen plasma should be administered (see Chap. 62). If these measures are not sufficient, firm petroleum-coated gauze packings need to be placed. Administration of an oral antibiotic such as trimethoprim-sulfamethoxazole or amoxicillin-clavulanic acid is usually recommended to prevent a secondary sinus infection, although efficacy has not been proven. In some cases of severe posterior bleeding, a "posterior pack" is required. This requires hospitalization and the administration of prophylactic intravenous antibiotics because of obstruction of the sinus ostia. Since the packing can cause hypoxemia secondary to a nasopulmonary reflex, careful monitoring of the arterial oxygen tension is necessary with pulse oximetry or arterial blood gas determination. Supplemental oxygen delivered by face mask may be required. Surgical management is reserved for patients who continue to bleed despite appropriate anterior and posterior packing, and patients who have severe recurrent bleeding after the removal of a posterior nasal pack.

NASAL DISCHARGE AND OBSTRUCTION Rhinitis Acute, self-limited nasal inflammation, or rhinitis, causing discharge and obstruction is usually due to acute viral upper respiratory tract infection. Chronic rhinitis may take several forms: *Vasomotor rhinitis* is characterized by an autonomic imbalance with increased parasympathetic tone involving the nasal mucosa. Usually there is no history of allergy and nasal smears may show nonspecific inflammatory cells; the etiology is unknown. Treatment includes decongestants and topical steroids and in severe cases may require surgical resection of the inferior turbinate or (rarely) interruption of the vidian nerve. *Allergic rhinitis* is often associated with a history of allergies. Nasal polyps may be present and in a small number of patients may be associated with hypersensitivity to aspirin. Medical treatment includes topical steroid sprays, oral decongestant and/or antihistaminic preparations, and desensitization to allergens (see Chap. 267). *Atrophic rhinitis* is characterized by foul odor and epistaxis with nasal obstruction. Examination reveals crusting, debris, and necrosis of the normal tissues and turbinates. Causes include excessive surgical resection of the turbinates, various types of infections, and granulomatous diseases such as Wegener's granulomatosis. Treatment requires management of the underlying disease, as well as nasal douches with saline. If the underlying cause is corrected, surgical reconstruction may be

accomplished. *Rhinitis medicamentosa* refers to reactive swelling of the nasal turbinates, nasal obstruction, and increased watery secretions caused by the imprudent use of topical decongestants, specifically imidazoles and sympathomimetics. Treatment consists of termination of topical decongestants and administration of oral decongestants and topical steroids. A short course of systemic steroids may be helpful.

Cerebrospinal fluid rhinorrhea CSF rhinorrhea may follow trauma to the nose or mid-face, blunt cranial injury (e.g., basal skull fracture) causing cribriform plate fracture, or complicated nasal or transphenoidal surgery. It is characterized by a clear nasal discharge and may be complicated by acute or recurrent bacterial meningitis (see Chap. 354). The diagnosis is often confirmed by testing the fluid for glucose. The use of antibiotics to prevent infection is controversial since it is not clear that they are effective and they may change the nature of the infecting organism. Surgical treatment is necessary if spontaneous closure of the leak does not occur. Prior to definitive surgery, intravenous metrizamide coupled with computed tomographic (CT) study or fluorescein injections may demonstrate the site of the leak.

Miscellaneous disorders Less common infections and granulomatous, neoplastic, or vasculitic disorders may cause persistent discharge, obstruction, or necrotizing lesions. The infections include nasal diphtheria (Chap. 102), tuberculosis, leprosy, syphilis [with "congenital snuffles" (Chap. 128)]; glanders (Chap. 112); infection with *Klebsiella rhinoscleromatis;* histoplasmosis, cryptococcosis, and blastomycosis (Chap. 151); and mucocutaneous leishmaniasis (Chap. 160). Neoplasms include squamous cell carcinoma, malignant melanoma, lymphoma, and mycosis fungoides. Granulomatous necrotizing lesions with nasal septal destruction include Wegener's granulomatosis (Chap. 276), sarcoidosis (Chap. 277) and midline granuloma (Chap. 279). Diagnosis of these various disorders is established by culture, and histologic characteristics of biopsy materials. Treatment is outlined in the individual chapters on these diseases.

Nasal septal perforation A septal perforation is commonly the result of trauma, including nasal septal surgery and transphenoidal surgery of the pituitary gland. Perforation may be self-induced by nose picking and by substance abuse, specifically cocaine. Various granulomatous diseases, heavy metal poisoning, syphilis, leprosy, and foreign bodies are additional causes. The size of the perforation determines the clinical symptomatology such as respiratory whistling. Foreign bodies cause local inflammation, nasal obstruction, secondary infection of either the skin or paranasal sinuses, and local necrosis of the nasal tissue that can lead to septal perforation.

NASAL POLYPS AND PAPILLOMAS *Nasal polyps* are the most common mass lesion in the nose or paranasal sinuses and may be confused with neoplasms. Most patients will have associated allergic rhinitis; rarely nasal polyps occur after trauma or in cystic fibrosis. Samter's triad is rare and consists of asthma, nasal polyps, and acute hypersensitivity reactions to aspirin or nonsteroidal anti-inflammatory agents. Patients with polyps may have few symptoms or have rhinorrhea, obstruction, and anosmia. The polyps are usually seen on direct intranasal examination, and in contrast to normal nasal tissue there is no innervation so that polyps are painless on probing or manipulation. Treatment consists of surgical removal and therapy of the underlying allergic rhinitis, including glucocorticoid nasal sprays or low doses of oral glucocorticoids.

Squamous papillomas are relatively common tumors in the nose and are usually found anteriorly to overlie the alar mucosa or the nasal vestibule. These lesions can cause nasal obstruction and hemorrhage and may involve the paranasal sinuses. Thorough surgical removal is required, as these tumors frequently recur. A subtype known as the *inverting papilloma* is usually unilateral and affects men predominantly. The inverting papilloma is histologically benign but may be locally aggressive. Approximately 10 percent of inverting papillomas are associated with malignant transformation into squamous cell cancers. Such tumors occur in older individuals, but it is not clear if these malignancies represent actual malignant degeneration or only occur in conjunction with the inverting papilloma.

ANOSMIA See Chap. 24.

THE PARANASAL SINUSES

ANATOMY AND DEVELOPMENT The paranasal sinuses are cavities within the facial skeleton that are lined by ciliated respiratory epithelium and drain into the nose. The maxillary and ethmoid sinuses are present at birth; the ethmoid labyrinth grows and expands with age, so that the anterior ethmoid cells usually project above the orbital rim to develop into the frontal sinuses. Unilateral agenesis of one of the frontal sinuses is common; 4 percent of normal individuals will have bilateral agenesis. The sphenoid sinuses are the last to develop and often do not mature until patients reach their early twenties. The pituitary is located posteriorly and superiorly and may often bulge into the superior wall of the sphenoid sinus.

SINUSITIS Acute sinusitis Acute sinusitis frequently follows a viral infection of the upper respiratory tract. Rhinovirus, adenovirus, influenza, and parainfluenza virus may be recovered with bacteria in about one-fifth of cases. *Streptococcus pneumoniae* and *Haemophilus influenzae* (usually unencapsulated) account for approximately half of the bacteria isolated by direct sinus puncture and aspiration. Group A *Streptococcus*, *Staphylococcus aureus*, and *Branhamella catarrhalis* are found less frequently. Anaerobic mouth flora (see Chap. 108) are isolated in approximately 5 percent of cases and may be associated with dental disease. Sinusitis that develops in hospitalized patients, particularly following prolonged nasotracheal intubation, and sinusitis in patients on immunosuppressive or antimicrobial treatment has a higher frequency of gram-negative enteric bacteria.

Symptoms include fever, local pain, obstruction of the nasal cavity, secondary anosmia, and a purulent nasal discharge. Point-tenderness may be present over the affected sinus and transillumination of light may be diminished. In ethmoid sinusitis orbital cellulitis or blepharitis may herald intraorbital complications. The white blood cell count is elevated, with a left shift in the differential count. CT scan is most useful for confirming ethmoid or sphenoid infection and can define the extent of involvement of other sinuses.

Maxillary sinusitis can generally be treated on an outpatient basis. Therapy consists of systemic decongestants and oral antibiotics. Amoxicillin-clavulanic acid, trimethoprim-sulfamethoxazole, or cefaclor are all reasonable choices and are replacing ampicillin or amoxicillin because of the increasing frequency of β-lactamase-producing *H. influenzae* and *B. catarrhalis*. More acutely ill patients and those with complicating medical disorders such as diabetes mellitus or immunosuppressive therapy may require intravenous antibiotics. Needle aspiration of the maxillary sinus may be indicated to determine the precise microbial etiology of sinusitis in patients with a poor response to antimicrobials, persisting air-fluid levels, and facial pain.

Frontal sinusitis can present in a manner similar to maxillary sinusitis. However, because of the proximity of the frontal sinuses to the anterior cranial fossa the use of intravenous antibiotics is recommended. Additionally, serial neurologic evaluations may be required. If symptoms do not improve within 48 h after beginning therapy, surgical drainage of the affected sinus is recommended. Acute *sphenoid sinusitis* presents classically with retroorbital pain. Air-fluid levels on standard radiographs or CT scans should be diagnostic. Acute *ethmoid sinusitis* may be more difficult to diagnose clinically, although upper eyelid swelling should raise the index of suspicion.

In acute bacterial sinusitis, topical decongestant sprays (oxymetazoline, phenylephrine), used sparingly, and systemic decongestants are useful adjuncts to antimicrobials in treating the infection and restoring proper drainage. Suspected intracranial complications from acute sinusitis require immediate surgical drainage (see below).

Chronic sinusitis This common disorder has several etiologies. It can be allergic in nature or secondary to anatomic abnormalities, such as a deviated nasal septum. Symptoms of chronic sinusitis may be more vague and transient compared to the acute processes. However, a chronic purulent discharge associated with postnasal drainage, facial pain, and the sensation of pressure within the face or eye are common. Thickening of the sinus mucosa is usually present on x-rays; air-fluid levels are absent except in the case of exacerbations of acute sinusitis. Chronic sinusitis is associated more often with anaerobic organisms than are acute infections. If antibiotics, topical decongestants, and oral decongestants fail to improve the symptoms, sinus lavage may be indicated. Intranasal steroids are used in patients with known allergies and allergic rhinitis. Some patients with chronic or recurring sinusitis will have disorders of immunoglobulin production (Chap. 263), dyskinetic cilia (Chap. 208), or Wegener's granulomatosis (Chap. 276). If symptoms still persist, sinus surgery may be required to establish proper ventilation and drainage of the affected sinuses.

Complications of bacterial sinusitis EXTRACRANIAL COMPLICATIONS These most often involve the orbit. The medial border of the orbit is also the lateral border of the ethmoid labyrinth. Acute ethmoiditis can result in infection traversing the separating thin plate of bone to cause an *orbital cellulitis*. Infection in the other sinuses may also lead to orbital cellulitis. Orbital cellulitis may be either *preseptal* or *postseptal*, is accompanied by pain and lid edema, and may be a major threat to vision or a means of extension into the central nervous system. Preseptal orbital cellulitis requires prompt hospitalization and intravenous antibiotic therapy. Urgent ophthalmologic examination is necessary to assess visual acuity. Postseptal orbital cellulitis results from infection traversing the orbital septum; it requires emergency *surgical* treatment. Signs of postseptal infection include chemosis, conjunctival infection, and proptosis. Extraocular movements may become impaired, ultimately progressing to a frozen globe with the rapid development of blindness.

The *superior orbital fissure syndrome* is a complication of infection of the sphenoid sinus. Patients usually present with a palsied abducens nerve (VI) followed by lesions of cranial nerves III, IV, and V, orbital pain, exophthalmos, and ophthalmoplegia. Treatment involves documentation of sphenoid sinusitis and rapid surgical exploration.

Frontal sinus infection may extend into the anterior table of the frontal bone and cause osteomyelitis. The presentation includes fever, frontal headache, leukocytosis, and cool doughy, tender edema over the affected frontal sinus (''Pott's puffy tumor''). CT scanning is indicated to document the extent of the infection and in particular potential intracranial involvement (epidural, subdural, or frontal lobe brain abscess).

INTRACRANIAL COMPLICATIONS These include meningitis; epidural, subdural, or brain abscess; and cavernous sinus thrombosis. They are discussed in Chap. 354.

Fungal sinusitis This disorder is discussed in Chap. 151.

SINUS NEOPLASMS Neoplastic diseases of the paranasal sinuses are rare. Benign osteomas most commonly involve the frontal bone and may be a complication of chronic sinus disease. Malignancies include carcinoma of the maxillary sinus and sarcoma. Woodworkers, nickel workers, and patients with chronic sinusitis are at increased risk for developing carcinoma of the maxillary sinuses. Symptoms of neoplasms can include repeated acute sinusitis and/or recurrent epistaxis. Sinus films and/or CT scans are used to establish their existence. Biopsies are necessary for diagnosis.

EAR

OTITIS MEDIA Acute otitis media Viral upper respiratory tract infection is the most common predisposing factor to acute otitis media. The hallmark of middle ear infection is pain. A sense of fullness, purulent otorrhea, hearing loss, vertigo or tinnitus, fever, and leukocytosis may be present. Otoscopic examination will confirm the diagnosis of acute otitis media, by demonstrating a red, dull, and bulging or perforated tympanic membrane. *S. pneumoniae* (approximately 35 percent) and *H. influenzae* (approximately 20 percent) are the most frequent bacteria in middle ear effusions in acute otitis media. The majority of *H. influenzae* infections are due to the nontypeable strains. In children, infection by *H. influenzae* type b (about 10 percent of cases) can cause severe systemic toxicity and may be associated with meningitis (see Chaps. 115 and 354). Other common bacteria include *B. catarrhalis,* group A *Streptococcus,* and *Staph. aureus.* Mixed anaerobic bacteria can occasionally cause acute otitis media. Respiratory viruses are implicated in the pathogenesis but are rarely cultured. Respiratory syncytial and influenza viruses are among the more frequently incriminated agents.

Treatment of acute otitis media includes the use of antibiotics such as: amoxicillin-clavulanic acid, trimethoprim-sulfamethoxazole, or cefaclor. Antihistamines are not effective. Occasionally tympanocentesis is required for bacteriologic diagnosis in refractory cases. In persistent infection, a myringotomy with or without the insertion of a ventilating tube may be necessary. Severe pain, infection in immunologically compromised patients, or failure of antibiotic therapy are indications for surgical drainage of the middle ear space.

OTITIS MEDIA WITH CHRONIC EFFUSION Serous otitis media with chronic effusion is a leading cause of hearing loss in children and occasionally in adults. Otoscopic examination will show a retracted tympanic membrane associated with fluid in the middle ear cavity. Standard audiometry and tympanometry can reveal a conductive hearing loss and flat tympanogram consistent with restrictive disease in the middle ear space.

Therapy can be divided into conservative and surgical approaches. Decongestants and antihistamines have been advocated in the treatment of serous effusions, although their usefulness is unproven. Glucocorticoids and antibiotics have been used as well as mechanical insufflation via the eustachian tube (politerization). Control of predisposing factors is also indicated: i.e., the treatment of allergy, nasal infection, or chronic sinus infection. Occasionally the use of ventilating tubes is required for treatment of a chronic effusion in the middle ear with or without infection. This provides drainage for a potentially infected middle ear and will improve a conductive hearing loss caused by the accumulation of serous fluid in the middle ear.

Chronic otitis media The bacterial flora in chronic otitis media is variable. *Pseudomonas aeruginosa* and *Staph. aureus* are the most commonly isolated organisms, followed by *Escherichia coli* and *Proteus* species. Chronic foul-smelling otorrhea is associated with anaerobic infection. Chronic suppuration of the middle ear may be associated with perforation of the tympanic membrane and cholesteatoma (predominantly keratin debris) formation. Imaging with conventional x-rays or CT will show signs of mucosal thickening in the middle ear space as well as in the mastoid cavity. Cholesteatoma may penetrate into the temporal bone and, rarely, the cranial cavity. Treatment is directed at eradicating the infection with a combination of local care, antibacterial ear drops, and often systemic antibiotics. Surgical removal of a cholesteatoma is required.

MASTOIDITIS The mastoid air cells are in direct continuity with the middle ear space unless blocked by an intervening mass. Cholesteatoma, either acquired or congenital, may obstruct the natural drainage of the mastoid air cells. Because of the direct communication between the two cavities, every otitis media is in the truest sense a mastoiditis. The organisms causing mastoid infections are generally the ones that cause acute middle ear infections. Radiographs of the mastoid air cells frequently demonstrate fluid or mucosal thickening within the honeycomb labyrinth of the mastoid. This indicates chronic infection, and treatment is similar to that of acute otitis media.

Emergent simple mastoidectomy is indicated when there is high fever and leukocytosis with radiographic evidence of destruction of trabeculae and the honeycomb of the mastoid air cells. Signs of acute otitis media are usually also present. A subperiosteal abscess may be associated, in which case examination will reveal an ear that is displaced inferiorly and laterally with a red fluctuant mass behind the pinna. When suspected clinically, CT scanning will usually confirm the diagnosis.

COMPLICATIONS OF OTITIS MEDIA AND MASTOIDITIS Extracranial complications include conductive, mixed, and sensorineural hearing loss. Labyrinthitis manifested by vertigo as well as weakness or complete paralysis of the ipsilateral facial nerve may be direct complications of a middle ear infection. A syndrome consisting of otalgia, a draining middle ear, and paralysis of the ipsilateral sixth cranial nerve reflects infection of the petrous apex of the temporal bone (Gradenigo's syndrome). Therapy is medical, with surgical intervention reserved for refractory cases. Intracranial complications of otitis media include meningitis, brain abscess, epidural abscess, lateral sinus thrombophlebitis, and otitic hydrocephalus (see Chap. 364).

EXTERNAL OTITIS The external auditory canals are lined by skin and are subject to the same diseases of skin as the rest of the body. Psoriasis may be the cause of an external otitis. Glands within the external auditory canal secrete cerumen, which acidifies the external auditory canal and minimizes the overgrowth of bacteria. *Otitis externa* (swimmer's ear) is most common in the summer months and is thought to arise from a change in the milieu of the external auditory canal by increased alkalinization. This leads to the overgrowth of bacteria, most commonly *Staphylococcus, Streptococcus,* and *Pseudomonas* species. Treatment includes topical antibacterial ear drops, although occasionally systemic antibiotics are required. Mycotic infections that cause otitis externa refractory to antibacterial treatment are diagnosed by smears and culture and are treated with topical antifungal ear drops. *Herpes zoster* in the external auditory canal can cause an associated loss of the sensory and motor functions of the nerve VII (Ramsay-Hunt syndrome) (see Chaps. 136 and 360).

Necrotizing (malignant) otitis externa This progressive necrotizing infection results in osteomyelitis of the temporal bone and is almost always caused by *P. aeruginosa.* Occasionally the soft tissues and the cartilage of the pinna are also involved. The disorder occurs most commonly in patients with insulin dependent diabetes mellitus. The diagnosis should be suspected in patients with severe refractory otorrhea and disproportional pain. Physical examination will often reveal granulation tissue in the posterior ear canal wall that is eroding into the temporal bone. The auricle and surrounding scalp may be swollen, tender, and necrotic. CT, bone, and occasionally indium 111 leukocyte scans are useful for making the diagnosis. Treatment consists of local care including debridement and antibacterial ear drops combined with intravenous antibiotics directed against *P. aeruginosa* (Chap. 111). Good control of coexisting *diabetes mellitus* may hasten recovery (Chap. 319). Occasionally radical debridement of the temporal bone is required.

Perichondritis Perichondritis is an infection or inflammation of the cartilage of the pinna. The most common organism found in infectious perichondritis is *P. aeruginosa.* The lobule is spared infection because it contains no cartilage. *Relapsing polychondritis* is an inflammatory disease of the external ear that initially may mimic infection and needs to be distinguished from perichondritis (see Chap. 284).

THE PHARYNX

ACUTE PHARYNGITIS The cause of acute pharyngitis is almost always infection, although for pharyngeal inflammation and ulceration it may be agranulocytosis or injury by chemicals or radiation. The major symptom of acute pharyngitis regardless of etiology is sore throat, with or without attendant difficulty in swallowing. Examination will reveal erythema and congestion of the mucosa with hypertrophy of the lymphoid tissue including the tonsils. Exudate if present is suggestive of infection by group A *Streptococcus.* The differential diagnosis of acute exudative pharyngitis is discussed in detail in Chap. 101. Exudate may be seen with a variety of viral infections, in particular those caused by Epstein-Barr virus (Chap. 137), herpes simplex virus (Chap. 135), or adenovirus (Chap. 140). Other organisms that produce an exudate include the gonococcus (Chap. 110), *Corynebacterium diphtheriae* (Chap. 102), *Mycoplasma pneumoniae* (Chap. 154), and the TWAR strains of *Chlamydia* (Chap. 155). Infection with respiratory syncytial virus and parainfluenza and influenza viruses may also cause sore throat without exudate, whereas in rhinovirus infections (Chap. 140) a "scratchy" throat may be a prominent feature. The diagnosis and treatment of the specific causes are covered in the individual chapters.

COMPLICATIONS   Chronic or acute infection of the naso- or oropharynx and its lymphoid tissue may lead to a variety of pyogenic complications that require emergent surgical drainage or removal. These include recurrent tonsillitis and peritonsillar and retropharyngeal abscesses and are discussed in Chaps. 91 and 101. Ludwig's angina, which is *not* a pharyngeal infection but rather a mixed bacterial infection of the sublingual or submandibular space, is discussed in Chaps. 91 and 108.

PHARYNGEAL TUMORS   The nasopharynx can be the site of a variety of neoplasms. These include lymphomas, lymphoepitheliomas (Schmenke's tumor), squamous cell carcinoma, and anaplastic carcinoma. Less common tumors include amelanotic melanoma, rhabdomyosarcoma, and extramedullary plasmacytomas (often associated with multiple myeloma). Pharyngitis and lymphoid hypertrophy may cause obstruction, particularly in children. In adults, symptoms of obstruction, particularly when chronic, should raise concern about a possible neoplasm. Voice changes may be present with hyponasality. A conductive hearing loss may be due to blockage of the distal eustachian tube.

The most common neoplasm of the oropharynx is a squamous cell carcinoma. Clinical signs and symptoms include dysphagia, odynophagia, halitosis, weight loss, and in advanced cases, respiratory obstruction. Risk factors include excessive alcohol intake and cigarette smoking. Endoscopy and biopsy are required for diagnosis and staging. Therapy may include surgery, radiation, or combined modality treatments depending on the stage of the tumor and the status of the lymph nodes in the neck. Benign and malignant tumors of the minor salivary glands can present in the pharynx. Lymphomas, including Hodgkin's disease, may cause unilateral tonsillar swelling (see Chap. 302).

ORAL CAVITY DISORDERS

Disorders of the oral cavity are reviewed in Chap. 41.

THE LARYNX

SIGNS AND SYMPTOMS OF LARYNGEAL DISEASE   Persistent unexplained change in the voice, i.e., hoarseness or weakness, is pathognomonic of laryngeal disorders. Other symptoms include cough that may be dry or associated with the production of clear, purulent, or blood-streaked sputum; pain that may refer to other branches of the vagus nerve, manifested by otalgia, and upper respiratory obstruction causing stridor. Dysphagia and odynophagia may be associated with neoplastic lesions of the larynx. Besides evaluation of the neck, oropharynx, and gag and swallowing reflexes, physical examination should include an indirect mirror examination and, if available, flexible fiberoptic endoscopy. Vocal cord dysfunction, mass lesions, mucosal ulceration, infection of the larynx, structural abnormalities, and occasionally subglottic lesions will be evident on these examinations. Definitive diagnosis requires biopsy usually under anesthesia.

DISORDERS OF VOCAL CORD FUNCTION (see Chap. 360)   The vagus nerve can be damaged at the nuclear level in the brainstem; in the neck, where it loops around either the aorta on the left or the subclavian artery on the right; or in the tracheo-esophageal groove as it proceeds superiorly to innervate the intrinsic laryngeal musculature. The superior laryngeal nerve branches from the vagus nerve relatively high in the neck as part of the neurovascular pedicle that contains the superior thyroid artery. A lesion distal to this branching will result in isolated recurrent laryngeal nerve damage that causes paralysis of the posterior cricoarytenoid muscle and fixes the vocal cord on the affected side in a paramedian position. With combined dysfunction of both the recurrent and superior laryngeal nerves the

vocal cord is paralyzed in an intermediate position, producing a faint, breathy voice, but a larger airway for the inspiration of air. With isolated superior laryngeal nerve dysfunction paralysis of the cricothyroid muscle occurs, the vocal cord on the affected side abducts, but the larynx is only slightly rotated and the vocal cord appears bowed.

Careful physical examination will help define the possible anatomic lesions causing either unilteral or bilateral vocal cord paralysis. Bilateral paramedian vocal cord paralysis is a surgical emergency. Although the voice may be preserved, stridor can be life-threatening. Emergency tracheotomy or endotracheal intubation is the usual treatment.

LARYNGEAL INFECTIONS   Acute epiglottitis   Rapidly progressive cellulitis of the epiglottis and surrounding tissues in the supraglottic airway can cause acute airway obstruction. In infants and children the causative agent is most commonly *H. influenzae* type b and bacteremia is frequent (see Chap. 115).

In adolescents and adults with acute bacterial epiglottitis, the clinical presentation may be less fulminant and other organisms have been implicated in some cases (e.g., *S. pneumoniae*, *Staph. aureus*). Frequently the patient complains of dysphagia, odynophagia, and fever that has progressed over one to two days. Depending on the degree of respiratory obstruction, stridor may or may not be present, but hoarseness and loss of voice power are almost universal findings. As in children, the adult with epiglottitis usually prefers to lean forward, drooling oral secretions. Because the caliber of the airway is larger in the adult, intubation or tracheotomy may not be necessary, but the possibility of complete airway obstruction dictates management. An edematous, cherry red epiglottis and surrounding pharyngeal mucosa are characteristic findings on fiberoptic examination, which in adults is the best way to confirm the diagnosis. In infants and children this approach is contraindicated because of the threat of acute airway obstruction (see Chap. 115). A lateral film of the neck may reveal an enlarged epiglottis—the so-called "thumb sign."

Until the possibility of airway obstruction has passed the adult patient is best managed by admission to an intensive care unit where adequate clinical monitoring is available. Fiberoptic examination in adults with a nasopharyngoscope should be performed only after preparations have been made to secure the airway by endotracheal intubation or, if necessary, tracheostomy. After blood and throat cultures are obtained, appropriate antibiotic treatment is initiated with either a combination of ampicillin and chloramphenicol, cefuroxime, or another third-generation cephalosporin, such as cefotaxime, administered intravenously (see Chaps. 85 and 115). Oxygen should be administered as dictated by O_2 saturations on pulse oximetry or arterial blood gas determination. Humidified air by face tent is advisable. If respiratory obstruction worsens, endotracheal intubation is required. Glucocorticoids have been administered as part of the treatment but with unproven benefit. Resolution of clinical manifestations usually occurs over 36 to 48 h. A child should not be extubated nor a patient removed from an intensive care setting unless the acute cellulitis has resolved, as confirmed by endoscopy.

Croup (laryngotracheobronchitis)   Croup is a syndrome produced by acute infection of the lower air passages and is most commonly seen in children below age 3. The most common pathogen is the *Parainfluenza* virus (Chap. 140), but a variety of respiratory viruses and *Mycoplasma pneumoniae* can produce acute laryngotracheobronchitis and the croup syndrome. The pathophysiology is primarily one of circumferential mucosal inflammation in the subglottic larynx and trachea with variable involvement and spasm of the vocal cords; the epiglottis is not involved. The clinical hallmarks, namely, a barking or brassy cough with or without stridor and hoarseness, are discussed in Chap. 140. Croup can be distinguished readily from epiglottitis by lateral films of the neck which show no epiglottal edema, or by careful direct examination. Management of severe croup requires hospitalization, close observation, humidification, oxygenation as dictated by pulse oximetry, and rarely intubation. Glucocorticoid administration has been advocated by some, but the benefits are questionable.

Tuberculous laryngitis Tuberculous laryngitis is usually associated with active pulmonary tuberculosis. Characteristic manifestations include hoarseness, cough, and blood-tinged sputum; because of the large number of organisms in the sputum it is usually highly contagious. The most common site of disease in the larynx is in the interarytenoid fold (in the posterior portion of the larynx). Because granulomas tend to be subepithelial, *deep submucosal biopsies* may be essential for diagnosis. Treatment is the same as for pulmonary tuberculosis (Chap. 125), and symptomatic measures include voice rest and analgesics for pain. Occasionally tracheostomy is needed to protect the airway.

Fungal infections of the larynx The most commonly found mycotic infections of the larynx are histoplasmosis, candidiasis, and blastomycosis. Symptoms can include hoarseness, cough, dyspnea, dysphagia, and odynophagia. Examination may reveal oral and esophageal thrush with candidiasis or nodules on the vocal cords with or without ulceration (histoplasmosis or blastomycosis). With the latter, diagnosis is confirmed by biopsy showing microabscesses in an epithelium infiltrated with giant cells, mononuclear cells, and yeast (Chap. 151). Treatment with systemic antifungal agents is necessary. While not a fungus, actinomycosis may involve the pharynx and larynx from adjacent mandibular or tonsillar infection. The diagnosis and treatment are discussed in Chap. 152.

Other laryngeal infections Other infections which may involve the larynx include tertiary syphilis (Chap. 128), lepromatous leprosy (Chap. 126), diphtheria (Chap. 102), and glanders (Chap. 112). Biopsy is usually required for the diagnosis of syphilis and leprosy, both of which may produce infiltrating nodular lesions. Other diagnostic measures and treatment are discussed in the individual chapters on these agents.

PERICHONDRITIS *Perichondritis* in the larynx due to pyogenic bacterial infection or an inflammatory process may be difficult to distinguish from traumatic injury, certain neoplasms, or injury induced by radiation. The thyroid cartilage is the most common cartilage affected and an abscess may form beneath the mucoperichondrium. Symptoms and signs include pain, tenderness, and swelling that are usually slowly progressive but occasionally very acute. Hoarseness, airway compromise, dysphagia, and odynophagia require prompt radiographic evaluation to exclude the possibility of a foreign body. The airway should then be secured in the operating room. Treatment may require antibiotics or glucocorticoids and debridement of laryngeal granulations.

INFLAMMATORY DISORDERS OF THE LARYNX Ulcers and granulomas of the true vocal cords may result from a variety of types of abuse, including excessive use of the voice. Reflux esophagitis may cause contact ulcers of the vocal cords over the posterior larynx and the arytenoids. Persistent hoarseness is the most common manifestation. In reflux eosophagitis, both throat and gastric pain are common, and a history of gastric ulcer disease is common. On physical examination the classical lesion involves ulceration of the mucosa over the arytenoid cartilages. Treatment requires management of the underlying esophageal or gastric disease (Chaps. 237 and 238). Treatment of the larynx is symptomatic, with voice rest and speech therapy.

Vocal cord nodules Vocal abuse can cause vocal cord or "singer's" nodules. Sinusitis, upper respiratory tract infections, and allergy are known precipitating factors. Tobacco and alcohol may add to irritation. The diagnosis is made by direct or indirect (mirror) laryngoscopy. Treatment for children consists of voice therapy and parental counseling, and for adults voice rest and treatment of precipitating disorders. Occasionally operative removal of the nodules is required.

Sarcoid Sarcoidosis may rarely cause granulomatous disease of the epiglottis and surrounding structures of the vocal cords with sparing of the cords. Hoarseness and airway obstruction may be present (see Chap. 277).

Cricoarytenoid joint arthritis The cricoarytenoid joint is an articular joint which may be involved by systemic arthritis such as gout and rheumatoid arthritis. With rheumatoid arthritis of the cricoarytenoid joint, pain, aggravated by speech, or dysphagia associated with hoarseness are the most common symptoms. On physical examination a bright red swelling of the arytenoid is a common finding, and the vocal cords may be fixed. Evidence of systemic rheumatoid arthritis is usually present (see Chap. 270). Besides treatment for systemic rheumatoid disease, tracheostomy may be required if airway obstruction occurs.

LARYNGEAL STENOSIS Stenosis of the larynx is typically divided into supraglottic, glottic, and subglottic types. Many patients have stenosis at more than one level. Stenosis can be caused by ingestion of caustic materials, endotracheal intubation, irradiation, inflammatory or granulomatous disease, or infection. The etiology is usually apparent by history but with infiltrative processes may require biopsy for diagnosis. Most patients have some hoarseness, and, if the stenosis is severe, stridor and significant airway obstruction may be present. Symptomatic subglottic stenosis following endotracheal intubation is more common in children and may be progressive. Useful diagnostic studies include lateral neck x-rays with linear tomography to determine the site and extent of the stenosis, and confirmation by direct laryngoscopy. Flow-volume-loop studies will reveal upper airway obstruction (see Chap. 201). Management ranges from manual dilatation to surgical reconstruction, depending on the location and degree of the stenosis. With acute severe respiratory obstruction tracheostomy can be lifesaving and is generally preferred over intubation.

FOREIGN BODIES Choking on foods and other foreign bodies causes over 2000 deaths per year in the United States, and is the sixth most common cause of accidental death. Most foreign body aspiration occurs in children under four years of age. The aspiration in such cases is infrequently observed and may not be suspected initially. Peanuts seem to be the most common foreign body aspirated by children, followed by other food stuffs and metallic objects. Most of the foreign bodies lodge within the bronchial tree and about 5 percent get stuck in the larynx. In adults aspiration of poorly chewed food (the so-called "cafe coronary," often associated with inebriation, poor dentition, or swallowing disorders) is the most common cause of acute obstruction. Symptoms can include "sticking" pain localized to the larynx, laryngeal spasm, change in voice quality up to complete aphonia, stridor, and dyspnea, or complete lack of air movement despite attempted respiratory excursions. Perforation of the larynx by sharp objects may lead to infection. For acute obstruction with aphonia and no air movement forced pressure to the epigastrium—the *Heimlich maneuver*—is indicated to dislodge the material. Foreign bodies retained in the trachcobronchial tree require prompt endoscopic removal.

NEOPLASMS OF THE LARYNX **Benign tumors** The most common type of benign laryngeal tumor is the papilloma. Other tumors include hemangioma, angiofibroma, chemodectoma, neurofibroma, chondroma, and granular cell myoblastoma. As with many other laryngeal disorders, the presentation is with hoarseness. Dyspnea, dysphagia, and pain are late findings. Fiberoptic endoscopy can be done in an outpatient setting to evaluate hoarseness. If a laryngeal tumor is seen, formal endoscopic evaluation and biopsy are necessary. The histopathology is generally diagnostic and dictates subsequent treatment.

PAPILLOMA The papilloma is a benign tumor of the larynx that is caused by the human papilloma virus (Chap. 150) of which three predominant serotypes are involved in laryngeal disease. At present there is some debate as to whether there are two clinical forms: an adult form and a juvenile form. Generally, the adult form tends to be unifocal and easier to treat. Juvenile laryngeal papillomatosis is often multifocal and occurs in preschool children. Extensive laryngeal and tracheal involvement may cause stridor, and routine examination can be difficult. Endoscopic evaluation in the operating room with biopsy is needed for diagnosis.

The proper treatment of laryngeal papillomatosis is controversial, and recurrence is common. The mainstay of therapy is the carbon dioxide laser and several operative procedures may be required in order to extirpate the lesions. Papillomas can also be removed by mechanical debridement with a cupped forceps, cryotherapy, wide surgical excision (which is more commonly performed in the oropharynx and the oral cavity), and by argon laser treatment after photosensitization. Children with laryngotracheal papillomatosis may require long-term tracheostomies. Systemic α-interferon increases the rate of remission and decreases that of recurrence within the first 6 months of treatment, but long-term remission is rare with interferon alone. Because of the possibility of malignant degeneration, radiation should be avoided.

Laryngeal malignancies Squamous cell carcinoma, the most common neoplasm of the larynx, usually presents after the fifth decade of life and is associated with tobacco and alcohol use. Less common malignancies include neuroendocrine tumors, tumors of the minor salivary glands, and neoplasms of mesodermal origin. Hoarseness is the most prominent manifestation of cancers of the vocal cords; origin from other laryngeal locations may be asymptomatic until late in the course, when stridor and/or dyspnea develop. Pain can be scratchy, vague, and nonspecific or it may present as ipsilateral otalgia referred by the vagus nerve. Dysphagia may be produced by laryngeal tumors that have spread out of the larynx to invade either the base of the tongue or the walls of the adjacent hypopharynx. Odynophagia, chronic cough, and hemoptysis may also occur. Halitosis from tumor necrosis, metastatic cervical adenopathy, and weight loss are late features of this disease.

Laryngeal cancer is diagnosed by direct laryngoscopy, pharyngoscopy, and biopsy. The extent of spread beyond the site of origin can be assessed by physical examination and radiographic studies including CT and MRI. A staging system that categorizes the location, size, and extent of spread of malignancies has been utilized to develop appropriate therapeutic approaches and for prognostic purposes. Small stage 1 lesions are localized to the vocal cord and can be cured by radiation in over 90 percent of cases. Partial laryngectomy may be curative for more extensive localized disease, with radiation reserved for recurrences. Total laryngectomy is employed for advanced cancer and is combined with radical neck dissection if the tumor has spread to draining lymph nodes. Radiation can be employed either as adjunctive initial treatment or reserved for recurrences. Decisions as to which therapeutic approach to employ are usually best made by a multidisciplinary tumor board. As with other squamous cell cancers, metabolic complications such as hypercalcemia or hyponatremia may complicate advanced disease (see Chap. 309). Extensive surgery and external beam irradiation may lead to hypoparathyroidism and/or hypothyroidism.

REFERENCES

BALLENGER JJ: Acquired ultrastructural alterations of respiratory cilia and clinical disease: A review. Ann Otol Rhinol Laryngol 97:253, 1988

ENGLISH GM (ed): *Otolaryngology*, revised edition. New York, Harper & Row, 1989

FRICK WE, BUSSE WW: Respiratory infections: Their role in airway responsiveness and pathogenesis of asthma. Clin Chest Med 9:539, 1988

GWALTNEY JM: Sinusitis, in *Principles and Practice of Infectious Diseases*, 3d ed, GL Mandell et al (eds). New York, Churchill Livingstone, 1990, pp 510–514

HEALY G et al: Treatment of recurrent respiratory papillomatosis with human leukocyte interferon. N Engl J Med 319:401, 1988

HUOVINEN P et al: Pharyngitis in adults; the presence and coexistence of viruses and bacterial organisms. Ann Intern Med 110:612, 1989

LUCENT FE, HYAMS VJ: Inflammatory and neoplastic disorders of the nasal mucosa. Clin Dermatol 5:35, 1987

NACLERIO RM: The pathophysiology of allergic rhinitis: Impact of therapeutic intervention. J Allergy Clin Immunol 82:927, 1988

Nasal obstruction. Otolaryngol Clin North Am 22: 2, 1989

PARSONS JT et al: Hyperfractionation for head and neck cancer. Int J Radiat Oncol Biol Phys 14:649, 1988

TOGIAS A et al: Studies on allergic and nonallergic nasal inflammation. J Allergy Clin Immunol 81:782, 1988

WENIG BM et al: Moderately differentiated neuroendocrine carcinoma of the larynx: A clinicopathologic study of 57 cases. Cancer 62:2658, 1988

215   NEOPLASMS OF THE LUNG

JOHN D. MINNA

Each year, primary carcinoma of the lung affects more than 100,000 males and 50,000 females in the United States, most of whom die within 1 year of diagnosis, making it the leading cause of cancer death. The peak incidence of lung cancer occurs between ages 55 and 65 years. The overall incidence is increasing, causing the age-adjusted lung cancer death rate to double every 15 years. However, the effects of antismoking efforts started 10 to 20 years ago have finally started to be seen in a flattening of the incidence rate of lung cancer in white males while, unfortunately, the rate in females is still increasing. At the time of diagnosis, only 20 percent of all lung cancer patients will have local disease, while 25 percent will have disease spread to regional lymph nodes, and 55 percent will have distant metastatic cancer. Even in those patients with supposedly localized disease, overall 5-year survival is only 30 percent for males and 50 percent for females, and this survival rate has not changed significantly over the past 20 years. Thus, primary carcinoma of the lung is a major health problem with a generally grim prognosis. However, an orderly approach to diagnosis, staging, and treatment based on knowledge of the clinical behavior of lung cancer allows selection of the best therapy for either potential cure or optimal palliation of individual patients. This approach should be multidisciplinary, involving interaction of internists, chest physicians, medical, radiation, and surgical oncologists, pathologists, and supportive care personnel.

PATHOLOGY

The histologic classification of primary lung neoplasms recommended by the World Health Organization in 1977 should be used. Four major cell types make up 95 percent of all primary lung neoplasms. These are squamous or epidermoid carcinoma, small cell (also called "oat cell") carcinoma, adenocarcinoma (including bronchioloalveolar), and large cell (also called large cell anaplastic) carcinoma. The remainder include combined epidermoid and adenocarcinomas, carcinoids, bronchial gland tumors (including cylindromas and mucoepidermoid tumors), and mesotheliomas, as well as rarer tumor types. The various cell types have different natural histories and responses to therapy, and thus a correct histologic diagnosis by an experienced pathologist is the first step to correct treatment. In the past 10 years, for unknown reasons, the incidence of adenocarcinoma is rising while that of epidermoid cancer is falling.

Major treatment decisions are made on the basis of the crucial distinction between histologic classification of a tumor as a small cell carcinoma or one of the "non-small cell" varieties (which include epidermoid, adenocarcinoma, large cell carcinoma, bronchioloalveolar carcinoma, and mixed versions of these). Some of these distinctions are summarized in Tables 215-1 and 215-2. In general, small cell carcinoma has spread beyond the bounds of resectional surgery at the time of presentation and is primarily managed with chemotherapy with or without radiotherapy. In contrast, non-small cell cancers found to be localized at the time of presentation should be considered for a curative attempt with either surgery or radiotherapy. However, the response of non-small cell cancers to chemotherapy usually is not dramatic, making such therapy less important in metastatic disease than it is in nearly all small cell lung cancer patients.

Ninety percent of patients with lung cancer of all histologic types are cigarette smokers, while the rare nonsmoking patient who develops lung cancer usually has adenocarcinoma. However, in nonsmokers with adenocarcinoma involving the lung, the possibility of other primary sites, particularly breast cancer in women, should be considered. Epidermoid and small cell cancers usually present as central

TABLE 215-1 Incidence, frequency of metastases, and surgical resectability of the major lung cancer histologic types

Cell type	Incidence in autopsy series, %	Necropsy frequency of distant metastases when clinically localized, %*	Resectability rate (AJC study), %†	5-Year survival after curative resection, %
Non-small cell carcinoma:				
Epidermoid	33	17	60	37
Adenocarcinoma	25	40	38	27
Large cell carcinoma	16	14	38	27
Small cell carcinoma	25	63	11	<1

* Determined from autopsy studies of patients dying of causes other than cancer within 30 days following an apparent curative surgical resection.
† AJC = American Joint Committee Study for Cancer Staging and End Results Reporting, indicating percentage of cases thought to undergo a curative resection.
SOURCE: Adapted from JD Minna et al, 1989.

masses with endobronchial growth, while adenocarcinomas and large cell cancers tend to present as peripheral nodules or masses with pleural involvement. Epidermoid and large cell cancers cavitate in 20 to 30 percent of cases. Bronchioloalveolar carcinoma can present as a single mass, a diffuse, multinodular lesion, or as a fluffy infiltrate.

ETIOLOGY

The large majority of lung cancers are caused by carcinogens and tumor promoters ingested via cigarette smoking. There is a dose-response relationship between the lung cancer death rate and the total amount (often expressed in "cigarette pack-years") of cigarettes smoked, such that the risk is increased sixty- to seventyfold for the man smoking two packs a day for 20 years compared to the nonsmoker. Conversely, the chance of developing lung cancer decreases with cessation of smoking but may never return to the nonsmoker level. The increase in lung cancer in women is also associated with a rise in female cigarette smoking. As a preventive measure, efforts to get persons to stop smoking should continue. However, this is extremely difficult as the smoking habit represents a powerful addiction to nicotine. Therefore, it is equally important to prevent people from starting to smoke. Probably there is a cocarcinogenic effect of smoking and industrial or environmental pollutants such as radon gas from natural sources in the ground.

The current poor prognosis for most patients with lung cancer requires the continued performance of well-designed clinical trials to test new forms of therapy. These include further adjuvant and neoadjuvant trials combined with surgery and radiotherapy; prospective testing of tumor sensitivity in vitro to drugs, radiation therapy, and biologic response modifiers; tests of anti-growth factor therapy; and application of newer methods using monoclonal antibodies for early detection. The key intervention remains prevention, and broad antismoking efforts must continue. However, the detection of genetic lesions predisposing to malignancy would be a major step forward in focusing preventive efforts, early diagnosis, and eventually targeting therapy at the products that make lung cancer cells malignant.

While human lung cancer is not thought of as a genetic disease, a variety of molecular genetic studies have shown that lung cancer cells have acquired a number of genetic lesions including activation of dominant oncogenes and inactivation of the newly discovered tumor suppressor or recessive oncogenes (Chap. 300). In fact, it appears that to become clinically evident, lung cancer cells have to accumulate a large number (perhaps 10 or more) of such lesions. For the dominant oncogenes these include: point mutations in the coding regions of the *ras* family of oncogenes (particularly in the K-*ras* gene in adenocarcinoma of the lung); amplification, rearrangement, and/or loss of transcriptional control of *myc* family oncogenes (c-, N-,

TABLE 215-2 Comparison between small cell and non-small cell lung cancers

	Small cell	Non-small cell
Histology	Scant cytoplasm; small hyperchromatic nuclei with fine chromatin pattern; nucleoli indistinct; diffuse sheets of cells	Abundant cytoplasm; pleomorphic nuclei with coarse chromatin pattern; nucleoli often prominent; glands or squamous architecture
General neuroendocrine properties:		
Dense core granules	Present	Absent*
L-Dopa decarboxylase activity	High	Absent
Chromogranin	Present	Absent
Synaptophysin	Present	Absent
Neuron-specific enolase	High	Low
Creatine kinase BB isozyme	High	Low
Leu-7, HNK-1 antigens	Present	Absent
Peptide hormone production:		
Gastrin releasing peptide gene products	Present	Absent
Other neuropeptides	ACTH, AVP, calcitonin, ANF	PTH
Other markers:		
HLA, β₂-microglobulin	Absent/low	Present
Intermediate filament pattern	"SCLC"	"Non-SCLC"
Neurofilaments	Present	Absent
EGF receptors	Low or absent	Present
Mucin	Absent	Present in adenocarcinomas
Surfactant associate proteins	Absent	Often present
Carcinoembryonic antigen	Present	Present
Cytogenetics:		
3p(14–23) deletion	Present 100%	Present in 40–50%
rb gene abnormality	Present in majority	Present in minority
Other deletions (e.g., 17p)	Present	Present
Response to radiotherapy	Objective shrinkage in 80–90%; often complete response	Objective shrinkage in 30–50%; uncommonly complete
Response to combination chemotherapy:		
Overall regression rate	90%	30–40%
Complete regression rate	50%	5%
Overall 5-year survival rates	5%	8%

*Ten percent of non-small cell lung cancers have populations of cells expressing neuroendocrine markers, and these are best demonstrated by immunohistochemical stains.

and L-*myc*), with changes in c-*myc* found in non-small cell cancers while changes in all *myc* family members are found in small cell lung cancer; high-level, deregulated expression of the c-*raf* serine-threonine kinase activity; and high-level, deregulated expression of members of the *jun* family of oncogenes, which act as transcription factors and mediate cellular responses to tumor promoters. For the recessive oncogenes, cytogenetic and restriction fragment length polymorphism (RFLP) analysis has shown a prominent deletion involving chromosome region 3p(14–23) present in all small cell and 40 to 50 percent of non-small cell lung cancers; other deletions involving chromosome region 17p in small cell lung cancer; and most specifically, abnormalities of the *rb* gene (in chromosome region

13q14) in small cell lung cancer. In fact, the *rb* gene exhibits abnormalities in DNA, RNA, or protein in perhaps all small cell lung cancers and some non-small cell lung cancers.

The large number of genetic lesions could be acquired by several mechanisms. Cell biologic studies have shown that lung cancer cells produce a large number of peptide hormones which can act to stimulate their growth in an "autocrine" fashion. These include gastrin releasing peptide and transferrin in small cell lung cancer and insulin-like growth factors in all types of lung cancer. The production of these factors, and in addition, the high level of expression of *jun* family oncogenes, provides a setting for tumor promotion (outgrowth of cells with genetic lesions) in bronchial epithelium after genetic lesions have been initiated by carcinogens in cigarette smoke or the environment. Other possible sources for these genetic lesions include familial inheritance or lesions acquired during development. While lung cancer does not have a clear pattern of Mendelian inheritance, there are several indications of a potential for familial association. These include the inheritance of the high-debrisoquine metabolic phenotype; studies that show that first-degree relatives of lung cancer probands have a significant (two- to threefold) excess risk of lung cancer or other cancers, many of which are not smoking-related; and the strong risk of developing lung cancer that has been shown to be linked with development of chronic obstructive pulmonary disease.

CLINICAL MANIFESTATIONS AND MODE OF PRESENTATION

Lung cancer gives rise to signs and symptoms from local tumor growth, invasion or obstruction of adjacent structures, growth in regional nodes via lymphatic spread, growth in distant metastatic sites after hematogenous dissemination, or as a remote effect (paraneoplastic syndrome) usually resulting from peptide hormone secretion by the tumor. Appropriate identification of these signs and symptoms as tumor-related will guide further evaluation and therapy and be of prognostic importance.

If programs screening asymptomatic patients are excluded, 5 to 15 percent of patients are detected while asymptomatic, usually on a routine chest radiograph, while the vast majority of patients present with some sign or symptom. Signs and symptoms secondary to central or endobronchial growth of the primary tumor include cough, hemoptysis, wheeze and stridor, dyspnea, and pneumonitis (fever and productive cough) from obstruction. Signs and symptoms secondary to the peripheral growth of the primary tumor include pain from pleural or chest wall involvement, cough, dyspnea on a restrictive basis, and symptoms of lung abscess resulting from tumor cavitation. Signs and symptoms related to the regional spread of tumor in the thorax by contiguity or by metastasis to regional lymph nodes include tracheal obstruction, esophageal compression with dysphagia, recurrent laryngeal nerve paralysis with hoarseness, phrenic nerve paralysis with elevation of the hemidiaphragm and dyspnea, and sympathetic nerve invasion and paralysis with Horner's syndrome. *Pancoast's*, or *superior sulcus tumor, syndrome* results from local extension of a tumor (usually epidermoid) growing in the apex of the lung with involvement of the eighth cervical and first and second thoracic nerves, with shoulder pain which characteristically radiates in the ulnar distribution of the arm, often with radiologic destruction of the first and second ribs. Often Horner's syndrome and Pancoast's syndrome will coexist. Other problems of regional spread include *superior vena cava syndrome* from vascular obstruction; pericardial and cardiac extension with resultant tamponade, arrhythmia, or cardiac failure; lymphatic obstruction with resultant pleural effusion; and lymphangitic spread through the lungs with hypoxemia and dyspnea. In addition, bronchioloalveolar carcinoma can spread transbronchially, producing tumor growing along multiple alveolar surfaces with resultant impairment of oxygen transfer, respiratory insufficiency, dyspnea, hypoxemia, and production of large amounts of sputum.

Extrathoracic metastatic disease is found at autopsy in over 50 percent of patients with epidermoid carcinoma, 80 percent of patients with adeno- and large cell carcinoma, and over 95 percent of patients with small cell cancer. These autopsy studies have found lung cancer metastases in virtually every organ system. Thus, the majority of lung cancer patients eventually need therapy to palliate symptoms. Common clinical problems related to extrathoracic metastatic lung cancer include brain metastases with neurologic deficits; bone metastases with pain and pathologic fractures; bone marrow invasion with cytopenias or leukoerythroblastosis; liver metastases causing biochemical liver dysfunction, anorexia, biliary obstruction, and pain; lymph node metastases in the supraclavicular region and occasionally in the axilla and groin that can be painful and ulcerate; and spinal cord compression syndromes from epidural or bone metastases.

Paraneoplastic syndromes are common in lung cancer patients and may be the presenting finding or first sign of recurrence. In addition, paraneoplastic syndromes may mimic metastatic disease and, unless detected, lead to inappropriate palliative rather than curative treatment. Often the paraneoplastic syndrome may be relieved with successful treatment of the tumor, and tumor treatment is the basis for correcting such syndromes. In some cases the pathophysiology of the paraneoplastic syndrome is known, particularly when a hormone with biologic activity is secreted by a tumor (Chap. 309). However, in many cases the pathophysiology is unknown. *Systemic symptoms* of anorexia, cachexia, and weight loss (seen in 30 percent of patients), with fever, and suppressed immunity, are paraneoplastic syndromes of unknown etiology. *Endocrine syndromes* are seen in 12 percent of patients and have the best understood pathophysiology, including hypercalcemia and hypophosphatemia resulting from ectopic parathyroid hormone or PTH-related peptide production by epidermoid cancer; hyponatremia with the syndrome of inappropriate secretion of antidiuretic hormone or possibly atrial natriuretic factor by small cell cancer; and ectopic secretion of ACTH by small cell cancer, which usually results in additional electrolyte disturbances, especially hypokalemia, rather than the changes in body habitus seen in Cushing's syndrome from a pituitary adenoma.

Skeletal connective tissue syndromes include clubbing in 30 percent (usually non-small cell) and hypertrophic pulmonary osteoarthropathy in 1 to 10 percent (usually adenocarcinomas) with periostitis and clubbing giving pain, tenderness, and swelling over the affected bones, and a positive bone scan. *Neurologic-myopathic syndromes* are seen in only 1 percent of patients but are dramatic and include the myasthenic *Eaton-Lambert syndrome* with small cell cancer, while peripheral neuropathies, subacute cerebellar degeneration, cortical degeneration, and polymyositis are seen with all lung cancer types. *Coagulation and thrombotic and hematologic manifestations* occur in 1 to 8 percent of patients and include migratory venous thrombophlebitis (*Trousseau's syndrome*); nonbacterial thrombotic (marantic) endocarditis with arterial emboli; disseminated intravascular coagulation with hemorrhage; and anemia, granulocytosis, and leukoerythroblastosis. *Cutaneous manifestations* such as dermatomyositis and acanthosis nigricans are uncommon (1 percent or less) as are the *renal manifestations* of nephrotic syndrome or glomerulonephritis (1 percent or less).

DIAGNOSIS AND STAGING

EARLY DIAGNOSIS Screening persons at high risk (males over 45 years of age smoking 40 or more cigarettes per day) for lung cancer with sputum cytologies and chest radiographs every 4 months has shown a prevalence rate of lung cancer in asymptomatic patients of four to eight cases per 1000 persons. With follow-up screening, four new cases of lung cancer are found per 1000 persons followed per year. These lung cancers are detected 72 percent of the time by radiographs alone, 20 percent by cytology alone, while 6 percent are detected by both methods. In contrast to nonscreened patients, 90 percent of these screened patients who develop lung cancer are asymptomatic, 62 percent have resectable lung cancer, and 53 percent of all the new cases are postsurgical stage I (see below) with a 5-year survival probability of 45 percent. However, in a large, multi-institutional, prospective randomized trial there was no difference in the survival rate between the screened and the nonscreened group of smoking males ≥45 years old. This was because of the presence of metastases in the majority of patients even when tumors were detected at a very early stage.

ESTABLISHING A TISSUE DIAGNOSIS OF LUNG CANCER Once signs, symptoms, or screening studies suggest lung cancer, it is necessary to establish a tissue diagnosis of malignancy, determine the histologic cell type, and stage the patient for appropriate treatment. In the initial evaluation of each patient, tumor tissue should be obtained so that a histologic diagnosis of cancer and tumor cell type can be firmly made. Distinction of small cell from non-small cell lung cancer is crucial and is often difficult in cytology preparations. Therefore, cytologic diagnoses from washings or needle aspirates should be reserved for very high risk patients or patients relapsing with cancer after initial treatment. Tumor tissue can be obtained from a bronchial biopsy or transbronchial forceps biopsy at fiberoptic bronchoscopy; from node biopsy at mediastinoscopy; from the operative specimen at the time of definitive surgical resection; from percutaneous biopsy of an enlarged lymph node, soft tissue mass, lytic bone lesion, bone marrow, or pleural lesion; or from an adequate cell block from a malignant pleural effusion.

STAGING PATIENTS WITH LUNG CANCER Lung cancer staging consists of two parts: first, a determination of the location of tumor (anatomic staging) and second, an assessment of a patient's ability to withstand various antitumor treatments (physiologic staging). For example, in a patient with non-small cell lung cancer it is crucial to determine if the tumor can be resected by a standard surgical procedure such as a lobectomy or pneumonectomy (determination of "resectability") based on the anatomic stage of the tumor and whether the patient could tolerate such a surgical procedure (determination of "operability") based on the cardiopulmonary condition of the patient.

Non-small cell lung cancer The TNM international stage system (ISS) developed by the American Joint Committee (AJC) on End Results Reporting, and modified by an international commission, should be used in non-small cell lung cancer, particularly in preparing patients for curative attempts with surgery or radiotherapy (Table 215-3). The various T (tumor size), N (regional node involvement), and M (presence or absence of distant metastasis) factors are combined to form different stage groups and, in addition, there is a group covering occult carcinoma detected on screening cytology exam with no other evidence of tumor (Table 215-3).

Small cell lung cancer A simple two-stage system adapted from the Veterans Administration Lung Cancer Study Group is used. In this two-stage system, *limited stage disease* (about 30 percent of all small cell cancer patients) is defined as disease confined to one hemithorax and regional lymph nodes (including mediastinal, contralateral hilar, and usually ipsilateral supraclavicular nodes), while *extensive stage disease* (about 70 percent of all patients) is defined as disease beyond this. Employed in staging are clinical studies such as physical examination, x-rays, scans, and bone marrow examination. In part, the definition of *limited stage* relates to whether the known tumor can be encompassed within a tolerable radiation therapy port. Thus, contralateral supraclavicular nodes, recurrent laryngeal nerve involvement, and superior vena caval obstruction can all be limited stage disease. However, cardiac tamponade, malignant pleural effusion, and bilateral pulmonary parenchymal involvement are generally scored as extensive stage disease because of the size of the radiation therapy port required to cover all known disease.

GENERAL STAGING PROCEDURES (Table 215-4) All lung cancer patients should have a complete history and physical examination, with evaluation of all other medical problems and a determination of performance status and weight loss, both of which have

TABLE 215-3   TNM classification of lung cancer using the new International Staging System (ISS)

PRIMARY TUMOR (T)

T0	No evidence of a primary tumor.
TX	Occult cancer seen in bronchial washing cytologies but not seen on x-ray or fiberoptic bronchoscopy.
TIS	Carcinoma in situ.
T1	Tumor ≤3 cm in greatest dimension, surrounded by lung or visceral pleura, and without evidence of invasion proximal to a lobar bronchus at bronchoscopy. (Uncommon superficial tumors of any size with invasive components limited to the bronchial wall that extend proximal to the main bronchus are also classified as T1.)
T2	Tumor >3 cm in greatest dimension *or* a tumor of any size that either invades the visceral pleura or has associated atelectasis–obstructive pneumonitis extending to the hilar region. At bronchoscopy, the proximal extent of demonstrable tumor must be within a lobar bronchus or at least 2 cm distal to the carina. Any associated atelectasis or obstructive pneumonitis must involve less than an entire lung.
T3	A tumor of any size with direct extension into the chest wall (including superior sulcus tumors), diaphragm, mediastinal pleura, or pericardium without involving heart, great vessels, trachea, esophagus, or vertebral body *or* a tumor in the main bronchus within 2 cm of the carina without involving the carina.
T4	A tumor of any size with invasion of the mediastinum or involving heart, great vessels, trachea, esophagus, vertebral body, or carina *or* the presence of a malignant pleural effusion. (Pleural effusions that are not bloody and not exudative with several negative cytopathologic examinations are not scored as a malignant effusion for staging purposes.)

REGIONAL LYMPH NODES (N)

N0	No demonstrable metastasis to regional lymph nodes.
N1	Metastasis to lymph nodes in the peribronchial or ipsilateral hilar region, or both, including direct extension.
N2	Metastasis to ipsilateral mediastinal or subcarinal lymph nodes.
N3	Metastasis to contralateral mediastinal, contralateral hilar, ipsilateral or contralateral scalene, or supraclavicular lymph nodes.

DISTANT METASTASIS (M)

M0	No known distant metastasis.
M1	Distant metastasis present with site specified (e.g., brain).

STAGE GROUPING USING THE NEW ISS

Occult carcinoma	TX	N0	M0
Stage 0	TIS	Carcinoma in situ	
Stage I	T1	N0	M0
	T2	N0	M0
Stage II	T1	N1	M0
	T2	N1	M0
Stage IIIa	T3	N0	M0
	T3	N1	M0
	T1–3	N2	M0
Stage IIIb	Any T	N3	M0
	T4	Any N	M0
Stage IV	Any T	Any N	M1

SOURCE: Adapted from CF Mountain.

great prognostic value. An ear, nose, and throat examination is also necessary because of the frequent occurrence of second cancers in this area. While not done in every patient, fiberoptic bronchoscopy remains a cornerstone of lung cancer staging and follow-up, providing material for pathologic examination, and information on tumor size, location, degree of bronchial obstruction, and recurrence.

Chest roentgenograms are needed to evaluate tumor size and nodal involvement, and it is very useful to obtain old x-ray films for comparison. Chest computed tomography (CT) scans are now widely used in the staging and follow-up of lung cancer patients. CT scans are of use in non-small cell lung cancer in preoperative staging to detect mediastinal nodes and pleural extension, and in the planning of curative radiation therapy to allow design of fields to encompass all known tumor volume while avoiding as much normal tissue as possible. However, definitive characterization of mediastinal nodal

TABLE 215-4   Pretreatment staging procedures for lung cancer patients

ALL PATIENTS

Complete history & physical examination
    Determination of performance status and weight loss
    Ear, nose, and throat examination
Complete blood count with platelet determination
Serum electrolytes, glucose, calcium, phosphorus, renal and liver function tests
Electrocardiogram
Skin test for tuberculosis
Chest x-ray
Computed tomography scan of brain, chest, abdomen, and radionuclide scan of bone if any of the above studies suggest presence of tumor metastasis in these organs
X-rays of suspicious bony lesions detected by scan or symptom
Barium swallow radiographic examination if esophageal symptoms exist
Pulmonary function studies and arterial blood gas measurements if signs or symptoms of respiratory insufficiency are present
Biopsy of accessible lesions suspicious for cancer if a histologic diagnosis is not yet made or if treatment or staging decisions would be based on whether or not a lesion contained cancer

PATIENTS PRESENTING WITH NO OBVIOUS CONTRAINDICATION TO CURATIVE SURGERY OR RADIOTHERAPY

All above and:

Fiberoptic bronchoscopy with washings, brushings, and biopsy of suspicious areas
Pulmonary function tests and arterial blood gas measurements
Coagulation tests
Computed tomographic scans of brain, chest, and abdomen
If surgical resection is planned: surgical evaluation of the mediastinum at mediastinoscopy or at thoracotomy
If the patient is a poor surgical risk or a candidate for curative radiotherapy: Transthoracic fine-needle aspiration biopsy or transbronchial forceps biopsy of peripheral lesions if material from routine fiberoptic bronchoscopy is negative.

PATIENTS PRESENTING WITH DISEASE THAT IS NOT CURABLE BY EITHER SURGERY OR RADIOTHERAPY*

For non-small cell lung cancer or unknown, all under "All Patients" and:

Fiberoptic bronchoscopy if indicated by hemoptysis, obstruction, pneumonitis, or no histologic diagnosis of cancer
Biopsy of accessible lesions suspicious for tumor to obtain a histologic diagnosis or if therapy would be altered by finding of tumor
Transthoracic fine-needle aspiration biopsy or transbronchial forceps biopsy of peripheral lesions if fiberoptic bronchoscopy is negative and no other material exists for a histologic diagnosis
Diagnostic and therapeutic thoracentesis if a pleural effusion is present

For proven small cell lung cancer, all under "All Patients" and:

Fiberoptic bronchoscopy with washings and biopsy
Chest, abdomen, and brain CT scans useful but not mandatory
Bone marrow aspiration and biopsy

---

* Patients with non-small cell lung cancer and extrathoracic metastatic disease, malignant pleural effusion, or intrathoracic disease beyond the bounds of a tolerable radiotherapy port.

---

involvement should depend upon histologic proof when planning curative treatment. In small cell lung cancer, CT scans are used for chest radiation treatment planning and assessing the response to chemotherapy and radiation therapy. In following patients after surgery or radiotherapy, procedures which can make interpretation of conventional chest x-rays difficult, CT scans can provide good evidence of tumor recurrence.

If signs or symptoms suggest organ involvement by tumor, appropriate CT or radionuclide scans (e.g., brain, liver, or bone) are performed, as well as radiographs of any suspicious bony lesions. Routine scans are not obtained in the asymptomatic patient because of the high frequency of false-positive and false-negative studies. Any accessible lesions suspicious for cancer should be biopsied if a histologic diagnosis has not already been made, or if treatment decisions would be based on whether or not the lesion contained cancer.

In patients presenting with a mass lesion on chest x-ray and no obvious contraindications to a curative approach with surgery or radiotherapy after the initial evaluation, the mediastinum must be investigated. Approaches vary between different centers and include: (1) performing chest CT scan, and if this is positive, mediastinoscopy; (2) proceeding directly to mediastinoscopy (right-sided tumors) or lateral mediastinotomy (left-sided lesions) on all patients; (3) proceeding directly to thoracotomy with staging of the mediastinum at this time. In patients presenting with disease confined to the chest but not resectable, thus making them candidates for curative radiotherapy, other tests are only done as indicated to evaluate specific symptoms. In patients presenting with non-small cell cancer that is not curable by either surgery, radiotherapy, or their combination, all of the general procedures are done plus fiberoptic bronchoscopy as indicated to evaluate hemoptysis, obstruction, or pneumonitis; as well as diagnostic-therapeutic thoracentesis with cytologic examination if fluid is present.

STAGING OF SMALL CELL LUNG CANCER Pretreatment staging for patients with histologically documented small cell lung cancer includes the initial general lung cancer evaluation as well as fiberoptic bronchoscopy with washings and biopsies to determine the tumor extent before therapy; brain CT scan, since 10 percent of patients have metastases; bone marrow biopsy and aspiration, since 20 to 30 percent of patients have tumor in the bone marrow; and CT or radionuclide scans of liver and bone if symptoms or other findings are suggestive of disease involvement in these areas. Chest and abdominal CT scans are very useful but not mandatory to evaluate and follow tumor response to therapy. Percutaneous or peritoneoscopy-directed liver biopsy may be performed if other findings are suggestive but not diagnostic of the presence of tumor in the liver, and if tumor involvement here would alter the planned therapy.

If signs or symptoms of spinal cord compression or leptomeningitis develop at any time in lung cancer patients of any histologic type, a myelogram or magnetic resonance scan and examination of the cerebrospinal fluid cytology are performed to determine the need for local therapy to the site of compression (usually with radiotherapy) and for intrathecal chemotherapy (usually with methotrexate) if malignant cells are detected. In addition, a brain CT scan is performed to search for brain metastases that are often associated with spinal cord or leptomeningeal metastases.

DETERMINATION OF RESECTABILITY AND OPERABILITY In patients with non-small cell lung cancer, the following are major contraindications to curative attempts by surgery or radiotherapy alone using standard treatment methods: extrathoracic distant metastases; superior vena cava syndrome; vocal cord and, in most cases, phrenic nerve paralysis; malignant pleural effusion; cardiac tamponade; tumor within 2 cm of the carina (not curable by surgery but potentially curable by radiotherapy); metastasis to the contralateral lung; bilateral endobronchial tumor (potentially curable by radiotherapy); metastasis to the supraclavicular lymph nodes; lymph node metastasis in the contralateral mediastinum (potentially curable by radiotherapy); involvement of the main stem pulmonary artery; and a histologic diagnosis of small cell lung cancer.

PHYSIOLOGIC STAGING Patients with lung cancer often have cardiopulmonary and other problems related to chronic obstructive pulmonary disease as well as other medical problems. To improve their preoperative condition, correctable problems (e.g., anemia, electrolyte and fluid disorders, infections, and arrhythmias) should be addressed, smoking stopped, and appropriate chest therapy instituted. Since it is not always possible to predict whether a lobectomy or pneumonectomy will be required until the time of operation, a conservative approach is to restrict resectional surgery to patients who could potentially tolerate a pneumonectomy. In addition to nonambulatory performance status, a myocardial infarction within the past 3 months is a contraindication to thoracic surgery because 20 percent of patients will die of reinfarction alone, while an infarction in the past 6 months is a relative contraindication. Other major contraindications include: uncontrolled major arrhythmias; maximum breathing capacities of less than 40 percent predicted; an FEV_1 less than 1 L; CO_2 retention (which is more serious than hypoxemia); and severe pulmonary hypertension. Recommending surgery when the FEV$_1$ is 1.1 to 2.4 L requires careful judgment, while an FEV$_1$ over 2.5 L will usually permit a pneumonectomy. In patients with borderline pulmonary status or a question of pulmonary hypertension, split pulmonary function testing by ventilation-perfusion lung scans can define physiologic operability. The activity from quantitative scans is summed for each lung in the anterior and posterior view, and the ratio of the normal to total lung activity multiplied by the FEV$_1$. Pneumonectomy is physiologically tolerable if this predicted value is greater than 1 L.

TREATMENT

After a histologic diagnosis is obtained and appropriate anatomic and physiologic staging studies are completed, the overall treatment approach to patients with lung cancer may be formulated (Table 215-5).

NON-SMALL CELL LUNG CANCER: LOCALIZED DISEASE In patients with non-small cell lung cancer of stages I and II (Table 215-3) who can tolerate operation, the treatment of choice is pulmonary resection. In stage IIIa cases with favorable age, cardiopulmonary function, and anatomy, resection should also be considered. If a complete resection is possible, the 5-year survival rate for N1 disease is about 50 percent, while it is about 30 percent for N2 disease. However, only 20 percent of all patients who have N2 disease are technically resectable, and in most cases these resectable patients are only discovered to have N2 disease at thoracotomy. Patients with contralateral or bilateral positive mediastinal (N3) nodes, extracapsular nodal involvement, or fixed nodes are not currently considered resectable. New approaches to convert patients from unresectable to resectable status include: chest wall resections for direct extension of tumor; tracheal sleeve pneumonectomy; and sleeve lobectomy for lesions near the carina. Neoadjuvant (preoperative) chemotherapy, while experimental, gives tumor response rates of 50 to 60 percent and converts many responding patients to resectability.

The extent of resection is a matter of surgical judgment based on findings at exploration. In general, conservative resection that en-

compasses all known tumor gives survival equal to that obtained with more extensive procedures. Thus, lobectomy is preferred to pneumonectomy, while wedge resections and segmentectomies are reserved for patients with poor pulmonary reserve and small peripheral lesions. Approximately 43 percent of all lung cancer patients will undergo thoracotomy. Of these, 76 percent will have a definitive resection, 12 percent will only be explored for disease extent, and 12 percent will have a palliative procedure with known disease left behind. The fraction of long-term survivors following definitive surgical therapy is remarkably consistent throughout major centers performing lung cancer surgery in the United States. Approximately 30 percent of all patients resected for cure survive 5 years, and 15 percent survive 10 years. The 30-day hospital mortality following pulmonary resection at major centers is also very consistent, 3 percent for lobectomy and 6 percent for pneumonectomy. As a function of postsurgical treatment stage the 5-year survival data are (1) epidermoid: stage I, 54 percent, stage II, 35 percent, stage IIIa N0–N1, 19 percent, stage IIIa N2, 13 percent; (2) adenocarcinoma and large cell carcinoma: stage I, 51 percent, stage II, 18 percent, stage IIIa N0–N1, 10 percent, stage IIIa N2, 2 percent. Thus, the majority of patients who were initially thought to have a "curative" resection ultimately died of metastatic disease (usually within 2 years of surgery).

MANAGEMENT OF OCCULT AND STAGE 0 CARCINOMAS When sputum cytology screening indicates malignant cells but a normal chest radiograph is found (TX tumor stage), the lesion must be localized. Over 90 percent can be localized by meticulous examination of the bronchial tree with a fiberoptic bronchoscope under general anesthesia and collection of a series of differential brushings and biopsies. Often carcinoma in situ or multicentric lesions are found in these patients. Current recommendations are for the most conservative surgical resection, allowing removal of the cancer and conservation of lung parenchyma even if the bronchial margins are positive for carcinoma in situ. The 5-year overall survival for these occult cancers is approximately 60 percent. Close follow-up of these patients is indicated because of the high incidence of second primary lung cancers (approximately 5 percent per patient per year). A new approach to in situ or multicentric lesions uses systemically administered hematoporphyrin (which localizes to tumors and sensitizes them to light) followed by bronchoscopic phototherapy.

SOLITARY PULMONARY NODULE When a patient presents with an asymptomatic, solitary pulmonary nodule (defined as an x-ray density completely surrounded by normal aerated lung, with circumscribed margins, of any shape, usually 1 to 6 cm in greatest diameter), a decision to resect or follow the nodule must be made. Approximately 35 percent of all such lesions in adults will be malignant, the majority being primary lung cancer, while less than 1 percent are malignant in nonsmoking patients under 35 years of age. A complete history, including a smoking history, physical examination, routine laboratory tests, fiberoptic bronchoscopy, and old chest x-rays are obtained. If no diagnosis is immediately apparent, the following risk factors would all argue strongly in favor of proceeding with resection to establish a histologic diagnosis: history of cigarette smoking; age 35 years or older; a relatively large-sized lesion; lack of calcification; chest symptoms; associated atelectasis, pneumonitis, or adenopathy; and growth of the lesion compared to old x-rays. At present, only two radiographic criteria are strongly reliable for benignity of a solitary pulmonary nodule: lack of growth over a period greater than 2 years and certain characteristic patterns of calcification. Calcification alone does not exclude malignancy. However, a dense central nidus, multiple punctate foci, "bull's eye" (granuloma), and "popcorn ball" (hamartoma) calcifications are all highly suggestive of a benign lesion.

When old x-rays are not available and the characteristic calcification patterns are absent, the following approach is reasonable: nonsmoking patients under 35 years can be followed with serial chest x-rays every 3 months for 1 year and then yearly. If any significant growth is found, a histologic diagnosis is needed. For patients over 35 and all patients with a smoking history, a histologic diagnosis must be made.

TABLE 215-5 Summary of treatment approach to lung cancer patients

NON-SMALL CELL LUNG CANCER

Resectable (stages I, II, IIIa, and selected T3, N2 lesions)
  Surgery
  Radiotherapy for "nonoperable" patients
  Postoperative radiotherapy for N2 disease
Nonresectable (N2 and M1)
  Confined to chest: high-dose chest radiotherapy (RT) if possible
  Extrathoracic: RT to symptomatic local sites; chemotherapy (CT) (for good-performance status patients, with evaluable lesions)

SMALL CELL LUNG CANCER

Limited stage (good performance status)
  Combination chemotherapy + chest RT
Extensive stage (good performance status)
  Combination chemotherapy
Complete tumor responders (all stages)
  Prophylactic cranial RT
Poor-performance-status patients (all stages)
  Modified dose combination chemotherapy
  Palliative RT

ALL PATIENTS

Radiotherapy for brain metastases, spinal cord compression, weight-bearing lytic bony lesions, symptomatic local lesions (nerve paralyses, obstructed airway, hemoptysis in non-small cell lung cancer and in small cell cancer not responding to chemotherapy)
Appropriate diagnosis and treatment of other medical problems and supportive care during chemotherapy
Encouragement to stop smoking

This can either occur at the time of nodule resection or, if the patient is a poor operative risk, via transthoracic fine-needle biopsy. Some institutions would use preoperative fine-needle aspiration on all such lesions; however, all positive lesions will have to proceed to resection, and negative cytologic findings will in most cases have to be confirmed by histology on a resected specimen. While much has been made of sparing patients an operation, the high probability of finding a malignancy (particularly in smokers over 35) and the excellent chance for surgical cure when the tumor is small, all suggest an aggressive approach to these lesions.

RADIOTHERAPY   Those patients who are stage III, as well as those with stages I and II disease who refuse surgery or appear not to be candidates for pulmonary resection for medical reasons, should be considered for radiation therapy with curative intent. The decision to administer high-dose and potentially curative radiotherapy is based upon the extent of disease and the volume of the chest that requires irradiation. Patients with distant metastases, positive supraclavicular nodes, pleural effusion, or cardiac involvement are generally not considered for such curative radiation treatment. The median survival for unresectable patients with non-small cell lung cancer localized to the chest undergoing primary radiotherapy with curative intent is less than 1 year. However, 6 percent of these patients are alive at 5 years and cured when treated with radiotherapy alone. In addition to potential cure, radiotherapy, by controlling the primary tumor, may increase the quality and length of life of noncured patients. Treatment usually involves midplane doses of 55,000 to 60,000 mGy (5500 to 6000 rad), and the major concern is the amount of lung parenchyma and other organs in the thorax included within the treatment plan, including the spinal cord, heart, and esophagus. Patients with a major degree of underlying pulmonary disease may have to have the treatment plan compromised because of the deleterious effect of radiation on pulmonary function. Either split course or continuous fraction radiotherapy can be given with similar survival results. The development of radiation pneumonitis is proportional to the dose of radiation and volume of lung incorporated within the radiation field. The full clinical syndrome (dyspnea, fever, and radiographic infiltrate corresponding to the treatment port) occurs in 5 percent of cases. Acute radiation esophagitis occurs during treatment but usually is self-limited, while spinal cord injury should be avoided by careful treatment planning.

COMBINED MODALITY THERAPY   Recent randomized trials have shown survival benefit for adjuvant chemotherapy given after surgical resection. However, this will have to be confirmed before adjuvant chemotherapy after surgery or radiotherapy is recommended for general use. Many centers give high-dose, postoperative radiation if postsurgical staging documents nodal disease. However, randomized trials of postoperative radiotherapy, while showing improved local tumor control, have not shown survival benefit.

Carcinomas of the superior pulmonary sulcus producing *Pancoast's syndrome* are often treated with combined radiotherapy and surgery. These patients should have the usual preoperative staging procedures, including mediastinoscopy as well as CT scans to determine tumor extent and neurologic examination with electromyography to document neurologic findings. Often a histologic diagnosis is not made, and with the constellation of tumor location and pain distribution the diagnostic accuracy for cancer is better than 90 percent. If mediastinoscopy is negative, two curative approaches may be used in treating a Pancoast's syndrome tumor. In the first, preoperative irradiation [30,000 mGy (3000 rad) in 10 treatments] is given to the area followed by an en bloc resection of the tumor and involved chest wall 3 to 6 weeks later. At 3 years, survival figures of 42 percent for epidermoid and 21 percent for adeno- and large cell carcinomas have been reported. The second approach involves radiotherapy alone in curative doses and standard fractionation with similar survival to combined modality therapy reported.

Data have now appeared suggesting a high frequency of brain metastases as isolated sites of relapse in patients with adenocarcinoma of the lung otherwise cured by surgery or radiotherapy. While there is no proven role for "prophylactic" cranial irradiation, it is not unreasonable to follow potentially cured, asymptomatic adenocarcinoma patients with frequent brain CT scans to detect such recurrence at the earliest possible time so that radiotherapy can be given.

DISSEMINATED NON-SMALL CELL LUNG CANCER   The 70 percent of patients who have unresectable non-small cell cancer have a poor prognosis. For example, median survivals of 34, 25, 17, 8, and 4 weeks are seen for patients with performance status scores of 0 (asymptomatic), 1 (symptomatic, fully ambulatory), 2 (in bed <50 percent of the time), 3 (in bed >50 percent of the time), and 4 (bedridden), respectively. Standard medical management, the judicious use of pain medications, and the appropriate use of radiotherapy form the cornerstone of management. Patients whose primary tumors are causing symptoms such as bronchial obstruction with pneumonitis, hemoptysis, or upper airway or superior vena caval (SVC) obstruction should, in general, have radiotherapy to the primary tumor. The case for prophylactic treatment of the asymptomatic patient is to prevent major symptoms from occurring within the thorax. However, if the patient can be followed closely, deferring treatment until the development of symptoms is appropriate. Usually a course of 30,000 to 40,000 mGy (3000 to 4000 rad) over 2 to 4 weeks is given to the tumor. The frequencies of relief by radiation therapy of intrathoracic symptoms are hemoptysis, 84 percent; SVC syndrome, 80 percent; dyspnea, 60 percent; cough, 60 percent; atelectasis, 23 percent; and vocal cord paralysis, 6 percent. Other symptoms of metastatic disease treated with radiotherapy include cardiac tamponade (treated with pericardiocentesis and radiation therapy to the entire cardiac silhouette); painful bony metastases (with relief in 66 percent of cases); brain or spinal cord compression; and brachial plexus involvement. Usually, with brain and cord compression, dexamethasone (25 to 100 mg total per day in four divided doses) is also given and then rapidly tapered to the lowest dosage which relieves neurologic symptoms. In all cases, the key to effective palliation is to detect the complication and begin radiotherapy at the earliest possible time. Pleural effusions are common and are usually treated with thoracentesis as needed, but without radiotherapy. If they recur and are symptomatic, chest tube drainage with a sclerosing agent such as intrapleural tetracycline is used. The chest is first completely drained. Then 1000 mg of tetracycline is dissolved in 100 mL of normal saline, and 50 mL of 1% xylocaine added, and this is injected via the chest tube. The chest tube is clamped and the patient rotated onto different sides to distribute the sclerosing agent. Then 24 to 48 h later the chest tube is pulled when there is little drainage (usually less than 100 mL per 12 h). Symptomatic intrabronchial lesions that recur after surgery or radiotherapy, or the development of such lesions in patients with severely compromised pulmonary function, are difficult to treat with conventional therapy. However, neodymium-YAG (yttrium-aluminum-garnet) laser therapy administered via a flexible fiberoptic bronchoscope (usually under general anesthesia) can provide palliation to 80 to 90 percent of patients even when the tumor has relapsed after radiotherapy. In addition, patients can be retreated with YAG laser therapy.

The use of chemotherapy for non-small cell lung cancer requires careful judgment to balance potential benefits and toxicity. However, recent results suggest modest survival benefit from such combination chemotherapy. Approximately 30 to 40 percent of patients will have objective tumor response to combination chemotherapy. However, a complete clinical regression of tumor (a "complete response") occurs in less than 5 percent of cases. Those patients whose tumors respond to chemotherapy have significantly longer survivals (around 30 to 40 weeks median survival) compared to those patients who do not respond to therapy (10 to 20 weeks median). The problem is that the responding patients also have better prognostic features (such as good performance status), and it is difficult to separate the effect of these on survival from that of chemotherapy. However, in patients with good performance status, response to chemotherapy is also associated with prolonged survival, and in some cases, relief of symptoms. Nevertheless, such combination chemotherapy can have severe side effects including treatment-related mortality. Thus, in those patients with non-small cell lung cancer who desire chemotherapy, it is reasonable to give chemotherapy if the patient is fully ambulatory, has an evaluable tumor mass (to follow response to therapy), has not received prior chemotherapy, and is able to understand and accept the potential benefits and toxicities from such therapy. The chemotherapy should be delivered by an experienced physician or medical oncologist, who should use one of the published standard regimens, such as "CAP" [cyclophosphamide, doxorubicin (Adriamycin), cisplatin]; etoposide + cisplatin; or mitomycin C + vinblastine + cisplatin.

SMALL CELL LUNG CANCER Untreated patients with small cell lung cancer have median survivals of only 6 to 17 weeks, while patients treated with combination chemotherapy have median survivals of 40 to 70 weeks. Thus, the correct integration of chemotherapy with or without radiotherapy or surgery is the cornerstone of the treatment of small cell cancer. The goal of treatment is to obtain a complete clinical regression of tumor documented by repeating the initial positive staging procedures, particularly fiberoptic bronchoscopy with washings and biopsy. The initial response, determined 6 to 12 weeks after the start of therapy, predicts both median and long-term survival and potential cure. Patients obtaining a complete clinical regression of tumor survive longer than patients with only partial regression (tumor shrinkage of more than 50 percent of visible disease with no sign of tumor progression elsewhere), who in turn survive longer than patients with no response. In addition, all long-term (over 3 years) survivors come from the complete response group.

Following initial staging, patients are grouped into the limited or extensive disease stages and classified as being physiologically able or not able to tolerate combination chemotherapy or combined modality chemoradiotherapy. The overall mortality rate from initial combination chemotherapy even in these selected patients is about 5 percent at major centers. This figure is comparable to the operative mortality rate for pulmonary resection and indicates the need for physiologic staging of patients before chemotherapy. Such therapy should be reserved for ambulatory patients, with no prior chemotherapy or radiotherapy, no other major medical problems, and adequate heart, liver, renal, and bone marrow function. The arterial P_{O_2} on room air should be above 6.6 kPa (50 mmHg), and there should be no CO_2 retention. All patients with some or more of these limitations must have their initial chemoradio- or chemotherapy modified to prevent undue toxicity. In all patients the chemoradiotherapy must be coupled with supportive care for infectious, hemorrhagic, and other medical complications. This induction period is best supervised by a medical oncologist. Meticulous attention to the details of therapy and the day to day management of the patient through the initial 6 to 12 weeks of treatment is essential if therapy-related mortality is to be kept low.

Chemotherapy A variety of effective combination chemotherapy regimens have been reported for small cell lung cancer, including CAV (cyclophosphamide + doxorubicin + vincristine); CAVP-16 (cyclophosphamide + doxorubicin + VP-16); and VP-16 (etoposide) + cisplatin. At present there is no evidence that any one regimen is better than another if adequate drug dose and schedules are used. The initial combination chemotherapy often results in moderate to severe granulocytopenia (e.g., granulocyte counts less than 500 to 1500 per microliter) and thrombocytopenia (platelets less than 50,000 to 100,000 per microliter). Following the initial "induction" therapy, patients should be restaged to determine if they have entered a "complete clinical remission," indicated by complete disappearance of all clinically evident lesions and paraneoplastic syndromes, or a "partial remission"; or have "no response" or tumor progression (seen in 10 percent of patients or less). Following this, "maintenance" chemotherapy is given to responding patients for periods of 6 to 12 months in 3-, 4-, or 6-week cycles, depending on the chemotherapy regimen used. Appropriate drug dose modifications are made to keep the white blood count above 2000 per microliter and the platelet count above 50,000 per microliter. The patients are restaged between 6 and 12 months, depending on the individual regimens; if they are still in a complete remission, chemotherapy is stopped. The value of more prolonged chemotherapy is not documented. Patients with a partial tumor regression are generally kept on chemotherapy until the time of objective tumor progression and then switched to new chemotherapy (either with known activity or on an experimental protocol). Patients not responding or with objective tumor progression should be switched to new chemotherapy, preferably with a non-cross-resistant combination in an attempt to get an objective tumor response.

High-dose [40,000 mGy (4000 rad)] radiotherapy to the whole brain should be given to patients with documented brain metastases. Prophylactic cranial irradiation (PCI) may be given to patients with complete responses, as this will significantly decrease the development of brain metastases (occurring in 60 to 80 percent of patients living 2 or more years who do not receive such prophylactic radiotherapy), but such prophylactic therapy has not been shown to prolong survival. Because some studies indicate possible deficits in cognitive ability that could be related to PCI, long-term quality of life after PCI needs to be further studied. In the case of symptomatic progressive lesions in the chest or at other critical sites, if radiotherapy has not yet been given to these areas, it may be administered in full doses [e.g., 40,000 mGy (4000 rad) to the chest tumor mass].

There are definite toxicities of both an acute and chronic nature that should be expected with combined modality chemoradiotherapy, particularly if chemo- and radiotherapy are given concurrently. However, retrospective analysis of long-term survivors and analysis of local failures in the chest following chemotherapy alone suggest that chest radiotherapy is of benefit, and thus it is currently recommended for limited stage patients. Patients should be selected (limited stage disease with PS 0–1 and initial good pulmonary function) such that radiotherapy can be given in full doses, by conventional fractionation, and in a manner that will not sacrifice too much lung. The radiation oncologist must be prepared to deliver tailored radiotherapy with shaping of fields during treatment, much the same as is done for Hodgkin's disease. In extensive stage disease, the routine use of initial chest radiotherapy usually is not advocated. However, in favorable patients (e.g., those with PS 0–1, good pulmonary function, and only one site of extensive disease) radiotherapy can be considered. In all patients, if chemotherapy is inadequate to relieve local tumor symptoms, a course of radiotherapy can be added.

Several centers around the world have reported potential cure rates of 15 to 25 percent for limited stage disease and 1 to 5 percent for extensive stage disease. Overall, approximately 50 percent of patients with limited stage and 30 percent with extensive stage disease will enter a complete remission, and 90 to 95 percent of all patients will have some objective tumor shrinkage (complete or partial response). These responses increase the median survival from 2 to 4 months for untreated patients to 10 to 12 months for extensive stage and 14 to 18 months for limited stage patients. In addition, most patients have relief of their tumor-related symptoms and improvement of performance status. However, the maintenance of good performance status by the patient while receiving outpatient chemotherapy requires judgment and skill on the part of the medical oncologist delivering the chemotherapy so as to avoid undue therapeutic toxicity. New treatments such as new drug combinations, very intensive initial or "reinduction" therapy with autologous bone marrow infusion, as well as novel forms of combining chemo- and radiotherapy and surgery should all be reserved for approved clinical protocols.

While surgical resection is not routinely recommended for small cell lung cancer, occasional small cell cancer patients will either meet the usual AJC requirements for resectability (stage I or II with negative mediastinal nodes) or only have a histologic diagnosis made on review of the resected surgical specimen. Such patients have been reported to have high cure rates (above 25 percent) if adjuvant combination chemotherapy is used. Thus, such uncommon, resectable small cell lung cancer patients are candidates for combined modality surgery and chemotherapy.

BENIGN LUNG NEOPLASMS

The benign neoplasms of the lung, representing less than 5 percent of all primary tumors, include bronchial adenomas and hamartomas (90 percent of such lesions) and a group of very uncommon neoplasms (chondromas, fibromas, lipomas, hemangiomas, leiomyomas, teratomas, pseudolymphomas, and endometriosis). The diagnostic and primary treatment approach is basically the same for all of these neoplasms. They can present as central masses causing airway obstruction, cough, hemoptysis, and pneumonitis with or without x-ray findings but be accessible to fiberoptic bronchoscopy. Alternatively, they can present without symptoms as solitary pulmonary nodules and thus will be evaluated as part of a solitary pulmonary nodule workup. In all cases, the extent of surgery must be determined at operation, and a conservative procedure with appropriate reconstructions is usually performed.

BRONCHIAL ADENOMAS Bronchial adenomas (80 percent of which are central) are slowly growing intrabronchial lesions that represent 50 percent of all benign pulmonary neoplasms. Eighty to ninety percent are carcinoids, 10 to 15 percent are adenocystic tumors (or cylindromas), and 2 to 3 percent are mucoepidermoid tumors. Adenomas present in patients 15 to 60 years old (average age 45) as intrabronchial lesions and are often symptomatic for several years. Patients may have chronic cough, recurrent hemoptysis, or obstruction with atelectasis, lobar collapse, or pneumonitis and abscess formation. Bronchial carcinoids, which usually follow a benign course, and small cell lung cancers, which are highly malignant, are both derived from the same normal bronchial epithelial component, the Kulchitsky cell. This cell is part of the amine precursor uptake and decarboxylation (APUD) system. Carcinoids, like small cell lung cancers, may secrete other hormones such as ACTH or arginine vasopressin and thus cause paraneoplastic syndromes which resolve with resection. In addition, bronchial carcinoids when metastatic (usually to the liver) may produce the carcinoid syndrome, with cutaneous flush, bronchoconstriction, diarrhea, and cardiac valvular lesions (see Chap. 262), which small cell lung cancer does not. Occasionally pathologists may have difficulty in distinguishing carcinoids from small cell lung cancers. Carcinoid tumors appearing more aggressive histologically (referred to as "atypical carcinoids") metastasize in 70 percent of cases to regional nodes, liver, or bone, compared to only a 5 percent metastasis rate of carcinoids with typical histology.

Bronchial adenomas of all types, because of their endobronchial and often central location, are usually visible via fiberoptic bronchoscopy, and tissue for histologic diagnosis is obtained in this manner. Because they are hypervascular, they can bleed profusely after bronchoscopic biopsy, and this should be anticipated. Bronchial adenomas must be dealt with as potentially malignant and thus require removal not only for symptom relief but also because they can be locally invasive or recurrent, potentially can metastasize, or may produce paraneoplastic syndromes. Surgical excision is the primary treatment for all types of bronchial adenomas. The extent of surgery is determined at operation and should be as conservative as possible. Often bronchotomy with local excision, sleeve resection, segmental resection, or lobectomy is sufficient. Five-year survival rates following surgical resection are 95 percent, decreasing to 70 percent if regional nodes are involved. The treatment of metastatic pulmonary carcinoids is currently unclear because they can either be indolent, growing slowly over several years, or behave more like small cell lung carcinoma. Assessment of the tempo and the histology of the disease in the individual patient is necessary to determine if and when chemotherapy or radiotherapy is indicated.

HAMARTOMAS Pulmonary hamartomas have a peak incidence at age 60 and are more frequent in men than in women. Histologically, they contain normal pulmonary tissue components (smooth muscle and collagen) in a disorganized fashion. They are usually peripheral, clinically silent, and benign in their behavior. While it would be advantageous to avoid thoracotomy in these older patients, unless the radiographic findings are pathognomonic of hamartoma with "pop-corn" calcification, the lesions will usually have to be resected for diagnosis, particularly if the patient is a smoker.

METASTATIC PULMONARY TUMORS

The lung is frequently the site of metastatic disease from primary cancers outside the lung. Usually such metastatic disease is considered incurable. However, two special situations may arise. First is the development of a solitary pulmonary shadow on chest x-ray in a patient known to have an extrathoracic neoplasm. This may represent a metastasis or a new primary lung cancer. Because the natural history of lung cancer is worse than for most other primary tumors, it is wise to approach the single pulmonary nodule in a patient with a known extrathoracic tumor as though the nodule were a primary lung cancer, particularly if the patient is over 35 years of age and a smoker. This means a vigorous evaluation looking for other sites of active cancer and, if none are found, surgical resection of the nodule. Second, multiple pulmonary nodules may be resected for cure as well. This is usually recommended if, after careful staging, (1) the patient can tolerate the contemplated pulmonary resection; (2) the primary tumor has been definitively and successfully treated; and (3) all known metastatic disease can be encompassed by the projected pulmonary resection. The key is selection and screening of patients to exclude patients with uncontrolled primary tumors and extrapulmonary metastases. Primary tumors whose pulmonary metastases have been successfully resected for cure include osteogenic and soft tissue sarcomas; colon, rectal, uterine, cervix, and corpus tumors; head and neck, breast, testis, and salivary gland cancer; melanoma; and bladder and kidney tumors. Five-year survival rates of 20 to 30 percent have been found in carefully selected patients, and the most dramatic results have been seen in osteogenic sarcomas, where resection of pulmonary metastases (sometimes requiring several thoracotomies) is becoming a standard curative treatment approach.

REFERENCES

Benowitz NL: Pharmacologic aspects of cigarette smoking and nicotine addiction. N Engl J Med 319:1318, 1988

Brutinel WM et al: A two-year experience with the neodymium-YAG laser in endobronchial obstruction. Chest 8:159, 1987

Bunn PA Jr: Lung cancer. Semin Oncol 15(1):318, 1988

Finkelstein DM et al: Long-term survivors in metastatic non-small cell lung cancer: An Eastern Cooperative Oncology Group Study. J Clin Oncol 4:702, 1986

Fontana RS: Screening for lung cancer, recent experience in the United States. Cancer Treat Res 28:91, 1986

Lung Cancer Study Group: Effects of postoperative mediastinal radiation on completely resected stage II and stage III epidermoid cancer of the lung. N Engl J Med 315:1377, 1986

Martini N et al: Comparative merits of conventional, computed tomographic, and magnetic resonance imaging in assessing mediastinal involvement in surgically confirmed lung carcinoma. J Thorac Cardiovasc Surg 90:639, 1985

Minna JD et al: Lung cancer, in *The Principles and Practice of Oncology*, 3d ed, VT DeVita et al (eds). Philadelphia, Lippincott, 1989

——— et al: Genetic changes involved in the pathogenesis of human lung cancer including oncogene activation, chromosomal deletions, and autocrine growth factor production, in *Accomplishments in Cancer Research 1987*, JG Fortner, JE Rhoads (eds). General Motors Cancer Research Foundation, Philadelphia, Lippincott, 1988, p 155

Mountain CF: Prognostic implications of the International Staging System for Lung Cancer: A new international staging system for lung cancer. Chest 89:225s, 1986; Semin Oncol 15:236, 1988

Ruckdeschel JC et al: A randomized trial of the four most active regimens for metastatic non-small cell lung cancer. J Clin Oncol 4:14, 1986

Seifter EJ, Ihde DC: Therapy of small cell lung cancer: A perspective on two decades of clinical research. Semin Oncol 15:278, 1988

216 DISORDERS OF THE PLEURA, MEDIASTINUM, AND DIAPHRAGM

DAVID J. PIERSON

THE PLEURA

STRUCTURE AND FUNCTION The visceral and parietal pleurae consist of single layers of mesothelial cells, along with blood vessels, lymphatics, and connective tissue, that are separated by the pleural space. The latter is one of the body's "potential spaces," meaning that its volume is essentially zero unless some disease process causes fluid or solid tissue to accumulate there. Parietal pleura lines the chest cavity—chest wall, diaphragm, and mediastinum—and contains sensory fibers; visceral pleura covers the entire surface of both lungs and contains no pain fibers. Pleural fluid is elaborated from both the parietal and visceral pleural membranes, which in humans are both supplied by systemic vessels. Absorption is principally (approximately 90 percent) by lymphatics, which also absorb particles, large proteins, and cells. The remainder is absorbed by convection across the mesothelium into the lung or chest wall.

The pleural space is like an interstitial space, and excessive fluid can collect there (pleural effusion) according to the Frank-Starling relationship among hydrostatic pressure, osmotic pressure, and capillary permeability: excessive back-pressure from the visceral surface (e.g., congestive heart failure), a profound decrease in serum proteins (e.g., nephrotic syndrome), and pulmonary inflammation or lymphatic obstruction (e.g., pneumonia or infiltrating tumor) can all be associated with pleural effusion.

CLINICAL MANIFESTATIONS OF PLEURAL DISEASE *Pleuritic pain* is caused by irritation of sensory fibers in the parietal pleura and is typically produced or worsened by deep inhalation, cough, or other movement of the thorax. It is most often unilateral, sharp, and felt over the involved area, although it can be referred to the shoulder, neck, or abdomen. Pleuritic pain is often associated with splinting of the chest wall and with rapid, shallow breathing. Malignant tumors involving the parietal pleura typically cause steady, dull pain rather than the intermittent, lancinating pain of acute pleural inflammation. Pleural inflammation is often accompanied by a friction rub, a scratchy, rubbing sound heard on auscultation over the affected area during both inspiration and expiration. Friction rubs are often transitory and typically disappear as fluid accumulates in the pleural space.

Pleural effusion causes compression of adjacent lung tissue, producing dyspnea in proportion both to its size and to the functional status of the underlying lung. When an effusion is very large and symptoms are severe, removal of only 300 to 500 mL by thoracentesis may markedly decrease the patient's dyspnea. Physical signs of pleural effusion include diminished chest excursion over the effusion (when large), reduced tactile fremitus, dullness to percussion, diminished or absent breath sounds over the effusion, and bronchial breath sounds, sometimes with *E-to-A change,* from the lung just superior to the fluid level.

Symptoms of *pneumothorax* include pleuritic pain and dyspnea, although these vary considerably among individuals and some are virtually asymptomatic. Physical examination is less helpful than with pleural effusion, and the classic physical signs of pneumothorax (enlargement and diminished motion of the affected hemithorax, hyperresonance to percussion, and distant breath sounds) are often demonstrable only after the examiner has seen the patient's chest radiograph. The exception is tension pneumothorax, in which severe respiratory distress, hypotension, and tracheal deviation away from the affected side are often present.

Pleural tumors produce a dull pain, localized percussion dullness, and, when very large, the characteristic signs of pleural effusion.

DIAGNOSTIC TECHNIQUES Detection of pleural effusion on the chest radiograph depends upon the size of the effusion, the patient's position, and the technique and quality of the film. Effusions of 250 mL or more may go undetected on an upright film, and much larger volumes can be inapparent in a supine film. A film taken in the lateral decubitus position, with the affected side down, can detect a much smaller effusion (100 to 150 mL). Blunting of the costophrenic angle is the most common radiographic sign on an upright film; others are an increase in the distance between stomach bubble and lower left lung margin, a meniscus-like tracking of fluid up the lateral borders of the lungfields, and wider than normal interlobar fissures.

Pleural effusions may produce a restrictive defect on pulmonary function testing (reduced total lung capacity and vital capacity with normal ratio of forced expiratory volume in one second to forced vital capacity; Chap. 201), and its severity is related to the degree to which the underlying lung is compressed.

Thoracentesis (needle aspiration of pleural fluid) is the primary means of evaluating pleural fluid; as discussed below, its findings are used in determining the most likely diagnosis and to guide further investigation. It should be performed in all cases of undiagnosed pleural effusion, and whenever unusual or atypical features are present in effusion of "known" cause (e.g., fever or leukocytosis in congestive heart failure). In acute pneumonia, pleural effusion more than 1 cm in thickness on lateral decubitus radiograph should be tapped promptly, or, if small, followed using frequent repeat films with thoracentesis if an increase in size occurs.

Closed pleural biopsy, using any of several needles designed for this purpose, is unnecessary if the fluid is a transudate but indicated in any undiagnosed exudative effusion (see next section). Sufficient fluid should be present to separate the two pleural surfaces in order to reduce the likelihood of lung puncture. Ultrasound guidance can be helpful when the effusion is small or loculated. Several specimens should be taken, and a repeat procedure may be necessary to document diagnoses such as tuberculosis and certain malignancies. In cases in which an exudative pleural effusion remains undiagnosed despite needle pleural biopsy, pleuroscopy (thoracoscopy) under general anesthesia may be helpful. In experienced hands this procedure can frequently obviate thoracotomy.

PLEURAL EFFUSION Clinical evaluation of a patient with pleural effusion relies heavily upon examination of fluid obtained by thoracentesis. Effusions are most conveniently separated into transudates (ultrafiltrates of plasma resulting from increased hydrostatic pressure or profoundly decreased serum oncotic pressure) and exudates (protein-rich effusions resulting from increased capillary permeability), as characterized further in Table 216-1. An exudate is present whenever the total fluid/serum protein ratio exceeds 0.5 or the pleural fluid lactic dehydrogenase level exceeds 60 percent of the serum level.

TABLE 216-1 Evaluation of pleural fluid

	Transudate	Exudate
Typical appearance	Clear	Clear, cloudy, or bloody
Protein		
Absolute value	<3.0 g/dL	>3.0 g/dL*
Pleural fluid/serum ratio	<0.5	>0.5
Lactic dehydrogenase		
Absolute value	<200 IU/L	>200 IU/L
Pleural fluid/serum ratio	<0.6	>0.6
Glucose	>60 mg/dL (usually same as in blood)	Variable; often <60 mg/dL
Leukocytes	<1000/mL	>1000/mL
Polymorphonuclear	<50%	Usually >50% in acute inflammation
Erythrocytes	<5000/mL†	Variable
Pleural biopsy indicated?	No	Parapneumonic/other acute inflammation: no; chronic/subacute or undiagnosed effusion: yes

*Less in hypoproteinemic states.
†Assuming atraumatic tap.

Differential diagnosis   Presence of a transudative pleural effusion generally denotes a systemic condition rather than pleural disease, whereas an exudate usually implies pathology involving the pleura itself. Aside from demonstration of organisms or malignant cells in the fluid, however, few findings are pathognomonic for specific diagnoses. Erythrocyte counts exceeding 100,000 per milliliter, when not associated with trauma, are most often seen in malignancy and pulmonary embolism. Pleural fluid eosinophilia (>10 percent of all cells) may be seen in resolving infection, hydropneumothorax, asbestos-related effusion, and other conditions. A low glucose concentration (<60 mg/dL) suggests empyema, malignancy, and tuberculosis, but this is variable; very low levels (<15 mg/dL) are characteristic of rheumatoid effusions.

Pleural fluid pH has enjoyed considerable popularity as a diagnostic aid. Its main use is in distinguishing complicated (e.g., infected) from benign parapneumonic effusions, and even here it has not proved as valuable as originally suggested. A value of <7.00 units in a patient with pneumonia indicates the presence of empyema, but nearly always when this occurs, the Gram stain is positive or the fluid is frankly purulent. Values of less than 7.20 units are often found in empyema, but do not always indicate the need for thoracostomy tube drainage. Pleural fluid pH is sufficiently variable and nonspecific in conditions other than pneumonia to be of dubious clinical value.

Table 216-2 lists the principal causes of pleural effusion, in roughly descending order of frequency, along with characteristics of the effusion in each. Congestive heart failure causes more effusions than any other condition, with parapneumonic effusion, malignancy-associated effusion, and effusion associated with pulmonary embolism next in frequency.

Pleural effusion in malignancy   Most malignancy-associated pleural effusions occur in patients with lung cancer (35 percent of such effusions), breast cancer (25 percent), or lymphoma (10 percent). Pleural effusion in patients with malignancy is usually due to a local effect of the tumor, such as lymphatic obstruction or bronchial obstruction with pneumonia or atelectasis. However, it can also be a result of systemic effects of tumor elsewhere (e.g., pulmonary embolism secondary to hypercoagulability) or of therapy. The presence of malignant cells in the pleural effusion of a patient with lung cancer signifies inoperability, and tumor-related effusion in other malignancies generally implies a poor prognosis. Therapy depends upon the patient's symptoms. If the patient is asymptomatic, treatment may not be necessary. For mild symptoms thoracentesis may suffice. However, recurrent, symptomatic effusions usually require more definitive therapy. Chemical pleurodesis with tetracycline hydrochloride (20 mg/kg, instilled after chest tube drainage of the effusion, with clamping of the tube for 1 to 2 h) is the procedure of choice in most cases and is often successful. Thoracotomy with pleurectomy or pleural abrasion has a high success rate but is a major procedure with significant mortality. Systemic chemotherapy is generally ineffective, as is radiotherapy unless mediastinal lymph node enlargement is causing the effusion.

Chylothorax   Pleural effusion due to leakage of chyle (thoracic duct lymph) into the pleural space is usually associated with lymphoma, lung cancer with mediastinal spread, or mediastinal fibrosis and may also be seen following trauma. The fluid is a milky-appearing exudate, usually with demonstrable fat globules on Sudan III staining and a total fat content of 1 to 4 g/dL. The cholesterol concentration is low. Therapy is usually unsuccessful in chylothorax associated with malignancy, although radiotherapy may be beneficial in some cases. Surgery becomes necessary in posttraumatic chylothorax if chyle drainage persists for more than 10 days.

Pseudochylothorax, a rare condition with similar gross appearance but high cholesterol content and demonstrable cholesterol crystals, is seen in long-standing benign effusions such as those due to tuberculosis or rheumatoid arthritis.

Hemothorax   This is defined as a grossly bloody pleural effusion, with hematocrit at least 25 percent of that in the peripheral blood. Its usual cause is penetrating or nonpenetrating chest trauma, but it may also be iatrogenic (following central line placement, thoracentesis, or pleural biopsy, especially in patients with coagulopathy) or may occur in association with spontaneous pneumothorax. Therapy consists of thoracostomy tube drainage, both to remove the blood and to monitor the rate of bleeding; massive or persistent blood loss

---

TABLE 216-2   Characteristics of pleural effusion in different disorders*

Condition	Typical findings
Congestive heart failure	Transudate; protein may increase with diuresis or chronicity; right side more frequent but often bilateral; may localize in fissure (pseudotumor)
Pneumonia	Exudate; bacterial infections: in ⅓ of patients (more with pneumococcus and gram-negatives), cells mainly polymorphonuclears; viral infections: less common, usually small, cells mainly mononuclear; may be eosinophilic (>10%) in either; designated an empyema when organisms or gross purulence present
Malignancy	Exudate: lymphocytic, often hemorrhagic, with malignant cells in fluid or on pleural biopsy; often large and symptomatic; frequency: lung > breast > lymphoma > others
Pulmonary embolism	Exudate (75%) or transudate (25%); may be hemorrhagic; occurs in ⅓ to ½ of patients
Tuberculosis	Exudate: lymphocyte-predominant, high-protein; eosinophilia (>10%) rare; unilateral; small to moderate in majority; usually no associated parenchymal abnormality on chest radiograph; tubercle bacilli demonstrable in 10% on smear, 25% on culture, 50–75% on pleural biopsy; presentation either acute (<1 week, fever, chest pain) or subacute; can be asymptomatic
Cirrhosis	Transudate; usually right-sided; can be massive and symptomatic, even without marked ascites
Rheumatoid arthritis	Exudate; leukocyte count variable; glucose often very low (<15 mg/dL); LDH may be very high; may contain high cholesterol level and/or crystals; effusion occurs in 5% of patients, more commonly in men; may persist for months and require repeated drainage
Systemic lupus erythematosus	Exudate; leukocyte count variable; glucose near serum level; fluid complement levels (C3, C4 components) typically low; LE cells may be present; effusion occurs in ⅓ to ½ of patients; often bilateral, usually small and of short duration
Drug-induced effusion	Exudate; in drug-induced lupus, characteristics are similar to those in naturally occurring lupus; uncommon otherwise; often eosinophilic
Dressler's syndrome	Exudate; in setting of pleuropericarditis following myocardial infarction, trauma, or surgery involving pericardium
Benign asbestos-related effusion	Exudate: cells variable, often serosanguineous; may be eosinophilic (>10%); sometimes bilateral; can recur; usually small to moderate in size; asymptomatic in ⅔; related to amount of exposure; shorter lag time than with other asbestos-related conditions
Pancreatitis	Exudate with high amylase (of pancreatic origin); usually small-to-moderate size; typically left-sided but may be bilateral
Intraabdominal abscess	Exudate; leukocyte count (polymorphonuclears) often very high; glucose >60 mg/dL; sterile
Esophageal perforation	Rapidly increasing exudate, often with air-fluid level; epithelial cells, sometimes with food particles; high amylase (of salivary origin); may be on either side or bilateral; usually acute presentation with severe pain, toxicity, prostration

*In roughly descending order of frequency in clinical practice.

(e.g., >200 mL/h for >4 to 6 h) generally indicates the need for thoracotomy.

Empyema Pleural empyema (empyema thoracis) consists of a pleural fluid collection that is infected and/or frank pus. It is usually due to contiguous bacterial infection of the lung, but can also occur following external contamination (penetrating trauma, chest tube placement, or other surgical procedure) or esophageal perforation. Empyema can also develop as a complication of bacteremia from a distant source. Successful therapy requires prompt, complete drainage in addition to appropriate antibiotics administered systemically. Although needle aspiration may be attempted in early empyema if it is small and the fluid is thin, repeated aspiration and at least daily radiographic examinations will be required until it is certain that this has been successful. Chest tube drainage should be the initial therapy in most instances. Promptness is important, as loculation of the fluid sometimes develops within hours. If this happens, or if the patient does not defervesce within a few days, early limited thoracotomy, with resection of a small section of rib and establishment of assured drainage, is the therapy of choice. This approach appears to decrease morbidity and length of hospitalization as compared to "conservative" management with the ever-present hazard of fibrothorax despite the use of multiple chest tubes, instillation of fibrinolytic agents, and repeated drainage of loculations.

PNEUMOTHORAX Lung inflation is maintained so long as the pleural surfaces remain in complete contact. However, if air enters the pleural space from any source (pneumothorax), the lung will collapse in proportion to its natural elastic recoil (less than normal in emphysema, more in pulmonary fibrosis) and the quantity of air that accumulates. Tension pneumothorax occurs when pleural air collects under pressure, as when a flap of tissue permits air to enter the pleural space during deep breathing, coughing, or positive-pressure breathing but prevents it from leaving. Intrapleural pressures of more than 15 to 20 cmH$_2$O displace the mediastinum and compromise venous return to the heart, creating a true medical emergency.

Primary (simple) spontaneous pneumothorax This is a disorder most commonly affecting tall, slender men between 20 and 40 years of age and is believed to occur when subpleural blebs at the lung apices rupture directly into the pleural space. Although the pathophysiology is uncertain, the blebs may be a consequence of the increased traction placed on the uppermost parts of the lung during maximal inflation. From 30 to 50 percent of affected individuals experience a recurrence (75 percent ipsilateral, 25 percent contralateral), and after one recurrence subsequent episodes are much more likely. Chest pain and dyspnea are the usual symptoms, the former often beginning abruptly while the patient is at rest and tending to lessen as the pneumothorax increases in size. Severe, incapacitating symptoms are rare, as is tension pneumothorax.

Management is designed both to reexpand the affected lung and to decrease the likelihood of a recurrence on that side. Whether and how to drain the pleural air collection depends upon the size of the pneumothorax. Very small primary spontaneous pneumothoraces (< 10 to 15 percent of the diameter of the hemithorax on chest radiograph) may be observed without treatment so long as the patient's symptoms are mild and stable, although it may take a week or more for the air to be resorbed. The air is absorbed significantly faster if the patient breathes O$_2$-enriched gas. For larger air collections the choice is between simple aspiration and tube thoracostomy. Simple aspiration of a first primary pneumothorax, using a standard polyethylene intravenous catheter or commercial kit prepackaged with catheter and one-way flutter valve, is favored by many clinicians and permits the patient to return to normal activity sooner than formal chest tube drainage. When the pneumothorax is a recurrence or occupies >50 percent of the hemithorax, tube thoracostomy is the treatment of choice, with connection to a water seal once the air has been evacuated by suction. The tube should be left in place for 24 h after the lung has fully reexpanded without further air leak, clamped for another 24 h, and then removed if there is no radiographic evidence of recurrence. Although it is not indicated in a first episode, patients with recurrent primary spontaneous pneumothorax should probably be treated with intrapleural instillation of tetracycline hydrochloride or another sclerosing agent in an attempt to produce pleurodesis. Open thoracotomy should be considered if air leak persists after several days of tube drainage under suction, or if the condition recurs despite an attempt at chemical pleurodesis.

Secondary (complicated) spontaneous pneumothorax Unlike primary spontaneous pneumothorax, a generally benign condition which occurs in otherwise healthy young individuals, development of pneumothorax in a patient with underlying pulmonary disease is more serious and frequently life-threatening. Virtually all patients have dyspnea, most experience chest pain, and cyanosis and hypotension occur in perhaps 10 percent. Chronic obstructive pulmonary disease is the most common associated condition, although secondary pneumothorax is also a recognized feature of asthma, cystic fibrosis, idiopathic pulmonary fibrosis, tuberculosis, sarcoidosis, lung abscess, *Pneumocystis carinii* pneumonia, and several rarer pulmonary diseases. It is also common in the adult respiratory distress syndrome. In each instance the primary event is believed to be overdistention and rupture of an alveolus with dissection of air into the pleural space. The rupture may be directly across the visceral pleura, or air may dissect into an adjacent bronchovascular sheath, with subsequent centripetal air dissection to the root of the lung, and thence into the mediastinum and pleural space. This diagnosis should be considered whenever a patient with chronic lung disease develops sudden clinical deterioration. Tube thoracostomy should be performed promptly in all cases. Failure of complete lung reexpansion and persistent bronchopleural air leak (bronchopleural fistula) are more common than with primary spontaneous pneumothorax. Sclerosis of the pleural surfaces using tetracycline or another agent should probably be done after the first episode, because of the seriousness of the condition.

Traumatic pneumothorax This may follow either penetrating or nonpenetrating chest trauma. The air may reach the pleural space by alveolar overdistention and rupture, direct laceration of the lung by fractured rib or foreign object, or by entry of air directly through the chest wall. Treatment is by tube thoracostomy. If there is a large air leak and the lung fails to reexpand with suction, injury to the trachea or main bronchus should be suspected. Hydropneumothorax after closed-chest injury may be a sign of esophageal rupture, a diagnosis further suggested if the fluid contains high levels of amylase.

Iatrogenic pneumothorax Probably more common than all forms of spontaneous pneumothorax combined, this develops as a result of direct puncture or laceration of the visceral pleura (during attempts at central line placement, percutaneous lung aspiration, thoracentesis, or closed pleural biopsy), transbronchial lung disruption (bronchoscopic forceps biopsy or brushing), or direct alveolar overdistention (anesthesia, cardiopulmonary resuscitation, or mechanical ventilation). The diagnosis should be suspected in a patient who develops respiratory distress or hemodynamic deterioration following any of the above procedures. It is also commonly detected for the first time on a postprocedure or routine chest radiograph. Treatment differs from that for spontaneous pneumothorax in that prevention of recurrence is not a concern. Pneumothorax developing in a patient on mechanical ventilation should always be treated with chest tube drainage if the patient cannot be removed from the ventilator. Other patients may be observed without treatment if the pneumothorax is small and asymptomatic, or the air may be aspirated using a small catheter as described for primary spontaneous pneumothorax. Tube thoracostomy may be required if the latter is unsuccessful.

Catamenial pneumothorax is a rare condition in which spontaneous pneumothorax (usually right-sided) occurs in women over 25 to 30 years of age in association with menstruation. Whether it is the result of minute endometrial implants or of passage of air from the peritoneal cavity via a small diaphragmatic rent is controversial. The diagnosis should be considered if spontaneous pneumothorax develops within 48 h of the onset of a menstrual period. Ovulation-suppressing drugs are the preferred treatment, as the condition characteristically recurs and otherwise requires surgical exploration. Pleurodesis may be the treatment of choice, especially if the woman wants to conceive.

TUMORS OF THE PLEURA Most neoplastic disease involving the pleura is metastatic. Less common but increasing in incidence is *primary pleural mesothelioma,* a tumor that may also occur in the peritoneum. Both benign localized and diffuse malignant pleural mesotheliomas occur. The rare benign form may be asymptomatic, produce chest pain and cough, or be associated with a rheumatic-like syndrome. It remains localized, has a smooth, rounded radiographic appearance, and resembles a fibroma histologically. Surgical resection is curative. *Malignant mesothelioma* is a highly malignant neoplasm associated in the great majority of cases with prior asbestos exposure (Chap. 206). The latter may have been brief, and the usual lag time between exposure and clinical onset exceeds 25 years. Mesothelioma causes dull, persistent chest pain, dyspnea, and cough, and there is often a bloody pleural effusion. While malignant cells in fluid or pleural tissue can usually be demonstrated, the precise identification of the tumor as a mesothelioma is much more difficult. The diagnosis can be made on cytologic examination of pleural fluid in only about 10 percent of cases, and from closed pleural biopsy in 25 to 30 percent; even with thoracotomy the diagnosis cannot always be made with certainty prior to autopsy. Survival from the time of diagnosis averages less than 1 year, and no clearly effective therapy exists. Radiotherapy, local or systemic chemotherapy, radical pleuropneumonectomy, and various combinations of these have failed to show convincing benefit.

THE MEDIASTINUM

Most clinicians divide the mediastinum into anterior, middle, and posterior compartments as seen on the lateral chest radiograph (Fig. 216-1). The anterior compartment consists of everything lying superior to and forward of the heart shadow. Its normal contents include the thymus gland, substernal extensions of thyroid and parathyroid glands,

FIGURE 216-1 Division of the mediastinum into anterior, middle, and posterior compartments, as visualized in the lateral projection. (*From Pierson.*)

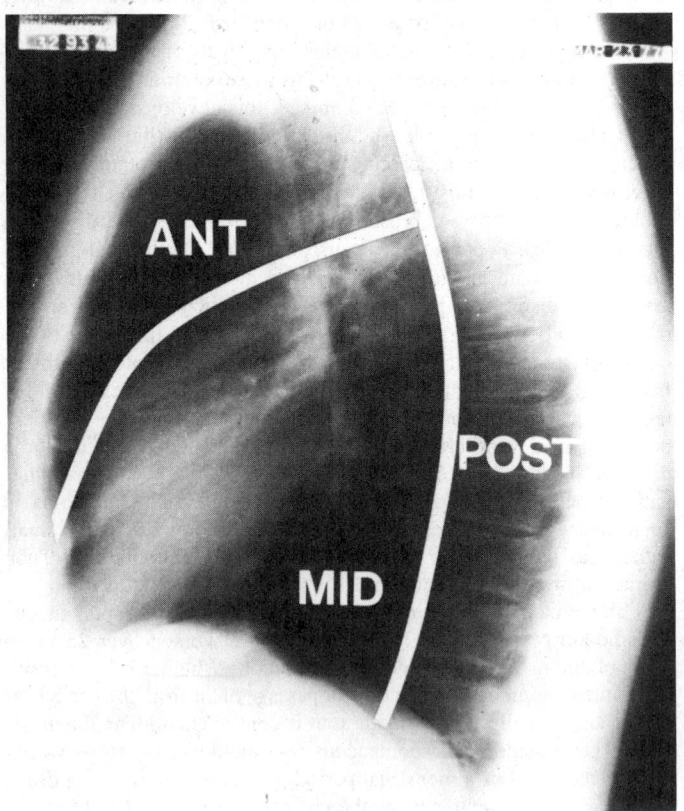

the aortic arch and its main branches, the innominate veins, and lymphatics and lymph nodes in addition to loose areolar tissue. Posterior and inferior to the anterior compartment is the middle mediastinum, which contains the heart, pericardium, trachea and main bronchi, the pulmonary hila, the phrenic and vagus nerves, and lymph nodes. The posterior mediastinum occupies the space seen within the margins of the thoracic vertebrae on lateral projection; it normally contains the esophagus, descending aorta, azygos and hemiazygos veins, thoracic duct, vagus nerve, sympathetic chains, and lymph nodes. Assigning these structures to the three compartments is in agreement with embryonic development, and helps to understand how disease processes involving the mediastinum are manifested clinically.

Methods of investigating the mediastinum include imaging by conventional radiography, computed tomography, magnetic resonance imaging, and radionuclide scanning. Techniques for obtaining mediastinal tissue, usually necessary for diagnosis of a mediastinal mass, include several procedures of varying invasiveness. Transbronchial needle aspiration of subcarinal or paratracheal lymph nodes via the fiberoptic bronchoscope may help to establish unresectability in patients with lung cancer. For many years the "gold standard" for mediastinal investigation has been suprasternal mediastinoscopy, which allows visualization and biopsy of lymph nodes and other masses in the superior portion of the anterior mediastinum. This procedure is complemented by anterior mediastinotomy, which permits access to structures in the subaortic fossa via an incision in the left second intercostal space. Although there are numerous possible complications, in experienced hands these procedures offer an alternative to formal surgical exploration with low morbidity and mortality.

MEDIASTINITIS Inflammation of the mediastinal structures is usually infectious in etiology and is best classified into "acute" and "chronic" categories.

Acute mediastinitis Once rare and invariably fatal, acute mediastinitis is more frequently encountered in the era of endoscopy and median sternotomy, and treatment is more often successful. There are several routes of infection. Perforation of the esophagus can occur, either "spontaneously" following forceful vomiting with a full stomach (*Boerhaave's syndrome*), as a result of penetrating trauma or instrumentation, or by an eroding carcinoma. The trachea can also be disrupted by any of the last three of these. Infection can also extend directly into the mediastinum from lung, pleura, and elsewhere both above and below the diaphragm. The onset of acute mediastinitis is typically sudden and dramatic, with chills, fever, apprehension, and prostration. Tachycardia, tachypnea, and systemic toxicity are prominent findings, and subcutaneous emphysema may be present. *Hamman's sign* (a crunching sound heard over the anterior chest in synchrony with cardiac systole) is characteristic but not invariably present. Radiographic hallmarks include mediastinal widening, air in the mediastinum and soft tissues, and pneumo- or hydropneumothorax. Therapy consists of prompt surgical drainage of both mediastinum and pleural cavities, along with appropriate antibiotics. Mortality may be as high as 75 percent when surgery is delayed, but can be reduced to 25 percent or less if drainage is achieved within 24 h of the precipitating event.

Mediastinitis following cardiac surgery has become an important entity during the last 20 years, occurring after 1 to 2 percent of procedures in several large series. It tends to be a less fulminating condition than acute mediastinitis in other settings. Most patients have drainage from the sternotomy incision and other localized signs of infection, and the diagnosis is generally made by reexploration of the wound. Treatment consists of surgical debridement and establishment of adequate drainage in addition to appropriate antibiotic therapy.

Chronic mediastinitis Granulomatous mediastinitis and mediastinal fibrosis represent the ends of a spectrum of chronic inflammation that causes varying degrees of host reaction and progresses in some cases to a largely acellular fibrosis. Granulomatous mediastinitis, most often due to histoplasmosis or tuberculosis, is usually asymptomatic and is detected as a mediastinal mass on chest radiograph. The end stage of mediastinal fibrosis can be caused not only by these infections but also by drugs (especially methysergide), so-called multisystem fibrosing disorder, silicosis, malignancy, syphilis, radiation, and other processes. Unlike the earlier form, this condition presents with symptoms, of which those of superior vena caval obstruction predominate. Compression of the esophagus, tracheo-bronchial tree, pulmonary vessels, and mediastinal nerves can also occur. Patients with chronic mediastinitis present with the superior vena caval syndrome (giddiness, headache, epistaxis, facial puffiness, cyanosis, and distended veins in face, neck, and arms), or with mediastinal widening detected on chest radiograph. Computed tomography reveals the extent of involvement but often cannot distinguish between benign and malignant processes, and in most cases flexible (fiberoptic) bronchoscopy, followed by surgical exploration, is required. No therapy is of definite help. Amphotericin and other specific therapies for presumed causes of chronic mediastinitis are generally ineffective, and the benefit of surgical "debulking" in areas of extensive fibrosis has not been shown.

PNEUMOMEDIASTINUM (MEDIASTINAL EMPHYSEMA) Air may appear within the tissue planes of the mediastinum spontaneously, in association with blunt or penetrating trauma, following instrumentation of the airways or esophagus, or because of disease above the thoracic outlet or below the diaphragm. Spontaneous pneumomediastinum occurs with sharply raised intrathoracic pressure, as in strenuous vomiting or coughing, or marked pressure swings from positive to negative, as in acute severe asthma. Alveolar overdistention and a pressure gradient from alveolus to bronchovascular sheath lead to dissection of air via the interstitium to the hila and mediastinum. From there, if it does not rupture into the pleural space and cause a pneumothorax, the air may spread into the subcutaneous tissue of the neck, chest, and elsewhere. Retrosternal pain and dyspnea are the usual symptoms, although there may be none, and physical examination may reveal Hamman's sign and subcutaneous emphysema. Chest radiographs in the posteroanterior and lateral positions confirm the diagnosis. Unlike spontaneous pneumothorax, spontaneous mediastinum does not recur and requires no treatment beyond reassurance and symptomatic relief of discomfort. Hemodynamic compromise and even cardiovascular collapse have been reported, but this is very rare. Fever and leukocytosis may occur, but do not require treatment if the patient otherwise feels well.

TUMORS AND CYSTS The most practical means of classifying mass lesions in the mediastinum is according to their location, as shown in Table 216-3. Overall, the most common etiologies for a

---

TABLE 216-3 Tumors and cysts of the mediastinum

Masses occurring in the anterior mediastinum
  Thymoma
  Germ cell tumors: teratoma; seminoma; embryonal cell carcinoma;
    choriocarcinoma
  Lymphoma
  Mesenchymal tumors: lipoma; fibroma; others
  Thyroid
  Parathyroid
Masses occurring in the middle mediastinum
  Lymph nodes: lymphoma; metastatic cancer; granulomatous disease
  Developmental cysts: pericardial; bronchogenic; enteric
  Vascular masses and enlargements
  Diaphragmatic hernias
Masses occurring in the posterior mediastinum
  Neurogenic tumors
    Arising from peripheral nerves: neurofibroma; neurilemmoma;
      neurosarcoma
    Arising from sympathetic ganglia: ganglioneuroma;
      ganglioneuroblastoma; neuroblastoma; sympathicoblastoma
    Arising from paraganglionic tissue: pheochromocytoma;
      paraganglioma (chemodectoma)
  Esophageal lesions: neoplasms; achalasia; hiatal hernia
  Diaphragmatic hernias
  Miscellaneous conditions: primary carcinoma or sarcoma; pancreatic
    pseudocyst; thoracic duct cyst; extramedullary hematopoiesis;
    meningocele

---

mediastinal mass in an adult are neurogenic tumors, thymomas, and developmental cysts, which together account for approximately 60 percent of all cases. Lymphomas and germ cell tumors such as teratoma and seminoma account for another 25 percent, and the other 15 percent is made up of a large number of reported lesions.

At least half of all mediastinal masses are asymptomatic, and of these some 90 percent prove to be benign. On the other hand, of masses that produce symptoms for which the patient consults a physician, at least half are malignant. Symptoms are usually those caused by invasion or compression of surrounding tissues or organs by the tumor. Such complaints frequently include cough, dyspnea, recurrent respiratory infections, dysphagia, and chest pain. Superior vena caval syndrome, hoarseness due to vocal cord paralysis, Horner's syndrome, phrenic nerve involvement, and spinal cord compression are other presentations. Unique to mediastinal tumors as a group is the frequency with which they are associated with systemic syndromes. These include myasthenia gravis (thymoma), pure red cell aplasia (thymoma), Cushing's syndrome (thymoma; carcinoid), gynecomastia (certain germ cell tumors), hypertension (pheochromocytoma, ganglioneuroma), and hypercalcemia (lymphoma, parathyroid adenoma), among others.

Aside from a very few circumstances, such as the demonstration of teeth in a teratoma or functioning thyroid tissue on radionuclide scan, none of the causes of a mediastinal mass is sufficiently specific in its features to permit a diagnosis to be made noninvasively. Thus, the main focus of diagnostic evaluation is an orderly preparation for obtaining a tissue diagnosis. Unless the diagnosis is discovered in the general evaluation of the patient, as in lymphoma or widespread carcinoma, tissue from the mass will have to be obtained. Needle aspiration or biopsy suffers from the limitations of sampling error in lesions that are frequently heterogeneous, and also from insufficient material for a definitive diagnosis in many cases. Because most lesions should be removed, even if benign, surgical exploration is considered by many to be the most expeditious approach.

THE DIAPHRAGM

A continuous sheet of muscle and tendon, normally broken only by openings for the principal structures passing from the thorax into the abdomen, the diaphragm is the main muscle of inspiration. The right and left halves are innervated separately, the motor supply exclusively via the phrenic nerves (C3 to C5), and the sensory input jointly from the phrenics and the lower intercostals. When the dome-shaped diaphragm contracts, it displaces the abdominal contents downward and the rib cage upward and outward, creating negative pressure in the chest and allowing air to flow passively into the lungs. The flattened diaphragm is characteristic of a hyperinflated condition; contraction of the diaphragm actually pulls the lower ribs inward. The principal disorders of the diaphragm are paralysis of one or both of its halves and hernias or eventrations producing localized bulges or masses.

DIAPHRAGMATIC PARALYSIS Unilateral diaphragmatic paralysis is caused by interruption of the phrenic nerve, occasionally by trauma but most commonly by invading tumor (chiefly bronchogenic carcinoma). Often it may prove to be idiopathic, despite extensive diagnostic evaluation. Unilateral diaphragmatic paralysis is usually asymptomatic, discovered on a routine film or during evaluation of lung cancer, although some patients complain of dyspnea. Pulmonary function is only mildly affected. The diagnosis is confirmed when an elevated hemidiaphragm is shown on fluoroscopy to move paradoxically (that is, upward) during the "sniff" maneuver. No treatment is known.

Although less common, bilateral diaphragmatic paralysis is a much more debilitating condition, and frequently leads to hypercapnic respiratory failure. It may occur because of cervical spinal cord trauma, cold cardioplegia during cardiac surgery, motor neuron disease, polyneuropathy, poliomyelitis, or mediastinal malignancy.

Most patients complain of severe dyspnea, worse when supine, and paradoxical (inward) motion of the abdomen is observed during inspiration when the patient is in the supine position. The vital capacity is severely reduced, more so in the supine position, but the "sniff test" under fluoroscopy may not reveal abnormal motion. Measurement of transdiaphragmatic pressure changes during inspiration, using esophageal and gastric balloons, can help to confirm the diagnosis. Assisted ventilation for all or part of each day is the treatment of choice; this may be accomplished without tracheostomy using a rocking bed, corset-type positive-pressure wrap, or negative-pressure ventilator. Electrophrenic respiration (diaphragm pacing), reported by a small number of investigators to be successful in long-term management, has proved to be ineffective, uncomfortable, or otherwise unsatisfactory for many patients.

DIAPHRAGMATIC HERNIAS AND EVENTRATIONS Herniation of the stomach or other viscera into the chest through the esophageal hiatus is by far the most common of the diaphragmatic hernias and eventrations (see Chap. 237). Hernias through the foramen of Bochdalek occur in the posterolateral chest, usually on the left, and are most often seen in infants. They may contain fat, the upper pole of the kidney, or occasionally the spleen. Anterior diaphragmatic hernias through the foramina of Morgagni occur most often in patients with increased intraabdominal pressure or marked obesity. Nearly always asymptomatic, they may contain omental fat, bowel, stomach, or even liver. Radiographically they appear as an anterior rounded density in the region of the right cardiophrenic angle. Diagnosis may be aided by radiographic contrast studies or by computed tomography. Although strangulation of the hernia's contents has been reported, both types of diaphragmatic hernia are nearly always asymptomatic and require no treatment. However, surgical exploration may become necessary to exclude other diagnoses. Eventration of the diaphragm is a localized elevation of a hemidiaphragm, evident on physical examination or chest radiograph, caused either by incomplete muscle development or localized atrophy. Most often seen in obese adults, it is typically asymptomatic.

REFERENCES

CELLI BR: Respiratory muscle function. Clin Chest Med 7:567, 1986

LIGHT RW: *Pleural Diseases.* Philadelphia, Lea & Febiger, 1983

——: Pneumothorax, in *Textbook of Respiratory Medicine*, JF Murray, JA Nadel (eds). Philadelphia, Saunders, 1988, pp 1745–1759

PIERSON DJ: Disorders of the mediastinum, in *Textbook of Respiratory Medicine*, JF Murray, JA Nadel (eds). Philadelphia, Saunders, 1988, pp 1781–1829

SAHN SA: Malignant pleural effusions, in *Pulmonary Diseases and Disorders*, 2d ed, AP Fishman (ed). New York, McGraw-Hill, 1988, pp 2159–2170

SARR MG et al: Mediastinal infection after cardiac surgery. Ann Thorac Surg 38:415, 1984

SILVERMAN NA, SABISTON DC: Mediastinal masses. Surg Clin North Am 60:757, 1980

TARVER RD et al: Imaging the diaphragm and its disorders. J Thorac Imag 4:1, 1989

WINTERBAUER RH: Nonneoplastic pleural effusions, in *Pulmonary Diseases and Disorders*, 2d ed, AP Fishman (ed). New York, McGraw-Hill, 1988, 2139–2157

217 DISORDERS OF VENTILATION

ELIOT A. PHILLIPSON

HYPOVENTILATION

DEFINITION AND ETIOLOGY Alveolar hypoventilation exists by definition when arterial P_{CO_2} (Pa_{CO_2}) increases above the normal range of 37 to 43 mmHg, but in clinically important hypoventilation syndromes Pa_{CO_2} is generally in the range of 50 to 80 mmHg. Hypoventilation disorders can be acute or chronic. The acute disorders, which represent life-threatening emergencies, are discussed in Chap. 218; this chapter deals with chronic hypoventilation syndromes.

TABLE 217-1 Chronic hypoventilation syndromes

Mechanism	Site of defect	Disorder
Impaired respiratory drive	Peripheral and central chemoreceptors	Carotid body dysfunction, trauma Prolonged hypoxia Metabolic alkalosis
	Brainstem respiratory neurons	Bulbar poliomyelitis, encephalitis Brainstem infarction, hemorrhage, trauma Brainstem demyelination, degeneration Chronic drug administration Primary alveolar hypoventilation syndrome
Defective respiratory neuromuscular system	Spinal cord and peripheral nerves	High cervical trauma Poliomyelitis Motor neuron disease Peripheral neuropathy
	Respiratory muscles	Myasthenia gravis Muscular dystrophy Chronic myopathy
Impaired ventilatory apparatus	Chest wall	Kyphoscoliosis Fibrothorax Thoracoplasty Ankylosing spondylitis Obesity-hypoventilation
	Airways and lungs	Laryngeal and tracheal stenosis Obstructive sleep apnea Cystic fibrosis Chronic obstructive pulmonary disease

SOURCE: Phillipson.

Chronic hypoventilation can result from numerous disease entities (Table 217-1), but in all cases the underlying mechanism involves a defect in either the metabolic respiratory control system, the respiratory neuromuscular system, or the ventilatory apparatus. Disorders associated with impaired respiratory drive, defects in the respiratory neuromuscular system, and upper airway obstruction produce an increase in Pa_{CO_2}, despite normal lungs, because of a reduction in overall minute volume of ventilation, and hence in alveolar ventilation. In contrast, disorders of the chest wall, lower airways, and lungs typically produce an increase in Pa_{CO_2}, often despite a normal or even increased minute volume of ventilation, because of severe ventilation-perfusion mismatching that results in net alveolar hypoventilation.

Several hypoventilation syndromes involve combined disturbances in two elements of the respiratory systems. For example, patients with chronic obstructive pulmonary disease may hypoventilate not simply because of impaired ventilatory mechanics but also because of a reduced central respiratory drive, which can be inherent or secondary to a coexisting metabolic alkalosis (related to diuretic and steroid therapy).

PHYSIOLOGICAL AND CLINICAL FEATURES Regardless of cause, the hallmark of all alveolar hypoventilation syndromes is an increase in alveolar P_{CO_2} (PA_{CO_2}) and therefore in Pa_{CO_2} (Fig. 217-1). The resulting respiratory acidosis eventually leads to a compensatory increase in plasma HCO_3^- concentration and a decrease in Cl^- concentration. The increase in PA_{CO_2} produces an obligatory decrease in PA_{O_2}, resulting in hypoxemia. If severe, the hypoxemia manifests clinically as cyanosis and can stimulate erythropoiesis and induce secondary polycythemia. The combination of chronic hypoxemia and hypercapnia may also induce pulmonary vasoconstriction, leading eventually to pulmonary hypertension, right ventricular hypertrophy, and congestive heart failure. The disturbances in arterial blood gases are typically magnified during sleep because of a further reduction in central respiratory drive. The resulting increased nocturnal hypercapnia may cause cerebral vasodilation leading to morning headache;

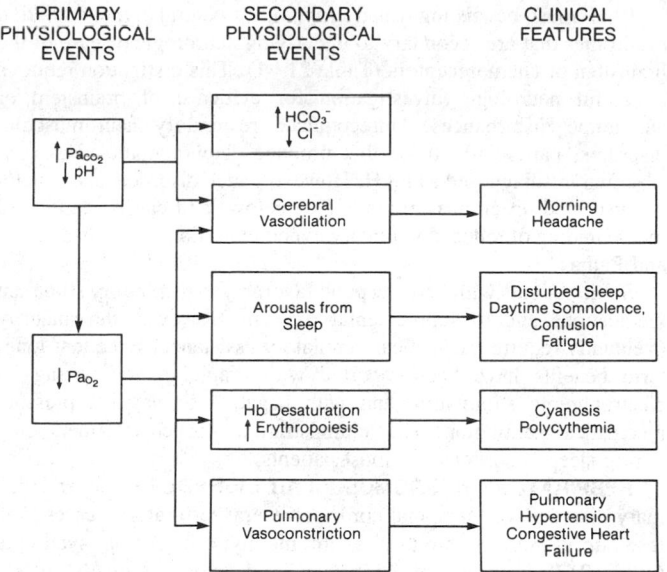

<table>
<tr><th>PRIMARY PHYSIOLOGICAL EVENTS</th><th>SECONDARY PHYSIOLOGICAL EVENTS</th><th>CLINICAL FEATURES</th></tr>
</table>

FIGURE 217-1 Physiologic and clinical features of alveolar hypoventilation. *(After EA Phillipson.)*

(EMGdi) responses. During sleep, hypoventilation is usually more marked, and central apneas and hypopneas are common. However, because the behavioral respiratory control system (which is anatomically distinct from the metabolic control system), the neuromuscular system, and the ventilatory apparatus are intact, such patients can usually hyperventilate voluntarily, generate normal inspiratory and expiratory muscle pressures (P_{Imax}, P_{Emax}, respectively) against an occluded airway, generate normal lung volumes and flow rates on routine spirometry, and have normal respiratory system resistance and compliance and a normal alveolar-arterial P_{O_2} [(A-a) P_{O_2}] difference. Patients with defects in the respiratory neuromuscular system also have impaired responses to chemical stimuli, but in addition are unable to hyperventilate voluntarily or to generate normal static respiratory muscle pressures, lung volumes, and flow rates. However, at least in the early stages of the disease the resistance and compliance of the respiratory system and the alveolar-arterial oxygen difference are normal.

In contrast to patients with disorders of the respiratory control or neuromuscular systems, patients with disorders of the chest wall, lungs, and airways typically demonstrate abnormalities of respiratory system resistance and compliance, and have a widened (A-a) P_{O_2}. Because of the impaired mechanics of breathing, routine spirometric tests are abnormal, as is the ventilatory response to chemical stimuli. However, because the neuromuscular system is intact, tests that are independent of resistance and compliance are usually normal, including tests of respiratory muscle strength and tests of respiratory control that do not involve airflow.

TREATMENT The management of chronic hypoventilation must be individualized to the patient's particular disorder, circumstances, and needs and should include measures directed to the underlying disease. Coexistent metabolic alkalosis should be corrected, including elevations of HCO_3^- that are inappropriately high for the degree of chronic hypercapnia. Administration of supplemental oxygen is effective in attenuating hypoxemia, polycythemia, and pulmonary hypertension, but can aggravate CO_2 retention and the associated

sleep quality may also be severely impaired, resulting in morning fatigue, daytime somnolence, mental confusion, and intellectual impairment. Other clinical features associated with hypoventilation syndromes are related to the specific underlying disease (Table 217-1).

DIAGNOSIS Investigation of the patient with chronic hypoventilation involves several laboratory tests that will usually localize the disorder to either the respiratory control system, the neuromuscular system, or the ventilatory apparatus (Fig. 217-2). Defects in the control system impair responses to chemical stimuli, including ventilatory, occlusion pressure, and diaphragmatic electromyographic

FIGURE 217-2 Pattern of laboratory test results in alveolar hypoventilation syndromes, based on the site of defect. Ventil = ventilation; P.1 = mouth pressure generated after 0.1 s of inspiration against an occluded airway; EMGdi = diaphragmatic EMG; P_{Imax}, P_{Emax} = maximum inspiratory or expiratory pressure that can be generated against an occluded airway; (A-a) P_{O_2} = alveolar-arterial P_{O_2} difference; N = normal. Defects in the metabolic control system impair central respiratory drive in response to chemical stimuli (CO_2 or hypoxia); therefore responses of EMGdi, P.1, and minute volume of ventilation are reduced and hypoventilation during sleep is aggravated. In contrast, tests of voluntary respiratory control, muscle strength, lung me-

chanics, and gas exchange [(A-a) P_{O_2}] are normal. Defects in the respiratory neuromuscular system impair muscle strength; therefore all tests dependent on muscular activity (voluntary or in response to metabolic stimuli) are abnormal, but lung resistance, lung compliance, and gas exchange are normal. Defects in the ventilatory apparatus usually impair gas exchange. Because resistance and compliance are also impaired, all tests dependent on ventilation (whether voluntary or in response to chemical stimuli) are abnormal; in contrast, tests of muscle activity or strength that do not involve airflow (that is, P.1, EMGdi, P_{Imax}, P_{Emax}) are normal. *(After EA Phillipson.)*

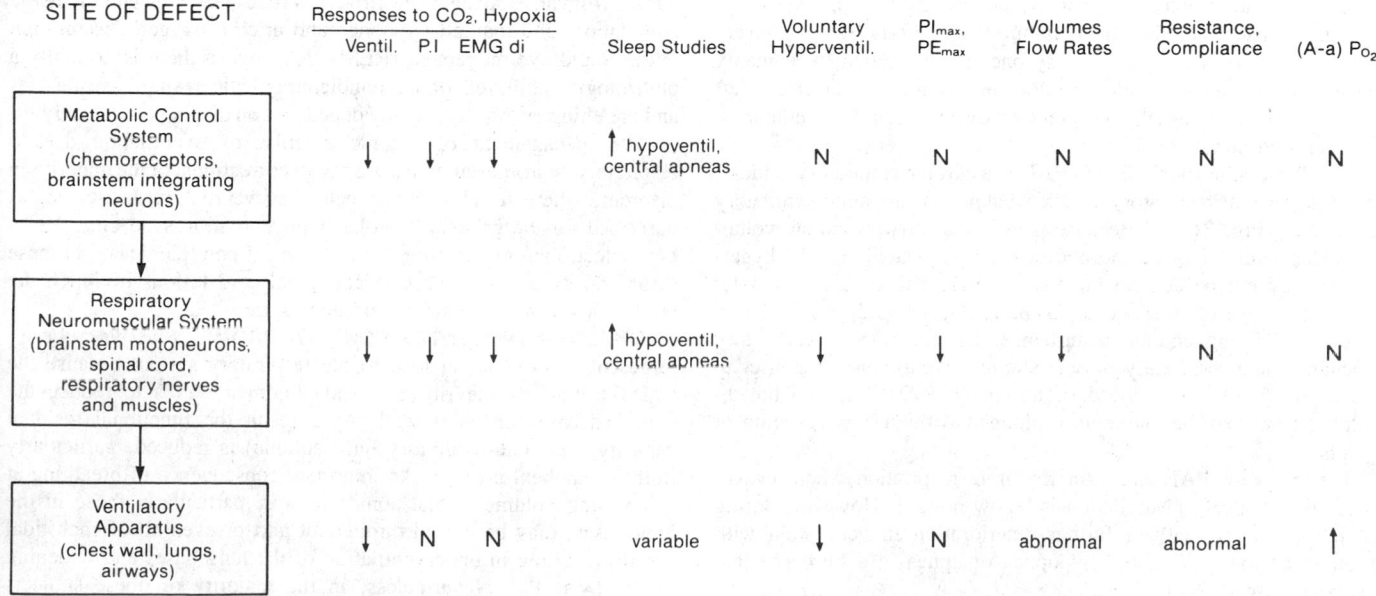

SITE OF DEFECT	Responses to CO₂, Hypoxia			Sleep Studies	Voluntary Hyperventil.	PI_{max}, PE_{max}	Volumes Flow Rates	Resistance, Compliance	(A-a) P_{O_2}
	Ventil.	P.I	EMG di						
Metabolic Control System (chemoreceptors, brainstem integrating neurons)	↓	↓	↓	↑ hypoventil, central apneas	N	N	N	N	N
Respiratory Neuromuscular System (brainstem motoneurons, spinal cord, respiratory nerves and muscles)	↓	↓	↓	↑ hypoventil, central apneas	↓	↓	↓	N	N
Ventilatory Apparatus (chest wall, lungs, airways)	↓	N	N	variable	↓	N	abnormal	abnormal	↑

neurologic symptoms. For this reason supplemental oxygen must be prescribed judiciously and the results monitored carefully. Pharmacologic agents that stimulate respiration (particularly progesterone) are of benefit in some patients, but generally results are disappointing.

Most patients with chronic hypoventilation related to impairment of respiratory drive or neuromuscular disease eventually require mechanical ventilatory assistance for effective management. When hypoventilation is severe, treatment may be required on a 24-h basis, but in many patients ventilatory assistance only during sleep produces dramatic clinical improvement and lowering of daytime Pa_{CO_2}. In patients with reduced respiratory drive but intact respiratory lower motor neurons, phrenic nerves, and respiratory muscles, diaphragmatic pacing through an implanted phrenic electrode can be very effective. However, for patients with defects in the respiratory nerves and muscles, electrophrenic pacing is contraindicated. Such patients can usually be managed effectively with either intermittent negative pressure ventilation in a cuirass, or intermittent positive pressure ventilation delivered through a tracheostomy or nosemask. For patients who require ventilatory assistance only during sleep, positive pressure ventilation through a nosemask is the preferred method because it obviates a tracheostomy and avoids the problem of upper airway occlusion that can arise in a negative pressure ventilator.

Hypoventilation related to restrictive disorders of the chest wall (Table 217-1) can also be managed effectively with nocturnal intermittent positive pressure ventilation through a nosemask or tracheostomy. Nocturnal ventilatory assistance has also been advocated for patients with hypercapnic chronic obstructive lung disease, as a means of alleviating possible chronic respiratory muscle fatigue, but the efficacy of such an approach has yet to be confirmed.

HYPOVENTILATION SYNDROMES

PRIMARY ALVEOLAR HYPOVENTILATION Primary alveolar hypoventilation (PAH) is a disorder of unknown cause, characterized by chronic hypercapnia and hypoxemia in the absence of identifiable neuromuscular disease or mechanical ventilatory impairment. The disorder is thought to arise from a defect in the metabolic respiratory control system, but few neuropathologic studies have been reported in such patients. Isolated PAH is relatively rare, and although it occurs in all age groups, the majority of reported cases have been in males aged 20 to 50 years. The disorder typically develops insidiously, and often first comes to attention when severe respiratory depression follows administration of standard doses of sedatives or anesthetics. As the degree of hypoventilation increases, patients typically develop lethargy, fatigue, daytime somnolence, disturbed sleep, and morning headaches; and eventually cyanosis, polycythemia, pulmonary hypertension, and congestive heart failure (Fig. 217-1). Despite severe arterial blood gas derangements, dyspnea is uncommon, presumably because of impaired chemoreception and ventilatory drive. If left untreated, PAH is usually progressive over a period of months to years and ultimately fatal.

The key diagnostic finding in PAH is a chronic respiratory acidosis in the absence of respiratory muscle weakness or impaired ventilatory mechanics (Fig. 217-2). Because patients can hyperventilate voluntarily and reduce Pa_{CO_2} to normal or even hypocapnic levels, hypercapnia may not be demonstrable in a single arterial blood sample, but the presence of an elevated plasma HCO_3^- should draw attention to the underlying chronic disturbance. Despite normal ventilatory mechanics and respiratory muscle strength, ventilatory responses to chemical stimuli are reduced or absent (Fig. 217-2), and breath-holding time may be markedly prolonged without any sensation of dyspnea.

Patients with PAH maintain rhythmic respiration when awake, although the level of ventilation is below normal. However, during sleep there is typically a further deterioration in ventilation with frequent episodes of central hypopnea or apnea, a disturbance that has been termed *Ondine's curse*.

PAH must be distinguished from other central hypoventilation syndromes that are secondary to underlying neurologic disease of the brainstem or chemoreceptors (Table 217-1). This distinction requires a careful neurologic investigation for evidence of brainstem or autonomic disturbances. Unrecognized respiratory neuromuscular disorders, particularly those that produce diaphragmatic weakness, are often misdiagnosed as PAH. However, such disorders can usually be suspected on clinical grounds (see below) and can be confirmed by the finding of reduced voluntary hyperventilation, as well as P_{Imax} and P_{Emax}.

Some patients with PAH respond favorably to respiratory stimulant medications and to supplemental oxygen. However, the majority eventually require mechanical ventilatory assistance. Excellent long-term benefits have been reported with diaphragmatic pacing by electrophrenic stimulation and with negative or positive pressure mechanical ventilation. The administration of such treatment only during sleep is sufficient in most patients.

RESPIRATORY NEUROMUSCULAR DISORDERS Several primary disorders of the spinal cord, peripheral respiratory nerves, and respiratory muscles produce a chronic hypoventilation syndrome (Table 217-1). Hypoventilation usually develops gradually over a period of months to years, and often first comes to attention when a relatively trivial increase in mechanical ventilatory load (such as mild airways obstruction) produces severe respiratory failure. In some of the disorders (such as motor neuron disease, myasthenia gravis, and muscular dystrophy) involvement of the respiratory nerves or muscles is usually a later feature of a more widespread disease. In other disorders respiratory involvement can be an early or even isolated feature, and hence the underlying problem is often not suspected. Included in this category are the postpolio syndrome [a form of chronic respiratory insufficiency that develops 20 to 30 years following recovery from poliomyelitis (Chap. 355)], the myopathy associated with adult acid maltase deficiency, and idiopathic diaphragmatic paralysis.

Generally respiratory neuromuscular disorders do not result in chronic hypoventilation unless there is significant weakness of the diaphragm. Distinguishing features of bilateral disphragmatic weakness include orthopnea, paradoxical movement of the abdomen in the supine posture, and paradoxical diaphragmatic movement under fluoroscopy. However, the absence of these features does not exclude diaphragmatic weakness. Important laboratory features are a rapid deterioration of ventilation during a maximum voluntary ventilation maneuver and reduced P_{Imax} and P_{Emax} (Fig. 217-2). More sophisticated investigations reveal reduced or absent transdiaphragmatic pressures, calculated from simultaneous measurement of esophageal and gastric pressures; reduced diaphragmatic EMG responses (recorded from an esophageal electrode) to transcutaneous phrenic nerve stimulation; and marked hypopnea and arterial oxygen desaturation during rapid eye movement (REM) sleep, when there is normally a physiologic inhibition of all nondiaphragmatic respiratory muscles and breathing becomes critically dependent on diaphragmatic activity.

The management of chronic alveolar hypoventilation due to respiratory neuromuscular disease involves treatment of the underlying disorder, where feasible, and mechanical ventilatory assistance, as described for the primary alveolar hypoventilation syndrome. However, electrophrenic diaphragmatic pacing is contraindicated in these disorders, except for high cervical spinal cord lesions in which the phrenic lower motor neurons and nerves are intact.

OBESITY-HYPOVENTILATION SYNDROME Massive obesity represents a mechanical load to the respiratory system because the added weight on the rib cage and abdomen serves to reduce the compliance of the chest wall. As a result the functional residual capacity (i.e., end-expiratory lung volume) is reduced, particularly in the recumbent posture. An important consequence of breathing at a low lung volume is that some airways, particularly those in the lung bases, may be closed throughout part or even all of each tidal breath, resulting in underventilation of the lung bases and widening of the (A-a) P_{O_2}. Nevertheless, in the majority of obese subjects

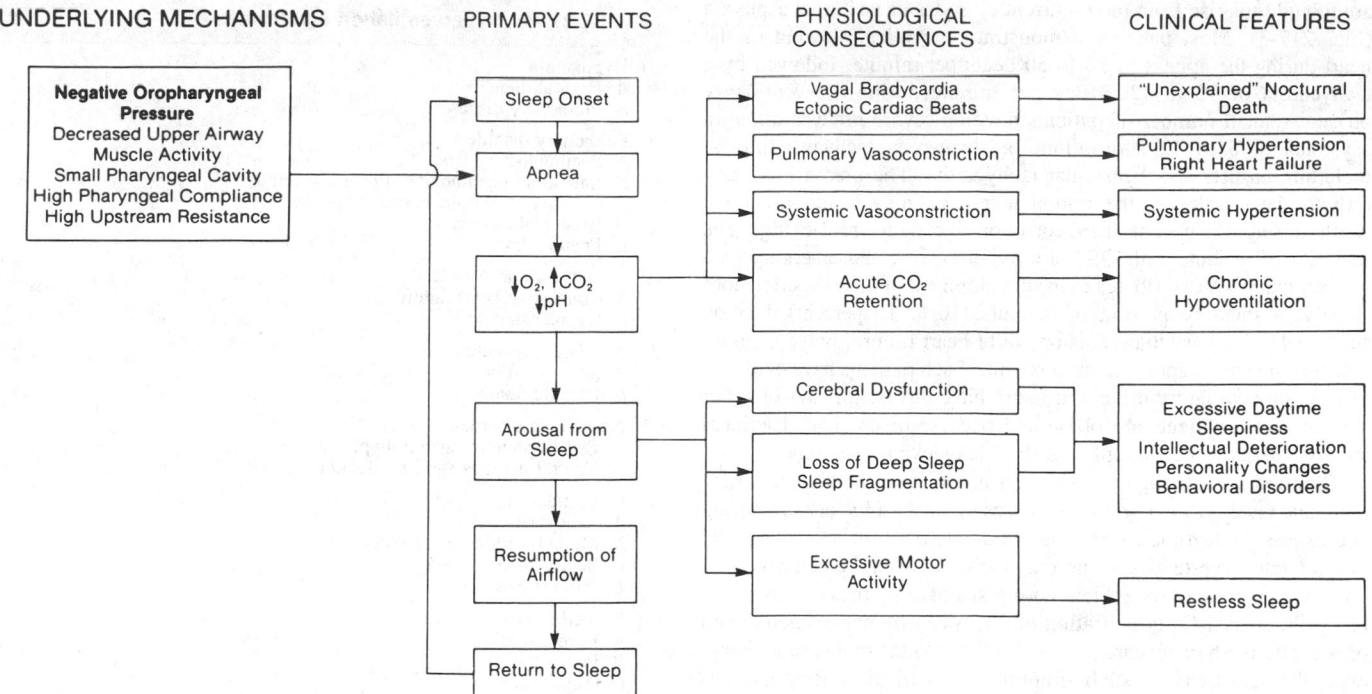

FIGURE 217-3 The primary sequence of events, underlying mechanisms, physiologic responses, and clinical features of obstructive sleep apnea. *(After EA Phillipson, Med North Am 23: 2314, 1982.)*

central respiratory drive is increased sufficiently to maintain a normal Pa_{CO_2}. However, a small proportion of obese subjects develop chronic hypercapnia, hypoxemia, and eventually polycythemia, pulmonary hypertension, and right heart failure. Those patients who also develop daytime somnolence have been designated as having the *Pickwickian syndrome* (see Chap. 34). In many such patients obstructive sleep apnea is a prominent feature, and even in those patients without sleep apnea, sleep-induced hypoventilation is an important element of the disorder and contributes to its progression. Most patients demonstrate a decrease in central respiratory drive which may be inherent or acquired, and many have mild to moderate degrees of airflow obstruction, usually related to smoking. Based on these considerations, several therapeutic measures can be of considerable benefit, including weight loss, cessation of smoking, elimination of obstructive sleep apnea, and enhancement of respiratory drive by medications such as progesterone.

SLEEP APNEA Sleep apnea is defined as an intermittent cessation of airflow at the nose and mouth during sleep. By convention apneas of at least 10 s duration have been considered important, but in most patients the apneas are 20 to 30 s in duration, and may be as long as 2 to 3 min. There is uncertainty as to the minimum number of apneas that should be considered clinically important, although by the time most patients come to attention they have at least 10 to 15 events per hour of sleep.

Sleep apneas have been classified into three types: central, obstructive, and mixed. In central sleep apnea (CSA) the neural drive to all the respiratory muscles is transiently abolished. In contrast, in obstructive sleep apnea (OSA) airflow ceases despite continuing respiratory drive because of occlusion of the oropharyngeal airway. Mixed apneas, which consist of a central apnea followed by an obstructive component, are a variant of OSA.

OBSTRUCTIVE SLEEP APNEA (OSA) Pathogenesis The definitive event in OSA is occlusion of the upper airway at the level of the oropharynx (Fig. 217-3). The resulting apnea leads to progressive asphyxia until there is a brief arousal from sleep, whereupon airway patency is restored and airflow resumes. The patient then returns to sleep and the sequence of events is repeated, often up to 400 to 500 times per night.

The immediate factor leading to collapse of the upper airway in OSA is the generation of a critical subatmospheric pressure during inspiration that exceeds the ability of the airway dilator and abductor muscles to maintain airway stability (Fig. 217-3). Sleep plays a permissive but crucial role by reducing the activity of the muscles of the upper airways. Alcohol is frequently an important cofactor because of its selective depressant influence on these muscles. In most patients the patency of the airway is also compromised structurally and therefore predisposed to occlusion. In a minority of patients the structural compromise is due to obvious anatomic disturbances, such as adenotonsillar hypertrophy, retrognathia, and macroglossia. However, in the majority of patients the structural defect is simply a subtle reduction in airway size that can often be appreciated clinically as "pharyngeal crowding" and that can usually be demonstrated by imaging or acoustic reflection techniques. Obesity frequently contributes to the reduction in size of the upper airways. More sophisticated studies also demonstrate a high airway compliance—i.e., the airway is "floppy" and therefore prone to collapse. In some patients a high upstream (i.e., nasal) resistance contributes to collapse of the upper airway by increasing the subatmospheric pressure generated in the pharynx during inspiration.

Pathophysiological and clinical features The narrowing of the upper airways during sleep, which predisposes to OSA, inevitably results in snoring. In most patients, snoring antedates the development of obstructive events by many years. However, the majority of snoring individuals do not have an OSA disorder; hence snoring alone does not warrant an investigation for OSA.

The recurrent episodes of nocturnal asphyxia and of arousal from sleep that characterize OSA lead to a series of secondary physiologic events, which in turn give rise to the clinical complications of the syndrome (Fig. 217-3). The most common manifestations are neuropsychiatric and behavioral disturbances that are thought to arise from the fragmentation of sleep and loss of slow-wave sleep induced by the recurrent arousal responses. The most pervasive manifestation is excessive daytime sleepiness. OSA is now recognized as a leading cause of daytime sleepiness and is being increasingly implicated as a risk factor for motor vehicle and industrial accidents. Other related symptoms include intellectual impairment, memory loss, personality disturbances, and impotence.

The other major manifestations are cardiorespiratory in nature and are thought to arise from the recurrent episodes of nocturnal asphyxia (Fig. 217-3). Most patients demonstrate a cyclical slowing of the heart during the apneas to 30 to 50 beats per minute, followed by a tachycardia of 90 to 120 beats per minute during the ventilatory phase. A small number of patients develop severe bradycardia with asystoles of 8 to 12 s duration, or dangerous tachyarrhythmias, including unsustained ventricular tachycardia. The presence of such arrhythmias has led to the notion that OSA may result in sudden death during sleep, but firm corroborative data are lacking. The majority of patients with OSA are hypertensive, and emerging data *suggest* that OSA contributes to the development of their hypertension. Finally, a small proportion of patients (10 to 15 percent) develop sustained pulmonary hypertension, right heart failure, polycythemia, and chronic hypercapnia and hypoxemia. Such patients have evidence of reduced ventilatory drive and many have diffuse airways obstruction. All such patients are obese and because of daytime sleepiness are considered to be examples of the Pickwickian syndrome.

Diagnosis Although OSA occurs at any age, the typical patient is a male aged 30 to 60 years who presents with a history of snoring and excessive daytime sleepiness, moderate obesity, and often mild to moderate hypertension. The diagnosis can often be confirmed by direct observation of the patient during sleep, or by the demonstration of cyclic arterial O_2 desaturation during sleep by ear oximetry, and of a cyclic brady/tachycardia by overnight Holter monitoring. However, the sensitivity of such simplified tests in diagnosing OSA is uncertain. Furthermore, while such tests can be helpful in diagnosing a sleep apnea disorder, they are not useful in identifying or excluding other possible causes of daytime sleepiness (narcolepsy, nocturnal myoclonus, nonrestorative sleep, phase-shifts syndromes). Therefore the definitive investigation for suspected OSA is polysomnography, a detailed overnight sleep study that includes recording of (1) electrographic variables that permit the identification of sleep and its various stages; (2) ventilatory variables that permit the identification of apneas and their classification as central or obstructive; (3) arterial O_2 saturation by ear oximetry; and (4) heart rate. The key diagnostic finding in OSA are episodes of airflow cessation at the nose and mouth despite evidence of continuing respiratory effort.

Treatment Several approaches to treatment of OSA have been advocated (Table 217-2). Patients with mild to moderate OSA can often be managed effectively by modest weight reduction if obese, avoidance of alcohol, improvement of nasal patency, and avoidance of sleeping in the supine posture. In some patients with more severe OSA, tricyclic medications, particularly protriptyline (20 to 30 mg at bedtime), have been beneficial in relieving daytime sleepiness and reducing the frequency of obstructive events. The role of nocturnal supplemental oxygen in managing OSA is uncertain. In some patients oxygen reduces the number of apneas, whereas in other patients it lengthens the duration of apneas. The most widely used treatments in severe OSA are uvulopalatopharyngoplasty and nasal continuous positive airway pressure (CPAP) during sleep. Uvulopalatopharyngoplasty is a surgical procedure designed to increase the pharyngeal lumen by resecting redundant soft tissue. When applied to unselected

TABLE 217-2 Management of obstructive sleep apnea (OSA)

Mechanism	Mild to moderate OSA	Severe OSA
↑ Upper airway muscle tone	Avoidance of alcohol, sedatives	Tricyclics
↑ Upper airway lumen size	Weight reduction Avoidance of supine posture	Uvulopalatopharyngoplasty
↓ Upper airway subatmospheric pressure	Improved nasal patency	Nasal continuous positive airway pressure
Bypass occlusion		Tracheostomy

SOURCE: Phillipson.

TABLE 217-3 Hyperventilation syndromes

I Hypoxemia
  A High altitude
  B Pulmonary disease

II Pulmonary disorders
  A Pneumonia
  B Interstitial pneumonitis, fibrosis, edema
  C Pulmonary emboli, vascular disease
  D Bronchial asthma
  E Pneumothorax

III Cardiovascular disorders
  A Congestive heart failure
  B Hypotension

IV Metabolic disorders
  A Acidosis (diabetic, renal, lactic)
  B Hepatic failure

V Neurologic disorders
  A Psychogenic or anxiety hyperventilation
  B Central nervous system infection, tumors

VI Drug-induced
  A Salicylates
  B Methylxanthine derivatives
  C Beta-adrenergic agonists
  D Progesterone

VII Miscellaneous
  A Fever, sepsis
  B Pain
  C Pregnancy

patients with OSA it produces long-term benefits in only about 50 percent of cases. More recent attempts to select patients based on the specific site of upper airway occlusion have yielded a higher success rate. Nasal CPAP, which prevents upper airway occlusion by splinting the pharyngeal airway with a positive pressure delivered through a nosemask, is currently the most successful approach to treatment, being well-tolerated and effective in over 80 percent of patients. For the few patients with severe OSA in whom all other treatment approaches fail, tracheostomy provides immediate relief.

CENTRAL SLEEP APNEA (CSA) Pathogenesis The definitive event in CSA is transient abolition of central drive to the ventilatory muscles. The resulting apnea leads to a primary sequence of events similar to those of OSA (Fig. 217-3). Several underlying mechanisms can result in cessation of respiratory drive during sleep. First are defects in the metabolic respiratory control system and respiratory neuromuscular apparatus. Such defects usually produce a chronic alveolar hypoventilation syndrome (in addition to CSA) which becomes more severe during sleep when the stimulatory effect of wakefulness on breathing is abolished. In contrast are CSA disorders that arise from transient instabilities in an otherwise intact respiratory control system. Common to all these disorders in a P_{CO_2} level during sleep that falls transiently below the critical P_{CO_2} required for respiratory rhythm generation. The most frequent instability of this type occurs at sleep onset, because the P_{CO_2} level of wakefulness is often lower than that required for rhythm generation in sleep; hence an apnea develops at sleep onset until P_{CO_2} rises to the critical level. However, if the central nervous system state fluctuates at sleep onset between "asleep" and "awake," a pattern of periodic breathing develops as respiration follows the changes in state. During each cycle the waning phase of ventilation includes an hypopnea or outright central apnea (Cheyne-Stokes respiration). Hypoxia, whether due to high altitude or to underlying cardiorespiratory disease, enhances the tendency to periodic breathing and CSA, because of the associated hyperventilation that may drive P_{CO_2} levels during wakefulness well below the critical value required for respiratory rhythm generation during sleep. Hyperventilation due to CNS disease produces periodic breathing and CSA by a similar mechanism. Circulatory slowing secondary to cardiac failure may also induce ventilatory instability by prolonging the time lag between changes in blood gas values by ventilation and the detection of those changes by the peripheral and central chemoreceptors (Chap. 182). Consequently the ventilatory system overshoots the mark before reversing direction, resulting in periodic breathing that frequently includes central apneas.

Pathophysiological and clinical features Many healthy individuals demonstrate a small number of central apneas during sleep, particularly at sleep onset and in REM sleep. These apneas are not associated with any physiologic or clinical disturbances. In patients with clinically important CSA, the primary sequence of events that characterizes the disorder leads to prominent physiologic and clinical consequences (Fig. 217-3). In those patients whose CSA is a component of an alveolar hypoventilation syndrome, daytime hypercapnia and hypoxemia are usually evident, and the clinical picture is dominated by a history of recurrent respiratory failure, polycythemia, pulmonary hypertension, and right heart failure. Complaints of sleeping poorly, morning headache, and daytime fatigue and sleepiness are also prominent. In contrast, in patients whose CSA results from an instability in respiratory drive, the clinical picture is dominated by features related to sleep disturbance, including recurrent nocturnal awakenings, morning fatigue, and daytime sleepiness.

Diagnosis Initially, many patients with CSA are suspected clinically of having OSA because of a history of snoring, sleep disturbance, and daytime sleepiness. However, obesity and hypertension are less prominent in CSA than OSA. Definitive diagnosis of CSA requires a polysomnographic study, with the *key observation being recurrent apneas that are not accompanied by respiratory effort*. Measurements of transcutaneous P_{CO_2} are particularly useful in CSA. Those patients with a defect in respiratory control or neuromuscular function typically demonstrate an elevated P_{CO_2} that tends to increase progressively during the night, particularly during REM sleep. In contrast, patients with instabilities in the respiratory control system often demonstrate a mild degree of hypocapnia, which is an integral pathogenetic feature of their disorder (see above).

Treatment The management of patients whose CSA is a component of an alveolar hypoventilation syndrome is essentially the same as the management of the underlying hypoventilation disorder. Management of patients whose CSA arises from an instability of respiratory drive is more problematic. Patients with hypoxemia usually respond favorably to nocturnal supplemental oxygen. Others have responded to acidification with acetazolamide, and recent reports indicate a good response to nasal CPAP (as for OSA) in some patients. The precise mechanism by which CPAP abolishes central apneas is not clear.

HYPERVENTILATION AND ITS SYNDROMES

DEFINITION AND ETIOLOGY Alveolar hyperventilation exists when P_{ACO_2} decreases below the normal range of 37 to 43 mmHg. Hyperventilation is not synonymous with hyperpnea, which refers to an increased minute volume of ventilation without reference to P_{ACO_2}. Although hyperventilation is frequently associated with dyspnea, patients who are hyperventilating do not necessarily complain of shortness of breath; and conversely, patients with dyspnea need not be hyperventilating.

Numerous disease entities can be associated with alveolar hyperventilation (Table 217-3), but in all cases the underlying mechanism involves an increase in respiratory drive. Thus hypoxemia drives ventilation by stimulating the peripheral chemoreceptors, and several pulmonary disorders and congestive heart failure drive ventilation by stimulating afferent vagal receptors in the lungs and airways. Low cardiac output and hypotension stimulate the peripheral chemoreceptors and inhibit the baroreceptors, both of which increase ventilation. Metabolic acidosis, a potent respiratory stimulant, excites both the peripheral and central chemoreceptors and increases the sensitivity of the peripheral chemoreceptors to coexistent hypoxemia. Hepatic failure can also produce hyperventilation, presumably as a result of metabolic stimuli acting on the peripheral and central chemoreceptors.

Several neurologic disorders are thought to drive ventilation through the behavioral respiratory control system. Included in this category are psychogenic or anxiety hyperventilation and severe cerebrovascular insufficiency, which may interfere with the inhibitory influence normally exerted by cortical structures on the brainstem respiratory neurons. Rarely, disorders of the midbrain and hypothalamus induce hyperventilation, and it is conceivable that fever and sepsis also cause hyperventilation through effects on these structures. Several drugs cause hyperventilation by stimulating the central or peripheral chemoreceptors or by direct action on the brainstem respiratory neurons. Chronic hyperventilation is a normal feature of pregnancy and results from the effects of progesterone and other hormones acting on the respiratory neurons.

PHYSIOLOGICAL AND CLINICAL FEATURES Because hyperventilation is associated with increased respiratory drive, muscle effort, and minute volume of ventilation, the most frequent symptom associated with hyperventilation is dyspnea. However, there is considerable discrepancy between the degree of hyperventilation, as measured by P_{ACO_2}, and the degree of associated dyspnea. In patients whose hypocapnia is associated with alkalemia, neurologic symptoms may be present, including dizziness, visual impairment, syncope, and seizure activity (secondary to cerebral vasoconstriction); paresthesias, carpopedal spasm, and tetany (secondary to decreased free serum calcium); and muscle weakness (secondary to hypophosphatemia). Severe alkalemia can also induce cardiac arrhythmias and evidence of myocardial ischemia. Patients with a primary respiratory alkalosis are also prone to periodic breathing and central sleep apnea.

DIAGNOSIS In most patients with a hyperventilation syndrome, the cause is readily apparent on the basis of history, physical examination, and knowledge of coexisting medical disorders (Table 217-3). In patients in whom the cause is not clinically apparent, investigation begins with arterial blood gas analysis, which establishes the presence of alveolar hyperventilation (decreased P_{ACO_2}) and its severity. Equally important is the arterial pH, which generally allows the disorder to be classified as either a primary respiratory alkalosis (elevated pH) or a primary metabolic acidosis (decreased pH). Also of importance is the Pa_{O_2} and calculation of the (A-a) P_{O_2} since a widened alveolar-arterial oxygen difference suggests a pulmonary disorder as the underlying cause. The finding of a reduced plasma HCO_3^- establishes the chronic nature of the disorder and points towards an organic cause. Measurements of ventilation and arterial or transcutaneous P_{CO_2} during sleep are very useful in suspected psychogenic hyperventilation, since such patients do not maintain the hyperventilation during sleep.

The disorders that most frequently give rise to unexplained hyperventilation are pulmonary vascular disease (particularly chronic or recurrent thromboembolism) and psychogenic or anxiety hyperventilation. Hyperventilation due to pulmonary vascular disease is associated with exertional dyspnea, a widened (A-a) P_{O_2} and maintenance of hyperventilation during exercise. In contrast, patients with psychogenic hyperventilation typically complain of dyspnea at rest and not during mild exercise, and of the need to sigh frequently. They are also more apt to complain of dizziness, sweating, palpitations, and paresthesias. During mild to moderate exercise their hyperventilation tends to disappear and (A-a) P_{O_2} is normal, but heart rate and cardiac output may be increased relative to metabolic rate.

TREATMENT Alveolar hyperventilation is usually of relatively minor clinical consequence and therefore is generally managed by appropriate treatment of the underlying cause. In the few patients in whom alkalemia is thought to be inducing significant cerebral vasoconstriction, parasthesias, tetany, or cardiac disturbances, inhalation of a low concentration of CO_2 can be very beneficial. For patients with disabling psychogenic hyperventilation, careful explanation of the basis of their symptoms can be reassuring and is often sufficient. Others have benefited from beta-adrenergic antagonists or an exercise program. Specific treatment for anxiety may also be indicated.

REFERENCES

CHERNIACK NS, LONGOBARDO GS: Abnormalities in respiratory rhythm, in *Handbook of Physiology*, section 3: *The Respiratory System*, vol 2, *Control of Breathing*, NS Cherniack, JG Widdicombe (eds). Bethesda, MD, Am Physiol Soc, 1986, pp 729–749

PHILLIPSON EA: Hypoventilation syndromes, in *Textbook of Respiratory Medicine*, JF Murray, JA Nadel (eds). Philadelphia, Saunders, 1988, chap 84, pp. 1831–1840

————: Sleep disorders, in *Textbook of Respiratory Medicine*, JF Murray, JA Nadel (eds). Philadelphia, Saunders, 1988, chap 85, pp 1841–1860

————, BOWES G: Control of breathing during sleep, in *Handbook of Physiology*, section 3: *The Respiratory System*, vol 2, *Control of Breathing*, NS Cherniack, JG Widdicombe (eds). Bethesda, MD, Am Physiol Soc 1986, pp 649–689

PLUM F, LEIGH RJ: Abnormalities of central mechanisms, in *Regulation of Respiration, Part 2*, TF Hornbein (ed), *Lung Biology in Health and Disease*, vol 17. New York, Marcel Dekker, 1981, pp 989–1067

THAWLEY SE (ed): Sleep apnea disorders. Med Clin North Am 69(6), 1985

218   ADULT RESPIRATORY DISTRESS SYNDROME

ROLAND H. INGRAM, JR.

Adult respiratory distress syndrome (ARDS) is a descriptive term that has been applied to many acute, diffuse infiltrative lung lesions of diverse etiologies when they are accompanied by severe arterial hypoxemia. The term was chosen because of several clinical and pathologic similarities between such acute illnesses in adults and the neonatal respiratory distress syndrome. However, in the neonatal form, immaturity of alveolar surfactant production and a highly compliant chest wall are primarily involved in the pathophysiology, whereas in the adult, alveolar surfactant changes are secondary to the primary process, and the chest wall is not compliant. Despite the large number of causes (Table 218-1), the clinical characteristics, respiratory pathophysiologic derangement, and current techniques for management of these acute abnormalities are remarkably similar. It has been argued that the "lumping" of such processes of different etiologies obscures the unique features of each in terms of pathogenesis, prevention, and specificity of treatment. The conditions listed do not always lead to respiratory failure and specific treatment of the underlying processes will often be different. Therefore, the reader is urged to refer to the appropriate sections of this text for the special characteristics of each condition and to recognize that only the common features at the onset of respiratory failure will be covered in this chapter. Moreover, many of the listed conditions are often present in combination and may come into play at different times in the clinical course of the adult respiratory distress syndrome.

PATHOPHYSIOLOGY   Regardless of the initiating process, ARDS is invariably associated with increased liquid in the lungs. It is a form of pulmonary edema, although distinct from cardiogenic pulmonary edema because pulmonary capillary pressure is not elevated (Chap. 36). Since hydrostatic pressures are not elevated, there is increased permeability of the alveolocapillary membranes that occurs via direct chemical injury in the case of inhaled toxic gases or aspirated acid or indirectly through activation and aggregation of formed elements of the blood within pulmonary capillaries in the case of septicemia and/or endotoxemia. Although platelet aggregation occurs, the major offenders appear to be monocytic phagocytes and polymorphonuclear leukocytes that adhere to endothelial surfaces and undergo a respiratory burst to inflict oxidant injury and release mediators of inflammation such as leukotrienes, thromboxanes, and prostaglandins. The monocytic phagocytes, mainly macrophages in the alveoli and those lining the vasculature, also release oxidants, mediators, and a series of degradative enzymes and peptides that directly damage endothelial and alveolar surfaces and cause polymorphonuclear leukocytes to release their lysosomal enzymes. Initially the injury to the alveolocapillary membrane results in leakage of liquid, macromolecules, and cellular components from the blood vessels into the interstitial space and, with increasing severity, into the alveoli. The increasing vascular permeability to proteins (decreased reflection coefficient σ, discussed in Chap. 36) leaves the hydrostatic gradient unopposed so that even mild elevations in capillary pressures greatly increase interstitial and alveolar edema. Alveolar collapse occurs secondary to the effect of the alveolar liquid, especially its fibrinogen, that interferes with normal surfactant activity and because of possible impairment of further surfactant production by injury to the granular pneumocytes. Though radiographically diffuse, the regional dysfunction is nonhomogeneous; it leads to severe ventilation-perfusion imbalance and the shunting of blood through regions in which alveoli are collapsed or filled with liquid. The lungs become less compliant—i.e., stiffen because of interstitial edema, alveolar collapse, and increase in surface forces. Because of the decreased compliance, large inspiratory pressures must be generated by the respiratory muscles so that the work of breathing is elevated. The large mechanical load may lead to fatigue of the muscles of breathing with resulting diminution in tidal volumes and worsening gas exchange. Both hypoxemia and the stimulation of receptors in the stiff lung parenchyma cause an increase in respiratory frequency, decrease in tidal volume, and deterioration in gas exchange.

PATHOLOGY   In the absence of specific demonstrable pathogens, the pathology is remarkably similar among the various conditions leading to ARDS, since the lung has a limited number of ways in which it reacts to a large number of injuries. Grossly, the lungs are heavy, edematous, and nearly airless with regions of hemorrhage, atelectasis, and consolidation. By light microscopy there is edema and cellular infiltration of interalveolar septa and interstitial spaces surrounding airways and blood vessels, atelectasis and hyaline membranes in many regions, engorgement of vessels with red blood cells, and aggregates of platelets and polymorphonuclear leukocytes along with interstitial and alveolar hemorrhage. In addition to loss of alveolar type I pneumocytes, both hyperplasia and dysplasia of the granular (type II) pneumocytes are often present.

If the illness has been prolonged beyond 10 days, there is often a surprising amount of fibrosis in addition to the acute changes. In instances of recovery and subsequent death from another cause, significant interstitial fibrosis and emphysematous changes may be found in the lung. Many patients, however, will recover completely and have normal pulmonary function with no respiratory symptoms. Hence aggressive clinical management is both indicated and often rewarding.

CLINICAL CHARACTERISTICS   At the time of initial injury and for several hours thereafter the patient may be free of respiratory symptoms or signs. The earliest sign often is an increase in respiratory frequency followed shortly by dyspnea. Arterial blood gas measurement in the earlier period will disclose a depressed P_{O_2} despite a decreased P_{CO_2} so that the alveolar-arterial difference for oxygen (Chap. 201) is increased. At this early stage, administration of oxygen results in a significant increase in the arterial P_{O_2}. The brisk rise in

---

TABLE 218-1   Conditions which may lead to the adult respiratory distress syndrome

1 Diffuse pulmonary infections (e.g., viral, bacterial, fungal, *Pneumocystis*)
2 Aspiration (e.g., gastric contents with Mendelson's syndrome, water with near drowning)
3 Inhalation of toxins and irritants (e.g., chlorine gas, NO_2, smoke, ozone, high concentrations of oxygen)
4 Narcotic overdose pulmonary edema (e.g., heroin, methadone, morphine, dextropropoxyphene)
5 Nonnarcotic drug effects (e.g., nitrofurantoin)
6 Immunologic response to host antigens (e.g., Goodpasture's syndrome, systemic lupus erythematosus)
7 Effects of nonthoracic trauma with hypotension
8 In association with systemic reactions to processes initiated outside the lung (e.g., gram-negative septicemia, hemorrhagic pancreatitis, amniotic fluid embolism, fat embolism)
9 Postcardiopulmonary bypass ("pump lung," "postperfusion lung")

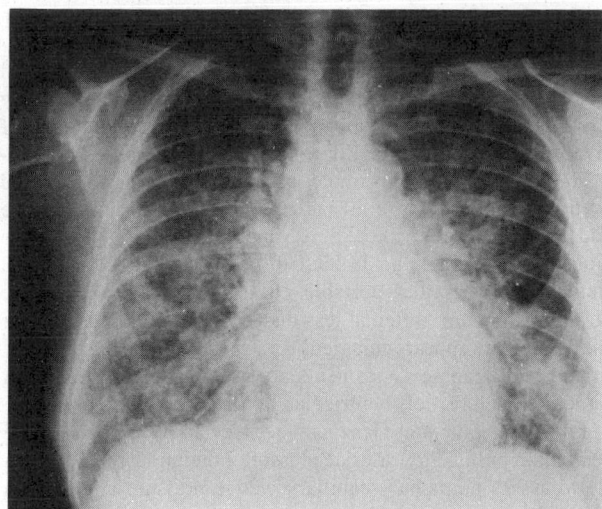

FIGURE 218-1 A standard posteroanterior chest radiograph from a patient with the adult respiratory distress syndrome secondary to a severe viral pneumonitis. Such a diffuse radiographic change is typical of all conditions listed in Table 218-1 when they are severe enough to cause acute hypoxemic respiratory failure. A similar radiographic picture is also seen in pulmonary edema due to left ventricular failure (Chap. 36). Often in such acutely ill patients, the radiograph must be taken with a portable unit and the film exposed from the anterior direction. Both the anteroposterior exposure and the failure to take a deep inspiration result in an apparent enlargement of the cardiac silhouette which further obscures the reliable detection of left ventricular failure.

P_{O_2} indicates that ventilation-perfusion mismatching and, possibly, diffusion impairment account for the widened alveolar-arterial P_{O_2} difference ($PA_{O_2} - Pa_{O_2}$) initially. Physical examination may be unremarkable, although a few fine inspiratory rales may be audible. Radiographically the lung fields may be clear or demonstrate only minimal and scattered interstitial infiltrates. With progression, the patient becomes cyanotic and increasingly dyspneic and tachypneic. Rales may become more prominent and easily heard throughout both lung fields along with regions of tubular breath sounds; the chest radiograph demonstrates diffuse, extensive bilateral interstitial and alveolar infiltrates (Fig. 218-1). At this point hypoxemia cannot be corrected simply by increasing the oxygen concentration of the inspired gas, and mechanical ventilatory support must be started. Right-to-left shunting of blood through collapsed or filled alveoli becomes the major mechanism for arterial hypoxemia at this more advanced stage. In contrast to ventilation-perfusion mismatching and diffusion impairment, with right-to-left shunts, $PA_{O_2} - Pa_{O_2}$ remains high with breathing of pure oxygen. Positive end-expiratory pressure (PEEP) serves to increase lung volume, which in turn opens collapsed alveoli and decreases shunting. With further progression, and if mechanical ventilator and PEEP therapy are delayed, the combination of increasing tachypnea and decreasing tidal volumes results in alveolar hypoventilation, a rising P_{CO_2}, and worsening hypoxemia; these represent an ominous constellation of findings.

MANAGEMENT OF HYPOXEMIC RESPIRATORY FAILURE The brief description given above contains the salient principles of management, integrated with the clinical events that lead to escalation of therapeutic interventions. Implicit in that description is that the simplest method and the lowest inspired fraction of oxygen (FI_{O_2}) should be used to give the desired result. The oxyhemoglobin dissociation curve gives some guide to the most desirable level of Pa_{O_2}. At a P_{O_2} of 60 mmHg hemoglobin is approximately 90 percent saturated. Therefore, a reasonable objective is to achieve that Pa_{O_2}, since higher levels add little to oxygenation and introduce the risk of oxygen toxicity to the lung. In contrast to respiratory failure complicating chronic airways obstruction (Chap. 210), depression

of ventilation is not an important factor in hypoxemic respiratory failure.

There are multiple means for delivering O_2, in order of increasing effectiveness: soft nasal prongs, simple face masks, and face masks with inspiratory reservoir bags. The effective FI_{O_2} (that is actually entering the trachea) will be determined by the concentration of O_2 delivered from the tank or wall device, its flow rate, and the minute ventilation of the patient. In the hypoxemic form of respiratory failure, it is reasonable to start with moderate flow rates (5 to 10 liters per minute of 100% O_2) and monitor arterial blood gases, adjusting flow rates and O_2 concentrations depending upon results.

If adequate oxygenation cannot be maintained with these less invasive measures, endotracheal intubation should be done and mechanical ventilatory support should be instituted (see Chap. 219). The rationale behind mechanical ventilatory support in a patient who is hyperventilating is *not* to increase ventilation but to increase mean lung volume, thereby opening previously closed airways and improving oxygenation. This is accomplished by using large tidal volumes (approximately 10 to 15 mL per kilogram of lean body weight) at a slower breathing rate (12 to 15 breaths per minute) than the spontaneous one of the patient. Most often, at this juncture, the respiratory system is sufficiently stiff that high inflation pressures are required and a volume-cycled ventilator (in contrast to the pressure-cycled ones) is needed. If the patient makes expiratory efforts during the inflation cycle, peak inspiratory pressures will increase, possibly enough to activate the high-pressure pop-off valve, which results in delivery to the patient of a smaller tidal volume than selected. Under these circumstances during controlled ventilation, consideration is often given to sedation and/or neuromuscular paralysis. However, an alternative is to institute synchronized intermittent mandatory ventilation (SIMV). In the SIMV mode, the patient is allowed to breathe spontaneously with periodic delivery of mandatory breaths that are synchronized with spontaneous inspiratory efforts. If the spontaneous breathing rate is so rapid that expiratory efforts occur before the mandatory breath is fully delivered, sedation and/or paralysis should be used with controlled ventilation.

Should the Pa_{O_2} be greater than 60 mmHg, the next step is to lower the FI_{O_2}. If the FI_{O_2} can be lowered to 0.6 or less with a Pa_{O_2} equal to or greater than 60 mmHg the mechanical ventilation should proceed at that FI_{O_2} as long as necessary. There are two indications for the addition of PEEP, the rationale for which is to increase lung volume further, thereby opening previously closed alveoli. First, if the FI_{O_2} cannot be lowered to or below 0.6, then PEEP should be added to allow a decrease of the FI_{O_2} below the toxic range. Second, if the Pa_{O_2} cannot be increased to or above 60 mmHg with an FI_{O_2} of 1.0, PEEP should be added. The optimal magnitude of the PEEP is determined by the response of the Pa_{O_2} and the extent of the cardiovascular alterations resulting from the higher pressure. The major alteration is a decrease in cardiac output due to two mechanisms. First, increased intrapleural pressures serve to impede venous return directly, an effect which is, to a variable extent, offset by peripheral venoconstriction. Second, increases in lung volume may increase pulmonary vascular resistance, leading to increased pressure and dilatation of the right ventricle, which in turn displaces the interventricular septum toward the left. This displacement decreases left ventricular diastolic compliance; hence less filling leads to smaller stroke volumes. An additional mechanism for decreased diastolic filling of the ventricles is direct compression of the heart by the stiffened lung. The optimal levels of PEEP are those associated with the greatest delivery of O_2 to the body; the latter is the product of cardiac output and arterial oxygen content.

Patients who are critically ill may simultaneously develop both deterioration of arterial oxygenation, due to increased lung fluid and/or a fall in mixed venous oxygen levels, and precarious hemodynamics, due to the pressure effects of mechanical ventilation and/or cardiac dysfunction with either a contracted or an expanded intravascular volume. Ventilator adjustments (see Chap. 219) are not often helpful because higher inflation pressures reflect worsening lung function. In this situation of falling blood pressure, urinary output, and arterial oxygenation, the decision to expand intravascular volume by infusion or to decrease it by diuresis is difficult. Body weight change is rarely a reliable indicator of blood volume since there is often fluid retention from positive intrathoracic pressures produced by the ventilator (see Chap. 219) plus "third space" fluid sequestration, especially with sepsis. Nor is physical examination of much help since rales are usual in any case and portable anteroposterior chest radiographs do not allow accurate assessment of subtle changes in cardiac size. Therefore a flow-directed right heart balloon-tipped (Swan-Ganz) catheter is often used for monitoring pulmonary arterial and capillary wedge pressures and measuring changes in cardiac output by the thermodilution technique. Recognition of over-damping and accelerative artifacts in the pulmonary arterial pressure signal and learning the criteria for true wedging are essential if serious misinterpretations are to be avoided. Even with accurate pressure measurements, there is an additional precaution that must be taken with regard to interpretation of intrathoracic vascular pressures referenced to atmosphere when PEEP is being used. If pleural pressure is greater than atmospheric, as is most often the case with PEEP, the transmural (i.e., intravascular minus pleural) pressure will be overestimated and could lead to errors in both assessment and management. Since the lungs are stiff only a portion of the applied PEEP is transmitted to the pleural space. A reasonable estimate of the transmural pressure is gained by examining vascular pressures just before inflation and subtracting from these pressures an amount equal to one-half the value of PEEP. In view of the leaky alveolocapillary membrane it is best to keep the pulmonary capillary wedge pressure as low as is compatible with a reasonable cardiac output, arterial pressure, and urinary output. Inotropic and selective vasoactive agents (e.g., dopamine, p. 387) have been used with some success to achieve this, but require careful monitoring to assess effects and adjust doses.

Mixed venous blood P_{O_2} values have long been considered to indicate the adequacy of oxygen delivery relative to demand. A low value (e.g., <20 mmHg) surely indicates that there is tissue hypoxemia irrespective of measured cardiac output and Pa_{O_2}. However, a high value does not exclude serious tissue hypoxemia, especially in gram-negative septicemia, in which systemic low-resistance shunts can develop and leave several capillary beds underperfused.

Body position may also affect the degree of arterial oxygenation. Although patients with ARDS have diffuse lung disease, there may be some regional variation in the extent of disease such that one side is more severely involved than the other. In this instance the less involved lung should be the more dependent one when the patient is in a lateral position. Since the distribution of pulmonary blood flow is so heavily determined by gravity (Chap. 201), having the more involved lung, with its minimal ventilation, in the more dependent position results in a measurable increase in intrapulmonary shunting which may be manifested by a striking fall in Pa_{O_2}. The possible contribution of a positional effect on arterial oxygenation should always be considered before escalating therapeutic interventions.

Occasionally PEEP must be gradually increased to levels in excess of 20 cmH$_2$O in an attempt to maintain arterial oxygenation. At these high levels of PEEP there may be a paradoxic decrease in Pa_{O_2}. The explanation for this paradox is as follows: high levels of PEEP may not open some of the closed airways but will overdistend those alveolar units already open. Overdistention of units increases the vascular resistance in these regions and results in more blood perfusing regions with closed airways, thereby increasing the degree of shunt. The only alternative is to decrease PEEP to a level associated with the greatest delivery of oxygen to the body (product of cardiac output and arterial oxygen content).

In the situations where maximal PEEP with $F_{I_{O_2}}$ of 1.0 does not supply sufficient oxygen, the possibility of utilizing extracorporeal membrane oxygenators (ECMO) has been both considered and tried. Despite the logical appeal of this form of supportive therapy, a randomized, large prospective study of ECMO therapy has demonstrated that, while it can support gas exchange, there is no effect on survival in acute hypoxemic respiratory failure.

COMPLICATIONS   Increasing severity of the clinical illness and continued radiographic progressions in association with the primary process often obscure complications that arise during the course of acute hypoxemic respiratory failure. The development of *left ventricular failure* is a good example of a common, easily missed complication. This is because all patients are likely to have diffuse rales and rhonchi, even without left ventricular failure, and these sounds also serve to make it difficult to detect gallop rhythms. An additional difficulty is that portable chest films are taken in the anteroposterior direction, often at less than full lung inflation, so that the cardiac silhouette appears enlarged. As a consequence, the ordinary physical and radiographic assessments are not always reliable. With deterioration, therefore, left ventricular failure should be suspected; it is helpful to insert a Swan-Ganz catheter (see above) which can be used to monitor pulmonary arterial pressure continuously and intermittently to assess pulmonary capillary wedge pressure and oxygen content of mixed venous blood.

With a diffuse radiographic pattern, a secondary bacterial infection is easily overlooked; therefore, frequent sputum smears and cultures should be obtained, especially when there is fever. With many conditions—e.g., gram-negative septicemia, acute hemorrhagic pancreatitis, and "shock lung"—there may be associated *disseminated intravascular coagulation,* which leads to gastrointestinal and intrapulmonary hemorrhage (Chap. 289). Frequent monitoring of platelet count, fibrinogen level, and partial thromboplastin and prothrombin times is helpful in the early detection of this complication and in guiding treatment.

Bronchial obstruction by endotracheal or tracheostomy tubes is common. When these tubes are too long or poorly anchored, they may slide into one main bronchus, usually the right one because of its less angulated origin from the trachea. The tube then blocks ventilation of the other main bronchus, and atelectasis may ensue. This event usually causes abrupt deterioration in the patient with respiratory failure. It is detected readily by physical examination, which reveals the absence of breath sounds over the occluded lung. The tube should immediately be pulled back slowly if this complication is suspected. In the course of treating ARDS with mechanical ventilators and high inflation pressures, *pneumothorax* or *pneumomediastinum* may develop and may be impossible to detect except radiologically. Occasionally the presence of subcutaneous emphysema provides a clinical clue. Any deterioration should lead to consideration of this complication, repetition of the chest radiograph, and immediate institution treatment of pneumothorax, if present. If deterioration is sudden, *tension pneumothorax* should be suspected; if physical signs are present, a pleural catheter should be inserted immediately without radiographic confirmation. High oxygen concentrations (>0.60) for prolonged periods can produce both the lesions and the clinical picture of ARDS. Therefore, the *minimal* oxygen concentration associated with acceptable arterial oxygenation should always be used.

Discontinuation of mechanical ventilatory support   The ability of the patient to maintain adequate gas exchange without the support of a mechanical ventilator is most often heralded by a decreasing $F_{I_{O_2}}$ requirement, smaller inflation pressures for mandatory or assisted breathing, and a fall in spontaneous respiratory rate (see Chap. 219).

PROGNOSIS   Given the diversity of the etiologies and the frequency of associated diseases, it is difficult, if not impossible, to give meaningful prognostic figures for ARDS. If all recently published series are taken together, the mortality rate is between 50 and 60 percent. This represents an improved survival rate over the nearly 100 percent mortality rate of a few years ago and is a result of the application of modern treatment techniques described above. If ARDS is due to drug overdose, the mortality rate is low; if associated with shock, the chances of a fatal outcome are much greater. It has become apparent that multiple organ system failure (e.g., renal, hepatic) supervenes when there is an extrapulmonic source of sepsis in need of surgical drainage and that almost all such patients die despite maximal support of the respiratory and cardiovascular systems. Other etiologies and associated diseases fall between these two extremes. The following factors appear to be associated with a poor outcome: an increase in $P_{A_{O_2}} - P_{a_{O_2}}$, requiring increasing inspired O_2 concentrations and PEEP; decreasing compliance, requiring greater inflation pressures; either low or falling colloid osmotic pressures; and the onset of systemic arterial hypotension not responding to intravascular volume replacement.

In survivors with previously normal lung function, the long-term prognosis for recovery appears to be remarkably good. Lung volumes and arterial blood gases have been shown to return to normal levels within 4 to 6 months after respiratory failure. There are instances, however, when the fibrotic residua are sufficiently great that complete recovery is unlikely.

REFERENCES

COHEN AB et al: A peptide from alveolar macrophages that releases neutrophil enzymes into the lungs in patients with the adult respiratory distress syndrome. Am Rev Respir Dis 137:1151, 1988

GLAUSER FL et al: Worsening oxygenation in the mechanically ventilated patient. Am Rev Respir Dis 138:458, 1988

HOGG JC: Neutrophil kinetics and lung injury. Physiol Rev 67(4):1249, 1987

MATTHAY MA, CHATTERJEE K: Bedside catheterization of the pulmonary artery: Risks compared with benefits. Ann Intern Med 109:826, 1988

MATUSCHAK GM, RINALDO JE: Organ interactions in the adult respiratory distress syndrome during sepsis. Chest 94(2):400, 1988

PETTY TL: The use, abuse, and mystique of positive end-expiratory pressure. Am Rev Respir Dis 138:475, 1988

PINGLETON SK: Complications of acute respiratory failure. Am Rev Respir Dis 137:1463, 1988

RAFFIN TA: ARDS: Mechanisms and management. Hosp Pract 22(11):65, 1987

REYNOLDS HY: Lung inflammation: Normal host defense or a complication of some diseases? Annu Rev Med 38:295, 1987

219 MECHANICAL VENTILATORY SUPPORT

PAUL N. LANKEN

TYPES OF MECHANICAL VENTILATORY SUPPORT

All types of mechanical ventilatory support share a common life-sustaining therapeutic goal: to support respiratory gas exchange as safely and comfortably as possible in patients with respiratory failure, while the underlying condition responds to therapy or resolves spontaneously.

POSITIVE PRESSURE VENTILATORS Positive pressure ventilators are characterized by positive inspiratory airway pressures, i.e., greater than atmospheric, and, as a rule, all are used with cuffed tracheal tubes in order to prevent excessive leak of tidal volume around the tube during inflation. Currently, most adult patients are supported by *volume-cycled* mechanical ventilators in which inspiration ceases after a certain tidal volume has been delivered. As a rule, this method of ventilation reliably delivers preset tidal volumes despite severe and/or fluctuating derangements of respiratory mechanics. All volume-cycled ventilators also have inspiratory pressure alarms that function as "pop-off" valves if peak airway pressures exceed a certain value; this results in decreased tidal volumes delivered in an effort to diminish the risk of barotrauma (injury of the lung from high pressure). Much less commonly used in adults are *pressure-cycled* mechanical ventilators in which inspiration ceases once a preset inspiratory pressure is reached. The major limitation of this type of ventilator is its inability to deliver constant tidal volume when the patient's respiratory mechanics change as discussed below.

NEGATIVE PRESSURE VENTILATORS Negative pressure mechanical ventilators mimic spontaneous inspiration by applying subatmospheric pressure to expand the chest cavity and to make alveolar pressure negative. Examples include the venerable iron lung, or Drinker respirator, as well as more comfortable current versions (cuirass respirators) that enclose just the patient's trunk. Most operate as pressure-cycled ventilators with the same limitations as noted above; on the other hand, they can be used with uncuffed tracheal tubes or, in selected cases, with no tracheal tubes at all.

PHYSIOLOGIC PRINCIPLES OF MECHANICAL VENTILATION

STATIC PRESSURE-VOLUME RELATIONSHIPS In positive pressure ventilation, tidal volumes distend both the lungs and their enclosing structure—the chest bellows (chest wall and diaphragm). The relationship between tidal volumes and their distending pressures at end-inspiration defines the static compliance (Cst) of the respiratory system, i.e., the lungs and chest wall, where Cst equals the ratio of the change in volume to change in pressure (Fig. 219-1A). The normal range of Cst is 50 to 100 mL per cmH_2O.

DYNAMIC PRESSURE-VOLUME RELATIONSHIPS During a positive pressure inflation, the pressure at the proximal end of the tube, i.e., proximal airway pressure, exceeds alveolar pressure and provides the pressure gradient for airflow into the lungs. Note that the proximal airway pressure has two components: (1) alveolar pressure which is determined by the *static* pressure volume curve (Fig. 219-1A) for any degree of lung inflation, and (2) the pressure drop due to resistance by the airways to airflow. The proximal airway pressure during inflation is described by the dynamic pressure-volume curve of the respiratory system (Fig. 219-1B).

High peak proximal airway pressures can result from excessively high resistance to airflow, as occurs in severe asthma (Fig. 219-1C), or from abnormally low static compliance, as occurs in pulmonary edema (Fig. 219-1D). From Fig. 219-1 one can also see how the same peak pressure may deliver markedly different tidal volumes depending on the type and degree of alteration in lung mechanics; for this reason pressure-cycled ventilators are used infrequently in adult patients with respiratory failure.

INDICATIONS FOR MECHANICAL VENTILATION

Specific indications for mechanical ventilation vary according to the underlying mechanism causing the patient's respiratory failure. The latter can result from impairment of the respiratory system which has traditionally been divided into four functional components: (1) central neural drive; (2) the chest bellows, including peripheral nervous system and the respiratory muscles; (3) airways; and (4) alveoli.

CENTRAL NEURAL DRIVE Examples of patients with impaired central neural drive are those with self-administered narcotic or sedative drug overdoses, with excessive iatrogenic sedative therapy, and, rarely, those with strokes involving the brainstem. The trachea should be intubated to prevent aspiration if there is a diminished or lost gag reflex. A mechanical ventilator can then be used to monitor the respiratory rate and spontaneous tidal volumes as well as for therapy of subsequent hypoventilation.

CHEST BELLOWS (INCLUDES PERIPHERAL NERVOUS SYSTEM AND RESPIRATORY MUSCLES) Patients with respiratory failure due to disorders of chest bellows commonly include those with neuromuscular weakness, caused, for example, by myasthenia gravis (Chap. 366) or the Guillain-Barré syndrome (Chap. 363), as well as those with chest wall problems such as flail chest or severe kyphoscoliosis. As a general rule, when the vital capacity is less than 1 L, or 15 mL/kg body weight, elective intubation should be done and mechanical ventilation begun. Lower vital capacities (<10 mL/kg) and/or an arterial P_{CO_2} (Pa_{CO_2}) above 45 mmHg are indications for immediate intubation and mechanical ventilation.

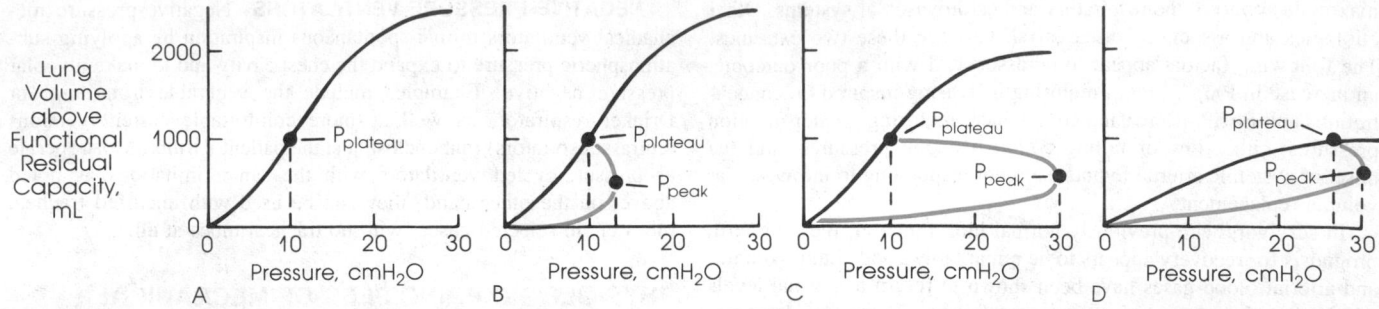

FIGURE 219-1 Schematic representations of pressure-volume curves of respiratory system (lungs and chest wall) during positive pressure mechanical ventilation. *A.* Static pressure-volume curve. $P_{plateau}$ is the alveolar pressure at end-inspiration after a 1000-mL tidal volume. It is measured by momentarily delaying the start of expiration after inflation by a tidal volume and allowing the gauge pressure to "plateau" at an end-inspiratory value. The slope of the curve from the origin to $P_{plateau}$ represents *static compliance*, which in this example is 100 mL per cmH_2O (Cst = change in volume ÷ change in pressure = 1000 mL ÷ 10 cmH_2O = 100 mL per cmH_2O). *B.* Dynamic pressure-volume curve added to the static pressure-volume curve. The peak proximal airway pressure (P_{peak}) is displayed during inspiration on the ventilator's pressure gauge. The pressure difference between the dynamic and static pressure-volume curves at the same lung volume represents the pressure drop due to resistance to airflow by the artificial and natural airways. P_{peak} is only 2 to 4 cmH_2O higher than $P_{plateau}$ in patients with normal airway resistance. *C.* Static and dynamic pressure-volume curves in a patient with severe asthma. Greatly increased P_{peak} is from airway obstruction. $P_{plateau}$ remains unchanged because static compliance is normal. *D.* Static and dynamic pressure-volume curves in a patient with pulmonary edema. Both P_{peak} and $P_{plateau}$ are increased because of decreased static compliance. In this disorder, because P_{peak} is only modestly elevated above $P_{plateau}$ (airway resistance being relatively normal), some clinicians have used P_{peak} instead of $P_{plateau}$ as the denominator in the ratio for respiratory system compliance. This latter ratio has been designated *dynamic compliance.* (*Adapted from Lanken.*)

AIRWAYS Indications for intubation and mechanical ventilation in patients with severe asthma (Chap. 204) depend on the level of Pa_{CO_2}: (1) Hypercapnia, i.e., $Pa_{CO_2} > 45$ mmHg, unresponsive to pharmacologic therapy almost always indicates the need for emergency intubation and mechanical ventilation; or (2) normocapnia, i.e., $Pa_{CO_2} = 40$ mmHg, may be associated with respiratory muscle fatigue or increasingly severe airways obstruction and is also an indication for intubation and mechanical ventilation. Since early in most asthmatic episodes the Pa_{CO_2} is low (30 to 33 mmHg) due to alveolar hyperventilation, a Pa_{CO_2} of 40 mmHg often represents a deteriorating clinical status with incipient respiratory failure. A normal Pa_{CO_2} in this situation has been termed *the cross-over point* to heighten clinicians' awareness of its ominous importance. In contrast, in patients with chronic obstructive pulmonary disease (COPD) (Chap. 210), initiation of mechanical ventilation should be for acute respiratory distress associated with a severe respiratory acidosis, e.g., arterial pH < 7.25, rather than for hypercapnia alone, since even quite high Pa_{CO_2} levels may be chronic and well tolerated.

ALVEOLI Examples of respiratory failure due to impairment of the alveolar component of the respiratory system include cardiogenic pulmonary edema, noncardiogenic pulmonary edema, also known as the adult respiratory distress syndrome (ARDS), extensive pneumonias, and diffuse alveolar hemorrhage syndromes. Diffuse alveolar flooding due to any cause results in an increased right-to-left shunt across the lungs, usually greater than 20 percent, and severe hypoxemic respiratory failure. Mechanical ventilation is urgently indicated in patients with these types of disorders if hypercapnia develops or if hypoxemia remains life-threatening, e.g., $Pa_{O_2} < 50$ mmHg, despite therapy with 100% oxygen delivered by a tight-fitting face mask. Positive end-expiratory pressure (PEEP) is often added to mechanical ventilation to decrease the right-to-left shunt and improve the hypoxemia. PEEP is also used in these patients to allow a reduction in fractional inspired oxygen Fi_{O_2} in order to avoid oxygen toxicity. The rationale for the use of PEEP is to increase the end-expiratory lung volume, i.e., functional residual capacity, with attendant opening of previously collapsed and unventilated alveoli that were the cause of the high right-to-left shunt.

CARE OF PATIENTS RECEIVING MECHANICAL VENTILATION

GENERAL MEDICAL CARE Patients receiving mechanical ventilation to treat acute respiratory failure of any cause are usually clinically unstable and may be critically ill. In such patients, undetected disconnection from the ventilator may be lethal. Because of these considerations, acutely ill patients needing mechanical ventilation are admitted routinely to an intensive care unit (ICU) or other suitable special care unit that meets the needs of these patients in terms of availability of appropriate equipment and properly trained professional personnel.

Medical care of acutely ill ventilator-dependent patients is as challenging as it is comprehensive, requiring a broad knowledge of general internal medicine as well as of critical care medicine. The patients' medical care should be closely integrated with specialized care provided by others on the ICU health care team: the nursing staff, respiratory therapists, physical and occupational therapists, and others. Such collaborative ICU care represents an holistic approach to patient care including medical, emotional, and social aspects.

Three specific components of general ICU care should be given to all ventilator-dependent patients and deserve special mention: (1) systemic or local therapy to prevent stress erosions of the gastric mucosa; (2) appropriate nutrition based on assessments of nutritional status, resting energy expenditures, and anticipated duration of mechanical ventilation; and (3) careful monitoring of fluid balance and body weight since positive pressure ventilation predisposes to water and sodium retention. The mechanism of the latter observation relates to reduced cardiac output and possibly to decreased secretion of atrial natriuretic peptide (ANP).

PATIENT MONITORING DURING MECHANICAL VENTILATION All patients on mechanical ventilators should have continuous ECG monitoring as well as frequent measurements of vital signs, serum electrolytes, urine output, and fluid balance. The ICU team should also follow closely the patient's mental and neurologic status, respiratory secretions, and the integrity of the patient's skin and mucous membranes. Ventilator parameters and tracheal cuff pressures should also be monitored frequently. Determinations of arterial pH, P_{CO_2} and P_{O_2} should be made at appropriate intervals to assess alveolar ventilation and arterial oxygenation. Continuous pulse oximetry and end-tidal P_{CO_2} monitoring are often useful in selected patients during periods of respiratory instability or during weaning trials.

PATIENT CARE PROBLEMS ARISING FROM MECHANICAL VENTILATION Artificial airways In most patients mechanical ventilation is begun via naso- or endotracheal tubes; some of these patients go on to have tracheostomies—usually when the mechanical ventilatory support is anticipated to be of long duration. Tracheostomies are done after 2 or 3 weeks of mechanical ventilation not to decrease tracheal complications, since both classes of artificial airways have comparable complication rates, but rather to improve patient comfort and provide a more secure airway for patients needing chronic ventilator support. This support may be carried out at home or in a long-term care facility. Either type of tube should be used with the now-standard high-volume "floppy" cuff, which should be inflated to a sufficient pressure to allow just a slight (~50 mL) leak during inflation (minimal leak technique) or to occlude the trachea just enough to prevent any leak (minimal occlusion technique) in order to try to prevent severe tracheal wall damage at the cuff site.

Adverse hemodynamic consequences Positive pressure ventilation raises pleural pressure during inspiration which, in turn, decreases systemic venous blood return to the right atrium and, therefore, cardiac output. This effect may cause significant hypotension in the presence of blood volume depletion or in situations in which the mean alveolar pressure (and hence pleural pressure) is relatively high over the entire respiratory cycle. The latter occurs frequently during mechanical ventilation when there is: (1) a high inspiration-to-expiration (I:E) ratio, e.g., 1:1 or more; (2) addition of therapeutic positive end-expiratory pressure (PEEP) (Fig. 219-2); or (3) the presence of occult (non-therapeutic) positive end-expiratory pressure, also called auto-PEEP (Fig. 219-2). Occult PEEP occurs frequently in patients with severe airways obstruction and may cause profound hypotension that should be treated by intravascular volume expansion, increasing the time for expiration, and/or changing from assist mode to intermittent mandatory ventilation (IMV) mode.

Barotrauma Injury to the lung by high distending pressures and volumes, i.e., barotrauma, not uncommonly occurs in ventilator-dependent patients, especially in those receiving high airway pressures. Barotrauma includes asymptomatic pneumothorax and tension pneumothorax with cardiovascular collapse, as well as the presence of air in the mediastinum (*pneumomediastinum*) or in the subcutaneous tissues in the neck or thorax (*subcutaneous emphysema*). Prevention of barotrauma is attempted by lowering peak airway pressures; this is achieved by decreasing tidal volume or inspiratory flow rates while maintaining alveolar ventilation. High peak airway pressures are often caused by poor synchrony between an anxious patient's spontaneous breathing efforts and the mechanical ventilator. This is treated as much as possible by reassurance and, if necessary, by sedation alone or sedation with pharmacologic paralysis.

The diagnosis of barotrauma can be elusive by clinical examination and, for this reason, daily chest radiographs of critically ill patients on mechanical ventilators are recommended. Therapy of severe barotrauma, e.g., tension pneumothorax, requires chest tube drainage and suction.

WEANING FROM MECHANICAL VENTILATORY SUPPORT

Success in weaning, the process of removing patients from mechanical ventilatory support, generally depends more on successful therapy or resolution of the precipitating cause of the respiratory failure than on the weaning technique utilized. For this reason, knowledge of the cause of the patient's respiratory failure, and whether the process has been reversed, is important in determining when to begin weaning. The weaning process should be done in steps as follows: (1) assessment prior to weaning; (2) trials of progressively less ventilator dependence, resulting in total ventilatory independence; and (3) removal of the tracheal tube, i.e., extubation.

ASSESSMENT PRIOR TO WEANING Preweaning physiologic assessment should address the basic question of whether the level of ventilation that patients can sustain (ventilatory supply) is equal to or greater than the ventilation that is needed to maintain their level of P_{CO_2} (ventilatory demand). Factors determining the balance between ventilatory supply and demand (Table 219-1) are reflected by a set of weaning parameters (Table 219-2) whose values have been found to be reasonably good predictors for success or failure in weaning. As a cautionary note, these weaning parameters should not be regarded as absolute criteria to predict weanability, but rather as one aspect of a preweaning assessment best understood in the context of the patient's overall clinical condition.

As noted above, the overall *clinical assessment* of the patient prior to weaning is equally as, if not more, important than the patient's weaning parameters. For example, it is imperative that the patient be relatively stable hemodynamically and not experiencing frequent life-threatening arrhythmias. In addition, the patient's neurologic status should be stable, with sufficient gag and cough reflexes to permit extubation. Other major organ system failure may preclude weaning through various mechanisms, e.g., metabolic acidosis in patients with renal failure, or a heightened drive to breathe in patients with hepatic failure.

TRIALS OF WEANING There are four commonly used weaning techniques: (1) "T-piece" trials; (2) the nearly equivalent ventilator

FIGURE 219-2 Schematic representations of theoretical alveolar pressure wave forms and the ventilator's pressure gauge (right-hand side of figure) displaying proximal airway pressure (pressure in the ventilator's tubing near the proximal end of the tracheal tube) during mechanical ventilation, showing the effect of therapeutic positive end-expiratory pressure (PEEP) and occult PEEP (auto-PEEP). At the start of inspiration (insp) the negative deflections (small arrows) indicate the patient's spontaneous inspiratory effort which initiates the assisted breath. *A.* In the assist mode with no therapeutic PEEP added and in the absence of auto-PEEP; note that alveolar pressure falls rapidly to zero (large arrow) during passive expiration. At end-expiration, both the alveolar pressure and proximal airway pressure are zero. *B.* In the assist mode after the addition of 10 cmH$_2$O of PEEP; note that alveolar pressure again falls rapidly (large arrow) during passive expiration but to a new stable baseline of 10 cmH$_2$O. At end-expiration both the alveolar and proximal airway pressures are 10 cmH$_2$O. *C.* In the assist mode, a patient with severe airways obstruction has 10 cmH$_2$O of occult PEEP (auto-PEEP) due to a prolonged time for alveolar emptying. Note that the alveolar pressure never falls to a stable baseline (large arrow) during passive expiration before the next inspiration starts. At end-expiration, alveolar pressure is 10 cmH$_2$O but the proximal airway pressure gauge displays 0 cmH$_2$O, reflecting atmospheric pressure due to the circuit's open exhalation valve and not the alveolar pressure—hence the term occult PEEP. However, if the expiratory tubing is abruptly occluded at end-expiration, the gauge would rise from 0 cmH$_2$O to 10 cmH$_2$O, indicating the presence and magnitude of the auto-PEEP.

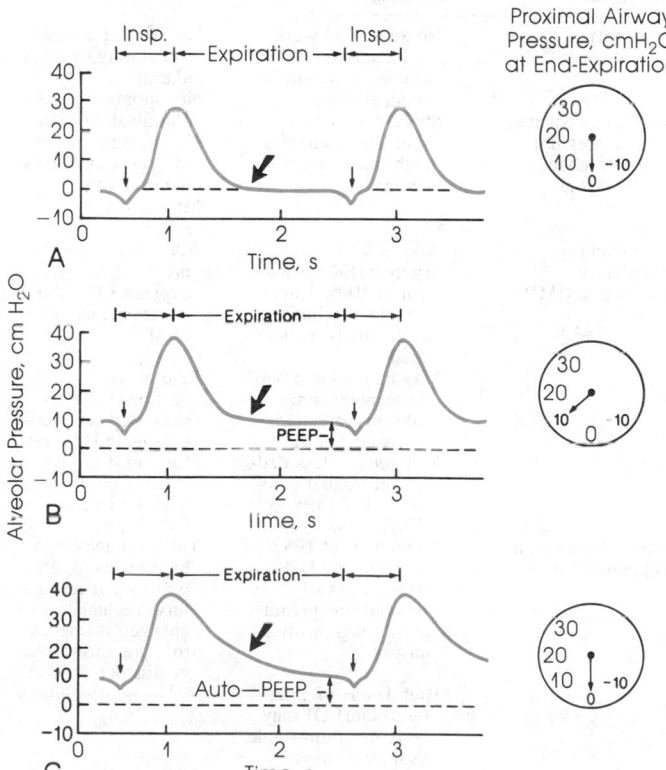

TABLE 219-1　Major factors determining the balance between ventilatory supply and demand

I Factors limiting ventilatory supply*
  A Respiratory muscle weakness (e.g., fatigue)
  B Unfavorable length-tension relationship (e.g., due to lung hyperinflation)
  C Airways obstruction (e.g., asthma)
  D Restricted lung volumes (e.g., pneumonia)
II Factors raising ventilatory demand†
  A High physiologic dead space-tidal volume ratio (V_D/V_T) (e.g., emphysema)
  B Elevated minute oxygen consumption and hence CO_2 production (e.g., sepsis)
  C Respiratory quotient (RQ) greater than 1.0 (e.g., excessive carbohydrate feeding)
  D Maintaining arterial P_{CO_2} below 36 mmHg (e.g., due to metabolic acidosis)

* The maximal sustainable ventilation (MSV) which is usually equal to ~½ maximal voluntary ventilation (MVV).
† The spontaneous minute ventilation ($\dot{V}_E$) needed to maintain a certain arterial P_{CO_2} set by the patient's central neuronal drive. If this $\dot{V}_E$ is greater than the patient's maximal sustainable ventilation, the patient will develop respiratory muscle fatigue at that $\dot{V}_E$.

TABLE 219-2　Various parameters useful for weaning from mechanical ventilators

Parameter	Value predicting failure	Value predicting success
I Respiratory muscle function		
A Maximal inspiratory pressure	< -20 mmHg	> -30 mmHg
II Ventilatory demand		
A Spontaneous respiratory rate	>35/min	<30/min
B Minute ventilation ($\dot{V}_E$)	>10 L/min	<10 L/min
C V_D/V_T*	≥0.6	<0.4
III Ventilatory ability		
A Vital capacity	<10 mL/kg	≥15 mL/kg
B Maximal voluntary ventilation	$<2 \times$ resting $\dot{V}_E$	$\geq 2 \times$ resting $\dot{V}_E$
IV Oxygenation		
A Intrapulmonary right-to-left shunt	>20%	<20%

* Physiologic dead space-tidal volume ratio.
SOURCE: Lanken.

mode of continuous positive airway pressure (CPAP) used without any PEEP, i.e., CPAP trials; (3) intermittent mandatory ventilation (Fig. 219-3); and (4) inspiratory pressure support ventilation (Fig. 219-3). Some major advantages and disadvantages of each of these four techniques are listed in Table 219-3. As a general rule, during any type of weaning trial the patients' clinical status needs to be assessed frequently; if patients become clinically unstable or acutely distressed, the trial should be stopped and the patients should be hand ventilated ("bagged") or returned to the ventilator.

FIGURE 219-3 Schematic representation of proximal airway pressure wave forms during assisted ventilation and two modes of weaning. *A.* During mechanical ventilation in the assist mode, the patient "triggers" each breath by a short inspiratory effort (T) preceding the ventilator breath (Assist) at a rate of 15 per min. *B.* During synchronized intermittent mandatory ventilation (SIMV), the patient breathes spontaneously (Spont) at a rate of 20 per min, also from the ventilator's demand valve, and also receives unassisted ventilator-delivered tidal volumes (IMV) at a preset rate of approximately 7 per min. The SIMV breaths are synchronized to avoid "stacking" a ventilator breath on top of a spontaneous breath. *C.* During inspiratory pressure support ventilation, the patient breathes spontaneously at a rate of 20 per min from the ventilator's demand valve, as in the example of SIMV above, but the inspiratory effort is aided by the ventilator maintaining the proximal airway pressure relatively constant at 10 cmH₂O during the entire inspiration (IPS).

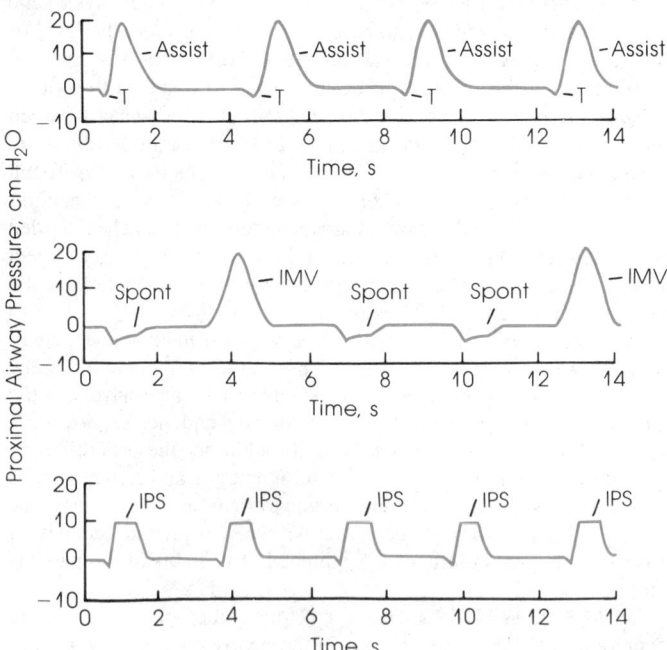

Preweaning patient education, encouragement, and similar measures to support the patient's psychological needs before and during weaning are important adjuncts to any weaning technique.

In a *T-piece trial*, the patient is disconnected from the mechanical ventilator and breathes spontaneously with the tracheal tube connected to a humidified gas source via a plastic connector called a T-piece. These periods of spontaneous breathing should be of a specific duration, and not to the point of fatigue; the periods are increased progressively depending on the patient's ventilatory capacity and endurance. Some newer ventilators have an additional mode that more closely resembles a T-piece trial by providing continuous gas flow through the inspiratory and expiratory circuits; patients inspire from this bias flow, rather than from a demand valve.

In a *CPAP trial* for weaning, commonly utilized without any

TABLE 219-3　Comparison of advantages and disadvantages of four commonly used weaning techniques

Technique	Major advantages	Major disadvantages
T-piece trial	No additional work of breathing needed to open ventilator's demand valve	No exhaled volume monitoring or other alarms No automatic sighs
Continuous positive airway pressure (CPAP) mode, i.e., a CPAP trial	Still connected to ventilator's circuits with full monitor's alarms	Additional work of breathing required to open ventilator's demand valve May lack sighs on some ventilators
Intermittent mandatory ventilation (IMV)	Allows for transition from 100% mechanical to 100% spontaneous ventilation as gradually as desired	Additional work of breathing to open demand valve during spontaneous breaths
	May be tolerated better hemodynamically by patients in left heart failure	Rate of weaning may be slower due to slow step-wise decreases in IMV rate
	May require less bedside personnel compared to T-piece or CPAP trials	May result in less bedside observations than T-piece or CPAP trials
Inspiratory pressure support (IPS)	Low levels of IPS (5–10 cmH₂O) decrease work of spontaneous breathing through artificial airway	Tidal volumes with high levels of IPS will vary if respiratory mechanics change (analogous to a pressure-cycled ventilator)
	High levels of IPS (≥20 cmH₂O) may be more comfortable than assist mode	

additional PEEP, the patient remains connected to the ventilator, which provides the safety of the ventilator's alarm systems as well as psychological reassurance to the patient.

In weaning by use of *intermittent mandatory ventilation* (IMV), the ventilator's tidal volumes are delivered at progressively lower rates. IMV weaning may be a rapid or slow process. In a typical "slow" wean the starting rate is usually just less than the rate during the assist mode, and at the completion of the weaning period, which may be several days to weeks in duration, the finishing rates are $\frac{1}{2}$ to 1 per min (which probably function mostly as sighs). These "mandatory" ventilatory tidal volumes are synchronized so as not to be given simultaneously with the patient's own tidal volume. In an IMV wean, patients can breathe spontaneously at their own tidal volume and rate (Fig. 219-3) and thus can take over their own ventilation at rates as gradually as appropriate.

In *inspiratory pressure support* (IPS) weaning, the patient's spontaneous tidal volumes are augmented by application of a certain level of positive pressure during spontaneous inspirations. In this mode, the volume-cycled ventilator functions analogously to a pressure-cycled ventilator in the assist mode. High levels (≥ 20 cmH_2O) of IPS in patients with unstable respiratory mechanics will result in variable tidal volumes because of the problems noted above with the use of pressure-cycled ventilators in this type of patient.

Extubation The final step in the weaning process is extubation of the tracheal tube from the patient. However, some patients may be totally weanable from the ventilator, i.e., they can breathe spontaneously, but cannot be extubated because of problems with upper airway obstruction or excessive airway secretions, or because of the need to protect the airway from massive aspiration in patients with poor or absent gag reflexes.

Following extubation, swallowing function may take from several hours to several days or longer to return to normal, and a slow, cautious approach to oral intake is advisable.

REFERENCES

Brochard L et al: Improved efficacy of spontaneous breathing with inspiratory pressure support. Am Rev Respir Dis 136:411, 1987

Lanken PN: Mechanical ventilation, in *Pulmonary Diseases and Disorders*, 2d ed, AP Fishman (ed). New York, McGraw-Hill, 1988, chap. 155

Luce JM et al: Intermittent mandatory ventilation. Chest 79:678, 1981

Pepe PE, Marini JJ: Occult positive end-expiratory pressure in mechanically ventilated patients with airflow obstruction. Am Rev Respir Dis 126:166, 1982

Pingleton SK: Complications of acute respiratory failure. Am Rev Respir Dis 137:1463, 1988

Tobin MJ: Respiratory monitoring in the intensive care unit. Am Rev Respir Dis 138:1625, 1988

PART EIGHT

220 IMPACT OF MOLECULAR BIOLOGY ON NEPHROLOGY

SETH L. ALPER / HARVEY F. LODISH

Molecular biology has had two major impacts on nephrology: the cloning and sequencing of cDNAs and genes encoding proteins that play key roles in electrolyte homeostasis has provided new insight into renal function in health and disease, and the chromosomal mapping of mutations affecting the kidney has made possible new approaches to the prevention and treatment of hereditary diseases of the kidney. In addition, new animal models of kidney disease have been created with single genetic lesions. It is now clear that the techniques of modern biology will recast our understanding of renal development, renal injury, and the progression of chronic renal disease.

PROTEIN SEQUENCES FROM DNA CLONING A partial list of proteins of importance to renal function is given in Table 220-1. Some of the proteins comprise isoforms encoded by families of related genes, while others are products of alternative RNA transcripts from single genes. Sequence analysis of these isoforms has uncovered greater protein diversity than had been suspected by biochemical or physiologic analysis. Some of the isoforms are expressed in specific cell types, specific subcellular compartments, at specific times during development, or in response to hormonal or metabolic stimuli. Individual, engineered mutations in single domains of multidomain, multifunctional proteins have allowed structure-function relationships to be addressed at the single amino acid level even for proteins of low abundance.

MOLECULAR GENETICS OF KIDNEY DISEASE The number of genetic diseases of the kidney and of electrolyte metabolism for which the molecular basis has been elucidated is small: diabetes insipidus in the Brattleboro rat, the salt-wasting form of congenital adrenal hyperplasia secondary to steroid 21-hydroxylase deficiency, and hypocalcemic vitamin D–resistant rickets (Table 220-2).

The Brattleboro rat lacks circulating vasopressin and is therefore a useful model of central diabetes insipidus (see Chap. 315). This deficiency in the rat arises from the deletion of a single guanosine residue in the neurophysin coding region of the vasopressin-neurophysin-glycoprotein precursor gene. The single base deletion shifts the reading frame by which RNA is transcribed from the gene and creates a novel carboxy-terminal amino acid sequence without a stop codon. The result is normal baseline RNA transcription and splicing, deficient enhancement of mRNA level by dehydration, and impaired accumulation of the altered hormone precursor. The latter defect may be due to failure of the ribosome to release the mRNA in the absence of a stop codon or to instability of the altered protein translation product.

Adrenal steroid 21-hydroxylase deficiency results in decreased synthesis of mineralocorticoids and glucocorticoids, ACTH-mediated adrenal hyperplasia, and androgen excess (see Chaps. 317 and 324). The 21-hydroxylase is a cytochrome P_{450} enzyme, encoded by a gene on chromosome 6. One or more copies of a pseudogene are located near the coding gene. The pseudogene sequence differs from the functional gene in an 8-bp deletion in exon 3, a single base insertion in exon 7, a point mutation in exon 8, and four base changes in the putative promoter region. The pseudogene is not transcribed. The deficiency syndrome can arise from unequal gene crossover, from conversion of the functional gene to a pseudogene, or from single amino acid substitutions in the enzyme.

Hypocalcemic vitamin D–responsive rickets (see Chap. 340) is an autosomal recessive disorder characterized by target organ resistance to the action of 1,25-dihydroxy vitamin D and caused by altered function of the 1,25-dihydroxy vitamin D_3 receptor. In two affected families the receptors exhibited a unique single base change, resulting in an amino acid substitution in one of the DNA-binding zinc finger structures of the vitamin D receptor. In other instances the disorder

---

TABLE 220-1 Selected cDNA clones encoding proteins of importance to renal function

Transport proteins
 Na^+-K^+ ATPases
 Ca^{2+} ATPases
 H^+-K^+ ATPase
 H^+ ATPase 31-kDa subunit
 Na^+-glucose symporter
 Glucose carriers
 Anion exchangers
 Na^+/H^+ antiporter
 K^+ channels
 Putative urea carrier
 Multiple drug carrier

Hormones and signal transducers
 EGF, EGF receptor
 PDGF receptor
 Insulin receptor
 TGF-β
 IL-1 receptor
 IL-2 receptors
 Catecholamine and muscarinic receptors
 1,25-$(OH)_2$ vitamin D receptor
 Aldosterone and glucocorticoid receptors
 Thyroxine and vitamin A receptors
 ANF and ANF receptor
 Vasopressin and oxytocin
 Parathyroid hormone-like protein
 Erythropoietin and erythropoietin receptor
 Renin
 Angiotensinogen and angiotensin receptor
 Kallikrein
 Protein kinases
 G proteins
 Phospholipases

Other proteins
 Carbonic anhydrases
 Angiotensin converting enzyme
 Tamm-Horsfall protein
 Fructose-1-P aldolase B
 28-kd Ca^{2+} binding protein
 Sm-D autoantigen
 gp330 Heymann nephritis antigen
 p30 nephritic antigen
 Heparan sulfate proteoglycan core protein
 Fibronectin and fibronectin receptor
 Laminin and laminin receptor

SOURCE: After Alper and Lodish.

TABLE 220-2 Some inherited diseases of renal function or electrolyte metabolism that have been mapped to chromosomal loci

Disease	Affected gene product	Locus
Renal Cell Carcinoma		3p21→
von Hippel-Lindau syndrome		3p25
Congenital adrenal hyperplasia	Cytochrome P_{450} 21-OHase*	6p21.3
Cystic fibrosis	Cl^- channel or its regulator	7q22.3-q23.1
Isolated aldosterone deficiency	Corticosterone methyl oxidase II (cytochrome P_{450} II-OHase)?*	
Osteopetrosis–renal tubular acidosis–cerebral calcification syndrome	Carbonic anhydrase II†	8q22
Familial Mediterranean fever		9
Tuberous sclerosis		9q11-q22
Fructose intolerance	Fructose-1-phosphate aldolase B*	9q22
Nail-patella syndrome		9q34
Wilms' tumor		11p13
Vitamin D-Responsive rickets	$1,25(OH)_2$ vitamin D receptor	12
Hemodialysis-related amyloidosis		15q21-q22
Adult polycystic kidney disease		16p13.31-p13.12
Urolithiasis (2,8-dihydroxyadenine)	Adenosine phosphoribosyl-transferase	16q24
Diabetes insipidus		20
Hypophosphatemia		Xp22
Hypomagnesemia		Xp22
Fabry disease		Xq22
Alport's disease		Xq22-q25
Lowe oculocerebrorenal syndrome		Xq25
Lesch-Nyhan syndrome	Hypoxanthine-guanine phosphoribosyl-transferase*	Xq26-q27.2
Nephrogenic diabetes insipidus		Xq28
Proximal renal tubular acidosis		X
Orofaciodigital syndrome		X
Gout type II		X
Pseudohypoparathyroidism		X

Symbols: * molecular basis for mutations(s) described; † normal gene has been cloned but molecular basis for mutation(s) not yet described.
SOURCE: Compiled from: McKusick VA, *The Morbid Anatomy of the Human Genome.* Howard Hughes Medical Institute, 1988. (After Alper and Lodish.)

appears to be due to the presence of a premature termination codon that causes the formation of a short and nonfunctional receptor protein.

The autosomal recessive syndrome of osteopetrosis with mixed renal tubular acidosis and cerebral calcification (see Chap. 345) is tightly linked to a deficiency of carbonic anhydrase II (CAII). The disease and CAII both map to chromosome band 8q22, where the gene is also tightly linked to the genes for two other carbonic anhydrase enzymes. CAII is the only one of these carbonic anhydrases expressed in kidney and in brain. The mouse with CAII deficiency, created by ethylnitrosourea mutagenesis of whole animals and detected by isozyme screening, is runted and has alkaline urine but lacks osteopetrosis and cerebral calcification. The molecular defect in both human and murine deficiencies remains to be determined. Table 220-2 lists several additional diseases in which the altered or deficient protein is known but in which the molecular genetic defect associated with disease has not been reported. In addition, several diseases are listed for which only an approximate chromosomal location of the affected gene is available.

LINKAGE ANALYSIS AND ADULT POLYCYSTIC KIDNEY DISEASE

It is possible in many instances to determine the chromosomal location of a disease locus and to clone the gene responsible in the absence of knowledge of the underlying biochemical defect

that causes the disease (see Chap. 6). The numerous differences in DNA sequence among individuals (polymorphisms) are most easily detected when they alter the length of a DNA restriction fragment, resulting in a restriction fragment length polymorphism (RFLP) in the population. The combination of family linkage studies with molecular cloning of these DNA markers has led to the construction of genetic linkage maps with cloned polymorphic DNA markers arrayed at intervals along the lengths of each chromosome. With a collection of these RFLP markers and a large, multigenerational family affected with an autosomal dominant disease or multiple families in which one or more members is affected by an autosomal recessive mutation, the chromosomal locus of the disease gene can be determined by establishing genetic linkage with markers residing close to it. The first autosomal disease mapped by linkage to RFLP markers was Huntington's disease on chromosome 4. Using the same approach, Reeders et al localized to the short arm of chromosome 16 the genetic locus whose mutation causes autosomal dominant adult polycystic kidney disease (see Chap. 231). This locus is closely linked to the α-globin gene cluster. The inheritance of the α-globin locus can be followed by means of a RFLP that is so polymorphic that only 1 percent of people are homozygous at that locus. Detection of this RFLP allows the inheritance of each parentally contributed copy of chromosome 16 (carrying its α-globin allele) to be followed individually. Figure 220-1 shows that in one Dutch family, allele C of this polymorphic locus cosegregates with polycystic disease while the other alleles, D, G, J, and H, segregate independently, consistent with close linkage of the polymorphic locus to polycystic disease.

Adult polycystic disease (APKD) in Northern Europe may be caused by a single genetic locus since 28 families from England, Scotland, the Netherlands, and Finland all displayed close linkage of the disease to the α-globin cluster. However, two families of Italian origin with adult polycystic disease have demonstrated no linkage of the mutant gene to the α-globin cluster. Thus, mutations in at least two different genes are capable of causing APKD.

TRANSGENIC MICE AND ANIMAL MODELS OF KIDNEY DISEASE

The development of the capacity to introduce foreign genes into the germ lines of mice has made it possible to construct animal models for several human diseases. A foreign gene can cause disease either by its own inappropriate expression or by disrupting an endogenous gene. Genes can be introduced into mice in several ways. Cloned DNA can be directly injected into a pronucleus of a fertilized mouse egg, or embryos at any of several developmental stages can

FIGURE 220-1 Autoradiograph of a Southern blot of restriction enzyme-digested genomic DNA from individuals of a single family cohort, displaying alleles C, D, G, J, and H of the polymorphic locus tightly linked to the α-globlin locus. Of these, only allele C cosegregates with polycystic disease (APKD). (*After ST Reeders et al.*)

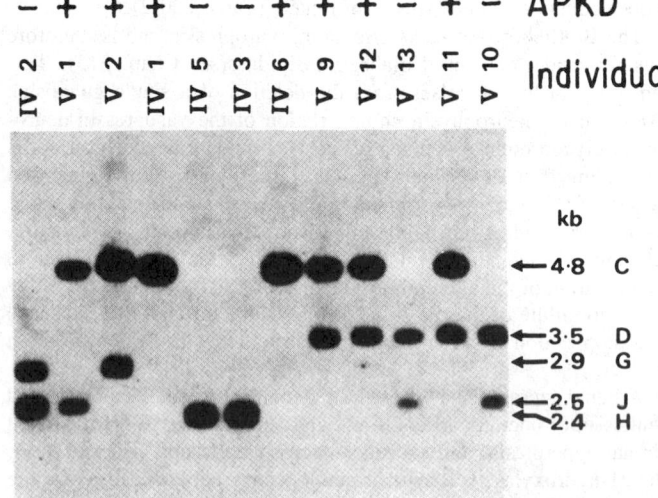

be infected by replication-deficient, integrating retroviruses. Alternatively, cultured embryonic stem cells can be injected into host blastocysts, where they colonize the embryo and contribute to the germ line of the resulting chimeric animals. The stem cells can be selected in cell culture for altered expression of the gene of interest before blastocyst injection.

Several lines of transgenic mice develop disorders of the kidney. Mice that carry the SV40 large T antigen (a viral oncogene) adjacent to SV40 viral enhancer sequences die from choroid plexus ependymoma at 5 months of age. The large T-antigen protein is expressed in the tumors and at lower level in kidney and thymus. Kidney tubules that express large T antigen develop epithelial cell proliferation with occasional cystic dilatation. Large T antigen was not clearly present in glomerular cells, but the mice developed progressive glomerular sclerosis with increasing proteinuria and nonspecific glomerular IgG deposits.

Ectopic expression of the Thy-1 surface protein member of the immunoglobulin superfamily in the kidneys of transgenic mice is also associated with glomerular disease. The function of the protein is unknown, but in some tissues it may play a role in cell-cell recognition or in proliferation. Though mouse kidney lacks Thy-1, it is present in human and rat kidney.

Mice that carry a chimeric Thy-1 gene whose 5′ flanking sequences and protein coding sequences are of murine origin and whose 3′ flanking sequence is of human origin expressed murine Thy-1 in glomerular podocytes. These mice develop severe proteinuria and segmental glomerulosclerosis with foot process swelling and vacuolation, mesangial and subendothelial deposits, occasional mesangial proliferation, and nonspecific deposits of IgG, IgM, and C3 in the mesangium. The onset of proteinuria coincided with an increase in Thy-1 mRNA expression in glomerular podocytes. These experiments suggest that a glomerular podocyte specific enhancer sequence in the 3′ flanking region of the human Thy-1 gene promotes expression of the Thy-1 gene in proximal tubule epithelium only when the sequence is removed from its normal context.

Retroviral infection of preimplantation embryos usually results in insertional inactivation of native genes for creation of mutant phenotypes. Once a phenotype of interest is found and a line of mice established, the inactivated gene can be cloned by screening a genomic library with a retroviral probe. One transgenic mouse line created in this way yielded homozygotes for the retroviral insertion, and these animals died at age 8 weeks with anemia, hypercholesterolemia, and proteinuric renal failure. At 5 to 6 weeks the mice developed a mesangioproliferative glomerulonephritis marked by mesangial thickening, fibrin deposition, and foot process fusion followed later by tubular dilatation, protein inspissation, and a monocytic interstitial infiltrate without evidence of vasculitis. The gene whose disruption leads to this pathology is under investigation.

UROLOGIC CANCER   Molecular biology has increased the understanding of urologic cancers in three principal areas: pathogenesis, hypercalcemia of malignancy, and resistance to chemotherapy. Two varieties of oncogenes are associated with malignant transformation, "dominant" and "recessive" (see also Chap. 10). Dominant oncogenes encode growth-promoting proteins. A single functional copy of a dominant oncogene confers some aspects of the malignant phenotype. H-*ras,* the first dominant oncogene to be discovered, was identified in a cell line derived from a human urinary bladder carcinoma. Recessive oncogenes are postulated to be "antioncogenes" or negative regulators of cell growth. The best example of a recessive oncogene is the retinoblastoma (*Rb*) gene on chromosome 13. Loss of function of both normal *Rb* alleles contributes to the formation of retinoblastoma and in some cases osteosarcoma. In sporadic retinoblastoma, these loss-of-function events are both somatic mutations. In hereditary retinoblastoma the germ line already carries an inactivating mutation of *Rb* on one copy of chromosome 13. Retinal cells in which the second copy of the *Rb* gene is inactivated give rise to retinoblastomas.

Hereditary Wilms' tumor may arise by a similar mechanism involving a putative antioncogene locus on chromosome 11. Antioncogenes have been proposed to play similar roles in nonfamilial tumors of the urinary tract. For example, somatic deletions of portions of chromosome 11 occur in some cases of transitional cell carcinoma, and most renal cell carcinomas contain deletions of chromosome 3, often in the setting of unbalanced translocations of a variety of other chromosome fragments to the same region of chromosome 3. A search for the smallest chromosomal deletions associated with Wilms' tumor and with renal cell carcinoma may lead to the cloning of genes that share some of the growth-inhibitory or tumor-suppressor properties of the retinoblastoma gene.

Renal cell carcinoma is often associated with paraneoplastic syndromes (see Chap. 309). The humoral hypercalcemia of renal cell carcinoma is mediated by the secreted peptide products of the parathyroid hormone-like peptide gene, PTH-LP. PTH-LP acts by binding to PTH receptors and activating adenylate cyclase. The PTH-LP cDNA has been cloned from a renal cell carcinoma cell line, and an alternatively spliced PTH-LP cDNA encoding a different *C*-terminal amino acid sequence was cloned from a lung carcinoma cell line. The PTH-LP *N*-terminal 13 amino acids share 62 percent identity with PTH, but the proteins are different in sequence thereafter and in length.

Renal cell carcinoma is generally insensitive to chemotherapeutic drugs, possibly because the kidney is a site of high-level expression of the multiple drug resistance gene (*mdr*-1). The *mdr*-1 protein is a plasma membrane glycoprotein of the proximal tubule brush border and functions in tumor cells as an ATP-dependent, efflux pump for a variety of pharmacologic agents. Several related *mdr* genes, which undergo alternative splicing, spontaneous point mutations, and gene amplification, contribute to variable resistance in different tumors.

Drug resistance in renal cell carcinoma is associated with high levels of expression of *mdr*-1 mRNA. This drug resistance is reversed by high-dose verapamil and quinidine, agents that block *mdr*-1. Thus, newer antagonists of drug efflux may make it possible to treat renal cell carcinoma with drugs such as adriamycin and vinca alkaloids that are ordinarily ineffective when the *mdr*-1 protein is functional.

REFERENCES

ALPER SL, LODISH HF: Molecular biology of renal function, in *The Kidney,* 4th ed, BM Brenner, FC Rector, Jr (eds). Philadelphia, in press

FOJO AT et al: Intrinsic drug resistance in human kidney cancer is associated with expression of a human multidrug-resistance gene. J Clin Oncol 5:1922, 1987

JAENISCH R: Transgenic animals. Science 240:1468, 1988

KOVACS G et al: Consistent chromosome 3p deletion and loss of heterozygosity in renal cell carcinoma. Proc Natl Acad Sci USA 85:1571, 1988

MACKAY K et al: Glomerulosclerosis and renal cysts in mice transgenic for the early region of SV40. Kidney Int 32:827, 1987

MALLOY PJ et al: Point mutations in the human vitamin D receptor gene associated with hypocalcemic rickets. Science 242:1702, 1988

MILLER WL: Gene conversions, deletions, and polymorphisms in congenital adrenal hyperplasia. Am J Hum Genet 42:4, 1988

REEDERS ST et al: A highly polymorphic DNA marker linked to adult polycystic kidney disease on chromosome 16. Nature 317:542, 1985

RICHTER D: Molecular events in expression of vasopressin and oxytocin and their cognate receptors. Am J Physiol 255:F207, 1988

SLY WS et al: Carbonic anhydrase II deficiency in 12 families with the autosomal recessive syndrome of osteopetrosis with renal tubular acidosis and cerebral calcification. N Engl J Med 313:139, 1985

221   APPROACH TO THE PATIENT WITH DISEASES OF THE KIDNEYS AND URINARY TRACT

FREDRIC L. COE / BARRY M. BRENNER

Diseases of the kidneys and urinary tract frequently give rise to consistent arrays or clusters of clinical signs, symptoms, and laboratory findings called *syndromes*. Syndromes are useful diagnostically because each has fewer causes than the individual clinical signs and symptoms it contains. For example, any injured capillary bed from glomerulus to the urethral meatus can cause hematuria, but only glomerular injury can also cause heavy albuminuria and erythrocyte casts (Chap. 49), and only a few of the diseases that injure the glomerular capillaries enough to cause hematuria and proteinuria also cause a rapid fall in glomerular filtration rate. Routine clinical evaluation is often sufficient to suggest that a particular syndrome may be present (Table 221-1), but additional laboratory measurements beyond the routine, as well as radiologic and/or urologic evaluation and sequential clinical observations, are usually required to establish the diagnosis. This chapter presents the general features of the syndromes and the clinical and laboratory data required for their recognition and outlines the diseases that cause them. Succeeding chapters in this section describe the diseases and their treatment in detail.

ACUTE (ARF) AND RAPIDLY PROGRESSIVE RENAL FAILURE (RPRF) Whether the glomerular filtration rate falls over a period of days (acute renal failure) or weeks (rapidly progressive renal failure) is a useful distinction, because the causes of these two syndromes are somewhat different (Tables 221-1 and 221-2). For example, acute tubular necrosis, from sepsis, nephrotoxic materials, shock, or other cause (see Chap. 223), presents itself as and is the usual cause of acute renal failure, whereas extracapillary proliferative (crescentic) glomerulonephritis, due to immunologic injury or to vasculitis, is an important cause of rapidly progressive, but not acute, renal failure (Chap. 227).

Proof for the existence of either syndrome requires serial determination of the glomerular filtration rate (GFR) or blood urea nitrogen or serum creatinine level. Anuria or oliguria (Chap. 49) strongly suggest acute renal failure, as life cannot be sustained for long with such inadequate renal function. Symptoms and signs of uremia of recent onset suggest rapidly progressive or acute renal failure, but could also result from chronic renal failure that has only recently become life-threatening. Although edema, hypertension, and abnormalities of electrolytes and the urine sediment (Table 221-1) are frequent in acute and rapidly progressive renal failure, they occur in other syndromes as well and are not specific.

The causes of these two important syndromes number about 36, but only 18 (indicated by T, Table 221-2) typically cause acute renal failure, and 8 cause rapidly progressive renal failure. Urinary obstruction, acute tubular necrosis, some forms of vasculitis, major renal vascular accidents, and endogenous and exogenous nephrotoxins are the usual causes of acute renal failure. Vasculitis and crescentic forms

---

TABLE 221-1 Initial clinical and laboratory data base for defining major syndromes in nephrology

Syndromes	Important clues to diagnosis	Findings which are common but not of diagnostic value	Location of discussion of diseases causing syndrome
Acute or rapidly progressive renal failure	Anuria Oliguria Documented recent decline in GFR	Hypertension, hematuria Proteinuria, pyuria Casts, edema	Chaps. 223, 227, 229, 230, 233
Acute nephritis	Hematuria, RBC casts Azotemia, oliguria Edema, hypertension	Proteinuria Pyuria Circulatory congestion	Chaps. 226 to 228
Chronic renal failure	Azotemia for > 3 months Prolonged symptoms or signs of uremia Symptoms or signs of renal osteodystrophy Kidneys reduced in size bilaterally Broad casts in urinary sediment	Hematuria, proteinuria Casts, oliguria Polyuria, nocturia Edema, hypertension Electrolyte disorders	Chaps. 222, 224
Nephrotic syndrome	Proteinuria > 3.5 g per 1.73 m² per 24 h Hypoalbuminemia Hyperlipidemia Lipiduria	Casts Edema	Chaps. 223, 228
Asymptomatic urinary abnormalities	Hematuria Proteinuria (below nephrotic range) Sterile pyuria, casts		Chap. 227
Urinary tract infection	Bacteriuria > 10⁵ colonies per milliliter Other infectious agent documented in urine Pyuria, leukocyte casts Frequency, urgency Bladder tenderness, flank tenderness	Hematuria Mild azotemia Mild proteinuria Fever	Chap. 95
Renal tubule defects	Electrolyte disorders Polyuria, nocturia Symptoms or signs of renal osteodystrophy Large kidneys Renal transport defects	Hematuria "Tubular" proteinuria Enuresis	Chaps. 229, 231
Hypertension	Systolic/diastolic hypertension	Proteinuria Casts Azotemia	Chaps. 39, 196, 230
Nephrolithiasis	Previous history of stone passage or removal Previous history of stone seen by x-ray Renal colic	Hematuria Pyuria Frequency, urgency	Chap. 232
Urinary tract obstruction	Azotemia, oliguria, anuria Polyuria, nocturia, urinary retention Slowing of urinary stream Large prostate, large kidneys Flank tenderness, full bladder after voiding	Hematuria Pyuria Enuresis, dysuria	Chap. 233

TABLE 221-2   Syndromes produced by diseases of the kidneys and urinary tract

Diseases (Chap.)	ARF	RPRF	AN	CRF	NS	AUA
Bilateral arterial occlusion (230)	T					
Acute tubular necrosis (223)	T					
Bilateral acute renal vein thrombosis (230)	T					
Acute uric acid nephropathy (229)	T					
Hypovolemia (223)	T					
Cardiovascular collapse (223)	T					
Acute bilateral upper tract obstruction (233)	T					
Hypercalcemic nephropathy (229)	T			O		
Hemolytic uremic syndrome (230)	T	O	O			
Acute urinary retention (233)						
Malignant nephrosclerosis (230)	T	O				
Essential mixed cyroimmunoglobulinemia (228)	T	O	O	O	O	
Nephrotoxic drugs and chemicals (223, 229)	T			O		
Oxalate nephropathy (229)	T			O		
Cortical necrosis (223)	T			O		
Postpartum glomerulosclerosis (223)	T			O		
Hypersensitivity nephropathy (229)	T		O			P,H,L
Scleroderma (230)	T					P
Idiopathic rapidly progressive GN (227)	O	T	T		R	
Goodpasture's syndrome (227)	O	T	T	O		P,H
Non-Goodpasture's anti-GBM disease (227)	O	T	T	O		P,H
Acute bacterial endocarditis or visceral sepsis (227)		T	T	O	O	
Microscopic polyarteritis nodosa (228, 230)		T	T			
Wegener's granulomatosis (228, 230)		T	T			
Allergic granulomatosis (276)		T	T			
Acute radiation nephritis (229)		T	T			P
Poststreptococcal glomerulonephritis (227)		R	T	O	R	P,H
Nonstreptococcal postinfectious GN (227)		R	T	R	R	P,H
Macroscopic polyarteritis nodosa (276, 228, 230)				T		P,H
Diffuse proliferative lupus nephritis (228)	R	O	R	T	O	P,H,L
Chronic radiation nephritis (229)				T	O	
Balkan nephropathy (229)				T		P*,H
Analgesic nephropathy (229)				T		L,H
Heavy metals (lead, cadmium, mercury) (229)				T		P*
Cystinosis (229)				T		P*
Chronic obstructive uropathy (233)				T		H
Adult polycystic renal disease (231)				T		H,P
Medullary cystic renal disease (231)				T		
Gouty nephropathy (229)				T		
Minimal change disease (227)					T	
Idiopathic membranous nephropathy (227)				O	T	P,H
Membranoproliferative glomerulonephritis (227)		R	O	O	T	P,H
Renal amyloidosis (228)				O	T	P
Membranous lupus nephropathy (228)				O	T	P
Renal vein thrombosis (230)	O			O	T	
Rheumatoid arthritis (228)				O	T	
Congenital nephrotic syndrome (228)				O	T	
Dermatomyositis (227)					T	
Dermatitis herpetiformis (227)				O	T	P
Medullary sponge kidney (231)						T:H
Nephrolithiasis (226)						T:H
Neoplasms (234)						T:H
Arteriolar nephrosclerosis (230)				O		T:P
Waldenström's macroglobulinemia (228)	O					T:P
Multiple myeloma (228)	O	O		O	O	T:P
Reflux nephropathy (95, 230)				O	O	T:P
Diabetic nephropathy (228, 327)				O	O	T:P
Toxemia of pregnancy (230)						T:P
Orthostatic proteinuria (227)						T:P
Sarcoid nephropathy (228)						T:P
Hypokalemic nephropathy (229)						T:P
Berger's (IgA) nephropathy (227)	R	R	O	O	O	T:H,P
Henoch-Schönlein purpura (228)		O	O	R	O	T:H,P
Fabry's disease (228)				O		T:H,P
Alport's syndrome (228)				O		T:H,P
Sickle cell nephropathy (228)				O	R	T:H,P
Subacute bacterial endocarditis (90)						T:H,P
Minimal and mesangial lupus nephritis (228)						T:P,H
Mesangial proliferative GN (227)				R	O	T:P,H
Mixed connective tissue disease (228)					R	T:P,H
Chronic glomerulonephritis (224)				O		T:P,H
Nail patella syndrome (228)				R		T:P,H
Focal glomerulosclerosis (227)		R	O	O	O	T:P,H,L
Focal and segmental lupus nephritis (228)				O	O	T:P,H,L
Sjögren's syndrome (228)						T:L,P
Urinary and renal infection (95)						T:L,H

NOTE: T, typical presentation; O, occurs frequently, but not invariably; R, occurs rarely; P*, tubular proteinuria; P, proteinuria; H, hematuria; L, leukocyturia; ARF, acute renal failure; RPRF, rapidly progressive renal failure; AN, acute nephritis; CRF, chronic renal failure; NS, nephrotic syndrome; AUA, asymptomatic urinary abnormality.

of glomerulonephritis are the main causes of rapidly progressive renal failure. Hemolytic-uremic syndrome, malignant nephrosclerosis, and essential mixed cryoimmunoglobulinemia occasionally present as rapidly progressive renal failure. Idiopathic rapidly progressive glomerulonephritis—the prototype of a disease that produces rapidly progressive renal failure—sometimes causes acute renal failure. Chronic renal failure may occur in some patients with diseases that typically cause acute renal failure. Nevertheless, despite some variability of disease presentations, the finding of acute or rapidly progressive renal failure narrows the range of causes.

ACUTE NEPHRITIS (AN)   A number of diseases involve the glomeruli and, to a generally lesser extent, the tubules in an acute but transient inflammatory process, manifested clinically by acute reduction in GFR, rapidly progressive renal failure, and salt and water retention. Expansion of the extracellular volume, if marked, causes hypertension, pulmonary vascular congestion, and facial and peripheral edema (Chap. 227). Since the causes of this syndrome all can damage the glomerular wall enough to permit red blood cells and plasma proteins to enter the urinary space and appear in the urine, gross or microscopic hematuria, red blood cell casts, and proteinuria are necessary for the diagnosis of acute nephritis, and their absence suggests other diagnostic possibilities. Acute nephritis itself is a transient inflammatory process, so its clinical and laboratory manifestations wax and wane over days to weeks. Many of the diseases that cause acute nephritis also cause acute or rapidly progressive renal failure (Table 221-2).

The fact that many diseases produce both acute nephritis and acute or rapidly progressive renal failure, some produce only acute nephritis, and some produce acute or chronic renal failure without acute nephritis is useful in diagnosis. Only two diseases, poststreptococcal glomerulonephritis and nonstreptococcal postinfectious glomerulonephritis, typically cause acute nephritis alone, and only three of the diseases that typically cause acute renal failure, idiopathic rapidly progressive glomerulonephritis, Goodpasture's syndrome, and non-Goodpasture's antiglomerular basement membrane (anti-GBM) disease, also cause acute nephritis (Table 221-2). On the other hand, most of the diseases that cause acute nephritis also cause rapidly progressive renal failure.

Acute glomerulonephritis following infection with group A streptococci is the prototype of a disease that causes acute nephritis alone (Chap. 227). Immune complexes deposit in the subepithelial region of the glomerular capillary wall, between the basement membrane and the visceral epithelial cells that separate the membrane from the urinary space, and provoke an intense but transient inflammatory process. GFR falls, but returns to normal within weeks to months in the vast majority of affected patients. Deposition of immune complexes is also believed to be the cause of acute nephritis following other bacterial and viral infections, and of lupus nephritis, membranoproliferative glomerulonephritis, Henoch-Schönlein purpura, and Berger's disease, i.e., IgA nephropathy. That the typical presentations of the last four diseases are chronic renal failure, nephrotic syndrome, and asymptomatic urinary abnormalities illustrates the weakness of relationships between pathogenesis and final clinical manifestations.

Renal biopsy is usually required for the evaluation of patients with acute nephritis, whether or not acute or rapidly progressive renal failure is also present. The usual histologic picture is proliferative glomerulonephritis, often with extracapillary crescent formation, but prognosis and treatment are influenced strongly by the precise histologic and ultrastructural pattern, as well as the types of immune complexes and immunoglobulins deposited in the renal tissues.

CHRONIC RENAL FAILURE (CRF)   Chronic renal failure is a syndrome which results from progressive and irreversible destruction of nephrons, regardless of cause (Chap. 224). This syndrome may be considered to exist when GFR is found to be reduced and is known to have been reduced for at least 3 to 6 months (Table 221-1). Often a gradual decline in GFR can be documented over a period of years. Proof of chronicity is also provided by the demonstration of bilateral reduction of kidney size by abdominal scout film, ultrasonography, intravenous pyelography, or tomography. Other

findings consistent with long-standing renal failure, such as renal osteodystrophy or signs and symptoms of uremia, also help to establish this syndrome. Several laboratory abnormalities are often regarded as reliable indicators of chronicity of renal disease, such as anemia, hyperphosphatemia, or hypocalcemia, but these are not specific and may be misleading (Chap. 222). In contrast, the finding of broad casts in the urinary sediment (Chap. 49) is specific for chronic renal failure, the wide diameters of these casts reflecting the compensatory dilatation and hypertrophy of surviving nephrons. Proteinuria is a frequent but nonspecific finding, as is hematuria. Chronic obstructive uropathy, polycystic and medullary cystic diseases, analgesic nephropathy, and the inactive end stage of any chronic tubulointerstitial nephropathy are excellent examples of conditions in which the urine often contains little or no protein, cells, or casts even though nephron destruction has progressed to the stage of chronic renal failure.

When ARF occurs and there is also clear evidence of CRF, the acute component must be evaluated as if CRF were not present, largely because the acute component is potentially reversible. In most instances, depletion of extracellular fluid volume accounts for the acute deterioration of renal function, but other factors such as urinary tract obstruction, drug-induced nephrotoxicity, or exacerbation of the underlying renal disease may also be responsible (Chap. 224).

NEPHROTIC SYNDROME (NS)   This syndrome is generally held to be present when a patient excretes more than 3.5 g protein per 1.73 m² surface area per 24 h that consists mainly of albumin (massive proteinuria) and has reduced serum albumin concentration, edema, and hyperlipidemia (Table 221-1). Massive proteinuria alone has come to define the syndrome since this finding connotes serious renal disease whether or not the protein losses lead to hypoalbuminemia, lipid disturbances, or edema (Chap. 49). Provided the proteins appearing in the urine are not abnormal paraproteins readily excreted by the normal kidney (e.g., immunoglobulin light chains in multiple myeloma), massive proteinuria is invariably a sign of injury to the glomeruli.

Common causes of the nephrotic syndrome include minimal change disease, idiopathic membranous glomerulopathy, focal glomerulosclerosis, and diabetic glomerulosclerosis (Chaps. 227 and 228). Because these diseases typically cause less inflammation than those that cause acute nephritis, the urine contains fewer cellular elements, and acute changes in GFR and urine volume are uncommon. Hematuria may be a frequent manifestation of some forms of nephrotic syndrome, however, especially chronic membranoproliferative glomerulonephritis (Chap. 227). The presence of many cellular or granular casts should suggest lupus nephritis (Chap. 228) or one of the other causes of acute nephritis associated with massive proteinuria such as essential mixed cryoimmunoglobulinemia, acute bacterial endocarditis, visceral sepsis, and Henoch-Schönlein purpura (Table 221-2).

ASYMPTOMATIC URINARY ABNORMALITIES (AUA)   As indicated in Table 221-2, mild degrees of microscopic hematuria, pyuria, casts, or less than 3.5 g protein per 1.73 m² surface area per 24 h may be present in the urine of a patient lacking concurrent evidence of other nephrologic syndromes. By exclusion, these patients are best considered to belong to the syndrome of asymptomatic urinary abnormalities. Isolated hematuria or proteinuria, or unexplained pyuria, are the most frequent abnormalities that occur in this syndrome.

Isolated hematuria, without proteinuria or casts, may be the sole clue to the presence of neoplasm, stone, or infection (e.g., tuberculosis) in any part of the urinary tract (Chaps. 49, 226, 232, and 234). Isolated hematuria may also arise from renal papillae in analgesic and sickle cell nephropathies (Chaps. 229 and 230). Persistent isolated hematuria often requires intravenous pyelography, cystoscopy, and, occasionally, renal arteriography to identify the source of bleeding. *Nephronal hematuria*, in which red blood cells or hemoglobin pigment is present in casts, indicates damage to the nephron (Chap. 49). It occurs without proteinuria, mainly in benign recurrent hematuria and Berger's disease (Chap. 227). *Nephronal hematuria and proteinuria* occur together in many specific renal diseases that may eventually lead to chronic renal failure (Chap. 224). In general, the combination of nephronal hematuria and proteinuria suggests a worse prognosis than either one alone.

Isolated proteinuria, without red blood cells or other formed elements in the urinary sediment, is characteristic of many renal diseases which manifest little or no inflammatory reaction within the glomeruli (e.g., diabetes mellitus, amyloidosis). Less than nephrotic-range proteinuria is common in mild forms of all the diseases that can cause overt nephrotic syndrome (Chaps. 227 and 228). "Tubular" proteinuria (Chap. 49) is the rule in cystinosis, in heavy metal intoxication from cadmium, lead, or mercury, and in the peculiar Balkan nephropathy localized to a small region along the Danube River (Chap. 229).

Pyuria (leukocyturia) may also be a sole urinary abnormality and frequently reflects infection or inflammation of the lower urinary tract rather than intrinsic parenchymal renal disease. Nevertheless, prominent pyuria can occur in any inflammatory disease of the kidneys, especially tubulointerstitial nephritis, lupus nephritis, pyelonephritis, and renal transplant rejection, but usually in association with mild proteinuria or hematuria. The finding of leukocyte casts (Chap. 49) establishes the kidney as the site of the inflammatory reaction.

Pyuria associated with urine that is sterile on routine bacteriologic culture presents a special problem. Certain causes of "sterile pyuria" that are clinically obvious include (1) recent bacterial urinary infection being treated with antibiotics, (2) glucocorticoid therapy, (3) acute febrile episodes, (4) cyclophosphamide administration, (5) pregnancy, (6) renal transplant rejection, (7) recent genitourinary trauma, and (8) prostatitis and cystourethritis. Leukocytes from vaginal secretions may contaminate the urine, so a midstream, clean-catch urine sample should be collected to substantiate a urinary origin. Pyuria associated with proteinuria, nephronal hematuria (Chap. 49), or casts probably signifies inflammatory disease of the renal glomeruli, tubules, interstitium, or microcirculation, and evaluation should focus not upon the pyuria but upon identifying the nature of the renal disease.

Persistent sterile pyuria that cannot be ascribed to any of the foregoing causes has a narrow differential diagnosis. Unusual infections, such as tuberculosis, fungi, atypical mycobacteria, *Haemophilus influenzae,* anaerobic bacteria, fastidious bacteria that grow only on enriched media, and L forms, all must be sought. Intravenous pyelography is needed to detect causes such as urinary tract calculi, papillary necrosis, and renal infiltration by lymphoma or myeloma cells. The latter is usually suspected because of other evidence of myeloma or lymphoma, for both rarely involve only the kidneys. If all tests are negative, cystoscopy may reveal cystitis or trigone inflammation.

URINARY TRACT INFECTION (UTI) This syndrome is defined by the demonstration in urine of pathogenic organisms, either bacteria, tubercle bacilli, or fungi (Chap. 95). When urine specimens are obtained for culture, the condition under which the urine is collected must minimize contamination from external genitourinary surfaces. Women should void into a wide-mouthed sterile container after preliminary cleansing of the vulva with a moist, sterile gauze pledget. In men, midstream collection is usually adequate. Bacterial colony counts of 10^5 organisms per milliliter or greater in urine generally indicate urinary tract colonization and infection. Levels above 10^2 colonies per milliliter are sufficient to indicate infection in symptomatic patients (Table 221-1) and in urine samples obtained by suprapubic aspiration or bladder catheter (Chap. 229). When the urinary tract is anatomically normal, *Escherichia coli* is the usual bacterial pathogen. After prolonged antibiotic treatment of persistent infections, particularly when urinary drainage is impaired or stones are present, *Klebsiella, Enterobacter,* and *Proteus* species predominate.

As discussed in Chap. 95, the presence of a positive urine culture need not imply that an organism is producing tissue inflammation or injury. In some patients, tissue effects may be trivial; in others, injury may be occurring even though symptoms or urinary abnormalities are not present at the time of evaluation. When bacteriuria is associated with tissue inflammation or injury, clinical manifestations usually

depend upon the site(s) involved. Dysuria, frequency, urgency, and suprapubic tenderness are common symptoms of bladder and urethral inflammation (Chap. 49 and Table 221-1). Prostatitis also leads to frequency, dysuria, and urgency, and the prostate may be boggy and tender on rectal examination. Flank pain, chills, fever, nausea and vomiting, hypotension from sepsis, and leukocyte casts all suggest true renal parenchymal infection, i.e., pyelonephritis; their absence, however, does not exclude pyelonephritis.

RENAL TUBULE DEFECTS (RTD) This syndrome encompasses a large number of acquired and hereditary disorders, all of which tend to affect tubules more than glomeruli. Hereditary anatomic defects, including such entities as polycystic renal disease, medullary cystic disease, and medullary sponge kidney, are readily detected by intravenous pyelography, which is usually performed because of hematuria, bacteriuria, flank pain, or unexplained azotemia (Chap. 231).

Defects in tubule transport functions, on the other hand, tend not to be associated with prominent renal anatomic defects and arise either as inherited traits (Chap. 231) or during the course of acquired renal disease (Chap. 229). In general, these functional defects impair secretion and/or reabsorption of electrolytes and organic solutes, or limit urinary concentrating and diluting ability (Table 221-1). Typical manifestations of such functional disturbances include polyuria and nocturia (Chap. 49), metabolic acidosis (Chap. 51), and various disorders of fluid and electrolyte balance (Chap. 50). Such defects are defined by direct physiologic measurements; their elucidation requires a sound understanding of normal renal physiology.

HYPERTENSION (H) Hypertension is considered to exist when the average of a series of reliable blood pressure measurements exceeds 140 mmHg systolic or 90 mmHg diastolic (Table 221-1). The pathogenetic mechanisms, clinical and laboratory manifestations, and therapeutic approaches are discussed in detail elsewhere (Chaps. 39 and 196). In addition, a number of renal complications of hypertension are reviewed in Chap. 230, as is the entity of renal artery stenosis, an infrequent but potentially curable cause of hypertension.

NEPHROLITHIASIS (N) This syndrome is established with certainty when a stone is passed, visualized by x-ray, or removed at surgery or cystoscopy (Table 221-1 and Chap. 232). Less certain, but highly suggestive, evidence of nephrolithiasis exists in the patient with renal colic, painful hematuria, or unexplained pyuria, dysuria, and urinary frequency (Chap. 49). Colic varies in its symptomatology but usually begins suddenly in one flank, radiates downward toward the groin, and is excruciatingly painful.

Most renal stones are composed of calcium, uric acid, cystine, or struvite (magnesium ammonium phosphate). All are radiopaque except for those composed solely of uric acid and are, therefore, visible by routine abdominal radiography. Uric acid stones appear as radiolucent filling defects and can be mistaken for tumor or blood clot.

URINARY TRACT OBSTRUCTION (UTO) Documentation of the various structural or functional causes of urinary tract obstruction usually requires radiologic or surgical visualization. The manifestations of obstruction, which initiate the search for its causes, are numerous (Table 221-1) and are reviewed in Chap. 233. Anuria in an adult is almost always due to obstruction of bladder outflow. Less commonly, blockage of upper urinary drainage from both kidneys, or from a solitary functioning kidney, accounts for total or near-total cessation of urine flow. A large bladder after voiding is a sign of outflow obstruction, usually due to urethral stricture, tumor, stone, neurogenic causes, or prostatic hypertrophy. Nocturia, frequency and overflow incontinence, and slowing or hesitancy of micturition are also suggestive of outflow obstruction (Chap. 49). Upper tract obstruction often produces few clinical manifestations. When it is incomplete or unilateral, urine volume may be normal, or even elevated because of a loss of renal concentrating ability. Urinary stasis secondary to obstruction commonly predisposes to recurrent urinary tract infection, chronic obstruction to progressive loss of renal function (Table 221-2).

REFERENCES

BLACK DAK: Diagnosis and renal disease, in *Renal Disease,* 4th ed, DAK Black (ed). St. Louis, Blackwell, 1980

CAMERON JS: The natural history of glomerulonephritis, in *Renal Disease,* 4th ed, DAK Black (ed). St. Louis, Blackwell, 1980, p 329

COE FL, BUSHINSKY DA: Clinical and laboratory assessment of patients with renal and urinary tract disease, in *Clinical Nephrology,* BM Brenner, F Coe, and FC Rector Jr (eds). Philadelphia, Saunders, 1987, p 1

222 DISTURBANCES OF RENAL FUNCTION

BARRY M. BRENNER / THOMAS H. HOSTETTER / STEVEN C. HEBERT

Near constancy of the composition of the internal environment, including the volume, tonicity, and compartmental distribution of the body fluids, is a state essential to survival. With day-to-day variations in amount as well as composition of food and fluids, preservation of the internal environment requires the continuous excretion of these substances (and/or their by-products) in amounts that balance the quantities acquired by ingestion and metabolic transformation. Although losses from skin, lungs, and intestine normally contribute to this excretory capacity, by far the greatest responsibility for solute and water excretion is borne by the kidneys.

The kidneys operate primarily to maintain the composition and volume of the *extracellular* fluid compartment. The continuous exchange of water and solutes across all cell membranes, however, permits the kidneys to contribute indirectly to the regulation of the volume, composition, and tonicity of the *intracellular* fluids as well. To accomplish these tasks, the kidney has evolved physiologic mechanisms that enable the individual to excrete any excesses of water and nonmetabolized solute contained in the diet, as well as the nonvolatile end products of nitrogen metabolism, such as urea and creatinine. By contrast, when faced with deficits of water and/or any of the other major constituents of the body fluids, renal excretion of these substances can be curtailed, reducing the likelihood of severe volume or solute depletion. The purpose of this chapter is to review the major excretory functions of the normal kidney and to examine the way these functions are affected by disorders that impair the operations of this organ in humans.

MECHANISMS OF RENAL EXCRETORY FUNCTION WITH NORMAL AND REDUCED NEPHRON MASS

The volume of urine excreted per day (about 1.5 L, or roughly 1 mL/min) is the small residuum of two very large, and in many ways opposing, processes—namely, *ultrafiltration* of 180 L or more fluid per day (approximately 125 mL/min) across glomerular capillaries on the one hand and, on the other, *reclamation* (or *reabsorption*) of more than 99 percent of this ultrafiltrate by transport processes operating in the renal tubules. The remarkable feat of the initial step in this process in humans is underscored by the fact that, under resting conditions, about 20 percent of the cardiac output passes through the kidneys, which comprise less than 1 percent of body weight. Hence, per unit weight of tissue, the rate of blood flow to the kidneys is greater than that to other solid organs, including heart, brain, and liver.

GLOMERULAR ULTRAFILTRATION Urine formation begins with the elaboration of a protein-free ultrafiltrate of plasma across the walls of the glomerular capillaries. The rate of ultrafiltration (glomerular filtration rate, GFR) is determined by three factors: (1) the

balance of pressures acting across the capillary wall (the glomerular capillary hydrostatic and Bowman's space oncotic pressures tend to favor filtration, while glomerular capillary oncotic and Bowman's space hydrostatic pressures tend to retard it), (2) the rate at which plasma flows through the glomeruli, and (3) the permeability and the total surface area of the filtering capillaries. A decrease in GFR can be expected when (1) glomerular hydrostatic pressure is reduced (as in hypotensive shock), (2) tubule (hence, Bowman's space) hydrostatic pressure is increased (ureteral or bladder neck obstruction), (3) plasma oncotic pressure rises to unusually high levels (hemoconcentration due to dehydration; multiple myeloma or other dysproteinemias), (4) renal (hence, glomerular) blood and plasma flow are decreased (circulatory collapse, profound heart failure), and (5) permeability and/or total filtering surface area is reduced (acute or chronic glomerulonephritis).

Despite the extraordinarily high rate of water movement across the glomerular capillary wall, all but the smallest of the circulating plasma proteins are normally excluded from passage through this barrier. Molecules the size of inulin (approximately 5200 mol wt) or smaller normally appear in glomerular urine in the same concentrations as in plasma water, whereas the transport of substances of increasingly greater size diminishes progressively, normally approaching very low values as the size of serum albumin is approached. The *glomerular capillary basement membrane* and the *slitlike diaphragms* that connect adjacent epithelial cell foot processes on the urinary aspect of the glomerular capillary wall (Fig. 49-1) serve as major barriers to protein filtration. In addition to these mechanical gates, *electrostatic factors* also serve to retard the filtration of plasma proteins, especially albumin. The albumin molecule behaves as a polyanion in physiologic solution, and is therefore retarded by the anionic glycoproteins in the various component layers of the glomerular wall. With disruption of these mechanical and electrostatic barriers, as seen in many forms of glomerular injury (see Chaps. 226 to 228), large quantities of plasma proteins gain access to the urine.

BIOLOGIC CONSEQUENCES OF SUSTAINED REDUCTIONS IN GFR Measurement of total GFR of both kidneys provides a sensitive and commonly employed index of overall renal excretory function. When renal excretory function is impaired, either acutely or chronically, one or more of the determinants of GFR in affected nephrons is altered unfavorably so that total GFR declines. The magnitude of the decline is determined by the sum of the impairments of function of individual glomeruli. Initially, the effect of such impairments in single-nephron GFR (SNGFR), no matter how small, is to reduce the total rate of excretion of water and those solutes normally contained in the glomerular ultrafiltrate. In the steady state, these reduced rates of filtration, when accompanied by comparably reduced rates of excretion, lead to *retention* and *accumulation* of the unexcreted substances in the body fluids. Further reduction in GFR augments the degree to which these substances are retained.

Figure 222-1 depicts the major patterns of response to these impairments in filtration. The degree of reduction in total GFR is plotted on the abscissa, expressed as a percentage of normal (100 percent). For the various solutes normally contained in glomerular filtrate, three general types of response are common, depicted by curves A, B, and C. Curve A describes the pattern seen with substances, such as creatinine and urea, which normally depend largely on glomerular filtration for their excretion into the urine; i.e., secretion fails to influence urinary excretion appreciably. Therefore, as GFR falls, plasma levels of creatinine, urea, and other substances normally excreted largely by filtration rise progressively, albeit in the nonlinear manner illustrated.

The clinical course of chronic renal failure (CRF) usually also conforms to the pattern described by curve A. Patients with CRF usually pass from a long asymptomatic period of "compensation" to a more accelerated and clinically symptomatic terminal phase. In other words, chronic forms of renal injury that lead to slow but inexorable destruction of nephron mass usually lead to progressive but modest elevations in creatinine and urea levels in plasma, but

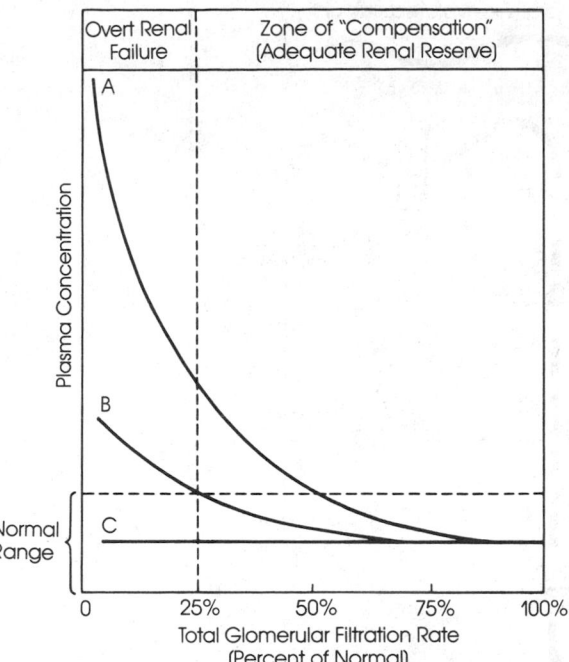

FIGURE 222-1 Representative patterns of adaptation for different types of solutes in body fluids in chronic renal failure. (*After NS Bricker et al, in Brenner and Rector, 3d ed.*)

not to levels beyond the range of normal, despite loss of as much as 50 percent of total GFR. With further loss of nephron mass, and further reduction in GFR, however (even though the rate of nephron destruction may not be accelerated), the limits of renal reserve are exceeded, and continued accumulation of curve A–type solutes leads to plasma concentrations clearly beyond the range of normal (Fig. 222-1). Because these retained solutes are believed to exert "toxic" effects on virtually all organ systems, manifestations of CRF now become overt. As a result, for patients with reduced renal mass, even small additional decrements in total GFR may spell the difference between "compensation" and overt uremia.

The accumulation of curve A–type solutes with progressive renal failure continues until external balance for these solutes is achieved, that is, until acquisition and/or production rates and excretion rates are exactly matched. In the case of creatinine, for example, assuming a constant rate of creatinine production, a 50 percent reduction in GFR results in an approximate doubling of the plasma creatinine concentration. The latter restores the filtered load of creatinine (that is, GFR × plasma creatinine concentration) to normal, and urinary excretion rate again becomes equivalent to the rate of creatinine production. Unfortunately, since no mechanism exists in human beings for augmenting creatinine excretion beyond this level, elimination of retained creatinine is not possible, and plasma concentration remains twice normal. With progressive reduction in GFR, plasma creatinine levels continue to rise, due both to the most recent loss of nephron excretory function and to the retention associated with earlier nephron destruction (Fig. 222-1). *In practice, so long as the net rates of acquisition and production (i.e., liver function and muscle mass) remain reasonably constant, the inverse relationship between plasma concentrations of solutes such as creatinine and urea and GFR is sufficiently reliable and predictable to allow plasma levels of the solutes to serve as useful clinical indexes of GFR.*

In contrast to solutes of the curve A type, plasma levels of substances such as phosphate, urate, and potassium (K^+) and hydrogen (H^+) ions usually fail to rise above the normal range until GFR falls to a small percentage of normal. With progressive renal failure this pattern of response, depicted by curve B in Fig. 222-1, reflects the participation of tubule transport mechanisms that contribute to the excretion of these substances. In other words, *as GFR declines, the*

tubules facilitate the excretion of progressively greater fractions of the filtered load of these solutes, either by enhancing their net secretion and/or by diminishing their net reabsorption. Plasma levels of curve B–type solutes, therefore, rise much less than do those of curve A because, with progressive reduction in GFR, *excretion rate per nephron* and, therefore, *fractional excretion* both increase. Eventually, however, enhanced fractional excretion can no longer offset the reduction in the filtered load of these solutes caused by a markedly diminished GFR, and plasma levels rise above the normal range (Fig. 222-1). For urate, phosphate, and K^+, at least, increased fractional excretion usually serves to maintain normal plasma levels until GFR falls to less than one-fourth of normal.

Finally, for certain solutes, such as sodium chloride (NaCl), concentrations in plasma remain virtually constant, and at normal levels, throughout the entire course of CRF, despite continued ingestion of these substances in normal amounts. Such solutes conform to the pattern described by curve C in Fig. 222-1. The extent of compensation is nearly complete and represents a fundamental adaptation to renal injury. To illustrate the magnitude of the adaptation involved, it is useful to compare the excretion of Na^+ in an individual with normal renal excretory function (GFR of 125 mL/min) with that in an individual with advanced renal insufficiency (GFR of 2 mL/min). Both subjects are allowed to ingest a diet containing 7 g salt per day (120 mmol Na^+). With a normal serum Na^+ concentration of 140 mmol/L, external Na^+ balance is achieved in the normal individual by excreting approximately 0.5 percent of the filtered load of Na^+. By contrast, for external balance to be maintained in the patient with CRF, fractional excretion of Na^+ must rise to 30 percent. *In other words, external balance for Na^+ demands that the same quantity of Na^+ (120 mmol) be excreted into the urine each day in the subject with CRF as in the normal subject.* Given the drastic reduction in GFR faced by the patient with CRF, external balance can be achieved only by a progressive transformation of the Na^+ reabsorptive processes in surviving tubules, so that a progressively larger fraction of the filtered load of Na^+ escapes reabsorption and appears in final urine. In short, *the rate of excretion of Na^+ per surviving nephron increases in inverse proportion to the composite GFR of surviving nephrons.*

MECHANISMS OF TUBULE TRANSPORT WITH NORMAL AND REDUCED NEPHRON MASS Loss of renal function with nearly all forms of progressive renal disease is usually attended by a progressive distortion of renal morphology and architecture. Despite this structural disarray, glomerular and tubule functions often remain as closely integrated (i.e., *glomerulotubular balance*) in the diseased kidney as they do in the normal organ, at least until the final stages of CRF. A fundamental feature of this *intact nephron hypothesis* is that following loss of nephron mass, residual renal function derives primarily from the operation of surviving healthy nephrons, while the diseased nephrons are believed to cease functioning. Despite progressive nephron destruction, there is considerable evidence to suggest that many of the mechanisms that contribute to the maintenance of solute and water balance differ only quantitatively, and not qualitatively, from those believed to govern fluid and solute homeostasis under normal physiologic conditions. The most important of these are considered below.

Tubule transport of sodium chloride and water in health Most of the filtered water and Na^+ salts are reabsorbed by the tubules, leaving small and variable amounts, equivalent on a day-to-day basis to the quantities ingested, to reach the final urine. About two-thirds of the glomerular ultrafiltrate is reabsorbed in the *proximal tubule* with little change in the osmolality or Na^+ concentration of the unreabsorbed fraction (Fig. 222-2). In other words, fluid reabsorption in the proximal tubule is nearly *isosmotic* and is coupled to the active transport of Na^+. Since Cl^- and HCO_3^- are the primary anions in the extracellular fluid, most of the filtered Na^+ is reabsorbed with these anions. In the early convoluted portion of the proximal tubule, bicarbonate is the principal anion accompanying the reabsorption of sodium. This process occurs via a Na^+/H^+ exchange mechanism at

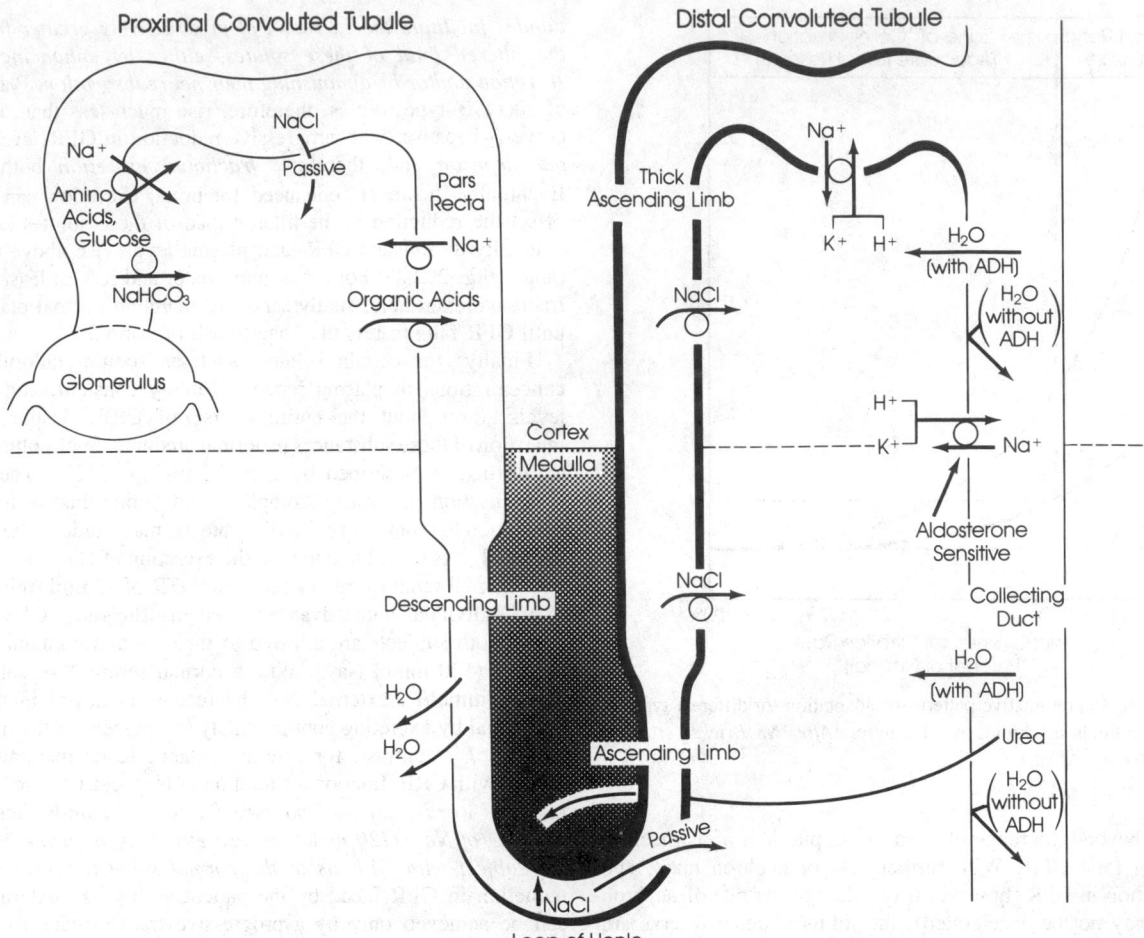

FIGURE 222-2 Transport functions of the various anatomic segments of the mammalian nephron. Fluid reabsorption across the proximal tubule is isosmotic and accounts for reabsorption of approximately two-thirds of the filtered Na^+ and H_2O. The major portions of the filtered HCO_3^-, amino acids, and glucose are reabsorbed in the early proximal convoluted tubule. Reabsorption of glucose and amino acids is coupled to Na^+ transport and thereby generates a negative potential difference within the tubule lumen. At the same time, HCO_3^- is reabsorbed by a nonelectrogenic mechanism, via H^+ secretion. The active transport of these solutes results in transepithelial concentration and effective osmotic pressure gradients promoting H_2O flow across the proximal tubule, into the peritubular capillaries. The rise in tubule fluid Cl^- concentration is a necessary reciprocal consequence of the decreased luminal HCO_3^- concentration. The resultant high concentration of Cl^- becomes an important force for the outward passive transport of Cl^- down its concentration gradient, resulting in a lumen-positive potential difference in the late proximal convoluted tubule. The pars recta of the proximal tubule is capable of active electrogenic transport of Na^+ independent of organic solute transport. Under normal conditions, approximately one-third of the glomerular filtrate enters the descending limb of Henle's loop. Because the thin descending limb is incapable of active outward NaCl transport and is characterized by low permeability to Na^+ but high H_2O permeability, H_2O is abstracted passively as the fluid approaches the bend of Henle's loop. Hypertonic

fluid with a greater NaCl concentration but lower urea concentration than the surrounding medullary interstitium thus enters the thin ascending limb of Henle. This segment differs from the descending limb in that it is largely impermeable to H_2O and urea but highly permeable to NaCl. These characteristics allow for passive diffusion of NaCl out of the ascending limb. Active electrogenic NaCl transport across the water-impermeable thick ascending limb of Henle allows for separation of solute and water. In consequence tubule fluid becomes dilute, and the medullary interstitium hypertonic. Irrespective of the final osmolality of the urine, the fluid that enters the distal convoluted tubule is always hypoosmotic. This segment exhibits active Na^+ reabsorption. All but the terminal portion of the distal convoluted tubule is water impermeable, even in the presence of ADH. Aldosterone exerts its effect in this segment by enhancing Na^+ reabsorption, which is variably coupled to K^+ and H^+ secretion. The cortical and papillary portions of the collecting duct are sites where ADH exerts its principal effect. The permeability of these segments to H_2O in the absence of ADH is very low but can be greatly enhanced in the presence of ADH. These segments are also characterized by active Na^+ reabsorption, which appears to depend on the presence of mineralocorticoid. In the absence of ADH, the collecting tubule is water impermeable so that hypotonic tubule fluid courses through it. However, in the presence of ADH, water is avidly reabsorbed here, resulting in hypertonic final urine.

the luminal brush border and is dependent upon both cystolic and brush border carbonic anhydrase. Glucose, amino acids, and other organic solutes (e.g., lactate) are also extensively reabsorbed in the proximal convoluted tubule by a cotransport process that links the cellular entry of these organic substrates with Na^+. Three processes appear to operate in parallel to couple water (i.e., volume) absorption with solute absorption in the proximal tubule. First, given the remarkably high water permeability of this nephron segment, very small transepithelial osmolality differences, that is, *luminal hypotonicity* on the order of 2 to 3 mosmol, produced by solute absorption, could drive volume absorption. Second, due to the *preferential*

absorption of HCO_3^- and organic solutes in the early portions of the proximal tubule, the concentrations of these substances decrease while that of Cl^- increases along the length of the proximal tubule. Volume absorption would occur if the rate of Na^+ and Cl^- diffusion down their respective electrochemical gradients were more rapid than the back diffusion of sodium bicarbonate into the lumen. Finally, an *effective osmotic gradient* would be established (despite equal macroscopic osmolalities of luminal and peritubular fluids) if the effective osmolality produced by Cl^- in the lumen were greater than that for bicarbonate in the peritubular fluid.

The rate of reabsorption of fluid from proximal convoluted tubules and peritubular interstitium is sensitive to the effects of *physical factors*, i.e., the hydrostatic and colloid osmotic (or oncotic) pressures acting across the walls of the peritubular capillaries. Because the plasma proteins in glomerular capillaries are concentrated by ultrafiltration, there is a marked rise in the oncotic pressure as plasma flows along the glomerular capillary network. This step-up in plasma oncotic pressure is transmitted largely unchanged to the peritubular capillaries, via the efferent arterioles. These resistance vessels cause a substantial drop in hydrostatic pressure, however, so that when the plasma reaches the peritubular capillaries, oncotic pressure greatly exceeds hydrostatic pressure. These *Starling forces* are therefore oriented in an *uptake mode*, in contrast to the *filtration mode* at the glomerulus, where hydrostatic pressure exceeds oncotic. The extent to which oncotic pressure exceeds hydrostatic pressure in the peritubular capillary network is thought to modulate the overall rate of reabsorption of fluid by the proximal tubules. Therefore, when peritubular oncotic pressure falls, or hydrostatic pressure rises, uptake of fluid by these capillaries is reduced. As a result, fluid is retained in the interstitial space, altering the hydrostatic pressure in the space, and ultimately retarding the egress of fluid from the lateral intercellular channels. Without an adequate route of drainage, fluid in the channels leaks back into the tubule lumen and diminishes *net fluid reabsorption* by this tubule segment. The opposite occurs in states in which peritubular oncotic pressure increases (increased filtration fraction) or hydrostatic pressure decreases (enhanced efferent arteriolar tone). Under these circumstances, peritubular capillary uptake of reabsorbate is augmented, leading ultimately to *enhanced net fluid reabsorption* by the proximal tubule.

In contrast to the proximal tubule, active outward transport of NaCl from tubule lumen to peritubular blood has not been established for the *thin limbs of Henle's loop*. However, passive outward salt transport does occur, as indicated in Fig. 222-2. In the next segment of the nephron, the *medullary thick ascending limb of Henle,* the concentration of NaCl is reduced below the level that prevails at the beginning of this segment. Here Cl^- absorption occurs by an active process involving a furosemide-sensitive $Na^+:K^+:2Cl^-$ cotransport mechanism in the luminal membrane, with one-half of Na^+ absorption proceeding passively, driven by the lumen-positive transepithelial voltage. Since the ascending limb of Henle is always impermeable to water, net NaCl reabsorption not only generates hypotonic tubule fluid, but also gives rise to the high NaCl concentration of the outer medullary interstitium (Fig. 222-2). In certain animals vasopressin (ADH) enhances NaCl absorption but not water permeability in the medullary portion of the thick ascending limb, but an effect of this hormone on this segment in human beings is uncertain.

The fluid leaving the thick ascending limb of Henle is normally low in NaCl concentration, a condition largely independent of the organism's diet or state of hydration. In the *distal convoluted tubule,* water reabsorption is variable, depending on the state of hydration or, more specifically, on the presence or absence of the ADH in plasma. In the absence of ADH, this and more distal nephron segments are impermeable to water, so that the hypotonic fluid entering this segment is excreted as *dilute urine*. Indeed, continued salt reabsorption along the distal convoluted tubule results in further dilution of the urine. In the presence of ADH, the permeability of the late portion of this segment to water increases, and as a result, the osmolality of the late distal tubule fluid rises to a value close to that of plasma. NaCl continues to be reabsorbed from the tubule lumen, against moderately steep chemical and electrical gradients. The reabsorptive process for NaCl at this site is enhanced by *aldosterone.*

The *cortical collecting tubule* possesses an extremely low permeability to water in the absence of ADH, whereas this permeability increases greatly in the presence of the hormone. The sensitivity of this segment to ADH appears to be more pronounced than that of the distal convoluted tubule. As with the distal convoluted tubule, the cortical collecting tubule is capable of further active reabsorption of NaCl.

The terminal segment of the distal nephron is the highly branched *papillary collecting duct.* Continued electrolyte transport in this segment results in the large ion concentration differences that normally exist between urine and plasma. As in the cortical collecting tubule, Na^+ transport appears to be active since reabsorption proceeds against sizable electrochemical gradients. The rate of Na^+ transport in this segment depends on the diet and on the load of Na^+ delivered from more proximal segments, and is affected by aldosterone. The permeability of this segment to water also increases markedly in the presence of ADH.

Effects of reduced nephron mass on sodium chloride transport in surviving nephrons With reductions in nephron mass the remaining healthy or less damaged nephrons may hypertrophy so that GFR is increased toward normal. For example, a patient who has a unilateral nephrectomy for renal cell carcinoma or for donation for transplantation loses one-half of the nephron mass, and GFR is reduced by 50 percent at the time of surgery. However, several months after the nephrectomy GFR may return to 80 percent of the preoperative value for two kidneys. This requires that the blood flow, GFR, and transport functions of individual remaining nephrons increase above normal values. This "compensatory hypertrophy" is evident by the large glomeruli and tubular structures observed on histologic sections of the kidney and by increases in many of the biochemical processes associated with tubule transport (e.g., Na^+, K^+-ATPase). Similar hypertrophic changes occur in nephrons from kidneys damaged by other processes (e.g., glomerulonephritis); however, as nephron damage progresses, the hypertrophy of single nephrons can no longer make up for the magnitude of nephron loss, and total GFR falls.

With progressive destruction of nephrons, *maintenance of external balance for NaCl requires that fractional salt excretion increase as GFR decreases.* Very likely several mechanisms contribute to this adaptive increase in fractional salt excretion. With losses of functioning nephron units, peritubular capillary hydrostatic and oncotic pressures are probably altered in directions that serve to suppress proximal tubule reabsorption of NaCl and water. For example, a rise in peritubular capillary hydrostatic pressure, which tends to inhibit net proximal fluid reabsorption, might be anticipated with arterial hypertension, a common feature of renal insufficiency. Similarly, peritubular oncotic pressure might be expected to decline with renal injury, owing both to reductions in filtration fraction and to hypoalbuminemia. While such alterations in peritubular factors clearly account for diminution in proximal fluid reabsorption in response to falling levels of GFR in animals, such alterations have not been established with certainty in humans. Aldosterone, normally an important determinant of Na^+ reabsorption in distal portions of the nephron, is probably not a major factor responsible for reducing fractional Na^+ reabsorption, since aldosterone levels in plasma are rarely reduced in CRF. Furthermore, external Na^+ balance is preserved in bilaterally adrenalectomized uremic dogs maintained on fixed doses of mineralocorticoid. Yet another factor contributing to the suppression of fractional NaCl reabsorption in CRF may relate to the retention of solutes as GFR declines. In addition to urea and creatinine, a host of *organic acids* (including *hippurates*) also accumulate. These substances are normally excreted by both filtration and tubule secretion; the latter process involves a carrier-mediated organic acid transport system in proximal tubule epithelia. When GFR is reduced and plasma levels of these organic acids increase, sufficient fluid may accompany the secretion of these organic anions into the proximal tubule lumen (by osmosis) to diminish net fluid reabsorption, and even favor net fluid secretion. Evidence in support of this mechanism derives from studies in which uremic sera were capable of inducing net fluid secretion in isolated proximal tubules of rabbits in vitro.

Several substances that regulate NaCl transport across the tubules may also participate in the enhanced fractional excretion of salt in renal insufficiency. Atrial natriuretic peptide is released from the cardiac atria in response to plasma volume expansion and atrial distention. This hormone effects a natriuresis by reducing net sodium reabsorption through its complementary actions on active collecting duct Na$^+$ transport and on physical factors within the adjacent vasa recta. Thus, atrial natriuretic peptide likely participates in the uremic adaptation to salt balance. In addition, prostaglandin E reduces NaCl reabsorption from the thick ascending limb. Since prostaglandin E production per nephron appears to rise in renal insufficiency, the local action of this prostaglandin may also contribute to natriuresis in the setting of reduced renal mass. Finally, other inhibitors of ion transport appear in uremic serum including an inhibitor(s) of the Na$^+$, K$^+$-ATPase. This factor(s) has not been fully characterized, and whether it represents an adaptation for maintenance of homeostasis or an unregulated accumulation of a toxin is also uncertain.

Serum and urine from patients and dogs with uremia contain factors capable of inhibiting NaCl transport across frog skin, toad bladder, and rat renal tubule. Accumulation of natriuretic factors in uremia may not be without cost; the "trade-off" for maintenance of external Na$^+$ balance is the possibility of abnormalities occurring in Na$^+$ transport across cell membranes, which often occurs in advanced renal insufficiency. This possibility is discussed in greater detail in Chap. 224.

The obligatorily high rate of solute excretion per surviving nephron (so-called osmotic diuresis due to urea and other retained solutes) may also contribute to enhancing fractional NaCl excretion, much as occurs in normal subjects following administration of nonreabsorbable solutes such as mannitol. Finally, certain forms of CRF tend to be associated with unusually pronounced salt losses in urine. These *salt-wasting nephropathies* include chronic pyelonephritis and other tubulointerstitial diseases (see Chap. 229) as well as polycystic and medullary cystic diseases. These disorders have in common greater destruction of medullary and interstitial than cortical and glomerular portions of the renal parenchyma. Preferential impairment of tubule reabsorptive function, rather than a primary reduction in GFR, may, therefore, underlie the salt-losing tendency in these disorders. A number of clinical derangements associated with the altered renal handling of NaCl in CRF (including hypo- and hypervolemia, hypertension, etc.) are considered in Chap. 224.

Effects of reduced nephron mass on water reabsorption in surviving nephrons   As with NaCl, there is a progressive increase in the fractional excretion of water with advancing renal insufficiency, so that even the patient with a total GFR of 5 mL/min or less can usually maintain external water balance. The adaptations in the handling of water by the tubules of the diseased kidney are of importance in the pathogenesis of the urinary concentrating defect and, hence, of the polyuria and nocturia seen commonly in CRF (see Chap. 49). To appreciate the mechanisms involved, the responses of a normal and a uremic subject in maintaining external water balance need to be compared. Assuming that both subjects ingest the same diet and also the same amount of fluid, total solute and volume excretion in each subject should be identical as well. If the *obligatory solute load* to be excreted in each is assumed to be 600 mosmol per day, and urine osmolality is 300 mosmol/kg, a urine volume of 2 L/d will be required to excrete the total solute load in each subject. If GFR in normal and uremic subjects is 180 and 4 L/d, respectively, urinary volume excretion of 2 L/d represents excretion of slightly more than 1 percent of the filtered water in the normal individual, compared with a much larger value, 50 percent, in the uremic subject. Since the range of urine osmolalities that the diseased kidney can achieve (250 to 350 mosmol/kg) is much narrower than in the normal (40 to 1200 mosmol/kg), the individual with normal function is able to excrete the obligatory daily solute load of 600 mosmol in as little as 500 mL urine per day or as much as 15 L/d, compared with the much narrower range in the patient with renal insufficiency, from about 1.7 to 2.4 L/d.

In CRF, the limited ability to concentrate the urine usually correlates closely with other measures of impaired renal function. Isosthenuria is, therefore, a nearly universal finding when GFR falls below 25 mL/min. At this level of GFR and below, urine osmolality does not rise even with supraphysiologic parenteral doses of vaso-

pressin, suggesting that the concentrating defect is related not only to loss of diseased nephrons but also to impaired concentrating ability in surviving nephrons. As has been discussed, with diminution in functioning nephron mass, there is a concurrent increase in fractional excretion of a number of solutes. As a consequence, solute diuresis per nephron obligates a nearly isosmotic amount of water and prevents the elaboration of either hypotonic or hypertonic urine. Disease-induced abnormalities of the architecture of the renal medulla (loops of Henle, vasa recta), aberrations in renal medullary blood flow, and defective transport of NaCl in the ascending limb of Henle undoubtedly also contribute to this defect in urine concentration. Finally, there is suggestive evidence that uremia per se may impair the responsiveness of terminal nephron segments to vasopressin.

Since patients with renal insufficiency are usually unable to excrete concentrated urine, they must have access to adequate amounts of water in order to ensure the excretion of total daily solute loads. For this reason, restriction of fluid intake may prove extremely hazardous in patients with CRF. Likewise, impairment of diluting capacity may prevent many patients from excreting large amounts of ingested fluids. The consequences of the abnormal water excretion patterns in CRF, including the tendencies to development of hypo- and hypernatremia, are considered in Chaps. 50 and 224.

Tubule transport of phosphate with normal and reduced nephron mass   Under normal physiologic conditions, about 80 to 90 percent of the filtered load of phosphate is reabsorbed, mainly in the proximal tubule. *Parathyroid hormone (PTH)*, by augmenting phosphate excretion via inhibition of this proximal reabsorptive process (Chap. 339), plays a key role in phosphate homeostasis. In normal humans, when dietary phosphate intake increases, a *transient* rise in plasma phosphate concentration is usually observed. This results in a similarly transient reduction in the plasma ionized calcium concentration (due largely to calcium phosphate deposition in bone), which, in turn, stimulates PTH secretion. By enhancing fractional phosphate excretion, PTH restores external phosphate balance and normophosphatemia. This then enables plasma ionized calcium levels to return to normal, thereby removing the stimulus to PTH release, and restoring all elements of the phosphate control system to the original steady state.

With advancing renal disease, and constant dietary intake of phosphate, external phosphate balance is achieved by progressive reduction in fractional phosphate reabsorption. Enhanced PTH secretion is an important determinant of this phosphaturic response to reduced nephron mass. With each succeeding decrement in GFR, the total amount of phosphate filtered by surviving glomeruli is reduced, leading to transient retention of phosphate and, therefore, a rise (albeit small) in the phosphate concentration in extracellular fluid, including plasma. This rise in plasma phosphate concentration leads to a reciprocal small decline in plasma ionized calcium concentration and a corresponding increase in PTH secretion. Although the phosphaturic response of surviving tubules to this elevation in circulating PTH is thought to restore plasma phosphate and, therefore, calcium levels to normal (at least in the "compensated" stage of CRF described by the relatively flat portion of curve B in Fig. 222-1), the biologic cost of this return to normophosphatemia and normocalcemia is a *persistent elevation in the plasma PTH level*. With successive decrements in GFR, each stage in this overall process is repeated, but at an ever-increasing cost, namely, *progressive elevation in the circulating level of PTH.*

Alterations in vitamin D metabolism also contribute to the elevated PTH levels in renal failure. The kidneys are normally the major site of *metabolic conversion of vitamin D to its active metabolites*. As discussed in Chap. 339, precursors of the active form of vitamin D, synthesized in skin or acquired from foods, undergo initial hydroxylation in the liver to form 25-hydroxyvitamin D [25(OH)D]. The kidney is the site of a second important hydroxylation step, formation of 1,25-dihydroxyvitamin D [1,25(OH)$_2$D]. This activated form of vitamin D acts directly on the parathyroid gland to suppress PTH secretion as well as to enhance intestinal calcium and phosphate absorption and promote resorption of these ions from bone. In addition, $1,25(OH)_2D$ probably opposes the phosphaturic action of PTH at the level of the renal tubule by augmenting, rather than diminishing, phosphate reabsorption. With advancing renal disease, reduction in renal mass causes vitamin D hydroxylation to be impaired; phosphate retention also suppresses this important hydroxylation reaction. Not only are the circulating levels of $1,25(OH)_2D$ diminished in uremia, but the receptors that mediate its action within the parathyroid cells are diminished. These two effects disinhibit parathyroid hormone secretion and thereby increase circulating PTH levels. Reduction in circulating $1,25(OH)_2D$ levels, by suppressing calcium absorption from gut, contributes further to the development of the hypocalcemia and PTH excess of CRF, the consequences of which are considered in Chap. 224.

At least two additional processes are thought to contribute to elevated PTH levels in renal failure. One relates to the skeletal resistance to the calcemic effect of PTH seen in uremia. This resistance necessitates a greater than normal level of circulating PTH to effect an increment in serum calcium concentration. The other derives from the finding that reductions in renal mass impair the ability of the kidneys to degrade circulating PTH. The fact that phosphate conforms more to a curve B– than curve C–type solute in Fig. 222-1 indicates that these forms of adaptation are limited; ultimately phosphate retention occurs when GFR falls below about 25 mL/min.

Since PTH exerts major biologic effects on bone, as well as renal tubules, the external balance of phosphate in CRF is achieved at the expense of elevated PTH levels, which, in turn, account for many of the bone changes of renal osteodystrophy (i.e., *secondary hyperparathyroidism*, Fig. 224-1). In support of this ingenious *trade-off hypothesis*, studies in animals with CRF suggest that when dietary phosphate intake is reduced in proportion to the reduction in GFR, external balance of phosphate no longer requires augmentation of fractional phosphate excretion in surviving nephrons. Accordingly, circulating PTH levels no longer rise, and the typical bone changes of secondary hyperparathyroidism are diminished, if not prevented.

Hydrogen and bicarbonate transport with normal and reduced nephron mass As discussed in Chap. 51, the pH of extracellular fluid is normally maintained within a narrow range, 7.36 to 7.44, despite day-to-day variations in the quantity of acids entering the body fluids from dietary and metabolic sources (approximately 1 mmol H^+ per kilogram of body weight per day). These acids consume both intracellular and extracellular buffers, of which bicarbonate (HCO_3^-) is the most important in the intracellular compartment. Such buffering minimizes the changes in pH that would otherwise occur. The HCO_3^- buffer system would be of little long-term benefit were it not for homeostatic mechanisms, however, since with unrelenting acquisition of nonvolatile acids from dietary and metabolic sources, buffering capacity would ultimately be exhausted, eventually culminating in fatal acidosis. The kidneys normally function to prevent this possibility by *regenerating* HCO_3^- and, thereby, maintaining the concentration of HCO_3^- in the plasma. In addition to generating HCO_3^-, the kidneys also *reclaim* essentially all the HCO_3^- present in the glomerular ultrafiltrate. This reabsorptive process takes place largely in the proximal tubule and is virtually complete below a critical serum HCO_3^- concentration—the threshold concentration—which in humans is normally about 26 mmol/L, identical to the concentration of HCO_3^- in plasma. As a consequence, urinary wastage of HCO_3^- is prevented. Alternatively, when plasma HCO_3^- concentration rises above this threshold level, reabsorption of HCO_3^- becomes less complete, and the excess HCO_3^- escapes into the final urine, returning the plasma HCO_3^- concentration to the threshold level. Despite reabsorption of all the filtered HCO_3^-, metabolic acidosis would still ensue if HCO_3^- consumed in buffering nonvolatile strong acids were not constantly regenerated.

The *reabsorption* of filtered HCO_3^- in the proximal tubule occurs by the following mechanism. In proximal tubule cells, H^+, formed by the splitting of water into H^+ and OH^-, is secreted into the tubule lumen, very likely in exchange for Na^+. The OH^- ion, under the influence of *carbonic anhydrase*, combines with CO_2 to form HCO_3^-, which moves across the peritubular cell membrane via an electrogenic $Na(HCO_3)_2$ cotransporter to enter the extracellular HCO_3^- pool. The H^+ secreted into the tubule lumen combines with a filtered HCO_3^-, forming H_2CO_3. Dehydration of the latter in the proximal tubule lumen leads to the formation of CO_2 which also diffuses from lumen to peritubular blood. As a result, *a filtered HCO_3^-* ion is reclaimed. Secreted H^+ ions are also free to combine with non-HCO_3^- buffers (e.g., phosphate or ammonia) in the tubule fluid and are excreted in these forms in the final urine. HCO_3^-, the other original product of the breakdown of H_2CO_3, formed within the tubule cell, enters the peritubular blood, and *an HCO_3^- ion is regenerated*.

Hydrogen ions in the urine are bound primarily to filtered buffers (e.g., phosphate) in an amount (the so-called titratable acid) equivalent to the amount of alkali required to titrate the pH of the urine to the pH of blood. It is usually not possible, however, to excrete all the daily acid load as titratable acid alone. To serve as an additional buffer, the cells of the renal tubules generate ammonia (NH_3), largely from the hydrolysis of glutamine. NH_3 diffuses from these cells into the tubule lumen, where it combines with H^+ to form NH_4^+. As noted above, each mole of NH_4^+ excreted into the urine is associated with the regeneration of 1 mol of HCO_3^-. *Ammoniagenesis*, a process which occurs within proximal tubule cells, is responsive to the acid-base needs of the individual. When faced with an acute acid burden and an increased need for HCO_3^- regeneration, the rate of renal ammonia synthesis increases sharply.

The quantity of hydrogen ions excreted as titratable acid and NH_4^+ is equal to the quantity of HCO_3^- regenerated in tubule cells and added to the plasma. Under steady-state conditions, the quantity of net acid excreted into the urine (the sum of titratable acid and NH_4^+ minus HCO_3^-) must equal the quantity of acid gained by the extracellular fluid from all sources. Metabolic acidosis and alkalosis result when this delicate balance is perturbed, the former the result of *insufficient* net acid excretion, the latter due to *excessive* acid excretion.

Progressive loss of renal function usually causes little or no change in arterial pH, plasma bicarbonate concentration, or arterial carbon dioxide tension (P_{CO_2}) until GFR falls below 50 percent of normal. Thereafter, all three quantities tend to decline as *metabolic acidosis* ensues. In general, the metabolic acidosis of CRF is not due to overproduction of endogenous acids, but is largely a reflection of the reduction in renal mass, which limits the amount of NH_3 (and therefore HCO_3^-) that can be generated. Although surviving nephrons are probably capable of generating supernormal quantities of NH_3 *per nephron*, the diminished nephron population causes overall NH_3 production to be reduced to an extent inadequate to permit sufficient buffering of H^+ in urine. Though patients with CRF may acidify the urine normally (i.e., urine pH as low as 4.5), the defect in NH_3 production limits total daily acid excretion to 30 to 40 mmol, or one-half to two-thirds the quantity of nonvolatile acid formed in the same time period. Metabolic acidosis is the inevitable consequence of this positive balance for H^+, which in most patients with stable CRF is relatively mild and nonprogressive (arterial pH of approximately 7.33 to 7.37).

Given this substantial daily accumulation of H^+, and the typically stable and nonprogressive nature of the resulting acidosis, including the observed relative constancy of the plasma HCO_3^- concentration (albeit at reduced levels of 14 to 20 mmol/L), it follows that some large tissue source of buffering must account for the stability of the acidosis in CRF. Bone is the most likely candidate, particularly in view of its large reservoir of alkaline salts (calcium phosphate and calcium carbonate). Dissolution of this buffer source probably contributes to the osteodystrophy of CRF (see Fig. 224-1).

Although the acidosis of CRF is a consequence of the reduction in total renal mass and is therefore tubular in origin, it nevertheless depends to a large extent on the level of GFR. When GFR is reduced to only a moderate extent (i.e., to about 50 percent of normal), retention of anions, principally sulfates and phosphates, is not pronounced, so that as the plasma HCO_3^- level falls owing to tubule dysfunction, retention of Cl^- by the kidneys leads to the development of *hyperchloremic acidosis*. At this stage, therefore, *the anion gap is normal*. With further reduction in GFR and more pronounced azotemia, however, retention of phosphates, sulfates, and other *unmeasured* anions is the rule, and plasma Cl^- concentration falls to normal levels despite the reduction in plasma HCO_3^- concentration. *A moderate to large anion gap therefore develops*.

Tubule potassium transport with normal and reduced nephron mass As with H^+, the concentration of K^+ in extracellular fluid is normally maintained within a relatively narrow range, 4 to 5 mmol/L. Ninety-five percent or more of total-body K^+ is in the intracellular fluid compartment, where the intracellular concentration is approximately 160 mmol/L. Normal individuals maintain external K^+ balance by excreting into the urine an amount of K^+ per day equivalent to the amount ingested, minus the relatively small amounts lost in stool and sweat. K^+ is freely filtered at the glomerulus, although the amount excreted usually represents no more than about 20 percent of the quantity filtered. The great bulk of the filtered K^+ is *reabsorbed* in the early portions of the nephron, about two-thirds in the proximal tubule, and an additional 20 to 25 percent in the loop of Henle. A K^+ *secretory process* operates in the distal tubule and terminal nephron segments. This process is largely dependent on Na^+ reabsorption and the accompanying lumen-negative voltage creating an electrical gradient across the tubule wall, favoring K^+ secretion into the lumen of distal tubule and collecting duct.

The ability to maintain external K^+ balance and normal plasma K^+ concentration as well, until relatively late in the course of CRF, is a consequence primarily of a progressive increase in fractional excretion of K^+. Greatly enhanced rates of K^+ secretion in distal portions of surviving tubules appear to underlie this adaptation. The augmented secretion rate of aldosterone is believed to contribute to enhanced tubule secretion of K^+. In addition both the increased distal tubule flow rates in residual functioning nephrons due to the osmotic diuresis and the enhanced luminal electronegativity created by the increased concentration of highly impermeable anions such as phosphate and sulfate enhance K^+ excretion. Aldosterone also stimulates net entry of K^+ into the lumen of the colon, a mechanism known to be enhanced in CRF. More detailed discussions of the abnormalities in K^+ homeostasis in acute and chronic forms of renal failure are given in Chaps. 223 and 224.

REFERENCES

BALLERMANN BJ, BRENNER BM: Biologically active atrial peptides. J Clin Invest 76:2041, 1985

BRENNER BM, RECTOR FC JR (eds): *The Kidney*, 3d ed. Philadelphia, Saunders, 1986

BRICKER NS: On the pathogenesis of the uremic state: An exposition of the "trade-off" hypothesis. N Engl J Med 286:1093, 1972

FEINFELD DA, SHERWOOD LM: Parathyroid hormone and 1,25(OH)₂D₃ in chronic renal failure. Kidney Int 33:1049, 1988

HAYSLETT JP: Functional adaptation to reduction in renal mass. Physiol Rev 59:137, 1979

HOSTETTER TH, BRENNER BM: Glomerular adaptations to renal injury, in *Contemporary Issues in Nephrology*, vol 8: *Chronic Renal Failure*. New York, Churchill Livingstone, 1981

KAJI D, KAHN T: Na⁺-K⁺ pump in chronic renal failure. Am J Physiol 252:F785, 1987

MAXWELL MH et al: *Clinical Disorders of Fluid and Electrolyte Metabolism*, 4th ed. New York, McGraw-Hill, 1987

ROSE BD: *Clinical Physiology of Acid-Base and Electrolyte Disorders*, 2d ed. New York, McGraw-Hill, 1984

WARNOCK DG: Uremic acidosis. Kidney Int 34:278, 1988

223 ACUTE RENAL FAILURE

ROBERT J. ANDERSON / ROBERT W. SCHRIER

Acute renal failure is defined as a rapid deterioration in renal function sufficient to result in accumulation of nitrogenous wastes in the body. Approximately 5 percent of all hospitalized patients develop acute renal failure. In some clinical settings such as intensive care units, acute renal failure occurs in up to 20 percent of patients. Development of acute renal failure increases the likelihood of a fatal outcome by eightfold in hospitalized patients, and mortality rates of oliguric and nonoliguric varieties of acute renal failure range from 20 to 90 percent. The high frequency and mortality demand a logical approach to early diagnosis and prompt therapy of acute renal failure.

PRESENTING MANIFESTATIONS Acute renal failure is usually recognized by finding a rising blood urea nitrogen and/or serum creatinine concentration during biochemical monitoring of the seriously ill patient. It is noteworthy that reductions in glomerular filtration rates of 20 to 40 percent occur before significant increases in serum creatinine concentrations can be detected. A falling urine output is also frequently associated with acute renal failure. However, many patients with acute renal failure are not oliguric, and the presence of urinary flow rates >20 to 30 mL/h does not exclude the presence of acute renal failure. Sometimes acute renal failure presents because of other clinical (e.g., abnormal mental status, gastrointestinal symptoms, fluid overload, pericarditis) or laboratory (e.g., anemia, hyperkalemia, metabolic acidosis, hypocalcemia, hyperphosphatemia, abnormal urinalysis) manifestations of loss of renal function.

DIFFERENTIAL DIAGNOSIS (See Table 223-1) Urine formation begins with glomerular ultrafiltration of blood delivered to the kidneys, proceeds through tubular processing of the ultrafiltrate by secretion and absorption, and ends by excretion of urine through the ureters, bladder, and urethra. It follows that acute renal failure can be due to decreased renal perfusion (prerenal azotomia), renal parenchymal disorders (renal azotemia), or obstruction to urine flow (postrenal azotemia).

Prerenal azotemia causes 40 to 80 percent of cases of acute renal failure. Prerenal azotemia, if appropriately treated, is readily reversible. Inadequately treated, prolonged renal hypoperfusion can lead to ischemic acute tubular necrosis with significant morbidity and mortality. A decrease in renal perfusion sufficient to lower glomerular capillary perfusion pressure usually occurs in the setting of either extracellular fluid volume loss (e.g., gastrointestinal hemorrhage, burns, diarrhea, diuretics) or sequestration (e.g., pancreatitis, peritonitis, muscle crush injury). Prerenal azotemia can also result from marked reduction in cardiac output (e.g., cardiogenic shock and severe congestive heart failure), peripheral vasodilation (e.g., sepsis), or profound renal vasoconstriction as occurs in severe liver disease (hepatorenal syndrome) and sepsis. A careful review of intake and output, serial weights, hemodynamic parameters, and clinical events is important for the recognition of prerenal azotemia. Physical examination including assessment of blood pressure and pulse rate, jugular venous pressure, cardiac function, skin turgor, and mucous membranes should be undertaken in all patients with acute renal failure.

Two types of commonly used pharmacologic agents can cause acute renal failure on a hemodynamic basis. Nonsteroidal anti-inflammatory agents decrease the synthesis of renal vasodilatory prostaglandins (e.g., prostacyclin, prostaglandin E_2). In settings of an increase in endogenous renal vasoconstrictors (e.g., circulating norepinephrine and angiotensin II) and increased renal adrenergic neural tone, a compensatory rise in renal vasodilatory prostaglandins occurs. Thus, in these settings, nonsteroidal anti-inflammatory agents can result in profound renal vasoconstriction and acute renal failure. Nonsteroidal anti-inflammatory agents should be used cautiously in any patient with diminished renal perfusion. Such states include

TABLE 223-1 Major causes of acute renal failure

Disorder	Example
PRERENAL FAILURE	
Hypovolemia	Skin, gastrointestinal, or renal volume loss; hemorrhage; sequestration of extracellular fluid (burns, pancreatitis, peritonitis)
Cardiovascular failure	Impaired cardiac output (infarction, tamponade); vascular pooling (anaphylaxis, sepsis, drugs)
POSTRENAL FAILURE	
Extrarenal obstruction	Urethral occlusion; bladder, pelvic, prostatic, or retroperitoneal neoplasms; prostatism; surgical accident; medications; calculi; pus; blood clots
Intrarenal obstruction	Crystals (uric acid, oxalic acid, sulfonamides, methotrexate)
Bladder rupture	Trauma
SPECIFIC RENAL DISEASES	
Vascular diseases	Vasculitis; malignant hypertension; thrombotic thrombocytopenic purpura; scleroderma; arterial and/or venous occlusion
Glomerulonephritis	Immune-complex disease; antiglomerular basement membrane disease
Interstitial nephritis	Drugs; hypercalcemia; infections, idiopathic
ACUTE TUBULAR NECROSIS	
Postischemic	All conditions listed above for prerenal failure
Pigment-induced	Hemolysis (transfusion reaction, malaria); rhabdomyolysis (trauma, muscle disease, coma, heat stroke, severe exercise, potassium or phosphate depletion)
Toxin-induced	Antibiotics; contrast material; anesthetic agents; heavy metals; organic solvents
Pregnancy-related	Septic abortion; uterine hemorrhage; eclampsia

volume depletion, shock, edematous disorders (such as cirrhosis of the liver, heart failure, and nephrotic syndrome), underlying renal insufficiency, and advanced age. Angiotensin-converting enzyme inhibitors can also decrease glomerular capillary perfusion pressure. With the agents, a decrease in systemic arterial, and thus renal perfusion, pressure combined with efferent glomerular arteriolar dilation can result in acute renal failure. These agents are particularly prone to induce acute renal failure in patients with bilateral renal artery stenosis, unilateral renal artery stenosis without a contralateral kidney, or other high-renin disorder states (e.g., volume depletion and edematous disorders).

Postrenal causes account for 10 percent or less of all cases of acute renal failure. Since obstruction to urine flow is usually amenable to treatment, it must be considered in every patient with deteriorating renal function. Bladder neck obstruction due to prostatic disease or denervation (e.g., neuropathy or anticholinergic medications) is a relatively common cause of postrenal azotemia and can be evaluated by suprapubic palpation and percussion for an enlarged bladder as well as by postvoid bladder catheterization to measure residual volume. Obstruction of the upper urinary tract is a less common cause of renal failure since it requires simultaneous obstruction of both ureters or unilateral ureteric obstruction with severe disease or absence of the contralateral kidney. Causes of bilateral urinary tract obstruction include retroperitoneal fibrosis and space-occupying processes such as tumor or abscess, surgical accident (e.g., ureteral ligation), or bilateral intraureteric occlusion (stones, papillary tissue, blood clots, or pus). A careful rectal and pelvic examination is essential in evaluation for postobstruction renal failure. A plain film of the

abdomen may reveal retroperitoneal disease or radiopaque calculi (90 percent of kidney stones). If obstruction of the upper urinary tract cannot be excluded by ultrasound, infusion pyelography, or computed tomographic scanning, investigation of the patency of the ureter(s) by retrograde pyelography may be required. Obstruction to urine flow can also occur within the kidney. Such intrarenal obstruction is usually due to intratubular precipitation of poorly soluble material such as uric acid (tumor chemotherapy), oxalic acid (ethylene glycol overdose, methoxyflurane anesthesia, small-bowel bypass surgery), methotrexate (insoluble metabolites), acyclovir, sulfonamides (outdated, long-acting insoluble compounds), or, perhaps, myeloma proteins.

After pre- and postrenal forms of azotemia have been excluded, it is appropriate to focus on renal causes of azotemia. Disorders of the large renal arteries such as thrombosis, emboli, and dissection and disorders of the smaller renal arterial vessels including vasculitis, malignant hypertension, hemolytic-uremic syndrome, thrombotic thrombocytopenic purpura, disseminated intravascular coagulation, and scleroderma can all present as acute renal failure. These disorders usually have prominent extrarenal manifestations and a microangiopathic pattern of red blood cell destruction evident on peripheral blood smear examination. Acute glomerulonephritis (discussed in Chap. 227) is another occasional cause of acute renal failure, particularly in younger patients. Acute interstitial nephritis in the setting of drug hypersensitivity can cause acute renal failure, usually associated with unexplained fever, skin rash, arthralgias, and peripheral eosinophilia. Commonly used therapeutic agents that can induce acute renal failure due to acute interstititial nephritis include furosemide, penicillin, phenytoin, sulfonamides, rifampin, nonsteroidal anti-inflammatory drugs, trimethoprim, cimetidine, and captopril.

ACUTE TUBULAR NECROSIS   After exclusion of renal vascular, glomerular, and interstitial causes of acute renal failure, there remains a large group of patients commonly referred to as having acute tubular necrosis. While overt tubular necrosis has not always been found on renal biopsy or autopsy of such patients, tubular dysfunction is a uniform hallmark of this form of acute renal failure.

Sixty percent of cases of acute tubular necrosis are related to surgery or trauma. Forty percent occur in a medical setting, and 1 to 2 percent are related to pregnancy. The most common cause is *renal ischemia*. Conditions associated with renal ischemia include severe hemorrhage, profound volume depletion, intraoperative hypotension, cardiogenic shock, sepsis, and operative procedures associated with interruption of renal circulation. The duration of the ischemia is important in the development of acute tubular necrosis. If ischemia is brief, then correction can restore renal function (i.e., prerenal azotemia). With longer duration of renal hypoperfusion, acute tubular necrosis may supervene.

Nephrotoxic agents can also cause acute tubular necrosis. In the past, heavy metals, organic solvents, and glycols were common factors. Although these toxins are now less frequent, their occasional occurrence illustrates the importance of seeking a history of occupational and environmental toxin exposure in each patient with acute renal failure. Aminoglycoside antibiotics and radiographic contrast agents are now the leading nephrotoxic causes of acute renal failure. Indeed, acute tubular necrosis occurs in 10 to 20 percent of patients receiving a course of an aminoglycoside. The renal failure associated with these drugs is enhanced by depletion of intravascular volume, advancing age, the presence of underlying renal disease, potassium depletion, and the concomitant use of other nephrotoxic agents or potent diuretics. Radiographic contrast agents have little nephrotoxicity in healthy individuals. However, in patients with underlying renal disease, particularly patients with diabetic nephropathy, contrast exposure is associated with a 10 to 40 percent frequency of acute tubular necrosis. Some anesthetic agents (methoxyflurane and enflurane) also may induce acute renal failure.

Release of large amounts of myoglobin into the circulation is another common cause of acute tubular necrosis. Rhabdomyolysis and myoglobinuria are often due to extensive trauma with crush injuries, but nontraumatic rhabdomyolysis can also be associated with increased muscle oxygen consumption (heat stroke, severe exercise, and seizures), decreased muscle energy production (hypokalemia, hypophosphatemia, and genetic enzymatic deficiencies), muscle ischemia (arterial insufficiency, drug overdosage with resultant coma and muscle compression, cocaine overdose), infections (influenza, Legionnaires' disease), and direct toxins (alcohol). Questioning of patients with acute renal failure for muscular symptoms as well as examination for tender, swollen muscles is therefore important, although many patients may have muscle necrosis without muscle symptoms. The exact mechanism whereby myoglobinuria results in acute renal failure is uncertain. Myoglobin is not directly nephrotoxic, but direct nephrotoxicity of other muscle breakdown products, as well as tubular obstruction due to myoglobin precipitation and cast formation, has been proposed as the mechanism of inquiry. Most patients with rhabdomyolysis-associated acute renal failure also have concomitant depletion of intravascular volume and renal hypoperfusion.

Intravascular hemolysis may also cause acute tubular necrosis. Although pure hemoglobin per se is not a potent nephrotoxin, toxic substances from red blood cell stroma and concomitant renal hypoperfusion may act synergistically to induce acute renal failure. Lastly, it is not always possible to establish a definite etiology for some cases of acute tubular necrosis. In many cases, multiple etiologies are likely, as in patients with shock who are volume-depleted, have received blood transfusions, are septic, and have received nephrotoxic antibiotics.

PATHOPHYSIOLOGY (Fig. 223-1)   Current pathogenic theories of acute tubular necrosis suggest either a tubular or a vascular basis for renal failure. One tubular theory suggests that casts and cellular debris obstruct tubular lumina with resultant increases in intratubular pressure sufficient to decrease net filtration pressure. Alternatively, some investigators feel that "back-leak" of glomerular filtrate across damaged renal tubular epithelium is responsible for azotemia in acute tubular necrosis. Proponents of a vascular basis for acute tubular necrosis suggest that marked decreases in renal perfusion pressure, severe afferent arteriolar constriction, or efferent arteriolar dilatation reduce glomerular plasma flow and hydrostatic pressure sufficiently to diminish glomerular filtration. This vascular theory has led some

proponents to suggest that *vasomotor nephropathy* might be the preferred term for such cases. Another theory of acute renal failure suggests that alterations in the permeability properties of the glomerular capillary wall are responsible for acute renal failure. Alternatively, some signal in the distal tubule at the macula densa may initiate a tubuloglomerular feedback mechanism leading to a fall in glomerular filtration pressure. On balance, it seems likely that both tubular and vascular events interact to cause acute renal failure. For example, ischemia may cause a lower glomerular capillary pressure, which then predisposes to slow tubular flow. Ischemic cellular necrosis with release of apical membrane into the tubular lumen may result in sludging debris and ultimately in secondary tubular obstruction. Additional studies are required to define the relative importance of such factors and to define mechanisms that are involved in the initiation (early) and maintenance (late) phases of acute renal failure.

PATHOLOGY   The histopathologic alterations in kidneys of patients with clinical features of acute tubular necrosis vary from no or minimal abnormalities on light microscopy to tubular necrosis with disrupted, necrotic, or regenerating tubular epithelium, intratubular casts, interstitial edema, and interstitial cellular infiltration. Tubular collapse and dilated tubules both may be present. Unless either disseminated intravascular coagulation or severe, prolonged ischemic lesions are present, intrarenal blood vessels and glomeruli are normal by light and electron microscopy. Microdissection studies demonstrate two general types of renal lesions. Direct nephrotoxic injury causes a uniform, diffuse necrosis of proximal tubular cells, especially of proximal convoluted and straight tubules. The tubular basement membrane is unaltered. In contrast, following renal ischemia, mild, patchy necrosis tends to be most marked in tubular segments at the corticomedullary junction. The juxtamedullary proximal straight tubule and medullary thick ascending limb of Henle appear particularly vulnerable. Disruption of tubular basement membrane is also observed. Despite these histologic differences, the clinical course of nephrotoxic and ischemic acute renal failure is similar. A lack of correlation between renal histopathologic changes and renal functional parameters is common. Renal biopsies performed after recovery from acute renal failure either demonstrate minor abnormalities or are normal.

DIAGNOSTIC APPROACH (See Table 223-1)   The diagnosis of acute tubular necrosis is one of exclusion since prerenal (renal hypoperfusion), postrenal (obstruction of urine flow), and other intrarenal disorders (glomerulonephritis, renal interstitial and vascular diseases) may all lead to deteriorating renal function. In contrast to acute tubular necrosis, however, prerenal, postrenal, and other intrarenal vascular, glomerular, or interstitial disorders may be specifically treatable.

The initial presentation of the patient with end-stage chronic renal failure may be confused with acute renal failure when there is no information about renal function prior to presentation. Under these circumstances, the presence of uremic osteodystrophy, uremic neuropathy, bilateral small kidneys on abdominal films or ultrasound, and unexplained anemia suggests chronic renal failure. However, some end-stage renal diseases, such as amyloidosis, polycystic kidney disease, diabetic glomerulosclerosis, scleroderma, and rapidly progressive glomerulonephritis, may present with normal-sized or enlarged kidneys, making it necessary for continued observation and sometimes renal biopsy to distinguish between potentially reversible forms of acute renal failure and end-stage chronic renal failure.

The pattern of urine flow may provide a diagnostic clue as to the cause of declining renal function. Complete anuria (no urine by catheterization) is rare in acute tubular necrosis. Potential causes of total anuria include complete bilateral ureteric obstruction, diffuse cortical necrosis, rapidly progressive glomerulonephritis, and bilateral renal artery occlusion. Wide fluctuations in daily urine output suggest intermittent obstructive uropathy. Polyuria (>3 L per day) can be a hallmark of partial urinary tract obstruction and is secondary to the accompanying defect in renal concentrating ability. Although oliguria (<400 mL per day) has been considered to be a cardinal feature of

FIGURE 223-1   Potential pathogenic schema in acute renal failure.

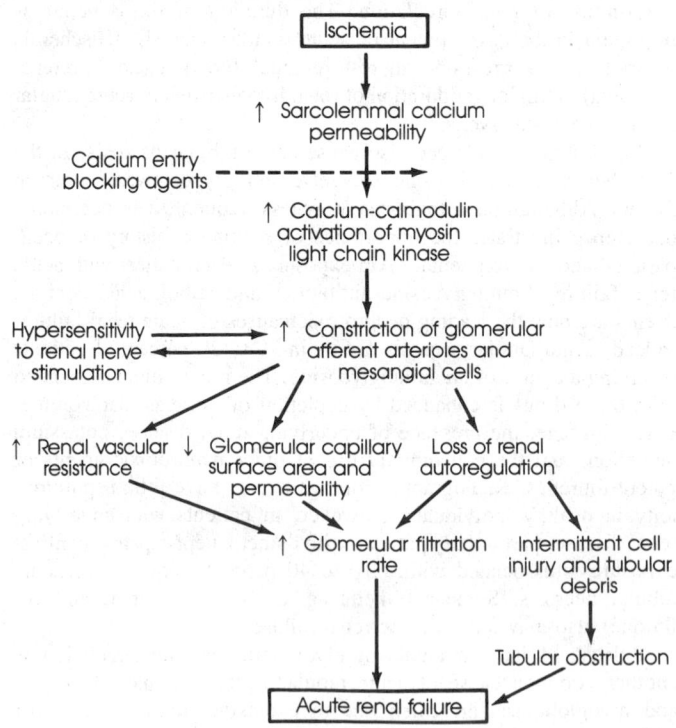

TABLE 223-2   Urine findings in prerenal azotemia and acute renal failure

Laboratory test	Prerenal azotemia	Acute renal failure
Urine osmolality (mosmol/kg)	>500	<400
Urine sodium (mmol/L)	<20	>40
Urine/plasma creatinine	>40	<20
Fractional excretion* of filtered sodium	<1	2
Urine sediment	Normal or occasional hyaline and granular casts	Brown granular casts, cellular debris

$$* \frac{\text{Urine Na/serum Na}}{\text{Urine creatinine/serum creatinine}} \times 100.$$

acute tubular necrosis, many patients have urine volumes of greater than 1 L per day. This situation is termed nonoliguric acute renal failure.

Examination of the urinary sediment is also of value in the differential diagnosis of acute impairment of renal function. Sediment containing few formed elements or only hyaline casts suggests prerenal azotemia or obstructive uropathy. With acute tubular necrosis, brownish pigmented cellular casts and renal tubular epithelial cells are present in over 75 percent of patients. Red blood cell casts suggest the presence of glomerular or vascular inflammatory diseases of the kidney and are rarely, if ever, present with acute tubular necrosis. The presence of large numbers of polymorphonuclear leukocytes, singly or in clumps, suggests acute diffuse interstitial nephritis or papillary necrosis. Eosinophilic casts on Hansel's stain of urine sediment support a diagnosis of acute hypersensitivity interstitial nephritis. The combination of brownish pigmented granular casts and positive occult blood tests on urine in the absence of hematuria indicates either hemoglobinuria or myoglobinuria. In acute renal failure, the finding in fresh, warm urine of large numbers of uric acid crystals may suggest a diagnosis of acute uric acid nephropathy, while large numbers of oxalic acid or hippuric acid crystals suggests ethylene glycol toxicity. The presence of large numbers of broad casts (greater than two to three white blood cells in diameter) suggests chronic renal disease.

Chemical analysis of urine composition is also helpful in differentiating acute tubular necrosis from prerenal azotemia in the oliguric patient (Table 223-2). Other disorders associated with abrupt deterioration in renal function and intact renal tubular integrity, such as glomerulonephritis, vasculitis, and early (few hours) obstructive uropathy, may cause urine chemical values similar to those encountered in prerenal azotemia. Prior administration of diuretic agents, osmotic diuresis due to mannitol, glycosuria, bicarbonaturia, and ketonuria may interfere with renal tubular reabsorption of sodium and water and thus alter urinary chemical indexes. A urinary uric acid/creatinine concentration ratio of greater than 1 is compatible with acute uric acid nephropathy as a cause of the acute renal failure.

The cause of declining renal function may not be readily apparent. In some cases, features considered atypical for acute tubular necrosis (gradual onset of renal failure; anuria in the absence of obstructive uropathy; the presence of marked hypertension, heavy proteinuria, significant hematuria, underlying systemic disease, and prolonged oliguria) will be present. Since such atypical features may indicate the presence of a potentially treatable form of renal parenchymal disease, e.g., Wegener's disease, systemic lupus erythematosus, Goodpasture's syndrome, or rapidly progressive glomerulonephritis, a diagnostic renal biopsy may be indicated when the cause of renal failure is not apparent or such atypical features are present.

CLINICAL COURSE   The clinical course in acute tubular necrosis can be divided into an initiating phase, a maintenance phase, and a recovery phase. The initiating phase is the period of time between the precipitating event and the appearance of acute renal failure which

is no longer reversible by alteration in extrarenal factors. Recognition of the initiating phase of acute renal failure is extremely important since early correction of the underlying cause of renal failure may theoretically prevent the development of the maintenance phase. However, the initiating phase of acute renal failure may be evident to the clinician only in retrospect because it lacks characteristic signs and symptoms.

Oliguria has been considered the cardinal feature of the initiating and maintenance phases of acute tubular necrosis. However, up to 40 to 50 percent of all patients with acute tubular necrosis are nonoliguric (urine volume >400 mL per day). Progressive acute renal failure without oliguria can result from any type of renal insult, including both ischemic and toxic insults, and this form of renal failure appears to be particularly frequent following nephrotoxic (e.g., aminoglycoside) drug injury. Progressive azotemia occurs in nonoliguric patients owing to the marked impairment in glomerular filtration rate and renal concentrating capacity. For example, maximal urine osmolality of the nonoliguric patient averages only 350 mosmol per kilogram of water. Therefore, with a urine output of 1000 mL per day, a maximum of 350 mosmol solute can be excreted daily. In acute renal failure, daily solute loads may be increased from normal values of 600 mosmol to values as high as 1000 mosmol. Thus, a positive solute (predominately urea and creatinine) balance and azotemia would occur despite a daily urine output of 1 L.

When oliguria occurs, it starts shortly following the inciting event and lasts an average of 10 to 14 days. However, the oliguric phase may be as short as a few hours or as long as 6 to 8 weeks in the elderly patient with underlying vascular disease. If oliguria persists for longer than 4 weeks, the diagnosis of acute tubular necrosis should be reconsidered; diffuse cortical necrosis, rapidly progressive glomerulonephritis, renal artery occlusion, renal vasculitis, renal emboli, and superimposed volume depletion may be present. Anuria is not characteristic of acute tubular necrosis, but severe oliguria with urine volume less than 100 mL per day may last for several days.

Urinary elimination of nitrogenous wastes, water, electrolytes, and acid is impaired in the initiating and maintenance phases of acute renal failure. The magnitude of resultant abnormalities in blood chemistry depends on whether the patient is oliguric or nonoliguric and on the patient's catabolic state. Nonoliguric patients have higher levels of glomerular filtration than do oliguric patients and thus excrete more nitrogenous waste, water, and electrolytes in their urine. Hence, abnormalities in blood chemistry are generally milder in nonoliguric than oliguric patients with acute renal failure. The complications, need for dialysis, and mortality are also less in nonoliguric patients.

In the afebrile, noncatabolic, oliguric patient with acute renal failure, the daily increments in blood urea nitrogen (BUN) and serum creatinine average 4 to 8 mmol/L (10 to 20 mg/dL) and 40 to 80 μmol/L (0.5 to 1.0 mg/dL), respectively. In catabolic patients with fever, sepsis, or extensive trauma, daily increments in BUN and serum creatinine may be much higher. In patients with acute renal failure due to rhabdomyolysis, the daily increment in serum creatinine may be disproportionately higher than the BUN. This is due to the release from muscle of creatine, which is converted by nonenzymatic hydrolysis to creatinine.

Salt and water overload with resultant hyponatremia, edema, and pulmonary congestion are ever-present dangers in patients with acute renal failure, particularly oliguric patients. Hyponatremia results from excessive water intake, and edema is due to excessive sodium and water intake. In contrast, if urinary losses are not replaced, the nonoliguric patient with a relatively high rate of urine flow and high concentration of urine sodium may develop intravascular volume depletion which can retard recovery of renal function.

Hyperkalemia due to decreased renal elimination of potassium and continued tissue potassium release is a frequent accompaniment of acute tubular necrosis. The usual rate of increase in serum potassium in the noncatabolic, oliguric patient is 0.3 to 0.5 mmol per day. Higher rates of rise in serum potassium concentration suggest the possibility of an endogenous (tissue destruction, hemolysis) or exogenous (medication, diet, blood transfusion) potassium load or of cellular shift of potassium due to acidemia. Generally, hyperkalemia is asymptomatic until serum potassium increases to values above 6.0 to 6.5 mmol/L. Then electrocardiographic abnormalities (bradycardia, recent appearance of left axis deviation, peaked T waves, prolonged QRS complexes, prolonged PR interval, and decreased amplitude of the P waves) and ultimately cardiac arrest can occur. Hyperkalemia can also cause muscle weakness and flaccid quadriparesis.

Hyperphosphatemia, *hypocalcemia*, and mild *hypermagnesemia* are usually present in acute tubular necrosis. Hyperphosphatemia results from decreased renal phosphorus elimination in the presence of continued release of phosphorus from tissues. The serum phosphorus is usually in the range of 2 to 2.3 mmol/L, but higher values may occur in the traumatized, catabolic patient or in the patient with rhabdomyolysis. Hypocalcemia often develops during acute renal failure. The reason is not clear, but resistance to parathyroid hormone may play a role. Increases in serum magnesium are mild (to levels of 0.8 to 1.2 mmol/L), unless magnesium-containing compounds such as antacids are ingested.

Metabolic acidosis is a regular accompaniment of acute tubular necrosis. The usual daily production of approximately 1 mmol per kilogram of body weight of nonvolatile acid from endogenous metabolic sources can no longer be eliminated by the damaged kidney. The retention of organic acids is sufficient to produce a daily decrease of 1 to 2 mmol/L in plasma bicarbonate and metabolic acidosis with an anion gap.

Mild hyperuricemia is due to decreased renal uric acid excretion. In catabolic patients with extensive tissue damage, higher values of serum uric acid may be observed. Elevation of serum amylase due to impaired renal amylase excretion may occur in the absence of evidence of pancreatitis. The elevations of amylase are usually less than twice the upper limit of normal.

Hematologic abnormalities are usually present in acute tubular necrosis. A normocytic normochromic anemia occurs shortly following the onset of significant azotemia. This anemia is due to impaired erythropoiesis as well as to a mild and variable shortened red blood cell survival. Additional factors that may contribute to anemia include hemodilution, gastrointestinal blood loss, and suppressed erythropoiesis due to infections or drug administration. White blood cell production is not severely disturbed in acute renal failure. However, mild leukocytosis is usually present. Leukocytosis persisting after the initial week of acute renal failure should suggest the possibility of infection. Mild degrees of thrombocytopenia due to reduction of bone marrow platelet production may be observed early in the course. Qualitative defects in platelet function occur and, in association with additional poorly defined coagulation disturbances, contribute to the bleeding tendency of acute renal failure. Acute renal failure may follow intravascular hemolysis and may also be a complication of several primary hematologic or vascular disorders that have major hematologic manifestations such as disseminated intravascular coagulation, thrombotic thrombocytopenic purpura, hemolytic uremic syndrome, and systemic lupus erythematosus.

Infections complicate 30 to 70 percent of all cases of acute tubular necrosis and are a leading cause of morbidity and mortality. The sites of infection include the respiratory tract, operative sites, and urinary tract. Resultant septicemia is frequent, and both gram-positive and gram-negative organisms are encountered. Operative site abscesses (especially intraabdominal) are associated with a poor prognosis if not recognized and treated promptly. Although the exact factors responsible for the high rate of infection remain to be determined, disruption of normal anatomic barriers with intravenous infusions and indwelling catheters may play a role. Host defenses including leukocyte function may be impaired in the setting of uremia. Minimization of use of catheters and intravenous lines, careful daily examination, and prompt thorough evaluation of fever are important. It is also important to emphasize that uremia may obscure fever associated with infections.

Cardiovascular complications include volume overload, hypertension, arrhythmias, and pericarditis. Volume overload is usually due to excessive sodium and water administration. Mild hypertension is seen in 15 to 25 percent of cases and usually appears in the second week of oliguria. This hypertension is usually also a manifestation of extracellular fluid volume overload; however, increased activity of the renin-angiotensin system may also be involved in some instances. Supraventricular arrhythmias may complicate 20 to 30 percent of cases of acute renal failure. Known causes for these arrhythmias include congestive heart failure, electrolyte abnormalities, digitalis intoxication, pericarditis, and anemia. Pericarditis currently occurs infrequently, probably because of prompt dialysis.

Neurologic abnormalities are common in acute renal failure. In undialyzed patients, lethargy, somnolence, confusion, disorientation, asterixis, agitation, myoclonic muscle twitching, and generalized seizures may be observed. These neurologic abnormalities are most often encountered in the elderly patient and generally respond well to dialysis. In addition to uremia per se, drug administration, metabolic and electrolyte abnormalities, and primary neurologic disease may cause neurologic disturbances in the patient with acute renal failure.

Gastrointestinal complications include anorexia, nausea, vomiting, ileus, and poorly defined abdominal complaints. The combination of stress of acute illness and bleeding disorders can lead to gastrointestinal hemorrhage in 10 to 30 percent of patients. Fortunately, the gastrointestinal hemorrhage is usually mild and easily controlled with conservative therapy. Intravenous desmopressin (0.4 μg/kg intravenously) lowers the bleeding time and improves hemostasis in some patients with acute renal failure. Cryoprecipitate can also be used especially in cases refractory to desmopressin.

The recovery phase of acute renal failure commences when the glomerular filtration rate increases so that the BUN and serum creatinine concentrations no longer continue to increase. In oliguric acute renal failure, the recovery phase is heralded by a progressive increase in urine volume. Generally, in the first days the urine volume may double daily, and in some cases a daily urine volume may be greater than 2 L for a few days. In nonoliguric patients, a marked diuretic phase is usually not observed. The duration of the recovery phase in patients with serum creatinine concentrations greater than 440 μmol/L (5 mg/dL) averages 10 to 25 days in oliguric patients and 5 to 10 days in nonoliguric patients. The major complications of acute renal failure, such as infections, gastrointestinal hemorrhage, fluid and electrolyte disturbances, and cardiovascular dysfunction, may persist or first appear during the recovery phase. In addition, persistent abnormalities in glomerular and tubular function during the recovery phase can lead to over- or underhydration or electrolyte disturbances unless careful daily weight, intake and output, biochemical, and clinical monitoring are continued. Hypercalcemia may occur during the recovery phase, especially in patients with rhabdomyolysis. The cause of this complication remains obscure, but mobilization of calcium from damaged muscle into extracellular fluid has been suggested.

Although the major improvement in renal function occurs within the first 1 to 2 weeks of the recovery phase, renal function continues to improve for up to a year following acute renal failure. Sensitive tests of glomerular and tubular function also suggest that some mild defects in renal function may persist indefinitely following acute tubular necrosis. However, the majority of patients achieve clinically normal renal function, and there is no evidence of late progression of renal dysfunction or of complications such as hypertension.

Mortality rates in large series of patients with acute renal failure vary from 20 to 90 percent. Mortality rates are highest in postoperative or traumatized patients, intermediate in patients with acute renal failure encountered in a medical setting, and lowest in acute renal failure observed in an obstetric setting. Advanced age, the presence of serious underlying illness, a catabolic state, and the development of multiple medical complications (especially concomitant acute respiratory failure) during the course are associated with higher mortality rates. Another determinant of outcome is the severity of

TABLE 223-3   General therapeutic approach to patient with acute renal failure

1 Exclude all specifically treatable causes of decreasing renal function including correction of prerenal and postrenal factors.
2 Attempt to establish a urine output.
3 Conservative therapy:
  a Decrease intake of nitrogen, water, and electrolytes to match output.
  b Provide adequate nutrition.
  c Alter medication therapy.
  d Maintain clinical monitoring (frequency of vital signs determined by patient status; intake and output, body weight, inspection of wound and intravenous sites, and physical examination required daily).
  e Maintain biochemical monitoring (frequency of BUN, creatinine, electrolytes, and blood counts will be dictated by patient status; in catabolic oliguric patients, daily determination will be needed; calcium, phosphorus, magnesium, and uric acid can often be determined less often).
4 Provide dialytic therapy.

the renal failure. As stated above, oliguric acute renal failure requiring dialysis is associated with three- to fivefold increases in mortality when compared with nonoliguric acute renal failure that usually does not require dialysis. Infections, complications resulting from fluid and electrolyte disturbances, gastrointestinal hemorrhage, and progression of the primary underlying disease are the major causes of mortality in acute renal failure.

MANAGEMENT (Table 223-3)   The first principle of therapy is to exclude causes of deterioration in renal function that are potentially remedial. A search for prerenal factors, obstructive uropathy, glomerulonephritis, renal vascular and interstitial disease, and intrarenal crystal precipitation should be performed. Once the diagnosis of acute tubular necrosis is made by exclusion, little specific therapy is available. Dialysis for the removal of nephrotoxins, such as carbon tetrachloride, ethylene glycol, and heavy metals following chelation therapy, may be indicated. Even in the presence of acute tubular necrosis, any prerenal abnormalities should be corrected both to improve the circulation and to avoid delay in the onset of the recovery phase. In the oliguric patient in whom prerenal factors have been corrected, it has become common clinical practice to administer either a potent loop diuretic or mannitol in an attempt to enhance urine flow. In patients who remain oliguric despite potent diuretics, low-dose infusions of dopamine (1 to 3 mg per kilogram body weight per minute) may increase renal blood flow and allow a diuretic response to potent diuretics. The rationale for such therapy is based on the thought that there is an early phase of renal failure during which the correction of prerenal factors and establishment of urine flow can prevent an oliguric state. Prospective studies have demonstrated lower morbidity and mortality rates in nonoliguric as compared with oliguric acute renal failure. However, a prospective controlled study of the utility of potent diuretics and dopamine in early acute renal failure to convert oliguric to nonoliguric renal failure is needed.

Conservative therapy is capable of controlling many of the manifestations of acute renal failure. After any defects in intravascular volume have been corrected, fluid intake should equal measured output plus estimated insensible losses. Sodium and potassium administration should not exceed measured losses. Daily monitoring of fluid balance and body weight allow assessment of the volume status. A daily weight loss of 0.2 to 0.3 kg occurs in the well-managed patient with acute renal failure. Greater weight loss suggests hypercatabolism or volume depletion, and lesser weight loss suggests excessive salt and water administration. Since most pharmacologic agents are eliminated at least in part by the kidney, careful attention to medication usage and dosage adjustment is needed. The serum sodium concentration provides a guideline for water administration. A decrease in serum sodium indicates a relative excess of total-body water, while an abnormally high concentration indicates a relative deficiency of body water as compared to total-body sodium.

To minimize catabolism, daily intake should include at least 100 g of carbohydrate. Some studies suggest in addition that intravenous administration of a mixture of amino acids and hypertonic glucose improves morbidity and mortality in patients with acute renal failure following surgical procedures or trauma (see Chap. 75). Since parenteral hyperalimentation may be associated with significant complications, this form of nutrition should be reserved for catabolic patients in whom the enteral routine of alimentation does not prove to be satisfactory. Additional means of minimizing catabolism include early removal or debridement of necrotic tissue, control of pyrexia, and early, specific antimicrobial therapy.

The mild metabolic acidosis associated with acute tubular necrosis is generally not treated unless serum bicarbonate falls to below 10 mmol/L. Rapid correction of acidemia by acute alkali administration may decrease ionized calcium concentrations and precipitate tetany. Hypocalcemia is usually asymptomatic and rarely requires specific therapy. Hyperphosphatemia should be controlled with 30 to 60 mL aluminum hydroxide administered orally four to six times per day, since a high calcium-phosphorus product may cause soft tissue calcification. For the occasional patient with profound hyperphosphatemia, early dialysis therapy may be warranted. Unless acute uric acid nephropathy is a diagnostic consideration, the secondary hyperuricemia of acute renal failure is usually not treated with allopurinol. Because of the decreased glomerular filtration rate, the filtered load of uric acid, and thus intratubular deposition, is low. Also, for unknown reasons, clinical gout rarely complicates acute renal failure, despite hyperuricemia. Careful observation of the hematocrit and stool for occult blood is important for the early detection of gastrointestinal blood loss. If a rapid decrease in hematocrit appears to be out of proportion to the degree of renal failure, alternative causes of anemia should be sought.

Congestive heart failure and hypertension indicate volume overload and should be treated accordingly, recognizing, of course, that many drugs such as digoxin are largely excreted by the kidneys. Continuous arteriovenous hemofiltration can remove large amounts of extracellular fluid in the setting of acute renal failure. This therapy is often utilized in patients with oliguric acute tubular necrosis who require large amounts of hyperalimentation fluid to maintain caloric and nitrogen balance. As suggested earlier, hypertension occasionally may persist in the absence of volume overload; thus factors such as hyperreninemia may contribute to the hypertension. Selective histamine-2-receptor blockade (cimetidine, ranitidine) therapy has been of benefit in preventing gastrointestinal bleeding in some seriously ill patients but has not yet been studied in acute renal failure. Avoidance and early detection of infection require minimization of interruption of normal anatomic barriers, including avoidance of long-term catheterization of the urinary bladder, provision of mouth and skin care, promotion of early mobilization, utilization of aseptic techniques for intravenous and tracheostomy sites, and close clinical monitoring. Fever and suspected infection should be promptly evaluated with careful inspection of lung, wounds, urinary tract, and intravenous sites.

Hyperkalemia is an ever-present threat in acute renal failure. Mild elevations of serum potassium (<6.0 mmol/L) can best be treated by withdrawal of all sources of potassium and by continued close laboratory observation. If serum potassium increases to values greater than 6.5 mmol/L and particularly if any electrocardiographic changes appear, active therapy should be instituted. Therapy of such hyperkalemia can be divided into emergent and nonemergent forms. Emergent therapy includes intravenous administration of calcium (5 to 10 mL of 10% calcium chloride solution intravenously over 2 min with electrocardiographic monitoring), bicarbonate (44 mmol intravenously over 5 min), and insulin and glucose (200 to 300 mL of 20% glucose with 20 to 30 units regular insulin given intravenously over 30 min). Nonemergent therapy includes administration of potassium-binding ion exchange resins such as sodium polystyrene sulfonate. This can be administered orally every 3 to 4 h in 25- to 50-g doses with 100 mL 20% sorbitol to avoid constipation. Alternatively, in the patient who cannot take oral medications, 50 g sodium polystyrene sulfonate and 50 g sorbitol in 200 mL water can be given as a retention enema at 1- to 2-h intervals. With refractory hyperkalemia, hemodialysis may be necessary.

Some patients with acute tubular necrosis, particularly those who are nonoliguric and noncatabolic, can be successfully managed with minimal or no dialytic therapy. There has been an increasing tendency to use dialysis therapy early in acute renal failure in an attempt to minimize the development of complications. Early (prophylactic) use of dialysis frequently simplifies management, allowing more liberal fluid and potassium intake and improvement of the general well-being of the patient. Absolute indications for dialysis include symptomatic uremia (usually manifested by central nervous system and/or gastrointestinal symptoms), development of resistant hyperkalemia, severe acidemia or fluid overload not responsive to medical therapy, and pericarditis. In addition, many centers attempt to keep predialysis levels of serum creatinine less than 700 to 900 μmol/L (8 to 10 mg/dL). Adequate prevention of uremic symptoms may require no or infrequent dialysis in the noncatabolic, nonoliguric patient or daily dialysis in the catabolic, traumatized patient. Often, peritoneal dialysis is an acceptable alternative to hemodialysis. Peritoneal dialysis may be especially useful in the patient with noncatabolic acute tubular necrosis when the need for infrequent dialysis is anticipated. Slow, continuous arteriovenous filtration using highly permeable filters has been advocated as a means of controlling extracellular volume. Currently available filters connected via an arteriovenous shunt allow for removal of 5 to 12 L of plasma ultrafiltrate per day without use of a pump. Thus, these devices appear particularly useful in the oliguric volume-overloaded patient with hemodynamic instability.

PREVENTION Because of the high mortality and morbidity of acute renal failure, prophylactic therapy deserves special mention. The first principle of prevention is aggressive resuscitation of the traumatized patient. A fivefold reduction in deaths secondary to acute renal failure occurred from the Korean War to the Vietnamese conflict. This reduction in mortality was probably due to earlier evacuation from the field and more rapid restoration of extracellular fluid volume. A second factor in prevention of acute renal failure is minimization of the use of potential nephrotoxins, particularly in high-risk patients. Finally, maintenance of normal extracellular fluid volume and high urinary flow and solute excretion rates may prevent and/or attenuate the development of acute renal failure in selected situations, such as open-heart surgery, following severe trauma, when rhabdomyolysis and/or intravascular hemolysis is present, and in association with some nephrotoxins including cisplatin, radiographic contrast agents, and amphotericin B. Maintenance of high urine flow and solute excretion rates also can preserve renal function in the setting of high renal loads of potentially insoluble crystalline material such as uric acid and methotrexate.

ACUTE RENAL FAILURE IN PREGNANCY When acute renal failure occurs during pregnancy, it is usually in either the earlier or later stages of gestation. During the first trimester, acute renal failure usually occurs in the setting of nontherapeutic, nonsterile abortion. In these cases, volume depletion, sepsis, and nephrotoxins contribute to the acute renal failure. This form of acute renal failure has markedly declined with the widespread availability of sterile abortion.

Acute renal failure late in pregnancy can occur from either excessive postpartum hemorrhage or preeclampsia. Most such patients generally recover total renal function, but for those who do not histologic evidence of diffuse cortical necrosis is found, which usually complicates the severe hemorrhage of abruptio placentae and is associated with clinical and laboratory evidence of intravascular coagulation.

A rare form of acute renal failure occurring 1 to 12 weeks following uncomplicated pregnancy has been described and termed postpartum glomerulosclerosis. This disorder is usually characterized by irreversible, rapidly progressive renal failure, although milder cases have been described. These patients have an associated microangiopathic hemolytic anemia. The renal histopathologic changes are indistinguishable from those associated with malignant hypertension or scleroderma. The pathophysiology of this disorder has not been defined. No therapy is consistently successful, although heparin therapy has been advocated.

HEPATORENAL SYNDROME The hepatorenal syndrome is a complication of advanced liver disease in which renal failure occurs in the absence of clinical, laboratory, or anatomic evidence of other causes of renal dysfunction. The renal failure is usually associated with oliguria, an unremarkable urinary sediment, and low urinary sodium concentrations (<10 mmol/L). Generally, the renal failure occurs in the setting of advanced hepatic cirrhosis complicated by jaundice, ascites, and hepatic encephalopathy. Occasionally, this syndrome may complicate fulminant hepatitis. The mechanism of the renal failure is not known. The lack of consistent histopathologic alterations in kidneys and the restoration of normal renal function when kidneys from donors with hepatorenal syndrome are transplanted into recipients without liver disease suggest a functional defect. The administration of nonsteroidal anti-inflammatory agents to patients with decompensated cirrhosis may cause a clinical picture identical to that seen with hepatorenal syndrome. With cessation of these drugs, renal function often improves.

Treatment of the hepatorenal syndrome is usually unsuccessful. Care should be taken in the cirrhotic patient not to induce major changes in intravascular volume by large paracentesis or aggressive diuresis, maneuvers that may precipitate hepatorenal syndrome. Since this syndrome mimics prerenal azotemia, a cautious trial of expansion of intravascular volume is warranted. In a few cases, recovery has followed portacaval shunting, insertion of an abdominal-venous (Leveen) shunt, or prolonged hemodialysis. These treatments have not been subjected to controlled trials. The abdominal-venous shunt may be associated with peritonitis, intravascular coagulation, and pulmonary congestion. Improvement in hepatic function often results in parallel improvement in renal function. Every effort should be made to ensure that more specifically treatable causes of concomitant liver and renal dysfunction, such as infections (leptospirosis, hepatitis with immune-complex disease), toxins (aminoglycosides, carbon tetrachloride), and circulatory disorders (severe heart failure, shock), are not present. It should also be recalled that jaundiced patients with liver disease may be particularly susceptible to acute tubular necrosis.

REFERENCES

ANDERSON RJ, SCHRIER RW: Acute tubular necrosis, in *Diseases of the Kidney*, RW Schrier, CW Gottschalk (eds). Boston, Little, Brown, 1988, p 1413

BADR KF, ICHIKAWA I: Prerenal failure: A deleterious shift from renal compensation to decompensation. N Engl J Med 319:623, 1988

BRENNER BM, LAZARUS JM (eds): *Acute Renal Failure*. Philadelphia, Saunders, 1987

MEYERS BD, MORAN SM: Hemodynamically mediated acute renal failure. N Engl J Med 314:97, 1986

SHUSTERMAN N et al: Risk factors and outcome of hospital-acquired acute renal failure. Am J Med 83:65, 1987

224 CHRONIC RENAL FAILURE

BARRY M. BRENNER / J. MICHAEL LAZARUS

In contrast to the remarkable capacity of the kidney to regain function following the various forms of acute renal injury discussed in the preceding chapter, renal injury of a more sustained nature is often not reversible but leads instead to progressive destruction of nephron mass. Despite successful treatment of hypertension, urinary tract obstruction and infection, and systemic disease, many forms of renal injury associated with permanent nephron loss progress inexorably to chronic renal failure (CRF). Reduction of renal mass causes structural and functional hypertrophy of remaining nephrons. This "compensatory" hypertrophy is due to adaptive hyperfiltration mediated by increases in glomerular capillary pressures and flows. Eventually these adaptations prove "maladaptive" in that they predispose to glomerular sclerosis, an enhanced functional burden on less affected glomeruli, leading in turn to their ultimate destruction.

Glomerulonephritis, in its several forms, was the most common initiating cause of chronic renal failure in the past. In recent years, possibly because of more aggressive treatment of glomerulonephritis and because of changing practices in patient acceptance of end-stage renal disease programs, diabetes mellitus and hypertension have become the leading causes of chronic renal failure (see Table 224-1). These and other progressive forms of renal disease are considered in detail in the remaining chapters of this section. Irrespective of cause, the eventual impact of severe reduction in nephron mass is an alteration in function of virtually every organ system in the body. *Uremia* is the term generally applied to the clinical syndrome in patients suffering from profound loss of renal function. Although the cause(s) of the syndrome remain unknown, the term *uremia* was adopted originally because of the presumption that the abnormalities seen in patients with CRF resulted from retention in the blood of urea and other end products of metabolism normally excreted in the urine. But the term *uremia* represents more than renal excretory failure alone. A host of metabolic and endocrine functions normally subserved by the kidney are also impaired in CRF, and the inexorable course to renal failure is often accompanied by severe malnutrition, impaired metabolism of carbohydrates, fats, and proteins, and defective utilization of energy. Therefore, the *uremia* no longer carries pathophysiologic meaning but instead refers generally to the constellation of signs and symptoms associated with CRF, regardless of cause.

The presentation and severity of signs and symptoms of uremia often vary greatly from patient to patient, depending, at least in part, on the magnitude of the reduction in functioning renal mass as well as the rapidity with which renal function is lost. As discussed in Chap. 222, in the relatively early stage of CRF [i.e., when total glomerular filtration rate (GFR) is reduced but not to levels below about 35 to 50 percent of normal], overall renal function is sufficient to maintain the patient symptom-free, although renal reserve may be diminished. At this stage of renal impairment baseline excretory, biosynthetic, and other regulatory functions of the kidney are generally well maintained. At a somewhat later stage in the course of CRF (GFR about 20 to 35 percent of normal), *azotemia* occurs, and initial manifestations of renal insufficiency usually appear. Although patients are relatively asymptomatic at this stage, renal reserve is diminished sufficiently that any sudden stress, such as intercurrent infection, urinary tract obstruction, dehydration, or administration of a nephrotoxic drug, may compromise renal function still further, often leading to signs and symptoms of overt uremia. With further loss of nephron mass (GFR below 20 to 25 percent of normal), the patient develops *overt renal failure*. Uremia may be viewed as the final stage in this inexorable process, when many of or all the untoward manifestations of CRF become evident clinically. In this chapter the causes and clinical characteristics of the disturbances of the various organ systems seen in patients with CRF will be considered.

PATHOPHYSIOLOGY AND BIOCHEMISTRY OF UREMIA

ROLE OF RETAINED TOXIC METABOLITES The finding that sera from patients with uremia exert toxic effects in a variety of biologic test systems has motivated a diligent search to identify the responsible toxin(s). The most likely candidates thought to qualify as toxins in uremia are the *by-products of protein and amino acid metabolism*. Unlike fats and carbohydrates, which are eventually metabolized to carbon dioxide and water, substances that are easily excreted even in uremic subjects via lungs and skin, the products of protein and amino acid metabolism depend largely on the kidneys for excretion. A vast number of such products have been identified, with urea being quantitatively the most important. *Urea* represents some 80 percent or more of the total nitrogen excreted into the urine in patients with CRF maintained on diets containing 40 or more

TABLE 224-1 Primary Diagnoses—Medicare End-Stage Renal Disease Program*

Diabetic nephropathy	27.7%
Hypertension	24.5%
Glomerulonephritis	21.2%
Polycystic kidney disease	3.9%
Other/unknown	22.7%

* Number of new patients in 1985, 28,944.
SOURCE: Health Care Financing Administration, Bureau of Data Management and Strategy.

grams of protein per day. The *guanidino compounds* are the next most abundant of the nitrogenous end products of protein metabolism and include substances such as guanidine, methyl- and dimethyl-guanidine, creatinine, creatine, and guanidinosuccinic acid. As with urea, guanidines are derived, at least in part, from urea cycle amino acids. Other metabolic products of amino acid and protein catabolism that have been implicated as possible uremic toxins include *urates and other end products of nucleic acid metabolism, aliphatic amines,* a variety of *peptides,* and, finally, several *derivatives of the aromatic amino acids tryptophan, tyrosine, and phenylalanine*. The role of these substances in the pathogenesis of the clinical and biochemical abnormalities seen in CRF is unclear. It is generally believed that uremic symptoms correlate only in a rough and inconsistent way with concentrations of urea in blood. Nevertheless, although urea is probably not a major cause of overt uremic toxicity, it may account for some of the clinical abnormalities, including anorexia, malaise, vomiting, and headache. On the other hand, elevated levels of plasma *guanidinosuccinic acid,* by interfering with activation of platelet factor III by adenosine diphosphate (ADP), contribute to the impaired platelet function seen in CRF. *Creatinine,* generally regarded as a nontoxic substance, may cause adverse effects following conversion to more toxic metabolites such as sarcosine and methylguanidine. Whether these substances, as well as *creatine,* a metabolic precursor of creatinine, and the other compounds cited above, are of clinical importance in the pathogenesis of uremic toxicity remains to be established.

Nitrogenous compounds of larger molecular weight are also retained in CRF. A toxic role for these substances has been suggested because of the impression that patients treated with intermittent peritoneal dialysis are less troubled with neuropathy than patients maintained on chronic hemodialysis, despite higher levels of urea and creatinine in blood in the former group. Since the clearance of small molecules depends mainly upon blood and dialysate flow rates, which are higher with hemodialysis, whereas clearance of larger molecules depends more on membrane surface area and time, which are greater with peritoneal dialysis, this latter form of therapy may be a more effective means of removing these substances of larger molecular weight. A multicenter study examining clearance of small vs. middle-sized molecular substances, dialysis time, and morbidity indicated that urea or other small-molecular-weight substances play a more important role. Evidence that removal of "middle" molecules is associated with objective improvement in clinical well-being is unsubstantiated. The role of middle molecules in the uremic syndrome remains speculative.

Not all these middle-sized molecules accumulate in uremic plasma because of decreased renal excretion alone. The kidney normally *catabolizes* a number of circulating plasma proteins and polypeptides; with reduced renal mass, this capacity may be impaired greatly. Furthermore, plasma levels of many polypeptide hormones [including parathyroid hormone (PTH), insulin, glucagon, growth hormone, luteinizing hormone, and prolactin] rise with advancing renal failure, often markedly so, not only because of impaired renal catabolism but also because of enhanced secretion. Of these, excessive parathyroid hormone (PTH) may be an important uremic "toxin" because of its adverse effect on several organ systems. The consequences of high circulating levels of PTH and other hormones in chronic renal failure are considered below and in Chap. 222.

EFFECTS OF UREMIA ON CELLULAR FUNCTIONS

Alterations in the composition of intracellular and extracellular fluids in CRF have long been recognized. Such abnormalities are believed to be a consequence, at least in part, of *defective ion transport* across cell membranes generally, with retained uremic toxins possibly mediating these alterations in transmembrane ion transport. Integrity of cellular volume and composition depends to a large extent on the active outward transport of Na^+ from cell interior to exterior, the resulting intracellular fluid being relatively low in Na^+ and high in K^+, whereas the reverse is true for extracellular fluid. Active Na^+ transport is a metabolically costly process, accounting for a major fraction of basal energy utilization and oxygen consumption. The consequences of this efflux of Na^+ from cells are many and include, most notably, (1) the generation of a resting electrical potential difference across the cell membrane (with this transcellular voltage oriented so that cell interior is electronegative to cell exterior), and (2) a mechanism for enhancing the influx of K^+ into cells.

In experimental animals, partial inhibition of this active efflux mechanism for Na^+ across cell membranes leads to alterations in body composition and cell functions similar to those demonstrable in erythrocytes, leukocytes, skeletal muscle, and other tissues obtained from uremic subjects. These include increased and decreased intracellular concentrations of Na^+ and K^+, respectively, and reduction in magnitude of the transcellular voltage. These alterations have been shown to be largely reversed by efficient hemodialysis and, for erythrocytes at least, to be recreated when cells from normal subjects are incubated in uremic serum. Other derangements in cellular function have also been implicated as causes for altered body composition in uremia. For example, *Na^+- and K^+-stimulated ATPase activity* is decreased in erythrocytes and brain from uremic patients and animals, respectively. Whether the "uremic toxins" that account for these derangements in cellular function represent abnormally retained products of metabolism which fail to be excreted or normal substances present in increased quantities in response to reduced renal mass remains unknown. *Parathyroid and natriuretic hormones*, examples of this category of substances, are discussed in this context in Chap. 222.

EFFECTS OF UREMIA ON WHOLE-BODY COMPOSITION

What is the impact of these disturbances in active transcellular Na^+ transport on the uremic organism as a whole? From the pathophysiologic considerations already discussed, CRF is likely to lead to abnormally high intracellular Na^+ concentrations, and hence to osmotically induced overhydration of cells generally, whereas these same cells are thought to be relatively deficient in K^+. With the inevitable onset of malaise, anorexia, nausea, vomiting, and diarrhea, patients with CRF may eventually develop protein-calorie malnutrition and negative nitrogen balance, often with profound losses of lean body mass and fat deposits. Owing to the concomitant tendency for salt and water retention, these losses often go unnoticed until the late stages of CRF. Whereas a large fraction of the increase in total-body water in uremia is the result of expansion of intracellular volume, extracellular volume expansion also is observed commonly. With initiation of intermittent hemodialysis or renal transplantation, there is often an immediate and substantial loss of body weight, due primarily to correction of this overhydration. With successful transplantation, the initial diuresis is followed by a period of weight gain, due to restoration of lean body mass and fat deposits to preillness levels. For patients on chronic dialysis, the anabolic response is less dramatic, even when therapy is regarded as optimal, involving mainly reaccumulation of fat deposits. The failure to restore lean body mass to normal with chronic dialysis may reflect insufficient intake of protein, which, in adequately dialyzed patients, should be maintained at levels of 0.8 to 1.4 g per kilogram of body weight per day.

Deficits in intracellular K^+ concentration in CRF have already been mentioned and may result from inadequate intake (poor diet or overzealous K^+ restriction by the physician), excessive losses (vomiting, diarrhea, diuretics), reduction of Na^+- and K^+-stimulated ATPase, or a combination of these. In addition to promoting losses of K^+ into urine (which may be substantial if urine volume remains relatively normal in uremic subjects), the high levels of plasma aldosterone often seen in CRF may also augment net secretion of K^+ into the colon, thereby contributing to marked K^+ losses in stool or diarrheal fluids. Despite deficits in intracellular K^+ concentration, serum K^+ is usually normal or high in CRF, owing most often to metabolic acidosis, which induces an efflux of K^+ from cells. Additionally, uremic patients are relatively resistant to the action of insulin (see below), which normally enhances K^+ uptake by skeletal muscle.

EFFECTS OF UREMIA ON METABOLISM

HYPOTHERMIA   In animals injections of urine, urea, or other retained toxic metabolites can induce hypothermia, and basal heat production diminishes soon after nephrectomy. Since active Na^+ transport across cell membranes accounts for a major proportion of basal energy production, the inverse relationship between body temperature and degree of azotemia is due, probably in part, to inhibition of the sodium pump by some retained toxin(s). Dialysis usually returns body temperature to normal.

CARBOHYDRATE METABOLISM   The ability to metabolize glucose is impaired in most patients with CRF. The defect largely involves a slowing of the rate at which blood glucose concentration declines to the normal range after administration of a glucose load. Fasting blood sugar levels are usually normal or only slightly elevated; severe hyperglycemia and/or ketosis is uncommon. Consequently, the *glucose intolerance of CRF* usually does not require specific therapy (hence the term *azotemic pseudodiabetes*). Because insulin depends to a large extent on the kidney for its removal from plasma and degradation, circulating insulin levels tend to be increased in uremia. Whereas insulin levels in plasma are only slightly to moderately increased in most fasting uremic subjects, levels in excess of normal are usually found in response to a glucose load. The response to intravenous insulin in patients with CRF is also abnormal, and the rate of utilization of glucose by peripheral tissues often is diminished. The glucose intolerance of uremia results largely from this peripheral resistance to the action of insulin. Other possible factors contributing to glucose intolerance include intracellular deficits of potassium, metabolic acidosis, increased levels of glucagon and other hormones including catecholamines, growth hormone, and prolactin, as well as the myriad of potentially toxic metabolites retained in CRF. In true insulin-dependent diabetics, there is often a decrease in insulin requirement with progressive azotemia, a phenomenon not related solely to decreased caloric intake.

NITROGEN AND LIPID METABOLISM   Since the capacity to eliminate the nitrogenous end products of protein catabolism is reduced, CRF may be regarded as a state of *protein intolerance*. As discussed above, retention of the end products of nitrogen metabolism is a dominant cause of the signs and symptoms of uremic toxicity.

Hypertriglyceridemia and decreased high-density lipoprotein cholesterol are common in uremia, whereas cholesterol levels in plasma are usually normal. Whether uremia accelerates triglyceride production by the liver and intestine is unknown. The well-known lipogenic effect of hyperinsulinism may contribute to increased triglyceride synthesis. The rate of removal of triglycerides from the circulation, which depends in large part on the enzyme *lipoprotein lipase*, is depressed in uremia, an effect not corrected appreciably by hemodialysis. The high incidence of premature atherosclerosis in patients on chronic dialysis (see "Cardiovascular and Pulmonary Abnormalities" below) may be related in part to these abnormalities in lipid metabolism.

CLINICAL ABNORMALITIES IN UREMIA

The diagnosis of chronic renal failure is based on recognition of a constellation of signs and symptoms with or without reduced urine output but always with elevation in serum urea nitrogen and creatinine concentrations. As pointed out in Chap. 222, elevation of serum urea nitrogen and creatinine occur late in the course of renal failure. Differentiation between acute and chronic renal failure can be difficult. The history is often most helpful, particularly if normal renal function existed prior to a sudden recent insult. The laboratory findings and physical examination may not be helpful in the differentiation. The hallmark of chronic renal failure is the presence of reduced kidney size on either ultrasound, abdominal scout film, or pyelogram. In the absence of small kidneys, renal biopsy may be necessary for diagnosis.

As noted earlier, CRF leads ultimately to disturbances in function of every organ system. With the application of chronic dialysis in the past three decades, the incidence and severity of these disturbances have been modified, so that where modern medicine is practiced, the overt and florid manifestations of uremia have largely disappeared. Unfortunately, however, even optimal dialysis therapy is not a panacea for the patient with CRF, because, as indicated in Table 224-2, some disturbances resulting from impaired renal function fail to respond fully, while others progress despite dialysis treatment. Furthermore, as with many complex therapeutic modalities, intermittent dialysis may be responsible for the appearance of unique abnormalities not seen prior to initiation of therapy; these abnormalities should be viewed as complications of dialysis.

FLUID, ELECTROLYTE, AND ACID-BASE DISORDERS (See also Chaps. 50 and 51) **Sodium and volume homeostasis** In most patients with stable CRF, modest increases in total body Na^+ and water content can be documented, although objective signs of extracellular fluid (ECF) volume expansion may not be apparent. With ingestion of excessive amounts of salt and water, however, control of excess volume becomes an important clinical and therapeutic consideration. In general, excessive *salt* ingestion contributes to, or aggravates, congestive heart failure, hypertension, ascites, and edema. On the other hand, hyponatremia and weight gain are the consequence of excessive ingestion of *water*, abnormalities which in most patients are relatively mild or asymptomatic. In most patients, daily intake of fluid equal in volume to urine volume per day plus about 500 mL usually maintains the serum Na^+ concentration at normal levels. Hypernatremia is relatively infrequent in CRF. In the edematous patient with CRF not on dialysis, diuretics and modest restriction of salt and water intake are the mainstays of therapy. In volume-expanded dialysis patients, management should include ultrafiltration and restriction of salt and water intake between dialyses.

Patients with CRF have impaired renal mechanisms for conserving Na^+ and water (see Chap. 222). When an *extrarenal* cause for increased fluid loss is present (e.g., vomiting, diarrhea, fever), these patients are prone to develop ECF volume depletion, with signs and symptoms of dry mouth and other mucous membranes, dizziness, syncope, tachycardia, decreased filling of jugular veins, orthostatic hypotension, and vascular collapse. Depletion of extracellular fluid volume typically results in deterioration of residual renal function and, in the previously stable and asymptomatic patient with mild CRF, signs and symptoms of overt uremia. Cautious fluid repletion usually restores extracellular and intravascular volumes to normal and often, but not always, returns renal function to previously stable levels.

Potassium homeostasis Derangements in K^+ balance (see Chaps. 50 and 222) are occasionally documented by laboratory analysis in patients with CRF but are rarely responsible for clinical symptoms unless GFR is below 5 mL/min or an endogenous (hemolysis, trauma, infection) or exogenous (stored blood, K^+-containing medications) K^+ load is administered. Despite progression of renal failure, most patients maintain normal serum K^+ concentrations until the final stages of uremia. This ability to sustain K^+ balance with

TABLE 224-2 Clinical abnormalities in uremia*

FLUID AND ELECTROLYTE DISTURBANCES

Volume expansion and contraction (I)
Hypernatremia and hyponatremia (I)
Hyperkalemia and hypokalemia (I)
Metabolic acidosis (I)
Hyperphosphatemia and hypophosphatemia (I)
Hypocalcemia (I)

ENDOCRINE-METABOLIC DISTURBANCES

Renal osteodystrophy (I or P)
Osteomalacia (D)
Secondary hyperparathyroidism (I or P)
Carbohydrate intolerance (I)
Hyperuricemia (I or P)
Hypothermia (I)
Hypertriglyceridemia (P)
Protein-calorie malnutrition (I or P)
Impaired growth and development (P)
Infertility and sexual dysfunction (P)
Amenorrhea (P)
Dialysis (amyloid, beta$_2$ microglobulin) arthropathy (D)

NEUROMUSCULAR DISTURBANCES

Fatigue (I)
Sleep disorders (P)
Headache (I or P)
Impaired mentation (I)
Lethargy (I)
Asterixis (I)
Muscular irritability (I)
Peripheral neuropathy (I or P)
Restless legs syndrome (I or P)
Paralysis (I or P)
Myoclonus (I)
Seizures (I or P)
Coma (I)
Muscle cramps (D)
Dialysis disequilibrium syndrome (D)
Dialysis dementia (D)
Myopathy (P or D)

CARDIOVASCULAR AND PULMONARY DISTURBANCES

Arterial hypertension (I or P)
Congestive heart failure or pulmonary edema (I)
Pericarditis (I)
Cardiomyopathy (I or P)
Uremic lung (I)
Accelerated atherosclerosis (P or D)
Hypotension and arrhythmias (D)

DERMATOLOGIC DISTURBANCES

Pallor (I or P)
Hyperpigmentation (I, P, or D)
Pruritus (P)
Ecchymoses (I or P)
Uremic frost (I)

GASTROINTESTINAL DISTURBANCES

Anorexia (I)
Nausea and vomiting (I)
Uremic fetor (I)
Gastroenteritis (I)
Peptic ulcer (I or P)
Gastrointestinal bleeding (I, P, or D)
Hepatitis (D)
Refractory ascites on hemodialysis (D)
Peritonitis (D)

HEMATOLOGIC AND IMMUNOLOGIC DISTURBANCES

Normocytic, normochromic anemia (P)
Microcytic (aluminum-induced) anemia (D)
Lymphocytopenia (P)
Bleeding diathesis (I or D)
Increased susceptibility to infection (I or P)
Splenomegaly and hypersplenism (P)
Leukopenia (D)
Hypocomplementemia (D)

* Virtually all the abnormalities contained in this table are completely reversed in time by successful renal transplantation. The response of these abnormalities to hemo- or peritoneal dialysis therapy is more variable. (I) denotes an abnormality that usually improves with an optimal program of dialysis and related therapy. (P) denotes an abnormality that tends to persist or even progress, despite an optimal program. (D) denotes an abnormality that develops only after initiation of dialysis therapy.

advancing renal failure is due to adaptations in the renal distal tubules and colon, sites where aldosterone and other factors serve to enhance K^+ secretion (see Chap. 222). Not surprisingly, oliguria, or disruption of key adaptive mechanisms, can lead to *hyperkalemia* and its potentially ominous effects on cardiac function. Antikaliuretic drugs such as spironolactone, triamterene, or amiloride should be used with extreme caution in chronic renal failure. Likewise, angiotensin-converting enzyme inhibitors and beta blockers may be a cause of hyperkalemia. In the transplanted patient, cyclosporin A is another common cause of increased serum potassium. Hyperkalemia in CRF may also be induced by abrupt lowering of arterial blood pH, since acidosis is associated with efflux of K^+ from intracellular to extracellular fluids. A useful index of the magnitude of this hydrogen-potassium exchange is that for every 0.1-unit change in blood pH, there will be a reciprocal change in serum K^+ concentration of approximately 0.6 mmol/L. Correction of acidosis-induced hyperkalemia with sodium bicarbonate is the treatment of choice. Intravenous insulin and dextrose are useful in lowering serum potassium acutely, while the ion exchange resin sodium polystyrene sulfonate is useful in longer-term control of hyperkalemia. When hyperkalemia persists in the absence of excessive K^+ intake, oliguria, or acute acidosis, the possibility of *hyporeninemic hypoaldosteronism* should be considered. Patients with this syndrome have reduced circulating levels of renin and aldosterone in the plasma and often also have diabetes mellitus.

Hypokalemia due to diminished ability of the kidneys to conserve K^+ is uncommon in most forms of CRF. When hypokalemia occurs in these patients, poor dietary K^+ intake, usually in association with excessive diuretic therapy or gastrointestinal losses, is likely to be the underlying cause. When hypokalemia occurs as a result of primary K^+ wasting in urine, it may represent a solitary renal reabsorptive defect or, more commonly, may be associated with other solute transport abnormalities, as in Fanconi's syndrome, renal tubular acidosis, or other forms of hereditary or acquired tubulointerstitial diseases (see Chaps. 229 and 231). A discussion of the clinical consequences and management of hypokalemia and hyperkalemia is given in Chap. 50.

Metabolic acidosis   With advancing renal failure, total daily acid excretion and buffer production fall below the level needed to maintain external balance of hydrogen ions. Metabolic acidosis is the inevitable result, and the mechanisms involved are considered in Chap. 222. In most patients with stable renal insufficiency, administration of 20 to 30 mmol sodium bicarbonate or sodium citrate per day usually corrects the acidosis. In response to a sudden acid challenge (whether from an endogenous or exogenous source), however, patients with CRF are susceptible to acidosis, which requires more substantial quantities of alkali for correction. Administration of sodium must be carried out with careful attention to the patient's volume status.

Phosphate, calcium, and bone   As discussed in detail in Chap. 222, hypocalcemia in chronic renal failure results from the impaired ability of the diseased kidney to synthesize 1,25-dihydroxyvitamin D [$1,25(OH_2)D$], the active metabolite of vitamin D (Fig. 224-1). Reabsorption of calcium in the gut is impaired when circulating levels of this active metabolite are low. Also serum phosphate concentration begins to rise when GFR falls below about 25 percent of normal. Calcium deposition in bone is dependent on the availability of phosphate; retention of phosphate in plasma, therefore, facilitates calcium entry into bone and contributes to the hypocalcemia and elevation of plasma PTH levels in CRF. Finally, in advanced CRF, the ability of PTH to mobilize calcium salts from bone may be altered. Despite these various causes of hypocalcemia, symptoms of tetany are rare unless patients are treated with large amounts of alkali.

Overproduction of parathyroid hormone, disordered vitamin D metabolism, chronic metabolic acidosis, and excessive fecal losses of calcium all contribute to the bone diseases in uremia (Fig. 224-1). *Renal* and *metabolic osteodystrophy* are imprecise terms that encompass a number of skeletal abnormalities, including osteomalacia, osteitis fibrosa cystica, osteosclerosis, and, in children especially, impaired bone growth. Although clinical symptoms of bone disease are uncommon, occurring in less than 10 percent of predialysis patients with advanced renal failure, radiologic and histologic abnormalities are observed in, respectively, about 35 and 90 percent. In patients treated by dialysis for several years, symptoms of bone disease are a major cause of morbidity. Renal osteodystrophy is more common in children than in adults, and especially in patients with congenital renal anomalies associated with slowly progressive renal insufficiency. On radiologic examination, three types of lesions can be identified: (1) changes analogous to those in children with nutritional rickets, namely, widened osteoid seams at the growth margin of

FIGURE 224-1   Pathogenesis of bone diseases in chronic renal failure.

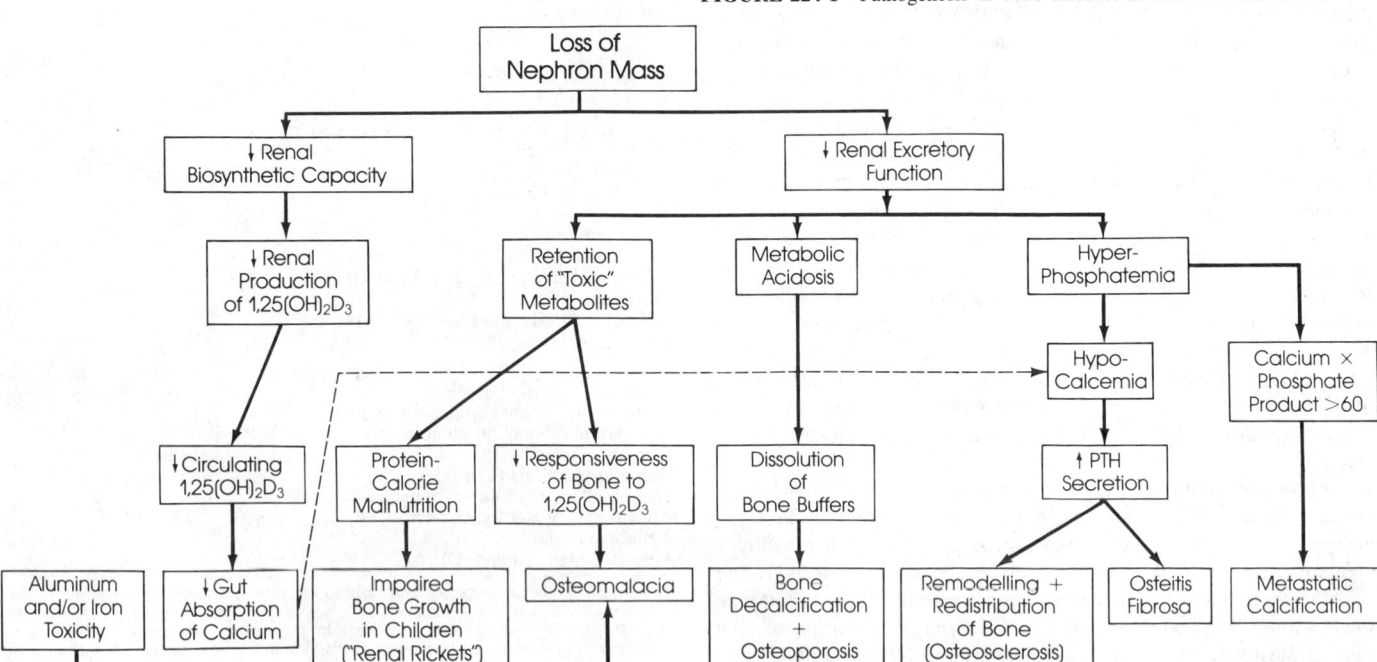

bones (so-called renal rickets); (2) the bone changes of *secondary hyperparathyroidism (osteitis fibrosa cystica)*, characterized by osteoclastic bone resorption and manifested by subperiosteal erosions, especially of the phalanges, long bones, and distal ends of the clavicles; and (3) *osteosclerosis,* often best evidenced by enhanced bone density in the upper and lower margins of vertebrae, producing the so-called rugger jersey spine.

Osteomalacia was initially thought to be secondary to decreased availability of 1,25(OH$_2$)D. There is now evidence that osteomalacia is also due to deposition of aluminum in the calcification fronts. The sources are aluminum in dialysate as well as aluminum-containing phosphate-binding agents. In aluminum-induced osteomalacia, the serum level of parathyroid hormone is usually low and that of calcium is often high. With osteitis fibrosa cystica and osteomalacia there is a tendency to spontaneous fractures which are often slow to heal. The ribs are most commonly involved. Painful joints may occur due to calcium deposition in bursa and other periarticular structures. Bone pain may be seen in the absence of fractures. When bone pain is severe, a proximal *myopathy* often coexists, giving rise to gait abnormalities and even leading to cessation of ambulation. The incidence of *aseptic necrosis of the hip* is increased in renal transplant recipients, probably related to chronic glucocorticoid therapy, secondary hyperparathyroidism, and altered vitamin D metabolism. In CRF there is often a tendency to *extraosseous,* or *metastatic, calcification,* especially when the calcium-phosphate product is very high. Medium-sized blood vessels; subcutaneous, articular, and periarticular tissues; myocardium; eyes; and lungs are common sites of metastatic calcification. An arthropathy in chronic dialysis patients is associated with deposition of amyloid or beta$_2$ microglobulin. The cause is unknown but may be related to chronic exposure of blood to certain dialysis membranes.

Management of renal osteodystrophy includes reduction in dietary phosphate available for absorption through the use of a restricted phosphate diet as well as phosphate-binding agents. Calcium carbonate is the preferred phosphate-binding agent, but in some circumstances a combination of aluminum hydroxide and calcium carbonate is necessary. Dialysate calcium, oral calcium, aluminum hydroxide, and calcitriol or dihydrotachysterol must be properly balanced to maintain the serum phosporus at approximately 1.4 mmol/L (4.5 mg/dL) and the serum calcium at approximately 2.5 mmol/L (10 mg/dL) in an attempt to improve osteitis fibrosa cystica, osteomalacia, and myopathy. Treatment should be initiated early in chronic renal failure so that secondary hyperparathyroidism and bone disease may be prevented. It is particularly important to keep the calcium-phosphorous product in the normal range to avoid metastatic calcification or any possible role of these substances in progressive renal insufficiency.

Other solutes Other derangements in CRF include *hyperuricemia* and *hypermagnesemia*. Uric acid retention is a common feature of CRF but rarely leads to symptomatic gout. Hypophosphatemia is usually a consequence of overzealous oral administration of phosphate-binding gels. Because serum magnesium levels tend to rise in CRF, magnesium-containing antacids and cathartics should be avoided.

CARDIOVASCULAR AND PULMONARY ABNORMALITIES Fluid retention in uremic patients often results in congestive heart failure and/or pulmonary edema. A unique form of pulmonary congestion and edema may occur even in the absence of volume overload and is associated with normal or mildly elevated intracardiac and pulmonary wedge pressures. This entity, characterized radiologically by perihilar vascular congestion giving rise to a "butterfly wing" distribution, is due to increased permeability of the alveolar capillary membrane. This low-pressure pulmonary edema, as well as cardiopulmonary abnormalities associated with circulatory overload, usually responds promptly to vigorous dialysis.

Arterial hypertension is the most common complication of end-stage renal disease. When it is not present, the patient either has a salt-wasting form of renal disease (e.g., polycystic or medullary cystic disease or chronic pyelonephritis), is receiving antihypertensive therapy, or is volume-depleted, the last condition usually being due to excessive gastrointestinal fluid losses or overzealous diuretic therapy. Since fluid overload is the major cause of hypertension in uremic subjects, the normotensive state can usually be restored by dialysis. Nevertheless, some patients remain hypertensive, despite rigorous salt and water restriction and ultrafiltration, because of hyperreninemia. In most cases, routine antihypertensive drug therapy is effective. A small minority of these patients develop *accelerated or malignant hypertension,* manifested by markedly elevated systolic and diastolic pressures, severe hyperreninemia, encephalopathy, seizures, retinal changes, and papilledema. Use of drugs such as diazoxide, minoxidil, captopril, enalapril and nitroprusside, along with control of extracellular volume, generally controls such hypertension.

Pericarditis, once a common complication of CRF, is now infrequent because of early initiation of dialysis. Retained metabolic toxins are thought to be the cause of *pericarditis.* The unusual occurrence of pericarditis in the well-dialyzed patient is usually due to viral infection or systemic disease.

The clinical presentation of pericarditis in uremic subjects is generally similar to that of other etiologies (Chap. 193), except that pericardiocentesis for effusions usually yields hemorrhagic fluid. Treatment with intensive dialysis is recommended, and systemic anticoagulation should be avoided to minimize the occurrence of hemorrhagic tamponade. In some patients, pericardiocentesis with intrapericardial instillation of air or glucocorticoids is effective for pericardial tamponade. Pericardiectomy should be considered only after more conservative treatment has failed.

Chronically dialyzed patients have a disturbingly high incidence of *accelerated atherosclerosis,* leading to development of significant coronary, cerebral, and peripheral vascular manifestations. There are ample causes for these complications, including hypertension, hyperlipidemia, glucose intolerance, chronic high cardiac output, and metastatic vascular and myocardial calcification.

HEMATOLOGIC ABNORMALITIES *Normochromic, normocytic anemia* occurs regularly in CRF and contributes to fatigability and listlessness in these patients. Erythropoiesis is depressed in CRF, due both to the effects of retained toxins on bone marrow and to diminished biosynthesis of erythropoietin by the diseased kidney or to the presence of erythropoietin inhibitors. The use of recombinant human erythropoietin results in a dramatic increase in hematocrit and hemoglobin suggesting that reduced serum erythropoietin is perhaps the more important of these factors. The anemia of chronic uremia may also be due in part to aluminum intoxication, which causes a microcytic anemia, fibrosis of the bone marrow due to hyperparathyroidism, and, occasionally, inadequate replacement of folic acid. *Hemolysis* also occurs and involves an extracorpuscular defect since survival of erythrocytes from normal subjects is reduced when these cells are transfused into uremic patients, and erythrocytes from patients with CRF have relatively normal survival times when transfused into normal individuals. Gastrointestinal and chronic dialyzer *blood loss* contributes to anemia, as does *hypersplenism* in the occasional patient. Blood loss is exaggerated in hemodialysis patients because of the need for heparin during dialysis. Transfusions may contribute to suppression of erythropoiesis in CRF and, due to increased risk of hepatitis and hemosiderosis, should be avoided unless anemia aggravates other underlying disorders (for example, coronary or cerebrovascular disease). Androgen therapy has been shown to improve erythropoiesis in some dialysis patients not previously subjected to nephrectomy. Parenteral or oral iron therapy is indicated only in patients with documented iron deficiency due to chronic blood loss. In those patients in whom multiple blood transfusions have been administered, one should consider the possibility of hemachromatosis. Folic and ascorbic acids and the soluble B vitamins should be given to offset chronic losses of these substances via dialysis. As indicated above, clinical trials with recombinant human erythropoietin show this agent to be extremely effective in correcting anemia. Commercial availability of erythropoietin is expected in the near future.

Abnormal hemostasis is another common derangement in CRF, characterized by a tendency to abnormal bleeding and bruising. Bleeding from the surgical wounds or spontaneously into the gastrointestinal tract, pericardial sac, and intracranial vault, in the form of subdural hematoma or intracerebral hemorrhage, is of greatest concern. Prolongation of bleeding time, decreased platelet factor III activity, abnormal platelet aggregation and adhesiveness, and impaired prothrombin consumption contribute to the clotting defects. The abnormality in factor III correlates with increased plasma levels of guanidinosuccinic acid and can largely be corrected by dialysis. Prolongation of the bleeding time is common even in the well-dialyzed patient. Abnormal bleeding times and coagulopathy in renal failure may be reversed with desmopressin, cryoprecipitate, conjugated estrogens, and blood transfusions, and possibly by use of recombinant human erythropoietin.

A wide variety of changes in leukocyte formation and function also occur in uremia leading to *enhanced susceptibility to infection.* Lymphocytopenia and atrophy of lymphoid structures occur in CRF, whereas neutrophil production is relatively unimpaired. Nevertheless, all leukocyte cell types may be affected adversely by uremic serum. Decreased chemotaxis is among the best documented of the defects occurring in uremic leukocytes, with resulting impairment of acute inflammatory response and decreased delayed hypersensitivity. There is a tendency for uremic patients to have less fever in response to infection. For these reasons, infections may be difficult to recognize in uremia. Leukocyte function may also be impaired in patients with CRF because of coexisting acidosis, hyperglycemia, protein-calorie malnutrition, and serum and tissue hyperosmolarity (due to azotemia). Mucosal barriers to infection may also be defective, and, in dialysis patients, vascular access devices are also common portals of entry for pathogens, particularly staphylococci. Glucocorticoids and immunosuppressive drugs add further to the risk of serious infection in many of these patients. Leukopenia is a common transient finding in patients exposed to cellophane-derived membranes during dialysis (Chap. 225).

NEUROMUSCULAR ABNORMALITIES Subtle disturbances of central nervous system function, including inability to concentrate, drowsiness, and insomnia, are among the earliest symptoms of uremia. Mild behavioral changes, loss of memory, and errors in judgment soon follow and often are associated with signs of neuromuscular irritability, including hiccups, cramps, and fasciculations and twitching of large muscle groups. Asterixis, myoclonus, and chorea are common in terminal uremia, as are stupor, seizures, and coma. Many of these neuromuscular complications of severe uremia resolve with dialysis, although nonspecific EEG abnormalities may persist.

Peripheral neuropathy is a common complication of advanced CRF. Initially, sensory nerve involvement exceeds motor, lower extremities are involved more than the upper, and the distal portions of the extremities more than proximal. The "restless legs syndrome," characterized by ill-defined sensations of discomfort in the feet and lower legs and frequent leg movement, is a disturbing complication. If dialysis is not instituted soon after onset of sensory abnormalities, motor involvement follows, often leading to loss of deep tendon reflexes, weakness, peroneal nerve palsy (foot drop), and, eventually, flaccid quadriplegia. Accordingly, early evidence of peripheral neuropathy is generally taken as a firm indication to initiate dialysis or transplantation.

Two types of neurologic disturbances appear to be unique to patients on chronic dialysis. One is the syndrome of *dialysis dementia,* seen in patients who have been on dialysis for a number of years. This syndrome is characterized by speech dyspraxia, myoclonus, dementia, and eventually seizures and death. Aluminum intoxication is probably a major contributor to this syndrome. Other factors (viral infection?) also likely play a role since only a small percent of patients with increased aluminum exposure develop the syndrome. The other disturbance, dialysis disequilibrium, occurs during the first few dialyses, in association with rapid reduction of blood urea levels.

Nausea, vomiting, drowsiness, headache, and even grand mal seizures have been attributed to the more rapid (dialysis-induced) pH change and reduction in osmolality of extracellular than intracellular fluids within the cranium, leading to cerebral edema and raised intracranial pressure.

GASTROINTESTINAL ABNORMALITIES Anorexia, hiccups, nausea, and vomiting are common and early manifestations of uremia. The use of carefully monitored protein restriction in the diet may be useful to slow progression of renal insufficiency if initiated early. Protein restriction is also useful in diminishing nausea and vomiting late in the course. Protein restriction should not, of course, be implemented in those patients with severe protein-calorie malnutrition. *Uremic fetor,* a uriniferous odor to the breath, derives from the breakdown of urea in saliva to ammonia and is often associated with unpleasant taste sensation. Mucosal ulcerations leading to blood loss can occur at any level of the gastrointestinal tract in very late stages of CRF—so-called uremic gastroenteritis. Peptic ulcer disease is particularly common, occurring in as many as one-fourth of uremic subjects. Whether this high incidence is related to increased gastric acidity, hypersecretion of gastrin, or secondary hyperparathyroidism is unknown. Most of the gastrointestinal symptoms, except those related to peptic ulcer disease, usually improve with dialysis. A syndrome of idiopathic ascites is seen rarely in patients on chronic dialysis, presumably secondary to fluid overload and/or chronic passive hepatic congestion. Patients with chronic renal failure, particularly those with polycystic kidney disease, have an increased incidence of diverticulosis. Hbs Ag hepatitis is more common in patients on chronic dialysis and is discussed in detail in Chap. 225.

ENDOCRINE-METABOLIC DISTURBANCES The common disturbances in parathyroid function, glucose, and insulin metabolism, as well as the lipid, protein-calorie, and other nutritional abnormalities of uremia have already been considered. In general, pituitary, thyroid, and adrenal gland functions are relatively normal, often despite abnormalities in circulating thyroxine, growth hormone, aldosterone, and cortisol levels. In women, estrogen levels are low, and amenorrhea and inability to carry pregnancies to term are early manifestations of uremia. While menses frequently reappear after chronic dialysis is initiated, successful pregnancies remain rare. In men with CRF, including those on chronic dialysis, impotence, oligospermia, and germinal cell dysplasia are common, as are reduced plasma testosterone levels. As with growth, sexual maturation is often impaired in adolescent children, even among those on chronic dialysis.

DERMATOLOGIC ABNORMALITIES The skin shows many abnormalities. This is not surprising in view of anemia (pallor), defective hemostasis (ecchymoses and hematomas), calcium deposition and secondary hyperparathyroidism (pruritus, excoriations), dehydration (poor skin turgor, dry mucous membranes), and the general cutaneous consequences of protein-calorie malnutrition. A sallow, yellow cast may reflect the combined influences of anemia and retention of a variety of pigmented metabolites, or *urochromes.* In advanced uremia urea concentrations in sweat may reach sufficiently high levels that, after evaporation, a fine white powder can be found on the skin surface—so-called uremic (urea) frost. Although many of these cutaneous abnormalities improve with dialysis, *uremic pruritus* is usually resistant to most systemic and topical therapies. Hemochromatosis causes a slate-gray–bronze discoloration of the skin and is common in the dialysis patient who has received multiple transfusions.

REFERENCES

ACCHIARDO SR et al: Malnutrition as the main factor in morbidity and mortality of hemodialysis patients. Kidney Int 24:S199, 1983

ANDERSON S, BRENNER BM: Effects of aging on the renal glomerulus. Am J Med 80:435, 1986

ANDRASSY K, RITZ E: Uremia as a cause of bleeding. Am J Nephrol 5:313, 1985

DEYKIN D: Uremic bleeding. Kidney Int 24:698, 1983

DUMBAULD S et al: Carbohydrate metabolism during fasting in chronic hemodialysis patients. Kidney Int 24:222, 1983

ESCHBACH JW et al: Correction of the anemia of end-stage renal disease with recombinant human erythropoietin: Results of a combined phase I and II clinical trial. N Engl J Med 316:73, 1987

GOKAL R et al: Iron metabolism in hemodialysis patients: A study of the management of iron therapy and overload. Q J Med 48:369, 1979

GOLDBLUM SE, REED WP: Host defenses and immunologic alterations associated with chronic hemodialysis. Ann Intern Med 93:597, 1980

JUBELIRER SJ: Hemostatic abnormalities in renal disease. Am J Kidney Dis 5:219, 1985

KLAHR S et al: Factors that may retard the progression of renal disease. Kidney Int 32:S35, 1987

KOPPLE JD, MASSRY SG: Uremic toxins: What are they? How are they identified? Semin Nephrol 3:263, 1983

LIM VS: Reproductive function in patients with renal insufficiency. Am J Kidney Dis 9:363, 1987

LIVIO M et al: Conjugated estrogens for the management of bleeding associated with renal failure. N Engl J Med 315:731, 1986

LUGER A et al: Abnormalities in the hypothalamic-pituitary-adrenocortical axis in patients with chronic renal failure. Am J Kidney Dis 9:51, 1987

MAHONEY C et al: Central and peripheral nervous system effects of chronic renal failure. Kidney Int 24:170, 1983

MASSRY SG: Neurotoxicity of parathyroid hormone in uremia. Kidney Int 28:S17, 1985
——— et al: Current status of the use of 1,25(OH)$_2$D$_3$ in the management of renal osteodystrophy. Kidney Int 18:409, 1980

SHERRARD DJ: Renal osteodystrophy. Semin Nephrol 6:56, 1986

SLATOPOLSKY E: The interaction of parathyroid hormone and aluminum in renal osteodystrophy. Kidney Int 31:842, 1987

225 DIALYSIS AND TRANSPLANTATION IN THE TREATMENT OF RENAL FAILURE

CHARLES B. CARPENTER / J. MICHAEL LAZARUS

Over the past four decades, dialysis and transplantation have become effective in prolonging the lives of patients with renal insufficiency. The approach to treatment in acute renal failure is different than in chronic renal failure because of the irreversible nature of the latter. Conservative medical management and dialysis are the mainstays of therapy for acute renal failure. Obviously, transplantation is not a treatment for this group of patients. Options for treatment of patients with *chronic* or *irreversible* renal failure are outlined in Fig. 225-1.

Initially patients are managed with conservative therapy, but eventually they require hemodialysis, peritoneal dialysis, or cadaver or related donor transplantation. Because of limited success with each of these treatment modalities, chronic renal failure should be approached with the concept of moving from one form of therapy to another as indicated by the degree of success and incidence of complications with each.

Therapy for renal failure should be initiated at a time when complications will be moderate, but not when the patient is completely asymptomatic. The advanced complications of uremia, as noted in Chaps. 222 and 224, should be avoided by early treatment. Early dialysis is especially applicable to patients with acute renal failure in whom resumption of renal function can be expected and to patients with chronic renal failure who have a good immunologic match with a related donor. In the latter group, early transplantation will likely

FIGURE 225-1 Options for patients with chronic or irreversible renal failure.

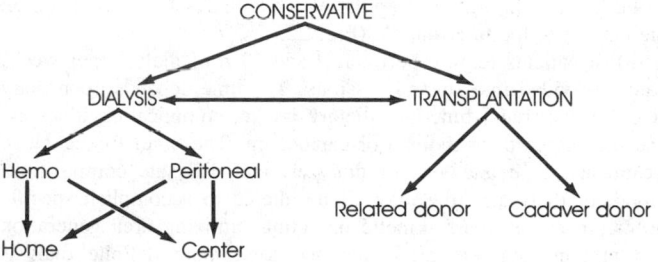

	TABLE 225-1 Contraindications to kidney transplantation

1 Absolute contraindications
  a Reversible renal involvement
  b Ability of conservative measures to maintain useful life
  c Advanced forms of major extrarenal complications (cerebrovascular or coronary disease, neoplasia)
  d Active infection
  e Active glomerulonephritis
  f Previous sensitization to donor tissue
2 Relative contraindications (see text)
  a Age
  b Presence of vesical or urethral abnormalities
  c Iliofemoral occlusive disease
  d Psychiatric problems
  e Oxalosis

lead to resumption of normal renal function. In the remainder of patients, the clinical judgment to move from conservative treatment to dialysis or transplantation is determined by the patient's quality of life and whether or not the benefits of treatment outweigh the risks. Treatment with dietary protein restriction and aggressive control of hypertension, as described in Chap. 224, may prolong the time before dialysis and/or transplantation are required, but should be carried out only if complications of such therapy do not worsen long-term morbidity and mortality.

Selection of patients to receive dialysis and/or transplantation is a matter of some debate. Because of the reversible nature of acute renal failure, *all* patients with this diagnosis should be supported with dialysis, at least for some period of time, to allow return of renal function. In patients with irreversible or chronic renal failure, criteria for selection for transplantation are generally more stringent than those for dialysis and are guided by the possibility of complications related to immunosuppressive therapy. Table 225-1 lists practical considerations in the selection of a recipient for a human renal allograft. Such a procedure should be undertaken only when conservative treatment has failed, when there are no reversible elements in the patient's renal failure, and when the patient is too ill to be maintained comfortably with the usual methods of treatment. However, morbidity is less if transplantation is performed before the patient is critically ill. Transplantation should not be utilized in an attempt to salvage patients from failure to thrive on dialysis.

The recipient should be free of life-threatening extrarenal complications such as cancer, severe coronary artery disease, and cerebrovascular disease. Provided that diffuse vascular involvement is not present, diabetes mellitus is not a contraindication. Oxalosis may recur in relatively short order in a transplanted kidney and is generally a contraindication for this procedure. Although age may be a limiting factor, it is advanced "physiologic" rather than chronologic age which contraindicates transplantation. In general, patients reach a "physiologic" limit at approximately age 60 to 65 years when the incidence of complications due to glucocorticoids becomes much higher than in younger patients. Although abnormalities of the bladder and urethra present additional hazards, successful renal allografts have been placed in individuals with these abnormalities by prior constitution of an artificial bladder (i.e., ileal conduit) into which the donor ureter is placed. Patients with any disease process that may be aggravated by glucocorticoids, cyclosporine, azathioprine, or other immunosuppressive agents, or any patient with medical complications so severe that the risks of operation and drug therapy are high, should not be offered transplantation. In evaluating potential exclusionary diseases, it should be kept in mind that quality of life and long-term results are superior in the *successful* renal transplantation.

Criteria for treatment with hemodialysis or peritoneal dialysis are more liberal since dialysis has less morbidity than transplantation in older patients and those with the aforementioned medical complications. Because of the cost of these programs, some have suggested that entry be restricted in those of advanced age. Such decisions based on moral, social, and economic issues continue to generate debate. In general, nearly all patients are accepted if they or their families desire prolongation of life. In most areas of the world, the cost of medical care for chronic renal failure is borne by government.

CONSERVATIVE TREATMENT

As discussed in Chap. 224, conservative (nondialytic, nontransplant) therapy should be instituted early to control symptoms, minimize complications, prevent long-term sequelae of uremia, and slow the progression of renal insufficiency. Every effort should be made to correct any of the reversible components which aggravate renal impairment. In patients with acute renal failure, prerenal factors, such as volume depletion, decreased cardiac output, or renal artery stenosis, or postrenal components, such as urethral or ureteral obstruction, must be sought and corrected. Such pre- and postrenal components may exacerbate underlying parenchymal disease in patients with chronic renal insufficiency and must be treated in this group as well. Most important is treatment of the underlying disease or complications of renal insufficiency which further hasten the loss of nephrons. Hypertension, urinary tract infections, nephrolithiasis, structural abnormalities of the urinary tract, or those forms of glomerulonephritis which may respond to therapy should be treated aggressively. Preventive aspects include avoidance of nephrotoxic drugs and radiopaque agents in the patient with already compromised renal insufficiency.

Modification of diet is an important aspect of conservative therapy. Early restriction of sodium and fluid may be important in the treatment of hypertension. As renal insufficiency progresses, restriction of foods high in phosphate and potassium is necessary. Reduction of protein content reduces anorexia, nausea, and vomiting and, if initiated early, may retard progression of the disease. Adult patients should receive no less than 0.6 g of protein per kilogram of body weight per day to avoid negative nitrogen balance. Supplementation of low-protein diets with essential ketoamino acid therapy may be useful in prolonging the period of conservative therapy by allowing utilization of urea as a source of nonessential nitrogen. Preliminary results from a study by the multicenter National Institutes of Health/Health Care Financing Administration suggest that control of hypertension may be as important as protein content of the diet. Correction of electrolyte imbalance, e.g., use of sodium bicarbonate or calcium carbonate to correct mild acidosis, or bicarbonate, dextrose and insulin, and potassium exchange resins for treatment of hyperkalemia, is necessary in more advanced states of uremia. Some chemical abnormalities of renal failure do not require or are not amenable to treatment; hypermagnesemia, hyperamylasemia, hypertriglyceridemia, or mild carbohydrate intolerance generally do not require therapy. Treatment of hyperuricemia may be in order if the patient suffers from gout. However, hyperuricemia alone may not be detrimental. Secondary hyperparathyroidism may accentuate progression of renal failure. Whether this is due to hyperphosphatemia, an elevated calcium-phosphorus product, or parathyroid hormone itself is not clear. Nonetheless, vigorous efforts using phosphate-binding agents and calcium supplements and vitamin D products (dihydrotachysterol or calcitriol) to maintain the serum calcium are effective in suppressing parathyroid stimulation, perhaps in slowing renal insufficiency, and likely avoiding severe bone disease later (see Chap. 340). To avoid visceral and vascular calcification, it is important to maintain the calcium-phosphorus product in the physiologic range. Fluid, sodium, potassium, phosphate, and protein restrictions offer the patient a very restricted and often unacceptable diet. This, coupled with the administration of multiple medications, often occurs at a time when the complications of uremia appear and consideration for dialysis and/or transplantation is in order.

While conservative measures are being carried out, it is necessary to prepare the patient with an intensive educational program to explain the possibilities of eventual renal failure and the various forms of therapy available. The more knowledgeable patients are concerning

hemodialysis, peritoneal dialysis, and transplantation, the easier and more appropriate will be their decisions at a later time. With hemodialysis, the major method of obtaining blood for treatment is from an arteriovenous fistula. Since these devices often take several months to develop, prophylactic placement of a fistula in a patient planning for hemodialysis is important in minimizing future complications of circulatory access. For those patients who select peritoneal dialysis (continuous ambulatory peritoneal dialysis—CAPD; or continuous cyclic peritoneal dialysis—CCPD), placement of the peritoneal catheter does not require preparation, and therapy can be instituted as soon as uremic signs and symptoms develop. In those patients who may perform home dialysis or undergo transplantation, early education of family members for selection and preparation as a home dialysis helper or a related donor for transplantation should occur well before the onset of symptomatic renal failure. In those patients who may have a good antigenic match with a willing donor, transplantation without intervening hemodialysis or peritoneal dialysis should be considered. In considering related donor transplantation, the risk of unilateral nephrectomy, including development of proteinuria and hypertension, should be considered. As discussed below, the success rate of cadaver donor transplantation has improved sufficiently that this form of therapy should be carefully considered both with the patient and with family members who are potential donors.

DIALYSIS

HEMODIALYSIS   Hemodialysis employs the process of diffusion across a semipermeable membrane (cellulose acetate, Cupraphane, polyacrilonitrile, polymethylmethacrylate, polysulfone) to remove unwanted substances from the blood while adding desirable components. A constant flow of blood on one side of the membrane and a cleansing solution–dialysate on the other allows removal of waste products in a fashion grossly similar to that of glomerular filtration. By altering the composition of the dialysate, the method of exposure of blood and dialysate (geometry of the dialyzer), the type and surface area of dialysis membrane, and the frequency and duration of exposure, patients without renal function can be maintained in a relatively healthy state. Hemodialysis equipment consists of three components—the blood delivery system, the composition and delivery system of the dialysate, and the dialyzer itself. Blood is pumped to the dialyzer by a roller pump through lines with appropriate equipment to measure flow and pressures within the system; blood flow should be approximately 300 to 350 mL/min. Hydrostatic pressure within the system can be manipulated to achieve desirable fluid removal, so-called ultrafiltration. The dialysate is delivered to the dialyzer from a storage tank or proportioning system which manufactures dialysate on line. In most systems dialysate passes once across the membrane, countercurrent to blood flow at a rate of 500 mL/min, or it may be recirculated multiple times at higher flow rates. The composition of the dialysate is similar to plasma water, but may be altered depending upon the patient's needs. The dialysate potassium is most often varied, but the sodium, calcium, and acetate or bicarbonate may be varied depending upon the situation. The principal type of dialyzer now in use in most dialysis units in the United States is the hollow fiber or capillary dialyzer, in which membrane material is spun into fine capillaries, thousands of which are packed into bundles with blood flowing through the capillaries while dialysate is circulated on the outside of the fiber bundle (Fig. 225-2).

Most patients require between 9 and 12 h of dialysis per week, equally divided into several sessions. The time depends upon body size, residual renal function, dietary intake, complicating illnesses, and the degree of anabolism or catabolism. The time, frequency of treatments, type and size of dialyzer, and dialysate composition, blood, or dialysate flow may all be altered to accomplish specific needs. In recent years, kinetic modeling, utilizing urea generation and protein catabolic rates, has led to a more definite dialysis

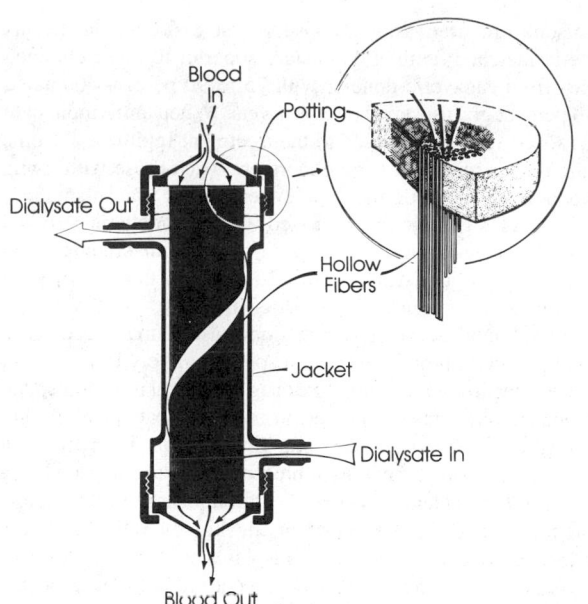

FIGURE 225-2 Hollow fiber or capillary dialyzer; the most commonly used artificial kidney.

prescription. The development of bicarbonate dialysis, variable sodium delivery, high flux or ultraefficient membranes, and urea kinetic modeling has allowed for significant reductions in dialysis time. Clinical trials of this so-called high flux, short-time dialysis are underway. Forms of treatment for the patient with acute renal failure include slow continuous ultrafiltration (SCUF) or continuous arteriovenous hemodialysis (CAVHD)—techniques that employ high efficiency dialyzers with very slow blood and/or dialysate flow rates. This therapy is useful in the unstable, acute renal failure patient and has essentially replaced acute peritoneal dialysis in the ICU and is often preferable to intermittent hemodialysis.

Many complications in the chronic dialysis patient are related to underlying disease or those uremic conditions not reversed by dialytic therapy. These and other related problems of hemodialysis are discussed in Chap. 224. The Achilles' heel of hemodialysis is access to the circulation. The development of the arteriovenous shunt made chronic dialysis possible. This device has had a high failure rate because of infection and thrombosis and led in 1966 to the development of the arteriovenous (AV) fistula. The fistula is preferably created from a native vein, but if not available, a prosthetic conduit (extended polytetrafluoroethylene) subcutaneously placed between an artery and a nearby vein may be utilized. Cannulation of arteriovenous fistulas with 15- to 16-gauge needles allows blood flow sufficient to carry out hemodialysis. Unfortunately, infection, thrombosis, and aneurysm formation also occur in the arteriovenous fistula, particularly in prosthetic devices. There is a relatively high incidence of septicemia and septic embolization associated with shunt and fistula infection; the most common infecting agent is *Staphylococcus aureus*.

In addition, failure of the AV fistula has a significant psychological impact. Depression and altered self-image are common psychiatric problems. The rapid flux in osmolality may cause a disequilibrium syndrome, while rapid changes in electrolytes (particularly potassium) may lead to arrhythmia during dialysis. Hypotension is a common phenomenon during hemodialysis and is due to many factors—the size of the extracorporeal circulation, degree of ultrafiltration, change in serum osmolality, presence of autonomic neuropathy, concomitant use of antihypertensive agents, removal of catecholamines, or infusion of acetate (used as the dialysate buffer) which is a cardiac depressant and vasodilator. Syndromes of dialysis dementia and osteomalacia may be secondary to aluminum contamination of dialysate water or from oral intake of aluminum hydroxide. An increased incidence of HBsAG (hepatitis B surface) antigenemia is related to decreased

immunologic integrity. Patients with chronic antigenemia are usually asymptomatic and have little derangement of liver function. There is a higher rate of non-A, non-B hepatitis and cytomegalovirus infection, but these, too, are usually of mild degree. Patients with AIDS often have renal failure terminally and have poor prognosis with or without dialysis. Because of the high incidence of AIDS in IV drug abusers who also have heroin nephropathy, the presence of HIV-positive patients is now common in dialysis units. There is little to suggest that multiple blood transfusions in dialysis patients have played a role in this incidence. Based on clinical experience and recommendations from the Centers for Disease Control, these patients are treated in dialysis units as are other patients with no special precautions. All patients should receive universal precautions for infection control. Mechanical and/or iatrogenic complications such as hemolysis, air embolus, blood leaks, and contaminated dialysate are less common with improved equipment. Membrane-induced adverse reactions may occur, as exemplified by complement-mediated leukopenia and hypoxemia. More prominent symptoms such as back and chest pain, bronchospasm, and anaphylaxis may rarely occur in this reaction. Heparin, necessary during the hemodialysis procedure, may lead to complications such as subdural hematoma and retroperitoneal, gastrointestinal, pericardial, and pleural hemorrhage. One of the major concerns in long-term dialysis patients is the high incidence of mortality related to myocardial infarction and cerebral vascular accidents. These are likely due to the preexistence and continuation of common risk factors in the uremic patient such as hypertension, hyperlipidemia, vascular calcification due to hyperparathyroidism, and high cardiac output due to anemia or other factors. The potential for complications should cause the physician to evaluate the risk/benefit ratio with dialysis treatment before proceeding in the individual patient. Advantages of hemodialysis are the relatively short treatment time and minimal interruption of life-style between treatments. It is more efficient than peritoneal dialysis, allowing rapid changes in abnormal serum values. Hemodialysis can be performed in the home, but the patient requires an assistant during treatment. It is the most widely utilized form of dialysis.

PERITONEAL DIALYSIS Peritoneal dialysis, like hemodialysis, may be performed in various settings and with a number of different techniques. In patients with acute renal failure, intermittent peritoneal dialysis has largely been displaced by intermittent hemodialysis or CAVHD. Chronic peritoneal dialysis was attempted in the late 1940s but was relatively unsuccessful until development of a permanent peritoneal catheter in 1968—the Tenckhoff catheter. Use of this indwelling catheter and closed continuous cycle dialysate delivery equipment led to treatment protocols with which patients were treated 2 to 3 times per week for a total of 30 to 40 h (intermittent peritoneal dialysis—IPD) to achieve clearances and fluid removal similar to those of hemodialysis. In 1978, the concept of constant peritoneal lavage with prolonged dwell times led to the development of CAPD, which differs from intermittent peritoneal dialysis in that patients instill fluid into the peritoneal cavity, seal the catheter, continue in an ambulatory mode, and every 4 to 6 h empty the peritoneal cavity and replace the dialysate. This technique utilizes 2-L containers of dialysate and obviates the need for dialysis equipment. Modification of the technique using a cyclic dialysate delivery device to exchange dialysate during the night and chronic dwelling of fluid during the waking hours (CCPD) is more acceptable to some patients.

IPD or CCPD may be performed in a center or at home (usually overnight), while CAPD can be performed anywhere. As with hemodialysis, the composition of the dialysate can be modified for ultrafiltration and clearance needs. The major difference in peritoneal dialysate formulas is in the amount of dextrose used as an osmotic agent. Advantages of peritoneal dialysis are avoidance of heparinization and vascular surgery and a slower clearance rate (helpful for some cardiovascular patients). It is more amenable to total self-treatment. Disadvantages include the longer treatment time (intermittently or continuous involvement). It should not be used in patients with extensive abdominal surgery or pulmonary compromise. Inadequate clearance may occur in patients with scleroderma, vasculitis, malignant hypertension, or peritoneal disease. Complications include catheter tunnel infection, peritonitis, moderate protein loss, hypertriglyceridemia, hypercholesterolemia, obesity, and inguinal and abdominal hernias. CAPD is the predominant peritoneal dialysis but requires greater patient compliance and has a higher rate of peritonitis than IPD because of multiple entries into the system.

RESULTS   At the end of 1987, approximately 98,400 patients were on chronic dialysis in the United States. Approximately 85 percent of patients are on hemodialysis, and 15 percent perform peritoneal dialysis. Over the past 20 years nearly 87,000 patients have undergone renal transplantation in this country. Approximately 1800 living related and 7000 cadaver renal transplants are performed in the United States per year. Of new patients with end-stage renal disease, approximately 35 to 50 percent are physically and psychologically suitable for transplantation. Many of these patients are on hemodialysis and peritoneal dialysis awaiting availability of a cadaver kidney. An acutely ill or medically complicated patient will likely undergo dialysis in a hospital dialysis unit or intensive care unit, while stable patients may be dialyzed as outpatients in the hospital dialysis unit, in an out-of-hospital dialysis center, or at home. Most centers attempt to have patients participate in their own care, so-called self-dialysis. Approximately 18,000 patients were performing home dialysis, either hemodialysis or peritoneal dialysis (CAPD or CCPD) at the end of 1987, this number representing 19 percent of all patients on dialysis. Home dialysis (either hemodialysis or peritoneal) is preferable for many because of self-reliance and freedom from hospital or center dialysis schedules. Patient motivation is the primary factor in selection of home or in-center self-dialysis. Dialysis performed in the hospital setting is most expensive, while home dialysis with a nonpaid family assistant or alone (peritoneal dialysis only) is somewhat less expensive than in-center dialysis. Despite absence of equipment, peritoneal dialysis is as expensive as home hemodialysis because of the cost of dialysate and of hospitalization related to an increased incidence of peritonitis. The total amount of Medicare payments for end-stage renal disease (covering hemodialysis, peritoneal dialysis, and transplantation) in the year 1987 was 2.5 billion dollars, substantially greater than anticipated at the initiation of the end-stage renal disease program in 1973. This cost reflects an increasing number of recipients and not an increasing cost per patient.

The mean age for patients on dialysis is the late fifties, partly because nephrosclerosis and eventual renal failure from other parenchymal diseases occur in older patients, but more likely because the selection process favors transplantation in younger patients.

Approximately 10 to 20 percent of patients with chronic renal failure are totally rehabilitated by dialysis, and another 30 to 40 percent of nondiabetic patients may be expected to be rehabilitated to a functional status even if not employed. Twenty percent of patients will be returned to a level of function not considered rehabilitated but able to care for themselves. The remainder (approximately 20 percent) are fully dependent on support from others. Diabetics, who have a rehabilitation rate and survival rate significantly lower than that of nondiabetic patients, make up much of the latter two groups. Determination of mortality rates is variable, related to the age of the patient and the disease process(es) involved. Mean mortality for the entire ESRD program is approximately 18 percent per year. This number has substantially increased over the past 10 years, probably in relation to the increased age and co-morbid complications of this population. In patients less than 45 years of age and with no complicating medical illnesses, mortality with hemodialysis, peritoneal dialysis, or transplantation is below 5 percent per year.

TRANSPLANTATION

Transplantation of the human kidney is frequently appropriate for the treatment of advanced chronic renal failure. Worldwide, tens of thousands of such procedures have been performed. When azathioprine

and prednisone are used as immunosuppressive drugs, the results with properly matched familial donors are superior to those obtained with organs from cadaveric donors, with 75 to 90 percent compared to 50 to 60 percent graft survival rates at 1 year. When antilymphocyte globulins (ALG) have been added to the treatment regimens in some centers, the results with cadaveric donors approach those with living related donors, at least for the first 2 years after transplantation. Cyclosporine has significantly improved 1-year cadaveric survival rates to the 80 percent range, when used along with prednisone in place of azathioprine and ALG. With all therapies, the rate of graft loss from rejection is much slower after the first year, although occasionally an acute irreversible rejection episode may occur after many months of good function. This is especially likely if the patient neglects to take the immunosuppressive drugs. Clinical renal transplant results in recent years have improved in regard to patient morbidity and mortality rates, the latter declining to less than 5 percent in a number of centers. These findings represent an increasing tendency on the part of transplant teams to decrease immunosuppressive therapy so that in the case of severe rejection the kidney rather than the patient is lost. Second and even third transplants are being performed, and the overall results show a 10 to 20 percent reduction in expected survival compared to first transplants; cyclosporine therapy does not erase the increased risk of rejecting subsequent transplants, however. Overall, transplantation returns the majority of patients to a near-normal life-style.

DONOR SELECTION   Donor sources are cadavers or volunteer blood-related living donors. Living volunteer donors should be normal on physical examination and of the same major ABO blood group, because there is good evidence that crossing major blood group barriers prejudices survival of the allograft. It is, however, possible to transplant a kidney of a type O donor into an A, B, or AB recipient. Selective renal arteriography should be performed on volunteer donors to rule out the presence of multiple or abnormal renal arteries, because the surgical procedure is difficult and the ischemic time of the transplanted kidney long when vascular abnormalities exist. Cadaveric donors should be free of malignant neoplastic disease because of the possible transmission of cancer to the recipient.

In the United States, a coordinated national system (United Network for Organ Sharing) of computerized information sharing and logistical support for the transportation of cadaver kidneys to suitable recipients is under development. It is now possible to remove cadaver kidneys and to maintain them for over 48 h on cold pulsatile perfusion or simple flushing and cooling. This permits adequate time for various typing, cross matching, transportation, and selection problems to be solved.

TISSUE TYPING AND CLINICAL IMMUNOGENETICS   Matching for antigens of the HLA major histocompatibility gene complex (Chap. 14) is the ideal criterion for selection of donors for renal allografts. Each mammalian species has a single chromosomal region that encodes the strong, or major, transplantation antigens, and the analogous sixth chromosomal region is called *HLA* in human beings. Other antigens, called "minor," may nevertheless play crucial roles, especially the ABH(O) blood groups and an endothelial antigen which is shared with blood monocytes, but not lymphocytes. Evidence for designation of HLA as the genetic region encoding strong transplantation antigens comes from the success rate in living related donor renal and bone marrow transplantation, with superior results in HLA-identical sibling pairs. Nevertheless, 5 to 10 percent of HLA-identical renal allografts are rejected, often within the first weeks after transplantation. It is likely, though not proved, that these failures represent states of prior sensitization to non-HLA antigens. Non-HLA antigens are relatively weak and therefore suppressible by conventional immunosuppressive therapy. Once priming has occurred, however, secondary responses are much more refractory to treatment. In fact, ABH incompatibilities are hazardous because of the presence of natural anti-A and anti-B antibodies in recipients and the normal expression of A and B blood group substances on endothelium.

Living related donors From 1962 to 1982 when azathioprine was the main immunosuppressive drug, living related donors provided superior graft survivals. Among first-degree relatives, the general level of expected graft success was in direct proportion to matching for 2,1, or no HLA haplotypes, as defined by HLA serologic typing and the presence or absence of a proliferative response in the mixed lymphocyte response (MLR) (Chap. 14). HLA-incompatible siblings did slightly better than the overall average with cadaveric donors (50 to 60 percent at 1 year), while HLA semi-identicals (haploidentical) were in the 70 to 75 percent range. Intrafamilial MLRs among haploidenticals were found to be a measure of responsiveness. Low responder donor-recipient pairs had a 1-year graft survival rate of 90 percent, while vigorous responders were at the level of 55 percent unless donor-specific blood transfusions were given to eliminate this disadvantage. The MLR is a relatively imprecise technique, but it has been repeatedly shown that for both living related and cadaveric donors, MLR reactivity with a specific donor is more predictive of graft outcome than serologic typing for HLA-A, -B, -C, or -DR antigens.

Cyclosporine has had a major impact upon the assumption that living related donors are generally superior to cadaveric donors, because in most recent series the improvement in cadaveric results rivals the 80 percent 1-year result previously attained only with haploidentical relatives. One must now weigh the choices in light of the availability of organs and waiting times on dialysis, rather than on the initial rate of graft success. Long-term survival rates, comparing the various donor types and treatment protocols, are not improved in the cyclosporine era, if one assesses graft survival over a decade in terms of half-lives. With azathioprine or cyclosporine, the half-life measured after the first year is 30 to 34 years with HLA-identical donors, 11 to 12 years with haploidentical donors, and 7 to 9 years with cadaveric donors. The major advantage of cyclosporine over azathioprine, therefore, is in the superior level of initial results at 1 to 2 years for cadaveric transplantation and not in the rate of graft loss thereafter.

There has been concern expressed regarding the potential risk to a volunteer kidney donor of premature renal failure after several years of increased blood flow and hyperfiltration per nephron in the remaining kidney. There are a few reports of development of hypertension, proteinuria, and even lesions of focal segmental sclerosis in donors under long-term followup. Documentation of difficulties in significant numbers of donors followed for 15 or more years is unusual, however, and it may be that having a single kidney becomes significant only when another condition, such as hypertension, is superimposed. In this regard, it is desirable to consider the risk of development of type I diabetes mellitus in a family member who is a potential donor to a diabetic renal failure patient. Measurements of anti-insulin and anti-islet antibodies should be made and glucose tolerance tests should be performed in such cases to rule out a prediabetic state. The acceptance of living unrelated donors (spouses, distant relatives, close friends) has been debated as a means to improve the supply of organs and to shorten the waiting period on dialysis. Since volunteer donors who are not matched for one or both HLA haplotypes present as strong a tissue barrier as randomly matched cadaveric donors, they cannot be expected to provide, on average, as reliable a source for long-functioning grafts as a well-matched cadaveric organ. It is illegal in the United States to purchase organs for transplantation.

HLA matching and cadaveric donors The question of whether matching of HLA antigens in unrelated donor-recipient pairs would approximate the high initial success rates and slow rates of subsequent graft loss found with HLA-identical sib pairs could not be answered until the 1980s when reliable class II histocompatibility (DR) typing became widely available. With the 1-year success rate now at 80 to 85 percent for first cadaveric grafts, it is difficult to see an early improvement related to matching when small series of cases are compiled, especially, as is often the case, when the reporting centers have a very small fraction of well-matched cases. Now that pooled data on several thousands of cadaveric renal transplants from all over the world are available, the HLA-matching effect can be clearly seen, especially in the long-term survival figures. Figure 225-3 shows data for 3 years and projections to 10 years, based on the exponential nature of the actuarial plot. Well-matched cases, compatible for HLA-A, -B, and -DR antigens show results comparable to those with HLA-identical sibs. Poorly matched cases, though starting off well at 1 to 2 years, are projected to lose 70 percent of grafts by the end of the first decade. Other analyses show that HLA-DR compatibility alone is the most powerful influence, followed by HLA-B, and to a lesser extent HLA-A. Repeat transplants, following rejection of first grafts, do less well by about 15 to 20 percent, and in these cases the benefits of HLA matching are even more striking, while cyclosporine adds relatively little. These results indicate that HLA antigens of various loci are not of equal strength in the immunosuppressed patient and that only 2 or 3 of them need to be matched to produce improved results. The likelihood of obtaining compatibility for HLA-B and -DR in a given case depends upon the relative frequencies of the recipient's antigens in the general population and upon the pool size of donors available. In addition, the chances depend upon how many

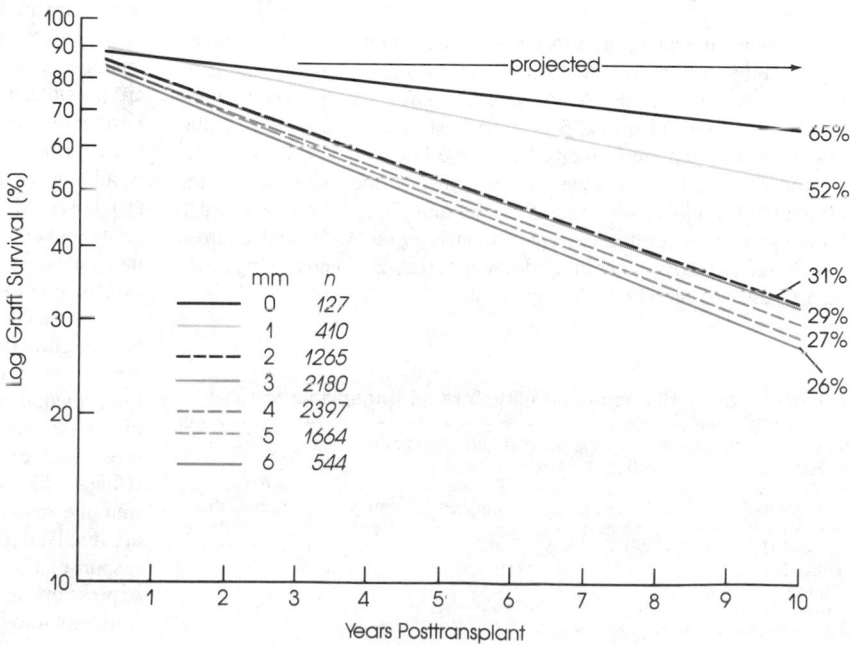

FIGURE 225-3 Survival of first cadaveric renal grafts in the cyclosporine era. The effects of mismatches (mm) for HLA-A, -B, -DR antigens (zero to 6) are shown through 3 years and projected to 10 years. *(From PI Terasaki.)*

mm	n
0	127
1	410
2	1265
3	2180
4	2397
5	1664
6	544

other potential recipients are waiting and upon the willingness of transplant centers to share organs on this basis. A 20 to 30 percent rate of DR-compatible cadaveric transplants has been achieved by some organ sharing systems. With the United Network for Organ Sharing waiting list of over 12,000 potential recipients and 8000 or more donors per year, levels approaching these rates and higher are possible.

Presensitization   A positive cross match of recipient serum with donor T lymphocytes representing anti-HLA class I is usually predictive of an acute vasculitic event termed *hyperacute* rejection. A few years ago it was thought that patients making such antibodies, tested against a surrogate panel of normal lymphocytes, were at high risk for accelerated, if not hyperacute, rejection, even when the donor-specific cross match was negative. That this is no longer so can be attributed to the greater efforts being made in monitoring patients on dialysis, defining not only the presence or absence of antibodies but also the HLA antigens to which they are directed. Patients with anti-HLA antibodies can be safely transplanted if careful cross matching is performed. Patients sustained by hemodialysis often show fluctuating antibody titers and specificity patterns, sometimes, but not always, temporally related to receipt of blood transfusions. At the time of assignment of a cadaveric kidney, cross matches are performed with more than one highly reactive serum, and the previously analyzed antibody specificities are also taken into account. Anti-HLA antibody responses do not necessarily recur several months later when the incompatible antigen is given in a blood product transfusion. Indeed, it seems relatively safe to ignore positive cross matches with sera kept in storage for several months as long as recent sera are negative. Data on this point are conflicting, showing either no risk or a 15 percent increased risk of early graft loss if only the stored serum samples older than 6 months are reactive with donor cells. The loss of anamnesis to HLA by chronic dialysis patients may result from development of specific unresponsiveness due to suppressor cell activation, or from anti-idiotypic immunity. Presensitization to antigens expressed on B lymphocytes, but not T lymphocytes, is not a contraindication to transplantation. Some of these antibodies are anti-DR, while others are non-HLA IgM antibodies active in the cold and at room temperature, but apparently not relevant to graft survival.

Endothelial-monocyte system   In some cases of unexpected accelerated rejection, antibodies with reactivity to renal endothelium and blood monocytes have been found, both in the circulation and in eluates from rejected grafts. Practical aspects of typing and cross matching for this non-HLA system are difficult. Second transplants following rapid loss of the first graft seem to be particularly at risk.

Overview of transplantation immunogenetics   In addition to the ABH(O) blood groups, the important histocompatibility antigens presently known are HLA-A, -B, -C, -DR, and the endothelial-monocyte system (Table 225-2). The best current data suggest that major primary immunogenicity lies in the DR antigens, while A, B, C, and endothelial-monocyte antigens provide the major targets for effector IgG, and in the case of A, B, and C, at least, for killer T lymphocytes. Hence the current emphasis is on A, B, and C cross matching and DR matching, although HLA-B compatibility adds significantly to the DR-matching effect.

Blood transfusions   At a time when it appeared that transfusion-induced sensitization against a random lymphocyte panel was predictive of a high graft failure rate, a number of transplantation units undertook a policy of withholding blood from as many dialysis patients as possible. The clinical need for blood was found to be less than originally thought, especially in nonnephrectomized patients, and avoidance of possible exposure to hepatitis was also a consideration. The overall experience with the nontransfused patients was a dramatic one, confirmed many times over: such patients were at the *highest risk* for graft failure. Since the early 1980s, however, there has been a progressive loss of the transfusion effect, with little or no detriment now remaining in the nontransfused patients. The loss of the transfusion effect cannot be directly attributed to the introduction of cyclosporine, as the transfusion effect had declined before large numbers of patients received this agent. It seems unlikely that worldwide changes in blood bank processing practices are involved. It is most likely that the overall level of clinical management, particularly in recognition and prompt treatment of rejection, has played a role. Indeed, when looked at carefully, some centers withholding transfusions have noted increased rejection activity in their nontransfused patients but have not had difficulty in treating them. One study shows, however, that graft survival is still decreased in that subset of nontransfused patients who also have an early clinically apparent rejection episode. The current practice to use little or no blood in preparation for transplantation comes at a propitious time because of concerns regarding HIV transmission. The efficacy of recombinant erythropoietin in sustaining red blood cell mass in chronic renal failure patients will further reduce the clinical need for blood transfusions.

IMMUNOLOGY OF REJECTION   Knowledge of the immunology of tissue transplantation stems largely from animal experimentation. However, enough evidence has accumulated in humans, particularly in kidney transplantation, to indicate that the evidence is similar though not identical for the different species. The immunologic mechanisms are not qualitatively different from those found in other areas of immunology (Chap. 13). The evidence is that early rejection is associated with T lymphocytes having direct specificity against donor antigens. These may be cytotoxic cells (CD8 + or CD4 +) or cells which mediate DTH (CD4 +); however, significant numbers of B lymphocytes, null cells, natural killer (NK) cells, and macrophages appear in the early infiltrate, and cells capable of mediating antibody-dependent cell-mediated cytotoxicity (ADCC) are also present (Fig. 225-4). Many of the B lymphocytes produce immunoglobulins. The spectrum of cellular and humoral response and graft injury is quite varied, depending upon specific genetic differences between donor and recipient and states of presensitization. The greater the degree of presensitization, the more likely it is that one will find antibody-mediated vascular lesions. All of the processes shown in Fig. 225-4 are possible, but their relative contribution varies from case to case. Further dissection of the heterogeneity of the human allograft response, utilizing newer techniques for identification of lymphocyte subsets, is adding to the value of graft biopsy as a guide to therapy and prognosis. Monitoring of peripheral blood lymphocyte subsets, utilizing monoclonal antibodies (Chap. 13) to functionally related surface molecules, such as CD4 (T-helper cells) and CD8 (T-suppressor/cytotoxic cells), has been related to the degree of rejection activity in some surveys, but the CD4/CD8 ratio has not always been clinically meaningful. Part of the problem may lie in the fact that these subsets are not as uniquely related to function as originally believed. Indeed, the principal role of the CD4 molecule appears to be the promotion of interaction of T cells with class II HLA molecules on antigen-presenting cells, and, similarly, CD8 interacts with class I HLA (Chaps. 13, 14). Finally, the cytokine mediators of the cellular immune response (IL-1, IL-2, IL-3, IL-4, IL-6, IFNγ) (Chap. 13) are involved in the control and expression of the alloimmune rejection response. For example, T-cell production of IFNγ causes increased expression of HLA antigens upon endothelial cells. In normal immunobiology this effect may be to promote more efficient pre-

---

TABLE 225-2   Histocompatibility in renal transplantation

RELATIVE IMPORTANCE OF TYPING AND CROSS MATCHING FOR SEROLOGICALLY DEFINED ANTIGENS

Antigens	Typing (antigen matching)	Cross matching
Class I (HLA-A, -B, -C)	+ +	+ + +
Class II (HLA-DR)	+ + +	−
Endothelial-monocyte (non-HLA)	? −	+ + +

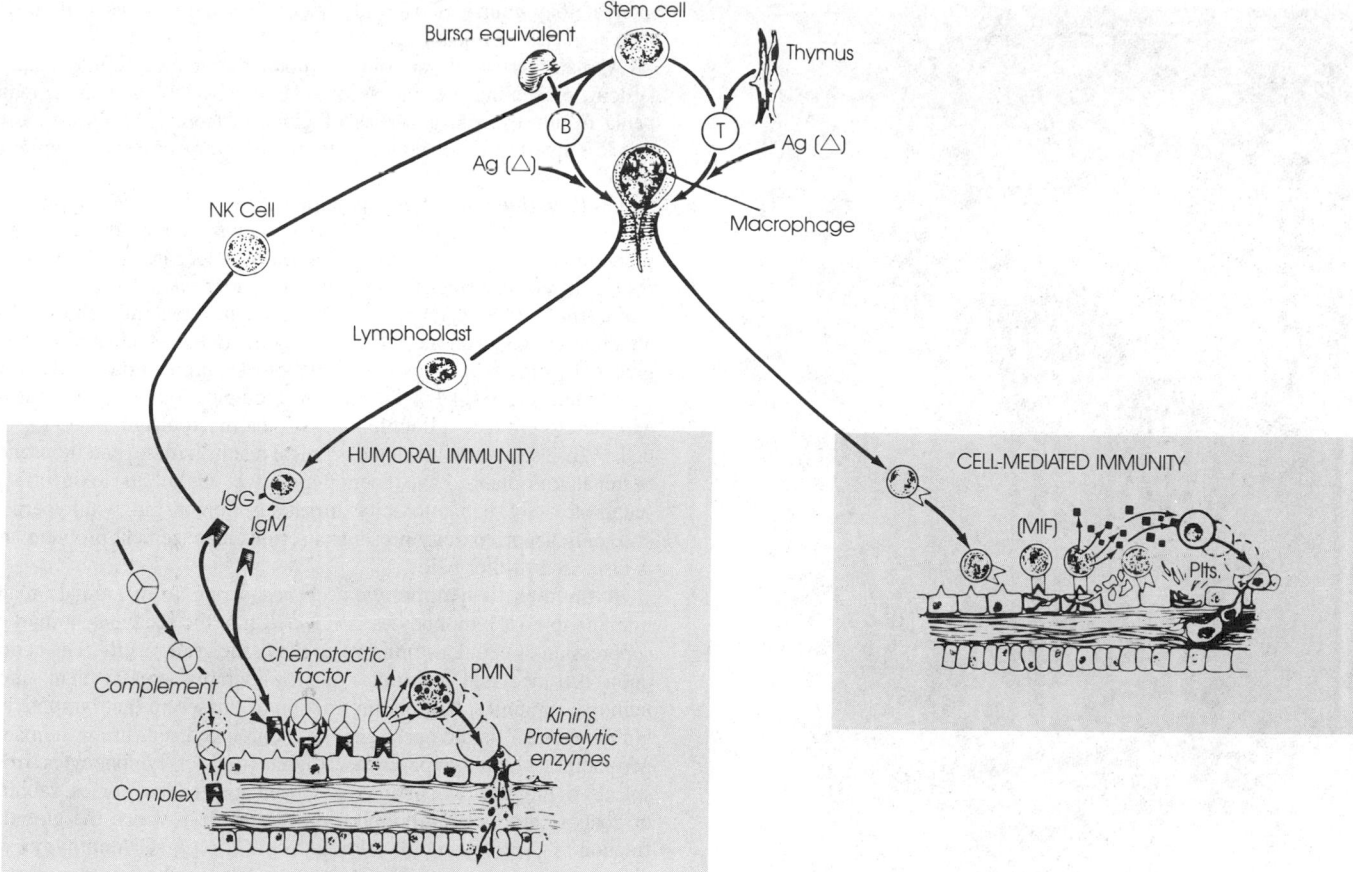

FIGURE 225-4 Overall scheme of the development of effector mechanisms in graft rejection. Bone marrow stem cells differentiate under the influence of the thymus gland into mature thymus-derived (T) lymphocytes, or under the influence of an equivalent to the avian bursa of Fabricius into mature bone marrow–derived (B) lymphocytes. Exposure to antigen (△) results in an interaction between T cells and B cells, and often involves macrophages. The sensitized B cells, after mitoses, develop into immunoglobulin-secreting cells (e.g., plasma cells), illustrated here by IgG and IgM. Such immunoglobulins may form immune complexes with antigen in the circulation which activate the complement sequence, or they may react directly with antigens on the blood vessel surface. Elaboration of secondary mediators, including the products of complement activation, results in vascular damage as illustrated. Sensitized T lymphocytes are the primary effector cells in cell-mediated immunity and may react directly with antigens in the graft to exert a cytotoxic effect. In addition, T cells release factors, such as macrophage migration inhibition factor (MIF), which may accelerate the rate of mononuclear cell infiltration. This process is similar to delayed-type hypersensitivity (DTH). It has also been shown that unsensitized non-T cells (NK cells) can be activated to exert cytotoxic effects by the fixation of IgG to target cells, followed by interaction of the IgG (Fc portion) with an Fc receptor on the NK cell. Finally, platelet aggregation and thrombosis can occur following the endothelial damage induced by any of these mechanisms. (See Fig. 13-1.)

sentation of foreign antigen, while in transplantation it enhances the immunogenicity of the vascularized transplant. Also, IL-2 is the major growth factor for expansion of effector T cells. It is the product of a major subset of CD4 cells, while other CD4 cells produce B-cell growth factors, such as IL-4.

The failure of transplanted kidneys after several years of adequate function is due to a form of "chronic rejection." In such kidneys the development of nephrosclerosis, with proliferation of the vascular intima of renal vessels, and intimal fibrosis, with marked decrease in the lumen of the vessels, takes place (Fig. 225-5). The result is renal ischemia, hypertension, widespread tubular atrophy, interstitial fibrosis, and glomerular atrophy with eventual renal failure. It is not established, however, whether slow deterioration of graft function over years is due to the same mechanisms in all cases. Except for the established influence of HLA incompatibility, little is known about the pathogenesis of progressive renal failure in the transplanted population.

IMMUNOSUPPRESSIVE TREATMENT When histocompatibility differences exist between donor and recipient, it is necessary to modify or suppress the immune response in order to enable the recipient to accept a graft. Immunosuppressive therapy, in general, suppresses all immune responses, including those to bacteria, fungi, and even malignant tumors. In the 1950s when clinical renal transplantation began, sublethal total-body irradiation was employed. Currently, immunosuppression is more safely induced pharmacologically. Agents used in humans to suppress the immune response are discussed in the following paragraphs.

Drugs *Azathioprine*, an analogue of mercaptopurine, is the keystone to immunosuppressive therapy in humans. This agent can inhibit synthesis of DNA, RNA, or both. Because cell division and proliferation are a necessary part of the immune response to antigenic stimulation, suppression by this agent may be mediated by the inhibition of mitosis of immunologically competent lymphoid cells, interfering with synthesis of DNA. Alternatively, immunosuppression may be brought about by blocking the synthesis of RNA (possibly messenger RNA), inhibiting processing of antigens prior to lymphocyte stimulation. This drug has little effect in suppressing a secondary immune response, however. Therapy with azathioprine is generally instituted 2 days prior to transplantation in the recipient of a living donor kidney and on the day of transplantation in the case of a cadaveric donor kidney recipient at a level of 4 mg/kg per day. The drug is later tapered to levels of 1.5 to 3 mg/kg per day, as long as the allograft functions. Because the drug is rapidly metabolized by the liver, its dosage need not be varied directly in relation to renal

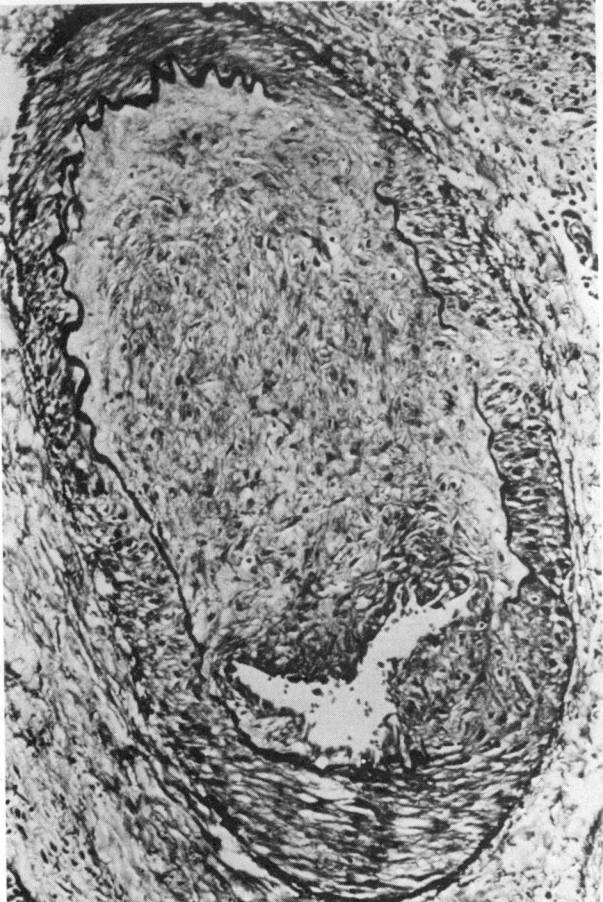

FIGURE 225-5 Biopsy of the renal cadaveric allograft illustrating obliterative endarteritis. Loss of the media is associated with intimal thickening. The elastic tissue shows dissolution of the elastica. The evidence for arteritis with subsequent thrombosis is typically the gaps in the elastica and media. The intimal thickening probably represents organization of a thrombus formed in response to the arteritis. [*From GJ Dammin, JP Merrill, in Structural Basis for Renal Disease, EL Becker (ed), New York, Hoeber-Harper, 1968.*]

function, even though renal failure results in retention of the metabolites of azathioprine. Some patients are unusually sensitive to this drug, particularly when renal function is compromised, and reduction in dosage is required because of leukopenia and occasionally thrombocytopenia. Excessive amounts of azathioprine may also cause jaundice, anemia, and alopecia. If it is essential to administer allopurinol concurrently, the azathioprine dose must be drastically reduced, since inhibition of xanthine oxidase delays degradation. This combination is best avoided.

The *glucocorticoids* are important adjuncts to immunosuppressive therapy. Of all the agents employed, prednisone has effects that are easiest to assess, and in large doses it is the most effective agent for the reversal of rejection. In general, 30 to 40 mg prednisone is given immediately prior to or at the time of transplantation, and the dosage is gradually reduced. The well-known side effects of the glucocorticoids, particularly impairment of wound healing and predisposition to infection, make it desirable to taper the dose as rapidly as possible in the immediate postoperative period. Customarily methylprednisolone, 0.5 to 1.0 g intravenously, is administered immediately upon diagnosis of beginning rejection and continued once daily for 3 days. When the drug is effective, the results are usually apparent within 96 h. Such "pulse" doses are less effective in the chronic rejection process. Most patients whose renal function is stable after 6 months or a year do not require large doses of prednisone; maintenance doses of 15 or 20 mg per day are the rule. Many patients tolerate an

alternate-day course of steroids better than daily doses without an increased risk of rejection.

A major effect of steroids is upon the monocyte-macrophage system, preventing the release of IL-6 and IL-1. Although lymphopenia results from large doses of glucocorticoids, this is primarily due to sequestration of recirculating blood lymphocytes to lymphoid tissue.

Cyclosporine A is a fungal peptide with potent immunosuppressive activity in animals and in in vitro systems. It appears to have a preferential effect upon early activation of helper-inducer T lymphocytes, thereby sparing suppressor T-cell responses. Assessment of this agent in human renal transplantation has generally shown that although it works alone, it is more effective in conjunction with glucocorticoids. Since cyclosporine blocks production of IL-2 by helper-inducer (CD4+) T cells, its combination with steroids is expected to produce a double block in the macrophage → IL-1 → T cell → IL-2 sequence. As noted, clinical results with several thousands of renal transplants have been impressive. Of all its toxic effects (nephrotoxicity, hepatotoxicity, hirsutism, tremor, gingival hyperplasia), only nephrotoxicity presents a serious management problem and is discussed further below.

Antibodies to lymphocytes　When serum from animals made immune to host lymphocytes is injected into the recipient, a marked suppression of cellular immunity to the tissue graft results. The action upon cell-mediated immunity is considerably greater than upon humoral immunity. A globulin fraction of the serum (antilymphocyte globulin, ALG) is the agent generally employed. For use in humans, peripheral human lymphocytes, thymocytes, or lymphocytes from spleens or thoracic duct fistulas have been injected into horses, rabbits, or goats to produce antilymphocyte serum, from which the globulin fraction is then separated. Although ALG, or ATG (antithymocyte globulin), is unquestionably effective in prolonging grafts in experimental animals, its efficacy in the transplantation of human tissue is less clear, as it varies from source to source. Heterologous antibody against defined T-lymphocyte subsets, in the form of mouse antihuman monoclonal antibody, may offer a more precise approach to this form of therapy. OKT3, in common clinical use, is such an antibody. It is directed to the CD3 molecules which form a portion of the T-cell antigen–receptor complex; hence, CD3 is expressed on all mature T cells. CD4 or CD8 molecules also form part of the fully activated cluster of molecules, and monoclonal antibodies to these offer the potential for more selective targeting of T-cell subsets. Another approach to more selective therapy already under clinical trial is to target the 55-kDa beta chain of the IL-2 receptor, expressed only on T cells that have been recently activated. When the antibody is administered during the first 10 days after transplantation, a powerful immunosuppression results, allowing marked reduction or elimination of cyclosporine during the first few days after graft placement.

Other techniques　Among other techniques of immunosuppression, thymectomy and splenectomy have not been widely accepted. Local irradiation of the transplanted kidney in two or three doses of 3500 mGy (350 rad) has also been utilized. This technique may result in fewer early rejection episodes in cadaveric transplants than in nonirradiated controls. Fractional total-lymph-node irradiation (TLI), as employed in the therapy of Hodgkin's disease, is continuing under investigation.

CLINICAL COURSE AND MANAGEMENT OF THE RECIPIENT

Bilateral nephrectomy at some point prior to transplantation is performed for a specific cause but not as a routine. Hypertension which is difficult to control or infection involving the end-stage kidneys are the two most common indications. Nephrectomized patients maintain a much lower hematocrit level, but this is no longer considered a disadvantage per se, because blood transfusions need not be avoided in preparation for transplantation. Difficulties do arise when these multiply transfused patients become sensitized and must remain on dialysis. Nephrectomy per se does not appear to affect the survival of subsequent renal allografts.

Adequate hemodialysis should be performed within 48 h of surgery, and care should be taken that the serum potassium level is not markedly elevated so that intraoperative cardiac arrhythmias can be averted. The diuresis that commonly occurs postoperatively must be carefully monitored; in many instances it may be massive, reflecting the inability of ischemic tubules to regulate sodium and water excretion. Massive potassium losses may occur and occasionally be symptomatic. Most chronically uremic patients have some excess of extracellular fluid, and some degree of negative balance should be accomplished, provided hemodynamics remain stable. Acute tubular necrosis (ATN) may cause immediate oliguria or may follow an initial short period of graft function. ATN is most likely to occur when cadaveric donors have been hypotensive, or if the interval between cessation of blood flow and organ harvest (warm ischemic time) has been more than a few minutes. Recovery usually occurs within 3 weeks, although periods as long as 6 weeks have been reported. Superimposition of rejection upon ATN is common, and the differential diagnosis may be difficult. Cyclosporine therapy prolongs ATN, and some patients do not diurese until they are switched to azathioprine. Many centers avoid starting cyclosporine for the first several days, using ALG or a monoclonal antibody along with azathioprine and prednisone until renal function is established.

The rejection episode Early diagnosis of rejection allows prompt institution of therapy to preserve renal function and prevent irreversible damage due to fibrosis. Clinical evidence of rejection may be characterized by fever, swelling, and tenderness over the allograft, and by significant reduction in urine volume. In patients whose renal function is good initially, oliguria may be accompanied by decreased urinary sodium concentration and increased osmolarity. These changes may not be present in the more chronic stages of rejection or when renal function is impaired at the onset of rejection.

Arteriography and radioactive iodohippurate sodium renograms of the transplanted kidney may be useful in ascertaining changes in the renal vasculature and in renal blood flow, even in the absence of urinary flow. Diagnostic ultrasound is the procedure of choice to rule out urinary obstruction or to confirm the presence of perirenal collections of urine, blood, or lymph. When renal function has been good initially, a rise in the serum creatinine level and a decrease in the creatinine clearance is the most sensitive and reliable indicator of possible rejection.

Cyclosporine may cause deterioration in renal function in a manner similar to a rejection episode. In fact, rejection processes tend to be more indolent with cyclosporine, and the only way to make a diagnosis may be by renal biopsy. Cyclosporine has an afferent arteriolar constrictor effect upon the kidney and, in addition, may produce permanent vascular and interstitial injury after sustained high-dose therapy. There is no universally accepted lesion(s) which makes a diagnosis of cyclosporine toxicity, although interstitial fibrosis and thickening of arteriolar walls have been noted by some. Basically, if the biopsy does not reveal moderate and active cellular rejection activity, the serum creatinine will most likely respond to a reduction in cyclosporine dose. Blood levels of drug can be useful if very high or very low but precise correlation with renal function does not exist. If rejection activity is present in the biopsy, appropriate therapy is indicated.

OKT3 monoclonal antibody, given intravenously for 10 to 14 days, is effective in more than 90 percent of first rejections, although it is less effective if methylprednisolone pulses have failed and in cases of severe recurrent rejection activity. A major problem with OKT3 is that severe systemic reactions may be produced during the first day or two of therapy. Chills, fever, hypotension, and headache are the direct result of the antibody effects upon the targeted T cells, most likely related to the known potential of OKT3 to activate T cells nonspecifically. If the antibody is administered to overhydrated oliguric patients, pulmonary edema may be induced. These reactions are not characteristic of other monoclonal antibodies, such as those to the IL-2 receptor. Recurrent or rebound rejection activity may require additional therapy. In such circumstances methylprednisolone may be effective even though it failed initially. Second courses of

OKT3 may be given in spite of anti-mouse antibodies generated in response to the first course, if the titers are low and the human antibodies are not directed to the combining site region (idiotype) of the OKT3.

Management problems Modification of the usual clinical manifestations of infection by immunosuppressive therapy is a major problem in the posttransplant period. The major toxic effect of azathioprine is bone marrow suppression, while cyclosporine has no marrow effects. They both may predispose to unusual opportunistic infections, however. The signs and symptoms of infection may be masked and distorted, and fever without obvious cause is common. Only after days or weeks will it become apparent that it has a viral or fungal origin. Bacterial infections are most common during the first month after transplantation. The importance of blood cultures in such patients cannot be overemphasized, because systemic infection without obvious foci is frequent, although wound infections with or without urinary fistulas are most common. Particularly ominous are rapidly occurring pulmonary lesions, which may result in death within 5 days of onset. When these become apparent, immunosuppressive agents should be discontinued except for maintenance doses of prednisone. Aggressive diagnostic procedures, including transbronchial and open lung biopsy, are frequently indicated. In the case of *Pneumocystis carinii* (Chap. 163) trimethoprim-sulfamethoxazole is the treatment of choice; amphotericin B has been used effectively in systemic fungal infections. Prophylaxis against *P. carinii* with daily low-dose trimethoprim-sulfamethoxazole is very effective. Involvement of the oropharynx with *Candida* (Chap. 151) may be treated with local nystatin. Small doses (a total of 300 mg) of amphotericin given over a period of 2 weeks may be effective in refractory oral candidiasis. *Aspergillus* (Chap. 151), *Nocardia* (Chap. 152), and cytomegalovirus (CMV) (Chap. 138) infections also occur. CMV is a common and dangerous infection in transplant recipients. It does not generally appear until the end of the first posttransplant month. Active CMV infection is sometimes associated, or occasionally confused, with rejection episodes. Patients at highest risk for severe CMV disease are those without anti-CMV antibodies who receive a graft from a CMV antibody–positive donor (15 percent mortality). Serial intravenous administration of high titer CMV immune globulin is effective in reducing this risk. Prophylactic use of acyclovir and other antiviral agents is under study. The complications of glucocorticoid therapy are well known and include gastrointestinal bleeding, impairment of wound healing, osteoporosis, diabetes, cataract formation, and hemorrhagic pancreatitis. The treatment of jaundice in transplant patients should include cessation of azathioprine or cyclosporine therapy, if hepatitis or drug toxicity is suspected. It is surprising that total cessation of azathioprine or cyclosporine therapy often does not result in rejection of a graft. Antiplatelet agents and anticoagulants, although effective in theory, have not been successful in the prevention of the chronic vascular lesion. Persistent elevation of serum creatinine levels above 220 μmol/L (2.5 mg/dL) in patients maintained on cyclosporine is an indication for dose reduction, but if rejection activity develops, addition of azathioprine is indicated. Some centers convert patients from cyclosporine to azathioprine after 6 to 12 months. Our own experience with such conversions between 4 and 8 months after transplantation has been satisfactory; however, 30 percent of patients had temporally related rejection episodes requiring additional steroid therapy. Subsequent follow-up showed improved renal function in most cases. The alternative to conversion is to use lower doses of cyclosporine. Since the question of long-term cumulative toxicity to the kidney remains open, lower doses are recommended for the long term. Reduction of cyclosporine is best accomplished by routine use of "triple therapy" in which the following dose levels are common for maintenance after 6 to 8 months: cyclosporine, 3 to 5 mg per kilogram of body weight per day; azathioprine, 1.0 to 1.5 mg/kg per day; prednisone, 0.15 to 0.20 mg/kg per day.

In spite of the potential teratogenic effects of immunosuppressive agents, both women and men have become parents after transplantation. The incidence of congenital abnormalities in the offspring is not unusual.

Glomerular lesions Even identical twins who do not require immunosuppression may develop glomerular lesions after transplantation. These represent recurrence of a glomerulonephritic process. Glomerular lesions may occur in 10 to 15 percent of allografts, even when the original disease was accidental removal of a solitary kidney. The pathogenesis is related to a chronic rejection process. In other cases the lesions resemble those of the patient's own original disease. The recurrence of the nephrotic syndrome with "nil disease" in transplanted kidneys whose recipient's original nil disease had progressed to renal failure with focal sclerosis, and the recurrence in renal allografts of the classic lesions of IgA nephropathy and of membranoproliferative glomerulonephritis with electron-dense deposit disease are classic examples. In the last of these, the incidence of recurrence has been reported to be as high as 30 to 40 percent. In most instances, however, the recurrence of the original renal lesions represents no threat to the patient's immediate prognosis, and a primary diagnosis of glomerulonephritis is rarely taken as a contraindication to transplantation.

Malignancy The incidence of tumors arising in patients on immunosuppressive therapy is 5 to 6 percent, or approximately 100 times greater than that observed in the general population in the same age range. The most common lesions are cancer of the skin and lips and carcinoma in situ of the cervix, as well as lymphomas, particularly reticulum cell sarcoma in the central nervous system and gastrointestinal tract.

Other complications *Hypercalcemia* after transplantation may indicate failure of hyperplastic parathyroid glands to regress. Aseptic necrosis of the head of the femur is probably due to preexisting hyperparathyroidism. With improved management of calcium and phosphorus metabolism during chronic dialysis, the incidence of parathyroid-related complications has fallen dramatically.

Hypertension may be caused by (1) native kidneys, (2) rejection activity in the transplant, (3) renal artery stenosis, if an end-to-end anastomosis was constructed with an iliac artery branch, and (4) renal vasoconstriction from cyclosporine toxicity. The latter may improve with reduction in cyclosporine dose. Whereas angiotensin-converting enzyme inhibitors may be useful, calcium channel blockers are frequently more effective in cyclosporine-treated patients.

Chronic hepatitis, particularly when due to hepatitis B virus, can be a progressive fatal disease over a decade or so. Patients who are persistently HBsAg positive are at higher risk, according to some studies, but the presence of non-A non-B disease is also a concern when one embarks upon a course of deliberate immunosuppression in a transplant recipient.

Both chronic dialysis and renal transplant patients have a higher incidence of death from myocardial infarction and stroke than in the population at large, and this is particularly true in diabetics. Contributing factors are hypertension and hypertriglyceridemia. Increased low density lipoprotein cholesterol and depressed high-density lipoprotein cholesterol concentrations may be exaggerated after transplantation and require treatment.

REFERENCES

CARPENTER CB, MILFORD EL: Renal transplantation: Immunobiology, in *The Kidney*, 3d ed, B Brenner, F Rector (eds). Philadelphia, Saunders, 1986, p 1907
——————: HLA matching in cadaveric renal transplantation, in *Transplantation Immunology*, PF Halloran (ed). Philadelphia, Saunders, Immunol Aller Clin North Am 9:1, 1989
COLLINS AJ, KESHAVIAH PR: Are there limitations to shortening dialysis treatment? Trans Am Soc Artif Intern Organs 34:1, 1988
GOTCH FA, SARGENT JA: A mechanistic analysis of the National Cooperative Dialysis Study (NCDS). Kidney Intern 28:526, 1985
HAKIM RM, LAZARUS JM: Medical aspects of hemodialysis, in *The Kidney*, 3d ed, B Brenner, F Rector (eds). Philadelphia, Saunders, 1986, p 1791
——————, ——————: Hemodialysis in acute renal failure, in *Acute Renal Failure*, B Brenner, JM Lazarus (eds). Philadelphia, Saunders, 1986, p 643
LOERTSCHER R et al: Postoperative management of the renal transplant recipient and long-term complications, in *Renal Transplantation, Contemporary Issues in Nephrol-ogy*, Vol 19, EL Milford, BM Brenner, JH Stein (eds). New York, Churchill Livingstone, 1989, p 197
NOLPH KD et al: Continuous ambulatory peritoneal dialysis in the United States: A three year study. Kidney Intern 28:198, 1985
RUBIN RH: Infection in the renal transplant recipient, in *Renal Transplantation, Contemporary Issues in Nephrology*, Vol 19, EL Milford, BM Brenner, JH Stein (eds). New York, Churchill Livingstone, 1989, p 147
SIGLER MH et al: Solute transport in continuous hemodialysis: A new treatment for acute renal failure. Kidney Intern 32:562, 1987
TERASAKI PI (ED): *Clinical Transplants 1987*. Los Angeles, UCLA Tissue Typing Laboratory, 1987

226 IMMUNOPATHOGENIC MECHANISMS OF RENAL INJURY

RICHARD J. GLASSOCK / BARRY M. BRENNER

Recognition of the important role played by immunologic processes in many forms of renal injury, especially those involving the glomerular circulation, constitutes one of the significant advances in the understanding of renal diseases. Through investigation of experimental models of disease in animals, the details of the immune processes responsible for renal injury have been evaluated; yet large gaps in our knowledge still exist regarding etiologic factors and pathogenetic events.

IMMUNOPATHOLOGY Immune renal injury may be divided into the initiating pathogenetic events and the processes that mediate the actual tissue injury. The general concepts of immunopathogenesis are presented in Chap. 13. One mechanism of injury involves the reaction of a circulating antibody with its respective renal antigen in situ. Thus, an immune complex is formed at the site of tissue injury rather than at a distant location. The antigen may either be an intrinsic, or native, constituent of the kidney or one that has been bound to the renal tissue by a particular biochemical or immunologic reaction. This mechanism is often referred to as *anti-tissue antibody-mediated disease*. The intrinsic antigens may be insoluble and slowly renewable components of the extracellular matrix (e.g., basement membrane or mesangial matrix glycoproteins) or soluble components of cells or cell membranes (e.g., epithelial, mesangial, or endothelial cells) associated with the matrix components. Bound or extrinsic antigens can be derived from a variety of sources. The mechanisms of binding of extrinsic antigens to the constituents of renal tissue can be quite diverse. The reactions of circulating antibody to the intrinsic or bound (planted) tissue antigens can give rise to distinctive structural alterations and immunohistochemical appearances, as discussed below.

Another pathogenetic category involves the localization of circulating macromolecular aggregates composed of antigens and antibodies (i.e., circulating immune complexes) within renal structures, principally glomeruli. This mechanism is referred to as *immune-complex-induced disease*. The immune complexes need not bear any special immunochemical relationships with renal structures, and the kidney is a passive participant, damaged by processes that originate elsewhere. The source of the antigen in immune-complex-induced disease may be either *endogenous* (autologous) or *exogenous* (environmental). Further, exogenous antigens may either be biologically inert or derived from an organism capable of self-replication (e.g., bacteria, viruses). Under special circumstances environmental agents may combine with autologous substances to result in new antigenic compounds (hapten-protein conjugates) that act in concert with antibodies to form immune complexes.

In contrast to the above mechanisms, which involve antibody, cell-mediated immune processes may also result in injury to glomerular, vascular, and tubulointerstitial regions of the kidney. A precise role for the cell-mediated immune processes in human renal disease is less well established than for certain experimental models.

Finally, certain human glomerular diseases are prominently associated with an abnormal activation of the alternative pathway of the complement cascade (see also Chap. 13), although such activation need not be directly involved in the pathogenesis of tissue injury.

ANTIBODY REACTION WITH INTRINSIC OR PLANTED RENAL ANTIGENS **Anti-basement membrane antibody disease** This form of renal injury is relatively uncommon in humans. By mechanisms that remain obscure, autoantibodies (usually of the IgG isotype) directed to epitopes on the noncollagen domains of type IV (basement membrane) collagen arise in the circulation. These autoantibodies deposit in the kidney glomerular basement membrane (GBM) and/or tubular basement membrane (TBM) and, on occasion, elsewhere (alveolar basement membrane, choroid plexus basement membrane). Since the epitope is part of a repeating subunit uniformly expressed in basement membranes, the deposits of IgG appear linear by immunofluorescent microscopy (Fig. 226-1A). Electron-dense lattices of antigen-antibody complexes are not seen by electron microscopy. The local interaction of the autoantibody with the fixed and native basement membrane antigen leads to a perturbation in the structural components and also to the local activation of mediator systems to be described below. Although activation of the complement cascade facilitates injury by virtue of chemotactic and cytolytic effects, glomerular injury may also occur independent of complement activation. Because the antigen-antibody interaction occurs within the lamina rara interna or on the capillary luminal side of the lamina densa, circulating polymorphonuclear leukocytes, monocytes, and platelets are frequently involved in the mediation of glomerular injury.

Proteinuria results from the loss of glomerular anionic residues (see Chap. 49) and by structural defects in the capillary wall brought about by the local release of cationic lysosomal enzymes within infiltrating inflammatory cells. The glomerular filtration rate may decline if the loss of filtering surface area is sufficient to overcome adaptive increases in capillary flows and pressures in remaining capillary channels or nephron units. Obstruction of individual capillary channels may be the consequence of local coagulation, infiltration by inflammatory cells, or endothelial disruption. Leakage of macromolecules and cells such as fibrinogen and monocytes into Bowman's space through gaps in the capillary wall may provoke extracapillary proliferation as fibrinogen is polymerized to fibrin and monocytes release monokines locally.

Renal disease due to anti-basement membrane antibody production is seen primarily in three circumstances: in connection with glomerulonephritis and pulmonary hemorrhage due to anti-GBM autoantibodies (Goodpasture's syndrome), in idiopathic glomerulonephritis due to anti-GBM antibodies without pulmonary hemorrhage, and in idiopathic tubulointerstitial nephritis due to anti-TBM antibody production. In all instances, characteristic findings serve to identify the pathogenetic mechanism: (1) circulating autoantibodies react with basement membrane antigens in vitro; (2) linear deposits of IgG are found in the involved tissue; and (3) eluates of disease tissue contain immunoglobulin reactive with normal, native basement membrane antigens in vivo and in vitro.

Antibodies reactive with non-GBM-related antigens The glomerular capillary wall and mesangium are composed of a number of potentially immunogenic glycoproteins in addition to the GBM glycoprotein mentioned above. These antigens are distributed throughout the basement membrane, mesangial matrix, and cell surfaces.

Binding in situ of passively administered heterologous antibody or actively induced antibody to these antigens produces differing patterns of immunoglobulin localization and functional and structural alteration of the capillary wall. If the antigen is localized in clusters in relationship to the epithelial aspect of the capillary wall, the reaction with antibody in situ may give rise to granular or beadlike deposits of IgG detected by immunofluorescence and to electron-dense subepithelial deposits (Fig. 226-1B).

While the number of possible antigen-antibody interactions in this category is large, few have been documented to be responsible for human glomerular or tubulointerstitial disease. Thus far, animal

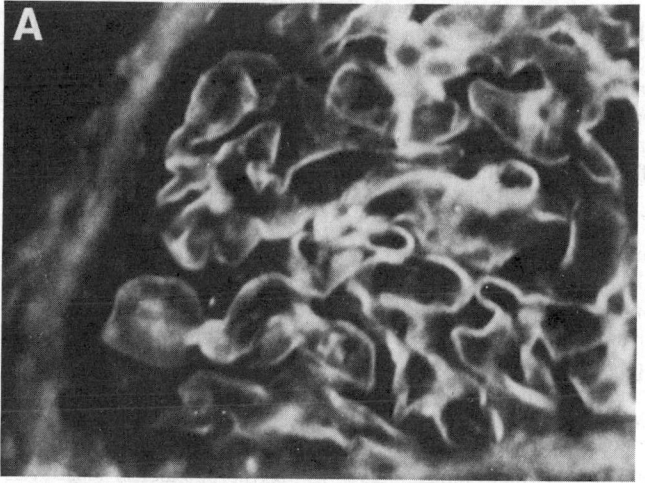

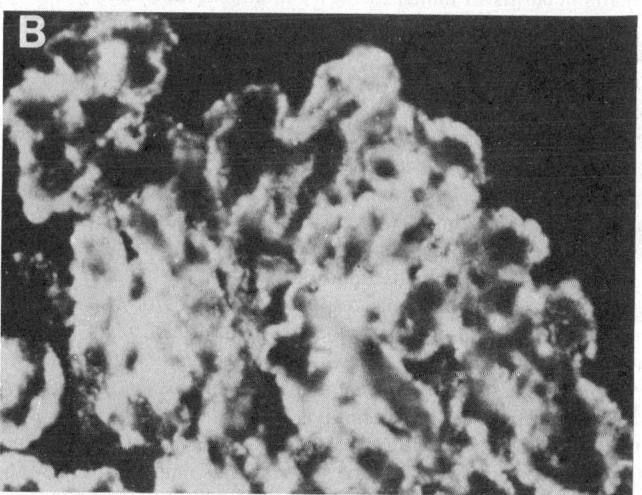

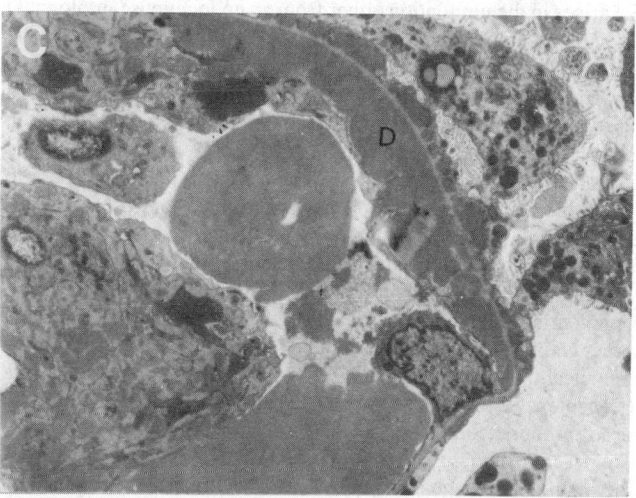

FIGURE 226-1 *A.* Immunofluorescence photomicrograph of a portion of a glomerulus from a patient with anti-glomerular basement membrane antibody-mediated glomerular injury. Note the linear deposits (fluorescein-labeled antihuman IgG). *B.* Immunofluorescence photomicrograph of a portion of a glomerulus from a patient with immune-complex-mediated (in situ or circulating) glomerular injury. Note the irregular, granular deposits (fluorescein-labeled antihuman IgG). *C.* Electron micrograph of a portion of a glomerular capillary from a patient with immune-complex-mediated glomerular injury. Note the electron-dense deposits, *D.*

experimentation has proceeded at a greater pace than understanding of human analogues of this mechanism. The best studied animal model is Heymann's nephritis, which is induced in rats by passive administration of a heterologous antibody to a particular glomerular capillary wall antigen or by active immunization with the antigen in complete Freund's adjuvant. The antigen-antibody interaction occurs in the subepithelial space in the glomerulus and at the brush border of the proximal tubule, where the antigen is synthesized as a component of endocytotic clathrin-coated pits on the surface of the glomerular visceral and proximal tubular epithelial cells. A granular pattern of IgG deposits and subepithelial electron-dense deposits are seen by immunofluorescence and electron microscopy, respectively. Localized activation of the complement cascade, including assembly of the membrane attack complex, may be responsible for altered glomerular permeability, but local variations in the basement membrane may also account for the changes in permselectivity. Since the antigen-antibody reactions occur on the epithelial side of the capillary wall, circulating cellular elements, such as polymorphonuclear leukocytes and monocytes, are not involved in glomerular injury. A similar mechanism might also be active in some idiopathic membranous glomerulonephritis in human beings. Additional reactions involving the binding of circulating antibody to intrinsic structural or self-surface antigens have been described in animals.

Antibodies reacting with planted glomerular antigens Circulating endogenous or environmental substances with special affinity for glomerular structures, including the glomerular capillary wall or mesangium, may deposit in these structures and thus act as a "planted" antigen. An antibody or cellular response to these planted nonglomerular or extrinsic antigens could result in disease as a result of the formation of antigen-antibody complexes in situ. The pattern of disease produced depends upon the sites of the planted antigen and the nature of the immune response. Examples of such planted antigens thus far described include certain drugs, plant lectins, cationized plasma proteins, aggregated immunoglobulins, and deoxyribonucleic acid. Experimental models of this sequence have been described, but there is little definitive information.

CIRCULATING IMMUNE-COMPLEX DISEASE (See Chap. 268)   The deposition in the kidney of immune complexes formed in the circulation accounts for many diseases of the kidney for which there is clear evidence of participation of some immunologic process. In this category an immunogenic replicating or nonreplicating substance arises in the circulation either from an endogenous (autologous) or exogenous (environmental) source. Antibody response to the antigen while the antigen remains in the circulation leads to the formation of an aggregate of antigen and antibody known as a *circulating immune complex*. The complement system plays an important role in the transport and removal of circulating immune complexes, and defects in the complement system may predispose to the deposition and accumulation of immune complexes at various tissue sites, including the glomerulus. Activated complement components, particularly C1q and C3b, interfere with the precipitation of immune complexes or solubilize preformed immune complexes, thus preventing their deposition as insoluble aggregates. Circulating immune complexes containing bound C3b are transported to the mononuclear phagocyte system (liver, spleen) via the erythrocyte CR1 receptor. Such transport and delivery favors uptake and degradation of immune complexes by the mononuclear phagocyte system. A small fraction of circulating immune complexes may escape removal by the mononuclear phagocyte system and instead be trapped by vascular structures including the glomeruli. Circulating immune complexes trapped in these sites have the capability of evoking inflammation utilizing many of the mediator systems described above. One of the best-studied examples of this circulating immune-complex disease involving a nonreplicating antigen is serum sickness, which results from the acute or chronic administration of an immunogenic, soluble, heterologous, foreign serum protein (see Fig. 268-1). A small portion of the immune complexes localize within the glomerular mesangium; in the walls of peripheral capillaries; and in joints, heart

valves, choroid plexus, splenic sinusoids, and larger blood vessels, particularly at sites of turbulent flow. Once deposited, these complexes evoke an inflammatory response at the site of deposition.

Although this formulation presupposes that immune complexes form within the circulation and then are deposited in vascular structures, immune complexes may form in the extravascular (interstitial) compartment by virtue of diffusion into this fluid compartment of cell-derived antigens and circulating antibody. Such a phenomenon may explain the deposition of immune complexes in the interstitial areas of the kidney, with relative sparing of the glomerular circulation. Regardless of the nature of the antibody or antigen or the particular circumstances surrounding the immunologic events, a valuable clue to the presence of immune-complex deposition or in situ formation is the morphologic pattern found when tissues are examined by immunofluorescence or electron-microscopic techniques. Granular, discontinuous, and irregular deposits of Ig, often in conjunction with complement components, are found by immunofluorescence (Fig. 226-1B), whereas electron-dense deposits are seen by electron microscopy (Fig. 226-1C). Sometimes these deposits acquire a definite substructure, but for the most part they are rather homogeneous. The deposits may develop in several locations within the glomerulus: beneath the epithelial cells (subepithelial), within the basement membrane (intramembranous), beneath the endothelium (subendothelial), and within the mesangial matrix. Immune complexes may also localize in the peritubular capillary network. The reason for localization at these differing sites may involve factors such as size or charge of the complexes, receptors for the Fc or complement components within glomerular structures, or local hemodynamic events. The deposits appear to increase in size by aggregation, and glomerular cells may participate in their removal. The persistence of deposits is related to the rate of formation balanced by the activity of removal systems. Ig itself in a circulating immune complex trapped in the glomerular circulation may behave as a planted antigen, either via the idiotypic determinants in the antigen-binding sites of antibody or via the Fc portions evoking an anti-immunoglobulin (rheumatoid factor) response. The roles played by anti-idiotype antibody or rheumatoid factor in the evolution of glomerular lesions in immune-complex-mediated disease is not clear. Once deposited in glomeruli, circulating immune complexes evoke local inflammatory and functional changes, which at least for the glomerular circulation may be relatively independent of complement or polymorphonuclear leukocytes. In situ formation of an immune complex in the subepithelial space may not be associated with the accumulation of inflammatory cells. Infiltrating monocytes may play a critical role in mediating glomerular injury. The morphologic lesions which result from immune-complex deposition may vary considerably, from diffuse proliferative to nonproliferative membranous or sclerosing lesions. Coagulation, platelet aggregation, activation of the complement cascade, and release of vasoactive amines may participate in determining the pattern of morphologic response.

The *exogenous* antigens involved in circulating immune-complex-mediated disease are derived chiefly from infectious agents such as bacteria, viruses, or parasites. Replication of the organism provides a continuing source of antigen. The best-studied examples of these in humans are *infective endocarditis, leprosy, syphilis, hepatitis B,* and *malaria.* The endogenous antigens involved in human disease vary considerably and include *DNA, thyroglobulin, autologous immunoglobulins, erythrocyte stroma, renal tubule antigens,* and *tumor-specific* or *tumor-associated* antigens.

CELL-MEDIATED IMMUNITY IN GLOMERULAR AND TUBULOINTERSTITIAL DISEASES   The roles of specifically sensitized cells acting independently of antibody (T cytotoxic cells), "armed" macrophages, and antibody-dependent cell-mediated cytotoxicity in the pathogenesis of glomerular and tubulointerstitial diseases have been difficult to establish. The glomerulus and probably the cortical interstitium possess the necessary elements to support a cell-mediated response to an autologous or heterologous antigen. Mononuclear cells capable of processing antigen and activating T helper-inducer cells in a major histocompatibility complex–restricted fashion are present in the glomerular mesangium and interstitium. A number of experimental diseases of the kidney, most notably tubulointerstitial nephritis, are the consequence of a cell-mediated immune response. However, relatively few human diseases can be ascribed to cell-mediated immune processes exclusively. The rejection of renal allografts in nonsensitized recipients is clearly a cell-mediated process (see Chap. 225).

By utilizing a variety of in vitro techniques cell-mediated hypersensitivity to both environmental and endogenous antigens is demonstrable in diseases of the kidney, including glomerulonephritis. The precise role such "sensitized" cells play in the actual tissue injury is unclear. It is likely that diseases that do not fit into an antibody- or immune-complex-mediated category will be explained as reactions of the cell-mediated variety. One likely candidate for this category is so-called minimal change disease, one of the subsets of idiopathic nephrotic syndrome. Furthermore, because of the prominence of lymphoid cell infiltration, various forms of chronic tubulointerstitial nephritis may also be cell-mediated reactions (see Chap. 229).

COMPLEMENT-ASSOCIATED GLOMERULAR INJURY Although there is little evidence that complement activation, independent of antitissue antibody or circulating immune complexes, can bring about glomerular injury, there are certain associations between complement and renal disease. The clinicopathologic entity known as *idiopathic mesangiocapillary glomerulonephritis* (see also Chap. 227) may be associated with serum complement deposition within glomeruli suggestive of involvement of the alternative pathway of complement activation, perhaps independent of immune-complex deposition. These patterns are not necessarily unique to this group of disorders since they may also be observed in postinfectious glomerulonephritides and in certain collagen-vascular diseases.

The activation of the complement cascade and the assembly of active cleaving enzymes is discussed more fully in Chap. 13. Briefly, the classical pathway of complement activation is initiated when antibodies (usually IgG or IgM) bind to their respective antigens and expose a C1q binding site on the Fc portion of the Ig molecule. Bound C1q activates C1r and C1s to form active C1qrs, which results in cleavage of C4 and C2 and leads to the assembly of the classical C3 and C5 convertases, C4b2a and C4b2a3b, respectively. The alternative pathway of complement is initiated when an active form of C3 in the fluid phase ($C3H_2O$) reacts with factors B, D, and properdin, forming a C3 convertase, C3Bb. IgA immune complexes, polysaccharides, or lipopolysaccharides have the potential of activating C3 via the alternative pathway. The resultant conversion of native C3 to C3b autocatalytically generates additional C3Bb. The amplification of C3Bb formation contributes to the generation of the C5 convertases, C42Bb3Bb from the classical pathway and C3bBGP from the alternative pathway. These C5 convertases cleave native C5 to C5a and C5b. The two pathways of complement activation thus converge upon C5, and with the interaction of the terminal complement components (C6, C7, C8, and C9) a lytic polymer of C5b6, 7, 8, 9 (n) is formed on the cell surface (the membrane attack complex). Several cleaved molecules (C3a, C5a) have potent proinflammatory and chemotactic properties. Inhibitor proteins control the activation of complement, including C1 inhibitor, factor H (β_1H), and factor I. As discussed previously, C1q and C3b have important functions relating to the aggregation and solubilization of immune complexes, and C3b participates in the transport of immune complexes to the removal sites in the mononuclear phagocyte system.

In *idiopathic mesangiocapillary glomerulonephritis*, particularly the subset known as *dense deposit disease*, serum C3 levels are depressed; C4, C1, and C2 levels tend to be normal; and C3 may be deposited in glomeruli without Ig (see also Chap. 227). In addition, an autoantibody (an immunoconglutinin) to alternative pathway C3 convertase is frequently found in the circulation. This autoantibody reacts with a conformational neoantigen of the alternative pathway C3 convertase and stabilizes this enzyme from the influence of C3b inactivator and β_1H in a fashion similar to properdin. As a result sera containing this autoantibody are capable of inducing C3 cleavage in

vitro by permitting the assembly of a stable fluid phase C3 convertase. This antibody is also known as C3 nephritic factor (C3NeF) and was first described in patients with glomerulonephritis and persistent depression of C3 levels.

The relationship between these aberrations in the complement pathway and glomerular injury is uncertain. No experimental models of persistent activation of the alternative pathway are associated with glomerulonephritis; thus, glomerular injury may be a closely associated but unrelated phenomenon, perhaps genetically determined. The recognition that certain structural genes for complement components (C2, C4) are closely associated with the major histocompatibility complex provides a potential explanation for the association of disease susceptibility with defects in biosynthesis of complement proteins. On the other hand, persistent hypocomplementemia may interfere with the normal removal processes for environmental antigens such as viruses. Such a defect might favor the persistence of these antigens in the circulation and enhance the likelihood of formation of circulating immune complexes. The discovery that C3 and its degradation product (primarily C3b) are able to solubilize aggregates of antigen and antibody may provide an additional explanation for the occurrence of immune-complex disease in association with defects of complement synthesis or activation.

Once initiated, immune injury is mediated by the interaction of humoral and cellular factors. Activation of the complement (C) cascade may lead to the cytolysis of the cellular constituents of the glomerulus or to the production of biologically active fragments capable of enhancing vascular permeability or attracting polymorphonuclear leukocytes and other cellular constituents. Coagulation may be initiated by alterations in the endothelial surface and exposure of collagen matrix, followed by localized platelet aggregation. Interactions between the complement cascade and the coagulation process are numerous and complex. Complement activation may trigger coagulation and vice versa. Activation of the Hageman factor can initiate the kallikrein-kinin system. Potent vasoactive peptides, prostaglandins, and leukotrienes may thus be released and play a role in alterations in local and systemic hemodynamics observed in conjunction with immunologically induced renal diseases. Polymorphonuclear leukocytes, eosinophils, monocytes (macrophages), and platelets can be called forth to participate in immune-mediated injury to varying degrees. Polymorphonuclear leukocytes and monocytes appear to participate in glomerular injury by virtue of their ability to release factors that degrade basement membrane glycoproteins and by facilitating the local production of toxic oxygen species (hydroxyl radical and superoxide anion). Activated monocytes may also express a membrane-bound procoagulant, thus fostering local fibrin deposition. Platelet deposition may be involved in the proliferation of glomerular cells via the release of a platelet-derived growth factor or may alter the anionic charge of the capillary wall by local release of cationic proteins, thus facilitating altered glomerular permselectivity. The composite result of these events is to alter the structural and functional integrity of the glomerular capillary and/or peritubular capillary wall, leading to reduced filtration capacity, enhanced permeability to plasma proteins, and migration of cellular elements (i.e., erythrocytes and leukocytes) outside the intravascular compartment.

REFERENCES

COUSER WG et al: Complement and the direct mediation of glomerular injury. A new perspective. Kidney Int 29:879, 1985

FRIES JWV et al: Determinants of immune complex–mediated glomerulonephritis. Kidney Int 34:333, 1988

SCHIFFERLI JA et al: The role of complement and its receptors in the elimination of immune complexes. N Engl J Med 315:488, 1986

SCHREINER GF JR et al: Macrophages and cellular immunity in experimental glomerulonephritis. Springer Semin Immunopathol 5:251, 1982

WILSON CB (guest ed): Immunopathology of renal disease, in *Contemporary Issues in Nephrology*, vol 18, BM Brenner, JH Stein (eds). New York, Churchill Livingstone, 1988

227 THE MAJOR GLOMERULOPATHIES

RICHARD J. GLASSOCK / BARRY M. BRENNER

Alterations of the structural and functional integrity of the glomerular capillary circulation are often associated with the findings, either singly or in combination, of hematuria, proteinuria, reduced glomerular filtration rate (GFR), and hypertension. Five major glomerulopathic syndromes are recognized: *acute glomerulonephritis, rapidly progressive glomerulonephritis, chronic glomerulonephritis,* the *nephrotic syndrome,* and *asymptomatic urinary abnormalities.* This chapter deals with diseases in which the kidney is either the sole or the predominant organ involved (i.e., the primary glomerulopathies) or is involved as a complication of infection or drug exposure. Glomerular injury associated with multisystem disorders or heredofamilial conditions is discussed in Chap. 228.

ACUTE GLOMERULONEPHRITIS

The causes of acute glomerulonephritis (AGN) are given in Table 227-1. The "acute nephritic syndrome" consists of the abrupt onset of *hematuria* and *proteinuria,* accompanied by evidence of *azotemia* (i.e., reduced GFR) and renal *salt and water retention.* If GFR is reduced markedly, oligoanuria may be present (see also Chap. 223). Salt and water retention leads to circulatory congestion, hypertension, and edema. Hematuria is most likely the consequence of migration of erythrocytes across damaged glomerular and/or peritubular capillary walls leading to the presence of erythrocytes in tubule fluid in the early part of the nephron. Proteinuria is the consequence of either a loss of anionic charges of the capillary wall (charge-selective defect) or the appearance of glomerular capillaries with larger-than-normal pore radius, permitting large plasma protein molecules to traverse the glomerular filter. Glomerular filtration rate is reduced presumably because of infiltration of the capillaries by inflammatory cells, which thereby reduce filtering surface area. Alternatively, the filtering surface area could be functionally decreased due to the local elaboration of vasoactive compounds capable of reversibly contracting mesangial cells (e.g., angiotensin II, leukotrienes), thereby leading to a reduction in the number of perfused glomerular capillaries. Extensive crescentic disease may obliterate Bowman's space, further impeding filtration. Fluid retention is due in part to decreased glomerular filtration rate but probably also to persistence of avid distal nephron salt and water reabsorption. Extracellular and intravascular fluid volumes are expanded by salt and fluid retention.

The edema of acute glomerulonephritis tends to appear initially in areas of low tissue pressure, such as the *periorbital* areas, but may subsequently progress to involve dependent portions of the body and

---

TABLE 227-1 Causes of acute glomerulonephritis

I Infectious diseases
  A Poststreptococcal glomerulonephritis*
  B Nonstreptococcal postinfectious glomerulonephritis
    1 Bacterial: infective endocarditis,* "shunt nephritis," sepsis,* pneumococcal pneumonia, typhoid fever, secondary syphilis, meningococcemia
    2 Viral: hepatitis B, infectious mononucleosis, mumps, measles, varicella, vaccinia, echovirus, and coxsackievirus
    3 Parasitic: malaria, toxoplasmosis
II Multisystem diseases: systemic lupus erythematosus,* vasculitis,* Henoch-Schönlein purpura,* Goodpasture's syndrome
III Primary glomerular diseases: mesangiocapillary glomerulonephritis, Berger's disease (IgA nephropathy),* "pure" mesangial proliferative glomerulonephritis
IV Miscellaneous: Guillain-Barré syndrome, irradiation of Wilms's tumor, self-administered diphtheria-pertussis-tetanus vaccine, serum sickness

* Most common causes.

---

lead to *ascites* and/or *pleural effusions. Circulatory congestion* is manifested by an increase in systemic and pulmonary vascular pressures, normal or increased cardiac output, and a shortened circulation time. In the absence of underlying valvular, myocardial, or coronary artery disease or severe diastolic hypertension there is little likelihood that true left ventricular congestive heart failure will develop. If pulmonary capillary pressure rises above the opposing plasma oncotic pressure, however, pulmonary edema may ensue. *Arterial diastolic hypertension* is the consequence of several factors, including extracellular fluid volume expansion, enhanced cardiac output, and modest increases in peripheral vascular resistance. Plasma renin activity, aldosterone, and the sympathetic nervous system are relatively suppressed. Hypertension may at times be accompanied by encephalopathy, particularly in young children.

The extent and severity of urinary abnormalities in AGN vary considerably. Gross (macroscopic) *hematuria* is the most common, and is often described by the patient as smoky-, coffee-, or cola-colored urine. Lesser degrees of hematuria may go unrecognized by the patient or parent; for this reason, the features of fluid retention and hypertension may be ascribed erroneously to other illnesses if examination of the urine sediment is omitted from the initial evaluation. Hematuria is often, but not invariably, accompanied by the excretion of *red cell casts.* The erythrocytes in the urinary sediment are characteristically small, distorted, fragmented, and hypochromic (dysmorphic hematuria). Leukocyturia and leukocyte casts may indicate the presence of inflammation in the glomerulus and interstitium. The degree of *proteinuria* varies according to the nature and severity of the underlying glomerular lesions. Rarely, protein excretion rates are within the normal range, but generally they are between 0.2 and 3 g/d. If proteinuria is marked and sustained, the nephrotic syndrome may appear (see below).

The short-term evolution of acute glomerulonephritis generally depends upon the nature of the underlying glomerular lesions and their treatment. For example, in infective endocarditis resolution of urinary findings and improved renal function may occur rapidly after control of the bacteremia by antimicrobials. Within a week or so of onset, most patients with poststreptococcal acute glomerulonephritis begin to experience spontaneous resolution of fluid retention and hypertension. Urinary abnormalities often take longer to resolve. A few patients with the acute nephritic syndrome in the ensuing weeks will develop a rapidly progressive form of renal failure (i.e., rapidly progressive glomerulonephritis, discussed below). The long-term outlook for patients with AGN is considered below in the context of treatment of specific lesions. Renal biopsy is useful in characterizing the nature of the underlying lesion but need not be done in every case.

ACUTE POSTSTREPTOCOCCAL GLOMERULONEPHRITIS
Clinical features and diagnosis This disorder can be viewed as the archetype of AGN. Poststreptococcal glomerulonephritis (PSGN) follows in the wake of *pharyngeal or cutaneous infection* with one of a limited number of strains of *group A β-hemolytic streptococci.* These potentially "nephritogenic" streptococci may be identified by serotyping of a cell wall antigen (M protein). Among outbreaks of infection with proved "nephritogenic" strains of streptococci the PSGN attack rate is relatively uniform, but because of variation in the nephritogenicity among group A streptococci, attack rates with outbreaks of infection vary considerably. Among families, asymptomatic episodes of PSGN exceed symptomatic episodes by a factor of 3 or 4 to 1. Immunity to M protein is type-specific, long-lasting, and protective. Repeated episodes of PSGN are therefore unusual. Outbreaks of pharyngeal infection–associated PSGN are commonest in children aged 6 to 10. AGN following cutaneous streptococcal infection is more commonly associated with poor personal hygiene, overcrowding, and concomitant cutaneous disease, such as scabies infestation. Seasonal and geographic variations in prevalence of PSGN are more marked for pharyngeal- than for cutaneous-associated disease.

An important feature of PSGN is the existence of a *latent period* between the earliest manifestations of infection and the onset of recognizable signs and symptoms of nephritis. Following pharyngeal infections the latent period usually is 6 to 10 days in duration. Cutaneous infections are associated with longer latent periods, averaging about 2 weeks. Definitive signs of glomerular inflammation occurring at the same time as, or shortly after, infection usually indicate an *exacerbation* of a preexisting chronic glomerular disease such as Berger's disease (IgA nephropathy) (see below).

The diagnosis of PSGN rests upon the demonstration of at least two of the following three features: (1) A group A β-hemolytic streptococcus of a potentially nephritogenic M-protein type is found in a throat or skin lesion. (2) An immune response to one or more of the streptococcal *exoenzymes,* including antistreptolysin O (ASO), antistreptokinase (ASK), anti-deoxyribonuclease B (ADNAase B), anti-nicotinyl adenine dinucleotidase (ANADase), or antihyaluronidase (AH), can be demonstrated. ASO responses are typically brisk in pharyngeal infections, but often absent in cutaneous infection, whereas AH, ADNAase, and ANADase responses occur after the latter. Testing for multiple antibody responses and serial determinations are necessary to achieve a diagnostic accuracy of 90 percent. Early antimicrobial therapy may prevent the antibody response to exoenzymes and render throat cultures negative but may not prevent the development of PSGN; this makes accurate serologic diagnosis difficult or impossible. (3) A transient decline in the serum concentration of the C3 component of complement, with a return to normal within 8 weeks after the first signs of renal disease, can be demonstrated. Other complement components (i.e., C1q and C4) are frequently less depressed. In addition to these laboratory features it is desirable to document a latent period appropriate to the nature of the infection. Furthermore, the patient should not have any known preexisting renal disease.

Other laboratory features commonly observed in PSGN include transient cryoimmunoglobulinemia and positive tests for circulating immune complexes. The erythrocyte sedimentation rate is usually elevated, while C-reactive protein and rheumatoid factor are generally normal or undetectable. Mild anemia and hypoalbuminemia, both largely dilutional in origin, may be present. Severe hypoalbuminemia may be encountered if heavy proteinuria is present and prolonged. Excretion rates of urinary protein in excess of 3.5 g/d occur in less than 20 percent of hospitalized patients. Proteinuria is usually of a nonselective character and frequently contains high concentrations of fibrin-degradation products and C3 protein, particularly during the diuretic phase. Hyponatremia, hyperchloremia, hyperkalemia, and metabolic acidosis may be seen in azotemic or oliguric patients, especially those with free access to water or potassium. Plasma renin activity and aldosterone secretion rates are low, reflecting suppression secondary to expanded plasma volume. Urinary sodium concentration is usually low, reflecting avid salt reabsorption in the distal nephron. Abdominal films reveal normal or enlarged kidneys. The chest x-ray may be normal or reveal a slightly enlarged heart, often accompanied by signs of pulmonary congestion. The electrocardiogram may reveal nonspecific T-wave abnormalities. Rheumatic fever rarely coexists with acute PSGN.

The differential diagnosis of PSGN includes other infectious or primary renal diseases which may produce an identical acute nephritic syndrome (Table 227-1). Multisystem diseases such as systemic lupus erythematosus, Henoch-Schönlein purpura, and vasculitis may present initially as acute nephritis (Chap. 228). Predominantly nonglomerular diseases, including thrombotic thrombocytopenic purpura, hemolytic-uremic syndrome, atheroembolic renal disease, and acute hypersensitivity interstitial nephritis may also present the features of the acute nephritic syndrome (Chaps. 229 and 230).

Pathology and pathogenesis Renal biopsies performed early in the course reveal *diffuse, endocapillary proliferative glomerulonephritis.* Infiltration of glomeruli with polymorphonuclear leukocytes and monocytes is common. The glomerular capillary walls are usually thin and delicate and free of necrosis. Occasional discrete proteinaceous deposits projecting from the outer aspects of the capillary wall

toward the urinary space (humps) may be recognized by light microscopy and coincide with the electron-dense deposits seen by electron microscopy. Segmental extracapillary proliferation (crescents) may involve a few glomeruli, but diffuse and extensive circumferential crescent formation is uncommon except among a subset of patients presenting with severe and rapidly progressive acute renal failure (see section below on rapidly progressive glomerulonephritis). Extraglomerular vessels and tubulointerstitial areas are usually normal. Red blood cells are frequently seen in the lumens of distal tubules, where they form red blood cell casts and dysmorphic erythrocytes.

By immunofluorescence microscopy, granular deposits of IgG are seen in peripheral capillary loops and mesangium, nearly always accompanied by C3 and properdin and less commonly by C1q and C4 (Chap. 226). Several patterns of Ig and/or C3 deposition have been described. Extensive involvement of the peripheral capillary loops with deposits may be associated with a poorer prognosis, while deposits exclusively involving the mesangium usually indicate a more benign outcome. The precise nature of the antigen-antibody systems involved remains unknown. Most likely the antigen is derived from the streptococcal organism itself, but this has been difficult to verify. The profile of altered serum complement components described above, and the prominent C3 and properdin deposition in glomeruli, are suggestive of involvement of the alternative pathway of complement activation (Chap. 226).

Course and treatment The ultimate *prognosis* for PSGN differs between sporadic and epidemic forms and between adults and children. *Epidemic* forms of the disease in *children* have a uniformly favorable short- and long-term prognosis. Few patients die of complications of renal failure (fewer than 1 percent), and nearly all experience a spontaneous resolution of clinical signs within a week after the onset of illness. Abnormalities in the urinary sediment and protein excretion subside slowly in the ensuing months; in a few cases, several years elapse before the urinary sediment is consistently normal. Among children with PSGN during epidemics of streptococcal infection, and in whom some form of preexisting chronic glomerular disease was absent, long-term follow-up has revealed little or no evidence of progression to chronic renal disease. A small percentage may develop extensive crescentic glomerulonephritis with its relentlessly progressive course. The site of the streptococcal infection, the type of M protein, the severity of abnormalities of complement or urinary sediment, or the extent of the rise in antibody response to exoenzymes have little or no bearing on the ultimate prognosis. Prolonged and persistent heavy proteinuria and/or abnormal GFR imply a more unfavorable outcome. *Sporadic* cases of PSGN among *children* may have more serious long-term consequences, although this remains controversial. After the subsidence of the acute disease, some children develop slowly progressive glomerular capillary obliteration (glomerulosclerosis), reduced GFR, and hypertension; after several decades, end-stage renal failure from chronic glomerulonephritis may result. The persistence of proteinuria is the rule in such cases.

The prognosis for *adults* with PSGN is less favorable than for children. The reason for this apparent difference is poorly understood. Although the overall prognosis for PSGN in *epidemics* seems good, *sporadic* PSGN in adults is associated with lasting and/or progressive deterioration in renal function in as many as one-third to one-half of cases. This may take the form of persistent proteinuria and/or hematuria or of slowly progressive glomerulosclerosis and renal failure, often accompanied by hypertension. This evolution seems more likely to occur when the initial disease is unusually severe. Whether milder forms of sporadic PSGN can lead to chronic disease is an unresolved issue (see "Chronic Glomerulonephritis" below).

The *treatment* of acute PSGN is supportive. It is reasonable to recommend bed rest until the signs of glomerular inflammation and circulatory congestion (primarily hypertension) subside, but prolonged periods of inactivity are of no demonstrable benefit in the healing process. Fluid retention, circulatory congestion, and edema may be treated with sodium and fluid restriction or loop diuretics. Diuresis alone often ameliorates mild to moderate hypertension. If severe hypertension is present, vasodilator drugs such as nitroprusside, nifedipine, hydralazine, or diazoxide may be useful. Encephalopathy and pulmonary congestion generally improve with lowering of blood pressure and the relief of circulatory overload. Digitalis should be avoided except in instances of well-documented organic heart disease with congestive failure. Treatment with ion exchange resins and/or dialysis may be required for cases of severe oliguria, fluid overload, and hyperkalemia. Mild protein restriction is desirable for azotemic patients. A 7- to 10-day course of antimicrobials (e.g., penicillin or erythromycin) should be given if streptococcal infection is documented. Long-term chemoprophylaxis is not indicated. Steroids and cytotoxic drugs are not of value.

NONSTREPTOCOCCAL ACUTE POSTINFECTIOUS GLOMERU-LONEPHRITIS Clinical features and diagnosis A wide variety of infectious illnesses other than those caused by group A β-hemolytic streptococci may also be associated with AGN (Table 227-1). These include *bacteremic states* and various *viral* and *parasitic* diseases. Ordinarily these diseases can be diagnosed by the presence of typical extrarenal clinical features or by bacteriologic or serologic findings. Infective endocarditis, sepsis of other types, typhoid fever, infectious mononucleosis, acute viral hepatitis (hepatitis B), falciparum malaria, and toxoplasmosis are examples of infectious diseases capable of evoking AGN. Circulating immune complexes play an important role in the pathogenesis of AGN in these diseases. Chronic or subacute bacteremic states are frequently associated with persistent depression of serum complement components C1q, C4, and C3, elevated levels of rheumatoid factor, circulating cryoimmunoglobulins, and strongly positive tests for circulating immune complexes. Control of infection usually results in the resolution of glomerular inflammation, although, in occasional instances, rapidly progressive or chronic glomerulonephritis may ensue.

RAPIDLY PROGRESSIVE GLOMERULONEPHRITIS

Transient azotemia, often associated with a brief period of oliguria, is common in AGN. A diuresis usually follows within days or a few weeks, and GFR returns to normal. On the other hand, some cases of AGN are characterized by a rapidly progressive form of renal failure, which often develops abruptly and displays little tendency for spontaneous or complete recovery. The clinical term *rapidly progressive glomerulonephritis (RPGN)* is often applied to this group to connote the development of renal failure in a period of weeks to months, rather than years or decades, as is typical of chronic glomerulonephritis (see below). Usually, but not invariably, extensive *extracapillary (crescentic) glomerulonephritis* is the pathologic lesion underlying the syndrome of RPGN, and the two terms are often used interchangeably.

RPGN can arise in four clinical settings (Table 227-2): (1) as a renal complication of an acute or subacute infectious disease, (2) as a renal complication of many multisystem diseases, (3) in association with the use of certain drugs, and (4) as a primary or idiopathic glomerular disease. In the latter circumstance the RPGN can arise de novo or be superimposed on another primary glomerular disease process. RPGN occurring as a primary glomerular disease will be discussed here, while that arising secondary to infectious diseases, multisystem diseases, or drugs will be considered in Chap. 228.

IDIOPATHIC RAPIDLY PROGRESSIVE GLOMERULONEPHRI-TIS Clinical features and diagnosis This disorder affects individuals in a broad age distribution and has a predilection for males. Wide geographic differences in the prevalence of the disease have been noted, and outbreaks ("miniepidemics") may occur. Some patients have had recent heavy exposure to volatile hydrocarbons, but there is little evidence to support a cause-and-effect relationship. While a flulike or viral prodrome may occur, frank arthritis, sinusitis, otitis, skin rash, neuritis, or encephalopathy are uncommon and are more in keeping with a multisystem disease. Symptoms of weakness,

TABLE 227-2 Causes of rapidly progressive glomerulonephritis

I Infectious diseases
  A Poststreptococcal glomerulonephritis*
  B Infective endocarditis*
  C Occult visceral sepsis
  D Hepatitis B infection (with vasculitis and/or cryoimmunoglobulinemia)
  E Human immunodeficiency virus infection (?)
II Multisystem diseases
  A Systemic lupus erythematosus*
  B Henoch-Schönlein purpura*
  C Systemic necrotizing vasculitis (including Wegener's granulomatosis)*
  D Goodpasture's syndrome*
  E Essential mixed (IgG/IgM) cryoimmunoglobulinemia
  F Malignancy
  G Relapsing polychondritis
  H Rheumatoid arthritis (with vasculitis)
III Drugs
  A Penicillamine*
  B Hydralazine
  C Allopurinol (with vasculitis)
  D Rifampin
IV Idiopathic or primary glomerular disease
  A Idiopathic crescentic glomerulonephritis*
    1 Type I—with linear deposits of Ig (anti-glomerular basement membrane antibody–mediated)
    2 Type II—with granular deposits of Ig (immune-complex–mediated)
    3 Type III—with few or no immune deposits of Ig ("pauci-immune")
    4 Anti-neutrophil cytoplasmic antibody–induced, ? "forme fruste" of vasculitis
  B Superimposed on another primary glomerular disease
    1 Mesangiocapillary (membranoproliferative glomerulonephritis)* (especially type II)
    2 Membranous glomerulonephritis*
    Berger's disease (IgA nephropathy)*

---

* Most common.

nausea, and vomiting (indicative of azotemia) usually dominate the clinical picture. Oliguria, abdominal or flank pain, and hemoptysis may also be present (see "Goodpasture's Syndrome," Chap. 228). The blood pressure is normal or modestly elevated. Urinalysis typically reveals dysmorphic hematuria and red cell casts, but relatively benign urine sediments may be present. Proteinuria is always present and may be massive. Other biochemical features of the nephrotic syndrome are uncommon, probably because of the concomitant reduction in GFR. Proteinuria is typically nonselective, and high concentrations of fibrin degradation products are found in urine. Azotemia develops early and tends to progress at a rapid rate. Other clinical and laboratory features relate to the underlying pathology and pathogenesis.

Pathology and pathogenesis Idiopathic RPGN is not a homogeneous disease. By light microscopy the characteristic abnormality in the kidneys is *extensive extracapillary proliferation*, i.e., crescents. The extent and degree of glomerular involvement varies; however, among patients with rapid deterioration of renal function it is usual for more than 70 percent of glomeruli to be involved with circumferential crescents. Endocapillary proliferation, if prominent, suggests the presence of infection. Segmental or diffuse endocapillary necrosis suggests underlying systemic necrotizing vasculitis. Fibrin-related antigens are nearly always demonstrable within the crescents by special stains or by immunofluorescence. Gaps or focal discontinuities in the glomerular basement membrane (GBM) and/or Bowman's capsule are observed in association with crescents.

Variations in the underlying pathogenetic mechanisms responsible for RPGN are illustrated by immunofluorescence studies of renal biopsies (Chap. 226). In approximately 5 to 20 percent of cases, *linear deposits* of IgG indicate involvement of *anti-GBM antibodies*. Circulating anti-GBM antibodies can be demonstrated by indirect immunofluorescence, hemagglutination, or radioimmunoassay techniques. Patients in this subgroup tend to have normal serum complement levels and a marked tendency to develop hemoptysis (see also "Goodpasture's Syndrome," Chap. 228). These patients frequently are HLA-DR2 antigen–positive. About 30 to 40 percent of cases will have findings of *immune-complex–mediated disease*, namely, *granular deposits* of immunoglobulin by immunofluorescence microscopy and electron-dense deposits by electron microscopy. This mechanism of RPGN tends to occur in older individuals, to produce more constitutional symptoms, and to result in more disturbances of the complement pathways than does anti-GBM antibody–mediated disease. Hemoptysis may also occur, but circulating anti-GBM antibodies are absent. C3 levels may be decreased. The remainder of cases of RPGN reveal scanty or no immunoglobulins or complement by immunofluorescence (''pauci-immune''); their pathogenesis is unknown. This group also tends to include older individuals, in whom serum complement concentrations are normal and anti-GBM antibodies are absent. Occasionally, mild hemoptysis may occur. This latter variation may represent a ''forme fruste'' of systemic necrotizing vasculitis with isolated renal involvement. Such patients often have detectable anti-neutrophil cytoplasmic antibody characteristic of systemic necrotizing vasculitis and Wegener's granulomatosis (see Chap. 228).

Lung hemorrhage may be observed in a variety of circumstances associated with RPGN. This subject is covered in greater detail in the section on Goodpasture's syndrome in Chap. 228. Uncommonly, other idiopathic (primary) glomerular diseases may be complicated by a superimposed rapidly progressive glomerulonephritis accompanied by extensive crescent formation. These primary glomerular diseases include mesangiocapillary (membranoproliferative) glomerulonephritis, Berger's disease (IgA nephropathy), and membranous glomerulonephritis (Table 227-2). The pathogenetic mechanisms underlying this complication vary.

Course and treatment   The prognosis for preservation of renal function in RPGN is poor. Patients with crescent formation in 70 percent or more of glomeruli or oliguria or severe reduction in GFR (less than 5 mL/min) at the time of presentation and those with an anti-GBM antibody–mediated process have the worst prognosis. Although advances in treatment are changing the outlook for patients with RPGN, as many as one-half require maintenance hemodialysis within 6 months of discovery of the illness. Exceptional patients with crescentic glomerulonephritis have a more protracted illness. Spontaneous resolution is uncommon, except among patients with infection as the basis for formation of antigen-antibody complexes, where removal of antigen can take place.

Glucocorticoids, in the form of ''pulses'' of parenteral methylprednisolone in high doses, and daily oral prednisone, often combined with *cytotoxic agents* (azathioprine or cyclophosphamide), have yielded varying degrees of success, particularly in the patients with granular or minimal Ig deposits in glomeruli, especially in association with vasculitis. Since no controlled studies have yet been conducted, however, it is difficult to ascertain the value of these regimens. Nonetheless, more than two-thirds of patients treated with several ''pulses'' of intravenous methylprednisolone have experienced improvement in renal function often sufficient to avoid the necessity of dialysis. The addition of *anticoagulants* (heparin or warfarin sodium) and antithrombotic agents (dipyridamole, sulfinpyrazone) seems rational on the basis of evidence for involvement of the coagulation process in the genesis of crescent formation. However, evidence of benefit from such therapies in animals with experimentally induced crescentic glomerulonephritis is inconsistent, in part because of variations in the severity of the disease models, the timing of treatment, and the nature of the anticoagulant or antithrombotic agent used. Anticoagulants may be hazardous in patients with advanced renal failure. *Ancrod,* a fibrinogenolytic agent not yet released in the United States, may also be an effective agent. *Intensive plasma exchange* (plasmapheresis—2 to 4 L of plasma daily or three times weekly), combined with steroids and cytotoxic agents, has been employed in patients with RPGN with very encouraging preliminary results, especially in patients revealing linear Ig deposits in glomeruli (anti-GBM antibody–mediated disease). A beneficial effect of intensive plasma exchange combined with immunosuppressive agents has also been claimed in patients with RPGN who do not demonstrate evidence of anti-GBM antibody production. Such benefit has been observed even when the patients have progressed to dialysis-dependent renal

failure. Some of these latter patients may have a forme fruste of systemic necrotizing vasculitis. Since few prospective studies comparing the efficacy of glucocorticoids plus immunosuppressive agents versus combined intensive plasma exchange, glucocorticoids, and immunosuppressive agents have been performed, the contribution of intensive plasma exchange to the observed improvements has not been established.

Beneficial effects appear to be greatest when such combined therapy is instituted early in the course of disease, before glomerular abnormalities are advanced. Renal biopsy assessment of the nature, severity, and potential reversibility of disease is a vital aspect of evaluation of patients suspected of having rapidly progressive glomerulonephritis. Such biopsies should be performed early in the course of disease. Despite aggressive therapy, many patients with oliguria do poorly. Treatment must be individualized, and because regular dialysis therapy and/or transplantation are available to most patients with RPGN, one should probably err on the side of a conservative approach, unless compelling evidence in support of potential reversibility is present.

RPGN may recur after renal transplant. It is difficult to be certain of the precise risk in individual cases. At present it seems prudent to recommend that, after initiating dialysis, a period of 3 to 6 months be allowed to elapse before undertaking renal transplantation in patients who have circulating anti-GBM antibodies. There is no convincing evidence that bilateral nephrectomy in advance of transplantation reduces the risk of recurrent disease in the transplant.

THE NEPHROTIC SYNDROME

In its overt form, the nephrotic syndrome (NS) is characterized by *albuminuria, hypoalbuminemia, hyperlipidemia,* and *edema.* These abnormalities are direct or indirect consequences of excessive glomerular leakage of plasma proteins into the urine (see also Chaps. 38 and 49). The defects in the charge- or size-selective barriers of the glomerular capillary wall that underline the excessive filtration of plasma proteins can arise as a consequence of a wide variety of disease processes, including immunologic disorders, toxic injuries, metabolic abnormalities, biochemical defects, and vascular disorders. Thus, nephrotic syndrome is a common end point of a variety of disease processes damaging the permeability properties of the glomerular capillary wall. *Heavy proteinuria* is the hallmark of the nephrotic state. Arbitrarily, protein excretion rates in excess of 3.5 g per 1.73 m^2 surface area per day [or urinary protein concentration of greater than 0.4 mg/mmol (3.5 mg/dL) creatinine] are considered to be in the nephrotic range, primarily because proteinuria of this magnitude is seldom observed in tubulointerstitial and vascular diseases of the kidney. Sustained heavy proteinuria is often, but not invariably, accompanied by *hypoalbuminemia.* Excessive urinary losses, increased renal catabolism, and inadequate hepatic synthesis of albumin all contribute to this depression of plasma albumin. The resulting decrease in plasma oncotic pressure leads to a disturbance in the Starling forces acting across peripheral capillaries. Intravascular fluid migrates into the interstitial tissue (i.e., *edema*), particularly in areas of low tissue pressure. These disturbances initiate a series of homeostatic adjustments designed to correct the resulting deficit in effective plasma volume. These include activation of the renin-angiotensin-aldosterone system, enhanced vasopressin secretion, stimulation of the sympathetic nervous system, and perhaps an alteration in the secretion or renal response to atrial natriuretic peptide. These and other poorly understood adjustments lead to renal sodium and water retention, primarily because of avid reabsorption in distal nephron segments, resulting in unrelenting edema. The severity of edema correlates with the level of serum albumin and with the extent of urinary protein losses. The extent and severity of edema are conditioned by factors such as heart disease or peripheral vascular disease. Profound hypoalbuminemia may occasionally be associated with severe plasma volume reduction, postural hypotension, syncope, and shock. Occasionally acute renal failure may occur. Although this formulation indicates that nephrotic syndrome is invariably accompanied by a significant deficit in intravascular volume and homeostatically appropriate renal salt and water retention, this pattern is not always observed. In fact, measurements of plasma volume, renin, and aldosterone, and determination of the events underlying renal salt and water reabsorption have documented heterogeneity in the pathophysiology of fluid volume homeostasis. Some have expanded intravascular fluid volume and suppressed renin-aldosterone axis, presumably mediated by primary, non-aldosterone-dependent renal salt and fluid retention, resembling the pathophysiology of acute nephritis (see above). These patients often, but not invariably, have some decrease in GFR and structural glomerular lesions. At the other end of the spectrum are patients with overt hypovolemia, hyperreninemia, and avid secondary renal salt retention. Serum albumin levels are low, extracellular fluid volume is expanded, and edema is usually present in both groups.

The diminished plasma oncotic pressure also appears to stimulate hepatic lipoprotein synthesis, and *hyperlipidemia* is a frequent accompaniment of the nephrotic state. Low-density lipoproteins and cholesterol are elevated most frequently, but as the plasma oncotic pressure falls further, very low density lipoproteins and triglycerides also increase. Excessive urinary losses of plasma protein factors regulating lipoprotein synthesis or disposal may also contribute to the hyperlipidemic state. Whether these lipid abnormalities contribute to accelerated atherosclerosis remains controversial. Lipid bodies (fatty casts, oval fat bodies) commonly appear in the urine.

Urine losses of plasma proteins other than albumin are also of importance. Loss of thyroxine-binding globulin may produce abnormalities in thyroid function tests, including a low thyroxine and an enhanced resin triiodothyronine uptake. Loss of cholecalciferol-binding protein may lead to a vitamin D deficiency state and secondary hyperparathyroidism and may contribute to the hypocalcemia and hypocalciuria seen commonly. Enhanced urinary excretion of transferrin may produce an iron-resistant microcytic, hypochromic anemia. Zinc and copper deficiency may result from urinary losses of metal-binding proteins. A hypercoagulable state frequently accompanies severe nephrotic syndrome [serum albumin less than 20 g/L (2 g/dL)]. A variety of factors contribute to the enhanced tendency to thrombosis in nephrotic patients including deficiencies in antithrombin III (due to urine losses), reduced levels or activity of protein C or protein S, hyperfibrinogenemia, enhanced platelet aggregation, and hyperlipidemia.

Some patients develop severe IgG deficiency, in part due to urinary losses and hypercatabolism. Low-molecular-weight complement components may also be lost in the urine and contribute to defects in the opsonization of bacteria. Various drug-binding proteins (chiefly albumin) may be decreased, altering the pharmacokinetics and toxicity of many drugs. Cellulose acetate electrophoresis of serum reveals, in addition to diminished albumin levels, increases of alpha and beta globulins.

COMPLICATIONS AND MANAGEMENT OF THE NEPHROTIC SYNDROME *Edema* should be managed cautiously and conservatively. Overly vigorous diuresis with potent loop diuretics (furosemide or ethacrynic acid) may result in an abrupt decline in effective plasma volume as the deficit in plasma oncotic pressure may preclude mobilization of the extracellular fluid into the intravascular compartment. This is more likely to occur if plasma volume is diminished and may lead to further reduction in GFR, worsening azotemia, and postural hypotension. Severe extracellular volume depletion may predispose to the development of acute renal failure. The temptation to administer concentrated salt-poor albumin should be resisted, as nearly all the administered protein will be excreted in 24 to 48 h, so that any beneficial effect on plasma oncotic pressure will be transient. However, such treatment may be necessary in severely hypoalbuminemic patients suffering from profound postural symptoms or very refractory anasarca.

The treatment of *hyperlipidemia* is frequently unsuccessful, and its influence on morbidity and mortality is uncertain. Colestipol, probucol, and lovastatin can all result in modest decrements in plasma total cholesterol in patients with nephrotic hyperlipidemia. Whether such treatment will be associated with a reduction in risk for atherosclerosis and ischemic heart or cerebral disease is not proven.

The *thromboembolic complications* of NS are reasonably common, including spontaneous peripheral venous and/or arterial, pulmonary arterial, and renal venous occlusions. *Renal vein thrombosis* (RVT), either unilateral or bilateral, is a particularly distressing complication. In the past, this was regarded as a cause rather than a consequence of NS, a conclusion no longer held. Certain glomerular lesions are more likely than others to be associated with RVT. These include membranous glomerulonephritis, mesangiocapillary glomerulonephritis, and amyloidosis. Features suggestive of *acute* RVT include unilateral or bilateral flank or loin pain, gross hematuria, left-sided varicocele, widely fluctuating GFR and urinary protein excretion rates, and asymmetry of renal size and/or function. Scalloping of the ureters (due to collateral circulation) and evidence of pulmonary emboli and/or infarction (Chap. 230) may occur in chronic RVT.

Chronic forms of RVT are commonly asymptomatic. Some advocate an aggressive approach in patients with nephrotic syndrome due to lesions associated with inherently high prevalence of RVT (e.g., membranous glomerulonephritis), routinely employing selective renal venous angiography. If RVT is detected, long-term (optimal duration unknown) anticoagulants are prescribed. Such an approach might prevent later development of serious embolic complications, but since the true risk of pulmonary embolism in this group of patients is not known, although probably low, the benefits-risk relationship of this approach cannot be determined. A more conservative approach has also been advocated in which renal venous angiography is performed only in those patients who have a pulmonary embolism (e.g., symptoms, compatible laboratory findings, and a high-probability ventilation-perfusion scan or pulmonary angiogram) and who have negative noninvasive studies directed toward detecting deep venous thrombosis in the lower extremities. Since such patients would receive anticoagulant therapy in any case, the value of localizing the site of thrombosis is not established. Positive ventilation-perfusion scans in asymptomatic nephrotic patients are likely to have limited value, since subsegmental defects in perfusion may be observed in nephrotic patients even in the absence of renal vein or lower extremity deep venous thrombosis. These changes could conceivably be due to in situ pulmonary arterial thrombosis. The risk of renal vein thrombosis or deep venous thrombosis is increased primarily in patients with nephrotic syndrome and a very low serum albumin level [e.g., less than 20 g/L (2 g/dL)]. The presence of a documented thromboembolic complication is usually regarded as a clear indication for long-term oral anticoagulation. The effectiveness of heparin may be impaired by concomitant antithrombin III deficiency, a factor required for the full expression of the heparin-induced antithrombin effect.

High-protein diets are frequently prescribed; however, the beneficial effect of this approach can be challenged since the main effect of increasing dietary protein is to increase urinary protein excretion rate and the effect on serum albumin levels is modest. Furthermore, such diets are difficult to manage with concomitant salt restriction and, at least theoretically, could aggravate the progression of an underlying structural glomerular lesion. An alternative approach is to prescribe modest protein restriction (e.g., 0.6 g/kg body weight per day), particularly in azotemic patients; some also advocate adding a supplementary amount of dietary protein equal to urinary protein losses. Dietary protein should be of high biologic value and can be supplemented with amino acids. Plasma albumin and transferrin concentrations as well as urinary protein excretion rates should be monitored to evaluate the effect of diet on overall nutritional status. Correction of transport protein deficiencies is not feasible. Supplemental vitamin D might be desirable if deficiency is present, but this has not been fully evaluated clinically. In rare circumstances, profound protein malnutrition or other complications of massive proteinuria may justify ablation of renal function by medical or surgical means.

TABLE 227-3 Causes of the nephrotic syndrome

I Primary glomerular diseases*
  A Minimal change disease*
  B Mesangial proliferative glomerulonephritis†
  C Focal and segmental glomerulosclerosis*
  D Membranous glomerulonephritis*
  E Mesangiocapillary glomerulonephritis*
    1 Type I
    2 Type II
    3 Other variants
  F Other uncommon lesions
    1 Crescentic glomerulonephritis
    2 Focal and segmental proliferative glomerulonephritis†
    3 Unclassifiable lesions
II Secondary to other diseases
  A Infections: poststreptococcal glomerulonephritis,* endocarditis, "shunt nephritis," secondary syphilis, leprosy, hepatitis B,* acquired immunodeficiency syndrome (AIDS), infectious mononucleosis, malaria, schistosomiasis, filariasis
  B Drugs: organic gold; inorganic, organic, and elemental mercury; penicillamine; "street" heroin,* probenecid; captopril; Tridione; mesantoin; perchlorate; antivenom; antitoxins; contrast media
  C Neoplasia: Hodgkin's disease, lymphomas, leukemia, carcinomas, melanoma, Wilms's tumor
  D Multisystem: systemic lupus erythematosus,* Henoch-Schönlein purpura,* vasculitis, Goodpasture's syndrome, dermatomyositis, dermatitis herpetiformis, amyloidosis,* sarcoidosis, Sjögren's syndrome, rheumatoid arthritis
  E Heredofamilial: diabetes mellitus,* Alport's syndrome, sickle cell disease, Fabry's disease, nail-patella syndrome, lipodystrophy, congenital nephrotic syndrome
  F Miscellaneous: preeclamptic toxemia, thyroiditis, myxedema, malignant obesity, renovascular hypertension, chronic interstitial nephritis with vesicoureteric reflux, chronic allograft rejection, bee stings

* Most common.
† Includes Berger's disease (IgA nephropathy).

A classification of the causes of nephrotic syndrome is provided in Table 227-3. The multisystemic, heredofamilial, neoplastic, and metabolic causes are discussed in Chap. 228. The primary (idiopathic) glomerular diseases associated with nephrotic syndrome, as well as the diseases secondary to infectious or drug etiologies, are considered below.

IDIOPATHIC NEPHROTIC SYNDROME This diagnosis is arrived at by exclusion of known causes of NS, such as infections, drug exposure, malignancy, multisystem disease, or hereditary disorders. The idiopathic forms of NS are further classified according to the morphologic features found on renal biopsy (Table 227-4). Performance of a renal biopsy, at least among adults, is required for the accurate diagnosis of idiopathic NS and for the formulation of a rational plan of treatment. Children need not always be subjected to renal biopsy since careful clinical study can often lead to accurate diagnosis.

Minimal change disease This is often referred to as *lipoid nephrosis, nil lesion,* or *foot process disease.* In this form of idiopathic NS, although little or no alterations of the glomerular capillaries are demonstrable by light microscopy (hence the designation "minimal change"), *diffuse epithelial foot process effacement*[1] is evident by electron microscopy. Immunofluorescence microscopy reveals absent or irregular and nonspecific deposits of immunoglobulin and complement components (chiefly IgM and C3). Minimal change disease is the most frequently encountered form of idiopathic NS in children, accounting for more than 70 to 80 percent of cases diagnosed before

[1] The term "fusion" is often used to describe these changes in foot processes, although true fusion of cell membranes does not occur.

TABLE 227-4 Idiopathic nephrotic syndrome

SELECTED FEATURES OF UNDERLYING PRIMARY GLOMERULAR LESIONS

Lesion	Morphology*			Approximate prevalence in children/ adults, %	Common clinical/ lab features	Response to therapy†	Likelihood of maintaining renal function‡
	LM	IFM	EM				
Minimal change	Normal or very mild proliferation	Negative–trace IgM	Foot process fusion, no deposits	70+/15–20	Highly selective proteinuria,§ *normal* C3, decreased IgG, increased IgM	Steroids + + Cytotoxic drugs + (cyclophosphamide, chlorambucil) Frequent relapses	95+
Mesangial proliferative	Diffuse proliferation	Negative or variable mesangial IgM, IgG, C3¶	Mesangial deposits	15–20/5–10	Hematuria, *normal* C3	Steroids ± Cytotoxic drugs (?)	80 (?)
Focal sclerosis	Focal and segmental sclerosis	Focal and segmental IgM, C3	Foot process fusion, sclerosis, hyaline	10/10–20	Hematuria, leukocyturia, poorly selective proteinuria, *normal* C3	Steroids + Cytotoxic drugs −	45–50
Membranous glomerulonephritis	Thick capillary wall, spikes of BM material	Diffuse granular capillary wall IgG	Subepithelial deposits	<5/30–40	Variable protein selectivity, *normal* C3, renal vein thrombosis	Steroids ± Cytotoxic drugs +	70+
Mesangial proliferative glomerulonephritis							
Type I	Mesangial interposition, lobular change	Diffuse C3; variable IgG, IgM	Subendothelial deposits	8/<5	Hematuria, *reduced* C3 (intermittent)	Steroids (?) Anticoagulants (?) Cytotoxic drugs (?) Antithrombotics +	60
Type II	Mesangial interposition	C3 capillary wall and mesangial nodules	Intramembranous deposits	3/<5	Hematuria, *reduced* C3 (persistent), +C3NF	Steroids − Cytotoxic drugs −	45

* LM = light microscopy, IFM = immunofluorescence microscopy, EM = electron microscopy, BM = basement membrane.
† Response to therapy: + + = highly responsive, + = variably responsive, ± = occasionally responsive, − = unresponsive.
‡ Percent of patients maintaining sufficient renal function to obviate need for chronic dialysis or transplantation within 5 years.
§ Protein selectivity = differential protein clearance, e.g., IgG/transferrin clearance ratio. Highly selective = <0.1, moderately selective = 0.11 to 0.20, poorly selective = >0.20.
¶ Ig deposits are seen in Berger's disease.
NOTE: C3NF = C3 nephritic factor.

the age of 8. This lesion is not rare in adults, representing 15 to 20 percent of cases of idiopathic NS in patients over the age of 16. There is a slight predilection for males. Typically patients present with overt NS, normal blood pressure, normal or slightly reduced GFR, and a "benign" urinary sediment. Varying degrees of microscopic hematuria are found in up to 20 percent of cases. Urinary protein is typically highly selective in children (e.g., it contains principally albumin and minimal amounts of high-molecular-weight plasma proteins such as IgG, alpha$_2$ macroglobulin, or C3) but is variable in adults. The pattern of protein excretion indicates a major "charge-selective" defect in permselectivity. Fibrin split products and C3 are absent in the urine. Serum levels of complement components are normal, except for a slight reduction in C1q. IgG concentrations are often quite depressed during relapse, whereas IgM levels are modestly increased, both during remission and relapse. Some cases may have associated allergic diathesis (e.g., to milk, pollens, etc.), a history of recent immunization, or upper respiratory infection. Circulating immune complexes may be found in some patients using certain assays. The histocompatibility antigen HLA-B12 is more prevalent when minimal change disease is associated with atopy, indicating a possible genetically based predisposition to this disease. Thromboembolic manifestations occur, but renal vein thrombosis is uncommon.

Spontaneous remissions and relapses of heavy proteinuria may occur. Interestingly, an identical lesion is encountered in patients with Hodgkin's disease in whom NS develops, suggesting a role for lymphocytes in its pathogenesis. Except for patients who develop focal and segmental sclerosing lesions (see below), a progressive decline in GFR does not occur. Acute renal failure is rare. In the preantibiotic era infection with encapsulated organisms (e.g., pneumococci) was a leading cause of death, but now the mortality rate is low, and most deaths are associated with complications of treatment rather than the disease itself. Rarely, acute renal failure may occur even without profound hypovolemia. The mechanism is obscure but could relate to tubular obstruction from heavy proteinuria or interstitial edema or severe glomerular epithelial cell effacement. The renal failure is often responsive to steroids and diuretics.

Since the etiology and pathogenesis are unknown, treatment is empirical and symptomatic. Glucocorticoids markedly enhance the natural tendency for this disease to undergo spontaneous remission. Daily or alternate-day oral steroid therapy seems to be equally effective; the latter is associated with fewer steroid-related complications. Daily prednisone (60 mg/m^2 surface area in children, 1 to 1.5 mg/kg body weight in adults) for 4 weeks, followed by alternate-day prednisone (35 to 40 mg/m^2 in children, 1 mg/kg in adults) for 4 additional weeks is a regimen often recommended for initial treatment of this disorder.

Over 95 percent of children (less than age 16) with minimal change disease respond with a complete disappearance of proteinuria within 8 weeks of the institution of prednisone therapy. Because of the high probability of minimal change disease in children, many pediatricians prefer to treat without an initial renal biopsy. A complete steroid response in such circumstances is highly indicative of underlying minimal change disease in children.

On the other hand, only about 30 to 70 percent of adults with minimal change disease respond within 8 weeks of instituting prednisone therapy, with a maximum response often not attained until 20 to 24 weeks from initiation of treatment. Patients over the age of 40 seem to be less responsive to steroids than those under the age of 40 when the disease is discovered. Ultimately the overall response rate in adults is only slightly less than that observed in children. The delayed response to glucocorticoids in adults could be due, in part, to the lower doses of prednisone relative to the doses used in children. Because of the likelihood of a lesion other than minimal change disease and the fact that some of these other lesions (e.g., focal sclerosis) may also sometimes respond to glucocorticoids, a steroid-responsive adult patient with idiopathic nephrotic syndrome cannot be assumed to have minimal change disease.

Among both adults and children, 50 to 60 percent of patients with minimal change disease relapse during the tapering phase of steroid withdrawal or at varying intervals after the cessation of therapy. Such relapses generally indicate a steroid-dependent patient. Frequent relapses (more than three per year) may require repetitive treatment with steroids and may be associated with exogenous Cushing's syndrome. Such patients can ordinarily be identified within 12 to 18 months after steroid treatment. Relapses may be treated with the initial regimen but with more gradual withdrawal of prednisone and with low maintenance doses of 5 to 10 mg daily or on alternate days for 3 to 6 months.

A steroid-dependent patient or one with multiple relapses may benefit by a brief course of cyclophosphamide 2 to 3 mg/kg body weight per day or chlorambucil 0.1 to 0.2 mg/kg body weight per day for 8 to 10 weeks. The steroid-dependent frequently relapsing patient has a lower likelihood of having a prolonged relapse-free interval after such therapy. Overall, only about half of frequently relapsing patients with minimal change disease treated with cyclophosphamide or chlorambucil remain free of disease after 5 years. Among children with minimal change disease the frequency of relapses declines with age. However, cytoxic agents have adverse effects on bone marrow and, in the case of cyclophosphamide, the gonads and urinary bladder. Careful monitoring of hematologic and urinary findings is mandatory. They may also be oncogenic. Azathioprine, previously believed to be ineffective in minimal change disease, will require reevaluation because of anecdotal reports of slow but eventual disappearance of proteinuria in patients with minimal change disease and steroid-sensitive or steroid-dependent nephrotic syndrome treated for 6 months to 1 year with azathioprine 2 to 2.5 mg/kg body weight per day. Cyclosporine in doses of 4 to 6 mg/kg body weight per day induces lasting remissions of nephrotic syndrome in as many as 50 percent of patients treated for 8 to 10 weeks. Further controlled trials are needed before this nephrotoxic agent can be recommended for routine use. Cyclosporine may yet prove to be valuable for steroid-dependent patients who continue to relapse despite cyclophosphamide or chlorambucil therapy or who become steroid unresponsive.

The use of cytotoxic agents should be reserved for patients who develop serious complications of multiple courses of steroid therapy. The long-term prognosis of patients with the minimal change lesion is excellent; a 10-year survival is in excess of 90 percent, but a few develop renal failure as a consequence of development of focal sclerosing glomerular lesions (see below) in association with acquired resistance to glucocorticoid therapy.

Mesangial proliferative glomerulonephritis   The lesion is characterized by a mild to moderate diffuse, but distinct, increase in the cellularity of the glomerular capillary bed. The peripheral glomerular capillary walls are thin and delicate, and extracapillary proliferation is not seen. The precise nature of the proliferating cells is not clearly understood but may represent combinations of proliferating mesangial cells, endothelial cells, and infiltrating mononuclear cells. Glomerular involvement is usually reasonably uniform, although there may be segmental accentuation of hypercellularity. Necrosis of glomerular tufts is absent. Deposits of proteinaceous material, if seen, are confined to the mesangial areas. Interposition of mesangial cells and cytoplasm into the periphery of the glomerular capillary wall is not seen. By immunofluorescence, a variety of patterns are observed. If granular IgA deposits in the mesangium predominate, accompanied by C3 and fibrin-reactive antigens but not the early acting components of the complement cascade, then the lesion is categorized as IgA nephropathy, or Berger's disease (see below). Other patterns of immunofluorescence include a predominance of IgM deposits in a granular pattern diffusely throughout the mesangium, isolated mesangial C3 deposits, scattered mesangial IgG deposits, and no immunoglobulin or complement deposits. Thus, mesangial proliferative glomerulonephritis represents a heterogeneous group of glomerular diseases. Some patients with this morphologic lesion may in fact represent instances of resolving postinfectious glomerulonephritis, hereditary nephritis, or other multisystem diseases such as Henoch-

Schönlein purpura, vasculitis, or systemic lupus erythematosus. Electron-microscopic findings are nonspecific. Occasionally small electron-dense paramesangial deposits may be observed.

The findings of large electron-dense deposits in the mesangium in association with the morphologic appearance of mesangial proliferative glomerulonephritis should heighten the suspicion of a multisystem disease or Berger's IgA nephropathy. This lesion accounts for approximately 10 percent of idiopathic nephrotic syndrome in adults and 15 percent in children. It is more common in older children and young adults. Males are affected slightly more often than females. Hematuria, either gross or microscopic, is common. Loin pain, bilateral or unilateral, may be seen in the idiopathic disorder but is more frequently observed in patients who have underlying IgA nephropathy. Laboratory features are not distinctive. Renal function may be modestly decreased or normal at the time of diagnosis. Complement component levels are most often normal. IgG levels may be modestly reduced, and IgA levels may be increased. Antistreptolysin O titers are usually normal. Proteinuria is most often nonselective. The pathogenesis of this lesion is unknown and almost certainly the result of diverse pathogenetic processes. The presence of mesangial immunoglobulin deposits and circulating immune complexes in some, but not all, patients suggests an immune-complex pathogenesis, although the antigen(s) is unknown.

Among adult patients with well-developed nephrotic syndrome and moderate to severe diffuse mesangial proliferation, there is a tendency for persistence of proteinuria and progression to renal insufficiency. This is particularly true if focal and segmental glomerular sclerosis are superimposed on the mesangial proliferative lesion at the time of the initial biopsy. Patients with milder forms of mesangial proliferative glomerulonephritis, particularly when unassociated with mesangial immunoglobulin deposition, may follow a more benign course. Some patients, particularly children, behave in a fashion similar to those with the minimal change lesion. Since renal biopsies from patients with the minimal change lesion may display mild degrees of glomerular hypercellularity, the benign course followed by these patients may indicate that they have the minimal change lesion with more prominent mesangial proliferation rather than a separate disorder under the heading of mesangial proliferative glomerulonephritis. Well-developed mesangial proliferative lesions, particularly in association with mesangial IgM deposits, tend to be unresponsive to glucocorticoid therapy and to evolve into focal and segmental glomerular sclerosis. Indeed, mesangial proliferative glomerulonephritis may be a predecessor of the lesion of focal and segmental glomerulosclerosis. Patients with mesangial proliferative glomerulonephritis who have complete remission of proteinuria following treatment with glucocorticoids similar to that for the minimal change lesion tend to do well, with little inclination toward progressive renal insufficiency. Exacerbations and remissions of proteinuria may occur. Steroid-unresponsive patients with persistent nephrotic syndrome progress at variable rates to renal insufficiency. The role of adjunctive cytotoxic therapy (cyclophosphamide, chlorambucil, or azathioprine) has not yet been established in this disorder.

Because of the variable pathogenesis and the relative rarity of this disorder, long-term prospective studies of natural history and therapy have not been conducted. Many patients, particularly those with mild degrees of proliferation and a remitting course following glucocorticoids, have a very benign prognosis. Other patients, particularly those with steroid unresponsiveness and superimposed focal and segmental glomerulosclerosis on the initial biopsy, have a poor prognosis, often developing end-stage renal failure 5 to 10 years after the diagnosis.

Focal and segmental glomerulosclerosis (focal sclerosis)   This lesion is characterized by sclerosis and hyalinization of some, but not all, glomeruli (hence the term *focal*). Among affected glomeruli, only a portion of the glomerular tuft is abnormal (hence, *segmental*). There is a predilection for these lesions initially to affect the *juxtamedullary glomeruli* and to be associated with progressive tubulointerstitial damage. By immunofluorescence, granular and

nodular deposits of IgM and C3 are found in the segmental sclerosing lesion. By electron microscopy, focal basement membrane collapse and denudation of epithelial surfaces are noted. All glomeruli reveal diffuse epithelial foot process effacement. This lesion accounts for 10 to 15 percent of cases of idiopathic NS among children and adults. Males are affected more often than females. Focal sclerosis may represent a stage in the evolution of a subgroup of patients with minimal change disease or "pure" mesangial proliferative glomerulonephritis (see above). In more than two-thirds of cases of focal sclerosis overt NS is present at diagnosis; the remainder have proteinuria in the nonnephrotic range. Hypertension, reduced GFR, abnormal tubule function, and abnormal urinary sediment occur commonly. Focal sclerosis may have features indistinguishable from either minimal change disease, mesangial proliferative glomerulonephritis, or membranous glomerulopathy (see below). Proteinuria is nearly always nonselective or becomes so on follow-up. Fibrin degradation products and C3 may be present in the urine. Serum levels of C3 are normal and IgG levels are reduced, but not as severely as in minimal change disease. Similar lesions may be seen in association with heroin abuse, vesicoureteral reflux, acquired immunodeficiency syndrome, solitary kidney, and renal allograft rejection and may complicate other primary glomerular diseases in the late stages. The occurrence of focal and segmental glomerulosclerosis in remnant glomeruli after extensive renal ablation has led to the suggestion that hyperfiltration (or some hemodynamic determinant thereof) may play a causative role in pathogenesis. The attendant lipid abnormalities (e.g., hypercholesterolemia) may also contribute to the progressive nature of the underlying lesion. Abnormalities in the prevalence of HLA antigens have not been consistently described. Renal vein thrombosis is uncommon.

There is little tendency for spontaneous remission, except among children. GFR declines, albeit at variable rates. A subset of patients with focal sclerosis, heavy proteinuria (i.e., greater than 15 to 20 g/d), and profound hypoalbuminemia progress quite rapidly to end-stage renal failure, occasionally in a period of only a few months.

The etiology and pathogenesis of focal sclerosis are unknown. Immune-complex–mediated disease has been postulated, primarily on the basis of immunofluorescence findings, and circulating immune complexes have been found in some cases.

Although few prospective trials have been conducted, a decline in the level of proteinuria concomitant with glucocorticoid therapy and a lowered risk of progressive renal failure among patients with complete or partial remission of proteinuria suggest that steroids exert a beneficial effect on the natural history of the disorder. Indeed, between 20 and 40 percent of patients treated with either alternate-day prednisone (100 to 200 mg) or daily prednisone in a fashion similar to that described for minimal change disease experience complete or partial remissions of proteinuria. If such remissions persist following reduction of steroid dosage, significant protection from progressive renal failure may be provided. The effect of cytotoxic drugs and anticoagulants requires further study. At least half of patients with persistent heavy proteinuria develop end-stage renal failure or die of intercurrent illnesses within 10 years of diagnosis. The rate at which renal failure develops is inversely related to the magnitude of proteinuria. Patients who consistently excrete more than 10 g/d develop end-stage renal failure in a median of approximately 3 years. The prognosis is worse for those patients with azotemia or hypertension at diagnosis. This lesion recurs in renal allografts, occasionally within a few hours of transplantation, suggesting as its cause a circulating glomerular permeability "toxin."

Membranous glomerulonephritis   This lesion is characterized by irregular, discontinuous proteinaceous deposits along the outer (or subepithelial) aspect of the glomerular capillary wall. These deposits contain IgG and appear dense by electron microscopy. Unlike focal sclerosis, *all glomeruli are involved uniformly.* At an early stage all glomeruli may appear normal by light microscopy, but as the disease progresses, immune deposits coalesce, and new basement membrane-like material is produced, causing the capillary wall to thicken.

Eventually, increased amounts of basement membrane material project toward the urinary space, giving the appearance of "spikes." There is little proliferation of capillary endothelial or mesangial cells, although mesangial sclerosis may occur in advanced cases. Tubulointerstitial atrophy and vascular lesions are other late manifestations.

This disorder accounts for 30 to 40 percent of cases of idiopathic NS in adults but is rare in children. In over 80 percent of cases the nephrotic syndrome is overt. In the remainder only isolated proteinuria is found. Men are affected more often than women. Blood pressure, GFR, and urinary sediment tend to be normal early in the course, making it difficult to distinguish membranous glomerulopathy from minimal change disease on clinical grounds. Urinary protein selectivity is quite variable. Serum complement components are normal, but IgG levels are modestly depressed. Membranous glomerulonephritis may develop in association with systemic lupus erythematosus (Chap. 228), certain chronic infections (e.g., malaria, hepatitis B), solid tumors (e.g., melanoma and cancer of the lung and colon), or exposure to heavy metals (gold, mercury) or drugs (penicillamine, captopril). A careful search for these causes is warranted in every case of membranous glomerulonephritis. Renal vein thrombosis is frequent in affected patients (see above).

Spontaneous complete remissions of NS are common in children and occur in 20 to 40 percent of adults. Steroid treatment does not greatly influence the development of lasting complete remissions, but may reduce proteinuria to nonnephrotic levels. A long-term beneficial effect of steroids is still a source of controversy. There is no agreement as to the optimal management. Retrospective surveys have often demonstrated no apparent difference in overall mortality or progression to renal failure. Prospective clinical trials have reported efficacy for short-term, high-dose, alternate-day prednisone and for combinations of intravenous methylprednisolone, oral prednisone, and chlorambucil and combinations of prednisone and cyclophosphamide, particularly in the subgroup with progressive renal failure and persistent heavy proteinuria.

Since the long-term prognosis for patients with idiopathic membranous glomerulonephritis is favorable, a conservative approach to treatment is generally recommended. Parameters to identify patients likely to develop progressive renal insufficiency include male sex, older age at onset, presence of hypertension, presence of elevated serum creatinine at discovery, presence of hypertension, and, possibly, severe hyperlipidemia and proteinuria greater than 10 g/d. Renal biopsy findings do not greatly aid in the determination of prognosis, but very advanced glomerular capillary wall alterations, segmental sclerosis, interstitial fibrosis, and tubular atrophy all augur a poor prognosis. Patients with several features associated with a poor prognosis may be candidates for a more aggressive therapeutic approach. Delay of such an aggressive approach to therapy (e.g., combined cytotoxic agents and glucocorticoids) until *after* renal impairment is progressive is advocated by some investigators. Nevertheless, many physicians treat patients with idiopathic membranous glomerulonephritis with a course of alternate-day prednisone as described above for 8 weeks followed by a week of tapering dosage. Such a regimen is seldom associated with adverse consequences unless some contraindication to steroid administration is present. Whether such treatment will prevent end-stage renal failure in patients so treated remains to be established. As indicated above, slowly progressive renal functional impairment occurs almost exclusively in those patients with persistent proteinuria in the nephrotic range. Such renal failure seldom develops within 3 to 4 years of diagnosis. However, on occasion patients may have a more rapidly progressive course. The rapid decline of renal function in a patient with membranous glomerulonephritis suggests a complicating drug-induced interstitial nephritis, acute renal vein thrombosis, or superimposed crescentic glomerulonephritis. Within 10 years of the time of the diagnosis, however, 20 to 30 percent of patients die of intercurrent illness or develop end-stage renal failure. The majority of survivors have complete or partial remission of proteinuria. A few patients have developed superimposed RPGN.

Mesangiocapillary glomerulonephritis This disorder is characterized by proliferation of mesangial cells, often with segmental or diffuse interposition of these cells or their cytoplasm into peripheral capillary loops. Mesangial matrix synthesis is increased as well. The glomerular capillary wall is irregularly thickened, by virtue of the mesangial extensions and the attendant synthesis of basement membrane–like material. This group of disorders is also known as *membranoproliferative* or *lobular glomerulonephritis*. Several immunofluorescence and electron-microscopic patterns are present and reflect heterogeneous mechanisms of pathogenesis. In the *type I* lesion, subendothelial electron-dense deposits are present, C3 is deposited in a granular pattern indicative of immune-complex pathogenesis, and IgG and the early components of complement may or may not be present. In the *type II* lesion the lamina densa of the GBM is transformed into an electron-dense character, giving rise to the term *dense deposit disease*. Basement membranes in Bowman's capsules and in tubules are similarly affected. C3 is found irregularly in the GBM and in granules or rings in the mesangium. Small amounts of Ig (typically IgM) are present, but the early acting complement components are absent from the deposits. Properdin deposition is variable. Additional ultrastructural variants, based upon location of deposit and basement membrane changes, have also been described.

Mesangiocapillary glomerulonephritis, types I and II, is found in 5 to 10 percent of idiopathic NS in children, particularly between the ages of 8 to 16 years, and somewhat less commonly in adults. Type I accounts for at least two-thirds of cases. Males and females are affected equally. In 50 to 75 percent of patients, a full-blown NS is present, often with features of AGN. In the remainder, proteinuria in the nonnephrotic range is nearly always accompanied by microscopic hematuria. Blood pressure and GFR are frequently abnormal, and the urinary sediment is active. Functional abnormalities of the renal tubules are common. Urinary protein selectivity is usually poor; fibrin degradation products and C3 are found in the urine. Serum C3 levels are reduced in the majority of cases. The early acting complement components C1q, C4, and C2 are often normal, especially in type II disease. This pattern may be indicative of activation of the alternate complement pathway (see Chap. 226). C3 nephritic factor (C3NF) is often found in the serum of patients with type II, especially if the C3 level is quite low. Circulating immune complexes are found in type I. Lesions similar to type I membranoproliferative glomerulonephritis may also be found in SLE, hemolytic-uremic syndrome, transplant rejection, chronic hepatitis B antigenemia, and "shunt" nephritis. Renal vein thrombosis may occur. Type II nephritis may be associated with partial lipodystrophy.

Spontaneous remissions are uncommon. Long-term, alternate-day prednisone therapy (0.3 to 0.5 mg/kg body weight every other day) may delay the progression of the disease. Treatment regimens that combine steroids and cytotoxic agents are not of proven value. Anticoagulants and inhibitors of platelet aggregation (acetylsalicylic acid plus dipyridamole) may have a beneficial effect. The course is progressive, and approximately half of patients die or develop end-stage renal failure within 10 years of the diagnosis. The prognosis for type II lesions seems somewhat worse than for type I. Type II disease almost invariably recurs in the transplanted kidney but does not always result in the premature loss of the allograft.

Other forms of idiopathic nephrotic syndrome In a small percentage of adults and children with idiopathic NS (i.e., 5 to 10 percent) other lesions are encountered on renal biopsy. These include *crescentic glomerulonephritis* and *focal* and *segmental proliferative glomerulonephritis*. The pathogenetic mechanisms for these lesions vary. For example, some cases of focal and segmental glomerulonephritis may have extensive mesangial IgA deposits and fit into the category of Berger's disease (see below). Serum C3 levels are usually normal. The clinical characteristics, natural history, and response to treatment of these lesions are not well defined. Hematuria is common and may be recurrent. Proteinuria tends to be nonselective. Spontaneous remissions of NS are uncommon. Since no controlled studies have been conducted, it is not possible to evaluate the effectiveness of treatment. Crescentic glomerulonephritis is likely to have a poor prognosis, whereas mesangial and focal and segmental proliferative glomerulonephritis have a more favorable long-term outlook.

NEPHROTIC SYNDROME CAUSED BY INFECTIOUS AGENTS, DRUGS, OR CHEMICALS   Table 227-3 lists the common infectious and drug-related etiologies of NS. In many instances, NS abates following cure of the infection or withdrawal of the offending medication. In patients receiving gold therapy for rheumatoid arthritis or in those exposed to inorganic, organic, or elemental mercury or to penicillamine, membranous glomerulonephritis is usually the lesion responsible for NS. NS is known to follow immunization and antiserum treatment of tetanus or snakebite and to occur in situations associated with atopy.

ASYMPTOMATIC URINARY ABNORMALITIES

This group of patients has *proteinuria in the nonnephrotic range and/ or hematuria,* unaccompanied by edema, reduced GFR, or hypertension. Abnormalities are often discovered incidentally and may be persistent or recurrent. In some this syndrome is a phase in the natural history of other glomerulopathic syndromes, especially nephrotic syndrome or chronic glomerulonephritis. Common glomerular disorders that present as asymptomatic proteinuria and/or hematuria are listed in Table 227-5. The heredofamilial and multisystem diseases are discussed in Chap. 228. The presence of dysmorphic erythrocytes and/or red cell casts indicates a glomerular cause for the hematuria.

IDIOPATHIC RENAL HEMATURIA (See also Chap. 49)   **Berger's disease (IgA nephropathy)**   This disorder was first described by Berger and Hinglais in 1968 and is characterized by recurrent episodes of gross or microscopic hematuria. The diagnosis depends on the finding of prominent IgA deposits in the mesangium by immunofluorescence microscopy. Berger's disease is the most common cause of recurrent hematuria of glomerular origin. It most commonly affects young adults, mostly men. Typically, episodes of macroscopic hematuria are associated with minor flulike illnesses or vigorous exercise. Vague constitutional symptoms may be present, but skin rash, arthritis, and abdominal pain are absent. Urine protein excretion rates are usually less than 3.5 g/d; protein excretion is normal or only mildly increased. The nephrotic syndrome develops occasionally. In some patients a self-limited and reversible form of acute renal failure may occur. Such episodes are frequently preceded by an upper respiratory infection and accompanied by bouts of macroscopic hematuria. Thus, these patients resemble those with acute poststreptococcal glomerulonephritis. Renal biopsy may reveal scattered noncircumferential crescentic glomerulonephritis, usually involving less than half of glomeruli, accompanied by marked tubular abnormalities, interstitial nephritis, and erythrocytes in tubular lumina. On rare occasions, patients present with the syndrome of malignant hypertension. Blood pressure, GFR, and serum albumin are usually normal early in the disease. Serum IgA levels are increased in about 50 percent of cases, while serum complement component levels remain normal. Biopsy of the skin of the volar surface of the forearm sometimes reveals dermal capillary deposits of IgA, C3, and fibrin but not early acting complement components or IgA secretory fragments. Similar skin biopsy findings are encountered in Henoch-Schönlein purpura (Chap. 228). Indeed, Berger's disease may be a monosymptomatic form of Henoch-Schönlein purpura.

Renal biopsy reveals a spectrum of changes, but diffuse mesangial proliferative or focal and segmental proliferative glomerulonephritis is found most often. In some cases glomerular morphology may be normal by light microscopy; uncommonly, crescents may be found (see above). The distinguishing feature is the finding by immunofluorescence microscopy of *diffuse mesangial deposition of IgA,* often accompanied by lesser amounts of IgG and nearly always by C3 and properdin, but not by C1q or C4. Fibrin reactive antigens are also common in the mesangium or in association with crescents if the latter are present. The pathogenesis of IgA nephropathy is unknown, but the systemic character of the IgA deposits (skin and glomerular capillaries), the presence of circulating IgG and IgA complexes in the majority of cases, and its similarity to Henoch-Schönlein purpura suggest that it is an immune-complex–mediated disease. The nature and source of the antigen are unknown.

The prognosis is variable, but the disease tends to progress slowly. Approximately 50 percent of patients develop end-stage renal failure within 25 years of the time of diagnosis. Azotemia, hypertension, or proteinuria in the nephrotic range at diagnosis are associated with a poor prognosis. At present, there is no evidence that therapy influences the natural history, although intermittent steroid therapy or broad-spectrum antibiotics may reduce the frequency of episodes of gross hematuria. Glucocorticoids may also result in remissions of proteinuria in those patients with nephrotic syndrome and mild glomerular abnormalities by light microscopy. IgA nephropathy recurs in the transplanted kidney in approximately 30 to 40 percent of cases. Such recurrences seldom result in loss of renal function but may be associated with hematuria.

Other primary renal hematurias   Some cases of recurrent hematuria do not reveal the typical immunofluorescence findings seen in Berger's disease. This group of patients is poorly defined, and the etiology and pathogenesis are varied. Some may represent resolving episodes of acute glomerulonephritis or early examples of mesangiocapillary or hereditary glomerulonephritis (Alport's syndrome, see Chap. 228). The common morphologic lesions are focal and segmental or diffuse mesangial proliferative glomerulonephritis, although mild and nonspecific glomerular changes may also be observed. Immunofluorescence studies reveal varying degrees of immunoglobulin and/or complement component deposition (principally IgM and/or C3) in the mesangium. Some cases show linear deposits of IgG, suggesting a possible anti-GBM antibody pathogenesis. Electron microscopy may reveal dense deposits in the mesangium or thin and attenuated glomerular basement membranes. Overall, these patients have an excellent prognosis, with frequent spontaneous permanent remissions of recurrent hematuria. Progressive renal insufficiency is unusual. Because of the benign prognosis no treatment is indicated.

ISOLATED NONNEPHROTIC PROTEINURIA OF GLOMERULAR ORIGIN (See also Chap. 49)   Mild to moderate degrees of proteinuria (i.e., greater than 150 mg but less than 2.0 g/d), unaccompanied by abnormalities in the urinary sediment or evidence of hypertension or reduced renal function, are common. Such patients may display other features of heredofamilial or multisystem diseases, including diabetes

---

TABLE 227-5   Glomerular causes of asymptomatic urinary abnormalities

I Hematuria with or without proteinuria
  A Primary glomerular diseases
    1 Berger's disease (IgA nephropathy)*
    2 Mesangiocapillary glomerulonephritis
    3 Other primary glomerular hematurias accompanied by "pure" mesangial proliferation, focal and segmental proliferative glomerulonephritis, or other lesions
    4 "Thin basement membrane" disease (? forme fruste of Alport's syndrome)
  B Associated with multisystem or heredofamilial diseases
    1 Alport's syndrome and other "benign" familial hematurias*
    2 Fabry's disease
    3 Sickle cell disease
  C Associated with infections
    1 Resolving poststreptococcal glomerulonephritis*
    2 Other postinfectious glomerulonephritides*
II Isolated nonnephrotic proteinuria
  A Primary glomerular diseases
    1 "Orthostatic" proteinuria*
    2 Focal and segmental glomerulosclerosis*
    3 Membranous glomerulonephritis*
  B Associated with multisystem or heredofamilial diseases
    1 Diabetes mellitus*
    2 Amyloidosis*
    3 Nail-patella syndrome

* Most common.

mellitus, amyloidosis, rheumatoid arthritis, or cancer. The abnormality may either be persistent or evanescent. Proteinuria may occur primarily in the upright posture (*orthostatic proteinuria*) or be present both in recumbent and erect positions (*constant proteinuria*). Fixed and reproducible orthostatic proteinuria has a benign prognosis and frequently disappears on long-term follow-up. Renal biopsies reveal normal glomeruli or trivial alterations of dubious significance. On the other hand, persistent and constant proteinuria may be indicative of a more serious disease, and renal biopsies often reveal definite evidence of a structural lesion. Some of the lesions have been discussed in the context of idiopathic nephrotic syndrome. Other patients have an unsuspected disease such as amyloidosis or diabetes mellitus. In the remainder, the lesions are usually trivial and nonspecific, and the long-term significance is uncertain. In primary glomerular diseases, so long as urinary protein excretion remains modest, the prognosis is excellent, and deterioration of renal function is uncommon. Renal biopsy is not commonly undertaken in patients with persistent and isolated nonnephrotic proteinuria, as determining underlying morphology seldom leads to specific therapy and adds information chiefly of a prognostic nature. Since patients with proteinuria more than 2.0 g/d are more likely to have lesions that will progress, many nephrologists limit renal biopsies to this latter group of patients.

CHRONIC GLOMERULONEPHRITIS

The syndrome of chronic glomerulonephritis (CGN) is characterized chiefly by *persistent urinary abnormalities* (e.g., proteinuria and/or hematuria) and by *slowly progressive impairment of renal function*, eventuating in hypertension, contracted, granular kidneys, and end-stage renal failure. With the possible exception of the minimal change lesion associated with idiopathic nephrotic syndrome (see above) all the disorders described in this chapter and in Chap. 228 can lead eventually to CGN. The pathophysiology of CGN in the context of renal failure is described in Chaps. 222 and 224.

The structural alterations in this syndrome may be categorized as *proliferative* (including mesangial, endo- and/or extracapillary proliferative glomerulonephritis, and focal and segmental proliferative glomerulonephritis), *sclerosing* (including focal and diffuse glomerular sclerosis), and *membranous*. Such lesions are found in most patients with CGN. In the remainder, the underlying lesions are not readily categorized morphologically, and they are often referred to as chronic "*nonspecific*" *glomerulonephritis*.

The clinical characteristics of the specific lesions are described in other sections of this chapter. The etiologic and pathogenetic origins of chronic nonspecific glomerulonephritis are undoubtedly heterogeneous. Complicating vascular disease contributes to the glomerular obliteration. Some of the patients categorized as having chronic nonspecific glomerulonephritis may have had an earlier unrecognized or undiagnosed episode of acute PSGN.

The detection of CGN usually occurs in one of several ways: (1) the incidental finding of abnormal urine, impaired renal function, or hypertension during multiphasic screening of asymptomatic individuals or evaluation of such individuals for an unrelated illness; (2) the result of the insidious onset of progressive symptoms or signs of advanced renal disease, especially anemia and hypertension; or (3) after an exacerbation of glomerulonephritis, usually during the course of a nonspecific viral or bacterial illness. In advanced stages, the clinical separation of CGN from other causes of renal failure may be difficult; however, the presence of symmetrically contracted kidneys, moderate to heavy proteinuria, abnormal urinary sediment (especially red blood cell casts), and x-ray evidence of normal pyelocalyceal systems are all suggestive of CGN.

The evolution of CGN varies, depending upon the nature of the underlying disease and the presence or absence of complications, especially hypertension. Ten, fifteen, twenty, or more years may elapse from the first discovery of an abnormal urine sediment until

the development of end-stage renal failure. Renal biopsy is necessary to define the precise nature of the underlying glomerular lesion. The principal advantage of a morphologic evaluation among patients presenting with the syndrome of CGN is to determine prognosis rather than therapy.

Treatment is supportive and symptomatic. Despite many years of controlled and uncontrolled trials, unequivocal evidence of a favorable effect of treatment with steroids, cytotoxic agents, nonsteroidal anti-inflammatory agents, and anticoagulants has yet to be provided. The management of specific lesions is discussed in greater detail in the relevant sections of this chapter. Hypertension and symptomatic urinary tract infections should be treated vigorously, taking care to avoid nephrotoxic agents. Diuretics should generally be employed only as adjuncts to antihypertensive management or to deal with debilitating degrees of edema. Rigorous salt restriction is usually unnecessary and may be hazardous. In the absence of congestive heart failure or marked hypoalbuminemia, severe edema is rare until the terminal phases of the illness. Potassium restriction is usually unnecessary. Protein and phosphate restriction may slow the rate of progression of renal failure.

REFERENCES

CAMERON JS, GLASSOCK RJ (eds): *The Nephrotic Syndrome*. New York, Dekker, 1988

EMANCIPATOR S, SCHENA FP (eds): Immunoglobulin A nephropathy. Semin Nephrol 7:275, 1987

GLASSOCK RJ et al: Primary glomerular diseases, in *The Kidney*, 3d ed, BM Brenner, FC Rector Jr (eds). Philadelphia, Saunders, 1986, p 929

KORBET SM et al: Minimal-change glomerulopathy of adulthood. Am J Nephrol 8:291, 1988

RODRIGUEZ-ITURBE B: Epidemic post-streptococcal glomerulonephritis. Kidney Int 25:129, 1984

SHORT CD, MALLICK N: Membranous glomerulopathy, in *Textbook of Nephrology*, 2d ed, S Massry, R Glassock (eds). Baltimore, Williams and Wilkins (in press)

228   GLOMERULOPATHIES ASSOCIATED WITH MULTISYSTEM DISEASES

RICHARD J. GLASSOCK / BARRY M. BRENNER

Glomerular injury may be a prominent feature of diseases that affect multiple organs and systems. By and large the etiologies of these diseases are unknown, but aberrant immunologic processes, neoplasia, metabolic disturbances, and biochemical abnormalities are believed to be dominant factors in their pathogenesis. These processes lead to alterations in glomerular structure and function. Some of the glomerular lesions are specific for the underlying disease (e.g., amyloidosis, nodular diabetic glomerulosclerosis); however, the majority are nonspecific. Proteinuria results from defects in the charge- and/or size-selective glomerular permeability barriers. Reductions in glomerular filtration rate develop because of loss of filtration surface area. Although the extrarenal manifestations are useful in establishing a diagnosis, some may present with predominant or exclusive renal involvement and only covert extrarenal manifestations.

IMMUNOLOGICALLY MEDIATED MULTISYSTEM DISEASES

SYSTEMIC LUPUS ERYTHEMATOSUS (See also Chap. 269) Systemic lupus erythematosus (SLE) is the archetype of an immunologically mediated disease and is representative of the multisystem diseases in which renal involvement is common. The etiology of SLE is unknown; however, viral infection, genetic factors, and abnormal immune responsiveness probably interact to produce the disease. The principal mechanism for tissue injury in SLE appears to be the deposition of circulating immune complexes, although other mechanisms may also play a role, including antitissue antibody and in situ immune-complex formation (see Chap. 226). The circulating immune complexes may be composed of a variety of endogenous antigens combined with autoantibodies. DNA (single-stranded and double-stranded) is a major antigenic component of immune complexes. The prevalence of clinical renal involvement in SLE ranges from as low as 35 percent to more than 90 percent in different series. Manifestations of renal disease range from mild abnormalities of the urinary sediment (predominantly hematuria) to massive proteinuria, and from chronic indolent glomerulonephritis to a fulminant inflammatory process leading to rapidly progressive renal failure.

The diagnosis and extrarenal manifestations of SLE are described in Chap. 269. This section will deal with the renal involvement. Although extrarenal features usually dominate the clinical picture, SLE may present initially with renal manifestations. Morphologic evidence of renal involvement may exist with or without clinical manifestations. If immunofluorescence and electron-microscopic studies of renal tissue are performed, abnormalities are present in virtually every patient with SLE. The abnormal glomerular morphologic lesions in SLE form a spectrum based upon correlative light- and electron-microscopic and immunofluorescence studies of renal biopsies.

Minimal lupus glomerular lesion This pattern is characterized by few or no changes by light microscopy. Immunofluorescence studies reveal moderate immunoglobulin (Ig) and complement deposits exclusively in mesangium. Scattered electron-dense deposits are found in mesangium by electron microscopy. Clinical manifestations may include mild proteinuria and microscopic hematuria. Nephrotic syndrome is uncommon. Glomerular filtration rate (GFR) is almost always normal. Serologic manifestations vary depending upon the activity of extrarenal disease. Antibodies to DNA are usually present in low titer, and levels of C3 and C4 may be decreased, especially if dermatitis is severe. Circulating immune complexes may also be detected in skin lesions.

Mesangial lupus glomerulonephritis This pattern is characterized by mild to moderate diffuse mesangial cell proliferation and/or mesangial sclerosis. Immunofluorescence studies reveal immunoglobulins (IgG, IgM, and IgA) and complement components (C1q, C4, and C3) deposited in a granular pattern principally in the mesangium. By electron microscopy, electron-dense deposits are also found to be confined to the mesangium. This morphologic appearance may be present in the absence of clinical renal disease or may be associated with minor abnormalities in the urinary sediment and modest proteinuria. Nephrotic syndrome and hypertension may occasionally be present. GFR is almost always normal. Mesangial lupus glomerulonephritis may be the initial renal involvement in SLE, from

which other patterns evolve. Associated serologic abnormalities depend upon the degree of extrarenal activity. These include increased levels of antibody to denatured, single-stranded DNA (ssDNA) or native, double-stranded DNA (dsDNA); depressed serum levels of C3, C4, and C1q; and detectable levels of circulating immune complexes (CIC) (Table 228-1).

Focal and segmental lupus glomerulonephritis This pattern is characterized by focal and segmental cellular proliferation, often associated with necrosis, superimposed on diffuse mesangial hypercellularity. Granular deposits of immunoglobulins and complement involve both the mesangium and occasional glomerular capillary loops. By electron microscopy, dense subendothelial deposits are found in the mesangium and in a few peripheral capillary loops. Clinical and laboratory evidence of renal injury is more common than in mesangial lupus glomerulonephritis. Nephrotic syndrome may occur in 10 to 20 percent of patients, but in general GFR is well preserved. This lesion may persist, resolve, or progress to diffuse proliferative lupus glomerulonephritis. Serologic features of active disease are often present in untreated patients.

Diffuse proliferative lupus glomerulonephritis This pattern is characterized by diffuse mesangial and endothelial cell proliferation that may include extensive peripheral capillary wall interposition of mesangial cells. In addition focal cellular necrosis, hematoxylinophilic bodies, fibrinoid necrosis, and "wire loops" (capillaries whose basement membranes are thickened markedly owing to subendothelial deposits) may be present. Extensive extracapillary proliferative (crescentic) glomerulonephritis, vasculitis, and interstitial nephritis may also be found. Varying degrees of chronic lesions may also be present. These include focal and segmental glomerulosclerosis, fibrocellular crescents, interstitial fibrosis, tubular atrophy, and nephroangiosclerosis. Granular deposits of immunoglobulins and complement components are extensive and involve the mesangium and nearly every capillary loop. Electron microscopy reveals extensive subendothelial and mesangial electron-dense deposits as well as occasional intramembranous or subepithelial deposits. Most patients have an active urinary sediment, heavy proteinuria, and progressive impairment of renal function; occasionally, clinical evidence of renal involvement is lacking. In the untreated patient evidence of serologic activity is usually present, including depressed serum C3 and C4 concentrations, high levels of precipitating and nonprecipitating complement-fixing antibody to dsDNA, cryoimmunoglobulinemia, and circulating immune complexes. This lesion is associated with an ominous prognosis, although vigorous treatment may modify the course (see below).

Membranous lupus glomerulonephritis This pattern is nearly identical with that described for idiopathic membranous glomerulonephritis (Chap. 227), except that mesangial deposits and mesangial proliferation are more frequent. There is thickening of the glomerular capillary wall due to the presence of immunoglobulin and complement-

TABLE 228-1 Serologic findings in selected multisystem diseases

Disease	C3	Ig	FANA	Anti-dsDNA	Anti-GBM	Cryo-Ig	CIC	ANCA
Systemic lupus erythematosus	↓ ↓	↑ IgG	+ + +	+ +	−	+ +	+ + +	±
Goodpasture's syndrome	−	−	−	−	+ + +	−	±	−
Henoch-Schönlein purpura	−	↑ IgA	−	−	−	±	+ +	−
Polyarteritis	↓ ↑	↑ IgG	+	±	−	+ +	+ + +	+ + +
Wegener's granulomatosis	↓ ↑	↑ IgA, IgE	−	−	−	±	+ +	+ + +
Cryoimmunoglobulinemia	↓	±	−	−	−	+ + +	+ +	−
Multiple myeloma	−	↓ ↑ IgG, IgA, IgD, IgE	−	−	−	+	±	−
Waldenström's macroglobulinemia	−	↑ IgM	−	−	−	−	−	−
Amyloidosis	−	± Ig	−	−	−	−	−	−

NOTE: C3 = C3 component of complement; Ig = immunoglobulin levels; FANA = fluorescent antinuclear antibody assay; anti-dsDNA = antibody to double-stranded (native) DNA; anti-GBM = antibody to glomerular basement membrane antigens; cryo-Ig = cryoimmunoglobulin; CIC = circulating immune complexes; ANCA = anti-neutrophil cytoplasmic antibody; − = normal; + = occasionally slightly abnormal; + + = often abnormal; + + + = severely abnormal.

containing electron-dense deposits in the subepithelial space, often associated with a spike-like basement membrane reaction. Nearly all patients have heavy proteinuria and the nephrotic syndrome. Although GFR may be normal initially, most patients ultimately develop progressive renal failure. A proliferative lesion may occasionally evolve, and the prognosis then assumes that of diffuse proliferative glomerulonephritis. Serologic features of SLE may or may not be present at the time of diagnosis of this nephropathy. Antibody to dsDNA tends to be nonprecipitating. Some patients with membranous lupus glomerulonephritis may be erroneously categorized as having idiopathic membranous glomerulopathy (see Chap. 227). Measurements of the level of antibody to dsDNA or ssDNA and circulating immune complexes and biopsies of skin for dermal-epidermal deposits of Ig (''lupus band test'') may be helpful for diagnosis in such cases.

Sclerosing or end-stage lupus glomerulonephritis   This pattern is characterized by obliterative and sclerosing lesions of the glomeruli and probably represents a late stage of proliferative lesions. Immunofluorescence studies may be only weakly positive for immunoglobulins; subendothelial deposits are infrequent. Hypertension and impaired renal function are common. Serologic parameters of activity of SLE may or may not be present.

Prognosis and treatment   The prognosis and treatment of SLE with renal involvement depends upon the nature of the underlying renal lesion especially with regard to the class and the activity of the morphologic disease and to the extent and severity of associated glomerulosclerosis and interstitial fibrosis. Patients with milder forms of renal disease (e.g., minimal, mesangial, or focal lupus glomerulonephritis) tend to do well if treatment is directed to control of the extrarenal manifestations of the disease. Glucocorticoids in modest doses, salicylates, or antimalarials are usually sufficient. Potent nonsteroidal, anti-inflammatory agents may cause functional depression of GFR and should be used with caution in patients with known renal involvement. Serologic parameters, including anti-dsDNA and complement components (C3, C4), should be followed serially. Fluorescent antinuclear antibody tests have little value in prognosis or in following the effectiveness of treatment. A return to normal values for antibody to dsDNA and/or complement components is a favorable sign; however, persistently abnormal serologic features do not necessarily indicate worsening or progressive renal involvement, especially in patients with active extrarenal manifestations. For patients with mild lesions, 85 percent or more can be expected to survive at least 10 years. Patients with membranous lupus glomerulonephritis who receive treatment directed primarily at the extrarenal features also have favorable long-term prognosis. On the other hand, patients with diffuse proliferative lupus glomerulonephritis do less well and, therefore, warrant a more aggressive approach toward ameliorating the renal disease. High-dose, long-term oral glucocorticoid therapy, although capable of improving extrarenal signs of active disease and reducing the acute inflammatory component of the renal lesions, is not an altogether satisfactory regimen for lupus nephritis. Such treatment is associated with a high prevalence of side effects and may not prevent progression of chronic lesions. High-dose, short-term intravenous methylprednisolone is effective in reducing signs of systemic activity of the disease, especially in patients with recent deterioration. Adjunctive use of cytotoxic agents (azathioprine, cyclophosphamide, or chlorambucil) exerts a steroid-sparing effect and may prevent progression of chronic lesions, particularly among those with mild chronic lesions prior to therapy. The optimal regimen has not yet been established; however, intermittent intravenous cyclophosphamide (500 to 1000 mg/m² surface area monthly for 6 to 12 months) plus low-dose oral prednisone (0.5 mg/kg body weight per day) and combinations of azathioprine, cyclophosphamide, and low-dose oral prednisone appear to be relatively safe and more effective. Because prospective randomized trials have involved only small numbers of patients, it is premature to adopt any particular regimen as the treatment of choice. Even combinations of azathioprine and low-dose prednisone may exert an overall beneficial effect in certain patients. Little is gained by using a combined steroid-cytotoxic approach in patients with advanced renal failure due to progressive glomerular capillary obliteration and sclerosis. These patients are best treated with dialysis and/or transplantation. Reports claiming efficacy of combined intensive plasma exchange and immunosuppressive therapy for severe glomerulonephritis have not been substantiated in a randomized prospective trial. Such treatment therefore cannot be recommended for the *routine* management of patients with severe and progressive glomerular disease. However, anecdotal reports of dramatic recovery from extrarenal manifestations (e.g., central nervous system lupus) consequent to the use of intensive plasma exchange plus immunosuppression have appeared. Since, from time to time, patients with systemic lupus erythematosus may develop a syndrome closely resembling thrombotic thrombocytopenic purpura, the beneficial effect of intensive plasma exchange may be the consequence of an alteration in thrombotic microangiopathy rather than control of an active immunologically mediated process.

Serologic studies, especially serial measurements of antibody to dsDNA, complement components, and circulating immune complexes, may be useful in assessing patients under therapy. Return of these parameters to normal usually indicates satisfactory control of disease and indicates that drug dosage can be safely diminished. These measurements can be monitored to guide more aggressive therapy when appropriate. However, too heavy reliance on serologic parameters of activity should be discouraged. The correlation between clinical activity and serologic disturbances is poor, at least among patients receiving therapy with steroids and immunosuppressive agents.

Overall, long-term prognosis for patients with SLE and renal involvement has greatly improved. Whether changes in methods of diagnosis, serologic monitoring, or treatment are responsible is unknown. Progression to end-stage renal disease is now relatively uncommon even for patients with diffuse proliferative glomerulonephritis. Cerebral involvement and infectious complications of therapy are now major causes of morbidity and mortality in SLE. Patients with SLE seem to do well on regular chronic dialysis; moreover, as uremia develops, some patients experience remissions of extrarenal activity. In transplanted patients, recurrence of SLE in the renal allograft is uncommon. Thus, patients with SLE and nephritis are satisfactory candidates for both dialysis and transplantation.

GOODPASTURE'S SYNDROME   There is a lack of agreement concerning the use of the term *Goodpasture's syndrome*. Some apply this eponym to clinical states and diseases having in common glomerulonephritis and pulmonary hemorrhage. Others restrict the use of the eponym to patients displaying the triad of *glomerulonephritis, pulmonary hemorrhage*, and *antibody to basement membrane antigens*. As was mentioned earlier (Chap. 227), pulmonary hemorrhage, covert or overt, can accompany many forms of glomerular disease including systemic necrotizing vasculitis, Wegener's granulomatosis, systemic lupus erythematosus, cryoimmunoglobulinemia, Henoch-Schönlein purpura, and several nonglomerular diseases associated with renal function abnormalities (e.g., *Legionella* infection, renal vein thrombosis with pulmonary embolus). This section will deal with Goodpasture's syndrome as mediated by antibody to basement membrane antigens. The etiology is unknown. Goodpasture's syndrome may appear at any age and typically affects young men. However, the frequency may be increasing in women.

Pulmonary hemorrhage may be mild and easily overlooked or severe and life-threatening. The initial manifestations of pulmonary involvement are cough, mild shortness of breath, and hemoptysis. Hilar pulmonary infiltrates may be seen by chest x-ray, and hypoxia is frequent. With marked intraalveolar hemorrhage pulmonary carbon monoxide uptake is increased, and the pulmonary clearance of radioactive carbon monoxide is depressed. Pulmonary iron sequestration may be documented by scanning of the lungs with ⁵⁹Fe. Hemosiderin-laden macrophages may be seen in the sputum, but this is a nonspecific finding. Iron-deficiency anemia may result if pulmonary bleeding is prolonged and severe. A history of recent inhalation of volatile hydrocarbons or of viral influenza may be obtained. Fever, arthralgias, and other systemic symptoms are mild or absent at the time of presentation. Other disorders in which renal disease is associated with pulmonary (alveolar) hemorrhage can ordinarily be differentiated from Goodpasture's syndrome by their extrarenal features and by typical serologic findings (Table 228-1).

The glomeruli in Goodpasture's syndrome range from normal or nearly normal to focal proliferative and necrotizing glomerulonephritis; most often there is extensive extracapillary proliferation (crescents). Rapidly progressive renal failure is the common feature, although patients may initially have normal renal function and mild microscopic abnormalities in the urinary sediment. Immunofluorescence studies of renal biopsy material reveal the typical *linear deposits* of anti-basement membrane antibody, often but not necessarily always accompanied by C3 deposition. Electron-microscopic studies do not reveal electron-dense deposits.

Circulating antibody to glycopeptide antigens related to the noncollagenous domains on type IV (basement membrane) collagen are found in over 90 percent of cases if sera are examined early in the course by immunofluorescence or radioimmunoassay (Table 228-1). The level of circulating antibody does not correlate well with the severity of the renal or pulmonary manifestations. Measurements of circulating antibody are of diagnostic value and have no prognostic significance. Serum complement components are nearly always normal, and circulating immune complexes, anti-neutrophil cytoplasmic antibodies, and cryoimmunoglobulins are absent. About 80 to 85 percent of patients are HLA-DR2 antigen–positive.

The course is variable. Patients surviving an initial bout of severe hemoptysis may undergo long-term remissions or may have repeated bouts of pulmonary hemorrhage. Mild forms of glomerular injury may not progress, and the principal clinical problems may be related to recurrent hemoptysis. The diagnosis in such patients may be confused with idiopathic pulmonary hemosiderosis. More commonly the renal disease is progressive, sometimes fulminant, leading to oliguric renal failure in a matter of a few weeks or months (i.e., rapidly progressive glomerulonephritis).

Life-threatening degrees of pulmonary hemorrhage may respond temporarily to high doses of parenteral methylprednisolone (10 to 15 mg/kg body weight) given over short periods. The effectiveness of such therapy in reversing extensive crescentic glomerular lesions is not established. Anticoagulants are contraindicated in the face of active pulmonary hemorrhage. Intensive plasma exchange (2 to 4 L/d plasma), in combination with cytotoxic drugs and modest doses of glucocorticoids, has been associated with dramatic remissions of pulmonary hemorrhage and improvement of the glomerular lesions. This is particularly true if treatment is initiated early in patients with relatively acute disease in whom oliguria has not yet developed. The duration and frequency of plasma exchanges depend upon the response of the patient and the changes in levels of circulating antibody to glomerular basement membrane antigens. Renal biopsy is helpful in guiding the management, but even in the presence of extensive crescent formation responses may be satisfactory. If irreversible glomerular obliteration, extensive interstitial fibrosis, and tubular atrophy are found, especially in the oliguric patient with long-standing disease, plasma exchange offers little hope for improving the renal lesion. Such patients are best managed by regular hemodialysis and/or transplantation. Although recurrences may occasionally develop, the diagnosis is not a contraindication to transplantation so long as the procedure is delayed until levels of circulating anti-basement membrane antibody decrease to undetectable levels.

HENOCH-SCHÖNLEIN PURPURA (See also Chap. 288) This disorder is characterized by nonthrombocytopenic purpura, arthralgias, abdominal pain, and glomerulonephritis. Renal involvement is common and is manifested chiefly by hematuria and proteinuria. In some instances renal involvement is severe, leading to rapidly progressive glomerulonephritis or nephrotic syndrome. The onset of the disease may resemble acute postinfectious glomerulonephritis. Serum complement component levels are usually normal. Serum IgA

levels are increased in about half the patients (Table 228-1). Renal biopsy reveals a spectrum of abnormalities. Mild diffuse mesangial cell proliferation and/or focal and segmental proliferative glomerulonephritis is most common when bouts of macroscopic hematuria and proteinuria are present. More severe and diffuse proliferative glomerulonephritis, sometimes accompanied by extracapillary proliferation (crescents), arises in patients with heavy proteinuria and/or rapidly diminishing GFR. Characteristically, immunofluorescence studies reveal mesangial and peripheral capillary granular deposits of IgA, IgG, C3, and fibrinogen but not C1q, C4, or IgA secretory piece. Similar immunofluorescence findings are present in the dermal capillaries of biopsies of involved and uninvolved skin. Electron microscopy reveals electron-dense deposits principally in the mesangium. These findings suggest that Henoch-Schönlein purpura is due to circulating IgA-containing immune complexes. Circulating cryoimmunoglobulins and immune complexes may be present, but the nature of the antigen and the antibody reactivity of the IgA are unknown. Although food allergies and upper respiratory infections may be present, there is no clear-cut etiologic relationship. *Berger's disease* (IgA nephropathy, Chap. 227) may represent a form of Henoch-Schönlein purpura.

The diagnosis is ordinarily not difficult when the typical clinical features are present. The differential diagnosis includes SLE, polyarteritis, infective endocarditis, postinfectious glomerulonephritis, and essential cryoimmunoglobulinemia.

The course is usually benign; however, progressive renal failure may occur. Renal biopsy is a useful prognostic tool. Patients with persistent urinary abnormalities may experience deterioration of renal function several years after diagnosis. Treatment is symptomatic. There is no convincing evidence that glucocorticoid or immunosuppressive therapy is beneficial for the renal lesion, although these treatments may ameliorate extrarenal features. Patients with rapidly progressive (crescentic) glomerulonephritis benefit from intensive plasma exchange combined with immunosuppressive drugs (see Chap. 227).

SYSTEMIC NECROTIZING VASCULITIS (See also Chap. 276) Glomerular involvement is common in the heterogeneous group of disorders that result from widespread inflammatory and necrotizing lesions of blood vessels. Several variations are recognized, including microscopic polyarteritis (hypersensitivity angiitis), macroscopic polyarteritis (periarteritis nodosa), Wegener's granulomatosis, allergic angiitis and granulomatosis, rheumatoid vasculitis, temporal arteritis, and Takayasu's arteritis. Henoch-Schönlein purpura and SLE can also be considered as examples of vasculitis. Many patients with glomerulonephritis accompanying systemic necrotizing vasculitis have characteristic extrarenal findings such as cutaneous palpable purpura, necrotizing skin lesions, pulmonary infiltrates, upper airway or sinus lesions, mononeuritis multiplex, fever, and wasting. Hypertension is frequent in polyarteritis nodosa but may be absent in hypersensitivity vasculitis and Wegener's granulomatosis. Necrotizing pulmonary infiltrates, upper airway disease, sinusitis, and otitis characterize the Wegener's granulomatosis variant. Laboratory findings, often nonspecific, include anemia, mild leukocytosis, eosinophilia, and markedly elevated erythrocyte sedimentation rate. Autoantibodies to a cytoplasmic antigen present in polymorphonuclear leukocytes have been reported in a high percentage of patients with Wegener's granulomatosis and possibly also systemic necrotizing vasculitis (Table 228-1). The detection of such autoantibodies may be helpful in establishing the nature of the underlying disease in patients suspected of having vasculitis. Renal biopsies are a poor means of establishing the diagnosis, since they frequently reveal segmental or diffuse necrotizing glomerulonephritis with or without crescents in the absence of any extraglomerular vascular involvement. Lung biopsies more frequently reveal the typical granulomatous necrotizing vasculitis characteristic of Wegener's granulomatosis. Sural nerve biopsies may be useful in establishing the diagnosis of vasculitis in patients presenting with mononeuritis multiplex.

The prognosis is generally poor for patients with systemic necrotizing vasculitis, especially in the absence of treatment; however, aggressive management with glucocorticoids combined with cyclophosphamide has been associated with improvement in overall prognosis. Treatment of patients with Wegener's granulomatosis with combined glucocorticoid-cyclophosphamide regimens for 6 to 12 months has resulted in long-term remissions. Some patients with fulminant glomerulonephritis secondary to systemic necrotizing vasculitis in which severe glomerular involvement is accompanied by extensive crescent formation and rapidly progressive renal failure may be benefited by combined therapy involving plasma exchange, glucocorticoids, and intravenous or oral cyclophosphamide. The long-term prognosis for such patients remains uncertain, since extrarenal involvement and/or complications of immunosuppressive treatment may ultimately be fatal.

MISCELLANEOUS IMMUNOLOGICALLY MEDIATED MULTISYS-TEM DISEASES   Mixed connective tissue disease (MCTD)   In this disorder (also see Chap. 272) renal disease is uncommon and, if present, mild. Clinical manifestations include hematuria and proteinuria and occasionally nephrotic syndrome. Pathologically, membranous glomerulonephritis or mesangiocapillary glomerulonephritis is seen. The prognosis is generally favorable, and treatment is directed at extrarenal manifestations. Glucocorticoid therapy often results in improvement of the glomerular lesions.

Rheumatoid arthritis   Several forms of glomerular injury may occur in rheumatoid arthritis (Chap. 270). Secondary amyloidosis is present in 5 to 10 percent of patients with long-standing arthritis. Nephrotic syndrome may arise as a complication of either gold or penicillamine therapy (see Chap. 227). In addition, the kidney may share in the vasculitis seen occasionally in severe rheumatoid arthritis. Finally, patients with rheumatoid arthritis (untreated with gold or penicillamine) may develop a mild proliferative glomerulitis or membranous glomerulonephritis which resembles lesions seen in SLE. Proteinuria, sometimes with nephrotic syndrome, is the principal clinical feature of such lesions. Prolonged and excessive use of analgesics may lead to renal papillary necrosis.

Other disorders   *Sjögren's syndrome* (Chap. 273) may be associated with nephrotic syndrome due to membranous or mesangiocapillary glomerulonephritis (type I) or, more frequently, interstitial nephritis. *Sarcoidosis* is rarely complicated by membranous glomerulonephritis. *Partial or total lipodystrophy* may be associated with mesangiocapillary glomerulonephritis (type II, dense deposit disease) (see Chaps. 227 and 336). Complement abnormalities consist of depressed C3 levels, normal C1q and C4 levels, and circulating C3 nephritic factor.

Chronic liver disease may be complicated by glomerular disease. The nephrotic syndrome may appear in the course of *chronic active hepatitis* associated with persistent hepatitis B surface antigenemia. Glomerular lesions include membranous glomerulonephritis or mesangiocapillary (type I) glomerulonephritis. Immunofluorescence studies in such patients reveal granular deposits of immunoglobulins, complement components, and hepatitis B viral antigens, indicating an immune-complex disease. Serum C3 levels are often reduced, and tests for circulating immune complexes and cryoimmunoglobulins are frequently positive. Occasionally patients with little clinical evidence of liver disease develop distinct glomerular lesions secondary to chronic hepatitis B infection. *Acute viral hepatitis* may be associated with transient hematuria or proteinuria and may resemble other postinfectious glomerulonephritides (see Chap. 227). Severe *chronic liver disease* (cirrhosis) may be associated with diffuse glomerulosclerosis. Few clinical manifestations of glomerular disease are found. Prominent mesangial IgA deposits, of unknown pathogenic significance, have been noted in patients with cirrhosis.

MULTISYSTEM DISEASES ASSOCIATED WITH PARAPROTEINEMIA AND NEOPLASIA

ESSENTIAL (MIXED) CRYOIMMUNOGLOBULINEMIA   This disorder is associated with circulating cold precipitable immunoglobulins (cryoimmunoglobulins), usually consisting of IgG and IgM; the latter possesses rheumatoid factor activity. Purpura, necrotizing skin lesions in cold-exposed areas, arthralgias, fever, and hepatosplenomegaly are common. Hepatitis B infection and other occult fungal, bacterial, or viral infections may be the cause of this syndrome. Circulating cryoimmunoglobulins are also found in chronic infections and probably represent circulating immune complexes with unusual physical properties. Glomerular disease results from the precipitation of the cryoimmunoglobulin in the glomerular capillaries and may result in acute renal failure, rapidly progressive (crescentic) glomerulonephritis, or the nephrotic syndrome. Serum complement components are depressed, and circulating immune complexes are present (Table 228-1). Pathologically, a diffuse proliferative glomerulonephritis may be seen with findings consistent with the deposition of the circulating cryoimmunoglobulin. Eradication of the underlying infection, if possible, is of value in treatment. Intensive plasma exchange, accompanied by the administration of glucocorticoids and cytotoxic agents, has been of some success in severe cases.

MONOCLONAL GAMMOPATHIES   *Multiple myeloma* (Chap. 265) may be associated with at least three types of glomerular injury. Amyloidosis (Chap. 266) (see below) occurs in 10 to 15 percent of patients with multiple myeloma. Lesions may resemble nodular diabetic glomerular sclerosis, and monoclonal cryoimmunoglobulins may be deposited in glomeruli. Proteinuria and the nephrotic syndrome are common. In addition, a tubulointerstitial lesion (myeloma kidney) consisting of large, laminated intratubular casts, tubule cell atrophy, interstitial fibrosis, and inflammation is common in patients with multiple myeloma and acute or chronic renal failure. *Waldenström's macroglobulinemia* may cause acute renal failure when the IgM paraprotein precipitates in glomerular capillaries as "thrombi." Intensive plasma exchange and therapy with alkylating agents may be beneficial. Hyperviscosity may cause functional alterations in GFR. Renal amyloidosis is uncommon. *Benign monoclonal gammopathies* are seldom associated with glomerular complications, except for mild asymptomatic proteinuria and, rarely, nephrotic syndrome. Excessive production of *light chains of Ig* (especially kappa type) may evoke glomerular alterations (nodular glomerulosclerosis, focal sclerosis) due to deposition of the protein in mesangium or along the subendothelial aspect of the glomerular capillary wall.

AMYLOIDOSIS (See also Chap. 266)   This disorder may occur in the absence of systemic disease (primary amyloidosis), may be secondary to chronic inflammatory processes (e.g., rheumatoid arthritis, osteomyelitis, paraplegia), multiple myeloma or other neoplastic diseases, or may occur in a hereditary form. All forms may affect the glomeruli.

Primary amyloidosis commonly affects the kidneys and usually occurs in older age groups. Proteinuria, often of nephrotic proportions, is the most common manifestation of renal involvement. The urine sediment tends to be benign. The degree of proteinuria is not necessarily related to the extent of glomerular deposition of amyloid. Enlarged kidneys may be present in patients with well-preserved renal function, but this is a nonspecific finding. The blood pressure is normal unless advanced uremia is present. Typical pathologic features include hypocellular glomeruli infiltrated with amorphous deposits that stain with Congo red and exhibit green birefringence under polarized light. The fibrillar nature of the amyloid deposits can be demonstrated by electron microscopy. Immunofluorescence studies reveal amorphous deposits of immunoglobulin and complement in glomeruli. Renal vein thrombosis may complicate the course of amyloidosis.

Renal amyloidosis is a progressive disease for which there is no established treatment. Remissions may occur in secondary amyloidosis if the cause can be eliminated. Remissions in primary amyloidosis are exceedingly rare; a few reports describe remissions following the use of cytotoxic agents. Overall the 5-year survival for patients with primary amyloidosis is less than 20 percent. Azotemia, persistent nephrotic syndrome, and myocardial involvement confer an even more ominous prognosis.

NEOPLASTIC DISEASE Glomerular alterations may develop with a variety of neoplastic diseases. *Carcinomas,* especially adenocarcinoma of lung, colon, stomach, and breast, may be accompanied by glomerular lesions resembling idiopathic membranous glomerulonephritis, although, on occasion, crescentic or focal and segmental proliferative glomerulonephritis or amyloidosis may be present. Nephrotic syndrome is the most common clinical renal manifestation, and approximately 3 to 10 percent of patients with idiopathic nephrotic syndrome associated with membranous glomerulonephritis harbor an underlying malignancy. Successful treatment of the tumor, especially by surgical means, may lead to a remission of the renal manifestation. Presumably the glomerular lesions arise because of the deposition of circulating immune complexes that are composed of tumor antigen and antitumor antibody. Amyloidosis may occasionally occur.

Lymphomas and leukemias may also give rise to glomerular abnormalities. Hodgkin's disease is commonly associated with the findings of idiopathic nephrotic syndrome (minimal change disease). Other glomerular lesions may include membranous glomerulonephritis, focal proliferative and sclerosing glomerulonephritis, and amyloidosis. The mechanism of the association of Hodgkin's disease with minimal change disease may involve an underlying T-cell abnormality. Proteinuria may wax and wane with fluctuations in the clinical activity of the Hodgkin's disease. Remissions may be produced by local irradiation of involved lymph nodes or by systemic chemotherapy.

METABOLIC, BIOCHEMICAL, AND HEREDITARY DISORDERS

DIABETIC NEPHROPATHY (See also Chap. 319) Diabetes mellitus affects the structure and function of the kidney in many ways. The term *diabetic nephropathy* encompasses all the lesions occurring in the kidneys of patients with diabetes mellitus. These lesions include *glomerulosclerosis* (diffuse or nodular), *arterionephrosclerosis, chronic interstitial nephritis, papillary necrosis,* and various tubular lesions. Diabetic nephropathy is associated with a variety of clinical syndromes, including mild asymptomatic proteinuria, nephrotic syndrome, progressive renal failure (acute, rapidly progressive, or chronic), and hypertension. Glomerular lesions are particularly common and account for the majority of abnormal clinical findings referable to the kidney. *Diffuse diabetic glomerulosclerosis* (diffuse intercapillary glomerulosclerosis) is the most common lesion and can be identified in the vast majority of diabetic patients regardless of the presence of abnormal clinical findings referable to the kidney. This lesion consists of a mild diffuse increase in mesangial matrix accompanied by an increased width of the glomerular basement membrane. Various exudative lesions, such as capsular drops and fibrin caps, may also be present. Hyaline arteriosclerosis, particularly of the efferent arteriole, is also common. Taken together, these lesions suggest the diagnosis of diabetes mellitus, but individually they are not specific. *Nodular glomerulosclerosis* (Kimmelstiel-Wilson lesion), on the other hand, is reasonably specific for juvenile onset (type I) diabetes mellitus. This lesion consists of PAS-positive, laminated, intercapillary nodules on a background of an increase in mesangial matrix. At the periphery of the nodules open glomerular capillary loops are found. The nodules are relatively acellular, in contrast to the cellular lesions of membranoproliferative glomerulonephritis (often referred to as *lobular glomerulonephritis*). A variable percentage of glomeruli may be affected. The pathogenesis of diffuse or nodular diabetic glomerulosclerosis is poorly understood.

The principal clinical manifestation of diabetic glomerular disease is proteinuria. Initially, only small amounts of albumin (20 to 40 μg/min) are excreted, particularly following exercise (microalbuminuria). This amount of albumin excretion is undetectable by routine screening methods. Under ordinary circumstances, microalbuminuria develops within 10 to 15 years from the onset of hyperglycemia and usually progresses within 3 to 7 years to overt proteinuria and clinical diabetic nephropathy. With "tight" control of hyperglycemia and/or rigorous control of elevated blood pressure, the development of microalbuminuria may be prevented or reversed. With time, the quantity of protein excreted usually increases and may progress to an overt nephrotic syndrome. Glomerular filtration rate is initially elevated and subsequently falls towards normal coincident with the onset of overt proteinuria. The urinary sediment is typically benign, although microhematuria and/or pyuria may also be present if a complicating urinary tract infection or papillary necrosis is present. Hypertension develops as GFR falls but is seldom of malignant proportions. When hypertension is severe or abrupt in onset, one should suspect a complicating atherosclerotic renal arterial stenosis. Typically, plasma renin activity is normal or decreased. Acquired hyporeninemic hypoaldosteronism with persistent hyperkalemia and mild hyperchloremic metabolic acidosis is common. Once azotemia develops, the disease progresses at variable rates. End-stage renal failure usually develops within 5 years of the onset of overt proteinuria and clinical nephropathy. Despite poor control of hyperglycemia, only about 50 to 60 percent of insulin-dependent diabetic patients develop clinical nephropathy. The factors that protect the remaining patients from renal failure are unknown. Patients with non-insulin-dependent diabetes mellitus may also develop clinical nephropathy.

Until the cause of diabetes mellitus is established, prevention of the glomerulopathy will not be feasible. If the abnormal diabetic milieu is responsible for the vascular complications (including glomerular disease), as some have suggested, then very precise regulation of blood sugar (e.g., meticulous attention to diet, exercise, and insulin dosage and servofeedback devices for insulin administration) may be effective in reducing the development of nephropathy. Once the nephropathy has reached a clinically recognizable stage, aggressive management of hypertension may slow the rate of loss of renal function, but strict control of blood sugar does not seem to retard the rate of progression once overt nephropathy (proteinuria >500 mg/d) has emerged. Patients with end-stage renal failure due to diabetic nephropathy are not ideal candidates for long-term dialysis because of concomitant multiple organ dysfunction secondary to widespread arteriovascular disease. Mortality rates among diabetics on chronic dialysis are about three times higher than among similarly treated nondiabetics of comparable age. Renal transplantation may be successful in the younger diabetic, especially if a living related donor is available. The success rate is somewhat less than in the nondiabetic population, due to the adverse effects of extrarenal vascular involvement (e.g., coronary artery disease), but transplantation is a viable alternative to dialysis in selected patients. Recurrence of typical diabetic glomerular lesions has been documented in renal allografts, but thus far, progressive loss of GFR secondary to recurrent disease has not been noted.

ALPORT'S SYNDROME This disorder consists of sensorineural deafness associated with hereditary nephritis. Renal disease manifests itself at an early age, principally as recurrent hematuria. Men are more frequently and more severely affected than women. Slowly progressive renal insufficiency in men commonly terminates in end-stage renal disease in the second to third decade. There is no clear-cut relationship between the onset or severity of the hearing abnormality and the extent of renal disease. Other associated abnormalities include two related ophthalmologic complications, spherophakia and lenticonus, as well as thrombopenia, hyperprolinemia, and cerebral dysfunction. Family studies have indicated autosomal dominant or X-linked modes of inheritance with variable expressivity. The pathogenesis may be due to defective synthesis of glycopeptide (noncollagenous) components of glomerular and tubular basement membranes.

The pathologic features detected by light microscopy are nonspecific, and a diagnosis cannot be established by optical microscopy alone. Both glomerular and interstitial lesions are present. Focal and diffuse glomerular proliferation, with segmental sclerosis, is common. Interstitial foam cells are nonspecific findings. Electron microscopy reveals thinning, splitting, and delamination of both glomerular and tubular basement membranes, thought by some to be specific for the syndrome. Immunofluorescence studies fail to reveal deposits of immunoglobulins or complement components. The autoantibody to basement membrane antigens found in patients with Goodpasture's syndrome does not react with the glomeruli of some patients with Alport's syndrome. Treatment is supportive; glucocorticoids and cytotoxic agents are ineffective. The disease is not known to recur following transplantation.

FABRY'S DISEASE (See also Chap. 331)   This disorder, angiokeratoma corporis diffusum, is an X-linked inborn error of glycosphingolipid metabolism that leads to the accumulation of neutral glycosphingolipids in many tissues including the kidney. A milder disease may develop in heterozygous females. Manifestations include angiokeratomas involving the lower trunk, scrotum, and buttocks; acroparesthesia; corneal opacities; tortuous retinal veins; and premature coronary and cerebral ischemic disease. Renal manifestations include hematuria and modest proteinuria, often associated with slowly progressive renal failure. Light-microscopic findings include foamy alterations of the epithelial cells of the glomerulus due to the accumulation of lipid. Electron microscopy reveals intracellular rounded laminated bodies ("myelin figures"). The disorder is untreatable unless replacement of the deficient enzyme can be ensured; successful renal transplantation may correct the enzyme deficiency.

NAIL-PATELLA SYNDROME   This autosomal dominant disease is characterized by dystrophic nails, absence of one or both patellae, iliac horns, and renal disease. The renal manifestations include isolated proteinuria and hematuria and occasionally the nephrotic syndrome. Progressive renal failure is uncommon. Glomerular lesions are nonspecific by light microscopy, but electron microscopy reveals a characteristic moth-eaten appearance of the glomerular basement membrane associated with intramembranous collagen fibrils. The prognosis is generally favorable. No treatment is known.

CONGENITAL NEPHROTIC SYNDROME   This autosomal recessive trait is characterized by the development of nephrotic syndrome at the time of or shortly after birth. It occurs with highest frequency in families of Finnish origin. Affected individuals have very large placentas, low birth weight, anasarca, polycythemia, and initially normal GFRs. Levels of alpha fetoprotein are increased in amniotic fluid and maternal serum. Proteinuria is marked and nonselective. Nephrotic syndrome appearing several months after birth is usually due to other causes, especially minimal change disease or focal glomerular sclerosis (Chap. 227). Congenital syphilis and congenital toxoplasmosis may produce similar syndromes and must be excluded. Pathologically, microcystic transformation of the cortical nephrons results in proximal tubular dilatation. Glomerular changes are nonspecific. The anionic charge density on glomerular basement membrane is reduced. Extensive effacement of the foot processes and sclerosis of the glomerular tufts are seen by electron microscopy. Immunofluorescence findings are nonspecific. The course is progressive, and few patients survive the first year of life. Treatment is ineffective. Death is usually due to inanition, infection, or renal failure. A few patients may survive long enough to be considered for renal transplantation.

SICKLE CELL DISEASE (See also Chap. 295)   This disorder is an autosomal trait characterized by an abnormal hemoglobin (hemoglobin S). Glomerular lesions occur occasionally in homozygous disease. The medulla is affected, leading to impairment of concentrating ability and acid excretion and, occasionally, to papillary necrosis. Rarely, patients develop mainly glomerular lesions, either membranous or mesangiocapillary glomerulonephritis, accompanied by proteinuria and a nephrotic syndrome. Immunofluorescence studies demonstrate renal deposition of immunoglobulin and complement in a granular pattern suggesting immune-complex–mediated disease. In a few instances, renal tubuloepithelial antigens are localized in these deposits, suggesting that ischemic damage of the kidney may release autologous antigens to provoke the immune-complex disease. The course in patients with the glomerulopathy of sickle cell disease is often relentless, leading to end-stage renal disease. No treatment is known to be effective. Transplantation is occasionally successful.

TABLE 228-2   Drugs associated with glomerular lesions
Elemental, inorganic, or organic mercury compounds
Organic gold compounds
Penicillamine
Captopril
Heroin
Amphetamines
Probenecid
Oxazoladinedione derivatives (e.g., trimethadione)
Antivenoms and antitoxins
Sulfonamides
Vaccinations
Allopurinol
Hydralazine
Rifampin
Nonsteroidal anti-inflammatory agents

LECITHIN:CHOLESTEROL ACYLTRANSFERASE DEFICIENCY (See also Chap. 326)   This autosomal recessive trait leads to absence in plasma of the enzyme that catalyzes the conversion of lecithin and cholesterol to lysolecithin and cholesteryl ester. Multiple lipoprotein abnormalities develop, including absence of α and pre-β lipoproteins, hypertriglyceridemia, accumulation of abnormal lipoproteins, and increased plasma-esterified cholesterol. Corneal opacities, anemia, hyperuricemia, proteinuria, and progressive renal failure are characteristic. Foam cells are present in bone marrow and glomeruli, and a picture resembling focal and segmental glomerulosclerosis may evolve. Treatment is generally ineffective, but plasma or blood transfusions may transiently correct the disorder. Renal failure has been corrected by renal transplantation, but recurrence of disease in allografts may occur.

DRUG-INDUCED GLOMERULAR DISEASE   Many drugs have been associated with the development of glomerular disease; however, it is usually difficult to establish a direct cause and effect relationship. In a few situations the association is clear-cut, and reexposure has led to recurrence of disease. A partial listing of these drugs is provided in Table 228-2. Certain *heavy metals* (Hg, Au) and their inorganic salts or organic compounds may produce membranous glomerulonephritis and nephrotic syndrome. Removal of the drug is not invariably associated with resolution. *Sulfhydryl compounds* (penicillamine, captopril) may also cause membranous or proliferative glomerulonephritis. The risk of developing a renal complication following penicillamine or gold therapy for rheumatoid arthritis is influenced by genes in the major histocompatibility complex. *Nonsteroidal anti-inflammatory agents* may produce nephrotic syndrome (minimal change disease), interstitial nephritis, and acute renal failure. *Probenecid, trimethadione,* or *paramethadione* may be associated with nephrotic syndrome and a variety of glomerular lesions, including minimal change disease and membranous glomerulonephritis. *Heroin* abuse may be associated with focal and segmental glomerulosclerosis that may progress to nephrotic syndrome and progressive renal failure. *Intravenous amphetamine abuse* may be associated with systemic necrotizing vasculitis. Chronic hepatitis B infection may be involved in the development of glomerular lesions in association with intravenous drug abuse. Allopurinol, hydralazine, and rifampin may be associated with vasculitis and/or crescentic glomerulonephritis.

REFERENCES

BALOW JE: Renal vasculitis. Kidney Int 27:954, 1985

——— et al: Effect of treatment on the evolution of renal abnormalities in lupus nephritis. N Engl J Med 311:491, 1984

GLASSOCK R et al: Secondary glomerular diseases, in *The Kidney*, 3d ed, BM Brenner, FC Rector Jr (eds). Philadelphia, Saunders, 1986, p 1014

GRUNFELD JP: The clinical spectrum of hereditary nephritis. Kidney Int 27:83, 1985

KYLE RA, GREIPP PR: Amyloidosis (AL): Clinical and laboratory features in 229 cases. Mayo Clin Proc 58:665, 1983

PONTICELLI C et al (eds): *Antiglobulins, Cryoglobulins and Glomerulonephritis*. Dodrecht, Martinus Nijhoff, 1986

SALANT D: Immunopathogenesis of crescentic glomerulonephritis and lung purpura. Kidney Int 32:408, 1987

229 TUBULOINTERSTITIAL DISEASES OF THE KIDNEY

BARRY M. BRENNER / THOMAS H. HOSTETTER

An etiologically diverse group of bilateral renal diseases can be distinguished from those considered in Chaps. 227 and 228 because the histologic and functional abnormalities involve the tubules and interstitium to a greater degree than the glomeruli and renal vasculature (see Table 229-1). Morphologically, acute forms of these disorders are characterized by interstitial edema, often associated with cortical and medullary infiltration by polymorphonuclear leukocytes and patchy areas of tubule cell necrosis. In more chronic forms, interstitial fibrosis predominates, inflammatory cells are typically mononuclear, and abnormalities of the tubules tend to be more widespread, as evidenced by atrophy, luminal dilatation, and thickening of tubule basement membranes. In the past, the diagnosis of chronic pyelonephritis (see Chap. 95) was almost universally applied when these chronic tubulointerstitial abnormalities were found. It is now apparent that only a small proportion of these lesions result from infection. Nonbacterial factors, including exogenous toxins and metabolic and immunologic derangements, constitute the major pathogenic mechanisms thought to be involved. Because of the nonspecific nature of the histology, particularly in chronic tubulointerstitial diseases, biopsy specimens rarely provide a specific diagnosis. The urine sediment is also unlikely to be diagnostic, except in allergic forms of acute tubulointerstitial disease in which eosinophils may predominate in the urinary sediment.

Defects in tubule function often accompany these alterations of

TABLE 229-1 Principal causes of tubulointerstitial disease of the kidney

I Toxins
   A Exogenous toxins
      1 Analgesic nephropathy
      2 Lead nephropathy (see Chap. 372)
      3 Miscellaneous nephrotoxins (e.g., antibiotics, cyclosporine, radiographic contrast media, heavy metals)
   B Metabolic toxins
      1 Acute uric acid nephropathy (see Chap. 329)
      2 Gouty nephropathy (see Chap. 329)
      3 Hypercalcemic nephropathy (see Chap. 340)
      4 Hypokalemic nephropathy (see Chap. 50)
      5 Miscellaneous metabolic toxins (e.g., hyperoxaluria, cystinosis, Fabry's disease)
II Neoplasia
   A Lymphoma (see Chap. 302)
   B Leukemia (see Chap. 296)
   C Multiple myeloma (see Chap. 265)
III Immune disorders
   A Hypersensitivity nephropathy
   B Sjögren's syndrome (see Chap. 273)
   C Amyloidosis (see Chap. 266)
   D Transplant rejection (see Chap. 225)
   E Tubulointerstitial abnormalities associated with glomerulonephritis (see Chaps. 227 and 228)
   F AIDS (see Chap. 264)
IV Vascular disorders (see Chaps. 223 and 230)
   A Arteriolar nephrosclerosis
   B Atheroembolic disease
   C Sickle cell nephropathy
   D Acute tubular necrosis
V Hereditary renal diseases
   A Hereditary nephritis (Alport's syndrome) (see Chap. 228)
   B Medullary cystic disease (see Chap. 231)
   C Medullary sponge kidney (see Chap. 231)
   D Polycystic kidney disease (see Chap. 231)
VI Infectious injury (see Chap. 95)
   A Acute pyelonephritis
   B Chronic pyelonephritis
VII Miscellaneous disorders
   A Chronic urinary tract obstruction (see Chap. 233)
   B Vesicoureteral reflux
   C Radiation nephritis

tubule and interstitial structure. Proximal tubule dysfunction may be manifested as selective reabsorptive defects leading to hypokalemia, aminoaciduria, glycosuria, phosphaturia, uricosuria, or bicarbonaturia (proximal or type II renal tubular acidosis, see Chap. 231). In combination these defects constitute the *Fanconi syndrome*. Protein excretion is usually modest, rarely exceeding 2 g/d. The excreted proteins are typically of low molecular weight and include beta$_2$ microglobulin, lysozyme, and immunoglobulin light chains. Defective proximal tubule reabsorption of these readily filtered small proteins accounts for their augmented excretion. Tubule sodium reabsorption may also be deranged in patients with advanced tubulointerstitial diseases, predisposing to salt wasting and hypovolemia. One or more of these reabsorptive defects are commonly encountered with heavy metal poisoning, multiple myeloma, and other diffuse tubulointerstitial processes.

Defects in urinary acidification and concentrating ability often represent the most troublesome of the tubule dysfunctions encountered in patients with tubulointerstitial disease. Hyperchloremic metabolic acidosis often develops at a relatively early stage in the course. Patients with this finding generally elaborate urine of maximal acidity (pH of 5.3 or less). In such patients the defect in acid excretion is usually caused by a reduced capacity to generate and excrete ammonia due to the reduction in renal mass. Preferential damage to the collecting ducts, as in amyloidosis or chronic obstructive uropathy, may also predispose to distal or type I renal tubular acidosis, characterized by high urine pH (>5.5) during spontaneous or NH_4Cl-induced metabolic acidosis. Patients with tubulointerstitial diseases affecting medullary and papillary structures predominantly may also evidence concentrating defects, with resultant nocturia and polyuria. The impairment in maximal concentration is typically unresponsive to the administration of vasopressin, and hence is a form of nephrogenic diabetes insipidus. Analgesic nephropathy and sickle cell disease are prototypes of this form of injury.

Although the major structural defects originate in the tubules and interstitium, progressive reduction in glomerular filtration rate (GFR) is a functional accompaniment of most, if not all, forms of tubulointerstitial damage, reflecting secondary injury to glomeruli and other elements of the renal microcirculation. Indeed oliguric, acute renal failure may be caused by acute forms of tubulointerstitial disease, and about a third of patients with chronic renal insufficiency suffer from a primary chronic tubulointerstitial disease.

TOXINS

A number of factors make the renal tubules and interstitium particularly prone to toxic injury. Although the kidneys constitute less than 1 percent of total body mass, they receive approximately 20 percent of the cardiac output, and 90 percent or more of renal blood flow is distributed to the renal cortex. Exposure of tubules and interstitium of the renal cortex to circulating toxins is, therefore, quantitatively greater than is that of most other tissues. Transport processes in renal tubules contribute further to the intrarenal accumulation of toxins, enhancing local concentrations of noxious agents. The urinary concentrating mechanism can also establish high levels of toxins within medullary and papillary portions of the kidney, predisposing these regions to chemical injury. Finally, the relatively acid pH of the fluid within most nephron segments may affect the ionization characteristics of potentially toxic compounds and thereby influence local concentration and solubility. Although these processes render the kidney vulnerable to toxic injury, the role of nephrotoxins in renal damage often goes unrecognized because the manifestations of such injury are usually nonspecific in nature and insidious in onset. Diagnosis largely depends upon a history of exposure to a certain toxin, a difficult matter since exposure may be occult. Particular attention should be paid to the occupational history, as well as to an assessment of exposure—current and remote—to drugs, especially antibiotics and analgesics. The recognition of a potential association between a patient's renal disease and exposure to a nephrotoxin is crucial, because, unlike many other forms of renal disease, progression of the functional and morphologic abnormalities associated with toxin-induced nephropathies may be prevented, and even reversed, by eliminating additional exposure.

EXOGENOUS TOXINS Analgesic nephropathy Individuals who ingest large quantities of analgesic drugs are particularly prone to develop tubulointerstitial damage and papillary necrosis. Indeed, in Australia, Switzerland, and Sweden, analgesic abuse is one of the most common causes of chronic renal failure, and it is an important cause of renal insufficiency in the United States as well. In animals *phenacetin* and *aspirin* can induce papillary necrosis when either of these drugs is given in quantities far in excess of usual therapeutic doses. However, these drugs are most likely to cause renal damage when ingested in combination. Epidemiologic studies leave no doubt that the chronic ingestion of mixtures of these analgesics can produce permanent and irreversible renal injury in humans.

Morphologically, analgesic nephropathy is characterized by papillary necrosis and tubulointerstitial inflammation. At an early stage, damage to the vascular supply of the inner medulla (vasa recta) leads to a local interstitial inflammatory reaction and, eventually, to papillary ischemia, necrosis, fibrosis, and calcification. Destruction of papillae usually precedes extension of the tubulointerstitial abnormalities to the renal cortex and, therefore, occurs before renal size and GFR are reduced significantly. Although papillary necrosis is a common finding in patients with the nephropathy of analgesic abuse, necrosis of papillae may also occur in patients with chronic pyelonephritis, diabetes mellitus, sickle cell disease, and obstructive uropathy. The susceptibility of the renal papillae to damage by phenacetin is believed to be related to the establishment of a renal gradient for the phenacetin metabolite *acetaminophen,* resulting in papillary tip concentrations tenfold higher than those in renal cortex. Hydration dissipates this gradient and may explain the protective effect of this maneuver in preventing phenacetin-induced papillary necrosis in animals. Aspirin in these analgesic compounds contributes to renal injury by uncoupling oxidative phosphorylation in renal mitochondria and by inhibiting the synthesis of renal prostaglandins, which are potent endogenous renal vasodilator hormones. Both effects of aspirin favor hypoxia in renal tissues and, therefore, enhance the susceptibility of the inner medulla to nephrotoxic injury.

Analgesic nephropathy occurs some three to five times more commonly in women than men. A direct relationship exists between the total amount of analgesic compounds ingested and the degree of renal impairment. The intake of 1.0 g phenacetin per day for 1 to 3 years or the total ingestion of 2 kg phenacetin in combination with other analgesics appear to represent minimum requirements for the development of analgesic nephropathy. In such patients, renal function usually declines gradually, in association with chronic necrosis of papillae and diffuse tubulointerstitial damage to the renal cortex. Occasionally, papillary necrosis may be associated with hematuria and even renal colic, due to obstruction of a ureter by necrotic tissue. More than half of patients with analgesic nephropathy have pyuria, which, if persistently associated with sterile urine, provides an important clue to the diagnosis. Nonetheless, active pyelonephritis may coexist in patients with analgesic nephropathy. Proteinuria, if present, is typically mild (less than 1 g/d). Patients with analgesic nephropathy are usually unable to generate maximally concentrated urine, reflecting the underlying medullary and papillary damage. An acquired form of distal renal tubular acidosis may contribute to the development of *nephrocalcinosis.* The occurrence of anemia out of proportion to the degree of azotemia may also provide a clue to the diagnosis of analgesic nephropathy. Occult gastrointestinal bleeding (usually secondary to analgesic-induced gastritis) and, in an occasional patient, hemolysis (particularly in those with glucose-6-phosphate dehydrogenase deficiency) contribute to the anemia. Vague abdominal complaints, nonspecific headaches, and arthralgias are common. Moderate hypertension is also common and progresses to a malignant phase in only a small minority. When analgesic nephropathy has progressed to renal insufficiency, the kidneys usually appear bilaterally

shrunken on intravenous pyelography, and the calyces are deformed. A "ring sign" on the pyelogram is pathognomonic of papillary necrosis and represents the radiolucent sloughed papilla surrounded by the radiodense contrast material in the calyx. Transitional cell carcinoma may develop in the urinary pelvis or ureters as a late complication of analgesic abuse.

Every effort must be made to convince the patient who ingests excessive analgesics to discontinue this hazardous practice. When renal damage is at an early stage, cessation of abuse usually arrests the progression of the nephrotoxic process; not infrequently, overall renal function improves with time. With continued abuse, however, progressive renal damage leads invariably to chronic renal failure.

Lead nephropathy (See also Chap. 375) Children and adults suffering from lead intoxication often develop a chronic tubulointerstitial renal disease. In children, lead poisoning usually results from ingestion of lead-based paints (pica). The oxide of lead liberated from paint, or present in the vapor arising from the welding of metals covered with lead-based paint, may be inhaled in substantial quantities, thereby constituting an industrial form of exposure in adults. Alcohol, illegally distilled in an apparatus constructed from automobile radiators (so-called moonshine), is another cause of lead poisoning. Tubule transport processes enhance the accumulation of lead within renal cells, particularly in the proximal convoluted tubule, leading to cell degeneration, mitochondrial swelling, and eosinophilic intranuclear inclusion bodies rich in lead. In addition to tubule degeneration and atrophy, lead nephropathy is associated with ischemic changes in the glomeruli, fibrosis of the adventitia of small renal arterioles, and focal areas of cortical scarring. Eventually, the kidneys become atrophic. In addition to progressive azotemia, abnormalities of tubule function may occur, particularly *renal glycosuria* and *aminoaciduria.* Urinary excretion of lead, bile pigments, and porphyrin precursors, such as δ-aminolevulinic acid, coproporphyrin, and urobilinogen, may be increased. Patients with chronic lead nephropathy are characteristically *hyperuricemic,* a consequence of enhanced reabsorption of filtered urate. Acute gouty arthritis (so-called saturnine gout) occurs in about 50 percent of patients with lead nephropathy, in striking contrast to other forms of chronic renal failure in which gout is rare (also see Chap. 329). Hypertension is also a complication. Therefore, in any patient with slowly progressive renal failure, atrophic kidneys, gout, and hypertension, the diagnosis of lead intoxication should be considered. In addition, patients with chronic lead poisoning often complain of abdominal colic and have evidence of anemia, peripheral neuropathy, and encephalopathy. The diagnosis may be suspected by finding elevated serum levels of lead. However, because blood levels may not be elevated even in the presence of a toxic total-body burden of lead, the quantitation of lead excretion following a standardized infusion of the chelating agent calcium disodium edetate is a more reliable indicator of serious lead exposure. Urinary excretion of more than 0.6 mg of lead per day is indicative of overt or potential toxicity. Treatment includes removing the patient from the source of exposure and augmenting lead excretion with a chelating agent such as calcium disodium edetate.

Miscellaneous nephrotoxins Therapeutic use of lithium salts for manic-depressive illness has been associated with tubulointerstitial disease. The most frequent clinical finding is a mild to moderate nephrogenic diabetes insipidus resulting in polyuria and polydipsia. It is unclear whether long-term lithium therapy produces irreversible chronic tubulointerstitial lesions and impairment of glomerular filtration rate. Though present evidence suggests that some patients develop histologic evidence of such injury, there are only rare reports of chronic renal insufficiency attributable to this agent. In any case, renal function should be followed in patients taking this drug, and caution should be exercised if lithium is employed in patients with underlying renal disease.

The immunosuppressant cyclosporine causes both acute and chronic renal injury. The acute injury and the use of cyclosporine in transplantation are discussed in Chap. 225. The chronic injury is a progressive decline in filtration rate with mild proteinuria and arterial hypertension. The histologic changes in renal tissue comprise patchy interstitial fibrosis and tubular atrophy. In addition, the intrarenal vasculature often demonstrates hyalinosis, and focal segmental glomerular sclerosis can be present as well. Indeed, renal vasoconstriction induced by the drug appears to be a major mechanism of the renal injury. In patients receiving this drug for renal transplantation, chronic rejection and recurrence of the primary disease may coincide with chronic cyclosporine injury, and on clinical grounds, distinction among these may be difficult. Whether the chronic injury can be prevented by dose reduction is uncertain. However, use of the lowest doses of cyclosporine consistent with adequate immunosuppression appears to mitigate nephrotoxicity. In addition, treatment of any associated arterial hypertension may lessen renal injury.

Many agents that commonly lead to acute renal failure are also capable of producing tubulointerstitial injury (see Chap. 223). These include antibiotics (e.g., aminoglycosides, amphotericin B), radiographic contrast agents, various hydrocarbons (e.g., carbon tetrachloride), and heavy metals (e.g., mercury, cadmium, and bismuth).

METABOLIC TOXINS Acute uric acid nephropathy (See also Chap. 329) Acute overproduction of uric acid and extreme hyperuricemia often lead to a rapidly progressive renal insufficiency, so-called acute uric acid nephropathy. This tubulointerstitial disease is usually seen in patients given cytotoxic drugs for the treatment of lymphoproliferative or myeloproliferative disorders but may also occur in these patients before such treatment is begun. The pathologic changes are largely the result of deposition of uric acid crystals in the kidneys and their collecting systems, leading to partial or complete obstruction of collecting ducts, renal pelvis, or ureter. Since obstruction is often bilateral, patients typically show the clinical course of acute renal failure, characterized by oliguria and rapidly rising serum creatinine concentration. In the early phase uric acid crystals can be found in urine, usually in association with microscopic or gross hematuria. Peak serum uric acid levels vary but are almost always above 1200 μmol/L (20 mg/dL) and may even exceed 3500 μmol/L (60 mg/dL).

Prevention of hyperuricemia in patients at risk by treatment with allopurinol in doses of 200 to 800 mg/d prior to cytotoxic therapy reduces the danger of acute uric acid nephropathy. Once hyperuricemia develops, however, efforts should be directed to preventing deposition of uric acid within the urinary tract. Increasing urine volume with potent diuretics (furosemide or mannitol) effectively lowers intratubular uric acid concentrations, and alkalinization of the urine to pH 7 or greater with sodium bicarbonate and/or a carbonic anhydrase inhibitor (acetazolamide) enhances uric acid solubility. If these efforts, together with allopurinol therapy, are ineffective in preventing acute renal failure, dialysis should be instituted to lower the serum uric acid concentration as well as to treat the acute manifestations of uremia. The combination of conservative therapy and hemodialysis allows most patients with acute uric acid nephropathy to survive acute renal failure and ultimately recover renal function.

Gouty nephropathy (See also Chap. 329) Patients with less severe but prolonged forms of hyperuricemia are predisposed to a more chronic tubulointerstitial disorder, often referred to as *gouty nephropathy*. Since other conditions associated with hyperuricemia, such as hypertension, nephrolithiasis, pyelonephritis, and even lead poisoning, may contribute to renal damage, the effect of chronic hyperuricemia per se on renal function is unclear. Nevertheless, the severity of renal involvement correlates with the duration and magnitude of the elevation of the serum uric acid concentration. Histologically, the distinctive feature of gouty nephropathy is the presence of crystalline deposits of uric acid and monosodium urate salts in kidney parenchyma. These deposits are believed to represent the primary pathogenic process in gouty nephropathy, with intraluminal crystallization of uric acid taking place in distal tubules and collecting ducts where urine pH is generally quite low and where uric acid concentrations are considerably in excess of levels in plasma. These deposits not only cause intrarenal obstruction, but also incite an inflammatory response, leading to lymphocytic infiltration, foreign-

body giant cell reaction, and eventual fibrosis, especially of medullary and papillary regions of the kidney. Bacteriuria and pyelonephritis occur in about one-fourth of cases, presumably as complications of intrarenal urinary stasis. Since patients with gout frequently suffer from hypertension and hyperlipidemia, degenerative changes of the renal arterioles may constitute a striking feature of the histologic abnormality, often out of proportion to other morphologic defects. Clinically, gouty nephropathy is an insidious cause of renal insufficiency. Early in its course, GFR may be near normal, often despite focal morphologic changes in medullary and cortical interstitium, proteinuria, and diminished urinary concentrating ability. Whether reducing serum uric acid levels with allopurinol exerts a beneficial effect on the kidney remains to be demonstrated. Although such undesirable consequences of hyperuricemia as gout and uric acid stones respond well to allopurinol, use of this drug in asymptomatic hyperuricemia has not been shown to improve renal function consistently. On the other hand, uricosuric agents such as probenecid, which may increase uric acid stone production, clearly have no role in the treatment of renal disease associated with hyperuricemia.

Hypercalcemic nephropathy (See also Chap. 340) Chronic hypercalcemia, as occurs in primary hyperparathyroidism, sarcoidosis, multiple myeloma, vitamin D intoxication, or metastatic bone disease, can cause tubulointerstitial damage and progressive renal insufficiency. The earliest renal lesion induced by hypercalcemia is a focal degenerative change in renal epithelia, primarily in collecting ducts, distal convoluted tubules, and loops of Henle. Tubule cell necrosis leads to nephron obstruction and stasis of intrarenal urine, favoring local precipitation of calcium salts and infection. Dilatation and atrophy of tubules eventually occur, as do interstitial fibrosis, mononuclear leukocyte infiltration, and interstitial calcium deposition (nephrocalcinosis). Calcium deposition may also occur in glomeruli and the walls of renal arterioles. Clinically, the most striking defect is an inability to concentrate the urine maximally, resulting in polyuria and nocturia. Defective transport of chloride in the ascending limb of Henle's loop is responsible, at least in part, for this concentrating defect. Additionally, reduced collecting duct responsiveness to vasopressin may contribute to this abnormality. Reductions in GFR and renal blood flow also occur, both in states of acute severe hypercalcemia and with prolonged hypercalcemia of lesser severity. Distal renal tubular acidosis and sodium and potassium wasting have also been described in these chronic states. Eventually, uncontrolled hypercalcemia leads to severe tubulointerstitial damage and overt renal failure. Urinalysis is rarely a clue to the presence of hypercalcemic renal failure, but abdominal x-rays may demonstrate nephrocalcinosis as well as nephrolithiasis, the latter due to the hypercalciuria which often accompanies hypercalcemia. Treatment for hypercalcemic nephropathy consists of reducing the serum calcium concentration toward normal and correcting the primary abnormality of calcium metabolism. The management of hypercalcemia is discussed in Chap. 340. Prognosis for recovery of renal function depends upon the severity of the renal lesion at the time hypercalcemia is corrected. Renal dysfunction of recent onset secondary to acute hypercalcemia may be completely reversible. Gradual, progressive renal insufficiency related to chronic hypercalcemia, however, may not improve with correction of the calcium disorder. Nonetheless, every effort should be made to return serum calcium concentration to normal in order to minimize further loss of renal function.

Hypokalemic nephropathy (See also Chap. 50) Disturbances of renal structure and function occur commonly in patients with moderate to severe potassium depletion of at least several weeks' duration. Histologically, renal epithelial cells are often seen to contain numerous vacuoles, most marked in proximal, and to a lesser extent, distal convoluted tubules. These findings usually disappear with potassium repletion. Glomeruli are reduced in size and may become sclerotic while larger blood vessels are usually uninvolved. Whether prolonged or recurrent potassium deficiency results in irreversible tubulointerstitial fibrosis, scarring, and atrophy is unresolved. Loss of urinary concentrating ability is the most commonly encountered functional defect. Studies in animals have shown that this urinary concentrating abnormality is preceded by a period of primary polydipsia. The reduced concentrating capacity which eventually develops is due, at least in part, to defective operation of the countercurrent multiplier system. Elevated rates of intrarenal prostaglandin synthesis may also contribute to this concentrating defect, since prostaglandins antagonize the hydroosmotic action of antidiuretic hormone on collecting-duct epithelium. Symptoms of nocturia, polyuria, and polydipsia are frequently encountered in patients with chronic potassium depletion, although, occasionally, patients with severe hypokalemia have no complaints referable to the urinary tract. Patients with hypokalemic nephropathy may have an enhanced susceptibility to pyelonephritis. The polydipsia is probably due to both the impaired renal concentrating ability and a primary disorder of the thirst mechanism, which is believed to be a common feature of chronic potassium depletion. Urinalysis often reveals no abnormalities except for mild proteinuria. Serum creatinine and urea nitrogen concentrations usually remain within normal limits. Treatment should be directed at repleting body potassium stores and correcting the primary process responsible for potassium loss. With correction of body potassium, functional and histologic abnormalities of the kidneys usually disappear, although maximal urinary concentrating ability may not return to normal for several months.

Miscellaneous metabolic toxins   Urinary oxalate, derived from the metabolism of glycine and, to a variable extent, from ingested oxalate, may deposit as insoluble intratubular calcium oxalate crystals and result in chronic tubulointerstitial damage in patients with hereditary or acquired forms of *hyperoxaluria*. *Cystinosis* and *Fabry's disease* are other hereditary depositional disorders affecting the renal tubules and interstitium (see Chaps. 228, 231, and 232).

RENAL PARENCHYMAL DISEASE ASSOCIATED WITH EXTRARENAL NEOPLASM

In addition to being the site of origin of several benign and malignant neoplasms (see Chap. 234), the kidneys are frequently affected by neoplasms arising outside the urinary tract. Except for the glomerulopathies associated with lymphomas and several solid tumors (see Chap. 228), the renal manifestations of primary extrarenal neoplastic processes are confined mainly to the interstitium and tubules. Although metastatic renal involvement by solid tumors is unusual, the kidneys are often invaded by neoplastic cells in various lymphomas and leukemias and in multiple myeloma. In postmortem studies of patients with *lymphoma*, renal involvement is found in approximately half. The involvement may be focal, in the form of multiple discrete nodules, or diffuse, with lymphomatous infiltration throughout the renal parenchyma. Diffuse infiltration is seen most commonly in lymphomas other than Hodgkin's disease. There may be flank pain related to massive renal infiltration, and x-rays may show enlargement of one or both kidneys. Renal insufficiency occurs in a minority of cases, and overt uremia is rare. Treatment of the primary disease may improve renal function in these cases.

The kidneys are also commonly involved in various forms of *leukemia*. At postmortem examination, bilateral renal involvement is present in approximately 50 percent of cases. As with lymphoma, uremia is rarely, if ever, a consequence of leukemic infiltration of the kidneys. The kidneys can also be involved in leukemias because of the associated high incidence of hyperuricemia, hypercalcemia, and lysozymuria. The myelogenous leukemias, particularly of the monocytic type, may be complicated by tubule defects involving potassium and magnesium wasting.

In contrast, infiltration of the kidneys with *myeloma* cells is infrequent (see Chap. 265). When it occurs, the process is usually focal, so that renal insufficiency from this cause is also uncommon. The more usual lesion is *myeloma kidney*, characterized histologically by atrophic tubules, many with eosinophilic intraluminal casts, and numerous multinucleated giant cells within tubule walls

and in the interstitium. The frequent occurrence of myeloma kidney in patients with Bence Jones proteinuria has suggested a causal relation. Bence Jones proteins are thought to cause myeloma kidney through direct toxicity to renal tubule cells. In addition, Bence Jones proteins may precipitate within the distal nephron where the high concentrations of these proteins and the acid composition of the tubule fluid favor intraluminal cast formation and intrarenal obstruction. Indeed, positive immunofluorescence staining for immunoglobulin light chains can often be demonstrated in casts found in myeloma kidneys. Occasionally, acute renal failure occurs after intravenous pyelography in patients with multiple myeloma and is believed to result from the further precipitation of Bence Jones proteins induced by dehydration prior to radiographic study. Dehydration of the patient with myeloma in preparation for intravenous pyelography should, therefore, be avoided. Multiple myeloma may also affect the kidneys indirectly. Hypercalcemia or hyperuricemia may lead to the nephropathies described above. Proximal tubule disorders are also seen occasionally, including type II proximal renal tubular acidosis and the Fanconi syndrome. Additionally, intrarenal deposits of *amyloid* (see below) may contribute to impaired excretory function.

IMMUNE DISORDERS

HYPERSENSITIVITY NEPHROPATHY   An acute diffuse tubulointerstitial reaction may result from hypersensitivity to a number of drugs. First reported after the use of sulfonamides, acute tubulointerstitial damage is now seen most often with the antibiotic *methicillin*, although *ampicillin, penicillin, cephalothin, phenindione, thiazides, furosemide,* and nonsteroidal anti-inflammatory drugs have also been implicated. Of note, the tubulointerstitial nephropathy which develops in some patients taking nonsteroidal anti-inflammatory drugs may be associated with nephrotic-range proteinuria and histologic evidence of minimal change glomerulopathy. Grossly, the kidneys are usually enlarged. Histologically, the glomeruli appear normal. The principal pathologic abnormalities are in the interstitium of the kidney, which reveals pronounced edema and infiltration with polymorphonuclear leukocytes, lymphocytes, plasma cells, and, in some cases, large numbers of eosinophils. If the process is severe, tubule cell necrosis and regeneration may also be apparent. Immunofluorescence studies either have been unrevealing or have demonstrated a linear pattern of immunoglobin and complement deposition along tubule basement membranes. In a few cases of methicillin-induced acute tubulointerstitial disease, circulating anti-tubule basement membrane antibodies have also been found, suggesting that autoantibody formation may have been induced by the penicilloyl hapten of methicillin (by conjugation of hapten with tubule basement membrane proteins, thereby altering the native antigenicity of the basement membrane). In cases associated with nonsteroidal anti-inflammatory drugs a role for cell-mediated immunity has been proposed, since renal infiltration by both T and B lymphocytes has been observed with a relative predominance of cytotoxic T cells. Evidence for an immunologic basis for these various drug-related nephropathies also derives from the facts that the onset of nephropathy does not appear to be dose-related, often follows a second exposure to the drug presumed to be responsible for the renal injury, and often is associated with increased levels of serum IgE. In the case of methicillin, the patients usually develop evidence of renal injury after about 2 weeks of drug administration. Hematuria, fever, skin rash, and eosinophilia are prominent. Many patients develop azotemia which typically resolves after withdrawal of the offending drug. Proteinuria and pyuria often accompany the hematuria, and occasionally eosinophils are found in the urine sediment. The clinical picture may be confused with acute glomerulonephritis, but when acute azotemia and hematuria are accompanied by eosinophilia, skin rash, and a history of drug exposure, a hypersensitivity reaction leading to acute tubulointerstitial nephritis should be regarded as the leading diagnostic possibility. Discontinuation of the drug usually results in complete reversal of the renal injury; rarely, renal damage may be irreversible. Glucocorticoids have been used, but their value has not been established.

SJÖGREN'S SYNDROME (See also Chap. 273) Keratoconjunctivitis sicca, or Sjögren's syndrome, is an immunologic disorder characterized by dryness of mucous membranes and mononuclear cell infiltration of salivary and lacrimal glands; it is often seen in patients with rheumatoid arthritis. When the kidneys are involved, the predominant histologic findings are those of chronic tubulointerstitial disease. Interstitial infiltrates are composed primarily of lymphocytes, causing the histology of the renal parenchyma in these patients to resemble that of the salivary and lacrimal glands. Renal functional defects associated with this disorder include diminished urinary concentrating ability and distal (type I) renal tubular acidosis. Urinalysis may show pyuria (predominantly lymphocyturia) and mild proteinuria.

AMYLOIDOSIS (See also Chaps. 228 and 266) Glomerular pathology usually predominates and leads to heavy proteinuria and azotemia. However, tubule function may also be deranged, giving rise to a nephrogenic diabetes insipidus and to distal (type I) renal tubular acidosis. In several cases these functional abnormalities correlated with peritubular deposition of amyloid, particularly in areas surrounding vasa rectae, loops of Henle, and collecting ducts. Bilateral enlargement of the kidneys, especially in a patient with massive proteinuria and tubule dysfunction, should raise the possibility of amyloid renal disease.

AIDS (See also Chap. 264) Tubulointerstitial and glomerular pathology in patients with acquired immunodeficiency syndrome (AIDS) causes proteinuria and renal insufficiency. Some of the abnormalities result from associated nephrotoxic insults including intravenous drug abuse and multiple exposure to nephrotoxic antibiotics. In addition, the accumulated effects of multiple septic episodes, such as infectious granulomatous cytomegalovirus inclusions, and Kaposi's sarcoma obviously are secondary to the compromised immune state and should not be considered AIDS-specific renal disease. However, glomerular sclerosis has been reported as a complication of AIDS without apparent other cause. The prevalence of a specific AIDS-related renal lesion appears to be variable with few if any such cases noted in some areas of the United States. The reason for this disparity is uncertain. Based on the limited available data, black patients with AIDS may be especially at risk for renal complications, and the variations in reported prevalence of renal disease in AIDS may, in part, reflect different racial distributions among the AIDS populations studied.

TUBULOINTERSTITIAL ABNORMALITIES ASSOCIATED WITH GLOMERULONEPHRITIS A number of primary glomerulopathies may also be associated with damage to tubules and interstitium. Pathogenetically, the extraglomerular component in these renal disorders often involves the same mechanisms that are responsible for the more pronounced glomerular injury. For example, in more than half of patients with the nephropathy of systemic lupus erythematosus, deposits of immune complexes can be identified in tubule basement membranes, usually accompanied by an interstitial mononuclear inflammatory reaction. Similarly, in many patients with glomerulonephritis associated with antiglomerular basement membrane antibody, the same antibody can be shown to be reactive against tubule basement membranes as well.

MISCELLANEOUS DISORDERS

VESICOURETERAL REFLUX (See also Chaps. 95 and 227) Normally, the junction of the terminal ureter with the urinary bladder provides a competent sphincter so that during micturition urine leaves the bladder only via the urethra. However, when the function of the ureterovesical junction is impaired, urine may reflux into the ureters due to the high intravesical pressure that develops during voiding. Clinically, reflux is often detected on the voiding

and postvoiding films obtained during intravenous pyelography, although voiding cystourethrography may be required for definitive diagnosis. Bladder infection may ascend the urinary tract to the kidneys through incompetent ureterovesical sphincters. Not surprisingly, therefore, reflux is often discovered in patients with acute and/or chronic urinary tract infections. In children particularly, reflux of minor degree may disappear with time and standard therapy of intercurrent urinary infection. With more severe degrees of reflux, characterized by marked dilatation of ureters and renal pelves, progressive renal damage often appears, and although active infection may also be present, uncertainty exists as to the necessity of infection in producing the scarred kidney of reflux nephropathy. In contrast to those with other forms of chronic tubulointerstitial disease, patients with renal insufficiency and scarring due to reflux often demonstrate substantial proteinuria. Indeed, in such cases glomerular lesions similar to those of idiopathic focal glomerulosclerosis (Chap. 227) are often present in addition to the usual changes of chronic tubulointerstitial disease. Surgical correction of reflux is usually necessary only with the more severe degrees of reflux since renal damage correlates with the extent of reflux. Obviously, if extensive glomerulosclerosis already exists, urologic repair may no longer be warranted.

RADIATION NEPHRITIS Renal dysfunction can be expected to occur if 23,000 Gy (2300 rad) or more of x-ray irradiation is administered to both kidneys during a period of 5 weeks or less. Histologic examination of the kidneys reveals hyalinized glomeruli, atrophic tubules, extensive interstitial fibrosis, and hyalinization of the media of renal arterioles. Radiation-induced renal ischemia is believed to be the main pathogenic factor responsible for the tubulointerstitial damage, which may not become evident clinically for months after completion of radiation. The presentation of acute radiation nephritis includes rapidly progressive azotemia, moderate to malignant hypertension, anemia, and proteinuria which may reach the nephrotic range. More than 50 percent of these cases progress to chronic renal failure. A more insidious form of radiation nephritis is characterized by slower development of azotemia, anemia, and nephrotic syndrome. Malignant hypertension may follow unilateral renal irradiation and resolve with ipsilateral nephrectomy. Radiation nephritis in recent years has all but vanished because of heightened awareness of its pathogenesis by radiotherapists.

REFERENCES

ADLER SG et al: Hypersensitivity phenomena and the kidney: Role of drugs and environmental agents. Am J Kidney Dis 5:75, 1985

BATUMEN V et al: The role of lead in gout nephropathy. N Engl J Med 304:520, 1981

BOTON R et al: Prevalence, pathogenesis, and treatment of renal dysfunction associated with chronic lithium therapy. Am J Kidney Dis 10:329, 1987

BUCKALEW VM JR, SCHEY HM: Analgesic nephropathy: A significant cause of morbidity in the United States. Am J Kidney Dis 7:164, 1986

COE FL, BUSHINSKY DA: Clinical and laboratory assessment on patients with renal and urinary tract disease, in *Clinical Nephrology*, BM Brenner et al (eds). Philadelphia, Saunders, 1987, p 1

COTRAN RS: Glomerulosclerosis in reflux nephropathy. Kidney Int 21:528, 1982

———— et al: Tubulointerstitial diseases, in *The Kidney*, 3d ed, BM Brenner, FC Rector Jr (eds). Philadelphia, Saunders, 1986, p 1143

HUMES HD, WEINBERG J: Toxic nephropathies, in *The Kidney*, 3d ed, BM Brenner, FC Rector Jr (eds). Philadelphia, Saunders, 1986, p 1491

HUMPHREYS MH, SCHOENFELD PY: AIDS and renal disease. Kidney 20:7, 1987

MURRAY T, GOLDBERG M: Chronic interstitial nephritis: Etiologic factors. Ann Intern Med 82:453, 1975

MYERS BD: Cyclosporine nephrotoxicity. Kidney Int 30:964, 1986

WILSON CB, DIXON FJ: Renal response to immunological injury, in *The Kidney*, 3d ed, BM Brenner, FC Rector Jr (eds). Philadelphia, Saunders, 1986, p 800

230   VASCULAR INJURY TO THE KIDNEY

KAMAL F. BADR / BARRY M. BRENNER

Adequate delivery of blood to the glomerular capillary network is crucial for glomerular filtration and overall salt and water balance. Thus, in addition to the threat to the viability of renal tissue, vascular injury to the kidney may compromise the maintenance of body fluid volume and composition. Involvement of the renal vessels by atherosclerotic, hypertensive, embolic, inflammatory, and hematologic disorders is usually a manifestation of generalized vascular pathology. The morphologic and clinical responses to these insults and the unique renal vasculopathy associated with the toxemias of pregnancy are considered in this chapter.

THROMBOEMBOLIC DISEASES OF THE RENAL ARTERIES

Thrombosis of the major renal arteries or their branches is an important cause of deterioration of renal function, especially in the elderly. It is often difficult to diagnose and therefore requires a high index of suspicion. Thrombosis may occur as a result of intrinsic pathology in the renal vessels (posttraumatic, atherosclerotic, or inflammatory) or as a result of emboli originating in distant vessels, most commonly fat emboli, emboli originating in the left heart (mural thrombi following myocardial infarction, bacterial endocarditis, or aseptic vegetations), or "paradoxical" emboli passing from the right side of the circulation via a patent foramen ovale or atrial septal defect. Emboli are bilateral in 15 to 30 percent of cases.

The clinical presentation is variable, depending on the time course and the extent of the occlusive event. Acute thrombosis and infarction, such as follows embolization, may result in sudden onset of flank pain and tenderness, fever, hematuria, leukocytosis, nausea, and vomiting. If infarction occurs, renal enzymes may be elevated, namely, aspartate transaminase (AST), lactic dehydrogenase (LDH) most reliable, and alkaline phosphatase, which rise and fall in the order listed. Urinary LDH and alkaline phosphatase may also increase after infarction. Renal function deteriorates acutely, leading in bilateral thrombosis to acute oliguric renal failure. More gradual (i.e., atherosclerotic) occlusion of a single renal artery may go undetected. A spectrum of clinical presentations lies between these two extremes (Table 230-1). Hypertension usually follows renal infarction and results from renin release in the peri-infarction zone. Hypertension is usually transient but may be persistent. Diagnosis is established by renal arteriography.

Management of *acute* renal arterial thrombosis includes surgical intervention, anticoagulant therapy, conservative and supportive therapy, and control of hypertension. The choice of treatment depends mainly on: (1) the condition of the patient, in particular the patient's ability to withstand major surgery, and (2) the extent of renovascular occlusion and amount of renal mass at risk of infarction. In general, supportive care and anticoagulant therapy are indicated in unilateral disease. In bilateral thrombosis, medical and surgical therapies yield comparable results. Twenty-five percent of patients die during the acute episode, usually from extrarenal complications. In *chronic* ischemic renal disease, surgical revascularization is more likely to preserve and improve renal function and to control the hypertension (see below).

ATHEROEMBOLIC DISEASE OF THE RENAL ARTERIES

Atheroembolic disease typically results from multiple showers of cholesterol-containing microemboli dislodged from atheromatous plaques in large arteries. Such emboli occlude small (150- to 200-μm diameter) vessels in the kidney and in other organs (retina, brain, pancreas, muscles, skin, and extremities). It usually occurs in an elderly individual with atherosclerotic disease elsewhere and usually follows aortic surgery or renal or coronary arteriography. Spontaneous atheroembolic disease has been reported. Manifestations include deterioration of renal function (sudden or gradual), mild proteinuria, microscopic hematuria, and leukocyturia. Urine volume may remain normal or fall to oliguric levels depending on severity. Renal ischemia can induce or exacerbate preexisting hypertension.

Antemortem diagnosis of atherosclerotic renal emboli is difficult. The demonstration of cholesterol emboli in the retina is helpful, but a firm diagnosis is established only by demonstration of cholesterol crystals in the smaller arteries and arterioles in renal biopsy or autopsy specimens. These may also be seen in asymptomatic skeletal muscle or skin. No specific treatment is available.

RENAL VEIN THROMBOSIS

Thrombosis of one or both main renal veins (RVT) occurs in a variety of settings (Table 230-2). The pathogenesis is not always clear, particularly when it occurs in so-called hypercoagulable states such as may develop in pregnant women, users of oral contraceptives, subjects with nephrotic syndrome, or dehydrated infants. Nephrotic syndrome accompanying membranous glomerulopathy and certain carcinomas seems to predispose to the development of RVT, which occurs in 10 to 50 percent of patients with these disorders. RVT may exacerbate preexisting proteinuria but is infrequently the cause of the nephrotic syndrome.

The clinical manifestations depend on the severity and abruptness of its occurrence. Acute cases occur typically in children and are characterized by sudden loss of renal function, often accompanied by fever, chills, lumbar tenderness (with kidney enlargement), leukocytosis, and hematuria. Hemorrhagic infarction and renal rupture may lead to hypovolemic shock. In young adults RVT is usually suspected from an unexpected and relatively acute or subacute deterioration of renal function and/or exacerbation of proteinuria and hematuria in the appropriate clinical setting (underlying nephrotic syndrome, trauma, pregnancy, oral contraceptive use). In cases of gradual thrombosis, usually occurring in the elderly, the only manifestation may be recurrent pulmonary emboli or development of hypertension. A Fanconi-like syndrome and proximal renal tubular acidosis have been described.

The definitive diagnosis can only be established through selective renal venography with visualization of the occluding thrombus. Treatment consists of anticoagulation, the main purpose of which is prevention of pulmonary embolization, although some authors have also claimed improvement in renal function and proteinuria. Encouraging reports have appeared concerning the use of streptokinase. Spontaneous recanalization with clinical improvement has also been observed. Anticoagulant therapy is more rewarding in the acute thrombosis seen in younger individuals. Nephrectomy is advocated in infants with life-threatening renal infarction. Thrombectomy is effective in some cases.

RENAL ARTERY STENOSIS

Stenosis of the main renal artery and/or its major branches accounts for 2 to 5 percent of hypertension. The common cause in the middle-aged and elderly is an atheromatous plaque at the origin of the renal artery. In younger women, stenosis is due to intrinsic structural abnormalities of the arterial wall caused by a heterogeneous group of lesions termed *fibromuscular dysplasia*.

TABLE 230-1   Clinical presentations of ischemic renal disease

1 Acute renal failure
2 Progressive azotemia in a patient with known renovascular hypertension (usually on medical therapy)
3 Unexplained progressive azotemia in an elderly patient with or without refractory hypertension
4 Hypertension and azotemia in a renal transplant patient

TABLE 230-2   Conditions associated with renal vein thrombosis

1 Trauma
2 Extrinsic compression (lymph nodes, aortic aneurysm, tumor)
3 Invasion by renal cell carcinoma
4 Dehydration (infants)
5 Nephrotic syndrome
6 Pregnancy or oral contraceptives

Renal artery stenosis should be suspected when hypertension develops in a previously normotensive individual over 50 years of age or in the young (under 30 years) with suggestive features: symptoms of vascular insufficiency to other organs, high-pitched epigastric bruit on physical exam, symptoms of hypokalemia secondary to hyperaldosteronism (muscle weakness, tetany, polyuria), and metabolic alkalosis. If renovascular hypertension is suspected, a positive captopril test, which has a sensitivity and specificity of greater than 95 percent, constitutes an excellent screening procedure to assess the need for more invasive radiographic evaluation. The test relies on the exaggerated increase in plasma renin activity (PRA) following administration of captopril to patients with renovascular hypertension as compared to those with essential hypertension. It is considered positive when all of the following criteria are satisfied: stimulated PRA of 12 (μg/L)/h; absolute increase in PRA of 10 (μg/L)/h or more; and increase in PRA of greater than 150 percent (or 400 percent if baseline PRA is less than 3 (μg/L)/h. In the appropriate clinical setting, particularly in the presence of a positive captopril test, digital subtraction renal arteriography should be performed. This procedure obviates the need for cannulation of the arterial system and has a low incidence of false-positive (5 percent) and false-negative (10 percent) results. The most definitive diagnostic procedure is bilateral arteriography with repeated bilateral renal vein and systemic renin determinations. If renal vein renin measurements from the two kidneys differ by a factor of 1.5:1 or more (higher value from the affected kidney) in a patient with radiographic unilateral renal artery stenosis, the chance of cure of hypertension by surgical reconstruction is almost 90 percent, particularly if renal vein renin from the unaffected kidney is equal to or less than systemic levels (suppressible). A ratio of less than 1.5:1, however, does not exclude the diagnosis of renovascular hypertension, particularly in the presence of bilateral disease.

The aims of treatment are control of the blood pressure and restoration of perfusion to the ischemic kidney. In general, it is now firmly established that interventional therapy (i.e., surgery or angioplasty) is superior to medical therapy, which, while controlling blood pressure, does little to salvage renal mass lost to ischemic injury. Success rates with percutaneous transluminal angioplasty in young patients with fibromuscular dysplasia are 50 percent cure and 30 percent improvement in blood pressure control. Due to its relative noninvasiveness as compared to surgery, therefore, angioplasty is the primary therapeutic option for patients with renal artery stenosis. Angioplasty is best suited for noncalcified segmental short lesions and is also useful in some elderly patients who are poor surgical risks. About half of elderly individuals with reduced renal function as a result of renal arterial stenosis improve following angioplasty or surgery, even when preintervention arteriography shows little evidence of cortical perfusion. If angioplasty fails, surgical reperfusion should be considered.

Renal artery stenosis, particularly if atherosclerotic, is a progressive disease that may lead to gradual and silent loss of renal functional tissue. Compensatory contralateral hypertrophy may maintain renal function until affected by superimposed pathologic processes, at which time azotemia supervenes. Even if angioplasty or surgery fail to return blood pressure to normal, these procedures usually render medical therapy easier.

HEMOLYTIC UREMIC SYNDROME (HUS) AND THROMBOTIC THROMBOCYTOPENIC PURPURA (TTP)

HUS and TTP, consumptive coagulopathies characterized by microangiopathic hemolytic anemia and thrombocytopenia, have a particular predilection for the kidney and the central nervous system, the latter especially in TTP. The kidneys of patients with HUS or TTP often exhibit a ''flea-bitten'' appearance, the result of multiple cortical hemorrhagic infarcts. The major sites of pathology are the small renal arteries and afferent arterioles, which are nearly occluded as a result of marked intimal hyperplasia (particularly in TTP) and fibrin deposits in the subintimal regions. When the vasoocclusive process is extensive, bilateral cortical necrosis may occur. In addition, arteriolar micro-

aneurysms, glomerular infarction, or nonspecific focal changes may be seen. In keeping with the focal nature of the vascular lesions, patchy areas of interstitial edema, tubular necrosis, and, eventually, fibrosis occur. By immunofluorescence staining, complement components and immunoglobulins may be demonstrated in the arterioles, and fibrinogen deposits are present in arteries, arterioles, and glomerular capillary loops.

Several mechanisms have been implicated in the etiology of the intravascular coagulopathy seen in HUS and TTP including induction of a generalized Shwartzman phenomenon by microorganisms or endotoxin, genetic predisposition, and deficiency of platelet antiaggregatory substance(s) (e.g., prostacyclin). Some patients improve following exchange transfusion or plasmapheresis, suggesting accumulation of an as yet unidentified toxin.

Renal failure is common in both HUS and TTP, usually manifested by oligoanuria (more severe in HUS), azotemia, mild proteinuria, microscopic and/or gross hematuria, and cylindruria. Patients with HUS have more severe renal failure, often marked by oligoanuria and hypertension and commonly progressing to chronic renal failure. The prognosis in HUS is better in children than adults. In TTP, the course of which may span days to months, renal failure is usually less severe. The overall prognosis, however, remains poor in view of the severe CNS involvement.

In the management of TTP, high-dose glucocorticoids and plasma exchange often provide complete remission or cure. Plasma exchange should be initiated as early as possible, and the treatment cycles can be repeated if thrombocytopenia recurs. Splenectomy and antiplatelet therapy have also been used with varying degrees of success in TTP patients. The success of plasma exchange in adult HUS is less well established than in TTP.

ARTERIOLAR NEPHROSCLEROSIS

Whether hypertension is ''essential'' or of known etiology, persistent exposure of the renal circulation to elevated intraluminal pressures results in development of intrinsic lesions of the renal arterioles (hyaline arteriolosclerosis) that eventually lead to loss of function (nephrosclerosis). Nephrosclerosis is divided into two distinct entities: ''benign'' and ''malignant'' (or accelerated).

Benign arteriolar nephrosclerosis Benign arteriolar nephrosclerosis is seen in patients who are hypertensive for an extended period of time (blood pressure more than 150/90) but whose hypertension has not progressed to a malignant form (described below). Such patients, usually in the older age group, are often discovered to be hypertensive on routine physical examination or as a result of nonspecific symptomatology (e.g., headaches, weakness, palpitations).

Kidney size is normal to reduced, with loss of cortical mass leading to a fine granularity. Although the larger arteries may show atherosclerotic changes, the characteristic pathology is in the afferent arterioles, which have thickened walls due to deposition of homogeneous eosinophilic material (hyaline arteriolosclerosis). This material is composed of plasma proteins and fats that have been deposited in the arteriolar wall due to injury to the endothelium, probably secondary to the elevated intraluminal hydraulic pressure. Narrowing of vascular lumina results, with consequent ischemic injury to glomeruli and tubules.

Nephrosclerosis accompanying long-standing systemic arterial hypertension is only one manifestation of a generalized process affecting the cardiovascular system. Physical examination, therefore, may reveal changes in retinal vessels (arteriolar narrowing and/or flame-shaped hemorrhages), cardiac hypertrophy, and possibly signs of congestive heart failure. Renal disease may manifest as a mild to moderate elevation of serum creatinine concentration, microscopic hematuria, and/or mild proteinuria. In general, clinical evaluation does not reveal significant renal abnormalities. More specialized examination may disclose elevated urinary albumin excretion, tapering and loss of caliber of intrarenal vessels on arteriography, and an exaggerated natriuresis in response to a fluid challenge. Patients with benign nephrosclerosis maintain a near-normal glomerular filtration rate despite a reduction in renal blood flow.

Malignant arteriolar nephrosclerosis   Patients with long-standing benign hypertension or patients not known to be hypertensive previously may develop malignant hypertension characterized by a sudden (accelerated) elevation of blood pressure (diastolic often above 130 mmHg) accompanied by papilledema, central nervous system manifestations, cardiac decompensation, and acute progressive deterioration of renal function. The absence of papilledema does not rule out the diagnosis in a patient with markedly elevated blood pressure and rapidly declining renal function. The kidneys are characterized by a flea-bitten appearance resulting from hemorrhages in surface capillaries. Histologically, two distinct vascular lesions can be seen. The first, affecting arterioles, is fibrinoid necrosis, i.e., infiltration of arteriolar walls with eosinophilic material including fibrin. There is thickening of vessel walls and, occasionally, an inflammatory infiltrate (necrotizing arteriolitis). The second lesion, involving the interlobular arteries, is a concentric hyperplastic proliferation of the cellular elements of the vascular wall with deposition of collagen to form a hyperplastic arteriolitis (onion-skin lesion). Fibrinoid necrosis occasionally extends into the glomeruli, which may also undergo proliferative changes or total necrosis. Most glomerular and tubule changes are secondary to ischemia and infarction. The sequence of events leading to the development of malignant hypertension is poorly defined. Two pathophysiologic alterations appear central in its initiation and/or perpetuation: (1) increased permeability of vessel walls to invasion by plasma components, particularly fibrin, which activates clotting mechanisms leading to a microangiopathic hemolytic anemia, thus perpetuating the vascular pathology; and (2) activation of the renin-angiotensin-aldosterone system at some point in the disease process, which contributes to the acceleration and maintenance of blood pressure elevation and, in turn, to vascular injury.

Malignant hypertension is most likely to develop in a previously hypertensive individual, usually in the third or fourth decade of life. There is a higher incidence among men, particularly black men. The presenting symptoms are usually neurologic (dizziness, headache, blurring of vision, altered states of consciousness, and focal or generalized seizures). Cardiac decompensation and renal failure appear thereafter. Renal abnormalities include a rapid rise in serum creatinine, hematuria (at times macroscopic), proteinuria, and red and white blood cell casts in the sediment. Nephrotic syndrome may be present. Elevated plasma aldosterone levels cause hypokalemic metabolic alkalosis in the early phase. Uremic acidosis and hyperkalemia eventually obscure these early findings. Hematologic indices of microangiopathic hemolytic anemia (i.e., schistocytes) are often seen.

Control of hypertension is the principal goal of therapy for both benign and malignant forms. The time of initiation of therapy, its effectiveness, and patient compliance are crucial factors in arresting the progression of benign nephrosclerosis. Untreated, most of these patients succumb to the extrarenal complications of hypertension. In contrast, malignant hypertension is a medical emergency; its natural course includes a death rate of 80 to 90 percent within 1 year of onset, almost always due to uremia. Supportive measures should be instituted to control the neurologic, cardiac, and other complications of acute renal failure, but the mainstay of therapy is prompt and aggressive reduction of blood pressure, which, if successful, can reverse all complications in the majority of patients. Presently, 5-year survival is 50 percent, and some patients have evidence of partial reversal of the vascular lesions and a return of renal function to near-normal levels.

SCLERODERMA (PROGRESSIVE SYSTEMIC SCLEROSIS)   Renal vascular involvement in scleroderma is characterized by a distinctive lesion of the small arteries (diameters of 150 to 500 μm) consisting of intimal proliferation, medial thinning, and increased collagen deposition in the adventitial layer. Fibrinoid changes in the walls of afferent arterioles and microinfarcts may occur. Glomerular changes are generally nonspecific and secondary to ischemic damage. Tubules are often atrophic. As part of a generalized increase in vasomotor tone, a vasospastic (Raynaud-like) phenomenon at the level of the renal vasculature contributes to the renal insufficiency. Reduction in renal blood flow is the major mechanism underlying the deterioration in kidney function, being present in 80 percent of patients, even in the absence of other clinical abnormalities. As vascular narrowing progresses, hypertension, azotemia, and proteinuria eventually develop. Plasma renin rises in response to sustained renal ischemia. The resulting hypertension causes further renal injury and may play a role in the intimate destruction of nephrons. As more and more nephrons are lost to the combined insults of ischemia and hypertension, development of azotemia heralds a particularly grim prognosis. Proteinuria, usually mild, is a consequence of ischemic and hypertensive glomerular injury.

Although the majority of patients with scleroderma present with extrarenal manifestations, renal involvement is eventually manifested in half of patients followed for up to 20 years. Renal involvement can present in one of two ways, depending on whether malignant hypertension is superimposed on the renal pathology: (1) *Persistent urinary abnormalities* with or without hypertension tend to follow an indolent course with mild proteinuria, occasional casts, cellular elements in the urinary sediment, and a propensity for development of hypertension. Azotemia is absent initially, but when it develops, dialysis is required within 1 year. (2) *Scleroderma renal crisis* is a rapid deterioration in renal function, usually accompanied by malignant hypertension, oliguria, fluid retention, microangiopathic hemolytic anemia, and central nervous system involvement. It may occur in patients with previously undemonstrable or slowly progressive renal disease. Untreated, it leads to chronic renal failure within days to months.

The prognosis of scleroderma renal disease is generally poor, particularly following the onset of azotemia. Aggressive antihypertensive therapy may be effective in delaying the progression of renal failure. In scleroderma renal crisis, prompt treatment with beta blockers, minoxidil, and particularly angiotensin I converting enzyme (ACE) inhibitors may reverse acute renal failure. The effect of these interventions on renal function over the long term is uncertain.

SICKLE CELL NEPHROPATHY   Sickle cell disease causes renal complications that arise mainly as a result of sickling of red blood cells in the microvasculature. The hypertonic and relatively hypoxic environment of the renal medulla, coupled with the slow blood flow in the vasa recta, favors the sickling of red blood cells, with resultant local infarction (papillary necrosis). Functional tubule defects in patients with sickle cell disease are likely the result of partial ischemic injury to the renal tubules.

In addition to the intrarenal microvascular pathology described above, young patients with sickle cell disease are characterized by renal hyperperfusion, glomerular hypertrophy, and hyperfiltration. Many of these individuals eventually develop a glomerulopathy leading to proteinuria (present in as many as 30 percent) and, in some, the nephrotic syndrome. Mild azotemia and hyperuricemia can also develop, but advanced renal failure and uremia are rare. Although an immunologic basis for the glomerulopathy of sickle cell disease has been proposed, hemodynamically mediated renal injury, resulting from intrarenal hyperperfusion and glomerular hyperfiltration, may be the major pathogenetic mechanism. Nephron loss secondary to ischemic injury also contributes to the development of azotemia in these patients.

The renal complications of sickle cell disease include the following: *Cortical infarcts* can cause loss of function, persistent hematuria, and perinephric hematomas. *Papillary infarcts*, demonstrated radiographically in 50 percent of patients with sickle trait, lead to an increased risk of bacterial infection in the scarred renal tissues and functional tubule abnormalities. Painless gross hematuria occurs with a higher frequency in sickle trait than in sickle cell disease and likely results from infarctive episodes in the renal medulla. *Functional tubule abnormalities* such as nephrogenic diabetes insipidus result from marked reduction in vasa recta blood flow, combined with ischemic tubule injury. This concentrating defect places these patients at increased risk of dehydration and, hence, sickling crises. The concentrating defect also occurs in individuals with sickle trait. Other tubule defects involve potassium and hydrogen ion excretion, occasionally leading to hyperkalemic, metabolic acidosis and a defect in uric acid excretion which, combined with increased purine synthesis in the bone marrow, results in hyperuricemia. Glomerulopathy is an established consequence of sickle cell disease and is due to a combination of hemodynamically mediated glomerular injury referred to earlier and an immune-complex glomerulonephritis in which tubule epithelial antigens, released into the circulation during episodes of ischemic injury, provoke an antibody response leading to immune-complex deposition in the glomeruli. Proteinuria is the chief manifestation of sickle cell glomerulopathy and may reach nephrotic proportions.

TOXEMIAS OF PREGNANCY Renal function is "reset" at a higher level during normal pregnancy. Renal plasma flow (RPF) and glomerular filtration rate (GFR) both increase by 30 to 50 percent. Therefore, serum creatinine levels above 70 μmol/L (0.8 mg/dL) or blood urea nitrogen (BUN) levels above 4.6 mmol/L (13 mg/dL) are abnormal in pregnant women and should be investigated. Systolic and diastolic blood pressures decrease by an average of 10 to 15 mmHg below pregravid values. A diastolic pressure above 75 mmHg during the second trimester or above 85 mmHg during the third trimester is therefore abnormal. Vasodilation in the uterine, renal, and cutaneous beds, vasodilator prostaglandin release from the uteroplacental unit, and a decrease in arteriolar sensitivity to angiotensin II all play a role in the decline of blood pressure during pregnancy.

Preeclampsia-eclampsia The toxemia syndrome, usually occurring in the third trimester of primigravidas, includes hypertension, proteinuria, edema, consumptive coagulopathy, sodium retention, hyperreflexia (preeclampsia), and, if uncontrolled, convulsions (eclampsia). In pure preeclampsia (i.e., not superimposed on previously existing hypertensive or renal disease) the primary sites of pathology are the glomerular endothelial cells. These cells show marked swelling due to an increase in cytoplasmic volume with vacuolization (endotheliosis) and encroach on the vascular lumen, rendering the enlarged glomeruli ischemic. The glomerular basement membrane and the extraglomerular blood vessels are intact. The pathogenesis is unknown. Coagulation abnormalities, hormonal factors, uteroplacental ischemia, and immune mechanisms have all been implicated. The mechanisms mediating the hypertension are also not understood. Despite sodium retention, intravascular volume is contracted as compared to pregravid values. An increased sensitivity to angiotensin II is the basis for the "roll-over test" (an increase in diastolic blood pressure of 20 mmHg or more upon changing the patient's position from lateral recumbent to supine, presumably due to alterations in circulating angiotensin levels). In the supine position, the reduction in venous return due to compression by the gravid uterus increases circulating levels of angiotension II. This results in a hypertensive response in preeclamptic patients, who are hyper-responsive to angiotensin II, but not in normal women, in whom pregnancy leads to a relative resistance to the pressor effects of this hormone.

A diagnosis of preeclampsia-related hypertension can be made when repeated measurements over a 4- to 6- h period show a blood pressure of 140/85 mmHg or more. The rise in blood pressure tends to be more severe at night. When preeclampsia occurs in a previously hypertensive patient, a rapid acceleration of the blood pressure elevation is accompanied by an increase in proteinuria, oliguria, edema, and coagulopathy. This is a life-threatening syndrome and tends to recur with future pregnancies. In addition to proteinuria, which correlates with the severity of the renal lesion, GFR and RPF are depressed. In view of the preexisting high levels, however, GFR in preeclamptic women often remains above nonpregnant levels. Uric acid clearance also falls, resulting in hyperuricemia. In the postpartum period, these patients are particularly susceptible to the development of "postpartum renal failure," which is thought to be a form of adult HUS.

Management consists of bed rest in a quiet environment and control of neurologic manifestations and blood pressure, the former with magnesium sulfate and the latter usually with vasodilators such as hydralazine and methyldopa. Diuretics are avoided. The ultimate "treatment" is delivery, which should be induced if fetal maturity is adequate or if life-threatening coagulopathy or renal failure occur. The long-term prognosis is generally favorable.

Bilateral cortical necrosis Acute bilateral cortical necrosis is associated with septic abortions, abruptio placentae, and preeclampsia. Coagulation in cortical vessels and arterioles leads to renal tissue necrosis. Anuria and renal failure ensue, and may be irreversible. In other cases renal function returns partially, but on long-term follow-up most patients slowly progress to uremia.

VASCULITIS The kidney is commonly involved in systemic disorders in which necrotizing inflammatory injury to vessels is a primary feature. Several lines of evidence point toward an immunologic pathogenesis for the vasculitides, the prototype of which is periarteritis nodosa (PAN).

Periarteritis nodosa In PAN, arcuate and intralobular arteries are primarily involved. Acute lesions are characterized by destruction of the internal elastic lamina, segmental fibrinoid necrosis of the intima and/or the entire vessel wall, intense intra- and periarterial leukocytic infiltration, and occasional aneurysmal dilatation of the vessel wall (demonstrable radiographically). Fibroblast proliferation leads eventually to occlusion and obliteration of vessel lumina. These vascular changes typically lead to glomerular ischemia, occasionally associated with proliferative changes in the glomerular tufts and juxtaglomerular apparatus. Progression to acute necrotizing crescentic glomerulonephritis may occur.

Clinically, renal involvement in PAN is often associated with hypertension (renin-mediated) which at times progresses to a severe or malignant form. Hematuria, microscopic or gross, can also occur as a result of ischemia, hypertensive renal injury, or glomerulonephritis. Proteinuria is usually mild, and the urinary sediment contains all of the formed elements (red and white blood cells, renal epithelial cells, and their respective casts). Nephrotic syndrome is uncommon. Acute renal failure occurs in approximately 10 percent of cases and is usually the result of malignant hypertension and/or the development of rapidly progressive, crescentic glomerulonephritis. The diagnosis of PAN can be established by documenting the typical arterial lesions in biopsy material from involved organs (testes, muscle, skin). Renal biopsy seldom shows the arterial lesions but may reveal focal or diffuse crescentic glomerulonephritis. Renal and celiac arteriography, however, frequently demonstrates characteristic aneurysmal dilatation of the involved arteries.

Untreated, PAN is generally progressive, causing death from renal failure, gastrointestinal bleeding, or other extrarenal catastrophes. Encouraging therapeutic results have been obtained with glucocorticoid therapy in combination with cytoxic agents (cyclophosphamide or azathioprine) and plasma exchange. In addition, hypertension should be controlled. Early initiation of antihypertensive therapy prolongs survival in more than 90 percent of patients and causes complete remission in 20 percent. Allergic granulomatosis (Churg-Strauss syndrome), a variant of PAN, is similar in its renal manifestations but also causes immediate-type hypersensitivity reactions, including primary pulmonary involvement, asthma, and eosinophilia.

Hypersensitivity angiitis (microscopic form of PAN) Hypersensitivity angiitis is an acute fulminant form of necrotizing vasculitis in which the characteristic pathologic finding is an intense leukocytic infiltration of the smaller renal vessels (arterioles, venules, capillaries) with or without fibrinoid necrosis. Thus, the pathology is more often limited to the glomerular vessels (including the afferent and postglomerular arterioles). The infiltrating leukocytes fragment as they invade the vessel walls giving rise to the term *leukocytoclastic angiitis*. Endothelial proliferative changes are also seen, and in severe cases the pathologic picture may be indistinguishable from crescentic (rapidly progressive) glomerulonephritis. Immunofluorescence staining may reveal IgG and IgM in the mesangium. In contrast to the subacute or chronic course of PAN, hypersensitivity angiitis is characterized by rapid onset of renal failure. Urinalysis reveals proteinuria (at times reaching nephrotic range), hematuria, and casts. Microangiopathic hemolytic anemia and systemic eosinophilia are often present. Hypertension, however, is characteristically absent or mild. Uremia leads to death in the majority. Treatment regimens are similar to PAN, but the response to glucocorticoids appears to be more favorable in this disease than in PAN.

Other vasculitides in which renal involvement is present include Wegener's granulomatosis (in which the renal lesion is primarily in the form of a necrotizing glomerulitis) and Takayasu's arteritis, which may involve the main renal arteries and their branches (see Chap. 276).

REFERENCES

BARRÉ P et al: Successful treatment with streptokinase of renal vein thrombosis associated with oral contraceptive use. Am J Nephrol 6:316, 1986

EKNOYAN G, RIGGS SA: Renal involvement in patients with thrombotic thrombocytopenic purpura. Am J Nephrol 6:117, 1986

HAKIM RM et al: Successful management of thrombocytopenia, microangiopathic anemia, and acute renal failure by plasmapheresis. Am J Kidney Dis 3:170, 1985

HOLLENBERG NK: The treatment of renovascular hypertension: Surgery, angioplasty, and medical therapy with converting enzyme inhibitors. Am J Kidney Dis 1(Suppl):52, 1987

JACOBSON HR: Ischemic renal disease: An overlooked clinical entity? Kidney Int 34:729, 1988

KASHGARIAN M: Pathology of small blood vessels in hypertension. Am J Kidney Dis 5:A104, 1985

LINDHEIMER MD, BAYLIS C (eds): Renal function and disease in pregnancy: An international symposium. Am J Kidney Dis 9:243, 1987

LLACH F: *Renal Vein Thrombosis.* New York, Futura, 1983

MATERSON BJ: Special uses for captopril. Am J Kidney Dis 1(Suppl):88, 1987

MULLER FB et al: The captopril test for identifying renovascular disease in hypertensive patients. Am J Med 80:6333, 1986

RATLIFFE N: Renal vascular disease: Pathology of large blood vessel disease. Am J Kidney Dis 5:A93, 1985

WORKING GROUP ON RENOVASCULAR HYPERTENSION: Final Report: Detection, evaluation, and treatment of renovascular hypertension. Arch Intern Med 147:820, 1987

231   HEREDITARY TUBULAR DISORDERS

FREDRIC L. COE / SATISH KATHPALIA

POLYCYSTIC RENAL DISEASE IN ADULTS

ETIOLOGY AND PATHOLOGY   This disease is found in 1 in 500 autopsies and 1 in 3000 hospital admissions and accounts for approximately 10 percent of end-stage renal failure. Inheritance is autosomal dominant and is linked in most families to the alpha-hemoglobin gene complex and the phosphoglycerate kinase genes on the short arm of chromosome 16. The cortex and medulla of both kidneys are usually filled with thin-walled, spherical cysts, ranging from millimeters to centimeters in diameter, that enlarge the organs and interfere with their function, presumably by compressing the nephrons and causing localized obstruction. The cysts, which are lined by a low cuboidal epithelium, contain straw-colored fluid that becomes hemorrhagic with trauma or infection. The intervening renal parenchyma may be normal or show changes of nephrosclerosis or interstitial nephritis.

CLINICAL FEATURES   Symptoms usually begin in the third or fourth decades. Flank pain is frequent. Other common symptoms include gross and microscopic hematuria, especially after trauma, and nocturia due to impaired concentrating ability. Ten percent of patients pass renal calculi whose composition and pathogenesis have not been well studied. Stones and blood clots both cause renal colic.

Usually the kidneys are palpable and asymmetric and have a knobby surface. Hypertension develops in 75 percent of patients, and progression to chronic renal failure usually occurs (Table 231-1).

Proteinuria is common but rarely exceeds 2 g/d. Urinary infection occurs at some time in most patients, especially as a consequence of instrumentation and renal calculi; women are infected more frequently than men. Erythrocytosis may occur because of high erythropoietin levels; in other patients blood loss anemia may result from the hematuria.

Acute renal failure can result from infection, ureteral obstruction due to clots or stone, or sudden angulation of a ureter by a nearby cyst. Azotemia progresses slowly in the absence of these complications. Patients with end-stage chronic renal failure tend to have higher hematocrits than their counterparts with other renal diseases. Fluid overload is infrequent because of a tendency for renal salt wasting.

Hepatic cysts are present in about 30 percent of patients. Hepatic function is usually normal, and the liver cysts can be asymptomatic or cause epigastric discomfort or biliary colic or become infected. Cysts also may occur in the spleen, pancreas, lungs, ovaries, testes, epididymis, thyroid, uterus, broad ligament, and bladder. Subarachnoid hemorrhage from intracranial aneurysm causes death or neurologic injury in about 9 percent of patients, but routine cerebral arteriography is not warranted. Mitral valve prolapse (26 percent) and mitral, aortic, and tricuspid valve incompetence occur more often than in control groups.

DIAGNOSIS   Palpable kidneys, hypertension, or abnormalities of urine in asymptomatic individuals are often the only manifestations. Excretory or retrograde urography typically shows large kidneys with elongated pelvises and flat calyces indented by cysts. Ultrasonography and radioisotopic renal scanning can both demonstrate the cysts quite well. Gray scale sonography is preferable to intravenous pyelography for screening individuals at risk, especially when genetic counseling is desired. Computed tomography may be useful.

TREATMENT   Superimposed renal damage such as is produced by analgesics, obstruction, urinary infection, nephrotoxic antibiotics, and hypertension must be guarded against. Dehydration and inadequate intake of sodium chloride (less than 100 mmol/d) should be avoided. The management of chronic renal failure is simplified because fluid overload is not a usual problem and the hypertension is usually amenable to treatment, but the cysts can cause special problems, such as pain, bleeding, infection, or ureteral obstruction. Puncture of cysts, and in some instances even nephrectomy, may be necessary.

POLYCYSTIC RENAL DISEASE IN INFANTS AND CHILDREN

CLINICAL FEATURES   The *infantile form* manifests itself at birth by diffusely enlarged kidneys, renal failure, and maldevelopment of intrahepatic bile ducts. The *childhood form* consists of medullary ductal ectasia which is usually asymptomatic, in association with congenital hepatic fibrosis and portal hypertension. Both conditions are rare, and both are inherited as autosomal recessive traits. Renal failure develops frequently in both forms, but death in the childhood form usually results as a consequence of hepatic disease.

MORPHOLOGY   In the infantile form, the distal tubules and collecting ducts are dilated into elongated cysts that are arranged in a radial fashion, particularly in the cortex, and make the kidneys large and spongy. In the childhood form, cysts are fewer in number, cortical collecting ducts are less involved, and the kidneys are not as large. Small intrahepatic bile ducts are irregularly dilated, and large interconnecting spaces, lined by hyperplastic epithelium, fill the portal areas. There is portal fibrosis rather than dilatation and proliferation of small bile ducts, and portal hypertension is the rule by late childhood.

DIAGNOSIS AND TREATMENT   Infantile polycystic kidneys may be large enough to cause dystocia. At birth they do not function and cause oliguric renal failure, respiratory distress, hypertension, and

TABLE 231-1 Renal tubule defects

Disease	Renal morphologic abnormalities	Functional abnormalities	Mode of Inheritance*	Associated abnormalities
Adult polycystic disease	Cortical and medullary cysts	Chronic renal failure	AD	Hepatic cysts, intracranial aneurysms
Infantile polycystic disease	Distal tubule and collecting duct cysts	Renal failure in the newborn	AR	Intrahepatic bile duct abnormalities
Childhood polycystic disease	Medullary ductal ectasia	Variable chronic renal failure	AR	Hepatic fibrosis and portal hypertension
Medullary sponge kidneys	Ectatic ducts of Bellini	Nephrocalcinosis	AD + S	None
Medullary cystic disease, recessive	Distal tubule and collecting duct cysts	Chronic renal failure, <20 yr salt wasting, polyuria	AR	Variable retinal degeneration (renal retinal dysplasia)
Medullary cystic disease, dominant	Same	Chronic renal failure, >20 yr salt wasting, polyuria	AD	None
Bartter's syndrome	Hyperplasia of juxtaglomerular and medullary interstitial cells	Hypokalemia, high renin and aldosterone levels, polyuria	AR	None
Liddle's syndrome	None	Hypokalemia, low aldosterone levels	AR	None
Familial nephrogenic diabetes insipidus	None	Vasopressin-resistant renal concentrating defect	XL	None
Renal tubular acidosis, type 1	Papillary nephrocalcinosis	Inability to lower urine pH normally, reduced acid excretion	AD	Periodic paralysis, hypokalemia, non-anion-gap metabolic acidosis, growth retardation, rickets
Renal tubular acidosis, type 2	None	Reduced bicarbonate reabsorption	AR AD XL	Non-anion-gap metabolic acidosis, growth retardation rickets, Fanconi syndrome
Renal tubular acidosis, type 4	Underlying renal disease	Reduced proton and potassium secretion	ACQ	Azotemia
X-linked vitamin D–resistant rickets	None	Reduced phosphate reabsorption, hypophosphatemia	XL	Rickets, osteomalacia, normal serum 1,25-D
Vitamin D–dependent rickets, type 1	None	Defective renal 1,25-D production	AR	Rickets, osteomalacia, low serum 1,25-D
Vitamin D–dependent rickets, type 2	None	Defective cell, 1,25-D receptors	AR	Rickets, osteomalacia, high serum 1,25-D, variable alopecia
Oncogenic osteomalacia	None	Reduced phosphate reabsorptions, hypophosphatemia	ACQ	Osteomalacia; mesenchymal tumors; cancer of the prostate or lung
Renal glucosuria	None	Reduced glucose reabsorption	AD	None
Isolated hypouricemia	None	Reduced urate reabsorption	AR	Variable hypercalciuria, bone demineralization
Cystinuria	Cystine stones	Reduced reabsorption of dibasic amino acids	AR	Short stature
Hartnup's disease	None	Reduced reabsorption of mono-amino and carboxylic amino acids	AR	Pellagra-like rash, ataxia, delirium
Iminoglycinuria	None	Reduced reabsorption of proline, hydroxyproline, and glycine	AR	None
Adult Fanconi syndrome	Swan neck deformity of the proximal tubule	Reduced proximal tubule reabsorption of bicarbonate, glucose, uric acid, phosphate, and amino acids	AR	Rickets, osteomalacia, acidosis, dwarfism, low serum potassium
Lowe's syndrome (oculo-cerebrorenal syndrome)	Same	Same	XL	Ocular and cerebral malformations

* AR, autosomal recessive; AD, autosomal dominant; XL, X-linked; ACQ, acquired; S, sporadic.

congestive heart failure. Intravenous pyelography may reveal a mottled nephrogram with variable retention of contrast material in cysts that correspond to dilated cortical and medullary collecting ducts. On retrograde urography the calyces are blunted, and pyelotubular reflux may be seen. In the childhood type the intravenous pyelogram may suggest medullary sponge kidney, because medullary tubular ectasia is prominent. Renal failure and chronic infection are common.

MEDULLARY SPONGE KIDNEY

PATHOLOGY The ducts of Bellini, i.e., the terminal collecting ducts that reach the ends of the papillae and drain the urine into the renal pelvis, are dilated to cystic proportions and frequently contain calcium oxalate calculi. The kidneys are asymmetric, and the more abnormal kidney is usually the larger. One or more medullary cysts are found near the tip of each involved papilla, and calculi form in the terminal collecting ducts in, or proximal to, the cysts (Fig. 231-1). Parenchymal alterations are secondary to intrarenal obstruction. The cysts are lined by cuboidal and, sometimes, by pseudostratified and stratified squamous epithelium.

CLINICAL DIAGNOSIS AND TREATMENT Medullary sponge kidney is present in 1 of 200 unselected intravenous pyelograms. Although most cases are sporadic, autosomal dominant inheritance has been described. The disease has a bimodal pattern of appearance, the first in adolescence and the second during the third and fourth

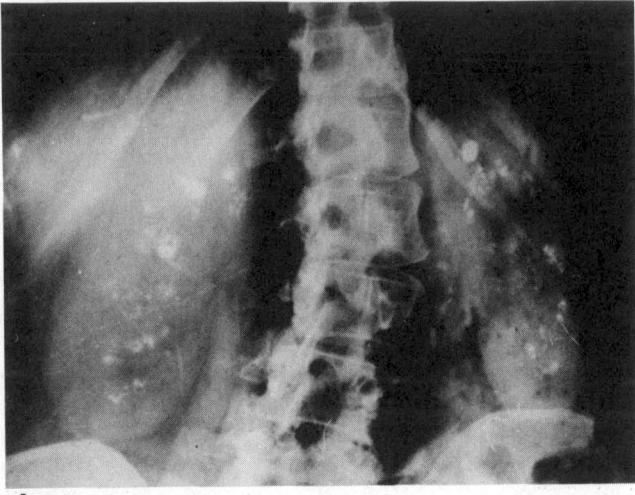
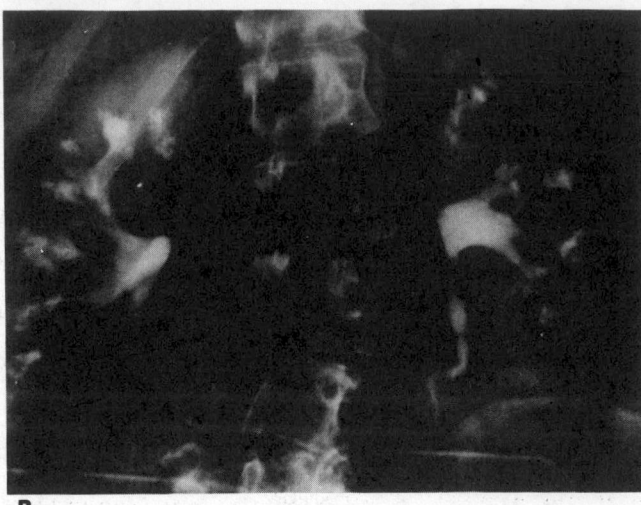

FIGURE 231-1 *A.* Radiographic appearance of medullary sponge kidney. Abdominal flat plate reveals multiple bilateral calcifications. *B.* Radiographic contrast material accumulates in the dilated and cystic terminal collecting ducts and obscures the calcifications.

decades. Calculi, infection, and hematuria occur in 60, 35, and 30 percent of patients, respectively. Papillary nephrocalcinosis due to clusters of stones in cysts is common. Hypercalciuria occurs in nearly half of stone-forming patients but is equally common in other forms of calcium stone disease (Chap. 232). Hypertension is no more common than in the general population. Renal failure is rare, unless nephrolithiasis and/or renal infections are severe.

The diagnosis is made by intravenous urography. The magnitude of pyelotubular backflow varies from a simple papillary blush to tubular ectasia at the tips of the papillae. Small pyramidal cysts and nephrocalcinosis are frequent, and papillary concretions are obscured by the urographic contrast medium. Ectatic collecting ducts are difficult to fill during retrograde pyelography, and the contrast material remains separate from papillary concretions in the cysts.

Asymptomatic patients require no treatment except advice to avoid dehydration and thereby reduce the risk of stone formation. The metabolic etiology of stones should be sought and treated conventionally, while infection and urologic consequences of stones should be treated as described in Chap. 232. Medullary sponge kidneys are vulnerable to infection, and urologic instrumentation should, therefore, be minimized.

MEDULLARY CYSTIC DISEASE (NEPHRONOPHTHISIS COMPLEX)

ETIOLOGY   Several hereditary medullary cystic diseases have similar morphology but different patterns of inheritance. The recessive form is associated with renal failure before 20 years of age (early-onset type), whereas the dominant form causes renal failure only after the second decade (adult-onset type). When renal disease is associated with retinal degeneration (renal retinal dysplasia), inheritance is always recessive, but renal failure occurs during adult life.

PATHOLOGY   In both forms, most of the cysts are in the medulla and the corticomedullary region and involve the collecting ducts and distal convoluted tubules. Cysts have a low, frequently atrophic, epithelium and range in size from microscopic dimensions to millimeters. The kidneys usually are asymmetrically scarred and shrunken. Both tubular atrophy and periglomerular fibrosis are present, but the former is more severe. In advanced cases, glomeruli become sclerotic and hyalinized, cortical fibrosis and cellular interstitial infiltration appear, and the histology is difficult to differentiate from that of chronic interstitial nephritis.

DIAGNOSIS AND TREATMENT   Concentrating ability, acid excretion, and sodium conservation are defective as might be expected from a lesion that damages distal segments of the nephron. The disease is marked by polyuria, progressive renal failure, stunted growth, severe anemia, hyperchloremic metabolic acidosis, and poor sodium conservation. In adults, the inability to conserve sodium may cause a salt-wasting syndrome that resembles adrenal insufficiency but is unresponsive to mineralocorticoids. Hypertension usually is a terminal event. The urinalysis is normal at first, but proteinuria may develop. On intravenous pyelography, the kidneys are small, scarred, and without calcification. The calyces are distorted by numerous cysts in the corticomedullary area.

High sodium and water intake and alkali replacement for acidosis are needed. Treatment of infections, anemia, hypertension, and other aspects of end-stage renal failure are as discussed in Chap. 224. Genetic counseling may be helpful in family planning and in selection of an unaffected related donor for renal transplantation.

BARTTER'S SYNDROME

Bartter's syndrome consists of hypokalemia due to renal potassium wasting, elevated plasma renin activity and aldosterone secretion, normal blood pressure, hyporesponsiveness of blood pressure to infused angiotensin II, and hyperplasia of the granular cells of the juxtaglomerular apparatus of the kidney. Weakness or periodic paralysis and polyuria occur because of chronic potassium depletion. Hypomagnesemia may be present. Hyperplasia of renal medullary interstitial cells, which produce prostaglandins PGE and PGF, has been described, along with elevated PGE_2 production. Inheritance is autosomal recessive, and manifestations commonly begin in childhood.

PATHOGENESIS   The main defect seems to be reduced NaCl reabsorption by the thick ascending limb of Henle's loop (TAHL). Volume depletion stimulates aldosterone production and raises serum aldosterone levels, and the combination of high aldosterone levels and increased delivery of NaCl and water to the distal nephron causes kaliuresis and hypokalemia. Magnesuria and hypomagnesemia occur, perhaps because TAHL is a main site for magnesium reabsorption and because hypomagnesemia worsens kaliuresis. Hypokalemia further increases aldosterone production by stimulating release of prostaglandins E_2 and I_2, which promote increased secretion of renin. Both angiotensin II and aldosterone increase renal kallikrein, which increases plasma bradykinin. The normal blood pressure reflects an interaction between the vasodepressor actions of PGE_2 and bradykinin and the elevated angiotensin II. Bartter's syndrome may be mimicked by magnesium deficiency, covert laxative use, or vomiting. Magnesium depletion causes kaliuresis; laxatives cause potassium and volume depletion; vomiting causes renal potassium wasting and volume depletion.

Excessive production of PGE_2 resulting from hypokalemia, a known stimulator of PGE_2 synthesis, may be a secondary consequence of the syndrome. In some cases blockade of PGE_2 production with indomethacin lowers renin levels and restores vascular response to angiotensin II infusion, but does not reduce potassium wasting.

TREATMENT The dietary intake of sodium chloride and potassium should be liberal; potassium supplements may be required. Pharmacologic blockade of aldosterone action on the distal tubules by spironolactone can prevent potassium wasting, though sodium intake must be increased. Inhibition of prostaglandin synthesis with indomethacin, ibuprofen, or aspirin has met with varying success, as indicated above. Beta-adrenergic blockade may lower renin production.

LIDDLE'S SYNDROME (PSEUDOHYPERALDOSTERONISM)

This rare inherited disorder is characterized by hypertension, hypokalemic alkalosis, and negligible aldosterone secretion. It appears to be due to an unusual tendency of distal tubules or collecting ducts to conserve sodium and excrete potassium despite the virtual absence of aldosterone. No other biochemical abnormalities have been described. However, transport rates of sodium in red blood cells are altered. These patients respond to 100 mg per day of triamterene (Chap. 182), a diuretic agent that blocks sodium and potassium exchange in the distal tubule.

FAMILIAL NEPHROGENIC DIABETES INSIPIDUS (DI)

In this disease the distal tubules and collecting ducts are unresponsive to vasopressin because of an X-linked recessive disorder, with variable expressivity in heterozygous females. Affected individuals excrete large volumes of hypotonic urine even when plasma osmolality and vasopressin concentration are both high. Polyuria, polydipsia, and hypertonic dehydration after restriction of fluid intake all result from renal tubular insensitivity to vasopressin (AVP) (also see Chap. 315). Unresponsiveness to vasopressin may be secondary to reduced production of cyclic adenosine 5'-monophosphate (cyclic AMP) in the epithelium of the collecting ducts, to the inability of cyclic AMP to increase the permeability of collecting duct luminal cell membranes to water, or to a combination of the two. Other hereditary tubular defects such as juvenile nephronophthisis, medullary cystic and polycystic diseases, cystinosis, and congenital or acquired chronic urinary tract obstruction can also cause vasopressin-resistant (nephrogenic) DI, but in these syndromes the characteristic features of the underlying disorder are present.

Affected infants easily become dehydrated, hypernatremic, and hyperthermic, and damage of the central nervous system, including mental retardation, may result. In the absence of dehydration, overall renal function is normal. On intravenous pyelography the renal pelvis, ureters, and bladder are dilated, as in any form of DI, because of massive diuresis.

Oral hydration usually is adequate treatment except during early infancy, when hypotonic parenteral fluids may be required. Vasopressin and its synthetic analogues are ineffective, but diuretic agents such as chlorothiazide reduce polyuria. This drug inhibits NaCl reabsorption in the cortical portions of the TAHL, thereby reducing production of free water. In addition, chlorothiazide produces a diuresis that causes contraction of extracellular fluid volume which, in turn, stimulates reabsorption of NaCl and water in the proximal tubule and limits their delivery to the TAHL. Sodium restriction enhances its effect.

RENAL TUBULAR ACIDOSIS (RTA)

In this group of disorders renal excretion of acid is reduced out of proportion to any reduction of glomerular filtration rate. Metabolic acidosis results, but in contrast to renal failure the anions that accompany surplus hydrogen ions in the blood, such as sulfate and phosphate, are excreted normally and are unavailable to balance the fall in serum bicarbonate. Therefore, the kidneys reabsorb chloride in unusually large amounts, and serum chloride rises to preserve electroneutrality in the extracellular fluid. The result is *hyperchloremic acidosis*, and the unmeasured anion gap is normal. There is general agreement that four types of RTA exist (Table 231-2). Types 1 and 2 are often hereditary. Type 3 is a rare mixture of types 1 and 2. Type 4 is acquired and is associated with either hyporeninemic hypoaldosteronism or tubular hyporesponsiveness to circulating mineralocorticoids.

TYPE 1 (DISTAL) RTA Sporadic cases occur, but autosomal dominant inheritance is usual. The kidney does not lower urine pH normally, either because the collecting ducts permit excessive back-diffusion of hydrogen ions from lumen to blood or because they fail to transport hydrogen ions against a steep pH gradient. Since titration of urine buffers and diffusion trapping of NH_4^+ in the tubules both depend upon a low intraluminal pH, excretion of acid is deficient. However, urine ammonium excretion is as high or higher than in normal people whose urine is equally alkaline. Urinary osmotic concentration and potassium conservation also tend to be impaired.

Chronic acidosis lowers tubule reabsorption of calcium, causing renal hypercalciuria and mild secondary hyperparathyroidism. The hypercalciuria, alkaline urine, and low levels of urine citrate—which normally complexes about 40 percent of urine calcium—cause calcium phosphate stones and nephrocalcinosis. Growth is stunted in children because of rickets; this growth defect responds to amelioration of the acidosis with sodium bicarbonate or other alkali. In the adult, bone disease takes the form of osteomalacia. In both children and adults, bone disease may result, in part, from acidosis-induced loss of bone mineral and from inadequate production of 1,25-dihydroxyvitamin D_3 [$1,25(OH)_2D_3$]. Since the kidney does not conserve potassium or concentrate the urine normally, polyuria and hypokalemia occur. Given the stress of an intercurrent illness, acidosis and hypokalemia can be life-threatening.

The diagnosis is suggested by osteomalacia or rickets, hyperchloremic acidosis associated with alkaline urine, and calcium phosphate stones or nephrocalcinosis. To prove that the urine pH cannot be lowered normally, the oral ammonium chloride (NH_4Cl) loading test should be carried out: 0.1 g (1.9 mmol) NH_4Cl per kilogram of body weight is administered, and the blood and urine pH are followed with time. Although systemic acidosis worsens, urine pH does not fall below 5.5. Urinary infection must not be present during this test because bacteria may possess urease, which hydrolyzes urea to ammonia and produces an alkaline urine. When hyperchloremic acidosis is severe and the urine is grossly alkaline, the test is unnecessary.

TABLE 231-2 Comparison of three types of renal tubular acidosis*

Finding	Type 1	Type 2	Type 4
Non-anion-gap acidosis	Yes	Yes	Yes
Minimum urine pH	>5.5	<5.5	<5.5
% filtered HCO_3 excreted	<10	>15	<10
Serum potassium	Low	Low	High
Fanconi syndrome	No	Yes	No
Stones/nephrocalcinosis	Yes	No	No
Daily acid excretion	Low	Normal	Low
Ammonium excretion	High for pH	Normal	Low for pH
Daily HCO_3 replacement needs	<4 mmol/kg	>4 mmol/kg	<4 mmol/kg

* HCO_3, bicarbonate. Type 3 renal tubular acidosis is a rare form of a mixture of types 1 and 2.

A confusing situation may occur when type 1 RTA results from nephrocalcinosis due to hereditary idiopathic hypercalciuria. In this circumstance, stones may be composed of calcium phosphate, but hypokalemia and metabolic acidosis are absent; urine pH is abnormally high and does not fall below 5.5 after NH_4Cl administration. Incomplete RTA is a common term for this circumstance. Other hereditary diseases that cause RTA, such as medullary sponge kidney, galactosemia, Ehler-Danlos syndrome, Fabry's disease, and hereditary elliptocytosis, can be excluded by clinical findings. The relatives of patients with type 1 RTA should be screened for this treatable cause of renal damage.

Treatment   Sodium bicarbonate tablets (10 grains = 7.2 mmol base) and Shohl's solution (1 mmol base per milliliter, as Na and K citrate) are both convenient for treatment; the dose should be 0.5 to 2.0 mmol/kg body weight in four or five divided doses daily. The total dose of alkali should be raised until acidosis and hypercalciuria are both eliminated, and the patients should be followed by measurements of serum chloride and CO_2 content and of urine calcium excretion approximately twice yearly. Potassium supplementation is normally not required. Requirements for alkali usually rise during intercurrent illnesses but are usually below 4 mmol/kg body weight per day. Incomplete RTA is best treated using thiazide diuretics as in ordinary idiopathic hypercalcemia (Chap. 232).

TYPE 2 (PROXIMAL) RTA   Proximal RTA usually occurs as part of a generalized disorder of proximal tubule function. It can be a transient disorder of infancy which usually disappears in childhood. An isolated form, i.e., without accompanying phosphaturia, aminoaciduria, and uricosuria, has been described in one family. The pathophysiology of proximal RTA is the same whether isolated or part of a generalized disorder. Bicarbonate reabsorption in the proximal tubule is defective, and renal bicarbonate wasting occurs at a normal concentration of plasma bicarbonate. As plasma bicarbonate falls, the filtered load drops to a level that the defective tubule can reabsorb. Then the urine is free of bicarbonate and has a low pH. Potassium wasting and hypokalemia occur, especially when supplementary alkali is given, because bicarbonate is excreted in the urine partly as the potassium salt. Hypercalciuria is moderate, and stone formation is rare. During the NH_4Cl loading test, urine pH falls below 5.5.

Treatment is often not required. When acidosis is severe, bicarbonate must be given in large amounts daily, often above 4 mmol/kg body weight, and even up to 10 mmol/kg per day, because bicarbonate is rapidly excreted in the urine. Another approach is to use a thiazide diuretic and a low-salt diet, which induce mild volume depletion and enhance proximal bicarbonate reabsorption, thereby reducing the required dose. Potassium supplements are needed during treatment because excessive sodium bicarbonate reaches the distal nephron, where much of the sodium is exchanged for potassium, which is then lost in the urine.

TYPE 4 RTA   Some patients have a form of renal tubular acidosis that differs from types 1 and 2 and has been called type 4. They have metabolic acidosis without an elevation of the anion gap but differ from type 1 patients in having an acid urine during periods of severe acidosis (Table 231-2), and from type 2 patients in having low urine excretion of bicarbonate and a daily replacement alkali requirement of <4 mmol/kg body weight. They differ from both types 1 and 2 in having a high serum potassium level and a low urine ammonia excretion rate. They have neither Fanconi syndrome nor stone disease. Because potassium and hydrogen excretion are abnormal, they are considered to have generalized distal nephron dysfunction that is due either to intrinsic renal disease or to abnormal aldosterone levels. Hyperkalemia worsens acidosis by suppressing renal production of ammonia, which is the most important urinary buffer, and thereby limiting acid excretion.

The most common patients with type 4 renal tubular acidosis have hyporeninemic hypoaldosteronism; plasma levels of renin and aldosterone are subnormal, even during extracellular volume depletion. Diabetic nephropathy, nephrosclerosis from hypertension, and chronic tubulointerstitial nephropathies are the usual causes. Hyperkalemia

and acidosis can be treated with replacement doses of a mineralocorticoid hormone such as fludrocortisone, 0.1 to 0.2 mg/d; some patients may require 0.3 to 0.5 mg/d, suggesting tubule unresponsiveness to the hormone. Furosemide can also improve the hyperkalemia and acidosis, provided salt intake is sufficient to prevent extracellular volume contraction.

A less common condition is *mineralocorticoid-resistant hyperkalemia;* hyperkalemia and acidosis do not improve despite mineralocorticoid hormone treatment. This occurs in occasional patients with underlying renal disease who also have severe salt wasting, as a consequence of distal nephron damage. Plasma renin and aldosterone levels are elevated, and extracellular fluid volume depletion may occur. Treatment requires salt and alkali, but mineralocorticoid supplements are not necessary. Other patients with mild acidosis have no evidence of renal disease and do not waste salt in the urine. Plasma renin and aldosterone levels are low, but hyperkalemia and acidosis do not respond to mineralocorticoid hormone treatment. The cause is thought to be abnormally high distal tubule permeability to chloride ion; sodium chloride reabsorption is elevated, the potential across the distal tubule epithelium is presumed to be below normal, potassium secretion is reduced because it is driven by the transepithelial voltage, hyperkalemia causes acidosis by suppressing ammonia production, and extracellular volume expansion from sodium chloride absorption suppresses renin and aldosterone levels and causes hypertension. The main evidence for this formulation is that infusion of sodium with anions such as bicarbonate or sulfate raises potassium excretion to normal or supranormal levels. Treatment of this rare condition is with thiazide diuretics or low-sodium diet.

Primary mineralocorticoid deficiency from diseases of the adrenals also causes hyperkalemia and acidosis. Evaluation and treatment of adrenal disorders is discussed in Chap. 317.

VITAMIN D DISORDERS

FAMILIAL X-LINKED HYPOPHOSPHATEMIC VITAMIN D–REFRACTORY RICKETS (See also Chap. 341)   Reduced tubular reabsorption of phosphate by the proximal tubule and hypophosphatemia occur in this X-linked dominant disease, which is also termed *renal phosphate leak*. Patients may be asymptomatic but are usually short and have rachitic bones; the legs are particularly short and deformed, and osteomalacia develops in adult life. Bone age and dentition are retarded, and the teeth are poorly developed. The skull becomes deformed, and the maxillofacial region may be abnormal. Overgrowth of bone at sites of muscular attachment can limit movement or compress nerves. Bony abnormalities are less common in women. Serum alkaline phosphatase is elevated, serum parathyroid levels are normal or high, serum calcium is usually normal, and urinary calcium excretion is normal or low.

The hypophosphatemia arises in part from decreased tubular reabsorption of phosphate and increased fractional excretion of phosphate. Intestinal absorption of calcium and phosphate may be decreased in untreated patients but increased during treatment with vitamin D. Although glycinuria and mild glucosuria may occur, most patients exhibit only a defect in excretion of phosphate. Absence of hyperchloremic acidosis and a normal serum calcium concentration help to exclude RTA, malabsorption, and nutritional rickets.

Treatment requires oral neutral phosphate, 1 to 4 g daily, in divided doses, and 10,000 to 50,000 units of vitamin D; one must watch for hypercalcemia. Combination of oral phosphate with calcitriol may be more beneficial. Bony deformities require orthopedic management, but corrective surgery, except for genu valgum, should be postponed until active growth is completed.

VITAMIN D–DEPENDENT RICKETS TYPE 1   (See also Chap. 341)   Also known as hereditary pseudovitamin D–deficiency rickets, this disease is inherited as an autosomal recessive trait. Defective production of $1,25(OH)_2D_3$ by the kidneys, perhaps because of a genetic defect in 25-hydroxycholecalciferol 1α-hydroxylase, has been proposed as the basis for the disease. However, the dose of calcitriol required to heal rickets is higher than that for vitamin D–deficiency rickets, suggesting an attenuated response to, or excessive degradation of, $1,25(OH)_2D_3$.

Rickets usually begins before 2 years of age. Serum calcium is low, parathyroid hormone concentration and alkaline phosphatase are high, and plasma phosphorus is variable. Urinary calcium is decreased, fecal calcium is increased, and tubular phosphate reabsorption is reduced. Serum levels of $1,25(OH)_2D_3$ are undetectable. Amino-aciduria and hyperchloremic acidosis can occur, but urinary cyclic AMP increases normally in response to PTH infusion.

The 1α-hydroxylated metabolites of vitamin D bypass the enzyme defect and produce a dramatic healing of rickets. Vitamin D_2, 10,000 to 40,000 units per day, is also effective, but oral calcium, 0.5 to 2.0 g/d, is needed as well. The need for vitamin D persists throughout life. Calcitriol, an ideal replacement therapy, is the drug of choice, but one must watch for hypercalcemia.

VITAMIN D–DEPENDENT RICKETS TYPE 2 Like type 1, this disease causes rickets, hypocalcemia, hypophosphatemia, and secondary hyperparathyroidism. Serum levels of $1,25(OH)_2D_3$ are elevated, and treatment with additional $1,25(OH)_2D_3$ does not increase the serum calcium level or heal the bone disease even though it can reduce serum levels of parathyroid hormone. Generalized alopecia is often present and may be either a linked defect or the result of the mineral disorder. The cause appears to be an autosomal recessive defect of the $1,25(OH)_2D_3$ receptor. Treatment with a high dose of calcitriol and mineral supplements may achieve healing of bone, but relapse may occur despite continued treatment.

ONCOGENIC OSTEOMALACIA Mesenchymal tumors, usually benign, can cause renal phosphate wasting similiar to that of X-linked hypophosphatemic rickets, with resulting osteomalacia. Carcinoma of the prostate and oat cell carcinoma of the lung also have caused this syndrome. The disease almost always occurs in adults and develops gradually, over years. The tumors occur mainly in the extremities, head, nose, and mandible, in close association with bone. Their removal cures the phosphate wasting and leads to healing of the osteomalacia.

RENAL GLUCOSURIA

See Chap. 336.

ISOLATED HYPOURICEMIA (See also Chap. 336)

This disorder, in which there is a defect in proximal tubular reabsorption of sodium urate, is inherited as an autosomal recessive trait. Hypouricemia can also occur in the Fanconi syndrome, Hartnup's disease, and Wilson's disease. Uric acid clearance is high, and urine oxypurine levels are normal, excluding hereditary xanthinuria. Patients are asymptomatic except for occasional uric acid nephrolithiasis. No specific treatment is needed except the avoidance of dehydration. Coexistent hypercalciuria and decreased bone density have been described in a few patients, who may have a related disease.

SELECTIVE DISORDERS OF AMINO ACID TRANSPORT

HARTNUP'S DISEASE (See also Chap. 336) In this rare autosomal recessive disorder, renal and intestinal transport of monoamino–monocarboxylic amino acids is defective. An erythematous, scaly, pellagra-like rash appears after exposure to sunlight, and episodic cerebellar ataxia, emotional instability, delirium, and aminoaciduria all occur. The prevalence is 1 in 15,000 newborns.

Dietary monoamino–monocarboxylic amino acids undergo bacterial degradation in the intestinal lumen. At the same time, they are lost in the urine. Inadequate tryptophan availability limits nicotinamide synthesis and leads to secondary pellagra (see Chap. 76). Decreased absorption and urine loss of the other monoamino–monocarboxylic amino acids can cause generalized malnutrition.

The diagnosis is based upon demonstration of massive urine losses of alanine, serine, threonine, asparagine, glutamine, valine, leucine, isoleucine, phenylalanine, tyrosine, tryptophan, histidine, glycine, and citrulline. Hypouricemia may occur. Renal function is otherwise normal. Most patients respond to treatment with oral nicotinamide, 40 to 200 mg/d, and a high-protein diet to compensate for amino acid malabsorption and loss. The ultimate prognosis is good, and the disease often improves with age.

FAMILIAL IMINOGLYCINURIA (See also Chap. 336) This autosomal recessive trait is characterized by excessive urinary excretion of proline, hydroxyproline, and glycine despite normal plasma levels of these amino acids, probably because of deletion or alteration of a membrane transport protein of the renal tubule cells. The patients are asymptomatic. Iminoglycinuria can occur in normal newborn infants up to 3 months of age.

FANCONI SYNDROME

Fanconi syndrome is a constellation of transport defects in the proximal tubule involving amino acids, monosaccharides, sodium, potassium, calcium, phosphate, bicarbonate, uric acid, and proteins. Generalized aminoaciduria, glucosuria, salt wasting, hypercalciuria, hypophosphatemia, proximal renal tubular acidosis, hypouricemia, and tubular proteinuria (Chap. 49) may result. Fanconi syndrome can be acquired secondary to diseases such as cystinosis, tyrosinemia, galactosemia, fructose intolerance, glycogen storage disease (type 1), Wilson's disease, familial nephrosis, and hereditary amyloidosis. Lowe's (or oculocerebrorenal) syndrome is an X-linked recessive form of the Fanconi syndrome associated with ocular and cerebral abnormalities.

An autosomal recessive disease, *adult Fanconi syndrome*, occurs in the absence of any systemic disorder. The term *adult* is misleading since cases are recognized in childhood, but no abnormalities are apparent at birth. Dwarfism and hypophosphatemic rickets occur along with the laboratory abnormalities of Fanconi syndrome. Renal failure is rare, and the prognosis is good when the systemic manifestations are treated. Typically, there is a "swan-neck" deformity and cellular atrophy of the initial portion of the proximal tubule which is probably the anatomic basis of this tubular disorder. The associated defects in the transport of water, sodium, potassium, acid, and phosphate excretion often require treatment. Water, sodium, and potassium intake must be liberal, and phosphate supplements may be needed. Metabolic acidosis can be corrected by the administration of alkali. Vitamin D helps promote bone healing. Glucosuria, uricosuria, and tubular proteinuria do not require treatment.

CYSTINURIA

See Chap. 336.

REFERENCES

AVIOLI LV: Vitamin D–resistant rickets, in *Diseases of the Kidney*, 3d ed, LE Earley, CW Gottschalk (eds). Boston, Little, Brown, 1979, p 1055

BERNSTEIN J, KISSANE JM: Hereditary disorders of the kidney. Part 1: Parenchymal defects and malformations. Perspect Pediatr Pathol 1:117, 1973

CANTANI A et al: Familial juvenile nephronophthisis: A review and differential diagnosis. Clin Pediatr 25:90, 1986

COE FL, PARKS JH: Calcium phosphate stones and renal tubular acidosis, in *Nephrolithiasis: Pathogenesis and Treatment*. Chicago, Year Book, 1988, chap 5

DEFRONZO FA, THIER SO: Inherited disorders of renal tubule function, in *The Kidney*, 3d ed, BM Brenner, FC Rector Jr (eds). Philadelphia, Saunders, 1986, p 1297

GABOW PA et al: Polycystic kidney disease: Prospective analysis of nonazulemic patients and family members. Ann Intern Med 101:238, 1984

GAMBLIN GT et al: Vitamin D–dependent rickets type 2. J Clin Invest 75:954, 1985

GARRICK R et al: Bartter's syndrome: A unifying hypothesis. Am J Nephrol 5:379, 1985

HUSSACK KF et al: Echocardiographic findings in autosomal dominant polycystic kidney disease. N Engl J Med 319:907, 1988

KIMBERLING WF et al: Linkage heterogeneity of autosomal dominant polycystic kidney disease. N Engl J Med 319:913, 1988

KUPIER JJ: Medullary sponge kidney, in *Cystic Diseases of the Kidney*, KD Gardner Jr (ed). New York, Wiley, 1976, p 151

LEVEY AS et al: Occult intracranial aneurisms in polycystic kidney disease. N Engl J Med 308:986, 1983

LEVY HL: Hartnup disorder, in *The Metabolic Basis of Inherited Disease*, 6th ed, CR Scriver et al (eds). New York, McGraw-Hill, 1989, chap 101, p 2515

LIBBER S et al: Treatment of nephrogenic diabetes insipidus with prostaglandin synthesis inhibitors. J Pediatr 108:35, 1986

LIDDLE GW et al: A familial renal disorder simulating primary aldosteronism but with negligible aldosterone secretion. Trans Assoc Am Phys 76:199, 1963

NARINS RG et al: Metabolic acid-base disorders, in *Fluid, Electrolyte and Acid-Base Disorders*, AI Arieff, RA DeFronzo (eds). NY, Churchill Livingstone, 1985, p 269

RASMUSSEN H, TENENHOUSE HT: Hypophosphatemias, in *The Metabolic Basis of Inherited Disease*, 6th ed, CR Scriver et al (eds). New York, McGraw-Hill, 1989, chap 105, p 2581

REEVES WB, ANDREOLI TE: Nephrogenic diabetes insipidus, in *The Metabolic Basis of Inherited Disease*, 6th ed, CR Scriver et al (eds). New York, McGraw-Hill, 1989, chap 78, p 1985

SCHWAB SJ et al: Renal infections in autosomal dominant polycystic kidney disease. Am J Med 82:714, 1987

SCRIVER CR: Familial renal iminoglycinuria, in *The Metabolic Basis of Inherited Disease*, 6th ed, CR Scriver et al (eds). New York, McGraw-Hill, 1989, chap 102, p 2529

SIRIS ES et al: Tumor-induced osteomalacia. Am J Med 82:307, 1987

TOFUKU Y et al: Hypouricemia due to renal urate wasting: Two types of tubular transport defects. Nephron 30:39, 1982

232 NEPHROLITHIASIS

FREDRIC L. COE / MURRAY J. FAVUS

TYPES OF STONES

Calcium salts, uric acid, cystine, and struvite ($MgNH_4PO_4$) are the basis of most kidney stones in the western hemisphere. Calcium oxalate and calcium phosphate stones make up 75 to 85 percent of the total (Table 232-1) and may be admixed in the same stone. Calcium phosphate in stones is usually hydroxyapatite [$Ca_5(PO_4)_3OH$] or, less commonly, brushite ($CaHPO_4 \cdot H_2O$).

Calcium stones are more common in men; the average age of onset is the third decade. Most persons who form a single calcium stone eventually form another, and the intervals between successive stones shorten or remain constant, suggesting that stone-forming activity usually does not wane with time. The average rate of new stone formation in patients who have previously formed a stone is about one stone every 2 or 3 years. Calcium stone disease is frequently familial.

In the urine, calcium oxalate monohydrate crystals (whewellite) usually grow as biconcave ovals that resemble red blood cells in shape and size but may occur in a larger, "dumbbell" form. In polarized light the crystals appear bright against a dark background with an intensity that is dependent upon orientation, a property known as *birefringence*. Calcium oxalate dihydrate crystals (weddellite) are bipyramidal and only weakly birefringent. Apatite crystals do not exhibit birefringence and appear amorphous, because the actual crystals are too small to be resolved by light microscopy. Brushite produces elongated lathlike (narrow, long, rectangular) crystals.

Uric acid stones (Table 232-1) are radiolucent and are also formed mainly by men. Half of patients with uric acid stones have gout; uric acid lithiasis is usually familial whether or not gout is present. In urine, uric acid crystals are red-orange in color because they adsorb the pigment uricine. Anhydrous uric acid produces small crystals that appear amorphous by light microscopy. They are indistinguishable from apatite crystals, except for their birefringence. Uric acid dihydrate tends to form teardrop-shaped crystals as well as flat, square plates; both are strongly birefringent. Uric acid gravel appears like red dust,

and the stones are also orange or red on some occasions. *Cystine stones* are uncommon (Table 232-1), are lemon yellow, and sparkle; they are radiopaque because they contain sulfur. Cystine crystals appear in the urine as flat, hexagonal plates.

Struvite ($MgNH_4PO_4$) *stones* are common (Table 232-1) and potentially dangerous. These stones, formed mainly by women, result from urinary tract infection with urease-producing bacteria, usually *Proteus* species. The stones can grow to a large size and fill the renal pelvis and calyces to produce a "staghorn" appearance. They are radiopaque and have a variable internal density. In urine, struvite crystals are rectangular prisms that have been likened to coffin lids.

MANIFESTATIONS OF STONES

As stones grow upon the surfaces of the renal papillae or within the collecting system, they need not produce symptoms. Accordingly, asymptomatic stones may be discovered during the course of abdominal radiographic studies undertaken for unrelated reasons. Sometimes stones cause gross or microscopic hematuria. In fact, stones rank, along with benign and malignant neoplasms, renal cysts, and genitourinary tuberculosis, as among the common causes of isolated hematuria. Much of the time, however, stones break loose and enter the ureter or occlude the ureteropelvic junction, causing pain and obstruction.

STONE PASSAGE A stone can traverse the ureter without symptoms, but most of the time passage produces pain and bleeding. The pain begins gradually, usually in the flank, but increases over the next 20 to 60 min to become so severe that narcotic drugs are often needed for its control. The pain may remain in the flank or spread downward and anteriorly toward the ipsilateral loin, testicle, or vulva. Pain that migrates downward always indicates that the stone has passed to the lower third of the ureter, but if the pain does not migrate, the position of the stone cannot be predicted. A stone in the portion of the ureter within the bladder wall causes frequency, urgency, and dysuria that may be confused with urinary tract infection. Hematuria is usual with passage of a stone.

OTHER SYNDROMES **Staghorn calculi** Struvite, cystine, and uric acid stones often grow too large to enter the ureter. They gradually fill the renal pelvis and may extend outward through the infundibula to the calyces themselves.

Nephrocalcinosis Calcium stones grow on the renal papillae. Most break loose and cause colic, but sometimes they remain in place so that multiple papillary calcifications are found by x-ray, a condition termed *nephrocalcinosis*. Papillary nephrocalcinosis is very common in hereditary distal renal tubular acidosis and in other states characterized by severe hypercalciuria. In medullary sponge kidney disease (Chap. 231) calcification may occur in dilated distal collecting ducts.

Sludge There can be enough uric acid or cystine in the urine to plug both ureters with precipitate. Calcium oxalate crystals do not do this because less than 100 mg oxalate usually is excreted daily in the urine even in severe hyperoxaluric states, compared with 1000 mg uric acid in patients with ordinary hyperuricosuria and 400 to 800 mg cystine in patients with cystinuria. Calcium phosphate crystals can render the urine milky but do not plug the urinary tract.

INFECTION Although urinary tract infection is not a direct consequence of stone disease, it can occur after instrumentation or surgery of the urinary tract, which are frequent in the treatment of stone disease. Stone disease and urinary infection can enhance the seriousness of one another and interfere with treatment. Obstruction of an infected kidney by a stone may lead to sepsis and extensive damage of renal tissue, since it converts the urinary tract proximal to the obstruction into a closed, or partially closed, space that can become an abscess. On the other hand, some forms of infection, those due to bacteria that possess the enzyme urease, can cause stones composed of struvite.

ACTIVITY OF STONE DISEASE *Active disease* means that new stones are forming or that preformed stones are growing. Sequential

TABLE 232-1 Major causes of renal stones

Stone type and causes	Percent of all stones*	Percent occurrence of specific causes*	Ratio of men to women	Etiology	Diagnosis	Treatment
Calcium stones	75–85		2:1 to 3:1			
Idiopathic hypercalciuria		50–55	2:1	Hereditary (?)	Normocalcemia, unexplained hypercalciuria†	Thiazide diuretic agents
Hyperuricosuria		20	4:1	Diet	Urine uric acid >750 mg per 24 h (women), >800 mg per 24 h (men)	Allopurinol or diet
Primary hyperparathyroidism		5	3:10	Neoplasia	Unexplained hypercalcemia	Surgery
Distal renal tubular acidosis		Rare	1:1	Hereditary	Hyperchloremic acidosis, minimum urine pH >5.5	Alkali replacement
Intestinal hyperoxaluria		~1–2	1:1	Bowel surgery	Urine oxalate >50 mg per 24 h	Cholestyramine or oral calcium loading
Hereditary hyperoxaluria		Rare	1:1	Hereditary	Urine oxalate and glycolic or L-glyceric acid increased	Fluids and pyridoxine
Idiopathic stone disease		20	2:1	Unknown	None of the above present	Oral phosphate, fluids
Uric acid stones	5–8					
Gout		~50	3:1 to 4:1	Hereditary	Clinical diagnosis	Alkali to raise urine pH
Idiopathic		~50	1:1	Hereditary (?)	Uric acid stones, no gout	Allopurinol if daily urine uric acid above 1000 mg
Dehydration		?	1:1	Intestinal, habit	History, intestinal fluid loss	Alkali, fluids, reversal of cause
Lesch-Nyhan syndrome		Rare	Men	Hereditary	Reduced hypoxanthine-guanine phosphoribosyltransferase level	Allopurinol
Malignant tumors		Rare	1:1	Neoplasia	Clinical diagnosis	Allopurinol
Cystine stones	1		1:1	Hereditary	Stone type; elevated cystine excretion	Massive fluids, alkali, D-penicillamine if needed
Struvite stones	10–15		2:10	Infection	Stone type	Antimicrobial agents and judicious surgery

* Values are percent of patients who form a particular type of stone and who display each specific cause of stones.
† Urine calcium above 300 mg per 24 h (men), 250 mg per 24 h (women), or 4 mg/kg per 24 h either sex. Hyperthyroidism, Cushing syndrome, sarcoidosis, malignant tumors, immobilization, vitamin D intoxication, rapidly progressive bone disease, and Paget's disease all cause hypercalciuria and must be excluded in diagnosis of idiopathic hypercalciuria.

radiographs of the renal areas are needed to document the growth or appearance of new stones and to ensure that stones which pass are actually newly formed, not preexistent ones.

PATHOGENESIS OF STONES

Urinary stones usually arise because of the breakdown of a delicate balance. The kidneys must conserve water, but they must also excrete materials that have a low solubility. These two opposing requirements must be balanced during adaptation to a particular combination of diet, climate, and activity. The problem is mitigated to some extent by the fact that urine contains substances that inhibit crystallization of calcium salts and others that bind calcium in soluble complexes. But these protective mechanisms are less than perfect. When the urine becomes supersaturated with insoluble materials, because excretion rates are excessive and/or because water conservation is extreme, crystals form and may grow and aggregate to form a stone.

SUPERSATURATION In a solution in equilibrium with crystals of calcium oxalate, the product of the chemical activities of the calcium and oxalate ions in the solution is termed the *equilibrium solubility product*, because it is the activity product that is unique to the equilibrium condition. If the crystals are removed, and if either calcium or oxalate ions are added to the solution, the activity product will increase, but the solution may remain clear; no new crystals form. Such a solution is considered to be *metastably supersaturated*. If new calcium oxalate seed crystals are now added, they will grow in size. Ultimately, the activity product reaches a critical value at which a solid phase begins to develop spontaneously. This value is called the *upper limit of metastability*, or the *formation product*. Stone growth in the urinary tract requires a urine that, on the average, is above the equilibrium solubility product. Persistence of a stone requires an average activity product at least equal to the solubility product. Excessive supersaturation is common in stone formation.

Calcium, oxalate, and phosphate form many stable soluble complexes among themselves and with other substances in urine, such as citrate. As a result, their free ion activities are considerably below their chemical concentrations and can be measured only by indirect techniques. Reduction in ligands such as citrate can increase ion activity without measurably changing total urinary calcium. Urine supersaturation can be increased by dehydration or by overexcretion of calcium, oxalate, or phosphate. Supersaturation of the urine with cystine or uric acid also occurs when overexcretion or low urine volume is present. Urine pH can also be an important factor; phosphate and uric acid are weak acids that dissociate readily over the physiologic range of urine pH. Alkaline urine contains more urate and dissociated phosphate, favoring deposits of sodium hydrogen urate, brushite, and apatite. Below a urine pH of 5.5, uric acid crystals (pK 5.47) predominate, whereas phosphate crystals are rare. The solubility of calcium oxalate, on the other hand, is not influenced by changes in urine pH. Measurements of supersaturation in a pooled 24-h urine sample are averages that probably underestimate the risk of precipitation. Transient dehydration or postprandial bursts of overexcretion may cause values that are considerably above the average.

NUCLEATION **Homogeneous nucleation** In urine that is supersaturated with respect to calcium oxalate, these two ions form clusters. The higher the supersaturation, the larger and more numerous the clusters become. Most small clusters eventually disperse because the internal forces that hold them together are too weak to overcome the random tendency of ions to move away. Clusters of over 100 ions can remain stable because attractive forces balance surface losses. Once they are stable, nuclei can grow at levels of supersaturation below that needed for their creation. The formation product marks the point at which stable nuclei become frequent enough to create a permanent solid phase.

Heterogeneous nucleation   If a supersaturated urine is seeded with preformed nuclei of a crystal that is similar in structure to calcium oxalate, calcium and oxalate ions in solution will bind to the crystal's surface as they would upon a seed crystal of calcium oxalate itself. The organized growth of one crystal on the surface of another is called *epitaxial growth*, and the seeding of a supersaturated solution by foreign nuclei is called *heterogeneous nucleation*. Sodium hydrogen urate, uric acid, and hydroxyapatite crystals can serve as heterogeneous nuclei that permit calcium oxalate stones to form even though urine calcium oxalate supersaturation never exceeds the metastable limit.

INHIBITORS OF CRYSTAL GROWTH AND AGGREGATION   Stable nuclei must grow and aggregate to produce a stone of clinical significance. Urine contains potent inhibitors of both of these processes for calcium oxalate and calcium phosphate but not for uric acid, cystine, or struvite. Inorganic pyrophosphate is a potent inhibitor that appears to affect calcium phosphate more than calcium oxalate crystals. Other urine components that appear to be glycoproteins inhibit the growth of calcium oxalate crystals. Slowing of crystal growth increases the apparent upper limit of metastability, because the critical growth of ion clusters into stable nuclei is hindered. As a consequence of the presence of these inhibitors, crystal growth in urine is slow compared with growth in simple salt solutions, and the upper limit of metastability is higher. Urine citrate may also inhibit crystal growth or nucleation.

EVALUATION AND TREATMENT OF PATIENTS WITH NEPHROLITHIASIS

A majority of patients with nephrolithiasis have remediable metabolic disorders that cause stones and can be detected by chemical analysis of the serum and urine. A practical outpatient evaluation consists of three 24-h urine collections, each with a corresponding blood sample; measurements of serum and urine calcium, uric acid and creatinine, urine oxalate and citrate, and serum electrolytes should be made. When possible, the composition of kidney stones should be determined because treatment depends on stone type (Table 232-1). No matter what disorders are found, every patient should be counseled to avoid dehydration and to drink six to eight glasses of water daily. Since treatment is prolonged, the use of medications must be justified by the activity and severity of stone disease and the importance of protection against new stones.

The management of stones that are already present in the kidneys or urinary tract requires a combined medical and surgical approach. The specific treatment for any individual depends upon the location of the stone, the extent of obstruction, the function of the affected and unaffected kidneys, the presence or absence of urinary tract infection, the progress of stone passage, and the risk of operation or anesthesia, given the overall clinical state of the patient. In general, severe obstruction, infection, intractable pain, or serious bleeding are indications for removal of a stone.

In the past, stones could be removed only by operation or by passing a flexible basket retrograde up the ureter from the bladder during cystoscopy. However, there now are three new alternatives. Extracorporeal lithotripsy causes the in situ fragmentation of stones in the kidney, renal pelvis, or proximal ureter by exposing them to extracorporeal shock waves. The patient is submerged in a water tank, the kidney with the stone is centered at the focal point of parabolic reflectors, and high-intensity shock waves are created by high-voltage discharge. The waves are focused by the reflectors so that they pass through the patient and fracture the stone as they pass. After multiple discharges, most stones are reduced to powder that moves through the ureter into the bladder. Larger fragments are removed by cystoscopy. Percutaneous ultrasonic lithotripsy requires the passage of a rigid cystoscope-like instrument into the renal pelvis through a small incision in the flank. Stones can be disrupted by a small ultrasound transducer, and fragments can be removed directly. The last method is endoscopic passage of an ultrasonic transducer

into the ureter via a cystoscope; ureteral stones that are inaccessible to extracorporeal or percutaneous lithotripsy can be fragmented and removed. These various forms of lithotripsy are replacing pyelolithotomy and ureterolithotomy.

CALCIUM STONES   Idiopathic hypercalciuria (See also Chap. 340)   This condition appears to be hereditary, and its diagnosis is straightforward (Table 232-1). In some patients, primary intestinal hyperabsorption of calcium causes transient postprandial hypercalcemia that suppresses secretion of parathyroid hormone. The renal tubules are deprived of the normal potent stimulus to reabsorb calcium at the same time that the filtered load of calcium is increased. In other patients, reabsorption of calcium by the renal tubules appears to be defective, and secondary hyperparathyroidism is evoked by urinary losses of calcium. Renal synthesis of 1,25-dihydroxyvitamin D is increased, producing intestinal hyperabsorption of calcium. In the past, the separation of "absorptive" and "renal" forms of hypercalciuria has been used to guide treatment. However, these may not be distinct entities but the extremes of a continuum of behavior. Hypercalciuria contributes to stone formation by raising urine saturation with respect to calcium oxalate and calcium phosphate.

Thiazide diuretics lower urine calcium in both types of hypercalciuria and are effective in preventing the formation of stones. The drug effect requires slight contraction of the extracellular fluid volume, and massive use of NaCl will reduce its therapeutic effect. Potassium citrate is useful to prevent hypokalemia and raise urine citrate; the latter lowers urine calcium ion levels.

Hyperuricosuria   About 20 percent of calcium oxalate stone formers are hyperuricosuric, primarily because of an excessive intake of purine from meat, fish, and poultry. The mechanism of stone formation probably is heterogeneous nucleation of calcium oxalate by crystals of sodium hydrogen urate or uric acid that lodge in the terminal ends of the collecting ducts and produce an anchored site on which calcium oxalate can deposit. A low purine diet is desirable but difficult for many patients to achieve. The alternative is allopurinol, usually 100 mg bid. Some patients eventually alter their diets so that allopurinol can be withdrawn.

Primary hyperparathyroidism (See also Chap. 340)   The diagnosis of this condition is established by documenting hypercalcemia that cannot be otherwise explained accompanied by inappropriately elevated serum concentrations of parathyroid hormone. Hypercalciuria, usually present, raises the urine supersaturation of calcium phosphate and/or calcium oxalate (Table 232-1). Prompt diagnosis is important since parathyroidectomy is effective treatment and should be carried out before renal damage has occurred.

Distal renal tubular acidosis (See also Chap. 231)   The defect in this condition seems to reside in the distal nephron, which cannot establish a normal pH gradient between urine and blood, leading to hyperchloremic acidosis. The minimum urine pH in response to an oral challenge with NH_4Cl, 1.9 mmol per kilogram of body weight, is above 5.5. Hypercalciuria, an alkaline urine, and a low urine citrate cause supersaturation with respect to calcium phosphate. Calcium phosphate stones form, nephrocalcinosis is common, and osteomalacia or rickets may occur. Renal damage is frequent, and glomerular filtration rate falls gradually. Treatment with supplemental alkali reverses hypercalciuria and limits the production of new stones. The usual dose of sodium bicarbonate is 0.5 to 2.0 mmol per kilogram of body weight per day, in four to six divided doses. An alternative is Shohl's solution, which contains citrate and citric acid. Incomplete renal tubular acidosis (RTA) is a form of the disorder in which systemic acidosis is absent but urine pH cannot be lowered below 5.5 after an exogenous acid load such as ammonium chloride. Incomplete RTA may develop in some patients who form calcium oxalate stones because of idiopathic hypercalciuria; the importance of the RTA in producing stones in this situation is uncertain, and thiazide treatment is a reasonable alternative. Some patients with incomplete RTA form calcium phosphate stones because of low urine citrate and an abnormally alkaline urine and are best treated with alkali as if RTA were complete.

Hyperoxaluria Overabsorption of dietary oxalate and consequent oxaluria, i.e., so-called intestinal oxaluria, is one consequence of fat malabsorption (Chap. 240). The latter can be caused by a variety of conditions, including bacterial overgrowth syndromes, chronic disease of the pancreas and biliary tract, jejunoileal bypass in treatment of obesity, or ileal resection for inflammatory bowel disease. With fat malabsorption, calcium in the bowel lumen is bound by fatty acids instead of oxalate, which is left free for absorption in the colon. Delivery of unabsorbed fatty acids and bile salts to the colon may injure the colonic mucosa and enhance oxalate absorption. Dietary excess of oxalate, ascorbic acid loading, and hereditary hyperoxaluric states are less common causes of hyperoxaluria. Ethylene glycol intoxication and methoxyflurane can also cause oxalate overproduction and hyperoxaluria. Hyperoxaluria from any cause can produce tubulointerstitial nephropathy (Chap. 229) and lead to stone formation.

The oxalate-binding resin cholestyramine, at a dose of 8 to 16 g per day, correction of fat malabsorption, and a low-fat diet are effective treatments for oxaluria secondary to intestinal absorption. Calcium lactate, 8 to 14 g per day, which precipitates oxalate in the gut lumen is an alternative form of therapy. There is no effective treatment for primary hyperoxaluria, the result of an enzymatic defect involving the metabolism of the precursor of oxalate that is inherited as an autosomal recessive (also see Chap. 335). A high fluid intake, phosphate, and pyridoxine (200 mg per day) are recommended, but irreversible renal failure secondary to recurrent stone formation usually occurs before age 20.

Idiopathic calcium lithiasis At least 20 percent of patients have no obvious cause for stones (Table 232-1). The best treatment appears to be a high fluid intake, so that the urine specific gravity remains at 1.005 or below throughout the day and night. Oral phosphate at a dose of 2 g phosphorus daily may lower urine calcium and increase urine pyrophosphate and thereby reduce the rate of recurrence. Orthophosphate causes mild nausea and diarrhea initially, but tolerance may improve with continued intake. Thiazide treatment to reduce calcium excretion and allopurinol to diminish uric acid output may also be helpful. There are no adequate studies to support the use of supplemental magnesium, pyridoxine, or methylene blue.

URIC ACID STONES These stones form because the urine becomes supersaturated with undissociated uric acid, uric acid that is protonated at its N-9 position. In gout, idiopathic uric acid lithiasis, and dehydration, the average pH is abnormally low, usually below 5.4, and often below 5.0. Undissociated uric acid therefore predominates and is soluble in urine only in concentrations of 100 mg per liter. Concentrations above this level represent supersaturation that causes crystals and stones to form. Hyperuricosuria, when present, increases supersaturation, and urine of low pH can be excessively supersaturated with undissociated uric acid even though the daily excretion rate is normal. Myeloproliferative syndromes, chemotherapeutic treatment of malignant tumors, and the Lesch-Nyhan syndrome cause such massive production of uric acid and consequent hyperuricosuria that stones and uric acid sludge occur even at a normal urine pH. The renal collecting tubules can be plugged by uric acid crystals with consequent acute renal failure.

The two goals of treatment are to raise urine pH and to lower excessive urine uric acid excretion to less than 1 g per day. Supplemental alkali, 1 to 3 mmol per kilogram of body weight per day, should be given in three or four evenly spaced, divided doses, one of which should be given at bedtime. The form of the alkali may be important. Potassium citrate may reduce the risk of calcium salts crystallizing when urine pH is increased, whereas sodium citrate or sodium bicarbonate may increase the risk. If the overnight urine pH is below 5.5, the evening dose of bicarbonate may be raised, or 250 mg acetazolamide added at bedtime. With massive overexcretion of uric acid, high doses of allopurinol, exceeding 300 mg daily, may be needed. Treatment with allopurinol should be instituted before chemotherapy of highly cellular tumors, since massive hyperuricosuria can be expected. Alkali treatment must be avoided if hypercalciuria is also present.

CYSTINURIA AND CYSTINE STONES (See also Chap. 336) In this disorder proximal tubular and jejunal transport of cystine and the other dibasic amino acids, lysine, arginine, and ornithine, are defective, and excessive amounts are lost in the urine. Clinical disease is due solely to the insolubility of cystine, which forms stones.

Pathogenesis Cystinuria probably occurs because of defective transport of amino acids by the brush borders of renal tubule and intestinal epithelial cells. Cystine, lysine, arginine, and ornithine appear to share a common renal transport pathway, since infusion of lysine decreases tubular reabsorption of the other three. But cystine is also transported by a separate transport mechanism, because cystinuria and dibasic aminoaciduria can each occur independently. The intestinal defects are not similar in all patients who are homozygous for cystinuria, and the extent of aminoaciduria in those relatives of cystinuric patients who are heterozygous carriers of the defect varies from family to family. Three types of inheritance have been described (see Chap. 336).

Diagnosis and treatment Cystine stones are formed only by patients with cystinuria, but 10 percent of stones formed by cystinuric patients do not contain cystine; therefore, every stone former should be screened for the disease. The sediment from a first morning urine specimen in many patients with homozygous cystinuria reveals typical flat hexagonal platelike cystine crystals. Cystinuria can also be detected using the urine sodium nitroprusside test. The test is positive with 75 to 125 mg cystine per gram of creatinine, a concentration lower than that in the urine of patients with cystinuria but above the levels in normal urine. Because the test is sensitive, it is positive in many asymptomatic heterozygotes for cystinuria. A positive nitroprusside test or the finding of cystine crystals in the urine sediment should be evaluated by measurement of daily cystine excretion. Normal adults excrete 40 to 60 mg cystine per gram of creatinine, heterozygotes usually excrete less than 300 mg/g, and patients with homozygous cystinuria almost always excrete above 250 mg/g.

Treatment consists of a high fluid intake, even at night. Daily urine volume should exceed 3 L. Raising urine pH with alkali is helpful, provided the urine pH exceeds 7.5. Because side effects are frequent, penicillamine, which forms the soluble disulfide cysteine-penicillamine, should be used only when fluid loading and alkali therapy are ineffective. Mercaptopropinylglycine has been used to dissolve renal calculi by perfusion of the renal pelvis and has been given by mouth to prevent stones. Low-methionine diets have not proved to be practical for clinical use.

STRUVITE STONES These stones are a result of urinary infection with bacteria, usually *Proteus* species, which possess urease, an enzyme that degrades urea to NH_3 and CO_2. The NH_3 hydrolyzes to NH_4^+ and raises pH, usually to 8 or 9. The CO_2 hydrates to H_2CO_3 and then dissociates to CO_3^{2-} which precipitates with calcium as $CaCO_3$. The NH_4^+ precipitates PO_4^{3-} and Mg^{2+} to form the triple salt $MgNH_4PO_4$. The result is a stone of calcium carbonate admixed with struvite. Struvite does not form in urine in the absence of infection, because NH_4^+ concentration is low in urine that is alkaline in response to physiologic stimuli. Chronic *Proteus* infection can occur because of impaired urinary drainage, urologic instrumentation or surgery, and especially with chronic antibiotic treatment, which can favor the dominance of *Proteus* in the urinary tract.

Treatment Methenamine mandelate, which lowers urine pH and liberates formaldehyde, is used for chronic suppression of infection when a stone is present. More extreme lowering of urine pH with chronic administration of NH_4Cl may retard stone growth but may also raise urine calcium level and promote the formation of calcium oxalate stones. Antimicrobial treatment is best reserved for dealing with acute infection and for maintenance of a sterile urine after surgery, in the hope of preventing recurrence or minimizing stone growth. Surgery may be appropriate for severe obstruction, pain, bleeding, or intractable urinary infection. Since stones can regrow from any infected fragment which is left behind, recurrences following operation are quite common. In some centers, it is possible to irrigate the renal pelvis and calyces with Renacidin, a solution that dissolves struvite, using a catheter passed through a cutaneous flank incision into the kidney.

REFERENCES

COE FL, PARKS JH: *Nephrolithiasis: Pathogenesis and treatment*. Chicago, Year Book, 1988

———— et al: Effect of low calcium diet on urine calcium excretion, parathyroid function, and serum 1,25(OH)$_2$D$_3$ levels in patients with idiopathic hypercalciuria and in normal subjects. Am J Med 72:25, 1982

FLEISCH H, FAVUS MJ: Disorders of stone formation, in *The Kidney*, 3d ed, BM Brenner, FC Rector Jr (eds). Philadelphia, Saunders, 1986, p 1403

NAKAGAWA Y et al: Purification and characterization of the principal inhibitors of calcium oxalate monohydrate crystal growth in human urine. J Biol Chem 258:12594, 1983

NEWMAN DM et al: Long-term follow-up of 1,900 ESWL treatments, in *Shock Wave Lithotripsy*, JE Lingeman, DM Newman (eds). New York, Plenum, 1988

PAK CYC (ed): Urolithiasis. Kidney Int 13:341, 1978

————: Kidney stones, in *Williams' Textbook of Endocrinology*, 7th ed, JD Wilson, DW Foster (eds). Philadelphia, Saunders, 1985, p 1256

SMITH LH: Urolithiasis, in *Diseases of the Kidney*, 4th ed, RW Schrier, CW Gottschalk (eds). Boston, Little, Brown, 1988, p 785

STRAUSS AL et al: Factors that predict relapse of calcium nephrolithiasis during treatment. Am J Med 72:25, 1982

WEBB DR et al: Extracorporeal shockwave lithotripsy, endourology and open surgery: The management and follow-up of 200 patients with urinary calculi. Ann R Coll Surg Engl 67:337, 1985

233 URINARY TRACT OBSTRUCTION

BARRY M. BRENNER / EDGAR L. MILFORD / JULIAN L. SEIFTER

Obstruction to the flow of urine, with attendant stasis and elevation in urinary tract pressure, impairs renal and urinary conduit functions and represents a common cause of acute and chronic renal failure. With early relief of obstruction, the defects in function usually disappear completely. However, chronic obstruction may produce profound and permanent loss of renal mass (renal atrophy) and excretory capability, as well as enhanced susceptibility to local infection and stone formation. Early and accurate diagnosis and prompt and appropriate therapy are, therefore, essential to minimize the otherwise devastating effects of obstruction on urinary tract structure and function.

ETIOLOGY Obstruction to urine flow can result from *intrinsic* or *extrinsic mechanical blockade* as well as from *functional defects* not associated with fixed occlusion of the urinary drainage system. Lesions causing mechanical obstruction can occur at any level of the urinary tract, from the renal calyces to the external urethral meatus. Normal points of narrowing, such as the ureteropelvic and uretero-vesical junctions, bladder neck, and urethral meatus, are common sites of obstruction. When blockage is above the level of the bladder, unilateral dilatation of the ureter (*hydroureter*) and renal pyelocalyceal system (*hydronephrosis*) occur; when the lesion is at or below the level of the bladder, bilateral involvement is the rule.

Common forms of obstruction are listed in Table 233-1. In childhood, *congenital malformations*, including marked narrowing of the ureteropelvic junction, anomalous (retrocaval) location of the ureter, and posterior urethral valves predominate. The latter defect is the most common cause of bilateral hydronephrosis in boys. Children may also have bladder dysfunction secondary to congenital urethral stricture, urethral meatal stenosis, or bladder neck obstruction. In adults, urinary tract obstruction is due mainly to *acquired defects*. Pelvic tumors, calculi, and urethral stricture predominate. Ligation of, or injury to, the ureter during pelvic or colonic surgery can lead to hydronephrosis which, if unilateral, may remain relatively silent and undetected. Obstructive uropathy may also result from extrinsic neoplastic (carcinoma of cervix or colon, retroperitoneal lymphoma)

TABLE 233-1 Common mechanical causes of urinary tract obstruction

Ureter	Bladder outlet	Urethra
CONGENITAL		
Ureteropelvic junction narrowing or obstruction	Bladder neck obstruction	Posterior urethral valves
Ureterovesical junction narrowing or obstruction	Ureterocele	Anterior urethral valves
Ureterocele		Stricture
Retrocaval ureter		Meatal stenosis
		Phimosis
ACQUIRED INTRINSIC DEFECTS		
Calculi	Benign prostatic hypertrophy	Stricture
Inflammation	Cancer of prostate	Tumor
Trauma	Cancer of bladder	Calculi
Sloughed papillae	Calculi	Trauma
Tumor	Diabetic neuropathy	Phimosis
Blood clots	Spinal cord disease	
Uric acid crystals		
ACQUIRED EXTRINSIC DEFECTS		
Pregnant uterus	Carcinoma of cervix, colon	Trauma
Retroperitoneal fibrosis	Trauma	
Aortic aneurysm		
Uterine leiomyomata		
Carcinoma of uterus, prostate, bladder, colon, rectum		
Retroperitoneal lymphoma		
Accidental surgical ligation		

or inflammatory disorders. One such inflammatory disorder is retroperitoneal fibrosis, a process of unknown cause seen most commonly in middle-aged men, which occasionally leads to bilateral ureteral obstruction. Occurring in some patients taking methysergide for relief of migraine, retroperitoneal fibrosis must be distinguished from other retroperitoneal causes of ureteral obstruction, particularly lymphomas and pelvic neoplasms.

Functional impairment of urine flow usually results from disorders that involve both the ureter and bladder. Common functional lesions include neurogenic bladder, often with adynamic ureter, and vesicoureteral reflux. Reflux of urine from bladder to ureter(s) is more common in children than adults and may result in severe unilateral or bilateral hydroureter and hydronephrosis. Abnormal insertion of the ureter into the bladder is the most common cause of vesicoureteral reflux in children. Reflux in the absence of urinary tract infection or bladder neck obstruction usually does not lead to renal parenchymal damage and often resolves spontaneously as the child matures. Surgical reinsertion of the ureter into the bladder is indicated if reflux is severe and unlikely to improve spontaneously, if renal function deteriorates, or if urinary tract infections recur despite chronic antimicrobial therapy.

CLINICAL FEATURES The pathophysiology and clinical features of urinary tract obstruction are summarized in Table 233-2. *Pain* is the symptom which most commonly provokes the need for medical attention. The pain of urinary tract obstruction is due to distention of the collecting system or renal capsule. The severity of the pain is influenced more by the rate at which distention develops than by the degree of distention. Acute supravesical obstruction, as from a stone lodged in a ureter (Chap. 232), is associated with excruciatingly severe pain, usually called *renal colic*. This pain is relatively steady and continuous, with little fluctuation in intensity, and often radiates to the lower abdomen, testes, or labia. By contrast, more insidious causes of obstruction, such as chronic narrowing of the ureteropelvic junction, may produce little or no pain yet result in total destruction of the affected kidney. Flank pain which comes on only with micturition is pathognomonic of vesicoureteral reflux.

TABLE 233-2 Pathophysiology of bilateral ureteral obstruction

Hemodynamic effects	Tubule effects	Clinical features
ACUTE		
↑ Renal blood flow ↓ GFR ↓ Medullary blood flow ↑ Vasodilator prostaglandins	↑ Ureteral and tubule pressures ↑ Reabsorption of Na^+, urea, water	Pain (capsule distention) Azotemia Oliguria
CHRONIC		
↓ Renal blood flow ↓ ↓ GFR ↑ Vasoconstrictor prostaglandins ↑ Renin-angiotensin production	↓ Medullary osmolarity ↓ Concentrating ability Structural damage; parenchymal atrophy ↑ Transport functions for Na^+, K^+, H^+	Azotemia Hypertension ADH-insensitive polyuria Natriuresis Hyperkalemic, hyperchloremic acidosis
RELEASE OF OBSTRUCTION		
Slow ↑ in GFR (variable)	↓ Tubule pressure ↑ Solute load per nephron (urea, NaCl) Natriuretic factors present	Postobstructive diuresis Potential for volume depletion and electrolyte imbalance (Na^+, K^+, PO_4^{2-}, Mg^{2+} excretion)

Azotemia develops in urinary tract obstruction when overall excretory function is impaired. This may occur in the setting of bladder outlet obstruction, bilateral renal pelvic or ureteric obstruction, or unilateral disease in a patient with a solitary functioning kidney. Complete bilateral obstruction should be suspected when acute renal failure is accompanied by anuria. Any patient with renal failure otherwise unexplained or with a history of nephrolithiasis, hematuria, prostatic enlargement, pelvic surgery, trauma, or tumor should be evaluated for urinary tract obstruction.

Symptoms of *polyuria* and *nocturia* commonly accompany chronic partial urinary tract obstruction and result from impaired renal concentrating ability. This defect usually does not improve with administration of vasopressin and is therefore a form of acquired nephrogenic diabetes insipidus. Disturbances in sodium chloride transport in the ascending limb of Henle and, in azotemic patients, the osmotic (urea) diuresis per nephron lead to decreased medullary hypertonicity and, hence, a concentrating defect. Partial obstruction, therefore, may be associated with increased rather than decreased urine output. Indeed, wide fluctuations in urinary output in a patient with azotemia should always raise the possibility of intermittent or partial urinary tract obstruction. If fluid intake is inadequate, severe dehydration and hypernatremia may develop. Hesitancy and straining to initiate the urinary stream, postvoid dribbling, urinary frequency, and (overflow) incontinence are common in patients with obstruction at or below the level of the bladder (see Chap. 49).

In addition to loss of urinary concentrating ability and azotemia, partial bilateral urinary tract obstruction often results in other derangements of renal function, including *acquired distal renal tubular acidosis, hyperkalemia,* and *renal salt wasting.* These defects in tubule function are often accompanied by evidence of widespread renal tubulointerstitial damage. Morphologic abnormalities appear early in the course of obstruction; initially the interstitium becomes edematous and infiltrated with mononuclear inflammatory cells. With continued obstruction, the interstitium becomes fibrotic; scarring and atrophy of the papillae and medulla occur and precede these processes in the cortex.

The possibility of urinary tract obstruction must always be considered in patients with urinary tract infections or urolithiasis. Urinary stasis encourages the growth of organisms as well as the formation of crystals, especially magnesium ammonium phosphate (struvite). *Hypertension* is seen frequently in acute and subacute

forms of unilateral obstruction and is usually a consequence of increased release of renin by the involved kidney. Chronic unilateral or bilateral hydronephrosis, in the presence of extracellular volume expansion or other forms of renal disease, may result in significant hypertension. *Polycythemia,* an infrequent complication of obstructive uropathy, is probably secondary to increased erythropoietin production by the obstructed kidney.

DIAGNOSIS A history of difficulty in voiding, pain, infection, or changes in urinary volume is common. Evidence for distention of the kidney or urinary bladder often can be obtained by palpation and percussion of the abdomen. A careful rectal examination may reveal enlargement or nodularity of the prostate, abnormal rectal sphincter tone, or a rectal or pelvic mass. The penis should be inspected for evidence of meatal stenosis or phimosis. In the female, vaginal, uterine, and rectal lesions responsible for urinary tract obstruction are usually revealed by inspection and palpation.

Urinalysis and examination of the urine sediment may reveal hematuria, pyuria, and bacteriuria. Often, however, the urine sediment is devoid of abnormal elements, even when obstruction leads to marked azotemia and extensive structural damage. An abdominal scout film should be obtained to evaluate the possibility of nephrocalcinosis or a radiopaque stone at any level of the urinary collecting system. As indicated in Fig. 233-1 if urinary tract obstruction is

FIGURE 233-1 Diagnostic approach for urinary tract obstruction in unexplained renal failure. Circles represent diagnostic procedures, and squares indicate clinical decisions based on available data. CT, computed tomography; IVP, intravenous pyelogram.

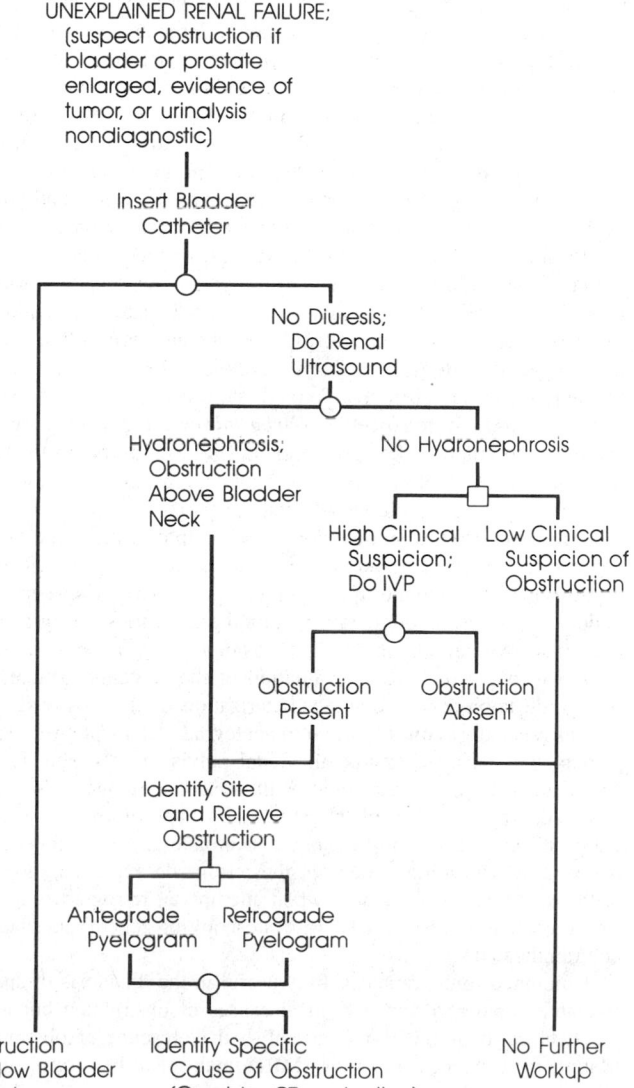

suspected, abdominal ultrasonography should be performed to evaluate renal and bladder size, as well as pyelocalyceal and ureteral contours. If distention of these structures is absent, functionally significant urinary tract obstruction can safely be excluded in differential diagnosis. Abdominal ultrasound may also detect an obstructing pelvic mass.

Intravenous pyelography is indicated if an obstructive abnormality is revealed by ultrasound. If the patient is not azotemic, a standard dose of contrast medium usually provides adequate information. With renal insufficiency, however, high-dose (drip-infusion) pyelography with nephrotomography is usually required for adequate visualization. In the presence of obstruction, the appearance time of the nephrogram is often delayed but eventually becomes more dense than normal because of slow tubular fluid flow rate which results in enhanced water reabsorption by the nephrons and greater concentration of contrast medium within tubules. The kidney involved by an acute obstructive process is usually slightly enlarged, and there is dilatation of the calyces, renal pelvis, and ureter above the obstruction. The ureter, however, is not tortuous, as is the case when the obstruction is chronic. In comparison with the nephrogram, the pyelogram may be extremely faint, especially if the dilated renal pelvis is voluminous, causing dilution of the contrast medium. The radiographic study should be continued until the site of obstruction is determined or the contrast medium is excreted. Delayed films taken as long as 48 h after contrast administration may be necessary to determine the exact site of obstruction. Radionuclide scans define less anatomic detail than intravenous pyelography and, like the pyelogram, are of limited value when renal function is poor. Nonetheless, such scans are sensitive in the detection of obstruction and provide a substitute test in some patients at high risk for reaction to intravenous contrast dyes.

Patients suspected of having intermittent ureteropelvic obstruction (whether functional or mechanical) should have radiologic evaluation while they are in pain, since a normal pyelogram is commonly seen during asymptomatic periods. Hydration or mannitol infusion often helps to provoke a symptomatic attack. Voiding cystourethrography is of great value in the diagnosis of vesicoureteral reflux and bladder neck and urethral obstructions. Patients with obstruction at or below the level of the bladder exhibit thickening, trabeculation, and diverticula of the bladder wall. Postvoiding films reveal residual urine. If these radiographic studies fail to provide adequate information for diagnosis, endoscopic visualization by the urologist often permits precise identification of lesions involving the urethra, prostate, bladder, and ureteral orifices. To facilitate visualization of a suspected lesion in a ureter or renal pelvis, *retrograde* or *antegrade pyelography* should be attempted. These diagnostic studies may be preferable to the intravenous pyelogram in the azotemic patient in whom poor excretory function precludes adequate visualization of the collecting system. Furthermore, intravenous pyelography carries the risk of contrast-induced renal failure in some patients with renal insufficiency, diabetes mellitus, and multiple myeloma, particularly when performed under conditions of dehydration. For these reasons retrograde and antegrade pyelography may offer advantages over the intravenous approach in the diagnostic evaluation of the azotemic patient. The retrograde approach involves catheterization of the involved ureter under cystoscopic control, while the antegrade technique necessitates placement of a catheter into the renal pelvis via a needle inserted percutaneously under ultrasonic or fluoroscopic guidance. While the antegrade approach carries the added advantage of providing immediate and certain decompression of a unilateral obstructing lesion, many urologists initially attempt the retrograde approach and resort to the antegrade method only when attempts at retrograde catheterization are unsuccessful or when cystoscopy or general anesthesia is contraindicated.

Computed tomography (CT) is useful in the diagnosis of specific intraabdominal and retroperitoneal causes of obstruction but is less practical as an initial test to establish the presence of obstruction. Magnetic resonance imaging (MRI) may also be useful in the identification of specific obstructive causes.

TREATMENT AND PROGNOSIS An individual with any form of urinary tract obstruction complicated by infection requires relief of obstruction as soon as possible to prevent development of generalized sepsis and progressive renal damage. On a temporary basis, depending on the site of obstruction, drainage is often satisfactorily achieved by nephrostomy, ureterostomy, or ureteral, urethral, or suprapubic catheterization. The patient with acute urinary tract infection and obstruction should be given appropriate antibiotics based on in vitro bacterial sensitivity and ability of the drug to concentrate in the kidney and urine. Treatment may be required for 3 to 4 weeks. Chronic or recurrent infections in an obstructed kidney with poor intrinsic function may necessitate nephrectomy. When infection is not present, immediate surgery often is not required, even in the presence of complete obstruction and anuria (because of the availability of dialysis), at least until acid-base, fluid and electrolyte, and cardiovascular status are restored to normal. Nevertheless, the site of obstruction should be ascertained as soon as feasible, in part because of the possibility that sepsis may occur and necessitate prompt urologic intervention. Elective relief of obstruction is usually recommended in patients with urinary retention, recurrent urinary tract infections, persistent pain, or progressive loss of renal function. Infrequently, mechanical obstruction can be alleviated by nonsurgical means, as with radiation therapy for retroperitoneal lymphoma. Likewise, functional obstruction secondary to neurogenic bladder may be decreased with the combination of frequent voiding and cholinergic drugs. The approach to obstruction secondary to renal stones is discussed in Chap. 232.

With relief of obstruction, the *prognosis* regarding return of renal function depends largely upon whether irreversible renal damage has occurred. When obstruction is not relieved, the course will depend mainly on whether the obstruction is complete or incomplete, bilateral or unilateral, and whether urinary tract infection is also present. Complete obstruction with infection can lead to total destruction of the kidney within days. Studies in dogs suggest that relief of complete obstruction of 1 and 2 weeks' duration restores glomerular filtration rate to 60 and 30 percent of normal, respectively; after 8 weeks of obstruction, recovery does not occur. Nevertheless, in the absence of definitive evidence of irreversibility, every effort should be made to decompress in the hope of restoring renal function at least partially.

In patients undergoing cystectomy for bladder cancer, the ileal conduit is the currently preferred urinary diversionary procedure. In benign disease a sigmoid conduit may result in less ureteral reflux and secondary chronic renal insufficiency. These approaches are preferable to ureterosigmoidostomy, a procedure complicated by a high incidence of ureteral obstruction, reflux, hypokalemic metabolic acidosis, pyelonephritis, and neoplasms developing at the ureteral anastomotic site.

POSTOBSTRUCTIVE DIURESIS Relief of bilateral, but not unilateral, complete urinary tract obstruction commonly leads to a postobstructive diuresis, characterized by polyuria, which may be massive. The urine is usually hypotonic and may contain a large amount of sodium chloride. The natriuresis is due, at least in part, to the excretion of retained urea, which acts as a poorly reabsorbable solute and diminishes salt and water reabsorption in the tubules (osmotic diuresis). The increase in intratubular pressure very likely also contributes to the impairment in net sodium chloride reabsorption, especially in the terminal nephron segments. Natriuretic factors (other than urea) may also accumulate during uremia induced by obstruction and depress salt and water reabsorption when urine flow is reestablished. In the majority of patients this diuresis is physiologic, resulting in the *appropriate* excretion of the excesses of salt and water retained during the period of obstruction. When extracellular volume and composition return to normal, the diuresis usually abates spontaneously. Therefore, replacement of urinary losses should serve only to prevent hypovolemia, hypotension, or disturbances in serum electrolyte concentrations. Occasionally, iatrogenic expansion of extracellular volume, secondary to administration of excessive quantities of intravenous fluids, is responsible for, or sustains, the diuresis observed in the postobstructive period. Replacement of no more than two-thirds of urinary volume losses per day is usually effective in avoiding this complication. In a rare patient, however, relief of obstruction may be followed by urinary salt and water losses severe enough to provoke profound dehydration and vascular collapse. In these patients, an intrinsic defect in tubule reabsorptive function is probably responsible for the marked diuresis. Appropriate therapy in such patients includes intravenous administration of large quantities of salt-containing solutions to replace sodium and volume deficits.

REFERENCES

HARRIS RH, YARGER WE: The pathogenesis of post-obstructive diuresis. J Clin Invest 56:880, 1975

KAYE AD, POLLACK HM: Diagnostic imaging approach to the patient with obstructive uropathy. Semin Nephrol 2:55, 1982

KLAHR S et al: Urinary tract obstruction, in *The Kidney*, 3d ed, BM Brenner, FC Rector Jr (eds). Philadelphia, Saunders, 1986, p 1443

WILSON DR: Renal function during and following obstruction. Ann Rev Med 28:329, 1977

———: Urinary tract obstruction, in *Diseases of the Kidney*, 4th ed, RW Schrier, SW Gottschalk (eds). Boston, Little, Brown, 1988, p 715

234 TUMORS OF THE URINARY TRACT

MARC B. GARNICK / BARRY M. BRENNER

TUMORS OF THE KIDNEY

RENAL CELL CARCINOMA Renal cell carcinoma (renal adenocarcinoma, formerly ''hypernephroma'') accounts for 85 percent of all primary renal neoplasms. Approximately 18,000 new cases are diagnosed annually with 8000 deaths in the United States. The peak age incidence is between 55 and 60 years; the male-to-female ratio is 2:1. Environmental risk factors include exposure to cigarette smoke and cadmium. Hereditary forms of renal cell carcinoma, which are commonly multifocal and bilateral, occur in a high proportion of patients with von Hippel–Lindau disease (retinal and central nervous system hemangiomas, autosomal dominant transmission). The genetic defect associated with the disease has been identified. Marker chromosomal translocations between chromosomes 3 and 8 and 3 and 11 have been found in several kindreds with familial renal cancer. Patients with end-stage renal disease on chronic dialysis may develop renal cystic disease and associated renal carcinomas. Renal cell carcinoma arises from the proximal convoluted tubular epithelium. The term ''hypernephroma'' for renal cell carcinoma (reflecting the previously held notion of cellular origin from adrenal ''rests'') should be abandoned.

Clinical features Renal cell carcinoma has been called the ''internist's tumor'' because the lesion is often diagnosed, even in the absence of metastases, by its *systemic* rather than by urologic manifestations. The triad of *gross hematuria, flank pain,* and a *palpable abdominal mass,* although considered classic evidence for the clinical diagnosis, is encountered in less than 10 percent of cases; however, many patients demonstrate at least one of these manifestations. The most common presenting abnormality is *hematuria,* which occurs in 60 percent of cases. Although microscopic hematuria is a consistent abnormality of the urinary sediment, bleeding is not usually evident grossly, allowing the tumor to grow to a large size before clinical manifestations such as flank pain and fullness appear. Contiguous extension to the renal capsule, perirenal fat, lymph nodes, renal vein, inferior vena cava, and ipsilateral adrenal gland is common. The most common sites of distant metastases include lung, mediastinum, bone, central nervous system, thyroid, and liver.

Systemic symptoms of fatigability, weight loss, and cachexia occur in about 50 percent of patients. Intermittent fever, unassociated with infection, occurs occasionally and may be the only presenting sign. Anemia is present at the onset in approximately 50 percent of cases. Erythrocytosis is seen in about 5 percent of patients and has been linked to elaboration of erythropoietin. Eosinophilia, leukemoid reactions, thrombocytosis, and increased erythrocyte sedimentation rate also occur. Renal cell carcinomas may produce hormones or hormone-like substances, including parathyroid hormone and prostaglandins (which may lead to hypercalcemia), prolactin (galactorrhea), renin (hypertension), gonadotropins (feminization and masculinization), and glucocorticoids (Cushing's syndrome). In vascular tumors, intrarenal arteriovenous fistulas may predispose to high-output congestive heart failure. Tumor invasion of the renal vein and inferior vena cava may result in the development of abrupt, symptomatic left varicocele and lower extremity edema, respectively. Hepatic vein occlusion by tumor, with or without vena caval obstruction, may lead to hepatosplenomegaly and ascites. Disturbances in liver function (elevated alkaline phosphatase, hypoalbuminemia, and prolonged prothrombin time) are sometimes found in patients without demonstrable liver metastases and are often reversed following removal of the primary tumor.

Diagnosis (See Fig. 234-1) Although intrarenal calcifications and/or alterations in renal contours seen on the abdominal scout film may suggest the presence of a renal cell carcinoma, *intravenous pyelography* (IVP) with *nephrotomography* is the primary examination by which most renal masses are detected and evaluated. The major task is to differentiate cystic lesions from renal neoplasms. Splaying, distortion or nonvisualization of the collecting system, and distorted renal outlines suggest cancer. Nephrotomography provides clear delineation of renal borders and further aids in distinguishing cystic from solid lesions. *Ultrasonography* has improved the ability to distinguish cysts from renal neoplasms. When combined with nephrotomography, the accuracy of ultrasonography in diagnosing a benign cyst approaches 97 percent. If a cystic lesion on IVP, combined with a benign-appearing sonolucent cystic lesion on ultrasound, is found in an asymptomatic patient without hematuria, cyst puncture is probably unnecessary. Repeat IVP or ultrasound should then be performed periodically, initially every year and then, if no change has occurred during the interval, less often.

If diagnostic accuracy beyond 97 percent is required or if there are changes on repeat IVP or ultrasound, needle aspiration with evaluation of the aspirated fluid for cytology can be performed. The finding of clear yellow fluid or negative cytology usually supports the diagnosis of a simple cyst. Aspiration of cloudy or bloody fluid usually demands a surgical diagnosis, even though the cytology may be negative for cancer. A renal cystogram following aspiration can sometimes provide additional valuable information. Although renal cell carcinoma may coexist within a simple cyst, this is rare.

If the IVP or ultrasound examination demonstrates a lesion which does not satisfy the criteria for a benign, simple cyst, *computed tomography* (CT) is the next modality employed. CT is comparable and possibly superior to selective renal arteriography in both diagnosing and staging renal cell carcinoma. In addition, CT is equivalent to selective renal arteriography in the determination of renal vein involvement and superior to arteriography in determining whether regional nodes are enlarged (representing either tumor or hyperplasia) and/or the liver is involved. CT is the preferred modality for the diagnosis and staging of renal cell carcinoma. Thus, selective renal arteriography is not necessarily needed preoperatively. If, however, the findings on CT are equivocal or additional definition of vascular anatomy is required, renal arteriography should complement CT studies. Magnetic resonance imaging (MRI) has also been used extensively in the evaluation of renal masses. Its role compared to CT scanning is being defined.

OTHER STUDIES Evaluation of urinary cytology is not useful in the diagnosis of renal adenocarcinomas. Retrograde pyelography may be a useful adjunct for opacifying the collecting systems that are not

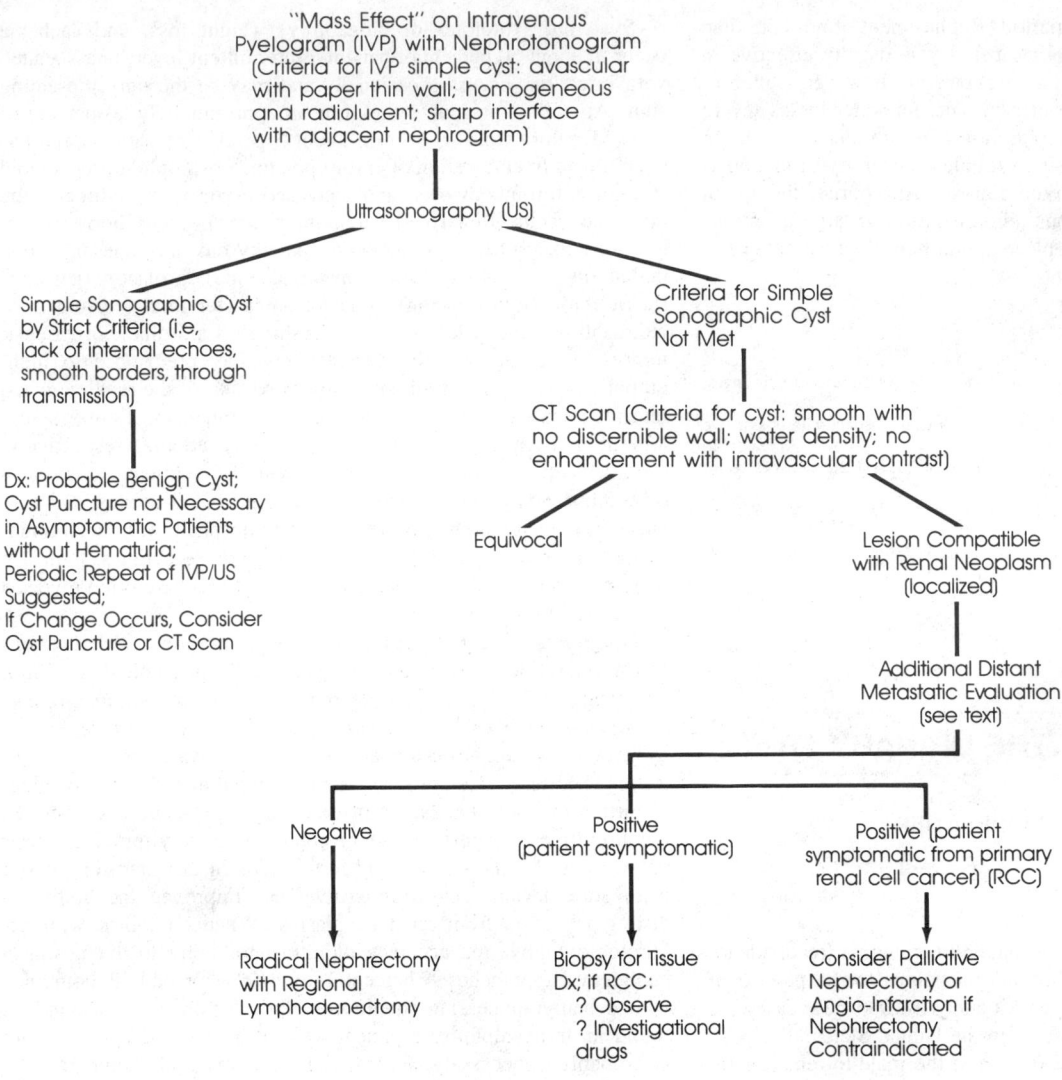

FIGURE 234-1   Diagnostic evaluation for renal mass.

filled by standard IVP and may suggest the diagnosis of transitional cell carcinoma of the renal pelvis. In patients who present with hematuria and a renal mass, cystoscopy is an important adjunct to exclude the coexistence of an unsuspected urothelial tumor, such as carcinoma of the bladder.

If the diagnosis of renal cell carcinoma is considered likely, the patient should then undergo routine chest x-ray, bone scan, and liver function studies, in addition to the abdominal CT, to evaluate other potential sites of tumor spread.

Staging, primary treatment, and prognosis   If there is no evidence of metastatic disease following the preoperative evaluation, the treatment of choice for renal cell carcinoma is radical nephrectomy. In addition to en bloc removal of the kidney with the surrounding Gerota's fascia, many urologic surgeons advocate regional lymphadenectomy to help determine prognosis. Preoperative arterial embolization of the main renal artery with a variety of agents may help to simplify the operative approach for large lesions. There is no role for localized pre- or postoperative radiation therapy.

Following surgical and pathologic evaluation, renal cell cancers are staged as follows: stage I, tumor confined within the kidney capsule; stage II, invasion through the renal capsule but confined within Gerota's fascia; stage III, involvement of regional lymph nodes, ipsilateral renal vein, or vena cava; stage IV, distant metastases. Five-year survival rates for stage I range from 60 to 75 percent; for stage II, 47 to 65 percent; for stage III without regional lymph node

involvement, 25 to 50 percent; with regional lymph node involvement, 5 to 15 percent; for stage IV, less than 5 percent.

Systemic therapy for metastatic disease   There is no standard chemotherapeutic, hormonal, or immunologic program for patients with metastatic renal cancer. Although early reports demonstrated a favorable effect using progestational or androgenic agents, there seems to be very little role for hormonal therapy of renal cell carcinoma. Commonly employed chemotherapy programs include the use of vinblastine sulfate, with or without the use of nitrosoureas. Interferons have been used with limited success. The use of interleukin 2 and lymphokine-activated killer cells (LAK cells) has been reported to be successful in selected patients. The management of patients with renal adenocarcinoma is investigational, and entry of patients into phase II clinical trials is encouraged.

Selected management of patients with metastatic disease There is little wisdom in hoping for spontaneous regression of metastases by removing the kidney of a patient who presents with stage IV renal cell carcinoma who is otherwise asymptomatic. If, however, the primary lesion is associated with pain, bleeding, or other paraneoplastic phenomena, it is sometimes useful to remove the primary tumor or to consider angioinfarction for local therapy despite the presence of metastatic disease. In patients who have had renal cell cancer in the past who then present with an isolated pulmonary or central nervous system metastasis, it is often useful to resect these metastases. Generally, patients selected for surgical nodulectomy have been disease-free for at least 1 year from the original diagnosis to the time of metastatic development and have tumors with a slow doubling time. On occasion, radiation therapy may offer palliation to painful bony lesions and may relieve an obstructed bronchus or ureter.

MISCELLANEOUS TUMORS OF THE KIDNEY In children, Wilms's tumor (nephroblastoma) is the most common cancer of the kidney. These tumors respond well to multimodality therapy including surgery, radiation, and combination chemotherapy, usually with dactinomycin and vincristine. Metastatic lesions to the kidney occur commonly in patients with lung and breast cancer and melanoma. Kidney involvement with malignant lymphoma, too, is common; however, functional renal abnormalities from parenchymal involvement are unusual.

Benign renal tumors are usually recognized as incidental findings at autopsy. However, on occasion, the lesion can cause persistent hematuria and, like the renal oncocytoma, can undergo malignant degeneration. These lesions are usually managed with nephrectomy when detected clinically. In newborns and infants, mesoblastic nephroma (fetal hamartoma) is the most common benign tumor and is successfully treated by simple nephrectomy.

TUMORS OF THE URINARY COLLECTING SYSTEM

The lining of the urinary collecting system from the renal pelvis to the urethra is made up of transitional cell epithelium or "urothelium." This entire lining is subject to carcinogenic influences which may explain the multicentric characteristics of urothelial neoplasms. Numerically, cancer of the bladder is the most common followed by tumors of the renal pelvis. Ureteral and urethral cancers are rare.

BLADDER CARCINOMA Approximately 40,000 new cases of bladder cancer are diagnosed annually with 11,000 deaths in the United States. Men are affected three times as frequently as women, and the disease is unusual in patients under 40 years of age. Epidemiology studies have demonstrated an increased incidence of transitional cell carcinoma following exposure to aromatic amines, particularly 2-naphthylamine. This probably accounts for the high incidence of urothelial cancers among cigarette smokers and workers in the dye, chemical, and certain rubber industries. Individuals with chronic, recurrent nephrolithiasis and recurrent upper urinary tract infections also have an increased incidence of urothelial cancers. Squamous carcinomas occur more frequently in patients with chronic infestation with *Schistosoma haematobium*. Squamous and adeno-carcinomas have a worse prognosis compared to transitional cell tumors. Long-term administration of the anticancer alkylating agent cyclophosphamide, which is metabolized to the active compounds acrolein and phosphoramide mustard, is associated with the development of urothelial neoplasms.

Clinical features Gross and microscopic hematuria are the most common presenting complaints (75 percent of patients); other features include dysuria, urinary frequency, and urgency (25 percent of patients), which may be the only manifestations of bladder cancer. Persistence of these symptoms in a previously asymptomatic patient deserves careful attention. Other manifestations, such as ureteral obstruction, pelvic pain, or symptoms from visceral or osseous metastases, occur in a minority of patients at presentation.

Diagnosis and staging Urinary cytology, obtained by examination of bladder washing, catheterized urine or voided urine, IVP, and cystoscopic evaluation with tumor biopsies and selected mucosal biopsies, as well as bimanual examination under anesthesia, are the mainstays for diagnosis of bladder cancer. Findings on IVP that suggest a bladder carcinoma include unilateral or bilateral ureteral obstruction with hydronephrosis, filling defect, or lack of distensibility of the bladder. Additional staging information may be obtained with abdominal or pelvic CT scanning. Following endoscopic resection of a bladder neoplasm, the depth of penetration into the bladder wall is

assessed. If additional staging workup, including physical examination, chest x-ray, and routine serum chemistries, are within normal limits, the patient is clinically staged, based upon the cystoscopic biopsy, as having either *superficial* or *invasive* disease. Additional information about perivesical extension or nodal metastases can be obtained at the time of cystectomy and indicates the true pathologic stage of disease. A substantial number of patients who are clinically staged endoscopically as having muscle-invasive disease will have occult lymphatic or distant metastases if surgically staged at the time of cystectomy. Such occult micrometastatic disease indicates systemic involvement and accounts for the high percentage of patients who eventually develop distant metastatic disease despite treatment of the primary bladder lesion.

Treatment Bladder cancer can be subdivided conceptually as being *superficial, invasive,* or *metastatic. Superficial carcinoma* of the bladder includes patients with carcinoma in situ, mucosal involvement (stage 0), or submucosal involvement (stage A). These patients are generally treated with endoscopic resection and selected bladder biopsies with repeat cystoscopic evaluations every 3 to 6 months. Approximately 50 to 70 percent of these patients have a superficial recurrence (limited to the mucosa or submucosa) within a period of 3 years following initial diagnosis. Patients with superficial recurrences are then often treated with intravesical therapies, including thiotepa, doxorubicin mitomycin, bacillus Calmette-Guérin (BCG) or interferons, in addition to cystoscopic resection. The use of intravesical therapy may decrease the number of superficial recurrences, but its effect on the natural history of the disease, in terms of preventing the development of invasive lesions, is unclear.

An additional 12 percent with initial superficial disease eventually develop progressive disease into the bladder muscularis (stage B), perivesical fat (stage C) or metastatic disease to lymph nodes (stage D1), bone, or other viscera (stage D2). Alternatively, patients may present initially with invasive or metastatic disease.

INVASIVE DISEASE These patients generally have extension of tumor into the muscle and/or perivesical fat. Traditional treatments are cystectomy (radical or simple), radiation therapy, or preoperative radiation therapy followed by cystectomy. Five-year survival rates are approximately 45 percent with such treatments. The majority of these patients die of distant metastatic disease despite radical surgery or radiation rather than from local recurrences. In addition, the use of multimodality therapy, including chemotherapy with radiation therapy, may spare individuals with invasive disease radical cystectomy. Surgical techniques, utilizing portions of the small bowel as bladder reservoirs, have enhanced the quality of life in individuals undergoing radical cystectomy. Such procedures allow continent urinary diversion (e.g., Koch pouch), thus eliminating the need for an external ostomy appliance.

METASTATIC DISEASE For patients who have distant metastatic disease in lymph nodes, viscera, or bone, the use of systemic chemotherapy has produced responses from 30 to 70 percent of patients, but usually not lasting more than 6 months. Following the development of metastatic disease, most patients die within 2 years. The most active agents include cisplatin, methotrexate, doxorubicin, cyclophosphamide, and vinblastine, and combinations of these agents have on occasion produced meaningful and durable remissions. One therapeutic strategy for patients with invasive disease consists of initiating chemotherapy followed by definitive local treatment to the bladder (surgery or radiation). The goal of such programs is to eradicate micrometastases that are commonly present in patients with invasive disease.

TRANSITIONAL CELL CANCER OF THE RENAL PELVIS Renal pelvic tumors account for approximately 10 percent of all primary renal cancer. Nearly 90 percent are transitional cell carcinomas. In addition to the etiologic associations implicated for bladder carcinoma, renal pelvic tumors also occur with analgesic abuse nephropathy. These patients are usually middle-aged women with a psychiatric history or chronic headaches who ingest >3 kg of analgesics over years. The exact amount and type of analgesic which induces transitional cell cancer of the renal pelvis is unknown, although aspirin and/or phenacetin can induce the disease experimentally.

Most patients present with painless, gross hematuria. Ureteral obstruction and pain secondary to clots are unusual. The diagnosis is suggested by IVP, which may demonstrate an obstructed, poorly functioning, or nonvisualized kidney or filling defects in a visualized kidney, and a positive urinary cytology. Cystoscopy and retrograde pyelography with brush biopsy generally establish the nature and location of the renal pelvic or ureteral tumor. For low-grade, low-stage tumors, conservative treatment with local excision and preservation of the kidney parenchyma is associated with favorable 5-year survival rates. For high-stage, high-grade lesions, the treatment of choice is radical nephroureterectomy and removal of the cuff of the bladder containing the ipsilateral ureteral orifice. This latter operative approach is dictated by the high likelihood of recurrence in the ureteral stump and orifice if not removed. In addition, routine follow-up with cystoscopies and urinary cytologies are mandatory to help detect the subsequent development of metachronous bladder carcinomas and/or contralateral ureteral and renal pelvic tumors. Five-year survival rates range from 10 to 50 percent. Although chemotherapy programs employed for bladder cancer have been used for patients with metastatic transitional cell carcinoma of the renal pelvis, the overall results are not as successful.

REFERENCES

Brodsky G, Garnick MG: Renal tumors in the adult patient, in *Renal Pathology*, CC Tisher, BM Brenner (eds). Philadelphia, Lippincott, 1989, p 1467

Chisholm GD, Roy RR: The systemic effects of malignant renal tumors. Br J Urol 43:687, 1971

Cronan J, Zeman RK: Renal mass imaging: The internist's role. Am J Med 81:1026, 1986

Cronin RE et al: Renal cell carcinoma: Unusual systemic manifestations. Medicine 55:291, 1976

Garnick MB (ed): Genitourinary cancer, in *Contemporary Issues in Clinical Oncology*, vol 5. New York, Churchill Livingstone, 1985

Hricak H: Detection and staging of renal neoplasms: A reassessment of MR imaging. Radiology 166:643, 1988

Kalish LA et al: A determination of appropriate endpoints in assessing efficacy of intravesical therapies in superficial bladder cancer. J Clin Oncol 5:2004, 1987

Rieselbach RE, Garnick MB (eds): *Cancer and the Kidney*. Philadelphia, Lea & Febiger, 1982

Sternberg CN et al: M-VAC (methotrexate, vinblastine, doxorubicin, and cisplatin) for advanced transitional cell carcinoma of urothelium. J Urol 139:461, 1988

West WH et al: Constant infusion recombinant interleukin-2 in adoptive immunotherapy of advanced cancer. N Engl J Med 316:898, 1987 section 1 **Disorders of the alimentary tract**

235 APPROACH TO THE PATIENT WITH GASTROINTESTINAL DISEASE

KURT J. ISSELBACHER / DANIEL K. PODOLSKY

BIOLOGIC CONSIDERATIONS The mucosal surface of the gastrointestinal tract comprises a remarkably dynamic population of epithelial cells that are highly developed in their capacity for transmembrane absorption and secretion. These secretory and absorptive abilities facilitate the essential role of the digestive tract in digestion and nutrient uptake, which must be accomplished while maintaining the barrier between the host and potentially harmful pathogens and mutagens in the lumen. The latter is accomplished through both the physical integrity of the intact mucosal surface and the extensive population of resident immune cells.

The intestinal surface itself also contains the distinctive M cells that serve to sample the antigenic milieu of the lumen. The predominance of suppressor lymphocytes within the surface epithelial layer (intraepithelial lymphocytes) suggests that dampening of the body's response to the enormous number of potentially antigenic substances in the lumen is necessary to prevent the constant and unrestrained activation of immune and inflammatory processes. Conversely, the presence of large numbers of helper lymphocytes as well as other cellular effectors of immune response in the lamina propria and submucosa attests to a large armamentarium ready to respond when surface defenses have been breached. No doubt the concentration of so many immune cells capable of attracting and activating inflammatory cells predisposes to the numerous inflammatory conditions to which the gastrointestinal tract is subject.

The mucosal surface of the gastrointestinal tract is also remarkable for the very rapid turnover of the epithelial cell population. It has been suggested that the surface epithelial cell populations turn over in their entirety every 24 to 72 h. This may permit rapid restitution of a functional cell population following an acute insult and may reduce the risk of malignancy through loss of cells affected by the many potential and actual mutagens in the luminal contents. Nevertheless, this proliferative potential must inherently create the setting for neoplastic disorders, which are so common to the gastrointestinal tract. Another fundamental feature of gastrointestinal mucosa is the spatial segregation of the proliferative compartment from the terminally differentiated cells. This is true throughout the gastrointestinal tract but is most apparent in the small intestine where a gradient of differentiation exists from the depths of the crypts of Lieberkühn to the villus tip. This organization is important in understanding the histology and pathophysiology of many mucosal disorders, e.g., nontropical sprue.

In view of the important secretory and absorptive activities of mucosal surface, diseases of the gastrointestinal tract may result in clinical consequences secondary to the physical disruption of the mucosal layer (e.g., blood loss, fluid loss, pathogenic invasion) or nutritional derangements due to impaired digestion and nutrient absorption. In focal or localized disease processes the former predominate, while the latter may be especially prominent in disorders that affect the gastrointestinal tract in a diffuse manner.

While the essential role of the gastrointestinal tract is the absorption of nutrients and excretion of the products is in large part accomplished at the luminal surface, these processes are also dependent on the deeper muscular layers for the coordinated propulsion of food through the lumen. The complexity of both local and distant neural and endocrine factors that contribute to the regulation of intestinal motility is only now becoming fully appreciated. Disruption of normal motility is quite common, with functional bowel complaints affecting as much as 15 percent of adult individuals. Alterations in frequency of bowel movements, abdominal distention, abdominal pain, and nausea, individually or in varying combinations, may result from dysmotility. In addition, structural lesions may also indirectly lead to symptoms through their impact on motility involving some or all regions of the gastrointestinal tract. These range from the *direct* effects of an obstructing lesion to the *indirect* actions of substances released by a primary mucosal disorder (e.g., inflammatory mediators such as arachidonic acid metabolites that also affect smooth-muscle activity).

Although valid unifying generalizations can be made about the gastrointestinal tract in its entirety, the spectrum of diseases affecting this system and their clinical manifestations are significantly related to the constituent organ(s) involved. Thus, esophageal disorders predominantly manifest through their relationship to swallowing, while gastric disorders are dominated by features relating to acid secretion, and disease of the small and large intestine by disruption of nutrition and alterations of bowel movements. Similarly, diseases of the related ancillary organs, the exocrine pancreas and the hepatobiliary system, present characteristic clinical challenges. Finally, it should be remembered that in addition to intrinsic disease, the gastrointestinal tract may be affected by systemic disorders. These include vascular, inflammatory, infectious, and neoplastic conditions leading to focal or diffuse structural lesions. Metabolic and endocrine abnormalities as well as drugs can disrupt normal bowel motility.

CLINICAL CONSIDERATIONS History A thorough clinical history is almost uniformly reliable in directing the clinician's attention to appropriate diagnostic considerations in the patient with gastrointestinal symptoms. The most common complaints resulting from disorders involving the gastrointestinal tract include pain, alteration in bowel habit, especially diarrhea and constipation, and indigestion. Among these, abdominal pain is the most frequent and variable and may reflect a broad spectrum of problems from the least threatening to the most urgent. Ascertaining the location (upper or lower, localized or diffuse), character (sharp, burning, cramping), and relationship of the pain to meals will often provide significant insight into the most important diagnostic considerations. If eating produces the symptom, the clinician should determine whether the discomfort occurs while eating (as in esophageal disorders and abdominal angina), shortly after the meal (as often occurs in biliary tract disease), or 30 to 90 min later (as typically seen in peptic disease). Pain that is not affected by eating suggests a process outside of the bowel lumen, such as an abscess, peritonitis, pancreatitis, and some malignancies. Conversely, identification of factors that relieve the symptom is also helpful, e.g., relief with eating or antacids is characteristic of peptic ulcer disease or gastritis. Relationship of the discomfort to bowel movement, especially in association with an altered bowel habit, should focus attention on a disorder of the small or large bowel such as inflammatory bowel disease.

Alterations in bowel habit can result either from disruption of normal intestinal motility or significant structural pathology. A thorough determination of the temporal evolution of the change and the nature of the alteration in conjunction with other constitutional symptoms such as weight loss, fever, or anorexia is important. Temporary variation in bowel habit in association with some life stress and in the absence of signs of systemic illness is suggestive of the common "irritable bowel syndrome," especially when the alteration varies between diarrhea and constipation. Small pellet-like stools are often described by the patient. Associated symptoms of bloating, nausea, and "gas" are also common. This diagnosis can essentially be made only on the basis of a thorough history and physical examination which exclude structural disease. In contrast, the onset of worsening constipation in an adult with previously regular habits, especially when accompanied by systemic symptoms such as weight loss, suggests the possible presence of an underlying obstructing process, particularly malignancy. If diarrhea is present, one should determine the average number of stools, their consistency, their pattern, and if any blood is present. Although *diarrhea* refers to an increased frequency of movements, patients will often use the term to describe loose or watery stools primarily. The occurrence of nocturnal or true bloody diarrhea almost always reflects structural rather than functional bowel disease. A pungent odor or the presence of undigested meat in the movement are suggestive of pancreatic insufficiency. An alteration in color can be seen in cholestasis or steatorrhea (light-colored) or hemorrhage (melenic to maroon or bright red). Mucus in the movement is usually a sign of functional bowel syndrome, while pus is more strongly suggestive of infectious or inflammatory disease. Less common but more dramatic are the symptoms of acute gastrointestinal bleeding, including hemetemesis, melena, and hematochezia, which usually leads to prompt efforts to find medical attention but should always be solicited by the clinician.

In the evaluation of male patients, especially those with diarrhea, a tactful inquiry into sexual activity is essential. Homosexual males are at increased risk for a large variety of gastrointestinal disorders as well as the acquired immunodeficiency syndrome, which may first manifest itself with gastrointestinal symptoms. Finally, careful attention must be given to a general medical history with an emphasis on any medications or nonprescription drugs that may have been used. Thyroid and other metabolic disorders, especially those affecting calcium metabolism, can cause a variety of gastrointestinal symptoms. Unless asked, patients may forget to mention that they take aspirin almost daily for headache, and this may account for occult blood found in the stool. The use of daily laxatives may explain chronic diarrhea.

Physical examination, endoscopy, and radiology All of the cardinal methods of examination are helpful in evaluating the patient with gastrointestinal symptoms. *Inspection* may disclose signs of cholestasis or nutritional deficiencies. An abnormal contour of the abdomen or inspection of the perianal region may manifest signs of a mass or a draining fistula. *Auscultation* is also important. A succussion splash can be elicited in the patients with symptoms of gastric outlet obstruction. The absence of bowel sounds or alteration

in pitch can lead to recognition of an evolving ileus or an obstructing process. A bruit may also be appreciated where there are symptoms of ischemic bowel disease. Careful *palpation* of the abdomen is especially important in detecting tenderness and masses, which in the appropriate clinical setting will lead to the recognition of cholecystitis, regional enteritis, periappendiceal abscess, and many other disorders. These findings will often be complemented by *percussion*, which is essential to assessing liver and spleen size. In addition to the examination of the abdomen, a carefully performed digital rectal examination is also essential. In the patient with complaints of incontinence the integrity of the sphincter can be assessed. Most importantly, masses intrinsic to the rectum as well as abnormalities in the pelvis or the pouch of Douglas may only be detected by this examination, and the presence or absence of frank or occult blood in the stool is always important diagnostic information. Sigmoidoscopy should be viewed as a routine extension of the physical examination in the patient with diarrhea or other alteration in bowel habit as well as in the patient with known or suspected blood loss from the lower bowel. This procedure, which can be performed with either the rigid sigmoidoscope or a flexible fiberoptic instrument, allows for direct inspection of the rectosigmoid mucosa permitting detection of cancers and polyps in this segment that may well be missed by barium x-rays. Inflammatory changes of the mucosa can help identify the patient with infectious dysentery or other forms of colitis, most notably ulcerative colitis. The findings of edema, granularity, and diffuse friability (easily induced mucosal bleeding) as well as superficial ulcerations are characteristic in the latter disorder. Fresh stool samples for microbiologic studies and superficial mucosal biopsies obtained at the time of sigmoidoscopy can also yield crucial diagnostic information.

Definitive demonstration or exclusion of structural lesions of the gastrointestinal tract, particularly the great majority of disorders that primarily affect mucosal surface, can often not be accomplished by physical examination alone. Many disorders of the upper or lower gastrointestinal tract are accessible to inspection through fiberoptic instruments. As a result, endoscopic studies are supplanting conventional contrast x-ray studies for many clinical problems, both because of the heightened precision of these diagnostic tools and the opportunity in some instances to accomplish a meaningful therapeutic intervention as an adjunct to the acquisition of diagnostic information. However, it should be emphasized that *no procedure should be considered routine* and used indiscriminately; there must be a rational basis for its use in the individual patient. These techniques are discussed in detail in Chap. 236. Upper gastrointestinal endoscopy permits evaluation of the esophagus, stomach, and duodenum and, with specially designed instruments, the proximal jejunum. When the clinical history warrants a diagnostic examination of the upper gastrointestinal tract for a structural lesion, endoscopic examination is preferable to radiologic study in most patients when the choice is available. Side-viewing scopes permit inspection and cannulation of the ampulla of Vater facilitating retrograde cholangiopancreatography. The colonoscope can be used to visualize the entire colon and often the terminal ileum, resulting in more accurate diagnosis of inflammatory bowel disease. Frequently colonic polyps can be removed at the time of initial colonoscopic identification.

While endoscopic techniques are relatively precise in defining many problems, the limitations of these tools as well as the continued advantages of x-ray studies in some situations should be recognized. Endoscopic tools are not useful in assessing gastrointestinal (GI) motility, which may be more accurately gauged by barium studies. In addition, some areas, notably the small intestine, remain relatively inaccessible to fiberoptic instruments. In hospitals where endoscopy is not feasible, the upper GI series and barium enema remain good diagnostic modalities for the upper and lower GI tract especially when air-contrast techniques are employed. However, they should generally be avoided in the patient with GI bleeding or suspected bowel obstruction. In addition the physician must exercise judgment in preparing the patient for these studies, recognizing that cathartics may markedly worsen the condition of a patient with obstructing lesions or colitis.

Although endoscopy has obviated the role for many conventional GI x-rays, other radiologic imaging modalities are assuming an increasingly crucial role in the approach to the patient with gastrointestinal symptoms. These techniques include ultrasound (US), computed tomography (CT), and magnetic resonance imaging (MRI). The application of these tools to the liver and biliary tract is discussed in Chap. 248. Both US and CT are useful in the delineation of abdominal masses. CT, though more expensive, is often more effective in the evaluation of the lower abdomen, where inflammatory masses in patients with Crohn's disease or complications of diverticular disease may be accurately imaged. MRI may permit exquisitely accurate information on the anatomic extent of invasive rectal cancers and blood flow in patients with vascular disorders, but the full range of its uses in GI disorders remains to be delineated.

Finally, one must emphasize that the optimal use of endoscopic and radiologic imaging techniques also depends on the recognition that each modality has inherent limitations. Only the clinician can determine whether the information is sufficient to establish or exclude a diagnosis in a patient with relevant historical and/or physical findings and a negative or nondiagnostic study. Was the preparation of the patient or the examination of sufficient quality to have detected an abnormality if present? Was the examiner aware of the important diagnostic considerations, and was the study adapted to address those concerns? Conversely only the physician can determine whether irregularities found in diagnostic studies are indeed causally related to the patient's symptoms. This judgment usually relies upon a sound understanding of the biologic basis of gastrointestinal disorders.

DIAGNOSTIC APPROACHES   Problems of swallowing   The approach should be as follows:

1 *Thorough determination of the nature of dysphagia.* Is the difficulty primarily in swallowing liquids, solids, or both? The location of the difficulty from the patient's perspective and presence or absence of accompanying odynophagia are important to ascertain. These historical clues are complemented by careful visual and neurologic examination of the oropharynx when appropriate.

2 *Routine esophageal x-rays* in the upright and lateral or Trendelenburg position. The horizontal views are essential for demonstration of the swallowing mechanism, unaided by gravity, and of the esophagogastric junction. For details of the pharyngoesophageal area cineradiography is necessary because of the rapidity with which the contrast medium passes through. Hiatus hernia is extremely common (in 15 to 35 percent of persons over 50) and often asymptomatic unless spontaneous reflux of gastric contents can be demonstrated to occur repeatedly. Careful attention is usually needed to detect lower esophageal rings or webs which may be visible as indentations in the barium column only from a limited angle.

3 *Esophagoscopy.* This procedure is desirable to describe lesions suggested by x-ray or, if the lesion is unsuspected, to obtain biopsies from masses or abnormal mucosa and to obtain washings for exfoliative cytologic study. The diagnoses of peptic esophagitis and Barrett's esophagus are made endoscopically. Endoscopy is the most sensitive technique for identifying esophageal or gastric varices, although they are seldom important in the absence of hemorrhage.

4 *Manometric studies* of the upper esophagus, particularly in conjunction with cineradiography. At present, this procedure offers the best differential between disorders primary in the central nervous system, primary pharyngeal muscular disease, and cricopharyngeal dystonia. Manometry of the lower esophagus is useful in the diagnosis of diffuse esophageal spasm, achalasia, and infiltrative diseases that can alter esophageal motility.

Peptic or digestive disorders   The approaches to these disorders include:

1 *Insertion of a nasogastric tube.* This is used to establish whether significant gastric retention (more than 75 mL of gastric contents in the fasting state) exists and whether there is acid, bile, blood, or other material in these contents. If pyloric obstruction or gastric atony is present, the tube is used to maintain suction while the patient's electrolyte and fluid balance is restored to normal; the stomach is kept as clean as possible so that reliable diagnostic investigation may be carried out.

2 *Upper intestinal endoscopy.* This procedure is most helpful in identifying the diffuse mucosa in gastritis or, together with biopsy and brushings for cytology, in differentiating between peptic and neoplastic ulcerating lesions. It may identify a specific bleeding site in clinical situations where several potential bleeding sites could exist, such as in the patient with portal hypertension. The significance of the described association of gastritis with *Campylobacter pylori* in patients with nonulcer dyspepsia, particularly the elderly, remains uncertain, but it can be detected by endoscopy and biopsy. Endoscopy can detect a number of potential sources of upper GI bleeding which are often missed by x-ray studies (e.g., erosive gastritis, Mallory-Weiss syndrome). Gastroscopy is also particularly helpful in inspecting the postoperative stomach, especially in detecting stomal ulceration or so-called alkaline reflux gastritis. The first and second portions of the duodenum can also be examined with the fiberoptic gastroscope, and important information about ulcers and other lesions can be obtained by this procedure. Radiologic studies may be useful when endoscopy is not readily available or in the assessment of suspected motility disorders (e.g., gastroparesis). In addition, radiologic examination may be preferred when there are contraindications to safe endoscopy.

3 *Gastric acid secretory studies.* These are useful in the diagnosis of the Zollinger-Ellison syndrome or atrophic gastritis and for determination of completeness of vagotomy. Suspected gastric carcinoma is better diagnosed directly through gastroscopy and biopsy than indirectly through acid secretory studies (achlorhydria). These studies should not be obtained for the routine diagnosis of uncomplicated duodenal ulcer. There is no convincing evidence that acid studies are useful in determining the type of surgery for duodenal ulcer.

Obstructive and vascular disorders of the small intestine   When intestinal problems present as obstructive syndromes, the plain x-ray of the abdomen is the most important diagnostic adjunct to careful physical examination. Patterns of dilatation of individual loops of intestine may be characteristic, as in volvulus or acute pancreatitis; erect and decubitus views will often show fluid levels in the affected segments. Motility disorders of the small intestine (temporary ileus or chronic intestinal pseudo-obstruction) may also present with obstructive symptoms and similar x-ray findings but must be managed medically without surgical intervention. Air under the diaphragm is diagnostic of a perforated viscus; air in the portal vein usually results from intestinal necrosis secondary to mesenteric vascular occlusion. The diagnostic accuracy of the plain x-ray in all types of intestinal obstruction is about 75 percent. In patients with symptoms of incomplete obstruction, the radiographic small-bowel series will often be diagnostic in defining the site and degree of obstruction. Infrequently, in this setting, all conventional x-ray studies are unremarkable. In such cases, the radiologist may perform a small-bowel enteroclysis study by passing a special tube into the proximal jejunum; the rapid instillation of barium through the tube will distend the intestine and often reveal subtle lesions missed by other tests.

Vascular diseases of the small intestine are among the most difficult diseases to diagnose. In chronic mesenteric ischemia, radiographic, endoscopic, and laboratory tests are usually normal. Early in the course of acute mesenteric ischemia, the plain film of the abdomen may be unremarkable despite complaints of severe abdominal pain. In these settings, prompt mesenteric angiography is essential in confirming the diagnosis of vascular disease.

Inflammatory and neoplastic diseases of small and large intestine   Patients with these conditions are usually identified by history, physical examination, and careful examination of the stools for exudate and blood. Examination of fresh stool samples for common bacterial pathogens and parasites by laboratories skilled in these techniques is important in identifying or excluding infectious causes of diarrhea, particularly in the patient with colitis. Sigmoidoscopy is valuable in identifying mucosal and neoplastic lesions of the lower 25 cm of the colon. The mucosal surface of the entire colon and terminal ileum can be examined directly and biopsied through the fiberoptic sigmoidoscope or colonoscope. The radiologic examination of the small intestine is highly reliable in identifying the prestenotic and stenotic lesions of Crohn's disease. In the colon a single barium enema examination in a well-prepared patient has a diagnostic accuracy of 80 to 85 percent; the addition of air-contrast technique brings the accuracy up over 90 percent, but none of these figures is meaningful if the patient is poorly prepared for the examination, and the cecal area is hard to examine adequately because of its anatomy. Colonoscopy may be preferable, if available, for its greater accuracy and the capability to remove the vast majority of polyps as well as to obtain preoperative tissue confirmation in the patient who probably has cancer. The immunologic assay for the carcinoembryonic antigen has not proved to be specific for colonic cancer; nevertheless, it does contribute to the detection of residual or recurrent disease in postoperative patients.

Peroral biopsy of the small intestine and forceps biopsy of the rectosigmoid are of considerable importance in revealing mucosal disease. Rectal biopsy is an excellent means of demonstrating amyloidosis, schistosomiasis, and amebiasis. Submucosal disease is not seen in these superficial biopsies. Hirschsprung's disease is histologically diagnosed by a deep surgical biopsy of the lower part of the rectum.

Malabsorption syndromes Malabsorption may be suspected on the basis of history and physical examination and is confirmed by examination of the stools. Radiologic examination is of general help in ruling out local lesions and suggesting motor and secretory dysfunction, but it is rarely diagnostic unless an abnormal small-bowel mucosa or fistulas between intestine and stomach are demonstrated.

The tests useful in the diagnosis of malabsorption are discussed in Chap. 240. A simple screening test for excessive fat in the stools can be accomplished by the microscopic examination of a stool specimen stained with Sudan. Chemical analysis of 3-day stool collection for fat, with the patient on a standard diet, is used to establish the diagnosis of steatorrhea. The D-xylose absorption test is about 90 percent accurate in separating mucosal disease from pancreatic insufficiency. Peroral biopsy of the small intestine is of value in the diagnosis of celiac disease, and it may show the less common infiltrations of the mucosa by amyloid or bacterial mucoproteins (Whipple's disease). Leakage of protein into the intestinal lumen may cause hypoproteinemia and can be demonstrated by the recovery in stools of the serum protein alpha$_1$ antitrypsin or intravenously administered markers such as albumin labeled with iodine or chromium isotopes.

Pancreas The pancreas is difficult to study directly because of its anatomic location and relative inaccessibility. Calcification of the pancreas on a plain abdominal film is highly suggestive of chronic pancreatitis and may be associated with fat malabsorption. Pancreatic exocrine insufficiency can be documented by intubation of the duodenum and collection of pancreatic juice after stimulation with secretin or a test meal. Abdominal ultrasound and CT are the best radiographic means of searching for pancreatic enlargement (see Chaps. 259 and 260). Both techniques may also be used to guide needle biopsies of the pancreas and may provide sufficient diagnostic information to obviate the need for exploratory surgery. The pancreatic duct can be cannulated via the fiberoptic duodenoscope and visualized by the injection of radiographic dye. Visualization of the duct may be helpful in the diagnosis of pancreatic pseudocysts, carcinoma, or chronic pancreatitis.

REFERENCES

Johnson LR et al: *Physiology of the Gastrointestinal Tract*, 2d ed. New York, Raven, 1987
Sleisenger MH, Fordtran JS: *Gastrointestinal Disease*, 4th ed. Philadelphia, Saunders, 1989

236 GASTROINTESTINAL ENDOSCOPY

MICHAEL B. KIMMEY / FRED E. SILVERSTEIN

Fiberendoscopes have revolutionized the examination of the gastrointestinal tract. Because of the flexibility of the fiberoptic bundles and because of controllability of the instrument tip, the operator can steer the instrument around multiple bends under visual control. A channel permits passage of a variety of endoscopic tools such as biopsy forceps, foreign-body forceps, cytology brushes, wash tubes, and electrocautery snares. The viewing window and the light at the instrument's distal end can be washed free of obscuring material. Fluid can be aspirated from hollow organs, and air can be insufflated as needed to improve visualization. The video endoscope is a modification of the fiberendoscope in which a charged coupled device on the distal tip of the instrument transmits the image onto a TV screen. This system is being increasingly used because it permits storage, analysis, and transmission of the endoscopic images.

The usefulness of fiberendoscopy in diagnosing gastrointestinal disease is well established. Shallow lesions such as erosions or healing ulcers are missed by single-contrast x-ray but not by endoscopy. The brilliant success of polypectomy via the colonoscope has led to the development of other endoscopic therapeutic techniques such as endoscopic sphincterotomy; endoscopic therapy is now a recognized alternative to surgery in many situations.

Although esophagogastroduodenoscopy (EGD) is not a procedure for the occasional operator, it should be available in every general hospital. It is a relatively easy procedure to perform technically, but training and continued experience are necessary for optimal diagnostic accuracy. Complications are most frequent when the operator is inexperienced. Before the procedure the competent endoscopist always takes a history and examines the patient. Particular attention to cardiac, pulmonary, and blood clotting functions is essential.

The more complex procedures such as colonoscopy and endoscopic retrograde cholangiopancreatography (ERCP) require special dexterity, a substantial investment of time for learning, and constant practice to maintain adequate skill; they are probably best accomplished by subspecialists.

UPPER GASTROINTESTINAL ENDOSCOPY Here forward-, oblique-, and side-viewing instruments may be used for EGD. After a careful explanation of the procedure to the patient, pharyngeal topical anesthesia with viscous lidocaine or various anesthetic sprays is followed by intravenous diazepam to the point of mild sedation. With small-caliber instruments less or no diazepam is needed. The tip of the endoscope is placed at the cricopharyngeal sphincter of the esophagus and the patient is encouraged to swallow while gentle pressure is exerted. Small amounts of air are passed through the endoscope to visualize the esophageal lumen. The endoscope is then passed under direct vision into the stomach. The gastric body and antrum are carefully examined. The instrument tip is retroflexed to view the gastric cardia, the fundus, and the whole lesser curvature. The pylorus is traversed, and the first and second portions of the duodenum are visualized. The examination is repeated as the instrument is withdrawn. Visualized lesions can be recorded on photographs or videotape. Biopsies and brush cytologic examinations can be obtained from suspicious areas.

EGD is a relatively safe procedure in experienced hands. Several large surveys suggest a risk of serious complications during diagnostic EGD of approximately 1 in 800 and a risk of death of approximately 1 in 5000. The risks are higher in emergency procedures and in the elderly or seriously ill. In a survey of patients examined by endoscopy during bleeding, 1 in 200 had serious complications and 1 in 700 died from the procedure. The main causes of mortality were cardiopulmonary complications and perforations by the instrument. Endoscopy is preferred over x-ray in the urgent diagnosis of gastrointestinal illness in women who might be pregnant.

Gastroesophageal reflux disease Esophagitis is one of the commonest diseases of the upper gastrointestinal tract (see Chap. 237). Esophageal pain may be confused with cardiac disease, or esophagitis may present as painless blood loss. Because esophagitis usually involves only the superficial mucosa, it cannot be diagnosed by routine single-contrast radiography. At endoscopy, friable mucosa, linear erosions, and ulcerations of erosive esophagitis are clearly visible. Not every patient with heartburn requires esophagoscopy, but the procedure is indicated if the patient complains of dysphagia, if an x-ray shows a stricture, a mass, or an ulcer, if symptoms persist despite therapy, or if antireflux surgery is contemplated.

The squamous mucosa of the esophagus is more vulnerable to peptic digestion than is the columnar epithelium of the stomach. Thus, esophagitis is located on the squamous side of the esophagogastric junction and is most severe in the distal esophagus where the squamous mucosa is most exposed to regurgitated acid and pepsin from the stomach. Discrete peptic ulceration of the esophagus is uncommon.

A short area of esophagitis or a stricture can be seen at levels as high as the arch of the aorta. This is explained by progressive replacement of distal eroded squamous mucosa with metaplastic epithelium, which is more resistant to peptic digestion (Barrett's epithelium). This finding can be documented by biopsy. Such epithelium is more prone to malignant transformation and, therefore, may merit regular surveillance with esophagoscopy and biopsy every 12 to 24 months. If dysplasia is present, more frequent surveillance may be indicated to detect carcinoma.

Esophagitis may progress to scarring and stricture formation. The endoscopic appearance of a benign stricture is characteristic but not diagnostic; a malignancy should be ruled out by biopsy and cytologic brushing before medical treatment is undertaken with dilation and antacids. The whole length of the stricture should be sampled. Endoscopy is also indicated to biopsy the rim of an esophageal ulcer to rule out cancer.

Dilations of difficult strictures are best initiated by passing a flexible-tipped guidewire via the biopsy channel of the endoscope through the stricture under direct vision. The endoscope can then be withdrawn over the wire, which serves as a guide for passage of progressively larger polyvinyl dilators through the stricture under fluoroscopic control. An alternative technique utilizes balloon catheters passed via the endoscope channel or over a guidewire through the stricture. The balloon is inflated under endoscopic and/or fluoroscopic guidance to dilate the stricture.

Peptic ulcer Esophagogastroduodenoscopy is more accurate than upper gastrointestinal x-ray in detecting ulcers. It has been suggested that x-ray be abandoned entirely in favor of endoscopy for detecting ulcers. This makes sense when the source of acute upper gastrointestinal bleeding is sought and urgent surgical intervention is being considered. However, in the workup of the patient with less pressing ulcer complaints, an upper gastrointestinal x-ray is still often used as the initial diagnostic test. As more radiologists routinely use air contrast to obtain better mucosal detail, diagnostic sensitivity for superficial lesions will increase. The greater expense and discomfort of endoscopy are justified if the x-ray is equivocal, or suggests that the ulcer is malignant, if the x-ray is negative but the clinical picture suggests peptic ulceration, or if the patient is about to be operated on for ulcer. Patients with duodenal ulcers shown by x-ray or with classic ulcer deformities of the duodenal bulb do not require endoscopy for diagnosis if the presenting symptoms are characteristic and if the symptomatic response to antiulcer treatment is good. Screening endoscopy using small-diameter endoscopes without sedation is a reasonable alternative to contrast x-rays as the initial diagnostic test in the symptomatic patient.

There are some situations in which x-ray reveals ulcers missed by endoscopy, e.g., ulcers in hourglass constrictions of the stomach or in small, incompletely visualized duodenal bulbs. Fiberendoscopy is especially useful in visualizing postbulbar ulcers, giant duodenal ulcers, and stomal ulceration after partial gastrectomy, all of which can be missed by x-ray. Endoscopy may be of use in determining the cause of gastric outlet obstruction. In most circumstances, patients with duodenal ulcers do not need follow-up endoscopy to see if the ulcer has healed.

In the enthusiasm for fiberendoscopy one must not forget that visual interpretation of gross pathology is subjective—one observer's ulcer is another's erosion. An erosion is confined to the mucosa and heals without a trace, whereas an ulcer is deeper and usually implies a chronic recurrent disease. Endoscopically, erosions are superficial, small, and multiple; ulcers are deeper and larger and tend to be solitary. In the future it is likely that lesions seen endoscopically will be easily recorded for review on videotape or disk, just as currently all lesions seen fluoroscopically are demonstrated in spot films.

Cancer The endoscopic appearance of upper gastrointestinal cancer may seem obvious, especially if there is a mass growing into the lumen. On the other hand, malignant ulcers, infiltrative carcinomas, or small early carcinomas are frequently impossible to diagnose by their gross appearance. Six to eight biopsies should be taken from the rim of a gastric ulcer to exclude malignancy. Experience and skill in choosing the biopsy site improves the accuracy. A cytologic examination of lavage or brush specimen adds to the diagnostic accuracy in all areas of the upper gastrointestinal tract (see Chap. 239).

In most patients gastric ulcers should be assessed for healing by endoscopy after 12 weeks of antiulcer therapy. Persistent ulcers should be biopsied if they were not biopsied at the time of the initial diagnosis. Some patients with a low likelihood of malignancy, for example, a young person taking anti-inflammatory drugs, can be assessed for healing radiographically.

Primary gastric lymphoma can mimic benign gastric ulcer or adenocarcinoma on gastroscopy or x-ray. It can be diagnosed by biopsy or cytology, although the accuracy is not as high as in adenocarcinoma. The 5-year survival for lymphoma is higher than for adenocarcinoma.

If a polypoid lesion of the stomach is covered by mucosa that appears normal by gastroscopy, the likelihood of malignancy is very small. Such lesions are often intramural, extramucosal benign tumors such as leiomyomas or pancreatic rests. Polyps covered by abnormal-appearing mucosa can be benign or malignant. Random biopsy can miss carcinoma within a polyp. If technically feasible, polyps should, therefore, be removed in their entirety by snare cautery for histologic examination. If over 2 cm in diameter, they are more likely to contain cancer (see Chap. 239). Large polyps may require surgical excision.

Ampullary carcinoma may be diagnosed by biopsy during duodenoscopy although a prior endoscopic sphincterotomy may increase diagnostic yield. Other primary duodenal malignancies are very rare. Extensions from pancreatic or biliary tract cancer are difficult to diagnose because the tumor may not have extended into the mucosa and may therefore not be accessible for endoscopic biopsy or cytologic examination. In these secondary tumors, diagnosis must depend upon some combination of echography, hypotonic duodenography, selective pancreatic angiography, and endoscopic retrograde cholangiopancreatography, with cytologic examination of ductal contents.

Upper gastrointestinal bleeding (See also Chap. 46) Endoscopy within the first 12 to 24 h of an upper gastrointestinal hemorrhage can be very helpful in planning rational therapy by visualizing the bleeding source. Shallow lesions not visible by x-ray may be seen (esophagitis, Mallory-Weiss tear, erosive gastritis, shallow stress ulcer, and telangiectasia). Lesions that are visible by x-ray may not be the source of bleeding. Only endoscopy can determine the actual bleeding site. For example, visualization of a spurting artery which is flooding the stomach indicates massive ongoing bleeding requiring prompt therapeutic intervention. Several studies have shown that the demonstration at endoscopy of any bleeding whatsoever or a non-bleeding vessel or sentinel clot in the ulcer base makes rebleeding more likely.

A conservative estimate of the diagnostic accuracy of emergency endoscopy in upper gastrointestinal bleeding is 80 to 85 percent. Endoscopic diagnosis of bleeding erosive gastritis may be made too frequently when blood from another unsuspected source spreads over the gastric mucosa or when trauma from overly vigorous antecedent lavage creates submucosal ecchymoses. To avoid overdiagnosis of erosive gastritis, portions of the gastric wall should be washed free of blood to determine the true appearance of the underlying gastric mucosa.

Every patient having endoscopy for upper gastrointestinal bleeding merits a complete endoscopic examination of the esophagus, stomach, and duodenum. Finding a potential bleeding lesion is not proof that this is the source of hemorrhage unless active bleeding is seen. Up to 50 percent of patients with esophageal varices can be shown endoscopically to be bleeding from another source such as erosive gastritis, duodenal ulcer, or gastric ulcer. Occasionally it is not possible to diagnose the exact lesion that is bleeding, but localizing the area of bleeding can be very helpful; for example, bright red arterial blood may be seen pouring into the stomach from the duodenum when the esophagus and stomach are relatively free of blood.

There are three controversial areas. First, *do all bleeders need endoscopy?* Endoscopy is indicated in all patients who may require surgery because of continual bleeding or rebleeding because selection of the type of operation depends on what lesion is bleeding. Although 85 percent of upper gastrointestinal bleeders stop spontaneously, it is impossible to predict which ones will; therefore, endoscopy is recommended for most bleeders. Second, *how early should endoscopy be performed in the acutely bleeding patient?* Most studies suggest that the diagnostic accuracy of esophagogastroduodenoscopy remains high for the first 12 to 24 h after the bleeding episode. All would agree that it is desirable to delay endoscopy until vital signs have been stabilized after adequate blood replacement. Upper endoscopy is usually performed during waking hours at a time during the first day of bleeding when the patient's vital signs are stable and when the full endoscopic team is available. Emergency endoscopy at night should be reserved for those patients with continued massive bleeding or rebleeding requiring an immediate decision regarding surgery or other treatment. If the patient is exsanguinating, endoscopy can follow induction of anesthesia just preceding surgery. Thus, the patient's airway is protected by an endotracheal tube. Finally, *does endoscopy affect the clinical outcome?* Earlier studies suggest that it does not. Recent studies of the endoscopic treatment of bleeding lesions with heater probes and bipolar probes suggest that these methods are safe and reduce blood requirements, need for surgery, and mortality in some patients with bleeding ulcers.

Injection therapy of bleeding lesions is another therapeutic modality used to stop bleeding. Injection of a dilute solution of epinephrine followed by injection of either alcohol or a sclerosing agent often stops active bleeding from peptic ulcers. Injection of various sclerosing solutions into or next to esophageal varices is currently the treatment of choice for stopping active variceal bleeding. Repeated injection sclerotherapy to achieve variceal eradication produces results comparable to portacaval shunting in terms of mortality, although rebleeding after sclerotherapy may necessitate further sclerotherapy or shunting.

Emergency and therapeutic endoscopy is not for the inexperienced. It requires considerable technical skill and interpretive experience and the best available instruments.

Percutaneous endoscopic gastrostomy The placement of feeding or decompression gastrostomy tubes can be facilitated with the use of an endoscope. Under sedation, the endoscope's light within the stomach is used to identify a suitable location for a gastrostomy in the left upper quadrant of the abdomen. A needle is introduced into the stomach percutaneously and then a snare passed through the endoscope is used to capture a wire or suture placed through the needle. A feeding tube is advanced over the wire into the stomach. Feedings are begun the following day. Hospitalization time and morbidity and mortality associated with operative gastrostomy is reduced.

Patients with transfer dysphagia secondary to strokes and degenerative neurologic disorders benefit the most from this procedure. Other indications for percutaneous endoscopic gastrostomy include dysphagia produced by head and neck neoplasms, and the inability to eat secondary to diffuse cerebral injury. Patients with severe gastroparesis can be fed through a jejunal feeding tube placed through the gastrostomy and then directed through the pylorus. Simultaneous gastric decompression is possible through a separate lumen in the gastrostomy.

Palliation of esophageal carcinoma Patients with dysphagia caused by malignant esophageal strictures usually cannot be cured by esophagectomy. Surgical resection and radiation therapy are often chosen for palliation of dysphagia in this situation. The endoscopist can also help palliate these patients when radiation therapy has failed or when surgical risks are too great.

Dilatation of malignant strictures is usually possible with polyvinyl dilators passed over an endoscopically placed guidewire. Dilatation may improve the patient's swallowing initially, but more definitive therapy is usually needed. This can be in the form of laser ablation or by placement of a prosthesis or stent. Tumor within the esophageal lumen can be destroyed by application of Nd:YAG laser energy using a laser waveguide placed through the biopsy channel of the endoscope. Alternatively, after stricture dilatation large-caliber stents can be placed over a dilator. When the dilator is removed, the stent lumen is available for the passage of food. Stenting is especially useful in the palliation of malignant tracheoesophageal fistulas.

Other indications Upper endoscopy is usually substituted for x-ray in the urgent diagnosis of gastrointestinal illness in *pregnancy.* Patients with *dysphagia* merit esophagoscopy because the cause is frequently organic and may be missed by x-ray. Dysphagia caused by esophageal spasm or dysrhythmia is best diagnosed by manometry or cineradiography in addition to endoscopy. *Painful swallowing* (odynophagia), especially in immunosuppressed or diabetic patients, may merit esophagoscopy because biopsy and brushings of the involved esophageal wall may reveal monilial, herpetic, or cytomegalic virus infections. Soon after ingestion of a corrosive agent, if there is no indication of wall necrosis, limited and gentle esophagoscopy is useful in evaluating the severity of injury. Many impacted foreign bodies can be removed from the esophagus or stomach with a snare or forceps; sharp foreign bodies are usually best removed by pulling them into the lumen of a rigid tubular esophagoscope or by pulling them into a protective overtube around a fiberoptic endoscope. Careful esophagoscopy after removal of an esophageal foreign body is important to determine whether there is an underlying lesion which caused the impaction (e.g., cancer, benign stricture, peptic esophagitis).

In the postoperative stomach, gastroscopy is especially useful in detecting carcinoma, recurrent ulceration, retrograde intussusception, and stomal stricture. Several European studies indicate a definite threat of carcinoma developing in the gastric stump 10 to 20 years after a Billroth II gastrectomy. The diagnosis of such postoperative carcinomas may require many biopsies of seemingly normal mucosa near the anastomosis. Studies of the natural history of this condition in the United States do not suggest a similar high incidence of postoperative carcinoma.

When the duodenal bulb shows reddening or nodularity, many endoscopists diagnose *duodenitis.* There is little evidence to suggest

COLOR ATLASES

Atlas 1   Atlas of common lesions encountered during the physical examination of the skin

Atlas 2   Atlas of infectious diseases

Atlas 3   Atlas of endoscopic findings

Atlas 4   Atlas of fundoscopic examination

Atlas 5   Atlas of hematology

The skin and mucous membrane may frequently contain a variety of lesions that are rarely a major complaint (see Fig. 47-1). They are, therefore, incidental findings in the general physical examination. The recognition of "bumps and blemishes" is a necessary first step for physicians inasmuch as they will be required to distinguish the trivial from the serious and important skin changes. For example, such a serious lesion as a malignant melanoma may be incidentally discovered during a routine physical examination (see Figs. A1-30 to A1-32 and the discussion in Chap. 302).

The common disorders of the skin that every physician should be able to recognize are presented in this series of color photographs (Figs. A1-1 to A1-23).

A1-1 **Dermatofibroma** is especially common in middle life and in women. The lesions, when pigmented, are occasionally confused with malignant melanoma. They appear as isolated, slightly elevated, hard, button-like nodules (*A*). In fair-skinned persons, the lesions are not usually skin color, but are pink or dark red, yellowish brown, or gray-black. They are usually less than 1 cm in diameter. A diagnostic sign is that a dermatofibroma dimples or becomes depressed (*B*) when it is laterally compressed; melanocytic nevus and melanoma, however, with which dermatofibroma may be easily confused, become elevated with lateral compression.

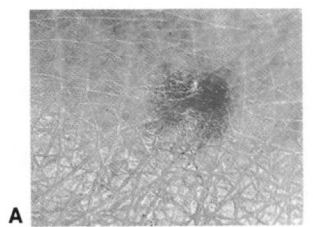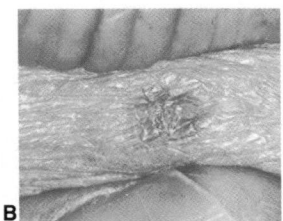

A   B

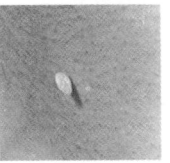

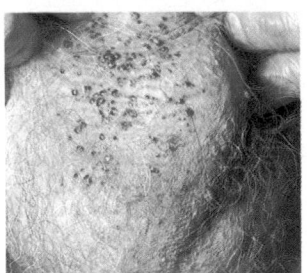

A1-2 **Acrochordon** (skin tag) is very common after middle life and appears on the neck, especially in women, in the axillae, and on the upper part of the trunk. The lesions are small (1 to 5 mm), soft, pedunculated papules, usually of normal skin color.

A1-3 **Angiokeratomas** are bizarre vascular dilatations that occur under the tongue and on the scrotum and consist of myriads of 2- to 3-mm purplish red papules. They are of no known significance. When they occur on the trunk and extremities, a biopsy is indicated to rule out glycolipid lipidosis or Fabry's disease.

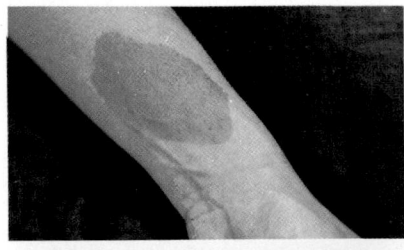

A1-4 **Café au lait macules** are found in about 10 percent of the normal population and, in fair-skinned persons, are light yellowish brown macules, which may also be markers of neurofibromatosis and polyostotic fibrous dysplasia (Albright's syndrome). The presence of six or more café au lait macules with a diameter of 1.5 cm or greater is diagnostic of neurofibromatosis.

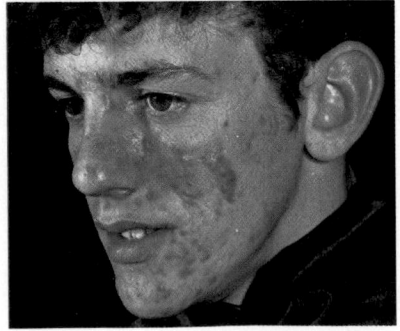

A1-5 **Acne** is a condition in which the most characteristic lesion is the comedo, or "blackhead," that later becomes a conical erythematous papule or pustule. A third type of lesion is the "blind boil," which is a dermal cyst without an orifice. This lesion is often associated with atrophic or hypertrophic scarring. Cystic acne may appear with only a very few comedones; also, comedo-like acne may occur with few cysts or erythematous papules.

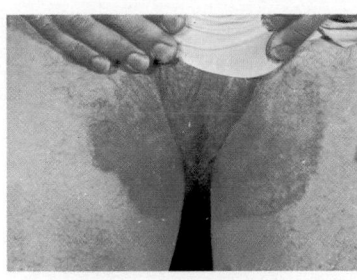

Al-6 **Dermatophytosis** is identified by the striking polycyclic, annular shape of the scaling, especially on the feet and hands, where there is often a scalloped pattern. A positive diagnosis of dermatophytosis is quickly established by direct examination of scales from the advancing border; the mycelia are revealed when the scales are immersed in 10% potassium hydroxide or Swartz stain.

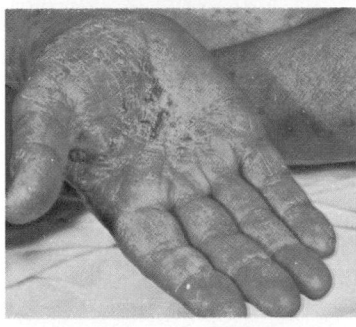

Al-7 **Eczematous dermatitis** is a very common cutaneous reaction that is localized to the hands of housewives, to the legs in patients with chronic venous insufficiency, and behind the ears in patients with seborrheic dermatitis. In subacute eczematous dermatitis, there are mild erythema, dry scales, and often small red papules, many of which are excoriated. In chronic eczematous dermatitis, lichenification is the most prominent feature.

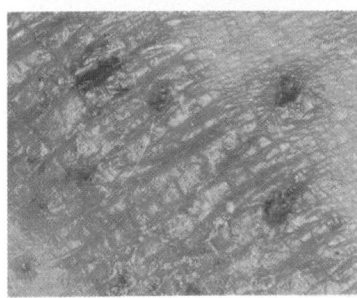

Al-8 **Localized lichenification** results from repeated rubbing of the skin and consists of isolated, circumscribed plaques. These single lesions vary in size from 2 to 10 cm and occur most often on the extensor aspect of the forearm and in the scrotal, nuchal, inguinal, and anogenital areas. The perianal and vulvar areas may become diffusely lichenified. Lichenification is thought to be more frequent in persons with an atopic background.

Al-9 **Melasma (chloasma)** is the so-called "mask" of pregnancy, but it also occurs in men and in women taking progestational agents. The pigmentation is uniform and is limited to the exposed areas of the face. There is no scaling or epidermal change. In fair-skinned persons, the pigment may be any shade from light tan to a very dark brown. It is most often seen on the cheek and upper lip, as here, and on the forehead.

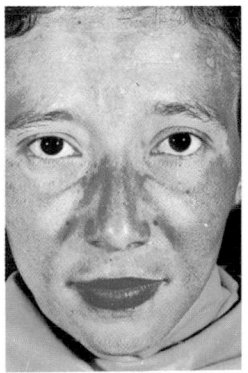

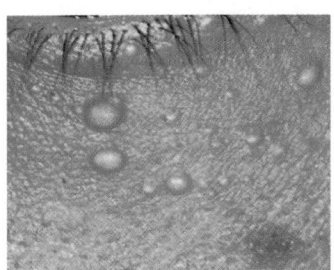

Al-10 **Milia** are a collection of lesions, occurring most commonly on the face, and consist of tiny (1 to 2 mm), white, hard, rounded, superficial papules. There is no orifice, and the keratinous contents are easily expressed by lateral compression after the making of a tiny incision in the dome of the lesion.

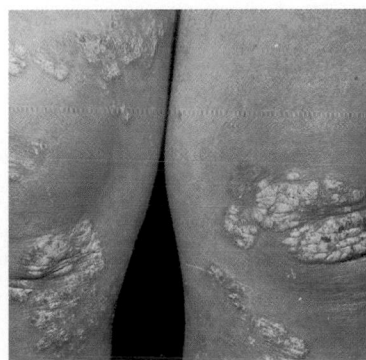

Al-11 **Psoriasis,** affecting more than 2 percent of the population, consists of isolated scaling papules or plaques and is quite commonly observed in the routine physical examination. The lesions occur most frequently on the scalp, elbows, and knees. The color and type of scales are the identifying features of the lesions. The scales are either dense and lamellated with peripherally detached edges or loose and branny. The plaques are pink to deep red, and the borders are distinct.

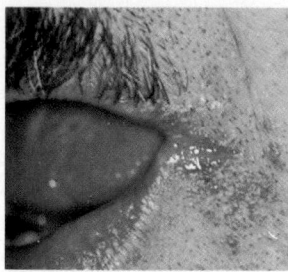

A1-12 **Perlèche** consists of painful small fissures at the angles of the mouth, often covered with yellow crusts. Perlèche most often occurs with poorly fitting dentures and in moniliasis and secondary syphilis.

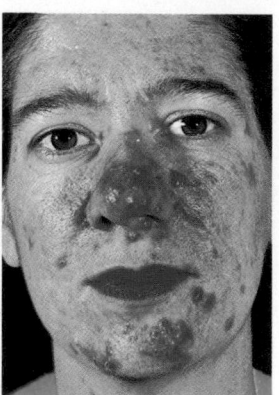

A1-13 **Rosacea,** usually limited to the face, consists of tiny, erythematous papules and pustules 1 to 5 mm in size. The pustules, often tiny and sometimes hardly visible, sit on the dome of the papules. The diffuse redness of the face is due to vasodilatation, as well as to myriad telangiectases. In men, rhinophyma, a disfiguring enlargement of the nose, may occur.

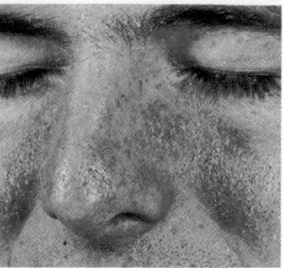

A1-14 **Seborrheic dermatitis,** a common disorder found in all age groups, occurs most frequently on the scalp, eyebrows, and nasolabial folds and behind the ears. Scaling is the prominent feature and is loose and branny; it may be yellow and oily or dry and white. The lesion may become exudative and crusted or eczematous.

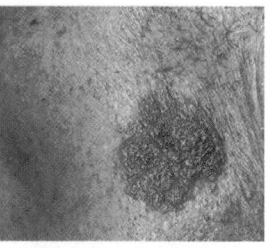

A1-15 **Seborrheic keratosis** appears in middle life and may occur on exposed or unexposed areas but is especially common on the trunk. The lesions are irregularly round or oval flat-topped papules or plaques that seem "stuck" on the skin. The margins are distinct, and the surface is often warty or consists of multiple tiny projections (vegetation). In fair-skinned persons, the lesions are light brown at first but, enlarging, become more heavily pigmented and may be confused with malignant melanoma.

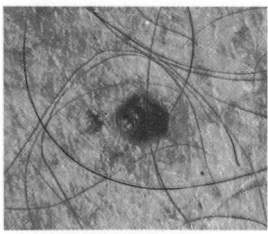

A1-16 **Senile angioma ("cherry red spot")** appears in the third decade. On the lip, the lesion is usually singular and consists of a bluish red round nodule. On the trunk, the lesions are small (2 to 3 mm), bright red, globular papules.

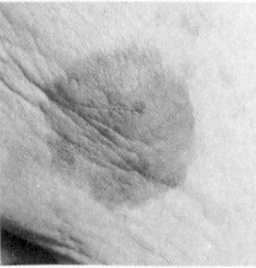

A1-17 **Senile lentigo** occurs as a single macule or as a group of isolated, sharply circumscribed macules on the exposed areas, especially on the dorsal surfaces of the hands and arms and on the forehead and cheeks. The macules are usually light yellowish brown, but may be dark brown; the color is somewhat variegated, rather than uniform as it is in a café au lait macule. Rarely, dark brown *papules* develop in these lesions, and then the condition is called *lentigo maligna,* which may slowly develop, over a period of years, into a melanoma (lentigo maligna melanoma).

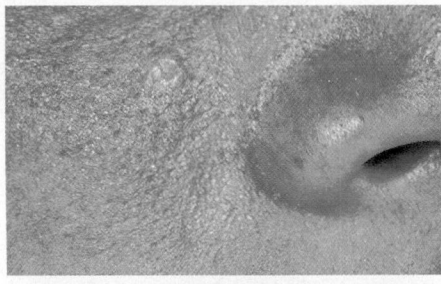

A1-18 **Senile sebaceous adenoma** occurs on the face in patients over 40 and is often diagnosed as basal-cell carcinoma. The lesions are soft, small, flat-topped papules, varying in size from 1 to 8 mm, and are characterized by a minute central depression from which sebaceous material can be exuded by lateral compression.

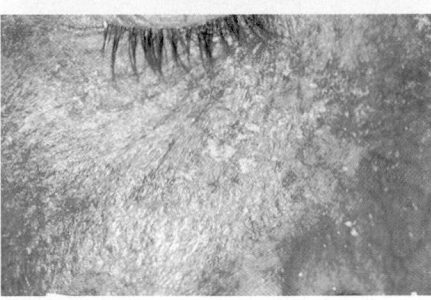

A1-19 **Solar keratosis** (1) occurs usually in persons with light skin prone to sunburn or with darker skin after chronic excessive exposure; (2) is strictly limited to exposed skin, especially on the face and dorsal surfaces of the hands; (3) is more easily felt than seen (gritty and sandpaperish); (4) in fair-skinned persons, consists of skin-colored or light brown macules or slightly raised papules with superficial adherent scales not easily removed; and (5) is associated with marked wrinkling, telangiectasia, and often diffuse, tiny, pale yellow papules indicating solar degeneration of connective tissue ("turkey skin").

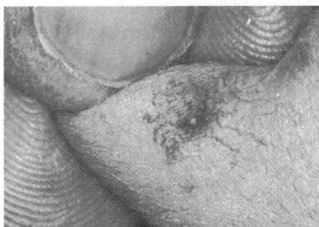

A1-20 **Spider nevus** consists of a central, punctate, bright red macule or papule (the body) from which fine red lines radiate like spider legs. There is often a red flare between the radiating vessels. On diascopy, the central body pulsates.

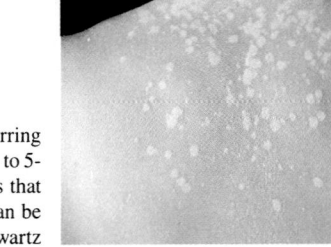

A1-21 **Tinea versicolor** is a relatively common disorder occurring primarily on the trunk and appearing in two forms: as scattered, 3- to 5-mm, very slightly scaling brown macules or as whitish macules that may be confused with vitiligo. The fungal spores and hyphae can be easily demonstrated on direct examination of the scales using Swartz stain.

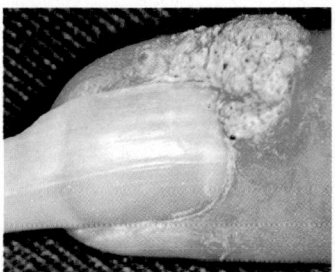

A1-22 **Verruca vulgaris** may occur at any age, but it is most common in children. The lesions, which vary in size from 0.5 to 2.0 cm, are round or oval, firm, skin colored papules with multiple tiny keratotic, rounded or filiform projections covering the surface (vegetation). They occur most frequently on the hands and soles.

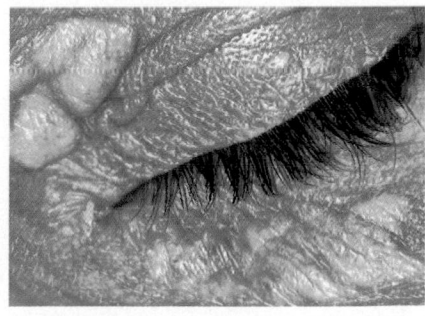

A1-23 **Xanthelasma** consists of one or more bright yellow, sharply marginated plaques with no epidermal change, usually occurring on the eyelids. All patients with xanthelasma should be investigated for evidence of plasma lipid abnormalities.

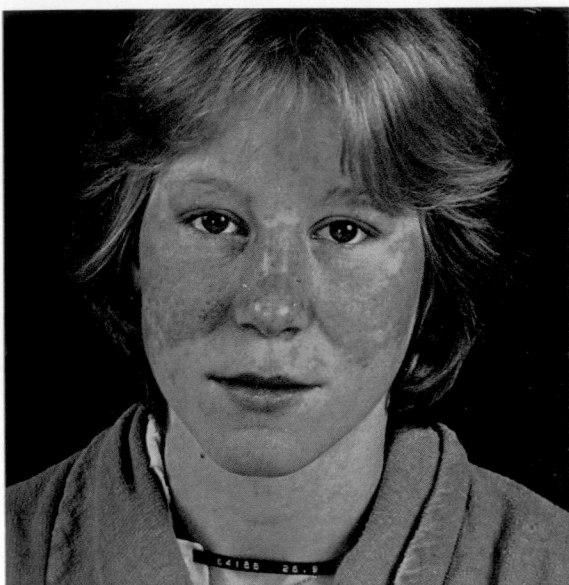

A1-24 **Systemic lupus erythematosus.** Erythematous, confluent, butterfly-like eruption with fine scaling.

A

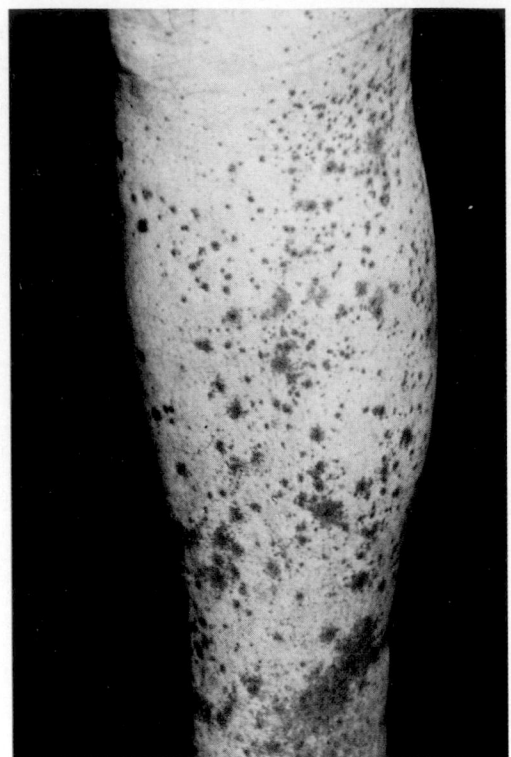

A1-25 **Necrotizing vasculitis syndrome.** Scattered discrete, purpuric eruption on the legs. The purpura is "palpable."

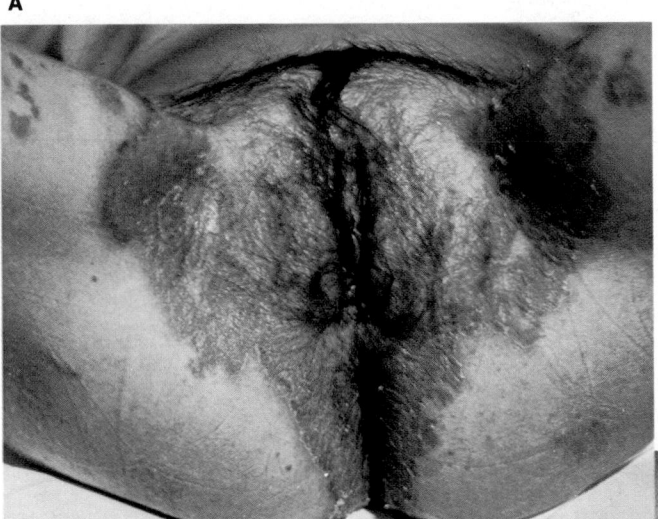

A1-26 **Glucagonoma** (*A*) and **acquired zinc deficiency** (*B*). Circinate and gyrate areas of blistering, erosion, and maceration. The eruption is often mistaken for psoriasis or mucocutaneous moniliasis.

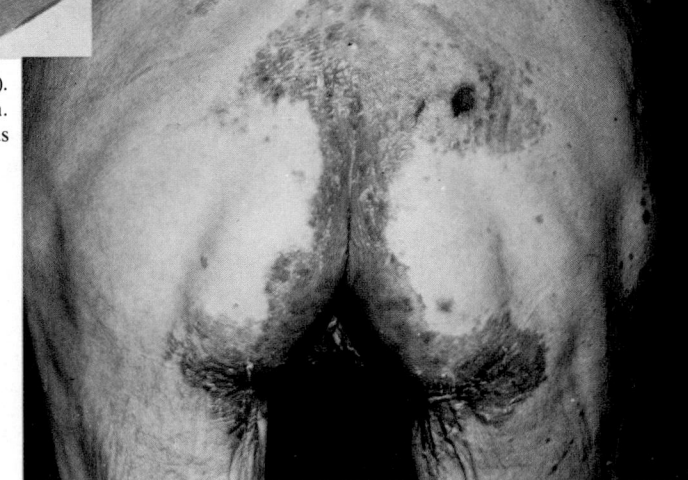

B

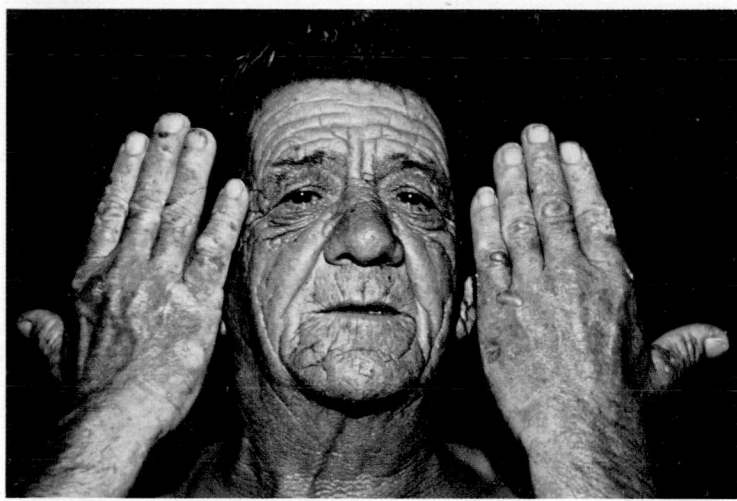

A1-27 **Porphyria cutanea tarda.** Violaceous suffusion in the periorbital skin is evident. There are erosions and pink atrophic scars at sites of previous bullae on the dorsa of the hands.

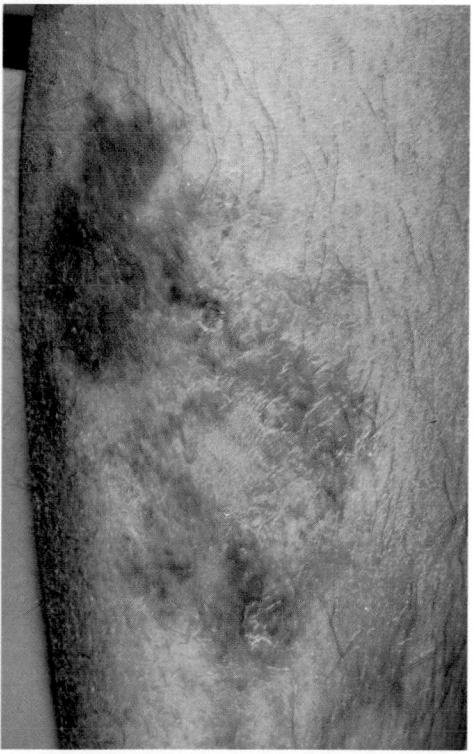

A1-28 **Necrobiosis lipoidica.** The lesion often begins as a small, dusky red, elevated nodule with a sharp border. It slowly enlarges, becomes flattened and eventually depressed as the dermis becomes atrophic. The color becomes brownish yellow except for the border, which may remain reddened. Delicate vessels can be seen through the atrophic epidermis.

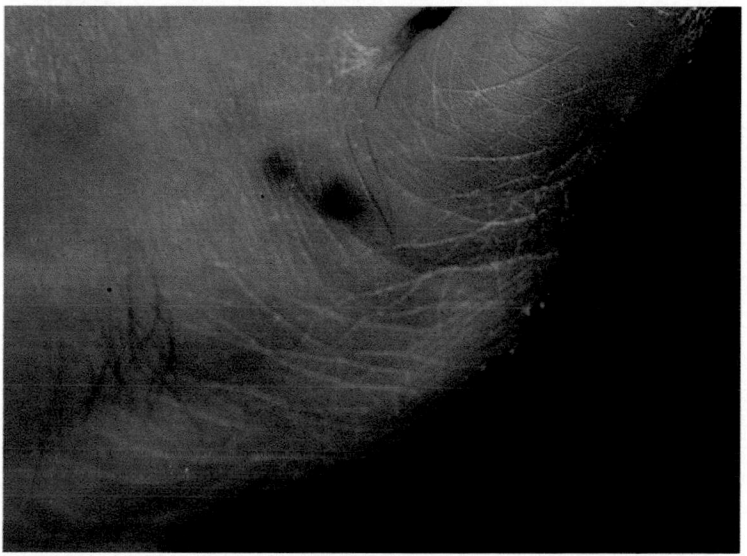

A1-29 Two purplish red nodules of **Kaposi's sarcoma** in a patient with AIDS.

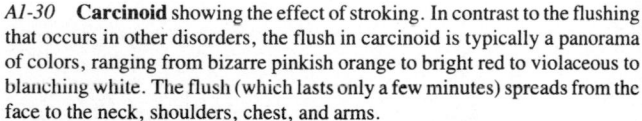

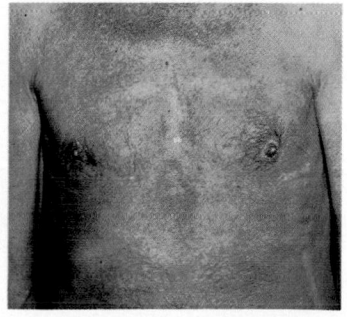

A1-30 **Carcinoid** showing the effect of stroking. In contrast to the flushing that occurs in other disorders, the flush in carcinoid is typically a panorama of colors, ranging from bizarre pinkish orange to bright red to violaceous to blanching white. The flush (which lasts only a few minutes) spreads from the face to the neck, shoulders, chest, and arms.

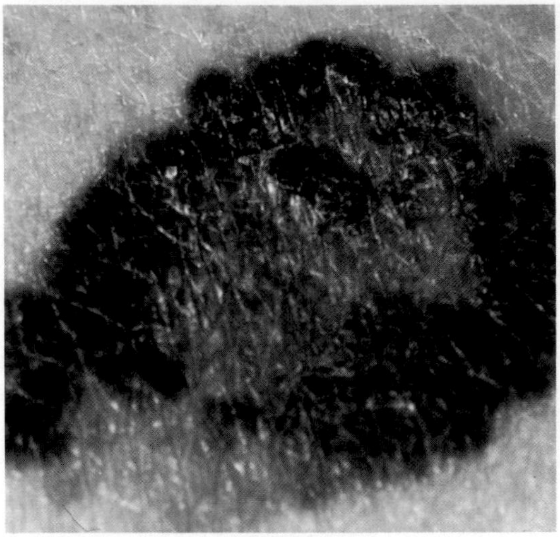

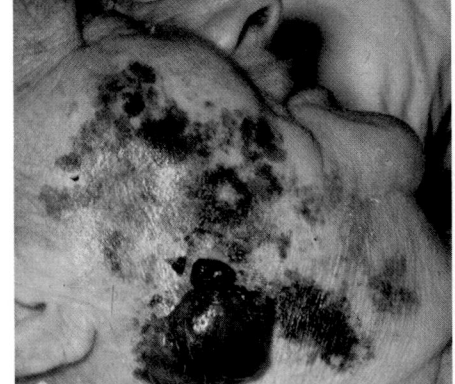

A1-31 **Malignant melanoma.** On close inspection melanomas shown are characterized by irregular surface (*A*), irregular border and notching (*B*), and nodularity (*C*). Also shown are a reniform melanoma (*D*), an extensive lentigo maligna on face of patient (*E*) and a regressive melanoma characterized by grayish color infiltrated with pink areas (*F*). (From Hospital Practice, January 1982, with permission.)

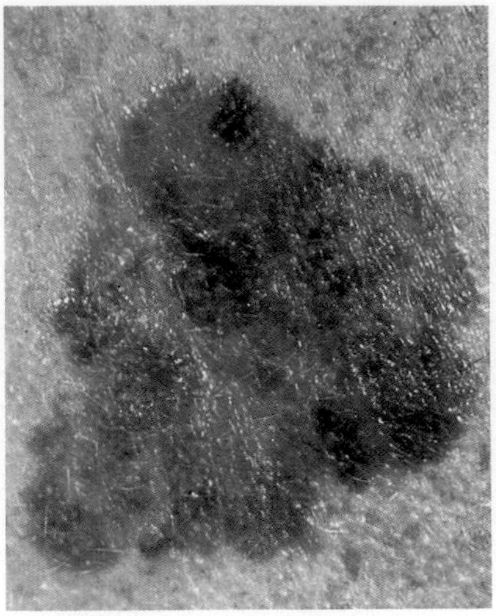

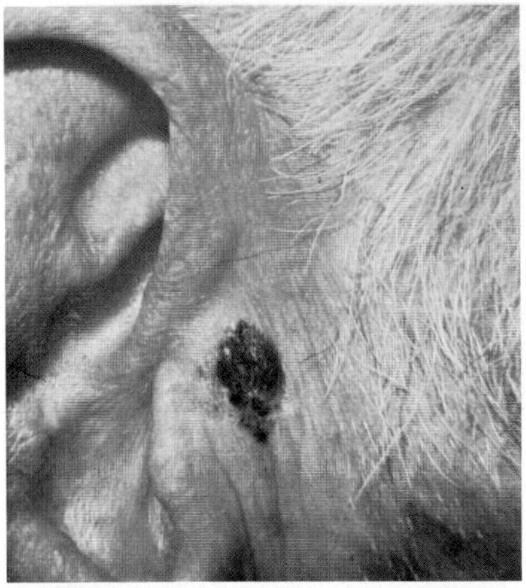

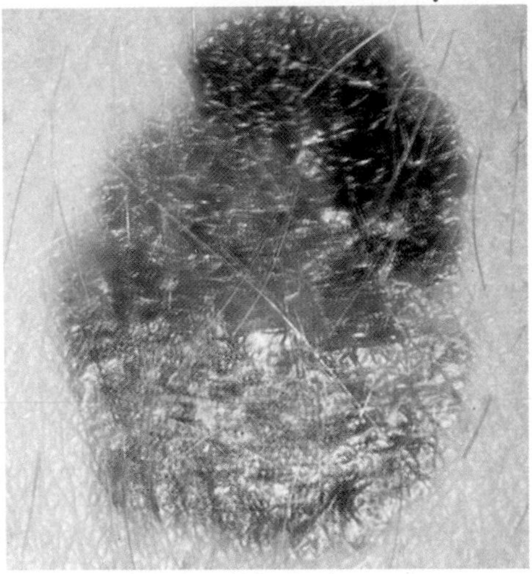

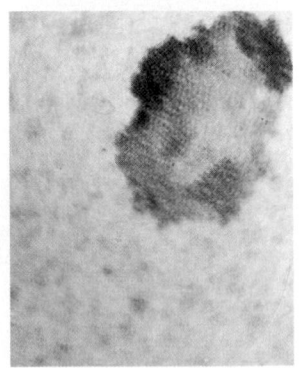

A

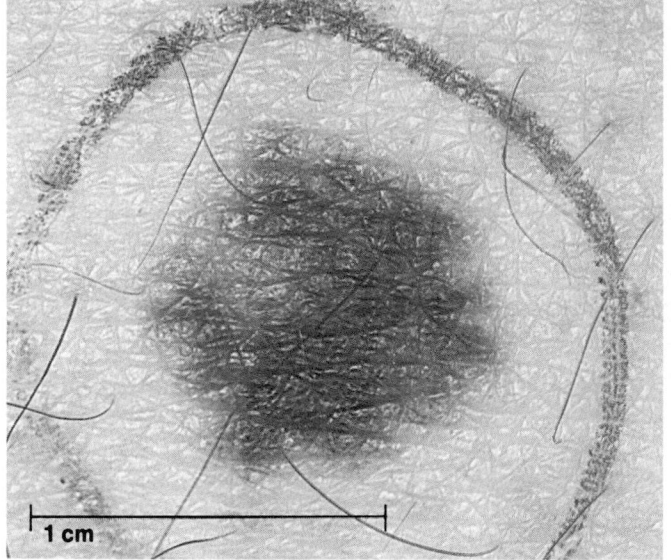

B

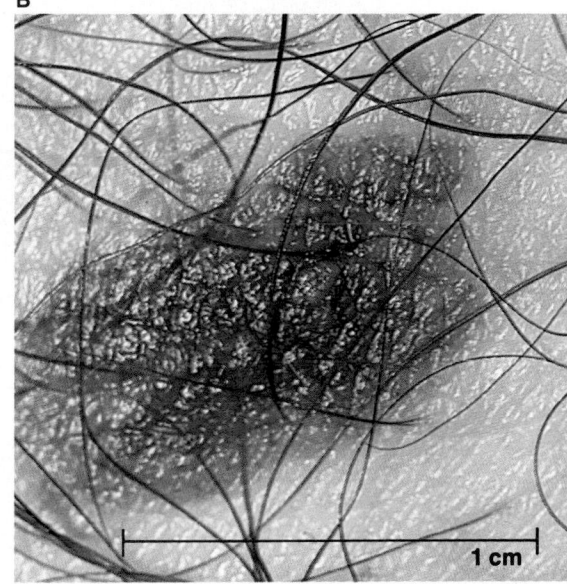

A1-32 **Dysplastic melanocytic nevi.** (*A*) Round, essentially macular lesions in which the slightly elevated area is present at 12:00 o'clock. The elevation is detectable only by oblique lighting. Note striking variegation of color with tan, brown, and pink areas. (*B*) This lesion is more obviously elevated in the central portion. Note "pebbly" surface. Both lesions have indistinct and irregular borders. (From Dermatologic Capsule & Comment 7(4):4, 1985, with permission.)

A1-33 **Malignant melanoma — dysplastic nevus syndrome.** This 28-year-old woman gave a history of a rapidly growing (3 to 6 months), asymptomatic lesion on her right scapular area. Her mother had melanoma and both mother and siblings had many dark "moles." Diagnosis: (1) Superficial spreading melanoma, level IV, 4.75 mm. (2) Regional nodes — of 32 removed, 1 was positive. (3) Dysplastic nevus syndrome with family history of melanoma. Note primary lesion and many dark "moles" on back (*A*) and dysplastic nevi on untanned areas under the bathing suit straps (*B*). (From Dermatologic Capsule & Comment 6(4):3, 1984, with permission.)

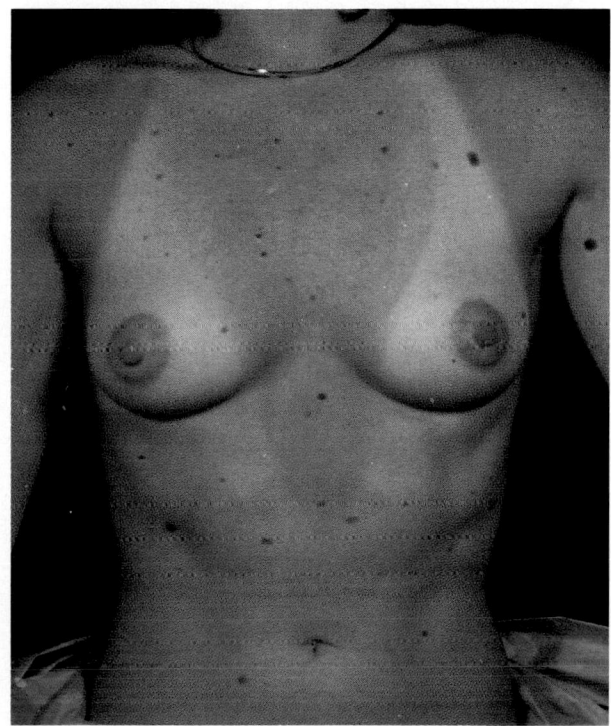

B

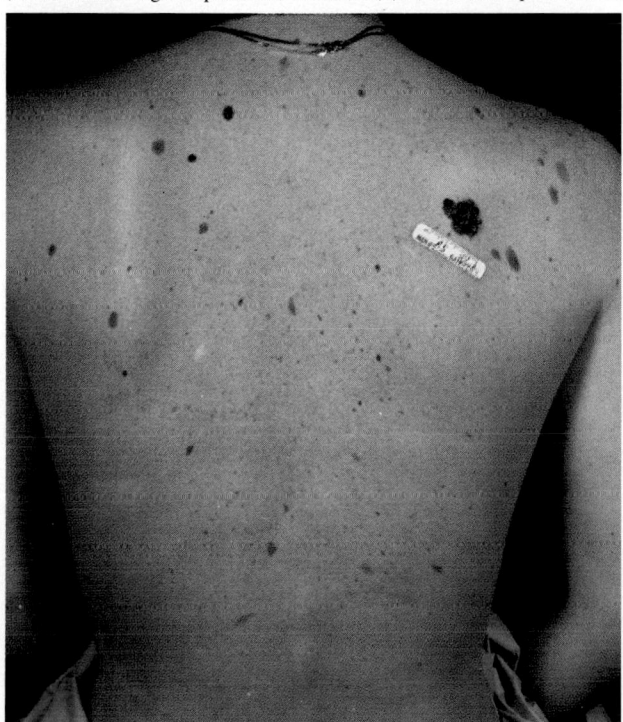

A

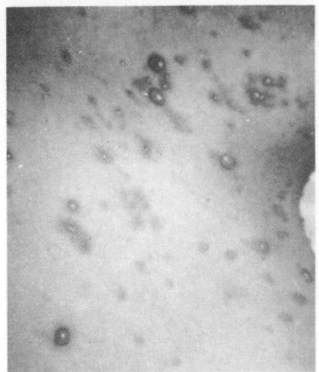

A2-1 **Varicella** (chickenpox).[3]

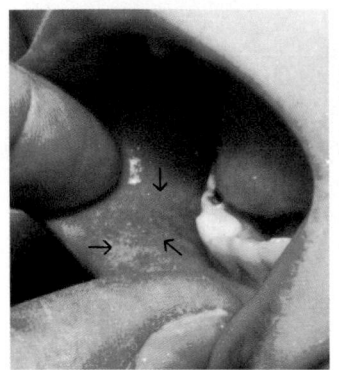

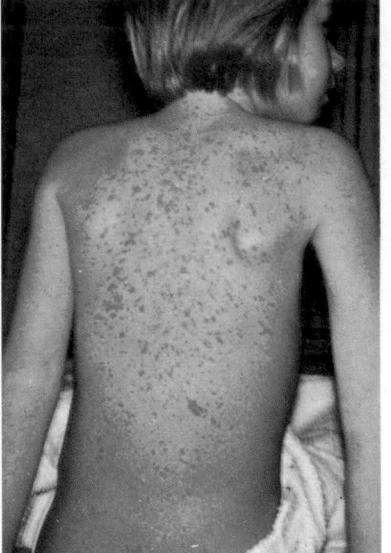

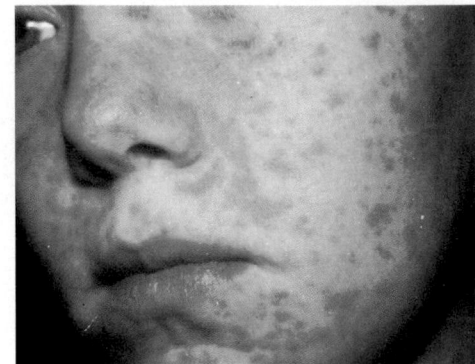

A2-2 **Measles** (rubeola).[3]

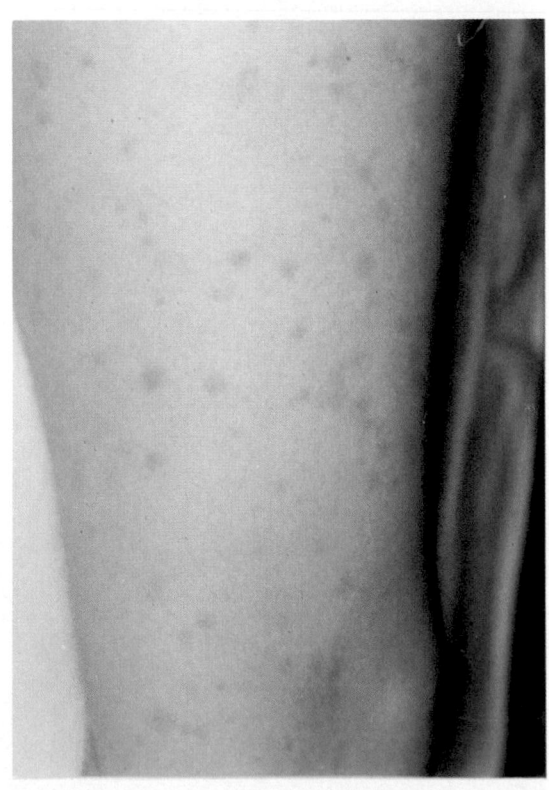

A2-3 **Rocky Mountain spotted fever** — early rash.[2]

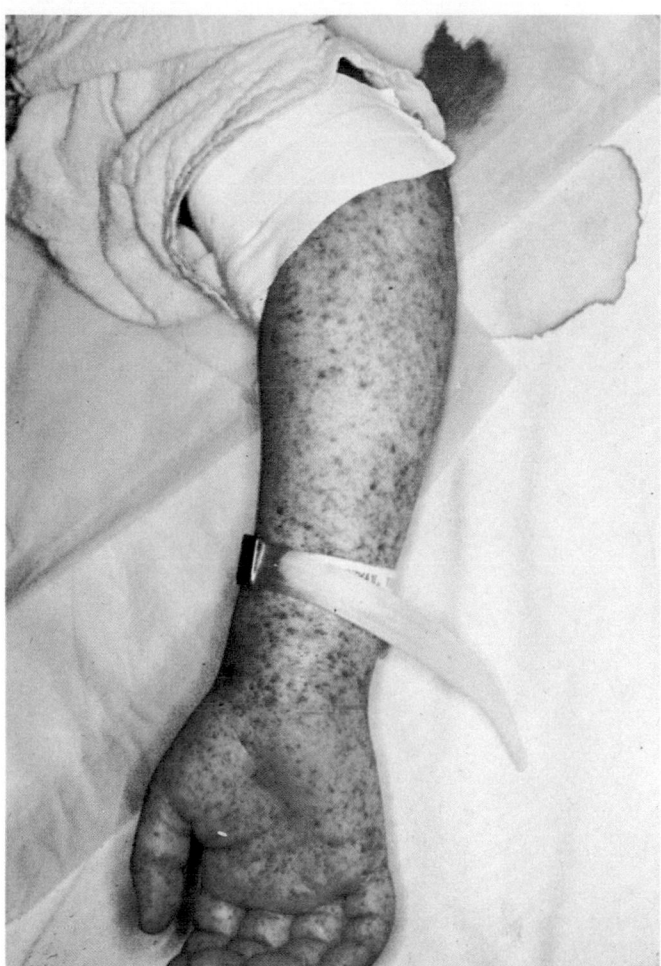

A2-4 **Rocky Mountain spotted fever** — late rash.[2]

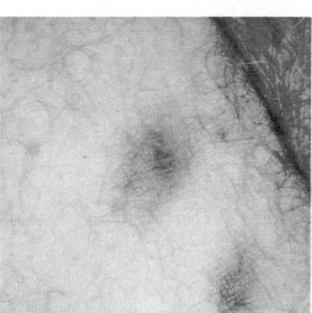

A2-7 **Pseudomonas septicemia.**[3]

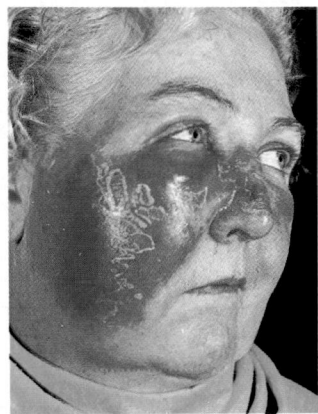

A2-8 **Facial erysipelas.**[3]

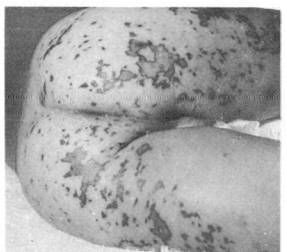

A2-5 **Meningococcemia.**[3]

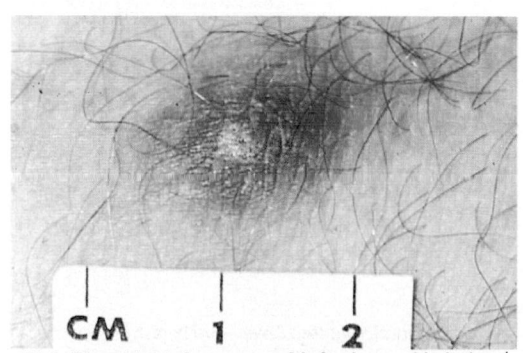

A2-6 **Disseminated gonococcal infection** — skin lesion.[4]

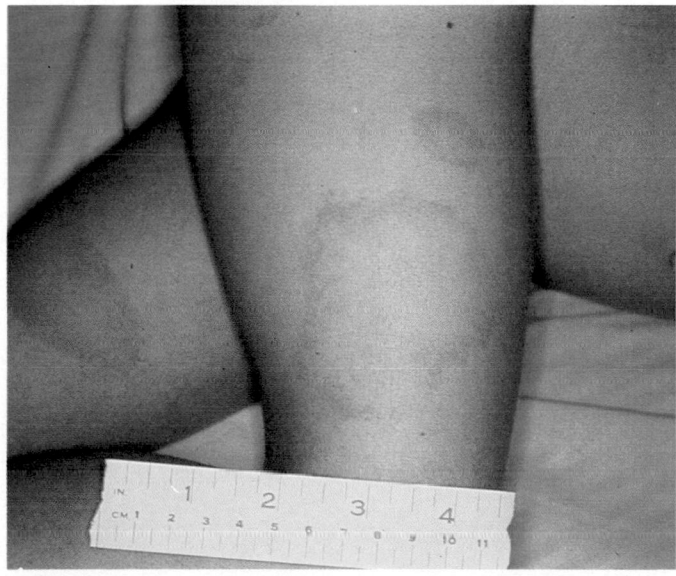

A2-9 **Lyme disease: erythema chronicum migrans** — secondary lesion.[5]

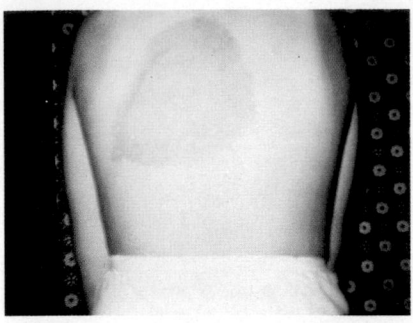

A2-10 **Lyme disease: erythema chronicum migrams** — primary lesion.[5]

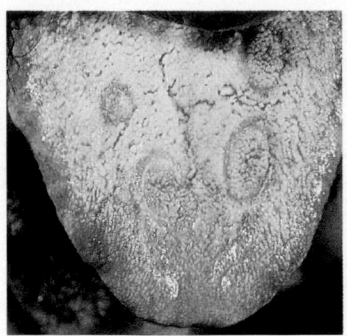

A2-11 Mucous patches involving the tongue in **secondary syphilis**.[4]

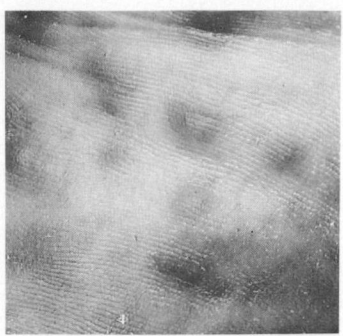

A2-12 **Papulosquamous lesions of secondary syphilis** on the sole of the foot.[4]

A2-13 **Macular syphilids** in early secondary syphilis.[4]

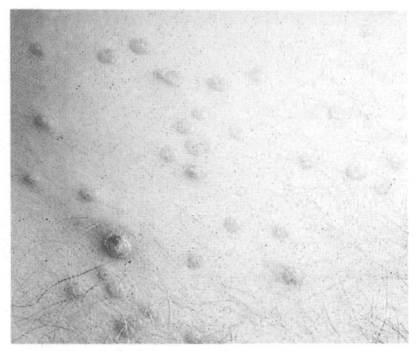

A2-14 **Molluscum contagiosum** of the lower abdomen in a patient with coexisting genital molluscum lesions. Note central umbilication and pale-salmon color.[4]

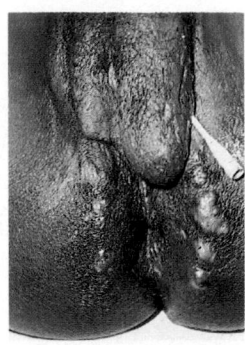

A2-15 **Esthiomene** due to lymphogranuloma venereum.[4]

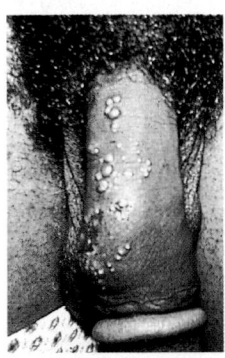

A2-16 **Severe primary HSV* infection** with extensive vesicles, ulcerations, and penile edema.[4]

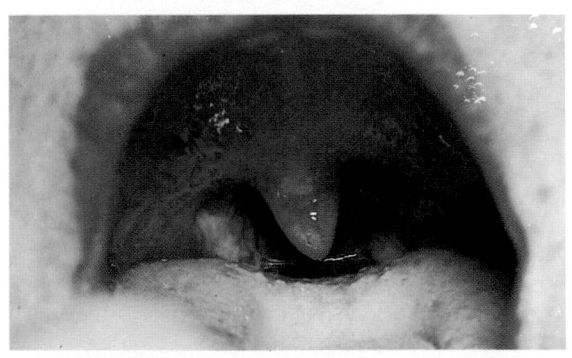

A2-17 **Primary HSV* pharyngitis** showing ulcerative lesions on the uvula and palate together with exudative tonsillitis. HSV-2 was recovered from pharyngeal and genital lesions.[4]

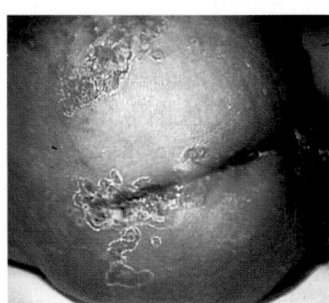

A2-18 **Neonatal HSV* infection.** Ulcers and crusting lesions on the buttocks.[4]

*Herpes Simplex Virus

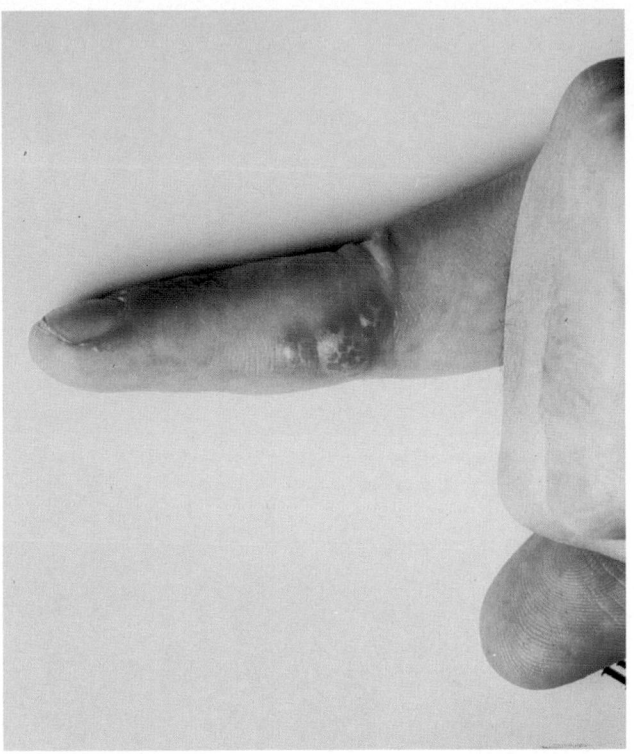

A2-19 **Herpetic whitlow**.[1]

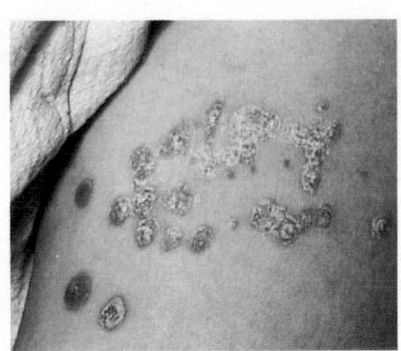

A2-20 **Keratodermia blenorrhagica** in Reiter's syndrome.[4]

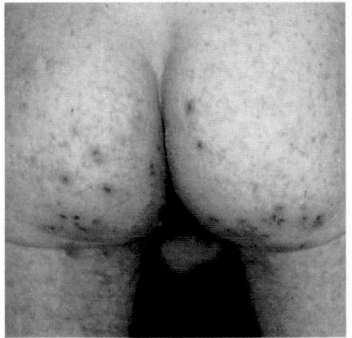

A2-21 Grouped excoriations due to **scabies** on the lower buttocks, simulating dermatitis herpetiformis.[4]

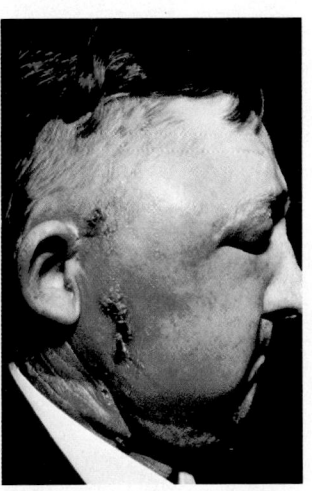

A2-22 **Cervicofacial actinomycosis**.[3]

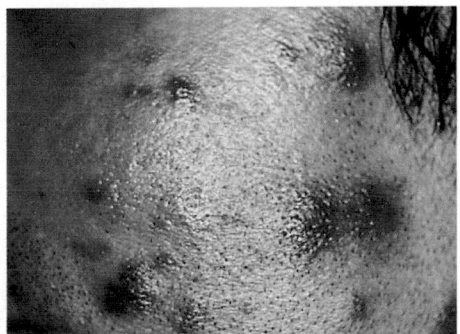

A2-23 Lesions of **Kaposi's sarcoma** on the cheek of a homosexually active man.[4]

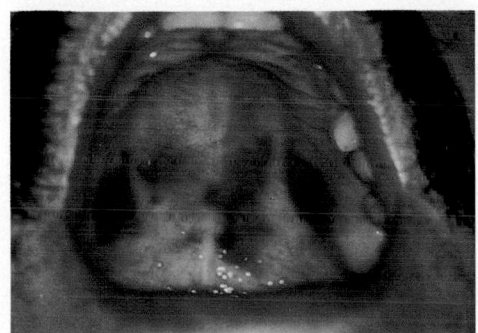

A2-24 **Kaposi's sarcoma** involving the palate of a homosexually active man.[4]

Sources

1 Courtesy of Lawrence Corey, M.D.

2 Courtesy of Theodore E. Woodward, M.D.

3 Fitzpatrick TB et al: *Dermatology in General Medicine,* 2nd ed. New York, McGraw-Hill, 1984

4 Holmes KK et al: *Sexually Transmitted Diseases.* New York, McGraw-Hill, 1984

5 Steere AC et al: Ann Intern Med 86:685, 1977 (reprinted with permission)

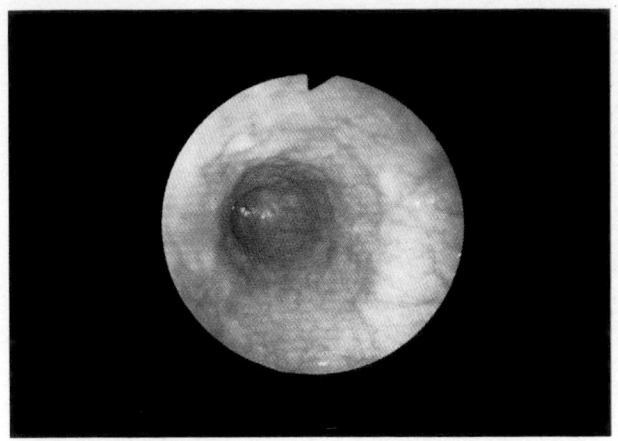

A3-1 **Normal esophagus;** normal fine vasculature can be seen.

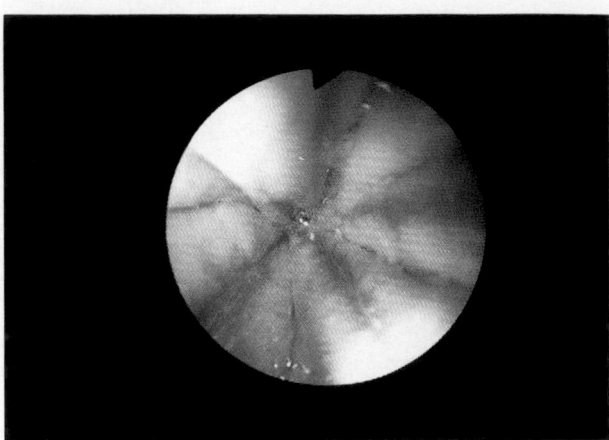

A3-2 **Peptic regurgitant esophagitis;** linear red streaks with a central white streak are noted extending up the esophagus.

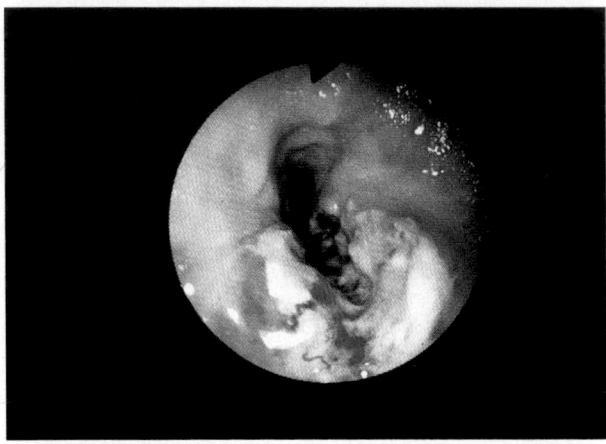

A3-3 **Ulcerated squamous cell carcinoma,** with a depressed center, involving one wall of the esophagus.

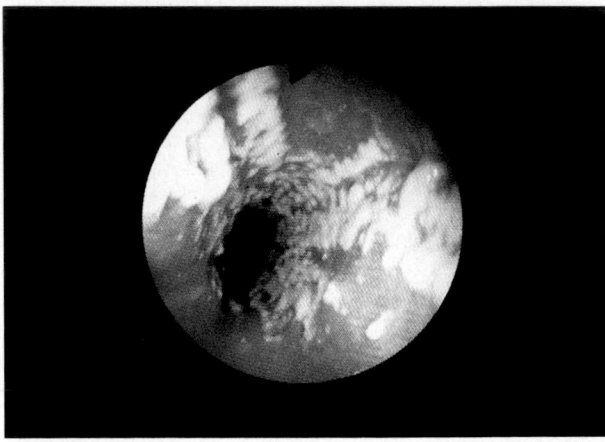

A3-4 **Moniliasis of the esophagus.** A white exudate is seen with underlying erythematous mucosa.

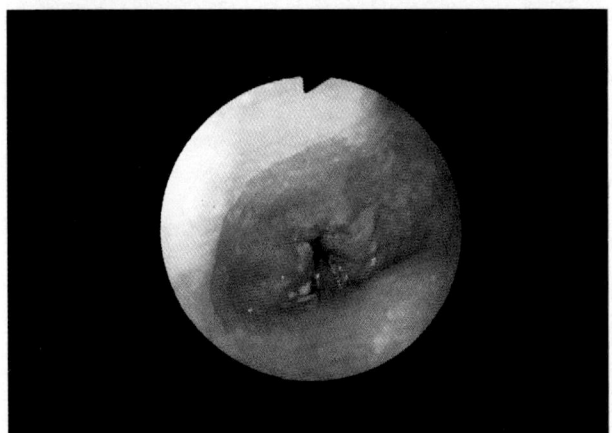

A3-5 **Barrett's metaplasia of the esophagus with an adenocarcinoma.** The squamo-columnar junction is noted in the proximal esophagus. A mucosal irregularity in the center of the photograph was an adenocarcinoma.

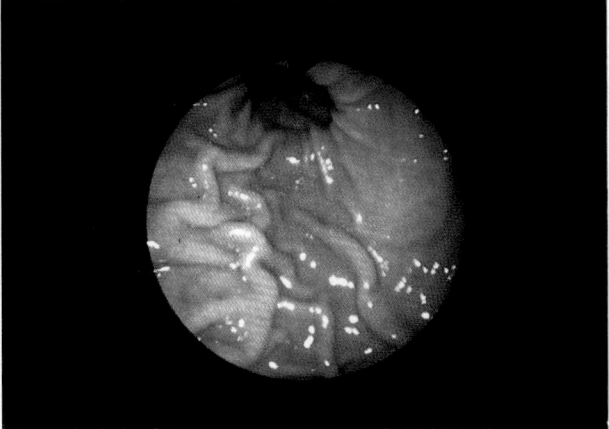

A3-6 **Normal body of the stomach with rugal folds.**

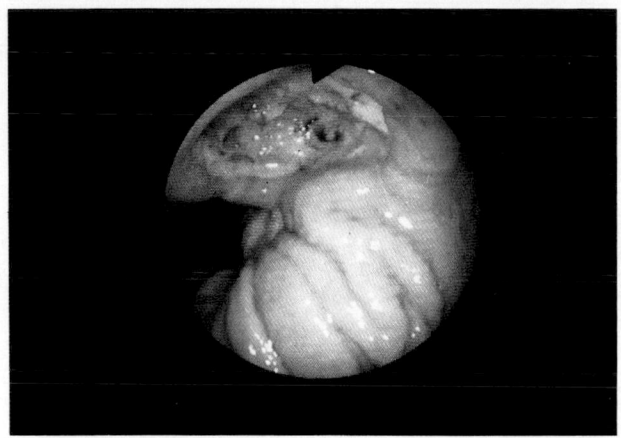

A3-7 **Large, benign, lesser curve, gastric ulcer.** The folds end at the ulcer margin.

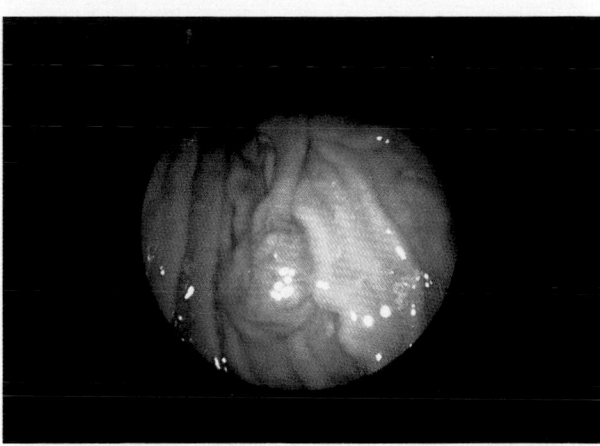

A3-8 **Gastric polyp.** The histologic type must be determined by excision and pathologic examination.

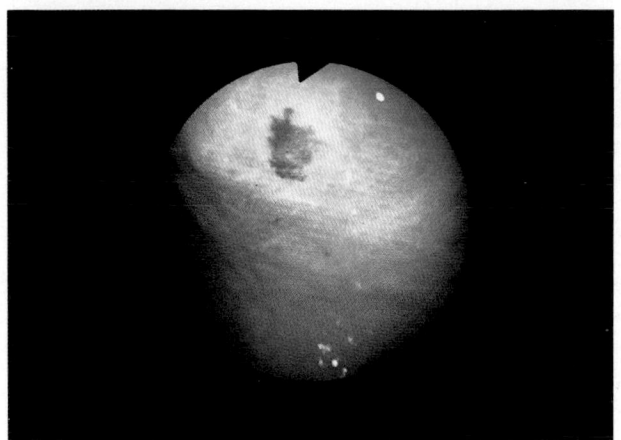

A3-9 **Arteriovenous malformation of the gastric mucosa.**

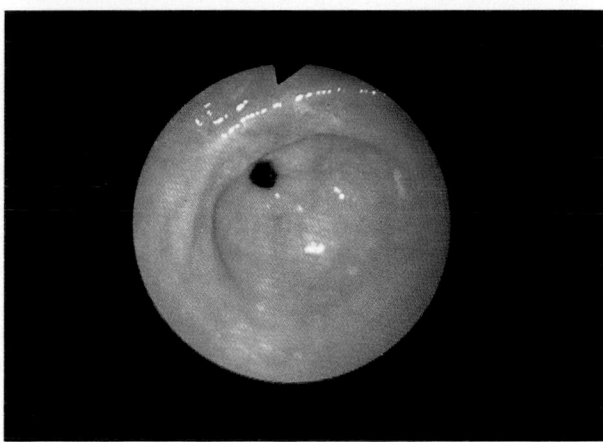

A3-10 **Normal pylorus.** Note the absence of gastric rugal folds in the antrum proximal to the pylorus.

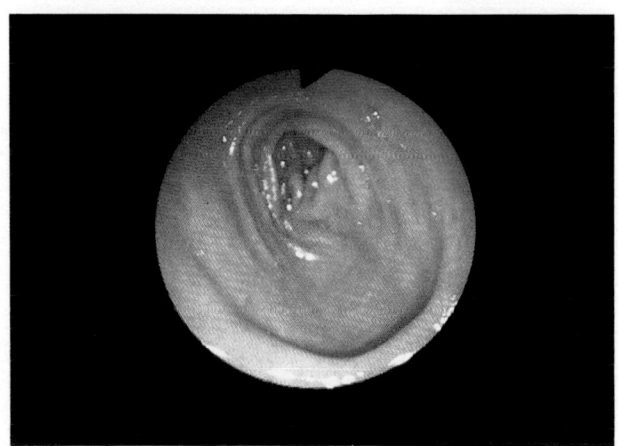

A3-11 **Normal duodenal bulb.**

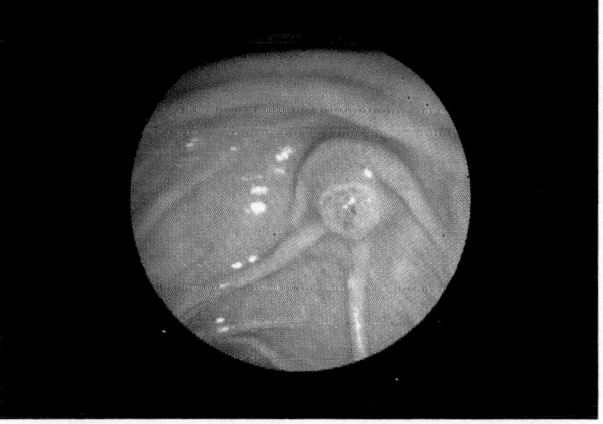

A3-12 **Normal papilla of Vater.** The fold pattern surrounding the papilla is normal; bile is seen adjacent to the papilla.

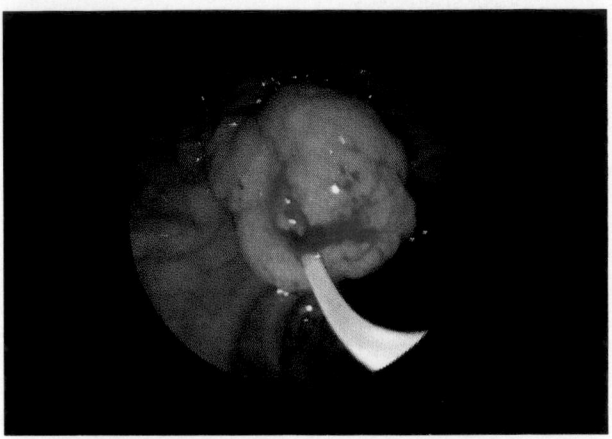

A3-13 **Periampullary carcinoma.** The mass at the papilla of Vater has been catheterized during ERCP.

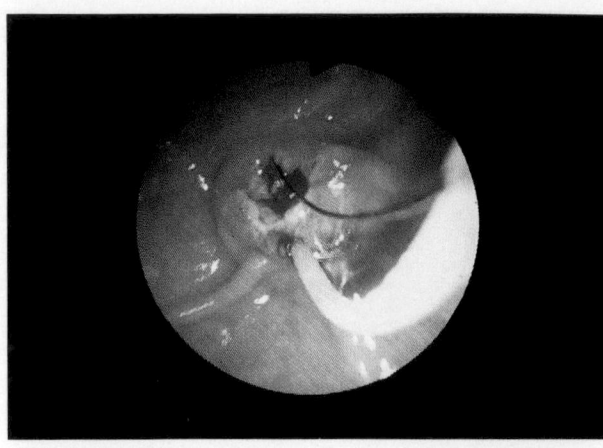

A3-14 **Endoscopic papillotomy.** A papillotome has been passed into the papilla, the wire bowed, and an incision made, with electrosurgical current, in the superior aspect of the papilla.

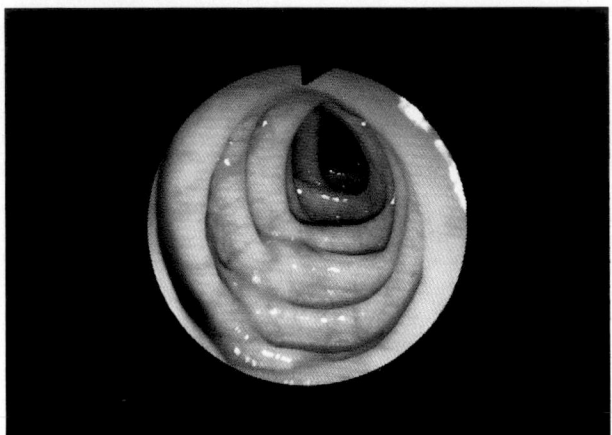

A3-15 **Normal colon;** typical haustral folds and a normal vascular pattern can be seen.

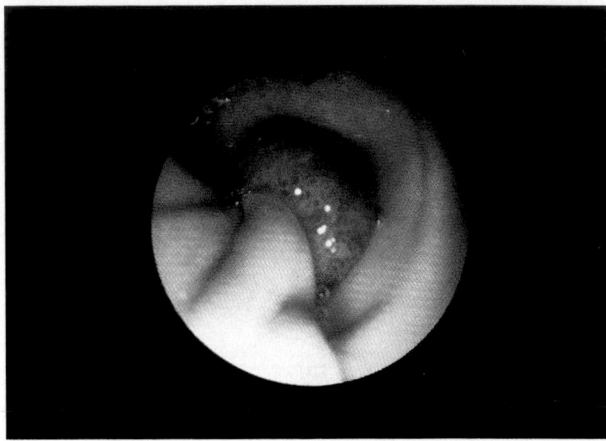

A3-16 **Colonic adenomatous polyp.** The polyp is erythematous; a stalk is seen covered with normal mucosa.

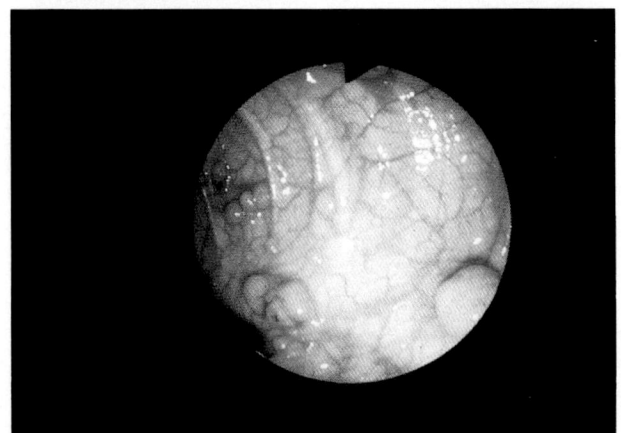

A3-17 **Multiple, small, colonic adenomatous polyps** in a case of familial polyposis coli. This colon must be removed to prevent the development of cancer.

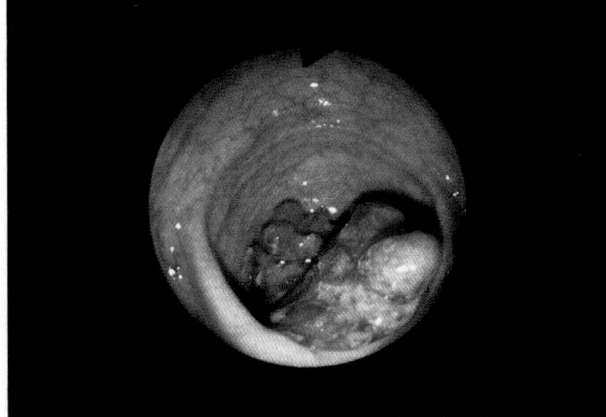

A3-18 **Colon adenocarcinoma.** The cancer is multilobed and growing into the lumen.

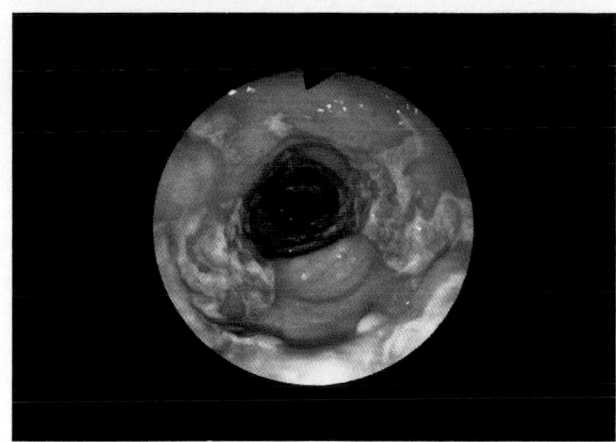

A3-19 **Crohn's colitis** with linear, serpiginous, white-based ulcers surrounded by colonic mucosa which is relatively normal.

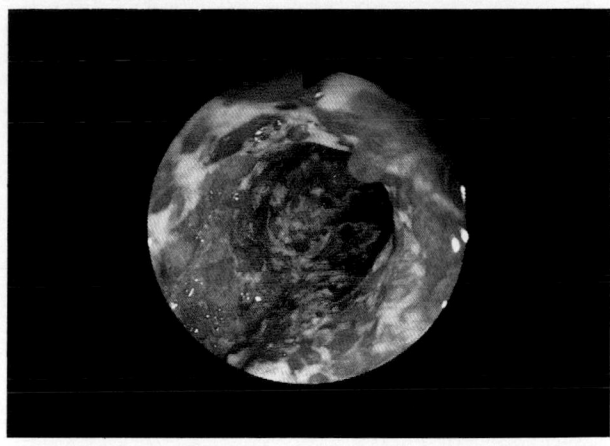

A3-20 **Severe ulcerative colitis** with diffuse ulceration, bleeding, and exudation.

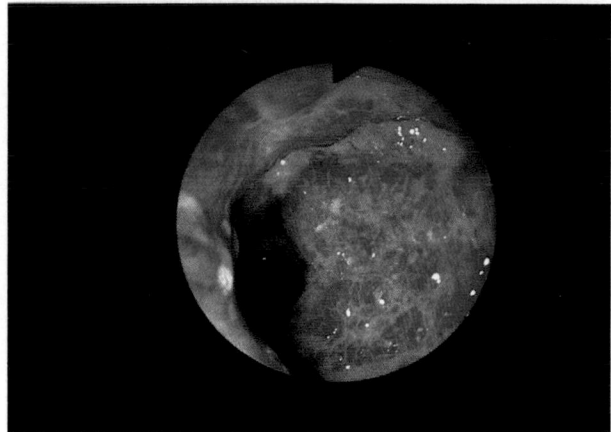

A3-21 **Kaposi's sarcoma involving the colon** in a patient with AIDS. The erythematous lesions involve most of the colonic mucosa in the photograph.

Source: Courtesy of FE Silverstein and GN Tytgat: *Atlas of Gastrointestinal Endoscopy.* Gower Medical Publishing, New York, 1987.

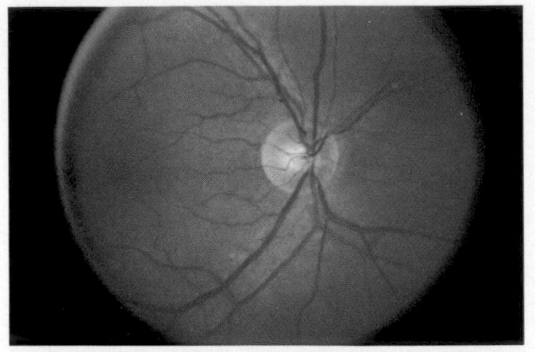

A4-1 **Normal optic nerve and retina.**

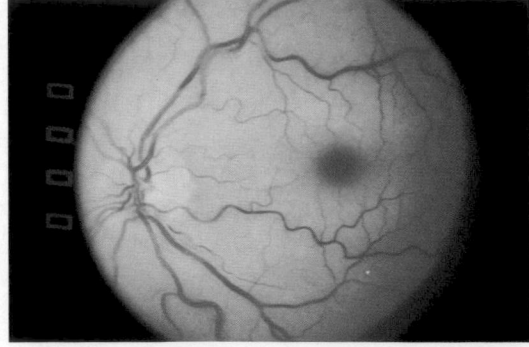

A4-2 **Central retinal artery occlusion.**

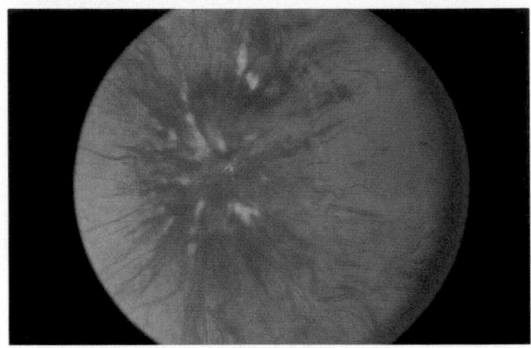

A4-3 **Central retinal vein occlusion.**

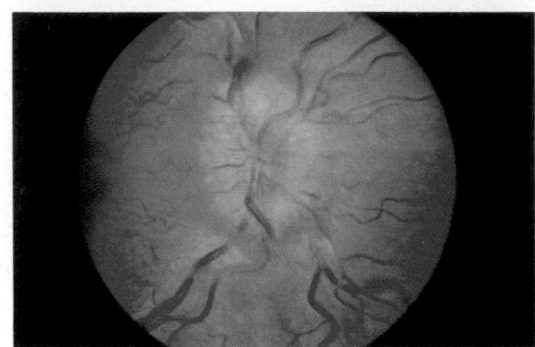

A4-4 **Early papilledema.**

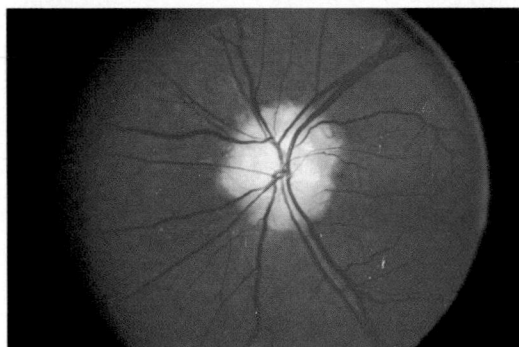

A4-5 **Drusen of the optic nerve head.**

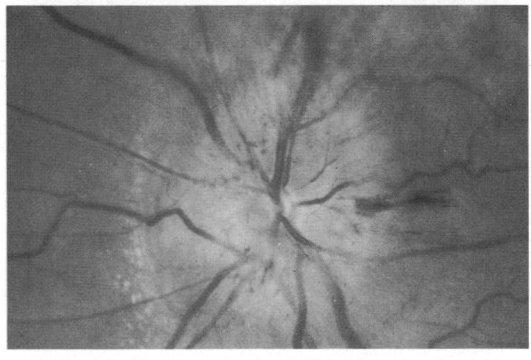

A4-6 **Anterior ischemic optic neuropathy.**

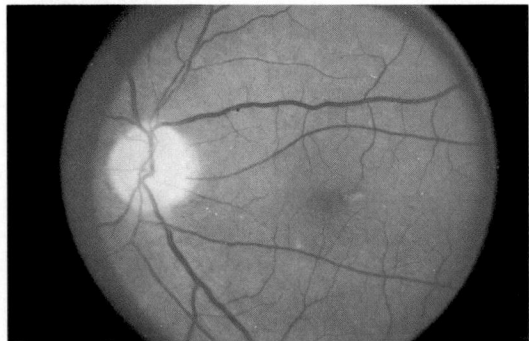

A4-7 **Primary optic atrophy.**

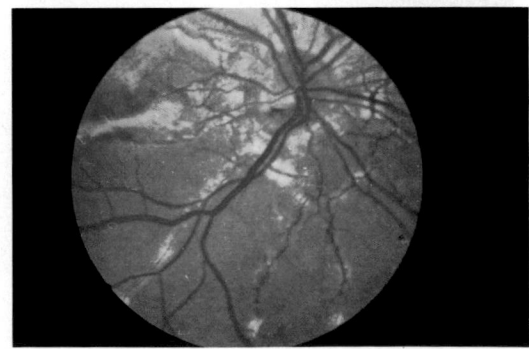

A4-8 **Angioid streaks.**

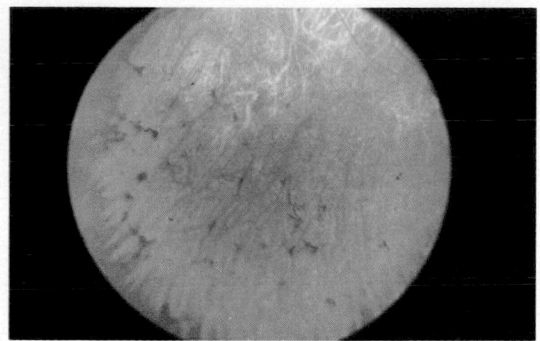

A4-9 **Retinitis pigmentosa.**

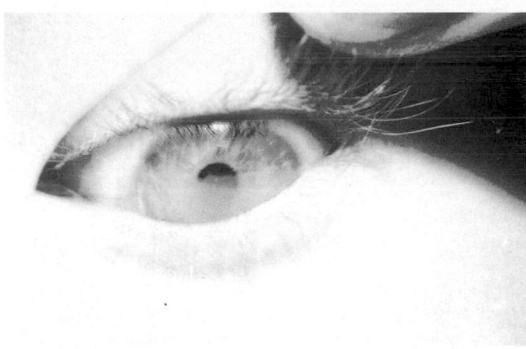

A4-10 **Band keratopathy.**

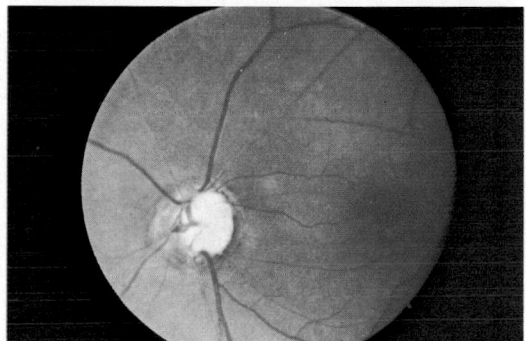

A4-11 **Glaucomatous optic disk with secondary atrophy.**

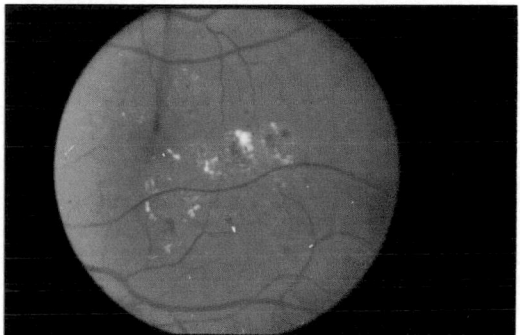

A4-12 **Diabetic retinopathy with microaneurysms.**

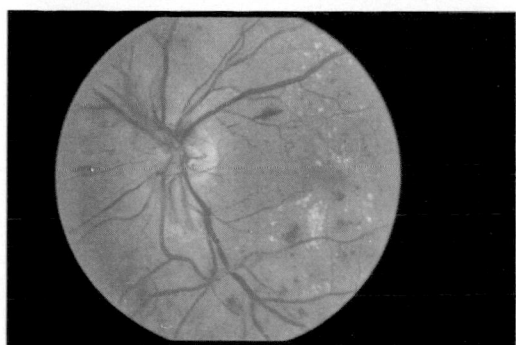

A4-13 **Proliferative diabetic retinopathy.**

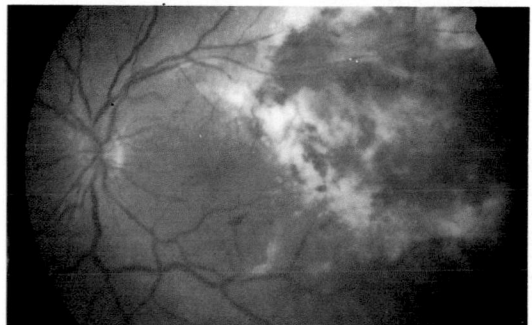

A4-14 **Cytomegalovirus retinitis in AIDS.**
(Courtesy of Donald J. D'Amico, M.D.)

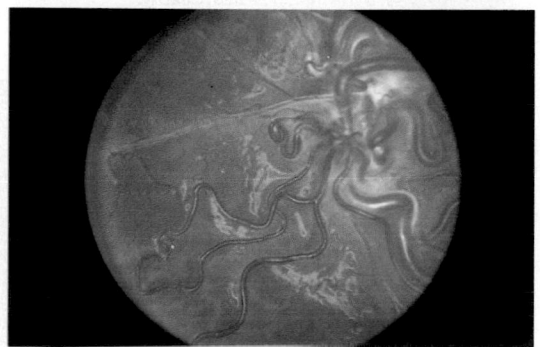

A4-15 **Retinal arteriovenous malformation in the Wyburn-Mason syndrome.**

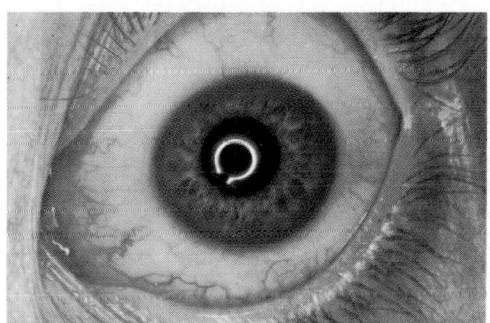

A4-16 **Kayser-Fleischer ring in Wilson's disease.**
(Note: The ring is the golden brown pigment at the periphery of the cornea and is characteristically broader superiorly and inferiorly than it is medially and laterally.)

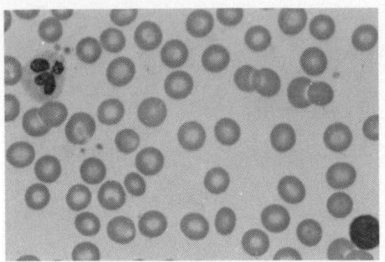

A5-1 **Normal blood smear.** Normal red blood cells are round, possess an area of central pallor, appear slightly smaller than the nucleus of a mature lymphocyte, and vary little in size (anisocytosis) or in shape (poikilocytosis).

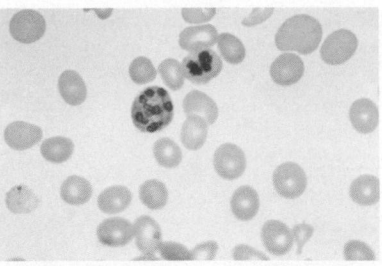

A5-2 **Megaloblastic anemia.** Oval macrocytes, well filled with hemoglobin, are admixed with lesser numbers of small teardrop-shaped red blood cells. Note also hypersegmented granulocyte.

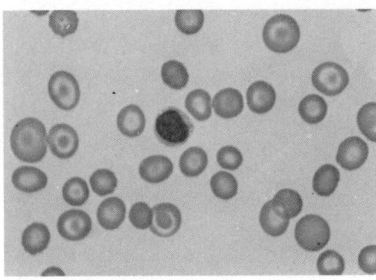

A5-3 **Liver disease.** Round macrocytes of rather uniform size are seen. Many of the macrocytes are also target cells.

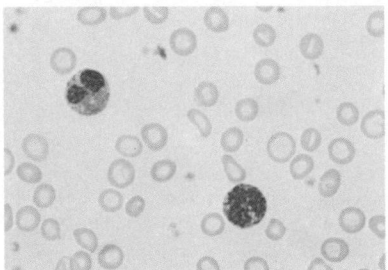

A5-4 **Iron-deficiency anemia.** In severe iron deficiency, the red blood cells are smaller than normal (microcytosis), and their central area of pallor is expanded (hypochromia) so that the cells appear to have only a thin rim of hemoglobin.

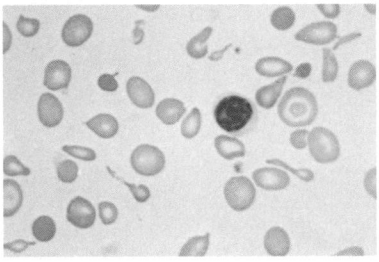

A5-5 **β thalassemia intermedia.** Microcytic and hypochromic red blood cells are seen that resemble the red blood cells of severe iron deficiency anemia shown in Fig. A5-4. Many elliptical and teardrop-shaped red blood cells are noted.

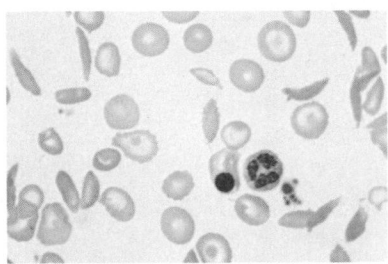

A5-6 **Sickle cell anemia.** The elongated and crescent-shaped red blood cells seen on this smear represent circulating irreversible sickled cells. Target cells and a nucleated red blood cell are also seen.

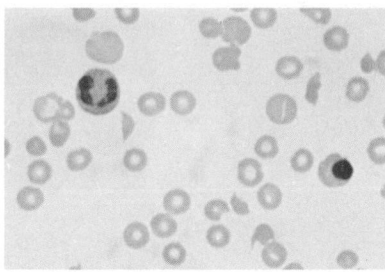

A5-7 **Traumatic hemolysis.** The helmet-shaped red blood cell and the small triangular-shaped red blood cells seen on this smear represent morphologic evidence of mechanical damage to red blood cells within the circulatory tree.

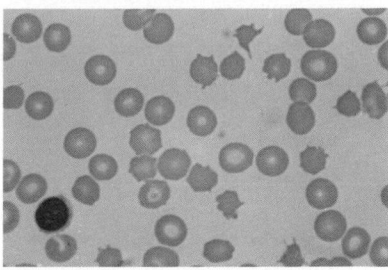

A5-8 **Spur cell anemia.** Spur cells are recognized as distorted red blood cells containing several irregularly distributed thornlike projections. Cells with this morphologic abnormality are also called acanthocytes.

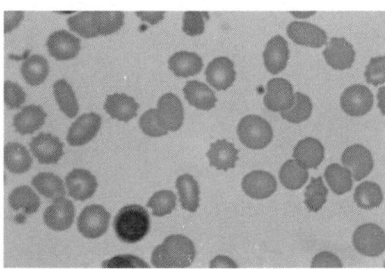

A5-9 **Uremia.** The red blood cells in uremia may acquire numerous, regularly spaced, small spiny projections. Such cells, called burr cells or echinocytes, are readily distinguishable from the irregularly spiculated acanthocytes shown in Fig. A5-8.

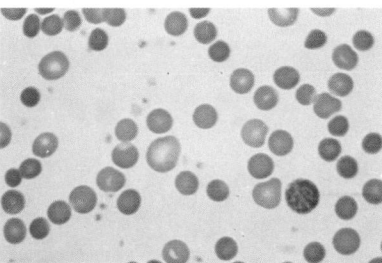

A5-10 **Hereditary spherocytosis.** Small, densely staining red blood cells are seen that have lost their central area of pallor (microspherocytes). Microspherocytes may also be found in other hemolytic disorders (Fig. A5-11).

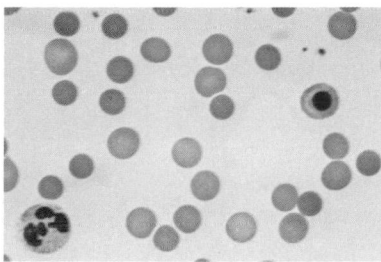

A5-11 **Immunohemolytic anemia.** Microspherocytes are seen on this blood smear along with several macrocytes with a slight purple tinge (polychromasia). The latter represent new red blood cells released early from the bone marrow. The microspherocytes seen in immunohemolytic anemia may be indistinguishable from the microspherocytes seen in hereditary spherocytosis (Fig. A5-10).

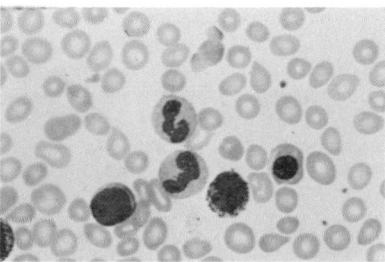

A5-12 **Myeloid metaplasia.** Teardrop-shaped red blood cells, a nucleated red blood cell, and immature myeloid cells are seen on this blood smear.

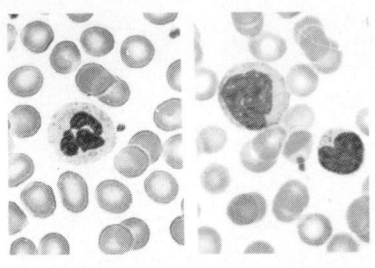

A   **B**

A5-13 A. **Normal granulocyte.** The normal granulocyte has a segmented nucleus with heavy, clumped chromatin; fine neutrophilic granules are dispersed throughout its cytoplasm. *B.* **Normal monocyte and lymphocyte.** The normal monocyte is a large cell with an indented or folded nucleus containing loose, strandlike chromatin; the cytoplasm is a blue-gray color and usually contains fine azurophilic granules. The normal lymphocyte is a smaller cell. Its nucleus is usually round but may be indented, as in the cell shown in this plate. The nuclear chromatin has a smudgy appearance; the cytoplasm is a blue color.

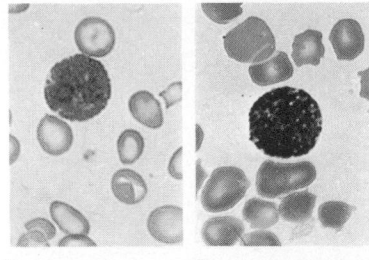

A   **B**

A5-14 A. **Normal eosinophil.** The eosinophil contains large, bright-orange granules; the nucleus is bilobed. *B.* **Basophil.** The basophil contains large purple-black granules which fill the cell and obscure the nucleus.

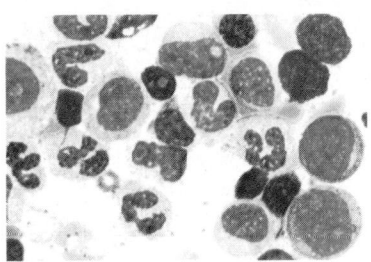

A5-15 **Normal granulocyte precursors in marrow.** The earliest granulocytic precursor (myeloblast) possesses a round nucleus with fine, punctate chromatin and one or more nucleoli; the cytoplasm is blue. As nuclear differentiation proceeds, the nucleoli disappear, the chromatin coarsens, and the nucleus becomes increasingly indented and finally segmented. As cytoplasmic differentiation proceeds, azurophilic granules appear and the cytoplasm changes color from blue to the yellow-pink-gray hue of the mature granulocyte, and as this occurs the azurophilic granules become obscured by fine neutrophilic granules.

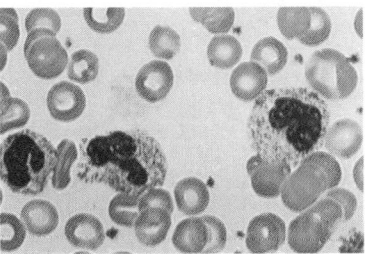

A5-16 **Neutrophils with toxic granulation.** In infection and other toxic states, azurophilic granules may become visible in mature granulocytes as coarse, dark-staining cytoplasmic granules.

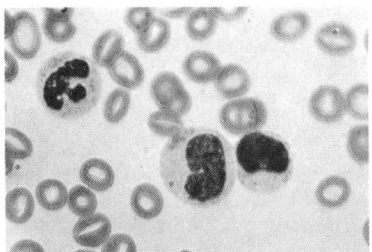

A5-17 **Band with Döhle body** (center). Döhle bodies are discrete, blue-staining, nongranular areas found in the periphery of the cytoplasm of the neutrophil in infections and other toxic states. They represent aggregates of rough endoplasmic reticulum.

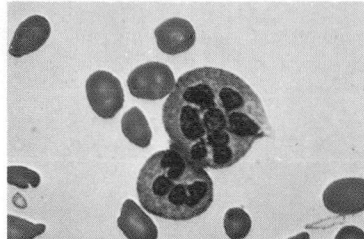

A5-18 **Hypersegmentation.** Frequent five-lobed granulocytes on a blood smear or granulocytes with more than five lobes are evidence of hypersegmentation, an important clue to the diagnosis of megaloblastic anemia.

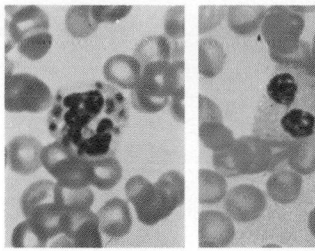

A   **B**

A5-19 A. **Chédiak-Higashi anomaly.** In this ultimately fatal disorder, the granulocytes contain huge cytoplasmic granules, formed from aggregation and fusion of azurophilic and specific granules. Large, abnormal granules are found in other granule-containing cells throughout the body. *B.* **Pelger-Hüet anomaly.** In this benign disorder, the majority of granulocytes are bilobed. The nucleus frequently has a spectacle-like or "pince-nez" configuration.

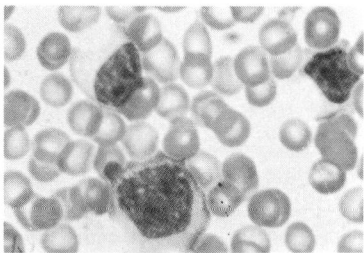

A5-20 **Reactive lymphocytes** (infectious mononucleosis). Reactive lymphocytes are usually large, cytoplasmic lymphocytes. The nucleus may be eccentrically placed and may have irregular borders and indentations (not seen on this plate). The cytoplasm contains areas that stain a darker blue due to their increased content of RNA. The cytoplasm may be indented where it abuts against a red blood cell.

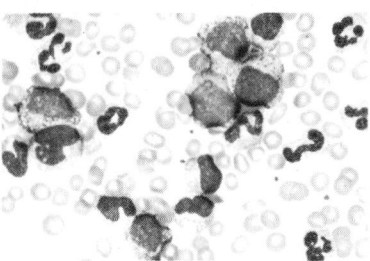

A5-21 **Chronic granulocytic leukemia.** The peripheral blood WBC count is high due to increased numbers of granulocytes and their precursors. The majority of the WBCs are segmented granulocytes or band forms, but as seen on this plate, myelocytes and promyeloblasts (not seen on this plate) may also be found on review of the blood smear.

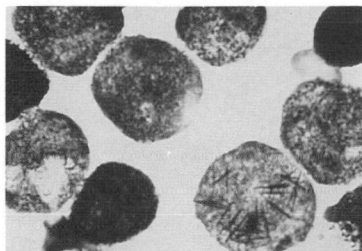

A5-22 **Leukemic cell in acute promyelocytic leukemia.** Note multiple Auer rods.

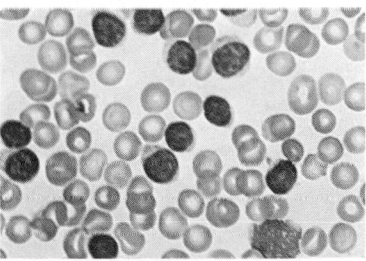

A5-23 **Chronic lymphocytic leukemia.** The peripheral blood WBC count is high due to increased numbers of small, well-differentiated lymphocytes. However, the leukemic lymphocytes are fragile, and substantial numbers of broken, smudged cells are usually also present on the blood smear.

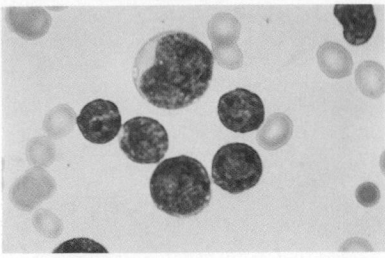

A5-24 **Leukemic cells in acute lympho-blastic leukemia** characterized by round or convoluted nuclei, high nuclear/cytoplasmic ratio and absence of cytoplasmic granules.

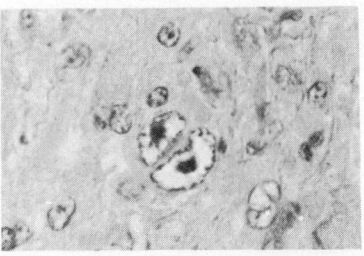

A5-25 **Hodgkin's disease:** Reed-Sternberg cell in marrow (center). The Reed-Sternberg cell is recognized by its bilobed, mirror-image nucleus, which contains in each lobe a giant, inclusion body–like nucleolus. The cytoplasmic borders of the cell cannot be identified on this plate.

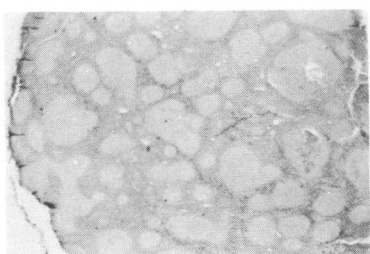

A5-26 **Non-Hodgkin's nodular lymphoma** (lymph node). This low-power view illustrates that a proliferative process has caused the normal architecture of the lymph node to be replaced by multiple nodules of varying size that extend throughout the entire lymph node.

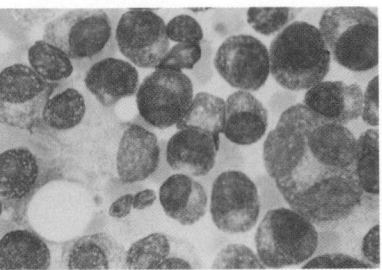

A5-27 **Multiple myeloma** (marrow). The cells bear the characteristic morphologic features of plasma cells, round or oval cells with an eccentric nucleus composed of coarsely clumped chromatin, a densely basophilic cytoplasm, and a perinuclear clear zone (hof) containing the Golgi apparatus. Binucleate and multinucleate malignant plasma cells can also be seen.

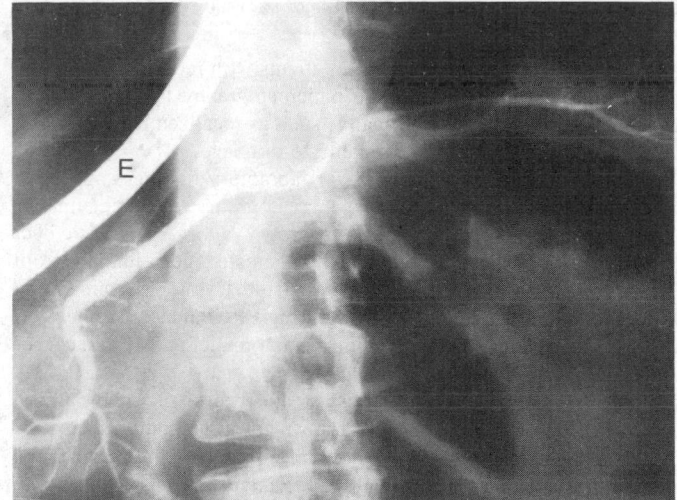

A

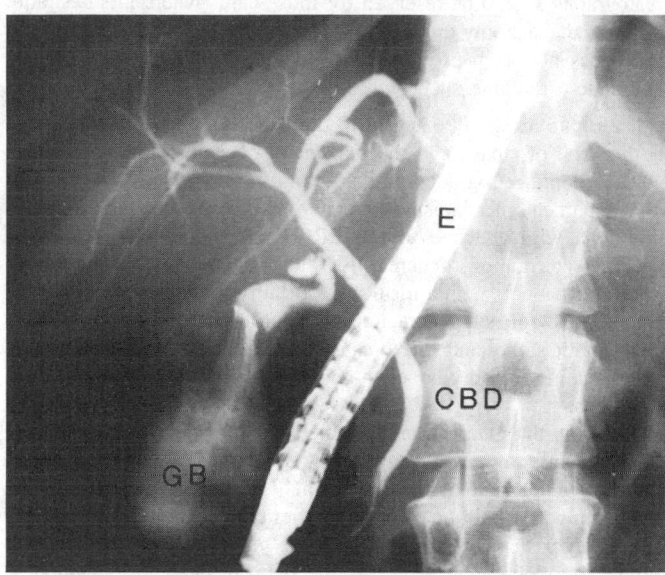

B

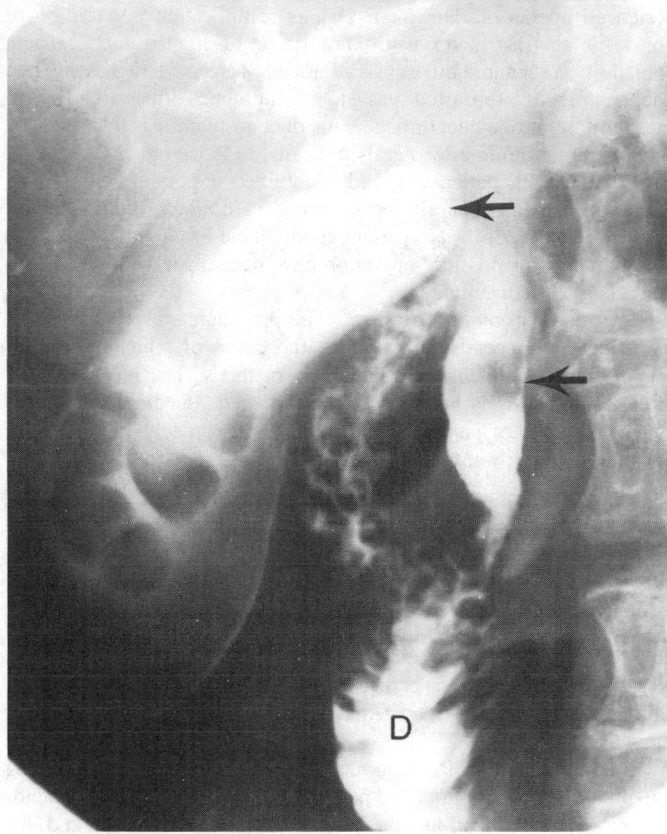

C

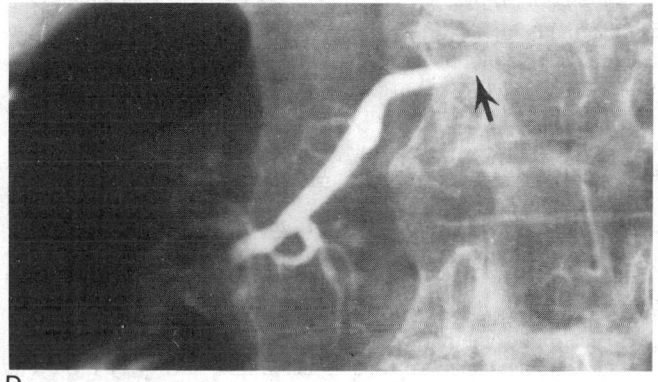

D

FIGURE 236-1 *A.* A tapering pancreatic duct of normal caliber is seen and may be compared to the endoscope (E) 1 cm in diameter. *B.* Normal cholangiogram. The diameter of the common duct (CBD) is normal. The intrahepatic ducts branch normally, and the gallbladder (GB) can be seen. The endoscope (E) is seen in the duodenum. *C.* Several stones (arrows) can be seen in an obstructed, dilated common duct. The gallbladder also contains several stones. Regurgitated contrast material is seen in the duodenum (D). *D.* The sharp cutoff (arrow) of the pancreatic duct is caused by a carcinoma of the body of the pancreas. *(Courtesy of Dr. Charles Rohrmann.)*

that this picture is of significance. On the other hand, diffuse and bleeding erosions of the duodenal bulb merit a diagnosis of *erosive duodenitis,* especially after ingestion of mucosal irritants such as aspirin. A nodular or narrow duodenum will occasionally yield granulomas on biopsy, indicative of Crohn's disease.

ENDOSCOPIC RETROGRADE CHOLANGIOPANCREATOGRA-PHY (ERCP) This endoscopic technique involves placing a side-viewing instrument in the descending duodenum. The papilla of Vater is cannulated, contrast medium is injected, and the pancreatic ducts and hepatobiliary tree are visualized radiographically. Skilled operators can visualize 90 to 95 percent of pancreatic ducts and 90 percent of biliary ducts.

ERCP is performed on an x-ray table. The oropharynx is usually anesthetized with topical lidocaine, and most endoscopists sedate the patient with intravenous diazepam. Atropine and glucagon are given intravenously to induce duodenal hypotonia. The pancreatic duct is

usually visualized first and gently filled throughout its entire length with 2 to 5 mL of contrast material with constant fluoroscopic monitoring (Fig. 236-1A). Injection is continued until the first side branches are seen or until the patient complains of pain. Overfilling is avoided. By insertion of the cannula at a more acute cephalad angle, the common bile duct and the whole biliary tract including the gallbladder are visualized (Fig. 236-1B).

ERCP is a safe procedure when performed by an experienced operator. Asymptomatic amylase elevations occur in 30 to 40 percent of patients after pancreatography and are rarely of clinical significance. Pancreatitis occurs in only 1 percent of patients but is usually benign and self-limited. By monitoring the pancreas during injection using a high-resolution TV screen, the force of injection can be limited to avoid filling of pancreatic acini. This probably minimizes the complication of pancreatitis. In a nationwide survey of complications, the morbidity rate was 3 percent and mortality rate 0.2 percent.

Morbidity and mortality rates were substantially higher with inexperienced operators. The main serious complication is retention of nonsterile contrast material proximal to an obstructed duct, causing cholangitis or pancreatic sepsis. Patients suspected of having bile duct obstruction are started on systemic antibiotics prior to the ERCP. Furthermore, if bile duct or pancreatic duct obstruction is first revealed by ERCP, antibiotic coverage is indicated to reduce the incidence of bacteremia; such patients should be drained if possible either with endoscopic therapy (papillotomy, stents, nasobiliary drains, etc.) or surgically within 36 h. No patient should have ERCP unless advance arrangements for possible operation have been made with the patient and a surgical consultant.

Retrograde cholangiography   This procedure is especially useful in patients with persistent jaundice the cause of which cannot be established by conventional diagnostic methods. The important differential diagnosis is between "surgical" and "medical" jaundice. When the cause of jaundice is unclear, approximately 15 percent of patients thought to have "medical" jaundice prove to have extrahepatic biliary obstruction requiring surgery or endoscopic therapy, and, conversely, the same percentage of patients thought to have "surgical" jaundice prove to have an open ductal system by ERCP and can be spared unnecessary intervention.

Remediable causes of obstructive jaundice which can be diagnosed by retrograde cholangiography include common duct stones (Fig. 236-1C) and benign and malignant strictures. In jaundiced patients with suspected primary liver disease, such as primary biliary cirrhosis, ERCP can relieve the worry that an operable obstruction is being missed.

In addition to ERCP, there are four other methods of visualizing the biliary tree in the jaundiced patient. Which test to use first depends on the clinical situation, the availability of equipment, and the experience of the specialists using the techniques. The first method is *percutaneous transhepatic cholangiography* (PTC), in which contrast material is injected from the exterior via a "skinny" needle into the intrahepatic bile ducts under fluoroscopic control; success in visualizing the ducts is 90 to 100 percent if the ducts are dilated, but only approximately 70 percent if they are not dilated. PTC is generally safe, but complications do occur (sepsis, bleeding, bile leak, etc.). The morbidity for this procedure is approximately 10 percent; the reported mortality varies from 0.1 to 0.9 percent. The three other methods, which are noninvasive, use *ultrasound, computed tomography* (CT scan), and radionuclide biliary scintigraphy. The first two techniques employ sound waves or x-rays to visualize organs and any stones, cysts, or solid masses within them. They can also be used to determine whether the biliary ducts or gallbladder are enlarged. The radionuclide scans are used to determine patency of the cystic and common ducts and to study gallbladder emptying after administration of cholecystokinin (CCK).

The relative usefulness of these five tests is not established. Many physicians first try ultrasound or CT scan to see whether the biliary ducts are dilated and to seek the cause of the patient's jaundice (stones, pancreatic mass, etc.). The radionuclide scan will determine if the cystic duct and bile ducts are patent. Direct visualization is undertaken if the diagnosis is not established. PTC is often attempted first if an intrahepatic or proximal bile duct obstruction is suggested by imaging tests. ERCP is used first if distal obstruction is suspected. Advantages of the endoscopic approach are that the papilla and the pancreatic duct are seen (in addition to the biliary ducts) and that therapy can be performed with endoscopic sphincterotomy or drainage when appropriate. In the event of a technical failure or incomplete information resulting from either ERCP or PTC, the other technique is tried. This approach detects most lesions requiring surgical intervention.

ERCP or PTC can also be useful in patients with biliary pain, cholangitis, or impaired liver function after previous biliary surgery. Remediable postoperative lesions such as strictures can be discovered and sometimes treated endoscopically. Should endoscopic therapy fail, their precise anatomy is outlined so that reoperation is less difficult.

Retrograde pancreatography   Patients with recurrent or chronic pancreatitis may merit retrograde pancreatography to seek a lesion which can be approached surgically, such as localized pancreatitis in the tail or ductal pathology amenable to drainage.

Patients with symptoms, signs, or laboratory findings suggesting pancreatic carcinoma may have pancreatograms suggesting malignancy with a narrowed, encased, or sharply "cutoff" pancreatic duct (Fig. 236-1D). Differentiation of such pancreatic ductal findings from benign inflammatory disease can be difficult. Cytologic examination of pancreatic duct contents obtained during ERCP may prove helpful. Unfortunately, most patients with symptomatic pancreatic cancer diagnosed by ERCP are inoperable.

Patients presenting with painless steatorrhea of pancreatic origin may be shown to have a ductal pattern suggesting chronic pancreatitis or pancreatic carcinoma. Pancreatography has not been useful in the study of obscure upper abdominal pain. Pancreatic cysts can be better diagnosed by noninvasive techniques such as ultrasound, and pancreatography should be reserved for those cases where it is desirable to outline the anatomy immediately prior to surgery. Pancreatography alone does not seem promising as a method of screening for early pancreatic carcinoma.

Therapeutic ERCP   Access to the pancreatic and biliary tree for the removal of stones and the placement of stents is made possible by endoscopic retrograde sphincterotomy (ERS). The pancreatic or biliary sphincter mechanism is cut using electrosurgical current passed through a wire attached to the ERCP catheter. Complications of bleeding, perforation, pancreatitis, and cholangitis occur in about 8 percent of patients with a resulting mortality rate of approximately 1 percent. The role of pancreatic sphincterotomy in the management of pancreatic stones and strictures is currently controversial; however, biliary sphincterotomy is now an established therapy for several conditions.

Common bile duct stones in patients with prior cholecystectomy are successfully removed from the bile duct after ERS by experienced operators 90 percent of the time. Small stones are pulled into the duodenum with a balloon catheter or after being captured by a basket. Stones larger than 1.5 cm in diameter may be difficult to extract without prior fragmentation by mechanical or other techniques. Common duct stones in younger patients with intact gallbladders are best removed at the time of cholecystectomy. Older patients with increased surgical risks can sometimes be managed with ERS and stone extraction alone; cholecystectomy can be delayed or avoided entirely. ERS is also assuming an increasing role in the initial treatment of patients with acute cholangitis and severe biliary pancreatitis.

Patients with benign and malignant bile duct strictures may benefit from the endoscopic placement of biliary stents after ERS. Benign strictures frequently remain dilated following removal of stents that have been left in place for several months. Patients with either pancreatic carcinoma or cholangiocarcinoma resulting in obstructive jaundice can be effectively palliated by placement of a biliary stent. Stents usually occlude after 3 to 6 months and must be exchanged if recurrent jaundice or cholangitis develops. Strictures involving the hilum of the liver (see Chap. 258) are difficult to palliate endoscopically because stents must be placed into both sides of the liver. These patients may be more effectively palliated with surgical or percutaneous radiologic techniques.

Other diagnostic techniques   Critical comparative studies are needed of the various approaches to biliary tree disorders and to pancreatic diseases (ERCP, PTC, angiography, CT scanning, and ultrasound). The role of magnetic resonance imaging in diseases of the pancreas and biliary tree is yet to be defined. Endoscopic ultrasound may also prove to be a valuable technique to image the intestinal wall and adjacent organs.

COLONOSCOPY The interior of the entire length of the colon from anus to cecum can be visualized by the experienced colonoscopist. This is one of the most significant diagnostic and therapeutic applications of fiberoptic endoscopy because it can diagnose potentially curable colonic cancers missed by other techniques and remove potentially precancerous adenomatous polyps.

Approximately 40 percent of colonoscopies are performed because of an abnormal barium enema showing a polyp or a narrowing or filling defect suggesting carcinoma. Approximately 40 percent of colonoscopies are done because of gastrointestinal bleeding. The ability to examine the whole colon is proving valuable in the management of some patients with inflammatory bowel disease.

Patients are prepared for colonoscopy with a liquid diet for 2 days, magnesium citrate laxation the evening before examination, and tap water enemas the morning of the procedure. Another increasingly utilized method of preparing the colon is a total-gut lavage with a nonabsorbable electrolyte solution. This method prepares the patient without laxatives or enemas and only requires a few hours. Immediately before the procedure patients are lightly sedated with intravenous diazepam and meperidine.

The main complications of colonoscopy are hemorrhage and perforation (morbidity rate is 0.5 to 1.3 percent; mortality rate is 0.02 percent). The complication rate for polypectomy is 1 to 2 percent. Diverticular or ischemic disease and prior irradiation make the procedure more difficult and hazardous. The risk of perforation is also increased in the patient with very active colitis, and colonoscopy should be avoided during the acute phase.

Polyps (See also Chap. 243) A polyp seen on barium enema merits colonoscopy for two reasons: it may be an artifact or a cancer, and a second polyp or cancer may have been missed. The polyp can usually be excised, with lower morbidity and mortality rates than with surgery. The best way to rule out cancer within a polyp is to remove it completely for histologic examination. Hyperplastic polyps do not become malignant; colonic polyps that show benign neoplasia histologically may become malignant (tubular and villous adenomas). The risk of neoplastic polyps being cancerous increases with their size. The risk is also higher in villous adenomas. Pedunculated polyps with cancer confined to the mucosa and with an uninvolved stalk can be cured by removal with an electrocautery snare during colonoscopy. Thus, most colonoscopists will remove all polyps more than 0.5 cm in diameter. It is more difficult to know what to do with polyps smaller than 0.5 cm in diameter because more than 50 percent may be adenomatous. A coagulating biopsy technique can be used to both biopsy and destroy even the smallest adenomatous polyp in the hope that the subsequent risk of developing colonic cancer will be reduced. The wisdom of this course of action is suggested by a sigmoidoscopic study in which the removal of all polyps reduced the expected incidence and invasiveness of subsequently developing cancers in the anatomic area screened. Most agree that the patient with adenomatous polyps is more likely to develop another polyp or cancer and therefore merits a regular screening program. The optimal frequency of follow-up examinations after polypectomy is not yet established. The current recommendation is a digital examination and stool test for occult blood yearly. When a polyp is discovered, the entire colon should be examined for synchronous polyps or cancer. This should probably be repeated at 1 year and, if negative, every 3 years thereafter. If stools are positive for occult blood or symptoms develop, immediate evaluation is indicated.

Cancer screening by x-ray All filling defects on barium enema merit evaluation by colonoscopy. If the lesion is a pedunculated polyp, it can be removed for histologic examination; if its appearance suggests a cancer, it can be biopsied and brushed for histologic and cytologic confirmation. When a polyp or a carcinoma is found, the remainder of the colon should be screened for additional polyps and synchronous carcinoma. This avoids multiple colotomies to search for a second lesion and reduces surgical morbidity. Approximately 40 percent of lesions diagnosed as a mass by x-ray are not present on colonoscopy or are found to be due to lesions such as a polyp rather than a cancer.

Narrowing by x-ray An etiologic diagnosis of segmental narrowing may be difficult by x-ray. Colonoscopy often determines the cause of segmental narrowing and differentiates adenocarcinoma from inflammation secondary to ischemia, irradiation, diverticular disease, or Crohn's colitis. Even the most classic "apple-core" lesion indicated by x-ray may be covered by normal mucosa at colonoscopy, suggesting an extrinsic inflammatory lesion. In 10 to 30 percent of patients, narrowed segments present on x-ray are not visualized during colonoscopy, probably because they are areas of temporary spasm. Such findings avoid unnecessary operations.

Chronic bleeding (x-ray and sigmoidoscopy negative) This condition leads to approximately 40 percent of colonoscopies. The x-ray is more likely to miss a lesion when single contrast is used rather than air contrast. The cause of bleeding is found in approximately 40 percent of such patients. The common bleeding sources are adenomatous polyp (20 percent), adenocarcinoma (10 percent), and Crohn's disease (7 percent). Many of these carcinomas are resectable, and this group may benefit most from colonoscopy. If no bleeding source is found, a search may be appropriate for an upper gastrointestinal source with an upper gastrointestinal x-ray and/or upper endoscopy.

Inflammatory bowel disease Colonoscopy is not routinely indicated in patients with inflammatory bowel disease. Colonoscopy may help in the initial diagnosis, especially in differentiating Crohn's colitis from ulcerative colitis. It can aid the surgeon in assessing the activity and extent of the disease before surgery. Colonoscopy can evaluate radiographic abnormalities suggesting cancer, such as strictures, polyps, or masses. Colonoscopy may be indicated in patients with ulcerative colitis of more than 10 years' duration because of the increased risk of carcinoma; it is hoped that repeated colonoscopies will serve to detect these malignancies earlier than x-ray and while the lesions are still curable. The frequency of colonoscopy and/or double-contrast barium enema examination in such patients is not yet established. If an expert gastrointestinal pathologist finds high-grade dysplasia in colonic biopsies in a patient with long-standing ulcerative colitis, most would consider this to be an indication for colectomy. Preparation for colonoscopy must often be modified for patients with inflammatory bowel disease. Colonoscopy is contraindicated in patients with toxic megacolon, very active disease, or a possible intestinal perforation.

Other indications The flexible sigmoidoscope is replacing the rigid 25-cm sigmoidoscope for routine screening because it can be passed to 40 to 60 cm with minimal preparation, less discomfort, and a higher diagnostic yield. After segmental colonic resection for carcinoma, colonoscopy may detect early mucosal recurrence and differentiate it from benign anastomotic strictures or bleeding suture granulomas. These patients must also be periodically screened for the development of polyps or additional carcinomas. Colonoscopy is occasionally used during laparotomy to assist the surgeon in ruling out other lesions. The colonoscope can be advanced to the cecum rapidly with the surgeon's assistance, and additional polyps removed without colotomy. Colonscopy is useful in the management of selected patients with lower gastrointestinal bleeding. Patients with severe active bleeding are best managed with radionuclide-labeled red blood cell scans followed immediately, if active bleeding is present, by selective angiography. Colonoscopic visualization in this setting is difficult because of excessive luminal blood. If the labeled red blood cell scan is negative, colonic lavage with a balanced electrolyte solution followed in several hours by colonoscopy may identify the bleeding site. Bleeding polyps may be removed by snare electrocautery. Endoscopic hemostatic therapy may be useful in other bleeding lesions such as angiodysplasia.

Colonoscopy detects some carriers of the dominant familial polyposis gene before diagnosis by barium enema and sigmoidoscopy. Carcinoma is a great threat in those familial polyposis syndromes which produce many adenomatous polyps (familial polyposis and Gardner's syndrome); in these conditions, polypectomy is useful for diagnosis, but colectomy is the only treatment which prevents development of carcinoma. These patients are also at risk of developing duodenal and periampullary cancer and should probably undergo periodic surveillance with a side-viewing duodenoscope.

CONTRAINDICATIONS   All types of fiberoptic endoscopy are contraindicated in certain patients, including those who are uncooperative or combative or who have perforation of the intestine. Patients with acute medical illness such as myocardial infarction have increased risks at endoscopy. The relative benefits and risks of the procedure must be carefully weighed in these situations.

CONSCIOUS LAPAROSCOPY   The potentials for laparoscopy in conscious patients have not been as fully appreciated in North America as they have been in other countries, where it has been used widely for over 20 years. This procedure has extremely low mortality and morbidity rates in experienced hands. The instrument usually used for laparoscopy is a stiff tube with a lens system that provides a superb view. Under local anesthesia pneumoperitoneum is gradually induced with air or nitrous oxide.

Much of the exterior of the liver, gallbladder, spleen, peritoneum, diaphragm, and pelvic organs can be clearly visualized. Portions of the colon and small bowel can also be seen. Lesions can be biopsied under direct vision and any resultant bleeding controlled by electrocoagulation. Furthermore, in centers with extensive experience contrast material can be injected into the liver to visualize vascular, lymphatic, and biliary systems.

Laparoscopy may permit one to make a difficult diagnosis without resorting to laparotomy by biopsying localized hepatic disease under direct vision. Laparoscopy can often help differentiate "medical" from "surgical" jaundice and may also enable staging of malignant disease without laparotomy.

REFERENCES

CELLO JP et al: Endoscopic sclerotherapy versus portacaval shunt in patients with severe cirrhosis and acute variceal hemorrhage: Long-term follow-up. N Engl J Med 316:11, 1987

COTTON PB: Endoscopic management of bile duct stones (apples and oranges). Gut 25:587, 1984

FLEISCHER D: Endoscopic therapy of upper gastrointestinal bleeding in humans. Gastroenterology 90:217, 1986

HAGGITT RC et al: Prognostic factors in colorectal carcinomas arising in adenomas: Implications for lesions removed by endoscopic polypectomy. Gastroenterology 89:328, 1985

JENSEN DM, MACHICADO GA: Diagnosis and treatment of severe hematochezia: The role of urgent colonoscopy after purge. Gastroenterology 95:1569, 1988

LAINE L: Multipolar electrocoagulation in the treatment of active upper gastrointestinal tract hemorrhage. N Engl J Med 316:1613, 1987

SILVERSTEIN FE, TYTGAT GNJ: Atlas of Gastrointestinal Endoscopy. Philadelphia, Saunders, 1987

SIVAK MV: Gastroenterologic Endoscopy. Philadelphia, Saunders, 1987

237   DISEASES OF THE ESOPHAGUS

RAJ K. GOYAL

The two major functions of the esophagus are the transport of the food bolus from the mouth to the stomach and the prevention of retrograde flow of gastrointestinal contents. The transport function is achieved by peristaltic contractions (see Chap. 42). Retrograde flow is prevented by the two esophageal sphincters, which remain closed between swallows. The upper esophageal sphincter remains closed by the elastic properties of its wall and by tonic contraction of the cricopharyngeus and inferior pharyngeal constrictor muscles due to continuous neural excitation of the lower motor neurons which innervate these muscles via motor end plates. The opening of the

upper sphincter is due to inhibition of contraction of the cricopharyngeus and inferior pharyngeal constriction and forward displacement of the larynx by the suprahyoid muscles. In contrast, the lower esophageal sphincter remains closed because of its intrinsic myogenic tone, and a neural pathway, consisting of preganglionic parasympathetic fibers in the vagus nerve and postganglionic myenteric inhibitory neurons, causes its relaxation. A reflex increase in the lower sphincter pressure occurs with an increase in intraabdominal pressure and ingestion of a protein meal. Fatty meals, smoking, and beverages with a high xanthine content (tea, coffee, cola) cause a reduction in sphincter pressure. Many hormones and neurotransmitters can modify lower sphincter pressure. Cholinergic muscarinic (M-2 receptor) agonists, alpha-adrenergic agonists, gastrin, pancreatic polypeptide, substance P, and prostaglandin $F_{2\alpha}$ cause contraction; in contrast, ganglionic stimulants, beta-adrenergic agonists, dopamine, cholecystokinin, secretin, vasoactive intestinal peptide (VIP), calcitonin-gene-related peptide (CGRP), ATP, and adenosine cause relaxation of the sphincter. These effects are mediated by actions on the inhibitory intramural neurons or on the sphincter muscle directly. Effects of many of these agents are pharmacologic rather than physiologic.

SYMPTOMS

DYSPHAGIA   See Chap. 42.

ESOPHAGEAL PAIN   *Heartburn,* or pyrosis, is characterized by burning retrosternal discomfort that may move up and down the chest like a wave. When severe, it may radiate to the sides of the chest, neck, and angles of the jaw. Heartburn is a characteristic symptom of reflux esophagitis and may be associated with regurgitation or a feeling of warm fluid climbing up the throat. It is aggravated by bending forward, straining, or lying recumbent and is worse after meals. It is relieved by upright posture, by swallowing of saliva or water, or, more reliably, by antacids. Heartburn appears to be produced by heightened mucosal sensitivity and can be reproduced by infusion of dilute (0.1 N) hydrochloric acid (Bernstein test) or neutral hyperosmolar solutions into the esophagus.

Odynophagia, or painful swallowing, is characteristic of nonreflux esophagitis, particularly monilial and herpes esophagitis. Odynophagia may also occur with peptic ulcer of the esophagus (Barrett's ulcer), carcinoma with periesophageal involvement, caustic damage of the esophagus, and esophageal perforation. Odynophagia is unusual in uncomplicated reflux esophagitis. Crampy chest pain associated with impaction of the small bowel should be distinguished from odynophagia.

Chest pain other than heartburn and odynophagia occurs when the esophageal muscle contracts with excessive force, for a long duration, and repetitively, as in diffuse esophageal spasm. This may occur spontaneously or during a meal. Chest pain due to periesophageal involvement caused by carcinoma or peptic ulcer may be constant and agonizing. Sometimes different types of esophageal pains exist together in the same patient, and frequently patients are not able to describe the pain accurately enough to allow its classification.

REGURGITATION   Regurgitation is the effortless appearance of gastric or esophageal contents in the mouth. In distal esophageal obstruction and stasis, as in achalasia or a large diverticulum, the regurgitated material consists of tasteless mucoid fluid or undigested food. Regurgitation of sour or bitter-tasting material occurs in severe gastroesophageal reflux and is associated with incompetence of both the upper and lower esophageal sphincters. Regurgitation may result in laryngeal aspiration, with spells of coughing and choking that awaken the patient from sleep, and aspiration pneumonia. Water brash is reflex salivary hypersecretion which occurs in response to peptic esophagitis; it should not be confused with regurgitation.

DIAGNOSTIC TESTS

RADIOLOGIC STUDIES   Barium swallow with fluoroscopy and esophagogram is the most widely used test for diagnosis of esophageal

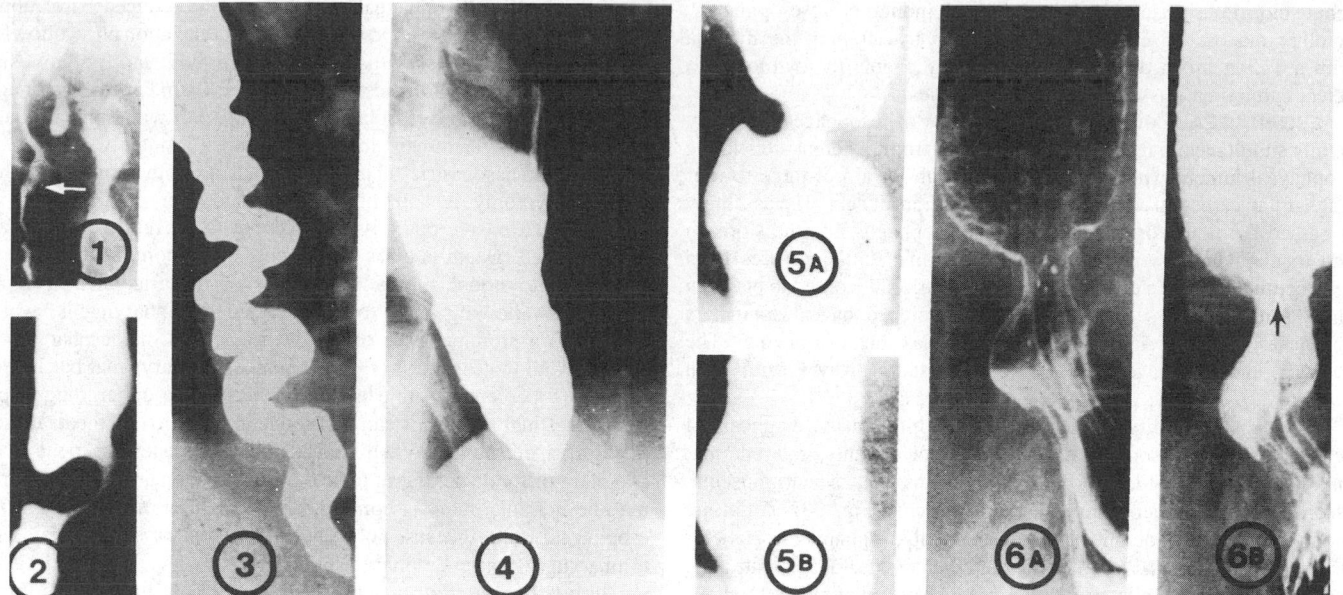

FIGURE 237-1 Radiographic appearance of some motor disorders of the pharynx and esophagus. (1) Pharyngeal paralysis with tracheal aspiration (arrow). (2) Cricopharyngeal achalasia. Note the prominent cricopharyngeus, which is recognized by its smoothness and location in the posterior wall. (3) Diffuse esophageal spasm. Note typical corkscrew appearance of the lower part of the esophagus. (4) Achalasia showing dilation of esophageal body with air-fluid level and closed lower esophageal sphincter. (5) Muscular (contractile) lower esophageal ring. Note a symmetric contraction in 5A that has disappeared in 5B, obtained during the same examination. (6) Scleroderma esophagus showing dilated esophagus with a stricture in 6A and reflux of barium from the stomach into the esophagus in 6B. *(Courtesy of Dr. Harvey Goldstein.)*

disease and can be used to evaluate both structural and motor disorders. The pharynx is examined to detect stasis of barium in the valleculae and pyriform sinuses and regurgitation of barium into the nose and tracheobronchial tree. Since the pharyngeal phase of swallowing lasts no more than a second, cineradiography may be necessary to permit detection and analysis of abnormalities of pharyngeal function. Spontaneous reflux of barium from the stomach into the esophagus should be sought in patients with suspected reflux esophagitis. Esophageal peristalsis is best studied in the recumbent position since in the upright position the passage of most of the barium occurs by gravity alone. A double-contrast esophagogram, obtained by coating the esophageal mucosa with barium and distending the esophageal lumen with air using effervescent granules, is particularly useful in demonstrating mucosal ulcers and early cancers. Figures 237-1 and 237-2 illustrate the radiographic appearance of some esophageal disorders.

ESOPHAGOSCOPY   Fiberoptic esophagogastroduodenoscopy is described in Chap. 236. Esophagoscopy is the direct method of establishing the cause of mechanical dysphagia and of identifying mucosal lesions, such as superficial ulcers and esophagitis, which may not be identified by the usual barium swallow. In the presence of marked luminal narrowing, examination can be achieved by using a smaller caliber endoscope, although on occasion a stricture must be dilated prior to a complete endoscopic examination. Transendo-

FIGURE 237-2   Selected structural lesions of the esophagus. (1) Carcinoma of the esophagus with typical annular narrowing with overhanging margins and destruction of the mucosa. (2) Leiomyoma of the esophagus with smooth filling defect and right angles of origin from the esophageal wall. (3) Esophageal ulcer in columnar-cell-lined esophagus (Barrett's esophagus). (4) Monilial esophagitis with irregular plaquelike filling defects. (5) Long stricture secondary to lye ingestion. (6) Peptic stricture, short and tubular, with associated hiatus hernia. (7) Mucosal lower esophageal mucosal (Schatzki) ring. Thin weblike annular constriction at the esophagogastric junction is associated with a small hiatal hernia. *(Courtesy of Dr. Harvey Goldstein.)*

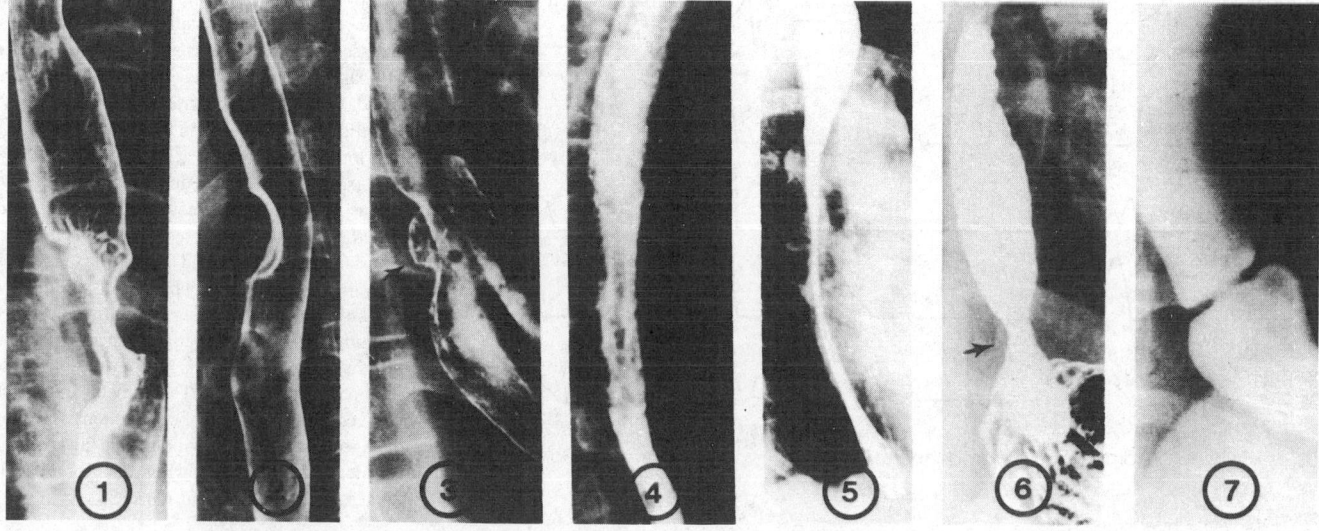

scopic biopsies are useful in diagnosing carcinoma, reflux esophagitis, or other mucosal diseases. Obtaining cells by scraping the mucosa with a Teflon brush during endoscopy may enable the cytologist to detect carcinoma missed by mucosal biopsies.

ESOPHAGEAL MOTILITY The study of esophageal motility entails simultaneous recording of pressures from different sites in the esophageal lumen. This is usually done with a train of three to four water-filled catheters connected to pressure transducers. The assembly is passed by mouth or nose through the esophagus into the stomach and then gradually withdrawn 1 cm at a time until pressures from each centimeter of the esophagus and pharynx are recorded in between and during swallows. The upper and lower esophageal sphincters appear as zones of high pressure that relax on swallowing. The pharynx and esophageal body show peristaltic waves with each swallow.

Esophageal motility studies are very helpful in the diagnosis of achalasia, diffuse esophageal spasm and its variants, scleroderma, and other motor disorders of the esophagus, as well as neuromuscular disorders of the upper esophagus and pharynx (Fig. 237-3) but are of no value in the diagnosis of mechanical dysphagia. In patients with reflux esophagitis, esophageal manometry is useful in quantitating lower esophageal competence and providing information on the status of the esophageal body motor activity. The information obtained by manometry is quantitative and cannot be obtained by barium swallow or endoscopy.

Special tests for the evaluation of reflux esophagitis are described later.

MOTOR DISORDERS

STRIATED MUSCLE Pharyngeal paralysis Pharyngeal paralysis is characterized by dysphagia, nasal regurgitation, and tracheobronchial aspiration during swallowing. It occurs in a variety of neuromuscular disorders (see Table 42-2). Some of these disorders may also involve laryngeal and orofacial muscles. When the suprahyoid muscles are also paralyzed, the upper sphincter does not open with swallowing, leading to paralytic achalasia of the upper esophageal sphincter and severe dysphagia.

Barium swallow, oropharyngography, and cineradiography reveal stasis of barium in the valleculae and pyriform sinuses, nasal and tracheobronchial aspiration, and closed upper sphincter (Fig. 237-1). Pharyngeal motility studies demonstrate reduced amplitude of pharyngeal and upper esophageal contractions and reduced basal upper esophageal sphincter pressure without further relaxation on swallowing (Fig. 237-3). Patients with myasthenia gravis and polymyositis respond to treatment for these diseases (see Chap. 366). Dysphagia in patients with cerebrovascular accident improves with time, although not completely. Treatment in most instances is mainly supportive, consisting of nasogastric tube feeding and physiotherapy. Cricopharyngeal myotomy is sometimes performed, but its usefulness is unproved. Extensive operative procedures to prevent aspiration are rarely needed. Death is often due to pulmonary complications.

Cricopharyngeal achalasia Failure of the cricopharyngeus to relax on swallowing leads to a contracted cricopharyngeus, which appears as a prominent bar on the posterior wall of the pharynx on barium swallow (Fig. 237-1). A transient cricopharyngeal bar is seen in up to 5 percent of subjects without dysphagia undergoing upper gastrointestinal studies; it can be produced in normal subjects during a Valsalva maneuver. When contraction is persistent, patients may complain of food sticking in their throats. Cricopharyngeal myotomy may be helpful, but it is contraindicated in the presence of gastroesophageal reflux because in such patients this procedure may lead to pharyngeal and pulmonary aspiration.

Globus hystericus A sensation of a constant lump in the throat but with no difficulty during swallowing occurs especially in subjects with emotional disorders, particularly in women. Barium studies are normal, but manometry shows a hypertensive upper sphincter. Treatment is primarily one of reassurance.

SMOOTH MUSCLE Achalasia Achalasia is a motor disorder of the esophageal smooth muscle in which the lower esophageal sphincter is hypertensive, does not relax properly with swallowing, and the normal peristalsis of the esophageal body is replaced by abnormal contractions. Based upon the changes in the esophageal body, achalasia can be of two types: in *classic achalasia* simultaneous contractions of small amplitude occur, while in *vigorous achalasia* contractions are simultaneous in onset, large in amplitude, and repetitive, resembling those seen in diffuse esophageal spasm.

PATHOPHYSIOLOGY The underlying abnormality is defective innervation of the smooth-muscle portion of the esophageal body and the lower esophageal sphincter. Pathologically, vigorous achalasia is associated with less severe neural damage than classic achalasia, which shows a marked reduction in myenteric neurons. Primary idiopathic achalasia accounts for most of the patients seen in the United States. Secondary achalasia may be caused by gastric carcinoma infiltrating the esophagus, lymphoma, Chagas' disease, neu-

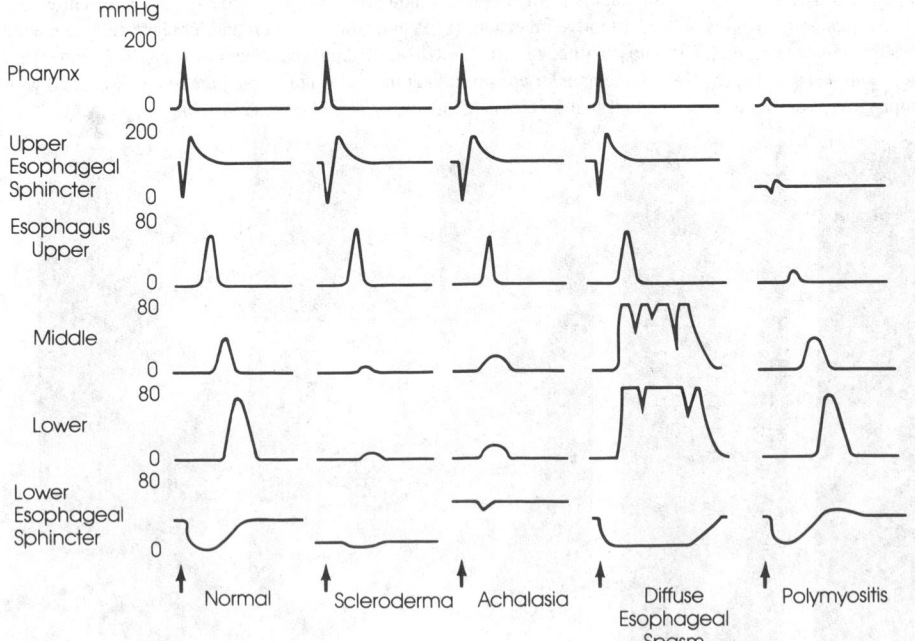

FIGURE 237-3 Motility patterns in selected esophageal and pharyngeal disorders. In normal subjects, the upper and lower esophageal sphincters appear as zones of high pressure. With a swallow (indicated by ↑), pressure in the sphincters falls and a contraction wave starts in the pharynx and progresses down the esophagus. In scleroderma, the lower part of the esophagus (smooth muscle) shows reduced amplitude of contractions, which may be peristaltic or simultaneous in onset, and hypotension of the lower sphincter. In achalasia, the lower part of the esophagus shows reduced amplitude of contractions that are simultaneous in onset. In contrast to scleroderma, the lower esophageal sphincter in achalasia is hypertensive and fails to relax in response to a swallow. In diffuse esophageal spasm, the lower part of the esophagus shows simultaneous onset, large amplitude, long duration, repetitive contractions. In polymyositis, the smooth-muscle part of the esophagus is normal. The skeletal muscle part shows reduced amplitude of contractions. The upper esophageal sphincter is hypotensive and may not relax normally on swallowing due to associated weakness of the suprahyoid muscles.

ropathic chronic intestinal pseudoobstruction syndrome, irradiation, and certain toxins and drugs. Hypertensive or hypercontracting lower esophageal sphincter may be considered as variants of achalasia.

CLINICAL FEATURES Achalasia affects patients of all ages and both sexes. Dysphagia, chest pain, and regurgitation are the main symptoms. Dysphagia occurs early with both liquids and solids and is worsened by emotional stress and hurried eating. Various maneuvers designed to increase intraesophageal pressure, including the Valsalva, may help passage of the bolus into the stomach. Chest pain is more pronounced in vigorous achalasia than in classic achalasia. Regurgitation and pulmonary aspiration occur because of retention of large volumes of saliva and ingested food in the esophagus. The presence of gastroesophageal reflux argues against achalasia, although some of these patients may describe their chest pain as heartburn. The overall course is usually chronic with progressive dysphagia and weight loss over months to years.

DIAGNOSIS Chest x-ray shows absence of the gastric air bubble and sometimes a tubular mediastinal mass beside the aorta. The presence of an air-fluid level in the mediastinum in the upright position represents unpassed food in the esophagus and is characteristic. Barium swallow shows esophageal dilatation, and in advanced cases the esophagus may become sigmoid. On fluoroscopy normal peristalsis is lost in the lower two-thirds of the esophagus. The terminal part of the esophagus shows a persistent beaklike narrowing representing the nonrelaxing lower esophageal sphincter [Fig. 237-1(2)]. In patients with vigorous achalasia, there may be pronounced nonperistaltic contractions without a dilated esophagus.

Manometry shows normal or elevated basal lower esophageal sphincter pressure and swallow-induced relaxation which is absent or reduced in degree, duration, and consistency (Fig. 237-3). The esophageal body shows elevated resting pressure. In response to swallows, primary peristaltic waves are replaced by simultaneous-onset contractions. These contractions may be of poor amplitude (classic achalasia) or of large amplitude and long duration (vigorous achalasia). Administration of the cholinergic muscarinic agonist mecholyl causes a marked increase in baseline esophageal pressure, and administration of cholecystokinin (CCK), which normally causes a fall in the sphincter pressure, paradoxically causes contraction of the lower esophageal sphincter. Endoscopy is helpful in excluding the secondary causes of achalasia, particularly gastric carcinoma.

TREATMENT Medical treatment using soft foods, sedatives, nitrates, and anticholinergic drugs is usually unsatisfactory. Calcium channel antagonists such as nifedipine have been used with some success. The best available therapy involves balloon dilation to reduce the basal lower esophageal sphincter pressure by tearing muscle fibers. In experienced hands this technique is effective in about 85 percent of patients. Perforation and bleeding are potential complications. Heller's extramucosal myotomy of the lower sphincter, in which the circular muscle layer is incised, is equally effective. Reflux esophagitis and peptic stricture may follow successful treatment of achalasia. However, this complication is more frequent with myotomy than with balloon dilation.

Diffuse esophageal spasm and related motor disorders Diffuse esophageal spasm is a motor disorder of the esophageal smooth muscle characterized by multiple spontaneous contractions and by swallow-induced contractions that are of simultaneous onset, large amplitude, long duration, and repetitive occurrence. Variants of diffuse esophageal spasm show some but not all of these motor abnormalities.

PATHOPHYSIOLOGY The pathogenesis of the various abnormalities of peristalsis in diffuse esophageal spasm is not known. Histopathologic studies show patchy neural degeneration localized to nerve processes rather than the prominent degeneration of nerve cell bodies seen in achalasia.

Variants of diffuse esophageal spasm, such as large amplitude but peristaltic contractions (sometimes called nutcracker esophagus) or normal amplitude but simultaneous contractions, frequently occur as a primary disease or in association with a variety of diseases as well as emotional stress and aging. Collagen vascular disease, diabetic neuropathy, reflux esophagitis, irradiation esophagitis, esophageal obstruction, and cholinergic and anticholinergic drugs can cause esophageal motor abnormalities. The relationship between reflux esophagitis and motor abnormalities is controversial. Overlapping features of diffuse esophageal spasm and achalasia occur in vigorous achalasia. The variant syndromes are more frequent in clinical practice than classic diffuse esophageal spasm.

CLINICAL FEATURES The symptomatic patient with diffuse spasm or its variants presents with chest pain, dysphagia, or both. Chest pain is particularly marked in patients with esophageal contractions of large amplitude and of long duration. Chest pain usually occurs at rest but may be brought on by swallowing or by emotional stress. The pain is retrosternal; it may radiate to the back, sides of the chest, both arms, or the sides of the jaw and may last for a few seconds to several minutes. It may be acute and severe, mimicking the pain of myocardial ischemia. Dysphagia for solids and liquids may occur with or without chest pain.

Diffuse esophageal spasm must be differentiated from other causes of chest pain, particularly ischemic heart disease with atypical angina. Often a complete cardiac workup is done before the esophageal etiology is seriously considered. The presence of dysphagia in association with pain should point to the esophagus as the site of disease. Symptoms of esophageal spasm should be carefully distinguished from those of reflux esophagitis; sometimes the two may coexist.

DIAGNOSIS Barium swallow shows that normal sequential peristalsis below the aortic arch is replaced by uncoordinated simultaneous contractions that produce the appearance of curling or multiple ripples in the wall, sacculations, and pseudodiverticula—the "corkscrew" esophagus [Fig. 237-1(3)]. Sometimes an esophageal contraction obliterates the lumen and barium is pushed away in both directions. The lower esophageal sphincter opens normally.

Manometry reveals the characteristic prolonged large amplitude and repetitive contractions of simultaneous onset in the lower part of the esophagus (Fig. 237-3). Only one or two of these abnormalities may be present in variants of diffuse spasm. Because the abnormalities may be episodic, manometry may be normal at the time of the study; therefore, several techniques are used in attempts to provoke esophageal spasm. Cold swallows produce chest pain but do not produce spasm on manometric studies. Solid boluses and pharmacologic agents, particularly edrophonium, induce both chest pain and motor abnormalities. However, there is a poor correlation between induction of pain and motility changes. Ergonovine may cause coronary artery spasm and should not be used. Overall, the usefulness of pharmacologic provocative tests is limited.

TREATMENT Anticholinergics are usually of limited value because the main nerves that mediate esophageal contractions are noncholinergic. Agents that relax smooth muscle such as sublingual nitroglycerin (0.3 to 0.6 mg) or longer acting agents such as isosorbide dinitrate (2.5 to 10 mg sublingually before meals) and nifedipine (10 to 20 mg before meals) may be helpful in some cases. Esophageal dilation with mercury-filled rubber dilators may produce symptomatic relief as a result of distention of the lower esophagus, but this is largely a placebo effect. Reassurance and tranquilizers are helpful in allaying patients' apprehension. Balloon dilation is sometimes attempted but can be hazardous in inexperienced hands. In severe cases resistant to all therapy, a longitudinal myotomy of esophageal circular muscle is performed; it relieves pain in up to two-thirds of patients.

Scleroderma involving the esophagus The esophageal lesions in systemic sclerosis consist of muscular atrophy of the smooth-muscle portion, with weakness of contraction in the lower two-thirds of the esophageal body and incompetence of the lower esophageal sphincter. The esophageal wall is thin and atrophic with or without areas of patchy fibrosis. Patients present with dysphagia to solids and to liquids in the recumbent position. They may also present with heartburn and regurgitation due to gastroesophageal reflux and esophagitis, which in turn may lead to stricture formation and more pronounced dysphagia. Barium swallow shows dilation and loss of peristaltic contractions in the middle and distal portions of the esophagus. The lower esophageal sphincter is patulous, and gastroesophageal reflux may occur freely (Fig. 237-1). Mucosal changes from esophageal ulceration may be detected, and esophageal stricture may be present. Motility studies show marked reduction in the amplitude of smooth-muscle contractions, which may be peristaltic or nonperistaltic. Lower esophageal sphincter resting pressure is subnormal, but relaxation is normal (Fig. 237-3). Currently, there is no effective treatment for the motor difficulty. Reflux esophagitis and its complications should be treated aggressively as described under reflux esophagitis.

INFLAMMATORY DISORDERS

GASTROESOPHAGEAL REFLUX AND ESOPHAGITIS Reflux esophagitis consists of esophageal mucosal damage resulting from reflux of gastric or intestinal contents into the esophagus. Depending on the causative agent, it is referred to as peptic, bile, or alkaline esophagitis.

Pathophysiology Three considerations involved in the pathophysiology of reflux esophagitis are (1) the pathogenesis of the esophageal reflux episode, (2) the cumulative, or net, esophageal reflux, and (3) the pathogenesis of esophagitis.

Two conditions must be met for a *reflux episode* to occur: the gastrointestinal contents must be ''ready'' to reflux, and the antireflux mechanism at the lower end of the esophagus must be compromised. Gastrointestinal contents are most likely to reflux (1) when gastric volume is increased (after meals, with pyloric obstruction or gastric stasis syndrome, and in acid hypersecretory states), (2) when the gastric contents are located near the gastroesophageal junction (due to recumbency or bending), and (3) when gastric pressure is increased (with obesity, pregnancy, ascites, or tight binders or girdles).

The normal antireflux mechanisms consist of the lower esophageal sphincter (LES) and the anatomic configuration of the gastroesophageal junction. Reflux occurs only when the LES–gastric pressure gradient is lost. It can be caused by increased intragastric pressure or a transient or sustained decrease in the sphincter tone itself. Most patients with reflux have lower than normal LES pressures. The incompetence of the LES may be primary or secondary. The secondary causes include scleroderma-like diseases, a myopathic type of chronic intestinal pseudoobstruction syndrome, pregnancy, female sex hormones, smoking, smooth-muscle relaxants (such as beta-adrenergics, aminophylline, nitrates, and calcium channel blockers), destruction of the sphincter by surgical resection, myotomy or balloon dilation, and esophagitis. Some patients have normal lower esophageal sphincter pressures but their sphincter relaxes inappropriately, allowing reflux to occur. The importance of the anatomic configuration of the esophagogastric junction is not fully known at present. However, the role of a sliding hiatal hernia in the impairment of the reflux barrier is not felt to be so important as was once thought.

The net or *cumulative esophageal reflux*, i.e., the amount and duration of refluxed material remaining in the esophagus, is dependent on (1) the amount of refluxed material per episode and frequency of episodes, (2) the clearing of the esophagus by gravity and peristaltic contraction, and (3) neutralization by salivary secretion.

Esophagitis is a complication of reflux, and it develops when the mucosal defenses that normally counteract the effect of injurious agents on the esophageal mucosa succumb to the onslaught of the refluxed acid pepsin or bile. *Mild esophagitis* shows microscopic changes of mucosal infiltration with granulocytes or eosinophils, hyperplasia of basal cells, and elongation of dermal pegs. It can occur with or without endoscopic abnormalities. *Erosive esophagitis* shows endoscopically visible damage to the mucosa in the form of marked redness, friability, bleeding, superficial linear ulcers, and exudates. *Peptic stricture* results from fibrosis that causes constriction of the esophageal lumen. The fibrosis is predominantly submucosal,

but it may involve the whole wall. Peptic strictures occur in about 10 percent of patients with reflux esophagitis. Short peptic strictures caused by spontaneous reflux are usually 1 to 3 cm long and are present in the distal esophagus near the squamocolumnar junction (Fig. 237-2). Long and tubular peptic strictures are the result of persistent vomiting or prolonged nasogastric intubation. Replacement of the squamous epithelium of the esophagus by columnar epithelium (*Barrett's esophagus*) may also result from reflux esophagitis. Columnar-cell-lined esophagus may be further complicated by peptic ulcer or peptic stricture high up in the lower or midesophagus, and adenocarcinoma in 2 to 5 percent.

Clinical features Heartburn is the characteristic symptom and is produced by the contact of refluxed material with the inflamed esophageal mucosa. Angina-like or atypical chest pain may occur in some patients, while others may experience no heartburn or chest pain. Dysphagia suggests development of peptic stricture. In peptic strictures, the usual history is of several years of heartburn preceding dysphagia. However, in one-third of patients dysphagia may be the presenting symptom. Progressive dysphagia and weight loss may indicate development of adenocarcinoma in Barrett's esophagus. Bleeding occurs due to mucosal erosions or Barrett's ulcer. Reflux in the absence of esophagitis is usually asymptomatic. Severe reflux may reach the pharynx and mouth and result in laryngitis, morning hoarseness, and pulmonary aspiration. Recurrent pulmonary aspiration can cause aspiration pneumonia, pulmonary fibrosis, or chronic asthma.

Diagnosis Evaluation of reflux esophagitis is designed to assess the presence and severity of reflux, nature of refluxant, presence and severity of esophagitis, and pathophysiology of reflux. History, barium swallow, esophagoscopy, mucosal biopsy, esophageal motility, and a variety of special tests are utilized.

The *presence of reflux* is suggested by history. Spontaneous reflux from the stomach into the esophagus on barium examination suggests advanced reflux. Reflux of barium induced by stressful maneuvers is not very helpful, however, because of a high incidence of false-positive and false-negative results. Recently, scintiscan using ^{99m}Tc-sulfur colloid has been used to quantitate gastroesophageal reflux. Several tests that utilize the recording of esophageal luminal pH with a small pH electrode have been proposed to detect and quantitate reflux of gastric acid. In these tests the pH electrode is swallowed, positioned in the stomach, gradually withdrawn across the LES, and then fixed at 5 cm above the sphincter. In the standard acid reflux test, a diagnosis of reflux can be made by failure of the pH to rise as the electrode enters the esophagus and by a decrease in esophageal pH with straining maneuvers. Quantitative information on the acid reflux is obtained by long-term (24-h) esophageal pH recording. The pH recordings are helpful only in the evaluation of acid reflux. The presence of bile or alkaline reflux is suggested by the occurrence of reflux symptoms in the absence of gastric acid and by the demonstration of bile in the aspirate of esophageal reflux.

The *presence and complications of reflux esophagitis* are assessed by barium swallow, esophagoscopy, mucosal biopsy, and the Bernstein test. Barium swallow is usually normal in uncomplicated esophagitis but may reveal the complication of stricture or ulcer formation. A high esophageal peptic stricture, deep ulcer, and adenocarcinoma suggest complications of Barrett's esophagus. Uncomplicated Barrett's esophagus is not diagnosed by barium studies. Esophagoscopy may reveal the presence of erosive esophagitis, distal peptic stricture, or columnar-cell-lined lower esophagus with or without a proximally located peptic stricture, ulcer, or adenocarcinoma. Esophagoscopy may be normal in many patients with esophagitis; in such patients mucosal biopsies and Bernstein tests are helpful. The mucosal biopsies should be obtained 5 cm above the LES because in the distal esophagus mucosal changes are quite frequent in normal subjects. False-positive and false-negative results occur in approximately 10 percent of biopsies. Patients with Barrett's esophagus will show columnar mucosa lining the esophagus which may be of gastric fundic, cardiac, or specialized type. The Bernstein test consists of an infusion of solutions of 0.1 N HCl and normal saline into the esophagus. It is useful in diagnosing reflux esophagitis which is not endoscopically obvious. In patients with reflux esophagitis, infusion of acid, but not of saline, reproduces the symptoms of heartburn. Infusion of acid in normal subjects produces no symptoms. Reflux esophagitis should be included in the differential diagnosis of chest pain, esophagitis, upper gastrointestinal bleeding, and dysphagia.

The *causative and predisposing factors* are assessed by history, esophageal motility, and esophageal clearance studies. Esophageal motility studies may provide useful quantitative information on the competence of the LES and of esophageal motor function. Barium swallow and scintiscans can be used to study esophageal clearance. An esophageal acid clearance test using a pH electrode quantifies the number of swallows necessary to clear the esophagus of 10 mL of instilled dilute 0.1 N HCl.

Full diagnostic evaluation is not necessary in every patient with reflux esophagitis. In transient and mild cases with a clear-cut history of reflux esophagitis, a therapeutic trial may be sufficient. In persistent cases, and when the diagnosis is not clear, barium swallow, esophagoscopy, and esophageal motility with pH monitoring are indicated.

Patients with angina-like chest pain in whom coronary artery disease has been excluded may be investigated by 24-h ambulatory esophageal pH and motility recording. Most of these patients are found to have reflux esophagitis, while a few have esophageal motor disorders. It should also be remembered that reflux esophagitis may frequently coexist with coronary artery disease.

Treatment The goals of treatment are to decrease gastroesophageal reflux, neutralize refluxate, improve esophageal clearance, and protect the esophageal mucosa. These goals can be achieved by certain general measures and specific drug treatments. The management of uncomplicated cases generally includes weight reduction, sleeping with elevation of the head of the bed, and elimination of factors that increase abdominal pressure. Patients should avoid smoking, fatty foods, coffee, chocolate, alcohol, mint, orange juice, ingestion of large quantities of fluids with meals, and certain medications (such as anticholinergic drugs, calcium channel blockers, and other smooth-muscle relaxants). Antacids (40 to 80 meq, 1 and 3 h after meals) or H-2-blocking agents (cimetidine 300 mg, ranitidine 150 mg, or famotidine 20 mg at bedtime) to neutralize acidity are usually successful.

In moderate to severe cases, the above measures are more strictly enforced. H-2 blockers are used in higher doses (cimetidine, 300 mg qid; ranitidine, 150 mg tid; famotidine, 20 mg tid). A protective agent such as sucralfate (1-g chewable tablet, 1 h before meals) is useful in many cases. If the patient does not respond fully, a prokinetic agent such as metoclopramide, 10 mg qid, domperidone, or cisapride is prescribed to raise sphincter pressure, hasten gastric emptying, and improve esophageal clearance. (Domperidone and cisapride have not yet been approved for use in the United States.) Inhibition of H^+,K^+-ATPase, the pump that is responsible for acid secretion, with omeprazole (currently undergoing clinical trials in the United States) may be very effective in resistant cases. Reflux esophagitis requires prolonged therapy for 3 to 6 months or longer if the disease recurs quickly. Patients with reflux esophagitis with complications such as Barrett's esophagus (with or without a deep ulcer) should be treated vigorously. Patients who have an associated peptic stricture are treated with dilators to relieve dysphagia in addition to vigorous treatment for reflux. Close follow-up with periodic endoscopic biopsies is indicated in patients with Barrett's esophagus to detect and treat high-grade dysplasia and early adenocarcinoma.

Antireflux surgery (Belsey repair, Nissen's fundoplication, and Hill repair), in which the gastric fundus is wrapped around the esophagus, increases the lower sphincter pressure and should be considered in resistant and complicated cases of reflux esophagitis that do not fully respond to medical therapy and when there is persistently inadequate lower sphincter pressure but normal peristaltic contractions in the esophageal body.

Patients with alkaline esophagitis are treated with general measures and neutralization of bile salts with cholestyramine, aluminum hydroxide, or sucralfate. Sucralfate is particularly useful in these cases, as it also serves as a surface protector.

INFECTIOUS ESOPHAGITIS With the recent increase in immunodeficiency states, infectious esophagitis has become increasingly important. Infectious esophagitis can be due to viral, bacterial, fungal, or parasitic organisms. In severely immunocompromised patients, multiple organisms may coexist.

Viral esophagitis (See also Chap. 135) *Herpes simplex virus* (HSV) type I may occasionally cause esophagitis in the immunocompetent person, but either type I or II may afflict patients who are immunosuppressed. These patients complain of the acute onset of chest pain, odynophagia, and dysphagia. Bleeding may occur in severe cases, and systemic manifestations such as nausea, vomiting, fever, chills, and mild leukocytosis may be present. The persistent infection may lead to superinfection of denuded esophageal mucosa with fungi or bacteria, and HSV pneumonia. Herpes blisters on the nose and lips provide a clue to the diagnosis. Barium swallow is inadequate to detect early lesions and cannot reliably distinguish HSV from other types of infections. Endoscopy shows vesicles and small, discrete, punched-out superficial ulcerations with or without fibrinous exudate. In later stages there is diffuse erosive esophagitis caused by enlargement and coalescence of the ulcers. Mucosal cells from biopsy of the edge of an ulcer or cytological smear show ballooning degeneration, ground glass change in the nuclei with eosinophilic intranuclear inclusions (Cowdry type A), and giant cell formation on routine stains. Culture becomes positive within days and is helpful in diagnosis. For prophylaxis in a severely immunocompromised host, acyclovir, 800 mg orally twice daily or 250 mg/m² body surface area every 12 h intravenously, is recommended. For treatment of esophagitis, intravenous therapy, 250 mg/m² every 8 h is usually initiated. As swallowing improves, the therapy is changed to 200 to 400 mg orally five times daily. Symptoms usually resolve in 1 week, but large ulcerations may take longer to heal. These patients may also have reflux esophagitis which may worsen the symptoms and add to complications.

Varicella-zoster virus (VZV) rarely produces esophagitis in children with chickenpox and adults with herpes zoster. Esophageal VZV can also be the source of disseminated VZV infection in the absence of skin involvement. In an immunocompromised host, VZV esophagitis causes vesicles and confluent ulcers and usually resolves spontaneously, but it may cause necrotizing esophagitis in a severely compromised host. On routine histology of mucosal biopsies or cytology specimens, VZV is difficult to distinguish from HSV, but the distinction can be made immunohistologically or on culture. Acyclovir is effective in prevention and treatment of esophagitis, but much higher doses are needed than those for HSV.

Cytomegalovirus (CMV) infections occur only in the immunocompromised patient. CMV is usually activated from a latent stage or may be acquired from blood product transfusions. CMV lesions initially appear as serpiginous ulcers in an otherwise normal mucosa. These may coalesce to form giant ulcers, particularly in the distal esophagus. The virus involves submucosal fibroblasts and endothelial cells of the blood vessels but not the epithelial cells.

Patients present with painful swallowing, chest pain, hematemesis, nausea, and vomiting. Barium swallow may show nonspecific abnormalities or large esophageal ulcers. Diagnosis requires endoscopy and biopsies of the center of the ulcer. Mucosal brushings are not useful. Routine histology shows intranuclear and small intracytoplasmic inclusions in large fibroblasts and endothelial cells of blood vessels. Immunohistology with monoclonal antibodies to CMV and in situ hybridization of CMV DNA can be performed on centrifugation culture and are useful for early diagnosis. Ganciclovir (DHPG) 5 mg/kg every 12 h intravenously and, more recently, Foscarnet are investigational drugs which are active against CMV. Therapy is continued until healing, which may take weeks to months.

Human immunodeficiency virus (HIV) may be associated with a self-limited syndrome of acute esophageal ulceration associated with oral ulcers and a maculopapular skin rash. This syndrome occurs in homosexual men coincident with both HIV seroconversion and the inversion of the T-lymphocyte helper/suppressor ratio. Electron microscopy of affected tissue reveals retrovirus-like particles that are different from CMV or HSV.

Bacterial esophagitis   *Bacterial esophagitis* is unusual, but esophagitis caused by *Lactobacillus* and beta-hemolytic streptococci has been described in the immunocompromised host. In profoundly granulocytopenic patients and in patients with cancer, bacterial esophagitis is often missed because it is commonly present with other organisms including viruses and fungi, and because bacteria are difficult to identify on routine histology. In patients with AIDS, infection with *Cryptosporidium* and *Pneumocystis carinii* may cause nonspecific inflammation of the distal esophagus.

Candida esophagitis   Many *Candida* species are normal in the throat but become pathogenic and produce esophagitis in immunodeficiency states. These include HIV; malignant neoplasms (particularly lymphoma and leukemia); treatment with immunosuppressive agents, glucocorticoids, and broad-spectrum antibiotics; diabetes mellitus; hypoparathyroidism; systemic lupus erythematosus; hemoglobinopathy; corrosive esophageal injury; and esophageal stasis. Occasionally, monilial esophagitis occurs in the absence of any of the above predisposing factors. Patients may be asymptomatic or complain of odynophagia and dysphagia. Oral thrush or other evidence of mucocutaneous candidiasis may be absent. Rarely, *Candida* esophagitis may be complicated by esophageal bleeding, perforation, and stricture or by systemic invasion. Barium swallow may be normal or may show multiple nodular filling defects of various sizes (Fig. 237-2). Large nodular defects may resemble clusters of grapes. Endoscopy shows small yellow-white raised plaques with surrounding erythema in mild disease. In extensive disease, confluent linear and nodular plaques are seen. Diagnosis is made by demonstration of yeast or hyphae forms in the smear of plaques and exudate stained with Gram's, periodic acid Schiff, or silver stains. Biopsies are usually not positive. Culture is not useful in diagnosis but may be helpful in confirming the species and, if needed, the drug sensitivities of the yeast (see Chap. 151). In normal or minimally immunocompromised patients, nystatin or clotrimazole is often successful. Nystatin is used as an oral suspension (100,000 units per milliliter) in doses of 10 to 20 mL every 6 h; clotrimazole (10-mg tablet) is to be sucked every 6 h. Ketoconazole (200 to 400 mg in a single oral dose) is considered the treatment of choice; the higher dose is used in the severely immunocompromised host. Poorly responsive patients are treated with amphotericin, 10 to 15 mg as an intravenous infusion for 6 h daily for a total dose of 300 to 500 mg. Miconazole and amphotericin lozenges are currently not available in the United States. The treatment is for 7 to 10 days followed by nystatin, clotrimazole, or ketoconazole for as long as the host resistance remains low.

OTHER TYPES OF ESOPHAGITIS   *Radiation esophagitis* is a common occurrence during radiation treatment for lung, mediastinal, or esophageal carcinoma. The frequency and severity of esophagitis increases with the amount of radiation to the area and the concomitant use of certain chemotherapeutic agents such as doxorubicin, bleomycin, cyclophosphamide, and cisplatin. Dysphagia and odynophagia are the main symptoms and may last several weeks to several months after the conclusion of therapy. The esophageal mucosa becomes erythematous, edematous, and friable. Superficial erosions coalesce to form larger superficial ulcers. Submucosal fibrosis and degenerative changes in the blood vessels, muscles, and myenteric neurons may be present. The treatment is relief of pain with viscous lidocaine during the acute phase, while indomethacin may lessen the radiation damage. Esophageal stricture may develop and require dilation. *Corrosive esophagitis* occurs following ingestion of caustic agents, such as strong alkalies or acids. When severe, corrosive injury may lead to esophageal perforation, bleeding, and death. Healing is usually associated with stricture formation. Caustic strictures are usually long and rigid (Fig. 237-2) and generally require dilation with dilators

passed over a guide-wire through the stricture. *Pill-induced esophagitis* is associated with the ingestion of certain pills and accounts for many cases of erosive esophagitis. Antibiotics such as doxycycline, tetracycline, and clindamycin account for over half of the cases. Other commonly prescribed pills that cause esophageal injury include aspirin, potassium chloride, ferrous sulfate, quinidine, alprenolol, and various steroidal and nonsteroidal anti-inflammatory agents. *Sclerotherapy* for bleeding esophageal varices usually produces transient retrosternal chest pain and dysphagia due to edema, inflammation, and deranged motility. Esophageal ulcer, stricture, hematoma, or perforation may occur. *Esophagitis associated with mucocutaneous and systemic diseases* is usually associated with blister and bulla formation, epithelial desquamation, and thin, weblike or dense esophageal strictures. Esophageal involvement is indicated by development of odynophagia and dysphagia. Pemphigus vulgaris and bullous pemphigoid form intraepithelial and subepithelial bullae, respectively, and can be distinguished by a specific immunohistology. They are both characterized by sloughing of epithelium or esophageal casts. Glucocorticoid treatment is usually effective. Dystrophic epidermolysis bullosa is an inherited disease that presents in childhood in which local trauma is associated with bulla formation and scarring. Cicatricial pemphigoid, Stevens-Johnson syndrome, and toxic epidermolysis bullosa can produce esophageal bullous lesions and strictures requiring gentle dilation. Graft-versus-host disease occurs in patients who have received allogeneic bone marrow transplants and is associated with generalized desquamation and esophageal strictures. Beçhet's disease may involve the esophagus and may respond to steroid therapy. Crohn's disease, ulcerative colitis, and an erosive lichen planus can also involve the esophagus. Crohn's disease and ulcerative colitis cause aphthous ulcers, and Crohn's disease may cause inflammatory strictures, sinus tract, filiform polyps, and fistulas in the esophagus.

OTHER ESOPHAGEAL DISORDERS

DIVERTICULA   Diverticula are outpouchings of the wall of the esophagus. *Zenker's diverticula* appear in the natural weakness in the posterior hypopharyngeal wall and cause halitosis and regurgitation of saliva and food particles consumed several days previously. When they become large and filled with food, they can compress the esophagus and cause dysphagia or complete obstruction. *Midesophageal diverticula* may be caused by traction from old adhesions or by propulsion associated with esophageal motor abnormalities. *Epiphrenic diverticula* may be associated with achalasia. Small or medium-sized diverticula and midesophageal and epiphrenic diverticula are usually asymptomatic. *Diffuse intramural diverticulosis* of the esophagus is due to dilation of the deep esophageal glands. This may lead to chronic candidiasis or a stricture high up in the esophagus. These patients may present with dysphagia. Symptomatic Zenker's diverticula are treated by cricopharyngeal myotomy with or without diverticulectomy. Very large symptomatic esophageal diverticula are removed surgically. When they are associated with motor abnormalities, distal myotomy is performed. Strictures associated with diffuse intramural diverticulosis are treated with rubber dilators.

WEBS AND RINGS   Weblike constrictions of the esophagus are usually congenital or inflammatory in origin. Asymptomatic hypopharyngeal webs are demonstrated in up to 10 percent of normal individuals. When concentric, they cause intermittent dysphagia to solids. Symptomatic hypopharyngeal webs with iron-deficiency anemia in middle-aged women constitute Plummer-Vinson syndrome. The clinical importance of this syndrome is uncertain. Midesophageal webs are rare. *Lower esophageal mucosal ring* (Schatzki ring) is a thin, weblike constriction located at the squamocolumnar mucosal junction at or near the border of the lower esophageal sphincter (Fig. 237-2). It invariably produces dysphagia when the diameter is less than 1.3 cm. The dysphagia to solids is the only symptom, and it is usually episodic. Asymptomatic rings may be present in about 10 percent of normal individuals. Lower esophageal ring is one of the common causes of dysphagia. Symptomatic webs and mucosal lower esophageal ring are easily treated by dilation. *Lower esophagitis muscular ring* (contractile ring) is located proximal to the site of mucosal rings and may represent the abnormal uppermost segment of the lower esophageal sphincter. These rings are characterized by a change in size and shape from one time to another (Fig. 237-1). They may also cause dysphagia and should be differentiated from peptic strictures, achalasia, and lower esophageal mucosal ring. They are treated by dilation.

HIATAL HERNIA Hiatal hernia is a herniation of a part of the stomach into the thoracic cavity through the esophageal hiatus in the diaphragm. *Sliding hiatal hernia* is one in which the gastroesophageal junction and fundus of the stomach slide upward. A sliding hernia may result from weakening of the anchors of the gastroesophageal junction to the diaphragm, longitudinal contraction of the esophagus, or increased intraabdominal pressure. Small sliding hernias can be demonstrated commonly during barium studies if intraabdominal pressure is increased. Their incidence increases with age; in the sixth decade of life the prevalence of such hernias is around 60 percent. It is unlikely that a small sliding hiatal hernia by itself produces any clinical symptoms, and its role in the pathogenesis of reflux esophagitis is uncertain. *Paraesophageal hernia* is one in which the esophago-gastric junction remains fixed in its normal location and a pouch of stomach is herniated beside the gastroesophageal junction through the esophageal hiatus. A paraesophageal or mixed paraesophageal and sliding hernia may become incarcerated and strangulate. This situation is manifested by acute chest pain, dysphagia, and a mediastinal mass, and requires prompt operative treatment. A herniated gastric pouch may cause dysphagia and may be the site of gastritis and ulceration causing chronic blood loss. A large paraesophageal hernia should be surgically repaired because of a high rate of complications.

MECHANICAL TRAUMA *Esophageal rupture* may be caused by (1) iatrogenic damage from instrumentation of the esophagus or external trauma; (2) increased intraesophageal pressure associated with forceful vomiting or retching (this is also called spontaneous rupture or Boerhaave's syndrome); or (3) diseases of the esophagus such as corrosive esophagitis, esophageal ulcer, and neoplasm. The site of perforation is variable and depends on the cause. Instrumental perforation usually occurs in the pharynx or in the lower esophagus. The esophageal perforation often occurs just above the diaphragm in the posterolateral wall. Esophageal perforation causes severe retrosternal chest pain that may be worsened by swallowing and breathing. Free air enters the mediastinum and spreads to neighboring structures and causes palpable subcutaneous emphysema in the neck, mediastinal crackling sounds on auscultation, and pneumothorax. With time, secondary infection supervenes, and mediastinal abscess and pleuropulmonary suppurative complications may develop. Esophageal perforation associated with vomiting usually deposits gastric contents in the mediastinum and causes severe mediastinal complications. On the other hand, instrumental perforation may be mild and free of severe complications. Spontaneous rupture of the esophagus may mimic myocardial infarction, pancreatitis, or ruptured abdominal viscus. Symptoms of chest pain may be mild, particularly in the elderly. Mediastinal emphysema may develop late. X-ray of the chest shows abnormalities in the majority of patients, and diagnosis is confirmed by swallow of radiopaque contrast material. Treatment includes esophageal and gastric suction and parenteral broad-spectrum antibiotics. Surgical drainage and repair of the laceration should be performed as soon as possible. In patients with terminal carcinoma, surgical repair may not be feasible, and those with minor instrumental perforation can be treated conservatively. Extensive corrosive damage may require esophageal diversion and subsequent excision of the damaged portion of the esophagus.

Mucosal tear (Mallory-Weiss Syndrome) This is usually caused by vomiting and retching, and it usually involves the gastric mucosa near the squamocolumnar mucosal junction but may also involve the esophageal mucosa. Patients present with upper gastrointestinal bleeding that may be severe. Most patients recover with only conservative management, but those with severe arterial bleeding require surgery.

Intramural hematoma Emetogenic injury, particularly in patients with bleeding abnormalities, can cause bleeding between the mucosa and muscle layers of the esophagus. The patients develop sudden dysphagia. Diagnosis is made by barium swallow and computed tomographic scan. Spontaneous resolution usually occurs.

FOREIGN BODIES Foreign bodies may lodge in the cervical esophagus just beyond the upper esophageal sphincter, around the aortic arch, or above the lower esophageal sphincter. Impaction of a bolus of food, particularly a piece of meat or bread, may occur when the esophageal lumen is narrowed due to stricture, carcinoma, or a lower esophageal ring. Acute impaction causes complete inability to swallow and severe chest pain. Both foreign bodies and food boluses may be removed endoscopically. Use of meat tenderizer to facilitate passage of an obstructed meat bolus is to be discouraged because of potential esophageal perforation and aspiration pneumonia.

REFERENCES

AGHA FP et al: Esophageal involvement in epidermolysis bullosa dystrophica: Clinical and roentgenographic manifestations. Gastrointest Radiol 8:111, 1983

BOTT S et al: Medication-induced esophageal injury: Survey of the literature. Am J Gastroenterol 82:758, 1987

CASTELL DO, JOHNSON LF (eds): *Esophageal Function in Health and Disease.* New York, Elsevier, 1983

CLOUSE R: Motor disorders (of the esophagus), in *Gastrointestinal Disease*, MH Sleisenger, JS Fordtran (eds). Philadelphia, Saunders, 1989, pp 559–593

CRIST J et al: Intramural mechanism of esophageal peristalsis: Roles of cholinergic and noncholinergic nerves. Proc Natl Acad Sci USA 81:3595, 1984

DODDS WJ The pathogenesis of gastroesophageal reflux disease. AJR 151:49, 1988

GOYAL RK, CRIST JR: Chest pain of esophageal etiology. Hosp Pract 23:15, 1988

McDONALD GB et al: Esophageal infections in immunosuppressed patients after marrow transplantation. Gastroenterology 88:1111, 1985

MELLOW MH et al: Esophageal acid perfusion in coronary artery disease: Induction of myocardial ischemia. Gastroenterology 85:306, 1983

SHAPIRO J, GOYAL RK: Disorders of the upper esophageal sphincter, in *The Larynx: A Multidisciplinary Approach*, M Fried (ed). Boston, Little, Brown, 1988, pp 293–317

SPECHLER SJ, GOYAL RK: Barrett's esophagus. N Engl J Med 315:362, 1986

SUBRAMANYAM K, PATTERSON M: Chronic esophageal ulceration after endoscopic sclerotherapy. J Clin Gastroenterol 8:58, 1986

WHEELER RR et al: Esophagitis in the immunocompromised host: Role of esophagoscopy in diagnosis. Rev Infect Dis 9:88, 1987

238 PEPTIC ULCER AND GASTRITIS

JAMES E. McGUIGAN

Peptic ulcer is a term used to refer to a group of ulcerative disorders of the upper gastrointestinal tract, involving principally the most proximal portion of the duodenum and the stomach, which have in common participation of acid-pepsin in their pathogenesis. The major forms of common peptic ulcer are duodenal ulcer and gastric ulcer, both of which are chronic diseases. Ulcer associated with the Zollinger-Ellison syndrome, caused by gastrin-releasing tumors (gastrinomas) usually located in the pancreas, is also considered a form of peptic ulcer.

Although our present knowledge of the etiology of peptic ulcer is incomplete, available information supports a crucial role for acid-pepsin. The development of ulcer or the resistance to ulceration is determined by the balance between *aggressive factors* (including secreted gastric acid and pepsin) and those factors that comprise *mucosal defense* or *mucosal resistance* to ulceration. Peptic ulcer results when the aggressive effects of acid-pepsin outweigh the protective effects of gastric or duodenal mucosal resistance. Considering the extraordinary corrosive character of acid-pepsin, why do not all humans develop peptic ulcer? The normal capacity of gastric and proximal duodenal mucosa to resist the corrosive effects of acid and pepsin is unique. This resistance is not shared by other tissues; hence the susceptibility of the esophageal mucosa to injury from refluxed gastric juice, the frequent ulceration of the small intestine when attached surgically to actively secreting gastric mucosa, and corrosion of the skin predictably produced with gastrocutaneous fistulas.

Much has been learned about mechanisms regulating gastric secretion and factors that appear important in development of peptic ulcer. Consideration of gastric physiology provides an understanding of some etiologic elements as well as a rational basis for treatment of peptic ulcer.

GASTRIC PHYSIOLOGY RELATED TO PEPTIC ULCER

AGGRESSIVE FACTORS: ACID AND PEPSINS The gastric mucosa possesses an extraordinary capacity to secrete acid. Parietal cells (oxyntic cells), interspersed along the course of mucosal glands of the body and fundus of the stomach, secrete hydrochloric acid by a process involving oxidative phosphorylation. Parietal cells secrete hydrogen ions at a concentration 3 million times that found in blood. The estimated concentration of HCl secreted directly by parietal cells is approximately 160 mM. Each secreted hydrogen ion (H$^+$) is accompanied by a chloride ion (Cl$^-$). With each increase in hydrogen ion secretion, there is a reciprocal decrease in sodium ion secretion. For each hydrogen ion secreted into the gastric lumen, one bicarbonate ion (HCO$_3^-$) is released into the gastric venous circulation, accounting for the *alkaline tide*, a direct reflection of the magnitude of gastric H$^+$ secretion. Bicarbonate is released from carbonic acid generated from carbon dioxide by parietal cell carbonic anhydrase. The final step in hydrogen ion secretion is accomplished by a proton pump mechanism involving a specific hydrogen-potassium adenosine triphosphatase (H$^+$,K$^+$-ATPase) located in the microvillus membrane of the parietal cells' secretory canaliculi. This H$^+$,K$^+$-ATPase exchanges hydrogen for potassium across the microvillus membrane. The two-component hypothesis for secretion of acid-containing gastric juice proposes that parietal cells secrete a virtually pure HCl solution, which is mixed (in various proportions) with nonparietal cell alkaline gastric glandular secretions that are similar in ionic composition to extracellular fluid.

Multiple *chemical*, *neural*, and *hormonal* factors participate in regulation of gastric acid secretion. *Acid secretion is stimulated* by gastrin and by vagal cholinergic postganglionic fibers via muscarinic receptors on parietal cells. Gastrin, the most potent known stimulant of gastric acid secretion, is contained in and released into the circulation from cytoplasmic secretory granules of gastrin cells (or G cells) which are scattered singly or in small clusters among the epithelial lining cells of the mid and deeper portions of the antral pyloric glands. Gastrin is present in tissues and body fluids in multiple molecular forms (Fig. 238-1). The principal form of gastrin in the gastric antral mucosa (or in gastrinoma) is heptadecapeptide gastrin (G-17), which contains 17 amino acid residues, the active site region being the carboxyl-terminal tetrapeptide amide (Try-Met-Asp-Phe-

NH$_2$). Gastrin II is the form of gastrin in which the tyrosyl residue at position 12 is sulfated, and gastrin I is the nonsulfated form. G-17 accounts for more than 90 percent of gastrin in antral mucosa. Approximately two-thirds of serum gastrin consists of a larger molecular species of gastrin, which contains 34 amino acids (G-34). The carboxyl-terminal 17 amino acids of G-34 are identical to those of G-17 and may also be sulfated (G-34 II) or nonsulfated (G-34 I). Although G-17 has a shorter half-life than G-34, circulating G-17 is approximately as potent as G-34 in stimulating gastric acid secretion.

Gastrin is also present in duodenal mucosa, with its highest concentration in the most proximal duodenum (approximately 10 percent of antral concentration). The mucosal concentration of gastrin and the proportion of G-17 decrease with progression down the duodenum. The effects of gastrin and vagal stimulation on gastric acid secretion are intimately interrelated. Vagal stimulation increases gastric acid secretion by cholinergic stimulation of parietal cell secretion, by stimulating release of gastrin into the circulation, and by lowering the parietal cell threshold for response to circulating gastrin concentrations. There is also some evidence suggesting that certain vagal branches or fibers may inhibit gastrin release.

Large amounts of histamine are present in mast cells, and in endocrine cells of some species, in the parietal cell–containing regions of the gastric mucosa. Mast cells are located in close proximity to parietal cells, with a ratio of one mast cell to every two or three parietal cells. For many years views differed on the importance of histamine in stimulating gastric acid secretion; some suggested that histamine was the "final common pathway" for cholinergic and gastrin stimulation of parietal cell acid secretion, while others were skeptical about any role for histamine in the acid secretory process. Interest in the role of histamine in acid secretion was renewed by the discovery of H-2-receptor antagonists which inhibited competitively the action of histamine on H-2 receptors (located on gastric parietal, cardiac atrial, and uterine smooth-muscle cells). These drugs were shown to exert negligible effect on H-1 receptors, which are inhibited readily by conventional antihistamines (H-1-receptor antagonists). H-2-receptor antagonists (e.g., cimetidine, ranitidine, famotidine, nizatidine) inhibit basal acid secretion as well as secretion in response to feeding, gastrin, histamine, hypoglycemia, or vagal stimulation. Most data support the conclusions that (1) histamine plays an important role in stimulating gastric acid secretion and (2) histamine acts in concert with gastrin and cholinergic activity on parietal cells, which bear receptors for histamine, gastrin, and acetylcholine, but that (3) there is still uncertainty as to whether histamine is the final common effector molecule in the stimulation of parietal cell secretion. Histamine stimulates gastric acid secretion by increasing parietal cell cyclic adenosine monophosphate (AMP), thereby activating cyclic AMP–dependent protein kinase(s). Gastrin and cholinergic agents, which do not stimulate cyclic AMP production, stimulate acid secretion by increasing parietal cell cytosolic calcium.

The major physiologic stimulus for gastric acid secretion is ingestion of food. Traditionally, regulation of gastric acid secretion has been classified into three phases—cephalic, gastric, and intestinal. This classification is of some value in analyzing factors that participate in regulation of gastric acid secretion. The *cephalic phase* encompasses the gastric acid secretory response to the sight, smell, taste, and anticipation of food. The *gastric phase* is induced by the presence

Big Gastrin (G34)	$\lceil$Glu-Leu-Gly-Pro-Gln-Gly-Pro-Pro-His-Leu-Val-Ala-Asp-Pro-Ser-Lys-Lys- -Gln-Gly-Pro-Trp-Leu-Glu-Glu-Glu-Glu-Glu-Ala-Tyr*-Gly-Trp-Met-Asp-Phe-NH$_2$
Heptadecapeptide Gastrin (G 17)	$\lceil$Glu-Gly-Pro-Trp-Leu-Glu-Glu-Glu-Glu-Glu-Ala-Tyr*-Gly-Trp-Met-Asp-Phe-NH$_2$
Minigastrin (G 14)	Trp-Leu-Glu-Glu-Glu-Glu-Glu-Ala-Tyr*-Gly-Trp-Met-Asp-Phe-NH$_2$
C-Terminal Pentapeptide	Gly-Trp-Met-Asp-Phe-NH$_2$

FIGURE 238-1 Amino acid sequences of selected gastrin peptides, all of which contain the common C-terminal pentapeptide amide. (*Tyrosyl is sulfated in gastrin II and nonsulfated in gastrin I molecules.)

of food in the stomach. The *intestinal phase* is due to the entry or presence of food within the lumen of the small intestine. Although these three phases are convenient for considering the diverse contributions to gastric acid secretion, each phase is complex and not necessarily due to a single stimulatory control mechanism.

The cephalic phase, which includes cortical and hypothalamic components, is considered to be mediated primarily by vagal activation, which increases gastric acid secretion principally by effecting stimulation of parietal cells and to lesser extent by promoting gastrin release. The gastric phase results from stimulation of chemical and mechanical receptors in the gastric wall by luminal contents. Mechanical distention of the stomach stimulates gastric acid secretion but results in little, if any, gastrin release; this mechanical effect is inhibited by atropine and appears to be mediated by vagal reflexes. Food in the stomach promotes gastric acid secretion by increasing gastrin release, principally due to the content of *protein* and especially the *products of protein digestion* contained in the meal; oral glucose and fat cause slight increases in serum gastrin but do not stimulate gastric acid secretion. Food in the proximal small intestine stimulates the intestinal phase of gastric acid secretion. A peptone meal (which contains partially hydrolyzed meat protein) introduced into the small intestine stimulates gastric acid secretion but not gastrin release. Food in the small intestine may induce release of an intestinal hormone(s) (distinct from gastrin) that stimulates gastric acid secretion. Increases in circulating amino acids, absorbed from the small intestine, may also contribute to the intestinal phase of gastric acid secretion. *Basal* or *interdigestive gastric acid secretion* can be considered to be a *fourth phase* of acid secretion. This phase is unrelated to feeding, it reaches its peak around midnight and its lowest point about 7 A.M., and neural pathways are probably most important in its regulation.

Ingestion of both caffeine-containing and caffeine-free *coffee* stimulates gastric acid secretion: both forms of coffee stimulate gastrin release. Ingestion of *ethanol* and ethanol-containing beverages stimulates gastric acid secretion. Specifically, ingestion of 5 or 10% ethanol solutions or 10% bourbon whiskey results in prompt gastric acid secretion without increasing gastrin release; however, white wine stimulates gastric acid secretion and gastrin release. Intravenous ethanol stimulates gastric acid secretion, suggesting that both systemic and local mechanisms are involved.

Intravenous *calcium* stimulates gastric acid secretion and produces minimal increases in serum gastrin levels. Oral calcium has been reported to stimulate gastric acid secretion directly, i.e., without an increase in serum calcium or gastrin concentrations. Except in patients who harbor gastrinomas, hypercalcemia is not usually associated with gastric acid hypersecretion or with increases in serum gastrin.

Inhibition of gastric acid secretion can be produced by several mechanisms. Acid secretion may be inhibited by acid in the stomach or duodenum, by hyperglycemia, or by hypertonic fluids or fat in the duodenum. Reduction of the intragastric pH to 3.0 produces partial inhibition of gastrin release; further reduction to pH 1.5 or below blocks completely release of gastrin to almost all stimuli. The precise mechanism by which this pH-dependent feedback control of gastrin release operates has not been defined. Cholinergic and noncholinergic intramural neurons have been proposed as potential mediators. *Somatostatin* appears to play an important role in inhibition of gastrin release produced by acid in the gastric lumen. Somatostatin-containing antral mucosal endocrine cells (D cells) have cytoplasmic processes which extend to neighboring gastrin cells. Somatostatin inhibits gastrin release by its local (paracrine) effects on gastrin cells. In addition, in the acid-secreting portion of the stomach cytoplasmic processes of somatostatin cells extend to intimate contact with parietal cells and other cells. Somatostatin reduces gastric acid secretion by inhibiting gastrin release and by directly inhibiting parietal cell secretion. Acid in the duodenum decreases acid secretion by the stomach, perhaps by promoting release into the circulation of intestinal peptides that then inhibit gastric acid secretion. *Secretin*, which is a linear polypeptide (27 amino acids) related structurally to glucagon, is capable of inhibiting gastric acid secretion. Secretin is released

from endocrine cells (S cells) in the mucosa of the small intestine in response to mucosal acidification. Fat in the duodenum also inhibits gastric acid secretion; gastric inhibitory peptide (GIP) has been proposed as a candidate for this enterogastrone action; however, this effect of GIP remains to be proved. The mechanisms by which hyperglycemia or intraduodenal hyperosmolality inhibit gastric acid secretion are not known. Additional peptides residing in the mucosa of the proximal small intestine which possess the capacity to inhibit gastric acid secretion include vasoactive intestinal peptide (VIP), enteroglucagon, neurotensin, peptide YY, and urogastrone. Vasoactive intestinal peptide, a neuropeptide and putative neurotransmitter, is restricted in its location to neurons; it is unlikely to inhibit gastric acid secretion as a circulating hormone since, although released in response to feeding, it is inactivated during its portal passage through the liver. Enteroglucagon is composed of oxyntomodulin (glucagon with an 8-amino acid carboxyl-terminal extension) and glicentin (oxyntomodulin with a 32-amino acid amino-terminal extension). Neurotensin, oxyntomodulin, and peptide YY are released from the small intestine in response to luminal lipid perfusion. Urogastrone is structurally and functionally identical to epidermal growth factor. The extent to which these numerous peptides in the mucosa of the small intestine contribute to the physiologic regulation of gastric acid secretion has not been defined.

The proteolytic effects of *pepsins* in concert with the corrosive properties of secreted gastric acid are integral components in the tissue injury which produces peptide ulceration. Gastric acid catalyzes the cleavage of inactive pepsinogen molecules, converting them to proteolytically active pepsins, and also provides the appropriate low pH required for pepsin activity. Pepsin activity, maximal in the range of pH 1.5 to 2.0, is reduced substantially above pH 4.0, and these enzymes are denatured and irreversibly inactivated at neutral or alkaline pH. A variety of pepsinogens and their respective pepsins are present in gastric juice. Pepsinogens (and their corresponding active pepsins) have been classified by immunochemical techniques as either PG I (pepsinogens 1 through 5) or PG II (pepsinogens 6 and 7). Pepsinogen I is found in chief and mucous cells in the body and fundus of the stomach. Pepsinogen II is located in cells of the pyloric glands, Brunner's glands of the duodenum, mucous cells of the gastric cardiac glands, and the same cells in which PG I is found. Both PG I and PG II are present in plasma, whereas only PG I can be detected in urine. In general, there is a direct correlation between PG I serum concentrations and maximal gastric acid secretion. Most agents which stimulate gastric acid secretion also stimulate pepsinogen secretion. Cholinergic action is particularly potent in promoting pepsinogen secretion. Although it inhibits gastric acid secretion, secretin stimulates pepsinogen secretion.

In addition to secretion of hydrochloric acid parietal cells also secrete *intrinsic factor*. Agents which stimulate gastric acid secretion also lead to secretion of intrinsic factor.

MUCOSAL DEFENSE The precise mechanisms whereby the normal stomach and duodenum resist the corrosive effects of acid-pepsin (i.e., *mucosal resistance* to injury or *mucosal defense*) have not been defined completely. However, a variety of factors have been advanced as potential contributors to mucosal defense. *Gastric mucus* is proposed to play an important role in mucosal defense and thereby in preventing peptic ulceration. Gastric mucus is secreted by gastric mucous cells located on the surface of the gastric mucosal epithelium and in gastric glands. Mucus secretion is enhanced by mechanical or chemical irritation and by cholinergic stimulation. Gastric mucus is present in gastric juice in a soluble phase and as an insoluble mucus gel layer, approximately 0.6 mm in thickness, which coats the mucosal surface of the stomach. Normally the mucus gel is secreted constantly by gastric mucous epithelial cells and is continuously solubilized by pepsins secreted into the gastric lumen. Gastric mucus is a large polymeric glycoprotein (2×10^6 mol wt) containing four subunits connected by disulfide bridges. Depolymerization of the glycoprotein subunits of mucus, by peptic digestion or disruption of disulfide bonds, renders the glycoprotein incapable of forming or maintaining the gel. When intact, this mucus gel serves as an unstirred water layer which slows ionic diffusion but is much more impermeable to penetration by macromolecules such as pepsins (34,000 mol wt). Pepsin molecules secreted into the gastric lumen are denied reentry by the intact mucus gel, thereby potentially protecting mucosal cells from proteolytic injury. *Bicarbonate ions*, secreted by nonparietal gastric epithelial cells, enter the mucus gel, contributing to the development of a microenvironment in the gel with a substantial hydrogen ion gradient between the zone of the gel facing the gastric lumen (more acid, approaching pH of 2) and the zone in contact with the gastric mucosal cells (more alkaline, approaching pH of 7). As an unstirred water layer the mucus gel slows hydrogen ion diffusion back toward the gastric mucosal surface, allowing buffering by bicarbonate within the gel. Gel thickness is increased by administration of prostaglandins of the E series and reduced by nonsteroidal anti-inflammatory drugs, including aspirin. Gastric bicarbonate secretion is stimulated by calcium, certain prostaglandins of the E and F series, cholinergic agents, and dibutyryl cyclic guanosine monophosphate. It is inhibited by NSAIDs including aspirin, and by acetazolamide, alpha-adrenergic agents, and ethanol.

Gastric mucus also contains antigenic determinants used to classify AB(H) blood group substances. Approximately three-fourths of the population secrete gastric juice containing these AB(H) substances, and those individuals are referred to as *secretors*.

Normally the gastric luminal epithelial cell surfaces and intercellular tight junctions provide an almost completely impermeable *gastric mucosal barrier* to back-diffusion of hydrogen ions from the lumen: this barrier may be an important component of mucosal resistance to acid-peptic injury. The barrier can be interrupted by bile acids, salicylates, ethanol, and weak organic acids, thereby permitting back-diffusion of hydrogen ions from lumen to gastric tissues. This may cause cell injury, release of histamine from mast cells, further stimulation of acid secretion, damage to small blood vessels, mucosal hemorrhage, and erosion or ulceration. Interruption of the gastric mucosal barrier appears to contribute to the hemorrhagic erosive gastritis associated with salicylate or ethanol ingestion and to other forms of gastric mucosal injury. Maintenance of normal *mucosal blood flow* is an essential component of mucosal resistance to injury. Decreased mucosal blood flow, accompanied by back-diffusion of luminal hydrogen ions, is important in producing gastric mucosal damage.

Prostaglandins are present in abundant quantities in the gastric mucoas. Various prostaglandins, particularly those of the E series, have been shown to inhibit gastric mucosal injury caused by a wide variety of agents. Endogenous prostaglandins appear to play several important roles in mucosal defense. Prostaglandins stimulate secretion of gastric mucus and gastric and duodenal mucosal bicarbonate. Prostaglandins participate in the maintenance of gastric mucosal blood flow, in the integrity of the gastric mucosal barrier, and in epithelial cell renewal in response to mucosal injury.

MEASUREMENT OF GASTRIC ACID SECRETION Since HCl secretion by the stomach appears to be important in the production of peptic ulcer disease, measurement of basal and stimulated gastric acid secretion may be of value in the assessment of some patients with peptic ulcer. The range of values for normal subjects is extremely broad and overlaps substantially with the values in patients with duodenal ulcer, gastric ulcer, and even the Zollinger-Ellison syndrome. Mean basal acid output (BAO) in normal males without known ulcer disease is about 1.5 to 2.0 mmol/h. In general, basal and stimulated acid outputs in females are approximately two-thirds to three-fourths those found in males. In duodenal ulcer patients mean basal acid output averages from 4 to 6 mmol/h, again, with a wide degree of variation. Patients with gastric ulcer tend to have gastric acid secretory rates that are normal or often slightly less than those for normal subjects.

Measurement of gastric acid output is not helpful in the diagnosis or exclusion of peptic ulcer and is clearly not necessary in most ulcer patients. However, it is of value in selected clinical situations.

Detection of gastric acid hypersecretion is important when the Zollinger-Ellison syndrome is suspected. Measurement of gastric acid output is useful to detect achlorhydria, as in patients with pernicious anemia. Since patients with benign gastric ulcer virtually always secrete some acid, pentagastrin-fast achlorhydria in a patient with a gastric ulcer is almost always associated with malignancy. Measurement of gastric acid secretion is indicated in the search for the cause of ulcer recurrence after peptic ulcer surgery; it is also of value in patients in whom hypergastrinemia has been identified, in order to distinguish between clinical conditions characterized by gastric acid hypersecretion or achlorhydria.

In order to measure gastric acid output, a radiopaque gastric tube is passed so that its tip is located in the most dependent portion of the stomach. With the patient reclining or in a semirecumbent position on the left side, the position of the tube is verified by fluoroscopy. Gastric contents are aspirated and discarded. Basal gastric acid secretions are then collected in four consecutive 15-min intervals to determine the 1-h basal acid output. Secretion volume and acid concentration (titrated with sodium hydroxide to pH 7.0 or calculated by formula from the pH of the aspirated gastric juice) are measured, and acid output is expressed in millimoles per hour.

A variety of substances have been used to stimulate maximal acid output (MAO) by the stomach. These have included *histamine*, *betazole* (Histalog)—a structural analogue of histamine, and *pentagastrin* (Peptavlon). Histamine, the first standard stimulant used for gastric acid secretory testing, requires the simultaneous administration of an antihistaminic agent (H-1-receptor antagonist) to inhibit untoward systemic side effects. Betazole possesses fewer undesired side effects than histamine and does not require concomitant administration of an antihistamine. Pentagastrin (N-tert-butyloxycarbonyl-β-Ala-Try-Met-Asp-Phe-NH$_2$) contains the biologically active carboxyl-terminal tetrapeptide amide portion of the gastrin molecule and is currently the preferred and most commonly used agent to induce maximal acid secretion. Following collection of basal acid secretion, gastric juice is collected for four additional consecutive 15-min periods after the subcutaneous injection of pentagastrin (6 μg/kg). MAO is expressed as millimoles of acid aspirated during the 1 h after pentagastrin administration. Peak acid output (PAO) is calculated by combining the two highest consecutive 15-min acid outputs following pentagastrin injection and multiplying by 2.

DUODENAL ULCER

Duodenal ulcer is characteristically a chronic and recurrent disease. Duodenal ulcers are usually deep and sharply demarcated. They tend to penetrate through the submucosa, often into the muscularis propria. This is in contrast to erosions which are limited to the mucosa. The ulcer floor contains no intact epithelium and usually consists of a zone of eosinophilic necrosis resting on a base of granulation tissue surrounded by variable amounts of fibrosis. The ulcer bed may be clear or may contain blood or a proteinaceous exudate with entrapped erythrocytes and acute and chronic inflammatory cells. More than 95 percent of duodenal ulcers occur in the first portion of the duodenum, and approximately 90 percent of those are located within 3 cm of the junction of the pyloric and duodenal mucosa. Duodenal ulcers are usually round or oval, but may be irregular or elliptic. They are usually less than 1 cm in diameter. Rarely, duodenal ulcers may be extremely large (3 to 6 cm in diameter) and may be mistaken radiographically for the entire duodenal bulb. These giant ulcers often escape radiologic detection and are usually identified by endoscopy, or at surgery or postmortem examination.

The absolute prevalence of duodenal ulcer in the population is not known. Estimates have ranged from 6 to 15 percent. This variation in estimates may be explained by differences in the populations examined, study designs, diagnostic methods (e.g., endoscopy vs. radiologic examination) and by actual changes occurring in the frequency of duodenal ulcer. During the past 40 years the frequency of duodenal ulcer (and its complications) has been decreasing in the United States and England, especially in males. The reasons for this reduction are not known. The best current estimates suggest that approximately 10 percent of the population have clinical evidence of duodenal ulcer at some time in their lives. The natural history of duodenal ulcer is spontaneous healing and recurrence: about 60 percent of healed duodenal ulcers recur within 1 year, and 80 to 90 percent recur within 2 years. Duodenal ulcer is slightly more common in males than in females and is approximately three times as frequent as clinically recognized gastric ulcer.

ETIOLOGY AND PATHOGENESIS Although much is now known concerning factors that contribute to the development of duodenal ulcer, we do not completely understand its pathogenesis. It is clear that acid secretion by the stomach is required for production of a duodenal ulcer, but the factors which render the acid-secreting subject susceptible to duodenal ulceration have not been defined completely. Though as a group duodenal ulcer patients secrete more acid than normal, from one-half to two-thirds of them have acid secretory rates (BAO and MAO) within the normal range. Duodenal ulcer patients have approximately 1.9 billion parietal cells, with a maximum capacity of approximately 42 mmol gastric acid secreted per hour; this is in contrast to 1.0 billion parietal cells and a 22 mmol/h secretion rate for nonduodenal ulcer subjects (mean approximate values). However, variations in both groups are so large that most duodenal ulcer patients fall within the normal range. As a group duodenal ulcer patients also have comparable increases in gastric secretion of pepsin and in serum pepsinogen I levels. Peptic ulcer develops when there is an unfavorable balance between acid-pepsin secretion and mucosal resistance: in the pathogenesis of duodenal ulcer, evidence favors the importance of absolute or, in most instances, relative gastric hypersecretion. In contrast, for gastric ulcer defective mucosal resistance appears to be the major contributing factor.

Fasting *serum gastrin* concentrations are normal in duodenal ulcer patients. However, in many duodenal ulcer patients more gastrin is released into the circulation in response to a protein-containing meal than by normal subjects. Duodenal ulcer patients also have greater gastric acid secretory responses to administered gastrin than do nonulcer subjects. In duodenal ulcer patients intragastric acid may be less effective in inhibiting gastrin release and further gastric acid secretion. Therefore, although fasting serum gastrin levels are in the normal range in patients with common duodenal ulcer, gastrin may still play an important role in their frequent, but not invariable, gastric acid hypersecretion. Duodenal ulcer patients tend to empty their stomachs more rapidly than do nonduodenal ulcer patients. This phenomenon, when coupled with gastric acid hypersecretion, may contribute to a greater rate of acid delivery to the first part of the duodenum (the primary location of ulceration) in patients with duodenal ulcer.

Genetic factors appear to be important. Duodenal ulcers are approximately three times as common in first-degree relatives of duodenal ulcer patients as in the general population. Patients with duodenal ulcers have an increased frequency of blood group O and of the nonsecretory status [those who do not secrete AB(H) blood group antigens in their gastric juice], but these associations are weak. An increased incidence of HLA-B5 antigen has been reported in white male subjects with duodenal ulcer. Elevated serum pepsinogen I (PG I) levels, inherited as an autosomal dominant trait, are found in about 50 percent of patients with duodenal ulcer. Individuals with this trait have a frequency of duodenal ulcer which is eight times greater than that of the general population.

Cigarette smoking has been associated with increased duodenal ulcer frequency, decreased response to therapy, and increased duodenal ulcer mortality. Cigarette smoking does not increase gastric acid secretion. It has been suggested that the increased incidence of duodenal ulcer among cigarette smokers may be due to inhibition of pancreatic bicarbonate secretion (an endogenous neutralizer of secreted gastric acid) by nicotine or cigarette smoking and/or by accelerated emptying of gastric acid into the duodenum.

The incidence of duodenal ulcer has also been reported to be increased in patients with chronic renal failure, alcoholic cirrhosis, renal transplantation, hyperparathyroidism, systemic mastocytosis, and chronic obstructive pulmonary disease.

Gastric colonization with *Helicobacter pylori* has been reported in 80 to 100 percent of patients with duodenal ulcer. This has been proposed as a potential contributing factor in the pathogenesis of duodenal ulcer. At present it is uncertain whether *H. pylori* plays a role in producing duodenal ulcer or if its presence reflects a commensal association. Antibodies to herpes simplex have been reported to be higher in titer and more frequent in sera of patients with duodenal ulcer than in normals.

The importance of *psychological factors* in the pathogenesis of duodenal ulcer remains controversial. Contrary to earlier views, there is no single, characteristic duodenal ulcer personality. Chronic anxiety and psychological stress may, however, be factors in exacerbation of ulcer activity. There is some evidence that patients with duodenal ulcer may view stress more negatively than nonulcer subjects. There have been no differences identified in the frequency of duodenal ulcer among different socioeconomic classes or occupation groups.

CLINICAL FEATURES Epigastric pain is by far the most frequent symptom of duodenal ulcer. The pain is often described as sharp, burning, or gnawing. Alternatively, the pain may be ill-defined, boring, or aching, or may be perceived as abdominal pressure or fullness, or as a hunger sensation. In approximately 10 percent of patients the pain is located to the right of the epigastrium. The pain of duodenal ulcer characteristically occurs from 90 min to 3 h after eating. It frequently awakens the patient at night. Pain on awakening before breakfast is sufficiently rare in patients with duodenal ulcer as to challenge the diagnosis. The pain is usually relieved within a few minutes by food or antacids. Symptoms tend to be recurrent and episodic. The severity of pain varies widely from patient to patient. Duodenal ulcers recur often in the absence of pain. Episodes of pain may persist for periods of several days to weeks or months. Periods of remission usually last from weeks to years and are almost always longer than the episodes of pain. In some patients the disease is more aggressive, with frequent and persistent symptoms and/or development of complications. Pain relief with antacids or food is believed to result from acid neutralization. Ingestion of food leads to transient partial neutralization of gastric acid, which is followed by gastrin release and resultant stimulation of acid secretion. With subsequent gastric emptying and increasing gastric acid secretion, a sufficiently low pH is achieved in the stomach and first portion of the duodenum that pain results. Acid-induced pain in patients with duodenal ulcer is believed to be due to (1) acid stimulation of chemical receptors and/or (2) alterations in gastric motility.

Changes in the character of ulcer pain may signal the development of complications. For example, ulcer pain which becomes constant, is longer relieved by food or antacids, or radiates to the back or to either upper quadrant may herald *penetration* of the ulcer (often posteriorly into the pancreas). Pain associated with duodenal ulcer which is accentuated, rather than relieved, by food and/or is accompanied by vomiting often indicates *gastric outlet obstruction*. Abrupt, severe, or generalized abdominal pain is characteristic of free ulcer *perforation* into the peritoneal cavity. Weight loss, in the absence of some degree of gastric outlet obstruction, is unusual. Duodenal ulcer may cause acute gastrointestinal *hemorrhage*, with vomiting of blood or coffee-grounds material, or with the passage of black, tarry stools or even frankly red blood, if the bleeding is massive. More commonly blood loss with duodenal ulcer is more subtle, with occult blood loss detected by stool examination or by variable degrees of anemia which may be accompanied by iron deficiency.

It is important to emphasize that *many patients with active duodenal ulcer have no ulcer symptoms*. This leads to a significant, although not precisely quantifiable, underestimate of duodenal ulcer frequency in the population. Prospective studies using upper gastrointestinal endoscopy suggest that approximately half of duodenal ulcers recur in the absence of symptoms. Endoscopic studies also show a lack of good correlation between ulcer activity, symptom resolution, and ulcer healing. The absence of prior ulcer-type pain does not exclude duodenal ulcer as a potential cause for acute or chronic gastrointestinal hemorrhage, gastric outlet obstruction, or abrupt ulcer perforation.

On *physical examination* epigastric tenderness is by far the most frequent abnormal finding. The area of tenderness is usually in the midline, often midway between the umbilicus and the xiphoid process. In approximately 20 percent of patients the tender area is to the right of the midline. Acute free ulcer perforation into the peritoneal cavity often produces a rigid, boardlike abdomen, usually with generalized rebound tenderness. Initially auscultation of the abdomen may reveal hyperactive bowel sounds which, with clinical progression, may diminish or disappear. Patients with gastric outlet obstruction caused by a duodenal or pyloric channel ulcer may have a "succussion splash" produced by fluid and air in the distended stomach. Tachycardia and/or hypotension, in some instances demonstrable only by orthostatic maneuvers, may result from acute duodenal ulcer hemorrhage. Cutaneous and mucosal pallor may reflect anemia from acute or chronic blood loss.

Only about 5 percent of duodenal ulcers are located distal to the duodenal bulb, and most of these are in the immediate postbulbar portion of the first part of the duodenum. Postbulbar ulcer pain may be located in the right upper quadrant or may radiate through the back. Obstruction and hemorrhage are more frequent with postbulbar ulcers than with those in the duodenal bulb. Most immediate postbulbar ulcers, i.e., within 2 cm of the duodenal bulb, are of the common duodenal ulcer variety. Ulceration, located in or beyond the second portion of the duodenum, suggests the Zollinger-Ellison syndrome.

The pyloric channel, which is 1 to 2 cm in length, is the narrowest portion of the gastric outlet. Because of their gastric acid secretory characteristics and clinical features, pyloric channel ulcers are classified with duodenal rather than with gastric ulcers. Ulcers in this location often produce symptoms similar to those of a duodenal ulcer; however, symptoms tend to be less responsive to food and antacids. In patients with pyloric channel ulcers, food may accentuate rather than relieve ulcer pain and may produce vomiting due to partial gastric outlet obstruction. In general, surgery is required more frequently for pyloric channel ulcers than for those in the duodenal bulb.

FIGURE 238-2   Deformed duodenal bulb with ulcer crater.

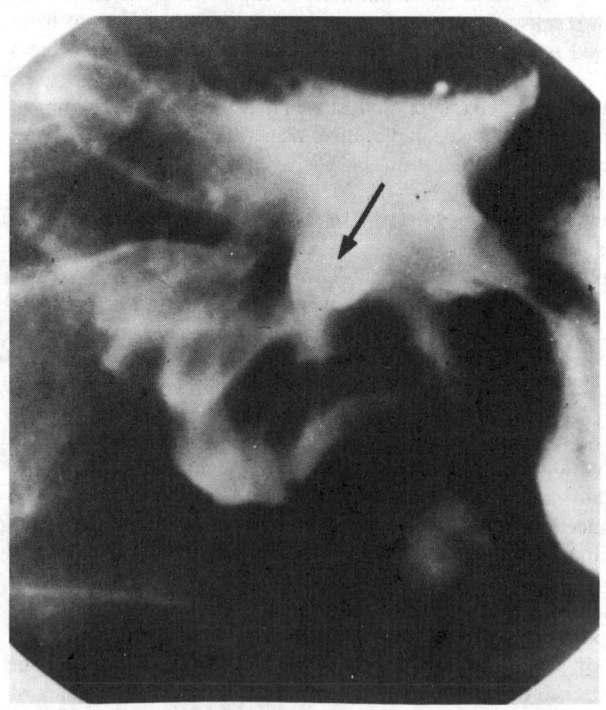

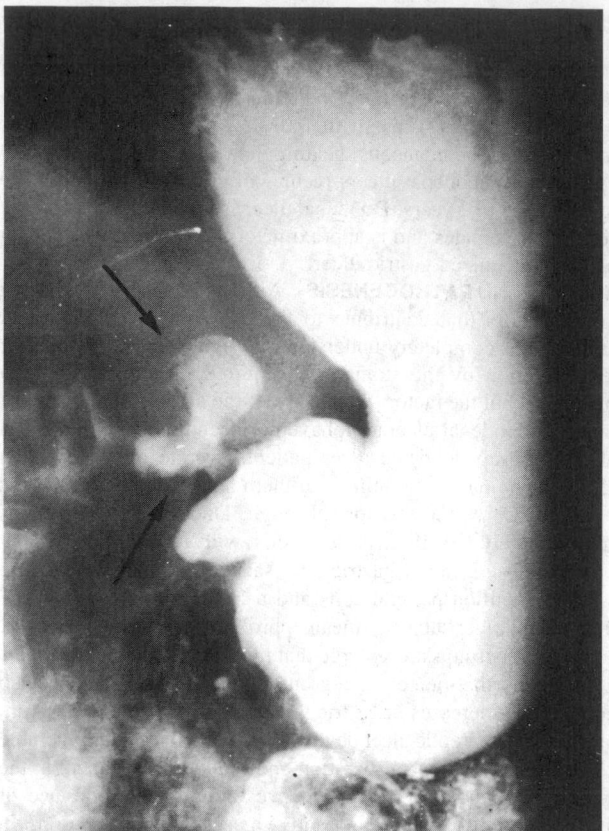

FIGURE 238-3   Distortion of the duodenal bulb with "cloverleaf" deformity.

DIAGNOSIS   Barium examination of the upper gastrointestinal tract is of value in identifying duodenal ulcer and is still the most common initial method used to establish the diagnosis. The proportion of ulcers identified radiographically depends on the skill, persistence, enthusiasm, and diagnostic criteria of the radiologist. Using conventional single-contrast barium techniques, 70 to 80 percent of duodenal ulcers found at endoscopy can be identified by x-ray examination. With double-contrast barium examinations, it is possible to detect about 90 percent of duodenal ulcers. On x-ray the typical duodenal ulcer appears as a discrete crater in the proximal portion of the duodenal bulb. Marked deformity of the duodenal bulb, common in patients with chronic recurrent duodenal ulcer, may make radiographic identification of the ulcer difficult or impossible (Figs. 238-2 and 238-3).

Use of fiberoptic endoscopic examination of the upper gastrointestinal tract has facilitated accurate diagnosis of duodenal ulcer. Duodenoscopy is not required for diagnosis of duodenal ulcer when it has been identified by barium radiographic examination. Endoscopy may be of greatest value, however, (1) in detecting duodenal ulcer suspected in the absence of a radiographically demonstrable ulcer, (2) in patients with radiographic deformity and uncertainty regarding ulcer activity, (3) in identifying ulcers too small or too superficial to be recognized by x-ray, and (4) in identifying (or excluding) an ulcer as the source of active gastrointestinal hemorrhage. Duodensocopy permits direct visualization and photographic documentation of the character of the ulcer—its size, shape, and location—and may provide a reference base for assessment of ulcer healing.

Measurement of gastric acid secretion is not necessary in the assessment of most patients with clinical features of typical duodenal ulcer. Determination of serum gastrin is recommended in those patients in whom surgery is planned or gastrinoma is suspected. Epigastric pain readily relieved by food or antacids strongly suggests duodenal ulcer. However, even after careful radiographic and endoscopic examination many patients with these ulcer-like symptoms have no evidence of ulcer: this has led to the term *nonulcer dyspepsia*. Although symptoms are similar, it is uncertain whether this entity is related to peptic ulcer.

MEDICAL TREATMENT Major objectives of duodenal ulcer therapy are relief of pain and acceleration of ulcer healing. Prevention of ulcer recurrence and complications are additional important objectives. In the past enthusiasm has been expressed for virtually every kind of treatment ever tried for duodenal ulcer. Conclusions regarding the effectiveness of therapy were obscured by spontaneous healing of duodenal ulcer, an intrinsic component of the natural history of the disease, and by imprecise methods used to assess ulcer activity. Specific effective agents currently available and recommended for consideration in treatment of duodenal ulcer are considered below.

Antacids For many decades antacids have been the major form of treatment for duodenal ulcer. Prospective endoscopic studies conducted only relatively recently have verified the effectiveness of antacids in accelerating duodenal ulcer healing. Many types of antacids are available for use in treatment of duodenal ulcer. The ideal antacid should be potent in neutralizing acid, inexpensive, not adsorbed from the gastrointestinal tract, and should contain negligible amounts of sodium. It should be sufficiently palatable to be tolerated with repeated dosage and should be free from side effects. Individual antacids differ substantially in their capacities to neutralize acid, their sodium contents, their absorption properties, and their potential adverse effects. Although the ideal antacid is yet to be developed, a number of preparations are available that can be used effectively in treatment of patients with duodenal ulcer.

The most widely used antacid preparations are mixtures of aluminum hydroxide and magnesium hydroxide, in some instances with additional agents. *Aluminum hydroxide* neutralizes hydrochloric acid with the production of aluminum chloride and water. Use of aluminum hydroxide tends to produce constipation. Aluminum binds phosphate within the gut lumen, thereby facilitating phosphate excretion. As a consequence, prolonged and regular use of aluminum hydroxide may induce systemic phosphate depletion with resultant weakness, malaise, and anorexia. Phosphate depletion is probably restricted to, and should be considered in, those patients with phosphate-poor diets, e.g., dietary deficiency with chronic alcoholism or other states of reduced dietary protein intake.

Magnesium hydroxide is a potent antacid which neutralizes hydrochloric acid, producing magnesium chloride and water. Magnesium hydroxide may produce loose stools. This laxative effect and the constipating effects of aluminum hydroxide can be overcome by using these agents in combination or by alternating their use. From 5 to 10 percent of magnesium in magnesium hydroxide is absorbed by the small intestine. Magnesium is excreted by the kidney, and hypermagnesemia, which is not a problem with normal renal function, does develop in a small number of patients with renal insufficiency who are treated with magnesium-containing antacids. *Magnesium trisilicate*, which is included in various antacid mixtures, is a slow-acting weak antacid.

Calcium carbonate is a potent and inexpensive antacid. In neutralizing acid, it is converted to calcium chloride in the stomach. Approximately 10 percent of calcium ingested as calcium carbonate is absorbed from the proximal small intestine. Calcium carbonate is unique among antacids in that its ingestion is followed by stimulation of gastric acid secretion ("acid rebound"). This is due to the direct action of calcium in stimulating parietal cell acid secretion and, perhaps to a lesser extent, to calcium-mediated stimulation of gastrin release. Chronic calcium carbonate adminstration may be associated with the milk-alkali syndrome, producing elevations of serum calcium, phosphate, urea nitrogen, creatinine, and bicarbonate. These patients may develop renal calcinosis and progressive renal insufficiency. Because of its potential adverse effects, calcium carbonate is not recommended for use as an antacid for treatment of patients with peptic ulcer.

Sodium bicarbonate is a potent, rapidly acting, inexpensive antacid. However, because of its tendency to induce systemic alkalosis and its high sodium content, it should not be used as an antacid in treatment of peptic ulcer.

Acceptance of the crucial role of acid in the pathogenesis of duodenal ulcer has provided a rational basis for the use of antacids in treatment of patients with duodenal ulcer. In a controlled endoscopic study, 4 weeks of treatment with a potent magnesium and aluminum hydroxide antacid mixture increased the rate of duodenal ulcer healing. Ulcer healing occurred in 45 percent of patients receiving placebo and in 78 percent of those treated with 30 mL antacid (144 mmol) given 1 and 3 h after meals and at bedtime. It has been proposed more recently that smaller and less frequent doses may also achieve satisfactory ulcer healing.

H-2-receptor antagonists It has been known for decades that conventional antihistamines, which readily block the actions of histamine on smooth muscle of blood vessels, the gut, or bronchi do not inhibit histamine-stimulated gastric acid secretion. The parietal cell receptor for histamine has been classified as an H-2 receptor and that blocked by classic antihistamines as an H-1 receptor. H-2-receptor antagonists are potent inhibitors of basal (unstimulated) and of stimulated gastric acid secretion. At the present time H-2-receptor antagonists are the therapeutic agents selected most frequently for the management of patients with duodenal ulcer.

Cimetidine was the first H-2-receptor antagonist developed and has been used most extensively in the treatment of duodenal ulcer. Cimetidine is related structurally to histamine (Fig. 238-4), sharing the same imidazole ring, but bearing an extended side chain which

FIGURE 238-4 Chemical structures of histamine and the H-2-receptor antagonists cimetidine, ranitidine, famotidine and nizatidine. Note the imidazole ring shared by histamine and cimetidine but absent in ranitidine, nizatidine, and famotidine.

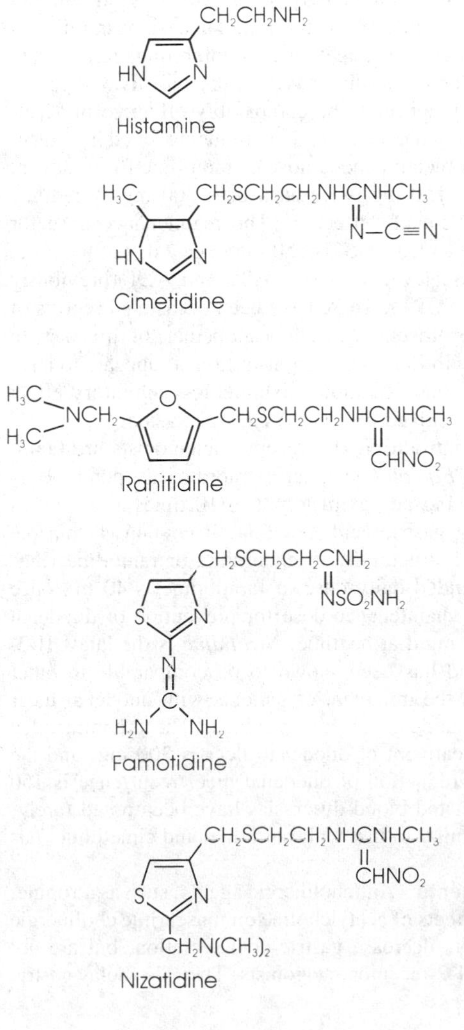

contains a cyanoguanidine group. Much of the information regarding the actions of H-2-receptor antagonist was obtained in the detailed characterization of the actions of cimetidine. Cimetidine (300 mg) was shown to inhibit basal acid secretion by more than 80 percent and meal-stimulated acid secretion by approximately 70 percent. It strikingly reduced acid secretory·responses to histamine, caffeine, insulin, hypoglycemia, and gastrin, Cimetidine has been shown to be effective in promoting endoscopically verified duodenal ulcer healing. Initially the oral dose of cimetidine recommended and used in treatment of duodenal ulcer was 300 mg four times daily, with meals and at bedtime. More recently 400 mg cimetidine twice each day or 800 mg once daily has been shown to be equally effective. Treatment of active duodenal ulcer with cimetidine is continued for periods from 4 to 8 weeks. In patients with healed duodenal ulcer prolonged administration of cimetidine (400 mg at bedtime) has been shown to reduce substantially the frequency of duodenal ulcer recurrence.

Considering the enormous number of patients who have been treated with cimetidine, few serious adverse effects have been experienced. Slight and reversible increases in serum transaminase and creatinine levels may occur. Central nervous system abnormalities have been reported in a small number of patients with substantial hepatic-renal functional impairment. Brief increases in serum prolactin have been found after intravenous and oral cimetidine. Cimetidine has been shown to inhibit the cytochrome P_{450} hepatic enzyme system, and therefore may increase blood levels, duration of action, and pharmacologic effects of drugs metabolized by this system. Tender gynecomastia due to the weak antiandrogenic effect of cimetidine may occur in patients with the Zollinger-Ellison syndrome, who require large doses for prolonged periods of time.

Ranitidine, the second H-2-receptor antagonist made available for use, is also prescribed widely in treatment of patients with duodenal ulcer. It is a substituted aminomethylfuran which is structurally unrelated to histamine (Fig. 238-4). On a molar basis, ranitidine is about six times as potent as cimetidine in inhibiting gastric acid secretion. Cimetidine and ranitidine have similar half-lives, approximately 120 min. They appear to be comparably effective in accelerating healing of duodenal ulcer and in reducing duodenal ulcer recurrence. The initial recommended dose of ranitidine for treatment of duodenal ulcer was 150 mg twice each day; 300 mg at bedtime has been found to be equally effective. The maintenance dose for reducing duodenal ulcer recurrence is 150 mg once a day at bedtime. Ranitidine may increase levels of serum AST and ALT (previously designated SGOT and SGPT). There have been occasional reports of reversible hepatitis, hepatocellular, hepatocanalicular, or mixed, with or without jaundice, with ranitidine adminstration. It appears to have no antiandrogen properties. Ranitidine exhibits less inhibitory effect on the cytochrome P_{450} mixed oxygenase enzyme system.

The most recently introduced H-2-receptor antagonists are famotidine and nizatidine. *Famotidine* is an extraordinarily potent H-2-receptor antagonist, being approximately 8 to 10 times as potent as ranitidine in inhibiting gastric acid secretion. It contains a thiazole ring and is not related structurally to cimetidine or ranitidine (Fig. 238-4). The recommended daily dose of famotidine is 40 mg once daily at bedtime. The maintenance dose for prevention of duodenal ulcer recurrence is 20 mg/d at bedtime. *Nizatidine* is the latest H-2-receptor antagonist and has been shown to be comparable to other agents in this class in the treatment of patients with duodenal ulcer and in reduction of duodenal ulcer recurrence. The recommended once daily dose for treatment of duodenal ulcer is 300 mg, and the maintenance dose for reduction of duodenal ulcer recurrence is 150 mg at bedtime. Associated blood dyscrasias have been noted rarely, and hepatotoxicity, similar to that with ranitidine and cimetidine, has also been reported.

Anticholinergic agents   Anticholinergic agents, such as atropine, act by inhibiting the effects of acetylcholine on muscarinic cholinergic receptors. These agents decrease gastric acid secretion, but are not nearly as effective as H-2-receptor antagonists. They also delay gastric emptying. Most studies have *not* shown that anticholinergic agents hasten healing or improve symptoms of duodenal ulcer; therefore, they are not recommended as primary agents for treatment for duodenal ulcer. Side effects include dryness of mouth, blurring of vision, cardiac arrhythmias, and urinary retention. They should not be used in patients with glaucoma, impaired gastric emptying, or history or symptoms of urinary retention. There are at least two classes of muscarinic cholinergic receptors (M-1 and M-2). *Pirenzepine* is a relatively selective anticholinergic agent, which is more specific in inhibiting gastric acid secretion, with fewer side effects, than other anticholinergic agents. Pirenzepine, not yet available for prescribing in the United States, has been shown to be effective in treatment of duodenal ulcer. It may prove useful as primary therapy or as adjunctive therapy in duodenal ulcer patients.

Coating agents   Several drugs that act neither by neutralization nor by inhibition of gastric acid secretion have been used in treatment of duodenal ulcer. Among these is *sucralfate*, a complex polyaluminum hydroxide salt of sucrose sulfate. Sucralfate becomes highly polar at acid pH and binds to the ulcer bed for up to 12 h, whereas relatively little binds to intact gastric or duodenal mucosa. It is believed that adherence of sucralfate to granulation tissue impedes diffusion of H^+ to the base of the ulcer. In addition sucralfate binds bile acids and pepsins and may, therefore, reduce their injurious effects. Sucralfate may increase endogenous tissue prostaglandins and thereby increase mucosal defense. It is only minimally absorbed, with less than 5 percent appearing in the urine. Sucralfate appears to be similar to antacids and H-2-receptor antagonists in its effectiveness in treatment of duodenal ulcer and in prevention of duodenal ulcer recurrence. The recommended dose of sucralfate is 1 g 1 h before each meal and at bedtime. *Colloidal bismuth* compounds also aid ulcer healing. They form (in an acid medium) a bismuth-protein coagulant which is believed to protect the ulcer from acid-peptic digestion. Bismuth-containing compounds may also be of value in treatment of duodenal ulcer because of their effects on *H. pylori*, a bacterium which appears important in the pathogenesis of some form(s) of gastritis (see below) and, as noted previously, which has been proposed as a potential pathogenetic factor in the etiology of duodenal ulcer. Several duodenal and gastric ulcer trials have shown good healing rates and reduced ulcer recurrence rates in patients treated with colloidal bismuth subcitrate. Colloidal bismuth compounds appear to be the only class of antiulcer drugs that eradicate *H. pylori* and the gastritis associated with its colonization. Some investigators have found lower relapse rates in patients with duodenal ulcer after treatment with colloidal bismuth compared with H-2-receptor antagonists.

Prostaglandins   A variety of *prostaglandins*, particularly those of the E series (PGE_1 and PGE_2), have been shown effective in clinical trials in treatment of duodenal ulcer, with healing rates comparable to those achieved with antacid therapy and H-2-receptor antagonists. Their action is believed to be twofold: (1) they reduce basal and stimulated gastric acid secretion, and (2) they enhance mucosal resistance to tissue injury. The principal mechanism by which exogenous prostaglandins enhance mucosal defense has not been clarified completely. However, they exert the following actions which appear important in mucosal defense to injury. PGEs (1) stimulate gastric mucus secretion, (2) stimulate gastric and duodenal bicarbonate secretion, (3) maintain gastric mucosal blood flow, (4) maintain the gastric mucosal barrier to back-diffusion of H^+, and (5) stimulate mucosal cellular renewal and regeneration.

Proton pump inhibition   The final phase of hydrogen ion secretion by parietal cells is accomplished by an enzyme (H^+,K^+-ATPase) which serves as a proton pump, exchanging potassium for hydrogen. *Omeprazole*, a specific inhibitor of parietal call H^+,K^+-ATPase, has been shown to be extraordinarily potent in decreasing gastric acid secretion. Omeprazole binds to the H^+,K^+-ATPase, irreversibly inactivating the enzyme. This drug, currently being evaluated in clinical trials, is very effective in accelerating healing of common duodenal ulcers and ulcers in patients with gastrinoma (see below). Omeprazole is not yet approved for prescribing.

Diet With little or no justification, many different diet programs have been used for treatment of patients with duodenal ulcer. There is no evidence that bland diets reduce gastric acid secretion, promote healing, or relieve symptoms of duodenal ulcer. Similarly, soft diets or diets free of spices or fruit juices have not been proven to be of benefit. Although traditionally milk and cream have been prescribed in treatment of ulcer patients, there is no evidence that they benefit ulcer healing. They may contribute to development of the milk-alkali syndrome and may accelerate atherogenesis. Many physicians recommend that patients with duodenal ulcer avoid coffee, with or without caffeine, and other caffeine-containing beverages because of their effects on gastric secretion. It may also be desirable to restrict alcohol intake in these patients. It is reasonable to suggest that if patients experience symptoms after ingestion of certain foods, these foods should be avoided.

General therapeutic considerations How does one integrate the large amount of available information concerning treatment of duodenal ulcer in selecting a therapeutic program for individual patients? There are several reasonable alternatives: effective therapy may be based on neutralization of gastric acid by antacids, on inhibition of gastric acid secretion by antisecretory agents, or on local actions of some other agents. There is no evidence that combinations of these drugs are required in treatment of duodenal ulcer. The various classes of agents appear to be comparably effective in accelerating duodenal ulcer healing and in reducing ulcer recurrence. In general, although side effects differ from group to group, these are all safe and effective drugs. Most duodenal ulcers will heal within 4 or 6 weeks of treatment with each of these groups of agents. It is seldom necessary to continue treatment of active duodenal ulcer for more than 8 weeks.

There is not yet general agreement concerning which patients should receive prolonged maintenance therapy to reduce the frequency of duodenal ulcer recurrence. Most physicians do not initiate maintenance treatment after the first (uncomplicated) episode of duodenal ulcer activity. Maintenance therapy is often recommended in patients with frequent, especially severe, duodenal ulcer recurrences, in those with previous, especially recurrent, duodenal ulcer complications, and perhaps in those with troublesome ulcer disease and other medical conditions which would make ulcer complication or surgery particularly hazardous. Maintenance therapy, when recommended, is usually continued for at least 1 year. Elimination of cigarette smoking, in most studies, appears to facilitate ulcer healing and may reduce duodenal ulcer recurrence. There is no evidence that dietary manipulation plays an important role in duodenal ulcer treatment.

GASTRIC ULCER

The peak incidence for gastric ulcer is in the sixth decade, approximately 10 years later than for duodenal ulcer. Slightly more than half of gastric ulcers occur in males. Gastric ulcers are deep, penetrating beyond the mucosa of the stomach and are similar histologically to duodenal ulcer, but often with more extensive gastritis surrounding the ulcer. Almost all benign gastric ulcers are found immediately distal to the junction of the antral mucosa with the acid-secreting mucosa of the body of the stomach. The location of this junction is variable, especially on the lesser gastric curvature. In general, the antrum extends approximately two-thirds of the way up the lesser curvature and one-third of the way up the greater curvature of the stomach. Benign gastric ulcers are rare in the fundus of the stomach. Benign gastric ulcers are virtually always accompanied by antral gastritis with variable amounts of mucosal atrophy. Gastritis may be present or absent with aspirin-associated gastric ulcers; they are usually located in the antrum, but they are not confined to the junction of the antral and parietal cell mucosa, as are common gastric ulcers.

ETIOLOGY AND PATHOGENESIS Acid-pepsin appears to be important in the pathogenesis of gastric ulcer; however, in contrast to duodenal ulcer, gastric ulcer patients generally have acid secretory rates that are normal or reduced compared with nonulcer subjects. Although many patients with gastric ulcer have reduced rates of acid secretion, true achlorhydria (in response to pentagastrin stimulation) almost never occurs in patients with benign gastric ulcer. Ten to twenty percent of patients with gastric ulcers also have duodenal ulcers. Patients with both duodenal and gastric ulcers tend to have acid secretory patterns that parallel those of duodenal ulcer. Patients with pyloric channel ulcers have acid secretory rates and clinical patterns similar to those found with common duodenal ulcer.

Most evidence supports the primary importance of defective gastric mucosal resistance and/or direct gastric mucosal injury as most important elements in the pathogenesis of gastric ulcer. Unlike duodenal ulcer, serum gastrin levels are increased in a significant proportion of gastric ulcer patients, but increases are limited to those with gastric acid hyposecretion. Gastric emptying has been shown to be delayed in gastric ulcer. It has been suggested that regurgitation of duodenal contents, especially those containing bile, may induce gastric mucosal injury and subsequent gastric ulceration by interruption of the gastric mucosal barrier with resultant back diffusion of secreted hydrogen ions.

CLINICAL FEATURES As with duodenal ulcer, epigastric pain is the most common symptom; however, it is less typical and predictable than in patients with duodenal ulcer. Some gastric ulcer patients experience no relief of pain with eating. Pain may actually be precipitated or accentuated by food, and relief of symptoms with antacids is less consistent than with duodenal ulcers. Gastric ulcers tend to heal, but then recur, often in the same location. Recognizable episodes of recurrent gastric ulcer activity are, in general, less frequent than those of duodenal ulcer. The precise incidence of gastric ulcer is not known, since many gastric ulcer patients are asymptomatic. Although duodenal ulcer is identified clinically more frequently than gastric ulcer, most autopsy studies show an equal or greater proportion of gastric ulcers. This may be due in part to acute preterminal events, but also may reflect the often asymptomatic clinical course of gastric ulcer. Whereas in duodenal ulcer patients nausea and vomiting almost always indicate gastric outlet obstruction, in patients with gastric ulcer they may occur in the absence of mechanical obstruction. Weight loss may occur due to anorexia or aversion to food due to discomfort produced by eating.

Hemorrhage is a common complication, occurring in approximately 25 percent. Mortality is greater in patients with gastric ulcer than with duodenal ulcer. Gastric ulcer perforation occurs less frequently than hemorrhage. Mortality with perforation of gastric ulcers is approximately three times that with duodenal ulcers. Increased mortality is due in part to the increased age of gastric ulcer patients, but also may result from uncertainty and delay in diagnosis and from greater soilage of the peritoneum with gastric ulcer perforation. Gastric outlet obstruction may develop when ulcers are in the pyloric channel or in the most distal antrum but is rare with ulcer in other parts of the stomach.

DIAGNOSIS The history is of value in suspecting gastric ulcer, but it is not as characteristic as in duodenal ulcer. The two major methods for diagnosis are barium examination and endoscopy. Gastric ulcer can usually be identified by standard barium examination with an accuracy that approaches 90 percent. Both benign and malignant gastric ulcers are more common on the lesser than on the greater curvature (Fig. 238-5). Radiation of gastric mucosal folds from the margin of the ulcer crater suggests a benign lesion. Large gastric ulcers, i.e., those greater than 3 cm in diameter, are more often malignant than smaller ones. An ulcer within a mass, as defined radiographically, also suggests malignancy. Approximately 4 percent of gastric ulcers which appear benign radiographically prove to be malignant (by endoscopic biopsy or at surgery). Because of false-positive and false-negative errors, radiographic appearance cannot be used as the sole criterion for the benign or malignant nature of a gastric ulcer.

Endoscopic visualization of the ulcer allows definition of its size,

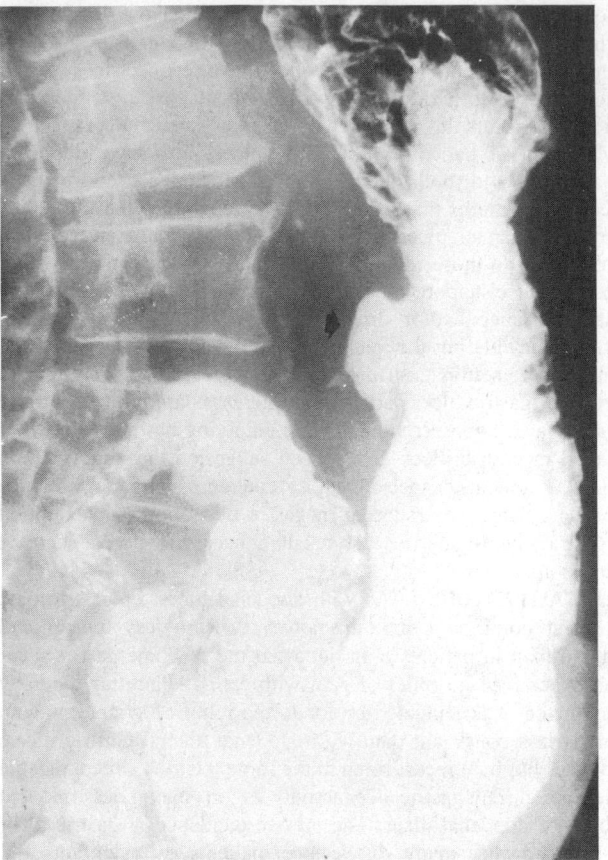

FIGURE 238-5   Benign lesser curvature gastric ulcer. Note ulceration beyond the projected margins of the stomach and the collar of edema.

location, and, by biopsy, its histologic characteristics. At gastroscopy a total of at least six biopsies should be obtained from the inner margin of the ulcer and from the ulcer bed. If accurate cytology is available, brushings of the ulcer should be obtained prior to biopsy. By application of combined radiographic, endoscopic, and histologic techniques, distinguishing a malignant from a benign gastric ulcer should be possible with substantially more than 95 percent confidence.

Gastric ulcer with pentagastrin-fast achlorhydria is rare. When it occurs it almost always indicates gastric carcinoma. However, most patients with gastric carcinoma (about two-thirds to three-fourths) are capable of secreting some gastric acid, although usually less than normal.

MEDICAL TREATMENT   In general, with whatever medical treatment modality is selected gastric ulcers tend to heal more slowly than duodenal ulcers, and the healing response rates are somewhat less than those for duodenal ulcer. *Antacids* are effective in gastric ulcer treatment. However, since acid hypersecretion is not characteristic of the disease, smaller doses of antacid may be required than for treatment of duodenal ulcer. *H-2-receptor antagonists* and *sucralfate* are approximately as effective as antacid therapy in the treatment of gastric ulcer. The dosage schedules used for these drugs are similar to those for patients with duodenal ulcer.

Anticholinergic agents have been recommended by some physicians. However, because of substantial side effects of anticholinergic drugs, their tendency to reduce gastric emptying which is already impaired in these patients, the fact that gastric ulcer patients are often older and, therefore, more susceptible to the complications of these agents, and the lack of evidence for their benefit, the use of anticholinergic drugs in gastric ulcer treatment does not appear justified. Some studies have suggested that hospitalization and/or cessation of smoking are of benefit in gastric ulcer healing.

Since salicylates and other nonsteroidal anti-inflammatory drugs (NSAIDs) have been associated with the development of gastric

ulcers, patients with gastric ulcer should not ingest these or should be treated with the lowest doses required. Alcohol, because of its injurious effects on the gastric mucosa, should probably also be avoided. Milk and cream, as well as bland or homogenized diets, have not been shown to be of value in treatment. In general, it is probably sufficient to recommend that patients consume a diet of their own choice. Since coffee (caffeine-containing or caffeine-free) and other caffeine-containing liquids stimulate gastric acid secretion, it may be desirable to avoid these beverages.

Carbenoxolone has been used in many countries (though it is not available in the United States) in the treatment of gastric ulcer. This drug is a hydrolytic produce of glycyrrhizic acid (derived from licorice) and has been shown to decrease symptoms and increase the rate of gastric ulcer healing. Carbenoxolone does not decrease gastric acid secretion but increases the life span of gastric mucosal epithelial cells and increases the secretion and viscosity of gastric mucus. Carbenoxolone possesses aldosterone-like effects, so sodium and water retention tend to occur. It is possible to inhibit the aldosterone-like effects of carbenoxolone by use of aldosterone antagonists; however, the latter also abolish the ulcer-healing effect of carbenoxolone. Problems with sodium and water retention and availability of alternative drugs have led to its decreased use worldwide.

Benign gastric ulcers should heal completely within 3 months of vigorous therapy. The failure of gastric ulcer to decrease satisfactorily in size and to heal with medical treatment has been used to suggest gastric malignancy. The following is suggested as one reasonable scheme to monitor gastric ulcer healing. Upper gastrointestinal barium examination or gastroscopy is suggested after 4 weeks of treatment, at which time definite healing of benign gastric ulcers should be demonstrable: the diameter of most ulcers should be reduced by more than 50 percent. If not, malignancy must be suspected and exfoliative cytology and biopsies of the ulcer should be performed. If no malignancy is identified, medical therapy should be continued. If the ulcer has not healed completely at 8 weeks, endoscopic examination should be repeated in another month, at which time most benign gastric ulcers should have healed. In general, large gastric ulcers heal more slowly than smaller ones. It is important to continue treatment to endoscopically verified complete ulcer healing. One must be alert, however, for the occasional "healing" of an ulcerating gastric carcinoma with treatment. Apparently complete healing does not guarantee the benign nature of a gastric ulcer, since approximately 70 percent of gastric ulcers eventually found to be malignant will undergo significant (albeit usually incomplete) healing with medical treatment.

COMPLICATIONS AND SURGERY FOR PEPTIC ULCER

Surgery is reserved for patients with complications of peptic ulcer and for those who do not respond to vigorous and attentive medical treatment. Complications include hemorrhage, obstruction, and perforation.

Hemorrhage occurs in approximately 15 percent of patients with duodenal ulcers; a recurrence of bleeding is estimated to occur in about 40 percent of patients with an initial hemorrhage. In most patients hemorrhage from peptic ulcer responds satisfactorily to medical management, including gastric suction and antacid or H-2-receptor antagonist administration.

Free *perforation* into the peritoneal cavity occurs in approximately 6 percent of patients with duodenal ulcer. Five to ten percent of these patients will have had no recognizable ulcer symptoms prior to perforation. Simultaneous hemorrhage occurs in approximately 10 percent of patients with duodenal ulcer perforation; mortality is greatly increased in this group. Duodenal ulcers, especially those located posteriorly, may penetrate into adjacent structures, most often the pancreas, frequently resulting in increased serum amylase levels. Less commonly, duodenal ulcers may penetrate into the liver, biliary tract, or colon.

Gastric outlet *obstruction* occurs in 2 to 4 percent of patients admitted to the hospital with duodenal or pyloric channel ulcers. Symptoms include abdominal bloating, nausea, vomiting, and weight loss. These patients usually have had ulcer symptoms for many years and often obstructive symptoms for several months.

Failure to respond satisfactorily to medical treatment requires consideration of surgery. The true incidence of lack of ulcer healing with vigorous medical programs is not known. It is clear that, especially with currently available drugs, the vast majority of patients with peptic ulcer can be treated successfully without surgery.

Decisions regarding surgery for patients with complications of peptic ulcer must be individualized. Risks of surgery must be balanced against risks of the disease. The patient's discomfort, costs of medical care and hospitalization, and time lost from work must be examined in relation to the morbidity and possible mortality associated with surgery and anesthesia, risks of recurrent ulcer, and long-term postoperative sequelae. The skill and experience of the surgeon must be weighed as major factors in considering operation.

SURGERY FOR DUODENAL ULCER No single surgical procedure has been accepted universally as the most satisfactory duodenal ulcer operation. At present the most commonly performed surgical procedures are *vagotomy with antrectomy, vagotomy with pyloroplasty, and parietal cell vagotomy* (also referred to as *proximal gastric or superselective vagotomy*) without a gastric drainage procedure.

With conventional (truncal) vagotomy and antrectomy, the vagal trunks are transected, the antrum is removed, and gastrointestinal continuity is reestablished by anastomosis of the remaining stomach with the proximal duodenum (Billroth I anastomosis) or with a loop of the jejunum (Billroth II anastomosis). Vagotomy and antrectomy is an effective procedure with a low recurrence rate (approximately 1 percent). Morbidity and mortality with vagotomy and antrectomy are variable, depending upon patient selection and the skill of the surgeon, but are probably slightly greater than with vagotomy and pyloroplasty.

When the procedure of vagotomy and pyloroplasty is selected, pyloroplasty is performed to facilitate gastric drainage after truncal or selective vagotomy. Vagotomy is performed to inhibit vagal stimulation of gastric acid secretion. Vagotomy does not inhibit gastrin release; in fact, release of gastrin is enhanced after vagal interruption. Three types of vagotomy are now used in the surgical treatment of duodenal or pyloric channel ulcer, namely, *truncal vagotomy, selective vagotomy*, and *parietal cell vagotomy*. Pyloroplasty with truncal vagotomy is associated with approximately 1 percent mortality. Ulcer recurrence during the 5 years after surgery is about 5 to 8 percent. With selective vagotomy only the branches of the vagus that supply the stomach are transected, preserving the vagal innervation of the other abdominal viscera. Selective vagotomy has been found by some surgeons to result in a more complete vagotomy, less ulcer recurrence, and fewer postvagotomy complications than truncal vagotomy. Parietal cell vagotomy denervates only the acid-secreting portion of the stomach, sparing the branches of the vagus that innervate the antrum, which makes a gastric drainage procedure (e.g., pyloroplasty) unnecessary. Both immediate and late postoperative complications are less common with parietal cell vagotomy than with truncal vagotomy, and reductions in acid secretion are similar to those achieved with truncal or selective vagotomy. Mortality with parietal cell vagotomy is less than 1 percent. Most studies indicate that with experience, recurrence is comparable to that of other forms of vagotomy with pyloroplasty. This procedure, which is being used with increasing frequency, appears to be a safe and effective surgical therapy.

SURGERY FOR GASTRIC ULCER Surgical treatment is required for gastric ulcer patients who do not respond satisfactorily to medical therapy or who develop complications similar to those described for duodenal ulcer. With the available diagnostic accuracy of careful radiographic examination, endoscopy, biopsy of the ulcer margins, and exfoliative cytology, it should rarely be necessary to operate because of remaining uncertainty regarding the malignant or benign nature of the ulcer. The recommended surgical procedure for the treatment of gastric ulcer is antrectomy with gastroduodenal (Billroth I) anastomosis. It is not necessary to perform a vagotomy when antrectomy is performed by gastric ulcer (not located in the pyloric channel).

CONSEQUENCES AND SYNDROMES AFTER PEPTIC ULCER SURGERY

Modern surgery for peptic ulcer is effective in the treatment of ulcer complications and in the prevention of ulcer recurrence. However, numerous postoperative sequelae and syndromes may occur.

RECURRENT ULCERATION Recurrent ulceration has been reported in approximately 5 percent of all patients after surgery for peptic ulcer. Approximately 95 percent of these recurrences follow surgery for duodenal ulcer disease. The risk of development of recurrent ulcer is 3 to 10 percent after surgery for duodenal ulcer and approximately 2 percent after gastric ulcer surgery. Recurrence is more common after vagotomy and pyloroplasty and after parietal cell vagotomy than after vagotomy and antrectomy. When ulcers occur after partial gastric resection, the ulcer is usually located at the anastomosis (stomal or marginal ulcer) or immediately distal to it in the small intestine. Abdominal pain is the most common symptom in patients with a stomal ulcer. The pain is usually epigastric but is often not characteristic of common duodenal ulcer. It is usually, but not always, relieved by meals or antacids and, in general, tends to be more persistent and progressive than that observed with unoperated duodenal ulcer. Hemorrhage or anemia due to blood loss, nausea and vomiting from obstruction, weight loss, or symptoms from perforation may occur. The development of a stomal ulcer after duodenal ulcer surgery usually indicates that an incomplete vagotomy was performed. Inadequate gastric resection, when performed without vagotomy, may also result in stomal ulceration. Additional causes for the development of recurrent ulcer include an excessively long jejunal afferent loop, and inadvertently performed gastroileal or gastrocolic anastomosis, poor gastric drainage, and ingestion of ulcerogenic drugs. Less commonly, a marginal ulcer may be caused by acid hypersecretion secondary to gastrinoma or a retained antrum.

Radiographic examination with barium is of limited diagnostic value and identifies only from 50 to 65 percent of stomal ulcerations. Surgical deformity at the anastomotic site often may mimic stomal ulcer in its absence or conceal it when present. When suspected, endoscopic examination is required to identify stomal ulceration. Medical treatment with antacids is almost always unsatisfactory in patients with stomal ulcer. H-2-receptor antagonists have been used successfully to induce healing of stomal ulcers. The long-term effectiveness of these agents on stomal ulcers and prevention of their recurrence remain to be established. Surgery is usually necessary for treatment of ulcer recurrence, and it is usually, but not invariably, successful. In patients with recurrent ulcer provocative testing with measurements of serum gastrin should be performed to identify or exclude gastrinoma (see below).

RECURRENT ULCER DUE TO RETAINED ANTRUM Recurrent ulcers have been described in a small number of patients after antrectomy with gastrojejunostomy (Billroth II anastomosis) in which the antral resection was not complete. In these patients the distal antrum, inadvertently not resected, remains in continuity with the duodenum after surgery. These patients usually develop or continue to have gastric acid hypersecretion due to gastrin release by the residual antral mucosa which is no longer in contact with gastric acid, the normal inhibitor of gastrin release. In these patients fasting serum gastrin levels may be normal to moderately increased. Patients with retained antrum can be distinguished from those with gastrinoma by intravenous injection of secretion with measurements of serum gastrin. Gastrinoma patients exhibit substantial increases in serum gastrin, whereas in those with retained antrum, serum gastrin levels

TABLE 238-1 Provocative gastrin tests

| Disorder | Serum gastrin response (change from basal levels) | |
	After IV secretion injection	After test meal
Zollinger-Ellison (gastrinoma)	Increase (greater than 200 pg/mL)	Little or no increase (increases less than 50%)
Common duodenal ulcer	No change, slight decrease, or small increase	Moderate increase (may be slightly more than normal, but less than in gastrin cell hyperplasia)
Antral gastrin cell hyperplasia	No change, slight decrease, or small increase	Striking increase (greater than 200%)
Achlorhydria (e.g., pernicious anemia, chronic gastritis)	No change, slight decrease, or small increase	Moderate increase

decrease after secretin adminstration (see Table 238-1). These patients can be treated successfully by surgical removal of the remaining antrum.

AFFERENT LOOP SYNDROMES Patients with partial gastric resection with gastrojejunostomy (Billroth II anastomosis) may experience abdominal bloating and pain 20 min to 1 h after eating, frequently followed by nausea and vomiting. The vomitus often contains large amounts of bile. Characteristically, the bloating and abdominal discomfort are relieved by vomiting. This type of afferent loop syndrome, which is uncommon, is believed to be caused by distention of an incompletely draining afferent intestinal loop by pancreatic and biliary secretions which are stimulated by eating. Serum amylase levels may be mildly or moderately increased. Because of partial obstruction it is often difficult to demonstrate the afferent loop by barium meal examination. Treatment is surgical correction of the incomplete afferent loop obstruction, and, in some instances, revision to a gastroduodenal anastomosis.

A second form of afferent loop dysfunction is that due to stasis with bacterial overgrowth within the afferent loop. These patients may exhibit the same characteristics as are found with other forms of small intestinal bacterial overgrowth or blind loop syndromes (see Chap. 240). These include malabsorption, especially of fat and vitamin B_{12}. Correction of the afferent loop bacterial overgrowth syndrome can be accomplished by surgical revision of the afferent loop.

BILE REFLUX GASTRITIS After peptic ulcer surgery a small proportion of patients experience early satiety, abdominal discomfort, and vomiting, which is believed due to reflux of duodenal contents into the stomach. Endoscopic examination usually reveals regurgitated bile in the stomach and diffuse gastritis, often involving the entire gastric remnant. Various terms assigned to this entity include *alkaline reflux gastritis*, *bile reflux gastritis*, *duodenogastric reflux*, and *bilious vomiting*. The mechanisms or materials contained in the refluxed intestinal contents accounting for these symptoms have not been defined. Although the term bile reflux gastritis has been used, there is no certainty that regurgitated bile is responsible for the syndrome. Administration of cholestyramine, intended to bind bile acids and facilitate their excretion, has not been of benefit in this disorder. Some surgeons have reported successful treatment of bile reflux gastritis by diversion of duodenal contents from proximity to the stomach with a Roux en Y anastomosis.

DUMPING SYNDROME Following peptic ulcer surgery some patients experience an assortment of vasomotor symptoms after eating. These include palpitation, tachycardia, lightheadedness, diaphoresis, and less frequently, postural hypotension. Abdominal discomfort and vomiting may also occur. The vasomotor symptoms, referred to as the *early dumping syndrome*, are usually experienced within 30 min after eating and are believed to result from rapid emptying of hyperosmolar gastric contents into the proximal small intestine. This leads to a shift of fluid into the gut lumen and produces intestinal distention and contraction of plasma volume. Additional proposed mechanisms for these symptoms include stimulation of autonomic reflexes secondary to small intestinal distention and/or release of hormones from the gut in response to rapid entry of gastric contents into the duodenum or jejunum.

The *late dumping syndrome* refers to a symptom complex comprising dizziness, lightheadedness, palpitation, diaphoresis, confusion, and, in rare instances, syncope, occurring 90 min to 3 h after eating. The symptoms can often be precipitated by meals rich in simple carbohydrates, especially sucrose. The syndrome appears to be caused by hypoglycemia due to insulin release stimulated by abrupt increases in blood glucose secondary to rapid emptying of sugar-containing meals into the proximal small intestine.

Both forms of the dumping syndrome are treated by dietary measures. These include limitation of simple sugar-continuing liquids and solids (sweets), elimination of liquids at mealtime, and frequent small meals. Most patients have not been benefited by surgical procedures such as creation of reversed jejunal loops and isoperistaltic jejunal interposition.

POSTVAGOTOMY DIARRHEA A significant number of patients experience diarrhea after peptic ulcer surgery, especially with a procedure including truncal vagotomy. Diarrhea usually occurs within 2 h of eating. Although the mechanism is not clear, interruption of vagal fibers to the abdominal viscera appears to play an important role in the production of the diarrhea. The surgical drainage procedure, pyloroplasty or antrectomy, which removes the pyloric regulatory emptying mechanism, may also contribute to the diarrhea. Diarrhea has been estimated to occur in 20 to 30 percent of patients after truncal vagotomy with drainage, in 10 to 20 percent with selective vagotomy and drainage, and in only 1 to 8 percent of those with parietal cell vagotomy (without drainage). Rapid emptying of gastric contents into the small intestine, resulting in increased fluid volume within the intestinal lumen, due to the osmotic action of the meal, may also contribute to the diarrhea.

HEMATOLOGIC COMPLICATIONS Intrinsic factor secreted by gastric parietal cells is necessary for active absorption of vitamin B_{12} by the distal ileum. Patients who have had total gastrectomy invariably will develop malabsorption of vitamin B_{12} and should receive monthly intramuscular injections of vitamin B_{12} (50 to 100 µg) indefinitely. Megaloblastic anemia due to vitamin B_{12} deficiency is rare after partial gastric resection; however, reduced serum vitamin B_{12} levels have been observed in about 14 percent of these patients. Even more rarely vitamin B_{12} deficiency may be produced by bacterial overgrowth in a stagnant afferent loop following Billroth II anastomosis. Gastritis in the remaining stomach develops in more than 60 percent of duodenal ulcer patients after vagotomy and antrectomy or vagotomy and pyloroplasty. This may result in decreased vitamin B_{12} absorption. Inasmuch as the stomach secretes intrinsic factor in excess of need by approximately 100 times, peptic ulcer patients treated with partial gastric resection do not develop vitamin B_{12} deficiency secondary to the amount of stomach resected. (In addition, the resected portion of the stomach is almost always principally antrum, which contains few parietal cells.) However, after peptic ulcer surgery patients may develop decreased serum vitamin B_{12} levels due to reduced absorption of food-bound vitamin B_{12}; these patients will often have normal absorption of free vitamin B_{12}, as used in the Schilling test. The precise mechanism of the malabsorption of food-bound vitamin B_{12} is not known. It may be due in part to rapid emptying of gastric contents, with reduced efficiency of intrinsic factor binding of vitamin B_{12}. Anemia after peptic ulcer surgery may also result from deficiency produced by malabsorption of iron or folate. A combined deficiency of vitamin B_{12}, iron, and folate is common in patients with anemia following partial or subtotal gastric resection. Iron deficiency is the most common single hematologic defect after peptic ulcer surgery and may result from either blood loss (e.g., with persistent or recurrent ulcers) or from iron malabsorption. Patients with gastric resection malabsorb dietary iron but have normal absorption of iron salts;

therefore they will respond favorably to treatment with therapeutic oral iron preparations. Folate deficiency may result from either reduced dietary intake or impaired folate absorption. Except for the anemia produced by blood loss in association with early recurrent ulcer disease, the development of anemia after peptic ulcer surgery is gradual, usually occurring several years postoperatively.

The nature of the anemia after ulcer surgery should be clarified by determination of the red blood cell morphology and by measurements of serum iron, folate, and vitamin B_{12}. Iron or folate deficiency may be treated by oral replacement. Vitamin B_{12} deficiency should be treated with monthly intramuscular injections of the vitamin.

OSTEOMALACIA AND OSTEOPOROSIS Osteoporosis and osteomalacia may develop after partial or complete gastrectomy but occur rarely after vagotomy and pyloroplasty. Osteomalacia is extremely frequent following gastrojejunostomy or Billroth II anastomosis. These bone changes are believed to result from malabsorption of calcium and vitamin D. Patients may develop bone pain and have pathologic fractures. The incidence of bone fractures in men following gastric resection has been estimated to be almost twice that of control subjects of similar age. Reduced bone density requires years to develop and can be identified by x-ray. Patients with osteomalacia usually have increased levels of serum alkaline phosphatase and may have reduced serum calcium concentrations. These patients should be treated by supplemental oral vitamin D and calcium. In fact, the frequency of osteoporosis and osteomalacia after partial or complete gastrectomy is sufficiently great that treatment with vitamin D and calcium should probably be instituted and continued indefinitely in these patients, especially females, following gastric resection.

GENERAL MALABSORPTION (See Chap. 240) Mild, chemically demonstrable steatorrhea is common in patients after ulcer surgery. Weight loss is more common after partial gastric resection than with vagotomy without resection and occurs in approximately 60 percent of patients in whom a portion of the stomach has been removed. The major cause of weight loss after peptic ulcer surgery is reduced food intake. On a 100-g fat diet, loss of stool fat seldom exceeds 15 g per day (normal individuals, less than 7 g per day). The causes of maldigestion and malabsorption after peptic ulcer surgery include rapid gastric emptying, reduced dispersion of food in the stomach, reduced bile concentrations in the gut lumen, increased rate of transit of the meal through the small intestine, and reduced or delayed pancreatic secretory responses to feeding. Steatorrhea and weight loss, sometimes accompanied by vitamin B_{12} malabsorption, may develop as a result of bacterial overgrowth, especially in patients with afferent loop bacterial stasis. Overt symptoms and other manifestations of malabsorption appearing after surgery for peptic ulcer may also be due to other preexisting conditions, including latent celiac sprue and chronic pancreatitis.

CARCINOMA AFTER PARTIAL GASTRECTOMY Several studies have documented an increased incidence of adenocarcinoma of the stomach in duodenal ulcer patients following partial gastric resection and after vagotomy and drainage without resection. This usually develops 10 or more years after ulcer surgery. The possibility of carcinoma of the stomach should be considered when abdominal symptoms, which may be similar to or distinct from those due to the original ulcer, appear many years after apparently successful surgery.

ZOLLINGER-ELLISON SYNDROME (GASTRINOMA)

In 1955 Zollinger and Ellison described the syndrome that bears their names, which consists of ulcer disease of the upper gastrointestinal tract, marked increases in gastric acid secretion, and nonbeta islet cell tumors of the pancreas.

ETIOLOGY AND PATHOGENESIS Zollinger and Ellison, in their original description of the syndrome, suggested that the ulcer disease in these patients resulted from release of a secretagogue from these tumors into the circulation which accounted for the often enormously increased rates of gastric acid secretion. Their proposal proved correct when in 1960 extracts of Zollinger-Ellison (Z-E) tumors were shown to stimulate gastric acid secretion. Subsequently, it was found that these pancreatic islet cell tumors contained gastrin and that there were large amounts of this hormone in the circulation producing the pathophysiologic characteristics of the syndrome. These gastrin-containing tumors are therefore now called *gastrinomas*.

Most gastrinomas are found within the pancreas. Pancreatic gastrinomas may vary in size from 2 mm to more than 20 cm in diameter. Multiple, apparently primary tumors are common. In from one-half to two-thirds of patients multiple gastrinomas are in the pancreas; however, more than half are not identified at surgery. Pancreatic gastrinomas are most common in the head of the pancreas. Approximately 13 percent of patients with this syndrome have tumors in the wall of the duodenum, especially in its second portion. Gastrinomas have also been located less commonly in other sites, including the hilum of the spleen and rarely in the stomach. Primary gastrinomas, surrounded by lymphoid tissue, have been found in proximity to the pancreas, proximal duodenum, and spleen. These may be confused with, but are distinct from, metastasis to regional lymph nodes. In rare instances, the Z-E syndrome has resulted from other gastrin-containing tumors, e.g., parathyroid and ovarian adenomas. About two-thirds are histologically or biologically malignant. Malignant gastrinomas usually grow slowly; however, a small portion may be rapidly invasive and may metastasize early and widely. Metastasis is most common to regional lymph nodes and liver; spread may also be to peritoneal surfaces, spleen, bone, skin, or mediastinum. Gastrinomas have light-microscopic similarities to carcinoid tumors and may be mistaken for carcinoid tumors, especially when they arise from the mucosa of the small intestine or stomach. Pancreatic islet cell hyperplasia occurs in approximately 10 percent of patients with the Z-E syndrome. Hyperplasia of the islets, accompanying recognized or unidentified gastrinoma, appears to be an association or a consequence, rather than a cause, of excess gastrin release, since gastrin is not present in the hyperplastic tissue.

In 20 to 25 percent of patients with the Z-E syndrome, the gastrinoma is a component of the multiple endocrine neoplasia type I (MEN I) syndrome, an autosomal dominant disorder with a high degree of penetrance and great variability in expressivity. Patients with MEN I may have hyperplasia, adenomas, or carcinoma involving, in order of frequency, the parathyroid glands, pancreatic islets, and pituitary. Hyperparathyroidism is present in 87 percent of patients with MEN I syndrome, and gastrinoma is present in approximately half of these patients (see Chap. 325).

In most gastrinomas approximately 80 to 95 percent of gastrin is in the form of heptadecapeptide gastrin (G-17), with most of the remainder being G-34. In contrast, approximately two-thirds of circulating gastrin in gastrinoma patients is G-34; most of the remainder is G-17. However, smaller amounts of even larger forms of gastrin and smaller gastrin fragments can be detected in the serum. When sought for, almost all gastrin secreting islet cell tumors are found to contain multiple hormones, which are usually clinically silent. These have included, among others, ACTH, glucagon, melanocyte-stimulating hormone, parathyroid hormone, growth hormone releasing factor (GRF), insulin, pancreatic polypeptide, and vasoactive intestinal peptide. Of these ACTH is the most common; it is found in approximately 30 percent of gastrin-secreting tumors in patients with the Z-E syndrome. Cushing's syndrome with increased serum ACTH levels has been reported in 8 percent of 75 Z-E patients. ACTH-releasing gastrinomas are often aggressively malignant. Alternatively, in patients with gastrinoma associated with MEN I, Cushing's syndrome may result from ACTH release from associated pituitary tumors; the symptoms of Cushing's syndrome are generally mild and the gastrinomas are usually not metastatic. Approximately one-third of patients with gastrinomas have increases in serum concentrations of *pancreatic polypeptide*.

The parietal cell mass is substantially expanded to from three to six times normal, secondary to the tropic effects of circulating gastrin on parietal cells. Small, multicentric, noninvasive carcinoid tumors have been identified in the gastric mucosa of patients with the Z-E syndrome. These tumors and associated focal areas of enterochromatin-like (ECL) cell hyperplasia are believed to represent consequences of substantial and sustained hypergastrinemia. They have also been found in the gastric mucosa of patients with pernicious anemia, in which substantial increases in serum gastrin are found in the absence of gastric acid secretion.

While the true incidence of the Z-E syndrome is not known, estimates are that it accounts for 0.1 to 1 percent of peptic ulcers. The Z-E syndrome may occur at any age, but initial manifestations are most common between ages 30 and 60.

CLINICAL FEATURES From 90 to 95 percent of patients with gastrinomas develop ulceration of the gastrointestinal tract at some point during the course of their disease. Profound gastric acid hypersecretion is found in most, but not all, patients. Especially early in the course of the disease symptoms are usually similar to those of patients with typical peptic ulcer. However, ulcer symptoms may be more fulminant, progressive, and persistent, and, in general, respond poorly to the usual medical and surgical peptic ulcer treatment programs. The anatomic site of the ulcers in patients with gastrinoma is similar, but not identical, to that of patients with common types of peptic ulcer. About 75 percent of gastrinoma patients have ulcers in the first portion of the duodenum or in the stomach; these are usually single, but may be multiple. When multiple ulcers occur, they are frequently located not only in the first portion of the duodenum, the site of common duodenal ulcer, but also in the remainder of the duodenum or even the jejunum. In one large series, 14 percent of the ulcers were in the duodenum beyond its first portion and 11 percent in the jejunum.

Diarrhea occurs in about 40 percent of patients, and about 7 percent of patients with gastrinoma have diarrhea in the absence of ulcer disease. The diarrhea is due to the outpouring of large amounts of hydrochloric acid into the proximal duodenum and can be reduced or eliminated by aspiration of gastric juice. The excessive acid has been shown to reduce the pH of the contents of the proximal and distal jejunum to as low as 1 and 3.6, respectively. Inflammatory changes may be produced in the mucosa of the small intestine, secondary to the injurious effect of large amounts of acid and pepsin. Steatorrhea, which is less common than diarrhea, results from inactivation of pancreatic lipase by large concentrations of acid in the proximal small intestine and from decreases in luminal bile acids. The decrease in intraluminal bile acid concentration is caused by precipitation of the major bile acids at low pH. This then leads to impaired micelle formation, which, in turn, reduces intestinal absorption of fatty acids and monoglycerides (see Chap. 240). Vitamin B_{12} malabsorption, not correctable by addition of intrinsic factor, has been detected in some patients with the Z-E syndrome. Although gastric secretion of intrinsic factor appears normal, the reduced pH within the gut interferes with intrinsic factor–mediated vitamin B_{12} absorption. This can be corrected by neutralization of the intestinal contents. The mechanism by which low pH in the gut interferes with intrinsic factor action is not known.

DIAGNOSIS The presence of gastrinoma should be suspected in patients with a compatible clinical history, especially in those with marked acid hypersecretion. Two-thirds of gastrinoma patients have basal gastric acid outputs (BAO) that exceed 15 mmol/h. In some instances the basal output may be greater than 100 mmol/h. However, there is substantial overlap in rates of gastric acid secretion among patients with gastrinoma and duodenal ulcer and normal subjects. Gastrinoma patients often have BAO rates that are greater than 60 percent of those induced by maximal stimulation (MAO). In most normal subjects and duodenal ulcer patients basal acid secretory rates are less than 60 percent of maximal secretion. However, because of frequent exceptions to these guidelines in patients with gastrinomas and common duodenal ulcers, the use of the BAO/MAO ratio is of no value in the certain identification of patients with gastrinoma.

Some radiographic features may suggest the diagnosis of the Z-E syndrome. Large mucosal folds may be demonstrated most promi-

nently in the stomach, but also in the duodenum, and, in some instances, the jejunum. The lumen of the stomach and small intestine often contains large amounts of fluid. Radiographic features of most ulcers in these patients, except when they are multiple and/or distal in location, are similar to those of common peptic ulcer. Gastrinomas are difficult to localize. In almost half of patients with clinical and laboratory evidence the tumors cannot be identified at surgery. Arteriography is of limited value in identifying gastrinomas; only from 20 to 30 percent of primary tumors or hepatic metastases found at surgery have been identified by arteriography. Computed tomography is of slightly greater value in identifying gastrinomas. Use of both selective arteriography and CT has been reported to identify 44 percent of gastrinomas in Z-E patients and 80 percent of those located at surgery. Endoscopic retrograde pancreaticoduodenography has not proved to be of assistance in the diagnosis or exclusion of pancreatic gastrinomas. A small number of duodenal wall gastrinomas have been identified and confirmed histologically by duodenoscopy.

The diagnosis in a patient with clinical features consistent with the Z-E syndrome depends upon the demonstration of *increased serum gastrin levels* by radioimmunoassay. Fasting serum gastrin levels in normal subjects and patients with typical duodenal ulcer average approximately 20 to 50 pg/mL and usually do not exceed 150 pg/mL. Patients with gastrinoma almost always have fasting serum gastrin levels that are greater than 200 pg/mL and have been found as high as 450,000 pg/mL. Approximately half of these patients have fasting serum gastrin levels that are less than 1000 pg/mL (an approximate mean value for serum gastrin for patients with gastrinoma).

Several provocative tests have been used to evaluate patients with possible gastrinoma, especially those who do not exhibit pronounced hypergastrinemia (i.e., serum gastrin > 1000 pg/mL). These tests utilize measurements of serum gastrin levels in response to intravenous secretin injection, calcium infusion, or ingestion of a standard test meal (see Table 238-1).

In the *secretin injection test,* secretin (Kabi secretin, 2 units per kilogram) is given intravenously over 30 to 60 s. Gastrin is measured in serum samples obtained before injection of secretin and at 5-min intervals thereafter for 30 min. In normal individuals and patients with common duodenal ulcer, secretin produces no change, small reductions, or small increases in serum gastrin levels. In contrast, in gastrinoma patients intravenous secretin induces substantial increases in serum gastrin. The gastrin levels increase promptly by at least 200 pg/mL, usually at 5 min (and virtually always by 10 min), then gradually decrease toward or to preinjection levels by 30 min. In the *calcium infusion test* serum samples for gastrin measurements are obtained before and at 30-min intervals for 4 h after initiation of a constant 3-h intravenous infusion of calcium gluconate (5 mg calcium per kilogram per hour). In gastrinoma patients serum gastrin concentrations usually increase above the basal serum gastrin by more than 400 pg/mL. The third provocative test involves the *feeding of a standard meal:* gastrin is measured in serum samples obtained before the meal and at 15-min intervals after it for 90 min. In gastrinoma patients serum gastrin levels increase little or not at all, seldom reaching values 50 percent greater than fasting levels (see Table 238-1).

The secretin injection test is by far the most valuable provocative test in identifying gastrinoma patients. Positive serum gastrin responses to intravenous secretin are found in more than 95 percent of patients with gastrinoma. Using the criteria suggested, substantial increases in serum gastrin following secretin injection have been detected only rarely in nongastrinoma patients. Reduced gastric acid secretion, achlorhydria or profound hypochlorhydria, is by far the most common cause of hypergastrinemia. For this reason gastric acid secretion should be measured before consideration of the secretin injection test. Exaggerated release of gastrin in response to calcium infusion is found in more than 80 percent of gastrinoma patients; however, this exaggerated response to calcium infusion occurs in some nongastrinoma patients with hypergastrinemia (e.g., with achlorhydria). Enhanced gastrin release with calcium infusion is not observed in gastrinoma patients in the absence of the abnormally large gastrin release in response to secretin. Since the calcium infusion test does not add to the sensitivity or specificity of the secretin injection test and since calcium infusion is potentially more hazardous, it is not now recommended.

In a very small proportion of duodenal ulcer patients (much less than 1 percent), gastric acid hypersecretion may be accompanied by increased serum gastrin levels due to hyperfunction and/or hyperplasia of antral gastrin cells (G cells). These patients can be distinguished from those with gastrinoma by the secretin and meal stimulation tests. In patients with this antral gastrin cell abnormality, intravenous secretin does not produce the large increases in serum gastrin characteristic of gastrinoma, but ingestion of the test meal does lead to generous increases in serum gastrin levels, frequently exceeding the fasting serum gastrin concentration by more than 200 percent (see Table 238-1).

TREATMENT In general, patients with Z-E syndrome are resistant to those medical therapies and surgical procedures designed for and usually effective in treating common peptic ulcer. Antacids may produce transient symptomatic relief but rarely, if ever, induce ulcer healing or sustained relief of symptoms. Incomplete gastric resection (with or without vagotomy) or pyloroplasty with vagotomy is frequently followed by prompt and often fulminant ulcer recurrence. Many patients with gastrinoma have had multiple surgical procedures, particularly in those instances in which the diagnosis was not established initially. Mortality was reported to be lowest in those patients with multiple gastric surgical procedures in whom gastrectomy was the initial gastric surgery for the Z-E syndrome: this led to the conclusion that when gastric surgery was required in gastrinoma patients, total gastrectomy was the surgical procedure of choice.

Recent development of more effective drugs to reduce acid secretion and more precise diagnostic techniques to locate the gastrinomas have increased substantially the therapeutic options. The key to management in these patients is individualization of treatment, since patients with the Z-E syndrome are highly heterogeneous with respect to clinical manifestations and extent of disease. As with many other predominantly malignant tumors, the ideal treatment is removal of the gastrinoma.

H-2-receptor antagonists are effective in reducing gastric acid secretion, producing symptom relief, and inducing ulcer healing in patients with the Z-E syndrome. They are indicated as initial treatment of gastrinoma patients, for prolonged treatment of those patients who are not candidates for tumor resection, and in those in whom total gastrectomy is not anticipated. *Cimetidine* was the first H-2-receptor antagonist used widely and successfully in the treatment of these patients. Improvement in clinical symptoms, decreases in gastric acid output, and ulcer healing were found in 80 to 85 percent. Administration of cimetidine has been required at 4- to 6-h intervals, with total daily doses usually four to eight times those used in the treatment of common duodenal ulcer. More recently, *ranitidine* and *famotidine* have been used effectively in treatment of patients with the Z-E syndrome. These H-2-receptor antagonists require comparable increases in dosage when compared with doses used in treatment of common duodenal ulcer. When instituted, H-2-receptor antagonist therapy must be continued indefinitely, since even temporary discontinuance is usually followed by ulcer recurrence. The dose of H-2-receptor antagonist required to maintain a satisfactory reduction in gastric acid secretion can be assessed by measuring the basal gastric acid output during the hour immediately prior to the next anticipated dose of the drug: the goal is to reduce gastric acid output to less than 10 mmol/h at that time.

The most effective drug in reducing gastric acid secretion and in inducing ulcer healing in patients with the Z-E syndrome is the H^+,K^+-ATPase inhibitor omeprazole. This drug is extremely potent in inhibiting gastric acid secretion, and, as a function of potency and dosage, its effectiveness can be prolonged and sustained. This drug is not yet available for prescribing in the United States. Some Z-E patients, in whom gastrinomas could not be identified or removed surgically, have been treated effectively with parietal cell vagotomy, which has reduced or, in a few instances, eliminated the doses of H-2-receptor antagonists required in these patients.

Treatment for patients with the Z-E syndrome should be individualized. In selecting the best therapy, the biologic behavior of these tumors and the clinical manifestations in each patient must be taken into consideration. Early studies indicated that morbidity and mortality in patients with the Z-E syndrome were due principally to complications of severe ulcer disease. However, with earlier diagnosis, effective antiulcer treatment, and longer follow-up, more frequent consequences of the malignant invasive properties of gastrinoma are now being recognized. Complete *surgical resection of the tumors*, when possible, represented *optimal treatment in patients with gastrinoma*. Complete surgical removal of gastrinoma, with cure, has been achieved in approximately 25 percent of patients with the Z-E syndrome. Successful tumor resection is rarely, if ever, achieved in gastrinoma patients with MEN I because of the overwhelming likelihood that multifocal tumors, often with metastasis though frequently indolent, are present at the time of diagnosis.

Therapeutic doses of H-2-receptor antagonists are indicated in the period during which the diagnosis is being established, while the location and extent of the tumor are being determined, and also as treatment prior to anticipated surgery. At present, H-2-receptor antagonists are certainly indicated for patients who are poor operative candidates, who refuse surgery, and in whom surgical removal of the tumor is not possible. Patients with aggressively invasive gastrinoma have been treated with streptozotocin and 5-fluorouracil, in some instances combined with adriamycin, in attempts to reduce tumor bulk and associated symptoms. Success with chemotherapy is limited, with only an approximate 40 percent initial response and no complete responses. When metastatic and/or otherwise nonresectable gastrinoma is present, control of the ulcer disease may be achieved in most instances by treatment with H-2-receptor antagonists, perhaps with parietal cell vagotomy, or rarely, when required, by total gastric resection. There is no convincing evidence that tumor progression is usually influenced by gastrectomy.

STRESS ULCERS AND EROSIONS

A variety of acute ulcerative lesions of the gastrointestinal tract are distinct clinically from chronic peptic ulcer. Among these are the acute upper gastrointestinal erosions and ulcers often observed in patients with shock, massive burns, sepsis, and severe trauma. These are often referred to as *stress erosions* and *ulcers*. These lesions, which are frequently multiple, are most common in the acid-secreting portion of the stomach, but they may also occur in the antrum and duodenum.

These erosions and superficial ulcers are extremely frequent and occur in about 90 percent of patients with massive injuries and burns. The most common clinical finding in these patients is painless gastrointestinal hemorrhage. Blood loss is usually minimal but may be substantial. Erosions develop most frequently approximately 24 h after trauma. Small amounts of blood loss may be detected in the first 24 to 48 h after trauma. However, when massive hemorrhage occurs, it is usually more than 2 or 3 days after the acute insult. The diagnosis is best established by upper gastrointestinal endoscopy. The erosions are most often too superficial to be recognized by barium examination of the upper gastrointestinal tract. Acute stress ulcers and erosions should be suspected when there is evidence of upper gastrointestinal bleeding in patients with severe injuries, burns, infections, and/or shock.

Many theories have been proposed to explain stress-associated acute mucosal ulceration. Mucosal ischemia and tissue injury from gastric acid appear to be important in the production of these acute stress erosions and ulcers. There is usually no evidence of acid hypersecretion; however, the lesions cannot be produced in experimental animals in the absence of acid. Most evidence supports the conclusion that mucosal ischemia is the most important element in the production of stress erosions and ulceration.

The treatment of acute stress ulcerations and erosions is principally preventive. In high-risk patients the frequency of stress ulcerations can be diminished by vigorous use of antacids to neutralize gastric contents and H-2-receptor antagonists to inhibit gastric acid secretion. When medical therapy fails to arrest bleeding, surgical approaches have included pyloroplasty and vagotomy and total gastrectomy.

The term *Cushing's ulcer* has been applied to acute ulcer of the upper gastrointestinal tract associated with intracranial injury or increases in intracranial pressure, e.g., with brain tumors or subdural hematoma. These ulcers may involve the stomach, proximal duodenum, or esophagus and frequently lead to hemorrhage or perforation. They do not differ histologically from acute stress ulceration. However, unlike stress ulcers, Cushing's ulcers are frequently associated with gastric acid hypersecretion. Treatment includes correction of increased intracranial pressure, when possible, and the usual measures for treatment of acute erosions and ulcerations, including vigorous therapy with antacids or H-2-receptor antagonists.

DRUG-ASSOCIATED ULCERS AND EROSIONS

Gastric and duodenal ulcers have been described following administration of many drugs. Aspirin ingestion has been shown to be associated with an increased incidence of gastric ulcer and, probably to a lesser extent, duodenal ulcer, and is a frequent cause of hemorrhagic erosive gastritis. Gastric mucosal injury, similar to that produced by aspirin, has also been observed in patients treated with a variety of other NSAIDs (e.g., indomethacin, ibuprofen, naproxen, tolmetin, sulindac, piroxicam, diflunisal, fenoprofen). The specific mechanism by which salicylates and other NSAIDs induce, or are associated with, gastric ulcer has not been established. Several mechanisms have been proposed, with most evidence favoring depletion of protective tissue prostaglandins by the well-recognized capacities of these agents to inhibit prostaglandin synthesis (see "Gastritis," below). They may contribute to development of gastric ulcer by interruption of the gastric mucosal barrier, permitting back-diffusion of hydrogen ions that may injure the gastric mucosa. Misoprostol, a prostaglandin E analogue, is effective in prevention of NSAID-induced gastric ulcers at dosage of 200 μg four times daily.

Administration of glucocorticoids has been reported and is commonly assumed to be associated with ulcer disease of the upper gastrointestinal tract. The subject remains controversial, since some data support and other data reject this association.

GASTRITIS

Gastritis is *inflammation of the gastric mucosa*. Gastritis is not a single disease. Rather, it is a group of disorders that have inflammatory changes in the gastric mucosa in common, but that have different clinical features, histologic characteristics, and pathogenesis. Several classifications have been used for consideration of gastritis. In general, these classifications have been based on (1) the acuteness or chronicity of the clinical manifestations, (2) the histologic features characterizing the gastritis, (3) the anatomic distribution of the gastritis, or, in some instances, (4) the proposed pathogenesis of each of the two principal forms of chronic gastritis. Based on the *clinical features* of the gastritis, the two principal forms, which constitute very different clinical entities, are *acute gastritis* and *chronic gastritis*. Different types of chronic gastritis exhibit histologic features which permit their classification according to the presence or absence of mucosal atrophy associated with the gastritis and the anatomic distribution of the gastritis or atrophy in the gastric mucosa.

In this section the major clinical forms of acute gastritis and chronic gastritis will be addressed, including reference to the histologic features of the major forms of gastritis. Attention will also be directed to additional specific forms of gastritis.

ACUTE GASTRITIS The principal, and certainly the most dramatic, form of acute gastritis is *acute hemorrhagic gastritis*, which is also referred to as *acute erosive gastritis*. These terms reflect the bleeding from the gastric mucosa almost invariably found in this form of gastritis and the characteristic loss of integrity of the gastric mucosa (erosion) that accompanies the inflammatory lesion. Gross examination in hemorrhagic gastritis shows edema, mucosal friability, erosions, and sites of bleeding with extravasation of blood into the mucosa and the lumen of the stomach. Gastric erosions and sites of hemorrhage may be distributed diffusely throughout the gastric mucosa or may be localized to the body or antrum of the stomach. They are often placed linearly on the crests of the gastric folds.

Histologic examination of the gastric mucosa reveals infiltration of the lamina propria with mononuclear cells and polymorphonuclear leukocytes with extravasation of blood in the mucosa, distorting the glandular structures. Proteinaceous exudate containing polymorphonuclear leukocytes may be present in gastric glands. Gastric erosions, by definition, are limited to the mucosa and do not extend beneath the muscularis mucosae. Acute erosive gastritis may accompany deeper, more focal lesions, which represent acute ulcers and may extend to and through all layers of the gastric wall.

Etiology and pathogenesis Acute erosive gastritis may develop without apparent explanation but is more likely to occur in several specific clinical circumstances. Erosive gastritis is usually associated with serious illness or with various drugs. Erosive gastritis has been estimated to occur in up to 80 to 90 percent of critically ill hospitalized patients. It is most often found in patients in medical or surgical intensive care units with severe trauma, major surgery, hepatic, renal, or respiratory failure, shock, massive burns, or severe infections with septicemia. Acute erosive gastritis associated with these severe illnesses is often referred to as *stress-induced gastritis*. The contributions of all mechanisms responsible for erosive gastritis in critically ill patients have not been defined completely. However, important participating elements appear to include ischemia of the gastric mucosa, acid diffusion from the gastric lumen into gastric mucosal tissues, and, perhaps in some forms, bile acids and/or other duodenal-pancreatic secretions refluxed into the gastric lumen. Mucosal ischemia and acid in the gastric lumen are clearly crucial elements in the etiopathogenesis of stress-induced gastritis. Septic shock with resulting mucosal ischemia produces gastric erosions in experimental animals. During such experimentally induced shock the intramural pH of the gastric mucosa falls precipitously when the gastric lumen is irrigated with HCl: this produces severe hemorrhagic lesions. The decrease in intramural pH results from diffusion of luminal hydrogen ions, which damage the gastric mucosa. With neutral pH irrigation the fall in intramural pH is much less and gastric lesions are minimal. Counteracting the effects of acid by vigorous and continuous treatment with antacids or by inhibiting secretion with H-2-receptor antagonists has been effective in reducing the incidence and the hemorrhagic complications of acute erosive gastritis in critically ill patients.

Various agents are known to injure the gastric mucosa. These include aspirin and other NSAIDs, bile acids, pancreatic enzymes, and ethanol. These agents disrupt the gastric mucosal barrier, which under normal conditions impedes the back-diffusion of hydrogen ions from the gastric lumen to the mucosa (despite and against an enormous H^+ concentration gradient). The most common and very important cause of drug-associated acute erosive gastritis is ingestion of aspirin or other NSAIDs. These drugs inhibit gastric mucosal cyclooxygenase activity, thereby reducing the synthesis and tissue levels of endogenous mucosal prostaglandins, which appear to play important roles in mucosal defense. This reduction in tissue prostaglandins is thought to be a principal, but perhaps not the exclusive, mechanism by which aspirin and other NSAIDs damage the gastric mucosa. It is possible that aspirin may injure small vessels in the gastric mucosa by inhibition of prostacyclin in the walls of small blood vessels or by inhibition of synthesis of thromboxane by platelets. An additional proposed mechanism for aspirin-induced gastrointestinal mucosal injury is via the effects of sodium salicylate, the product of aspirin metabolism found in the circulation, which is toxic to mitochondrial respiration and oxidative phosphorylation of cells. This may produce endothelial and epithelial cell injury with hemorrhage into the tissues or vascular thrombosis by endothelial cell disruption. Acid in the gastric lumen appears crucial to the production of salicylate-associated injury to the gastric mucosa.

Ethanol damage to the gastric mucosa is associated principally with subepithelial hemorrhages with surrounding edema and only slight to moderate increases in mucosal inflammatory cells. The mechanism by which alcohol injures the gastric mucosa is uncertain. Proposals have included cell injury due to its inherent lipophilic and lipolytic properties and/or interruption of the gastric mucosal barrier or direct damage to small mucosal blood vessels.

Clinical features   Bleeding from the gastric mucosa with acute gastritis may range from abrupt and dramatic upper gastrointestinal hemorrhage to the most subtle blood loss, perhaps detected only by the presence of occult blood in the stool or development of mild, asymptomatic, and unexplained anemia. Patients with acute erosive gastritis may have hematemesis and/or melena as well as less apparent forms of gastrointestinal blood loss. Except for possible consequences of blood loss, erosive gastritis is usually asymptomatic. However, less common symptoms may include epigastric or upper abdominal pain, nausea, and vomiting. Pain is much less common with erosive gastritis than with ulcer disease, with painless gastrointestinal hemorrhage more commonly the only clinical manifestation. Physical examination is often normal in patients with acute hemorrhagic gastritis. However, they may have upper abdominal tenderness or evidence of blood loss such as pallor, tachycardia, and hypotension. When they occur, abnormalities of white blood cell count, such as leukocytosis or leukopenia, more often reflect the associated serious illness than the gastritis.

Diagnosis   The presence of erosive gastritis is usually first suspected by detection of blood in the stool or in the gastric aspirate. The diagnosis is best established by upper gastrointestinal endoscopic examination, which reveals mucosal hemorrhages, friability and congestion, erosions, and, in some instances, superficial or deep ulcerations which, when present, are usually in the fundus or body of the stomach. Radiographic examination is much less reliable in detecting acute hemorrhagic-erosive gastritis.

Treatment   Treatment should be directed to prevention of erosive gastritis, treatment of the associated disease, withdrawal of the offending agent, and general supportive measures, as required, including maintenance of oxygen, blood volume, and fluid and electrolyte requirements. In the past, iced-saline lavage has been used in treatment of patients with hemorrhagic gastritis. However, this has never been shown to be effective in reducing gastrointestinal hemorrhage in these patients. Hourly antacid administration (e.g., 30 mL of an aluminum-magnesium hydroxide liquid preparation) and/or administration of an H-2-receptor antagonist (usually intravenously) have been shown to be effective in reducing the frequency of hemorrhagic gastritis in critically ill patients. These drugs should be used in doses and frequency sufficient to maintain the pH of gastric contents above 4. Although proven of value in prevention, it is less certain that they are effective in treatment of acute hemorrhagic gastritis. However, a similar therapeutic program with antacids or H-2-receptor antagonists does seem reasonable and generally is advised. Sucralfate has also been used in treatment of these patients. Misoprostol is effective in prevention of hemorrhagic gastritis, erosions, or gastric ulceration associated with ingestion of aspirin and other nonsteroidal agents.

Most patients respond favorably during vigorous treatment by the measures indicated. Acute hemorrhagic gastritis tends to improve as the patient's clinical condition improves. Because of the rapid cell renewal and restitutive properties of the gastric mucosa, lesions of acute hemorrhagic gastritis may return to normal, both endoscopically

and histologically, within 48 h of an acute event. However, occasionally further measures are required in attempts to arrest persistent life-threatening blood loss. These have included embolization or vasopressin infusion of the left gastric artery. Uncommonly, surgery is required for relentless hemorrhage. Vagotomy and pyloroplasty with oversewing of focal bleeding ulcerations has been used with limited success, and, rarely, total gastrectomy may be required. Morbidity and mortality with surgery in these patients is very great, usually reflecting the severity of their associated illnesses. Surgical treatment should not be performed unless absolutely necessary.

Enteropathic erosive gastritis   Enteropathic erosive gastritis is a rare clinical entity with multiple erosions of the gastric mucosa found in the absence of recognized precipitating factors. These patients may have anorexia, nausea, vomiting, or poorly defined upper abdominal discomfort. Less commonly they show evidence of gastrointestinal blood loss or weight loss. Endoscopic examination is usually required to establish the diagnosis. Erosions, which may be few or numerous, are usually located on the crests of the folds, but may be found in any portion of the gastric mucosa. Gastric biopsies are performed primarily to exclude other abnormalities, e.g., gastric lymphoma, carcinoma, and Crohn's disease. Erosions usually heal completely and may or may not return. The etiology is not known, nor are there accepted principles for specific recommendations for therapy.

Acute gastritis associated with *Helicobacter pylori*   *Helicobacter pylori* (previously called *Campylobacter pylori*) is a short (0.2 to 0.5 μm in length), spiral-shaped, microaerophilic gram-negative bacillus which has been suggested as a potential cause of certain forms of acute and chronic gastritis. Gastric colonization has also been associated with duodenal and gastric ulcer (see ''Peptic Ulcer,'' above). With gastric colonization *H. pylori* are found in the deep portions of the mucus gel layer that coats the gastric mucosa and between the mucus gel layer and the apical surfaces of the gastric mucosal epithelial cells. They also may be located in the regions of the tight junctions between adjacent mucosal epithelial cells. They do not invade the gastric mucosa. *H. pylori* is associated with inflamed gastric mucosal epithelium in the stomach as well as with metaplastic gastric epithelium found elsewhere, e.g., in the duodenal bulb of most patients with duodenal ulcer.

There is evidence that *H. pylori* is the cause, or at least a principal cause, of a form of gastritis that has been designated *active chronic gastritis*. Active chronic gastritis is characterized by dense infiltration of the lamina propria of the gastric mucosa with invasion of the epithelial cell layer by polymorphonuclear leukocytes. The mucosal surface is usually intact, without erosions or hemorrhagic lesions. When erosions do occur, they are usually small and limited to the superficial epithelial cell layer. There is poor correlation between the histologic abnormalities and the endoscopic appearance of the mucosa: endoscopy may reveal subtle abnormalities, or, more often, the endoscopic appearance is totally normal. Histologic abnormalities are associated with positive culture for *H. pylori,* and the degree of histologic abnormality, in general, parallels the number of organisms that can be identified. In addition, the more active the gastritis, reflected by infiltration of the mucosa with polymorphonuclear leukocytes, the greater the likelihood that *H. pylori* will be found. Healing of the gastritis occurs when cultures become negative. Spontaneous disappearance of *H. pylori* has not been noted. It has been observed to persist in gastric mucosal biopsies of untreated patients for more than 2 years.

H. pylori has been identified in gastric samples by histologic examination, culture, urease activity, and by endonuclease analysis. On stained tissue sections *H. pylori* is Giemsa-positive and faintly hematoxylin-positive. It can be cultured successfully from biopsy material, but usually not from gastric secretions. *H. pylori* produce large amounts of urease. The rapid urease test of gastric biopsy material is a relatively simple and reliable method for presumptive identification of the presence of *H. pylori*. The test is inexpensive with good sensitivity and specificity. A urea breath test using ^{13}C or

^{14}C has also been developed for identifying *H. pylori*. Antibodies (IgG and IgA) to *H. pylori* have been identified in sera of individuals with *H. pylori* colonization. There is a high degree of correlation between these serum antibodies and histologic gastritis.

H. pylori synthesizes a protease that hydrolyzes gastric mucous glycoproteins, which may therefore disrupt the gastric mucus gel layer, contributing to mucosal injury. There is evidence that this form of acute gastritis with *H. pylori* is associated with reductions in gastric acid secretion. By retrospective examination, *H. pylori* were demonstrated in gastric mucosal biopsy specimens described from volunteers participating in gastric secretory studies who developed epidemic gastritis, with concurrent reductions in rates of gastric acid secretion.

When sought for, *H. pylori* has been identified in a large proportion of gastric biopsies of patients with several upper gastrointestinal diseases. It has been cultured from antral biopsy specimens in 90 to 100 percent of patients with duodenal ulcer, 70 percent with gastric ulcer, 80 percent with chronic gastritis involving the antral mucosa, and in 50 percent of patients with nonulcer dyspepsia.

H. pylori is also frequent in asymptomatic individuals considered to be otherwise well. Histologic gastritis has long been recognized as common in healthy asymptomatic individuals; recently it has been shown to be associated strongly with gastric *H. pylori* colonization. *H. pylori* with associated gastritis was found in the gastric biopsy samples of from 20 to 25 percent of healthy volunteer subjects. When these asymptomatic individuals were examined, there was no relationship between the histologic and endoscopic appearances of the gastric mucosa. Endoscopic examination usually appeared normal, in spite of the histologic evidence of gastritis and *H. pylori*.

Colloidal bismuth compounds have been shown to eradicate *H. pylori* from gastric mucosa. It is uncertain by what mechanism. Eradication may be due to antibacterial effects or perhaps to binding or coating of the organism. Amoxicillin (50 mg tid or qid), bismuth subsalicylate (30 mL qid), and metronidazole (500 mg tid) have each been used singly or in combination for periods of from 1 week to 2 months to eradicate *H. pylori*. Eradication of *H. pylori* results in disappearance of inflammatory changes in the gastric mucosa. Recolonization of the organism after treatment, usually with the same bacterial subtype, with recurrence of gastritis is very frequent and usually occurs within 1 month after initial eradication and discontinuance of treatment.

CHRONIC GASTRITIS The inflammatory cell infiltrate in chronic gastritis is composed principally of chronic inflammatory cells, predominantly lymphocytes and plasma cells. Polymorphonuclear leukocytes and eosinophils may be present in small numbers, but do not predominate. Chronic gastritis is often patchy and irregular in distribution.

Histologic classification Chronic gastritis has been classified descriptively on the basis of several characteristic histologic abnormalities. In its evolution chronic gastritis initially involves the superficial and glandular areas of the gastric mucosa and progresses to glandular destruction, which may be followed by a profound reduction in gland number (atrophy) and/or gland metaplasia.

Superficial gastritis is that form of gastritis with inflammatory changes in the lamina propria of the superficial mucosa, with cellular infiltration and edema separating the gastric glands. Superficial gastritis appears to represent the initial stage in the development of chronic gastritis. With superficial gastritis the inflammatory cell infiltrate is limited to the lamina propria of the upper (epithelial) half of the gastric mucosa and the glands are preserved. There may be a decrease in mucus in glandular mucous cells and in mitotic figures in cells of the glands.

Atrophic gastritis is the next stage in the developmental chronology of chronic gastritis. In atrophic gastritis the inflammatory infiltrate extends to the deep portions of the mucosa. There is progressive distortion and destruction of the glands, which become separated by the inflammatory process. Atrophic gastritis is followed by the development of the final stage of chronic gastritis, which is *gastric atrophy*. With gastric atrophy there is a profound loss of the glandular structures, which are now separated widely by connective tissue, with a greatly reduced or absent inflammatory infiltrate. The mucosa is thin, often revealing the prominence of its underlying vessels by endoscopic examination.

As chronic gastritis progresses, there may be changes in the morphology of the gastric glandular elements. *Intestinal metaplasia* is the term used to describe the conversion of gastric glands to the appearance of small-intestinal mucosal glands containing goblet cells. Intestinal metaplasia may be patchy or extensive in the gastric mucosa. With *pseudopyloric gland metaplasia* the glands of the body of the stomach assume the appearance of antral pyloric glands. Pseudopyloric metaplasia may occur with either atrophic gastritis or gastric atrophy.

Chronic gastritis: types A and B The two major forms of chronic gastritis have been classified as types A and B based on their distributions in the gastric mucosa coupled with some implications regarding their pathogenesis. *Type A gastritis* is the less common form of chronic gastritis: it characteristically involves the body and fundus of the stomach with relative sparing of the antrum. This is the form of gastritis that may lead to pernicious anemia. The frequent presence of antibodies to parietal cells and antibodies to intrinsic factor in sera of patients with type A gastritis and pernicious anemia has suggested an immune or autoimmune pathogenesis for this form of gastritis. Antibodies to parietal cells have been shown to be cytotoxic for gastric mucosal cells. Cell-mediated immune mechanisms have also been proposed to participate in gastric mucosal cell injury in pernicious anemia and related forms of type A gastritis. Antibodies to parietal cells have been found in sera of approximately 90 percent of patients with pernicious anemia and in more than half of other patients with type A gastritis. Relatives of patients with pernicious anemia have a higher than normal frequency of serum antibodies to parietal cells, atrophic gastritis, and reduced gastric acid secretion. In control populations parietal cell antibodies may be found in up to 20 percent of individuals over age 60 and in approximately 20 percent of all patients with hypoparathyroidism, Addison's disease, and vitiligo. About 50 percent of patients with pernicious anemia have antibodies to thyroid antigens, and approximately 30 percent of patients with thyroid disease have circulating antibodies to parietal cells. Serum antibodies to intrinsic factor are more specific than parietal cell antibodies and are present in about 40 percent of patients with pernicious anemia.

In patients with pernicious anemia the gastric parietal cell–containing glands are invariably destroyed, accounting for their inability to secrete gastric hydrochloric acid. Since, in human beings, parietal cells also secrete intrinsic factor, there is failure to absorb vitamin B_{12} actively with resulting hematologic and/or neurologic consequences characteristic of pernicious anemia. It has been estimated that the risk of cancer of the stomach in patients with type A gastritis and pernicious anemia is approximately three times that of the general population.

Type B gastritis is much the more common form of chronic gastritis. In younger patients type B gastritis principally involves the antrum, whereas in older patients the entire stomach is affected. This transition is estimated to require about 15 to 20 years. The incidence of chronic gastritis, most of it type B gastritis, increases with age, reaching 78 percent in individuals over age 50 and virtually 100 percent after age 70.

A large number of studies from various parts of the world have shown a strong association of *H. pylori* with type B gastritis. Chronic gastritis with *H. pylori* infection and/or persistence is associated with reduced gastric acid secretion. Eradication of *H. pylori* produces improvement in histologic findings; when treatment is stopped, inflammatory changes recur, and organisms reappear. These observations have favored the proposal that type B gastritis is caused by chronic bacterial infection by *H. pylori*. Chronic reflux of pancreatic-biliary secretions, bile acids and lysolecithin, in particular, has also been proposed as a potential factor in the production of type B chronic gastritis.

Gastric acid secretion is reduced in both type A and type B chronic gastritis. In general, the reduction in gastric acid secretion, which is complete in patients with pernicious anemia, is proportionate to the severity of parietal cell destruction and mucosal atrophy in the body and fundus of the stomach. Serum gastrin levels are usually elevated substantially in patients with pernicious anemia and are in approximately the same range as those of patients with the Z-E syndrome (gastrinoma). Since the antral mucosa is relatively spared, the antral gastrin-containing cells, deprived of feedback control normally exercised by acid in the stomach, release gastrin continuously. Serum gastrin levels are also often similarly elevated in patients with type A gastritis with achlorhydria or profound hypochlorhydria who do not have pernicious anemia. Patients with type B gastritis have serum gastrin levels that are highly variable, not consistently elevated and often in the normal range. A small portion of patients with type B gastritis have serum antibodies to gastrin, leading some to propose an autoimmune mechanism for this form of gastritis. Alternatively, and probably more likely, these antibodies represent responses to the inflammatory process rather than contributing factors.

There is no persuasive evidence that acute gastric mucosal injury associated with stress or with ethanol or aspirin or other NSAIDs progresses to chronic gastritis. Acute gastritis caused by *H. pylori* may be a form of gastritis in which there is sufficient information to suspect progression to a chronic form of gastritis, i.e., type B chronic gastritis.

Diagnosis Biopsy of the gastric mucosa provides the most reliable means of identifying and classifying gastritis. Caution must be exercised in the interpretation of a single gastric mucosal biopsy in a patient with suspected acute or chronic gastritis. The patchy and irregular distribution of the gastritis may lead to substantial sampling error. Therefore, several biopsies of suspected areas, when safe and possible, are recommended.

Treatment No specific treatment is required for type A or type B chronic gastritis with or without mucosal atrophy. The only form of chronic gastritis that requires specific treatment is pernicious anemia, the most complete expression of type A gastritis. Vitamin B_{12} deficiency in these patients, resulting from malabsorption of vitamin B_{12} secondary to destruction of parietal cells in the body and fundus of the stomach, requires indefinite regular parenteral vitamin B_{12} administration.

Ménétrier's disease *Ménétrier's* disease is a clinical entity characterized by large tortuous gastric mucosal folds. The abnormalities in Ménétrier's disease may be localized or diffused throughout the stomach. Prominent mucosal folds are often most conspicuous in the gastric body and fundus. Histologic inflammation is not a component of this disease. Therefore, it is not a form of gastritis. The primary pathologic feature is thickening of the gastric mucosa due to hyperplasia of surface and glandular mucous cells, which replace most of the chief and parietal cells. Pits of the gastric glands elongate and may become extremely tortuous. The lamina propria may contain an increased number of lymphocytes. Intestinal metaplasia may be present.

The most common symptom is epigastric pain. Anorexia, nausea, vomiting, and weight loss are less frequent. Gastric bleeding is unusual and, when present, is due to superficial mucosal erosions. Uncommonly, gastric ulcer or gastric carcinoma may develop in these patients. Patients often develop a protein-losing gastropathy resulting in hypoalbuminemia and edema. Gastric acid secretion is usually reduced or may be absent. Barium examination of the upper gastrointestinal tract reveals the large gastric folds, which are readily confirmed by endoscopic examination. The diagnosis is best established by deep mucosal biopsy (and cytology) to exclude gastric malignancy. The depth of these lesions and the disconcerting prominence of the folds may require a surgical full-thickness biopsy to exclude lymphoma or infiltrating carcinoma.

Anticholinergic agents and H-2-receptor antagonists have been reported to decrease protein loss in patients with Ménétrier's disease. Treatment includes a high-protein diet to replace protein losses. If present, ulcers should be treated as described previously for common gastric ulcer. Severe disease with persistent substantial protein loss may require total gastrectomy.

Gastritis due to corrosive agents Ingestion of a variety of corrosive chemicals can cause severe damage to the gastric mucosa. Because of its anatomic location, the antrum is a frequent site for such injury. Ingested substances which are particularly injurious to the gastric mucosa include strong acids (e.g., hydrochloric acid, sulfuric acid) or strong alkali (e.g., sodium hydroxide). Depending on dose and concentration these agents can cause injury ranging from mild inflammation to extensive tissue necrosis. With alkali ingestion (especially lye) the esophagus is particularly susceptible to severe injury, necrosis, and potential subsequent stricture. The stomach, especially the antrum, is more susceptible to acute injury by ingestion of strong acid. With ingestion of these corrosive substances patients may describe burning of the mouth, throat, and retrosternal area. Epigastric pain and vomiting often signal gastric injury. Hemorrhage and/or perforation may occur. Treatment of strong acid ingestion includes dilution with water, followed by antacids and supportive therapy as required. Neutralization of ingested lye by administrated acid is not recommended.

Infectious gastritis Infectious causes of gastritis, other than gastritis associated with gastric *H. pylori* colonization, are unusual. *Phlegmonous gastritis,* a rare form of bacterial gastritis, is a life-threatening disease with extensive infiltration of the gastric wall, tissue necrosis, and manifestations of generalized sepsis. Responsible infectious agents include, among others, streptococci, staphylococci, *Proteus* species, and *Escherichia coli.* Treatment includes appropriate intravenous antibiotics and necessary supportive care including fluid and electrolyte replacement as required. Lack of response to therapy may require gastrectomy. Additional infectious causes of gastritis may be found in immunocompromised patients. Gastric erosions may be produced by herpes simplex virus. Typical intranuclear inclusions of cytomegalovirus, with positive cultures, have been found by endoscopic gastric biopsy in some immunocompromised patients. This has been interpreted to represent disseminated cytomegalovirus infection.

Eosinophilic gastritis *Eosinophilic gastritis* may occur as isolated involvement of the stomach or as a component of eosinophilic gastroenteritis. Eosinophilic gastritis is characterized by extensive eosinophilic infiltration of the wall of the stomach, usually with circulating eosinophilia. Biopsy reveals extensive eosinophilic infiltration which may involve all coats of the stomach or may be limited to mucosa, submucosa, or muscular regions of the gastric wall. The antrum is involved more frequently than the gastric body or fundus. There may be prominent antral mucosal folds with edema and mucosal thickening, uncommonly leading to gastric outlet obstruction. Epigastric pain, which may be accompanied by nausea and vomiting, is the most frequent symptom. These patients usually respond favorably to treatment with glucocorticoids. Rarely surgery is required to establish the diagnosis or for relief of obstructive symptoms.

Granulomatous gastritis A variety of generalized diseases, some of which are infectious, can involve the stomach, producing *granulomatous gastritis.* Crohn's disease, as in the small intestine, may produce ulceration, granulomatous infiltration, and/or scarring with stricture formation. Its distinction from other gastric lesions requires biopsy at the time of endoscopic examination. Less common infectious causes of granulomatous disease of the stomach include, among others, histoplasmosis, candidiasis, syphilis, and tuberculosis. Rarely, idiopathic granulomatous gastritis and eosinophilic granulomas also involve the stomach. In patients with granulomatous disease of the stomach multiple biopsies and cytology are usually required to establish the diagnosis and to exclude malignancy. If the diagnosis is not established by biopsy at endoscopy, surgical exploration may be required.

Gastritis and prior gastric surgery Variable amounts of gastritis almost always occur in the remaining stomachs of patients treated surgically by partial gastrectomy and, to a somewhat lesser extent, after vagotomy and pyloroplasty. Gastritis is especially common and often severe after gastrojejunal (Billroth II) anastomosis.

Gastric surgery appears to accelerate the development of gastritis, with progressive loss of parietal cells in the gastric remnant after surgery. Most patients are asymptomatic; however, a small proportion develop mild or severe symptoms, most commonly epigastric pain, nausea, and vomiting. This form of gastritis been referred to as *alkaline gastritis* or *bile reflux gastritis*. It has been assumed, but not proven, that gastritis results from reflux of pancreaticobiliary secretions. Endoscopic examination often reveals a beefy red and sometimes friable gastric mucosa. Abnormalities may be limited to mucosa in the region of the anastomosis or may involve all the remaining gastric mucosa. Bile is often seen in the gastric remnant. Biopsies of involved mucosa at endoscopy show variable degrees of acute and/or chronic gastritis. Gastric acid secretion is usually decreased.

Managing patients with severe symptoms is very difficult. Various therapeutic approaches have been used with limited, if any, success. These have included cholestyramine, H-2-receptor antagonists, sucralfate, antacids, and pancreatic enzyme replacement. Surgery, which is sometimes successful, is Roux-en-Y, which diverts pancreaticobiliary secretions away from the gastric remnant. Nonsurgical modalities should be exhausted before proceeding with attempts to treat this disease by surgery.

REFERENCES

Peptic ulcer

BARDHAN KD et al: Double blind comparison of cimetidine and placebo in the maintenance and healing of chronic duodenal ulceration. Gut 20:158, 1979

DOOLEY CP, COHEN H: The clinical significance of *Campylobacter pylori*. Ann Intern Med 108:70, 1988

FRUCHT H et al: Secretin and calcium provocative tests in the Zollinger-Ellison syndrome: A prospective study. Ann Intern Med 111:713, 1989

KLOPPEL G et al: Pancreatic lesions and hormonal profile of pancreatic tumors in multiple endocrine neoplasia type I: An immunocytochemical study of nine patients. Cancer 57:1824, 1986

MATON PN et al: Cushing's syndrome in patients with the Zollinger-Ellison syndrome. N Engl J Med 315:1, 1986

McARTHUR KE et al: Treatment of acid-peptic diseases by inhibition of gastric H^+,K^+-ATPase. Annu Rev Med 37:97, 1986

McGUIGAN JE, TRUDEAU WL: Differences in rates of gastrin release in normal persons and patients with duodenal ulcer. N Engl J Med 288:64, 1973

PEURA DA, JOHNSON LF: Cimetidine for prevention and treatment of gastroduodenal lesions in patients in an intensive care unit. Ann Intern Med 103:173, 1985

RATHBONE BJ et al: *Campylobacter pyloridis*—a new factor in peptic ulcer disease? Gut 27:635, 1986

RICHARDSON CT: Sucralfate. Ann Intern Med 97:269, 1982

——— et al: Treatment of Zollinger-Ellison syndrome with exploratory laparotomy, proximal gastric vagotomy, and H₂-receptor antagonists: A prospective study. Gastroenterology 89:357, 1985

TAKEUCHI KD: Role of pH gradient in mucus in protection of gastric mucosa. Gastroenterology 84:331, 1983

VINAYEK R: et al: Famotidine in the therapy of gastric hypersecretory states. Am J Med 81:49, 1986

VON SCHRENK T et al: Prospective study of chemotherapy in patients with metastatic gastrinoma. Gastroenterology 94:1326, 1988

WOLFE MM, SOLL AH: The physiology of gastric acid secretion. N Engl J Med 319:1707, 1988

Gastritis

BARTHEL JS et al: Gastritis and *Campylobacter pylori* in healthy, asymptomatic volunteers. Arch Intern Med 148:1149, 1988

Campylobacter pylori becomes *Helicobacter pylori* (editorial). Lancet 2:1019, 1989

DOOLEY CP, COHEN H: The clinical significance of *Campylobacter pylori*. Ann Intern Med 108:70, 1988

LAINE L, WEINSTEIN WM: Histology of alcoholic hemorrhagic "gastritis": A prospective evaluation. Gastroenterology 94:1254, 1988

PEURA DA, JOHNSON LF: Cimetidine for prevention and treatment of gastroduodenal lesions in patients in an intensive care unit. Ann Intern Med 103:173, 1985

RAUWS EAJ et al: *Campylobacter pyloridis*–associated chronic active antral gastritis: A prospective study of its prevalence and the effects of antibacterial and antiulcer treatment. Gastroenterology 94:33, 1988

ROBERT A: Cytoprotection by prostaglandins. Gastroenterology 77:761, 1979

SEARCY CM, MALAGELADA J-R: Ménétrier's disease and idiopathic hypertrophic gastropathy. Ann Intern Med 100:565, 1984

SLOMIANY BL et al: *Campylobacter pyloridis* degrades mucin and undermines gastric mucosal integrity. Biochem Biophys Res Commun 144:307, 1987

TAKEUCHI KD: Role of pH gradient of mucus in protection of gastric mucosa. Gastroenterology 84:331, 1983

VANE JR: Inhibition of prostaglandin synthesis as a mechanism for aspirin-like drugs. Nature 23:232, 1971

239   NEOPLASMS OF THE ESOPHAGUS AND STOMACH

ROBERT J. MAYER

ESOPHAGEAL CANCER

Incidence and etiology   In the United States, cancer of the esophagus is a relatively uncommon but extremely lethal malignant condition. It is estimated that the diagnosis was made in 10,100 Americans in 1989, leading to 9400 deaths. Worldwide, the incidence of esophageal cancer varies strikingly. It occurs frequently within a so-called Asian esophageal cancer belt extending from the southern shore of the Caspian Sea on the west to northern China on the east and encompassing parts of Iran, Soviet Central Asia, Afghanistan, Siberia, and Mongolia. Additionally, high incidence "pockets" of the disease are present in such disparate locations as Finland, Iceland, Curaçao, southeastern Africa, and northwestern France. In North America and western Europe, the disease is far more common in blacks than whites, greater in males than females, appearing most frequently after age 50, and appearing to be an illness associated with lower socioeconomic classes.

A variety of causative factors have been implicated in the development of the disease (Table 239-1). In the United States, 80 to 90 percent of esophageal cancer cases are believed attributable to excess consumption of alcohol and/or a long-standing history of cigarette smoking. The relative risk increases with either the amount of tobacco smoked or alcohol consumed. The consumption of whiskey is seemingly linked to a higher incidence than the consumption of wine or beer. The development of esophageal cancer has also been associated with the ingestion of other carcinogens such as nitrites, smoked opiates, and fungal toxins in pickled vegetables, as well as with mucosal damage caused by such physical insults as long-term exposure to extremely hot tea, the ingestion of lye, radiation-induced strictures, and chronic achalasia. The presence of an esophageal web in association with glossitis and iron deficiency (i.e., Plummer-Vinson or Paterson-Kelly syndrome) and congenital hyperkeratosis and pitting of the palms and soles (i.e., tylosis palmaris et plantaris) have each been linked with esophageal cancer, as have dietary deficiencies of

TABLE 239-1   Some etiologic factors believed to be associated with esophageal cancer

I	Excess alcohol consumption
II	Cigarette smoking
III	Other ingested carcinogens
	A Nitrates (converted to nitrites)
	B Smoked opiates
	C Fungal toxins in pickled vegetables
IV	Mucosal damage from physical agents
	A Hot tea
	B Lye ingestion
	C Radiation-induced strictures
	D Chronic achalasia
V	Host susceptibility
	A Esophageal web with glossitis and iron deficiency (i.e., Plummer-Vinson or Paterson-Kelly syndrome)
	B Congenital hyperkeratosis and pitting of the palms and soles (i.e., tylosis palmaris et plantaris)
VI	? Dietary deficiencies—molybdenum, zinc, vitamin A
VII	? Celiac sprue
VIII	Chronic gastric reflux (i.e., Barrett's esophagus)—for adenocarcinoma

molybdenum, zinc, and vitamin A. The risk for esophageal cancer may be slightly greater in individuals with celiac sprue and is definitely increased in the presence of chronic gastric reflux (i.e., Barrett's esophagus).

Clinical features Approximately 15 percent of esophageal cancers occur in the upper third of the esophagus ("cervical esophagus"), 50 percent in the middle third, and 35 percent in the lower third. More than 85 percent of esophageal tumors are squamous cell carcinomas, arising from the squamous epithelium which lines the lumen of the esophagus. Adenocarcinomas, while far less frequent, develop more commonly from columnar epithelium which may appear in the distal esophagus in association with chronic gastric reflux (i.e., Barrett's esophagus). These malignancies have the biologic behavior of gastric rather than esophageal cancers. Attempts at endoscopic and cytologic screening for carcinoma in patients with Barrett's esophagus have not yet proved successful. It should be noted that squamous cell carcinomas and adenocarcinomas of the esophagus cannot be distinguished radiographically or endoscopically.

Progressive dysphagia and weight loss of short duration are the initial symptoms in the vast majority of patients. Dysphagia initially occurs with solid foods and gradually progresses to include semisolids and liquids. By the time these symptoms develop, the disease is usually incurable since difficulty in swallowing does not occur until 60 percent or more of the esophageal circumference is infiltrated with cancer. Dysphagia may be associated with pain on swallowing (odynophagia), pain radiating to the chest and/or back, regurgitation or vomiting, and aspiration pneumonia. The disease most commonly spreads to adjacent and supraclavicular lymph nodes, liver, lungs, and pleura. Tracheoesophageal fistulas may develop as the disease advances, leading to severe suffering. As with other squamous cell carcinomas, hypercalcemia may occasionally occur in the absence of osseous metastases. This is believed to result from a tumor-secreted protein structurally analogous to a portion of parathyroid hormone.

Diagnosis Routine, contrast radiographs effectively identify esophageal lesions of sufficient size to cause symptoms. In contrast to benign esophageal leiomyomata which result in esophageal narrowing with preservation of a normal mucosal pattern, esophageal carcinomas characteristically cause ragged, ulcerating changes in the mucosa in association with deeper infiltration, producing a picture resembling achalasia. Smaller, potentially resectable tumors are often poorly visualized despite technically adequate esophagograms. Because of this, esophagoscopy should be performed in all patients suspected of having an esophageal abnormality in order to visualize the tumor and to obtain histopathologic confirmation of the diagnosis. Since the same population of patients at risk for esophageal carcinoma (i.e., smokers and drinkers) also has a high rate of cancers of the lung and head and neck region, endoscopic inspection of the larynx, trachea, and bronchi should also be carried out. A thorough examination of the fundus of the stomach (by retroflexing the endoscope) is imperative as well. Endoscopic biopsies of esophageal tumors fail to recover malignant tissue in one-third of cases because the biopsy forceps cannot penetrate deeply enough through normal mucosa pushed in front of the carcinoma. Cytologic examination of tumor brushings frequently complements standard biopsies and should be performed routinely. The extent of tumor spread to the mediastinum and paraaortic lymph nodes should also be assessed by computed tomography (CT) scans of the chest and abdomen.

Treatment The prognosis for patients with esophageal carcinoma is poor. Less than 5 percent of patients are alive 5 years after the initial diagnosis, leading many physicians to focus management efforts solely on symptomatic control. Surgical resection of all gross tumor (i.e., total resection) is feasible in only 40 percent of cases, with residual tumor cells frequently present at the resection margins. Such esophagectomies are associated with a postoperative mortality rate in excess of 20 percent due to anastomotic fistulas, subphrenic abscesses, and respiratory complications. Less than 20 percent of patients who survive a total resection can be expected to be alive after 5 years. The therapeutic outcome following the administration

of primary radiation therapy [55 to 60 Gy (5500 to 6000 rad)] is not dissimilar to that of radical surgery, sparing patients perioperative morbidity but often resulting in less satisfactory palliation of obstructive symptoms. The evaluation of chemotherapeutic agents in patients with esophageal carcinoma has been hampered by ambiguity in the definition of "response" (i.e., benefit) and the debilitated physical condition of many treated individuals. Nonetheless, significant reductions in the size of measurable tumor masses have been reported in 15 to 25 percent of patients given single-agent treatment and in 30 to 60 percent of patients treated with drug combinations which include cisplatin. Recent therapeutic efforts have been directed at utilizing combination chemotherapy and radiation therapy as the initial therapeutic approach, either alone or followed by an attempt at operative resection. It remains to be determined whether such an intensive multimodality approach will increase the cure rate.

For the incurable, surgically unresectable patient with esophageal cancer, dysphagia, malnutrition, and the management of trachoesophageal fistulas loom as major issues. Approaches to palliation of these cancer-related complications include repeated endoscopic dilatation, the surgical placement of a gastrostomy or jejunostomy for hydration and feeding, and the surgical insertion of a polyvinyl prosthesis to bypass the tumor. Endoscopic fulguration of the obstructing tumor with lasers appears to be the most promising of these techniques.

TUMORS OF THE STOMACH

GASTRIC ADENOCARCINOMA **Incidence and epidemiology** For reasons which remain uncertain, the incidence and mortality rates for gastric cancer have decreased markedly during the past 60 years. In 1930, gastric cancer represented the leading cause of cancer-related deaths among American men by a factor of two, while the disease in women ranked just behind tumors of the uterine cervix and breast. During the ensuing years, the mortality rate from gastric cancer in the United States has dropped in men from 28 to 7.8 per 100,000 population, while in women, the rate has decreased from 27 to 3.7 per 100,000. Nonetheless, it was estimated in 1989 that 20,000 new cases of stomach cancer were diagnosed in the United States and that 13,900 Americans died of the disease. The decreased incidence in gastric cancer in the United States is also reflected worldwide. The incidence of gastric cancer varies widely among different countries, being comparatively high in Japan, China, Chile, and Ireland; however, a decrease in both incidence and mortality has occurred in these areas as well.

Epidemiologic surveys have suggested the risk of gastric cancer to be greater among lower socioeconomic classes. Furthermore, migrants from high- to low-incidence nations appear to maintain their susceptibility to gastric cancer while the risk for their offspring more closely approximates that of the new homeland. These findings suggest that an environmental exposure, probably beginning early in life, is related to the development of gastric cancer with dietary carcinogens considered the most likely factor(s).

Pathology Approximately 90 percent of stomach cancers are adenocarcinomas with 10 percent due to non-Hodgkin's lymphomas and leiomyosarcomas. Gastric adenocarcinomas may be subdivided into two categories: a *diffuse type* in which cell cohesion is absent, resulting in individual cells infiltrating and thickening the stomach wall without forming a discrete mass; and an *intestinal type* characterized by cohesive neoplastic cells forming glandlike tubular structures. The diffuse carcinomas occur more often in younger patients, develop throughout the stomach including the cardia, result in a loss of distensibility of the gastric wall (so-called linitis plastica or "leather bottle" appearance), and are associated with a far more ominous prognosis. Intestinal-type lesions are frequently ulcerative, more commonly appear in the antrum and lesser curvature of the stomach, and are often preceded by a prolonged precancerous process. While the incidence of diffuse carcinomas is similar in most populations,

TABLE 239-2 Dietary factors as a cause of gastric carcinoma*

Sources of nitrate-converting bacteria

I   Exogenous
    A   Bacterially contaminated food
    B   Frequent in lower socioeconomic classes who have higher incidence
       of the disease
    C   Diminished by improved food preservation and refrigeration
II   Endogenous
    A   Decreased gastric acidity
    B   Prior gastric surgery (antrectomy)—15 to 20 year latency period
    C   Atrophic gastritis and/or pernicious anemia
    D   ? Prolonged exposure to histamine-2-receptor antagonists

*HYPOTHESIS: Dietary nitrates are converted to carcinogenic nitrites by bacteria

the intestinal type tends to predominate in the high-risk geographic regions mentioned earlier and is less likely to be found in areas where the frequency of gastric cancer is declining. Thus, different etiologic factor(s) may be involved in these two subtypes. In the United States, the distal stomach is the site of origin of about half of gastric cancers. Approximately 20 percent of these tumors arise in the lesser curvature, 25 percent in the cardia, and only 3 to 5 percent in the greater curvature. More than 10 percent of gastric carcinomas involve the entire stomach.

Etiology The relationship between dietary patterns and the development of gastric carcinoma has been extensively investigated. The long-term ingestion of high concentrations of nitrates in dried, smoked, and salted foods appears to be associated with a higher risk. The nitrates are thought to be converted to carcinogenic nitrites by bacteria (Table 239-2). Such bacteria may be introduced exogenously through the ingestion of the partially decayed foods which are consumed in abundance worldwide by the lower socioeconomic classes. Bacteria may also appear endogenously as a result of a lack or loss of gastric acidity. This may occur when acid-producing cells of the gastric antrum have been surgically removed 15 to 20 years previously at the time of a partial gastrectomy to control benign peptic ulcer disease or when achlorhydria, atrophic gastritis, and even pernicious anemia develop in the elderly. Serial endoscopic examinations of the stomach in patients with atrophic gastritis have documented replacement of the usual gastric mucosa by intestinal-type cells. This process of intestinal metaplasia may lead to cellular atypia and eventual neoplasia. Since the declining incidence of gastric cancer in the United States is primarily a reflection of a decline in distal, ulcerating, intestinal-type lesions, it is conceivable that better food preservation and the availability to all socioeconomic classes of refrigeration for food storage have resulted in a decrease in the dietary ingestion of exogenous bacteria. It remains uncertain whether the iatrogenic achlorhydria induced by the widespread, prolonged use of parietal cell histamine antagonists will result in a future increase in intestinal-type gastric cancer.

Several additional etiologic factors have been associated with gastric carcinoma. Gastric ulcers and adenomatous polyps have occasionally been so linked, but data regarding a cause-and-effect relationship are unconvincing. The inadequate clinical distinction between benign gastric ulcers and small ulcerating carcinomas may, in part, account for this presumed association. The presence of extreme hypertrophy of gastric rugal folds (i.e., Ménétrier's disease), giving the impression of polypoid lesions, has been associated with a striking frequency of malignant transformation; such hypertrophy, however, does not represent the presence of true adenomatous polyps. Individuals with blood group A have been reported to have a higher incidence of gastric cancer than persons with blood group O; it is possible that this observation is related to differences in the mucous secretion of the various ABO blood groups, thereby leading to greater or lesser mucosal protection from carcinogens. No association has been identified between duodenal ulcers and gastric cancer.

Clinical features Gastric cancers, when superficial and surgically curable, usually produce no symptoms. As the tumor becomes more extensive, patients may complain of an insidious upper abdominal discomfort varying in intensity from a vague, postprandial fullness to a severe, steady pain. Anorexia, often with slight nausea, is very common but is not the usual presenting complaint. Weight loss may eventually be observed and nausea and vomiting are particularly prominent with tumors of the pylorus; dysphagia may be the major symptom caused by lesions of the cardia. There are no early physical signs of the disease, and the finding of a palpable abdominal mass generally indicates long-standing growth and, all too often, regional extension.

Gastric carcinomas spread by direct extension through the gastric wall to the perigastric tissues, occasionally adhering to adjacent organs such as the pancreas, colon, or liver. The disease also spreads via lymphatics or by seeding of peritoneal surfaces. Metastases to intraabdominal and supraclavicular lymph nodes may occur frequently as may metastatic nodules to the ovary (Krunkenberg's tumor) or to the peritoneal cul-de-sac (Blumer's shelf); malignant ascites may also develop. The liver is the most common site for hematogenous spread of tumor.

The presence of iron-deficiency anemia in men and occult blood in the stool of both sexes should mandate a search for an occult lesion in the gastrointestinal tract. Such a careful assessment is of particular importance in patients having atrophic gastritis or pernicious anemia. Unusual clinical features associated with gastric adenocarcinomas include migratory thrombophlebitis, microangiopathic hemolytic anemia, and acanthosis nigricans.

Diagnosis A double-contrast radiographic examination is the simplest diagnostic procedure for the evaluation of a patient with epigastric complaints. The use of double-contrast techniques helps to detect small lesions by improving mucosal detail. The stomach should be distended at some time during every radiographic examination since decreased distensibility may be the only indication of a diffuse infiltrative carcinoma. Although gastric ulcers can be detected fairly early, it may be impossible to distinguish benign from malignant lesions. The anatomic location of an ulcer is not in itself an indication of the presence or absence of a cancer.

The x-ray demonstration of a benign-appearing gastric ulcer presents special problems. Some physicians believe that gastroscopy is not mandatory if the radiographic features are typically benign, if complete healing can be visualized by x-ray within 6 weeks, and if a follow-up contrast radiograph several months later is normal. However, many feel that gastroscopic biopsy and brush cytology are required for all patients with a gastric ulcer in order to exclude a malignancy. The identification of malignant gastric ulcers prior to their penetration into surrounding tissues is crucial since the curability of such early lesions when limited to the mucosa or submucosa, even in the United States, is greater than 80 percent. Since gastric carcinomas are difficult to distinguish clinically or radiographically from gastric lymphomas, endoscopic biopsies should be made as deeply as possible due to the submucosal location of lymphoid tumors.

Treatment Surgical removal of the complete tumor with resection of adjacent lymph nodes offers the only chance for cure. However, this is possible in less than one-third of patients. In general, a subtotal gastrectomy represents the treatment of choice for patients with distal carcinomas while total or near-total gastrectomies are required for more proximal tumors. The prognosis following complete surgical resection is adversely influenced by the degree of tumor penetration into the stomach wall, regional lymph node involvement, and vascular invasion, characteristics found in the vast majority of American patients. As a result, the probability of survival after five years for the 25 to 30 percent of patients in the United States able to undergo a complete resection of a gastric cancer is approximately 25 percent for distal tumors and less than 10 percent for proximal tumors, with continued tumor recurrences being observed for at least 8 years following surgery. In the absence of ascites or extensive hepatic or peritoneal metastases, however, even the patient who is believed to be surgically incurable should be offered an attempt at resecting the primary lesion since the reduction of residual tumor offers the best form of palliation and may possibly enhance the probability for subsequent benefit if chemotherapy and/or radiation therapy are administered.

Gastric adenocarcinoma is a relatively radioresistant tumor, requiring doses of external beam irradiation in excess of the tolerance of surrounding structures such as bowel mucosa and spinal cord if adequate control of the primary tumor is to be achieved. As a result, the major role of radiation therapy in patients with gastric cancer has been limited to palliation of pain. Controlled trials have not been conducted to determine whether radiation therapy after a complete resection can prolong survival. In the setting of surgically unresectable disease limited to the epigastrium, comparative studies have shown that patients treated with 35 to 40 Gy (3500 to 4000 rad) did not live longer than similar patients not receiving radiotherapy; however, survival was prolonged slightly when 5-fluorouracil (5-FU) was given concomitantly with radiation therapy. In this clinical setting, the 5-FU may well be functioning as a radiosensitizer.

The administration of combinations of cytotoxic drugs to patients with advanced gastric carcinoma has been associated with reductions of greater than 50 percent in measurable tumor masses ("partial responses") in 30 to 50 percent of cases, providing significant benefit to individuals who respond to treatment. Such drug combinations have generally included 5-FU and doxorubicin together with mitomycin-C, cisplatin, or semustine (methyl-CCNU). Despite this encouraging response rate for a malignant condition once thought untreatable, complete disappearances of tumor masses remain uncommon, the partial responses are transient, and the overall impact of such multidrug therapy on survival has been a source of debate. The use of prophylactic (i.e., adjuvant) chemotherapy following the complete resection of a gastric cancer as a means of eradicating clinically undetectable micrometastases and improving the potential for cure has led to conflicting results; the role of adjuvant treatment remains an unsettled issue and such therapy should continue to be considered investigational.

PRIMARY GASTRIC LYMPHOMA Primary lymphoma of the stomach is relatively uncommon, comprising about 7 percent of gastric malignancies and about 2 percent of all lymphomas. It is, however, the most frequent extranodal location for lymphoma. The disease is difficult to distinguish clinically from gastric adenocarcinoma; both tumors are most often detected during the sixth decade of life, present with epigastric pain, early satiety, and generalized fatigue, and are usually characterized by ulcerations with a ragged, thickened mucosal pattern demonstrated by contrast radiographs. The diagnosis of lymphoma of the stomach may occasionally be made through cytologic brushings of the gastric mucosa, but usually requires a biopsy at the time of gastroscopy or laparotomy. The failure of gastroscopic biopsies to detect lymphoma should not be interpreted as being conclusive since superficial biopsies may miss the more deeply situated lymphoid infiltrate. The macroscopic pathology of gastric lymphoma may also mimic adenocarcinoma, either as a bulky ulcerated lesion localized in the corpus or antrum or as a diffuse process spreading throughout the entire gastric submucosa and even extending into the duodenum. Microscopically, the vast majority of gastric lymphoid tumors are non-Hodgkin's lymphomas of B-cell origin; Hodgkin's disease involving the stomach is extremely uncommon. Gastric lymphomas spread initially to regional lymph nodes (often to Waldeyer's ring) and may then disseminate.

Primary gastric lymphoma is a far more treatable disease than adenocarcinoma of the stomach, underscoring the need for making the correct diagnosis. All detectable tumor can be removed in over two-thirds of patients by some type of a subtotal gastrectomy. The prognosis in such patients is encouraging with 5-year survival rates of 40 to 60 percent having been reported. The best prognosis seems to be associated with those gastric lymphomas having small, single lesions, more differentiated histologies, and absence of spread to adjacent lymph nodes. While postoperative radiation therapy to the abdomen has been employed in the past, even when all obvious disease has been resected, the value of such a practice is open to serious question since the majority of recurrences develop in anatomic sites distant from the epigastrium and outside the fields of radiation treatment. Combination chemotherapy, which has proved to be highly effective in the management of disseminated non-Hodgkin's lymphoma including the diffuse large cell subtype, has recently gained increased favor as an adjunct to surgery, particularly when regional lymph node involvement is present. In the past, such drug therapy was not considered to be a substitute for surgery, even if the lymphoma were localized, since the rapid destruction of lymphoma masses by chemotherapy occasionally led to life-threatening hemorrhage. The results of recent clinical trials, however, have suggested that the probability for such bleeding may be relatively small and that drug treatment alone may be adequate to eradicate the lymphoma. If widespread disease is discovered at the time of laparotomy, combination chemotherapy should be utilized.

GASTRIC (NONLYMPHOID) SARCOMA Leiomyosarcomas are the most common of this group of gastric malignancies and comprise approximately 1 to 3 percent of all gastric neoplasms. They most frequently involve the anterior and posterior walls of the gastric fundus and often ulcerate and bleed. Even those lesions which appear benign on histologic examination may behave in a malignant fashion. Leiomyosarcomas rarely invade adjacent viscera and characteristically do not metastasize to lymph nodes but may spread to the liver and lungs. The treatment of choice is surgical resection. Combination chemotherapy should be reserved for patients with metastatic disease.

REFERENCES

Esophageal cancer

BOYCE HW: Palliation of advanced esophageal cancer. Semin Oncol 11:186, 1984

COIA LR ET AL: Nonsurgical management of esophageal cancer: Report of a study of combined radiotherapy and chemotherapy. J Clin Oncol 5:1783, 1987

KELSEN D: Chemotherapy of esophageal cancer. Semin Oncol 11:159, 1984

LIGHTDALE CJ, WINAWER SJ: Screening diagnosis and staging of esophageal cancer. Semin Oncol 11:101, 1984

POPLIN E ET AL: Combined therapies for squamous-cell carcinoma of the esophagus, a Southwest Oncology Group Study (SWOG - 8037). J Clin Oncol 5:622, 1987

REID BJ et al: Barrett's esophagus. Correlation between flow cytometry and histology in detection of patients at risk for adenocarcinoma. Gastroenterology 93:1, 1987

SCHOTTENFELD D: Epidemiology of cancer of the esophagus. Semin Oncol 11:92, 1984

SKINNER DB: Surgical treatment for esophageal carcinoma. Semin Oncol 11:136, 1984

Gastric tumors

ALLUM WH et al: Adjuvant chemotherapy in operable gastric cancer. Lancet 1:571, 1989

ANTONIOLI DA, GOLDMAN H: Changes in the location and type of gastric adenocarcinoma. Cancer 50:775, 1982

BEDIKIAN AY et al: The natural history of gastric cancer and prognostic factors influencing survival. J Clin Oncol 2:305, 1984

CORREA P: Clinical implications of recent developments in gastric cancer pathology and epidemiology. Semin Oncol 12:2, 1985

DOUGLASS HO, NAVA HR: Gastric adenocarcinoma—management of the primary disease. Semin Oncol 12:32, 1985

GOHMANN JJ, MACDONALD JS: Chemotherapy of gastric cancer. Cancer Invest 7:39, 1989

HABER DA, MAYER RJ: Primary gastrointestinal lymphoma. Semin Oncol 15:154, 1988

KURTZ RC, SHERLOCK P: The diagnosis of gastric cancer. Semin Oncol 12:11, 1985

LANGMAN MJS: Antisecretory drugs and gastric cancer. Br Med J 290:1850, 1985

LICHT JD et al: Gastrointestinal sarcomas. Semin Oncol 15:181, 1988

LIST AF et al: Non-Hodgkin's lymphoma of the gastrointestinal tract: An analysis of clinical and pathologic features affecting outcome. J Clin Oncol 6:1125, 1988

LUNDEGARDH G et al: Stomach cancer after partial gastrectomy for benign ulcer disease. N Engl J Med 319:195, 1988

240 DISORDERS OF ABSORPTION

NORTON J. GREENBERGER / KURT J. ISSELBACHER

MECHANISMS OF ABSORPTION

Diseases of the small intestine are frequently accompanied by alterations in intestinal function, and clinically this impaired function is seen as the malabsorption syndrome. In order to obtain a better appreciation of the derangements which occur in the many disorders of intestinal function, the processes of normal absorption will first be reviewed.

It is important to distinguish between digestion and absorption, since an increased loss of nutrients in the stool may be a reflection of a derangement of either process. Digestion involves the breakdown or hydrolysis of nutrients to smaller molecules in order to prepare the ingested substances for absorption, or transport across the intestinal cell. It will be recalled that most of the digestive process is initiated in the stomach by acid and pepsin and is continued in the upper small intestine primarily by the action of pancreatic enzymes such as lipase, amylase, and trypsin. As a result of these digestive actions carbohydrates are broken down to monosaccharides and disaccharides, proteins to peptides and amino acids, and fats to monoglycerides and fatty acids. In the adult it is in this form that nutrients are, to a large extent, transported across the epithelial surface of the intestinal cell.

ANATOMIC AND PHYSIOLOGIC FACTORS The intestine has an enormous surface area. This can be attributed in large part to its length, which in the adult is more than 4 m, and to the foldings of the surface plicae. At the light microscopic level, the villi of the small intestine provide additional surface area, which is further augmented by the presence of microvilli (approximately 2×10^8 per square centimeter) on the outer, or brush border, region of epithelial cells. Thus the total absorptive area of the small intestine is enormous.

Motility (contractility) of the bowel is an important process which permits nutrients to remain in intimate contact with the intestinal cells and possibly influences the continued movement of the nutrients *into* and along the absorbing channels, such as the lymphatics. Two types of motility aid in this process: the gross motility of the intestine itself and the motility of individual villi. Entrance of the nutrients into the general circulation is achieved via the capillaries into the portal system or via the lacteals into the intestinal lymphatics.

TYPES OF ABSORPTION Four mechanisms have been considered to be important in the transport of substances across the intestinal cell membrane, namely, active transport, passive diffusion, facilitated diffusion, and endocytosis.

Active transport involves the transport of a substance across the cell against an electric or chemical gradient; this process requires energy, is carrier-mediated, and is subject to competitive inhibition. *Passive diffusion* is the opposite of this process; energy is not required, transport is with (rather than against) the electric or chemical gradient, the process is not carrier-mediated, and it does not show properties of competitive inhibition. Thus active transport may be viewed as "uphill" transport, whereas passive diffusion is equivalent to "downhill" transport. *Facilitated diffusion* is similar to passive diffusion except that such a process shows evidence of being carrier-mediated and frequently subject to competitive inhibition.

Endocytosis is a process akin to phagocytosis. By this mechanism nutrients (soluble or particulate) upon entering the cell are surrounded by the components of the outer plasma cell membrane. In the intestinal tract endocytosis occurs in the neonatal period and, contrary to earlier belief, also occurs to a limited extent in the adult organism. While quantitatively limited, it appears to account, for example, for uptake of antigens.

SITES OF ABSORPTION While many substances are absorbed throughout the length of the small intestine, certain nutrients tend to be absorbed more in one region than in others. The proximal intestine is a major area for the absorption of iron, calcium, water-soluble vitamins, and fat (monoglycerides and fatty acids). Sugars are absorbed in the proximal intestine and also the midintestine. While the amino acids appear to be absorbed primarily in the middle of the small intestine, or jejunum, some absorption also occurs in the upper and lower areas. The distal small intestine appears to be the *major* absorptive area for bile salts and vitamin B_{12}. As is emphasized below, this factor is of clinical significance in circumstances where there has been removal or disease of the ileum.

The colon is important for the absorption of water and electrolytes, a process which occurs predominantly in the cecum. Although the rectum is not a usual site for absorption of ingested foodstuffs, drugs introduced by rectum may be absorbed there. Thus drugs introduced by this route, such as salicylates or steroids, may have systemic as well as local effects.

ABSORPTION OF SPECIFIC NUTRIENTS Carbohydrate absorption Much of the carbohydrate we ingest is in the form of starch, a complex polysaccharide consisting of many hexose units (attached either in a 1,4 or 1,6 linkage). By the action of salivary and pancreatic amylase, starch is hydrolyzed to oligosaccharides and then to disaccharides (mostly maltose). While monosaccharides such as glucose are readily absorbed, disaccharides are not. Disaccharides are split enzymatically into their component sugars by disaccharidases (or oligosaccharidases) located on or within the microvilli of intestinal epithelial cells. The two types of disaccharidases are β-galactosidases (lactase) and α-glucosidases (sucrase, maltase). By the action of these enzymes, lactose is split into glucose and galactose, sucrose into glucose and fructose, and maltose into two molecules of glucose. The resultant monosaccharides are then transported through the cell into the portal circulation. Most disaccharides are hydrolyzed so rapidly by brush border enzymes that the capacity of the transport mechanism is exceeded and some monosaccharides diffuse back into the intestinal lumen. Lactose, however, is hydrolyzed at a slower rate, and thus lactose hydrolysis is the rate-limiting step in lactose absorption.

Sugars such as glucose and galactose are absorbed by an active transport mechanism. The transport rate of sugars can be related to the substrate concentration by the expression K_t, where K_t stands for the monosaccharide substrate concentration that produces half the maximal transport rate. Published K_t values for glucose transport have varied widely, partly because of failure to consider the unstirred water layer, which constitutes a diffusion barrier for solutes.

Glucose (and galactose) entry into the cell is largely coupled to sodium ions (so-called symport); both sodium and glucose appear to bind to the hexose carrier in the microvillus membrane. Energy is required for the movement of glucose into the cell, which seems largely to come from the sodium pump and the Na^+,K^+-ATPase of the basolateral membrane (see below).

Protein and amino acid absorption Dietary proteins are initially subject to degradation in the stomach by pepsin. However, complete hydrolysis is largely achieved by the action of the pancreatic enzymes trypsin and chymotrypsin as well as by other endopeptidases and exopeptidases such as carboxypeptidase. By these enzymatic processes oligopeptides, dipeptides, and amino acids are formed. Just as there are disaccharidases in mucosal cells to digest disaccharides, there are also oligopeptidases to split small peptides. Dipeptidases are located in the cytoplasm as well as on the microvilli. Dipeptides are absorbed more rapidly than amino acids, and presumably their uptake involves a separate mechanism. Thus, digestion of proteins to amino acids occurs in three locations: intestinal lumen, brush border, and cytoplasm of mucosal cells. As indicated above, contrary to earlier beliefs proteins can also be absorbed by the adult intestine. Although quantitatively limited, protein absorption probably is immunologically significant.

Most naturally occurring amino acids are L-amino acids, and these are subject to a number of different transport processes. *Neutral* amino acids seem to share a common carrier mechanism; thus amino acids such as tryptophan and alanine show competitive inhibition. Among the *dibasic* amino acids which appear to have a distinct transport mechanism are arginine, ornithine, and lysine. The neutral amino acid cystine shares this mechanism. There is also a separate transport system for *glycine* and the *imino acids* proline and hydroxy-proline. There is also a transport system for *dicarboxylic* acids such as glutamic and aspartic acids. Therefore, in genetic disorders, such as cystinuria, one will find impaired absorption not only of cystine but also of arginine, ornithine, and lysine. Similarly in Hartnup disease, a defect in the transport of neutral amino acids (especially of tryptophan, phenylalanine, histidine) is found. In these genetic disorders uptake and absorption of dipeptides is normal.

Absorption of amino acids is rapid in the duodenum and jejunum but slow in the ileum. The actual mechanism of the absorption of amino acids by the intestine has not been elucidated. As in the case of carbohydrates, sodium ions appear to be required for the entry of these acids and the energy needed for their concentration within the cell. Some amino acids have affinity for more than one mechanism. For example, glycine may be transported by both the neutral and imino acid transport systems.

Fat absorption (Fig. 240-1) Most of the ingested dietary fats are in the form of long-chain triglycerides. These triglycerides contain both saturated fatty acids (such as palmitic and stearic) and unsaturated fatty acids (such as oleic and linoleic). The particle size of the fat is decreased largely by the churning action of the stomach. The entry of fat into the duodenum plus the presence of acid causes release of secretin and pancreozymin-cholecystokinin, which in turn leads to a stimulation of the flow of bile and pancreatic juice.

ROLE OF PANCREATIC LIPASE The hydrolysis of triglycerides by pancreatic lipase is a complex process involving lipase, colipase, and bile salts. Pancreatic lipase is an enzyme that binds to the oil-water interface of an emulsified triglyceride substrate. The detergent properties of bile salts permit pancreatic lipase to gain access to water-insoluble lipids. One of the important functions of bile salts is to clear the oil-water interface of dietary fat from proteins of exogenous and endogenous origin, thus making it available for pancreatic lipolysis. Colipase, a protein present in pancreatic juice, is also essential for the action of lipase; its function is to anchor the lipase close to the surface of the triglyceride droplet. All three components, i.e., pancreatic lipase, colipase, and bile salts, form a *ternary complex,* which generates lipolytic products that diffuse away from the complex and are absorbed. With colipase present, lipase remains at the interface and forms 2-monoglycerides and fatty acids, which are the major end products of triglyceride hydrolysis. Less than 5 percent of ingested fat remains in the form of diglycerides and triglycerides. Without colipase, bile acids would actually wash pancreatic lipase away from the interface, and the hydrolytic rate of triglycerides would be reduced.

ROLE OF BILE SALTS (Fig. 240-2) Bile salts play an important role in the digestion and absorption of fat. They are synthesized in the liver (approximately 200 to 600 mg daily) from cholesterol and excreted in the bile in the form of their glycine or taurine conjugates. In humans the principal bile acids excreted are conjugates of cholic and chenodeoxycholic acid. Bile salts are good detergents, because they have both polar (hydrophilic) and nonpolar (hydrophobic) groups. During digestion the concentration of conjugated bile salts in the lumen is in the range of 5 to 15 μmol/mL, and at these concentrations the bile salts aggregate to form *micelles*. Fatty acids and monoglycerides enter these micelles, forming mixed micelles. An emulsion of triglyceride is turbid; mixed micelles containing bile salts, fatty acids, and monoglycerides are clear solutions. The formation of *mixed micelles* and hence the solubilization of fatty acids and monoglycerides is much more effectively achieved with *conjugated bile salts* at the pH which normally exists in the intestinal lumen (Fig. 240-2).

Most conjugated bile salts are absorbed in the ileum and after entering the portal vein are subject to an enterohepatic circulation. By this process about 90 percent of the conjugated bile salts reaching the ileum is reabsorbed. As a consequence only about 200 to 600 mg bile salts is excreted in the feces per day, while, as part of the enterohepatic circulation, the 3- to 4-g bile salt pool circulates many times each day so that actually 20 to 30 g of bile salts may enter the duodenum each day. When the enterohepatic circulation is intact, the size of the bile salt pool is largely determined by the frequency of the enterohepatic circulation, i.e., the number of cycles per day (see also Chap. 258). If the ileum is diseased or removed, absorption of bile salts is impaired, and a significant fecal loss of bile salts will occur. As a consequence of this bile salt depletion, the concentration of bile salts in the intestinal lumen will also decrease, leading to further impairment of fat absorption. A similar result will occur if bile salt reabsorption is prevented by chelating agents, such as cholestyramine (see ''Regional Enteritis'' below). Diarrhea per se may result in increased fecal excretion of bile salts. This has been demonstrated both in normal subjects in whom diarrhea has been induced and in patients with chronic idiopathic diarrhea.

INTRAMUCOSAL ASPECTS OF FAT ABSORPTION (Fig. 240-1) After the hydrolysis of fatty acids to monoglycerides and their interaction with bile salts to form mixed micelles, the lipids pass through an ''unstirred'' water layer covering the cell surface. The mixed micelles apparently do not enter the cell, but instead the component fatty acids and monoglycerides are released from the micellar phase and then enter the cell by diffusion. In aqueous duodenal contents, large bile salt mixed micelles saturated with products of lipolysis coexist with larger liquid crystal liposomes of the same lipids saturated with free fatty acids and mixed bile salts. These phases are interconvertible and both may be important in fat digestion and absorption. Upon

FIGURE 240-1 Scheme of intestinal digestion, absorption, esterification, and transport of dietary triglycerides. TG = triglycerides; FA = fatty acids; MG = monoglycerides; BS = bile salts.

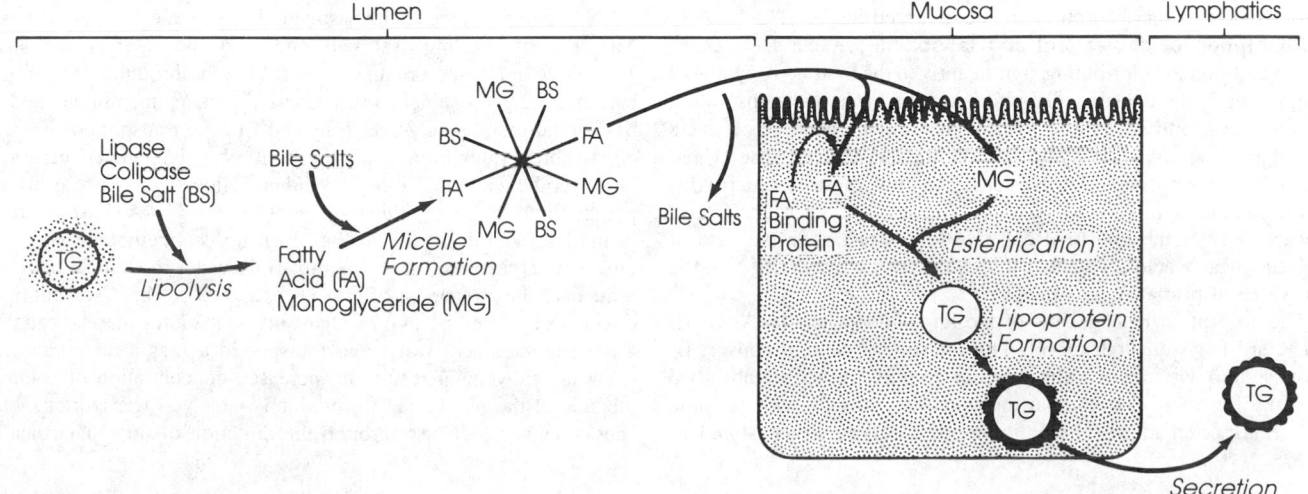

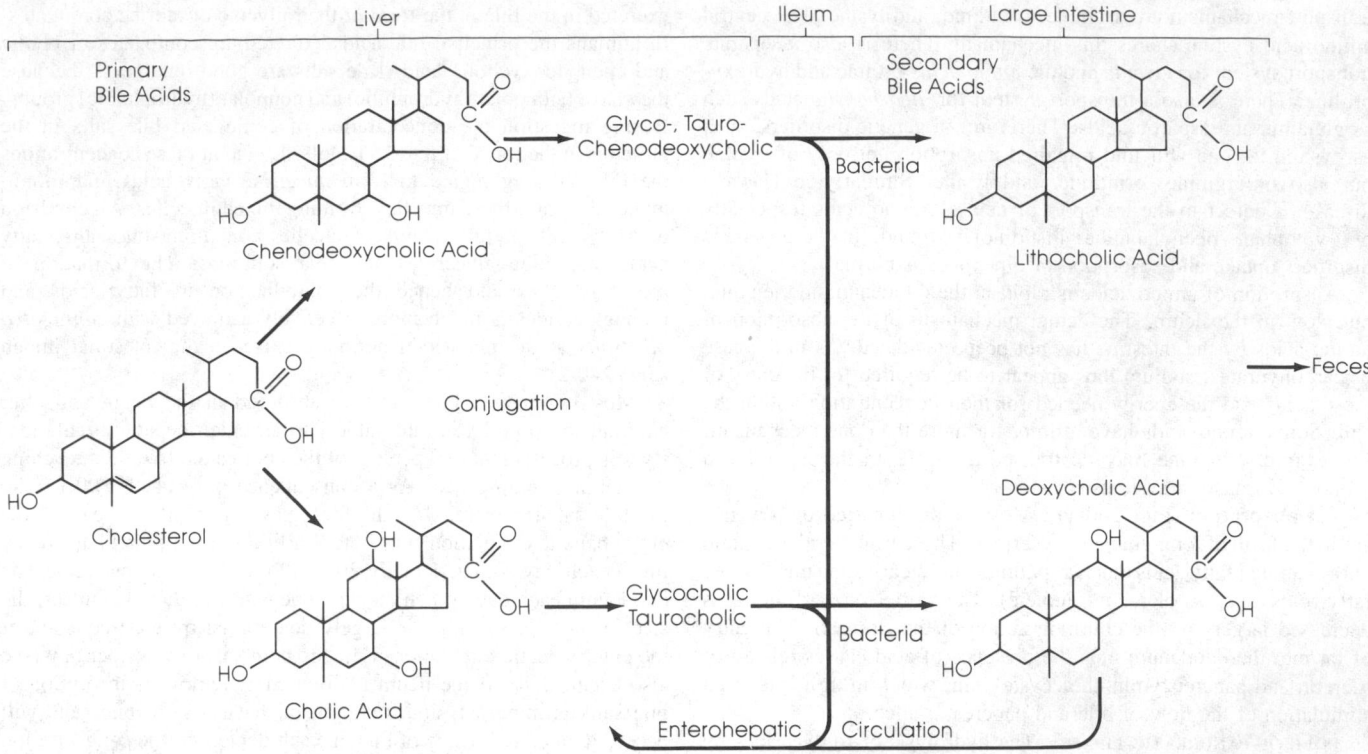

FIGURE 240-2   Scheme of hepatic and intestinal metabolism of bile salts and the enterohepatic circulation (from ileum to liver). Note that bacteria lead to the formation of secondary bile acids; of the latter, only deoxycholic acid is absorbed to any appreciable extent.

entry into the mucosal cell, fatty acids may interact with specific binding proteins. The subsequent fate of the intracellular lipid is strongly influenced by the fatty acid chain length. Fatty acids and monoglycerides derived from long-chain triglycerides (i.e., containing C-16 to C-18 fatty acids) are promptly *reesterified to triglycerides* by enzymes of the endoplasmic reticulum. These triglycerides then interact with specific apolipoproteins plus cholesterol and phospholipid to form chylomicrons and very low density lipoproteins. These initially accumulate in the Golgi region of the cell and then are secreted into the lacteals and the intestinal lymph. There are thus four major steps in the absorption of long-chain fatty acids and monoglycerides: (1) mucosal uptake and interaction with binding proteins, (2) reesterification to triglycerides, (3) lipoprotein formation, and (4) secretion into lymph.

By contrast, fatty acids derived from medium-chain triglycerides (i.e., containing C-8 and C-12 fatty acids) are *not reesterified* to any significant extent within the cell and are not incorporated into lipoproteins. Instead, they rapidly enter the portal venous system, where they are transported as fatty acids bound to albumin. The major aspects of fat absorption are summarized in Fig. 240-1.

Absorption of cholesterol and fat-soluble vitamins (A, D, E, K)   In addition to contributing significantly to the total-body synthesis of cholesterol, the intestine also plays an active role in the absorption of cholesterol and its esters. Within the lumen, cholesterol esters from the bile and diet are hydrolyzed by a pancreatic esterase. There is also a separate cholesterol esterase in the intestinal microvilli, which completes this hydrolysis. As a result, only free cholesterol appears to enter the intestinal cell. However, just as in the case of long-chain fatty acids, much of the cholesterol is reesterified and is then secreted primarily into lymph.

The absorption mechanisms of the fat-soluble vitamins A, D, E, and K are not well understood. The intestine is able to convert β-carotene into vitamin A. The vitamin A thus formed or absorbed from the lumen is esterified in the mucosa primarily with palmitic acid, transported in the chylomicrons of the lymph, and stored as retinol palmitate in the liver. The other lipid-soluble vitamins also appear in lymph chylomicrons, but esterification with fatty acids does not appear to be necessary for their transport.

Water and sodium absorption   In spite of extensive investigations the main mechanisms of water and electrolyte transport are not well understood. The mechanisms responsible for fluid absorption differ in the jejunum, ileum, and colon. There are two pathways by which water and ions cross the intestinal mucosa: the paracellular and transcellular pathways. Individual intestinal mucosa cells are joined near their apex by a "tight junction," and ions and water traverse this *paracellular* pathway during absorption and secretion. It is believed that the tight junction pathway contains aqueous-filled channels or pores. Such intercellular spaces are closed in the resting state and dilated during absorption. Considerable evidence has accumulated indicating that pumps and carriers are involved in intestinal water and solute transport. For example, in the ileum, Na^+ enters in exchange for H^+, and Cl^- enters in exchange for HCO_3^-. Sodium entry into the cell also occurs coupled with glucose via the glucose-sodium carrier in the microvillus membrane. Inside the cell, the Na^+ pump located in the basolateral membrane actively transports Na^+ out of the mucosal cell and into the intercellular space. *Transcellular* transport requires passage of ions through two membrane barriers, i.e., the apical brush border plasma membrane and the basolateral membrane. After Na^+ and Cl^- are transported across the brush border membrane into the cell, Na^+ is pumped across the basolateral membrane and Cl^- either follows passively or is also pumped into the intercellular space. The Na^+,K^+-ATPase is present in the basolateral but not in the brush border membrane and is the biochemical mediator of this pump. Bulk water movement obviously influences the movement of Na^+, K^+, and Cl^-. This "solvent drag" effect is explained by two mechanisms: (1) solutes may be caught in a moving stream of water and transported across a membrane, and (2) water movement results in increased concentration of solute on the side of the membrane from which water was transported, which causes solute to diffuse through the direction of flow. Diarrhea can

TABLE 240-1 Some mechanisms in the production of diarrhea

I Secretory diarrhea
  A Secretory agents associated with adenylate cyclase system
    1 Enterotoxin-producing bacteria (*Vibrio cholerae, Escherichia coli*)
    2 Methylxanthines (caffeine, theophylline)
    3 Prostaglandins
    4 Vasoactive intestinal peptide (VIP)
    5 Dihydroxy bile acids (affect colon primarily; effects seen after ileal resection)
  B Secretory agents *not associated* with adenylate cyclase system
    1 Glucagon, secretin, cholecystokinin-pancreozymin, serotonin, calcitonin, gastrin inhibitory polypeptide (GIP)
    2 Some laxatives* (ricinoleic acid, bisacodyl, phenolphthalein, dioctyl sodium sulfosuccinate)
    3 Bacterial enterotoxins (*Shigella, Staphylococcus aureus, Clostridium perfringens*)
  C Mucosal injury, altered cell permeability
    1 *Salmonella, Shigella*, invasive *E. coli*, gastroenteritis viruses
    2 Celiac sprue
    3 Inflammatory bowel disease (ulcerative colitis, regional enteritis)
  D Neoplasms with or without hormone production
    1 Gastrinoma (gastrin)
    2 Carcinoid syndrome (serotonin, prostaglandins)
    3 Medullary carcinoma of thyroid (calcitonin, prostaglandins)
    4 Pancreatic cholera syndrome (? VIP)
    5 Villous adenoma
II Osmotic diarrhea
  A Impaired carbohydrate absorption
    1 Disaccharidase deficiency (lactose or sucrose-isomaltose intolerance)
    2 Glucose-galactose malabsorption
  B Laxative ingestion or abuse
    1 Nonabsorbable osmotically active agents (lactulose, sorbitol, mannitol)
    2 Saline purgatives (magnesium phosphate, magnesium hydroxide–containing antacids)
  C Postsurgical disorders
    1 Vagotomy and pyloroplasty*
    2 Gastrojejunostomy* (Billroth I and II)
III Motility disorders
  A Laxative abuse*
  B Irritable bowel syndrome
  C Diverticular disease of the colon
  D Diabetic diarrhea with visceral neuropathy

* Multiple mechanisms involved in production of diarrhea.

be simply defined as impaired net absorption of water and electrolytes by the small intestine or colon. Some mechanisms producing diarrhea are listed in Table 240-1.

Calcium absorption Calcium is actively transported by the small intestine, and this process is intimately linked to the active form of vitamin D_3, namely, 1,25-dihydroxycholecalciferol. The role of two other intestinal cell proteins, calcium-binding protein and calmodulin, in the absorption of calcium remains unclear. Recent studies indicate that calcium is absorbed to the same extent from various calcium salts (carbonate, citrate, gluconate, lactate, and acetate) and from milk in healthy subjects; an average of 32 percent of the ingested calcium was absorbed from the various sources.

Iron absorption The formation of soluble iron complexes is important for maintaining intraluminal iron in an absorbable form. Gastric acid facilitates the chelation of inorganic iron with substances such as ascorbic acid, sugars, amino acids, and bile; these macromolecular complexes then remain soluble in the more alkaline duodenum and jejunum. With the average western diet the iron intake averages 15 to 25 mg per day; iron absorption averages 0.5 to 1.0 mg per day in men and 1.0 to 2.0 mg per day in women during their reproductive years. A regulatory mechanism for the absorption of inorganic iron appears to exist within the small-intestinal mucosal cells. Iron is actively transported by the small intestine, and the duodenum is the principal site of iron absorption. The absorption of elemental iron in humans and animals involves at least two distinct steps: (1) mucosal uptake of iron from the lumen and (2) mucosal transfer of iron to the plasma. Much of the iron entering the mucosal cell is not transferred to the plasma but remains trapped within the cell and is excreted into the lumen when the cell is shed. Iron lost by this mechanism seems to vary inversely with body iron stores.

However, this mucosal regulatory mechanism can be overcome when pharmacologic doses of iron are ingested. Hemoglobin iron is also absorbed by human subjects, depending upon body requirements for iron; the heme is split from globin in the lumen and absorbed as an intact metalloporphyrin. Organic iron in the form of hemoglobin is absorbed more effectively than iron from cereals and vegetables. The absorption of inorganic iron is increased by ascorbic acid. Similarly, the presence of anemia, liver injury, pregnancy, idiopathic hemochromatosis, or a portacaval shunt may result in increased iron absorption. Conversely, the prior ingestion of large doses of iron and the presence in the lumen of phosphates, carbonates, and phytates may lead to decreased absorption of inorganic iron. Impaired absorption of iron is frequent in disorders (such as nontropical sprue) which involve the duodenal mucosa.

Water-soluble vitamins *Vitamin B_{12} absorption* is discussed in Chap. 292. In the case of *folic acid absorption*, it should be emphasized that folates exist in food conjugated with glutamyl peptides. These *polyglutamates* must be deconjugated (by folic deconjugase) to monoglutamates for absorption to occur. Certain drugs (such as oral contraceptives, sulfasalazine, diphenylhydantoin, trimethoprim, and pyrimethamine) inhibit the absorption of dietary folate and hence can cause folate deficiency. Sulfasalazine, for example, competitively inhibits three enzymes important in the intestinal metabolism of folate, i.e., dihydrofolate reductase, methylene tetrahydrofolate reductase, and serine transhydroxymethylase. Thiamine and riboflavin appear to be absorbed by passive diffusion.

TESTS USEFUL IN THE DIAGNOSIS OF MALABSORPTION
Most of the tests useful in the diagnosis of malabsorption indicate the presence of abnormal absorptive or digestive function, and only a few tests may suggest a specific diagnosis. Accordingly, it is frequently necessary to employ a combination of tests to establish a diagnosis. To illustrate the use of various tests, the characteristic findings in nontropical sprue, an example of a primary malabsorptive disorder, and pancreatic insufficiency, an example of impaired digestion, are compared in Table 240-2.

Stool fat The qualitative examination of the stool for undigested muscle fibers, neutral fat, and split fat is a simple and reliable screening test for steatorrhea. The finding of an increased number of muscle fibers indicates impaired intraluminal digestion. Properly performed, the qualitative microscopic examination of a stool specimen with the Sudan III stain is of value and correlates well with the quantitative determination of fecal fat by the Van de Kamer method. The latter remains the most reliable measurement of steatorrhea. A normal fecal fat excretion is less than 6 g for 24 h, or greater than 94 percent coefficient of fat absorption.

Oral [^{14}C]triolein can also be used as an effective test for fat absorption. During the digestive process the triolein is hydrolyzed, and the labeled glycerol is absorbed and metabolized by the liver. The $^{14}CO_2$ produced is exhaled and can then be measured hourly (for 6 h) in the expired air. Normally more than 3.5 percent of the administered label [0.185 MBq (5 μCi)] appears in the breath per hour.

Xylose absorption In the most commonly employed test of carbohydrate absorption, the patient ingests 25 g D-xylose. A 5-h urine xylose excretion of 26 mmol (4.0 g) or greater is considered normal. Low values may be obtained in patients with ascites, intestinal bacterial overgrowth, or renal insufficiency, after administration of certain drugs (e.g., aspirin, indomethacin), and most commonly if the urine collection is incomplete. To prevent difficulties in interpreting the test, it is advisable to determine the blood xylose level 2 h after ingestion of xylose. A blood xylose level of 2 mmol/L (30 mg/dL) or greater indicates normal absorption of D-xylose. An abnormal D-xylose absorption test is found most frequently in disorders affecting the mucosa of the proximal small intestine, such as nontropical and tropical sprue.

Gastrointestinal x-ray studies All patients with malabsorption should have radiographic examinations of the small intestine and, in

TABLE 240-2 Tests useful in the diagnosis of malabsorptive disorders

Test	Normal values	Typical findings — Malabsorption (nontropical sprue)	Typical findings — Maldigestion (pancreatic insufficiency)	Comment
I Quantitative determination of stool fat	<6 g per 24 h; >95% coefficient of fat absorption	>6 g per 24 h	>6 g per 24 h	Best test for establishing presence of steatorrhea
II Carbohydrate absorption				
A D-Xylose absorption (25-g oral dose)	5-h urinary excretion 26 mmol (>4.5 g); peak blood level >2.0 mmol/L (>30 mg/dL)	↓	Normal	A good screening test for carbohydrate absorption
III Small-intestine x-rays		Malabsorption pattern	Normal or minimal malabsorption pattern; occasionally pancreatic calcification	
IV Blood tests				
A Serum calcium	2.2–2.7 mmol/L (9–11 mg/dL)	Frequently ↓	Usually normal	
B Serum albumin	35–55 g/L (3.5–5.5 g/dL)	Frequently ↓	Usually normal	Decreased levels of both serum albumin and globulins should raise the question of protein-losing enteropathy
C Serum cholesterol	3.90–6.45 mmol/L (150–250 mg/dL)	↓	Frequently ↓	Usually decreased in disorders associated with significant steatorrhea
D Serum iron	14–24 μmol/L (80–150 μg/dL)	Frequently ↓	Normal	Low values may reflect decreased body iron stores
E Serum magnesium	0.6–1.0 mmol/L (1.2–2.0 meq/liter)	Frequently ↓	Usually normal	
F Serum zinc	12–20 μmol/liter	Frequently ↓	Usually normal	Decreased levels common in malnutrition, cirrhosis, and malabsorption
G Serum carotenes	>100 IU/dL	↓	Usually ↓	Fairly satisfactory screening tests for malabsorption
H Serum vitamin A	>100 IU/dL	↓		
I Prothrombin time	70–100%; 12–15 s	Frequently ↓	Frequently ↓	
V Small intestinal mucosal biopsy		Abnormal	Normal	A specific diagnosis can be established in a small number of disorders (see text)
VI Urine tests				
A Vitamin B_{12} absorption	>8% urinary excretion in 48 h	Frequently ↓	Frequently ↓	Useful in determining whether vitamin B_{12} malabsorption is due to gastric or small-intestinal disorders
B Urine 5-hydroxyindole-acetic acid (5-HIAA)	10–47 μmol per 24 h (2–9 mg per 24 h)	↑	Normal	Slightly increased level (12–16 mg per 24 h) characteristically found in nontropical sprue
VII Breath tests				
A Breath H_2 (after 50 g lactose)	Minimal breath H_2	May be ↑	Normal	Secondary to lactase deficiency (see text)
B Breath H_2 (after 10 g lactulose)	Minimal breath H_2	May be normal or ↓	Normal	Early peak in bacterial overgrowth; can be used to determine intestinal transit time
C Breath $^{14}CO_2$ (after ^{14}C xylose)	Minute amounts $^{14}CO_2$	May be ↓	Usually normal	Increased in bacterial overgrowth
D Glycocholic acid metabolism (oral glycine-1-[^{14}C]glycocholate)	<1% of dose excreted $^{14}CO_2$ in 4 h	Normal	Normal	Increased $^{14}CO_2$ excretion with bacterial overgrowth or bile acid malabsorption (due to ileal resection or inflammatory disease)
	<4% of dose excreted in stools	Normal	Normal	Increased fecal excretion of ^{14}C in bile acid malabsorption
E [^{14}C]Triolein absorption (breath test)	>3.5% of dose as breath $^{14}CO_2$ per hour	Decreased	Decreased	Correlates well with chemical stool fat; recently introduced test
VIII Miscellaneous				
A Bacteria (culture)	<10^3 organisms per milliliter	Normal	Normal	>10^5 organisms per milliliter indicates bacterial overgrowth
B Secretin test	Volume >1.8 (mL/kg)/h Bicarbonate concentration >80 mmol/liter	Normal	Abnormal	See discussion of pancreatic insufficiency in Chaps. 259 and 260
C Bentiromide test	Urine excretion arylamines ≥50%	May be abnormal	Abnormal	See discussion of pancreatic disease in Chaps. 259 and 260

many cases, of the esophagus, stomach, and colon as well. Occasionally, the latter two examinations may provide important clues to the presence of such disorders as gastroileostomy, scleroderma, Zollinger-Ellison syndrome, ulcerative colitis, and intestinal fistulas. Traditional radiographic findings suggesting a diagnosis of malab-

sorption include flocculation of barium within fluid-filled loops causing fragmentation and segmentation of the barium column. However, these patterns are no longer demonstrated reliably in small-bowel series because of widespread use of barium products that contain a nonflocculating suspension of micropulverized barium sulfate. In

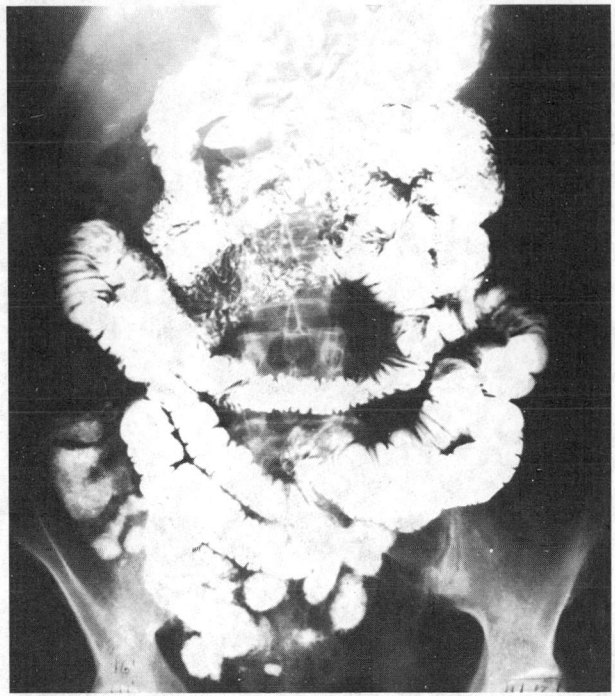

A

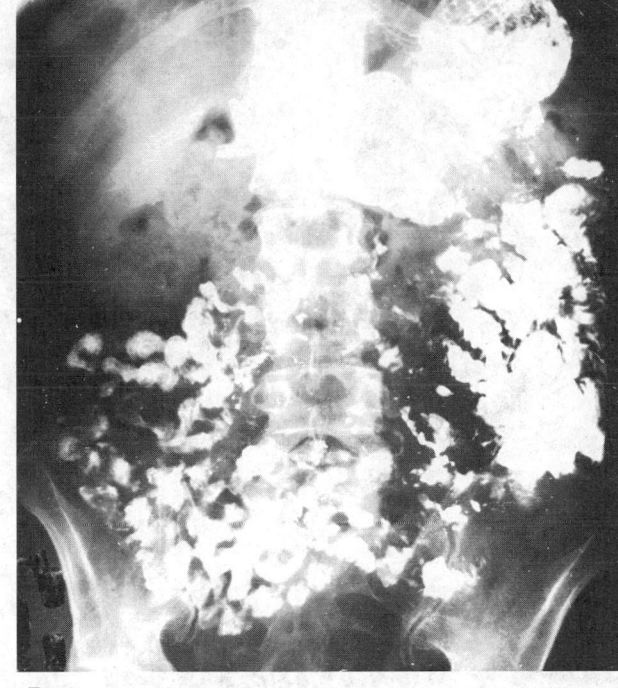

B

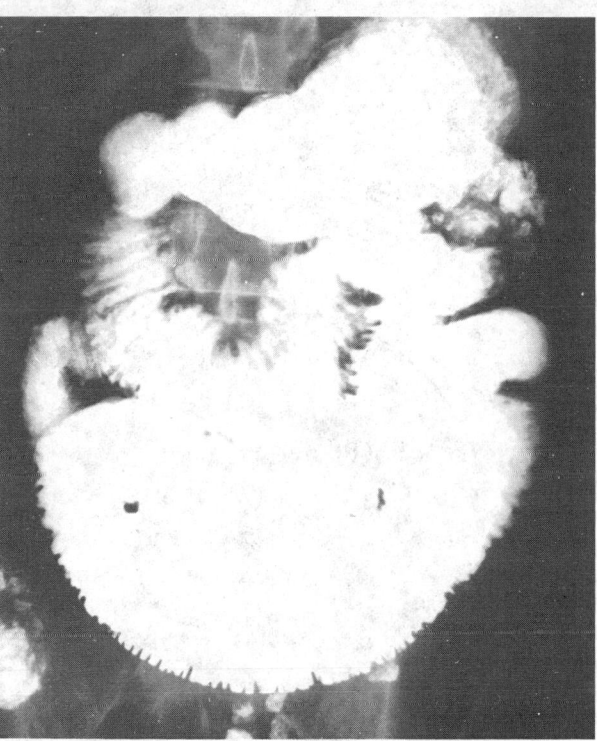

C

FIGURE 240-3 *A*. X-ray of a normal small intestine showing good mucosal pattern. *B*. Intestinal x-ray of a patient with nontropical sprue. Note dilatation of small bowel, lack of mucosal markings, and segmentation and clumping of barium. *C*. Intestinal x-ray of patient with obstructed lymphatics due to Köhlmeier-Degos disease, with "accordion-pleated" pattern (lower edge)

nontropical sprue, the most consistent abnormalities are thickened and nodular duodenal folds and dilatation of the small bowel. However, these findings are nonspecific and may be found in several of the disorders listed in Table 240-3. Some representative examples of abnormal small-bowel radiographs are shown in Fig. 240-3.

Small-intestinal biopsy The most commonly used instruments for obtaining peroral biopsy specimens from the small intestine

include the Rubin tube, the Crosby, Carey, and Ross-Moore capsules, and the upper gastrointestinal endoscope. Examination of small-bowel biopsy specimens has proved to be of considerable value in the differential diagnosis of malabsorptive disorders. Table 240-3 lists disorders associated with abnormalities in intestinal biopsies, and Fig. 240-4 depicts some illustrative lesions.

Schilling test for vitamin B$_{12}$ absorption The Schilling test is valuable in the differential diagnosis of malabsorption and is frequently carried out in three stages: (1) without intrinsic factor, (2) with intrinsic factor, and (3) after a course of treatment with antibiotics or anti-inflammatory drugs. Since vitamin B$_{12}$ is absorbed primarily

---

TABLE 240-3 Disorders associated with abnormalities in small-bowel biopsy specimens

I Disorders in which biopsy is of diagnostic value (diffuse lesions)
   A Whipple's disease: Lamina propria infiltrated with macrophages containing PAS-positive glycoproteins
   B Abetalipoproteinemia: Villus structure normal; epithelial cells vacuolated due to excess fat
   C Agammaglobulinemia: Flattened or absent villi; increased lymphocyte infiltration; absence of plasma cells
II Disorders in which biopsy may be of diagnostic value (patchy lesions)
   A Intestinal lymphoma: Infiltration of lamina propria and submucosa with malignant cells
   B Intestinal lymphangiectasia: Dilated lacteals and lymphatics in lamina propria; clubbed villi
   C Eosinophilic enteritis: Diffuse or patchy eosinophilic infiltration in lamina propria and mucosa
   D Amyloidosis: Presence of amyloid confirmed by special stains
   E Regional enteritis: Noncaseating granulomas
   F Parasitic infestations: Parasitic invasion of mucosa; adherence of trophozoites to mucosal surface, as in giardiasis
   G Systemic mastocytosis: Mast cell infiltration of lamina propria
III Disorders in which biopsy is abnormal but not diagnostic
   A Celiac sprue: Shortened or absent villi; hypertrophied crypts; damaged surface epithelium; mononuclear infiltrate
   B "Collagenous" sprue: Indistinguishable from celiac sprue; extensive subepithelial collagen deposition
   C Tropical sprue: Lesion similar to celiac sprue with shortened or absent villi; lymphocyte infiltration
   D Folate deficiency: Shortened villi; megalocytosis; decreased mitoses in crypts
   E Vitamin B$_{12}$ deficiency: Similar to folate deficiency
   F Acute radiation enteritis: Similar to folate deficiency
   G Systemic scleroderma: Fibrosis around Brunner's glands
   H Bacterial overgrowth syndromes: Patchy damage to villi and increased lymphocyte infiltration

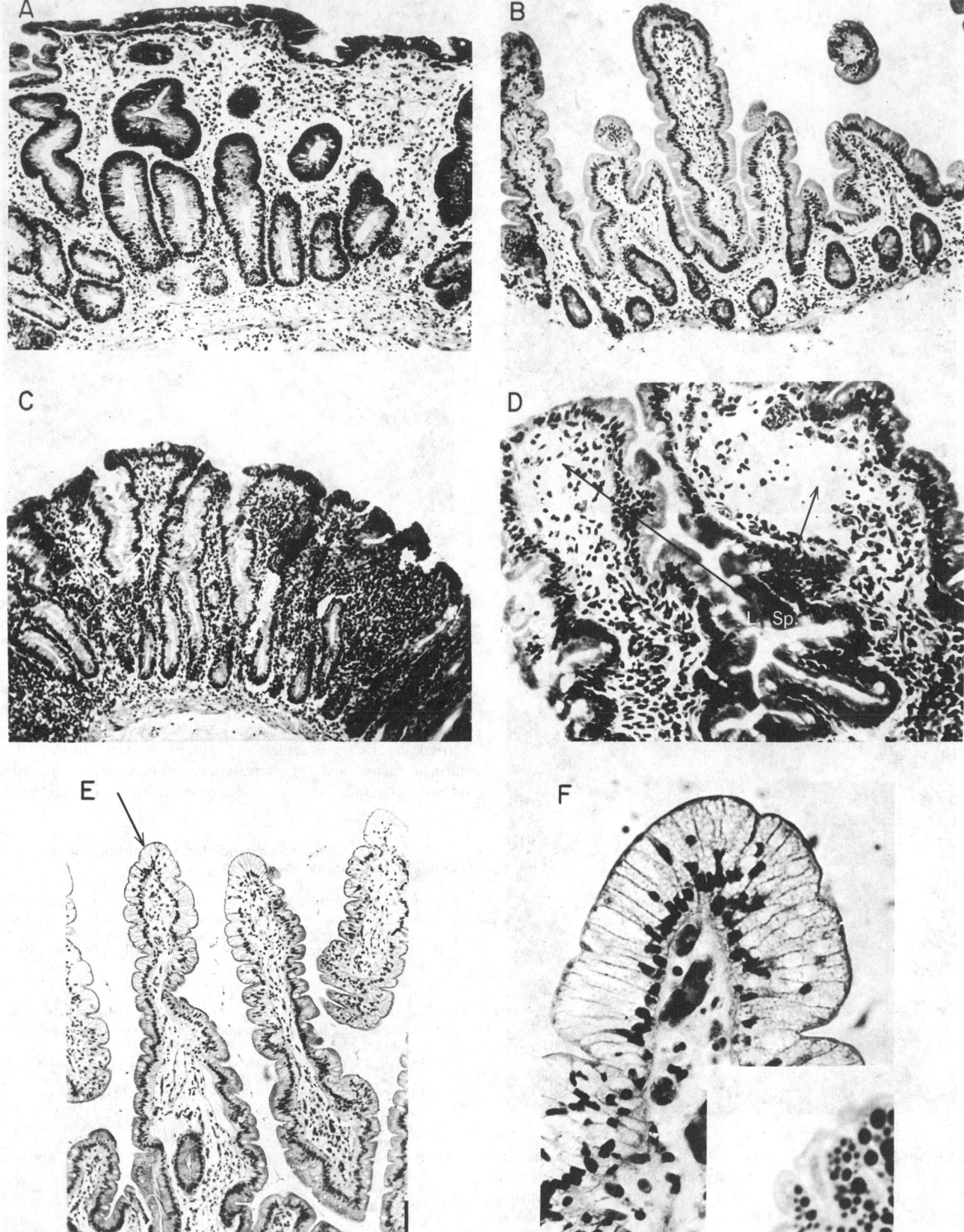

FIGURE 240-4   Typical peroral intestinal biopsies. *A.* Jejunal mucosa of patient with nontropical sprue. Note virtual absence of villi, elongated crypts (some cut in cross section), mononuclear infiltrate, cuboidal instead of columnar epithelium on top of villi (300×). *B.* Biopsy from the same patient as in *A*, after 9 months on a gluten-free diet. Note reappearance of villi with normal-appearing columnar cells and reduction in infiltrate and crypt height (300×). *C.* Biopsy from patient with agammaglobulinemia. The features bear a striking resemblance to those of nontropical sprue. There is a marked mononuclear infiltration, some of it in aggregates (200×). *D.* Close-up of villi of patient with protein-losing enteropathy. Note broadened and dilated tips, and lymphatic spaces (arrows). (450×). *E.* Intestinal biopsy from patient with abetalipoproteinemia. The villus tips have a "lacy" appearance (arrow) due to retained fat (300×). *F.* High-power micrograph of villus in *E.* Vacuoles are filled with lipid (750×). Insert shows dark-staining (osmium) lipid droplets in mucosal cells (osmium counterstained with Giemsa; 800×).

in the distal ileum, an abnormal Schilling test may indicate a pathologic condition of the distal small bowel. In disorders affecting the terminal ileum, such as regional enteritis and lymphomas, the first- and second-stage Schilling test are frequently abnormal. The ileal receptor site appears to be damaged in these disorders, and the impaired absorption of B_{12} is not corrected by the addition of intrinsic factor or the use of antibiotics. However, the Schilling test may normalize after treatment with prednisone or sulfasalazine. The Schilling test may also be useful in establishing a diagnosis of abnormal bacterial overgrowth of the small bowel, which may be present in disorders such as blind loop syndrome, scleroderma, and multiple small-bowel diverticula (see below). In the blind loop syndrome, for example, the bacteria can actually take up vitamin B_{12} with resultant impaired absorption of B_{12}. Under these conditions the first-stage Schilling test is frequently abnormal, as is the second stage. After appropriate antibiotic treatment the Schilling test usually returns to normal. Vitamin B_{12} absorption is frequently abnormal in patients with exocrine pancreatic insufficiency (see Chap. 260).

Secretin and other pancreatic tests The secretin test, secretin cholecystokinin test, intraduodenal perfusion with essential amino acids, and bentiromide test, which may be useful in establishing a diagnosis of pancreatic insufficiency, are discussed in detail in Chap. 259.

Serum calcium, albumin, cholesterol, magnesium, and iron Abnormal serum calcium, albumin, cholesterol, magnesium, and iron values may be found in several malabsorptive disorders. The primary value of such tests is to suggest that abnormal intestinal absorptive function may be present. These tests are usually of limited value in the *differential diagnosis* of malabsorption, but if abnormal, may be helpful in supporting this diagnosis.

Serum carotenes, vitamin A, and prothrombin time Absorption of the fat-soluble vitamins A, D, K, and E is frequently impaired in patients with steatorrhea. Measurements of serum carotene and vitamin A levels are useful as screening tests for malabsorption. However, other tests not only are more sensitive but often give more specific information than the serum carotene and vitamin A levels. The blood prothrombin time is an important test, since patients with malabsorption may present with abnormal bleeding due to vitamin K deficiency. If the decreased prothrombin activity is due to malabsorption, it should be readily correctable with parenteral vitamin K.

Breath tests The bile acid breath test utilizing [^{14}C]cholylglycine is a reasonably reliable screening test for bacterial overgrowth syndromes. Approximately two-thirds of patients with a positive small-bowel culture will have an abnormal bile acid breath test. However, in patients with suspected malabsorption of bile acids the test is rather insensitive without the additional determination of fecal bile acid excretion. The excretion of breath hydrogen after ingestion of lactose is a sensitive, specific, and noninvasive test for detecting lactase deficiency. Lactulose and [^{14}C]xylose breath tests for bacterial overgrowth have also been found helpful.

PATHOPHYSIOLOGIC BASIS FOR SYMPTOMS AND SIGNS IN MALABSORPTIVE DISORDERS The common symptoms and signs found in malabsorptive disorders are listed in Table 240-4. The most frequent symptoms are those of malnutrition, weight loss, and diarrhea. However, in each of the clinical settings listed in Table 240-4, it is important to consider the cause of the malabsorption.

DISORDERS OF MALABSORPTION
(See Table 240-5)

INADEQUATE DIGESTION   Liver and biliary tract disease It is not generally appreciated that patients with acute or chronic liver disease may develop malabsorption due to impaired intraluminal digestion. Steatorrhea has been described in acute viral hepatitis, chronic extrahepatic biliary tract obstruction, primary biliary cirrhosis, and postnecrotic and nutritional cirrhosis. Absorption of D-xylose and vitamin B_{12} are usually normal, and small-intestinal mucosal biopsy

TABLE 240-4   Pathophysiologic basis for symptoms and signs in malabsorptive disorders

Symptom or sign	Pathophysiology
GASTROINTESTINAL	
Generalized malnutrition and weight loss	Malabsorption of fat, carbohydrate, and protein → loss of calories
Diarrhea	Impaired absorption or increased secretion of water and electrolytes; unabsorbed dihydroxy bile acids and fatty acids → decreased absorption of water and electrolytes; excess load of fluid and electrolytes presented to the colon may exceed its absorptive capacity
Flatus	Bacterial fermentation of unabsorbed carbohydrate
Glossitis, cheilosis, stomatitis	Deficiency of iron, vitamin B_{12}, folate, and other vitamins
GENITOURINARY	
Nocturia	Delayed absorption of water, hypokalemia
Azotemia, hypotension	Fluid and electrolyte depletion
Amenorrhea, ↓ libido	Protein depletion and "caloric starvation" → secondary hypopituitarism
HEMATOPOIETIC	
Anemia	Impaired absorption of iron, vitamin B_{12}, and folic acid
Hemorrhagic phenomena	Vitamin K malabsorption → hypoprothrombinemia
MUSCULOSKELETAL	
Bone pain	Protein depletion → impaired bone formation → osteoporosis; Calcium malabsorption → demineralization of bone → osteomalacia
Osteoarthropathy	Cause uncertain
Tetany, paresthesias	Calcium malabsorption → hypocalcemia; magnesium malabsorption → hypomagnesemia
Weakness	Anemia; electrolyte depletion (hypokalemia)
NERVOUS SYSTEM	
Night blindness	Impaired absorption vitamin A → vitamin A deficiency
Xerophthalmia	Vitamin A deficiency
Peripheral neuropathy	Vitamin B_{12}, thiamine deficiency
SKIN	
Eczema	Cause uncertain
Purpura	Vitamin K deficiency
Follicular hyperkeratosis and dermatitis	Deficiency of vitamin A, zinc, essential fatty acids, and other vitamins

specimens are generally unremarkable. The steatorrhea associated with liver and biliary tract disease is thought to be due to impaired hepatic synthesis or excretion of conjugated bile salts, resulting in impaired formation of micellar lipid. In addition to steatorrhea, patients with liver disease may have impaired absorption of vitamin D and calcium, resulting in severe metabolic bone disease. This is particularly common in patients with primary biliary cirrhosis. Skeletal roentgenograms may show increased porosity of bone, cortical thinning, vertebral compression, and spontaneous pathologic fractures. Patients with alcohol-induced liver disease may also have exocrine pancreatic insufficiency. Accordingly, pancreatic function should be evaluated in patients with liver disease and malabsorption.

TABLE 240-5   Classification of the malabsorption syndromes

I Inadequate digestion
  A Postgastrectomy steatorrhea*
  B Deficiency or inactivation of pancreatic lipase
    1 Exocrine pancreatic insufficiency
      a Chronic pancreatitis
      b Pancreatic carcinoma
      c Cystic fibrosis
      d Pancreatic resection
    2 Ulcerogenic tumor of the pancreas (Zollinger-Ellison syndrome, gastrinoma)*
II Reduced intestinal bile salt concentration (with impaired micelle formation)
  A Liver disease
    1 Parenchymal liver disease
    2 Cholestasis (intrahepatic or extrahepatic)
  B Abnormal bacterial proliferation in the small bowel
    1 Afferent loop stasis
    2 Strictures
    3 Fistulas
    4 Blind loops
    5 Multiple diverticula of the small bowel
    6 Hypomotility states (diabetes, scleroderma, intestinal pseudoobstruction)
  C Interrupted enterohepatic circulation of bile salts
    1 Ileal resection
    2 Ileal inflammatory disease (regional ileitis)
  D Drugs (by sequestration or precipitation of bile salts)
    1 Neomycin
    2 Calcium carbonate
    3 Cholestyramine
III Inadequate absorptive surface
  A Intestinal resection or bypass
    1 Mesenteric vascular disease with massive intestinal resection
    2 Regional enteritis with multiple bowel resections
    3 Jejunoileal bypass
  B Gastroileostomy (inadvertent)
IV Lymphatic obstruction
  A Intestinal lymphangiectasia
  B Whipple's disease*
  C Lymphoma
V Cardiovascular disorders
  A Constrictive pericarditis
  B Congestive heart failure
  C Mesenteric vascular insufficiency
  D Vasculitis
VI Primary mucosal absorptive defects
  A Inflammatory or infiltrative disorders
    1 Regional enteritis*
    2 Amyloidosis
    3 Scleroderma*
    4 Lymphoma*
    5 Radiation enteritis
    6 Eosinophilic enteritis
    7 Tropical sprue
    8 Infectious enteritis (e.g., salmonellosis)
    9 Collagenous sprue
    10 Nonspecific ulcerative jejunitis
    11 Mastocytosis
    12 Dermatologic disorders (e.g., dermatitis herpetiformis)
  B Biochemical or genetic abnormalities
    1 Nontropical sprue (gluten-induced enteropathy); celiac sprue
    2 Disaccharidase deficiency
    3 Hypogammaglobulinemia
    4 Abetalipoproteinemia
    5 Hartnup disease
    6 Cystinuria
    7 Monosaccharide malabsorption
VII Endocrine and metabolic disorders
  A Diabetes mellitus*
  B Hypoparathyroidism
  C Adrenal insufficiency
  D Hyperthyroidism
  E Ulcerogenic tumor of the pancreas (Zollinger-Ellison syndrome, gastrinoma)*
  F Carcinoid syndrome

* Malabsorption caused by multiple defects.

Postgastrectomy malabsorption   The presence of a malabsorption syndrome has been documented frequently in patients after subtotal gastrectomy. Steatorrhea is more common with a Billroth II than a Billroth I type of anastomosis. Usually the fat loss is minimal, ranging from 7 to 10 g per 24 h. Patients with gross steatorrhea usually have impaired intraluminal fat digestion due to several factors: (1) With a Billroth II anastomosis the duodenum is bypassed, and

there is a decreased entry of stomach contents into the proximal duodenum (i.e., afferent loop). This leads to a decreased stimulus for the release of *secretin* and *cholecystokinin-pancreozymin* from the duodenum and may result in a depressed pancreatic enzyme response. (2) There may be *inadequate mixing* of the pancreatic enzymes and bile salts secreted into the proximal duodenum with the gastric contents entering the jejunum. (3) There may be *stasis* of intestinal contents in the afferent loop, resulting in abnormal bacterial proliferation in the proximal small bowel. This in turn may lead to abnormalities in bile salt metabolism (see "Malabsorption Due to Bacterial Overgrowth of the Small Bowel, Pathophysiology" below). (4) The presence of maldigestion may lead to *protein depletion*, which in turn may produce further impairment in pancreatic function. (5) The *loss of the reservoir function of the stomach* may result in decreased intestinal transit time. Perhaps the most important factor is rapid gastric emptying, which results in low luminal concentrations of digestive secretions for the first 60 to 80 min after a meal. Such a disorder has been described in patients with subtotal gastrectomy and duodenostomy (Billroth I), gastrojejunostomy (Billroth II), and truncal vagotomy and pyloroplasty (V&P). That gastric emptying rates are somewhat slower in patients with V&P may account for the overall less severe nutritional deficiencies in such patients. In some patients treatment with pancreatic enzymes may lead to significant improvement. Specimens of duodenal or jejunal fluid should be obtained for culture of both aerobic and anaerobic organisms and appropriate antibiotic therapy instituted if there is evidence of abnormal bacterial overgrowth (colony count of greater than 10^7 per milliliter of jejunal fluid). Because the duodenum is the principal site of absorption of iron and calcium, in patients with a Billroth II anastomosis impaired absorption of calcium and iron may also develop. Occult metabolic bone disease occurs frequently in this setting.

INADEQUATE ABSORPTIVE SURFACE (SHORT BOWEL SYNDROME)   Extensive intestinal resection often results in the short bowel syndrome. The most common disorders resulting in short bowel syndrome are (1) massive intestinal resection following a vascular insult to the small intestine, (2) regional enteritis with multiple bowel resections, and (3) jejunoileal bypass for morbid obesity. In general, the absorption of nutrients will be influenced by the extent and site of small bowel resected, the presence of the ileocecal valve, and adaptation of the remaining small bowel. Resection of 40 to 50 percent of the small bowel is usually well tolerated, provided the proximal duodenum, the distal half of the ileum, and the ileocecal valve are spared. By contrast, resection of the ileum and the ileocecal valve alone may induce severe diarrhea and malabsorption, even though less than 30 percent of the small intestine is resected.

Several measures are important in the management of short bowel syndrome: (1) The diet should contain at least 2500 kcal and consist primarily of carbohydrate and protein with fat restricted to less than 40 g per day. A fat-restricted diet is effective in reducing diarrhea, presumably because there is decreased production of hydroxy fatty acids from long-chain fats. Such hydroxy fatty acids, in essence, are cathartics and increase net secretion of water and electrolytes by the colon as well as the small bowel. (2) It is often necessary to provide vitamin and mineral supplements, which usually include K^+, Cl^-, Mg^{2+}, Ca^{2+}, trace metals (Zn, Cd, Mn), iron, folate, vitamin B_{12}, other vitamins (A, D, E, K, B_1, B_2, B_6, biotin), and essential fatty acids. (3) Specific drugs (for example, belladonna alkaloids, diphenoxylate, loperamide, and codeine), which decrease intestinal motility and prolong mucosal contact time, are helpful in controlling diarrhea. These agents also decrease ileostomy outputs. (4) A bile salt–sequestering agent such as cholestyramine blunts the effects of bile salts, which stimulate net secretion of water and electrolytes by the colon. (5) Patients with short-bowel syndrome may have gastric acid hypersecretion, which is often transient, and which results in dilution of pancreatic secretions as well as inactivation of pancreatic enzymes. Under these conditions, a histamine H-2 receptor antagonist is useful because it will suppress gastric acid secretion and decrease the volume of fluid entering the proximal small bowel, thus leading to an increased concentration of pancreatic enzymes. In addition, supplemental pancreatic enzyme therapy may be required. (6) A bypassed colon can be used to receive infusions of fluid and electrolytes since a portion of the colon can still absorb 1000 to 1500 mL fluid per day. Finally, (7) total parenteral nutrition is frequently required during the first 6 months after massive intestinal resection until some degree of adaptation has occurred. Such patients may also require long-term parenteral hyperalimentation with a silicone rubber catheter in the superior vena cava, and this can be done at home.

For a discussion of regional enteritis see Chap. 241.

MALABSORPTION DUE TO BACTERIAL OVERGROWTH OF THE SMALL BOWEL The proximal small intestine is usually bacteriologically sterile because of three factors: (1) the acid milieu of the stomach; (2) intestinal peristalsis, which sweeps bacteria to the distal small bowel; and (3) secretion into the lumen of the intestine of immunoglobulins, which may serve as coproantibodies. When bacteria are isolated from the upper small bowel, they are frequently contaminants transported from the mouth and upper respiratory tract, and the colony count rarely exceeds 10^4 per milliliter of jejunal fluid. The major mechanism limiting the growth of bacteria in the small intestine is normal peristalsis. Any disorder leading to impaired intestinal motility may result in abnormal stasis of intestinal contents with ineffective mechanical cleansing of bacteria. This in turn may lead to abnormal bacterial proliferation and malabsorption. Several malabsorptive disorders have been associated with bacterial overgrowth of the small bowel, and these are listed in Table 240-6.

Pathophysiology Bacterial overgrowth may result in changes in bile salt metabolism, and these are believed directly and indirectly to account for the steatorrhea. First, bacteria (especially anaerobic gram-positive bacteria) may lead to the intraluminal deconjugation of bile salts with a consequent production of free bile acids. In contrast to conjugated bile salts, unconjugated bile salts may be absorbed in the proximal small bowel by nonionic diffusion, resulting in decreased intraluminal concentrations of bile salts in the jejunum. Second, the decreased bile salt concentrations, the increase of unconjugated bile salts, and the decrease of the conjugated salts all serve to contribute to impaired intraluminal micelle formation and hence fat malabsorption. In addition to abnormalities in bile salt metabolism, intestinal mucosal lesions have been demonstrated in patients with intestinal stasis. Such lesions are often patchy in distribution, and the histologic appearance ranges in severity from minimal changes in villous architecture to severe lesions with virtual absence of villi. The etiology of these lesions is unclear; possible causes include damage caused by bacterial invasion, bacterial toxins, or metabolic products such as unconjugated bile salts. In this regard, certain bacteria such as *Bacteroides* elaborate proteases which solubilize brush border proteins and destroy disaccharidases such as sucrase and maltase. The impaired absorption of vitamin B_{12} is not related to the disturbed bile salt metabolism but appears to be due to uptake of vitamin B_{12} by microorganisms.

Many of the above abnormalities in bile salt metabolism may be reversed by appropriate antibiotic therapy. When such treatment is instituted, unconjugated bile salts in the jejunal fluid decrease, an increase in the micellar lipid phase will occur, and steatorrhea diminishes or disappears. In addition, significant improvement in the absorption of vitamin B_{12} will occur with broad-spectrum antibiotics such as tetracycline.

Clinical manifestations Breath tests, i.e., tests with [^{14}C]-labeled bile acid, [^{14}C]xylose, and lactulose, are useful screening tests for malabsorption syndrome due to abnormal bacterial overgrowth of the small intestine. A definitive diagnosis is established by demonstrating larger numbers of microorganisms (greater than 10^5 per milliliter) and a polymicrobial flora in cultures of duodenal or jejunal fluid. Other clinical features include the following: (1) steatorrhea of a moderate degree, usually in the range of 15 to 30 g fecal fat per 24 h; (2) macrocytic anemia with a megaloblastic bone marrow; (3) impaired absorption of vitamin B_{12} which is not corrected by intrinsic factor; and (4) correction of steatorrhea and impaired vitamin B_{12} absorption by antibiotic therapy. Absorption of D-xylose, peroral small-intestinal biopsy specimens, and other tests of absorptive function (Table 240-2) may be normal in these patients. A single course or intermittent courses (2 to 3 weeks per month) of therapy with antibiotics such as tetracycline, ampicillin, or trimethoprim-sulfamethoxazole are usually given.

Chronic intestinal pseudoobstruction (See also Chap. 243) Chronic intestinal pseudoobstruction is a heterogeneous syndrome with a variety of causes (Table 240-7). Primary or idiopathic intestinal pseudoobstruction is a chronic illness characterized by recurrent episodes of intestinal obstruction in which all known causes of mechanical obstruction and other illnesses known to produce intestinal pseudoobstruction have been excluded. In addition to abnormalities in small-bowel motility, derangements in esophageal, gastric, and colonic motility have also been described. The primary clinical manifestations are nausea and vomiting, abdominal pain, distention, constipation, diarrhea, and urinary tract symptoms. Patients typically exhibit prolonged transit of chyme along the gastrointestinal tract, especially the small bowel where pressure activity patterns are markedly disordered. Oral cisapride accelerates gastric emptying, normalizes intestinal transit, and improves propulsive small-bowel activity in patients with pseudoobstruction. Malabsorption, secondary to stasis of intestinal contents with resultant abnormal bacterial proliferation in the small bowel, is frequently present.

TABLE 240-6 Causes of intestinal bacterial overgrowth (intestinal colonization)

I Structural abnormalities producing stasis of intestinal contents
  A Multiple small-bowel diverticula
  B Strictures
    1 Regional enteritis*
    2 Radiation enteritis*
    3 Occlusive vascular disease; vasculitis
  C Billroth II subtotal gastrectomy with afferent loop stasis*
  D Multiple laparotomies resulting in adhesions and partial small-bowel obstruction
II Fistulas
  A Gastrocolic, gastroileal, jejunoileal, jejunocolic
III Motor abnormalities resulting in intestinal hypomotility
  A Scleroderma*
  B Amyloidosis*
  C Diabetes mellitus*
  D Hypothyroidism
  E Vagotomy
  F Intestinal pseudoobstruction (see Table 240-7)
IV Miscellaneous
  A Hypogammaglobulinemia*
  B Nodular lymphoid hyperplasia
  C Pernicious anemia
  D Pancreatic insufficiency
V No underlying disorder detected

* Multiple mechanisms may contribute to malabsorption in these disorders

---

TABLE 240-7 Causes of chronic intestinal pseudoobstruction

I Primary: Idiopathic
II Secondary
  A Collagen vascular disease
    1 Scleroderma
    2 Dermatomyositis/polymyositis
    3 Systemic lupus erythematosus
  B Amyloidosis
  C Endocrine disorders
    1 Myxedema
    2 Diabetes mellitus
  D Neurologic diseases
    1 Chagas' disease
  E Others
    1 Jejunoileal bypass
    2 Jejunal diverticulosis
    3 Drugs (tricyclic antidepressants, clonidine, etc.)

Tropical sprue   Tropical sprue is a malabsorptive disorder of unknown cause affecting residents of or visitors to tropical regions. Both epidemic and endemic forms of the disease have been recognized. Tropical sprue may have its onset months or even years after a patient has returned from the tropics. The etiology of the disorder has not been elucidated, but it might well result from one or more of the following: (1) a nutritional deficiency, (2) a transmissible infectious microorganism, and (3) a toxin elaborated by a microorganism or contained in the diet. It is of interest that coliform organisms, shown to produce an enterotoxin causing fluid secretion, have been isolated from the jejunum of tropical sprue patients but not from other patients with bacterial overgrowth of the proximal small bowel. Anorexia, diarrhea, weight loss, symptoms of anemia, sequelae of nutritional deficiency (Table 240-4), and abdominal distention are common findings. Patients are frequently deficient in iron as well as vitamin B_{12} and folate. Laboratory studies usually reveal anemia (megaloblastic in 60 percent of cases) and impaired absorption of fat, xylose, and vitamin B_{12}. Malabsorption of at least two nutrients is considered essential for the diagnosis. Jejunal biopsy classically reveals shortened and thickened villi, increased crypt depth, and increased infiltration of mononuclear cells in the lamina propria and epithelium (Table 240-3). However, these biopsy findings are not specific, and the lesion may be patchy; in addition, interpretation is difficult because "control" biopsies from asymptomatic residents in the same tropical region are often considered abnormal when compared with normal biopsies from patients in temperate zones. Such histologic findings have been termed *tropical jejunitis*. Treatment with vitamin B_{12}, folate, and antibiotics have all been effective in inducing a remission. A short course, i.e., 2 to 4 weeks, of therapy with a sulfonamide or tetracycline is usually given. Occasional patients require more prolonged antibiotic therapy.

Scleroderma   Although there are numerous reports of small-intestinal involvement in scleroderma, frank malabsorption has been reported infrequently. It has been suggested that malabsorption may be due to several factors: (1) lymphatic obstruction; (2) reduced arterial blood supply to the gut; (3) impaired intestinal motility leading to relative stasis of intestinal contents and hence bacterial overgrowth; and (4) involvement of the intestinal wall by the disease. At present there is little evidence to support the first two postulated mechanisms. In some cases abnormal bacterial proliferation in the upper small bowel has been documented, and in these patients antibiotic therapy has resulted in decrease in steatorrhea, gain in weight, and increased absorption of vitamin B_{12}. In the intestinal wall there may also be extensive deposition of collagen, especially in the muscular mucosa, submucosa, and muscularis externa, with significant muscle atrophy. Studies of duodenal myoelectric activity in scleroderma revealed normal slow-wave frequency and propagation velocity but decreased excitability of the bowel to mechanical stimuli such as distention and humoral stimuli such as pentagastrin and secretin. This motor dysfunction may be an important factor in the dilatation, atony, and stasis of intestinal contents in scleroderma.

Malabsorption in the acquired immunodeficiency syndrome   Diarrhea and weight loss occur frequently in patients with the acquired immunodeficiency syndrome (AIDS). These symptoms are often due to enteric infections or small-intestinal Kaposi's sarcoma. However, such symptoms can be due to malabsorption, which has been well-documented in patients with AIDS in whom identifiable enteric infections and intestinal involvement with Kaposi's sarcoma have been excluded. The presence of malabsorption in these patients has been documented by steatorrhea and abnormal D-xylose absorption tests. Serum zinc levels may be decreased. In addition, small-bowel biopsy specimens have revealed dense infiltration of mononuclear cells and histiocytes. Microorganisms have also been identified in the mucosa.

DISORDERS ASSOCIATED WITH LYMPHATIC OBSTRUCTION
Whipple's disease   This is a rare disorder characterized clinically by arthralgia, abdominal pain, diarrhea, progressive weight loss, dilated lacteals in the bowel wall, and impaired intestinal absorption.

Wasting, low-grade fever, increased skin pigmentation, and peripheral lymphadenopathy are frequently present. In addition, central nervous system manifestations including confusion, memory loss, focal cranial nerve signs, nystagmus, and ophthalmoplegia may be present. Laboratory examination usually reveals the presence of steatorrhea, impaired xylose absorption, abnormal small-bowel x-rays, hypoalbuminemia, and anemia. Hypoalbuminemia is due to excessive loss of serum albumin into the gastrointestinal tract as well as impaired synthesis of albumin.

The diagnosis is established by demonstrating the presence in the mucosa of macrophages containing large cytoplasmic granules which give a brilliant magenta stain with the periodic acid Schiff reagent (PAS). Such macrophages may also be seen in other tissues such as lymph nodes, spleen, or liver. The finding of PAS-positive macrophages in the lamina propria is not specific for Whipple's disease, but virtual replacement of most cellular elements in the lamina propria by these macrophages has been seen only in this disorder. In addition to the PAS-positive macrophages, jejunal biopsies frequently show dilated lymphatics and some degree of blunting of the intestinal mucosal villi.

Electron-microscopic studies have revealed the presence of rod-shaped structures (or bacilliform bodies) 0.3 by 1.5 to 2.5 μm within and adjacent to the macrophages in the lamina propria as well as within epithelial cells and polymorphonuclear leukocytes. The ultrastructural features of these bacilliform bodies suggest that they are microorganisms. It is of particular interest that after treatment of the patient with antibiotics the bacilliform bodies decrease or disappear together with a decrease in the number of PAS-positive macrophages. In addition, the reappearance of the bacteria often heralds the onset of a clinical relapse after antibiotics have been withdrawn.

Whipple's disease at one time was thought to be invariably fatal. However, it is now clear that therapy with antibiotics will usually induce a clinical remission. In a few cases there has been complete reversal of the histologic abnormalities in the jejunal mucosa, and some of these cases have been followed for 10 years. Patients with Whipple's disease should be treated with antibiotics such as trimethoprim-sulfamethoxazole for at least 1 year. Treatment with tetracycline alone or penicillin alone is not adequate initial therapy; relapse rates with these drugs are approximately 40 percent. The most important parameter for following the disease and predicting its course is the presence or absence of bacilli in sections of small-bowel biopsies.

Intestinal lymphoma   Steatorrhea is a manifestation of *primary* intestinal lymphoma. The disease occurs predominantly in men, and the mean age of onset of symptoms is about 50 years. The diagnosis should be suspected in patients with malabsorption with the following findings: (1) a malabsorption syndrome in which clinical and biopsy features resemble those of nontropical sprue but in which there is an incomplete response to a gluten-free diet, (2) the presence of *abdominal pain* and *fever*, and (3) signs and symptoms of intestinal obstruction. The usual stigmata of generalized lymphoma are frequently absent. Hepatomegaly, splenomegaly, palpable abdominal masses, and peripheral adenopathy are usually not found. Lymphangiography and CT scanning may reveal abnormal intraabdominal nodes. The diagnosis can be established by laparotomy and often may be made by thorough examination of multiple mucosal biopsy specimens obtained perorally. There may be a total absence of villi or lesser degrees of blunting and shortening of the villi. In contrast to nontropical sprue, the lamina propria is usually massively infiltrated with lymphoid cells. Malignancy may be diagnosed by demonstrating lymphoid cells with the cytologic features of malignancy, the presence of reticulum cells outside germinal centers, and infiltration and destruction of crypts by pleomorphic lymphoid cells. Some patients elaborate or secrete a fragment of the heavy chain of IgA immunoglobulins (α-*chain disease*). The latter is probably a variant of intestinal lymphoma.

The mechanism of malabsorption in intestinal lymphoma may be related to several factors: (1) diffuse involvement of the small-intestinal mucosa; (2) involvement of the bowel wall with lymphatic obstruction; and (3) localized stenosis with stasis of intestinal contents and bacterial overgrowth. It should be emphasized that it is often difficult, by clinical and morphologic features alone, to distinguish nontropical sprue from intestinal lymphoma. Indeed, there is evidence to suggest that lymphoma may develop as a late complication of nontropical sprue.

The course of intestinal lymphoma has ranged from 4 months to 4 years from the onset of symptoms. Perforation, bleeding, and intestinal obstruction are common terminal complications. There is insufficient evidence to determine whether radiation therapy, chemotherapy, or localized surgical resection modify the natural course of the disease.

CARDIOVASCULAR DISORDERS Steatorrhea has been described in patients with chronic congestive heart failure, superior mesenteric artery insufficiency, and constrictive pericarditis. Abnormal dilated mucosal lymphatics and excessive enteric loss of protein have been demonstrated in patients with constrictive pericarditis. The mechanism of steatorrhea in patients with chronic heart failure remains uncertain. It might be due to congestion and edema of the mucosa, mucosal hypoxia, or abnormalities in pancreatic function. Although pronounced steatorrhea is uncommon in congestive heart failure, these patients are frequently anorectic, and a low fat intake could mask a latent steatorrhea. Steatorrhea is quite infrequent in patients with vasculitis and is thought to be due to segmental infarction of the small bowel in addition to intestinal ischemia.

DEFECTS IN MUCOSAL FUNCTION

INFLAMMATORY OR INFILTRATIVE DISORDERS Regional enteritis The clinical features of regional enteritis are described in Chap. 241. Malabsorption in regional enteritis may result from several factors: (1) interruption of the enterohepatic circulation of bile salts by ileal disease or resection; (2) deconjugation of bile salts due to bacterial overgrowth, in turn related to strictures and/or fistulas; (3) active inflammatory bowel disease causing impaired mucosal cell function; (4) inadequate absorptive surface resulting from intestinal resection or fistulas; and (5) severe protein depletion producing impaired exocrine pancreatic function. Active ileal disease and/or ileal resection resulting in an interrupted enterohepatic circulation of and deficiency of conjugated bile salts appears to be the major factor responsible for steatorrhea as well as impaired absorption of vitamin B_{12}. Small-bowel absorptive function has been correlated with the extent of ileal disease or resection. When the length of ileal dysfunction exceeds 90 to 100 cm, virtually all patients will have steatorrhea and vitamin B_{12} malabsorption. After intestinal resection, the functional capacity of the remaining small bowel will depend on the site and extent of resection as well as the presence of residual inflammatory disease. Massive intestinal resection usually results in impaired absorption of all food constituents. When the malabsorption is due to strictures and blind loops as a result of previous surgical therapy, antibiotic therapy may be helpful, but surgical removal of these areas is usually necessary for long-term improvement. With diffuse inflammatory disease a florid malabsorption syndrome may occur with steatorrhea, hypocalcemia, impaired vitamin B_{12} absorption, and hypoalbuminemia due to increased enteric protein loss. Treatment with sulfasalazine and glucocorticoids drugs may be beneficial (see Chap. 241).

After *ileal resection*, patients frequently have bothersome diarrhea. This appears to be due to *interruption of the enterohepatic circulation* whereby increased amounts of bile salts reach the colon, where they interfere with water and electrolyte absorption and thus have a cathartic effect. The *bile salt–induced diarrhea* after ileal resection may respond to treatment with cholestyramine, an exchange resin which binds bile salts and causes them to lose their biochemical effect on the bowel. Patients with ileal resection of less than 100 cm and fecal fat excretion less than 20 g per day show the best symptomatic response to cholestyramine.

Chronic nongranulomatous ulcerative jejunoileitis This disorder is characterized by abdominal pain, weight loss, fever, diarrhea, steatorrhea, hypoalbuminemia, and protein-losing enteropathy. Clinical features mimic those found in both regional enteritis and celiac sprue. Indeed, the intestinal lesion may be indistinguishable from celiac sprue. However, exclusion of gluten from the diet does not result in any benefit. Glucocorticoid treatment has resulted in transient improvement, but long-term effects are unpredictable.

Amyloidosis This disorder is discussed in detail in Chap. 266.

Radiation injury to the small bowel Extensive morphologic damage of the small-intestinal mucosa often follows normal or excessive abdominal irradiation. These changes include a decrease in crypt mitoses, marked shortening of the villi, megalocytosis of epithelial cells, and inflammatory cell infiltration of the lamina propria. This may be associated with transient diarrhea and impaired intestinal absorption. However, restoration of normal intestinal architecture is usually complete within 2 weeks after cessation of therapy. Persistent diarrhea and malabsorption may develop shortly after x-ray therapy, or there may be a latent period of several years before the onset of diarrhea. Steatorrhea, ranging from 10 to 40 g per day, has been frequently observed, but impaired absorption of calcium, iron, D-xylose, or vitamin B_{12} is less common. In some patients intestinal strictures due to vasculopathy and ischemia may develop following irradiation, and thus stasis of intestinal contents and abnormal bacterial proliferation may occur. In others, intestinal lymphangiectasia, presumably due to lymphatic obstruction, has been documented. Diarrhea and malabsorption may be refractory to all methods of management. Treatment with antibiotics, pancreatic enzymes, gluten-free diet, adrenal glucocorticoids, and opiates has met with but limited success.

Eosinophilic enteritis Eosinophilic gastroenteritis is a disorder of the stomach, small bowel, and colon of unknown etiology characterized by peripheral blood eosinophilia and eosinophilic infiltration of the gut wall but without evidence of vasculitis. The clinical manifestations, usually recurrent, are protean and relate to the site of gastrointestinal tract involvement. Three main patterns have been identified: (1) Predominant mucosal disease manifested by iron-deficiency anemia, hypoalbuminemia due to protein-losing enteropathy, and mild steatorrhea. Patients in this group often present with a malabsorption syndrome and a history of intolerance to specific foods. (2) Predominant muscle layer disease characterized by marked thickening and rigidity of the stomach and proximal small bowel with obstructive symptoms and radiologic features of pyloric narrowing and obstruction. The obstructive form of eosinophilic gastroenteritis accounts for half of the cases reported since 1970. Accordingly, eosinophilic enteritis should be considered in the differential diagnosis of gastric outlet obstruction, diffuse small-bowel disease, and ileocolitis. Indeed, eosinophilic enteritis often mimics regional enteritis. (3) Predominant subserosal disease in which the cardinal manifestation is ascites with marked eosinophilia in the ascitic fluid. Although the above classification based on tissue layer of major involvement is useful in understanding the principal manifestations, it should be emphasized that multiple clinical forms, e.g., ascites (serosal involvement) and obstruction (muscular involvement), also occur.

Previous reports have emphasized food allergy and mucosal features of this disease. However, food sensitivity is related to symptoms in less than 20 percent of patients. In such patients fasting serum IgE levels are often elevated, and challenge with offending foods frequently evokes symptoms of abdominal pain and diarrhea in addition to a marked increase in serum IgE levels. In most patients with eosinophilic enteritis, however, immunologic studies including serum immunoglobulins, serum complement, lymphocyte quantitation, and lymphocyte response to nonspecific mitogens reveal no abnormalities. Thus, both IgE-mediated and IgE-dependent mechanisms may be operative in different patients with eosinophilic gastroenteritis. Several nonreaginic factors influence peripheral blood and tissue eosinophilia. It seems clear that evidence of allergy or food sensitivity is often absent and is not required for the diagnosis of eosinophilic enteritis. In addition, even in patients with food allergies, elimination diets are frequently ineffective and such patients may require prolonged glucocorticoid therapy to remain well. Surgical treatment for relief of obstructive symptoms and glucocorticoids are the mainstays of therapy.

Dermatitis and malabsorption   A malabsorption syndrome, usually mild, has been reported in patients with a variety of dermatologic disorders, including psoriasis, eczematoid dermatitis, and dermatitis herpetiformis. Proximal intestinal mucosal abnormalities are almost invariably found in patients with dermatitis herpetiformis. In one study 21 of 22 patients had lesions ranging in severity from a completely "flat" to an almost normal intestinal mucosa. The mucosal lesions were often patchy in distribution. Clinical and laboratory evidence of significant malabsorption was infrequent, possibly due to the limited length of small intestine involved in this skin disorder. While the skin lesions of dermatitis herpetiformis respond to sulfone, the gut lesions do not. By contrast, in some patients with blunted and flattened intestinal mucosal lesions, and steatorrhea, there may be a striking improvement in villous architecture and regression of steatorrhea after withdrawal of gluten from the diet without improvement in the skin lesions. Further, in patients with dermatitis herpetiformis and a morphologically normal small-intestinal mucosa, administration of a high-gluten diet may result in blunted and flattened mucosal lesions indistinguishable from those of nontropical sprue. As in the latter disease, an increased frequency of HLA-A1 and HLA-B8 are also seen. These observations raise the interesting question as to whether certain patients with dermatitis herpetiformis and a malabsorption syndrome have latent nontropical sprue.

BIOCHEMICAL OR GENETIC ABNORMALITIES Nontropical sprue   Nontropical sprue is a disorder characterized by malabsorption, abnormal small-bowel structure, and intolerance to gluten, a protein found in wheat and wheat products. It has been appropriately referred to as *gluten-induced enteropathy.* Celiac disease in children and nontropical sprue of the adult are probably one and the same disorder with the same pathogenesis.

There are insufficient data to provide an accurate estimation of the incidence of nontropical sprue in any population. This is largely because the severity of the disease varies greatly and individuals may have typical mucosal change and yet have no overt symptoms. Seventy percent of the cases in most reported series are women. The incidence in siblings appears to be many times higher than that in the general population, and it has been suggested that sprue may be inherited through a dominant gene of incomplete penetrance. Celiac sprue patients have an increased frequency of serum histocompatibility antigens, particularly of the HLA-B8 and HLA-Dw3 types. The HLA-B8 phenotype has been found in 85 to 90 percent of sprue patients as compared with 20 to 25 percent in normal subjects. The HLA-B8 antigen may be linked to immune response genes which may determine the immunologic recognition of certain substances. It has been suggested that such genetic factors may predispose to immunologic tolerance of dietary proteins such as the peptides in gluten or to the production of pathogenic antigluten antibodies which could result in binding of gluten to epithelial cells with subsequent tissue damage.

PATHOPHYSIOLOGY   Gluten and the related substance gliadin are high-molecular-weight proteins found especially in wheat. These proteins, as well as the larger peptide hydrolysis products (containing glutamine), are toxic when administered to patients with sprue in remission. The exact mechanism for this effect is not clear, but two theories have been proposed, namely, a "toxic" and an immunologic theory. One possible mechanism is that patients with sprue lack a specific mucosal peptidase, so that gluten or its larger glutamine-containing peptides are not effectively hydrolyzed to smaller peptides (i.e., dipeptides or amino acids). As a consequence "toxic" peptides might accumulate in the mucosa. It has been demonstrated that patients with sprue in remission will develop steatorrhea and typical mucosal changes when they are given gluten. Similar results will occur with the administration of peptide hydrolysates containing at least eight amino acids with a terminal glutamine residue. It has

been shown that when gluten is instilled into the *ileum* of sprue patients, histologic changes begin to occur within hours. This does not occur in the *upper jejunum,* suggesting that the effect is immediate and local rather than systemic. After noxious gluten fractions damage surface absorptive cells, the damaged cells are sloughed rapidly from the mucosal surface into the gut lumen. To compensate for this, cell proliferation increases, crypts undergo hypertrophy, and cell migration accelerates to replace the damaged and sloughed epithelial cells. This more rapid than normal epithelial cell renewal can be reversed by a gluten-free diet. The intestinal mucosa of patients with sprue shows many enzyme alterations, including decreased levels of disaccharidases, alkaline phosphatase, and peptide hydrolases, as well as impaired ability to digest gluten peptides. However, these abnormalities usually revert toward normal after successful treatment with a gluten-free diet. There is additional evidence supporting the concept of toxicity of gluten and gluten breakdown products in sprue. First, gliadin, especially the A-gliadin moiety, is toxic to sprue mucosa maintained in organ culture, causing ultrastructural changes and depression of disaccharidase activity. Second, sprue mucosa hydrolyzes a specific fraction of a gliadin digest (i.e., fraction 9) in a defective manner, and fraction 9 is selectively toxic to sprue mucosa. Third, specific fractions of gluten fed to sprue patients cause transient alterations in mucosal histology and depression of disaccharidase activity, but full recovery is observed in 72 h. The rapid onset of these changes and prompt recovery are consistent with a direct toxic effect. Despite intensive study, however, no persistent, specific, or selective peptidase deficiency has been demonstrated.

It has also been suggested that gluten or gluten metabolites may initiate an *immunologic reaction* in the intestinal mucosa. The presence of a mononuclear inflammatory cell infiltrate in the lamina propria of the mucosa, the beneficial response to glucocorticoid drugs, the finding of abnormal antibodies to gliadin in the serum of sprue patients, the synthesis of increased amounts of antigliadin antibody by sprue mucosa maintained in organ culture, and the elaboration of lymphokines such as migration inhibitory factor (MIF) by sprue mucosa incubated with gliadin have all been cited as evidence in support of this hypothesis. However, the evidence indicating that an abnormal (immune) mechanism is important in initiating or perpetuating this disease process remains to be determined.

A possible role for adenovirus serotype 12 (Ad12) in the pathogenesis of celiac sprue has been proposed based on two observations: (1) homology of amino acid sequences between a portion of A-gliadin and a viral-encoded protein (E1b) produced by Ad12; and (2) patients with untreated celiac sprue have a much higher frequency of antibodies to Ad12 compared to treated celiac patients and controls. These observations are in accord with the hypothesis that there must be an *environmental* factor as well as a *genetic predisposition* to explain why only certain people develop celiac sprue.

Jejunal biopsy specimens from patients with nontropical sprue usually show a characteristic lesion. There is blunting and flattening of the mucosal surface, with villi either absent or broad and short. The crypts are elongated, and there is generally a dense infiltration of inflammatory cells in the lamina propria. The surface epithelium is altered with a sparse brush border, cuboidal rather than the normal columnar cells, and infiltration of inflammatory cells in the epithelial layer. These changes are usually most severe in the proximal small bowel, presumably because this area of the bowel is exposed to the highest gluten concentration. The typical morphologic changes illustrated in Fig. 240-4 are characteristic of nontropical sprue but are not specific. Similar changes have been described in other conditions, including lymphoma, tropical sprue, and hypogammaglobulinemia associated with malabsorption. Many biochemical abnormalities have been demonstrated in mucosal biopsy specimens from nontropical sprue patients. Impaired esterification of fatty acids to triglycerides, decreased uptake of amino acids, and decreased activity of intestinal disaccharidases (especially lactase) have been well documented. The latter observation may account for the high incidence of milk intolerance in untreated sprue patients or those in relapse. However, the greater abundance of undifferentiated crypt cells may be important, since crypt cells normally have a lower capacity for nutrient uptake than do villus cells.

Since the mucosa is damaged and altered in patients with nontropical sprue, there may be *decreased release of pancreato-tropic hormones* (secretin and cholecystokinin, i.e., CCK). This results in decreased stimulation of the pancreas with lower than normal intraluminal levels of pancreatic enzymes in response to a meal. In addition, the gallbladder appears to be resistant to the action of cholecystokinin, resulting in absent or minimal contractions of the gallbladder, in turn leading to sequestration of bile salts in an inert gallbladder. These two defects may result in impaired intraluminal digestion of fat and protein, which will be superimposed on the defect in intestinal transport caused by a damaged mucosa.

Diarrhea is common in sprue patients and is due to a number of factors, including *impaired absorption* of salt and water by duodenum and jejunum, net *secretion* of water and electrolytes by an abnormally permeable jejunal mucosa, and net colonic secretion of water and electrolytes induced by unabsorbed fatty acids and hydroxy fatty acids. However, the distal small intestine in sprue has the ability to adapt to the damage and loss of absorptive capacity in the proximal small intestine. Indeed, increased ileal absorption of sodium, chloride, and water has been demonstrated in sprue patients.

CLINICAL FEATURES   Most patients with nontropical sprue will have a typical malabsorption syndrome characterized by weight loss, abdominal distention and bloating, diarrhea, steatorrhea, and abnormal tests of absorptive function. The characteristic alterations in tests of intestinal absorption are outlined in Table 240-2. It should be emphasized, however, that some sprue patients may present with isolated abnormalities which initially do not suggest the diagnosis of nontropical sprue. Thus, a patient may be admitted for investigation of iron-deficiency anemia without apparent blood loss or of abnormal bleeding due to hypoprothrombinemia but may not have diarrhea or overt steatorrhea. Likewise, sprue patients may present with puzzling metabolic bone disease without diarrhea or steatorrhea. Such patients usually complain of bone pain and tenderness and frequently are found to have extensive demineralization of bone, compression deformities, kyphoscoliosis, and Milkman's fractures. Emotional disturbances are common in these patients, and many individuals with a diagnosis of weight loss initially considered related to severe anxiety and depression are subsequently found to have nontropical sprue. In each of the above clinical settings, the diagnosis of sprue should be considered in the differential diagnosis.

Since there is no specific diagnostic test, three criteria should be met in order to establish a definite diagnosis of nontropical sprue: (1) evidence of malabsorption; (2) an abnormal small-bowel (jejunal) biopsy showing blunting and flattening of the villi along with changes in the surface epithelium; and (3) clinical, biochemical, and histologic improvement after institution of a gluten-free diet. In equivocal cases, the patient can be challenged with 30 to 50 g gluten orally, and if this promptly results in increased diarrhea and steatorrhea, the diagnosis of gluten-induced enteropathy is established. It should be emphasized that tests of intestinal absorption may reveal abnormalities which range from very minimal alterations to severe changes. Abnormalities in absorption tests have been shown to correlate reasonably well with the length of small-bowel involvement and to a lesser extent with the severity of the proximal lesion. A possible variant of celiac sprue is *collagenous* sprue. In this disorder small-bowel biopsy specimens characteristically reveal a blunted and flattened mucosa and large masses of eosinophilic hyalin material in the lamina propria. In one study of 349 jejunal biopsy specimens from 145 patients with celiac sprue, 45 (31 percent) showed basement membrane thickening often associated with collagen deposition, but dense collagen deposition was found in only 11 patients. Fatal, unremitting malabsorption developed in four of the latter patients. These observations suggest that collagenous membrane thickening is a fairly frequent finding in jejunal biopsies from patients with sprue

but that dense collagen deposits are an unusual feature and may indicate a poor prognosis.

TREATMENT   Despite the uncertainties concerned with the diagnosis of nontropical sprue, approximately 80 percent of the patients improve after institution of a *gluten-free diet*. Symptomatic improvement usually occurs within a few weeks, but improvement in tests of absorptive function and small-bowel histologic characteristics may not occur for months. It has been repeatedly demonstrated that strict adherence to a gluten-free diet more consistently results in improvement than does suboptimal gluten restriction. Nevertheless, even with strict diet adherence some cases show little improvement in intestinal histologic features. Patients with nontropical sprue treated with glucocorticoids but continuing a normal gluten-containing diet have shown symptomatic improvement as well as improvement in intestinal histology and tests of intestinal absorptive function. The mechanism by which glucocorticoids protect the mucosa from the effects of gluten is not clear.

If a patient with nontropical sprue does not respond to a gluten-free diet, other possibilities or complicating factors must be considered: (1) the diagnosis is incorrect; (2) the patient is not adhering strictly to the diet; (3) there may be another concurrent disease, such as pancreatic insufficiency; (4) the patient may have ulceration of the jejunum or ileum; (5) lactase deficiency may be present with resultant milk intolerance; (6) the patient may have collagenous sprue; or (7) he or she may have developed intestinal lymphoma, a disease which appears to occur more frequently in patients with sprue than in the general population. Finally, it should be emphasized that a small number of patients show a markedly delayed response to a gluten-free diet, with significant improvement occurring only after 24 to 36 months of therapy. Approximately 50 percent of patients with refractory sprue respond to glucocorticoids; such patients may also require parenteral hyperalimentation.

Systemic mastocytosis   Some evidence of malabsorption occurs in 30 percent of patients with systemic mastocytosis. Malabsorption is usually not severe and is manifested primarily as minimal or moderate steatorrhea and impaired absorption of D-xylose and vitamin B_{12}. Small-bowel biopsy specimens typically show moderate blunting of villi and mast cell infiltration.

Disaccharidase deficiency syndromes   As indicated above, the hydrolysis of disaccharides occurs on or within the brush border (microvilli) of intestinal epithelial cells by specific disaccharidases located there. As would be anticipated, both primary (genetic or familial) and secondary (acquired) deficiencies of these disaccharidases have been observed.

LACTASE DEFICIENCY IN THE ADULT   Instances of isolated deficiency of mucosal lactase occur; they are associated with symptoms of lactose intolerance. Since lactose is the principal carbohydrate of milk, such individuals show milk intolerance with symptoms of abdominal cramps, bloating or distention, and diarrhea. Similar symptoms will occur following the ingestion of lactose. The symptoms are due to the fact that lactose when not hydrolyzed is not absorbed, and its osmotic effect in the lumen leads to shifts of fluid into the intestinal tract. The pH of the stool will also decrease because of the production of lactic acid and short-chain fatty acids from the fermentation of lactose by colonic bacteria. Although primary intestinal lactase deficiency seems to be hereditary, lactose or milk intolerance may not become clinically evident until puberty or late adolescence. There are significant racial differences in the incidence of this entity. It would appear that about 5 to 15 percent of the adult white population shows intestinal lactase deficiency, but in black Americans, Bantus, and Orientals, the incidence has been reported as high as 80 to 90 percent.

The diagnosis may be suspected when one obtains a history of gastrointestinal symptoms following milk ingestion. It should be emphasized that the ingestion of only moderate amounts of lactose, e.g., 5 to 12 g or the amount contained in 100 to 240 mL milk, often results in symptoms. Bloating, cramps, and flatulence, but not diarrhea, are usually produced with ingestion of small to moderate amounts of lactose. The vast majority of lactose-intolerant patients are aware that they are milk-intolerant and avoid milk. That these symptoms are not due to allergic reactions to the proteins in milk (i.e., milk allergy or hypersensitivity) can be demonstrated by performing a lactose tolerance test. This test consists of administering an oral dose of lactose (usually from 0.75 to 1.5 g per kilogram of body weight) and obtaining serial blood samples for measurements of blood glucose. In a positive test, intestinal symptoms occur, and the blood glucose increases less than 1.1 mmol/L (20 mg/dL) above the fasting level. However, false-positive and false-negative tests occur in 20 percent of normal subjects because the test is influenced by gastric emptying and glucose metabolism. Measurement of breath hydrogen after ingestion of 50 g lactose is a more sensitive and specific test. The rationale for this test is that hydrogen is released from unabsorbed lactose by colonic bacteria and breath hydrogen excretion subsequently rises. The test is noninvasive and is not influenced by gastric emptying or metabolic factors. Approximately 70 percent of patients with primary lactose intolerance will respond to a lactose-restricted diet while the remaining 30 percent will not because of an underlying irritable bowel syndrome.

Acquired lactase deficiency is often seen in association with a variety of gastrointestinal diseases, in many of which there is histologic evidence of mucosal damage. The disorders in which lactose intolerance and lactase deficiency may occur include nontropical and tropical sprue, regional enteritis, viral and bacterial infections of the intestinal tract, giardiasis, abetalipoproteinemia, cystic fibrosis, and ulcerative colitis. Patients with both primary and acquired (secondary) lactase deficiency are often able to tolerate yogurt because the latter contains bacterial-derived lactases.

DEFICIENCY OF OTHER DISACCHARIDASES   Damage to the intestinal mucosa may produce decreased levels of other disaccharidases, such as sucrase-isomaltase, but usually these are not as depressed as lactase, and symptoms of specific intolerance, such as sucrose intolerance, are uncommon. There are instances of primary and apparently hereditary sucrose intolerance, but these always occur in association with sucrase-isomaltase deficiency. Sucrase-isomaltase deficiency, while not as frequent as lactase deficiency, is nonetheless an important cause of diarrhea, bloating, and cramping abdominal pain in children. Such patients are often unable to adhere to a low-sucrose diet. Thus, the observation that the symptoms of sucrose malabsorption can be ameliorated by the simple expedient of ingesting viable yeast cells is of considerable practical importance.

Hypogammaglobulinemia   Malabsorption may be associated with hypogammaglobulinemia or agammaglobulinemia. The hypogammaglobulinemia may be of the congenital or the acquired type, with the onset either in childhood or adulthood. When malabsorption has been noted, it has included impaired absorption of fat, D-xylose, and vitamin B_{12}. Peroral intestinal biopsy may reveal changes comparable to those seen in nontropical sprue, but often one finds a more striking mononuclear infiltrate giving a nodular appearance to the mucosa both microscopically and macroscopically. Diarrhea and steatorrhea may precede or follow the development of hypogammaglobulinemia, and these may worsen during infections and subside after the infection is controlled with antibiotics. Intestinal infestation with *Giardia lamblia* is common in hypogammaglobulinemic patients. Meticulous collection and culture of intestinal fluids have revealed excessive numbers of anaerobic bacteria in the small bowel of some patients with hypogammaglobulinemia. However, the relationship between such overgrowth with anaerobes and diarrhea and steatorrhea remains to be clarified. Arthritis, resembling rheumatoid arthritis, and thymoma have also been described in patients with this syndrome. In some patients improvement in diarrhea and malabsorption may occur spontaneously, whereas in others improvement may follow treatment with a gluten-free diet, glucocorticoids, antibiotics, injections of gammaglobulin, and cholestyramine. These forms of therapy have not been uniformly successful. Although transient improvement is common, complete cessation of symptoms is distinctly unusual.

The relationship between hypogammaglobulinemia and malab-

sorption remains obscure. There is no evidence to date indicating that excessive enteric loss of gammaglobulin or alteration of the intestinal microflora occurs, but abnormalities in IgA metabolism may be important in this syndrome. This immunoglobulin is the predominant one in the intestinal mucosa and is found in many exocrine secretions, including tears, saliva, gastric juice, and intestinal juice. A few patients have been described with malabsorption and selective deficiency of IgA.

Abetalipoproteinemia   See Chap. 326.

Hartnup disease, cystinuria   See Chap. 336.

ENDOCRINE AND METABOLIC DISORDERS Diabetes mellitus   The occurrence of diarrhea and steatorrhea in patients with diabetes mellitus has been well documented. When steatorrhea accompanies diabetes, it may be due to the presence of (1) exocrine pancreatic insufficiency, (2) coexistent nontropical sprue, (3) abnormal bacterial proliferation in the proximal small bowel, or (4) severe and uncontrolled diabetes per se (e.g., so-called diabetic diarrhea). Patients falling into the first three categories will usually respond in a satisfactory manner to treatment with pancreatic extracts, a gluten-free diet, and antibiotics, respectively. The pathogenesis of diarrhea and steatorrhea in patients in the fourth category remains poorly understood, and the response to various forms of therapy has been quite variable. It has been demonstrated that patients with diabetic diarrhea and steatorrhea may have involvement of the autonomic nervous system with degenerative changes in the sympathetic and parasympathetic nerves and ganglia. In some patients bacterial overgrowth in the stomach and proximal small bowel may occur and contribute to the diarrhea and steatorrhea.

The clinical features in patients with diarrhea and steatorrhea due to diabetes per se seem to be fairly uniform. Diabetes usually develops at a young age and is often severe and difficult to control. There is a distinct predominance of males. Several signs of autonomic neuropathy are usually present, including postural hypotension, anhydrosis, impotence, and bladder irregularities. Peripheral vascular disease and peripheral neuropathy are also common. Gastrointestinal x-rays may show delayed gastric emptying and disordered transit through the small bowel. Peroral small-bowel biopsy specimens are normal. Tests of intestinal absorptive function are normal except for steatorrhea and azotorrhea. There has been no consistent response to therapy with pancreatic extracts, gluten-free diet, or glucocorticoids. When bacterial overgrowth is present, broad-spectrum antibiotics may be helpful. Clonidine has proved useful in patients with large volume diarrhea not responding to dietary measures and anticholinergics.

Hypoparathyroidism   Steatorrhea has been documented in several patients with idiopathic hypoparathyroidism. In addition to hypocalcemia, impaired absorption of D-xylose and vitamin B_{12}, decreased serum iron values, and abnormal small-intestinal roentgenograms have been demonstrated in some cases. In such patients the serum phosphorus level is elevated (due to the hypoparathyroidism) rather than low (as in primary malabsorption). The cause of malabsorption in this disorder is unclear.

Adrenal insufficiency   Although there are few studies on fat excretion in adrenal insufficiency in human beings, malabsorption, especially of fat, appears to occur more frequently than has been generally appreciated. Patients with adrenal insufficiency have been found to have steatorrhea which is corrected by therapy with adrenal glucocorticoids.

Hyperthyroidism   There are few detailed studies on intestinal absorptive function in patients with hyperthyroidism. Mild to moderate steatorrhea and hypoalbuminemia have been reported, but absorption of D-xylose and vitamin B_{12} is frequently normal. Steatorrhea usually remits after successful treatment of hyperthyroidism. Clinical studies suggest that steatorrhea in hyperthyroidism is not due to any defect of pancreatic, biliary, or small-intestinal mucosal function but is a result of hyperphagia with ingestion of unusually large amounts of fat occurring in association with rapid gastric emptying and intestinal transit.

Ulcerogenic tumor of the pancreas (Zollinger-Ellison syndrome)
The clinical features of ulcerogenic tumor of the pancreas are described in Chap. 238. Malabsorption is frequently found in this disease. The acidification and dilution of intestinal contents caused by gastric acid hypersecretion leads to major disturbances in fat digestion and absorption. Impaired formation of micellar lipid due to inactivation of pancreatic lipase is probably the major factor in the production of steatorrhea. Other factors contributing to fat malabsorption in this disorder include (1) precipitation of glycine-conjugated bile salts due to low intraluminal pH, (2) alteration of the intestinal mucosa with ulceration and metaplasia, and (3) impaired fatty acid esterification and chylomicron formation.

Carcinoid syndrome (See Chap. 262) Although diarrhea is common in the carcinoid syndrome, malabsorption with significant steatorrhea is unusual. In many of the cases of carcinoid syndrome with steatorrhea there has been a prior intestinal resection (usually ileal), and in these cases the resection is the important factor in the causation of steatorrhea. However, direct involvement of the bowel wall and mesentery by the carcinoid tumor have been well documented. That abnormalities in serotonin metabolism may also be important is suggested from the decrease in the steatorrhea observed in some of these patients when treated with the antiserotonin drug methysergide. Although side effects may occur, for control of diarrhea and steatorrhea patients may be given a trial of 8 to 12 mg methysergide per day.

PROTEIN-LOSING ENTEROPATHY The gastrointestinal tract has been shown to play a significant role in the metabolism and physiologic degradation of plasma proteins. The exact magnitude of the normal gastrointestinal protein loss in human beings has remained unclear, but studies with labeled albumin have suggested that between 10 and 20 percent of the normal turnover of albumin may be accounted for by enteric protein loss. However, under certain pathologic conditions, excessive gastrointestinal protein loss may develop. An extensive number of disorders have been found to be associated with intestinal protein loss. Some of these are listed in Table 240-8.

Pathophysiology Several mechanisms have been proposed for the passage of plasma proteins across the gastrointestinal mucosa, both normally and in certain disease states. First, plasma proteins may pass into the gastrointestinal tract through an inflamed or ulcerated mucosa and account for the protein loss occasionally seen in regional enteritis and ulcerative colitis. Second, plasma protein loss may occur as a result of disordered mucosal cell structure. For example, patients with nontropical sprue have abnormal villous structure and surface epithelium, and these changes could facilitate the diffusion of plasma protein between the cells. Third, in the presence of increased lymphatic pressure, there may be increased passage of plasma proteins into the lumen via the intercellular spaces of the mucosal epithelium. This might be expected to occur in disorders in which there is granulomatous or neoplastic involvement of lymphatics. Fourth, dilated lymph vessels in the mucosa may rupture through the surface epithelium, discharging their contents into the intestinal lumen. This is thought to be important in the pathogenesis of steatorrhea and hypoproteinemia in patients with idiopathic intestinal lymphangiectasia (see "Intestinal Lymphangiectasia" below).

Several techniques have been developed for the detection and quantitation of gastrointestinal protein loss. In the past these have primarily involved the use of intravenously administered radiolabeled macromolecules such as ^{125}I-labeled serum albumin, ^{51}CrCl$_3$, ^{51}Cr-labeled albumin, and indium 111. ^{111}In-labeled transferrin and ^{51}CrCl$_3$ (which rapidly become attached to circulating transferrin) are the compounds available commercially for clinical use. After the intravenous administration of 0.93 to 1.11 MBq (25 to 30 μCi) of the labeled compound to normal subjects, between 0.1 and 0.7 percent of the administered radioactivity is recovered in the stool over a 4-day period. Patients with excessive enteric protein loss may excrete from 2 to 40 percent of the injected radioactive label. False-positive results may be obtained if the stool specimen is contaminated with urine. There is also a reliable and sensitive nonisotopic method to measure intestinal protein loss which involves the measurement of α$_1$-antitrypsin (AT). This serum enzyme, which has the same molecular weight as albumin (50,000), is resistant to proteolysis and when leaked into the intestinal lumen is not degraded. One can easily measure AT in serum and stool by radial immunodiffusion in order to obtain AT loss in stool (normal loss is less than 2.6 mg per gram of stool) or intestinal clearance of AT (normal is less than 13 mL/day). Results using AT as a marker of intestinal protein loss correlate well with the more cumbersome and costly isotopic methods. Random fecal AT assays can also be used as a simple screening method for enteric protein loss.

The rate of albumin synthesis and degradation can be determined using intravenously administered radioiodinated albumin and measuring the decline in radioactivity in the serum. Such studies carried out in patients with protein-losing enteropathies have demonstrated a reduced circulating (intravascular) and total-body pool of albumin, a normal or increased rate of albumin synthesis, markedly shortened albumin survival, and increased fecal protein loss. Whereas normal subjects catabolize 5 to 10 percent of their intravascular albumin pool each day (the fractional catabolic rate), patients with excessive enteric protein loss may have fractional catabolic rates of 50 to 60 percent.

Studies utilizing radioiodinated immunoglobulins have demonstrated a decreased intravascular globulin pool and increased fractional catabolic rate. However, the synthesis of IgG is usually normal, suggesting that a decreased level of IgG and increased enteric protein loss is not a potent stimulus for IgG synthesis. The increase in fractional catabolic rate is comparable for albumin, IgG, and IgM immunoglobulins, further suggesting that there is bulk loss of plasma proteins into the intestinal tract and not a selective loss of certain proteins. The finding of decreased globulins often is an ancillary aid in excluding renal, cardiac, and hepatic cases of hypoalbuminemia.

Abnormalities in albumin and globulin metabolism in patients with a protein-losing enteropathy may be reversed or diminished within a few months after the institution of appropriate therapy. It is obviously important that a specific etiologic diagnosis should be established in all patients with treatable disorders, who may be expected to have a remission induced by the appropriate therapy for the underlying disease. The intestinal protein loss in patients with nontropical sprue, Whipple's disease, constrictive pericarditis, re-

---

TABLE 240-8 Disorders associated with protein-losing enteropathy

I Stomach
  A Gastric carcinoma
  B Giant hypertrophy of the gastric mucosa
  C Atrophic gastritis
  D Postgastrectomy syndrome
II Small intestine
  A Intestinal lymphangiectasia
  B Nontropical sprue
  C Tropical sprue
  D Regional enteritis
  E Whipple's disease
  F Lymphoma
  G Intestinal tuberculosis
  H Acute infectious enteritis
  I Scleroderma
  J Jejunal diverticulosis
  K Allergic gastroenteropathy
III Colon
  A Colonic neoplasm
  B Ulcerative colitis
  C Granulomatous colitis
  D Megacolon
IV Heart
  A Congestive heart failure
  B Constrictive pericarditis
  C Interatrial septal defect
  D Primary cardiomyopathy
V Miscellaneous
  A Esophageal carcinoma
  B Gastrocolic fistula
  C Agammaglobulinemia
  D Nephrosis

gional enteritis, ulcerative colitis, and Ménétrier's disease has been ameliorated by therapy appropriate to the underlying disorder.

Intestinal lymphangiectasia PATHOPHYSIOLOGY The disorder intestinal lymphangiectasia is characterized by increased enteric loss of protein, hypoproteinemia, edema, lymphocytopenia, malabsorption, and abnormal dilated lymphatic channels in the small intestine. The high incidence of chylous effusions and abnormal peripheral, retroperitoneal, and thoracic lymphatics indicates that intestinal lymphangiectasia is part of a generalized congenital disorder of the lymphatic system. It has been suggested that the hypoplastic visceral lymphatic channels result in obstruction to lymph flow, with the subsequent development of increased intestinal lymphatic pressure. This in turn may lead to dilated lymphatic vessels throughout the small-bowel wall and mesentery. Hypoproteinemia and steatorrhea are thought to be due to rupture of the dilated lymphatic vessels with discharge of lymph into the bowel lumen. In adults approximately 1500 mL lymph, containing 70 g fat and 50 g albumin, passes through the thoracic duct each day. The leakage of a small amount of this lymph might be expected to result in considerable loss of protein and fat into the intestinal lumen. In addition, absorption of dietary long-chain triglycerides stimulates lymph flow, and this may increase further the retrograde leakage of intestinal lymph into the lumen. Three lines of evidence support the concept of intestinal leakage of lymph in intestinal lymphangiectasia: (1) chylous fluid has been recovered from the duodenum in these patients; (2) retrograde passage of contrast material from retroperitoneal lymphatics into the duodenum and jejunum has been documented; and (3) significant steatorrhea may persist in patients after institution of a completely fat-free diet, suggesting an increased enteric loss of endogenous fat present in lymph.

CLINICAL FEATURES The disease affects primarily children and young adults. All patients have edema, which may be asymmetric because of hypoplastic peripheral lymphatics. Chylous effusions and diarrhea are common symptoms. The primary laboratory finding is hypoproteinemia with decreased serum levels of albumin, immunoglobulins IgG, IgA, and IgM, transferrin, and ceruloplasmin. Despite moderate to severe hypogammaglobulinemia there does not appear to be an increased incidence of pyogenic bacterial infections. In addition, circulating antibody response to challenge with *Brucella* and typhoid antigens is normal. Steatorrhea is usually mild, although in some instances fat loss may be as much as 40 g per day. Some patients have hypocalcemia and impaired absorption of vitamin B_{12}. Lymphocytopenia (due to the loss of lymphocytes in lymph) is common, with lymphocyte counts ranging from 400 to 1000 per milliliter (normal: 1500 to 4000 per milliliter). This is associated with abnormal delayed hypersensitivity, as evidenced by prolonged homograft survival and impaired cutaneous responsiveness to antigens such as mumps and monilia.

Small-bowel roentgenograms are frequently abnormal, showing changes of mucosal edema and a malabsorption pattern. Lymphangiograms may demonstrate hypoplastic peripheral and visceral lymphatics with the absence of groups of retroperitoneal lymph nodes. Specimens of jejunal mucosa characteristically reveal dilated and telangiectatic lymphatic vessels in the lamina propria and submucosa. The villi may be club-shaped because of distortion from grossly dilated lymphatics (Fig. 240-4). Such changes in the intestinal mucosa may be reversed after appropriate therapy. The diagnosis of intestinal lymphangiectasia is therefore established by (1) small-intestinal biopsy and (2) demonstration of increased enteric protein loss using radioactive macromolecules.

TREATMENT A low-fat diet, by decreasing lymph flow, usually results in significant improvement with decreased fecal fat excretion, decreased enteric protein loss, increased serum calcium and albumin levels, and an increased half-life of injected ^{125}I-labeled albumin. Similar results may be obtained by the substitution of medium-chain triglycerides (MCT) for dietary long-chain triglycerides, since MCT are transported as medium-chain fatty acids by the portal vein rather than via the lymph.

REFERENCES

CALDWELL JH et al: Eosinophilic gastroenteritis with obstruction. Immunological studies of seven patients. Gastroenterology 74:825, 1978

CHERNER JA et al: Gastrointestinal dysfunction in systemic mastocytosis. A prospective study. Gastroenterology 95:657, 1988

CHUNG YC et al: Protein digestion and absorption in human small intestine. Gastroenterology 76:1415, 1979

COOPER BT et al: Celiac disease and malignancy. Medicine (Baltimore) 59:249, 1980

FLORENT C et al: Intestinal clearance of α_1-antitrypsin: A sensitive method for the detection of protein-losing enteropathy. Gastroenterology 81:777, 1981

GASKIN KJ et al: Colipase and maximally activated pancreatic lipase in normal subjects and patients with steatorrhea. J Clin Invest 69:368, 1982

GILLIN JS et al: Malabsorption and mucosal abnormalities of the small intestine in the acquired immunodeficiency syndrome. Ann Intern Med 102:619, 1985

HARMS HK: Enzyme substitution therapy with the yeast saccharomyces cerevisial in congenital sucrase-isomaltase deficiency. N Engl J Med 316:1306, 1987

HOWDLE PDet al: Cell-mediated immunity to gluten within the small intestinal mucosa in coeliac disease. Gut 23:115, 1982

KAGNOFF M et al: Evidence for the role of human intestinal adenovirus in the pathogenesis of coeliac disease. Gut 28:5, 1987

KEINATH RD et al: Antibiotic treatment and relapse in Whipple's disease. Long term followup of 88 patients. Gastroenterology 88:1867, 1985

KHOURI MR et al: Sudan stain of fecal fat: New insight into an old test. Gastroenterology 96: 421, 1989

KERLID P, WONG L: Breath hydrogen testing in bacterial overgrowth of the small intestine. Gastroenterology 95:982, 1988

KLIPSTEIN FA: Tropical sprue in travelers and expatriates living abroad. Gastroenterology 80:590, 1981

LOUGHRAN TP et al: T-cell intestinal lymphoma associated with celiac sprue. Ann Intern Med 104:44, 1986

LUBY LD et al: Lactulose/mannitol test: An ideal screen for celiac disease. Gastroenterology 96:79, 1989

MACGREGOR I et al: Gastric emptying of liquid meals and pancreatic and biliary secretion after subtotal gastrectomy or truncal vagotomy and pyloroplasty in man. Gastroenterology 72:195, 1977

MARA CS et al: Duodenal manifestations of nontropical sprue. Gastrointest Radiol 11:30, 1986

PETERS TJ, BJARNASON I: Coeliac syndrome: Biochemical mechanisms and the missing peptidase hypothesis revisited. Gut 25:913, 1984

SCHILLER LR et al: Studies on the prevalence and significance of radiolabeled bile acid malabsorption in a group of patients with idiopathic chronic diarrhea. Gastroenterology 92:151, 1987

SLEIKH MS et al: Gastrointestinal absorption of calcium from milk and calcium salts. N Engl J Med 317:532, 1987

STANGHELLINI V: Chronic idiopathic intestinal pseudo-obstruction: Clinical and intestinal manometric findings. Gut 28:5, 1987

241 INFLAMMATORY BOWEL DISEASE
Ulcerative colitis and Crohn's disease

ROBERT M. GLICKMAN

DEFINITION *Inflammatory bowel disease* (IBD) is a general term for a group of chronic inflammatory disorders of unknown etiology involving the gastrointestinal tract. Since there are no pathognomonic features or specific diagnostic tests, in a strict sense, these disorders remain diagnoses of exclusion. Their features are sufficiently characteristic, however, to permit accurate diagnosis in the majority of cases. Chronic IBD may be divided into two major groups, chronic nonspecific *ulcerative colitis* and *Crohn's disease*. The original description of the disease by Crohn, Ginzberg, and Oppenheimer in 1932 localized the disease to segments of ileum. However, the same process may involve the buccal mucosa, esophagus, stomach, and duodenum as well as the jejunum and ileum. Crohn's disease of the small bowel is also known as *regional enteritis*. In addition, a similar inflammatory picture may occur in the colon, either alone or with accompanying small-intestinal involvement. In most instances, this form of colitis can be distinguished clinically and pathologically from ulcerative colitis and is also referred to as *Crohn's disease of the colon*. Granulomatous colitis is a less accurate term since only a portion of cases exhibit granulomas. Clinically these disorders are characterized by recurrent inflammatory involvement of intestinal segments with diverse clinical manifestations often resulting in a chronic, unpredictable course.

EPIDEMIOLOGY The epidemiologic and etiologic considerations in ulcerative colitis and Crohn's disease share many features in common and will be discussed together. These diseases are more common in whites than in blacks and orientals with an increased incidence (three- to sixfold) in Jews compared to non-Jews. Both sexes are equally affected.

The incidence and prevalence of the two diseases differ slightly with most studies showing ulcerative colitis to be more common. When analyzed in western Europe and the United States, ulcerative colitis (including ulcerative proctitis) has an incidence of approximately 6 to 8 cases per 100,000 population and an estimated prevalence of approximately 70 to 150 cases per 100,000 population. Estimates of the incidence of Crohn's disease (colonic plus small bowel) are approximately 2 cases per 100,000 population; the prevalence is estimated at 20 to 40 per 100,000 population. Many believe the incidence of Crohn's disease (especially colonic) to be increasing.

While peak occurrence of both diseases is between ages 15 and 35, it has been reported in every decade of life. A familial incidence of IBD has been recorded with estimates that 2 to 5 percent of persons with Crohn's disease or ulcerative colitis will have one or more relatives affected. There is no specificity, however, for a given form of IBD within a given family. Such epidemiologic clustering of cases could argue for either genetic or common environmental influences on the development of these diseases (see below). It has been suggested that there is a probable hereditary basis for these disorders plus a strong environmental component.

ETIOLOGY AND PATHOGENESIS While the cause of ulcerative colitis and Crohn's disease remains unknown, certain features of these diseases have suggested several areas of possible etiologic importance. These include familial or genetic, infectious, immunologic, and psychological factors.

Inflammatory bowel disease is more common in whites, occurs with an increased frequency in Jews, and exhibits some familial clustering. This suggests that there may be a *genetic* predisposition to the development of the disease. In addition, the disease has been described in monozygotic twins. A search for genetic markers which might be of value in identifying susceptible individuals has not identified any single marker (i.e., histocompatibility antigen) in patients with inflammatory bowel disease.

The chronic inflammatory nature of these diseases has prompted a continuing search for a possible *infectious etiology*. In spite of numerous attempts to find known bacterial, fungal, or viral agents, no etiologic agent has thus far been isolated. Preliminary reports of isolates of cell wall variants of *Pseudomonas* or of transmissible agents producing cytopathic effects in tissue culture have yet to be confirmed. Efforts to produce specific granulomatous tissue reactions with filtrates from Crohn's disease tissue have yielded conflicting and nonreproducible results. As discussed below, many infectious agents can produce *acute* colitis or ileitis; however, there is no evidence that these agents are involved in *chronic* inflammatory bowel disease.

The theory that an *immune* mechanism may be involved is based on the concept that the extraintestinal manifestations which may accompany these disorders (e.g., arthritis, pericholangitis) may represent autoimmune phenomena and that therapeutic agents, such as glucocorticoids and azathioprine, may exert their effects via immunosuppressive mechanisms. Patients with inflammatory bowel disease may have *humoral antibodies* to colon cells, bacterial antigens such as *Escherichia coli*, lipopolysaccharide, and foreign proteins such as cow milk protein. In general, the presence and titer of these antibodies do not correlate with disease activity. It is likely that these antigens gain access to immunocompetent cells secondary to epithelial damage. In addition, IBD has been described in association with agammaglobulinemia as well as IgA deficiency, casting further doubt on the pathogenetic role of humoral antibodies. *Immune complexes* have also been invoked to explain extraintestinal manifestations of IBD. While there are well-defined examples of tissue injury resulting from immune complexes, studies utilizing specific detection techniques have failed to demonstrate an increased frequency of immune complexes in patients with IBD.

Associated abnormalities of *cell-mediated immunity* include cutaneous anergy, diminished responsiveness to various mitogenic stimuli, and decreases in the number of peripheral T cells. Since many of these changes may revert to normal when the disease is quiescent, it is likely that they are secondary phenomena. Experimental colitis has been produced in laboratory animals by prior sensitization with dinitrochlorobenzene, suggesting a T-cell–dependent mechanism of tissue injury. It remains to be determined whether the regulation of immune function (e.g., suppressor T cells) is of pathogenic importance in the etiology of IBD. Thus far, none of the altered immunologic findings have been specific for either ulcerative colitis or Crohn's disease.

The *psychological* features of patients with inflammatory bowel disease have also been stressed. It is not uncommon for these diseases to present initially or to flare in association with major psychological stresses such as the loss of a family member. It has been suggested that patients with IBD have a characteristic personality which renders them susceptible to emotional stresses which in turn may precipitate or exacerbate their symptoms. While there is little evidence directly relating possible emotional factors to the etiology of inflammatory bowel disease, there is little doubt that a chronic disease of unknown etiology affecting individuals in the prime of their life often results in feelings of anger, anxiety, and some degree of depression. These reactions are undoubtedly important factors in modifying the course of these diseases and in the response to therapy.

PATHOLOGY In ulcerative colitis there is an inflammatory reaction primarily involving the colonic mucosa. Grossly, the colon appears ulcerated, hyperemic, and usually hemorrhagic (Fig. 241-1). A striking feature of the inflammation is that it is *uniform* and *continuous* with no intervening areas of normal mucosa. The rectum is usually involved (95 percent of cases) and the inflammation extends proximally in a continuous fashion but for a variable distance. When there is involvement of the entire colon, there may be minimal involvement of a few centimeters of the terminal ileum, referred to as "backwash ileitis." This involvement never leads to the thickening and narrowing characteristic of Crohn's disease. The surface mucosal cells as well as the crypt epithelium and submucosa are involved in an inflammatory reaction with neutrophilic infiltration (Fig. 241-2A). This progresses to epithelial damage with loss of surface epithelial cells resulting in multiple ulcerations. Infiltration of the crypts with

FIGURE 241-1 Ulcerative colitis. Resected colon with portion of terminal ileum. The specimen showed uniform inflammation, erythema, and hemorrhage and a normal terminal ileum.

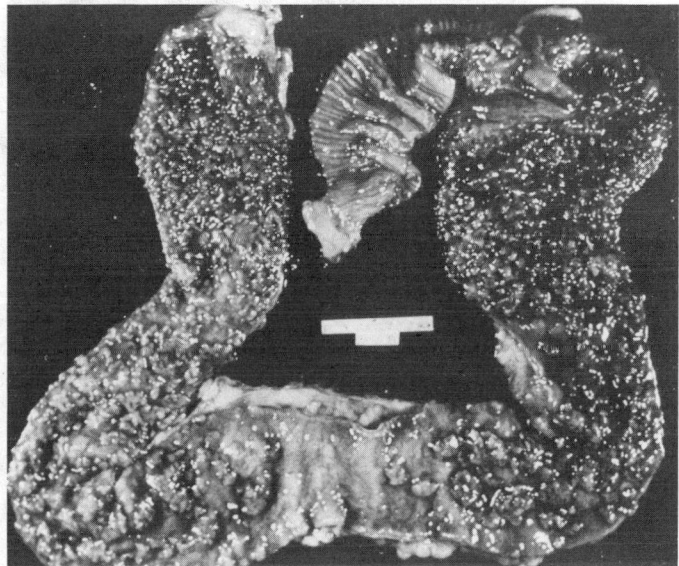

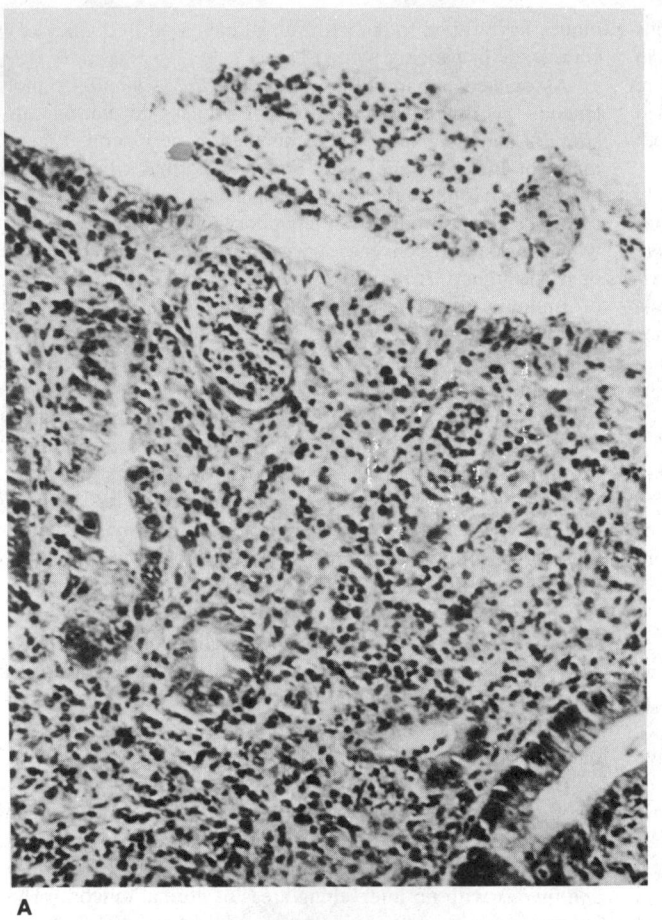

A

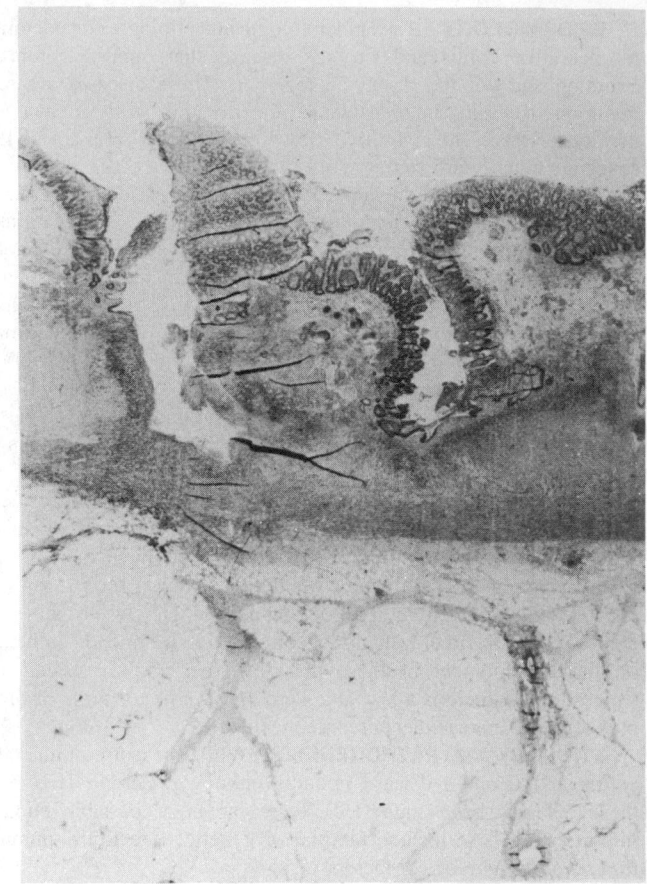

B

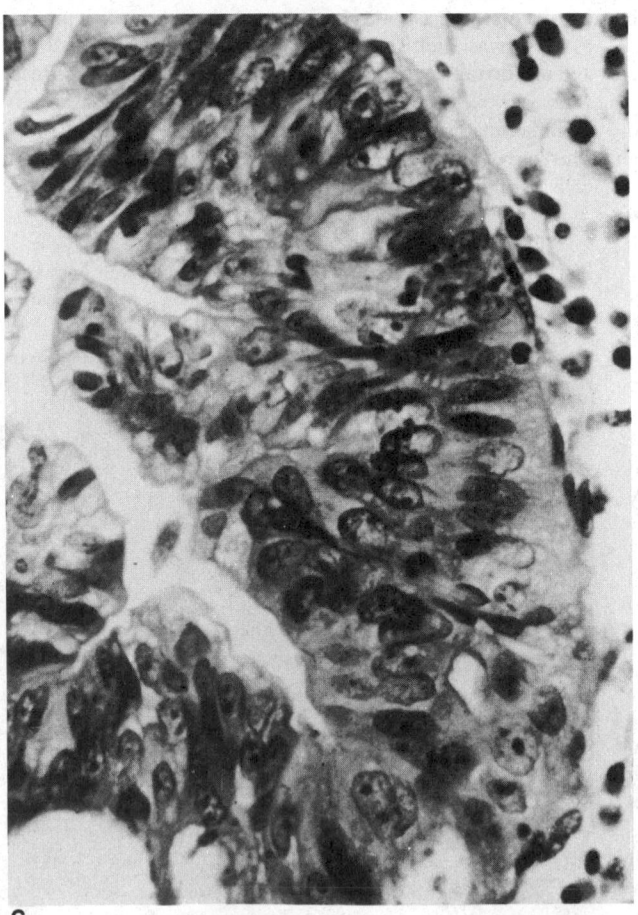

C

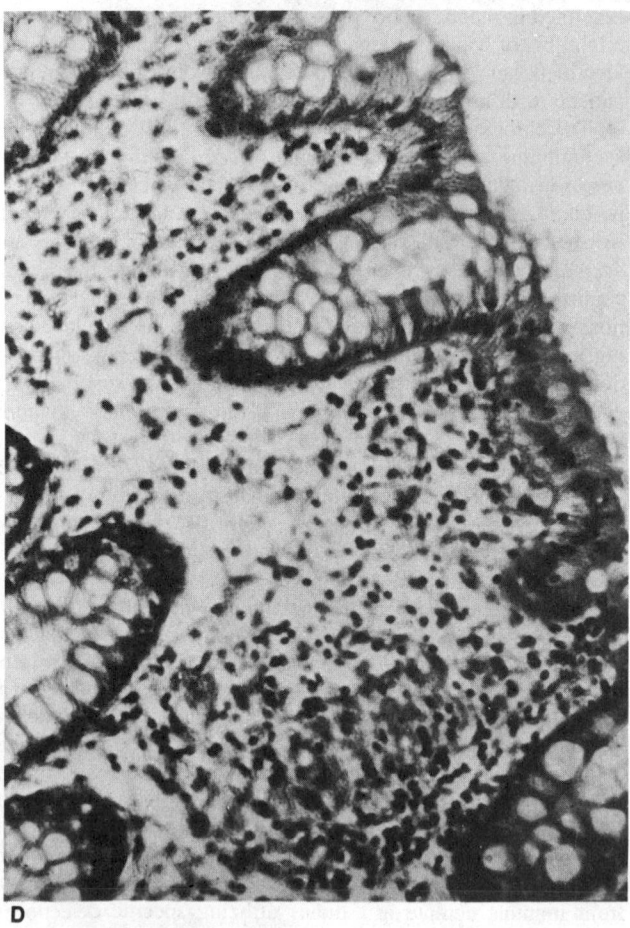

D

neutrophils results in characteristic (but not specific) small crypt abscesses and their eventual destruction. There may also be loss of crypt epithelium with a loss of goblet (mucus-producing) cells and submucosal edema. With repetitive cycles of inflammation, mild submucosal fibrosis develops. Regenerative activity is evidenced by irregular crypt epithelium often showing bifurcation at the base of the crypts. It is important to stress that, unlike Crohn's disease, deeper layers of the bowel beneath the submucosa usually are not involved. In severe ulcerative colitis, as seen with toxic megacolon, the bowel wall may become extremely thin, the mucosa denuded with inflammation extending to the serosa leading to dilatation and subsequent perforation.

Recurrent inflammation may lead to characteristic features of chronicity. Fibrosis and longitudinal retraction result in shortening of the colon. Loss of the normal haustral pattern leads radiologically to a smooth, "lead-pipe" appearance of the colon. Regenerating islands of mucosa surrounded by areas of ulceration and denuded mucosa appear as "polyps" protruding into the lumen of the colon. However, these protrusions are inflammatory in nature and not neoplastic and are therefore called pseudopolyps (Fig. 241-2*B*).

With long-standing ulcerative colitis, the surface epithelium may show features of *dysplasia*. Changes of nuclear and cellular atypia are thought to represent a premalignant change occurring in the setting of long-standing ulcerative colitis. Marked dysplasia in colonic biopsies in the setting of long-standing colitis is associated with a significant risk of a coexistent carcinoma elsewhere in the colon and may influence the decision to advise colectomy.

Crohn's disease, in contrast to ulcerative colitis, is characterized by chronic inflammation extending through *all layers of the intestinal wall* and involving the mesentery as well as regional lymph nodes. Whether or not the small bowel or colon is involved, the basic pathologic process is the same.

The earliest pathologic changes in Crohn's disease are poorly defined since surgery is usually not electively undertaken early in the course of the disease. At laparotomy, the terminal ileum appears hyperemic and boggy, with mesentery and mesenteric lymph nodes swollen and reddened. At this early stage, the bowel wall, although edematous, is usually pliable. While some patients with this initial presentation will subsequently develop typical regional enteritis, a significant number will recover completely. This acute form of ileitis will undoubtedly be shown to have diverse etiologies. Indeed, approximately 80 percent of patients with this presentation have been shown to be infected with *Yersinia enterocolitica,* an organism capable of producing a self-limited, acute inflammatory ileitis.

As the disease progresses, the gross appearance assumes a characteristic picture. The bowel appears greatly thickened and leathery with the lumen narrowed (Fig. 241-3). This characteristic stenosis can occur in any portion of the intestine and may be associated with varying degrees of intestinal obstruction. The mesentery appears greatly thickened, fatty, and often extends over the serosal surface of the bowel in characteristic fingerlike projections. The appearance of the mucosa is variable, depending on the severity and stage of the disease, but may appear relatively normal in sharp contrast to ulcerative colitis. In more advanced cases, the mucosa has a nodular, "cobblestoned" look. This is the result of submucosal thickening and mucosal ulceration, often linear in the long axis of the bowel at the base of mucosal folds. These ulcerations may penetrate into the submucosa

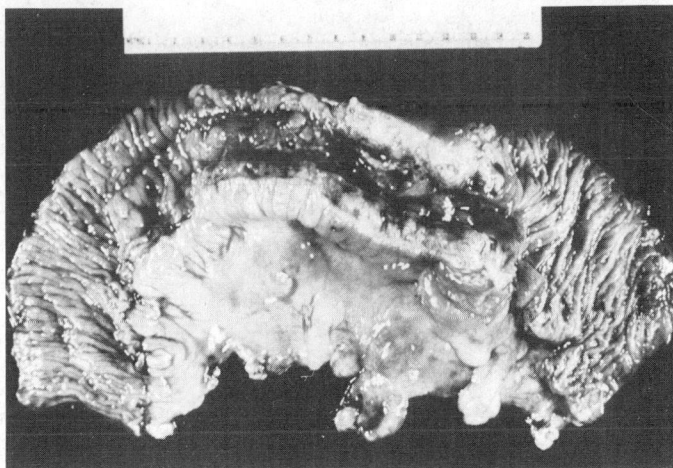

FIGURE 241-3 Regional enteritis. Resected specimen of terminal ileum demonstrates thickened bowel wall and chronically inflamed mucosa. Note the relatively sharp demarcation of the diseased segment with grossly normal mucosa on either side.

and muscularis and coalesce to form intramural channels which become manifested as fistulas and fissures.

There are other morphologic features distinguishing Crohn's disease from ulcerative colitis. In Crohn's disease, the disease is often *discontinuous;* severely involved segments of bowel are separated from each other with intervening segments of apparently normal bowel, producing "skip areas." In approximately 50 percent of Crohn's disease of the colon, the rectum may be spared. In sharp contrast, in ulcerative colitis the involvement is contiguous and the rectum is almost always involved. In addition, in Crohn's disease the transmural inflammatory process, involving serosa and mesentery, also accounts for the characteristic fistula and abscess formation. As a result of serosal inflammation, adjacent loops of small intestine may become adherent and matted together by a fibrinous peritoneal reaction, leading to palpable mass, most often in the right lower quadrant. Fistula formation may occur between adherent loops of intestine, colon, or other adjacent organs such as the bladder or vagina. Fistulous tracts may also lead to the skin or end blindly within the peritoneum or retroperitoneum, surrounded by adherent loops of bowel and inflammatory tissue. Fistula formation is not seen in ulcerative colitis.

Microscopically, granulomas are most helpful in distinguishing Crohn's disease from other forms of inflammatory bowel disease; they do not occur in ulcerative colitis. They may be seen in rectal or colonoscopic biopsies (Fig. 241-2*D*). While granulomas are a helpful finding when present, it is the chronic inflammation involving all layers of the intestinal wall which is most characteristic.

In most series reporting the distribution of Crohn's disease, approximately 30 percent will involve the small intestine (usually the terminal ileum) without colonic disease, 30 percent with only colonic involvement, and 40 percent with ileocolic involvement usually of the ileum and right colon. In a small number of patients (mostly children and adolescents) there may be diffuse and extensive ulceration of the jejunum and ileum.

While there often are sufficient features to permit distinction between ulcerative colitis and Crohn's disease of the colon (Table 241-1), in 10 to 20 percent of cases this distinction may not be possible.

CLINICAL FEATURES

ULCERATIVE COLITIS The major symptoms of ulcerative colitis are bloody diarrhea and abdominal pain, often with fever and weight loss in more severe cases. With mild disease, there may be one or two semiformed stools containing little blood and with no systemic

FIGURE 241-2 Colonic biopsies in inflammatory bowel disease. *A.* Ulcerative colitis. The surface mucosa is destroyed and the submucosa is diffusely infiltrated with polymorphonuclear leukocytes. Crypt abscesses are also present. *B.* Pseudopolyp. Regenerating island of mucosa with adjacent area of ulceration. *C.* Ulcerative colitis. Severe dysplasia occurring in long-standing chronic ulcerative colitis. Note atypical changes in the nuclei and marked palisading of nuclei of the crypt epithelium. *D.* Crohn's disease of the colon. Note the relatively intact mucosa with a solitary granuloma in the lamina propria.

TABLE 241-1 Pathologic and clinical features of IBD

	Ulcerative colitis	Crohn's disease
PATHOLOGIC		
Segmental	0	+ +
Transmural involvement	+/−	+ +
Granulomas	0	+/+ + (50%)
Fibrosis	+	+ +
Fissuring, fistulas	+/−	+ +
Mesenteric fat, lymph node involvement	0	+ +
CLINICAL		
Diarrhea	+ +	+ +
Rectal bleeding	+ +	+
Abdominal pain	+	+ +
Palpable mass	0	+ +
Fistulas	+/−	+ +
Strictures	+	+ +
Small bowel involvement	+/− ("backwash ileitis")	+ +
Rectal involvement	+ + (95%)	+/+ + (50%)
Extracolonic disease	+	+
Toxic megacolon	+	+/−
Recurrence after colectomy	0	+
Malignancy (with long-standing disease)	+	+/−

NOTE: 0 = never; +/− = rare; + = occasional; + + = frequent, common.

manifestations. In contrast, the patient with severe disease may have frequent liquid stools containing blood and pus, complain of severe cramps, and demonstrate symptoms and signs of dehydration, anemia, fever, and weight loss. With predominantly rectal involvement, constipation rather than diarrhea may be present, and tenesmus may be a major complaint. On occasion, intestinal symptoms may be overshadowed by fever, weight loss, or one of the extracolonic manifestations of the disease (see below).

The physical findings in ulcerative colitis are usually nonspecific; there may be some abdominal distention or tenderness along the course of the colon. In mild cases, the general physical examination will be normal. Extracolonic manifestations include arthritis, skin changes, or evidence of liver disease. Fever, tachycardia, and postural hypotension are usually associated with more severe disease. The laboratory findings are often nonspecific and usually reflect the degree and severity of bleeding and inflammation. There may be anemia which reflects chronic disease as well as iron deficiency from chronic blood loss. Leukocytosis with a left shift and an elevated sedimentation rate are often seen in the severely ill, febrile patient. Electrolyte abnormalities, especially hypokalemia, reflect the degree of diarrhea. Hypoalbuminemia is common with extensive disease and usually represents luminal protein loss through an ulcerated mucosa. An elevated alkaline phosphatase may indicate associated hepatobiliary disease (see below).

The clinical course of ulcerative colitis is variable. The majority of patients will suffer a relapse within 1 year of the first attack, reflecting the recurrent nature of the disease. There may, however, be prolonged periods of remission with only minimal symptoms. In general, the severity of symptoms reflects the extent of colonic involvement and the intensity of the inflammation. At one end of the spectrum are patients who present with limited involvement of the rectum (ulcerative proctitis) or rectum and sigmoid (ulcerative proctosigmoiditis). Consistent with this limited colonic involvement, the disease is usually mild, with minimal systemic or extracolonic manifestations. The major symptoms are rectal bleeding and tenesmus. Most of these patients, especially those with only rectal involvement, will not develop more extensive disease. In the remainder, the disease

may extend proximally with variable involvement. Most patients with ulcerative colitis (perhaps 85 percent) will have mild to moderate disease of an intermittent nature and can be managed without hospitalization. In approximately 15 percent of patients, the disease assumes a more fulminant course, involves the entire colon, and presents with severe bloody diarrhea and systemic signs and symptoms. The patients are at risk to develop toxic dilatation and perforation of the colon (described below) and represent a medical emergency.

CROHN'S DISEASE As discussed above, the basic pathologic features of Crohn's disease are the same whether the disease involves the small bowel or colon. The clinical presentation, however, will largely reflect the anatomic location of the disease and to some degree will predict which complications of the disease may develop. The clinical features of ulcerative colitis and Crohn's disease are compared in Table 241-1.

The major clinical features of Crohn's disease are fever, abdominal pain, diarrhea often without blood, and generalized fatigability. There may be associated weight loss. With *colonic involvement* diarrhea and pain are the most frequent symptoms. Rectal bleeding is distinctly less common than with ulcerative colitis and reflects (1) sparing of the rectum in many patients, and (2) the transmural nature of the disease with only irregular mucosal involvement. There may be associated severe anorectal complications such as fistulas, fissures, and perirectal abscess. Such features may antedate the clinical onset of colitis and should always raise the suspicion of associated Crohn's disease. With recurrent perirectal inflammation the anal canal may be thickened, and perianal fistulas or scarring may be present. With extensive colonic involvement, dilatation of the colon may occur. However, since Crohn's disease often results in a thickened colonic wall, this is less common with Crohn's disease than with ulcerative colitis. Extracolonic manifestations (discussed below), particularly arthritis, are seen more commonly with colonic than with small bowel Crohn's disease (regional enteritis).

With involvement of the *small bowel* there may be additional presenting signs and symptoms. Typically, the disease has its onset in a young adult with a history of fatigue, variable weight loss, right lower quadrant discomfort or pain, and diarrhea. Low-grade fever, anorexia, nausea, and vomiting may also be present. The abdominal pain may be steady and localized to the right lower quadrant or may assume a colicky or crampy pattern, reflecting variable degrees of intestinal stenosis. The diarrhea is often moderate, usually without gross blood; if there is no rectal involvement, tenesmus is absent. Physical examination at this time often reveals right lower quadrant tenderness with an associated fullness or mass reflecting adherent loops of bowel. At this time the patient may have mild anemia, mild to moderate leukocytosis, and an elevated sedimentation rate.

Since acute ileitis may have an abrupt onset with fever, leukocytosis, and right lower quadrant pain, the clinical picture may be indistinguishable from acute appendicitis. The diagnosis can be made only at laparotomy, when the characteristic beefy red terminal ileum, boggy mesenteric fat, and succulent mesenteric lymph nodes indicate that appendicitis alone could not produce this picture.

While the symptoms of diarrhea and abdominal pain will usually alert the clinician to the possibility of regional enteritis, other symptoms may dominate the clinical presentation. In children and the aged, fever of undetermined origin and unexplained weight loss may be prominent and initially may cause one to suspect underlying malignancy. In some patients, the first manifestation of the disease may be intestinal obstruction; in others the disease may present with fistula formation in the form of perianal sepsis or urinary tract infection resulting from an enterovesical fistula. Similarly, right ureteral obstruction and hydronephrosis may occur due to external compression of the ureter by a right lower quadrant inflammatory mass. On occasion, often in the setting of extensive small-bowel involvement, features of malabsorption may be prominent. These features, along with anorexia and the catabolic effects of the chronic inflammatory process, may combine to produce striking degrees of weight loss.

The complications of the disease are often local, resulting from intestinal inflammation and involvement of adjacent structures.

Intestinal obstruction is a frequent complication, occurring in 20 to 30 percent of patients during the course of the disease. In the initial stages, the obstruction usually is due to the acute inflammation and edema of the involved intestinal segment, usually the terminal ileum. However, as the disease progresses and fibrosis develops, obstruction may be due to a fixed narrowing of the bowel.

Fistula formation is a frequent complication of chronic regional enteritis as well as Crohn's disease of the colon. Fistulas may occur between contiguous segments of intestine; they may also burrow into the retroperitoneal spaces and present as cutaneous fistulas or indolent abscesses. In a significant number of patients, the first indication of the disease may be the presence of persistent rectal fissures, a perirectal abscess, or a rectal fistula. Although uncommon, pneumaturia should raise the suspicion of enterovesical fistula and is often associated with a persistent urinary tract infection.

Since Crohn's disease is a transmural disease with the bowel wall greatly thickened, free *intestinal perforation* is uncommon. In a small number of cases, however, it may be the presenting feature, and the disease is first discovered at the time of laparotomy for a perforated viscus. The passage per rectum of bright red blood should alert one to the possible coexistence of rectal involvement (i.e., ileocolitis). Crohn's disease may also involve the *stomach* and *duodenum*. The involvement is usually of the antrum and/or the first and second portions of the duodenum. Symptoms may include pain mimicking peptic ulcer disease. Later in the course of the disease, chronic scarring may produce gastric outlet or duodenal obstruction.

There are increasing reports of *small-bowel* and *colonic malignancy* developing in the setting of long-standing Crohn's disease. Although the risk of developing malignancy is statistically increased, the complication is uncommon when compared with the frequency of malignancy in ulcerative colitis (see below). As in other chronic inflammatory diseases, patients with long-standing Crohn's disease may rarely develop secondary *amyloidosis,* which may manifest itself with hepatosplenomegaly or significant proteinuria. The presence of extensive ileal disease, resulting in *bile salt malabsorption,* is associated with a decreased bile salt pool and an increased lithogenicity of bile (see Chap. 240). Up to 30 percent of patients with extensive ileal disease will develop gallstones. Also, in the setting of ileal disease and an intact colon there is increased colonic absorption of dietary oxalate with resultant hyperoxaluria and the development of *urinary oxalate stones.* Dehydration due to diarrhea is an additional predisposing factor in renal stone formation.

DIAGNOSIS

The diagnosis of IBD should be entertained in all patients presenting with diarrhea or bloody diarrhea, persistent perianal sepsis, and abdominal pain. There may be atypical presentations such as fever of unexplained origin in the absence of bowel symptoms or with extracolonic manifestations such as arthritis or liver disease antedating or overshadowing the bowel involvement. Since Crohn's disease may also involve the small intestine, it should be considered in the differential diagnosis of all types of malabsorption syndromes, intermittent intestinal obstruction, and abdominal fistulas.

The laboratory examination is usually nonspecific and reflects the extent and severity of the inflammatory reaction. In addition, when Crohn's disease involves the small bowel, laboratory features of malabsorption may be present. There may be a variable degree of anemia, from occult blood loss or the effect of chronic inflammation on the bone marrow. Folate or vitamin B_{12} malabsorption may also contribute to the anemia. While the Schilling test may be abnormal in patients with extensive ileal disease, frank macrocytic anemia due to vitamin B_{12} malabsorption alone is unusual, attesting to the marked efficiency of ileal absorption of the vitamin. When there is significant diarrhea, electrolyte abnormalities (hypokalemia, hypomagnesemia) may be prominent. Hypocalcemia may reflect extensive mucosal involvement and malabsorption of vitamin D. Hypoalbuminemia may result from amino acid malabsorption as well as from protein-losing enteropathy. Variable degrees of steatorrhea may result from bile salt depletion and mucosal damage. Mild abnormalities of liver function (especially an increased serum alkaline phosphatase) may reflect the development of a fatty liver in the malnourished patient or a coexisting pericholangitis. Significant jaundice is unusual. Proteinuria may reflect secondary amyloidosis, a rare complication.

Sigmoidoscopy and *radiologic* studies of the bowel are most important in establishing the diagnosis of inflammatory bowel disease. Sigmoidoscopy must be performed in all patients presenting with chronic diarrhea and in all instances of rectal bleeding. While meticulous air-contrast barium enema examination of the perfectly prepared colon may disclose the earliest mucosal changes in either ulcerative colitis or Crohn's disease (see below), a conventional barium enema examination is often "normal" in early disease. Direct visualization of the colonic mucosa combined with biopsy is the most sensitive way of determining whether rectal inflammation is present. It can often be performed without prior enema preparation in the patient actively having diarrhea. The goal of sigmoidoscopy is to establish *whether* mucosal inflammation is present and not necessarily to determine its full *extent* at the initial examination. Thus, if sigmoidoscopic changes are encountered within the first 8 to 10 cm, it is not necessary to pass the instrument to its full length which may cause discomfort when the bowel is acutely inflamed. In ulcerative colitis, findings include a loss of mucosal vascularity, diffuse erythema, friability of the mucosa, and often an exudate consisting of mucus, blood, and pus. The most characteristic feature is mucosal friability, best demonstrated by lightly wiping the surface of the mucosa with a cotton swab and observing the mucosa for the appearance of diffuse, small bleeding points. Equally characteristic is the uniformity of involvement. Once diseased mucosa is encountered (usually in the rectum), there are no areas of intervening normal mucosa before the proximal extent of the disease is reached. Ulceration is shallow, may be small or confluent, but invariably occurs in segments of active colitis. Rectal biopsy may corroborate mucosal inflammation. With more chronic disease, the mucosa may show a granular appearance and pseudopolyps may be present.

Endoscopic examination of the colon is also of value in the diagnosis of colonic Crohn's disease. The findings are of ulcerations which may be tiny, aphthous erosions or deep, longitudinal fissures. They usually occur in segments of otherwise normal mucosa. Since the mucosa is not uniformly involved, friability and diffuse granularity, which are hallmarks of ulcerative colitis, are not characteristic of Crohn's colitis. Rather a cobblestone appearance, which is a coarse irregularity of the mucosal surface, reflects submucosal inflammation and is characteristic of Crohn's disease. Pseudopolyps, edema, and strictures may be seen in Crohn's colitis as well as in ulcerative colitis. Colonic mucosal biopsy reveals granulomas in 30 to 50 percent of specimens taken from involved areas. Features such as crypt abscesses, infiltration with inflammatory cells, or ulcerations are nonspecific but compatible features. Since skip areas and rectal sparing are characteristic of Crohn's disease, colonoscopy may be superior to sigmoidoscopy in the evaluation of Crohn's disease. Colonoscopic examination is also indicated when Crohn's disease appears only to involve the small bowel. Ileal biopsy may be feasible, and coexisting colonic involvement occurs in a significant number of cases. Perianal inflammatory lesions as well as areas of rectal disease seen at endoscopy will often show granulomatous inflammation. Rectal biopsy of seemingly "uninvolved" areas may also show microscopic evidence of granulomatous inflammation in only 5 to 15 percent of patients.

The *radiologic evaluation* of the bowel provides essential information in the diagnosis of IBD. Barium enema, in ulcerative colitis, may reveal the extent of the disease and help define associated features such as stricture, pseudopolyposis, or carcinoma. The earliest features seen in ulcerative colitis are irritability and incomplete filling

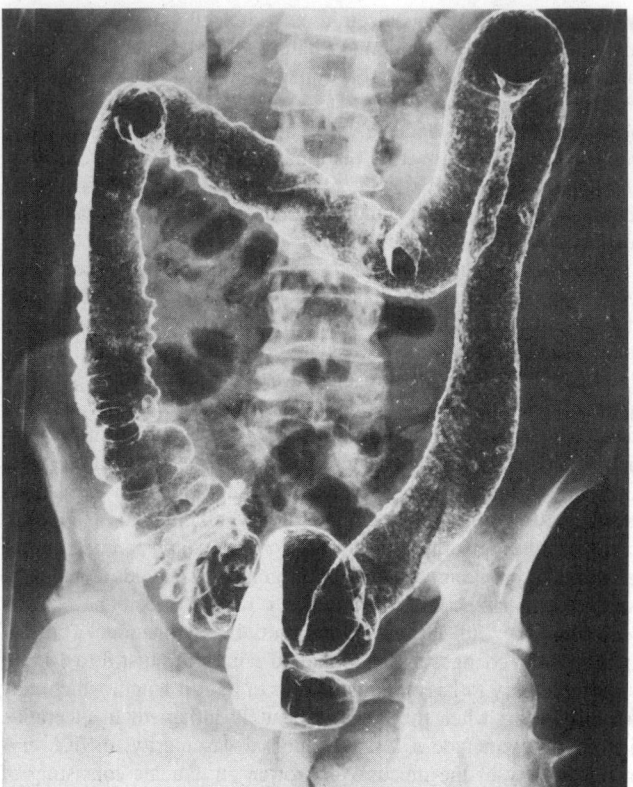

FIGURE 241-4 Acute ulcerative colitis, air-contrast study. Note the diffuse fine ulceration of the entire colon, producing serration along the contour of the bowel. *(Courtesy of R Gold, Columbia Presbyterian Medical Center.)*

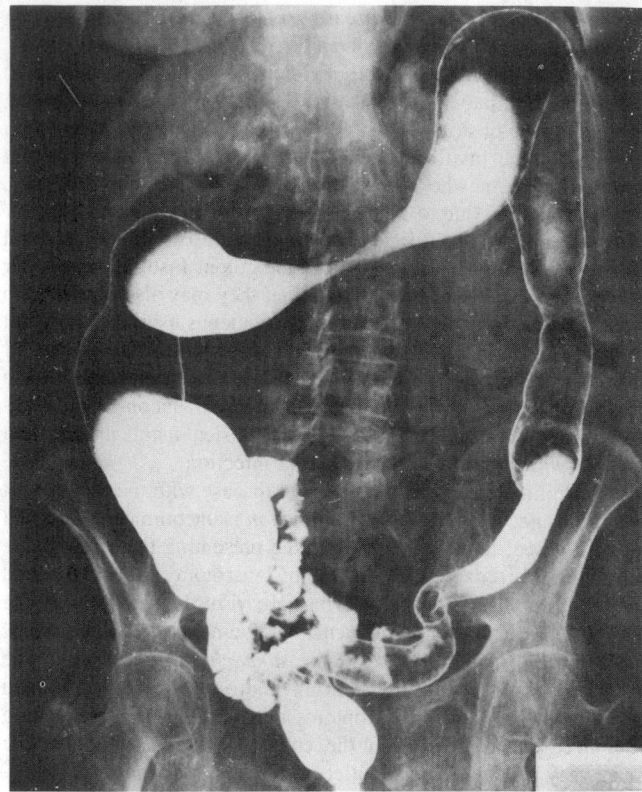

FIGURE 241-5 Chronic ulcerative colitis. Note the loss of haustrations and the fusiform stricture in the transverse colon. *(Courtesy of R Gold, Columbia Presbyterian Medical Center.)*

due to associated inflammation. Fine ulcerations may be seen at this time as serrations along the contour of the bowel producing a hazy margin (Fig. 241-4). The ulcerations may become deeper and with more fulminant disease produce a grossly ragged and irregular contour. Polypoid defects appear as a result of edematous mucosa between ulcerations. The diffuse pattern of ulceration is best seen on the evacuation film or on air-contrast barium enema. In the chronic stage of the disease (Fig. 241-5), the characteristic features are shortening of the bowel, depression of the flexures, narrowing of the bowel lumen, and rigidity. The bowel has a symmetric, ahaustral, tubular appearance with a decreased mucosal pattern. Although strictures are uncommon, when they occur they have a concentric lumen with fusiform tapering margins. Eccentricity should raise the suspicion of an associated carcinoma.

Barium enema examination in Crohn's disease of the colon has features which usually distinguish it from ulcerative colitis. Features characteristic of Crohn's disease include rectal sparing, the presence of skip lesions, and the finding of small ulcerations occurring on small irregular nodules. The small ulcerations often extend to produce longitudinal ulcers (Fig. 241-6) and transverse fissures which in reality are limited sinus tracts. These may extend into adjacent tissues to produce fistulas. Irregular thickening and fibrosis may lead to stricture formation which may be multiple. In 10 to 15 percent of cases the disease may uniformly involve the entire colon, making differentiation from ulcerative colitis more difficult. Reflux of barium into the terminal ileum during barium enema may reveal characteristic ileal changes of regional enteritis.

When Crohn's disease involves the small intestine, the terminal ileum is most characteristically involved with features similar to colonic involvement. Careful x-ray examination of the small bowel may demonstrate loss of mucosal detail and rigidity of involved segments resulting from submucosal edema or stenosis. The submucosal inflammation may lead to the characteristic radiologic cobblestoned appearance of the mucosa (Fig. 241-7), and fistulous tracts may be seen, especially in the ileocecal area (Fig. 241-8). Involvement of the stomach and duodenum usually appears radiologically as stiffening and infiltration of the mucosa and can mimic an infiltrative tumor. If such an appearance is due to regional enteritis, there is almost always coexistent involvement of either the jejunum or ileum. In Crohn's disease computed tomography (CT) imaging of the abdomen may be of value in the evaluation of thickened, separated bowel loops and to help distinguish thickened, matted loops (phlegmon) from intraabdominal abscess.

While barium studies often provide information on the pattern and extent of inflammatory bowel disease, caution must be exercised in obtaining these studies in the acutely ill patient with severe colitis in whom barium study and the bowel cleansing which precedes it may result in a worsening of the disease and can precipitate toxic dilatation of the colon.

Fiberoptic colonoscopy has added greatly to the diagnosis of colonic inflammatory bowel disease. Areas formerly beyond the reach of the sigmoidoscope can now be directly visualized and biopsy material obtained. Early in the course of colonic inflammation, endoscopic examination and biopsy are the most sensitive techniques to demonstrate mucosal involvement. Polypoid lesions, strictures, and unclear x-ray features can usually be fully defined. Periodic colonoscopic examination and biopsy are being increasingly used in cancer surveillance in patients with long-standing inflammatory bowel disease (see below).

DIFFERENTIAL DIAGNOSIS

Many entities must be considered in the differential diagnosis in IBD. The focus of the differential diagnosis will in large measure be determined by the presenting features of the disease. When *rectal bleeding* is the presenting complaint, a colonic source should be considered. While *hemorrhoids* are commonly found, they must be

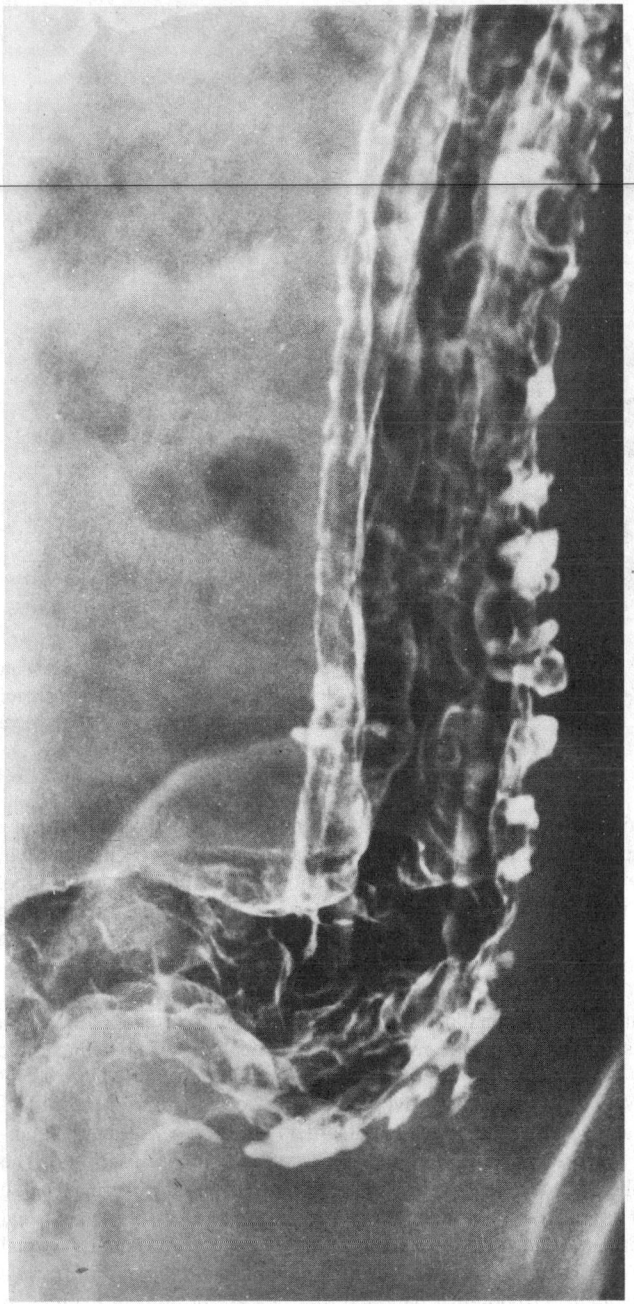

FIGURE 241-6 Crohn's colitis. Air-contrast study.

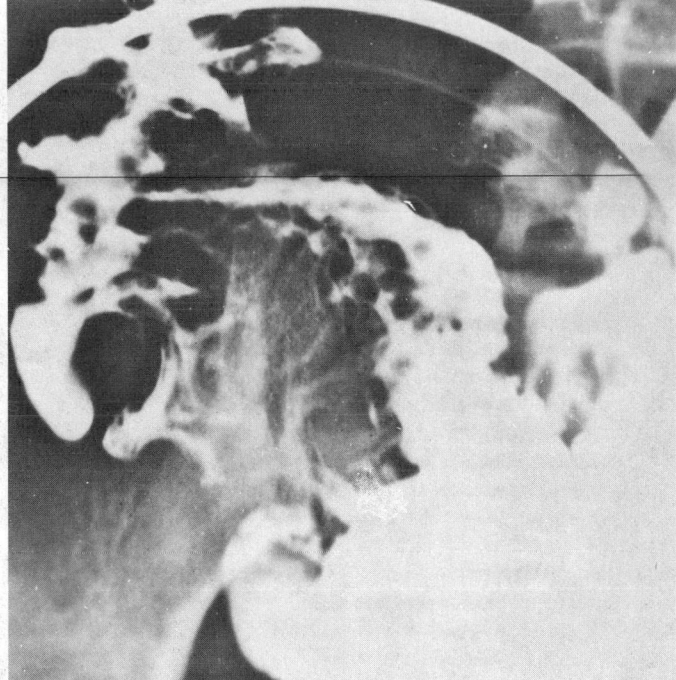

FIGURE 241-7 Crohn's ileocolitis. Note the nodularity and ulceration of the terminal ileum and the deformity of the cecum.

considered a tentative source of bleeding until sigmoidoscopy and barium enema have eliminated other colonic lesions. Colonic *neoplasms* (carcinoma, adenomatous polyps) may also present with rectal bleeding and can usually be diagnosed by barium enema with subsequent sigmoidoscopic or colonoscopic biopsy. It should be remembered that carcinoma may complicate long-standing colitis. Rectal bleeding from *colonic diverticula* or *arteriovenous malformations* usually present no problem in differential diagnosis since radiologic and endoscopic features of inflammatory bowel disease are absent. *Radiation proctitis*, which may present as a localized area of colitis, is usually found in the setting of pelvic irradiation. The onset may, however, occur at variable (months to years) periods of time after irradiation. Characteristic features on sigmoidoscopy include mucosal atrophy and telangiectasia along with friability and small ulcerations. A colitis sometimes indistinguishable from ulcerative colitis may occur in Behçet's syndrome and is associated with aphthous oral ulceration, uveitis, and urethritis.

Acute colitis may be caused by a variety of *infectious* agents (Chap. 92). Often presenting with bloody diarrhea, infectious colitis may be difficult to distinguish from IBD at initial presentation. Rectal biopsy in infectious colitis shows marked polymorphonuclear infiltration with pronounced edema and relative sparing of the crypts, features which may distinguish it from idiopathic inflammatory bowel disease. A listing of these agents is given in Table 241-2.

Amebiasis may present with bloody diarrhea and at sigmoidoscopy be indistinguishable from idiopathic ulcerative colitis. A history of recent foreign travel or homosexual exposure should always be sought. Since specific amebicidal therapy is necessary to eradicate this infection and corticosteroids may be detrimental, every effort should be made to exclude this diagnosis in appropriate individuals. Acute *bacillary dysentery* may be caused by *Shigella* and *Salmonella* or *Campylobacter*, all easily diagnosed by stool culture. *Yersinia enterocolitis*, which often presents as acute ileitis, can also produce a self-limited colitis, sometimes with granulomatous reaction. Infectious agents may cause acute proctitis indistinguishable from idiopathic ulcerative proctitis. Such infections, often seen in homosexuals, may be due to herpes simplex virus, *gonorrhea*, or *lymphogranuloma venereum* (LGV) as well as *amebiasis*. Recently, in homosexual men, non-LGV strains of *Chlamydia* have been shown to produce a granulomatous proctitis closely resembling Crohn's disease of the rectum.

Pseudomembranous colitis (antibiotic-associated colitis) is caused by a necrolytic toxin elaborated by *Clostridium difficile*, which under certain circumstances proliferates within the bowel. Most often the

TABLE 241-2 Microbiologic causes of colitis

Shigella
Salmonella
Amebiasis
Yersinia
Campylobacter
Lymphogranuloma venereum (LGV)
"Non-LGV" *Chlamydia*
Gonorrhea
Pseudomembranous colitis (*Clostridium difficile* toxin)
Tuberculosis

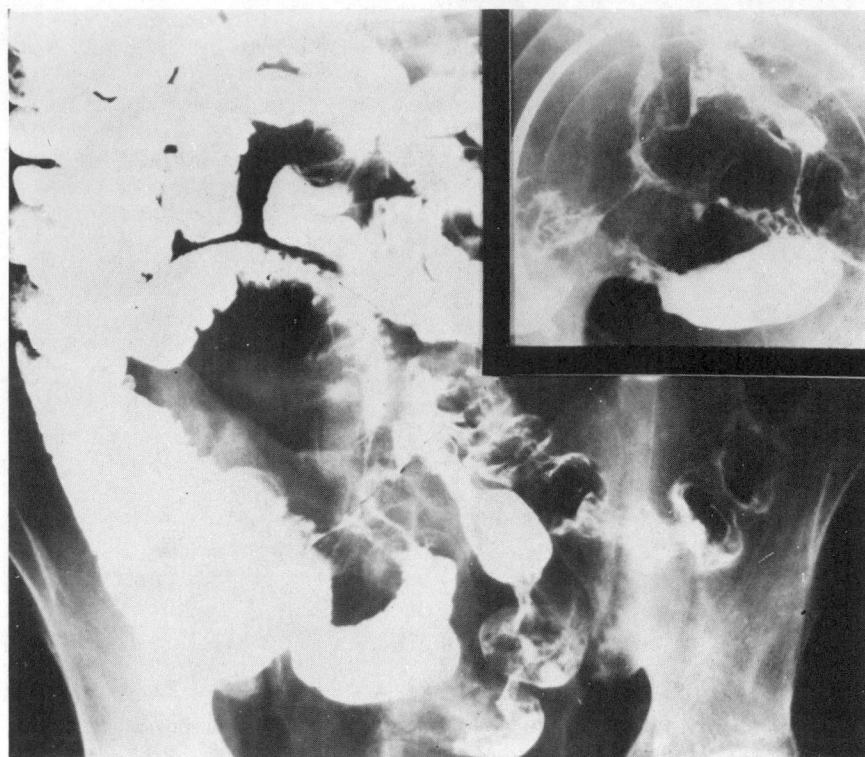

FIGURE 241-8 Regional enteritis. X-ray showing fistulas between loops of bowel. Insert is a compression film of this area; note fistulas between adjacent loops of bowel.

disease is a result of antibiotic therapy which presumably upsets the normal ecologic balance of the bowel flora permitting *C. difficile* to proliferate. Almost every antibiotic has been implicated, although cases related to the use of vancomycin or aminoglycosides are rare. Most often diarrhea is profuse and watery, although bloody diarrhea occurs in 5 percent of cases. Characteristic lesions are seen on sigmoidoscopy and appear as multiple, discrete yellowish plaques which on biopsy show features of acute inflammation and ulceration with a pseudomembrane of fibrin and necrotic material. On occasion lesions may be beyond reach of the sigmoidoscope and require colonoscopy. Diagnosis is best made by detecting *C. difficile* toxin in the stool. Treatment is either directed at binding the toxin or at eradicating the *C. difficile* organisms. Anion exchange resins such as cholestyramine (4 g PO qid for 5 days) will bind the toxin and may be used in mild cases. Vancomycin (250 mg PO qid for 7 to 14 days) is the treatment of choice for more severely ill patients and should produce clinical improvement within 5 days. Since vancomycin therapy is expensive, alternative therapies have been proposed. Metronidazole (500 mg PO tid) or bacitracin (25,000 units PO qid) have been suggested as alternative therapies. With all forms of therapy, relapse rates (15 to 30 percent) have been observed and may require a subsequent course of therapy to eradicate the organism. On occasion, infectious causes of colitis will be superimposed on ulcerative colitis or Crohn's disease. In this case, once the acute infection has subsided, symptoms and inflammatory mucosal changes may persist, raising the possibility of associated idiopathic IBD. Similar considerations apply to the patient with IBD who uncommonly may develop associated *pseudomembranous* colitis. The finding of *C. difficile* toxin in the stool and subsequent treatment will serve to clarify this presentation.

Abdominal pain in association with rectal bleeding, especially in the older age group, may be due to *ischemic colitis*. Because of an excellent collateral circulation, the rectum is usually spared. Radiologic features are often characteristic.

Inflammatory bowel disease may be difficult to distinguish from functional diarrhea early in the course of disease. The presence of constitutional symptoms such as fatigue, fever, and weight loss, coupled with laboratory features of anemia, elevated erythrocyte sedimentation rate, or occult blood in the stool should alert the clinician to the possibility of IBD. Similarly, finding leukocytes in a stained stool specimen points to an inflammatory basis for the diarrhea. In all cases, stool cultures and parasitologic examination of the stool are required to rule out enteric bacterial pathogens or amebiasis. In the *irritable bowel syndrome* sigmoidoscopy, rectal biopsy, and barium enema examination are all normal.

Once the diagnosis of idiopathic IBD has been established, the distinction between ulcerative colitis and Crohn's disease of the colon is usually possible. Differential diagnostic features are shown in Table 241-1.

With small-intestinal involvement (regional enteritis) the differential diagnosis should include disorders presenting with intraabdominal abscesses, fistulas, intestinal obstruction, and malabsorption. The finding of associated colonic involvement in patients with ileal disease will often serve to distinguish Crohn's disease from other ileal disorders. With diffuse involvement of the jejunum and ileum, regional enteritis must be distinguished from *nongranulomatous ulcerative jejunoileitis*. Abdominal pain and diarrhea are prominent features of this disorder, and weight loss, malabsorption, and hypoproteinemia tend to be more prominent than in regional enteritis. Small-bowel biopsy shows a more diffuse lesion with flattened villi (similar to celiac sprue), infiltration of the lamina propria, and mucosal ulceration. *Abdominal lymphoma* may likewise present with clinical and radiologic features difficult to distinguish from regional enteritis. Hepatosplenomegaly and peripheral adenopathy, when present, are helpful clues, but often disease is confined to the intestine. In such cases, laparotomy is usually required to make the definitive histologic diagnosis.

The advanced presentation of regional enteritis with areas of stenosis and draining fistulas may also be confused with *chronic fungal infection of the bowel,* including actinomycosis, aspergillosis, and blastomycosis. These infections often are seen in debilitated patients with impaired host defenses. Fungal skin tests and examination of fistula drainage and biopsy material for characteristic granules and fungi are helpful in making the diagnosis.

Intestinal tuberculosis characteristically produces stenotic lesions, usually in the terminal ileum, also often involving the contiguous cecum and ascending colon. Unlike regional enteritis, "skip areas" are unusual. Histologically, the granulomatous inflammation seen with *Mycobacterium* tuberculosis may be indistinguishable from regional enteritis; acid-fast stains and cultures are required. Fortunately in western countries primary intestinal tuberculosis is now rare; when intestinal involvement does occur, it invariably is associated with pulmonary tuberculosis.

COMPLICATIONS OF INFLAMMATORY BOWEL DISEASE

The complications of IBD may be classified as local, which are a direct reflection of mucosal inflammation and its extension, or systemic complications (Table 241-3). Local complications of IBD such as fistulas, abscesses, and strictures have been described above. In addition, perforation, toxic dilatation, and the development of carcinoma may complicate both ulcerative colitis and Crohn's disease.

PERFORATION Intestinal perforation can occur in severe ulcerative colitis since with extensive ulceration the bowel wall may become extremely thin. The clinical features are those of acute peritonitis with signs of peritoneal inflammation and the demonstration of free air under the diaphragm on upright film of the abdomen. These are an indication for immediate colectomy.

Toxic dilatation of the colon may occur in Crohn's colitis but is more common in ulcerative colitis. This complication can best be considered as a severe form of ulcerative colitis with the additional feature of colonic dilatation. It is thought that the neuromuscular tone of the bowel is affected by the severe inflammation resulting in dilatation. Injudicious use of hypomotility agents (codeine, diphenoxylate, loperamide, paregoric, anticholinergic agents) to treat diarrhea in the setting of acute colitis can precipitate this complication. Similarly, cathartic preparation and barium enema examination as well as superimposed hypokalemia may be contributing factors. Clinically, features of severe colitis are present with high fever, tachycardia, volume depletion, electrolyte imbalance, and abdominal pain. On examination, the patient appears toxic, and colonic dilatation may be evident. There is abdominal tenderness and if perforation has already occurred, peritoneal signs are present. Diarrhea may actually decrease markedly due to colonic atony, creating the false impression that the colitis is clinically improved. Plain film of the abdomen will show colonic dilatation with the colonic diameter more than 6 cm.

TABLE 241-3 Some systemic complications of inflammatory bowel disease

1 Nutritional and metabolic
  a Weight loss, ↓ muscle mass, growth retardation (children)
  b Electrolyte deficiency (K^+, Ca^{2+}, Mg^{2+})
  c Hypoalbuminemia (↓ nutrition, protein-losing enteropathy)
  d Anemia (chronic disease, iron deficiency; rarely folate or vitamin B_{12} deficiency in Crohn's disease)
  e Bile salt deficiency with ileal disease (steatorrhea and fat-soluble vitamin deficiency; ↑ colonic oxalate absorption → renal stones; ↑ lithogenicity of bile → gallstones)
2 Musculoskeletal
  a Peripheral arthralgia, arthritis
  b Ankylosing spondylitis, sacroileitis
  c Granulomatous myositis (rare)
3 Hepatobiliary disease
  a Fatty liver
  b Cholelithiasis
  c Pericholangitis, biliary cirrhosis (rare)
  d Sclerosing cholangitis
  e Bile duct carcinoma
  f Chronic active hepatitis and cirrhosis
4 Skin and mucous membrane
  a Erythema nodosum
  b Pyoderma gangrenosum
  c Aphthous stomatitis
  d Crohn's disease of buccal mucosa, gingiva, vagina
5 Eye
  Iritis, uveitis, episcleritis
6 Venous thrombosis and thromboembolism (hypercoagulability, dehydration, stasis)

There may be air in the wall of the colon, and irregular, ulcerated islands of mucosa may be silhouetted against the air shadow. While the transverse colon is the most common site of dilatation, this is probably largely positional, since with the patient supine, this is the highest portion of the colon. This presentation of colitis represents a true medical emergency and is associated with a mortality of greater than 30 percent if perforation has occurred. Appropriate therapy is discussed below.

CARCINOMA AND INFLAMMATORY BOWEL DISEASE There is an increased incidence of carcinoma in patients with chronic IBD when compared to the general population, especially in patients who have more extensive mucosal involvement (i.e., pancolitis) and those who have had their disease for extended periods of time. Cumulative risk of cancer rises steadily with the duration of disease. It has been estimated that with pancolitis there is a risk of cancer of 12 percent at 15 years, 23 percent at 20 years, and 42 percent at 24 years, although estimates in community-based practices have been lower. In children, the risk of cancer appears to rise more sharply after the first 10 years of disease, perhaps reflecting the higher incidence of pancolitis in children. Limited involvement of the colon (i.e., proctitis) has a low risk of malignant degeneration. Malignancy developing in Crohn's disease of the colon or small bowel is less well documented, but the incidences of both small- and large-bowel malignancies are increased compared to the general population. The incidence, however, is less than in ulcerative colitis.

The development of colon carcinoma arising in the setting of IBD demonstrates important differences when compared to carcinoma arising in a noncolitic population. Clinically, many of the earlier warning signs of a colonic neoplasm (i.e., rectal bleeding, change in bowel habits) will be difficult to interpret in the setting of colitis. In colitic patients the distribution of carcinomas is more uniform throughout the colon than in noncolitic patients; in the latter the majority of carcinomas are in the rectosigmoid within reach of the sigmoidoscope. In colitis patients the tumors are more often multiple, flat, and infiltrating and appear to have a higher grade of malignancy. There is some evidence to suggest that these features may reflect the younger age at which they occur rather than the associated colitis. Further adding to the difficulty in diagnosis is the frequent occurrence of mucosal irregularities, ulcerations, and pseudopolyps, making a small carcinoma difficult to diagnose radiologically or endoscopically.

Efforts have been directed to devise effective screening procedures to detect carcinoma developing in the setting of IBD. Carcinoembryonic antigen (CEA) may be elevated nonspecifically in ulcerative colitis and therefore is of limited value. Periodic barium enemas and/or sigmoidoscopy or colonoscopy have been suggested, but interpretation is sometimes hampered by abnormalities related to the colitis itself. The addition of colonic mucosal biopsy may add a significant dimension. It was originally suggested that a generalized precancerous lesion may be present in high-risk patients with colitis who either harbor an occult malignancy or who will develop cancer. Subsequent studies of rectal biopsies in patients with long-standing colitis showed that if dysplasia was present, there was approximately a 50-percent chance that an associated malignancy was present in those patients who subsequently came to colectomy. Complicating these findings was the fact that dysplastic changes were only found in rectal biopsies 60 percent of the time, making colonoscopy with multiple biopsies desirable. In addition, in some patients not undergoing colectomy, dysplasia was not a consistent finding on subsequent biopsies. While more information is needed on the prognostic significance and reproducibility of finding dysplastic changes on mucosal biopsy, it seems prudent to examine patients with colonic IBD of greater than 8 to 10 years' duration with colonoscopy and multiple mucosal biopsies at regular intervals. The frequency of such examinations has not been established, with recommendations varying from 6 months to 2 years. If severe dysplasia is found, then confirmation at less than 6-month intervals seems prudent. While most authorities would not advise "prophylactic" colectomy in the patient with long-standing colitis, the finding of severe dysplasia may well identify a subgroup who already harbor an occult carcinoma or who are at high risk of its development. There can be no uniform recommendation for this small group of patients, but many physicians will advise colectomy in this setting.

EXTRAINTESTINAL MANIFESTATIONS OF INFLAMMATORY BOWEL DISEASE

There are a variety of nonintestinal symptoms and signs which may be associated with IBD and occur in both ulcerative colitis and Crohn's disease (Table 241-3). Since some of these manifestations may not coincide with, or may overshadow, the underlying bowel disease, they may on occasion pose difficult diagnostic problems. Their etiology is currently unknown.

Joint manifestations are common in patients with IBD (~25 percent incidence). These may range from arthralgia only to an acute arthritis with painful, swollen joints.

The nondeforming arthritis is mono- or polyarticular and often migratory. Knees, ankles, and wrists are most commonly involved, but any joint may be affected. Joint fluid, if aspirated, reveals findings of an acute arthritis without crystals or evidence of infection. Tests for specific forms of arthritis (rheumatoid factor, antinuclear antibody, and LE factor) are negative. Typically, the arthritis correlates with activity of the underlying bowel disease. Rarely, peripheral arthritis may truly antecede clinical bowel symptoms. Arthritis is more commonly found in patients with colonic than with small-bowel involvement alone (regional enteritis).

In contrast, the central arthritis or ankylosing spondylitis associated with IBD is unrelated to the activity of the underlying bowel disease. It may antedate the bowel disease by years and persist after surgical or medical remission of the disease has been achieved. Symptoms are of low backache and stiffness with eventual limitation of motion. This may be associated with sacroileitis as well. X-rays usually reveal characteristic changes. In contrast to the peripheral arthritis, there is a strong association of HLA-B27 with ankylosing spondylitis, whether or not IBD is present.

Like the peripheral arthritis *skin manifestations* are more common with colonic disease. They occur in about 15 percent of patients, and when present the severity correlates with activity of the bowel disease. *Erythema nodosum* may be seen and heals without scarring. *Pyoderma gangrenosum,* an ulcerating lesion often occurring on the trunk, is relatively painless and may heal with scarring. In the rare patient, the lesion may persist even after colectomy for ulcerative colitis. *Aphthous ulcers* resemble "canker sores" of the mouth, and in approximately 5 to 10 percent of patients they are present during periods of active disease and then resolve. Their etiology is unknown and they are treated symptomatically. *Ocular manifestations* such as episcleritis, recurrent iritis, and uveitis occur in approximately 5 percent of patients and may represent a severe manifestation of the disease. In general, their activity parallels the course of the bowel disease, and the lesions may respond dramatically when colectomy is done for other indications.

Abnormalities of *liver function* are common in IBD. In the severely ill, malnourished patient, mild abnormalities of serum aminotransferases and alkaline phosphatase are often seen and represent nonspecific focal hepatitis or fatty infiltration. Factors favoring fatty infiltration of the liver in the severely ill patient are poor nutrition and often concomitant steroid therapy. The lesion is not progressive and resolves with disease remission. *Pericholangitis* is characterized histologically by portal tract inflammation, some bile ductular proliferation, and concentric fibrosis around bile ductules. Some authorities feel that this lesion represents the intrahepatic form of sclerosing cholangitis. Most often, the lesion is clinically insignificant, and its sole manifestation is an elevated serum alkaline phosphatase. It is usually nonprogressive and requires no therapy. Rarely, there may be an apparent progression to cirrhosis of either the postnecrotic or biliary type. Uncommonly, patients with IBD may develop *sclerosing cholangitis* (Chap. 258), a chronic inflammation of unknown etiology involving the extrahepatic and intrahepatic bile ducts which may produce varying degrees of extrahepatic biliary obstruction. Corticosteroids and immunosuppressive therapy are not beneficial. Reversal of the disease after colectomy is an inconsistent result and should not form the sole indication for colectomy. Cholangiocarcinoma, arising in the extrahepatic biliary tree, has an increased incidence in patients with chronic ulcerative colitis. Such patients will present with extrahepatic biliary obstruction which must be distinguished from sclerosing cholangitis. Finally, *chronic active hepatitis* which may progress to *cirrhosis* may be seen in IBD, although the exact relationship between these disorders is unknown. The evaluation and therapy are similar to the disease occurring in noncolitic patients. There is no clear evidence that colectomy influences the course of this form of liver disease.

TREATMENT

In general, the treatment of ulcerative colitis and Crohn's disease shares certain common principles. Initial treatment of all forms of uncomplicated IBD is primarily medical, and the principles of medical therapy are similar. Surgery is reserved for (1) specific complications and (2) intractability of disease. There are certain important differences, however, between ulcerative colitis and Crohn's disease; namely, the response to drug therapy may differ, complications often differ, and the prognosis after surgical therapy is not the same.

ULCERATIVE COLITIS   Medical therapy   Once the diagnosis is established, the severity of the disease must be assessed. Mild ulcerative colitis, including ulcerative proctitis, can usually be treated on an ambulatory basis. More severe disease, especially at initial presentation, is best treated in a hospital setting. The disease can rapidly worsen, and the course of a given attack cannot be predicted at the outset. The aims of therapy are to control the inflammatory process and replace nutritional losses. A certain degree of improvement usually follows intravenous correction of fluid and electrolyte disturbances. Blood transfusions may be required in severe anemia, especially when there is continued active bleeding. Agents to control diarrhea (diphenoxylate, loperamide, codeine, anticholinergics) should be used with extreme caution for fear of precipitating colonic dilatation and toxic megacolon. The decision to institute specific nutritional replacement therapy will be determined by the nutritional status of the patient and whether a protracted clinical course can be anticipated. In the severely ill patient, even clear liquids orally may stimulate colonic activity, and it is often wise to give the patients nothing by mouth. In this setting, intravenous alimentation, either peripheral or central, has been used as interim nutritional replacement therapy (see Chap. 75). While there is no evidence that intravenous alimentation is effective as primary therapy, it is an important component of a treatment program. In the less severely ill patients able to tolerate fluids by mouth, the use of elemental oral diets may be beneficial providing supplemental nutrition with low fecal volume. While milk is not contraindicated in ulcerative colitis, diarrhea will be exacerbated if there is an associated lactase deficiency.

The principal drugs used in the therapy of ulcerative colitis are the *anti-inflammatory agents, sulfasalazine* (Azulfidine) and *adrenal glucocorticoids* or ACTH. Sulfasalazine consists of a sulfonamide (sulfapyridine) moiety chemically bound to a salicylate (5-aminosalicylate); it undergoes bacterial cleavage in the colon. The liberated sulfapyridine is efficiently absorbed and largely excreted in the urine; the liberated 5-aminosalicylate believed to be the active component remains largely in the colon and is excreted in the stool. The salicylate moiety is thought to exert its action through inhibition of prostaglandin synthesis. While most physicians are familiar with the use of sulfasalazine to prevent recurrences of ulcerative colitis, it is less well appreciated that this agent is effective in the therapy of acute ulcerative colitis of mild to moderate severity. Therapeutic doses of 4 to 6 g daily are required. The drug is usually started at a dose of

500 mg bid and then increased daily or every other day by 1 g until the therapeutic dose is achieved.

In the severely ill patient who may not tolerate oral medication and for whom a more rapid time frame of therapy is often desired, initial therapy is begun with glucocorticoids or ACTH. While some physicians still prefer ACTH to corticosteroids, these agents appear equally effective when given in equivalent dosages and by comparable routes of administration. The choice is one of individual preference; however, oral prednisone (45 to 60 mg daily) is often employed initially. Alternatively, intravenous ACTH may be given (40 to 60 units) over an 8-h drip infusion. In the severely ill patient, parenteral administration of corticosteroids (i.e., intravenous hydrocortisone 300 to 400 ng daily) is preferable to avoid the uncertainty of adequate oral absorption. Improvement is usually noted after 7 to 10 days of such therapy by a reduction in fever, decreased bloody diarrhea, and an improvement in appetite.

After initial improvement low-roughage oral feedings can be resumed. At this point the dose of steroids can be tapered, or if ACTH was used initially, oral prednisone at reduced dosage can be started. There is no specific schedule for tapering glucocorticoids. The guiding principle, however, is that once clinical remission is achieved, there is no evidence that chronic steroid administration favorably influences the long-term outlook of the disease or that recurrences can be prevented by chronic steroid therapy. In practice, steroid therapy can be tapered and discontinued over a 2- to 3-month period after discharge. In some patients (10 to 15 percent) efforts to completely eliminate steroids may be associated with a flare of the disease, and low to moderate steroids (10 to 15 mg of prednisone daily) may be required to suppress disease activity. This should not be confused with the prophylactic administration of steroids to patients in remission, but rather represents incompletely responsive disease. Once the acutely ill patient is taking oral feedings, sulfasalazine should be added as described above in a daily dose of 2 g. Controlled trials have shown that this dose of sulfasalazine, when administered chronically to patients with ulcerative colitis, is effective in decreasing the frequency of relapses and should be continued chronically after glucocorticoids have been discontinued. Patients with glucose phosphate dehydrogenase deficiency or those exhibiting severe allergic reactions to the drug unfortunately cannot be maintained on it. Patients who exhibit intolerance for the drug (headache, nausea) or mild skin allergic reactions can be "desensitized" by gradually reintroducing the drug in small doses. Sulfasalazine is discontinued for 1 to 2 weeks and then is restarted at a dose of 0.125 to 0.25 g per day for 1 week with a gradual increase by 0.125 g per week to a maintenance dose of 2 g per day. The knowledge that the 5-aminosalicylate portion of the molecule is therapeutically efficacious has led to formulations of this compound without the sulfa moiety responsible for allergic reactions. 5-Aminosalicylate incorporated into enemas, enteric coated 5-ASA, or oral azodisalicylate (consisting of two molecules of 5-aminosalicylate joined by an azo bond) have shown encouraging results in the treatment of mild to moderate ulcerative colitis.

The use of immunosuppressive therapy with drugs such as azathioprine is less well established in ulcerative colitis. As a single agent in the therapy of acute ulcerative colitis, the drug is ineffective. However, the drug may be added to the regimen at a dose of 1.5 to 2.0 mg/kg when glucocorticoids fail or when the steroid dose needed to reduce inflammation is too high. It is desirable to monitor the blood count and observe the patient carefully for infection. Azathioprine may also have a limited role as a "steroid-sparing agent" in the patient with chronic ulcerative colitis who must be maintained on corticosteroids to control disease activity.

Toxic megacolon is a major complication of severe ulcerative colitis which requires rapid, intensive management best carried out jointly by the internist or gastroenterologist and surgeon. Once the diagnosis is established, prompt and vigorous use of intravenous fluids, electrolyte replacement therapy, and blood transfusions are indicated. Because of the fear of perforation and high likelihood that bacteremia and occult perforation have occurred, many physicians will institute broad-spectrum antibiotic coverage after appropriate cultures have been obtained. The patient is given nothing by mouth, and nasogastric suction is often instituted. Full intravenous corticosteroid therapy is also begun. Majority opinion favors an initial period of medical stabilization for the first 24 to 48 h. If significant objective improvement has not occurred and if perforation seems imminent, emergency colectomy should be carried out. While it is certainly true that some patients, under maximal medical therapy, may slowly improve and thus avoid colectomy, the risk of this course of action must be carefully considered. If perforation occurs, mortality rates rise sharply, approaching 50 percent in those who subsequently go on to colectomy.

At the other end of the spectrum is the patient with mild ulcerative colitis, limited to the rectum or rectosigmoid, who is managed on an ambulatory basis. Therapy is started with sulfasalazine, 0.5 to 1.0 g four times a day with meals. If rectal symptoms such as tenesmus are prominent, topical steroids in the form of small enemas may produce marked improvement. The equivalent of 100 mg hydrocortisone (20 mg prednisone) in 60 to 100 mL saline is used as a bedtime enema. On occasion the use of steroid foam preparations may be better tolerated in the patient with severe tenesmus. Retention enemas have been shown to deliver medication as far as the descending colon, and absorption of steroid is small (~10 to 20 percent). If large doses of rectal steroids are required for control, it is preferable to use oral prednisone at a moderate dosage (20 mg daily).

Psychotherapy The elements of trust and mutual understanding combined with the compassion and expertise of the physician are essential in the therapy of any chronic disease and are particularly important in the long-term management of patients with inflammatory bowel disease. Often these patients are intelligent young adults who are frequently resentful of a disease affecting them during the most productive years. Through the vigorous participation of the physician many patients are able to lead reasonably stable and productive lives. More formal psychiatric assistance may be required in the chronically ill patient, in particular children or adolescents, or in the elderly where severe depressive reactions are common. This is particularly true when colectomy is being advised and in the emotional adjustment which must be made after colectomy.

Pregnancy and ulcerative colitis While many physicians are apprehensive about the management and prognosis of ulcerative colitis in the pregnant patient, the outcome for the patient and the fetus is excellent. In general, the pregnancy is not threatened by coexistent colitis, with no increase in stillbirths or premature deliveries when compared to the general population. When patients with inactive colitis become pregnant, approximately 50 percent may have an exacerbation of their disease with some clustering of these flares during the first trimester and in the postpartum period. The therapy of ulcerative colitis during pregnancy is largely the same as in the nonpregnant patient. Sulfasalazine is used to treat mild to moderate disease since there is no evidence that the drug is harmful to the fetus or leads to increased incidence of fetal malformations. Women with inactive colitis who enter a pregnancy on maintenance sulfasalazine should be continued on the drug. Since sulfapyridine appears in breast milk, in the newborn with unconjugated hyperbilirubinemia from other causes, breast feeding should be discontinued or the drug stopped if the colitis is inactive. In most situations, however, the drug should be continued to protect the mother during the postpartum period from a relapse of disease. Corticosteroids should be used in the same dosage and for the same indications as in the nonpregnant patient.

Thus, it is clear that the patient with colitis can realistically plan to have a family. It is prudent, however, to bring active disease under control before pregnancy is undertaken to ensure the most optimal physical and emotional setting for the pregnancy. Similar conclusions apply to the management of Crohn's disease during pregnancy.

Surgical therapy Approximately 20 to 25 percent of patients with ulcerative colitis will require colectomy during the course of their disease. A major indication for colectomy is failure to respond to intensive medical management. Such patients, although not showing colonic dilatation, may fail to improve after 7 to 10 days of optimal medical therapy. Fever, persistent bloody diarrhea, and severe fatigue may persist, and consideration should be given to semielective colectomy. Elective colectomy may be performed in patients whose disease remains chronically active and who require continuous corticosteroid administration. Such patients are at risk of developing the complications of chronic steroid therapy. After colectomy these patients often feel more energetic and usually gain back weight to their preillness level. As discussed above, the patient with long-standing colitis is at high risk for colonic cancer. While most authorities do not advise ''prophylactic'' colectomy in the patient with quiescent disease, the finding of marked dysplasia on colonoscopic biopsies done as a part of a surveillance program should make the physician think seriously about advising colectomy.

The decision to advise colectomy in other than emergency circumstances is difficult for both patient and physician. Many patients have an understandable reluctance to undergo colectomy and have difficulty in conceptualizing life with an ileostomy. In most metropolitan centers there are ileostomy groups who visit patients preoperatively and can provide answers to many practical questions. It is also desirable for the patient to be visited by a nurse familiar with stoma care to instruct the patient on the practical aspects of handling the ileostomy.

While total proctocolectomy with permanent ileostomy is the procedure of choice for almost all patients undergoing colectomy, several alternative approaches have been suggested. The *continent ileostomy* is an ileal loop reservoir fashioned under the skin with a nipple valve to prevent spilling of ileal contents. Ileal effluent collects in this reservoir which must be emptied with a soft rubber catheter. Only a small stoma is externally visible, thus eliminating an external ileostomy appliance. Problems with this procedure include a failure of continence, irritation of the mucosa of the ileal reservoir from stasis (''pouchitis''), and bacterial overgrowth which may lead to mild malabsorption. Repeat operations are common, and this procedure should only be done by skilled surgeons familiar with the technique. *Ileorectal anastomosis* with *mucosal stripping* of the rectal segment is sometimes done in children who require colectomy. Newer forms of surgical therapy include ileoanal anastomosis with internal reservoirs thus preserving sphincteric function. These approaches are recent and not generally available.

CROHN'S DISEASE   The medical management of colonic Crohn's disease is similar in most respects to that of ulcerative colitis. In a multicenter study (National Cooperative Crohn's Disease Study), sulfasalazine was shown to be effective in the therapy of active colonic disease. Glucocorticoids also were efficacious but less so than with small-bowel involvement. The indications and dosages of these medications are similar to those for ulcerative colitis. Since in Crohn's disease, intraabdominal sepsis can result from fistula or abscess formation, corticosteroids must be used with caution and constant attention is required to detect evidence of sepsis, which can be masked by these agents. In general, the disease is less explosive in onset, and although toxic dilatation and perforation can occur, they are less common than in ulcerative colitis. The principles of management are the same. Because of the indolent nature of the disease, the response to therapy is often less complete than in ulcerative colitis, and the disease tends to progress despite apparent clinical inactivity. It may be more difficult to achieve a clinical remission and to withdraw steroids completely. As in ulcerative colitis, controlled studies have shown no benefit to continuing steroids after remission since the frequency of recurrence is not altered by prophylactic steroid therapy. Disappointingly, sulfasalazine did not decrease recurrence rates in Crohn's disease.

While response to therapy of the initial attack of Crohn's colitis may be satisfactory, many patients continue to have persistently active disease. This may express itself as progressive weight loss, diarrhea, and deterioration of general health. Perianal disease with predominantly left-sided colonic involvement (fistula formation and

perirectal abscesses) may constitute a recurrent problem. In one controlled study, *metronidazole* (20 mg/kg per day in divided dosage) resulted in marked improvement in 10 of 18 patients with chronic perineal fistulas associated with Crohn's disease. It is not clear whether the drug is active because of its antibacterial properties or through another mechanism. It is possible that this drug may prove to be of value in the therapy of the perineal complications of Crohn's disease before surgical therapy is attempted. The role of immuno-suppressive therapy such as azathioprine has been controversial in Crohn's disease. The multicenter United States study (National Cooperative Study) found azathioprine to be ineffective as a single agent in the therapy of active Crohn's disease. Yet there have been reports of dramatic improvement in a small percentage of patients when azathioprine (1.5 to 2 mg/kg) is added to a maximal program in the nonresponding patient. Some investigators have found 6-mercaptopurine (the active metabolite of azathioprine) effective in controlling disease activity when added to corticosteroids and sulfasalazine. However, a beneficial response may take 6 to 8 months in some patients.

The management of Crohn's disease of the small intestine (regional enteritis) is similar to that for colonic Crohn's disease, and as noted many patients have concomitant small- and large-bowel disease. Several additional considerations are pertinent, however. *Intestinal obstruction* is not uncommonly a presenting feature with ileal involvement. Initially, this may be secondary to acute inflammation and will respond to corticosteroids. With recurrent involvement and the development of fibrosis, steroid therapy is less effective and surgical decompression is required. *Nutritional problems* often are more severe with involvement of the small intestine than with colonic involvement alone. Added to the general catabolic nature of the disease may be loss of absorptive surface which may result from progressive involvement or because of surgical resection. Refinements in the technique of parenteral alimentation have made it possible to provide a patient's total daily caloric intake intravenously for a period of weeks or even months (see Chap. 75). Parenteral alimentation has been employed with increasing frequency in the severely ill patient as a means of placing the gastrointestinal tract ''at rest'' and in preparing the malnourished patient for surgery. With this approach the disease may become quiescent, and the drainage from fistulas may decrease. However, disease activity frequently recurs when oral feedings are resumed. On occasion, prolonged intravenous alimentation, administered at home, may be required when oral feedings are not effective or in children exhibiting severe growth failure associated with Crohn's disease. Most often it is possible to design a dietary program of oral supplementation to nourish the patient adequately.

In patients with extensive small-bowel involvement or in those with a short bowel resulting from extensive intestinal resection, supplementation of electrolytes, minerals, and vitamins will be required. Extensive ileal disease or resection often results in diarrhea induced by bile salts and in malabsorption; cholestyramine may be needed to control the diarrhea and medium-chain triglycerides added to reduce fat malabsorption (see Chap. 240). In patients with stenotic segments of intestine, a low-residue (low-fiber) diet should be recommended. A lactose-free diet should be instituted if there is an associated lactase deficiency. Other dietary modifications have not been shown to have any beneficial effect on the primary disease process. Patients should be encouraged to eat a nutritious, appealing diet of their own choosing. *Surgical therapy* is generally reserved for the complications of Crohn's disease rather than as a primary form of therapy. In contrast to ulcerative colitis, more patients with Crohn's disease will require surgery in the chronic management of the disease. Approximately 70 percent of patients will require at least one operation during the course of their disease. Although each case and situation must be individualized, in general, surgery may be required (1) for persistent or fixed bowel narrowing or obstruction; (2) for symptomatic fistula formation to the bladder, vagina, or skin; (3) for persistent anal fistulas or abscesses; and (4) for intraabdominal abscesses, toxic dilatation of the colon, or perforation. In contrast to ulcerative colitis, where colectomy is curative, in Crohn's disease surgical resection of the small or large intestine is followed by a high rate of recurrence. With resection of segments of small bowel or ileum and reanastomosis a recurrence rate of 50 to 75 percent over a 5-year period is not unusual. Recurrence of disease is invariably proximal to the created anastomosis. When total colectomy and ileostomy are performed for Crohn's disease of the colon without significant small-intestinal involvement, recurrence rates are lower, varying from 10 to 30 percent. Despite these recurrences, most patients do not develop a short-bowel syndrome and usually can expect significant improvement. Faced with the possibility of recurrent disease many physicians are reluctant to advise surgery in Crohn's disease, except for the type of clear-cut complications described above. Alternatively, patients with persistently active disease may require chronic maintenance on unacceptably high levels of corticosteroids and with the appreciable risk of steroid side effects. Just as a failure of medical therapy should lead to colectomy in ulcerative colitis, it should be the conclusion in the patient with Crohn's colitis without major small-bowel involvement. While in this setting there is also a definite rate of recurrence, such recurrences are often not disabling. When extensive small-bowel disease is present, surgical therapy is often not feasible and should only be reserved for specific disease complications.

The therapy of Crohn's disease in children presents special problems since normal growth and development may be retarded in the presence of active disease. In addition to conventional drug therapy, intensive nutritional therapy or the judicious use of surgery may be required.

PROGNOSIS

The overall prognosis of IBD has been favorably affected by the use of corticosteroids and sulfasalazine, as well as by supportive techniques such as intravenous alimentation. In *acute* ulcerative colitis these therapeutic modalities can result in a remission in almost 90 percent of patients. The mortality of an initial acute attack is approximately 5 percent. Poor prognostic factors and an increased mortality rate are likely when there is total colonic involvement, when the onset occurs over age 60, and when toxic megacolon develops.

The long-term prognosis of *chronic* ulcerative colitis is more difficult to assess due to the variable and intermittent nature of the disease and improvements in therapy. Left-sided colitis and ulcerative proctitis have a very favorable prognosis and probably no increase in mortality; similarly the long-term prognosis for extensive colitis has improved greatly. Older studies suggested a poor prognosis for extensive colitis, with less than 50 percent of patients surviving 15 years after onset. More recent observations (longest follow-up 11 years) show a 10-year mortality rate of between 5 and 10 percent for severe first attacks (excluding toxic megacolon). Approximately 75 percent of patients will experience relapses, and 20 to 25 percent will require colectomy. The problem of carcinoma developing in the setting of long-standing chronic ulcerative colitis is an important factor in determining the long-term prognosis of ulcerative colitis. As discussed above, periodic surveillance with colonoscopy and multiple biopsies to detect dysplastic changes is indicated to detect a high-risk group for which to advise colectomy.

The prognosis for Crohn's disease is not as favorable as for ulcerative colitis. An exception is *acute regional enteritis*, often discovered during laparotomy for suspected appendicitis; this has an excellent prognosis. More than two-thirds of such patients may show no subsequent evidence of regional enteritis, and this form of acute ileitis may well be due to *Yersinia* infection (see above). Prevailing surgical opinion favors a conservative approach in this situation, and in most instances operative resection is not advised.

In the majority of patients with Crohn's disease the course is chronic and intermittent regardless of the site of involvement. The disease responds less well to medical therapy with time, and over two-thirds of patients develop complications requiring surgery at some point in their disease. In contrast to ulcerative colitis, where mortality appears greatest early in the disease, in Crohn's disease the mortality rate increases with the duration of the disease, and probably ranges from 5 to 10 percent. Most deaths occur from peritonitis and sepsis. As indicated above, following surgery patients with Crohn's disease often have recurrence and relapses. Nevertheless, the therapy of Crohn's disease will result in reasonably stable and productive lives for most Crohn's disease patients.

REFERENCES

General

KIRSNER JB, SHORTER RG (eds): *Inflammatory Bowel Disease*, 2d ed. Philadelphia, Lea & Febiger, 1980

———, ———: Recent developments in "nonspecific" inflammatory bowel disease. N Engl J Med 306:775, 837, 1982

SLEISENGER MH, FORDTRAN JS (eds): *Gastrointestinal Diseases*, 4th ed. Philadelphia, Saunders, 1989

Etiology and diagnostic aspects

BLASER MJ, RELLER LB: *Campylobacter* enteritis. N Engl J Med 305:1444, 1981

CHAPMAN RW et al: Serum antibodies, ulcerative colitis, and sclerosing cholangitis. Gut 27:86, 1986

GOLDBERG HI et al: Computed tomography in the evaluation of Crohn's disease. Am J Roent 140:277, 1983

GREENSTEIN AJ et al: The extraintestinal complications of ulcerative colitis and Crohn's disease: A study of 700 patients. Medicine 55:401, 1976

JESS P: Acute terminal ileitis: A review of recent literature on the relationship to Crohn's disease. Scand J Gastroenterol 16:321, 1981

QUINN TC et al: *Chlamydia trachomatis* proctitis. N Engl J Med 305:195, 1981

SURAWICZ CM, BELIC L: Rectal biopsy helps to distinguish acute self limited colitis from idiopathic inflammatory bowel disease. Gastroenterology 86:104, 1984

TRNKA YM, LaMONT JT: Association of *Clostridium difficile* toxin with symptomatic relapse of chronic inflammatory bowel disease. Gastroenterology 80:693, 1981

VAN TRAPPEN G et al: *Yersinia* enteritis and enterocolitis: Gastroenterological aspects. Gastroenterology 72:220, 1977

Therapy of inflammatory bowel disease

AZAD KHAN AK et al: Optimum dose of sulphasalazine for maintenance treatment in ulcerative colitis. Gut 12:232, 1980

BERNSTEIN LH et al: Healing of perineal Crohn's disease with metronidazole. Gastroenterology 79:357, 1980

FARMER RG et al: Long-term follow-up of patients with Crohn's disease. Relationship between clinical pattern and prognosis. Gastroenterology 88:1818, 1985

KELTS DG et al: Nutritional basis of growth failure in children and adolescents with Crohn's disease. Gastroenterology 76:720, 1979

LENNARD JONES JE et al: Cancer in colitis: Assessment of the individual risk by clinical and histological criteria. Gastroenterology 73:1280, 1977

PEPPERCORN MA: Sulfasalazine. Ann Intern Med 3:377, 1984

PRESENT DH et al: 6-Mercaptopurine in the management of inflammatory bowel disease: short- and long-term toxicity. Ann Intern Med 111:641, 1989

RIDDELL RH et al: Dysplasia in inflammatory bowel disease. Hum Pathol 14:931, 1983

SCHROEDER KW et al: Coated oral 5-aminosalicylate acid therapy for mild to moderately active ulcerative colitis. A randomized study. N Engl J Med 317:1625, 1987

SUMMERS RW et al: National cooperative Crohn's disease study: Results of drug treatment. Gastroenterology 77:849, 1979

URSING B et al: A comparative study of metronidazole and sulfasalazine for active Crohn's disease. The Cooperative Crohn's Disease Study in Sweden. Gastroenterology 83:550, 1982

242 DISEASES OF THE SMALL AND LARGE INTESTINE

J. THOMAS LaMONT / KURT J. ISSELBACHER

SYMPTOMS OF INTESTINAL DISEASE

SYMPTOMS OF DISEASES OF THE SMALL INTESTINE The major clinical manifestations of small-bowel disease are *motility disturbances*, abdominal *pain* and *distention*, gastrointestinal *bleeding*, and *malabsorption*.

Altered intestinal peristalsis is a common manifestation of a variety of diseases. The presentation may be one of decreased motility, such as paralytic ileus resulting from metabolic disturbance or peritonitis, or intestinal obstruction caused by tumors, adhesions, volvulus, or intussusception (Chap. 244). Diarrhea frequently accompanies small-bowel disease (Chap. 44) resulting from direct mucosal involvement by inflammatory or infiltrative lesions (sprue, regional enteritis). The associated malabsorption of fat and bile salts is an important factor in the pathogenesis of diarrhea in these conditions (Chaps. 44 and 240).

Abdominal pain due to small-intestinal disease is usually periumbilical or supraumbilical and often poorly localized. With obstruction, pain is classically described as intermittent or colicky. Visceral pain arises from distention or stretching of the intestinal wall, or from inflammation of the overlying parietal peritoneum. As the intestine becomes progressively dilated with loss of muscular tone, the colicky nature of the pain may become less apparent. Acute inflammation of the small intestine which involves the visceral or parietal peritoneum is associated with steady, aching pain, usually located directly over the inflamed area, and may be accompanied by guarding and rebound tenderness if the parietal peritoneum is involved. *Gastrointestinal bleeding* due to small-bowel disease may be detected as occult bleeding or, less commonly, brisk hemorrhage. In general, bleeding from the stomach or small intestine causes black or tarry stool (melena), while bleeding from the colon causes passage of red blood or clots. Obviously, the appearance of blood in the stool depends not only on site of bleeding but also on the rate of the hemorrhage and the rapidity of transit; thus localization of the bleeding site by stool appearance alone may be misleading.

An important clue to the presence of small-bowel disease is the demonstration of malabsorption of fat. With extensive mucosal damage or lymphatic obstruction, the presenting symptoms may relate to any of the features of a malabsorption syndrome or protein-losing enteropathy (Chap. 240) and should direct attention to the small intestine.

SYMPTOMS OF COLONIC DISEASE The major symptoms of colonic disease are *alteration in bowel habit*, *rectal bleeding*, and *pain*. Alteration in bowel habit implies a change from previous patterns of defecation; hence a detailed history is important. Most normal individuals have one to three movements of well-formed stools each day. *Diarrhea* means the passage of watery or loose stools usually with increased frequency, while *constipation* implies infrequent passage of hard, dry stools; *obstipation* is the absence of spontaneous bowel movements. A persistent change in bowel habit, particularly in older individuals with no previous irregularity, is usually an important early symptom of organic disease of the colon and should never be labeled *functional* unless a thorough diagnostic evaluation is negative. The appearance of the stool may also provide important diagnostic clues. Blood coating the exterior of a formed stool implies a lesion in the anal canal or rectum, while blood admixed with the feces indicates a bleeding source higher in the colon. Brisk hemorrhage from the colon or distal small intestine results in passage of fresh blood, called *hematochezia*. This may appear as fresh blood and clots if the lesion is in the left colon, or darker maroon-colored blood if the bleeding source is in the right colon.

Pain resulting from colonic disease is usually localized to either of the lower abdominal quadrants, as opposed to pain of small-intestinal origin, which is localized to the periumbilical area or higher. Rectal pain is often felt deep in the pelvis, while pain in the anal canal is accurately localized to the perineum. The mechanisms of colonic pain are similar to those in other intestinal viscera (see Chap. 17). Distention from gas or fluid causes crampy or colicky pain from stretching of the muscle layers and resulting contraction or spasm. Pain of this type is often relieved by passage of flatus or stool. Pain may also result if the colonic wall is inflamed or infiltrated by tumor. Acute colonic inflammation which involves the visceral or parietal peritoneum produces sharply localized pain, which may be accom-

panied by abdominal guarding and rebound tenderness. An important symptom of rectal disease is *tenesmus*, or painful straining at stool, with a sensation of incomplete emptying after defecation. This symptom can be caused by retention of stool in the rectum, by tumors of the rectum which simulate retained stools, or by colonic inflammation.

DIAGNOSTIC PROCEDURES

PHYSICAL EXAMINATION Careful *examination* of the abdomen may disclose a mass or fistula associated with inflammatory or neoplastic disease, localized tenderness, or abdominal distention resulting from ileus or intestinal obstruction. The physical examination and findings in the patient with acute abdominal pain are discussed in Chap. 17.

Thorough examination may also reveal extraintestinal findings associated with small-intestinal diseases. Thus buccal pigmentation or telangiectasia may indicate coexistent small-bowel polyposis or intestinal telangiectasia and may clarify episodes of abdominal pain or chronic bleeding. Similarly, evidence of iritis, arthritis, or erythema nodosum may suggest the presence of inflammatory bowel disease.

Perhaps the most important part of the physical examination in the diagnosis of colonic diseases is the *digital rectal examination*. This procedure should never be omitted for reasons of modesty or fear of embarrassment because it is essential in the diagnosis of perianal, sphincteric, and ampullary lesions; prostatic and uterine abnormalities; and even small rectal masses. A metastatic tumor may be felt in the perirectal tissues as a shelf-like deformity (Blumer's shelf), especially anteriorly above the prostate. The fecal material on the glove should be immediately tested with guaiac-impregnated cards for occult blood. Approximately one-half of all rectal carcinomas lie within reach of the index finger, and omission of the rectal examination may delay diagnosis and worsen the prognosis.

STOOL EXAMINATION Abnormal stools constitute important objective evidence of colonic disease. Stools should be examined by the physician as soon as possible after defecation for the presence of visible blood on the surface or within the specimen. A small sample should be tested for occult blood. Microscopic examination of fresh stool is important in the diagnosis of parasitic diseases, particularly in amebic colitis when motile trophozoites can be seen in fresh, warm stool suspensions. Stool suspensions can also be stained with a drop of methylene blue for polymorphonuclear leukocytes, which indicate the presence of an acute inflammatory exudate as occurs in ulcerative colitis, amebic colitis, and bacillary dysentery. Fixed and stained slides of stool may also reveal amebas and other parasites, while stool culture is essential for the diagnosis of bacillary dysentery. Sudan III stain of stool is a useful screening test for steatorrhea.

BARIUM STUDIES The considerable length of the small intestine (some 4 to 7 m in the adult) makes *radiologic studies* of the small bowel of prime importance and usually forms the basis for the diagnosis of small-bowel diseases. *Small-bowel x-rays* are not usually part of a routine upper gastrointestinal series and must be specifically requested. In view of the length of the small bowel and wide variations in transit time, it is essential to provide the radiologist with as much information as possible, since the precise nature of the problem may determine various technical aspects of the examination. Enteroclysis is a specialized small-bowel barium study during which barium is infused rapidly via a nasogastric tube into the jejunum. This technique allows distention of bowel loops and rapid filling of the entire small intestine, thus avoiding the problems of inadequate distention and poor transit sometimes encountered in routine small-bowel barium studies. Enteroclysis is indicated in patients with suspected small-bowel lesions not visualized by ordinary barium studies.

Barium enema is a useful diagnostic tool for the identification of certain colonic diseases, including diverticulosis and its complications, motility disturbances, and displacement of the colon by extrinsic lesions. Barium enema is also useful for detection of loss of haustral markings in chronic ulcerative colitis, and for diagnosis of intestinal fistulas. Fiberoptic colonoscopy is more accurate for the diagnosis of early changes of inflammatory bowel disease, or for detection of colonic neoplasms. Colonoscopy offers the additional advantage of allowing biopsy of suspicious lesions, and removal of most polyps.

SIGMOIDOSCOPY The technique of fiberoptic sigmoidoscopy is not difficult to master, and with practice the discomfort to the patient is minimal. The availability of flexible fiberoptic sigmoidoscopes now makes it possible to examine the lower 40 to 60 cm of the colon, compared to the 25-cm limit of the rigid sigmoidoscope. Flexible sigmoidoscopy is generally less painful than rigid sigmoidoscopy. Because approximately half of all colorectal neoplasms lie in the distal 50 cm of the bowel, sigmoidoscopy is an important diagnostic tool. It should be stressed that a rectal carcinoma can be missed on routine barium enema yet easily visualized and biopsied through the sigmoidoscope. Furthermore, the earliest changes of ulcerative colitis may not be demonstrated radiographically but may be obvious through the sigmoidoscope. Rectal biopsy is easily and painlessly accomplished through the instrument and is associated with minimal morbidity except in the presence of bleeding disorders.

COLONOSCOPY See Chap. 236.

MESENTERIC ANGIOGRAPHY Angiography is helpful in the diagnosis of two conditions: intestinal ischemia and gastrointestinal hemorrhage. Patients suspected of having acute intestinal ischemia from arterial embolus as well as chronic ischemia (intestinal angina) should undergo angiography to locate the site of blockage. Angiography may be diagnostic in some patients with acute gastrointestinal blood loss, especially when bleeding exceeds 0.5 mL/min.

RADIONUCLIDE BLEEDING SCAN Bleeding from the small or large bowel can be localized in certain circumstances by radionuclide scanning of the abdomen after intravenous injection of technetium 99m sulfur colloid or autologous red cells labeled with the same agent (Fig. 242-1). If the patient is bleeding at a rate of 0.1 to 0.5 mL/min or greater, the location of radioactivity in the abdomen may indicate the source of bleeding. This diagnostic approach usually requires confirmation by another diagnostic modality such as angiography or endoscopy. The radionuclide bleeding scan is noninvasive, a particular advantage in older patients with bleeding from the small bowel or colon. The bleeding scan is not recommended in patients with suspected bleeding from the esophagus, stomach, or duodenum, who are best studied by upper endoscopy.

FIGURE 242-1 Radionuclide bleeding scan using intravenous injection of technetium-labeled autologous red cells. Ten minutes after injection, a blush appears in the right abdomen over the cecum (arrow). Thirty minutes after injection, the blush has increased in intensity. The cardiac blood pool is noted at the top. Surgery revealed a bleeding diverticulum in the cecum.

DISORDERS OF INTESTINAL MOTILITY

A major function of the intestinal tract is to propel the intestinal contents (food, secretions, chyme, feces) from stomach toward anus. Abnormalities of motility comprise the most common intestinal diseases: diverticulosis, megacolon, constipation, and irritable bowel syndrome. Although these conditions share a common abnormality, i.e., dysmotility, their clinical features are quite diverse.

DIVERTICULOSIS Diverticula may be either congenital or acquired and may affect either the small or large intestine. Congenital diverticula are herniations of the entire thickness of intestinal wall, while the more common acquired diverticula consist of herniations of the mucosa through the muscularis, generally at the site of a nutrient artery.

Small-intestinal diverticula Diverticula may occur in any portion of the small intestine; however, with the exception of Meckel's diverticulum, the most common locations are in the duodenum and jejunum. Most often diverticula are asymptomatic and discovered incidentally on upper gastrointestinal x-rays. On occasion, however, they may cause symptoms either because of their anatomic proximity to other structures or rarely from inflammation or bleeding.

Duodenal diverticula arise singly from the medial surface of the second portion of the duodenum. In most patients, they cause no symptoms. Rarely, they may present as acute diverticulitis with abdominal pain, fever, gastrointestinal bleeding or, most rarely, perforation. Adjacent structures, such as the bile or pancreatic ducts, may become involved; cases of common-duct obstruction and pancreatitis have been reported. Jejunal diverticula, while less common, may also be the site of acute inflammation, bleeding, or perforation with resulting abscess or peritonitis.

Multiple jejunal diverticula may be associated with a malabsorption syndrome related to bacterial overgrowth within the diverticula, similar to other situations where intestinal stasis (i.e., blind loops) permits bacterial proliferation. The consequences of bacterial proliferation with resultant mucosal damage, deconjugation of bile salts, and vitamin B_{12} malabsorption are discussed in Chap. 240.

Meckel's diverticulum, a persistent omphalomesenteric duct, is the most frequent congenital anomaly of the digestive tract, occurring in approximately 2 percent of autopsied adults. The diverticulum is wide-mouthed, about 5 cm long, and arises from the antimesenteric border of the ileum, usually within 100 cm of the ileocecal valve. The sac may be lined with normal ileal mucosa (approximately 50 percent) or contain gastric, duodenal, pancreatic, or colonic mucosa. While rarely symptomatic after age 5, Meckel's diverticulum may produce hemorrhage, inflammation, and obstruction in children and teenagers.

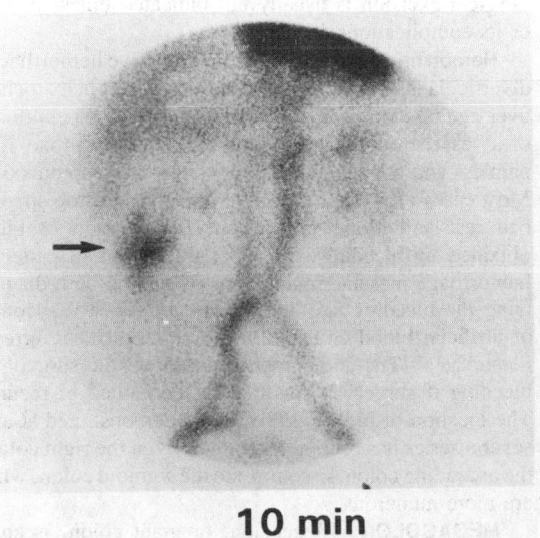

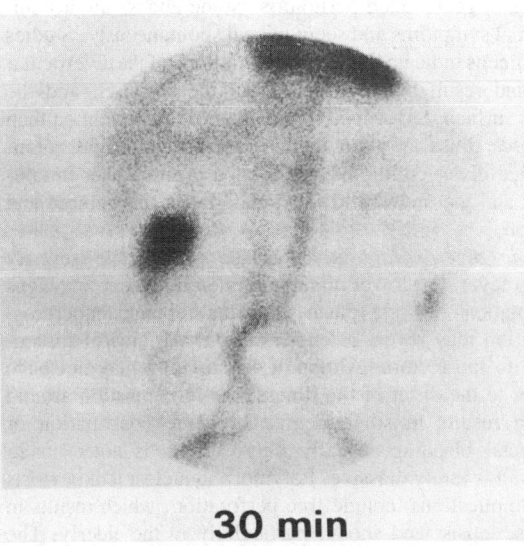

10 min   **30 min**

Hemorrhage occurs almost exclusively before age 10 and invariably results from peptic ulceration of ileal mucosa adjacent to a Meckel's diverticulum lined with gastric mucosa. The diagnosis may be established by isotope scanning of the abdomen after injection of technetium, which is taken up by the ectopic gastric mucosa in the diverticulum. False-negative and false-positive Meckel's scans are not uncommon; thus other clinical and laboratory features must be carefully assessed before recommending surgery. In older children and young adults inflammation of the diverticulum may mimic acute appendicitis. Mechanical obstruction may also occur if the diverticulum intussuscepts into the lumen of the bowel or twists on a fibrous remnant of the omphalomesenteric duct which extends from the diverticulum to the abdominal wall. The treatment of any of these complications of Meckel's diverticulum is surgical excision.

Colonic diverticula   Diverticula of the colon are herniations or saclike protrusions of the mucosa through the muscularis, at the point where a nutrient artery penetrates the muscularis. Diverticula occur most commonly in the sigmoid colon and decrease in frequency in the proximal colon. They increase with age, and the incidence ranges between 20 and 50 percent in western populations over age 50. The exact mechanism for their formation is unknown but may be related to an increase in intraluminal pressure. Thickening of the muscle coat of the colon in most patients with diverticula suggests that herniations of mucosa are caused by increased pressure produced by colonic muscle contractions. The rarity of colonic diverticula in underdeveloped nations in contrast to their frequent occurrence in western countries has led to the speculation that diverticula result from the highly refined western diet, which is deficient in dietary fiber or roughage. It is proposed that such diets result in decreased fecal bulk, narrowing of the colon, and an increase in intraluminal pressure in order to move the smaller fecal mass. The role of dietary fiber in the etiology and treatment of diverticular disease remains to be determined.

Colonic diverticula are usually asymptomatic and are an incidental finding on barium enema performed for other reasons. The major complications of inflammation, both acute and chronic, and hemorrhage occur in only a small percentage of individuals with diverticulosis. Since diverticulosis is quite common in older patients, one must avoid the temptation of attributing symptoms to the diverticula unless other conditions, especially colonic neoplasm, have been excluded.

Diverticulitis   Inflammation can occur in or around the diverticular sac. The cause of diverticulitis is probably mechanical, related to retention in the diverticula of undigested food residues and bacteria, which may form a hard mass called a *fecalith*. This compromises the blood supply to the thin-walled sac (made up solely of mucosa and serosa) and renders it susceptible to invasion by colonic bacteria. The inflammatory process may vary from a small intramural or pericolic abscess to generalized peritonitis. Some attacks are accompanied by minimal symptoms and seem to heal spontaneously. Studies of resected specimens indicate that most perforations of the diverticular sac are small and result in inflammation of the sac itself and the adjacent serosal surface. Diverticulitis occurs more often in men than women, and three times as often in the left as in the right colon. This suggests that diverticulitis may be related to the higher intraluminal pressures and the more solid fecal material in the sigmoid and descending colon.

Acute colonic diverticulitis is a disease of variable severity characterized by fever, left lower quadrant abdominal pain, and signs of peritoneal irritation—muscle spasm, guarding, rebound tenderness. Rectal examination may reveal a tender mass if the area of inflammation is close to the rectum. Although constipation may not have been noted prior to the onset of the illness, the inflammation around the colon often results in some degree of acute constipation or obstipation. Rectal bleeding, usually microscopic, is noted in 25 percent of cases; it is rarely massive. Polymorphonuclear leukocytosis is common. Complications include free perforation, which results in acute peritonitis, sepsis, and shock, particularly in the elderly. The

perforation may be walled off by adherent omentum or neighboring structures such as the bladder or small bowel. Abscess formation or fistulas then occur as the inflammatory mass burrows into other organs. Severe pericolitis may cause a dense, fibrous reaction or stricture around the bowel which can be associated with colonic obstruction.

DIFFERENTIAL DIAGNOSIS   In the less acute situation differential diagnosis is principally that of a neoplasm in the area of the diverticulosis. During the acute phase of diverticulitis, barium enema and sigmoidoscopy may be hazardous, since contrast material or air under pressure may lead to rupture of an inflamed diverticulum and convert a walled-off inflammatory lesion to a free perforation. These examinations are usually safe after adequate treatment and healing of the diverticulitis. The radiologic findings on barium enema suggestive of diverticulitis are leakage of barium from a diverticular sac, stricture formation, and the presence of a pericolic inflammatory mass. In many patients, the distortion caused by inflammation prevents a clear distinction between cancer and diverticulitis. In these cases colonoscopy or surgical excision may be required for accurate diagnosis.

TREATMENT   For the mild case without signs of perforation, treatment consists of bed rest, stool softeners, liquid diet, and a wide-spectrum antibiotic such as tetracycline or ampicillin. Repeated attacks of diverticulitis in the same area generally require surgical resection. Severe attacks with acute peritoneal signs, suspected abscess, or perforation require intravenous antibiotics directed against gram-negative anaerobic bacteria, followed by surgical drainage or resection. The usual procedure is a diverting colostomy with resection of the involved colon; reanastomosis is then performed at a second operation.

Painful diverticular disease without diverticulitis   Some patients with diverticulosis develop recurrent left lower quadrant colicky pain without clinical or pathologic evidence of acute diverticulitis. They often have bouts of alternating constipation and diarrhea, and the pain may be relieved by defecation or passage of flatus. These features suggest the coexistence of the irritable bowel syndrome (see below). Examination during a bout of pain reveals tenderness of the sigmoid colon, but signs of peritoneal inflammation such as rebound tenderness, muscle guarding, fever, and leukocytosis are absent. Barium enema shows typical diverticula without evidence of inflammation and stricture, plus a "sawtooth" irregularity of the lumen reflecting muscle hypertrophy and spasm. In some patients the pain is severe enough to warrant observation in a hospital and restriction of food since feeding aggravates the pain by causing colonic contraction. Anticholinergics, which reduce sigmoid contractions, and mild sedation are usually all that is required. After recovery the patient should be started on a high-residue diet or given a bulk laxative such as hemicellulose, unprocessed bran, or psyllium extract. Surgical excision is usually not indicated unless acute diverticulitis or its complications occur.

Hemorrhage from diverticula   Massive hemorrhage from colonic diverticula is one of the commonest causes of hematochezia in patients over age 60. This complication of diverticulosis is caused by erosion of a vessel by a fecalith within the diverticular sac. The bleeding is painless and not accompanied by signs or symptoms of diverticulitis. Most cases of mild or moderate hemorrhage stop spontaneously with bed rest and blood transfusion. Localization of bleeding can be obtained by bleeding scan or angiography. In patients with severe hemorrhage mesenteric angiography can be both diagnostic in localizing the bleeding site and therapeutic since vasoconstrictive drugs or artificial blood clot infused intraarterially can effectively control hemorrhage. The angiographer can direct the surgeon to the area of bleeding if surgery is required for continued or recurrent bleeding. The location of bleeding diverticula demonstrated at angiography on several series has been more commonly in the right colon, particularly the ascending colon, in contrast to the sigmoid colon, where diverticula are more numerous.

MEGACOLON   Megacolon, or giant colon, is characterized by massive distention of the colon usually accompanied by severe constipation or obstipation. This condition can be either congenital or acquired and is seen in all age groups. Acute toxic megacolon is a severe complication of chronic ulcerative colitis (see Chap. 241).

Aganglionic megacolon (Hirschsprung's disease) This is a congenital disorder which becomes manifest in early infancy, occurring more frequently in males, and is often familial. These infants have massive abdominal distention, absent bowel movements, and impaired nutrition due to chronic obstruction of the colon. In some individuals with less severe symptoms the disease may not be diagnosed until adolescence or early adulthood. The inability to defecate is caused by the absence of ganglion cells (Meissner's and Auerbach's plexuses) in a small segment of the distal colon, usually near the anus. This aganglionic segment is unable to relax to permit passage of stool, causing the normal colon proximal to it to become greatly dilated. On rectal examination the ampulla is empty of feces and the anal sphincter is normal. Barium enema reveals a narrowed segment in the rectosigmoid area, with massive dilatation above. Diagnosis is made by full-thickness surgical biopsy under anesthesia and demonstration of absent ganglion cells in the diseased segment. In most patients the aganglionic segment is in the rectosigmoid colon; in rare instances the lesion may involve more proximal bowel or even the entire colon. The treatment of choice is surgery which restores normal defecation. The most effective operation is a pull-through procedure in which normally innervated colon is anastomosed to the distal rectum just above the internal sphincter, thus bypassing the contracted aganglionic segment.

Chronic idiopathic megacolon This condition, also called *psychogenic megacolon,* has its onset later in childhood, usually at the time toilet training begins. It is characterized by severe chronic constipation and distention and, in contrast to Hirschsprung's disease, digital examination reveals the rectal ampulla to be invariably distended with feces. Barium enema shows the entire colon to be distended with stools, no narrowed segment is seen, and rectal biopsy discloses the normal complement of ganglion cells in Auerbach's plexus. Treatment is based on education in normal bowel habits, but a long course of enemas or large doses of mineral oil may be required until the patient acquires more normal bowel movements.

Acquired megacolon In Central and South America infection with *Trypanosoma cruzi* (Chagas' disease) can result in destruction of the ganglion cells of the colon, producing a clinical picture similar to congenital megacolon, except that the onset is in adult life rather than childhood. A number of other diseases are associated with megacolon in adults. Patients with schizophrenia or depression, particularly institutionalized patients, may have obstipation and massive colonic dilatation. Severe neurologic disorders including cerebral atrophy, spinal cord injury, and parkinsonism may also cause megacolon. Myxedema, infiltrative diseases such as amyloidosis, and scleroderma can also reduce colonic motility and produce marked colonic distention. Narcotic drugs, particularly morphine and codeine, can cause severe constipation, especially when administered to bedridden patients. Digital rectal examination of adults with acquired megacolon reveals a rectum distended with feces, as opposed to the empty rectum in aganglionic megacolon. Treatment is aimed at the underlying disease as well as the careful use of enemas and cathartics.

INTESTINAL PSEUDOOBSTRUCTION Intestinal pseudoobstruction is an acute or chronic motility disorder characterized by distention or dilatation of the small and large intestine. Abdominal pain, nausea, and vomiting may lead to diagnostic confusion with mechanical obstruction, but as the name of this condition implies, the underlying cause is not obstruction but rather a severe dysmotility resulting in distention. Pseudoobstruction may be primary or secondary and acute or chronic. In primary or idiopathic pseudoobstruction no other contributing condition can be identified, and the motility disorder is attributed to abnormalities of sympathetic innervation or of the muscle layers of the intestine. Secondary pseudoobstruction may result from scleroderma, diabetes, amyloidosis, neurologic diseases, drugs, or sepsis.

Chronic or intermittent secondary pseudoobstruction Numerous medical conditions can cause chronic dilatation of the large and small bowel. Some of these may involve the intestinal smooth muscle such as scleroderma, dermatomyositis, amyloidosis, or muscular dystrophy. Endocrine disorders, including myxedema and diabetes mellitus, may result in chronic distention which in the diabetic results from autonomic visceral neuropathy. Chronic neurologic diseases including Parkinson's disease and stroke may be complicated by chronic pseudoobstruction; in these patients drugs and relative immobility are contributing features. Finally, psychotic patients (especially those who are institutionalized) may suffer from prolonged megacolon.

The symptoms of chronic secondary pseudoobstruction are chronic or intermittent constipation, crampy abdominal pain, anorexia, and bloating. Gastric distention and disordered swallowing may be present. Abdominal x-rays reveal gaseous distention of the large and small bowel, and occasionally of the stomach. Air fluid levels are unusual and should raise the possibility of mechanical obstruction. Upper gastrointestinal series and barium enema do not reveal specific abnormalities of the intestine such as tumor, stricture, or volvulus. The presence of an autoimmune disorder or endocrinopathy may require confirmation by serologic or blood tests; biopsy may be needed as in amyloidosis or muscular dystrophy.

The treatment of chronic intestinal pseudoobstruction is made difficult due to the complexity and chronicity of the underlying systemic disease. Patients with scleroderma may respond to broad-spectrum antibiotics if intestinal bacterial overgrowth is suspected. Metoclopramide may benefit gastric dysmotility in the diabetic. Discontinuation of psychotropic or anti-Parkinson drugs may occasionally result in improvement. Cathartics and enemas may be required to relieve fecal impaction, and the regular use of stool softeners and a high-fiber diet may help prevent recurrences.

Idiopathic intestinal pseudoobstruction This term encompasses patients with signs and symptoms of pseudoobstruction in whom no systemic disease can be identified. The typical patient has recurrent attacks of abdominal pain and distention with nausea and vomiting. The small intestine is primarily involved, and chronic constipation is much less frequent than in secondary pseudoobstruction. Steatorrhea secondary to bacterial overgrowth of the small intestine is common and may lead to chronic diarrhea and malnutrition. Many patients exhibit abnormalities of motility in the esophagus and urinary bladder, in addition to the small and large intestine. Various defects have been described in patients with this syndrome, including abnormalities of the mesenteric plexus and myopathy of the intestinal and urinary bladder smooth muscle (so-called hollow visceral myopathy). Elevated prostaglandin E levels have been reported in some patients. Treatment of idiopathic pseudoobstruction is unsatisfactory. Surgery to relieve "obstruction" is to be avoided, since the condition is often worsened by abdominal surgery. Medical therapy with metoclopramide and cholinergic agents has been unsuccessful. Nutritional support in the form of low-residue elemental diets or parenteral hyperalimentation may be helpful. Unfortunately the lack of effective therapy and the progressive nature of the illness make the prognosis of idiopathic pseudoobstruction rather unfavorable. Death from malnutrition and steatorrhea are common. The long-term impact of total parenteral nutrition on this disease is not yet clear.

Acute intestinal pseudoobstruction This entity, sometimes referred to as Ogilvie's syndrome, is characterized by acute intestinal dilatation, involving primarily the colon but occasionally also the small intestine. As in other forms of pseudoobstruction, the clinical features are difficult to distinguish from mechanical obstruction. The patient may complain of colicky lower abdominal pain and acute constipation. Examination reveals a distended, tympanitic abdomen, with reduced or absent bowel sounds. Localized tenderness over the distended colon is common, but diffuse abdominal tenderness, rigidity, or rebound tenderness are unusual. Abdominal films reveal massive dilatation of the colon and small intestine, occasionally with the presence of air fluid levels. The cecum, being the most capacious part of the colon, is often massively dilated and tender. The onset of these symptoms usually occurs in patients who have recently undergone severe surgical or medical stress such as major surgery, myocardial infarction, sepsis, or respiratory failure. Patients with acute pseudoobstruction are frequently on respirators, have received narcotics or sedatives, and have metabolic and electrolyte disturbances.

Management of acute pseudoobstruction requires careful correction of fluid and electrolyte abnormalities, intubation of the stomach or small intestine for decompression, and avoidance of drugs which depress intestinal motility. Barium enema may be hazardous because of the risk of perforating the already dilated bowel. Some authorities recommend cecostomy when the diameter of the colon exceeds 8 cm to avoid ischemic necrosis and perforation. Decompressive colonoscopy is beneficial in some patients. The outcome depends in large part on the prognosis of the associated medical or surgical conditions. Patients who recover from the underlying medical or surgical conditions usually have a return of normal colonic function.

IRRITABLE BOWEL SYNDROME   The irritable bowel syndrome (IBS) is the most common gastrointestinal disease in clinical practice, and although not a life-threatening illness, it causes great distress to those afflicted and feelings of helplessness and frustration for the physician attempting to treat it. The patient with irritable bowel syndrome may present with one of *three clinical variants*. Patients with so-called spastic colitis complain primarily of chronic abdominal pain and constipation. A second group has chronic intermittent diarrhea, often without pain. Some patients have both features and complain of alternating constipation and diarrhea.

The basic pathophysiologic abnormality in the irritable bowel syndrome is an alteration of intestinal motility. Patients with the spastic colon variant (pain and constipation) have *increased* resting colonic motility; in contrast, those presenting primarily with diarrhea have *decreased* resting colonic motility. Both groups have an increase in colonic motility after injection of cholinergic drugs or cholecystokinin; motility may also be increased in association with psychological stress. It has been suggested that cholecystokinin may be a normal stimulus of intestinal motility and that the spastic colon may result from an exaggerated response to the normal release of cholecystokinin after eating.

Patients with the irritable bowel syndrome also exhibit an abnormal basic electrical rhythm in the colon, characterized by an increase in 3-cycle-per-minute slow-wave activity. It is not certain, however, whether these abnormalities of smooth-muscle contraction are primary or secondary to another underlying abnormality of intestinal neuromuscular function.

Evidence of significant psychological disturbances may be seen in some patients with irritable bowel syndrome. Depression, hysteria, and obsessive-compulsive traits are common, and psychological stress frequently triggers an exacerbation of symptoms. It should be noted, however, that increased intracolonic pressure has been observed in normal volunteers during acute stress. This suggests that psychological stress may be a nonspecific trigger of symptoms in the irritable bowel syndrome, as is the case in many other illnesses of diverse etiology.

Clinical features   The irritable bowel syndrome is a disease of young or middle-aged adults; female/male ratio is 2:1. The predominant feature is a history of chronic constipation, diarrhea, or both. The typical patient describes watery diarrhea occurring *intermittently* for months or years. The diarrhea is usually worse in the morning upon arising or after breakfast. After the passage of three or four loose stools with excessive mucus the patient may feel well for the remainder of the day. Diarrhea throughout the day or especially nocturnal diarrhea is most unusual. The diarrhea may last for weeks or months and then disappear spontaneously for variable periods of time. Some patients describe "pencil-like" pasty stools rather than diarrhea.

Another typical presentation is that of chronic abdominal pain with constipation, or with alternating constipation and diarrhea. These patients describe intermittent crampy lower abdominal pain, often

over the sigmoid colon, which is usually relieved by passage of flatus or stool. The patient may describe excessive bloating which is not discernible to the physician. A variety of other complaints, such as heartburn, excessive bloating, back pain, weakness, faintness, and palpitations, are frequent in patients with irritable bowel syndrome. The pain may occasionally be in the right upper quadrant or midepigastrium, leading to diagnostic confusion with biliary tract or peptic ulcer disease.

Physical examination reveals these patients to be anxious but otherwise normal. During intense pain, the abdomen may be distended, but no visible peristalsis is noted; the abdominal musculature is relaxed, and a tender sigmoid full of feces may be palpated in the left lower quadrant. Characteristically, the rectal ampulla is empty of feces. Sigmoidoscopy may reveal a prominent vascular pattern, muscle spasm, or excess mucus. The mucosa itself is normal.

The *diagnosis* of the irritable colon syndrome is suggested by the chronic intermittent nature of symptoms without obvious signs of physical deterioration, the relation of symptoms to environment or emotional stress, and the exclusion of other conditions. The evaluation should include a careful history, complete physical examination, and stool examination for occult blood, parasites, and pathogenic bacteria. In some patients colonoscopy will be necessary to exclude inflammation or neoplasia. Barium enema may reveal spasticity of the sigmoid, accentuated haustra, and a tubular appearance to the descending colon. Lactase deficiency may masquerade as irritable colon syndrome and should be excluded by a trial of milk restriction, a lactose tolerance test, or a lactose breath hydrogen test (see Chap. 240). Thyrotoxicosis is easily confused with irritable bowel syndrome and should be excluded by appropriate laboratory studies.

Treatment of the irritable colon syndrome requires both skill and patience. It is important that the patient be reassured that this condition normally does not lead to the development of chronic inflammatory bowel disease (i.e., ulcerative colitis) or colonic malignancy. It is also important for both the patient and the physician to realize that the condition is chronic, and while it may be alleviated, it cannot be cured. The patient should be encouraged to adapt to the symptoms so as to minimize their impact on life-style. The physician should not imply that the symptoms are largely emotional or psychological in origin, since this is usually rejected by the patient. It is appropriate, however, to emphasize the relationship between psychological stress and the onset of severity of symptoms, as this may allow the patient to better deal with the disease. After the diagnosis is established, frequent x-rays and endoscopies are not necessary; general physical examinations, hemograms, and stool examinations for occult blood, however, should be carried out at regular intervals.

Drug treatment is aimed at altering the abnormal colonic motility in this disease. Patients with constipation may respond to an increase in dietary bulk in the form of unprocessed bran or psyllium bulk laxatives. Mild sedation with phenobarbital or tranquilizers may be indicated, and anticholinergic drugs are useful in some patients. Troublesome diarrhea may respond to diphenoxylate (Lomotil) or paregoric. Unfortunately, no specific drug or dietary regimen affords good relief in all patients, and thus a number of therapeutic maneuvers need to be tried.

CHRONIC CONSTIPATION   In Chap. 44 the mechanism of defecation is discussed. Disorders involving the sensory or motor components of this mechanism may arise from destruction of the nerves subserving these functions, from invasion or inflammation of the rectosigmoid itself, or from central nervous system lesions. Most cases of chronic constipation arise from habitual neglect of afferent impulses, failure to initiate defecation, and accumulation of large, dry fecal masses in the rectum. This voluntary suppression of the call to stool may arise during the period of toilet training in childhood, or later in life because of a sense of social impropriety, unaccustomed surroundings, uncomfortable toilet facilities, or illnesses which require confinement to bed. Chronic constipation is much more common in women, with onset typically in late adolescence or early adulthood. As constant distention of the rectum with feces becomes chronic, the patient grows less aware of rectal fullness. Bowel movements become progressively more difficult, and painful hemorrhoids or anal fissures reinforce suppression of the urge to defecate. To avoid these problems, the patient begins the chronic use of laxatives or enemas, without which defecation becomes impossible.

Treatment The physician should make every attempt to educate the patient about the chain of events which has led to chronic constipation. Attempts should be made to alter patterns of many years' duration, and the patient must recognize the importance of responding to, rather than suppressing, the urge to defecate. It is helpful to initiate a routine whereby defecation is attempted at a given time each day. In most individuals the call to stool occurs in the morning after breakfast. Physical exercise such as a brisk walk just before attempts at defecation may be helpful. Patients are instructed to increase dietary bulk with foods rich in fiber, such as green vegetables and unprocessed cereal grains, or by the regular use of bulk laxatives, such as hemicellulose, psyllium extract, and powdered unprocessed bran. The success of such a regimen depends to some extent on the duration of symptoms. Elderly patients with long-standing constipation and reliance on enemas or laxatives are more resistant to these measures than younger patients whose bowel patterns are less established. Moreover, poor muscle tone, reduced physical activity, and increased incidence of other medical conditions make the problem more difficult in the older age group. Bedridden elderly patients often develop severe constipation and even fecal impaction unless preventive measures are taken. This applies not only to patients with previous constipation but also to those with regular bowel movements prior to their confining illness. Regular administration of stool softeners, bulk laxatives, or mild cathartics is necessary until full ambulation and a normal diet are resumed. The onset of fecal impaction in bedridden patients is heralded by a feeling of rectal distention, urgency of defecation, or tenesmus. Occasionally the fecal impaction will result in low-grade chronic obstruction with dilatation and increased fluid content proximal to the impaction; "paradoxical diarrhea" may thus occur as fluid moves past the obstructing fecal mass. This situation will be aggravated if antidiarrheal drugs are given because the underlying constipation will be worsened. The appropriate maneuver is to disimpact the rectum manually or to administer gentle enemas if the impaction is beyond the reach of the finger.

VASCULAR DISORDERS OF THE INTESTINE

Ischemia is the end result of interruption or reduction of the blood supply of the intestine. However, the clinical manifestations of intestinal ischemia range from mild chronic symptoms to catastrophic episodes, depending on the segment involved, the degree of involvement, and the rapidity of the process, and the clinician should be aware of this spectrum of manifestations (Table 242-1). The gut derives its arterial blood supply from the celiac axis and the superior and inferior mesenteric arteries. The small intestine is supplied by the celiac and superior mesenteric arteries; the colon is supplied by

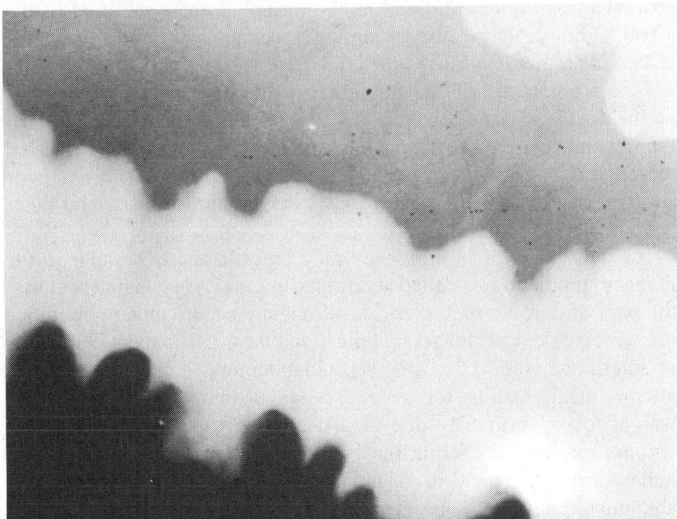

FIGURE 242-2 Barium enema showing "thumbprinting" or submucosal edema of the inferior margin of the transverse colon, in a patient with acute ischemic colitis.

branches of the superior and inferior mesenteric arteries. A rich network of anastomotic vessels and the possible development of collateral circulation determine the clinical picture of acute or chronic intestinal arterial insufficiency.

MESENTERIC ISCHEMIA AND INFARCTION Acute small-intestinal ischemia may be classified as *occlusive* or *nonocclusive*. Occlusion may result from arterial thrombus or embolus of the celiac or superior mesenteric arteries, or from venous occlusion in the same distribution. Arterial embolus occurs most commonly in patients with chronic or recurrent atrial fibrillation, artificial heart valves, or valvular heart disease, while arterial thrombosis is associated with extensive atherosclerosis or low cardiac output. Venous occlusion is quite rare and is occasionally seen in women taking oral contraceptives. Approximately one-half of patients with mesenteric ischemia do not have a definite occlusion of a major vessel, a condition referred to as *nonocclusive* ischemia. The exact cause of nonocclusive disease is obscure; systemic arterial hypotension, cardiac arrhythmias, prolonged heart failure, digitalis therapy, dehydration, and endotoxemia have been suggested as contributing factors.

The outstanding clinical feature of acute mesenteric ischemia is severe abdominal pain, often colicky and periumbilical at the onset, later becoming diffuse and constant. Vomiting, anorexia, diarrhea, and constipation are also frequent but of little diagnostic help. Examination of the abdomen may reveal tenderness and distention. Bowel sounds are often normal even in the face of severe infarction. Some patients have a surprisingly normal abdominal examination in spite of severe pain. Mild gastrointestinal bleeding is often detected by guaiac examination of stool, but gross hemorrhage is unusual except in ischemic colitis (see below). A typical laboratory finding is a pronounced polymorphonuclear leukocytosis. Late in the course of the disease (24 to 72 h) gangrene of the bowel occurs with diffuse peritonitis, sepsis, and shock. Abdominal plain films in patients with mesenteric ischemia may reveal air fluid levels and distention. Barium study of the small intestine reveal nonspecific dilatation, poor motility, and evidence of thick mucosal folds ("thumbprinting") (Fig. 242-2).

Acute mesenteric ischemia is a grave condition with a high morbidity and mortality. Patients suspected of having acute arterial embolus should undergo immediate celiac and mesenteric angiography to localize the embolus, followed by embolectomy. Restoration of normal circulation may allow complete recovery if performed before irreversible necrosis or gangrene has occurred. Unfortunately infarction and transmural necrosis are frequently found at surgery, necessitating resection. Arterial or venous thrombosis is not generally

TABLE 242-1 Patterns of intestinal ischemia

Condition	Etiology	Clinical features	Management
Mesenteric artery embolus	Arterial embolus associated with atrial fibrillation or rheumatic heart disease	Acute central abdominal pain, shock, peritonitis	Immediate angiography and embolectomy if possible
Abdominal angina	Atherosclerosis of celiac and superior mesenteric arteries	Chronic postprandial pain, weight loss	Angiography and surgery in selected cases
Ischemia colitis	Low-flow state	Acute lower abdominal pain, rectal bleeding	Sigmoidoscopy; surgery only for peritonitis

amenable to surgical removal of the thrombus, and resection of the affected bowel is required. Similarly, patients with nonocclusive ischemia are not candidates for corrective vascular surgery (as major vessels are patent). These individuals often have extensive necrosis of the small or large intestine because of the widespread nature of the ischemic event. The decision to operate on patients with suspected mesenteric ischemia is a difficult one as the typical patient is a poor surgical risk owing to advanced age, dehydration, sepsis, and other serious medical conditions.

Chronic arterial insufficiency may precede acute vascular insufficiency, producing so-called abdominal angina. As in angina pectoris, the pain of chronic mesenteric insufficiency occurs under conditions of increased demand for splanchnic blood flow. The patient complains of intermittent dull or cramping midabdominal pain 15 to 30 min after a meal, lasting for several hours postprandially. Significant weight loss is primarily due to a decreased food intake; however, chronic intestinal ischemia may also produce mucosal damage and malabsorption, which in turn aggravates the weight loss. Since abdominal angina may progress to bowel infarction, serious consideration should be given to performing arteriographic studies to confirm the diagnosis in those patients who are candidates for abdominal vascular surgery. The only definitive treatment is surgical removal of the arterial obstruction or the construction of bypass arterial grafts to the ischemic bowel.

A variety of systemic conditions are associated with *vasculitis* of the large and small arteries supplying the intestine. Most often, these disorders can be recognized by the associated extraintestinal manifestations as in polyarteritis nodosa, lupus erythematosus, dermatomyositis, Henoch-Schönlein purpura (allergic vasculitis), and rheumatoid vasculitis. When larger arteries are involved, as in polyarteritis nodosa, the picture of acute intestinal infarction is similar to embolic or atherosclerotic vascular occlusion. Often the involvement of smaller vessels leads to areas of intramural hemorrhage and edema leading to abdominal pain, variable degrees of intestinal obstruction, and bleeding. Barium enema may show "thumbprinting" and "spiculation" due to localized edema, hemorrhage, and ulceration. In many instances, treatment of the underlying disorder may lead to regression of symptoms. If signs of an acute abdomen develop, surgical exploration is usually indicated.

Intramural small-intestinal hemorrhage may occur with vasculitis, trauma, or impaired coagulation, especially in patients receiving anticoagulants. The clinical and radiologic features resemble those seen with vasculitis and local mucosal hemorrhage.

ISCHEMIC COLITIS Ischemia of the colon most often affects the elderly population because of the greater frequency of vascular disease in that group. Ischemic colitis is almost always a nonocclusive disease, that is, obstruction of major arteries is not seen. Shunting of blood away from the mucosa may contribute to this condition, but the mechanism of ischemia is not known.

The clinical picture depends upon the degree of ischemia and the rate of its development. In *acute fulminant ischemic* colitis the major manifestations are severe lower abdominal pain, rectal bleeding, and hypotension. Dilatation of the colon and physical signs of peritonitis are seen in severe cases. Plain abdominal films may reveal thumbprinting from submucosal hemorrhage and edema. Barium enema is hazardous in the acute situation because of the risk of perforation. Sigmoidoscopy or colonoscopy may detect ulcerations, friability, and bulging folds from submucosal hemorrhage. Angiography is not helpful in the management of patients with presumed ischemic colitis since a remedial occlusive lesion is very rarely found. Surgical resection may be required in some patients with fulminant ischemic colitis to remove gangrenous bowel; others with lesser degrees of ischemia may respond to conservative medical management.

Subacute ischemic colitis, the most common clinical variant of ischemic colonic disease, produces lesser degrees of pain and bleeding, often occurring over several days or weeks. The left colon may be involved, but the rectum is usually spared because of collateral blood flow, a distinguishing feature from acute ulcerative colitis. Barium enema reveals edema, cobblestoning, thumbprinting, and occasionally superficial ulceration. Angiography is not indicated as almost all cases are nonocclusive. Occasionally *stricture formation* may follow a bout of ischemic colitis or may present de novo without a history of antecedent pain or bloody diarrhea. Most cases of nonocclusive ischemic colitis resolve in 2 to 4 weeks and do not recur. Surgery is not required except for obstruction secondary to postischemic stricture.

ANGIODYSPLASIA OF THE COLON These are vascular ectasias (not neoplasms) which occur in the right colon of many older individuals and may cause bleeding (see Chap. 46). Angiodysplasia is a degenerative lesion consisting of dilated, distorted, thin-walled vessels lined by vascular endothelium. Angiodysplasia may result from partial obstruction of the submucosal venous plexus by the tension generated in the cecal wall during muscular contraction. Aortic stenosis occurs in some patients, and may cause chronic ischemia of the colon that leads to angiodysplasia. Grossly angiodysplasias look similar to spider angiomas of the skin and appear as star-shaped branching vessels in the submucosa measuring from 2 mm to 1 cm in diameter. The lesions are usually multiple and are found primarily in the cecum and ascending colon.

Cecal angiodysplasia is important because of the likelihood of bleeding, either massively or chronically. In patients over 60 approximately one-quarter of colonic bleeding episodes are secondary to angiodysplasia. The diagnosis requires careful angiography showing extravasation of contrast material into the lumen, or colonoscopy with visualization of bleeding lesions. Hemorrhage from angiodysplasia may be controlled by embolization during arteriography or by electrocautery through the colonoscope. Some patients with massive uncontrolled bleeding or multiple sites of angiodysplasia may require right hemicolectomy.

ANORECTAL PROBLEMS

HEMORRHOIDS The internal hemorrhoidal plexus of veins is located in the submucosal space above the valves of Morgagni. The anal canal separates it from the external hemorrhoidal venous plexus, but the two spaces communicate under the anal canal, the submucosa of which is attached to underlying tissue to form the interhemorrhoidal depression. Whenever the internal hemorrhoidal plexus is enlarged, there is associated increase in supporting tissue mass, and the resultant venous swelling is called an *internal hemorrhoid*. When veins in the external hemorrhoidal plexus become enlarged or thrombosed, the resultant bluish mass is called an *external hemorrhoid*.

Both types of hemorrhoids are very common and are associated with increased hydrostatic pressure in the portal venous system, such as during pregnancy, straining at stool, or with cirrhosis. When internal hemorrhoids enlarge, pain is not a usual feature until the situation is complicated by thrombosis, infection, or erosion of the overlying mucosal surface. Most persons complain of bright red blood on the toilet tissue or coating the stool, with a feeling of vague anal discomfort. The discomfort is increased when the hemorrhoid enlarges or prolapses through the anus; prolapse is often accompanied by edema and sphincteric spasm. Prolapse, if not treated, usually becomes chronic as the muscularis stays stretched, and the patient complains of constant soiling of underclothing with very little pain. Prolapsed hemorrhoids may become infected or thrombosed; the overlying mucous membrane may bleed profusely as the result of the trauma of defecation.

External hemorrhoids, because they lie under the skin, are quite often painful, particularly if there is a sudden increase in their mass. These episodes result in a tender blue swelling at the anal verge due to thrombosis of a vein in the external plexus and need not be associated with enlargement of the internal veins. Since the thrombus usually lies at the level of the sphincteric muscles, anal spasm often occurs.

The diagnosis of internal and external hemorrhoids is made by inspection, digital examination, and direct vision through the anoscope and proctoscope. Since such lesions are very common, they must not be regarded as the cause of rectal bleeding or chronic hypochromic anemia until a thorough investigation has been made of the more proximal gastrointestinal tract. Acute blood loss can occasionally be attributed to internal hemorrhoids. Chronic anemia in the presence of large but not definitely bleeding hemorrhoids should provoke a search for a polyp, cancer, or ulcer.

Most hemorrhoids respond to conservative therapy such as sitz baths or other forms of moist heat, suppositories, stool softeners, and bed rest. Internal hemorrhoids which remain permanently prolapsed are best treated surgically; milder degrees of prolapse or enlargement with pruritus ani or intermittent bleeding can be successfully handled by banding or injection of sclerosing solutions. External hemorrhoids which become acutely thrombosed are treated by incision, extraction of the clot, and compression of the incised area following clot removal. No surgical procedure should be carried out in the presence of acute inflammation of the anus, ulcerative proctitis, or ulcerative colitis. Both proctoscopy and barium enema should always be performed before a patient is subjected to hemorrhoidectomy.

ANAL INFLAMMATION Perianal inflammatory lesions may be primary or may be associated with inflammatory bowel disease or diverticular disease as mentioned above. Anal *fissures* are superficial erosions of the anal canal which usually heal rapidly with conservative therapy. Anal *ulcers* are more chronic and deep and give symptoms largely as the result of painful spasm of the external anal sphincter during and after defecation. Bleeding may occur with either fissure or ulcer; healing of the ulcer often is associated with a hypertrophied anal papilla and some degrees of anal contracture. *Fistula in ano*, a tract leading from the rectal lumen to the perianal skin, usually results from local crypt abscesses; fewer than 5 percent of such lesions found in medical practice in the United States are due to tuberculosis or cancer. The fistula is a chronically inflamed canal made up of fibrous tissue surrounding granulation tissue, the lumen of which may be difficult to demonstrate. Perirectal *abscesses* often represent the tracking down into the anal area of purulent material escaping from the rectosigmoid; diverticulitis, Crohn's disease, ulcerative colitis, or previous surgery may be the underlying cause. Fistulas between the rectum and vagina or the rectum and bladder represent serious complications of granulomatous, septic, or malignant disorders and require the patient to be hospitalized for definitive diagnostic and therapeutic procedures.

REFERENCES

Disorders of motility

BODE WE et al: Colonoscopic decompression for acute dilatation of the colon. Am J Surg 147:243, 1984

SCHUFFLER MD et al: Chronic intestinal pseudo-obstruction. Medicine 60:173, 1981

TROTMAN IF, MISEWICZ JJ: Sigmoid motility in diverticular disease and the irritable bowel syndrome. Gut 29:218, 1988

Diverticular diseases

BRIAN JE, STAIR JM: Non-colonic diverticular disease. Surg Gynecol Obstet 161:189, 1985

THOMPSON WG, PATEL DG: Clinical picture of diverticular disease of the colon. Clinics Gastrol 15:903, 1986

Intestinal ischemia and angiodysplasia

SANTOS JC et al: Angiodysplasia of the colon: Endoscopic diagnosis and treatment. Br J Surg 75:256, 1988

WILLIAMS L: Mesenteric ischemia. Surg Clin North Am 68:331, 1988

243 TUMORS OF THE LARGE AND SMALL INTESTINE

ROBERT J. MAYER

COLORECTAL CANCER

INCIDENCE Cancer of the large bowel is second only to lung cancer as a cause of cancer death in the United States. Approximately 151,000 new cases were anticipated in 1989, resulting in 61,300 deaths. The incidence and mortality rates for this extremely common malignant condition have not changed substantially in males during the past 40 years, although, for some reason, a slight decrease in the mortality rate has appeared in females. Colorectal cancer generally occurs in individuals 50 years of age or older.

ETIOLOGY AND RISK FACTORS (Table 243-1) **Diet** The etiology for most cases of large-bowel cancer appears to be related to environmental factors. The disease occurs more often in upper socioeconomic populations who live in urban areas. Epidemiologic studies in various countries have documented a direct correlation between mortality from colorectal cancer and per capita consumption of calories, meat protein, and dietary fat and oil as well as elevations in the serum cholesterol concentration and mortality from coronary artery disease. Any geographic variations in incidence do not appear to be related to genetic differences, since migrant groups tend to assume the large-bowel cancer incidence rates of their adopted countries. Furthermore, population groups such as Mormons and Seventh Day Adventists, whose lifestyle and dietary habits differ somewhat from those of their neighbors, have significantly lower-than-expected incidence and mortality rates for colorectal cancer, while the appearance of colorectal cancer has increased in Japan since that nation has adopted a more "western" diet. It is therefore assumed that dietary patterns influence the development of colorectal cancer. At least two hypotheses have been proposed to explain this relationship, neither of which is fully satisfactory.

ANIMAL FATS Based on the association of colorectal cancer with hypercholesterolemia and coronary artery disease as well as the increased incidence of large-bowel tumors in geographic areas where meat is a dietary staple, it has been suggested that the ingestion of animal fats leads to an increased proportion of anaerobes in the gut microflora, resulting in the conversion of normal bile acids into carcinogens. This provocative hypothesis is supported by several reports of increased amounts of fecal anaerobes in the stools of patients with colorectal cancer. However, there are conflicting data from population studies relating fat intake to the risk for colon cancer and from unsuccessful attempts at altering the profile of fecal microflora through short-term alterations in diet. Any definitive assessment of the animal fat concept must await a prospective survey of a defined population, correlating carefully obtained and periodically updated dietary histories with quantitative cultures of stool microflora, and determining the incidence of colorectal cancer in these individuals over a 10 to 20 year period of time.

FIBER The observation that South African Bantus ingest a diet far higher in roughage, produce more frequent, bulkier stools, and

TABLE 243-1 Risk factors for the development of colorectal cancer

Diet
  ? Animal fat
  ? Fiber
Hereditary syndromes (autosomal dominant inheritance)
  Polyposis coli
  Non-polyposis syndrome
Inflammatory bowel disease
Streptococcus bovis bacteremia
Ureterosigmoidostomy

have a lower incidence of large-bowel cancer than their American and European counterparts led to the proposal that the higher rate of colorectal cancer in western society is in large part the result of a low intake of dietary fiber. This theory suggests that dietary fiber accelerates intestinal transit time, thereby reducing the exposure of colonic mucosa to potential carcinogens and diluting these carcinogens because of enhanced fecal bulk. Such a proposition appears somewhat simplistic when subjected to careful scrutiny. Although an enhanced fiber intake increases fecal bulk, there has been no consistent evidence that a high fiber intake actually shortens the transit time of stool. Additionally, despite the generally higher fiber intake in low-incidence countries, the environmental differences between developing and industrialized nations are myriad and include such other important dietary variables as meat and fat consumption. Finally, a diet low in fiber may lead to chronic constipation and such associated conditions as diverticulosis. If a low fiber diet were a significant factor in the etiology of colorectal cancer, individuals having diverticulosis should be at higher risk for the development of large-bowel tumors; this does not appear to be the case.

OTHER   Emerging data suggest that the risk for the development of colorectal cancer may be diminished by the addition of calcium supplements to the diet. It is thought that such dietary calcium may inactivate bowel carcinogens through the formation of insoluble soaps. In support of this concept are (1) the finding that supplementary dietary calcium reduced the proliferation of colonic epithelial cells in familial colon cancer kindreds and (2) the results of a survey of the dietary habits of a cohort of about 2000 men over a 19-year period, suggesting that the risk of colonic cancer decreased with increased oral intake of calcium.

Thus, while the weight of epidemiologic evidence implicates diet as being the major etiologic factor for colorectal cancer, no single foodstuff has been sufficiently identified as being a causative or protective agent to justify specific recommendations for widespread changes in eating habits.

Hereditary factors and syndromes   As many as 25 percent of patients with colorectal cancer may have a family history of the disease, suggesting a hereditary predisposition. Such inherited large-bowel cancers can be divided into two main groups: the well-studied but uncommon polyposis syndromes and the less well defined non-polyposis syndromes (Table 243-2).

Polyposis coli (i.e., familial polyposis of the colon) is a rare condition characterized by the appearance of thousands of adenomatous polyps throughout the large bowel. The condition is transmitted in an autosomal dominant manner, although occasional patients with no family history are thought to have developed the polyposis due to a spontaneous mutation. Molecular studies have recently associated polyposis coli with a deletion in the long arm of chromosome 5. It has been hypothesized that the loss of this genetic material (i.e., allelic loss) results in the absence of tumor-suppressor genes whose protein products would normally inhibit neoplastic growth. The presence of soft tissue and bony tumors in addition to the colonic polyps characterizes a subset of polyposis coli known as *Gardner's syndrome*, while the appearance of malignant tumors of the central nervous system accompanying polyposis coli defines *Turcot's syndrome*. The colonic polyps in all these conditions are rarely present prior to puberty but are generally evident in affected individuals by age 25. If left surgically untreated, colorectal cancer will develop in almost all patients prior to age 40. Polyposis coli has been studied intensively and appears to result from a defect in the colonic mucosa leading to an abnormal proliferative pattern and an impaired ability for cellular repair following exposure to radiation or ultraviolet light. Once the multiple polyps that constitute polyposis coli are detected, patients should have a total colectomy. It remains unclear whether the optimal operative approach in such a clinical setting is to resect the entire colon and rectum, requiring the young patient to have a permanent ileostomy, or to perform an ileoproctostomy. While the latter procedure retains the distal rectum and anal sphincter, it places the patient at continued risk for the development of cancer in the rectal remnant and necessitates semiannual or annual proctoscopic surveillance. The offspring of patients with polyposis coli, who are often prepubertal when the diagnosis is made in the parent, have a 50 percent risk for the eventual development of this premalignant disorder and should be carefully screened on a periodic basis until age 35. Such screening should include endoscopic and/or contrast radiographic examinations. Testing for occult blood in the stool is an inadequate screening maneuver. Unfortunately, no disease-specific screening technique is generally available for the children of polyposis coli patients, although radioautographic measurements of colonic mucosal proliferation have been utilized with apparent efficacy in a small number of patients at highly specialized medical centers. Conceivably, molecular probes for the chromosome 5 deletion will prove to be useful in this regard in the future.

The hereditary predisposition for colorectal cancer in families having no history of polyposis coli has received increased attention since the identification of several kindreds who displayed risks as high as 50 percent for the development of a colonic malignancy. These colorectal lesions involve the proximal large bowel in an unusually high frequency. Such families frequently include patients having multiple primary cancers, with the association of colorectal and endometrial adenocarcinomas being especially prominent in women. The trait for cancer appears to be transmitted in an autosomal dominant manner and the median age for the appearance of an adenocarcinoma is under age 50, 10 to 15 years below the usual age for the general population. The offspring of such predisposed patients should undergo intensive screening beginning by age 25, and the screening should include triannual colonoscopies or double-contrast barium enemas.

Inflammatory bowel disease (See also Chap. 241)   Large-bowel cancer represents a not infrequent complication in patients with long-standing inflammatory bowel disease. The development of a neoplasm appears to occur more commonly in patients with ulcerative colitis than in those with granulomatous colitis, but such an impression may result in part from the occasional difficulty in differentiating these two conditions. The risk of colorectal cancer in a patient with inflammatory bowel disease is relatively small during the initial 10 years following the onset of the disease, but then appears to increase at a rate of approximately 0.5 to 1.0 percent per year. Actuarially derived cumulative cancer rates in such symptomatic patients have ranged from 8 to 30 percent after 25 years. The risk is generally considered to be higher in younger patients with pancolitis.

TABLE 243-2   Hereditable (autosomal dominant) gastrointestinal polyp syndromes

Syndrome	Distribution of polyps	Histologic type	Malignant potential	Associated lesions
Familial colonic polyposis	Large intestine	Adenoma	Common	None
Gardner's syndrome	Large and small intestines	Adenoma	Common	Osteomas, fibromas, lipomas, epidermoid cysts
Turcot's syndrome	Large intestine	Adenoma	Common	Brain tumors
Non-polyposis syndrome	Large intestine	Adenoma	Common	Endometrial tumors
Peutz-Jeghers syndrome	Small and large intestines, stomach	Hamartoma	Rare	Mucocutaneous pigmentation; tumors of the ovary, breast, pancreas, endometrium
Juvenile polyposis	Large and small intestines, stomach	Hamartoma rarely progressing to adenoma	Rare	Various congenital abnormalities

Cancer surveillance in patients with inflammatory bowel disease is unsatisfactory. Symptoms such as bloody diarrhea, abdominal cramping, and obstruction, which may signal the appearance of a tumor, are similar to the complaints of patients whose underlying disease is flaring. In patients with a history of inflammatory bowel disease lasting 15 years or more who continue to experience exacerbations, the surgical removal of the colon can significantly reduce the risk for cancer and also eliminate the target organ for the underlying chronic gastrointestinal disorder. The value of such surveillance techniques as colonoscopy with mucosal biopsies and brushings for less symptomatic individuals with chronic inflammatory bowel disease is uncertain. The purpose of such procedures has been the identification of premalignant mucosal dysplasia, thereby justifying surgical intervention. The lack of uniformity regarding the pathologic criteria that characterize dysplasia and the absence of data that such surveillance reduces the development of lethal cancers, however, has made this costly practice an area of controversy.

Other high-risk conditions *STREPTOCOCCUS BOVIS* BACTEREMIA For unknown reasons, individuals who develop endocarditis or septicemia from this fecal bacteria seem to have a high incidence of occult colorectal tumors. Endoscopic or radiographic screening for such patients appears advisable.

URETEROSIGMOIDOSTOMY   There is a 5 to 10 percent incidence of colon cancer 15 to 30 years after ureterosigmoidostomy to correct congenital extrophy of the bladder. Neoplasms characteristically are found at a site distal to the ureteral implant where colonic mucosa is chronically exposed to both urine and feces.

POLYPS The majority of colorectal cancers, regardless of etiology, are believed to arise from adenomatous polyps. A polyp is a grossly visible protrusion from the mucosal surface and may be classified pathologically as a nonneoplastic hamartoma *(juvenile polyp)*, a hyperplastic mucosal proliferation *(hyperplastic polyp)*, or an adenomatous polyp. Only adenomas are clearly premalignant and only a minority of such lesions ever develop into cancer. Population-screening studies and autopsy surveys have revealed that adenomatous polyps may be found in the colons of about 30 percent of middle-aged or elderly people. Based on this prevalence and the known incidence of colorectal cancers, it appears that less than 1 percent of polyps ever become malignant. Most polyps produce no symptoms and remain clinically undetected. Occult blood in the stool may be found in less than 5 percent of patients with such lesions.

A number of molecular changes have been described in the DNA obtained from adenomatous polyps, dysplastic lesions, and polyps containing microscopic foci of tumor cells (i.e., *carcinoma in situ*). Consistent with the multistep process leading to cancer, a series of alterations has been observed, often beginning with a specific mutation in the *ras* proto-oncogene followed by deletions in chromosomes 5, 18, and 17. The loss of genetic material on the short arm of chromosome 17 appears to be associated with activation of a gene leading to the production of transformation-associated protein p53. Thus, the altered proliferative pattern of the colonic mucosa (which results in the progression to a polyp and then to a carcinoma) may involve the mutational activation of an oncogene followed by and coupled with the loss of genes which normally suppress tumorigenesis. Based on this model, it is believed that neoplasia develops only in those polyps in which all of these mutational events take place.

Clinically, the probability of an adenomatous polyp becoming a cancer is dependent upon the gross appearance of the lesion and its histologic features. Adenomatous polyps may be pedunculated (i.e., extending from adjacent bowel on a stalk) or sessile (i.e., flat). Cancers develop more frequently in sessile polyps, with the probability being directly related to the size of the lesion. Histologically, adenomatous polyps may be tubular, villous (i.e., papillary), or tubulovillous. Villous adenomas, which are predominantly sessile in appearance, become malignant more than three times as often as tubular adenomas.

Following the detection of an adenomatous polyp, the entire large bowel should be visualized endoscopically or radiographically since synchronous lesions are present in approximately one-third of cases. Colonoscopy should then be repeated periodically, even in the absence of a previously documented malignancy, since such patients have a 30 to 50 percent probability of developing another adenoma and are at a higher-than-average risk for developing a colorectal carcinoma. Adenomatous polyps are thought to require more than 5 years of growth before becoming clinically significant; therefore, colonoscopy need not be carried out more frequently than every 3 years.

SCREENING The rationale for colorectal cancer screening programs is that the earlier detection of localized, superficial neoplasms in asymptomatic individuals will increase the surgical cure rate. Screening strategies have been based on the assumption that more than 60 percent of such early lesions are located in the rectosigmoid, making them accessible to rigid proctosigmoidoscopy. For unexplained reasons, however, there has been a consistent decrease during the past several decades in the proportion of large-bowel cancers arising in the rectum with a corresponding increase in the more proximal descending colon. As such, the potential for rigid proctosigmoidoscopy to detect a sufficient number of occult neoplasms to make the procedure cost-effective has been questioned. The availability of flexible, fiberoptic sigmoidoscopes, permitting trained operators to visualize the colon for up to 60 cm, should enhance cancer detection. Whether this added detection justifies the expenses of the device and the examination remains to be determined.

Most programs directed at the early detection of colorectal cancers have focused on digital rectal examinations and testing stool for the presence of occult blood. The digital examination should be part of any routine physical evaluation in adults older than age 40, serving as the best screening test for prostate cancer in men, a component of the pelvic examination in women, and as an inexpensive maneuver for the detection of masses in the rectum. The development of the Hemoccult test has greatly facilitated the potential to detect occult fecal blood. Unfortunately, even when performed optimally, the Hemoccult test has major limitations as a screening technique. Between 35 to 50 percent of patients with documented colorectal cancers have a negative fecal Hemoccult test, consistent with the intermittent bleeding pattern of these tumors. When random cohorts of asymptomatic persons have been tested, 3 to 6 percent have Hemoccult-positive stools. Colorectal cancers have been found in only 5 to 10 percent of these "test-positive" cases, with benign polyps being detected in an additional 20 to 30 percent. Consequently, a colorectal neoplasm will *not* be found in the majority of asymptomatic individuals with occult blood in their stool. Nonetheless, persons found to have Hemoccult-positive stool routinely undergo further medical evaluation that includes sigmoidoscopy, barium enema, and/or colonoscopy—procedures that not only are uncomfortable and expensive, but also are associated with a low but finite risk for significant complications. The added cost of these studies would appear justifiable, if the minority of patients found to have occult neoplasms because of Hemoccult screening could be shown to have an improved prognosis and prolonged survival. Prospectively controlled trials addressing this issue are ongoing.

Therefore, screening techniques for large-bowel cancer in asymptomatic persons remain unsatisfactory. Thus far, no controlled clinical study has demonstrated any screening maneuver that enhances the likelihood for cure. As a result, recommendations from governmental and private agencies are conflicting, and the issue remains unresolved.

CLINICAL FEATURES   Presenting symptoms Symptoms vary with the anatomic location of the tumor.

Since stool is relatively liquid as it passes through the ileocecal valve into the right colon, neoplasms arising in the cecum and ascending colon may become quite large, significantly narrowing the bowel lumen, without resulting in any obstructive symptoms or noticeable alterations in bowel habits. Lesions of the right colon commonly ulcerate, leading to chronic, insidious blood loss without a change in the appearance of the stool. Consequently, patients with tumors of the ascending colon often present with symptoms such as fatigue, palpitations, and even angina pectoris and are found to have

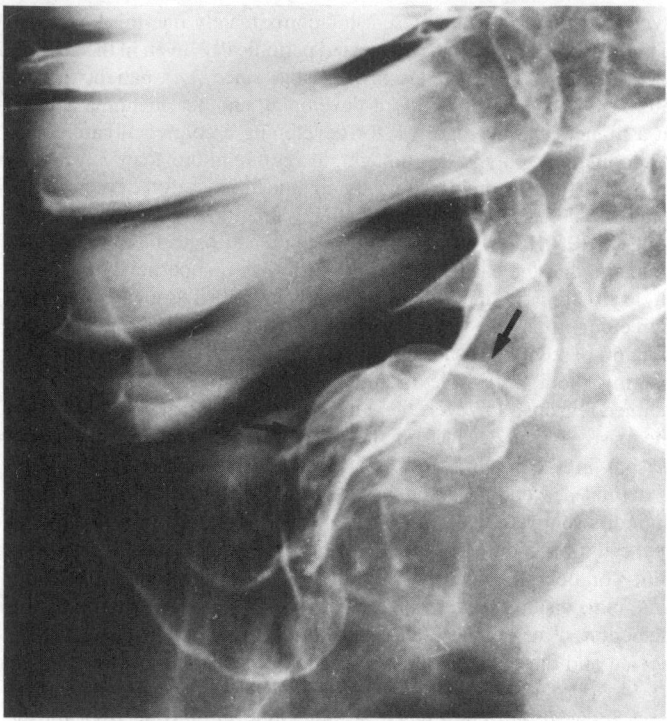

FIGURE 243-1   Double-contrast air-barium enema revealing a sessile tumor of the cecum in a patient with iron-deficiency anemia and guaiac-positive stool. The lesion at surgery was a stage B adenocarcinoma.

FIGURE 243-2   Annular, constricting adenocarcinoma of the descending colon. This radiographic appearance is referred to as an "apple-core" lesion and is always highly suggestive of malignancy.

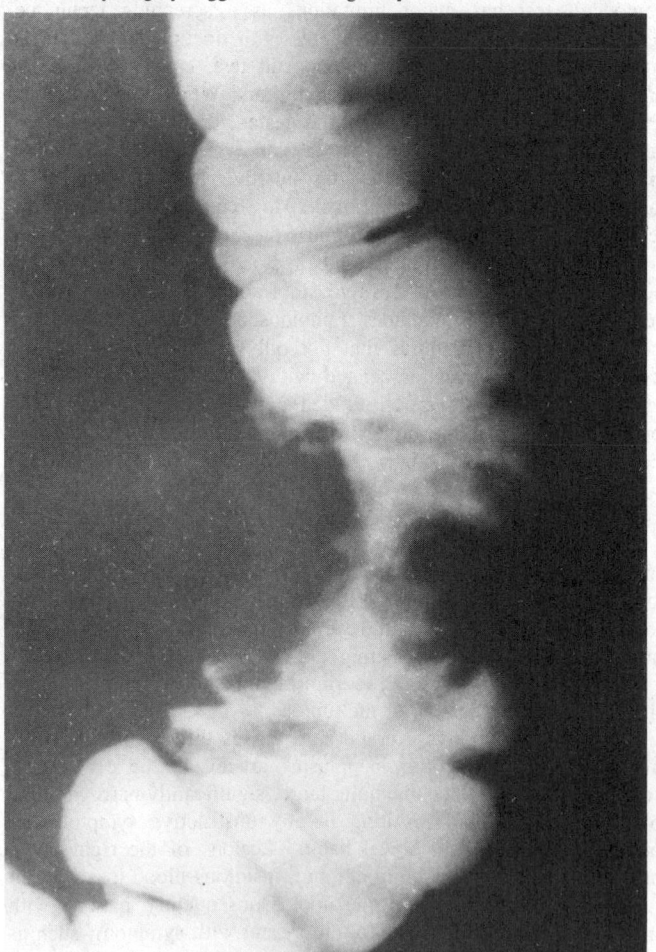

a hypochromic, microcytic anemia indicative of iron deficiency. Since the cancer may bleed intermittently, however, a random test for the presence of occult blood in the stool may be negative. As a result, the unexplained presence of iron-deficiency anemia in any adult (with the possible exception of a premenopausal, multiparous woman) mandates a thorough endoscopic and/or radiographic visualization of the entire large bowel (Fig. 243-1).

Since stool becomes more concentrated as it passes into the transverse and descending colon, tumors arising there tend to impede the passage of stool, resulting in the development of abdominal cramping, occasional obstruction, and even perforation. Radiographs of the abdomen often reveal characteristic annular, constricting lesions ("apple-core" or "napkin-ring") (Fig. 243-2).

Neoplasms arising in the rectosigmoid often are associated with hematochezia, tenesmus, and narrowing in the caliber of stool; nonetheless, anemia is an infrequent finding. While these symptoms may lead patients and their physicians to suspect the presence of hemorrhoids, the development of rectal bleeding and/or altered bowel habits demands a prompt digital rectal examination and proctosigmoidoscopy.

Staging, prognostic factors, patterns of spread   The prognosis for individuals having colorectal cancer is closely related to the depth of tumor penetration into the bowel wall and the presence of both regional lymph node involvement and distant metastases. These variables are incorporated into the staging system introduced by Dukes (Table 243-3). Patients with superficial lesions not penetrating into the muscularis or involving regional lymph nodes are designated as having *stage A* disease; those individuals whose tumors penetrate more deeply but without spread to lymph nodes are termed as having *stage B* disease; regional lymph node involvement defines *stage C* disease; and metastatic spread to sites such as liver, lung, or bone indicates *stage D* disease. Unless gross evidence of metastatic disease is present, it is impossible to accurately determine disease stage prior to surgical resection and pathologic analysis of the operative specimens.

Most recurrences after a surgical resection of a large-bowel cancer occur within the first 4 postoperative years, making the 5-year mark a fairly reliable indicator of cure. The likelihood for 5-year survival in patients with colorectal cancer is closely associated with their Dukes' stage (Table 243-3). That likelihood has appeared to improve during the past several decades when similar surgical stages have been compared. The most plausible explanation for this improvement appears to be more thorough intraoperative and pathologic staging. In particular, more exacting attention to pathologic detail has revealed that the prognosis following the resection of a colorectal cancer is not related merely to the presence or absence of regional lymph node involvement but may be more precisely assessed by the number of involved lymph nodes (i.e., 1 to 4 lymph nodes versus >5 lymph nodes). Other predictors of a poor prognosis after a total surgical resection include tumor penetration through the bowel wall into pericolic fat, poorly differentiated histology, perforation and/or tumor adherence to adjacent organs (increasing the risk for an anatomically adjacent recurrence), and venous invasion by tumor (Table 243-4). Regardless of the clinicopathologic stage, a preoperative elevation of the plasma carcinoembryonic antigen (CEA) titer is suggestive of eventual tumor recurrence. The presence of abnormal DNA content

TABLE 243-3   Dukes' classification of colorectal cancer

Stage	Pathologic description	Approximate 5-year survival, %
A	Cancer limited to mucosa and submucosa	>90
B	Cancer extends into muscularis or serosa	70–85
C	Cancer involves regional lymph nodes	30–60
D	Distant metastases (i.e., liver, lung, etc.)	5

TABLE 243-4 Poor prognostic predictors following total surgical resection

Tumor spread to regional lymph nodes
Number of regional lymph nodes involved
Tumor penetration through the bowel wall
Poorly differentiated histology
Perforation
Tumor adherence to adjacent organs
Venous invasion
Preoperative elevation of CEA titer (>5.0 ng/mL)
? Aneuploidy
? Specific chromosomal deletion (allelic loss)

(i.e., aneuploidy) and specific chromosomal deletions (i.e., so-called allelic loss) in tumor cells, as determined by flow cytometry and restriction fragment length polymorphism analysis respectively, appears to predict a higher risk for metastatic spread. In contrast to most other carcinomas and sarcomas, the prognosis in individuals with colorectal cancer is *not* influenced by the size of the primary lesion when adjusted for nodal involvement and histologic differentiation.

Cancers of the large bowel generally spread to regional lymph nodes or to the liver via the portal venous circulation. The liver represents the most frequent visceral site of metastatic dissemination; it is the initial site of distant spread in one-third of recurring colorectal cancers and eventually becomes involved in greater than two-thirds of such patients at the time of death. In general, colorectal cancer rarely metastasizes to the lungs, supraclavicular lymph nodes, bone, or brain without prior spread to the liver. A major exception to this rule occurs in patients having primary tumors in the distal rectum, from where tumor cells may spread through the paravertebral venous plexus, escaping the portal venous system and thereby reaching the lungs or supraclavicular lymph nodes without hepatic involvement. The median survival after the detection of distant metastases may range from 6 to 9 months (hepatomegaly, liver abnormalities) to 20 to 24 months (small liver nodule initially identified by elevated CEA level and subsequent CT scan).

TREATMENT Total resection of tumor represents optimal management when a malignant lesion is endoscopically or radiographically detected in the large bowel. An evaluation for the presence of metastatic disease, including a thorough physical examination, a chest x-ray, biochemical assessment of liver function, and a plasma CEA level, should be performed prior to surgery. When possible, a colonoscopy of the entire large bowel should be performed to identify synchronous neoplasms and/or polyps. The detection of metastases should not preclude surgery in patients with tumor-related symptoms such as gastrointestinal bleeding or obstruction, but may often result in a less radical operative procedure being carried out. At the time of laparotomy, the entire peritoneal cavity should be examined with the liver, pelvis, and hemidiaphragm being thoroughly inspected and the full length of the large bowel being carefully palpated. Following recovery from a complete resection, patients should be carefully observed for 5 years by semiannual physical examinations and yearly blood chemistries. If a complete colonoscopy was not performed preoperatively, this should be carried out within the first several postoperative months. Some authorities favor obtaining plasma CEA levels at 3-month intervals because of the sensitivity of this test as a marker for otherwise undetectable tumor recurrence. Subsequent endoscopic or radiographic surveillance of the large bowel, probably at triannual intervals, is indicated, since patients who have been cured of one colorectal cancer have a 3 to 5 percent probability of developing an additional bowel cancer during their lifetime and a risk in excess of 15 percent for the development of adenomatous polyps. Anastomotic (i.e., "suture-line") recurrences are infrequent in colorectal cancer patients, if the surgical resection margins were adequate and free of tumor.

Radiation therapy to the pelvis is generally recommended for patients with rectal cancer because of the 30 to 40 percent probability of regional recurrences following complete surgical resection of stages

B and C tumors, especially if they have penetrated through the serosa. This alarmingly high rate of local disease recurrence is believed to be due to the fact that the contained anatomic space within the pelvis limits the extent of the resection and because the rich lymphatic network of the pelvic side wall immediately adjacent to the rectum facilitates the early spread of malignant cells into surgically inaccessible tissue. Prospectively randomized trials have indicated that the prophylactic use of radiation therapy, either pre- or postoperatively, reduces the likelihood of pelvic recurrences but does not appear to prolong survival. Preoperative radiotherapy is clearly indicated for patients with large, potentially unresectable rectal cancers, since such anatomically fixed lesions may shrink sufficiently to permit subsequent surgical removal.

Chemotherapy in patients with advanced colorectal cancer has proven to be of only marginal benefit. Since its introduction into clinical trials more than 25 years ago, 5-fluorouracil (5-FU) remains the most effective treatment for this disease. It is as useful when given alone as when combined with other drugs, but is associated with only a 15 to 20 percent likelihood of reducing measurable tumor masses by 50 percent or more (i.e., partial response). While the probability for tumor response appears to be somewhat greater for patients with liver metastases when such chemotherapy is infused directly into the hepatic artery as compared to a peripheral vein, intraarterial treatment is costly and toxic and does not appear to prolong survival. The results of recent studies have suggested that the concomitant administration of folinic acid (also known as leucovorin or citrovorum factor) will improve the efficacy of 5-FU in patients with advanced colorectal cancer, presumably by enhancing the binding of 5-FU to its target enzyme, thymidylate synthetase, thereby increasing the suppression of DNA synthesis and accompanying cytotoxicity. The majority of randomized trials have indicated a threefold improvement in the likelihood of partial response when folinic acid is combined with 5-FU; however, the effect on survival is uncertain and the optimal dose-schedule remains to be defined.

The value of postoperative chemotherapy and/or radiation therapy has been assessed in patients with stages B and C cancers as a means of eradicating clinically undetectable micrometastases and thereby increasing the probability for cure. The weight of evidence from more than 12 prospectively randomized trials in patients who have undergone the resection of a colon cancer suggests that the use of such prophylactic chemotherapy (i.e., including 5-FU given alone or in combination with other cytotoxic drugs) does not reduce the recurrence rate or prolong survival. However, the results of two clinical studies have indicated that the administration of adjuvant 5-FU with an anthelmintic agent, levamisole, to patients with stage C cancers leads to a decrease in the likelihood of recurrence and a modest improvement in survival. The levamisole is thought to act in this therapeutic setting as a nonspecific immunomodulator. In contrast, in patients who have undergone the resection of a rectal cancer, data from controlled studies indicate that postoperative radiation therapy when combined with chemotherapy appears to reduce the likelihood of regional recurrences and increase the potential for cure. It has been postulated that the chemotherapy, ineffective when given prophylactically for patients with colon lesions, acts as a radiation sensitizer when given to individuals who have been operated upon for rectal cancer, thereby enhancing the biologic effect of the radiotherapy.

TUMORS OF THE SMALL INTESTINE

Small-bowel tumors comprise only 3 to 6 percent of gastrointestinal neoplasms. Because of their rarity, a correct diagnosis is often delayed. Abdominal symptoms are usually vague and poorly defined, and conventional radiographic studies of the upper and lower intestinal tract are often normal. Small-bowel tumors should be considered in the following situations: (1) recurrent, unexplained episodes of crampy abdominal pain; (2) intermittent bouts of intestinal obstruction, especially in the absence of inflammatory bowel disease or prior abdominal surgery; (3) intussuception in the adult; and (4) evidence of chronic intestinal bleeding in the presence of negative conventional radiographs. A careful small-bowel barium study is the diagnostic procedure of choice; the diagnostic accuracy may be improved by infusing barium through a nasogastric tube placed into the duodenum (enteroclysis).

BENIGN TUMORS In general, the histology of benign small-bowel tumors is difficult to predict on clinical and radiologic grounds alone. The symptomatology of benign tumors is not distinctive, with pain, obstruction, and hemorrhage being the most frequent symptoms. These tumors are usually discovered during the fifth and sixth decades of life, more often in the distal rather than the proximal small intestine. The most common benign tumors are adenomas, leiomyomas, lipomas, and angiomas.

Adenomas These tumors include those of the islet cells and Brunner's glands as well as polypoid adenomas. *Islet cell adenomas* are occasionally located outside the pancreas, and the associated syndromes are discussed in Chap. 320. *Brunner's gland adenomas* are not truly neoplastic but represent a hypertrophy or hyperplasia of submucosal duodenal glands. These appear as small nodules in the duodenal mucosa that secrete a highly viscous alkaline mucus. Most often this is an incidental radiographic finding not associated with any specific clinical disorder.

Polypoid adenomas (See Table 243-2) Approximately 25 percent of benign small-bowel tumors are polypoid adenomas. They may present as single polypoid lesions or, less commonly, as papillary villous adenomas. As in the colon, the sessile or papillary form of the tumor is sometimes associated with a coexistent carcinoma. Occasionally, patients with Gardner's syndrome (a variant of polyposis coli) may develop premalignant adenomas in the small bowel; such lesions are generally in the duodenum. Multiple polypoid tumors may occur throughout the small bowel (and occasionally the stomach and colorectum) in the Peutz-Jeghers syndrome. The polyps are usually hamartomas (juvenile polyps) having a low potential for malignant degeneration. Mucocutaneous melanin deposits as well as tumors of the ovary, breast, pancreas, and endometrium are also associated with this autosomal dominant condition.

Leiomyomas These neoplasms arise from smooth-muscle components of the intestine and are usually intramural, affecting the overlying mucosa. Ulceration of the mucosa may cause gastrointestinal hemorrhage of varying severity.

Lipomas These tumors occur with greatest frequency in the distal ileum and at the ileocecal valve. They have a characteristic radiolucent appearance, are usually intramural and asymptomatic, but may on occasion be associated with bleeding.

Angiomas While not true neoplasms, these lesions are important because they frequently cause intestinal bleeding. They may take the form of telangiectasia or hemangiomas. Multiple intestinal telangiectasia occur in a nonhereditary form confined to the gastrointestinal tract or as part of the hereditary Osler-Rendu-Weber syndrome. Vascular tumors may also take the form of isolated hemangiomas, most commonly in the jejunum. Angiography, especially during bleeding, is the procedure of choice in evaluating these lesions.

MALIGNANT TUMORS While infrequent in appearance, small-bowel malignancies occur in patients with long-standing regional enteritis and celiac sprue as well as in individuals with the acquired immunodeficiency syndrome (AIDS). In contrast to benign tumors, malignant tumors of the small bowel are frequently associated with fever, weight loss, anorexia, bleeding, and a palpable abdominal mass. After ampullary carcinomas (many of which arise from biliary or pancreatic ducts), the most frequently occurring small-bowel malignancies are adenocarcinomas, lymphomas, carcinoid tumors, and leiomyosarcomas.

Adenocarcinomas The most common primary cancers of the small bowel are adenocarcinomas, which account for about 50 percent of the malignant tumors. These neoplasms occur with highest frequency in the distal duodenum and proximal jejunum, where they tend to ulcerate and cause hemorrhage or obstruction. Radiologically,

they may be confused with chronic duodenal ulcer disease or with Crohn's disease if the patient has long-standing regional enteritis. The diagnosis is best made by endoscopy and biopsy under direct vision. Surgical resection is the treatment of choice.

Lymphomas Lymphomatous involvement of the small bowel may be primary or secondary. A diagnosis of a primary intestinal lymphoma requires histologic confirmation of a lymphoproliferative neoplasm in a clinical setting in which palpable adenopathy and hepatosplenomegaly are absent and there is no evidence of lymphoma on a chest radiograph, CT scan, peripheral blood smear, or on bone marrow aspiration and biopsy. In general, symptoms referable to the small bowel are present, usually accompanied by an anatomically discernible lesion. Secondary lymphoma of the small bowel refers to involvement of the intestine by a lymphoid malignancy extending from involved retroperitoneal lymph nodes and hence is a manifestation of a generalized systemic neoplasm (see Chap. 300).

Primary intestinal lymphoma comprises 25 percent of malignancies of the small bowel. Essentially all these neoplasms are non-Hodgkin's lymphomas, most frequently having a diffuse, large-cell (i.e., "high-grade") histology. Intestinal lymphoma involves the ileum more frequently than the jejunum, which, in turn, is more commonly affected than the duodenum, a pattern which mirrors the relative amount of normal lymphoid cells in these anatomic areas. The risk of small-bowel lymphoma is increased in patients with a prior history of malabsorptive conditions (e.g., celiac sprue), regional enteritis, and depressed immunologic function due to congenital immunodeficiency syndromes, prior organ transplantation, autoimmune disorders, or AIDS.

The development of localized or nodular masses that narrow the lumen results in periumbilical pain (made worse by eating) as well as weight loss, vomiting, and occasional intestinal obstruction. The diagnosis of small-bowel lymphoma may be suspected by the appearance on contrast radiographs of patterns such as infiltration and thickening of mucosal folds, mucosal nodules, areas of irregular ulceration, or stasis of contrast material. The diagnosis can be confirmed by surgical exploration and resection of involved segments. Intestinal lymphoma may occasionally be diagnosed by peroral intestinal mucosal biopsy, but since the disease mainly involves the lamina propria, full-thickness surgical biopsies are usually required.

Resection of the tumor constitutes the initial treatment modality. While postoperative radiation therapy has been offered to some patients following such a total resection, most authorities favor short-term systemic treatment with combination chemotherapy. The frequent presence of widespread intraabdominal disease at the time of diagnosis and the occasional multicentricity of the tumor often make a total resection impossible. Combination chemotherapy would appear to be appropriate management for these patients as well. The probability of sustained remission or cure is approximately 75 percent in patients with localized disease, but 25 percent or less in individuals with unresectable lymphoma.

A unique form of small-bowel lymphoma, diffusely involving the entire intestine, was first described in oriental Jews and Arabs and is referred to as immunoproliferative small intestinal disease (IPSID), Mediterranean lymphoma, or alpha-heavy chain disease. The typical presentation includes chronic diarrhea and steatorrhea associated with vomiting and abdominal cramps; clubbing of the digits may be observed as well. A curious feature in many patients with IPSID is the presence in the blood and intestinal secretions of an abnormal IgA which contains a shortened alpha-heavy chain and is devoid of light chains. It is suspected that the abnormal alpha chains are produced by plasma cells infiltrating the small bowel. The clinical course of patients with IPSID is generally one of exacerbations and remissions, with death frequently resulting from either progressive malnutrition and wasting or the development of an aggressive lymphoma. Chemotherapy and radiation therapy have been ineffective.

Carcinoid tumors Among the more common epithelial tumors of the small intestine are carcinoid tumors. They arise from argentaffin cells of the crypts of Lieberkühn and are found from the distal duodenum to the ascending colon, areas embryologically derived from the midgut. More than 50 percent of intestinal carcinoids are found in the distal ileum, with the majority congregating in close proximity to the ileocecal valve. Most intestinal carcinoids are asymptomatic and of low malignant potential, but invasion and metastases may occur, leading to the carcinoid syndrome (Chap. 262).

Leiomyosarcomas   Large, bulky tumors, leiomyosarcomas often are greater than 5 cm in diameter and may be palpable on abdominal examination. Bleeding, obstruction, and perforation are common.

CANCERS OF THE ANUS

Cancers of the anus account for 1 to 2 percent of the malignant tumors of the large bowel. The majority of such lesions arise in the anal canal which is defined as the anatomic area extending from the anorectal ring to a zone approximately halfway between the pectinate (or dentate) line and the anal verge. Carcinomas arising proximal to the pectinate line (i.e., in the transitional zone between the glandular mucosa of the rectum and the squamous epithelium of the distal anus) are known as basaloid, cuboidal, or cloacogenic tumors; approximately one-third of anal cancers have this histologic pattern. Malignancies arising distal to the pectinate line have a squamous cell histology, ulcerate more frequently, and represent approximately 55 percent of anal cancers. The prognosis for patients with basaloid and squamous cell cancers of the anus is identical when corrected for tumor size and the presence or absence of nodal spread.

Anal cancers occur most commonly in individuals with a prior history of chronic anal irritation. Such irritation may result from condylomata accuminata (i.e., viral lesions thought to be caused by papilloma virus infection), perianal fissures and/or fistulas, chronic hemorrhoids, and leukoplakia. The risk for anal cancer appears to be increased among homosexual males, presumably due to trauma related to anal intercourse. There presently are no data to indicate that anal cancers are AIDS-related tumors associated with infection by the human immunodeficiency virus. Anal cancers occur most commonly in middle-aged individuals, develop more frequently in women than men, and are most often associated with bleeding, pain, the sensation of a perianal mass, and perianal pruritus at the time of diagnosis.

Until recently, radical surgery (abdominal-perineal resection with lymph node sampling and a permanent colostomy) was the treatment of choice for this tumor type. The probability of survival 5 years following such a procedure ranged from 55 to 70 percent in the absence of spread to regional lymph nodes and decreased to less than 20 percent if nodal involvement was present. However, an alternative therapeutic approach combining external beam radiation with concomitant chemotherapy has resulted in biopsy-proven disappearance of all tumor in more than 80 percent of patients whose initial lesion was less than 5 cm in size. Tumor recurrences have occurred in less than 10 percent of these patients. Thus, it appears that more than 80 percent of patients with anal cancers can be cured with nonoperative treatment and that disfiguring surgery should be reserved for the minority of individuals who are found to have residual tumor after being managed initially with radiation combined with chemotherapy.

REFERENCES

Colorectal cancer

Etiology and risk factors

COLLINS RH JR et al: Colon cancer, dysplasia, and surveillance in patients with ulcerative colitis. N Engl J Med 316:1654, 1987
HAGGITT RC, REID BJ: Hereditary gastrointestinal polyposis syndromes. Am J Surg Path 10:871, 1986
LIPKIN M, NEWMARK H: Effect of added dietary calcium on colonic epithelial cell proliferation in subjects at high risk for familial colonic cancer. N Engl J Med 313:1381, 1985
VOGELSTEIN B et al: Genetic alterations during colorectal-tumor development. N Engl J Med 319:595, 1988
ZARIDZE DG: Environmental etiology of large bowel cancer. J Natl Cancer Inst 70:389, 1982

Polyps

CANNON-ALBRIGHT LA et al: Common inheritance of susceptibility to colonic adenomatous polyps and associated colorectal cancers. N Engl J Med 319:533, 1988
FENOGLIO-PREISER CM, HUTTER RVP: Colorectal polyps: Pathologic diagnosis and clinical significance. Cancer 35:322, 1985

Screening

GROSSMAN S et al: Colonoscopic screening of persons with suspected risk factors for colon cancer: II Past history of colorectal neoplasms. Gastroenterology 96:299, 1989
KNIGHT KK et al: Occult blood screening for colorectal cancer. JAMA 261:586, 1989
NEUGUT AI, PITA S: Role of sigmoidoscopy in screening for colorectal cancer: A critical review. Gastroenterology 95:492, 1988
SELBY JV, FRIEDMAN GD: Sigmoidoscopy in the periodic health examination of asymptomatic adults. JAMA 261:594, 1989
SIMON JB: Occult blood screening for colorectal carcinoma: A critical review. Gastroenterology 88:820, 1985

Clinical features

GASTROINTESTINAL TUMOR STUDY GROUP: Adjuvant therapy of colon cancer—results of a postoperatively randomized trial. N Engl J Med 310:737, 1984
KERN SE et al: Allelic loss in colorectal carcinoma. JAMA 261:3099, 1989
WANEBO JH et al: Preoperative carcinoembryonic antigen level as a prognostic indicator in colorectal cancer. N Engl J Med 229:448, 1978

Treatment

GASTROINTESTINAL TUMOR STUDY GROUP: Prolongation of the disease-free interval in surgically treated rectal carcinoma. N Engl J Med 312:1465, 1985
MAYER RJ et al: The status of adjuvant therapy for colorectal cancer. J Natl Cancer Inst 81:1359, 1989
MOERTEL CG et al: Levamisole and fluorouracil for adjuvant therapy of resected colon carcinoma. N Engl J Med 322:352, 1990

Tumors of the small intestine

HABER DA, MAYER RJ: Primary gastrointestinal lymphoma. Semin Oncol 15:154, 1988
LEVIN B: Neoplasms of the small bowel, in *Medical Oncology. Basic Principles and Clinical Management of Cancer*, P Calabresi et al (eds). New York, Macmillan, 1985, pp 875–883

Anal cancer

DALING JR et al: Sexual practices, sexually transmitted diseases, and the incidence of anal cancer. N Engl J Med 317:973, 1987
LEICHMAN L et al: Cancer of the anal canal: Model for preoperative adjuvant combined modality therapy. Am J Med 78:211, 1985

244   ACUTE INTESTINAL OBSTRUCTION

WILLIAM SILEN

ETIOLOGY AND CLASSIFICATION   Intestinal obstruction may be *mechanical* or *nonmechanical* (resulting from neuromuscular disturbances which produce either *adynamic* or *dynamic ileus*). The causes of mechanical obstruction of the lumen are conveniently divided into (1) lesions *extrinsic* to the intestine, e.g., adhesive bands, internal and external hernias; (2) lesions *intrinsic* to the wall of the intestine, e.g., diverticulitis, carcinoma, regional enteritis; and (3) obturation of the lumen, e.g., gallstone obstruction, intussusception. From the clinical standpoint, however, it is most useful to consider whether the obstructive mechanism involves the small or large intestine, because the causes, symptoms, and treatment are different (see below). Adhesions and external hernias are the most common causes of obstruction of the small intestine, constituting 70 to 75 percent of cases of this type. Adhesions, however, almost never produce obstruction of the colon, while carcinoma, sigmoid diverticulitis, and volvulus, in that order, are the most common etiologies and together account for about 90 percent of the cases.

Adynamic ileus is probably the most common overall cause of obstruction. Recent studies indicate that the development of this condition is mediated via the hormonal component of the sympathoadrenal system. Adynamic ileus will occur after any peritoneal insult, and its severity and duration will be dependent to some degree on the type of peritoneal injury. Hydrochloric acid, colonic contents, and pancreatic enzymes are among the most irritating substances, whereas blood and urine are less so. Adynamic ileus occurs to some degree after any abdominal operation, and its severity varies directly with the amount of intestinal handling and the length of the operation; it usually lasts 2 to 3 days after most operative procedures. Retroperitoneal hematomas, particularly associated with vertebral fracture, commonly cause severe adynamic ileus, and the latter may occur with other retroperitoneal conditions such as ureteral calculus or severe pyelonephritis. Thoracic diseases including lower-lobe pneumonia, fractured ribs, and myocardial infarction frequently produce adynamic ileus, as do electrolyte disturbances, particularly potassium depletion. Finally intestinal ischemia, whether the result of vascular occlusion or intestinal distention itself, may perpetuate an adynamic ileus. Spastic or dynamic ileus is very uncommon and results from extreme and prolonged contraction of the intestine. It has been observed in heavy metal poisoning, uremia, porphyria, and extensive intestinal ulcerations.

PATHOPHYSIOLOGY Distention of the intestine is caused by the accumulation of gas and fluid proximal to and within the obstructed segment. Seventy to eighty percent of intestinal gas consists of swallowed air, and because this is composed mainly of nitrogen, which is poorly absorbed from the intestinal lumen, removal of air by continuous gastric suction is a useful adjunct in the treatment of intestinal distention. The accumulation of fluid proximal to the obstructing mechanism results not only from ingested fluid, swallowed saliva, gastric juice, and biliary and pancreatic secretions but also from interference with normal sodium and water transport. During the first 12 to 24 h of obstruction there is a marked depression of flux from lumen to blood of sodium and consequently water in the distended proximal intestine. After 24 h, there is also movement of sodium and water into the lumen, contributing further to the distention and fluid losses. Intraluminal pressure rises from a normal of 2 to 4 cmH$_2$O to 8 to 10 cmH$_2$O. During peristalsis, when simple obstruction or a "closed loop" is present, pressures reach 30 to 60 cmH$_2$O. Closed-loop obstruction of the small intestine results when the lumen is occluded at two points by a single mechanism such as a hernial ring or adhesive band, thus producing a closed loop whose blood supply is often obstructed at the same time. Strangulation of the loop itself is thus common in association with marked distention proximal to the involved loop. A form of closed-loop obstruction is encountered when complete obstruction of the colon exists in the presence of a competent ileocecal valve (85 percent of individuals). Although the blood supply of the colon is not entrapped within the obstructing mechanism, distention of the cecum is extreme because of its greater diameter (LaPlace's law), and impairment of the intramural blood supply is considerable with consequent gangrene of the cecal wall, usually anteriorly. Necrosis of the small intestine may occur by the same mechanism of interference with intramural blood flow when distention is extreme, but this sequence is uncommon in the small intestine. Once impairment of blood supply occurs, bacterial invasion supervenes and peritonitis develops. The systemic effects of extreme distention include elevation of the diaphragm with restricted ventilation and subsequent atelectasis. Venous return via the inferior vena cava may also be impaired.

The loss of fluids and electrolytes may be extreme, and unless replacement is prompt, leads to hemoconcentration, hypovolemia, renal insufficiency, shock, and death. Vomiting, accumulation of fluids within the lumen by the mechanisms described above, and the sequestration of fluid into the edematous intestinal wall and peritoneal cavity as a result of impairment of venous return from the intestine all contribute to massive loss of fluid and electrolytes. As soon as significant impedance to venous return is present, the intestine becomes severely congested, and blood begins to seep into the intestinal lumen. Blood loss may reach significant levels when long segments of intestine are involved.

SYMPTOMS *Mechanical small-intestinal obstruction* is characterized by cramping midabdominal pain which tends to be more severe the higher the obstruction. The pain occurs in paroxysms, and the patient is relatively comfortable in the intervals between the pains. Audible borborygmi are often noted by the patient simultaneously with the paroxysms of pain. The pain may become less severe as distention progresses, probably because motility is impaired in the edematous intestine. When strangulation is present, the pain is usually more localized and may be steady and severe without a colicky component, a fact which often causes delay in diagnosis of obstruction. Vomiting is almost invariable, and it is earlier and more profuse the higher the obstruction. The vomitus initially contains bile and mucus and remains as such if the obstruction is high in the intestine. With low ileal obstruction, the vomitus becomes feculent, i.e., orange-brown in color with a foul odor, which results from the overgrowth of bacteria proximal to the obstruction. Singultus is common. Obstipation and failure to pass gas by rectum are invariably present when the obstruction is complete, although some stool and gas may be passed spontaneously or after an enema shortly after onset of the complete obstruction. Diarrhea is occasionally observed in partial obstruction. Blood in the stool is rare, even in the completely obstructed patient, but does occur in cases of intussusception. Other than some minor but inconsistent differences in pain patterns noted above, the symptoms of strangulating obstructions cannot be distinguished from those of nonstrangulating obstructions.

Mechanical colonic obstruction produces colicky abdominal pain similar in quality to that of small-intestinal obstruction but of much lower intensity. Complaints of pain are occasionally absent in stoic elderly patients. Vomiting occurs late, if at all, particularly if the ileocecal valve is competent. Paradoxically, feculent vomitus is very rare. A history of recent alterations in bowel habits and blood in the stool is common because carcinoma and diverticulitis are the most frequent causes. Constipation becomes progressive, and obstipation with failure to pass gas ensues. Acute symptoms may develop over a period of a week.

In *adynamic ileus,* colicky pain is absent, and only discomfort from distention is evident. Vomiting may be frequent but is rarely profuse. It usually consists of gastric contents and bile and is almost never feculent. Complete obstipation may or may not occur. Singultus is very common.

PHYSICAL FINDINGS *Abdominal distention* is the hallmark of all forms of intestinal obstruction. It is least marked in cases of obstruction high in the small intestine and most marked in colonic obstruction. Early in the course of the disease, especially in closed-loop strangulating small-bowel obstruction, distention may be barely perceptible or absent. Tenderness and rigidity are usually minimal; the temperature is rarely above 37.8°C (100°F) in nonstrangulating obstruction of the small and large intestine. Contrary to popular belief the same is true of strangulating obstruction until very late in the course of the disease, a fact which has often resulted in unfortunate delay in treatment. Signs and symptoms of shock also occur *very late* in strangulating obstruction. The appearance of shock, tenderness, rigidity, and fever often means that there has been contamination of the peritoneum with infected intestinal content. The presence of a palpable abdominal mass usually signifies a closed-loop strangulating small-bowel obstruction because the tense fluid-filled loop is the palpable lesion. Auscultation may reveal loud high-pitched borborygmi coincident with the colicky pain, but this classic finding is often not present late in strangulating or nonstrangulating obstruction. A quiet abdomen does not eliminate the possibility of obstruction, nor does it necessarily establish the diagnosis of adynamic ileus.

LABORATORY AND X-RAY FINDINGS Leukocytosis, with shift to the left, usually occurs when strangulation is present, but a normal white blood cell count does not exclude strangulation. Elevation of the serum amylase is encountered occasionally in all forms of intestinal obstruction, especially the strangulating variety.

The x-ray is extremely valuable but under certain circumstances may also be misleading. In nonstrangulating complete small-bowel obstruction, x-rays are almost completely reliable. Distention of fluid- and gas-filled loops of small intestine usually arranged in a "step-

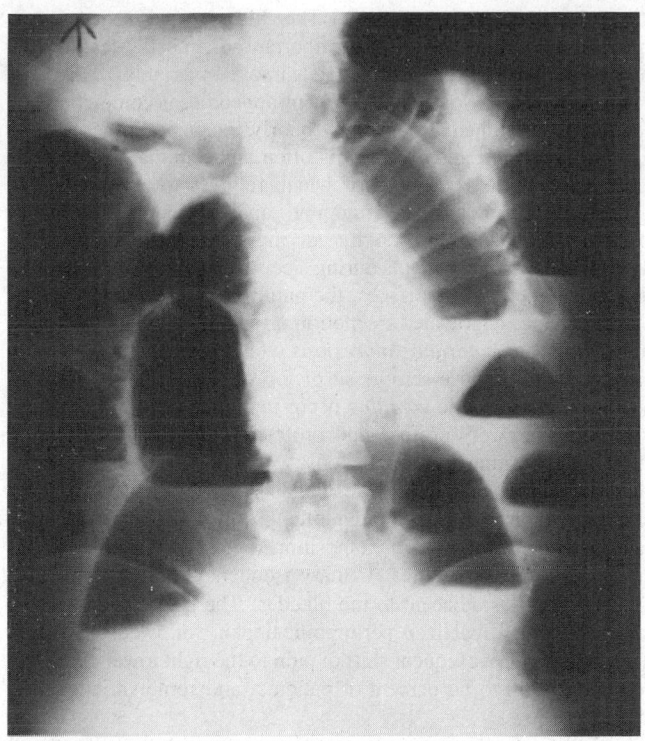

FIGURE 244-1 Acute mechanical obstruction of small intestine (upright film). Note air-fluid levels, marked distention of bowel loops, and absence of colonic gas.

ladder'' pattern with air-fluid levels and an absence or paucity of colonic gas are pathognomonic (Fig. 244-1). These findings, however, are absent in slightly over half the cases of strangulating small-bowel obstruction, especially early in the disease. A general haze due to peritoneal fluid and sometimes a ''coffee-bean''-shaped mass are seen in strangulating obstruction. Occasionally the films are normal, but when symptoms are consistent with obstruction of the small intestine, a normal film should suggest strangulation. Roentgenographic differentiation of partial mechanical small-bowel obstruction from adynamic ileus may be impossible since gas is present in both small and large intestine; however, colonic distention is usually more prominent in adynamic ileus. A radiopaque dye given by mouth is useful in making this distinction.

Colonic obstruction with a competent ileocecal valve is easily recognized because distention with gas is mainly confined to the colon. Barium enema, sigmoidoscopy, or colonoscopy, depending upon the suspected site of obstruction, are usually advisable to determine the nature of the lesion except when concomitant perforation is suspected, a rare occurrence. Sigmoidoscopy may be therapeutic in cases of sigmoid volvulus. When the ileocecal valve is incompetent, the films resemble those of partial small-bowel obstruction or adynamic ileus, and barium enema or colonoscopy is necessary to establish the correct diagnosis. Barium given by mouth is perfectly safe when obstruction is in the small intestine since the barium sulfate does not become inspissated in this location. *Barium should never be given by mouth to a patient with possible colonic obstruction* until that possibility has been excluded by barium enema.

PROGNOSIS AND TREATMENT Small-intestinal obstruction
The overall mortality rate for obstruction of the small intestine is about 10 percent, even under the most optimal conditions. While the mortality rate for nonstrangulating obstruction is as low as 5 to 8 percent, that for strangulating obstruction has been reported to be between 20 and 75 percent. Well over half of the deaths from small-bowel obstruction occur in those with strangulation; however, the latter constitute only one-fourth to one-third of the cases. Careful studies indicate that the clinical, laboratory, and x-ray findings are not reliable in distinguishing strangulating from nonstrangulating

obstruction when obstruction is complete. Complete obstruction is suggested when there has been a total cessation in the passage of gas or stool per rectum and when gas is absent in the distal intestine by x-ray. Since strangulating small-bowel obstruction is always complete, operation should always be undertaken in such patients after suitable preparation. Prior to operation, fluid and electrolyte balance should be restored, and decompression instituted by means of a nasogastric tube. Six to eight hours of preparation may be necessary. During this period broad-spectrum antibiotics are indicated if strangulation is felt to be likely, but operation should not be delayed unless there is unequivocal clinical and roentgenographic evidence of resolution of the obstruction during the period of preparation. Attempts to pass a long tube into the small intestine usually fail while putting the patient through uncomfortable unproductive manipulations which delay appropriate fluid replacement and decompression. *There are probably few if any indications for the use of a long intestinal tube.* Procrastination of operation because of improvement in well-being of the patient during resuscitation and gastric decompression usually leads to unnecessary and hazardous delay in proper treatment. Purely nonoperative therapy is safe only in the presence of incomplete obstruction and is best utilized in patients with (1) repeated episodes of partial obstruction, (2) recent postoperative partial obstruction, and (3) partial obstruction following a recent episode of diffuse peritonitis.

Colonic obstruction The mortality rate for colonic obstruction is about 20 percent. As in small-bowel obstruction, nonoperative treatment is contraindicated unless the obstruction is incomplete. Occasionally, but not always, when the obstruction is incomplete, nonoperative therapy may result in sufficient decompression that a definitive operative procedure can be undertaken at a later date. This can usually be accomplished by discontinuation of all oral intake and perhaps by nasogastric suction, although attempts to decompress a *completely* obstructed colon by intubation are almost invariably futile. A long intestinal tube will not decompress an obstructed colon with a competent ileocecal valve. When obstruction is complete, early operation is mandatory, especially when the ileocecal valve is competent; cecal gangrene is likely if the cecal diameter exceeds 10 cm on plain abdominal film. For obstruction on the left side of the colon, the most common site, preliminary operative decompression by cecostomy or transverse colostomy followed by definitive resection of the primary lesion is the treatment of choice. For a lesion of the right or transverse colon, primary resection and anastomosis can safely be performed because distention of the ileum with consequent discrepancy in size and hazard in suture are not present.

Adynamic ileus This type of ileus usually responds to nonoperative continuous decompression and adequate treatment of the primary disease. The prognosis is usually good. Recently, successful decompression of severe colonic ileus has been accomplished by colonoscopy, but this should be avoided if tenderness in the right lower quadrant suggests possible cecal gangrene. Rarely, adynamic colonic distention may become so great that cecostomy is required if cecal gangrene is feared. Spastic ileus usually responds to treatment of the primary disease.

REFERENCES

BECKER WF: Acute adhesive ileus: A study of 412 cases with particular reference to the abuse of tube decompression in treatment. Surg Gynecol Obstet 95:472, 1952
BULKLEY GB et al: Intraoperative determination of small intestinal viability following ischemic injury: Prospective controlled trial of two adjuvant methods (Doppler and fluorescein) compared with standard clinical judgement. Ann Surg 193:628, 1981
COHN I, ATIK M: Strangulation obstruction: Closed loop studies. Ann Surg 153:94, 1961
DUBOIS A et al: Postoperative ileus: Physiopathology, etiology and treatment. Ann Surg 178:781, 1973
GOUGH IR: Strangulating adhesive small bowel radiographs. Br J Surg 65:431, 1978
HOFSETTER SR: Acute adhesive obstruction of the small intestine. Surg Gynecol Obstet 152:141, 1981
JACKSON BR: The diagnosis of colonic obstruction. Dis Colon Rectum 25:603, 1982
NOLAN DJ: Barium examination of the small intestine. Gut 22:682, 1981

SHIELDS R: The absorption and secretion of fluid and electrolytes by the obstructed bowel. Br J Surg 52:774, 1965

SILEN W: *Cope's Early Diagnosis of the Acute Abdomen,* 17th ed. London, Oxford, 1987

245   ACUTE APPENDICITIS

WILLIAM SILEN

INCIDENCE AND EPIDEMIOLOGY   The maximum incidence of acute appendicitis occurs in the second and third decades of life. While the disease may be encountered at any time of life, it is relatively rare at the extremes of age. Males and females are equally affected except between puberty and age 25, when males predominate in a 3:2 ratio. Perforation is relatively much more common in infancy and in the aged, during which periods mortality rates are highest. The mortality rate has decreased steadily in Europe and the United States from 8.1 per 100,000 of the population in 1941 to less than 1 per 100,000 in 1970 and subsequently. The absolute incidence of the disease also decreased by about 40 percent between 1940 and 1960 but since then has remained unchanged. Although various factors such as changing dietary habits, altered intestinal flora, and better nutrition and intake of vitamins have been suggested to explain the reduced incidence, the exact reasons have not been elucidated. Of interest is that the overall incidence of appendicitis is much lower in underdeveloped countries, especially parts of Africa, and in lower socioeconomic groups.

PATHOGENESIS   The primary pathogenetic hallmark has always been thought to be luminal obstruction. While obstruction can be identified by careful examination in 30 to 40 percent of cases, recent studies have shown that ulceration of the mucosa is the initial event in the majority. The causation of the ulceration is unknown, although a viral etiology has been postulated. Recently, it has been suggested that infection with *Yersinia* organisms may cause the disease since careful study has shown that high complement fixation titers have been found in as many as 30 percent of cases of proven appendicitis 1 week after operation. Whether the inflammatory reaction attendant with ulceration is sufficient to obstruct the tiny appendiceal lumen even transiently is also not clear. Obstruction, when present, is most commonly caused by a fecalith, which results from accumulation and inspissation of fecal matter around vegetable fibers. Enlarged lymphoid follicles associated with viral infections (e.g., measles), inspissated barium, worms (e.g., pinworms, *Ascaris,* and *Taenia*), and tumors (e.g., carcinoid or carcinoma) may also obstruct the lumen. Secretion of mucus distends the organ, which has a capacity of only 0.1 to 0.2 mL, and luminal pressures rise as high as 60 cmH$_2$O. Luminal bacteria multiply and invade the appendiceal wall as venous engorgement and subsequent arterial compromise result from the high intraluminal pressures. Finally, gangrene and perforation occur. If the process evolves slowly, adjacent organs such as the terminal ileum, cecum, and omentum may wall off the appendiceal area so that a localized abscess will develop, whereas rapid progression of vascular impairment may cause perforation with free access to the peritoneal cavity. Subsequent rupture of primary appendiceal abscesses may produce fistulas between the appendix and bladder, small intestine, sigmoid, or cecum. Occasionally, acute appendicitis may be the first manifestation of Crohn's disease. While chronic infection of the appendix with tuberculosis, amebiasis, and actinomycosis may occur, a useful clinical aphorism states that *chronic appendiceal inflammation is not usually the cause of prolonged abdominal pain of weeks' or months' duration.* In contrast, it is clear that recurrent acute appendicitis does occur, often with complete resolution of inflammation and symptoms between attacks. Recurrent acute appendicitis may become more frequent as antibiotics are dispensed more freely.

CLINICAL MANIFESTATIONS   The history and sequence of symptoms are among the most important diagnostic features of appendicitis. The initial symptom is almost invariably *abdominal pain* of the visceral type, resulting from appendiceal contractions or distention of the lumen. It is usually poorly localized in the periumbilical or epigastric regions. There is often an accompanying urge to defecate or pass flatus, neither of which relieves the distress. This visceral pain is mild, often cramping, and rarely catastrophic in nature, usually lasting 4 to 6 h, but may not be noted by stoic individuals or by some patients during sleep. As inflammation spreads to the parietal peritoneal surfaces, the pain becomes somatic, steady, and more severe, aggravated by motion or cough and usually located in the *right lower quadrant. Anorexia* is so frequent that the presence of hunger should arouse serious suspicion of the diagnosis of acute appendicitis. *Nausea* and *vomiting* occur in 50 to 60 percent of cases, but vomiting is rarely profuse and protracted. The development of nausea and vomiting before the onset of pain is extremely rare. Change in bowel habit is of little diagnostic value since any or no alteration may be observed, although the presence of diarrhea caused by an inflamed appendix in juxtaposition to the sigmoid may cause serious diagnostic difficulties. Urinary frequency and dysuria occur if the appendix lies adjacent to the bladder. The typical sequence of symptoms (poorly localized periumbilical pain followed by nausea and vomiting with subsequent shift of pain to the right lower quadrant) occurs in only 50 to 60 percent of patients, and some variations are considered below.

Physical findings vary with time after onset of the illness and according to the location of the appendix, which may be situated deep in the pelvic cul-de-sac, in the right lower quadrant in any relation to the peritoneum, cecum, and small intestine, in the right upper quadrant, or even in the left lower quadrant. *The diagnosis cannot be established unless tenderness can be elicited.* While tenderness is sometimes absent in the early visceral stage of the disease, it ultimately always develops and is found in any location corresponding to the position of the appendix. Abdominal tenderness may be completely absent if a retrocecal or pelvic appendix is present, in which case the sole physical finding may be tenderness in the flank or on rectal or pelvic examination. Percussion, rebound tenderness, and referred rebound tenderness are often, but not invariably, present; they are most likely to be absent early in the illness. Flexion of the right hip and guarded movement by the patient are due to parietal peritoneal involvement. Hyperesthesia of the skin of the right lower quadrant and a positive psoas or obturator sign are often late findings and are rarely of diagnostic value. When the inflamed appendix is in close proximity to the anterior parietal peritoneum, muscular rigidity is present, yet is often minimal early. The temperature is usually normal or slightly elevated [37.2 to 38°C (99 to 100.5°F)], but a temperature above 38.3°C (101°F) should always suggest the presence of perforation. Tachycardia is commensurate with the elevation of the temperature. Rigidity and tenderness become more marked as the disease progresses to perforation and localized or diffuse peritonitis. Distention is rare unless severe diffuse peritonitis has developed. The alleged disappearance of pain and tenderness just prior to perforation is extremely unusual. A mass may develop if localized perforation has occurred but usually will not be detectable before 3 days after onset of the disease. Earlier presence of a mass suggests carcinoma of the cecum or Crohn's disease. Perforation is rare before 24 h after onset of symptoms, but the rate may be as high as 80 percent after 48 h.

Laboratory examination does not establish the diagnosis since the latter is based primarily on clinical grounds. Although moderate leukocytosis of 10,000 to 18,000 cells per microliter is frequent (with a concomitant shift to immature cells), the absence of leukocytosis does not eliminate the possibility of acute appendicitis. Leukocytosis of greater than 20,000 cells per microliter should alert the clinician to the probability of perforation. Anemia and blood in the stool suggest a primary diagnosis of carcinoma of the cecum, especially in elderly individuals. The urine may contain a few white or red blood cells without bacteria if the appendix lies close to the right ureter or bladder.

Urinalysis is most useful, however, in excluding genitourinary conditions which may mimic acute appendicitis. X-rays are rarely of value except when an opaque fecalith (5 percent of patients) is observed in the right lower quadrant (especially in children) together with other clinical findings consistent with appendicitis. Consequently there is no routine need to obtain films of the abdomen unless there is a possibility of other conditions such as intestinal obstruction or ureteral calculus. In some cases in which symptoms are either recurrent or more prolonged, a careful barium enema may disclose an extrinsic defect on the medial wall of the cecum or a calcified fecalith. The diagnosis may also be established by the ultrasonic demonstration of an enlarged and thick-walled appendix, but if the appendix cannot be seen, the diagnosis cannot be excluded.

While the typical historical sequence and physical findings are present in 50 to 60 percent of cases, it is obvious that a wide variety of atypical patterns of disease are encountered, especially at the age extremes and during pregnancy. The 70 to 80 percent incidence of perforation and generalized peritonitis in infants under 2 years of age is dramatic testimony to the importance of the history in the early detection of the disease. Any infant or child with diarrhea, vomiting, and abdominal pain is highly suspect. Fever is much more common in this age group, and abdominal distention is often the only physical finding. In the elderly, pain and tenderness are often obtunded, and thus the diagnosis is frequently delayed. A 30 percent incidence of perforation in patients over 70 attests to the importance of this delay. Elderly patients often present themselves initially with a slightly painful mass (a primary appendiceal abscess), or sometimes appear with adhesive intestinal obstruction 5 or 6 days after a previously undetected perforated appendix. Appendicitis occurs about once in every 1000 pregnancies and is the most common extrauterine condition requiring abdominal operation. The diagnosis may be missed or delayed because of the frequent occurrence of mild abdominal discomfort and nausea and vomiting during pregnancy. During the last trimester when the mortality rate from appendicitis is highest, uterine displacement of the appendix to the right upper quadrant and laterally leads to confusion in diagnosis.

DIFFERENTIAL DIAGNOSIS A listing of the differential diagnoses of acute appendicitis would produce an encyclopedic compendium of all conditions which cause abdominal pain since appendicitis may simulate any of these diseases. Diagnostic accuracy is about 75 to 80 percent for experienced clinicians and must be based solely on the clinical criteria outlined above. It is probably better to err slightly in the direction of overdiagnosis since delay is associated with perforation and increased morbidity and mortality. In unperforated appendicitis the mortality rate is 0.1 percent, little more than that associated with general anesthesia; for perforated appendicitis there is an overall mortality of 3 percent, a figure which increases to 15 percent in the elderly. In doubtful cases 4 to 6 h of observation is always more beneficial than harmful, however. The most common conditions discovered at operation when acute appendicitis is erroneously diagnosed are, in rough order of frequency, mesenteric lymphadenitis, no organic disease, acute pelvic inflammatory disease, ruptured graafian follicle or corpus luteum cyst, and acute gastroenteritis. In addition, acute cholecystitis, perforated ulcer, acute pancreatitis, acute diverticulitis, strangulating intestinal obstruction, ureteral calculus, and pyelonephritis frequently present diagnostic difficulties.

It is useful to consider separately some of the more common and difficult diagnostic possibilities, especially in the female. Differentiation of *pelvic inflammatory disease* from acute appendicitis may be virtually impossible. Gram-negative intracellular diplococci on cervical smear are not pathognomonic unless *Neisseria gonorrhea* can be cultured. Pain on movement of the cervix is not specific and may occur in appendicitis if perforation has occurred or if the appendix lies adjacent to the uterus or adnexa. *Rupture of a graafian follicle* (mittelschmerz) occurs at midcycle with spill of blood and fluid to produce pain and tenderness more diffuse and usually of a less severe degree than in appendicitis. Fever and leukocytosis are usually absent. *Rupture of a corpus luteum cyst* is identical clinically to rupture of a graafian follicle but develops about the time of menstruation. The presence of an adnexal mass and evidence of blood loss help differentiate *ruptured tubal pregnancy. Twisted ovarian cyst* and *endometriosis* occasionally are difficult to distinguish from appendicitis. In all of these female conditions, ultrasonic examination of the pelvis and laparoscopy may be of great value.

Acute mesenteric lymphadenitis is the appellation usually given when enlarged, slightly reddened lymph nodes at the root of the mesentery and a normal appendix are encountered at operation in a patient who usually has right lower quadrant tenderness and a somewhat higher temperature than most patients with acute appendicitis. Whether this is a single, discrete entity is unclear since the causative factor is not known. It has been recognized recently that some of these patients have infection with *Yersinia pseudotuberculosis* or *Y. enterocolytica* in which case the diagnosis can be established by culture of the mesenteric nodes or by serologic titers (Chap. 121). The diagnosis is essentially impossible clinically, although retrospectively there often appears to have been more diffuse pain and tenderness. Children seem to be affected more frequently than adults. Operation should be undertaken unless there is rapid resolution of all symptoms and findings. *Acute gastroenteritis* usually causes profuse watery diarrhea, often with nausea and vomiting but without localized findings. Between cramps, the abdomen is completely relaxed. In salmonella gastroenteritis the abdominal findings are similar, although the pain may be more severe and more localized, and fever and chills are common. The occurrence of similar symptoms among other members of the family may be helpful. When the diagnosis of acute pelvic appendicitis with perforation has been missed, gastroenteritis is the most common previous working diagnosis. Persistent abdominal or rectal tenderness should eliminate the diagnosis of gastroenteritis. *Regional enteritis* (Crohn's disease) is usually associated with a more prolonged history, often with previous exacerbations regarded by the patient or physician as episodes of gastroenteritis unless the diagnosis has been established previously. *Meckel's diverticulitis* usually cannot be distinguished from acute appendicitis but is very rare.

TREATMENT Cathartics and frequent enemas should be avoided if appendicitis is under consideration, and antibiotics should not be administered when the diagnosis is in question, as they will only mask the presence or development of perforation. The treatment is early operation and appendectomy as soon as the patient can be prepared. Preparation rarely takes more than 1 to 2 h in early appendicitis but may require 6 to 8 h in cases of severe sepsis and dehydration associated with late perforation. The *only* circumstance in which operation is *not* indicated is the presence of a palpable mass 3 to 5 days after the onset of symptoms. Should operation be undertaken at that time, a phlegmon rather than a definitive abscess will be found, and complications from dissection of such a phlegmon are frequent. Such patients treated with broad-spectrum antibiotics, parenteral fluids, and rest usually show resolution of the mass and symptoms within 1 week. *Interval appendectomy* can and should be done safely 3 months later. Should the mass enlarge or the patient become more toxic, drainage of the abscess is necessary. The complications of subphrenic, pelvic, or other intraabdominal abscesses usually follow perforation with generalized peritonitis and can be avoided by early diagnosis of the disease.

REFERENCES

BOLTON JP: Assessment of the value of the white cell count in management of suspected acute appendicitis. Br J Surg 62:906, 1975
BUSUTTIL RW et al: Effect of prophylactic antibiotics in acute nonperforated appendicitis: A prospective, randomized double-blind clinical study. Ann Surg 194:502, 1981
BUTLER C: Surgical pathology of acute appendicitis. Hum Pathol 12:870, 1981
JULIEN BCM et al: A prospective study of ultrasonography in the diagnosis of appendicitis. N Engl J Med 317:666, 1987

KOEPSELL TD et al: Factors affecting perforation in acute appendicitis. Surg Gynecol Obstet 153:508, 1981

RAVAL B et al: Use of computed tomography in appendicitis: Technique, findings, and pitfalls. J Comput Tomogr 11:17, 1987

SCHWERK WB et al: Ultrasonography in the diagnosis of acute appendicitis: A retrospective study. Gastroenterology 97:630, 1989

VANTRAPPEN G et al.: *Yersinia* enteritis and enterocolitis: Gastroenterological aspects. Gastroenterology 72:220, 1977

246   DISEASES OF THE PERITONEUM AND MESENTERY

KURT J. ISSELBACHER / J. THOMAS LaMONT

ACUTE PERITONITIS   Peritonitis is a localized or generalized inflammatory process of the peritoneum that may appear in both acute and chronic forms. In the acute form the motor activity of the intestine is decreased, and the intestinal lumen becomes distended with gas and fluid. Fluid accumulates as a result of failure to reabsorb the 7 or 8 liters normally secreted daily into the lumen and absorbed from the distal small bowel and colon. There is also accumulation of fluid in the peritoneal cavity as well as decreased oral intake. These combined losses can lead to rapid depletion of the plasma volume with impaired cardiac and renal function.

Etiology   Peritonitis may be due to entry of bacteria into the peritoneal cavity from a perforation in the gastrointestinal tract or from an external penetrating wound. It may be secondary to severe chemical reactions from the release of pancreatic enzymes, the digestive juices of the upper gastrointestinal tract, or bile as a result of injury or perforation of the intestine or biliary tract. Patients with systemic lupus erythematosus may have bouts of sterile peritonitis during attacks of their disease.

The most common causes of bacterial peritonitis are appendicitis, perforations associated with diverticulitis, peptic ulcer, gangrenous gallbladder, and gangrenous obstruction of the small bowel from adhesive bands, incarcerated hernia, or volvulus. Any lesion leading to the escape of intestinal bacteria may be a source, including a perforating carcinoma, foreign body, and ulcerative colitis. The peritoneal cavity is remarkably resistant to contamination, and unless continuing contamination occurs, the disease process becomes localized. Patients with alcoholic cirrhosis and ascites have an increased susceptibility to spontaneous bacterial peritonitis, usually from enteric pathogens. This complication occurs in the absence of recognizable perforation of a viscus, and may be due to leakage of bacteria through the intestinal wall.

Clinical features   These usually consist of increasing abdominal pain, distention, nausea and vomiting, inability to pass feces or flatus, fever, hypotension, tachycardia, thirst, and oliguria. On physical examination the patient appears acutely ill and febrile and has a variable degree of abdominal distention. The abdomen is usually acutely tender and tympanitic, often with rebound tenderness. The location of the pain and tenderness depends on the underlying cause and whether the inflammation is localized or generalized. In *localized* peritonitis, as seen in uncomplicated appendicitis or diverticulitis, the physical findings are limited to the area of inflammation. With widespread peritoneal inflammation there is *generalized* peritonitis with diffuse abdominal tenderness and rebound. Rigidity of the abdominal wall is a common finding in peritonitis and may be localized or generalized.

Peristalsis may be present initially but usually disappears as the illness progresses. Hypotension is common, as is leukocytosis, which often is greater than 20,000 cells per microliter. Plain abdominal films may reveal dilatation of the large and small bowel with edema of the small-bowel wall as evidenced by the distance between adjacent loops of gas-filled small intestine. Diagnostic paracentesis is sometimes valuable in determining the nature of the exudate as well as

whether bacteria can be demonstrated or cultured. Diabetic ketoacidosis, lead colic, gastric crises of syphilis, and acute porphyria may cause severe abdominal symptoms that resemble the picture of acute peritonitis.

GONOCOCCAL PERITONITIS   This usually involves an extension of gonococcal infection from a primary focus in the female reproductive tract. The signs of inflammation usually are limited to the pelvis, but there may be findings of a mild generalized peritonitis. Occasionally the patient has right upper quadrant pain and tenderness caused by gonococcal perihepatitis involving the liver capsule and adjacent peritoneum (Fitz-Hugh–Curtis syndrome; see also Chap. 110).

STARCH PERITONITIS   An acute granulomatous peritonitis can develop in some patients as a foreign-body reaction to cornstarch used to powder surgical gloves. The clinical picture is that of acute abdominal pain and fever 10 to 30 days after an abdominal operation. The diagnosis can be made by paracentesis and demonstration of starch granules in monocytes. However, most patients are reexplored because of the fear of abscess or bacterial peritonitis, with the finding of foreign-body granuloma studding the peritoneum.

PSEUDOMYXOMA PERITONEI   This is a rare condition resulting from rupture of a mucocele of the appendix or of a mucinous ovarian cyst. The abdomen becomes filled with masses of jelly-like material. Occasionally, with removal of the mucocele or the ovarian cyst and most of the myxomatous material, a cure may ensue. In other cases, however, the mucoid material recurs, leading to progressive wasting and eventual death. Colloid carcinoma arising from the stomach or colon with peritoneal implants may resemble pseudomyxoma at laparotomy. The course of this type of highly malignant tumor is one of rapid cachexia and early death. The diagnosis can usually be made by the appearance of many highly malignant cells in the peritoneal implants.

CANCER OF THE PERITONEUM   Aside from mesothelioma, which in most patients is caused by previous exposure to asbestos, cancer of the peritoneum is usually secondary to a neoplasm within the abdomen, most commonly of the stomach and ovary. This type of metastatic malignancy is invariably associated with progressive ascites with a high specific gravity and high protein content, often with large numbers of red blood cells or even gross blood. The diagnosis is established by demonstrating malignant cells in the fluid. The clinical progress of this malignant spread can sometimes be arrested by installations of radioactive gold, nitrogen mustard, or chloroquine.

FAMILIAL MEDITERRANEAN FEVER   See Chap. 278.

PNEUMATOSIS CYSTOIDES INTESTINALIS   This is a condition in which multiple gas-filled blebs or cysts accumulate in the intestinal wall beneath the serosal surface of the bowel. The exact source of the gas has not been explained satisfactorily. In some instances, this disease is associated with specific ulceration of the intestinal mucosa, in particular peptic ulcer with outlet obstruction. Cysts in the wall of the small bowel are seen as an occasional complication of mesenteric vascular occlusion. In the large bowel, these cysts are usually benign, may be seen with a variety of other disorders, and usually disappear in time.

There are no specific physical findings secondary to the pneumatosis, and the diagnosis is made either by x-ray or at laparotomy. Occasionally the subserosal cysts may rupture, resulting in pneumoperitoneum.

CHYLOUS ASCITES   This term refers to the accumulation of chyle (intestinal lymph) in the peritoneal cavity. The condition is sometimes associated with chylothorax. The fluid in the peritoneal cavity appears milky or creamy because of the presence of chylomicrons. This fat may be demonstrated microscopically by staining with Sudan III and may be removed by acidification of the fluid followed by extraction with ether. The chyle (lipid) will then go into the ether phase. Many conditions may be associated with the cloudy or milky-appearing peritoneal fluid, so-called pseudochylous ascites. The milky or turbid appearance is usually due to the presence of protein and desquamated cells. The turbidity of this fluid will not be removed with the ether but will clear with addition of alkali.

The causes of chylous ascites include (1) penetrating or nonpenetrating trauma that damages the main duct in the lymphatic system within the abdomen, (2) intestinal obstruction if it is associated with rupture of a major lymphatic channel, (3) congenital lymphangiectasia, (4) malignant disease or tuberculous infection that obstructs the intestinal lymphatics, (5) filariasis, or (6) cirrhosis.

The sudden accumulation of chyle in the peritoneal cavity often results in abdominal pain, signs of peritoneal irritation, and leukocytosis. These symptoms gradually subside, leaving the patient with a distended but nontender, fluid-filled abdomen. Lymphangiography is of value in determining the location of the leak or site of obstruction to the lymphatic channels. The course depends upon the underlying etiologic factors.

MESENTERIC LIPODYSTROPHY This is a rare disorder usually affecting middle-aged women and characterized pathologically by infiltration of the mesentery with lipid-laden macrophages and fibrous tissue. These patients present with ill-defined abdominal pain and occasionally an abdominal mass. The diagnosis is made at laparotomy by demonstration of thick fibrofatty masses at the root of the mesentery with retraction and distortion of the bowel loops.

REFERENCES

KIPFER RE et al: Mesenteric lipodystrophy. Ann Intern Med 80:582, 1974
LIMBER GK et al: Pseudomyxoma peritonei. Ann Surg 1978:587, 1973
PRESS OW et al: Evaluation and management of chylous ascites. Ann Intern Med 96:358, 1982
SCHWARTZ SI et al: *Principles of Surgery*, 5th ed. New York, McGraw-Hill, 1989
TITO L et al: Spontaneous bacterial peritonitis. Hepatology 8:27, 1988
WARSHAW AL: Diagnosis of starch peritonitis by paracentesis. Lancet 2:1054, 1972

section 2 Liver and biliary tract disease

247 BIOLOGIC AND CLINICAL APPROACHES TO LIVER DISEASE

KURT J. ISSELBACHER / DANIEL K. PODOLSKY

BIOLOGIC CONSIDERATIONS An understanding of diseases of the liver and their clinical manifestations can be derived from an understanding of fundamental hepatic structure and function. An appreciation of anatomic aspects of the liver and biliary tree from the gross level to that of the individual hepatocyte and other cellular constituents is needed to understand the spectrum of clinical manifestations of liver disease. The dual blood supply, unique to the liver and including the portal venous system, makes the liver an intermediate filter for most of the venous drainage of the abdominal viscera. This often leads to secondary hepatic involvement in a number of extrahepatic diseases and makes the liver a relatively common site of solid tumor metastases. Furthermore, an appreciation of the relevant anatomy, especially that of the portal venous system, is important in understanding clinically important manifestations of portal hypertension, a common complication of chronic liver disease when scarring and regeneration lead to distortion of the intrahepatic microvasculature. These anatomic considerations lead the clinician to look for evidence of splenic enlargement and hypersplenism, gastrointestinal bleeding, accumulation of ascites, and signs of portal-systemic encephalopathy. Certainly an understanding of the anatomy of the biliary tract from canaliculus to common bile duct is integral to understanding the basis and sequelae of obstructive jaundice. While inflammation of the gallbladder may lead to fever and pain, choledocholithiasis will cause biliary colic as well as jaundice. Diffuse processes affecting the intrahepatic ducts, such as primary sclerosing cholangitis, will lead to cholestasis and its attendant symptoms while a focal process affecting a single branch of the biliary tree, such as a neoplasm, usually will not.

The structural organization at a level intermediate between the gross anatomic and the cellular also contributes to the clinical patterns seen with disorders of the liver. While various concepts have been offered, most useful is that of the traditional liver lobule. Blood emanates from the portal venules at the periphery and passes through the hepatic sinusoids to the central vein. The portal venules, terminal bile ductules, and hepatic arterioles are arranged in a *triad*. Appreciation of this organization and the presence of concentric zones of function within the lobule explain distinct patterns of injury such as the centrilobular injury resulting from ischemia. These structural features no doubt also provide the basis for the relative preservation of hepatocellular function in many disorders that can lead to significant portal hypertension, such as schistosomiasis and biliary cirrhosis.

As important as the anatomic features are in understanding liver disease, many liver disorders and their manifestations can only be appreciated in the context of the functional complexity of the liver at the cellular level. As detailed in Chap. 250, the hepatocyte plays an important role in diverse general metabolic processes that may be deranged as a consequence of liver disease. In addition this metabolic diversity leads to hepatic involvement in many inborn errors of metabolism, including a wide variety of storage diseases, and less well-understood disorders of iron metabolism (hemosiderosis and hemochromatosis) and copper homeostasis (Wilson's disease).

Some other functional aspects should also be emphasized. The hepatocyte modifies numerous endogenous (e.g., bilirubin) and exogenous (e.g., alcohol, acetaminophen) potentially toxic compounds through oxidation, reduction, and conjugation carried out by several enzymes of the endoplasmic reticulum. Conjugation of substrates generally facilitates their hepatic excretion, converting water-insoluble substances to water-soluble derivatives. It is therefore not surprising that parenchymal liver disease may lead to either conjugated or unconjugated hyperbilirubinemia and jaundice. Metabolic modifications may significantly alter the pharmacologic activity of drugs through formation of derivatives with either decreased or enhanced activity. These metabolic processes may create intermediates which are toxic to the liver itself. This explains the selective susceptibility of the liver to the toxicity of carbon tetrachloride, acetaminophen, and, most importantly, alcohol, which is converted to acetaldehyde.

Additional functions of the hepatocyte that may have significant clinical ramifications include the production of a variety of soluble proteins for secretion into the circulation and the presence of receptors specific for various circulating ligands. The latter is a property shared with the Kupffer cell which fulfills much of its function as a constituent of the reticuloendothelial system by clearing a number of serum glycoproteins through asialoglycoprotein receptor–mediated endocytosis. There is evidence to suggest that some of the substances taken up by this endocytotic mechanism may subsequently pass to and through the hepatocyte to complete an enterohepatic circulation. Carcinoembryonic antigen (CEA) is a glycoprotein and putative tumor marker which is handled in this manner, leading to artifactual elevations in hepatobiliary disease. In contrast to the Kupffer cell, the spectrum of ligands taken up by hepatocytes via specific receptors is much broader. In addition to ligands targeted for lysosomal degradation, the hepatocyte possesses receptors for ligands which are metabolically active after their uptake and dissociation from their receptors. These include transferrin-bound iron and, most important, low-density lipoprotein (LDL) which contributes to regulation of overall body cholesterol metabolism. Disruption of lysosomal degradation of specific ligands in hereditary storage disease leads to hepatomegaly and to a variety of infiltrative disorders. Disruption of the nonlysosomal endocytotic pathway ligands can lead to systemic disorders. It is not clear whether specific receptors or other hepatocyte membrane components play a role in the relative or absolute tropism of infectious agents (particularly the hepatitis viruses) which account for a large proportion of both acute and chronic liver disease. However, the relative selectivity of the hepatitis viruses (A, B, non-A, non-B, and indirectly D) for the hepatocyte is essential in understanding the clinical features, which derive from the extent of hepatocyte destruction, of the illnesses caused by these agents. At the same time the hepatocyte may be infected by less strictly organotropic agents including other viruses (e.g., Epstein-Barr virus) and a wide variety of bacterial and parasitic organisms. The vascular supply of the liver leads to its frequent involvement in disseminated infections.

A final feature of hepatocyte cell biology that contributes to the expression of liver disease is the potential for proliferation and regeneration. Although few mitotic figures are seen in normal hepatic parenchyma, rapid regeneration involving both proliferation and cellular hypertrophy occurs following hepatic resection in experimental animals and humans. The capacity for hepatocellular regeneration is evident in the complete recovery which usually occurs following fulminant hepatitis (due either to viral or toxic agents) if the patient can be sustained through the period of acute injury. Architecturally disordered regeneration in concert with fibrosis is an essential factor in the development of cirrhosis and leads both to disruption of blood flow through the hepatic parenchyma and to uneven hepatocellular function due to distortion of normal lobular structure. Although the mechanisms which control hepatocyte proliferation after hepatocellular loss are incompletely understood, evidence suggests that a complex balance of various peptide growth factors plays an important role.

CLINICAL CONSIDERATIONS   In approaching the patient with known or suspected liver disease, consideration of the patient's problem in the context of a few salient questions permits the clinician to focus on the most important diagnostic possibilities and the severity of the illness. Is the problem primarily hepatocellular or cholestatic? Was the onset of the illness abrupt or gradual? Has the problem led to clinically significant impairment of normal hepatocellular function such as signs of altered mentation or coagulopathy? Are there signs or symptoms of portal hypertension? Important and reliable clues which address these questions may often be obtained from a careful history and physical examination.

Clinical History   A number of historic features may distinguish cholestatic and hepatocellular disease processes. A history of marked right upper quadrant pain or previous indigestion suggests cholelithiasis, cholecystitis, or choledocholithiasis, whereas vague nagging discomfort suggests hepatocellular or infiltrative disease with hepatomegaly causing pain due to distention of Glisson's capsule. Additional important symptoms which should be elicited include pruritus, jaundice, anorexia, weight loss, and fever. Complaints of easy bruising or mental confusion by the patient (or family) should be regarded as ominous signs of either fulminant acute or advanced chronic liver disease.

Family history is important with respect to jaundice, anemia, splenectomy, or cholecystectomy; a positive history may be helpful in diagnosing hemolytic anemia, congenital or familial hyperbilirubinemia, or gallstones. In Wilson's disease (hepatolenticular degeneration), there may be a family history of tremor or neurologic abnormalities. *Occupation* should be reviewed in detail, and *environmental factors* need to be examined. Note should be made of the use of any medications or exposure to known or putative toxins such as carbon tetrachloride, beryllium, or vinyl chloride. The patient should be asked about travel to other countries, especially to areas where hepatitis may be endemic. Careful questioning regarding alcohol intake is important in most cases. Since the alcoholic often denies or understates the amounts consumed, it may be desirable to check the validity of the history with relatives or close friends.

Contact with jaundiced patients (especially intimate or sexual relations) should be noted. If the patient has had any *injections,* hepatitis B or non-A, non-B infection may be the underlying disease. Injections include blood tests, blood or plasma transfusions, tattooing, and dental treatment. Postoperative jaundice may be due to the anesthetic, especially after multiple uses of halothane, or to impaired hepatic excretory function resulting from relative hypoxemia of liver cells during the operative or postoperative period.

As suggested, the *onset of the illness* should be noted. The relatively abrupt onset of nausea, anorexia, and aversion to smoking followed by progressive jaundice suggests viral hepatitis. A gradual development of jaundice associated with pruritus suggests cholestasis. Intermittent right upper quadrant abdominal pain followed by cholestatic jaundice points to gallstone disease, while the gradual onset of painless jaundice with weight loss is suggestive of tumor, such as carcinoma of the head of the pancreas. Jaundice associated with fever and chills makes cholangitis and extrahepatic biliary obstruction likely possibilities. The awareness of progressive abdominal swelling, perhaps first noticed because of tightness of clothing, suggests ascites which may be due to malignancy or an insidious first manifestation of cirrhosis. The patient with hepatitis generally feels ill, and dark urine and light stools occur before the appearance of scleral or skin icterus. In cholestatic hepatitis, the patient may feel relatively well and complain only of symptoms due to the obstruction, such as pruritus.

Physical examination   Jaundice is looked for in the sclera as well as the skin. Pallor indicative of anemia may be a reflection of hemolysis, cirrhosis, or neoplasm. Significant cachexia, especially of the extremities, may be associated with cancer or cirrhosis. In the cirrhotic patient, one should look for stigmas of alcohol abuse such as parotid and lacrimal gland enlargement and Dupuytren's contracture, as well as other features of cirrhosis such as gynecomastia, testicular atrophy, and diminished axillary or pubic hair.

The *skin examination* may reveal ecchymoses due to prothrombin deficiency, or purpura due to thrombocytopenia. *Palmar erythema* or *spider angiomas* may reflect acute or chronic liver disease. Spider angiomas are usually found above the umbilicus and especially on the face, neck, shoulders, forearms, and dorsum of the hands. The presence of a few spider angiomas is not abnormal in women, especially during pregnancy. However, their appearance in men is always abnormal and should be carefully searched for. In chronic cholestasis, *scratch marks, finger clubbing,* and *xanthoma* of the eyelids and extensor surfaces of the tendons of the wrists and ankles may be found. A *slate color* to the skin due to increased melanin should suggest the presence of hemochromatosis.

Evaluation of the *mental state* and *neurologic function* is important. Slight deterioration of the intellect and minimal personality changes may suggest hepatocellular disease or the presence of portal-systemic venous shunts, but care must be taken to exclude other causes such as neurologic disease. The presence of flapping tremor of the hands (asterixis) may be found in association with portal-systemic encephalopathy or impending hepatic coma.

Abdominal examination may reveal ascites, which, together with dilated periumbilical veins, suggests cirrhosis and extensive portal collateral circulation. If additional features of liver disease are lacking, malignancy must be more seriously considered. A very large nodular and rock-hard liver suggests the presence of hepatoma or hepatic metastases. Careful percussion is necessary to evaluate the size of a nonpalpable liver. A small liver may indicate cirrhosis (especially postnecrotic); a small liver which diminishes in size suggests severe hepatitis or massive hepatic necrosis. In the alcoholic, fatty infiltration and cirrhosis often produce a uniform enlargement of the liver. The liver edge is tender in hepatitis, in congestive heart failure, and occasionally in malignant disease and with alcoholism (especially "alcoholic hepatitis").

A palpable and sometimes visibly enlarged gallbladder (Courvoisier's sign) suggests extrahepatic biliary obstruction often due to pancreatic cancer. A tender gallbladder and positive Murphy's sign suggest cholelithiasis or choledocholithiasis. A palpable spleen may indicate hepatitis or cirrhosis; significant splenomegaly may be a reflection of portal hypertension.

Abdominal auscultation may reveal the presence of a venous hum over dilated collateral veins radiating from the umbilicus, the so-called caput medusae. In advanced cirrhosis this venous hum is virtually diagnostic of significant portal hypertension. A bruit may sometimes be heard over large regenerating nodules in cirrhosis and occasionally over hepatomas and metastatic nodules in the liver. A friction rub may occasionally be heard over hepatomas and metastatic liver nodules.

Serum assays for biochemical markers of liver disease are an integral part of the proper evaluation of liver and biliary tract disease. In general, the serum bilirubin is measured to confirm the presence and severity of jaundice and determine the extent of bilirubin conjugation. Aminotransferase (transaminase) elevations reflect the severity of active hepatocellular damage, while alkaline phosphatase elevations are found with cholestasis and hepatic infiltrates. Serum albumin and the prothrombin time are used as indexes of hepatic synthetic function. These and other tests are reviewed in Chaps. 47 and 249.

The further evaluation of patients with hepatobiliary disease should be individualized depending on the history, physical findings, and initial screening laboratory tests. Hepatocellular disease such as hepatitis is often sufficiently clear so that only serologic tests are needed. Nonetheless in many patients, computed tomography (CT), ultrasound, scintiscans, or liver biopsy may be needed to determine the nature of the liver disease. When hepatic tumors are suspected, CT, ultrasound, or scintiscan may be performed followed by liver biopsy or laparoscopy for a more specific diagnosis. When biliary obstruction is suspected, the first examination is usually an ultrasound study to determine the size of the bile ducts, whether gallstones are present, or whether there is the suggestion of a mass in the head of the pancreas. Frequently more information is needed and thus a cholangiogram, performed through the endoscope or through percutaneous puncture under ultrasound or CT guidance, should be obtained.

CLASSIFICATION OF LIVER DISEASE No single classification of the various types of liver disease is entirely satisfactory because in many instances the etiology and pathogenetic mechanism are obscure. As a consequence, one finds an abundance of labels and names applied to hepatic disorders. Some individuals use the term *hepatitis* to imply viral infection, others simply to connote evidence of hepatic inflammation. The often used words *acute, subacute,* and *chronic* are ambiguous. *Chronicity* should refer to continuing or recurrent disease (i.e., duration). *Activity* should refer to evidence of the presence of perpetuation of liver cell injury; this is most readily identified by serum transaminase elevations and by the degree of hepatocellular necrosis on biopsy.

Because of the difficulties involved in defining the etiology of many types of liver disease, in most instances the process is best defined and described by an examination of the morphologic character of the lesion. Therefore, a *morphologic classification* of liver disease, as outlined in Table 247-1, appears at present more practical than one based on etiology.

REFERENCES

Schiff L, Schiff ER: *Diseases of the Liver,* 6th ed. Philadelphia, Lippincott, 1987
Sherlock S: *Diseases of the Liver and Biliary System,* 8th ed. Oxford, Blackwell, 1989
Wright R et al: *Liver and Biliary Disease,* 2d ed. Philadelphia, Saunders, 1985

TABLE 247-1 Classification of liver disease

I Parenchymal
  A Hepatitis (viral, drug-induced, toxic)
    1 Acute
    2 Chronic (persistent or active)
  B Cirrhosis
    1 Alcoholic (portal, nutritional, Laennec's cirrhosis)
    2 Postnecrotic
    3 Biliary
    4 Hemochromatosis
    5 Rare types (e.g., Wilson's disease, galactosemia, cystic fibrosis of pancreas, alpha₁-antitrypsin deficiency)
  C Infiltrations
    1 Glycogen
    2 Fat (neutral fat, cholesterol, gangliosides, cerebrosides)
    3 Amyloid
    4 Lymphoma, leukemia
    5 Granuloma (e.g., sarcoidosis, tuberculosis, idiopathic)
  D Space-occupying lesions
    1 Hepatoma, metastatic tumor
    2 Abscess (pyogenic, amoebic)
    3 Cysts (polycystic disease, *Echinococcus*)
    4 Gummas
  E Functional disorders associated with jaundice
    1 Gilbert's syndrome
    2 Crigler-Najjar syndrome
    3 Dubin-Johnson and Rotor syndromes
    4 Cholestasis of pregnancy and benign recurrent cholestasis
II Hepatobiliary
  A Extrahepatic biliary obstruction (by stone, stricture, or tumor)
  B Cholangitis
III Vascular
  A Chronic passive congestion and cardiac cirrhosis
  B Hepatic vein thrombosis (Budd-Chiari syndrome)
  C Portal vein thrombosis
  D Pylephlebitis
  E Arteriovenous malformations

---

248 HEPATOBILIARY IMAGING

LAWRENCE S. FRIEDMAN / LAURENCE NEEDLEMAN

Selection of appropriate imaging techniques for the liver and biliary tract in a given patient depends on the particular clinical problem and on an understanding of the uses and limitations of each technique; in many situations, two or more imaging methods may provide complementary and useful information. In determining the optimal studies, communication between the clinician and the radiologist is essential.

PLAIN ABDOMINAL RADIOGRAPHS AND BARIUM STUDIES OF THE GASTROINTESTINAL TRACT Standard plain films of the abdomen provide little diagnostic information about the hepatobiliary system. They may permit a rough estimation of hepatic size and detection of splenic enlargement or gross ascites. Their major value is in demonstrating *calcified lesions,* including gallstones (about 15 percent are radiopaque) and intrahepatic lesions such as echinococcal cysts, calcified granulomas due to previous tuberculosis or histoplasmosis, or, rarely, tumors or vascular lesions. Plain abdominal x-rays may also demonstrate *air in the biliary tract,* as may occur after endoscopic papillotomy or with a biliary-enteric fistula, either surgical or as a result of inflammation or erosion of a stone from the gallbladder into the intestine. Emphysematous cholecystitis is associated with air in the wall of the gallbladder as a result of severe inflammation. Air seen in a branching pattern extending to the periphery of the liver is usually within portal venous branches and associated with serious inflammatory processes in the intestine.

A barium swallow may demonstrate large esophageal varices in patients with portal hypertension, although endoscopy is more sensitive for the detection of varices.

ULTRASONOGRAPHY   Ultrasonography has the advantages of relatively low cost, potential portability, and safety, as ionizing radiation is not required. Ultrasound imaging depends on small differences in the acoustic properties of soft tissue. Short pulses (1 μs) of high-frequency sound (3 to 10 million Hz) are transmitted into the patient; at each interface between tissues of different acoustic properties, a small portion of the energy is reflected back to the transducer, which also acts as a receiver. With *B-mode*, or *gray-scale*, ultrasound scanning, ultrasound reflections are displayed as shades of gray; cross-sectional, transverse, longitudinal, or oblique images of organs can be produced depending on the orientation of the transducer. With *real-time* ultrasonography, scanning is so rapid that a continuously changing ("real time") image is displayed, thus permitting a survey of the abdominal anatomy in a short period of time and demonstration of physiologic tissue movements, such as arterial pulsations. The major limitation of ultrasonography is its inability to penetrate bone or air, including bowel gas, which may limit complete examination of abdominal organs. In general, tissue penetration of ultrasound decreases as resolution increases.

Ultrasonography is the preferred initial method for imaging the gallbladder and biliary tree (Fig. 248-1). It is sensitive and specific (>95 percent) for the detection of *cholelithiasis*, and, unlike oral cholecystography, is not limited by the presence of jaundice or dye allergy in the patient. Ultrasonography is also highly sensitive for detecting a *dilated biliary tract* in patients with cholestasis and may indicate whether the site of obstruction is in the intra- or extrahepatic ducts. The cause of biliary obstruction, such as a mass lesion in the head of the pancreas or porta hepatis, may also be detected by ultrasonography, although the area around the distal common bile duct may be obscured by bowel gas.

FIGURE 248-1   Sonogram showing dilated bile ducts due to pancreatic carcinoma. The diameter of the extrahepatic bile ducts is 1.2 cm measured anterior to the portal vein (between asterisks). The site of maximal dilatation is 2.0 cm in the distal common bile duct (between arrows).

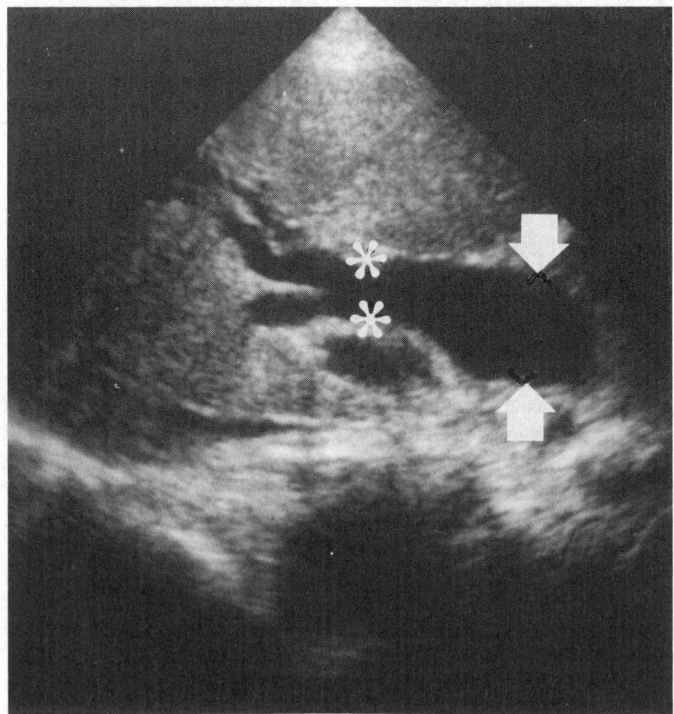

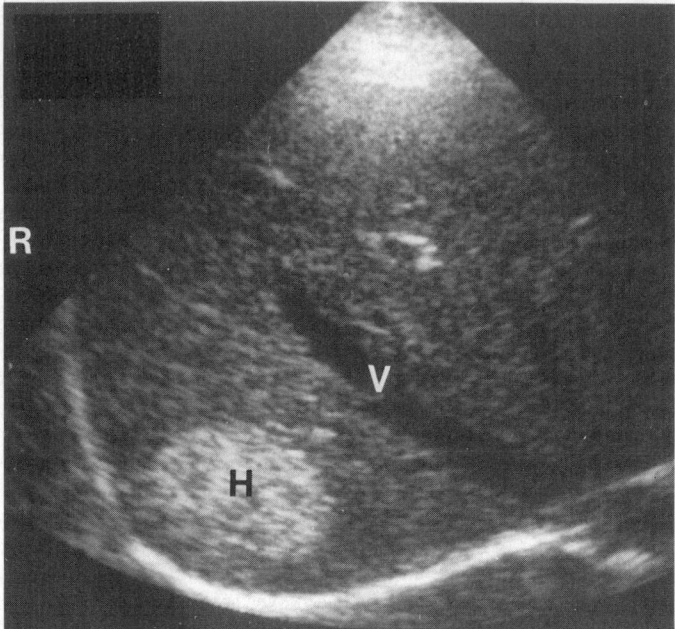

FIGURE 248-2   Sonogram showing an echogenic mass which represents a hemangioma (H) in the posterior right lobe of the liver lateral to the right hepatic vein (V). R = right side of the patient.

Ultrasonography is also a primary screening examination for hepatic disease, which may be suspected because of symptoms, hepatomegaly, abnormal liver function tests, jaundice, or the suspicion of a mass lesion (Fig. 248-2). In general, *focal hepatic lesions* are better visualized than diffuse parenchymal disease such as fatty liver, hepatitis, or cirrhosis. Hepatic masses as small as 1 cm may be detected, and cystic lesions or abscesses can be distinguished from solid lesions, although the nature of a solid hepatic mass (adenoma, hepatocellular carcinoma, metastasis, hemangioma, etc.) may not be identified. Nevertheless, a specific diagnosis may be facilitated by percutaneous "thin"-needle biopsy of hepatic lesions under ultrasound guidance, and insertion of a catheter under ultrasound guidance may permit nonoperative drainage of an abscess. Other uses of ultrasonography include detection of ascites when the physical examination is equivocal, demonstration of portal vein thrombosis in patients with bleeding gastroesophageal varices, and evaluation of patency of portosystemic shunts in patients with recurrent variceal bleeding after shunt surgery. Ultrasonography is usually the first imaging study performed in patients with hepatic dysfunction after liver transplantation to look for a biliary leak or vascular occlusion.

Doppler ultrasonography allows detection of the presence and direction of blood flow based on changes in the frequency of back-scattered ultrasound waves caused by the movement of blood. *Intraoperative ultrasonography* involves the application of the ultrasound transducer to the exposed liver at surgery, thereby increasing the sensitivity of detecting occult hepatic metastases. *Endosonography* involves the attachment of an ultrasound transducer to the tip of an endoscope to permit ultrasonographic imaging from within the bowel lumen, thereby minimizing the obscuring effects of bowel gas. Compared to conventional imaging techniques, endosonography permits more precise determination of the depth of tumor invasion through the bowel wall and improved detection of early pancreatic lesions.

COMPUTED TOMOGRAPHY   Because computed tomographic (CT) scans can detect very small differences in the attenuation of x-rays, structures not visible on conventional radiographs can be identified. With current CT scanning techniques, the radiation dose received by the patient is similar to that of diagnostic procedures such as barium enema. The identification of anatomic structures can be facilitated by the administration of an oral contrast agent to define

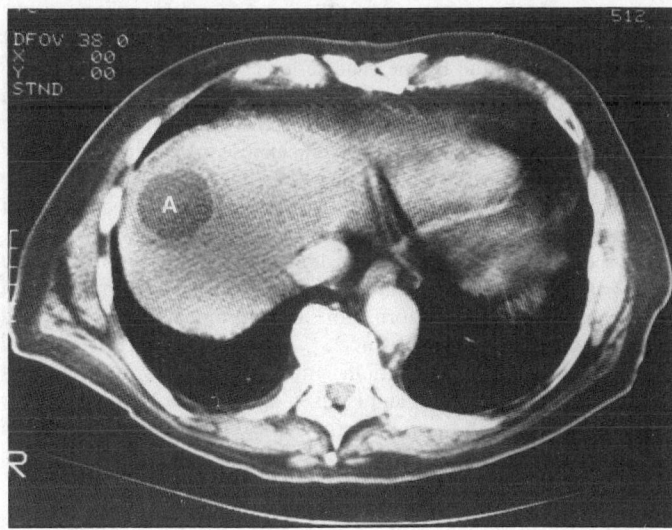

FIGURE 248-3 CT scan with contrast showing a low attenuation mass (*A*) in the dome of the liver, which represents an amebic abscess. R = right side of the patient.

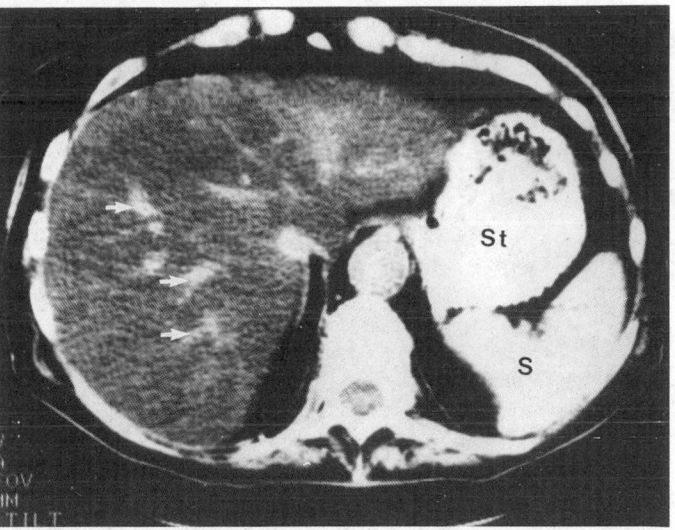

FIGURE 248-4 CT scan showing fatty infiltration of the liver. Note that the attenuation of the liver is lower than that of the spleen (S). The more highly attenuated linear structures of the liver (arrows) are the intrahepatic vessels. St = stomach filled with orally administered barium contrast agent.

the bowel lumen or an intravenous contrast agent to enhance blood vessels and tissues. In general, anatomic definition is more complete with CT scanning than with ultrasonography, and CT scanning has the additional advantage that obesity and intestinal gas do not reduce the quality of the examination. However, a paucity of fat in malnourished patients or children may limit the resolution of the CT image. The disadvantages of CT scanning are radiation exposure and cost. In many instances, CT scanning is reserved for patients in whom ultrasonography is technically difficult or inconclusive.

CT scanning before and after intravenous administration of a contrast agent is an excellent method of evaluating *hepatic masses.* Cystic lesions are readily identified, and abscesses can usually be distinguished from tumors (Fig. 248-3). Masses as small as 1 cm can usually be identified by CT scanning, and, as with ultrasonography, the lesions can be biopsied under CT guidance. Intravenous administration of a contrast agent may result in enhancement of a primary or secondary tumor relative to the surrounding liver, and certain lesions, such as a cavernous hemangioma, may show a pattern of enhancement that is characteristic enough to confirm the diagnosis. Invasion of blood vessels by tumor may also be demonstrated in this way. CT scanning has a more limited role in the evaluation of diffuse liver disease, such as cirrhosis, in which the density of the liver remains in the normal range. However, characteristic CT findings may be associated with *fatty infiltration* of the liver, in which the density of the liver is significantly reduced (Fig. 248-4), and *hemochromatosis,* or *secondary iron overload,* in which the density of the liver is increased, and an estimate of hepatic iron concentration may be made.

Although CT scanning is nearly as accurate as ultrasonography in detecting cholelithiasis or dilated bile ducts, ultrasonography is usually the preferred initial test because of its availability, lack of risk, and lower cost. However, CT scanning is more accurate than ultrasonography in identifying the level and cause of biliary obstruction. CT scanning may be used to define the extent of carcinoma of the gallbladder.

MAGNETIC RESONANCE IMAGING   Magnetic resonance (MR) imaging detects the density of protons in tissue water and lipids and their relaxation times. Since hydrogen nuclei (protons) have an odd number of particles, they behave like magnets when placed in a strong magnetic field. In MR imaging, protons aligned in a magnetic field are subjected to a brief pulse of weak radio waves, the frequency of which (termed the *resonant frequency*) is related mathematically to the externally applied magnetic field. The pulse of radio waves

causes the protons to change their direction of spin and alignment. After the radio wave pulse, the protons return to their original orientation and emit energy with the same radio frequency as that absorbed. Imaging may be accomplished by the detection and analysis of proton density, the T1 relaxation time (a measure of the rate at which the nuclei realign themselves in the magnetic field), or the T2 relaxation time (a measure of the rate at which the emitted radio frequency energy decays). Each method produces a slightly different type of image. The choice of imaging technique depends on the contrast resolution needed for a particular organ. In general, because the magnetic environments of protons in fat, intracellular water, and extracellular water differ, MR imaging provides sharp contrast differentiation of tissues containing varying amounts of water or fat.

In addition to excellent contrast resolution between normal and abnormal tissues, advantages of MR imaging include the lack of ionizing radiation and the ability to image in transverse, longitudinal, coronal, or even oblique planes. Its disadvantages include cost, slow imaging time that results in blurred images due to respiration and peristalsis, and limitations imposed by a strong magnetic field, such as the inability to study patients with pacemakers and other metallic devices.

The range of applications of MR imaging and its role relative to other imaging modalities are under evaluation. MR imaging of *mass lesions* of the liver appears to have greater sensitivity than CT scanning; however, like CT scanning, MR imaging cannot reliably distinguish primary from metastatic tumors (Fig. 248-5). Hepatic abscesses can be detected readily, although on occasion, it may be difficult to distinguish abscesses from tumors with necrotic centers. MR imaging is sensitive in the detection of hemangiomas, which often have an appearance sufficiently characteristic to permit differentiation from hepatic malignancy. Whereas its value in diffuse parenchymal liver disease such as hepatitis or cirrhosis is uncertain, MR imaging can serve as a useful noninvasive method for the diagnosis and monitoring of iron and copper deposition in hemochromatosis, secondary iron overload, or Wilson's disease. Similarly, a modification of MR imaging (*proton spectroscopic imaging*), in which the image of fat is subtracted from the image of water, shows promise in identifying fatty liver and quantifying hepatic fat content. Since rapidly flowing blood is often signal-free on MR imaging, blood vessels can be distinguished without the need for a contrast agent in most cases; thus, MR imaging may be useful in assessing the surgical resectability of vascular tumors.

The gallbladder and bile ducts can be demonstrated by MR

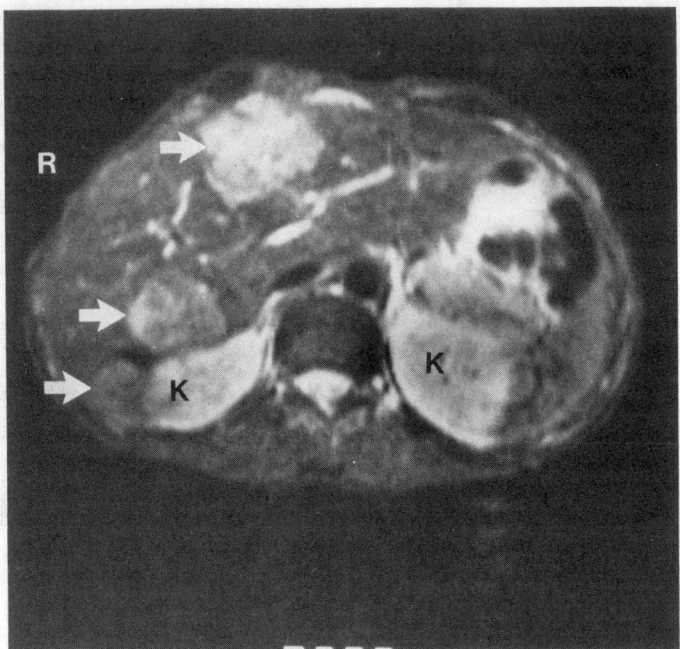

FIGURE 248-5 Magnetic resonance (MR) image of the liver showing three hepatic metastases (arrows) with higher signal than the surrounding liver. R = right side of the patient, K = kidney.

imaging, and cholelithiasis and cholecystitis can be detected; however, MR imaging currently offers no advantages over other imaging techniques. Although gallstones in the common bile duct are not detected by MR imaging, other causes of bile duct obstruction, such as pancreatitis or pancreatic carcinoma, may be identified.

Currently, MR imaging is based on hydrogen, which is the most abundant nucleus in the body and very sensitive to MR. *MR spectroscopy* also permits imaging based on other isotopes, such as phosphorus 31, with the ability to permit study of the metabolic state of normal and diseased organs.

RADIOISOTOPE SCANNING A variety of radioisotopes can be used to study the anatomy and function of the liver and biliary system. After injection into a peripheral vein, the radioisotope is extracted by the liver and excreted in the bile. A scintillation (gamma) camera produces an image by detecting the radiation emitted during the decay of the radioisotope. Depending on the information desired, radioisotopes can be chosen that are taken up by hepatic parenchymal cells, Kupffer cells, or neoplastic and inflammatory cells or that are rapidly excreted in bile. Because radioisotope scanning of the liver seldom provides a precise diagnosis, it has largely been replaced by ultrasonography and CT scanning for first-line imaging. However, radioisotope scanning of the biliary tract is an important tool in the investigation of acute cholecystitis.

Technetium 99m–labeled sulfur colloid scanning The most commonly used radiopharmaceutical for anatomic evaluation of the liver is ^{99m}Tc-labeled sulfur colloid, which is taken up by reticuloendothelial (Kupffer) cells in the liver. Such scanning can be used to assess the size and shape of the liver. Any disease process that results in replacement of Kupffer cells, including *primary and metastatic tumors, cysts,* and *abscesses,* produces a "cold" area in the hepatic scintigram. Lesions greater than 2 to 3 cm in diameter can be reliably detected. The resolution of ^{99m}Tc-sulfur colloid scanning is nearly equivalent to that of ultrasonography, CT scanning, and MR imaging, but it is not as specific as these techniques in determining the nature of the lesion. Because of impaired blood flow and reticuloendothelial function, *diffuse hepatic disease,* such as hepatitis and cirrhosis, may result in decreased or patchy uptake of radiocolloid with preferential uptake by the bone marrow and spleen, particularly when portal hypertension is present. Occasionally, the irregular uptake of radiocolloid in cirrhosis results in the falsely

positive appearance of hepatic filling defects. *Obstruction of the hepatic veins* (Budd-Chiari syndrome) may result in preferential uptake of radiocolloid by the caudate lobe of the liver.

Gold (^{198}Au)- and indium (^{111}In)-labeled colloids are also taken up by Kupffer cells and may be used to image the liver but are more expensive than ^{99m}Tc-sulfur colloid and expose the patient to a greater radiation dose. Newer scintigraphic techniques designed to improve the sensitivity of liver imaging include *single photon emission computed tomography* (SPECT), which permits visualization of the cross-sectional distribution of a radioisotope, and *positron emission tomography* (PET), which utilizes isotopes that decay by positron emission and provides information about regional blood flow and alterations in tissue metabolism.

Gallium scanning ^{67}Gallium citrate accumulates in tissues actively synthesizing protein and is taken up by *tumors and abscesses;* ^{75}selenomethionine has similar properties. On scanning, the lesion appears as an area of increased activity, or "hot spot." Imaging with this agent may be useful in detecting hepatocellular carcinomas, Hodgkin's disease, some non-Hodgkin's lymphomas, and melanomas, although nonspecific uptake of gallium by the liver, bone marrow, and gastrointestinal tract limit the reliability of gallium scanning.

Tagged blood cell scanning Intravenous injection of *autologous white blood cells* labeled with ^{111}In increases the specificity of radioisotope scanning for the detection of hepatic (and abdominal) *abscesses.* Similarly, *autologous red blood cells* or circulating proteins such as albumin or transferrin labeled with ^{111}In or ^{99m}Tc provide a sensitive method of identifying *hemangiomas* that are detected as mass lesions by ultrasonography or CT scanning (Fig. 248-6).

Biliary scanning A variety of radiopharmaceuticals are rapidly cleared by hepatocytes and excreted in the bile, thus permitting scintigraphic evaluation of the biliary tract. The earliest agent used for this purpose was ^{131}I-rose bengal, which, because of its high radiation dose, has been replaced by agents that can be labeled with ^{99m}Tc. The most widely used agents are *N*-substituted iminoacetic acids (HIDA, PIPIDA, DISIDA), which concentrate in the bile even when serum bilirubin levels are elevated. Biliary scanning is used most often in evaluating patients with suspected *acute cholecystitis,* in whom visualization of the gallbladder excludes obstruction of the cystic duct and hence acute cholecystitis (Fig. 248-7). Persistent nonvisualization of the gallbladder over several hours with normal visualization of the liver, bile ducts, and intestine indicates a diagnosis of acute cholecystitis with 95 percent accuracy. False-positive results may occur in patients receiving parenteral nutrition or narcotics and those with hepatitis. Biliary scanning is less accurate in patients with chronic cholecystitis, in whom delayed visualization of the gallbladder is frequent. However, biliary scanning may be useful in identifying

FIGURE 248-6 ^{99m}Tc-labeled autologous red blood cell scan of the hemangioma shown in Fig. 248-2. S = spleen, K = kidney.

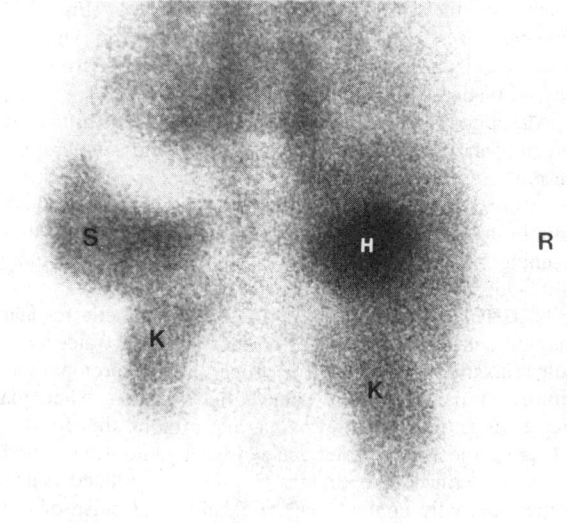

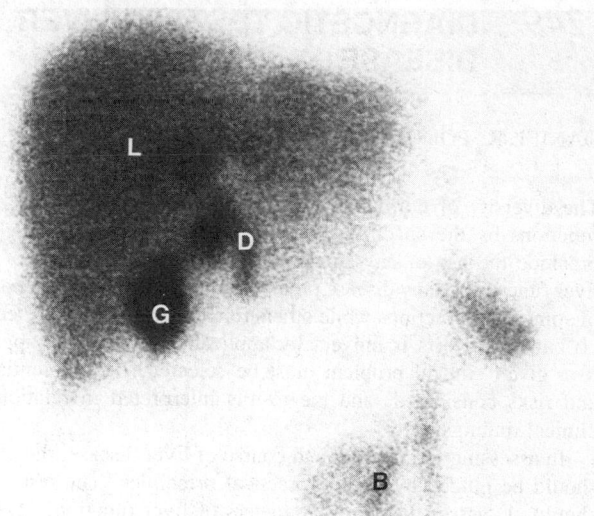
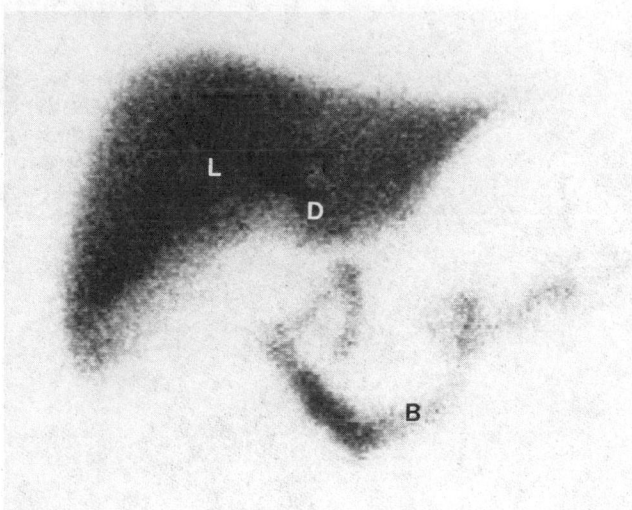

FIGURE 248-7 *A.* Hepatobiliary scan using ⁹⁹ᵐTc-DISIDA in a normal person showing uptake in the liver (L), gallbladder (G), bile ducts (D), and bowel (B) with patency of the cystic duct and biliary system. *B.* Abnormal hepatobiliary scan showing radioisotope in the liver (L), bile ducts (D), and bowel (B) but not in the gallbladder. This is due to an obstructed cystic duct (with a patent common bile duct) due to acute cholecystitis.

cholestasis, acute and chronic biliary obstruction, bile leaks, biliary-enteric fistulas, and *choledochal cysts.*

ORAL CHOLECYSTOGRAPHY Although the use of oral cholecystography declined markedly with the advent of ultrasonography, the recent development of nonsurgical approaches to the treatment of cholelithiasis (e.g., extracorporeal shock wave lithotripsy and oral dissolution therapy with chenodeoxycholic or ursodeoxycholic acid) had led to a resurgence of interest in oral cholecystography. The test is simple and inexpensive. It involves radiographic assessment of gallbladder opacification 14 to 16 h after oral administration of iopanoic acid or 10 to 12 h after oral administration of sodium tyropanoate, both of which are concentrated in the gallbladder after intestinal absorption and hepatic excretion. A second dose of dye may need to be administered to as many as 15 to 25 percent of persons in whom gallbladder opacification is not achieved after a single dose.

Nonvisualization of the gallbladder indicates *gallbladder disease* with nearly 95 percent certainty, whereas normal visualization excludes gallbladder disease with 97 percent certainty. Failure of the gallbladder to opacify may also result from patient noncompliance, intestinal malabsorption, and liver disease; the gallbladder will not visualize when the serum direct bilirubin level is greater than 34 μmol/L (2 mg/dL). Oral cholecystography is as sensitive as ultrasonography in the overall detection of gallbladder disease (stones, polyps, adenomyomatosis, cholesterolosis, cholecystitis), although ultrasonography is more sensitive in detecting stones per se. However, oral cholecystography is more accurate in determining the *number and size of stones* and, unlike ultrasonography, can demonstrate *cystic duct patency,* factors that are important in determining a patient's suitability for nonoperative gallstone therapy.

CHOLANGIOGRAPHY In the past, *intravenous cholangiography,* in which contrast dye is administered as a bolus by peripheral vein, was the principal radiographic technique to visualize the bile ducts. Because of a high rate of serious reactions to the dye, the lack of bile duct visualization when the serum bilirubin level was above 42 μmol/L (2.5 mg/dL), and the development of more effective radiologic techniques to visualize the bile ducts, intravenous cholangiography has become obsolete.

Percutaneous transhepatic cholangiography (THC) This technique involves the direct percutaneous injection, via a "thin" (22-gauge) needle, of contrast dye into bile ducts in the liver under fluoroscopic guidance. When intrahepatic ducts are dilated, the success rate of duct opacification approaches 100 percent, but when the intrahepatic ducts are not dilated, as in primary sclerosing cholangitis,

the success rate is around 90 percent and multiple attempts may be required. Serious complications occur in no more than 3 percent of cases and include hemorrhage, bile peritonitis, and sepsis.

THC may be used to determine the cause of *biliary obstruction* or *cholestasis* and is of particular value in evaluating the potential surgical resectability of proximal cholangiocarcinomas. In addition, biliary biopsies and cytologic brushings may be obtained and strictures may be balloon-dilated via a catheter inserted through the THC tract. In patients with biliary obstruction who are poor operative risks, an external drain may be left in place to permit biliary decompression or an internal stent (endoprosthesis) may be placed to relieve obstruction.

Endoscopic retrograde cholangiopancreatography (ERCP) (See Chap. 236) This technique uses fiberoptic endoscopy to visualize the ampulla of Vater and guide the insertion of a catheter through the ampulla for the selective injection of contrast material into the common bile and pancreatic ducts, which are then imaged radiologically (see Chap. 236). The success rate for cannulation depends on the experience of the endoscopist and can approach 95 percent or more; unlike THC, successful biliary cannulation does not depend on a dilated bile duct. Serious complications may occur in about 5 percent of cases and include pancreatitis and cholangitis.

Using THC, ERCP, or both, the biliary system can be visualized in nearly all patients. ERCP is preferable when the bile ducts are not dilated and when an *ampullary, pancreatic, or distal bile duct lesion* is suspected. In patients with *choledocholithiasis,* ERCP permits sphincterotomy and stone extraction. Additionally, ERCP may permit ampullary biopsy, pancreatic or biliary ductal brushings for cytologic examination, balloon dilation of a stricture, placement of a nasobiliary drain to decompress an obstructed biliary system, and insertion of a stent to relieve biliary obstruction caused by tumors. ERCP can also be used for *manometric measurements of the sphincter of Oddi,* a potentially valuable technique in the diagnosis of papillary stenosis and ampullary spasm.

ANGIOGRAPHY Angiography is required less often now than in the past for evaluating the hepatobiliary system. Nevertheless, newer contrast agents, improved techniques of vascular catheterization, and the development of therapeutic applications make angiography of value in certain situations. Selective cannulation of the hepatic artery or one of its branches may be helpful in distinguishing certain *vascular lesions* of the liver, including hemangiomas, adenomas, focal nodular hyperplasia, hemangioendotheliomas, and hepatocellular carcinomas (Fig. 248-8). Angiography may be particularly valuable in assessing the *surgical resectability* of an isolated hepatic lesion or in identifying

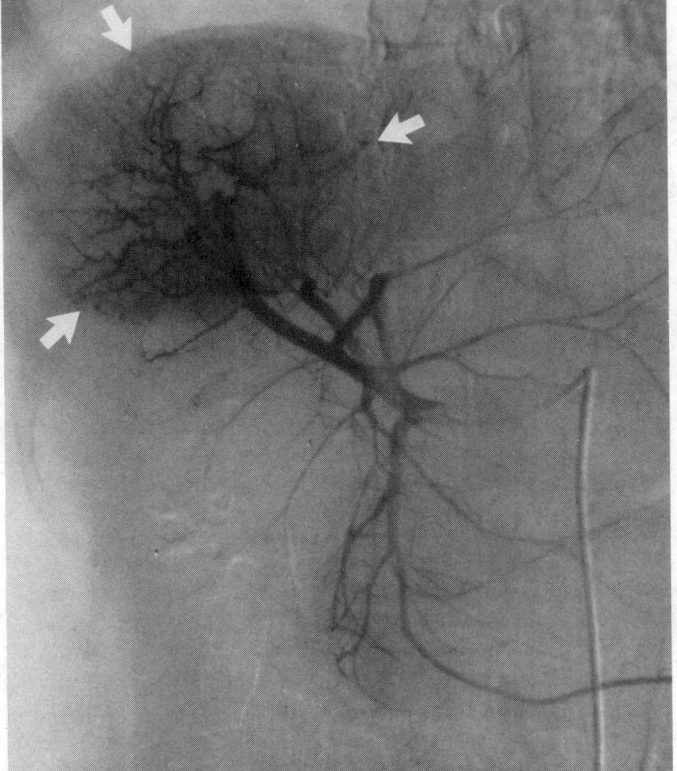

FIGURE 248-8 Arterial phase of a selective hepatic angiogram showing a hepatocellular carcinoma as a hypervascular mass (outlined by arrows) with many irregular and corkscrew-shaped tumor vessels in the right lobe of the liver.

a vascular occlusion after liver transplantation. In planning portosystemic shunt surgery, angiography is the best imaging technique to define portal venous anatomy and assess the patency of the vessels to be used. The portal venous system may be examined on the venous phase of celiac and superior mesenteric arteriography or after direct injection of contrast into the portal venous system via a splenic or transhepatic route. Hepatic venography and hemodynamic measurements, including wedged hepatic venous pressures, can be obtained concurrently (see Chap. 254). Therapeutic applications of angiography include *embolization* of bleeding vessels, arteriovenous fistulas, and certain highly vascular or inoperable tumors.

REFERENCES

COOPERBERG PL, GIBNEY RG: Imaging of the gallbladder, 1987. Radiology 163:605, 1987

COUNCIL ON SCIENTIFIC AFFAIRS, AMERICAN MEDICAL ASSOCIATION: Magnetic resonance imaging of the abdomen and pelvis. JAMA 261:420, 1989

FERRUCCI JT et al: Advances in hepatobiliary radiology. Radiology 168:3198, 1988

MARTON KI, DOUBILET P: How to image the gallbladder in suspected cholecystitis. Ann Intern Med 109:722, 1988

ROTHSCHILD MA, ORATZ M: Hepatic imaging. Semin Liv Dis 9:1, 1989

SHERLOCK S: *Diseases of the Liver and Biliary System*, 8th ed. Oxford, Blackwell, 1989

TAYLOR KJW et al: Noninvasive imaging of the hepatobiliary system, in *Diseases of the Liver*, 6th ed, L Schiff, ER Schiff (eds). Philadelphia, Lippincott, 1987, pp 261–309

WRIGHT R et al: *Liver and Biliary Disease: Pathophysiology, Diagnosis, Management*, 2d ed. London, Saunders, 1985

249   DIAGNOSTIC TESTS IN LIVER DISEASE

DANIEL K. PODOLSKY / KURT J. ISSELBACHER

The diversity of normal liver functions and the disruption of these functions by the spectrum of disorders which may affect the liver preclude the use of any single test as a reliable measure of overall liver function. Many disease processes may lead to severe impairment of some liver functions while others remain entirely unaffected. Since no battery of tests is universally applicable, those most appropriate to a given clinical problem must be selected, their potential value and risks considered, and the results interpreted in relation to the clinical findings.

In assessing the severity and course of liver disease, the physician should be guided by several practical principles. The tests selected should (1) assess different parameters of liver function, (2) be used *serially* in order to evaluate the evolution or course of the disease, and (3) be interpreted within the total clinical context, with recognition that any single laboratory test may be fallible.

BLOOD TESTS OF LIVER FUNCTION (See Table 249-1)

BILIRUBIN   Bilirubin metabolism and its assessment are discussed in detail in Chaps. 47 and 251. Spectrophotometric determinations of serum bilirubin in the clinical laboratory measure two pigment fractions: (1) the water-soluble conjugated fraction that gives a *direct reaction* with the diazo reagent and consists largely of conjugated bilirubin (as the mono- and diglucuronide), and (2) the lipid-soluble *indirect-reaction* fraction (total minus direct) that represents primarily unconjugated bilirubin. The serum of normal adults (when measured by the van den Bergh reaction) contains less than 4.2 µmol/L (0.25 mg/dL) direct-reacting bilirubin and 17 µmol/L (1 mg/dL) or less of total bilirubin. Studies with high-performance liquid chromatography (HPLC) suggest that even these levels may be artifactually high in normal persons (see Chap. 47).

Conjugated hyperbilirubinemia with elevated direct- and indirect-reacting material indicates impairment of secretion into the bile, while unconjugated hyperbilirubinemia reflects impaired conjugation. The latter is found in a limited number of processes including such nonhepatic conditions as hemolytic anemia and ineffective erythropoiesis (increased pigment load) and a few hepatic disorders, principally Gilbert's syndrome or the relatively rare Crigler-Najjar syndrome. Although measurement of both the direct and total serum bilirubin will determine whether the patient has predominantly unconjugated or conjugated hyperbilirubinemia, this distinction is of limited usefulness since the majority of hepatobiliary disorders lead to conjugated hyperbilirubinemia. In most instances, fractionation of serum bilirubin does not distinguish cholestasis due to parenchymal disease from that arising from biliary tract processes.

TABLE 249-1   Abnormalities shown by tests of liver function

Test	Type of liver disease	
	Obstructive	Parenchymal
AST and ALT (SGOT and SGPT)	↑	↑ – ↑↑↑
Alkaline phosphatase	↑↑↑	↑
Albumin	N	↓ – ↓↓↓
Prothrombin time	N– ↑ *	↑ – ↑↑↑
Bilirubin	N– ↑↑↑	N– ↑↑↑
γ-Glutamyl transpeptidase (GGT)	↑↑↑	N– ↑↑↑
5′-Nucleotidase	↑ – ↑↑↑	N– ↑

* Correctable with parenteral vitamin K if elevated.
NOTE: N, normal; ↑, elevated; ↓, decreased.

Bilirubin appears in the urine only after it is converted to a water-soluble form; generally this involves conjugation with polar glucuronide groups which enhance water solubility. Rapid assessment of bilirubinuria is possible using commercially available dipsticks and may be helpful as an initial screening measure. Bilirubinuria occurs with even minimal degrees of jaundice and may be detected before jaundice is evident. Its usefulness is otherwise quite limited. Urobilinogen, a product of luminal bacterial metabolism of bilirubin, is reabsorbed from the bowel and secreted in the urine. Complete bile duct obstruction blocks excretion of bilirubin into the gut and results in disappearance of urobilinogen from the urine. Assessment of urobilinogen in a freshly collected 2-h urine specimen by the Watson method (normal values 0.2 to 1.2 units) may distinguish biliary tract obstruction from parenchymal dysfunction, but this test has been largely superseded by newer methods.

SERUM ENZYME ASSAYS A number of serum enzymes have been used to distinguish and assess hepatocellular injury and biliary tract dysfunction or obstruction. All have inherent limitations in sensitivity and specificity, and none truly distinguish these processes definitively. Elevations in enzyme activities may also be seen in association with nonhepatic disorders. Nevertheless, with proper and careful interpretation, a number of serum enzymes provide important clinical tools.

Aminotransferases (transaminases) Assays of many serum enzymes have been proposed as indicators of hepatocellular damage. Of these, aspartate aminotransferase (AST,SGOT) and alanine aminotransferase (ALT,SGPT) activities have proven most useful. These enzymes catalyze the transfer of the γ-amino groups of aspartate and alanine, respectively, to the γ-keto group of ketoglutarate, leading to the formation of oxaloacetic acid and pyruvic acid. In contrast to ALT, which is found primarily in the liver, AST is present in many tissues including heart, skeletal muscle, kidney, and brain and is thus somewhat less specific as an indicator of liver function. The source of serum AST and ALT in the normal person [less than 0.58 µkat/L (35 U/L)] is unclear, and the mechanism responsible for clearance of these enzymes is uncertain. In the hepatocyte, ALT is found exclusively in the cytosol, while different isoenzymes of AST exist in mitochondria and the cytosol. Although elevated serum levels of AST or ALT may be observed in a variety of nonhepatic diseases, notably in myocardial infarction and skeletal muscle disorders, these disorders can usually be clinically distinguished from liver disease. Conversely, uremia may lead to spuriously low aminotransferase values.

Serum AST and ALT are elevated to some extent in nearly all liver disorders. Highest levels are found in association with conditions causing extensive hepatic necrosis, such as severe viral hepatitis, toxin-induced liver injury, or prolonged circulatory collapse. Lesser elevations are encountered in mild acute viral hepatitis as well as in both diffuse and focal chronic liver diseases (e.g., chronic active hepatitis, cirrhosis, and hepatic metastases). However, the absolute levels of aminotransferases correlate poorly with severity of liver injury or prognosis, and serial determinations are usually most helpful. Thus in the patient with massive hepatic necrosis, there may be marked elevations in the early phase (i.e., 24 to 48 h), but by the time the patient is tested 3 to 5 days later the levels may be in the range of 3.34 to 5.8 µkat/L (200 to 350 U/L). It is noteworthy that in severe alcoholic hepatitis one commonly finds only modest increases in these enzymes (generally less than 5.0 µkat/L). Minimal elevations of AST and ALT (less than 1.67 µkat/L) may also be found in association with biliary tract obstruction; higher levels suggest the development of cholangitis with resultant hepatic cell necrosis.

In general AST and ALT levels parallel each other, with one exception. In alcoholic hepatitis the AST/ALT ratio may be greater than 2; this appears to result from a reduction in hepatic ALT content due to a deficiency in the cofactor pyridoxine-5-phosphate.

Alkaline phosphatase Human serum contains several forms of alkaline phosphatase, a plasma membrane–derived enzyme of uncertain physiologic function which hydrolyzes synthetic phosphate esters

at pH 9. These activities arise from bone, intestine, liver, and placenta. A number of different assays have been developed which utilize different substrates.

In the absence of bone disease or pregnancy, elevated levels of alkaline phosphatase activity usually reflect impaired biliary tract function. The increased levels reflect increased synthesis of the enzyme by hepatocytes and biliary tract epithelium rather than regurgitation of enzyme due to obstruction. Bile acids may play a role both by inducing synthesis and by promoting solubilization of the membrane-associated enzyme activity.

Slight to moderate increases in alkaline phosphatase (1 to 2 times normal) occur in many patients with parenchymal liver disorders such as hepatitis and cirrhosis; transient increases may occur in all types of liver disease. However, the most striking increases in alkaline phosphatase (3 to 10 times normal) occur with extrahepatic biliary tract (mechanical) obstruction or with intrahepatic (functional) cholestasis, as in drug-induced cholestasis or primary biliary cirrhosis. Conversely, it is unusual for the serum alkaline phosphatase to remain normal when there is obstructive jaundice, and a normal enzyme level argues strongly against the presence of cholestasis. The alkaline phosphatase is usually mildly elevated in metastatic or infiltrative liver disease (e.g., leukemia, lymphoma, and sarcoid). The enzyme may be elevated in the presence of incomplete biliary obstruction or when there is obstruction of only one hepatic duct, conditions in which the serum bilirubin is often normal or only slightly elevated. Serum alkaline phosphatase is also elevated in nonhepatic disorders, most notably in some bone disorders (e.g., Paget's disease, osteomalacia, and metastases to bone) and sometimes with malignancy. Occasionally tumors produce an alkaline phosphatase which is identical or similar to the placental form, the so-called Regan isoenzyme.

Although one can usually make a reasonable assessment as to whether an elevation of the alkaline phosphatase is of hepatic or nonhepatic origin, several methods can distinguish the different isoenzymes facilitating resolution of any uncertainty. In contrast to that derived from bone, the hepatic isozyme is stable to treatment with heat (56°C for 15 min) or urea. These enzymes can also be separated by electrophoresis, but this is usually impractical. Parallel determination of serum 5'-nucleotidase activity is also helpful; an increase of both 5'-nucleotidase and alkaline phosphatase is consistent with an hepatobiliary source of the enzyme elevation. Even after correction for age and sex (higher levels being found in the young and in older women), isolated elevations in alkaline phosphatase may occasionally be encountered in adults with no apparent disease.

5'-Nucleotidase, leucine aminopeptidase, and γ-glutamyltranspeptidase 5'-Nucleotidase catalyzes the hydrolysis of phosphate from the 5' position of the pentose component of the nucleotide. Although tissue distribution is widespread, elevations are generally associated with hepatobiliary disease. The principal value of the 5'-nucleotidase measurement is to confirm the hepatic origin of an elevated alkaline phosphatase level in children, pregnant women, or in those settings where coincident bone disease may be present. However, 5'-nucleotidase levels do not always parallel alkaline phosphatase in liver disease, and lack of elevation does not exclude an hepatic source of elevated serum alkaline phosphatase.

Despite a widespread tissue distribution, *leucine aminopeptidase,* a protease which cleaves amino-terminal amino acids from peptides, is significantly elevated only in diseases of the pancreas and hepatobiliary system. There is considerable overlap in values of the peptidase levels found in patients with hepatocellular disease and in those with cholestatic jaundice; thus, in general, its measurement is of little clinical value.

γ-Glutamyltranspeptidase GGT catalyzes the transfer of the γ-glutamyl group from peptides such as glutathione to other amino acids and may play a role in amino acid transport. It is found throughout the hepatobiliary system as well as in other tissues. In liver disease, GGT correlates with alkaline phosphatase levels and is the most sensitive indicator of biliary tract disease. However, elevations of GGT are nonspecific and may be associated with pancreatic, cardiac, renal, and pulmonary disorders as well as with diabetes and alcoholism. This enzyme may be increased by agents which induce microsomal enzymes, and it has been suggested as a potential marker of alcoholism. However, overall lack of specificity has limited its clinical usefulness.

Other enzymes Measurement of total serum lactic dehydrogenase (LDH) or its isoenzymes is usually not helpful in diagnosis of liver disease because of this enzyme's nearly ubiquitous body distribution. Moderate LDH elevations are common in acute viral hepatitis, cirrhosis, and metastatic carcinoma to the liver. Biliary tract disease may also produce slight elevations. Numerous other dehydrogenases (e.g., isocitrate dehydrogenase, sorbitol dehydrogenase, and glutamate dehydrogenase) have been used or proposed as markers of liver disease, but none appear to offer significant diagnostic improvement over standard aminotransferase determinations. Elevation of serum ornithine carbamyl transferase (OCT), a urea cycle enzyme present only in liver and intestine, occurs primarily in liver disease, but its lack of association with any specific type of liver disease has limited its diagnostic usefulness also.

SERUM PROTEINS Extensive liver injury may lead to *decreased* blood levels of albumin, prothrombin, fibrinogen, and other proteins synthesized exclusively by hepatocytes. In contrast to measurements of serum enzymes, serum protein levels reflect liver synthetic function rather than just cell injury. Three important caveats should be remembered regarding interpretation of serum protein levels: (1) they are neither early nor sensitive indicators of liver disease (because of the extent of hepatic reserve and their half-life, see below), (2) they are of little value in the differential diagnosis of liver disease, and (3) decreases in their serum levels are not specific for liver disease.

Albumin and globulin Albumin is quantitatively the most important serum protein synthesized by the liver; the normal serum value ranges from 35 to 55 g/L (see Chap. 250). Albumin has a fairly long half-life (14 to 20 days) with less than 5 percent turnover daily; it is therefore not a good indicator of acute or mild liver injury. Furthermore, there is a substantial reserve of hepatic albumin synthesis; thus, adequate synthesis may continue until there is extensive hepatocellular injury. Serum levels are influenced by a variety of nonhepatic factors, most notably nutritional status, hormonal factors, and plasma oncotic pressure. Routes of degradation in health remain undefined, but nonhepatic conditions may lead to depressed serum albumin levels mainly due to excessive loss despite adequate synthetic function (e.g., nephrotic syndrome or protein-losing enteropathy). Nonetheless, reduction in the serum albumin levels provides an excellent indication of the severity of chronic liver disease. In the patient with ascites, an increased volume of distribution as well as an absolute reduction in protein synthesis may contribute to hypoalbuminemia.

Serum globulins are a heterogeneous group of proteins whose production in a variety of tissues is influenced by a number of factors. Serum globulins (normal: 20 to 35 g/L) include alpha and beta globulins as well as serum immunoglobulins, the latter largely accounting for the gamma fraction. Serum globulins are often diffusely elevated in association with chronic liver disease and in other nonhepatic disorders. In cirrhosis varying degrees of hyperglobulinemia may occur; this may reflect increased stimulation of the peripheral reticuloendothelial compartment due to shunting of antigens past the liver and impaired clearance by hepatic Kupffer cells. Although some have suggested that elevations in different globulin fractions as assessed by electrophoretic or other means may have a differential diagnostic value, this remains a largely unfulfilled promise. Similarly, the albumin/globulin ratio has no physiologic significance.

Clotting factors The liver synthesizes six coagulation factors: fibrinogen (factor I), prothrombin (factor II), and factors V, VII, IX, and X. With the exception of factor V, production of functional proteins requires the presence of the cofactor, vitamin K. Because most of these factors are normally present in excess, impaired coagulation is usually seen only in severe liver disease. Abnormalities

of these factors can be most efficiently determined by the one-stage *prothrombin time*, which measures the rate of prothrombin conversion to thrombin in the presence of thromboplastin and calcium and requires the integrity of most of the vitamin K–dependent clotting factors (see Chap. 62). Factor VII is the rate-limiting factor in this pathway and thus has the greatest influence on the prothrombin levels. The prothrombin time is dependent on normal hepatic synthesis of clotting factors and sufficient intestinal uptake of vitamin K. Absorption of this fat-soluble vitamin itself requires adequate dietary intake and normal function of intestinal mucosa and biliary secretion. Severe acute or chronic parenchymal liver injury may lead to prolongation of the prothrombin time due to impaired synthesis of the clotting proteins. Because these proteins have a shorter half-life than that of albumin, the prothrombin time may be an earlier indicator than serum albumin of severe liver injury. In both acute and chronic hepatocellular injury, an increase in the prothrombin time serves as an ominous prognostic sign. Because it is a fat-soluble vitamin, prolongation of the prothrombin time may result from vitamin K malabsorption which may occur with cholestasis due to biliary tract disease or due to fat malabsorption (steatorrhea) of any cause (e.g., pancreatic insufficiency). Poor dietary intake, antibiotic therapy, or use of warfarin-type anticoagulants are additional causes of a prolonged prothrombin time, owing to deficiencies of active vitamin K. These processes can be distinguished from hepatic synthetic failure by demonstrating normalization of the prothrombin time (within 24 to 48 h) after parenteral injections of vitamin K. The *partial thromboplastin time*, which reflects the activities of fibrinogen, prothrombin, and factors V, VIII, IX, X, XI, and XII, may also be prolonged in severe liver disease. Clotting functions should be assessed in all patients with liver disease prior to any surgical procedure, including liver biopsy (see Chaps. 62 and 288).

BLOOD AMMONIA Ammonia is elevated in the blood of some patients with either acute or chronic liver disease. Although influenced by a number of factors (summarized in Chap. 250), elevations in blood ammonia reflect disruption of the pathways of urea synthesis by which the liver detoxifies amine groups. A markedly elevated blood ammonia usually reflects severe hepatocellular necrosis. Cirrhotic patients, especially those with endogenous or surgically created portal-systemic shunting, often have varying degrees of hyperammonemia and hepatic encephalopathy. However, there is only a rough correlation between blood ammonia levels and the degree of hepatic encephalopathy; some patients will function normally with a twofold elevation, while others will be stuporous at the same concentration. Ammonia levels may increase before the onset of coma; similarly, they may return to normal some 48 to 72 h before improvement of the neurologic status.

SERUM LIPIDS AND LIPOPROTEINS AND BILE ACIDS Abnormalities in serum lipids and lipoproteins are sensitive but nonspecific indicators of liver diseases. Acute parenchymal liver disease is commonly associated with increased plasma triglycerides, decreased cholesterol esters, and abnormal lipoproteins. The absence of alpha and prebeta bands with a concomitant increase in the beta fraction is typical of acute viral hepatitis. Less marked but more persistent abnormalities are found in patients with chronic parenchymal disease reflecting deficiencies in lecithin:cholesterol acyltransferase (LCAT) and hepatic triglyceride lipase. Either intra- or extrahepatic cholestasis may lead to an increase in unesterified cholesterol and in serum phospholipids. Lipoprotein X, a distinctive lipoprotein encountered in cholestasis, consists of equimolar amounts of unesterified cholesterol and lecithin which is regurgitated from the biliary tract. Although characteristically seen in patients with extrahepatic biliary obstruction, lipoprotein X may be found in any cholestatic condition.

Removal of bile acids from portal blood is impaired in liver disease because of parenchymal damage and portal-systemic shunts; there may also be reentry of bile acids into blood from injured hepatocytes or an obstructed biliary tract. Although there are a variety of techniques for measuring serum bile acids, these determinations are not yet of proven value for routine clinical use.

IMMUNOLOGIC AND OTHER TESTS

A number of immunologic derangements may be seen in liver disease. Antimitochondrial antibodies are found in 85 to 90 percent of patients with primary biliary cirrhosis. In this test, serum is incubated with rabbit hepatocytes. The presence of antimitochondrial antibodies can then be assessed after subsequent staining with a fluorescein-tagged second antibody. However, this marker is not entirely specific and is occasionally found in patients with chronic active hepatitis and drug-induced hepatitis. Its primary value is in helping to distinguish primary biliary cirrhosis from extrahepatic biliary obstruction. In chronic active hepatitis the *lupus erythematosus–cell test* (LE-cell test) may be positive, and *antinuclear antibodies* as well as *anti-smooth-muscle antibodies* may be present (see Chap. 269). Alpha fetoprotein is of value in the diagnosis of hepatocellular carcinoma (see Chap. 255). Measurements of serum alpha$_1$-antitrypsin and ceruloplasmin should be performed in infants with cirrhosis or hepatitis since they may reflect alpha$_1$-antitrypsin deficiency or Wilson's disease, respectively (see Chaps 256 and 330).

OTHER DIAGNOSTIC PROCEDURES

PERCUTANEOUS NEEDLE BIOPSY OF THE LIVER Percutaneous needle biopsy is a safe, simple, and valuable method for the diagnostic evaluation of liver disease. *Diffuse parenchymal disorders* such as cirrhosis, hepatitis, and drug reactions may be diagnosed with remarkable accuracy. In *disseminated focal diseases* (such as granulomas or tumor infiltrates) serial sections may demonstrate characteristic lesions.

Biopsy is performed under local anesthesia, usually with the Menghini (aspiration), Klatskin, or Vim-Silverman (cutting) needle, by either a transpleural or subcostal approach. If the operator is skillful and patients carefully selected, morbidity should be quite low and limited to occasional postbiopsy pain or vasovagal reactions.

Some of the most frequent indications for needle biopsy are (1) unexplained hepatomegaly or hepatosplenomegaly; (2) cholestasis of uncertain cause; (3) persistently abnormal liver function tests; (4) suspected systemic or infiltrative diseases such as sarcoidosis, miliary tuberculosis, or fever of unknown origin; and (5) suspected primary or metastatic liver tumor. Percutaneous liver biopsy may be performed either for diagnostic purposes or to evaluate the extent and severity of a known disease process. However, other new and improved noninvasive diagnostic methods have obviated the need for biopsy in many circumstances, and thus biopsy should be performed only when information from these other techniques is inadequate.

Needle biopsy should not be performed if (1) the patient is unable to cooperate; (2) clinical or laboratory evidence indicates impaired hemostasis (prothrombin time prolonged by 3 s or more over control, thrombocytopenia less than 80 to 100 $\times$ 10^9 platelets per liter, or partial thromboplastin time or bleeding time prolonged); (3) there is infection of the right pleural space or septic cholangitis; (4) tense ascites is present, with risk of continued leakage of ascitic fluid; (5) compatible blood is not available for transfusion in case of hemorrhage; or (6) high-grade biliary obstruction is suspected and there is an increased risk of bile peritonitis. With the increasing use of CT scan and ultrasonography, it is possible to perform "directed" aspiration biopsies of isolated lesions with very thin needles. Aspirated material can be used for cytology (tumors) and culture (abscesses) but is often inadequate for assessment of liver architecture.

LAPAROSCOPY AND LAPAROTOMY (PERITONEOSCOPY) See Chap. 236.

REFERENCES

BRENSILVER HL, KAPLAN MM: Significance of elevated liver alkaline phosphatase in serum. Gastroenterology 68:1556, 1975
FERRUCCI JT JR et al (eds): *Interventional Radiology of the Abdomen*, 2d ed. Baltimore, Williams and Wilkins, 1985

KEMENY MM et al: A projected analysis of laboratory tests and imaging studies to detect hepatitic lesions. Ann Surg 195:163, 1982
MOSS, AA et al Hepatic tumors: Magnetic resonance and CT appearance. Radiology 150:191, 1984
ROTHSCHILD MA et al: Serum albumin. Hepatology 8:385, 1988
SABESIN SM: Cholestatic lipoproteins—Their pathogenesis and significance. Gastroenterology 83:704, 1982

250   DERANGEMENTS OF HEPATIC METABOLISM

DANIEL K. PODOLSKY / KURT J. ISSELBACHER

The liver plays a central role in the maintenance of metabolic homeostasis. It is therefore not surprising that the development of clinically important liver disease is accompanied by diverse systemic manifestations of disordered metabolism. The liver has considerable reserve capacity, so minimal or even moderate cell injury may not be reflected by measurable changes in its metabolic function. However, some functions of the liver are more sensitive than others, and a variety of defects may be seen, depending on the nature and extent of the initial insult.

The biochemical functions in which the liver plays a major role include (1) the intermediate metabolism of amino acids and carbohydrates, (2) synthesis and degradation of proteins and glycoproteins, (3) metabolism and degradation of drugs and hormones, and (4) regulation of lipid and cholesterol metabolism. The derangements of these functions are discussed in connection with their occurrence in various forms of parenchymal liver disease. Alterations of bilirubin, bile salt, and porphyrin metabolism are discussed elsewhere (Chaps. 46, 240, 328).

Metabolic derangements are most evident in the patient with advanced liver disease, and the manifestations are similar regardless of the initial etiologic insult. To a varying degree similar abnormalities are observed in patients with severe chronic hepatitis, micronodular cirrhosis, and postnecrotic cirrhosis. Since the many functions of the liver may be affected to varying degrees in individual patients, no single test effectively measures the overall state of liver function. The proper interpretation of liver function tests is discussed in Chap. 249.

CARBOHYDRATE METABOLISM The liver functions to maintain normal levels of blood sugar by a combination of glycogenesis, glycogenolysis, glycolysis, and gluconeogenesis. These pathways are regulated by a number of hormones including insulin, glucagon, growth hormone, and certain catecholamines. Although it has been presumed that exquisite sensitivity of the hepatocytes to insulin is responsible for the uptake of an oral glucose load by the liver, there are also data that have challenged the importance of insulin-mediated glucose uptake by the hepatocyte. In the fasting state, the liver contributes to glucose homeostasis by glycogenolysis and gluconeogenesis in response to hypoinsulinemia and hyperglucagonemia. Maintenance of normal blood glucose levels through gluconeogenesis is ultimately related to catabolism of muscle protein, which provides the necessary amino acid precursors, especially alanine. In a complementary fashion, in the postprandial state, the liver directs alanine and branched-chain amino acids to the peripheral tissues, where they are then incorporated into muscle protein. These reciprocal pathways form a glucose-alanine shuttle which is modulated by ambient changes in the hormones mentioned above (Fig. 250-1). While it has been presumed that synthesis of glycogen and fatty acid in the postprandial state arises from direct conversion of glucose, there are data to suggest that, in fact, these pathways are *indirect* with products deriving from 3-carbon metabolites of glucose or other gluconeogenic compounds such as lactate, fructose, and alanine.

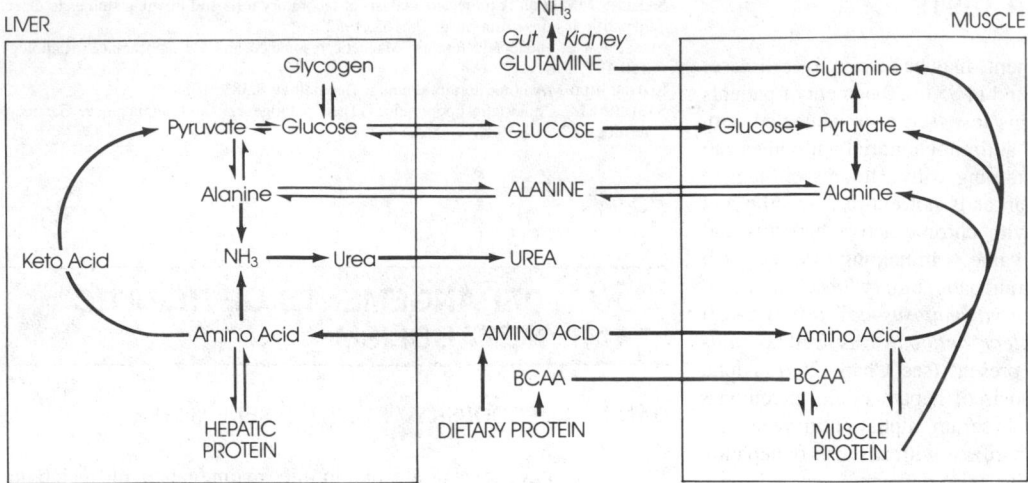

FIGURE 250-1 Carbohydrate-protein exchange between muscle and liver. After an overnight fast there is net release of amino acids by muscle (predominantly alanine and glutamine). These are derived from transamination of pyruvate, degraded amino acids, and glucose. Branched-chain amino acids (BCAA) are particularly important as a source of nitrogen for alanine synthesis. Alanine is utilized for gluconeogenesis by the liver, and urea is formed as a by-product. The main sites of glutamine uptake are the kidney and gut, where it is used for ammonia production and as a possible source of energy, respectively. Following ingestion of dietary protein, skeletal muscle goes into an anabolic phase; there is selective hepatic escape and muscle uptake of dietary BCAA, reduced muscle output of alanine and glutamine, and a reduced rate of hepatic gluconeogenesis. Hepatic tissue protein also goes into an anabolic phase following protein ingestion. (*Modified with permission from AS Tavill in Wright et al.*)

Abnormalities of glucose homeostasis are common in cirrhosis (Table 250-1). Most frequently hyperglycemia and glucose intolerance are observed. Glucose intolerance is associated with normal or increased levels of plasma insulin (except in patients with hemochromatosis), suggesting that insulin resistance rather than insulin deficiency may be responsible. One of the factors that may play a role in the apparent insulin resistance is an absolute decrease in the liver's ability to metabolize a glucose load because of a decrease in functioning hepatocellular mass. There is also evidence that response to insulin is diminished due to both receptor and postreceptor defects in hepatocytes of patients with cirrhosis. In addition, both hyperinsulinemia and hyperglucagonemia may be present due to decreased hepatic clearance of this hormone resulting from portal-systemic shunting. In patients with hemochromatosis, insulin levels, however, may indeed be low due to pancreatic iron deposition and sometimes concomitant genetic diabetes mellitus. Patients with cirrhosis may also have elevated serum lactate levels reflecting the decreased capacity of the liver to utilize lactate for gluconeogenesis.

Hypoglycemia, although more common in acute fulminant hepatitis, may also be seen with end-stage cirrhosis. Glycogen in the liver accounts for 5 to 7 percent of the normal tissue weight. Because the capacity of the liver to store glycogen is limited (approximately 70 g) and glucose consumption continues at a constant rate (approximately 150 g per day), hepatic glycogen stores are depleted after 1 day of fasting. Hypoglycemia in end-stage cirrhosis may be due to decreased hepatic glycogen stores, diminished glucagon responsiveness, or decreased capacity to synthesize glycogen due to extensive parenchymal destruction.

AMINO ACID AND AMMONIA METABOLISM Through a variety of anabolic and catabolic processes, the liver is the major site of amino acid interconversion. Amino acids utilized for hepatic protein synthesis are derived from dietary protein, metabolic turnover of endogenous protein (primarily from muscle), and direct synthesis in the liver. Most of the amino acids entering the liver via the portal vein are catabolized to urea (except for the branched-chain amino acids leucine, isoleucine, and valine). A lesser amount is released into the general circulation as free amino acids, and these may play an important role in the glucose-alanine cycle mentioned above. In addition, amino acids are utilized for the synthesis of liver intracellular proteins, plasma proteins, and special compounds such as glutathione, glutamine, taurine, carnosine, and creatine. Disruption of normal amino acid metabolism may be reflected in altered plasma amino acid concentrations. In general, levels of aromatic amino acids normally metabolized by the liver (as well as methionine) are elevated, while those of the branched-chain amino acids, largely utilized by skeletal muscle, tend to be normal or depressed. It has been suggested that an alteration in the ratio of these two types of amino acids plays a role in the development of hepatic encephalopathy (see below), but there is not agreement on this concept.

Hepatic catabolism or degradation of amino acids involves two major reactions: transamination and oxidative deamination. In transamination an amino group of an amino acid is transferred to a keto acid. This process is catalyzed by aminotransferases which are found in very high amounts in liver but are also present in other tissues, such as kidney, muscle, heart, lung, and brain. Glutamic-oxaloacetic acid transaminase (aspartate aminotransferase, AST) has been studied most extensively, and increased levels are found in the serum secondary to various types of liver injury (e.g., acute viral and drug-induced hepatitis). As a result of transamination, amino acids can enter the citric acid cycle and then function in the intermediary metabolism of carbohydrates and lipids. Most of the nonessential amino acids are also synthesized in the liver by transamination. Oxidative deamination, which results in conversion of amino acids to keto acids (and ammonia), is catalyzed by L-amino-acid oxidase with two exceptions: glycine oxidation is catalyzed by glycine oxidase, and glutamic oxidation is catalyzed by glutamic dehydrogenase. With severe liver damage (e.g., massive hepatic necrosis), utilization of

TABLE 250-1 Alteration of glucose metabolism in cirrhosis

Factors leading to hyperglycemia:
  Decreased hepatic glucose uptake
  Decreased hepatic glycogen synthesis
  Hepatic resistance to insulin
  Portal-systemic glucose shunting
  Peripheral insulin resistance
  Hormonal abnormalities (serum)
    ↑ Glucagon
    ↓ Cortisol
    ↑ Insulin (↓ in hemochromatosis)
Factors leading to hypoglycemia:
  Decreased gluconeogenesis
  Decreased hepatic glycogen content
  Hepatic resistance to glucagon
  Poor oral intake
  Hyperinsulinemia secondary to portal-systemic shunting

amino acids is impaired, free amino acids in the bloodstream increase, and an "overflow" type of aminoaciduria may occur.

Urea production is intimately related to the metabolic pathways outlined above, providing a means for disposal of ammonia, the toxic product of nitrogen metabolism. Disruption of this process is of particular clinical importance in the patient with severe acute and chronic liver disease. The fixation of amino acid–derived NH_3 in the form of urea is carried out via the Krebs-Henseleit cycle. The final step of this cycle, the formation of urea by arginase, is irreversible. In advanced liver disease urea synthesis is often depressed, leading to an accumulation of NH_3, usually with a significant reduction in blood urea nitrogen (BUN), an ominous sign of liver failure. This finding may be obscured by superimposed renal impairment, which often develops in patients with severe hepatic failure. Urea is mostly excreted by the kidney, but approximately 25 percent will diffuse into the intestine where it is converted to NH_3 by bacterial urease. The intestinal production of ammonia also occurs from the bacterial deamination of unabsorbed amino acids and of protein derived from the diet, exfoliated cells, or blood in the gastrointestinal tract.

Gut NH_3 is absorbed and transported to the liver via the portal vein, where it is again converted to urea. The kidney also produces varying amounts of NH_3, largely by the deamination of glutamine. The contributions of the gut and kidney to ammonia synthesis have important implications for the management of the hyperammonemic state frequently seen in patients with advanced liver disease usually in association with portal-systemic shunting of blood.

While the exact chemical mediators of hepatic encephalopathy remain unknown, elevated levels of blood NH_3 generally correlate with the degree of encephalopathy, although approximately 10 percent of such patients have normal levels of blood ammonia. In addition, therapeutic measures that reduce serum NH_3 levels also usually lead to clinical improvement. The several mechanisms known to lead to increased blood NH_3 levels in patients with cirrhosis are illustrated in Fig. 250-2 and include the following: (1) If there is excessive nitrogenous material in the intestine (from bleeding or dietary protein), excessive amounts of NH_3 will be formed by bacterial deamination of amino acids. (2) If renal function declines (as in the hepatorenal syndrome), blood urea nitrogen rises, leading to increased diffusion of urea into the intestinal lumen, where bacterial urease converts it to NH_3. (3) If hepatic function is significantly depressed, diminished

urea synthesis may occur with a resultant decrease in the removal of NH_3. (4) If alkalosis (often due to central hyperventilation) and hypokalemia accompany hepatic decompensation, there may be a decrease in the renal availability of H^+ ions; as a result, the NH_3 produced from glutamine by the action of renal glutaminase is permitted to enter the renal vein (rather than being excreted as NH_4^+) leading to increased peripheral blood NH_3 levels. In addition hypokalemia itself leads to increased NH_3 production. (5) If portal hypertension is present and anastomoses exist between the portal vein and systemic venous channels, these portal-systemic shunts will allow NH_3 from the gut to bypass hepatic detoxification, leading to elevated blood NH_3 levels. Thus, with portal-systemic shunting of blood, elevated NH_3 levels may develop even with relatively little hepatocellular dysfunction. It is unclear what effects these same factors may have on other compounds which may play a role in the development of hepatic encephalopathy.

An additional factor important in determining whether a given NH_3 level in the blood will be detrimental to the central nervous system is the blood pH. The more alkaline the pH, the more toxic a given level of NH_3 is likely to be. At 37°C the pK of NH_3 is 8.9; this is close enough to the pH of blood that minor changes in pH can affect the NH_4^+/NH_3 ratio. Because un-ionized NH_3 crosses membranes more readily than NH_4^+ ions, alkalosis favors the entry of ammonia into the brain (with subsequent changes in cell metabolism) by shifting the equilibrium of the following reaction to the right

$$NH_4^+ + OH^- \rightleftharpoons NH_3 + HOH$$

As a result, alkalosis not only increases peripheral blood NH_3 levels by renal mechanisms but also increases tissue levels by influencing the diffusion of NH_3 across membranes.

PROTEIN SYNTHESIS AND DEGRADATION The liver is an important site of protein synthesis and degradation. Although the body muscle mass produces the greatest total amount of protein, the liver has the highest rate of synthesis per gram of tissue. The liver synthesizes not only the proteins it needs, but also and perhaps more importantly it produces numerous export proteins. Among the latter, albumin is the most important; *it is produced at a rate of approximately 12 g per day*, representing 25 percent of total hepatic protein synthesis and half of all exported protein. The average normal half-life of serum albumin is 17 to 20 days. The proportion of hepatocytes carrying out active albumin synthesis varies from 10 to 60 percent depending on the body's requirements. Approximately 60 percent of albumin is found in the extravascular spaces, but plasma albumin is still the most abundant circulating protein.

Albumin contributes significantly to the plasma oncotic pressure. In addition, it is the principal binding and transport protein for numerous substances including some hormones, fatty acids, trace metals, tryptophan, bilirubin, and other organic anions of both endogenous and exogenous origin. Despite the many important functions of albumin, rare individuals with congenital analbuminemia appear to have no major physiologic derangements other than the excessive accumulation of extravascular fluid. While many of the less hydrophobic ligands may be transported in the unbound form, this suggests that other serum proteins may also play a role in binding and transport.

Much has been learned about the mechanisms involved in the synthesis of secretory proteins, especially of albumin (see Fig. 250-3). Polyribosomes bound to the rough endoplasmic reticulum (RER) of the hepatocyte are the principal site of translation of messenger ribonucleic acid (mRNA) coding for export proteins; in contrast proteins destined for intracellular use, such as ferritin, are synthesized on free rather than bound polyribosomes in the cytoplasm. After a short-term fast, there is a decrease in the amount of albumin mRNA associated with the RER; instead more mRNA is found in the cytosol and in a state dissociated from polyribosomes. Albumin, like secretory proteins produced by other organs, appears to be synthesized initially as a larger precursor, preproalbumin. This precursor molecule contains an additional 24 extra amino acid residues

FIGURE 250-2 Major factors (steps 1 to 4) influencing the level of blood ammonia. In cirrhosis with portal hypertension, venous collaterals allow ammonia to bypass the liver (step 5), permitting the entry of ammonia into the systemic circulation (portal-systemic shunting).

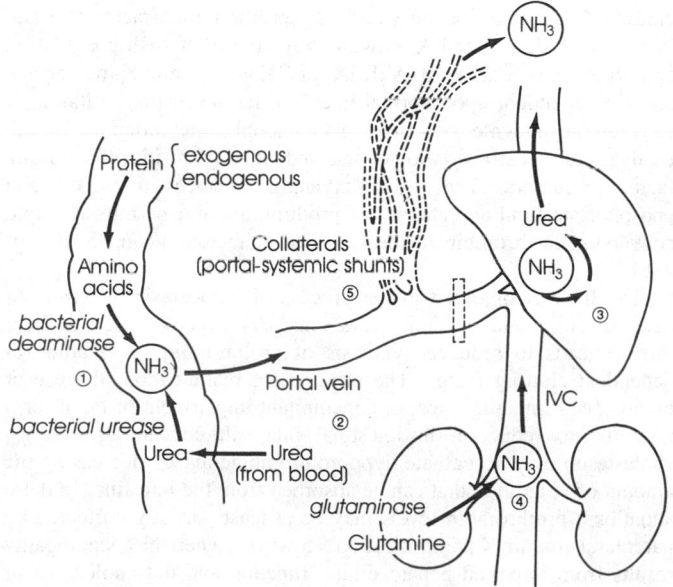

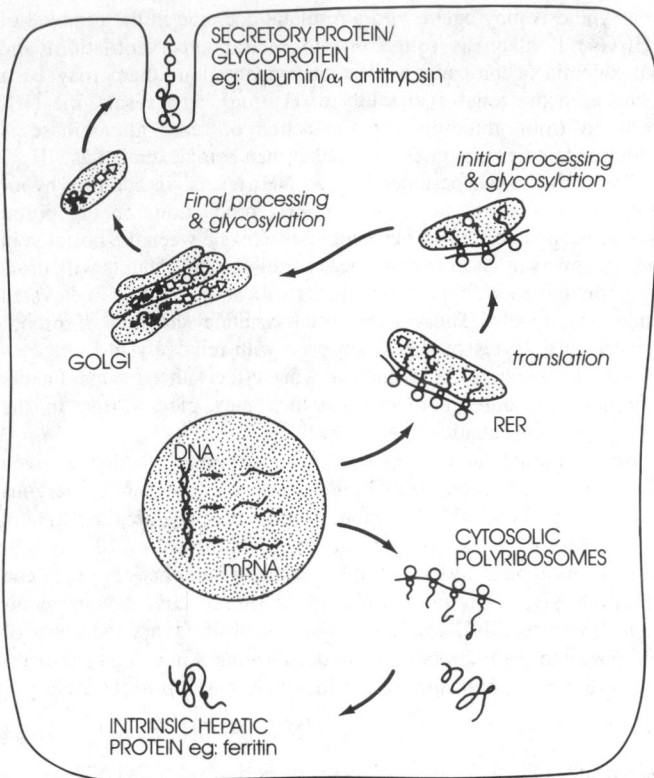

FIGURE 250-3 Schematic diagram illustrating major steps in synthesis, processing, and secretion of proteins and glycoproteins by the liver. Ribosomal subunits and mRNA form polysome complexes to initiate protein synthesis. Polyribosomes synthesizing proteins destined for export (e.g., albumin) associate with membranes to form membrane-bound polysomes [i.e., the rough endoplasmic reticulum (RER)]. Synthesis of precursor molecule (e.g., "preproalbumin") occurs and is followed by stepwise proteolytic cleavage and secretion from the cell. Other export proteins (e.g., α_1-antitrypsin) are first glycosylated in the RER and Golgi prior to secretion. Proteins produced for intracellular use (e.g., ferritin) are synthesized on non-membrane-bound cytosolic polyribosomes and processed by stepwise proteolytic cleavage and secretion from the cell.

on the *N* terminus, referred to as a "signal peptide," which undergoes two sequential cleavages (or "processing"); the molecule is then transported to the Golgi apparatus prior to secretion. The "pre" portion of preproalbumin is cleaved within the RER even before protein synthesis is completed; the "pro" segment is removed within the lumen of the ER. Once synthesis and processing are completed, albumin is transported from the Golgi vesicles to the hepatocyte surface by mechanisms which are unclear but almost certainly involve the microfilaments and microtubule apparatus of the cell. Although the hepatic lymph space of Disse provides a potential avenue for the newly released albumin, most secreted proteins enter the plasma.

Albumin synthesis is subject to a number of regulatory influences. These include the rate of transcription of specific mRNAs and the availability of the substrate tRNA (transfer RNA). At the translational level, the integrity of polyribosomes and their synthetic abilities is modified by factors affecting initiation, elongation, and release of peptides and proteins as well as by the availability of ATP, GTP, and magnesium ions. The rate of albumin synthesis is also influenced by the availability of amino acid precursors, especially tryptophan, the scarcest of the essential amino acids. Indeed in patients with large carcinoid tumors albumin synthesis may decrease precipitously when tryptophan is consumed by carcinoid cells in the production of 5-hydroxytryptophan (serotonin) (see Chap. 262). The rate of albumin synthesis is also affected by colloid oncotic pressure with increased production occurring in response to falling oncotic pressure. Finally, influences of hormones such as insulin and glucagon on hepatic

protein metabolism are closely integrated with the nutritional factors discussed above.

The liver also produces a wide variety of other secretory proteins, most of which have a synthetic pathway and processing procedure similar to that of albumin (Fig. 250-3). The presence of a *signal peptide*, such as the "prepro" segment of albumin, which is subsequently removed during protein maturation appears to be a general mechanism for orienting proteins in the membranes of the endoplasmic reticulum and directing them for export rather than for intracellular use or degradation. Most proteins undergo even further modification in the form of sequential *glycosylation* in the RER and Golgi apparatus. The carbohydrate moieties of these glycoproteins appear to be important in determining their site of action and their rate of tissue uptake after secretion. Some of the clinically important secretory glycoproteins include ceruloplasmin, α_1-antitrypsin, and most other alpha and beta globulins. While the site of albumin catabolism is uncertain, the removal of terminal sialic acid residues after secretion and the resultant exposure of penultimate galactose or *N*-acetylglucosamine residues appears to result in receptor-mediated uptake of "aged" proteins by hepatocytes and Kupffer cells, followed by their subsequent degradation. Reduced amounts of the hepatic receptor for asialoglycoproteins appear to result in elevated serum concentrations of these glycoproteins in patients with severe and chronic liver disease.

One of the clinically most important derangements in protein metabolism is the development of hypoalbuminemia, which results largely from reduced synthetic activity. Decreased synthesis may be caused by a decrease in the number as well as the function of hepatocytes. A decrease in the dietary supply of amino acids can also contribute to deficient synthesis. To some extent the body attempts to compensate for decreased albumin synthesis by reducing the rate of degradation. Attempts to raise the serum albumin level by intravenous infusions are often futile because this compensatory mechanism can be blunted and the decrease in albumin degradation may not occur. The reduced degradation of albumin is not a general phenomenon in chronic liver disease because other proteins such as fibrinogen are degraded more rapidly than normal. The degree of hypoalbuminemia is also augmented in the patient with ascites, in which large amounts of the body's albumin are present in the ascitic fluid. When there is increased hepatic venous pressure (as in postsinusoidal or hepatic vein outflow block), there may be increased hepatic lymph production with extravasation into the peritoneal cavity. In contrast to intestinal lymph, the protein content of hepatic lymph appears to be relatively uninfluenced by ascitic oncotic pressure, most likely reflecting the lack of tight junctions between sinusoidal endothelial cells.

Other proteins produced by the liver include many of the blood-clotting factors: fibrinogen (factor I), prothrombin (factor II), and factors V, VII, IX, and X as well as inhibitors of both coagulation and fibrinolysis. Factors II, VII, IX, and X are vitamin K–responsive and are dependent upon normal intestinal fat absorption. Vitamin K activates an enzyme system in liver endoplasmic reticulum which catalyzes the γ carboxylation of selected glutamyl residues in clotting factor precursors. The γ carboxylation enhances the Ca^{2+} and phospholipid binding capacity of prothrombin and permits its rapid conversion to thrombin in the presence of factors V and X (Chap. 288).

The liver is involved in the process of hemostasis by virtue of both anabolic and catabolic functions. As expected, severe liver disease leads to reduced synthesis of prothrombin, a vitamin K–dependent clotting factor. The presence of malnutrition, the use of broad-spectrum antibiotics, or concomitant impairment of fat absorption due to reduction in intestinal bile salt concentration (e.g., cholestasis) may accentuate hypoprothrombinemia by decreasing the amount of vitamin K that can be absorbed from the intestine. In these situations, prothrombin levels may be at least partially corrected by parenteral vitamin K administration. However, when the coagulopathy results from impaired hepatocellular function and not cholestasis or intestinal factors, exogenous vitamin K is unlikely to correct or improve prothrombin synthesis. The vitamin K–dependent clotting proteins have a substantially shorter serum half-life than albumin; therefore, hypoprothrombinemia usually precedes the development of hypoalbuminemia, especially in the patient with acute hepatocellular disease. In cirrhosis, coagulopathy may be further aggravated by the thrombocytopenia resulting from hypersplenism.

Since the liver is also the site of production of non-vitamin K–dependent clotting factors, severe liver disease injury may lead to decreased plasma concentrations of factor V in addition to factors II, VII, IX, and X. It is unusual for fibrinogen to be reduced significantly, unless there is an associated disseminated intravascular coagulation (DIC). For unclear reasons, the damaged liver may actually produce increased amounts of fibrinogen as well as other proteins collectively designated acute-phase reactants (C-reactive proteins, haptoglobin, ceruloplasmin, and transferrin). The latter are produced both in response to liver injury (e.g., severe chronic active hepatitis) and in association with systemic illnesses such as cancer, rheumatoid arthritis, bacterial infections, burns, and myocardial infarctions. However, while the diseased liver may produce normal or increased amounts of fibrinogen, the molecules themselves may be qualitatively abnormal (i.e., structurally and functionally), reflecting more subtle derangements in protein synthesis. These functionally abnormal fibrinogen molecules may contribute to the altered hemostasis frequently found in patients with chronic liver disease.

DETOXIFICATION MECHANISMS Water-soluble drugs and endogenous substances usually are excreted unchanged in the urine or bile. However, lipid-soluble compounds tend to accumulate in the body and affect cellular processes, unless they are converted to less active compounds or to more water-soluble metabolites which are more easily excreted. Hepatic blood flow, protein binding, and the intrinsic capacity of the liver to eliminate a drug are all primary determinants of hepatic drug clearance. The liver has an important role in the metabolism of many exogenous drugs and endogenous hormones by virtue of several enzyme systems involved in biochemical transformation. The relative importance of these various factors differs depending on how well a drug is extracted by the liver. There are two major types of reactions. The first, *phase I reactions,* result in chemical modification of reactive groups by oxidation, reduction, hydroxylation, sulfoxidation, deamination, dealkylation, or methylation. Such modifications usually involve one of several enzymatic systems, including the mixed-function oxidases, cytochromes b_5 and P_{450} (microsomal), and the glutathione S-acyltransferases (cytoplasmic). These biochemical reactions usually lead to *inactivation* of drugs such as barbiturates and benzodiazepines. However, *activation* may also occur. For example, cortisone is activated to cortisol and prednisone to prednisolone (both products being more potent than the parent compounds); imipramine, a depressant, is converted to desmethylimipramine, an antidepressant. In the same manner, phase I reactions may even convert a nontoxic compound to a toxic one as in the metabolism of isoniazid and acetaminophen. Similarly, some carcinogens may be activated by formation of highly reactive epoxide intermediates in the liver, while other carcinogens may be detoxified.

The enzymes responsible for phase I reactions, especially those involving the cytochrome P_{450} system, can be induced by drugs such as ethanol, barbiturates, haloperidol, and glutethimide. Conversely, hepatic microsomal enzymes may be inhibited by agents such as chloramphenicol, cimetidine, disulfiram, dextropropoxyphene, allopurinol, and, paradoxically, by ethanol. The concomitant administration of two drugs metabolized by the same microsomal enzyme may result in modification, potentiation, or diminution of the pharmacologic efficacy of either or both drugs. Activity of phase I reactions may also change with aging.

Phase II reactions may follow phase I reactions or proceed independently; these involve the conversion of substances to their glucuronide, sulfate, acetyl, taurine, or glycine derivatives, thereby converting lipophilic substances to water-soluble derivatives and permitting their excretion in bile or urine. Conjugation catalyzed by

microsomal UDP (uridine diphosphate)-glucuronyltransferases to form glucuronide derivatives is one of the most common phase II reactions. In general, the conjugates are more soluble than the parent compound and are pharmacologically inactive.

An awareness that there may be varying degrees of impairment in the hepatic uptake, detoxification, and excretion of certain drugs is important in the clinical management of patients with chronic liver disease. Portal-systemic shunting of blood may decrease the "first-pass effect" of drugs absorbed from the gut. In cirrhosis, altered intrahepatic hemodynamics due to a disordered liver architecture may also reduce the rates of hepatic drug clearance. Hypoalbuminemia will permit drugs usually bound to albumin to be present in increased concentrations of their unbound form in the circulation and extracellular spaces; this may result in an increased activity of such drugs. Most importantly, a decrease in the amount of function of microsomal enzymes responsible for phase I and phase II reactions will result in slower rates of drug inactivation and elimination. Drugs for which there may be a decreased clearance in patients with liver disease include anticonvulsants (e.g., phenytoin, phenobarbital), anti-inflammatory agents (e.g., acetaminophen, phenylbutazone, glucocorticoids), minor tranquilizers, cardioactive drugs (e.g., lidocaine, quinidine, propranolol), and antibiotics (e.g., nafcillin, chloramphenicol, tetracyclines, clindamycin, trimethoprim, rifampin, pyrazinamide). This will lead to decreased dosage requirements and a narrowing of the range between therapeutic and toxic drug levels. Finally, the patient with chronic liver disease may demonstrate alterations in the pharmacologic effects of drugs in addition to or independent of changes in their pharmacokinetics such as an increased central nervous system sensitivity to opiates and other sedatives.

The difficulties in safely administering pharmacologic agents to patients with both acute and chronic liver disease are underscored by the frequency with which administration of benzodiazepines is cited as precipitating hepatic coma. It may be very difficult clinically to determine whether agitation, confusion, and irrational behavior are due to early hepatic encephalopathy or are related to the concurrent use of benzodiazepines, opiates, barbiturates, and other depressants. It should be recognized that there is great variation of drug clearance in patients with liver disease; although data on average clearances may provide a reasonable estimate for initial dosages, subsequent adjustments in dose need to be individualized in order to attain the desired plasma drug concentration.

The mechanism by which some agents exert a hepatotoxic effect may involve the same metabolic pathways responsible for normal drug detoxification. The mechanism of acetaminophen toxicity is particularly illustrative. Acetaminophen is metabolized and detoxified by the hepatic mixed-function oxygenase system, but one of the intermediate products is a potent free radical (postulated metabolite N-acetylimidoquinone) which can inactivate many enzymes and proteins by binding irreversibly to their sulfhydryl groups. Normally this interaction can be prevented by reduced glutathione. In the presence of excessive amounts of the acetaminophen free radical (e.g., from overdosage or underlying liver disease), the glutathione levels of the hepatocytes are readily exhausted and the excess free radicals can lead to inactivation of cellular proteins and produce widespread hepatocellular necrosis. In the case of acetaminophen overdosage, the very early administration of sulfhydryl groups in the form of N-acetylcysteine can often prevent this drug-induced liver injury.

HORMONE METABOLISM In addition to its role in the metabolism of diverse pharmacologic agents, the liver is also responsible for inactivation or modification of several endogenous hormones; therefore, chronic liver disease may be accompanied by signs of apparent hormonal imbalance. Some hormones (e.g., insulin and glucagon) are inactivated in the liver by proteolysis or deamination. Thyroxine and triiodothyronine are metabolized in the liver by reactions involving deiodination. Steroid hormones, such as glucocorticoids and aldosterone, are first inactivated to their tetrahydro derivative (by reduction of the Δ^4 double bond and the 3-keto group), followed by conjugation, mostly with glucuronic acid. Testosterone is metabolized to the isomeric 17-ketosteroids androsterone and etiocholanolone and excreted in the urine mostly as sulfate conjugates. Estrogens, such as estradiol, may be converted to estriol and estrone and then conjugated with glucuronic acid or sulfate. Abnormalities in estrogen (and testosterone) metabolism are believed to be involved in the development of the spider angiomas, loss of axillary or pubic hair, and testicular atrophy frequently seen in patients with chronic liver disease. In addition, increased portal-systemic shunting of testosterone and androstenedione secondary to portal hypertension may lead to the development of gynecomastia in cirrhotic males due to increased peripheral conversion to estradiol and estrone, especially in patients with alcoholic cirrhosis. In patients with alcoholic liver disease, feminization may also be related to the direct toxic effects of alcohol on the gonadal-pituitary-hypothalamic axis which lead to the overall reduction in serum testosterone found in patients with cirrhosis. Similar effects are also seen in patients with hemochromatosis due to deposition of iron in these sites. However, gynecomastia is often lacking in the latter, apparently due to a coincident reduction in plasma concentration of androstenedione, a major precursor for estrogen synthesis.

Estrogens also act directly on the liver to impair hepatic secretory activity. Estradiol and related estrogens, such as those present in contraceptive pills, interfere with sodium sulfobromophthalein and bile salt excretion and worsen the preexisting defect in secretion of conjugated bilirubin in patients with Dubin-Johnson syndrome; they may also elevate plasma alkaline phosphatase levels (see Chap. 249). Related steroids such as etiocholanolone and pregnanediol have been shown to stimulate δ-aminolevulinic acid (ALA) synthetase activity leading to increased porphobilinogen excretion. Since these steroids exert these effects only in their unconjugated form, the increased hepatic levels of δ-aminolevulinic acid synthetase in patients with alcoholic cirrhosis may be secondary to the action of gonadal steroids.

LIPID METABOLISM: FATTY ACIDS AND TRIGLYCERIDES

Under normal conditions, most of the fatty acids taken up by the liver and esterified to triglyceride are derived from adipose tissue or the diet. Some fatty acids (especially saturated ones) are synthesized in the liver from acetate. The fatty acids may then be converted enzymatically to triglyceride, esterified with cholesterol, incorporated into phospholipids, or oxidized to CO_2 or ketone bodies. Most of the triglyceride is produced for export, but in order to be secreted it must be converted to lipoproteins by combining with relatively specific apoprotein moieties. This emphasizes the importance of protein synthesis for the release and secretion of triglyceride from the liver. It should be noted that the liver plays a major role in regulating lipoprotein levels by virtue of both its degradative and synthetic functions. Thus, the liver is quantitatively the major site of low-density lipoprotein (LDL) catabolism with dual high- and low-affinity receptor-mediated pathways playing a role. In addition chylomicron remnants are removed and degraded by the liver, where their constituents have a number of metabolic effects. The liver is not only the primary site of very low density lipoprotein (VLDL) secretion but also accounts for a major portion of its subsequent degradation by mechanisms similar to that of chylomicron remnant degradation and conversion to LDL via the action of hepatic lipase. The liver may also play a role in high-density lipoprotein (HDL) catabolism. It is noteworthy that with the exception of cholestatic disease (see below), clinically significant alterations in lipoprotein and cholesterol metabolism are usually not found in patients with chronic liver disease.

Studies on the production of fatty liver have shown that singly or in combination, one or more of the steps depicted in Fig. 250-4 may be involved. An increased influx of fatty acids mobilized from adipose tissue due to drugs (e.g., ethanol or glucocorticoids) or secondary to diabetic ketosis may lead to a fatty liver. Similarly, increased levels of fatty acids in the liver, either from enhanced fatty acid synthesis or from decreased fatty acid oxidation, may lead to increased triglyceride formation. In some instances (e.g., ethanol excess) there

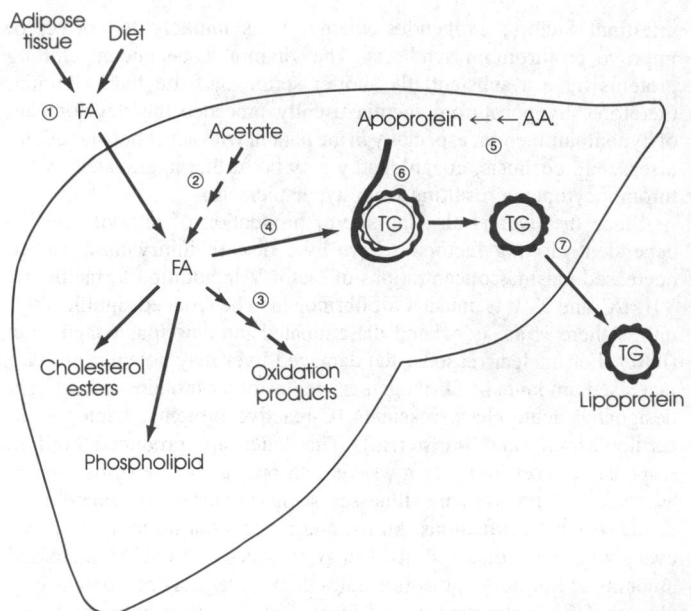

FIGURE 250-4 Factors in the uptake and esterification of fatty acids to triglyceride by the liver, including the formation and release of triglyceride as lipoprotein. The numbers refer to steps, which, if altered, may result in increased liver triglyceride (i.e., fatty liver).

may also be increases in the carbohydrate backbone, α-glycerophosphate, involved in fatty acid esterification to triglyceride. Since release of triglyceride involves the formation of lipoproteins, lipid accumulation may occur because of decreased apoprotein synthesis. This appears to be the case in fatty livers seen in patients with protein-calorie malnutrition (kwashiorkor) and due to toxins such as carbon tetrachloride, phosphorus, or ethionine, as well as following excessive doses of antibiotics like tetracycline that can inhibit protein synthesis. Finally, there may be impaired lipoprotein secretion from the liver. Alcohol is perhaps the most common agent leading to a fatty liver, but the mechanism(s) whereby alcohol leads to increased liver triglyceride is not clear. Depending on factors such as dose or duration, alcohol ingestion may affect any of the seven steps shown in Fig. 250-4; however, the primary factor for the production of the alcohol-induced fatty liver remains to be determined. The alterations in the redox state due to excessive accumulation of NADH resulting from oxidation of alcohol may also contribute.

In addition to the changes leading to fatty liver, there are many metabolic alterations which may be found in the blood of patients following the ingestion of large amounts of alcohol. These include, among others, *increased* plasma levels of lactate, proline, urate, and triglycerides and *decreased* plasma levels of glucose, magnesium, phosphate, and triiodothyronine (T_3).

CHOLESTEROL Cholesterol and bile acid synthesis is carried out primarily by the liver. Cholesterol synthesis is subject to a number of metabolic controls, most of them mediated via the rate-limiting biosynthetic enzyme 3-hydroxy-3-methylglutaryl coenzyme A reductase (HMG-CoA reductase). Cholesterol exists either free or combined with fatty acids in the form of cholesterol esters; in the plasma both are found primarily in association with β-lipoproteins. The plasma and liver also contain lecithin–cholesterol acyltransferase (LCAT), an enzyme involved in the conversion of free cholesterol to its esterified form. Since there is exchange of free cholesterol between tissues, changes in plasma cholesterol levels reflect changes in total body cholesterol. However, decreases in plasma cholesterol esters may reflect hepatic damage and impaired hepatic cholesterol esterification.

Severe liver injury often leads to a decrease in *total* serum cholesterol levels, including both free and esterified fractions. This may be due to decreased synthesis of cholesterol and cholesterol esters, decreased apoprotein synthesis, or both. In cholestasis (either intra- or extrahepatic) total serum cholesterol often increases strikingly. Disorders of cholestasis are associated with marked abnormalities of lipoprotein metabolism. In primary biliary cirrhosis there are pronounced elevations in serum free cholesterol and LDL; conversely, serum HDL is reduced and may disappear from the serum in patients with long-standing disease. Similar but less marked changes are seen in other cholestatic conditions.

The increase in serum free cholesterol (and phospholipid) and the concomitant decrease in esterified cholesterol in cholestasis may be related to a decrease in the hepatic production of LCAT. Reduced levels of LCAT are also correlated with the appearance of an abnormal LDL, referred to as lipoprotein X (LP-X). Although LP-X, which has a high content of free cholesterol and triglyceride, was originally thought to be a specific indicator of biliary tract obstruction, it is evident that it appears in any cholestatic condition. While the depressed hepatic production of LCAT may be responsible for altered lipid content and composition of lipoproteins, the factors leading to the overall increase in total serum cholesterol are not clear. In experimental animals, bile duct ligation results in a net increase in hepatic cholesterol synthesis, and in "regurgitation" of bile salts, cholesterol, and LP-X into venous radicals. However, it is difficult to translate these experimental findings to the patient with primary biliary cirrhosis unless any insult to cells lining the biliary canaliculi and ductules can impair the delicate balance of lipid synthesis and removal.

Most of the derangements of hepatic metabolism discussed above are evident only in patients with severe or long-standing liver disease. Indeed, in all but the most severe cases of acute viral hepatitis, hepatic metabolic functions are remarkably well preserved, and in most cases of mild to moderate acute viral hepatitis, it is uncommon to observe clinically important alterations in carbohydrate, protein, and lipid metabolism. However, in the patients with severe or fulminant hepatitis, whether from a viral or toxic agent, the metabolic derangements may be similar to those seen in more chronic disease. For example, in fulminant hepatitis there may be pronounced hypoprothrombinemia and impaired coagulation, hypoalbuminemia, and the relatively acute development of ascites, as well as hyperammonemia and encephalopathy. However, in contrast to patients with cirrhosis, abnormalities in carbohydrate metabolism are more likely to lead to profound hypoglycemia than to hyperglycemia. This hypoglycemia appears to reflect both a marked decrease in hepatic glycogen stores and a diminished glucagon responsiveness. There may also be poor oral intake due to nausea and anorexia together with increased glucose utilization secondary to hyperinsulinemia (due to portal-systemic shunting and decreased insulin degradation).

REFERENCES

ARIAS IM et al: *The Liver: Biology and Pathophysiology,* 2d ed. New York, Raven, 1988

CAVALLO-PERIN P et al: Mechanism of insulin resistance in human liver cirrhosis. Evidence of a combined receptor and post-receptor defect. J Clin Invest 75:1659, 1985

COOPER AD: Role of the liver in the degradation of lipoproteins. Gastroenterology 88:192, 1984

FLANNERY DB et al: Current status of hyperammonemic syndromes. Hepatology 2:495, 1982

HOYUMPA AM et al: Hepatic encephalopathy. Gastroenterology 77:803, 1979

KLEG HK et al: Conversion of androgens to estrogens in idiopathic hemochromatosis: Comparison with alcoholic liver disease. J Clin Endocrin Metab 61:1, 1985

OWEN OE et al: Hepatic, gut and renal substrate flux rates in patients with hepatic cirrhosis. J Clin Invest 68:240, 1981

ROTHSCHILD MA et al: Serum albumin. Hepatology 8:355, 1988

SHERLOCK S: *Diseases of the Liver and Biliary System,* 8th ed. Oxford, Blackwell, 1989

SMITH AR et al: Alteration in plasma and CSF amino acids, amines and metabolites in hepatic coma. Ann Surg 187:343, 1978

WILLIAMS RC: Drug administration in hepatic disease. N Engl J Med 309:1616, 1983

WRIGHT R et al: *Liver and Biliary Disease,* 2d ed. Philadelphia, Saunders, 1985

251 BILIRUBIN METABOLISM AND HYPERBILIRUBINEMIA

KURT J. ISSELBACHER

The normal metabolism of bilirubin and the approach to the patient with jaundice have been presented in Chap. 47. With a consideration of these pathways, the disorders of bilirubin metabolism can be divided into four major categories, namely, those due to (1) increased pigment production, (2) reduced hepatic uptake of bilirubin, (3) impaired hepatic conjugation, and (4) decreased excretion of the conjugated pigment from the liver into bile. The first three of these disorders are associated with predominantly unconjugated hyperbilirubinemia. The fourth group, defective excretion, is associated with predominantly conjugated hyperbilirubinemia and bilirubinuria.

DISORDERS CAUSING PREDOMINANTLY UNCONJUGATED HYPERBILIRUBINEMIA

The plasma concentration of unconjugated bilirubin is determined by (1) the rate at which newly synthesized bilirubin enters the plasma (bilirubin turnover) and (2) the rate of removal of bilirubin by the liver (hepatic bilirubin clearance). Disturbances of the latter can result from derangements of hepatic bilirubin uptake, conjugation, or both. Measurements of these variables, although not routinely available, permit a classification of patients into those with *increased bilirubin turnover* (e.g., hemolysis), those with *decreased bilirubin clearance* (e.g., Gilbert's syndrome), and those in whom both mechanisms operate.

OVERPRODUCTION OF BILIRUBIN (INCREASED TURNOVER) Increased destruction of circulating erythrocytes (intravascular and extravascular hemolysis) In disorders associated with hemolysis, most commonly the hemolytic anemias, the rate of bilirubin production is increased and may even exceed the amount that can be removed by a normal liver. The resulting jaundice is primarily an unconjugated hyperbilirubinemia. There is often also a small increase in the serum conjugated bilirubin (see Chap. 47). If significant anemia or other adverse factors are present (e.g., fever, sepsis, hypoxemia, or vascular collapse), the ability of the liver to handle the pigment load will be compromised, and the degree of jaundice will be greater.

The clinical and diagnostic features of the various hemolytic anemias are described in Chap. 294. The presence of reticulocytosis, shortened red blood cell survival, and increased fecal urobilinogen, in the absence of clinical and laboratory evidence of liver disease, strongly suggest hemolysis and overproduction of bilirubin as the cause of the jaundice. It is obvious, however, that in some cases (e.g., cirrhosis, tumors, and sepsis), hemolysis *plus* deranged liver function may be present. In most cases of uncomplicated hemolytic states, the mean serum bilirubin level will be in the range of 51 to 86 μmol/L (3 to 5 mg/dL); rarely, higher levels may be seen.

Jaundice due to increased pigment production may also be seen as a consequence of *tissue infarction* (e.g., pulmonary infarcts) and large *collections of blood in tissues* (e.g., leakage from blood vessels after catheterization studies, rupture of an aortic aneurysm). If hypotension and hypoxemia also supervene, jaundice is usually more pronounced, and the resulting impairment of liver function may also lead to a significant increase in the serum conjugated bilirubin level (see "Postoperative Jaundice" below).

Except in early infancy, elevations of serum unconjugated bilirubin levels are not generally harmful per se, and the prognosis is that of the hemolytic process itself. However, in the neonatal state and infancy, unconjugated bilirubin levels above 340 μmol/L (20 mg/dL) may lead to *kernicterus* due to bilirubin deposition in the lipid-rich basal ganglia (see Chap. 358). Chronic overproduction of bilirubin may result in the formation of gallstones composed predominantly of bilirubin (''pigment stones''). In this situation, all the potential complications of calculus disease of the biliary tract (Chap. 258) may be superimposed on the chronic hemolytic state which produced it.

Increased production of bilirubin from sources other than circulating erythrocytes   As indicated in Chap. 47, about 15 to 20 percent of the circulating bilirubin is normally derived from sources other than the destruction of circulating red blood cells. This represents the so-called early-labeled fraction; it includes the synthesis of bilirubin from nonhemoglobin heme in the liver and from hemoglobin heme in the marrow.

In some conditions, jaundice results from an increased destruction of red blood cells or their precursors in the marrow—a process referred to as *ineffective erythropoiesis* (see Chaps. 47 and 61). In patients with thalassemia, pernicious anemia, and congenital erythropoietic porphyria, such an increased rate of formation of the early-labeled bilirubin fraction has been demonstrated. It is possible that some cases of unexplained unconjugated hyperbilirubinemia may be caused by an increased hepatic production of bilirubin from nonhemoglobin heme, but this phenomenon has not yet been demonstrated clinically.

IMPAIRED HEPATIC UPTAKE OF BILIRUBIN   Drugs   Only a few drugs have been definitely shown to influence the uptake of bilirubin by the liver. Flavaspidic acid, used in the treatment of tapeworm infestation, may cause unconjugated hyperbilirubinemia, as well as impairment of sodium sulfobromophthalein (BSP) clearance, during its administration. The jaundice readily subsides following treatment. Flavaspidic acid competes with bilirubin for binding to ligandin, leading thereby to unconjugated hyperbilirubinemia. The jaundice which may occur with novobiocin and some cholecystographic dyes is also apparently due to an interference in bilirubin uptake.

Gilbert's syndrome   Some cases of this syndrome of chronic unconjugated hyperbilirubinemia may be due to a defect in hepatic uptake (as reflected by alteration in BSP kinetics). In most cases, however, a deficiency of bilirubin glucuronyl transferase can be demonstrated. Hence this syndrome is best considered as a defect in bilirubin conjugation (see below).

IMPAIRED BILIRUBIN CONJUGATION (DECREASED ACTIVITY OF BILIRUBIN GLUCURONYL TRANSFERASE)   Neonatal jaundice (physiologic jaundice of the newborn)   Almost every infant exhibits some transient unconjugated hyperbilirubinemia between the second and fifth days of life. While during gestation the placenta serves to clear bilirubin from the fetus, after birth infants must detoxify the pigments themselves. However, at this stage the hepatic enzyme glucuronyl transferase is still ''immature'' and inadequate for the task. As a result, unconjugated bilirubinemia develops, usually not exceeding 86 µmol/L (5 mg/dL). The activity of glucuronyl transferase increases within several days to 2 weeks after birth, and concomitantly the serum bilirubin returns to normal. In the premature infant the glucuronyl transferase activity is less, and the neonatal jaundice may be more pronounced. The ''maturation'' of the fetal and neonatal liver may be enhanced by treatment of the pregnant mother or the newborn infant with phenobarbital or related drugs. This results in a clear-cut reduction of the degree and duration of unconjugated hyperbilirubinemia in the newborn. In infants with a superimposed hemolytic process (e.g., erythroblastosis), the excessive pigment load leads to more pronounced jaundice, and bilirubin levels may exceed 340 µmol/L (20 mg/dL). It should be emphasized that neonatal jaundice is not present at the time of delivery; if jaundice is present at birth, other causes must be considered.

The cytoplasmic liver cell protein ligandin binds bilirubin in the hepatocyte and may assist in the transfer of bilirubin to the endoplasmic reticulum for conjugation (Chap. 47). It has been proposed that deficiency of ligandin may contribute to neonatal jaundice.

An additional facet of the ''immature'' liver is a concomitant defect in the excretion of *conjugated* bilirubin. Rarely this defect persists beyond the time needed for the development of adequate glucuronide conjugation and may explain the occasional presence of

conjugated hyperbilirubinemia in infants with erythroblastosis (*inspissated bile syndrome*).

When in the neonatal state unconjugated bilirubin levels approach or exceed 340 µmol/L (20 mg/dL), the infants may develop and die of *kernicterus* (bilirubin encephalopathy). This condition results from unconjugated bilirubin deposition in the lipid-rich basal ganglia. In the past treatment consisted of exchange transfusions, and albumin infusions were used to increase binding of bilirubin in the circulation and diminish its entry into the brain. The current approach is *phototherapy;* intense illumination of these patients with strong white or blue light leads to the photoisomerization of bilirubin to water-soluble isomers that are rapidly excreted in the bile without the prior need of conjugation. However, another novel approach involves decreasing bilirubin production from heme by inhibitors of the enzyme, heme oxygenase. Synthetic protoporphyrins, such as tin protoporphyrin, have been successfully administered to patients with neonatal hyperbilirubinemia with marked reduction in the serum bilirubin and with no major side effects.

Hereditary glucuronyl transferase deficiency   There are currently three syndromes that fall into this category. As indicated in Table 251-1, they reflect progressive decreases in the activity of glucuronyl transferase and thus may be part of a spectrum, i.e., from minimal deficiency to complete absence of bilirubin glucuronyl transferase.

GILBERT'S SYNDROME   Since the original report by Gilbert in 1907, there has been an increased recognition of this benign but chronic disorder characterized by mild, persistent, unconjugated hyperbilirubinemia. The patient usually does not manifest this disorder until after the second decade and is often unaware of the jaundice until it is detected by physical examination or routine laboratory testing. The total serum bilirubin level usually ranges and fluctuates from 21 to 51 µmol/L (1.2 to 3 mg/dL) and rarely exceeds 86 µmol/L (5 mg/dL). With the van den Bergh diazo reaction, less than 20 percent of the bilirubin gives a direct reaction; however, studies using more accurate methods (such as high-pressure liquid chromatography) show that the serum bilirubin in patients with Gilbert's syndrome is almost all unconjugated. Typically the jaundice fluctuates and is exacerbated following prolonged fasting (see below), surgery, fever or infection, and excessive exertion or alcohol ingestion. Liver function tests are normal, and the liver cells usually appear normal by light microscopy.

With the exception of hemolytic anemias, this disorder is probably the most common cause of mild unconjugated hyperbilirubinemia. Detailed studies show these patients to have a partial deficiency of bilirubin glucuronyl transferase. Some patients also manifest decreased bilirubin uptake and increased hemolysis. Decreased glucuronyl transferase alone or together with a decrease in bilirubin uptake

TABLE 251-1   Hereditary unconjugated hyperbilirubinemias with deficiency of glucuronyl transferase

Features	Mild (Gilbert's syndrome)	Moderate (Crigler-Najjar syndrome type II)	Severe (Crigler-Najjar syndrome type I)
Inheritance	Unclear*	Dominant†	Recessive
Serum bilirubin, µmol/L (mg/dL)	17–102 (1–6)	102–340 (6–20)	340–770 (20–45)
Kernicterus	No	Rare	Yes
Conjugated bilirubin in bile	Yes (↑ monoconjugates)	Yes (↑ ↑ monoconjugates)	No
Response to phenobarbital	Yes	Yes	No
Bilirubin conjugation	↓ ‡	↓ ↓	Absent

* Many cases are without familial incidence.
† Variable expressivity.
‡ Other defects such as occult hemolysis and ↓ bilirubin uptake may coexist.

appears to account for the observed *decrease in hepatic bilirubin clearance*. A decreased clearance and hepatic uptake of bile salts has also been shown.

Previously Gilbert's syndrome was traditionally defined as mild, chronic, unconjugated hyperbilirubinemia occurring in the absence of hemolysis. However, with the use of radiobilirubin kinetics and erythrocyte half-life studies, at least two forms of Gilbert's syndrome have been described. One group includes patients with decreased bilirubin clearance and *no hemolysis*. A second group includes those who also have *evidence of hemolysis* (often occult) and hence increased bilirubin turnover. The simultaneous presence of both derangements appears to be a chance occurrence of two not uncommon disorders in the same patient and does not imply a causal relationship. There is additional evidence of the heterogeneity of patients with Gilbert's syndrome. Some patients have an increase in hepatocyte lipofuscin and an increase in the smooth endoplasmic reticulum (SER); others show an increase in hepatic lysosomal enzymes.

A feature of Gilbert's syndrome which can be useful diagnostically is the increase in serum bilirubin following prolonged fasting or calorie deprivation. Patients with this disorder, when placed on 1255 kJ (300 kcal) per day for 2 days, will increase their serum bilirubin by 26 μmol/L (1.5 mg/dL) or more, the major increase being in the unconjugated fraction. It appears that a decrease in glucuronyl transferase activity is needed in order to obtain this effect. Patients with hemolysis do not show an increase in serum bilirubin with fasting. As a reflection of the mild decrease in glucuronyl transferase in Gilbert's syndrome (1) serum bilirubin levels will decrease when the enzyme activity is enhanced following phenobarbital administration, and (2) the bile shows a modest increase in monoconjugates of bilirubin (see Table 251-1).

In general, the diagnosis of this benign but not uncommon disorder is made by exclusion. The syndrome is suspected in a patient with low-grade unconjugated hyperbilirubinemia with (1) no systemic symptoms, (2) *no overt* or clinically recognizable hemolysis, (3) normal tests of routine liver function, and (4) a liver biopsy (although usually not necessary) that is normal by light microscopy.

CRIGLER-NAJJAR SYNDROME (TYPES I AND II) This disorder is known to exist in two forms. Type I is the clinically *severe* form (originally described by Crigler and Najjar) and is due to *absence of glucuronyl transferase*. Type II has more *moderate* clinical findings due to *partial deficiency of glucuronyl transferase*. The major differences between the two variants are summarized in Table 251-1.

Type I (Crigler-Najjar) is a rare disorder. Infants develop high unconjugated bilirubin levels in the serum [340 to 770 μmol/L (20 to 45 mg/dL)]. Absence of the enzyme can be demonstrated in the liver. Routine liver function tests are normal, as is liver histology. Because of the absence of glucuronyl transferase no conjugated bilirubin is formed by the liver; hence no bilirubin is secreted by the liver, and the bile is colorless.

Phototherapy may temporarily and transiently reduce the unconjugated bilirubin level. Phenobarbital has no effect since the enzyme defect is complete and no drug "induction" is therefore possible. Affected infants usually die within the first year of life, although some patients have survived to the second or third decade of life. Death is usually from kernicterus. A strain of rats (Gunn rat) with the type I defect exists and is widely used as an animal model of the Crigler-Najjar syndrome (type I).

Type II patients have a *partial deficiency* of glucuronyl transferase, and their disorder is less severe. Serum unconjugated bilirubin levels are lower [103 to 340 μmol/L (6 to 20 mg/dL)], jaundice may not appear until adolescence, and neurologic complications are uncommon. The bile contains variable amounts of conjugated bilirubin with a significant increase in monoconjugates. Phenobarbital is effective in lowering the serum bilirubin level in type II patients. However, the disorder is relatively benign in those patients whose bilirubin is less than 308 to 340 μmol/L (18 to 20 mg/dL).

Acquired deficiency of glucuronyl transferase As with any enzyme, glucuronyl transferase is susceptible to inhibition by a variety

of agents, and because of the decreased activity of the enzyme in the neonatal state, such inhibition may be more evident at that time. Neonatal jaundice may be aggravated or prolonged in infants treated with *drugs* such as chloramphenicol or novobiocin, or with *vitamin K*. In some breast-fed infants jaundice has been ascribed to the presence in *breast milk* of pregnane-3β,20α-diol, an inhibitor of glucuronyl transferase. When the infant is removed from the breast, the "breast-milk jaundice" subsides.

Hypothyroidism delays the normal "maturation" of glucuronyl transferase. In cretins, neonatal jaundice may be prolonged for weeks or months. In fact, the presence of prolonged unconjugated hyperbilirubinemia after birth may be a clue to an underlying hypothyroidism.

In the infant, as well as in the adult, *liver cell damage* leads to impairment in glucuronide conjugation as a result of decreased transferase activity. However, since excretion is probably the rate-limiting step in bilirubin metabolism and since this step is always interfered with to a greater extent than conjugation in parenchymal liver disease, the pigment which accumulates in the blood is predominantly conjugated bilirubin.

DISORDERS CAUSING COMBINED CONJUGATED AND UNCONJUGATED HYPERBILIRUBINEMIA

In jaundice due to primary liver disease, the plasma usually exhibits elevated levels of both conjugated and unconjugated bilirubin, and *urine contains bilirubin*. The relative proportions of the two pigments are highly variable. In many familial hepatic abnormalities (described below) and in some forms of liver injury, the jaundice is largely due to increases in conjugated bilirubin. Such a serum pigment pattern is also seen with extrahepatic biliary obstruction. One *cannot differentiate* intrahepatic and extrahepatic causes of jaundice from either the levels or proportions of unconjugated and conjugated bilirubin in serum. Thus the main purpose of the initial fractionation of the serum bilirubin is to distinguish hepatic parenchymal and biliary obstructive disease from the disorders associated with predominantly unconjugated hyperbilirubinemia.

FAMILIAL DEFECTS IN HEPATIC EXCRETORY FUNCTION
Dubin-Johnson syndrome This disorder, also called *chronic idiopathic jaundice*, is a benign, autosomally inherited hyperbilirubinemia characterized by the presence of a dark pigment in the centrilobular region of the liver cells. Functionally there exists a *defect in biliary excretion* of bilirubin, cholephilic dyes, and porphyrins. Using the diazo method for measuring bilirubin, the serum pigment in these patients typically has been observed to be in the range of 51 to 257 μmol/L (3 to 15 mg/dL) and predominantly of the conjugated type. However, with the newer and more accurate method (alkaline methanolysis and high-pressure liquid chromatography), homozygous patients with the Dubin-Johnson syndrome have been shown to have significant levels of serum *unconjugated bilirubin*. This finding may in part reflect pigment which, after conjugation by the liver, is deconjugated in the hepatobiliary system and refluxed into the plasma. Moreover, the serum contains more diconjugated than monoconjugated bilirubin, just the reverse of what is seen in acquired hepatobiliary disease and Rotor syndrome. This reversed ratio is believed to be characteristic and diagnostic for homozygous patients.

Patients with Dubin-Johnson syndrome may be asymptomatic or have vague constitutional or gastrointestinal symptoms. Not infrequently the liver is slightly enlarged; in about one-fourth of the cases there is mild hepatic tenderness. Oral and intravenous cholangiography fails to visualize the biliary tract. There is typically and characteristically a late rise in the plasma BSP elimination curve at *90 min*. This is caused by the reflux from the liver of the conjugated dye and reflects the defect in the hepatic excretory transport maximum (T_m). It is noteworthy that there is no such secondary rise in plasma when dyes which are not conjugated by the liver are given, such as indocyanine green. When bile salts such as ursodeoxycholic acid are given, these patients show a decreased hepatic uptake and clearance. In the liver the striking feature is the presence of a brown or black pigment in the hepatocytes. Some findings suggest that this unique pigment is "melanin-like"; others indicate it to be a polymer of epinephrine metabolites.

These patients also show an abnormality in coproporphyrin excretion. Normal urine contains mostly coproporphyrin III and small amounts of coproporphyrin I; Dubin-Johnson patients show a reversal of this pattern, i.e., they excrete predominantly coproporphyrin I. Heterozygotes show an intermediate excretory pattern.

There is impaired excretion of many metabolites, including conjugated bilirubin, BSP, and iodinated dyes. Excretion of bile acids, however, is normal. Oral contraceptive agents may accentuate hyperbilirubinemia or may produce jaundice for the first time. Features of cholestasis such as pruritus or steatorrhea are usually lacking, and, specifically, serum alkaline phosphatase levels are *not* elevated. The overall prognosis of the disorder is excellent.

Rotor syndrome This is similar in many respects to the Dubin-Johnson syndrome. However, *there is no pigment in the liver cells,* and the serum conjugated bilirubin has more monoconjugates than diglucuronide conjugates. The gallbladder is usually visualized on cholecystography, and there is an increase in the *total* urinary coproporphyrins but *not* an increased percentage in excretion of coproporphyrin I. The BSP excretion pattern does *not* show a secondary rise at 90 min. The impairment in excretion which is typical of Dubin-Johnson syndrome is not present; instead in most cases of the Rotor syndrome there is impairment of *hepatic storage capacity* (S). This rare syndrome is inherited as an autosomal recessive trait and is genetically distinct from Dubin-Johnson syndrome.

Benign familial recurrent cholestasis This is a relatively rare syndrome characterized by recurrent attacks of pruritus and jaundice. During an attack the serum alkaline phosphatase and bile acid levels are markedly elevated, and liver biopsy shows the morphologic features of cholestasis. However, there is no mechanical biliary obstruction, with cholangiography revealing a patent biliary tree. Remissions are the rule, and at such times hepatic function tests and liver morphologic features are usually normal. The cause of the disorder is unknown; cirrhosis does not develop, and the disorder is benign. A congenital origin has been postulated on the basis of the early age of onset and familial incidence.

Recurrent jaundice of pregnancy This form of jaundice is also known as *intrahepatic cholestasis of pregnancy.* During a normal pregnancy some derangements in liver function occur, especially during the last trimester. Usually these consist of slight increases in BSP retention and in serum alkaline phosphatase. This mild increase in alkaline phosphatase during pregnancy is normally of placental rather than of hepatic origin. With a normal pregnancy elevations of serum bilirubin either do not occur or are less than 34 μmol/L (2 mg/dL).

In a small number of pregnant women an intrahepatic cholestasis may appear. This usually occurs in the third trimester but may develop any time after the seventh week of gestation. The clinical features consist primarily of pruritus and jaundice. Serum bilirubin levels are usually less than 103 μmol/L (6 mg/dL). The serum alkaline phosphatase and cholesterol levels are elevated significantly, while other liver function tests are only mildly deranged. Histologically the liver shows varying degrees of cholestasis but only a few parenchymal cell changes. The clinical and laboratory abnormalities subside promptly after delivery and are usually normal within 7 to 14 days.

This condition has been seen more frequently in Scandinavia and Europe than in the United States. Since steroid hormones and specifically estrogens can induce changes in hepatic excretory function in normal individuals (see Chap. 250), these patients probably have an increased susceptibility or sensitivity to the hepatic effects of estrogenic and progestational hormones. The intrahepatic cholestasis is usually termed *recurrent*, since the syndrome often (but not always)

reappears in subsequent pregnancies. The process is benign and self-limited, and treatment is usually not needed, but cholestyramine administration will diminish the pruritus. This disorder must be distinguished from the many other causes of jaundice not unique to pregnancy, such as viral hepatitis. It must also be distinguished from the idiopathic *acute fatty liver of pregnancy* and the *tetracycline-induced* fatty liver. The latter two conditions are rare, occur in the last trimester, and have a high fatality rate; however, in these disorders there is evidence of diffuse parenchymal damage and not just cholestasis.

ACQUIRED DEFECTS OF HEPATIC EXCRETORY FUNCTION
Drug-induced cholestasis A condition entirely analogous to the intrahepatic cholestasis of pregnancy may occur in some women following the use of oral contraceptive agents. In some, mild cholestatic jaundice may occur, liver function returns to normal when the drugs are withdrawn, and chronic liver disease does not appear to result. It is relevant that one-third of the reported patients with jaundice due to oral contraceptives also have a history of recurrent intrahepatic cholestasis of pregnancy.

The nature of these changes produced by the natural and synthetic female sex hormones is very similar to those resulting from the administration of certain testosterone analogues, especially those with α substitutions at the 17 position of the steroid nucleus. These agents (such as methyltestosterone and norethandrolone) commonly cause BSP retention and less commonly cause jaundice or significant changes in other liver functions. However, unlike the female hormones, these agents have been implicated as a cause of chronic liver disease, especially biliary cirrhosis.

Because of these phenomena, synthetic steroid sex hormones should not be used in patients with liver disease. Conversely, in individuals using these agents the appearance of jaundice or elevations in serum aminotransferase (transaminase) levels or alkaline phosphatase contraindicates their further use. However, mild to moderate increases in BSP retention alone are probably not of clinical significance, although liver function tests should be carried out periodically.

As is discussed in detail in Chap. 252, there are many drugs which may produce not only cholestasis but liver injury resembling acute hepatitis or cholestatic hepatitis. In contrast to the jaundice produced by the steroid hormones, the clinical features are those of fever, rash, arthralgia, and eosinophilia, with the liver showing a pronounced inflammatory reaction. These features suggest that such reactions are *allergic* or *toxic* in nature and therefore differ from the effects caused by the steroid hormones, which probably represent an exaggerated response by the liver to the normal action of these hormones.

Postoperative jaundice The occurrence of postoperative jaundice is a problem of increasing importance. It is perhaps seen more frequently now than in earlier years, because patients are able to undergo more major surgical procedures (i.e., cardiac surgery, repair of ruptured aneurysms) and survive. In approaching this problem the possible pathogenic mechanisms listed in Table 251-2 need to be considered. The patient may have *pigment overload,* especially from blood transfusions (with hemolysis of stored blood), from resorption of blood in extravascular spaces, and less commonly from hemolytic anemia. *Hepatocellular damage* and decreased liver cell function may occur due to concurrent use of hepatotoxic drugs (Chap. 252) or anesthetics such as halothane. Hepatocellular necrosis may follow profound shock; with lesser degrees of hypotension or hypoxemia, morphologic damage may be slight, but significant impairment of function may occur. Hence, prior shock or hypotension plus pigment overload may produce significant jaundice. Extensive sepsis can also produce jaundice, often of a cholestatic type. Concurrent renal impairment due to hypotension and hypoxemia may enhance the degree of jaundice because the renal excretion of conjugated bilirubin is decreased. *Extrahepatic obstruction* due to surgical damage or stones needs to be considered, and may be excluded by ultrasound studies.

A form of jaundice referred to as *benign postoperative intrahepatic*

TABLE 251-2 Conditions causing or contributing to postoperative jaundice

I Increased pigment load
  A Hemolytic anemia
  B Transfusions (especially of stored blood)
  C Resorption of hematomas, blood in extravascular spaces
II Impaired hepatocellular function
  A Hepatitis-like picture
    1 Halothane anesthesia
    2 Drugs
    3 Shock
    4 Infection with hepatitis viruses
  B Cholestatic picture
    1 Hypotension, hypoxemia
    2 Drugs
    3 Sepsis
III Extrahepatic obstruction
  A Bile duct injury
  B Choledocholithiasis

cholestasis may be seen. In the typical case the patient has had major and prolonged surgery for a catastrophic event such as a ruptured aortic aneurysm complicated by hypotension and hypoxemia, extensive blood loss into tissues, and massive blood replacement. Jaundice may be noted on the second or third postoperative day, and the serum bilirubin, predominantly conjugated, may reach 340 to 680 μmol/L (20 to 40 mg/dL) by the eighth to tenth day. Serum alkaline phosphatase levels may be elevated three- to tenfold. Typically the serum aspartate aminotransferase (AST, SGOT) is only mildly elevated. The liver morphology is striking in that necrosis is not seen, only cholestasis and erythrophagocytosis.

The cause of this type of postoperative cholestatic jaundice is uncertain. However, it probably reflects (1) increased pigment load,

(2) decreased liver function due to hypoxemia and hypotension, and (3) decreased renal bilirubin excretion due to varying degrees of tubular necrosis as a result of shock. This diagnostic possibility must be considered in the postoperative patient with marked cholestatic jaundice. The course of the jaundice is self-limited and will subside if the other systemic complications do not predominate and lead to death.

Hepatitis and cirrhosis These disorders, discussed in detail in Chaps. 252 to 254, constitute the *most common disorders associated with jaundice*. As has been stated previously, when the liver cell is damaged, as in viral hepatitis, there is often impairment in all three major hepatic phases of bilirubin metabolism, namely, uptake, conjugation, and excretion. Since the excretory step is the one which is rate-limiting and most readily affected by injury, significant amounts of conjugated bilirubin reenter the systemic circulation. There are also usually lesser increases in the serum unconjugated bilirubin. This phenomenon is probably a reflection of the impaired uptake and conjugation, and is due in part to the shortened life span of red blood cells often found in liver disease. In most patients with hepatitis and cirrhosis, the total serum bilirubin levels tend not to exceed 860 μmol/L (50 mg/dL). (For a summary of laboratory features in icteric states, see Table 251-3.)

EXTRAHEPATIC BILIARY OBSTRUCTION Anatomic or mechanical obstruction of the bile ducts is most commonly due to stones, tumors, or strictures. The clinical picture is quite similar to that of intrahepatic cholestasis with pronounced elevations of the serum conjugated bilirubin and alkaline phosphatase levels. Usually, but not always, fever, pain, and chills may be present. In contrast to hepatitis and cirrhosis, the serum bilirubin level often tends to plateau and rarely exceeds levels of 600 μmol/L (35 mg/dL). The reason for this plateau is not clear but may be related to renal excretion of

TABLE 251-3 Laboratory features in icteric states

Bilirubin disorder	Serum bilirubin Unconjugated	Serum bilirubin Conjugated	Urine bilirubin	Comments
I Overproduction				
A Hemolysis (intra- and extravascular)	↑	N	0	↑ Bilirubin turnover; serum bilirubin rarely exceeds 68 μmol/L (4 mg/dL)
B Ineffective erythropoiesis	↑	N	0	Splenomegaly; normal RBC survival; normoblasts in marrow
II Defective hepatic uptake				
A Some drugs (e.g., flavaspidic acid, novobiocin)	↑	N	0	Normal liver biopsy
B Gilbert's syndrome (some cases)				
III Defective conjugation				
A Neonatal jaundice	↑	Low	0	↓ Glucuronyl transferase; ? ↓ ligandin
B Gilbert's syndrome	↑	Low	0	↓ Glucuronyl transferase and ↓ bilirubin uptake; some may have ↑ hemolysis; bile contains ↑ monoconjugates
C Crigler-Najjar syndrome (types I and II)	↑	Low	0	Type I = absence of transferase; Type II = deficiency of transferase; bile contains ↑↑ monoconjugates
IV Defective excretion				
A Intrahepatic obstruction				
1 Familial syndromes				
a Dubin-Johnson	↑	↑	+	Abnormal BSP curve, hepatic lipochrome pigment; ↑ urinary coproporphyrin type I
b Rotor	↑	↑	+	No liver pigment; ↑ total urinary coproporphyrin
2 Drugs (e.g., chloramphenicol, methyltestosterone)	↑	↑	+	↑ Alkaline phosphatase but other function tests usually normal
3 Benign recurrent cholestasis	↑	↑	+	↑ Alkaline phosphatase
4 Recurrent jaundice of pregnancy (third trimester)	↑	↑	+	↑ Alkaline phosphatase; may be reproduced in afflicted subjects by estrogens or progesterone
B Extrahepatic obstruction (tumors, stone, stricture of bile duct)				↑↑ Alkaline phosphatase (often > fourfold)
1 Partial	↑	↑	+	
2 Complete	↑	↑	+	
V Hepatocellular disease*				
A Hepatitis	↑	↑	+	Conjugated/total serum bilirubin >50–70%; liver biopsy important for diagnosis
B Cirrhosis: Same as hepatitis	↑	↑		

* Note that in hepatocellular disease there is generally an interference in all pathways of bilirubin metabolism (i.e., impaired uptake, conjugation, and excretion).

conjugated bilirubin or alternative pathways of bilirubin catabolism in obstructive jaundice.

REFERENCES

Benign familial recurrent cholestasis

DePagter AGF et al: Familial benign intrahepatic cholestasis. Gastroenterology 71:202, 1976

Endo T et al: Bile acid metabolism in benign recurrent intrahepatic cholestasis. Gastroenterology 76:1002, 1979

Dubin-Johnson and Rotor syndromes

Berk PD et al: Inborn errors of bilirubin metabolism. Med Clin North Am 59:803, 1975

Rosenthal P et al: Homozygous Dubin-Johnson syndrome exhibits a characteristic serum bilirubin pattern. Hepatology 1:540, 1981

Swartz HM et al: On the nature and excretion of the hepatic pigment in the Dubin-Johnson syndrome. Gastroenterology 76:958, 1979

Wolkoff AW et al: Hereditary jaundice and disorders of bilirubin metabolism, in The Metabolic Basis of Inherited Disease, 6th ed. CR Scriver et al (eds). New York, McGraw, 1989, pp 1367–1408

Wolpert E et al: Abnormal sulfobromophthalein metabolism in Rotor's syndrome and obligate heterozygotes. N Engl J Med 206:1099, 1977

Glucuronyl transferase deficiency states

Berthelot P, Dhumeaus D: New insights into the classification and mechanisms of hereditary, chronic, non-hemolytic hyperbilirubinemia. Gut 19:474, 1978

Dawson J et al: Gilbert's syndrome: Evidence of morphologic heterogeneity. Gut 20:848, 1979

Felsher BF, Carpio NM: Caloric intake and unconjugated hyperbilirubinemia. Gastroenterology 69:42, 1975

Fevery J et al: Unconjugated bilirubin and an increased proportion of bilirubin monoconjugates in the bile of patients with Gilbert's syndrome and Crigler-Najjar disease. J Clin Invest 60:970, 1977

Ohkubo H et al: Ursodeoxycholic acid oral tolerance test in patients with constitutional hyperbilirubinemias and effect of phenobarbital. Gastroenterology 81:126, 1981

———— et al: Effects of corticosteroids on bilirubin metabolism in patients with Gilbert's syndrome. Hepatology 1:168, 1981

Olsson R et al: Gilbert's syndrome: does it exist? A study of the prevalence of symptoms in Gilbert's syndrome. Acta Med Scand 224:485, 1988

Postoperative jaundice

Hootegem PV et al: Serum bilirubins in hepatobiliary disease: Comparison with other liver function tests and changes in the postobstructive period. Hepatology 5:112, 1985

Koff RS: Postoperative jaundice. Med Clin North Am 59:823, 1975

LaMont JT, Isselbacher KJ: Postoperative jaundice, in Liver and Biliary Disease, 2d ed, R Wright et al (eds). Philadelphia, Saunders, 1985

252   ACUTE HEPATITIS

JULES L. DIENSTAG / JACK R. WANDS / KURT J. ISSELBACHER

ACUTE VIRAL HEPATITIS

Acute viral hepatitis is a systemic infection affecting the liver predominantly. Five categories of viral agents have been implicated: hepatitis A virus (HAV), hepatitis B virus (HBV), two types of non-A, non-B hepatitis agents, one bloodborne, the other enterically transmitted, and the HBV-associated delta agent. Although these agents can be distinguished by their antigenic properties, all five types produce clinically similar illnesses. These range from asymptomatic and inapparent to fulminant and fatal acute infections common to all five types, on the one hand, and from subclinical persistent infections to rapidly progressive chronic liver disease with cirrhosis and even hepatocellular carcinoma, common to the bloodborne types (HBV, delta, and bloodborne non-A, non-B), on the other.

VIROLOGY AND ETIOLOGY Hepatitis A Hepatitis A virus (HAV) is a nonenveloped 27-nm, heat-, acid-, and ether-resistant RNA virus in the picornavirus family; it has been classified as enterovirus type 72 (Fig. 252-1). Its virion is composed of four polypeptides designated VP1 to VP4. Inactivation of viral activity can be achieved by boiling for 1 min, by contact with formaldehyde and chlorine, or by ultraviolet irradiation. All strains of this virus identified to date are immunologically indistinguishable and belong to one serotype. Hepatitis A has an incubation period of approximately 4 weeks. The virus is present in the liver, bile, stools, and blood during the late incubation period and acute preicteric phase of illness. Despite persistence of virus in the liver, viral shedding in feces, viremia, and infectivity diminish rapidly once jaundice becomes apparent. Unlike other hepatitis viruses, hepatitis A virus can be grown readily in tissue culture. In addition, its 7500-nucleotide genome has been cloned and characterized.

Antibodies to HAV (anti-HAV) can be detected during acute illness when serum aminotransferase activity is elevated and fecal HAV shedding is still occurring. This early antibody response is predominantly of the IgM class and persists for several months. During convalescence, however, anti-HAV of the IgG class becomes the predominant antibody (Fig. 252-2). Therefore, the diagnosis of hepatitis A is made during acute illness by demonstrating high-titer anti-HAV of the IgM class. Following acute illness, anti-HAV of the IgG class remains detectable indefinitely, and patients with serum anti-HAV are immune to reinfection. Indeed, the IgG anti-HAV present in immune globulin accounts for the protection it affords against HAV infection.

Hepatitis B This viral infection is unique in that concentrations of viral antigen and viral particles in the blood may reach 500 μg/mL and 10 trillion particles per milliliter, respectively. Electron-microscopic studies have demonstrated three particulate forms (Table 252-1) of HBV (see Fig. 252-1). The most numerous are the 22-nm particles which appear as spherical or long filamentous forms; these are antigenically identical with the outer surface or coat of HBV, and they are thought to represent excess viral coat protein. Outnumbered in serum by a factor of 100 or 1000 to 1 compared to the spheres and tubules are large 42-nm spherical particles, which represent the intact hepatitis B virion. These large particles consist of an outer coat and an inner icosahedral nucleocapsid core measuring 27 nm in diameter. Previous studies have shown that antiserum obtained from hemophiliacs, who had presumably been exposed repeatedly to hepatitis viruses through multiple blood transfusions, would form a precipitin line by diffusion in agar gel with an antigen present in hepatitis serum. This antigen, identified in the serum of an Australian aborigine, was originally called Australia antigen or hepatitis-associated antigen and is now referred to as hepatitis B surface antigen (HBsAg). The discovery of this antigen provided the first serologic test to distinguish hepatitis B from other types of hepatitis. HBsAg consists primarily of two major polypeptides, one of 24,000 mol wt and its glycosylated counterpart of 28,000 mol wt. A number of different HBsAg subdeterminants have been identified. There is a common group-reactive antigen, a, shared by all HBsAg isolates. In addition, HBsAg may contain one of several subtype-specific antigens, namely, d or y, w or r, as well as other more recently characterized specificities. These HBsAg subtypes provide additional epidemiologic markers in evaluating the transmission of hepatitis B infection in that subtypes "breed true." For example, studies of hepatitis outbreaks have shown that index cases and their contacts have identical HBsAg subtypes. Clinical course and outcome, however, are independent of subtype.

The intact 42-nm virion can be disrupted by mild detergents and the 27-nm nucleocapsid core particle isolated. Naked core particles do not circulate in serum. The antigen expressed on the surface of the nucleocapsid core is referred to as hepatitis B core antigen (HBcAg), and the corresponding antibody is anti-HBc. HBcAg does not cross-react with HBsAg. A third antigen associated with hepatitis B is hepatitis B e antigen (HBeAg). HBeAg is a soluble, nonparticulate antigen which is found only in HBsAg-positive serum and is immunologically and biochemically distinct from HBsAg and intact HBcAg but appears to be an internal component or degradation

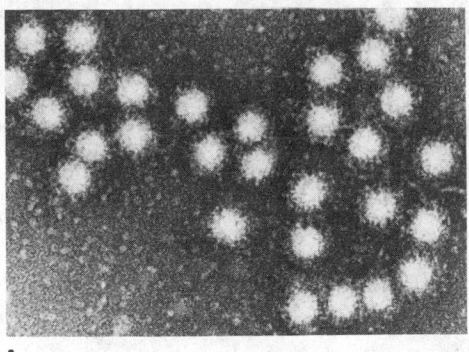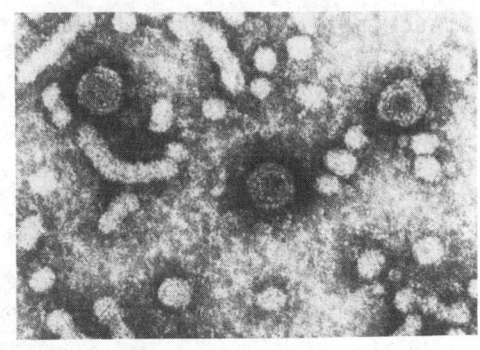

FIGURE 252-1 *A.* Electron micrograph of 27-nm hepatitis A virus particles purified from stool of a patient with acute hepatitis A virus infection and aggregated by hepatitis A antibody. *B.* Electron micrograph of concentrated serum from a patient with acute hepatitis B infection, demonstrating the 42-nm virions, tubular forms, and spherical 22-nm particles of hepatitis B surface antigen. 132,000×.

A   **B**

product of the core of HBV. HBsAg-positive serum containing HBeAg is more likely to be highly infectious and to be associated with the presence of hepatitis B virions (and DNA polymerase and HBV DNA, see below) than HBeAg-negative or anti-HBe-positive serum. For example, HBsAg carrier mothers who are HBeAg-positive almost invariably transmit hepatitis B infection to their offspring, while HBsAg carrier mothers with anti-HBe rarely infect their offspring.

In every individual with acute hepatitis B infection, HBeAg develops transiently, early in the course of illness, but persistent HBeAg positivity correlates with ongoing viral replication and may be associated with continuing disease actvity in chronic hepatitis; its disappearance may be a harbinger of biochemical improvement and potential resolution of infection. Unfortunately HBeAg is not a sufficiently discriminating marker to support prognostic predictions or to substitute for morphologic evaluation of severity in patients with chronic hepatitis.

Within the nucleocapsid core, in addition to HBeAg, is a predominantly double-stranded, but partially single-stranded, DNA genome measuring 3200 nucleotides as well as a DNA polymerase, which directs replication and repair of HBV DNA. In vitro, the polymerase can repair the single-stranded gap and render it double-stranded. Once thought to be unique among viruses, HBV is now recognized as one of a family of animal viruses, hepadnaviruses (hepatotropic DNA viruses), and is classified as hepadnavirus type 1. Viruses similar to HBV infect certain species of woodchucks, ground squirrels, and Pekin ducks, to mention the most carefully characterized. Like HBV, all have the same distinctive three morphologic forms, have counterparts to the virus antigens of HBV, replicate within the liver, contain their own, endogenous DNA polymerase, have partially double-stranded, partially single-stranded genomes, and, for the most part, are associated with acute and chronic hepatitis and hepatocellular carcinoma. Evidence suggests that hepadnaviruses rely on replicative strategies typical of retroviruses. Instead of DNA replication directly

from a DNA template, hepadnaviruses rely on reverse transcription (effected by the DNA polymerase) of minus-strand DNA from an RNA intermediate. Although HBV has not been cultivated in vitro, its genome has been cloned in bacterial, yeast, and mammalian cell vectors and has been completely characterized. Four segments of the genome have been characterized: (1) the pre-S and S gene, which code for HBsAg and several other poorly characterized pre-S gene products, including receptors on the HBV surface for polymerized human serum albumin and hepatocyte receptors; (2) the C gene, which codes for HBcAg and HBeAg; (3) the P gene, which codes for DNA polymerase; and (4) the X gene, which codes for a recently identified protein seen more frequently in patients with chronic hepatitis and hepatocellular carcinoma but which remains to be further characterized. The pre-S region consists of both pre-S1 and pre-S2. The protein product of the S gene is HBsAg ("major protein"); the product of the pre-S2 plus S gene region is the "middle protein"; and the product of the pre-S1 plus pre-S2 plus S regions is the "large protein." Compared to the smaller spherical and tubular particles of HBV, complete virions are enriched in "large protein." Both pre-S proteins and their respective antibodies can be detected during HBV infection. Not only has the HBV genome been cloned but its gene products have been expressed by recombinant vectors. In addition, the delineation of the gene and amino acid maps of HBV has led to the production in the laboratory of synthetic HBsAg polypeptides. Although HBV cannot be cultivated from clinical material in in vitro systems, several cell lines have been transfected with HBV DNA. Such transfected cells support in vitro replication of the intact virus and its component proteins.

After infection with HBV, the first virologic marker detectable in serum is HBsAg (Fig. 252-3). Circulating HBsAg precedes elevations of serum aminotransferase activity and clinical symptoms and remains detectable during the entire icteric or symptomatic phase of acute hepatitis B and beyond. In typical cases, HBsAg becomes undetectable 1 to 2 months following the onset of jaundice and rarely persists beyond 6 months. After HBsAg disappears, antibody to HBsAg (anti-HBs) becomes detectable in serum and remains detectable indefinitely thereafter. Because HBcAg is sequestered within an HBsAg coat, HBcAg is not detectable routinely in the serum of patients with HBV infection. On the other hand, antibody to HBcAg (anti-HBc) is readily demonstrable in serum, beginning within the first 1 to 2 weeks after the appearance of HBsAg and preceding detectable levels of anti-HBs by weeks to months. Because variability exists in the time of appearance of anti-HBs following HBV infection, occasionally a gap of several weeks or longer may separate the disappearance of HBsAg and the appearance of anti-HBs. During this "gap" or "window" period, anti-HBc may represent serologic evidence of current or recent HBV infection, and blood containing anti-HBc in the absence of HBsAg and anti-HBs has been implicated in the development of transfusion-associated hepatitis B. In part because the sensitivity of immunoassays for HBsAg and anti-HBs has increased, however, this window period is rarely encountered. In some persons, years after HBV infection, anti-HBc may persist in the circulation longer than anti-HBs. Therefore, isolated anti-HBc does not necessarily indicate

FIGURE 252-2 Scheme of typical clinical and laboratory features of viral hepatitis type A.

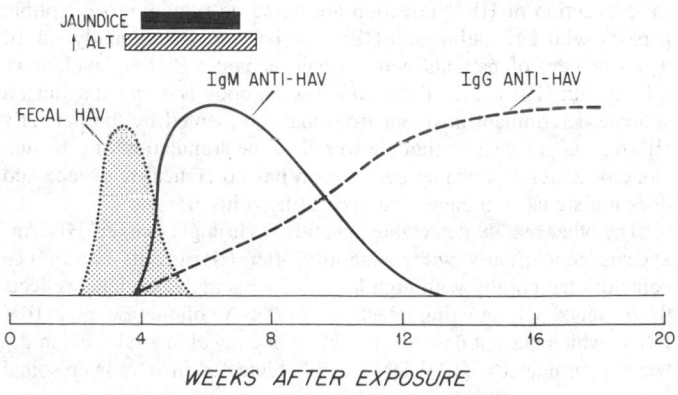

WEEKS AFTER EXPOSURE

TABLE 252-1   Nomenclature and features of hepatitis antigens and antibodies

Hepatitis type	Particle diameter, nm	Description	Antigen	Corresponding antibody	Remarks
A	27	Icosahedral virus particle	Hepatitis A virus (HAV)	Hepatitis A antibody (anti-HAV)	RNA virus; present in stool and serum early in course of hepatitis A
B	42	Intact virion (surface and core); spherical	Hepatitis B surface antigen (HBsAg) Hepatitis B core antigen (HBcAg)	Hepatitis B surface antibody (anti-HBs) Hepatitis B core antibody (anti-HBc)	DNA virus; found in serum
	27	Nucleocapsid core of virion, icosahedral	HBcAg	Anti-HBc	Core contains DNA and DNA polymerase; present in hepatocyte nuclei but not in serum Anti-HBc detected in serum during and after acute infection
	22	Appear as spherical and filamentous forms; both have same antigenic properties as surface of virion; represent excess viral coat material	HBsAg	Anti-HBs	HBsAg detectable in > 90% of patients with acute hepatitis B; found in serum, body fluids, and hepatocyte cytoplasm Anti-HBs appears following B infection; protective antibody
	Nonparticulate	Soluble protein, internal component of nucleocapsid	Hepatitis B e antigen (HBeAg)	Hepatitis B e antibody (anti-HBe)	HBeAg found in HBsAg-positive serum only, correlates with infectivity and presence of intact virus particles
C	(presumed 30–60 nm)	Particle not identified	HCAg	Anti-HCV	10,000 nucleotide single-stranded RNA virus; cause of bloodborne non-A, non-B hepatitis; antibody appears after 1 to 3 months
D	35–37	Hybrid particle with HBsAg coat and delta nucleocapsid core	Hepatitis delta antigen (HDAg)	Hepatitis delta antibody (anti-HD)	Defective RNA virus, requires helper function of HBV
E	27–32 nm	Icosahedral virus particle	HEAg	Anti-HEV	RNA virus present in stool; cause of enteric non-A, non-B hepatitis

active virus replication; most instances of isolated anti-HBc represent hepatitis B infection in the remote past. Distinction between recent and remote HBV infection can be accomplished by determination of the immunoglobulin class of anti-HBc. Anti-HBc of the IgM class (IgM anti-HBc) predominates during the first approximately 6 months after acute infection, whereas IgG anti-HBc is the predominant class of anti-HBc beyond 6 months. Therefore, patients with current or recent acute hepatitis B, including those in the anti-HBc window,

FIGURE 252-3 Scheme of typical clinical and laboratory features of acute viral hepatitis type B.

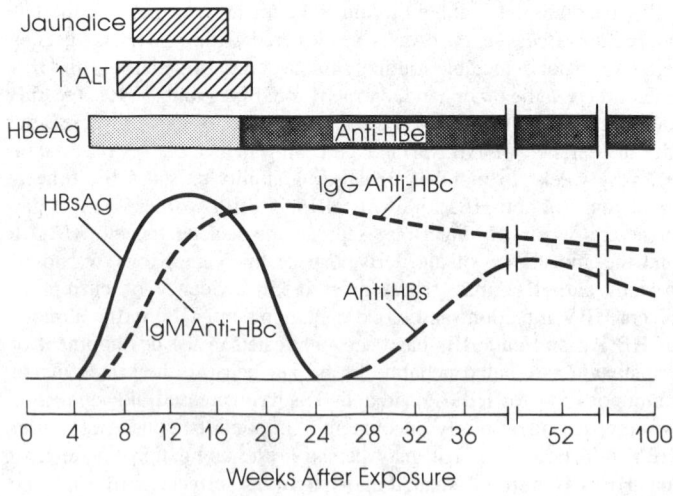

have IgM anti-HBc in their serum. In patients who have recovered from hepatitis B in the remote past as well as those with chronic HBV infection, anti-HBc is predominantly of the IgG class. Infrequently, in no more than 1 to 5 percent of patients with acute HBV infection, levels of HBsAg are too low to be detected; in such cases, the presence of IgM anti-HBc establishes the diagnosis of acute hepatitis B. Similarly, isolated anti-HBc may occur in the rare patient with chronic hepatitis B whose HBsAg level is below the sensitivity threshold of contemporary immunoassays (a low-level carrier); in such cases, the anti-HBc is of the IgG class. Generally, in persons who have recovered from hepatitis B, anti-HBs and anti-HBc persist indefinitely.

The temporal association between the appearance of anti-HBs and resolution of HBV infection as well as the observation that persons with anti-HBs in serum are protected against reinfection with HBV suggest that *anti-HBs is the protective antibody.* Therefore, strategies for prevention of HBV infection are based on providing susceptible persons with circulating anti-HBs (see below). Occasionally, in 10 to 20 percent of patients with chronic hepatitis B, low-level, low-affinity anti-HBs can be detected. This antibody is directed against a subtype determinant different from that represented by the patient's HBsAg; its presence is thought to reflect the stimulation of a related clone of antibody forming cells, but it has no clinical relevance and does not signal imminent clearance of hepatitis B.

The other readily detectable hepatitis B virologic marker, HBeAg, appears concurrently with or shortly after HBsAg. Its appearance coincides temporally with high levels of virus replication and reflects the presence of circulating intact virions, DNA polymerase, and HBV DNA, which are not detected routinely in clinical laboratories; in the hepatocyte nucleus, HBV DNA can be detected in free or episomal form. This *replicative* stage of HBV infection is the time of maximal infectivity. In self-limited HBV infections, HBeAg becomes undetectable shortly after peak elevations in aminotransferase activity, before the disappearance of HBsAg, and anti-HBe then becomes detectable, coinciding with a period of relatively lower infectivity (Fig. 252-3). In protracted HBV infection, HBeAg may remain detectable, indicating persistent replicative infection. When HBeAg is absent and anti-HBe present in chronic hepatitis B, infection is usually *nonreplicative*. In this phase of chronic infection, when HBV DNA is demonstrable in hepatocyte nuclei, it tends to be integrated into the host genome. In the nonreplicative phase, only spherical and tubular forms of HBV, *not intact virions,* circulate. Occasionally, nonreplicative HBV infection converts back to replicative infection. Such spontaneous reactivations are accompanied by reexpression of HBeAg and HBV DNA as well as by exacerbations of liver injury.

Hepatitis B antigens and DNA have been identified in extrahepatic tissues, such as lymph nodes, bone marrow, circulating lymphocytes, spleen, and pancreas. The clinical relevance of these findings remains obscure.

Delta hepatitis The delta hepatitis agent, hepatitis D virus (HDV), is a defective RNA virus which coinfects with and requires the helper function of HBV for its replication and expression. Slightly smaller than HBV, delta is a formalin-sensitive, 35- to 37-nm virus with a hybrid structure. Its nucleocapsid expresses delta antigen, which bears no antigenic homology with any of the HBV antigens, and contains a small, 1700-nucleotide RNA genome that is nonhomologous with HBV DNA but that has features of plant satellite viruses or viroids. This delta core is "encapsidated" by an outer coat of HBsAg. Thus, delta can either infect a person simultaneously with HBV ("coinfection") or superinfect a person already infected with HBV ("superinfection"); when delta infection is transmitted from a donor with one HBsAg subtype to an HBsAg-positive recipient with a different subtype, the delta agent assumes the HBsAg subtype of the recipient, rather than the donor. Because delta relies absolutely on HBV, the duration of delta infection is determined by the duration of and cannot outlast HBV infection. Delta antigen is expressed primarily in hepatocyte nuclei and is occasionally detectable in serum. During acute delta infection, anti-delta of the IgM class predominates; in self-limited infection, anti-delta is low-titer and transient, rarely remaining detectable beyond the clearance of HBsAg and delta antigen. In chronic delta infection, anti-delta circulates in high titer, and both IgM and IgG anti-delta can be detected. Delta antigen in the liver and delta RNA in serum and liver can be detected during HDV replication.

Non-A, non-B hepatitis Sensitive serologic tests for identifying both types A and B hepatitis have led to the identification of hepatitis cases with incubation periods and modes of transmission consistent with an infectious disease but without serologic evidence of hepatitis A or B infection. Identified initially among recipients of transfused blood, these cases of so-called non-A, non-B hepatitis have not been associated serologically with Epstein-Barr virus or cytomegalovirus (except in rare instances) or with other viruses known to involve the liver. Long before a non-A, non-B hepatitis virus had been identified definitively, cross-challenge studies in chimpanzees suggested that there are at least two different bloodborne non-A, non-B hepatitis agents. One has been isolated from clotting factor VIII concentrates, is chloroform-sensitive, and induces ultrastructural cytoplasmic tubular changes in hepatocytes. The other has been isolated from clotting factor IX concentrates, is chloroform-resistant, and does not induce cytoplasmic tubular changes in hepatocytes. The former type appears to be the most frequently encountered after blood transfusion.

An almost 15-year quest to identify an agent of non-A, non-B viral hepatitis ended in 1988 with the identification of an RNA virus with immunologic specificity for transfusion-associated non-A, non-B hepatitis. Among complementary DNA (cDNA) fragments cloned in *Escherichia coli* from the pellet of a chimpanzee plasma with unusually high infectivity, one clone expressed a protein that reacted with antibody in convalescent serum but not preillness serum from

chimpanzees with experimentally induced non-A, non-B hepatitis. This viral antigen was found as well in the livers of infected, but not uninfected-control, chimpanzees. Most chimpanzees and humans studied with well-pedigreed transfusion-related non-A, non-B hepatitis acquire antibody to this virus between 1 and 3 months after the onset of acute illness. Validation of an immunoassay for antibody to this agent came most convincingly from its ability to distinguish, in panels of coded serum samples, between pedigreed non-A, non-B hepatitis cases and pedigreed negative, noninfectious samples as well as other-disease controls. The virus appears to be a single-stranded RNA virus with a genome of approximately 10,000 nucleotides. It has *no homology with HBV*, retroviruses, or other hepatitis viruses; however, its genome, size, and stability are consistent with its inclusion in the togavirus family of lipid-enveloped agents that includes the arboviruses (such as yellow fever and dengue viruses) and rubella virus. Only one continuous open reading frame (gene) has been identified. This agent has been named *hepatitis C virus (HCV)*. The question remains whether this is the only agent of "bloodborne" non-A, non-B hepatitis or whether another agent will be identified, as suggested by the chimpanzee cross-challenge studies cited above. Because the titer of this agent in serum is so low, practical diagnostic tests for virus antigen remain to be developed.

In addition, a distinct type of waterborne non-A, non-B hepatitis has been identified in India, Asia, and Central America (so-called epidemic or enteric non-A, non-B hepatitis), which, because of its epidemiologic resemblance to hepatitis A, has been labeled by some "non-A hepatitis" and has been classified provisionally as "hepatitis E" (for enteric) virus (HEV). Enteric non-A, non-B hepatitis is caused by a 27- to 32-nm HAV-like virus; however, there is no genomic or antigenic homology between the enteric non-A, non-B agent and HAV or other picornaviruses. This virus has been detected in stools from patients with epidemic non-A, non-B hepatitis and has been transmitted serially in chimpanzees. Fecal excretion of the virus and immune responses to it have been documented in experimentally infected chimpanzees. Routine tests for clinical purposes, however, have not yet been developed. Details of virologic events and humoral immune responses remain to be described.

PATHOGENESIS While data on the pathogenesis of hepatitis A, non-A, non-B hepatitis, and delta hepatitis are very limited, evidence suggests that the clinical manifestations of and outcomes following acute liver injury associated with HBV infection are determined by the immunologic responses of the host. The existence of asymptomatic hepatitis B carriers with normal liver histology and function suggests that the virus is not directly cytopathic. The facts that lymphoid cells are juxtaposed with necrotic hepatocytes in the livers of patients with liver injury and that patients with defects in cellular immune competence are more likely to remain chronically infected rather than to clear the virus are cited to support the role of cellular immune responses in the pathogenesis of hepatitis B–related liver injury. To date, however, because adequate animal and laboratory models are lacking, support for this hypothesis remains circumstantial. Still, the model that has the most experimental support involves cytolytic T cells sensitized specifically to recognize host and hepatitis B viral antigens on the liver cell surface. Although HBsAg was initially thought to be the most likely viral target antigen on the hepatocyte surface, recent laboratory observations suggest that HBcAg, present on the cell membrane in minute quantities, is the viral target antigen that, with host antigens, invites cytolytic T cells to destroy HBV-infected hepatocytes. Debate does continue, however, over the relative importance of viral and host factors in the pathogenesis of liver injury associated with hepatitis B and its outcome.

Although the mechanism of HBV-induced liver injury remains uncertain, immune complex–mediated tissue damage appears to play a major pathogenetic role in the extrahepatic manifestations of acute hepatitis B. The occasional prodromal serum sickness–like syndrome observed in acute hepatitis B appears to be related to the deposition in tissue blood vessel walls of circulating immune complexes leading to activation of the complement system. The clinical consequences are urticarial rash, angioedema, fever, and arthritis. During the early prodrome of hepatitis B in these patients, HBsAg in high titer in association with small amounts of anti-HBs leads to the formation of soluble, circulating immune complexes (in antigen excess). Complement components in the serum are depressed during the arthritic phase of the illness and are also detectable in the circulating immune complexes. In addition to complement components, these complexes contain HBsAg, anti-HBs, IgG, IgM, IgA, and fibrin. After the patient recovers from the serum sickness–like syndrome, these immune complexes disappear.

In patients who become carriers of HBsAg following acute hepatitis, other types of immune-complex disease may be seen. Glomerulonephritis with the nephrotic syndrome is occasionally observed; HBsAg, immunoglobulin, and C3 deposition has been found in the glomerular basement membrane. While polyarteritis nodosa develops in considerably fewer than 1 percent of patients with hepatitis B, 20 to 30 percent of patients with polyarteritis nodosa have HBsAg in serum. In these patients, the affected small and medium-sized arterioles have been shown to contain HBsAg, immunoglobulins, and complement components.

PATHOLOGY   The typical morphologic lesions of hepatitis A, B, delta, and non-A, non-B are often similar and consist of panlobular infiltration with mononuclear cells, hepatic cell necrosis, hyperplasia of Kupffer cells, and variable degrees of cholestasis. Hepatic cell regeneration is present, as evidenced by numerous mitotic figures, multinucleated cells, and "rosette" or "pseudoacinar" formation. The mononuclear infiltration consists primarily of small lymphocytes, although plasma cells and eosinophils are occasionally seen. Liver cell damage consists of hepatic cell degeneration and necrosis, cell dropout, ballooning of cells, and acidophilic degeneration of hepatocytes (forming so-called Councilman-like bodies). Large hepatocytes with a ground glass appearance of the cytoplasm may be seen in chronic but not in acute hepatitis B; these cells have been shown to contain HBsAg and can be identified histochemically with orcein or aldehyde fuchsin. In uncomplicated viral hepatitis, the reticulin framework is preserved.

In bloodborne non-A, non-B hepatitis, the histologic lesion is often remarkable for a relative paucity of inflammation, a marked increase in activation of sinusoidal lining cells, the presence of fat, and occasionally bile duct lesions in which biliary epithelial cells appear to be piled up without interruption of the basement membrane.

In enteric non-A, non-B hepatitis, a common histologic feature is marked cholestasis.

A more severe histologic lesion, *bridging hepatic necrosis,* also termed *subacute* or *confluent necrosis,* is occasionally observed in some patients with acute hepatitis. "Bridging" between lobules results from large areas of hepatic cell dropout, with collapse of the reticulin framework. Characteristically, the bridge consists of condensed reticulum, inflammatory debris, and degenerating liver cells that span adjacent portal areas, portal to central veins, or central vein to central vein. This lesion has been thought to have prognostic significance; in many of the originally described patients with this lesion, a subacute course terminated in death within several weeks to months, or chronic active hepatitis and postnecrotic cirrhosis developed. More recent investigations have failed to uphold the association between bridging necrosis and such a poor prognosis in patients with acute hepatitis. Although the frequency of bridging may be higher among hospitalized patients with severe acute hepatitis, and although cirrhosis, chronic hepatitis, and even death have been observed in this group, the frequency of bridging necrosis in uncomplicated acute viral hepatitis is probably on the order of 1 to 5 percent. Prospective studies have failed to demonstrate a difference in prognosis between patients with acute hepatitis who have bridging necrosis and those who do not. Therefore, although demonstration of this lesion in patients with chronic hepatitis has prognostic significance (see Chap. 253), its demonstration during acute hepatitis is less meaningful, and liver biopsies to identify this lesion are no longer undertaken routinely in patients with acute hepatitis. In *massive*

hepatic necrosis (fulminant hepatitis, acute yellow atrophy), the striking feature at postmortem examination is the finding of a small, shrunken, and soft liver. Histologic examination reveals massive necrosis and dropout of liver cells of most lobules with extensive collapse and condensation of the reticulin framework.

Immunofluorescence and immunoperoxidase antibody studies have been instrumental in localizing HBsAg to the cytoplasm and plasma membrane of infected liver cells. In contrast, HBcAg predominates in the nucleus, but, occasionally, scant amounts are also seen in the cytoplasm and on the cell membrane. Electron-microscopic studies of liver biopsy material have demonstrated the presence of HBsAg particles in the cytoplasm and HBcAg particles in the nucleus of liver cells during hepatitis B infection. These morphologic observations suggest that DNA is synthesized and packaged within core particles in the nucleus, while the surface coat is assembled in the cytoplasm, resulting in the formation of intact hepatitis B virus. Delta antigen is localized to the hepatocyte nucleus, while HAV antigen is localized to the cytoplasm.

EPIDEMIOLOGY   Prior to the availability of serologic tests for hepatitis viruses, all viral hepatitis cases were labeled either as "infectious" or "serum" hepatitis. Modes of transmission overlap, however, and *a clear distinction among the different types of viral hepatitis cannot be made solely on the basis of clinical or epidemiologic features* (Table 252-2). The most accurate means to distinguish the various types of viral hepatitis involves specific serologic testing.

Hepatitis A   *This agent is transmitted almost exclusively by the fecal-oral route.* Spread of HAV is enhanced by poor personal hygiene and overcrowding, and large outbreaks as well as sporadic cases have been traced to contaminated food, water, milk, and shellfish. Intrafamily and intrainstitutional spread are also common. Early epidemiologic observations suggested that there is a predilection for hepatitis A to occur in late fall and early winter. In temperate zones, epidemic waves have been recorded every 5 to 20 years as new segments of nonimmune population appeared; however, in developed countries, the incidence of type A hepatitis has been declining, presumably as a function of improved sanitation, and these cyclic patterns are no longer being observed. No HAV carrier state has been identified after acute type A hepatitis; perpetuation of the virus in nature depends presumably on nonepidemic, inapparent subclinical infection.

In the general population, anti-HAV, an excellent marker for previous HAV infection, increases in prevalence as a function of increasing age and of decreasing socioeconomic status. Serologic evidence of prior hepatitis A infection occurs in about 40 percent of urban populations in the United States, fewer than 5 percent of whom recall having had a symptomatic case of hepatitis. In developing countries, exposure, infection, and subsequent immunity are almost universal in childhood. As the frequency of subclinical childhood infections declines in developed countries, a susceptible cohort of adults emerges. Hepatitis A tends to be more symptomatic in adults; therefore, paradoxically, as the frequency of HAV infection declines, the likelihood of clinically apparent, even severe, HAV illnesses increases in the susceptible adult population. Travel to endemic areas is a common source of infection for adults from nonendemic areas.

Hepatitis B   It has long been recognized that a major route of hepatitis B transmission is percutaneous, but the outmoded designation "serum hepatitis" is an inaccurate label for the epidemiologic spectrum of HBV infection recognized today. As detailed below, most of the hepatitis transmitted by blood transfusion is not caused by HBV; moreover, in approximately half of patients with acute type B hepatitis, there is no history of an identifiable percutaneous exposure. We now recognize that many cases of type B hepatitis result from less obvious modes of nonpercutaneous or covert percutaneous transmission. HBsAg has been identified in almost every body fluid from infected persons—saliva, tears, seminal fluid, cerebrospinal fluid, ascites, breast milk, synovial fluid, gastric juice, pleural fluid and urine and even rarely in feces. Although there is abundant evidence to suggest that feces are not infectious, at least some of these body fluids—most notably semen and saliva—have been shown

TABLE 252-2 Comparisons of type A, type B, and non-A, non-B hepatitis

Feature	Hepatitis A	Hepatitis B*	Non-A, non-B hepatitis Bloodborne (hepatitis C)	Enteric (hepatitis E)
Incubation	15–45 days (mean 30)	30–180 days (mean 60–90)	15–160 (mean 50)	14–60 (mean 40)
Onset	Acute	Often insidious	Insidious	Acute
Age preference	Children, young adults	Any age	Any age but more common in adults	Young adults (20–40 years)
Transmission route:				
Fecal-oral	+ + +	–	Unknown	+ + +
Other nonpercutaneous†	+/–	+ +	+ +	+/–
Percutaneous	Unusual	+ + +	+ + +	–
Severity	Mild	Often severe	Moderate	Mild
Prognosis	Generally good	Worse with age, debility	Moderate	Good
Progression to chronicity	None	Occasional (5–10%)	Occasional (10–50%)	None
Prophylaxis	IG	Standard IG (not documented) HBIG, hepatitis B vaccine	?	?
Carrier	None	0.1–30%‡	Approximately 1%	None

* Concomitant delta hepatitis is similar in these features to hepatitis B, but more severe outcomes are favored.
† For example, sexual or maternal-neonatal contact.
‡ Varies considerably throughout the world, see text.

to be infectious, albeit less so than serum, when administered percutaneously or nonpercutaneously to experimental animals. Among the nonpercutaneous modes of HBV transmission, oral ingestion has been documented as a potential route of exposure but one whose efficiency is quite low. On the other hand, the two nonpercutaneous routes considered to have the greatest impact are intimate (especially sexual) contact and perinatal transmission.

In sub-Saharan Africa, intimate contact among toddlers is considered instrumental in contributing to the maintenance of the high frequency of HBsAg in the population. Perinatal transmission occurs primarily in infants born to HBsAg carrier mothers or mothers with acute hepatitis B during the third trimester of pregnancy or during the early postpartum period. Perinatal transmission is uncommon in North America and western Europe but occurs with great frequency and is the most important mode of HBV perpetuation in the Far East and developing countries. Although the precise mode of perinatal transmission is unknown, and although approximately 10 percent of infections may be acquired in utero, epidemiologic evidence suggests that most infections occur approximately at the time of delivery and are not related to breast feeding. Likelihood of perinatal transmission of HBV correlates with the presence of HBeAg; 90 percent of HBeAg-positive mothers but only 10 to 15 percent of anti-HBe-positive mothers transmit HBV infection to their offspring. In most cases, acute infection in the neonate is clinically asymptomatic, but the child is very likely to become an HBsAg carrier.

The more than 200 million HBsAg carriers in the world constitute the main reservoir of hepatitis B in human beings. Serum HBsAg is infrequent (0.1 to 0.5 percent) in normal populations in the United States and western Europe; however, a prevalence of up to 5 to 20 percent has been found in the far east and in some tropical countries, and as high as 30 percent in persons with Down's syndrome, lepromatous leprosy, leukemia, Hodgkin's disease, polyarteritis nodosa, patients with chronic renal disease on hemodialysis, and needle-using drug addicts.

Other groups with high rates of HBV infection include spouses of acutely infected persons, sexually promiscuous persons (especially promiscuous homosexual men), health care workers exposed to blood, persons who require repeated transfusions especially with pooled blood product concentrates (e.g., hemophiliacs), residents and staff of custodial institutions for the mentally retarded, prisoners, and, to a lesser extent, family members of chronically infected patients. In volunteer blood donors, the prevalence of anti-HBs, a reflection of previous HBV infection, ranges from 5 to 10 percent, but the prevalence is higher in lower socioeconomic strata, older age groups, and persons—including those mentioned above—exposed to blood products.

Prevalence of infection, modes of transmission, and human

behavior conspire to mold geographically different epidemiologic patterns of HBV infection. In the Far East and Africa, hepatitis B, a disease of the newborn and young children, is perpetuated by a cycle of maternal-neonatal spread. In North America and western Europe, hepatitis B is primarily a disease of adolescence and early adulthood, the time of life when intimate sexual contact as well as recreational and occupational percutaneous exposures tend to occur.

Delta hepatitis Infection with the delta agent has a worldwide distribution, but two epidemiologic patterns exist. In Mediterranean countries (northern Africa, southern Europe, the Middle East), delta infection is endemic among those with hepatitis B, and the disease is transmitted predominantly by nonpercutaneous means, especially close personal contact. In nonendemic areas, such as the United States and northern Europe, delta infection is confined to persons exposed frequently to blood and blood products, primarily drug addicts and hemophiliacs. Delta hepatitis can be introduced into a population through drug addicts or by migration of persons from endemic to nonendemic areas. Thus, patterns of population migration and human behavior facilitating percutaneous contact play important roles in the introduction and amplification of delta infection. Occasionally, the migrating epidemiology of delta hepatitis is expressed in explosive outbreaks of severe hepatitis, such as those that have occurred in remote South American villages as well as in urban centers in the United States. Ultimately, such outbreaks of delta hepatitis—either of coinfections with acute hepatitis B or of superinfections in those already infected with HBV—may blur the distinctions between endemic and nonendemic areas.

Non-A, non-B hepatitis (hepatitis C) Routine screening of blood donors for HBsAg and the elimination of commercial blood sources have markedly decreased the frequency of hepatitis B after transfusion, but posttransfusion hepatitis still remains an important medical problem. The likelihood of posttransfusion hepatitis has been reported to be from 0.3 to 9 cases per 1000 units transfused, and the risk of anicteric hepatitis following transfusion is much greater than that of clinical hepatitis with jaundice. The risk of viral hepatitis after transfusion of blood derivatives is dependent on the methods by which these products are processed. The *greatest risk* follows the use of multiple pooled donor products such as concentrates of factors II, VII, VIII, IX, and X. Hepatitis has developed in 20 to 30 percent of individuals receiving these pooled products for the first time. Blood products associated with an *average risk* include whole blood, packed red blood cells, single donor platelets, and plasma. Products such as albumin and immune and hyperimmune globulin, because of prior treatment of these substances by heating to 60°C or by cold ethanol extraction, involve *no risk*. It had been suggested that frozen, glycerol-treated, washed red blood cells may carry a reduced risk of hepatitis, but this has been disproved.

Currently, hepatitis B accounts for only 5 to 10 percent of posttransfusion hepatitis. More of a problem is the occurrence of non-A, non-B hepatitis, which, prior to the development of a virus-specific screening test, accounted for approximately 90 to 95 percent or more of posttransfusion hepatitis cases following transfusion of voluntarily donated blood prescreened for HBsAg. The fact that non-A, non-B hepatitis is transmitted by transfused blood from asymptomatic donors (Table 252-2) and that it can be transmitted to chimpanzees by blood from patients with chronic hepatitis suggests that there is a carrier state for it. The frequency of posttransfusion non-A, non-B hepatitis approaches 5 to 10 percent of blood recipients, especially recipients of multiple units of blood products. Now that there is a serologic screening test to identify the major agent of this hepatitis, reduction and even elimination of infection due to transfusion may be possible.

In addition to being transmitted by transfusion, non-A, non-B hepatitis cases have been observed in other settings of percutaneous and nonpercutaneous exposure, e.g., intrafamily contact, intravenous drug abuse, occupational contact, nosocomial infection, use of hemodialysis units, and intrainstitutional contact. Special attention is merited by non-A, non-B hepatitis in hemophiliacs, in whom the incubation period may be as brief as 1 to 4 weeks, and in renal transplant recipients, up to 20 percent of whom have chronic liver disease. In the early years after transplantation, the death rate in patients with hepatitis is higher, as a result not of liver failure but of severe infections outside the hepatobiliary tree. However, 5 to 10 years after transplantation complications of chronic liver disease account for increased morbidity and mortality.

In western countries, non-A, non-B hepatitis accounts for approximately 15 to 30 percent of sporadic cases of viral hepatitis presenting for medical evaluation. Occurrence of multiple bouts of among drug abusers and hemophiliacs reinforces cross-challenge studies in chimpanzees that suggest that there is more than one such bloodborne agent. Eight percent of patients with transfusion-associated non-A, non-B hepatitis and 50 to 60 percent with the sporadic form have detectable anti-HCV; whether a more sensitive test for anti-HCV will raise these frequencies, or whether another non-A, non-B virus accounts for the residual cases, remains to be seen.

Non-A, non-B hepatitis (hepatitis E) Enteric non-A, non-B hepatitis identified in India, Asia, Africa, and Central America resembles hepatitis A in its primarily enteric mode of spread. The commonly recognized cases occur after contamination of water supplies as after monsoon flooding, but sporadic, isolated cases occur. Infections arise in populations that are immune to HAV, and favor young adults. It is not known if the E form occurs outside of recognized endemic areas, for example, in the United States, or if it accounts for any of the sporadic non-A, non-B cases in nonendemic areas. Cases imported from endemic areas have been found in the United States.

CLINICAL AND LABORATORY FEATURES Symptoms and signs The *prodromal symptoms* of acute viral hepatitis are systemic and quite variable. Constitutional symptoms of anorexia, nausea and vomiting, fatigue, malaise, arthralgias, myalgias, headache, photophobia, pharyngitis, cough, and coryza may precede the onset of jaundice by 1 to 2 weeks. The nausea, vomiting, and anorexia are frequently associated wth alterations in olfaction and taste. A low-grade fever between 38 and 39°C/(100 to 102°F) is more often present in hepatitis A than in non-A, non-B or B, except when hepatitis B is heralded by a serum sickness–like syndrome; rarely, a fever of 39.5 to 40°C/(103 to 104°F) may accompany the constitutional symptoms. Dark urine and clay-colored stools may be noticed by the patient from 1 to 5 days prior to the onset of clinical jaundice.

With the onset of *clinical jaundice* the constitutional prodromal symptoms usually diminish, but in some patients mild weight loss (2.5 to 5 kg) is common and may continue during the entire icteric phase. The liver becomes enlarged and tender and may be associated with right upper quadrant pain and discomfort. Infrequently, patients present with a cholestatic picture, suggesting extrahepatic biliary obstruction. Splenomegaly and cervical adenopathy are present in 10 to 20 percent of patients with acute hepatitis. Rarely, a few spider angiomas appear during the icteric phase and disappear during convalescence. During the *recovery phase,* constitutional symptoms disappear, but usually some liver enlargement and abnormalities in biochemical tests of hepatic function are still evident. The duration of the posticteric phase is variable, ranging from 2 to 12 weeks, and usually is more prolonged in acute hepatitis B and in non-A, non-B hepatitis. Complete clinical and biochemical recovery is to be expected 1 to 2 months after all cases of hepatitis A and E and 3 to 4 months after the onset of jaundice in three-quarters of uncomplicated cases of hepatitis B and C. In the remainder biochemical recovery may be delayed. A substantial proportion of patients with viral hepatitis never become icteric.

Infection with the delta agent (HDV) can occur in the presence of acute or chronic HBV infection; the duration of HBV infection determines the duration of delta infection. When acute delta and HBV infection occur simultaneously, clinical and biochemical features may be indistinguishable from those of HBV infection alone. As opposed to patients with *acute* HBV infection, patients with *chronic* HBV infection can support HDV replication indefinitely. This can happen when acute HDV infection occurs in the presence of a nonresolving acute HBV infection. More commonly, acute HDV infection becomes chronic when it is superimposed on an underlying chronic HBV infection. In such cases, the delta superinfection appears as a clinical exacerbation or an episode resembling acute viral hepatitis in someone already chronically infected with HBV. In the past, events resembling acute hepatitis in a HBV carrier or a patient with chronic hepatitis B were attributed to superimposed non-A, non-B hepatitis or to the natural history of the disease. A proportion of such episodes, however, represent acute superinfection with HDV. Delta superinfection in a patient with chronic hepatitis B often leads to clinical deterioration (see below).

In addition to superinfections with other hepatitis agents, acute hepatitis-like clinical events in persons with chronic hepatitis B may accompany spontaneous HBeAg–to–anti-HBe seroconversion or spontaneous reactivation, i.e., reversion from nonreplicative to replicative infection. Such reactivations can occur as well in therapeutically immunosuppressed patients with chronic HBV infection when cytotoxic-immunosuppressive drugs are withdrawn; in these cases, restoration of immune competence is thought to allow resumption of previously checked cell-mediated cytolysis of HBV-infected hepatocytes.

Laboratory features The serum aminotransferases AST and ALT (previously designated SGOT and SGPT) show a variable increase during the prodromal phase of acute viral hepatitis and precede the rise in bilirubin level (see Figs. 252-2 and 252-3). The acute level of these enzymes, however, does not correlate well with the degree of liver cell damage. Peak levels vary from 400 to 4000 IU or more; these levels are usually reached at the time the patient is clinically icteric and diminish progressively during the recovery phase of acute hepatitis. The diagnosis of anicteric hepatitis is difficult and requires a high index of suspicion; it is based on clinical features and on aminotransferase elevations, although mild increases in conjugated bilirubin may also be found.

Jaundice is usually visible in the sclera or skin when the serum bilirubin value exceeds 43 μmol/L (2.5 mg/dL). When jaundice appears, the serum bilirubin typically rises to levels ranging from 85 to 340 μmol/L (5 to 20 mg/dL). The serum bilirubin may continue to rise despite falling serum aminotransferase levels. In most instances the total bilirubin is equally divided between the conjugated and unconjugated fractions. Bilirubin levels above 340 μmol/L (20 mg/dL) extending and persisting late into the course of viral hepatitis are more likely to be associated with severe disease. In certain patients with underlying hemolytic anemia, however, such as glucose-6-phosphate dehydrogenase deficiency and sickle cell anemia, high serum bilirubin is common, resulting from superimposed hemolysis. In such patients bilirubin levels greater than 513 μmol/L (30 mg/dL) have been observed and are not necessarily associated with a poor prognosis.

Neutropenia and lymphopenia are transient and are followed by a relative lymphocytosis. Atypical lymphocytes (varying between 2 and 20 percent) are common during the acute phase. These atypical lymphocytes are indistinguishable from those seen in infectious mononucleosis. Measurement of the prothrombin time (PT) is important in patients with acute viral hepatitis, for a prolonged value may reflect a severe synthetic defect, signify extensive hepatocellular necrosis, and indicate a worse prognosis. Occasionally a prolonged PT may occur with only mild increases in the serum bilirubin and aminotransferase levels. Prolonged nausea and vomiting, inadequate carbohydrate intake, and poor hepatic glycogen reserves may contribute to hypoglycemia noted occasionally in patients with severe viral hepatitis. Serum alkaline phosphatase may be normal or only mildly elevated, while a fall in serum albumin is uncommon in uncomplicated acute viral hepatitis. In some patients mild and transient steatorrhea has been noted as well as slight microscopic hematuria and minimal proteinuria.

A diffuse but mild elevation of the gamma globulin fraction is common during acute viral hepatitis. Serum IgG and IgM are elevated in about one-third of patients during the acute phase of viral hepatitis, but serum IgM elevation is seen more characteristically during acute hepatitis A. During the acute phase of viral hepatitis, antibodies to smooth muscle and other cell constituents may be present, and low titers of rheumatoid factor, antinuclear antibody, and heterophil antibody can also be found occasionally. These antibodies are nonspecific and can also be associated with other viral and systemic diseases. In contrast, virus-specific antibodies, which appear during and after hepatitis virus infection, are serologic markers of diagnostic importance.

As described above, serologic tests are available with which to establish a diagnosis of hepatitis A, B, delta, and C. Tests for fecal or serum HAV are not routinely available. Therefore, a diagnosis of type A hepatitis is based on detection of IgM anti-HAV during acute illness (Fig. 252-2). Rheumatoid factor can give rise to false-positive results in this test.

A diagnosis of HBV infection can usually be made by detection of HBsAg in serum. Infrequently, levels of HBsAg are too low to be detected during acute HBV infection even with the current generation of highly sensitive immunoassays. In such cases, the diagnosis can be established by the presence of IgM anti-HBc. Alternatively, de novo appearance of anti-HBc and anti-HBs during illness and convalescence may support the diagnostic impression.

The titer of HBsAg bears little relation to the severity of clinical disease. Indeed, there may be an inverse correlation between the serum concentration of HBsAg and the degree of liver cell damage.

For example, titers are highest in immunosuppressed patients, lower in chronic liver disease (but higher in chronic persistent than in chronic active hepatitis), and very low in acute fulminant hepatitis. These observations suggest that in hepatitis B the degree of liver cell damage and the clinical course are probably related to variations in the patient's immune response to HBV rather than to the amount of circulating HBsAg. In immunocompetent persons, however, there is a correlation between markers of HBV *replication* and liver injury (see below).

Another serologic marker which may be of value in patients with hepatitis B is HBeAg. Its principal clinical usefulness is as an indicator of relative infectivity. Because HBeAg is invariably present during early acute hepatitis B, HBeAg testing is indicated primarily during follow-up of chronic infection.

In patients with hepatitis B surface antigenemia of unknown duration, e.g., blood donors whose blood is found to be HBsAg-positive and who are referred to a physician for evaluation, testing for IgM anti-HBc may be useful to distinguish between acute or recent infection (IgM anti-HBc-positive) and chronic HBV infection (IgM anti-HBc-negative, IgG anti-HBc-positive). A false-positive test for IgM anti-HBc may be encountered in patients with high-titer rheumatoid factor.

Anti-HBs is rarely detectable in the presence of HBsAg in patients with *acute* hepatitis B, but 10 to 20 percent of persons with *chronic* HBV infection may harbor low-level anti-HBs. This antibody is directed not against the common group determinant, *a*, but against the heterotypic subtype determinant (e.g., HBsAg of subtype *ad* with anti-HBs of subtype *y*). In most cases, this serologic pattern cannot be attributed to infection with two different HBV subtypes, and the presence of this antibody is not a harbinger of imminent HBsAg clearance. When such antibody is detected, its presence is of no recognized clinical significance.

After immunization with hepatitis B vaccine, which consists of HBsAg alone, anti-HBs is the only serologic marker to appear. A summary of the commonly encountered serologic patterns of hepatitis B and their interpretations appears in Table 252-3. Tests for the detection of HBV DNA in liver and serum or DNA polymerase in serum are available in a limited number of research laboratories. Like HBeAg, serum HBV DNA and DNA polymerase are indicators of HBV replication, but they are more sensitive. These markers are useful in following the course of HBV replication in patients with chronic hepatitis B receiving experimental antiviral chemotherapy, with interferon for example. In immunocompetent persons a general correlation does appear to exist between the level of HBV replication, as reflected by the level of HBV DNA in serum, and the degree of liver injury. High serum HBV DNA levels, increased expression of viral antigens, and necroinflammatory activity in the liver go hand

TABLE 252-3   Commonly encountered serologic patterns of hepatitis B infection

HBsAg	Anti-HBs	Anti-HBc	HBeAg	Anti-HBe	Interpretation
+	−	IgM	+	−	Acute HBV infection, high infectivity
+	−	IgG	+	−	Chronic HBV infection, high infectivity
+	−	IgG	−	+	Late-acute or chronic HBV infection, low infectivity
+	+	+	+/−	+/−	1 HBsAg of one subtype and heterotypic anti-HBs (common)
					2 Process of seroconversion from HBsAg to anti-HBs (rare)
−	−	IgM	+/−	+/−	1 Acute HBV infection
					2 Anti-HBc window
−	−	IgG	−	+/−	1 Low-level HBsAg carrier
					2 Remote past infection
−	+	IgG	−	+/−	Recovery from HBV infection
−	+	−	−	−	1 Immunization with HBsAg (after vaccination)
					2 Remote past infection (?)
					3 False-positive

in hand unless immunosuppression interferes with cytolytic T-cell responses to virus-infected cells; reduction of HBV replication with antiviral drugs, such as interferon, tends to be accompanied by an improvement in liver histology.

Before the availability of reliable serologic tests for hepatitis C, a diagnosis of non-A, non-B hepatitis was made by serologic exclusion of HAV and HBV infection in the setting of a compatible history. Now that a specific antibody test is available, the potential exists for making a specific serologic diagnosis; however, delays of 1 to 3 months before the appearance of detectable antibody may interfere with serodiagnosis during acute illness. Furthermore, the level of antibody appears to be quite low. A helpful clinical clue is the episodic pattern of aminotransferase elevation seen frequently in non-A, non-B hepatitis. A diagnosis of acute non-A, non-B hepatitis can be entertained if tests for HBsAg, IgM anti-HBc, and IgM anti-HAV are negative. If follow-up samples are obtained 1 or more months after the onset of acute illness, a specific serologic diagnosis of bloodborne non-A, non-B hepatitis ("hepatitis C") may be made. If the specific antibody test remains negative, infection with a second bloodborne or an enteric non-A, non-B hepatitis agent ("hepatitis E") should be considered. A diagnosis of non-A, non-B hepatitis may be more difficult to establish in patients with chronic hepatitis who have anti-HBc in their blood. The anti-HBc in such cases will almost invariably be of the IgG class; it represents either HBV infection in the remote past or current HBV infection with low-level virus carriage.

The presence of HDV infection can be identified by demonstrating intrahepatic delta antigen or, more practically, an antidelta seroconversion (a rise in titer of anti-HD or de novo appearance of IgM anti-HD). Circulating HDAg, also diagnostic of acute infection, is detectable only briefly, if at all. Because IgM anti-HD is transient and IgG anti-HD is often undetectable once HBsAg disappears, retrospective serodiagnosis of acute self-limited, simultaneous HBV and HDV infection is difficult.

When a patient presents with acute hepatitis and has HBsAg and anti-HD in the serum, determination of the class of anti-HBc is helpful in establishing the relationship between infection with HBV and HDV. Although IgM anti-HBc does not distinguish *absolutely* between acute and chronic HBV infection, its presence is a reliable indicator of recent infection and its absence a reliable indicator of infection in the remote past. In simultaneous acute HBV and HDV infections, IgM anti-HBc will be detectable, while in acute HDV infection superimposed upon chronic HBV infection, anti-HBc will be of the IgG class.

In the future, tests for the presence of HDV-associated RNA will be useful for determining the presence of ongoing HDV replication and relative infectivity. Currently, probes for this marker are restricted to a limited number of research laboratories. Similarly, diagnostic tests for the enteric non-A, non-B hepatitis agent are cumbersome and remain limited to a small number of research laboratories.

Liver biopsy is rarely necessary or indicated in acute viral hepatitis, except when there is a question about the diagnosis or when there is clinical evidence suggesting a diagnosis of chronic active hepatitis.

Little agreement exists over routine diagnostic algorithms to be applied in the evaluation of cases of acute viral hepatitis. One potential approach is to test every patient with three serologic tests, HBsAg, IgM anti-HAV, and IgM anti-HBc (Table 252-4). The presence of HBsAg, with or without IgM anti-HBc, represents HBV infection. If IgM anti-HBc is present, the HBV infection is considered acute; if IgM anti-HBc is absent, the HBV infection is considered chronic. A diagnosis of acute hepatitis B can be made in the absence of HBsAg when IgM anti-HBc is detectable. A diagnosis of acute hepatitis A is based on the presence of IgM anti-HAV. If IgM anti-HAV coexists with HBsAg, a diagnosis of simultaneous HAV and HBV infections can be made; if IgM anti-HBc (with or without HBsAg) is detectable, the patient has simultaneous acute hepatitis A and B, and if IgM anti-HBc is undetectable, the patient has acute hepatitis A superimposed on chronic HBV infection. Absence of all

TABLE 252-4 Simplified diagnostic approach in patients presenting with acute hepatitis

Test patient's serum for

HBsAg	IgM anti-HAV	IgM anti-HBc	Diagnostic conclusion
+	−	+	Acute hepatitis B
+	−	−	Chronic hepatitis B
+	+	−	Acute hepatitis A superimposed on chronic hepatitis B
+	+	+	Acute hepatitis A and B
−	+	−	Acute hepatitis A
−	+	+	Acute hepatitis A and B (HBsAg below detectable level)
−	−	+	Acute hepatitis B (HBsAg below detectable level)
−	−	−	Compatible with non-A, non-B hepatitis*

* Confirm with follow-up test for antibody to non-A, non-B hepatitis agent.

serologic markers is consistent with a diagnosis of non-A, non-B hepatitis. A follow-up test for antibody to hepatitis C can be done to confirm the diagnosis serologically.

If a serologic diagnosis of chronic hepatitis B is made, testing for HBeAg and anti-HBe is indicated to evaluate relative infectivity. Testing for HBV DNA in such patients provides a more quantitative and sensitive test for the level of virus replication and, therefore, is very helpful during antiviral therapy (see Chap. 253). In patients with hepatitis B, testing for anti-HD is useful under the following circumstances: severe and fulminant cases, severe chronic cases, cases of acute hepatitis-like exacerbations in patients with chronic hepatitis B, persons with frequent percutaneous exposures, and persons from areas where delta infection is endemic.

PROGNOSIS Virtually all previously healthy patients with hepatitis A recover completely from their illness with no clinical sequelae. Similarly in acute hepatitis B, 90 percent of patients have a favorable course and recover completely. There are, however, certain clinical and laboratory features which suggest a more complicated and protracted course. Patients of advanced age and with serious underlying medical disorders such as congestive heart failure, severe anemia, and diabetes mellitus may have a prolonged course and are more likely to experience severe hepatitis. Initial presenting features such as ascites, peripheral edema, and symptoms of hepatic encephalopathy suggest a poorer prognosis. In addition, a prolonged prothrombin time, low serum albumin, hypoglycemia, and very high serum bilirubin values suggest severe hepatocellular disease. Patients with these clinical and laboratory features deserve prompt hospital admission. The case fatality rate in hepatitis A and B is very low (approximately 0.1 percent) but is increased by advanced age and underlying debilitating disorders. Among patients ill enough to be hospitalized for acute hepatitis B, the fatality rate is 1 percent. Non-A, non-B hepatitis occurring after transfusion is less severe during the acute phase than type B hepatitis and is more likely to be anicteric; fatalities are rare, but the precise case fatality rate is not known. In outbreaks of the waterborne type of non-A, non-B hepatitis (hepatitis E) in India and Asia, the case fatality rate is 1 to 2 percent, and up to 10 percent in pregnant women. Patients with simultaneous acute hepatitis B and delta hepatitis do not necessarily experience a higher mortality rate than do patients with acute hepatitis B alone; however, in several recent outbreaks of acute simultaneous HBV and HDV infection among drug addicts, the case fatality rate has approximated 5 percent. In the case of delta superinfection of a person with chronic hepatitis B, the likelihood of fulminant hepatitis and death is increased substantially. Although the case fatality rate for delta hepatitis has not been defined adequately, in outbreaks of severe delta superinfection in isolated populations with a high hepatitis B carrier rate, the mortality rate has been recorded as in excess of 20 percent.

COMPLICATIONS AND SEQUELAE   A small proportion of patients with hepatitis A experience *relapsing hepatitis* weeks to months after apparent recovery from acute hepatitis. Relapses are characterized by recurrence of symptoms, aminotransferase elevations, occasionally jaundice, and fecal excretion of HAV. Another unusual variant of acute hepatitis A is *cholestatic hepatitis,* characterized by protracted cholestatic jaundice and pruritus. Even when these complications occur, hepatitis A remains self-limited and does not progress to chronic liver disease. During the prodromal phase of acute hepatitis B, a serum sickness–like syndrome characterized by arthralgia or arthritis, rash, angioedema, and rarely hematuria and proteinuria may develop in some patients. This syndrome occurs prior to the onset of clinical jaundice, and these patients are often erroneously diagnosed as having rheumatoid arthritis or other rheumatologic diseases such as systemic lupus erythematosus. This syndrome occurs in about 5 to 10 percent of patients with acute hepatitis B. The diagnosis can be established by measuring serum aminotransferase levels, which are almost invariably elevated, and serum HBsAg.

The most feared complication of viral hepatitis is *fulminant hepatitis* (massive hepatic necrosis); fortunately this is a rare event. This is primarily seen in hepatitis B and delta hepatitis as well as enteric non-A, non-B hepatitis. Hepatitis B accounts for more than 50 percent of fulminant hepatitis cases, a sizeable proportion of which are associated with delta infection. Participation of the delta agent can be documented in approximately one-third of patients with acute fulminant hepatitis B and two-thirds of patients with fulminant hepatitis superimposed on chronic hepatitis B. Fulminant hepatitis is seen less frequently in bloodborne non-A, non-B hepatitis, and only occasionally in hepatitis A. Patients usually present with signs and symptoms of encephalopathy that may evolve to deep coma. The liver is usually small, and the prothrombin time excessively prolonged. The combination of rapidly shrinking liver size, rapidly rising bilirubin level, and marked prolongation of the prothrombin time, together with clinical signs of confusion, disorientation, somnolence, ascites, and edema, indicates that the patient has hepatic failure with encephalopathy. Cerebral edema is common; brainstem compression, gastrointestinal bleeding, sepsis, respiratory failure, cardiovascular collapse, and renal failure are terminal events. The mortality is exceedingly high (greater than 80 percent in patients with deep coma), but patients who survive may have a complete biochemical and histologic recovery.

It is particularly important to document the disappearance of HBsAg following apparent clinical recovery from acute hepatitis B. Before laboratory methods were available to distinguish between acute and acute hepatitis–like exacerbations ("spontaneous reactivations") of chronic hepatitis B, observations suggested that approximately 10 percent of patients remained HBsAg-positive for longer than 6 months after the onset of clinically apparent acute hepatitis B. Half of these persons were found to clear the antigen from their circulations during the next several years, but the other 5 percent remained chronically HBsAg-positive. More recent observations suggest that the true rate of chronic infection after clinically apparent acute hepatitis B is as low as 1 to 2 percent in normal, immunocompetent, young adults. Earlier, higher estimates may have been biased by inadvertent inclusion of acute exacerbations in chronically infected patients; these patients, chronically HBsAg-positive before exacerbation, were unlikely to seroconvert to HBsAg-negative thereafter. Whether the rate of chronicity is 10 or 1 percent, such patients have anti-HBc in serum; anti-HBs is either undetected or detected at low titer against the opposite subtype specificity of the antigen (see "Laboratory Features" above). These patients may (1) be asymptomatic carriers, (2) have low-grade chronic persistent hepatitis, or (3) have chronic active hepatitis with or without cirrhosis. The likelihood of becoming an HBsAg carrier after acute HBV infection is especially high among neonates, persons with Down's syndrome, chronically hemodialyzed patients, and immunosuppressed patients, including persons with human immunodeficiency virus infection.

Chronic active hepatitis is a major late complication of acute hepatitis B occurring in a small proportion of acute cases but more common in those with chronic infection (see Chap. 253). Certain clinical and laboratory features suggest progression of acute hepatitis to chronic active hepatitis: (1) lack of complete resolution of clinical symptoms of anorexia, weight loss, and fatigue and the persistence of hepatomegaly; (2) the presence of bridging or multilobular hepatic necrosis on liver biopsy during protracted, severe acute viral hepatitis; (3) failure of the serum aminotransferase, bilirubin, and globulin levels to return to normal within 6 to 12 months following the acute illness; and (4) the continued presence of HBsAg 6 months or more after acute hepatitis, suggesting chronic viral infection of the liver.

Although acute delta hepatitis infection does not increase the likelihood of chronicity of simultaneous acute hepatitis B, delta hepatitis has the potential for contributing to the severity of chronic hepatitis B. Delta hepatitis superinfection can transform asymptomatic or mild chronic hepatitis B into severe, progressive chronic active hepatitis and cirrhosis; it can also accelerate the course of chronic active hepatitis B. Some delta superinfections in patients with chronic hepatitis B lead to fulminant hepatitis. After transfusion-associated acute non-A, non-B hepatitis, as many as 50 percent of patients have abnormal biochemical liver tests for more than a year. In a majority of such patients, liver histology is consistent with chronic active hepatitis. Although many of these patients have no symptoms and a nonprogressive course, ultimately, cirrhosis develops in as many as 20 percent of those with *chronic* posttransfusion non-A, non-B hepatitis within 10 years of acute illness. The likelihood of chronic hepatitis is also approximately 50 percent after sporadic non-A, non-B hepatitis occurring in the absence of identifiable percutaneous inoculation with blood products or contaminated needles. In contrast, neither HAV nor enteric non-A, non-B hepatitis causes chronic liver disease.

Rare complications of viral hepatitis include pancreatitis, myocarditis, atypical pneumonia, aplastic anemia, transverse myelitis, and peripheral neuropathy. *Carriers* of HBsAg, particularly those infected in infancy or early childhood, have an enhanced risk of hepatocellular carcinoma (see Chap. 255). In children, hepatitis B may present rarely with anicteric hepatitis, a nonpruritic papular rash of the face, buttocks, and limbs, and lymphadenopathy (papular acrodermatitis of childhood or Gianotti-Crosti syndrome).

DIFFERENTIAL DIAGNOSIS   Viral diseases such as infectious mononucleosis; those due to cytomegalovirus, herpes simplex, and coxsackieviruses; and toxoplasmosis may share certain clinical features with viral hepatitis and cause elevation in serum aminotransferase and less commonly in serum bilirubin levels. Tests such as the differential heterophil and serologic tests for these agents may be helpful in the differential diagnosis if HBsAg, anti-HBc, and IgM anti-HAV determinations are negative. A complete drug history is particularly important, for many drugs and certain anesthetic agents can produce a picture of either acute hepatitis or cholestasis (see below). Equally important is a past history of unexplained "repeated episodes" of acute hepatitis. This should alert the physician to the possibility that the underlying disorder is chronic active hepatitis. Alcoholic hepatitis must also be considered, but usually the serum aminotransferase levels are not as markedly elevated and other stigmata of alcoholism may be present. The finding on liver biopsy of fatty infiltration, a neutrophilic inflammatory reaction, and "alcoholic hyaline" would be consistent with alcohol-induced rather than viral liver injury. Because acute hepatitis may present with right upper quadrant abdominal pain, nausea and vomiting, fever, and icterus, it is often confused with acute cholecystitis, common duct stone, or ascending cholangitis. Patients with acute viral hepatitis may tolerate surgery poorly; therefore, it is important to exclude this diagnosis, and in confusing cases, a percutaneous liver biopsy may be necessary prior to laparotomy. Viral hepatitis in the elderly is often misdiagnosed as obstructive jaundice resulting from a common duct stone or carcinoma of the pancreas. Because acute hepatitis in the elderly may be quite severe and the operative mortality high, a thorough evaluation including biochemical tests, radiographic studies of the biliary tree, and even liver biopsy may be necessary to exclude primary parenchymal liver disease. Another clinical constellation that may mimic acute hepatitis is right ventricular failure with passive hepatic congestion or hypoperfusion syndromes, such as those associated with shock, severe hypotension, and severe left ventricular failure. Clinical features are usually sufficient to distinguish between the two entities. Very rarely, malignancies metastatic to the liver can mimic acute or even fulminant viral hepatitis. Occasionally, genetic or metabolic liver disorders (e.g., Wilson's disease, alpha$_1$ antitrypsin deficiency) are confused with viral hepatitis.

MANAGEMENT   Treatment of acute attack   There is no specific treatment for *typical acute viral hepatitis.* Although hospitalization may be required for clinically severe illness, most patients do not require hospital care. Forced and prolonged bed rest is not essential for full recovery, but many patients will feel better with restricted physical activity. A high-calorie diet is desirable, and because many patients may experience nausea late in the day, the major caloric intake is best tolerated in the morning. Intravenous feeding is necessary in the acute stage if the patient has persistent vomiting and cannot maintain oral intake. Drugs capable of producing adverse reactions such as cholestasis and drugs metabolized by the liver should be avoided. If severe pruritus is present, the use of the bile salt–sequestering resin cholestyramine will usually alleviate this symptom. Glucocorticoid therapy has no value in acute viral hepatitis. Even in severe cases associated with *bridging necrosis,* controlled trials have failed to demonstrate the efficacy of steroids. In fact, such therapy may be hazardous.

Physical isolation of patients with hepatitis to a single room and bathroom is rarely necessary except in the case of fecal incontinence for hepatitis A and E or uncontrolled, voluminous bleeding for hepatitis types B (with or without concomitant delta hepatitis) and bloodborne non-A, non-B. Because most patients hospitalized with hepatitis A excrete little if any HAV, the likelihood of HAV transmission from these patients during their hospitalization is low. Therefore, burdensome *enteric precautions are no longer recommended.* Although gloves should be worn when the bedpans or fecal material of patients with hepatitis A are handled, these precautions do not represent a departure from sensible procedure for all hospitalized patients. For patients with types B and bloodborne non-A, non-B hepatitis, emphasis should be placed on blood precautions, i.e., avoiding direct, ungloved hand contact with blood and other body fluids. Enteric precautions are unnecessary. The importance of simple hygienic precautions, such as hand washing, cannot be overemphasized.

Hospitalized patients may be discharged when there is substantial symptomatic improvement, a significant downward trend in the serum aminotransferase and bilirubin values, and a return to normal of the prothrombin time. Mild aminotransferase elevations should not be considered contraindications to the gradual resumption of normal activity.

In *fulminant hepatitis,* the goal of therapy is to support the patient by maintenance of fluid balance, support of circulation and respiration, control of bleeding, correction of hypoglycemia, and treatment of other complications of the comatose state in anticipation of liver regeneration and repair. Protein intake should be restricted and oral lactulose or neomycin administered. Massive doses of glucocorticoids have been administered, but such therapy has been shown in controlled trials to be ineffective. Likewise, exchange transfusion, plasmapheresis, human cross-circulation, porcine liver cross-perfusion, and hemoperfusion have not been proven to enhance survival. Meticulous intensive care is the one factor that does appear to improve survival. Orthotopic liver transplantation is resorted to with increasing frequency, with excellent results, in patients with fulminant hepatitis (see Chap. 257).

HAZARDS TO MEDICAL AND PARAMEDICAL PERSONNEL Health care workers exposed frequently to blood, body tissues, and fluids have an increased risk of viral hepatitis, primarily hepatitis B. Approximately 15 percent of health workers have one or more serologic markers of HBV infection, and 1 percent are HBsAg-positive. The risk is higher in surgeons, pathologists, laboratory technologists who process blood specimens, technologists who draw blood and insert intravenous cannulas, hemodialysis staff, and others who perform invasive procedures. Transmission of HBV infection in health care settings, however, appears to be unidirectional, from patients to staff. With rare exceptions, HBsAg-positive health personnel do not increase the risk of HBV infection for their patients. Asymptomatic HBsAg carriers represent the greater risk to health personnel, because there are no readily identifiable clinical features that allow their recognition. Approximately 1 percent of all patients admitted to large metropolitan hospitals are HBsAg-positive, but 90 percent of these are not identified routinely. Patients with a past history of hepatitis or multiple transfusions, patients from countries where hepatitis B is endemic, sexually active homosexual men, intravenous drug abusers, and patients with chronic liver disease, chronic renal failure, polyarteritis nodosa, and Down's syndrome should have routine HBsAg determinations because of the high frequency of HBsAg positivity in these groups. If positive, they are potentially infectious, and appropriate precautions should be taken during operative or other acute-care procedures. In hemodialysis units, introduction of patient and staff education, routine periodic screening for HBsAg and aminotransferase elevations, and segregation of HBsAg-positive patients from susceptible patients have reduced dramatically the incidence of new HBV infections in both patients and medical personnel. Immunization with hepatitis B vaccine is another important measure in limiting the spread of hepatitis B to health workers (see below).

PROPHYLAXIS   Because therapy for viral hepatitis is limited, emphasis is placed on prevention through immunization. The prophylactic approach differs for each of the types of viral hepatitis. In the past, immunoprophylaxis relied exclusively on passive immunization with antibody-containing globulin preparations purified by cold ethanol fractionation from the plasma of hundreds of normal donors. Currently, for hepatitis B, active immunization with a vaccine is available as well.

Hepatitis A   All preparations of immune globulin (IG) contain anti-HAV. Although the titers may vary, all IG preparations appear to have an antibody concentration sufficient to be protective. When administered before exposure or during the early incubation period, IG is effective in preventing clinically apparent type A hepatitis. In some cases, IG does not abort infection but, by attenuating it, renders it inapparent. As a result long-lasting "passive-active" immunity occurs; however, this is now considered to be the exception rather than the rule. For intimate contacts (household, institutional) of persons with hepatitis A, administration of 0.02 mL/kg is recommended as early after exposure as possible; it may be effective even when administered as late as 2 weeks after exposure. Prophylaxis is not necessary for casual contacts (office, factory, school, or hospital), for most elderly persons, who are very likely to be immune, or for those known to have anti-HAV in their serum. In day-care centers, recognition of hepatitis A cases in children or staff should provide a stimulus for immunoprophylaxis in the center and in the children's family members. By the time most common-source outbreaks of type A hepatitis are recognized, it is usually too late in the incubation period for IG to be effective; however, prophylaxis may limit the frequency of secondary cases. For travelers to tropical countries, developing countries, and other areas outside of standard tourist routes, IG prophylaxis is recommended. When such travel lasts less than 3 months, 0.02 mL/kg is given; for longer travel or residence in these areas, a dose of 0.06 mL/kg every 4 to 6 months is recommended. Administration of plasma-derived globulin is safe; it has not been associated with transmission of AIDS to recipients, and the AIDS virus (human immunodeficiency virus, HIV) is inactivated by 25 percent alcohol, to which plasma is subjected during the cold ethanol fractionation process. Killed, live attenuated, and genetically engineered hepatitis A vaccines are being developed.

Hepatitis B   Until recently, prevention of hepatitis B was based on *passive* immunoprophylaxis either with standard IG, containing modest levels of anti-HBs, or hepatitis B immune globulin (HBIG), containing high-titer anti-HBs. The efficacy of standard IG has never been established and remains questionable; even the efficacy of HBIG, demonstrated in several clinical trials, has been challenged, and its contribution appears to be in reducing the frequency of clinical *illness*, not in preventing *infection*. Although HBV cannot be cultivated in vitro in the classical sense, a vaccine for *active* immunization has been prepared from purified, noninfectious 22-nm spherical forms of HBsAg derived from the plasma of healthy HBsAg carriers. The vaccine is subjected to three different chemical inactivation steps which, cumulatively, destroy the infectivity of every known virus, including HIV. In controlled clinical trials among high-risk persons, this plasma-derived vaccine was shown to be immunogenic, highly effective in preventing HBV infection, and, despite its unconventional source, very safe. In addition, a genetically engineered vaccine derived from recombinant yeast has been introduced. The latter vaccine consists of HBsAg particles that are nonglycosylated but are otherwise indistinguishable from natural HBsAg; this second-generation vaccine is comparable in immunogenicity, protective efficacy, and safety to the first-generation, plasma-derived vaccine. Current recommendations can be divided into those for preexposure and postexposure prophylaxis.

For *preexposure* prophylaxis against hepatitis B in settings of frequent exposure (health workers exposed to blood, hemodialysis patients and staff, residents and staff of custodial institutions for the developmentally handicapped, intravenous drug abusers, promiscuous homosexual men as well as promiscuous heterosexuals, persons such as hemophiliacs who require long-term, high-volume therapy with blood derivatives, household and sexual contacts of HBsAg carriers, and persons living in or traveling extensively in endemic areas), three intramuscular (deltoid, not gluteal) injections of hepatitis B vaccine are recommended at 0, 1, and 6 months. Pregnancy is *not* a contraindication to vaccination. The recommended dose for each injection of plasma-derived vaccine is 20 μg for immunocompetent adults, 40 μg for immunosuppressed patients (hemodialysis patients, transplant recipients, and oncology patients receiving chemotherapy), and 10 μg for infants and children under the age of 10. One of the available recombinant vaccines is formulated to contain 10 μg for normal adults and 5 μg for children; another contains 20 μg and 10 μg for adults and children, respectively.

For unvaccinated persons sustaining an exposure to HBV, *postexposure* prophylaxis with a combination of HBIG (for rapid achievement of high-titer circulating anti-HBs) and hepatitis B vaccine (for achievement of long-lasting immunity as well as its apparent efficacy in attenuating clinical illness after exposure) is recommended. For *perinatal* exposure of infants born to HBsAg-positive mothers, a single dose of HBIG, 0.5 mL, should be administered intramuscularly in the thigh *immediately after birth*, followed by a complete course of three 10-μg injections of plasma-derived hepatitis B vaccine (or 5 μg of recombinant vaccine) to be started within the first 12 h to 1 week of life. For those experiencing a direct percutaneous inoculation or transmucosal exposure to HBsAg-positive blood or body fluids (e.g., accidental *needle stick*, other mucosal penetration, or ingestion), a single intramuscular dose of HBIG, 0.06 mL/kg, administered as soon after exposure as possible, is followed by a complete course of hepatitis B vaccine to begin within the first week. For those exposed by *sexual* contact to a patient with acute hepatitis B, the Immunization Practices Advisory Committee of the United States Public Health Service recommends a single intramuscular dose of HBIG, 0.06 mL/kg, within 14 days of exposure, to be followed by either a second HBIG injection or, only when HBsAg positivity in the index case persists beyond 3 months, a complete course of hepatitis B vaccine. Other authorities, however, recommend a combination of HBIG followed by a complete course of hepatitis B vaccine injections for all sexual contacts of patients with acute hepatitis B, regardless of the duration of HBsAg positivity in the index case. When both HBIG and hepatitis B vaccine are recommended, they may be given at the same time but at separate sites.

The precise duration of protection afforded by hepatitis B vaccine

is unknown; however, approximately 80 to 90 percent of immunocompetent vaccinees retain protective levels of anti-HBs for at least 5 years. Thereafter and even after anti-HBs becomes undetectable, protection persists against clinical hepatitis B, hepatitis B surface antigenemia, and chronic HBV infection. Currently *booster* immunizations are not recommended routinely, except in immunosuppressed persons who have lost detectable anti-HBs or immunocompetent persons who sustain percutaneous HBsAg-positive inoculations after losing detectable antibody.

Delta hepatitis Infection with the delta hepatitis agent can be prevented by vaccinating susceptible persons with hepatitis B vaccine. No product is available for immunoprophylaxis to prevent delta superinfection in HBsAg carriers; for them, avoidance of percutaneous exposures and limitation of intimate contact with persons who have delta infection are recommended.

Non-A, non-B hepatitis For transfusion-associated non-A, non-B hepatitis, the effectiveness of IG prophylaxis has not been demonstrated consistently and is not recommended. The most effective measure for reducing the frequency of posttransfusion non-A, non-B hepatitis is the elimination of commercially obtained donor blood and reliance exclusively on volunteer blood donors. The presence of elevated ALT and/or anti-HBc in donor blood was found to correlate with the risk of non-A, non-B hepatitis in recipients. Both of these markers appear to identify segments of the blood donor population with an increased risk of bloodborne viral infections. In the late 1980s, screening of donor blood for these surrogate markers was introduced. At the same time, exclusion of blood donors in high-risk groups for AIDS and screening of blood donors for anti-HIV were introduced. These measures, introduced to limit transfusion-associated AIDS, have the potential to lower the risk of infection with other bloodborne agents, like non-A, non-B hepatitis virus, as well. Finally, the recent introduction of blood donor screening for antibody to hepatitis C is expected to reduce further the risk of non-A, non-B hepatitis after transfusion. Another approach, chemical treatment of blood products and concentrates to inactivate non-A, non-B hepatitis virus infectivity, is also being pursued. Studies to test the efficacy of standard IG after needle stick, sexual, or perinatal exposure to non-A, non-B hepatitis have not been done. Because the inoculum is considerably smaller in these settings than that associated with transfusion, and because of its safety and low cost, some authorities do recommend postexposure prophylaxis with a single dose of IG, 0.06 mL/kg (or 0.5 mL for neonatal exposure), in these situations. The efficacy of IG for prevention of enteric non-A, non-B hepatitis remains to be evaluated.

TOXIC AND DRUG-INDUCED HEPATITIS

Liver injury may follow the inhalation, ingestion, or parenteral administration of a number of pharmacologic and chemical agents. These include industrial toxins (e.g., carbon tetrachloride, trichloroethylene, and yellow phosphorus), the heat-stable toxic bicyclic octapeptides of certain species of *Amanita* and *Galerina* (hepatotoxic mushroom poisoning), and more commonly, pharmacologic agents used in medical therapy. It is essential that any patient presenting with jaundice or impaired liver function be questioned carefully about exposure to chemicals used in work or at home and drugs taken by prescription or bought "over the counter." In general, two major types of chemical hepatotoxicity have been recognized: (1) direct toxic type and (2) idiosyncratic type.

As shown in Table 252-5, direct toxic hepatitis occurs with predictable regularity in individuals exposed to the offending agent and is dose-dependent. The latent period between exposure and liver injury is usually short (often several hours), although clinical manifestations may be delayed for 24 to 48 h. Agents producing toxic hepatitis are generally systemic poisons or are converted in the liver to toxic metabolites. The direct hepatotoxins result in morphologic abnormalities which are reasonably characteristic and reproducible

TABLE 252-5   Some features of toxic and drug-induced hepatic injury

Features	Direct toxic effect		Idiosyncratic			Other
	(Carbon tetrachloride, e.g.)	(Acetaminophen, e.g.)	(Halothane, e.g.)	(Isoniazid, e.g.)	(Chlorpromazine, e.g.)	(Oral contraceptive agents, e.g.)
Predictable and dose-related toxicity	+	+	0	0	0	+
Latent period	Short	Short	Variable	Variable	Variable	Variable
Arthralgia, fever, rash, eosinophilia	0	0	+	0	+	0
Liver morphology	Necrosis, fatty infiltration	Centrilobular necrosis	Similar to viral hepatitis	Similar to viral hepatitis	Cholestasis *with* portal inflammation	Cholestasis *without* portal inflammation, vascular lesions

for each toxin. For example, carbon tetrachloride and trichloroethylene characteristically produce a centrilobular zonal necrosis, whereas yellow phosphorus poisoning typically results in periportal injury. The hepatotoxic octapeptides of *Amanita phalloides* usually produce massive hepatic necrosis. The lethal dose of the toxin is about 10 mg, the amount found in a single deathcap mushroom. Tetracycline, when administered in intravenous doses greater than 1.5 g daily, leads to microvesicular fat deposits in the liver. Liver injury, which is often only one facet of the toxicity produced by the direct hepatotoxins, may go unrecognized until jaundice appears.

In idiosyncratic drug reactions the occurrence of hepatitis is usually infrequent and unpredictable, the response is not dose-dependent, and it may occur at any time during or shortly after exposure to the drug. Extrahepatic manifestations of hypersensitivity, such as rash, arthralgias, fever, leukocytosis, and eosinophilia occur in about one-quarter of patients with idiosyncratic hepatotoxic drug reactions; this observation and the unpredictability of idiosyncratic drug hepatotoxicity contributed to the hypothesis that this category of drug reactions is immunologically mediated. More recent evidence, however, suggests that even idiosyncratic reactions represent direct hepatotoxity but are caused by drug metabolites rather than by the intact compound. Even the prototype of idiosyncratic hepatoxicity reactions, halothane hepatitis, and isoniazid hepatotoxicity, associated frequently with hypersensitivity manifestations, are now recognized to be mediated by toxic metabolites which damage liver cells directly. Currently, idiosyncratic reactions are thought to result from differences in metabolic reactivity to specific agents; host susceptibility is mediated by the kinetics of toxic metabolite generation, which differs among individuals. Idiosyncratic reactions lead to a morphologic pattern that is more variable than those produced by direct toxins; a single agent is often capable of causing a variety of lesions, although certain patterns tend to predominate. Depending on the agent involved, idiosyncratic hepatitis may result in a clinical and morphologic picture indistinguishable from viral hepatitis (e.g., halothane) or may simulate extrahepatic bile duct obstruction clinically with morphologic evidence of cholestasis and minimal hepatocellular damage (e.g., chlorpromazine). Morphologic alterations may also include bridging hepatic necrosis (e.g., methyldopa), or, infrequently, hepatic granulomas (e.g., sulfonamides).

Not all adverse hepatic drug reactions can be classified as either toxic or idiosyncratic in type. For example, oral contraceptives, which combine estrogenic and progestational compounds, may result in impairment of hepatic function and occasionally in jaundice. However, they do not produce necrosis or fatty change, manifestations of hypersensitivity are generally absent, and susceptibility to the development of oral contraceptive–induced cholestasis appears to be genetically determined.

Because drug-induced hepatitis is often a presumptive diagnosis and many other disorders produce a similar clinicopathologic picture, evidence of a causal relationship between the use of a drug and subsequent liver injury may be difficult to establish. The relationship is most convincing for the direct hepatotoxins, which lead to a high frequency of hepatic impairment after a short latent period. Idiosyn-

cratic reactions may be reproduced, in some instances, when rechallenge, after an asymptomatic period, results in a recurrence of signs, symptoms, and morphologic and biochemical abnormalities. Rechallenge, however, is often ethically unfeasible, because severe reactions may occur.

Treatment of toxic and drug-induced hepatic disease is largely supportive, as in acute viral hepatitis. Withdrawal of the suspected agent is indicated at the first sign of an adverse reaction. In the case of the direct toxins, liver involvement should not divert attention from renal or other organ involvement which may also threaten survival.

In Table 252-6 several classes of chemical agents are listed, together with examples of the pattern of liver injury produced by them. Certain drugs appear to be responsible for the development of chronic as well as acute hepatic injury. For example, oxphenisatin, alpha methyldopa, and isoniazid have been associated with chronic active hepatitis, and halothane and methotrexate have been implicated in the development of cirrhosis. A syndrome resembling primary biliary cirrhosis has been described following treatment with chlorpromazine, methyl testosterone, tolbutamide, and other drugs. Portal hypertension in the absence of cirrhosis may result from alterations in hepatic architecture produced by vitamin A or arsenic intoxication, industrial exposure to vinyl chloride, or administration of thorium dioxide. The latter three agents have also been associated with

TABLE 252-6   Principal alterations of hepatic morphology produced by some commonly used drugs and chemicals

Principal morphologic change	Class of agent	Example
Cholestasis	Anabolic steroid	Methyl testosterone*
	Antithyroid	Methimazole
	Chemotherapeutic	Erythromycin estolate
	Oral contraceptive	Norethynodrel with mestranol
	Oral hypoglycemic	Chlorpropamide
	Tranquilizer	Chlorpromazine*
Fatty liver	Chemotherapeutic	Tetracycline
	Anticonvulsant	Sodium valproate
	Antiarrhythmic	Amiodarone
Hepatitis	Anesthetic	Halothane†
	Anticonvulsant	Phenytoin
	Antihypertensive	Methyldopa†
	Chemotherapeutic	Isoniazid†
	Diuretic	Chlorothiazide
	Laxative	Oxyphenisatin†
Toxic (necrosis)	Hydrocarbon	Carbon tetrachloride
	Metal	Yellow phosphorus
	Mushroom	*Amanita phalloides*
	Analgesic	Acetaminophen
	Solvent	Dimethylformamide
Granulomas	Anti-inflammatory	Phenylbutazone
	Chemotherapeutic	Sulfonamides
	Xanthine oxidase inhibitor	Allopurinol

* Rarely associated with primary biliary cirrhosis-like lesion.
† Occasionally associated with chronic active hepatitis or bridging hepatic necrosis or cirrhosis.

angiosarcoma of the liver. Oral contraceptives have been implicated in the development of hepatic adenoma and, rarely, hepatocellular carcinoma and occlusion of the hepatic vein (Budd-Chiari syndrome). Another unusual lesion, peliosis hepatis (blood cysts of the liver), has been observed in some patients treated with oral contraceptives or anabolic steroids. The existence of these hepatic disorders expands the spectrum of liver injury induced by chemical agents and emphasizes the need for a thorough drug history in all patients with liver dysfunction.

The following are the patterns of adverse hepatic reactions for some prototypic agents.

ACETAMINOPHEN HEPATOTOXICITY (DIRECT TOXIN)   Acetaminophen, an analgesic and antipyretic that is available without a prescription, has caused severe centrolobular hepatic necrosis when ingested in large amounts in suicide attempts or accidentally by children. A single dose of 10 to 15 g, occasionally less, may produce clinical evidence of liver injury. Fatal fulminant disease is usually (although not invariably) associated with ingestion of 25 g or more. Blood levels of acetaminophen correlate with the severity of hepatic injury (levels above 300 μg/mL 4 h after ingestion are predictive of the development of severe damage, while levels below 150 μg/mL suggest that hepatic injury is highly unlikely). Nausea, vomiting, diarrhea, abdominal pain, and shock are early manifestations occurring 4 to 12 h after ingestion. Then 24 to 48 h later, when these features are abating, hepatic injury becomes apparent. Maximal abnormalities and hepatic failure may not be evident until 4 to 6 days after ingestion. Renal failure and myocardial injury may be present.

Acetaminophen hepatotoxicity is mediated by a toxic reactive metabolite formed from the parent compound by the cytochrome P_{450} mixed-function oxidase system of the hepatocyte. This metabolite is detoxified by binding to glutathione. When excessive amounts of the metabolite are formed, glutathione levels in liver fall, and the metabolite is covalently bound to nucleophilic hepatocyte macromolecules. This process is believed to lead to hepatocyte necrosis; the precise sequence and mechanism are unknown. Hepatic injury may be potentiated by prior administration of alcohol or other drugs, by conditions which stimulate the mixed-function oxidase system, or by conditions such as starvation which reduce hepatic glutathione levels. In chronic alcoholics, the toxic dose of acetaminophen may be as low as 2 g.

Treatment of acetaminophen overdosage includes gastric lavage, supportive measures, and oral administration of activated charcoal or cholestyramine to prevent absorption of residual drug. Neither of the latter agents appears to be effective if given more than 30 min after acetaminophen ingestion; if they are used, the stomach lavage should be done before other agents are administered orally. In patients with high acetaminophen blood levels (>200 μg/mL measured at 4 h or >100 μg/mL at 8 h after ingestion) the administration of sulfhydryl compounds (e.g., cysteamine, cysteine, or N-acetylcysteine) appears to reduce the severity of hepatic necrosis. These agents appear to act by providing a reservoir of sulfhydryl groups to bind the toxic metabolites or by stimulating synthesis and repletion of hepatic glutathione. Therapy should be begun within 8 h of ingestion but may be effective even if given as late as 24 h after overdose. Later administration of sulfhydryl compounds is of uncertain value.

Survivors of acute acetaminophen overdose usually have no evidence of hepatic sequelae. In a few patients prolonged or repeated administration of acetaminophen in therapeutic doses appears to have led to the development of chronic active hepatitis and cirrhosis.

HALOTHANE HEPATOTOXICITY (IDIOSYNCRATIC REACTION)   Halothane, a nonexplosive fluorinated hydrocarbon anesthetic agent that is structurally similar to chloroform, has been reported to result in severe hepatic necrosis in a small number of individuals, many of whom have previously been exposed to this agent. The failure to produce similar hepatic lesions reliably in animals, the rarity of hepatic impairment in human beings, and the delayed appearance of hepatic injury suggest that halothane is not a direct hepatotoxin but may be a sensitizing agent. However, manifestations of hypersensitivity are seen in fewer than 25 percent of cases. A genetic predisposition leading to an idiosyncratic metabolic reactivity has been postulated and appears to be the most likely mechanism of halothane hepatotoxicity. Supporting this postulate is the demonstration in patients with halothane hepatitis and their family members of increased lymphocyte susceptibility to damage in vitro by electrophilic drug metabolites. Adults (rather than children), obese people, and women appear to be particularly susceptible. Fever, moderate leukocytosis, and eosinophilia may occur in the first week following halothane administration. Jaundice usually is noted 7 to 10 days after exposure but may occur earlier in previously exposed patients. Nausea and vomiting may precede the onset of jaundice. Hepatomegaly is often mild, but liver tenderness is common. The serum aminotransferase levels are elevated. The pathologic changes at autopsy are indistinguishable from massive hepatic necrosis resulting from viral hepatitis. The case fatality rate of halothane hepatitis is not known but may vary from 20 to 40 percent in cases with severe liver involvement. In rare instances cirrhosis has been observed following repeated bouts of halothane hepatitis; however, in most patients who recover, the liver returns to normal. It is strongly suggested that patients in whom unexplained spiking fever, especially delayed fever, or jaundice develops after halothane anesthesia not receive this agent again. Because cross-reactions between halothane and methoxyfluorane have been reported, the latter agent should not be used after halothane reactions. Later-generation halogenated hydrocarbon anesthetics are felt to be associated with a lower risk of hepatotoxicity; however, rare cases have been observed.

METHYLDOPA HEPATOTOXICITY (TOXIC AND IDIOSYNCRATIC REACTION)   Minor alterations in liver tests are reported in about 5 percent of patients treated with this antihypertensive agent. These trivial abnormalities typically resolve despite continued drug administration. In less than 1 percent of patients, acute liver injury resembling viral hepatitis, or chronic active hepatitis, or rarely a cholestatic reaction is seen 1 to 20 weeks after methyldopa is started. In 50 percent of cases the interval is shorter than 4 weeks. A prodrome of fever, anorexia, and malaise may be noted for a few days before the onset of jaundice. Rash, lymphadenopathy, arthralgia, and eosinophilia are rare. Serologic markers of autoimmunity are infrequently detected, and fewer than 5 percent of patients have a Coombs-positive hemolytic anemia. In about 15 percent of patients with methyldopa hepatotoxicity the clinical, biochemical, and histologic features are those of chronic active hepatitis with or without bridging necrosis and macronodular cirrhosis. With discontinuation of the drug, the disorder usually resolves, although progression has been seen in a few patients.

ISONIAZID HEPATOTOXICITY (TOXIC AND IDIOSYNCRATIC REACTION)   In approximately 10 percent of adults treated with the antituberculosis agent isoniazid, elevated serum aminotransferase levels develop during the first few weeks of therapy; this appears to represent an adaptive response to a toxic metabolite of the drug. Whether or not isoniazid is continued, these values (usually below 200 units) return to normal in a few weeks. In about 1 percent of treated patients, an illness develops which is indistinguishable from viral hepatitis; approximately half of these cases occur within the first 2 months of treatment, while in the remainder, clinical disease may be delayed for many months. Liver biopsy reveals morphologic changes similar to those of viral hepatitis or bridging hepatic necrosis. The disease may be severe, with a case fatality rate of 10 percent. Important liver injury appears to be age-related, increasing substantially in frequency after age 35; the highest frequency is in patients over age 50, the lowest under the age of 20. Fever, rash, eosinophilia, and other manifestations of drug allergy are distinctly unusual. A reactive metabolite of acetylhydrazine, a metabolite of isoniazid, may be responsible for liver injury. A picture resembling chronic active hepatitis has been observed in a few patients.

SODIUM VALPROATE HEPATOTOXICITY (TOXIC AND IDIOSYNCRATIC REACTION)   Sodium valproate, an anticonvulsant useful in the treatment of petit mal and other seizure disorders, has been associated with the development of severe hepatic toxicity and, rarely, fatalities in both children and adults. Asymptomatic elevations of serum aminotransferase levels have been recognized in as many as 45 percent of treated patients. These "adaptive" changes, however, appear to have no clinical importance, for major hepatotoxicity is not seen in the majority of patients despite continuation of drug therapy. In those rare patients in whom jaundice, encephalopathy, and evidence of hepatic failure are found, examination of liver tissue reveals microvesicular fat and bridging hepatic necrosis predominantly in the centrolobular zone. Bile duct injury may also be apparent. It seems likely that sodium valproate is not directly hepatotoxic but that its metabolite, 4-pentenoic acid, may be responsible for hepatic injury.

PHENYTOIN HEPATOTOXICITY (IDIOSYNCRATIC REACTION) Phenytoin, diphenylhydantoin, a mainstay in the treatment of seizure disorders, has been associated in rare instances with the development of severe hepatitis-like liver injury leading to fulminant hepatic failure in some instances. In many patients the hepatitis is associated with striking fever, lymphadenopathy, rash (Stevens-Johnson syndrome or exfoliative dermatitis), leukocytosis, and eosinophilia, suggesting an immunologically mediated hypersensitivity mechanism. Despite these observations, there is also evidence that metabolic idiosyncrasy may be responsible for hepatic injury. In the liver, phenytoin is converted by the cytochrome P_{450} system to metabolites which include the highly reactive electrophilic arene oxides. These metabolites are normally metabolized further by epoxide hydrolases. A defect (genetic or acquired) in epoxide hydrolase activity would permit covalent binding of arene oxides to hepatic macromolecules, thereby leading to hepatic injury. Regardless of the mechanism, hepatic injury is usually manifest within the first 2 months after beginning phenytoin therapy. With the exception of an abundance of eosinophils in the liver, the clinical, biochemical, and histologic picture resembles that of viral hepatitis. In rare instances, bile duct injury may be the salient feature of phenytoin hepatotoxicity with striking features of intrahepatic cholestasis. Asymptomatic elevations of aminotransferase and alkaline phosphatase levels have been observed in a sizeable proportion of patients receiving long-term phenytoin therapy. These liver changes are believed by some authorities to represent the potent hepatic enzyme–inducing properties of phenytoin and are accompanied histologically by swelling of hepatocytes in the absence of necroinflammatory activity or evidence of chronic liver disease.

CHLORPROMAZINE HEPATOTOXICITY (CHOLESTATIC IDIOSYNCRATIC REACTION) In about 1 percent of patients receiving chlorpromazine, intrahepatic cholestasis with jaundice develops after 1 to 4 weeks of treatment. In rare instances, jaundice has been reported after a single exposure. Anicteric reactions are frequent. The onset may be abrupt with fever, rash, arthralgias, lymphadenopathy, nausea, vomiting, and epigastric or right upper quadrant pain. Pruritus may precede the appearance of jaundice, dark urine, and light stools. Eosinophilia with or without mild leukocytosis may be present, and conjugated hyperbilirubinemia, moderately elevated serum alkaline phosphatase, and mildly elevated serum aminotransferase levels (100 to 200 units) are noted. Liver biopsy reveals cholestasis, bile plugs in dilated bile canaliculi, and a dense portal infiltrate of polymorphonuclear, eosinophilic, and mononuclear leukocytes. Occasionally, scattered foci of hepatic parenchymal necrosis may be evident. Jaundice and pruritus usually subside within 4 to 8 weeks following cessation of therapy, without sequelae, and fatalities are rare. Cholestyramine may be of value in relieving severe pruritus. In a small number of patients, jaundice is prolonged for several months to years; rarely, a disorder resembling but distinct from primary biliary cirrhosis may develop.

AMIODARONE HEPATOTOXICITY (TOXIC AND IDIOSYNCRATIC REACTION) Therapy with this potent antiarrhythmic drug is accompanied in 15 to 50 percent of patients by modest elevation of serum aminotransferase levels that may remain stable or diminish despite continuation of the drug. Such abnormalities may appear days to many months after beginning therapy. A proportion of those with elevated aminotransferase levels have detectable hepatomegaly, and clinically important liver disease develops in fewer than 5 percent of patients. Features that represent a direct effect of the drug on the liver and that are common to the majority of long-term recipients are ultrastructural phospholipidosis, unaccompanied by clinical liver disease, and interference with hepatic mixed-function oxidase metabolism of other drugs. The relatively common elevations in aminotransferase levels are also considered a predictable, dose-dependent, direct hepatotoxic effect. On the other hand, in the rare patient with clinically apparent, symptomatic liver disease, liver injury resembling that seen in alcoholic liver disease is observed. The so-called pseudoalcoholic liver injury can range from steatosis, to alcoholic hepatitis–like neutrophilic infiltration and Mallory's hyaline, to cirrhosis. Electron-microscopic demonstration of phospholipid-laden lysosomal lamellar bodies can help to distinguish amiodarone hepatotoxicity from typical alcoholic hepatitis. This category of liver injury appears to be a metabolic idiosyncracy which allows hepatotoxic metabolites to be generated. Rarely, an acute idiosyncratic hepatocellular injury, resembling viral hepatitis or cholestatic hepatitis, occurs. Hepatic granulomas have occasionally been observed. Because amiodarone has a long half-life, liver injury may persist for months after the drug is stopped.

ERYTHROMYCIN HEPATOTOXICITY (CHOLESTATIC IDIOSYNCRATIC REACTION) The most important adverse effect associated with erythromycin is the infrequent occurrence of a cholestatic reaction. Although most of these reactions have been associated with erythromycin estolate, other erythromycins may also be responsible. The reaction usually begins during the first 2 or 3 weeks of therapy and includes nausea, vomiting, fever, right upper quadrant abdominal pain, jaundice, leukocytosis, and moderately elevated aminotransferase levels. The clinical picture can resemble acute cholecystitis or bacterial cholangitis. Liver biopsy reveals variable cholestasis, portal inflammation comprising lymphocytes, polymorphonuclear leukocytes, and eosinophils, and scattered foci of hepatocyte necrosis. Symptoms and laboratory findings usually subside within a few days of drug withdrawal, and evidence of chronic liver disease has not been found on follow-up. The precise mechanism remains ill-defined.

ORAL CONTRACEPTIVE HEPATOTOXICITY (CHOLESTATIC REACTION) The administration of oral contraceptive combinations of estrogenic and progestational steroids results in significant bromsulphthalein (BSP) retention in a high proportion of patients, and, to a far lesser extent, elevation of serum alkaline phosphatase. Weeks to months after taking these agents, intrahepatic cholestasis with pruritus and jaundice is noted in a small number of patients. Especially susceptible seem to be patients with recurrent idiopathic jaundice of pregnancy, severe pruritus of pregnancy, or a family history of these disorders. Laboratory studies, with the exception of liver biochemical tests, are normal, and extrahepatic manifestations of hypersensitivity are absent. Liver biopsy reveals cholestasis with bile plugs in dilated canaliculi and striking bilirubin staining of liver cells. In contrast to chlorpromazine-induced cholestasis, portal inflammation is absent. The lesion is reversible on withdrawal of the agent, and sequelae have not been reported. The two steroid components appear to act synergistically on hepatic function, although the estrogen may be primarily responsible. Oral contraceptives are contraindicated in patients with a history of recurrent jaundice of pregnancy. Primarily benign but, rarely, malignant neoplasms of the liver, hepatic vein occlusion, peliosis hepatis, and peripheral sinusoidal dilatation have also been associated with oral contraceptive therapy.

17,α-ALKYL-SUBSTITUTED ANABOLIC STEROIDS (CHOLESTATIC REACTION) In the majority of patients receiving these agents, used therapeutically mainly in the treatment of bone marrow failure but used surreptitiously and without medical indication by athletes to improve their performance, mild hepatic dysfunction develops. Impaired excretory function is the predominant defect, but the precise mechanism is uncertain. Jaundice, which appears to be dose-related, develops in only a minority of patients and may be the sole clinical manifestation of hepatotoxicity, although anorexia, nausea, and malaise are described in some patients. Pruritus is not a prominent feature. Serum aminotransferase levels are usually under 100 units, and serum alkaline phosphatase levels are normal, mildly elevated, or, in less than 5 percent of patients, three or more times the upper limit of normal. Examination of liver tissue reveals cholestasis without inflammation or necrosis. Hepatic sinusoidal dilatation and peliosis hepatis have been found in a few patients. The cholestatic disorder is usually reversible on cessation of treatment, although fatalities have been linked to peliosis. An association with hepatic adenoma and hepatocellular carcinoma has been reported.

TRIMETHOPRIM-SULFAMETHOXAZOLE HEPATOTOXICITY (IDIOSYNCRATIC REACTION) This antibiotic is used routinely for urinary tract infections in immunocompetent persons and for prophylaxis against and therapy of *Pneumocystis carinii* pneumonia in immunosuppressed persons (transplant recipients, patients with AIDS). With its increasing use, its occasional hepatotoxicity is being recognized with growing frequency. Its likelihood is unpredictable but, when it occurs, trimethoprim-sulfamethoxazole hepatotoxicity follows a relatively uniform latency period of several weeks and is often accompanied by eosinophilia, rash, and other features of a hypersensitivity reaction. Biochemically and histologically, acute hepatocellular necrosis predominates, but cholestatic features are quite frequent. Occasionally, cholestasis without necrosis occurs, and, very rarely, a severe cholangiolytic pattern of liver injury is observed. In most cases, liver injury is self-limited, but rare fatalities have been recorded. The hepatotoxicity is attributable to the sulfamethoxazole component of the drug and is similar in features to that seen with other sulfonamides; tissue eosinophilia and granulomas may be seen.

REFERENCES

Viral hepatitis

ALTER HJ et al: Detection of antibody to hepatitis C virus in prospectively followed transfusion recipients with acute and chronic non-A, non-B hepatitis. N Engl J Med 321:1494, 1989
——— (ed): Viral hepatitis. Semin Liver Dis 6:1, 1986
BRADLEY DW et al: Enterically transmitted non-A, non-B hepatitis: Serial passage of disease in cynomolgus macaques and tamarins and recovery of disease-associated 27- to 34-nm viruslike particles. Proc Natl Acad Sci USA 84:6277, 1987
DAVIS GL, HOOFNAGLE, JH: Reactivation of chronic type B hepatitis presenting as acute viral hepatitis. Ann Intern Med 102:762, 1985
DIENSTAG JL, ISSELBACHER KJ: Therapy of acute and chronic hepatitis. Arch Intern Med 141:1419, 1981
———: Non-A, non-B hepatitis. I. Recognition, epidemiology, and clinical features. II. Experimental transmission, putative virus agents and markers, and prevention. Gastroenterology 85:439 and 743, 1983
GERETY RJ (ed): Non-A, Non-B Hepatitis. New York, Academic 1981
——— (ed): Hepatitis A. Orlando, Academic, 1984
——— (ed): Hepatitis B. Orlando, Academic, 1985
IMMUNIZATION PRACTICES ADVISORY COMMITTEE: Recommendations for protection against viral hepatitis. Ann Intern Med 103:391, 1985
———: Update on hepatitis B prevention. Ann Intern Med 107:353, 1987
JACOBSON IM, DIENSTAG JL: Viral hepatitis vaccines. Annu Rev Med 36.241, 1985
KUO G et al: An assay for circulating antibodies to a major etiologic virus of human non-A, non-B hepatitis. Science 244:362, 1989
LEMON SM: Type A viral hepatitis: New developments in an old disease. N Engl J Med 313:1059, 1985
RIZZETTO M: The delta agent. Hepatology 3:729, 1983
——— et al (eds): The Hepatitis Delta Virus and Its Infection. New York, Alan R Liss, 1987
——— et al: Hepatitis delta virus infection of the liver: Progress in virology, pathobiology, and diagnosis. Semin Liver Dis 8:350, 1988
SEEFF LB, HOOFNAGLE JH: Immunoprophylaxis of viral hepatitis. Gastroenterology 77:161, 1979
———, KOFF R: Passive and active immunoprophylaxis of hepatitis B. Gastroenterology 86:958, 1984
——— et al: A serologic follow-up of the 1942 epidemic of post-vaccination hepatitis in the United States Army. N Engl J Med 316:765, 1987
SEEGER C et al: Biochemical and genetic evidence for the hepatitis B virus replication strategy. Science 232:477, 1986
SZMUNESS W et al: Hepatitis B vaccine: Demonstration of efficacy in a controlled clinical trial in a high-risk population in the United States. N Engl J Med 303:833, 1980
——— et al (eds): Viral Hepatitis: 1981 International Symposium. Philadelphia, Franklin Institute Press, 1982
THEILMANN L et al: Detection of pre-S1 proteins in serum and liver of HBsAg-positive patients: A new marker for hepatitis B virus infection. Hepatology 6:186, 1986

VERME G et al (eds): Viral Hepatitis and Delta Infection. New York, Alan R. Liss, 1983
VYAS GN et al (eds): Viral Hepatitis and Liver Disease. Orlando, Grune & Stratton, 1984
ZUCKERMAN AJ (ed): Viral Hepatitis and Liver Disease. New York, Alan R Liss, 1988

Drug-induced hepatitis

BLACK M et al: Isoniazid-associated hepatitis in 114 patients. Gastroenterology 69:389, 1975
ISHAK KG, IREY NS: Hepatic injury associated with the phenothiazines: Clinicopathologic and follow-up study of 36 patients. Arch Pathol 93:283, 1972
LUDWIG J, AXELSEN R: Drug effects on the liver: An updated tabular compilation of drugs and drug-related hepatic diseases. Dig Dis Sci 28:651, 1983
MITCHELL JR, JOLLOW DJ: Metabolic activation of drugs to toxic substances. Gastroenterology 68:392, 1975
RIGAS B et al: Amiodarone hepatotoxicity. Ann Intern Med 104:348, 1986
SHERLOCK S: Hepatic reactions to drugs. Gut 20:634, 1979
SMILKSTEIN MJ et al: Efficacy of N-acetylcysteine in the treatment of acetaminophen overdose. N Engl J Med 319:1557, 1988
ZAFRANI ES et al: Cholestatic and hepatocellular injury associated with erythromycin esters: Report of nine cases. Am J Dig Dis 24:38, 1979
ZIMMERMAN HJ: Hepatotoxicity. New York, Appleton-Century-Crofts, 1978
——— (ed): Drug-induced liver disease. Semin Liver Dis 1:91, 1981
———, ISHAK KG: Valproate-induced hepatic injury: Analysis of 23 fatal cases. Hepatology 2:591, 1982

253 CHRONIC HEPATITIS

JACK R. WANDS / KURT J. ISSELBACHER

Chronic hepatitis refers to three related disorders—chronic persistent hepatitis, chronic lobular hepatitis, and chronic active hepatitis. These are characterized by a combination of hepatocyte necrosis and inflammation of varying severity persisting for more than 6 months. The clinically most important disorder, chronic active hepatitis, may lead to hepatic failure and death or result in the development of cirrhosis and its sequelae. While all three forms of chronic hepatitis share some common histopathologic features and appear to be incited by similar etiologic factors, their pathogeneses, clinical presentations, natural histories, prognoses, and therapies are different.

CHRONIC PERSISTENT AND CHRONIC LOBULAR HEPATITIS Definition and etiology Chronic persistent and chronic lobular hepatitis result from infections with hepatitis B virus (HBV) and non-A, non-B hepatitis viruses. Other etiologies may exist but are poorly defined. In general, these are both nonprogressive disorders; hepatic failure is not seen and evolution into cirrhosis is exceedingly rare. Occasionally, however, patients with chronic active hepatitis may be seen during spontaneous remission, at which time the histopathologic findings may suggest chronic persistent or chronic lobular hepatitis. Under these circumstances relapses and progression to the more serious underlying chronic active hepatitis may occur. Another exception to the nonprogression of chronic persistent and lobular hepatitis occurs in patients positive to hepatitis B surface antigen (HBsAg), in whom superinfection with delta agent (HDV) may lead to the development of chronic active hepatitis (see Chap. 252). Indeed, the clinical presentation of rapidly progressive liver injury in a known chronic HBsAg carrier should suggest infection with HDV.

Pathology In typical chronic persistent hepatitis there is infiltration of the portal areas with mononuclear cells, but there is no erosion of the limiting plate (so-called piecemeal necrosis) or extension of the inflammation into the liver lobule. A "cobblestone" arrangement of liver cells, indicative of hepatic regenerative activity, is a common feature. Minimal fibrosis may be observed, but *cirrhosis is characteristically absent*. In chronic lobular hepatitis, in addition to the portal inflammatory changes, lobular inflammation and focal hepatocellular necrosis are prominent features during clinically active phases. The morphologic features of chronic persistent, lobular, and active hepatitis are compared in Table 253-1.

Clinical and laboratory features Most patients with chronic persistent and/or lobular hepatitis are asymptomatic, although some may complain of anorexia, fatigue, and occasionally of nausea and

TABLE 253-1   Some distinguishing features of chronic persistent, chronic lobular, and chronic active hepatitis

Features	Chronic persistent hepatitis	Chronic lobular hepatitis	Chronic active hepatitis
CLINICAL			
Onset like acute hepatitis	≈70%	≈90%	≈30%
Recurrent acute episodes	Infrequent	Common	Common
Extrahepatic involvement	Rare	Rare	Common
Prognosis	Good	Good	Variable
LIVER HISTOLOGY			
Piecemeal necrosis	Inconstant	Inconstant	Typical
Site of inflammation	Portal	Portal/lobular in active phase	Portal, extending into lobule
Lobular architecture	Preserved	Preserved	Distorted
Fibrosis	Slight	Slight	Common
Progression to cirrhosis	Rare	Rare	Common

vomiting. Physical findings are usually normal, but the liver may be slightly enlarged and tender. Laboratory data show mild elevations of aminotransferase and alkaline phosphatase levels and these abnormalities may persist for months to years. During active phases of chronic lobular hepatitis, aminotransferase levels may resemble those seen in acute viral hepatitis.

Management   Once the diagnosis of chronic persistent or lobular hepatitis has been established by liver biopsy, no specific therapy is required since such patients generally do not develop fibrosis and cirrhosis. Follow-up examination is recommended every 6 to 12 months until aminotransferase values have returned to normal and to identify the rare patient who may progress to chronic active hepatitis.

CHRONIC ACTIVE HEPATITIS   Definition   Chronic active hepatitis is a disorder of diverse etiologies characterized by continuing hepatic necrosis, active inflammation, and fibrosis which may lead to or be accompanied by liver failure, cirrhosis, and death. The prominence of extrahepatic features and seroimmunologic abnormalities has led to the use of a variety of terms to describe this disorder. These terms include autoimmune hepatitis, lupoid hepatitis, subacute hepatitis, and chronic active liver disease. *Chronic active hepatitis* seems to be the most appropriate designation for this clinicopathologic entity, regardless of the etiology and the clinical variations.

Pathology   Although chronic active hepatitis may be suspected from the clinical history and the physical findings, *liver biopsy is necessary to establish the diagnosis*. The cardinal histopathologic features observed in the liver include (1) a dense mononuclear and plasma cell infiltration of the portal zones which greatly expands into the liver lobule; (2) destruction of the hepatocytes at the periphery of the lobule (piecemeal necrosis) with erosion of the limiting plate surrounding the portal triads; (3) connective tissue septa extending from the portal zones into the lobule, isolating parenchymal cells into clusters and enveloping bile ducts; and (4) evidence of hepatic regeneration with "rosette" formation, thickened liver cell plates, and regenerative "pseudolobules." This process may be patchy, and individual liver lobules may remain uninvolved. Councilman-like bodies, which represent necrosis of single liver cells, may be seen in the periportal areas. The lesion of bridging hepatic necrosis may be seen in some patients with chronic active hepatitis. This lesion or its more extensive variant, multilobular bridging hepatic necrosis, suggests the presence of severe disease.

There is substantial morphologic evidence that in some instances chronic active hepatitis will progress to or is accompanied by the development of cirrhosis. On liver biopsy, cirrhosis can be demon-

strated in 20 to 50 percent of patients, even early in the course of the disease, and at autopsy postnecrotic cirrhosis may be found. It is also possible that many cases of so-called cryptogenic cirrhosis are the result of chronic active hepatitis after inflammation and necrosis have subsided. In other patients fibrosis is not progressive and morphologic evidence of cirrhosis cannot be found.

Etiology   Multiple etiologic agents may initiate chronic active hepatitis. Probably the most important and common triggering factors are infection with hepatitis B virus or the non-A, non-B hepatitis viruses. In about one-third of patients the disease begins abruptly following an illness typical of acute viral hepatitis. Persistence of HBsAg in the serum is found in 20 to 30 percent of patients with chronic active hepatitis, suggesting that persistent hepatitis B virus infection may be related to the development of this disease. Many of these HBsAg-positive patients also have positive tests for the hepatitis B e antigen (HBeAg) and have high levels of HBV-DNA in serum, indicating active viral replication (see Chap. 252). Superinfection with delta hepatitis agent in HBsAg-positive individuals may lead to the development of chronic active hepatitis and in general leads to a more serious clinical course than HBV infection alone. Similarly, persistent non-A, non-B hepatitis virus infections may be responsible for cases of chronic active hepatitis following transfusion-associated and sporadic non-A, non-B hepatitis. Drugs are involved in the pathogenesis of some cases. For example, features typical of chronic active hepatitis have been found in some patients in association with the administration of methyldopa. In these patients challenge with methyldopa has led to increased activity of the disease, while discontinuance has resulted in clinical, biochemical, and histologic improvement. Oxyphenisatin, isoniazid, nitrofurantoin, and other drugs have also been incriminated as etiologic agents in patients with chronic active hepatitis. Thus, chemical as well as viral agents may play a role in the production of chronic active hepatitis. The existence of other triggering factors seems likely, but their nature and mechanisms of action remain to be determined.

Immunopathogenesis   There is increasing evidence that the progressive parenchymal cell destruction in patients with chronic active hepatitis involves an interaction with the immune system conditioned or controlled by genetic factors. Evidence to support this concept includes the following facts: (1) In the liver the histopathologic lesions are composed predominantly of thymus-derived or T lymphocytes and plasma cells in association with progressive liver cell destruction and replacement by fibrous tissue. (2) A variety of circulating "autoantibodies" are frequently detected, such as anti-smooth-muscle, antimitochondrial, and antithyroid antibodies. (3) The persistence of HBsAg in the serum and the hepatitis B core antigen (HBcAg) in the liver cell following an attack of acute hepatitis B is frequently associated with the development of chronic active or chronic persistent hepatitis. (4) Other "autoimmune" diseases such as thyroiditis, diabetes mellitus, ulcerative colitis, Coombs-positive hemolytic anemia, proliferative glomerulonephritis, and Sjögren's syndrome may be associated with chronic active hepatitis or may occur in relatives of affected patients. (5) Histocompatibility antigens HLA-B1 or -B8 and -DRw3 and -DRw4 are more prevalent than expected in patients with chronic active hepatitis without HBsAg. (6) Finally, the use of glucocorticoids, believed to be effective in a variety of immunologic and autoimmune disorders, is often beneficial in the treatment of severe chronic active hepatitis.

There is increasing evidence that cellular immune reactions may be important in the pathogenesis of chronic active hepatitis. It has been suggested that lymphocytes become sensitized to altered or new antigens present on the surface membranes of hepatocytes. This hypothesis is supported in part by studies demonstrating that circulating and liver-derived lymphocytes may have the capability of causing liver cell damage in vitro.

Humoral immune mechanisms may be responsible for some of the clinical manifestations of chronic active hepatitis. In particular, extrahepatic features such as arthralgias, arthritis, rash, and glomerulonephritis appear to be mediated by the deposition of circulating immune complexes. Furthermore, complement activation, as demonstrated by low serum complement levels, and the presence of complement components in immune complexes suggest that circulating immune complexes may be involved in mediating extrahepatic inflammation and tissue damage.

Clinical features The clinical spectrum of chronic active hepatitis ranges from asymptomatic illness at one end to fatal hepatic failure at the other. All age groups are affected. In approximately two-thirds of patients the disease has an *insidious onset* over a period of several weeks to months, or the disease is discovered incidentally, and the duration of the illness is uncertain. In the remainder an abrupt onset similar to that in acute viral hepatitis is seen, but features of chronic active hepatitis usually develop during the ensuing 12 to 24 months. The clinical and laboratory features suggesting progression from acute hepatitis to chronic active hepatitis are discussed in Chap. 252. *Fatigue* is a common symptom. Persistent or recurrent *jaundice* is a common feature in severe disease. Intermittent deepening of jaundice and recurrent symptoms of *malaise, anorexia,* and *low-grade fever,* suggestive of a superimposed acute hepatitis, are common throughout the course of the illness. In some patients complications of cirrhosis, such as ascites, variceal bleeding, encephalopathy, coagulopathy, or hypersplenism, may first bring the patient to medical attention. In others the extrahepatic features dominate the clinical picture, and liver disease is entirely unsuspected. Extrahepatic presenting features may include amenorrhea, bloody diarrhea (due to associated ulcerative colitis), abdominal pain, arthralgia or arthritis, macular or papular eruptions, acne, erythema nodosum, pleurisy, pericarditis, anemia, azotemia, and sicca syndrome (of keratoconjunctivitis and xerostomia). These extrahepatic features and abnormal serologic reactions tend to be more frequent in women than men and in patients without serologic evidence of preceding hepatitis B.

The *course* of chronic active hepatitis is variable, and the disease may persist for long periods without clinically overt liver disease. This appears to be particularly true of chronic active hepatitis associated with hepatitis B virus or non-A, non-B hepatitis viruses. The condition may on occasion spontaneously remit into a clinically inactive phase, although continuing hepatocellular necrosis or progression to cirrhosis is usually the rule. The histologic lesion may reverse itself completely before the development of cirrhosis in some HBsAg-positive patients after their antigenemia has spontaneously cleared or following the loss of viral replication as measured by disappearance of HBV-DNA from serum and seroconversion of HBeAg from positive to negative and the development of anti-HBe. If untreated, the case fatality rate may be high during the first few years of illness, especially in patients with clinically and histologically severe disease. Death usually occurs as a result of liver failure and hepatic coma. Later death is often due to a complication of cirrhosis—variceal hemorrhage or intercurrent infection. Primary hepatocellular carcinoma is an uncommon complication of HBsAg-negative chronic active hepatitis even when the disease has progressed to postnecrotic cirrhosis. This finding is in contrast to long-term HBsAg carriers with chronic active hepatitis and/or cirrhosis in whom the incidence of liver carcinoma is high (see Chap. 252).

Laboratory findings Liver function tests are invariably abnormal but may not correlate with the clinical severity or histopathologic findings in the individual case. Many patients have normal serum bilirubin, alkaline phosphatase, and globulin levels with only minimal aminotransferase elevations or HBsAg positivity and yet have a liver biopsy consistent with severe chronic active hepatitis. Serum aspartate aminotransferase (SGOT) and alanine aminotransferase (SGPT) levels are increased and fluctuate in the range of 100 to 1000 units in most cases. In severe cases the serum bilirubin is moderately elevated [51.3 to 171 μmol/L (3 to 10 mg/dL)]. Mild hypoalbuminemia occurs in patients with active disease or in those with advanced cirrhosis. Serum alkaline phosphatase levels may be moderately elevated or near normal. The prothrombin time is often prolonged, particularly late in the disease or during active phases.

Hypergammaglobulinemia (greater than 2.5 g/dL) is common,

particularly in patients with extensive plasma cell infiltration of the liver. A variety of abnormal serologic reactions and circulating autoantibodies are found in chronic active hepatitis. Some of these serologic reactions are nonspecific and may be seen in other viral diseases. Circulating autoantibodies against DNA, IgG, smooth muscle, and mitochondria support the concept that chronic active hepatitis is indeed a systemic disease. HBsAg may be found in 20 to 30 percent of patients with chronic active hepatitis, more commonly in men than women.

Differential diagnosis Early in the course of chronic active hepatitis the disease may resemble typical *acute viral hepatitis.* However, the persistence of symptoms, including biochemical abnormalities such as elevated serum aminotransferase and bilirubin levels or circulating HBsAg over the ensuing months indicates that a chronic liver disorder is present. The major entities which must be distinguished from chronic active hepatitis are *chronic persistent and lobular hepatitis.* As indicated in Table 253-1, in chronic persistent and lobular hepatitis the onset of the illness frequently resembles acute hepatitis. The aminotransferase enzyme values are variably elevated, and HBsAg may be present in serum. Fatigue, anorexia, malaise, right upper quadrant discomfort, and hepatomegaly may be associated with all three forms of chronic hepatitis. Thus, a definitive diagnosis can only be established by liver biopsy since a *differentiation between chronic active, chronic persistent, and lobular hepatitis cannot be made by clinical and biochemical criteria.* This distinction is important because chronic persistent and lobular hepatitis are not progressive disorders, rarely if ever result in cirrhosis, and require no therapy.

The presence of extrahepatic manifestations in chronic active hepatitis such as pleuritis, arthritis, and arthralgias may cause confusion with *connective tissue disorders* such as rheumatoid arthritis and systemic lupus erythematosus. The existence of clinical and biochemical features suggestive of progressive liver disease clearly distinguishes chronic active hepatitis from these disorders. In adolescence, *Wilson's disease* may present with features of chronic active hepatitis before the neurologic manifestations become apparent; serum ceruloplasmin, serum and urinary copper determination, and measurement of the liver copper levels will establish the diagnosis. Late in the course of chronic active hepatitis some patients may present with *postnecrotic cirrhosis* without evidence of active hepatitis. This lesion, termed cryptogenic cirrhosis, may also represent an end stage of other destructive liver diseases (e.g., primary biliary cirrhosis). *Primary biliary cirrhosis* may share histologic similarities with chronic active hepatitis, particularly early in the disease. However, in primary biliary cirrhosis the prominence of pruritus plus markedly elevated serum alkaline phosphatase and cholesterol levels, the presence of high titers of antimitochondrial antibodies (in contrast to the low levels seen in chronic active hepatitis), and the pattern of histologic progression will usually permit differentiation from chronic active hepatitis.

Management In chronic active hepatitis *not* associated with hepatitis B virus or non-A, non-B viruses glucocorticoid therapy is the treatment of choice. Glucocorticoids have been shown to be effective in prolonging survival of these patients during the first few years of illness when the mortality rate is high. A therapeutic response characterized by a complete clinical, biochemical, and histologic remission is to be expected in 60 to 80 percent of patients. Either prednisone or prednisolone therapy should be initiated at a dose of 20 to 40 mg daily. This dose can usually be gradually tapered within 2 to 3 months to 10 to 20 mg daily. The beneficial effects of glucocorticoid treatment on the course and prognosis of patients with mild or asymptomatic chronic active hepatitis has not been established.

Improvement of fatigue and anorexia is usually noted within days to several weeks. Biochemical improvement is to be expected over several weeks to months, with a fall in serum bilirubin and globulin levels and a rise in serum albumin. The serum aminotransferase level usually drops promptly, but the absolute value of the aminotransferase *alone* does not appear to be a useful marker of recovery in the individual patient. Histologic improvement, characterized by a decrease in mononuclear infiltration and subsequent improvement in the extent of hepatocellular necrosis, may be delayed for 6 to 24 months. After a favorable clinical and biochemical response, repeat liver biopsy may show features consistent with chronic persistent hepatitis. Despite this histologic improvement, relapses are common when glucocorticoids are discontinued.

Reduction of the suppressive glucocorticoid doses should be performed cautiously, particularly at lower prednisone levels, since even small decrements in therapy may be associated with clinical worsening, and increasing dosage may be needed for control of spontaneous exacerbation. Unless major complications require discontinuation of glucocorticoids, they should be prescribed for at least 12 months or longer in order to reduce the risk of relapse.

Other therapeutic approaches have been used in the treatment of severe chronic active hepatitis, particularly in the elderly and in patients with major side effects from glucocorticoids. An initial prednisone dosage of 30 mg, tapered down to 10 to 20 mg, in combination with 50 to 75 mg azathioprine has been demonstrated to be effective; this treatment avoids the adverse effects of high dosage of glucocorticoids. However, *azathioprine alone is not effective* in the treatment of chronic active hepatitis. Alternate-day prednisone therapy diminishes steroid side effects but usually does not provide adequate therapy.

Glucocorticoids have little if any beneficial effect on the natural course of HBsAg-positive chronic active hepatitis. Treatment of *asymptomatic* HBsAg carriers who only have evidence of chronic active hepatitis on liver biopsy is not justified. In *symptomatic* HBsAg-positive patients with severe chronic active hepatitis, glucocorticoids have not been shown to be of value either in short- or long-term therapy. Similarly, in chronic active hepatitis caused by non-A, non-B viruses long-term glucocorticoid therapy is not beneficial and may be detrimental. Other therapeutic modalities have been used in the treatment of chronic active hepatitis associated with hepatitis B virus or non-A, non-B viruses including azathioprine, D-penicillamine, cyclophosphamide, interleukin 2, acyclovir, adenine arabinoside, and adenine arabinoside monophosphate. These agents have not yet been shown to be effective in the majority of patients. Randomized controlled studies on a limited number of patients with chronic active hepatitis caused by hepatitis B virus or non-A, non-B viruses using alpha interferon showed some promise in reducing or eliminating viral replication. In those patients who responded, improvement in serum alanine aminotransferase values and liver histopathology has been observed. These and other therapeutic strategies (e.g., combination of different interferons, glucocorticoid therapy and withdrawal followed by interferon, and others) are currently undergoing controlled clinical trials. While none of these therapeutic strategies can be recommended for general use at present, patients with chronic active viral hepatitis may benefit from referral to medical centers participating in therapeutic trials.

REFERENCES

CASELMANN WH et al: β and γ interferon in chronic active hepatitis: A pilot trial of short term combination therapy. Gastroenterology 96:449, 1989

CZAJA AJ et al: Laboratory assessment of severe chronic active liver disease during and after corticosteroid therapy. Correlation of serum transaminase and gamma globulin levels with histologic features. Gastroenterology 80:667, 1981

HODGES JR et al: Chronic active hepatitis: The spectrum of disease. Lancet 1:550, 1982

HOOFNAGEL JH et al: Randomized, control trial of recombinant alpha interferon in patients with chronic active hepatitis B. Gastroenterology 95:1318, 1988

JACYNA MR et al: Randomized controlled trial of interferon alpha (lymphoblastoid interferon) in chronic non-A, non-B hepatitis. Br Med J 298:80, 1989

LAM KC et al: Deleterious effect of prednisolone in HBsAg-positive chronic active hepatitis. N Engl J Med 304:380, 1981

MACKAY IR, TAIT BD: HLA associations with autoimmune-type chronic active hepatitis: Identification of B8-DRw3 haplotypes by family studies. Gastroenterology 79:95, 1980

SEEF LB, KOFF RS: Therapy for chronic active hepatitis. Adv Intern Med 29:109, 1984

WEISSBERG JI et al: Survival in chronic hepatitis B. An analysis of 379 patients. Ann Intern Med 101:613, 1984

WELLER IVD et al: Effects of prednisone/azathioprine in chronic hepatitis B viral infection. Gut 23:650, 1982

254   CIRRHOSIS OF THE LIVER

DANIEL K. PODOLSKY / KURT J. ISSELBACHER

Cirrhosis is a pathologically defined entity which is associated with a spectrum of characteristic clinical manifestations. The cardinal pathologic features reflect irreversible chronic injury of the hepatic parenchyma and include extensive fibrosis in association with the formation of regenerative nodules. These features result from hepatocyte necrosis, collapse of the supporting reticulin network with subsequent connective tissue deposition, distortion of the vascular bed, and nodular regeneration of remaining liver parenchyma. The pathologic process should be viewed as a final common pathway of many types of chronic liver injury. Clinical features of cirrhosis derive from the morphologic alterations and often reflect the severity of hepatic damage rather than the etiology of the underlying liver disease. Loss of functioning hepatocellular mass may lead to jaundice, edema, coagulopathy, and a variety of metabolic abnormalities; fibrosis and distorted vasculature lead to portal hypertension and its sequelae, including gastroesophageal varices and splenomegaly. Ascites and hepatic encephalopathy result from both hepatocellular insufficiency and portal hypertension.

Classification of the various types of cirrhosis based solely on etiology or morphology is unsatisfactory. A single pathologic pattern may result from a variety of insults, while the same insult may produce several morphologic patterns. Nevertheless most types of cirrhosis may be usefully classified by a mixture of etiologically and morphologically defined entities as follows: (1) alcoholic; (2) cryptogenic and postviral or postnecrotic; (3) biliary; (4) cardiac; (5) metabolic, inherited, and drug-related; and (6) miscellaneous. This chapter considers first the various types of cirrhosis and then the major clinical complications of chronic liver disease and cirrhosis.

ALCOHOLIC LIVER DISEASE AND CIRRHOSIS

Definition Alcoholic cirrhosis, historically referred to as Laennec's cirrhosis, is the most common type of cirrhosis encountered in North America and many parts of western Europe and South America. It is usually characterized by diffuse fine scarring, fairly uniform loss of liver cells, and small regenerative nodules, and therefore, it is sometimes referred to as micronodular cirrhosis. However, micronodular cirrhosis may also result from other types of liver injury (e.g., following jejunoileal bypass), and thus alcoholic cirrhosis and micronodular cirrhosis are not necessarily synonymous. Conversely alcoholic cirrhosis may progress to macronodular cirrhosis with time.

Alcoholic cirrhosis is only one of many consequences resulting from chronic alcoholic ingestion, and it often accompanies other forms of alcohol-induced liver injury. The three principal alcohol-induced hepatic lesions are designated: (1) alcoholic fatty liver, (2) alcoholic hepatitis, and (3) alcoholic cirrhosis. These morphologic categories are rarely found in a pure form, and features of each may be present to varying degrees in an individual patient.

Etiology Although chronic alcoholism is the most common cause of cirrhosis, the quantity and duration of drinking necessary to cause cirrhosis remain unclear. The typical alcoholic patient with cirrhosis has had a daily consumption of a pint or more of whiskey, several quarts of wine, or an equivalent amount of beer for at least 10 years. The amount and duration of ethanol ingestion, rather than the type of alcoholic beverage or the pattern of ingestion, appear to be the important determinants of liver injury. In general, the latent period preceding the development of cirrhosis is inversely related to the level of daily alcohol intake. Rates of ethanol metabolism are under genetic control, but no metabolic defect has been identified in cirrhotic patients or their families to suggest a unique "susceptibility" to ethanol or its toxic effects. Although malnutrition per se does not appear to lead to cirrhosis, it is possible that nutritional factors may augment the detrimental effects of chronic alcohol ingestion on the liver. The finding that only 10 to 15 percent of alcoholics develop cirrhosis suggests that other factors may affect the impact of alcohol on the liver. Women, on average, appear to develop alcohol-induced liver injury at lesser levels of consumption than men, suggesting that hormonal factors may play a role in susceptibility.

Alcoholic fatty liver occurs in most heavy drinkers but is reversible on cessation of alcohol consumption and is not thought to be an inevitable precursor of alcoholic hepatitis or cirrhosis. In contrast, alcoholic hepatitis, an inflammatory lesion characterized by infiltration of the liver with leukocytes, liver cell necrosis, and alcoholic hyaline, is thought to be the major precursor of cirrhosis. Subsequent healing accompanied by fibrosis distorts the normal lobular architecture. Indeed, *deposition of collagen in perivenular spaces* may be the earliest manifestation of the process which ultimately leads to cirrhosis.

Pathology and pathogenesis ALCOHOLIC FATTY LIVER The liver is enlarged, yellow, greasy, and firm. Hepatocytes are distended by large cytoplasmic fat vacuoles which push the hepatocyte nucleus against the cell membrane. Accumulation of fat in the liver of the alcoholic results from the combination of impaired fatty acid oxidation, increased uptake and esterification of fatty acids to form triglycerides, and diminished lipoprotein biosynthesis and secretion.

ALCOHOLIC HEPATITIS Morphologic features include hepatocyte degeneration and necrosis, often with ballooned cells, and an infiltrate of polymorphonuclear leukocytes and lymphocytes. The polymorphonuclear cells may encircle damaged hepatocytes which contain *Mallory bodies*, or *alcoholic hyaline*. These are clumps of perinuclear, deeply eosinophilic material believed to represent aggregated intermediate filaments. Mallory bodies are highly suggestive of, but *not specific* for, alcoholic hepatitis, since morphologically similar material has been seen in association with morbid obesity, jejunoileal bypass surgery, poorly controlled diabetes mellitus, and a variety of other disorders including Wilson's disease and Indian childhood cirrhosis. Deposition of collagen around the central vein and in perisinusoidal areas, often termed central hyaline sclerosis, may be associated with an increased likelihood of progression to cirrhosis.

ALCOHOLIC CIRRHOSIS With continued alcohol intake and destruction of hepatocytes, fibroblasts (including myofibroblasts with contractile properties) appear at the site of injury and stimulate collagen formation. Weblike septa of connective tissue appear in periportal and pericentral zones and eventually connect portal triads and central veins. This fine connective tissue network surrounds small masses of remaining liver cells which regenerate and form nodules. Although regeneration occurs within the small remnants of parenchyma, cell loss generally exceeds replacement. With continuing hepatocyte destruction and collagen deposition, the liver shrinks in size, acquires a nodular appearance, and becomes hard as "end-stage" cirrhosis develops. Although alcoholic cirrhosis is usually a progressive disease, appropriate therapy and strict avoidance of alcohol may arrest the disease at most stages and permit functional improvement.

Clinical features SIGNS AND SYMPTOMS Clinical manifestations of *alcoholic fatty liver* are often minimal or entirely absent, and the disorder may not be recognized unless another illness (frequently alcohol-related) brings the patient to medical attention. Hepatomegaly, at times accompanied by tenderness, may be the only finding. Jaundice, ascites, and edema are only seen with more serious liver injury.

The clinical severity of *alcoholic hepatitis* varies enormously, ranging from asymptomatic or mild illness to fatal hepatic insufficiency. Typically, the clinical features of alcoholic hepatitis resemble those of viral or toxic liver injury. Patients often experience anorexia, nausea and vomiting, malaise, weight loss, abdominal distress, and jaundice. Fever as high as 39.4°C (103°F) may be seen in about half of cases. On physical examination, tender hepatomegaly is common, and splenomegaly is found in about one-third of patients. The patient may have cutaneous arterial "spider" angiomas and jaundice. More severe cases may be complicated by ascites, edema, bleeding, and

encephalopathy. At the time of initial presentation, the central nervous system findings may be difficult to distinguish from manifestations of concurrent alcohol intoxication or withdrawal (see below).

Although jaundice, ascites, and encephalopathy may subside with abstinence, continued alcohol excess and poor dietary habits usually lead to repeated acute episodes of hepatic decompensation. Some patients die during these acute exacerbations, but most recover after several weeks or months. Even after complete abstinence, clinical recovery may be protracted, and histologic abnormalities can persist up to 6 months or longer. Cholestatic jaundice mimicking biliary tract obstruction may also develop in some cases of acute alcoholic hepatitis.

Alcoholic cirrhosis may also be clinically silent; in fact 10 percent of cases are discovered incidentally at laparotomy or autopsy. In many cases symptoms are insidious in onset, occurring usually after 10 or more years of excessive alcohol use and progressing slowly over subsequent weeks and months. Anorexia and malnutrition lead to weight loss and a reduction in skeletal muscle mass. The patient may experience easy bruising, increasing weakness, and fatigue. Eventually the clinical manifestations of hepatocellular dysfunction and portal hypertension ensue, including progressive jaundice, bleeding from gastroesophageal varices, ascites, and encephalopathy. The abrupt onset of one of these complications may be the first event prompting the patient to seek medical attention. In other cases, cirrhosis first becomes evident when the patient requires treatment of symptoms related to alcoholic hepatitis.

A firm, nodular liver may be an early sign of disease; the liver may be either enlarged, normal, or decreased in size. Other frequent findings include jaundice, palmar erythema, spider angiomas, parotid and lacrimal gland enlargement, clubbing of fingers, splenomegaly, muscle wasting, and ascites with or without peripheral edema. Men may have decreased body hair and/or gynecomastia and testicular atrophy, which, like the cutaneous findings, result from disturbances in hormonal metabolism, including increased peripheral formation of estrogen due to diminished hepatic clearance of the precursor androstenedione. Testicular atrophy may reflect hormonal abnormalities or the toxic effect of alcohol on the testes. In women, signs of virilization or menstrual irregularities may occasionally be encountered. Dupuytren's contractures resulting from fibrosis of the palmar fascia with resulting flexion contracture of the digits are associated with alcoholism but are not specifically related to cirrhosis.

Over a period of 3 to 5 years, the cirrhotic patient typically becomes emaciated, weak, and chronically jaundiced. Ascites and other signs of portal hypertension become increasingly prominent. Most patients with advanced cirrhosis die in hepatic coma, commonly precipitated by hemorrhage from esophageal varices or intercurrent infection. Progressive renal dysfunction often complicates the terminal phase of the illness.

LABORATORY FINDINGS Routine hematologic and biochemical blood tests are usually normal in patients with alcoholic fatty liver, except for minimal elevations of the serum AST (aspartate aminotransferase, SGOT); occasionally alkaline phosphatase and bilirubin levels are also elevated. In more advanced alcoholic liver disease, abnormalities of laboratory tests are more common. Anemia may result from acute and chronic gastrointestinal blood loss, coexistent nutritional deficiency (notably of folic acid and vitamin B_{12}), hypersplenism, and a direct suppressive effect of alcohol on the bone marrow. Hemolytic anemia presumably due to effects of hypercholesterolemia on erythrocyte membranes resulting in unusual spurlike projections (acanthocytosis) has been described in some alcoholics with cirrhosis. Leukocytosis is often present in severe alcoholic hepatitis; however, some patients with this disorder may have leukopenia and thrombocytopenia due to hypersplenism or an inhibitory effect of alcohol on the bone marrow. Mild or pronounced hyperbilirubinemia may be found, usually in association with varying elevations of serum alkaline phosphatase levels. Frequently elevated are levels of serum AST, but levels greater than 5 μkat (300 units) are unusual and should prompt one to look for other coincident or complicating factors. In contrast to viral hepatitis, the serum AST is usually disproportionately elevated relative to alanine aminotransferase (AST/ALT ratio > 2).* This discrepancy may result from the proportionally greater inhibition of ALT synthesis by ethanol, which may be partially reversed by pyridoxal phosphate.

The serum prothrombin time is frequently prolonged, reflecting reduced synthesis of clotting proteins, most notably the vitamin K–dependent factors (see "Coagulopathy" below). The serum albumin level is usually depressed, while serum globulins are increased. Hypoalbuminemia reflects in part overall impairment in hepatic protein synthesis, while hyperglobulinemia is thought to result from nonspecific stimulation of the reticuloendothelial system. Elevated blood ammonia levels in patients with hepatic encephalopathy reflect diminished hepatic clearance because of impaired liver function and shunting of portal venous blood around the cirrhotic liver into the systemic circulation (see below and Chap. 250).

A variety of metabolic disturbances may be detected. Glucose intolerance due to endogenous insulin resistance may be present; however, clinical diabetes is uncommon. Central hyperventilation may lead to respiratory alkalosis in patients with cirrhosis. *Dietary deficiency* and *increased urinary losses* lead to hypomagnesemia and *hypophosphatemia*. In patients with ascites and dilutional hyponatremia, hypokalemia may occur from increased urinary potassium losses due in part to hyperaldosteronism. Prerenal azotemia is also observed in such patients.

Diagnosis   *Alcoholic fatty liver* should be suspected in alcoholic patients with hepatomegaly and normal or minimally deranged liver function tests. Alcoholic fatty liver may be seen in combination with alcoholic hepatitis or established cirrhosis. *Alcoholic hepatitis* should be considered in an alcoholic who has been drinking heavily and demonstrates jaundice, fever, an enlarged, tender liver, or ascites. The clinical impression is often supported by the deranged results of tests of liver function and other laboratory abnormalities described above. Alcoholic hepatitis or fatty liver may be present in association with alcoholic cirrhosis.

Alcoholic cirrhosis should be strongly suspected in patients with a history of prolonged or excessive alcohol intake and physical signs of chronic liver disease. The clinical features and laboratory findings are usually sufficient to provide reasonable indication of the presence and extent of hepatic injury. Although a percutaneous needle biopsy of the liver is not usually necessary to confirm the typical findings of alcoholic hepatitis or cirrhosis, it may be helpful in distinguishing patients with less advanced liver disease from those with cirrhosis and in excluding other forms of liver injury such as viral hepatitis. Biopsy may also be helpful as a diagnostic tool in evaluating patients with clinical findings suggestive of alcoholic liver disease who deny alcohol intake. In patients with features of cholestasis, ultrasonography may be appropriate to exclude the presence of extrahepatic biliary obstruction. When the clinical status of an otherwise stable cirrhotic patient deteriorates without an obvious explanation, complicating conditions, such as infection, portal vein thrombosis, and hepatocellular carcinoma, should be sought.

Prognosis   The patient with an alcoholic fatty liver and no complications has a good prognosis; rapid and complete resolution usually follows cessation of alcohol intake. In patients with alcoholic hepatitis, the presence of marked hyperbilirubinemia, rising serum creatinine, marked prolongation of the prothrombin time (> 1.5 times control), ascites, and encephalopathy are associated with a poor short-term prognosis; the in-hospital mortality in these patients may exceed 50 percent. In milder cases, clinical recovery may be complete, but repeated bouts of alcoholic hepatitis usually lead to irreversible and progressive chronic liver injury. Abstinence from alcohol as well as early and appropriate medical care can decrease long-term morbidity and mortality, and delay or prevent the appearance of further complications. Patients who have had a major complication of cirrhosis and who continue to drink, have a 5-year survival of less than 50

* ALT = alanine aminotransferase, SGPT.

percent. However, those patients who remain abstinent have a substantially better prognosis. In general, overall outlook in patients with advanced liver disease remains poor; most of these patients eventually die as a result of massive variceal hemorrhage and/or profound hepatic encephalopathy.

Treatment   Alcoholic hepatitis and cirrhosis are serious illnesses that require long-term medical supervision and careful management. Therapy of the underlying liver disease is largely supportive. Specific treatment is directed at particular complications such as variceal bleeding and ascites (see below). Some studies suggest that administration of prednisone or prednisolone in moderately large doses may be helpful in patients with severe alcoholic hepatitis and encephalopathy. However, the use of glucocorticoids in acute alcoholic hepatitis remains controversial and is not recommended. Although a number of studies have supported the use of propylthiouracil in the management of acute alcoholic hepatitis, the way it works is as yet undefined, and its efficacy has not been unequivocally established. More recently maintenance therapy with colchicine (0.6 mg PO bid) in the patient has been shown to slow progression and increase longevity of alcoholic liver disease in one long-term study. Other agents, such as penicillamine and intravenous infusion of insulin and glucagon, have been used experimentally, but their therapeutic efficacy and safety remain to be demonstrated.

In the absence of signs of impending hepatic coma, the patient should be placed on a diet containing at least 1 g protein per kilogram of body weight and 8500 to 12,500 kJ (2000 to 3000 kcal) per day. Use of diets enriched in branched-chain amino acids has been advocated in patients predisposed to hepatic encephalopathy, but the value of these diets in patients with compensated cirrhosis is unproven. Daily multivitamin supplements should be prescribed, with the addition of large parenteral doses of thiamine in patients with Wernicke-Korsakoff disease (see Chap. 357). The patient should be made to realize that there is no medication that will protect the liver against the effects of further alcohol ingestion. Therefore, alcohol should be absolutely forbidden. An important component of the complete care of such patients is encouragement to become involved in an appropriate alcohol counseling program.

All medicines must be administered with caution in the patient with cirrhosis, especially those eliminated or modified through hepatic metabolism or biliary pathways. In particular, care must be taken to avoid overzealous use of drugs that may directly or indirectly precipitate complications of cirrhosis. For example, vigorous treatment of ascites with diuretics may result in electrolyte abnormalities or hypovolemia which can lead to coma. Similarly, even modest doses of sedative can lead to deepening encephalopathy.

POSTNECROTIC CIRRHOSIS, POSTVIRAL CIRRHOSIS

Definition   Postnecrotic cirrhosis represents the final common pathway of many types of advanced liver injury. *Coarsely nodular, posthepatitic,* and *multilobular cirrhosis* are terms synonymous with postnecrotic cirrhosis. The term *cryptogenic cirrhosis* has been used interchangeably with postnecrotic cirrhosis, but this designation should be reserved for those cases in which the etiology of cirrhosis is unknown (approximately 10 percent of all patients with cirrhosis).

Postnecrotic cirrhosis is characterized morphologically by (1) extensive confluent loss of liver cells, (2) stromal collapse and fibrosis resulting in broad bands of connective tissue containing the remains of many portal triads, and (3) irregular nodules of regenerating hepatocytes, varying in size from microscopic to several centimeters in diameter.

Etiology   Postnecrotic cirrhosis is a morphologic term referring to a defined stage of advanced chronic liver injury of both specific and unknown (cryptogenic) causes. Epidemiologic and serologic evidence suggests that viral hepatitis (hepatitis B or non-A, non-B) may be an antecedent factor in at least one-fourth of cases of apparently cryptogenic postnecrotic cirrhosis. In areas where hepatitis B virus infection is endemic (e.g., southeast Asia, sub-Saharan Africa), up to 15 percent of the population may acquire the infection in early childhood, and cirrhosis may ultimately develop in one-fourth of these chronic carriers. Although hepatitis B infection is much less prevalent in the United States, it is relatively common among certain high-risk groups (e.g., promiscuous homosexual men, intravenous drug abusers), and contributes to an increased incidence of cirrhosis. In the United States non-A, non-B hepatitis agents appear to account for many cases of cirrhosis following blood transfusions. It is estimated that non-A, non-B hepatitis occurs in up to 10 percent of blood recipients, of whom as many as 5 to 10 percent may ultimately develop postnecrotic cirrhosis. Because reliable serologic markers for non-A, non-B hepatitis are not yet available, the number of cases of postnecrotic cirrhosis attributable to this agent (or agents) is difficult to determine but may be substantial (see Chap. 252). Postnecrotic cirrhosis may also develop in patients with chronic active hepatitis of the autoimmune type (see Chaps. 252 and 253).

Other probable causes of postnecrotic cirrhosis, including drugs and toxins, are listed in Table 254-1. In some instances, advanced alcoholic liver disease and primary biliary cirrhosis may lead to postnecrotic cirrhosis.

Pathology   The postnecrotic liver is typically shrunken in size, distorted in shape, and composed of nodules of liver cells separated by dense and broad bands of fibrosis. The microscopic picture is consistent with the gross impression: nodules are highly variable in size with large amounts of connective tissue separating the disorganized islands of regenerating parenchyma.

Clinical features   In patients with cirrhosis of known etiology in whom there is progression to a postnecrotic stage, the clinical manifestations are an extension of those resulting from the initial disease process. Usually clinical symptoms are related to portal hypertension and its sequelae, such as ascites, splenomegaly, hypersplenism, encephalopathy, and bleeding esophageal varices. The hematologic and liver function abnormalities resemble those seen with other types of cirrhosis. In a few patients with postnecrotic cirrhosis the diagnosis may be made incidentally at operation, at postmortem, or by a needle biopsy of the liver performed to investigate asymptomatic hepatosplenomegaly.

Diagnosis and prognosis   Postnecrotic cirrhosis should be suspected in patients with signs and symptoms of cirrhosis or portal hypertension. Needle or operative liver biopsies confirm the diagnosis, although nonuniformity of the pathologic process may result in sampling errors. The diagnosis of cryptogenic cirrhosis is reserved for those patients in whom no known etiology can be demonstrated. About 75 percent of patients have progressive disease despite supportive therapy and die within 1 to 5 years from complications including exsanguinating variceal hemorrhage, hepatic encephalopathy, or superimposed hepatocellular carcinoma.

Treatment   Management is usually limited to treatment of the complications of portal hypertension, including control of ascites, avoidance of drugs or excessive protein intake that may induce hepatic coma, and prompt treatment of infections (see below). In patients with asymptomatic cirrhosis, expectant management alone is appropriate. In those patients in whom postnecrotic cirrhosis has developed as a result of a treatable condition, therapy directed at the primary disorder may limit further progression (e.g., Wilson's disease, hemochromatosis).

BILIARY CIRRHOSIS

Biliary cirrhosis results from injury to or prolonged obstruction of either the intrahepatic or extrahepatic biliary system. It is associated with impaired biliary excretion, destruction of hepatic parenchyma, and progressive fibrosis. Primary biliary cirrhosis is characterized by chronic inflammation and fibrous obliteration of intrahepatic bile ductules. Secondary biliary cirrhosis is the result of long-standing obstruction of the larger extrahepatic ducts. Although primary and secondary biliary cirrhosis are separate pathophysiologic entities with respect to the initial insult, many clinical features are similar.

PRIMARY BILIARY CIRRHOSIS   Etiology and pathogenesis   The cause of primary biliary cirrhosis remains unknown. Several observations suggest that a disordered immune response may be involved. Primary biliary cirrhosis is frequently associated with a variety of disorders presumed to be autoimmune in nature, such as the CRST syndrome (calcinosis, Raynaud's phenomenon, sclerodactyly, telangiectasia), the sicca syndrome (dry eyes and dry mouth), autoimmune thyroiditis, and renal tubular acidosis. Most importantly, a circulating IgG antimitochondrial antibody is detected in more than 95 percent of patients with primary biliary cirrhosis and only rarely in other forms of liver disease. In addition, elevated serum levels of IgM and cryoproteins consisting of immune complexes capable of activating the alternate complement pathway are found in 80 to 90 percent of patients. Lymphocytes are prominent in the portal regions and surround damaged bile ducts. These histologic findings resemble those noted in graft-versus-host disease following liver and bone marrow transplantation and suggest that damage to bile ducts may be immunologically mediated, perhaps reflecting a defect in a suppressor cell population.

Pathology   Primary biliary cirrhosis is often divided into four stages based on morphologic findings. The earliest recognizable lesion (stage I), termed *chronic nonsuppurative destructive cholangitis*, is a necrotizing inflammatory process of the portal triads. It is characterized by destruction of medium and small bile ducts, a dense infiltrate of acute and chronic inflammatory cells, mild fibrosis, and occasionally bile stasis. At times, periductal granulomas and lymph follicles are found adjacent to affected bile ducts. Subsequently, the inflammatory infiltrate becomes less prominent, the number of bile ducts is reduced, and smaller bile ductules proliferate (stage II). Progression over a period of months to years leads to a decrease in interlobular ducts, loss of liver cells, and expansion of periportal fibrosis into a network of connective tissue scars (stage III). Ultimately, cirrhosis, which may be micronodular or macronodular, develops (stage IV).

TABLE 254-1   Cirrhosis and/or liver disease associated with infectious, metabolic, hereditary, drug-related, and other types of disorders

1 Infectious diseases
  a Viral hepatitis [hepatitis B, non-A, non-B, hepatitis D, cytomegalovirus (Chaps. 138, 326, and 333)]
  b Toxoplasmosis (Chap 162)
  c Schistosomiasis (Chap. 170)
  d Ecchinococcus (Chap. 171)
  e Brucellosis (Chap. 119)
2 Inherited and metabolic disorders (see also Chap. 256)
  a Hemochromatosis (Chap. 327)
  b Wilson's disease (Chap. 330)
  c Alpha₁-antitrypsin deficiency (Chap. 208)
  d Galactosemia (Chap. 337)
  e Glycogen storage disease (Chap. 332)
  f Gaucher's disease (Chap. 331)
  g Hereditary fructose intolerance (Chap. 337)
  h Hereditary tyrosinemia (Chap. 334)
  i Fanconi's syndrome (Chap. 331)
3 Drugs and toxins (Chap. 252)
  a Methyldopa
  b Methotrexate
  c Isoniazid
  d Perhexilene maleate
  e Oxyphenisatin
  f Arsenicals
  g Pyrrolidizine alkaloids (venoocclusive disease)
  h Oral contraceptives (Budd-Chiari)
4 Other or unproven causes
  a Sarcoidosis (Chap. 252)
  b Graft-versus-host disease
  c Chronic inflammatory bowel disease (Chap. 241)
  d Cystic fibrosis (Chap. 209)
  e Jejunoileal bypass (Chap. 45)
  f Diabetes mellitus (Chap. 319)

Clinical features SIGNS AND SYMPTOMS Many patients with primary biliary cirrhosis are asymptomatic, and the disease is initially detected on the basis of elevated serum alkaline phosphatase levels during routine screening. The majority of such patients remain asymptomatic and do not develop progressive liver injury.

Among patients with symptomatic disease 90 percent are women ages 35 to 60. The earliest symptom is usually pruritus, which may be either generalized or limited initially to the palms and soles. After several months or years, jaundice and gradual darkening of the exposed areas of the skin (melanosis) may ensue. Other early clinical manifestations of primary biliary cirrhosis reflect impaired bile excretion. These include steatorrhea and the malabsorption of lipid-soluble vitamins often resulting in easy bruising (vitamin K deficiency), bone pain due to osteomalacia (vitamin D deficiency), occasionally night blindness (vitamin A deficiency), and dermatitis (possibly vitamin E and/or essential fatty acid deficiency). Protracted elevation of serum lipids, especially cholesterol, leads to subcutaneous lipid deposition around the eyes (xanthelasmas) and over joints and tendons (xanthomas). Over a period of months to years, the itching, jaundice, and hyperpigmentation slowly worsen. Eventually signs of hepatocellular failure and portal hypertension develop and ascites appears. Death due to hepatic insufficiency usually occurs within 5 to 10 years after the first signs of the illness and is often precipitated by uncontrolled variceal hemorrhage or infection.

Physical examination may be entirely normal in the early phase of the disease, when patients are asymptomatic or pruritus is the sole complaint. Later there may be jaundice of varying intensity, hyperpigmentation of the exposed skin areas, xanthelasmas and tendinous and planar xanthomas, moderate to striking hepatomegaly, splenomegaly, and clubbing of the fingers. Bone tenderness, signs of vertebral compression, ecchymoses, glossitis, and dermatitis may all be noted. Clinical evidence of the sicca syndrome can be found in as many as 75 percent of patients, and serologic evidence of autoimmune thyroid disease in 25 percent. Other conditions encountered with increased frequency include rheumatoid arthritis, CRST syndrome, scleroderma, pernicious anemia, and renal tubular acidosis.

LABORATORY FINDINGS Primary biliary cirrhosis is increasingly diagnosed at a presymptomatic stage, prompted by the finding of a two- to fivefold elevation of the serum alkaline phosphatase during routine screening. Serum 5'-nucleotidase activity is also elevated. In this setting, serum bilirubin and aminotransferase levels are usually normal, but the diagnosis is supported by a positive antimitochondrial antibody test (titer > 1:40). The latter is both *relatively* specific and sensitive; a positive test is found in over 90 percent of symptomatic patients. As the disease evolves, the serum bilirubin level rises progressively and may reach 510 μmol/L (30 mg/dL) or more in the final stages. Serum aminotransferase values rarely exceed 2.5 to 3.3 μkat (150 to 200 units). Hyperlipidemia is common, and a striking increase of the serum unesterified cholesterol is often noted. An abnormal serum lipoprotein (lipoprotein X) may be present in primary biliary cirrhosis but is not specific and appears in other cholestatic conditions. A deficiency of bile salts in the intestine leads to moderate steatorrhea and impaired absorption of the fat-soluble vitamins and hypoprothrombinemia. Patients with primary biliary cirrhosis have elevated liver copper levels, but this finding is not specific and is found in all disorders in which there is prolonged cholestasis.

Diagnosis Primary biliary cirrhosis should be considered in middle-aged women with unexplained pruritus or an elevated serum alkaline phosphatase and in whom there may be other clinical or laboratory features of protracted impairment in biliary excretion. Although a positive serum antimitochondrial antibody determination provides important diagnostic evidence, false-positive results do occur, and therefore liver biopsy should be performed to confirm the diagnosis. In most cases the biliary tract should be evaluated to exclude remediable extrahepatic biliary tract obstruction especially in view of the frequent presence of coexisting cholelithiasis.

Treatment There is no specific therapy for primary biliary cirrhosis. Corticosteroids are ineffective and may actually worsen the bone disease. D-Penicillamine has been tried because of its ability to chelate copper and because of its possible antifibrotic and immunomodulating activities. However, the drug appears to be ineffective and has a high incidence of unacceptable side effects. While some have suggested that azathioprine may be helpful in slowing the progression of disease, this has not been established. Colchicine has been shown to have some effect in slowing the progression of disease in symptomatic patients and should be tried (0.6 mg PO bid) unless gastrointestinal intolerance is limiting. Although not yet confirmed, treatment with low-dose methotrexate has been reported to halt or reverse progression of primary biliary cirrhosis.

Treatment is generally directed toward the relief of symptoms. Although the mechanism of the protracted pruritus is not entirely clear, cholestyramine, an oral bile salt–sequestering resin, may be helpful in doses of 8 to 12 g per day to decrease both the pruritus and the hypercholesterolemia. Steatorrhea can be reduced by a low-fat diet and substituting medium-chain triglycerides for dietary long-chain triglycerides. Fat-soluble vitamins A and K should be given by parenteral injection at regular intervals to prevent or correct night blindness and hypoprothrombinemia, respectively. Zinc supplementation may be necessary if night blindness is refractory to vitamin A therapy. Osteomalacia may be ameliorated by dietary calcium supplements in conjunction with oral vitamin D. In advanced disease, $25(OH)D_3$ or $1,25(OH_2)D_3$ may be preferred to vitamin D since poor hepatic function may limit conversion of vitamin D to the active metabolites. The management of ascites, variceal hemorrhage, and encephalopathy is described below. The role of hepatic transplantation for patients with primary biliary cirrhosis is under study; this may offer the best, and only, hope for survival in patients with end-stage disease.

SECONDARY BILIARY CIRRHOSIS Etiology Secondary biliary cirrhosis results from prolonged partial or total obstruction of the common bile duct or its major branches. In adults, obstruction is most frequently caused by postoperative strictures or gallstones, usually with superimposed infectious cholangitis. Chronic pancreatitis may lead to biliary stricture and secondary cirrhosis. Secondary biliary cirrhosis may also develop in patients with pericholangitis or idiopathic sclerosing cholangitis. Patients with malignant tumors of the common bile duct or pancreas rarely survive long enough to develop secondary biliary cirrhosis. In children, congenital biliary atresia and cystic fibrosis are common causes of secondary biliary cirrhosis. Choledochal cysts if unrecognized may also be a rare cause of secondary biliary cirrhosis.

Pathology and pathogenesis Unrelieved obstruction of the extrahepatic bile ducts leads to (1) bile stasis and focal areas of centrilobular necrosis followed by periportal necrosis, (2) proliferation and dilatation of the portal bile ducts and ductules, (3) sterile or infected cholangitis with accumulation of polymorphonuclear infiltrates around bile ducts, and (4) progressive expansion of portal tracts by edema and fibrosis. Extravasation of bile from ruptured interlobular bile ducts into areas of periportal necrosis leads to the formation of "bile lakes" surrounded by cholesterol-rich pseudoxanthomatous cells. As in other forms of cirrhosis injury is accompanied by regeneration in residual parenchyma. These changes gradually lead to a finely nodular cirrhosis. In general, at least 3 to 12 months is required for biliary obstruction to result in cirrhosis. Relief of the obstruction is frequently accompanied by biochemical and morphologic improvement.

Clinical features SIGNS AND SYMPTOMS The signs and symptoms of secondary biliary cirrhosis are similar to those of primary biliary cirrhosis. Jaundice and pruritus are usually the most prominent features. In addition, fever and/or right upper quadrant pain, reflecting bouts of cholangitis or biliary colic, are typical. The manifestations of portal hypertension are found only in advanced cases.

LABORATORY TESTS Elevation in serum alkaline phosphatase and conjugated hyperbilirubinemia are nearly always present. There is a moderate increase in serum aminotransferases. When the disease is complicated by cholangitis, elevations in aminotransferase levels and leukocytosis are more pronounced. As in primary biliary cirrhosis, there are abnormalities in serum lipids (including the presence of lipoprotein X) and laboratory findings consistent with steatorrhea. However, the antimitochondrial antibody test is usually negative.

Diagnosis Secondary biliary cirrhosis should be considered in any patient with clinical and laboratory evidence of prolonged obstruction to bile flow, especially when there is a history of previous biliary tract surgery or gallstones, bouts of ascending cholangitis, or right upper quadrant pain. Cholangiography (either percutaneous or endoscopic) usually demonstrates the underlying pathologic process. Liver biopsy, although not always necessary from a clinical standpoint, can document the development of cirrhosis.

Treatment Relief of obstruction to bile flow, by either surgical or endoscopic means, is the most important step in the prevention and therapy of secondary biliary cirrhosis. Effective decompression of the biliary tract results in a significant improvement in both symptoms and survival, even in patients with established cirrhosis. When obstruction cannot be relieved, as in sclerosing cholangitis, antibiotics may be helpful acutely in controlling superimposed infection or, when administered on a chronic basis, as prophylactic therapy in suppressing recurring episodes of ascending cholangitis. Without relief of obstruction, there is a steady progression to end-stage cirrhosis and its terminal manifestations.

CARDIAC CIRRHOSIS

Definition Prolonged, severe right-sided congestive heart failure may lead to chronic liver injury and cardiac cirrhosis. The characteristic pathologic features of fibrosis and regenerative nodules distinguish cardiac cirrhosis from both reversible passive congestion of the liver due to acute heart failure and acute hepatocellular necrosis ("ischemic hepatitis" or "shock liver") resulting from systemic hypotension and hypoperfusion of the liver.

Etiology and pathology In right-sided heart failure, retrograde transmission of elevated venous pressure via the inferior vena cava and hepatic veins leads to congestion of the liver. Hepatic sinusoids become dilated and engorged with blood, and the liver becomes tensely swollen. With prolonged passive congestion and ischemia from poor perfusion secondary to reduced cardiac output, necrosis of centrilobular hepatocytes ensues and leads to fibrosis in these central areas. Ultimately centrilobular fibrosis develops with collagen extending outward in a characteristic stellate pattern from the central vein. Gross examination of the liver shows alternating red (congested) and pale (fibrotic) areas, a pattern often referred to as "nutmeg liver." Improvement in management of cardiac disorders, particularly advances in surgical treatment, has reduced the frequency of cardiac cirrhosis.

Clinical features In acute passive congestion, the liver becomes enlarged and tender, and the patient may complain of severe right upper quadrant pain due to stretching of Glisson's capsule. The serum bilirubin is usually only mildly increased and may be predominantly either conjugated or unconjugated. The AST level is mildly elevated but may be transiently very high following a period of marked systemic hypotension (shock liver), when the clinical picture can mimic acute viral or drug-induced hepatitis. The serum albumin and prothrombin are usually normal, but may become abnormal in shock liver or with the development of cirrhosis. In cases of tricuspid insufficiency the liver may be pulsatile, but this finding disappears as cirrhosis develops. With prolonged right-sided heart failure the liver is enlarged, firm, and usually nontender. The signs and symptoms of heart failure usually overshadow the liver disease. Bleeding from esophageal varices is rare, but chronic encephalopathy may be prominent with a waxing and waning course reflecting variations in the severity of right-sided heart failure. Ascites and peripheral edema, often primarily related to the underlying cardiac dysfunction, may be worsened by the superimposed liver disease.

Diagnosis The presence of a firm, enlarged liver with signs of chronic liver disease in a patient with valvular heart disease, con-

TABLE 254-2 Some causes of noncirrhotic hepatic fibrosis

1 Idiopathic portal hypertension (noncirrhotic portal fibrosis, Banti's syndrome); three variants:
  a Intrahepatic phlebosclerosis and fibrosis
  b Portal and splenic vein sclerosis
  c Portal and splenic vein thrombosis
2 Schistosomiasis ("pipe-stem" fibrosis with presinusoidal portal hypertension)
3 Congenital hepatic fibrosis (may be associated with polycystic disease of liver and kidneys)

strictive pericarditis, or cor pulmonale of long duration (>10 years) should suggest cardiac cirrhosis. Liver biopsy can confirm the diagnosis but is usually contraindicated because of coagulopathy or ascites. Coexistent chronic heart and liver disease should also raise the possibility of hemochromatosis, amyloidosis, or other infiltrative diseases.

Budd-Chiari syndrome resulting from the occlusion of the hepatic veins or inferior vena cava may be confused with acute congestive hepatomegaly. In this condition the liver is grossly enlarged and tender, and severe intractable ascites is present. However, signs and symptoms of heart failure are notably absent. The most common cause is thrombosis of the hepatic veins, often in the setting of polycythemia rubra vera, myeloproliferative syndromes, paroxysmal nocturnal hemoglobinuria, or other hypercoagulable states; it may also result from invasion of the inferior vena cava by tumor, such as renal cell or primary hepatocellular carcinoma. Idiopathic membranous obstruction of the inferior vena cava is the most common cause of this syndrome in Japan. Hepatic venography or liver biopsy showing centrilobular congestion and sinusoidal dilatation in the absence of right-sided heart failure establishes the diagnosis of Budd-Chiari syndrome. Venoocclusive disease affecting the sublobular branches of the hepatic veins and the hepatic venules may result from hepatic irradiation, treatment with some antineoplastic agents, use of oral contraceptives, or ingestion of pyrrolidizine alkaloids present in some herbal teas ("bush tea disease") and can mimic congestive hepatomegaly.

Treatment Prevention or treatment of cardiac cirrhosis depends on the diagnosis and therapy of the underlying cardiovascular disorder. Improvement in cardiac function frequently results in improvement of liver function and stabilization of the liver disease.

METABOLIC, HEREDITARY, DRUG-RELATED, AND OTHER TYPES OF CIRRHOSIS (See Table 254-1). Cirrhosis or hepatitis may result from a wide variety of other processes encompassing the spectrum of etiologic factors listed in Table 254-2. Although some of these disorders have distinctive clinical or morphologic features, the manifestations of cirrhosis are largely independent of the underlying pathogenic mechanism.

NONCIRRHOTIC FIBROSIS OF THE LIVER Several diseases, either congenital or acquired, may be associated with localized or generalized hepatic fibrosis. They are distinguished from cirrhosis by the absence of hepatocellular damage and the lack of nodular regenerative activity. The clinical manifestations in such cases are largely secondary to portal hypertension. The different types of these disorders are indicated in Table 254-2; with the exception of schistosomiasis, all these conditions are relatively rare.

MAJOR SEQUELAE OF CIRRHOSIS

The clinical course of patients with advanced cirrhosis is usually complicated by a number of important sequelae which are independent of the etiology of the underlying liver disease. These include portal hypertension and its consequences (i.e., gastroesophageal varices and splenomegaly), ascites, hepatic encephalopathy, spontaneous bacterial peritonitis, hepatorenal syndrome, and hepatocellular carcinoma.

PORTAL HYPERTENSION Definition and pathogenesis Normal pressure in the portal vein is low (10 to 15 cm saline; 7 to 10 mmHg) because vascular resistance in the hepatic sinusoids is minimal. Portal hypertension (>30 cm saline) most commonly results from increased resistance to portal blood flow. Because the portal venous system lacks valves, resistance at any level between the heart and splanchnic vessels results in retrograde transmission of an elevated pressure. Increased resistance can occur at three levels relative to the hepatic sinusoids: (1) presinusoidal, (2) sinusoidal, and (3) postsinusoidal. Obstruction in the *presinusoidal* venous compartment may be anatomically outside of the liver (e.g., portal vein thrombosis) or within the liver itself but at a functional level proximal to the hepatic sinusoids so that the liver parenchyma is not exposed to the elevated venous pressure (e.g., schistosomiasis). *Postsinusoidal* obstruction may also occur outside the liver at the level of the hepatic veins (e.g., Budd-Chiari syndrome), the inferior vena cava, or, less commonly, within the liver (e.g., venoocclusive disease in which the central hepatic venules are the primary site of injury). When cirrhosis is complicated by portal hypertension, the increased resistance is usually sinusoidal. While distinctions between pre-, post-, and sinusoidal processes are conceptually appealing, functional resistance to portal flow in a given patient may occur at more than one level. Portal hypertension may also arise from increased blood flow (e.g., massive splenomegaly or arteriovenous fistulas), but the low-outflow resistance of the normal liver makes this a rare clinical problem.

Cirrhosis is the most common cause of portal hypertension in the United States. Clinically significant portal hypertension is present in greater than 60 percent of patients with cirrhosis. *Portal vein obstruction* is the second most common cause; it may be idiopathic or occur in association with cirrhosis, infection, pancreatitis, or abdominal trauma. *Hepatic vein thrombosis* (Budd-Chiari syndrome) and hepatic venoocclusive disease are relatively infrequent causes of portal hypertension (see above). Portal vein occlusion may result in massive hematemesis from gastroesophageal varices, but ascites is usually found only with cirrhosis. Noncirrhotic portal fibrosis accounts for only a few patients with portal hypertension.

Clinical features The major clinical manifestations of portal hypertension include hemorrhage from gastroesophageal varices, splenomegaly with hypersplenism, ascites, and acute and chronic hepatic encephalopathy. All of these features are related, at least in part, to the development of portal-systemic collateral channels. The absence of valves in the portal venous system facilitates retrograde (hepatofugal) blood flow from the high-pressure portal venous system to the lower-pressure systemic venous circulation. Major sites of collateral flow involve the veins around the rectum (hemorrhoids), cardioesophageal junction (esophagogastric varices), retroperitoneal space, and the falciform ligament of the liver (periumbilical or abdominal wall collaterals). Abdominal wall collaterals appear as tortuous epigastric vessels that radiate from the umbilicus toward the xiphoid and rib margins (caput medusae).

Diagnosis In patients with known liver disease, the development of portal hypertension usually becomes evident by the appearance of splenomegaly, ascites, encephalopathy, and/or esophageal varices. Conversely, the finding of any of these features should lead one to evaluate the patient for the presence of underlying portal hypertension and liver disease. Varices may be documented by either barium swallow or fiberoptic esophagoscopy and lend indirect support to the diagnosis of portal hypertension. Although rarely necessary, portal venous pressure may be measured directly by percutaneous transhepatic "skinny needle" catheterization or indirectly through transjugular cannulation of the hepatic veins. Both free and wedged hepatic vein pressure (WHVP) should be measured. While WHVP is elevated in sinusoidal and postsinusoidal portal hypertension including cirrhosis, this measurement is usually normal in presinusoidal portal hypertension. In patients in whom additional information is necessary (e.g., preoperative evaluation before portal-systemic shunt surgery) or percutaneous catheterization is not feasible, mesenteric and hepatic angiography may be helpful. Particular attention should be directed to the venous phase to assess the patency of the portal vein and the direction of portal blood flow.

Treatment Although treatment is usually directed toward a specific complication of portal hypertension, attempts are sometimes made to reduce the pressure in the portal venous system. Surgical decompression procedures have been used for many years to lower portal pressure in patients with bleeding esophageal varices (see below). However, portal-systemic shunt surgery does not result in improved survival rates in patients with cirrhosis. There are also reports that beta-adrenergic receptor blockers, such as propranolol, may reduce portal venous pressure. Treatment of patients with clinically significant sequelae of portal hypertension, especially variceal bleeding, with doses of propranolol titrated to reduce the resting pulse by 25 percent is reasonable if no contraindications exist.

Vigorous treatment of patients with alcoholic hepatitis and cirrhosis, chronic active hepatitis, and other liver diseases may lead to a fall in portal pressure and to a reduction in variceal size. In general, however, portal hypertension due to cirrhosis is not reversible. In selected patients hepatic transplantation may be beneficial (e.g., end-stage primary biliary cirrhosis).

VARICEAL BLEEDING Pathogenesis While vigorous hemorrhage may arise from any portal-systemic venous collaterals, bleeding is most common from varices in the region of the gastroesophageal junction. The factors contributing to bleeding from gastroesophageal varices are not entirely understood but include the degree of portal hypertension and the size of the varices. Esophagitis with erosion of underlying varices does not appear to play an important role.

Clinical features and diagnosis Variceal bleeding often occurs without obvious precipitating factors and usually presents with painless but massive hematemesis with or without melena. Associated signs range from mild postural tachycardia to profound shock, depending on the extent of blood loss and degree of hypovolemia. Because patients with varices may bleed from other gastrointestinal lesions (e.g., peptic ulcer, gastritis), exclusion of other bleeding sources is important even in patients with prior variceal hemorrhage. Fiberoptic endoscopy is the best choice for evaluating upper gastrointestinal hemorrhage in patients with known or suspected portal hypertension.

Treatment Variceal bleeding is a life-threatening emergency. Prompt estimation and vigorous replacement of blood losses to maintain intravascular volume are essential and take precedence over diagnostic studies and more specific intervention to stop the bleeding. Replacement of clotting factors with fresh frozen plasma is important in patients with coagulopathy. Patients are best managed in an intensive care unit and often require close monitoring of central venous or pulmonary capillary wedge pressures, urine output, and mental status. Only when the patient is hemodynamically stable should attention be directed toward specific diagnostic studies (especially endoscopy) and other therapeutic modalities to prevent further or recurrent bleeding.

About half of all episodes of variceal hemorrhage cease without intervention, although the risk of rebleeding is very high. The medical management of acute variceal hemorrhage includes the use of vasoconstrictors (vasopressin), balloon tamponade, and endoscopic sclerosis of varices (sclerotherapy). Intravenous infusion of *vasopressin* at a rate of 0.1 to 0.9 units per minute results in generalized vasoconstriction leading to diminished blood flow in the portal venous system. Intravenous infusion of vasopressin has been shown to be as effective as selective intraarterial administration. Control of bleeding can be achieved in up to 80 percent of cases, but bleeding recurs in more than half after the vasopressin is tapered and discontinued. Furthermore, a number of serious side effects, including cardiac and gastrointestinal tract ischemia, acute renal failure, and hyponatremia, may be associated with vasopressin therapy. If bleeding is too vigorous or endoscopy is not available, *balloon tamponade* of the bleeding varices may be accomplished with a triple-lumen (Sengstaken-Blakemore) or four-lumen (Minnesota) tube with esophageal and gastric balloons. After the tube is introduced into the stomach, the gastric balloon is inflated and pulled back into the cardia of the stomach. If bleeding does not stop, the esophageal balloon is inflated for additional tamponade. Careful monitoring for complications such as esophageal rupture is essential. Where available, *endoscopic sclerosis* of esophageal varices should be employed to control bleeding acutely. In this procedure, the varices are injected with one of several sclerosing agents (e.g., sodium morrhuate) via a needle-tipped catheter passed through the endoscope. After initial endoscopic identification of varices as the presumed source of bleeding, such "sclerotherapy" controls acute bleeding in up to 90 percent of cases. In addition, repeated sclerotherapy until obliteration of all varices is accomplished should be performed in an effort to prevent recurrent bleeding. While available data support the efficacy of sclerotherapy in controlling bleeding acutely, further studies are needed to define the technique and the overall role of sclerotherapy in the management of variceal bleeding. Prophylactic sclerosis of esophageal varices in the absence of proven bleeding is not indicated. Although beta-adrenergic blocking agents (e.g., propranolol) have no role in the management of acute variceal bleeding, a number of studies suggest they may be of value in reducing the risk of recurrent upper gastrointestinal hemorrhage in the patient with portal hypertension.

Surgical therapy of portal hypertension and variceal bleeding involves the creation of a portal-systemic shunt to permit decompression of the portal system. Two types of portal systemic shunts have been used: *nonselective shunts* to decompress the entire portal system and *selective shunts* intended to decompress only the varices while maintaining blood flow to the liver itself. Nonselective shunts include end-to-side or side-to-side portacaval and proximal splenorenal anastomoses; selective shunts include the distal splenorenal shunt. Nonselective shunts are more likely to be complicated by encephalopathy than selective shunts. Emergency portal-systemic nonselective shunts may control acute hemorrhage, but such surgery is usually used only as a last resort because early operative mortality is greater than 30 percent. The role of portal-systemic shunt surgery after initial control of bleeding by nonoperative means is also uncertain. Surgically created shunts effectively reduce the risk of recurrent hemorrhage, but the overall mortality of patients undergoing such surgery is comparable to that of unoperated patients. Although patients who have undergone portal-system surgery succumb to recurrent bleeding less commonly than unoperated patients, this improvement is counterbalanced by increased morbidity from encephalopathy and death from progressive liver failure. Prophylactic shunt surgery should not be performed in patients with nonbleeding varices. Increasingly, therapeutic portal-systemic shunt has been reserved for patients who experience further bleeding despite serial endoscopic sclerotherapy. Other surgical procedures (e.g., esophageal transection) have also been advocated for the management of acute variceal bleeding although their efficacy remains unproven.

SPLENOMEGALY **Definition and pathogenesis** Congestive splenomegaly is common in patients with severe portal hypertension. Rarely, massive splenomegaly from nonhepatic disease leads to portal hypertension due to increased blood flow in the splenic vein.

Clinical features Although usually asymptomatic, splenomegaly may be massive and contribute to the thrombocytopenia or pancytopenia of cirrhosis. In the absence of cirrhosis, splenomegaly in association with variceal hemorrhage should suggest the possibility of splenic vein thrombosis.

Treatment Splenomegaly usually requires no specific treatment, although massive enlargement of the spleen may occasionally necessitate splenectomy at the time of shunt surgery. Splenectomy may also be indicated if splenomegaly is the cause rather than the result of portal hypertension. Thrombocytopenia alone is rarely severe enough to necessitate removal of the spleen.

ASCITES **Definition** Ascites is the accumulation of excess fluid within the peritoneal cavity. It is most frequently encountered in patients with cirrhosis and other forms of severe liver disease, but a number of other disorders may lead to either transudative or exudative ascites (see Chap. 48).

Pathogenesis The accumulation of ascitic fluid represents a state of total-body sodium and water excess, but the event that initiates this imbalance is unclear. Two theories have been proposed

(see Fig. 254-1). The "underfilling" theory suggests that the primary abnormality is inappropriate sequestration of fluid within the splanchnic vascular bed due to portal hypertension and a consequent decrease in effective circulating blood volume. According to this theory, an apparent decrease in intravascular volume (underfilling) is sensed by the kidney, which responds by retaining salt and water. The "overflow" theory suggests that the primary abnormality is inappropriate renal retention of salt and water in the absence of volume depletion.

Regardless of the initiating event, a number of factors contribute to accumulation of fluid in the abdominal cavity (see Fig. 254-1). *Portal hypertension* plays an important role in the formation of ascites by raising hydrostatic pressure within the splanchnic capillary bed. *Hypoalbuminemia* and *reduced plasma oncotic pressure* also favor the extravasation of fluid from plasma to peritoneal cavity, and thus ascites is infrequent in patients with cirrhosis unless both portal hypertension and hypoalbuminemia are present. *Hepatic lymph* may weep freely from the surface of the cirrhotic liver due to distortion and obstruction of hepatic sinusoids and lymphatics and contribute to ascites formation. In contrast to the contribution of transudative fluid from the portal vascular bed, hepatic lymph may weep into the peritoneal cavity even in the absence of marked hypoproteinemia because the endothelial lining of the hepatic sinusoids is discontinuous. This mechanism may account for the high protein concentration present in the ascitic fluid of some patients with the Budd-Chiari syndrome.

Renal factors also play an important role in perpetuating ascites. Patients with ascites fail to excrete a water load in a normal fashion. They have increased renal sodium reabsorption by both proximal and distal tubules, the latter due largely to secondary hyperaldosteronism and increased plasma renin activity. Renal vasoconstriction, perhaps

FIGURE 254-1 Multiple factors involved in development of ascites. Current concepts suggest that initiating factor may be either primary sodium retention ("overflow") or diminished effective intravascular volume ("underfilling").

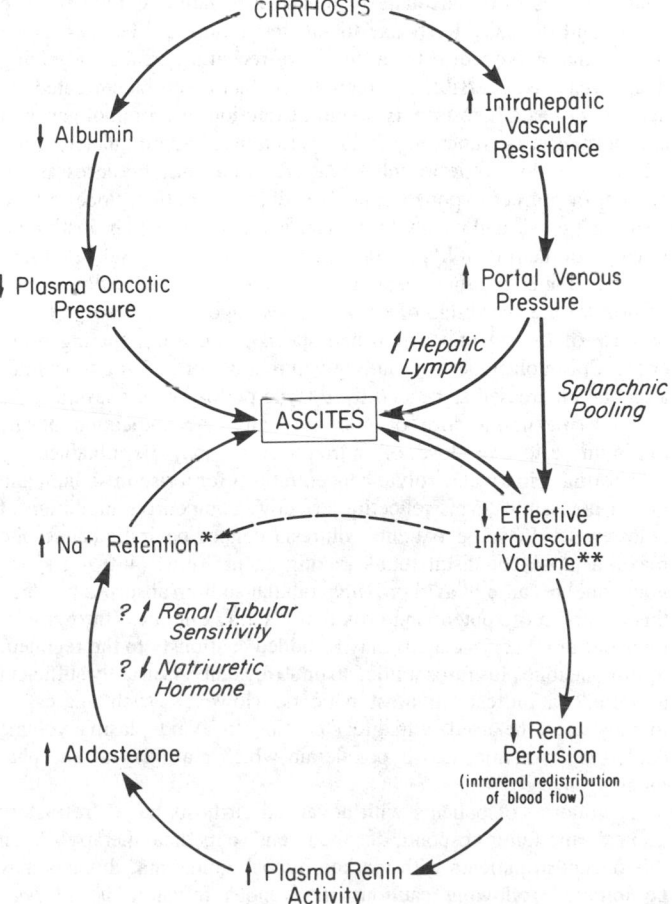

resulting from increased serum prostaglandin or catecholamine levels, may also contribute to sodium retention.

Clinical features and diagnosis   Usually ascites is first noticed by the patient because of increasing abdominal girth. More pronounced accumulation of fluid may cause shortness of breath because of elevation of the diaphragm. When peritoneal fluid accumulation exceeds 500 mL, ascites may be demonstrated on physical examination by the presence of shifting dullness, a fluid wave, or bulging flanks. Ultrasound examination can detect smaller quantities of ascites and should be performed when physical examination is equivocal. Paracentesis should usually be performed with a small-gauge needle at the time of initial evaluation or at the time of any clinical deterioration of a cirrhotic patient. A small amount of fluid (less than 200 mL) should be obtained and examined for evidence of infection, tumor, or other possible causes and complications of ascites.

Treatment   When ascites develops in the setting of severe, acute liver disease, resolution of ascites is likely to follow improvement in liver function. More commonly, ascites develops in patients with stable or steadily worsening liver function. Therapeutic intervention is indicated both to prevent potential complications and to control progressive increase in ascites, which may become pronounced enough to cause physical discomfort. However, overzealous attempts to reduce ascites may deplete the intravascular volume faster than fluid can be mobilized from the ascitic compartment and may precipitate renal failure. Thus, therapy aimed at reducing ascites should be gentle and incremental (see below). The goal is the loss of no more than 1.0 kg daily if both ascites and peripheral edema are present and no more than 0.5 kg daily in patients with ascites alone. To initiate therapy it may be desirable to hospitalize the patient so that daily weights and frequent serum electrolyte levels can be monitored and compliance ensured. Although abdominal girth measurements are frequently used as an index of fluid loss, they tend to be unreliable.

Strict bed rest is often recommended because of improved renal clearance in the supine position. However, salt restriction is the most important cornerstone of therapy. A diet containing 800 mg sodium (2 g NaCl) is often adequate to induce a negative sodium balance and permit diuresis. Response to salt restriction and bed rest alone is more likely to occur if the ascites is of recent onset, the underlying liver disease is reversible, a precipitating factor can be corrected, or the patient has a high urinary sodium excretion (~ 25 mmol per day) and normal renal function. Fluid restriction of approximately 1500 mL per day does little to enhance diuresis but may be necessary to prevent or correct hyponatremia. If sodium restriction alone fails to result in diuresis and weight loss, diuretic therapy should be instituted. Because of the role of hyperaldosteronism in sustaining salt retention, spironolactone or other distal tubule–acting diuretics (triamterene, amiloride) are the drugs of choice. These agents are also preferred because of their gentle action and specific potassium-sparing properties. Spironolactone is initially given in a dose of 25 mg four times a day and increased as needed by 100 mg per day every several days up to a maximum dose of 400 mg daily. An indication of the minimum effective dose of spironolactone may be obtained by monitoring urinary electrolyte concentrations for a rise in sodium and fall in potassium levels reflecting effective competitive inhibition of aldosterone. In some patients, diuresis cannot be initiated despite maximal doses of distal tubule–acting agents (e.g., 400 mg spironolactone) because of avid proximal tubular sodium absorption. When this occurs, more potent and proximally acting diuretics (furosemide, thiazide, or ethacrynic acid) may be added cautiously to the regimen. Spironolactone plus furosemide, 40 or 80 mg daily, is usually sufficient to initiate a diuresis in most patients. However, such aggressive therapy must be used with great caution to avoid plasma volume depletion, azotemia, and hypokalemia which may lead to encephalopathy.

A minority of patients with advanced cirrhosis have "refractory ascites" and fail to respond, despite intensive medical therapy. When this occurs in patients with marked hypoalbuminemia, diuresis may be initiated following cautious intravenous infusion of *salt-poor albumin*. Because of the short half-life of infused albumin, this approach is of short-term benefit and may, in fact, precipitate variceal hemorrhage due to expansion of the intravascular volume. In some patients a side-to-side *portacaval shunt* may result in improvement in ascites although generally these patients are extremely poor surgical risks. Intractable ascites can also be treated with the surgical implantation of a plastic *peritoneovenous shunt* which has a pressure-sensitive, one-way valve allowing ascitic fluid to flow from the abdominal cavity to the superior vena cava. However, the usefulness of this technique is limited by a high rate of complications such as infection, disseminated intravascular coagulation, and thrombosis of the shunt. Although clinical experience has long led to caution in removing large volumes of ascites by paracentesis for fear of precipitating progressive renal failure, recent studies have demonstrated the safety of this approach when combined with concomitant intravenous infusion of albumin in amounts proportional to those removed. Removal of up to 5 L of fluid using this approach has been found to speed reduction of ascites safely in the patient with tense ascites.

SPONTANEOUS BACTERIAL PERITONITIS   Patients with ascites and cirrhosis may develop acute bacterial peritonitis without an obvious primary source of infection. Typical features include abrupt onset of fever, chills, generalized abdominal pain, and rebound abdominal tenderness accompanied by cloudy ascitic fluid with a high white cell count and usually positive bacterial cultures. However, the clinical symptoms *may be minimal,* and some patients manifest only worsening jaundice or encephalopathy in the absence of localizing abdominal complaints. The diagnosis is based on careful examination of the ascitic fluid. An ascitic fluid leukocyte count of greater than 500 cells per cubic millimeter or more than 250 polymorphonuclear leukocytes should suggest the possibility of bacterial peritonitis while results of bacterial cultures of ascitic fluid are pending. Empiric therapy with ampicillin and an aminoglycoside or cefotaximene should be initiated when the diagnosis is first suspected because enteric gram-negative bacilli are found in the majority of cases; less frequently the infection is caused by pneumococci and other gram-positive bacteria. Specific antibiotic therapy can be selected once the specific organism is identified. Therapy is usually administered for 10 to 14 days.

HEPATORENAL SYNDROME   Definition and pathogenesis   Hepatorenal syndrome is a serious complication in the patient with cirrhosis and ascites, and is characterized by worsening azotemia with avid sodium retention and oliguria in the absence of identifiable specific causes of renal dysfunction. The exact basis for this syndrome is not clear, but altered renal hemodynamics appear to be involved. The kidneys are structurally intact; urinalysis and pyelography are usually normal. Renal biopsy although rarely needed is also normal, and in fact kidneys from such patients have been successfully used for renal transplantation. There are indications that an imbalance in certain metabolites of arachidonic acid (prostaglandins and thromboxane) may play a pathogenetic role.

Clinical features and diagnosis   Worsening azotemia, hyponatremia, progressive oliguria, and hypotension are the hallmarks of the hepatorenal syndrome. This syndrome, which is distinct from prerenal azotemia, may be precipitated by severe gastrointestinal bleeding, sepsis, or overly vigorous attempts at diuresis or paracentesis; it may also occur without an obvious cause. The diagnosis is supported by the demonstration of avid urinary sodium retention. Typically the urine sodium concentration is less than 5 mmol per liter, a concentration lower than that generally found in uncomplicated prerenal azotemia. The urinary sediment is unremarkable.

Treatment   Treatment is usually unsuccessful. Although some patients with hypotension and decreased plasma volume may respond to infusions of salt-poor albumin, volume expansion must be undertaken with caution to avoid precipitating variceal bleeding. Vasodilator therapy, including intravenous infusion of dopamine, is not effective.

HEPATIC ENCEPHALOPATHY   Definition   Hepatic (portal-systemic) encephalopathy is a complex neuropsychiatric syndrome characterized by disturbances in consciousness and behavior, personality changes, fluctuating neurologic signs, asterixis or "flapping tremor," and distinctive electroencephalographic changes. Encephalopathy may be *acute* and reversible or *chronic* and progressive. In severe cases, irreversible coma and death may occur. Acute episodes may recur with variable frequency.

Pathogenesis The specific cause of hepatic encephalopathy is unknown. The most important factors in the pathogenesis are severe hepatocellular dysfunction and/or intrahepatic and extrahepatic shunting of portal venous blood into the systemic circulation, so that the liver is largely bypassed. As a result of these processes, various toxic substances absorbed from the intestine are not detoxified by the liver and lead to metabolic abnormalities in the central nervous system. Ammonia is the substance most often incriminated in the pathogenesis of encephalopathy. Many, but not all, patients with hepatic encephalopathy have elevated blood ammonia levels, and recovery from encephalopathy is often accompanied by declining blood ammonia levels. Other compounds and metabolites which may contribute to the development of encephalopathy include mercaptans (derived from intestinal metabolism of methionine), short-chain fatty acids, and phenol. Several observations suggest that excessive concentrations of gamma-aminobutyric acid (GABA), an inhibitory neurotransmitter, in the CNS are important in the reduced levels of consciousness seen in hepatic encephalopathy. Increased CNS GABA may reflect failure of the liver to efficiently extract precursor amino acids. False neurochemical transmitters (e.g., octopamine), resulting in part from alterations in plasma levels of aromatic and branched-chain amino acids, may also play a role. An increase in the permeability of the blood-brain barrier to some of these substances may be an additional factor involved in the pathogenesis of hepatic encephalopathy.

In the patient with otherwise stable cirrhosis, hepatic encephalopathy often follows a clearly identifiable precipitating event (see Table 254-3). Perhaps the most common predisposing factor is *gastrointestinal bleeding*, which leads to an increase in the production of ammonia and other nitrogenous substances which are then absorbed. Similarly, *increased dietary protein* may precipitate encephalopathy as a result of increased production of nitrogenous substances by colonic bacteria. *Electrolyte disturbances*, particularly hypokalemic alkalosis secondary to overzealous use of diuretics, vigorous paracentesis, or vomiting, may precipitate hepatic encephalopathy. Systemic alkalosis causes an increase in the amount of nonionic ammonia (NH_3) relative to ammonium ions (NH_4^+). Only nonionic (uncharged) ammonia readily crosses the blood-brain barrier and accumulates in the central nervous system. Hypokalemia also directly stimulates renal ammonia production. Hypoxia, injudicious use of central nervous system–depressing drugs (e.g., barbiturates, benzodiazepines), and acute infection may trigger or aggravate hepatic encephalopathy, although the mechanisms involved are not clear. Other potential precipitating factors include superimposed acute viral hepatitis, al-

coholic hepatitis, extrahepatic bile duct obstruction, surgery, and other coincidental medical complications.

Clinical features and diagnosis Hepatic encephalopathy has protean manifestations, and any neurologic abnormality, including focal deficits, may be encountered. In patients with acute encephalopathy, neurologic deficits are completely reversible upon correction of underlying precipitating factors and/or improvement in liver function, but in patients with chronic encephalopathy the deficits may be irreversible and progressive. Cerebral edema is frequently present and contributes to the clinical picture and overall mortality in patients with both acute and chronic encephalopathy.

The diagnosis of hepatic encephalopathy should be considered when four major factors are present: (1) acute or chronic hepatocellular disease and/or extensive portal-systemic collateral shunts (the latter may be either spontaneous, e.g., secondary to portal hypertension, or surgically created, e.g., portacaval anastomosis); (2) disturbances of awareness and mentation which may progress from forgetfulness and confusion to stupor and finally coma; (3) shifting combinations of neurologic signs, including asterixis, rigidity, hyperreflexia, extensor plantar signs, and rarely, seizures; and (4) a characteristic (but nonspecific) symmetric, high-voltage, slow-wave (2 to 5 per second) pattern on the electroencephalogram. Asterixis ("liver flap," "flapping tremor") is a nonrhythmic asymmetric lapse in voluntary sustained position of the extremities, head, and trunk. It is best demonstrated by having the patient extend the arms and dorsiflex the hands. Because elicitation of asterixis depends on sustained voluntary muscle contraction, it is not present in the comatose patient. Asterixis is nonspecific and also occurs in patients with other forms of metabolic brain disease. Alterations in personality, mood disturbances, confusion, deterioration in self-care and handwriting, and daytime somnolence are additional clinical features of encephalopathy. *Fetor hepaticus*, a unique musty odor of the breath and urine believed to be due to mercaptans, may be noted in patients with varying stages of hepatic encephalopathy. Some patients may develop spastic paraparesis or *chronic progressive hepatocerebral degeneration*, the latter a clinical variant of hepatic encephalopathy characterized by a slow decline in intellectual function, tremor, cerebellar ataxia, choreoathetosis, and psychiatric symptoms.

Grading or classifying the stages of hepatic encephalopathy is often helpful in following the course of the illness and assessing response to therapy. One useful classification is shown in Table 254-4.

The diagnosis of hepatic encephalopathy is usually one of exclusion. There are no diagnostic liver function test abnormalities, although an elevated serum ammonia level in the appropriate clinical setting is highly suggestive of the diagnosis. Examination of the cerebrospinal fluid is unremarkable, and computed tomography of the brain shows no characteristic abnormalities. A number of conditions, particularly disorders related to acute and chronic alcoholism, can mimic the clinical features of hepatic encephalopathy. These include acute alcohol intoxication, sedative overdose, delirium tremens, Wernicke's encephalopathy, and Korsakoff's psychosis (see Chap. 357). Subdural hematoma, meningitis, and hypoglycemia or other metabolic encephalopathies must also be considered, especially in patients with

---

TABLE 254-3 Common precipitants of hepatic encephalopathy

1 Increased nitrogen load
  a Gastrointestinal bleeding
  b Excess dietary protein
  c Azotemia
  d Constipation
2 Electrolyte imbalance
  a Hypokalemia
  b Alkalosis
  c Hypoxia
  d Hypovolemia
3 Drugs
  a Narcotics, tranquilizers, sedatives
  b Diuretics (see 2)
4 Miscellaneous
  a Infection
  b Surgery
  c Superimposed acute liver disease
  d Progressive liver disease

TABLE 254-4 Clinical stages of hepatic encephalopathy

Stage	Mental status	Asterixis	EEG
I	Euphoria or depression, mild confusion, slurred speech, disordered sleep	+/−	Usually normal
II	Lethargy, moderate confusion	+	Abnormal
III	Marked confusion, incoherent speech, sleeping but arousable	+	Abnormal
IV	Coma; initially responsive to noxious stimuli, later unresponsive	−	Abnormal

alcoholic cirrhosis. In young patients with liver disease and neurologic abnormalities, Wilson's disease should be excluded.

Treatment Early recognition and prompt treatment of hepatic encephalopathy are essential. Patients with acute, severe hepatic encephalopathy (stage IV) require the usual supportive measures for the comatose patient. Specific treatment of hepatic encephalopathy is aimed at (1) elimination or treatment of precipitating factors and (2) lowering of blood ammonia (and other toxin) levels by decreasing the absorption of protein and nitrogenous products from the intestine. In the setting of acute gastrointestinal bleeding, blood in the bowel should be promptly evacuated with enemas and laxatives in order to reduce the nitrogen load. Protein should be excluded from the diet, and constipation should be avoided. Ammonia absorption can be decreased by the administration of lactulose, a nonabsorbable disaccharide that acts as an osmotic laxative. Metabolism of lactulose by colonic bacteria may also result in an acid pH that favors conversion of ammonia to the poorly absorbed ammonium ion. In addition lactulose may actually diminish ammonia production through its direct effects on bacterial metabolism. Lactulose syrup can be administered in a dose of 30 to 50 mL every hour until diarrhea occurs; thereafter the dose is adjusted (usually 15 to 30 mL three times daily) so that the patient has two to four soft stools daily. Intestinal ammonia production by bacteria can also be decreased by oral administration of the antibiotic neomycin, at a dose of 0.5 to 1.0 g every 6 h. Although poorly absorbed, neomycin may reach sufficient concentrations in the bloodstream to cause renal toxicity. The use of agents such as levodopa, bromocriptine, keto-analogues of essential amino acids, and intravenous amino acid formulations rich in branched-chain amino acids in the treatment of acute hepatic encephalopathy remain of unproven benefit. Hemoperfusion to remove toxic substances and therapy directed primarily toward coincident cerebral edema in acute encephalopathy are also of unproven value.

Chronic encephalopathy may be effectively controlled by administration of lactulose. Management of patients with chronic encephalopathy should include dietary protein restriction, sometimes to levels as low as 40 g daily, in combination with low doses of lactulose or neomycin. Nephrotoxicity or ototoxicity may be limiting in prolonged usage of neomycin. There are suggestions that vegetable protein may be preferable to animal protein.

OTHER SEQUELAE OF CIRRHOSIS Coagulopathy Patients with cirrhosis often demonstrate a variety of abnormalities in both cellular and humoral clotting function. Thrombocytopenia may result from hypersplenism. In the alcoholic patient, there may be direct bone marrow suppression by ethanol. Diminished protein synthesis may lead to reduced production of fibrinogen (factor I), prothrombin (factor II), and factors V, VII, IX, and X. Reduction in levels of all factors except factor V may be worsened by the coincident malabsorption of the fat-soluble cofactor vitamin K due to cholestasis (see Chap. 240). Recent reports have documented the appearance of normal factor VIII levels following liver transplantation in patients with classical hemophilia probably as a result of production by nonhepatocellular components of the donor organ.

Hepatocellular carcinoma (See Chap. 255.)

REFERENCES

Alcoholic and postnecrotic cirrhosis

BARRY RE, McGIVAN JD: Acetaldehyde alone may initiate hepatocellular damage in acute alcoholic liver disease. Gut 26:1065, 1985

BASKIN B et al: Ethanol and liver regeneration. Hepatology 8: 408, 1988

CARITHERS RL et al: Methylprednisolone therapy in patients with severe alcoholic hepatitis: A randomized multicenter trial. Ann Intern Med 110:685, 1989

GLUUD C et al: Prognostic indicators in alcoholic cirrhotic men. Hepatology 8:222, 1988

ORREGO H et al: Long-term treatment of alcoholic liver disease with propylthiouracil. N Engl J Med 317: 1421, 1987

SATO S et al: Liver fibrosis in alcoholics: Detection by FAB radioimmunoassay of serum procollagen III peptides. JAMA 256: 1471, 1986

SØRENSEN TIA et al: Prospective evaluation of alcohol abuse and alcoholic liver injury in man as predictors of development of cirrhosis. Lancet 2:241, 1984

Biliary cirrhosis

BABB C et al: Type III procollagen peptide: A marker of disease activity and prognosis in primary biliary cirrhosis. Lancet 1,1021, 1988

BESWICK DR et al: Asymptomatic primary biliary cirrhosis: A progress report on long-term follow-up and natural history. Gastroenterology 89:267, 1985

BODENHEIMER H JR et al: Evaluation of colchicine therapy in primary biliary cirrhosis. Gastroenterology 95:124, 1988

CHRISTENSEN E et al: Beneficial effects of azathioprine and predictor of prognosis in primary biliary cirrhosis: Final results of an international trial. Gastroenterology 89:1084, 1985

ESQUIVEL CO et al: Transplantation for primary biliary cirrhosis. Gastroenterology 94: 1207, 1988

KAPLAN MM et al: Primary biliary cirrhosis treated with low dose oral pulse methotrexate. Ann Int 109:429, 1988

NEUBERGER J et al: Double-blind controlled trial of D-penicillamine in patients with primary biliary cirrhosis. Gut 26:114, 1985

YEAMAN SJ et al: Primary biliary cirrhosis: Identification of two major M2 mitochondrial autoantigens. Lancet 1:1067, 1988

Hepatic encephalopathy

BASSETT ML et al: Amelioration of hepatic encephalopathy by pharmacologic antagonism of the GABA-Benzodiazepene receptor complex in a rabbit model of fulminant hepatic failure. Gastroenterology 93:1069, 1987

DUDLEY FJ et al: Hepatorenal syndrome without avid sodium retention. Hepatology 6:248, 1986

FRASER CL, ARIEFF AI: Hepatic encephalopathy. N Engl J Med 313:865, 1985

JONES EA et al: The neurobiology of hepatic encephalopathy. Hepatology 4:1235, 1984

MORGAN MY, HAWLEY KE: Lactitol vs. lactulose in the treatment of acute hepatic encephalopathy in cirrhotic patients: A double blind randomized study. Hepatology 7:1278.

SCHAFER DF: Hepatic coma: Studies on the target organ. Gastroenterology 93: 1131, 1987

SKOLNICK P: The γ-aminobutyric acid A (GABA$_A$)-benzodiazepine receptor complex, pp 534–536, in: Jones EA, moderator. The γ-aminobutyric A (GABA$_A$) receptor complex and hepatic encephalopathy: some recent advances. Ann Intern Med 110:532, 1989

Portal hypertension and ascites

CELLO JP et al: Endoscopic sclerotherapy versus portacaval shunt in patients with severe cirrhosis and variceal hemorrhage. N Engl J Med 311:1589, 1984

CROSSLEY JR, WILLIAMS R: Spontaneous bacterial peritonitis. Gut 26:325, 1985

EPSTEIN M: The sodium retention of cirrhosis: A reappraisal. Hepatology 6:312, 1986

GINÉS P et al: Comparison of paracentesis and diuretics in the treatment of cirrhotics with tense ascites: Results of a randomized study. Gastroenterology 93:234, 1987

MILLIKAN WJ et al: The Emory prospective randomized trial: Selective versus nonselective shunt to control variceal bleeding. Ann Surg 201:712, 1985

NICHOLLS KM et al: Sodium excretion in advanced cirrhosis: Effect of expansion of central blood volume and suppression of plasma aldosterone. Hepatology 6:235, 1986

PASTA L et al: Propranolol for prophylaxis of bleeding in cirrhotic patients with large varices: A multicenter randomized clinical trial. Hepatology 8:1, 1988

PINTO PC et al: Large-volume paracentesis in nonedematous patients with tense ascites: Its affect on intravascular volume. Hepatology 8: 207, 1988

PINZANI M et al: Altered furosemide pharmacokinetics in chronic alcoholic liver disease with ascites contributes to diuretic resistance. Gastroenterology 92:294, 1987

TERBLANCHE J et al: Controversies in the management of bleeding esophageal varices. N Engl J Med 320:1394, 1469, 1989

255 NEOPLASMS OF THE LIVER

KURT J. ISSELBACHER / JACK R. WANDS

PRIMARY CARCINOMA Tumors of hepatocytes or hepatocellular carcinomas account for 80 to 90 percent of liver carcinomas; but there are also bile duct cell carcinomas (cholangiocarcinomas) or those of mixed origin. There is, however, little practical purpose in distinguishing between the two types, since both may be found in different parts of the same tumor and the clinical courses are similar.

Epidemiology and etiology In North and South America and Europe primary liver cancers account for only 1 to 2 percent of malignant tumors found at autopsy. However, in parts of Africa and Asia they may account for up to 20 to 30 percent of all types of malignancy. Liver cell carcinoma is up to four times more common in men than in women. The peak incidence occurs in the fifth and sixth decades of life in western countries, but one to two decades earlier in Africa and Asia, areas with a high prevalence of liver carcinoma. Cirrhosis, usually macronodular or postnecrotic, is found in 60 to 75 percent of autopsied patients with primary liver cell carcinoma in all parts of the world. In view of the wide geographic variation in the incidence of hepatocellular carcinoma, different etiologic factors appear to be involved.

1 *Chronic liver disease* of any type predisposes to the development of carcinoma. A variety of metabolic, alcoholic, viral, or idiopathic chronic liver diseases can lead to liver cell carcinoma. Thus, α_1-*antitrypsin deficiency* and hereditary tyrosinosis, with active liver disease since birth, has a high incidence of developing into carcinoma. In the adult age group, *hemochromatosis* has the highest risk of malignant degeneration, presumably owing to the long duration of the chronic liver inflammation and cirrhosis. Alcoholic and postnecrotic cirrhosis are the most common forms of underlying liver disease in patients with liver carcinoma in western countries.

2 *Hepatitis B (HBV)* is endemic in many areas of Africa and Asia. The prevalence of HBV antigenemia in the normal population is up to 10 to 15 percent in some parts of Africa and the Far East. In these areas, most patients with hepatocellular carcinoma (90 to 95 percent) will have serologic evidence of recent or past HBV infection (see Chap. 252). Approximately 60 to 70 percent of these patients will have chronic hepatitis and/or cirrhosis at the time of clinical presentation. In most instances HBV-DNA integration has been found in the genome of tumor cells as well as in the adjacent uninvolved hepatocytes. HBV-DNA integration appears to occur most commonly in long-term chronic carriers and in those individuals who acquire infection at birth. The relative risk of developing a primary hepatocellular carcinoma in an HBV chronic carrier as compared to an uninfected individual is approximately 100:1. It is recommended that known chronic HBV carriers have biannual alpha fetoprotein (AFP) determinations to screen for subclinical hepatocellular carcinoma (see below).

3 *Mycotoxins*, metabolites of saprophytic fungi, including certain known hepatic carcinogens (e.g., aflatoxins), are continuously ingested in foodstuffs in small amounts and are found in high concentrations in foods in parts of Africa and Asia, where liver cell carcinoma is found more frequently. Ingested mycotoxins and viral inflammation and cirrhosis as the result of HBV infection may act synergistically to increase the risk of liver cell cancer.

4 *Hormonal factors* may be important in view of the male predominance in liver cancer and the effect of sex hormones on experimental carcinogenesis. Hepatocellular carcinoma has been reported in some patients on long-term androgenic therapy. Long-term use of *oral contraceptives* rarely leads to development of hepatic cell adenoma, a benign neoplasm, but malignant transformation into carcinoma has been reported.

Clinical features Cancers of the liver may escape clinical recognition during life because they often occur in patients with underlying cirrhosis, and the symptoms and signs may initially suggest a progression of the underlying liver disease. *Hepatomegaly,* with *pain* or *tenderness,* usually moderate in degree and localized to the upper abdomen or the right upper quadrant, is often the major complaint. Other important clinical features which should alert the clinician to the diagnosis include a *mass* in the liver, particularly if tender; the presence of a *friction rub* or *bruit* over the liver; and *blood-tinged ascites* (hemoperitoneum) which occurs in about 20 percent of cases. However, all such signs and symptoms reflect far advanced and usually inoperable disease and this underscores the value of early detection by AFP screening or ultrasound determinations. Jaundice is characteristic of cholangiocarcinoma but is relatively uncommon in hepatocellular carcinoma in the absence of active liver disease.

Anemia and *elevated alkaline phosphatase* and *AFP* levels are common laboratory findings. In a patient with cirrhosis, a disproportionately high serum alkaline phosphatase in relation to other abnormal liver function tests is often a clue to an infiltrating or partially obstructing liver carcinoma.

Diagnosis The clinical features outlined above should suggest the possibility of primary liver carcinoma. A number of imaging procedures are used to detect liver tumors including ultrasound, CT scanning, MRI, or hepatic artery angiography (see Chap. 248). Ultrasound is frequently used to screen high-risk populations and should be the first procedure used when hepatocellular carcinoma is suspected; it is relatively sensitive and can detect most tumors greater than 3 cm. MRI is also being used with increasing frequency. Celiac axis angiography is sensitive and indispensable before surgery.

AFP, a unique fetal α_1-globulin, is found in the serum of many patients with hepatocellular carcinoma. Very high levels, greater than 500 μg/L, occur in about 70 percent of patients. The serum AFP may be *slightly elevated* in about 5 to 10 percent of patients with large hepatic metastases from gastrointestinal tumors, and in about one-third of patients with acute or chronic viral hepatitis; only rarely do levels over 500 μg/L occur in these conditions. Minimally elevated levels of AFP may persist in some patients with chronic hepatitis. AFP is also elevated up to 500 μg/L in maternal sera during normal pregnancy. The detection and persistence of *high levels* of serum AFP (over 500 or 1000 μg/L) in an adult with liver disease and without an obvious gastrointestinal tract tumor strongly suggest the presence of primary liver carcinoma. However, gradually increasing AFP levels even when starting at a low (<50 μg/L) serum level may signal the development of a small (<3 cm) subclinical hepatocellular carcinoma, particularly in the high-risk HBV carrier group with and without chronic hepatitis and cirrhosis.

Percutaneous *liver biopsy* can be diagnostic, especially if the biopsy is taken in the area of a palpable nodule or mass localized by ultrasound or CT scans. False negatives may occur in as many as one-fourth of patients if the biopsy is performed in a routine, blind manner with the intercostal approach, and well-differentiated hepatocellular carcinoma may be difficult to diagnose by aspiration cytology or even needle biopsy. Cytologic examination of ascitic fluid is invariably negative for tumor cells. *Laparoscopy* or *laparotomy* with open liver biopsy may be required for diagnosis. This direct approach has the additional advantage of identifying the occasional patient with localized resectable tumor who may be suitable for partial hepatectomy.

Course and management The course of the disease is fatal and usually rapid. Most patients die within 3 to 6 months from gastrointestinal hemorrhage, progressive cachexia, or hepatic failure.

Surgical resection offers the only chance of cure but the 5-year survival is low and only a few patients have resectable tumors at presentation. However, with AFP and ultrasound screening programs to identify subclinical hepatocellular carcinoma in high-risk populations, it is likely that 5-year survival rates will be substantially improved.

If the patient is young, in good general health, and has no obvious extrahepatic involvement, solitary hepatic lesions may be excised with *partial hepatectomy,* but the 5-year survival rate is low. Persistently high or rising levels of AFP after excision of the tumor are suggestive of residual or recurrent tumor. Hepatocellular carcinoma may respond for brief periods to systemic or intraarterial chemotherapy. However, the results are still poor, and further trials of combined drug therapy are in progress. Liver transplantation can now be considered a therapeutic option, but recurrence of tumor and frequent appearance of metastases after transplantation have limited the usefulness of this procedure (see Chap. 257). Aggressive surgery or transplantation may prove to be of value in the treatment of small, localized tumors if diagnosed early or in the slower-growing fibrolamellar type of liver cell carcinoma. Other approaches which are of limited usefulness include hepatic artery embolization and hepatic artery perfusion (via implanted pumps) with fluorouracil and doxorubicin. Monoclonal antibodies tagged with radioactive or cytotoxic agents are also being investigated as potentially effective approaches.

OTHER BENIGN AND MALIGNANT TUMORS These tumors are very rare. Hepatoblastomas are histologically distinct primary malignant tumors of the liver occurring only in infancy and early childhood and characteristically have very high levels of serum AFP. They are usually solitary masses, may be resectable and have a higher 5-year survival rate than hepatocellular carcinoma. *Hemangiomas,* the most common benign tumors, are usually single and small, but may present as a large hepatic nodule. Percutaneous needle liver biopsy is contraindicated if the diagnosis is suspected because of the danger of hemorrhage. The diagnosis can be made by angiography. Surgical excision is usually not indicated unless the tumors are large and symptomatic or a malignant lesion cannot be excluded. *Hemangioendotheliomas* or *angiosarcomas* are rare malignant vascular tumors. They can be caused by chronic *vinyl chloride* exposure and may appear 15 to 20 years after the administration of thorium dioxide.

Hepatic adenomas, although rare, are particularly prone to occur in women taking oral contraceptives for long periods. These benign neoplasms may regress when the pill is discontinued. Focal nodular hyperplasia, a nonneoplastic hamartoma, may also become more vascular with long-term use of oral contraceptives leading to increased risk of pain or hemorrhage. Other rare tumors include benign cholangiomas, rhabdomyomas, rhabdomyosarcomas, and a number of other benign and malignant tumors arising from various mesenchymal elements. These tumors usually present as a palpable mass in the liver or with intraabdominal hemorrhage. They can be visualized and their extent defined by angiography. Surgical exploration and open biopsy or resection are usually required for definitive diagnosis.

METASTATIC TUMORS   Metastatic malignant tumors of the liver are common in clinical practice, ranking second only to cirrhosis as a cause of fatal liver disease. In the United States the incidence of clinically significant metastatic carcinoma is at least 20 times greater than that of primary carcinoma. Hepatic metastases have been reported at autopsy in 30 to 50 percent of patients dying from malignant disease.

Pathogenesis   The liver is uniquely vulnerable to invasion by tumor cells. Its size, high rate of blood flow, and double perfusion by hepatic artery and portal vein combine to make it the most common site of metastases except for the lymph nodes. In addition, local tissue factors or endothelial membrane characteristics appear to enhance metastatic implants. Virtually all types of neoplasms except those primary in the brain may metastasize to the liver. The most common primary tumors are those of the gastrointestinal tract, lung, breast, and melanomas. Less common are metastases from tumors of the thyroid, prostate, and skin.

Clinical features   Most patients with metastatic malignancy of the liver present with (1) symptoms referable only to the primary tumor, with asymptomatic hepatic involvement discovered in the course of clinical evaluation; (2) nonspecific symptoms of weakness, weight loss, fever, sweating, and loss of appetite; or rarely, with (3) features indicating active hepatic disease, especially abdominal pain, hepatomegaly, or ascites.

Patients with widespread metastatic liver involvement usually have suggestive clinical signs of cancer and hepatic enlargement. Some have localized induration or tenderness, and occasionally a friction rub may be found over tender areas of the liver.

Abnormal liver function tests are frequent but often mild and nonspecific. They reflect the effects of fever and wasting, as well as the infiltrating neoplastic process itself. An increase in serum alkaline phosphatase is the most common and frequently the only abnormality noted. Hypoalbuminemia, anemia, and occasional mild elevation of transaminase levels may also be found with more widespread disease. Greatly elevated serum levels of carcinoembryonic antigen (CEA) are usually found when the metastases are from primary malignancies in the gastrointestinal tract, breast, or lung.

Diagnosis   Evidence of metastatic invasion of the liver should be sought actively in any patient with a primary malignancy, especially of the lung, gastrointestinal tract, or breast, before resection of the primary lesion is undertaken. Abnormal liver function tests, particularly an elevated alkaline phosphatase, or demonstration of a mass by liver scintiscan, ultrasound, or CT may provide a presumptive diagnosis. Blind percutaneous needle biopsy of the liver will result in a positive diagnosis of metastatic disease in only 60 to 80 percent of cases with hepatomegaly and elevated alkaline phosphatase levels. Serial sectioning of specimens, two or three repeat biopsies, or

cytologic examination of biopsy smears may increase the diagnostic yield by 10 to 15 percent. The yield is greatly increased when biopsies are directed by ultrasound or CT or obtained by laparoscopy.

Treatment   Most metastatic carcinomas respond poorly to all forms of treatment, which is usually only palliative. Surgical removal of a single large metastasis is rarely feasible. Systemic chemotherapy with combinations of different chemotherapeutic agents briefly may slow tumor growth and reduce symptoms in some patients but does not significantly alter the prognosis. It remains to be determined whether newer drugs or combination chemotherapy eventually will prove to be more effective.

REFERENCES

BEASLEY RP et al: Hepatocellular carcinoma and hepatitis B virus. Lancet 2:1129, 1981
BRECHOT C et al: Evidence that hepatitis B virus has a role in liver cell carcinoma in alcoholic liver disease. N Engl J Med 306:1384, 1982
DIBICEGLIE AM: Hepatocellular carcinoma. Ann Intern Med 108:390, 1988
LIAW Y-F et al: Early detection of hepatocellular carcinoma in patients with chronic type B hepatitis. A prospective study. Gastroenterology 90:263, 1986
LOTZE MT: Surgical management of hepatocellular carcinomas. Gastroenterology Clin North Am 16:613, 1987
MALT RA: Surgery for hepatic neoplasms. N Engl J Med 313:1591, 1985
OKUDA K et al: Natural history of hepatocellular carcinoma and prognosis in relation to treatment. Study of 850 patients. Cancer 56:918, 1985
OMATA M et al: Hepatocellular carcinoma in the USA: Etiologic considerations. Localization of hepatitis B antigens. Gastroenterology 76:279, 1979
ORDER SE et al: Iodine 131 antiferritin, a new treatment modality in hepatoma. A radiation therapy oncology group study. J Clin Onc 3:1573, 1985
POPPER H et al: Relationship of the hepatitis B virus carrier state to hepatocellular carcinoma. Hepatology 7:764, 1987
SHAFRITZ DA et al: Integration of hepatitis B virus DNA into the genome of liver cells in chronic liver disease and hepatocellular carcinoma. N Engl J Med 305:1067, 1981
TANG ZHAO-YON: *Subclinical Hepatocellular Carcinoma*. New York, Springer, 1985
ZAMAN SN et al: Risk factors in development of carcinoma in cirrhosis: Prospective study of 613 patients. Lancet 1:1357, 1985

256   INFILTRATIVE AND METABOLIC DISEASES AFFECTING THE LIVER

KURT J. ISSELBACHER / DANIEL K. PODOLSKY

Many disseminated, systemic, or metabolic diseases involve the liver in a diffuse manner by the infiltration of abnormal cells or the accumulation of chemical substances or metabolites. Chemical accumulation may be extracellular or intracellular and may involve hepatocytes, Kupffer cells, or other elements of the reticuloendothelial system. Although infiltrative diseases may vary widely in their etiology and extrahepatic manifestations, the findings in the liver may be quite similar. Generalized enlargement and firmness of the liver, gradual and nonspecific deterioration of liver function, and, less often, signs of portal hypertension or ascites are typical features of this group of diseases. Differential diagnosis by clinical means may be difficult on occasion, but in patients in whom ancillary clinical findings do not establish the diagnosis, the diffusely infiltrated liver provides an excellent source of tissue for diagnostic purposes.

As discussed in Chap. 6, the tools of molecular biology, especially recombinant DNA probes and restriction fragment length polymorphism will undoubtedly play a significant role in arriving at the molecular basis for many of these disorders. Some diseases will reflect the manifestation of mutant structural genes causing absent or reduced amounts of a gene product (e.g., phenylalanine hydroxylase deficiency leading to classic phenylketonuria), or a structurally *altered* gene which is functionally inactive (e.g., alpha, antitrypsin). In other instances the mutation may affect *gene regulation* as in Menke's syndrome, a rare disorder of zinc metabolism that affects the liver, which appears to result from faulty regulation of metallothionein gene expression.

LIPID INFILTRATIONS

FATTY LIVER   Slight to moderate enlargement of the liver due to diffuse infiltration of liver cells by neutral fat (triglyceride) is a common clinical and pathologic finding. Although minimal fatty changes are often transient and have no clinical significance, persistent or extensive fatty infiltration may produce dysfunction and symptoms that require careful evaluation.

Etiology   The major causes of fatty liver encountered in clinical practice depend on the age, geographic location, and metabolic-nutritional status of the patient population. *Chronic alcoholism* is the most common cause of fatty liver in this country and in other countries with a high alcohol intake. The severity of fatty involvement is roughly proportional to the duration and degree of alcoholic excess. *Protein malnutrition*, especially in infancy and early childhood, accounts for most cases of severe fatty liver in the tropical zones of Africa, South America, and Asia. The hepatic changes may be associated with other clinical and pathologic features of kwashiorkor. Patients with adult-onset *diabetes mellitus*, especially those who are overweight and are poorly controlled, often have fatty livers. *Obesity* is commonly associated with fatty infiltration of the liver; this recedes as weight reduction occurs. However, *jejunoileal bypass* for surgical treatment of morbid obesity is sometimes associated with severe fatty liver and hepatic failure that may be fatal. In patients with Cushing's syndrome and in those receiving large doses of corticosteroids, fatty infiltration of the liver may occur. In many *chronic illnesses*, especially those complicated by impaired nutrition or malabsorption, increased fat is found in liver cells. For example, patients with ulcerative colitis, chronic pancreatitis, or protracted heart failure frequently have moderately fatty livers at the time of death. Patients maintained on prolonged *intravenous hyperalimentation* may also develop fatty livers.

Acute fatty liver is caused by a number of hepatotoxins and is frequently accompanied by signs and symptoms of liver failure. Carbon tetrachloride intoxication, DDT poisoning, and ingestion of substances containing yellow phosphorus result in severe fatty liver. Acute and prolonged alcohol ingestion may also be considered in this category and may be associated with a rapidly enlarging and fat-laden liver. *Acute fatty liver of pregnancy* is a rare but often fatal condition seen during the third trimester of pregnancy which is characterized by nausea, vomiting, abdominal pain, renal failure, and coma. It should be distinguished from the benign cholestasis more frequently encountered during the third trimester of pregnancy. *Massive tetracycline therapy*, in amounts of 3 to 12 g intravenous, is a rare cause of acute fatty liver and fatal hepatic coma. Other drugs (e.g., valproic acid) have also been associated with the development of a fatty liver.

Pathogenesis   The hepatic lipid deposits, which consist largely of triglycerides and lesser amounts of phospholipid and cholesterol, appear as vacuoles of varying size within the cytoplasm of liver cells. In extreme cases, every liver cell is involved, and lipids comprise up to 30 to 40 percent of the total liver weight.

The biochemical mechanisms leading to hepatic triglyceride accumulation are described in Chap. 250. Fatty infiltration has been produced in experimental animals by a variety of toxic agents and drugs, such as alcohol, carbon tetrachloride, and orotic acid. Deficiencies, such as choline deficiency, readily lead to increased fat in the liver in the rat. Many of these factors appear to disrupt synthesis of proteins, including the apoproteins needed for transport of triglycerides out of the liver as lipoproteins. However, with few exceptions experimental studies do not explain the pathogenesis of fatty liver in clinical disease. Moderate doses of ethanol may produce both acute and chronic fatty changes in human subjects, probably by its direct effects on hepatic triglyceride and fatty acid metabolism (Chap. 250).

Protein deficiency seems to account for the fatty liver of kwashiorkor, and impaired protein synthesis for the fat accumulation following tetracycline and carbon tetrachloride administration. In diabetes mellitus and in starvation, increased mobilization of fatty acids from adipose tissue may be involved. Fatty infiltration during hyperalimentation appears to be derived from the high concentration of dextrose rather than from any lipid infusions.

Clinical features   The signs and symptoms of fatty liver are related to the degree of fat infiltration, the time course of its accumulation, and the underlying cause. The obese or diabetic patient with chronic fatty liver is usually asymptomatic and has only mild tenderness over the enlarged liver. The liver function tests are normal or show mild elevations of alkaline phosphatase, transaminases, or aminotransferases. In contrast, the rapid accumulation of fat seen in the setting of hyperalimentation may lead to marked tenderness, presumably resulting from stretching of Glisson's capsule. Similarly, alcoholic patients with acute fatty liver following a bout of heavy drinking may have right upper quadrant pain and tenderness often with laboratory evidence of cholestasis. The clinical presentation of acute fatty liver of pregnancy or fatty liver from hepatotoxins is similar to that of fulminant hepatic failure arising from any cause, with evidence of hepatic encephalopathy, marked elevations of prothrombin time and transaminases, and variable degrees of jaundice.

Diagnosis   The findings of a firm, nontender, and generally enlarged liver with minimal hepatic dysfunction in a patient with chronic alcoholism, malnutrition, poorly controlled diabetes mellitus, or obesity should suggest a fatty liver. When diagnostic uncertainty exists, needle biopsy of the liver will demonstrate the increased fatty content and possibly the underlying primary disorder. In acute fatty liver of pregnancy and in most cases of Reye's syndrome (see below), fat accumulates in small vacuoles (microvesicular fat) rather than in the large cytoplasmic droplets encountered in other disorders. The reason for the morphologic appearance of the fat in these two disorders is unclear.

Treatment   Adequate nutritional intake, removal of alcohol or offending toxins, and correction of any associated metabolic disorders usually result in recovery. There is no clinical rationale for the use of lipotropic agents such as choline. When indicated, attention should be directed to abstinence from alcohol, careful control of diabetes, weight loss, or correction of intestinal absorptive defects. In the alcoholic fatty liver there is gradual disappearance of fat from the liver after 4 to 8 weeks of adequate diet and abstinence from alcohol. Similarly, fatty infiltration usually resolves within 2 weeks after discontinuation of parenteral hyperalimentation. However, restitution of intestinal continuity may not prevent progression of disease in patients who have had extensive intestinal bypass surgery.

REYE'S SYNDROME (FATTY LIVER WITH ENCEPHALOPATHY)   This acute illness is encountered exclusively in children below 15 years of age. It is characterized clinically by vomiting, and signs of progressive central nervous system damage, signs of hepatic injury, and hypoglycemia. Morphologically there is extensive fatty vacuolization of the liver and renal tubules. The cause is unknown, although viral and toxic agents, especially salicylates, have been implicated. Increased aspirin use and much higher serum salicylate levels in children with this illness than in the general population have been described during outbreaks of Reye's syndrome. However, it seems clear that this illness may also occur in the absence of exposure to salicylates. In fatal cases, the liver is enlarged and yellow with striking diffuse fatty microvacuolization of cells. Peripheral zonal hepatic necrosis has also been present in some cases. Fatty changes of the renal tubular cells, cerebral edema, and neuronal degeneration of the brain are the major extrahepatic changes. Electron microscopic studies show structural alterations of mitochondria in liver, brain, and muscle.

The onset usually follows an upper respiratory tract infection, especially influenza or chickenpox. Within 1 to 3 days persistent vomiting occurs, together with stupor, which usually progresses rapidly to generalized convulsions and coma. The liver is enlarged, but *jaundice is characteristically absent or minimal.* Elevations in serum aminotransferases and prothrombin time, hypoglycemia, metabolic acidosis, and elevated serum ammonia levels are the major laboratory findings. The mortality rate in Reye's syndrome is approximately 50 percent. Therapy consists of infusions of glucose and fresh frozen plasma, as well as intravenous mannitol to reduce the cerebral edema. Chronic liver disease has not been reported in survivors.

NIEMANN-PICK DISEASE (See Chap. 331)   This rare heritable disorder, of which there are five types, is found mainly in Jewish infants and is characterized by the accumulation of sphingomyelin and cholesterol in reticuloendothelial cells of the liver, spleen, bone marrow, and brain due to deficiency of sphingomyelinase. Hepatomegaly and splenomegaly are present, together with elevations in serum aminotransferase and alkaline phosphatase levels, but jaundice and other evidence of hepatic dysfunction are rare. The liver, which is typically large, yellow, and fatty, shows clusters of lipid-filled, foamy Kupffer cells. Diagnosis is made by lipid analysis of the tissue obtained from bone marrow aspiration.

GAUCHER'S DISEASE (See Chap. 331)   Accumulations of large reticuloendothelial cells containing the cerebroside glucosylceramide (Gaucher's cells) in the liver and spleen account for the characteristic moderate to massive hepatosplenomegaly found in patients with the juvenile and adult forms of this disorder. Rarely, ascites or portal hypertension is produced by compression of the intrahepatic vasculature. The diagnosis may be made readily by liver biopsy and demonstration of the Gaucher's cells but should be confirmed by demonstration of a deficiency of the enzyme glucosylceramide β-glucosidase in peripheral leukocytes.

WOLMAN'S AND CHOLESTEROL ESTER STORAGE DISEASES Wolman's disease is a rare and fatal familial lipidosis of infancy producing hepatosplenomegaly and stippled calcification of the adrenal glands. Liver biopsy shows clusters of foam cells (reticuloendothelial cells filled with cholesterol ester and triglycerides), hepatocytes containing fat, and patchy fibrosis. A related but less severe genetic disorder is cholesterol ester storage disease. In this condition there is hypercholesterolemia and accumulation of both cholesterol esters and triglycerides in hepatic lysosomes. Both of these storage disorders are associated with hepatic deficiencies of cholesterol ester hydrolase and triglyceride lipase.

Other rare lipid disorders associated with hepatomegaly and increased fat in the liver include abetalipoproteinemia, Tangier disease, Fabry's disease, and types I and V hyperlipoproteinemia. (See Chap. 326 for details.)

HEPATIC GLYCOGEN ACCUMULATION

DIABETIC GLYCOGENOSIS   Hepatic enlargement caused by distention of liver cells with glycogen is present in some poorly controlled diabetic patients and often in juvenile diabetic patients (see Chap 319). More often, however, hepatomegaly is related to fatty infiltration (see above). Ketoacidosis and vigorous insulin therapy may further enhance hepatic enlargement and glycogen deposition. In the absence of cirrhosis, hepatomegaly usually decreases with careful control of the diabetes.

GLYCOGEN STORAGE DISEASE (See Chap. 332)   The normal liver contains 1 to 5 percent glycogen (by weight). Except for types V and VII, the liver is involved in all genetically determined glycogen storage diseases. There is disruption of glucose homeostasis due to an inability to mobilize hepatic glycogen stores. In types I, II, and VI hereditary glycogen storage diseases, increased amounts of glycogen (and fat) are found. Types III and IV are associated with derangements of glycogen structure, and cirrhosis may be present. Fasting hypoglycemia is present in all these diseases. Enzymatic and chemical analysis of liver tissue is usually needed for diagnosis.

Hepatic changes are common in patients with unrecognized or untreated galactosemia. In early weeks of life fatty infiltration and cholestasis may be noted in acutely ill infants. If the disease goes unrecognized for months or years, cirrhosis may develop. (See also Chap. 337.)

HEPATIC MINERAL ACCUMULATION

WILSON'S DISEASE (See Chap. 330)   This rare disease, predominantly of young people, is characterized by cirrhosis, softening and degeneration of the basal ganglia, and pigmentation of the cornea (Kayser-Fleischer rings). Increased copper deposition in the tissues seems to be responsible for the liver and basal ganglia changes. Liver cells are ballooned and show increased glycogen with glycogen vacuolization in the nuclei. The liver shows all grades of changes, from minimal to severe periportal or macronodular cirrhosis.

HEMOCHROMATOSIS (See Chap. 327)   This relatively common genetically determined disorder involves accumulation of abnormal amounts of iron due to inappropriate absorption in the intestine. The liver, as a primary site of iron storage, is most directly affected. There is diffuse deposition of excess iron in hepatocytes, in contrast to the characteristic accumulation of iron in the reticuloendothelial compartment typical of secondary iron overload and hemosiderosis. Hepatic iron overload commonly results in hepatomegaly. Although liver function is initially well preserved, if the disease is untreated, progressive impairment is followed by the development of cirrhosis.

OTHER INFILTRATIVE DISEASES

HURLER'S SYNDROME (See Chap. 333)   This is an uncommon hereditary disease that is characterized by the widespread tissue deposition of mucopolysaccharide (chondroitin sulfate B and heparin sulfate) in many tissues. The liver is frequently enlarged and firm. Microscopically, Kupffer cells and other macrophages are enlarged and filled with metachromatic granular material. Cirrhosis may be a late complication.

ALPHA₁ ANTITRYPSIN DEFICIENCY (See also Chap. 210)   Patients with homozygous deficiency of serum alpha₁ antitrypsin (α1AT) are prone to develop emphysema in adult life. The disease is suggested by the absence of alpha₁ globulin on serum electrophoresis (α1AT makes up 90 percent of this fraction normally) and confirmed by direct measurement of α1AT. The exact phenotype can then be determined by starch electrophoresis. Although there are 16 recognized alleles, only PiZ and PiS are associated with clinical disease. The molecular bases of these altered products have been related to single nucleic acid substitutions, e.g., PiZ is caused by a G (guanine) to A (adenine) transposition which results in a substitution of a glutamic acid for lysine at residue 292 in the α1AT protein. Hepatocytes of some patients with this deficiency contain globules positive to the periodic acid Schiff (PAS) reaction. Approximately 10 percent of children with homozygous deficiency (PiZZ phenotype) of α1AT will develop significant liver disease including neonatal hepatitis and progressive cirrhosis. It has been suggested that 15 to 20 percent of all chronic liver disease in infancy may be attributed to α1AT deficiency. In adults, the most common manifestation of α1AT deficiency is asymptomatic cirrhosis, which may progress from a micronodular to a macronodular state and may be complicated by the development of hepatocellular carcinoma. The occurrence of liver disease in these patients is not dependent upon the development of lung disease.

RETICULOENDOTHELIAL DISORDERS (See also Chaps. 63 and 302)

Moderate to massive hepatomegaly and splenomegaly occur frequently in the various types of leukemia and lymphoma. Jaundice, when present, is usually slight and results from hemolysis. Deep and protracted jaundice is distinctly rare and is caused by obstruction of the intrahepatic or extrahepatic bile ducts by tumor. Liver biopsy specimens reveal portal and sinusoidal infiltrates in most cases of leukemia, but the cellular pattern may be mixed and nonspecific. Liver biopsy is diagnostic in only 5 percent of patients with Hodgkin's disease. This percentage is increased in those with advanced disease or splenomegaly. Directed biopsy at laparoscopy or laparotomy is more likely to be positive than "blind" needle biopsy. Nonspecific histologic changes in the liver have been described in patients with lymphoma and may contribute to the abnormal liver function tests.

Myeloid metaplasia and other myeloproliferative disorders associated with extramedullary hematopoiesis produce hepatomegaly which may reach huge proportions, especially following splenectomy. Serum alkaline phosphatase elevations are often found. Ascites and portal hypertension, resulting from diffuse involvement of portal venules and lymphatics, are rare complications.

GRANULOMATOUS INFILTRATIONS

Perhaps as a result of the large population of mononuclear phagocytes, a number of systemic granulomatous diseases involve the liver, including sarcoidosis, miliary tuberculosis, histoplasmosis, brucellosis, schistosomiasis, berylliosis, and drug reactions. In addition, isolated granulomas of no diagnostic importance may be found occasionally in patients with various forms of cirrhosis and hepatitis. The liver infiltrated by granulomas may be slightly enlarged and firm, but hepatic dysfunction is usually limited and manifested only by mild increases in serum alkaline phosphatase and occasionally aminotransferase levels. In a few patients with sarcoidosis or brucellosis, portal hypertension may develop, and extensive postnecrotic scarring or postnecrotic cirrhosis may follow healing of the granulomatous lesions as in schistosomiasis.

Needle biopsy of the liver reveals granulomas and often provides the first definite evidence of a systemic or disseminated granulomatous disease. In patients with sarcoidosis who have neither clinical nor laboratory evidence of hepatic involvement, needle biopsy is positive in about 80 percent of cases. In cases of suspected miliary tuberculosis a portion of the biopsy should be cultured and stained for mycobacteria. The organism can be detected in the majority of cases, particularly when caseating granulomas are present. Serial sections of the biopsy specimen should be examined if granulomas are not apparent. Individual granulomas are rarely specific in their microscopic appearance, and final diagnosis usually requires other clinical, laboratory, or histologic data.

In approximately 20 percent of patients it is not possible to identify a cause for the granulomatous infiltration. When these infiltrates are accompanied by fever of unknown etiology, the diagnosis of granulomatous hepatitis should be considered. This is an uncommon disorder of unknown etiology and is diagnosed by exclusion. While granulomatous hepatitis invariably responds to moderate doses of corticosteroids, relapses are frequent, and such therapy should never be undertaken unless tuberculous disease or other causes of granulomatous infiltration have been excluded. This may include an initial empiric trial of antituberculous therapy.

AMYLOIDOSIS (See also Chap. 266)

Systemic amyloidosis, whether primary and idiopathic, familial, or secondary to chronic inflammatory or neoplastic diseases, often involves the liver. Grossly, the liver infiltrated with amyloid is enlarged and pale and rubbery in consistency. Microscopically, the birefringent amyloid deposits appear as homogeneous waxy material within the space of Disse, often being concentrated in the periportal areas and associated with atrophy of adjacent liver cell plates. Selective involvement of the walls of blood vessels, especially of the hepatic arterioles, may be a striking feature of primary amyloidosis. With this possible exception, however, the hepatic lesions are the same in all forms of amyloidosis and are present in 60 to 90 percent of cases.

An enlarged and firm liver is found in about 60 percent of patients, and ascites occurs in advanced stages of the disease in about 20 percent. Jaundice, portal hypertension, and other signs of chronic liver disease are usually absent. Liver function changes, although frequent, correlate poorly with the extent of liver infiltration. Hypoalbuminemia and elevated serum alkaline phosphatase are common. Hypoalbuminemia, however, may be related to the nephrotic syndrome owing to renal involvement; the prothrombin time is usually normal. The diagnosis is established by biopsy of rectum, skin, liver, or other involved organs and demonstration of the characteristic Congo red–staining deposits by polarizing microscopy.

REFERENCES

BOVE KE: Reye's syndrome, in *Hepatology, A Textbook of Liver Disease*, D Zakim, TD Boyer (eds). Philadelphia, Saunders, 1982, pp 1212–1220

GISHAN FK, GREENE HL: Liver disease in children with PIZZ α_1-antitrypsin deficiency. Hepatology 8:307, 1988

GLENNER GG: Amyloid deposits and amyloidosis. The β-fibrilloses. N Engl J Med 302:1283, 1980

HEUBI JE et al: Grade I Reye's syndrome: Outcome and predictors of progression to deeper coma grades. N Engl J Med 311:1539, 1984

HURWITZ ES et al: Public Health Service Study on Reye's syndrome and medications. N Engl J Med 313:842, 1985

KIDD VJ, WOO SLC: Recombinant DNA probes used to detail genetic disorders of the liver. Hepatology 4:731, 1984

REYNOLDS TB et al: Hepatic granulomas, in *Hepatology, A Textbook of Liver Disease*, D Zakim, TD Boyer (eds). Philadelphia, Saunders, 1982, pp 995–1009

RILEY C et al: Acute fatty liver of pregnancy: A reassessment based on observations in nine patients. Ann Intern Med 106:703, 1987

SCHIFF L, SCHIFF ER: *Diseases of the Liver*, 6th ed. Philadelphia, Lippincott, 1987

SPECHLER SJ, KOFF RS: Wilson's disease: Diagnostic difficulties in the patient with chronic hepatitis and hyperceruloplasminemia. Gastroenterology 78:103, 1980

SCRIVER CR et al (eds): *The Metabolic Basis of Inherited Disease*, 6th ed. New York, McGraw-Hill, 1989

257 LIVER TRANSPLANTATION

RUDI SCHMID

Orthotopic liver transplantation, i.e., replacement of a diseased liver by a healthy organ recovered from a recently brain-dead individual, is surgically difficult, requires a full array of supporting services usually available only in large tertiary medical centers, and carries a considerable operative and postoperative mortality. However, the risk-versus-benefit ratio has improved to an extent where liver transplantation has become a promising approach for selected patients whose liver disease is progressive, life-threatening, and beyond the reach of traditional therapy.

The first orthotopic liver transplantation in a human was performed by Starzl and associates in 1963 at the University of Colorado in Denver, but the survival of this patient and several subsequently transplanted patients was less than 1 month. The following years brought refinements in both surgical technique and postoperative management that improved survival rates, but by 1976 only 24 percent of adults and 33 percent of children who underwent liver transplantation survived for more than 1 year. Until the 1970s, performance of the operation remained almost entirely limited to the Denver center and to another liver transplantation facility established by Calne in 1968 in Cambridge, England. Since 1980, however, the prospect for prolonged survival with good quality of life has improved owing largely to development of better techniques for organ preservation, improvements in surgical techniques including the development of a pump-driven venovenous bypass system, and advances in immunosuppression, particularly the use of cyclosporine in combination with steroids. As a result, an increasing number of transplant centers are being established, and the total number of successful liver transplants exceeded 3,000 by the end of 1986. Over 1200 liver transplantations were performed in the United States in 1988.

INDICATIONS FOR LIVER TRANSPLANTATION   In the absence of absolute or relative contraindications (see below), potential candidates for liver transplantation are children and adults who suffer from severe, irreversible liver disease for which alternative medical or surgical treatments have been exhausted. Timing of the operation is of critical importance; the disease should be in a late enough stage to allow the patient all opportunity for spontaneous stabilization or recovery but early enough to give the surgical procedure a fair chance of success. As a general rule, transplantation should be considered in patients with end-stage liver disease who are experiencing or have experienced life-threatening complications of hepatic failure, whose quality of life has deteriorated to unacceptable levels, or whose liver disease predictably will result in irreversible damage to the central nervous system. The decision to transplant requires the combined judgment of an experienced team of hepatologists, transplant surgeons, anesthesiologists, and specialists in supporting services; the well-informed consent of the patient or the patient's family or authorized representative must also be obtained.

TRANSPLANTATION IN CHILDREN   Biliary atresia   The most common indication for transplantation in children is biliary atresia, which results in progressive distortion of intrahepatic bile ducts and cirrhosis, leading to hepatic insufficiency and death. Hepatoportoenterostomy (Kasai procedure) performed in the first two months of life may provide substantial, albeit usually transient, improvement, but in a small percentage of patients this procedure has been reported to result in prolonged stabilization obviating further surgery. In the majority of patients, however, progressive liver disease eventually requires transplantation, but the operation preferably should be delayed as long as possible to permit the child optimal development.

Metabolic disorders   Genetically transmitted diseases associated with progressive liver failure constitute another major indication in children and adolescents. In progressive cirrhosis due to α_1-antitrypsin deficiency, transplantation results in appearance of the donor α_1-antitrypsin phenotype and return of the plasma enzyme level toward normal. In Wilson's disease presenting with acute hepatic failure or with progressive neurologic deficiency that is unresponsive to chelation therapy, liver transplantation is the treatment of choice. Improvement in neurologic function and return of plasma ceruloplasmin concentration to normal have been reported. Liver failure in Byler's, Alagille's, and Wolman's disease and in protoporphyria, tyrosinemia, and some types of glycogenosis have been indications for transplantation. In Crigler-Najjar disease type I and in certain hereditary disorders of the urea cycle and of amino acid or lactate-pyruvate metabolism, transplantation may be the only way to prevent impending deterioration of central nervous system function, despite the fact that the replaced liver is structurally normal. Combined heart and liver transplantation have yielded dramatic improvement in cardiac function and plasma cholesterol level in children with homozygous familial hypercholesterolemia. In hereditary oxalosis, improvement has been reported after combined liver and kidney transplantation.

TRANSPLANTATION IN ADULTS   Nonalcoholic cirrhosis   Chronic active hepatitis due to presumed autoimmunity and cirrhosis of nonviral etiology with liver failure are important indications for transplantation. From the mid-1970s to 1985, the actuarial 1-year survival of 275 patients transplanted for these conditions progressively rose from 31 percent to approximately 70 percent.

Primary biliary cirrhosis   Because primary biliary cirrhosis has an indolent and often fluctuating course, liver transplantation is indicated only in patients who have progressed to an end stage of the disease or whose quality of life has deteriorated to an unacceptable level. Survival is similar to that in nonalcoholic cirrhosis. In the posttransplantation period, it may be difficult to distinguish between homograft rejection and potential recurrence of the original disease because the clinical, laboratory, and histologic features of the two conditions are similar.

Sclerosing cholangitis   Transplantation has been successful in patients with primary sclerosing cholangitis or with Caroli's disease in whom surgical drainage procedures failed to prevent progressive deterioration of hepatic function. Recurrent infections with sepsis are frequent indications for transplantations in these patients.

Hepatic vein thrombosis   Transplantation has been reported in 17 patients with Budd-Chiari syndrome with an actuarial 3-year survival of 60 percent. Because spontaneous recannulation of the obstructed hepatic veins occasionally occurs, the operation should be reserved for patients with progressive hepatic decompensation or irreversible hepatorenal syndrome. Postoperative anticoagulation is essential in these patients. Although many patients with Budd-Chiari syndrome have underlying polycythemia vera or a covert myeloproliferative disorder, this usually is no contraindication for liver transplantation.

Hepatobiliary cancer   Overall survival of patients who undergo transplantation for primary hepatocellular carcinoma or cholangiocarcinoma is significantly less than that for other categories of liver disease because the majority of patients succumb to disseminated carcinomatosis. Moreover, because the results have improved only slightly in recent years, the proportion of transplanted patients who received homografts for primary liver cancer has progressively decreased since 1980. The most promising approach to primary liver cancer clearly is early detection when the tumor is small and amenable to total resection. Several experimental protocols including lethal irradiation of the cancer-containing liver followed by resection and orthotopic transplantation are currently being evaluated.

CONTRAINDICATIONS FOR TRANSPLANTATION   Absolute contraindications for transplantation include life-threatening systemic diseases, infections, preexisting cardiovascular or pulmonary disease, metastatic malignancies, and therapy-resistant arterial hypotension. Preexisting renal disease is a relative contraindication; successful concomitant renal transplantation has been reported. Portal vein thrombosis is another relative contraindication; successful thrombectomy or construction of a venous bypass with subsequent liver transplantation have been performed. In alcohol-related liver disease, the outcome of transplantation generally has been disappointing; only 27 out of 819 patients reported up to August 1984 were transplanted for this condition. In patients with advanced alcohol-related cirrhosis who, despite abstinence for at least 6 months and adequate nutritional state, develop hepatic decompensation, transplantation may be contemplated when all other means of therapy have failed; relatively few patients, however, fulfill these qualifications. Patients with chronic viral hepatitis B, particularly those positive for HBsAg and HBeAg and those with non-A, non-B hepatitis, although the infection usually recurs in the homograft, increasingly are transplanted with acceptable survival results. Information is inadequate to determine whether recurrent infection also occurs in chronic hepatitis B without evidence of active viral replication. Patients with delta hepatitis are poor risks for transplantation. In fulminant hepatitis of all etiologies associated with encephalopathy and/or hepatorenal syndrome, results of transplantation generally have been discouraging. Interpretation of available results is difficult because most reports fail to distinguish between hepatic coma stages III and IV, which have strikingly different prognoses with conservative management.

RESULTS OF TRANSPLANTATION   Survival   Since 1983, the survival rate of patients undergoing liver transplantation has steadily improved. In 1985, the overall prospect for 1-year survival was about

70 percent, with children faring slightly better than adults. Of 152 patients who underwent liver transplantation at various centers between January 1980 and April 1983 and who survived the initial three postoperative months, the 3-year survival rate was 79 percent in adults with nonalcoholic cirrhosis and 92 percent in children with biliary atresia; in 102 patients transplanted after April 1983 who survived the initial three postoperative months, 1-year survival rates reached 89 percent in adults and 96 percent in children.

Posttransplantation quality of life In patients who have undergone transplantation for life-threatening chronic liver disease, objective evaluation of the quality of life after surgery is inherently difficult, and reliable information is sparse. Nonetheless, full rehabilitation seems to have been achieved in the majority of those who survived the first three postoperative months and escaped chronic rejection or unmanageable infection. Immunosuppressive medication in reduced doses is continued indefinitely. Several women who underwent transplantation and received immunosuppressive therapy have conceived and carried the pregnancy to term without demonstrable damage to the infants.

TECHNICAL AND MANAGEMENT ASPECTS Surgical techniques Liver donors commonly are procured from accident victims 2 months to 45 years of age who are brain-dead and without detectable hepatic dysfunction. Cardiovascular and respiratory functions are sustained artificially until the liver can be removed. Prolonged periods of hypotension or hypoxia preclude donation, and compatibility of ABO blood type and organ size are important considerations in donor selection, although successful ABO-incompatible or reduced donor organ transplants have been performed successfully. A recent report suggests that implantation of a female liver into a male recipient results in reduced homograft survival. Multiple-organ procurement (including the liver, heart, and kidneys, but not the pancreas) is technically feasible. Following perfusion with cold electrolyte solution the donor liver is packed in ice; a new perfusion solution recently developed by Belzer at the University of Wisconsin allows for at least 20 h of preservation without significant impairment of graft viability.

Removal of the recipient's liver is technically difficult, particularly in the presence of varices or scarring from previous abdominal operations. After the portal vein and inferior vena cava are dissected, a pump-driven bypass system is applied that reroutes blood from the portal vein and inferior vena cava to the superior vena cava, thereby preventing congestion of visceral organs. In implanting the new liver, meticulous attention must be directed to reestablishment of the portal venous and hepatic arterial circulations and to reconstruction of biliary drainage. The latter usually is achieved by anastomosis of the common bile ducts or by choledochojejunostomy to a Roux en Y limb, if the common bile duct of the recipient cannot be used for reconstruction.

A transplant operation requires 8 to 12 h. Because of excessive bleeding associated with portal hypertension and liver failure, large volumes of blood, blood products, and volume expanders may be required during surgery.

POSTOPERATIVE COURSE AND MANAGEMENT Postoperative complications Patients who undergo liver transplantation are frequently malnourished, so that attention to multiple organ failure is of primary importance. Because of the fluids administered during surgery, patients may become overloaded during the immediate postoperative period, necessitating continuous monitoring of cardiovascular and pulmonary function. Cardiovascular instability also may result from electrolyte imbalance during reperfusion of the donor liver. Pulmonary function may be further compromised by paralysis of the right hemidiaphragm caused by phrenic nerve injury. The hyperdynamic state with increased cardiac output frequently occurring in patients with liver failure rapidly reverses after successful liver transplantation. Postoperative jaundice is almost invariable and reflects the large administered pigment load and variable degrees of ischemic or mechanical injury sustained by the liver during harvesting, preservation, and implantation. Prerenal azotemia, acute kidney injury due to hypotension, or renal toxicity caused by antibiotics or cyclosporine are frequently encountered in the postoperative period and sometimes require dialysis. Other postoperative complications related to technical difficulties include stenosis or leakage of the anastomosed common bile duct, intraperitoneal hemorrhage, and thrombosis of the reconstructed hepatic artery or of the portal or hepatic vein. Acute upper gastrointestinal hemorrhage or unexplained transient hemolytic anemia, with or without thrombocytopenia, may occur.

Bacterial, viral, or fungal infections related to the required immunosuppressive therapy may be life-threatening in the postoperative period. These infections may involve the biliary tree, liver, upper gastrointestinal tract, or lungs, and they demand early recognition and prompt management. *Candida, Nocardia, Pneumocystis carinii*, and cytomegalovirus are frequent infective agents, but viruses of the herpes group, other mycoses, or gram-negative bacteria may also be pathogens. In most transplant centers, patients routinely are given antibiotic and antifungal therapy prophylactically. Routine use of sulfamethoxazole with trimethoprim decreases the incidence of postoperative *P. carinii* infection.

Immunosuppression The introduction in 1980 of cyclosporine as an immunosuppressive agent contributed substantially to the improvement in transplant survival. The drug depresses both humoral and cell-mediated immunity via inhibition of interleukin 2 production without affecting rapidly dividing cells in the bone marrow, which may account for the reduced incidence of systemic posttransplantation infection. Unfortunately, cyclosporine causes dose-related renal tubular injury and direct renal artery vasospasm, which usually can be managed by reducing the dose. Other adverse effects of long-term cyclosporine use are hypertension, hyperkalemia, tremor, hirsutism, and hyperplasia of the gums. Because of these side effects, combinations of cyclosporine and prednisone or cyclosporine, prednisone, and azathioprine are preferable regimens for immunosuppressive treatment during the initial postoperative months. For long-term management, renal toxicity may make it necessary to reduce cyclosporine to very low doses. In many centers, cyclosporine treatment is initiated prior to or on the day of surgery and is continued by intravenous route through the operation and the immediate postoperative period until oral administration can be resumed.

Transplant rejection Despite the use of cyclosporine in various combinations, homograft rejection still occurs in the majority of patients 1 to 6 weeks after surgery. To date no clinically documented "hyperacute" rejections have been observed in humans although a reproducible animal model has now been developed. Early signs suggesting liver rejection are leukocytosis, increase in serum bilirubin level, and rise in aminotransferase and alkaline phosphatase activity; these may be followed by fever, tenderness in the right upper abdomen, diarrhea, ascites, and progressive deterioration of hepatic function. Because of the lack of specificity of these manifestations, differential diagnosis between homograft rejection, biliary obstruction, viral hepatitis, and recurrence of the original liver disease frequently is difficult. Radiographic visualization of the biliary tree and/or percutaneous liver biopsy often are helpful in establishing the correct diagnosis. Early morphologic features of rejection characteristically include portal infiltration with small lymphocytes and variable numbers of polymorphonuclear leukocytes, centrolobular bile stasis, selective injury to bile duct epithelium associated with polymorphonuclear infiltration, and, at times, endothelial inflammation of portal or central veins and occasionally of hepatic arterioles. These findings are similar to those in graft-versus-host disease and may be indistinguishable from those of primary biliary cirrhosis. As soon as transplant rejection is suspected, it is treated with intravenous methylprednisolone in repeated boluses; if this fails to reverse the rejection processes, many centers are also using antilymphocyte antibodies, either as polyclonal antilymphocyte globulin or the monoclonal agent OKT-3.

Chronic rejection is a relatively rare event that appears to be unrelated to the occurrence of preceding acute rejection episodes. It is associated with progressive cholestasis, bile duct proliferation, focal parenchymal necrosis, mononuclear infiltration, and fibrosis. These morphologic findings may be so similar to those of chronic viral hepatitis that differentiation between the two may be difficult. In some patients with therapy-resistant chronic rejection, retransplantation has yielded encouraging results.

REFERENCES

BUSUTTIL RW, Moderator: Liver transplantation today. Ann Intern Med 104:377, 1986

DEMETRIS AJ et al: Pathologic analysis of liver transplantation for primary biliary cirrhosis. Hepatology 8:939, 1988

MADDREY WC (ed): *Transplantation of the Liver.* New York, Elsevier, 1988

O'GRADY TG, WILLIAMS R: Present position of liver transplantation and its impact on hepatologic practice. Gut 29:566, 1988

POLSON RJ et al: Evidence for disease recurrence after liver transplantation for primary biliary cirrhosis. Clinical and histologic follow-up studies. Gastroenterology 97:7P5,1989

SCHARSCHMIDT BF: Human liver transplantation: An analysis of 819 patients from 8 centers, in *Recent Advances in Hepatology*, HC Thomas, EA Jones (eds). London, Churchill-Livingstone, 1985, vol 2

STARZL TE et al: Liver transplantation. N Engl J Med 321:1014, 1092, 1989

258   DISEASES OF THE GALLBLADDER AND BILE DUCTS

NORTON J. GREENBERGER / KURT J. ISSELBACHER

PHYSIOLOGY OF BILE PRODUCTION AND FLOW   Bile secretion and composition   Bile formed in the hepatic lobules is secreted into a complex network of canaliculi, small bile ductules, and larger bile ducts which run with lymphatics and branches of the portal vein and hepatic artery in portal tracts situated between hepatic lobules. These interlobular bile ducts coalesce to form larger septal bile ducts that join to form the right and left hepatic ducts, which in turn unite to form the common hepatic duct. The common hepatic duct is joined by the cystic duct of the gallbladder to form the common bile duct which enters the duodenum (often after joining the main pancreatic duct) through the ampulla of Vater.

Hepatic bile is a pigmented isotonic fluid with an electrolyte composition resembling blood plasma. The electrolyte composition of gallbladder bile differs from that of hepatic bile since most of the inorganic anions, chloride and bicarbonate, have been removed by reabsorption across the basement membrane.

Major components of bile by weight include water (82 percent), bile acids (12 percent), lecithin and other phospholipids (4 percent), and unesterified cholesterol (0.7 percent). Other constituents include conjugated bilirubin, proteins (IgA, by-products of hormones, and other proteins metabolized in the liver), electrolytes, mucus, and, often, drugs and their metabolic by-products.

The total daily basal secretion of hepatic bile is approximately 500 to 600 mL. The metabolic products of hepatocyte uptake and synthesis are secreted into the bile canaliculi, which are lined by microvillus membrane components associated with microfilaments of actin, microtubules, and other contractile elements. Within the hepatocyte, conjugation of many of the bile constituents may occur, while other components of bile such as primary bile acids, lecithin, and some cholesterol are synthesized de novo. Three mechanisms are important in regulating bile flow: (1) active transport of bile acids from hepatocytes into the canaliculi, (2) bile acid–independent ATPase-mediated transport of sodium, and (3) ductular secretion. The last is a secretin-mediated and cyclic AMP–dependent phenomenon which appears to result from the active transport of sodium and bicarbonate into the ductule with resulting passive movement of water across the cell membrane.

The bile acids   The primary bile acids, cholic and chenodeoxycholic acids, are synthesized from cholesterol in the liver, conjugated with glycine or taurine, and excreted into the bile. Secondary bile acids, including deoxycholate and lithocholate, are formed in the colon as bacterial metabolites of the primary bile acids. However, lithocholic acid is much less efficiently absorbed from the colon than deoxycholic acid. Other secondary bile acids, found in trace amounts, which include ursodeoxycholic acid (a stereoisomer of chenodeoxycholate) and a variety of other unusual or "aberrant" bile acids, may be produced in increased amounts in patients with chronic cholestatic syndromes. In normal bile, the ratio of glycine to taurine conjugates is about 3:1, while in patients with cholestasis, increased concentrations of sulfate and glucuronide conjugates of bile acids are often found.

Bile acids are detergents which in aqueous solutions and above a critical concentration of about 2 mM form molecular aggregates called *micelles.* Cholesterol alone is poorly soluble in aqueous environments, and its solubility in bile depends upon both the lipid concentration and the relative molar percentages of bile acids and lecithin. Normal ratios of these constituents favor the formation of solubilizing "mixed micelles," while abnormal ratios promote the precipitation of cholesterol crystals in bile.

In addition to facilitating the biliary excretion of cholesterol, bile acids are necessary for the normal intestinal absorption of dietary fats via a micellar transport mechanism (see Chap. 240). Bile acids also serve as a major physiologic driving force for hepatic bile flow and aid in water and electrolyte transport in the small bowel and colon.

Enterohepatic circulation   Bile acids are efficiently conserved under normal conditions. Conjugated and unconjugated bile acids are absorbed by *passive diffusion* along the entire gut. Quantitatively much more important for bile salt recirculation, however, is the *active transport* mechanism for conjugated bile acids in the distal ileum (see Chap. 240). The reabsorbed bile acids enter the portal bloodstream and are taken up rapidly by hepatocytes, reconjugated, and resecreted into bile (enterohepatic circulation).

The normal bile acid pool size is approximately 2 to 4 g. During digestion of a meal, the bile acid pool undergoes at least one or more enterohepatic cycles depending upon the size and composition of the meal. Normally the bile acid pool circulates approximately 5 to 10 times daily. Intestinal absorption of the pool is about 95 percent efficient, so that fecal loss of bile acids is in the range of 0.3 to 0.6 g/d. This fecal loss is compensated by an equal daily synthesis of bile acids by the liver, and thus the size of the bile salt pool is maintained. Bile acids returning to the liver suppress de novo hepatic synthesis of primary bile acids from cholesterol by inhibiting the rate-limiting enzyme 7α-hydroxylase. While the loss of bile salts in stool is usually matched by increased hepatic synthesis, the maximum rate of synthesis is approximately 5 g/d, which may be insufficient to replete the bile acid pool size when there is pronounced impairment of intestinal bile salt reabsorption.

Gallbladder and sphincteric functions   In the fasting state, the sphincter of Oddi offers a high-pressure zone of resistance to bile flow from the common bile duct into the duodenum. This tonic contraction serves to (1) prevent reflux of duodenal contents into the pancreatic and bile ducts, and (2) promote bile filling of the gallbladder. The major factor controlling the evacuation of the gallbladder is the peptide hormone cholecystokinin, which is released from the duodenal mucosa in response to the ingestion of fats and amino acids. Cholecystokinin produces (1) powerful contraction of the gallbladder, (2) decreased resistance of the sphincter of Oddi, (3) increased hepatic secretion of bile, and thus (4) enhanced flow of biliary contents into the duodenum.

Hepatic bile is "concentrated" within the gallbladder by energy-dependent transmucosal absorption of water and electrolytes. Almost the entire bile acid pool may be sequestered in the gallbladder following an overnight fast for delivery into the duodenum with the first meal of the day. The normal capacity of the gallbladder is 30 to 75 mL of bile.

DISEASES OF THE GALLBLADDER

CONGENITAL ANOMALIES Anomalies of the biliary tract may be found in 10 to 20 percent of the population, including abnormalities in number, size, and shape (e.g., agenesis of the gallbladder, duplications, rudimentary or oversized "giant" gallbladders, and diverticula). Phrygian cap is a clinically innocuous entity in which a partial or complete septum (or fold) separates the fundus from the body. Anomalies of position or suspension are not uncommon and include left-sided gallbladder, intrahepatic gallbladder, retrodisplacement of the gallbladder, and "floating" gallbladder. The latter condition predisposes to acute torsion, volvulus, or herniation of the gallbladder.

GALLSTONES **Pathogenesis of gallstones** Gallstones are quite prevalent in most western countries. In the United States, autopsy series have shown gallstones in at least 20 percent of women and in 8 percent of men over the age of 40. It is estimated that 16 to 20 million persons in the United States have gallstones and that approximately 1 million new cases of cholelithiasis develop each year.

Gallstones are crystalline structures formed by concretion or accretion of normal or abnormal bile constituents. These stones are divided into three major types; cholesterol and mixed stones account for 80 percent of the total, with pigment stones comprising the remaining 20 percent. Mixed and cholesterol gallstones usually contain more than 70 percent cholesterol monohydrate plus an admixture of calcium salts, bile acids and bile pigments, proteins, fatty acids, and phospholipids. Pigment stones are primarily composed of calcium bilirubinate; they contain less than 10 percent cholesterol.

CHOLESTEROL AND MIXED STONES AND BILIARY SLUDGE Cholesterol is relatively water insoluble and requires aqueous dispersion into either micelles or vesicles, both of which require the presence of a second lipid to "liquify" the cholesterol. When the cholesterol content of bile exceeds the amount which can be solubilized by bile salt and bile salt–lecithin micelles, the excess is dispersed in larger lipid vesicles (Fig. 258-1). Vesicles are spherical particles composed of lecithin and cholesterol and contain only traces of bile salts. Vesicles and micelles are important cholesterol-solubilizing and -transport agents in bile supersaturated with cholesterol.

There are several important mechanisms in the formation of lithogenic (stone-forming) bile. The most important is increased biliary secretion of cholesterol. This may occur in association with obesity, high-caloric diets, or drugs (e.g., clofibrate) and may result from increased activity of hydroxymethylglutaryl-coenzyme A (HMG-CoA) reductase, the rate-limiting enzyme of hepatic cholesterol synthesis. In some patients, impaired hepatic conversion of cholesterol to bile acids may also occur, resulting in an increase of the lithogenic cholesterol/bile acid ratio. Lithogenic bile also results from decreased hepatic secretion of bile salts and phospholipids which may follow impaired hepatic synthesis (e.g., rare inborn errors of metabolism such as cerebrotendinous xanthomatosis) or conditions affecting the enterohepatic circulation of these constituents (e.g., prolonged parenteral alimentation or ileal disease or resection). In addition, most patients with gallstones appear to have reduced activity of hepatic cholesterol 7α-hydroxylase, the rate-limiting enzyme for primary bile acid synthesis.

A second important abnormality is defective vesicle formation because the vesicles have too little phospholipid and an excess of cholesterol. While cholesterol saturation of bile is an important prerequisite for gallstone formation, it is not sufficient by itself to produce cholesterol precipitation in vivo.

A third important mechanism is *nucleation* of cholesterol monohydrate crystals, which is greatly accelerated in human lithogenic bile; it is this feature rather than the degree of cholesterol supersaturation that distinguishes lithogenic from normal gallbladder bile. Accelerated nucleation of cholesterol monohydrate in bile may be due to either an *excess* of *pronucleating factors* or a *deficiency* of *antinucleating* factors. Nonmucin and mucin glycoproteins and lysine

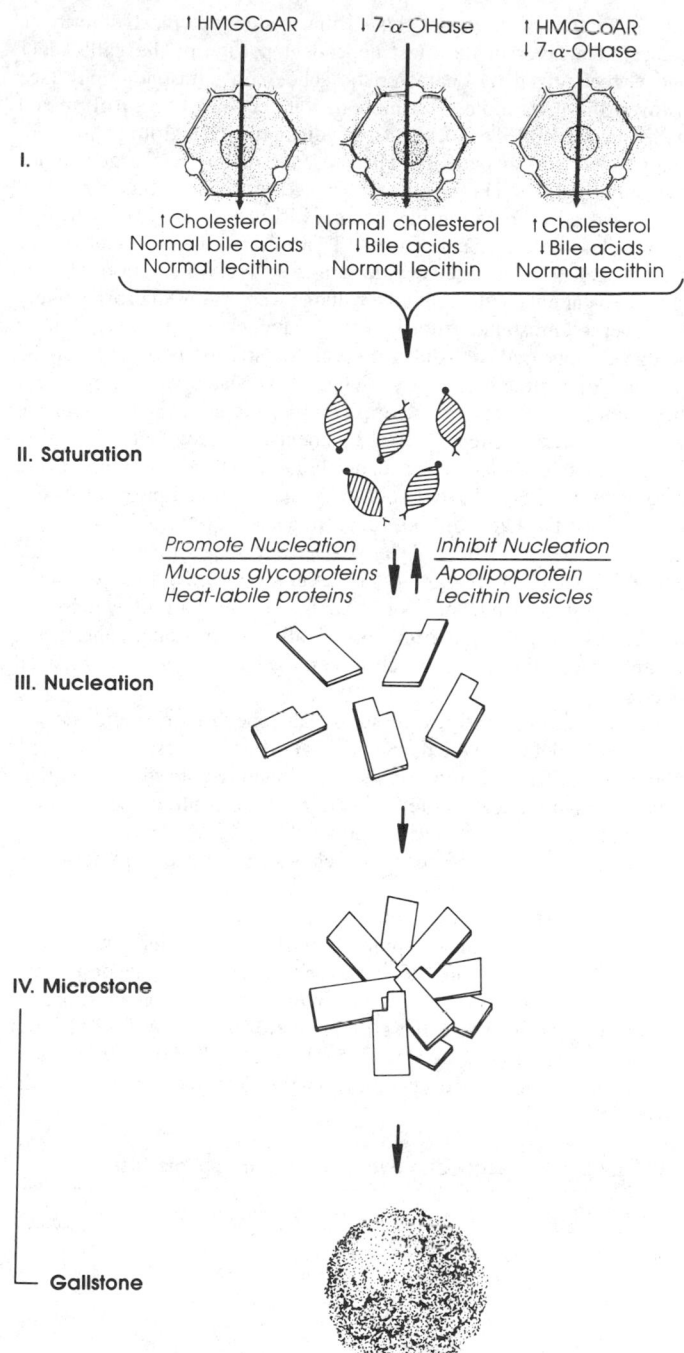

FIGURE 258-1 Scheme showing pathogenesis of gallstone formation. Conditions or factors that increase the ratio of cholesterol to bile acids and lecithin favor gallstone formation. (HMG CoAR = hydroxymethylglutaryl-coenzyme A reductase; 7-α-OHase = 7α-hydroxylase.)

phosphatidylcholine appear to be pronucleating factors while apolipoproteins AI and AII appear to be antinucleating factors. However, the characterization of additional pronucleating and antinucleating factors remains incomplete. Cholesterol monohydrate crystal nucleation and crystal growth probably occur within the mucin gel layer. Vesicle fusion leads to liquid crystals which in turn nucleate into solid cholesterol monohydrate crystals. Continued growth of the crystals occurs by direct nucleation of cholesterol molecules from supersaturated unilamellar biliary vesicles.

A fourth important mechanism in cholesterol gallstone formation concerns *biliary sludge*. Biliary sludge is a thick mucous material which upon microscopic examination reveals lecithin-cholesterol crystals, cholesterol monohydrate crystals, calcium bilirubinate, and mucin thread or mucous gels. Biliary sludge typically forms a crescentlike layer in the most dependent portion of the gallbladder and is recognized by characteristic echoes on ultrasonography (see below). In vitro, cholesterol monohydrate crystals (>50 μm) mixed with mucus produce echoes that are indistinguishable from gallbladder sludge observed in patients. The presence of biliary sludge implies two abnormalities: (1) the normal balance between gallbladder mucin secretion and elimination has become deranged; and (2) nucleation from biliary solutes has occurred. That biliary sludge is a precursor form of gallstone disease is evident from several observations. In one study, 96 patients with gallbladder sludge were followed prospectively by several ultrasound studies. In 17 patients (18 percent), biliary sludge disappeared and did not recur for at least two years. In 58 patients (60 percent), biliary sludge disappeared and reappeared. Importantly, gallstones developed in 14 patients in 8 of whom the gallstones were "silent." In 12 patients, cholecystectomies were performed, 6 for gallstone-associated biliary pain and 3 in symptomatic patients with sludge but without gallstones who had prior attacks of pancreatitis; the latter did not recur after cholecystectomy. It should be emphasized that biliary sludge can develop with disorders that cause gallbladder hypomotility, i.e., surgery, burns, total parenteral nutrition, pregnancy, and oral contraceptives—all of which are associated with gallstone formation. Finally, biliary sludge can account for the observation that most cholesterol gallstones have a pigmented center.

To summarize briefly, cholesterol gallstone disease occurs because of several defects which include: (1) bile supersaturation with cholesterol; (2) nucleation of cholesterol monohydrate with subsequent crystal retention and stone growth; and (3) abnormal gallbladder motor function with delayed emptying and stasis. Other important factors known to predispose to cholesterol stone formation are summarized in Table 258-1.

PIGMENT STONES Gallstones composed largely of calcium bilirubinate are much more common in the orient than in western countries. The presence of increased amounts of unconjugated, insoluble bilirubin in bile results in the precipitation of bilirubin which may aggregate to form pigment stones or may fuse to form the nidus for growth of mixed cholesterol gallstones. In western countries, chronic hemolytic states (with increased conjugated bili-

TABLE 258-1 Predisposing factors for cholesterol and pigment gallstone formation

1 Cholesterol and mixed stones
  a Demography: northern Europe and North and South America greater than orient; probable familial, hereditary aspects
  b Obesity, high-calorie diet (↑ cholesterol output)
  c Clofibrate therapy (↑ cholesterol output)
  d Malabsorption of bile acids (e.g., ileal disease or resection) (↓ bile salt secretion)
  e Female sex hormones: women > men after puberty; oral contraceptives and other estrogens (↓ bile salt secretion)
  f Age, especially among males
  g Other factors: pregnancy, diabetes mellitus, dietary polyunsaturated fats (↑ cholesterol output)
  h Prolonged parenteral alimentation
2 Pigment stones
  a Demographic/genetic factors: orient, rural setting
  b Chronic hemolysis
  c Alcoholic cirrhosis
  d Chronic biliary tract infection, parasite infestation
  e Increasing age

rubin in bile) or alcoholic liver disease are associated with an increased incidence of pigment stones. Deconjugation of soluble bilirubin mono- and diglucuronide may be mediated by the enzyme β-glucuronidase, which is sometimes produced when bile is chronically infected by bacteria. Pigment stone formation is especially prominent in Asians and is often associated with infections in the biliary tree (see Table 258-1).

Diagnosis of gallstones Procedures of potential use in the diagnosis of cholelithiasis and other diseases of the gallbladder are detailed in Table 258-2. The plain abdominal film may detect gallstones containing sufficient calcium to be radiopaque (10 to 15 percent of cholesterol and mixed stones and approximately 50 percent of pigment stones). Plain radiography may also be of use in the diagnosis of emphysematous cholecystitis, porcelain gallbladder, limey bile, and gallstone ileus.

Ultrasonography of the gallbladder is very accurate in the identification of cholelithiasis and has several advantages over oral cholecystography (see Fig. 258-2A). The gallbladder is easily visualized with the technique, and, in fact, failure to image the gallbladder

TABLE 258-2 Diagnostic evaluation of the gallbladder

Procedure	Diagnostic advantages	Diagnostic limitations	Comment

Plain abdominal x-ray	Low cost
	Readily available
		Relatively low yield
		?Contraindicated in pregnancy
			Pathognomonic findings in:
			  Calcified gallstones
			  Limey bile, porcelain GB
			  Emphysematous cholecystitis
			  Gallstone ileus

Oral cholecystogram (OCG)	Low cost
	Readily available
	Accurate identification of gallstones (90–95%)
	Identification of GB anomalies, hyperplastic cholecystoses
	Identification of chronic GB disease after nonvisualization on double dose
		?Contraindicated in pregnancy
		?Contraindicated with history of reaction to iodinated contrast
		Nonvisualization with:
		  Serum bilirubin >34–68 μmol/L (2–4 mg/dL)
		  Failure to ingest or absorb tablets
		  Impaired hepatic excretion
		Very small stones may be undetected
		More time-consuming than GBUS
			A useful procedure in identification of gallstones if diagnostic limitations prevent GBUS

Gallbladder ultrasound (GBUS)	Rapid Accurate identification of gallstones (>95%) Simultaneous scanning of GB, liver, bile ducts, pancreas "Real-time" scanning allows assessment of GB volume, contractility Not limited by jaundice, pregnancy May detect very small stones	Bowel gas Massive obesity Ascites Recent barium study	Procedure of choice for detection of stones
Radioisotope scans (HIDA, DISIDA, etc.)	Accurate identification of cystic duct obstruction Simultaneous assessment of bile ducts	?Contraindicated in pregnancy Serum bilirubin >103–205 μmol/L (6–12 mg/dL) Cholecystogram of low resolution	Indicated for confirmation of suspected cholecystitis

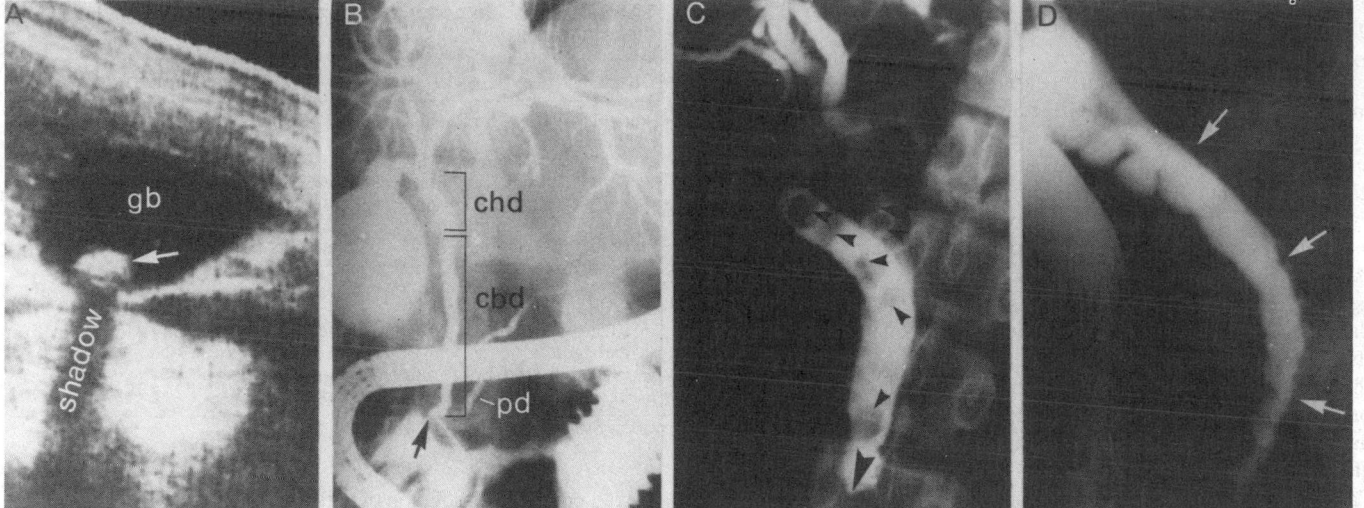

FIGURE 258-2 Examples of ultrasound and radiologic studies of the biliary tract. *A*. An ultrasound study showing a distended gallbladder containing a single large stone (arrow) which casts an acoustic shadow. *B*. Endoscopic retrograde cholangiopancreatogram (ERCP) showing normal biliary tract anatomy. In addition to the endoscope and large vertical gallbladder filled with contrast dye, the common hepatic duct (chd), common bile duct (cbd), and pancreatic duct (pd) are shown. The arrow points to the ampulla of Vater.

C. Percutaneous transhepatic cholangiogram (PTHC) showing choledocholithiasis. The biliary tract is dilatated and contains multiple radiolucent calculi (small arrows). The dilatation is due to obstruction by a large stone in the distal portion of the duct (large arrow). *D*. ERCP showing sclerosing cholangitis. The common bile duct is to the right of the endoscope. Following retrograde cholangiography, the common bile duct shows thickening of the wall with a narrow, beaded lumen typical of sclerosing cholangitis.

successfully in a fasting patient correlates well with the presence of underlying gallbladder disease. Stones as small as 2 mm in diameter may be confidently identified provided that firm criteria are used [e.g., acoustic "shadowing" of opacities that are within the gallbladder lumen and that change with the patient's position (by gravity)]. In major medical centers the false-negative and false-positive rates for ultrasound in gallstone patients are about 2 to 4 percent. Biliary sludge is material of low echogenic activity that typically forms a layer in the most dependent position of the gallbladder. This layer shifts with postural changes but fails to produce acoustic shadowing; these two characteristics distinguish sludges from gallstones.

Oral cholecystography (OCG) is a useful procedure for the diagnosis of gallstones but has been largely replaced by ultrasound. False-positive results are rare, but the oral cholecystogram may be falsely negative (when good opacification is achieved) in approximately 5 to 10 percent of patients with gallstones. Factors which may produce nonvisualization of the OCG are summarized in Table 258-2. When these can be excluded, nonvisualization of the gallbladder following a second dose of oral contrast agent is highly correlated with underlying cystic duct obstruction or chronic inflammation of the gallbladder.

Radiopharmaceuticals such as ^{99m}Tc-labeled *N*-substituted iminodiacetic acids (HIDA, DIDA, DISIDA, etc.) are rapidly extracted from the blood and are excreted into the biliary tree in high concentration even in the presence of mild to moderate serum bilirubin elevations. Failure to image the gallbladder in the presence of biliary ductal visualization may indicate cystic duct obstruction, acute or chronic cholecystitis, or surgical absence of the organ. Such scans have their greatest application in the diagnosis of acute cholecystitis.

Symptoms of gallstone disease Gallstones usually produce symptoms by causing inflammation or obstruction following their migration into the cystic duct or common bile duct. The most specific and characteristic symptom of gallstone disease is biliary colic. Obstruction of the cystic duct or common bile duct by a stone produces increased intraluminal pressure and distention of the viscus which cannot be relieved by repetitive biliary contractions. The resultant visceral pain is characteristically a severe, steady aching or pressure in the epigastrium or right upper quadrant of the abdomen with frequent radiation to the interscapular area, right scapula, or shoulder.

Biliary colic begins quite suddenly and may persist with severe intensity for 1 to 4 h, subsiding gradually or rapidly. An episode of biliary pain is sometimes followed by a residual mild ache or soreness in the right upper quadrant which may persist for 24 h or so. Nausea and vomiting frequently accompany episodes of biliary colic, and mild elevations of serum bilirubin [not exceeding 85.5 μmol/L (5 mg/dL)] occur in 25 percent of patients. Persistence of a high serum bilirubin level suggests common duct stones. Fever or chills (rigors) with biliary colic usually imply an underlying complication, i.e., cholecystitis, pancreatitis, or cholangitis. Complaints of vague epigastric fullness, dyspepsia, eructation, or flatulence, especially following a fatty meal, should not be confused with biliary colic. Such symptoms are frequently elicited from patients with gallstone disease but are not specific for biliary calculi. Biliary colic may be precipitated by eating a fatty meal, by consumption of a large meal following a period of prolonged fasting, or by eating a normal meal.

Natural history of gallstones Gallstone disease discovered in an asymptomatic patient or in a patient whose symptoms are not referable to cholelithiasis is a common clinical problem. The natural history of "silent" or asymptomatic gallstones has occasioned much debate. In contrast to previous reports, a study of predominantly male silent gallstone patients suggests that the cumulative risk for the development of symptoms or complications requiring surgery is relatively low—10 percent at 5 years, 15 percent at 10 years, and 18 percent at 15 years. Patients remaining asymptomatic for 15 years were found to be unlikely to develop symptoms during further follow-up, and most patients who did develop complications from their gallstones experienced *prior* warning symptoms. Similar conclusions apply to diabetics with silent gallstones. Decision analysis has suggested that (1) the cumulative risk of death due to gallstone disease while on expectant management is small; and (2) prophylactic cholecystectomy is not warranted.

Complications requiring cholecystectomy appear to be much more common in gallstone patients who have developed symptoms of biliary colic. Patients found to have gallstones at a young age are more likely to develop symptoms from cholelithiasis than are patients older than 60 years at the time of initial diagnosis. Patients with diabetes mellitus and gallstones may be somewhat more susceptible to septic complications, but the magnitude of risk of septic biliary complications in diabetic patients is incompletely defined. In addition, asymptomatic gallstone patients with nonvisualization of the gallbladder on OCG appear to have an increased tendency to develop symptoms and complications.

Treatment of gallstones SURGICAL THERAPY Although the management of silent gallstones remains controversial, the risk of developing symptoms or complications requiring surgery is quite small (in the range of 1 to 2 percent per year) in most asymptomatic gallstone patients. Thus, a recommendation for prophylactic cholecystectomy in a patient with gallstones should probably be based on assessment of three factors: (1) the presence of symptoms which are frequent enough or severe enough to interfere with the patient's general routine; (2) the presence of a prior complication of gallstone disease, i.e., history of acute cholecystitis, pancreatitis, gallstone fistula, etc.; or (3) the presence of an underlying condition predisposing the patient to increased risk of gallstone complications (e.g., calcified or porcelain gallbladder, cholesterolosis, adenomyomatosis, nonvisualizing gallbladder on oral cholecystography, and/or a previous attack of acute cholecystitis regardless of current symptomatic status). Patients with very large gallstones (over 2 cm in diameter) and patients having gallstones in a congenitally anomalous gallbladder might also be considered for prophylactic cholecystectomy. Although age under 50 years is a worrisome factor in asymptomatic gallstone patients, few authorities would now recommend routine cholecystectomy in all young patients with silent stones.

MEDICAL THERAPY—GALLSTONE DISSOLUTION Treatment with oral chenodeoxycholic acid (CDCA, chenic acid) or its 7β-epimer, ursodeoxycholic acid (UDCA), to dissolve cholesterol or mixed gallstones has resulted in complete or partial dissolution of such stones in approximately 50 to 60 percent of patients with radiolucent gallstones. Biliary secretion of these agents following oral bile acid administration alters the bile acid/cholesterol/lecithin ratio in bile (the lithogenic index). The major therapeutic effect of CDCA, however, is thought to be secondary to a decrease in HMG-CoA reductase activity, which in turn results in decreased hepatic cholesterol synthesis. UDCA administration appears to produce a lamellar liquid crystalline phase in bile which allows dispersion of cholesterol from stones by physical-chemical means.

Oral bile acid therapy is essentially ineffective in dissolving (1) pigment gallstones, which represent approximately 20 percent of radiolucent stones; (2) radiopaque or calcified gallstones; (3) gallstones greater than approximately 1.5 cm in diameter; and (4) gallstones in gallbladders poorly opacified following oral cholecystography. In patients with multiple, small, radiolucent gallstones in a functioning gallbladder, success rates for CDCA therapy of up to 80 percent have been reported if daily doses of 10 to 15 mg/kg of CDCA are used over a 1- to 3-year treatment period. However, lower daily doses of CDCA, i.e., 5 to 10 mg/kg, have resulted in much lower complete dissolution (5 to 15 percent) as well as lower partial dissolution rates (40 percent). Further, some massively obese patients may require doses as high as 20 to 25 mg/kg per day of CDCA to achieve cholesterol desaturation of bile. Ultrasound appears to be more sensitive than oral cholecystography in following patients during and after stone dissolution therapy (Table 258-3).

Chenodeoxycholic acid therapy is usually associated with self-limited diarrhea in most patients given an optimal therapeutic dose. In addition, approximately 25 percent of patients treated with CDCA acid develop mild (two- to threefold) and transient (less than 6 months) elevations of serum aminotransferase levels. Although hepatic injury has been described, biopsy and liver function studies in humans have shown serious CDCA-related hepatotoxicity in less than 1 to 2 percent of patients.

Ursodeoxycholic acid is therapeutically effective at lower doses (5 to 10 mg/kg per day) than chenodeoxycholic acid and has not been associated with the relatively high incidence of diarrhea and serum aminotransferase elevations seen in CDCA-treated patients. On the other hand, UDCA treatment has been associated with calcification of previously uncalcified gallstones in more than 10 percent of patients.

TABLE 258-3   Chenodeoxycholic acid (CDCA) and gallstone dissolution

RESULTS OF U.S. NATIONAL COOPERATIVE GALLSTONE STUDY

1 Patients—916 with radiolucent stones, treated 24 months
   a Placebo
   b Low-dose CDCA; 375 mg per day
   c High-dose CDCA; 750 mg per day
2 Results—best with high dose
   a Complete dissolution, 13.5%
   b Partial dissolution, 27.3%; complete plus partial, 40.8%
   c Best results—women, thin patients, small stones
3 Side effects
   a Mild diarrhea
   b Changes in hepatic structure, function; 3% clinically significant liver damage
   c Elevation (10%) of serum LDL cholesterol
4 Recurrence—likely when CDCA stopped

SOURCE: *Schoenfield et al.*

After complete dissolution of gallstones by either CDCA or UDCA and withdrawal of such treatment, current information suggests a recurrence rate of 30 to 55 percent over 3 to 12 years of follow-up. There appears to be an approximately linear increase in gallstone recurrence of 10 to 15 percent per annum over the first 3 to 5 years after which there may be a plateau with no further recurrence. The recurrence rate is lower in patients who had a single gallstone compared to those with multiple stones. In clinical trials designed to prevent recurrences, UDCA in doses of 3 mg/kg or 200 to 300 mg/d may delay and/or reduce recurrence.

Direct dissolution of gallstones within a period of hours using methyl tertiary butyl ether or other solvents through percutaneously placed biliary catheters has also been reported. Such solvent dissolution of gallbladder or ductal stones by continuous perfusion appears promising.

GALLSTONE LITHOTRIPSY Electrohydraulic extracorporeal shock wave lithotripsy, combined with medical litholytic therapy, is a safe and effective treatment in selected patients with radiolucent gallbladder calculi. The usual criteria for selection of patients include: (1) history of biliary colic; (2) radiolucent stones; (3) gallbladder visualization by oral cholecystography; (4) 1 to 4 stones with the diameter of the largest <30 mm; and (5) absence of acute cholecystitis, cholangitis, biliary obstruction, acute pancreatitis, and pregnancy. Approximately 30 percent of patients referred for lithotripsy meet the selection criteria. In one study of 175 patients, gallstones disintegrated in all but one patient; with concurrent litholytic therapy (oral CDCA and UDCA) gallstones completely disappeared in 30 percent of the patients at 2 months, 48 percent at 2 to 4 months, 63 percent at 4 to 8 months, 78 percent at 8 to 12 months, and 91 percent at 12 to 18 months. Side effects include biliary colic (35 percent), cutaneous petechiae (14 percent), transient hematuria (37 percent), and pancreatitis (1.5 percent). Important issues to be addressed with future studies are: (1) What is the recurrence rate after complete disappearance of stones? (2) Is lithotripsy effective in patients with calcified stones? (3) What is the efficacy of other types of lithotripters i.e., ultrasound waves generated by piezoelectric devices?

ACUTE AND CHRONIC CHOLECYSTITIS   Acute cholecystitis Acute inflammation of the gallbladder wall usually follows obstruction of the cystic duct by a stone. Inflammatory response can be evoked by three factors: (1) *mechanical inflammation* produced by increased intraluminal pressure and distention with resulting ischemia of the gallbladder mucosa and wall; (2) *chemical inflammation* caused by the release of lysolecithin (due to the action of phospholipase on lecithin in bile) and other local tissue factors; and (3) *bacterial inflammation,* which may play a role in 50 to 85 percent of patients with acute cholecystitis. The organisms most frequently isolated by culture of gallbladder bile in these patients include *Escherichia coli, Klebsiella* species, group D *Streptococcus, Staphylococcus* species, and *Clostridium* species.

Acute cholecystitis often begins as an attack of biliary colic which progressively worsens. Approximately 60 to 70 percent of patients report having experienced prior attacks which resolved spontaneously. As the episode progresses, however, the pain of acute cholecystitis becomes more generalized in the right upper abdomen. As with biliary colic, the pain of cholecystitis may radiate to the interscapular area, right scapula, or shoulder. Peritoneal signs of inflammation such as increased pain with jarring or on deep respiration may be apparent. The patient is anorectic and often nauseated. Vomiting is relatively common and may produce symptoms and signs of vascular and extracellular volume depletion. Jaundice is unusual early in the course of acute cholecystitis but may occur when edematous inflammatory changes involve the bile ducts and surrounding lymph nodes.

A low-grade fever is characteristically present, but shaking chills or rigors are not uncommon. The right upper quadrant of the abdomen is almost invariably tender to palpation. An enlarged, tense gallbladder is palpable in one-quarter to one-half of patients. Deep inspiration or cough during subcostal palpation of the right upper quadrant usually produces increased pain and inspiratory arrest (Murphy's sign). A light blow delivered to the right subcostal area may elicit a marked increase in pain. Localized rebound tenderness in the right upper quadrant is common, as are abdominal distention and hypoactive bowel sounds from paralytic ileus, but generalized peritoneal signs and abdominal rigidity are usually lacking, absent perforation.

The diagnosis of acute cholecystitis is usually made on the basis of a characteristic history and physical examination. The triad of sudden onset of right upper quadrant tenderness, fever, and leukocytosis is highly suggestive. Typically, leukocytosis in the range of 10,000 to 15,000 cells per microliter with a left shift on differential count is found. The serum bilirubin is mildly elevated [(less than 85.5 μmol/L (5 mg/dL)] in 45 percent of patients, while 25 percent have modest elevations in serum aminotransferases (usually less than a fivefold elevation). The radionuclide (e.g., HIDA) biliary scan may be confirmatory if bile duct imaging is seen without visualization of the gallbladder. Ultrasound will demonstrate calculi in 90 to 95 percent of cases.

Approximately 75 percent of patients treated medically have remission of acute symptoms within 2 to 7 days following hospitalization. In 25 percent, however, a complication of acute cholecystitis will occur despite conservative treatment (see below). In this setting, prompt surgical intervention is required. Of the 75 percent of patients with acute cholecystitis who undergo remission of symptoms, approximately one-quarter will experience a recurrence of cholecystitis within 1 year, and 60 percent will have at least one recurrent bout within 6 years. In view of the natural history of the disease, acute cholecystitis is best treated by early surgery whenever possible.

ACALCULOUS CHOLECYSTITIS   In 5 to 10 percent of patients with acute cholecystitis, calculi obstructing the cystic duct are not found at surgery. In over 50 percent of such cases an underlying explanation for acalculous inflammation is not found. An increased risk for the development of acalculous cholecystitis is especially associated with serious trauma or burns, with the postpartum period following prolonged labor, and with orthopedic and other nonbiliary major surgical operations in the postoperative period. Other precipitating factors include vasculitis, obstructing adenocarcinoma of the gallbladder, diabetes mellitus, torsion of the gallbladder, "unusual" bacterial infections of the gallbladder (e.g., *Leptospira, Streptococcus, Salmonella,* or *Vibrio cholerae*), and parasitic infestation of the gallbladder. Acalculous cholecystitis may also be seen with a variety of other systemic disease processes (sarcoidosis, cardiovascular disease, tuberculosis, syphilis, actinomycosis, etc.) and may possibly complicate periods of prolonged parenteral hyperalimentation.

Although the clinical manifestations of acalculous cholecystitis are indistinguishable from those of calculous cholecystitis, the setting of acute gallbladder inflammation complicating severe underlying illness is characteristic of acalculous disease. Ultrasound, CT scanning, or radionuclide examinations demonstrating a large, tense, static gallbladder without stones and with evidence of poor emptying over a prolonged period may be diagnostically useful in some cases.

The complication rate for acalculous cholecystitis exceeds that for calculous cholecystitis. Successful management of acute acalculous cholecystitis appears to depend primarily upon early diagnosis and surgical intervention with meticulous attention to postoperative care.

EMPHYSEMATOUS CHOLECYSTITIS   So-called emphysematous cholecystitis is thought to begin with acute cholecystitis (calculous or acalculous) followed by ischemia or gangrene of the gallbladder wall and infection by gas-producing organisms. Bacteria most frequently cultured in this setting include anaerobes such as *Clostridium welchii,* or *perfringens,* and aerobes such as *E. coli.* This condition occurs most frequently in elderly men and in patients with diabetes mellitus. The clinical manifestations are essentially indistinguishable from those of nongaseous cholecystitis. The diagnosis is usually made on plain abdominal film by the finding of gas within the gallbladder lumen, dissecting within the gallbladder wall to form a gaseous ring, or in the pericholecystic tissues. The morbidity and mortality rates with emphysematous cholecystitis are considerable. Prompt surgical intervention coupled with appropriate antibiotics is mandatory.

Chronic cholecystitis   Chronic inflammation of the gallbladder wall is almost always associated with the presence of gallstones and is thought to result from repeated bouts of subacute or acute cholecystitis or from persistent mechanical irritation of the gallbladder wall. The presence of bacteria in the bile occurs in more than one-quarter of patients with chronic cholecystitis. Although the presence of infected bile in a patient with *chronic* cholecystitis undergoing elective cholecystectomy probably adds little to the operative risk, intraoperative Gram's staining and routine culturing of bile has been advocated to identify those patients whose gallbladder is colonized with *Clostridium* species. Appropriate antibiotics intra- and postoperatively are recommended in such patients because colonization with these organisms may be associated with devastating septic complications following surgery. Chronic cholecystitis may be asymptomatic for years, may progress to symptomatic gallbladder disease or to acute cholecystitis, or may present with complications (see below).

Complications of cholecystitis   EMPYEMA AND HYDROPS   Empyema of the gallbladder usually results from progression of acute cholecystitis with persistent cystic duct obstruction to superinfection of the stagnant bile with a pus-forming bacterial organism. The clinical picture resembles that of cholangitis with high fever, severe right upper quadrant pain, marked leukocytosis, and, often, prostration. Empyema of the gallbladder carries a high risk of gram-negative sepsis and/or perforation. Emergency surgical intervention with proper antibiotic coverage is required as soon as the diagnosis is suspected.

Hydrops or mucocele of the gallbladder may also result from prolonged obstruction of the cystic duct, usually by a large solitary calculus. In this instance, the obstructed gallbladder lumen is progressively distended, over a period of time, by mucus (mucocele) or by a clear transudate (hydrops) produced by mucosal epithelial cells. A visible, easily palpable, nontender mass often extending from the right upper quadrant into the right iliac fossa may be found on physical examination. The patient with hydrops of the gallbladder frequently remains asymptomatic, although chronic right upper quadrant pain also may occur. Cholecystectomy is indicated since empyema, perforation, or gangrene may complicate the condition.

GANGRENE AND PERFORATION   Gangrene of the gallbladder results from ischemia of the wall and patchy or complete tissue necrosis. Underlying conditions often include marked distention of the gallbladder, vasculitis, diabetes mellitus, empyema, or torsion resulting in arterial occlusion. Gangrene usually predisposes to perforation of the gallbladder, but perforation may also occur in chronic cholecystitis without premonitory warning symptoms. *Localized perforations* are usually contained by the omentum or by adhesions produced by recurrent inflammation of the gallbladder. Bacterial superinfection of the walled-off gallbladder contents results in abscess formation. Most patients are best treated with cholecystectomy, but some seriously ill patients may be managed with cholecystostomy and drainage of the abscess. *Free perforation* is less common but is associated with a mortality rate of approximately 30 percent. Such patients may experience a sudden transient relief of right upper quadrant pain as the distended gallbladder decompresses; this is followed by signs of generalized peritonitis.

FISTULA FORMATION AND GALLSTONE ILEUS   *Fistulization* into an adjacent organ adherent to the gallbladder wall may result from inflammation and adhesion formation. Fistulas into the duodenum are most common, followed in frequency by those involving the hepatic flexure of the colon, stomach or jejunum, abdominal wall, and renal pelvis. Clinically "silent" biliary-enteric fistulas occurring as a complication of chronic cholecystitis have been found in up to 5 percent of patients undergoing cholecystectomy. Asymptomatic cholecystoenteric fistulas may sometimes be diagnosed by finding gas in the biliary tree on plain abdominal films. Barium contrast studies or endoscopy of the upper gastrointestinal tract or colon may demonstrate the fistula, but oral cholecystography will almost never result in opacification of either the gallbladder or the fistulous tract. Treatment in the symptomatic patient usually consists of cholecystectomy, common bile duct exploration, and closure of the fistulous tract.

Gallstone ileus refers to mechanical intestinal obstruction resulting from the passage of a large gallstone into the bowel lumen. The stone customarily enters the duodenum through a cholecystoenteric fistula at that level. The site of obstruction by the impacted gallstone is usually at the ileocecal valve, provided that the more proximal small bowel is of normal caliber. The majority of patients do not give a history of either prior biliary tract symptoms or complaints suggestive of acute cholecystitis or fistulization. Large stones over 2.5 cm in diameter are thought to predispose to fistula formation by gradual erosion through the gallbladder fundus. Diagnostic confirmation may occasionally be found on the plain abdominal film (e.g., small-intestinal obstruction with gas in the biliary tree and a calcified, ectopic gallstone) or following an upper gastrointestinal series (cholecystoduodenal fistula with small-bowel obstruction at the ileocecal valve). Early laparotomy is indicated with enterolithotomy and careful palpation of the more proximal small bowel and gallbladder to exclude other stones.

LIMEY (MILK OF CALCIUM) BILE AND PORCELAIN GALLBLADDER Calcium salts may be secreted into the lumen of the gallbladder in sufficient concentration to produce calcium precipitation and diffuse, hazy opacification of bile or a layering effect on plain abdominal roentgenography. This so-called limey bile or milk of calcium bile is usually clinically innocuous, but cholecystectomy is recommended since limey bile most often occurs in an hydropic gallbladder. In the entity called porcelain gallbladder, calcium salt deposition within the wall of a chronically inflamed gallbladder may be detected on the plain abdominal film. Cholecystectomy is advised in all patients with porcelain gallbladder since in a high percentage of cases this finding appears to be associated with the development of carcinoma of the gallbladder.

Treatment of cholecystitis MEDICAL THERAPY   Although surgical intervention remains the mainstay of therapy for acute cholecystitis and its complications, a period of in-hospital stabilization may be required before cholecystectomy. Oral intake is eliminated, nasogastric suction is initiated, and extracellular volume depletion and electrolyte abnormalities are repaired. Meperidine or pentazocine are usually employed for analgesia since they may produce less spasm of the sphincter of Oddi than drugs such as morphine. Intravenous antibiotic therapy is usually indicated in patients with severe acute cholecystitis even though bacterial superinfection of bile may not have occurred in the early stages of the inflammatory process. Postoperative complications of wound infection, abscess formation, or sepsis are reduced in antibiotic-treated patients. Effective single-agent antibiotics include ampicillin, cephalosporins, chloramphenicol, or aminoglycosides, but in diabetic or debilitated patients and in those with signs of gram-negative sepsis, combination antibiotic treatment may be preferable (see also Chap. 83).

SURGICAL THERAPY   The optimal timing of surgical intervention in patients with acute cholecystitis remains controversial. Urgent (emergency) cholecystectomy or cholecystostomy is probably appropriate in most patients in whom a complication of acute cholecystitis such as empyema, emphysematous cholecystitis, or perforation is suspected or confirmed. In uncomplicated cases of acute cholecystitis up to 30 percent of patients fail to resolve their symptoms on appropriate medical therapy, and progression of the attack or a supervening complication leads to the performance of early operation (within 24 to 72 h). The technical complications of surgery are not increased in patients undergoing early as opposed to delayed cholecystectomy. Delayed surgical intervention is probably best reserved for (1) patients in whom the overall medical condition imposes an unacceptable risk for early surgery, and (2) cases in which the diagnosis of acute cholecystitis is in doubt. Early cholecystectomy is the treatment of choice for most patients with acute cholecystitis. Mortality figures for emergency cholecystectomy in most centers approach 3 percent, while the mortality risk for elective or early cholecystectomy approximates 0.5 percent in patients under age 60. Of course, the operative risks increase with age-related diseases of other organ systems and with the presence of long-term or short-term complications of gallbladder disease. Seriously ill or debilitated patients with cholecystitis may be managed with cholecystostomy and tube drainage of the gallbladder. Elective cholecystectomy may then be done at a later date.

Postcholecystectomy complications   Early complications following cholecystectomy include atelectasis and other pulmonary disorders, abscess formation (often subphrenic), external or internal hemorrhage, biliary-enteric fistula, and bile leaks. Jaundice may indicate absorption of bile from an intraabdominal collection following a biliary leak, or mechanical obstruction of the common bile duct by retained calculi, intraductal blood clots, or extrinsic compression. Routine performance of intraoperative cholangiography during cholecystectomy has helped to reduce the incidence of these early complications.

Overall, cholecystectomy is a very successful operation which provides total or near-total relief of presurgical symptoms in 75 to 90 percent of patients. The most common cause of persistent postcholecystectomy symptoms is an overlooked extrabiliary disorder (e.g., reflux esophagitis, peptic ulceration, postgastrectomy syndrome, pancreatitis, or irritable bowel syndrome). In a small percentage of patients, however, a disorder of the extrahepatic bile ducts may result in persistent symptomatology. These so-called postcholecystectomy syndromes may be due to (1) biliary strictures, (2) retained biliary calculi, (3) cystic duct stump syndrome, (4) stenosis or dyskinesia of the sphincter of Oddi, or (5) bile salt–induced diarrhea or gastritis.

CYSTIC DUCT STUMP SYNDROME   In the absence of cholangiographically demonstrable retained stones, symptoms resembling biliary colic or cholecystitis in the postcholecystectomy patient have frequently been attributed to disease in a long (>1 cm) cystic duct remnant (cystic duct stump syndrome). Careful analysis, however, reveals that postcholecystectomy complaints are attributable to other causes in almost all patients in whom the symptom complex was originally thought to result from the existence of a long cystic duct stump. Accordingly, considerable care should be taken to investigate the possible role of other factors in the production of postcholecystectomy symptoms before attributing them to cystic duct stump syndrome.

PAPILLARY DYSFUNCTION, PAPILLARY STENOSIS, SPASM OF THE SPHINCTER OF ODDI, AND BILIARY DYSKINESIA   Symptoms of biliary colic accompanied by signs of recurrent, intermittent biliary obstruction may be produced by papillary stenosis, papillary dysfunction, spasm of the sphincter of Oddi, and biliary dyskinesia. Papillary stenosis is thought to result from acute or chronic inflammation of the papilla of Vater or from glandular hyperplasia of the papillary segment. Five criteria have been used to define papillary stenosis: (1) upper abdominal pain, usually right upper quadrant or epigastric; (2) abnormal liver tests; (3) dilatation of the common bile duct upon endoscopic retrograde cholangiopancreatogram (ERCP) examination;

(4) delayed (longer than 45 min) drainage of contrast material from the duct; and (5) increased basal pressure of the sphincter of Oddi, a finding that may be of only minor significance. A useful alternative to ERCP is hepatobiliary scintigraphy using ^{99m}Tc-diisopropyl iminodiacetic acid, especially if ERCP and/or biliary manometry are either unavailable or not feasible. In patients with papillary stenosis, quantitative hepatobiliary scintigraphy has revealed delayed transit from the common bile duct to the bowel, ductal dilatation, and abnormal time-activity dynamics. This technique can also be used before and after sphincterotomy to document improvement in biliary emptying. Treatment consists of endoscopic or surgical sphincteroplasty to ensure wide patency of the distal portions of both the bile and pancreatic ducts. The greater the number of the above criteria present, the greater the likelihood that a patient does have a degree of papillary stenosis sufficient to justify correction. The factors usually considered as indications for sphincterotomy include: (1) prolonged duration of symptoms; (2) lack of response to symptomatic treatment; (3) presence of severe disability; and (4) the patient's choice of sphincterotomy over surgery (given a clear understanding on his or her part of the risks involved in both procedures).

Criteria for diagnosing dyskinesia of the sphincter of Oddi are even more controversial than those for papillary stenosis. Proposed mechanisms include spasm of the sphincter, denervation sensitivity resulting in hypertonicity, and abnormalities of the sequencing or frequency rates of sphincteric contraction waves. When thorough evaluation has failed to demonstrate another cause for the pain, and when cholangiographic and manometric criteria suggest a diagnosis of biliary dyskinesia, medical treatment with nitrites or anticholinergics to attempt pharmacologic relaxation of the sphincter has been proposed. Endoscopic sphincterotomy or surgical sphincteroplasty may be indicated in patients who fail to respond to a 2 to 3 month trial of medical therapy, especially if basal sphincter of Oddi pressures are elevated.

BILE SALT–INDUCED CATHARSIS AND GASTRITIS Postcholecystectomy patients may develop symptoms and signs of gastritis, which has been attributed to duodenogastric reflux of bile. However, firm data linking an increased incidence of bile gastritis with surgical removal of the gallbladder are lacking. Similarly, the occurrence of cholestyramine-responsive diarrhea in a small number of patients following cholecystectomy has been attributed to an alteration of the enterohepatic circulation of bile acids induced or unmasked by removal of the gallbladder.

THE HYPERPLASTIC CHOLECYSTOSES The term *hyperplastic cholecystoses* is used to denote a group of disorders of the gallbladder characterized by excessive proliferation of normal tissue components.

Adenomyomatosis is characterized by a benign proliferation of gallbladder surface epithelium with gland-like formations, extramural sinuses, transverse strictures, and/or fundal nodule ("adenoma" or "adenomyoma") formation. Outpouchings of mucosa termed Rokitansky-Aschoff sinuses may be seen on oral cholecystography in conjunction with hyperconcentration of contrast medium. Characteristic dimpled filling defects may also be seen.

Cholesterolosis is characterized by abnormal deposition of lipid, especially cholesterol esters, in the lamina propria of the gallbladder wall. In its diffuse form ("strawberry gallbladder"), the gallbladder mucosa is brick red and speckled with bright yellow flecks of lipid. The localized form shows solitary or multiple "cholesterol polyps" studding the gallbladder wall. Cholesterol stones of the gallbladder are found in nearly half the cases. Cholecystectomy is indicated in both adenomyomatosis and cholesterolosis when symptomatic or when cholelithiasis is present.

CANCER OF THE GALLBLADDER Most cancers of the gallbladder develop in conjunction with stones rather than polyps. In patients with gallstones, the risk for developing gallbladder cancer, while increased, is still quite low. In one study, gallbladder cancer developed in only 5 of 2583 patients with gallstones followed for a median of 13 years. In the United States, adenocarcinomas comprise the vast majority of the estimated 6500 new cases of gallbladder

cancer diagnosed each year. The female/male ratio is 4:1 and the mean age at diagnosis is approximately 70 years. The clinical presentation is most often one of unremitting right upper quadrant pain associated with weight loss, jaundice, and a palpable right upper quadrant mass. Cholangitis may supervene. The gallbladder is rarely visualized on OCG, and preoperative diagnosis of the condition is rare. Once symptoms have appeared, spread of the tumor outside the gallbladder by direct extension or by lymphatic or hematogenous routes is almost invariable. Over 75 percent of gallbladder carcinomas are unresectable at the time of surgery, the exceptions being tumors discovered incidentally at laparotomy. The 1-year mortality rate for unresectable disease is approximately 95 percent, and only 5 percent of patients survive 5 years or more from the time of diagnosis. Radical operative resection does not appear to improve survival. Results of trials with radiation and chemotherapy of primary gallbladder cancer have also been disappointing.

DISEASES OF THE BILE DUCTS

CONGENITAL ANOMALIES Biliary atresia and hypoplasia Atretic and hypoplastic lesions of the extrahepatic and major intrahepatic bile ducts are the most common biliary anomalies of clinical relevance encountered in infancy. The clinical picture is one of severe obstructive jaundice during the first month of life, with pale stools. The diagnosis is confirmed by surgical exploration with operative cholangiography. Approximately 10 percent of cases of biliary atresia are treatable with Roux en Y choledochojejunostomy, with the Kasai procedure (hepatic portoenterostomy) being attempted in the remainder in an effort to restore some bile flow. Most patients, even those having successful biliary-enteric anastomoses, eventually develop chronic cholangitis, extensive hepatic fibrosis, and portal hypertension.

Choledochal cysts Cystic dilatation may involve the free portion of the common bile duct, i.e., choledochal cyst, or may present as diverticulum formation in the intraduodenal segment. In the latter situation chronic reflux of pancreatic juice into the biliary tree can produce inflammation and stenosis of the extrahepatic bile ducts leading to cholangitis or biliary obstruction. Because the process may be gradual, approximately 50 percent of patients present with onset of symptoms after age 10. The diagnosis may be made by ultrasound, abdominal computed tomography (CT), or cholangiography. Surgical treatment involves excision of the "cyst" and biliary-enteric anastomosis. Patients with choledochal cysts are at increased risk for the subsequent development of cholangiocarcinoma.

Congenital biliary ectasia Cystic dilatation of the intrahepatic bile ducts may involve either the major intrahepatic radicles (Caroli's disease) or the inter- and intralobular ducts (congenital hepatic fibrosis) or both. In Caroli's disease, clinical manifestations include recurrent cholangitis, abscess formation in and around the affected ducts, and, sometimes, gallstone formation within portions of ectatic intrahepatic biliary radicles. The CT scan and cholangiographic patterns are usually diagnostic, and treatment with ongoing antibiotic therapy is usually undertaken in an effort to limit the frequency and severity of recurrent bouts of cholangitis. Progression to secondary biliary cirrhosis with portal hypertension, amyloidosis, extrahepatic biliary obstruction, cholangiocarcinoma, or recurrent episodes of sepsis with hepatic abscess formation is common.

CHOLEDOCHOLITHIASIS Pathophysiology and clinical manifestations Passage of gallstones into the common bile duct occurs in approximately 10 to 15 percent of patients with cholelithiasis. The incidence of common duct stones increases with increasing age of the patient, so that up to 25 percent of elderly patients may have calculi in the common duct at the time of cholecystectomy. Undetected duct stones are left behind in approximately 1 to 5 percent of cholecystectomy patients. The overwhelming majority of bile duct stones are cholesterol or mixed stones formed in the gallbladder which then migrate into the extrahepatic biliary tree through the cystic duct. Primary calculi arising de novo in the ducts are usually pigment stones developing in patients with (1) chronic hemolytic diseases; (2) hepatobiliary parasitism or chronic, recurrent cholangitis; (3) congenital anomalies of the bile ducts (especially Caroli's disease); or (4) dilated, sclerosed, or strictured ducts. Common duct stones may remain asymptomatic for years, may pass spontaneously into the duodenum, or (most often) may present with biliary colic or a complication.

Complications CHOLANGITIS Cholangitis may be acute or chronic, and symptoms result from inflammation which usually requires at least partial obstruction to the flow of bile. Bacteria are present on bile culture in approximately 75 percent of patients with acute cholangitis early in the symptomatic course. The characteristic presentation of acute cholangitis involves biliary colic, jaundice, and spiking fevers with chills (Charcot's triad). Blood cultures are frequently positive and leukocytosis is typical. *Nonsuppurative* acute cholangitis is most common and may respond relatively rapidly to supportive measures and to treatment with antibiotics (see Chap. 83). In *suppurative* acute cholangitis, however, the presence of pus under pressure in a completely obstructed ductal system leads to symptoms of severe toxicity—mental confusion, bacteremia, and septic shock. Response to antibiotics alone in this setting is relatively poor, multiple hepatic abscesses are often present, and the mortality rate approaches 100 percent unless prompt surgical correction of the obstructing lesion and drainage of infected bile is carried out.

OBSTRUCTIVE JAUNDICE Gradual obstruction of the common bile duct over a period of weeks or months usually leads to initial manifestations of jaundice or pruritus without associated symptoms of biliary colic or cholangitis. Painless jaundice may occur in patients with choledocholithiasis, but this manifestation is much more characteristic of biliary obstruction secondary to malignancy of the head of pancreas, bile ducts, or ampulla of Vater.

In patients whose obstruction is secondary to choledocholithiasis, associated chronic calculous cholecystitis is very common and the gallbladder in this setting may be relatively indistensible. The absence of a palpable gallbladder in most patients with biliary obstruction from duct stones is the basis for *Courvoisier's law,* i.e., that the presence of a palpably enlarged gallbladder suggests that the biliary obstruction is secondary to an underlying malignancy rather than to calculous disease. Biliary obstruction causes progressive dilatation of the intrahepatic bile ducts as intrabiliary pressures rise. Hepatic bile flow is suppressed, and regurgitation of conjugated bilirubin into the bloodstream leads to jaundice accompanied by dark urine (bilirubinuria) and light-colored (acholic) stools.

Common bile duct stones should be suspected in any patient with cholecystitis whose serum bilirubin level exceeds 85.5 μmol/L (5 mg/dL). The maximum bilirubin level is seldom over 256.5 μmol/L (15.0 mg/dL) in patients with choledocholithiasis unless concomitant hepatic disease or another factor leading to marked hyperbilirubinemia exists. Serum bilirubin levels of 342.0 μmol/L (20mg/dL) or more should suggest the possibility of neoplastic obstruction. The serum alkaline phosphatase level is almost always elevated in biliary obstruction. A rise in alkaline phosphatase often precedes clinical jaundice and may be the only abnormality in routine liver function tests. There may be a two- to tenfold elevation of serum aminotransferases, especially in association with acute obstruction. Following relief of the obstructing process, serum aminotransferase elevations usually return rapidly to normal, while the serum bilirubin level may take 1 to 2 weeks to return to normal. The alkaline phosphatase usually falls slowly, lagging behind the decrease in serum bilirubin.

PANCREATITIS The most common associated entity discovered in patients with nonalcoholic acute pancreatitis is biliary tract disease. Biochemical evidence of pancreatic inflammation complicates acute cholecystitis in 15 percent of cases and choledocholithiasis in over 30 percent, and the common factor appears to be the passage of gallstones through the common duct. Coexisting pancreatitis should be suspected in patients with symptoms of cholecystitis who develop (1) back pain or pain to the left of the abdominal midline, (2)

prolonged vomiting with paralytic ileus, or (3) a pleural effusion, especially on the left side. Surgical treatment of gallstone disease is usually associated with resolution of the pancreatitis.

SECONDARY BILIARY CIRRHOSIS Secondary biliary cirrhosis may complicate prolonged or intermittent duct obstruction with or without recurrent cholangitis. Although this complication may be seen in patients with choledocholithiasis, it is more common in cases of prolonged obstruction from stricture or neoplasm. Once established, secondary biliary cirrhosis may be progressive even after correction of the obstructing process, and increasingly severe hepatic cirrhosis may lead to portal hypertension or to hepatic failure and death. Prolonged biliary obstruction may also be associated with clinically relevant deficiencies of the fat-soluble vitamins A, D, and K.

Diagnosis and treatment The diagnosis of choledocholithiasis is usually made by cholangiography (see Table 258-4), either preoperatively or intraoperatively at the time of cholecystectomy. The incidence of coexisting common duct stones in patients with cholelithiasis is relatively high. Operative cholangiography should be performed routinely during surgical procedures on the biliary tract. Preoperative indications for common duct exploration include (1) cholangiographic demonstration of ductal stones, (2) jaundice or cholangitis preceding operation, (3) a history of gallstone-related pancreatitis, and (4) cholangiographic evidence of a markedly enlarged common bile duct. Operative indications for exploration of the duct include (1) manual palpation of stones in the common bile duct, (2) positive intraoperative cholangiogram, (3) enlargement of the common bile duct or cystic duct at operation, (4) multiple small stones or "sand" in the gallbladder, and (5) a gallbladder empty of stones at surgery in a patient with previously documented gallstones.

In most cases of choledocholithiasis, the treatment of choice is cholecystectomy with choledocholithotomy and T-tube drainage of the bile ducts. A T-tube cholangiogram is usually performed prior to T-tube removal on or before the tenth postoperative day. Retained calculi seen on T-tube cholangiography may be removed percutaneously by placement of a steerable basket catheter under radiographic guidance through the matured T-tube sinus tract. Endoscopic sphincterotomy followed by spontaneous or basket stone extraction is an additional nonsurgical alternative in the management of patients with common duct stones, especially in elderly or poor-risk patients.

TRAUMA, STRICTURES, AND HEMOBILIA Benign strictures of the extrahepatic bile ducts result from surgical trauma in approximately 95 percent of cases and occur in about 1 in 500 cholecystectomies. Strictures may present with bile leak or abscess formation in the immediate postoperative period or with biliary obstruction or cholangitis as long as 2 years or more following the inciting trauma. The diagnosis is established by percutaneous or endoscopic cholangiography. Successful operative correction by a skillful surgeon with duct-to-bowel anastomosis is usually possible, although mortality rates from surgical complications, recurrent cholangitis, or secondary biliary cirrhosis are high.

Hemobilia may follow traumatic or operative injury to the liver or bile ducts, intraductal rupture of a hepatic abscess or aneurysm of the hepatic artery, biliary or hepatic tumor hemorrhage, or mechanical complications of choledocholithiasis or hepatobiliary parasitism. Diagnostic procedures such as liver biopsy, percutaneous transhepatic cholangiography (PTHC), and transhepatic biliary drainage catheter placement may also be complicated by hemobilia. Patients often present with a classic triad of biliary colic, obstructive jaundice, and melena or occult blood in the stools. The diagnosis is sometimes made by cholangiographic evidence of blood clot in the biliary tree, but selective angiographic verification may be required. Although minor episodes of hemobilia may resolve without operative intervention, surgical ligation of the bleeding vessel is frequently required.

EXTRINSIC COMPRESSION OF THE BILE DUCTS Partial or complete biliary obstruction may sometimes be produced by extrinsic compression of the ducts. The most common cause of this form of obstructive jaundice is carcinoma of the head of the pancreas. Biliary obstruction may also occur as a complication of either acute or

TABLE 258-4 Diagnostic evaluation of the bile ducts

Procedure	Diagnostic advantages	Diagnostic limitations	Contraindications	Complications	Comment
Hepatobiliary ultrasound (HBUS)	Rapid Simultaneous scanning of GB, liver, bile ducts, pancreas Accurate identification of dilated bile ducts Not limited by jaundice, pregnancy Guidance for fine-needle biopsy	Bowel gas Massive obesity Ascites Barium Partial bile duct obstruction Poor visualization of distal CBD	None	None	Initial procedure of choice in investigating possible biliary obstruction
Computed body tomography (CT)	Simultaneous scanning of GB, liver, bile ducts, pancreas Accurate identification of dilated bile ducts, masses Not limited by jaundice, gas, obesity, ascites High-resolution image Guidance for fine-needle biopsy	Extreme cachexia Movement artifact Ileus Partial bile duct obstruction High cost May not be readily available	Pregnancy	Reaction to iodinated contrast, if used	Indicated for evaluation of hepatic or pancreatic masses Procedure of choice in investigating possible biliary obstruction if diagnostic limitations prevent HBUS
Percutaneous transhepatic cholangiogram (PTHC)	Extremely successful when bile ducts dilated Best visualization of proximal biliary tract Possible separate visualization of obstructed left ductal system Bile cytology/culture Percutaneous transhepatic drainage	Nondilated or sclerosed ducts	Pregnancy Uncorrectable coagulopathy Massive ascites ? Hepatic abscess	Bleeding Hemobilia Bile peritonitis Bacteremia, sepsis	Usually, initial cholangiogram of choice when bile ducts are dilated

Endoscopic retrograde cholangiopancreatogram (ERCP)	Simultaneous pancreatography
	Visualization/biopsy of ampulla and duodenum
	Best visualization of distal biliary tract
	Bile or pancreatic cytology
	Endoscopic sphincterotomy and stone removal
	? Biliary manometry
	Not limited by ascites, coagulopathy, abscess
		Gastroduodenal obstruction
		? Roux en Y biliary-enteric anastomosis
			Pregnancy
			? Acute pancreatitis
			? Severe cardiopulmonary disease
				Pancreatitis
				Cholangitis, sepsis
				Infected pancreatic pseudocyst
				Perforation (rare)
				Hypoxemia, aspiration
					Cholangiogram of choice in:
					  Absence of dilated ducts
					  ? Pancreatic, ampullary or gastroduodenal disease
					  Prior biliary surgery
					  PTHC contraindicated or failed
					  Endoscopic sphincterotomy a treatment possibility

NOTE: Intravenous cholangiography (IVC) is an obsolete technique because 40% of common duct stones are missed and there is poor resolution even with tomography. There are few indications for its use especially since other cholangiographic techniques are usually available.

chronic pancreatitis or involvement of lymph nodes in the porta hepatis by lymphoma or metastatic carcinoma. The latter should be distinguished from cholestasis resulting from massive replacement of the liver by tumor.

HEPATOBILIARY PARASITISM Infestation of the biliary tract by adult helminths or their ova may produce a chronic, recurrent pyogenic cholangitis with or without multiple hepatic abscesses, ductal stones, or biliary obstruction. This condition is relatively rare but does occur in inhabitants of southern China and elsewhere in southeast Asia. The organisms most commonly involved are trematodes or flukes, including *Clonorchis sinensis*, *Opisthorchis viverrini* or *felineus*, and *Fasciola hepatica*. The biliary tract may also be involved by intraductal migration of adult *Ascaris lumbricoides* from the duodenum or by intrabiliary rupture of hydatid cysts of the liver produced by *Echinococcus* species. The diagnosis is made by cholangiography and the presence of characteristic ova on stool examination. When obstruction is present, the treatment of choice is laparotomy under antibiotic coverage, with common duct exploration and a biliary drainage procedure. It should be emphasized that in the orient, one also sees cholangiohepatitis associated with pigment lithiasis, which may, in fact, be more common than cholangitis due to parasites.

SCLEROSING CHOLANGITIS Primary or idiopathic sclerosing cholangitis is a disorder characterized by a progressive, inflammatory, sclerosing and obliterative process affecting the extrahepatic and, often, the intrahepatic bile ducts. The lesion may appear as an isolated entity or may occur in association with inflammatory bowel disease, especially ulcerative colitis, or with multifocal fibrosclerosis syndromes such as retroperitoneal, mediastinal, and/or periureteral fibrosis, Riedel's struma, or pseudotumor of the orbit. Papillary stenosis and sclerosing cholangitis are also important complications of the acquired immunodeficiency syndrome (AIDS); cytomegalovirus and cryptosporidia infections have been observed frequently in such patients, raising the question whether these microbes may be a pathogenetic factor in primary sclerosing cholangitis. Secondary sclerosing cholangitis may occur as a long-term complication of choledocholithiasis, cholangiocarcinoma, operative or traumatic biliary injury, or contiguous inflammatory processes.

Patients with sclerosing cholangitis often present with signs and symptoms of chronic or intermittent biliary obstruction: jaundice, pruritus, right upper quadrant abdominal pain, or acute cholangitis. Late in the course, complete biliary obstruction, secondary biliary cirrhosis, hepatic failure, or portal hypertension with bleeding varices may occur. The diagnosis is usually established by finding thickened ducts with narrow, beaded lumina on cholangiography (see Fig. 258-2D). The cholangiographic technique of choice in suspected cases is probably ERCP since intrahepatic ductal involvement may make PTHC difficult or impossible. When a diagnosis of sclerosing cholangitis has been established, a search for associated diseases, especially for chronic inflammatory bowel disease, should be carried out.

Therapy with cholestyramine may help control symptoms of

pruritus, and antibiotics are useful when cholangitis complicates the clinical picture. Vitamin D and calcium supplementation may help prevent the loss of bone mass frequently seen in patients with chronic cholestasis. Glucocorticoids have not been shown to be efficacious. In cases where complete or high-grade biliary obstruction has occurred, surgical intervention may be appropriate. Efforts at biliary-enteric anastomosis or stent placement may, however, be complicated by recurrent cholangitis and further progression of the stenosing process. The role of colectomy in patients with sclerosing cholangitis complicating chronic ulcerative colitis is uncertain. The prognosis is unfavorable, with a mean survival of 4 to 10 years following the diagnosis, regardless of therapy. Primary sclerosing cholangitis is one of the most common indications for liver transplantation. In one study, the mean follow-up time from the diagnosis of primary sclerosing cholangitis to the time of liver transplantation was 5.8 years.

CHOLANGIOCARCINOMA Benign tumors of the extrahepatic bile ducts are extremely rare causes of mechanical biliary obstruction. The majority of these are papillomas, adenomas, or cystadenomas which present with obstructive jaundice or hemobilia. Adenocarcinoma of the extrahepatic ducts is relatively more common. There is a slight male preponderance (60 percent), and the peak age incidence is in the fifth to seventh decades. Apparent predisposing factors include (1) some chronic hepatobiliary parasitic infestations, (2) congential anomalies with ectactic ducts, (3) sclerosing cholangitis and chronic ulcerative colitis, and (4) occupational exposure to possible biliary tract carcinogens (workers in rubber or automotive plants). Cholelithiasis is not clearly associated with cholangiocarcinoma as a predisposing factor. The lesions may be diffuse or nodular; the latter often arise at the confluence of the hepatic ducts (Klatskin tumors). This tumor is usually associated with a *collapsed* gallbladder and such a finding mandates that the proximal hepatic ducts be optimally visualized by cholangiography.

Patients with cholangiocarcinoma usually present with biliary obstruction, painless jaundice, pruritus, weight loss, and acholic stools. A deep-seated, vaguely localized right upper quadrant pain may be an associated complaint. Hepatomegaly and a palpable, distended gallbladder are frequent accompanying signs. Fever is unusual unless associated with ascending cholangitis. Because the obstructing process is gradual, the cholangiocarcinoma is often far advanced by the time it presents clinically. The diagnosis is most frequently made by cholangiography following ultrasound demonstration of dilated intrahepatic bile ducts. Any focal strictures of the bile ducts should probably be considered malignant until proved otherwise. Long-term palliation of the tumor is possible in some cases when radiation and/or chemotherapy are combined with palliative drainage of the biliary tree.

CARCINOMA OF THE PAPILLA OF VATER The ampulla of Vater may be involved by extension of tumor arising elsewhere in the duodenum or may itself be the primary site of origin of sarcomas, carcinoid tumors, or adenocarcinomas. Papillary adenocarcinomas are associated with slow growth and a more favorable clinical prognosis than diffuse, infiltrative cancers of the ampulla, which are more frequently widely invasive. The presenting clinical manifestation is usually obstructive jaundice. ERCP is probably the preferred diagnostic technique when ampullary carcinoma is suspected, because it allows for direct endoscopic inspection and biopsy of the ampulla as well as for performance of pancreatography to exclude a diagnosis of pancreatic malignancy. Cancer of the papilla is usually treated by wide, often radical, surgical excision. Lymph node or other metastases are present at the time of surgery in approximately 20 percent of cases, and the 5-year survival rate following surgical therapy in this group is only 5 to 10 percent. In the absence of metastases, however, radical pancreaticoduodenectomy (Whipple procedure) is associated with 5-year survival rates as high as 40 percent, and several long-term survivors have been reported.

REFERENCES

BISMUTH H, MALT RA: Carcinoma of the biliary tract. N Engl J Med 301:704, 1979

CAREY MC et al: Whither biliary sludge? Gastroenterology 95:508, 1988

DOWLING RH et al: Gallstone recurrence and post dissolution management, in *Enterohepatic circulation of Bile Acids and Sterol Metabolism*, G Paumgartren, A Stichl, W Gersk (eds). Lancaster, PA, MTP Press, 1985, pp 361–369

FERRUCCI JT JR, MUELLER PR: Interventional radiology of the biliary tract. Gastroenterology 82:974, 1982

GRACIE WA, RANSOHOFF DF: The natural history of silent gallstones. The innocent gallstone is not a myth. N Engl J Med 307:798, 1982

HOLZBACH RT et al: Biliary proteins: Unique inhibitors of cholesterol crystal nucleation in human gallbladder bile. J Clin Invest 72:35, 1984

HOOD K et al: Prevention of gallstone recurrence by non-steroidal antiinflammatory drugs. Lancet 2:1223, 1988

LEE SP et al: Origin and fate of biliary sludge. Gastroenterology 94:170, 1988

LEVY PF et al: Human gallbladder mucin accelerates nucleation of cholesterol in artifical bile. Gastroenterology 87:270, 1984

MARINGHINI A et al: Gallstones, gallbladder cancer, and other gastrointestinal malignancies: An epidemiologic study in Rochester, Minnesota. Ann Intern Med 107:30, 1987

MATON PN et al: Outcome of chenodeoxycholic acid (CDCA) treatment in 125 patients with radiolucent gallstones. Medicine 61:86, 1982

MESSIN B et al: Does total parenteral nutrition induce gallbladder sludge formation and lithiasis? Gastroenterology 84:1012, 1983

PALME KR, HOFMANN AF: Intraductal monooctanoin for the direct dissolution of bile duct stones: Experience in 343 patients. Gut 27:196, 1986

PODDA M et al: Efficacy and safety of a combination of dienodeoxycholic acid and ursodeoxycholic acid for gallstone dissolution. Gastroenterology 96:222, 1989

RANSOHOFF DF: Assessment of prophylactic cholecystectomy and medical therapy for diabetics with silent gallstones. Gastroenterology 92:1588, 1987

SACKMAN M et al: Shock wave lithotripsy of gallbladder stones. The first 175 patients. N Engl J Med 318:393, 1988

SAUERBRUCH T et al: Fragmentation of bile duct stones by extracorporeal shock waves. Gastroenterology 96:222, 1989

SCHNEIDERMON D et al: Papillary stenosis and sclerosing cholangitis in the acquired immunodeficiency syndrome. Ann Intern Med 106:546, 1987

SHAFFER EA et al: Cholescintigraphic detection of functional obstruction of the sphincter of Oddi: Effect of papillotomy. Gastroenterology 90:728, 1986

SILVIS SE et al: What is the post-cholecystectomy pain syndrome? Gastrointestinal Endoscopy 31:401, 1985

SMITH BF, LAMONT JT: The central issue of cholesterol gallstones. Hepatology 6:529, 1986

THISTLE JL et al: Dissolution of cholesterol gallbladder stones by methyl-tert-butyl ether administered by percutaneous transhepatic catheter. N Engl J Med 320:633, 1989

WIESNER RH et al: Comparison of clinicopathologic features of primary sclerosing cholangitis and primary biliary cirrhosis. Gastroenterology 88:108, 1985 section 3 **Disorders of the pancreas**

259 APPROACH TO THE PATIENT WITH PANCREATIC DISEASE

NORTON J. GREENBERGER / PHILLIP P. TOSKES

GENERAL CONSIDERATIONS

Inflammatory disease of the pancreas may be acute or chronic. Although good data exist concerning the frequency of acute pancreatitis (about 5000 new cases per year in the United States with a mortality rate of about 10 percent), the number of patients who suffer with relapsing pancreatitis or chronic pancreatitis is largely undefined. The relative inaccessibility of the pancreas to direct examination and the nonspecificity of the abdominal pain associated with pancreatitis make the diagnosis of pancreatitis difficult and usually dependent on elevation of blood amylase levels. Many patients with chronic pancreatitis do not have elevated blood amylase levels. Some patients with chronic pancreatitis develop signs and symptoms of pancreatic exocrine insufficiency, and thus objective evidence for pancreatic disease can be demonstrated. However, greater than 90 percent of the pancreas must be damaged before maldigestion of fat and protein is manifested. Obviously there is a very large reservoir of pancreatic exocrine function, and the signs and symptoms usually associated with exocrine insufficiency are late manifestations, depending on virtually complete destruction of the gland. Even the secretin stimulation test, which is the most sensitive method of assessing pancreatic exocrine function, is probably abnormal only when greater than 70 percent of exocrine function has been lost. Thus, the number of patients who have subclinical exocrine dysfunction (i.e., less than 90 percent loss of function) is unknown.

The clinical manifestations of acute and chronic pancreatitis and pancreatic insufficiency are protean. Thus, patients may present with hyperlipidemia, vitamin B_{12} malabsorption, hypercalcemia, hypocalcemia, hyperglycemia, ascites, pleural effusions, and chronic abdominal pain with normal amylase levels. Indeed, if the clinician considers pancreatitis as a possible diagnosis only when presented with a patient having classic symptoms (i.e., severe, constant epigastric pain that radiates through to the back, along with an elevated blood amylase level), only a minority of the patients with pancreatitis will be correctly diagnosed.

As emphasized in Chap. 260, the etiologies as well as the clinical manifestations are quite varied. Although it is well appreciated that *pancreatitis* is frequently secondary to alcohol abuse and biliary tract disease, pancreatitis is also caused by drugs, trauma, and viral infections, and is associated with metabolic and connective tissue disorders. In addition, in approximately 15 percent of patients with acute pancreatitis and 25 percent of patients with chronic pancreatitis, the etiology is obscure.

TESTS USEFUL IN THE DIAGNOSIS OF PANCREATIC DISEASE

Several tests have proved of value in the evaluation of pancreatic exocrine function. Examples of specific tests and usefulness in the diagnosis of acute and chronic pancreatitis are summarized in Table 259-1.

PANCREATIC ENZYMES IN BODY FLUIDS The serum amylase is widely used as a screening test for acute pancreatitis in the patient with acute abdominal or back pain. A value greater than 150 Somogyi units per deciliter should raise the question of acute pancreatitis. Levels greater than 300 units make the diagnosis more likely, and values greater than three times normal virtually clinch the diagnosis if gut perforation or infarction is excluded. In acute pancreatitis the serum amylase is usually elevated within 24 h and remains so for 1 to 3 days. Levels return to normal within 3 to 5 days unless there is extensive pancreatic necrosis, incomplete ductal obstruction, or pseudocyst formation. Approximately 70 to 75 percent of patients with acute pancreatitis will have an elevated serum amylase. Normal values, however, may occur if (1) there is a delay (2 to 5 days) in obtaining blood samples, (2) the underlying disorder is chronic pancreatitis rather than acute pancreatitis, and (3) hypertriglyceridemia is present. Patients with hypertriglyceridemia and proven pancreatitis have been found to have spuriously low levels of amylase activity. Importantly, serum lipase and urinary amylase levels may be abnormal in this setting, thus facilitating the diagnosis of acute pancreatitis.

The serum amylase is often elevated in other conditions (Table 259-2), in part because the enzyme is found in many organs in addition to the pancreas (salivary glands, liver, small intestine, kidney, fallopian tube) and can be produced by various tumors (carcinoma of the lung, esophagus, breast, and ovary). Isoenzymes of amylase fall into two general categories, those arising from the pancreas (P isoamylases) and those from nonpancreatic sources (S isoamylases). The measurement of serum isoamylases is of clinical importance. Isoamylase analysis of normal serum shows that about 35 to 45 percent of the amylase is of pancreatic origin. For example, in patients with acute pancreatitis, the total serum amylase returns to normal more rapidly than pancreatic isoamylase. Thus, in patients seen after the first day, the pancreatic isoamylase is a more sensitive indicator of pancreatitis than the total serum amylase. In addition, in certain conditions, such as the postoperative state, acute alcohol intoxication, and diabetic ketoacidosis, it had been assumed that elevations in serum amylase indicated acute pancreatitis. However, the elevation of serum amylase in such conditions has been shown to actually be of the S type. The general availability of a simple assay that employs a protein which selectively inhibits nonpancreatic amylase has led to more widespread use of isoamylase determinations.

Urine amylase is increased in acute pancreatitis and may be elevated after serum values have returned to normal. The finding that the renal clearance of amylase is increased in acute pancreatitis has led to the suggestion that the amylase/creatinine clearance ratio (C_{am}/C_{cr}) may be a more sensitive and specific test for the diagnosis of acute pancreatitis.

However, experience with the C_{am}/C_{cr} has demonstrated that it is no more sensitive than the serum amylase. In addition, the specificity of the C_{am}/C_{cr} has been seriously questioned because the ratio is also increased in a number of other disorders, e.g., diabetic ketoacidosis, burns, pancreatic neoplasms, renal failure, and the postoperative state. The mechanism of increased renal amylase clearance in acute pancreatitis is secondary to a reversible renal tubular defect which results in decreased amylase reabsorption.

Elevation of ascitic fluid amylase occurs in acute pancreatitis as well as (1) in pancreatogenous ascites due to disruption of the main pancreatic duct of a leaking pseudocyst and (2) in other abdominal disorders which simulate pancreatitis (e.g., intestinal obstruction, intestinal infarction, and perforated peptic ulcer). Elevation of pleural

TABLE 259-1 Tests useful in the diagnosis of acute and chronic pancreatitis and pancreatic tumors

Test	Principle	Comment
I Pancreatic enzymes in body fluids		
A Amylase		
1 Serum	Pancreatic inflammation leads to increased enzyme levels	Simple; 20–40% false-negatives and -positives; reliable if test results are two to three times the upper limit of normal
2 Urine	Renal clearance of amylase is increased in acute pancreatitis	May be abnormal when serum levels normal; false-negatives and -positives
3 Amylase/creatinine clearance ratio (C_{am}/C_{cr})	Renal clearance of amylase greater than clearance of creatinine	No more sensitive than the serum amylase; many false-positives
4 Ascitic fluid	Disruption of gland or main pancreatic duct leads to increased amylase concentration	Can establish diagnosis of pancreatitis; false-positives with intestinal obstruction and perforated ulcer
5 Pleural fluid	Exudative pleural effusion with pancreatitis	False-positives with carcinoma of the lung and esophageal perforation
6 Isoenzymes	P isoamylases arise from the pancreas; S isoamylases are from other sources	More sensitive than total serum amylase in diagnosis of acute pancreatitis; useful in identifying nonpancreatic causes of hyperamylasemia
B Serum lipase	Pancreatic inflammation leads to increased enzyme levels	New methods of determination greatly simplified; positive in 70–85% of cases; excellent specificity; normal in nonpancreatic hyperamylasemic conditions
C Serum trypsin-like immunoreactivity (TLI)	Pancreatic inflammation leads to increased levels	*Elevated* in acute pancreatitis and renal failure; *decreased* in chronic pancreatitis *with* steatorrhea; normal in chronic pancreatitis *without* steatorrhea and steatorrhea with normal pancreatic function
D Pancreatic polypeptide (PP)	PP confined almost totally to the pancreas; release stimulated by nutrients and hormones; such release parallels pancreatic enzyme secretion	Basal, meal-simulated, and hormone (secretin CCK)-stimulated PP levels *decreased* in chronic pancreatitis; fasting PP levels >125 pg/mL argues against chronic pancreatitis and pancreatic cancer
II Studies pertaining to pancreatic structure		
A Radiologic and radionuclide tests		
1 Plain film of the abdomen	Abnormal in acute and chronic pancreatitis	Simple; normal in >50% of both acute and chronic pancreatitis
2 Upper gastrointestinal x-rays	Abnormally thickened duodenal folds; displacement of stomach or widening of duodenal loop suggests a pancreatic mass (inflammatory, neoplastic, cystic)	Simple; frequently normal; largely superseded by US and CT scanning
3 Ultrasonography (US)	Can provide information on edema, inflammation, calcification, pseudocysts, and mass lesions	Simple, noninvasive; sequential studies quite feasible; useful in diagnosis of pseudocyst
4 CT scan	Permits detailed visualization of pancreas and surrounding structures	Useful in the diagnosis of pancreatic calcification, dilated pancreatic ducts, and pancreatic tumors; may not be able to distinguish between inflammatory and neoplastic mass lesions
5 Selective angiography	Can identify pancreatic neoplasms (1) by sheathing of celiac or superior mesenteric branches by tumor or (2) by tumor staining; displacement of vessels by tumor	Indicated (1) in suspected islet cell tumors and (2) prior to pancreatic or duodenal resection; most reliable features reflect nonresectable pancreatic cancer
6 Endoscopic retrograde cholangiopancreatography (ERCP)	Cannulation of pancreatic and common bile duct permits visualization of pancreatic-biliary ductal system	Provides diagnostic data in 60–85% of cases; differentiation of chronic pancreatitis from pancreatic carcinoma may be difficult
B Pancreatic biopsy with US or CT guidance	Percutaneous biopsy with skinny needle and localization of lesion by US	High diagnostic yield; laparotomy avoided; requires special technical skills
III Tests of exocrine pancreatic function		
A Direct stimulation of the pancreas with analysis of duodenal contents		
1 Secretin-pancreozymin (CCK) test	Secretin leads to increased output of pancreatic juice and HCO_3^-; CCK leads to increased output of pancreatic enzymes; pancreatic secretory response related to functional mass of pancreatic tissue	Sensitive enough to detect occult disease; involves duodenal intubation and fluoroscopy; poorly defined normal enzyme response; overlap in chronic pancreatitis; large secretory reserve capacity of the pancreas
B Indirect stimulation of pancreas with measurement of pancreatic enzymes		
1 Lundh test meal	Test meal (fat, carbohydrate, and protein) causes increased release of CCK, which causes increased enzyme output; trypsin concentration measured	Useful in pancreatic exocrine insufficiency; false-negatives with delayed gastric emptying; false-positives in primary mucosal disease of the gut and choledocholithiasis; does not measure secretory capacity
2 Benzoyl-tyrosyl-*p*-aminobenzoic (Bz-Ty-PABA, bentiromide) test	Synthetic peptide (Bz-Ty-PABA) specifically cleaved by chymotrypsin, liberating PABA which is absorbed and PABA metabolite excreted in the urine	Simple and reliable test of pancreatic exocrine function
C Measurement of intraluminal digestion products		
1 Microscopic examination of stool for undigested meat fibers and fat	Lack of proteolytic and lipolytic enzymes causes decreased digestion of meat fibers and triglycerides	Simple, reliable; not sensitive enough to detect milder cases of pancreatic insufficiency
2 Quantitative stool fat determination	Lack of lipolytic enzymes brings about impaired fat digestion	Reliable, reference standard for defining severity of malabsorption; does not distinguish between maldigestion and malabsorption

TABLE 259-1 Tests useful in the diagnosis of acute and chronic pancreatitis and pancreatic tumors (*continued*)

Test	Principle	Comment
3 Fecal nitrogen	Lack of proteolytic enzymes leads to imparied protein digestion, causing increase in stool nitrogen	Does not distinguish between maldigestion and malabsorption; low sensitivity
D Measurement of pancreatic enzymes in feces		
1 Chymotrypsin	Pancreatic secretion of proteolytic enzymes	May be useful in cystic fibrosis; tedious; 10% false-positives and false-negatives

fluid amylase occurs in acute pancreatitis, chronic pancreatitis, carcinoma of the lung, and esophageal perforation.

In the past, serum lipase levels were not frequently performed because of methodological problems. However, newer methods are now available and development of automated lipase assays should lead to their routine use and obviate present reliance on total amylase measurements in the diagnosis of acute pancreatitis. In two representative studies, lipase determinations exhibited good *sensitivity* and excellent *specificity;* lipase levels were elevated in 70 to 85 percent of patients with acute pancreatitis, and the specificity was 99 percent. An obvious advantage of the lipase assay is that this enzyme is normal in several disorders associated with hyperamylasemia (e.g., macroamylasemia, diabetic ketoacidosis, renal failure, salivary gland lesions).

Assay for trypsinogen (or trypsin-like immunoreactivity) has a theoretical advantage over amylase and lipase determinations in that the pancreas is the only organ that contains this enzyme. The test appears to be useful in the diagnosis of both acute and chronic pancreatitis. Sensitivity and specificity are comparable to amylase and lipase determinations. Since trypsinogen is also excreted by the kidney, elevated values are found in renal failure.

A recent study evaluated the sensitivity and specificity of five

TABLE 259-2 Causes of hyperamylasemia and hyperamylasuria

I Pancreatic disease
  A Pancreatitis
    1 Acute
    2 Chronic: ductal obstruction
    3 Complications of pancreatitis
      a Pancreatic pseudocyst
      b Pancreatogenous ascites
      c Pancreatic abscess
  B Pancreatic trauma
  C Pancreatic carcinoma
II Nonpancreatic disorders
  A Renal insufficiency
  B Salivary gland lesions
    1 Mumps
    2 Calculus
    3 Irradiation sialadenitis
    4 Maxillofacial surgery
  C "Tumor" hyperamylasemia
    1 Carcinoma of the lung
    2 Carcinoma of the esophagus
    3 Breast carcinoma, ovarian carcinoma
  D Macroamylasemia
  E Burns
  F Diabetic ketoacidosis
  G Pregnancy
  H Renal transplantation
  I Cerebral trauma
  J Drugs: morphine
III Other abdominal disorders
  A Biliary tract disease: cholecystitis, choledocholithiasis
  B Intraabdominal disease
    1 Perforated or penetrating peptic ulcer
    2 Intestinal obstruction or infarction
    3 Ruptured ectopic pregnancy
    4 Peritonitis
    5 Aortic aneurysm
    6 Chronic liver disease
    7 Postoperative hyperamylasemia

SOURCE: After WB Salt II, S Schenker, Medicine 55:269, 1976.

assays used to diagnose acute pancreatitis: two amylase assays, one lipase, one trypsinlike immunoreactivity (TLI), and one pancreatic isoamylase. The data obtained show that (1) if the best cutoff level is used, all assays have similar specificities and suggest that (2) total serum amylase is as good an indicator of acute pancreatitis as any of the others. However, inherent in many such studies is the problem that the recognition and diagnosis of acute pancreatitis hinges upon the finding of an elevated serum amylase. The question arises as to whether any diagnostic test result can be proved superior to the total serum amylase level if hyperamylasemia is required for the diagnosis. In other studies, when "objective" confirmation of the clinical diagnosis of pancreatitis was required (ultrasonography, CT, laparotomy), the sensitivity of the serum amylase has been as low as 68 percent. With these limitations in mind, the recommended screening tests for acute pancreatitis are *total serum amylase and serum lipase activities*. Serum amylase values greater than three times normal are highly specific.

STUDIES PERTAINING TO PANCREATIC STRUCTURE Radiologic tests Plain films of the abdomen provide useful information in 30 to 50 percent of patients with acute pancreatitis. The most frequent abnormalities include (1) a localized ileus usually involving the jejunum ("sentinel loop"); (2) a generalized ileus with air-fluid levels; (3) the "colon cutoff sign," which results from isolated distention of the transverse colon; (4) duodenal distention with air-fluid levels; and (5) a mass, which is frequently a pseudocyst. In chronic pancreatitis, an important radiographic finding is pancreatic calcification, which characteristically is localized adjacent to and superimposed on the second lumbar vertebra (see Fig. 260-1).

Upper gastrointestinal x-rays may reveal displacement of the stomach by the retroperitoneal mass (see Fig. 260-2A) or widening and effacement of the duodenal C loop, which also suggests the presence of a pancreatic mass that could be an inflammatory, cystic, or neoplastic process. However, their use has been largely superceded by ultrasound.

Ultrasonography (echography) can provide important information in patients with acute pancreatitis, chronic pancreatitis, pancreatic calcification, pseudocyst, and pancreatic carcinoma. It is a useful procedure in the evaluation of the patient with acute pancreatitis. Echographic appearances can indicate the presence of edema, inflammation, and calcification (not obvious on plain films of the abdomen), as well as pseudocysts, mass lesions, and gallstones (see Figs. 260-1 to 260-3). In acute pancreatitis the pancreas is characteristically enlarged. In pancreatic pseudocyst the usual appearance is that of an echo-free, smooth, round fluid collection. Pancreatic carcinoma distorts the usual landmarks, and mass lesions greater than 3.0 cm are usually detected as localized, echo-free solid lesions. Ultrasound is often the initial investigation for most patients with suspected pancreatic disease. However, obesity, excess small- and large-bowel gas, and recently performed barium-contrast examinations can interfere with ultrasound studies, which are often technically unsatisfactory.

Computed tomography is the best imaging study for initial evaluation of a suspected chronic pancreatic disorder. It is especially useful in the detection of pancreatic tumors, fluid-containing lesions such as pseudocysts and abscesses, and calcium deposits. Most lesions are characterized by (1) enlargement of the pancreatic outline, (2) distortion of the pancreatic contour, or (3) fluid-containing lesions that have different attenuation coefficients than normal pancreas. However, it is occasionally difficult to distinguish between inflammatory and neoplastic lesions. Oral water-soluble contrast agents may be used to opacify the stomach and duodenum during CT scans; this permits more precise delineation of various organs as well as mass lesions.

Selective catheterization of the celiac and superior mesenteric arteries combined with superselective catheterization of others such as the hepatic, splenic, and gastroduodenal arteries permits visualization of the pancreas and detection of pancreatic neoplasms and pseudocysts. Pancreatic neoplasms can be identified by the sheathing of blood vessels by a mass lesion (see Fig. 260-3). Hormone-producing pancreatic tumors are especially likely to exhibit increased vascularity and tumor staining. Angiographic abnormalities are noted in many patients with pancreatic carcinoma but are uncommon in patients without pancreatic disease. Angiography complements ultrasonography and endoscopic retrograde cholangiopancreatography (ERCP) in the study of a patient with a suspected pancreatic lesion and may be carried out if ERCP is either unsuccessful or nondiagnostic.

Endoscopic retrograde cholangiopancreatography   ERCP may provide useful information on the status of the pancreatic ductal system and thus aid in the differential diagnosis of pancreatic disease (see Figs. 260-2 and 260-3). Pancreatic carcinoma is characterized by stenosis or obstruction of either the pancreatic duct or common bile duct; both ductal systems are often abnormal. In chronic pancreatitis ERCP abnormalities include (1) luminal narrowing; (2) irregularities in the ductal system with stenosis, dilatation, sacculation, and ectasia; and (3) blockage of the pancreatic duct by calcium deposits. Differentiation from carcinoma may be difficult because of similar overlapping features, i.e., ductal stenosis and irregularity. Elevated serum and/or urine amylase levels following ERCP have been reported in 25 to 75 percent of patients, but clinical pancreatitis is uncommon. In a series of 300 patients pancreatitis occurred in only five patients following ERCP. If no lesion is found within the biliary and/or pancreatic ducts in a patient with repeated attacks of acute pancreatitis, manometric studies of the sphincter of Oddi may be indicated.

Pancreatic biopsy with radiologic guidance   Percutaneous aspiration biopsy of a pancreatic mass often distinguishes between a pancreatic inflammatory mass and a pancreatic neoplasm.

TESTS OF EXOCRINE PANCREATIC FUNCTION

Pancreatic function tests (Table 259-1) can be divided into the following:

1 *Direct stimulation of the pancreas* by intravenous infusion of secretin or secretin plus cholecystokinin (CCK) followed by collection and measurement of duodenal contents
2 *Indirect stimulation of the pancreas* utilizing nutrients or amino acids, fatty acids, and synthetic peptides followed by assay of proteolytic, lipolytic, and amylolytic enzymes
3 Study of *intraluminal digestion products* such as undigested meat fibers, stool fat, and fecal nitrogen
4 *Measurement of fecal pancreatic enzymes* such as chymotrypsin

The secretin test, used to detect diffuse pancreatic disease, is based on the physiologic principle that the pancreatic secretory response is directly related to the functional mass of pancreatic tissue. In the standard assay, secretin is given intravenously in a dose of 1 clinical unit (CU) per kilogram, either as a bolus or continuous infusion. Obviously, results will vary with the secretin preparation used, dose, mode of administration, and completeness of collection of duodenal contents. Normal values for the standard secretin test are (1) volume output >2.0 mL/kg per hour, (2) bicarbonate (HCO_3^-) concentration >80 meq/L, and (3) HCO_3^- output >10 meq in 1 h. The most reproducible measurement having the highest level of discrimination between normal subjects and patients with chronic pancreatitis appears to be the maximal bicarbonate concentration.

The *combined secretin-CCK test* permits measurement of pancreatic amylase, lipase, trypsin, and chymotrypsin. Although there is overlap in the distribution of enzyme output in normal subjects and patients with pancreatitis, markedly decreased enzyme outputs suggest advanced damage and destruction of acinar cells. With frank exocrine pancreatic insufficiency there is usually an overall reduction in both HCO_3^- concentration and output of several enzymes. However, with lesser degrees of pancreatic damage there may be a dissociation between HCO_3^- concentration and enzyme output. There may also be a dissociation between the results of the secretin test and other tests of absorptive function. For example, patients with chronic pancreatitis often have abnormally low outputs of HCO_3^- after secretin but have normal fecal fat excretion. Thus, the secretin test measures the secretory capacity of ductular epithelium, while fecal fat excretion indirectly reflects intraluminal lipolytic activity. Steatorrhea does not occur until intraluminal levels of lipase are markedly reduced, underscoring the fact that only small amounts of enzymes are necessary for intraluminal digestive activities. An abnormal secretin test should suggest only that chronic pancreatic damage is present; it will not consistently distinguish between chronic pancreatitis and pancreatic carcinoma.

Another test of exocrine pancreatic function, which indirectly reflects intraluminal chymotrypsin activity, has been evaluated in patients with pancreatic disease. This test (the *tripeptide hydrolysis* or *bentiromide* test) utilizes a synthetic peptide, *N*-benzoyl-L-tyrosyl-p-aminobenzoic acid (Bz-Ty-PABA), that is specifically cleaved by chymotrypsin to Bz-Ty and PABA. Normally, after oral administration, the peptide reaches the small intestine, where it is hydrolyzed by chymotrypsin with the liberation of PABA, which is rapidly absorbed and excreted in the urine. Results in several hundred patients with chronic pancreatitis and other disorders indicate that PABA excretion is significantly lower in chronic pancreatitis compared with controls. Depending on the severity of pancreatic exocrine impairment, the overall sensitivity is 60 percent (range 46 to 74 percent), and the specificity if coupled with a D-xylose test approximates 90 percent.

Measurement of *intraluminal digestion products*, i.e., undigested muscle fibers, stool fat, and fecal nitrogen, is discussed in Chap. 240. Measurement of chymotrypsin in stool reflects pancreatic output of this proteolytic enzyme. Decreased chymotrypsin activity in stool has been reported in patients with chronic pancreatitis and cystic fibrosis. However, normal values may occur in patients with pancreatic insufficiency, and false-positive results have been reported in up to 10 percent of normal individuals.

Tests useful in the diagnosis of exocrine pancreatic insufficiency and the differential diagnosis of malabsorption are also discussed in Chaps. 240 and 260.

260   ACUTE AND CHRONIC PANCREATITIS

NORTON J. GREENBERGER / PHILLIP P. TOSKES /
KURT J. ISSELBACHER

BIOCHEMISTRY AND PHYSIOLOGY OF PANCREATIC EXOCRINE SECRETION

GENERAL CONSIDERATIONS   The pancreas secretes 1500 to 3000 mL isosmotic alkaline (pH > 8.0) fluid per day containing about 20 enzymes and zymogens. The pancreatic secretions provide the enzymes needed to effect the major digestive activity of the gastrointestinal tract and provide an optimum pH for the function of these enzymes.

REGULATION OF PANCREATIC SECRETION   Hormonal and neural mechanisms

The exocrine pancreas is under both hormonal and neural control, with hormonal control being of primary importance. *Gastric acid* is the stimulus for the release of secretin, a peptide with 27 amino acids. Sensitive radioimmunoassay studies for secretin suggest that the pH threshold for the release of secretin from the duodenum and jejunum is 4.5. Secretin stimulates the secretion of pancreatic juice rich in *water and electrolytes*. Release of cholecystokinin (CCK) from duodenum and jejunum is largely produced by long-chain fatty acids, certain essential amino acids (tryptophan, phenylalanine, valine, methionine), and gastric acid itself. CCK evokes an *enzyme-rich secretion from the pancreas*. Gastrin, although it shares an identical terminal tetrapeptide with CCK, is a weak stimulus for pancreatic enzyme output. The *parasympathetic nervous system* (via the vagus) exerts some control over pancreatic secretion. Part of this is mediated by the release of gastrin, and part is secondary to a direct effect of acetylcholine on the pancreatic acinar cell. Also, vagal stimulation effects release of vasoactive intestinal peptide (VIP), a secretin agonist. Vagal control of pancreatic secretion seems to be most important following a truncal vagotomy, but even in such patients severe maldigestion does not ensue. Bile salts also stimulate pancreatic secretion, thereby integrating the functions of the biliary tract, pancreas, and small intestine.

Pancreatic secretion at the cellular level   There appear to be two functionally distinct pathways by which secretagogues can stimulate pancreatic secretion. Studies with isolated pancreatic acinar cells indicate that secretin, VIP, and cholera toxin interact with receptors on the acinar cell, leading to an increase in cellular cyclic adenosine monophosphate (cyclic AMP). CCK, acetylcholine, gastrin, and various other peptides (e.g., bombesin, caerulein) react with other receptors on the acinar cell to cause an increased turnover of phosphatidylinositol and the release of membrane calcium and induce changes in the electrical properties of the pancreatic acinar cell surface and junctional membranes. When a secretagogue that increases cyclic AMP is added to a secretagogue that increases calcium outflux, potentiation of enzyme secretion occurs.

WATER AND ELECTROLYTE SECRETION   Although sodium, potassium, chloride, calcium, zinc, phosphate, and sulfate are found within pancreatic secretion, *bicarbonate is the ion of primary physiologic importance*. In the acini and in the ducts, secretin causes the cells to add water and bicarbonate to the fluid. In the ducts an exchange occurs between bicarbonate and chloride. There is a good correlation between the maximal bicarbonate output after stimulation with secretin and the pancreatic mass. The bicarbonate output of 120 to 300 mmol/d helps neutralize gastric acid production and creates the appropriate pH for the activity of the pancreatic enzymes.

ENZYME SECRETION   The pancreas secretes amylolytic, lipolytic, and proteolytic enzymes. Amylolytic enzymes such as amylase hydrolyze starch to oligosaccharides and to the disaccharide maltose. The *lipolytic enzymes* include lipase, phospholipase A, and cholesterol esterase. Bile salts *inhibit* lipase, but colipase, another constituent of pancreatic secretion, binds to lipase and prevents this inhibition. Bile salts *activate* phospholipase A and cholesterol esterase. *Proteolytic enzymes* include *endopeptidases* (trypsin, chymotrypsin), which act on the internal peptide bonds of proteins and polypeptides; *exopeptidases* (carboxypeptidases, aminopeptidases), which act on the free carboxyl-terminal end and free amino-terminal end of peptides, respectively; and elastase. The proteolytic enzymes are secreted as inactive precursors (zymogens). Ribonucleases (deoxyribonucleases, ribonuclease) are also secreted. While parallel secretion of pancreatic enzymes usually occurs, nonparallel secretion can occur as a result of exocytosis from heterogeneous sources within the pancreas. *Enterokinase*, an enzyme found within the duodenal mucosa, cleaves the lysine-isoleucine bond of trypsinogen to form trypsin. Trypsin then activates the other proteolytic zymogens in a cascade phenomenon. All pancreatic enzymes have pH optima in the alkaline range.

AUTOPROTECTION OF THE PANCREAS   Autodigestion of the pancreas is prevented by the packaging of proteases in precursor form and by the synthesis of protease inhibitors. These protease inhibitors are found within the acinar cell, the pancreatic secretions, and the alpha$_1$- and alpha$_2$-globulin fractions of plasma.

EXOCRINE-ENDOCRINE RELATIONSHIPS   Pancreatic glucagon (29 amino acid residues) has a high degree of structural similarity to secretin. It decreases volume and enzyme secretion by the pancreas but not bicarbonate secretion. Glucose, in large concentrations, may also inhibit pancreatic exocrine secretion. The choleretic and insulinotropic effects of secretin are shared by glucagon.

ENTEROPANCREATIC AXIS AND FEEDBACK INHIBITION   Pancreatic enzyme secretion in human beings is controlled, at least in part, by a negative feedback mechanism induced by the presence of active serine proteases in the duodenum. To illustrate, intraduodenal perfusion with phenylalanine causes a prompt increase in plasma CCK levels as well as increased secretion of chymotrypsin. However, simultaneous perfusion with trypsin blunts both responses. Conversely, duodenal perfusion with protease inhibitors actually leads to enzyme hypersecretion. It appears that serine proteases inhibit pancreatic secretion by acting upon a CCK-releasing peptide found within the lumen of the small intestine.

ACUTE PANCREATITIS

GENERAL CONSIDERATIONS   Pancreatic inflammatory disease may be classified as follows: (1) acute pancreatitis and (2) chronic pancreatitis. This classification is based primarily on clinical criteria with the obvious difference between the acute and chronic varieties being restoration of normal function in the former and permanent residual damage in the latter. The pathologic spectrum of acute pancreatitis varies from *edematous pancreatitis*, which is usually a mild and self-limited disorder, to *necrotizing pancreatitis*, in which the degree of pancreatic necrosis correlates with the severity of the attack and its systemic manifestations. The term *hemorrhagic pancreatitis* is less meaningful in a clinical sense because variable amounts of interstitial hemorrhage can be found in pancreatitis as well as in other disorders such as pancreatic trauma, pancreatic carcinoma, and severe congestive heart failure.

The incidence of pancreatitis varies in different countries and depends upon etiologic factors, e.g., alcohol, gallstones, metabolic factors, and drugs (Table 260-1). In the United States, for example, acute pancreatitis is related to alcohol ingestion more commonly than to gallstones; in England the opposite obtains. Epidemiologic data based on autopsy data indicate that in the United States the overall prevalence of acute pancreatitis is approximately 0.5 percent. An upward trend has been noted in the crude death rate from 1.0 per 100,000 in 1955 to 1.3 in 1965.

ETIOLOGY AND PATHOGENESIS   There are many causative factors in the pathogenesis of acute pancreatitis (Table 260-1), but the mechanisms by which these conditions trigger pancreatic inflammation have not been identified. Alcoholic patients with pancreatitis may represent a special subset, since most alcoholics do not develop pancreatitis. The list of identifiable causes is growing, and it is likely that pancreatitis related to viral infections, drugs, and as yet undefined factors is more common than heretofore recognized.

Autodigestion is one pathogenetic theory which proposes that proteolytic enzymes (e.g., trypsinogen, chymotrypsinogen, proelastase, and phospholipase A) are activated within the pancreas rather than in the intestinal lumen. A variety of factors (such as endotoxins, exotoxins, viral infections, ischemia, anoxia, and direct trauma) are believed to activate these proenzymes. Activated proteolytic enzymes, especially trypsin, not only digest pancreatic and peripancreatic tissues but also can activate other enzymes such as elastase and phospholipase. The active enzymes then digest cellular membranes and cause proteolysis, edema, interstitial hemorrhage, vascular damage, coagulation necrosis, fat necrosis, and parenchymal cell necrosis. Cellular injury and death result in the liberation of activated enzymes. In addition, activation and release of bradykinin peptides and vasoactive substances (e.g., histamine) are believed to produce vasodilatation,

TABLE 260-1   Causes of acute pancreatitis

I Alcohol ingestion (acute and chronic alcoholism)
II Biliary tract disease (gallstones)
III Postoperative (abdominal, nonabdominal)
IV Postendoscopic retrograde cholangiopancreatography (ERCP)
V Trauma (especially blunt abdominal type)
VI Metabolic
  A Hypertriglyceridemia
  B Apolipoprotein CII deficiency syndrome
  C Hypercalcemia, e.g., hyperparathyroidism
  D Renal failure
  E After renal transplantation*
  F Acute fatty liver of pregnancy†
VII Hereditary pancreatitis
VIII Infections
  A Mumps
  B Viral hepatitis
  C Other viral infections (coxsackievirus, echovirus)
  D Ascariasis
  E Mycoplasma
IX Drug-associated
  A Definite association
    1 Azathioprine
    2 Sulfonamides
    3 Thiazide diuretics
    4 Furosemide
    5 Estrogens (oral contraceptives)
    6 Tetracycline
    7 Valproic acid
    8 Pentamidine
  B Probable association
    1 Chlorthalidone
    2 Ethacrynic acid
    3 Procainamide
    4 Iatrogenic hypercalcemia
    5 L-Asparaginase
X Connective tissue disorders with vasculitis
  A Systemic lupus erythematosus
  B Necrotizing angiitis
  C Thrombotic thrombocytopenic purpura
XI Penetrating peptic ulcer
XII Obstruction of the ampulla of Vater
  A Regional enteritis
  B Duodenal diverticulum
XIII Pancreas divisum
XIV Recurrent bouts of acute pancreatitis without obvious cause
  A Consider
    1 Occult disease of the biliary tree or pancreatic ducts
    2 Drugs
    3 Hypertriglyceridemia
    4 Pancreas divisum
XV Other

---

* Pancreatitis occurs in 3 percent of renal transplant patients and is due to many factors including surgery, hypercalcemia, drugs (corticosteroids, azathioprine, L-asparaginase, diuretics), and viral infections.
† Pancreatitis also occurs in otherwise uncomplicated pregnancy and is most often associated with cholelithiasis.

increased vascular permeability, and edema. There is thus a cascade of events culminating in the development of acute necrotizing pancreatitis.

The autodigestion theory has largely eclipsed two older theories. First, the "common channel" theory holds that such an anatomic arrangement facilitates reflux of bile into the pancreatic duct, and this results in activation of pancreatic enzymes. (Actually, a common channel with free communication between the common bile duct and main pancreatic duct is infrequently encountered.) The second theory is that obstruction and hypersecretion are pivotal in the development of pancreatitis. Obstruction of the main pancreatic duct, however, produces pancreatic edema but not pancreatitis.

A recent hypothesis to explain the intrapancreatic activation of zymogens is that they become activated by *lysosomal hydrolases* within the pancreatic acinar cell itself. In two different types of experimental pancreatitis, it has been demonstrated that digestive enzymes and lysosomal hydrolases become admixed; as a result the former can be activated within the acinar cell by the latter. *In vitro*, lysosomal enzymes such as cathepsin B can activate trypsinogen, and trypsin can activate the other protease precursors.

CLINICAL FEATURES *Abdominal pain* is the major symptom of acute pancreatitis. Pain may vary from a mild and tolerable discomfort to severe, constant, and incapacitating distress. Characteristically, the pain, which is steady and boring in character, is located in the epigastrium and periumbilical region and often radiates to the back as well as to the chest, flanks, and lower abdomen. The pain is frequently more intense when the patient is supine, and patients often obtain relief by sitting with the trunk flexed and knees drawn up. Nausea, vomiting, and abdominal distention due to gastric and intestinal hypomotility and chemical peritonitis are also frequent complaints.

Physical examination frequently reveals a distressed and anxious patient. Low-grade fever, tachycardia, and hypotension are fairly common. Shock is not unusual and may result from (1) hypovolemia secondary to exudation of blood and plasma proteins into the retroperitoneal space, i.e., a "retroperitoneal burn"; (2) increased formation and release of kinin peptides which cause vasodilatation and increased vascular permeability; and (3) systemic effects of proteolytic and lipolytic enzymes released into the circulation. Jaundice occurs infrequently; when present it usually is due to edema of the head of the pancreas with compression of the intrapancreatic portion of the common bile duct. Erythematous skin nodules due to subcutaneous fat necrosis may occur. In 10 to 20 percent of patients there are pulmonary findings, including basilar rales, atelectasis, and pleural effusion, the latter most frequently left-sided. Abdominal tenderness and muscle rigidity are present to a variable degree, but compared with the intense pain, these signs may be unimpressive. Bowel sounds are usually diminished or absent. A pancreatic pseudocyst may be palpable in the upper abdomen. A faint blue discoloration around the umbilicus (Cullen's sign) may occur as the result of hemoperitoneum, and a blue-red-purple or green-brown discoloration of the flanks (Turner's sign) reflects tissue catabolism of hemoglobin. The latter two findings, which are uncommon, indicate the presence of a severe necrotizing pancreatitis.

LABORATORY DATA The diagnosis of acute pancreatitis is usually established by the presence of an increased serum amylase. Values elevated threefold above normal virtually clinch the diagnosis if overt salivary gland disease and gut perforation or infarction are excluded. However, there appears to be no definite correlation between the severity of pancreatitis and the degree of serum amylase elevation. After 48 to 72 h, even with continuing evidence of pancreatitis, total serum amylase values tend to return to normal. However, pancreatic isoamylase and lipase levels may remain elevated for 7 to 14 days. It will be recalled that amylase elevations in serum and urine occur in many conditions other than pancreatitis (see Table 259-2). Importantly, patients with *acidemia* (arterial pH ≤ 7.32) may have spurious elevations in serum amylase. In one study, 12 of 33 acidemic patients had an elevated serum amylase but only one had an elevated lipase value; 9 had salivary-type amylase as the predominant serum isoamylase. This explains why patients with diabetic ketoacidosis may have marked elevations in serum amylase without any other evidence to support a diagnosis of acute pancreatitis. The urine amylase C_{am}/C_{cr} ratio is usually elevated in patients with severe pancreatitis; this ratio usually is not increased in patients with normal serum amylase. Serum lipase activity increases in parallel with amylase activity, and measurement of both enzymes increases the diagnostic yield. An elevated serum lipase or trypsin value is usually diagnostic of acute pancreatitis; these tests are especially helpful in patients with nonpancreatic causes of hyperamylasemia (see Table 259-4). Markedly increased levels of peritoneal or pleural fluid amylase [>1500 nmol/L (>5000 units per deciliter)] are also helpful, if present, in establishing the diagnosis.

Leukocytosis (15,000 to 20,000 leukocytes per microliter) occurs frequently. More severe cases may show hemoconcentration with hematocrit values exceeding 50 percent because of loss of plasma into the retroperitoneal space and peritoneal cavity. *Hyperglycemia* is common and is due to multiple factors that include decreased insulin release, increased glucagon release, and increased output of adrenal glucocorticoids and catecholamines. *Hypocalcemia* occurs in approximately 25 percent of cases, and its pathogenesis is incompletely understood. While earlier studies suggested that the parathyroid gland response to a decrease in serum calcium is impaired, subsequent observations have failed to confirm this. Intraperitoneal saponification of calcium by fatty acids in areas of fat necrosis occurs occasionally with large amounts (up to 6.0 g) dissolved or suspended in ascitic fluid. Such "soap formation" also may be significant in patients with pancreatitis, mild hypocalcemia, and little or no obvious ascites. *Hyperbilirubinemia* [serum bilirubin >68 μmol/L (>4.0 mg/dL)] occurs in approximately 10 percent of patients. However, jaundice is transient and serum bilirubin levels return to normal in 4 to 7 days. Serum alkaline phosphatase and aspartate aminotransferase (AST) levels are also transiently elevated and parallel serum bilirubin values. When markedly elevated [i.e., >8.5 μmol/L (>500 units per deciliter)], serum lactic dehydrogenase (LDH) levels suggest a poor prognosis. Serum albumin is decreased to ≤30 g/L (≤3.0 g/dL) in about 10 percent of cases and is associated with more severe pancreatitis and an increased mortality rate (Table 260-2). Methemalbumin, a circulating heme metabolite attached to albumin, has been considered as a useful index of severe necrotizing pancreatitis. Its usefulness, however, has been limited by its nonspecificity for pancreatitis (it occurs, for example, in abdominal trauma, bone fractures, soft-tissue trauma, and retroperitoneal hematoma) and its absence in the majority of cases of severe necrotizing pancreatitis. *Hypertriglyceridemia* occurs in 15 to 20 percent of cases, and serum amylase levels in such patients are often spuriously normal (see Chap. 259). Most patients with hypertriglyceridemia and pancreatitis, when subsequently examined, show evidence of an underlying derangement in lipid metabolism which probably antedated the pancreatitis. Approximately 25 percent of patients have *hypoxemia* (arterial P_{O_2} ≤ 60 mmHg), which may herald the onset of adult respiratory distress syndrome. Finally, the electrocardiogram is occasionally abnormal in acute pancreatitis with ST-segment and T-wave abnormalities simulating myocardial ischemia.

Radiologic studies useful in the diagnosis of acute pancreatitis are listed in Table 259-1 and discussed in Chap. 259. Although one or more of the abnormalities are found in over 50 percent of patients, the findings are inconstant and nonspecific. The chief value of conventional x-rays [chest; kidney, ureter, and bladder (KUB)] in acute pancreatitis is to help exclude other diagnoses, especially a perforated viscus. Upper gastrointestinal tract x-rays have been superseded by ultrasonography and CT scanning. A CT scan may confirm the clinical impression of acute pancreatitis even in the face of normal serum amylase levels. Importantly, CT is quite helpful in indicating the severity of acute pancreatitis and its expected morbidity and mortality. Sonography and radionuclide scanning (PIPIDA, HIDA) are useful in acute pancreatitis to evaluate the gallbladder and biliary tree.

DIAGNOSIS Any severe acute pain in the abdomen or back should suggest acute pancreatitis. The diagnosis is usually entertained when a patient with a possible predisposition to pancreatitis presents with severe and constant abdominal pain, nausea, emesis, fever, tachycardia, and abnormal findings on abdominal examination. Laboratory studies frequently reveal leukocytosis, abnormal x-rays of the abdomen and chest, hypocalcemia, and hyperglycemia. The diagnosis is usually confirmed by finding an elevated serum amylase and/or lipase. Obviously, not all the above features have to be present for the diagnosis to be established.

The *differential diagnosis* should include consideration of the following disorders: (1) perforated viscus, especially peptic ulcer; (2) acute cholecystitis and biliary colic; (3) acute intestinal obstruction; (4) mesenteric vascular occlusion; (5) renal colic; (6) myocardial infarction; (7) dissecting aortic aneurysm; (8) connective tissue disorders with vasculitis; (9) pneumonia; and (10) diabetic ketoacidosis. A penetrating duodenal ulcer can usually be identified by upper gastrointestinal x-rays and/or endoscopy. A perforated duodenal ulcer is readily diagnosed by the presence of free intraperitoneal air. It may be difficult to differentiate acute cholecystitis from acute pancreatitis since an elevated serum amylase may be found in both disorders. Pain of biliary tract origin is more right-sided and gradual in onset, and ileus is usually absent; sonography and radionuclide scanning are helpful in establishing the diagnosis of cholelithiasis and cholecystitis. Intestinal obstruction due to mechanical factors can be differentiated from pancreatitis by the history of colicky pain, findings on abdominal examination, and x-rays of the abdomen showing characteristic changes of mechanical obstruction. Acute mesenteric vascular occlusion is usually evident in elderly debilitated patients with brisk leukocytosis, abdominal distention, and bloody diarrhea, in whom paracentesis shows sanguinous fluid and arteriography shows vascular occlusion. Serum as well as peritoneal fluid amylase levels are increased, however, in patients with intestinal infarction. Systemic lupus erythematosus and polyarteritis nodosa may be confused with pancreatitis, especially since pancreatitis may develop as a complication of those diseases. Diabetic ketoacidosis is often accompanied by abdominal pain and elevated total serum amylase levels, thus closely mimicking acute pancreatitis. However, the serum lipase and pancreatic isoamylase are not elevated in diabetic ketoacidosis.

COURSE OF THE DISEASE AND COMPLICATIONS There is an increased mortality rate with three or more risk factors identifiable either at the time of admission to hospital or during the initial 48 h of hospitalization (see Table 260-2). It is important to identify the patient with acute pancreatitis with an increased risk of dying. This subgroup is characterized by the following features: (1) respiratory failure with an arterial P_{O_2} <60 mmHg; (2) shock; (3) massive colloid replacement; (4) serum calcium <2.0 mmol/L (<8 mg/dL); and (5) the presence of "toxic broth" or dark (hemorrhagic) fluid on abdominal paracentesis. The presence of any one factor constitutes a severe attack. In one large series characterized by at least three of the first four features, the survival rate was only 29 percent in the patients treated with medical measures but increased to 64 percent with operative treatment. In another series, the mortality rate was 0.9 percent in patients with zero to two factors (Table 260-2), 16 percent in patients with three to four factors, and 40 percent with five to six factors present. The high mortality rate of such severely ill patients is due in large part to infection and warrants intensive radiologic intervention and monitoring and/or a combination of radiologic and surgical means as discussed in detail below.

The local and systemic complications of acute pancreatitis are listed in Table 260-3. Patients frequently develop an inflammatory mass in the first 2 to 3 weeks after pancreatitis. These may be phlegmons, abscesses, or pseudocysts (see below). Systemic complications include pulmonary, cardiovascular, hematologic, renal, metabolic, and central nervous system abnormalities. Pancreatitis, hypertriglyceridemia, and alcoholism constitute a triad in which cause and effect remain incompletely understood. However, several reasonable conclusions can be drawn. First, hypertriglyceridemia can precede and apparently cause the development of pancreatitis. Second,

---

TABLE 260-2 Factors adversely influencing survival in acute pancreatitis*

I Risk factors identifiable upon admission to hospital
  A Increasing age
  B Hypotension
  C Abnormal pulmonary findings
  D Abdominal mass
  E Hemorrhagic or discolored peritoneal fluid
  F Increased serum LDH levels
  G Leukocytosis
  H Hyperglycemia
  I First attack of pancreatitis
II Risk factors identifiable during initial 48 h of hospitalization
  A Fall in hematocrit > 10 percent with hydration and/or hematocrit < 30 percent
  B Necessity for massive fluid and colloid replacement
  C Hypocalcemia
  D Hypoxemia with or without adult respiratory distress syndrome
  E Hemorrhagic brown peritoneal fluid, i.e., "toxic broth"
  F Hypoalbuminemia
  G Azotemia

* Increased mortality with three or more risk factors.

TABLE 260-3   Complications of acute pancreatitis

I Local
  A Pancreatic phlegmon
  B Pancreatic abscess
  C Pancreatic pseudocyst
    1 Pain
    2 Rupture
    3 Hemorrhage
    4 Infection
    5 Obstruction of gastrointestinal tract (stomach, duodenum, colon)
  D Pancreatic ascites
    1 Disruption of main pancreatic duct
    2 Leaking pseudocyst
  E Involvement of contiguous organs by necrotizing pancreatitis
    1 Massive intraperitoneal hemorrhage
    2 Thrombosis of blood vessels
    3 Bowel infarction
  F Obstructive jaundice
II Systemic
  A Pulmonary
    1 Pleural effusion
    2 Atelectasis
    3 Mediastinal abscess
    4 Pneumonitis
    5 Adult respiratory distress syndrome
  B Cardiovascular
    1 Hypotension
      a Hypovolemia
      b Hypoalbuminemia
    2 Sudden death
    3 Nonspecific ST-T changes in electrocardiogram simulating myocardial infarction
    4 Pericardial effusion
  C Hematologic
    1 Disseminated intravascular coagulation (DIC)
  D Gastrointestinal hemorrhage*
    1 Peptic ulcer disease
    2 Erosive gastritis
    3 Hemorrhagic pancreatic necrosis with erosion into major blood vessels
    4 Portal vein thrombosis, variceal hemorrhage
  E Renal
    1 Oliguria
    2 Azotemia
    3 Renal artery and/or renal vein thrombosis
  F Metabolic
    1 Hyperglycemia
    2 Hypertriglyceridemia
    3 Hypocalcemia
    4 Encephalopathy
    5 Sudden blindness (Purtscher's retinopathy)
  G Central nervous system
    1 Psychosis
    2 Fat emboli
  H Fat necrosis
    1 Subcutaneous tissues (erythematous nodules)
    2 Bone
    3 Miscellaneous (mediastinum, pleura, nervous system)

* Aggravated by coagulation abnormalities (DIC).

the vast majority (>80 percent) of patients with acute pancreatitis do not have hypertriglyceridemia. Third, almost all patients with pancreatitis and hypertriglyceridemia are *either* alcoholics who have been drinking shortly before the onset of pancreatitis *or* patients with preexistent hypertriglyceridemia. Fourth, many of the patients with this triad have persistent hypertriglyceridemia after recovery from pancreatitis and abstention from alcohol. Finally, patients with a deficiency of apolipoprotein CII have an increased incidence of pancreatitis; apolipoprotein CII activates lipoprotein lipase, which is important in clearing chylomicrons from the bloodstream.

Purtscher's retinopathy, a relatively unusual complication, refers to the sudden and severe loss of vision in patients with acute pancreatitis. It is characterized by a peculiar funduscopic appearance with cotton-wool spots and hemorrhages confined to an area limited by the optic disk and macula; it is believed to be due to posterior retinal artery occlusion with aggregated granulocytes.

TREATMENT   In most patients (approximately 85 to 90 percent) with acute pancreatitis, the disease is self-limited and subsides spontaneously, usually within 3 to 7 days after treatment is instituted. Medical therapy is aimed at reducing pancreatic secretion and, in

essence, "putting the pancreas at rest." Conventional measures include (1) analgesics for pain, (2) intravenous fluids and colloids to maintain normal intravascular volume, (3) no oral alimentation, and (4) nasogastric suction to decrease gastrin release from the stomach and prevent gastric contents from entering the duodenum. Recent controlled trials, however, have shown that nasogastric suction offers no clear-cut advantages in the treatment of mild to moderately severe acute pancreatitis. Its use, therefore, must be considered elective rather than mandatory.

It has been demonstrated that CCK-stimulated pancreatic secretion is almost abolished in four different experimental models of acute pancreatitis. This probably explains why drugs to block pancreatic secretion in acute pancreatitis have failed to have any therapeutic benefit. For this and other reasons, anticholinergic drugs are not indicated in acute pancreatitis. Although antibiotics have been used in the treatment of acute pancreatitis, three recent randomized prospective trials have shown no benefit from the use of antibiotics in acute pancreatitis of mild to moderate severity. However, because secondary infection of necrotic pancreatic tissue (phlegmon, abscess, pseudocyst) or obstructed biliary passages (ascending cholangitis, complicating choledocholithiasis) contributes to much of the late mortality, appropriate *antibiotic therapy of established infection* is obviously quite important. Previous reports suggested that glucagon was useful in acute pancreatitis, but controlled trials have not provided convincing evidence of effectiveness. Similarly, a protease inhibitor such as aprotinin (Trasylol) and cimetidine have not proved effective.

A CT scan provides valuable information on the severity and prognosis of acute pancreatitis (Fig. 260-1). The following classification is in widespread use: grade A, normal; grade B, focal or diffuse pancreatic edema; grade C, extension of inflammatory changes to the peripancreatic fat; grade D, phlegmon or a single ill-defined fluid collection in or around the pancreas and often extending to the lesser sac and/or pararenal space; grade E, two or more fluid collections *or* presence of gas in or adjacent to the pancreas. Recent studies suggest that the likelihood of prolonged pancreatitis or serious complications is negligible when CT scans are either grade A or B; possible although unlikely with a grade of C; and most likely to occur with grades D and E. The patient with mild to moderate pancreatitis usually requires treatment with intravenous fluids, fasting, and possibly nasogastric suction for 2 to 4 days. A clear liquid diet is frequently started on the third to sixth day and a regular diet by the fifth to seventh day. The patient with unremitting *fulminant pancreatitis* usually requires inordinate amounts of fluid and close attention to complications such as cardiovascular collapse, respiratory insufficiency, and pancreatic infection. The latter should be managed by a combination of radiologic and surgical means (see below). While earlier uncontrolled studies suggested that *peritoneal lavage* via a percutaneous dialysis catheter is helpful in severe pancreatitis, recent studies indicate that such treatment does not influence the outcome of such attacks. Laparotomy with adequate drainage and removal of necrotic tissue should be considered if conventional therapy does not halt the patient's deterioration. The use of parenteral nutrition makes it possible to give nutritional support to patients with severe, acute, or protracted pancreatitis who are unable to eat normally. Finally, patients with severe gallstone-induced pancreatitis may improve dramatically if papillotomy is carried out within the first 36 to 72 h of the attack.

PANCREATIC PHLEGMON, ABSCESS, AND PSEUDOCYST   The *phlegmon* is a solid mass of swollen, inflamed pancreas often containing patchy areas of necrosis; it may be present for 1 to 2 weeks. This prolonged inflammatory process should not be confused with a pseudocyst, a differentiation which is usually accomplished by sonography. A phlegmon should be suspected if abdominal pain, fever, leukocytosis, and hyperamylasemia persist for more than 5 days and especially if an abdominal mass is also present. Differentiation from an abscess may be difficult even with a CT scan. Occasionally, extensive areas of pancreatic necrosis develop in phlegmons and require incision and drainage. Phlegmons may also

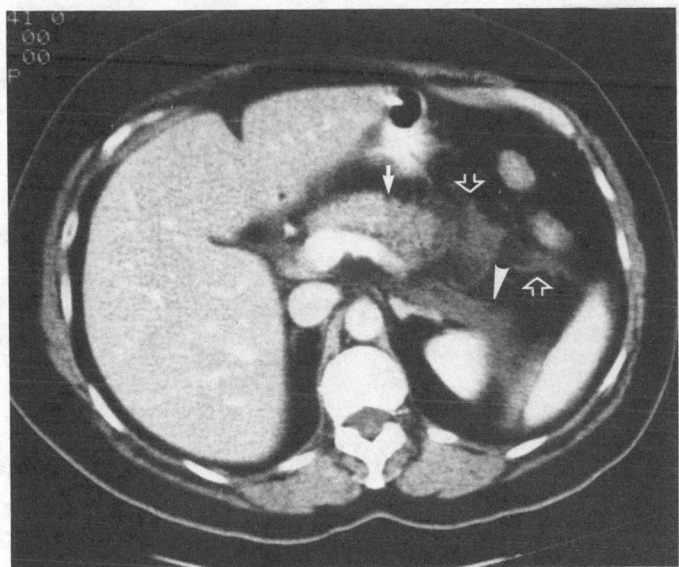

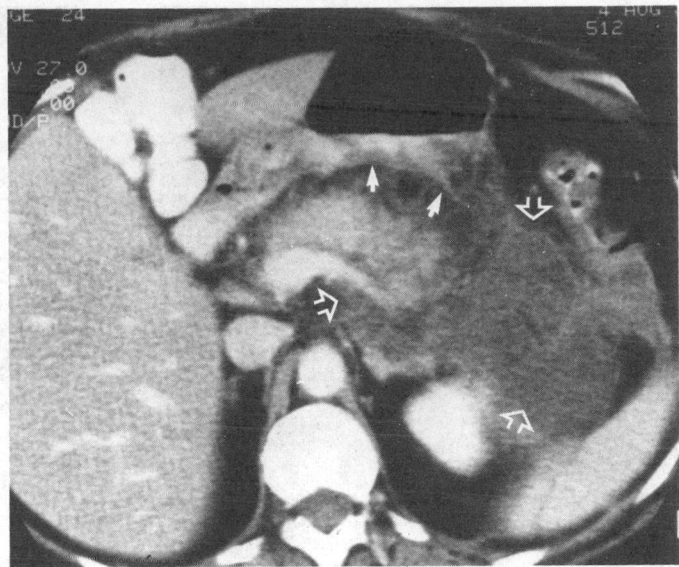

A

B

FIGURE 260-1 Acute pancreatitis: CT evolution. *A*. This contrast-enhanced CT scan of the abdomen was performed on the day of admission on a patient with clinical evidence of acute pancreatitis. Note the mildly decreased density of the body of the pancreas to the left of the midline (arrow). There are a few linear strands in the peripancreatic fat, suggesting inflammation (open arrows). A small amount of fluid is seen in the anterior pararenal space (arrowhead). *B*. Nine days after admission, there is a marked worsening with severe inflammation of the pancreas evidenced by anterior displacement of the posterior gastric wall (arrows), increased inflammation of the peripancreatic fat, and increased pancreatic effusion in the anterior perirenal space and around the splenic vein (open arrows). (*Courtesy of Dr. P.R. Ros, University of Florida College of Medicine.*)

be secondarily infected, resulting in abscess formation. The latter occurs in 10 percent of patients with acute pancreatitis. The early diagnosis of pancreatic infection can be accomplished by CT-guided needle aspiration. In one study, 60 patients, representing 5 percent of all admissions for acute pancreatitis, were suspected of harboring a pancreatic infection on the basis of fever, leukocytosis, and an abnormal CT scan (phlegmon, pseudocyst, or extrapancreatic fluid collection). Importantly, 36 of 60 patients (60 percent) had a pancreatic infection with 20 of the 36 (55 percent) developing infection within the first 2 weeks. This study suggests that only guided aspiration can reliably distinguish sterile from infected pancreatitis. The following are guidelines for patients meeting the above selection criteria: (1) pseudocysts and phlegmons should be aspirated promptly because more than half could be infected; (2) extrapancreatic fluid collections need not be aspirated promptly as most are sterile; (3) if a phlegmon is found initially to be sterile but fever and leukocytosis persist, allow several days of observation before considering reaspiration, as clinical improvement frequently occurs; and (4) if fever and leukocytosis recur after an interval of well-being, consider reaspiration.

Severe pancreatitis with the presence of three or more risk factors, postoperative pancreatitis, early oral feeding, early laparotomy, and perhaps injudicious use of antibiotics predispose to the development of pancreatic abscess. Pancreatic abscess may also develop because of communication of a pseudocyst with the colon, after inadequate surgical drainage of a pseudocyst, or after needling of a pseudocyst. The characteristic signs of abscess are fever, leukocytosis, ileus, and rapid deterioration in a patient initially recovering from pancreatitis. However, the only manifestations may be persistent fever and signs of continuing pancreatic inflammation. Drainage of pancreatic abscesses by nonsurgical percutaneous catheter techniques, using CT guidance, has been only moderately successful (resolution in 50 to 60 percent of patients). Accordingly, laparotomy with radical sump drainage and possibly resection of necrotic tissue is usually required because the mortality rate for undrained pancreatic abscess approaches 100 percent. Multiple abscesses are common and reoperation is frequently required.

Pseudocysts of the pancreas are collections of tissue, fluid, debris, pancreatic enzymes, and blood, which develop over a period of 1 to 4 weeks after the onset of acute pancreatitis in approximately 15 percent of patients. In contrast to true cysts, pseudocysts do not have epithelial lining and the walls consist of necrotic tissue, granulation tissue, and fibrous tissue. Disruption of the pancreatic ductal system is common. However, the subsequent course of this disruption varies widely, namely, from spontaneous healing to continuous leakage of pancreatic juice causing tense ascites. Pseudocysts are preceded by pancreatitis in 90 percent of cases and by trauma in 10 percent. Approximately 85 percent are located in the body or tail of the pancreas and 15 percent in the head. Some patients have two or more pseudocysts. Abdominal pain, with or without radiation to the back, is the usual presenting complaint. A palpable, tender mass may be found in the middle or left upper abdomen. The serum amylase is elevated in 75 percent of patients some time during their illness and may fluctuate markedly.

Pseudocysts often displace some portion of the gastrointestinal tract on x-ray examination in 75 percent of cases (Fig. 260-2). Sonography, however, is reliable in detecting pseudocysts. Sonography also permits differentiation between an edematous and an inflamed pancreas (pancreatic phlegmon), which can give rise to a palpable mass and an actual pseudocyst. Furthermore, serial ultrasound studies will indicate whether a pseudocyst has resolved. CT scanning complements the use of ultrasound in the diagnosis of pancreatic pseudocyst (Fig. 260-2), especially when it is infected.

The management of pseudocysts is compromised by incomplete knowledge of the natural history of this disorder. In studies utilizing sonography, pseudocysts resolved in 25 to 40 percent of patients. However, pseudocysts that are greater than 5 cm and that persist for greater than 6 weeks rarely disappear. In others, serious complications may occur such as (1) pain caused by expansion of the lesion and pressure on other viscera, (2) rupture, (3) hemorrhage, and (4) abscess. Rupture of a pancreatic pseudocyst is a particularly serious complication. Shock almost always supervenes and mortality rates range from 14 percent if the rupture is not associated with hemorrhage to over 60 percent if hemorrhage has occurred. Rupture and hemorrhage are the prime causes of mortality in pancreatic pseudocyst. A triad of findings, e.g., increase in size of the mass, localized bruit over the mass, and a sudden decrease in hemoglobin and hematocrit levels without obvious signs of external blood loss, should alert one to the diagnosis of hemorrhage from a pseudocyst. Thus, in pseudocyst

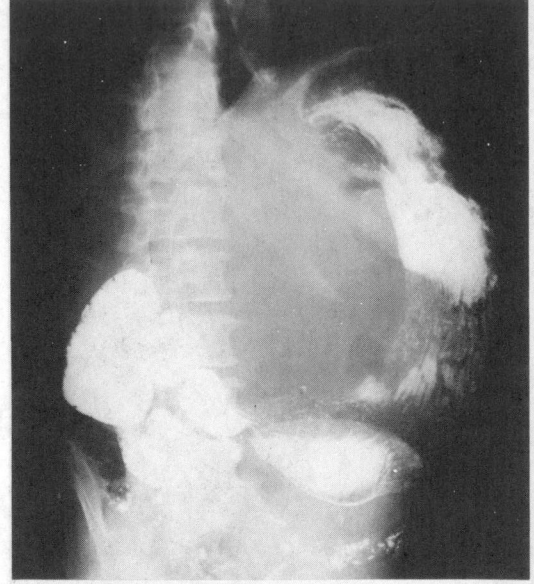

A

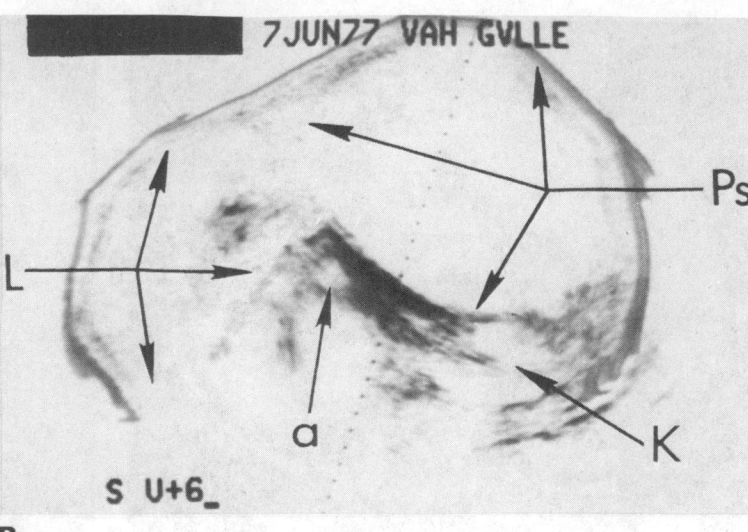

B

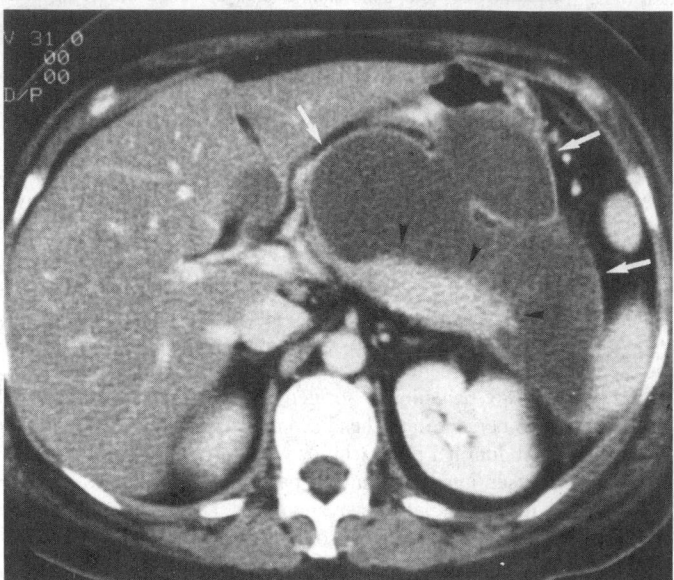

C

FIGURE 260-2   Pseudocyst of the pancreas. *A.* Upper gastrointestinal x-ray showing displacement of stomach by pseudocyst. *B.* Sonogram showing pseudocyst (Ps). K = kidney; a = aorta; L = liver. *C.* CT scan showing pseudocyst. Note a large lobulated fluid collection (arrows) surrounding the tail of the pancreas (arrowheads). Note the dense, thin rim in the periphery representing the fibrous capsule of the pseudocyst. (*Courtesy of Dr. P. R. Ros, University of Florida College of Medicine.*)

demonstrate passage of contrast material from a major pancreatic duct or a pseudocyst into the peritoneal cavity. As many as 15 percent of patients with pseudocysts have concurrent pancreatic ascites. The differential diagnosis should include intraperitoneal carcinomatosis, tuberculous peritonitis, constrictive pericarditis, and Budd-Chiari syndrome.

If the pancreatic duct disruption is posterior, an internal fistula may develop between the pancreatic duct and pleural space producing a pleural effusion, which is usually left-sided and often massive. This often requires thoracentesis or chest tube drainage.

Treatment usually involves placing the patient on nasogastric suction and parenteral alimentation to decrease pancreatic secretion. In addition, paracentesis is performed to keep the peritoneal cavity free of fluid and, it is hoped, effect sealing of the leak. If ascites continues to recur after 2 to 3 weeks of medical management, the patient should be operated on following pancreatography to define the anatomy of the abnormal duct.

patients who are stable and uncomplicated and in whom serial ultrasound studies show a decreasing pseudocyst, conservative therapy is indicated. Conversely, patients with a pseudocyst which is expanding and which is complicated by rupture, hemorrhage, and abscess should be operated on. Using ultrasound or CT guidance, sterile chronic pseudocysts can be treated safely with single or repeated needle aspiration or more prolonged catheter drainage with an expected success rate of 45 to 75 percent. The success rate with infected pseudocysts is considerably less, i.e., 40 to 50 percent. Patients not responding to drainage require surgical therapy. Therapy consists of internal or external drainage of the cyst. Prolonged observation of a nonresolving pancreatic pseudocyst exposes the patient to increased risks which exceed those of elective surgery.

PANCREATIC ASCITES AND PANCREATIC PLEURAL EFFU-SIONS Pancreatic ascites is usually due to disruption of the main pancreatic duct, often associated with an internal fistula between the duct and the peritoneal cavity or a leaking pseudocyst (see also Chap. 48). The diagnosis of pancreatic ascites is suggested in a patient with an elevated serum amylase who also has increased levels of albumin [>30 g/L (>3.0 g/dL)] and amylase in the ascitic fluid. In addition, endoscopic retrograde cholangiopancreatography (ERCP) will often

CHRONIC PANCREATITIS AND PANCREATIC EXOCRINE INSUFFICIENCY

GENERAL AND ETIOLOGIC CONSIDERATIONS Chronic inflammatory disease of the pancreas may present as episodes of acute inflammation superimposed upon a previously injured pancreas or as chronic damage with persistent pain or malabsorption. The causes of relapsing chronic pancreatitis are similar to those of acute pancreatitis (Table 260-2), except that frequently there is an appreciable incidence of cases of undetermined origin. In addition, the pancreatitis associated with gallstones is predominantly acute or relapsing acute in nature. A cholecystectomy is almost always performed in patients after the first or second attack of gallstone-associated pancreatitis. Patients with chronic pancreatitis may present with persistent abdominal pain, with or without steatorrhea, and some may present with steatorrhea and no pain.

Patients with chronic pancreatitis who develop extensive destruction of the pancreas (i.e., less than 10 percent of exocrine function remaining) will demonstrate steatorrhea and azotorrhea. In the adult in the United States, alcoholism is the most common cause of clinically apparent pancreatic exocrine insufficiency, while cystic

TABLE 260-4 Causes of pancreatic exocrine insufficiency

 I Alcohol, chronic alcoholism
 II Cystic fibrosis
 III Severe protein calorie malnutrition with hypoalbuminemia
 IV Pancreatic and duodenal neoplasms
 V Pancreatic resection
 VI Gastric surgery
   A Subtotal gastrectomy with Billroth II anastomosis
   B Subtotal gastrectomy with Billroth I anastomosis
   C Truncal vagotomy and pyloroplasty
 VII Gastrinoma (Zollinger-Ellison syndrome)
 VIII Hereditary pancreatitis
 IX Traumatic pancreatitis
 X Hemochromatosis
 XI Shwachman's syndrome (pancreatic insufficiency and bone marrow dysfunction)
 XII Trypsinogen deficiency
 XIII Enterokinase deficiency
 XIV Isolated deficiencies of amylase, lipase, or proteases
 XV Alpha$_1$-antitrypsin deficiency
 XVI Idiopathic pancreatitis

fibrosis is the most frequent cause in children. In up to 25 percent of adults in the United States with chronic pancreatitis, the cause is not known, i.e., they have idiopathic chronic pancreatitis. In other parts of the world, severe protein calorie malnutrition is a common etiology. Table 260-4 lists other causes of pancreatic exocrine insufficiency, but they are relatively uncommon.

PATHOPHYSIOLOGY Unfortunately, the events that initiate an inflammatory process within the pancreas are still not well understood, and the many hypotheses will not be reviewed. In the case of alcohol-induced pancreatitis, however, it has been suggested that the primary defect may be the precipitation of protein (inspissated enzymes) within the ducts. The resulting ductal obstruction can lead to duct dilatation, diffuse atrophy of the acinar cells, fibrosis, and eventual calcification of some of the protein plugs. While patients with alcohol-induced pancreatitis generally consume large amounts of alcohol, some consume very little (i.e., 50 g or less per day). Thus, prolonged consumption of "socially acceptable" amounts of alcohol is compatible with the development of pancreatitis. In addition, the finding of extensive pancreatic fibrosis in patients who have expired during their first attack of clinical acute alcohol-induced pancreatitis supports the concept that such patients already have chronic pancreatitis.

CLINICAL FEATURES Patients with relapsing chronic pancreatitis may present with symptoms identical with those found in acute pancreatitis, but their pain may be continuous or intermittent, or pain may be absent. The pathogenesis of this pain is poorly understood. Although the classic description is that of epigastric pain radiating through the back, the pain pattern is often atypical. The pain may be maximal in the right or left upper quadrants in the back or diffuse throughout the upper abdomen; it may even be referred to the anterior chest or flank. Characteristically, the pain is persistent, deep-seated, and unresponsive to antacids. It often is increased by alcohol and ingestion of heavy meals (especially foods rich in fat). Often the pain is so severe as to require the frequent use of narcotics.

Weight loss, abnormal stools, and other signs of symptoms suggestive of malabsorption (see Table 240-5) are common in chronic pancreatitis. However, clinically apparent deficiencies of fat-soluble vitamins are surprisingly rare. The physical findings in these patients are usually not impressive such that there is a disparity between the severity of the abdominal pain and the paucity of physical signs (save some abdominal tenderness and mild temperature elevation).

DIAGNOSTIC EVALUATION (See Chap. 259) In contrast to patients with relapsing acute pancreatitis, the serum amylase and lipase levels are usually not elevated. Elevations of the serum bilirubin and alkaline phosphatase may indicate cholestasis secondary to chronic inflammation around the common bile duct (Fig. 260-3). Many patients demonstrate impaired glucose tolerance, and some may have an elevated fasting blood glucose level.

The classic triad of pancreatic calcification, steatorrhea, and diabetes mellitus usually establishes the diagnosis of chronic pancreatitis and exocrine pancreatic insufficiency but is found in less than one-third of chronic pancreatitis patients. Accordingly, it is often necessary to perform an intubation test such as the *secretin stimulation test*, which usually becomes abnormal when 70 percent or more of pancreatic exocrine function has been lost. Approximately 40 percent of patients with chronic pancreatitis have *cobalamin (vitamin B$_{12}$) malabsorption* which is corrected by the administration of oral pancreatic enzymes. There is usually a marked excretion of fecal fat (see Chap. 240), which can be reduced with the administration of oral pancreatic enzymes. A fecal fat concentration ≥9.5 percent is characteristic of pancreatogenous steatorrhea (see Table 259-1). The bentiromide test (Chap. 259) and D-xylose urinary excretion test are useful in patients with "pancreatic steatorrhea," since the bentiromide test will be abnormal and the D-xylose excretion usually normal. A decreased serum trypsinogen strongly suggests pancreatic exocrine insufficiency.

The radiographic hallmark of chronic pancreatitis is the presence of scattered calcification throughout the pancreas (Fig. 260-3). Diffuse pancreatic calcification indicates that significant damage has occurred and obviates the need for a secretin test. Alcohol is by far the most common cause of pancreatic calcification, but it may also be seen in severe protein-calorie malnutrition, hereditary pancreatitis, posttraumatic pancreatitis, hyperparathyroidism, islet cell tumors, and idiopathic chronic pancreatitis. An ongoing prospective study of 107 patients has shown convincingly that pancreatic calcification may decrease or even disappear either following ductal decompression or spontaneously in one-third of patients with severe chronic pancreatitis. Pancreatic calcification is a dynamic process that is incompletely understood.

Special techniques such as sonography, CT scanning, and ERCP have added new dimensions to the diagnosis of pancreatic disease. In addition to excluding pseudocysts and pancreatic cancer, sonography may show calcification or dilated ducts associated with chronic pancreatitis (Fig. 260-4). Similar benefits can be derived from CT scans. ERCP is the only nonoperative technique which provides a direct view of the pancreatic duct. In patients with alcohol-induced pancreatitis, ERCP may reveal a pseudocyst missed by sonography or CT scan.

COMPLICATIONS OF CHRONIC PANCREATITIS The complications of chronic pancreatitis are protean. *Cobalamin (vitamin B$_{12}$) malabsorption* occurs in 40 percent of patients with alcohol-induced chronic pancreatitis and in virtually all with cystic fibrosis. The cobalamin malabsorption is consistently corrected by the administration of pancreatic enzymes (containing proteases). The cobalamin malabsorption may be due to excessive binding of cobalamin by nonintrinsic factor cobalamin-binding proteins. The latter are ordinarily destroyed by pancreatic proteases, but with pancreatic insufficiency the nonspecific binding proteins escape degradation and compete with intrinsic factor for cobalamin binding. Although the majority of patients show *impaired glucose tolerance*, the development of diabetic ketoacidosis and coma is uncommon. Similarly, end organ damage (retinopathy, neuropathy, nephropathy) is also uncommon, and the appearance of these complications should raise the question of concomitant genetic diabetes mellitus. A nondiabetic retinopathy, peripheral in location and secondary to vitamin A and/or zinc deficiency, is common in these patients. High-amylase-containing *effusions* occur within the pleura, pericardium, or peritoneum. *Gastrointestinal bleeding* may occur from a peptic ulcer, gastritis, a pseudocyst eroding into the duodenum, or from ruptured varices secondary to splenic vein thrombosis due to inflammation of the tail of the pancreas. *Icterus* may occur, owing to either edema of the head of the pancreas compressing the common bile duct or chronic cholestasis secondary to chronic inflammatory reaction around the intrapancreatic portion of the common bile duct (Fig. 260-3). This chronic obstruction may lead to cholangitis and ultimately biliary cirrhosis. *Subcutaneous fat necrosis* may appear as tender red nodules on the lower extremities. *Bone pain* may be secondary to intramedullary fat necrosis. Inflammation of the large and small joints of the

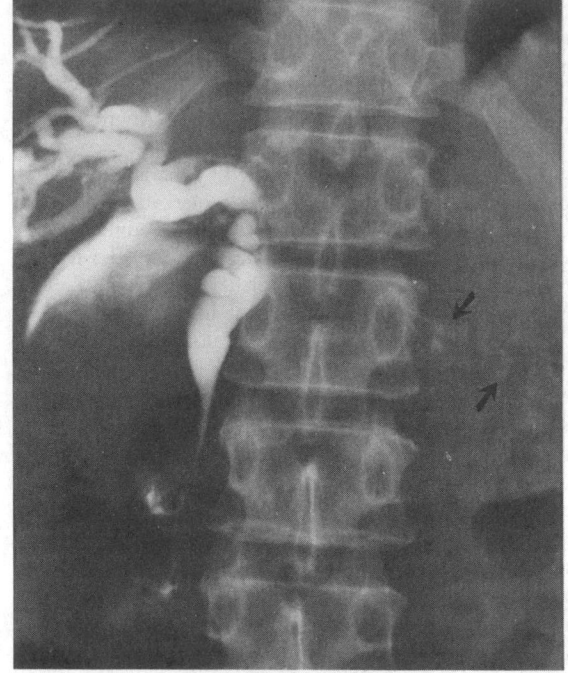

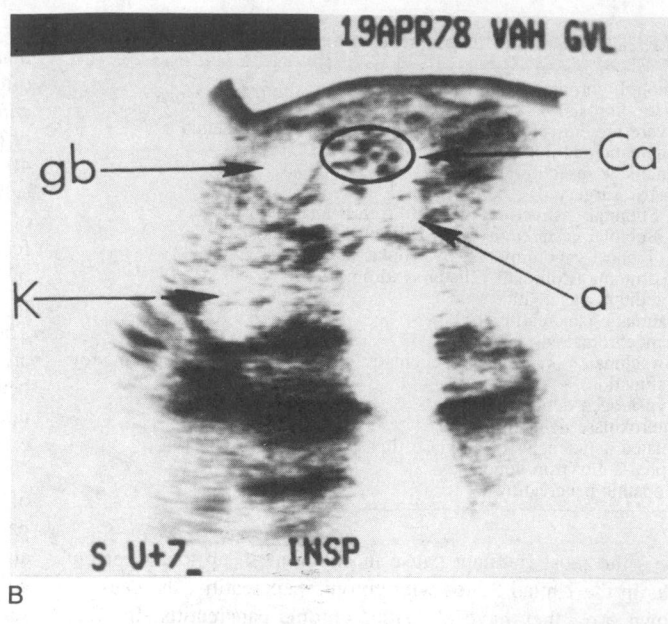

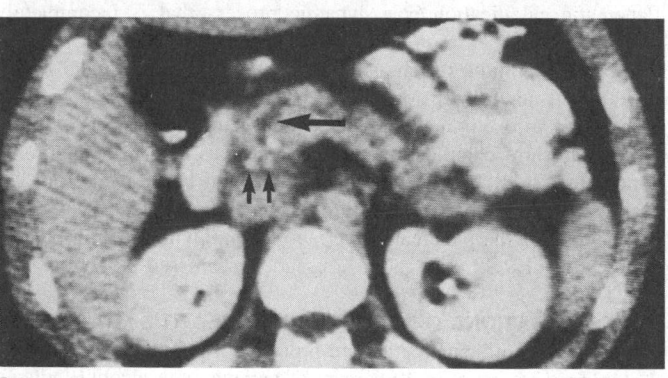

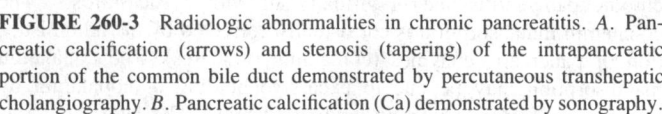

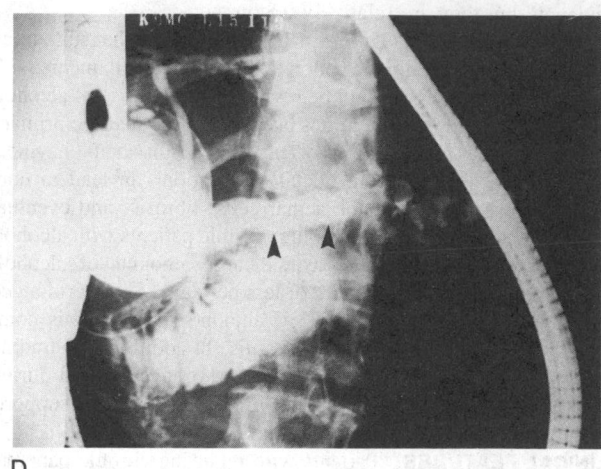

FIGURE 260-3 Radiologic abnormalities in chronic pancreatitis. *A*. Pancreatic calcification (arrows) and stenosis (tapering) of the intrapancreatic portion of the common bile duct demonstrated by percutaneous transhepatic cholangiography. *B*. Pancreatic calcification (Ca) demonstrated by sonography. gb = gallbladder; K = kidney; a = aorta. *C*. Pancreatic calcification (vertical arrows) and dilated pancreatic duct (horizontal arrow) demonstrated by CT scan. D. Endoscopic retrograde cholangiopancreatogram shows grossly dilated pancreatic ducts (arrows) in a patient with long-standing pancreatitis.

upper and lower extremities may occur. The incidence of pancreatic carcinoma is probably increased in patients with diffuse calcification. Perhaps the most common and troublesome complication is addiction to narcotics.

TREATMENT AND APPROACH TO MANAGEMENT Therapy for patients with chronic pancreatitis is directed to two major problems, namely, pain and malabsorption. Patients with intermittent attacks of pain are essentially treated like those with acute pancreatitis (see above). Patients with severe and persistent pain should avoid alcohol completely and avoid large meals rich in fat. Since the pain is often severe enough to require frequent use of narcotics (and hence addiction), a number of surgical procedures have been developed for pain relief. ERCP allows the surgeon to plan the operative approach. If there is a stricture of the pancreatic duct, then a *local resection* may ameliorate the pain. Unfortunately isolated localized strictures are not common. In most patients with alcohol-induced disease, the pancreas is diffusely involved and surgically correctible localized ductal disease is rare. When there is primary ductal obstruction and dilatation, ductal decompression may provide effective pain palliation. Short-term pain relief may be achieved in up to 80 percent of patients,

while long-term pain relief occurs in approximately 50 percent. In some of these patients, however, pain relief can be achieved only by resecting 50 to 95 percent of the gland. Although pain relief is achieved in three-quarters of these patients, they tend to develop pancreatic endocrine and exocrine insufficiency and must be on pancreatic enzyme replacement therapy. It is important to screen the patients carefully, for such radical surgery is contraindicated in those who are severely depressed or suicidal or continue to drink. Procedures such as sphincteroplasty, splanchnicectomy and celiac ganglionectomy, and nerve blocks usually bring only temporary relief and are not recommended.

Two double-blind controlled trials have demonstrated that large doses of conventional pancreatic enzymes (eight tablets with each meal and at bedtime) decrease the abdominal pain in patients with chronic pancreatitis. The patients most likely to respond to such therapy with amelioration of pain are those with mild to moderate exocrine pancreatic dysfunction as evidenced by an abnormal secretin test, normal fat absorption, and minimal abnormalities upon ERCP examination. These clinical observations seem to fit in with data in human beings and experimental animals which demonstrate a negative

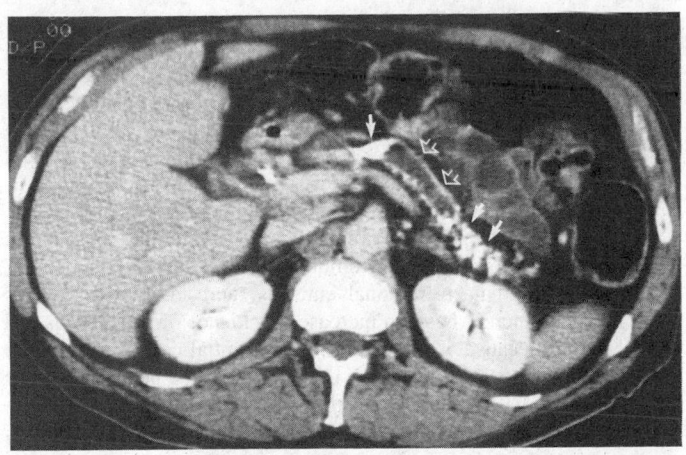

A

FIGURE 260-4 Chronic pancreatitis and pancreatic calculi: CT scan and ERCP appearance. *A.* In this contrast-enhanced CT scan of the abdomen, there is evidence of an atrophic pancreas with multiple calcifications (arrows). Note a markedly dilated pancreatic duct seen in this section through the body and tail (open arrows). *B.* ERCP in the same patient demonstrates the dilated pancreatic duct as well as an intrapancreatic duct calculus (arrows). These findings correlate nicely with the CT scan appearance.

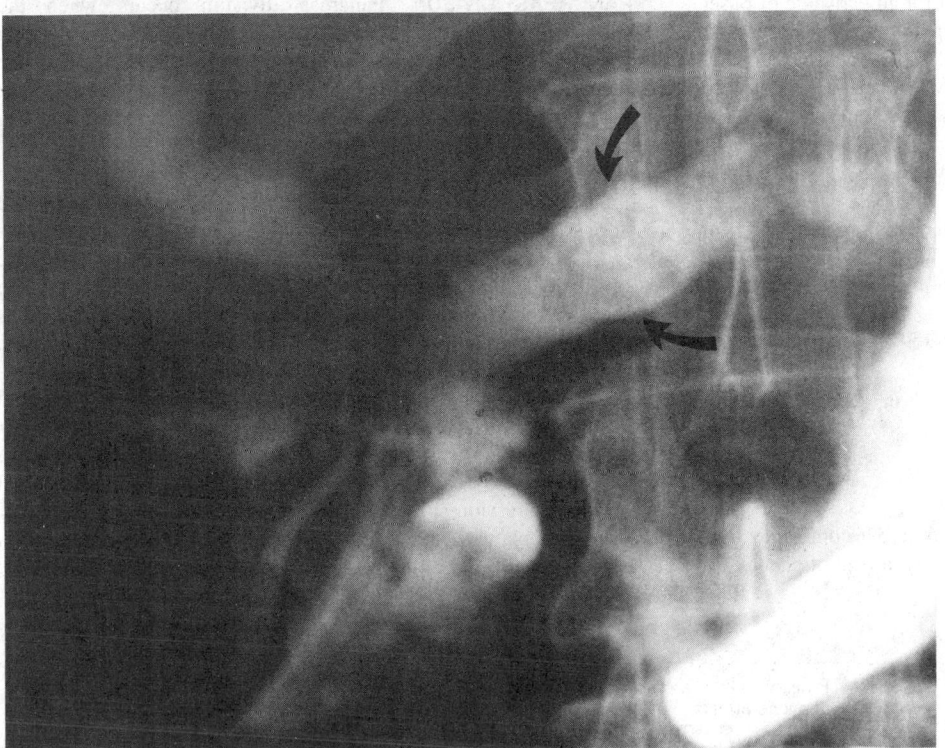

B

feedback regulation for pancreatic exocrine secretion controlled by the amount of proteases within the lumen of the proximal small intestine. It seems reasonable to approach the patient with severe persistent or continuous abdominal pain thought to be secondary to chronic pancreatitis in the following manner. After other causes of abdominal pain (peptic ulcer, gallstones, etc.) have been appropriately excluded, a pancreatic *sonogram* should be done. If no mass is found, a *secretin test* may be performed, since with chronic pancreatitis and pain this test usually will be abnormal. If the secretin test is abnormal (i.e., decreased bicarbonate concentration or volume output), a 3- to 4-week *trial of pancreatic enzymes* is appropriate. Eight conventional tablets or three enteric-coated capsules are taken at meals and at bedtime. If no relief is obtained, and especially if the volume secreted during the secretin test is very low, ERCP should be performed. If a pseudocyst or a localized ductal obstruction is found, appropriate surgery should be considered. A provocative study from South Africa questions the significance of the relationship of dilated ducts and/or strictures to pain. The finding of an appreciable obstruction or stricture in 65 percent of the patients who were pain-free more than 1 year, compared with 79 percent of the group with pain, suggests that factors other than duct obstruction or narrowing may be important in the pathogenesis of pain. It may be that the most important factors

in the relief of pain are abstinence from alcohol and progressive pancreatic dysfunction rather than the surgical procedure per se. If no surgically remedial lesion is found and severe pain continues despite abstinence from alcohol, subtotal pancreatic resection may be necessary.

The treatment of malabsorption rests upon the use of pancreatic enzyme replacement therapy. Although diarrhea and steatorrhea are usually improved, the results are frequently less than satisfactory. The major problem is delivery of enough active enzyme into the duodenum. Steatorrhea can be abolished if 10 percent of the normal amount of lipase could be delivered into the duodenum at the proper time. This concentration of lipase cannot be achieved with the presently available preparations of pancreatic enzymes, even if the latter are given in large doses. These poor results may be due to inactivation of lipase by gastric acid, food emptying from the stomach more rapidly than the exogenously administered pancreatic enzymes, and variation in the enzyme activity of various batches of commercially available pancreatic extracts.

For the usual patient three to eight tablets or capsules of a potent enzyme preparation should be administered with meals. Some patients on conventional tablets require adjuvant therapy to improve enzyme replacement treatment. Although initially cimetidine was considered an effective adjuvant, studies have failed to confirm this. Sodium bicarbonate (1.3 g with meals) is effective and inexpensive. Antacids containing calcium carbonate or magnesium hydroxide are not effective and may actually result in increased steatorrhea. Adjuvant therapy should not be given with enteric-coated microsphere preparations because such therapy may increase the gastric pH such that these preparations would release their enzymes into the stomach rather than the small intestine.

Patients with severe exocrine pancreatic insufficiency secondary to alcohol who continue to drink have a high mortality (in one series 50 percent were dead when followed for 5 to 12 years) and significant morbidity (weight loss, lassitude, vitamin deficiency, and narcotic addiction). Pain may abate if progressive severe exocrine insufficiency continues. If abstinence is pursued and vigorous replacement therapy is utilized for the maldigestion-malabsorption, the patients do reasonably well.

HEREDITARY PANCREATITIS   Hereditary pancreatitis is a rare disease similar to chronic pancreatitis except for an early age of onset and evidence of hereditary factors (involving an autosomal dominant gene with incomplete penetrance). These patients have recurring attacks of severe abdominal pain which may last from a few days to a few weeks. The serum amylase and lipase levels may be elevated during acute attacks but are usually normal. Patients frequently develop pancreatic calcification, diabetes mellitus, and steatorrhea, and in addition, they have an increased incidence of pancreatic carcinoma. Such patients often require ductal decompression to obtain pain relief. Abdominal complaints in relatives of patients with hereditary pancreatitis should raise the question of pancreatic disease.

PANCREATIC ENDOCRINE TUMORS

Pancreatic endocrine tumors are summarized in Table 260-5 and discussed in Chap. 262.

OTHER CONDITIONS

ANNULAR PANCREAS   When there is a failure in communication of the ventral and dorsal anlage of the pancreas, a ring of pancreatic tissue encircles the duodenum. Such an annular pancreas may cause intestinal obstruction in the neonate or the adult. Symptoms of postprandial fullness, epigastric pain, nausea, and vomiting may be present for years before the diagnosis is entertained. The radiographic findings are symmetric dilatation of the proximal duodenum with bulging of the recesses on either side of the annular band, effacement of the duodenal mucosa without destruction of the mucosa, accentuation of the findings in the right anterior oblique position, and the lack of change on repeated examinations. The differential diagnosis should include duodenal webs, tumors of the pancreas or duodenum, postbulbar peptic ulcer, regional enteritis, and adhesions. Patients with annular pancreas have an increased incidence of pancreatitis and peptic ulcer. Because of these and other potential complications, the treatment is surgical even though the condition has been present for years. Retrocolic duodenojejunostomy is the procedure of choice, although some surgeons advocate Billroth II gastrectomy, gastroenterostomy, and vagotomy.

PANCREAS DIVISUM   Pancreas divisum occurs when the embryologic ventral and dorsal parts of the pancreas fail to fuse so that pancreatic drainage is accomplished mainly through the accessory papilla. Pancreas divisum is the most common congenital anatomic variant of the human pancreas. Current evidence indicates that this anomaly is not a predisposing factor to the development of pancreatitis in the great majority of patients with this anomaly. However, the combination of pancreas divisum and a small accessory orifice could result in dorsal duct obstruction. The challenge is to identify this subset of patients with dorsal duct pathology. Cannulation of the dorsal duct by ERCP is not as easily done as is cannulation of the ventral duct (Fig. 260-5). Patients with pancreatitis and pancreas divisum demonstrated by ERCP should be treated with conservative measures including pancreatic enzyme therapy. Many of these patients have idiopathic pancreatitis unrelated to the pancreas divisum and will respond well to pancreatic enzyme therapy. Endoscopic or surgical intervention is indicated only when the above methods fail. If marked dilation of the dorsal duct can be demonstrated, surgical ductal decompression should be performed. The appropriate therapy for those patients without dilation of the dorsal duct is not yet defined. It should be stressed that the ERCP appearance of pancreas divisum,

TABLE 260-5   Pancreatic endocrine tumors

Syndrome	Hormone(s) produced	Primary hormone effects	Pathologic features	Clinical features
Zollinger-Ellison	Gastrin	Gastric acid hypersecretion with basal acid outputs usually >15 mmol/h (>15 meq/h)	Delta cell islet tumors; 10% aberrant (duodenal); 60% malignant	Severe peptic ulcer disease often refractory to therapy; ectopic ulcers; diarrhea; multiple endocrine adenomas (parathyroid, pituitary, adrenal, thyroid)
Insulinoma	Insulin	Hypoglycemia with inappropriately increased serum insulin levels	Beta cell islet tumors; 80–90% benign	Hypoglycemic symptoms
Glucagonoma	Glucagon; pancreatic polypeptide	Hyperglucagonemia →glucose intolerance	Alpha cell islet tumors; 60% malignant	Slow-growing pancreatic tumor; hyperglycemia; bullous and eczematoid dermatitis, weight loss; anemia; gastric and intestinal motor abnormalities
Somatostatinoma	Somatostatin; pancreatic polypeptide	Somatostatin inhibits insulin, gastrin and pancreatic enzyme secretion; decreased bile flow	Delta cell islet tumor	Pancreatic tumor; diarrhea; steatorrhea; gallstones; diabetes mellitus; anemia
Pancreatic cholera	Vasoactive intestinal peptide (VIP) ? Gastric inhibitory polypeptide ? Prostaglandin E ? Pancreatic peptide	Net secretion of salt and water by gut	? Delta cell tumor; >50% malignant	Pancreatic tumor with severe watery diarrhea; flushing; weight loss; hypokalemia; hypercalcemia; hypochlorhydria; hyperglycemia; inordinate fecal water and electrolyte losses
Carcinoid	Serotonin; prostaglandins	Altered gut motility; diarrhea	Enterochromaffin cells; non-beta cell islet tumors	Carcinoid syndrome with flushing; wheezing; diarrhea; alcohol intolerance; hepatomegaly

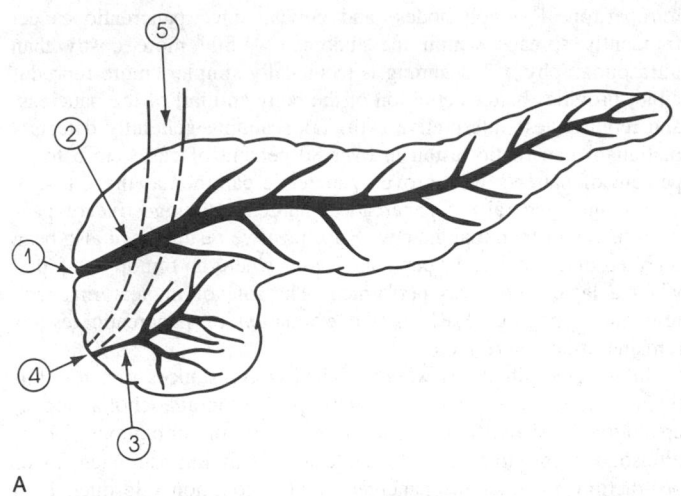

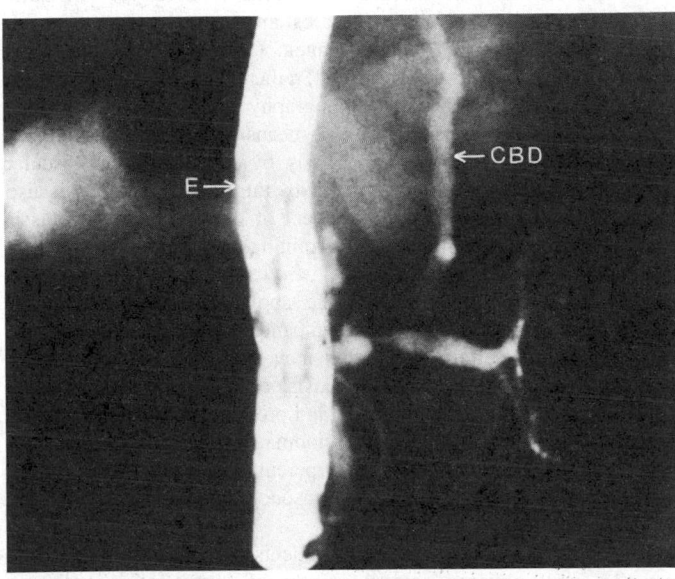

FIGURE 260-5 Illustration of the pancreatic ducts and typical ERCP of pancreas divisum. *A.* Diagram of the ventral and dorsal structures of the pancreas: (1) duct of Santorini; (2) pancreatic duct from the dorsal anlage; (3) pancreatic duct from the ventral anlage; (4) duct of Wirsung; and (5) common bile duct. *B.* ERCP showing filling only of the ventral component of the pancreatic duct and the common bile duct (CBD) from cannulization of the duct of Wirsung. Failure to fill the pancreatic duct of the body and tail of the pancreas is diagnostic of ventral pancreas or pancreas divisum. E = endoscope.

i.e., a small-caliber ventral duct with an arborizing pattern, may be confused with an obstructed main pancreatic duct secondary to a mass lesion.

MACROAMYLASEMIA Macroamylasemia is a condition whereby amylase is circulating in the blood in a polymer form too large to be easily excreted by the kidney. The patient with this condition will demonstrate an elevated serum amylase value, a low urinary amylase, and a C_{am}/C_{cr} of less than 1 percent. The presence of macroamylase can be documented by chromatography of the serum. The prevalence of macroamylasemia is 1.5 percent of the nonalcoholic general adult hospital population. Usually macroamylasemia is an incidental finding and is not related to disease of the pancreas or other organs. It is important to be aware of this condition so that patients with macroamylasemia will not be needlessly evaluated and treated for pancreatic disease.

REFERENCES

AMMANN RW et al: Evolution and regression of pancreatic calcification in chronic pancreatitis. A prospective long-term study of 107 patients. Gastroenterology 95:1018, 1988

BALTHAZAR EJ et al: Acute pancreatitis: Prognostic value of CT. Radiology 156:767, 1985

BLOCK H et al: Identification of pancreas necrosis in severe acute pancreatitis: Imaging procedures versus clinical staging. Gut 227:1035, 1986

CERZOF SG et al: Early diagnosis of pancreatic infection by computed tomography guided aspiration. Gastroenterology 93:1315, 1987

CHOI TK et al: Somatostatin in the treatment of acute pancreatitis: A prospective randomized trial. Gut 30:223, 1989

COTTON PB: Pancreas divisum. Pancreas 3:245, 1988

ECKFELDT JH et al: High prevalence of hyperamylasemia in patients with acidemia. Ann Intern Med 104:362, 1986

GARDNER JD, JENSEN RT: Gastrointestinal peptides: The basis of action at the cellular level, in *Recent Progress in Hormone Research*, vol 39. New York, Academic, 1983

GULLO L et al: Effect of cessation of alcohol use on the course of pancreatic dysfunction in alcoholic pancreatitis. Gastroenterology 95:1063, 1988

JACOBSON DG et al: Trypsin-like immunoreactivity as a test for pancreatic insufficiency. N Engl J Med 310:1307, 1984

KOLARS JC et al: Comparison of serum amylase, pancreatic isoamylase and lipase in patients with hyperamylasemia. Dig Dis Sci 29:289, 1984

LIENER IE et al: Effect of trypsin inhibitor from soybeans (Bowman-Birk) on the secretory activity of the human pancreas. Gastroenterology 94:419, 1988

MOOSSA AR: Surgical treatment of chronic pancreatitis: An overview. Br J Surg 74:661, 1987

NEOPTOLEMOS JP et al: Control trial of urgent endoscopic retrograde cholangiopancreatography and endoscopic sphincterotomy versus conservative treatment for acute pancreatitis due to gallstones. Lancet 2:979, 1988

NIEDERAU C, GRENDELL JH: Diagnosis of chronic pancreatitis. Gastroenterology 88:1973, 1985

RANSON JH-C: Risk factors in acute pancreatitis. Hosp Pract 20:69, 1985

SLAFF J et al: Protease specific suppression of pancreatic exocrine secretion. Gastroenterology 87:44, 1984

STEER ML et al: Pancreatitis. The role of lysosomes. Dig Dis Sci 29:934, 1984

STEWART AF et al: Hypocalcemia associated with calcium soap formation in a patient with a pancreatic fistula. N Engl J Med 315:496, 1986

TOSKES PP, GREENBERGER NJ: Acute and chronic pancreatitis. DM, vol 24, 1983

VAN DYKE JA et al: Pancreatic imaging. Ann Intern Med 102:212, 1985

VENTRUCCI M et al: Role of serum pancreatic assays in the diagnosis of pancreatic disease. Dig Dis Sci 34:39, 1989

261 PANCREATIC CANCER

ROBERT J. MAYER

INCIDENCE AND ETIOLOGY The incidence of pancreatic carcinoma in the United States has increased significantly as the median life expectancy of the American population has been prolonged. The tumor results in the death of more than 95 percent of afflicted patients. Approximately 25,000 individuals died of pancreatic cancer in 1989, making it the fifth most common cause of cancer-related mortality. The disease appears to occur somewhat more frequently in males than in females and in blacks than in whites. It rarely develops prior to the age of 50.

Little is known about the causes of pancreatic cancer. Cigarette smoking represents the most consistently observed risk factor for the development of the tumor, with the disease being two to three times more common in heavy smokers than in nonsmokers. It is uncertain whether this apparent association reflects a direct carcinogenic effect of metabolites of cigarette smoke on the pancreas or whether an as yet undefined exposure occurring more frequently in cigarette smokers is responsible for the enhanced risk. There are no convincing data to link such epidemiologic factors as alcohol abuse, chronic pancreatitis, cholelithiasis, or preexisting diabetes mellitus with the development of pancreatic cancer. Furthermore, the weight of clinical data has failed to support any association between coffee consumption and pancreatic cancer.

CLINICAL FEATURES More than 90 percent of pancreatic cancers are ductal adenocarcinomas, with islet cell tumors constituting

TABLE 261-1   Presenting signs and symptoms of pancreatic carcinoma

Frequent:
   Abdominal pain
   Weight loss
   Jaundice (lesions of pancreatic head only)
Infrequent:
   Glucose intolerance
   Palpable gallbladder
   Migratory thrombophlebitis
   Gastrointestinal hemorrhage
   Splenomegaly

the remaining 5 to 10 percent. Pancreatic cancers occur twice as frequently in the pancreatic head (about 70 percent of cases) as in the body (about 20 percent) or tail (about 10 percent) of the gland.

With the exception of jaundice, the initial symptoms associated with pancreatic cancer are often insidious in nature and are usually present for longer than 2 months prior to the time the cancer is diagnosed (Table 261-1). Pain and weight loss are present in more than 75 percent of patients. The pain typically has a gnawing, visceral quality, occasionally radiating from the epigastrium to the back, and generally representing a more severe problem in lesions arising in the body or tail since such tumors may become quite large prior to being detected. Characteristically, the pain improves somewhat on bending forward. The development of significant pain is suggestive of retroperitoneal invasion and infiltration of the splanchnic nerves, indicating the primary lesion to be far advanced and surgically unresectable. The weight loss observed in the majority of patients having pancreatic carcinoma is primarily the result of anorexia, although in the initial period of the disease, subclinical malabsorption may also be a contributing factor.

Jaundice due to biliary obstruction is found in more than 80 percent of patients having tumors in the pancreatic head and is typically accompanied by darkening of urine, a claylike appearance of stool, and pruritus. In contrast to the "painless jaundice" sometimes observed in patients having carcinomas of the bile ducts, duodenum, or periampullary regions, the majority of icteric individuals having ductal carcinomas of the pancreatic head will complain of significant abdominal discomfort. Although the gallbladder is usually enlarged in patients with carcinoma of the head of the pancreas, it is palpable in less than 50 percent of cases (Courvoisier's sign). The presence, however, of an enlarged gallbladder in a jaundiced patient without biliary colic should suggest malignant obstruction of the extrahepatic biliary tree.

The vast majority of patients with pancreatic cancer do not develop clinical diabetes mellitus; in one study, glucose intolerance was found in only 6 percent of a group of 924 patients whose presenting symptoms were carefully analyzed. Other uncommon initial manifestations include venous thrombosis and migratory thrombophlebitis, gastrointestinal hemorrhage resulting from varices due to tumor compression of the portal venous system, and splenomegaly caused by cancerous encasement of the splenic vein.

DIAGNOSTIC PROCEDURES (Fig. 261-1) Despite the availability of serologic tests for tumor-associated antigens such as the carcinoembryonic antigen (CEA) and CA 19-9 and noninvasive imaging techniques such as CT scanning and ultrasonography, the early diagnosis of a potentially resectable pancreatic carcinoma remains extremely difficult. The nonspecificity of the initial symptoms and the poor sensitivity of both serologic assays and noninvasive techniques have frustrated the development of effective screening procedures. When the disease is clinically suspected in a patient having vague, persistent abdominal complaints, an ultrasound to visualize the gallbladder as well as the pancreas should be performed as well as upper GI contrast radiographs to rule out the presence of a hiatal hernia or a peptic ulcer. If these studies fail to provide an explanation for the symptoms, a CT scan should be considered. Such a scan should encompass not only the pancreas but also the liver,

retroperitoneal lymph nodes, and pelvis, since pancreatic cancer frequently spreads within the abdomen. While more costly than ultrasonography, CT scanning is technically simpler, more reproducible, provides better definition of the body and tail of the pancreas, and requires less interpretive skill. CT scanning generally detects a malignant pancreatic lesion in over 80 percent of cases; in 5 to 15 percent of patients with proven pancreatic carcinoma, the CT scan shows only generalized pancreatic enlargement suggestive of pancreatitis rather than malignancy. False-positive results have also been reported in about 5 to 10 percent of cases where no tumor was found when a laparotomy was performed. The role of nuclear magnetic resonance imaging (MRI) in the evaluation of pancreatic lesions remains to be determined.

In selected situations where clinical circumstances dictate additional diagnostic evaluation, endoscopic retrograde cholangiopancreatography (ERCP) may clarify the cause of ambiguous CT or ultrasonographic findings. The characteristic findings are stenosis or obstruction of either the pancreatic or the common bile duct; both duct systems are abnormal in over half the cases. The differentiation between carcinoma and chronic pancreatitis by ERCP can be quite difficult, particularly if both diseases are present. False-negative results with ERCP are quite infrequent (less than 5 percent) and usually occur in the setting of islet cell, rather than ductal, carcinomas.

Selective and superselective angiography may be of value in some patients. Angiography is an effective means of detecting carcinomas in the body and tail of the pancreas by demonstrating vascular narrowing, displacement, or occlusion by tumor. Angiography is also useful in assessing whether encasement of peripancreatic vessels is present; this is of importance in determining the potential for surgical resection.

Regardless of the results of the above diagnostic studies, a histologic confirmation of a presumed pancreatic cancer is mandatory to be absolutely certain that malignancy exists and to rule out the presence of such other neoplasms as an islet cell tumor or a lymphoma, for which the therapeutic approach and prognosis differ significantly from those for the usual ductal carcinoma. Such tissue confirmation may often be obtained through a percutaneous needle aspiration biopsy of the pancreas with CT or ultrasonographic guidance, thereby obviating surgical exploration.

It should be emphasized that patients with carcinoma of the pancreas may undergo several months of investigation before a diagnosis is established. In the past, this period of diagnostic delay and accompanying emotional uncertainty erroneously led to an impression that the pain and weight loss might not have had an organic cause, resulting in an association of pancreatic cancer and depression. The availability of CT scans has resulted in a prompter diagnosis and dispelled this incorrect notion. Unfortunately, however, even laparotomy may not provide a definitive diagnosis, because chronic pancreatitis may also produce a hard mass in the head of the pancreas, making it indistinguishable from carcinoma by palpation. Furthermore, a superficial biopsy of such a mass may not show neoplastic tissue, revealing only evidence of pancreatitis since the cancer itself is often surrounded by edematous, inflamed, and fibrotic tissue (i.e., changes associated with chronic pancreatitis).

TREATMENT Complete surgical resection of pancreatic tumors offers the only effective treatment for this disease. Unfortunately, such "curative" operations are only possible in 10 to 15 percent of patients with pancreatic cancer and are limited, for all practical purposes, to those individuals having tumors in the pancreatic head in whom jaundice was the initial symptom. Patients considered for such a procedure should have no evidence of metastatic spread on a chest radiogram and abdominal-pelvic CT scan, should undergo preoperative celiac angiography (to exclude evidence of surgical unresectability such as vascular invasion by tumor), and should involve care by an experienced surgeon, since mortality rates of greater than 15 percent have been associated with this procedure. Although the potential for cure in patients with pancreatic cancer is restricted to those few who are able to undergo a complete surgical

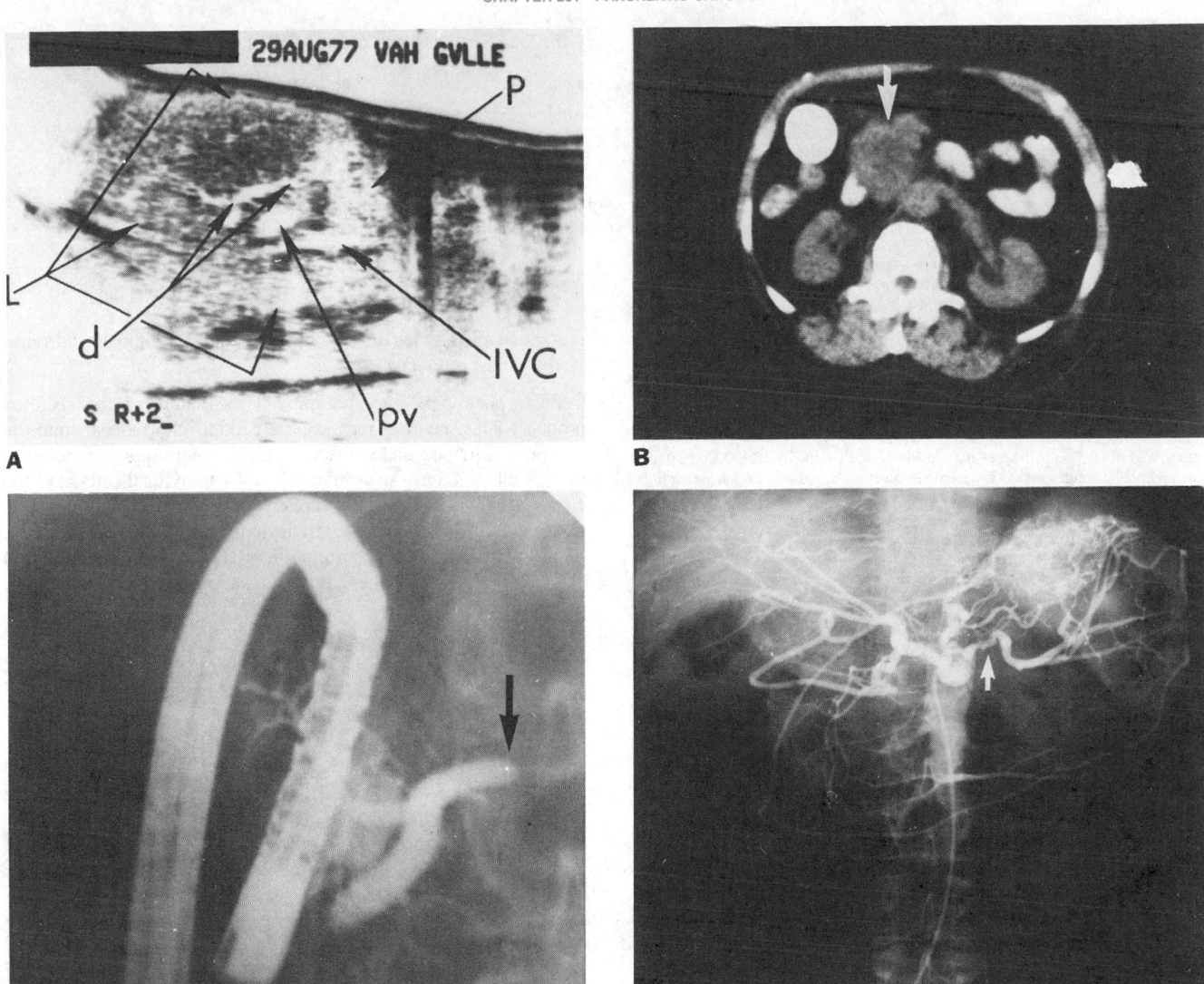

FIGURE 261-1 Carcinoma of the pancreas. *A.* Sonogram showing pancreatic carcinoma (P), dilated intrahepatic bile ducts (d), dilated portal vein (pv), and inferior vena cava (IVC). *B.* CT scan showing pancreatic carcinoma (arrow). *C.* ERCP showing abrupt cut off of the duct of Wirsung (arrow). *D.* Arteriogram showing sheathing of splenic artery by tumor encasement (arrow).

resection, the 5-year survival rate following such operations is only 10 percent. Nonetheless, an attempt at the procedure merits strong consideration, particularly for lesions in the pancreatic head, since ductal carcinomas often cannot be distinguished preoperatively from ampullary, duodenal, and distal bile duct tumors or pancreatic cyst adenocarcinomas, all of which have far higher resectability and cure rates. Furthermore, survival is prolonged three- to fourfold in those patients who eventually experience disease recurrence following pancreatic resection than in those whose tumor is not excised, indicating that such operations have a palliative as well as curative potential. The risk for tumor recurrence is unaffected by the type of operative procedure [i.e., total pancreatectomy versus pancreaticoduodenectomy ("Whipple resection")] but is increased by the presence of lymph node metastases or tumor invasion into adjacent viscera.

The median survival for patients whose pancreatic cancers are surgically unresectable is approximately 5 months. Management of such individuals should be directed at symptomatic palliation. Ambulatory patients having tumors in the pancreatic head should be considered for surgical diversion of the biliary system. If jaundice has already developed, therapeutic options include either nonoperative biliary decompression by endoscopic or percutaneous, transhepatic

biliary drainage or surgical biliary bypass. External beam radiation in patients with unresectable tumors which have not spread beyond the pancreas does not appear to prolong survival, although a sufficient reduction in tumor size may lead to palliation of pain. However, the addition of 5-fluorouracil (5-FU) chemotherapy to external beam irradiation has increased the survival time for these patients, perhaps by acting as a radiosensitizing agent. A similar combination of radiation therapy and 5-FU appears to have prolonged the survival and increased the cure rate when compared to a prospectively randomized nontreatment control group of patients who had a complete surgical resection of their pancreatic cancer. This observation has been made in a small patient population and thus demands confirmation prior to the general acceptance of the efficacy of postoperative ("adjuvant") treatment.

The experience utilizing chemotherapy in the management of patients with widely metastatic pancreatic cancer has been disappointing. No presently available drug regimen can be considered as being "standard." Newer forms of therapy must be developed and should constitute the initial treatment for consenting, ambulatory patients.

Pancreatic endocrine tumors are discussed in Chap. 262.

REFERENCES

BERG RJ, CONNELLY RR: Updating the epidemiologic data on pancreatic cancer. Semin Oncol 6:275, 1979

CANCER OF THE PANCREAS TASK FORCE: Staging of cancer of the pancreas. Cancer 47:1631, 1981

CONNOLLY MM et al: Survival in 1001 patients with carcinoma of the pancreas. Ann Surg 206:366, 1987

GASTROINTESTINAL TUMOR STUDY GROUP: Pancreatic cancer. Adjuvant combined radiation and chemotherapy following curative resection. Arch Surg 120:899, 1985

GUDJONSSON B et al: Cancer of the pancreas. Diagnostic accuracy and survival statistics. Cancer 42:2494, 1978

MOERTEL CT et al: Therapy of locally unresectable pancreatic adenocarcinoma: A randomized comparison of high dose (6,000 rads) radiation alone, moderate dose radiation (4,000 rads) + 5-fluorouracil, and high dose radiation + 5-fluorouracil. The Gastrointestinal Tumor Study Group. Cancer 48:1705, 1981

MOOSA AR, LEVIN B: The diagnosis of "early" pancreatic cancer: The University of Chicago experience. Cancer 47:1688, 1981

O'CONNELL MJ: Current status of chemotherapy for advanced pancreatic and gastric cancer. J Clin Oncol 3:1031, 1985

SPEER AG et al: Randomized trial of endoscopic versus percutaneous stent insertion in malignant obstructive jaundice. Lancet 2:57, 1987

STEINBERG WM et al: Comparison of the sensitivity and specificity of the CA 19-9 and carcinoembryonic antigen assays in detecting cancer of the pancreas. Gastroenterology 90:343, 1986

WARSHAW AL, SWANSON RS: Pancreatic cancer in 1988: Possibilities and probabilities. Ann Surg 208:541, 1988

262 ENDOCRINE TUMORS OF THE GASTROINTESTINAL TRACT AND PANCREAS

LEE M. KAPLAN

Tumors arising from neuroendocrine cells of the gastrointestinal tract and pancreas present special challenges in diagnosis and therapy. Unlike other gastrointestinal neoplasms, these tumors may cause symptoms from excess hormone secretion rather than from growth, invasion, or local anatomic effects. Frequently slow growing, they may nonetheless be life-threatening because of uncontrolled release of specific hormones and neurotransmitters. These neoplasms arise from within the gastrointestinal mucosa and pancreatic islets in cells that normally secrete monoamines and peptide hormones. For example, gastrin-secreting G cells within the gastric and duodenal mucosa regulate gastric acid secretion, and insulin-secreting β cells within the pancreatic islets serve a crucial role in the homeostatic control of glucose metabolism. Overall, more than 30 distinct secretory products have been identified within neuroendocrine cells of the gut.

BIOLOGIC CONSIDERATIONS

A striking feature of neuroendocrine tumors is the preservation of highly differentiated cell function. Tumor cells contain secretory granules and maintain the capacity for *a*mine *p*recursor *u*ptake and *d*ecarboxylation (APUD), a process essential for the production of monoamine neurotransmitters such as serotonin, dopamine, and histamine. This characteristic has fostered the term *APUDomas* for neoplasms derived from these cells, which can be located in the thyroid (C cells), adrenal medulla, lung (neuroendocrine cells), skin (melanocytes), and nervous system (glial cells and neuroblasts), as well as the gastrointestinal tract and pancreas. These cells also synthesize and secrete peptide hormones by a separate mechanism. Several of the known APUDomas are listed in Table 262-1. It was postulated that this specialized capability implies a common embryologic origin for these diverse cells, but in fact cells of *varied* heritage can acquire the APUD phenotype during differentiation.

Studies of neuroendocrine cell physiology have revealed several

TABLE 262-1 Distribution of APUD tumors

Origin	Tumors
Gastrointestinal tract	Carcinoid tumor
Pancreas	Islet cell carcinoma
Central nervous system	Ganglioneuroblastoma, neuroblastoma, chemodactoma, paraganglionoma
Thyroid	Medullary thyroid carcinoma
Skin	Melanoma
Adrenal medulla	Pheochromocytoma
Lung	Carcinoid tumor, small cell carcinoma

important characteristics of secretory cells and the clinical syndromes caused by their products:

1 Cellular phenotype does not predict the nature of the secreted product. Thus, neurons may secrete peptide "hormones" into the synaptic cleft, and endocrine cells may secrete monoamines previously classified as "neurotransmitters." Individual cells have the capacity to synthesize and secrete both peptide and monoamine transmitters, which may coexist in individual secretory granules. Many symptoms of enterochromaffin cell tumors (carcinoid tumors) appear to arise from the combined actions of monoamine and peptide products.

2 Transmitter secretion by neuroendocrine cells is frequently episodic or pulsatile. Although the regulation of secretion is poorly understood, the temporal pattern of hormone release may vary depending on the hormonal milieu, physiologic state, or stage of development. Thus, symptoms produced by abnormal secretion of hormones from neuroendocrine tumors may be intermittent, especially in early stages when tumor cells may behave more like their normal counterparts.

3 Individual cells have the *potential* to secrete a wide array of transmitters. This feature is particularly evident for the peptide hormones. Depending on the stage of development, cellular environment, and other as-yet-unidentified factors, neuroendocrine cells can change secretory profiles dramatically. For example, in cell culture, clonal populations may suddenly change from the secretion of insulin to cholecystokinin, gastrin, or even glucagon. Endocrine tumors may contain heterogeneous populations of cells so that within individual tumors a single cell type may predominate, or there may be multiple cell types in varying proportions. In addition, the secretory profile of a tumor may vary with time, producing a dramatic alteration of symptoms. Individual metastatic implants can also display different phenotypes from the primary tumor and from each other.

4 Individual hormones and transmitters secreted by neuroendocrine cells may regulate physiologic activity (e.g., secretion, absorption, or contractility), stimulate or inhibit growth, or affect the development of target cells. Thus, the humoral activity of gut neuroendocrine tumors can cause a wide variety of effects, including gastric acid hypersecretion, abnormal intestinal motility, gastric epithelial hyperplasia, gallstone formation, mesenteric and cardiac fibrosis, and necrosis of the skin.

5 Hormone production by neuroendocrine cells is tightly regulated at many levels, including RNA transcription, precursor peptide processing, and secretion. These cells in addition may be subject to control by neighboring secretory cells (*paracrine regulation*). Thus, multiple cell types may act in concert to control the growth, secretory characteristics, and thus the clinical manifestations of individual tumors. Abnormal secretion by the tumors themselves may disrupt the normal regulated function of neighboring neuroendocrine cells, and neoplastic transformation may disturb hormone secretion by these cells. Cells may secrete partially processed hormone precursors, leading to unpredictable effects, or display altered susceptibility to regulation by exogenous stimuli. Occasionally, such characteristics can be exploited to permit specific diagnostic tests for individual tumors.

TABLE 262-2   Gastrointestinal endocrine tumor syndromes

Syndrome	Cell type	Clinical features	Percentage malignant	Major products
Carcinoid syndrome	Enterochromaffin, entero-chromaffin-like	Flushing, diarrhea, wheezing, hypotension	~100	Serotonin, histamine, miscellaneous peptides
Zollinger-Ellison, gastrinoma	Non-β islet cell, duodenal G cell	Peptic ulcers, diarrhea	~70	Gastrin
Insulinoma	Islet β cell	Hypoglycemia	~10	Insulin
Verner-Morrison, WDHA, VIPoma, pancreatic cholera	Islet D_1 cell	Diarrhea, hypokalemia, hypochlorhydria	~60	Vasoactive intestinal peptide
Glucagonoma	Islet A cell	Mild diabetes mellitus, erythema necrolytica migrans, glossitis	>75	Glucagon
Somatostatinoma	Islet D cell	Diabetes mellitus, diarrhea, steatorrhea, gallstones	~70	Somatostatin
GRFoma	Non-β islet cell	Acromegaly	—	Growth hormone–releasing hormone (GRF)
CRFoma	Non-β islet cell	Cushing's syndrome	—	Corticotropin-releasing hormone (CRF)
PPoma	Islet PP cell	Rare necrolytic erythema	—	Pancreatic polypeptide (PP)
Neurotensinoma	Non-β islet cell	None	—	Neurotensin
Miscellaneous tumors	Non-β islet cell	Hypercalcemia	—	Parathyroid hormone
		Inappropriate ADH	—	Vasopressin
		Hyperpigmentation	—	Melanocyte-stimulating hormone

Neuroendocrine tumors of the gastrointestinal tract can be classified by cell type, major hormone secreted, and site of origin. These characteristics, alone or in combination, correlate well with the observed clinical syndromes. Table 262-2 lists the important tumors in this category, along with their clinical presentations, major secreted products, cells of origin, and biologic behavior.

DIAGNOSTIC CONSIDERATIONS

Several distinct syndromes of hormone excess have been described in which symptoms may suggest the presence of an endocrine tumor of the gastrointestinal tract or pancreas. Moreover, these tumors may present as part of the type I multiple endocrine neoplasia (MEN I) syndrome (see Chap. 325). MEN I patients frequently develop parathyroid and pituitary adenomas that may produce symptoms of hypercalcemia, hyperprolactinemia, hyperthyroidism, or growth hormone excess. Diagnosis is suggested by history, physical findings, elevated blood levels of the relevant peptide hormone(s), or elevated urinary levels of the major metabolites of monoamine transmitters. Further confirmation of hormone-producing tumors may be provided by provocative tests that reveal abnormalities in the regulation of hormone secretion. For example, tolbutamide may enhance somatostatin secretion from somatostatinoma cells. Normal somatostatin-secreting D cells do not show this effect. Other examples of *abnormal* regulation in tumor cells include enhancement by secretin of gastrin secretion in gastrinomas, and pentagastrin stimulation of calcitonin secretion in medullary thyroid (C cell) tumors.

Anatomic definition for pancreatic tumors should be sought by computed tomography (CT), and endoscopic visualization or barium contrast studies should be obtained for suspected mucosal and submucosal tumors. In cases where tumors are too small to be visualized by these noninvasive methods, angiography or selective venous sampling for hormone determination may provide anatomic localization. CT and magnetic resonance imaging are the preferred means of assessing metastatic spread, since the liver and lymph nodes are the initial sites of tumor metastasis.

THERAPEUTIC CONSIDERATIONS

Therapy of endocrine tumors has two goals: (1) to decrease or reverse the growth and spread of the tumor, and (2) to relieve the symptoms of hormone overproduction. When the tumor is localized, both goals may be accomplished by surgical excision. However, most of these tumors are malignant and have spread by the time of diagnosis, and control of growth in such malignant tumors has proven difficult. Thus far, the greatest benefit has been seen with chemotherapeutic regimens that include streptozocin, alone or in combination with fluorouracil or doxorubicin. Control of hepatic metastases has been achieved with hepatic artery embolization, although this approach is palliative rather than curative.

Several approaches are used to control the effects of excess hormone production by these tumors. The most common is to block the function of the target tissue. For example, gastric acid hypersecretion induced by gastrin-producing tumors may be reversed by medications that inhibit acid secretion (e.g., H-2-receptor blockers or proton pump blockers) or by surgical resection of the stomach. Diazoxide is used to help reverse the effects of hyperinsulinemia, and hypomotility agents may ameliorate the diarrhea caused by hypersecretion of vasoactive intestinal peptide (VIP), gastrin, somatostatin, neurotensin, or serotonin.

A second approach is to block release of the transmitter from the tumor cells. The success of this approach depends upon the continued ability of the tumor cells to respond to such physiologic or pharmacologic stimuli. Initial trials used somatostatin, a peptide hormone that inhibits the release of numerous hormones and amine transmitters. While somatostatin controls the symptoms of many of these tumors, it has a short half-life and must be given intravenously. These limitations have been largely overcome by the use of octreotide, a longer-acting analogue of somatostatin with similar actions that can be administered subcutaneously. The chemical structures of somatostatin and octreotide are shown in Fig. 262-1 (see also Chap. 313). Octreotide frequently relieves the symptoms of several endocrine tumors that are inadequately controlled by tumor resection or ablation. In addition, tumor regression occurs in occasional patients, suggesting that the hormone agonist may have some growth-inhibiting effects. The major known side effects of octreotide are dose-dependent and are similar to symptoms of somatostatin excess, including steatorrhea, mild hyperglycemia, nausea, and abdominal pain. The clinical disorders that respond to therapy with octreotide are summarized in Table 262-3.

CARCINOID TUMORS

Carcinoid tumors are the most protean and the most common gastrointestinal endocrine tumors, accounting for approximately 55

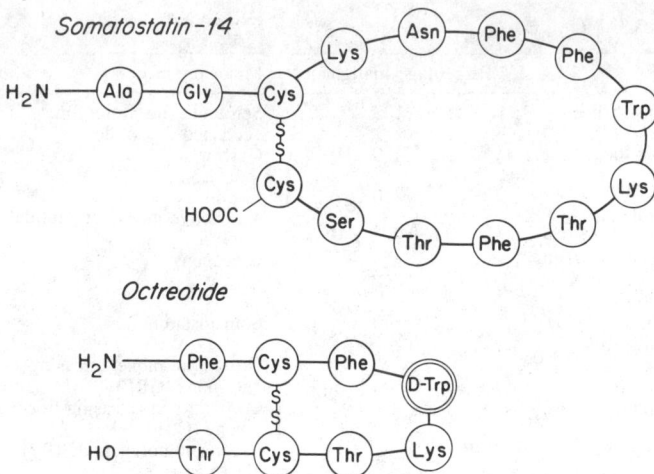

FIGURE 262-1 Structures of somatostatin-14 and octreotide. The double circle denotes the substitution of D-tryptophan for the naturally occurring L-tryptophan. This substitution inhibits peptide degradation and prolongs serum half-life.

percent of such neoplasms. They may present with gastrointestinal bleeding, abdominal pain, obstruction from tumor growth or tumor-induced mesenteric fibrosis, or symptoms arising from tumor-secreted hormones. The name *carcinoid* was applied to these tumors because slow growth and the homogeneous appearance of tumor cells led early investigators to underestimate their malignant potential. They pursue an indolent course and the interval between onset of symptoms and diagnosis averages 4.5 years. Carcinoid tumors arise from neuroendocrine cells throughout the body but are most prevalent in the gastrointestinal tract, pancreas, and pulmonary bronchi. Ninety percent of these tumors arise in the enterochromaffin or Kulchitsky cells within the gastrointestinal tract. The tumors can be found anywhere from the stomach to the rectum and are most common in the appendix, rectum, and ileum. Gastrointestinal carcinoids frequently cause abdominal pain, bleeding, or intestinal obstruction. Although they are rarely large, the tumors may become the leading point for intussusception. In addition, mesenteric spread stimulates a local fibrous reaction, causing intestinal kinking, obstruction, and vascular compromise. Rare sites of carcinoid tumors include the

thymus, esophagus, biliary duct, Meckel's diverticulum, breast, and ovary. No risk factors have been clearly defined for these tumors, although the incidence of gastric carcinoids may be increased in patients with pernicious anemia, achlorhydria, and Hashimoto's thyroiditis. Carcinoids of the bronchus and small intestine may occur in association with MEN I. Thymic carcinoids may be associated with hyperparathyroidism or Cushing's syndrome.

Appendiceal tumors comprise nearly half of all carcinoid tumors and are incidental findings in 0.3 to 0.7 percent of routine appendectomy specimens. They are usually small, solitary, and benign. Local invasion is common but metastatic spread is rare, and the presence of tumor does not necessarily confer appreciable morbidity or mortality. Colorectal carcinoids have a similarly benign course and are usually asymptomatic. In contrast, small-bowel and bronchial carcinoids have a more malignant course. Local transmural invasion, early metastasis to lymph nodes and liver, and symptoms from hormone secretion are common. Other sites of metastatic spread include bone, and less commonly, heart, breast, and eye. The risk of metastatic spread is dependent on tumor size. Metastases are found in fewer than 2 percent of tumors less than 1 cm in diameter, but in nearly 100 percent of tumors greater than 2 cm. Additional primary tumor implants within the gastrointestinal tract are found in 40 percent of patients.

CARCINOID SYNDROME Enterochromaffin cells secrete a variety of hormones and are embryologically related to thyroid C cells, adrenal medullary cells, and melanocytes. Tumors of each of these cell types may produce syndromes of hormone excess. Hormone secretion by carcinoid cells can cause distinctive and debilitating effects (carcinoid syndrome) long before local growth or metastatic spread is apparent. Manifestations of the carcinoid syndrome include the triad of cutaneous flushing, diarrhea, and valvular heart disease and, less commonly, telangiectasias, wheezing, and paroxysmal *hypo*tension. Early in the course, symptoms are usually episodic and may be provoked by stress, catecholamines, and ingestion of food or alcohol. During acute paroxysms, systolic blood pressure typically falls 20 to 30 mmHg. Diarrhea may result from several mechanisms. The most common type is mixed secretory and hypermotility-induced, producing watery stools unresponsive to fasting. Other causes include partial mechanical obstruction from tumor or fibrosis, and mesenteric vascular insufficiency from local fibrosis. Endocardial fibrosis can cause valvular heart disease, usually affecting the proximal side of the tricuspid and pulmonary valves and leading to tricuspid insufficiency, pulmonary stenosis, and secondary right-sided heart failure. Left-sided valvular disease may occur in association with bronchial carcinoids, presumably because venous effluent from these tumors passes directly into the pulmonary veins, avoiding inactivation of the hormone mediators in the lung.

Approximately 5 percent of all patients with carcinoid tumors experience one or more symptoms of the carcinoid syndrome. The likelihood of developing symptoms is strongly dependent on the origin and behavior of the tumor. While 30 to 60 percent of small-bowel carcinoids are associated with systemic manifestations, only 3.5 percent of lung, 1 percent of appendix, and virtually no rectal carcinoids produce the syndrome. In patients with intestinal carcinoids, the humoral symptoms only develop in the setting of metastatic disease to the liver. Bronchial and other extraintestinal carcinoids, whose hormone products are not immediately cleared by the liver, may produce the carcinoid syndrome in the absence of metastasis.

Carcinoid tumors may be classified on the basis of embryonic origin (Table 262-4). Clinical features, secreted hormones, diagnostic evaluation, and prognosis vary according to whether a carcinoid arises in foregut, midgut, or hindgut structures. For example, carcinoid syndrome is less common in patients with foregut carcinoids than midgut tumors, but the syndrome, when it occurs, is more likely to include wheezing. Patients with foregut carcinoid syndrome more often have dramatic cutaneous flushing involving the whole body than those with tumors of midgut or hindgut organs. The flush of bronchial carcinoids may be prolonged (lasting hours to days);

TABLE 262-3   Clinical uses of octreotide in gastrointestinal disease

Hormone-secreting tumors	
Carcinoid tumor	Inhibits cutaneous flushing, controls diarrhea, reverses hypotension, aids perioperative management, ?inhibits growth
VIPoma	Controls diarrhea
Insulinoma	Controls hypoglycemia acutely, aids perioperative management
Gastrinoma	Perioperative management, ?controls diarrhea
Glucagonoma	Controls necrolytic erythema
Dumping syndrome	Controls diarrhea, vasomotor symptoms
Diarrhea	Inhibits intestinal secretion, motility
Short-bowel syndrome	
Ileostomy	
Diabetic neuropathy	
Acquired immunodeficiency syndrome	
Fistulas	Inhibits fluid and enzyme secretion, promotes healing
Pancreatic	
Enteric	
Crohn's disease	
Gastrointestinal bleeding	
Portal hypertensive gastropathy	Reduces portal pressure, splanchnic blood flow
Esophageal and gastric varices	Reduces portal pressure, splanchnic blood flow

TABLE 262-4   Characteristics of carcinoid tumors

Embryonic origin	Site of primary tumor	Frequency, %	Carcinoid syndrome Characteristics	Monoamines
Foregut	Bronchus	3.5	Intense flush, lasting up to several hours; associated lacrimation, salivation, facial edema; wheezing; diarrhea; left- and right-sided cardiac lesions	5-HT, ± Histamine
	Stomach	~5	Intense, patchy, whole body flush, with defined borders, wheals, usually lasting several minutes; pruritus; wheezing; diarrhea	5-HTP, Histamine, ± 5-HT
	Duodenum, jejunum	~40	Diarrhea	5-HT
	Pancreas, gallbladder	Rare	Occasional necrolytic erythema	
Midgut	Ileum	~40	Facial flush, usually lasting seconds to minutes; telangiectasias; cardiac lesions; peritoneal fibrosis; diarrhea	5-HT, ± Histamine
	Appendix	~1		
Hindgut	Colon	Rare	Mild facial flush	5-HT
	Rectum	0	Diarrhea	

NOTE: 5-HT = 5-hydroxytryptamine (serotonin); 5-HTP = 5-hydroxytryptophan.

associated with excessive lacrimation, salivation, and facial edema; and occasionally producing significant hypotension. The cutaneous manifestations of gastric carcinoids, though lasting only minutes, are frequently well-circumscribed and associated with wheals, pruritus, and high levels of histamine secretion. Midgut carcinoids commonly cause the carcinoid syndrome. Acute episodes of flushing tend to be less severe than those associated with foregut tumors, but facial telangiectasias may develop late in the course. Midgut tumors are more frequently associated with cardiac manifestations and peritoneal fibrosis. Hindgut tumors rarely cause the carcinoid syndrome. A rare variant syndrome associated with ovarian carcinoids causes severe peritoneal fibrosis.

Serotonin (5-hydroxytryptamine, 5-HT) is the most common secretory product of carcinoid tumors. As shown in Fig. 262-2,

carcinoid tumors synthesize serotonin by enzymatic modification of circulating tryptophan. Up to 50 percent of the dietary intake of tryptophan can be converted to serotonin by these cells, which may leave inadequate substrate for incorporation into proteins and conversion to niacin. As a result, patients with widely metastatic carcinoid tumors may suffer symptoms of protein malnutrition (see Chap. 71) or mild pellagra (see Chap. 76). Serotonin induces intestinal secretion, inhibits intestinal absorption, and stimulates intestinal motility. High serotonin levels are likely the cause of diarrhea in most cases of carcinoid syndrome. Serotonin also stimulates fibroblast growth and fibrogenesis and thus may mediate or accelerate the peritoneal and cardiac valvular fibrosis in this disease. Excess serotonin secretion alone does not account for cutaneous flushing. Multiple monoamine and peptide factors contribute to the vasomotor changes; the relative contributions of each mediator may vary from patient to patient.

Carcinoid tumors elaborate multiple monoamines and peptide hormones, including histamine, catecholamines, bradykinins, tachykinins, enkephalins and endorphins, vasopressin, gastrin, adrenocorticotrophin, and prostaglandins (Table 262-5). Many secrete somatostatin, neurotensin, substance P, neurokinin A, and motilin. The elevated circulating levels of these substances mediate many of the pathophysiologic changes of carcinoid syndrome, although the relative contributions of each remain to be identified.

DIAGNOSIS The diagnosis of carcinoid tumors is influenced by the presenting features of the tumor. Patients with nonfunctional tumors (i.e., without the carcinoid syndrome) usually present with symptoms due to the direct effects of the tumor in the gastrointestinal tract, including abdominal pain or tenderness, nausea, malaise, weight loss, intestinal or biliary obstruction, or gastrointestinal bleeding. Depending on the location of the tumor and whether metastases are

FIGURE 262-2 Metabolic pathway of serotonin in the carcinoid syndrome.

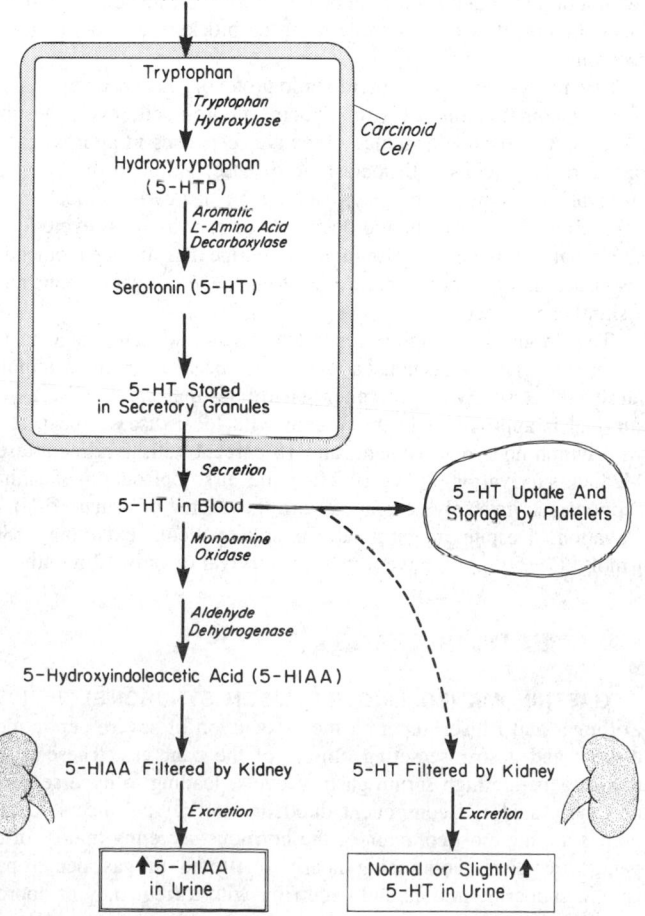

TABLE 262-5   Hormone mediators of carcinoid syndrome

Clinical feature	Frequency, %	Candidate mediators
Diarrhea	78	5-HT, histamine, prostaglandins, VIP, glucagon, gastrin, calcitonin
Cutaneous flushing	94	5-HT, 5-HTP, kallikrein, NKA, histamine, SK, SP, prostaglandins
Telangiectasia	25	Unknown
Wheezing	18	5-HT, histamine
Abdominal pain	51	Tumor, hepatic enlargement, bowel ischemia (fibrosis)
Heart disease		5-HT
Right-sided	40	
Left-sided	13	
Pellagra dermatosis	7	Tryptophan depletion (5-HT synthesis)

NOTE: 5-HT = 5-hydroxytryptamine (serotonin); 5-HTP = 5-hydroxytryptophan; NKA = neurokinin A; SK = substance K; SP = substance P; VIP = vasoactive intestinal peptide.
SOURCE: After W Creutzfeldt and F Stockmann, Am J Med 82:4, 1987.

present, endoscopy, barium studies, or CT may allow anatomic localization. Radiographic studies should include small-bowel follow-through or direct instillation of radiographic contrast material into the small bowel (enteroclysis) to identify tumors in the jejunum and ileum. Despite the improved detection of tumors, however, their pathologic identity is usually not suspected before resection or liver biopsy.

Evaluation of patients with clinical features of carcinoid syndrome is based on the observation that serotonin is secreted by the large majority of functional carcinoid tumors. As shown in Fig. 262-2, serotonin is metabolized in the blood to 5-hydroxyindoleacetic acid (5-HIAA), which is cleared by the kidneys. Plasma and platelet serotonin and urinary 5-HIAA levels are usually elevated in the setting of carcinoid syndrome. Measurement of urinary 5-HIAA excretion is the most useful diagnostic test, and approximately 75 percent of patients excrete more than 80 μmol/d (15 mg/d). Specificity of this test approaches 100 percent after exclusion of ingested substances known to elevate 5-HIAA levels; these include bananas, plantain, pineapple, kiwi fruit, walnuts, plums, pecans, avocados, guaifenesin, and acetaminophen. Conversely, aspirin and levodopa ingestion can cause a falsely depressed 5-HIAA level. In some patients with carcinoid syndrome and normal urinary 5-HIAA, documentation of elevated plasma or platelet serotonin concentrations may establish the diagnosis. However, many gastric carcinoid tumors lack the aromatic L-amino acid decarboxylase and convert 5-hydroxytryptophan (5-HTP) serotonin with low efficiency. Since 5-HTP is not metabolized to 5-HIAA, urinary studies may be misleading. These patients may have elevated urinary serotonin levels, since renal cells contain aromatic L-amino acid decarboxylase. Diagnosis in these cases may be confirmed by demonstrating elevated plasma 5-HTP, histamine, or peptide hormone levels, although it frequently rests on the anatomic detection of the tumor itself. Attempts to provoke cutaneous flushing are helpful for documenting flushing in cases when the clinical history is equivocal. Ethanol, pentagastrin, or microgram quantities of epinephrine can be used for this purpose. Abdominal ultrasonography, CT, and selective angiography are the most sensitive tests for detecting metastatic disease in the liver. Since most patients with the humoral syndrome have metastases, liver biopsy is the most common access to histologic diagnosis. Additional information about bone metastases and cardiac sequelae may be obtained with bone scans and echocardiography, respectively. In patients in whom a tumor cannot be detected, imaging with radiolabeled metaiodobenzyl guanidine may be helpful. This agent is concentrated by neuroendocrine cells and accumulates in many carcinoid tumors.

TREATMENT   Effective treatment of the carcinoid syndrome may require more than one approach. Therapy should be selected according to the severity of symptoms. Since nearly all patients with carcinoid syndrome have metastatic disease, resection is rarely curative. Mild diarrhea may be controlled with hypomotility agents such as loperamide or diphenoxylate/atropine. In patients who have undergone ileal resection, diarrhea can be exacerbated by bile salt malabsorption and frequently responds to cholestyramine. Flushing, if rare and mild, may not require therapy. Combination therapy with histamine H-1- and H-2-receptor antagonists (e.g., diphenhydramine and ranitidine) can inhibit the cutaneous flush associated with foregut carcinoids. Phenoxybenzamine may provide additional benefit by inhibiting the release of bradykinin. Methyl xanthine bronchodilators and glucocorticoids are helpful in relieving the dyspnea and wheezing associated with bronchial carcinoids. β-Adrenergic agonists should be avoided since they may provoke acute exacerbations. Serotonin antagonists, including cyproheptadine and methysergide, have been used to provide relief of diarrhea. Unfortunately, these agents have little effect on flushing and other vasomotor symptoms and methysergide can induce fibrosis similar to that caused by the carcinoid itself. ICS 205-930, an investigational agent that selectively blocks the 5-HT$_3$ subset of neuronal serotonin receptors, inhibits diarrhea in the carcinoid syndrome.

Octreotide is a potent inhibitor of hormone secretion by carcinoid cells. Indeed, this agent provides effective control of diarrhea, flushing, and wheezing in more than 75 percent of cases. Octreotide is effective in the management of acute manifestations of the carcinoid syndrome such as hypotension or resulting angina, as well as the transient exacerbation caused by hepatic artery embolization or the induction of general anesthesia. However, octreotide must be administered in two or three subcutaneous injections each day. It is not yet known whether octreotide can prevent the observed cardiac (or mesenteric) fibrosis. Established valvular heart disease is not reversed by any form of medical therapy.

Surgery, hepatic artery embolization, and chemotherapy have been used to reduce the burden of tumor tissue. Surgery is the treatment of choice for small (<2-cm diameter) carcinoid tumors of the appendix or large bowel. Patients with carcinoid syndrome from isolated bronchial or other extraintestinal carcinoids may also be amenable to curative resection. Most patients with carcinoid syndrome, however, have gross metastatic disease. Hepatic resection generally provides only transient amelioration of symptoms and no improvement in survival. In isolated cases, however, long-term palliation has been achieved by resection of a *single* hepatic metastasis after removal of the primary tumor. Several less-invasive approaches have been tried to limit the hepatic tumor burden and control humoral symptoms, including selective hepatic artery infusion of chemotherapy, local irradiation, and hepatic arterial occlusion. Unfortunately, carcinoid tumors are generally radioresistant and respond weakly to chemotherapy. Arterial occlusion by gel foam embolization provides transient relief of symptoms in approximately 90 percent of patients. Its success derives in part from the fact that the hepatic artery supplies less than half of the blood supply of normal liver tissue but nearly all the blood supply of the tumor. Side effects of therapy include pain, fever, and occasional synthetic liver dysfunction. Effectiveness of therapy can be monitored with serum transaminase levels, which should rise substantially over the first 24 to 48 h after embolization. Patients undergoing embolization may experience acute exacerbation of carcinoid symptoms provoked by the sudden release of hormones from the tumor. Although such effects are rarely life-threatening, prophylactic treatment with histamine-receptor blockers and octreotide is recommended.

Several systemic chemotherapeutic protocols have been evaluated. Various combinations of streptozocin, fluorouracil, cyclophosphamide, and doxorubicin induce objective responses in approximately one-third of patients with metastatic disease, although the effect on survival is minimal. Leukocyte interferon decreases tumor size in approximately 20 percent and decreases urinary 5-HIAA excretion in about half of patients. Although octreotide has induced objective responses in a few cases, controlled trials have not yet demonstrated a significant effect.

The prognosis is highly dependent on the site and stage of the disease at diagnosis. As noted above, appendiceal and rectal carcinoids rarely affect survival. For other gastrointestinal carcinoids, 5-year survival is approximately 95 percent with local disease, 65 percent with lymph node involvement, and 18 percent with liver metastases. Median survival is 2½ years after the first episode of flushing. Prognosis is inversely correlated with the degree of urinary 5-HIAA elevation. Despite attempts at therapy, patients excreting >800 μmol/d (>150 mg/d) have a median survival of only 13 months.

PANCREATIC ISLET-CELL TUMORS

GASTRINOMA (ZOLLINGER-ELLISON SYNDROME)   In 1955, Zollinger and Ellison reported the association of severe peptic ulcer disease and gastrin-secreting tumors of the pancreas. These gastrinomas generate high serum gastrin levels, leading to hypersecretion of gastric acid and consequent duodenal and jejunal ulcers. Gastrinomas are the most common of the hormone-secreting tumors of the pancreatic islets, comprising nearly one-tenth of gastroenteropancreatic endocrine tumors and occurring with a frequency of approximately 4×10^{-7} in an unselected population in Ireland. Zollinger-Ellison syndrome may account for up to 0.1 percent of patients with duodenal ulcer disease in the United States. Ulcer disease develops in almost all patients with gastrinoma and is the presenting problem in approximately 70 percent. More than half of patients experience diarrhea (either watery stools or steatorrhea), and approximately 30 percent present with diarrhea alone. Radiologic and endoscopic examinations frequently reveal increased gastric fluid and thickened rugal folds. The age distribution of patients with gastrinoma is similar to that in ordinary acid peptic disease, with a broad peak in the fifth to eighth decades. Gastrinoma should be considered in all patients with recurrent or refractory ulcer disease, ulcers associated with gastric hypertrophy, ulcers in the distal duodenum or jejunum, ulcers in patients with diarrhea, kidney stones, hypercalcemia, or pituitary disease, or a strong family history of duodenal ulcer disease or endocrine tumors.

In patients with ulcer disease or diarrhea, serum fasting gastrin levels of greater than 200 ng/L (200 pg/mL) suggest the diagnosis. However, since gastric acid exerts a negative feedback on the *normal* G-cell secretion of gastrin, inhibition of acid secretion can also lead to elevated gastrin levels in this range. Thus, the serum gastrin level does not reliably predict gastrinoma in the presence of atrophic gastritis, partial gastric resection, histamine-receptor blockers such as cimetidine or ranitidine, or proton pump blockers such as omeprazole. The *sine qua non* of Zollinger-Ellison syndrome is hypergastrinemia in the presence of gastric acid hypersecretion. More than 90 percent of patients have a basal acid output (BAO) greater than 15 mmol/h. In the setting of ulcer disease without gastric outlet obstruction, this level of hyperchlorhydria is diagnostic of gastrinoma. In patients who have previously undergone gastric surgery, BAO >5 mmol/h is diagnostic. Secretin infusion provides a second means of distinguishing gastrinoma from other causes of hypergastrinemia. Secretin has little effect on gastrin secretion from normal G cells (causing a modest increase or decrease in serum gastrin levels) but usually stimulates gastrin secretion by gastrinoma cells. This provocative test is particularly useful in the 50 percent of gastrinoma patients with modest elevations in serum gastrin. Zollinger-Ellison syndrome is predicted by an *increase* in serum gastrin of at least 200 ng/L (200 pg/mL) within 15 min of a single intravenous injection of secretin (2 units per kg body weight). Approximately 90 percent of patients with gastrinoma will demonstrate a diagnostic rise in serum gastrin at 2, 5, 10, or 15 min after secretin injection.

Between one-fourth and one-half of gastrinomas occur in association with the MEN I syndrome (see Chap. 325). Hyperparathyroidism is the most common component of MEN I and occurs in about 80 percent of patients with this form of Zollinger-Ellison syndrome. All gastrinoma patients should be screened for possible MEN I by measurement of serum calcium, phosphorus, cortisol, and prolactin levels and imaging of the sella turcica. First-degree relatives of patients with MEN I also should be similarly screened.

Approximately 80 percent of gastrin-secreting tumors arise in pancreatic islets, including nearly all of those associated with MEN I, and most are located in the pancreatic head. Another 10 to 15 percent arise from G cells in the duodenum, and the remainder are scattered in the distal small bowel, stomach, spleen, liver, lymph nodes, and ovary (mucinous cystadenoma). The tumors are usually small and are frequently multifocal, especially when associated with MEN I. The biologic behavior may be variable. In most reported series, one-half to two-thirds of these tumors are malignant, with metastases in lymph nodes and liver and less frequently in bone. However, the prevalence of metastatic disease at the time of diagnosis appears to have decreased, perhaps owing to the more widespread consideration and earlier detection of these tumors. Such observations have important therapeutic implications since isolated tumors are more likely to be cured by resection. Gastrinomas, like most other islet-cell tumors, are generally slow-growing, but growth patterns vary widely and metastases may be more aggressive than the primary tumor itself.

Treatment of Zollinger-Ellison syndrome is directed at the sequelae of excess gastrin secretion and at the tumor itself. The availability of potent inhibitors of gastric acid secretion has reduced the need for gastric surgery in these patients. Reduction of BAO to <10 mmol/h is usually sufficient to control symptoms. H-2-receptor blockers, including cimetidine, ranitidine, famotidine, and nizatidine, are effective, although optimal therapy may require two to three times the standard daily dose for ordinary peptic ulcer disease and more frequent administration for control of acid output and symptoms. Omeprazole, which inactivates the parietal cell H^+,K^+-ATPase, is a more potent inhibitor of gastric acid secretion and controls symptoms of Zollinger-Ellison syndrome in nearly all patients. With each of these medical regimens, control of symptoms and acid secretion frequently requires increasing doses over time. Basal acid output or gastric pH should be measured yearly to evaluate the continued efficacy of therapy, and the rare patient who fails to respond to medical therapy should be treated surgically. However, patients with coexistent hyperparathyroidism should undergo parathyroid resection before a decision is made about gastric surgery, since resolution of hypercalcemia may permit better medical control of gastric acid secretion. In most cases, parietal cell vagotomy reduces acid secretion sufficiently to permit effective medical therapy. In rare cases, uncontrollable gastric acid secretion or complications of the ulcer disease mandate total gastrectomy.

Because of the effective control of hormone-mediated symptoms, morbidity and mortality from gastrinoma is increasingly related to the growth and spread of tumor itself. Curative resection of the gastrinoma is possible in 15 to 20 percent of cases and is favored by extrapancreatic location and inability to detect the tumor mass preoperatively. Gastrinomas in association with MEN I syndrome are not amenable to surgical cure, although these tumors generally have a benign natural history. Preoperative evaluation with CT and selective angiography is used to exclude multiple primary tumors and metastases. Treatment of unresectable gastrinoma includes chemotherapy, hormonal therapy, and hepatic artery embolization. Chemotherapeutic regimens including streptozocin and fluorouracil, with or without doxorubicin, commonly induce partial responses. Leukocyte interferon may also cause objective response, but octreotide does not appear to be effective. Hepatic artery embolization may decrease hepatic tumor burden and ameliorate pain. Unfortunately, none of these approaches prolongs survival of patients with metastatic disease, which approximates 25 percent at 10 years.

INSULINOMA (β CELL TUMOR) The hallmark of pancreatic β cell tumors is the development of symptomatic hypoglycemia from unregulated insulin hypersecretion (see also Chap. 320). Insulinomas are the second most common functioning islet cell tumors and have a reported prevalence of approximately 8×10^{-7} in an unselected Irish population. They arise most frequently in the fifth to seventh decades although cases have been reported at all ages. In infants and children, insulinoma must be distinguished from diffuse β cell adenomatosis or nesidioblastosis. Whipple's triad describes the classic presentation of insulinoma and includes fasting hypoglycemia, *symptoms* of hypoglycemia, and immediate relief after intravenous glucose administration. Weight gain may result from increased food ingested to combat symptoms of hypoglycemia. In the current era, the diagnosis of insulinoma is made by demonstrating fasting hypoglycemia in the presence of normal or elevated plasma insulin levels. Symptoms related to the hypoglycemia include headache, slurred speech, psychologic alterations, visual disturbances, confusion, and, ultimately, coma and death. Hypoglycemia also induces the secondary release of catecholamines, leading to tremulousness, diaphoresis, pallor, palpitations, cardiac arrhythmias, and behavioral irritability. Because of the episodic release of insulin, symptoms early in the course may be intermittent or occur only after somewhat prolonged periods of fasting. However, symptoms do develop early so that tumors are usually small and solitary at the time of diagnosis. Multiple primary tumors are found in approximately 10 percent of patients. An additional 10 percent are malignant, with spread to the local lymph nodes and the liver. As with gastrinomas, insulinomas are frequently associated with MEN I (see Chap. 325) and such tumors are more likely to be multifocal. Extrapancreatic insulin-secreting tumors are rare and usually arise in ectopic pancreatic tissue.

Diagnosis is made by demonstrating fasting hypoglycemia and an inadequate response of insulin to the hypoglycemia. Patients are fasted under close supervision for up to 72 h, followed, if necessary, by an exercise tolerance test. Serum glucose, insulin, and cortisol levels are determined every 1 to 2 h or at any time that symptoms appear. Approximately 75 percent of patients with insulinoma develop hypoglycemia within 24 h, as evidenced by a serum glucose less than 2.8 mmol/L (50 mg/dL) in men or 2.5 mmol/L (45 mg/dL) in women. However, there is no absolute glucose level which defines hypoglycemia, so the diagnosis of insulinoma depends on demonstrating inadequate insulin suppression in the face of falling glucose levels. Because hypoglycemia inhibits insulin secretion from normal β cells, the ratio of plasma insulin (in μU/mL) to serum glucose (in mg/dL) is maintained at less than 0.3. In patients with insulinoma, the ratio is usually >0.4 and increases with fasting. Documentation of rising cortisol levels excludes hypoglycemia secondary to hypothalamic-pituitary-adrenal dysfunction. It is also necessary to exclude other causes of fasting hypoglycemia, including administration of exogenous insulin, sulfonylurea ingestion, severe liver failure, and tumors that secrete insulinlike growth factors (e.g., fibrosarcoma, mesothelioma, and hemangiopericytoma). Exogenous insulin administration can be excluded by measuring levels of the C peptide of proinsulin, which normally vary in parallel with the plasma insulin concentrations. Since insulin administration suppresses endogenous insulin secretion, detection of normal or elevated C-peptide levels is inconsistent with insulin abuse. In addition, because insulinoma cells often process proinsulin incompletely, the serum often has an increased ratio of proinsulin to insulin. A ratio greater than 20 percent in the appropriate clinical setting is suggestive of insulinoma. Serum levels of sulfonylureas should be elevated if hyperinsulinemic hypoglycemia is caused by these agents. Normal glucose/insulin ratios exclude liver failure and tumors which secrete insulinlike growth factors. (Refer to Chap. 320 for a more complete discussion of hypoglycemia syndromes.)

Once a diagnosis of insulinoma is established, acute treatment is supportive with intravenous glucose infusion as required to maintain plasma levels within the normal range. Hyperglycemic agents, including diazoxide, beta-adrenergic-receptor blockers, and phenytoin can be used to support serum glucose levels but their effects are variable and may last only a short time. Octreotide is a potent inhibitor of insulin secretion by these tumors and may be the most effective agent for acute management. Definitive therapy is accomplished by surgical resection. Because insulinomas are usually small (90 percent are <2 cm in diameter), only half are detected by CT. Angiography with selective venous sampling for insulin levels is about 80 percent sensitive and palpation at laparotomy detects 80 to 90 percent of tumors. At surgery, detectable tumors should be resected. The effectiveness of intervention is monitored by determination of intraoperative blood glucose levels. If no detectable tumors are found, stepwise distal pancreatectomy is performed until frozen sections of resected specimens and/or blood glucose measurements indicate that all tumor has been removed. If no tumor is found, or if multiple tumors are present, pancreatectomy is limited to 70 to 80 percent to preserve digestive and endocrine pancreatic function.

Patients with metastatic disease and those whose insulinomas are not removed by partial pancreatectomy can frequently be managed with hyperglycemic agents such as diazoxide or octreotide. In one study, all of the seven patients with metastatic insulinoma showed a response to octreotide, although the degree of response was variable. However, hypoglycemia may be worsened by octreotide administration, perhaps owing to inhibition of glucagon or growth hormone by this agent. Diazoxide, though frequently effective, can cause troubling side effects, including salt and fluid retention, hypertrichosis, and gastrointestinal upset. The combination of streptozocin and fluorour-

acil is the mainstay of chemotherapy for metastatic disease. These agents induce objective remission in approximately half of patients and are associated with a modest but significant increase in survival. Patients with residual tumor should be followed carefully for changes in secretory profile which may affect therapy. Such changes may include development of hyperglycemia as a result of glucagon-secreting metastases.

VIPOMA [VERNER-MORRISON SYNDROME; WATERY DIARRHEA HYPOKALEMIA ACHLORHYDRIA (WDHA) SYNDROME; PANCREATIC CHOLERA] Verner and Morrison described a syndrome of watery diarrhea, hypokalemia, and renal failure in association with non-β cell tumors of the pancreatic islets. The clinical features of this syndrome are caused by the high levels of vasoactive intestinal peptide (VIP) secreted by the tumors. VIPomas comprise approximately 2 percent of gastroenteropancreatic tumors and have a prevalence of approximately 1×10^{-7} in the Irish population studied. The manifestations of VIPoma include secretory diarrhea, profound weakness, hypokalemia, and hypochlorhydria. Stool volume is greater than 3 L/d in 80 percent of patients, and nonanion gap acidosis usually occurs as a result of bicarbonate losses in the stool. Other electrolyte abnormalities include hypercalcemia in approximately two-thirds of patients and hypophosphatemia. Approximately half of patients develop hyperglycemia, which results from hypokalemia- and VIP-induced glycogenolysis in the liver, and a fifth of patients experience cutaneous flushing. Although most symptoms can be reproduced by infusion of exogenous VIP, these tumors also contain other peptide hormones, including the VIP-related peptide histidine-methionine (PHM), somatostatin, helodermin, and neurotensin, each of which may contribute to clinical features exhibited by individual patients. Diagnosis rests on the demonstration of high plasma VIP levels in the setting of a stool volume of at least 1 L/d. Lesser increases in VIP levels occur in patients with hepatic failure and intestinal ischemia.

VIPomas are most commonly pancreatic tumors. Unlike gastrinomas and insulinomas, however, VIPomas frequently grow to a large size before becoming clinically apparent. On average, the size of these tumors at the time of diagnosis is second only to the nonfunctioning pancreatic islet cell tumors. Although they are slow-growing, these tumors are usually malignant. Approximately three-fifths are metastatic at the time of diagnosis. Eighty percent of VIPomas are located in the body or tail of the pancreas. A few cases have been seen in association with MEN I. However, there is no constant relation between the two syndromes. Between 10 and 15 percent of VIP-secreting tumors arise from neuroendocrine cells in the intestinal mucosa, and a few are ganglioneuroblastomas, mastocytomas, pheochromocytomas, or small cell carcinomas of the lung.

Treatment is surgical extirpation whenever possible. However, metastases may preclude this approach. Preoperative evaluation should include CT to localize the tumor and any metastases that may be present. In addition to supportive therapy with fluids and electrolytes, prednisone is frequently effective in reducing the volume of diarrhea, despite its inability to alter serum VIP levels. Octreotide inhibits the secretion of VIP and ameliorates symptoms in approximately 80 percent of patients. VIPomas often produce symptoms related to the large size of the tumor itself. Surgery may be indicated to relieve local effects or to remove a single large primary tumor. For patients with symptomatic metastatic disease, chemotherapy and hepatic artery embolization have the greatest benefit on tumor burden. Regimens containing streptozocin and fluorouracil are the most effective chemotherapy, inducing objective partial remission in up to 90 percent of cases.

GLUCAGONOMA In 1966, McGovern described a rare syndrome of diabetes mellitus and necrolytic migratory erythema in association with a pancreatic islet cell tumor. To date, fewer than 200 cases have been reported, most presenting in middle age. The observation that these tumors secrete high levels of glucagon suggested a cause for the diabetes and that the peptide may have a role in the other clinical features. Although these tumors frequently synthesize and secrete additional peptides, including pancreatic polypeptide, somatostatin, insulin, and gastrin, the common link is hyperglucagonemia. Glucagonomas are characteristically single, large, and slow-growing. More than 75 percent have metastasized at the time of diagnosis, most commonly to the liver and bones. Glucagonoma has been reported in association with MEN I. A fasting plasma glucagon of >1000 ng/L (>1000 pg/mL) establishes the diagnosis. More modest elevations of plasma glucagon levels may occur in diabetic ketoacidosis, renal failure, hepatic failure, sepsis, prolonged fasting, and gluten-sensitive enteropathy. Hypocholesterolemia and hypoaminoacidemia are common, with alanine, glycine, and serine levels usually less than 25 percent of normal. Glucagonoma may be distinguished from other hyperglucagonemic syndromes by the failure of glucose to suppress and the failure of arginine to enhance serum glucagon concentrations.

The characteristic glucagonoma skin rash is erythematous, raised, scaly, sometimes bullous, sometimes psoriatic, and ultimately crusted. It is located primarily on the face, abdomen, perineum, and distal extremities. After resolution, the regions of the acute eruption usually remain indurated and hyperpigmented. Patients may also experience glossitis, stomatitis, angular cheilitis, dystrophic nails, and hair-thinning. The diabetes is usually mild or asymptomatic and may manifest only as an abnormality on an oral glucose tolerance test. Ketoacidosis has not been reported. Weight loss, hypoaminoacidemia, anemia, and thromboembolic disease also occur in association with this syndrome. A causal association between hyperglucagonemia and skin disease has been difficult to prove, leading to speculation that the rash may result from nutritional deficiency. In some patients, the rash responds to oral zinc or intravenous amino acid therapy. Octreotide therapy has also yielded good results. However, dermatologic symptoms frequently recur after each of these therapies.

Because the tumor is usually large and found only in the pancreas, it is easily identified by CT, ultrasound, or angiography. Surgical therapy is curative in approximately 30 percent of patients. Resection is more frequently aimed at decreasing tumor burden. Despite occasional objective responses, attempts at chemotherapy with combinations of streptozocin, fluorouracil, doxorubicin, and dacarbazine have little impact. Fortunately, the slow-growing nature of the tumor allows for prolonged survival even in many cases of metastatic disease.

SOMATOSTATINOMA Somatostatin-secreting tumors are the most recent group to be identified with a defined clinical syndrome. The classic triad of somatostatinoma includes diabetes mellitus, steatorrhea, and cholelithiasis. These symptoms derive from the widespread inhibitory actions of somatostatin, including inhibition of insulin release, pancreatic enzyme and bicarbonate secretion, and gallbladder motility, respectively. The diabetes is usually mild, and in a few cases, *hypo*glycemia has been seen, perhaps from the cosecretion of other peptides. Individual somatostatinomas have been shown to secrete insulin, calcitonin, gastrin, VIP, adrenocorticotrophin, prostaglandins, substance P, motilin, and glucagon. Patients with somatostatinomas may also develop hypochlorhydria, weight loss, and paroxysmal hypertension.

Approximately 60 percent of reported somatostatinomas are located in the pancreas. The second most common site is in the small intestine, although intestinal tumors are associated with lower plasma somatostatin levels and are more commonly asymptomatic. Like glucagonomas and VIPomas, these tumors are usually single, large, and metastatic at the time of diagnosis. Somatostatinomas have not been reported in association with MEN I. Curiously, the occasional coincidence of pheochromocytoma, café au lait spots, and neurofibromatosis suggests a possible association with MEN type IIb (see Chap. 325). Small cell lung carcinomas, medullary thyroid carcinomas, pheochromocytomas, and paragangliomas that secrete somatostatin have also been described.

MISCELLANEOUS FUNCTIONAL ISLET CELL TUMORS In addition to the diseases described above, islet cell tumors have been associated with several other syndromes of hormone excess, including acromegaly (growth hormone or growth hormone–releasing hormone), hypercalcemia (parathormone-like peptide), diarrhea and diabetes mellitus (neurotensin), and Cushing's syndrome (corticotropin-releasing factor or adrenocorticotropin).

NONFUNCTIONING ISLET CELL TUMORS (See also Chap. 261) More than 15 percent of pancreatic islet cell tumors are not associated with any definable hormone-mediated syndrome. Nonetheless, many of these nonfunctioning islet cell tumors synthesize and secrete one or more regulatory peptides, including pancreatic polypeptide, substance P, and motilin. With increasing availability of radioimmunoassay and immunohistochemical reagents, protein products will probably be defined for more and more of these tumors. Nonetheless, most of these tumors behave in a similar fashion. They arise most commonly in the head and tail of the pancreas and are frequently large (5 to 10 cm in diameter) at the time of diagnosis. The most common clinical manifestations are abdominal pain, jaundice, a palpable mass, malaise, and bleeding esophageal or gastric varices (from splenic vein compression). Though slow-growing, at least half of these tumors present with metastases to the liver or lymph nodes. Surgical cure is achieved in approximately 20 percent. The remainder are poorly responsive to chemotherapy. Streptozocin with or without fluorouracil induces objective responses in approximately 60 percent of patients. Five-year survival for patients with these tumors is approximately 40 percent, with many long-term survivors despite known metastatic disease.

REFERENCES

Carcinoid tumors and syndrome

FELDMAN JM: Carcinoid tumors and syndrome. Semin Oncol 14:237, 1987
FELDMAN JM, O'DORISIO TM: Role of neuropeptides and serotonin in the diagnosis of carcinoid tumors. Am J Med 81 (Suppl 6B):41, 1986
GODWIN JD: Carcinoid tumors: An analysis of 2837 cases. Cancer 36:560, 1975
KVOLS LK et al: Treatment of the malignant carcinoid syndrome: Evaluation of a long-acting somatostatin analogue. N Engl J Med 315:663, 1986
MARTENSSON H et al: Bronchial carcinoids: An analysis of 91 cases. World J Surg 11:356, 1987
MOERTEL CG et al: Carcinoid tumor of the appendix: Treatment and prognosis. N Engl J Med 317:1699, 1987
NORHEIM I et al: Malignant carcinoid tumors: An analysis of 103 patients with regard to tumor localization, hormone production, and survival. Ann Surg 206:115, 1987
OBERG K et al: Treatment of malignant carcinoid tumors with human leukocyte interferon: Long-term results. Cancer Treatment Rep 70:1297, 1986
THORSON A et al: Malignant carcinoid of the small intestine with metastases to the liver, valvular disease of the right side of the heart, peripheral vasomotor symptoms, bronchoconstriction, and an unusual type of cyanosis: A clinical and pathologic syndrome. Am Heart J 47:795, 1954

Islet cell tumors

BLOOM SR, POLAK JM: Glucagonoma syndrome. Amer J Med 82 (Suppl 5B):25, 1987
BOSTWICK DG et al: Expression of opioid peptides in tumors. N Engl J Med 317:1439, 1987
BRANDI ML et al: Familial multiple endocrine neoplasia type I: A new look at pathophysiology. Endocrine Rev 8:391, 1987
GORDEN P et al: Somatostatin and somatostatin analogue (SMS 201-995) in treatment of hormone-secreting tumors of the pituitary and gastrointestinal tract and non-neoplastic diseases of the gut. Ann Intern Med 110:35, 1989
KENT RB et al: Nonfunctioning islet cell tumors. Ann Surg 193:185, 1981
KREJS GJ: VIPoma syndrome. Amer J Med 82 (Suppl 5B):37, 1987
KVOLS LK et al: Treatment of metastatic islet cell carcinomas with a somatostatin analogue (SMS 201-995). Ann Intern Med 107:162, 1987
VINIK AI et al. Somatostatinomas, PPomas, neurotensinomas. Semin Oncol 14:263, 1987
WOLFE MM, JENSEN RT: Zollinger-Ellison syndrome. N Engl J Med 317:1200, 1987
WYNICK D et al: Symptomatic secondary hormone syndromes in patients with established malignant pancreatic endocrine tumors. N Engl J Med 319:605, 1988

section 1 Disorders of the immune system

263 PRIMARY IMMUNE DEFICIENCY DISEASES

MAX D. COOPER / ALEXANDER R. LAWTON III

INTRODUCTION Immunologic functions are mediated by two developmentally independent, but functionally interacting, families of lymphocytes. The activities of B and T lymphocytes, and their products, in host defense are closely integrated with the functions of other cells of the reticuloendothelial system. Macrophages, dendritic cells, and the Langerhans' cells in the skin play an important role in the trapping and presentation of antigens to T and B cells to initiate the immune response. Macrophages also become effector cells, especially when activated by products of lymphocytes. The scavenger activity of polymorphonuclear leukocytes is directed and made specific by antibodies in concert with products of the complement system (see Chap. 13). Natural killer (NK) cells, a population of granular lymphocytes, may spontaneously kill tumor and virus-infected cells, activities that are enhanced by the interferon products of immune and inflammatory cells. Killing by NK cells can also be targeted by IgG antibodies for which NK cells have cell-surface receptors. The interaction of basophils and tissue mast cells with IgE antibodies in causation of immediate-type hypersensitivity is discussed in Chap. 267. Consideration of these interrelationships is an important part of the analysis of patients with suspected immune deficiency.

CLINICAL DISEASE FEATURES COMMON TO IMMUNE DEFICIENCY Immunodeficiency syndromes, whether congenital, spontaneously acquired, or iatrogenic, are characterized by unusual susceptibility to infection and not infrequently to autoimmune disease and lymphoreticular malignancies. The types of infection often provide the first clue to the nature of the immunologic defect.

Patients with *defects in humoral immunity* have recurrent or chronic sinopulmonary infection, meningitis, and bacteremia, most commonly caused by pyogenic bacteria such as *Haemophilus influenzae, Streptococcus pneumoniae*, and staphylococci. These and other pyogenic organisms also cause frequent infections in individuals who have either neutropenia or a deficiency of the pivotal third component of complement (C3). The tripartite collaboration of antibody, complement, and phagocytes in host defense against pyogenic organisms makes it important to assess all three systems in individuals with unusual susceptibility to bacterial infections.

Antibody-deficient patients in whom cell-mediated immunity is intact have an interesting response to viral infections. The clinical course of primary infection with viruses such as varicella zoster or rubeola, unless complicated by bacterial infection, does not differ significantly from that of the normal host. However, long-lasting immunity may not develop, and as a result multiple bouts of chickenpox and measles may occur. Such observations suggest that intact T cells may be sufficient for control of established viral infections, while antibodies play an important role in limiting the initial dissemination of virus and in providing long-lasting protection. Exceptions to this generalization are becoming more widely recognized. Agammaglobulinemic patients fail to clear hepatitis B virus from their circulation and have a progressive, and often fatal, course. Poliomyelitis has occurred following live-virus vaccination in some patients. Chronic encephalitis, which may progress over a period of months to years, is being observed with apparently increasing frequency. Echoviruses and adenoviruses have been isolated from brain, spinal fluid, or other sites in such patients; in others no agent has been detected.

The occurrence of an unusually serious infection, for example, *H. influenzae* meningitis in an older child or adult, warrants consideration of humoral immune deficiency. Bacterial infections in certain sites may also suggest this possibility. Chronic otitis media occurs frequently in patients with hypogammaglobulinemia, and is significant because of its relative rarity in normal adults. Pansinusitis, although almost invariably present in immunoglobulin deficiency, is a less helpful finding because it is not rare in apparently normal people. Bacterial infections of the skin or urinary tract are less frequent problems in hypogammaglobulinemic patients.

Infestation with the intestinal parasite *Giardia lamblia* is a frequent enough cause of diarrhea in antibody-deficient patients to warrant diagnostic duodenal aspiration and intestinal biopsy when the organism cannot be demonstrated in the stool.

Abnormalities of cell-mediated immunity predispose to disseminated virus infections, particularly with latent viruses such as herpes simplex (see Chap. 135), varicella zoster (see Chap. 136), and cytomegalovirus (see Chap. 138). In addition, patients so affected almost invariably develop mucocutaneous candidiasis and frequently acquire widely disseminated fungal infections. Pneumonia caused by the protozoan *Pneumocystis carinii* is also common (see Chap. 163).

T-cell deficiency is probably always accompanied by some abnormality of antibody responses (see Fig. 263-1), although this may not be reflected by hypogammaglobulinemia. This may explain in part why patients with primary T-cell defects are also subject to overwhelming bacterial infection.

The most severe form of immune deficiency occurs in individuals, often infants, who lack both cell-mediated and humoral immune functions. Individuals with severe combined immunodeficiency are susceptible to the whole range of infectious agents including organisms not ordinarily considered pathogenic. Multiple infections with viruses, bacteria, and fungi occur, often simultaneously. Because donor

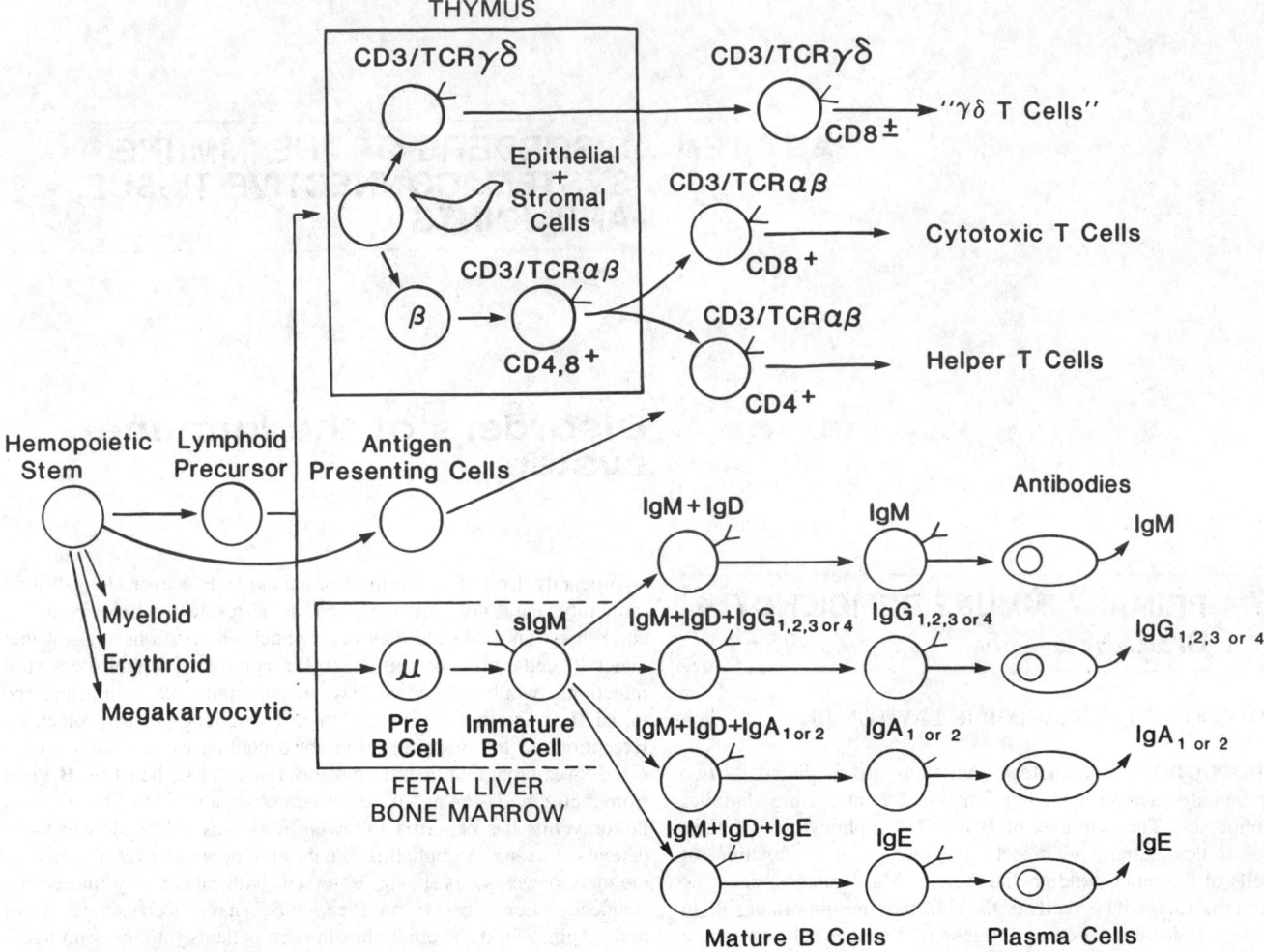

FIGURE 263-1 Hypothetical model outlining the differentiation of hemopoietic stem cells along T- and B-cell lineages. Failure to develop T and B cells may result from defective stem cells or from inborn metabolic errors affecting both cell types. Rarely, other hematopoietic cell lines are also absent. Absence of either T or B cells suggests malfunction of central lymphoid tissues, including the thymus and the fetal liver–bone marrow complex. B-cell deficiency may result from failure to generate pre-B cells from their stem cell precursors or from failure of pre-B cells to give rise to their B-lymphocyte progeny. Similarly, differentiation may be arrested at several levels within the T-cell lineage; arrests at the thymocyte level and failure to develop the helper subset have been observed in immunodeficient patients. Agammaglobulinemia and deficiencies of some T-cell functions may occur despite the presence of normal numbers of B or T cells in the circulation. Failure of B lymphocytes to differentiate to plasma cells can be due to intrinsic cellular abnormalities or to faulty T-cell regulation.

lymphocytes cannot be rejected by the recipients, blood transfusions can produce fatal graft-versus-host disease.

DIFFERENTIATION OF T AND B CELLS   The functional deficits which occur in both congenital and acquired immunodeficiencies are usefully viewed as being caused by defects at various points along the differentiation pathways of immunocompetent cells. For this reason certain features of the development and differentiation of T and B cells that are especially relevant to the analysis of immunodeficiency are briefly presented here; Chap. 13 provides a general account of their roles in cellular and humoral immunity.

A subpopulation of hematopoietic stem cells may become restricted to lymphoid differentiation prior to migration to the thymus, where T cells are generated, or to the fetal liver and adult bone marrow, where B-cell development begins (Fig. 263-1). A major function of central lymphoid tissues is to generate the clonal diversity characteristic of the immune system. Each T or B lymphocyte is induced to express surface receptor molecules of a unique specificity for antigen. The receptors of B lymphocytes are immunoglobulin molecules which are formed by paired heavy and light chains of either κ or λ type. The heavy chain gene loci are on the long arm of chromosome 14; the 5'-3' order of these is V_H (variable), D (diversity), and J_H (joining) minigene families followed by the C_H (constant region) genes, C_μ, C_δ, $C_{\gamma3}$, $C_{\gamma1}$, $C_{\alpha1}$, $C_{\gamma2}$, $C_{\gamma4}$, C_ϵ, and $C_{\alpha2}$. The κ gene family, consisting of V_κ, J_κ, and C_κ genes, is located on chromosome 2, and the homologous λ gene loci on chromosome 22.

The T-cell receptors are related cell surface molecules with antigen-binding specificity. The receptor on most T cells is composed of two polypeptide chains, called α and β. The β-chain family is located on chromosome 7, and consists of V_β, D_β, J_β, and C_β minigene loci. The α-chain family on chromosome 14 similarly consists of a series of V_α, D_α, J_α, and C_α genes. A smaller subpopulation of T cells express a T-cell receptor composed of γ and δ polypeptide chains. The γ-chain gene family is located on chromosome 7, and the δ-chain family is located in the midst of the α gene locus on chromosome 14.

The genetic strategy for creating functional gene complexes encoding antigen receptors is similar for T and B cells. For example, a functional V region gene of the immunoglobulin heavy chain is formed by productive rearrangement of one each of the V_H, D, and J_H genes and deletion of the intervening DNA to generate a contiguous coding structure which is then transcribed together with the nearest C_H gene. Functional light chain genes are formed by a V-J rearrangement in either the κ or λ gene loci. The V_β gene is similarly composed of a rearranged set of V_β, D_β, and J_β genes forming a contiguous coding structure, which the T cell then transcribes along with the nearest C_β gene. Because there are many different V, D, and J genes, they can be put together in various combinations to encode a large number of receptor molecules having different antigen-binding specificities.

Generation of clonal diversity requires cellular proliferation, such that each of the different receptor specificities encoded in the genome comes to be uniquely expressed by individual cells. A clone consists of all cells that express the identical antigen-binding receptors. Estimates for the total number of B-cell clones usually vary between 10 and 100 million. T-cell clonal diversity may be equally extensive. The initial step in clonal development is independent of antigen and reflects a genetically programmed sequence of differentiation analogous to that of primary erythropoiesis or myelopoiesis. This phase, termed *primary differentiation*, begins early in human fetal development and may continue into adult life.

The most primitive morphologically identifiable cell in the B lineage is called a pre-B cell. These cells have undergone a productive V_HDJ_H rearrangement and express cytoplasmic μ chains (the heavy chain of IgM). Since light chain gene rearrangement and expression occurs later, pre-B cells lack the membrane-bound immunoglobulin receptors which characterize B lymphocytes. Pre-B cells are generated in fetal liver and in the bone marrow of adults. Pre-B cells proliferate in response to growth factors made by neighboring stromal cells and, after undergoing a productive rearrangement of light chain VJ genes, become immature B lymphocytes that express surface IgM receptors. These B lymphocytes differ from their more mature counterparts in an important physiologic characteristic; they are highly susceptible to inactivation when their receptors bind antigen. Consequently, immature B cells encountering self-antigens may be eliminated or rendered anergic.

The developmental sequence for expression of diverse immunoglobulin classes by human B lymphocytes begins with expression of IgM. The expression of IgD on IgM-bearing cells occurs later. Lymphocytes committed to synthesis of IgG, IgA, and IgE are derived from IgM-bearing precursors through a genetic switch mechanism. Each of the heavy chain constant region genes except C_δ is preceded by a switch region composed of repetitive nucleotide sequences. The heavy chain class switch is accomplished by splicing of the switch region of μ with the switch region in front of the downstream heavy chain gene to be expressed next.

T-lineage cells also undergo sequential rearrangements of the minigene families encoding their antigen receptors. On entering the epithelial thymus, lymphoid precursor cells may follow one of two T-cell pathways. The first involves rearrangement of V_γ and J_γ genes to express γ chains and rearrangement of V_δ, D_δ, and J_δ genes to express δ chains. These associate with the CD3 proteins to form the CD3/γδ T-cell receptor (TCR) complex of γδ T cells. Pre-T cells beginning development along the second differentiation pathway in the thymus rearrange one each of the V_β, D_β, and J_β genes prior to the expression of a complete β chain. At a later differentiation stage, similar rearrangements of V_α and J_α genes occur in the α-chain family, and then the completed antigen receptor molecule of one α chain and one β chain is expressed together with the CD3 protein complex on the cell surface of an immature αβ T cell. Initially the αβ T cells express both the CD4 and CD8 accessory molecules on their surface. Later, as these cells mature under the influence of a self-antigen selection process, they either down-regulate the CD8 molecule to become CD4+ T cells with helper cell potential or they cease to express the CD4 molecule to become CD8+ T cells with cytotoxic potential. The CD4+ αβ T cells leaving the thymus have been selected to recognize peptide fragments presented in the groove of class II major histocompatibility (MHC) molecules of antigen-presenting cells. The CD8+ αβ T cells migrating from the thymus have been selected to recognize peptide fragments in the cleft of class I MHC molecules expressed by virtually all types of nucleated cells. The CD4 and CD8 molecules are called accessory molecules because they have binding affinity for class II or class I MHC molecules, respectively. While the γδ T cells express neither CD4 nor CD8 molecules during their intrathymic development, they may

express CD8 molecules as mature T cells in peripheral lymphoid tissues. The expression of these cell surface molecules, called differentiation antigens, can be defined by their reactivity with monoclonal antibodies. This provides a powerful tool for elucidating the developmental relationships of both T and B lymphocytes (Fig. 263-1).

The γδ T cells constitute a minor population of peripheral T cells and their function is presently unknown. The αβ T cells bearing the CD4 markers constitute approximately 70 percent of circulating T cells and function as helper-inducer cells, necessary for expression of effector functions of both T and B cells. The αβ T cells expressing CD8 molecules constitute 20 to 30 percent of circulating T cells, mediate cytotoxic reactions, and may be responsible for suppression of immune responses. Developmental arrests or failure of function of one or more of these T-cell subsets may be responsible for immunodeficiency or autoimmune diseases.

The events designated *secondary differentiation* follow stimulation of specific clones of lymphocytes by antigen. These processes are synonymous with the immune response (see Chap. 13). Particularly important in consideration of immunodeficiencies are the collaborative interactions among macrophages, T cells, and B cells. While B lymphocytes may differentiate to IgM-secreting plasma cells when stimulated by thymus-independent antigens, such as lipopolysaccharides, most antibody responses, particularly those of the IgA and IgG classes, require intimate collaboration between T and B cells. Antigens bound to the antibody receptors on B cells are internalized, partially digested, and recycled to the cell surface, where they are presented on class II molecules to the T cell. The activated T cell in turn produces soluble factors that promote growth and differentiation of the B cell. These factors include the interleukins IL-2, IL-4, IL-5, IL-6, and γ interferon.

Differentiation of T or B cells may be arrested at either the primary or secondary stages. Reflecting the complex cellular interactions involved in immune responses and the pivotal role played by T lymphocytes, immune deficiencies primarily involving T cells are usually also associated with abnormal B-cell function. Conversely, immunodeficiencies manifested primarily by inability to produce antibodies may be caused by T-cell defects not associated with abnormal cell-mediated immunity.

EVALUATION OF IMMUNODEFICIENT PATIENTS   A careful history and physical examination will usually indicate whether the major problem involves the antibody-complement-phagocyte system or cell-mediated immunity. A history of a normal response to smallpox vaccination or of contact dermatitis due to poison ivy suggests intact cellular immunity. Persistent mucocutaneous candidiasis suggests deficient cell-mediated immunity. Lymphopenia and the absence of palpable lymph nodes may be important findings. However, patients with profound immunodeficiency may have diffuse lymphoid hyperplasia. Most immunodeficiencies may be diagnosed by thoughtful use of tests available in local or regional clinical laboratories. More precise evaluation of immunologic functions and treatment may require referral to specialized centers. Table 263-1 presents a résumé of widely available laboratory investigations.

Humoral immunity   With rare exceptions, deficiency of humoral immunity is accompanied by diminished serum concentration of one or more classes of immunoglobulin. Normal values vary with age, and adult concentrations of IgM (0.8 g/L) are reached at about 1 year, of IgG (8.0 g/L) at 5 to 6 years, and of IgA (1.0 g/L) at puberty (see Chap. 13). Also, the wide range of values among normal adults creates difficulty in defining the lower limits of normal. Reasonable estimates for low normal values are 0.4 g/L for IgM, 5 g/L for IgG, and 0.5 g/L for IgA. In the presence of borderline hypogammaglobulinemia, assessing the patient's capacity to produce specific antibodies becomes particularly important. Most hospital laboratories can measure isohemagglutinins, anti-streptolysin O, and "febrile agglutinins." Typhoid H and O agglutinins can be measured before and after immunization with standard typhoid vaccine. State public health laboratories and private specialty laboratories can perform titrations

TABLE 263-1 Laboratory evaluation of host defense status

I Initial screening assays*
  A Complete blood count with differential smear
  B Serum immunoglobulin levels: IgM, IgG, IgA, IgD, IgE
II Other readily available assays
  A Quantification of blood mononuclear cell populations by immunofluorescence assays employing monoclonal antibody markers†
    T cells: CD2, CD3, CD4, CD8
    B cells: CD20, CD21, μ, δ, γ, α, κ, λ immunoglobulin determinants
    NK cells: CD16
    Monocytes: CD15
    Activation markers: HLA-DR, CD25
  B T-cell functional evaluation
    1 Delayed hypersensitivity skin tests (PPD, Candida histoplasmin, tetanus toxoid)
    2 Proliferative response to mitogens (phytohemagglutinin, concanavalin A) and allogeneic cells (mixed lymphocyte response)
  C B-cell functional evaluation
    1 Natural or commonly acquired antibodies: isohemagglutinins; antibodies to common viruses (influenza, rubella, rubeola) and bacterial toxins (diphtheria, tetanus)
    2 Response to immunization with protein (tetanus toxoid) and carbohydrate (pneumococcal vaccine, *H. influenza B* vaccine) antigens
    3 Quantitative IgG subclass determinations
  D Complement
    1 CH$_{50}$
    2 C3, C4
  E Phagocyte function
    1 Reduction of nitroblue tetrazolium
    2 Chemotaxis assays
    3 Bactericidal activity

* Together with a history and physical examination, these tests will identify more than 95 percent of patients with primary immunodeficiencies.
† The menu of monoclonal antibody markers may be expanded or contracted to focus on particular clinical questions.

for antibodies to common viral agents and bacterial toxins, such as diphtheria and tetanus.

Since antibody deficiency may be mimicked clinically by deficiency of complement components, measurement of total hemolytic complement (CH$_{50}$) should be a part of the evaluation of host defense. Measurement of C3 alone is inadequate for screening, since deficiencies of both early and late complement components may predispose to bacterial infection (see Chap. 13). Estimation of numbers of circulating B lymphocytes has been of great value in determining the pathogenesis of certain types of immune deficiency. B lymphocytes are identified by the presence of membrane-bound immunoglobulins; additional markers include HLA-DR antigens, receptors for aggregated IgG (Fc receptor), and receptors for the d fragment of the third complement component (CR2) which also binds the Epstein-Barr virus. Following activation, B cells express increased levels of several cell surface antigens, some of which serve as receptors for soluble growth and differentiation-promoting factors that are made by T cells. Most of these molecules on the B-cell surface can be identified and enumerated by specific monoclonal antibodies.

Pokeweed mitogen (PWM), an extract of the plant *Phytolacca americana*, has the capacity to induce primed B lymphocytes to proliferate and differentiate to plasma cells. This activity requires the presence of T lymphocytes, which also proliferate in response to PWM. Thus, this in vitro assay can measure not only the capacity of B lymphocytes to differentiate but also the "helper" function of patients' T lymphocytes.

Cellular immunity Human T lymphocytes may be enumerated by their expression of the TCR/CD3 complex of surface molecules. The CD2 antigenic molecule is also expressed by almost all of the T cells, and a few non-T-lineage lymphocytes. This molecule can bind to the LFA-3 molecule present on sheep erythrocytes and on antigen-presenting cells. The CD4 molecule serves as a marker for helper T cells, but macrophages also express this molecule in relatively low levels. Conversely, the CD8 molecule is expressed by cytotoxic T cells. This cell surface molecule may also be expressed by subpopulations of γδ T cells and non-T-lineage lymphocytes with natural killer activity.

Normal levels of serum immunoglobulins and antibody responsiveness are reliable indices of intact helper T-cell function. T-lymphocyte function can be measured directly by delayed hypersensitivity skin testing, using a variety of antigens to which the majority of older children and adults have been sensitized. The most generally useful skin test antigen is a 1:5 dilution of tetanus toxoid injected intradermally, since almost all individuals will have been sensitized. Purified protein derivative (PPD), histoplasmin, mumps antigen, and extracts of *Candida* or *Trichophyton* may also be used.

T-lymphocyte function may be estimated in vitro by the capacity of cells to proliferate in response to antigens to which the patient has been sensitized, to lymphocytes from an unrelated donor, to antibodies that cross-link the CD3/TCR complex, or to the T-cell mitogens, which include phytohemagglutinin, concanavalin A, and pokeweed mitogen. The response is usually quantified by measurement of incorporation of radioactive thymidine into newly synthesized DNA. It is also possible to measure the production of lymphokines (or interleukins) by activated T cells. Finally, the ability of T cells activated in mixed lymphocyte culture to lyse target cells can be measured.

The capacity of T lymphocytes from immunologically normal persons to be activated in vitro with antigens or mitogens may be markedly diminished by acute febrile illness, treatment with corticosteroids, or stress. Caution should be exercised in interpreting abnormal results in these circumstances.

CLASSIFICATION Primary immunodeficiencies may be either congenital or acquired, and are currently classified according to mode of inheritance and whether the defect involves T cells, B cells, or both (Table 263-2). In general, this classification will be followed in the following discussion, which emphasizes three related concepts; first, that immunodeficiencies are most logically viewed as defects of cellular differentiation; second, that these defects may involve either primary development of T or B cells or the antigen-dependent phase of their differentiation; and third, that defects of secondary B-cell differentiation may in some instances reflect T-cell abnormalities resulting from faulty T-B collaboration.

Secondary immunodeficiencies are those not caused by intrinsic abnormalities in development or function of T and B cells. The best known of these is the acquired immunodeficiency syndrome (AIDS) which may follow infection with the human immunodeficiency virus (HIV) (see Chap. 264). Other examples are immune deficiency associated with malnutrition, protein-losing enteropathy, and intestinal lymphangiectasia. Also considered secondary are immunodeficiencies resulting from hypercatabolic states such as occur in myotonic dystrophy, immunodeficiency associated with lymphoreticular malignancy, and immunodeficiency resulting from treatment with x-rays, antilymphocyte serum, or cytotoxic drugs.

Incidence As a group, the primary immunodeficiencies are relatively common. Isolated IgA deficiency may occur in approximately 1 in 600 individuals. While no other specific category approaches this frequency, the cumulative total is approximately 1 in 400 individuals in North America.

The more severe forms of primary immunodeficiency have their onset early in life and all too frequently result in death during childhood. Immunodeficiencies may become apparent at any age, however, and a substantial number of patients with congenital hypogammaglobulinemia survive to middle age or beyond. In a referral center for patients with immunodeficiency diseases, approximately two-thirds of the immunodeficient patients will be adults. Improved methods of diagnosis and treatment may increase this ratio in the future.

Severe combined immunodeficiency (SCID) This syndrome is characterized by gross functional impairment of both humoral and cell-mediated immunity and by susceptibility to devastating fungal, bacterial, and viral infections. It is usually congenital, may be inherited either as an X-linked or autosomal recessive defect, or may occur sporadically. Affected infants rarely survive beyond 1 year without treatment. This syndrome has been associated with a diversity

TABLE 263-2 WHO classification of primary immunodeficiencies

A Combined immunodeficiencies
  1 Severe combined immunodeficiency (SCID):
    a X-linked
    b Autosomal recessive ("Swiss-type agammaglobulinemia")
  2 Adenosine deaminase (ADA) deficiency
  3 Purine nucleoside phosphorylase (PNP) deficiency
  4 MHC class II deficiency
  5 Reticular dysgenesis
B Predominantly antibody deficiencies
  1 X-linked agammaglobulinemia
  2 X-linked hypogammaglobulinemia with growth hormone deficiency
  3 Ig deficiency with increased IgM ("Hyper-IgM syndrome")
  4 Ig heavy chain–gene deletions
  5 κ-chain deficiency
  6 IgA deficiency
  7 Selective deficiency of IgG subclasses (with or without IgA deficiency)
  8 Common variable immunodeficiency (CVID)
  9 Transient hypogammaglobulinemia of infancy
C Other well-defined immunodeficiency syndromes
  1 Wiskott-Aldrich syndrome
  2 Ataxia telangiectasia
  3 3d and 4th pouch/arch syndrome (DiGeorge)
D Syndromes associated with immunodeficiency
  1 Chromosome abnormalities:
    a Bloom syndrome
    b Fanconi anemia
    c Down syndrome
  2 Multiple organ system abnormalities:
    a Partial albinism
    b Short-limbed dwarfism
    c Cartilage hair hypoplasia
    d Agenesis of the corpus callosum
  3 Hereditary metabolic defects:
    a Transcobalamin II deficiency
    b Acrodermatitis enteropathica (zinc deficiency)
    c Type I orotic aciduria
    d Biotin-dependent carboxylase deficiency
  4 Hypercatabolism of Ig:
    a Familial hypercatabolism of Ig
    b Myotonic dystrophy
    c Intestinal lymphagiectasia
  5 Other:
    a Hyper-IgE syndrome
    b Chronic mucocutaneous candidiasis
    c Thymoma
    d Immunodeficiency following hereditarily-determined susceptibility to Epstein-Barr virus

of defects in development of immunocompetent cells, some of which may be related to specific enzymatic abnormalities.

The classic example of SCID, *Swiss-type agammaglobulinemia*, is characterized by severe lymphopenia involving both T and B cells, and is inherited with an autosomal recessive pattern. Rarely, other hematopoietic cell lines fail to develop in a variant form of SCID called *reticular dysgenesia*. About half of patients with autosomal recessive SCID are deficient in an enzyme involved in purine metabolism, adenosine deaminase (ADA). Studies of the pathophysiologic relationship of ADA deficiency to abortive lymphoid differentiation suggest that intracellular accumulation of adenosine and deoxyadenosine triphosphate, by inhibiting ribonucleotide reductase enzymes, interferes with DNA synthesis. Improvement of both clinical status and immunologic function has occurred in patients treated with a source of exogenous ADA. The cellular defect in the lymphopenic forms of SCID logically rests with the precursor cells for both T and B lineages. The immunologic defects in all of these types of SCID patients have been repaired following transplantation of bone marrow or fetal liver as a source of stem cells, confirming the hypothesis that the stromal microenvironments of the thymus and bone marrow of these patients are capable of supporting T- and B-cell differentiation of normal stem cells.

SCID may also occur with an X-linked inheritance pattern. Affected boys may not have severe lymphopenia; most have normal numbers of B lymphocytes with few or no circulating T lymphocytes. This developmental disorder can also be repaired by transplantation of bone marrow stem cells from a histocompatible sibling. Transplants

of haploidentical bone marrow, depleted of donor T cells to prevent graft-versus-host disease, may also correct the T-cell deficit, but the antibody deficiency may persist for years in this instance.

Treatment of SCID patients should probably be attempted only in centers with a strong research interest in this problem. It is crucial that these patients be recognized early and not be given blood transfusions which may cause fatal graft-versus-host disease.

T-cell immunodeficiency Reflecting the diversity of T-cell functions, abnormalities of T-cell development may be responsible for a wide spectrum of immune deficiencies including severe combined immunodeficiency, selective defects in cell-mediated immunity, and syndromes presenting as antibody deficiency with apparently normal cell-mediated immunity. These defects may be acquired (see Chap. 264) as well as congenital. Until recently, laboratory assays of T-lymphocyte function were limited to correlates of cell-mediated immunity; no means were available for studying T-cell regulatory functions. Quantification of T-cell subsets and of their growth factor receptors using monoclonal antibodies, accompanied by functional measurements of helper and cytotoxic activity, are expanding the spectrum of immunodeficiencies primarily related to T-cell abnormalities. The genes for the T-cell receptors, the CD3 protein complex, other surface molecules involved in signal reception and transduction, and T-cell-derived interleukins have all been cloned. Assays for their products are also becoming available. The availability of these assays and DNA probes will also allow more precise definition of T-cell disorders, the numbers of which will increase with the use of these sophisticated tools for T-cell analysis.

DI GEORGE'S SYNDROME This is the classic example of isolated T-cell deficiency which results from maldevelopment of thymic epithelial elements derived from the third and fourth pharyngeal pouches. Defective development of other organs formed in part by cells of embryonic neural crest origin is also seen in these patients. Affected infants usually present with congenital cardiac defects, particularly those involving the great vessels, hypocalcemic tetany due to failure of parathyroid development, and absence of a normal thymus. Associated abnormalities may include abnormal ears, shortened philtrum, micrognathia, and hypertelorism. Serum immunoglobulin concentrations are frequently normal, but antibody responses, particularly of IgG and IgA isotypes, are usually impaired. Lymphocyte counts may be near normal, but most of the lymphocytes are B cells. Carefully performed autopsies have often revealed a tiny, histologically normal thymus, usually in an ectopic location. With time, most patients develop functional T cells. A few patients with Di George's syndrome transplanted with fetal thymus have rapidly developed immunocompetent T cells of host origin. However, it is difficult to be certain whether long-term improvement is the result of a small thymus gland in an ectopic location or due to grafted thymus epithelium.

Children lacking the congenital anomalies associated with Di George's syndrome may present with severe impairment of cell-mediated immunity. Some have normal or even increased immunoglobulin levels, while others have selective deficiencies of one or more immunoglobulin classes. Specific antibody responses are usually impaired even in patients with normal concentrations of immunoglobulins. This ill-defined entity has been called the *Nezelof's syndrome*.

Inherited deficiency of the enzyme purine nucleoside phosphorylase (PNP) is associated with an often severe and selective deficiency of T-lymphocyte function. This enzyme functions in the same purine salvage pathway as ADA; toxic effects of the *PNP deficiency* may be related to intracellular accumulation of deoxyguanosine triphosphate (GTP).

ATAXIA-TELANGIECTASIA This is an autosomal recessive genetic disorder characterized by cerebellar ataxia, oculocutaneous telangiectasia, and immunodeficiency. The responsible gene appears to be closely linked to the thy-1 gene on chromosome 11. Onset of truncal ataxia usually occurs in infancy and is progressive. Immunodeficiency may be clinically manifest by recurrent and chronic sinopulmonary infection leading to bronchiectasis. However, not all patients have immunodeficiency. The two most frequent causes of death are chronic pulmonary disease and malignancy. Lymphomas are most common, although carcinomas have also occurred.

The immunologic abnormalities seem to be related to maldevelopment of the thymus. The thymus is markedly hypoplastic and similar in appearance to an embryonic thymus. The peripheral T cell pool is frequently reduced in size, especially in lymphoid tissue compartments. Cutaneous anergy and delayed rejection of skin grafts are common. Although the number and class distribution of B lymphocytes are usually normal, most patients are deficient in serum IgE and IgA, and a smaller number have reduced serum levels of IgG, particularly of the IgG2, IgG4 subclasses. IgM and IgD are usually normal.

There is circumstantial evidence that ataxia-telangiectasia may involve a generalized defect in cellular differentiation related to the defects in DNA repair mechanisms which have been identified in these patients. Cultured cells from these patients are highly susceptible to radiation-induced chromosomal damage. Defective DNA repair mechanisms may account for the high incidence of malignancies in these patients. Ovarian agenesis also occurs frequently. Persistence of very high serum levels of oncofetal proteins, including alpha-fetoprotein and carcinoembryonic antigen, may be of diagnostic value.

Only symptomatic treatment is available. Unless a severe IgG deficiency is present, therapy with gamma globulin is not indicated. Unusual sensitivity to x-irradiation should be kept in mind in planning therapy for patients who develop cancer.

Immunoglobulin deficiency syndromes X-LINKED AGAMMA-GLOBULINEMIA Males with this syndrome often begin to have recurrent bacterial infections late in the first year of life, when maternally derived immunoglobulins have disappeared. Affected individuals have very few immunoglobulin-bearing B lymphocytes in their circulation and lack primary and secondary lymphoid follicles. However, pre-B cells are found in normal frequency in their bone marrow. This developmental block at the pre-B to B cell level contrasts with earlier and later arrests in B-cell differentiation characterizing other immunodeficiencies (see below and Fig. 263-1). The gene defect has been mapped to the Xq 21.3–22 region. B cells from obligate carriers utilize the normal X chromosome exclusively, while T cells and myeloid cells express either X chromosome. *X-linked agammaglobulinemia with growth hormone deficiency* is a rare disorder that maps to a different region of the X chromosome.

Agammaglobulinemia is a misnomer, as most patients with this and other forms of severe panhypogammaglobulinemia synthesize some immunoglobulins. Within the same family some affected males have had substantial levels of IgM, IgG, and IgA, while others have been nearly agammaglobulinemic. All these patients were markedly deficient in circulating B lymphocytes. This observation suggests that the few B lymphocytes which escape the block in differentiation are fully capable of plasma cell maturation and immunoglobulin synthesis. However, antibody replacement therapy is needed in all of these patients because of the limited number of B-cell clones that are generated.

A form of arthritis with some of the features of rheumatoid disease occurs in some of these patients. *Mycoplasma* organisms are sometimes the cause of the arthritis. Chronic encephalitis of viral etiology appears to be an increasingly frequent terminal complication. Some of these patients have also had an associated dermatomyositis. The frequency with which these complications occur is reduced by adequate treatment with gamma globulin.

TRANSIENT HYPOGAMMAGLOBULINEMIA OF INFANCY This is a reversible syndrome in which normal physiologic hypogammaglobulinemia of infancy is unusually prolonged and severe. IgG levels of normal-term infants commonly drop to levels of 3.0 to 4.0 g/L between 3 and 6 months of age as maternally derived IgG is catabolized; levels subsequently rise reflecting the infants' increased synthetic capacity. Periodic immunologic assessment is needed to

differentiate transient hypogammaglobulinemia from other forms of antibody deficiency. Antibody replacement therapy is recommended only in rare instances of severe or recurrent infections.

ISOLATED DEFICIENCY OF IgA This immunodeficiency occurs with a frequency of approximately 1 in 600 individuals of European origin. IgA deficiency is much less common in people of Asian and African origin. In Japan, for example, the incidence is approximately 1 in 18,500. While the precise genetic basis for this difference in incidence is unknown, IgA deficiency is frequently associated with certain MHC haplotypes in caucasians. The defective gene(s) predisposing to IgA deficiency may be in the class III region of the MHC genes on chromosome 6.

With rare exceptions, IgA1 and IgA2 subclasses are both deficient in serum and in mucous secretions. Many adults with isolated IgA deficiency do not seem to have unusual problems with infection. Nevertheless, this condition is not benign. As a group, individuals with IgA deficiency have an increased number of respiratory infections of varying severity, and a few have had severe pulmonary disease such as bronchiectasis. Chronic diarrheal disease also occurs. The incidence of asthma and other atopic diseases among IgA-deficient patients is high, and, conversely, the incidence of IgA deficiency among atopic children has been found to be 20 to 40 times that in the normal population. IgA deficiency is also significantly associated with autoimmune diseases such as rheumatoid arthritis and systemic lupus erythematosus. Selective reductions in the IgG2 and IgG4 subclasses have been associated with the increased infections seen in some IgA-deficient individuals. Finally, some IgA-deficient patients develop significant levels of antibodies to IgA. These patients may have severe anaphylactic reactions when transfused with normal blood or blood products.

IgA deficiency is often familial, but can also occur in association with congenital intrauterine infections, such as toxoplasmosis, rubella, and cytomegalovirus infection. IgA deficiency sometimes follows treatment with phenytoin or penicillamine. Most commonly, the syndrome appears as a sporadic defect.

The pathogenesis of IgA deficiency, whether genetic or induced by environmental insult, involves a block in terminal differentiation of B lymphocytes. Virtually all patients have detectable IgA-bearing B lymphocytes, although their numbers may be reduced. In normal children and adults, most of the B lymphocytes bearing IgA have only that immunoglobulin class on their surface, while in IgA-deficient patients and normal neonates, IgA-bearing lymphocytes also bear surface IgM. This immature phenotype is associated in most patients with failure of their cultured lymphocytes to secrete IgA when stimulated by pokeweed mitogen. While there is as yet no generally accepted pathogenic mechanism, suspicion remains high that many of these patients have a primary defect in essential regulatory interactions between T and B cells.

Treatment of IgA deficiency is essentially symptomatic. IgA cannot be effectively replaced by exogenous gamma globulin or plasma, and use of either can increase the risk of development of antibodies to IgA. IgA-deficient patients in need of transfusion should be screened for the presence of antibodies to IgA, and ideally should be given blood only from IgA-deficient donors. Treatment with immune globulin may benefit the exceptional IgA-deficient person in whom IgG2 and IgG4 subclass deficiencies are associated with severe infections. The risk of anaphylactic reactions to contaminating IgA must always be considered in treating IgA-deficient patients.

X-LINKED IMMUNODEFICIENCY WITH INCREASED LEVELS OF IgM This is a specific syndrome only because of its inheritance pattern. IgG and IgA levels are usually very low or undetectable, while IgD levels may be high. The number and distribution of B lymphocytes bearing IgM and IgD have been normal, while IgG and IgA B lymphocytes are often undetectable, suggesting a defect in isotype switching. The clinical patterns of infection are similar to those occurring with other hypogammaglobulinemic states. Neutropenia often occurs in affected males and can increase their vulnerability to infections. Adequate antibody replacement by immune globulin administration may both reverse the neutropenia and reduce the frequency of infections

ISOLATED DEFICIENCY OF IgM   This syndrome has been reported rarely in this country but was detected frequently in a British population. Approximately 20 percent of these patients were asymptomatic while 60 percent had severe recurrent infections, often with bacteremia. Pneumococcal pneumonia and meningococcal meningitis have been noted in IgM-deficient patients. Other associated conditions included gastrointestinal disease, atopy, splenomegaly, and development of malignancy. The condition was frequently familial, and was four times more common in males than females. The number of circulating B lymphocytes has varied from very low to normal.

IgG SUBCLASS DEFICIENCIES   Selective deficiencies in one or more of the four IgG subclasses are seen in some patients with repeated infections. The IgG subclass deficiency may easily go undetected when the total serum IgG level is measured, because IgG2, IgG3, and IgG4 together account for only 30 to 40 percent of the IgG antibodies, and even a deficiency in IgG1 may be masked by increases in the remaining IgG isotypes. However, the current availability of subclass-specific monoclonal antibodies allows precise measurement of IgG subclass levels.

Homozygous deletions of genes encoding the constant region of the different γ chains is the basis for the IgG subclass deficiency in some individuals. For example, deletion of the $C_{\alpha 1}$, $C_{\gamma 2}$, $C_{\gamma 4}$, and C_ϵ was responsible for one individual's inability to make IgA1, IgG2, IgG4, and IgE. Interestingly, individuals with this and other patterns of C_H-gene deletions often do not have unusual infections.

Most of the IgG subclass–deficient individuals with repeated infections appear to have regulatory defects which prevent normal B-cell differentiation. The defect may extend to other isotypes. IgA deficiency may accompany IgG2 and IgG4 subclass deficiencies (see the section on IgA deficiency, above), and an inability to produce IgM antibodies to polysaccharide antigens often reflects a broader defect in antibody responsiveness. This subgroup of patients may benefit from administration of gamma globulin. However, a thorough immunologic assessment is needed to identify the relatively few patients with IgG subclass deficiency who need this therapy.

COMMON VARIABLE IMMUNODEFICIENCY   This represents a heterogeneous group of syndromes which may be congenital or acquired, sporadic or familial, and which occur in both males and females. These patients have in common the clinical manifestations of antibody deficiency associated with panhypogammaglobulinemia. The majority of these patients have normal numbers of B lymphocytes. These are clonally diverse, but have an immature phenotype. In the few patients studied, B lymphocytes capable of binding specific antigens were present, and these increased in frequency following immunization. Consistent with the evidence that B lymphocytes in these patients are able to recognize antigens and proliferate but fail to differentiate to plasma cells is the frequent occurrence of nodular lymphoid hyperplasia, including splenomegaly and intestinal lymphoid hyperplasia.

By use of assays capable of measuring B-lymphocyte differentiation to plasma cells in vitro, three major types of defects have been tentatively identified. First, and most common, is an intrinsic abnormality of B lymphocytes. B lymphocytes from these patients can be activated via their immunoglobulin receptors to express functional receptors for T cell–derived growth factors, but they fail to differentiate into immunoglobulin-secreting plasma cells even when provided with differentiation factors from normal T cells. Second, there is evidence that in some patients the T cells, or their products, may actively suppress terminal differentiation of autologous or normal B lymphocytes. The increase in suppressor activity could be either a primary or secondary abnormality. Finally, quantitative deficiency of helper T-cell function has been observed in some patients, usually also in association with defective B-cell function. This functional defect may or may not be associated with reduced numbers of CD4 + T cells.

It is important to consider the diagnosis of common variable immunodeficiency in adults with chronic pulmonary infections, some of whom will present with unexplained bronchiectasis. Intestinal diseases, including chronic giardiasis, intestinal malabsorption, and atrophic gastritis with pernicious anemia, are common in this group of patients. Patients with common variable immunodeficiency may also present with signs and symptoms highly suggestive of lymphoid malignancy, including fever, weight loss, splenomegaly, generalized lymphadenopathy, and lymphocytosis. Routine histologic examination of lymphoid tissues usually reveals germinal center hyperplasia which may be difficult to distinguish from nodular lymphoma (see Chap. 302). Demonstration of a normal distribution of immunoglobulin isotypes and light chain classes on circulating and tissue B lymphocytes can serve to distinguish these patients from those having a monoclonal B-cell malignancy with secondary hypogammaglobulinemia. The monthly administration of immune gamma globulin in adequate doses (see below) is an essential part of the treatment of all of these complications.

IMMUNODEFICIENCY WITH THYMOMA   The association of hypogammaglobulinemia with spindle cell thymoma usually occurs relatively late in adult life. Bacterial infections and severe diarrhea often reflect the antibody deficiency, whereas fungal and viral infections are infrequent complications. T-cell numbers and cell-mediated immunity are usually intact, but these patients are very deficient in circulating B lymphocytes and pre-B cells in the bone marrow. They also frequently have eosinopenia, and may develop erythroid aplasia. Complete bone marrow failure has occurred in a few immunodeficient patients with thymoma. The relationship between the thymoma and apparent abnormalities of hematopoietic stem cells remains conjectural.

WISKOTT-ALDRICH SYNDROME   This is an X-linked genetic disease characterized by eczema, thrombocytopenia, and repeated infections. Affected boys often present with bleeding in infancy. Most do not survive childhood, dying of complications of bleeding, infection, or lymphoreticular malignancy. The immunologic defects in this disease are well characterized but poorly understood. Serum concentrations of IgM are usually decreased, while IgA and IgG are normal and IgE is frequently increased. However, synthetic rates for all three classes may be elevated, indicating a significant element of hypercatabolism. The number and class distribution of B lymphocytes are usually normal. Functionally, these boys are consistently unable to make antibodies to polysaccharide antigens normally; responses to protein antigens are often not impaired early in the course of the disease. While most patients acquire a diminished number of T cells, serial appraisal of affected males suggests that the T-cell defects are secondary. They frequently become anergic, and their T cells do not respond normally to challenge with ubiquitous antigens. The nature of the primary defect is still unknown.

Transplantation of histocompatible bone marrow from a sibling donor has corrected both hematologic and immunologic abnormalities in several patients. In patients lacking a suitable donor, splenectomy may improve platelet counts and reduce the risk of serious hemorrhage. Because of the increased risk of pneumococcal bacteremia, splenectomized patients should probably receive prophylactic penicillin.

Miscellaneous immunodeficiency syndromes   Infection with *Candida albicans* is the almost universal accompaniment of severe deficiencies in cell-mediated immunity. The syndrome of *chronic mucocutaneous candidiasis* is different because superficial candidiasis is usually the only major manifestation of immunodeficiency. These patients rarely develop systemic infection with *Candida* or other fungal agents and are not unusually susceptible to virus or bacterial disease. The syndrome is often congenital and may be associated with single or multiple endocrinopathies as well as iron deficiency. Treatment of associated conditions may lead to improvement or even cure of *Candida* infection.

No uniformity of immunologic defects has been identified in these patients, although defects of antibody formation have been detected occasionally. Humoral immunity, including ability to make specific anti-*Candida* antibodies, is usually normal. Many patients are anergic, some to a variety of antigens and some only to *Candida*; anergy in some patients has been related to inability of their lymphocytes to produce migration inhibition factor.

Results of treatment with antifungal agents, such as amphotericin B, have been variable. In some patients, intensive treatment with amphotericin B coupled with surgical removal of infected nails has led to sustained improvement. Ketoconazole, an oral antifungal agent, is reported to be quite effective.

X-LINKED LYMPHOPROLIFERATIVE SYNDROME   This is an X-linked recessive disease in which there appears to be a selective impairment in immune elimination of Epstein-Barr virus (EBV). Infectious mononucleosis in affected males may have a fulminant and fatal outcome, may be associated with development of B-cell malignancies, or may result in acquired hypogammaglobulinemia, aplastic anemia, or agranulocytosis. Antibodies to EBV have been detected in some patients but are often absent in the face of infection. Generation of cytotoxic T cells appears to be the primary mechanism of control of EBV infection in normal persons, and natural killer cells may also play a role in eliminating EBV-infected B cells. While the gene defect has been mapped to the Xq 24–27 region, the nature of the cellular defect which prevents a normal response to EBV in patients with the X-linked lymphoproliferative syndrome has not been defined.

Metabolic abnormalities associated with immunodeficiency   The relation of deficiencies of the purine salvage enzymes, adenosine deaminase and purine nucleoside phosphorylase, to immunodeficiency was discussed earlier. Other inherited metabolic defects should be briefly mentioned because of their potential importance in understanding the molecular basis of immunologic function. Inherited *deficiency of transcobalamin II,* the serum carrier molecule responsible for transport of vitamin B_{12} to tissues, is associated with failure of immunoglobulin production as well as megaloblastic anemia, leukopenia, thrombocytopenia, and severe malabsorption. All abnormalities are reversed by administration of pharmacologic doses of vitamin B_{12}. The syndrome of *acrodermatitis enteropathica* includes severe desquamating skin lesions, intractable diarrhea, bizarre neurologic symptoms, variable combined immunodeficiency, and an often fatal outcome. This disease is apparently caused by an inborn error of metabolism resulting in malabsorption of dietary zinc, and can be effectively treated by parenteral or large oral doses of zinc. Zinc deficiency might in part account for the immunodeficiency which accompanies severe malnutrition.

TREATMENT OF IMMUNODEFICIENCIES   Most immunodeficiency diseases involving severe abnormalities of T-cell function, with or without hypogammaglobulinemia, are treated with bone marrow transplants. Histocompatible marrow from a sibling donor is preferred but haploidentical marrow may be used after removal of T cells. This therapy is complex and is best done by experienced research teams.

The increasing availability of purified gamma interferon, lymphocyte growth factors, and other biologically active cytokines promises to be important in the therapy of certain immunologic disorders. Genetic engineering also holds promise for future therapy of certain genetic defects of the immune system.

Replacement therapy with human gamma globulin should be used in patients who have recurrent bacterial infections and are deficient in IgG. Maintenance of serum IgG levels between 3.0 and 5.0 g/L is sufficient to prevent most serious infections, although chronic sinusitis, otitis media, and bronchitis may persist. These serum levels usually can be achieved by intravenous administration of IgG, 300 to 400 mg/kg, at monthly intervals. Alternatively, intramuscular injections of 100 mg/kg, at two- to four-week intervals, may suffice in some hypogammaglobulinemic patients.

The advantage of intravenous immune globulin is that higher amounts of antibodies can be given with less discomfort. Since higher levels of serum antibodies afford better protection from infections, intravenous antibody replacement is currently considered the treatment of choice for hypogammaglobulinemia. In patients with mild to moderate IgG deficiency (3.0 to 4.0 g/L), the decision to treat should be based on clinical symptoms and response to antigenic challenge.

Gamma globulin treatment is of no value in patients with deficiencies of immunoglobulins other than IgG. This form of treatment is not benign. Some patients develop symptoms of diaphoresis, tachycardia, flank pain, and hypotension during or immediately following injections. This reaction may be mediated by aggregates of IgG in the intramuscular preparations of gamma globulin but also may occur as a consequence of antibodies produced by the patient against donor immunoglobulins, particularly IgA.

Infusion of fresh plasma, 10 to 20 mL/kg at intervals of 3 to 4 weeks, has the advantage of replacing IgM and IgA as well as IgG. However, both IgM and IgA have a half-life of only a few days, and this source of antibodies can be recommended only in rare cases in which IgM antibodies may be needed to control an unusually resistant infection. The major disadvantage of plasma is the risk of transmitting hepatitis virus or other viruses, which can be particularly devastating in immunodeficient patients. This risk can be minimized by use of selected donors, usually family members, carefully screened for the absence of HIV and hepatitis virus infections.

Use of plasma or immune globulin selected on the basis of a high titer of antibodies to a particular agent may be indicated in certain situations. For example, antibodies to the causative echovirus may dramatically improve encephalitis in immunodeficient patients.

Therapy with exogenous IgG may not suffice to eliminate the chronic sinopulmonary inflammation and its progression to pulmonary fibrosis and bronchiectasis. Therefore, maintenance of good pulmonary toilet with regular postural drainage can be an especially important part of patient management. The principles of antibiotic therapy are not different in these than other patients, except that the index of suspicion of bacterial infection should remain very high.

REFERENCES

BURKS WA, STEEL RW: Selection IgA deficiency. Ann Allergy 57:3, 1986
COOPER MD: B lymphocytes: Normal development and function. N Engl J Med 317:1452, 1987
EIBL M et al: Primary immunodeficiency diseases—Report of a WHO Scientific Group. Immunodeficiency Rev 2:1, 1989
GOOD RA: Bone marrow transplantation for immunodeficiency diseases. Am J Med Sci 294:68, 1987
HANSON LA et al: Immunoglobulin subclass deficiency. Pediatr Infect Dis J 7:S17, 1988
PAUL WE: *Fundamental Immunology*, 2d ed. New York, Raven, 1989
ROIFMAN CM, GELFAND EW: Replacement therapy with high dose intravenous gammaglobulin improves sinopulmonary disease in patients with hypogammaglobulinemia. Pediatr Infect Dis J 7:S92, 1988
ROSEN FS et al: The primary immunodeficiencies. N Engl J Med 311:235, 300, 1984
ROYER HD, REINHERZ EL: T lymphocytes: Ontogeny, function, and relevance to clinical disorders. N Engl J Med 274:1171, 1987

264   THE ACQUIRED IMMUNO-DEFICIENCY SYNDROME (AIDS)

ANTHONY S. FAUCI / H. CLIFFORD LANE

DEFINITION   The acquired immunodeficiency syndrome was originally defined for surveillance purposes by the Centers for Disease Control (CDC) as the presence of a reliably diagnosed "opportunistic" disease that is at least moderately indicative of an underlying defect in cell-mediated immunity in the absence of known causes of underlying immune defects such as iatrogenic immunosuppression or malignant neoplasms. Following the demonstration in 1984 that the human immunodeficiency virus (HIV) is the etiologic agent of AIDS, reliable tests for HIV antibody as well as for the virus itself became available. Since that time the case definition of AIDS has undergone several revisions with regard to inclusion and exclusion criteria. Despite this complexity the simple common denominator of AIDS is infection with HIV and subsequent development of persistent constitutional symptoms and/or AIDS-defining diseases such as secondary infections, neoplasms, and neurologic disease (see below). It is appropriate to think in terms of the spectrum of HIV-related disease rather than the presence or absence of AIDS according to a strict definition. This concept has been reinforced by prospective, natural history studies of HIV-infected individuals. In those studies, the risk for developing a typical AIDS-defining opportunistic infection (*Pneumocystis carinii* pneumonia) within 1 year was 15 percent in individuals with less than 0.200×10^9 CD4+ T lymphocytes per liter (200 cells per microliter) in the absence of prior symptoms of HIV infection, and as high as 47 percent in individuals with two or more symptoms of HIV infection. Thus, the risk of serious outcome of HIV infection, particularly with regard to opportunistic infections, is predictable on the basis of the degree of immunosuppression as measured by the level of circulating CD4+ T cells. Since, in the absence of therapy (see below), most HIV-infected individuals experience progressive diminution of circulating CD4+ T cells, HIV infection itself is part of the spectrum of HIV-related disease.

ETIOLOGY AIDS is caused by HIV, a human retrovirus of the lentivirus group. The four recognized human retroviruses belong to two distinct groups: the human T lymphotropic (or leukemia) retroviruses, HTLV-I and HTLV-II, and the human immunodeficiency viruses, HIV-1 and HIV-2. The former are transforming viruses, and the latter are cytopathic viruses (see Chap. 134). The most common cause of AIDS throughout the world is HIV-1. HIV-2 has about 40 percent sequence homology with HIV-1 and is more closely related to some members of a group of simian immunodeficiency viruses (SIV). It has been identified predominantly in western African countries, is much less common, and is felt to be less pathogenic than HIV-1. HIV has the usual retroviral genes (*env, gag,* and *pol*) and six extra genes involved in the replication and other biologic activities of the virus (see Chap. 134). Various isolates of HIV-1 manifest heterogeneity, particularly in the region of the envelope gene.

INCIDENCE AND PREVALENCE AIDS was first recognized in the United States in the summer of 1981 when the CDC reported the unexplained occurrence of *Pneumocystis carinii* pneumonia in 5 previously healthy homosexual men in Los Angeles and Kaposi's sarcoma in 26 previously healthy homosexual men in New York and Los Angeles. By mid-1990, approximately 120,000 cases among adults and adolescents and approximately 2000 cases among children less than 13 years old had been reported in the United States. It is estimated that between 1 and 1.5 million people are infected in the United States, and in the absence of effective therapy (see below) it is projected that by 1992 there will have been 365,000 reported cases.

AIDS is a global epidemic with virtually every country in the world reporting cases. In addition to the United States, areas of the world with the highest incidence include western Europe, central Africa, South America (particularly Brazil), and Canada.

Sexual contact is the major mode of transmission of HIV worldwide. The virus can also be transmitted by blood or blood products both in individuals who share contaminated needles for intravenous drug use and in those who receive transfusions of blood or blood products. Infected mothers efficiently (30 to 40 percent) transmit the virus to their infants perinatally and as early as the first and second trimesters of pregnancy. Virus can also be transmitted from mother to infant via breast feeding. There is absolutely no evidence that HIV can be transmitted by casual contact or that the virus can be spread by insects such as by a mosquito bite.

Among the adult cases reported in the United States, approximately 60 percent are in homosexual or bisexual men who do not use intravenous drugs. The next largest number of cases (20 percent) is seen among heterosexual men and women intravenous drug users and is related to the sharing of needles and other drug paraphernalia. Seven percent of cases are in men who are homosexual or bisexual and who also use intravenous drugs. Approximately 1 percent of cases are in hemophiliacs with no history of other risk factors. These individuals were exposed to HIV because of the large quantities of factor VIII and/or plasma concentrates that they received intravenously as replacement for deficient clotting factors. An additional 2 percent of cases are in nonhemophiliacs who have received transfusions of blood or blood products. Five percent of cases are in persons who have had heterosexual contact with an individual known to be infected or one belonging to a known risk category for HIV infection. Approximately half of these individuals with heterosexually acquired AIDS were infected by having sex with an intravenous drug user, and an additional 30 percent of such patients have had heterosexual contact with a person born in a country (such as certain central African countries) with a high incidence of heterosexually acquired HIV infection. Despite the fact that the majority of cases of AIDS have occurred among homosexual or bisexual men, the rate of new cases of AIDS is now higher among intravenous drug users than among homosexual men in cities, such as New York, where there are high concentrations of intravenous drug users. This has led to a progressive increase in the proportion of heterosexually acquired AIDS since intravenous drug users can infect their sexual partners. Furthermore, this pattern has also led to a dramatic increase in HIV-infected infants and new cases of pediatric AIDS. Approximately 80 percent of all pediatric (<13 years of age) AIDS cases have infection from their mothers, and of these the vast majority of infants were born of mothers who were either intravenous drug users themselves or the sexual partners of intravenous drug users. The remainder of pediatric cases have occurred among blood transfusion recipients (11 percent) and hemophiliacs (5 percent).

The epidemic of HIV infection and the epidemic of HIV disease in the United States are somewhat discordant. Although the figures vary widely from city to city, the prevalence of HIV infection among homosexual men is extremely high; approximately 50 to 60 percent of homosexual men attending sexually transmitted diseases clinics in high-incidence cities, such as San Francisco and New York, are HIV seropositive. However, a saturational effect and, more importantly, behavior modification together have brought the epidemic of new infection among homosexual men in the United States to a peak. This is indicated by the fact that the rate of new infection among homosexual men in San Francisco in 1982 to 1983 was approximately 19 percent per year, while it is now less than 1 percent per year. Nonetheless, the epidemic of disease among homosexual men has far from peaked. In the absence of effective therapy that can prevent disease in infected individuals (see below), the majority of new cases within the next few years will still be among homosexual men. Likewise, despite the fact that over 70 percent of persons with hemophilia A are HIV seropositive, screening of blood donors and heat treatment of factor VIII concentrates has resulted in a virtual halt in the new infections among hemophiliacs. Yet those infected will continue to develop disease. The same holds true for infections acquired via blood transfusions among nonhemophiliacs. Rare infections will continue to occur by transfusion of contaminated blood, since a very small percentage of individuals who are infected may escape detection by screening tests conducted among blood donors (see below). The chance of a single unit of donated blood containing HIV is estimated to range from 1 in 40,000 to 1 in 250,000.

The situation is somewhat different among intravenous drug users. The prevalence of HIV infection among intravenous drug users is high, especially among inner-city minority populations in the United States; in New York City the HIV seroprevalence in this group approximates 55 to 60 percent. Furthermore, there is no evidence that the epidemic of new infections has peaked among this group. Seroprevalence studies of emergency room patients in a hospital in inner-city Baltimore indicated that approximately 5 percent of all emergency room admissions were HIV-seropositive, a reflection of the high incidence of intravenous drug use of that population and of spread to heterosexual partners of intravenous drug users. Likewise, studies of approximately 5000 patients attending two inner-city sexually transmitted disease clinics in Baltimore indicated that approximately 5 percent of patients were infected with HIV. Of HIV-infected patients 25 years of age or younger, 46 percent of men and 72 percent of women denied high-risk behavior other than heterosexual activity, adding further credence to the concept that substantial secondary spread of HIV is occurring through heterosexual contact, predominantly with infected intravenous drug users. In this regard, there is a significant association of HIV infection with syphilis (see Chap. 128) in accord with the correlation of genital ulcers and heterosexual transmission of HIV noted in other studies (see below).

Although the precise prevalence of HIV infection in the general population in the United States is unknown, it is felt to be quite low. This belief is based on data collected from millions of blood donors that indicate that among this group, which voluntarily excludes individuals who knowingly practice high-risk behavior, less than 0.04 percent of people are HIV-seropositive. This is in contrast to the central African country of Zaire in which as many as 3 to 5 percent of the general population may be positive. Surveys of new military recruits in the United States have shown that approximately 0.15 percent are HIV-seropositive. The discrepancy between this group and the blood donor population likely reflects the fact that military recruits are younger, are more sexually active, and contain a higher proportion of inner-city minorities (see above). Broad seroprevalence studies designed to be representative of the entire population of the United States are currently being undertaken by the CDC.

There is a small but real occupational risk of HIV infection among health care workers who are exposed to the virus through penetrating injuries and, to a much lesser extent, through mucosal splash incidents involving large amounts of blood. Of the several hundred health care workers who have sustained penetrating injuries with instruments contaminated with HIV-infected blood, less than 0.5 percent have become infected.

PATHOPHYSIOLOGY AND IMMUNOPATHOGENESIS   The common denominator of AIDS is a profound immunosuppression, predominantly of cell-mediated immunity, that leads to a variety of opportunistic diseases, particularly certain infections and neoplasms. Other features of AIDS, such as Kaposi's sarcoma and neurologic abnormalities, cannot be explained directly by the immunosuppressive effects of HIV since these complications may occur prior to the development of severe immunologic impairment.

The main cause of the immune defect in AIDS is a quantitative and qualitative deficiency in the subset of thymus-derived (T) lymphocytes termed the *T4 population*. This subset of cells is defined phenotypically by the presence of the CD4 surface molecule, which is the cellular receptor for HIV. Although the T4 cell is the major cell type infected with HIV, virtually any human cell that expresses the CD4 molecule on its surface is capable of binding to and being infected with HIV. Of particular importance are cells of the monocyte-macrophage lineage.

HIV binds specifically and with high affinity, via a stretch of amino acids in the viral envelope (gp 120), to a portion of the V1 region of the CD4 molecule located near its *N*-terminus. Following binding, the virus fuses with the target cell membrane and is internalized. It then utilizes the enzyme reverse transcriptase to transcribe its genomic RNA to DNA, which is integrated into the cellular DNA where it exists for the life of the cell as a "provirus" (see Chap. 134). The provirus may remain latent or be activated to transcribe mRNA and genomic RNA, leading to protein synthesis, assembly, new virion formation, and budding of virus from the cell surface. Although the precise mechanism by which the virus induces cell death has not been established, it is felt that the major mechanism is massive viral budding from the cell surface, which leads to disruption of the plasma membrane and resulting osmotic disequilibrium. Other mechanisms that might contribute to the diminution of T4 cells are: infection of a T4-cell precursor leading ultimately to reduction by attrition of T4 cells; selective depletion of CD4+ lymphoid or nonlymphoid cells that serve T4 cells, such as by supplying an essential cytokine; formation of syncytia between uninfected cells and infected cells expressing viral envelope proteins on their surface, leading to the "innocent bystander" death of uninfected cells from fusion with infected cells; autoimmune phenomena whereby virus-specific cellular or humoral immune responses

eliminate infected cells expressing viral proteins or uninfected cells that have bound or expressed viral proteins on their surface; and secretion of substances toxic to T4 cells by HIV-infected cells.

Functional abnormalities of uninfected T4 cells have been well documented in HIV-infected individuals. This is particularly true of the antigen-responsive T4-cell subset, which is defective early in the course of HIV infection. The precise mechanism of this defect is unclear. However, it may be related to a variety of factors including the selective infection of the memory subset of T4 cells, which leads to their early elimination and results in defective responses to recall antigens in the remaining cells. In addition, HIV proteins can interfere in vitro with the interaction between the CD4 molecule and its natural ligand, the major histocompatibility (MHC) class II molecule, which is critical to the monocyte-T4 cell interactions essential for specific immune responses to soluble antigen. Furthermore, antibodies to the HIV envelope protein may cross-react with class II MHC molecules and interfere with immune function.

Following initial infection with HIV, there is generally an abrupt, slight-to-moderate decrease in circulating T4 lymphocytes, which usually levels off with counts remaining stable for years. This sequence may reflect containment of the virus by immune responses. After variable periods, the T4 cells usually insidiously and progressively decrease in number, likely reflecting a gradual escape from immune containment. However, the course of infection in certain individuals may be punctuated by abrupt and dramatic decreases in T4 counts. Once the T4-lymphocyte count drops to 0.200×10^9 per liter (200 cells per microliter) or less, the chances of developing an opportunistic infection such as *Pneumocystis carinii* pneumonia are high, and this level of T4 cells is prognostic of a serious clinical complication.

In the early phases of HIV infection, the suppressor-cytotoxic subset of T cells, phenotypically defined by the CD8 surface molecule, is sometimes initially elevated. The T8 subset is believed to be responsible for the containment of HIV infection in T4 cells. As infection progresses, T8-cell numbers may be normal or, in many cases, become decreased late in the course of infection.

Although only 1 in 10,000 to 1 in 1000 T4 cells in the peripheral blood of AIDS patients actively expresses virus at any given time (the figure is lower during the asymptomatic phase), the number of cells that harbor latent HIV provirus is as high as 1 in 100 to 1 in 10. The viral burden per constant number of T4 cells increases as the T4-cell number is depleted and as disease progresses. Factors that induce the conversion of latent infection to actively replicating virus are potentially important in the pathogenesis of HIV disease. Mitogens, antigens, and transfected heterologous viral genes have been demonstrated to induce virus expression in vitro. Furthermore, cytokines such as tumor necrosis factor alpha (TNF-α), IL-6, and granulocyte-macrophage colony stimulating factor (GM-CSF) can also induce virus expression in infected cells. Since TNF-α is secreted in response to a number of infections, many of which occur as opportunistic infections in HIV-infected individuals, a cycle of progressive induction of HIV from latently infected cells may occur as disease progression occurs, and more secondary infections ensue. Thus, certain cytokines involved in the regulation of the normal immune response may serve as cofactors (see below) in the in vitro induction of virus expression in cells already infected with HIV.

The relationship between the depletion of T4 lymphocytes and profound immunosuppression is clear. Since the T4-lymphocyte subset is responsible for the induction and/or regulation of virtually the entire immune system, the selective defect in this subset results in global impairment of components of immunity that depend, at least in part, on inductive signals from the T4 cell. These include defects in natural killer cells, virus-specific cytotoxic T cells, B cells, and monocytes. Some of these defects can be corrected in vitro by supplying inductive signals in the form of lymphokines derived from T4 cells.

B lymphocytes from AIDS patients are polyclonally activated, resulting in hypergammaglobulinemia and circulating immune complexes. The consequences of B-cell abnormalities are most obvious in children with AIDS, in whom there is an increase in bacterial infections with organisms against which an intact humoral immune response is required for protection. It is felt that the nonspecific polyclonal activation of B cells interferes with the ability to mount an adequate de novo humoral immune response. The mechanism of the polyclonal hyperactivity of B cells in HIV-infected individuals is unclear, but may relate to activation of Epstein-Barr virus (EBV) in the absence of the normal regulatory T-cell influences, the elaboration of factors derived from T cells and monocytes that can trigger B cells, or the possible direct triggering of B cells by HIV itself. There is no evidence that HIV can infect B cells in vivo.

Circulating monocytes are normal in number in HIV-infected individuals; however, a number of monocyte functional abnormalities have been reported including defects in chemotaxis, secretion of interleukin 1, certain cytotoxic functions, and the ability to present antigen to T cells. Infection of circulating monocytes cannot explain these functional abnormalities, since in vivo infection of circulating monocytes occurs rarely and in very low frequency, whereas infection of tissue macrophages and of macrophage lineage cells in the brain (see below) and other organs is easily demonstrable. The reported abnormalities of circulating monocytes are likely related in part to the activation of these cells in vivo by cytokines. Infection of monocyte precursors in bone marrow with HIV may directly or indirectly be responsible for certain of the hematologic abnormalities in HIV-infected individuals. Given the fact that HIV can persist in macrophages without causing a cytopathic effect, macrophages may serve as reservoirs of HIV and may contribute to the dissemination of virus in the body.

HIV has been demonstrated in the brains of infected individuals with neuropsychiatric abnormalities (see below). In addition, the virus can be isolated from the cerebrospinal fluid (CSF) of a high percentage of infected individuals without detectable neuropsychiatric findings. The predominant brain cells infected with HIV are of the monocyte-macrophage lineage such as microglial cells. There is no convincing evidence that neurons can be infected with HIV. Although the mechanisms of nervous system tissue damage by HIV are unknown, it is felt that release of toxic cytokines from HIV-infected monocyte-macrophage lineage cells may play a role. In addition, products of HIV may impair neuron function.

HIV-infected individuals have an increased incidence of neoplasms such as Kaposi's sarcoma, some B-cell lymphomas, Hodgkin's disease, and certain carcinomas. The mechanism of this diathesis is unknown, and immunosuppression is not the only factor involved. For example, EBV has been implicated in some of the B-cell lymphomas that occur with HIV infection. HIV does not cause these tumors directly since viral sequences have not been demonstrated in the DNA from the tumor cells. HIV may contribute to the development of Kaposi's sarcoma by inducing the secretion of a growth factor from infected CD4+ cells which in turn induces endothelial cells to secrete a number of cytokines that cause the proliferation of the mixed cell types characteristic of Kaposi's sarcoma (see Chap. 134).

The pathogenesis of the hypercatabolic wasting syndrome seen in many HIV-infected individuals is unclear, but may be due in part to increased levels of cytokines such as TNF-α, also termed *cachetin*, which causes cachexia in animals (see Chap. 20).

A variety of potential cofactors may play a role in the transmission of and susceptibility to HIV infection and in the development of disease in infected individuals. For example, there is a strong association between genital ulcerations and susceptibility to HIV infection through sexual contact. In addition, cytokines such as TNF-α may be important cofactors in the induction of expression of virus in already infected cells (see above). Furthermore, coinfection with HTLV-I or human herpesvirus 6 enhances the expression of HIV in vitro.

The precise role of the immune system in the prevention or slowing of progression of disease in HIV-infected individuals is unclear. Such individuals make antibodies directed against a number of viral proteins, and neutralizing antibodies can be demonstrated in most infected persons. However, studies of the relationship between the presence and level of neutralizing antibodies and clinical outcome have produced conflicting results. Likewise, HIV-specific, MHC-restricted, cytotoxic T cells have been demonstrated in HIV-infected persons, but their relationship to protection is also unclear. Other immune mechanisms, such as antibody-dependent cellular cytotoxicity and natural killer cell activity, have been demonstrated in vitro against the virus; their role, if any, in protection remains to be determined.

CLINICAL MANIFESTATIONS   The clinical consequences of HIV infection form a spectrum ranging from the asymptomatic state to severe disease (Table 264-1). The majority of individuals experience no recognizable symptoms or signs at the time of initial infection, but some patients develop an *acute illness* (group I) approximately 3 to 6 weeks following primary infection. It is characterized by nonspecific signs and symptoms including fevers, rigors, arthralgias, myalgias, maculopapular rash, urticaria, abdominal cramps, diarrhea, and aseptic meningitis. The syndrome lasts 2 to 3 weeks and resolves spontaneously. Seroconversion usually occurs 8 to 12 weeks after presumed exposure.

Although the length of time from initial infection to the development of clinical disease varies greatly, the mean period is estimated to be between 8 and 10 years. During that period of time, individuals are classified as having *asymptomatic infection* (group II). Approximately 75 percent of individuals will develop some degree of symptoms, including full-blown AIDS (36 percent), within 7 years of initial infection, and up to 80 to 90 percent of infected persons develop some degree of deterioration of immune function within 3 years of infection, usually in the absence of symptoms.

Certain patients, otherwise asymptomatic, develop *persistent generalized lymphadenopathy* (group III). This syndrome is defined as palpable lymphadenopathy (lymph node enlargement of ≥ 1 cm) at two or more extrainguinal sites that persists for more than 3 months in the absence of a concurrent illness or condition, other than HIV infection, to explain the findings. It has been postulated that this phenomenon in the absence of other symptoms represents a state of immunologic containment of the virus and is a favorable sign. However, patients at this stage frequently go on to disease progression, and so any viral containment that occurs is only transient.

The stage of HIV infection that has defied precise clinical classification is that of nonspecific signs or symptoms with or without a substantial decrease in T4 cells (<200 T4 cells per microliter). This has generally been referred to empirically as early *AIDS-related complex* (ARC) if individuals manifest one or two signs or symptoms such as fatigue, fever, weight loss, persistent skin rash, oral hairy leukoplakia, herpes simplex, and oral thrush, and advanced ARC if more than two of these manifestations are present. The line between advanced ARC and full-blown AIDS is not clear, and a certain level of *constitutional disease* (group IV, subgroup A) should be considered as AIDS. This latter group is defined as consisting of one or more of the following: fever persisting for more than 1 month, involuntary weight loss of greater than 10 percent of baseline, or diarrhea persisting for more than 1 month in the absence of another cause to explain the findings. Patients may develop a hypercatabolic wasting syndrome in the absence of any other signs or symptoms of HIV infection and may be categorized as group IV, subgroup A patients,

TABLE 264-1   Classification system for HIV infection

Group I	Acute infection
Group II	Asymptomatic infection
Group III	Persistent generalized lymphadenopathy
Group IV	Other disease:
Subgroup A	Constitutional disease
Subgroup B	Neurologic disease
Subgroup C	Secondary infectious diseases
Subgroup D	Secondary neoplasms
Subgroup E	Other conditions

SOURCE: Modified from Centers for Disease Control, 1986 and 1987.

or more frequently this syndrome may occur in patients who already have developed another AIDS-defining condition such as opportunistic infections or neoplasms (see below). In any case, in the majority of patients no underlying direct cause of the wasting syndrome is identified.

Neurologic disease is common in HIV-infected individuals; 40 to 60 percent of patients with AIDS manifest neurologic dysfunction and 80 to 90 percent manifest neuropathologic abnormalities at autopsy. The most common neurologic disorder is HIV encephalopathy, also referred to as the AIDS dementia complex. If this syndrome or myelopathy or peripheral neuropathy occur in the absence of a concurrent condition or illness other than HIV infection, it constitutes in itself an AIDS-defining illness (group IV, subgroup B). Other neurologic complications of AIDS include cryptococcal meningitis,

central nervous system (CNS) toxoplasmosis, primary CNS lymphoma, progressive multifocal leukoencephalopathy, cytomegalovirus (CMV) infection, peripheral neuropathies, vacuolar myelopathy, and aseptic meningitis. CNS mass lesions in an HIV-infected individual should be considered either toxoplasmosis or primary CNS lymphoma until proven otherwise. The former gives a typical "ring-enhancing" appearance on computed tomography (CT) with contrast (see Chap. 162).

The most common clinical manifestation of AIDS is opportunistic infection (group IV, subgroup C). It is not unusual for an AIDS patient to have more than one opportunistic infection simultaneously (Table 264-2). *Pneumocystis carinii* pneumonia (see Chap. 163) is the most common opportunistic infection, occurring in approximately 80 percent of patients at some point during the course of their illness.

TABLE 264-2 Commonly encountered opportunistic infections in AIDS and their treatments

Infecting agent	Reference chapters*	Manifestations	Treatment	Toxicities of treatment	Comment
Pneumocystis carinii	163	Pneumonia (usually interstitial); rarely dissemination	Trimethoprim/sulfamethoxazole, 15–20/75–100 mg/kg per day PO or IV in 3–4 divided doses for 2–3 weeks *or*	Skin rash, neutropenia, megaloblastosis, thrombocytopenia	Trimethoprim (5 mg/kg q 6 h) and dapsone 100 mg/d may be as effective as trimethoprim/sulfamethoxazole.
			Pentamidine isethionate, 3–4 mg/kg per day by slow IV; 2–3 weeks duration of therapy	Hypoglycemia, hyperglycemia, hypocalcemia, azotemia, hepatic dysfunction, hypotension	After episode of *P. carinii* pneumonia or in patients with CD4+ lymphocytes <0.200 × 10⁹/L (<200 cells/μL) prophylaxis is recommended with aerosolized pentamidine isethionate, 300 mg monthly, or trimethoprim/sulfamethoxazole 320/1600 mg bid.
Cytomegalovirus	138	Retinitis, enteritis, cerebritis, pneumonitis, esophagitis, adrenalitis	Ganciclovir [9-(1,3-dihydroxy-2 propoxymethyl) guanine (DHPG)] 5 mg/kg IV bid for 2–3 weeks, then 5 mg/kg IV qd maintenance *or*	Bone marrow suppression	Bone marrow toxicity of ganciclovir may be additive with that of zidovudine. Maintenance therapy should be continued indefinitely; reinductions required often with both drugs. Foscarnet still in clinical trials.
			Foscarnet (phosphonoformate) 60 mg/kg tid for 2–3 weeks, then 90 mg/kg qd maintenance, IV	Azotemia, seizures, hypomagnesemia	
Candida albicans	151,87	Oral thrush	Clotrimazole troches, 5 times daily *or*	Generally free of toxicity	
			Nystatin suspension 5 mL swish and swallow, qid *or*	Generally free of toxicity	
			Ketoconazole, 200–400 mg/d PO	Hepatitis, adrenal insufficiency	
		Esophagitis	Mild: Swallow nystatin suspension, sucking clotrimazole troches *or*		
			Ketoconazole 200–400 mg/d PO	Hepatitis, adrenal insufficiency	
			Severe: Amphotericin B, 0.3 mg/kg per day IV for 5–10 d	Fever, chills, nausea, vomiting, thrombophlebitis, azotemia, hypokalemia, anemia, hypomagnesemia	
		Rarely disseminated	Amphotericin B, 0.4–0.5 mg/kg per day or as a double dose on alternate days for several weeks		
Mycobacterium avium-intracellulare	127,85	Disseminated, particularly in bone marrow, lung, lymph node, liver	No recognized therapy; 3 to 5 drugs chosen from among isoniazid, ethambutal, rifampin, ethionamide, pyrazinamide, cycloserine, streptomycin, amikacin, clofazimine, ansamycin	See Chaps. 85 and 127	No regimen yet shown to be reliably effective.

TABLE 264-2 Commonly encountered opportunistic infections in AIDS and their treatments *(continued)*

Infecting agent	Reference chapters*	Manifestations	Treatment	Toxicities of treatment	Comment
Mycobacterium tuberculosis	125,85	Pulmonary; disseminated (frequent)	2 or 3 drugs chosen from among isoniazid, rifampin, ethambutol, pyrazinamide, streptomycin and others (see Chap. 125)	See Chaps. 85 and 125	Short-course regimens not recommended. Initial response to therapy generally good. Role for long-term maintenance therapy remains unclear.
Cryptococcus neoformans	151	Meningitis; pulmonary; disseminated	Amphotericin 8, 0.5–0.6 mg/kg per day IV when used alone or 0.3 mg/kg per day when used in combination with 5-fluorocytosine (5FC, flucytosine) *or in combination with* 5-Fluorocytosine, 150 mg/kg per day in 4 divided doses q 6 h PO	See above for *Candida albicans* treatment Rash, myelosuppression, hepatitis	Requires indefinite maintenance therapy; ketoconazole or fluconazole may be effective. Fluconazole (still in clinical trials) may also be effective as initial therapy.
Toxoplasma gondii	162	Encephalitis; intracerebral mass; ocular disease (rare)	Pyrimethamine loading dose of 100–200 mg PO in 2 divided doses for 2 days; maintenance dose of 25 mg/d in single dose *plus* Sulfadiazine loading dose of 50–75 mg/kg PO; thereafter maintenance dose of 75–100 mg/kg per day in 4 divided doses q 6 h PO *plus* Folinic acid, 10 mg/d PO in single dose	Anemia, neutropenia, thrombocytopenia, rash Usual for sulfonamides (see Chap. 85), especially crystalluria, hematuria, rash	Initial response in patients who recover usually occurs within 2 to 3 weeks. Requires indefinite maintenance therapy.
Herpes simplex	135,86	Severe mucocutaneous disease including perianal skin Esophagitis; pneumonia; disseminated (rare)	Acyclovir, 250 mg/m^2 q 8 h for 7 d IV; *or* 200 mg PO, 5 times daily for 10 d Acyclovir, 10 mg/kg q 8 h for 10 d IV	Generally free of toxicity Azotemia, CNS changes, rash, mild hepatitis	May recur, but maintenance therapy usually not indicated
Herpes zoster	136,86	Severe cutaneous disease; dissemination (rare)	Acyclovir, 500 mg/m^2 q 8 h IV for 7 d	Azotemia, CNS changes, rash, mild hepatitis	
Cryptosporidium	166	Prolonged, severe diarrhea; malnutrition, wasting	None proven; spiramycin in clinical trials Supportive care including antimotility agents.		Protracted diarrhea, unresponsive to therapy, may lead to inanition.
Isospora belli	166	Severe diarrhea; may be indistinguishable from cryptosporidiosis	Trimethoprim/sulfamethoxazole, 160/800 mg qid PO for 10 d, then bid for 3 weeks	See above for *Pneumocystis carinii*	Prophylaxis using trimethoprim/sulfamethoxazole 160/800 mg 3 times weekly or sulfadoxine/pyramethamine 500/25 mg once per week has been effective.
Salmonella sp.	113	Septicemia, diarrhea	Ampicillin, trimethoprin/sulfamethoxazole, quinolones, or chloramphenicol depending on microbial sensitivities; see Chap. 85 for details	See Chap. 85	Ciprafloxacin may also be effective.

* The reader is referred to the indicated chapter for detailed discussion of infection, treatment, and treatment toxicities.

Patients may present with typical findings such as fever, dyspnea, and hypoxia. However, in contrast to the presentation in immunosuppressed patients without AIDS in whom the onset is usually abrupt and explosive, patients with AIDS often have an indolent presentation with symptoms gradually accelerating over weeks prior to the establishment of the diagnosis. The chest x-ray may be normal, show an interstitial infiltrate or, in the case of patients receiving aerosolized pentamidine, reveal upper lobe cavitary disease. Because of the large number of microorganisms in AIDS patients, the diagnosis can usually be made by histochemical staining of induced sputum, or if that fails by bronchoscopy with staining of material from transbronchial biopsy or bronchial lavage. It is unusual to have to resort to thoracotomy and lung biopsy to establish the diagnosis. Extrapulmonary disseminated *P. carinii* may occur more frequently in individuals receiving aerosolized pentamidine isethionate as prophylaxis against pulmonary infection (see below).

Cytomegalovirus infections (see Chap. 138) are common in AIDS patients and appear as fever and disseminated organ system involvement. CMV chorioretinitis can result in serious visual impairment and even blindness. CMV can cause enteritis with intractable diarrhea, interstitial pneumonitis, and adrenalitis. CMV infection of the CNS is an uncommon cause of neurologic complications.

Candida albicans (see Chap. 151) is an extremely common infection in AIDS patients and is usually manifested as oral thrush or esophagitis. Detectable candidemia and disseminated candidiasis are unusual. Oral candidiasis in an HIV-infected individual without other opportunistic infections indicates ARC and is prognostic of progression to AIDS.

Mycobacterium avium-intracellulare (see Chap. 127) is uncommon in individuals without HIV infection but can exist as a localized or disseminated infection in AIDS patients and is readily isolated from bone marrow, lymph nodes, liver biopsies, and blood of infected individuals. It generally occurs as a smoldering infection, is rarely the primary cause of death, but is associated with wasting syndromes. Active infection with *M. tuberculosis* (see Chap. 125) occurs in as many as 10 percent of AIDS patients. The risk of active tuberculosis is particularly high among HIV-infected nonwhites and intravenous drug users and has led to a resurgence of tuberculosis in some cities. Although the prevalence and incidence of *M. tuberculosis* infection are similar in HIV-infected and non-HIV-infected intravenous drug users, the risk of active tuberculosis is elevated only for HIV-seropositive subjects. As in non-AIDS patients, the lungs are the most frequent site of disease, but more than half of AIDS patients with tuberculosis have at least one extrapulmonary site. As a consequence, the CDC includes extrapulmonary tuberculosis as an AIDS-defining diagnosis in HIV-infected individuals.

Cryptococcus neoformans infection (see Chap. 151) occurs in approximately 10 percent of AIDS patients as meningitis (approximately 75 percent of infections) or as disseminated disease with the lungs being the predominant organ involved. In patients with meningitis, CSF leukocyte count and protein and glucose levels may be normal. Diagnosis is established on the basis of CSF cultures and CSF cryptococcal antigen levels, with the latter usually reaching extremely high titers. Serum crytococcal antigen may be positive in these patients.

Toxoplasma gondii (see Chap. 162) is one of the most common CNS infections in AIDS patients. It occurs as an encephalitis or as an intracerebral mass lesion. Manifestations include focal neurologic changes or diffuse signs and symptoms such as mental status abnormalities and seizures. CT scans with contrast usually show multiple lesions with ring enhancement. Ocular disease occurs rarely. Serologic studies that suggest recrudescence rather than primary infection are not reliable for diagnosis, and microbiologic confirmation is often required on tissue obtained by stereotactic needle biopsy or at craniotomy. If these latter approaches are not feasible because of the location of lesions deep in the cerebral cortex, empiric treatment may be indicated in some patients in the absence of a confirmed diagnosis.

Herpes simplex virus infection (see Chap. 135) in patients with AIDS or ARC may be manifest as severe mucocutaneous disease, including perianal involvement and esophagitis; pneumonitis has been reported. Herpes zoster infection (see Chap. 136) can involve a single or several dermatomes and rarely disseminates beyond the skin.

Persistent diarrhea is frequent in AIDS patients, and in fact diarrhea that persists for longer than 1 month without an obvious cause in an HIV-infected individual establishes the diagnosis of AIDS (Table 264-1; group IV, subgroup A). The enteric pathogen *Cryptosporidium* (see Chap. 166) is an important cause of prolonged or recurrent diarrhea and may lead to malabsorption and wasting. In an immunocompetent host cryptosporidia usually cause an explosive, profuse, watery diarrhea accompanied by abdominal cramping that lasts for 5 to 11 days and abates spontaneously. In AIDS patients cryptosporidiosis is usually indolent in onset and prolonged in duration with abdominal cramping and systemic manifestations similar to those seen in normal hosts. However, prolonged and often intractable diarrhea may lead to inanition. *Isospora belli* (see Chap. 167) also causes a severe diarrhea in AIDS patients and may be indistinguishable clinically from that caused by cryptosporidia. Diarrheal syndromes can also occur secondary to CMV enteritis, Kaposi's sarcoma in the gastrointestinal tract, or other intestinal parasites and microbes.

Bacterial infections, in particular infections with encapsulated organisms, occur more commonly in children with AIDS. Even among adults, *Salmonella* infections (see Chap. 113) are a relatively common cause of diarrhea and bacteremia. Other pyogenic bacterial infections include *Haemophilus influenza* (see Chap. 115) and *Streptococcus pneumoniae* (see Chap. 99). Because of the frequent use of indwelling venous catheters in AIDS patients, infections around these devices and septicemia with *Staphylococcus aureus* and *Staph. epidermidis* (see Chap. 100) are common.

Less common infections in AIDS patients include *coccidioidomycosis* (see Chap. 151), *aspergillosis* (Chap. 151), *histoplasmosis* (Chap. 151), and *nocardiosis* (Chap. 152), and disseminated cat-scratch disease (Chap. 98).

Kaposi's sarcoma (group IV, subgroup D) is characterized histopathologically by proliferation of a mixed cell population including endothelial cells. It is often the presenting clinical manifestation of AIDS. HIV is not the direct cause of Kaposi's sarcoma, and there is no evidence of malignant transformation of cells. Furthermore, the presence and extent of Kaposi's sarcoma is not necessarily related to the degree of HIV-induced immunosuppression. The role of HIV in Kaposi's sarcoma may be the induction of growth factors that cause proliferation of the cells composing the tumor (see Chap. 134). Kaposi's sarcoma occurs in approximately 34 percent of male homosexuals with AIDS and in less than 10 percent of heterosexual AIDS patients. The reason for this discrepancy is unclear; there has been speculation that one or more cofactors present in the homosexual population accounts for the relatively higher prevalence of Kaposi's sarcoma among this group. However, such cofactors have not been identified.

Kaposi's sarcoma presents clinically as multifocal vascular nodules in the skin and viscera. The course ranges from indolent, with only skin manifestations, to fulminant, with extensive visceral involvement. The pattern of Kaposi's sarcoma in AIDS patients differs significantly from that of non-HIV-infected patients. In elderly men in the United States and Europe and in organ transplant recipients who are pharmacologically immunosuppressed, the disease is generally indolent, and extracutaneous involvement occurs in only 10 percent of patients. In non-HIV-infected children and young adults with Kaposi's sarcoma in central Africa, there is a 20 percent incidence of extracutaneous spread of disease. In contrast, extracutaneous involvement occurs in over 70 percent of AIDS patients with Kaposi's sarcoma.

The skin lesions of Kaposi's sarcoma generally present as papules or plaques that ultimately evolve into nodules. Lesions can occur in any location, but the face is a common site, especially the tip of the nose and pinnae of the ears. In advanced cases, involvement of lymphatics can cause facial edema. Oral mucous membranes are also involved frequently as are the lower extremities, particularly the soles of the feet. In the early stages, the lesions are usually painless, but some patients experience considerable pain, especially in lower extremities. Significant edema can occur with lower extremity disease. The skin and mucous membrane lesions are red or purple, do not blanch on pressure, and turn a brownish color if they resolve on therapy.

Although any organ system can be involved in the disseminated form of Kaposi's sarcoma, lymph nodes, gastrointestinal tract, and lungs are most commonly involved. Kaposi's sarcoma in the lungs often leads to extensive interstitial disease with severe impairment of diffusing capacity and may result in massive pulmonary hemorrhage. Pulmonary Kaposi's sarcoma must be differentiated from *P. carinii* pneumonia since both can present with fever and interstitial patterns on chest x-ray. Pleural effusions and bilateral lower lobe infiltrates are much more common in Kaposi's sarcoma.

Certain *lymphoid neoplasms* (see Chap. 302) are associated with HIV infection. There is an increased incidence of high-grade non-Hodgkin's lymphoma of a B-cell type, including primary B-cell lymphoma of the brain. In fact, non-Hodgkin's lymphoma occurring in an HIV-infected individual constitutes a diagnosis of AIDS (group IV, subgroup D, Table 264-1). In addition to the brain, common extranodal sites of lymphoma include bone marrow, gastrointestinal tract, liver, skin, and mucous membranes. The lymphomas are particularly aggressive, and mortality rates are high. Hodgkin's disease in HIV-infected individuals usually follows an atypically aggressive clinical course with involvement of multiple extranodal sites. The histopathologic types are usually nodular sclerosing and of mixed cellularity. The relationship between the lymphomas and HIV infection is unclear; there is no evidence that HIV directly transforms the tumor cells (see Chap. 134).

Thrombocytopenia may occur as the initial presenting sign of HIV infection. Various mechanisms of thrombocytopenia have been reported including the nonspecific deposition of complement and immune complexes on platelets, resulting in their clearance from the circulation, as well as the presence of an antibody against a 25-kD platelet protein. Platelet counts are usually 20 to 50 $\times$ 10^9 per liter (20,000 to 50,000 per microliter), but may be much lower; severe purpura has been reported. In some patients the thrombocytopenia has resolved spontaneously, but most require therapy such as glucocorticoid administration, which generally results in temporary remissions but further suppresses the immune system; splenectomy has also induced remissions (see Chap. 287). Treatment of HIV infection with zidovudine (see below) has resulted in remissions of HIV-associated thrombocytopenia.

Nonspecific interstitial pneumonitis accounts for approximately 30 percent of all episodes of clinical pneumonitis in AIDS patients. It must be distinguished from pulmonary Kaposi's sarcoma and microbial pneumonitis, particularly that caused by *P. carinii* (see above). Nonspecific interstitial pneumonitis should be suspected in patients with a clinical pneumonitis whose CD4 + lymphocyte count is >0.200 $\times$ 10^9 per liter (>200 cells per microliter). *Lymphocytic interstitial pneumonia* occurs rarely in adults with AIDS, but is found in 30 to 50 percent of children. It is felt to be an EBV-associated lymphoproliferative disease of the lungs.

DIAGNOSIS   The diagnosis of AIDS is made in an HIV-infected individual who falls within the classification level of group IV disease in Table 264-1 (see above). However, it is more appropriate to think of HIV infection as a continuous spectrum of disease rather than a strict AIDS versus non-AIDS type of categorization (see Table 264-1).

Laboratory detection of HIV infection is accomplished by a number of diagnostic tests. The most widely used is a test for HIV antibody employing the enzyme-linked immunosorbent assay (ELISA). This extremely sensitive technique has been useful in screening large numbers of individuals for HIV infection. Its major disadvantage is a relatively high incidence of false-positive reactions when used to screen people at low risk of infection. The rate of false-positive reactions with first-generation ELISAs, which employ lysates from HIV-infected cells as a source of antigen, has been reduced with second-generation tests, which use recombinant DNA proteins or synthetic peptides of the virus as antigens. All positive ELISA reactions should be repeated, and if the repeat determination is also reactive, the results should be confirmed by a more specific test for antibody. The most commonly employed confirmatory test is a western blot test that identifies antibodies to specific viral proteins. Other confirmatory tests are the immunofluorescence assay (IFA) and the radioimmunoprecipitation assay (RIPA).

Detectable antibodies to HIV usually do not appear for weeks or months following infection. Ninety-five percent of infected individuals develop detectable antibodies within 5 months of infection. However, patients may rarely be infected for 3 to 4 years before antibody is detectable. Under these circumstances, demonstration of the virus is necessary to make the diagnosis of HIV infection. Virus can be detected by assays for circulating viral protein (antigenemia), particularly the p24 core antigen. The disadvantage of this test is that although p24 antigenemia may be present prior to the development of antibodies, the antigen may not be detectable in a substantial proportion of healthy HIV-infected antibody-positive patients. In experienced laboratories, virus can be isolated in a high proportion of cases by coculture of infected patient cells with mitogen-activated peripheral blood blast cells from normal subjects. A research tool that may ultimately be a highly sensitive clinical test for detecting virus is the polymerase chain reaction (Chap. 6), which selectively amplifies viral genes allowing detection of HIV DNA present at very low frequencies in infected cells.

TREATMENT AND PROGNOSIS   The period between infection and development of symptoms is long, but variable. Mathematical models suggest that the mean incubation period for adults is approximately 8 to 10 years, whereas children under 5 years of age generally develop symptoms within 2 years. Prospective studies of a large cohort of homosexual and bisexual men indicated that after approximately 7 years of infection, 36 percent had progressed to AIDS and another 40 percent had other manifestations of infection; only 20 percent remained symptom-free. It is currently believed that virtually all infected individuals will ultimately develop progressive disease. Consequently, the therapeutic approach is to treat the HIV infection with antiretroviral drugs when indicated (see below), to treat prophylactically to prevent certain opportunistic infections when appropriate (see below), and to treat opportunistic infections and neoplasms as they occur.

Patients with AIDS or ARC should be treated with the nucleoside analogue zidovudine (3'-azido-3'-deoxythymidine; AZT) at a dose of 200 mg, orally every 4 h. If this dose cannot be tolerated, it should be reduced to 100 mg every 4 h. One report indicates that the lower dose is as effective as the higher dose and is accompanied by considerably less toxic side effects. HIV-infected individuals who have one or two symptoms and levels of CD4 + lymphocytes <0.500 $\times$ 10^9 per liter (<500 cells per microliter) benefit from zidovudine, 200 mg every 4 h, as evidenced by delay of progression to advanced ARC or AIDS. In addition, asymptomatic individuals with similar CD4 + cell counts have benefited from zidovudine, 100 mg every 4 h while awake for a total daily dose of 500 mg, because the progression to advanced ARC or AIDS is likewise delayed. Dramatic improvements in HIV-related neurologic manifestations have also been reported after administration of zidovudine. The most common toxic side effects are bone marrow suppression, resulting in anemia (often requiring transfusions) and neutropenia, and gastrointestinal intolerance. These toxicities are dose-dependent and often resolve upon reduction of the dose. Other nucleoside analogues such as dideoxyinosine (ddI) are currently being evaluated.

Treatments of the most common opportunistic infections encountered in AIDS patients are listed in Table 264-2 and in the individual chapters dealing with each infection. All of these infections have high rates of recurrence to varying degrees. For example, infections causes by CMV, *Toxoplasma gondii*, and *Cryptococcus neoformans* require maintenance treatment for life. In addition, continuous treatment or prophylaxis for other infections may be required. It is recommended that *aerosolized pentamidine isethionate*, 300 mg once per month, or trimethoprim/sulfamethoxazole, 320/1600 mg twice daily, be given to individuals who have had a previous bout of *P. carinii* pneumonia or whose CD4 + lymphocyte level is ≤0.200 $\times$ 10^9 per liter (≤200 cells per microliter).

Kaposi's sarcoma that is cosmetically acceptable to the patient, does not interfere with function, and is without significant symptoms should not be treated. When indicated, radiation therapy in the form of superficial photon or electron beam [200 cGy (200 rad) for 10 treatments] to the involved cutaneous areas or high-energy megavoltage irradiation [1500 to 3500 cGy (1500 to 3500 rad) depending on the tissue involved] may palliate localized cutaneous and extracutaneous disease. Alternatively, in patients with Kaposi's sarcoma and CD4 + -lymphocyte levels >0.150 $\times$ 10^9 per liter (>150 cells per microliter) interferon alpha (5 to 35 $\times$ 10^6 units per day adjusted for toxicity) may induce complete or partial responses in tumors in 30 to 40 percent of patients. In addition, inferferon alpha has a significant antiretroviral effect that may be helpful in combination with other antiretroviral agents. Other single agents, such as vinblastine or doxorubicin, and combinations of drugs, including etoposide (VP-16), doxorubicin, vinblastine, and bleomycin (see Chap. 301), have resulted in transient improvement in advanced disease. A major difficulty with chemotherapy is the compounding of the immunosuppressed state and the increase in risk of opportunistic infections.

Treatment of the lymphoid neoplasms should follow guidelines of therapy for non-AIDS patients (see Chap. 302). Since these tumors generally follow a more aggressive course in AIDS patients, response rates and duration of responses are less favorable than in a non-AIDS population.

A number of attempts at immune reconstitution have been undertaken. These have included bone marrow transplantation, especially between identical twins when one of the pair has AIDS; infusion of histocompatible lymphocytes; and administration of soluble mediators such as interleukin 2 and interferon gamma. Temporary partial reconstitution of the immune response has been noted in some cases.

There is no cure for AIDS, and no antiretroviral regimen is capable of eliminating HIV completely from infected individuals. As a consequence, the prognosis for infected individuals, particularly those that have advanced to symptomatic disease, is grave. Nonetheless, at least one drug (zidovudine) causes limited prolongation of survival in AIDS patients and a delay in the progression of disease in infected individuals. It is generally felt that the ultimate chemotherapeutic regimen for HIV infection, which it is hoped will lead to it becoming a chronic manageable disease, will be a combination of several antiretroviral agents acting at different phases of the HIV life cycle together with an immunoenhancing agent.

PREVENTION   Education, counseling, and behavior modification are the cornerstones of prevention of HIV infection. Widespread voluntary testing for HIV infection together with counseling of infected individuals should prove helpful in behavioral modification programs among infected individuals who would otherwise be unaware of their HIV status and who could potentially infect sexual partners. In addition, infected individuals may benefit from early therapeutic intervention even if they are asymptomatic. The incidence of new infections per year among homosexual and bisexual men in certain high-prevalence cities such as San Francisco has decreased dramatically from the early years of the epidemic. This has resulted, at least in part, from behavioral modifications regarding the number of sex partners and safe sexual practices. Several studies indicate that condom use decreases the risk of HIV transmission.

Screening of the blood supply for antibodies to HIV has almost eliminated infections among transfusion recipients and hemophiliacs who require replacement of plasma components. Continuing high rates of new infections among intravenous drug users, their heterosexual partners, and children born to intravenous drug users or to the female sexual partners of intravenous drug users will require intensive efforts aimed at treatment of drug abuse together with behavioral modification.

Health care workers should practice universal precautions when handling blood and body fluids and follow all guidelines for the prevention of transmission of HIV and hepatitis B virus that have been issued by the Centers for Disease Control (see Chap. 83).

The development of a vaccine to prevent infection and/or disease with HIV will be an important tool in the strategy for world-wide containment of the AIDS epidemic. Several candidate vaccines are undergoing early phase I testing in humans. In the monkey model of simian immunodeficiency virus (SIV), immunization with whole killed SIV is effective in protecting animals from challenge with live virus by preventing either infection or the development of disease following infection. These studies lend optimism to the feasibility of developing a safe and effective vaccine for HIV in the future.

REFERENCES

CENTERS FOR DISEASE CONTROL: Classification system for human T-lymphotropic virus type III/lymphadenopathy-associated infections. Morb Mort Week Rep 35:334, 1986
————: Revision of the CDC surveillance case definition for acquired immunodeficiency syndrome. Morb Mort Week Rep 36:1S, 1987
————: Guidelines for prevention of transmission of human immunodeficiency virus and hepatitis B virus to health-care and public safety workers. Morb Mort Week Rep 38:S-6, 1989
CURRAN JW et al: Epidemiology of HIV infection and AIDS in the United States. Science 239:610, 1988

FAUCI AS: The human immunodeficiency virus: Infectivity and mechanisms of pathogenesis. Science 239:617, 1988
FISCHL MA et al: The efficacy of azidothymidine (AZT) in the treatment of patients with AIDS and AIDS-related complex. A double-blind, placebo-controlled trial. N Engl J Med 317:185, 1987
GALLO RC, MONTAGNIER L: AIDS in 1988. Sci Am 259:41, 1988
HO DD et al: The acquired immunodeficiency syndrome (AIDS) dementia complex. Ann Intern Med 111:400, 1989
KNOWLES DM et al: Lymphoid neoplasia associated with the acquired immunodeficiency syndrome (AIDS). Ann Intern Med 108:744, 1988
LANE HC et al: Anti-retroviral effects of interferon-α in AIDS-associated Kaposi's sarcoma. Lancet 2:1218, 1988
PHAIR J et al: The risk of *Pneumocystis carinii* pneumonia among men infected with human immunodeficiency virus type 1. N Engl J Med 322:161, 1990
PIZZO PA et al: Acquired immune deficiency syndrome in children. Current problems and therapeutic considerations. Am J Med 85:(Suppl 2A) 195, 1988
PRICE RW et al: The brain in AIDS: Central nervous system HIV-1 infection and AIDS dementia complex. Science 239:586, 1988
ROSENBERG ZF, FAUCI AS: The immunopathogenesis of HIV infection. Adv Immunol 46:377, 1989
SELWYN PA et al: A prospective study of the risk of tuberculosis among intravenous drug users with human immunodeficiency virus infection. N Engl J Med 320:545, 1989

265   PLASMA CELL DISORDERS

DAN L. LONGO

GENERAL PRINCIPLES   The plasma cell disorders are monoclonal neoplasms related to each other by virtue of their development from common progenitors in the B-lymphocyte lineage. Multiple myeloma, Waldenström's macroglobulinemia, primary amyloidosis (see Chap. 266), and the heavy chain diseases comprise this group and may be designated by a variety of synonyms such as monoclonal gammopathies, paraproteinemias, plasma cell dyscrasias, and dysproteinemias. A schema for the normal development of B lymphocytes is depicted in Fig. 265-1. Mature B lymphocytes destined to produce IgG, bear surface immunoglobulin molecules of both M and G heavy chain isotypes with both isotypes having identical idiotypes (variable regions). Under normal circumstances, maturation to antibody-secreting plasma cells is stimulated by exposure to the antigen for which the surface immunoglobulin is specific; however, in the plasma cell disorders the control over this process is lost. The clinical manifestations of all the plasma cell disorders relate to the expansion of the neoplastic cells, to the secretion of cell products (immunoglobulin molecules or subunits, lymphokines), and to some extent to the host's response to the tumor.

There are three categories of structural variation among immunoglobulin molecules that form antigenic determinants, and these are used to classify immunoglobulins (Chap. 13). *Isotypes* are those determinants that distinguish among the main classes of antibodies of a given species and are the same in all normal individuals of that species. Therefore, isotypic determinants are by definition recognized by antibodies from a distinct species (heterologous sera) but not by antibodies from the same species (homologous sera). There are five heavy chain isotypes (M, G, A, D, E) and two light chain isotypes (kappa, lambda). *Allotypes* are distinct determinants that reflect regular small differences between individuals of the same species in the amino acid sequences of otherwise similar immunoglobulins. These differences are determined by allelic genes, and by definition they are detected by antibodies made in the same species. *Idiotypes* are the third category of antigenic determinants. They are unique to the molecules produced by a given clone of antibody-producing cells. Idiotypes are formed by the unique structure of the antigen binding portion of the molecule.

Antibody molecules (see Fig. 265-2) are composed of two heavy chains (mol wt ~ 50,000) and two light chains (mol wt ~ 25,000). Each chain has a constant portion (limited amino acid sequence variability) and a variable region (extensive sequence variability).

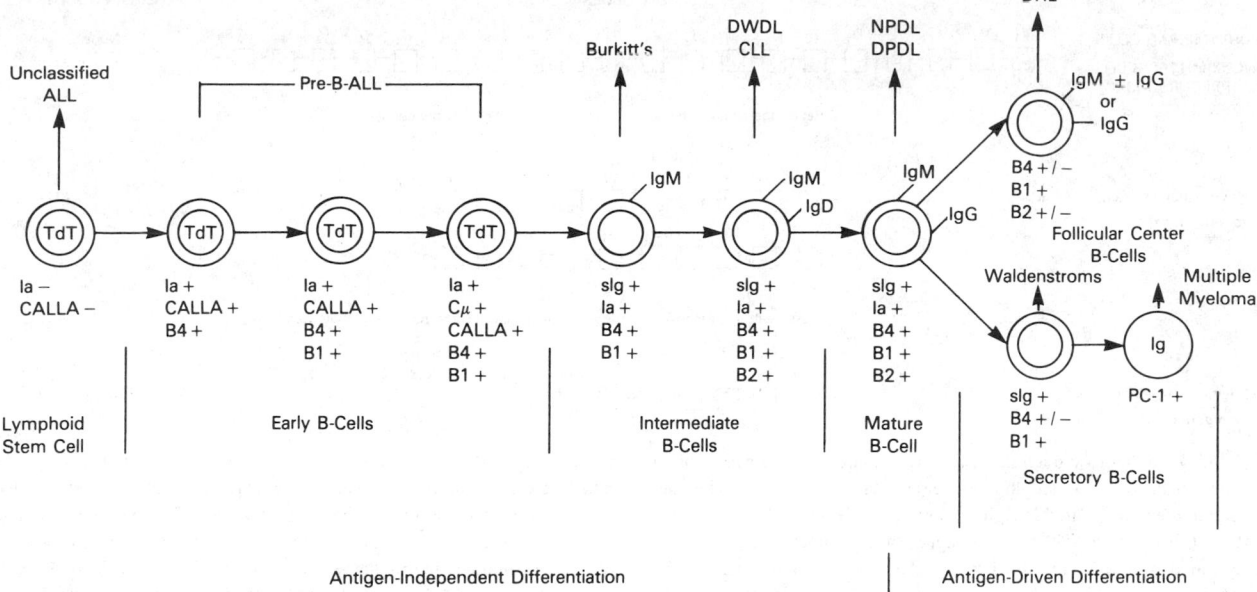

FIGURE 265-1 Schematic representation of the pathway of differentiation of normal B cells. CALLA, B1, B2, B4, Ia, PC-1, and sIg (surface immunoglobulin) are cell markers used to distinguish discrete stages of development. Terminal transferase (TdT) is a cellular enzyme. The stage of differentiation arrest for each lymphoproliferative disorder is shown. The following abbreviations are used: ALL, acute lymphoblastic leukemia; DWDL, diffuse well-differentiated lymphocytic lymphoma; CLL, chronic lymphocytic leukemia; NPDL, nodular poorly differentiated lymphocytic lymphoma; DPDL, diffuse poorly differentiated lymphocytic lymphoma; DHL, diffuse histiocytic or large-cell lymphoma.

The light and heavy chains are linked by disulfide bonds and are aligned so their variable regions are adjacent to one another. This variable region forms the antigen recognition site of the antibody molecule; its unique structural features form a particular set of determinants called idiotypes that are reliable markers for a particular clone of cells because each antibody is formed and secreted by a single clone. Each chain is specified by distinct genes, synthesized separately, and assembled into an intact antibody molecule after translation (see Fig. 265-3). Because of the mechanics of the gene rearrangements necessary to specify the immunoglobulin variable regions (VDJ joining for the heavy chain, VJ joining for the light chain; see Fig. 265-3), a particular clone rearranges only one of the two chromosomes to produce an immunoglobulin molecule of only one light chain isotype and only one allotype (allelic exclusion).

After exposure to antigen, the variable region may become associated with a new heavy chain isotype (class switch). Each clone of cells performs these sequential gene arrangements in a unique way. This results in each clone producing a unique immunoglobulin molecule. In most cells, light chains are synthesized in slight excess, are secreted as free light chains by plasma cells, and are cleared by the kidney, but less than 10 mg of such light chains is excreted per day.

Electrophoretic analysis of components of the serum proteins permits determination of the amount of immunoglobulin in the serum (Fig. 265-4). The variety of immunoglobulins move heterogeneously in an electric field and form a broad peak in the gamma region. The gamma globulin region of the electrophoretic pattern is usually increased in the serum of patients and animals with plasma cell tumors. There is a sharp spike in this region called an M component

FIGURE 265-2 Schematic depiction of an IgG molecule. Each molecule consists of two heavy and two light chains linked by disulfide bonds. There are two types of light chains, kappa (genes on chromosome 2) and lambda (chromosome 22), each containing two domains. There are 10 types of heavy chains: 4 types of G (G1 to G4), 2 of A (A1, A2), 2 of M (M1, M2), and 1 each of D and E (all on chromosome 14), each with four domains. A domain is 100 to 110 amino acids in length. Within each domain is an intrachain disulfide bond that produces a loop. V_H (variable domain of the heavy chain) and V_L (variable domain of the light chain) form an antigen binding site whose unique determinants form an idiotype. Immunoglobulins of the same isotype (e.g., IgG1κ) differ between individuals. The determinants that distinguish them are called allotypic determinants and are located on C_L (constant domain of the light chain) and C_{H2} (second constant domain of the heavy chain). C_{H2} is also the main site of glycosylation (CHO) and complement binding. Papain cleaves the molecule into antigen-binding (Fab) and crystallizable (Fc) components. The portion of the heavy chain in an Fab fragment is called the Fd piece. Fc receptors on cells bind to the C_{H3} domain. IgM and IgA occur as polymers and each unit of two heavy and two light chains is connected by a J (joining) chain. The heavy chain isotypes determine the function of the antibody.

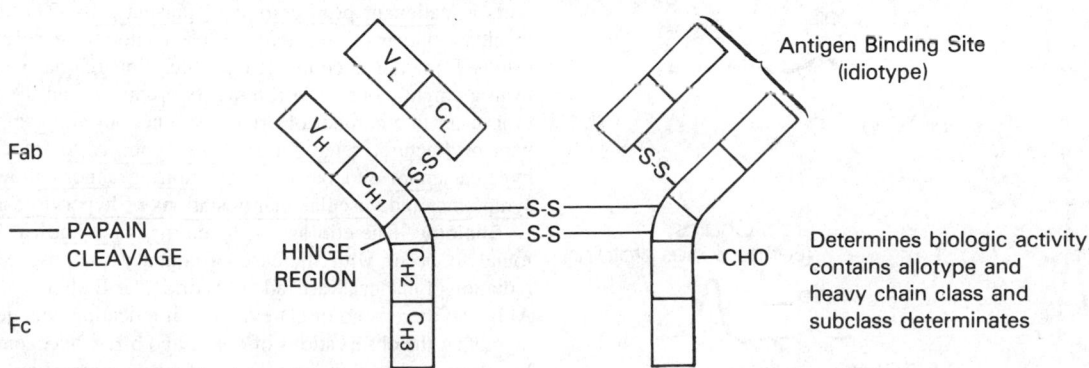

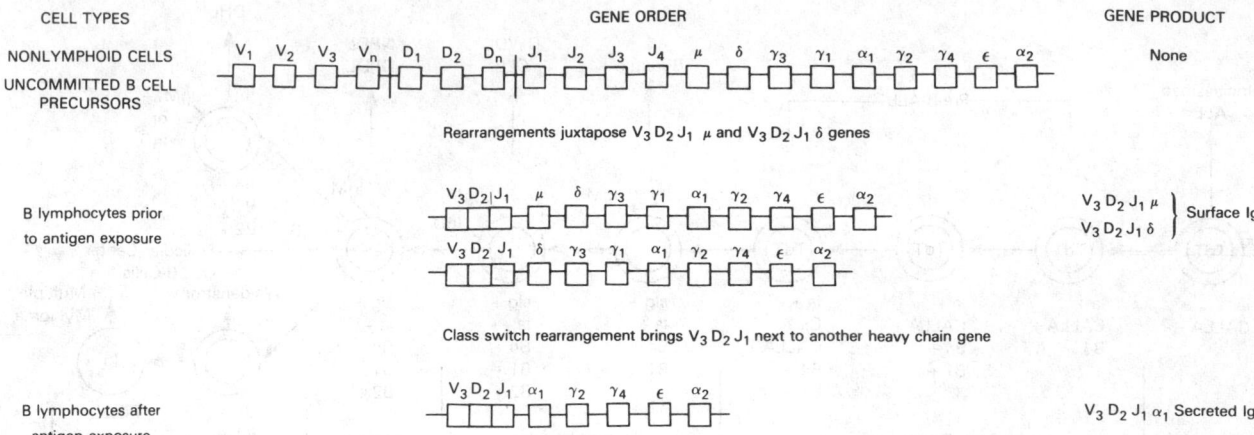

FIGURE 265-3 Schematic diagram of the organization and translocation of immunoglobulin genes. Immunoglobulin heavy chains are encoded by four distinct genetic elements, variable (Igh-V), diversity (Igh-D), joining (Igh-J), and constant (Igh-C) genes. The variable region of the immunoglobulin heavy chain is encoded by the V, D, and J genes. The same variable region may be associated with any of the 10 heavy chain constant region genes. In the germline genome (all cells except B cells) the V, D, and J genes are widely separated and there are numerous forms of each. Once a cell becomes committed to B-cell differentiation, a single V gene and a single D gene translocate to a single J gene, and the intervening genetic material is excised. This is called VDJ joining. The newly formed VDJ gene is transcribed into a single message along with either an M or D isotype C gene. Upon exposure to antigen, another rearrangement may occur so that the VDJ gene may be associated with a G, A or E isotype C gene. In light chain genes, there appear to be no D genes, and thus, light chain variable regions are formed by VJ joining.

(M for monoclonal). Less commonly the M component may appear in the beta$_2$ or alpha$_2$ globulin region. The antibody must be present at a concentration of at least 5g/L (0.5 g/dL) to be detectable by this method. This corresponds to approximately 10^9 cells producing the antibody. Confirmation that such an M component is truly monoclonal relies on the use of immunoelectrophoresis that shows a single light and heavy chain type. Hence, immunoelectrophoresis and electrophoresis provide qualitative and quantitative assessment of the M component, respectively. Once the presence of an M component has been confirmed, electrophoresis provides the more practical information for managing patients with monoclonal gammopathies. In a given patient, the amount of M component in the serum is a reliable measure of the tumor burden. This makes the M component an excellent tumor marker; yet it is not specific enough to be used to screen asymptomatic patients. In addition to the plasma cell disorders, M components may be detected in other lymphoid neoplasms such as chronic lymphocytic leukemia and lymphomas of B- or T-cell origin; nonlymphoid neoplasms such as chronic myelogenous leukemia, breast and colon cancer; a variety of nonneoplastic conditions such as cirrhosis, sarcoidosis, parasitic diseases, Gaucher's disease, and pyoderma gangrenosum; and a number of autoimmune conditions, including rheumatoid arthritis, myasthenia gravis, and cold agglutinin disease. A very rare skin disease known as lichen myxedematosus or papular mucinosis is associated with a monoclonal gammopathy. Highly cationic IgGλ is deposited in the dermis of patients with this disease. It is unclear whether this organ specificity reflects the specificity of the antibody for some antigenic component of the dermis. The nature of the M component is variable. It may be an intact antibody molecule of any heavy chain subclass, or it may be an altered antibody or fragment. Isolated light or heavy chains may be produced. In some plasma cell tumors such as extramedullary or solitary bone plasmacytomas, less than a third of patients will have an M component. In about 20 percent of myelomas, only light chains are produced and in most cases are secreted in the urine as Bence Jones proteins. The frequency of myelomas of a particular heavy chain class is roughly proportional to the serum concentration, so that IgG myelomas are more common than IgA and IgD myelomas. In some cases, the antigen specificity of the monoclonal antibody is known.

MULTIPLE MYELOMA **Definition** Multiple myeloma represents a malignant proliferation of plasma cells. The terms multiple myeloma and myeloma may be used interchangeably. The disease results from the uncontrolled proliferation of plasma cells derived from a single clone. The tumor, its products, and the host response to it result in a number of organ dysfunctions and symptoms of bone pain or fracture, renal failure, susceptibility to infection, anemia, hypercalcemia, and occasionally clotting abnormalities, neurologic symptoms, and vascular manifestations of hyperviscosity.

Etiology The etiology of myeloma is not known. Myeloma was found to occur with increased frequency in those exposed to the radiation of nuclear warheads in World War II after a 20-year latency. Although there is no direct evidence implicating oncogenes in human myeloma, the observations of c-*myc* and b-*lym* oncogenes in Burkitt's lymphoma, the high incidence of chromosomal translocations in

FIGURE 265-4 Representative electrophoretic patterns of serum and urine. The upper panel illustrates the normal pattern of serum and urine protein on electrophoresis. Since there are many different immunoglobulins in the serum, their differing mobilities in an electric field produce a broad peak. The lower panel illustrates the patterns of serum and urine proteins in a patient with myeloma. The predominance of a product of a single cell is reflected by a "church spire" sharp peak. The presence of free light chains in the urine is reflected in a peak, as well.

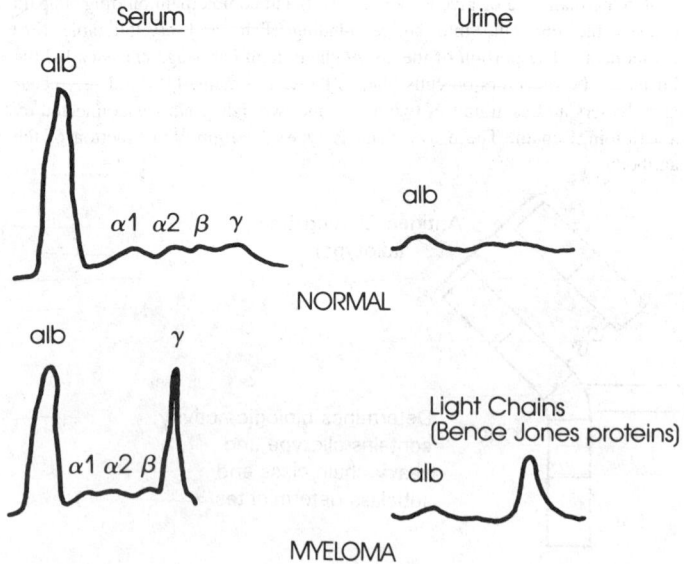

human B-cell tumors, and the role of type C RNA viruses in murine plasmacytoma formation suggest that cells of the B-cell lineage may be susceptible to growth deregulation by such stimuli. The murine plasmacytoma models are particularly interesting in that there is evidence that the induction of plasmacytomas may require exposure to foreign antigens as well as a cellular event. This suggests that chronic antigenic stimulation may play a role in the transformation of a particular B-cell clone. There is also some evidence for a genetic predisposition to myeloma in humans. Patients with myeloma have a significantly higher incidence of expressing the Glm(x) heavy chain allotype marker, and there is a weak but significant linkage disequilibrium that shows the HLA-B5 determinant being expressed more commonly than expected in myeloma patients. There is the possibility that the neoplastic event in myeloma may involve cells earlier in B-cell differentiation than the plasma cell. Circulating B cells bearing surface immunoglobulin that share the idiotype of the M component are present in myeloma patients. It is possible that the malignant clone escapes normal control mechanisms at a pre-plasma cell stage of differentiation and the chronic exposure to a particular antigenic stimulus drives the cell to terminal differentiation. It remains difficult to distinguish benign from malignant plasma cells on the basis of morphologic criteria in all but a few cases.

Incidence and prevalence Myeloma is primarily a disease of the elderly and increases in incidence with age. The median age at diagnosis is 64 years. The disease is rare under age 40. The yearly incidence is around 3 per 100,000 and remarkably similar in a variety of countries throughout the world. Males are slightly more commonly affected than females and blacks have nearly twice the incidence of whites. In the age group over 25 years of age the incidence is 30 per 100,000.

Pathogenesis and clinical manifestations (Table 265-1) Bone pain is the most common symptom in myeloma and is present in nearly 70 percent of patients. The pain usually involves the back and ribs, and unlike the pain of metastatic carcinoma which often is worse at night, the pain of myeloma is precipitated by movement. Persistent localized pain in a patient with myeloma usually signifies a pathologic fracture. The bone lesions of myeloma are caused by the proliferation

of the tumor cells and the activation of osteoclasts which destroy the bone. The osteoclasts respond to osteoclast activating factors (OAF) made by the myeloma cells (OAF activity can be mediated by several cytokines including interleukin 1, lymphotoxin, and tumor necrosis factor). However, production of these factors stops following administration of corticosteroids or interferon-gamma. The bone lesions are lytic in nature and are rarely associated with osteoblastic new bone formation; therefore, radioisotopic bone scanning is less useful in diagnosis than plain radiography. The bony lysis results in substantial mobilization of calcium from bone, and serious acute and chronic complications of hypercalcemia may dominate the clinical picture (see below). Localized bone lesions may expand to the point that mass lesions may be palpated, especially on the skull (Fig. 265-5), clavicles, and sternum, and the collapse of vertebrae may lead to symptoms of spinal cord compression.

The next most common clinical problem in patients with myeloma is susceptibility to bacterial infections. The most common infections are pneumonias and pyelonephritis, and the most frequent pathogens are *Streptococcus pneumoniae*, *Staphylococcus aureus*, and *Klebsiella pneumoniae* in the lungs and *Escherichia coli* and other gram-negative organisms in the urinary tract (Chap. 82). In about 25 percent of patients recurrent infections are the presenting features, and over 75 percent of patients will have a serious infection at some time in their course. The susceptibility to infection has several contributing causes. First, patients with myeloma have diffuse hypogammaglobulinemia if the M component is excluded. The hypogammaglobulinemia is related to both decreased production and increased destruction of normal antibodies. Moreover, some patients generate a population of circulating regulatory cells in response to their myeloma that can suppress normal antibody synthesis. In the case of IgG myeloma, normal IgG antibodies are broken down more rapidly than normal because the catabolic rate for IgG antibodies varies directly with the serum concentration. The large M component results in fractional catabolic rates of 8 to 16 percent instead of the normal 2 percent. These patients have very poor antibody responses, especially to polysaccharide antigens such as those on bacterial cell walls. Such responses are normally T-cell-independent. Most measures of T-cell function in myeloma are normal but a subset of CD4+ cells may be decreased. Granulocyte lysozyme content is low and granulocyte migration is not as rapid as normal in patients with myeloma, probably

TABLE 265-1 Pathogenesis and clinical manifestations of multiple myeloma

Clinical finding	Underlying cause	Pathogenic mechanism
Hypercalcemia, pathologic fractures, cord compression, lytic bone lesions, osteoporosis, bone pain	Skeletal destruction	Tumor expansion; production of osteoclast activating factors (OAF) by tumor cells
Renal failure	Light chain proteinuria, hypercalcemia, urate nephropathy, amyloid glomerulopathy (rare)	Toxic effects of tumor products; light chains, OAF, DNA breakdown products
	Pyelonephritis	Hypogammaglobulinemia
Anemia	Myelophthisis, decreased production, increased destruction	Tumor expansion; production of inhibitory factors and autoantibodies by tumor cells
Infection	Hypogammaglobulinemia, decreased neutrophil migration	Decreased production due to tumor-induced suppression; increased IgG catabolism
Neurologic symptoms	Hyperviscosity, cryoglobulins, amyloid deposits	Products of tumor; properties of M component; light chains
	Hypercalcemia, cord compression	OAF
Bleeding	Interference with clotting factors, amyloid damage of endothelium, platelet dysfunction	Products of tumor; antibodies to clotting factors; light chains; antibody coating of platelets
Mass lesions		Tumor expansion

FIGURE 265-5 Bony lesions in multiple myeloma. The skull demonstrates the typical "punched out" lesions characteristic of multiple myeloma. The lesion represents a purely osteolytic lesion with little or no osteoblastic activity. *(Courtesy of Dr. Geraldine Schechter.)*

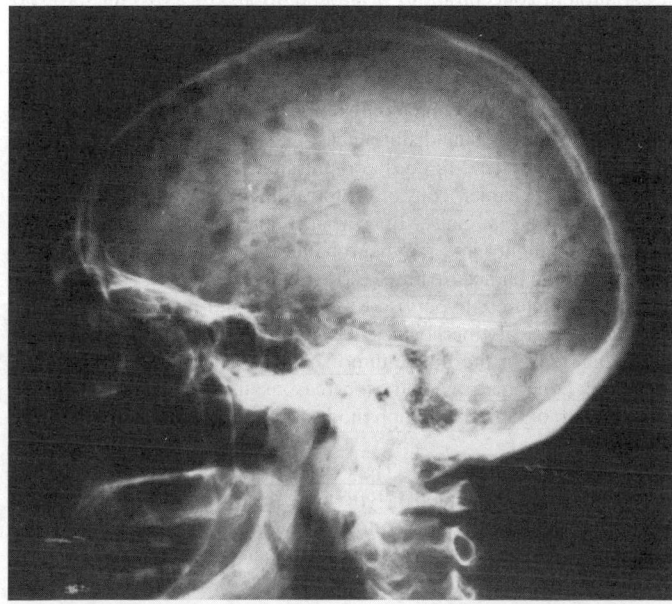

the result of a product of the tumor. There are also a variety of abnormalities in complement functions in myeloma patients. All of these factors contribute to the immune deficiency of these patients.

Renal failure occurs in nearly 25 percent of myeloma patients, and some renal pathology is noted in over half. There are many contributing factors. Hypercalcemia is the most common cause of renal failure. Glomerular deposits of amyloid, hyperuricemia, recurrent infections, and occasional infiltration of the kidney by myeloma cells all may contribute to renal dysfunction. However, tubular damage associated with the excretion of light chains is almost always present. Normally, light chains are filtered, reabsorbed in the tubules and catabolized. With the increase in amount of light chains presented to the tubule, the tubular cells become overloaded with these proteins, and tubular damage results either directly from light chain toxic effects or indirectly from the release of intracellular lysosomal enzymes. The earliest manifestation of this tubular damage is the adult Fanconi syndrome (a type 2 proximal renal tubular acidosis) with increased loss of glucose, amino acids, and defects in the ability of the kidney to acidify and concentrate the urine. The proteinuria is not accompanied by hypertension, and the protein is nearly all light chains. Generally, there is very little albumin in the urine because glomerular function is usually normal. When the glomeruli are involved, the proteinuria is nonselective. Patients with myeloma also have a decreased anion gap [i.e., sodium minus (chloride plus bicarbonate)] because the M component is cationic, resulting in retention of chloride. This is often accompanied by hyponatremia that is felt to be artificial (pseudohyponatremia) because each volume of serum has less water as a result of the increased protein.

Anemia occurs in about 80 percent of myeloma patients. It is usually normocytic and normochromic and related both to the replacement of normal marrow by expanding tumor cells and to the inhibition of hematopoiesis by factors made by the tumor. In addition, mild hemolysis may contribute to the anemia. A larger than expected fraction of patients may have megaloblastic anemia due to either folate or vitamin B_{12} deficiency. Granulocytopenia and thrombocytopenia are very rare. Clotting abnormalities may be seen due to the failure of antibody-coated platelets to function properly or to the interaction of the M component with clotting factors I, II, V, VII, or VIII. Raynaud's phenomenon and impaired circulation may result if the M component forms cryoglobulins, and hyperviscosity syndromes may develop depending on the physical properties of the M component (most common with IgM, IgG3, and IgA paraproteins). Hyperviscosity is defined on the basis of the relative viscosity of serum as compared to water. Normal relative serum viscosity is 1.8 (i.e., serum is normally almost twice as viscous as water). Symptoms of hyperviscosity occur at a level of 5 to 6, a level usually reached at paraprotein concentrations of around 40 g/L (4 g/dL) for IgM, 50 g/L (5 g/dL) for IgG3, and 70 g/L (7 g/dL) for IgA.

Although neurologic symptoms occur in a minority of patients, they may have many causes. Hypercalcemia may produce lethargy, weakness, depression, and confusion. Hyperviscosity may lead to headache, fatigue, visual disturbances, and retinopathy. Bony damage and collapse may lead to cord compression, radicular pain, and loss of bowel and bladder control. Infiltration of peripheral nerves by amyloid can be a cause of carpal tunnel syndrome and other sensorimotor mono- and polyneuropathies.

Many of the clinical features of myeloma, e.g., cord compression, pathologic fractures, hyperviscosity, sepsis, and hypercalcemia, can present as medical emergencies. Despite the widespread distribution of plasma cells in the body, tumor expansion is dominantly within bone and bone marrow and, for reasons unknown, rarely causes enlargement of spleen, lymph nodes, or gut-associated lymphatic tissue.

Diagnosis and staging   The classic triad of myeloma is marrow plasmacytosis (>10 percent), lytic bone lesions, and a serum and/or urine M component. The diagnosis may be made in the absence of bone lesions if the plasmacytosis is associated with a progressive increase in the M component over time or if extramedullary mass

lesions develop. There are two important variants of myeloma, solitary bone plasmacytoma and extramedullary plasmacytoma. These lesions are associated with an M component in less than 30 percent of the cases, they may affect younger individuals, and both are associated with median survivals of 10 or more years. Solitary bone plasmacytoma is a single lytic bone lesion without marrow plasmacytosis. Extramedullary plasmacytomas usually involve the submucosal lymphoid tissue of the nasopharynx or paranasal sinuses without marrow plasmacytosis. Both tumors are highly responsive to local radiation therapy. If an M component is present, it should disappear after treatment. Solitary bone plasmacytomas may recur in other bony sites or evolve into myeloma. Extramedullary plasmacytomas rarely recur or progress.

The most difficult differential diagnosis in patients with myeloma involves their separation from people with benign monoclonal gammopathies or monoclonal gammopathies of uncertain significance (MGUS). MGUS is vastly more common than myeloma, occurring in 1 percent of the population over age 50 and in up to 10 percent over age 75. Patients with MGUS usually have fewer than 20 g/L (2 g/dL) of M components, no urinary Bence Jones protein, less than 5 percent marrow plasmacytosis, and no anemia, renal failure, lytic bone lesions, or hypercalcemia. When bone marrow cells are exposed to radioactive thymidine in order to quantitate dividing cells, patients with MGUS always have a labeling index less than 1 percent and patients with myeloma always have a labeling index greater than 1 percent. Other discriminators include plasma cell acid phosphatase and β-glucuronidase, both of which are low in MGUS patients, and the salmon calcitonin stimulation test, which is positive only in patients with active ongoing bone destruction. Only about 11 percent of patients with MGUS go on to develop myeloma. Typically, patients with MGUS require no therapy.

The clinical evaluation of patients with myeloma includes a careful physical examination searching for tender bones and masses. It is paradoxic that only a small minority of patients have an enlargement of the spleen and lymph nodes, the physiologic sites of antibody production. Chest and bone radiographs may reveal lytic lesions or diffuse osteopenia. A complete blood count with differential may reveal anemia. Erythrocyte sedimentation rate is elevated. Very rare patients (~2 percent) may have plasma cell leukemia with more than 2000 plasma cells per microliter. This may be seen in disproportionate frequency in IgD (~12 percent) and IgE (~25 percent) myelomas. Serum calcium, urea nitrogen, creatinine, and uric acid may be elevated. Protein electrophoresis and measurement of serum immunoglobulins are useful for detecting and characterizing M spikes, supplemented by immunoelectrophoresis, which is especially sensitive for identifying low concentrations of M components not detectable by protein electrophoresis. A 24-h urine specimen is necessary to quantitate protein excretion and a concentrated aliquot is used for electrophoresis and immunological typing of any M component. Serum alkaline phosphatase is usually normal even with extensive bone involvement because of the absence of osteoblastic activity. It is also important to quantitate serum beta₂ microglobulin (see below).

The serum M component will be IgG in 53 percent of patients, IgA in 25 percent, IgD in 1 percent, and 20 percent of patients will have only light chains in serum and urine. Dipsticks for detecting proteinuria are not reliable at identifying light chains, and the heat test for detecting Bence Jones protein is falsely negative in about 50 percent of patients with light chain myeloma. Fewer than 1 percent of patients have no identifiable M component, and these are usually light chain myelomas in which renal catabolism has made them undetectable in the urine. About two-thirds of patients with serum M components also have urinary light chains. The light chain isotype may have an impact on survival. Patients secreting lambda light chains have a significantly shorter overall survival than those secreting kappa light chains. It is not clear whether this is due to some genetically important determinant of cell proliferation or because lambda light chains are more likely to cause renal damage and form amyloid than are kappa light chains. The heavy chain isotype may have an impact on patient management as well. About half of patients with IgM paraproteins develop hyperviscosity compared to only 2 to 4 percent of patients with IgA and IgG M components. Among IgG myelomas, it is the IgG3 subclass that has the highest tendency to form both concentration- and temperature-dependent aggregates, leading to hyperviscosity and cold agglutination at lower serum concentrations.

The staging system for patients with myeloma is a functional system for predicting survival and is based on a variety of clinical and laboratory tests, unlike the anatomic staging systems for solid tumors. Details of the staging system are given in Table 265-2. Based upon the hemoglobin, calcium, M component, and degree of skeletal involvement, the total-body tumor burden is estimated to be low (stage I, $<0.6 \times 10^{12}$ cells per square meter), intermediate (stage II, 0.6 to 1.2×10^{12} cells per square meter), or high (stage III, $>1.2 \times 10^{12}$ cells per square meter), and the stages are further subdivided on the basis of renal function (A if serum creatinine <2 mg/dL, B if >2). Patients in stage IA have a median survival of more than 5 years and those in stage IIIB about 15 months. Beta$_2$ microglobulin is a protein of 11,000 mol wt with homologies with the constant region of immunoglobulins that is the light chain of the class I major histocompatibility antigens (HLA-A, -B, -C) on the surface of every cell. Serum beta$_2$ microglobulin is the single most powerful predictor of survival and can substitute for staging. Patients with beta$_2$ microglobulin levels less than 0.004 g/L have a median survival of 43 months and those with levels higher than 0.004 g/L only 12 months. It is also felt that once the diagnosis of myeloma is firm, histologic features of atypia may also exert an influence on prognosis.

Treatment and course   About 10 percent of patients with myeloma will have an indolent course demonstrating only very slow progression of disease over many years. Such patients only require antitumor therapy when the serum myeloma protein rises above 50 g/L (5 g/dL) or progressive bone lesions develop. Patients with solitary bone plasmacytomas and extramedullary plasmacytomas may

be expected to enjoy prolonged, disease-free survival after local radiation therapy to a dose of around 40 Gy. There is a low incidence of occult marrow involvement in patients with solitary bone plasmacytoma. Such patients are usually detected because their serum M component falls slowly or disappears initially only to return after a few months. These patients respond well to systemic chemotherapy.

The vast majority of patients with myeloma require therapeutic intervention. In general, such therapy is of two sorts: systemic chemotherapy to control the progression of myeloma and symptomatic supportive care to prevent serious morbidity from the complications of the disease. All patients with stage II or III disease and stage I patients exhibiting Bence Jones proteinuria, progressive lytic bone lesions, vertebral compression fractures, recurrent infections, or rising serum M component should be treated with systemic combination chemotherapy. Although there are no reported cases of long-term disease-free survival (i.e., cured patients), there is no doubt that therapy can prolong and improve the quality of life for myeloma patients.

The standard treatment has consisted of intermittent pulses of an alkylating agent [L-phenylalanine mustard (L-PAM, melphalan), cyclophosphamide, or chlorambucil] and prednisone administered for 4 to 7 days every 4 to 6 weeks. The alkylating agents appear to be roughly equally active, but resistance to one agent is often accompanied by resistance to the others. The usual doses are as follows: melphalan, 8 mg/m² body surface area per day; cyclophosphamide, 200 mg/m² per day; chlorambucil, 8 mg/m² per day; prednisone, 25 to 60 mg/m² per day. Because of their near equivalence in antitumor efficacy, we favor cyclophosphamide as the alkylating agent because it is less toxic to the marrow stem cell compartment and results in a lower incidence of acute myelodysplastic syndromes than do the other alkylating agents. Doses may need adjustment based on marrow tolerance. However, there are few constraints on the dose of the steroid pulse and it appears that more is better. Recent evidence suggests that higher dose-intensity of the steroid (i.e., mg/m² per week) is associated with significantly longer survival. Patients responding to therapy generally have a prompt and gratifying reduction in bone pain, hypercalcemia, and anemia, and often have fewer infections. The serum M component lags substantially behind the symptomatic improvement, often taking 4 to 6 weeks to fall. This fall depends upon the rate of tumor kill and the fractional catabolic rate of immunoglobulin, which in turn depends upon the serum concentration (for IgG). Light chain excretion, with a functional half-life of approximately 6 h, may fall within the first week of treatment. However, since urine light chain levels may relate to renal tubular function, they are not a reliable measure of tumor cell kill. Calculations of tumor cell kill are made by extrapolation of the serum M-component level and rely heavily on the assumption that every tumor cell produces immunoglobulin at a constant rate. The data on which this assumption is based are reasonable, but recently it has been possible to alter the rate of immunoglobulin production of a myeloma in vitro with calcium channel blockers, a finding that may have clinical utility, for example, in patients with hyperviscosity. Thus, it is possible that a treatment might affect immunoglobulin production without killing the tumor cell, a situation that would result in an overestimation of the antitumor effects of the treatment if current criteria for response were applied. About 60 percent of patients will achieve at least a 75 percent reduction in serum M-component level and tumor cell mass in response to an alkylating agent and prednisone. Although this is a tumor reduction of less than one log, clinical responses may last many months. Efforts to improve the fraction of patients responding and the degree of response have involved adding other active chemotherapeutic agents to the treatment program. Patients with more advanced disease may benefit most from such an approach, but 3- to 5-drug therapy is experimental at this time.

The ideal duration of therapy has not been determined. Most physicians treat every 4 to 6 weeks for 1 or 2 years. Cessation of therapy is followed by relapse, usually within a year. Retreatment may be associated with a second response in up to 80 percent of

TABLE 265-2 Myeloma staging system

Stage	Criteria	Estimated tumor burden ($\times 10^{12}$ cells/m²)

I	All of the following:
	1 Hemoglobin >100 g/L (10 g/dL)
	2 Serum calcium <12 mg/dL
	3 Normal bone x-ray or solitary lesion
	4 Low M-component production
	  a IgG level <50 g/L (<5 g/dL)
	  b IgA level <30 g/L (<3 g/dL)
	  c Urine light chain <4 g/24 h
		<0.6 (low)

II	Fitting neither I nor III	0.6–1.20 (intermediate)

III	One or more of the following:
	1 Hemoglobin <85 g/L(<8.5 g/dL)
	2 Serum calcium (>12 mg/dL)
	3 Advanced lytic bone lesions
	4 High M-component production
	  a IgG level >70 g/L (>7 g/dL)
	  b IgA level >50 g/L (>5 g/dL)
	  c Urine light chains >12 g/24 h
		>1.20 (high)

SUBCLASSIFICATION BASED ON SERUM CREATININE LEVELS

Level	Stage	Median survival, months
A <2 mg/dL	IA	61
B >2 mg/dL	IIA,B	55
	IIIA	30
	IIIB	15

ALTERNATIVE STAGING BASED ON SERUM BETA$_2$ MICROGLOBULIN LEVELS

Level	Stage	Median survival, months
<4 µg/mL	I	43
>4 µg/mL	II	12

patients. Maintenance therapy may prolong the duration of response, but no study has demonstrated this to result in prolonged survival. The regrowth rate of the tumor during relapse accelerates with each relapse. Patients primarily resistant to initial therapy have a median survival of less than a year. High-dose pulsed steroids used alone (200 mg prednisone every other day or 1 g/m² per day methylprednisolone for 5 days) or VAD combination chemotherapy (vincristine, 0.4 mg per day 4-day continuous infusion; doxorubicin, 9 mg/m² per day in a 4-day continuous infusion; dexamethasone, 40 mg per day for 4 days per week for 3 weeks) may offer useful palliation in patients resistant to primary therapy.

About 15 percent of patients die within the first 3 months after diagnosis, and subsequently the death rate is about 15 percent per year. The disease usually follows a chronic course for 2 to 5 years before developing an acute terminal phase usually marked by the development of pancytopenia with a cellular marrow that is refractory to treatment. Widespread organ infiltration by myeloma cells occurs and survival is less than 6 months. About 46 percent of patients die in the chronic phase of disease from progressive myeloma (16 percent) and renal failure (10 percent), sepsis (14 percent), or both (6 percent). Death in the acute terminal phase (26 percent) is chiefly from progressive myeloma (13 percent) and sepsis (9 percent). Five percent of patients die of acute leukemia, myeloblastic or monocytic, and although it has been debated that this is related to the primary disease, it appears more likely to be the result of chronic therapy with alkylating agents. Nearly 23 percent of patients die of myocardial infarction, chronic lung disease, diabetes, or strokes, all intercurrent illnesses related more to the age of the patient group than the tumor.

Supportive care directed at the anticipated complications of the disease may be as important as primary antitumor therapy. The hypercalcemia generally responds well to corticosteroid therapy, hydration, and natriuresis. Calcitonin may add to the inhibitory effects of steroids on bone resorption. Dichloromethane diphosphonate has also been shown to reduce osteoclastic bone resorption. Treatments aimed at strengthening the skeleton, like fluorides, calcium, and vitamin D with or without androgens, have been suggested but are not of proven efficacy. Iatrogenic worsening of renal function may be prevented by the use of allopurinol during chemotherapy to avoid urate nephropathy and by maintaining a high fluid intake to help excrete light chains and calcium. In the event of acute renal failure, plasmapheresis is approximately 10 times more effective at clearing light chains than peritoneal dialysis, and acutely reducing the protein load may result in functional improvement. Urinary tract infections should be watched for and treated early. Chronic dialysis probably should not be initiated in patients who have failed to respond to antitumor therapy. Plasmapheresis may be the treatment of choice for hyperviscosity syndromes. Although the pneumococcus is a dreaded pathogen in myeloma patients, they do not respond to pneumococcal polysaccharide vaccines. The advent of intravenous gamma globulin preparations raises some hope that prophylactic administration may prevent some serious infections, but this has not been tested. Chronic oral antibiotic prophylaxis is probably not warranted. Patients developing neurologic symptoms in the lower extremities, severe localized back pain, or problems with bowel and bladder control may need emergency myelography and radiation therapy for palliation. Most bone lesions respond to analgesics and chemotherapy, but certain painful lesions may respond most promptly to localized radiation. The chronic anemia may respond to hematinics (iron, folate, cobalamin) and some have responded to androgens. The pathogenesis of the anemia should be established and specific therapy instituted, where possible.

WALDENSTRÖM'S MACROGLOBULINEMIA In 1948, Waldenström described a malignancy of lymphoplasmacytoid cells that secreted IgM. In contrast to myeloma, the disease was associated with lymphadenopathy and hepatosplenomegaly, but the major clinical manifestation was the hyperviscosity syndrome. The disease resembles the related diseases chronic lymphocytic leukemia, myeloma, and lymphocytic lymphoma. Waldenström's macroglobulinemia and IgM

myeloma both follow a similar clinical course. The diagnosis of IgM myeloma is usually reserved for patients with lytic bone lesions and is important only because of the hazard of pathologic fractures.

The etiology of macroglobulinemia is unknown. The disease is similar to myeloma in being slightly more common in men and occurring with increased incidence with age (median, 64 years). There have been reports that the IgM in some patients with macroglobulinemia may have specificity for myelin-associated glycoprotein (MAG), a protein that has been associated with demyelinating disease of the peripheral nervous system and may be lost earlier and to a greater extent than the better known myelin basic protein in patients with multiple sclerosis. There is a surface antigen on natural killer cells that is cross-reactive with the MAG, and coincidentally, natural killer cells are decreased in multiple sclerosis. Sometimes patients with macroglobulinemia develop a peripheral neuropathy before the appearance of the neoplasm. There is speculation that the whole process begins with a viral infection that may elicit an antibody response that cross-reacts with a normal tissue component.

Like myeloma, the disease involves the bone marrow, but unlike myeloma, it does not cause bone lesions or hypercalcemia. Like myeloma, a serum M component is present in the serum in excess of 30 g/L (3 g/dL), but unlike myeloma, the size of the IgM paraprotein results in little renal excretion and only around 20 percent of patients excrete light chains. Therefore, renal disease is not common. The light chain isotype is kappa in 80 percent of the cases. Patients present with weakness, fatigue, and recurrent infections, similar to myeloma patients, but epistaxis, visual disturbances, and neurologic symptoms like peripheral neuropathy, dizziness, headache, and transient paresis are much more common in macroglobulinemia. Physical examination reveals adenopathy and hepatosplenomegaly, and ophthalmoscopic examination may reveal vascular segmentation and dilatation of the retinal veins characteristic of hyperviscosity states. Patients may have a normocytic, normochromic anemia, but rouleaux formation and a positive Coombs' test are much more common than in myeloma. Malignant lymphocytes are usually present in the peripheral blood. About 10 percent of macroglobulins are cryoglobulins. These are pure M components and are not the mixed cryoglobulins seen in rheumatoid arthritis and other autoimmune diseases. Mixed cryoglobulins are composed of IgM or IgA complexed with IgG, for which they are specific. In both cases, Raynaud's phenomenon and serious vascular symptoms precipitated by the cold may occur, but mixed cryoglobulins are not commonly associated with malignancy. Patients suspected of having a cryoglobulin based on history and physical examination should have their blood drawn into a warm syringe and delivered to the laboratory in a container of warm water to avoid errors in quantitating the cryoglobulin.

Control of serious hyperviscosity symptoms like an altered state of consciousness or paresis can be achieved acutely by plasmapheresis because 80 percent of the IgM paraprotein is intravascular. Aside from this, management is identical to that of myeloma. About 80 percent of patients respond to chemotherapy and their median survival is over 3 years. The absence of other serious organ toxicities results in a longer life span of patients with macroglobulinemia compared to those with myeloma.

HEAVY CHAIN DISEASES The heavy chain diseases are rare lymphoplasmacytic malignancies. Their clinical manifestations vary with the heavy chain isotype. They secrete a defective heavy chain that usually has an intact Fc fragment and a deletion in the Fd region. Gamma, alpha, and mu heavy chain diseases have been described, but no reports of delta or epsilon heavy chain diseases have appeared. Molecular biologic analysis of these tumors has revealed structural genetic defects that may account for the aberrant chain secreted.

Gamma heavy chain disease (Franklin's disease) This disease affects people of widely different age groups and countries of origin. It is characterized by lymphadenopathy, fever, anemia, malaise, hepatosplenomegaly, and weakness. Its most distinctive symptom is palatal edema, resulting from node involvement of Waldeyer's ring, and this may progress to produce respiratory compromise. The diagnosis depends upon the demonstration of an anomalous serum M component [often <20 g/L (<2 g/dL)] that reacts with anti-IgG but not anti-light chain reagents. The M component is typically present in *both serum* and *urine*. Most of the paraproteins have been of the gamma$_1$ subclass, but other subclasses have been seen. The patients may have thrombocytopenia, eosinophilia, and nondiagnostic bone marrow. Patients usually have a rapid downhill course and die of infection; however, some patients have survived 5 years with chemotherapy.

Alpha heavy chain disease (Seligmann's disease)   This is the commonest of the heavy chain diseases. It is closely related to a malignancy known as Mediterranean lymphoma, a disease that affects young people in parts of the world such as the Mediterranean, Asia, and South America in which intestinal parasites are common. The disease is characterized by an infiltration of the lamina propria of the small intestine with lymphoplasmacytoid cells that secrete truncated alpha chains. Demonstrating alpha heavy chains is difficult because the alpha chains tend to polymerize and appear as a smear instead of a sharp peak on electrophoretic profiles. Despite the polymerization, hyperviscosity is not a common problem in alpha heavy chain disease. Without J-chain–facilitated dimerization, viscosity does not increase dramatically. Light chains are absent from serum and urine. The patients present with chronic diarrhea, weight loss, and malabsorption and have extensive mesenteric and paraaortic adenopathy. Respiratory tract involvement occurs rarely. Patients may vary widely in their clinical course. Some may develop diffuse aggressive histologies of malignant lymphoma. Chemotherapy may produce long-term remissions. Rare patients appear to have responded to antibiotic therapy, raising the question of the etiologic role of antigenic stimulation perhaps by some chronic intestinal infection.

Mu heavy chain disease   The secretion of isolated mu heavy chains into the serum appears to occur in a very rare subset of patients with chronic lymphocytic leukemia. The only features that may distinguish patients with mu heavy chain disease are the presence of vacuoles in the malignant lymphocytes and the excretion of kappa light chains in the urine. The diagnosis requires ultracentrifugation or gel filtration to confirm the nonreactivity of the paraprotein with the light chain reagents because some intact macroglobulins fail to interact with these serums. The tumor cells seem to have a defect in the assembly of light and heavy chains because they appear to contain both in their cytoplasm. There is no evidence that such patients should be treated differently from other patients with chronic lymphocytic leukemia.

REFERENCES

ALEXANIAN R et al: Prognosis of asymptomatic multiple myeloma. Arch Intern Med 148: 1963, 1988

BELCH A et al: A randomized trial of maintenance versus no maintenance melphalan and prednisone in responding multiple myeloma patients. Br J Cancer 57:94, 1988

CHAK LY et al: Solitary plasmacytoma of bone: Treatment, progression and survival. J Clin Oncol 5:1811, 1987

DURIE BGM et al: Pretreatment tumor mass, cell kinetics and prognosis in multiple myeloma. Blood 55:364, 1980

FARHANGI M (cd): Plasma cell myeloma and the myeloma proteins. Semin Oncol 13:259, 1986

GRIEPP PR et al: Value of beta-2-microglobulin level and plasma cell labeling indices as prognostic factors in patients with newly diagnosed myeloma. Blood 72:219, 1988

KYLE RA: Monoclonal gammopathy of undetermined significance. Natural history in 241 cases. Am J Med 64:814, 1978

KYLE RA (ed): Myeloma and related disorders, in *Neoplastic Diseases of the Blood*, New York, Churchill Livingstone, 1985, pp 385–676

PALMER M et al: Dose-intensity analysis of melphalan and prednisone in multiple myeloma. J Natl Cancer Inst 80:414, 1988

PILARSKI LM et al: Pre-B cells in peripheral blood of multiple myeloma patients. Blood 66:416, 1985

SALMON SE et al: Alternating combination chemotherapy and levamisole improves survival in multiple myeloma: A Southwest Oncology Group study. J Clin Oncol 1:453, 1983

SHEEHAN T et al. The efficacy and toxicity of VAD in the treatment of myeloma and related disorders. Scand J Haematol 37:426, 1986

266   AMYLOIDOSIS

ALAN S. COHEN

DEFINITION AND CLASSIFICATION   Amyloidosis may be defined as the extracellular deposition of the fibrous protein amyloid in one or more sites of the body. It was named by Virchow in 1854 on the basis of its color after staining with iodine and sulfuric acid. This protein has unique ultrastructural, x-ray diffraction, and biochemical characteristics. It can be deposited locally where it has no clinical consequences or may involve virtually any organ system of the body leading to severe pathophysiologic changes, or the disease may fall between these two extremes. The natural history of amyloidosis is poorly understood, and the clinical diagnosis is often not made until the disease is far advanced. It is now clear that there are multiple clinically and biochemically different forms of amyloid, that are so classified because of the unique fibrous structure that they all possess. The following classification is clinically the most useful: (1) primary (AL type) amyloidosis (no evidence for preexisting or coexisting disease); (2) amyloid associated with multiple myeloma (also AL type); (3) secondary or reactive (AA type) amyloidosis associated with chronic infectious diseases (e.g., osteomyelitis, tuberculosis, leprosy) or chronic inflammatory diseases (e.g., rheumatoid arthritis); (4) heredofamilial amyloidosis, a variety of neuropathic [AF transthyretin (prealbumin) type], renal, cardiovascular, and other syndromes, plus the amyloidosis associated with familial Mediterranean fever (AA type); (5) local amyloidosis (focal, often tumorlike, deposits which occur in isolated organs, often endocrine, without evidence of systemic involvement); (6) amyloidosis associated with aging, especially in the heart and in the brain, and (7) amyloid associated with long-term hemodialysis. These clinical forms and their current biochemical classification are listed in Table 266-1.

PATHOLOGY AND STRUCTURE   Amyloid is amorphous, eosinophilic, extracellular, and ubiquitous in distribution. The involved organs may have a rubbery consistency and a waxy, pink or gray appearance. Organ enlargement, especially of the liver, kidney, spleen, and heart, may be prominent.

Microscopically, amyloid stains pink with the hematoxylin-eosin stain and shows metachromasia with crystal violet. The Congo red stain imparts a unique green birefringence when sections are viewed in the polarizing microscope. This is the single most useful procedure for establishing the presence of amyloid. Amyloid deposits may be focal in almost any area of the body but are most often perivascular.

The heart may show focal or diffuse interstitial deposits in the myocardium, endocardium, or pericardium. In the aged heart, the atrium is usually focally involved or there may occur more diffuse lesions of the atria and ventricles. In the kidney, the glomerulus is primarily affected, although interstitial, peritubular, and vascular amyloid occur. In early lesions, small nodular or diffuse deposits appear near the basement membrane and, as the disease progresses, the glomerulus may be massively laden with amyloid, and its capillary bed will be occluded. In the gastrointestinal tract, there may be perivascular deposits only, or irregular or diffuse deposits may be found in the submucosa, in the muscularis mucosa, or subserosa. The amyloid may appear at any level or portion of the gastrointestinal tract including the gallbladder and pancreas. In the nervous system, amyloid has been described along peripheral nerves, in autonomic ganglia, and in senile plaques, in neurofibrillary tangles, as well as in blood vessels ("congophilic angiopathy") of the central nervous system. It may be found in any portion of the orbit including the vitreous humor and cornea. In summary, there is virtually no area of the body that is spared. This ubiquitous distribution elicits a wide variety of clinical symptoms and signs.

All types of human amyloid consist of fine, nonbranching rigid fibrils that in tissue sections measure approximately 10×10^9 m (100 Å) in diameter. Isolated amyloid fibrils have a delicate, thin,

TABLE 266-1 Biochemical and clinical classification of amyloid

Biochemical type	Clinical form	Comment
AL	1 Primary	Homologous to N-terminal residue of variable region of kappa or lambda light chain (or rarely whole chain). Varied molecular weight.
	2 Multiple myeloma-associated	
AA	3 Secondary (reactive)	Serum protein SAA is putative precursor; Arg-Ser-Phe-Phe-Ser sequence to 76 amino acids.
AF$_{transthyretin}$	4 Heredofamilial* especially familial amyloid polyneuropathy (Portuguese, Japanese, Swedish, Greek, Italian)	Many with single amino substitution of methionine for valine at position 30; multiple other variants exist.
AE	5 Local Focal skin, lung, etc. amyloid Focal endocrine-related amyloid i.e., thyroid (medullary carcinoma)	Calcitonin precursor; other endocrine-related forms of amyloid exist.
AS	6 Senile (aging) Heart	Two types: (1) transthyretin; (2) atrial natriuretic peptide.
	Brain	Beta protein (A4) of Alzheimer's disease
AH	7 Chronic hemodialysis-related amyloid	Beta$_2$ microglobulin

* The sole hereditary recessive amyloid is that associated with familial Mediterranean fever. This amyloid is biochemically of the AA type.

nonbranching fibrous character. The individual fibril (or filament) has a diameter of about 7×10^9 m (70 Å) and tends to aggregate laterally. Each fibril (filament) has subunit protofibrils of 3 to 3.5 $\times$ 10^9 m (30 to 35 Å) diameter. X-ray diffraction of isolated amyloid fibrils reveals a cross beta pattern, the "pleated sheet" of Pauling and Corey, indicating that the polypeptide chain runs transversely to the long axis of the fibril specimen.

A second component, the plasma component or pentagonal unit (P component or AP) with a different ultrastructure, x-ray diffraction pattern, and chemical characteristics, has also been isolated from amyloid and is identical with a serum alpha globulin (SAP). It has many similarities to C-reactive protein, but it does not behave in humans as a classic acute phase protein. It is not responsible for the characteristic tinctorial properties or ultrastructure of amyloid.

BIOCHEMISTRY OF AMYLOID FIBRILS The bulk of amyloid deposits consists of fibrils. Purified amyloid derived from the fibril is a protein. The chemical composition of the different clinical forms of amyloid are distinct and allow for more precise diagnosis (Table 266-1). The homology of the fibril of primary and myeloma amyloid to the N-terminal region of the variable fragment of an immunoglobulin light chain and subsequently, in a limited number of cases, to a homogeneous light polypeptide chain, has been demonstrated. These light chain–related proteins range in size from about 5000 to 25,000 Da and are now termed amyloid light chain (AL) or AL$_\kappa$ or AL$_\lambda$ (Table 266-1). Amino acid sequence analysis indicates that most primary amyloid proteins contain the N-terminal amino acid residue identical to the variable regions of the light chain (Asp-Ile-Gln-Ser-Pro-Ser-Ser-Leu- . . .).

Another protein that is unrelated to any known immunoglobulin has been described in the secondary amyloid deposits. This protein, amyloid A (AA) protein, can be isolated from the amyloid of patients with secondary amyloidosis and from that associated with familial Mediterranean fever. It is a unique protein with a molecular weight of about 8500 Da made up of 76 amino acid residues arranged in a single chain, and an amino acid sequence beginning with Arg-Ser-Phe. . . . Some heterogeneity has been demonstrated (i.e., AAs of different molecular weights).

Antisera to alkali-degraded amyloid fibrils of the AA protein have detected an antigenically related serum component, SAA. Amino acid analysis, peptide maps, and sequence studies suggest that AA protein is an amino terminal fragment of SAA and is derived from it by proteolysis. SAA behaves as an acute phase reactant and is elevated in infection and inflammation. In addition, SAA is elevated in amyloid-resistant animals suggesting that the appearance of amyloid is not solely determined by the level of SAA. SAA associates with the HDL$_3$ subclass of serum lipoproteins and is often referred to as apoSAA. It is likely that humans have a three-gene family for SAA. Human SAA$_1$ and SAA$_2$ are similar by restriction mapping and SAA$_3$ is different in the region of exon 3. An SAA inducing factor (now known to be interleukin 1) is released from stimulated macrophages and causes the release of SAA from hepatocytes, the site of SAA synthesis. The precise regulation of the conversion of SAA to the insoluble AA protein of amyloidosis is not understood.

Familial amyloid polyneuropathy (FAP) is a dominant hereditary disease affecting kinships originating in Portugal, Japan, Sweden, and elsewhere. A 14,000-Da protein has been isolated from the tissues of patients from each of the above-noted geographically distributed kinships. Immunologic and amino acid sequence analysis has identified it as transthyretin (prealbumin), the first association of this molecule with a disease. It has also been shown that in many kinships there is a single amino acid substitution, methionine for valine at position 30 in the transthyretin isolated from the amyloid. Multiple other variants have also been shown to exist (Table 266-2).

A number of other amyloid proteins have been isolated and characterized. These include several from focal endocrine-related amyloid lesions such as precalcitonin from the amyloid of medullary carcinoma of the thyroid and insulinoma amyloid polypeptide (IAPP) of the pancreas that is related to calcitonin gene-related peptide. Transthyretin has also been isolated from senile cardiac amyloid and atrial natriuretic peptide has been isolated as a distinct and separate

TABLE 266-2 Amino acid variations in hereditary amyloidoses

Clinical geography	Mutant position	Normal amino acid	Mutant amino acid
Familial amyloid polyneuropathy: amyloid protein = transthyretin			
1 Portugal; Sweden; Japan; Greece; Italy	30	Val	Met
2 Poland (Israel)	33	Phe	Ile
3 U.S.A.—West Virginia (Appalachia)	60	Thr	Ala
4 U.S.A.—Illinois (German)	77	Ser	Tyr
5 U.S.A.—Indiana (Swiss)	84	Ile	Ser
Familial amyloid cardiopathy: amyloid protein = transthyretin			
1 Denmark	111	Leu	Met
Familial amyloid cerebral hemorrhage			
1 Iceland: abnormal protein = cystatin C (gamma trace)	?58	?Gln	NK*
2 Netherlands: abnormal protein = ?beta protein			

* NK = Not known

protein from these lesions. Beta₂ microglobulin has been identified as the protein from the amyloid associated with chronic hemodialysis.

Of great interest is confirmation that the lesions known as senile plaques (which contain amyloid) and the meningeal vascular amyloid of Alzheimer's disease consist of a newly described protein, beta protein (or A4 protein).

P component of amyloid In addition to the characteristic fibrils described above, a second component, the P component, has been noted in most amyloid deposits. P component (AP) has been recognized by electron microscopy as a pentagonal-shaped structured unit having an outside diameter of about 9×10^9 m (90 Å) and an inside diameter of about 4×10^9 m (40 Å). On immunoelectrophoresis it migrates as an alpha globulin, and it possesses antigenic identity with a constituent of normal human plasma (SAP). The amino acid sequence is distinct from that of the amyloid fibrils. Its pentagonal ultrastructure is similar to C-reactive protein (CRP), but the latter is one-half the molecular weight of AP and has other well-defined differences despite a 50 to 60 percent homology on amino acid sequence. AP binds to amyloid fibrils in a calcium-dependent fashion almost universally and has been used as a marker of amyloid.

IMMUNOBIOLOGY OF AMYLOID The precise etiology and pathogenesis of amyloidosis are unknown. Experimentally, the induction of AA amyloidosis has been shown to be a multifactorial process that is contributed to by the type of inflammatory stimulation, the nature of the SAA isotype, and the genetic background of the host. During inflammation, the mediator, interleukin 1, stimulates hepatic cells to produce increased SAA. SAA is partially degraded by monocyte or leukocyte surface enzymes to form AA. It is likely that macrophages play a role in the SAA degradation. Related abnormalities such as altered connective tissue glycosaminoglycans, altered macrophage enzymes, or enzyme inhibitors have all been postulated.

In AL amyloid, a monoclonal population of bone marrow plasma cells appears to be present and either consistently produces small lambda or kappa fragments or clones of immunoglobulins that are processed (cleaved) in an abnormal fashion by macrophage enzymes to produce the partially degraded light chains responsible for AL amyloidosis.

The formation of amyloid may also be determined in part by the intrinsic beta configuration of at least a portion of the polypeptide chain such as in transthyretin, beta₂ microglobulin, and other amyloidogenic proteins. Clearly in the hereditary amyloidoses the substitution of a single amino acid variant contributes to the overall pathogenesis.

It has also been demonstrated that a new substance known as amyloid enhancing factor (AEF), possibly a cytokine, contributes at least to the accelerated formation of secondary and probably other forms of amyloid.

CLINICAL MANIFESTATIONS The clinical manifestations of amyloidosis are varied and depend entirely on the area of the body which is involved.

Kidney Renal involvement may consist of mild proteinuria or frank nephrosis. In some cases, the urinary sediment may show only a few red blood cells. The renal lesion is usually not reversible and in time leads to progressive azotemia and death. The prognosis does not appear to be related to the degree of the proteinuria; when azotemia finally develops, the prognosis is grave. In one series the mean survival of patients with renal amyloid from the time of biopsy was 29 months, but in a few cases there was presumptive evidence of regression of the renal amyloid. The utilization of chronic hemodialysis and of kidney transplantation will clearly improve the prognosis of renal amyloid. Hypertension is rare except in longstanding amyloidosis. Renal tubular acidosis or renal vein thrombosis may occur. Localized accumulation of amyloid may be noted in the ureter, bladder, or other parts of the genitourinary tract.

Liver While hepatic involvement is common, liver function abnormalities are minimal and occur late in the disease. The two tests most useful in indicating hepatic amyloid are the Bromsulphalein (BSP) extraction and serum alkaline phosphatase activity; however,

no liver function tests are truly specific or sensitive for amyloid. Liver scans produce variable and nonspecific results. Portal hypertension occurs but is uncommon. Intrahepatic cholestasis has been noted in about 5 percent of patients with AL (primary) amyloidosis. In a series of 38 patients in whom liver tissue was available for examination, all 38 had some amyloid present, irrespective of the type of amyloidosis (primary or secondary), and contrary to previous notions, parenchymal amyloid was more extensive in the AL cases. Hepatomegaly is common, and AL hepatic amyloid is usually accompanied by the nephrotic syndrome and by congestive heart failure. Prognosis is poor, and one group of 80 patients with proven AL hepatic amyloid had a median survival of 9 months. Amyloidosis of the spleen characteristically is not associated with leukopenia and anemia.

Heart Cardiac manifestations consist primarily of congestive failure and cardiomegaly (with or without murmurs) and a variety of arrhythmias. Although the cardiac manifestations predominantly reflect diffuse myocardial amyloid, the endocardium, valves, and pericardium may be involved as well. Pericarditis with effusion is rare, although the differential diagnosis of constrictive pericarditis versus restrictive cardiomyopathy frequently arises. Echocardiography has demonstrated symmetric thickening of the left ventricular wall, hypokinesia and decreased systolic contraction and thickening of the interventricular septum and left ventricular posterior wall, and left ventricular cavities of small to normal size. Two-dimensional echocardiography produces the characteristic findings of thickened right and left ventricles, a normal left ventricular cavity, and especially a diffuse hyperrefractile "granular sparkling" appearance. Hearts which are heavily infiltrated with amyloid may or may not show an enlarged silhouette. Fluoroscopy usually shows decreased mobility of the ventricular wall; angiographic studies usually demonstrate thickened ventricular wall, decreased ventricular mobility, and absence of rapid ventricular filling in early diastole. Cardiac amyloidosis can present as intractable heart failure. Electrocardiographic abnormalities include a low-voltage QRS complex and abnormalities in atrioventricular and intraventricular conduction, often resulting in varying degrees of heart block. Owing to their propensity to develop conduction defects and arrhythmias, patients with cardiac amyloidosis appear to be especially sensitive to digitalis, and this drug should be used with caution. Radionuclide techniques utilizing technetium 99 pyrophosphate for cardiac scanning are often positive, especially in patients with amyloid-related congestive heart failure.

Skin Involvement of the skin is one of the most characteristic manifestations of primary amyloidosis. The lesions may consist of slightly raised, waxy papules or plaques which usually are clustered in the folds of the axillae, anal, or inguinal regions, the face and neck, or mucosal areas such as ear or tongue. Periorbital ecchymoses ("black eye syndrome") have been reported. The lesions are seldom pruritic. Involvement of the skin or mucosa may not be apparent clinically but may be demonstrated by biopsy. Gentle rubbing of the skin may induce bleeding into the skin, leading to purpura. Cutaneous involvement also can occur in secondary amyloidosis; in one series it was found in 42 percent of such patients, in 55 percent of a group of patients with primary disease, and in all 11 patients with hereditary amyloid neuropathy.

Gastrointestinal tract Gastrointestinal symptoms are common in amyloidosis. They may result from direct involvement of the gastrointestinal tract at any level or from infiltration of the autonomic nervous system with amyloid. The symptoms include those of obstruction, ulceration, malabsorption, hemorrhage, protein loss, and diarrhea. Infiltration of the tongue occasionally leads to macroglossia. When not enlarged, the tongue may become stiffened and firm to palpation. While infiltration of the tongue is characteristic of primary amyloidosis or amyloidosis accompanying multiple myeloma, it is occasionally seen in the secondary form of the disease.

Gastrointestinal bleeding may occur from any of a number of sites, notably the esophagus, stomach, or large intestine, and may be severe. Amyloid infiltration of the esophagus may lead to an incompetent or nonrelaxing lower esophageal sphincter, nonspecific motility disorders of the esophageal body, or rarely achalasia. Small-bowel lesions may lead to clinical and x-ray changes of obstruction. A malabsorption syndrome is seen at times. Amyloidosis may develop in association with other entities involving the gastrointestinal tract, especially tuberculosis, granulomatous enteritis, lymphoma, and Whipple's disease; differentiation of these conditions, which give rise to secondary amyloidosis, from diffuse primary amyloidosis of the small bowel may be difficult. Similarly, amyloidosis of the stomach may closely mimic gastric carcinoma, with obstruction, achlorhydria, and the radiologic appearance of tumor masses.

Nervous system Neurologic manifestations may include peripheral neuropathy, postural hypotension, inability to sweat, Adie's pupil, hoarseness, and sphincter incompetence. These manifestations are especially prominent in the heredofamilial amyloidoses. The cranial nerves are generally spared except for those involving the pupillary reflexes. Carpal tunnel syndrome may be caused by several amyloidoses, especially primary (AL) and chronic hemodialysis (B_2M) amyloid. Peripheral neuropathy is frequent in the former type. Amyloid occurs in the central nervous system as a component of senile plaques, neurofibrillary tangles, and in blood vessels ("congophilic angiopathy"). The protein concentration in the cerebral spinal fluid may be increased. Infiltrates of the cornea or vitreous body may be present in hereditary amyloid syndromes. Certain of these syndromes are characterized by a bilateral scalloping appearance of the pupil.

Endocrine Amyloid may infiltrate the thyroid or other endocrine glands but rarely causes endocrine dysfunction. Local amyloid deposits almost invariably accompany medullary carcinoma of the thyroid. Amyloid is often found in the adrenal gland, pituitary gland, and pancreas. Little if any clinical dysfunction is present unless there is massive replacement of the gland by amyloid.

Joints Amyloid can directly involve articular structures by its presence in the synovial membrane and synovial fluid or in the articular cartilage. Amyloid arthritis can mimic a number of rheumatic diseases because it can present as a symmetric arthritis of small joints with nodules, morning stiffness, and fatigue. Most patients with amyloid arthropathy eventually are found to have multiple myeloma. The synovial fluid usually has a low white blood cell count, a good to fair mucin clot, a predominance of mononuclear cells, and no crystals. Studies of surgical specimens suggest a significant incidence of amyloid in cartilage, capsule, and synovium in osteoarthritis. Amyloid infiltration of muscle may lead to a pseudomyopathy.

Respiratory system The nasal sinuses, larynx, and trachea may be involved by accumulations of amyloid which block the ducts, in the case of the sinuses, or the air passages. Amyloidosis of the lung involves the bronchi and alveolar septa diffusely. The lower respiratory tract is affected most frequently in primary amyloidosis and in the disease associated with dysproteinemia. Pulmonary symptoms attributable to amyloid are present in about 30 percent of these patients and in some are the most serious manifestations of the disease. In secondary amyloidosis, pulmonary disease is a frequent histopathologic accompaniment but seldom gives rise to clinically significant symptoms. Amyloid may also be localized in the bronchi or pulmonary parenchyma and may resemble a neoplasm. In these cases, local excision should be attempted and, when successful, may be followed by prolonged remissions.

Hematopoietic system Hematologic changes may include fibrinogenopenia, increased fibrinolysis, and selective deficiency of clotting factors. Deficient factor X seems to be due to nonspecific calcium-dependent binding to the polyanionic amyloid fibrils. Splenectomy in the patient with such a factor-X deficiency can relieve the deficiency and the associated bleeding disorder, since factor X has been shown to bind to the large masses of splenic amyloid.

HEREDOFAMILIAL AMYLOIDOSIS There is no generally accepted nosology for the heredofamilial amyloid syndromes. Some reports emphasize the site of predominant organ involvement as neuropathic, nephropathic, or cardiopathic amyloidosis, while others

stress the genetic aspects. To date, virtually all analyses of pedigrees have shown that, with one major exception, the mode of inheritance is autosomal dominant. The exception is amyloidosis of familial Mediterranean fever (FMF), which is inherited as an autosomal recessive disorder and is an AA type of amyloid. Even in FMF amyloid, however, several kinships with autosomal dominant inheritance have been reported. The recognizable clinical patterns still form the basis for classification, although serum abnormalities (decreased serum prealbumin in several types of familial amyloid polyneuropathy) have been reported. Table 266-3 proposes a tentative classification and is based largely on the major site of organ involvement, in addition to genetic data and ethnic background. Specific single amino acid mutations have already been listed in Table 266-2.

The heredofamilial amyloidoses include a group primarily involving the nervous system. Among these are lower limb neuropathy [familial amyloid polyneuropathy (FAP)], first described in Portugal, which has a poor prognosis and is characterized by progressively severe neuropathy including marked autonomic nervous system involvement. This variety also has been described in Japan, Sweden, and in families of Greek, of Swedish and of Italian origin. In some of these individuals, bilateral "scalloped" pupils are pathognomonic of the disease. The second type of neuropathy has been found in families of Swiss origin in Indiana and of German origin in Maryland. It is a milder disease and is often associated with a carpal tunnel syndrome and vitreous opacities. A more severe variety of generalized neuropathy associated with renal amyloidosis has been described in Iowa in a family of English-Irish-Scottish ancestry.

Several types of severe familial renal disease in association with amyloid have been described. Possibly the most remarkable is FMF, a disorder subdivided into phenotype I, with irregularly occurring fever and abdominal, chest, or joint pain, preceding or accompanying renal amyloid, and phenotype II, in which renal amyloidosis is the first or only manifestation of the disease. Colchicine treatment prevents attacks of FMF and appears to prevent subsequent deposition of amyloid as well. Sporadically, other hereditary forms of renal amyloidosis have been described, including the curious association of urticaria, deafness, and renal amyloid.

Severe familial amyloid heart disease has been described in a Danish family, and familial persistent atrial standstill with amyloid in a family of Mexican-American origin. Hereditary cerebral amyloid with hemorrhage in an Icelandic family appears to be due to gamma trace protein (cystatin C) deposits and is associated with a decrease of these proteins in the cerebrospinal fluid. A similar disorder has been reported from the Netherlands. Miscellaneous hereditary amyloid syndromes include hereditary multiple endocrine neoplasms type II (including medullary carcinoma of the thyroid with amyloid) as well as others listed in Table 266-3.

DIAGNOSIS The specific diagnosis of amyloidosis depends upon obtaining a tissue specimen by biopsy and the demonstration of amyloid with appropriate stains. First, of course, the disease must be suspected. When a patient with a chronic disorder predisposing to amyloid such as rheumatoid arthritis, tuberculosis, paraplegia, multiple myeloma, bronchiectasis, or leprosy develops hepatomegaly, splenomegaly, malabsorption, cardiac disease, or, most importantly, proteinuria, amyloid should come to mind. In addition, in any heredofamilial syndromes, especially those which have a dominant autosomal mode of inheritance and are characterized by peripheral neuropathy, nephropathy, or cardiopathy, the diagnosis of amyloid should be considered. Finally, primary systemic amyloid should be considered in any individual with a diffuse noninflammatory infiltrative disease involving either mesenchymal tissues—blood vessels, heart, gastrointestinal tract—or parenchymal tissues—kidney, liver, spleen, adrenal.

When the diagnosis is suspected, it is good practice to perform an abdominal subcutaneous fat pad aspirate or a rectal biopsy. If there is a specific reason for not carrying out these procedures, other sites including skin, gums, or the suspected organ—kidney, liver—

TABLE 266-3 Classification of heredofamilial amyloidoses

Types	Forms
Familial amyloid polyneuropathy	
Type I Portuguese (Andrade)	*1* Portuguese
	2 Swedish
	3 Japanese
	4 Greek
	5 English
	6 German
	7 Italian
Type II Indiana (Rukavina)	*1* Swiss
	2 German
Type III Iowa (Van Allen)	*1* Scottish-English-Irish
(possibly same as type I)	
Type IV Cranial neuropathy and	*1* Finnish
corneal lattice dystrophy	*2* Danish
(Meretoja)	*3* Dutch
Familial oculoleptomeningeal amyloid	*1* German
	2 Dutch
	3 Japanese
Hereditary cerebral amyloid with hemor-	*1* Icelandic
rhage	*2* Dutch
Familial nephropathy	
Type I Familial Mediterranean fever	*1* Sephardic Jewish
(Heller)(recessive)	*2* Armenian
	3 Turkish
Type II Fever and abdominal pain	*1* Swedish
	2 Sicilian
Type III Urticaria, deafness, renal	
disease	
Familial cardiopathy	
Type I Progressive heart failure	*1* Danish
Type II Hereditary atrial standstill	*1* Mexican-American

may be biopsied. All tissues obtained must be stained with Congo red and examined in the polarizing microscope for green birefringence. A modified potassium permanganate stain will allow reasonably accurate differentiation of the AA type from AL amyloid. In the former, pretreatment with permanganate, followed by the standard Congo red stain, abolishes the green birefringence (i.e., the tissue is permanganate-sensitive). Beta$_2$ microglobulin amyloid is also permanganate-sensitive. The AL and AF prealbumin types are permanganate-resistant.

In order to establish the relationship of immunoglobulin-related amyloid to multiple myeloma, electrophoretic and immunoelectrophoretic studies on serum or urine should be performed when the biopsy reveals amyloid deposition. Most of these patients will have only relatively small paraprotein components and only a few will have frank multiple myeloma.

PROGNOSIS AND TREATMENT The course of amyloidosis is difficult to document since dating the time of origin of the disease is rarely possible. When amyloidosis develops in patients with rheumatoid arthritis, it seldom becomes evident when the arthritis is less than 2 years in duration. The mean duration of arthritis before amyloidosis was detected was 16 years in one series. When amyloidosis develops in patients with multiple myeloma, manifestations leading to initial hospitalization are more apt to be related to amyloid disease than to myeloma. In these cases prognosis is very poor, and life expectancy is usually less than 6 months.

Instances have been reported of amyloidosis accompanying treatable infections, such as osteomyelitis, in which at least partial remission has occurred following treatment of the primary disease. There have been similar experiences following successful treatment of tuberculosis or drainage of chronic empyema. However, many such reports are not substantiated by biopsy proof of resorption.

Generalized amyloidosis is usually a slowly progressive disease and leads to death in several years, but it may have a better prognosis than was suspected in the past. The average survival in most large series is 1 to 4 years, but a number of individuals with amyloid have been followed 5 to 10 years and longer.

The major cause of death is renal failure. Sudden death, presumably due to arrhythmias, is also quite common. Occasionally, gastrointestinal hemorrhage, respiratory failure, intractable heart failure, and superimposed infections are the terminal events.

There is no specific therapy for any variety of amyloidosis. Rational therapy should be directed at (1) decreasing chronic antigenic stimuli that produce amyloid, (2) inhibition of the synthesis and extracellular deposition of amyloid fibrils, and (3) promoting lysis or mobilization of existing amyloid deposits.

A variety of agents have been used to treat amyloidosis. Proof of their efficacy is not available. The finding that a portion of the immunoglobulin light chain is incorporated in the amyloid of patients with primary amyloidosis and its presumed synthesis by plasma cells has led to the use of alkylating agents. However, these agents cause bone marrow depression, and there are reports of acute leukemia developing in amyloidosis patients receiving melphalan. Moreover, there is experimental evidence that immunosuppressive agents may enhance the deposition of preexisting amyloid. Hence, conservative and supportive measures have been the mainstay of management. Recent trials have indicated that a prednisone/melphalan regimen or a prednisone/melphalan/colchicine program prolongs life. Studies in several centers are underway to compare these programs to each other and to colchicine alone (see below).

Patients with severe renal amyloidosis and azotemia have been subjected to bilateral nephrectomy and renal transplantation followed by immune therapy. One of two patients died of infection 5 months after surgery. The donor kidney showed no evidence of amyloidosis. The second patient achieved a 10-year clinical remission after receiving a transplanted kidney. Notwithstanding the hazards of operating upon patients with systemic amyloidosis who may have cardiac involvement, carefully selected azotemic patients clearly benefit from transplantation.

Colchicine has been shown to be effective in preventing acute attacks in patients with FMF, and two groups of investigators independently have reported the inhibition of amyloid deposition in the mouse model by colchicine. It is conceivable, therefore, that colchicine is effective in blocking amyloid deposition. One large study has shown it to be effective in prolonging life in primary (AL) amyloidosis using a life-table survivorship analysis. However, the exact mechanism of its action is unknown. The use of dimethylsulfoxide (DMSO) in the treatment of amyloid has had variable results.

REFERENCES

COHEN AS: Amyloidosis. N Engl J Med 277:522, 1967

———, SKINNER M: Diagnosis of amyloidosis, in *Laboratory Diagnostic Procedures in the Rheumatic Diseases,* 3d ed, AS Cohen (ed). Orlando, Fla, Grune & Stratton, 1985

——— et al: Amyloid proteins, precursors, mediator, and enhancer. Lab Invest 48:1, 1983

GLENNER GG et al: Amyloid fibril proteins: Proof of homology with immunoglobulin light chains. Science 172:1150, 1971

——— et al: *Amyloid and Amyloidosis.* New York, Excerpta Medica, 1980

HUSBY G, SLETTEN K: Chemical and clinical classification of amyloidosis, 1985. Scand J Immunol 23:253, 1986

KISILEVSKY R: From arthritis to Alzheimer's disease: Current concepts on the pathogenesis of amyloidosis. Can J Physiol Pharm 65:1805, 1987

KYLE RA, GREIPP PR: Amyloidosis (AL): Clinical and laboratory features in 229 cases. Mayo Clin Proc 58:665, 1983 section 2 **Disorders of immune-mediated injury**

267 DISEASES OF IMMEDIATE TYPE HYPERSENSITIVITY

K. FRANK AUSTEN

The term *atopic allergy* implies a familial tendency to manifest alone or in combination such conditions as asthma, rhinitis, urticaria, and eczematous dermatitis (atopic dermatitis). However, individuals without an atopic background may also develop hypersensitivity reactions, particularly urticaria and anaphylaxis, associated with the same class of antibody, IgE, found in atopic individuals. The designation *diseases of immediate type hypersensitivity* presents a more suitable framework than the broad term *allergy* or the restrictive definition of atopy.

The fixation of IgE to human basophils has been demonstrated by radioautography and electron microscopy and to intraepithelial and perivenular mast cells in tonsils, adenoids, and nasal polyps of humans by immunofluorescence. IgE-dependent mediator generation and release also occur in the mast cells of human lung slices, nasal polyps, or skin and have been observed in those tissues most involved in diseases of immediate type hypersensitivity.

Studies with purified rat peritoneal mast cells have indicated that the IgE receptor is transmembrane-linked and that stereospecific receptor perturbation activates a polyphosphatidyl inositol–selective phospholipase C to elaborate 1,2-diacylglycerols (1,2-DAG) and inositol-1,4,5-*bis*-phosphate (IP$_3$), which in turn activate protein kinase C and mobilize intracellular calcium ions, respectively. These events may be augmented by the formation of calcium ion channels and attenuated by the activation of adenylate cyclase with formation of cyclic 3',5'-adenosine monophosphate (cyclic AMP) and activation of cyclic AMP–dependent protein kinase. The calcium ion-dependent activation of phospholipases cleaves membrane phospholipids to generate lysophospholipids, which like 1,2-DAG, are fusogenic and may facilitate the fusion of the secretory granule perigranular membrane with the cell membrane, a step which releases the membrane-free granule containing the preformed or primary mediators of mast cell effects. The arachidonic acid generated simultaneously by phospholipase action is processed oxidatively into secondary mediators of the prostaglandin and leukotriene (Fig. 267-1) classes. The lysophospholipid formed from release of arachidonic acid from 1-*0*-alkyl-2-acyl-*sn*-glyceryl-3-phosphorylcholine can be acetylated in the second position to form platelet activating factor (PAF) (Fig. 267-2). The secretory granule of the human mast cell has a crystalline structure, unlike mast cells of lower species, and IgE-dependent cell activation can be characterized morphologically by solubilization and swelling of the granule contents within the first minute of receptor perturbation; this reaction is followed by the ordering of intermediate filaments about the swollen granule, movement toward the cell surface, and fusion of the perigranular membrane with that of other granules and with the plasmalemma to form extracellular channels for mediator release while maintaining cell viability.

Important insight into the diversity of mast cells within a species has been gained from studies of serosal mast cells considered to be connective tissue mast cell (CTMC) and mucosal mast cell (MMC) populations from rats infected with *Nippostrongylus brasiliensis*. The CTMC secretory granules stain with alcian blue and counterstain with safranin, contain large amounts of histamine, heparin proteoglycan, chymotryptic protease termed neutral protease I, and carboxypeptidase A, generate prostaglandin D$_2$ upon IgE-Fc–dependent activation, and remain viable ex vivo in coculture with fibroblasts in the absence of added T-cell factors. The MMC secretory granules stain with alcian blue but not safranin, contain small amounts of histamine and a distinct chymotryptic protease termed neutral protease II, generate leukotriene C$_4$ in preference to prostaglandin D$_2$ (PGD$_2$) during activation-secretion, and are T-cell factor–dependent for appearance in vivo or generation from progenitors in vitro. Upon stimulus-specific activation in vitro, the membrane-derived lipid mediators such as leukotrienes, PGD$_2$, and PAF along with histamine and selected secretory granule–associated acid hydrolases are solubilized, whereas the neutral proteases, which are cationic, remain largely complexed to the anionic proteoglycans. It is speculated that the macromolecular complex serves to deliver the neutral proteases so that the endo- and exoproteases can function in concert at the substrate site.

Histamine and the various lipid mediators alter venular permeability, and the cysteinyl leukotrienes constrict both vascular and nonvascular smooth muscle. Leukotrienes C$_4$ and D$_4$ (LTC$_4$ and

FIGURE 267-1 Metabolism of phospholipids to arachidonic acid and cyclooxygenase-derived products. Cleavage of arachidonic acid from membrane phospholipids during cellular activation proceeds either by the action of phospholipase A$_2$ (PLase A$_2$) or by the sequential action of phospholipase C (PLase C) and diacylglycerol lipase (DAG lipase). Biosynthesis of prostaglandins is depicted with the structure of PGD$_2$, which is the predominant product from mast cells via the terminal action of a PGD$_2$ synthetase. The η-lipoxygenase family of monolipoxygenases; includes 5-lipoxygenase, which initiates the pathway to leukotriene generation. Abbreviations: PGG$_2$, PGH$_2$, PGI$_2$, PGE$_2$, PGF$_{2\alpha}$, PGD$_2$, prostaglandins G$_2$, H$_2$, I$_2$, E$_2$, F$_{2\alpha}$, and D$_2$, respectively; TxA$_2$, TxB$_2$, thromboxane A$_2$ and B$_2$, respectively; 6-k-PGF$_{1\alpha}$, 6-keto-prostaglandin F$_{1\alpha}$; HHT, 12-hydroxy-heptadecatrienoic acid. (*Modified from Schwartz and Austen, Immunological Diseases, 4th ed.*)

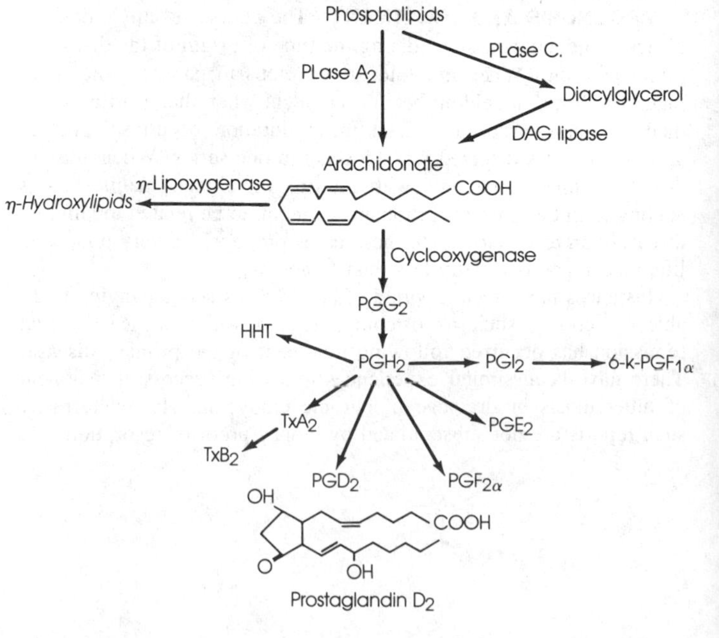

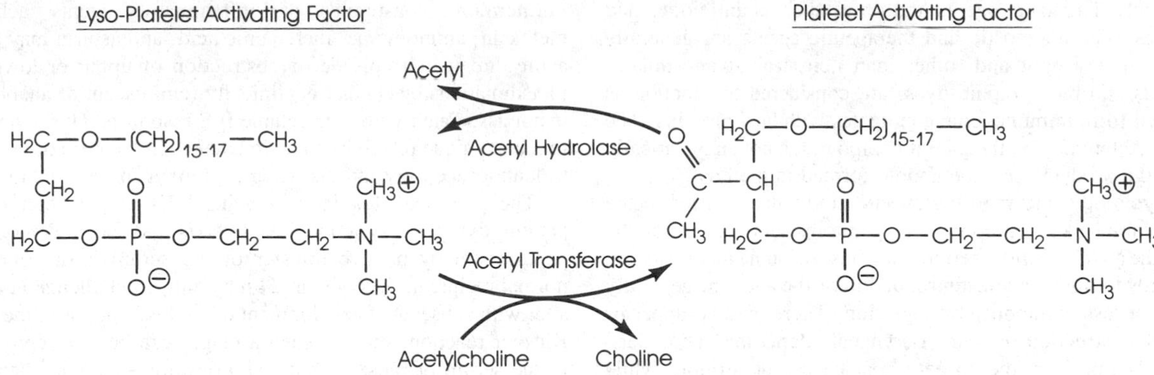

Lyso-Platelet Activating Factor   Platelet Activating Factor

FIGURE 267-2 Synthesis and degradation of platelet activating factor. *(From Schwartz and Austen, Immunological Diseases, 4th ed.)*

LTD$_4$) are logs more potent than histamine in constricting human airway smooth muscle when administered by aerosol, and leukotriene E$_4$ (LTE$_4$), the most stable member of the family, is also somewhat more potent than histamine. The 5-lipoxygenation of arachidonic acid to 5S-hydroperoxy-6-*trans*-8,11,14-*cis*-eicosatetraenoic acid (5-HPETE) and then to 5,6-*trans*-oxido-7,9-*trans*-11,14-*cis*-eicosatetraenoic acid (LTA$_4$) is followed by the adduction of glutathione via a microsomal LTC$_4$ synthase to yield 5S-hydroxy-6R-S-glutathionyl-7,9-*trans*-11,14-*cis*-eicosatetraenoic acid (LTC$_4$); upon transport across the membrane to the extracellular environment LTC$_4$ undergoes sequential cleavage of the glutathione portion to yield the cysteinyl-glycyl (LTD$_4$) and cysteinyl (LTE$_4$) derivatives. Alternatively, a cytosolic LTA$_4$ epoxide hydrolase converts LTA$_4$ into 5S-12R-dihydroxy-6,14-*cis*-8,10-*trans*-eicosatetraenoic acid (LTB$_4$), which mediates leukocyte margination and directed (chemotactic) migration in human sites.

The evidence for diversity of mast cells within the human is more subtle than in the rat, but nonetheless is sufficient to suggest possible functional implications. Mast cells of human lung, intestine, and skin each stain with alcian blue but not safranin and have a similar histamine content. Dispersed partially purified human lung and intestinal mast cells respond to activation by IgE-Fc–dependent mechanisms with generation of LTC$_4$ and PGD$_2$; are not activated by various peptide agonists; are enriched for the secretory granule neutral protease tryptase; and exhibit secretory granules with a scroll and crystalline ultrastructure. In the lung they synthesize heparin proteoglycan in a 2:1 ratio to chondroitin sulfate E proteoglycan, and in the intestine they are T-cell-dependent, as revealed by their absence from mucosal sites in patients with T-cell deficiencies. The skin mast cells are readily stimulated for exocytosis by diverse peptides such as C5a anaphylatoxin, substance P, and f-Met-Leu-Phe; elaborate PGD$_2$ with IgE-Fc receptor–dependent activation; are much enriched for the secretory granule neutral proteases—tryptase, chymase, and carboxypeptidase A—and for heparin proteoglycan; exhibit secretory granules with a lattice and crystalline ultrastructure; and are present in the intestinal submucosa of patients with T-cell deficiencies. Whether mast cell diversity is determined entirely by the microenvironment or is dictated in part by different progenitors derived from a common marrow precursor is not established.

In any event, mast cells bearing specific recognition units are distributed at cutaneous and mucosal surfaces and in deeper tissues about venules, are an expansile population during T-cell stimulation, and could regulate the entry of foreign substances by their rapid response capability. A local increase in venular permeability via the action of histamine and membrane-derived lipid mediators could introduce critical plasma proteins such as complement and immunoglobulin. Phagocytic cells such as eosinophils would be elicited by PAF and specific peptides, while LTB$_4$ would recruit neutrophils and, in time, monocyte-macrophages. The secretory granule exo- and endoproteases might function to clear damaged connective tissue elements and facilitate tissue repair. There is even evolving evidence that mast cells via their constituents can regulate fibroblast proliferation

and/or angiogenesis. Local and subclinical regulation of the tissue microenvironment would represent an initial and homeostatic physiologic response, while an intense or continuous stimulus would result in inflammation and tissue injury which could be either beneficial or detrimental (hypersensitivity) depending upon the appropriateness of the immunologic specificity.

Consideration of the mechanism of immediate type hypersensitivity diseases in the human has focused largely on the IgE-dependent recognition of otherwise nontoxic substances. Support for this thesis has come from the finding that clinical atopic allergy is associated with elevated total levels of IgE and in some instances with an immune response that is specifically linked to the histocompatibility locus. Populations of allergic whites have a significantly higher total serum level of IgE than nonallergic individuals, and highly atopic persons with asthma have significantly higher serum levels of IgE than those with fewer allergic manifestations. IgE distribution in normal families is consistent with the dominant inheritance of the low-IgE phenotype. As a result of the action of a single IgE regulator gene, the majority of family members would have elevated IgE levels as a possible basis for their atopic state. The association between HLA histocompatibility type and the immediate hypersensitivity response has been noted in persons of the low-IgE phenotype who were studied with highly purified allergens, generally of small size. Such presumptive evidence of immune response (Ir) genes by linkage disequilibrium, that is, the association of the hypersensitivity response with a particular histocompatibility haplotype, represents an additional element in the polygenic atopic allergic state. Nonetheless, all the studies taken together, both of families and of populations, seem to indicate that the genetically determined elevated IgE levels found in about three-fourths of atopic allergic subjects exert the predominant influence on most specific IgE responses. It is also likely that diseases of immediate type hypersensitivity may occur because of deficient intracellular controls of mediator generation or release, or both, or that the extracellular controls directed against mediator inactivation may be impaired.

ANAPHYLAXIS **Definition** The life-threatening anaphylactic response of a sensitized human appears within minutes after administration of specific antigen and is manifested by respiratory distress often followed by vascular collapse or by shock without antecedent respiratory difficulty. Cutaneous manifestations exemplified by pruritus and urticaria with or without angioedema are characteristic of such systemic anaphylactic reactions. Gastrointestinal manifestations include nausea, vomiting, crampy abdominal pain, and diarrhea.

Predisposing factors and etiology There is no convincing evidence that age, sex, race, occupation, or geographic location predisposes a human to anaphylaxis except through exposure to some immunogen. According to most studies, atopy does not predispose individuals to penicillin anaphylaxis.

The materials capable of eliciting the systemic anaphylactic reaction in the human include the following: heterologous proteins in the form of antiserum, hormones, enzymes, Hymenoptera venom, pollen extracts, and foods; polysaccharides such as iron dextran; and most commonly diagnostic agents and drugs such as antibiotics and even vitamins. The diagnostic and therapeutic agents are generally of low molecular weight and, other than nonsteroidal anti-inflammatory agents and radiographic dyes, are considered to function as haptens which form immunogenic conjugates with host proteins. The conjugating hapten may be the parent compound, a nonenzymatically derived storage product, or a metabolite formed in the host.

Pathophysiology and manifestations Individuals differ in the time of appearance of perception of symptoms and signs, but the hallmark of the anaphylactic reaction is the onset of some manifestation within seconds to minutes after introduction of the antigen, generally by injection or less commonly by ingestion. There may be upper or lower airway obstruction or both. Laryngeal edema may be experienced as a "lump" in the throat, hoarseness, or stridor, while bronchial obstruction is associated with a feeling of tightness in the chest or audible wheezing. A particularly characteristic feature is the eruption of well-circumscribed, discrete cutaneous wheals with erythematous, raised, serpiginous borders and blanched centers. These urticarial eruptions are intensely pruritic and may be localized or distributed. They may coalesce to form giant hives, and seldom persist beyond 48 h. A localized, nonpitting, deeper edematous cutaneous process, angioedema, may also be present. It may be asymptomatic or cause a burning or stinging sensation.

In fatal cases with clinical bronchial obstruction, the lungs show marked hyperinflation on gross and microscopic examination. The microscopic findings in the bronchi, however, are limited to luminal secretions, peribronchial congestion, submucosal edema, and eosinophilic infiltration, and the acute emphysema is attributed to intractable bronchospasm which subsides with death. The angioedema resulting in death by mechanical obstruction occurs in the epiglottis and larynx, but the process is also evident in the hypopharynx and to some extent the trachea; on microscopic examination there is wide separation of the collagen fibers and the glandular elements; vascular congestion and eosinophilic infiltration are also present. Patients dying of vascular collapse without antecedent hypoxia from respiratory insufficiency have visceral congestion but no major shift in the distribution of blood volume. The associated electrocardiographic abnormalities, with or without infarction, noted in some patients could reflect a primary cardiac event or be secondary to a critical reduction in plasma volume.

The angioedematous and urticarial manifestations of the anaphylactic syndrome have been attributed to release of endogenous histamine. A role for the cysteinyl leukotrienes in altering pulmonary mechanics by causing marked bronchiolar constriction seems likely. Vascular collapse without respiratory distress in response to experimental challenge with the sting of a hymenopteran was associated not only with marked and prolonged elevations in blood histamine but also with evidence of intravascular coagulation and kinin generation. Based upon the findings that patients with systemic mastocytosis and episodic hypotension proceeding to vascular collapse excrete large amounts of PGD_2 in addition to histamine and are controlled by administration of a nonsteroidal agent but not by antihistamines alone, it may be that PGD_2 is also of importance in the hypotensive anaphylactic reactions. Because of the marked coronary arterial constrictor action of the cysteinyl leukotrienes upon administration to experimental animals, these substances may be involved in the disease process of patients with myocardial ischemia without or with infarction.

Diagnosis The diagnosis of an anaphylactic reaction depends largely upon an accurate history revealing the onset of the appropriate symptoms and signs within minutes after the responsible material is encountered. When only a portion of the full syndrome is present, such as isolated urticaria, sudden bronchospasm in an asthmatic patient, or vascular collapse after intravenous administration of an agent, it is difficult to exclude a nonimmunologic, toxicologic or idiosyncratic response. For example, intravenous administration of a chemical mast cell–degranulating agent may elicit generalized urticaria, angioedema, and a sensation of retrosternal oppression with or without clinically detectable bronchoconstriction or hypotension.

Furthermore, nonsteroidal anti-inflammatory agents such as indomethacin, aminopyrine, mefenamic acid, and aspirin may precipitate a life-threatening episode of obstruction of upper or lower airways in asthmatic subjects that is clinically reminiscent of anaphylaxis but is not associated with a detectable IgE response. This syndrome may reflect a unique reactivity to an imbalance in the ratio of prostaglandin to leukotriene biosynthesis when cyclooxygenase is inhibited.

The presence of a labile reagin (IgE) in the heart blood of a patient dying of systemic anaphylaxis has been demonstrated at postmortem by passive transfer of the serum intradermally into a normal recipient, followed in 24 h by antigen challenge into the same site, with subsequent development of a wheal and flare, the Prausnitz-Küstner reaction. Indeed, such a reagin can be transiently identified in the serum of most patients who develop systemic anaphylaxis to a variety of different agents. In order to avoid the hazards of transferring hepatitis to the recipient in the Prausnitz-Küstner reaction, it is preferable to employ the less sensitive monkey recipient or a human leukocyte suspension enriched with basophils for subsequent antigen challenge. It is presumed that the activity responsible for most cases of systemic anaphylaxis resides with the IgE class, since the Prausnitz-Küstner activity in the serums of patients with systemic reactions to Hymenoptera venom or human seminal plasma protein can be removed by IgE immunosorbent columns. Furthermore, radioimmunoassays have demonstrated specific IgE antibodies in patients with anaphylactic reactions to insulin and to parathormone, but such approaches require purified antigens. In the transfusion anaphylactic reaction that occurs in patients with IgA deficiency, the responsible specificity resides in IgG anti-IgA rather than in IgE; the mechanism of the reaction is presumed to be complement activation with secondary mast cell participation.

Treatment and prevention Early recognition of an anaphylactic reaction is mandatory, since death occurs within minutes to hours after the first symptoms. Mild symptoms such as pruritus and urticaria can be controlled by administration of 0.2 to 0.5 mL of 1:1000 epinephrine subcutaneously, with repeated doses as required at 3-min intervals for a severe reaction. If the antigenic material was injected into an extremity, the rate of absorption may be reduced by prompt application of a tourniquet proximal to the reaction site, administration of 0.2 mL of 1:1000 epinephrine into the site, and removal without compression of an insect stinger, if present. An intravenous infusion should be initiated to provide a route for administration of epinephrine, diluted 1:50,000, volume expanders, and vasopressor agents if intractable hypotension occurs. Epinephrine most likely acts to reverse the action of mediators on target tissues, and its early administration appears critical. When epinephrine fails to control the situation, hypoxia due to airway obstruction or related to a cardiac arrhythmia, or both, must be considered. Oxygen via a nasal catheter or intermittent positive pressure breathing of oxygen with 0.5 mL isoproterenol diluted 1:200 in saline may be helpful, but either endotracheal intubation or a tracheostomy is mandatory if progressive hypoxia exists. Ancillary agents such as the antihistamine diphenhydramine, 50 to 80 mg intramuscularly or intravenously, and aminophylline, 0.25 to 0.5 g intravenously, are appropriate for urticaria-angioedema and bronchospasm, respectively. Intravenous corticosteroids are not effective for the acute event but may be considered for persistent bronchospasm and hypotension.

Prevention of anaphylaxis must take into account the sensitivity of the recipient, the dose and character of the diagnostic or therapeutic agent, and the effect of the route of administration on the rate of absorption. If there is a definite history of a past anaphylactic reaction, even though mild, it is advisable to select another agent or procedure. A skin test should be performed before the administration of certain materials producing a high incidence of anaphylactic reactions, such as horse serum or allergenic extracts, or when the nature of the past adverse reaction is unknown. Since even a skin or conjunctival test can produce a serious reaction, a scratch test should precede these tests in a high-risk situation. With regard to penicillin, two-thirds of patients with a positive reaction history and positive intradermal skin tests to benzylpenicilloyl-polylysine (BPL) and/or the minor determinant mixture (MDM) of benzylpenicillin products experience allergic reactions with treatment, and these are almost uniformly of the anaphylactic type in those patients with minor determinant reactivity. Even patients without a history of previous clinical reactions have a 6 percent incidence of positive skin tests to the two test materials, and about 3 per 1000 with a negative history experience anaphylaxis with therapy with a mortality of about 1 per 100,000. The value of skin testing is both to permit therapy with the agent in question when the risk does not exist and to emphasize the hazards where the sensitivity is confirmed. In the event that an agent must be used despite a positive history, a positive skin test, or both, the following precautionary measures should be taken: An intravenous infusion should be started, with intubation equipment and a tracheostomy set at hand; the material should be given intradermally, then subcutaneously, and then intramuscularly in increasing doses at 20- to 30-min intervals so that the initial dose by the next route does not exceed the final dose by the previous route. It is difficult to be certain that the mediator-containing cells have been exhausted, and therapeutic use of the agent may be accompanied by untoward consequences. It may be critical to give the therapeutic agent at regular intervals to prevent the reestablishment of a sensitized cell pool of large size. A different form of protection involves the development of blocking antibody of the IgG class which is protective against Hymenoptera venom–induced anaphylaxis by interacting with antigen so that less reaches the sensitized tissue mast cells; to be effective this immunotherapy requires the use of specific or cross-reacting Hymenoptera venom rather than whole-insect-body extracts.

URICARIA AND ANGIOEDEMA Definition Urticaria and angioedema may appear separately or together as cutaneous manifestations of localized nonpitting edema; a similar process may occur at mucosal surfaces of the upper respiratory or gastrointestinal tract. *Urticaria* involves only the superficial portion of the dermis presenting as well-circumscribed wheals with erythematous raised serpiginous borders with blanched centers which may coalesce to become giant wheals. *Angioedema* is a well-demarcated localized edema involving the deeper layers of the skin including the subcutaneous tissue. Recurrent episodes of urticaria and/or angioedema of less than 6 weeks' duration are considered acute, while attacks persisting beyond this period are designated chronic.

Predisposing factors and etiology The occurrence of urticaria and angioedema is probably more frequent than usually described because of the evanescent, self-limited nature of such eruptions, which seldom require medical attention when limited to the skin. Although persons in any age group may experience acute or chronic urticaria and/or angioedema, these lesions increase in frequency after adolescence, with the highest incidence occurring in persons in the third decade of life; indeed, one survey of college students indicated that some 15 to 20 percent had experienced a pruritic wheal reaction.

The classification of urticaria-angioedema presented in Table 267-1 focuses on the different mechanisms for eliciting clinical disease. Only the IgE-dependent and the IgG-mediated reactions in IgA-deficient persons should be considered immediate hypersensitivity. However, the other mechanisms are important for differential diagnosis, and most cases of chronic urticaria are idiopathic. The appearance of urticaria and angioedema in atopic persons in the absence of a specific exposure is attributed to the atopic diathesis and implies an IgE mechanism. Urticaria and/or angioedema occurring during the appropriate season in patients with seasonal respiratory allergy or as a result of exposure to animals or molds is attributed to inhalation of pollens, animal dander, and mold spores, respectively. However, urticaria and angioedema secondary to inhalation are relatively uncommon compared with ingestion of fresh fruits, shellfish, chocolate, nuts, tomatoes, and various drugs, including penicillin-contaminated milk products, which may elicit not only the anaphylactic syndrome with prominent gastrointestinal complaints but also chronic urticaria. Additional etiologies include physical stimuli such as cold, solar rays, exercise, and mechanical irritation (dermographism).

TABLE 267-1 Classification of urticaria with angioedema

1 IgE-dependent
  a Atopic diathesis
  b Specific antigen sensitivity (pollens, foods, drugs, fungi, molds, Hymenoptera venom, helminths)
  c Physical: dermographism; cold; light; cholinergic; vibratory; exercise-related
2 Complement-mediated
  a Hereditary angioedema: type 1; type 2
  b Acquired angioedema: type 1; type 2
  c Necrotizing vasculitis
  d Serum sickness
  e Reactions to blood products
3 Nonimmunologic
  a Direct mast cell–releasing agents: opiates; antibiotics; curare, D-tubocurarine; radiocontrast media
  b Agents which presumably alter arachidonic acid metabolism: aspirin and nonsteroidal anti-inflammatory agents; azo dyes and benzoates
4 Idiopathic

Angioedema without urticaria occurs with C$\bar{1}$ inhibitor (C$\bar{1}$INH) deficiency that can be inborn as an autosomal dominant characteristic or can be acquired in association with lymphoproliferative disorders. The urticaria and angioedema associated with classical serum sickness or with idiopathic cutaneous necrotizing angiitis is believed to be an immune-complex disease when hypocomplementemia is a concomitant. The idiosyncratic drug reactions to mast cell granule-releasing agents and to nonsteroidal anti-inflammatory drugs, resembling anaphylaxis, or limited to cutaneous sites.

Pathophysiology and manifestations Urticarial eruptions are distinctly pruritic, involve any area of the body from the scalp to the soles of the feet, and appear in crops of 24- to 72-h duration with old lesions fading as new ones appear. The most common sites are the extremities, external genitalia, and face, particularly the region of the eyes and lips. Although self-limited in duration, angioedema of the upper respiratory tract may be life-threatening due to laryngeal obstruction, while gastrointestinal involvement may present with abdominal colic, with or without nausea and vomiting, and may precipitate unnecessary surgical intervention. No residual discoloration occurs with either urticaria or angioedema unless there is an underlying process leading to superimposed extravasation of erythrocytes.

The pathology of urticaria and angioedema is usually characterized by massive edema of the dermis in urticaria, and of the subcutaneous tissue as well as the dermis in angioedema. Collagen bundles in affected areas are widely separated, and the venules are sometimes dilated. The perivenular infiltrate may consist of lymphocytes, eosinophils, and neutrophils that are present in varying combination and number throughout the dermis. Allergen-induced wheal-and-flare reactions are characterized by mast cell degranulation and an accumulation of eosinophils over hours to days. The elicitation of a wheal-and-flare response upon injection of the relevant allergen into a patient with urticaria and/or angioedema, or into a site in a normal recipient prepared with serum from the patient, the Prausnitz-Küstner reaction, indicates an IgE-dependent, mast cell–mediated reaction.

Perhaps the best-studied example of mast cell–mediated urticaria and angioedema is *cold urticaria*. Acquired cold urticaria is a disorder in which patients exposed to cold experience an urticarial eruption that may evolve into angioedema and be associated with syncope. Cryoglobulins, cryofibrinogens, cold agglutinins, or hemolysins may be recognized, but not in the majority of patients. The finding in a number of patients of a serum factor, characterized as being of the IgE class, that is capable of transferring the cold urticaria reaction to a skin site of a normal recipient has focused attention upon the mast cell in this condition. Immersion of an extremity in an ice bath precipitates angioedema of the distal portion with urticaria at the air interface within minutes of the challenge. Histologic studies reveal marked mast cell degranulation with associated edema of the dermis and subcutaneous tissues. The venous effluent of the cold-challenged and angioedematous extremity reveals a marked rise in plasma content of histamine, low-molecular-weight eosinophilotactic activity, and high-molecular-weight neutrophil chemotactic activity, which are presumably of mast cell origin, whereas the venous effluent of the contralateral normal extremity contains none of these mediators. Elevations of plasma histamine with biopsy-proven mast cell degranulation have also been demonstrated with systemic attacks of *cholinergic urticaria* and *exercise-induced erythema-angioedema* precipitated experimentally by exercise on a treadmill while wearing a wet suit.

Diagnosis The rapid onset and self-limited nature of urticarial and angioedematous eruptions are distinguishing features. Additional characteristics are the occurrence of the urticarial crops in various stages of evolution and the asymmetric distribution of the angioedema. Urticaria and/or angioedema involving IgE-dependent mechanisms are often appreciated by historical considerations implicating specific allergens, by seasonal incidence, by exposure to certain environments, or by physical stimuli such as cold, exercise, sunlight (solar urticaria), or trauma (dermographism). Direct reproduction of the lesion with physical stimuli is particularly valuable because it so often establishes the cause of the lesion. The diagnosis can be confirmed by careful testing with the putative foreign substance to determine if a local wheal and flare results, and by passive transfer of such a reaction with serum of the patient to a skin site in a normal recipient, the Prausnitz-Küstner phenomenon. Passive transfer to the skin of a nonhuman primate or in vitro to human basophils may also be attempted. IgE-mediated urticaria and/or angioedema may or may not be associated with an elevation of total IgE or with peripheral eosinophilia. Fever, leukocytosis, or an elevated sedimentation rate are characteristically absent.

The classification of urticarial and angioedematous states noted in Table 267-1 in terms of possible mechanisms necessarily includes some differential diagnostic points. Hypocomplementemia is not observed in IgE-mediated mast cell disease and can reflect either an acquired abnormality generally attributed to the formation of immune complexes or a genetic deficiency of $C\overline{1}INH$. Chronic recurrent urticaria, generally in females, associated with arthralgias, an elevated sedimentation rate, and normo- or hypocomplementemia suggests an underlying cutaneous necrotizing angiitis. Confirmation depends upon a biopsy which reveals cellular infiltration, nuclear debris, and fibrinoid necrosis of the venules.

Hereditary angioedema is an autosomal dominant state associated with the absence of functional $C\overline{1}INH$. The diagnosis is suggested not only by family history but also by the lack of urticarial lesions, the prominence of recurrent gastrointestinal attacks of colic, and episodes of laryngeal edema. Laboratory diagnosis depends upon demonstrating the antigenic lack of $C\overline{1}INH$ (type 1) in most kindreds, but some kindreds have an antigenically intact nonfunctional protein (type 2) and require a functional assay to establish the diagnosis. The natural substrates of uninhibited $C\overline{1}$, C4, and C2 are chronically depleted but fall further during attacks due to the activation of additional C1 to $C\overline{1}$. An acquired form of $C\overline{1}INH$ deficiency, associated with lymphoproliferative disorders, has the same clinical manifestations and differs in the lack of a familial element; in the reduction of $C1/C\overline{1}$ as well as $C\overline{1}INH$, C4, and C2; and in the presence of an anti-idiotypic antibody to the monoclonal immunoglobulin expressed on the B cells (type 1). In a second acquired form of $C\overline{1}INH$ deficiency with angioedema due to appearance of IgG anti-$C\overline{1}INH$ (type 2) B cell malignancy has not been prominent.

Urticaria and angioedema must be differentiated from contact sensitivity, an acute vesicular eruption that progresses to chronic thickening of the skin with continued allergenic exposure. They must also be differentiated from atopic dermatitis, a condition that may present as erythema, edema, papules, vesiculation, and oozing proceeding to a subacute and chronic stage in which vesiculation is less marked or absent, and in which scaling, fissuring, and lichenification predominate in a distribution that characteristically involves the flexor surfaces. In cutaneous mastocytosis the reddish-brown macules and papules, characteristic of urticaria pigmentosa, urticate with pruritus upon trauma, and in systemic mastocytosis, without or with urticaria pigmentosa, there is an episodic systemic flushing with or without urticaria but no angioedema.

Prevention and treatment Identification of the etiologic factor(s) and their elimination provide the most satisfactory therapeutic program; this approach is feasible to varying degrees with IgE-mediated reactions to allergens or physical stimuli. Topically applied steroids are of no benefit in the management of urticaria and/or angioedema, and while systemic steroids have no general value, they are helpful in an occasional patient with necrotizing cutaneous angiitis, pressure urticaria, or even ordinary urticaria and angioedema. Antihistamines of the H1 class and sympathomimetic agents often provide symptomatic relief; cyproheptadine, hydroxyzine, and a combination of H1 and H2 antihistamines are held to be even more beneficial. The therapy of inborn $C\overline{1}INH$ deficiency has been simplified by the finding that attenuated androgens correct the biochemical defect and afford prophylactic protection. Since the affected individuals are heterozygous, with the depletion of $C\overline{1}INH$ being due to a combination of deficient synthesis and excessive utilization of the normal gene product, the efficacy of the attenuated androgens is attributed to production by the normal gene of an amount of functional $C\overline{1}INH$ sufficient to control the spontaneous activation of C1 to $C\overline{1}$. Since the use of such agents for children and pregnant women is not yet accepted, the antifibrinolytic agent ϵ-aminocaproic acid may be used occasionally to control spontaneous attacks or for preoperative prophylaxis in some patients.

ALLERGIC RHINITIS Definition Allergic rhinitis is characterized by sneezing, rhinorrhea, obstruction of the nasal passages, conjunctival and pharyngeal itching, and lacrimation. Although commonly seasonal because of its relation to airborne pollens, other patterns and etiologies occur. The use of the term "hay fever" to describe seasonal allergic rhinitis is a common convention but is literally inappropriate because the symptom complex is neither produced by hay nor associated with fever.

Predisposing factors and etiology Allergic rhinitis generally presents in atopic individuals, that is, in persons with a family history of a similar or related symptom complex and a personal history of collateral allergy expressed as eczematous dermatitis, urticaria, and/or asthma (see Chap. 204). Symptoms generally appear before the fourth decade of life and tend to diminish gradually with aging, although complete spontaneous remissions are uncommon. A relatively small number of weeds which depend upon wind rather than insects for cross-pollination, as well as certain grasses and trees, produce sufficient quantities of pollen suitable for wide distribution by air currents to elicit seasonal allergic rhinitis. The dates of pollination of these species generally vary little from year to year in a particular locale but may be quite different in another climate. Molds, which are widespread in nature because they occur in soil or decaying organic matter, may propagate spores in a pattern dependent upon climatic conditions. Perennial allergic rhinitis occurs in response to allergens that are present throughout the year such as in desquamating epithelium in animal dander, the processed materials or chemicals utilized in an industrial setting, or the dust accumulating at work or at home. Dust has a diverse content including mites, and many patients with perennial rhinitis are sensitive only to house dust. Moreover, in many patients with perennial rhinitis, no clear-cut allergen can be demonstrated. The ability of allergens to cause rhinitis rather than lower respiratory symptoms may be attributed to their size, 10 to 100 μm, and retention within the nose. However, even when the allergen penetrates to the lower respiratory tract, whether it elicits a bronchoconstrictor response resulting from mediator release depends on the presence of chronically hyperirritable airways.

Pathophysiology and manifestations Episodic rhinorrhea, sneezing, and obstruction of the nasal passages with lacrimation and pruritus of the conjunctiva, nasal mucosa, and oropharynx are the hallmarks of allergic rhinitis. The nasal mucosa is pale and boggy, but the nares are not reddened or excoriated. The conjunctiva may be congested and edematous; the pharynx is generally unremarkable but may appear injected. Swelling of the turbinates and mucous membranes with obstruction of the sinus ostia and eustachian tubes precipitates secondary infections of the sinuses and middle ear, respectively, commonly in perennial but rarely in seasonal disease. Nasal polyps often arise concurrently with edema and/or infection within the sinuses and increase obstructive symptoms.

The nose presents a large mucosal surface area through the folds of the turbinates and serves to adjust the temperature and moisture content of inhaled air and to filter out particulate materials. The convoluted nasal passages readily filter out particles above 10 μm in size by impingement in a mucous blanket at bends in their course; ciliary action then moves the entrapped particles toward the pharynx. Entrapment of pollen and digestion of the outer coat by mucosal enzymes such as lysozymes release protein allergens generally of 10,000 to 40,000 molecular weight. Although the initial interaction occurs between the allergen and intraepithelial mast cells sensitized with specific IgE, the bulk of the mast cells are located beneath the mucosal surface and are recruited secondarily. During the symptomatic season when the mucosa are already swollen and hyperemic, there is enhanced adverse reactivity to the seasonal pollen as well as to antigenically unrelated pollens for which there is underlying hypersensitivity. This priming effect is attributed to improved penetration of the allergens to the deeper perivenular mast cells. Biopsy specimens of nasal mucosa during an episodic allergic reaction show profound submucosal edema with infiltration predominantly by eosinophils, although some neutrophil polymorphonuclear leukocytes are present. Polyps, a feature in perennial rhinitis, are mucosal protrusions containing chiefly edema fluid with variable degrees of eosinophilic infiltration.

The mucosal surface fluid contains not only IgA that is present preferentially because of its secretory piece, but also IgE, which apparently arrives by diffusion from plasma cells distributed in proximity to mucosal surfaces. IgE fixes to mucosal and submucosal mast cells, and the intensity of the clinical response to inhaled allergens is quantitatively related to the naturally occurring or experimentally defined pollen dose. Specific IgE is distributed not only to tissue mast cells but also to circulating basophilic leukocytes; patients with more severe clinical disease have basophils which release histamine in response to lesser concentrations of allergen in vitro than do cells from patients with milder disease. Human nasal polyps from ragweed-sensitive patients release histamine, eosinophilotactic peptides, and spasmogenic leukotrienes upon challenge with ragweed allergen in vitro. In sensitive individuals, the introduction of allergen into the nose is associated with sneezing, "stuffiness," and discharge, and the fluid contains histamine, PGD_2, and leukotrienes. Thus, the mast cells of nasal polyp tissue, and of the nasal mucosa and submucosa, generate and release mediators through IgE-dependent reactions which are capable of producing tissue edema and eosinophilic infiltration.

Diagnosis The diagnosis of seasonal allergic rhinitis depends largely upon an accurate history of occurrence coincident with the pollination of the offending weeds, grasses, or trees. The continuous character of perennial allergic rhinitis due to contamination of the home or place of work makes historical analysis difficult, but there may be a variability in symptoms that can be related to animal exposure or work habits. Patients with perennial rhinitis commonly develop the problem in adult life, are more often women than men, and manifest nasal polyps and thickening of the sinus membranes by x-ray. The term *vasomotor rhinitis* designates a symptom complex resembling perennial allergic rhinitis without an established allergic basis. Other entities to be excluded are exposure to irritants, upper respiratory infection, pregnancy with prominent nasal mucosal edema, prolonged topical use of alpha-adrenergic agents in the form of nose drops, and the use of certain therapeutic agents such as rauwolfia. Nasal polyps are a characteristic of perennial allergic rhinitis and are often associated with sinus infection.

The nasal secretions of allergic patients are rich in eosinophils, and peripheral eosinophilia with elevations in relation to clinical exacerbations is a common feature. Local or systemic neutrophilia implies infection. Total serum IgE is frequently elevated, but the demonstration of immunologic specificity for IgE is critical to an etiologic diagnosis. Some normal individuals will exhibit a wheal-and-flare skin response to intracutaneous inoculation of high concentrations of common airborne allergens. The diagnosis rests not only on the skin test alone, but also on the correlation of the clinical history with skin reactivity to concentrations of allergen selected by controlled testing. This provides the best balance of selectivity with specificity. Scratch tests with food allergens are unreliable, while intracutaneous testing may be dangerous, and elimination diets are the best approach to the diagnosis. Regardless of method of testing, food allergy is uncommon as a significant cause of allergic rhinitis.

Although standard radioimmunodiffusion techniques can be used to screen for patients with markedly elevated levels of IgE, their sensitivity of less than 1000 ng/mL is insufficient to detect the elevations in most atopic allergic patients. A commonly employed technique, sensitive to about 50 ng/mL, is known as the competitive radioimmunosorbent test (RIST). In this procedure, the IgE of the serum competes with radiolabeled IgE for solid-phase-bound anti-IgE; the displacement of radiolabeled IgE is compared to a standard curve to yield the IgE concentration of the serum. Other assays, such as the noncompetitive RIST, in which the anti-IgE immunosorbent is exposed to a series of standard IgE preparations before introducing the unknown, and double-antibody radioimmunoprecipitin test (RIP), have greater sensitivity and reproducibility, respectively, and, like the competitive RIST, establish a normal geometric mean serum IgE for nonallergic whites of less than 120 ng/mL. Even more useful is the measurement of specific anti-IgE in serum by its binding to a solid-phase allergen and quantitation by the subsequent uptake of radiolabeled anti-IgE. This radioallergosorbent technique (RAST) correlates satisfactorily with the bioassay of specific IgE by skin test or histamine release from peripheral blood leukocytes and is convenient for the patients; however, it requires defined allergens and full standardization. Further, neither the immunochemical nor bioassay detection of a previous immune response to a foreign material mandates a therapeutic intervention, unless there is relevant concomitant evidence of a significant clinical problem.

Prevention and treatment Avoidance of exposure to the offending allergen is the most effective means of controlling allergic diseases; removal of pets from the home to avoid animal danders, utilization of air filtration devices to minimize the concentrations of airborne pollens, travel to nonpollinating areas during the critical periods, and even a change of domicile to eliminate a mold spore problem may be necessary. *Immunotherapy*, often termed *hyposensitization*, consists of repeated subcutaneous injections of gradually increasing concentrations of the allergen(s) considered to be specifically responsible for the symptom complex. Controlled studies in ragweed and grass allergic rhinitis have established that patients are partially relieved of their symptoms by such treatments applied over a period of years. Improvement appears to be dose-related, and the end point is based either on severe adverse local or systemic reactions to the allergen injection or on satisfactory relief of symptoms. The immunologic characteristics of a response include a rise in antibodies of the IgG class, a small increase in specific IgE early in the treatment course followed by a plateau or decline, and a decline in the percentage of histamine released from peripheral blood basophilic leukocytes challenged with a fixed concentration of the allergen. The antibodies of the IgG class might well reduce or neutralize the quantity of allergen available for interaction with the tissue mast cells but, more importantly, could modify the seasonal booster response in specific IgE synthesis. None of the individual parameters of the response to immunotherapy correlates well with the assessments of clinical efficacy, suggesting that benefit is derived from a complex of effects. Immunotherapy should be reserved for clearly documented seasonal diseases that cannot be managed with drugs because of their side effects.

Management with pharmacologic agents offers a diverse approach. Antihistamines are the only specific end-organ antagonists available for control of a mast cell–derived reaction and are limited to competition with but one mediator. Nonetheless, antihistamines are very effective for some patients, and the side effects such as drowsiness and gastrointestinal distress, which limit the dosage of a particular preparation, can sometimes be circumvented by use of an agent of different structure. An orally active agent with alpha-adrenergic activity is often employed for its decongestant effects and to partially counteract the drowsiness produced by antihistamines. Topical administration of alpha-adrenergic agents may be helpful but has the immediate disadvantage of rebound vasodilatation, and prolonged usage may produce a chronic rhinitis. The topically active steroids of the beclomethasone class ameliorate symptoms of both seasonal and perennial rhinitis without detectable adrenal suppression and represent a major advance in therapy. Cromolyn sodium inhaled nasally has also given encouraging prophylactic results and is of particular merit because it acts to prevent mast cell activation.

REFERENCES

AUSTEN KF: Biologic implications of the structural and functional characteristics of the chemical mediators of immediate-type hypersensitivity. The Harvey Lectures, Series 73, 1977–1978, p 93

CAULFIELD JP et al: Secretion in dissociated human pulmonary mast cells. Evidence for solubilization of granule contents before discharge. J Cell Biol 85:299, 1980

CRETICOS PS et al: Peptide leukotriene release after antigen challenge in patients sensitive to ragweed. N Engl J Med 310:1626, 1984

GREEN GR et al: Evaluation of penicillin hypersensitivity: Value of clinical history and skin testing with penicilloyl-polylysine and penicillin G. J Allerg Clin Immunol 60:339, 1977

ISHIZAKA T, ISHIZAKA K: Activation of mast cells for mediator release through IgE receptors. Progr Allergy 34:188, 1984

LEWIS RA, AUSTEN KF: The biologically active leukotrienes: Biosynthesis, metabolism, receptors, functions, and pharmacology. J Clin Invest 73:889, 1984

MARSH DG et al: Genetics of the human immune response to allergens. J Allerg Clin Immunol 65:322, 1980

SCHWARTZ LB, AUSTEN KF: The mast cells and mediators of immediate hypersensitivity, in Immunological Diseases, 4th ed, M Samter et al (eds). Boston, Little, Brown, 1988, p 157

SOTER NA et al: Urticaria and arthralgias as manifestations of necrotizing angiitis (vasculitis). J Invest Dermatol 63:485, 1974

————: Release of mast cell mediators and alterations in lung function in patients with cholinergic urticaria. N Engl J Med 302:604, 1980

268   IMMUNE-COMPLEX DISEASES

THOMAS J. LAWLEY / MICHAEL M. FRANK

DEFINITION   The term *immune-complex disease* refers to a group of diseases thought to be mediated by the deposition of immune complexes in specific organ or tissue sites including the glomerulus of the kidney and blood vessel walls. In general these immune deposits are thought to arise from antigen-antibody complexes formed in the circulation. Once deposited in tissues, the complexes activate a variety of potent soluble mediators of inflammation, such as the complement proteins, causing an influx of polymorphonuclear neutrophils and monocytes. These activated cells release toxic products of oxygen metabolism as well as various proteases and other enzymes, ultimately causing tissue damage. While the specific etiology of these diseases is variable, they share a common pathophysiology. The clinical features of these diseases are quite diverse, ranging from mild cutaneous eruptions to severe organ involvement with pericarditis, glomerulonephritis, and vasculitis.

PATHOPHYSIOLOGY   The introduction of foreign or noxious materials into an individual is often followed by an immune response. Specific antibody produced in the course of this response binds to antigen, forming immune complexes. In general, these complexes are phagocytosed and destroyed by macrophages of the reticuloendothelial system. However, at times these complexes are deposited in tissues, causing inflammation and tissue damage. In recent years, there has been a concerted effort to understand the mechanisms underlying this damage.

The biologic activity of the complexes has been studied in detail. It has been shown that the isotype of antibody affects biologic activity. Thus IgG- and IgM-containing complexes activate the classic complement pathway, and IgA-containing complexes may activate the alternative complement pathway. In contrast, cell surface IgE complexes are capable of mediating the degranulation of mast cells by a noncytotoxic, complement-independent mechanism.

The size of the immune complexes in the circulation is an important parameter of toxicity. In general the larger (>19 S) complexes cause more tissue damage than the smaller complexes. The size is related to the concentration and molar ratio of antibody and antigen, as well as to the avidity of the antibody for the antigen. The ratio of antigen to antibody may range from antibody excess through antigen-antibody equivalence to antigen excess. In marked antibody excess, antigen valences are saturated and in general the complexes are small. Under conditions of marked antigen excess, antibody-combining sites are saturated, chances for lattice formation are limited, and, again, the complexes are small. At equivalence or mild antigen excess, lattice formation is facilitated, and large complexes can form. Immune complexes formed at moderate antigen excess are thought to be most pathogenic, perhaps because they are most efficient at activating the various mediator systems like the complement cascade.

Net charge of antigen and antibody also appears to be important in determining the pathophysiologic effect of the complexes. It has been shown that positively charged immune complexes tend to deposit in renal glomeruli, while complexes containing similar antigen with neutral charge tend to penetrate glomeruli slowly. This is presumably due to the fact that the glomerulus presents a negatively charged surface to the circulation. Similarly, there is a relationship between the degree of binding of immune complexes to the basement membrane of skin, which is also negatively charged, and the degree of positive charge of the complexes.

The first human disease in which circulating immune complexes were thought to play a pathogenic role was serum sickness. In their classic monograph, "Die Serumkrankheit," Clemens von Pirquet and Bela Schick described in great detail their experiences with the use of horse antidiphtheria toxin in children. They found that a reproducible reaction pattern occurred 8 to 13 days following the subcutaneous injection of horse serum protein. The patients developed fever, malaise, cutaneous eruptions, arthralgias, leukopenia, lymphadenopathy, and albuminuria. The authors suggested that this reaction pattern was caused by the interaction of host antibody, formed in the 8 days following the injection of the horse serum, with horse serum protein. They believed that this interaction led to the deposition of antigen-antibody complexes in tissue with resulting tissue damage, but the technology necessary to pursue this hypothesis was not available.

Numerous large retrospective studies of human serum sickness confirmed the observations of von Pirquet and Schick, but it was not until the studies of Germuth and Dixon that evidence for the role of circulating immune complexes in serum sickness was obtained. These investigators utilized rabbit models of serum sickness.

In the acute serum sickness model, the injection of antigen is followed by a period of intravascular equilibration and then by intravascular-extravascular equilibration lasting several days. The equilibration period is followed by a progressive decline in the level of antigen in the circulation, representing the normal degradation of the injected serum protein. Following this period of decay, there is a sudden acceleration in the clearance of the antigen from the circulation, usually beginning at about 7 to 8 days. The period of rapid decline in the level of antigen in the circulation is due to the development of an immune response in the recipient animal. This

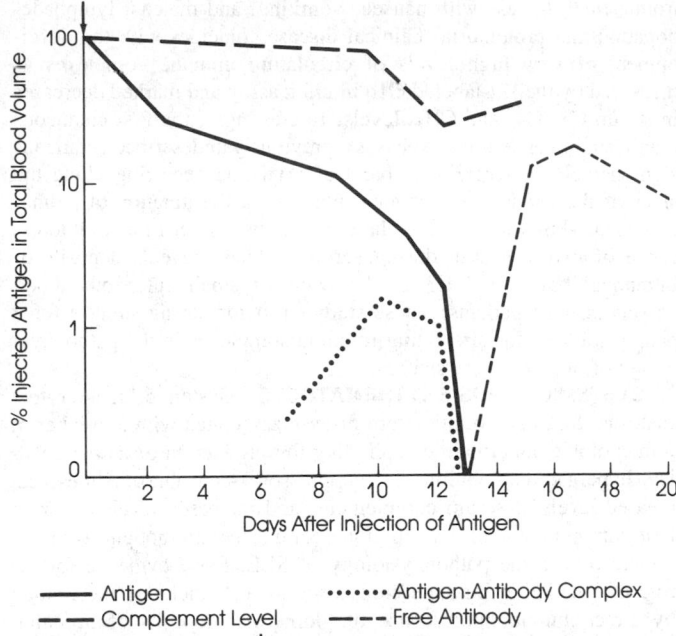

FIGURE 268-1 The rabbit model of acute serum sickness. Radiolabeled antigen is injected at day 0. After a period of equilibration of antigen between the intravascular and extravascular space, there is progressive elimination of antigen from the circulation. With the onset of the animal's immune response there is rapid elimination of antigen from the circulation. Coincident with the phase of rapid elimination is the appearance of antigen-antibody complexes in the circulation and a fall in serum complement. Complete antigen clearance is associated with the appearance of free antibody in the circulation. At the time when antigen-antibody complexes are seen in the circulation, immunopathologic findings are maximal.

results in the formation of antigen-antibody complexes and subsequent clearance of the complexes from the circulation by the cells of the reticuloendothelial system (RES) (Fig. 268-1). During the period in which the complexes are being formed in the circulation, there is a fall in the animal's serum complement levels. At this time pathologic changes occur in large arteries, renal glomeruli, joints, and cardiac vessels. The glomerulonephritis noted during this period has been studied extensively. It is characterized by swelling of the endothelial cells and marked proteinuria with little hematuria; an infiltrate of monocytes but very few granulocytes is found in the renal glomeruli. Immunofluorescence studies have shown that antigen, host immunoglobulin, and C3 are deposited along the glomerular basement membrane in a typical granular pattern. On electron-microscopic examination of kidney sections, few abnormalities are seen except swelling of endothelial cells. Late in the reaction subepithelial deposits of electron-dense material are noted in some animals; however, at this time fluorescent antibody examination is negative for immunoglobulin and complement in the glomeruli. The deposits may represent immunologically altered immunoglobulin or complement.

There is also a very high incidence of arteritis in the coronary artery outflow tract and at branching points of the aorta in the acute serum sickness model. The arteritis is characterized by marked intimal proliferation of endothelium. This is followed by degradation of the internal elastic lamina and adventitia with resulting fibrinoid necrosis of the vessel. On immunofluorescence microscopy, host immunoglobulin, antigen, and C3 are found roughly in the region of the internal elastic lamina, but these immunoreactive materials are rapidly removed and are gone in several days. It has been suggested that the polymorphonuclear neutrophils present in the lesions phagocytize these complexes. In contrast to the findings in glomerulonephritis, materials which decrease complement activity or inhibit the polymorphonuclear leukocytic response diminish or block the development of arteritis.

At the time of the development of serum sickness in this animal model, there are high-molecular-weight immune complexes in the circulation; the animals that become sick regularly have complexes that are greater than 19 S in their sedimentation characteristics. Acute serum sickness is present only as long as these circulating immune complexes persist and resolves rapidly once the antigen is cleared from the circulation and the immune complexes are gone.

It is possible to induce chronic glomerulonephritis in animals by the repeated intravenous injection of the antigen. The dose of antigen injected is critical to the development of the disease. Antigen excess must be produced after each antigen administration, and immune complexes must circulate in the animals. These animals develop glomerulonephritis but not the arteritis characteristic of acute serum sickness.

Other animal models of immune-complex disease closely resemble systemic lupus erythematosus. The most widely studied and best characterized is the disease that occurs spontaneously in the F_1 hybrid of New Zealand black (NZB) and New Zealand white (NZW) mice. These animals develop antibodies to nucleic acids including double-stranded DNA and have decreased numbers of suppressor T cells. They also develop circulating immune complexes and an immune-complex-mediated glomerulonephritis that eventuates in renal insufficiency and death. Direct immunofluorescence microscopy of the kidneys in these animals reveals deposits of DNA, antibodies to DNA, and C3 in the glomerular basement membrane. The female NZB-NZW mice develop these changes before the males, and this sex difference may be related to a switch in the class of antibodies to DNA from IgM to IgG that occurs much earlier in the females than in the males.

Over the years a great deal of attention has been paid to the fate of immune complexes in animal models. Injection of antigens into immunized animals is followed by the deposition of the antigen in the liver, spleen, and lung, all elements of the RES. Detailed studies have examined the fate of preformed immune complexes of carefully determined size in a variety of animals. In general, the findings of these studies have paralleled those reported in the animal models of serum sickness. The very large insoluble complexes are rapidly removed from the circulation. Soluble complexes that are greater than 19 S in their sedimentation characteristics are removed by the liver and persist in the circulation for only a matter of minutes. The major factor appearing to govern the rate of clearance of these large, preformed complexes from the circulation is the rate of hepatic blood flow. In some studies complement activation by complexes is also important in their metabolism, and injected complexes go through a complex series of processing steps. Large-lattice-size complexes appear to be dissociated by complement into smaller entities. Following injection, complexes containing complement components become associated with cells with complement receptors. Human erythrocytes have complement receptors, and these cells appear to be particularly important in the processing of complexes. It is believed that complement-coated complexes associate with complement receptors on red cell surfaces and that the complexes are stripped from these cells as they course through the sinusoids of the liver. They are then metabolized. Fc receptors for IgG also play a prominent role in the removal of IgG-containing immune complexes from the circulation, and any manipulation that affects the interaction of Fc receptors and the Fc fragment of IgG in the complexes predisposes to failure to clear the complexes and to tissue deposition. It is possible to measure RES Fc-receptor functional activity in patients and normal individuals by intravenously injecting IgG-sensitized autologous radiolabeled erythrocytes and then monitoring the rate of disappearance of these immune particles from the bloodstream. In those diseases with tissue deposition of immune complexes there tends to be an associated RES Fc-receptor defect and delayed clearance of the antibody-sensitized cells from the circulation. Another form of immune-complex-mediated tissue damage follows local formation of immune complexes in tissues such as the kidney. Glomerular subepithelial immune-complex deposits are thought to form often on an in-site basis. This may occur as a result of antibody binding to fixed glomerular antigens or antibody binding to "planted" nonglomerular antigens. In the latter instance it is believed that certain cationic antigens can bind to the laminae rarae of the capillary wall in a glomerulus through charge-dependent mechanisms. This "planted" antigen is then recognized by antibody, and local tissue damage results.

DETECTION OF CIRCULATING IMMUNE COMPLEXES Many different assays are available for the detection of soluble immune complexes in various biologic fluids. Although these assays vary in their sensitivity and reproducibility, they have expanded our understanding of circulating immune complexes and their role in various disease states. In general, early tests for the detection of circulating immune complexes relied on physical characteristics of the immune complexes, such as their high molecular weight or cold insolubility. These rather insensitive techniques have been replaced by assays for immunologic components or biologic activities of immune complexes. Although there are now sensitive radioimmunoassays for the detection of circulating immune complexes containing IgG, IgM, and IgA, these tests are not antigen-specific. In fact, in most cases in which circulating immune complexes are demonstrable, the component antigen(s) is (are) unknown. As with most laboratory tests, immune-complex assays may be influenced by other factors. Anticoagulants, endotoxin, and free DNA as well as immunoglobulin aggregates formed after the sample is obtained may result in false-positive results. The impact of these factors can be reduced by the selection of immune-complex assays that are unaffected by these variables and by the use of two or more different assays in situations in which critical evaluation of circulating immune complexes is desired. Several of the most sensitive and commonly used immune-complex assays will be described briefly: (1)C1q binding, or solid-phase radioassays, (2)Raji cell assays, and (3)conglutinin assays. *C1q* is a subcomponent of the first component of complement and will bind to immune complexes containing IgG subclasses 1 to 3 or IgM via noncovalent attachment to a specific site on the Fc portion of immunoglobulin. *Raji cells* are a lymphoblastoid cell line with cell surface receptors for complement, especially C3. The assays are based on the ability of circulating immune complexes that contain bound complement components in their lattices to bind to the surface of the Raji cells via the complement receptors. The bound complexes are easily detected. *Conglutinin* is a 750-kDa nonimmunoglobulin protein found in certain bovine sera that will bind to a cleavage fragment of human C3 known as iC3b. Immune complexes containing iC3b will bind to conglutinin attached to a solid-phase substrate and can be detected.

SERUM SICKNESS Drug hypersensitivity reactions are the most common cause of serum sickness today. It is hypothesized that the drug acting as a hapten binds to a plasma protein. The drug-protein complex is seen as foreign and induces typical serum sickness. Commonly occurring signs and symptoms of serum sickness include fever, cutaneous eruptions (morbilliform and/or urticarial), arthralgias, lymphadenopathy, and albuminuria. Less common manifestations are arthritis, nephritis, neuropathy, and vasculitis. The time required for primary sensitization to an offending agent is approximately 1 to 3 weeks. However, clinical manifestations may develop within 12 to 36 h if there is a history of a previous immunizing exposure. Drug-induced serum sickness usually abates within days after withdrawal of the causative agent. Reactions may persist for longer intervals, particularly if repository or long-acting agents are responsible for the problem. Drugs responsible for serum sickness include penicillin, sulfonamides, thiouracils, hydantoins, *p*-aminosalicylic acid, phenylbutazone, thiazides, and streptomycin. Foreign antisera and blood products may also induce serum sickness reactions.

Recent studies of patients receiving intravenous infusions of horse antithymocyte globulin (ATG) as therapy for bone marrow failure have confirmed and expanded the immunologic findings in animal models of serum sickness in humans. The patients develop signs and symptoms of serum sickness 8 to 13 days after beginning therapy with ATG (Fig. 268-2). These include fever; malaise; cutaneous eruptions; arthralgias and arthritis, mainly of the large joints; gas-

trointestinal distress with nausea, vomiting, and melena; lymphadenopathy; and proteinuria. Clinical disease coincides with the development of very high levels of circulating immune complexes as measured by the ^{125}I-labeled C1q binding assay and marked decreases in serum C3, C4, and CH$_{50}$ levels. Interestingly, the first cutaneous manifestation of serum sickness is a previously undescribed cutaneous sign, namely, a serpiginous band of erythema occurring along the sides of the hands, feet, fingers, and toes at the junction of palmar or plantar skin with the dorsolateral surface. Direct immunofluorescence of involved skin during serum sickness reveals deposits of immunoglobulins and C3 in the walls of small cutaneous blood vessels in most patients. These studies provide strong support for a pathogenic role for circulating immune complexes in the pathophysiology of human serum sickness.

SYSTEMIC LUPUS ERYTHEMATOSUS Systemic lupus erythematosus (SLE) is a multisystem disease associated with a number of immunologic abnormalities including the production of autoantibodies, hypergammaglobulinemia, suppressor-T-cell abnormalities, decreased levels of serum complement, and increased levels of circulating immune complexes. Immune complexes are thought to play a critical role in the pathophysiology of SLE. Early evidence for the role of circulating immune complexes in SLE included the finding by direct immunofluorescence of glomerular deposits of immunoglobulin, complement, and DNA in kidney biopsies. Mixed IgM-IgG cryoglobulins were found in the sera of a substantial number of SLE patients, and when the antibody specificity of these cryoprecipitates was examined, reactivity was found against single- and double-stranded DNA as well as ribonucleoprotein. Utilizing the newer, more sensitive assays, circulating immune complexes have been found in a high percentage of patients with SLE. An explanation for the continued circulation of immune complexes in patients with SLE has been provided by the demonstration of defective function of the reticuloendothelial system (RES) in these patients. Patients with SLE have been shown to have delayed clearance of autologous red blood cells coated with IgG from the circulation, suggesting an impaired function of RES Fc-IgG receptors. The prolonged RES clearance in these patients was found to be correlated with increased levels of circulating immune complexes as measured by the C1q binding assay and with clinical disease activity. Studies in the same patients after their disease improved with treatment revealed a significant correlation between clinical improvement, improvement of Fc-mediated clearance, and decreased levels of circulating immune complexes. Individuals with SLE also have decreased numbers of C3b receptors on their erythrocytes. Whether the decreased number of receptors is primary or secondary remains to be established. Nonetheless, abnormalities of both Fc-IgG and C3b receptors which are responsible for phagocytosis of circulating immune complexes are present in patients with SLE.

VASCULITIS There is strong circumstantial evidence for the role of circulating immune complexes in the various forms of hypersensitivity or necrotizing vasculitis. Features of the classic "palpable purpura" of cutaneous necrotizing vasculitis closely resemble the clinical, histopathologic and immunopathologic features of the Arthus reaction. The Arthus reaction is a model for immune-complex-mediated vascular damage in which antigen is injected intradermally into an animal which possesses circulating antibody against that antigen. In both vasculitis and the Arthus reaction, deposits of immunoglobulin and complement are found in the walls of blood vessels in early lesions. The histopathology of both consists of infiltrates of polymorphonuclear neutrophils, leukocytoclasis, endothelial cell damage and necrosis, hemorrhage, and perivascular deposits of fibrin. Electron microscopy of lesions of cutaneous necrotizing vasculitis reveals subendothelial electron-dense deposits compatible with immune complexes. The available evidence indicates the presence of immune complexes at the site of tissue damage in necrotizing vasculitis. In accord with these findings is the demonstration of circulating immune complexes in a high percentage of patients with this disease.

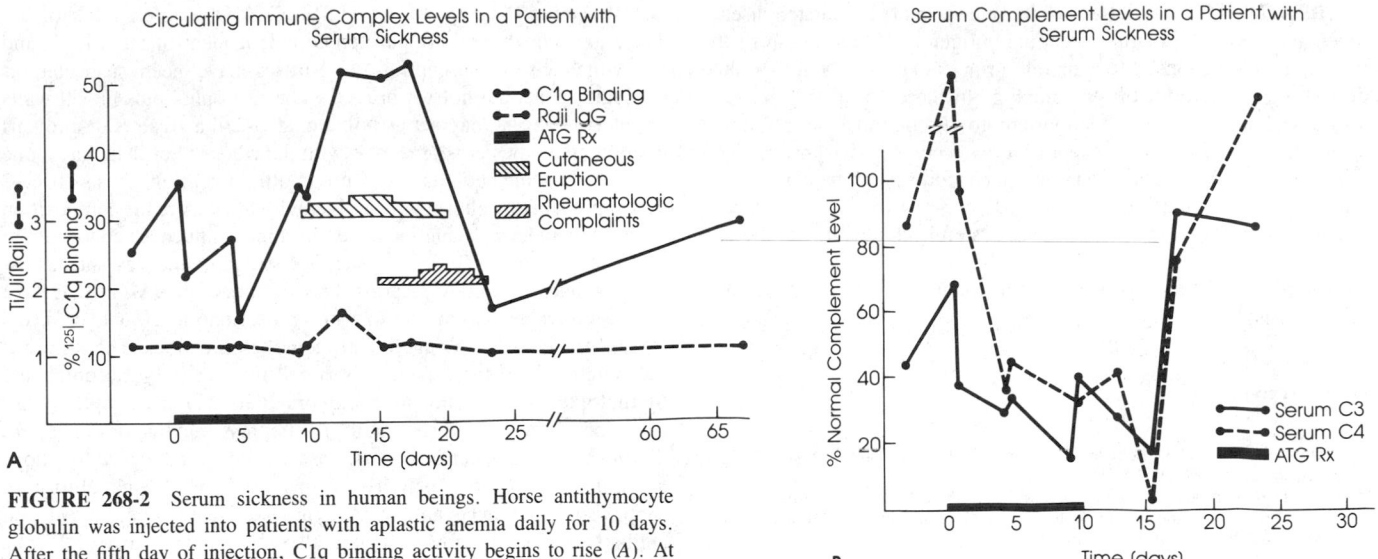

FIGURE 268-2 Serum sickness in human beings. Horse antithymocyte globulin was injected into patients with aplastic anemia daily for 10 days. After the fifth day of injection, C1q binding activity begins to rise (*A*). At the same time there is a dramatic fall in plasma levels of C3 and C4 and onset of clinical symptoms (*B*).

LABORATORY FINDINGS In theory the essential feature of immune-complex disease would be the finding of circulating immune complexes. In practice there is great variability from disease to disease in the frequency of positive immune-complex assays. In some diseases, such as SLE, there is a high frequency of positive immune-complex assays. In others, like membranoproliferative glomerulonephritis, the frequency of positive assays is much lower. Part of the reason for this has to do with the stage of disease under study. In some cases immunologic phenomena are responsible for the initiation of the disease and the initial tissue insult. However, subsequent injury is caused by scarring, inflammation, and repair mechanisms that result in more extensive tissue damage. Thus, progression of disease may occur at a time when immunologic injury is no longer occurring. A second reason for the failure to detect circulating immune complexes in diseases thought to be mediated by them has to do with technical difficulties in the measurement of such complexes. There are many types of assays for immune complexes. Most are indirect and rely on a biologic or biochemical property of the complexes such as the binding of complement components. The pattern of positive reaction clearly varies from disease to disease. Clearly each assay recognizes a different type of complex with maximal efficiency. Since multiple assays are rarely performed on one specimen, complexes, although present, may not be detected. Finally, although a disease is classified as immune-complex-related because of the finding of immune deposits in affected tissues or because of the similarity of its pathologic findings to those of animal models of immune-complex disease, the disease may not be actually caused by circulating immune complexes. For example, antibody may be formed to a tissue component, bind to it in a tissue site, and induce damage. Such is thought to be the case in Goodpasture's disease. For all of these reasons, assays for the detection of circulating immune complex, while often useful, are rarely critical for diagnosis or patient management.

Examination of tissues using immunofluorescent techniques to detect immune deposits is also of great interest in establishing the diagnosis of immune-complex disease. Immune complexes deposited in tissues may be evanescent. For example, in cutaneous vasculitis, lesions must be biopsied within 12 h of their appearance. Although helpful in diagnosis and in establishing pathogenesis, testing for immune deposits in tissue is rarely required for diagnosis.

Another test commonly used to infer the presence of immune complexes is the measurement of serum complement. Decreased levels are taken to indicate the presence of complexes. In fact, it has been suggested that the levels of serum C4 and C3 are the most sensitive indexes of disease activity in SLE. However, the correlation between disease activity and complement levels is rough at best, and some patients with active SLE may have relatively normal complement levels for several reasons. The normal range of complement component levels is wide, and a given patient may have depressed levels with serum concentrations falling from high-normal levels to low-normal levels. In general complement components act as acute phase reactants, and the lowering of serum complement may be masked by increased synthesis. Moreover, under many circumstances activation of complement may mediate profound pathophysiologic effects, although few molecules of complement are actually involved. For example, complement binding to red cells may be responsible for much of the red cell destruction that occurs with ABO-mismatched transfusions; yet serum complement levels may be unchanged because too few molecules are used in erythyrocyte destruction to detect a fall in titer. Finally, all types of complexes do not activate complement in the same way. Massive antigen release from red cells occurring during the course of vivax malaria infection leads to the rapid formation of antigen-antibody complexes in the circulation. For unknown reasons these complexes only interact with the early components of the classic complement pathway, while C3 and the later complement components are not recruited. Thus, if one measures levels of C3, no fall in titer is noted, although complexes are present and massive complement activation has taken place. The complexes formed in SLE activate optimally the classic pathway; presumably those involved in IgA glomerulonephritis activate the alternative pathway. Therefore, the complement test chosen for examination may be important.

Other tests may suggest indirectly the presence of immune-complex disease. For example, a finding of mixed IgG-IgM cryoprecipitates suggests the presence of immune complexes. The presence of antinuclear antibodies suggests autoimmunity, as does the presence of a number of tissue-component-specific antibodies. Similarly, the presence of specific antigen such as hepatitis B surface antigen in the circulation together with appropriate clinical symptoms may suggest an immune-complex disease. Most patients with active immune-complex-mediated disease have an elevated erythrocyte sedimentation rate, although this is not invariably the case. Patients with Takayasu's arteritis may have a normal erythrocyte sedimentation rate during the later phases of the evolution of lesions when most pathology is caused by scarring, fibrosis, and repair within vessel walls. Finally, specific laboratory test findings such as red cell casts in the urine in glomerulonephritis or mild cerebrospinal fluid pleocytosis in the presence of cerebritis are discussed in the chapters concerning those diseases.

TREATMENT The therapy of immune-complex-mediated disease relies upon removal of the offending antigen and interruption of the inflammatory response. In general serum sickness is a self-limited disease that is seldom life-threatening. In the case of drug-induced serum sickness it is most important to discontinue the offending agent. In many instances, supportive care combined with antihistamines for urticaria and acetaminophen for fever, myalgias, and arthralgias is adequate. If serious renal, vascular, or central nervous system involvement occurs, the use of systemic glucocorticoid therapy is indicated.

The therapy of SLE is discussed in Chap. 269 and the therapy of vasculitis is discussed in Chap. 276.

REFERENCES

COCHRANE CB, KOFFLER D: Immune complex disease in experimental animals and man. Adv Immunol 16:185, 1963

DIXON F: The role of antigen-antibody complexes in disease. Harvey Lect 52:21, 1963

FRANK MM et al: Immunoglobulin G–Fc receptor mediated clearance in autoimmune diseases. Ann Intern Med 98:206, 1983

GERMUTH FC JR.: A comparative histologic and immunologic study in rabbits of induced hypersensitivity of the serum sickness type. J Exp Med 97:257, 1953

LAWLEY TJ et al: A prospective clinical and immunologic analysis of patients with serum sickness. N Engl J Med 311:1407, 1984

MANNIK M, AREND WP: Fate of preformed immune complexes in rabbits and rhesus monkeys. J Exp Med 134:19s, 1971

VON PIRQUET C, SCHICK B: Serum Sickness. Baltimore, Williams & Wilkins, 1951

THEOFILOPOULOS AN, DIXON FJ: The biology and detection of immune complexes. Adv Immunol 28:89, 1979

269 SYSTEMIC LUPUS ERYTHEMATOSUS

BEVRA HANNAHS HAHN

DEFINITION AND PREVALENCE Systemic lupus erythematosus (SLE) is a disease of unknown etiology in which tissues and cells are damaged by deposition of pathogenic autoantibodies and immune complexes. Ninety percent of cases are in women, usually of child-bearing age, but children, men, and the elderly can be affected. In the United States, the prevalence of SLE in urban areas varies from 15 to 50 per 100,000; it is more common and more severe in blacks than in whites. Hispanic and Asian populations are also susceptible.

PATHOGENESIS AND ETIOLOGY Production of pathogenic antibodies and immune complexes, coupled with failure to suppress them, are the basic abnormalities underlying SLE. These antibodies are listed in Table 269-1. Not all antibodies or immune complexes are pathogenic. Some antibodies cause disease because of their antigen specificity. Examples are antibodies to erythrocyte surface antigens or to coagulation factors. Others cause disease because of their immunoglobulin (Ig) isotype, ability to fix complement (C'), avidity, and/or electrical charge. For example, complement-fixing cationic antibodies bind to the polyanions in glomerular basement membrane, bind antigen, and cause damage.

The pathogenesis of SLE includes genetic, environmental, and sex hormonal factors. These result in abnormal humoral and cellular immune responses and inadequate clearing of antibodies and immune complexes. Genetic predisposition is indicated by higher concordance for clinical disease in monozygotic than in dizygotic twins, a 10 percent frequency of patients with more than one affected individual in the family; and the fact that 6 percent of SLE patients have inherited deficiencies of complement components. Several genes in the HLA class II and III regions increase the relative risk (RR) for SLE as follows: DR2 (RR3), DR3 (RR3), and null alleles for C4, as in C4A.Q0 (RR3), and C4A.Q0.Q0 (RR17). Combinations of these

genes increase RR even further: DR2, C4A.Q0 confers a RR of 25. There are probably additional genes, independent of HLA I, II, and III, which confer susceptibility. Viruses have been suspected as etiologic agents but not yet proven to be. Phospholipids in cell walls of enteric bacteria may act as polyclonal B-cell activators or antigens to elicit antibodies cross-reactive with the ribose phosphate backbone in DNA. In some patients, exposure to ultraviolet light causes disease flares, probably by altering the antigenicity of DNA or the composition of dermal-epidermal junctions. Sex hormone influences contribute to the pathogenesis of SLE. In general, estrogen enhances and testosterone reduces antibody responses. Men and women with SLE have increased hydroxylation of estrogen and estrone to 16 α-hydroxyestrone, producing prolonged estrogenic stimulation. The ultimate outcome of all of these factors is B-cell hyperactivity, accompanied by multiple abnormalities in immunoregulation. For example, quantities of T helper-inducer and T suppressor-cytotoxic cells are diminished during periods of disease activity, and many functions are abnormal. Helper activity is increased, while the ability of suppressors to reduce anti-DNA synthesis is impaired. Direct and antibody-mediated cytotoxicity are also abnormal. Ability of T cells to secrete interleukin 2 is suppressed, and abnormal interferons are produced. Failure to suppress antibody production also results from abnormalities in the humoral idiotype–anti-idiotype network. Finally, immune complexes are cleared more slowly than normal, related in part to both inherited and acquired deficiencies of complement (CR1) receptors on cell surfaces.

Clinical manifestations of the disease are determined by which antibody subpopulations and immune complexes are present in the patient's repertoire; which organs, cells, or cell products are their targets; and the ability of the patient to correct the abnormalities.

CLINICAL MANIFESTATIONS At onset, SLE may involve only one organ system (with additional manifestations occurring later) or may be multisystemic. Clinical manifestations are listed in Table 269-2. Autoantibodies are usually detectable on the patient's initial visit. Disease severity varies from mild and intermittent to persistent and ultimately fatal. Most patients experience exacerbations interspersed with periods of relative quiescence. Fewer than 10 percent have long-lasting, symptom-free remissions. *Systemic symptoms* are usually prominent and include fatigue, malaise, fever, anorexia, weight loss, and nausea.

Musculoskeletal Almost all SLE patients experience arthralgias and myalgias; most develop arthritis. Pain is often out of proportion to physical findings, which include symmetric fusiform swelling of joints [most frequently proximal interphalangeal (PIP) and metacarpophalangeal (MCP) joints of the hands, wrists, and knees], diffuse puffiness of hands and feet, and tenosynovitis. Joint deformities are unusual, although 10 percent of patients develop swan-neck deformities and ulnar drift at the MCP joints. Erosions are rare, but subcutaneous nodules over elbows and fingers occur. Myopathy can be inflammatory and related to active disease or iatrogenic, secondary to hypokalemia or to glucocorticoids or hydroxychloroquine. Ischemic necrosis of bone also causes "joint" pain and is a common cause of hip, knee, and shoulder pain in these patients.

Cutaneous The *malar* ("butterfly") *rash* is a fixed erythematous rash, flat or raised, over the cheeks and bridge of the nose, often involving the chin and ears. It is usually exacerbated by ultraviolet light. Scarring is absent, but telangiectases may develop. A more diffuse maculopapular rash, predominant in sun-exposed areas, is also common. Its presence usually indicates disease flare. Loss of scalp hair (which often heralds a flare) is usually patchy but can be extensive; the hair will regrow except in discoid lupus erythematosus (DLE). *Vasculitic skin lesions* include subcutaneous nodules, ulcers (usually on the legs), purpura, and infarcts of skin or digits. *DLE lesions* occur in some patients with SLE and can be disfiguring. They are circular with an erythematous rim, raised, and scaly with follicular plugging and telangiectasia. Central scarring produces depigmentation and permanent loss of appendages. They occur over the scalp, ears, face, and sun-exposed areas of the arms, back, and chest. Only 5

TABLE 269-1 Autoantibodies in patients with SLE

	Incidence, %	Antigen detected	Clinical importance
Antinuclear antibodies	95	Multiple nuclear and cytoplasmic antigens	Human cell line substrates are more sensitive than standard murine tissues. A repeatedly negative test on both makes SLE diagnosis unlikely. Multiple antibodies are detected.
Anti-DNA	70	DNA	Anti-dsDNA is relatively disease specific; anti-ssDNA is not. Associated with nephritis and clinical activity.
Anti-Sm	30	Protein complexed to 6 species of small nuclear RNA	Specific for SLE.
Anti-RNP	40	Protein complexed to U1RNA	High titer seen in syndromes with features of polymyositis, scleroderma, lupus, and mixed connective tissue disease. If present in SLE without anti-DNA, risk for nephritis is low.
Anti-Ro (SSA)	30	Protein complexed to Y_1–Y_5 RNA	Associated with Sjögren's syndrome, DR3 haplotype, subacute cutaneous lupus, inherited complement deficiencies, ANA-negative lupus, lupus in the elderly, neonatal lupus, congenital heart block in infants. Can cause nephritis.
Anti-La (SSB)	10	Phosphoprotein complexed with RNA pol III transcripts	Always associated with anti-Ro; risk for nephritis is low if present in SLE. Associated with Sjögren's syndrome.
Antihistone	70	Histones	More frequent in drug-induced LE (95%) than in spontaneous SLE.
Anticardiolipin	50	Phospholipid	Increases risk for venous or arterial thrombosis, thrombocytopenia, and spontaneous abortion. Associated with prolonged PTT (lupus anticoagulant) and false-positive VDRL.
Antierythrocyte	60	Erythrocyte surface antigens	A small proportion of these patients develop overt hemolysis.
Antiplatelet	—	Platelet surface	Associated with thrombocytopenia.
Antilymphocyte	70	Lymphocyte surface antigens	Probably associated with leukopenia and abnormal T-cell function.
Antineuronal	60	Neuronal and lymphocyte surface antigens	In CSF, high IgG titers correlate with diffuse CNS lupus.

percent of individuals with DLE progress to SLE; however, 20 percent of SLE patients have DLE lesions. Less frequent SLE skin lesions include urticaria, periorbital edema, bullae, erythema multiforme, lichen planus–like lesions, and panniculitis ("lupus profundus").

Patients with *subacute cutaneous lupus* (SCLE) are a distinct subset with recurring extensive skin lesions. Arthritis and fatigue are frequent; central nervous system and renal involvement are not. Some patients are antinuclear antibody (ANA)–negative. The majority have antibodies to Ro (SS-A) or to single-stranded (ss) DNA and carry the HLA-DR3 phenotype. The skin lesions are photosensitive polycyclic annular or papulosquamous psoriasiform lesions over the arms, trunk, and face; they become hypopigmented but not scarred.

Mucous membrane lesions are usually small, shallow, painless ulcers in the mouth and nose.

Renal manifestations Although almost all patients with SLE have deposits of immunoglobulin in glomeruli, only one-half have clinical nephritis, defined by persistent proteinuria. At presentation, most patients are asymptomatic (unless already uremic), except those with edema of the nephrotic syndrome. Urinalysis shows hematuria, cylindruria, and proteinuria. As discussed under "Pathology" (see below), most patients with mesangial or mild focal glomerulonephritis do not develop deterioration of renal function. In patients with more severe active or chronic lesions, renal failure is a major cause of death. Since mild lesions may not require aggressive therapy with glucocorticoids and/or cytotoxic drugs whereas severe lesions do, renal biopsy may provide information that will affect therapeutic decisions over the subsequent several months. Patients with deteriorating renal function and active urine sediment also require prompt, aggressive therapy; biopsy is not necessary unless they fail to respond. However, patients with a high proportion of sclerotic glomeruli on biopsy, usually with a serum creatinine of >265 μmol/L (>3 mg/dL), are unlikely to respond to immunosuppressive therapy. In

these cases, dialysis or transplantation should be planned. Patients with persistently abnormal urinalyses associated with high titers of antibodies to double-stranded (ds) DNA and hypocomplementemia are also at risk for severe nephritis; kidney biopsy is useful in these cases if the results are likely to have an impact on therapeutic decisions.

Nervous system Any region of the brain can be involved in SLE, as can the meninges, spinal cord, and cranial and peripheral nerves. Central nervous system (CNS) events may be isolated, single or multiple, but they usually occur in the setting of active disease in other systems. Mild mental dysfunction is the most frequent manifestation. Seizures are frequent and may be grand mal, petit mal, or focal. Other manifestations include psychosis, organic brain syndromes, headache (including migraine), focal infarcts with resultant deficits, extrapyramidal disorders, cerebellar dysfunction, hypothalamic dysfunction with inappropriate antidiuretic hormone (ADH) secretion, pseudotumor cerebri, subarachnoid hemorrhage, aseptic meningitis, transverse myelitis with paraplegia or quadriplegia, optic neuritis, cranial nerve palsies, and peripheral sensorimotor neuropathy resulting either in mononeuritis multiplex or glove-and-stocking deficits. Depression and anxiety are frequent.

Laboratory diagnosis of CNS disease can be difficult. Abnormal electroencephalograms are found in about 70 percent of patients and usually show diffuse slowing or focal abnormalities. The cerebrospinal fluid (CSF) shows elevated protein levels in 50 percent and an elevated number of mononuclear cells in 30 percent of patients. Lumbar puncture should be performed whenever CNS symptoms could result from infection, especially in patients receiving immunosuppressive therapy. Brain scans (including CT) and angiograms are most likely to be positive when focal neurologic deficits are present and are less helpful in cases with diffuse, nonfocal manifestations. Magnetic resonance imaging is the most sensitive radiographic technique to

TABLE 269-2 Clinical manifestations of SLE

	Percent of patients positive during course of disease
Systemic	95
Fatigue, malaise, fever, anorexia, nausea, weight loss	
Musculoskeletal	95
Arthralgias/myalgias	95
Nonerosive polyarthritis*	60
Hand deformities	10
Myopathy/myositis	40/5
Ischemic necrosis of bone	15
Cutaneous	80
Malar rash*	50
Discoid rash*	15
Photosensitivity*	40
Oral ulcers*	40
Other rashes—maculopapular, urticarial, bullous, subacute cutaneous lupus	40
Alopecia	40
Vasculitis	20
Panniculitis	5
Hematologic	85
Anemia (of chronic disease)	70
Hemolytic anemia	10
Leukopenia (<4000/mm³)	65 }*
Lymphopenia (<1500/mm³)	50
Thrombocytopenia (<100,000/mm³)	15
Circulating anticoagulant	15
Splenomegaly	10–20
Lymphadenopathy	15
	20
Neurologic	60
Organic brain syndromes	35
Psychosis	10 }*
Seizures	20
Other CNS (see text)	15
Peripheral neuropathy	15
Cardiopulmonary	60
Pleurisy	50
Pericarditis	30 }*
Myocarditis	10
Endocarditis (Libman-Sachs)	10
Pleural effusions	30
Lupus pneumonitis	10
Interstitial fibrosis	5
Pulmonary hypertension	<5
ARDS/hemorrhage	<5
Renal	50
Proteinuria >500 mg/24 h	50
Cellular casts	50 }*
Nephrotic syndrome	25
Renal failure	5–10
Gastrointestinal	45
Nonspecific (anorexia, nausea, mild pain, diarrhea)	30
Vasculitis with bleeding or perforation	5
Ascites	<5
Abnormal liver enzymes	40
Thrombosis	15
Venous	10
Arterial	5
Fetal loss	30 (of pregnancies)
Ocular	15
Retinal vasculitis	5
Conjunctivitis/episcleritis	10
Sicca syndrome	15

* In addition to two positive laboratory tests [positive ANA plus one or more of (1) positive LE cells, (2) anti-dsDNA, (3) anti-Sm, or (4) false-positive VDRL], a combination of these clinical and laboratory manifestations totalling four meet American Rheumatism Association criteria for classifying patients as SLE. Bracketed features count as one, even if more than one are present, e.g., leukopenia plus thrombocytopenia = one criterion.

TABLE 269-3 Laboratory manifestations of SLE

Tests that help *confirm the clinical diagnosis and predict severity*	Tests that may be helpful in *following the clinical course**

Relatively specific for SLE:
  anti-dsDNA
  anti-Sm
	Titer of anti-dsDNA
	Serum complement levels
	Westergren erythrocyte sedimentation rate

Not specific:
  ANA (most sensitive)
  THC, C3, C4
  Anti-Ro
  Direct Coombs' test
  VDRL
  PTT
  Anticardiolipin
  Hematocrit
  Leukocyte count
  Platelet count
  Urinalysis
  Serum creatinine
	Hematocrit
	Leukocyte count
	Platelet count
	Urinalysis
	Serum creatinine

* For each patient, the pattern of laboratory abnormalities (if any) associated with a disease flare should be established and only those tests used subsequently as adjuncts to clinical assessment.

detect structural abnormalities; however, it may be normal in certain SLE patients with CNS disease. Standard laboratory measures of disease activity (Table 269-3) often do not correlate with neurologic manifestations. Neurologic problems usually improve (with the exception of deficits related to infarcts) with therapy and/or time; recurrences are common.

Vascular Thrombosis in capillaries, small vessels, and medium-sized veins and arteries can be a major problem. Although vasculitis may play a role in the thrombotic process, there is increasing evidence that antibodies against phospholipids (anticardiolipin) are associated with clotting. These antibodies may be the "lupus anticoagulant." In addition, degenerative vascular changes associated with years of immune-complex deposition in vessel walls may predispose to symptomatic coronary artery disease in relatively young individuals with SLE. Anticoagulation with warfarin sodium is usually effective in reducing recurrences of venous clots; it is unclear whether any therapies reduce the incidence of arterial clotting.

Hematologic abnormalities The lupus anticoagulant usually binds to phospholipids in the prothrombin activator complex. It prolongs the partial thromboplastin time, an abnormality not corrected by addition of normal plasma. Three clinical sequelae may be associated with it. First, some patients experience repeated episodes of either venous or arterial clotting; these are often serious, especially if associated with pulmonary emboli, strokes, or occlusion of major arteries. Second, if the anticoagulant is associated with thrombocytopenia or hypoprothrombinemia, significant bleeding can occur. Third, in the absence of clotting or bleeding disorders, it may be a benign laboratory abnormality; biopsies and surgery can be performed without increased risk of bleeding. Antibodies to clotting factors (VIII, IX) are often associated with bleeding. Bleeding syndromes usually respond to glucocorticoids.

Anemia of chronic disease occurs in most patients during periods of disease activity. Frank hemolysis occurs in a small proportion of those with positive Coombs' tests; that syndrome is usually responsive to high-dose glucocorticoids. Splenectomy is often effective in steroid-resistant patients.

Leukopenia is common and usually reflects lymphopenia. In general, it is not associated with recurrent infections and does not require treatment.

Mild thrombocytopenia is common. Severe thrombocytopenia with bleeding and purpura occurs in 5 percent of patients and should be treated with high-dose glucocorticoids. If the platelet count has not risen to a safe range in 5 to 14 days, splenectomy should be considered.

Cardiopulmonary Pericardial pain is the most frequent symptom of cardiac lupus; effusions can occur. Tamponade has been reported and constrictive pericarditis occurs, but is rare. Myocarditis can cause arrhythmias and/or cardiac failure. Endocarditis of the Libman-Sachs verrucous type, a diagnosis made at autopsy, is usually not clinically significant; however, it can cause aortic or mitral regurgitation. Rarely, myocardial infarcts result from vasculitis of coronary arteries; more often they are associated with degenerative arterial disease.

Pleurisy and pleural effusions are common manifestations of SLE. Lupus pneumonitis causes recurrent episodes of fever, dyspnea, and cough; x-rays show infiltrates which come and go over a period of days or weeks, and/or areas of platelike atelectasis; this syndrome responds to glucocorticoids. However, *the most common cause of pulmonary infiltrates in patients with SLE is infection*. Interstitial pneumonitis leading to fibrosis occurs in a small proportion of patients; the inflammatory phase may respond to treatment, while the fibrosis does not. Occasionally, patients develop pulmonary hypertension. Infrequent but often fatal pulmonary manifestations include adult respiratory distress syndrome (ARDS) and massive intraalveolar hemorrhage.

Gastrointestinal Nonspecific gastrointestinal symptoms are common, but vasculitis of the intestine is the most dangerous manifestation. It causes acute or subacute crampy pain, vomiting, and diarrhea and can lead to intestinal perforation and death. Vasculitis is usually present simultaneously in other systems. Another gastrointestinal manifestation of SLE is a pseudoobstruction in which patients present with acute crampy abdominal pain; x-rays show dilated loops of small bowel which may be edematous. Surgery should be avoided unless true obstruction is present. Patients generally respond to glucocorticoid therapy. Acute pancreatitis occurs and can be severe; it may result from active SLE or from glucocorticoid therapy. Elevated serum levels of liver enzymes, especially transaminases, are common in patients with active SLE but are not associated with significant hepatic damage; they return to normal as the disease is treated.

Ocular The most important ocular manifestation of SLE is retinal vasculitis with infarcts; blindness can develop over a period of days. Examination of the retina shows areas of sheathed, narrow arterioles, and cytoid bodies (white exudates) adjacent to vessels. Other ocular abnormalities include conjunctivitis, episcleritis, and optic neuritis. The sicca syndrome is frequent.

PATHOLOGY Cutaneous lesions Acute systemic discoid (DLE) and subacute cutaneous LE skin lesions show similar histopathology. Characteristic changes include degeneration of the basal layer of the epidermis with disruption of the dermal-epidermal junction (DEJ) and scattered mononuclear cell infiltrates around vessels and appendages in the upper dermis. In DLE follicular plugging and hyperkeratosis are prominent. Deposits of immunoglobulin (Ig) and C′ are seen in the DEJ in 80 to 100 percent of lesional and 50 percent of nonlesional skin in patients with active SLE; the proportions are lower during remissions. Active subacute cutaneous lesions are positive for deposits of Ig and C′ only 50 percent of the time. Ig deposition in the DEJ *is not specific* for *LE*. Vasculitic lesions usually show leukocytoclastic angiitis.

Renal lesions Most renal lesions are caused by in situ immune-complex formation or deposition of circulating complexes in glomeruli. In mild nephritis, histology shows either no changes or proliferation confined to the mesangium. When Ig deposits are found solely in the mesangium, prognosis is good and renal failure is rare. If Ig and C′ extend outside the mesangium into capillary loops, the prognosis worsens. Associated glomerular histologic changes in ascending order of severity are (1) focal proliferative, (2) membranoproliferative, and (3) diffuse proliferative (see Chap. 228). Membranous changes without proliferation occur. In addition to those histologic categories, *active disease* and *increased risk of progression to renal failure* are associated with glomerular necrosis, cellular epithelial crescents, hyaline thrombi, leukocytic or mononuclear cell infiltrates in the tubular interstitium, and necrotizing vasculitis. In

addition, measures of *chronicity* are important, as they are associated with a *high incidence of renal failure*. They include glomerular sclerosis, fibrous crescents, interstitial fibrosis, and tubular atrophy. Focal proliferative and membranous changes are associated with 85 percent 5-year survival; diffuse proliferative glomerulonephritis is associated with 70 percent 5-year survival. Progression from focal to diffuse lesions can occur.

LABORATORY MANIFESTATIONS The presence of characteristic antibodies (Table 269-1) confirms the diagnosis of SLE. Antinuclear antibodies are the best screening test. If the test substrate is living human nuclei, as in WIL-2 or HEP-2 cells, more than 95 percent of lupus patients will have positive tests. Rodent liver or kidney substrates do not detect as wide a range of ANA or anticytoplasmic antibodies; approximately 85 percent of SLE serums are positive on those substrates. A positive ANA is not specific for SLE; ANA occur (usually in low titer) in some normal individuals; the frequency increases with aging. Furthermore, other autoimmune diseases, acute viral infections, chronic inflammatory processes, and several drugs may cause ANA positivity. Therefore, a positive ANA supports a diagnosis of SLE but *is not specific*; a negative ANA makes the diagnosis unlikely but not impossible. Antibodies to dsDNA and to Sm are relatively specific for SLE; other autoantibodies listed in Table 269-1 are not. High serum levels of ANA and anti-DNA and low levels of complement usually reflect disease activity, especially in patients with nephritis. Serum levels of cryoglobulins or other immune complexes occasionally correlate with disease activity. Total functional hemolytic complement (CH_{50}) levels are the most sensitive measure of complement activation but are also most subject to laboratory error. Quantitative levels of C3 and C4 are widely available. Very low levels of CH_{50} with normal levels of C3 suggest inherited deficiency of a complement component.

Hematologic abnormalities are common and include anemia (usually normochromic, normocytic but occasionally hemolytic), leukopenia, lymphopenia, and thrombocytopenia. In some patients the Westergren erythrocyte sedimentation rate correlates with disease activity.

Urinalysis and serum creatinine should be measured periodically in patients with SLE. When active nephritis is present, the urinalysis usually shows proteinuria, microscopic hematuria, and cellular or granular casts. Renal biopsy is indicated when results would influence therapeutic decisions. (See discussion under "Clinical Manifestations.")

Other tests that may be abnormal in SLE include false-positive tests for syphilis and abnormal coagulation tests, especially a prolonged partial thromboplastin time. Both are related to antibodies to cardiolipin, discussed under "Clinical Manifestations." Rheumatoid factors are present in 30 to 50 percent of patients.

The tests which are useful for diagnosis and for following the clinical course of patients with SLE are listed in Table 269-3.

PREGNANCY Since SLE is a disease of young women, pregnancy is a frequent occurrence. Fertility rates are normal in patients with SLE, but the rate of spontaneous abortion and stillbirths is high (30 to 50 percent), especially in women with lupus anticoagulant and/or antibodies to cardiolipin. A debate has arisen regarding treatment of pregnant women with SLE and these antibodies who have experienced fetal loss. Some authorities recommend no intervention; others have reported high rates of successful births if mothers are treated with high daily doses of glucocorticoids plus low doses of aspirin or with anticoagulating doses of subcutaneous heparin.

There may be increased flares of SLE during the first trimester (SLE may begin during pregnancy) and especially during the first 6 weeks postpartum. If severe renal or cardiac disease is absent and SLE is controlled, the majority of patients complete pregnancy safely and deliver normal infants. Glucocorticoids (except dexamethasone and betamethasone) are inactivated by placental enzymes and do not cause fetal abnormalities except for low birth weights. Neonatal lupus (related to the presence of anti-Ro in maternal serum) occurs in infants but is rare. A transient DLE-like rash, congenital heart block, and thombocytopenia can occur.

DIFFERENTIAL DIAGNOSIS The American Rheumatism Association has developed diagnostic criteria for SLE. Manifestations included are indicated by asterisks in Table 269-2. Any four of those, or a total of four when combined with certain autoantibodies, establish a diagnosis of definite SLE. Disease confined to one or two systems may be more difficult to classify. The disorders with which SLE can be confused include rheumatoid arthritis; skin disorders such as urticaria, erythema multiforme, rosacea, lichen planus; neurologic disorders such as idiopathic epilepsy or multiple sclerosis; hematologic disorders such as idiopathic thrombocytopenic purpura; and psychiatric disorders. It may also be difficult to distinguish SLE from other autoimmune disorders such as dermatomyositis and overlap syndromes. Some authorities classify patients with features of SLE, rheumatoid arthritis, polymyositis, and scleroderma, accompanied by high titers of anti-RNP, under the rubric "mixed connective tissue disease" (Chap. 272) and report a low incidence of nephritis and CNS disease and a high incidence of pulmonary disease and evolution into scleroderma. It is impossible to put some patients into a definite category; therapy should be directed toward the dominant manifestations. The possibility of drug-induced lupus should always be considered.

DRUG-INDUCED LUPUS Several drugs can cause a syndrome resembling SLE in individuals without any obvious predisposition to the disease. The most common offender is procainamide, which induces ANA in 50 to 75 percent of individuals within a few months; 20 percent of patients receiving the drug develop clinical drug-induced LE. Hydralazine induces ANA in 25 to 30 percent of individuals, and lupus-like symptoms in 10 percent. Both procainamide and hydralazine-induced lupus are more likely to occur in individuals who acetylate the drug slowly. The clinical syndrome consists of polyarthralgias and systemic symptoms in most patients. Polyarthritis occurs in 25 to 50 percent and pleuropericarditis occurs in 30 percent of patients with hydralazine-induced lupus and in 50 percent of patients with procainamide-induced lupus. Other manifestations typical of idiopathic SLE are unusual, including nephritis and CNS involvement. All patients with drug-induced lupus are ANA-positive; most have antibodies to histones. Antibodies to dsDNA and hypocomplementemia are rarely present—a helpful point in distinguishing drug-induced from idiopathic lupus. Anemia, leukopenia, lupus anticoagulant, thrombocytopenia, cryoglobulins, rheumatoid factors, false-positive VDRL, and positive direct Coombs' tests can occur. The initial therapeutic approach should be discontinuation of the suspect drug; most patients improve in days or a few weeks. In patients with severe symptoms, a short course (2 to 10 weeks) of glucocorticoids is indicated. Clinical symptoms rarely persist more than 6 months; ANA may remain positive for years. Other drugs which infrequently induce lupus-like illness include isoniazid, chlorpromazine, *d*-penicillamine, practolol, methyldopa, oral contraceptives, and possibly hydantoins and ethosuximide. Most lupus-inducing drugs can be used safely in patients with idiopathic lupus if there are limited alternatives.

PROGNOSIS The overall survival in patients with SLE is approximately 71 percent over 10 years. Patients with severe involvement of brain, lungs, heart, or kidney have the worst outcomes in terms of survival and disability. Infections and renal failure are the leading causes of death.

TREATMENT There is no cure for SLE. Complete remissions occur but are rare; therefore, patient and physician should plan, first, to control acute, severe flares and, second, to develop maintenance therapies in which symptoms are suppressed to an acceptable level, usually at the cost of some drug side effects. From 20 to 30 percent of SLE patients have mild disease with no life-threatening manifestations. However, their disease may be disabling because of pain and fatigue. These patients should be managed without glucocorticoids. Arthralgias, arthritis, myalgias, fever, and mild serositis may improve on nonsteroidal anti-inflammatory drugs (NSAIDs) including salicy-

lates. However, some NSAID toxicities such as hepatitis, aseptic meningitis, and renal impairment are especially frequent in SLE patients. The dermatitides of SLE (including DLE) and, occasionally, lupus arthritis may respond to antimalarials. Doses of 400 mg hydroxychloroquine daily may be associated with improvement of skin lesions in a few weeks. Side effects include retinal toxicity, rash, myopathy, and neuropathy. Regular ophthalmologic examinations should be performed at least every 6 months, since retinal toxicity is related to cumulative dose. Other therapies for skin rash include use of sunscreens (an SPF rating of 15 or higher is recommended) to prevent rashes and topical or intralesional glucocorticoids if rashes develop. Systemic glucocorticoids should be reserved for patients with disabling, severe lesions.

Life-threatening and severely disabling manifestations of SLE are treated with high doses of *glucocorticoids* (1 to 2 mg/kg per day). When the disease is active, glucocorticoids should be given in divided doses every 8 to 12 h. After the disease has been controlled for several days, doses should be consolidated to one morning dose; thereafter, the daily dose should be tapered as rapidly as clinical disease permits. Ideally, patients should be slowly converted to alternate-day therapy with a single morning dose of short-acting glucocorticoid (prednisone, prednisolone, methylprednisolone) to minimize side effects. However, the disease may flare on alternate days, in which case the lowest single daily dose that suppresses symptoms and major organ damage should be used. Undesirable side effects of chronic glucocorticoid therapy include cushingoid habitus, weight gain, hypertension, infection, capillary fragility, acne, hirsutism, accelerated osteoporosis, ischemic necrosis of bone, cataracts, glaucoma, diabetes mellitus, myopathy, hypokalemia, irregular menses, irritability, insomnia, and psychosis. Prednisone doses of 15 mg daily (or less) given before the hour of noon usually do not significantly suppress the hypothalamic pituitary axis. Some side effects can be minimized if one is alert for them; hyperglycemia, hypertension, edema, and hypokalemia should be treated. The physician should identify infections early and treat promptly. Immunizations with influenza and pneumococcal vaccines are safe and generally effective in patients with stable disease. Supplemental calcium (1000 to 1500 mg daily) with vitamin D (50,000 U weekly) in carefully selected patients (with normal 24-h urine calcium and normal serum calcium; ambulatory) receiving stable doses of glucocorticoids may help maintain bone mass. Some acutely ill lupus patients, including those with diffuse nephritis, have been treated with 3 to 5 days of 1000-mg intravenous "pulses" of methylprednisolone, followed by maintenance daily or alternate-day glucocorticoids. It is unclear whether there are any special advantages or toxicities to this regimen.

The use of *cytotoxic agents* (azathioprine, chlorambucil, cyclophosphamide) in SLE is somewhat controversial. Their use in lupus nephritis is probably associated with a lower rate of renal failure and fewer disease flares, and it permits faster tapering and lower maintenance doses of glucocorticoids. Undesirable side effects include bone marrow suppression, irreversible ovarian failure, hepatotoxicity (azathioprine), bladder toxicity (cyclophosphamide), and an increased risk for malignancies. If a lupus patient has life-threatening disease unresponsive to glucocorticoids or requires an unacceptably high maintenance dose of glucocorticoids, it is appropriate to consider cytotoxic drugs. Azathioprine is the least toxic; it may be given in a dose of 2 to 3 mg/kg per day orally. Cyclophosphamide is probably the most effective and the most toxic. Intravenous pulse doses (10 to 15 mg/kg) given once every 4 weeks have less urinary bladder toxicity and more rapid onset of action (5 to 15 days) than daily oral doses, but bone marrow suppression can be severe. Cyclophosphamide can also be used in daily oral doses (1.5 to 2.5 mg/kg per day) or in combination with low doses of azathioprine (0.5 to 1 mg/kg per day of each). After disease activity has been controlled for several months, tapering of cytotoxic agents and attempts to discontinue them are appropriate.

Several experimental therapies are being studied, including plasmapheresis, total-lymph-node irradiation, cyclosporine, sex hormone therapy, and intravenous gamma globulin.

Patients with nephrotic syndrome often maintain stable renal function in spite of persistent edema and hypoalbuminemia; hypertension is usually a concomitant problem. Such patients should be treated with 3 to 6 months of high-dose glucocorticoid therapy; if proteinuria does not diminish, the drug should be tapered and discontinued and treatment directed toward control of hypertension and hyperlipidemia.

It is appropriate in patients with end-stage nephritis to plan for dialysis or transplantation; their survival is similar to that of patients with other immune nephritides.

In the subsets of patients with SLE who do not have progressive, severe disease, patients should be informed that although SLE is a chronic, potentially serious disease, some patients can lead relatively normal lives if their disease is appropriately managed.

REFERENCES

AUSTIN HA III et al: Prognostic factors in lupus nephritis. Am J Med 75:382, 1983

BALOW JE et al: NIH conference: Lupus nephritis (includes treatment). Ann Intern Med 106:79, 1987

EBLING FM, HAHN BH: Pathogenic subsets of antibodies to DNA, in *International Reviews in Immunology*, H Kohler and C Bona (eds) 5:7995, 1989

GINZLER E et al: A multi-center study of outcome in systemic lupus erythematosus. I. Entry variables as predictors of prognosis. Arthritis Rheum 25:601, 1982

HARRIS EN et al: Thrombosis, recurrent fetal loss, thrombocytopenia: Predictive value of the anticardiolipin test. Arch Intern Med 146:2153, 1986

HOWARD PF et al: Relationship between C4 null genes, HLA-D region antigens and genetic susceptibility to systemic lupus erythematosus in Caucasian and Black Americans. Am J Med 81:187, 1986

LEAKER B et al: Lupus nephritis: Clinical and pathological correlation. Q J Med 62:163, 1987

REICHLIN M: *Antibodies to Cytoplasmic Antigens in Systemic Lupus Erythematosus*, R G Lahita (ed). New York, Wiley, 1987, chap 8, pp 257–269

ROTHFIELD N: Systemic lupus erythematosus: Clinical aspects and treatment, in *Arthritis and Allied Conditions*, 11th ed, DJ McCarty (ed). Philadelphia, Lea & Febiger, 1989, chap 67, pp 1022–1048

TAN EM: Systemic lupus erythematosus: Immunological aspects, in *Arthritis and Allied Conditions*, 11th ed, DJ McCarty (ed). Philadelphia, Lea & Febiger, 1989, chap 68, pp 1049–1054

——— et al: The 1982 revised criteria for the classification of systemic lupus erythematosus. Arthritis Rheum 25:1271, 1982

270 RHEUMATOID ARTHRITIS

PETER E. LIPSKY

Rheumatoid arthritis (RA) is a chronic, multisystem disease of unknown etiology. Although there are a variety of systemic manifestations, the characteristic feature of RA is persistent inflammatory synovitis, usually involving peripheral joints in a symmetric distribution. The potential of the synovial inflammation to cause cartilage destruction and bone erosions and subsequently joint deformities is the hallmark of the disease. Despite its destructive potential, the course of RA can be quite variable. Some patients may experience only a mild oligoarticular illness of brief duration with minimal joint damage, while others will have a relentless progressive polyarthritis with marked joint deformity. Most patients will experience an intermediate course.

EPIDEMIOLOGY AND GENETICS The prevalence of RA is approximately 1 percent of the population (range 0.3 to 2.1 percent); women are affected approximately three times more often than men. The prevalence increases with age, and sex differences diminish in the older age group. RA is seen throughout the world and affects all races. The onset is most frequent during the fourth and fifth decade of life, with 80 percent of all patients developing the disease between the ages of 35 and 50.

Family studies indicate a genetic predisposition. For example,

severe RA is found at approximately four times the expected rate in first-degree relatives of individuals with seropositive disease. Moreover, 30 percent of monozygous twins are concordant for RA, whereas only 5 percent of dizygous twins are concordant. The role of genetic influences in the etiology of RA was established by the demonstration of an association with the class II major histocompatibility complex gene product, HLA-DR4. As many as 70 percent of whites or Japanese with classic or definite RA express HLA-DR4 compared with 28 percent of control individuals. An association with HLA-DR4 has also been noted in blacks, Latin Americans, and Chippewa Indians, although the incidence of HLA-DR4 positivity in individuals with RA in these groups is not as great as in whites. In a number of groups, including Israeli Jews and Asian Indians, however, there is no association between the development of RA and HLA-DR4. In these individuals, there is an association between RA and HLA-DR1. Molecular analysis of HLA-DR antigens has provided insight into these apparently disparate findings. Thus, HLA-DR4 consists of a family of closely related antigens, including HLA-Dw4, Dw10, Dw13, Dw14, and Dw15, that differ structurally in the amino acids that surround position 70 of the third hypervariable region of the β chain of the molecule. Different members of the HLA-DR4 family of molecules are found to predominate in different ethnic groups. Thus, for example, in HLA-DR–positive North American whites, HLA-Dw4 and Dw14 are the most frequent subtypes, whereas HLA-Dw15 is most frequent in Japanese, and HLA-Dw10 is most common in Israeli Jews. Moreover, only some HLA-DR4 subtypes are associated with the development of RA. Thus, HLA-Dw4, Dw14, and Dw15, but not Dw10 or Dw13, are associated with the development of RA. The amino acids surrounding position 70 of the third hypervariable region of the HLA-DR β chain are very similar in HLA-Dw4, Dw14, and Dw15, whereas there are significant differences in HLA-Dw10 and Dw13. Of note, the amino acid sequence of the third hypervariable region of HLA-DR1 is identical to that of Dw14. These results suggest that this particular amino acid sequence in this region of the HLA-DR molecule may be a major genetic element conveying susceptibility to RA, regardless of whether it occurs in HLA-DR4 or HLA-DR1. Since this region of the HLA-DR molecule is involved in binding foreign peptides and thereby facilitating their presentation to specific T lymphocytes, it is possible that the association between particular HLA-DR molecules and RA may be explained by the capacity of individuals expressing these HLA-DR determinants to recognize an antigen that initiates the disease process.

Additional genes in the HLA-D complex may also convey susceptibility to RA. The haplotype HLA-DR4, DQw3.1 appears to be associated with more severe manifestations of RA, including Felty's syndrome, whereas pulmonary involvement in RA is associated with HLA-DR4. Finally, genes outside the HLA complex, such as those controlling the expression of the antigen receptor on T cells have also been associated with the development of RA.

To date, genetic risk factors cannot fully account for the incidence of RA, suggesting that environmental factors also play a role in the etiology of the disease. This is emphasized by epidemiologic studies in Africa that have indicated that climate and urbanization have a major impact on the incidence and severity of RA in groups of similar genetic background.

Besides an association between the development of RA and genes of the major histocompatibility complex, there appears to be a genetic predisposition for the development of certain toxic reactions induced by drugs used to treat RA. For example, the presence of the HLA-DR3 allele is highly associated with the development of side effects to gold therapy, including proteinuria, thrombocytopenia, and perhaps skin rash. Similarly, the presence of this allele appears to predispose to the development of proteinuria following therapy with D-penicillamine. In general, no association has been noted between HLA type and the response to therapy.

CLINICAL MANIFESTATIONS **Onset** Characteristically, RA is a chronic polyarthritis. In approximately two-thirds of patients, it begins insidiously with fatigue, anorexia, generalized weakness, and vague musculoskeletal symptoms until the appearance of synovitis becomes apparent. This prodrome may persist for weeks or months and defy diagnosis. Specific symptoms usually appear gradually as several joints, especially those of the hands, wrists, knees, and feet, become affected in a symmetric fashion. In approximately 10 percent of individuals, the onset is more acute with a rapid development of polyarthritis often accompanied by constitutional symptoms including fever, lymphadenopathy, and splenomegaly. In approximately one-third of patients, symptoms may initially be confined to one or a few joints. Although the pattern of joint involvement may remain asymmetric in a few patients, a symmetric pattern is more typical.

Signs and symptoms of articular disease   Pain, swelling, and tenderness may initially be poorly localized to the joints. Pain in affected joints, aggravated by movement, is the most common manifestation of established RA. It corresponds in pattern to the joint involvement but does not always correlate with the degree of apparent inflammation. Generalized stiffness is frequent and is usually greatest after periods of inactivity. Morning stiffness of greater than 1-h duration is an almost invariable feature of inflammatory arthritis and serves to distinguish it from various noninflammatory joint disorders. The length and intensity of the stiffness can be used as a crude assessment of disease activity. The majority of patients will experience constitutional symptoms such as weakness, easy fatigability, anorexia, and weight loss. Although fever to 40°C occurs on occasion, temperature elevation in excess of 38°C is unusual and suggests the presence of an intercurrent problem such as infection.

Clinically, synovial inflammation causes swelling, tenderness, and limitation of motion. Warmth is usually evident on examination, especially of large joints such as the knee, but erythema is infrequent. Pain originates predominantly from the joint capsule, which is abundantly supplied with pain fibers and is markedly sensitive to stretching or distention. Joint swelling results from accumulation of synovial fluid, hypertrophy of the synovium, and thickening of the joint capsule. Initially, motion is limited by pain. The inflamed joint is usually held in flexion to maximize joint volume and minimize distention of the capsule. Later, fibrous or bony ankylosis, or soft tissue contractures lead to fixed deformities.

Although inflammation can affect any diarthrodial joint, RA most often causes symmetric arthritis with characteristic involvement of certain specific joints such as the proximal interphalangeal and metacarpophalangeal joints. The distal interphalangeal joints are rarely involved. Synovitis of the wrist joints is a nearly uniform feature of RA and may lead to limitation of motion, deformity, and median nerve entrapment (carpal tunnel syndrome). Synovitis of the elbow joint often leads to flexion contractures that may develop early in the disease. The knee joint is commonly involved with synovial hypertrophy, chronic effusion, and frequently ligamentous laxity. Pain and swelling behind the knee may be caused by extension of inflamed synovium into the popliteal space (Baker's cyst). Arthritis in the forefoot, ankles, and subtalar joints can produce severe pain with ambulation as well as a number of deformities. Axial involvement is usually limited to the upper cervical spine. Involvement of the lumbar spine is not seen, and lower back pain cannot be ascribed to rheumatoid inflammation. On occasion, inflammation from the synovial joints and bursae of the upper cervical spine leads to atlantoaxial subluxation. This usually presents as pain in the occiput but on rare occasions may lead to compression of the spinal cord.

With persistent inflammation, a variety of characteristic deformities develop. These can be attributed to a number of pathologic events including laxity of supporting soft tissue structures; destruction or weakening of ligaments, tendons, and the joint capsule; cartilage destruction; muscle imbalance; and unopposed physical forces associated with the use of affected joints. Characteristic deformities of the hand include (1) radial deviation at the wrist with ulnar deviation of the digits often with palmar subluxation of the proximal phalanges (''Z'' deformity); (2) hyperextension of the proximal interphalangeal joints, with compensatory flexion of the distal interphalangeal joints

(swan-neck deformity); (3) flexion deformity of the proximal interphalangeal joints and extension of the distal interphalangeal joints (boutonnière deformity); and (4) hyperextension of the first interphalangeal joint and flexion of the first metacarpophalangeal joint with a consequent loss of thumb mobility and pinch. Typical deformities may also develop in the feet, including eversion at the hindfoot (subtalar joint), plantar subluxation of the metatarsal heads, widening of the forefoot, hallux valgus, and lateral deviation and dorsal subluxation of the toes.

Extraarticular manifestations   RA is a systemic disease with a variety of extraarticular manifestations. Although these occur frequently, not all of them have clinical significance. However, on occasion, they may be the major evidence of disease activity and source of morbidity and require management per se. As a rule, these manifestations take place in individuals with high titers of autoantibodies to the Fc component of immunoglobulin G (rheumatoid factors).

Rheumatoid nodules develop in 20 to 30 percent of persons with RA. They are usually found on periarticular structures, extensor surfaces, or other areas subjected to mechanical pressure, but they can develop elsewhere including the pleura and meninges. Common locations include the olecranon bursa, the proximal ulna, the Achilles tendon, and the occiput. Nodules vary in size and consistency and are rarely symptomatic, but on occasion they break down as a result of trauma or become infected. They are found almost invariably in individuals with circulating rheumatoid factor. Histologically, rheumatoid nodules consist of a central zone of necrotic material including collagen fibrils, noncollagenous filaments, and cellular debris, a midzone of palisading macrophages that express HLA-DR antigens, and an outer zone of granulation tissue. Examination of early nodules has suggested that the initial event may be a focal vasculitis.

Clinical weakness and atrophy of skeletal muscle are common. Muscle atrophy may be evident within weeks of the onset of RA and usually is most apparent in musculature approximating affected joints. Muscle biopsy may show type II fiber atrophy and muscle fiber necrosis with or without a mononuclear cell infiltrate.

Rheumatoid vasculitis which can affect nearly any organ system is seen in patients with severe RA and high titers of circulating rheumatoid factor. Rheumatoid vasculitis is very uncommon in blacks. In its most aggressive form, rheumatoid vasculitis can cause polyneuropathy and mononeuritis multiplex, cutaneous ulceration and dermal necrosis, digital gangrene, and visceral infarction. While such widespread vasculitis is very rare, more limited forms are not uncommon, especially in white patients with high titers of rheumatoid factor. Neurovascular disease presenting either as a mild distal sensory neuropathy or as mononeuritis multiplex may be the only signs of vasculitis. Cutaneous vasculitis usually presents as crops of small brown spots in the nail beds, nail folds, and digital pulp. Larger ischemic ulcers, especially in the lower extremity, may also develop. Myocardial infarction secondary to rheumatoid vasculitis has been reported as has vasculitic involvement of lungs, bowel, liver, spleen, pancreas, lymph nodes, and testes. Renal vasculitis is rare.

Pleuropulmonary manifestations, which are more commonly observed in men, include pleural disease, interstitial fibrosis, pleuropulmonary nodules, pneumonitis, and arteritis. Evidence of pleuritis is found commonly at autopsy, but symptomatic disease during life is infrequent. Typically, the pleural fluid contains very low levels of glucose in the absence of infection. Pleural fluid complement is also low compared with the serum level when these are related to the total protein concentration. Pulmonary fibrosis can produce impairment of the diffusing capacity of the lung. Pulmonary nodules may appear singly or in clusters. When they appear in individuals with pneumoconiosis, a diffuse nodular fibrotic process (Caplan's syndrome) may develop. On occasion, pulmonary nodules may cavitate and produce a pneumothorax or bronchopleural fistula. Rarely pulmonary hypertension secondary to obliteration of the pulmonary vasculature occurs. In addition to pleuropulmonary disease, upper airway obstruction from cricoarytenoid arthritis or laryngeal nodules may develop.

Clinically apparent heart disease attributed to the rheumatoid process is rare, but evidence of asymptomatic pericarditis is found at autopsy in 50 percent of cases. Pericardial fluid has a low glucose level and is frequently associated with the occurrence of pleural effusion. Although pericarditis is usually asymptomatic, on rare occasions death has occurred from tamponade. Chronic constrictive pericarditis may also occur.

RA tends to spare the central nervous system directly, although vasculitis can cause peripheral neuropathy. *Neurologic manifestations* may also result from atlantoaxial or midcervical spine subluxations. Nerve entrapment secondary to proliferative synovitis or joint deformities may produce neuropathies of median, ulnar, radial (interosseous branch), or anterior tibial nerves.

The rheumatoid process involves the *eye* in less than 1 percent of patients. Affected individuals usually have long-standing disease and nodules. The two principal manifestations are episcleritis, which is usually mild and transient, and scleritis, which involves the deeper coats of the eye and is a more serious inflammatory condition. Histologically, the lesion is similar to a rheumatoid nodule and may result in thinning and perforation of the globe (scleromalacia perforans). Fifteen to twenty percent of persons with RA may develop Sjögren's syndrome with attendant keratoconjunctivitis sicca.

Felty's syndrome consists of chronic RA, splenomegaly, neutropenia, and on occasion anemia and thrombocytopenia. It is most common in individuals with long-standing disease. These patients frequently have high titers of rheumatoid factor, subcutaneous nodules, and other manifestations of systemic rheumatoid disease. Felty's syndrome is very uncommon in blacks. It may develop after joint inflammation has regressed. Circulating immune complexes are often present, and evidence of complement consumption may be seen. The leukopenia is a selective neutropenia with polymorphonuclear leukocyte counts of less than 1500 per microliter, and sometimes less than 1000 per microliter. Bone marrow examination usually reveals moderate hypercellularity with a paucity of mature neutrophils. However, the bone marrow may be normal, hyperactive, or hypoactive; maturation arrest may be seen. Hypersplenism has been proposed as one of the causes of leukopenia, but splenomegaly is not invariably found and splenectomy does not always correct the abnormality. Excessive margination of granulocytes caused by antibodies to these cells, complement activation, or binding of immune complexes may contribute to granulocytopenia. Patients with Felty's syndrome have increased frequency of infections usually associated with neutropenia. The cause of the increased susceptibility to infection is related to defective function of polymorphonuclear leukocytes as well as the decreased number of cells.

Osteoporosis secondary to rheumatoid involvement is common and may be aggravated by corticosteroid therapy and immobilization. Osteopenia involves both juxtaarticular bone and long bones distant from involved joints.

LABORATORY FINDINGS No tests are specific for diagnosing RA. However, rheumatoid factors, which are autoantibodies reactive with the Fc portion of IgG, are found in more than two-thirds of adults with the disease. Widely utilized tests largely detect IgM rheumatoid factors. The presence of rheumatoid factor is not specific for RA. Rheumatoid factors are found in 5 percent of healthy persons. The frequency of rheumatoid factor in the general population increases with age, and 10 to 20 percent of individuals over 65 years old have a positive test. In addition, a number of conditions besides RA are associated with the presence of rheumatoid factor. These include systemic lupus erythematosus, Sjögren's syndrome, chronic liver disease, sarcoidosis, interstitial pulmonary fibrosis, infectious mononucleosis, hepatitis B, tuberculosis, leprosy, syphilis, subacute bacterial endocarditis, visceral leishmaniasis, schistosomiasis, and malaria. In addition, rheumatoid factor may appear transiently in normal individuals after vaccination or transfusion and may also be found in relatives of individuals with RA.

The presence of rheumatoid factor does not establish the diagnosis of RA but can be of prognostic significance because patients with high titers tend to have more severe and progressive disease with extraarticular manifestations. Rheumatoid factor is uniformly found in patients with nodules or vasculitis. The predictive value of the presence of rheumatoid factor in determining a diagnosis of RA is poor. Thus, less than one-third of unselected patients with a positive test for rheumatoid factor will be found to have RA. The test is not useful as a screening procedure but can be employed to confirm a diagnosis in individuals with a suggestive clinical presentation and, if present in high titer, to designate patients at risk for severe systemic disease.

Normochromic, normocytic anemia is frequently present in active RA. It is thought to reflect ineffective erythropoiesis; large stores of iron are found in the bone marrow. In general, anemia and thrombocytosis correlate with disease activity. The white blood cell count is usually normal, but a mild leukocytosis may be present. Leukopenia may also exist without the full-blown picture of Felty's syndrome. Eosinophilia, when present, usually reflects severe systemic disease.

The erythrocyte sedimentation rate is increased in nearly all patients with active RA. A variety of other acute phase reactants including ceruloplasmin and C-reactive protein are also elevated, and generally such elevations correlate with disease activity and the likelihood of progressive joint damage.

Synovial fluid analysis confirms the presence of inflammatory arthritis, although none of the findings is specific. The fluid is usually turbid, with reduced viscosity, increased protein content, and a slightly decreased or normal glucose concentration. The white cell count varies between 5 and 50,000 per microliter; polymorphonuclear leukocytes predominate. Total hemolytic complement, C3, and C4 are markedly diminished in synovial fluid relative to total protein concentration as a result of activation of the classic complement pathway by locally produced immune complexes.

When monoclonal antibodies specific for T-lymphocyte subsets are used to examine peripheral blood mononuclear cells of patients with RA, no specific changes in the numbers of circulating CD4+ (helper-inducer) or CD8+ (suppressor-cytotoxic) T cells are noted. However, an increased number of circulating T cells expressing HLA-DR, an indication of T-cell activation, can be observed. This finding is most frequent in patients with active joint disease.

RADIOGRAPHIC EVALUATION Early in the disease, roentgenograms of the affected joints are usually not helpful in establishing a diagnosis. They reveal only that which is apparent from physical examination, namely, evidence of soft tissue swelling and joint effusion. As the disease progresses, abnormalities become more pronounced, but none of the radiographic findings is diagnostic of RA. The diagnosis, however, is supported by a characteristic pattern of abnormalities including the tendency toward symmetric involvement. Juxtaarticular osteopenia may become apparent within weeks of onset. Loss of articular cartilage and bone erosions develop after months of sustained activity. The primary value of radiography is to determine the extent of cartilage destruction and bone erosion produced by the disease, particularly when one is considering therapy with disease-modifying drugs or surgical intervention.

CLINICAL COURSE AND PROGNOSIS The course of RA is quite variable and difficult to predict in an individual patient. Most patients experience persistent but fluctuating disease activity, accompanied by a variable degree of joint deformity. After 10 to 12 years, fewer than 20 percent of patients will have no evidence of disability or deformity. Features of patients that predict the development of disability include older age, female sex, more severe radiographic involvement, and the presence of rheumatoid nodules or elevated titers of rheumatoid factor. Neither pattern of disease onset nor currently available therapies appear to have an impact on the development of disabilities. Approximately 15 percent of patients with RA will have a short-lived inflammatory process that remits without major deformity.

Several features of patients with RA appear to have prognostic significance. Remissions of disease activity are most likely to occur during the first year. White females tend to have more persistent synovitis and progressively erosive disease than males. Persons who present with high titers of rheumatoid factor, C-reactive protein, and haptoglobin also have a worse prognosis, as do individuals with subcutaneous nodules or radiographic evidence of erosions at the time of initial evaluation. Although sustained disease activity of more than 1 year's duration portends a poor outcome, the rate of progression of joint abnormalities is not constant; the greatest progression takes place during the first 6 years of disease and at a much slower rate thereafter.

The median life expectancy of persons with RA is shortened by 3 to 7 years. Of the 2.5-fold increase in mortality rate, RA itself is a contributing feature in 15 to 25 percent. The increased mortality rate seems to be limited to patients with more severe articular disease and can be attributed largely to infection and gastrointestinal bleeding. Drug therapy may also play a role in the increased mortality rate seen in these individuals.

DIAGNOSIS   The diagnosis of RA is easily made in persons with typical established disease. In a majority of patients, the disease assumes its characteristic clinical features within 1 to 2 years of onset. The typical picture of bilateral symmetric inflammatory poly- arthritis involving small and large joints in both the upper and lower extremities with sparing of the axial skeleton except the cervical spine suggests the diagnosis. Constitutional features indicative of the inflammatory nature of the disease, such as morning stiffness, support the diagnosis. Demonstration of subcutaneous nodules is a helpful diagnostic feature. Additionally, the presence of rheumatoid factor, inflammatory synovial fluid with increased numbers of polymorpho- nuclear leukocytes, and radiographic findings of juxtaarticular bone demineralization and erosions of the affected joints substantiate the diagnosis.

The diagnosis is somewhat more difficult early in the course when only constitutional symptoms or intermittent arthralgias or arthritis in an asymmetric distribution may be present. A period of observation may be necessary before the diagnosis can be established. A definitive diagnosis of RA depends predominantly on characteristic clinical features and the exclusion of other inflammatory processes. The isolated finding of a positive test for rheumatoid factor or an elevated erythrocyte sedimentation rate, especially in an older person with joint pains, should not itself be used as evidence of RA.

Recently, the American Rheumatism Association has developed revised criteria for the classification of rheumatoid arthritis (Table 270-1). The newer criteria are simpler to apply than the previous ones and demonstrate a sensitivity of 91 to 94 percent and a specificity of 89 percent when used to classify patients with RA compared with control subjects with rheumatic diseases other than RA. The major differences between the new and old criteria are that results of invasive procedures such as biopsies are not included, the classifications of probable, definite, and classic RA have been eliminated, and patients with more than a single diagnosis are not eliminated by exclusion criteria. Although these criteria were developed as a means of disease classification for epidemiologic purposes, they are useful as guidelines for establishing the diagnosis. Failure to meet these criteria, however, especially during the early stages of the disease, does not exclude the diagnosis.

PATHOLOGY AND PATHOGENESIS   Microvascular injury and an increase in the number of synovial lining cells appear to be the earliest lesions in rheumatoid synovitis. The nature of the insult causing this response is not known. Subsequently, an increased number of synovial lining cells is seen along with perivascular infiltration with mononuclear cells. As the process continues, the synovium becomes edematous and protrudes into the joint cavity as villous projections.

Light-microscopic examination discloses a characteristic constel- lation of features which include hyperplasia and hypertrophy of the synovial lining cells, focal or segmental vascular changes, including microvascular injury, thrombosis and neovascularization, edema, and

---

TABLE 270-1   The 1987 revised criteria for the classification of rheumatoid arthritis

1 Guidelines for classification
   a Four of seven criteria are required to classify a patient as having rheumatoid arthritis.
   b Patients with two or more clinical diagnoses are not excluded.
2 Criteria*
   a Morning stiffness: Stiffness in and around the joints lasting 1 h before maximal improvement.
   b Arthritis of 3 or more joint areas: At least 3 joint areas, observed by a physician simultaneously, have soft tissue swelling or joint effusions, not just bony overgrowth. The 14 possible joint areas involved are right or left proximal interphalangeal, metacarpophalangeal, wrist, elbow, knee, ankle, and metatarsophalangeal joints.
   c Arthritis of hand joints: Arthritis of wrist, metacarpophalangeal joint, or proximal interphalangeal joint.
   d Symmetric arthritis: Simultaneous involvement of the same joint areas on both sides of the body.
   e Rheumatoid nodules: Subcutaneous nodules over bony prominences, extensor surfaces, or juxtaarticular regions observed by a physician.
   f Serum rheumatoid factor: Demonstration of abnormal amounts of serum rheumatoid factor by any method for which the result has been positive in less than 5% of normal control subjects.
   g Radiographic changes: Typical changes of RA on posteroanterior hand and wrist radiographs which must include erosions or unequivocal bony decalcification localized in or most marked adjacent to the involved joints.

* Criteria *a–d* must be present for at least 6 weeks. Criteria *b–e* must be observed by a physician.

---

infiltration with mononuclear cells often collected into aggregates around small blood vessels. Although this pathologic picture is typical of RA, it can also be seen in a variety of other chronic inflammatory arthritides. The mononuclear cell collections are variable in compo- sition and size. The predominant infiltrating cell is the T lymphocyte. T4 (helper-inducer) cells predominate over T8 (suppressor-cytotoxic) cells and are frequently found in close proximity to HLA-DR+ macrophages and dendritic cells. Analysis of T cells in synovial fluid has documented an enrichment in CD29-expressing memory T4 cells and a marked reduction in the number of CD45R-expressing naive T4 cells. In addition, the T8 cells are largely of the cytotoxic and not the suppressive phenotype.

Although the etiologic stimuli have not been identified, established rheumatoid synovitis is characterized by persistent immunologic activity. The infiltrating T cells appear to be activated, since they express activation antigens such as HLA-DR. In addition, they express an increased density of molecules, such as leukocyte function associated antigen 1 (LFA-1, CD11a/CD18) that have been implicated in a variety of cell-to-cell interactions, including binding of circulating cells to postcapillary venules just prior to entry into sites of tissue inflammation. Finally, the T cells appear to have proliferated locally in the synovial tissue, perhaps in response to sequestered antigen, since they express determinants such as very late antigen (VLA-1) that appears on T cells only after prolonged proliferation. Evidence of B-cell activation can also be found in the inflamed synovium, and plasma cells producing immunoglobulin and rheumatoid factor are characteristic features of rheumatoid synovitis. Large numbers of macrophages with an activated phenotype are also found in rheumatoid synovium.

The rheumatoid synovium is characterized by the presence of a number of secreted products of activated lymphocytes, macrophages, and other cell types. The local production of these cytokines appears to account for many of the pathologic and clinical manifestations of RA. Table 270-2 lists cytokines that have been identified in rheumatoid synovial fluid and indicates their putative role in the rheumatoid inflammatory process. These cytokines include those that are derived from T lymphocytes such as interleukin 2 (IL-2), IL-6, granulocyte- macrophage colony stimulating factor (GM-CSF), tumor necrosis factor α, and transforming growth factor β; those originating from activated macrophages, including IL-1, tumor necrosis factor α, IL-6, GM-CSF, macrophage CSF, platelet-derived growth factor, insulin-like growth factor, and transforming growth factor β; as well

TABLE 270-2 Cytokines in rheumatoid inflammation

Manifestation	Cytokine involved
1 Synovial tissue inflammation	
a Increased adherence of postcapillary venules	IL-1, TNFα, IFN-γ
b T-cell activation and proliferation	IL-1, TNFα, IL-6, IL-2
c B-cell differentiation and antibody formation	IL-1, TNFα, IL-6, IL-2, IFN-γ
d Increased expression of HLA antigens	IFN-γ, TNFα
e Macrophage activation	IFN-γ, GM-CSF, M-CSF, IL-2
2 Synovial fluid inflammation	
a Increased adherence of postcapillary venules	IL-1, TNFα, IFN-γ
b Chemotactic for PMN	TNFα
c Activation of PMN	TNFα, GM-CSF
3 Synovial proliferation	
a Fibroblast growth	PDGF, IL-1, IGF, FGF, TGFβ, EGF
b Neovascularization	TNFα, FGF, TGFβ
4 Cartilage and bone damage	
a Activation of chondrocytes	IL-1, TNFα
b Activation of fibroblasts	IL-1, TNFα
c Activation of osteoblasts-osteoclasts	IL-1, TNFα
5 Systemic manifestations	
a Fever, constitutional symptoms	IL-1, TNFα
b Acute phase reactants	IL-1, TNFα, IL-6

NOTE: IL-1, interleukin 1; IL-2, interleukin 2; IL-6, interleukin 6; TNFα, tumor necrosis factor α; IFN-γ, interferon γ; GM-CSF, granulocyte-macrophage colony stimulating factor; M-CSF, macrophage-colony stimulating factor; PDGF, platelet-derived growth factor; PMN, polymorphonuclear cells; IGF, insulin-like factor; FGF, fibroblast growth factor; TGFβ, transforming growth factor β; EGF, epidermal growth factor.

as those secreted by other cell types in the synovium, such as fibroblasts and endothelial cells, including IL-1, IL-6, GM-CSF, and macrophage CSF. The activity of these cytokines appears to account for many of the features of rheumatoid synovitis including the synovial tissue inflammation, synovial fluid inflammation, synovial proliferation, and cartilage and bone damage as well as the systemic manifestations of RA. In addition to the production of cytokines that propagate the inflammatory process, local factors are produced that tend to slow the inflammation including specific inhibitors of cytokine action and additional cytokines, such as transforming growth factor β, which inhibits many of the features of rheumatoid synovitis including T-cell activation and proliferation, B-cell differentiation, and migration of cells into the inflammatory site.

These findings have suggested that the propagation of RA is an immunologically mediated event, although the original initiating stimulus has not been characterized. One view is that the inflammatory process in the tissue is driven by the T4 helper-inducer cells infiltrating the synovium. Evidence for this includes (1) the predominance of T4 cells in the synovium; (2) the increase in soluble IL-2 receptors, a product of activated T cells, in blood and synovial fluid of patients with active RA; and (3) amelioration of the disease by removal of T cells by thoracic duct drainage or suppression of their function by total lymphoid irradiation. T lymphocytes produce a number of cytokines, including gamma interferon and GM-CSF, that can lead to activation of macrophages and also increased expression of HLA molecules. Moreover, T lymphocytes produce a variety of cytokines that promote B-cell proliferation and differentiation into antibody-forming cells and, therefore, may also promote local B cell stimulation. The resultant production of immunoglobulin and rheumatoid factor can lead to immune-complex formation with consequent complement activation and exacerbation of the inflammatory process by the production of the anaphylatoxins, C3a and C5a, and the chemotactic factor, C5a. The tissue inflammation is reminiscent of delayed-type hypersensitivity reactions occurring in response to soluble antigens or microorganisms. It is, however, unclear whether this represents a response to a persistent exogenous antigen or to altered autoantigens such as collagen, or immunoglobulin. Alterna-

tively, it could represent persistent responsiveness to activated autologous cells such as might occur as a result of Epstein-Barr virus infection. Also, the persistent inflammation could result from deranged immunoregulatory mechanisms that are either primary abnormalities or develop as a result of the local inflammatory response.

Overriding the chronic inflammation in the synovial tissue is an acute inflammatory process in the synovial fluid. The exudative synovial fluid contains a large number of polymorphonuclear leukocytes and relatively few mononuclear cells. A number of mechanisms play a role in stimulating the exudation of synovial fluid. Locally produced immune complexes can activate complement and generate anaphylatoxins and chemotactic factors. Local production by mononuclear phagocytes of factors such as IL-1, tumor necrosis factor α, and leukotriene B$_4$ can stimulate the endothelial cells of postcapillary venules to become more efficient at binding circulating cells, whereas tumor necrosis factor α and leukotriene B$_4$ stimulate the migration of polymorphonuclear leukocytes into the synovial site. In addition, vasoactive mediators such as histamine produced by the mast cells that infiltrate the rheumatoid synovium may also facilitate the exudation of inflammatory cells into the synovial fluid. Finally, the vasodilatory effects of locally produced prostaglandin E$_2$ may also facilitate entry of inflammatory cells into the inflammatory site. Once in the synovial fluid, the polymorphonuclear leukocytes can ingest immune complexes, with the resultant production of reactive oxygen metabolites and other inflammatory mediators, further adding to the inflammatory milieu. Locally produced cytokines such as tumor necrosis factor α and GM-CSF can additionally stimulate polymorphonuclear leukocytes. The production of large amounts of cyclooxygenase and lipoxygenase pathway products of arachidonic acid metabolism by cells in the synovial fluid and tissue further accentuates the signs and symptoms of inflammation.

The precise mechanism by which bone and cartilage destruction occurs has not been completely resolved. Although the synovial fluid contains a number of enzymes potentially able to degrade cartilage, the majority of destruction occurs in juxtaposition to the inflamed synovium, or pannus, that spreads to cover the articular cartilage. This vascular granulation tissue is composed of proliferating fibroblasts, small blood vessels, and a variable number of mononuclear cells. The cytokines IL-1 and tumor necrosis factor α play an important role by stimulating the cells of the pannus to release collagenase and other neutral proteases. These same two cytokines also activate chondrocytes in situ, stimulating them to produce proteolytic enzymes that can degrade cartilage locally. Finally, these two cytokines may contribute to the local demineralization of bone by activating osteoclasts. Prostaglandin E$_2$ produced by fibroblasts and macrophages may also contribute to bone demineralization.

TREATMENT **General principles** The goals of therapy of RA are: (1) relief of pain; (2) reduction of inflammation; (3) preservation of functional capacity; (4) resolution of the pathologic process; and (5) facilitation of healing. Currently available medications are capable of providing pain relief and some reduction in inflammation. Since the etiology of RA is unknown and the pathogenesis speculative, therapy remains empirical. None of the therapeutic interventions are curative, and, therefore, all must be viewed as palliative, aimed at relieving the signs and symptoms of the disease. The various therapies employed are directed at nonspecific suppression of the inflammatory process in the hope of ameliorating symptoms and preventing progressive damage to articular structures.

Management of patients with RA involves an interdisciplinary approach which attempts to deal with the various problems that these individuals have with functional as well as psychosocial interactions. A variety of physical therapies may be useful in decreasing the symptoms of RA. Rest ameliorates symptoms and can be an important component of the total therapeutic program. In addition, splinting to reduce unwanted motion of inflamed joints may be useful. Exercise directed at maintaining muscle strength and joint mobility without exacerbating joint inflammation is also an important aspect of the therapeutic regimen. A variety of orthotic devices can be helpful in supporting and aligning deformed joints to reduce pain and improve function.

Medical management of RA involves three general approaches. The first is the use of aspirin and other nonsteroidal anti-inflammatory drugs, simple analgesics, and if necessary, low-dose glucocorticoids to control the symptoms and signs of the local inflammatory process. These agents are rapidly effective at mitigating signs and symptoms, but they appear to exert little effect on the progression of the disease. A second group of drugs includes a variety of agents that have been classified as the disease-modifying drugs. These agents appear to have the capacity to decrease elevated levels of acute phase reactants in treated patients and, therefore, are thought to modify the destructive capacity of the disease. A third class of agents includes the immunosuppressive and cytotoxic drugs that have been shown to ameliorate the disease process in some patients.

A number of experimental approaches such as total-lymphoid irradiation, lymphoplasmapheresis, and the administration of the immunosuppressive agent cyclosporin have also been used to treat RA. Although some show potential for ameliorating disease, none has been shown to be a safe and cost-effective way to treat patients on a long-term basis. Recently, substitution of dietary omega-6 essential fatty acids with omega-3 fatty acids such as eicosapentaenoic acid found in certain fish oils has also been shown to provide symptomatic improvement in patients with RA. A variety of nontraditional approaches have also been claimed to be effective in treating RA, including diets, plant and animal extracts, vaccines, hormones, and topical preparations of various sorts. Many of these are costly, and none has been shown to be effective. However, belief in their efficacy ensures their continued use by some patients.

Nonsteroidal anti-inflammatory drugs Besides aspirin, there are now several additional nonsteroidal anti-inflammatory drugs (NSAIDs) available to treat RA. These include fenoprofen, ibuprofen, indomethacin, naproxen, meclofenamate, piroxicam, sulindac, tolmetin, dicloferac, and flurbiprofen. As a result of the capacity of these agents to block the activity of the enzyme cyclooxygenase and therefore the production of prostaglandins, prostacyclin, and thromboxanes, they have analgesic, anti-inflammatory, and antipyretic properties. These agents are all associated with a wide spectrum of toxic side effects. Some, such as gastric irritation, azotemia, platelet dysfunction, and exacerbation of allergic rhinitis and asthma, are related to the inhibition of cyclooxygenase activity, while a variety of others, such as rash, liver function abnormalities, and bone marrow depression, may not be. Elderly patients on diuretics may be at higher risk for certain toxic effects. None of the NSAIDs has been shown to be more effective than aspirin in the treatment of RA. However, these nonaspirin drugs are associated with a lower incidence of gastrointestinal intolerance. None of the newer NSAIDs appears to show significant therapeutic advantages over the other available agents. In addition, there is no consistent advantage of any of these newer agents over the others with respect to the incidence or severity of toxic manifestations.

Disease-modifying drugs Clinical experience has delineated a number of agents that appear to have the capacity to alter the course of RA. This group of agents includes gold compounds, D-penicillamine, the antimalarials, and sulfasalazine. In practice, these agents share a number of characteristics. They exert minimal direct nonspecific anti-inflammatory or analgesic effects, and therefore NSAIDs must be continued during their administration, except in a few cases when true remissions are induced with them. The appearance of benefit from disease-modifying drug therapy is usually delayed for weeks or months. As many as two-thirds of patients develop some clinical improvement as a result of therapy with any of these agents, although the induction of true remissions is unusual. In addition to clinical improvement, there is frequently an improvement in serologic evidence of disease activity, and titers of rheumatoid factor and the erythrocyte sedimentation rate frequently decline. Despite this, there is minimal evidence that disease-modifying drugs actually retard the development of bone erosions or facilitate their healing.

Each of these drugs is associated with considerable toxicity, and therefore, careful patient monitoring is necessary. Which disease-modifying drug should be the drug of first choice remains controversial, and trials have failed to demonstrate a consistent advantage of one over the other. Toxicity of the various agents thus becomes important in determining the drug of first choice. Failure to respond or development of toxicity to one agent does not preclude responsiveness to another. For example, a similar percentage of RA patients who have failed to respond to gold will respond to D-pencillamine when it is given as the second disease-modifying drug. No characteristic features of patients have emerged that predict responsiveness to a disease-modifying drug. Moreover, the indications for the initiation of therapy with one of these agents are not well defined.

Glucocorticoid therapy Although systemic glucocorticoid therapy can provide effective symptomatic therapy in patients with RA, these drugs should be avoided if possible because they do not alter the course of the disease and the potential toxicity of long-term therapy is substantial. Low-dose (less than 7.5 mg per day) prednisone has been advocated as useful additive therapy to control symptoms, but trials have not provided convincing evidence of efficacy and even low-dose therapy may promote osteoporosis.

Immunosuppressive therapy The immunosuppressive drugs azathioprine and cyclophosphamide have been shown to be effective in the treatment of RA and to exert therapeutic effects similar to those of the disease-modifying drugs. However, these agents are no more effective than the disease-modifying drugs. Moreover, they cause a variety of toxic side effects, and cyclophosphamide appears to predispose the patient to the development of malignant neoplasms. Therefore, these drugs have been reserved for patients who have clearly failed therapy with disease-modifying drugs. On occasion, extraarticular disease such as rheumatoid vasculitis may require cytotoxic immunosuppressive therapy.

The folic acid antagonist methotrexate, given in an intermittent low-dose (7.5 to 15 mg once weekly), also may be useful in the treatment of RA. Recent trials have documented the efficacy of methotrexate and have indicated that its onset of action is more rapid than that of disease-modifying drugs. Long-term trials have indicated that methotrexate does not induce remission, but rather suppresses symptoms while it is being administered. Maximal improvement is observed after 6 months of therapy with little additional improvement thereafter. Major toxicity includes gastrointestinal upset and liver function abnormalities that appear to be dose-related and hepatic fibrosis that can be quite insidious, requiring liver biopsy for detection in its early stages.

Surgery Surgery plays a role in the management of patients with severely damaged joints. Although arthroplasties and total joint replacements can be done on a number of joints, the most successful procedures are carried out on hips and knees. Realistic goals of these procedures are relief of pain, correction of deformity, and modest functional improvement. Reconstructive hand surgery may lead to cosmetic improvement and some functional benefit. Open or arthroscopic synovectomy may be useful in some patients with persistent monarthritis, especially of the knee. In addition, early tenosynovectomy of the wrist may prevent tendon rupture.

Approach to the patient with RA At the onset of disease it is difficult to predict the natural history of an individual patient's illness. Therefore, the usual approach is to attempt to alleviate the patient's symptoms with nonsteroidal anti-inflammatory drugs. Some patients may have mild disease that requires no additional therapy. Since the disease-modifying drugs are potentially toxic and not universally effective, their use is usually delayed until it is apparent that symptoms cannot be controlled adequately with nonsteroidal anti-inflammatory drugs.

At some time during most patients' course, the possibility of initiating disease-modifying drug therapy is entertained. With aggressive disease this might occur sooner, often within 3 to 6 months of disease onset, whereas in patients with more indolent disease, smoldering activity may not require such therapy for many years.

The development of bone erosions or radiographic evidence of cartilage loss is clear-cut evidence of the destructive potential of the inflammatory process and indicates the need for disease-modifying drug therapy. The other indications such as persistent pain, joint swelling, or functional impairment are much more subjective, however. The decision to begin use of a disease-modifying drug requires careful monitoring of joint swelling and functional activity, as well as an understanding of the patient's pain tolerance and expectation of therapy. In this setting, the fully informed patient must play an active role in the decision to begin disease-modifying drug therapy, after careful review of the therapeutic and toxic potential of the various drugs.

If a patient responds to a disease-modifying drug, therapy is continued with careful monitoring to avoid toxicity. All disease-modifying drugs provide a suppressive effect and therefore require prolonged administration. Even with successful therapy, local injection of glucocorticoids may be necessary to diminish inflammation that may persist in a limited number of joints. In addition, nonsteroidal anti-inflammatory drugs may be necessary to mitigate symptoms. Even after inflammation has totally resolved, symptoms from loss of cartilage and supervening degenerative joint disease or deformities may require additional treatment. Surgery may also be necessary to relieve pain or diminish the functional impairment secondary to deformity. Only when patients have persistent inflammatory disease or severe extraarticular manifestations is the use of cytotoxic immunosuppressive drugs or experimental procedures justified.

REFERENCES

ARNETT FC et al: The American Rheumatism Association 1987 revised criteria for the classification of rheumatoid arthritis. Arthritis Rheum 31:315, 1988

ATHANASON NA et al: Immunohistology of rheumatoid nodules and rheumatoid synovium. Ann Rheum Dis 47:398, 1988

CLELAND LG et al: Clinical and biochemical effects of dietary fish oil supplements in rheumatoid arthritis. J Rheum 15:10, 1988

CUSH JJ, LIPSKY PE: Phenotypic analysis of synovial tissue and peripheral blood lymphocytes isolated from patients with rheumatoid arthritis. Arthritis Rheum 31:1230, 1988

EMERY P et al: Deficiency of the suppressor-inducer subset of T lymphocytes in rheumatoid arthritis. Arthritis Rheum 30:849, 1987

FEIGENBAUM SL et al: Prognosis in rheumatoid arthritis: A longitudinal study of newly diagnosed younger adult patients. Am J Med 66:377, 1979

FIRESTEIN G, ZVAIFLER N: The pathogenesis of rheumatoid arthritis, in Immunology of Rheumatic Diseases, DS Pisetsky et al (eds). Rheumatic Dis Clin North Am 13:447, 1987

GOTO M et al: T cytotoxic and helper cells are markedly increased and T suppressor and inducer cells are markedly decreased in rheumatoid synovial fluids. Arthritis Rheum 30:737, 1987

HOCHBERG MC: Adult and juvenile rheumatoid arthritis: Current epidemiologic concepts. Epidemiol Rev 3:27, 1981

KEYSTONE EC et al: Elevated soluble interleukin-2 receptor levels in the sera and synovial fluids of patients with rheumatoid arthritis. Arthritis Rheum 31:844, 1988

KREMER JM, LEE JK: A long-term prospective study of the use of methotrexate in rheumatoid arthritis. Update after a mean of fifty-three months. Arthritis Rheum 31:577, 1988

LIPSKY PE: Gold, penicillamine and antimalarials, in Inflammation: Basic Principles and Clinical Correlates, JI Gallin et al (eds). New York, Raven Press, 1988, pp 897–910

MITCHELL DM et al: Survival, prognosis and causes of death in rheumatoid arthritis. Arthritis Rheum 29:706, 1986

NEPOM GT et al: The molecular basis for HLA class II associations with rheumatoid arthritis. J Clin Immunol 7:1, 1987

PINALS RS: Sulfasalazine in the rheumatic diseases. Semin Arthritis Rheum 17:246, 1988

PINCUS T et al: Severe functional declines, work disability, and increased mortality in seventy-five rheumatoid arthritis patients studied over nine years. Arthritis Rheum 27:864, 1984

SCHNEIDER HA et al: Rheumatoid vasculitis: Experience with 13 patients and review of the literature. Semin Arthritis Rheum 14:280, 1985

SCOTT TE et al: HLA-DR4 and pulmonary dysfunction in rheumatoid arthritis. Am J Med 82: 765, 1987

SHERRER YS et al: The development of disability in rheumatoid arthritis. Arthritis Rheum 29:494, 1986

UTSINGER DD et al (eds): Rheumatoid Arthritis. Philadelphia, Lippincott, 1985

271 SYSTEMIC SCLEROSIS (SCLERODERMA)

BRUCE C. GILLILAND

DEFINITION Systemic sclerosis (SSc) is a multisystem disorder of unknown etiology characterized by fibrosis of the skin, blood vessels, and visceral organs including the gastrointestinal tract, lungs, heart, and kidneys. The degree and rate of skin and internal organ involvement vary among patients. Two subsets, however, can be identified, even though there is some overlap. One subset is referred to as *diffuse cutaneous scleroderma* and is characterized by the rapid development of symmetric skin thickening of proximal and distal extremity, face, and trunk. These patients are at greater risk for developing kidney and other visceral disease early in their course. The other subset is *limited cutaneous scleroderma*, which is defined by symmetric skin thickening limited to fingers or distal extremity and to the face. This subset frequently has features of CREST syndrome, an acronym standing for calcinosis, Raynaud's phenomenon, esophageal dysmotility, sclerodactyly, and telangiectasia. The prognosis in limited cutaneous scleroderma is better except for the occasional patient who, after many years, develops pulmonary arterial hypertension or biliary cirrhosis. Systemic sclerosis of visceral organs also may occur in the absence of any skin involvement. Survival is determined by the severity of visceral disease, especially involving the heart, lungs, and/or kidneys.

Scleroderma can also occur in a localized form limited to the skin, subcutaneous tissue, and muscle, and without systemic involvement. The two localized forms are morphea, which occurs as single or multiple plaques of skin induration, and linear scleroderma, which involves an extremity or face.

SSc also occurs in association with features of other connective tissue diseases. The term *overlap syndrome* has been used to describe such patients. *Undifferentiated connective tissue disease* has been suggested as a designation for patients who do not have diagnostic criteria for any one connective tissue disease. *Mixed connective tissue disease* is a syndrome involving features of systemic lupus erythematosus, systemic sclerosis, polymyositis, and rheumatoid arthritis and very high titers of circulating antibody to nuclear ribonucleoprotein antigen (see Chap. 272). *Eosinophilic fasciitis* is a scleroderma-like illness and will be discussed in this chapter.

EPIDEMIOLOGY SSc has a worldwide distribution and affects all races. The onset of disease is usually in the third to fifth decade, and the incidence increases with age. Women are affected approximately three times as often as men, and even more often during the childbearing years. The onset of scleroderma in childhood is unusual. The annual incidence has been estimated to be 14.1 cases per million population based on a 20-year study performed in Allegheny County, Pennsylvania. The role of heredity has not been clarified. Several examples of familial SSc have been reported, and the finding of other connective tissue diseases and autoantibodies in relatives of involved patients suggests a hereditary predisposition.

Several environmental factors have been associated with the development of SSc and scleroderma-like illnesses. SSc appears to be more common in coal and gold miners, especially in those with more extensive exposure, suggesting that silica dust may be a predisposing factor. Workers exposed to polyvinyl chloride may develop Raynaud's phenomenon, acroosteolysis, scleroderma-like skin lesions, and nailfold capillary abnormalities similar to those observed in SSc. These workers may also develop hepatic fibrosis and angiosarcoma. The development of scleroderma has been associated with exposure to vinyl chloride, epoxy resins, and aromatic hydrocarbons such as benzine and toluene. In 1981, in Spain, a multisystem disease resembling scleroderma occurred following the ingestion of adulterated cooking oil (rapeseed oil). Approximately 20,000 people were affected. The patients initially develop interstitial pneumonitis, eosinophilia, arthralgias, arthritis, and myositis, followed subsequently by joint contractures, skin thickening, Raynaud's phenomenon, pulmonary hypertension, sicca syndrome, and resorption of the distal fingertips. Extensive sclerosis of the dermis and subcutaneous tissue has been noted in patients receiving pentazocine, a nonnarcotic analgesic agent. Bleomycin, an anticancer agent, produces fibrotic skin nodules, linear hyperpigmentation, alopecia, gangrene of fingers, and pulmonary fibrosis affecting mainly the lower lobes. In Japan, the use of paraffin or silicone for breast augmentation has been associated with the development of SSc.

PATHOGENESIS   The outstanding feature of SSc is the overproduction of collagen that is qualitatively normal. The increased collagen production is thought to be due to aberrant regulation of fibroblast cell growth and/or to increased biosynthesis of connective tissue. While etiology for this abnormal production is unknown, immunologic and vascular mechanisms are thought to play a role in the development of fibrosis and other features of SSc.

Numerous immunologic abnormalities have been noted in patients with SSc. Antinuclear antibodies are found in approximately 95 percent of patients and hypergammaglobulinemia in at least one-third of patients. Systemic sclerosis is also found in association with other connective tissue diseases suspected to be of autoimmune origin. Abnormalities of T-cell population have been noted, and include decreased CD8-suppressor-cell activity and increased CD4-helper-cell activity. The CD4/CD8 ratio is increased in peripheral blood and in early skin lesions of SSc due to decreased number of CD8 lymphocytes. CD4 cells have been shown to produce more interleukin 2 than cells from normal subjects. Natural killer (NK) cell activity is also reduced in the peripheral blood of patients, particularly in those with diffuse cutaneous disease early in their course. NK cells are a subpopulation of lymphocytes which participate in surveillance against certain microbes and neoplasms as well as in the control of the immune system. They have been shown to produce a number of immunomodulary proteins that inhibit B-cell differentiation, suppress immunoglobulin production, and lyse antigen-processing cells. The number of NK cells is normal in SSc patients, suggesting that the loss of function represents an intrinsic cellular defect.

Lymphocytes and monocytes are found in close proximity to fibroblasts in active skin disease of patients with SSc, which suggests a role for cell-mediated immunity in stimulating increased collagen production. These lymphocytes are mostly T cells. Studies have shown the number of circulating T cells in SSc patients to be normal or decreased; the latter finding may indicate attraction of T cells to sites of active disease in skin and other organs. Supernatants from activated normal peripheral lymphocytes contain lymphokines that can stimulate cultured fibroblasts to produce collagen. Crude extracts from skin of SSc patients or normals have been observed to stimulate patients' lymphocytes as measured by the macrophage migration inhibition test. Interleukin 1, a product of activated monocytes, also can stimulate fibroblast proliferation, but its importance in SSc is uncertain since studies have shown increased as well as decreased interleukin 1 production. Additional support for involvement of cell-mediated immunity in the pathogenesis of SSc is the appearance of scleroderma-like lesions in patients with graft-versus-host disease (GVHD) after bone marrow transplantation and in a murine model of chronic GVHD, conditions known to be associated with activated T cells. More recently, mast cells have been implicated in the development of fibrosis. Increased numbers of mast cells are found in the deeper layer of dermis in the early phase of disease. On interaction with T lymphocytes, mast cells release products that stimulate fibroblasts to secrete increased amounts of collagen. Further studies are required to better understand the role of altered immunity in the pathogenesis of SSc.

Vascular damage is also involved in the pathogenesis of SSc. Vascular abnormalities are noted before the appearance of fibrosis. Fibrosis is initially often perivascular, suggesting that vascular inflammatory events may subsequently affect the surrounding connective tissue. The initial event is postulated to be endothelial cell injury, which subsequently leads to intimal thickening, narrowing of the lumen, decreased distensibility, and eventual obliteration of blood vessels. The cause of endothelial damage is not known. The finding of a serum nonimmunoglobulin cytotoxic factor for endothelial cells in some patients has not been confirmed in other studies. The sera of some patients mediate antibody-dependent cellular cytotoxicity (ADCC) directed against human microvascular endothelial cells. Endothelial cell damage is reflected by elevated plasma levels of von Willebrand factor in SSc patients. The binding of von Willebrand factor to exposed subendothelium permits adhesion and activation of platelets. Activated platelets release platelet derived growth factor (PDGF), which has been demonstrated to be chemotactic and mitogenic for both smooth-muscle cells and fibroblasts. PDGF may be one of several factors stimulating intimal fibrosis and with its passage through the injured endothelium could also account for adventitial and perivascular fibrosis. Intravascular fibrin deposits appear in small arteries and arterioles and may cause the microangiopathic hemolytic anemia observed in some patients. The number of small arteries, arterioles, and capillaries in skin and other organs is eventually reduced. The remaining capillaries in skin dilate and proliferate to become visible telangiectatic lesions.

Chromosomal abnormalities have been noted in greater than 90 percent of SSc patients. These acquired abnormalities include chromatid breaks, acentric fragments, and ring chromosomes and are found in approximately 30 percent of mitotic cells. A chromosomal breakage factor has been found in the serum of SSc patients. The significance of these chromosomal abnormalities is unknown.

PATHOLOGY   In the skin, a thin epidermis overlies compact bundles of collagen which lie parallel to the epidermis. Fingerlike projections of collagen extend from the dermis into the subcutaneous tissue and bind the skin to the underlying tissue. Dermal appendages are atrophied, and rete pegs are lost. In early stages of disease, increased numbers of T cells, monocytes, plasma cells, and mast cells are found, particularly in the lower dermis of involved skin.

In the lower two-thirds of the esophagus, the histologic findings consist of a thin mucosa and increased collagen in the lamina propria, submucosa, and serosa. The degree of fibrosis is less than in the skin. Atrophy of the muscularis in the esophagus and throughout the involved portions of the gastrointestinal tract is more prominent than the amount of fibrotic replacement of muscle. Ulceration of the mucosa is often present and may be due to either SSc or superimposed peptic esophagitis. Striated muscles in the upper one-third of the esophagus are relatively spared. Similar changes may be found throughout the gastrointestinal tract, especially in the second and third portions of the duodenum, jejunum, and large intestine. Atrophy of the muscularis of the large intestine may lead to the development of large-mouth diverticula. In the later stages of the disease, the involved portions of the gastrointestinal tract become dilated. Infiltration of lymphocytes and plasma cells in the lamina propria is also present.

With pulmonary involvement, diffuse interstitial fibrosis, thickening of the alveolar membrane, and peribronchial fibrosis are observed. Bronchiolar epithelial proliferation accompanies the pulmonary fibrosis. Rupture of septa produces small cysts and areas of bullous emphysema. Small pulmonary arteries and arterioles show intimal thickening, fragmentation of the elastica, and muscular hypertrophy; this may occur without interstitial pulmonary fibrosis and produce pulmonary hypertension.

The synovium in patients with arthritis is similar to that seen in early rheumatoid arthritis and shows edema with infiltration of lymphocytes and plasma cells. A characteristic finding is a thick layer of fibrin overlying and within the synovium. Later in the disease the synovium may become fibrotic. Fibrinous deposits appear on the surfaces of tendon sheaths and in the overlying fascia and may lead to audible creaking over moving tendons.

Histologic features of primary myopathy consist of interstitial and perivascular lymphocytic infiltrations, degeneration of muscle fibers, and interstitial fibrosis. Arterioles may be thickened, and capillaries may be decreased in number. Pathologic and electrophysiologic findings of polymyositis in proximal muscles are present in the few patients who are considered to have the overlap syndrome of SSc and polymyositis.

Cardiac involvement consists of degeneration of myocardial fibers and irregular areas of interstitial fibrosis that is most prominent around blood vessels. Fibrosis also involves the conduction system, leading to atrioventricular conduction defects and arrhythmias. The wall of smaller coronary arteries may be thickened. Fibrinous pericarditis and pericardial effusions are found in some patients.

Renal involvement is found in over half the patients and consists of intimal hyperplasia of the interlobular arteries, fibrinoid necrosis of the afferent arterioles, including the glomerular tuft, and thickening of the glomerular basement membrane. Small cortical infarctions and glomerulosclerosis may be present. The renal pathologic change is often indistinguishable from that observed in malignant hypertension. Renal vascular lesions, however, may be present in the absence of hypertension. Immunofluorescence studies of kidney have shown IgM, complement components, and fibrinogen in the walls of affected vessels. Angiographic renal studies in patients with SSc may show constriction of the intralobular arteries, a finding that simulates the vasospasm of the digital arteries observed in Raynaud's phenomenon. Cold-induced Raynaud's phenomenon has been shown to decrease renal blood flow.

Primary liver involvement is not common. Primary biliary cirrhosis occurs in some patients, particularly in those with the limited cutaneous form of SSc. Fibrosis of the thyroid gland may develop in the presence or absence of autoimmune thyroiditis.

Thickening of the periodontal membrane with replacement of the lamina dura is demonstrated radiographically as widening of the periodontal space and rarely causes loosening of the teeth.

Pathologic changes in small arteries and arterioles consist of concentric subintimal proliferation and periadventitial fibrosis, with narrowing or occlusion of the lumen. These vascular abnormalities have been described in digits, skin, muscle, lung, kidney, and other viscera. Arteritis with fibrinoid necrosis is occasionally observed.

CLINICAL MANIFESTATIONS Systemic sclerosis usually begins insidiously; the first symptoms are frequently Raynaud's phenomenon and puffy fingers. Ninety-five percent of patients will experience Raynaud's phenomenon, which is defined as episodic vasoconstriction of small arteries and arterioles of fingers, toes, and sometimes the tip of the nose and the earlobes. Episodes are brought on by cold exposure, vibration, or emotional stress. Patients experience pallor and/or cyanosis followed by rubor on rewarming. Pallor and/or cyanosis are usually associated with coldness and numbness of fingers and/or toes, and rubor with pain and tingling. Raynaud's phenomenon may precede skin changes by several months or even years in those patients who subsequently develop the limited cutaneous form of SSc. After 2 or more years of Raynaud's phenomenon, few patients who have this as their only symptom will subsequently develop SSc.

In early disease, fingers and hands are swollen. Swelling may also involve forearms, feet, lower legs, and face. However, lower extremities are relatively spared. This edematous phase may last for a few weeks, months, or even longer. The edema may be pitting or nonpitting. The skin gradually becomes firm, thickened, and eventually tightly bound to underlying subcutaneous tissue (indurative phase). In patients with diffuse cutaneous scleroderma, skin changes will become generalized and involve the extremities, face, and trunk. Rapid progression of these changes over a 2- to 3-year period is associated with a greater risk of visceral disease, particularly of the lungs, heart, or kidneys. On the other hand, patients with limited cutaneous scleroderma will usually have a more gradual progression of skin changes which are restricted to fingers or distal extremity and face. After many years of disease, the skin may soften and return to normal thickness or become thin and atrophic.

In the extremity, the taut skin over fingers gradually limits full extension, and flexion contractures develop. Ulcers may appear on the volar pads of the fingertips and over bony prominences such as elbows, malleoli, and the extensor surface of the proximal interphalangeal joints of the hands. These ulcers may become secondarily infected. The soft tissue of fingertips is lost. In some instances, resorption of the terminal phalanges occurs. Skin over the extremities, face, and trunk may become darkly pigmented, even without exposure to the sun. Pigmentation of the skin may occur over superficial blood vessels and tendons. The skin loses hair, oil, and sweat glands and so becomes dry and coarse.

In some patients, particularly those with the limited cutaneous form of disease, calcific deposits develop in intracutaneous and subcutaneous tissue. The sites commonly involved are periarticular tissue, digital pads, olecranon and prepatellar bursae, and skin along the extensor surface of the forearms. The overlying skin may break down, with drainage of calcific material. Involvement of the face results in loss of skin wrinkles and facial expression, as well as microstomia, which may make eating and dental hygiene difficult. The capillary bed of nailfolds of the fingers may show enlargement of capillaries with little or no capillary loss, usually indicative of limited cutaneous scleroderma. In diffuse cutaneous scleroderma, there is disorganization of the capillary bed and decreased numbers of capillaries. These capillary changes, which are observed by wide angle microscopy or with an ophthalmoscope used as a magnifier, are not found in patients who have only Raynaud's phenomenon.

More than half the patients with SSc complain of pain, swelling, and stiffness of the fingers and knees. A symmetric polyarthritis, resembling rheumatoid arthritis, may be seen. In more advanced stages of the disease, leathery crepitation can be palpated over moving joints, especially the knee. Extensive fibrotic thickening of the tendon sheaths in the wrist can produce a carpal tunnel syndrome. Muscle weakness usually is present in patients with severe skin involvement and, in most cases, is due to disuse atrophy. There is a distinctive histologic myopathy that accompanies SSc which is not associated with muscle enzyme abnormalities. A few patients develop a myositis characterized by proximal muscle weakness and muscle enzyme elevations that are identical to polymyositis (overlap syndrome). In addition to terminal phalanges, resorption of bone may involve ribs, clavicle, and angle of mandible.

Symptoms attributable to esophageal involvement are present in more than 50 percent of patients and include epigastric fullness, burning pain in the epigastric or retrosternal regions, and regurgitation of gastric contents. These symptoms, most noticeable when the patient is lying flat or bending over, are due to the reduced tone of the gastroesophageal sphincter and to dilatation of the distal esophagus. Peptic esophagitis frequently occurs and may lead to strictures and narrowing of the lower esophagus. However, it seldom results in bleeding. Dysphagia, particularly of solid foods, may occur independent of other esophageal symptoms and is caused by the loss of esophageal motility due to neuromuscular dysfunction. Manometry or cineradiography reveals decreased amplitude or disappearance of peristaltic waves in the lower two-thirds of the esophagus. Raynaud's phenomenon in the absence of a connective tissue disease is also associated with esophageal dysmotility. Later in the course of the illness, dilatation and atony of the lower portion of the esophagus as well as reflux are seen. With gastric involvement, barium studies show dilatation, atony, and delayed gastric emptying.

Hypomotility of the small intestine produces symptoms of bloating and abdominal pain, and may suggest an intestinal obstruction or paralytic ileus (pseudoobstruction). Malabsorption syndrome with weight loss, diarrhea, and anemia is due to bacterial overgrowth in the atonic intestine or possibly to obliteration of lymphatics by fibrosis. Roentgenographic features of the second and third portions of the duodenum and of the jejunum include dilatation, loss of the usual feathery pattern, and delayed disappearance of barium. Pneumatosis intestinalis occasionally occurs and appears as radiolucent cysts or linear streaks within the wall of the small intestine. Benign pneumoperitoneum may result from the rupture of these cysts. Involvement of the large intestine may cause chronic constipation and fecal impaction with episodes of bowel obstruction. Barium studies of the large intestine may show dilatation, atony, and large-mouth diverticula. Some patients may have gastrointestinal features of SSc with little or no cutaneous or other organ involvement.

The lungs are affected in SSc in at least two-thirds of the patients. The most common symptom is exertional dyspnea, often accompanied by a dry, nonproductive cough. Symptoms may occur in the absence of pulmonary fibrosis, and patients with pulmonary fibrosis can be relatively asymptomatic. Bilateral basilar rales may be present. Restriction of chest movement caused by extensive skin involvement of the thorax rarely occurs. Aspiration pneumonia may result from gastric reflux due to lower esophageal atony. Superimposed bacterial or viral pneumonia can be a serious complication in patients with pulmonary fibrosis. There is an increased frequency of alveolar cell and bronchogenic carcinoma in patients with pulmonary fibrosis. Pulmonary function tests are frequently abnormal and show a reduction in vital capacity and decreased lung compliance. Impairment of gas exchange is reflected by a low diffusing capacity and low P_{O_2} with exercise. These abnormalities may be present even when the chest radiograph is normal. Chest film may show a pattern of linear densities, mottling, and honeycombing involving most prominently the lower two-thirds of the lung. In the absence of significant interstitial fibrosis, a severe form of pulmonary arterial hypertension develops after many years of disease in patients with limited cutaneous scleroderma. Less than 10 percent of patients will develop this complication, which is caused by narrowing and obliteration of pulmonary arteries and arterioles by intimal fibrosis and medial hypertrophy. Pulmonary hypertension is manifested by progressive worsening of dyspnea and eventually by appearance of right-sided heart failure. Electrocardiographic evidence of pulmonary hypertension is usually present. The prognosis is extremely poor with the development of pulmonary hypertension; the mean duration of survival is approximately 2 years.

Primary cardiac involvement in SSc includes pericarditis with or without effusions, heart failure, and varying degrees of heart block or arrhythmias. Cardiomyopathy attributable to myocardial fibrosis appears in fewer than 10 percent of patients, and involves primarily those patients with diffuse cutaneous scleroderma. Radionuclide studies have shown abnormalities of left ventricular function due to myocardial fibrosis. Cold-induced vasospasm of the hands produces defects in myocardial thallium perfusion. The characteristic pathologic feature of contraction band necrosis results from cardiac muscle damage caused by intermittent vasospasm of coronary vessels. Patients may experience angina pectoris even though coronary angiograms are normal. Patients can also develop left ventricular failure secondary to systemic hypertension or cor pulmonale secondary to pulmonary arterial hypertension.

Renal failure is the leading cause of death in SSc, accounting for almost half of the deaths. Significant renal disease occurs mostly in those patients with diffuse cutaneous scleroderma. A high risk of renal crisis is present in those patients who have rapidly progressive widespread skin thickening early in their course. Renal crisis is characterized by malignant hypertension, which can rapidly progress to renal failure. These patients manifest hypertensive encephalopathy, severe headache, retinopathy, seizures, and left ventricular failure. Hematuria and proteinuria are followed by oliguria and renal failure. The mechanism for the hypertensive crisis is activation of the renin-angiotensin system. Before the advent of effective antihypertensive drugs, the majority of these patients died within 6 months. Renal failure can also develop insidiously later in the course of disease in the setting of mild to moderate hypertension and proteinuria. In these patients or those with clinically unrecognized renal disease, reduction of renal plasma flow secondary to heart failure or volume depletion resulting from overdiuresis may precipitate renal crisis. An indicator

of impending renal failure is microangiopathic anemia, which may occur in a normotensive patient. The presence of a chronic pericardial effusion may also herald subsequent renal failure.

Symptoms of dry eyes and/or dry mouth are frequently present in patients with SSc. Lip biopsy may show lymphocytic infiltration of minor salivary glands characteristic of Sjögren's syndrome or intraglandular or periglandular fibrosis. Antibodies to SS-A (Ro) and/or SS-B (La) are found in those patients with lip biopsies consistent with Sjögren's syndrome and not in those with salivary gland fibrosis.

Hypothyroidism occurs in a significant number of patients and may be associated with high levels of antithyroid antibodies. Fibrosis of the thyroid gland may be present, but also occurs in the absence of autoimmune thyroiditis. Other manifestations of SSc include trigeminal neuralgia and male impotence secondary to decreased penile tumescence. These men have normal serum levels of testosterone and gonadotropins. Pathogenesis of this abnormality has been considered to be due either to vascular and/or autonomic nervous system abnormalities.

LABORATORY FINDINGS   The erythrocyte sedimentation rate may be elevated. Hypoproliferative anemia related to chronic inflammation is the most common cause of anemia in SSc. Anemia may also be caused by iron deficiency secondary to gastrointestinal bleeding. Bacterial overgrowth due to atony of the small bowel may lead to vitamin B_{12} and/or folic acid–deficiency anemia. Microangiopathic hemolytic anemia is most often associated with renal involvement and is caused by the presence of intravascular fibrin in renal arterioles. Hypergammaglobulinemia, consisting mostly of IgG, is found in approximately half the patients. Rheumatoid factor, in low titer, is present in 25 percent of patients. Antinuclear antibodies detected by using a cultured human laryngeal carcinoma cell line (HEp-2) substrate are present in 95 percent of patients. Antinuclear antibodies that have a high specificity for SSc are antitopoisomerase 1 (Scl-70), antinucleolar, and anticentromere. Antitopoisomerase 1, originally called anti-Scl-70, recognizes the nuclear enzyme DNA topoisomerase 1. These antibodies are found in about 20 percent of patients, and are associated with diffuse cutaneous involvement and interstitial pulmonary disease. They are seldom present in other disorders or in conjunction with anticentromere antibodies. Antinucleolar antibodies are relatively specific for SSc and are present in approximately 20 to 30 percent of patients. Anticentromere antibodies react with protein antigens located in the kinetochore region of chromosomes and are strongly associated with limited cutaneous scleroderma or CREST syndrome. Anticentromere antibodies are found in only about 10 percent of patients with diffuse cutaneous scleroderma and rarely in other connective tissue diseases. They are occasionally found in patients with only Raynaud's phenomenon and may indicate subsequent development of limited cutaneous disease. High titers of anti-RNP are present in those patients with features of mixed connective tissue disease. Anti-PM-Scl, formerly referred to as anti-PM1, may be found in SSc patients with polymyositis and renal involvement. Anti-SS-A and/or anti-SS-B are present in those patients with overlap syndrome of SSc and Sjögren's syndrome.

DIAGNOSIS   The diagnosis of SSc presents no difficulty in the presence of Raynaud's phenomenon, with typical skin lesions and visceral involvement. Although Raynaud's phenomenon may be the first symptom of SSc, most patients with Raynaud's phenomenon alone do not develop a connective tissue disease. Other causes of Raynaud's phenomenon include thoracic outlet (scalenus anticus and cervical rib) syndromes, shoulder-hand syndrome, trauma (jackhammer or vibratory machine operators), previous cold injury, vinyl chloride exposure, and circulating cryoglobulins or cold agglutinins. Linear scleroderma and morphea are localized forms of scleroderma that can usually be distinguished clinically. In early disease, SSc may initially be confused with rheumatoid arthritis, systemic lupus erythematosus, or polymyositis when articular or muscle involvement is prominent. SSc without cutaneous involvement should be considered in patients with unexplained pulmonary fibrosis, pulmonary hypertension, cardiomyopathies, heart block, dysphagia, or malabsorption syndrome. Several conditions have scleroderma-like features but lack the visceral involvement. Scleredema (scleredema adultorum of Buschke) occurs predominantly in children and is characterized by painless edematous induration involving the face, scalp, neck, trunk, and proximal portions of the extremities. Involvement of the hands and feet usually does not occur. Scleredema may be associated with previous streptococcal infection and is usually self-limited, resolving in 6 to 12 months. Histology reveals accumulation of mucopolysaccharides in the dermis and skeletal muscle. A rare entity, scleromyxedema (lichen myxedematosus), is manifested by yellowish or pale red papules in association with diffuse skin thickening which may involve the face and hands. Acid mucopolysaccharide deposits are found in the dermis. Monoclonal IgG may be detected in some of these patients. Primary amyloidosis may involve the skin of the extremities and face diffusely to give the appearance of scleroderma. Biopsy will clearly differentiate these entities.

COURSE AND PROGNOSIS The course of SSc is quite variable. Until disease differentiates into recognizable subsets, prognosis in early disease is difficult to predict. Patients with limited cutaneous scleroderma, especially those with anticentromere antibodies, have a good prognosis, with the notable exception of those few patients, less than 10 percent, who after 10 to 20 years or longer develop pulmonary arterial hypertension. Malabsorption syndrome and primary biliary cirrhosis are the causes of morbidity and mortality in some patients with limited cutaneous disease. On the other hand, the prognosis is generally worse in patients with diffuse cutaneous disease, particularly when the onset occurs at an older age. In addition, males have a worse prognosis. Renal and other visceral organ disease may develop early in the course of those patients with rapidly progressive generalized skin thickening. Death occurs most often from cardiac, renal, or pulmonary involvement. In one study the 10-year cumulative survival of patients with only renal involvement was 30 percent and of patients with only lung involvement, 50 percent. In patients without heart, lung, or kidney involvement, survival was 71 percent.

Skin may spontaneously soften after years of disease. Softening occurs in the reverse order of original skin involvement beginning with the trunk and followed by the proximal and then the distal extremities. Sclerodactyly may persist. Skin thickness may eventually approach normal.

TREATMENT Even though SSc cannot be cured, treatment of involved organ systems can relieve symptoms and improve function. The doctor-patient relationship is extremely important in caring for patients with this chronic debilitating illness. Once the diagnosis of SSc has been made, the patient and family should be instructed about this disorder. The patient will need repeated explanations and reassurances throughout his or her illness. Depending on the severity of illness, the patient will require monitoring of blood pressure, blood counts, urinalysis, and renal and pulmonary function on a regular basis.

Effectiveness of drug therapy in SSc is difficult to evaluate because of the variable course and severity of the disease. Many drugs have been used in the treatment of SSc without any consistent or prolonged benefit. In uncontrolled studies D-penicillamine has been reported to reduce skin thickening and prevent development of significant organ involvement. This drug interferes with inter- and intramolecular cross-linking of collagen and is also immunosuppressive. Its immunosuppressive activity may also lead to decrease of collagen production. Penicillamine is better tolerated when started at a low dose, usually 250 mg per day, and then increased at 1- to 3-month intervals up to 1.5 g per day as tolerated. Although a few patients can tolerate higher doses, most patients are maintained on a dose between 0.5 and 1 g per day. For optimal absorption, it is important to give this drug 1 h before or 2 h after a meal. This drug can be quite toxic; its more serious complications include glomerulonephritis with nephrotic syndrome, aplastic anemia, leukopenia, thrombocytopenia, and myasthenia gravis. Other side effects are fever, rash, anorexia, nausea,

and loss of taste. Patients should have monthly complete blood counts (including platelet count) and urinalysis. Azathioprine and other immunosuppressives have also been used in SSc, and should be reserved for those patients with rapidly progressive and life-threatening disease. Control studies are lacking. A trial of treatment with recombinant γ-interferon is currently in progress. This agent has been shown to inhibit collagen production.

Antiplatelet therapy may play a role in the treatment of SSc since the biologic products of platelets affect blood vessels. Low doses of aspirin block the formation of thromboxane A_2, a powerful vasoconstrictor and platelet aggregator. In addition, dipyridamole 200 to 400 mg in divided daily doses also decreases platelet adhesion to damaged vessel walls. While these drugs have a reasonable therapeutic rationale, a 2-year double-blind study did not show any benefit from their use. Reports of beneficial effects of colchicine or chlorambucil have not been documented in controlled studies.

Glucocorticoids are indicated in those patients with inflammatory myositis or pericarditis. The initial dose is 40 to 60 mg per day and is tapered based on clinical improvement. Prednisone 10 mg per day or less may be beneficial in treating arthritis refractory to nonsteroidal anti-inflammatory drugs and in reducing edema associated with the edematous phase of early skin involvement. Glucocorticoids are not otherwise indicated in the long-term treatment of SSc. High doses of glucocorticoids may play a role in precipitating acute renal failure. However, this association remains unclear.

The management of Raynaud's phenomenon is directed at control of vasospasm. Patients should be advised to dress warmly and wear mittens and socks, not to smoke, to remove causes of external stress, and to avoid drugs such as amphetamine and ergotamine. Beta blocking drugs may make Raynaud's phenomenon worse. Warmth of the central body induces peripheral vasodilatation. Drugs that block sympathetic vasoconstriction, such as reserpine, α-methyldopa, phenoxybenzamine, and prazosin may be useful in the treatment of Raynaud's phenomenon, but their side effects often curtail extended use. Calcium channel blockers, nifedipine and diltiazam, can be effective in alleviating Raynaud's phenomenon, but side effects of light-headedness and palpitations may limit their use. The dose of nifedipine is 10 to 20 mg tid. Ketanserin, an oral serotonin antagonist, has also been shown to be effective. Techniques of biofeedback have also been used with variable success for teaching patients to control the temperature of their hands. Surgical sympathectomy usually provides only temporary improvement, and it, along with other forms of therapy, does not prevent progression of the vascular lesion. The response to any therapy for Raynaud's phenomenon is limited by the degree of existing structural narrowing of digital arteries. Gangrene of distal digits may occur and require surgical amputation.

Numerous drugs have been claimed to soften the hidebound skin, but documentation in controlled studies is lacking. These drugs include D-penicillamine, colchicine, p-aminobenzoic acid, and vitamin E. Dryness of the skin may be reduced by avoiding frequent use of detergent soaps and by applying regularly hydrophilic ointments and bath oils. Regular exercise helps to maintain flexibility of extremities and pliability of skin. Massaging the skin several times a day may also be beneficial. Fingertip ulcerations can be protected by applying a guard or cage over the end of the finger. The use of an occlusive dressing over a noninfected ulcer may promote healing and protect the finger. Skin ulcers should be kept clean by soaking or by surgical or chemical debridement. Sympatholytic drugs or local nitroglycerine paste applied to the ulcer may be beneficial in promoting healing. Infected ulcers can usually be treated with topical antibiotics but may require systemic antibiotics especially when there is a question of underlying osteomyelitis.

Patients with reflux esophagitis are treated with small frequent meals, antacids between meals, and elevation of the head of the bed. Patients should be advised not to lie down for a few hours after a meal, and to avoid coffee, tea, and chocolate, which reduce the pressure of the lower esophageal sphincter. Cimetidine or ranitidine may be beneficial in some patients. Metoclopramide can also be of help in some patients. Patients with dysphagia should be instructed to chew their food thoroughly and wash it down with fluids. Malabsorption syndrome due to duodenal hypomotility and bacterial overgrowth may improve with intermittent use of appropriate antibiotics. Patients with severe debilitating malabsorption may benefit from parenteral hyperalimentation. Stool softeners and mild laxatives are usually adequate for treating constipation due to hypomotility of the colon.

Acute myositis is usually responsive to glucocorticoids; these drugs should not be used for the indolent primary form of muscle disease of SSc. Articular symptoms are treated with aspirin or other nonsteroidal anti-inflammatory agents.

Pulmonary fibrosis is not reversible, and therefore treatment is directed at symptoms or complications. Pulmonary infection requires prompt treatment with antibiotics. Hypoxia necessitates giving low concentrations of oxygen. The role of glucocorticoids in preventing progression of interstitial lung disease is not clear. Patients should receive Pneumovax and yearly influenza immunizations.

Recognition of early renal failure is important in order to preserve remaining function. Renal involvement is often accompanied by hypertension and mild to moderate proteinuria. An occasional patient may be normotensive. Antihypertensive agents are often effective in lowering blood pressure and stabilizing or reversing renal failure. These drugs include propranolol, clonidine, and minoxidil. Particularly effective are the angiotensin-converting enzyme inhibitors, which include captopril and enalapril. Dialysis may be required in patients with progressive renal failure. Some patients, however, have a slow return of renal function after several months and may no longer require dialysis.

Patients with cardiac failure require careful monitoring of digitalis and diuretic administration. Pericardial effusions may also improve with diuretics. Care should be taken to avoid overdiuresis which may lead to decreased renal blood flow, decreased cardiac output, and renal failure.

EOSINOPHILIC FASCIITIS   Eosinophilic fasciitis is a scleroderma-like syndrome characterized by inflammation followed later by sclerosis of the dermis, subcutis, and deep fascia. The disease affects adults, and often occurs after strenuous physical activity. Patients do not have Raynaud's phenomenon or internal organ involvement. Several immunologic abnormalities have been associated with eosinophilic fasciitis and include aplastic anemia, myelodysplastic syndrome, and thrombocytopenia. Patients usually have the abrupt onset of symmetric tenderness and swelling of the extremities which is rapidly followed by induration of the skin and subcutaneous tissue. The skin takes on a cobblestone or puckered appearance. Carpal tunnel syndrome appears early in the course, and flexion contractures develop later. A marked eosinophilia is found in the early stage of disease and subsequently decreases. Increased levels of polyclonal IgG and immune complexes are often present in the serum. A full-thickness biopsy consisting of skin, fascia, and superficial muscle shows perivascular infiltration of histiocytes, eosinophils, lymphocytes, and plasma cells. Biopsies later in the course show sclerosis. Spontaneous improvement and occasionally complete remission may occur after 2 to 5 years of disease. Some patients have persistent disease while others are left with flexion contractures. Administration of glucocorticoids may provide symptomatic improvement and will decrease the eosinophilia. Improvement has been reported with the use of the H-2 blocker cimetidine.

REFERENCES

EARNSHAW W et al: Three human chromosomal autoantigens are recognized by sera from patients with anti-centromere antibodies. J Clin Invest 77:426, 1986

HAWKINS RA et al: Increased dermal mast cell populations in progressive systemic sclerosis: A link in chronic fibrosis? Ann Intern Med 102:182, 1985

MARICQ HR et al: Microvascular abnormalities as possible predictors of disease subsets in Raynaud phenomenon and early connective tissue disease. Clin Exp Rheumatol 1:195, 1983

MEDSGER TA: Systemic sclerosis (scleroderma), localized scleroderma, eosinophilic fasciitis, and calcinosis, in *Arthritis and Allied Conditions*, 11th ed, McCarty DJ (ed). Philadelphia, Lea & Febiger, 1989, p 1118

MILLER EB et al: Reduced natural killer cell activity in patients with systemic sclerosis: Correlation with clinical disease type. Arthritis Rheum 31:1515, 1988

SEIBOLD JR: Scleroderma (systemic sclerosis), in *Textbook of Rheumatology*, 3d ed, WN Kelly et al (eds). Philadelphia, Saunders, 1989

SHULMAN LE: Diffuse fasciitis with eosinophilia: A new syndrome. Arthritis Rheum 20:S205, 1977

SILVER RM, LEROY EC: Systemic sclerosis (scleroderma), in *Immunological Diseases*, 4th ed, Samter M et al (eds). Boston, Little, Brown, 1988, p 1459

STEEN VD et al: D-Penicillamine therapy in progressive systemic sclerosis (scleroderma). Ann Intern Med 97:652, 1982

WEINER ES et al: Clinical associations of anti-centromere antibodies and antibodies to topoisomerase I. Arthritis Rheum 31:378, 1988

WHITESIDE TL et al: Soluble mediators from mononuclear cells increase the synthesis of glycosaminoglycan by dermal fibroblast cultures derived from normal subjects and progressive systemic sclerosis patients. Arthritis Rheum 28:188, 1985

272   MIXED CONNECTIVE TISSUE DISEASE

GORDON C. SHARP

DEFINITION   Mixed connective tissue disease (MCTD) is a syndrome characterized by a combination of clinical features similar to those of systemic lupus erythematosus (SLE), scleroderma, polymyositis, and rheumatoid arthritis and unusually high titers of circulating antibody to a nuclear ribonucleoprotein (RNP) antigen.

ETIOLOGY, PATHOGENESIS, AND PATHOLOGY   The etiologic and pathogenic mechanisms of MCTD remain unknown, but a number of clues point to the involvement of immune aberrations: (1) persistence of extremely high titers of antibody to nuclear RNP and a marked polyclonal hypergammaglobulinemia indicative of B-cell hyperactivity; (2) a suppressor T-cell defect; (3) circulating immune complexes during active disease; (4) deposition of IgG, IgM, and complement within vascular walls and along sarcolemmal and glomerular basement membranes; and (5) widespread lymphocytic and plasma cell infiltration of numerous tissues. One of the chief underlying pathologic findings in some adults and children with MCTD is a proliferative intimal and/or medial vascular lesion resulting in narrowing of the lumen of large vessels (e.g., pulmonary, renal, and coronary vessels and aorta) and of small arterioles of many organs. Such lesions in the lungs may contribute to pulmonary hypertension and abnormalities of pulmonary function.

CLINICAL MANIFESTATIONS   The age range in published reports of MCTD is from 4 to 80 years, with a mean of 37 years. Approximately 80 percent of patients have been female. Typical clinical features include Raynaud's phenomenon, polyarthritis, swollen hands or sclerodactyly, esophageal dysfunction, pulmonary involvement, and inflammatory myopathy. Malar rash, alopecia, lymphadenopathy, and cardiac and renal disease are less frequent manifestations.

Cutaneous manifestations of MCTD include the swollen, sausage-like appearance of the fingers, nonscarring alopecia, lupus-like rashes, heliotrope eyelids, erythematous patches over the knuckles, periungual telangiectasia, and "squared" telangiectasia over the hands and face. Scleroderma-like changes may be present but only occasionally become extensive.

Musculoskeletal abnormalities occur in most patients. Arthritis is usually nondeforming but may resemble rheumatoid arthritis. Proximal muscle weakness is frequent and may be severe. Serum levels of creatine phosphokinase and aldolase are often markedly elevated, electromyograms are typical of inflammatory myopathy, and biopsies show degeneration of muscle fibers and interstitial and perivascular infiltrates of lymphocytes and plasma cells.

Esophageal dysfunction has been demonstrated in 80 percent of all patients, including 70 percent of asymptomatic patients. Characteristic abnormalities include reduced upper and lower esophageal sphincter pressures and decreased amplitude of peristalsis in the distal two-thirds of the esophagus.

Pulmonary involvement occurs in 85 percent of patients with MCTD but may be clinically silent until far advanced. The most common clinical finding is exertional dyspnea, followed by pleuritic pain and bibasilar rales. Reduced diffusing capacity for carbon monoxide is the most frequent functional abnormality.

Cardiac disease is less common than pulmonary involvement in adults with MCTD but may be more frequent in children. Pericarditis is the most common cardiac finding; other findings have included mitral valve prolapse, myocarditis, congestive heart failure, and aortic insufficiency.

Renal disease in children and adults with MCTD has a combined prevalence of about 28 percent. Progressive renal failure is uncommon, and clinical and histologic findings suggest that vascular lesions may represent a more serious problem than immune complex nephritis in MCTD.

Other less frequent clinical manifestations include fever, lymphadenopathy, neurologic abnormalities, Sjögren's syndrome, hepatosplenomegaly, and intestinal involvement similar to that seen in scleroderma.

LABORATORY FINDINGS Almost all patients have positive fluorescent antinuclear antibody tests at high titers (usually greater than 1:1000) with a speckled pattern and very high titers of antibodies directed against the ribonuclease-sensitive nuclear RNP component of extractable nuclear antigen (ENA). Elevated anti–native DNA antibody titers and antibodies to the ribonuclease-resistant Sm component of ENA are uncommon in MCTD; their presence is usually associated with a severe flare-up of lupus-like features. High titers of circulating RNP antibodies usually persist for years, but antibody levels may decline significantly or become undetectable in patients who are in prolonged remission.

Recent studies have further elucidated the nature of the RNP and Sm antigens. Antibodies to RNP immunoprecipitate U1 snRNA-protein complexes and react with proteins designated 68K, A, and C, whereas Sm antibodies immunoprecipitate snRNA-protein complexes containing U1, U2, U4, U5, and U6 snRNAs and react with proteins designated B/B' and D. Furthermore, these antigenic complexes have been shown to have important biologic roles in the processing of messenger RNA. Several reports indicate that antibodies to the 68K protein are associated with anti-U1 RNP antibodies in MCTD, but rarely occur in SLE. Other preliminary studies have revealed that U1 68K-positive MCTD patients have disease associated with HLA-DR4 but not with HLA-DR3 as is found in patients with SLE.

Rheumatoid factor is found, often at very high titers, in over half of the patients with MCTD. Diffuse hypergammaglobulinemia is frequently noted and may be elevated to a level of 50 g per liter. A mild to moderate reduction in serum complement levels occurs in about 30 percent of patients. Other less frequent laboratory findings include leukopenia, anemia, and thrombocytopenia (mainly in children).

DIAGNOSIS The diagnosis of MCTD is based on a combination of typical overlapping clinical findings and high titers of circulating antibody to nuclear RNP antigen. In some patients, all the clinical manifestations may be present on initial evaluation. However, as clinicians have become more aware of the syndrome and tests for RNP antibody are being performed more frequently, MCTD is being recognized in an earlier phase in patients presenting with minimal symptoms (e.g., Raynaud's phenomenon, arthralgias, myalgias, and swollen hands). In some this mild "undifferentiated connective tissue disease" syndrome may persist for years, but a recent prospective, long-term study showed that the majority of patients with high titers of RNP antibodies and limited clinical manifestations ultimately developed signs and symptoms consistent with a diagnosis of MCTD.

TREATMENT AND PROGNOSIS Lacking controlled studies, specific treatment recommendations for MCTD are based on anecdotal

information. Salicylates, other nonsteroidal anti-inflammatory agents, hydroxychloroquine, vasodilators, and/or low doses of glucocorticoids are used to treat mild disease. In general, mild disease is quite responsive to low-dose glucocorticoids. If the disease is more severe and significantly involves major organ systems, higher doses of glucocorticoids (e.g., 1 mg/kg per day of prednisone) are usually required. As with SLE, a cytotoxic agent may be added in steroid-resistant or -dependent cases. However, the efficacy of this latter therapeutic regimen has not been substantiated by controlled clinical trials. The prognosis for MCTD is generally similar to that of SLE and somewhat better than for scleroderma.

REFERENCES

PETTERSSON I et al: The use of immunoblotting and immunoprecipitation of (U) small nuclear ribonucleoproteins in the analysis of sera of patients with mixed connective tissue disease and systemic lupus erythematosus. Arthritis Rheum 29:986, 1986

SHARP GC, SINGSEN BH: Mixed connective tissue disease, in *Arthritis and Allied Conditions*, 11th ed, DJ McCarty (ed). Philadelphia, Lea & Febiger, 1988, p 1080

SULLIVAN WD et al: A prospective evaluation emphasizing pulmonary involvement in patients with mixed connective tissue disease. Medicine 63:92, 1984

TAKEDA Y et al: Enzyme-linked immunosorbent assay using isolated (U) small nuclear ribonucleoprotein polypeptides as antigens to investigate the clinical significance of autoantibodies to these polypeptides. Clin Immunol Immunopathol 50:213, 1989

273 SJÖGREN'S SYNDROME

H. CLIFFORD LANE / ANTHONY S. FAUCI

DEFINITION Sjögren's syndrome is an immunologic disorder characterized by progressive destruction of the exocrine glands leading to mucosal and conjunctival dryness (sicca syndrome) accompanied by a variety of autoimmune phenomena. The disease can occur either by itself, in which case it is referred to as primary Sjögren's syndrome, or in association with other autoimmune diseases (see Chaps. 269 and 270), in which case it is referred to as secondary Sjögren's syndrome. In addition, some authors have divided the disease into two forms: glandular, when the only clinical manifestations are within the exocrine system, and extraglandular, when other tissues are involved as well.

INCIDENCE AND PREVALENCE The disease predominantly affects women in the third or fourth decades of life. Although precise incidence figures are not known, it has been suggested that Sjögren's syndrome is the second most common rheumatologic disease in the United States. Up to 30 percent of patients with rheumatoid arthritis, 10 percent of patients with systemic lupus erythematosus, and 1 percent of patients with scleroderma have been reported as having secondary Sjögren's syndrome. Immunogenetic predisposition appears to play an important role in the incidence of Sjögren's syndrome. The frequency of the HLA B8, the HLA-DRw3, and the MT-2 histocompatibility antigens is significantly increased in patients with primary Sjögren's syndrome.

PATHOPHYSIOLOGY AND IMMUNOPATHOGENESIS The two main mechanisms of tissue destruction in Sjögren's syndrome are lymphocytic infiltration and immune-complex deposition. In addition, approximately 10 percent of these patients develop a lymphoproliferative process known as *pseudolymphoma*. This disorder has many histologic features of lymphoma but is associated clinically with a benign course.

Virtually any organ system of the body may be affected in the patient with Sjögren's syndrome. The disease process is most striking in the salivary and lacrimal glands, where there is a progressive mononuclear cell infiltrate which generally leads to complete scarring. Renal disease may result from a lymphocytic interstitial nephritis or an immune-complex glomerulonephritis. Pulmonary involvement is most frequently due to interstitial pneumonitis caused by an infiltration of mononuclear cells, although discrete mass lesions due to pseudolymphoma may occur. Patients with Sjögren's syndrome may also develop an immune-complex vasculitis, at times associated with cryoglobulinemia. Thromboangiitis obliterans has also been seen, usually in patients with preexisting Raynaud's phenomena. Both the peripheral and the central nervous system manifestations of this disease are felt to be due to blood vessel inflammation.

Patients with Sjögren's syndrome exhibit two main types of immunoregulatory defects. The first of these is an abnormally active cellular immune system. This is evident by the intense inflammatory mononuclear cell infiltrates seen in the salivary glands of these patients. These infiltrates are made up predominantly of activated T cells; however, activated B lymphocytes can be detected as well. These mononuclear cell infiltrates are responsible for many of the clinical manifestations of Sjögren's syndrome, including the profound dryness of conjunctival and mucosal surfaces, interstitial nephritis, interstitial pneumonitis, and meningoencephalitis. The second immunoregulatory defect seen in patients with Sjögren's syndrome is oligoclonal B-cell activation. This results in hypergammaglobulinemia, oligoclonal spikes on protein electrophoresis, elevated levels of circulating immune complexes, and the production of autoantibodies. Among the autoantibodies seen are rheumatoid factor, SSA (anti-Ro), and SSB (anti-La). While the precise clinical significance of these and other serologic markers is unclear, it does appear that most patients with the more serious systemic manifestations of Sjögren's syndrome are SSA-positive.

CLINICAL MANIFESTATIONS AND LABORATORY ABNORMALITIES   The most common clinical manifestations of Sjögren's syndrome are keratoconjunctivitis sicca and xerostomia. Patients often complain initially of a gritty sensation in the eyes or severe dryness of the mouth. The lack of saliva may be associated with an increased rate of dental caries. Mucosal dryness may extend into the upper airway, in which case patients may complain of a persistent cough or hoarseness that is worse in cold weather. Corneal dryness may be so severe as to result in corneal ulcerations.

Renal involvement is seen in approximately 40 percent of patients with primary Sjögren's syndrome. This generally presents clinically as a mild interstitial nephritis that may result in renal tubular acidosis. This form of kidney disease rarely leads to chronic renal failure; however, it may be associated with a 50 percent reduction in creatinine clearance. A minority of patients with renal disease demonstrate an immune-complex glomerulonephritis. This is seen usually in the context of systemic vasculitis.

Twenty-five percent of patients with primary Sjögren's syndrome develop vasculitis (Chap. 276). This usually takes the form of a cutaneous palpable purpura or hypersensitivity vasculitis of the lower extremities. Patients with Sjögren's syndrome may also develop a severe, systemic vasculitis. This is often seen in the setting of cryoglobulinemia and may result in fever, skin rash, and bowel infarction. The vasculitic syndromes seen in patients with Sjögren's syndrome are generally episodic rather than chronic.

A variety of neurologic conditions have been described in patients with Sjögren's syndrome. The most common nervous system presentation is that of a sensory polyneuropathy and/or mononeuritis multiplex. Central nervous system involvement has been reported in this illness and may be focal or diffuse in its presentation. Patients have also been noted to develop a diffuse proximal myositis.

Pulmonary involvement generally takes the form of an interstitial pneumonitis which is usually of little clinical significance. Pulmonary mass lesions may occur that may be infectious, inflammatory, or neoplastic.

Approximately 10 percent of patients with Sjögren's syndrome develop pseudolymphoma. This unusual lymphoproliferative disorder may present as lymphadenopathy, parotid gland enlargement, or pulmonary nodules. Approximately 10 percent of the Sjögren's syndrome patients with pseudolymphoma may go on to develop a lymphocytic (non-Hodgkin's) lymphoma.

Autoimmune thyroid disease resembling Hashimoto's thyroiditis is a common accompaniment of Sjögren's syndrome. Approximately 50 percent of patients with Sjögren's syndrome have some evidence of biochemical hypothyroidism, and 10 percent of patients require thyroid supplement.

Pregnant women with anti-Ro (SSA) antibodies are at an increased risk of delivering infants with cardiac conduction defects. Thus, pregnancies need to be carefully monitored in this group of patients.

A variety of laboratory abnormalities may be seen in patients with Sjögren's syndrome. Among the serologic and hematologic abnormalities are elevated levels of circulating immune complexes, autoantibodies, leukopenia, thrombocytosis, and an elevation in the erythrocyte sedimentation rate. In addition, patients often have a high urine pH.

While the presence of these abnormalities may increase one's level of suspicion of a diagnosis of Sjögren's syndrome, they are not diagnostic by themselves.

DIAGNOSIS   A diagnosis of Sjögren's syndrome is made when the triad of keratoconjunctivitis sicca, xerostomia, and mononuclear cell infiltration of the salivary gland is noted. This latter finding is made by a lower lip biopsy. The differential diagnosis of Sjögren's syndrome includes sarcoidosis, lymphoma, primary amyloidosis, HIV infection, and graft-versus-host disease.

TREATMENT AND PROGNOSIS   Treatment is geared toward symptomatic relief of mucosal dryness and meticulous oral hygiene, and includes artificial tears, ophthalmologic lubricating ointments, nasal sprays of normal saline, moisturizing skin lotions, frequent sips of water, and oral fluoride treatments. There is currently no effective treatment for the ongoing exocrine gland destruction. Glucocorticoids have been used with varying degrees of success in the management of glomerulonephritis, interstitial pneumonitis, and pseudolymphoma. They have not proved to be effective in the management of the cutaneous vasculitis. Patients with systemic vasculitis associated with cryoglobulinemia may benefit from brief courses of immunosupressive therapy (Chap. 276). It should be stressed that this form of systemic vasculitis is episodic, and therefore, in contrast to most forms of systemic necrotizing vasculitis, does not require chronic immunosuppressive therapy. Therapy of pseudolymphoma should be reserved for those cases in which vital organ function is threatened. Because cytotoxic therapy may predispose to the transition from pseudolymphoma to true lymphoma, this form of immunosuppressive therapy should be reserved for potentially life-threatening situations.

The overall prognosis for patients with Sjögren's syndrome is quite good. Patients with secondary Sjögren's syndrome generally have less severe manifestations of Sjögren's than those with the primary form. Patients with primary disease are best managed with ocular and mucosal lubricants, attention to oral hygiene, frequent monitoring of thyroid function, and the reassurance that their disease, while a substantial source of morbidity, generally does not shorten life.

REFERENCES

Fox RI et al: Primary Sjögren's syndrome: Clinical and immunopathologic features. Semin Arthritis Rheum 14:77, 1984

Malinoiv KL et al: Neuropsychiatric dysfunction in primary Sjögren's syndrome. Ann Intern Med 103:344, 1985

Talal N et al (eds): *Sjögren's Syndrome: Clinical and Immunological Aspects.* New York, Springer-Verlag, 1987, p 299

Tsokos M et al: Vasculitis in primary Sjögren's syndrome. Histologic classification and clinical presentation. Am J Clin Pathol 88:26, 1987

274   ANKYLOSING SPONDYLITIS AND REACTIVE ARTHRITIS

JOEL D. TAUROG / PETER E. LIPSKY

ANKYLOSING SPONDYLITIS

Ankylosing spondylitis (AS) is an inflammatory disorder of unknown etiology that primarily affects the axial skeleton; peripheral joints and extraarticular structures may also be involved. The disease usually begins in the second or third decade; the prevalence in men is approximately three times that in women. It is considered the prototype of the group of disorders collectively referred to as the *spondyloarthropathies,* which includes ankylosing spondylitis, reactive arthritis, psoriatic arthritis and spondylitis, and enteropathic arthritis and spondylitis. In Europe, ankylosing spondylitis is often referred to by the eponyms Marie-Strümpell disease or Bekhterev's disease.

EPIDEMIOLOGY   Ankylosing spondylitis shows a striking correlation with the presence of the histocompatibility antigen HLA-B27. The disease occurs throughout the human populations of the world in proportion to the prevalence of this antigen. In North American Caucasians, the prevalence of HLA-B27 in the general population is 7 percent, whereas over 90 percent of patients with AS have inherited this antigen. The association with HLA-B27 is independent of disease severity.

In large population surveys, 1 to 2 percent of adults inheriting HLA-B27 have been found to have AS. In contrast, in families of patients with AS, 10 to 20 percent of adult first-degree relatives inheriting HLA-B27 have been found to have the disease. The concordance rate in identical twins is estimated to be 60 percent or less. These epidemiologic findings indicate that both genetic and environmental factors play a role in the pathogenesis of the disease and that the genetic factors may include allelic genes in addition to HLA-B27.

PATHOLOGY   Sacroiliitis is usually, but not invariably, one of the earliest manifestations of AS. The early lesion consists of subchondral granulation tissue containing lymphocytes, plasma cells, mast cells, macrophages, and chondrocytes. Usually, the thinner iliac cartilage is eroded first, then the thicker sacral cartilage. The irregularly eroded, sclerotic margins of the joint are gradually replaced by fibrocartilage regeneration and ultimately by ossification, so that in the end stage the joint may be totally obliterated. Radiographically, this progression is evident as erosion of the cortical margins of the joint with subchondral bony sclerosis, followed by apparent widening of the joint space caused by extensive erosion of the cortical margins, bony bridging, then fusion.

In the spine, the initial lesion consists of inflammatory granulation tissue at the junction of the annulus fibrosus of the disk cartilage and the margin of vertebral bone. The outer annular fibers are eroded and eventually replaced by bone, forming the beginning of a bony excrescence called a *syndesmophyte,* which then grows by continued enchondral ossification, ultimately bridging the adjacent vertebral bodies. Ascending progression of this process leads to the "bamboo spine" observed radiographically. Other lesions in the spine include diffuse osteoporosis, erosion of vertebral bodies at the disc margin (Romanus lesion), "squaring" of vertebrae, and inflammation and destruction of the disc-bone border. Inflammatory arthritis of the apophyseal joints is common; early, there is pannus eroding cartilage, often followed by bony ankylosis.

The pathology of arthritis in peripheral joints in AS can show synovial hyperplasia, lymphoid infiltration, and pannus formation, but the process lacks the exuberant synovial villi, fibrin deposits, ulcers, and plaques of plasma cells seen in rheumatoid arthritis. Furthermore, central cartilaginous erosions due to proliferation of subchondral granulation tissue are common in AS but rarely found in rheumatoid arthritis.

The enthesis, the site of tendinous or ligamentous attachment to bone, is another common site of pathology in AS, especially at sites localized around the spine and pelvis. Enthesitis is characterized by erosive, inflammatory lesions that may eventually undergo ossification.

Approximately 20 percent of patients with AS are affected by acute anterior uveitis. Few cases have been studied histologically, and none at an early stage. After recurrent attacks, the iris shows nonspecific inflammatory changes, scarring, increased vascularity, and many macrophages laden with pigment.

Aortic insufficiency develops in a small percentage of cases. There is thickening of the aortic valve cusps and the aorta near the sinuses of Valsalva, with dense adventitial scar tissue and intimal fibrous proliferation, the scar tissue often extending into the ventricular septum with resultant heart block.

Recently, microscopic inflammatory lesions of the colon and ileocolonic valve were reported in patients with AS lacking any clinical evidence of inflammatory bowel disease.

PATHOGENESIS   The pathogenesis of AS is poorly understood. A number of features of the disease implicate immune-mediated mechanisms, including elevated serum levels of IgA and acute phase reactants, inflammatory histology, and close association with HLA-B27. No specific event or exogenous agent that triggers the onset of the disease has been identified, although overlapping features with reactive arthritis and inflammatory bowel disease suggest that enteric bacteria may play a role. Evidence has been obtained suggesting antigenic interrelatedness between HLA-B27 and certain enteric bacteria, but it is not yet known whether this contributes to the pathogenesis of AS. There is also some evidence both in AS patients and in animal models for an association between spondylitis and immunity to cartilage proteoglycan.

CLINICAL MANIFESTATIONS   The symptoms of the disease are usually first noticed in late adolescence or early adulthood; onset after age 40 is unusual. In the majority of patients, the initial symptom is dull pain, insidious in onset, felt deep in the lower lumbar or gluteal region. Characteristically, this is accompanied by low-back morning stiffness of up to a few hours' duration that improves with activity. The stiffness may return following prolonged periods of inactivity. Within a few months of onset, the pain usually has become persistent and bilateral, and nocturnal exacerbation of the pain that forces the patient to get up and move around may be frequent.

In some patients, bony tenderness may accompany back pain or stiffness, while in others, it may be the predominant complaint. Common sites include the costosternal junctions, spinous processes, iliac crests, greater trochanters, ischial tuberosities, tibial tubercles, and heels. Occasionally, chest pain is the presenting complaint, because of involvement of the thoracic spine and chest wall articulations. Arthritis in the hips and shoulders occurs at some stage in 25 to 35 percent of all patients, and can lead to early symptoms. Arthritis of peripheral joints other than the hips and shoulders has been reported in up to 30 percent of patients and can occur at any stage of the disease. Peripheral arthritis is usually asymmetric. Neck pain and stiffness, indicating involvement of the cervical spine, is usually a relatively late manifestation. Occasional patients, especially those with a juvenile onset, present with predominantly constitutional symptoms such as fatigue, anorexia, fever, weight loss, or night sweats.

The most common extraarticular manifestation is acute anterior uveitis, which can antedate the onset of the joint disease. Attacks are typically unilateral and tend to recur, causing pain, photophobia, and increased lacrimation. Aortic insufficiency, sometimes producing symptoms of congestive heart failure, occurs in a few percent of patients and occasionally occurs early in the course of the spinal disease.

Initially, the physical findings reflect the manifestations of the inflammatory process. The most specific findings involve loss of spinal mobility, with limitation of anterior flexion, lateral flexion, and extension of the lumbar spine, and limitation of chest expansion.

Limitation of motion is usually out of proportion to the degree of bony ankylosis, reflecting spasm secondary to pain and inflammation. Pain in the sacroiliac joints may be elicited either with direct pressure or with maneuvers that stress the joints. In addition, there is commonly tenderness upon palpation at the sites of symptomatic bony tenderness mentioned above, and paraspinous muscle spasm is often present.

The Schober test is a useful measure of forward flexion of the lumbar spine. The patient stands erect, with heels together, and marks are made directly over the spine 5 cm below and 10 cm above the lumbosacral junction (identified by a horizontal line between the posterior superior iliac spines). The patient then bends forward maximally, while not bending the knees, and the distance between the two marks is measured. The distance between the two marks increases 5 cm or more in the case of normal lumbar mobility and less than 4 cm in the case of decreased lumbar mobility. Chest expansion is measured as the difference between maximal inspiration and maximal forced expiration in the fourth intercostal space in males, or just below the breasts in females. Normal chest expansion is 5 cm or greater.

Limitation or pain with motion of the hips or shoulders is usually present if either of these joints is involved. Careful examination is also necessary to detect inflammatory disease of peripheral joints. It should be emphasized that early in the course of mild cases, symptoms may be mild and nonspecific, and the physical examination may be completely normal.

The course of the disease is extremely variable, ranging from the individual on one end of the spectrum with mild stiffness and radiographically evident disease confined to the sacroiliac joints to the patient on the other end of the spectrum with a totally fused spine, severe bilateral hip arthritis and ankylosis, possibly accompanied by severe peripheral arthritis and extraarticular manifestations. Pain tends to be persistent early in the disease and then to become intermittent, with alternating exacerbations and quiescent periods. In a typical severe case with progression of the spondylitis to syndesmophyte formation, the patient's posture undergoes characteristic changes. The lumbar lordosis is obliterated with accompanying atrophy of the buttocks. The thoracic kyphosis is accentuated. If the cervical spine is involved, there may be a forward stoop of the neck. Hip involvement with ankylosis may lead to flexion contractures, compensated by flexion at the knees. The progression of the disease may be followed by measuring the patient's height, chest expansion, Schober test, and the distance between the occiput and the wall when the patient stands erect with the heels and back flat against the wall (occiput-to-wall test).

Onset of the disease in adolescence correlates with both a worse prognosis and more severe hip involvement. The disease in women tends to be milder than in men, with less frequent progression to total spinal ankylosis, although there is some evidence for an increased prevalence of isolated cervical ankylosis and of peripheral arthritis in women with AS.

The most serious complication of the spinal disease is spinal fracture, which can occur with even minor trauma to the rigid, osteoporotic spine. Most commonly, the cervical spine is involved, often leading to quadriplegia. Cauda equina syndrome is another infrequent complication of long-standing spinal disease in AS. Pulmonary involvement, characterized by slowly progressive upper lobe fibrosis, is a rare complication of long-standing AS; eventually the lesions can cavitate and become colonized by *Aspergillus*. Although cardiovascular involvement can occur early in the course of the disease, the prevalence of aortic insufficiency and of cardiac conduction disturbances, including third-degree heart block, increases with prolonged disease. Amyloidosis, especially involving the kidney, was found in 6 percent of one autopsy series, but the true prevalence appears to be considerably lower. Prostatitis has been reported to have an increased prevalence in men with AS.

Despite the persistence of the disease, most patients with AS do not experience disabling symptoms and are able to remain gainfully employed. Only in uncommon instances does the disease appear to shorten life, these being due largely to spinal trauma, aortic insufficiency, respiratory failure, amyloid nephropathy, or complications of therapy such as upper gastrointestinal hemorrhage. An excess mortality from leukemia was noted in patients treated with deep x-ray therapy to the spine, a common mode of therapy for AS until effective anti-inflammatory medications became available in the mid-1950s.

LABORATORY FINDINGS   There is no laboratory test that is diagnostic of AS. In most ethnic groups, the HLA-B27 gene is present in approximately 90 percent of patients with AS; American blacks appear to represent an exception, since the prevalence of B27 in this group has been reported to be only 50 percent. Most patients with active disease have an elevated erythrocyte sedimentation rate and an elevated C-reactive protein. A mild normochromic normocytic anemia may be present. Patients with severe disease may show an elevated alkaline phosphatase. Elevated serum IgA levels are common. Rheumatoid factor and antinuclear antibodies are uniformly absent unless caused by a coexistent process unrelated to AS. Synovial fluid from inflamed peripheral joints in AS is not distinctly different from that of other inflammatory joint diseases. In cases with restriction of chest wall motion, pulmonary function tests may demonstrate decreased vital capacity and increased functional residual capacity, but airflow measurements are normal and ventilatory function is usually well maintained.

RADIOGRAPHIC FINDINGS   Radiographically demonstrable sacroiliitis is usually present in AS. The earliest changes in the sacroiliac joints demonstrable by plain x-ray radiography show blurring of the cortical margins of the subchondral bone, followed by erosions and sclerosis. Progression of the erosions leads to "pseudowidening" of the joint space; as fibrous and then bony ankylosis supervene, the joints may become obliterated radiographically. The changes and progression of the lesions are usually symmetric.

In mild cases, years may elapse before unequivocal sacroiliac abnormalities are evident on plain radiographs. Although computed tomography and magnetic resonance imaging have been shown to detect abnormalities reliably at an earlier stage than plain radiography, these techniques are not generally used for routine diagnostic purposes.

Roentgenographic abnormalities generally appear in the sacroiliac joints before appearing elsewhere in the spine. In the lumbar spine, progression of the disease leads to straightening caused by loss of lordosis and reactive sclerosis caused by osteitis of the anterior corners of the vertebral bodies with subsequent erosion, leading to "squaring" of the vertebral bodies. Progressive ossification of the superficial layers of the annulus fibrosus leads to eventual formation of marginal syndesmophytes, visible on plain films as bony bridges connecting successive vertebral bodies on the anterior and lateral sides.

DIAGNOSIS   The diagnosis of early AS before the development of irreversible deformity can be difficult to establish. Criteria for the diagnosis of AS were formulated in 1961 (Rome criteria) and revised in 1966 (New York criteria). For definite AS, the New York criteria require the presence of advanced radiographic sacroiliitis and at least one of three clinical findings (limitation of motion of the lumbar spine in all three planes, pain at the thoracolumbar junction or in the lumbar spine, or chest expansion limited to ≤2.5 cm).

In 1984, modifications to the New York criteria were proposed, which, although not yet formally adopted, have been shown to be comparably specific but more sensitive than the original New York criteria, especially in diagnosing the disease at an earlier stage. The modified criteria consist of the following: (1) a history of inflammatory back pain (see below); (2) limitation of motion of the lumbar spine in both the sagittal and frontal planes; (3) limited chest expansion, relative to standard values for age and sex; and (4) definite radiographic sacroiliitis. Under the proposed modified New York criteria, the presence of radiographic sacroiliitis plus any one of the other three criteria is sufficient for a diagnosis of definite AS. The increased sensitivity of these modified criteria is largely the result of the inclusion of earlier stages of radiographic sacroiliitis than are permitted under the original New York criteria.

Several studies have identified a sizeable population of B27-positive individuals with symptoms typical of AS who lack definite radiographic sacroiliitis. However, when followed over time, most of these patients eventually develop radiographic changes. These studies indicate that diagnostic criteria based on radiographic findings may in some cases be too insensitive for the diagnosis of early AS. The B27 test is useful only as a diagnostic adjunct, since the presence of B27 is neither necessary nor sufficient for the diagnosis.

AS must be differentiated from numerous other causes of low back pain. The inflammatory back pain of AS is usually distinguished by the following five features: (1) age of onset below 40; (2) insidious onset; (3) duration greater than 3 months before medical attention is sought; (4) morning stiffness; and (5) improvement with exercise or activity. The most common causes of back pain other than AS are primarily mechanical or degenerative rather than inflammatory and do not show these features. Less common metabolic, infectious, and malignant causes of back pain must also be differentiated from AS.

TREATMENT There is no definitive treatment for AS. The principal goal of management is the conscientious participation of the patient in an exercise program designed to maintain functional posture and to preserve range of motion. Most patients require anti-inflammatory agents to achieve sufficient symptomatic relief to be able to remain functional and carry out the exercise program. It is not known whether drug treatment alone can alter the progression of the disease.

Worldwide, the most commonly used drug therapy for AS is indomethacin, although several other nonsteroidal anti-inflammatory drugs (NSAIDs) have also been proven to be effective in reducing pain and stiffness and are commonly used. Indomethacin is particularly effective as a 75-mg slow-release preparation taken once or twice daily. Although phenylbutazone at doses of 200 to 400 mg/d has been considered by several authorities to be the most effective agent in AS, because of its greater potential for serious side effects such as aplastic anemia and agranulocytosis, its use in the United States is confined to patients with severe disease whose symptoms do not respond well to other agents. Recent controlled trials suggest that sulfasalazine[1] in doses of 2 to 3 g/d may be useful in reducing axial and peripheral joint symptoms as well as in reversing laboratory evidence of inflammation. No therapeutic role for gold, penicillamine, immunosuppressive drugs, or systemic corticosteroids has been documented in AS. Occasionally, intralesional or intraarticular corticosteroid injections may be beneficial in patients with persistent enthesopathy or synovitis unresponsive to anti-inflammatory agents.

The most common indication for surgery in patients with AS is severe hip joint arthritis, the pain and stiffness of which are often dramatically relieved by total hip arthroplasty. A smaller number of patients may benefit from surgical correction of extreme flexion deformities of the spine or of atlantoaxial subluxation.

Attacks of acute anterior uveitis are usually effectively managed with local corticosteroid administration in conjunction with mydriatic agents. Coexistent cardiac disease may require pacemaker implantation or aortic valve replacement.

REACTIVE ARTHRITIS

Reactive arthritis refers to acute nonpurulent arthritis complicating an infection elsewhere in the body. In recent years, the term has been used primarily to refer to spondyloarthropathies following enteric or urogenital infections and occurring predominantly in individuals with the histocompatibility antigen HLA-B27. Included in this category is the constellation of clinical findings often referred to as *Reiter's syndrome.* Other forms of reactive arthritis not associated with HLA-B27 and showing a different spectrum of clinical features, such as rheumatic fever, are discussed elsewhere in this volume.

HISTORICAL BACKGROUND In 1916, Reiter described a patient who, following an episode of bloody diarrhea, developed a systemic illness with polyarthritis, conjunctivitis, and nongonococcal urethritis. Although similar cases had previously been described, this report served to focus attention on the triad of arthritis, urethritis, and conjunctivitis which subsequently was referred to as Reiter's syndrome. Additional clinical featues, particularly mucocutaneous lesions, were later recognized to be frequent accompaniments of the syndrome.

In recent years, the identification of several bacterial species capable of triggering the clinical syndrome, as well as the finding that three-fourths of the patients possess the HLA-B27 antigen, have led to the unifying concept of reactive arthritis as a clinical syndrome triggered by a specific etiologic agent in a genetically susceptible host. It is now recognized that a similar spectrum of clinical manifestations can be triggered by enteric infection with any of several *Shigella, Salmonella, Yersinia,* and *Campylobacter* species or with *Clostridium difficile,* by genital infection with *Chlamydia trachomatis,* and possibly by other agents as well. Although Reiter's syndrome can be said to represent one part of the spectrum of the clinical manifestations of reactive arthritis, it can be reasonably argued that the term is now largely of historical interest.

EPIDEMIOLOGY Like ankylosing spondylitis, reactive arthritis occurs predominantly in individuals who have inherited the HLA-B27 gene; in most series, 60 to 85 percent of the patients are B27-positive. In epidemics of arthritogenic bacterial infection, e.g., *Shigella flexneri,* it has been estimated that reactive arthritis develops in ~20 percent of the B27-positive individuals at risk. Some studies of families with multiple cases of AS or reactive arthritis have suggested that the two conditions tend to "breed true"; whether this is caused by genetic or environmental factors is not known. The disease is most common in individuals 18 to 40 years of age, but it is well-recognized both in children over 5 years of age and in older adults.

Although Reiter's syndrome has long been described as a disease predominantly of men, this conclusion is probably overstated and related to the ascertainment of cases. The sex ratio in reactive arthritis following enteric infection is nearly 1:1, whereas venereally acquired reactive arthritis is predominantly a male disease. The overall prevalence and incidence of reactive arthritis are difficult to assess because of the variable prevalence of the triggering infections and genetic susceptibility factors in different populations. Certain populations, such as the Navajo Indians of the southwestern United States and the Inuit Eskimos of Greenland, show a very high occurrence of reactive arthritis, whereas the disease is quite uncommon in certain other populations, such as the Haida Indians, with an equally high prevalence of HLA-B27. The reasons for these differences are not clear.

A particularly severe form of reactive arthritis has been described in patients with the acquired immunodeficiency syndrome. Most of these patients are HLA-B27-positive. From the incidence figures it can be inferred that B27-positive individuals with human immunodeficiency virus infection develop reactive arthritis at a higher than expected frequency.

PATHOLOGY Synovial histology is similar to that of other inflammatory arthropathies, including rheumatoid arthritis. Enthesitis is a common clinical finding in reactive arthritis; the histology of this lesion resembles that of ankylosing spondylitis. Microscopic histopathologic evidence of inflammation has been noted in the colon and ileum of patients with postvenereal as well as postenteritic reactive arthritis. The skin lesions of keratoderma blennorrhagica are histologically indistinguishable from psoriatic lesions.

ETIOLOGY AND PATHOGENESIS The first bacterial infection to be causally related to reactive arthritis was *Shigella flexneri.* An outbreak of shigellosis among Finnish troops in 1944 resulted in numerous cases of reactive arthritis. Of the four species of *Shigella, sonnei, boydii, flexneri,* and *dysenteriae, S. flexneri* has most often been implicated in cases of reactive arthritis, both sporadic and epidemic. *S. sonnei*, although responsible for the majority of cases of shigellosis in the United States, has only rarely been implicated in cases of reactive arthritis.

Other bacteria that have been definitively identified as triggers of reactive arthritis include several *Salmonella* species, *Yersinia enterocolitica*, and *Campylobacter jejuni*. There is suggestive evidence implicating several other microorganisms, including *Brucella*, *Yersinia pseudotuberculosis*, *Clostridium difficile*; the genitourinary pathogens *Chlamydia trachomatis*, *Neisseria gonorrhoeae*, and *Ureaplasma urealyticum*; and *Streptococcus pyogenes*. There are also numerous isolated reports of acute arthritis preceded by other bacterial, viral, or parasitic infections, but whether the microorganisms involved are actual triggers of reactive arthritis remains to be determined.

It has not been determined whether reactive arthritis occurs by the same pathogenetic mechanism following infection with each of these microorganisms, nor has the mechanism been fully elucidated in the case of any one of the known bacterial triggers. The immune response is presumed to play a principal role, but there is not yet general agreement on the relative importance of humoral versus cellular mechanisms. Most, if not all, of the triggering organisms share a capacity to invade host cells and survive intracellularly.

The largest body of data regarding the immune response in reactive arthritis has been generated by studies of *Y. enterocolitica*, particularly serotypes O:3 and O:9 in Finland, where these organisms frequently cause enteric infection in a population in which the prevalence of HLA-B27 is 14 percent. In comparison with individuals who fail to develop reactive arthritis following enteric infection with *Yersinia*, patients with *Yersinia*-triggered reactive arthritis show far fewer gastrointestinal symptoms attributable to the infection, a smaller initial IgM response, stronger and more persistent IgA and IgG responses, higher levels of IgA anti-*Yersinia* antibodies with a secretory component, and reduced T-cell proliferative responses to *Yersinia* antigens. These findings suggest an unusual persistence of the immune response to the infecting organism in those individuals in whom reactive arthritis develops. Circulating immune complexes containing *Yersinia* antigens have been found in a higher proportion of arthritic than nonarthritic individuals, and occasionally in the inflamed joints, but the significance of these findings is not clear.

It is not known to what extent reactive arthritis represents an autoimmune response against host tissues, as opposed to an immune response against antigens of the triggering organism that have disseminated to the target tissues. Both mechanisms appear to operate in animal models. Chlamydial antigens have been demonstrated in the synovium of a few patients with venereally acquired reactive arthritis, but it is not known whether they are the inciting antigenic stimulus. Similarly, *Yersinia enterocolitica* antigen has been detected in synovial fluid cells in patients with *Y. enterocolitica*–induced reactive arthritis, but the significance of this is unclear.

The role of HLA-B27 in reactive arthritis has yet to be fully elucidated. At present, the evidence favors some form of molecular mimicry, or the sharing of antigenic determinants between the HLA-B27 molecule and molecules encoded by the inciting microbial agent. Several reports have documented antigenic cross-reactivity between the B27 molecule and envelope glycoproteins of arthritogenic bacteria, including *Shigella flexneri* and *Yersinia pseudotuberculosis*, but the pathogenetic significance of this is not known. Many but not all B27-negative individuals with reactive arthritis possess HLA-B alleles that are antigenically cross-reactive with HLA-B27, notably HLA-B7.

CLINICAL FEATURES The clinical manifestations of reactive arthritis constitute a spectrum that ranges from an isolated, transient monarthritis to a more severe multisystem disease. In the majority of cases, a careful history will elicit some evidence of an antecedent infection 1 to 4 weeks before the onset of symptoms of the reactive disease. However, in a sizeable minority, particularly in cases of relapse, no clinical or laboratory evidence of an antecedent infection can be found. In many cases of presumed venereally acquired reactive disease, there is a history of a recent new sexual partner, even in the absence of laboratory evidence of infection.

Constitutional symptoms are common, including fatigue, malaise, fever, and weight loss. The musculoskeletal symptoms are usually acute in onset. Arthritis is usually asymmetric and additive, with involvement of new joints occurring over a period of a few days to 1 or 2 weeks. The joints of the lower extremities, especially the knee, ankle, and subtalar, metatarsophalangeal, and toe interphalangeal joints, are the most common sites of involvement, but the wrist and fingers can be involved as well. The arthritis is usually quite painful, and tense joint effusions are not uncommon, especially in the knee. Dactylitis, or "sausage digit," a diffuse swelling of a solitary finger or toe, is a distinctive feature of both reactive arthritis and psoriatic arthritis. Tendinitis and fasciitis are particularly characteristic lesions, producing pain at multiple insertion sites, especially the Achilles insertion, the plantar fascia, and sites along the axial skeleton. Spinal and low back pain are quite common, and may be caused by insertional inflammation, muscle spasm, acute sacroiliitis, or presumably, arthritis in intervertebral articulations.

Urogenital lesions may occur throughout the course of the disease. In males, urethritis may be marked or relatively asymptomatic, and may be either an accompaniment of the triggering infection or a result of the reactive phase of the disease. Prostatitis is also common. Similarly, in females cervicitis or salpingitis may be caused either by the infectious trigger or the sterile reactive process.

Ocular disease is common, ranging from transient, asymptomatic conjunctivitis to an aggressive anterior uveitis that occasionally proves refractory to treatment and results in blindness.

Mucocutaneous lesions are frequent. Oral ulcers tend to be superficial, transient, and often asymptomatic. The characteristic skin lesion, keratoderma blennorrhagica, consists of vesicles that become hyperkeratotic, ultimately forming a crust before disappearing. It is most common on the palms and soles, but may occur elsewhere as well. In patients with HIV infection, these lesions are often extremely severe and extensive, dominating the clinical picture. Lesions on the glans penis (*circinate balanitis*) are common; these consist of vesicles that quickly rupture to form painless superficial erosions, which in circumcised individuals can form crusts similar to those of keratoderma blennorrhagica. Nail changes are common and consist of onycholysis, distal yellowish discoloration, and/or heaped up hyperkeratosis.

Less frequent or rare manifestations of reactive arthritis include cardiac conduction defects, aortic insufficiency, central or peripheral nervous system lesions, and pleuropulmonary infiltrates.

Long-term follow-up studies suggest that some joint symptoms persist in many, if not most, patients with reactive arthritis. Recurrences of the acute syndrome are common, and as many as 25 percent of patients either become unable to work or are forced to change occupations because of persistent joint symptoms. Chronic heel pain is often a particularly distressing symptom. Ankylosing spondylitis is also a common sequela. In most studies, HLA-B27-positive patients have a worse outcome than B27-negative patients. The extent to which the long-term prognosis varies with different inciting agents is not known. However, patients with *Yersinia*-induced arthritis appear to have less chronic disease than those whose initial episode follows epidemic shigellosis.

LABORATORY AND RADIOGRAPHIC FINDINGS The erythrocyte sedimentation rate is elevated during the acute phase of the disease. Mild anemia may be present, and acute phase reactants tend to be increased. Synovial fluid is nonspecifically inflammatory, showing an elevated white cell count with a predominance of neutrophils. In most ethnic groups, three-fourths of the patients possess the HLA-B27 antigen. Although it is unusual for the triggering infection to persist through the time of onset of the reactive disease, it may occasionally be possible to culture the organism, for example, in the case of *Shigella*- or *Chlamydia*-induced disease. Serologic evidence of a recent infection may be present, such as a marked elevation of antibodies to *Yersinia* or *Chlamydia*.

In early or mild disease, radiographic changes may be absent or confined to juxtaarticular osteoporosis. With long-standing persistent disease, marginal erosions and loss of joint space can be seen in affected joints. Periostitis with reactive new bone formation is characteristic of the disease, as it is with all of the spondyloarthropathies. Spurs at the insertion of the plantar fascia are common.

Sacroiliitis and spondylitis similar to those described for ankylosing spondylitis may be seen as late sequelae. However, sacroiliitis is more commonly asymmetric than in AS, and the spondylitis, rather than ascending symmetrically from the lower lumbar segments, can begin anywhere along the lumbar spine. The syndesmophytes may be coarse and nonmarginal, arising from the middle of a vertebral body, a pattern rarely seen in primary AS.

DIAGNOSIS Reactive arthritis is a clinical diagnosis, there being no definitively diagnostic laboratory test or radiographic finding. The diagnosis should be entertained in any patient with an acute inflammatory, asymmetric, additive arthritis or tendinitis. The evaluation of such a patient should include careful questioning regarding possible antecedent triggering events such as an episode of diarrhea or dysuria. On physical examination, careful attention must be paid to the distribution of the joint and tendon involvement and to possible sites of extraarticular involvement, such as the eyes, mucous membranes, skin, nails, and genitalia. Synovial fluid aspiration and analysis may be helpful in excluding septic or crystal-induced arthritis.

Although typing for B27 is not needed to secure the diagnosis in clear-cut cases, it has prognostic significance in terms of severity, chronicity, and the propensity for spondylitis and uveitis. Furthermore, it can be helpful diagnostically in atypical cases, a positive test increasing and a negative test decreasing the probability that the diagnosis of reactive arthritis is correct.

It is particularly important to differentiate reactive arthritis from disseminated gonococcal disease, both of which can be venereally acquired and associated with urethritis. Gonococcal arthritis and tenosynovitis tend to involve both upper and lower extremities equally, whereas in reactive arthritis the symptoms usually predominate in the lower extremities. Back pain is common in reactive arthritis but is not a feature of gonococcal disease, whereas the vesicular skin lesions characteristic of disseminated gonococcal disease are not found in reactive arthritis. A positive gonococcal culture from the urethra or cervix does not exclude a diagnosis of reactive arthritis; however, culturing gonococci from blood, skin lesion, or synovium establishes the diagnosis of disseminated gonococcal disease. Occasionally, the only definitive way to distinguish the two is through a therapeutic trial of antibiotics.

Reactive arthritis shares many features with psoriatic arthropathy, including the asymmetry of the arthritis, a propensity for sausage digits and nail involvement, an association with uveitis, and skin lesions of similar histology. However, psoriatic arthritis is usually gradual in onset, the arthritis tends to affect primarily the upper extremities, and there is far less associated periarthritis. Psoriatic arthritis is not associated with mouth ulcers, urethritis, or bowel symptoms; and there is a female predominance. Although psoriatic arthropathy shows some distinctive radiographic features that are not found in reactive arthritis, these only occur late in the disease and are of little help diagnostically. Only psoriatic spondylitis, not the peripheral arthritis, is associated with HLA-B27, about 50 percent of the patients being positive. Occasional patients, usually B27-positive, following what appears to be a typical episode of reactive arthritis, will develop typical psoriasis and persistent arthritis, such that the two entities become indistinguishable.

TREATMENT Most patients with reactive arthritis are benefitted to some degree by nonsteroidal anti-inflammatory drugs, although rarely are symptoms of the acute arthritis completely ameliorated and some patients fail to respond at all. Indomethacin, 75 to 150 mg/d in divided doses, is the initial treatment of choice, with phenylbutazone, 100 mg tid or qid, being the NSAID of last resort because of its potentially serious side effects.

Patients with debilitating symptoms refractory to NSAID therapy may respond to cytotoxic agents such as azathioprine, 1 to 2 mg/kg per day, or methotrexate, 7.5 to 15 mg per week. Recent studies have suggested that sulfasalazine, up to 3 g/d in divided doses, also

may be beneficial to patients with persistent reactive arthritis.[2] There appears to be no place for systemic corticosteroids, antimalarials, gold, or penicillamine in the treatment of reactive arthritis. Although many clinicians routinely administer courses of antibiotics to patients with reactive arthritis, there is little evidence that this is beneficial.

Tendinitis and other enthesitic lesions occasionally may benefit from intralesional corticosteroids. Uveitis may require aggressive treatment with corticosteroids to prevent serious sequelae. Skin lesions ordinarily require only symptomatic treatment. In patients with HIV infection and reactive arthritis, many of whom have severe skin lesions, the skin lesions in particular appear to respond dramatically to systemic treatment with azidothymidine. Cardiac complications are managed conventionally; management of neurologic complications is symptomatic.

Patients need to be educated with regard to the nature of the disease and the factors that predispose to its recurrence. Comprehensive management includes counseling of patients in the use of condoms, avoidance of sexual promiscuity, and exposure to enteropathogens. Appropriate use of physical therapy, vocational counseling, and continued surveillance for long-term complications such as ankylosing spondylitis are also part of comprehensive care.

REFERENCES

CALABRO JJ, DICK C (eds): *Ankylosing Spondylitis—New Clinical Applications in Rheumatology.* Lancaster, UK, MTP Press, 1987

CALIN A (ed): *Spondylarthropathies.* Orlando, Grune & Stratton, 1984

GRANFORS K et al: *Yersinia* antigens in synovial fluid cells from patients with reactive arthritis. N Engl J Med 320:216, 1989

KEAT A: Reiter's syndrome and reactive arthritis in perspective. N Engl J Med 309:1606, 1983

KHAN MA et al: Spondylitic disease without radiographic evidence of sacroiliitis in relatives of HLA-B27-positive ankylosing spondylitis patients. Arthritis Rheum 28:40, 1985

LEIRISALO M et al: Ten-year follow-up study of patients with *Yersinia* arthritis. Arthritis Rheum 31:533, 1988

MIELANTS H et al: HLA antigens in seronegative spondylarthropathies. Reactive arthritis and arthritis in ankylosing spondylitis: Relation to gut inflammation. J Rheumatol 14:466, 1987

NISSILA M et al: Sulfasalazine in the treatment of ankylosing spondylitis: A twenty-six week, placebo-controlled clinical trial. Arthritis Rheum 31:1111, 1988

TOIVANEN A, TOIVANEN P (eds): *Reactive Arthritis.* Boca Raton, CRC Press, 1988

VAN DER LINDEN SM et al: Evaluation of diagnostic criteria for ankylosing spondylitis: A proposal for modification of the New York criteria. Arthritis Rheum 27:361, 1984

WINCHESTER R et al: The co-occurrence of Reiter's syndrome and acquired immunodeficiency. Ann Intern Med 106:19, 1987

275 BEHÇET'S SYNDROME

HARALAMPOS M. MOUTSOPOULOS

BEHÇET'S SYNDROME Behçet's syndrome is a multisystem disorder presenting with recurrent oral and genital ulcerations as well as uveitis often leading to blindness.

PREVALENCE, PATHOGENESIS, AND PATHOLOGY The disease has a worldwide distribution. The prevalence of Behçet's syndrome ranges from 1:1000 in Japan to 1:500,000 in North America and Europe. In the Mediterranean countries the prevalence might be higher. It affects mainly young adults, with men having more severe disease than females.

The etiology and pathogenesis of this syndrome remain obscure. Bacteria and viruses have been suggested as the causative agents, but there is no convincing proof. Today, Behçet's syndrome is considered an autoimmune disease because of the common denominator of vasculitis in most patients. Circulating autoantibodies to human oral mucous membrane and immune complexes are found in

---

[2]Azathioprine, methotrexate, and sulfasalazine have not been approved for this purpose by the Food and Drug Administration at the time of publication.

approximately 50 percent of the cases. Familial occurrence has been reported, and in patients from eastern Mediterranean countries and Japan, the disease appears to be linked to HLA-B5 and HLA-DR5 alloantigens.

CLINICAL FEATURES   The recurrent aphthous ulcerations are a sine qua non for the diagnosis. The ulcers are usually painful with a diameter ranging from 2 to 10 mm. They can be shallow or deep with a central yellowish necrotic base; appear singly or in crops; and are located on the lips, gums, buccal mucosa, and tongue. The palate, tonsils, and larynx are rarely involved. The ulcers persist for 1 to 2 weeks and subside without leaving scars. The genital ulcers resemble the oral ones in both appearance and course. Vaginal ulcers are usually painless and may be detected during routine pelvic examination. Painful genital ulcers may occur on the external genitalia.

Skin involvement includes folliculitis, erythema nodosum, and an acne-like exanthem. Severe dermal vasculitis is an infrequent event. Nonspecific skin inflammatory reactivity to any scratches, needle pricks, and intradermal saline injection (pathergy test) is a common and specific manifestation in Japanese and eastern Mediterranean patients.

Eye involvement is the most dreaded complication, as it occasionally progresses rapidly to blindness. The eye disease is usually present at the onset but also may develop within the first few years. In addition to iritis, posterior uveitis, retinal vessel occlusions, and optic neuritis can be seen in some cases of the syndrome. Hypopyon uveitis, which is considered the hallmark of Behçet's syndrome, is in fact a rare manifestation.

The arthritis of Behçet's syndrome is not deforming and affects the knees and ankles.

Superficial or deep peripheral vein thrombosis is seen in one-fourth of the patients. Pulmonary emboli, however, appear to be an exceptionally rare complication. The superior vena cava is obstructed occasionally, producing a dramatic clinical picture. Arterial involvement occurs infrequently and presents with aortitis or peripheral arterial aneurysm and arterial thrombosis.

The prevalence of central nervous system involvement differs geographically. High figures are quoted from northern Europe and the United States. The most common lesions are benign intracranial hypertension, a multiple sclerosis-like picture, and pyramidal involvement. Psychiatric disturbances are frequent.

Gastrointestinal involvement is reported in patients from Japan and include mucosal ulcerations of the gut.

Laboratory findings are mainly nonspecific indices of inflammation such as leukocytosis and elevated erythrocyte sedimentation rate as well as C-reactive protein levels; antibodies to human oral mucosa are also found.

PROGNOSIS AND TREATMENT   The severity of the syndrome usually abates with time; male sex and younger age at onset seem to predispose for severe illness. Apart from the cases with neurologic complications, the life expectancy seems to be normal, and the only serious complication is blindness.

Treatment of Behçet's syndrome is symptomatic and empirical. Mucous membrane involvement may respond to topical corticosteroids in the form of mouthwash or paste. The arthritis responds to rest and analgesics. Thrombophlebitis is treated with aspirin, 500 mg/d, and dipyridamole, 250 mg/d. Colchicine can be beneficial in the mild forms of the syndrome. The serious manifestations of Behçet's syndrome, i.e., uveitis and central nervous system involvement, require systemic corticosteroid therapy (prednisone, 1 mg/kg per day) and/or cytotoxic agents (chlorambucil, 0.1 mg/kg per day; azathioprine, 1 to 2 mg/kg per day; or cyclophosphamide, 1 to 2 mg/kg per day). There are early reports of the beneficial use of cyclosporin A in the uveitis of Behçet's syndrome.

REFERENCES

Nussenblatt RB et al: Effectiveness of cyclosporin therapy for Behçet's disease. Arthritis Rheum 28:671, 1985

O'Duffy JD et al: Summary of the Third International Conference on Behçet's disease. J Rheumatol 10:154, 1983

Shimizu T et al: Behçet's disease (Behçet's syndrome). Semin Arthritis Rheum 8:223, 1979

Yazici H, Moutsopoulos HM: Behçet's disease, in Current Therapy in Allergy and Immunology, LM Lichtenstein, AS Fauci (eds). Philadelphia, Decker, 1985

276   THE VASCULITIS SYNDROMES

ANTHONY S. FAUCI

DEFINITION   Vasculitis is a clinicopathologic process characterized by inflammation of and damage to blood vessels. The vessel lumen is usually compromised, and this is associated with ischemia of the tissues supplied by the involved vessel. A broad and heterogeneous group of syndromes may result from this process since any type, size, and location of blood vessel may be involved. Vasculitis and its consequences may be the primary or sole manifestation of a disease; alternatively, vasculitis may be a secondary component of another primary disease. Vasculitis may be confined to a single organ such as the skin, or it may simultaneously involve several organ systems.

PATHOPHYSIOLOGY AND PATHOGENESIS   Generally, most of the vasculitic syndromes are assumed to be mediated at least in part by immunopathogenic mechanisms. However, evidence to this effect is for the most part indirect. Deposition of immune complexes in tissues (see Chap. 268) is the most widely accepted pathogenic mechanism of vasculitis. Nonetheless, the causal role of immune complexes has not been clearly established in most of the vasculitic syndromes. Circulating immune complexes need not result in deposition of the complexes in blood vessels with ensuing vasculitis, and many patients with active vasculitis do not have demonstrable circulating or deposited immune complexes. This situation may result from an inadequacy of the techniques for detecting certain types of immune complexes or from the rapidity with which complexes may be cleared from the circulation. The actual antigen contained in the immune complex has only rarely been identified in vasculitic syndromes. In this regard, hepatitis B antigen has been identified in both the circulating and deposited immune complexes in a subset of patients with systemic vasculitis, most notably within the polyarteritis nodosa group (see below).

The mechanisms of tissue damage in immune-complex–mediated vasculitis resemble those described for serum sickness (Chap. 268). In this model, antigen-antibody complexes are formed in antigen excess and are deposited in vessel walls whose permeability has been increased by vasoactive amines such as histamine, bradykinin, and leukotrienes released from platelets or from mast cells as a result of IgE-triggered mechanisms. The deposition of complexes results in activation of complement components, particularly C5a, which is strongly chemotactic for neutrophils. These cells then infiltrate the vessel wall, phagocytose the immune complexes, and regurgitate their intracytoplasmic enzymes, which damage the vessel wall. As the process becomes subacute or chronic, mononuclear cells infiltrate the vessel wall. The common denominator of the resulting syndrome is compromise of the vessel lumen with ischemic changes in the tissues supplied by the involved vessel.

In addition to the classic immune-complex–mediated mechanisms of vasculitis, other immunopathogenic mechanisms may be involved in damage to vessels. The most prominent of these is cell-mediated immune injury as reflected in the histopathologic feature of granulomatous vasculitis. However, immune complexes themselves may induce granulomatous responses, and the presence of granulomas in or around blood vessels may be indicative of immune-complex mechanisms, delayed hypersensitivity or cell-mediated immune responses, or both. Vascular endothelial cells can express HLA class

II molecules following activation by cytokines such as interferon gamma. This allows these cells to participate in immunologic reactions such as interaction with T4 lymphocytes in a manner similar to antigen-presenting macrophages. In addition, endothelial cells can secrete interleukin 1 which may activate T lymphocytes and initiate or propagate in situ immunologic processes within the blood vessel. Other mechanisms such as direct cellular cytotoxicity or antibody directed against vessel components or antibody-dependent cellular cytotoxicity have been suggested in certain types of vessel damage. However, there is no convincing evidence to support their contribution to the pathogenesis of any of the recognized vasculitic syndromes.

It is unclear why certain individuals develop vasculitis in response to certain antigenic stimuli whereas others do not. However, it is likely that a number of factors are involved in the ultimate expression of a vasculitic syndrome. These include the genetic predisposition, the regulatory mechanisms associated with immune response to certain antigens, and the ability of the reticuloendothelial system to clear circulating complexes from the blood. The size and physicochemical properties of immune complexes, the relative degree of turbulence of blood flow, the intravascular hydrostatic pressure in different vessels, and the preexisting integrity of the vessel endothelium likely explain why only certain types of immune complexes cause vasculitis and why the vasculitic process is selective for only certain vessels in individual patients.

CLASSIFICATION OF VASCULITIC SYNDROMES A major feature of the vasculitic syndromes as a group is the fact that there is a great deal of heterogeneity at the same time as there is considerable overlap among them. This has led to both difficulty and confusion with regard to the categorization of these diseases. The classification scheme listed in Table 276-1 takes into account this heterogeneity and overlap, and will serve as a matrix to emphasize the fact that certain syndromes are predominantly systemic in nature and almost invariably lead to irreversible organ system dysfunction and even death if untreated, while others are usually localized to the skin and rarely result in irreversible dysfunction of vital organs. The distinguishing and overlapping features of the diseases listed in Table 276-1, which justify this classification scheme, will be discussed below.

SYSTEMIC NECROTIZING VASCULITIS

CLASSIC POLYARTERITIS NODOSA **Definition** Polyarteritis nodosa (PAN) in its classic form was described in 1866 by Kussmaul and Maier. It is a multisystem, necrotizing vasculitis of small- and medium-sized muscular arteries in which involvement of the renal and visceral arteries is characteristic. Classic PAN does not involve pulmonary arteries, although bronchial vessels may be involved; granulomas, significant eosinophilia, and an allergic diathesis are not part of the classic syndrome.

Incidence and prevalence It is difficult to establish an accurate incidence of this disease because of the fact that many reports of PAN actually have included diseases other than the classic syndrome. It is clearly an uncommon, but not a rare, disease. The mean age at onset is 45 years and the male to female ratio is 2.5:1.

Pathophysiology and pathogenesis The vascular lesion in classic PAN is a necrotizing inflammation of small- and medium-sized muscular arteries. The lesions are segmental and tend to involve bifurcations and branchings of arteries. They may spread circumferentially to involve adjacent veins. However, involvement of venules is not seen in classic PAN, and if present, suggests the polyangiitis overlap syndrome (see below). In the acute stages of disease, polymorphonuclear neutrophils infiltrate all layers of the vessel wall and perivascular areas, which results in intimal proliferation and degeneration of the vessel wall. Mononuclear cells infiltrate the area as the lesions progress to the subacute and chronic stages. Fibrinoid necrosis of the vessels ensues with compromise of the lumen, thrombosis, infarction of the tissues supplied by the involved vessel, and, in some cases, hemorrhage. As the lesions heal, there is collagen deposition, which may lead to further occlusion of the vessel lumen. Aneurysmal dilatations up to 1 cm in size along the involved arteries are characteristic of classic PAN. Granulomas and substantial eosinophilia with eosinophilic tissue infiltrations are not characteristically found and suggest allergic angiitis and granulomatosis (see below).

Multiple organ systems are involved, and the clinicopathologic findings reflect the degree and location of vessel involvement and the resulting ischemic changes (Table 276-2). As mentioned above, pulmonary arteries are not involved in classic PAN, and bronchial artery involvement is uncommon. The pathology in the kidney is predominantly that of arteritis; however, glomerulitis occurs in up to 30 percent of patients. In patients with significant hypertension, typical pathologic features of glomerulosclerosis may be seen alone or superimposed on lesions of glomerulonephritis. In addition, pathologic sequelae of hypertension may be found elsewhere in the body.

The presence of hepatitis B antigenemia in approximately 30 percent of patients with systemic vasculitis, particularly of the classic PAN type, together with the isolation of circulating immune complexes composed of hepatitis B antigen and immunoglobulin, as well as the demonstration by immunofluorescence of hepatitis B antigen, IgM, and complement in the blood vessel walls, strongly suggest the role of immunologic phenomena in the pathogenesis of this disease.

TABLE 276-1 Classification of the vasculitic syndromes

Systemic necrotizing vasculitis
  Classic polyarteritis nodosa
  Allergic angiitis and granulomatosis of Churg-Strauss
  Polyangiitis overlap syndrome
Hypersensitivity vasculitis:
  Exogenous stimuli proved or suspected
    Henoch-Schönlein purpura
    Serum sickness and serum sickness–like reactions
    Other drug-induced vasculitides
    Vasculitis associated with infectious diseases
  Endogenous antigens likely involved
    Vasculitis associated with neoplasms
    Vasculitis associated with connective tissue diseases
    Vasculitis associated with other underlying diseases
    Vasculitis associated with congenital deficiencies of the complement system
Wegener's granulomatosis
Giant cell arteritis
  Temporal arteritis
  Takayasu's arteritis
Other vasculitic syndromes
  Mucocutaneous lymph node syndrome (Kawasaki's disease)
  Isolated central nervous system vasculitis
  Thromboangiitis obliterans (Buerger's disease)
  Miscellaneous vasculitides

TABLE 276-2 Classic PAN: Organ system involvement at autopsy

Organ system	Percent
Kidney	85
Heart	76
Liver	62
Gastrointestinal tract:	51
Jejunum	37
Ileum	27
Mesentery	24
Colon	20
Duodenum	10
Gallbladder	10
Rectosigmoid	10
Appendix	7
Muscle	39
Pancreas	35
Testes	33
Peripheral nerves	32
Central nervous system	27
Skin	20

SOURCE: Cupps and Fauci, 1981, p 32.

TABLE 276-3 Clinical manifestations related to organ system involvement in classic PAN

Organ system	Percent incidence	Clinical manifestations
Renal	60	Renal failure, hypertension
Musculoskeletal	64	Arthritis, arthralgia, myalgia
Peripheral nervous system	51	Peripheral neuropathy, mononeuritis multiplex
Gastrointestinal tract	44	Abdominal pain, nausea and vomiting, bleeding, bowel infarction and perforation, cholecystitis, hepatic infarction, pancreatic infarction
Skin	43	Rash, purpura, nodules, cutaneous infarcts, livedo reticularis, Raynaud's phenomenon
Cardiac	36	Congestive heart failure, myocardial infarction, pericarditis
Genitourinary	25	Testicular, ovarian, or epididymal pain
Central nervous system	23	Cerebral vascular accident, altered mental status, seizure

SOURCE: Cupps and Fauci, 1981, p 29.

Clinical and laboratory manifestations Nonspecific signs and symptoms are the hallmarks of classic PAN. Fever, weight loss, and malaise are present in over one-half of cases. Patients usually present with vague symptoms such as weakness, malaise, headache, abdominal pain, and myalgias. Specific complaints related to the vascular involvement within a particular organ system may also dominate the presenting clinical picture as well as the entire course of the illness (Table 276-3). Renal involvement most commonly manifests as ischemic changes in the glomeruli; however, glomerulonephritis is seen in approximately 30 percent of patients. Hypertension may be related to both the renal polyarteritis as well as the glomerulitis and may dominate the clinical picture. Classic PAN may involve any organ system; the clinical manifestations related to specific organ system involvement are listed in Table 276-3.

There are no diagnostic serologic tests for classic PAN. In over 75 percent of patients the leukocyte count is elevated with a predominance of neutrophils. Eosinophilia is only rarely seen and, when present at high levels, suggests the diagnosis of allergic angiitis and granulomatosis. The anemia of chronic disease may be seen, and an elevated erythrocyte sedimentation rate (ESR) is invariably present. Other common laboratory findings reflect the particular organ involved. Hypergammaglobulinemia may be present, and up to 30 percent of patients have a positive test for hepatitis B surface antigen. Arteriograms may demonstrate characteristic abnormalities such as aneurysms in the small- and medium-sized muscular arteries of the kidneys and abdominal viscera.

Diagnosis The diagnosis of classic PAN is based on the demonstration of characteristic findings of vasculitis on biopsy material of involved organs. In the absence of easily accessible tissue for biopsy, the angiographic demonstration of involved vessels, particularly in the form of aneurysms of small- and medium-sized arteries in the renal, hepatic, and visceral vasculature, is sufficient to make the diagnosis. Aneurysms of vessels are not pathognomonic of classic PAN; furthermore, aneurysms need not always be present, and angiographic findings may be limited to stenotic segments and obliteration of vessels. Biopsy of symptomatic organs such as nodular skin lesions, painful testes, and muscle groups provides the highest diagnostic yields, while blind biopsy of asymptomatic organs is frequently negative. In cases associated with hepatitis B antigenemia, the demonstration of circulating hepatitis B antigen serves as important circumstantial evidence in support of the diagnosis.

Treatment and prognosis The prognosis of untreated classic PAN is extremely poor. The usual clinical course is characterized either by fulminant deterioration or by relentless progression associated with intermittent acute flare-ups. Death usually results from renal failure; from gastrointestinal complications, particularly bowel infarcts

and perforation; and from cardiovascular causes. Intractable hypertension often compounds dysfunction in other organ systems such as the kidneys, heart, and central nervous system leading to additional late morbidity and mortality. The 5-year survival rate of untreated patients has been reported to be 13 percent, while glucocorticoid treatment may increase this figure to over 40 percent. Extremely favorable therapeutic results have been reported in classic PAN with the combination of prednisone, 1 mg/kg per day, and cyclophosphamide, 2 mg/kg per day (see section on "Wegener's Granulomatosis" for a detailed description of this therapeutic regimen). This regimen has been reported to result in up to a 90 percent long-term remission rate even following the discontinuation of therapy. Isolated reports have indicated favorable therapeutic responses in classic PAN using plasmapheresis together with corticosteroids and cytotoxic agents.

ALLERGIC ANGIITIS AND GRANULOMATOSIS (CHURG-STRAUSS DISEASE) Definition Allergic angiitis and granulomatosis was described in 1951 by Churg and Strauss and is a disease characterized by granulomatous vasculitis of multiple organ systems, particularly the lung. It is similar in many respects to classic PAN except that the former has a high frequency of lung involvement, vasculitis of blood vessels of various types or sizes including veins and venules, intra- and extravascular granuloma formation together with eosinophilic tissue infiltration, and a strong association with severe asthma and peripheral eosinophilia.

Incidence and prevalence Allergic angiitis and granulomatosis is an uncommon disease whose exact incidence, similar to classic PAN, is difficult to determine due to the grouping of multiple types of vasculitic syndromes in many reported series. The disease can occur at any age with the possible exception of infants. The mean age of onset is 44 years with a male to female ratio of 1.3:1.

Pathophysiology and pathogenesis The vasculitis which is characteristic of allergic angiitis and granulomatosis is similar to that of classic PAN (see above) with certain notable exceptions. In addition to small- and medium-sized muscular arteries, capillaries, veins, and venules can be involved in the former disease. The characteristic histopathologic features of allergic angiitis and granulomatosis are granulomatous reactions that may be present in the tissues or even within the walls of the vessels themselves. These are usually associated with infiltration of the tissues with eosinophils. This process can occur in any organ in the body; however, in sharp contrast to classic PAN, lung involvement is predominant, with skin, cardiovascular system, kidney, peripheral nervous system, and gastrointestinal tract also commonly involved. Although the precise pathogenesis of this disease is uncertain, its strong association with asthma, its clinicopathologic manifestations which strongly suggest hypersensitivity phenomena, and its close similarity to classic PAN point to aberrant immunologic phenomena.

Clinical and laboratory manifestations Patients with allergic angiitis and granulomatosis exhibit nonspecific manifestations such as fever, malaise, anorexia, and weight loss similar to patients with classic PAN. In contrast to the latter disease, the pulmonary findings in allergic angiitis and granulomatosis clearly dominate the clinical picture with severe asthmatic attacks and the presence of pulmonary infiltrates. Skin lesions occur in approximately 70 percent of patients and include purpura in addition to cutaneous and subcutaneous nodules. Apart from the characteristic pulmonary findings, the multisystem involvement in this disease is quite similar to that of classic PAN (see above); an important exception is the fact that the renal disease in allergic angiitis and granulomatosis is less common and generally less severe than that of classic PAN.

The characteristic laboratory finding in virtually all patients with allergic angiitis and granulomatosis is a striking eosinophilia which reaches levels greater than 1000 cells per microliter in more than 80 percent of patients. The other laboratory findings are similar to those of classic PAN and reflect the organ systems involved.

Diagnosis Similar to classic PAN, the diagnosis of allergic angiitis and granulomatosis is made by biopsy, demonstrating vasculitis in a patient with the characteristic clinical manifestations. The biopsy findings are distinctive in the latter disease in that granulomatous vasculitis with eosinophilic tissue involvement together with peripheral eosinophilia are typical. Furthermore, pulmonary involvement is extremely common and is usually manifested by severe asthma associated with pulmonary infiltrates that may be fleeting in nature.

Treatment and prognosis The prognosis of untreated allergic angiitis and granulomatosis is poor with a reported 5-year survival of 25 percent. Unlike classic PAN, the cause of death is more likely to be related to pulmonary and cardiac disease as opposed to renal or gastrointestinal involvement. Glucocorticoid therapy has been reported to increase the 5-year survival to more than 50 percent. In glucocorticoid failures or in patients who present with fulminant multisystem disease, the treatment of choice is a combined regimen of cyclophosphamide and alternate-day prednisone which has resulted in a high rate of complete remission similar to the experience with classic PAN (see above).

POLYANGIITIS OVERLAP SYNDROME Many patients with systemic vasculitis manifest clinicopathologic characteristics which do not fit precisely into any classification, but which have overlapping features of classic PAN, allergic angiitis and granulomatosis, Wegener's granulomatosis, Takayasu's arteritis, or the hypersensitivity group of vasculitides. This subgroup has been referred to as the "polyangiitis overlap syndrome" and is part of the major grouping of systemic necrotizing vasculitis. It is clear that this entity does exist, and it has been designated with a distinct classification in order to avoid confusion in attempting to fit such overlap syndromes into one or other of the more classic vasculitic syndromes. This subgroup is truly a systemic vasculitis with the same potential for resulting in irreversible organ system dysfunction as the other systemic necrotizing vasculitides. The diagnostic and therapeutic considerations as well as the prognosis for this subgroup are the same as those for classic PAN and allergic angiitis and granulomatosis.

HYPERSENSITIVITY VASCULITIS

DEFINITION The term hypersensitivity vasculitis has been used to designate a heterogeneous group of disorders which are characterized by a vasculitic syndrome presumed to be associated with a hypersensitivity reaction following exposure to an antigen such as an infectious agent, a drug, or other foreign or endogenous substances. The common denominator of this group of diseases is the involvement of small vessels. Although any organ can be involved with this type of vasculitis, skin involvement generally dominates the clinical picture and the extracutaneous involvement is usually much less severe than that of the systemic vasculitides. There are multiple subgroups within the larger category of hypersensitivity vasculitis.

INCIDENCE AND PREVALENCE Although the exact incidence of this group of vasculitic syndromes is uncertain, it is clearly more common than the systemic necrotizing vasculitis group. The disease can occur at any age and in both sexes; however, different subgroups have a higher incidence in certain age groups and some are more common in males than females, or vice versa.

PATHOPHYSIOLOGY AND PATHOGENESIS The typical histopathologic feature of the hypersensitivity vasculitides is the presence of vasculitis of small vessels. Postcapillary venules are the most commonly involved vessels; capillaries and arterioles may be involved less frequently. This vasculitis is characterized by a leukocytoclasis which refers to the nuclear debris remaining from the neutrophils which have infiltrated in and around the vessels during the acute stages. In the subacute or chronic stages, mononuclear cells predominate; in certain subgroups, eosinophilic infiltration is seen. Erythrocytes often extravasate from the involved vessels, leading to palpable purpura.

Immune-complex deposition is generally considered to be the immunopathogenic mechanism of this type of vasculitis; however, formal proof that this is the case has not been established for all subgroups (see above). The hypersensitivity vasculitides can be broken down into two major categories depending on the type of putative antigen involved in the hypersensitivity reaction. In the originally described group, the antigen was foreign to the host, i.e., a drug, microbe, or foreign protein. In the second category, the antigen is felt to be endogenous to the host. Examples of these are the "self" proteins such as DNA or immunoglobulin which form immune complexes with their respective antibodies and lead to vasculitic complications in systemic lupus erythematosus and rheumatoid arthritis, respectively; other examples are the tumor antigens which form immune complexes with antibody and lead to vasculitis associated with certain neoplasms.

CLINICAL AND LABORATORY MANIFESTATIONS The hallmark of the broad group of hypersensitivity vasculitides is the predominance of skin involvement. Skin lesions may appear typically as palpable purpura; however, other cutaneous manifestations of the vasculitis may occur, including macules, papules, vesicles, bullae, subcutaneous nodules, ulcers, as well as recurrent or chronic urticaria. Despite the fact that skin lesions predominate, other organ systems may be involved to varying degrees and the extent to which this occurs may define a relatively distinct subgroup. Even in patients with isolated cutaneous involvement, the disease may be characterized by systemic signs and symptoms such as fever, malaise, myalgia, and anorexia. The skin lesions may be pruritic or even quite painful with a burning or stinging sensation. Lesions most commonly occur in the lower extremities in ambulatory patients or in the sacral area in bedridden patients due to the effects of hydrostatic forces on the postcapillary venules. Edema may accompany certain lesions, and hyperpigmentation often occurs in areas of recurrent or chronic lesions.

There are no specific laboratory tests which are diagnostic of hypersensitivity vasculitis. A mild leukocytosis with or without eosinophilia is characteristic as is an elevated ESR. Cryoglobulins and rheumatoid factor may be seen in certain cases, and serum complement levels follow no definite pattern. Laboratory abnormalities related to specific organ dysfunction reflect the involvement of these organs in the particular syndrome in question.

Henoch-Schönlein purpura The most distinctive subgroup of the hypersensitivity vasculitides is Henoch-Schönlein purpura, also referred to as anaphylactoid purpura, which is characterized by palpable purpura, most commonly distributed over the buttocks and lower extremities; arthralgias; gastrointestinal signs and symptoms; and glomerulonephritis. The disease is usually seen in children; however, individuals of any age may be affected. It has a remarkable tendency to resolve and recur several times over a period of weeks or months, usually ending in spontaneous resolution. A small percentage of patients progress to chronic disease. A number of antigens have been implicated in the immunopathogenesis of this disease, including infectious agents, drugs, certain foods, insect bites, and immunizations. IgA is the antibody class most often seen in the immune complexes of these patients. The typical palpable purpura is seen in virtually all patients; most patients develop polyarthralgias in the absence of frank arthritis. Gastrointestinal involvement, which is seen in almost 70 percent of pediatric patients, is characterized by colicky abdominal pain usually associated with nausea, vomiting, diarrhea, or constipation, which is frequently accompanied by the passage of blood and mucus per rectum; bowel intussusception may occur rarely. The renal involvement is usually characterized by a mild glomerulitis leading to hematuria with red blood cell casts (see also Chap. 228). Most patients recover completely and some do not require therapy. When glucocorticoid therapy is required, it is usually administered as 1 mg/kg per day of prednisone and tapered according to the clinical response.

Serum sickness and serum sickness–like reactions These reactions are characterized by the occurrence of fever, urticaria, polyarthralgias, and lymphadenopathy 7 to 10 days after primary exposure and 2 to 4 days after secondary exposure to a heterologous protein (classic serum sickness) or a nonprotein drug such as penicillin or sulfa (serum sickness–like reaction). Most of the manifestations are not due to a vasculitis; however, occasional patients will have typical cutaneous venulitis which may progress rarely to a systemic vasculitis. This disorder is discussed in detail in Chap. 268.

Vasculitis associated with other underlying primary diseases A number of diseases have vasculitis as a secondary manifestation of the underlying primary process. Foremost among these are the connective tissue diseases, particularly systemic lupus erythematosus (Chap. 269), rheumatoid arthritis (Chap. 270), and Sjögren's syndrome (Chap. 273). The most common form of vasculitis in these conditions is the small vessel venulitis isolated to the skin and clinically indistinguishable from the hypersensitivity vasculitides noted in response to an exogenous antigen. However, certain patients may develop a fulminant systemic necrotizing vasculitis indistinguishable from the polyarteritis nodosa group. Cryoglobulinemia may be seen in a number of the diverse vasculitic syndromes. Essential mixed cryoglobulinemia may present as a typical hypersensitivity vasculitis confined to the skin. However, typically it is associated with glomerulonephritis, arthralgias, hepatosplenomegaly, and lymphadenopathy in addition to skin involvement. The cryoglobulins usually consist of cryoprecipitable IgM rheumatoid factor directed against normal endogenous IgG.

Vasculitis can be associated with certain malignancies, particularly lymphoid or reticuloendothelial neoplasms. Leukocytoclastic venulitis confined to the skin is the most common finding; however, widespread systemic vasculitis may occur. Of particular note is the association of hairy-cell leukemia (Chap. 296) with classic PAN.

A leukocytoclastic vasculitis predominantly involving the skin with occasional involvement of other organ systems may be a minor component of many other diseases. These include subacute bacterial endocarditis, Epstein-Barr virus infection, chronic active hepatitis, ulcerative colitis, congenital deficiencies of various complement components, retroperitoneal fibrosis, and primary biliary cirrhosis. Association of hypersensitivity vasculitis with alpha₁ antitrypsin deficiency, intestinal bypass surgery, and relapsing polychondritis have been reported.

DIAGNOSIS The diagnosis of hypersensitivity vasculitis is made by the demonstration of vasculitis on biopsy. Given the predominance of cutaneous involvement, biopsy material is generally readily available. Patients who present with what appears to be isolated cutaneous vasculitis should undergo a systemic (usually noninvasive) workup of other organ systems since skin involvement is often the presenting feature of systemic vasculitis.

TREATMENT AND PROGNOSIS Most cases of hypersensitivity vasculitis resolve spontaneously, and others, such as Henoch-Schönlein purpura, remit and relapse before finally remitting completely. In those patients in whom persistent cutaneous disease evolves or in whom extracutaneous organ system involvement occurs, a variety of therapeutic regimens have been tried with variable results. In general, the treatment of this type of vasculitis has not been satisfactory. This is in contrast to the systemic necrotizing vasculitis group (see above) and Wegener's granulomatosis (see below) which generally are much more serious diseases than hypersensitivity vasculitis, but usually respond dramatically to the combination of prednisone and cyclophosphamide. Fortunately, since the disease is generally limited to the skin, this lack of consistent response to therapy usually does not lead to a life-threatening situation. When an antigenic stimulus is recognized as the precipitating factor in the vasculitis, it should be removed; if this is a microbe, appropriate antimicrobial therapy should be instituted. If the vasculitis is associated with another underlying disease, treatment of the latter often results in resolution of the former. In situations where disease is apparently self-limited, no therapy, except possibly symptomatic therapy, is indicated. When disease persists or results in progressive organ system dysfunction such as renal failure in Henoch-Schönlein purpura, glucocorticoid therapy should be instituted, usually as prednisone, 1 mg/kg per day, in a regimen aimed at rapid tapering where possible, either directly to discontinuation or by conversion to an alternate-day regimen

followed by ultimate discontinuation. In cases that prove refractory to glucocorticoids in which irreversible organ system dysfunction is likely, a trial of a cytotoxic agent such as cyclophosphamide in the regimen described above for systemic vasculitis is warranted. Patients with chronic vasculitis isolated to cutaneous venules rarely respond dramatically to any therapeutic regimen, and cytotoxic agents should be used only as a last resort in these patients. Plasmapheresis has been used with some success in fulminant cases. Dapsone has been tried in a number of patients with isolated cutaneous vasculitis with rare anecdotal reports of success. However, this drug has been consistently beneficial as therapy for cutaneous vasculitis only in patients with erythema elevatum diutinum (see below).

WEGENER'S GRANULOMATOSIS

DEFINITION Wegener's granulomatosis is a distinct clinicopathologic entity characterized by granulomatous vasculitis of the upper and lower respiratory tracts together with glomerulonephritis. In addition, variable degrees of disseminated vasculitis involving both small arteries and veins may occur.

INCIDENCE AND PREVALENCE Wegener's granulomatosis is an uncommon disease whose true incidence is difficult to determine. It is extremely rare in blacks compared to whites; the male to female ratio is 1.3:1. The disease can be seen at any age but is infrequent among preadolescents; the mean age of onset is approximately 40 years.

PATHOPHYSIOLOGY AND PATHOGENESIS The histopathologic hallmarks of Wegener's granulomatosis are necrotizing vasculitis of small arteries and veins together with granuloma formation which may be either intravascular or extravascular. Lung involvement typically appears as multiple, bilateral, nodular cavity infiltrates which on biopsy almost invariably reveal the typical necrotizing granulomatous vasculitis. Endobronchial disease either in its active form or as a result of fibrous scarring may lead to obstruction with atelectasis. Upper airway lesions, particularly those in the sinuses and nasopharynx, typically reveal inflammation, necrosis, and granuloma formation with or without vasculitis.

It its earliest form, renal involvement is characterized by a focal and segmental glomerulitis which may evolve into a rapidly progressive crescentic glomerulonephritis. Granuloma formation is only rarely seen on renal biopsy. In addition to the classic triad of upper and lower respiratory tracts and kidney disease, virtually any organ can be involved with vasculitis, granuloma, or both.

The immunopathogenesis of this disease is unclear, although the involvement of upper airways and lung suggests an aberrant hypersensitivity response to an exogenous or even endogenous antigen that enters through or resides in the upper airway. The demonstration of circulating and deposited immune complexes in certain patients together with granulomatous reactivity suggests either an overlap of delayed hypersensitivity and immune-complex–mediated mechanisms or a granulomatous response to the immune complexes themselves. Antibodies to a protein contained in the intracytoplasmic azurophil granules of neutrophils have been demonstrated in a high percentage of patients with active Wegener's granulomatosis. The pathophysiologic significance of these findings is unclear at present.

CLINICAL AND LABORATORY MANIFESTATIONS A typical patient presents with severe upper respiratory tract findings such as paranasal sinus pain and drainage, and purulent or bloody nasal discharge with or without nasal mucosal ulceration. Nasal septal perforation may follow, leading to saddle nose deformity. Serous otitis media may occur as a result of eustachian tube blockage.

Pulmonary involvement may be manifested as asymptomatic infiltrates or may be clinically expressed as cough, hemoptysis, dyspnea, and chest discomfort. It is present in approximately 95 percent of patients. Subglottic stenosis resulting from active disease or scarring may result in severe airway obstruction.

Eye involvement (60 percent of patients) may range from a mild conjunctivitis to episcleritis, scleritis, granulomatous sclerouveitis, ciliary vessel vasculitis, and retroorbital mass lesions leading to proptosis.

Skin lesions (45 percent of patients) appear as papules, vesicles, palpable purpura, ulcers, or subcutaneous nodules; biopsy reveals vasculitis, granuloma, or both. Cardiac involvement (12 percent of patients) manifests as pericarditis, coronary vasculitis, or, rarely, cardiomyopathy. Nervous system manifestations (22 percent of patients) include cranial neuritis, mononeuritis multiplex, or, rarely, cerebral vasculitis and/or granuloma.

Renal disease (85 percent of patients) generally dominates the clinical picture and, if left untreated, accounts directly or indirectly for most of the mortality in this disease. Although it may smolder in some cases as a mild glomerulitis with proteinuria, hematuria, and red blood cell casts, it is clear that once clinically detectable renal functional impairment occurs, rapidly progressive renal failure usually ensues unless appropriate treatment is instituted.

While the disease is active, most patients have nonspecific symptoms and signs such as malaise, weakness, arthralgias, anorexia, and weight loss. Fever may indicate activity of the underlying disease, but more often reflects secondary infection, usually of the upper airway.

Characteristic laboratory findings include a markedly elevated ESR, mild anemia and leukocytosis, mild hypergammaglobulinemia, particularly of the IgA class, and mildly elevated rheumatoid factor. Thrombocytosis may be seen as an acute phase reactant; hypocomplementemia is not seen despite the presence of circulating immune complexes in some patients. Antineutrophil cytoplasmic autoantibodies are seen in the majority of patients with active disease (see above).

DIAGNOSIS The diagnosis of Wegener's granulomatosis is a clinicopathologic one made by the demonstration of necrotizing granulomatous vasculitis on biopsy of appropriate tissue in a patient with the clinical findings of upper and lower respiratory tract disease together with evidence of glomerulonephritis. Pulmonary tissue, preferably obtained by open thoracotomy, offers the highest diagnostic yield, almost invariably revealing granulomatous vasculitis. Biopsy of upper airway tissue usually reveals granulomatous inflammation with necrosis but may not show vasculitis. Renal biopsy confirms the presence of glomerulonephritis.

In its typical presentation, the classic clinicopathologic complex of Wegener's granulomatosis usually provides ready differentiation from other disorders. However, if all of the typical features are not present at once, it needs to be differentiated from the other vasculitides, particularly allergic angiitis and granulomatosis, Goodpasture's syndrome (Chap. 228), tumors of the upper airway or lung, and infectious or noninfectious granulomatous diseases. Of particular note is the differentiation from idiopathic midline granuloma (see Chap. 279) which frequently erodes through the skin of the face, a feature never seen in Wegener's granulomatosis.

Of particular importance in the differential diagnosis is a disease called *lymphomatoid granulomatosis*. It is characterized by lung, skin, central nervous system, and kidney involvement in which atypical lymphocytoid and plasmacytoid cells infiltrate tissue in an angioinvasive manner. In this regard, it clearly differs from Wegener's granulomatosis in that it is not an inflammatory vasculitis in the classic sense, but an infiltration of vessels with atypical mononuclear cells; granuloma may be present in involved tissues. Approximately 50 percent of patients develop a true malignant lymphoma.

TREATMENT AND PROGNOSIS Wegener's granulomatosis was formerly universally fatal, usually within a few months after the onset of clinically apparent renal disease. Glucocorticoids alone led to some symptomatic improvement with little effect on the ultimate course of the disease. It has been well established that the treatment of choice in this disease is cyclophosphamide given in doses of 2 mg/kg per day orally. The leukocyte count should be closely monitored during therapy and the dosage adjusted in order to maintain the count above 3000 per cubic millimeter, which generally maintains the neutrophil count at approximately 1500 per microliter. With this approach, clinical remission can usually be induced and maintained without causing severe leukopenia with its associated risk of infection. Cyclophosphamide should be continued for 1 year following the induction of complete remission and gradually tapered and discontinued thereafter. Patients who cannot tolerate cyclophosphamide or who develop serious toxicity such as severe cystitis may be treated with azathioprine in similar doses.

At the initiation of therapy, glucocorticoids should be administered together with cyclophosphamide. This can be given as prednisone, 1 mg/kg per day initially (for the first month of therapy) as a daily regimen with gradual conversion to an alternate-day schedule followed by tapering and discontinuation after approximately 6 months.

Using the above regimen, the prognosis of this disease is excellent and long-term remission is achieved in over 90 percent of patients. A number of patients who developed irreversible renal failure, but who achieved subsequent remission on appropriate therapy, have undergone successful renal transplantation.

Because of anecdotal reports of some success with an intermittent, intravenous bolus of cyclophosphamide (1 gm/m^2 per month) in the treatment of Wegener's granulomatosis and other systemic vasculitides, prospective studies using this regimen are currently underway. In addition, recent reports have indicated a potential role for trimethoprim/sulfamethoxazole in the treatment of Wegener's granulomatosis. However, controlled prospective clinical trials are needed to substantiate these claims. Chronically administered cyclophosphamide in the regimen indicated above is still clearly the treatment of choice for Wegener's granulomatosis.

TEMPORAL ARTERITIS

DEFINITION Temporal arteritis, also referred to as cranial or giant cell arteritis, is an inflammation of medium- and large-sized arteries. It characteristically involves one or more branches of the carotid artery, particularly the temporal artery, hence the name cranial or temporal arteritis. However, it is a systemic disease and can involve arteries in multiple locations.

INCIDENCE AND PREVALENCE Temporal arteritis is an uncommon disease estimated to occur in 24 per 100,000 people. It is a disease of the elderly, occurring almost exclusively in individuals older than 55 years; however, well-documented cases have occurred in patients 40 years old or younger. It is more common in women than in men and is rare in blacks. Familial aggregation of this disease has been reported.

PATHOPHYSIOLOGY AND PATHOGENESIS Although the temporal artery is most frequently involved in this disease, patients often have a systemic vasculitis of multiple medium- and large-sized arteries which may go undetected. Histopathologically, the disease is a panarteritis with inflammatory mononuclear cell infiltrates within the vessel wall with frequent giant cell formation. There is proliferation of the intima and fragmentation of the internal elastic lamina. Pathophysiologic findings in organs result from the ischemia related to the involved vessels. Immunopathogenic mechanisms, particularly cell-mediated immunity, are felt to be involved in this disease, although the etiology is entirely unknown.

CLINICAL AND LABORATORY MANIFESTATIONS The disease is characterized clinically by the classic complex of fever, anemia, high ESR, and headaches in an elderly patient. Other manifestations include malaise, fatigue, anorexia, weight loss, sweats, and arthralgias. Temporal arteritis is closely associated with the polymyalgia rheumatica syndrome, which is characterized by stiffness, aching, and pain in the muscles of the neck, shoulders, lower back, hips, and thighs.

In patients with involvement of the temporal artery, headache is the predominant symptom and may be associated with a tender, thickened, or nodular artery which may pulsate early in the disease but may become occluded later. Scalp pain and claudication of the jaw and tongue may occur. A well-recognized and dreaded complication of temporal arteritis, particularly in untreated patients, is ocular involvement due primarily to ischemic optic neuritis, which may lead to serious visual symptoms, even sudden blindness in some patients. However, most patients have complaints relating to the head or eyes for months before objective eye involvement. Claudication of the extremities, strokes, myocardial infarctions, aortic aneurysms and dissections, and infarctions of visceral organs have been reported.

Characteristic laboratory findings in addition to the elevated ESR include a normochromic or slightly hypochromic anemia. Liver function abnormalities are common, particularly increased alkaline phosphatase levels. Increased levels of IgG and complement have been reported as have increased levels of circulating immune complexes.

DIAGNOSIS   The diagnosis of temporal arteritis and its associated clinicopathologic syndrome can often be made clinically by the demonstration of the classic picture of fever, anemia, and high ESR with or without symptoms of polymyalgia rheumatica in an elderly patient. The diagnosis is confirmed by biopsy of the temporal artery. Since involvement of the vessel may be segmental, the diagnosis may be missed on routine biopsy. Dramatic response to a trial of glucocorticoid therapy can confirm the diagnosis.

TREATMENT AND PROGNOSIS   Temporal arteritis and its associated symptoms are exquisitely sensitive to glucocorticoid therapy. Treatment should begin with prednisone, 40 to 60 mg per day followed by a gradual tapering to a maintenance dose of 7.5 to 10 mg per day. When ocular signs and symptoms occur, it is important that therapy be initiated or adjusted to control them. Because of the possibility of relapse, therapy should be continued for at least 1 to 2 years. The prognosis is generally good, and most patients achieve complete remission that is often maintained after withdrawal of therapy.

TAKAYASU'S ARTERITIS

DEFINITION   Takayasu's arteritis is an inflammatory and stenotic disease of medium- and large-sized arteries characterized by a strong predilection for the aortic arch and its branches. For this reason, it is often referred to as the aortic arch syndrome.

INCIDENCE AND PREVALENCE   Takayasu's arteritis is an uncommon disease, much less common than temporal arteritis. It is most prevalent in adolescent girls and young women. Although it is more common in the Orient, it is neither racially nor geographically restricted. An association of the disease has been described with HLA-DR2, MB1 in Japan and HLA-DR4, MB3 in the United States.

PATHOPHYSIOLOGY AND PATHOGENESIS   The disease involves medium- and large-sized arteries with a strong predilection for the aortic arch and its branches; the pulmonary artery may also be involved. The most commonly affected arteries seen by angiography are the subclavians, followed by the aortic arch, ascending aorta, carotids, and femorals. The involvement of the major branches of the aorta is much more marked at their origin than distally. Partial renal artery occlusion with resulting hypertension is common. The disease is a panarteritis with inflammatory mononuclear cell infiltrates and occasionally giant cells. There is marked intimal proliferation and fibrosis, scarring and vascularization of the media, and disruption and degeneration of the elastic lamina. Narrowing of the lumen occurs with or without thrombosis. The vasa vasorum are frequently involved. Pathologic changes in various organs reflect the compromise of blood flow through the involved vessels.

Immunopathogenic mechanisms, the precise nature of which is uncertain, are suspected in this disease.

CLINICAL AND LABORATORY MANIFESTATIONS   Takayasu's arteritis is a systemic disease with generalized as well as local symptoms. The generalized symptoms include malaise, fever, night sweats, arthralgias, anorexia, and weight loss which may occur months before vessel involvement is apparent. These symptoms may merge into those related to pain over the involved vessels followed

by symptoms of ischemia in organs supplied by the compromised vessels. Pulses are commonly absent in the involved vessels, particularly the subclavian artery. Aortic regurgitation may occur; hypertension is seen in almost 50 percent of cases. Cardiomegaly and cardiac failure secondary to aortic or pulmonary hypertension occur commonly; the coronary arteries themselves are rarely involved. Carotid artery involvement leads to a variety of central nervous system signs and symptoms with over one-half of patients experiencing syncopal episodes; stroke, which occurs in 15 percent of patients, may represent the first sign of disease; ocular signs and symptoms are present in 60 percent of patients.

The clinical course may be fulminant, may progress gradually, or may stabilize. Complications are related to the distribution of the involved vessels. Death usually occurs from congestive heart failure or cerebrovascular accidents.

Characteristic laboratory findings include an elevated ESR, mild anemia, leukocytosis, and elevated immunoglobulin levels.

DIAGNOSIS   The diagnosis of Takayasu's arteritis should be suspected strongly in a young woman who develops a decrease or absence of peripheral pulses, discrepancies in blood pressure, and arterial bruits. The diagnosis is confirmed by the characteristic pattern on arteriography which includes irregular vessel walls, stenosis, poststenotic dilatation, aneurysm formation, occlusion, and evidence of increased collateral circulation. Histopathologic demonstration of inflamed vessels adds confirmatory data; however, tissue is rarely readily available for examination.

TREATMENT AND PROGNOSIS   The course of the disease is variable, and spontaneous remissions may occur. Reported mortality statistics range from less than 10 percent to 75 percent, likely reflecting duration of follow-up. Although glucocorticoid therapy in doses of 40 to 60 mg prednisone per day alleviates symptoms, there are no convincing studies which indicate that they alone increase survival. However, recent studies suggest that glucocorticoid therapy can induce remissions in a high percentage of individuals. In addition, surgery and/or angioplasty may remarkably improve survival by decreasing the risk of stroke and correcting hypertension due to renal artery stenosis. A few patients who were refractory to glucocorticoid therapy responded favorably to cyclophosphamide, 2 mg/kg per day. However, long-term studies will be needed to confirm this.

MUCOCUTANEOUS LYMPH NODE SYNDROME (KAWASAKI'S DISEASE)

Mucocutaneous lymph node syndrome is an acute, febrile, multisystem disease of children. It is characterized by unresponsiveness to antibiotics; nonsuppurative cervical adenitis; and changes in the skin and mucous membranes such as edema, congested conjunctivae, erythema of the oral cavity, lips, and palms, and desquamation of the skin of the fingertips. Although the disease is generally benign and self-limited, it is associated with coronary artery aneurysms in 17 to 31 percent of cases, with an overall case fatality rate of 0.5 to 2.8 percent. These complications usually occur between the third and fourth week of illness during the convalescent stage. Vasculitis of the coronary arteries is seen in almost all of the fatal cases which have been autopsied. There is typical intimal proliferation and infiltration of the vessel wall with mononuclear cells. Beadlike aneurysms and thromboses may be seen along the artery. Most investigators agree that many of the cases of PAN formerly reported in children were actually arteritic complications of unrecognized mucocutaneous lymph node syndrome. Other manifestations include pericarditis, myocarditis, myocardial ischemia and infarction, and cardiomegaly.

Apart from the up to 2.8 percent of patients who develop fatal complications, the prognosis of this disease for uneventful recovery is excellent. High-dose intravenous gamma globulin (400 mg/kg per day for 4 consecutive days) together with aspirin (100 mg/kg per day for 14 days followed by 3 to 5 mg/kg per day for several weeks) have been shown to be effective in reducing the prevalence of coronary artery abnormalities when administered early in the course of the disease.

ISOLATED VASCULITIS OF THE CENTRAL NERVOUS SYSTEM

Isolated vasculitis of the central nervous system is an uncommon clinicopathologic entity characterized by vasculitis restricted to the vessels of the central nervous system without other apparent systemic vasculitis. Although the arteriole is most commonly affected, vessels of any size can be involved. The inflammatory process is usually composed of mononuclear cell infiltrates with or without granuloma formation. Cases have been associated with cytomegalovirus, syphilis, pyogenic bacterial and varicella-zoster infections, as well as with Hodgkin's disease and amphetamine abuse; however, in several cases no underlying disease process has been identified.

Patients may present with severe headaches, altered mental function, and focal neurologic defects. Systemic symptoms are generally absent. Devastating neurologic abnormalities may occur depending on the extent of vessel involvement. The diagnosis is generally made by demonstration of characteristic vessel abnormalities on arteriography and confirmed by biopsy of the brain parenchyma and leptomeninges. The prognosis of this disease is poor; however, some reports indicate that glucocorticoid therapy alone or together with cyclophosphamide in steroid-resistant patients administered as described above for the systemic vasculitides has induced sustained clinical remissions in a small number of patients.

THROMBOANGIITIS OBLITERANS (BUERGER'S DISEASE)

Thromboangiitis obliterans is an inflammatory occlusive peripheral vascular disease of unknown etiology which affects arteries and veins. Thrombosis of the vessels is likely the primary event, and so this disease is not a classic vasculitis. However, it is considered among the vasculitides because of the intense inflammatory response within the thrombus and the fact that there is often a vasculitis of the vasa vasorum in the arterial wall. The disease is discussed in detail in Chap. 198.

MISCELLANEOUS VASCULITIDES

A variety of disorders, many of which are uncommon, are characterized by varying degrees of inflammatory responses involving blood vessels. *Behçet's syndrome* is a clinicopathologic entity characterized by recurrent episodes of oral and genital ulcers, iritis, and cutaneous lesions. The underlying pathologic lesion is a leukocytoclastic ven ulitis, although vessels of any size and in any organ can be involved. This disorder is described in detail in Chap. 275.

Cogan's syndrome is a disease characterized by nonsyphilitic interstitial keratitis together with vestibuloauditory symptoms. It may be associated with a systemic vasculitis involving vessels of different sizes as well as the aortic valve.

Erythema nodosum is a common disease which is recognized as a hypersensitivity manifestation of a number of other disorders. It is a painful nodular process of the dermis and subcutaneous tissues. However, histopathologically, there is a vasculitis of small venules (see Chap. 56).

Erythema elevatum diutinum is a rare, chronic skin disorder of unknown etiology characterized by persistent red, purple, and yellowish papules, plaques, and nodules usually distributed symmetrically over the extensor surface of the limbs which on biopsy demonstrate a leukocytoclastic venulitis together with a marked dermal inflammatory infiltrate. The disease responds dramatically to dapsone therapy.

Eales' disease is a retinal vasculitis which predominantly affects males in the second and third decade of life and which produces a syndrome of recurrent hemorrhages into the retina and vitreous.

REFERENCES

ALARCON-SEGOVIA D: The necrotizing vasculitides. Med Clin North Am 61:240, 1977

CUPPS TR, FAUCI AS: *The Vasculitides*. Philadelphia, Saunders, 1981

——— et al: Chronic, recurrent small-vessel cutaneous vasculitis. Clinical experience in 13 patients. JAMA 247:1994, 1982

——— et al: Isolated angiitis of the central nervous system. Prospective diagnostic and therapeutic experience. Am J Med 74:97, 1983

FAUCI AS: Vasculitis, in *Clinical Immunology*, CW Parker (ed). Philadelphia, Saunders, 1980, pp 475–519

———: Vasculitis. J Allergy Clin Immunol 72:211, 1983

——— et al: The spectrum of vasculitis. Clinical, pathologic, immunologic, and therapeutic considerations. Ann Intern Med 89:660, 1978

——— et al: Wegener's granulomatosis: Prospective clinical and therapeutic experience with 85 patients for 21 years. Ann Intern Med 98:76, 1983

FAUCI AS, LEAVITT RY: Vasculitis, in *Arthritis and Allied Conditions: A Textbook of Rheumatology*, 11th ed, DJ McCarty (ed). Philadelphia, Lea & Febiger, 1989, pp 1166–118

KADISON P, HAYNES BF: Vasculitis: Mechanisms of vessel damage, in *Inflammation: Basic Principles and Clinical Correlates*. JI Gallin et al. New York, Raven, 1988, pp 703–717

LEAVITT RY, FAUCI AS: Polyangiitis overlap syndrome. Am J Med, 1986

SHELHAMER JH et al: Takayasu's arteritis and its therapy. Ann Intern Med 103:121, 1985

277 SARCOIDOSIS

RONALD G. CRYSTAL

DEFINITION Sarcoidosis is a chronic, multisystem disorder of unknown etiology characterized in affected organs by an accumulation of T lymphocytes and mononuclear phagocytes, noncaseating epithelioid granulomas, and derangements of the normal tissue architecture. Although there are usually skin anergy and depressed cellular immune processes in the blood, sarcoidosis is characterized at the sites of disease by exaggerated helper-T-lymphocyte immune processes. All parts of the body can be affected, but the organ most frequently affected is the lung. Involvement of the skin, eye, and lymph nodes is also common. The disease is often acute or subacute and self-limiting, but in many individuals it is chronic, waxing and waning over many years.

ETIOLOGY The etiology of sarcoidosis is unknown. A variety of infectious and noninfectious agents have been implicated, but there is no proof that any specific agent is responsible. However, all available evidence is consistent with the concept that the disease results from an exaggerated cellular immune response (acquired, inherited, or both) to a limited class of antigens or self-antigens.

INCIDENCE AND PREVALENCE Sarcoidosis is a relatively common disease affecting individuals of both sexes and almost all ages, races, and geographic locations. Females appear to be slightly more susceptible than males. Cases of sarcoid have been described in all of the major races, and the disease is found throughout the world. It has been suggested that sarcoid is more common in certain geographic areas such as the southeastern part of the United States, but when case-matched controls have been used, these geographic differences are less convincing. There is a remarkable diversity of the prevalence of sarcoidosis among certain ethnic and racial groups. The prevalence of sarcoidosis is from 10 to 40 per 100,000 in the United States and Europe. In the United States, the majority of patients are black, with a ratio of blacks to whites ranging from 10:1 to 17:1. In Europe, however, the disease affects mostly whites. Furthermore, while the prevalence per 100,000 in Sweden is 64, in France it is 10, in Poland 3, yet for Irish females living in London it is 200. In contrast, the disease is very rare among Eskimos, Canadian Indians, New Zealand Maoris, and southeast Asians.

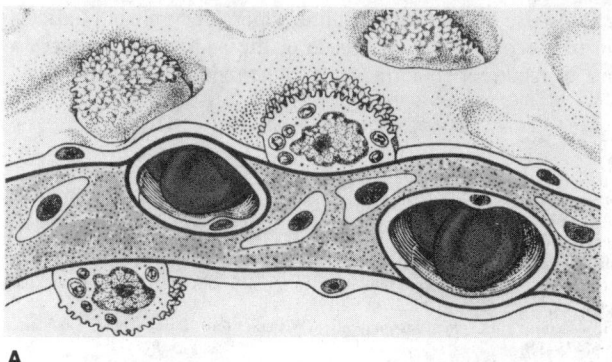

A

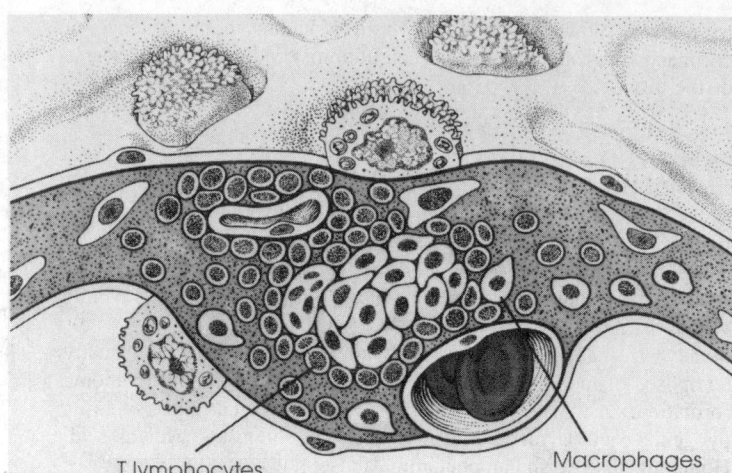

T lymphocytes   Macrophages

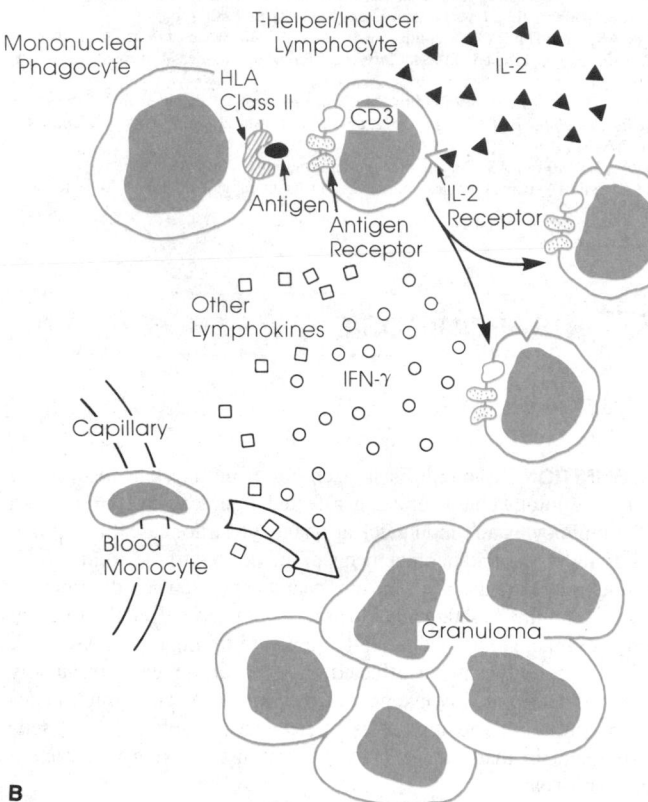

B

FIGURE 277-1 Pathogenesis of sarcoidosis. *A*. Histologic abnormalities. Normal alveoli *(left)* and alveoli in active sarcoidosis *(right)*. The latter are distorted by the accumulated T helper-inducer lymphocytes, alveolar macrophages, and macrophages aggregated into granulomas. There is mild damage to alveolar epithelial and endothelial cells. *B*. The exaggerated processes of T helper-inducer lymphocytes in affected organs result in the accumulation of these cells along with macrophages and macrophages aggregated into granulomas. The trigger for the T helper-inducer cells is unknown. It may be a limited class of antigens or self-antigens presented in the context of class II HLA surface molecules by mononuclear phagocytes to the T helper-inducer lymphocyte. The antigen class II HLA complex is identified by the T-cell antigen receptor, the CD3 signal transducing complex is triggered, and the T cell is activated. Consequent to this process the immune response is exaggerated and skewed to produce activated T helper-inducer cells that release interleukin 2, which drives the accumulation of more T helper cells. The activated T helper-inducer cells also release γ-interferon (IFN-γ) and other lymphokines, mediators that contribute to the recruitment and activation of blood monocytes and hence to granuloma formation.

Most patients present with sarcoidosis between the ages of 20 and 40, but it can occur in children and in the elderly. Several hundred kindred groups with familial sarcoidosis have been described, and the disease has been observed in twins, more commonly in monozygotic than in dizygotic pairs. There have also been several instances of husband-wife pairs identified, and geographic foci of sarcoid among unrelated individuals living closely within a community, arguing for some environmental factors in the pathogenesis of the disease. Although the histocompatibility locus HLA-B8 has been suggested to confer certain responses to sarcoidosis, no clear patterns in any HLA locus have emerged. Unlike many diseases in which the lung is involved, sarcoidosis favors nonsmokers.

PATHOPHYSIOLOGY AND IMMUNOPATHOGENESIS The first manifestation of the disease is an accumulation of mononuclear inflammatory cells, mostly T helper lymphocytes and mononuclear phagocytes, in affected organs. This inflammatory process is followed by the formation of granulomas, aggregates of macrophages and their progeny, epithelioid cells, and multinucleated giant cells. The typical sarcoid granuloma is a compact structure composed of an aggregate of mononuclear phagocytes surrounded by a rim of T helper-inducer lymphocytes and, to a far lesser extent, B lymphocytes. The overall structure is relatively discrete and is interspersed with fine collagen

fibrils, presumably remnants of the underlying connective tissue matrix. The giant cells within the granuloma can be of the Langhans' or foreign-body variety and often contain inclusions such as Schaumann bodies (conch-like structures), asteroid bodies (stellate-like structures), and residual bodies (refractile calcium-containing inclusions).

Together, the accumulated T cells, mononuclear phagocytes, and granulomas represent the active disease. Other than the fact that they take up space and thus their bulk modifies the local architecture, there is no evidence that the mononuclear inflammatory cells either alone or in the granuloma injure the affected organ by releasing mediators that damage the normal parenchymal cells or the extracellular matrix. Rather, organ dysfunction in sarcoid results from the accumulated inflammatory cells distorting the architecture of the affected tissue; if a sufficient number of structures vital to the function of the tissue are involved, the disease becomes clinically apparent in that organ. Thus, while autopsy series show that, to some extent, sarcoidosis involves most organs in the majority of patients, the disease manifests clinically only in organs where it affects function (such as the lung and eye) or in organs where it is readily observed (such as the skin or, by x-ray, the hilar nodes). For example, in the lung the inflammatory cells and granulomas distort the walls of the alveoli, bronchi, and blood vessels (Fig. 277-1*A*), thus altering the intimate relationships between air and blood necessary for normal gas exchange. When a sufficient amount of pulmonary tissue is involved, it is sensed by the individual as dyspnea. In contrast, most individuals with sarcoidosis have granulomatous mononuclear cell inflammation in the liver but usually do not have symptoms or functional derangements referable to that organ, likely because the disease process does not modify the local structures sufficiently to affect function.

If the disease is suppressed, either spontaneously or with therapy, the mononuclear inflammation is reduced in intensity and the number of granulomas is reduced. The granulomas resolve either by dispersion of the cells or by centripetal proliferation of fibroblasts from the periphery of the granuloma inward, to form a small scar. In chronic cases, the mononuclear cell inflammation persists for years. If the intensity of the inflammation is sufficiently high for a sufficiently long period, the derangements to the affected tissues result in extensive damage, the development of fibrosis, and permanent loss of organ function.

All available evidence suggests that active sarcoidosis results from an exaggerated cellular immune response to a variety of antigens or self-antigens, in which the process of T-lymphocyte triggering, proliferation, and activation is skewed in the direction of helper-inducer-T-lymphocyte processes (Fig. 277-1B). The result is an exaggerated helper-inducer-T-cell response, and thus the accumulation of large numbers of activated T cells in the affected organs. Since the activated helper-inducer T lymphocyte releases mediators that attract and activate mononuclear phagocytes, it is likely that the process of granuloma formation is a secondary phenomenon which is a consequence of the exaggerated helper-inducer-T-cell process. In this context, the current hypotheses of the cause of sarcoidosis, not mutually exclusive, include: (1) the disease is caused by a class of antigens, nonself or self, that trigger only the helper-inducer-T-cell arm of the immune response; (2) the disease results from an inadequate suppressor arm of the immune response, such that helper-inducer-T-cell processes cannot be shut down in a normal fashion; or (3) the disease results from inherited (and/or acquired) differences in immune response genes, such that the response to a variety of antigens is an exaggerated, helper-inducer-T-cell process.

Independent of the inciting agent(s) or the reason why there is an exaggerated helper-inducer-T-cell response, there is a general understanding of the processes responsible for the maintenance of the inflammation and the development of the granuloma. The T helper-inducer lymphocytes accumulate at the sites of disease, at least in part, because they proliferate in these sites at an exaggerated rate. This T-cell proliferation is maintained by the spontaneous release of interleukin 2 (IL-2), the T-cell growth factor, by activated T helper-inducer cells in the local milieu. In this regard, sarcoidosis is a remarkable example of compartmentalization of the immune system and a dramatic illustration of why disease activity of sarcoidosis cannot be assessed by evaluating the immune system only in the blood. Whereas the T helper-inducer cells in the involved organs are releasing IL-2 and proliferating at an enhanced rate, the T cells in other sites, such as blood, are quiescent. Furthermore, while there is a marked enhancement of the number of T helper-inducer cells at the sites of disease, the numbers of T helper-inducer cells in the blood are normal or slightly reduced. In the involved organs, the ratio of helper-inducer to suppressor-cytotoxic T cells may be as high as 10:1 compared to the ratio of 2:1 found in normal tissues or in the blood of affected individuals.

In addition to driving other T helper-inducer cells in the affected organs to proliferate, the T helper-inducer cells at the sites of disease are activated and release mediators that both recruit and activate mononuclear phagocytes. The T helper-inducer cells accomplish this by releasing a variety of mediators (lymphokines) including proteins capable of recruiting blood monocytes to the local milieu of the activated T cells and γ-interferon, a protein that, among its many actions, activates mononuclear phagocytes. Together, these mediators recruit blood monocytes to the affected organs and activate them, providing the building blocks for the formation of the granuloma.

In addition to these exaggerated cellular immune processes, active sarcoid is also characterized by hyperglobulinemia. Included among the immunoglobulins are antibodies against a variety of infectious agents as well as IgM anti-T-cell antibodies. However, there is no evidence that any of these antibodies plays a role in the pathogenesis of the disease, and they are thought to result from the nonspecific polyclonal stimulation of B cells by the activated T cells at the site of disease.

If the damage in the affected organs is sufficiently extensive so that the remaining parenchymal cells cannot reestablish the normal tissue architecture, the usual result is fibrosis, the proliferation of mesenchymal cells and deposition of their connective tissue products. There is convincing evidence that the fibroblast proliferation is directed by tissue macrophages spontaneously releasing growth signals for fibroblasts, including platelet-derived growth factor, fibronectin, and insulin-like growth factor 1. It is not known, however, why this fibrotic process occurs only in a relatively small proportion of individuals with sarcoidosis.

CLINICAL MANIFESTATIONS   Sarcoidosis is a systemic disease, and thus the clinical manifestations may be generalized or focused on one or more organs. However, because the lung is almost always involved, most patients have symptoms referable to the respiratory system. Independent of the site, the clinical manifestations of the disease relate directly to the exaggerated helper-inducer T cell–mononuclear phagocyte granulomatous inflammatory process itself, or to the sequela resulting from the permanent damage caused by this process.

Sarcoidosis is occasionally discovered in a completely asymptomatic individual, but more commonly it presents abruptly over 1 to 2 weeks or the affected individual develops symptoms insidiously over several months. Independent of the mode of presentation, about 75 percent of all cases present when the individual is less than 40 years of age.

The asymptomatic form is usually detected by a routine examination, such as a chest film. In the United States, this represents about 10 to 20 percent of all cases, but in countries where chest films are mandatory in preemployment screening programs, the proportion of asymptomatic patients is higher.

So-called acute or subacute sarcoidosis develops abruptly over a period of a few weeks and represents 20 to 40 percent of all cases. These individuals usually have constitutional symptoms such as fever, fatigue, malaise, anorexia, or weight loss. These symptoms are usually mild, but in approximately 25 percent of the acute cases, the constitutional complaints are extensive. Many patients have respiratory symptoms, including cough, dyspnea, or a vague retrosternal chest discomfort. Two syndromes have been identified in the acute group. Löfgren's syndrome, frequent in Scandinavian, Irish, and Puerto Rican females, includes the complex of erythema nodosum and x-ray findings of bilateral hilar adenopathy, often accompanied by joint symptoms. The Heerfordt-Waldenstrom syndrome describes individuals with fever, parotid enlargement, anterior uveitis, and facial nerve palsy.

The insidious form of sarcoidosis develops over months and is associated usually with respiratory complaints without constitutional symptoms. In the United States, 40 to 70 percent of all sarcoid patients are in this category. About 10 percent of these individuals have symptoms referable to organs other than the lung. It is the individuals who present with the insidious form of sarcoidosis who most commonly go on to develop chronic sarcoidosis, with permanent damage to the lung and other organs.

Despite the fact that sarcoidosis is a systemic disease and some evidence of inflammation can be detected in most organs in the majority of patients, sarcoidosis is important clinically because of the pulmonary abnormalities and, to a lesser extent, lymph node, skin, and eye involvement. Far less commonly, other organs are involved significantly.

Lung   Of individuals with sarcoidosis, 90 percent have an abnormal chest x-ray at some time during their course. Overall, approximately 50 percent develop permanent pulmonary abnormalities and 5 to 15 percent have progressive fibrosis of the lung parenchyma. Sarcoidosis of the lung is primarily an interstitial lung disease (see Chap. 211) in which the inflammatory process involves the alveoli, small bronchi, and small blood vessels. These individuals typically have symptoms of dyspnea, particularly with exercise, and a dry cough. In acute and subacute cases, physical examination usually reveals dry rales. Hemoptysis is rare, as is production of sputum.

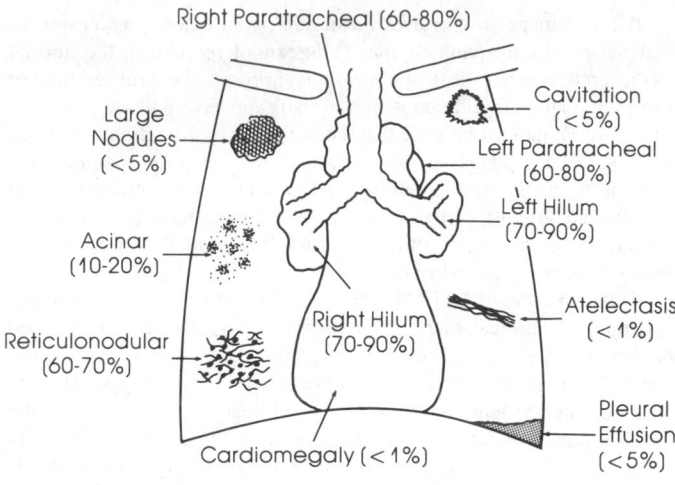

A

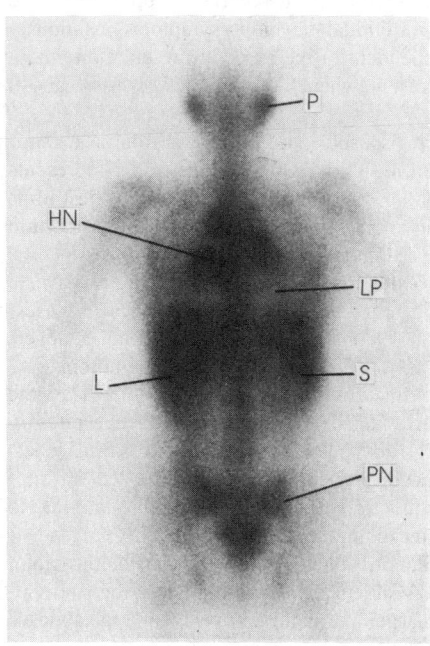

B

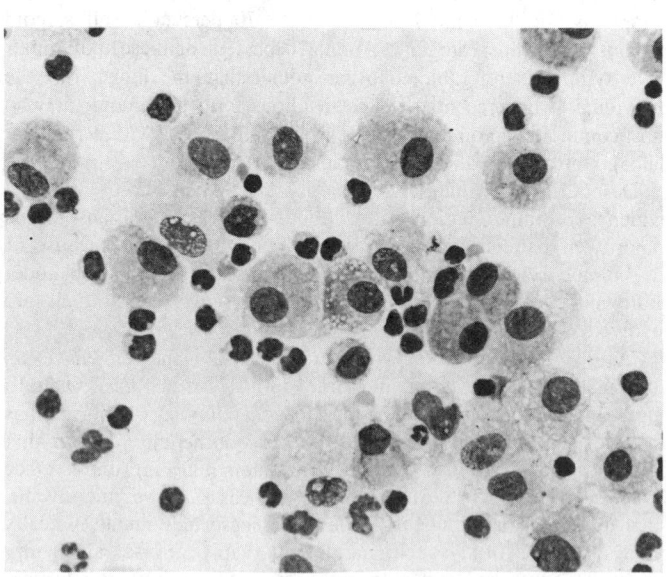

C

Occasionally, the large airways are involved to a degree sufficient to cause dysfunction. Distal atelectasis can result from endobronchial sarcoidosis or from external compression from enlarged intrathoracic nodes. Rarely, wheezing is heard, incorrectly suggesting asthma. Large-vessel pulmonary granulomatous arteritis is common, but it rarely causes major problems. If it dominates the pulmonary lesions, it is sometimes called "necrotizing sarcoidal granulomatosis." The pleura is involved in 1 to 5 percent of cases, almost always manifesting as a unilateral pleural effusion with characteristics of an exudate containing lymphocytes. The effusions usually clear within a few weeks, but chronic pleural thickening can result. Pneumothorax is very rare.

Lymph nodes   Lymphadenopathy is very common in sarcoidosis. Intrathoracic nodes are enlarged in 75 to 90 percent of all patients; usually this involves the hilar nodes, but the paratracheal nodes are commonly involved (Fig. 277-2A). Less frequently, there is enlargement of subcarinal, anterior mediastinal, or posterior mediastinal nodes. Peripheral lymphadenopathy is very common, particularly involving the cervical, axillary, epitrochlear, and inguinal nodes. The nodes in the retroperitoneal area and in the mesenteric chain can also enlarge. All of these nodes are nonadherent, with a firm, rubbery texture. Palpation causes no pain. Unlike nodes in tuberculosis, the nodes do not ulcerate. The lymphadenopathy rarely causes a problem for the affected individual; however, if it is massive, it can be disfiguring and can impinge on other organs and lead to functional impairment.

Skin   Sarcoidosis involves the skin in about 25 percent of cases. The most common lesions are erythema nodosum, plaques, maculopapular eruptions, subcutaneous nodules, and lupus pernio. Erythema nodosum, comprising bilateral, tender red nodules on the anterior surface of the legs, is not specific for sarcoidosis but is common, particularly in acute sarcoidosis, in combination with systemic symptoms and polyarthralgias. Treatment is not required since the lesions resolve spontaneously in 2 to 4 weeks. Erythema nodosum is much more common among sarcoid patients in Europe than in the United States. Skin plaques associated with sarcoid are purple, indolent lesions, often raised, and usually occur on the face, buttocks, and extremities. The maculopapular eruptions occur on the face around the eyes and nose, on the back, and on the extremities. These are elevated lesions less than 1 cm in diameter with a flat, waxy top. Subcutaneous nodules are most common on the trunk and extremities. Lupus pernio is characterized by indurated blue-purple, swollen, shiny lesions on the nose, cheeks, lips, ears, fingers, and knees. The lesions on the tip of the nose cause a bulbous appearance, sometimes associated with varicosities. The nasal mucosa is usually involved, and underlying bone can be destroyed. Sarcoidosis can also involve old surgical scars and tattoos. Although it may be disfiguring, cutaneous sarcoidosis rarely causes major problems. Clubbing of the fingers is occasionally observed in sarcoidosis if there is extensive pulmonary fibrosis.

Eye   Eye involvement occurs in approximately 25 percent of patients with sarcoidosis, and it can cause blindness. The usual lesions involve the uveal tract, iris, ciliary body, and choroid. Of those cases with eye involvement, approximately 75 percent have anterior uveitis and 25 to 35 percent have posterior uveitis. There is blurred vision, tearing, and photophobia. The uveitis can develop

FIGURE 277-2   Common laboratory findings of sarcoidosis. *A.* Schematic view of the abnormal findings on the chest x-ray. Shown are changes observed with the average frequency of occurrence. *B.* Typical gallium 67 scan of an individual with active sarcoidosis. The isotope has accumulated in the lung parenchyma (LP), liver (L), spleen (S), parotid (P), hilar nodes (HN), and pelvic nodes (PN). *C.* Cells recovered by bronchoalveolar lavage of an individual with active pulmonary sarcoidosis. The lavage analysis reflects the inflammation in the tissue. Shown are alveolar macrophages (large cells) and lymphocytes (small cells). The cell population is dominated by lymphocytes, in contrast to normals, in whom lymphocytes represent <20 percent of the cell population.

rapidly and may clear spontaneously over a 6- to 12-month period. It can also develop insidiously and be chronic. Conjunctival involvement is also common, usually with small, yellow nodules. When the lacrimal gland is involved, a keratoconjunctivitis sicca syndrome, with dry, sore eyes, can result.

Upper respiratory tract The nasal mucosa is involved in up to 20 percent of patients, usually presenting with nasal stuffiness. Any of the structures of the mouth can be involved, particularly the tonsils. Sarcoidosis involves the larynx in about 5 percent of cases. The epiglottis and areas around the true vocal cords are usually involved, but the cords themselves are not. These individuals are usually hoarse and they have dyspnea, wheezing, and stridor; complete obstruction can occur.

Bone marrow and spleen Sarcoidosis of the marrow is reported in 15 to 40 percent of cases, but it rarely causes hematologic abnormalities other than a mild anemia, neutropenia, and eosinophilia, and occasionally thrombocytopenia. Although splenomegaly occurs in only 5 to 10 percent of patients, celiac angiography or splenic biopsy reveals involvement in 50 to 60 percent of cases. The presentation and complications of splenomegaly in sarcoidosis are similar to those of splenomegaly in general.

Liver Although liver biopsy reveals liver involvement in 60 to 90 percent of cases, usually it is not important clinically. Sarcoidosis involves generally the periportal areas. Approximately 20 to 30 percent have hepatomegaly and/or biochemical evidence of liver involvement. Usually these changes reflect a cholestatic pattern and include an elevated alkaline phosphatase level; the bilirubin and aminotransferases are only mildly elevated, and jaundice is rare. Rarely, portal hypertension can occur, as can intrahepatic cholestasis with cirrhosis.

Kidney Clinically apparent primary renal involvement in sarcoidosis is rare, although tubular, glomerular, and renal artery disease have been reported. More commonly, but still in only 1 to 2 percent of all cases, there is a disorder of calcium metabolism with hypercalciuria, with or without hypercalcemia. If chronic, nephrocalcinosis and nephrolithiasis can result. It is believed that the calcium abnormalities are associated with enhanced calcium absorption in the gut, which is related to an abnormally high level of circulating 1,25-dihydroxyvitamin D produced by mononuclear phagocytes in the granulomas.

Nervous system All components of the nervous system can be involved in sarcoidosis. Neurologic findings are observed in about 5 percent of patients. Seventh nerve involvement with unilateral facial paralysis is most common. It occurs suddenly and is usually transient. Other common manifestations of neurosarcoid include optic nerve dysfunction, papilledema, palate dysfunction, hearing abnormalities, hypothalamic and pituitary abnormalities, chronic meningitis, and occasionally, space-occupying lesions. Psychiatric disturbances have been described, and seizures can occur. Rarely, multiple lesions which mimic multiple sclerosis, spinal cord abnormalities, and peripheral neuropathy can occur.

Musculoskeletal system The bones, joints, and/or muscles can be involved in sarcoidosis. Bone lesions are observed in 5 percent of patients and include variable-sized cysts in areas of expanded bone, well-defined round punched-out lesions, or lattice-like changes. Hand and foot bones are the common sites, but most bones can be involved. Occasionally, the bone lesions are tender and painful. Joint involvement is more common, with an incidence of 25 to 50 percent in known cases of sarcoidosis. Arthralgias and frank arthritis occur mostly in large joints; they can be migratory and are usually transient, but can be chronic and result in deformities. Although muscle biopsy frequently demonstrates granulomatous inflammation, muscle dysfunction is rare. However, nodules, polymyositis, and chronic myopathy have been described.

Heart Approximately 5 percent of patients have significant heart involvement, with clinical evidence of cardiac dysfunction. Left ventricular wall involvement is common. Arrhythmias are frequent, and serious conduction disturbances, including complete heart block, can occur. Papillary muscle dysfunction, pericarditis, and congestive heart failure are also observed. Cor pulmonale secondary to chronic pulmonary fibrosis may occur but is uncommon.

Endocrine and reproductive system The hypothalamic-pituitary axis is the part of the endocrine system most commonly involved; this usually presents as diabetes insipidus. Anterior pituitary dysfunction is also seen, manifesting as a deficiency in one or more pituitary hormones. Complete hypopituitarism is rare. Much less frequently, sarcoidosis can cause primary dysfunction of other endocrine glands. Adrenal cortical involvement resulting in Addison's syndrome has been described. Involvement of the reproductive organs occurs, but infertility is rare. Pregnancy is not affected by sarcoidosis, and patients with sarcoidosis who become pregnant usually improve during pregnancy. However, the disease may flare post partum; presumably this variation results from fluctuations in endogenous glucocorticoid production.

Exocrine glands Parotid enlargement is a classic feature of sarcoidosis, but clinically apparent parotid involvement occurs in less than 10 percent of patients. Bilateral involvement is the rule. The gland is usually nontender, firm, and smooth. Xerostomia can occur; other exocrine glands are affected only rarely.

Gastrointestinal tract Although sarcoidosis involvement of the gastrointestinal tract is found occasionally at autopsy, it rarely has clinical importance. Occasionally, patients have esophageal or gastric symptoms.

COMPLICATIONS The respiratory tract abnormalities cause most of the morbidity and mortality associated with sarcoidosis. The major problems are those characteristic of interstitial lung disease (see Chap. 211), particularly dyspnea and insufficient oxygen delivery to vital organs. Respiratory failure with carbon dioxide retention is rare. In some patients, lung destruction results in formation of bullae that may harbor mycetomas, which are usually aspergillomas; erosion into the parenchyma can result in massive bleeding. The most common complications apart from the lung are associated with the eye; however, with therapy blindness is rare. Complications of other organs include a gamut of abnormalities. The most serious are central nervous system lesions or cardiac involvement leading to congestive heart failure or sudden death.

LABORATORY ABNORMALITIES Common abnormalities in the blood include lymphocytopenia, an occasional mild eosinophilia, an increased erythrocyte sedimentation rate, hyperglobulinemia, and an elevated level of angiotensin-converting enzyme. Hypercalcemia is rare. Other serum abnormalities relate to involvement of specific organs such as liver, kidney, or endocrine glands.

Because the lung is involved so commonly, the routine chest film is almost always abnormal (Fig. 277-2A). The three classic x-ray patterns of pulmonary sarcoidosis are type I—bilateral hilar adenopathy with no parenchymal abnormalities; type II—bilateral hilar adenopathy with diffuse parenchymal changes; and type III—diffuse parenchymal changes without hilar adenopathy. The type III pattern is sometimes split into two categories with films that show fibrosis and upper lobe retraction classified separately. Although patients with type I x-rays tend to have the acute or subacute, reversible form of the disease while those with types II and III often have the chronic, progressive disease, these patterns do not represent the "stages" of sarcoidosis. Thus, except for epidemiologic purposes, this x-ray categorization is mostly of historic interest. The hilar adenopathy is almost always bilateral, but unilateral node enlargement can be seen. Nodes are also common in the paratracheal region. The diffuse parenchymal changes are typically reticulonodular infiltrates, but an acinar pattern is observed occasionally. Large nodules, similar to those of metastatic disease, are unusual but can occur. When there is massive fibrosis, the hila are pulled upward and there are conglomerate masses in the midlung zones. Some of the unusual chest x-ray findings in sarcoidosis include "egg shell" calcification of hilar nodes, pleural effusions, cavitation, atelectasis, pulmonary hypertension, pneumothorax, and cardiomegaly.

The lung function abnormalities of sarcoidosis are typical for interstitial lung disease (see Chap. 211) and include decreased lung volumes and diffusing capacity with a normal or supernormal ratio of the forced expiratory volume in 1 s to the forced vital capacity. Occasionally there is evidence of airflow limitation. There is usually mild hypoxemia and a mild, compensated hypocarbia.

The gallium 67 lung scan is usually abnormal, showing a pattern of diffuse uptake. If present, enlarged nodes are detected in these scans, as is inflammation in a variety of extrathoracic sites that usually have no clinical importance (Fig. 277-2*B*). Bronchoalveolar lavage demonstrates typically an increased proportion of lymphocytes, most of which are activated helper-inducer T lymphocytes (Fig. 277-2*C*). The remainder of the cells are mostly alveolar macrophages. In patients with significant fibrosis, a small number of neutrophils are also found. Eosinophils are rare.

The other laboratory features of sarcoidosis depend on the specific organ involved.

DIAGNOSIS   For a typical case, the diagnosis of sarcoidosis is made by a combination of clinical, radiographic, and histologic findings. In a young adult with constitutional complaints, respiratory symptoms, erythema nodosum, blurred vision, and bilateral hilar adenopathy, the diagnosis is almost always sarcoidosis. Commonly, however, the findings are more subtle. Furthermore, because sarcoidosis can occur in almost any place in the body, like tuberculosis or syphilis, it can be confused with many other disorders. In this context, the differential diagnosis of sarcoidosis must cover a wide range. However, it is confused most commonly with neoplastic diseases such as lymphoma or with disorders characterized also by a mononuclear cell granulomatous inflammatory process, such as the mycobacterial and fungal disorders.

The presence of skin anergy is typical but not diagnostic of sarcoidosis. The Kveim-Siltzbach skin test, the intradermal injection of a heat-treated suspension of a sarcoidosis spleen extract which is biopsied 4 to 6 weeks later, yields sarcoidosis-like lesions in 70 to 80 percent of individuals with sarcoidosis with less than 5 percent false-positives. However, the material is not widely available, and with the use of the transbronchial biopsy to obtain lung parenchyma for diagnostic purposes, the Kveim-Siltzbach test is not in general use.

No blood findings are diagnostic of the disease. Angiotensin-converting enzyme is elevated in the serum in approximately two-thirds of patients with sarcoidosis, but false-positives and false-negatives are common. An elevated 24-h urine calcium level is consistent with the diagnosis, but is not specific.

The chest x-ray cannot be used as the sole criterion for the diagnosis of sarcoidosis. While the finding of bilateral hilar adenopathy is the hallmark of this disease, a similar pattern is occasionally observed in lymphoma, tuberculosis, coccidioidomycosis, brucellosis, and bronchogenic carcinoma.

The pattern of the gallium 67 scan is not diagnostic for sarcoidosis nor is the finding of an increased proportion of lymphocytes among the cells recovered by bronchoalveolar lavage. However, the typical patterns of these tests (Fig. 277-2*B* and *C*) put the diagnosis in the general category of granulomatous lung disorders.

Whether or not the presentation is "classic," biopsy evidence of a mononuclear cell granulomatous inflammatory process is mandatory in order to make a definitive diagnosis of sarcoidosis. Because the lung is involved so frequently, it is the most common site to be biopsied, usually through a fiberoptic bronchoscope. Less common, but acceptable, sites for biopsy are the hilar nodes (by mediastinoscopy), the skin, conjunctiva, or lip. Rarely, the spleen, intraabdominal nodes, muscle, parotid or other salivary glands, upper respiratory tract, or the heart are biopsied for diagnostic purposes. At any of these sites, the findings must include the typical noncaseating granulomas. However, although histologic evidence is mandatory for a definitive diagnosis of sarcoidosis, the histologic findings are not sufficiently specific to make the diagnosis by themselves, as noncaseating granulomas are found in a number of other diseases, including infections and malignancy. Furthermore, although the liver or scalene nodes often reveal "positive" biopsies in cases of sarcoidosis, noncaseating granulomas from other causes are so frequent in these sites that they are not considered acceptable sites for establishing the diagnosis. Thus, the definitive diagnosis of sarcoidosis is based on the biopsy in the context of the history, physical examination, blood tests, x-ray, lung function, and, if available, gallium 67 scan and bronchoalveolar lavage. Patients with immunodeficiency virus (HIV) infection commonly have lymphocytopenia, chest x-ray abnormalities, positive gallium 67 chest scans, increased proportions of lavage lymphocytes (early in the course of the disease), and can have lung granulomas, and thus serologic testing for HIV infection should always be done in individuals suspected of having sarcoidosis.

PROGNOSIS   Overall, the prognosis in sarcoidosis is good. Most individuals who present with the acute disease are left with no significant sequela. Approximately half of all patients have some permanent organ dysfunction, but for most, this is mild, stable, and progresses rarely. In approximately 15 to 20 percent of cases, the disease remains active or recurs intermittently. Death is attributable directly to the disease in about 10 percent of all those affected.

TREATMENT   The therapy of choice for sarcoidosis is glucocorticoids. A variety of other drugs have been tried, including indomethacin, oxyphenbutazone, chloroquine, methotrexate, *p*-aminobenzoate, allopurinol, levamisole, and cyclophosphamide, but there is no evidence, apart from anecdotal, uncontrolled reports, to support their efficacy. Cyclosporine is ineffective for the pulmonary manifestations of the disease; anecdotal reports suggest it may be useful in extrathoracic sarcoid not responding to glucocorticoids.

The major problem in treating sarcoidosis is in deciding when to treat. Because the disease clears spontaneously in about 50 percent of patients, and because the permanent organ derangements often do not improve with glucocorticoids, there is controversy among clinicians as to the criteria for treatment. However, there is no question that glucocorticoids suppress effectively the activated T-helper-inducer-cell processes occurring at the sites of disease. Thus the major problem in making decisions concerning therapy in sarcoidosis is to determine the extent and activity of the inflammatory process in the organs at greatest risk, such as the lung, eye, heart, and central nervous system.

For the lung, this is based on a combination of history, physical findings, chest x-ray, and pulmonary function tests. Centers that see large numbers of these individuals also use criteria based on gallium 67 lung scans and bronchoalveolar lavage findings. The serum level of the angiotensin-converting enzyme has been suggested as a criterion for disease activity, but it is not specific for the lung. Unless the respiratory impairment is devastating, active pulmonary sarcoidosis is observed usually without therapy for 2 to 3 months; if the inflammation does not subside spontaneously, therapy is instituted. For the eye, decisions concerning therapy are based on slit-lamp examination and tests for visual acuity. For the heart and central nervous system, decisions are based on an estimate of the severity of the involvement; patients with minor dysfunction are usually observed, while patients with significant cardiac or neurologic abnormalities are treated. Usually, it is not necessary to treat the systemic symptoms, but occasionally the extent of the fevers, fatigue, and/or weight loss will necessitate therapy.

The usual therapy for sarcoidosis is prednisone, 1 mg/kg, for 4 to 6 weeks followed by a slow taper over 2 to 3 months. This is repeated if the disease again becomes active. Alternate-day therapy is used by some clinicians, but there is no evidence that it is as effective. High-dose bolus intravenous glucocorticoids are used occasionally, but are probably not as effective as oral therapy. Inhaled glucocorticoids are not efficacious. Mild ocular disease responds usually to local therapy but suppression of the uveitis often requires systemic glucocorticoids.

REFERENCES

CRYSTAL RG Interstitial lung disease of unknown etiology: Disorders characterized by chronic inflammation of the lower respiratory tract. N Engl J Med 310:154, 235, 1984

FANBURG BL, PITT EA: Sarcoidosis, in *Textbook of Respiratory Medicine*, JF Murray, JA Nadel (eds). Philadelphia, Saunders, 1988, pp 1486–1500

GRASSI C et al: *Sarcoidosis and Other Granulomatous Disorders, Proceedings of the XI World Congress.* Amsterdam, Excerpta Medica, 1988

HUNNINGHAKE GW et al: Maintenance of granuloma formation in pulmonary sarcoidosis by T-lymphocytes within the lung. N Engl J Med 302:594, 1980

JOHNS CJ: Sarcoidosis, in *Pulmonary Diseases and Disorders*, AP Fishman (ed). New York, McGraw-Hill, 1988, pp 645–666

MOLLER DR et al: Bias toward use of a specific T-cell receptor β-chain variable region in a subgroup of individuals with sarcoidosis. J Clin Invest 82:1183, 1988

PINKSTON P et al: Spontaneous release of interleukin-2 by lung T-lymphocytes in active pulmonary sarcoidosis. N Engl J Med 208:793, 1983

ROBINSON BWS et al: Gamma interferon is spontaneously released by alveolar macrophages and lung T-lymphocytes in patients with pulmonary sarcoidosis. J Clin Invest 75:1488, 1985

SALTINI C et al: Spontaneous release of interleukin-2 by lung T-lymphocytes in active pulmonary sarcoidosis is primarily from the Leu3 + DR + T-cell subset. J Clin Invest 77:1962, 1986

SHARMA OP: *Sarcoidosis: Clinical Management.* London, Butterworth, 1984

VENET A et al: Enhanced alveolar macrophage-mediated antigen-induced T-lymphocyte proliferation in sarcoidosis. J Clin Invest 75:293, 1985

278 FAMILIAL MEDITERRANEAN FEVER (FAMILIAL PAROXYSMAL POLYSEROSITIS)

SHELDON M. WOLFF

DEFINITION Familial Mediterranean fever (FMF) is an inherited disorder of unknown etiology, characterized by recurrent episodes of fever, peritonitis, and/or pleuritis. Arthritis, skin lesions, and amyloidosis are seen in some patients.

TERMINOLOGY The variety of names given to FMF has led to confusion concerning its clinical features. None of the names, including FMF, is completely satisfactory. Such terms as *periodic disease* and *periodic peritonitis* are inaccurate because the disease usually is not cyclical. *Benign paroxysmal peritonitis* is inappropriate because many of the patients have involvement of serosal surfaces other than the peritoneum, and some die of amyloidosis. *Familial paroxysmal polyserositis* is an acceptable alternative for the term *familial Mediterranean fever*.

ETHNOLOGY AND GENETICS FMF occurs predominantly in patients of non-Ashkenazi (Sephardic) Jewish, Armenian, and Arabic ancestry. However, the disease is not restricted to these groups, and has been seen in patients of Italian, Ashkenazi Jewish, and Anglo-Saxon descent as well as others.

The best studies of the genetics of FMF have been done in Israel, where the disease appears to be inherited as an autosomal recessive. Nevertheless, approximately 50 percent of patients give no family history of the disease. Consanguinity among the parents of FMF patients is as high as 20 percent, a figure which may be an underestimate. Approximately 60 percent of patients are male.

ETIOLOGY Although numerous pathogenetic mechanisms have been suggested, the etiology of FMF is unknown. Fever and inflammation are such prominent signs that frequent attempts have been made to implicate infectious agents and/or their products. However, extensive studies have failed to implicate these or any other specific infectious agents. Recently it has been suggested that FMF is caused by an abnormality of catecholamine metabolism. Others have suggested defects in complement, thus implicating alterations in the immune system. Substantiation of such potential pathogenic mechanisms is awaited.

It has been suggested that FMF may be a pathologic exaggeration of normal periodic temperature rhythmicity. However, extensive studies of temperature and other circadian rhythms in FMF patients have failed to demonstrate alterations from normal.

Because many FMF patients note that certain emotional or environmental changes may have profound effects on the frequency with which episodes of their disease occur, a psychosomatic basis has been suggested for the illness. There is no question that most patients eventually have transient or even permanent psychological alterations, which probably reflect their reaction to a chronic recurring illness that is forever threatening their social, economic, and personal well-being, but there is no evidence for a functional etiology for FMF.

The demonstration that FMF is inherited as an autosomal recessive disorder has led to the thesis that it is another inborn error of metabolism. Despite extensive studies, no such error has been found. Reported instances of excessive urinary excretion of porphyrins in FMF are probably examples of true porphyria and not FMF.

It has been reported that blood levels of unconjugated etiocholanolone were elevated during fever in six patients with FMF. Subsequent studies, however, showed no correlation between levels of etiocholanolone and fever.

PATHOLOGY Despite the striking clinical manifestations during an acute attack of FMF, no specific pathologic alterations have been found. At laparotomy, only acute peritoneal inflammation in which the exudate contains a predominance of polymorphonuclear leukocytes is found to be present. A disproportionately large number of male patients develop gallbladder disease with and without cholelithiasis, but extensive histopathologic examination has failed to reveal any specific pathologic changes. Pleural and joint inflammation are also nonspecific.

In the amyloidosis which accompanies FMF, amyloid is deposited in the intima and media of the arterioles, the subendothelial region of venules, the glomeruli, and the spleen. Aside from their vessels, the heart and liver are uninvolved.

MANIFESTATIONS In the majority of patients, the symptoms of FMF begin between the ages of 5 and 15, although attacks sometimes commence during infancy, and onset has occurred as late as age 52. The duration and frequency of attacks vary greatly in the same patient, and there is no set rhythm or periodicity to their occurrence. The usual acute episode lasts 24 to 48 h, but some may be prolonged for 7 to 10 days. The attacks range in frequency from twice weekly to once a year, but 2 to 4 weeks is the commonest interval. Spontaneous remissions lasting years have been seen. In the majority of cases, pregnancy is associated with an absence of acute episodes, and many patients note less frequent attacks in the summer than in the winter. There may be a decrease in the severity and frequency of the attacks with age or with development of amyloidosis.

Fever Fever is a cardinal manifestation of FMF and is present during most but not all attacks. Rarely, fever may be present without serositis. The temperature may be preceded by a chill and will peak in 12 to 24 h. Defervescence is often accompanied by diaphoresis. The fever ranges from 38.5 to 40°C but is quite variable.

Abdominal pain Abdominal pain occurs in more than 95 percent of patients, and may vary in severity in the same patient. Minor premonitory discomfort may precede an acute episode by 24 to 48 h. The pain usually starts in one quadrant and then spreads to involve the whole abdomen. The initial site is usually very tender. Tenderness may remain localized with referred pain in other areas, and there may be radiation to the back. There may be splinting of the chest and pain in one or both shoulders, typical of diaphragmatic irritation. Nausea and vomiting sometimes occur. The abdomen is usually distended, and may become rigid with decreased or absent bowel sounds. On x-ray, the wall of the small intestine may appear edematous, transit of barium is slowed, and fluid levels may be seen. An abdominal operation may precipitate an acute attack of FMF which may be confused with other postoperative complications.

Chest pain Most patients with abdominal attacks have referred chest pain at one time or another, and 75 percent also develop acute pleuritic pain with or without abdominal symptoms. In 30 percent, the attacks of pleuritis precede the onset of abdominal attacks by varying periods of time, and a small number of patients never develop abdominal attacks. Chest pain is usually unilateral and is associated with diminished breath sounds, a friction rub, or a transient pleural effusion.

Joint pain In Israel, 75 percent of patients report at least one episode of acute arthritis. Arthritis can be distinct from abdominal or pleural attacks, can be acute or, rarely, chronic, and may involve one or several joints. Effusions are common and the large joints are involved most frequently. Radiologic findings are nonspecific. Despite careful search, frank arthritis rarely has been seen in the United States. Some patients have a history of rheumatic fever–like illness in childhood, but in a large series of patients, including 30 from the Middle East, acute arthritis was not observed. Mild arthralgia is common during acute attacks but is nonspecific.

Skin manifestations Skin involvement is reported by 25 to 35 percent of patients. These lesions consist of painful, erythematous areas of swelling from 5 to 20 cm in diameter, usually located on the lower legs, the medial malleolus, or the dorsum of the foot. They may occur without abdominal or pleural pain and subside within 24 to 48 h.

Other signs and symptoms Involvement of other serosal membranes has been reported, but pericarditis and meningitis are rare. Hematuria, splenomegaly, and small white dots called *colloid bodies* in the ocular fundus are among the findings of questionable significance. Rarely migraine-like headaches accompany acute abdominal attacks, and some patients have become somewhat irrational or show extreme emotional lability during attacks. Whether these are primary manifestations of FMF or secondary effects of pain and fever is not known.

Complications A serious, but increasingly uncommon, complication of FMF is drug addiction or habituation. Obviously, efforts should be made to avoid use of narcotics. Depression and lack of motivation are common, and patients with FMF require considerable encouragement and support. A striking number of patients in one American series have developed gallbladder disease.

Amyloidosis has been reported in Israel, North Africa, and elsewhere in the Middle East, but there have been only rare reported instances of amyloidosis complicating FMF in the United States. These findings are even more striking because there are probably as many known FMF patients in the United States as in Israel. These differences are unexplained and suggest that environmental or nutritional, as well as genetic, factors may play a role in the development of amyloidosis in FMF.

LABORATORY FINDINGS Polymorphonuclear leukocytosis ranging from 10,000 to 30,000 cells per microliter is almost invariable during acute attacks. The erythrocyte sedimentation rate is elevated during attacks but returns to normal between attacks. Plasma fibrinogen, serum haptoglobin, ceruloplasmin, and C-reactive protein increase during the episodes. Increased levels of plasma dopamine beta-hydroxylase activity have been reported in FMF patients (see below). Plasma lipids are normal, and there are no consistent abnormalities of hepatic or renal function. When amyloidosis is present, laboratory findings are typical of a nephrotic syndrome followed by renal insufficiency. Electrocardiographic and electroencephalographic changes are inconstant and nonspecific.

DIAGNOSIS When the typical acute attacks of FMF occur in an individual of appropriate ethnic background who has a family history of FMF, the diagnosis is easy. When a patient is seen for the first time, a variety of other febrile illnesses must be excluded by appropriate study or observation. These include acute appendicitis, acute pancreatitis, porphyria, cholecystitis, intestinal obstruction, and other major abdominal catastrophes.

Some of the inherited forms of the hyperlipidemias may mimic the clinical picture of FMF, but lipid analysis will eliminate them from consideration. The patient with FMF is not immune to other diseases, and when an attack differs from the usual pattern or is more prolonged, consideration should be given to other diagnostic possibilities. The pleural form of the disease is sometimes difficult to differentiate from acute pulmonary infection or infarction, but the rapid disappearance of signs and symptoms resolves the problem. The joint manifestations may be more prolonged than other forms of FMF, and differentiation from septic arthritis, gout, and acute rheumatoid disease may be necessary. The erythema is sometimes difficult to differentiate from superficial thrombophlebitis or cellulitis.

Whether or not the patient is of the appropriate ethnic group, the most difficult diagnostic problem in FMF is the patient who presents with fever alone. In this situation, an extensive diagnostic workup for fever of unknown origin may be required. Fortunately, such patients are rare, and all eventually develop serosal involvement. Until specific diagnostic tests for FMF are available, patients with recurrent fever but without signs of inflammation of one of the serosal membranes should not be categorized as having FMF.

Recently it has been reported that FMF patients have increased levels of plasma dopamine beta-hydroxylase (RHP) activity and that these levels returned to normal during colchicine treatment. Confirmation of these findings should provide the basis for the first diagnostic test for FMF.

PROGNOSIS Despite the severity of the symptoms during some acute attacks, most patients are remarkably free of any debilitation during the intervals between attacks. With encouragement and an understanding of their disease, most FMF patients lead fairly normal lives. The greatest hazard to patients is prolonged periods of hospitalization due to erroneous diagnoses or failure to understand the disease. In the United States, the prognosis of patients with FMF does not seem to be different from that of patients with other chronic nonfatal illnesses. Death usually results from causes unrelated to the underlying disease.

The complication of amyloidosis in Israel, parts of North Africa, Turkey, and other parts of the Middle East makes the prognosis quite different from that in America. In the past, approximately 25 percent of FMF patients in Israel were known to have amyloidosis, and this complication usually led to death. However, the widespread use of colchicine has resulted in dramatically decreasing the incidence of amyloidosis.

TREATMENT Among the therapies tried have been antibiotics, hormones (including estrogens and adrenal corticosteroids), antipyretic drugs, immunotherapy, psychotherapy, elimination and low-fat diets, chloroquine, and phenylbutazone. When carefully studied and followed up, none of these therapies proved effective.

During the past 15 years, the outlook of patients with FMF has been altered dramatically. Goldfinger reported in 1972 that the prophylactic use of colchicine in five patients dramatically reduced the number of attacks. Subsequently, controlled trials in the United States and Israel have shown that chronic administration of colchicine will greatly reduce the number of acute attacks of FMF. It is recommended that 0.6 mg colchicine be taken by mouth three times a day. Patients often develop gastrointestinal side effects with this dose, however, in which case the dose should be reduced to 0.6 mg taken twice a day. Although an occasional patient will respond to 0.6 mg taken only once a day, this amount is less likely to be beneficial. Most FMF patients will respond favorably to colchicine prophylaxis.

In some patients, intermittent therapy may be beneficial. The patient should take 0.6 mg colchicine by mouth every hour for 4 h, then every 2 h for 4 h, and every 12 h thereafter for 48 h. The colchicine should be given at the first premonitory sign of an attack. If both acute and prophylactic colchicine therapy fail, supportive therapy is all that can be offered. Except for unusual circumstances, narcotics should not be given to FMF patients.

REFERENCES

BARAKAT MH et al: Plasma dopamine beta-hydroxylase: Rapid diagnostic test for recurrent hereditary polyserositis. Lancet 2:1280, 1988

DINARELLO CA et al: Colchicine therapy for familial Mediterranean fever. A double-blind trial. N Engl J Med 291:934, 1974

MATZNER Y et al: C5a-Inhibitor deficiency in peritoneal fluids from patients with familial Mediterranean Fever. N Engl J Med 314:1001, 1986

MEYERHOFF J: Familial Mediterranean fever: Report of a large family, review of the literature, and discussion of the frequency of amyloidosis. Medicine 59:66, 1980

ZEMER D et al: Colchicine in the prevention and treatment of the amyloidosis of familial Mediterranean fever. N Engl J Med 314:1001, 1986

279 MIDLINE GRANULOMA

SHELDON M. WOLFF

DEFINITION Midline granuloma is an uncommon disease characterized by localized inflammation, destruction, and often mutilation of the tissues of the upper respiratory tract and face. This condition has also been referred to as *lethal midline granuloma, malignant granuloma,* and *granuloma gangrenescens,* none of which is an appropriate term.

ETIOLOGY The etiology of midline granuloma is unknown. In view of the intense granulomatous inflammation, the disease is thought to represent a localized hypersensitivity reaction which leads to tissue destruction and mutilation. However, the responsible antigen(s) is unknown, and there is no immunologic evidence supporting this hypothesis. A variety of microorganisms have been considered as possible causative agents, but detailed microbiologic investigations have failed to detect the consistent presence of pathogenic organisms. In view of the clinical and pathologic features of the illness as well as the fact that some tumors, such as malignant reticulosis (or polymorphic reticulosis), can elicit a similar intense inflammatory response, some authors have suggested a neoplastic basis for midline granuloma. However, when malignant tissue is found in the lesions, the diagnosis of midline granuloma is no longer tenable.

It is possible that midline granuloma is part of the spectrum of what has been recently termed *angiocentric immunoproliferative lesions.* The latter are considered to represent a spectrum of postthymic T-cell proliferative lesions. In fact, the association of malignant reticulosis and also of lymphomatoid granulomatosis with this group seems justified. Whether "idiopathic" midline granuloma is an early or arrested form of angiocentric immunoproliferative lesions awaits the kind of sophisticated immunocytologic studies that have been performed in patients with T-cell lymphoproliferative diseases.

PATHOLOGY The most characteristic pathologic finding is acute or chronic inflammation with necrosis. Superimposed pyogenic infection of the involved tissues, including the sinuses, may contribute to nonspecific histologic findings. The pathologic hallmark, noncaseating granulomas, with or without giant cells, may be obscured by the inflammatory reaction, but when present this is strong evidence in favor of the diagnosis. Primary vasculitis is seen rarely; when it occurs, a search for other causes, most notably Wegener's granulomatosis, should be made (see Chap. 276). The presence of malignant cells makes the diagnosis of midline granuloma unacceptable. Until an etiology is established, the diagnosis of midline granuloma will rest on the characteristic clinical features outlined below.

CLINICAL FEATURES The disease may occur at any age, but the majority of patients are in the fifth and sixth decades. It is more common in women than men and has been reported in all races. Many patients report recurrent "sinus" problems, and some have histories of allergic rhinitis, although the significance of these features is unknown.

The major symptoms are usually related to the nose. Patients frequently complain of nasal stuffiness and occasionally of discharge. The first symptom in a smaller percentage of patients relates to ulceration of the mucosa of the nose, the buccal mucosa, or the gums. This has led to loosening of the teeth, and dentists are often consulted first by these patients. Rarely, patients will present first with eye findings related to conjunctival inflammation or even ulceration. Although the progression of symptoms in some patients may be slow, all too often the disease steadily, and sometimes rapidly, progresses. The characteristic symptoms of nasal discharge, difficulty in breathing through the nose, and pain over the sinuses, nose, or eye become more prominent with time. Once ulceration begins, the disease often progresses rapidly. The ulcers frequently involve the nasal septum and will lead to the characteristic septal perforation and a saddlenose deformity. The majority of patients develop ulceration and eventually perforations of the soft and hard palates. Untreated, the disease can lead to massive destruction and mutilation of the tissues involved, including the skin of the face and the eyes. Frequently, the necrotic tissue becomes infected, and systemic symptoms such as fever and anorexia appear. The destructive lesions can become very malodorous. The disease extends to involve local tissues and does not progress below the neck; if this happens, other diseases should be considered. As the necrotic process progresses and involves vital organs, patients may lose sight in the affected eye, experience dysphagia, and have difficulty in speech. Although spontaneous temporary remissions have been reported, untreated midline granuloma is fatal. The progression of the disease can be rapidly accelerated by surgical procedures in the affected areas. The patient usually dies from secondary infection, although erosion by the process into a major blood vessel or penetration into the central nervous system with superimposed meningitis can also cause death.

Aside from the granulomatous inflammation, necrosis, and destruction, no other specific clinical or pathologic findings are associated with midline granuloma. Occasionally, with superimposed infection, local lymphadenopathy may be noted, but it is not characteristic of the disease per se.

LABORATORY FINDINGS With progression of the disease, a variety of nonspecific abnormalities may be noted. These changes are characteristic of inflammatory processes in general or of secondary infections. For example, mild anemia, leukocytosis, elevated sedimentation rate, and hyperglobulinemia are common in these patients. Radiographic examination reveals pansinusitis, and as the disease advances, destruction of bone in the involved areas is characteristic.

DIFFERENTIAL DIAGNOSIS The diagnosis of midline granuloma is made by finding the characteristic histologic lesions in biopsies of the affected tissues. When the specimens show only inflammatory tissue, a presumptive diagnosis of midline granuloma can be made only when the characteristic clinical picture is present and other diseases with similar presentation have been excluded. The diagnosis of Wegener's granulomatosis is ruled out by the absence of vasculitis in the biopsy specimens and the localized nature of midline granuloma (i.e., no pulmonary or renal involvement). In addition, Wegener's granulomatosis rarely, if ever, causes erosion through facial tissues. It is often difficult to differentiate true midline granuloma from neoplasms of the upper airways such as malignant reticulosis and certain lymphomas. These may be clinically similar to midline granuloma and are often associated with granulomatous inflammation. Careful examination of generous biopsy material as well as concomitant workup for disseminated neoplasm often provides the clinicopathologic distinction. Other diseases to be excluded by appropriate laboratory techniques are histoplasmosis, blastomycosis, coccidioidomycosis, leprosy, tuberculosis, syphilis, mucocutaneous leishmaniasis, rhinoscleroma, and pseudotumor of the orbit. Occasional patients who inhale cocaine develop septal perforations with inflammation that may be difficult to differentiate from midline granuloma (if the patients deny cocaine abuse).

TREATMENT The complications of midline granuloma such as superimposed infections can be treated specifically. Although adrenal glucocorticoids are often used in the therapy of midline granuloma, they are of no value and probably are contraindicated if infection is present. Sporadic reports of therapy with cytotoxic agents are difficult to interpret, since some of the patients reported clearly had lymphoma or Wegener's granulomatosis, diseases where such agents are of definite value. However, some patients appear to respond to cytotoxic chemotherapy. Surgical removal of the involved tissue has been attempted but is useless and may, in fact, cause rapid progression of the disease.

The treatment of choice is radiotherapy to the local lesion. Although low dosages [10,000 mGy (1000 rad) and below] have been reported to be effective, many patients relapse after such therapy. Radiotherapy should be given in a dose of 50,000 mGy (5000 rad) to the involved areas. Where such a regimen is employed, long-lasting remissions (more than 20 years) and probable cures have been achieved. Following irradiation and after an appropriate period to allow for

tissue healing (usually 1 year), reconstructive and plastic surgery, which may be of enormous cosmetic and functional value, can be undertaken.

REFERENCES

FAUCI AS et al: Radiation therapy of midline granuloma. Ann Intern Med 84:140, 1976
FECHNER RE, LAMPPIN DW: Midline malignant reticulosis. Arch Otolaryngol 95:467, 1972
LIPFORD EH JR: Angiocentric immunoproliferative lesions: A clinicopathologic spectrum of post-thymic T-cell proliferation. Blood 72:1674, 1988

section 3 Disorders of the joints

280 APPROACH TO ARTICULAR AND MUSCULOSKELETAL DISORDERS

JOHN J. CUSH / PETER E. LIPSKY

Musculoskeletal complaints account for nearly 10 percent of all outpatient evaluations in general medical practice. Many of the musculoskeletal complaints that cause patients to seek medical attention are related to self-limited conditions requiring minimal evaluation and only symptomatic therapy and reassurance. However, some patients with similar symptoms may require additional laboratory testing to confirm a suspected diagnosis or document the extent and nature of the pathologic process. The initial goal of the clinician is to diagnose accurately and provide timely therapy while avoiding excessive diagnostic testing and unnecessary treatment.

Individuals with musculoskeletal complaints should be evaluated in a uniform, logical manner with a thorough history, a comprehensive physical examination, and appropriate laboratory testing. With such an approach and an understanding of the pathophysiologic processes underlying musculoskeletal complaints, an adequate diagnosis can be made in the vast majority of individuals. However, some patients will not fit immediately into an established diagnostic category. Many musculoskeletal disorders resemble each other at the outset and may take months or even years to evolve fully into a specific, recognizable syndrome. Such knowledge should temper the desire to establish a definitive diagnosis at the first encounter.

A paramount objective during the initial encounter is to determine whether the condition requires additional evaluation or immediate therapy. To make this decision, a knowledge of the particular anatomic sites of involvement (articular, periarticular, or extraarticular) and the nature of the pathologic processes (inflammatory or noninflammatory) is important (Table 280-1). Information derived from the patient's symptoms and signs allows the clinician to narrow the diagnostic considerations and assess the need for immediate diagnostic testing, therapeutic intervention, or continued observation over a period of time.

CLINICAL HISTORY Historic features of the disorder are important in establishing the nature and extent of the pathologic process and may also provide important clues to the diagnosis. Aspects of the patient profile including age, sex, race, and family history can provide important information. Certain diagnoses are more frequent

in different age groups. Systemic lupus erythematosus and Reiter's syndrome occur more frequently in the young, whereas fibrositis is most frequent in middle age and osteoarthritis and polymyalgia rheumatica are more prevalent among the elderly. Diagnostic clustering is also evident when *sex* and *race* are considered. Gout and the spondyloarthropathies are more common in men, whereas rheumatoid arthritis and fibrositis are more frequent in women. Racial predilections are noted with disorders such as polymyalgia rheumatica and giant cell arteritis (whites) and sarcoidosis (blacks). *Familial aggregation* may be seen in disorders such as ankylosing spondylitis, gout, rheumatoid arthritis, and Heberden's nodes of osteoarthritis.

The type of clinical presentation also provides important diagnostic clues. The *mode of onset* is characteristically acute in septic arthritis or gout, whereas osteoarthritis and fibrositis may have more indolent presentations.

Precipitating events such as trauma, drug administration, or antecedent illnesses should be sought. The *number and pattern* of involved structures often provide useful information. Disorders such as trauma and gout are typically focal, whereas others, such as polymyositis and fibrositis, are more diffuse in their involvement. Rheumatoid arthritis tends to be symmetric, whereas the spondyloarthropathies are asymmetric. The upper extremities are frequently involved in rheumatoid arthritis, whereas lower extremity arthritis is characteristic of Reiter's syndrome and gout at their onsets. Involvement of the axial skeleton is common in ankylosing spondylitis but is infrequent in rheumatoid arthritis with the notable exception of the

TABLE 280-1 Musculoskeletal disorders

I Anatomic sites of involvement	II Pathologic processes
A Articular	A Inflammatory
1 Synovium	1 Infectious
2 Articular cartilage	2 Crystal-induced
3 Juxtaarticular bone	3 Immunologic
4 Other—menisci, capsule	4 Reactive
B Periarticular	5 Idiopathic
1 Ligaments	B Noninflammatory
2 Tendons	1 Traumatic
3 Bursae	2 Mechanical or degenerative
C Extraarticular	3 Neoplastic
1 Muscle	4 Functional
2 Fascia	5 Other
3 Bone	
4 Nerve	
5 Skin and subcutaneous tissue	

cervical spine. The *chronology and evolution* of the patient's complaints may also be useful in suggesting diagnostic possibilities. Chronic (osteoarthritis), intermittent (gout), migratory (rheumatic fever), and additive (Reiter's syndrome) patterns are suggestive of certain disease processes. The duration of signs and symptoms alters the diagnostic considerations. Thus, the musculoskeletal signs and symptoms of hepatitis B virus infection may be identical with those of early rheumatoid arthritis, but rarely persist beyond 2 to 3 weeks.

Associated features outside the musculoskeletal system may also provide useful diagnostic information. A variety of musculoskeletal disorders may be associated with systemic features such as fever (systemic lupus erythematosus, infection), rash (systemic lupus erythematosus, Reiter's syndrome, rheumatic fever), or morning stiffness (inflammatory arthritis). In addition, some are associated with involvement of other organs including the eyes (Behçet's disease, sarcoid, Reiter's syndrome), the organs of the gastrointestinal tract (scleroderma, inflammatory bowel disease), the genitourinary tract (Reiter's syndrome, gonococcemia), or the nervous system (rheumatoid arthritis, vasculitis).

PHYSICAL EXAMINATION   The goal of the physical examination is to ascertain the structures involved, the nature of the disorder, the extent and functional consequences of the process, and the presence of systemic manifestations. A knowledge of topographic anatomy is necessary to identify the primary site(s) of involvement and differentiate between articular, periarticular, and extraarticular disease. The musculoskeletal evaluation is largely dependent on careful inspection, palpation, and a variety of specific physical maneuvers to elicit diagnostic signs.

Examination of involved and uninvolved joints will determine the absence or presence of *warmth, erythema,* or *swelling.* The examination should distinguish true articular swelling caused by synovial effusion or synovial proliferation from periarticular involvement which usually extends beyond the normal joint margins. Synovial effusion can be distinguished from synovial hypertrophy or bony hypertrophy by palpation. Bursal effusions (i.e., olecranon, prepatellar) overlie bony prominences and are fluctuant with sharply defined borders. Joint *stability* can be assessed by palpation and by the application of manual stress. Subluxation or dislocation, which may be secondary to traumatic, mechanical, or inflammatory causes, can be assessed by inspection and palpation. Joint *volume* can be assessed by palpation. Distention of the articular capsule by various processes causes pain. The patient will attempt to minimize the pain by maintaining the joint in the position of greatest volume and least intraarticular pressure, usually partial flexion. Clinically, this may be reflected as obvious swelling, voluntary or eventually fixed flexion deformities, or diminished range of motion, especially on extension when joint volumes are decreased. Active and passive *range of motion* should be assessed in all planes and is best quantified by a goniometer with contralateral comparison. Joint *crepitus* may be felt during these maneuvers and may be prominent in degenerative disorders. Limitation of motion is frequently caused by effusion, pain, deformity, or contracture. Contractures may be an indication of antecedent synovial inflammation. Joint *deformity* usually indicates a long-standing pathologic process. Deformities may result from ligament destruction, soft tissue contracture, bony enlargement, ankylosis, erosive disease, or subluxation. Examination of the musculature will document strength and the presence of atrophy, and also will elicit pain or spasm. The examiner should assess carefully for periarticular involvement, especially when articular complaints are not supported by objective findings referable to the joint capsule. The identification of musculoskeletal pain of soft tissue origin (periarticular or extraarticular) will prevent unwarranted and often expensive further evaluations.

ADDITIONAL INVESTIGATIONS   The vast majority of musculoskeletal disorders can be easily diagnosed by a complete history and physical examination. However, in a number of circumstances, additional investigations may be required to establish the diagnosis or confirm a suspected etiology. A number of features indicate the

need for additional evaluation. Patients with *acute monarticular* conditions require additional evaluation, as do those who present with *traumatic* or *inflammatory* conditions or those with *neurologic changes* or *systemic manifestations* of serious disease. Finally individuals with *chronic (>6 weeks)* symptoms, even of minor severity, are candidates for additional evaluation. The extent and nature of the additional investigation should be dictated by the pattern of the involvement and suspected pathologic process. Broad batteries of diagnostic tests and radiographic procedures are rarely a useful or cost-effective means to establish a diagnosis.

Besides a complete blood count, including a white blood cell and differential count, the routine evaluation should include a determination of the erythrocyte sedimentation rate, and C-reactive protein, which can be useful in discriminating inflammatory from noninflammatory musculoskeletal disorders.

Synovial fluid aspiration and analysis is always indicated in acute monarthritis or when a septic or crystal-induced arthropathy is suspected. Synovial fluid can be classified according to its appearance, cell count, glucose level, and viscosity. Noninflammatory synovial fluid is clear, amber-colored, with a white blood cell count of <3000 cells per microliter and a mononuclear cell predominance. The glucose concentration is normal and is usually within 0.55 to 0.83 mmol/L (10 to 15 mg/dL) of serum values. Synovial fluid viscosity is assessed by expressing fluid from the syringe one drop at a time. Normally there is a stringing effect, with a long tail behind each synovial drop. Such effusions are typical of osteoarthritis and trauma. Inflammatory fluid is turbid and yellow with an increased white cell count (3000 to 50,000 cells per microliter) and a polymorphonuclear leukocyte predominance. The protein is elevated, the glucose is normal or low, and the viscosity is poor, reflected by a short or nonexistent tail following each drop of synovial fluid. Such effusions are found in rheumatoid arthritis, gout, other inflammatory arthritides, and occasionally septic arthritis. Infectious fluid is turbid and opaque, with a white cell count >50,000 cells per microliter, and a polymorphonuclear leukocyte predominance. The protein is elevated, the glucose is low, and viscosity is poor. Such effusions are typical of septic arthritis but may rarely occur with sterile inflammatory arthritides such as rheumatoid arthritis or gout. Additionally, hemorrhagic synovial fluid may be seen with hemarthrosis or trauma. Synovial fluid should be analyzed immediately for crystals using a polarizing microscope. Monosodium urate, seen in gouty effusions, appears as long, needle-shaped, negatively birefringent, usually intracellular crystals, whereas calcium pyrophosphate dihydrate found in chondrocalcinosis and pseudogout is usually seen as short, rhomboid-shaped, positively birefringent crystals. When infection is suspected, synovial fluid should be Gram-stained and cultured appropriately. Whenever gonococcal arthritis is suspected, immediate plating of the fluid on appropriate culture medium is indicated. It should be noted that on occasion both crystal-induced arthritis and infection may occur in the same joint.

Serologic tests for rheumatoid factor (antibodies to IgG), antinuclear antibodies, complement levels, or antistreptolysin O titers should only be carried out when there is clinical evidence to suggest a specific diagnosis, as these have poor predictive value as screening tests.

DIAGNOSTIC IMAGING IN JOINT DISEASES   Historically, *conventional radiography* has played an integral part in the diagnosis and staging of articular disorders. Plain films are most appropriate when there is a history of prior trauma, suspected chronic infection, progressive disability, monarticular involvement, when therapeutic alterations are considered, or as a baseline assessment for what appears to be a chronic process. However, in most inflammatory disorders, early radiography is rarely helpful in establishing a diagnosis and often reveals only soft tissue swelling and juxtaarticular demineralization. As the disease progresses, calcification (soft tissue, cartilage, or bone), joint space narrowing, erosions, bony ankylosis, new bone formation (sclerosis, osteophytes, or periostitis), or subchondral cysts may develop and provide diagnostic information. The

TABLE 280-2 Application of diagnostic imaging techniques to musculoskeletal disorders

Method	Cost	Conditions evaluated	Indications
Ultrasound	+*	Focal	Synovial (Baker's) cyst Rotator cuff tears Tendon injury
Radionuclide scintigraphy			
⁹⁹ᵐTc	+ +	Diffuse	Metastatic bone survey Evaluation of Paget's disease Quantitative joint assessments Early polymyalgia rheumatica
¹¹¹In-WBC	+ +	Diffuse	Acute infections Prosthetic infections Osteomyelitis
⁶⁷Ga	+ +	Diffuse	Acute and chronic infections Osteomyelitis
Computed tomography	+ + +	Focal	Herniated intervertebral disks Sacroiliitis Spinal stenosis Osteoid osteoma Spinal trauma
Magnetic resonance imaging	+ + + +	Focal	Avascular necrosis Osteomyelitis Derangements of axial skeleton and spinal cord

* +, Arbitrary cost of ultrasound compared to other modalities.

use of high-quality films and proper positioning can eliminate the need for further studies.

The advent of additional imaging techniques has enhanced diagnostic sensitivity and can facilitate the early diagnosis of certain articular disorders. In selected circumstances, the appropriate use of these modalities is indicated when conventional radiography cannot provide adequate information (Table 280-2). *Ultrasonography* is useful in the detection of soft tissue abnormalities that cannot be fully appreciated by clinical eximination. There are a limited number of circumstances wherein ultrasound is the preferred method of evaluation. These include the assessment of synovial (Baker's) cysts, rotator cuff tears, and various tendon injuries. *Radionuclide scintigraphy* of the musculoskeletal disorders is useful to provide information regarding the metabolic status of bone and, along with radiography, is well suited for total-body assessment of the extent and distribution of musculoskeletal involvement. Scintigraphy, using ⁹⁹ᵐTc, ⁶⁷Ga, and ¹¹¹In-labeled white blood cells (In-WBC), has been applied to a variety of articular disorders with variable success. The proper application of these radioisotope techniques is dependent upon knowledge of their distribution and uptake about the joint under normal and diseased states. [*⁹⁹ᵐTc*] *pertechnate* is bound to albumin and accumulates in areas of increased vascularity; hence, the increased uptake observed with synovitis, infection, or neoplasia and the decreased uptake seen in early osteonecrosis. By contrast, [*⁹⁹ᵐTc*] *phosphate* is utilized as a bone-seeking radionuclide, whose distribution is dependent upon blood flow and uptake during new bone formation. Increased uptake is seen with inflammation, increased blood flow, bone remodeling, and heterotopic bone formation (Fig. 280-1). The nonspecificity of ⁹⁹ᵐTc scanning has limited its use to investigational and serial assessments of joint/bone involvement or metastatic bone surveys. *Gallium 67* binds to serum and cellular transferrin and lactoferrin and is preferentially taken up by neutrophils and tumor tissue (lymphoma) and is thus useful in the identification of infection and malignancies. Scanning with *¹¹¹In-WBC* has been

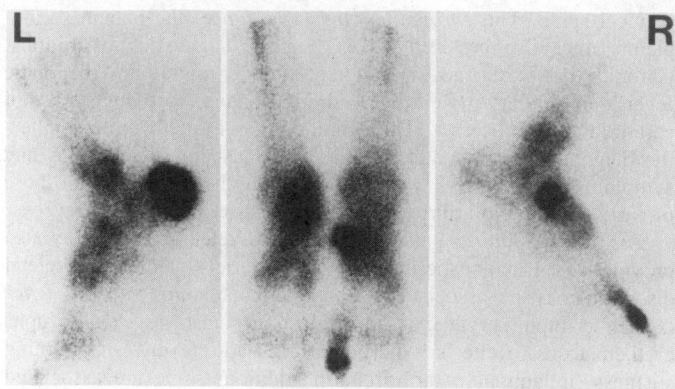

FIGURE 280-1 [⁹⁹ᵐTc] phosphate scintigraphy of the feet of a 33-year-old black male with Reiter's syndrome, manifested by sacroiliitis, urethritis, uveitis, asymmetric oligoarthritis, and enthesitis. This bone scan demonstrates increased uptake indicative of enthesitis involving the insertions of the left Achilles tendon and plantar aponeurosis and the right tibialis posterior tendon and arthritis of the right first interphalangeal joint.

used to detect both infectious and inflammatory arthritis. Although both have been used with success, ¹¹¹In-WBC scanning is more sensitive than use of ⁶⁷Ga in the early diagnosis of osteomyelitis and infected arthroplasties. Prior treatment with antibiotics reduces the diagnostic sensitivities of both ⁶⁷Ga and ¹¹¹In-WBC scintigraphy.

Computed tomography (CT) provides the physician with rapid reconstruction of sagittal, coronal, and axial images and spatial relationships among anatomic structures. It has proved to be most useful in the assessment of the axial skeleton because of its ability to visualize in the axial plane. Articulations previously considered difficult to visualize using conventional radiography, such as the zygoapophyseal, sacroiliac, sternoclavicular, and hip joints, can be effectively evaluated using CT. CT has been demonstrated to be

FIGURE 280-2 Superior sensitivity of magnetic resonance imaging in the diagnosis of osteonecrosis of the femoral head. A 25-year-old white male taking high-dose glucocorticoids for idiopathic thrombocytopenic purpura developed bilateral hip pain. Conventional x-ray films (*A*) demonstrated abnormalities only in the right hip consistent with stage II osteonecrosis (arrow). A bone scan (*B*) revealed increased uptake in the right hip only (arrow). MRI using spin echo proton density images (*C* and *D*) demonstrated low-density signals from both femoral heads (arrows), indicative of bilateral osteonecrosis.

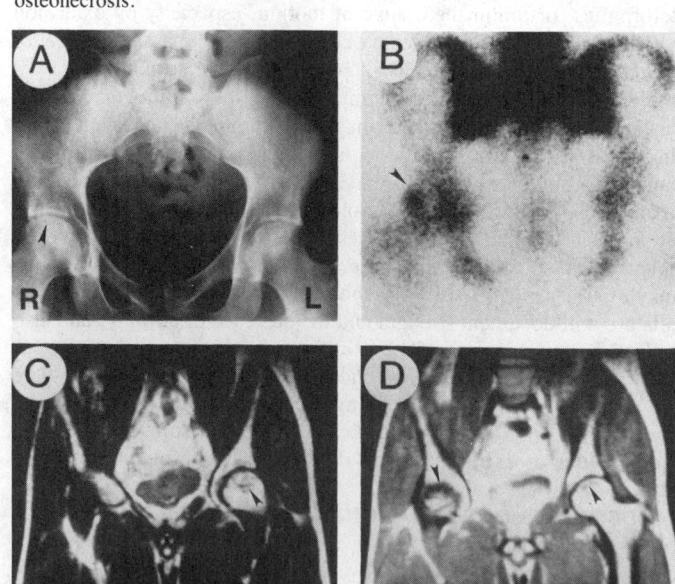

TABLE 280-3 Common musculoskeletal disorders in the elderly

I Inflammatory
   Polymyalgia rheumatica
   Temporal (giant cell) arteritis
   Gout
   Calcium pyrophosphate dihydrate deposition disease
II Mechanical
   Degenerative joint disease
   Spinal stenosis
III Metabolic
   Osteoporosis
   Myxedema
   Paget's disease
IV Associated with neoplastic disease
   Carcinomatous arthropathy or neuromyopathy
   Dermatomyositis
   Hypertrophic osteoarthropathy
V Drug-induced
   Diuretics (gout)
   Drug-induced lupus
   Corticosteroids (osteopenia, myopathy)

HUGHES GRV: Autoantibodies in lupus and its variants: Experience in 1000 patients. Br Med J 289:339, 1984

KEAN W: Arthritis in the elderly. Clin Rheum Dis 12:1, 1986

NAMEY TC: Nuclear medicine and special radiologic imaging and technique in the diagnosis of rheumatic disease, in *Textbook of Rheumatology*, WN Kelley et al (eds). Philadelphia, Saunders, 1985, p 608

POLLEY HF, HUNDER GG: *Rheumatologic Interviewing and Physical Examination of the Joints*. Philadelphia, Saunders, 1978

TAN EM: Antinuclear antibodies in diagnosis and management. Hosp Pract 18:79, 1983

WILSON FC: Principles of diagnosis and treatment of musculoskeletal trauma, in *The Musculoskeletal System: Basic Processes and Disorders*, FC Wilson (ed). Philadelphia, Lippincott, 1983, p 270

281 OSTEOARTHRITIS

KENNETH D. BRANDT / KAREN KOVALOV–ST. JOHN

Osteoarthritis (OA), also termed degenerative joint disease (DJD), represents failure of the diarthrodial (movable, synovial-lined) joint. In idiopathic (primary) OA, the most common form of the disease, no predisposing factor is apparent. Secondary OA appears pathologically indistinguishable from idiopathic OA but is attributable to an obvious underlying cause (Table 281-1).

EPIDEMIOLOGY OA is the most common joint disease of human beings and the leading cause of disability in the elderly; it has been estimated that 100,000 people in this country are unable to walk independently from bed to bathroom because of OA. A progressive increase in prevalence of OA is seen with increasing age. In a radiographic survey of women less than 45 years of age, only 2 percent had OA; between the ages of 45 to 64 years, however, the prevalence was 30 percent while for those older than 65 years it was 68 percent. The figures were similar in males but somewhat lower in the older age groups. OA is rare in children and young adults.

Under the age of 55 years the joint distribution of OA in men and women is similar; in older individuals hip OA is more common in men, while OA of interphalangeal joints and the thumb base is more common in women. The pattern of joint involvement is markedly influenced by prior vocational or avocational overload. Thus, OA is common in ankles of ballet dancers and metacarpophalangeal joints of prize fighters, although it is uncommon in these sites in the general population.

There are racial differences in both the prevalence of OA and the pattern of joint involvement. The Chinese in Hong Kong have a lower incidence of OA of the hip than do whites; OA is more frequent in Native Americans than in whites. Whether these differences are genetic or relate to cultural differences in joint usage is unknown.

Hereditary factors also underlie development of OA. For example, the mother of a woman with OA in distal interphalangeal joints (Heberden's nodes) is twice as likely to exhibit OA in these joints, and her sister three times as likely, as the mother and sister of an unaffected woman.

PATHOLOGY The earliest gross pathologic finding in OA is softening of the articular cartilage in habitually loaded areas of the joint surface (Fig. 281-1). With progression of OA the integrity of the surface is lost and the articular cartilage thins. Vertical clefts (fibrillation) extend into the depth of the cartilage. With joint motion, shards of fibrillated cartilage are shed, unmasking bone, which undergoes eburnation (sclerosis into a substance resembling ivory) with wear. Subchondral cysts develop. Some are filled with fibromyxomatous tissue; others communicate with the surface and contain synovial fluid. The fluid, under pressure during joint loading, may expand the cysts into large geodes. Beneath the damaged articular cartilage and at the joint margins osteophytes (bone spurs) form. Some may severely restrict joint movement. Blood vessels, arising from the subchondral marrow, infiltrate the calcified cartilage, leading to fragmentation and duplication of the tidemark. Endochondral ossification results in new bone at these sites.

useful in the diagnosis of low back pain syndromes, sacroiliitis, avascular necrosis, osteoid osteoma, tarsal coalition, osteomyelitis, and intraarticular osteochondral fragments.

In recent years, *magnetic resonance imaging* (MRI) has emerged as a useful method of musculoskeletal imaging. MRI has the advantages of providing greater anatomic detail and contrast resolution (Fig. 280-2). However, the cost and limited availability of MRI have thus far constrained its application to the evaluation of musculoskeletal disorders. MRI is capable of imaging muscle, cartilage, ligaments, tendons, pannus, synovial effusions, and bone. MRI has been shown to be a sensitive and effective means to detect soft tissue injuries (meniscal and rotator cuff tears), ischemic osteonecrosis of bone, and osteomyelitis and to assess the cervical spinal cord following cervical injury, subluxation, and/or arthritis.

EVALUATION OF THE ELDERLY FOR RHEUMATIC DISEASES
Musculoskeletal disorders in geriatric patients are often not diagnosed since complaints in the elderly may be insidious in onset and chronic in nature. In addition, older individuals frequently possess multiple interactive variables, including other medical conditions and therapies that may obscure the nature of the problem. This is compounded by the diminished reliability of laboratory testing in the elderly, owing to the wider range of nonpathologic serologic variability, including elevated erythrocyte sedimentation rates and low titers of rheumatoid factor or antinuclear antibodies. Although nearly all rheumatic disorders can afflict the elderly, certain diseases and drug-induced disorders are more common in this age group (Table 280-3). The elderly should be approached in the same manner used for all patients with musculoskeletal complaints, with additional inquiry to exclude common geriatric musculoskeletal disorders. An emphasis on identifying intercurrent medical conditions and therapies is extremely important. Drug-induced lupus erythematosus, gout, and chronic salicylate toxicity are all more common in the elderly. The physical examination should emphasize coexistent disease that may influence subsequent diagnosis and treatment.

REFERENCES

BELTRAN J et al: Rheumatoid arthritis: MR imaging manifestations. Radiology 165:153, 1987

BROWER AC: Imaging techniques and modalities, in *Arthritis in Black and White*, AC Brower (ed). Philadelphia, Saunders, 1988, p 1

ETTINGER WH: Approach to the diagnosis and management of musculoskeletal disease. Clin Geriatr Med 4:269, 1988

FRIES JF, MITCHELL DM: Joint pain or arthritis. JAMA 235:199, 1976

GATTER RA: *Practical Handbook of Joint Fluid Analysis*. Philadelphia, Lea & Febiger, 1984

GAYLIS NB: Initial evaluation of the arthritic patient: Piecing together the diagnostic clues. Postgrad Med 80(5):65, 1986

HALL H: Examination of the patient with low back pain. Bull Rheum Dis 33:1, 1983

TABLE 281-1 Classification of OA

I Idiopathic
  A Localized
    1 Hands: Heberden's and Bouchard's nodes (nodal), erosive interphalangeal arthritis (nonnodal), carpal–1st metacarpal
    2 Feet: hallux valgus, hallux rigidus, contracted toes (hammer/cockup toes), talonavicular
    3 Knee:
      (*a*) Medial compartment
      (*b*) Lateral compartment
      (*c*) Patellofemoral compartment
    4 Hip:
      (*a*) Eccentric (superior)
      (*b*) Concentric (axial, medial)
      (*c*) Diffuse (coxae senilis)
    5 Spine:
      (*a*) Apophyseal joints
      (*b*) Intervertebral joints (disk)
      (*c*) Spondylosis (osteophytes)
      (*d*) Ligamentous (hyperostosis, Forestier's disease, diffuse idiopathic skeletal hyperostosis
    6 Other single sites, e.g., glenohumoral, acromioclavicular, tibiotalar, sacroiliac, temporomandibular
  B Generalized OA includes 3 or more of the areas listed above (Kellgren-Moore)
II Secondary
  A Trauma
    1 Acute
    2 Chronic (occupational, sports)
  B Congenital or developmental
    1 Localized diseases: Legg-Calvé-Perthes, congenital hip dislocation, slipped epiphysis
    2 Mechanical factors: unequal lower extremity length, valgus/varus deformity, hypermobility syndromes
    3 Bone dysplasias: epiphyseal dysplasia, spondyloapophyseal dysplasia, osteonychodystrophy
  C Metabolic
    1 Ochronosis (alkaptonuria)
    2 Hemochromatosis
    3 Wilson's disease
    4 Gaucher's disease
  D Endocrine
    1 Acromegaly
    2 Hyperparathyroidism
    3 Diabetes mellitus
    4 Obesity
    5 Hypothyroidism
  E Calcium deposition diseases
    1 Calcium pyrophosphate dihydrate deposition
    2 Apatite arthropathy
  F Other bone and joint diseases
    1 Localized: fracture, avascular necrosis, infection, gout
    2 Diffuse: rheumatoid (inflammatory) arthritis, Paget's disease, osteopetrosis, osteochondritis
  G Neuropathic (Charcot joints)
  H Endemic
    1 Kashin-Beck
    2 Mseleni
  I Miscellaneous
    1 Frostbite
    2 Caisson's disease
    3 Hemoglobinopathies

SOURCE: From Mankin et al, 1986.

In the face of this breakdown of the extracellular matrix, the chondrocytes undergo mitotic division. Clones of new cells appear. Later in the disease, however, the cartilage becomes hypocellular. In many areas fibrocartilage replaces hyaline cartilage. The synovium shows foci of mononuclear cell infiltration, although pannus does not develop. Shards of cartilage which have broken off the articular surface may become embedded in the synovium, where they incite an inflammatory reaction. Marked fibrosis of the joint capsule may develop, further restricting joint motion.

PATHOGENESIS In normal joints articular cartilage serves two essential mechanical functions: First, it provides a smooth weight-bearing surface, so that one bone is able to glide effortlessly over the other within the joint. Secondly, it transmits load from one bone to the next so that the bones do not shatter with loading of the joint. Articular cartilage is made up of two major macromolecules, proteoglycans and collagen. Proteoglycans (PGs) provide elasticity and stiffness on compression; collagen provides tensile strength.

In OA, the earliest physicochemical change in the cartilage is an increase in water content, due to disruption of the collagen network which normally constrains the densely packed PGs and maintains them in an underhydrated state. Although no biochemical abnormalities have been detected in the type II collagen fiber itself, an abnormality in cross-linking of adjacent fibers may exist. Type IX collagen, a minor collagen of articular cartilage which is covalently linked to type II and present on the surface of the type II fiber, may function as a ''cross-linker.'' With the increase in cartilage water the PG concentration falls. The cartilage softens (chondromalacia) and offers diminished resistance to compression.

Levels of matrix-degrading enzymes, e.g., collagenase and proteoglycanases (PGases), are increased in OA cartilage. These enzymes are not derived from the synovial membrane or joint fluid but are secreted by the chondrocytes themselves in a latent form, which is converted to active enzyme by physiologic activator(s) (e.g., plasminogen activator/plasmin or other proteases). Normal articular cartilage contains inhibitors of matrix-degrading enzymes. In OA cartilage a stoichiometric imbalance appears to exist between the levels of degradative enzymes and of inhibitors.

The basis for the increased synthesis and secretion of matrix-degrading enzymes by the OA chondrocyte is unclear. Interleukin 1 and tumor necrosis factor, which are released by mononuclear cells in the OA synovium, may stimulate chondrocytes to synthesize and release degradative enzymes. Whether mechanical factors may directly stimulate enzyme release from the chondrocyte is unclear.

In addition to the increase in matrix degradation in OA, evidence exists of a marked synthetic response by the chondrocyte. Rates of synthesis of PGs, collagen, noncollagenous proteins, DNA, and RNA all are severalfold greater than normal, reflecting a very active ''repair'' effort by the OA chondrocyte. In some cases this may maintain a biomechanically adequate matrix. With progression of OA, however, the chondrocyte ''fails,'' the rate of PG synthesis falls, and the articular surface is lost.

Not only the articular cartilage but also the subchondral bone is metabolically active in OA. Appositional growth results in the subchondral sclerosis seen radiographically. Stiffening of the subchondral bone, which reduces its ability to absorb the energy of joint loading, may lead to mechanical breakdown of the overlying cartilage.

The pathogenesis of OA can be related to an abnormality in the geometry of the involved joint, in the material properties of the cartilage or bone, or in the supporting structures (e.g., ligaments or neuromuscular apparatus). Idiopathic primary OA of the hip appears to be related in most cases to incongruity of joint surfaces due, for example, to subtle degrees of acetabular dysplasia or slipped femoral capital epiphysis.

Ochronosis may be cited as an example of a condition in which OA is caused by an abnormality in the biomaterials of the joint. Congenital deficiency of the enzyme homogentisic acid oxidase leads to accumulation of homogentisic acid polymers in articular cartilage, where they bind to type II collagen and stiffen the tissue. The shock-absorbing properties of cartilage become compromised, and the risk of cartilage fibrillation is increased. Clinically, most patients with ochronosis develop severe generalized OA by the age of 40. Osteopetrosis, which leads to stiffening of the bone, is similarly associated with generalized OA in most patients who survive to middle age. In contrast, osteoporosis, which results in an abnormal softening of bone, bears an inverse relationship to OA.

That abnormalities in the ligamentous support of joints may be important in the pathogenesis of OA is suggested by the increased frequency of OA in Ehlers-Danlos syndrome. Neuropathic joint disease (Charcot arthropathy) is a severe form of degenerative joint disease seen in patients with a severe neurosensory disorder.

CLINICAL FEATURES OA usually affects a single joint or only a few joints. While the early stages are painless, joint pain eventually leads the patient to seek medical attention. This is often described as a deep ache, localized to the involved joint. Typically, the pain is aggravated by use and relieved by rest. As the disease progresses,

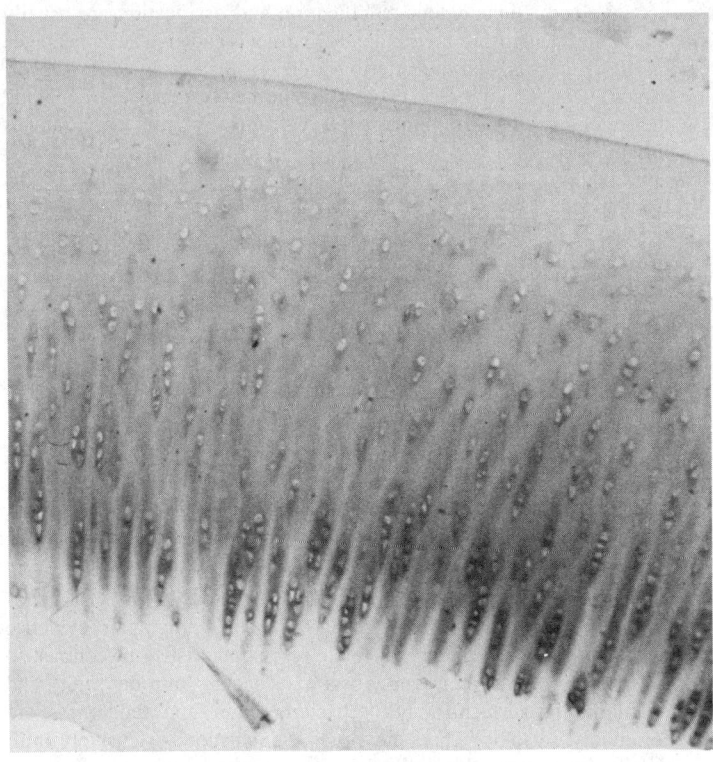
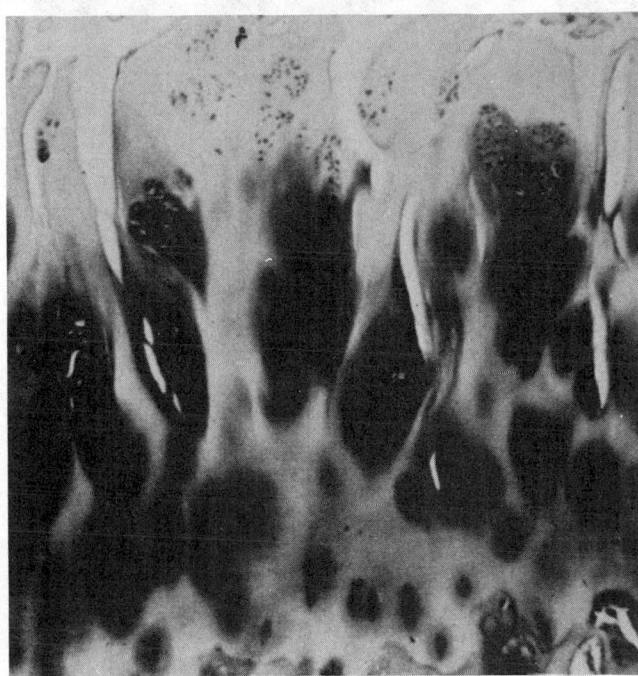

FIGURE 281-1 *A.* Normal articular cartilage. Note the intact surface and even distribution of chondrocytes. Mitotic figures are not present in normal adult articular cartilage. *B.* Osteoarthritic cartilage. Note the disruption of surface integrity, with vertical fissues (fibrillation) and irregular distribution of cells. Many of the chondrocytes have replicated and exist in clusters. Stained with Safranin-O, which binds to the sulfated glycosaminoglycan chains of proteoglycans. Note areas of diminished staining (pale extracellular matrix) due to patchy proteoglycan depletion.

the pain may become persistent. Stiffness of the involved joint upon arising in the morning or after immobility (e.g., following an automobile ride or an evening in a theater seat) may be prominent, but usually lasts less than 20 min. Systemic manifestations are not associated with primary OA.

Although the most striking structural changes in OA occur in the cartilage, joint pain in OA must arise from other structures since cartilage is aneural. In some patients pain may be due to stretching of nerve endings in the periosteum covering osteophytes. In others it may arise from microfractures in subchondral bone or from medullary hypertension caused by distortion of blood flow by hypertrophic subchondral trabeculae. Indeed, OA pain may be relieved temporarily by medullary core decompression, emphasizing the importance of hydraulic factors in some cases. Muscle spasm and joint instability leading to capsular stretching also may cause pain in OA.

In some patients with OA, joint pain may be due to synovitis. In patients with advanced OA marked synovial inflammation may be present. This may be due to phagocytosis of pieces of cartilage and bone derived from the abraded joint surface or to release from the cartilage of soluble matrix macromolecules, e.g., glycosaminoglycans or PGs. Synovitis may be due also to crystals of calcium pyrophosphate or calcium hydroxyapatite, which have been demonstrated in most synovial effusions from patients with OA. In other cases immune complexes, containing antigens derived from cartilage matrix, may be sequestered in collagenous tissue of the joint, leading to low-grade chronic immune synovitis. In the earlier stages of OA synovial inflammation may be absent. However, even in the absence of synovitis joint pain may be relieved by a nonsteroidal anti-inflammatory drug (NSAID) suggesting that these drugs have analgesic actions independent of their anti-inflammatory effects.

Physical examination of the OA joint may reveal localized tenderness and bony or soft tissue swelling. Bony crepitus (the sensation of bone rubbing against bone, evoked by joint movement) is characteristic. Synovial effusions are relatively uncommon and,

when present, usually small in volume. Palpation may reveal some warmth over the joint. Disuse, secondary to pain, can lead to periarticular muscle atrophy, suggesting even greater bony enlargement than actually exists. In advanced stages, gross deformity, bony hypertrophy, subluxation, and marked loss of joint motion may be striking. Although it is a common impression that OA is inevitably progressive, in many patients the disease stabilizes. In some, regression of symptoms, and even of radiographic changes, occurs.

Interphalangeal joints *Heberden's nodes,* bony enlargements of the distal interphalangeal joints, represent the most common form of idiopathic OA (Fig. 281-2). A similar process at the proximal interphalangeal joints leads to *Bouchard's nodes.* Often Heberden's nodes develop gradually, with little discomfort. However, they may present acutely with pain, redness, and swelling, sometimes triggered by minor trauma. Gelatinous dorsal cysts, filled with hyaluronic acid, may develop at the insertion of the digital extensor tendon into the base of the distal phalanx.

The second most frequent area of involvement in OA is the thumb base. Swelling, tenderness, and marked crepitus on movement of the joint are typical. Osteophytes may lead to a "squared" appearance of the thumb base.

The hip Congenital or developmental defects (e.g., acetabular dysplasia, Legg-Calvé-Perthes disease, slipped capital epiphysis) may be implicated in as many as 80 percent of cases of hip OA. Twenty percent of patients will develop bilateral involvement. Pain from hip OA is generally referred to the inguinal area but may be referred to the buttock or proximal thigh. Less commonly, hip OA presents as knee pain. Pain can be evoked by putting the involved hip through its range of motion; initially, flexion may be painless but internal rotation will exacerbate pain. Loss of internal rotation occurs early, followed by loss of extension, adduction, and flexion due to capsular fibrosis and/or buttressing osteophytes.

The knee OA of the knee may involve medial or lateral femorotibial compartments and/or the patellofemoral compartment. Palpation may reveal bony hypertrophy (osteophytes) and tenderness.

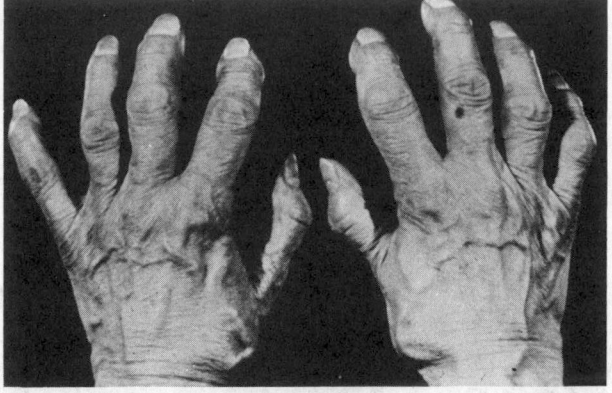

A

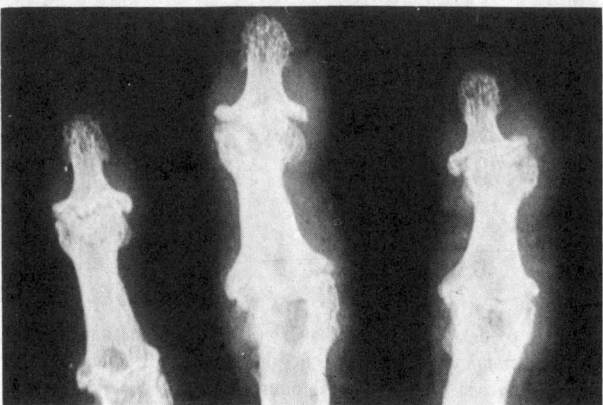

B

FIGURE 281-2 Osteoarthritis. *A.* Heberden's nodes of the distal interphalangeal joints and Bouchard's nodes of the proximal interphalangeal joints are present. The carpometacarpal joint is radially subluxed giving the hand a squared appearance. There is also angulation of the distal and proximal interphalangeal joints. *B.* Radiograph of the second, third, and fourth proximal and distal interphalangeal joints. Loss of joint space, osteophytes, and subchondral sclerosis and cysts are evident.

Effusions, if present, are generally small. Joint movement commonly elicits bony crepitus. OA in the medial compartment may result in a varus (bow-legged) deformity; in the lateral compartment it produces a valgus (knock-knee) deformity. A "shrug" sign (pain when the patella is compressed manually against the femur during quadriceps contraction) may be a sign of OA in the patellofemoral joint.

Chondromalacia patellae, which also is characterized by knee pain and a positive shrug sign, is a syndrome of patellofemoral pain, often bilateral, occurring in teenagers and young adults. It is more common in females than in males. It may be caused by a variety of factors (e.g., abnormal quadriceps angle, patella alta, trauma). Although exploration of the knee may reveal softening and fibrillation of cartilage on the posterior aspect of the patella, this is usually not progressive. In most cases chondromalacia patellae is not a precursor of OA. Usually, analgesics or NSAIDs and physical therapy are effective. In other cases, pain may be relieved by correction of patellar malalignment.

The spine Degenerative disease of the spine can involve the apophyseal joint, intervertebral disks, and/or paraspinous ligaments. *Spondylosis* refers to degenerative *disk* disease. The term *OA of the spine* should be reserved for degeneration of the apophyseal joints (true diarthrodial joints). Symptoms of spinal OA include localized pain and stiffness. Nerve root compression by an osteophyte blocking a neural foramen, prolapse of a degenerated disk, or subluxation of an apophyseal joint may cause radicular pain and motor weakness.

Marked calcification and ossification of paraspinous ligaments occur in *diffuse idiopathic skeletal hyperostosis* (DISH). Although DISH is often categorized as a variant of OA, diarthrodial joints are not involved. Ligamentous calcification and ossification are usually most prominent in the anterior spinal ligaments and give the appearance of "flowing wax" on the anterior bodies of the vertebrae. However, a radiolucency may be seen between the newly deposited bone and the vertebral body, differentiating DISH from the marginal osteophytes in spondylosis. Intervertebral disk spaces are preserved, and sacroiliac and apophyseal joints appear normal, helping to differentiate DISH from spondylosis and ankylosing spondylitis, respectively.

DISH occurs in middle age and in the elderly and is more common in men than in women. Patients are frequently asymptomatic, but may have musculoskeletal stiffness. Radiographic changes are generally much more severe than might be predicted from the mild symptoms caused by DISH.

Generalized OA Generalized OA is characterized by involvement of three or more joints or groups of joints (distal interphalangeal and proximal interphalangeal joints are counted as one group each). Heberden's and Bouchard's nodes are prominent. Symptoms may be episodic, with "flare-ups" of inflammation marked by soft tissue swelling, redness, and warmth. The erythrocyte sedimentation rate may be elevated, but serum rheumatoid factor tests are negative.

Erosive OA In erosive OA distal and/or proximal interphalangeal joints of the hands are most prominently affected. Erosive OA tends to be more destructive than typical OA, and radiographic evidence of collapse of the subchondral plate is characteristic. In contrast to other forms of OA, bony ankylosis may occur. Joint deformity and functional impairment may be severe. Pain and tenderness are commonly episodic. The synovium is much more extensively infiltrated with mononuclear cells than in other forms of OA.

LABORATORY AND RADIOGRAPHIC FEATURES The diagnosis of OA is usually based on clinical and radiographic features. In the early stages radiographs may be normal, but joint space narrowing becomes evident as articular cartilage is lost. Other characteristic radiographic findings include subchondral bone sclerosis, subchondral cysts, and marginal osteophytes. A change in joint contours, due to bony remodeling, and subluxation may be seen. In OA, great disparity often exists between the severity of radiographic findings, severity of symptoms, and functional ability. Thus, while more than 90 percent of people over the age of 40 have some radiographic changes of OA in weight-bearing joints, only 30 percent of these will have symptoms.

No laboratory studies are diagnostic of OA, but specific laboratory testing may help in identifying one of the underlying causes of secondary OA. Since primary OA is not systemic, the erythrocyte sedimentation rate, serum chemistry determinations, blood counts, and urinalysis are normal. Analysis of synovial fluid reveals mild leukocytosis (<2000 white blood cells per microliter), with a predominance of mononuclear cells.

Prior to the appearance of radiographic changes clinical diagnosis of OA without an invasive procedure (e.g., arthroscopy, arthrotomy) is limited. Approaches such as magnetic resonance imaging (MRI) and ultrasonography are expensive and not widely available, and the limits of resolution do not justify their routine clinical use for diagnosis of OA or for monitoring disease progression. Much effort is currently being devoted to evaluation of serologic tests for these purposes. The approach depends upon detection in synovial fluid and/or serum of macromolecules (e.g., PGs, glycosaminoglycans) released from degenerating cartilage or bone. None of these tests has yet proved suitable for clinical use.

TREATMENT No cure exists for OA. Treatment is aimed at reducing pain, maintaining mobility, and minimizing disability. The vigor of the therapeutic intervention should be dictated by the condition in the individual patient. For those with only mild disease, reassurance, instruction in joint protection, and an occasional analgesic may be all that is required.

Drug therapy Drug therapy in OA today is symptomatic. Often the joint pain can be controlled with only a simple analgesic (e.g., acetaminophen). For more severe pain dextrapropoxyphene hydrochloride may be used. Narcotics are rarely indicated in OA.

NSAIDs often decrease pain and improve mobility in OA. However, it is unclear whether this is due to their anti-inflammatory effect or to an analgesic action independent of their effect on inflammation. As indicated above, patients with OA may obtain symptomatic benefit from an NSAID even when evidence of synovitis is lacking. The superiority of NSAIDs over compounds providing comparable analgesia but without anti-inflammatory effect has not yet been adequately demonstrated in OA. Nonetheless, if signs of joint inflammation are present or simple analgesics are inadequate, it is reasonable to prescribe an NSAID for the patient with OA.

Claims have been made that some agents, such as polysulfated glycosaminoglycans, retard the progression of OA in human beings; it has been suggested that some NSAIDs also may have a "chondroprotective" effect. However, adequately controlled long-term clinical trials in human beings to support such claims have not been performed.

Systemic glucocorticoids have no place in the treatment of OA. However, intra- or periarticular injection of a depot glucocorticoid preparation may provide marked symptomatic relief. The injection should not be repeated in a given joint more often than every 4 to 6 months, since too frequent injections may accelerate cartilage breakdown. Temporary reduction of usage of the joint after the steroid injection may prolong the therapeutic response.

Reduction of joint loading OA may be caused or aggravated by poor body mechanics. Correction of poor posture and a support for excessive lumbar lordosis can be helpful. Excessive loading of the involved joint should be avoided. Overloading of the knee due to pronated feet or varus or valgus knee deformities may be corrected by orthotics or osteotomy. Running shoes may be helpful in cushioning load.

Patients with OA of the knee or hip should seek alternatives to prolonged standing, kneeling, and squatting. Obese patients should be counseled to lose weight, but this may be difficult to accomplish since caloric expenditure may be reduced due to the inactivity imposed by the painful joint.

Rest periods during the day may be of benefit, but complete immobilization of the painful joint is rarely indicated. For unilateral OA of the hip or knee a cane, held in the contralateral hand, is often useful. Bilateral disease may necessitate the use of crutches or a walker.

Physical therapy Heat applied to joints prior to exercise reduces pain and stiffness. A variety of modalities are available. Often the least expensive and most convenient is a hot shower or bath. Occasionally, better analgesia may be obtained with ice than with heat. Transcutaneous electrical nerve stimulation (TENS) may be helpful, especially for low back pain due to OA of the lumbar spine.

Disuse of the OA joint because of pain leads to muscle atrophy. Since muscles play a major role in protecting articular cartilage from stress, strengthening periarticular muscles is important. The atrophy of joint cartilage and bone which develops with disuse of a limb is due chiefly to reduction in loading of the joint by contraction of periarticular muscles (e.g., hamstrings and quadriceps for the knee). Exercises should be designed to maintain range of motion and strengthen muscles surrounding the joint. Isometric exercises are generally preferable to isotonic exercises, since they minimize joint stress.

Orthopedic surgery Joint replacement surgery should be reserved for patients with advanced OA in whom aggressive medical management has been unsuccessful. Arthroplasty may relieve pain and increase mobility. Osteotomy, which is surgically more conservative, may eliminate abnormal dynamic loading by correcting malalignment. In patients with hip or knee OA it may provide effective pain relief; it is of greatest benefit when the disease is only moderately advanced. Arthroscopic removal of loose cartilage fragments can prevent locking and also may relieve pain. Lavage of the joint with large quantities of Ringer's lactate, to flush out fibrin, cartilage shards, and other debris, may provide several months of comfort for patients whose joint pain has been refractory to analgesics and

NSAIDs, but controlled studies that support the efficacy of this procedure have not been published.

Chondroplasty (abrasion arthroplasty) has gained some popularity as treatment for OA. Well-controlled studies of its efficacy are lacking, however, and the fibrocartilaginous tissue which resurfaces the abraded bone is inferior to normal hyaline cartilage in its ability to withstand compressive and shear stresses.

REFERENCES

BRANDT KD: Osteoarthritis: Clinical patterns and pathology, in *Textbook of Rheumatology*, 2d ed, WN Kelley et al (eds). Philadelphia, Saunders, 1985, pp 1432–1448
———: Osteoarthritis. Clin Geriatr Med 4:279, 1988
———: Management of osteoarthritis, in *Textbook of Rheumatology*, 3d ed, WN Kelley et al (eds). Philadelphia, Saunders, 1989, pp 1501–1512
———, RADIN E: The physiology of articular stress: Osteoarthrosis. Hosp Practice 22:103, 1987
CIOMS: The epidemiology of chronic rheumatism, in *Atlas of Standard Radiographs of Arthritis*. Oxford, Blackwell, 1963
LAWRENCE JS et al: Osteoarthritis prevalence in the population and relationship between symptoms and x-ray changes. Ann Rheum Dis 25:1, 1966
MANKIN HJ, BRANDT KD: Pathogenesis of osteoarthritis, in *Textbook of Rheumatology*, WN Kelley et al (eds). Philadelphia, Saunders, 1989, pp 1469–1479
——— et al: Workshop on etiopathogenesis of osteoarthritis. J Rheumatol 13:1127, 1986

282 ARTHRITIS DUE TO DEPOSITION OF CALCIUM CRYSTALS

GARY S. HOFFMAN

CRYSTALLOGRAPHY AND ARTHRITIS The use of polarizing microscopy to identify sodium urate crystals in synovial fluid of patients with gout was described in 1961. Since then, application of this relatively simple technique and research tools such as electron microscopy, energy-dispersive elemental analysis, and x-ray diffraction have established the role of additional types of microcrystals, including calcium pyrophosphate dihydrate (CPPD), calcium hydroxyapatite (HA), and calcium oxalate (CaOx), in other forms of arthritis. Each of these materials may cause acute or chronic arthritis or periarthritis. In spite of differences in crystal morphology, chemistry, and physical properties, the clinical events that result from deposition and release of sodium urate, CPPD, HA, and CaOx may be indistinguishable. Prior to the use of crystallographic techniques in rheumatology, much of what was considered to be gouty arthritis, in fact, was not. The great frequency (at least 60 percent) with which either HA or CPPD are found in chronic effusions from osteoarthritic joints has raised many questions about their role in causing or enhancing arthritis in the elderly. Patients with the most severe osteoarthritis appear to have the highest incidence of concurrent HA and/or CPPD synovitis, implying an additive or synergistic relationship. The occasional coexistence of sodium urate, CPPD, HA, or CaOx in the same joint further emphasizes the importance of crystallographic analysis for these potentially difficult diagnostic problems. In the setting of acute articular or periarticular inflammation, aspiration and analysis of effusions are most important to assess the possibility of infection. Polarization microscopy, alone, may identify most typical crystals and allow diagnosis. HA, however, represents an exception. Because these crystals are not birefringent and may be extremely small, more sophisticated techniques would be required to confirm their presence. Apart from the identification of specific microcrystalline materials or organisms, synovial fluid characteristics are not pathognomonic. Chronic monarticular or pauciarticular effusions of uncertain etiology should be approached with an inquisitiveness similar to that given to the acute effusion. Although chronicity makes septic arthritis far less likely, it remains part of the differential diagnosis, as does microcrystalline arthropathy.

CALCIUM PYROPHOSPHATE DIHYDRATE (CPPD) DEPOSITION DISEASE **Pathogenesis**

CPPD crystal deposition in articular cartilage, synovium, and periarticular ligaments and tendons is most common in the elderly, affecting 10 to 15 percent of persons 65 to 75 years old and 30 to 60 percent of those more than 85 years old. In most cases this process is asymptomatic and the cause of CPPD deposition is uncertain. Because over 80 percent of patients are more than 60 years old, and 70 percent have preexisting joint damage from other conditions, it is likely that physical and chemical changes in aging cartilage favor crystal nucleation. Examples of such chemical alterations include the following: (1) Increased production of inorganic pyrophosphate and decreased levels of pyrophosphatases in cartilage extracts from patients with CPPD arthritis. The increase in pyrophosphate appears related to enhanced activity of ATP pyrophosphohydrolase, which catalyzes the reaction of ATP to AMP and pyrophosphate. (2) Diminution of cartilage glycoproteins that normally inhibit and regulate crystal nucleation and impair the ability of crystals to trigger the release of enzymes from neutrophils. Such inhibitors are probably chemically unique for different types of crystals. Inhibitor deficiencies may thus lead to increased crystal deposition, and at a later time, crystal shedding may be associated with an inadequately inhibited inflammatory response. The release of CPPD crystals in the joint space is followed by neutrophil phagocytosis of crystals and the release of inflammatory substances. In addition, neutrophils release a glycopeptide that is chemotactic for other neutrophils, thus augmenting inflammatory events. The same substance is present in gout. In both gout and CPPD arthritis, production of this glycopeptide can be suppressed by colchicine.

A minority of patients with CPPD arthropathy have an increased incidence of metabolic abnormalities or hereditary CPPD disease. These associations suggest that a variety of different metabolic products may enhance CPPD deposition. Included among these conditions are hyperparathyroidism, hemochromatosis, gout, hypophosphatasia, hypomagnesemia, hypothyroidism, ochronosis, Wilson's disease, and amyloid. Hemochromatosis is a good example. Ferrous ions may either directly alter cartilage or inhibit inorganic pyrophosphatases, leading to enhanced susceptibility to CPPD deposition. The presence of CPPD arthritis in individuals less than 50 years old should lead to consideration of these metabolic disorders and evaluation of serum calcium, phosphorus, alkaline phosphatase, iron, iron-binding capacity, magnesium, thyroxine, and thyroid-stimulating hormone. However, the likelihood of discovering these diseases, as occult conditions, in older persons with CPPD deposition is very small.

Clinical manifestations CPPD arthropathy may be asymptomatic, acute, subacute, or chronic or cause acute synovitis superimposed upon chronically involved joints. Acute CPPD arthritis was originally termed "pseudogout" by McCarty and coworkers because of its striking similarity to gout. He and others have since recognized that the clinical sequelae of CPPD deposition include: (1) induction or enhancement of some forms of osteoarthritis; (2) induction of severe resorptive disease that may radiographically mimic neuropathic arthritis; and (3) production of symmetric proliferative synovitis, clinically similar to rheumatoid arthritis.

The knee is the most frequently affected joint in CPPD arthropathy. Other sites include the wrist, shoulder, ankle, elbow, and hands. Rarely the temporomandibular joint and ligamentum flavum of the spinal canal may be involved. Clinical and radiographic evidence indicates that CPPD deposition is polyarticular in at least two-thirds of patients. When acute synovitis occurs, diagnosis is made by identification of rod- or rhomboid-shaped weakly positively birefringent crystals (Fig. 282-1) that stain with alizarin red S in synovial fluid. When the clinical picture resembles that of slowly progressive osteoarthritis, diagnosis may be more difficult. Joint distribution may provide important clues, suggesting a nonosteoarthritic process. For example, primary osteoarthritis almost never involves the metacar-

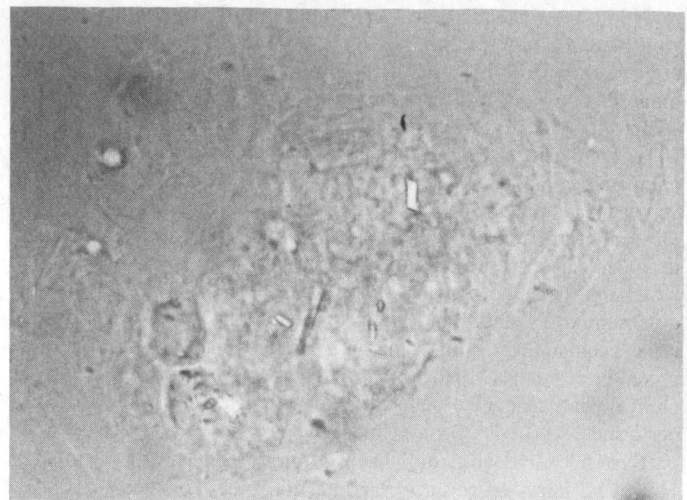

FIGURE 282-1 Calcium pyrophosphate dihydrate crystals, in a fragment of connective tissue, illustrate positive birefringence of rods and rhomboids (compensated polarized light microscopy). ×400. (*Courtesy of Ralph Schumacher.*)

pophalangeal, wrist, elbow, shoulder, or ankle joint. If radiographs reveal punctate and/or linear radiodense deposits in fibrocartilaginous joint menisci or articular hyaline cartilage (chondrocalcinosis), the diagnostic certainty of CPPD is further enhanced. *Definitive diagnosis* requires demonstration of typical crystals in synovial fluid or articular tissue. In the absence of joint effusion or indications to obtain a synovial biopsy, chondrocalcinosis is presumptive of CPPD deposition. One exception is chondrocalcinosis due to CaOx in some patients with chronic renal failure.

Acute attacks of CPPD arthritis may be precipitated by trauma, such as physical injury to an extremity, joint surgery, a sprain, or even a long walk. These events are believed to cause cartilaginous abrasion and microcrystal shedding into the joint space. Rapid diminution of serum calcium concentration, as may occur in severe medical illness or after surgery (especially parathyroidectomy), can also lead to pseudogout. How transient calcium disequilibrium may facilitate CPPD release is unclear.

In as many as 50 percent of cases, CPPD pseudogout may be associated with low-grade fever and on occasion temperature as high as 40°C. Whether or not radiographic proof of chondrocalcinosis is evident in the involved joint(s), synovial analysis with microbial stains and cultures is essential to rule out the possibility of infection. In fact, infection in a joint with any microcrystalline deposition process can lead to crystal shedding and subsequent synovitis from both crystals and microorganisms. Synovial fluid in uncomplicated pseudogout has inflammatory qualities. The WBC count can range from several thousand cells to 100,000 per milliliter, the mean being about 24,000 per milliliter and the predominant cell being the neutrophil. Polarization microscopy usually reveals weakly positively birefringent crystals in the extracellular fluid and within neutrophils.

Untreated, acute attacks may last a few days to as long as a month. *Treatment* by joint aspiration (to decrease intraarticular pressure) and nonsteroidal anti-inflammatory agents or intraarticular glucocorticoid injection may result in return to prior status within 10 days or less. For patients with frequent recurrent attacks of pseudogout, daily prophylactic treatment with low doses of colchicine may be helpful. Unfortunately, effective treatment does not exist to remove CPPD deposits from cartilage and the joint capsule. As a result, CPPD tends to cause progressive forms of arthritis.

CALCIUM HYDROXYAPATITE DEPOSITION DISEASE **Pathogenesis**

Calcium hydroxyapatite is the primary mineral of bone and teeth. Abnormal accumulation can occur in areas of tissue damage (dystrophic calcification), in hypercalcemic or hyperparathyroid states (metastatic calcification), and in certain conditions of unknown cause, such as tumoral calcinosis and periarticular calcification leading to acute and chronic tendinitis and/or bursitis. HA-induced tendinitis and bursitis are most common in the setting of overuse of an extremity. In chronic renal failure, hyperphosphatemia enhances HA deposits within as well as around joints. It was not until 1976 that HA was clearly established as a cause of arthritis.

HA and other basic calcium phosphates may be released from exposed bone and cause the acute synovitis occasionally seen in chronic stable osteoarthritis (e.g., the "hot" Heberden's node). HA deposition is also an important factor in an extremely destructive chronic arthropathy of the elderly that occurs most often in knees and shoulders. Joint destruction is associated with attenuation or rupture of supporting structures, leading to instability and deformity. Progression tends to be indolent, and synovial fluid WBC counts are usually less than 1000 cells per milliliter. Symptoms range from minimal to severe pain and disability that may lead to joint replacement surgery. Whether severely affected patients merely represent an extreme synovial tissue response to HA crystals that are so common in osteoarthritis is uncertain. Observations that favor articular HA deposition and joint destruction being a unique entity, rather than just a sequel of osteoarthritis, include the following: (1) Primary osteoarthritis of the shoulders is infrequent. (2) High levels of activated collagenase and neutral protease, as well as fragments of collagen, have been found in the noninflammatory synovial fluids of patients with severe HA arthropathy; the concentration of these enzymes exceeded those for rheumatoid arthritis and uncomplicated osteoarthritis. (3) Synovial membrane tissue cultures, exposed to HA crystals (or CPPD), markedly increased release of these enzymes, underscoring the destructive potential of abnormally stimulated synovial lining cells. (4) Although rare, HA crystals have been isolated from individuals less than 30 years old who have no evidence of osteoarthritis.

Clinical manifestations Periarticular and articular deposits may coexist and be associated with acute and/or chronic damage to the joint capsule, tendons, bursa, or articular surfaces. The most common sites of HA deposition include those in and/or around the knees, shoulders, hips, and fingers. Clinical manifestations include asymptomatic radiographic abnormalities, acute synovitis or tendinitis, and chronic destructive arthropathy. Most patients with HA arthropathy are elderly. Although the true incidence of HA arthritis is not known, 30 to 50 percent of patients with osteoarthritis have HA microcrystals in their synovial fluid. Such crystals can frequently be identified in clinically stable osteoarthritic joints, but are more likely to come to attention in persons experiencing acute or subacute worsening of joint pain and swelling. The synovial fluid WBC count in HA arthritis is usually low (<2000 per milliliter), but may at times have as many as 50,000 per milliliter. Most synovial fluid analyses reveal a predominance of mononuclear cells. Occasionally neutrophils may dominate.

Diagnosis Radiographic findings in HA arthropathy are not diagnostic. Intra- and/or periarticular calcifications with or without erosive, destructive, or hypertrophic changes may be present. X-ray films may also be normal.

Definitive diagnosis of HA arthropathy depends on identification of crystals from synovial fluid or tissue (Fig. 282-2). Individual crystals are very small, non-birefringent, and can only be seen by electron microscopy. Clumps of crystals may appear as 1- to 20-μm shiny intra- or extracellular globules that stain purplish on Wright's stain and bright red with alizarin red S. Absolute identification depends on electron microscopy with energy dispersive elemental analysis, x-ray diffraction, or infrared spectroscopy.

Treatment of HA arthritis is nonspecific. Acute attacks of synovitis may be selflimiting within days to several weeks. Aspiration of effusions, plus the use of nonsteroidal anti-inflammatory agents for 2 weeks or intraarticular injection of glucocorticoid salts appear to shorten the duration and intensity of symptoms. In patients with underlying severe destructive articular changes, response to medical therapy is usually less rewarding.

CALCIUM OXALATE (CaOx) DEPOSITION DISEASE **Pathogenesis** *Primary oxalosis* is a rare hereditary metabolic disorder (Chap. 335). Enhanced production of oxalic acid may result from at least two different enzyme defects, leading to hyperoxalemia and deposition of calcium oxalate crystals in tissues. Nephrocalcinosis, renal failure, and death usually occur prior to 20 years of age. Acute and/or chronic CaOx arthritis and periarthritis may complicate primary oxalosis during later years of illness.

Secondary oxalosis is more common than the primary disorder. It is one of the many metabolic abnormalities that complicate end-stage renal disease (ESRD). In ESRD calcium oxalate deposits have long been recognized in visceral organs, blood vessels, bones, and even cartilage. However, it was not until 1982 that such deposits were demonstrated to be one of the causes of arthritis in chronic renal failure. Thus far, reported patients have been dependent on long-term hemodialysis or peritoneal dialysis (see also Chap. 225), and many had received vitamin C (ascorbic acid) supplements. Ascorbic acid is metabolized to oxalate, which is inadequately cleared in uremia and by dialysis. Such supplements are now usually avoided in dialysis programs because of the risk of enhancing hyperoxalosis and its sequelae.

Clinical manifestations and diagnosis As was noted for the other calcium salts, CaOx aggregates can be found in articular cartilage, synovium, and periarticular tissues. From these sites,

FIGURE 282-2 *A*. Apatite rods from synovial fluid (electron microscopy). ×105,000. *B*. An electron micrograph demonstrates a cluster of dark apatite crystals within a synovial fluid mononuclear cell. (*Courtesy of Ralph Schumacher.*)

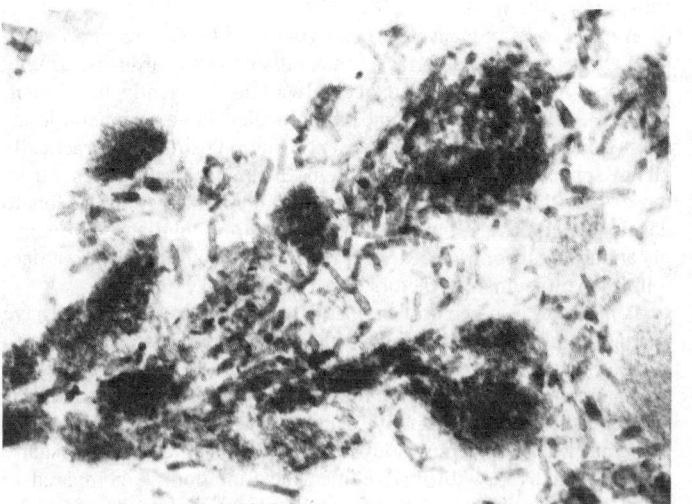

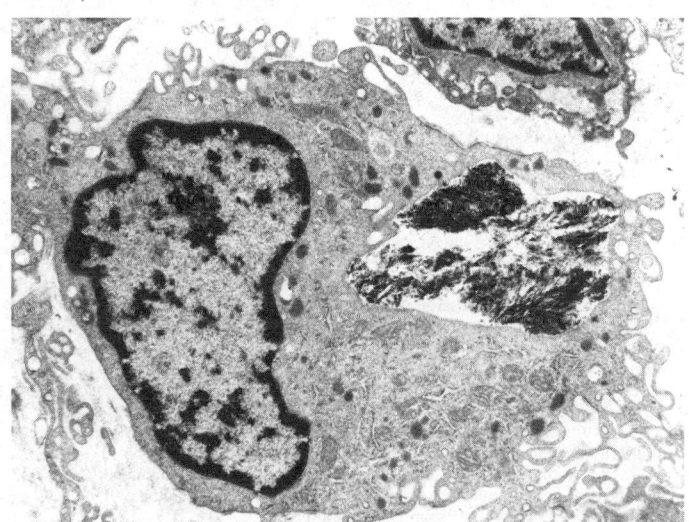

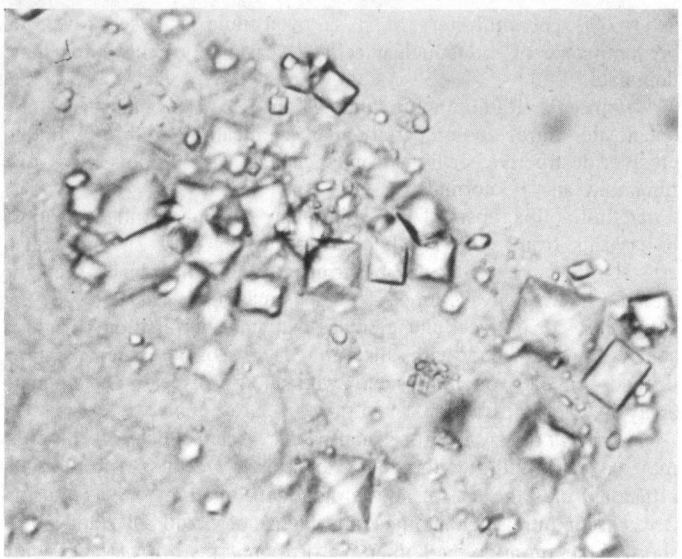

FIGURE 282-3 Calcium oxalate crystals demonstrate typical bipyramidal morphology (regular light microscopy). ×400. (*Courtesy of Ralph Schumacher.*)

crystals may be shed, causing acute synovitis. Persistent aggregates of CaOx may, like HA and CPPD, stimulate synovial proliferation and enzyme release, resulting in progressive articular destruction. Few well-studied cases have been reported. Deposits have been documented in fingers, wrists, elbows, knees, ankles, and feet. Any articular site could potentially be involved.

Each of the known microcrystalline arthropathies may be a complication of ESRD, and rare patients may have more than one type of crystal present in a joint effusion. The advent of crystallographic techniques has made it clear that most arthritic problems in ESRD are not, as was once believed, due to gout. Clinical features of acute CaOx arthritis may not be distinguishable from those due to sodium urate, CPPD, or HA. Radiographs may reveal chondrocalcinosis, a feature of either CPPD or CaOx deposition. CaOx-induced synovial effusions are usually noninflammatory, with less than 2000 leukocytes per milliliter. Predominant cell types have varied from being either neutrophils or mononuclear cells. In most instances, crystals are extracellular, although CaOx has been identified within neutrophils. Synovial membranes show modest signs of inflammation. CaOx has a variable shape and variable birefringence to polarized light. The most easily recognized forms are bipyramidal and strongly positively birefringent (Fig. 282-3).

Treatment of CaOx arthropathy with nonsteroidal anti-inflammatory agents, colchicine, intraarticular glucocorticoids, and increased frequency of dialysis has produced only slight improvement.

REFERENCES

ALVARELLOS A, SPILBERG I: Colchicine prophylaxis in pseudogout. J Rheumatol 13:804, 1986

DIEPPE PA et al: Apatite deposition disease. A new arthropathy. Lancet 1:266, 1976

———: Pyrophosphate arthropathy: A clinical and radiological study of 105 cases. Ann Rheum Dis 41:371, 1982

DOHERTY M, DIEPPE P: Crystal deposition disease in the elderly. Clin Rheum Dis 12:97, 1986

HALVERSON PB et al: Milwaukee shoulder syndrome: Eleven additional cases with involvement of the knee in seven (basic calcium phosphate crystal deposition disease). Semin Arthritis Rheum 14:36, 1984

HOFFMAN GS et al: Calcium oxalate microcrystalline-associated arthritis in end-stage renal disease. Ann Intern Med 97:36, 1982

MASUDA I, ISHIKAWA K: Clinical features of pseudogout attack. A survey of 50 cases. Clin Orthop 229:173, 1988

McCARTY DJ et al: The significance of calcium phosphate crystals in the synovial fluid of arthritic patients: The "pseudogout syndrome." Ann Intern Med 56:711, 1962

———: "Milwaukee shoulder"—association of microspheroids containing hydroxyapatite crystals, active collagenase, and neutral protease with rotator cuff defects. I. Clinical aspects. Arthritis Rheum 24:464, 1981

MOSKOWITZ R: Diseases associated with the deposition of calcium pyrophosphate or hydroxyapatitie, in *Textbook of Rheumatology*, 3d ed, WN Kelly et al (eds). Philadelphia, Saunders, 1989, chap 79

REGINATO AJ et al: Arthropathy and cutaneous calcinosis in hemodialysis oxalosis. Arthritis Rheum 29:1387, 1986

SCHUMACHER HR JR: Crystals, inflammation, and osteoarthritis. Am J Med 83 (Suppl 5A):11, 1987

TERKELTAUB RA et al: Serum and plasma inhibit neutrophil stimulation by hydroxyapatite crystals. Arthritis Rheum 31:1081, 1988

283 PSORIATIC ARTHRITIS AND ARTHRITIS ASSOCIATED WITH GASTROINTESTINAL DISEASES

PETER H. SCHUR

PSORIATIC ARTHRITIS Psoriatic arthritis is an inflammatory arthritis that occurs in patients with psoriasis. While psoriasis occurs in about 1 to 2 percent of the general population, psoriatic arthritis occurs in about 0.1 percent. Between 2.6 and 7 percent of people with arthritis have psoriasis; 0.5 to 40 percent of people with psoriasis have some form of arthritis (5 to 7 percent have "psoriatic arthritis").

Etiology and pathogenesis The etiology and pathogenesis are unknown. Indirect evidence has suggested that (viral) infections, trauma, increased cellular immunity to streptococci, decreased suppressor cell activation, immune complexes, and abnormal polymorphonuclear leukocyte (PMN) function may each play a role. Familial aggregation suggests the influence of genetic factors. Although HLA-B13, B17, CW6, and perhaps DR7 are increased in frequency in patients with psoriasis, most studies have observed an increased frequency of HLA-B17 and B27 in patients with psoriatic arthritis. The increase in HLA-B27 is noted especially in those with psoriatic spondylitis, while B27, B38, B39, and DR7 have been noted in association with peripheral arthritis in different studies.

Clinical manifestations Three major types of psoriatic arthritis have been recognized. A mean of 47 percent of patients (range 16 to 70 percent) have an asymmetric inflammatory arthritis. The psoriasis tends to precede the arthritis by many years. Disease appears equally in men and women. The proximal and distal interphalangeal (PIP, DIP) joints are most frequently involved (with characteristic sausage-shaped digits) and knees, hips, ankles, and wrists less frequently involved. Many have morning stiffness. Most patients have onychodystrophy (onycholysis, ridging, pitting), whose course does not parallel that of the synovitis. The prognosis is good, with only one-fourth of the patients developing progressive destructive disease; one-third develop inflammatory occular complications (conjunctivitis, iritis, episcleritis).

A mean of 25 percent of patients (range 15 to 39 percent) develop symmetric arthritis. Psoriasis and inflammatory arthritis usually develop simultaneously, and occur twice as frequently in women. The DIP, PIP, MCP, MTP, and, in particular, large peripheral joints are involved. Most patients experience morning stiffness. Practically all have onychodystrophy, which helps distinguish these patients from those with rheumatoid arthritis. Over half of this group go on to develop destructive arthritis, including arthritis mutilans. Eye complications are uncommon. None have subcutaneous nodules, but one-fourth have rheumatoid factors.

A mean of 23 percent of the patients (range 5 to 33 percent) have psoriatic "spondylitis," with or without peripheral joint involvement. Psoriasis tends to precede the arthritis by a few years and is twice as common in men. About half of this group have ankylosing spondylitis and the other sacroiliitis. Low back pain with morning stiffness is common. Many have onychodystrophy. The back disease is usually slowly progressive with little clinical deterioration; as compared to ankylosing spondylitis, the peripheral disease also tends not to be destructive except for the occasional patient with arthritis mutilans. Few patients have inflammatory ocular complications.

Some authors have described additional subsets of psoriatic arthritis: predominant DIP joint involvement (6 percent of cases), arthritis mutilans (5 percent), and juvenile psoriatic arthritis (2 percent).

The pathology is quite similar to that seen in rheumatoid arthritis: synoviocytic hyperplasia, early PMN infiltration and later mononuclear cell infiltration, cartilage erosion, and pannus formation. Fibrosis of the joint capsule and marrow is prominent in many.

Laboratory findings There are few laboratory abnormalities. Elevated erythrocyte sedimentation rates and complement levels reflect inflammation. Rheumatoid factors are uncommon and are more likely to be observed in those with symmetric arthritis. Immunoglobulin levels are normal. Uric acid levels are often elevated and parallel the extent and severity of the psoriasis. Sodium urate crystals in joint fluids suggest gout.

Radiologic investigation reveals findings quite similar to those of rheumatoid arthritis: soft tissue swelling, loss of the cartilage space, erosions, bony ankylosis, subluxations, subchondral cysts, but less demineralization. More unique, and suggestive of psoriatic arthritis are: erosions at DIP joints; expansion of the base of the terminal phalanx; whittling of the distal middle phalanx; cuplike erosions of the proximal terminal phalanx—"pencil-in-cup" appearance; proliferation of bone about osseous erosions; sacroiliitis, spondylitis; terminal phalangeal osteolysis; bone proliferation and periostitis (especially of phalanges); and telescoping of one bone into its neighbor, leading to the "opera-glass" deformity.

Diagnosis The diagnosis of psoriatic arthritis should be considered in individuals with arthritis and psoriasis. Psoriasis should be distinguished from seborrheic dermatitis and eczema. Psoriatic lesions may be quite small peripherally, or often hidden in the scalp, umbilicus, and gluteal folds. Fungal infection of nails can be distinguished from psoriasis, for the latter will demonstrate pitting and onycholysis. Furthermore, onychodystrophy is uncommon (20 percent) in uncomplicated psoriasis. It is often difficult to distinguish Reiter's syndrome from psoriatic arthritis since both manifest sausage toes. Reiter's syndrome usually presents in younger individuals, especially males; is less frequently progressive or destructive; and more likely associated with characteristic skin lesions (keratoderma blenorrhagica), urethritis, and conjunctivitis. Gout can be distinguished by the presence of intraarticular sodium urate crystals. Psoriasis in association with Heberden's nodes or Bouchard's nodes of the DIP and PIP joints, respectively, does not suggest psoriatic arthritis. Psoriatic arthritis differs from rheumatoid arthritis by the relevant lack of rheumatoid factors, the tendency to asymmetry, the frequent presence of nail lesions (onychodystrophy), and the high frequency of HLA-B27, especially in patients with axial skeletal involvement.

Treatment The treatment of psoriatic arthritis begins with patient education and physical and occupational therapy to maintain muscle strength and joint and muscle function. Orthotics and occasional intraarticular glucocorticoids for isolated acutely and severely inflamed joints may be added as needed. The mainstay, however, is the use of nonsteroidal anti-inflammatory drugs (NSAIDs) including salicylates. They will reduce inflammation and alleviate pain in the majority of patients. Aspirin and indomethacin are particularly useful. Oral colchicine has been reported to be of benefit. For those patients with more severe involvement, a disease-modifying antirheumatic drug should be utilized. While hydroxychloroquin is often successful in either causing amelioration or remission it carries a significant risk of exacerbation of psoriasis. Oral and intramuscular gold salts have caused remission in over 50 percent of patients, with few side effects. For the more severe cases, especially with extensive skin involvement, methotrexate is recommended. A total of three doses of 2.5 to 5 mg given 12 h apart once a week is recommended. Most patients respond well with respect to both skin lesions and arthritis. Patients who are resistant to oral therapy may respond to intravenous therapy. Renal

and liver function and a CBC should be monitored frequently, and abnormalities should prompt withholding of the drug until tests normalize. Liver biopsies are recommended after a total of 1.5 g of methotrexate and then every 2 years to identify patients with fibrosis and cirrhosis, which necessitates withdrawal of the drug. This is rare. However, patients are advised to avoid nephrotoxic and hepatotoxic (viz., ethanol) drugs. If methotrexate cannot be tolerated, 6-mercaptopurine and azathioprine have been proven successful. The arthritis of few patients responds to the psoriasis therapy known as PUVA (psoralen with UV-A radiation). Advanced forms of therapy should be provided only in consultation with, or by, persons expert in their use.

ARTHRITIS ASSOCIATED WITH GASTROINTESTINAL DISEASE

Inflammatory bowel disease (IBD) Arthritis has been observed to be associated with inflammatory bowel disease. Peripheral arthritis occurs in 9 to 20 percent of patients with IBD (e.g., ulcerative colitis, Crohn's disease). Arthritis is somewhat more likely to occur in patients with large-bowel disease and in those patients with complicatons such as abscesses, pseudomembranous polyposis, perianal disease, massive hemorrhage, erythema nodosum, stomatitis, uveitis, and pyoderma gangrenosum. Males and females are affected equally. The arthritis tends to be acute, is associated with flares of the bowel disease, occurs early in the course of the bowel disease, is self-limiting (90 percent under 6 months), and does not result in destruction. Involved joints are swollen, erythematous, warm, and painful. The majority of patients (90 percent) have polyarticular disease with knees, ankles, elbows, and wrists more commonly affected than PIP, MCP, and MTP joints. Half of patients have migratory arthritis. Granulomas, associated with Crohn's disease, can cause an erosive arthritis. Rarely a psoas abscess can result from bowel perforation, even resulting in (septic) hip arthritis. Rheumatoid factor tests are negative. In those persons who have only peripheral arthritis, there is no increase in frequency in HLA-B27. Synovial fluids have 5000 to 12,000 white blood cells per microliter, mostly PMNs. Radiographs demonstrate soft-tissue swelling and effusions without erosions or destruction. Pathologic examination of synovial biopsies reveals only nonspecific inflammation. The arthritis responds to successful treatment of the bowel disease such as colectomy (for ulcerative colitis), glucocorticoids, or sulfasalazine. NSAIDs are useful to relieve pain and inflammation, but should be used with caution because of possible gastrointestinal side effects.

Spondylitis occurs in 1.1 to 26 percent of patients with Crohn's disease or ulcerative colitis. Males and females are equally affected. Patients will typically complain of stiffness in the back and/or buttocks in the morning or after rest. Stiffness and associated pain are often relieved by exercise. Back symptoms are unrelated to those of the gastrointestinal disease. Physical examination reveals limited spinal flexion and reduced chest expansion. Some patients may have peripheral arthritis, especially of the hips and/or shoulders. Iritis is a frequent complication. Radiographs of the back show the typical findings of ankylosing spondylitis and bilateral sacroiliitis. HLA-B27 is found in 53 to 75 percent of these patients. Treatment includes NSAIDs, gluococorticoids for the bowel disease, and physical therapy. The axial disease progresses in a slow manner akin to ankylosing spondylitis.

Asymptomatic sacroiliitis detected by radiography occurs in 4 to 25 percent of patients with Crohn's disease or ulcerative colitis. By contrast, 52 percent of patients with IBD have abnormal technetium pyrophosphate bone scans of the sacroiliac joint. There is no increased frequency of HLA-B27. This "disease" does not necessarily progress to spondylitis.

Other complications of chronic IBD include: (1) finger clubbing (observed in 4 to 13 percent of patients with Crohn's disease, especially those with small bowel involvement) that may regress after surgery; (2) development of amyloid, especially in association with Crohn's disease; and (3) osteoporosis resulting from inactivity, malabsorption, and/or treatment with glucocorticoids. Osteomalacia can result from malabsorption. In this setting, acutely increased back pain should make compression fracture suspect.

Intestinal bypass arthritis Intestinal bypass surgery was developed for the treatment of obesity in 1952; 11 years later arthritis was recognized as a postoperative complication. Polyarthralgia and sometimes arthritis may occur weeks, even years following surgery in 8 to 36 percent of patients. Pain and tenderness exceed objective findings in most; others have noted episodes of abrupt onset of pain and inflammation. Tenosynovitis is common. Episodes may last for days and even months; tend to affect the knee, wrist, ankle, shoulder, and finger joints; and cause pain in the neck and back. The syndrome occurs more likely after jejunocolic than after jejunoileal surgery and more in females than males. There is often an associated urticarial, vesicular, pustular, macular, or nodular eruption. Raynaud's symptoms appear in one-third of the patients. X-rays generally show no joint damage, except marginal erosions in patients with persistent arthritis. Synovial fluids generally have white blood cell counts of 500 to 27,000 per microliter of mostly PMNs. Synovial biopsies show chronic synovitis with lymphocytes but without lymphoid follicles. Tests for rheumatoid factors, antinuclear antibodies, and HLA-B27 are usually negative, while immune complexes (and cryoglobulins) are often present. They contain bacterial antigens, their antibodies, IgA secretory component, and various complement components. These observations suggest that the syndrome has the following pathogenesis: bacteria proliferate in intestinal blind loops; bacterial antigens are absorbed; antibodies to these antigens develop and combine with them to form immune complexes which deposit in synovial tissue to cause arthritis. NSAIDs and glucocorticoids can relieve the joint symptoms but more lasting results can be achieved by tetracycline therapy to decrease bacteria; even better is reanastomosis of the bowel.

Whipple's disease (intestinal lipodystrophy) Whipple's disease is rare and occurs mostly in middle-aged Caucasian males who develop arthritis, prolonged diarrhea, malabsorption, and weight loss. Up to 90 percent of patients develop arthritis, usually prior to other symptoms. Knees and ankles and, to a lesser extent, fingers, hips, shoulders, elbows, and wrists are involved. The arthritis is acute in onset and is characterized by tender, red swollen joints. Symptoms are migratory, usually lasting just a few days, and are rarely chronic or cause permanent joint damage. Associated symptoms may include fever (54 percent), edema, serositis (pleurisy, pericarditis, endocarditis), pneumonia, hypotension, lymphadenopathy (54 percent), hyperpigmentation (54 percent), subcutaneous nodules, clubbing, and uveitis. Central nervous system (43 percent) involvement may develop with loss of memory, confusion, depression, headache, diplopia, and papilledema. Laboratory abnormalities include anemia (75 percent), low serum carotene (95 percent) and albumin levels (93 percent), and HLA-B27 (30 percent) in those patients with axial arthritis. Synovial fluids have been reported to contain 450 to 36,000 white blood cells per microliter (30 to 95 percent neutrophils) or a mild monocytosis. Joint x-rays rarely show erosions but may show a sacroiliitis in those occasional patients who have axial skeletal symptoms; abdominal x-rays, or CT scans, may reveal lymphadenopathy. The diagnosis is generally established by the detection of PAS-staining bacilliform structures in the lamina propria and/or in foamy macrophages in the small intestine. These inclusion-containing foamy macrophages have also been detected in the synovium, synovial fluid, abdominal and peripheral lymph nodes, pericardium, myocardium, liver, spleen, kidney, brain, and other tissues. Electron microscopy reveals rod-shaped organisms in the lamina propria of the small intestine. Although bacteria have not been isolated or cultured from these patients, the syndrome responds well to long-term antibiotic therapy: viz., penicillin, tetracycline, or erythromycin 0.5 g qid for one year. Some have recommended an initial 2-week course of penicillin and streptomycin. Trimethoprim-sulfamethoxazole benefits in the event of CNS involvement.

Reactive arthritis A Reiter's-like syndrome of arthritis 2 to 3 weeks following diarrhea caused by either *Shigella*, *Salmonella*, *Yersinia*, or *Campylobacter* organisms has been described (see Chap. 274). The term *Reiter's syndrome* applies if patients also have ocular, mucocutaneous, and/or urethral lesions. Synovial fluid cultures are typically negative. Most (90 percent) of these individuals are HLA-B27 positive. One group of investigators has demonstrated that an anti-*Klebsiella* antiserum reacted with cells from B27-positive spondylitic patients, but not from normal B27-positive individuals; the reaction could be inhibited by extracts of the above organisms as well as certain *Klebsiella*. These observations have suggested that a plasmid in these bacteria affect certain B27-positive individuals and may be involved in the pathogenesis of Reiter's syndrome and related spondyloarthropathies.

REFERENCES

FLEMING JL et al: Whipple's disease: Clinical, biochemical, and histopathologic features and assessment of treatment in 29 patients. Mayo Clin Proc 63:539, 1988

GRAVALLESE EM, KANTROWITZ GF: Arthritic manifestations of inflammatory bowel disease. Am J Gastroenterol 83:703, 1988

KAMMER GM et al: Psoriatic arthritis: A clinical, immunologic and HLA study of 100 patients. Semin Arthritis Rheum 9:75, 1979

KERR R, RESNICK D: Radiology of the seronegative spondyloarthropathies. Clin Rheum Dis 11:113, 1985

LAURENT MR: Psoriatic arthritis. Clin Rheum Dis 11:61, 1985

WOLHEIM FA: Enteropathic arthritis, in *Textbook of Rheumatology*, 3d ed, WN Kelley et al (eds). Philadelphia, Saunders, 1989, 62, pp 1064–1073

WOODROW JC: Genetic aspects of the spondyloarthropathies. Clin Rheum Dis 11:1, 1985

284 RELAPSING POLYCHONDRITIS AND MISCELLANEOUS ARTHRITIDES

BRUCE C. GILLILAND

RELAPSING POLYCHONDRITIS

Relapsing polychondritis is an episodic and often progressive inflammatory disorder affecting predominately the cartilage of the ears, nose, and tracheobronchial tree, as well as internal structures of the eyes and ears. Other manifestations include polyarthritis and aortic insufficiency. It is most common between the ages of 40 to 60 years but may affect children and the elderly. Relapsing polychondritis is an uncommon disorder which has been found in all races. Both sexes are equally affected, and no familial tendency is apparent. The etiology is unknown.

PATHOLOGY AND PATHOPHYSIOLOGY The earliest abnormality of cartilage noted histologically is a focal or diffuse loss of basophilic staining indicating depletion of acid mucopolysaccharides from the cartilage matrix. Inflammatory infiltrates are found adjacent to involved cartilage and consist of predominantly mononuclear cells and occasional plasma cells. In acute disease, polymorphonuclear white cells may also be present. Destruction of cartilage begins at the outer edges and advances centrally. There is lacunar breakdown and loss of chondrocytes. Degenerating cartilage is replaced by granulation tissue and later by fibrosis and focal areas of calcification. Small sites of cartilage regeneration may be present. Immunofluorescence studies have shown immunoglobulins and complement at sites of involvement. Fine granular material observed in the degenerating cartilage matrix by electron microscopy has been interpreted to be enzymes or immunoglobulins.

In the eye, lymphocytes and plasma cells have been found around episcleral vessels, as well as in the corneal stroma and iris. In the proximal aorta, mononuclear cells have been noted in the media along with loss of elastic and muscle tissue.

Immunologic mechanisms play a role in the pathogenesis of relapsing polychondritis. Immunoglobulin and complement deposits are found at sites of inflammation. In addition, antibodies to type II collagen and immune complexes are detected in the sera of some patients. The possibility that an immune response to type II collagen may be important in the pathogenesis is supported experimentally by the occurrence of auricular chondritis in rats immunized with type II collagen. Antibodies to type II collagen are found in the sera of these animals, and immune deposits are detected at sites of ear inflammation. Cell-mediated immunity may also be operative in causing tissue injury since lymphocyte transformation can be demonstrated when lymphocytes of patients are exposed to cartilage extracts.

Dissolution of cartilage matrix can be induced by the intravenous injection of crude papain, a proteolytic enzyme, into young rabbits, which results in collapse of their normally rigid ears within 4 h. Reconstitution of the matrix occurs in about 7 days. In relapsing polychondritis, loss of cartilage matrix also most likely results from action of proteolytic enzymes released from chondrocytes and monocytes that have been activated by inflammatory mediators.

CLINICAL MANIFESTATIONS Auricular chondritis is the most frequent presenting manifestation of relapsing polychondritis and eventually affects about 90 percent of patients. Usually both ears are involved. Patients experience the sudden onset of pain, tenderness, and swelling of the cartilaginous portion of the ear. Earlobes are spared since they do not contain cartilage. The overlying skin has a beefy red or violaceous color. Prolonged or recurrent episodes result in a flabby or droopy ear. Swelling may close off the external auditory meatus or the eustachian tube to cause otitis media, either of which can impair hearing. Inflammation of the internal auditory artery or its cochlear branch produces hearing loss, vertigo, ataxia, nausea, and vomiting. The cartilage of the nose becomes inflamed during the first or subsequent attacks. Approximately 80 percent of patients will eventually have nose involvement. The bridge of the nose becomes red, swollen, and tender, and may collapse, producing a saddle deformity. In some patients, the saddle deformity develops insidiously without overt inflammation.

Arthritis is the presenting manifestation in relapsing polychondritis in approximately one-third of patients and may be present for several months before other features appear. The arthritis is usually asymmetric, oligo- or polyarticular, and involves both large and small peripheral joints. An episode of arthritis lasts from a few days to several weeks and resolves spontaneously without residual joint deformity. Attacks of arthritis may not be temporally related to other manifestations of relapsing polychondritis. The joints are warm, tender, and swollen. Joint fluid has been reported to be noninflammatory. In addition to peripheral joints, inflammation may involve the costochondral and sternoclavicular cartilages. Destruction of these cartilages may result in a flail anterior chest wall.

Eye manifestations occur in greater than half of the patients and include conjunctivitis, episcleritis, iritis, and keratitis. Ulceration and perforation of the cornea may occur and cause blindness. Other manifestations include cataracts, proptosis, optic neuritis, and extraocular muscle palsies.

Laryngotracheal involvement occurs in approximately 70 percent of patients. Symptoms include hoarseness, a nonproductive cough, and tenderness over the larynx and proximal trachea. Mucosal edema, strictures, and/or collapse of laryngeal or tracheal cartilage may cause stridor and life-threatening airway obstruction necessitating tracheostomy. Collapse of cartilage in bronchi leads to pneumonia and, when extensive, to respiratory insufficiency.

Aortic regurgitation occurs in about 15 percent of patients and is due to progressive dilatation of the aortic ring or to destruction of the valve cusps. Other heart values can be affected. Aneurysmal dilatation of the proximal aorta as well as other medium to large vessels may also occur. Segmental necrotizing glomerulonephritis and renal vasculitis have been noted in some patients.

The course of disease is highly variable, with episodes lasting from a few days to several weeks and then subsiding spontaneously. In other patients, disease may have a chronic, smoldering course. In one study the 5-year estimated survival rate was 74 percent and the 10-year survival rate 55 percent. In contrast to earlier series, only

about half of the deaths could be attributed to relapsing polychondritis or complications of treatment. Pulmonary complications accounted for only 10 percent of all fatalities. In general, patients with more widespread disease have a worse prognosis.

LABORATORY FINDINGS Mild leukocytosis and normocytic normochromic anemia are often present. The erythrocyte sedimentation rate is usually elevated. Rheumatoid factor and antinuclear antibody tests are occasionally positive in low titer. Circulating immune complexes may be detected, especially in patients with early active disease. Elevated levels of gamma globulin may be present. Tracheal stenosis can be demonstrated by regular tomograms or computed tomography of the neck. Bronchography is performed for demonstrating bronchial narrowing. On a chest film, narrowing of main bronchi and, when aortic insufficiency is present, cardiomegaly can be observed. Radiographs may show calcification at previous sites of cartilage damage involving ear, nose, larynx, or trachea.

DIAGNOSIS Diagnosis is based on the recognition of the typical clinical features. Biopsies of the involved cartilage from the ear, nose, or respiratory tract will confirm the diagnosis but are only necessary when clinical features are not typical. Patients with Wegener's granulomatosis may have a saddle nose and pulmonary involvement but can be distinguished by the absence of auricular involvement and the presence of granulomatous lesions in the tracheobronchial tree. Patients with Cogan's syndrome have interstitial keratitis and vestibular and auditory abnormalities, but this syndrome does not involve the respiratory tract or ears. Reiter's syndrome may initially resemble relapsing polychondritis because of oligoarticular arthritis and eye involvement, but it is distinguished in time by the appearance of urethritis and typical mucocutaneous lesions and the absence of nose or ear cartilage involvement. Rheumatoid arthritis may initially suggest relapsing polychondritis because of arthritis and eye inflammation. The arthritis in rheumatoid arthritis, however, is erosive and symmetric. In addition, rheumatoid factor titers are usually high compared to relapsing polychondritis. Bacterial infection of the pinna may be mistaken for relapsing polychondritis, but differs by usually involving only one ear including the earlobe. Auricular cartilage may also be damaged by trauma or frostbite.

Relapsing polychondritis may develop in patients with a variety of autoimmune disorders including systemic lupus erythematosus, rheumatoid arthritis, Sjögren's syndrome, and vasculitis. In most cases, these disorders antedate the appearance of polychondritis usually by months or years. It is likely that these patients have an immunologic abnormality that predisposes them to development of this group of autoimmune disorders.

TREATMENT Prednisone, 40 to 60 mg/d, is often effective in suppressing disease activity and is tapered gradually once disease is controlled. In some patients, prednisone can be stopped, while in others low doses in the range of 10 to 15 mg/d are required for continued suppression of disease. Immunosuppressive drugs such as cyclophosphamide or azathioprine should be reserved for patients who fail to respond to prednisone.

MISCELLANEOUS ARTHRITIDES

NEUROPATHIC JOINT DISEASE Neuropathic joint disease (Charcot's joint) is a severe form of osteoarthritis associated with loss of pain sensation, proprioception, or both. In addition, normal muscular reflexes that modulate joint movement are decreased. Without these protective mechanisms, joints are subjected to repeated trauma, resulting in progressive cartilage damage. The distribution of joint involvement depends on the underlying neurologic disorder. In tabes dorsalis, knees, hips, and ankles are most commonly affected; in syringomyelia, the glenohumeral joint, elbow, and wrist; and in diabetes mellitus, the tarsal and tarsometatarsal joints. Resorption of metatarsals and phalanges is also seen in diabetic patients. In children, neuropathic joint disease is caused by congenital indifference to pain or meningomyelocele. Neuropathic joint disease is also observed in patients with amyloidosis and leprosy or following repeated intraarticular glucocorticoid injections. The mechanism of injury in the latter situation is thought to be an analgesic effect of steroids leading to overuse of a previously damaged joint which results in accelerated cartilage deterioration.

Neuropathic joint disease usually begins in a single joint and then progresses to involve other joints, depending on the underlying neurologic disorder. The involved joint progressively becomes enlarged from bony overgrowth and synovial effusion. Loose bodies may be palpated in the joint cavity. Joint instability, subluxation, and crepitus occur as the disease progresses. Charcot's joints may develop rapidly, and a totally disorganized joint with multiple bony fragments may evolve in a patient within weeks or months. The amount of pain experienced by the patient is less than would be anticipated based on the degree of joint involvement. Patients may experience sudden joint pain from intraarticular fractures of osteophytes or condyles. Initially, radiographs show early features of osteoarthritis followed subsequently by marked destructive and hypertrophic changes. Large, bizarre-shaped osteophytes and intraarticular bone fragments are observed. The radiographic findings of the diabetic Charcot's foot may be difficult to distinguish from those of osteomyelitis. Osteomyelitis is often suspected when the diabetic patient has an infected cutaneous ulcer on the foot. The Charcot's joint radiographically shows osteopenia, sharp cortical margins, and severe disruption and disorganization of the midtarsal and tarsometatarsal joints. In osteomyelitis, the bone margins are indistinct. The synovial fluid from a neuropathic joint is usually noninflammatory, may be bloody or xanthochromic, and may contain fragments of synovium, cartilage, and/or bone.

The primary focus of treatment is to provide stabilization of the joint. Treatment of the underlying disorder, even if successful, usually does not alter the joint disease. Braces and splints are helpful. Their use requires close surveillance since patients may be unable to appreciate pressure from a poorly adjusted brace. Fusion of a very unstable joint may improve function, but nonunion is frequent especially when immobilization of the joint is inadequate.

HYPERTROPHIC OSTEOARTHROPATHY Hypertrophic osteoarthropathy (HOA) is characterized by clubbing of digits, periosteal new bone formation, and arthritis. HOA occurs in a primary or familial form beginning usually in childhood. The secondary form of HOA is associated with intrathoracic malignancies, suppurative lung disease, congenital heart disease, and a variety of other disorders, and is more common in adults. Clubbing is almost always a feature of HOA but can occur as an isolated manifestation. It is unclear whether clubbing alone represents a partial expression of HOA or is a separate entity. The presence of only clubbing in a patient usually has the same clinical significance as HOA.

Pathology and pathophysiology In HOA, the periosteum becomes elevated and new bone is deposited beneath the periosteum while endosteal bone is resorbed. These changes occur primarily at the distal ends of metacarpals, metatarsals and long bones of the extremities. Occasionally, scapulae, clavicles, ribs, and pelvic bones are also affected. Mononuclear cell infiltration may be present in the adjacent soft tissue. Proliferation of connective tissue occurs in the nail bed and volar pad of digits, giving the distal phalanges a clubbed appearance. Small blood vessels in the clubbed digits are dilated and have thickened walls. In addition, the number of arteriovenous anastomoses is increased. The synovium of involved joints is edematous and may have an infiltration of lymphocytes and plasma cells.

The pathogenesis of HOA is not known. Both neurogenic and humoral theories have been proposed. In support of a neurogenic mechanism is the observation that the disorders most often associated with HOA involve sites innervated by the vagus nerve. Also, vagotomy may result in resolution of symptoms. A neural reflex initiated by vagal stimulation from the site of disease is thought to lead to vasodilatation and other features of HOA. The humoral theory postulates that a substance produced by the underlying disease and normally inactivated or removed by its passage through the lung reaches the systemic circulation in an active form and induces the changes of HOA. Several humoral substances, including immunoreactive growth hormone, estrogens, prostaglandins, and ferritin, have been suggested as but not proven to be mediators of HOA.

Clinical manifestations Primary HOA, also referred to as *pachydermoperiostitis* or *Touraine-Solente-Golé syndrome,* usually begins insidiously at puberty. It is inherited as an autosomal dominant with variable expression and is more common in boys than in girls. The skin of the face and scalp thickens, producing deep nasolabial folds, furrowed forehead and corrugated scalp which give the face a leonine appearance. The skin of the face and scalp is usually greasy, and there is excessive sweating, particularly of the palms and soles. The distal extremities are thickened due to proliferation of new bone and soft tissue, and when the process is extensive, they may resemble elephant feet. Marked clubbing of hands and feet produces a spade-like deformity and clumsiness. Acrolysis of the terminal phalanges of feet and hands may occur. Symptoms of bone and joint pain are usually seen only in those who have had their disease for two decades or longer.

HOA secondary to an underlying disease occurs more frequently than primary HOA. It accompanies a variety of disorders and may precede clinical features of the associated disorder by months. The progression of HOA tends to be more rapid when associated with malignancies, most notably bronchogenic carcinoma. Patients experience a burning or deep-seated aching pain in the distal extremities due to periostitis. The pain can be quite incapacitating, and is aggravated by dependency and relieved by elevation of the affected limbs. Joint manifestations vary from arthralgias to very painful arthritis, most often affecting the metacarpal-phalangeal and metatarsal-phalangeal joints, wrists, ankles, and knees. The involved joints are warm, tender, and swollen. Joint effusions are usually small, and the fluid is noninflammatory, containing only a few white cells. The distal extremities may be swollen and the overlying skin warm and erythematous. Pressure applied over the distal end of the forearms and lower legs may be quite painful. Clubbing is usually asymptomatic except for occasional warmth or burning of the fingertips. Clubbing usually evolves over months and often is first noted by the physician and not the patient. Patients, especially those with lung tumor, may experience severe skeletal pain prior to the appearance of clubbing. Clubbing is characterized by widening of the fingertips, enlargement of the distal volar pad, convexity of the nail contour, and the loss of the normal 15° angle between the proximal nail and cuticle. The thickness of the digit at the base of the nail is greater than the thickness at the distal interphalangeal joint. The base of the nail feels spongy when compressed and the nail can be easily rocked on its bed. Marked periungual erythema is usually present. When clubbing is advanced, the finger may have a drumstick appearance. Excessive sweating, oiliness of the skin, and thickening of the facial skin are uncommon in secondary HOA.

HOA occurs in 5 to 10 percent of patients with intrathoracic malignancies, the most common being bronchogenic carcinoma and pleural tumors. Lung metastases infrequently cause HOA. HOA is also seen in patients with intrathoracic infections including lung abscesses, empyema, bronchiectasis, chronic obstructive lung disease, and pulmonary tuberculosis. HOA may also accompany chronic interstitial pneumonitis, sarcoidosis, and cystic fibrosis. In the latter, clubbing is more common than the full syndrome of HOA. Other cases of clubbing include congenital heart disease with right-to-left shunts, Crohn's disease, ulcerative colitis, sprue, and neoplasms of the esophagus, liver, small and large bowel. In patients with congenital heart disease with right-to-left shunts, clubbing alone occurs more often than the full syndrome of HOA.

Unilateral clubbing has been found in association with aneurysms of the aorta, subclavian, or innominate artery and with arteriovenous fistula of brachial vessels. Clubbing of the toes but not fingers has been associated with an infected abdominal aortic aneurysm. Clubbing of a single digit may follow trauma, and has been reported in tophaceous gout and sarcoidosis.

Hyperthyroidism (Graves' disease), treated or untreated, may occasionally be associated with clubbing and periostitis of the bones of the hands and feet. This condition is referred to as *thyroid acropachy*. Periostitis is asymptomatic and occurs in the midshaft and diaphyseal portion of the metacarpal and phalangeal bones. The long bones of the extremities are seldom affected. Elevated levels of long-acting thyroid stimulator (LATS) are found in the serum of these patients.

Laboratory The laboratory abnormalities reflect the underlying disorder. The synovial fluid of involved joints has less than 500 white cells per microliter, and they are predominantly mononuclear. Radiographs show a faint radiolucent line beneath the new periosteal bone along the shaft of long bones at their distal end. These changes are most frequently observed at the ankles, wrists, and knees. The ends of the distal phalanges may show osseous resorption. Radionuclide studies show pricortical linear uptake along the cortical margins of long bones that may be present before any radiographic changes.

Treatment The treatment of hypertrophic osteoarthropathy is to identify the associated disorder and treat it appropriately. The symptoms and signs of hypertrophic osteoarthropathy may disappear completely with removal or effective chemotherapy of a tumor or with antibiotic therapy and drainage of a chronic pulmonary infection. Vagotomy or percutaneous block may lead to symptomatic relief in some patients. Aspirin, other nonsteroidal anti-inflammatory drugs, or analgesics may help control symptoms of hypertrophic osteoarthropathy.

FIBROSITIS Fibrositis, also termed *fibromyalgia*, is a commonly encountered disorder characterized by musculoskeletal pain, stiffness, and easy fatigability which affects predominantly women between the ages of 25 and 45 years. The term *fibrositis* is a misnomer, since this is not an inflammatory disorder of connective tissue. The etiology and pathogenesis of fibrositis are not known. A disturbance of normal stage 4 (non-REM) sleep has been suggested as playing a role in the development of fibrositis. Symptoms of fibrositis were produced in normal subjects by disturbing stage 4 sleep with a buzzer without wakening them. Sleep studies in patients with fibrositis have shown an alpha intrusion pattern superimposed on slow wave sleep. Muscle abnormalities have been found at sites of tenderness in some patients. Psychological abnormalities may also contribute to symptoms. A better understanding of fibrositis awaits further studies.

Symptoms are generalized aching and stiffness of the trunk, hip, and shoulder girdles. Other patients complain of generalized aching and muscle weakness. Patients perceive that their joints are swollen; however, joint examination is normal. Stiffness is usually present on arising in the morning and improves during the day, but may last all day in some patients. Patients complain of exhaustion and wake up tired. They also awake frequently at night and have trouble falling back asleep. Symptoms are made worse by stress or anxiety, cold, damp weather, and overexertion. Patients often feel better during warmer weather and vacations. Disorders commonly associated with fibrositis include irritable bowel syndrome, irritable bladder, headaches, and dysmenorrhea. Symptoms of fibrositis also occur in patients who carry the diagnosis of chronic fatigue syndrome.

The characteristic physical feature is the demonstration of specific tender sites which are exquisitely more tender than adjacent areas. Tender sites should be distinguished from the trigger points found in myofascial pain syndromes. Pressure over trigger points causes pain to be referred to a nearby site, while pressure over tender sites causes pain only at that site. The patient may suddenly jump or withdraw when the tender site is palpated. The sites of tenderness are remarkably constant in location. Common sites of tenderness are over the midpoint of the upper border of the trapezius, lateral epicondyles, supraspinatus, lower cervical spine, lumbar spine, posterior iliac spine, costochondral junctions, especially the second, gluteus maximus, and medial fat pad of the knee. Skinfold tenderness may be present, particularly over the upper scapular region. Subcutaneous nodules may be felt at sites of tenderness. Nodules in similar locations are present in normal persons but are not tender.

The diagnosis of fibrositis is made by recognizing the clinical manifestations. The joint and muscle examination is normal, and there are no laboratory abnormalties. Symptoms suggesting fibrositis are seen in patients with rheumatoid arthritis or other connective tissue diseases, and tender sites may be present. It is not clear whether this is part of the connective tissue disease or should be considered as fibrositis complicating the connective tissue disease.

Patients should be informed that they have a treatable condition which is not a crippling, deforming, or degenerative process. Salicylates or other nonsteroidal anti-inflammatory drugs only partially improve symptoms. Glucocorticoids have been of little benefit and should not be used in these patients. Local measures such as heat, massage, injection of tender sites with steroids or lidocaine, and acupuncture provide only temporary relief of symptoms. The use of tricyclics such as amitriptyline, 10 to 25 mg, doxepin, 10 to 25 mg, and cyclobenzaprine, 10 to 20 mg, at bedtime will give the patient restorative sleep resulting in clinical improvement. Higher doses of these medications may be necessary. Patients should improve their physical fitness by regular exercise and decrease the stress in their lives.

PSYCHOGENIC RHEUMATISM Patients may experience severe joint pain involving a few to several joints without physical findings of arthritis. These patients are often convinced that they have rheumatoid arthritis, systemic lupus erythematosus, or another connective tissue disease. This disorder is recognized by the inconsistencies, exaggerations, and emotional lability of the patient during the history and physical examination. Laboratory studies are normal. Organic disease needs to be excluded, which requires seeing the patient at regular intervals. This condition also needs to be distinguished from fibrositis. Anti-inflammatory or other drugs are not helpful.

CARPAL TUNNEL SYNDROME Carpal tunnel syndrome is an entrapment neuropathy of the median nerve at the wrist producing paresthesias and weakness of the hands. The syndrome is caused by pressure on the median nerve where it passes in company with the flexor tendons of the fingers through the tunnel formed by carpal bones and the transverse carpal ligament.

Compression of the median nerve is produced by any process that encroaches on the carpal tunnel. Localized tenosynovitis of the flexor tendons of the fingers is a frequent cause of carpal tunnel syndrome, particularly in middle-aged women. Premenstrual edema or edema occurring in pregnancy may also cause these symptoms. Symptoms can be precipitated by activities which require repeated flexion, pronation, and supination of the wrist, for example, sewing, driving, and operating computers. Other causes of carpal tunnel syndrome, often bilateral, are rheumatoid arthritis, acromegaly, hypothyroidism, and amyloidosis. Unilateral carpal tunnel syndrome is more likely due to trauma, physical activities involving one wrist, tuberculosis, gout, or calcium pyrophosphate deposition disease.

Patients experience numbness or paresthesias of the palmar surface of the thumb, index and middle fingers, and radial half of the ring finger. Numbness or paresthesias of the whole hand may occur. Pain may be referred to the forearm and less commonly to the shoulder and neck regions. Pain or tingling of the fingers often occurs at night and is relieved by shaking or exercising the hand. Weakness and atrophy of the thenar muscles usually appear later and can occur without significant sensory symptoms.

Thenar muscle weakness is manifested by decreased strength of abduction, opposition, and flexion of the thumb. On examination, symptoms of paresthesia or pain in the fingers may be reproduced by percussion over the volar surface of the wrist (Tinel's sign) or by full flexion of the wrist for 1 min (Phalen's maneuver). Decreased touch or hyperpathia to pinprick may be demonstrated over the fingers supplied by the median nerve. Nerve conduction studies of the median nerve show delayed latency across the wrist, confirming the diagnosis.

Treatment of patients with only sensory symptoms and minor

nerve conduction abnormalities consist of a wrist splint to be worn mainly at night, anti-inflammatory drugs, and local injection with steroids. If symptoms persist or motor abnormalities are present, surgical decompression of the carpal tunnel with release of the transverse carpal ligament and debridement is indicated.

TARSAL TUNNEL SYNDROME   Tarsal tunnel syndrome is an entrapment neuropathy of the posterior tibial nerve at the ankle producing aching, burning, tingling, and numbness of the plantar surface of the foot and toes. The syndrome is caused by compression of the posterior tibial nerve and its branches as they pass through the tunnel beneath the flexor retinaculum on the medial side of the ankle inferior and posterior to the medial malleolus. Also passing through this tunnel are the flexor tendons of the toes, vascular bundle, and the medial and lateral plantar branches of the posterior tibial nerve. Compression of the nerve in the tunnel may be caused by tenosynovitis resulting from overuse or trauma and by inflammatory arthritis such as rheumatoid arthritis. Other causes include pregnancy, myxedema, and amyloidosis.

Patients experience paresthesias of the plantar surface of the foot and toes which may radiate up the calf. Symptoms often occur at night and after standing, and may be relieved by movement of the foot and ankle. On examination, there may be loss of sensation over the plantar surface of the foot, but this is variable. Symptoms may be reproduced by percussion over the flexor retinaculum (Tinel's sign) or by applying firm pressure to this area. Diagnosis is confirmed by nerve conduction studies that show prolonged latency across the tunnel. Treatment consists of anti-inflammatory drugs and local injection of steroids. If symptoms persist, surgical decompression is indicated.

REFLEX SYMPATHETIC DYSTROPHY SYNDROME   The reflex sympathetic dystrophy syndrome (RSDS) is characterized by pain and tenderness usually of a distal extremity accompanied by signs and symptoms of vasomotor instability, trophic skin changes, and the rapid development of bony demineralization. A precipitating event can be identified in two-thirds of the cases. These include local trauma, myocardial infarction, strokes, and peripheral nerve injuries. RSDS is observed most often in individuals over the age of 50, reflecting the frequency of the accompanying disorder. The sex distribution is equal. An entire hand or foot is usually affected. Occasionally, RSDS will involve an isolated site such as the patella, hip, or one or two rays of a foot or hand. The contralateral side may be affected in up to 50 percent of patients, and subclinical disease may be present in virtually all patients. The pathogenesis of RSDS is poorly understood. The vasomotor manifestations are thought to be caused by abnormal stimulation of the sympathetic nervous system.

RSDS evolves through three clinical phases. The clinical manifestations of the first phase are pain and swelling of a distal extremity, which develop weeks to months following the precipitating event. The pain has an intense, burning quality. The involved extremity is warm, edematous, and tender especially around joints. Increased sweating and hair growth occur. In 3 to 6 months, the skin gradually becomes thin, shiny, and cool (second phase). Clinical features of the first two phases overlap. In another 3 to 6 months, the skin and subcutaneous tissue become atrophic, and irreversible flexion contractures of the hand or foot develop (third phase). Motion of the shoulder on the affected side is frequently painful and greatly restricted, a condition referred to as shoulder-hand syndrome (see "Adhesive Capsulities," below).

The laboratory abnormalities are those of the associated disorder. Radiographs of the involved distal extremity demonstrate mottled osteopenia referred to as Sudeck's atrophy. Later in the course, diffuse osteopenia develops. Similar changes, however, are observed in an immobilized limb following a fracture or paralysis. Bone scan in the early phase shows asymmetric and increased blood flow followed subsequently by increased radionuclide uptake in the periarticular bone of the involved side. Uptake may also be increased on the contralateral side indicating subclinical involvement.

Early recognition and treatment are important to prevent permanent disability. RSDS may be reversible in its early phases. Appropriate mobilization of the patient following a myocardial infarction, stroke, or injury may help to prevent this syndrome. Pain should be properly controlled. Application of heat or cold along with exercises are useful. Sympathetic nerve block may be effective and, if it is, can be followed by surgical sympathectomy. The response, however, may not be sustained. A short course of high-dose prednisone in conjunction with physical therapy has been beneficial in some patients. Prednisone is started at 60 mg/d for 4 days and gradually tapered over a 3-week period.

TSIETZE'S SYNDROME AND COSTOCHONDRITIS   Tsietze's syndrome is manifested by painful swelling of one or more costochondral articulations. Age of onset is usually before 40, and both sexes are equally affected. Most patients have only one joint involved, usually the second or third costochondral joint. The onset of anterior chest pain may be sudden or gradual. The pain may radiate to the arms or shoulder and is aggravated by sneezing, coughing, deep inspirations, or twisting motions of the chest. The term *costochondritis* is often used interchangeably with Tsietze's syndrome, but some restrict the former term to pain of the costochondral articulations without swelling. Costochondritis is observed in patients over age 40, tends to affect the third, fourth, and fifth costochondral joints, and occurs more often in women. Both syndromes may mimic cardiac or upper abdominal causes of pain. Rheumatoid arthritis, ankylosing spondylitis, or Reiter's syndrome may involve costochondral joints but are distinguished easily by their other clinical features. Other skeletal causes of anterior chest wall pain are xiphoidalgia and the slipping rib syndome, which usually involves the tenth rib. Analgesics, anti-inflammatory drugs, or local steroid injections usually relieve symptoms.

MUSCULOSKELETAL DISORDERS ASSOCIATED WITH HYPER-LIPIDEMIA   Musculoskeletal manifestations may be the first indication of a hereditary disorder of lipoprotein metabolism. Patients with type II hyperlipoproteinemia may have recurrent migratory polyarthritis involving knees and other large peripheral joints and, to a lesser degree, peripheral small joints. The involved joints can be warm, erythematous, and swollen. Arthritis usually has a sudden onset, lasts from a few days to 2 weeks, and does not cause joint damage. Several attacks occur a year. Synovial fluid from involved joints is not inflammatory, and contains few white cells and no crystals. Joint involvement may actually represent inflammatory periarthritis or peritendinitis and not intraarticular disease. The recurrent transient nature of the arthritis may suggest rheumatic fever, especially since patients with lipoproteinemia have an elevated erythrocyte sedimentation rate and a falsely elevated antistreptolysin O titer. Furthermore, patients may have aortic valvular disease secondary to atherosclerosis. Patients with type II hyperlipoproteinemia also have tendinous xanthomas in the Achilles, patellar, and extensor tendons of the hands and feet. These are located within tendon fibers and appear in childhood in homozygous patients and after the age of 30 in heterozygous patients. Tuberous xanthomas appear only in patients homozygous for type II hyperlipoproteinemia. They are located over the extensor surfaces of the elbows, knees and hands, and also on the buttocks. Patients with type IV hyperlipoproteinemia may also have a mild inflammatory arthritis affecting large and small peripheral joints, usually in an asymmetric pattern with only a few joints involved at a time. Arthritis may be persistent or recurrent with episodes lasting a few days. Joint fluid is noninflammatory. Periarticular hyperesthesia may be present. Large juxtaarticular bone cysts have been noted in a few patients. The pathogenesis of arthritis in both types of hyperlipoproteinemia is not well understood. Salicylates, other NSAIDs, or analgesics usually provide relief of symptoms.

PERIARTICULAR DISORDERS   Bursitis   Bursitis is inflammation of a bursa, which is a thin-walled sac lined with synovial tissue. The function of the bursa is to facilitate movement of tendons and muscles over bony prominences. Excessive frictional forces, trauma, systemic disease (e.g., rheumatoid arthritis, gout), or infection may cause bursitis. Subacromial bursitis (subdeltoid bursitis) is the most common form of bursitis. Another is trochanteric bursitis, which involves the bursa around the insertion of the gluteus medius to the greater trochanter of the femur. Patients experience pain over the lateral aspect of the hip and upper thigh and are tender over the posterior aspect of the greater trochanter. External rotation and resisted abduction of the hip elicit pain. Olecranon bursitis occurs over the posterior elbow, and when the area is acutely inflamed, infection should be excluded by aspirating and culturing fluid from the bursa. Achilles bursitis involves the bursa located above the insertion of the tendon to the calcaneus and results from overuse and wearing tight shoes. Retrocalcaneal bursitis involves the bursa which is located between the calcaneus and posterior surface of the Achilles tendon. The pain is experienced at the back of the heel, and swelling appears on the medial and/or lateral side of the tendon. It occurs in association with spondyloarthropathies, rheumatoid arthritis, gout and trauma. Ischial bursitis (weaver's bottom) affects the bursa separating the gluteus medius from the ischial tuberosity and develops from prolonged sitting on hard surfaces. Iliopsoas bursitis affects the bursa that lies between the iliopsoas muscle and hip joint and is lateral to the femoral vessels. Pain is experienced over this area and made worse by hip extension and flexion. Bursitis results from trauma or overuse and can be seen in patients with rheumatoid arthritis. Anserine bursitis is an inflammation of the sartorius bursa located over the medial side of the tibia just below the knee and is manifested by pain on climbing stairs. Tenderness is present over the insertion of the conjoint tendon of the sartorius, gracilis, and semitendinosus. Prepatellar bursitis (housemaid's knee) occurs in the bursa situated between the patella and overlying skin and is caused by kneeling on hard surfaces. Treatment of bursitis consists of prevention of the aggravating condition, rest of the involved part, a nonsteroidal anti-inflammatory drug, and local steroid injection.

Rotator cuff tendinitis Tendinitis of the rotator cuff is the major cause of a painful shoulder. Of the tendons forming the rotator cuff, the supraspinatus tendon is most often affected, probably because of its repeated impingement between the acromion and humeral head as well as its reduced blood supply occurring with abduction of the arm. The process evolves through inflammation, fibrosis, and tears of the tendon. Subacromial bursitis may also be present. Symptoms usually occur after injury or overuse, particularly in individuals over age 40. Patients complain of a dull aching in the shoulder that may interfere with sleep. Severe pain is experienced when the arm is actively abducted into an overhead position. Tenderness is present over the lateral aspect of the humeral head just below the acromion. Nonsteroidal anti-inflammatory drugs, local steroid injection, and physical therapy may relieve symptoms.

Patients may tear the supraspinatus tendon acutely by falling on an outstretched arm or lifting a heavy object. Symptoms are pain, along with weakness of abduction and external rotation of the shoulder. Atrophy of the supraspinatus muscles develops. The diagnosis is established by arthrogram. Surgical repair may be necessary in patients who fail to respond to conservative measures.

Calcific tendinitis This is characterized by deposition of calcium salts, primarily hydroxyapatite, within a tendon. The exact mechanism for calcification is not known but may be due to ischemia or degeneration of the tendon. The supraspinatus tendon is most often affected because of its frequent impingement and reduced blood supply when the arm is abducted. It usually develops after age 40. Calcification within the tendon may evoke acute inflammation, producing sudden and severe pain in the shoulder. Tendon calcification, however, may be asymptomatic or not related to the patient's symptoms.

Bicipital tendinitis and rupture Bicipital tendinitis, or tenosynovitis, is produced by friction on the tendon of the long head of the biceps as it passes through the bicipital groove. When the inflammation is acute, patients experience anterior shoulder pain which radiates down the biceps into the forearm. Abduction and external rotation of the arm are painful and limited. The bicipital groove is very tender

to palpation. Pain may be elicited along the course of the tendon by resisting supination of the forearm with the elbow at 90° (Yergason's supination sign). Acute rupture of the tendon may occur with vigorous exercise of the arm and is often painful. In a young patient, it should be repaired surgically. Rupture of the tendon in an older person may be associated with little or no pain and is recognized by the presence of persistent swelling of the biceps ("Popeye" muscle). Surgery is usually not necessary in this setting.

Adhesive capsulitis Often referred to as "frozen shoulder," adhesive capsulitis is characterized by pain and restricted movement of the shoulder usually in the absence of intrinsic shoulder disease. Adhesive capsulitis, however, may follow bursitis or tendinitis of the shoulder or be associated with systemic disorders such as chronic pulmonary disease, myocardial infarction, and diabetes mellitus. Prolonged immobility of the arm contributes to the development of adhesive capsulitis, and reflex sympathetic dystrophy is thought to be a pathogenic factor. The capsule of the shoulder is thickened, and a mild chronic inflammatory infiltrate and fibrosis may be present.

Adhesive capsulitis occurs more commonly in women after age 50. Pain and stiffness usually develop gradually over several months to a year, but may progress rapidly in some patients. Pain may interfere with sleep. The shoulder is tender to palpation, and both active and passive movement are restricted. Radiograph of the shoulder shows osteopenia. The diagnosis is confirmed by arthrogram, in that only a limited amount of contrast material, usually less than 15 mL, can be injected under pressure into the shoulder joint.

The majority of patients improve spontaneously 12 to 18 months after the onset of disease, but some may have permanent restriction of movement. Early mobilization of the arm following an injury to the shoulder may prevent the development of this disease. Slow but forceful injection of contrast material into the joint may lyse adhesions and stretch the capsule, resulting in improvement of shoulder motion. Manipulation under anesthesia may be helpful in some patients. Once established, therapy may have little effect on the natural course of the disease. Local injections of corticosteroids, nonsteroidal anti-inflammatory drugs, and physical therapy may provide relief of symptoms.

TUMORS OF JOINTS Primary tumors and tumorlike disorders of synovium are uncommon but should be considered in the differential diagnosis of monarticular joint disease. In addition, metastases to bone and primary bone tumors adjacent to a joint may produce joint symptoms.

Pigmented villonodular synovitis is characterized by exuberant proliferation of synovial cells usually involving a single joint. It occurs most often in young adults and affects both sexes equally. The etiology of this disorder is unknown.

The synovium is a brownish color and has numerous large, fingerlike villi which fuse to form pedunculated nodules. There is marked hyperplasia of synovial cells within the stroma of the villi. Hemosiderin granules and lipids are found in the cytoplasm of macrophages and in the interstitial tissue. Multinucleated giant cells may be present. The proliferative synovium grows into the subsynovial tissue and invades adjacent cartilage and bone.

The clinical picture of pigmented villonodular synovitis is characterized by the insidious onset of swelling and pain in one joint, most commonly the knee. Other joints affected include the hips, ankles, calcaneocuboid joints, elbows, and small joints of the fingers or toes. The disease may also involve the common flexor sheath of the hand. Symptoms may be mild, intermittent, and present for years before the patient seeks medical attention. Radiographs may show joint space narrowing, erosions, and subchondral cysts. The joint fluid contains blood and is dark-red or almost black in color. Lipid containing macrophages may be present in the fluid. The joint fluid may be clear if hemorrhages have not occurred.

The treatment of pigmented villonodular synovitis is complete synovectomy. With incomplete synovectomy, the villonodular synovitis recurs, and the rate of tissue growth may be faster than occurred originally. Irradiation of the involved joint has been successful in some patients.

Synovial chondromatosis is a disorder characterized by multiple focal metaplastic growths of normal-appearing cartilage in the synovium or tendon sheath. Segments of cartilage break loose and continue to grow as loose bodies. When calcification and ossification of loose bodies occur, the disorder is referred to as synovial osteochondromatosis. The disorder is usually monarticular and affects young to middle-aged individuals. The knee is most often involved, followed by hip, elbow, and shoulder. Symptoms are pain, swelling, and decreased motion of the joint. Radiographs may show several rounded calcifications within the joint cavity. Treatment is synovectomy; however, the tumor may recur.

Hemangiomas occur in synovium and in tendon sheaths. The knee is affected most commonly. Recurrent episodes of joint swelling and pain usually begin in childhood. The joint fluid is bloody. Treatment is excision of the lesion. *Lipomas* occur most often in the knee, originating in the subsynovial fat on either side of the patellar tendon. Lipomas also appear in tendon sheaths of the hands, wrists, feet, and ankles.

Synovial sarcoma (malignant synovioma) is a neoplasm of connective origin arising from tissue adjacent to large joints and seldom from the joint itself. It occurs most often in young adults and is more common in men. The tumor presents as a slowly growing mass near a joint, without much pain. The tumor spreads along tissue planes. The most common site of visceral metastasis is lung. The diagnosis is made by biopsy. Treatment is wide resection of the tumor including adjacent muscle and regional lymph nodes. Amputation of the involved distal extremity may be required. Chemotherapy may be beneficial in some patients with metastatic disease.

Synovial chondrosarcoma may arise in the synovium, tendon sheath, or bursa and is very rare. Treatment is radical excision or amputation.

REFERENCES

ALTMAN RD, TENENBAUM J: Hypertrophic osteoarthropathy, in *Textbook of Rheumatology*, WN Kelley et al (eds). Philadelphia, Saunders, 1989, chap 95, pp 1666–1673

BENNETT RM, GOLDENBERG DL (eds): *Rheumatic Disease Clinics of North America: The Fibromyalgia Syndrome*. Philadelphia, Saunders, 1989

ELLMAN MH: Neuropathic joint disease (Charcot joints), in *Arthritis and Allied Conditions*, DJ McCarty (ed). Philadelphia, Lea & Febiger, 1989, chap 81, pp 1255–1272

HERMAN JH: Polychondritis, in *Textbook of Rheumatology*, WN Kelley et al (eds). Philadelphia, Saunders, 1989, chap 83, pp 1513–1522

KOZIN F: Painful shoulder and the reflex sympathetic dystrophy syndrome, in *Arthritis and Allied Conditions*, DJ McCarty (ed). Philadelphia, Lea & Febiger, 1989, chap 97, pp 1509–1544

MICHET CJ JR et al: Relapsing polychondritis: Survival and predictive role of early disease manifestations. *Ann Intern Med* 104:74–78, 1986

NEER CS II: Impingement lesions. *Clin Orthop* 173:70–77, 1983

SCHILLER AL: Tumors and tumor-like lesions involving joints, in *Textbook of Rheumatology*, WN Kelly et al (eds). Philadelphia, Saunders, 1989, chap 100, pp 1775–1797

WEISMAN MH: Arthritis associated with hematologic disorders, storage diseases, disorders of lipid metabolism, and dysproteinemias, in *Arthritis and Allied Conditions*, DJ McCarty (ed). Philadelphia, Lea & Febiger, 1989, chap 84, pp 1312–1315

PART ELEVEN

HEMATOLOGY AND ONCOLOGY

285 IMPACT OF MOLECULAR BIOLOGY ON HEMATOLOGY

STUART H. ORKIN

Phenotypic variation is the essence of genetics, whether reflected as normal polymorphism or as inherited disease. Differences between individuals are encoded in cellular DNA (the genome), the reservoir of genetic information for the individual as well as the species. Until recently the precise relationship between a given phenotype (a trait or a disease) and a specific alteration in cellular DNA could only be inferred. For example, where a specific protein was known to be structurally abnormal in a clinical condition, demonstration of an amino acid replacement in the mutant product allowed one to predict a substitution in the DNA on the basis of the genetic code. Thus, the substitution of glutamic acid by valine at the sixth amino acid of the β chain of sickle hemoglobin could be accounted for by a change in a single nucleotide in cellular DNA (Chap. 5).

The past decade has witnessed a revolution in biomedical sciences with the introduction of the extraordinarily powerful methods of recombinant DNA that permit isolation of genes in pure form and their precise characterization. In many spheres of medicine recombinant DNA technology offers great promise, only one tangible consequence of which is the commercial production of new proteins such as growth factors, hormones, and enzymes. Nowhere has the impact of recombinant DNA been more immediate than in the understanding, diagnosis, and potential treatment of hematologic diseases.

RECOMBINANT DNA TECHNOLOGY AND THE NEW GENETICS (See also Chap. 6) With the tools of recombinant DNA, the relationship between a specific gene, an alteration in that gene, and a phenotype (or disease) can be established with certainty. This new capability rests on relatively simple procedures to isolate genes, determine their nucleotide sequences, and put genes back into cells to assess their function. Isolating a pure gene among the approximately 10^5 other genes in a cell is impossible by traditional biochemical means. Recombinant DNA methods, however, permit doing so by molecular cloning. In this context, cloning refers to the process by which one DNA molecule is joined to another (termed a *vector*) that can replicate autonomously in a specially chosen host, usually a bacterium or yeast. A common feature of cloning methods is the use of *restriction enzymes,* reagents that recognize specific sequences in double-stranded DNA and generate cleavages at or near those sites. As cloning methods were devised, techniques also were developed to permit rapid determination of the nucleotide sequence of cloned DNA and assessment of its function in cells. Ultimately direct correlations can be made between gene structure and gene function.

In parallel with the introduction of techniques to examine individual genes, methods were developed that utilize naturally occurring variation in DNA sequence as markers for the inheritance of disease genes and for the mapping of genes to specific chromosomes and subchromosomal regions. These methods are restriction enzyme digestion, electrophoresis, and molecular hybridization (the Southern blot procedure). The variations in DNA sequence they detect are commonly referred to as *restriction fragment length polymorphisms* (RFLPs). RFLPs may be used as markers for specific genes or gene regions in families affected with a disorder (see below). More broadly, RFLPs help determine the relative distance of one marker from another or of a marker from a disease locus to which it is linked (linkage analysis). While linkage analysis is beyond the scope of this chapter (see Chap. 6), it should be noted that sufficient RFLPs have been identified to permit construction of a low-resolution map of the human genome. With such a map, study of the correlation of RFLPs and disease phenotypes in families can be employed to position genes for inherited phenotypes on specific chromosomes. As noted below, the genes involved in inherited disorders can now be located and cloned by such approaches without prior knowledge of the protein product of the normal gene or even its cellular origin ("reverse genetics").

Until very recently cloning methods were the only means by which suitable amounts of pure gene DNA could be obtained for laboratory study. Now, a method termed the *polymerase chain reaction* (PCR) provides a simple technique for the acquisition of sufficient quantities of specific gene regions, if nucleotide sequence information exists regarding the gene itself. The use of specific synthetic DNA primers on either side of a target DNA region and repetitive enzymatic extension and denaturation on the template DNA allow for the in vitro synthesis of pure gene regions. Although PCR may seem unduly specialized or technical, it is remarkably efficient and convenient even for clinical laboratories. As such, its widespread use will probably revolutionize genetic diagnosis.

IMMEDIATE IMPACT OF THE NEW GENETICS ON HEMATO-LOGIC DISEASE The application of recombinant DNA technology to the analysis of disease has expanded greatly since its introduction in about 1978; therefore discussion of its impact on hematologic disease must of necessity be selective. In forging an understanding of the molecular basis of disease and testing new approaches to diagnosis based on genetic criteria, consideration of the hemoglobinopathies, particularly thalassemia syndromes, is particularly instructive.

Determining the molecular basis of disease For nearly three decades it has been appreciated that thalassemia syndromes result from unbalanced synthesis of globin chains (Chap. 295). Prior to recombinant DNA methods, reduced (or absent) synthesis of specific globin polypeptides in various thalassemia syndromes was established, as was deficiency of specific messenger RNAs. Whether deficiency was secondary to mutations in globin genes per se or in genes that regulate their expression, and how specific mutations led to reduced mRNA synthesis or function, were largely unknown. This changed with the advent of procedures that permitted isolation of globin genes from patients with thalassemias, determination of their nucleotide sequences, and analysis of expression of the cloned genes upon reintroduction into cells. It became possible to elucidate the precise molecular basis of these syndromes. Rather than representing a single type of mutation, thalassemia syndromes reflected the entire spectrum of molecular defects that might be predicted to interfere with gene expression. Lesions included gross gene deletions, but more commonly consisted of *single base substitutions* in globin genes that adversely affected gene transcription, proper removal of intervening sequences during RNA splicing, mRNA polyadenylation, translatability, or stability. Taken together, the thalassemia syndromes were the first genetic disorders to be described in detail at the molecular level.

The comprehensive dissection of the thalassemia syndromes relied on combining gene cloning with RFLP haplotype analysis. The latter method takes advantage of RFLPs to characterize the chromosome vicinity of the globin genes. In a given chromosomal region, the pattern of restriction site differences constitutes an RFLP haplotype, much as differences at the histocompatibility loci form a haplotype. It was reasoned that haplotype differences surrounding the human β-globin gene might provide a signature for different chromosomal backgrounds upon which mutations in the β-globin gene producing thalassemia might have arisen. It thus became possible to group potentially identical mutant alleles together and focus attention on those among them that differ from the others. Therefore, examination of cloned β-globin genes (representing different chromosome haplotypes) revealed a comprehensive picture of mutations in thalassemia with high efficiency and speed.

Impact on diagnosis At the clinical level, the new genetic methods have had their greatest impact on diagnosis. This has resulted from the development of techniques for the detection of specific gene defects in uncloned DNA samples. The feasibility of assigning specific defects in small DNA samples permits examination of the distribution of mutations in populations, carrier detection in families at risk (or those possibly at risk), and prenatal diagnosis as early as the first trimester by chorionic villus biopsy sampling and later by amniocentesis.

Although extensive DNA deletion, insertion, or rearrangement may often be the molecular basis of an inherited disorder, most gene mutations in inherited disorders are single nucleotide changes that cannot be detected by gross examination of gene structure. To diagnose such defects, highly sensitive assays are required that distinguish mutant from normal DNA sequences in a specific region of a gene. With a catalog of clinically relevant gene mutations for which individuals may be surveyed (as is available for the thalassemia syndromes), these procedures may be applied with great precision. The detection of the sickle cell mutation is already a classic demonstration of the application of recombinant DNA methods to diagnosis. A substitution of T for A in the sixth codon of the β-globin gene, which directs the replacement of valine for glutamic acid, is the underlying basis for sickle cell anemia. Quite fortuitously, this single change abolishes a recognition site in the gene for a restriction enzyme (Mst II) and, thereby, alters the fragments of the gene generated upon digestion of total DNA by this enzyme. With the procedure of Southern, in which DNA fragments are electrophoretically separated in gels and then probed for specific sequences by molecular hybridization (see Fig. 6-2, p. 34), the relevant β-globin gene fragments may be visualized. In this manner a molecular diagnosis of normal, sickle trait, or sickle cell anemia can be achieved accurately and reliably with a small DNA sample from blood cells or fetal material. This approach has been used in the prenatal diagnosis of sickle cell anemia with considerable success (Chap. 295).

Applications of polymerase chain reaction The newer and simpler PCR method was also first applied in the analysis of the sickle cell mutation. With synthetic DNA primers flanking the sickle mutation, the critical DNA segment can be amplified in vitro more than a millionfold to provide material sufficient for analysis by restriction enzyme digestion, molecular hybridization, or even direct DNA sequencing (see Fig. 6-3, p. 34). Since the method requires only minute samples, takes a matter of hours rather than days, and is readily adapted for automated handling, PCR is very rapidly finding its way into clinical as well as research laboratories.

The extraordinary power of PCR methodology is perhaps best exemplified by its application to the analysis of minimal residual disease in hematologic malignancies. In many forms of cancer very specific cytogenetic alterations occur (Chap. 300). Often these involve breakage and union of ordinarily separate chromosomal regions; typical examples are the translocations found in chronic myelogenous leukemia (Chap. 296). To the extent that such translocations are found within a limited target region, these chromosomal abnormalities may be detected with PCR primers flanking the breakpoints. An especially informative example is follicular lymphoma, in which there is frequently a chromosome 14;18 translocation. The 14;18 breakpoints connect one of six immunoglobin heavy chain joining (J_h) regions on chromosome 14 to a small breakpoint region on the BCL2 gene on chromosome 18. With PCR (using primers flanking the junctures), a single abnormal cell among more than 10^6 normal cells is detectable. Therefore, PCR presents the means to identify the subclinical presence of residual neoplastic cells. Although the precise clinical significance of small numbers of residual leukemic cells in patients in apparent remission remains to be determined, it is highly likely that correlations of the residual neoplastic cell burden with clinical outcome and treatment will be important for management of hematologic malignancies.

Detection of clonality in cell populations A related application of recombinant DNA methods to hematologic malignancies is the detection of *clonality in cell populations*. The clonal expansion of lymphoid cells is generally taken to reflect proliferation of malignant cells, whereas polyclonal expansion is not. Rearrangements of immunoglobulin genes and T-cell receptor loci normally accompany differentiation of B- and T-cells, respectively. In light of this, Southern blot analysis of lymphoid cell DNA with appropriate molecular probes can provide evidence regarding the clonality of cell populations. Taken together with other findings, such information can make clinical diagnoses more precise.

Using DNA probes that detect RFLPs, the cellular DNAs of virtually any two (or more) individuals can be distinguished, particularly if highly polymorphic probes (called *fingerprinting probes*) are employed. The capability of distinguishing the genotypes of cells has also found an application in the management of patients following bone marrow transplantation. Analysis of RFLPs following allogeneic transplantation enables assessing the relative contribution of host and donor hematopoietic cells. Engraftment of donor marrow, reemergence of host elements, and mixed cell chimerism can be evaluated with RFLP analysis.

Selected applications of recombinant DNA methods in clinical diagnosis are summarized in Table 285-1.

IMPACT ON THE UNDERSTANDING OF DISEASE AND NORMAL BIOLOGY Some diseases reflect a disturbance of normal cellular physiology. An understanding of their biochemical basis can often provide novel insights into normal biology. Until very recently, the analysis of inherited human disorders required identification and characterization of specific proteins and their corresponding genes. Many conditions, however, including those affecting the hematopoietic system, display phenotypes for which adequate biochemical explanations are lacking. In general, animal models that faithfully mimic human disorders are not available. However, using an approach that combines classical genetics and recombinant DNA methods, the gene affected in a disorder can now be identified without specific

TABLE 285-1   Recombinant DNA analysis in clinical diagnosis

Application	Examples
Detection of specific mutations in populations and families at risk	Carrier detection of sickle cell anemia Estimation of specific β-thalassemia mutations in populations
Prenatal diagnosis of disease	β Thalassemia, sickle cell anemia
Detection of minimal residual disease in malignancy	Chromosome 14;18 translocation in follicular lymphoma
Detection of clonality in cell populations	Rearrangement of Ig and T-cell receptor gene loci in lymphomas
Distinguishing genotypes of hematopoietic cells	Assessment of host/donor cell contributions following allogeneic bone marrow transplantation

knowledge of the protein product. With DNA probes that recognize RFLPs within families at risk for an inherited condition, markers that are very closely linked to a particular disease locus may be identified. By a variety of methods, the region of the relevant gene may be further delimited by additional linkage mapping or by use of patient samples bearing DNA deletions or chromosomal translocations. Ultimately, a region of DNA that gives rise to an mRNA that is structurally or quantitatively deranged in the disease defines the gene itself. This approach to the identification and characterization of the affected gene and its product is often termed *reverse genetics*.

Impact of reverse genetics Examples of the impact of this approach to disease are just emerging. One of the first involved the analysis of an inherited hematologic disorder, the X-linked variety of chronic granulomatous disease (X-CGD). In this disease activated phagocytic white blood cells of affected males fail to produce superoxide anion, an important chemical component of the host defense system against microorganisms. The cellular biochemistry of superoxide generation and its derangement in X-CGD had been actively studied since the first description of the rare disorder more than thirty years ago. Nonetheless, considerable controversy existed regarding the nature of the essential cellular proteins and the X-chromosome–encoded locus in the disease. Although the details are beyond the scope of this chapter, the molecular cloning of the gene involved in X-CGD rapidly demonstrated the requirement for a usual cytochrome molecule in white blood cell superoxide production. In addition, further work has provided useful biochemical and molecular reagents with which to pursue dissection of superoxide production in greater depth. Reverse genetics has also elucidated the genetic defects in Duchenne muscular dystrophy and in retinoblastoma.

The tremendous promise of the reverse-genetics approach to the understanding of inherited disorders relates to the extraordinary power of recombinant DNA methods, where in rapid succession (1) the protein product of a gene can be determined from a DNA sequence; (2) specific reagents to that protein can be generated either by immunization with synthetic peptides deduced from the sequence or with material manufactured in bacteria; and (3) the normal versions of the involved genes can be introduced into mammalian cells to analyze protein function. This approach will facilitate understanding of normal cellular physiology as well as efforts to correct disease phenotypes.

IMPACT OF THE NEW GENETICS ON TREATMENT OF HEMATOLOGIC DISORDERS In at least four areas recombinant DNA technology has had a major impact on clinical hematology. First, as noted above, identification of the specific gene mutations leading to thalassemia syndromes has led to effective and efficient prenatal diagnosis of disease. In geographic areas where these conditions are prevalent, programs for prenatal diagnosis, coupled with routine hematologic screening and genetic counseling, have already reduced the incidence of births of newly affected individuals. This is a significant achievement in public health management of a genetic disorder. Second, as also noted above, the development of new methods for the detection of specific DNA abnormalities in only a few cells among many allows better assessment of residual disease in hematologic malignancies. Correlation of clinical outcome with residual disease status and treatment is likely to lead to improved therapy. Third, the availability of new hematopoietic growth factors through molecular cloning and gene expression is beginning to change the clinical management of several conditions. For example, the use of erythropoietin constitutes a major new approach to the treatment of the anemia of chronic renal disease. Abnormalities of white blood cell production, particularly the transient neutropenia accompanying cancer chemotherapy, may be more effectively managed by administration of growth factors (colony stimulating factors) for myelomonocytic cells. Fourth, production of blood clotting factors by recombinant DNA methods provide a promising approach to the treatment of hemophilias.

Other applications of recombinant DNA technology in clinical hematology are more speculative, but two warrant discussion.

Since the production of fetal hemoglobin generally reduces the consequences of sickle cell anemia or thalassemia, studies have focused on the pharmacologic stimulation of fetal hemoglobin production in adults. Based on the observation that the modification of cellular DNA by methylation is often associated with gene inactivity, 5-azacytidine, a drug that causes widespread demethylation, has been tested for its effects on fetal hemoglobin production in patients with thalassemia or sickle cell anemia. While an augmentation in production has been observed, the molecular basis for the effect remains controversial. Nonetheless, this research has led to the testing of a variety of cytotoxic agents, such as hydroxyurea, that appear to exert a similar effect on fetal hemoglobin production. Although the precise mechanisms by which such drugs exert their effect is unclear, increases in fetal hemoglobin production are often in the range believed to be of clinical benefit.

Another attempt to modulate expression of genes in the treatment of an inherited disorder is the recent administration of the lymphokine *γ-interferon* to patients with chronic granulomatous disease. This lymphokine, previously known as macrophage activating factor, augments cellular killing of microbes by phagocytic cells. In part, this phenomenon may relate to the capacity of the γ-interferon to up-regulate expression of genes encoding some of the essential components of the superoxide-generating system of phagocytes. Limited clinical trials suggest that administration of γ-interferon may significantly enhance cellular function in selected patients with chronic granulomatous disease. From these two examples, it is already apparent that knowledge of the molecular biology of specific gene systems will generate novel therapies for the management of severe inherited hematologic disorders.

Somatic gene therapy A potential application of recombinant DNA technology to clinical hematology yet to be explored is *somatic genetic therapy*. The ability to clone genes and reintroduce them into cells offers prospects for correcting inherited disease by genetic means. The intent of such an approach would be to treat only somatic cells of the affected individual (somatic gene therapy), rather than attempting to correct the germline. At present, somatic gene therapy is being contemplated only for severe, life-threatening disorders for which conventional medical management is unsatisfactory. Many methods for the introduction of the normal version of a gene into a cell bearing defective versions have been considered. At present, the most promising avenue would appear to be the use of modified, recombinant RNA viruses (retroviruses) to achieve efficient transfer of new genetic material into hematopoietic stem cells.

In principle, the hematopoietic system is an attractive target for gene therapy as pluripotent stem cells self-renew and also give rise to cell progenitors and mature blood cells. Furthermore, extensive experience in bone marrow transplantation provides a strong base for management of the host, the handling of marrow cells, and the reconstitution of the hematopoietic system by infusion of donor cells. In somatic therapy, genetically modified cells of the affected patient, rather than stem cells from another individual, would be used for cellular reconstitution. The inherited disorders that seem most appropriate for this approach include immunodeficiencies, such as severe combined immunodeficiency due to lack of adenosine deaminase (Chap. 263), hemoglobinopathies (thalassemia and sickle cell anemia), storage disorders (such as Gaucher's disease), and coagulation factor deficiencies (such as hemophilia A). Although considerable progress in the methodologies required for somatic gene therapy has been made, efficient infection of sufficient numbers of stem cells by recombinant retroviruses and adequate expression of the introduced gene in hematopoietic stem cells and their progeny remain formidable problems preventing clinical use. Because correction of a mutant gene in the chromosome (rather than introduction of a normal gene copy randomly into the host cell genome) would be preferable since regulated expression would be guaranteed, attention is also being directed to the use of targeted gene insertion.

Current and potential applications of recombinant DNA methods

TABLE 285-2   Recombinant DNA and management of hematologic disease

Application	Examples
Current	
Prenatal diagnosis of inherited disorders	β Thalassemia and sickle cell anemia
Detection of minimal residual disease in malignancy	Translocation in follicular lymphoma
	Ig or T-cell receptor gene rearrangements
Administration of hematopoietic growth factors	Erythropoietin for anemia of chronic renal disease
Administration of clotting factors	Factor VIII for hemophilia A
Under study	
Modulation of gene expression to ameliorate severity of clinical disease	Stimulation of fetal hemoglobin production in sickle cell anemia
	Use of γ-interferon in chronic granulomatous disease
Possible for future	
Somatic therapy for the correction of inherited disease	Candidates
	Hemoglobinopathies
	Adenosine deaminase deficiency
	Storage disorders
	Coagulation deficiencies

in the management of hematologic disease are summarized in Table 285-2.

Disorders of the hematopoietic system have proved to be a fruitful arena for the application of recombinant DNA methods to clinical medicine. Progressively greater impact of these methods on diagnosis and on the understanding of pathophysiology is virtually assured. Sensitive diagnostic approaches to clonality and minimal residual disease are likely to guide future management of malignant disease. Finally, we can be cautiously optimistic about the potential of recombinant DNA technology to provide novel approaches to treatment, including pharmacologic manipulation of gene expression and somatic genetic therapy.

REFERENCES

ERLICH HA (ed): *PCR Technology: Principles and Applications for DNA Amplification.* New York, Stockton Press, 1989

Nichols EK: *Human Gene Therapy.* Cambridge, MA, Harvard, 1989

ORKIN SH: Reverse genetics in human disease. Cell 47:845, 1986

———: Molecular genetics and inherited human disease, in *The Metabolic Basis of Inherited Disease,* 6th ed, CR Scriver et al (eds). New York, McGraw-Hill, 1989, vol 1

———, KAZAZIAN HH JR: Mutation and polymorphism of the human beta-globin gene and its surrounding DNA. Ann Rev Genet 18:131, 1984

286   BLOOD GROUPS AND BLOOD TRANSFUSION

ELOISE R. GIBLETT

BLOOD GROUP ANTIGENS AND ANTIBODIES

Human red blood cell membranes contain over 300 different antigenic determinants, the molecular structure of which is dictated by genes at an unknown number of chromosomal loci. The term *blood group* is applied to any well-defined system of red blood cell antigens controlled by a locus having a variable number of allelic genes, such as *A*, *B*, and *O* in the ABO system. Over twenty blood group systems are currently recognized. The term *blood type* refers to the antigen phenotype, which is the serologic expression of the inherited blood group genes.

Alloantibodies specific for the blood group antigens may occur "naturally" (i.e., in the absence of known stimulus by foreign red blood cells) or in response to transfusion or pregnancy. Naturally occurring antibodies tend to be IgM molecules, and many of them (notably excepting anti-A and anti-B) react poorly at body temperature but readily agglutinate red blood cells at 5 to 20°C. Antibodies formed in response to exposure to another person's red blood cells or soluble blood group substances initially belong to the IgM class but usually change to the IgG class within a few weeks or months. In general, these "immune" antibodies react best at body temperature, and special laboratory procedures are required for their detection.

BLOOD GROUP SYSTEMS   ABO system: Genes and antigens There are four major allelic genes in this system: A^1, A^2, B, and O. The locus for these alleles is on the long arm of chromosome 9. The actual products of the first three genes are glycosyltransferases which select specific sugars, N-acetyl-D-galactosamine (GalNAc) by the A^1 and A^2 transferases and D-galactose (Gal) by the B transferase, attaching them by alpha-linkage to short (oligo) saccharide chains. These chains comprise the carbohydrate moiety of glycolipid and glycoprotein molecules on the red blood cells or in other tissues and fluids. Although the A^1 and A^2 transferases perform the same function, they have different rate constants, so people who inherit an A^1 gene have more A-reactive sites than those with an A^2 gene. The O gene product is a protein which cross-reacts immunologically with the A and B transferase molecules but has no detectable enzyme activity; thus it is functionally "silent."

Nearly all individuals produce "naturally occurring" antibodies against the A or B antigens not present on their own red blood cells, as shown in Table 286-1. This fact is used as the basis for confirming the red blood cell type. Most of the major phenotypes represent more than one genotype. In the absence of family studies, it is possible to infer the genotype from only three phenotypes: A_1B, A_2B, and O. In routine practice, the ABO type is determined by testing the red blood cells with anti-A and anti-B and by testing the serum against A, B, and O red blood cells. Under special circumstances, a further distinction between A and AB types is made by using anti-A_1, an antiserum prepared by absorbing anti-A typing serum with A_2 red blood cells. The remaining unabsorbed antibodies have A_1 specificity, reacting with A_1 and A_1B, but not with A_2 and A_2B cells. (Alternatively, anti-A_1 is prepared as a lectin from extracts of certain seeds.) The frequencies of the various phenotypes in two American blood donor populations are also given in Table 286-1.

Red blood cells of types O and A_2 have large amounts of another antigen, called H, which is the immediate precursor to A and B. H specificity depends on the presence of a fucose (Fuc) residue attached to the oligosaccharides by a transferase that is the product of a very common gene called *H*. (The H and ABO loci are not genetically linked.) In very rare individuals who fail to inherit an *H* gene from either parent (i.e., they are homozygous for its allele, *h*), the H transferase is not made, and the H-determining fucose is not attached. This prevents the addition of specific sugars by the *A* and *B* transferases. As a result, even if an *A* or *B* gene has been inherited, the red blood cells are not agglutinated by anti-A, anti-B, or anti-H, while the serum contains all three antibodies. When a patient requiring transfusion has this so-called O_h (or Bombay) phenotype, special arrangements are necessary to obtain blood of the same rare type from a source such as the Red Cross.

About 80 percent of people are either homozygous or heterozygous for the "secretor," or *Se*, gene, which has no effect on the formation of antigens intrinsic to red blood cells but which governs the production of a fucosyltransferase in secretory tissues. Homozygotes for the apparently inactive allele *se* are called *nonsecretors* because their secretory cells produce a very weakly reactive fucosyl transferase, so their body fluids virtually lack H, A, and B antigen activities.

Antibodies in ABO system   Red blood cells of newborn infants have a decreased number of H, A, and B reactive sites, and their

TABLE 286-1 Blood types of the ABO system (including Hh)

Genotype*	Phenotype	Antigens on red blood cells†	Antibodies in serum‡	Phenotype frequencies in Americans, %	
				Western European descent	African descent
A^1A^1 A^1A^2 A^1O	A_1	A_1, (H)	Anti-B (anti-H)	35	23
A^2A^2 A^2O	A_2	A_2, H	Anti-B (anti-A_1)	10	6
BB BO	B	B, (H)	Anti-A, -A_1	8	17
A^1B	A_1B	A, A_1, B	(Anti-H)	3	3
A^2B	A_2B	A, B, H	(Anti-A_1)	1	1
OO	O	H	Anti-A, -A_1 Anti-B	43	50
hh	O_h	None	Anti-A, -A_1 Anti-B Anti-H	Very rare	Very rare

* In all types except the last, the *H* allele is present as *HH* or *Hh*.
† (H) indicates occasional presence of weakly reacting H antigen.
‡ Antibodies in parentheses are, if present, weak cold agglutinins.
SOURCE: Race and Sanger.

plasma normally contains very little anti-A or anti-B. This finding is due to the fact that fetal immunoglobulin production is minimal, while most of the anti-A and anti-B produced in the mother are IgM molecules which cannot cross the placenta. However, in some type O adults, much of the anti-A, anti-B, and anti-AB (a cross-reacting antibody sometimes called anti-C) are of the IgG class and reach the infant's bloodstream. For this reason, ABO hemolytic disease of the newborn usually occurs in A (or B) infants of O mothers.

It is not acceptable medical practice to transfuse A, B, or AB blood into patients whose red blood cells lack the corresponding antigens, since their plasma contains incompatible antibodies. However, it is acceptable to give A or B blood (preferably as packed red blood cells) to AB recipients, or to give O packed red blood cells (*not* whole blood, except in severe emergencies) to patients of type A, B, or AB when the transfusion requirement exceeds the supply of type-specific blood. Although antibodies with A_1 specificity frequently occur in the plasma of A_2 and A_2B subjects, they are almost always weak cold agglutinins. Therefore, if anti-A_1 has been identified in a transfusion patient, it can be ignored unless it reacts in vitro with A_1 red blood cells at 37°C.

Lewis system Antigens in the Lewis system are not produced by red blood cells but are taken up as glycosphingolipid molecules from the surrounding plasma. There are two well-defined Lewis antigenic determinants, Le^a and Le^b, both of which are structurally related to the H, A, and B antigens.

Anti-Le^a and anti-Le^b are fairly common naturally occurring antibodies, produced mainly by subjects of phenotype O, Le(a−b−). Nearly all examples of these antibodies are of the IgM class, so they rarely, if ever, can cross the placenta during pregnancy. Were they to do so, destruction of the infant's red blood cells would be highly unlikely, since the Lewis glycosphingolipids are very poorly developed during fetal life.

Lewis antibodies (particularly anti-Le^a) are complement-binders; anti-Le^a in very rare instances causes transfusion reactions with intravascular hemolysis. However, the plasma of Le(a+) donors usually contains enough soluble Le^a antigen to neutralize the patient's anti-Le^a before it can attack the vulnerable red blood cells. Nevertheless, patients whose plasma contains anti-Le^a that strongly hemolyzes Le(a+) red blood cells or agglutinates them at temperatures above 30°C should be given blood from either Le(a−b+) or Le(a−b−) donors. Anti-Le^b is virtually never a transfusion hazard.

P system Several structurally related antigens are considered together under the heading of a single system called P. As in the ABO and Lewis systems, the gene products are glycosyltransferases,

attaching either D-galactose, N-acetyl-D-galactosamine, or N-acetyl-D-glucosamine to glycosphingolipids on the red blood cell membrane. P_1 and P, the major antigenic determinants, were previously thought to represent the expression of two allelic genes at the same locus, analogous to A^1 and A^2 in the ABO system. However, these two antigens represent quite different sugar sequences, and the genetic interpretation is complex.

Anti-P_1, which occurs frequently, almost never causes red blood cell destruction—the exceptions being those rare examples which react strongly with P_1 red blood cells in vitro at 37°C. In patients with paroxysmal cold hemoglobinuria, the so-called Donath-Landsteiner autoantibodies frequently react with globoside, a very common red blood cell glycosphingolipid with P specificity.

I system The I and i antigenic determinants are structurally heterogeneous, biochemically related to the H, A, B, Le, and P antigens. Most people inherit a gene associated with I antigen production, but the red blood cells of newborn infants react very weakly with anti-I and strongly with anti-i. A gradual reversal occurs during the first year or two, representing the development of I antigen in association with branching of carbohydrate chains on the cell membrane. In patients with certain kinds of "marrow stress," particularly thalassemia and hypoplastic anemia, red blood cell i activity is increased.

Anti-I is a common antibody, frequently found as a weak cold agglutinin of no clinical concern. In patients with the cold type of autoimmune hemolytic anemia, autoantibodies usually have anti-I or anti-I plus i specificity, and most of them belong to the IgM class (see Chap. 294). Anti-i production is associated mainly with lymphoid cell diseases, especially infectious mononucleosis and lymphosarcoma. A patient already having a "marrow-stressing" disorder such as thalassemia may develop an intense autoimmune hemolytic anemia due to anti-i. When transfusions are required, finding compatible blood poses no problem, since the red blood cells of most adults are i-negative. Even patients with strong cold-reacting anti-I antibodies are usually not difficult to transfuse safely if they are kept warm during the infusion. However, since anti-I often fixes complement, washed red cells may be preferable for transfusion to prevent exposure to additional complement components.

MNS system Closely linked genes on chromosome 4 determine the MN and Ss antigens, respectively. There are four inherited haplotypes: MS, Ms, NS, and Ns. Glycophorin A carries M and N specificity, while S and s are on glycophorin B. Absence of these sialoglycoproteins is associated with rare phenotypes such as En(a-), S^u, and M^k, but there are no accompanying hematologic abnormalities.

Anti-M and anti-N are usually naturally occurring IgM agglutinins with little capability of destroying red blood cells. Patients on long-term renal dialysis tend to form anti-N as either an auto- or alloantibody. These N-specific autoantibodies have no hemolytic potential, but they are alleged to cause rejection of kidneys kept refrigerated before transplantation.

Formation of anti-S or anti-s usually requires the stimulus of transfusion or pregnancy, and accordingly these antibodies often belong to the IgG class. A third antibody, anti-U, behaves serologically somewhat like anti-S plus anti-s, being formed in sensitized black subjects whose red blood cells have the S^u phenotype lacking S and s antigens. All three of these antibodies can hemolyze incompatible red blood cells in vivo, but they are readily detectable by adequate compatibility testing.

Rh system   The Rh locus is on chromosome 1. Rh antigenic determinants appear to be dependent on interaction between red blood cell membrane protein and phospholipid molecules. Many Rh phenotypes have been described serologically. While the underlying biochemical genetics is not well defined, recent evidence indicates that there are probably at least three tandem Rh loci, somewhat analogous to the complex HLA and immunoglobulin loci. The Rh alleles dictate the structure of a set of epitopes that are usually antithetical: C or c, E or e, and D or d (the latter having no corresponding antibody and therefore being simply the absence of D). These sets are inherited from each parent as a haplotype, such as CDe, cde, cDE, and so forth.

The $D(Rh_o)$ antigen is by far the most immunogenic of this or any other blood group system (except for those previously described systems in which the formation of antibodies does not depend on exposure to foreign red blood cells). About 15 percent of Caucasians lack the $D(Rh_o)$ antigen and are Rh-negative. When transfused only once with Rh-positive blood, these Rh-negative persons have about a 50 percent chance of forming anti-$D(Rh_o)$ antibodies, which could cause destruction of any subsequently transfused Rh-positive red blood cells. For this reason, Rh-negative patients are always given Rh-negative blood except when the transfusion requirements of a male or postmenopausal female exceed the available supply. Giving Rh-positive blood to Rh-negative premenopausal females is a very serious matter, because, unless adequate amounts of Rh immunoglobulin are given to prevent immunization, any subsequent pregnancy with an Rh-positive infant will almost always stimulate a secondary immune response, resulting in hemolytic disease of the newborn.

The Rh antigens C, c, E, and e are considerably less immunogenic than D, and it is impractical to match these antigens in donors and recipients. Of course, when previously sensitized patients form the corresponding antibodies, it is necessary to find donor blood lacking the specific antigens. The difficulty of this search varies. For example, about 20 percent of the population lack the c antigen and thus are compatible donors for a patient whose plasma contains anti-c. However, only 2 percent lack the e antigen, so patients with anti-e pose serious problems, especially when large amounts of blood are required. Blood banks often maintain donor calling lists or frozen red blood cells for use in such cases, and autologous transfusion is especially desirable for nonemergency procedures.

A large proportion of patients with acquired hemolytic anemia of the warm type have IgG autoantibodies which react with one or more Rh-associated antigens. In some instances, the specificity is clear-cut (for example, anti-e), but more often the antibodies react with all red blood cells except those of the rare type known as Rh_{null}. These cells lack all known Rh antigens, and the cell membrane is defective, reinforcing the belief that in normal red blood cells, molecules bearing the Rh determinants are an intrinsic part of the membrane protein structure.

Kidd, Kell, Duffy, and Lutheran systems   In the Kell and Duffy systems, anti-K and anti-Fy^a are frequently encountered antibodies capable of marked alloimmune red blood cell destruction. Even more dangerous are the antibodies in the Kidd system, anti-Jk^a and anti-Jk^b, which are notoriously difficult to detect. Whenever a patient has

a hemolytic transfusion reaction after transfusion of blood found to be compatible by the usual laboratory tests, the most likely cause is anti-Jk^a. Antibodies in the Lutheran system have only rarely been reported to cause red blood cell destruction.

Other blood group antigens   Many other red blood cell antigens have been described. The Xg^a antigen is of considerable scientific importance, since its locus is on the X chromosome. Other antigens are of clinical interest because they occur on the red blood cells of 95 percent or more of most populations, making it difficult to find compatible blood when their antibodies are present in patients requiring transfusion. Fortunately many of these antibodies have little ability to destroy red blood cells, even though they consist of IgG molecules and react in vitro at 37°C. Included in this category are most examples of anti-Sd^a (Sid), anti-Yt^a (Cartwright), anti-Yk^a (York), and many others. Nevertheless, both caution and experience are necessary when considering the transfusion of serologically incompatible blood, particularly when the antibodies react in vitro at body temperature. Antibodies with Chido (Ch^a) and Rodgers (Rg^a) specificity are incapable of causing hemolysis. Their respective antigenic determinants are located on the C4d fragment of the fourth component of complement and are thereby taken up from the plasma by red cells.

BIOLOGIC SIGNIFICANCE OF BLOOD GROUPS   **Immune reactions**   The relationship of blood group antigens and antibodies to alloimmune red blood cell destruction has been briefly discussed in the previous sections. Because antigens in the ABO system are present in other tissues, they play a role in determining histocompatibility, so that transplantation of ABO-incompatible kidneys and other organs carries a risk of rejection (see Chap. 225). However, successful grafting of ABO-incompatible bone marrow is possible when the patient is immunosuppressed and either given exchange transfusions of plasma compatible with the donor's red blood cells or the patient's own plasma is passed over a column containing oligosaccharides with A and/or B specificity.

Infertility and early fetal loss   Both of these effects have been ascribed to ABO incompatibility, although in some instances the data are of marginal significance. Nevertheless, many population geneticists believe that this factor plays a significant role in the processes of natural selection.

Disease-related phenotype changes   A and, to a lesser extent, B determinants are subject to certain biochemical changes, such as those caused by bacterial glycosidases, acetylases, and other enzymes. As a result, the red blood cells may develop new specificities, becoming either "polyagglutinable" or having "pseudo-B" characteristics. Another acquired alteration in ABO type occurs in some patients with acute myelocytic leukemia whose original type is A_1 or B. This change in phenotype, with partial or complete loss of agglutinability by anti-A or anti-B, can occasionally be a diagnostic aid in the early hypoplastic phase of leukemia. The changes in Ii specificity associated with "marrow stress" are described above (see "I System").

Other disease relationships   The incidence of certain diseases is related to blood type. For example, type O "nonsecretors" have about twice the incidence of duodenal ulcer than do secretors of types A or B. On the other hand, type A carries a higher incidence of tumors of salivary glands, stomach, and pancreas than does type O. Persons with the rare Rh_{null} type, whose red cells lack all the Rh antigens, have some degree of increased hemolysis, as do people with the McLeod phenotype. McLeod red blood cells react only weakly with antibodies against antigens of the autosomally controlled Kell system because they lack Kx, a very common X-linked Kell precursor antigen. Some boys with the X-linked form of chronic granulomatous disease also have the McLeod phenotype due to deletion of both genes, which are closely linked on the X chromosome. Individuals (mainly of African origin) who lack both Fy^a and Fy^b—the major antigens in the Duffy system—are protected against infestation by the malarial parasite, *Plasmodium vivax*, presumably because Fy^a and Fy^b act as specific recognition or acceptor sites for the merozoites.

Chromosome mapping Blood genetic markers, including the red and white blood cell allotypes as well as the plasma and blood cell enzyme phenotypes, are very useful for mapping the human chromosomes. Some of these markers are genetically linked to loci for genes causing metabolic diseases, and it is possible to predict the development of inherited malfunctions from specimens obtained in utero or from newborn infants. For example, the secretor gene locus is closely linked to the locus of the gene causing myotonic dystrophy, and a determination of the secretor status of a baby at risk can be used to predict the likelihood of its developing this disease, since both characters are inherited as autosomal dominants. In addition, tests for the restriction fragment length polymorphisms (RFLPs) can be performed on any tissue containing cellular DNA, including blood and amniotic fluid. The very large number of these genetic markers adds greatly to our potential ability to predict the occurrence of inherited diseases.

Medicolegal applications When the red blood cell antigens are combined with HLA, RFLPs, and the other genetic markers in blood, the probability of distinguishing one person from another is over 1 billion to 1. This high degree of individuality promotes the usefulness of genetic markers for ruling out paternity, maternity, and monozygosity in nearly all cases where those relationships do not exist.

BLOOD TRANSFUSION

INTRODUCTION Considerable morbidity and, to a lesser extent, mortality are associated with blood transfusion therapy. Responsible medical practice dictates that physicians have sufficient background information to make soundly reasoned judgments concerning the risks as well as the benefits of this procedure. They must decide not only what blood components (if any) are indicated but also what quantities are needed.

WHOLE BLOOD A unit of whole blood consists of approximately 450 mL blood collected into a plastic bag containing 63 mL of either citrate-phosphate-dextrose (CPD) or citrate-phosphate-dextrose–adenine (CPD-A) solution as anticoagulant and preservative. Blood collected in CPD has a refrigerated storage life of only 3 weeks, while CPD-A blood may be kept 5 weeks. At the end of these periods, about 70 to 80 percent of red blood cells are still viable, white blood cells and platelets are nonviable, and clotting factors V and VIII have low levels of activity. The storage time for packed red blood cells harvested from blood collected in CPD or CPD-A can be increased to 49 days by the addition of preservative solutions that contain mannitol.

Virtually the only reason to transfuse whole blood is to restore blood volume lost through recent hemorrhage, as with gastrointestinal bleeding, major surgery, or trauma. For assessing blood loss, routine laboratory tests are misleading for several hours after hemorrhage. Both hemoglobin and hematocrit measurements reflect the ratio of red blood cell mass to blood volume, rather than indicating the total circulating red blood cells. Since the compensatory vasoconstriction evoked by hemorrhage initially prevents extravascular fluids from replacing intravascular fluid loss, both laboratory measurements may be falsely high. Clinically, postural hypotension provides a warning that blood transfusion may be required. Pallor, syncope, tachycardia, thirst, and air hunger are useful indicators of massive blood loss (i.e., 1500 mL or more in adults), sometimes requiring immediate transfusion of type O red blood cells that have not been cross-matched. In less severe cases, maintaining the blood volume with saline or plasma expanders provides time for accurate blood typing and compatibility testing.

During surgery, blood loss can be measured quite accurately, and there is a tendency to "keep up" or even to "stay ahead" of lost volume by transfusion. Such practices lead to unwarranted use of blood with its attendant hazards. In most adult subjects, blood loss of 500 mL is easily tolerated, being equivalent to the amount given by a blood donor. Judicious use of crystalloid infusions is frequently all that is required to circumvent blood transfusion, even with blood losses up to a liter. In modern medicine, ordering "fresh" blood at any time is not acceptable practice, since proper component therapy is both safer and more scientifically based.

PACKED RED BLOOD CELLS The preparation of packed red blood cells from whole blood involves sedimentation or centrifugation followed by removal of plasma into a satellite bag, all in a closed system. Such packed cells have the same storage periods as whole blood. Removal of the plasma provides protection against circulatory overload as well as against excessive loads of sodium, potassium, citrate, ammonia, and antibodies (particularly anti-A) which might be harmful to the patient. Furthermore, the removed plasma can be used for preparing such products as cryoprecipitate, albumin, and immunoglobulins.

In the absence of recent blood loss, most transfusions are given to patients who need replacement of oxygen-carrying capacity. Packed red blood cells are much preferred to whole blood for this purpose, since the plasma serves no useful purpose and may be detrimental, especially in hypervolemic subjects. Diagnoses most frequently associated with the need for packed red blood cells fall into two major categories of anemia, hypoplastic and hemolytic.

Red blood cell hypoplasia Chronic bone marrow depression not responding to medical therapy may, under favorable circumstances, be treated by bone marrow transplantation (see Chap. 299). However, some patients are either unsuitable candidates or have no access to a marrow donor (although the increasing use of unrelated donors is shrinking the number of such subjects). The red blood cell mass of these patients can be maintained at functional levels for long periods, provided they do not develop multiple antibodies against red blood cell antigens. These patients are in general more liable to become immunologically refractory to platelets and white blood cells than to red blood cells. Patients whose red blood cell hypoplasia is secondary to marrow invasion by malignancy and/or to various chemo- or radiotherapeutic agents also require red blood cell transfusions. Again, sensitization to transfused platelets and white blood cells creates a greater problem than red blood cell immunization.

Hemolytic anemia In severe cases of inherited nonimmune hemolysis due to intrinsic red blood cell defects (e.g., sickle cell anemia, thalassemia, or severe deficiencies of glucose-6-phosphate dehydrogenase), the only hope of maintaining oxygen-carrying capacity through a crisis is the careful use of red blood cell transfusion. Patients with other forms of nonimmune hemolysis or ineffective erythropoiesis (e.g., vitamin B_{12}, folate, or iron deficiencies) are candidates for transfusion only if they are severely anemic and if the cause cannot be corrected by specific replacement therapy. Whenever any infusion is given to a patient with severe anemia, the possibility of precipitating heart failure must be recognized and circumvented by careful monitoring.

Patients with autoimmune hemolytic anemia are not good candidates for red blood cell transfusion. Not only are they liable to develop new alloantibodies, but they may have already formed such antibodies as the result of earlier transfusion or pregnancy. In the presence of circulating *auto*antibodies, alloantibodies are often difficult to detect, and transfused red blood cells may be rapidly destroyed. Consultation with a blood transfusion expert is desirable in cases where severe anemia with hypoxemia or cardiac failure poses an immediate threat to life.

PLATELETS Platelet concentrates are prepared by centrifugation of platelet-rich plasma to yield at least 5×10^{10} platelets from each donor unit. More porous plastic bags and gentle agitation facilitate gas transport across the container walls during storage at room temperature. A continuous supply of oxygen maintains aerobic platelet metabolism and prevents harmful drops in pH due to lactic acid production and CO_2 retention. These factors permit platelet storage for up to 5 days with posttransfusion survivals of 6 to 7 days. In adult thrombocytopenic patients without consumptive coagulopathy or platelet-specific antibodies, 1 unit of platelet concentrate raises the platelet count by about 10,000 per microliter.

Patients with idiopathic thrombocytopenic purpura produce auto-antibodies which react with all human platelets (see Chap. 287), and therefore derive little or no benefit from platelet transfusion. Similarly, in patients with thrombocytopenia due to a consumptive coagulopathy (as in infection or metastatic malignancy) the usefulness of platelet therapy is limited, unless its purpose is to keep the patient from bleeding while the primary cause is being treated.

The most rational use of platelets is to control bleeding in patients either with a temporary loss of platelets not due to immunity (e.g., massive blood replacement, prolonged surgery) or with suppressed platelet production (leukemia, lymphoma, treatment with radio- or chemotherapy). Since platelets are very immunogenic, and typing and cross-matching techniques are not yet practical, this blood component should not be given in the absence of clear indication. Most nonbleeding patients with platelet counts above 10,000 per microliter can maintain adequate hemostasis. However, patients in the immediate postoperative period may need to have their platelet counts elevated to as high as 100,000 per microliter. In other bleeding situations, a platelet count of 50,000 per microliter or more suggests other causes for hemorrhage, especially if there is no recent history of ingestion of aspirin or other drugs that interfere with platelet function, which would be reflected by a prolonged bleeding time. The effectiveness of platelet transfusion is assessed by comparing the platelet count before the infusion with counts obtained about 1 and 24 h later.

Choice of blood type Ideally, donors of platelets should have the same ABO and Rh types as the patient, since it is impossible to remove all red blood cells and plasma from the platelet concentrate. When it is necessary to use O donors for A, B, or AB recipients, the plasma may contain sufficient anti-A (or anti-B) to destroy some of the patient's red blood cells. Although this possibility is small, it deserves consideration in children or in adults receiving large numbers of platelet concentrates. When platelets of A, B, or AB donors are given to patients of unlike ABO type, the posttransfusion platelet increment may be somewhat diminished, although this is rarely a major problem. However, it is important that the number of red blood cells in such ABO-incompatible preparations be kept as small as possible.

Since some red blood cells are inevitably present in platelet concentrates, Rh-negative patients should receive platelets from Rh-negative donors whenever feasible, particularly if there is a possibility of subsequent pregnancy. However, lack of platelets from Rh-negative donors should not preclude transfusing Rh-positive donor platelets in a life-threatening situation. Patients who have the potential of becoming mothers can be protected against Rh alloimmunization by an injection of Rh immunoglobulin, about 20 μg for each milliliter of Rh-positive red blood cells present in the infusion. In other Rh-negative patients given platelets from Rh-positive donors, Rh-antibody formation can be expected to occur with a high frequency, but these antibodies do not interfere with the survival of subsequently transfused Rh-positive donor platelets, since they do not themselves contain Rh antigens.

Refractory state Patients who receive random donor platelets on more than one or two occasions frequently develop alloantibodies with either HLA or platelet antigen specificities. Such refractory patients can often be maintained with concentrates prepared by plateletpheresis from family members or HLA-compatible community pheresis donors. Failure to achieve a good response to histocompatible platelets suggests the presence of platelet-specific alloantibodies, nonimmune causes of platelet refractoriness, or hypersplenism.

PREVENTION OF PLATELET ALLOIMMUNIZATION Several approaches to preventing platelet alloimmunization have been tested in limited trials. Platelets express only class I, and not class II, HLA antigens, and may therefore not stimulate antibody production. It is thus possible that removal of white blood cells from platelet and red cell preparations can minimize antibody formation. Unfortunately, conflicting results have been reported from the use of leukocyte-poor preparations, probably reflecting the presence of variable numbers of contaminating white blood cells as well as nonstandard criteria for diagnosing alloimmunization. Efforts to settle this important question are in progress. An alternative method of preventing immunization is to reduce antigen exposure by using single-donor platelets obtained by pheresis rather than by using pooled platelet concentrates. This strategy probably delays but usually does not prevent eventual immunization.

WHITE BLOOD CELL TRANSFUSIONS Since it is now possible with platelet transfusions to control bleeding in many patients with hematologic malignancies, hemorrhage has been supplanted by infection as the most frequent cause of death. In general, neutrophil transfusion therapy should be considered in patients with severe neutropenia who have documented bacterial infections not responsive to appropriate antibiotic therapy. A course of neutrophil support usually consists of daily transfusion of 10 to 30 × 10⁹ neutrophils, obtained from normal donors by leukapheresis. Problems of maintaining patients for long periods in this way are even more difficult than those associated with platelets. Neutrophils have a very short life span in the bloodstream, and many questions remain unanswered about the best dosage schedules, the feasibility of neutrophil storage, the efficacy of neutrophils for fungal infections, and the recognition and management of alloimmunization. Hazards include alloimmunization to HLA and other antigens, pulmonary damage and other transfusion reactions, as well as graft-versus-host reactions and transmission of infection, particularly cytomegalovirus (CMV), to immunosuppressed recipients, including immunoincompetent infants. Irradiated and leukocyte-poor preparations reduce these risks, and are routinely used in patients undergoing marrow transplantation. The possibility of CMV infection is further reduced by selecting CMV-negative donors for these patients and those receiving transfusions of white blood cells if they are CMV negative.

PLASMA COMPONENT THERAPY Fresh frozen plasma and cryoprecipitate are major blood component preparations because they are necessary for the care of patients with coagulation disorders (see Chap. 288). Plasma can be used for expanding intravascular volume, but it carries the risk of viral transmission. Commercially prepared albumin solutions are preferable as volume expanders, as they have been heated to inactivate viruses. They are useful in special cases, such as nephrosis, certain gastroenteropathies, and severe malnutrition. Immunoglobulin preparations are also commercially made, including specific hyperimmune globulin for preventing the development of certain infectious diseases and for blocking the immune response to Rh antigen. Special clotting factor concentrates for the treatment of bleeding disorders and antithrombin III for coronary artery occlusion are discussed in appropriate chapters of this book.

PLASMAPHERESIS The introduction of cell separators has made plasmapheresis a simple procedure wherein as much as one to two plasma volumes may be exchanged in 1 to 3 h. The procedure has generally been used to reduce the plasma concentration of proteins, lipids, protein-bound hormones or toxins, antibodies, antigens, or immune complexes. While the number of different diseases that have been managed by this procedure is considerable, there are only a few in which the role of plasmapheresis is generally accepted. Even then, there is controversy regarding the frequency and volume of exchange as well as the nature of replacement fluids.

The most established indication is symptomatic hyperviscosity syndrome; plasmapheresis in this setting reproducibly results in clinical improvement. Plasmapheresis can also be used successfully in selected patients with myasthenia gravis, Goodpasture's syndrome, thrombotic thrombocytopenic purpura, and immune-complex-mediated vasculitis.

COMPLICATIONS OF BLOOD TRANSFUSION Transfusion reactions are classified as immune or nonimmune. The immunologically mediated reactions may be directed against red or white blood cells, platelets, or at least one of the immunoglobulins, IgA. Other less well defined hypersensitivity reactions also occur. The major nonimmune reactions are due to circulatory overload, massive transfusion, or transmission of an infectious agent.

Reactions due to red blood cells   Hemolysis due to red blood cell alloantibodies may occur within the circulation or extravascularly. The very rapid cell destruction associated with *intravascular hemolysis* is usually due to incompatibility within the ABO system, since both anti-A and anti-B fix complement, regardless of whether they are IgM or IgG molecules. Other possibilities to consider are anti-Jk^a, anti-Fy^a, and rarely anti-Le^a. Rh antibodies are usually not associated with hemoglobinemia. Symptoms include restlessness, anxiety, flushing, chest or lumbar pain, tachypnea, tachycardia, and nausea, followed by the typical findings of shock and renal failure. In comatose or anesthetized patients, the first sign of danger is often oozing of blood from the mucous membranes or operative site, due to intravascular coagulation.

Extravascular hemolysis is most commonly caused by antibodies of the Rh system, but several other antibodies, especially of the Kell, Duffy, and Kidd systems, are among the offenders. The clinical manifestations are usually milder, consisting of malaise and fever. Shock and renal complications rarely occur. Some patients have delayed reactions in which the transfused red blood cells have normal survival initially, but about a week later they are rapidly destroyed in the reticuloendothelial system. Such delayed reactions are commonly due to an anamnestic rise in antibodies previously stimulated by transfusion or pregnancy. Rarely, patients are found to have destroyed all the transfused cells in the absence of demonstrable antibodies.

LABORATORY INVESTIGATION   Of first importance in the investigation of a hemolytic transfusion reaction is a careful check on the identity of both the donor and the recipient, since clerical errors, especially mistakes in identity, are most frequently involved. Then the necessary steps include demonstrating that red blood cell destruction has occurred, investigating its cause, and determining the status of the patient's renal and coagulation mechanisms.

With recent *intravascular* lysis, the hemoglobin level is elevated in both plasma and urine (blood must be drawn cautiously to avoid red blood cell rupture). Also, depending on the number of red blood cells destroyed, there may be methemalbuminemia accompanied by marked reduction of serum haptoglobin and hemopexin. (Measuring the latter two substances is rarely necessary, and to be meaningful, both tests require knowledge of the pretransfusion levels for comparison.) The best indicator of *extravascular* lysis is a rise in unconjugated bilirubin, accompanied by failure of the hematocrit to reach the expected posttransfusion level.

Having a *pretransfusion* specimen of the patient's blood is very helpful, so that determination of both donor and recipient blood types can be repeated, along with the compatibility test. If antibodies are detected, this pretransfusion specimen is also valuable for determining specificity, aided by knowledge of the full antigen composition, since alloantibodies are formed only against antigens not present on the patient's own cells. The *posttransfusion* specimen may not contain the offending antibodies, since they could have been completely absorbed by the donor's incompatible red blood cells. However, it is desirable to examine the red blood cells in the posttransfusion sample, both microscopically for agglutinates and by the direct antiglobulin (Coombs) test. A positive result usually means that some of the donor's red blood cells, coated by the patient's antibodies, were still present when the blood was drawn. But it is also possible that the *donor's* plasma contained antibodies, missed during the donor screening procedure, which reacted with the red blood cells of the patient. Thus, if the direct antiglobulin test on the posttransfusion specimen is positive, the plasma of both donor and recipient should be examined for the responsible antibodies. In the absence of ABO incompatibility, significant destruction of a patient's red blood cells by a donor's alloantibodies is distinctly rare. More typically, the antibody-coated red blood cells survive well in vivo, but their presence can lead to a misdiagnosis of acquired hemolytic anemia.

TREATMENT   The care of patients with extravascular hemolysis should be conservative, avoiding additional transfusion unless the patient's life is otherwise threatened. Intravascular hemolysis is a far greater hazard, since shock and renal failure can occur. Immediate treatment with an osmotic diuretic is indicated unless acute tubular necrosis has already occurred. Renal blood flow can be increased with appropriate agents, shock controlled symptomatically, and disseminated intravascular coagulation treated appropriately. Management of the coagulopathy is discussed in Chap. 289, and treatment of renal shutdown in Chap. 223.

Other immunologically related reactions   In the absence of red blood cell destruction, most febrile reactions can be ascribed to immunity against white blood cell, platelet, or plasma antigens. Further laboratory workup is required only when the reaction is unusually severe. For example, patients with antibodies against IgA molecules sometimes undergo severe shock upon exposure to the blood of other human subjects. Such individuals must be transfused only with blood that lacks IgA or with repeatedly washed red blood cells. Patients with antibodies against white blood cells or platelets can usually be given packed red blood cells from which leukocytes have been removed after centrifugation or by filtration. Some centers use frozen and thawed red blood cells for transfusing patients sensitized to white blood cells, or to retard the occurrence of such sensitization in candidates for bone marrow transplantation. However, in patients who are candidates for renal transplantation, prior transfusions with white cell–containing products are often associated with improved prognosis—especially if the blood donor is subsequently used as the kidney donor.

Nonimmune transfusion reactions   Included in this category are circulatory overload, adverse effects of massive transfusion, infections, metabolic shock, air and fat embolisms, thrombophlebitis, and siderosis. The first three are by far the most common.

CIRCULATORY OVERLOAD   Patients with renal or cardiac insufficiency are liable to develop circulatory failure and pulmonary edema with even modest amounts of intravenous infusion. Infants are also vulnerable, since their vasculature does not accommodate rapidly to infusions. The onset may be immediate or delayed for up to 24 h after transfusion, with dyspnea and chest pain progressing to the full-blown picture of pulmonary edema. Susceptible patients should be transfused in a sitting position, with the rate of red blood cell flow not exceeding 2 mL/min, depending on body size and degree of impairment. A rise in central venous pressure heralds the danger of administering more red blood cells unless they are exchanged with whole blood removed from the patient.

MASSIVE TRANSFUSION   When the amount of stored blood transfused to bleeding patients greatly exceeds their normal blood volume, dilutional thrombocytopenia can occur, requiring infusion of platelet concentrates. Fresh frozen plasma is only rarely useful, but if the factor 8 level or fibrinogen content is low, infusing an appropriate amount of cryoprecipitate should be considered.

INFECTION   Many diseases, such as hepatitis, cytomegalovirus infection, syphilis, malaria, toxoplasmosis, brucellosis, and the acquired immunodeficiency syndrome (AIDS) can be transmitted by transfusion. In addition, blood that becomes infected during handling and storage can cause very severe shock, owing to toxic bacterial metabolites. Testing donated blood for evidence of transmissible infection is increasingly important to reduce transfusion risks. Tests for hepatitis B virus antigen and syphilis, as well as for the antibody to HIV (the AIDS-associated virus), are routinely performed on all donor units. In addition, many laboratories are now including "surrogate" tests for the hepatitis B core antibody and measurements of the plasma level of alanine–amino transferase. The current risk of hepatitis transmission by transfusion is not known, because these tests have only recently been introduced, and a test for non-A, non-B hepatitis will soon be available.

As mentioned earlier, CMV-negative immunocompromised patients, including low birthweight neonates, are candidates to receive blood products found negative for the CMV antibody. To reduce the risk of AIDS transmission, patients at high risk for the disease are instructed not to serve as donors. In addition, all blood is tested for the HIV antibody using an ELISA technique. Confirmatory tests, such as the Western blot technique, are performed before the donor is informed of a positive result, but blood found positive by the ELISA test is discarded. Transmission of AIDS by transfusion is now very rare, although sporadic cases may still occur when high-risk donors fail to be detected, especially during the early period after their exposure to the virus. The popularity of autologous transfusion has increased considerably in recent years and is a good procedure to consider, especially in patients who are candidates for elective surgery.

REFERENCES

ANSTEE DJ: Blood group active components of the human red cell membrane, in *Red Cell Antigens and Antibodies*, G Garratty (ed). Arlington, VA, American Association of Blood Banks, 1986, p 1

BARNES DM: HTLV-I: To test or not to test. Science 242:372, 1988

BEAL RW, ISBISTER JB: *Blood Component Therapy in Clinical Practice*. New York, Blackwell, 1988

BLOY C et al: Determination of the N-terminal sequence of human red cell Rh(D) polypeptide and demonstration that the Rh(D), (c), and (E) antigens are carried by distinct polypeptide chains. Blood 72:661, 1988

BOVE JR: Transfusion-transmitted diseases: Current problems and challenges, in *Progress in Hematology XIV*, EB Brown (ed). New York, Grune and Stratton, 1986, p 123

DAHR W: Immunochemistry of sialoglycoproteins in human red blood cell membranes, in *Recent Advances in Blood Group Biochemistry*, V Vengelen-Tyler and WJ Judd (eds). Arlington, VA, American Association of Blood Banks, 1986, p 23

GIBLETT ER: Blood group alloantibodies: An assessment of some laboratory practices. Transfusion 17:299, 1977

GIBLETT ER: Erythrocyte antigens and antibodies, in *Hematology*, 3d ed, WJ Williams et al (eds). New York, McGraw-Hill, in press, 1989

HAKOMORI S: Blood group ABH and li antigens of human erythrocytes: Chemistry, polymorphism and their developmental change. Semin Hematol 18:39, 1981

ISSITT PD: *Applied Blood Group Serology*, 3d ed. Miami, Montgomery Scientific Publications, 1985

KORETZ RL et al: Non-A, non-B transfusion hepatitis—a decade later. Gastroenterology 88:1251, 1985

MARSH WL, REDMAN CM: Recent developments in the Kell blood group system. Transf Med Rev 1:4, 1987

MOLLISON PL et al: *Blood Transfusion in Clinical Medicine*, 8th ed. Oxford, Blackwell, 1987

PITTIGLIO DH: Genetics and biochemistry of A, B, H and Lewis antigens, in *Blood Group Systems: ABH and Lewis*. Arlington, VA, American Association of Blood Banks, 1986, p 1

PETZ LD, SWISHER SN (eds): *Clinical Practice of Blood Transfusion*. New York, Churchill Livingston, 1981

RACE RR, SANGER R: *Blood Groups in Man*, 6th ed. Oxford, Blackwell, 1975

SLICHTER SJ: Transfusion and bone marrow transplantation. Transf Med Rev 2:1, 1988

WATKINS WM: Biochemistry and genetics of the ABO, Lewis, and P blood group systems, in *Advances in Human Genetics*, H Harris, K Hirschhorn (eds). New York, Plenum, 1980, vol 10, pp 1–136, 379–385

section 1 Clotting disorders

287 DISORDERS OF THE PLATELET AND VESSEL WALL

ROBERT I. HANDIN

Patients with platelet or vessel wall disorders usually bleed into superficial sites such as the skin, mucous membranes, genitourinary or gastrointestinal tract. Bleeding begins immediately after trauma and either responds to simple measures like pressure and packing, or requires systemic therapy with glucocorticoids, plasma fractions, or platelet concentrates. The most common platelet/vessel wall disorders are (1) various forms of thrombocytopenia, (2) von Willebrand's disease, and (3) drug-induced platelet dysfunction. This chapter reviews the diagnosis and treatment of quantitative and qualitative platelet disorders as well as vessel wall defects which cause bleeding. The physiology of normal hemostasis and the cardinal manifestations of bleeding arising from hemostatic disorders have been reviewed in Chap. 62.

PLATELET PRODUCTION AND KINETICS Platelets arise from the fragmentation of megakaryocytes, which are very large, polyploid bone marrow cells produced by several cycles of chromosomal duplication without cytoplasmic division. After leaving the marrow space, approximately one-third of the platelets are sequestered in the spleen, while the other two-thirds circulate for 7 to 10 days. Normally, only a small fraction of the platelet mass is consumed in the process of hemostasis, so that most platelets circulate until they become senescent and are removed by phagocytic cells. The normal blood platelet count is maintained between 150,000 and 450,000 per microliter. Although the regulatory signals are not well-defined, a decrease in platelet mass stimulates an increase in the number, size, and ploidy of megakaryocytes releasing additional platelets into the circulation.

The platelet count varies during the menstrual cycle, rising following ovulation and falling at the onset of menses. It is also influenced by the patient's nutritional state and can be decreased in severe iron, folic acid, or vitamin B_{12} deficiency. Platelets are *acute phase reactants* and patients with systemic inflammation, tumors, bleeding, and mild iron deficiency may have an increased platelet count, a benign condition called *secondary or reactive thrombocytosis*. In contrast, the increase in platelet count that is characteristic of the myeloproliferative disorders such as polycythemia vera, chronic myelogenous leukemia, myeloid metaplasia, and essential thrombocytosis can cause either severe bleeding or thrombosis.

MECHANISM OF THROMBOCYTOPENIA Thrombocytopenia is caused by one of three mechanisms—decreased bone marrow production, increased splenic sequestration, or accelerated destruction of platelets. In order to determine the etiology of thrombocytopenia, each patient should have a careful examination of the peripheral blood film, an assessment of marrow morphology by examination of an aspirate or biopsy, and an estimate of splenic size by bedside palpation. A scheme for classifying patients with thrombocytopenia based on these clinical observations and laboratory tests is outlined in Fig. 287-1.

Impaired production Disorders that injure stem cells or prevent their proliferation in marrow frequently cause thrombocytopenia. They usually affect multiple hematopoietic cell lines so that thrombocytopenia is accompanied by varying degrees of anemia and leukopenia. Diagnosis of a platelet production defect is readily established by examination of a bone marrow aspirate or biopsy, which should show a reduced number of megakaryocytes. The most common causes of decreased platelet production are marrow aplasia, fibrosis, or infiltration with malignant cells, all of which produce highly characteristic marrow abnormalities. Occasionally, thrombocytopenia is the presenting laboratory abnormality in these disorders. Cytotoxic drugs, which are frequently used in cancer chemotherapy, impair megakaryocyte proliferation and maturation and frequently cause thrombocytopenia. There are also rare marrow disorders like congenital amegakaryocytic hypoplasia and thrombocytopenia with absent radii (TAR syndrome), which selectively decrease megakaryocyte production.

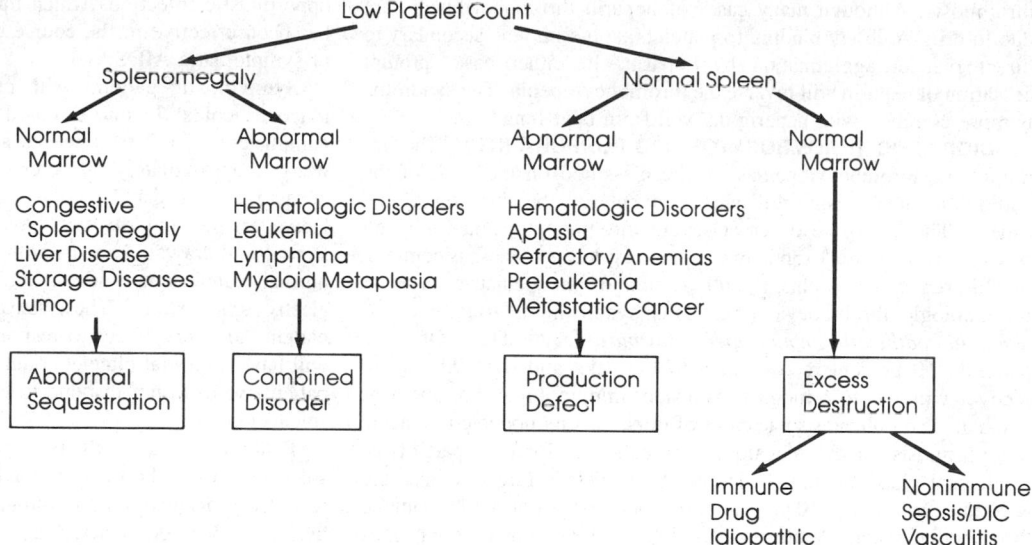

FIGURE 287-1 The clinical evaluation of patients with thrombocytopenia [*Modified from RI Handin, in W Beck (ed). Hematology, 4th ed, MIT Press, Cambridge, MA, 1985.*]

Splenic sequestration Since one-third of the platelet mass is normally sequestered in the spleen, splenectomy will increase the platelet count by 30 percent. In contrast, when the spleen enlarges, the fraction of sequestered platelets increases, lowering the platelet count. The most common causes of splenomegaly are portal hypertension secondary to liver disease, splenic infiltration with tumor cells in myeloproliferative or lymphoproliferative disorders, or with macrophages in storage disorders like Gaucher's disease. Isolated splenomegaly is rare and, in most patients, splenomegaly is accompanied by other clinical manifestations of the underlying disease. Many patients with leukemia, lymphoma, or a myeloproliferative syndrome have both marrow infiltration and splenomegaly and develop thrombocytopenia from a combination of impaired marrow production and splenic sequestration of platelets.

Accelerated destruction Abnormal vessels, fibrin thrombi, or intravascular prostheses can all shorten platelet survival and cause *nonimmunologic thrombocytopenia*. For example, thrombocytopenia is common in patients with vasculitis, the hemolytic uremic syndrome, thrombotic thrombocytopenic purpura (TTP), as one manifestation of disseminated intravascular coagulation (DIC), and in patients with prosthetic cardiac valves. In addition, platelets coated with antibody, immune complexes, or complement are rapidly cleared by mononuclear phagocytes in the spleen or other tissues inducing *immunologic thrombocytopenia*. The most common causes of immunologic thrombocytopenia are viral or bacterial infections, drugs, and a chronic autoimmune disorder referred to as idiopathic thrombocytopenic purpura (ITP). Patients with immunologic thrombocytopenia do not usually have splenomegaly and have an active bone marrow with an increased number of megakaryocytes.

DRUG-INDUCED THROMBOCYTOPENIA Many common drugs can cause thrombocytopenia (see Table 287-1). As previously mentioned, many chemotherapeutic agents are cytotoxic and depress megakaryocyte production. Ingestion of large quantities of alcohol has a similar marrow-depressing effect leading to transient thrombocytopenia. The syndrome is particularly common in binge drinkers. Thiazide diuretics, which are commonly used to treat hypertension or congestive heart failure, impair megakaryocyte production and can produce mild thrombocytopenia (50,000 to 100,000 per microliter), which may persist for several months after the drug is discontinued.

Most drugs induce thrombocytopenia by eliciting an immune response in which the platelet is an innocent bystander. The platelet is damaged by complement activation following the formation of drug-antibody complexes. Current laboratory tests can identify the causative agent in 10 percent of patients with clinical evidence of drug-induced thrombocytopenia. The best proof of a drug-induced etiology is a prompt rise in the platelet count when the suspected drug is discontinued. Patients with drug-induced platelet destruction may also have a secondary increase in megakaryocyte number without other marrow abnormalities.

Although most patients recover within 7 to 10 days and do not require therapy, occasional patients with platelet counts below 10,000 to 20,000 per microliter have severe hemorrhage and may require temporary support with glucocorticoids, plasmapheresis, or platelet transfusions while waiting for the platelet count to rise. A patient who has recovered from drug-induced immunologic thrombocytopenia should be instructed to avoid the offending drug in the future since only minute amounts of drug are needed to set up subsequent immune reactions. Certain drugs like phenytoin and gold salts may induce prolonged thrombocytopenia, since the drugs are cleared from body storage depots quite slowly. Heparin deserves special mention as it is a common cause of thrombocytopenia in hospitalized patients. It is estimated that 10 percent of patients receiving therapeutic doses of heparin develop thrombocytopenia and, occasionally, may have severe bleeding or intravascular platelet aggregation and paradoxical

---

TABLE 287-1 Drugs implicated in thrombocytopenia

I Suppression of platelet production
  A Myelosuppressive drugs
    1 Severe: cytosine arabinoside, daunorubicin
    2 Moderate: cyclophosphamide, busulfan, methotrexate, 6-mercaptopurine
    3 Mild: vinca alkaloids
  B Thiazide diuretics
  C Ethanol
  D Estrogens
II Immunologic platelet destruction
  A Clinical suspicion plus convincing experimental evidence
    1 Antibiotics: sulfathiazole, novobiocin, *p*-aminosalicylate
    2 Cinchona alkaloids: quinidine, quinine
    3 Foods: beans
    4 Sedatives, hypnotics, anticonvulsants: apronalide, carbamazepine
    5 Arsenical drugs used to treat syphilis
    6 Digitoxin
    7 Methyldopa
    8 Stibophen
  B Clinical suspicion (major drugs implicated)
    1 Aspirin
    2 Chlorpropamide
    3 Chloroquine
    4 Chlorothiazide and hydrochlorothiazide
    5 Gold salts
    6 Insecticides
    7 Sulfadiazine, sulfisoxazole, sulfamerazine, sulfamethazine, sulfamethoxypyridazine, sulfamethoxazole, sulfatolamide

thrombosis. Although many cases of heparin thrombocytopenia are due to drug-antibody binding to platelets, some may be secondary to direct platelet agglutination by heparin. In either case, prompt cessation of heparin will reverse the thrombocytopenia. The syndrome is more common with heparin derived from beef lung.

IDIOPATHIC THROMBOCYTOPENIC PURPURA (ITP)   The immunologic thrombocytopenias can be classified on the basis of the pathologic mechanism, the inciting agent, or the duration of the illness. The explosive onset of severe thrombocytopenia following recovery from a viral exanthem or upper respiratory illness is common in children and accounts for 90 percent of the pediatric cases of immunologic thrombocytopenia. This syndrome is usually called *acute idiopathic thrombocytopenic purpura* (acute ITP). Of these patients, 60 percent recover in 4 to 6 weeks and over 90 percent recover within 3 to 6 months. Transient immunologic thrombocytopenia also complicates some cases of infectious mononucleosis, acute toxoplasmosis, or cytomegalovirus infection and can be part of the prodromal phase of viral hepatitis. Acute ITP is rare in adults and accounts for less than 10 percent of postpubertal patients with immune thrombocytopenia. Acute ITP is caused by immune complexes containing viral antigens which bind to platelet Fc receptors or by antibodies produced against viral antigens which cross react with the platelet. In addition to the viral disorders described above, the differential diagnosis should include atypical presentations of aplastic anemia, acute leukemias, or metastatic tumor. A bone marrow examination is essential to exclude these disorders, which can occasionally mimic acute ITP.

Most adults present with a more indolent form of thrombocytopenia which may persist for many years and is referred to as *chronic ITP*. Women aged 20 to 40 are most commonly afflicted and outnumber men by a ratio of 3:1. They may present with an abrupt fall in platelet count and bleeding similar to patients with acute ITP. More often they have a prior history of easy bruising or menometrorrhagia. These patients have an autoimmune disorder with antibodies directed against target antigens on the glycoprotein IIb-IIIa complex or glycoprotein Ib (see Fig. 62-2). Although most antibodies function as opsonins and accelerate platelet clearance by phagocytic cells, occasional antibodies bind to epitopes on critical regions of these glycoproteins and impair platelet function.

Since a low platelet count may be the initial manifestation of systemic lupus erythematosus (SLE) or the first sign of a primary hematologic disorder, all patients with chronic ITP should have a bone marrow examination and an antinuclear antibody determination. In addition, patients with hepatic or splenic enlargement, lymphadenopathy, or atypical lymphocytes should have serologic studies for hepatitis, cytomegalovirus, Epstein-Barr virus, toxoplasma, and HIV. HIV infection has rapidly become a common cause of immunologic thrombocytopenia and should be considered in the differential diagnosis of thrombocytopenia in high-risk groups—homosexuals, hemophiliacs, and intravenous drug abusers. Thrombocytopenia can be (1) the initial symptom of HIV infection, (2) a manifestation of the AIDS-related complex (ARC), or (3) a complication of fully developed AIDS.

Treatment of patients with ITP must take into account the age of the patient, the severity of the illness, and the anticipated natural history. Although adults have a higher incidence of intracranial bleeding than children, specific therapy may not be necessary unless the platelet count is under 20,000 per microliter or there is extensive bleeding. Hemorrhage in patients with either acute or chronic ITP can usually be controlled with glucocorticoids but, in rare cases, may require plasmapheresis to reduce the antibody or immune complex level, or temporary phagocytic blockade with intravenous gamma globulin. Emergency splenectomy is usually reserved for patients with acute or chronic ITP who are desperately ill and have not responded to any medical measures designed to improve hemostasis. The treatment of symptomatic thrombocytopenia in patients with HIV infection presents a special problem because the administration of glucocorticoids or splenectomy may increase susceptibility to the opportunistic infections which threaten these patients. Splenectomy has been effective in the course of HIV infection prior to the onset of symptomatic AIDS.

Symptomatic patients with chronic ITP are usually placed on glucocorticoids. In one standard regimen, 60 mg of prednisone is administered for 2 to 4 weeks and rapidly decreased over another week. Approximately 50 percent of patients with chronic ITP will normalize their platelet count on these high doses of prednisone. However, the majority will have a fall in platelet count following steroid withdrawal. Patients with chronic ITP who fail to maintain a normal platelet count after 2 to 3 weeks of steroids are eligible for elective splenectomy. These steroid-responsive but steroid-dependent patients are very likely to respond to splenectomy, and 70 percent will have a normal platelet count within 1 week after surgery. Some patients who do not respond to glucocorticoids may still respond to splenectomy.

Patients who are still thrombocytopenic after steroid therapy or splenectomy or who relapse months to years after initial therapy have received a variety of immunosuppressive drugs including azathioprine, cyclophosphamide, vincristine, and vinblastine. More recently danazol, an impeded androgen, has been used with some success. Although each of these drugs may be beneficial, it is important to use some restraint as they have serious side effects. If a patient is not bleeding and maintains a platelet count over 20,000 per microliter, consideration should be given to withholding therapy, since there are many patients with severe chronic thrombocytopenia who have lived with their disease for two or three decades.

VON WILLEBRAND'S DISEASE   Von Willebrand's disease (vWD) is the most common inherited bleeding disorder and may occur in as many as 1 in 800 to 1000 individuals. The von Willebrand factor (vWF) is a heterogeneous multimeric plasma glycoprotein with two major functions. It facilitates platelet adhesion under conditions of high shear stress by linking platelet membrane receptors to vascular subendothelium; it also serves as the plasma carrier for factor VIII, the antihemophilic factor, a critical blood coagulation protein. The normal plasma vWF level is 10 mg/L. The vWF activity is distributed among a series of plasma multimers with estimated molecular weights ranging from 400,000 to over 20 million. A single large vWF precursor subunit is synthesized in endothelial cells and megakaryocytes, where it is cleaved and assembled into the disulfide-linked multimers present in plasma, platelets, and vascular subendothelium. A modest reduction in plasma vWF concentration, or a selective loss in the high-molecular-weight multimers, decreases platelet adhesion and causes clinical bleeding.

Although vWD is heterogeneous, there are certain clinical features which are common to all the syndromes. With one exception (type III disease), all forms are inherited as autosomal dominant traits and affected patients are heterozygous with one normal and one abnormal vWF allele. In mild cases, bleeding occurs only after surgery or trauma. More severely affected patients have spontaneous epistaxis or oral mucosal, gastrointestinal, or genitourinary bleeding. The laboratory findings are variable. The most diagnostic pattern is the combination of (1) a prolonged bleeding time, (2) a reduction in plasma vWF concentration, (3) a parallel reduction in ristocetin cofactor activity, and (4) reduced factor VIII activity. The variability in laboratory tests is related both to the heterogeneous nature of the defects in vWD and the fact that vWF synthesis or release is increased by ABO blood group type, central nervous disorders, systemic inflammation, or pregnancy. Since vWD is an autosomal dominant disorder, some vWF is produced by the remaining normal allele. Thus, patients with mild defects may have laboratory values that fluctuate over time and may occasionally be within the normal range.

The cDNA for vWF has been cloned and the gene localized to chromosome 12. Information is now appearing regarding the molecular genetics of the von Willebrand syndromes. There are three major types of vWD. Patients with *type I disease,* the most common abnormality, have a mild to moderate decrease in plasma vWF. In the milder cases, although hemostasis is clearly impaired, the vWF level is just below the lower limit of normal (50 percent activity, or 5 mg/L). In type I disease there is a parallel decrease in vWF antigen, factor VIII activity, and ristocetin cofactor activity, with a normal spectrum of multimers detected by sodium dodecyl sulfate–agarose (SDS-agarose) gel electrophoresis. Cultured endothelial cells derived from the umbilical cords of patients with vWD synthesize and secrete reduced quantities of vWF multimer and have a two- to fourfold reduction in vWF mRNA.

The variant forms of vWD (*type II disease*), which are much less common, are characterized by normal or near-normal levels of a dysfunctional protein. Patients with the *type IIa variant* of vWD have a deficiency in the high- and medium-molecular-weight forms of vWF multimer detected by SDS-agarose electrophoresis. This is due either to an inability to assemble the high-molecular-weight multimers or to premature catabolism after they leave the endothelial cell and enter the circulation. vWF protein derived from type IIa endothelial cells is unusually susceptible to proteolysis, in keeping with the observations of in vivo proteolytic degradation and rapid catabolism. The quantity of vWF antigen and the amount of associated factor VIII are usually normal. In the *type IIb variant*, there is also a loss in high-molecular-weight multimers. However, in type IIb cases, it is due to the inappropriate binding of vWF to platelets. This forms intravascular platelet aggregates which are rapidly cleared from the circulation causing mild, cyclic thrombocytopenia. Levels of total vWF antigen and factor VIII usually remain normal.

Approximately 1 in 1 million individuals have a very severe form of vWD that is phenotypically recessive (*type III disease*). Type III patients are usually the offspring of two parents with mild type I disease. However, in many cases, the parents are very mildly affected or are asymptomatic. Type III patients may inherit a different abnormality from each parent (a doubly heterozygous state) or be homozygous for a single defect. Type III patients have severe mucosal bleeding, no detectable vWF antigen or activity, and may have sufficiently low factor VIII levels to have occasional hemarthroses like mild hemophiliacs. Several type III families have been described with major deletions in the vWF gene that were detected by Southern blotting with vWF cDNA.

Appropriate therapy of vWD depends on the symptoms and the underlying type of disease. There are two therapeutic options. One involves the use of cryoprecipitate, which is a plasma fraction enriched in vWF and is appropriate treatment for all the inherited forms of vWD. During surgery, or after major trauma, patients should receive ten bags of cryoprecipitate twice daily. This regimen should be continued twice daily for 48 to 72 h to ensure optimal hemostasis. Minor bleeding episodes such as prolonged epistaxis or severe menorrhagia may respond to a single transfusion of cryoprecipitate. Recurrent menorrhagia, a major problem for women with severe vWD, can be effectively treated with oral contraceptive agents that suppress menses.

A second therapeutic option, which avoids the use of plasma and its attendant risk of serious viral infections, is the use of 1-desamino-8-D-arginine vasopressin (DDAVP), a vasopressin analogue which has minimal blood pressure–elevating and fluid-retaining properties and raises the plasma vWF level in normal individuals and patients with mild vWD. Patients with type I disease are the best candidates for DDAVP therapy. However, they must be tested for an adequate response prior to anticipated surgery, and vWF levels must be closely monitored during therapy since the patient may develop tachyphylaxis when therapy is continued for more than 48 h. DDAVP should not be given to patients with variant forms of vWD without prior testing, since it may not improve multimer pattern or hemostasis in type IIa patients, and it may actually worsen the defect or cause thrombotic complications in type IIb patients, since it increases the number of platelet-vWF aggregates and the degree of thrombocytopenia. It is also ineffective therapy for most patients with the severe form (type III) of vWD.

Although most cases of vWD are inherited, there are also acquired forms of vWD caused by antibodies which inhibit vWF function or by lymphoid or other tumors which selectively adsorb vWF multimers onto their surfaces. Anti-vWF antibodies have developed in patients with severe vWD following multiple transfusions, as well as in patients with autoimmune and lymphoproliferative disorders. Adsorption of vWF to tumor surfaces has been documented in patients with Waldenstrom's macroglobulinemia and Wilm's tumor and inferred in other patients with lymphoma. Treatment of acquired vWD should focus on controlling the underlying disease, since cryoprecipitate and DDAVP are usually not effective and the disorder can be fatal.

PLATELET MEMBRANE DEFECTS Receptors which modulate platelet adhesion and aggregation are located on the two major platelet surface glycoproteins. As previously discussed (see Chap. 62), vWF facilitates platelet adhesion by binding to glycoprotein Ib, while fibrinogen links platelets into aggregates via sites on the glycoprotein IIb-IIIa complex. There are two rare but well-defined platelet defects characterized by the loss of these glycoprotein receptors. Patients with the *Bernard-Soulier syndrome* have markedly reduced platelet adhesion and cannot bind vWF to their platelets owing to a deficiency in glycoprotein Ib complex. They also have reduced levels of several other membrane proteins, mild thrombocytopenia, and extremely large, lymphocytoid platelets. Platelets from patients with *Glanzmann's disease* or *thrombasthenia* are missing or markedly deficient in the glycoprotein IIb-IIIa complex. Their platelets do not bind fibrinogen and cannot form aggregates. The platelets undergo shape change and secretion and are of normal size.

Both of these disorders are inherited as autosomal recessive traits and are characterized by markedly impaired hemostasis and recurrent episodes of severe mucosal hemorrhage. In keeping with the selective nature of the defects, Bernard-Soulier platelets react normally to all stimuli except ristocetin. In contrast, thrombasthenic platelets adhere normally and will agglutinate with ristocetin but will not aggregate with any of the agonists which require fibrinogen binding, such as adenosine diphosphate (ADP), thrombin, or epinephrine.

The only effective therapy for hemorrhagic episodes in these two disorders is transfusion with normal platelets. This is usually effective, although alloimmunization will eventually limit the lifespan of infused platelets. In addition, a few patients have developed inhibitor antibodies with specificity for the missing protein. These antibodies bind to the protein which is expressed on the transfused normal platelets and impair their function.

PLATELET RELEASE DEFECTS The most common mild bleeding disorders arise from the ingestion of aspirin and other nonsteroidal anti-inflammatory drugs (NSAIDs) which inhibit platelet production of thromboxane A_2, an important mediator of platelet secretion and aggregation (see Figs. 62-3, 62-4). These drugs inhibit platelet cyclooxygenase, which converts arachidonic acid to a labile endoperoxide intermediate that is critical for thromboxane formation. Aspirin is the most potent agent, since it irreversibly acetylates the platelet enzyme so that a single dose impairs hemostasis for 5 to 7 days. The other agents are competitive and reversible inhibitors with more transient effects. Blocking thromboxane A_2 synthesis partially inhibits platelet release and aggregation with weak agonists such as ADP and epinephrine and produces a mild hemostatic defect. The administration of high doses of certain antibiotics, particularly penicillin, can coat the platelet surface, block platelet release, and impair hemostasis.

Patients generally have minimal symptoms such as easy bruising, and bleeding is usually confined to the skin. Occasional patients will have prolonged oozing after surgery, particularly with procedures involving mucous membranes such as periodontal, oral, or reconstructive plastic surgery. Not surprisingly, the antiplatelet effect of drugs like aspirin is more dramatic when they are administered to patients with underlying defects like vWD or hemophilia. Patients with drug-induced cyclooxygenase deficiency have a prolonged bleeding time, and their platelets fail to aggregate when incubated with arachidonic acid, epinephrine, or low doses of ADP. Platelet responses to collagen and thrombin are impaired at low doses, but normal at higher doses. Symptomatic patients should be encouraged to use drugs like acetaminophen which do not impair platelet function. Although most cases of cyclooxygenase deficiency are drug-induced, occasional patients have inherited disorders in platelet cyclooxygenase activity which impair thromboxane production or receptor level defects which prevent platelets from responding to thromboxane A_2. Although a number of metabolic disorders can perturb hemostasis, uremic platelet dysfunction is clinically the most important. The mechanism by which uremia impairs platelet function is not well understood, and retention of phenolic and guanidinosuccinic acids, excess prostacyclin production, or impaired vWF-platelet interactions have all been implicated. There is a good correlation between the degree of uremia and bleeding symptoms, and bleeding can usually be reversed by dialysis. In addition, the administration of cryoprecipitate or DDAVP, which raise plasma vWF levels, can also improve hemostasis.

STORAGE POOL DEFECTS Platelet granules have considerable amounts of adenine nucleotides, calcium, and adhesive glycoproteins like thrombospondin, fibronectin, and vWF, all of which promote platelet adhesion and aggregation. Thus, it is not surprising that patients with defective platelet granules have a mild bleeding disorder. Platelet storage pool defects may be inherited as an isolated disorder or be part of systemic granule packaging defects such as oculocutaneous albinism, the Hermansky-Pudlak, or the Chediak-Higashi syndromes. Clinically, these patients cannot be distinguished from those with other functional platelet disorders since they all have easy bruising, mucosal bleeding, and a prolonged bleeding time. They can be differentiated from patients with the cyclooxygenase defects since their platelets will usually aggregate in response to arachidonic acid. In addition, their platelets have decreased levels of specific granule constituents like ADP and serotonin and abnormalities in granule morphology that are best visualized by electron microscopy.

Occasionally, patients with acute and chronic leukemia or one of the myeloproliferative disorders develop an acquired storage pool disorder due to dysplastic megakaryocyte development. In addition, patients with liver disease and some patients with systemic lupus or other immune complex–mediated disorders may have circulating platelets which have degranulated prematurely. Platelet degranulation and a transient storage pool disorder have also been described following prolonged cardiopulmonary bypass.

VESSEL WALL DISORDERS Bleeding from vascular disorders (nonthrombocytopenic purpura) is usually mild and confined to the skin and mucous membranes. The pathogenesis of bleeding is poorly defined in many of the syndromes, and classical tests of hemostasis, including the bleeding time and tests of platelet function, are usually normal. Vascular purpura arise from damage to capillary endothelium, abnormalities in the vascular subendothelial matrix or extravascular connective tissues which support blood vessels, or from the formation of abnormal blood vessels. There are also several idiopathic disorders which involve the vessel wall and which can cause more severe bleeding and organ dysfunction.

Thrombotic thrombocytopenic purpura Thrombotic thrombocytopenic purpura (TTP) is a fulminant, often lethal disorder that may be initiated by endothelial injury and subsequent release of vWF and other procoagulant materials from the endothelial cell. In addition, some patients with TTP may have a unique circulating protein which induces platelet aggregation. Characteristic findings include the microvascular deposition of hyaline thrombi which stain for fibrin, thrombocytopenia, microangiopathic hemolytic anemia, fever, renal failure, fluctuating levels of consciousness, and evanescent focal neurologic deficits. The presence of hyaline thrombi in arterioles, capillaries, and venules without any inflammatory changes in the vessel wall is diagnostic. Gingival biopsies are positive in 30 to 40 percent of patients, and marrow biopsies are occasionally helpful. The presence of a severe Coombs negative hemolytic anemia with schistocytes or fragmented red blood cells in the peripheral blood smear, coupled with thrombocytopenia, and minimal activation of the coagulation system help to confirm the clinical suspicion of TTP.

This disorder should be distinguished from vasculitis and systemic lupus erythematosus, which can predispose patients to TTP and ITP. Levels of platelet-associated IgG and complement are usually normal in TTP.

The treatment of acute TTP has changed radically in the past few years. Steroids and heparin or emergency splenectomy have been abandoned, and the enthusiasm for antiplatelet therapy has diminished. Increasingly, treatment has focused on the use of exchange transfusion or intensive plasmapheresis coupled with infusion of fresh frozen plasma. With this therapeutic approach, the overall mortality has been markedly reduced, and over half the patients with TTP are recovering from this formerly fatal disorder. Most patients surviving the acute illness recover completely with no residual renal or neurologic disease. Occasional patients with a chronic relapsing form of TTP require maintenance plasmapheresis and plasma infusion, and a few patients are only controlled with glucocorticoids.

Hemolytic-uremic syndrome Hemolytic-uremic syndrome (HUS) is a disease of infancy and early childhood which closely resembles TTP. Patients present with fever, thrombocytopenia, microangiopathic hemolytic anemia, hypertension, and varying degrees of acute renal failure. In many cases, onset is preceded by a minor febrile or viral illness, and an infectious or immune complex–mediated etiology has been proposed. As in TTP, there is no evidence of disseminated intravascular coagulation. In contrast to TTP, the disorder remains localized to the kidney where hyaline thrombi are seen in the afferent arterioles and glomerular capillaries. Such thrombi are not present in other vessels, and neurologic symptoms, other than those associated with uremia, are uncommon. There is no effective therapy; however, with dialysis for acute renal failure, the initial mortality is only 5 percent. Between 10 and 50 percent of patients are left with some chronic renal impairment.

Henoch-Schönlein purpura Henoch-Schönlein or anaphylactoid purpura is a distinct, self-limited type of vasculitis which occurs in children and young adults. Patients have an acute inflammatory reaction in capillaries, mesangial tissues, and small arterioles which leads to increased vascular permeability, exudation, and hemorrhage. Vessel lesions contain IgA and complement components. The syndrome may be preceded by an upper respiratory infection or streptococcal pharyngitis or be associated with food or drug allergies. Patients develop a purpuric or urticarial rash on the extensor surface of the arms and legs and on the buttocks; they also have polyarthralgias or arthritis, colicky abdominal pain, and hematuria from focal glomerulonephritis. Despite the hemorrhagic features, all coagulation tests are normal. A small number of patients may develop fatal acute renal failure, and 5 to 10 percent develop chronic nephritis. Glucocorticoids provide symptomatic relief of the joint and abdominal pains but do not alter the course of the illness.

Metabolic and inflammatory disorders A number of acute febrile illnesses cause capillary fragility and skin bleeding. Immune complexes containing viral antigens, or the viruses themselves, may damage endothelial cells. In addition, certain pathogens such as the rickettsiae which cause Rocky Mountain spotted fever replicate in endothelial cells and damage them. Thrombocytopenia is also a frequent finding in acute infectious disorders and may contribute to skin bleeding. In addition, whenever the platelet count falls below 10,000 per microliter, gaps which develop between endothelial cells allow the diapedesis of red cells into the dermis leading to the formation of petechiae. Drugs such as the sulfonamides, penicillin, and allopurinol may cause vascular inflammation resulting in maculopapular or urticarial rashes. Some of these mechanisms are additive, and drug reactions in thrombocytopenic individuals cause an intensely hemorrhagic rash.

Occasionally, patients with diffuse polyclonal hyperglobulinemia will develop purpuric lesions on the lower limbs—a benign condition referred to as *hyperglobulinemic purpura*. Vascular purpura may occur in patients with various monoclonal plasma protein abnormalities including Waldenström's macroglobulinemia, multiple myeloma, and cryoglobulinemia. These proteins markedly increase serum viscosity and may impair blood flow through capillaries. Thus, retinal hemorrhage, central nervous system dysfunction, and skin necrosis have all been described in these syndromes due to the marked elevation in viscosity. In addition, the globulins may impair platelet aggregation and adhesion and interfere with fibrin polymerization. Patients with mixed cryoglobulinemia develop a more extensive maculopapular lesion due to immune complex–mediated damage to the vessel wall. The mixed cryoglobulinemia (usually IgG and anti-IgG) may be associated with arthralgias, diffuse weakness, and unexplained nephritis. Plasmapheresis will temporarily lower the level of globulins, remove immune complexes, and improve symptoms in these patients. However, long-term management must include control of the underlying disease which produces the abnormal globulins or immune complexes.

Patients with *scurvy* (vitamin C deficiency) develop painful episodes of perifollicular skin bleeding as well as bleeding into muscles and, occasionally, into the gastrointestinal and genitourinary tracts. The diagnosis is confirmed by the presence of hyperkeratosis of skin, gum swelling, and low levels of the vitamin in leukocytes. Vitamin C–deficient patients have markedly defective collagen synthesis, since ascorbic acid is needed to synthesize hydroxyproline, an essential constituent of collagen. Patients with *Cushing's syndrome,* which is characterized by excess production of glucocorticoids, or patients on large doses of glucocorticoids develop generalized protein wasting and may show skin bleeding or easy bruising due to atrophy of the supporting connective tissue around blood vessels. Aging causes a similar atrophy of perivascular connective tissue on the extensor surface of the hands and arms, leading to "senile purpura." These patients develop dark purple, irregularly shaped hemorrhagic areas due to abnormal skin mobility which tears small blood vessels.

Patients with inherited disorders of the connective tissue matrix such as *Marfan's syndrome, Ehlers-Danlos syndrome,* and *pseudoxanthoma elasticum* also have easy bruising. In addition to having fragile skin vessels and easy bruising, patients with Ehlers-Danlos syndrome may develop aneurysms in intraabdominal vessels and apoplectic rupture and hemorrhage due to defects in the vascular collagen network. Primary vascular abnormalities can also lead to bleeding. Patients with *Osler-Weber-Rendu disease* (hereditary hemorrhagic telangiectasia), an inherited autosomal dominant disorder, have frequent episodes of nasal and gastrointestinal bleeding from abnormal telangiectatic capillaries; patients with *angiodysplasia* of the colon have increased incidence of gastrointestinal bleeding. In the *Kasabach-Merritt syndrome* patients may have very extensive and progressively enlarging vascular malformations which may involve large portions of their extremities. Bleeding is secondary to disseminated intravascular coagulation triggered by stagnant blood flow through the tortuous abnormal vessels.

REFERENCES

HANDIN RI, WAGNER DD: Molecular and cellular biology of von Willebrand factor, in *Progress in Hemostasis and Thrombosis*, vol 9, BS Coller (ed). Philadelphia, Saunders, 1989, pp 233–259

MAJERUS P: Platelets, in *The Molecular Basis of Blood Diseases*, G Stamatoyanopoulis et al (eds). Philadelphia, Saunders, 1987, pp 689–722

SADLER JE, DAVIE EW: Hemophilia A, hemophilia B, and von Willebrand's disease, in *The Molecular Basis of Blood Diseases*, G Stamatoyanopoulis et al (eds). Philadelphia, Saunders, 1987, pp 575–630

STUART MJ, KELTON JG: The platelet: Quantitative and qualitative abnormalities, in *Hematology of Infancy and Childhood*, 3d ed, DG Nathan, FA Oski (eds). Philadelphia, Saunders, 1987, p 1343–1479

WILLIAMS WJ: et al (eds): *Hematology*, 4th ed. New York, McGraw-Hill, 1990

288 DISORDERS OF COAGULATION AND THROMBOSIS

ROBERT I. HANDIN

Patients with congenital plasma coagulation defects characteristically bleed into muscles, joints, and body cavities, hours or days after an injury. Most of the *inherited* plasma coagulation disorders are due to defects in single coagulation proteins, with the two X-linked disorders, factors VIII and IX deficiency, accounting for the majority of the congenital coagulation disorders. These patients merit special attention since they may have severe bleeding and chronic disability and require specialized medical therapy. With the exception of factor XIII deficiency, each of the known disorders prolongs either the prothrombin time (PT), partial thromboplastin time (PTT), or both of these important laboratory screening tests. If they are abnormal, quantitative assays of specific coagulation proteins are then carried out using the PT or PTT tests and plasma from congenitally deficient individuals as substrate. The corrective effect of varying concentrations of patient plasma is measured and expressed as a percentage of a normal pooled plasma standard. The interval range for most coagulation factors is from 50 to 150 percent of this average value, and the minimal level of most individual factors needed for adequate hemostasis is 25 percent.

Acquired coagulation disorders are both more frequent and more complex, arising from deficiencies of multiple coagulation proteins, and simultaneously affecting both primary and secondary hemostasis. The most common acquired hemorrhagic disorders are (1) disseminated intravascular coagulation, (2) the hemorrhagic diathesis of liver disease, and (3) vitamin K deficiency and complications of anticoagulant therapy.

Although congenital and acquired bleeding disorders are relatively rare, venous and arterial thrombosis and embolism are common medical disorders which have been recognized for over a hundred years. Although risk factors such as atherosclerotic vascular disease, congestive heart failure, malignancy, and immobility predispose patients to thrombosis, specific coagulation defects have not yet been identified in most patients with thromboembolism. Several inherited coagulation abnormalities have now been described which induce a hypercoagulable or prethrombotic state and predispose patients to thrombosis. These disorders merit special attention since they affect young people, cause recurrent episodes of thromboembolism, and may involve multiple members of a single family. An understanding of the biochemical basis of thromboembolism is also important since anticoagulant and antithrombotic regimes are based on the premise that modifying critical coagulation reactions will reduce the incidence of thrombosis. This chapter will review the diagnosis, natural history, and therapy of congenital and acquired plasma coagulation disorders, as well as the inherited prethrombotic disorders. The physiology of normal hemostasis and the cardinal manifestations of the hemorrhagic and thrombotic disorders are described in Chap. 62.

FACTOR VIII DEFICIENCY—HEMOPHILIA A Pathogenesis and clinical manifestations The antihemophilic factor (AHF) or factor VIII coagulant protein is a large (265,000-Da), single-chain protein which regulates the activation of factor X by proteases generated in the intrinsic coagulation pathway (see Figs. 62-4, 62-6). It is synthesized in liver parenchymal cells and circulates complexed to the von Willebrand protein (vWF). Previous efforts to purify and characterize the factor VIII molecule were limited by its low concentration (10 μg/L) and susceptibility to proteolysis. However, the cloning and sequencing of complementary DNA (cDNA) encoding the factor VIII molecule and the mapping of the factor VIII gene on the X chromosome have provided the first detailed picture of its structure and have resulted in improved methods for carrier detection and prenatal diagnosis.

One in 10,000 males is born with deficiency or dysfunction of the factor VIII molecule. The resulting disorder, hemophilia A, is characterized by bleeding into soft tissues, muscles, and weight-bearing joints. Although normal hemostasis requires 25 percent factor VIII activity, symptomatic patients usually have factor VIII levels below 5 percent, with a close correlation between the clinical severity of hemophilia and plasma AHF level. Patients with <1 percent factor VIII activity have *severe* disease; they bleed frequently even without discernible trauma. Patients with levels between 1 and 5 percent have *moderate* disease with less frequent bleeding episodes. Those with levels over 5 percent have *mild* disease with infrequent bleeding that is usually secondary to trauma. Occasional patients with factor VIII levels as high as 25 percent are discovered when they bleed after major trauma or surgery, although the vast majority of patients with hemophilia A have factor VIII levels below 5 percent.

Hemophilic bleeding occurs hours or days after injury, can involve any organ, and, if untreated, may continue for days or weeks. This can result in large collections of partially clotted blood putting pressure on adjacent normal tissues and can cause necrosis of muscle (compartment syndromes), venous congestion (pseudophlebitis), or ischemic damage to nerves. For example, hemophiliacs often develop femoral neuropathy due to pressure from an unsuspected retroperitoneal hematoma. They can also develop large calcified masses of blood and inflammatory tissue that are mistaken for soft tissue sarcomas (pseudotumor syndrome).

Patients with severe hemophilia are usually diagnosed shortly after birth because of an extensive cephalhematoma or profuse bleeding at circumcision. However, patients with moderate disease may not bleed until they begin to walk or crawl, and mild hemophiliacs may not be diagnosed until they are adolescents or young adults. Typically, a hemophiliac patient presents with pain followed by swelling in a weight-bearing joint, like the hip, knee, or ankle. The presence of blood in the joint (hemarthrosis) causes synovial inflammation, and repetitive bleeding erodes articular cartilage and causes osteoarthritis, articular fibrosis, joint ankylosis, and eventually muscle atrophy. Although bleeding may occur into any joint, after a joint has been damaged it may become a site for subsequent bleeding episodes.

Hematuria, in the absence of any genitourinary pathology, is also common. It is usually self-limited and may not require specific therapy. The most feared complications of hemophilia are oropharyngeal and central nervous system bleeding. Patients with oropharyngeal bleeding may require emergency intubation to maintain an adequate airway. Central nervous system bleeding can occur without antecedent trauma or without evidence of a specific lesion.

Patients suspected of having hemophilia should have screening tests of hemostasis including a platelet count, bleeding time, PT, and PTT. Typically, the patient will have a prolonged PTT with all other tests normal. Because of the similarity clinically of factors VIII and IX deficiency, any male with an appropriate bleeding history and a prolonged PTT should have specific assays for factor VIII and factor IX.

Therapy There are several tenets regarding the treatment of bleeding in hemophiliac patients: (1) Symptoms often precede objective evidence of bleeding. (2) Signs of bleeding may not appear until several days after well-documented trauma. Physicians caring for these patients have learned to rely on their patients to inform them of early symptoms, usually pain, and to begin treatment at that time. Early treatment is more effective, less costly, and can be lifesaving. (3) It is critical to avoid the use of aspirin or aspirin-containing drugs which impair platelet function and may cause severe hemorrhage.

Plasma products enriched in factor VIII have revolutionized the care of hemophilia patients, reduced the degree of orthopedic deformity, and permitted virtually any form of elective and emergency surgery. The widespread use of factor VIII concentrates has also produced serious complications including viral hepatitis, chronic liver disease, and the acquired immunodeficiency syndrome (AIDS). The standard therapeutic products are cryoprecipitate and factor VIII concentrate. *Cryoprecipitate*, which contains about half the factor VIII activity of fresh frozen plasma in one-tenth the original volume,

is simple to prepare and is produced in hospital or regional blood banks. It must be stored frozen and is thawed and pooled prior to administration. However, most patients utilize partially purified *factor VIII concentrate* which is prepared from multiple donors and supplied as a lyophilized powder. It can be refrigerated and reconstituted just prior to use.

There are three recent developments which have increased the safety of factor VIII therapy. First, heating of lyophilized factor VIII concentrates under carefully controlled conditions can inactivate human immunodeficiency virus (HIV) without destroying factor VIII coagulant activity. Second, highly purified factor VIII can be produced by adsorbing and eluting factor VIII from monoclonal antibody columns. Third, recombinant factor VIII is now undergoing clinical trials and may soon be marketed. All patients with hemophilia should receive either heat-treated or monoclonal purified factor VIII, and newly diagnosed hemophiliacs should only receive the monoclonal preparations to minimize viral infections and exposure to irrelevant proteins.

Each unit of factor VIII, which is the amount present in 1 mL of normal plasma, will raise the plasma level of the recipient by 2 percent per kilogram of body weight. Factor VIII has a half-life of 8 to 12 h, making it necessary to infuse it continuously or at least twice daily to sustain a chosen factor VIII level. In patients with mild hemophilia an alternative to the use of plasma products is desmopressin, which transiently increases the factor VIII level.

An uncomplicated episode of soft tissue bleeding, or an early hemarthrosis, can be treated with one infusion of cryoprecipitate or factor VIII concentrate sufficient to raise the factor VIII level to 15 or 20 percent. A more extensive hemarthrosis or retroperitoneal bleeding requires twice-daily or continuous infusions in order to keep the factor VIII level between 25 and 50 percent for at least 72 h. Life-threatening bleeding into the central nervous system, or major surgery, may require therapy for 2 weeks with levels kept at a minimum of 50 percent of normal. In addition to the prompt infusion of factor VIII–enriched plasma products, patients need skilled orthopedic care with immobilization of inflamed joints to promote healing and to prevent contractures, and physical therapy to strengthen muscles and maintain joint mobility. Prior to surgery every patient should be screened for the presence of an inhibitor to factor VIII.

Patients with hemophilia who do not have an inhibitor should receive factor VIII infusions just prior to surgery and will require daily monitoring so that the factor VIII level is maintained above 50 percent for 10 to 14 days after surgery. When patients undergo joint replacement or other major orthopedic surgery, therapy should be continued for 3 weeks. This permits adequate wound healing and the institution of necessary joint mobilization and physical therapy.

Hemophiliacs also require treatment prior to dental procedures. Filling of a carious tooth can be managed by a single infusion of cryoprecipitate or factor VIII concentrate coupled with the administration of 4 to 6 g of ε-aminocaproic acid (EACA) four times daily for 72 to 96 h after the dental procedure. EACA is a potent antifibrinolytic agent which will inhibit plasminogen activators present in oral secretions and stabilize clot formation in oral tissue. For major oral and periodontal surgery and extractions of permanent teeth, patients should be hospitalized and treated with factor VIII. Therapy should begin just prior to surgery and be continued for a minimum of 48 to 72 h.

Many centers have organized home care programs so that patients can administer their own factor VIII infusions with the onset of symptoms. Occasional patients with very frequent bleeding receive regularly scheduled infusions. However, the expense and inconvenience usually limit the use of "prophylactic" infusions. Concern regarding transmission of AIDS has complicated therapy of hemophilia, and some patients are reluctant to treat themselves.

Complications Most hemophiliacs have had multiple episodes of hepatitis, and a majority have elevated hepatocellular enzyme levels and abnormalities on liver biopsy. Ten to twenty percent of hemophiliacs also have hepatosplenomegaly, and a small number develop chronic active or persistent hepatitis or cirrhosis. Recently, a few patients with hemophilia and end-stage liver disease have received liver transplants with cure of both diseases. Along with homosexuals and intravenous drug abusers, hemophiliacs are at high risk for AIDS since they frequently receive blood products. Hemophiliacs can also present with the full range of AIDS-related syndromes including diffuse lymphadenopathy and immune thrombocytopenia. Although as many as 80 percent of multiply transfused hemophiliacs are HIV-positive and some have progressed to AIDS-related complex (ARC) or AIDS, recent advances in factor VIII concentrate preparation should prevent future HIV infection.

Despite frequent bleeding, severe iron-deficiency anemia is uncommon since most of the bleeding is internal and iron is effectively recycled. Mild iron deficiency from chronic epistaxis or gastrointestinal bleeding has been noted in some hemophiliacs. In addition, after receiving large doses of factor VIII concentrate, some patients develop a mild Coombs'-positive hemolytic anemia due to small amounts of anti-A and anti-B antibody present in commercial concentrates which bind to red cells and cause hemolysis.

Following multiple transfusions, between 10 and 20 percent of patients with severe hemophilia develop inhibitors to factor VIII. Inhibitors are, generally, IgG antibodies which rapidly neutralize factor VIII activity and prevent effective transfusion therapy. There are two types of inhibitors which have different biologic characteristics and lead to different clinical presentations. Patients with type I inhibitors have a typical anamnestic response and raise their antibody titer following exposure to factor VIII. Patients with a type II inhibitor have a low antibody titer which cannot be stimulated by factor VIII infusion. Patients with the type I inhibitor should not receive factor VIII. In an emergency, control of bleeding may require intensive plasmapheresis, or infusion of prothrombin complex concentrates which contain trace quantities of activated coagulation factors and can bypass the block in coagulation produced by the inhibitor. Patients with low-titer type II antibodies may respond to higher than normal doses of factor VIII.

Genetic counseling and carrier detection Until recently, carrier detection required biologic and immunologic assays which compared the ratio of factor VIII to vWF (von Willebrand factor) protein and were predictive in only 70 to 80 percent of cases. It is now possible to trace the most defective allele in some families by examining the inheritance of restriction fragment length polymorphisms (RFLPs) linked to the factor VIII gene. In addition, certain families have been identified with specific mutations and deletions in the factor VIII gene that can be detected by restriction enzyme digestion of their DNA. Previously, prenatal diagnosis required sampling fetal blood for coagulant activity. Now, in families with an identifiable RFLP linked to the gene or a gene deletion or rearrangement, precise diagnosis is possible early in pregnancy from either chorionic villus biopsy or amniocentesis. The amount of material required has decreased, and the rapidity of diagnosis has increased with the introduction of the polymerase chain reaction to amplify desired segments of genomic DNA.

Most women carriers of hemophilia produce sufficient factor VIII for normal hemostasis from the factor VIII allele on their normal X chromosome. However, occasional hemophilia carriers will have factor VIII levels far below 50 percent due to random inactivation of normal X chromosomes in tissue producing factor VIII. These symptomatic carriers may bleed with major surgery or bleed occasionally with menses. Rarely, true female hemophiliacs arise from consanguinity within families with hemophilia, or from concomitant Turner's syndrome or XO mosaicism in a carrier female.

FACTOR IX DEFICIENCY—HEMOPHILIA B Factor IX is a single-chain, 55,000-Da proenzyme which is converted to an active protease (IXa) by factor XIa or by the tissue factor–VIIa complex. Factor IXa then activates factor X in conjunction with activated factor VIII. Factor IX is one of a group of six proteins, synthesized in the liver, which require vitamin K for biologic activity. As previously discussed (see Chap. 62), vitamin K is a cofactor for a unique posttranslational modification which inserts a second carboxyl group onto certain glutamic acid residues on factor IX. This modification permits calcium binding and adsorption onto phospholipid surfaces. Factor IX cDNA has been cloned, the gene mapped on the X chromosome, linked RFLPs identified, and patients with deletions and mutations in the IX gene have been discovered.

Factor IX deficiency or dysfunction (hemophilia B, Christmas disease) occurs in 1 in 100,000 male births. Accurate laboratory diagnosis is critical, since it is clinically indistinguishable from factor VIII deficiency (hemophilia A) but requires treatment with a different plasma fraction. Either fresh frozen plasma or a plasma fraction enriched in the prothrombin complex proteins is used. In addition to the expected complications of hepatitis, chronic liver disease, and AIDS, the therapy of factor IX deficiency has a special hazard. Trace quantities of activated coagulation factors in prothrombin complex concentrates may activate the coagulation system and cause thrombosis and embolism. This is particularly common in immobilized surgical patients and patients with liver disease. As a result, some centers have returned to fresh frozen plasma for factor-IX–deficient surgical patients while others have recommended the addition of small doses of heparin to the concentrate to activate antithrombin III during the infusion and reduce hypercoagulability.

FACTOR XI DEFICIENCY Factor XI is a 160,000-Da, dimeric protein which is activated via the intrinsic coagulation pathway. It is converted to an active protease (XIa) by factor XIIa, in conjunction with high-molecular-weight kininogen and kallikrein (see Figs. 62-4 and 62-5). Factor XI deficiency is inherited as an autosomal recessive trait and is especially common in Ashkenazi Jews. In contrast to factors VIII and IX deficiency, the correlation between factor level and propensity to bleed is not as precise, there is less spontaneous bleeding, and hemarthroses are rare. Many patients with factor XI deficiency present with posttraumatic bleeding or with bleeding in the perioperative period, and occasional factor XI–deficient women have menorrhagia. Daily infusions of fresh frozen plasma are sufficient since the half-life of factor XI is approximately 24 h.

OTHER FACTOR DEFICIENCIES Deficiencies in factors V, VII, X, and prothrombin (factor II) are all exceedingly rare autosomal recessive disorders. Although spontaneous or posttraumatic musculoskeletal bleeding or menorrhagia can occur with these deficiencies, hemarthroses are uncommon. Fresh frozen plasma is the appropriate therapy, although prothrombin concentrates may be employed for patients with severe prothrombin or factors VII and X deficiency as long as the risks of hepatitis and thrombosis are recognized.

Defects in the contact activation pathway involving Hageman Factor (factor XII), high-molecular-weight kininogen, and prekallikrein cause laboratory abnormalities but no clinical bleeding. Despite dramatic prolongation of the PTT, which is often greater than 100 s, deficient individuals have normal hemostasis and can undergo major surgery without plasma replacement therapy. It is important to recognize and diagnose these disorders since the patients should neither be inappropriately treated with plasma nor denied indicated surgery on the basis of these laboratory abnormalities. As discussed in Chap. 62, there may be as yet undefined alternative pathways to activate factor XI in vivo which bypass this apparent defect in coagulation.

AFIBRINOGENEMIA AND DYSFIBRINOGENEMIA Fibrinogen is a 340,000-Da dimeric molecule made up of two sets of three covalently linked polypeptide chains. Thrombin sequentially cleaves fibrinopeptides A and B from the Aα and Bβ chains of fibrinogen to produce fibrin monomer, which then polymerizes to form a fibrin clot. Although fibrinogen is needed for platelet aggregation and fibrin formation, severe fibrinogen deficiency, paradoxically, does not usually cause serious bleeding except after surgery. Patients with afibrinogenemia, who have no detectable fibrinogen in plasma or platelets, may have infrequent, mild bleeding episodes. Preliminary genetic analyses do not show any deletion or structural changes in the genes encoding the α, β, and γ chains of fibrinogen despite the total absence of plasma fibrinogen.

Fibrinogen is an abundant plasma protein (2.5 g/L) that has been purified and completely sequenced. Mutations have been identified which alter the release of fibrinopeptides from the Aα and Bβ chains of fibrinogen, the rate of polymerization of fibrin monomers, and the sites for fibrin cross-linking. These dysfibrinogenemias are almost always inherited as autosomal dominant traits, so that patients have approximately equal concentrations of normal and mutant fibrinogen in their plasma. Patients with dysfibrinogenemia have a slightly prolonged PT and PTT, a prolonged thrombin time, and a disparity between the quantity of fibrinogen measured with functional and immunologic assays. Despite these abnormalities most patients have no symptoms while other patients have moderate bleeding. A few dysfibrinogenemias induce a hypercoagulable state and increase the risk of thrombosis, and others have been associated with an increased incidence of abortion (see Chap. 289).

FACTOR XIII DEFICIENCY AND DEFECTIVE FIBRIN CROSS-LINKING Factor XIII is a transglutaminase which stabilizes fibrin clots by forming ε-amino-γ-glutamyl cross-links between adjacent α and γ chains of fibrin. Factor XIII deficiency is an extremely rare inherited syndrome with only a few hundred documented cases. Patients usually bleed in the neonatal period from their umbilical stump or circumcision. In addition to hemorrhage, these patients may have poor wound healing, a high incidence of infertility among males, abortion among affected females, and a high incidence of intracerebral hemorrhage. These observations suggest that the enzyme may be important in other physiologic and pathologic processes beyond hemostasis, including placental implantation, spermatogenesis, and wound healing. Several drugs, including isoniazid, may bind to cross-linking sites on fibrinogen and mimic factor XIII deficiency by blocking enzyme activity. Normal hemostasis requires only 1 percent of normal enzyme activity, which can be achieved with small amounts of fresh frozen plasma.

VITAMIN K DEFICIENCY Vitamin K is a fat-soluble vitamin which plays a critical role in hemostasis. Dietary vitamin K is absorbed in the small intestine and stored in the liver. The vitamin is also synthesized by endogenous bacterial flora resident in the small intestine and colon; however, there is controversy regarding the quantity of endogenous vitamin K that is absorbed from the large intestine. Following absorption and transport, vitamin K is converted to an active epoxide in liver microsomes, and serves as a cofactor in the enzymatic carboxylation of glutamic acid residues on prothrombin complex proteins (Fig. 288-1).

There are three major causes of vitamin K deficiency—inadequate dietary intake, intestinal malabsorption, and loss of storage sites due to hepatocellular disease. Neonatal vitamin K deficiency, which causes hemorrhagic disease of the newborn, has disappeared from western countries with the routine administration of vitamin K to all newborn infants. Although there is, theoretically, a 30-day store of vitamin K in the normal liver, acutely ill patients can become deficient within 7 to 10 days. Acute vitamin K deficiency is particularly common in patients recovering from biliary tract surgery who have no dietary intake of vitamin K, have T-tube drainage of bile, and are on broad-spectrum antibiotics. Vitamin K deficiency is also seen in chronic liver disease, particularly primary biliary cirrhosis, and in some malabsorption states (see Chaps. 240 and 254).

With the onset of vitamin K deficiency, plasma levels of all the prothrombin complex proteins (factors II, VII, IX, X; protein C and protein S) decrease. Factor VII and protein C, which have the shortest half-lives, decrease first. Because of the rapid fall in factor VII, patients with mild vitamin K deficiency may have a prolonged PT and a normal PTT. Later, as the levels of the other factors fall, the PTT will also become prolonged. Parenteral administration of 10 mg of vitamin K rapidly restores vitamin K levels in the liver and permits normal production of prothrombin complex proteins within 8 to 10 h. Severe hemorrhage can be treated with fresh frozen plasma, which immediately corrects the hemostatic defect. If the cause of vitamin K deficiency cannot be eliminated, patients may need monthly injections. Purified prothrombin complex concentrates should be avoided as they contain trace quantities of activated forms of the prothrombin complex proteins and can cause thrombosis in patients with liver disease. They will also expose patients to an increased risk of hepatitis.

DISSEMINATED INTRAVASCULAR COAGULATION Disseminated intravascular coagulation (DIC) may be an explosive and life-threatening bleeding disorder. Although there is a long list of diseases complicated by DIC, it is most frequently associated with obstetrical catastrophes, metastatic malignancy, massive trauma, and bacterial sepsis (Table 288-1). In each case, a tentative triggering mechanism has been identified. For example, tumors and traumatized or necrotic tissue release materials resembling tissue factor into the circulation, while endotoxin from gram-negative bacteria activates several steps in the coagulation cascade. In addition to a direct effect on the activation of Hageman factor (factor XII), endotoxin induces the expression of tissue factor activity on the surface of monocytes and endothelial cells. These cell surfaces then accelerate coagulation reactions. This combination of potent thrombogenic stimuli causes the deposition of small thrombi and emboli throughout the microvasculature. This early thrombotic phase of DIC is then followed by a phase of procoagulant consumption and secondary fibrinolysis. Continued fibrin formation and fibrinolysis lead to hemorrhage from the depletion of coagulation proteins and platelets and the antihemostatic effects of fibrin degradation products (see Fig. 288-2).

The clinical presentation varies with the stage and severity of the syndrome. Most patients have extensive skin and mucous membrane bleeding and hemorrhage from multiple sites—usually surgical inci-

FIGURE 288-1 The mechanism of action of vitamin K, which is a cofactor in the formation of di-γ-carboxyglutamic acid residues on coagulation proteins, is depicted. Vitamin K is converted to an epoxide in liver microsomes. The epoxide is the active form and is reduced back to vitamin K by a liver membrane reductase. Warfarin blocks the action of the reductase and competitively inhibits the effects of vitamin K.

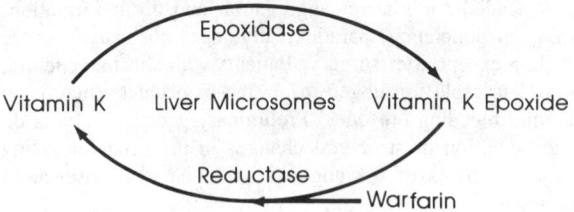

TABLE 288-1 Etiologic factors and disorders causing disseminated intravascular coagulation

Liberation of tissue factors	Obstetrical syndromes—abruptio placentae, amniotic fluid embolism, retained dead fetus, second trimester abortion
	Hemolysis
	Neoplasms, particularly mucinous adeno-carcinomas, acute promyelocytic leukemia
	Intravascular hemolysis
	Fat embolism
	Tissue damage—burns, frostbite, head injury, gunshot wounds
Endothelial damage	Aortic aneurysm
	Hemolytic uremic syndrome
	Acute glomerulonephritis
	Rocky Mountain spotted fever
Vascular malformation and decreased blood flow	Kasabach-Merritt syndrome
Infections	Bacterial: staphylococci, streptococci, pneumococci, meningococci, gram-negative bacilli
	Viral: arboviruses, varicella, variola, rubella
	Parasitic: malaria, kala-azar
	Rickettsial: Rocky Mountain spotted fever
	Mycotic: acute histoplasmosis

SOURCE: Modified from RI Handin, RD Rosenberg, in Hematology, 4th ed, WS Beck (ed), Cambridge, MA, MIT Press, 1985.

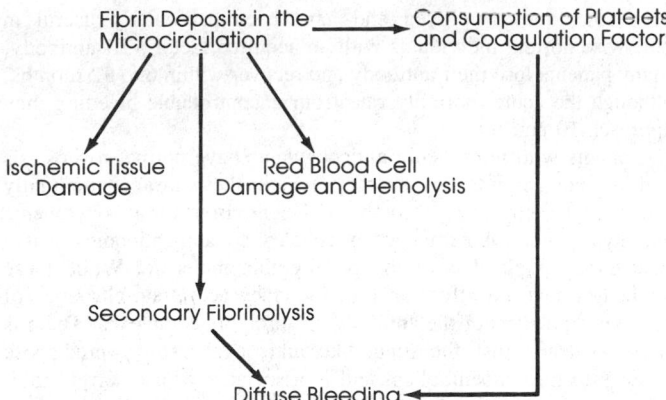

FIGURE 288-2 The pathophysiology of disseminated intravascular coagulation (DIC). Shown are the interactions between coagulation and fibrinolytic pathways which result in bleeding in patients with DIC.

sions, venipuncture, or catheter sites. Less often, patients present with peripheral acrocyanosis, thrombosis, and pregangrenous changes in digits, genitalia, and nose—areas where blood flow is markedly reduced by vasospasm or microthrombi. Occasional patients, particularly those with chronic DIC secondary to malignancy, have laboratory abnormalities without any evidence of thrombosis or hemorrhage.

The laboratory manifestations include thrombocytopenia, and the presence of schistocytes or fragmented red blood cells which arise from cell trapping and damage within fibrin thrombi; prolonged PT and PTT and thrombin time, and a reduced fibrinogen level from depletion of coagulation proteins; and elevated fibrin degradation products (FDPs) from intense secondary fibrinolysis. The cardinal manifestation of DIC, which correlates most closely with bleeding, is the plasma fibrinogen level.

Treatment DIC can cause life-threatening hemorrhage and requires prompt treatment. This should include: (1) an attempt to correct any reversible cause of DIC; (2) measures to control the major symptom, either bleeding or thrombosis; and (3) a prophylactic regimen to prevent recurrence in cases of chronic DIC. Treatment will vary with the clinical presentation. In patients with an obstetric complication like abruptio placentae or acute bacterial sepsis, the underlying disorder is easy to correct, and prompt delivery of the fetus and placenta or treatment with appropriate antibiotics will reverse the DIC syndrome. In patients with metastatic tumor causing DIC, control of the primary disease may not be possible and long-term prophylaxis may be necessary.

Patients with bleeding as a major symptom should receive fresh frozen plasma to replace depleted clotting factors, and platelet concentrates to correct thrombocytopenia. Those with acrocyanosis and incipient gangrene or thrombosis need immediate anticoagulation with intravenous heparin. The use of heparin in the treatment of bleeding is still controversial, although it is a logical way to reduce thrombin generation and prevent further consumption of clotting proteins. It should be reserved for patients with thrombosis or those who continue to bleed despite vigorous treatment with plasma and platelets.

Patients with mild DIC, who may not be symptomatic, may begin to bleed following stresses like surgery or chemotherapy. For example, mild DIC, without clinical bleeding, has been documented during saline- or prostaglandin-induced midtrimester abortions. Prophylactic treatment of patients with heparin may prevent progression of the DIC syndrome and has been used in the treatment of patients with acute promyelocytic leukemia and in some patients with a retained dead fetus who require surgical extraction. However, most patients with low-grade DIC can be managed simply with plasma and platelet replacement and do not require heparin. Chronic DIC does not respond to oral warfarin anticoagulants, but it can be controlled with long-

term heparin infusion. Occasional patients with indolent tumors and severe DIC have been maintained on heparin administered by intermittent subcutaneous injection or continuous infusion with portable pumps.

Despite our detailed understanding of the pathophysiology of DIC and a vigorous approach to therapy, there is little evidence that its treatment will change the natural history of the underlying disorder. Therapy will only stabilize the patient, prevent exsanguination or massive thrombosis, and permit institution of definitive therapy.

COAGULATION DISORDERS IN LIVER DISEASE Since the liver plays a central role in the synthesis and metabolism of coagulation proteins, liver dysfunction is frequently accompanied by a hemostatic defect. The major causes of hemorrhage in patients with liver disease are outlined in Table 288-2. It is important to recognize that bleeding is usually due to an anatomic lesion, which is then exacerbated by the hemostatic defects. Most patients bleed from complications of portal hypertension such as esophageal varices, or from gastritis and peptic ulceration of the gastrointestinal tract. Portal hypertension also causes splenomegaly, with splenic sequestration of platelets and thrombocytopenia, which contributes to the hemostatic defect (see Chap. 254).

Patients with hepatocellular liver disease cannot store vitamin K optimally and may have some degree of vitamin K deficiency. Cholestasis, which is a frequent feature of liver disease, impairs vitamin K absorption and further decreases liver vitamin K stores. They may also have decreased production of other coagulation proteins including fibrinogen and factor V. The liver also produces inhibitors of coagulation such as antithrombin III and proteins C and S and is the clearance site for activated coagulation factors and fibrinolytic enzymes. Thus, patients with liver disease are "hypercoagulable" and predisposed to developing DIC and may develop systemic fibrinolysis. For these reasons, coagulation defects in advanced liver failure are often difficult to distinguish from those of DIC.

Each patient with hemorrhage and liver disease should have a PT, PTT, platelet count, and fibrinogen determination, although it is not always possible to determine the major hemostatic abnormality from a single set of laboratory values. It is helpful to have previous laboratory data available for patients with chronic liver disease who develop an acute complication. Most patients present with moderate prolongation of the PT and PTT, mild thrombocytopenia, and a normal fibrinogen level. However, they may present with a more complex defect combining defective synthesis, abnormal clearance, and active consumption of coagulation proteins. Since vitamin K deficiency is so common, it is advisable to administer a single parenteral dose of vitamin K after initial laboratory studies have been obtained, even though this may only partially correct the laboratory abnormalities. The presence of severe thrombocytopenia or a low

TABLE 288-2 Causes of bleeding in liver disease

I Anatomic factors
  A Portal hypertension
    1 Varices
    2 Splenomegaly and secondary thrombocytopenia
  B Peptic ulceration
  C Gastritis
II Hepatic function abnormalities
  A Decreased synthesis of procoagulant proteins: fibrinogen, prothrombin, factors V, VII, IX, X, XI
  B Decreased synthesis of coagulation inhibitors: protein C, protein S, antithrombin III
  C Impaired absorption and metabolism of vitamin K
  D Failure to clear activated coagulation proteins leading to
    1 Disseminated intravascular coagulation
    2 Systemic fibrinolysis
III Complications of therapy
  A Dilution of platelets and coagulation proteins from massive transfusions
  B Infusion of activated coagulation proteins in prothrombin complex concentrates
  C Bleeding from heparin; thrombosis from ε-aminocaproic acid (EACA)

fibrinogen level suggests the additional complication of DIC and may require further studies and therapy.

The safest replacement therapy for a patient with liver disease is fresh frozen plasma since it supplies all known coagulation factors. However, even this form of therapy has drawbacks since large quantities of plasma may precipitate hepatic encephalopathy and cause fluid and sodium overload. Prothrombin complex concentrates should be avoided since they only replace the vitamin K–dependent factors, may be contaminated with hepatitis and AIDS virus, and contain trace quantities of activated coagulation proteins. Similarly, fibrinogen concentrates, or cryoprecipitate, which are rich in factor VIII and fibrinogen should not be used without additional fresh frozen plasma. Anticoagulation with heparin has been advocated to control DIC, but this is particularly hazardous and not recommended in cirrhosis since heparin is metabolized erratically and may thus lead to severe bleeding.

FIBRINOLYTIC DEFECTS Bleeding can also occur from defects in the fibrinolytic system. Patients with alpha$_2$ plasmin inhibitor deficiency have excess fibrinolysis following fibrin deposition after trauma or surgery and so may experience recurrent hemorrhage. Similarly, patients with cirrhosis have an impaired clearance of tissue plasminogen activator and systemic fibrinolysis which may contribute to their hemorrhagic defect. Rarely, patients with tumors such as metastatic prostatic carcinoma may develop diffuse bleeding from primary fibrinolysis rather than DIC. Clues to the diagnosis include a disproportionately low fibrinogen with a relatively normal PT and PTT and the presence of a normal or nearly normal platelet count. However, at times it is difficult or impossible to differentiate primary fibrinolysis from the secondary fibrinolysis accompanying DIC. Patients with clearly established primary fibrinolysis should not receive heparin; they do require plasma therapy and, occasionally, fibrinolytic inhibitors like EACA. However, EACA should not be given to patients suspected of having DIC unless they are also receiving heparin, since EACA can cause massive, often fatal, thrombosis in a patient with DIC.

CIRCULATING ANTICOAGULANTS Circulating anticoagulants, or inhibitors, are usually IgG antibodies which interfere with coagulation reactions. Specific inhibitors inactivate individual coagulation proteins and may cause severe hemorrhage. As discussed above, they arise in 15 to 20 percent of patients with factors VIII or IX deficiency who have received plasma infusions. *Specific* inhibitors also occur in previously normal individuals. Although the most common target protein is factor VIII, inhibitors have been described with a specificity for each of the coagulation proteins. Anti-factor VIII antibodies in nonhemophiliacs are seen in postpartum females, in patients on various drugs, as part of the spectrum of autoantibodies in systemic lupus erythematosus patients, and in normal elderly individuals. *Nonspecific* (lupus-like) inhibitors prolong coagulation tests by binding to phospholipids; they do not perturb hemostasis in vivo, unless associated with thrombocytopenia or prothrombin deficiency. While they are most often encountered in patients with systemic lupus erythematosus, nonspecific inhibitors have also been noted in patients with many other disorders and also in otherwise normal individuals.

The critical laboratory feature, which identifies the presence of either type of inhibitor, is the failure of normal plasma to correct a prolonged PT, PTT, or both. Plasma from patients with a specific inhibitor will progressively inactivate a coagulation protein and thus prolong whichever of these screening tests requires the participation of that clotting factor. This effect persists after dilution. Nonspecific inhibitors immediately prolong the PT and PTT and, at low dilution, block multiple coagulation reactions. However, these effects can be overcome by altering the quantity or type of phospholipid or by diluting the plasma.

Hemorrhage in patients with specific inhibitors may require treatment with massive plasma or concentrate infusion, the use of activated prothrombin complex concentrates to bypass the antibodies against factors VIII or IX, and plasmapheresis or exchange transfusion to lower antibody titer. Chronic immunosuppressive regimens have been sometimes employed and have been particularly useful in otherwise normal individuals with an acquired factor VIII antibody. Many patients lose their antibody and recover within 6 to 12 months, although the acute mortality rate from uncontrollable bleeding may approach 10 percent.

Patients with nonspecific anticoagulants have normal hemostasis and do not require any therapy unless they are concomitantly thrombocytopenic or prothrombin-deficient. Both thrombocytopenia and hypoprothrombinemia are secondary to autoantibodies which bind either to platelets or the prothrombin molecule. While these antibodies have no effect on function, they accelerate clearance of the coated platelets or the antibody-prothrombin complexes. There is some evidence that the lupus-like anticoagulant may predispose patients to thromboembolism and is associated with recurrent mid-trimester abortions in women. However, many of these women can successfully carry their fetuses to term following therapy with glucocorticoids.

INHERITED PRETHROMBOTIC DISORDERS As previously discussed (see Chap. 62), coagulation is carefully regulated by a series of inhibitors which limit thrombin generation and fibrin formation and by the fibrinolytic system which effectively removes fibrin thrombi (see Figs. 62-5 and 62-7). Inherited defects in the natural coagulation inhibitors (i.e., antithrombin, protein C, and protein S), abnormalities in the fibrinolytic system, and certain dysfibrinogenemias predispose patients to thrombosis (see Table 288-3). Although they are an important and rapidly expanding group of disorders, they account for less than 10 percent of patients with recurrent thromboembolism. The known disorders are all inherited as autosomal dominant traits, so that heterozygous individuals, who have a 50 percent reduction in protein concentration or a mixture of mutant and normal molecules, will have an increased risk of thrombosis. The patients all have similar clinical presentations with a strong family history of thrombosis, episodes of recurrent venous thromboembolism, and symptoms by their early twenties. Any patient with this distinctive history should be tested for the molecular abnormalities described below.

ANTITHROMBIN DEFICIENCY Antithrombin complexes with activated coagulation proteins and blocks their biologic activity (see Fig. 62-5). The rate of this reaction is enhanced by heparin-like molecules within the vessel wall or on endothelial cells. Plasma antithrombin III content varies from 5 to 15 mg/L (50 to 150 percent), with values only slightly below normal increasing the risk of thrombosis. For optimal screening, it is important to assess both the antithrombin III concentration by immunoassay and the plasma antithrombin and heparin cofactor activity with functional assays. The most common defect is mild (heterozygous) antithrombin defi-

---

TABLE 288-3 Prethrombotic disorders

INHERITED FORMS

Antithrombin III deficiency
Protein C deficiency
Protein S deficiency
Dysplasminogenemia
Dysfibrinogenemia
Defective release of plasminogen activator
Diminished venous content of plasminogen activator
Excessive release of plasminogen activator inhibitor
Heparin cofactor II deficiency
Homocystinuria

ACQUIRED DISORDERS

Chronic congestive heart failure
Metastatic tumor
Metastatic malignancy
Extensive trauma or major surgery
Myeloproliferative disorders
Behçet's syndrome
Kawasaki's disease
Ingestion of oral contraceptives or L-asparaginase

ciency, which occurs in 1 out of 2000 individuals. In addition, dysfunctional antithrombin molecules, with mutations affectng either the serine protease–binding site or the heparin-binding site, or activation of inhibitor by heparin have been described. Some investigators have suggested that another molecule called heparin cofactor II may also be a clinically important thrombin inhibitor. Some patients with thrombosis have been described who are heparin cofactor II–deficient.

Patients with antithrombin deficiency who develop acute thrombosis or embolism can be treated with intravenous heparin, since there is usually sufficient normal antithrombin to act as a heparin cofactor. Following their first episode of thromboembolism, patients should be placed on oral anticoagulants for life to prevent recurrent thrombosis. Family studies should be conducted when an antithrombin-deficient individual is discovered, since up to half the members of a kindred may be affected. Asymptomatic individuals with antithrombin deficiency should receive prophylactic anticoagulation with heparin or plasma infusions to raise their antithrombin level prior to medical or surgical procedures which may increase their risk of thrombosis. Chronic oral anticoagulation is not recommended until individuals at risk have a clinical thrombotic episode.

DEFICIENCIES OF PROTEINS C AND S Protein C is a vitamin K–dependent hepatic protein which binds to the endothelial cell surface protein thrombomodulin and is converted to an active protease by thrombin (Fig. 62-5). Activated protein C, in conjunction with protein S, proteolyzes factors Va and VIIIa, which shuts off fibrin formation. Activated protein C may also stimulate fibrinolysis and accelerate clot lysis. Deficiencies of proteins C and S are autosomal dominant disorders which may be more common than antithrombin deficiency and cause identical problems—recurrent venous thrombosis and pulmonary embolism. Dysfunctional molecules have also been definitely identified in patients with thrombosis. In addition, protein S activity may be reduced when there is an excess of C4b binding protein.

Heterozygous patients with acute thrombosis and moderate proteins C or S deficiency should be heparinized and then placed on oral anticoagulants. There are, however, two potential problems with the use of coumarin anticoagulants in these patients. First, these vitamin K antagonists (see Fig. 288-1 and Fig. 62-5), which lower the level of the procoagulant factors II, VII, IX, and X, may also reduce the concentration of proteins C and S and nullify the desired antithrombotic effect. In addition, there are patients with coumarin-induced skin necrosis who have protein C deficiency, suggesting that this defect may predispose patients to a rare but serious complication of oral anticoagulants.

Homozygous protein C deficiency, which is very rare, can cause fulminant intravascular coagulation in the neonatal period. Patients with homozygous protein C deficiency may require periodic plasma infusions rather than oral anticoagulants to prevent recurrent intravascular coagulation and thrombosis.

DYSFIBRINOGENEMIAS AND FIBRINOLYTIC DEFECTS Several families have now been described with recurrent venous thrombosis and embolism due to defects in fibrinogen or plasminogen or with decreased synthesis or release of tissue plasminogen activator. While the majority of dysfibrinogenemias cause bleeding, one variant, fibrinogen New York, is characterized by excessively rapid release of fibrinopeptides and recurrent thromboembolism. Patients with this disorder as well as those with an abnormal plasminogen which resists activation by streptokinase and urokinase have been successfully treated with heparin and oral anticoagulants. Defects in tissue plasminogen activator content or release have not been completely characterized. One group of patients with recurrent venous thrombosis and embolism failed to increase venous blood fibrinolytic activity when challenged with local ischemia or physical exercise. The other group had impaired fibrinolytic activity in extracts prepared from biopsied veins. The recent cloning of cDNA for tissue plasminogen activator (tPA) and the availability of immunoassays for tPA should facilitate more detailed studies of this class of defects. There is also recent evidence that young patients with acute myocardial infarction may have impaired fibrinolysis due to increased plasma levels of plasminogen activator inhibitor (PAI), a serine protease inhibitor which binds to tPA and is derived from endothelial cells.

In addition to the inherited disorders which predispose patients to thromboembolism, many common illnesses are associated with an increased risk of thrombosis (see Table 288-3). These patients are said to have a "hypercoagulable" or "prethrombotic" state. This increased risk is seen in patients with chronic congestive heart failure and metastatic malignancy and in patients undergoing major surgery. In these patients, the generation of tissue factor activity in damaged or ischemic tissue or metastatic tumor, coupled with venous stasis and endothelial injury, induce the formation of venous and, more rarely, arterial thrombi. There are also several hematologic disorders including paroxysmal nocturnal hemoglobinuria, essential thrombocythemia, and polycythemia vera in which poorly defined abnormalities in circulating leukocytes and platelets, or changes in blood flow and viscosity, predispose patients to venous and arterial thrombosis. Diseases which affect the endothelial cell, such as Behçet's syndrome, Kawasaki's disease, and homocystinuria, or the administration of drugs like the oral contraceptives, which lower antithrombin III levels, or L-asparaginase, which inhibits production of multiple coagulation factors, may also predispose patients to thrombosis.

REFERENCES

ANTONARAKIS SE: The molecular genetics of hemophilia A and B in man. Factor III and factor IX deficiency. Adv Hum Genet 17:17, 1988

GIDDINGS JC, PEAKE IR: Laboratory support in the diagnosis of coagulation disorders. Clin Haematol 14:571, 1985

KANE WH, DAVIE EW: Blood coagulation factors V and VIII: Structural and functional similarities and their relationship to hemorrhagic and thrombotic disorders. Blood 71:539, 1988

KASPER CK, DIETRICH SL: Comprehensive management of haemophilia. Clin Haematol 14:489, 1985

LAWN R: The molecular genetics of hemophilia. Sci Am 254:48, 1986

MAMMEN E: Congenital coagulation disorders. Semin Thromb Hemost 9:1, 1983

PIERCE GF et al: The use of purified clotting factor concentrates in hemophilia. Influence of viral safety, cost and supply on therapy. JAMA 261:3434, 1989

WHITE GC, SHOEMAKER CB: Factor VIII gene and hemophilia A. Blood 73:1, 1989

289 ANTICOAGULANT, FIBRINOLYTIC, AND ANTIPLATELET THERAPY

ROBERT I. HANDIN

ANTICOAGULANT AND FIBRINOLYTIC THERAPY

Anticoagulation with heparin, followed by treatment with oral vitamin K antagonists, is the standard treatment for acute venous thrombosis and pulmonary embolism. In addition, chronic oral anticoagulation is used to prevent cerebral arterial embolism from cardiac sources such as ventricular mural thrombi, atrial thrombi, or from an atherosclerotic, partially stenosed carotid or vertebral artery. Anticoagulants are also used, less successfully, to treat peripheral or mesenteric arterial thrombosis. These agents retard fibrin deposition on established thrombi and prevent the formation of new thrombi. The induction of a fibrinolytic state by the infusion of recombinant tissue plasminogen activator (rtPA) or pharmacologic agents such as streptokinase (SK) and urokinase (UK) has become an accepted mode of therapy for some thromboembolic disorders. This approach has been advocated for some patients with massive pulmonary embolism and systemic hypotension and to restore the patency of acutely occluded peripheral and coronary arteries. Prompt fibrinolytic therapy may reduce myocardial damage following acute coronary occlusion (see Chap. 189).

TABLE 289-1 Anticoagulant therapy with heparin

Clinical indication	Dose, U.S.P. units	Route
Prophylaxis in general surgery	5000 q 12 h	SC
Prophylaxis in medical patients with congestive heart failure, cardiomyopathy, or myocardial infarction	10,000 q 12 h	SC
Venous thromboembolism (acute)	5000 (bolus) 1000 qh	IV
Venous thromboembolism (prophylaxis in pregnancy, warfarin failures, or chronic DIC)	1000 qh	SQ (pump)

ACUTE ANTICOAGULATION WITH HEPARIN Heparin is a naturally occurring mucopolysaccharide polymer with tetrasaccharide sequences that bind to and activate antithrombin III. It is an extremely potent anticoagulant that can reduce thrombin generation and fibrin formation in patients with acute venous and arterial thrombosis or embolism (Table 289-1). Heparin is administered to patients with acute thrombosis or embolism by continuous intravenous infusion at a rate sufficient to raise the activated partial thromboplastin time (APTT) to 1.5 to 2 times the control value. This usually requires 1000 U.S.P. units per hour and is continued while patients are begun on oral anticoagulants and achieve appropriate prolongation of the prothrombin time. The usual duration of combined heparin-warfarin therapy is 5 to 7 days. Heparin is then discontinued, and the patient is maintained on warfarin. Alternatives include the administration of 5000 U.S.P. units of heparin four times a day either subcutaneously or intravenously. Long-term heparin administration via portable external or implantable pumps is occasionally needed for recurrent thromboembolism that is refractory to oral anticoagulants, for pregnant women with thromboembolism, and for patients with chronic disseminated intravascular coagulation (DIC). Lower doses of heparin (5000 U.S.P. units every 12 h) have also been used to prevent deep venous thrombosis in high-risk surgical and medical patients. Patients with congestive heart failure, myocardial infarction, or cardiomyopathy may require 10,000 U.S.P. units every 12 h for similar protection.

The major complication of heparin therapy is bleeding—especially from surgical sites and into the retroperitoneum. Aspirin or aspirin-containing drugs impair platelet function, and intramuscular injections in these patients may cause significant bleeding. Heparin's anticoagulant effect can be rapidly reversed by the administration of protamine sulfate. However, this is usually not necessary, and reduction or omission of heparin improves hemostasis and stops bleeding. Thrombocytopenia occurs in about 10 percent of heparin recipients, can be severe, and may be accompanied by intravascular platelet agglutination and arterial thrombosis. Recognition of this rare complication—thrombocytopenia and paradoxical thrombosis—is critical, since discontinuing heparin can reverse the syndrome and may be lifesaving. Heparin administration for longer than 2 months also carries a risk of osteoporosis. Commercial heparin preparations are heterogeneous and only about 20 percent of the infused material has anticoagulant activity. Low molecular weight heparin fractions, which retain anticoagulant activity, are the treatment of choice for patients with heparin-dependent thrombocytopenia who require additional heparin therapy. These fractions do not interact with platelets and may not cause thrombocytopenia.

CHRONIC ORAL ANTICOAGULATION The coumarin anticoagulants, which include warfarin and dicumarol (dicoumarol), prevent the reduction of vitamin K epoxides in the liver microsomes and induce a state analogous to vitamin K deficiency (see Fig. 288-1). They slow thrombin generation and clot formation by impairing the biologic activity of the prothrombin complex proteins and are used to prevent the recurrence of venous thrombosis and pulmonary embolism. Although regimens employing loading doses of drug have been advocated, the simplest way to induce anticoagulation is to administer a single dose of a coumarin compound and monitor the prothrombin time (PT) until the desired prolongation is achieved. For example, treatment can be initiated with 5 to 10 mg/d of warfarin or equivalent, with the goal of prolonging the PT to 1.5 to 2 times the control value. Although the PT may reach this value after a few days of therapy, effective anticoagulation, with stable reduction of all the prothrombin complex proteins, requires at least 1 week of warfarin administration. Most patients require a daily maintenance dose of 2.5 to 7.5 mg of warfarin to remain anticoagulated. As discussed above, patients should remain on heparin until the appropriate dose of a coumarin anticoagulant like warfarin is established.

Although warfarin anticoagulants reduce the recurrence of deep venous thrombosis and pulmonary or cerebral embolism, they may also cause bleeding. Any patient who takes oral anticoagulants requires frequent monitoring of the PT. Despite the most careful management, fluctuations in PT can occur. Various drugs that alter liver microsomal metabolism of coumarins or compete for albumin binding sites can increase or decrease the potency of warfarin (Table 289-2).

There is a direct relation between the duration of anticoagulation and the risk of recurrent thrombosis. Although recommendations vary somewhat, most patients with a single uncomplicated thromboembolic event have maximal benefit after 3 to 6 months of anticoagulation. About 10 percent of patients on an oral anticoagulant for 1 year have a serious complication requiring medical supervision, and 0.5 to 1 percent have a fatal hemorrhagic event despite careful medical management. The anticoagulant effects of coumarins can be reversed by infusion of fresh frozen plasma or by the administration of vitamin K. In many cases, reduction or omission of several doses improves hemostasis and stops hemorrhage. Despite the risk of bleeding, patients with prosthetic heart valves, severe mitral stenosis, cardiomyopathy, chronic congestive heart failure, recurrent or persistent atrial fibrillation, or an inherited "prethrombotic" disorder may require lifelong anticoagulation.

One devastating complication of oral anticoagulation is hemorrhagic skin necrosis. Some patients with this complication are deficient in protein C, a natural anticoagulant protein whose activity is reduced by vitamin K antagonists. Patients with suspected protein C deficiency should not begin oral anticoagulant therapy unless they simultaneously receive heparin or plasma infusions to restore protein C levels to normal. Patients with an inherited trait that causes coumarin resistance may require extremely high doses to get an anticoagulant effect. Psychologically disturbed patients may surreptitiously ingest coumarin and present with unexplained bleeding and a prolonged PT. Plasma coumarin levels can be measured to confirm such ingestion.

TABLE 289-2 Effect of drugs and metabolic changes on oral anticoagulant potency

I Factors leading to enhanced potency and increased prothrombin time
 A Reduced coumarin clearance
  1 Disulfiram (Antabuse)
  2 Metronidazole (Flagyl)
  3 Trimethoprim-sulfamethoxazole (Bactrim, Septra)
 B Reduced albumin binding
  1 Phenylbutazone
 C Additive hemostatic effect of certain drugs or disorders
  1 Aspirin
  2 Heparin
  3 Liver disease
  4 Thrombocytopenia
  5 Vitamin K deficiency
 D Increased turnover of vitamin K
  1 Clofibrate
  2 Hypermetabolism (e.g., hyperthyroidism)
II Factors leading to diminished potency and decreased prothrombin time
 A Accelerated coumarin clearance—induction of hepatic metabolizing enzymes
  1 Barbiturates
  2 Rifampin
 B Reduced absorption
  1 Cholestyramine
 C Impaired metabolism
  1 Genetic coumarin resistance

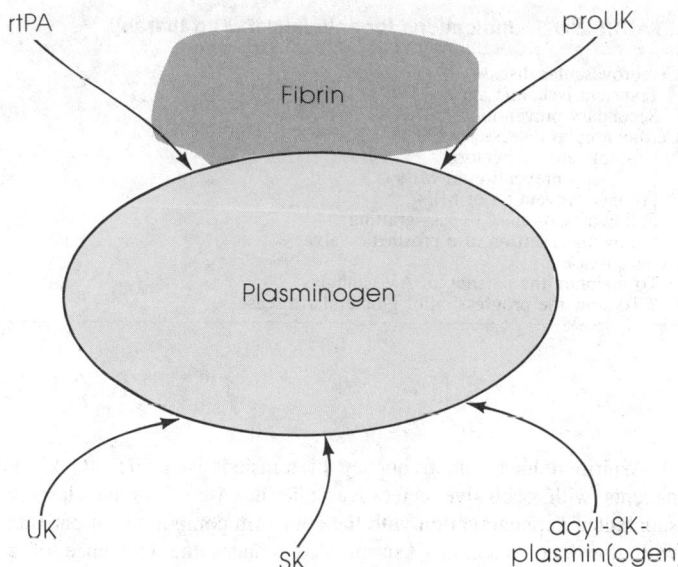

FIGURE 289-1 The mechanism of action of various plasminogen activators used for thrombolytic therapy. Recombinant tissue plasminogen activator (rtPA) and pro-urokinase (proUK) preferentially activate plasminogen bound to fibrin and are called "fibrin-specific" activators. Urokinase (UK), streptokinase (SK), and acylated streptokinase-plasminogen conjugates activate both free and fibrin-bound plasminogen.

FIBRINOLYTIC THERAPY Fibrinolysis, an important part of the normal hemostatic process, is initiated by the release of either tPA or pro-urokinase (proUK) from endothelial cells. These agents preferentially activate plasminogen, which is adsorbed onto fibrin clots. This serves to direct and localize the lytic process to sites that contain fibrin thrombi. Although fibrinolysis begins immediately after vascular injury, clot lysis and vessel recanalization may not be complete for 7 to 10 days. As previously discussed (see Chap. 62), the fibrinolytic pathway is important in normal hemostasis, as defects can predispose patients to either hemorrhage or recurrent thrombosis (see Chap. 288). In addition, activators of the fibrinolytic system are frequently employed to accelerate clot lysis in patients with thromboembolism (see Fig. 289-1, Table 289-3).

Several pharmacologic agents can accelerate clot lysis. These drugs are either naturally occurring products or chemically modified derivatives and differ with respite to fibrin specificity and complications (see Table 289-3). The cloning of the cDNA encoding tPA permitted the large-scale production of rtPA. This and proUK are relatively "fibrin-specific" agents that activate plasminogen more effectively in the presence of fibrin thrombi. This makes it theoretically possible to achieve more selective clot lysis without inducing the systemic lytic state that accompanies the infusion of urokinase (UK) or streptokinase (SK). In practice, some systemic fibrinolysis always

TABLE 289-3 Fibrinolytic activators

Product	Source	MW	Fibrin	Complications
Recombinant tissue plasminogen activator (rtPA)	Recombinant	70,000	+	Bleeding
Pro-urokinase (proUK)	Melanoma cell cultures	55,000	+	Bleeding
Urokinase (UK)	Renal tubular cell cultures	33,000	+	Bleeding
Streptokinase (SK)	β-Hemolytic streptococci	47,000	−	Immune reactions Bleeding
Acyl-SK-plasmin(ogen)	Chemical synthesis	139,00	+/−	Immune reactions Bleeding

TABLE 289-4 Indications for fibrinolytic therapy

Acute coronary occlusion/infarction
Acute peripheral arterial occlusion
Massive pulmonary embolism
Axillary vein thrombosis
Massive iliofemoral vein thrombosis

accompanies the infusion of effective doses of the fibrin-specific agents. In addition, all fibrinolytic agents can cause hemorrhage by attacking essential hemostatic plugs as well as pathologic thrombi. Thus, lytic therapy is not recommended for patients with recent surgery, indwelling cannulas, or a history of neurologic lesions, gastrointestinal bleeding, or hypertension.

Current indications for fibrinolytic therapy are listed in Table 289-4. Fibrinolytic therapy is now recommended for patients with acute myocardial infarction and with massive pulmonary embolism complicated by hypotension, severe hypoxemia, and right heart strain or failure. In addition, fibrinolytic agents have been successfully administered to patients with acute peripheral arterial embolism or occlusion and to patients with extensive iliofemoral thrombophlebitis. While such therapy may hasten lysis of venous thrombi, the long-term benefit remains unproven. There is no firm evidence that lytic therapy reduces postphlebitic complications. In contrast, fibrinolytic therapy may be of distinct benefit for thrombosis of the axillary vein, which does not respond well to conventional anticoagulation.

SK and UK are the oldest and most extensively studied fibrinolytic agents. SK is a bacterial enzyme, and UK is a product of renal tubular epithelial cells. These agents cannot discriminate between free and fibrin-bound plasminogen. When administered systemically for clot lysis, they also cause hypofibrinogenemia and a systemic lytic state. SK is an indirect plasminogen activator that interacts with circulating plasminogen to form an equimolar complex with proteolytic activity. The SK-plasminogen complex then activates additional plasminogen molecules that initiate fibrinolysis. In contrast, UK has intrinsic proteolytic activity and can activate plasminogen directly.

In the case of SK, one usually administers a loading dose of 250,000 units irrespective of body weight. Since patients may have antistreptococcal antibodies, the loading dose may need to be repeated. In addition, patients may develop acute allergic symptoms including urticaria and, occasionally, serum sickness reactions. With UK, a loading dose of 4400 units per kg body weight is administered over 10 to 30 min. Both regimens induce an intense lytic state as evidenced by a drop in fibrinogen, prolongation of the thrombin time, and a prolongation of the euglobulin lysis time—an in vitro measure of fibrinolytic activity, predominantly plasminogen activated. After the initial loading dose, 100,000 units of SK or 4400 units of UK per kg body weight are administered hourly for 24 to 72 h. At the desired time, the lytic state is reversed by discontinuing UK or SK and by administering heparin for 7 to 10 days. Heparin can be started 6 h after the fibrinolytic agent has been stopped. To enhance the likelihood of success, fibrinolytic therapy should be initiated as soon as possible after the onset of thrombosis or embolism.

The majority of myocardial infarcts are due to acute coronary occlusion, and fibrinolytic therapy has been tried extensively for acute coronary events. Initially, the nonspecific agents SK or UK were administered via a catheter placed in the diseased coronary artery in an attempt to achieve localized clot lysis. Fibrin-specific agents such as rtPA or proUK are now being administered intravenously; the former has been studied most extensively. Systemic infusion of 100 mg rtPA over 6 h restores vessel patency in approximately 75 percent of patients. Patients are then maintained on heparin for several days. ProUK given in a similar manner has almost identical effects. As discussed in Chap. 189, it is imperative to begin the therapy within a few hours of the onset of symptoms. Systemic fibrinogen levels fall 25 percent with this regimen. Bleeding is a major complication as rtPA cannot discriminate between pathologic intracoronary thrombi, which are undesirable, and vitally important hemostatic plugs; both contain fibrin and may coexist in the same patient. The most serious complication of fibrinolytic therapy, intracranial hemorrhage, is relatively rare but has devastating and sometimes fatal consequences. Thus, the same stringent contraindications discussed for systemic lytic therapy should be employed with fibrin-specific agents.

ANTIPLATELET DRUG THERAPY

Antiplatelet drugs have a role to play in the management of patients with arterial vascular disease and thromboembolism (see Table 289-5). Aspirin is the most widely studied of these drugs because of its unique pharmacology. A single dose of aspirin irreversibly acetylates and inactivates the enzyme cyclooxygenase and thereby inhibits platelet production of thromboxane A_2. Although aspirin may also inactivate cyclooxygenase in some tissues, including endothelial cells, such cells recover rapidly by synthesizing new enzyme. Platelets, which are anucleate, cannot synthesize new enzyme and remain inactive for the rest of their lifespan. As little as one 160 mg tablet of aspirin daily or a 325 mg tablet every other day inhibits platelet thromboxane production and aggregation.

Many antithrombotic regimens have employed dipyridamole, which inhibits phosphodiesterase and raises intracellular cyclic AMP in vitro. The usual dose of 50 to 100 mg four times daily has no discernible effect on platelet function. Dipyridamole has usually been administered in combination with aspirin; it is not clear that dipyridamole adds benefits when added to aspirin.

Patients with coronary artery disease who have unstable angina are at high risk for myocardial infarction (Chap. 189). In two large clinical trials, the prompt administration of aspirin dramatically reduced the progression to myocardial infarction in this group, although aspirin had no effect on the frequency, intensity, or duration of chronic angina. Aspirin also reduces the incidence of second infarction by 25 percent when administered to men who have had a myocardial infarct. In a large study of asymptomatic physicians, daily aspirin therapy also reduced the incidence of first infarcts and is now widely used for prevention of myocardial infarction. The combination of aspirin and dipyridamole, when begun prior to surgery, may also increase the patency of coronary bypass grafts, and the same combination reduces the incidence of cerebral emboli in patients on warfarin who have prosthetic intracardiac valves.

TABLE 289-5 Indications for antiplatelet drug therapy

Cerebrovascular disease
  Transient ischemic attacks
  Secondary prevention of CVA's
Cardiovascular disease
  Unstable angina pectoris
  Secondary prevention of MI's
  Primary prevention of MI's
  Following coronary bypass grafting
  Following insertion of a prosthetic valve
Renal disease
  To maintain the patency of AV cannulas
  ? To slow the progression of glomerular disease

Aspirin reduces the frequency of transient ischemic attacks in patients with occlusive cerebrovascular disease. This has largely supplanted anticoagulation with the coumarin compounds in patients with transient ischemia. Aspirin also reduces the incidence of a second stroke by 25 percent when administered to men following the first cerebrovascular accident. Aspirin is also effective in maintaining the patency of arteriovenous cannulas inserted into patients with renal failure who require hemodialysis. Aspirin plus dipyridamole may also slow the progression of some forms of glomerulonephritis, although these drugs are not widely used in the treatment of renal disease. However, aspirin appears not to be effective in maintaining the patency of vessels following percutaneous angioplasty.

REFERENCES

CLOUSE LJ, COMP PC: The regulation of hemostasis: The protein C system. N Engl J Med 314:1298, 1986
GOLLER BS: Platelets and thrombolytic therapy. N Engl J Med 322:33, 1990
LEE TH et al: Candidates for thrombolysis among Emergency Room patients with acute chest pain: Potential true- and false-positive rates. Ann Intern Med 110:957, 1989
LEVINE MN, HIRSH J: Hemorrhagic complications of anticoagulation therapy. Semin Thromb Hemost 12L:39, 1986
LOSCALZO J, BRAUNWALD E: Tissue plasminogen activator. N Engl J Med 319:925, 1988
SAOUR JN et al: Trial of different intensities of anticoagulation in patients with prosthetic heart valves. N Engl J Med 322:428, 1990

section 2 Disorders of the hematopoietic system

290 PATHOPHYSIOLOGY OF THE ANEMIAS

H. FRANKLIN BUNN

There is a large and coherent body of information on the birth, life, and death of red cells. A thorough familiarity with erythropoiesis and erythrocyte structure and function is necessary to understand the pathogenesis of the various anemias as well as to develop an orderly approach to diagnosis and management. Conversely, investigation of specific red cell disorders has provided unique insights into normal erythroid physiology.

RED CELL PRODUCTION   Red cells are derived from an undifferentiated progenitor cell in the bone marrow called the *pluripotent stem cell* (Fig. 290-1). A stem cell is one which is capable of both self-renewal and differentiation. *Pluripotent* implies that granulocytes, monocytes, and platelets also evolve from this ancestor cell. The pluripotent stem cell has the morphologic characteristics of a mature lymphocyte. The control of proliferation into differentiated cell lines is beginning to be understood owing in part to the isolation and characterization of hematopoietic stem cells and growth factors. As Fig. 290-1 shows, the most primitive erythroid progenitor which has been cultured from both bone marrow and peripheral blood is called the *erythroid burst-forming unit* (BFU_e). After 10 to 15 days in tissue culture it produces a large colony of recognizable red cell precursors. The BFU_e is responsive to high doses of the erythroid-promoting hormone erythropoietin, which acts synergistically with other growth

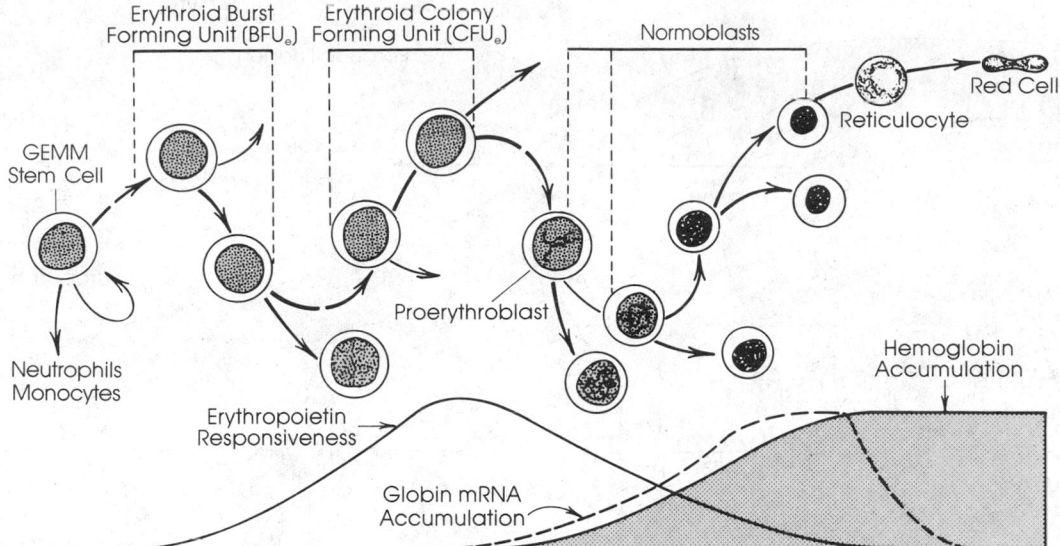

FIGURE 290-1 Differentiation and morphologic maturation of erythroid cells. Erythroid cells are derived from GEMM stem cells (shown on left) which are also capable of differentiating into neutrophils, monocytes (macrophages), and megakaryocytes. Under the influence of erythropoietin, ery-

throid precursor cells (BFU$_e$ → CFU$_e$) differentiate into proerythroblasts, the earliest recognizable erythroid cells in the bone marrow. During further maturation, globin mRNA accumulates, directing the cell to synthesize hemoglobin.

factors derived from lymphocytes, monocytes, and cells of the marrow stroma (fibroblasts, adipocytes, endothelial cells, etc.). A more mature cell, the *erythroid colony-forming unit* (CFU$_e$), produces a smaller clone of erythroid cells after 4 to 7 days in culture and is very sensitive to erythropoietin. Well-designed experiments involving incubation of uniform hematopoietic and stromal cell populations with purified growth factors should provide considerably more information about the mechanisms underlying the differentiation and maturation of erythroid cells in vivo, as well as insights into certain disorders of erythropoiesis.

Erythropoietin, a glycoprotein having a molecular weight of 34,000, has been purified to homogeneity. The cloning of the erythropoietin gene has made possible the synthesis of large amounts of biologically active hormone. Erythropoietin is produced, primarily by the kidneys, in response to hypoxia and is secreted into the plasma. Levels of this hormone are increased in direct proportion to the degree of hypoxia.

Erythropoietin interacts with a specific receptor on the surfaces of committed erythroid stem cells, inducing them to differentiate into proerythroblasts, the earliest red cell precursor that can be recognized on examination of the bone marrow. Normally the transition from the proerythroblast to the most mature normoblast involves three or four cell divisions over a 4-day period (Fig. 290-1). During this time, the nucleus becomes smaller, and an increasing amount of hemoglobin is produced in the cytoplasm. Following the last division, the pyknotic nucleus is removed from the normoblast, forming the reticulocyte which stays in the bone marrow for 2.5 to 3 days. The reticulocyte is then released into the general circulation, where it remains for another 24 h before it loses its mitochondria and ribosomes and assumes the morphologic appearance of a mature red cell.

Erythroid precursor cells ranging from the pronormoblast to the reticulocyte possess a specific surface receptor for the iron-transferrin complex, enabling them to incorporate sufficient iron for hemoglobin production (Fig. 290-2). The use of a radioactive iron label such as

FIGURE 290-2 Erythrocyte production, circulation, and destruction. Circulating iron-bound transferrin (TF) is bound to specific receptors on the surface of red blood cell precursors in the marrow. Most of this iron is incorporated into hemoglobin; the remainder is stored as ferritin. Following maturation of the erythroid precursor, the nucleus is shed and the red blood cell emerges from the marrow into the plasma where it circulates for approximately 120 days. The senescent red blood cell is taken up by the mononuclear phagocyte system and is destroyed. The heme iron is initially incorporated into ferritin. This storage iron is available for transport to the marrow via transferrin.

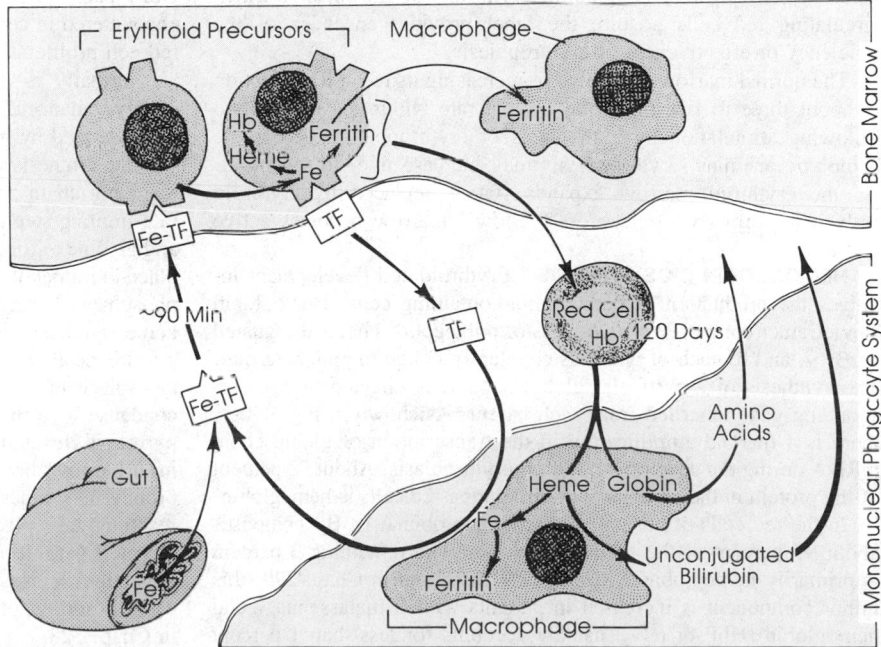

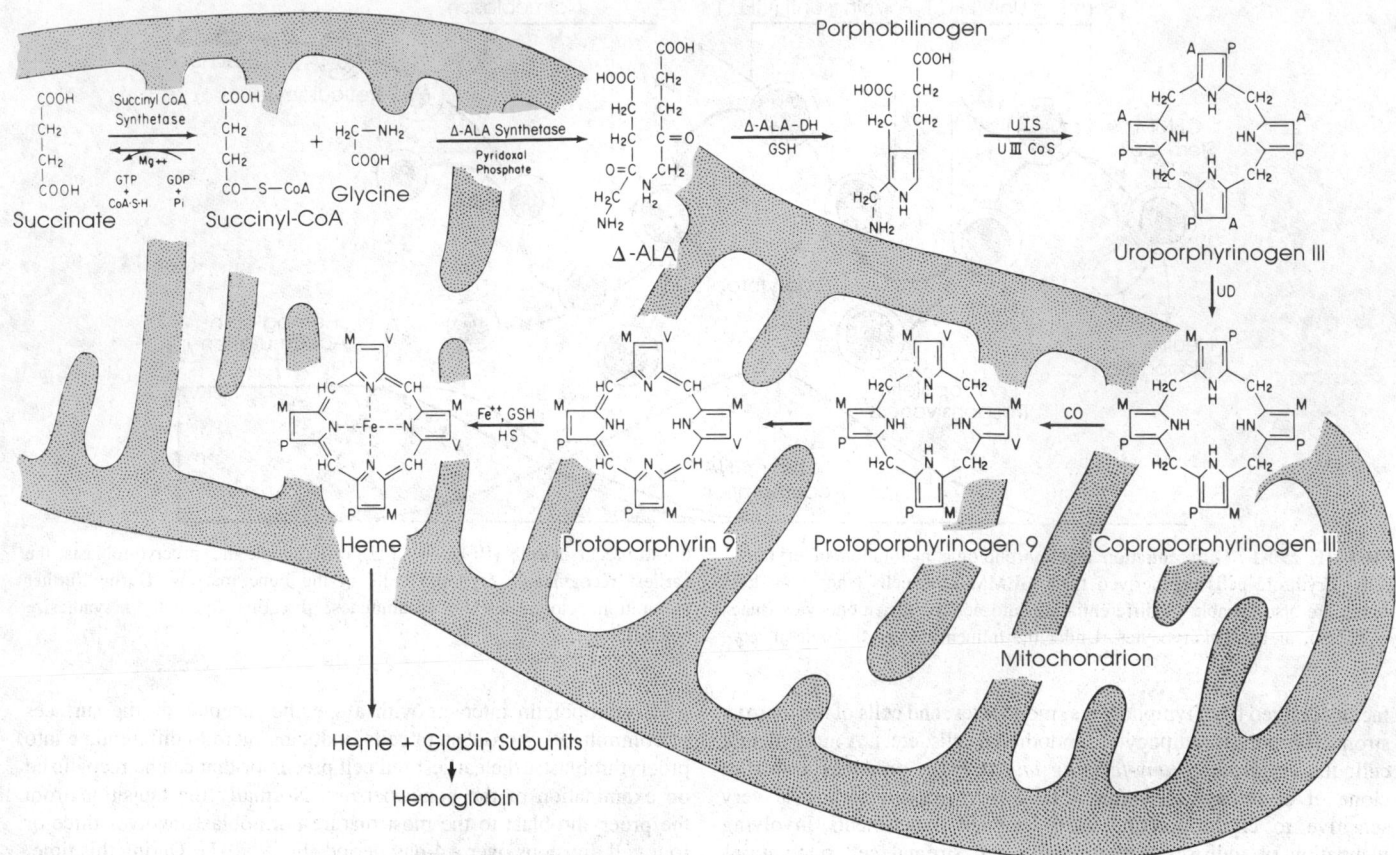

FIGURE 290-3   The biosynthesis of heme. The following abbreviations are used: CoA, coenzyme A; GTP, guanosine triphosphate; GDP, guanosine diphosphate; Pi, inorganic phosphorus; GSH, glutathione; δ-ALA-DH, δ-aminolevulinate dehydrase; UIS, uroporphyrinogen I synthetase; UIII CoS, uroporphyrinogen III cosynthetase; UD, uroporphyrinogen decarboxylase; CO, coproporphyrinogen oxidase; HS, heme synthetase; A, acetate; P, proprionate; M, methyl; V, vinyl. Enzymatic steps that occur in mitochondria are shown.

^{59}Fe permits a quantitative assessment of erythropoiesis. From the rate at which injected ^{59}Fe-labeled transferrin disappears from the plasma, plasma iron turnover can be calculated. This parameter is generally proportional to the total developing erythroid cell mass. Normally, about 80 percent of ^{59}Fe bound to plasma transferrin goes to erythroid cells in the marrow (Fig. 290-3*B*). After 4 to 6 days the labeled iron reappears in circulating erythrocytes. The extent to which circulating red cells acquire the label provides an index of the efficiency or effectiveness of erythropoiesis.

The normal marrow is capable of increasing its red cell production to about three to five times the normal rate within a week or two following stimulation by high levels of erythropoietin. In chronic hemolytic anemias, erythropoiesis may increase five- to sevenfold. As the erythroid marrow expands, fat is replaced by erythroid cells, and formerly inactive or "yellow" marrow becomes active or "red."

HEMOGLOBIN BIOSYNTHESIS   Erythroid cell development involves the production of hemoglobin-containing cells. Hemoglobin is a tetramer composed of two pairs of polypeptide chains designated α, β, γ, and δ, each of which is covalently linked to a heme group. The synthesis of a particular globin subunit is directed by a corresponding gene inherited from each parent. As shown in Fig. 290-1, there is a marked amplification in the transcription of globin chain mRNA during the development of proerythroblasts. About 98 percent of the protein in the cytoplasm of circulating red cells is hemoglobin.

In the red cells of normal adults, hemoglobin A ($\alpha_2\beta_2$) composes about 97 percent of the total hemoglobin. The remaining 3 percent is primarily hemoglobin A_2 ($\alpha_2\delta_2$). As discussed in Chap. 295, this minor component is increased in patients with β thalassemia. Fetal hemoglobin (HbF or $\alpha_2\gamma_2$) usually accounts for less than 1 percent of total hemoglobin in normal adult red cells. HbF is localized to 1 to 7 percent of red cells. In contrast, it is the main hemoglobin component of fetal red cells. During the last 3 months of gestation, γ-chain synthesis switches to β-chain synthesis. However, in certain types of congenital hemolytic anemias such as the β thalassemias and sickle cell anemia, the production of γ chains (and therefore of HbF) persists. In addition, increased levels of HbF may also be encountered in certain acquired anemias in which there is disordered red cell proliferation.

Normally α- and β-chain synthesis in erythroid precursors is evenly balanced. In contrast, the thalassemias (Chap. 295) are characterized by imbalance in globin chain synthesis.

The synthesis of *heme* in red cell precursors is closely matched to globin chain production. As shown in Fig. 290-3 the initial and rate-limiting step is the condensation of succinyl coenzyme A (CoA) and glycine to form δ-aminolevulinic acid. This reaction, which takes place in mitochondria, requires that glycine be activated by pyridoxal phosphate. Accordingly, patients with sideroblastic anemia in whom heme synthesis is usually defective may sometimes respond to pyridoxine therapy (Chap. 291). The next steps of heme synthesis take place in the cytosol. Two molecules of δ-aminolevulinic acid condense to form a ring structure, prophobilinogen. This colorless pyrrole is elevated in acute intermittent porphyria and can be detected in urine by the Watson-Schwartz test. The subsequent steps in prophyrin synthesis are also shown in Fig. 290-3. The last three reactions take place in mitochondria. Iron is inserted into protoporphyrin IX to form heme. In iron deficiency, as well as in lead poisoning, increased levels of protoporphyrin can be detected in red cells. Disorders of porphyrin synthesis and metabolism are discussed in Chap. 328.

HEMOGLOBIN STRUCTURE AND FUNCTION The primary role of red cells is to transport oxygen from lungs to tissues and to transport carbon dioxide in the reverse direction. Both of these functions are assumed by hemoglobin. The three-dimensional structure of human hemoglobin has been determined from x-ray crystallographic analysis. The important functional properties of hemoglobin such as heme-heme interaction, the pH dependency of oxygen affinity (the Bohr effect), and the interaction with 2,3-diphosphoglycerate can now be understood in stereochemical terms. This structural information has also been useful in explaining the abnormal functional properties of a number of human hemoglobin variants which are associated with clinical and hematalogic manifestations (see Chap. 295).

During the circulation through the lungs, hemoglobin becomes almost fully saturated with oxygen (1.34 mL O_2 per gram of hemoglobin). As red cells perfuse the capillary beds, oxygen is extracted. Efficient unloading of oxygen at relatively high oxygen tensions is possible because of the sigmoid shape of the oxygen dissociation curve (heme-heme interaction) (see Fig. 290-4). The affinity of hemoglobin for oxygen is modified by three intracellular cofactors: hydrogen ion, carbon dioxide, and 2,3-diphosphoglycerate (2,3-DPG). Increasing the concentrations of each of these three effectors results in a "shift to the right" in the oxygen dissociation curve. In human red cells, 2,3-DPG appears to be an important regulator of hemoglobin function. One molecule of 2,3-DPG binds to the β chains of deoxyhemoglobin, thereby decreasing oxygen affinity. Elevated levels of 2,3-DPG have been noted in various states of hypoxia. The resulting decrease in oxygen affinity permits enhanced oxygen release. The oxygenation of a particular organ or tissue depends on three main factors (depicted in Fig. 290-5): blood flow, oxygen-carrying capacity of the blood (hemoglobin concentration), and the affinity of the hemoglobin for oxygen. Patients with a primary abnormality of one of these three factors depend on adjustments in one or both of the other two in order to maintain optimal tissue oxygenation. For example, patients with anemia have two available modes of compensation: enhanced blood flow and decreased oxygen affinity, mediated by increased levels of 2,3-DPG. Conversely, individuals with a hemoglobin variant having increased oxygen affinity have a primary defect in oxygen unloading. As discussed in Chap. 295, such patients compensate by developing secondary erythrocytosis.

FIGURE 290-4 The oxyhemoglobin dissociation curve of normal blood. The major factors influencing the position of the curve are pH, temperature, and the intracellular concentration of 2,3-DPG. An increase in plasma pH or a decrease in temperature and 2,3-DPG causes an increase in oxygen affinity (shift to the left) and a relative decrease in oxygen unloading when going from an arterial P_{O_2} of 12.7 kPa (95 mmHg) to a venous P_{O_2} of 5.3 kPa (40 mmHg). Conversely, a decrease in pH or an increase in temperature and 2,3-DPG causes a decrease in oxygen affinity (shift to the right) and a relative increase in oxygen unloading.

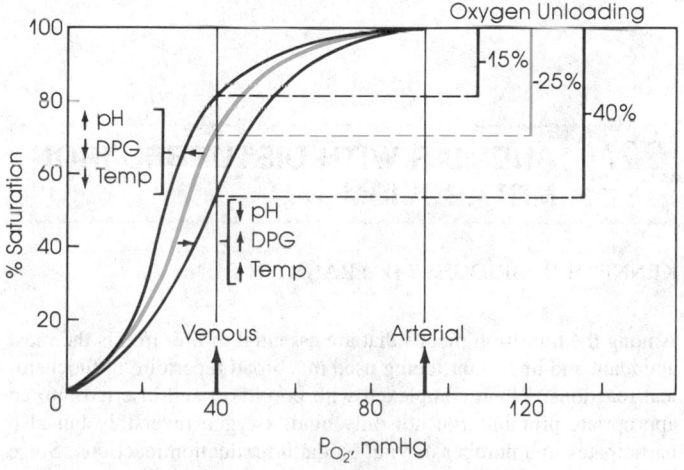

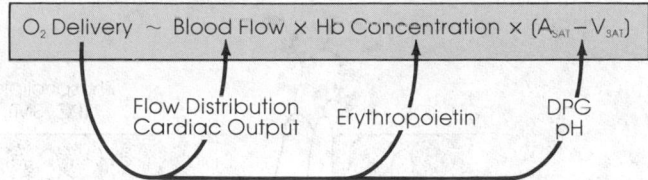

FIGURE 290-5 Oxygen delivered to an organ or tissue is directly proportional to (1) blood flow, (2) hemoglobin concentration, and (3) the difference in oxygen saturation of the arterial and venous blood. Patients with various types of hypoxia may compensate in the following ways: (1) The distribution of blood flow is altered to maintain oxygenation of vital organs; total cardiac output increases when hypoxia is severe. (2) Increased erythropoietin production stimulates erythropoiesis. (3) Oxygen unloading is enhanced by a shift to the right in the oxygen dissociation curve, mediated by an increase in red cell 2,3-DPG.

RED BLOOD CELL METABOLISM As the red cell emerges from the bone marrow, it loses its nucleus, ribosomes, and mitochondria and therefore all capability for cell division, protein synthesis, and oxidative phosphorylation. Compared with other cells, the erythrocyte has a rather simple scheme of intermediary metabolism. Glucose is virtually the only fuel utilized by the red cell. It readily enters the red cell by facilitated diffusion and is then converted to glucose-6-phosphate. There are two major pathways available for glucose-6-phosphate (Fig. 294-2). About 80 to 90 percent of this intermediate is converted to lactate by means of the glycolytic (or Embden-Meyerhof) pathway. Two moles of adenosine triphosphate (ATP) are generated for every mole of glucose that is metabolized. The intracellular mediator of hemoglobin function, 2,3-diphosphoglycerate, is synthesized in a side reaction shown in Fig. 294-2. About 10 percent of intracellular glucose-6-phosphate undergoes oxidation by means of the hexose-monophosphate shunt. This pathway maintains glutathione in the reduced form, thereby protecting sulfhydryl groups in hemoglobin and the red cell membrane from oxidation by peroxides and superoxide as well as by certain drugs and toxins. Such oxidant stress can compromise red cell function and viability in patients with a deficiency in glucose-6-phosphate dehydrogenase, the first enzymatic step in the hexose-monophosphate shunt (see Chap. 294). Less commonly, individuals may have a deficiency in one of the enzymes of the glycolytic pathway or in one of the other enzymes of the hexose-monophosphate shunt.

The red cell has rather modest metabolic obligations in keeping with its simplified structure. A significant portion of the ATP generated by glycolysis is spent in operating the sodium-potassium pump, necessary to preserve the ionic milieu in the cytoplasm and prevent colloid osmotic lysis. In addition, some metabolic energy is expended on maintenance and repair of the red cell membrane. Certain proteins in the membrane become phosphorylated by means of ATP and protein kinases, but the physiologic significance of this process is not yet understood. Finally, a small amount of metabolic currency is spent on maintaining hemoglobin iron atoms in the reduced form (Fe^{2+}).

The 120-day survival of the circulating red cell is dependent on preservation of the pliability of its membrane. The red cell membrane is composed of 50 percent protein, 40 percent lipid, and 10 percent carbohydrate. It is a bilayer consisting of molecules of phospholipid and cholesterol in a 1.2:1 molar ratio oriented in a stacked array so that the hydrophobic portions of the molecules are oriented toward the interior while the polar side groups are either on the external surface of the cell (the plasma membrane) or on the inner cytoplasmic surface (see Fig. 290-6). The distribution of phospholipids differs significantly in the two portions of the bilayer. The outer surface is relatively rich in lecithin and sphingomyelin while the inner surface has relatively more phosphatidyl serine and phosphatidyl ethanolamine. The lipids on the outer surface exchange freely with plasma lipids.

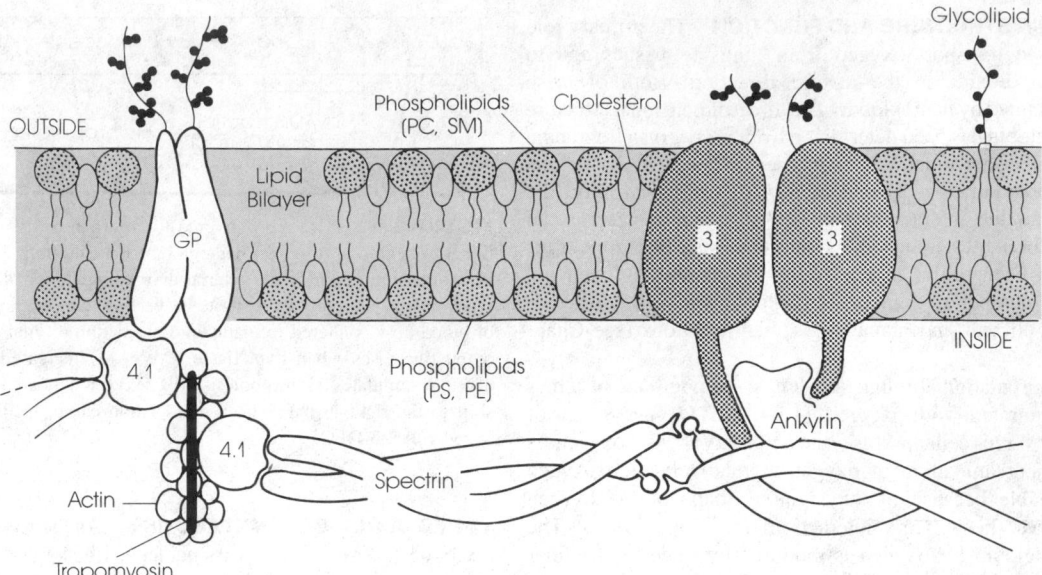

FIGURE 290-6 Diagram of a cross section of the red blood cell membrane. Spectrin, actin, tropomyosin, and protein 4.1 form a meshwork which laminates the inner surface of the membrane. In contrast, other proteins such as the glycophorins (GP) and protein 3 (the anion transport channel) traverse the lipid bilayer. Long polysaccharide chains are covalently attached to these proteins on the outer surface of the cell and also to glycolipid. The protein ankyrin forms a bridge between spectrin and a fraction of the anion transport proteins. Protein 4.1 binds to GP. Phospholipids in the lipid bilayer include phosphatidylcholine (PC) and sphingomyelin (SM), which are located primarily on the outer surface of the membrane, and phosphatidyl serine (PS) and phosphatidyl ethanolamine (PE), which are located primarily on the inner surface of the membrane.

The red cell membrane contains about eight major proteins depicted in Fig. 290-6 and a large number of minor components. These proteins can be divided into two groups. A few span the lipid bilayer so that one end of the polypeptide is on the external cell surface and the other is on the inner surface. Examples include glycophorin, which contains a number of polysaccharide blood group antigens, and band 3, which serves as a channel for the passage of anions in and out of the red cell. Other proteins bind only to the inner surface of the red cell membrane. These include several enzymes as well as structural proteins such as spectrin and actin, which interact to form a meshwork that laminates the cytoplasmic surface of the membrane.

It is likely that the physiologic demise of 120-day-old red cells is due to a loss of membrane flexibility preventing them from negotiating the narrow-bore channels of the microcirculation, including the sinusoids of the spleen. The factors responsible for red cell senescence are poorly understood. Experimental evidence indicates that deterioration of the red cell's metabolic machinery, sufficient to deplete it of ATP, can cause the cell to become spiculated (ecchinocytic) and lose its normal pliability. Depletion of ATP disrupts the spectrin and actin meshwork lining the inner membrane surface, resulting in aggregation of these proteins. Other factors such as enhanced rigidity and, perhaps, coating with immunoglobulin may also contribute to the recognition of the senescent red cell by the mononuclear phagocyte system. In contrast to normal red cells, there is a large and well-documented body of information on the mechanisms responsible for red cell destruction in various hemolytic anemias. These are discussed in Chap. 294.

Once the senescent red cell is sequestered (Fig. 290-2), hemoglobin is readily catabolized. Amino acids are released by proteolytic digestion and subsequently metabolized. The heme group is catabolized by a microsomal oxidizing system. The porphyrin ring is converted to bile pigments which are excreted almost quantitatively by the liver. One mole of carbon monoxide is formed per mole of heme that is broken down. Endogenous carbon monoxide production correlates directly with erythroid cell destruction. As Fig. 290-2 shows, the iron that is released during heme catabolism is initially incorporated into the storage protein ferritin, but it is eventually transported to marrow erythroid precursors by transferrin, the plasma iron–binding protein.

If red cell production is disordered, there may be significant destruction of erythroid cells within the bone marrow. A number of anemias are characterized by *ineffective erythropoiesis*, particularly those in which erythroid maturation is morphologically abnormal and the circulating red cells are abnormal in size. Examples discussed in detail elsewhere include megaloblastic anemias, sideroblastic anemias, and β thalassemia major. Such disorders are characterized by erythroid hyperplasia in the bone marrow and rapid uptake of labeled iron into the marrow but a low recovery of the labeled iron in circulating red cells. Endogenous carbon monoxide production and plasma levels of unconjugated bilirubin are generally elevated in ineffective erythropoiesis.

REFERENCES

Babior BM, Stossel TP: *Hematology: A Pathophysiological Approach*. New York, Churchill Livingston, 1984

Beck WS (ed): *Hematology*, 5th ed. Boston, MIT Press, 1990

Bennett V: The membrane skeleton of human erythrocytes and its implications for more complex cells. Ann Rev Biochem 54:273, 1985

Bunn HF, Forget BG: *Hemoglobin: Molecular, Genetic and Clinical Aspects*. Philadelphia, Saunders, 1986

Erslev AJ, Gabuzda TG: *Pathophysiology of Blood*, 3 ed. Philadelphia, Saunders, 1985

Jandl JH: *Blood, Textbook of Hematology*. Boston, Little, Brown, 1987

Spivak JL: Erythropoietin: A brief review. Nephron 52:289, 1989

291 ANEMIAS WITH DISTURBED IRON METABOLISM

KENNETH R. BRIDGES / H. FRANKLIN BUNN

Among the transition metals that are essential to life, iron is the most abundant and important, being used in a broad repertoire of biochemical reactions. When complexed with porphyrin and inserted into an appropriate protein, iron not only binds oxygen reversibly but also participates in a number of vital oxidation-reduction reactions. Since inorganic iron is highly toxic, specific processes have evolved for its assimilation, transport, and storage. Under normal circumstances, iron homeostasis is precisely maintained but can go awry in a variety of clinical settings, leading either to iron deficiency or iron overload.

PHYSIOLOGY OF IRON

IRON ABSORPTION This occurs predominantly in the duodenum and upper jejunum. Inorganic iron salts exist in either of two valence states, Fe^{2+} (ferrous) or Fe^{3+} (ferric). Most dietary iron consists of ferric salts, which form insoluble ferric hydroxide precipitates at physiologic pH. Absorption is aided by stomach acidity which maintains ferric iron in a soluble form. Normally about 10 percent of the 10 to 20 mg of iron ingested per day in an average diet is absorbed. Heme is much more readily absorbed than inorganic iron. Unfortunately, a dearth of meat in the diets of many people throughout the world limits the availability of this excellent iron source.

The absorption of inorganic iron is greatly influenced by dietary compounds which may chelate the element. Citrate and ascorbate, for example, increase iron absorption by forming soluble complexes which readily enter the epithelial cells lining the upper gastrointestinal tract. Other compounds such as tannates, which are found in teas, plant phytates, and phosphates form very tight complexes with iron and significantly inhibit absorption. The metabolic machinery involved in iron absorption is shared with several heavy metals, including lead, cadmium, and strontium. Increased iron absorption as occurs, for instance in iron deficiency, enhances the uptake of these elements.

TRANSPORT AND STORAGE The precise mechanism by which iron is translocated across the epithelial barrier in the intestine is unknown. Once this task is accomplished, however, the element is coupled to transferrin, an 80-kDa serum glycoprotein which delivers iron to tissues throughout the body (Fig. 291-1). Each transferrin molecule can bind two iron atoms. The aggregate binding sites of all the transferrin in the circulation comprise the total iron-binding capacity (TIBC) of plasma. Normally, 20 to 45 percent of the iron-binding sites are filled. Specific receptors on the plasma membranes of cells recognize transferrin, leading to the internalization of the protein and the release of iron into the cell cytoplasm. As might be expected, erythroid precursor cells in the bone marrow, which have a high requirement for iron, have a correspondingly high density of transferrin receptors.

Excess iron is stored in the body as ferritin or as hemosiderin. The iron in ferritin is enclosed within a protein shell, apoferritin, which can take up Fe^{2+} and oxidize it so that Fe^{3+} is deposited within the iron core. The synthesis of apoferritin is stimulated by iron. Small quantities of ferritin can be measured in serum. Under normal conditions there is a close correlation between serum ferritin concentration and body iron stores, with 1 µg/L serum ferritin equivalent to approximately 10 mg of storage iron. With time, ferritin is engulfed by lysosomes and catabolized to hemosiderin, a nonspecific mixture of partially degraded protein, lipid, and iron. Iron enters and leaves the ferritin molecule in a metabolically controlled fashion, making it available for the normal physiologic functions of the cell. In contrast, iron which is trapped in the hemosiderin meshwork is returned to the metabolic mainstream of the cell in a slow and unregulated fashion.

Body iron stores are assiduously conserved. In fact, no physiologic pathway of iron removal exists. A small daily loss of 1 to 2 mg of the element results from the shedding of senescent cells along the gastrointestinal and genitourinary tracts and from desquamation of skin (Fig. 291-1). Normally, this loss closely balances daily absorption. When the demand for iron is increased by depletion of body reserves due to growth spurts, pregnancy, or menstrual and pathologic hemorrhage, the efficiency of iron absorption can increase up to about 20 percent. With iron deficiency, absorption of the element can increase to between 30 and 40 percent of the amount ingested. In contrast, with iron overload no effective counterbalancing mechanism exists.

Iron kinetics Between 80 and 90 percent of absorbed iron is delivered to the bone marrow for erythropoiesis. The dynamics of iron utilization by the peripheral tissues can be monitored by loading plasma transferrin with the radioisotope ^{59}Fe and injecting the labeled protein back into the circulation. Such ferrokinetic studies reveal an exponential loss of label from the plasma, with a half-life of about 75 min. The plasma iron turnover (PIT) is the absolute amount of iron released from transferrin per unit of time, and is determined largely by the rate of erythropoiesis. Effective erythropoiesis results in the incorporation of 80 to 90 percent of iron into hemoglobin in circulating erythrocytes. With some anemias, such as the thalassemias, the megaloblastic anemias, and sideroblastic anemia, there is intramedullary destruction of nascent red cells. The result is a high PIT reflecting the increase in erythropoietic activity, but a diminished incorporation of the labeled iron into circulating erythrocytes. This combination is termed ineffective erythropoiesis. When erythropoiesis is diminished because of marrow hypoplasia, the PIT is correspondingly reduced.

LABORATORY INVESTIGATION OF IRON STORES *Direct assays* for evaluating iron stores require biopsy specimens. Most storage iron is found in the reticuloendothelial cells of the bone marrow, liver, and spleen or in hepatic parenchymal cells. The liver is a homogeneous tissue and therefore an excellent source by which to gauge iron stores. Prussian blue staining of liver biopsies, a commonly used technique, provides only a semiquantitative estimation of iron stores whereas atomic absorption spectroscopy furnishes accurate quantitative data. Formalin-fixed samples can be evaluated by this technique, allowing for transport and later testing. Liver biopsy with atomic absorption spectroscopic measurements is the gold standard for quantitative evaluation of iron overload. Bone marrow specimens do not provide a reliable estimation of iron excess but are useful in the evaluation of iron deficiency. Because of the cellular heterogeneity of bone marrow, histologic evaluation of iron deposits must focus on storage in macrophages. An absence of Prussian blue staining reliably reflects a deficiency in iron stores.

The simplest *indirect assay* of iron stores is the measurement of the ratio of serum iron to TIBC (Fig. 291-2). Iron deficiency depresses serum iron levels and boosts the TIBC. Therefore the transferrin is generally less than 10 percent saturated. Iron loading increases the serum iron with little effect on the TIBC, leading to greater than 80 percent saturation of transferrin. The ratio of iron to TIBC must be viewed with the patient's total clinical picture in mind. For example, serum iron and transferrin levels are depressed by conditions such as inflammation, cancer, and liver disease, leading at times to skewed ratios.

FIGURE 291-1 The distribution of iron in normal adults and internal iron kinetics. Bold arrows indicate major pathways of iron movement.

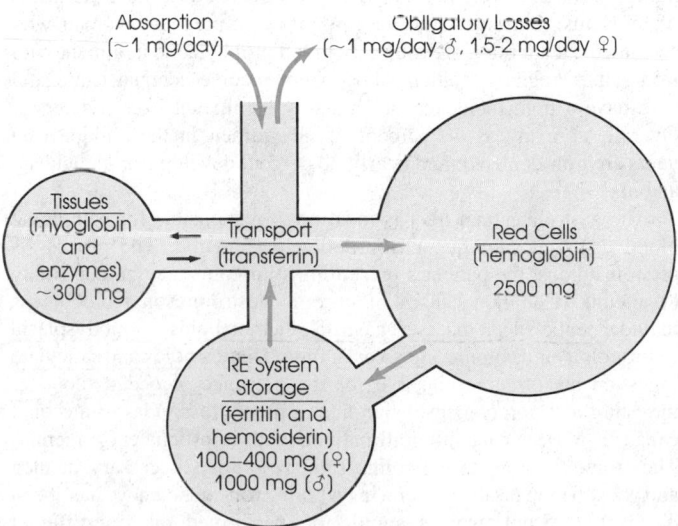

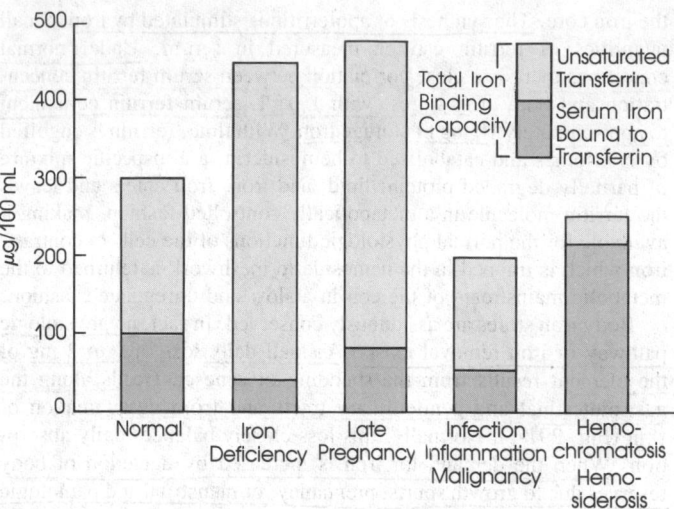

FIGURE 291-2 Serum iron and total iron-binding capacity in various disorders.

Iron stores are also reflected by *serum ferritin* levels. Ferritin in the circulation is a secretory form of the protein which is glycosylated and differs in subunit composition from the storage form found in cells. The physiologic function of serum ferritin is presently unknown. The protein normally contains very little iron. The concentration of serum ferritin rises with iron loading and declines with depletion of tissue iron stores. The serum ferritin level also increases with inflammation, cancer, and liver disease. In addition, the normal ranges for serum ferritin vary with age and sex. Therefore corrections for these factors should be made when values on a specific patient are interpreted.

In patients with iron deficiency, protoporphyrin IX accumulates in the red cell because there is insufficient iron to convert it to heme (see Fig. 290-3). The fluorometric assay of free erythrocyte protoporphyrin (FEP) is a reliable and cost-effective way of screening large groups of individuals such as schoolchildren for iron deficiency.

Computed tomography (CT) of the liver provides an excellent assessment of body iron stores, particularly with iron overload. The iron content of liver biopsy samples correlates well with determination by dual energy CT scanning. Another sensitive noninvasive technique for evaluating liver iron deposition is magnetic resonance imaging. Both instruments permit longitudinal evaluation and are valuable adjuncts in monitoring and treating patients with iron overload.

IRON-DEFICIENCY ANEMIA

ETIOLOGY Iron deficiency occurs when the rate of loss or utilization of the element exceeds its rate of assimilation. The stages of iron deficiency are shown in Table 291-1. Utilization is greatest during the rapid growth spurts of infancy and adolescence (Table 291-2). Depleted iron stores, if not frank anemia, are commonly seen

TABLE 291-1   Stages in the development of iron deficiency

	Normal	Mild	Moderate	Severe
Hemoglobin:	150 g/L	130 g/L	100 g/L	50 g/L
MCV	N	↓	↓	↓↓
MCHC	N	N	↓	↓↓
Marrow Fe stores	Present	Absent	Absent	Absent
Serum Fe/TIBC, μg/L	1000/3000	~750/3000	~500/4500	~250/6000

NOTE: MCV = mean corpuscular volume; MCHC = mean corpuscular hemoglobin concentration; TIBC = total iron-binding capacity; N = normal; ↓ = decreased.

TABLE 291-2   Causes of iron deficiency

I	Increased iron utilization
	A Postnatal growth spurt
	B Adolescent growth spurt
II	Physiologic iron loss
	A Menstruation
	B Pregnancy
III	Pathologic iron loss
	A Gastrointestinal bleeding
	B Genitourinary bleeding
	C Pulmonary hemosiderosis
	D Intravascular hemolysis
IV	Decreased iron intake
	A Cereal-rich, meat-poor diets
	B Food faddists
	C Elderly and indigent
	D Malabsorption

in children in these two age groups. Neonates born to iron-deficient women are rarely anemic, but do have low body iron stores. These infants lack the reserves needed for the swift growth which occurs after birth. The iron content of breast milk is comparable to that of cow's milk, but the bioavailability of iron is greater in breast milk. Iron deficiency during childhood has a number of deleterious consequences, including impaired cognition. Therefore, infants should receive iron supplementation.

In western countries, the increased demand for iron during adolescence is often accompanied by voluntary consumption of foods with low iron content. Among the elderly and the poor, financial constraints often produce a similar pattern of inadequate iron intake. Large numbers of people throughout the world have become inured to diets consisting largely of grains or cereals, which are inadequate sources of iron. The added burden of blood loss due to parasites such as hookworm makes iron deficiency a problem of staggering proportions.

Decreased absorption of iron This can occur in many clinical settings. After partial or total gastrectomy, the assimilation of dietary iron is impaired, owing primarily to increased motility and bypass of the proximal intestine, which is the primary site of iron absorption. Achlorhydria also contributes to decreased iron absorption. Patients with chronic diarrhea or intestinal malabsorption may also develop iron deficiency, particularly if the duodenum and proximal jejunum are involved. Sometimes iron-deficiency anemia is a harbinger of nontropical (celiac) sprue.

Iron loss This loss may be physiologic or pathologic. Examples of physiologic iron loss include menstruation and pregnancy. Menstrual blood loss doubles the daily iron requirement. With a term pregnancy, about 500 mg of iron are transferred from the mother to the fetus. Some of this iron is derived from increased gastrointestinal absorption of the element by the mother. In the absence of supplemental iron, however, her stores will be depleted to meet the needs of the fetus. Currently, the vast majority of pregnant women who seek medical attention are routinely given prophylactic treatment with iron salts. Pregnant women who do not receive adequate antenatal care have a high incidence of clinically significant iron deficiency. Overall, as many as 40 percent of all women in the childbearing years are iron-depleted, and nearly 20 percent develop iron-deficiency anemia.

The gastrointestinal tract is most often responsible for pathologic blood loss and subsequent iron-deficiency anemia. The process is often insidious; the patient's presenting symptoms may be due solely to anemia. Common causes of chronic gastrointestinal blood loss include peptic ulcer disease, gastritis, hemorrhoids, angiodysplasia of the colon, and colonic adenocarcinoma. Hemorrhoids and salicylate ingestion are often responsible for the presence of occult blood in the stool but rarely cause significant blood loss. Gastrointestinal cancer is a specter haunting all patients with iron-deficiency anemia. Therefore, a complete gastrointestinal workup is necessary in men and postmenopausal women in whom iron deficiency has been discovered. Stool guaiacs should be performed on six different occasions along with a digital rectal examination. Radiologic examination of the gastrointestinal tract and/or endoscopic procedures are obligatory. The patient must be assumed to have a gastrointestinal malignancy until proven otherwise.

In about 15 percent of patients with documented gastrointestinal bleeding, no source can be determined, even after extensive radiologic and endoscopic investigation. In tropical areas, parasitic infestations, particularly hookworm, are a major cause of blood loss. Occasionally, as in patients with hereditary telangiectasia or in those with a bleeding diathesis, gastrointestinal bleeding arises from multiple sites. Thrombocytopenia, qualitative platelet disorders, and von Willebrand's disease are more apt to cause gastrointestinal bleeding than are deficiencies of the soluble coagulation factors.

Blood loss from other sources rarely produces iron-deficiency anemia. Bleeding in the genitourinary tract usually is sufficiently alarming that medical attention is sought early in the process. Intravascular hemolysis with hemoglobin loss in the urine, e.g., paroxysmal nocturnal hemoglobinuria, is very unusual. Pulmonary hemorrhage, secondary to bronchiectasis or idiopathic pulmonary hemosiderosis, may also cause iron-deficiency anemia.

CLINICAL CONSEQUENCES OF IRON DEFICIENCY Cell growth and proliferation are impaired by iron deficiency. The production of red blood cells is in particular jeopardy owing to their high requirement for iron. Many aspects of the presentation of iron-deficiency anemia including weakness, lassitude, palpitations, and sometimes exertional dyspnea are common to all forms of chronic anemia. No definite link between these symptoms and tissue depletion of iron-dependent enzymes and cofactors has been established.

After the cells of the bone marrow, those of the gastrointestinal tract have the highest level of proliferative activity. Consequently many of the signs and symptoms of iron deficiency are localized to this organ system. Glossitis characterized by a reddened, swollen, smooth, shiny, and tender tongue occurs sporadically. Angular stomatitis involves erosion, tenderness, and swelling at the corners of the mouth. Gastric atrophy with achlorhydria occurs occasionally. A postcrycoid web (Plummer-Vinson syndrome) may develop with long-standing iron deficiency. Koilonychia, or spoon-shaped nails, result from slowing in the rate of growth of the nail plate. Menorrhagia is a common symptom in iron-deficient women. Both menorrhagia and gastric atrophy (mentioned above) may be a consequence as well as a cause of iron deficiency.

One peculiar symptom which is quite characteristic of iron deficiency is pica. Patients develop cravings for substances such as starch (amylophagia), ice (pagophagia), and clay (geophagia). Some of these materials, such as starch and clay, bind iron in the gastrointestinal tract, worsening the deficiency. The basis of this bizarre behavior is unknown. A particularly invidious consequence of iron deficiency is increased intestinal absorption of lead. Children from impoverished families, who often have both iron deficiency and pica, are at greatest risk of developing lead poisoning. The toxicity of lead is due at least in part to a disruption of heme synthesis in neural tissues, a process abetted by iron deficiency. These unfortunate children are thereby placed in double jeopardy.

Laboratory findings A variety of laboratory tests can be used to assess varying degrees of iron deficiency. The development of iron deficiency progresses in stages (Table 291-1), each of which correlates with clinical laboratory abnormalities. *Storage iron depletion* occurs first, during which iron reserves are lost without compromise of the iron supply for erythropoiesis. At this stage, a bone marrow aspirate stained with Prussian blue will show markedly reduced or absent deposits of iron in macrophages. This finding is accompanied by a decrease in the level of serum ferritin. The next stage is *iron-deficient erythropoiesis*, during which the erythroid iron supply is reduced without the development of anemia. The iron-binding capacity of the serum (TIBC) first rises, followed by a drop in serum iron. As a result, the fractional saturation of transferrin falls markedly. The circulating red cells become microcytic and hypochromic. This is accompanied by an increase in FEP. The final stage is the development

TABLE 291-3 Differential diagnosis of microcytic, hypochromic anemia

	Iron-deficiency anemia	β-Thalassemia trait	Anemia of chronic disease	Sideroblastic anemia
Serum iron	↓	N	↓	↑
TIBC	↑	N	↓	N
Serum ferritin	↓	N	↑	↑
Red cell protoprophyrin	↑	N	↑	↑ or N
Hb A$_2$	↓	↑	N	↓

NOTE: ↑ = increased; ↓ = decreased, N = normal; TIBC = total iron-binding capacity.

of frank *iron deficiency anemia*, wherein the red cells become more severely hypochromic and microcytic (Fig. A5-4). Often, only a thin rim of cytoplasm appears on the periphery of the red cell. Small fragments and bizarre poikilocytes are also seen. Such misshapen red cells have shortened survival in the circulation. The percentage of reticulocytes is usually normal but may increase temporarily following an acute episode of blood loss. The white count is usually normal, while the platelet count is normal or increased. The bone marrow displays moderate erythroid hyperplasia. Many of the late normoblasts appear to have scanty cytoplasm.

Differential diagnosis In a patient with hypochromic microcytic anemia, the major diagnostic possibilities are iron deficiency, thalassemia, anemia of chronic inflammation, and sideroblastic anemia. Several laboratory tests (shown in Table 291-3) are useful in the differential diagnosis. Mild iron deficiency may be readily confused with β-thalassemia trait or with the two-deletion forms of α thalassemia ($\alpha-/\alpha-$ or $--/\alpha\alpha$) (Chap. 295). In these mild forms of thalassemia, microcytosis is much more marked than hypochromia; accordingly the mean corpuscular hemoglobin concentration (MCHC) is usually normal. The red cell size distribution is more uniform than that in iron deficiency. Target cells and basophilic stippling are usually more prominent in thalassemia than in iron deficiency. Hemoglobin A$_2$ is elevated in β-thalassemia trait and decreased in iron deficiency and α thalassemia. If a patient with β-thalassemia trait develops iron deficiency, the level of Hb A$_2$ may fall to normal. The serum iron is normal or elevated in the thalassemias, and decreased in both iron deficiency and in the anemia of chronic disease. However, as Fig. 291-2 shows, the transferrin level is also decreased in the latter. The laboratory tests shown in Table 291-3 are not very helpful in determining whether a patient with a chronic inflammatory disease, such as rheumatoid arthritis, has become iron-deficient. The finding of a low serum ferritin level or absent iron stores in a bone marrow aspirate would be diagnostic of iron deficiency. A trial of iron therapy may be necessary to settle the issue. The diagnosis of *sideroblastic anemia* (see below) rests on the demonstration of ringed sideroblasts in the bone marrow. These patients often have a population of hypochromic microcytic red cells, even though the red cell indexes are usually normal.

THERAPY Iron deficiency responds very effectively to the administration of oral iron salts such as ferrous sulfate. One 325-mg tablet (60 mg of elemental iron) should be administered three times daily. Iron is best absorbed when taken between meals. The most common side effect is abdominal discomfort, characterized by bloating, fullness, and, on occasion, pain. Switching to ferrous gluconate or ferrous lactate may bring relief. Moreover, iron salts may be better tolerated if taken at mealtime. Iron-containing vitamin cocktails generally should be avoided since these preparations are costly and contain suboptimal amounts of iron.

A reticulocytosis occurs 3 to 4 days after the initiation of iron therapy, with a peak at about 10 days. Patients may not respond to iron replacement due to (1) an incorrect diagnosis; (2) noncompliance; (3) blood loss exceeding the rate of replacement; (4) bone marrow suppression by tumor, chronic inflammation, etc.; or (5) malabsorption. Malabsorption of iron is an infrequent problem, but requires parenteral iron replacement when it occurs. Iron-dextran complex may be administered as intramuscular injections following a 50-mg dose to test for allergic reactions. A total of about 2 g of iron-dextran may be administered in this fashion. A Z-tract should be used for the injections to prevent oozing of the compound into the dermis, which can produce intractable skin discoloration. In occasional patients so emaciated that they cannot tolerate intramuscular injections, iron-dextran can be given intravenously. The most convenient approach is to dilute 500 mg of the compound into 50 mL of sterile water and to infuse a test dose of 1 mL. If no adverse reaction is noted, the remainder of the solution can be delivered over several hours. The intravenous administration of up to 2 g of iron at a single sitting is generally well-tolerated. Occasionally patients experience arthralgias, chills, and fever which may persist for several days after the infusion. Long-term deleterious consequences are rare. The amount of iron required for replacement can be calculated from the deficit in the red cell mass, with an additional 1000 mg to replace the body stores. Blood transfusions are rarely necessary except for patients in whom severe iron-deficiency anemia threatens cardiovascular or cerebrovascular function.

ANEMIAS WITH SECONDARY IRON LOADING

Iron overload in individuals with chronic anemias may result either from multiple transfusions or from increased gastrointestinal absorption of the element owing to ineffective erythropoiesis.

SIDEROBLASTIC ANEMIAS These comprise a group of disorders of diverse cause (Table 291-4) characterized by ringed sideroblasts in the nucleated erythroid percursors in the bone marrow. Greater than 10 percent of the normoblasts contain iron-laden mitochondria which surround the nucleus and appear as pathognomonic "rings" with Prussian blue staining. A number of metabolic abnormalities have been noted in the sideroblastic anemias, including defects in one or more steps in heme synthesis. Since the initial and final steps of heme synthesis are located in the mitochondria (Fig. 290-3), it is difficult to know whether such abnormalities are the cause or the result of iron loading. In addition to the presence of ringed sideroblasts, these disorders share certain other features: bone marrow erythroid hyperplasia with decreased red cell production (ineffective erythropoiesis); a population of hypochromic, microcytic red cells reflecting defective heme synthesis; a marked increased in serum iron and transferrin saturation, sometimes accompanied by generalized iron overload.

Hereditary sideroblastic anemia is a rare X-linked disorder associated with defective activity of δ-aminolevulinic acid synthetase, the initial and rate-limiting enzyme in heme biosynthesis. Affected males have anemia of variable severity that often responds to treatment with large doses of pyridoxine.

Acquired sideroblastic anemias may be caused by a variety of insults including ethanol and isoniazid, which produce abnormalities in pyridoxine metabolism, and lead, which inhibits several steps in the heme synthetic pathway (Table 294-4). Ringed sideroblasts are found in about 30 percent of patients hospitalized for alcohol abuse, particularly in the setting of coexistent folate deficiency and malnutrition. This morphologic abnormality disappears within several days following cessation of alcohol ingestion. Secondary sideroblastic anemia has also been observed in a variety of inflammatory and neoplastic states. A particularly intractable form of the disorder sometimes occurs following treatment of malignancy, especially multiple myeloma, with alkylating chemotherapeutic agents.

Most commonly, however, acquired sideroblastic anemia is idiopathic, appearing spontaneously in older individuals. Disturbed growth and maturation occurs in all the lines which emanate from the hematopoietic stem cells. Chromosomal abnormalities are commonly observed in bone marrow cells. Neutropenia develops in a significant number of patients, as does thrombocytopenia. Some individuals have normal numbers of platelets which are, however, dysfunctional. A bleeding diathesis often results. About 10 percent of individuals with sideroblastic anemia will develop acute myelogenous leukemia. This proportion appears to be higher in cases arising from therapy with alkylating agents.

The treatment of secondary sideroblastic anemia focuses primarily on withdrawal of the offending agent. No specific treatment is presently available for idiopathic cases. Since pyridoxine is innocuous and inexpensive, all patients should be given a trial of the vitamin at 200 mg per day for 2 to 3 months, despite the low probability of response in the acquired disorder. Occasionally, an improvement in hematocrit occurs with androgen therapy. This therapy should be used cautiously in patients with liver disease, diabetes, or benign prostatic hypertrophy. Ongoing clinical trials are attempting to define the role of recombinant cytokines such as erythropoietin, granulocyte-monocyte colony stimulating factor (GM-CSF) and interleukin 3 in the treatment of sideroblastic anemia. Supportive therapy, sometimes including blood transfusions, is indicated in all patients.

TRANSFUSIONAL HEMOCHROMATOSIS Repeated blood transfusion is the most common cause of iron overload in patients with anemia. One unit of blood contains 200 to 250 mg iron. Therefore a patient who requires 3 units of blood per month will accumulate about 8 g of iron over the course of a year, enough to cause early clinical sequelae of iron loading. In order for the consequences of iron loading to play a major clinical role, a requirement for chronic transfusions must be coupled with a relatively long survival. The disorders which fulfill these criteria at present include (1) thalassemia major, (2) myeloproliferative and myelodysplastic syndromes (including sideroblastic anemia), and (3) aplastic anemia of moderate severity. Patients with chronic renal failure who are on dialysis also fall under this rubric at present. However, this last indication will be obviated by the recent availability of recombinant erythropoietin.

Transfusional iron overload produces a spectrum of problems similar to those seen with idiopathic hemochromatosis (Chap. 327). Of these, the most serious result from myocardial and hepatic iron deposition. Cardiac siderosis leads to arrhythmias, conduction defects, and congestive failure. The radionuclide ventriculogram is a reliable means of detecting early myocardial dysfunction. Iron deposition in the liver injures hepatocytes, leading to necrosis, fibrosis, and ultimately, cirrhosis. Serum transaminase levels are usually only modestly elevated, even in patients with heavy hepatic iron deposition. Disturbed glucose metabolism occurs commonly, although an oral glucose tolerance test is sometimes needed to demonstrate the defect. Gonadal dysfunction and ACTH deficiency are much less frequent. Hyperpigmentation reflects increased melanin production due to dermal iron deposition, but may not occur in fair-skinned patients. In the assessment of these patients, liver biopsy provides the greatest yield of information since iron content as well as the pathologic state of the organ can be determined. Liver CT scanning or magnetic resonance imaging are the most reliable noninvasive methods of estimating iron deposition. The iron/TIBC ratio and serum ferritin level are both elevated with transfusional hemochromatosis, but do not accurately establish the degree of iron overload in an individual.

The only treatment presently available for transfusional hemochromatosis is chelation therapy. Deferoxamine (deferrox) is the only agent which has been extensively evaluated and shown to prevent or reverse the complications of iron overload. The drug must be given parenterally over a period of 12 to 16 h. Generally, deferoxamine is

---

TABLE 291-4 The sideroblastic anemias

I Hereditary or congenital sideroblastic anemias
II Acquired sideroblastic anemias
   A Associated with drugs and toxins (e.g., alcohol, lead, isoniazid, chloramphenicol)
   B Associated with neoplastic and inflammatory disease (e.g., carcinoma, leukemia, lymphoma, rheumatoid arthritis)
   C Alkylating agent chemotherapy (e.g., cyclophosphamide)

delivered by subcutaneous infusion with a portable syringe pump. Considerable effort is being devoted to the development of a safe and effective oral iron chelating agent. Oral ascorbic acid supplementation markedly enhances iron excretion in patients on deferoxamine therapy. The vitamin increases the availability of storage iron to the chelator, by slowing the degradation of ferritin to hemosiderin. Cardiac toxicity has occurred in patients with hemochromatosis who consumed excessive amounts of ascorbic acid. The generation of injurious free radicals by iron released from storage sites is the probable mechanism of this effect. Further investigation into the basis of cellular injury in patients with hemochromatosis treated with ascorbic acid is needed to clarify the possible therapeutic utility of this vitamin.

REFERENCES

Bridges KR: Transfusion hemochromatosis, in *Transfusion Medicine*, WH Churchill, S Kurtz (eds). Cambridge, MA, Blackwell, 1988, pp 129–144

Gibson RS, MacDonald AC: Serum ferritin and dietary iron parameters in a sample of Canadian preschool children. J Can Dietetic Assoc 49:23, 1988

Huebers HA, Finch CA: The physiology of transferrin and transferrin receptors. Physiol Rev 67:520, 1987

Jacobs A, Clark RE: Pathogenesis and clinical variations in the myelodysplastic syndromes. Clin Haematol 15:925, 1986

Kontoghiorghes GJ et al: Effective chelation of iron in β-thalassemia with the oral chelator 1,2-dimethyl-3-hydropyrid-4-one. Br Med J 295:1509, 1987

Lanzkowsky P: Problems in diagnosis of iron deficiency anemia. Pediatr Ann 14:618, 1985

Piomelli S et al: Lead-induced abnormalities of porphyrin metabolism. The relationship with iron deficiency. Ann NY Acad Sci 514:278, 1987

Wolfe LC et al: Prevention of cardiac disease by subcutaneous deferoxamine in patients with thalassemia major. N Engl J Med 312:1600, 1985

292 MEGALOBLASTIC ANEMIAS

BERNARD M. BABIOR / H. FRANKLIN BUNN

The megaloblastic anemias are disorders caused by impaired DNA synthesis. Cells primarily affected are those having a relatively rapid turnover, especially hematopoietic precursors and gastrointestinal epithelial cells. Cell division is sluggish, but cytoplasmic development progresses normally, so megaloblastic cells tend to be large, with an increased ratio of RNA to DNA. Megaloblastic erythroid cells tend to be destroyed in the marrow in excessive numbers, an abnormality termed *ineffective erythropoiesis* (Chaps. 61 and 290).

Most megaloblastic anemias are due to a deficiency of cobalamin (vitamin B_{12}) and/or folic acid. The various clinical entities associated with megaloblastic anemia are listed in Table 292-1. This classification is easier to comprehend if the physiologic and biochemical principles discussed below are kept in mind.

PHYSIOLOGIC CONSIDERATIONS

FOLIC ACID Folic acid is the common name for pteroylmonoglutamic acid. It is synthesized by many different plants and bacteria. Fruits and vegetables constitute the primary dietary source of the vitamin. Some forms of dietary folic acid are labile and may be destroyed by cooking. The minimum daily requirement is normally about 50 μg but may be increased severalfold during periods of enhanced metabolic demand such as pregnancy.

The assimilation of adequate amounts of folic acid is dependent on the nature of the diet and its means of preparation. Folates in various foodstuffs are largely conjugated to polyglutamic acid. This highly polar side chain impairs the intestinal absorption of the vitamin. However, conjugases (γ-glutamyl carboxypeptidases) in the lumen

TABLE 292-1 Classification of the megaloblastic anemias

I Cobalamin deficiency
  A Inadequate intake: vegetarians (rare)
  B Malabsorption
    1 Inadequate production of intrinsic factor (IF)
      a Pernicious anemia
      b Gastrectomy
      c Congenital absence or functional abnormality of IF (rare)
    2 Disorders of terminal ileum
      a Tropical sprue
      b Nontropical sprue
      c Regional enteritis
      d Intestinal resection
      e Neoplasms and granulomatous disorders (rare)
      f Selective cobalamin malabsorption (Imerslund's syndrome) (rare)
    3 Competition for cobalamin
      a Fish tapeworm
      b Bacteria: blind loop syndrome
    4 Drugs: *p*-aminosalicylic acid, colchicine, neomycin
  C Other
    1 Nitrous oxide
    2 Transcobalamin II deficiency (rare)
II Folic acid deficiency
  A Inadequate intake: unbalanced diet (common in alcoholics, teenagers, some infants)
  B Increased requirements
    1 Pregnancy
    2 Infancy
    3 Malignancy
    4 Increased hematopoiesis (chronic hemolytic anemias)
    5 Chronic exfoliative skin disorders
    6 Hemodialysis
  C Malabsorption
    1 Tropical sprue
    2 Nontropical sprue
    3 Drugs: Phenytoin, barbiturates, (?) ethanol
  D Impaired metabolism
    1 Inhibitors of dihydrofolate reductase: methotrexate, pyrimethamine, triamterene, pentamidine, etc.
    2 Alcohol
    3 Rare enzyme deficiencies: dihydrofolate reductase, others
III Other causes
  A Drugs which impair DNA metabolism
    1 Purine antagonists: 6-mercaptopurine, azathioprine, etc.
    2 Pyrimidine antagonists: 5-fluorouracil, cytosine arabinoside, etc.
    3 Others: procarbazine, hydroxyurea, acyclovir, zidovudine
  B Metabolic disorders (rare)
    1 Hereditary orotic aciduria
    2 Others
  C Megaloblastic anemia of unknown etiology
    1 Refractory megaloblastic anemia
    2 Di Guglielmo's syndrome*
    3 Congenital dyserythropoietic anemia

* A form of acute nonlymphocytic leukemia with atypical, dysplastic changes in erythroid series.

of the gut convert polyglutamates to mono- and diglutamates, which are readily absorbed in the proximal jejunum.

There are binding proteins in plasma for folates, but their physiologic significance is unclear. Plasma folate is primarily in the form of N^5-methyltetrahydrofolate, a monoglutamate. N^5-Methyltetrahydrofolate is transported into cells by a carrier which is specific for the tetrahydro forms of the vitamin. Once in the cell, the folate is reconverted to the polyglutamate form, after removal of the N^5-methyl group in a cobalamin-requiring reaction (see below). The polyglutamate form may be useful for retention of folate by the cell.

Normal individuals have about 5 to 20 mg folic acid in various body stores, half in the liver. In light of the minimum daily requirement, it is not surprising that a deficiency will occur within months if dietary intake or intestinal absorption is curtailed.

COBALAMIN This vitamin is a complex organometallic compound in which a cobalt atom is situated within a corrin ring, a structure similar to the porphyrin from which heme is formed (Fig. 290-3). Unlike heme, however, cobalamin cannot be synthesized in the human body and must be supplied in the diet. The only dietary source of cobalamin are animal products: meat and dairy foods. The minimum daily requirement for cobalamin is about 2.5 μg.

During gastric digestion, cobalamin in food is released and forms

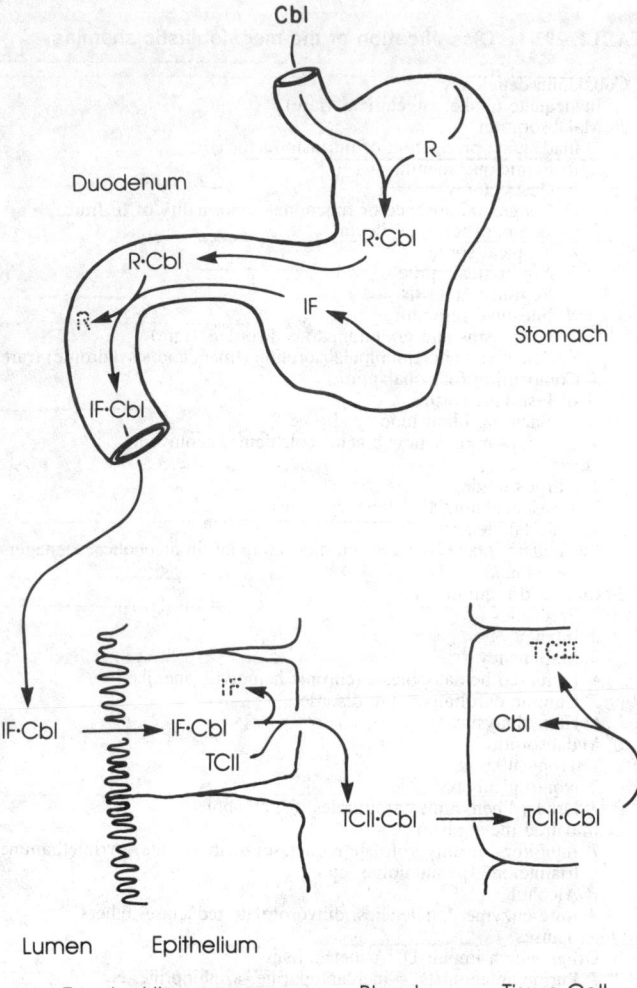

FIGURE 292-1 The assimilation of cobalamin. On entering the stomach dietary cobalamin (Cbl) forms a complex with R binding protein. As this protein is digested, cobalamin is transferred to intrinsic factor (IF). This complex passes through the intestine until it reaches specific receptors on the mucosa of the distal ileum. The internalized Cbl is then transferred to transcobalamin II (TCII) which circulates in the plasma until it is binds to receptors on cells throughout the body and is internalized.

a stable complex with gastric R binder, one of a group of closely related glycoproteins of unknown function which are found in secretions (e.g., saliva, milk, gastric juice, bile), phagocytes, and plasma. On entering the duodenum, the cobalamin–R binder complex is digested, releasing the cobalamin, which then binds to intrinsic factor (IF). This glycoprotein of molecular weight 50,000 is produced by the parietal cells of the stomach. The secretion of intrinsic factor generally parallels that of hydrochloric acid. The cobalamin-IF complex is resistant to proteolytic digestion and travels to the distal ileum, where specific receptors on the mucosal brush border bind the cobalamin-IF complex, thereby enabling the vitamin to be absorbed. Thus, intrinsic factor like transferrin (see Chap. 291) serves as a cell-directed carrier protein. The receptor-bound cobalamin-IF complex is taken into the ileal mucosal cell, where over the course of several hours the IF is destroyed and the cobalamin is transferred to another transport protein, transcobalamin II (TC II). The cobalamin–TC II complex is then secreted into the circulation, from which it is rapidly taken up by the liver, the bone marrow, and other cells. The pathway of cobalamin absorption is shown in Fig. 292-1. Normally, about 2 mg cobalamin is stored in the liver, and another 2 mg is stored elsewhere in the body. In view of the minimum daily requirement, about 3 to 6 years would be required for a normal individual to become deficient in cobalamin if absorption were to cease abruptly.

Although TC II is the acceptor for newly absorbed cobalamin, most circulating cobalamin is bound to transcobalamin I (TC I), a glycoprotein closely related to gastric R binder. TC I appears to be derived in part from leukocytes. The paradox that most circulating cobalamin is bound to TC I rather than TC II, even though TC II initially carries all the cobalamin that is absorbed by the intestine, is explained by the fact that cobalamin bound to TC II is rapidly cleared from the blood ($t_{1/2}$ about 1 h), while clearance of cobalamin bound to TC I requires many days. The function of TC I is unknown.

BIOCHEMICAL CONSIDERATIONS

FOLATE The *prime function* of this vitamin is to transfer 1-carbon moieties such as methyl and formyl groups to various organic compounds (see Fig. 292-2). The source of these 1-carbon moieties is usually serine, which reacts with tetrahydrofolate to produce glycine and $N^{5,10}$-methylenetetrahydrofolate. An alternative source is formiminoglutamic acid, an intermediate in histidine catabolism, which gives up its formimino group to tetrahydrofolate to yield N^5-formiminotetrahydrofolate and glutamic acid. These derivatives provide entry into an interconvertible donor pool consisting of tetrahydrofolate derivatives carrying various 1-carbon moieties (see Fig. 292-2). The constituents of this pool can donate their 1-carbon moieties to appropriate acceptor compounds to form metabolic intermediates which are ultimately converted to building blocks used in the synthesis of biologic macromolecules. The most important building blocks are (1) purines, in which the C-2 and C-8 atoms are introduced in folate-dependent reactions; (2) deoxythymidylate monophosphate (dTMP), synthesized from $N^{5,10}$-methylenetetrahydrofolate and deoxyuridylate monophosphate (dUMP); and (3) methionine, formed by the transfer of a methyl group from N^5-methyltetrahydrofolate to homocysteine. Cobalamin is also required for the formation of methionine from homocysteine (see below).

In all but one of the 1-carbon transfer reactions, tetrahydrofolate is produced. It can immediately accept a 1-carbon moiety and reenter the donor pool. The single exception is the thymidylate synthetase reaction (dUMP → dTMP), in which dihydrofolate is the product (Fig. 292-2). This must be reduced to tetrahydrofolate by the enzyme dihydrofolate reductase before it can reenter the donor pool. A number of drugs are able to inhibit dihydrofolate reductase, thereby diverting folate from the donor pool and producing what amounts to a state of folate deficiency in the face of normal tissue folate concentrations.

COBALAMIN In humans there are two metabolically active forms of cobalamin, identified by the alkyl group attached to the sixth coordination position of the cobalt atom: methylcobalamin and adenosylcobalamin. The vitamin preparation which is used therapeutically is cyanocobalamin (also called vitamin B_{12}). Cyanocobalamin

FIGURE 292-2 Scheme of folate metabolism.

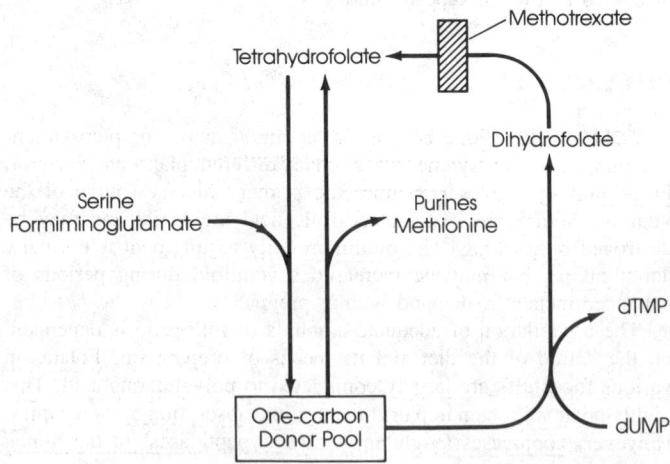

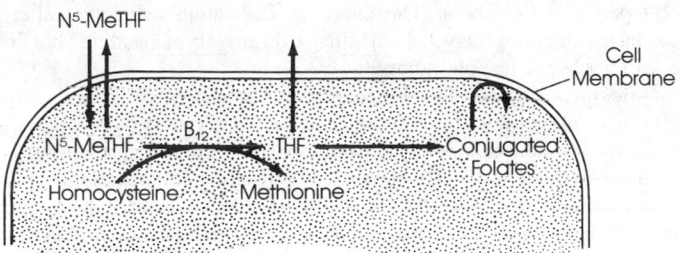

FIGURE 292-3 Diagram showing the interrelationship between cobalamin (methylcobalamin) and folate metabolism within the cell.

has no known physiologic role and must be converted to a biologically active form before it can be used by tissues.

Methylcobalamin is an essential cofactor in the conversion of homocysteine to methionine (Fig. 292-3). When this reaction is impaired, folate metabolism is deranged, and it is this derangement which is thought to underlie the defect in DNA synthesis and the megaloblastic maturation pattern in patients who are deficient in cobalamin (see Fig. 292-3). What appears to happen in cobalamin deficiency is that the unconjugated N^5-methyltetrahydrofolate newly taken from the bloodstream cannot be converted to other forms of tetrahydrofolate by methyl transfer. This is the so-called folate trap hypothesis. Since N^5-methyltetrahydrofolate is a poor substrate for the conjugating enzyme (this has been shown in rats and pigs but has not yet been demonstrated in humans), it largely remains in the unconjugated form and slowly leaks from the cell. Tissue folate deficiency therefore develops, and this results in megaloblastic hematopoiesis. This hypothesis explains the fact that tissue folate stores in cobalamin deficiency are substantially reduced, with a disproportionate reduction in conjugated as compared with unconjugated folates, despite normal or supranormal serum folate levels. It also explains why large doses of folate can produce a partial hematologic remission in patients with cobalamin deficiency.

Impairment in the conversion of homocysteine to methionine may also be partly responsible for the neurologic complications of cobalamin deficiency (see below). The methionine formed in this reaction is needed for the production of choline and choline-containing phospholipids as well as for the methylation of myelin basic protein. Nervous system damage is thought to result from interference with these processes due to decreased methionine production in cobalamin deficiency.

Adenosylcobalamin is required for the conversion of methylmalonyl coenzyme A (CoA) to succinyl CoA. Lack of this cofactor leads to large increases in the tissue levels of methylmalonyl CoA and its precursor, propionyl CoA. As a consequence, nonphysiologic fatty acids containing an odd number of carbon atoms are synthesized and incorporated into neuronal lipids. This biochemical abnormality may also contribute to the neurologic complications of cobalamin deficiency (see below).

CLINICAL DISORDERS

CLASSIFICATION OF MEGALOBLASTIC ANEMIAS (Table 292-1) The etiology of megaloblastic anemia varies in different parts of the world. In temperate zones, folate deficiency in alcoholics and pernicious anemia are the common types of megaloblastic anemias. In certain areas close to the equator, tropical sprue is endemic and an important cause. In Scandinavia, megaloblastic anemia is sometimes secondary to infestation by the fish tapeworm *Diphyllobothrium latum.*

The dietary intake of cobalamin is more than adequate for the body's requirements, except in true vegetarians (individuals who live on a purely vegetable diet) and their breast-fed infants. Thus, deficiency of cobalamin is almost always due to malabsorption. As explained in the section above, the absorption of cobalamin depends

upon a specific binding protein produced in the stomach and uptake by a specific receptor in the mucosa of the distal ileum. Accordingly, several steps in this process can go awry and lead to malabsorption. In contrast, the dietary intake of folic acid is marginal in many parts of the world. Furthermore, since the body's stores of folate are relatively low, folic acid deficiency can arise rather suddenly during periods of decreased dietary intake or increased metabolic demand. Finally, folic acid deficiency may be due to malabsorption. Often two or more of these factors coexist in a given patient.

Combined deficiencies of cobalamin and folic acid are not uncommon. Patients with tropical sprue are often deficient in both vitamins. The biochemical lesion that results in megaloblastic maturation of bone marrow cells also causes structural and functional abnormalities of the rapidly proliferating epithelial cells of the intestinal mucosa. Thus, severe deficiency of one vitamin can lead to malabsorption of the other. Furthermore, as discussed above, a deficiency of cobalamin causes a secondary reduction in cellular folic acid.

Finally, megaloblastic anemias may occasionally be induced by factors unrelated to a vitamin deficiency. Most such cases are caused by one or more of the many drugs which interfere with DNA synthesis. Less commonly, megaloblastic maturation is encountered in certain acquired defects of hematopoietic stem cells. Rarest of all are specific congenital enzyme deficiencies in which megaloblastic anemia is characteristically encountered.

COBALAMIN DEFICIENCY There are many conditions in which cobalamin deficiency may develop. Although each has its own characteristic manifestations, certain clinical features are common to all. These clinical features involve the blood, the gastrointestinal tract, and the nervous system.

The hematologic manifestations are almost entirely the result of anemia although very rarely purpura may appear, due to thrombocytopenia. Symptoms of anemia may include weakness, lightheadedness, vertigo, and tinnitus, as well as palpitations, angina, and the symptoms of congestive failure. On physical examination, the patient with florid cobalamin deficiency is pale, with slightly icteric skin and eyes. The pulse is rapid, and the heart may be enlarged; auscultation will reveal a systolic flow murmur. The spleen and liver may be somewhat enlarged. There may be a slight fever.

The gastrointestinal manifestations reflect the effect of cobalamin deficiency on the rapidly proliferating gastrointestinal epithelium. The patient sometimes complains of a sore tongue, which on inspection will be smooth and beefy red. Anorexia with moderate weight loss may also be evident, possibly accompanied by diarrhea and other gastrointestinal symptoms. These latter manifestations may be in part caused by megaloblastosis of the small-intestinal epithelium, which results in malabsorption.

The neurologic manifestations are the most worrisome of all, because they often fail to remit fully on treatment. They begin pathologically with demyelination, followed by axonal degeneration and eventual neuronal death; the final stage, of course, is irreversible. Sites of involvement include peripheral nerves, the spinal cord, where the posterior and lateral columns undergo demyelination, and the cerebrum itself. Signs and symptoms include numbness and paresthesias in the extremities (the earliest neurologic manifestations), weakness, ataxia, and poor finger coordination. There may be sphincter disturbances. Reflexes may be diminished or increased. The Romberg and Babinski signs may be positive, and position sense and vibration sense are usually diminished. Disturbances of mentation will vary from mild irritability and forgetfulness to severe dementia or frank psychosis. It should be emphasized that occasionally *neurologic disease may occur in a patient with a normal hematocrit and* normal red blood cell indexes.

In the usual patient, in whom hematologic problems predominate, the blood and bone marrow show characteristic megaloblastic changes which are described under "Diagnosis" below. The anemia may be very severe—hematocrits of 15 to 20 are not infrequent—but is surprisingly well tolerated by the patient because it develops so slowly.

Pernicious anemia   The most common cause of cobalamin deficiency in temperate climates is pernicious anemia, in which intrinsic factor secretion ceases owing to atrophy of the gastric mucosa. It is most frequently seen in individuals of northern European descent and American blacks and is much less common in southern Europeans and Orientals. Men and women are equally affected. It is a disease of the elderly, the average patient presenting near age 60; it is rare under 30, although typical pernicious anemia can be seen in children under 10 (juvenile pernicious anemia). Inherited conditions in which a histologically normal stomach secretes either an abnormal intrinsic factor or none at all will induce cobalamin deficiency in infancy or early childhood.

On the basis of incomplete evidence, pernicious anemia is currently thought to be caused by an autoimmune reaction against gastric parietal cells. There is considerable evidence for immunologic abnormalities in pernicious anemia. The incidence of pernicious anemia is substantially increased in patients with other diseases thought to be of immunologic origin, including Graves' disease, myxedema, thyroiditis, idiopathic adrenocortical insufficiency, vitiligo, and hypoparathyroidism. Patients with pernicious anemia also have abnormal circulating antibodies related to their disease: 90 percent have antiparietal cell antibody while 60 percent have anti-intrinsic factor antibody. Antiparietal cell antibody is also found in 50 percent of patients with gastric atrophy without pernicious anemia as well as in 10 to 15 percent of an unselected patient population, but anti-intrinsic factor antibody is usually absent from these patients. Relatives of patients with pernicious anemia have an increased incidence of the disease, and even clinically unaffected relatives may have anti-intrinsic factor antibody in their serum. A final point supporting an immunologic basis for pernicious anemia is the fact that corticosteroids have been reported to reverse the disease both pathologically and clinically.

The destruction of parietal cells in pernicious anemia is thought to be mediated by complement-fixing antibodies against the parietal cell surface. The observation that pernicious anemia is unusually common in patients with agammaglobulinemia, however, suggests that the cellular immune system may also play a role in its pathogenesis.

Pathologically, the most characteristic finding in pernicious anemia is gastric atrophy affecting the acid- and pepsin-secreting portion of the stomach; the antrum is spared. Other pathologic changes are secondary to the deficiency of cobalamin; these include megaloblastoid alterations in the gastric and intestinal epithelium and the neurologic changes described above. The abnormalities in the gastric epithelium appear as cellular atypia in gastric cytology specimens, a finding which must be carefully distinguished from the cytologic abnormalities seen in gastric malignancy.

The *clinical manifestations* are primarily those of cobalamin deficiency, as described above. The disease is of insidious onset and progresses slowly. Laboratory examination will reveal hypergastrinemia and pentagastrin-fast achlorhydria as well as the hematologic and other laboratory abnormalities discussed below in "Diagnosis."

Through appropriate replacement therapy, patients with pernicious anemia should experience complete and lifelong correction of all abnormalities which are due to cobalamin deficiency, except to the extent that irreversible changes in the nervous system may have occurred prior to treatment. These patients, however, are unusually subject to gastric polyps and have about twice the normal incidence of cancer of the stomach. In view of the latter complication, patients should be followed with frequent stool guaiac examinations together with further diagnostic studies when indicated.

Postgastrectomy   Following total gastrectomy or extensive damage to gastric mucosa as, for example, by ingestion of corrosive agents, megaloblastic anemia may develop because the source of intrinsic factor has been removed. In such patients the absorption of orally administered cobalamin is impaired. Megaloblastic anemia may also follow partial gastrectomy, but the incidence is lower than after total gastrectomy, in which cobalamin malabsorption occurs in 100 percent of patients. The cause of cobalamin deficiency after partial gastrectomy may be intestinal overgrowth of bacteria, but it does not always respond to antibiotics.

Intestinal organisms   Megaloblastic anemia may occur with intestinal stasis due to anatomic lesions (strictures, diverticula, anastomoses, "blind loops") or pseudoobstruction (diabetes mellitus, scleroderma, amyloid). This anemia is caused by colonization of the small intestine by large masses of bacteria which divert cobalamin from the host. Steatorrhea may also be seen under these circumstances, because bile salt metabolism is disturbed when the intestine is heavily colonized with bacteria. Hematologic responses have been observed after administration of oral antibiotics such as tetracycline and ampicillin.

Megaloblastic anemia is seen, in Scandinavia especially, in persons harboring the fish tapeworm *D. latum*. The anemia has been attributed to competition by the worm for cobalamin. Destruction of the worm eliminates the problem.

Ileal abnormalities   Cobalamin deficiency is commonly found in tropical sprue, while it is an unusual complication of nontropical sprue (gluten-sensitive enteropathy; see Chap. 240). Virtually any disorder which compromises the absorptive capacity of the distal ileum can result in cobalamin deficiency. Specific entities include regional enteritis, Whipple's disease, and tuberculosis. Segmental involvement of the distal ileum by disease can cause megaloblastic anemia without any other manifestations of intestinal malabsorption such as steatorrhea. Cobalamin malabsorption is also seen after ileal resection. The Zollinger-Ellison syndrome (intense gastric hyperacidity due to a gastrin-secreting tumor) may cause cobalamin malabsorption by acidifying the small intestine. This will retard the transfer of the vitamin from R binder to intrinsic factor and will impair the binding of the cobalamin–IF complex to the ileal receptors. Chronic pancreatitis may also cause cobalamin malabsorption by impairing the transfer of the vitamin from R binder to intrinsic factor. This abnormality can be detected by tests of cobalamin absorption (see below, Schilling test), but it is invariably mild and never causes clinical cobalamin deficiency. Finally, there is a rare congenital disorder, Imerslund-Gräsbeck disease, in which a selective defect in cobalamin absorption is accompanied by proteinuria.

FOLIC ACID DEFICIENCY   Patients with folic acid deficiency are more apt to be malnourished than those with cobalamin deficiency. Accordingly, they are likely to appear wasted. The gastrointestinal manifestations are similar to, but may be more widespread and more severe than those of, pernicious anemia. Diarrhea is often present, and cheilosis and glossitis are also encountered. However, in contrast to cobalamin deficiency, neurologic abnormalities do not occur.

The hematologic manifestations of folic acid deficiency are the same as those of cobalamin deficiency. Folic acid deficiency can generally be attributed to one or more of the following factors: increased demand for folate, inadequate intake, and malabsorption.

Inadequate intake   Folic acid malnutrition is commonly encountered among a number of groups. Alcoholics frequently become folate-deficient because their main source of caloric intake is alcoholic beverages. Distilled spirits are virtually devoid of folic acid, while beer and wine do not contain enough of the vitamin to satisfy the daily requirement. In addition, alcohol may interfere with folate metabolism. Narcotic addicts are also prone to become folate-deficient because of malnutrition. Many indigent and elderly individuals who subsist primarily on canned foods or "tea and toast" and occasional teenagers whose diet consists of "junk food" develop folate deficiency.

Increased demand   Tissues with a relatively high rate of cell division such as the bone marrow or gut mucosa have a large requirement for folate. Therefore, patients with chronic hemolytic anemias or other causes of very active erythropoiesis may become deficient if their high folate requirement is not met by dietary intake. Likewise, a pregnant woman may become deficient in folic acid because of the high demand of the developing fetus. Folate deficiency may also occur during the growth spurts of infancy and adolescence.

Malabsorption Folic acid deficiency is a common accompaniment of tropical sprue. Both the gastrointestinal symptoms and malabsorption are improved by the administration of either folic acid or antibiotics by mouth. Patients with nontropical sprue (gluten-sensitive enteropathy) may also develop significant folic acid deficiency which parallels other parameters of malabsorption. Similarly, alcohol-related folate deficiency may be due in part to malabsorption. In addition, other primary small-bowel disorders are sometimes associated with vitamin deficiency. These entities are all discussed in Chap. 240.

DRUGS Next to deficiency of folate or cobalamin, the most common cause of megaloblastic anemia is drug ingestion. Drugs which cause megaloblastic anemia do so by interfering with DNA synthesis, either directly or by antagonizing the action of folate. They can be classified as follows:

1 Direct inhibitors of DNA synthesis. The drugs in this category are used in the treatment of malignancy. Their efficacy depends on their ability to disrupt DNA synthesis. They include purine analogues (6-thioguanine, azathioprine, 6-mercaptopurine), pyrimidine analogues (5-fluorouracil, cytosine arabinoside), and other drugs which interfere with DNA synthesis by a variety of mechanisms (hydroxyurea, procarbazine).

The antiviral agents acyclovir, used in herpes simplex and herpes zoster infections, and zidovudine (AZT), used against the human immunodeficiency virus (HIV), can cause megaloblastic anemia. Megaloblastic anemia is only rarely seen with acyclovir, but it occurs regularly with zidovudine, representing the major toxicity of this drug.

2 Folate antagonists. The most toxic of these is methotrexate, an exceedingly powerful inhibitor of dihydrofolate reductase which is used in the treatment of certain malignancies. Much less toxic, but still capable of inducing a megaloblastic anemia, are several weak dihydrofolate reductase inhibitors that are used to treat a variety of nonmalignant conditions. These include pentamidine, trimethoprim, triamterene, and pyrimethamine.

The megaloblastic changes in methotrexate poisoning appear to result from the following sequence of events. In methotrexate-poisoned cells, the methylation of dUMP to dTMP is grossly impaired. As a consequence, the phosphorylation of dUMP to dUTP, normally a very minor reaction, becomes a major route of dUMP metabolism. The capacity of a highly specific dUTP pyrophosphatase to degrade dUTP back to dUMP is overwhelmed under these conditions, and dUTP accumulates in the cell. This dUTP is incorporated into newly synthesized DNA, because DNA polymerase cannot distinguish between dUTP and the closely related normal substrate, dTTP. As a result, defective strands of DNA are produced in which T is partly replaced by U. The U-containing regions of these defective strands are recognized by a specific repair system, which excises them and attempts to replace them with normal DNA. In methotrexate-poisoned cells, however, there is so much dUTP and so little dTTP that the new DNA is also likely to be defective. It is this futile cycle of faulty replication, error excision, faulty repair, etc., which explains the megaloblastic pattern of DNA synthesis in methotrexate-poisoned cells.

3 Nitrous oxide. Nitrous oxide inhalation causes the destruction of endogenous cobalamin. As ordinarily used, this anesthetic does not destroy enough cobalamin to cause clinical manifestations. Repeated or protracted exposure, however, may lead to a megaloblastic anemia. Fatal megaloblastic anemia has been reported in patients with tetanus who were given nitrous oxide continuously for weeks.

4 Others. A number of drugs antagonize folate by mechanisms which are poorly understood but are thought to involve an effect on absorption of the vitamin by the intestine. In this category are the anticonvulsants phenytoin (Dilantin) and primidone (Mysoline) and phenobarbital (Luminal). Megaloblastic anemia induced by these agents is mild.

ACUTE MEGALOBLASTIC ANEMIA Occasionally, a full-blown megaloblastic state can develop over the course of just a few days. This is usually seen following nitrous oxide anesthesia, but may occur in any patient with a serious illness requiring intensive care, especially a patient receiving multiple transfusions, dialysis, or total parenteral nutrition. An acute megaloblastic state can also be precipitated by the administration of a weak antifolate (e.g., trimethoprim) to a patient with marginal tissue folate stores.

The condition resembles an immune cytopenia, with a rapidly developing thrombocytopenia and/or leukopenia in the absence of anemia. The blood smear may be completely normal, but the marrow is always floridly megaloblastic. Acute megaloblastic anemia responds rapidly to treatment with folate plus cobalamin in the usual therapeutic doses.

OTHER Hereditary Megaloblastic anemia may be seen in several hereditary disorders. It is a regular feature of orotic aciduria, a deficiency of orotidylic decarboxylase and phosphorylase, leading to a defect in pyrimidine metabolism and characterized by retarded growth and development as well as by the excretion of large amounts of orotic acid. Megaloblastic anemia has been reported in a single case of the Lesch-Nyhan syndrome, a condition resulting from a deficiency of hypoxanthine-guanine phosphoribosyltransferase whose clinical manifestations include gout, mental retardation, and self-mutilation. It has also been described in methylmalonic aciduria due to a defect in the biosynthesis of the two metabolically active alkyl cobalamins, though it is not seen in methylmalonic aciduria due to methylmalonyl CoA mutase deficiency. Congenital folate malabsorption causes megaloblastic anemia, accompanied by ataxia and mental retardation. Megaloblastic anemia has been reported to accompany the congenital deficiency of two other folate-metabolizing enzymes: dihydrofolate reductase and N^5-methyltetrahydrofolate:homocysteine methyltransferase. These deficiencies are less well documented than is congenital folate malabsorption. A thiamine-responsive megaloblastic anemia accompanied by nerve deafness and diabetes mellitus has been reported in several children. Megaloblastic changes as well as multinuclearity of red blood cell precursors are seen in the marrow of certain patients with congenital dyserythropoietic anemia, a group of inherited disorders characterized by mild to moderate anemia presenting at any age and pursuing a benign course.

Transcobalamin II deficiency, like the congenital abnormalities in cobalamin absorption described previously, causes pronounced deficiency in cobalamin in infancy or early childhood, with all the accompanying manifestations. Megaloblastic anemia is not seen in hereditary transcobalamin I deficiency.

Refractory megaloblastic anemia This is a form of myelodysplasia in which megaloblastic erythropoiesis may sometimes be seen. Megaloblastic changes are restricted to the red blood cell series; large granulocyte precursors and giant metamyelocytes are not seen (see below). Like other forms of myelodysplasia, acquired sideroblastic anemia is associated with an increased incidence of acute leukemia.

Megaloblastic changes are seen in erythremic myelosis and acute erythroleukemia (di Guglielmo) where red blood cell precursors are prominently involved. Here, the marrow is characterized by bizarre erythroid maturation, with multinuclearity and multipolar mitotic figures in the red blood cell precursors. Erythremic myelosis is discussed further in Chap. 296.

DIAGNOSIS The finding of significant macrocytosis [mean corpuscular volume (MCV) > 100 fL] suggests the presence of a megaloblastic anemia. Other causes of macrocytosis include hemolysis, liver disease, alcoholism, hypothyroidism, and aplastic anemia. If the macrocytosis is marked (MCV > 110 fL), the patient is much more likely to have a megaloblastic anemia. The reticulocyte count is low, and the leukocyte and platelet count may also be decreased, particularly in severely anemic patients. The blood smear (Fig. A5-2) demonstrates marked anisocytosis and poikilocytosis, together with macroovalocytes, which are large, oval, fully hemoglobinized erythrocytes typical of megaloblastic anemias. There is some basophilic stippling, and an occasional nucleated red blood cell may be seen.

Hypokalemia
Salt Retention

In the white blood cell series, the neutrophils show hypersegmentation of the nucleus. This is such a characteristic finding that a single cell with a nucleus of six lobes or more should raise the immediate suspicion of a megaloblastic anemia. A rare myelocyte may also be seen. Bizarre, misshapen platelets are also observed. The bone marrow examination is very helpful in the diagnosis of megaloblastic anemia. The marrow is hypercellular with a decreased myeloid/erythroid ratio and abundant stainable iron. Red blood cell precursors are abnormally large and have nuclei that appear much less mature than would be expected from the development of the cytoplasm (nuclear-cytoplasmic asynchrony). The nuclear chromatin is more dispersed than it should be and consequently stains less intensely than normal. To the extent that it is aggregated, it condenses in a peculiar fenestrated pattern which is very characteristic of megaloblastic erythropoiesis. Abnormal mitoses may be seen. Granulocyte precursors are also affected, many being larger than normal, including giant bands and metamyelocytes. Megakaryocytes are decreased and show abnormal morphology.

Megaloblastic anemias are characterized by ineffective erythropoiesis (Chap. 290). In a severely megaloblastic patient as many as 90 percent of the red blood cell precursors may be destroyed before they are released into the bloodstream, compared with 10 to 15 percent in the normal subject. Enhanced intramedullary destruction of erythroblasts results in an increase in unconjugated bilirubin and lactic acid dehydrogenase (isoenzyme 1) in plasma. Abnormalities in iron kinetics also attest to the presence of ineffective erythropoiesis, with increased iron turnover but low incorporation of labeled iron into circulating red blood cells.

In evaluating a patient with megaloblastic anemia, it is important to determine whether there is a specific vitamin deficiency by measuring serum cobalamin and folate levels. The normal range of cobalamin in serum is 200 to 900 pg/mL; values less than 100 pg/mL indicate clinically significant deficiency. The normal serum concentration of folic acid ranges from 6 to 20 ng/mL; values of 4 ng/mL or less are generally considered to be diagnostic of folate deficiency. Unlike serum cobalamin, serum folate levels may reflect recent alterations in dietary intake. Measurement of red blood cell folate occasionally provides useful information since it is not subject to short-term fluctuations in folate intake and is, therefore, a better index of tissue folate stores than serum folate.

Once cobalamin deficiency has been established, its pathogenesis can be delineated by means of a Schilling test. A patient is given radioactive cobalamin by mouth followed shortly thereafter by an intramuscular injection of unlabeled cobalamin. The proportion of the administered radioactivity excreted in the urine during the next 24 h provides an accurate measure of absorption of cobalamin, assuming that a complete urine sample has been collected. Since cobalamin deficiency is almost always due to malabsorption (Table 292-1), this first stage of the Schilling test should be abnormal. The patient is then given labeled cobalamin bound to intrinsic factor. Absorption of the vitamin will now approach normal if the patient has pernicious anemia or some other type of intrinsic factor deficiency. If cobalamin absorption is still decreased, the patient may have bacterial overgrowth (blind loop syndrome) or ileal disease (including an ileal absorptive defect secondary to the cobalamin deficiency itself). Cobalamin malabsorption due to bacterial overgrowth can frequently be corrected by the administration of antibiotics. The Schilling test can provide equally reliable information after the patient has had adequate therapy with parenteral cobalamin.

Low serum cobalamin levels are sometimes found in patients who are hematologically normal and have normal Schilling tests. Many of these patients absorb cobalamin poorly when the vitamin is mixed with food. The question has been raised whether the neurologic and psychiatric abnormalities often seen in these patients may be due to a chronic state of cobalamin deficiency. If so—and this question is far from answered—symptomatic cobalamin deficiency in the absence of anemia may be far more widespread than is currently recognized.

TREATMENT

COBALAMIN DEFICIENCY Apart from specific therapy related to the underlying disorder (e.g., antibiotics for intestinal overgrowth with bacteria), the mainstay of treatment for cobalamin deficiency is replacement therapy. Since the defect is one of absorption, replacement should be administered parenterally, specifically in the form of intramuscular cyanocobalamin. (If intramuscular administration is contraindicated or refused, cobalamin deficiency can be managed by oral replacement therapy, but at doses of 300 to 1000 μg daily, it is an expensive mode of treatment which requires very close medical supervision to avoid relapse.) Treatment should be started with 100 μg cobalamin per day for a week. The frequency of administration of the vitamin may then be decreased, the goal being to give a total of 2000 μg during the first 6 weeks. The patient may then be placed on 100 μg cyanocobalamin intramuscularly every month, a regimen that must be maintained for the rest of the patient's life. If necessary, larger doses may be given at less frequent intervals (e.g., 1 mg every 2 to 4 months), but the risk of relapse is substantially greater than if the vitamin is given monthly.

The response to treatment is gratifying. Shortly after treatment is begun, and several days before a hematologic response is evident in the peripheral blood, the patient will experience an increase in strength and an improved sense of well-being. Marrow morphology begins to revert toward normal within a few hours after treatment is initiated. Reticulocytosis begins 4 to 5 days after therapy is started and peaks at about day 7 (Fig. 292-4), with subsequent remission of the anemia over the next several weeks. If a reticulocytosis does not occur, or if it is less brisk than expected from the level of the hematocrit, a search should be made for other factors contributing to the anemia (e.g., infection, coexisting folate deficiency, or hypothyroidism). Hypokalemia and salt retention may occur early in the course of therapy; usually these developments are of no consequence, but occasionally they may lead to severe illness or even death.

In most cases, replacement therapy is all that is needed for the treatment of cobalamin deficiency. Occasionally, however, a patient with a severe anemia will have such a precarious cardiovascular status that emergency transfusion is necessary. This must be done with great care, since it is very easy to precipitate florid congestive failure in such patients by fluid overload. Blood must be administered slowly in the form of packed cells, with very close observation, giving as an initial dose no more than 100 mL. This small volume will frequently be enough to ameliorate the cardiovascular problems sufficiently that further therapy can be restricted to cobalamin replacement. If necessary, blood may be administered by exchanging patient blood (mostly plasma) for packed cells.

With lifelong treatment, patients should experience no further manifestations of cobalamin deficiency. As previously stated, neu-

FIGURE 292-4 Hematologic response of a patient with pernicious anemia to an intramuscular injection of 100 μg cobalamin on day 0. (*From A Erslev, TG Gabuzda, Pathophysiology of Blood, Philadelphia, Saunders, 1975.*)

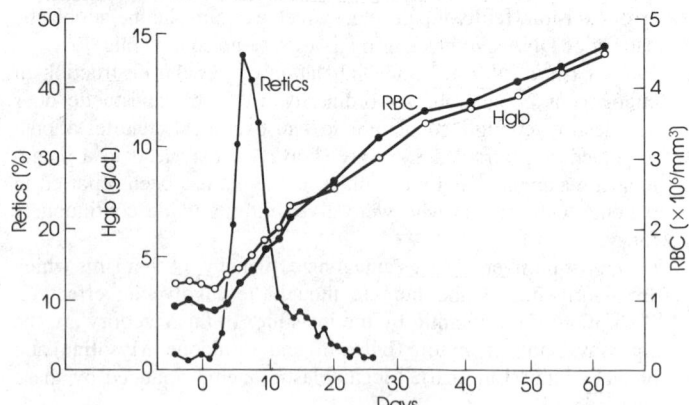

rologic symptoms may not be fully corrected even by optimal therapy. The potential for late development of gastric carcinoma in pernicious anemia necessitates careful follow-up of the patient.

FOLATE DEFICIENCY Like cobalamin deficiency, folate deficiency is treated by replacement therapy. The usual dose of folate is 1 mg per day, by mouth, but higher doses (up to 5 mg per day) may be required for folate deficiency due to malabsorption. Parenteral folate is rarely necessary. The hematologic response is similar to that seen after replacement therapy for cobalamin deficiency—that is, a brisk reticulocytosis after about 4 days, followed by correction of the anemia over the next 1 to 2 months. The duration of therapy depends on the basis of the deficiency state. Patients with a continuously increased requirement (such as patients with hemolytic anemia) or those with malabsorption or chronic malnutrition should continue to receive oral folic acid indefinitely. In addition, the patient should be encouraged to maintain an optimal diet containing adequate amounts of folate.

Folate, particularly in large doses, can correct the megaloblastic anemia of cobalamin deficiency without altering the neurologic abnormalities. The neurologic manifestations may even be aggravated by folate therapy. Cobalamin deficiency can thus be masked in patients who for one reason or another are taking large doses of folate. For this reason, a hematologic response to folate must never be used to rule out cobalamin deficiency in a given patient; cobalamin deficiency can be excluded only by appropriate laboratory evaluation.

OTHER CAUSES OF MEGALOBLASTIC ANEMIA Megaloblastic anemia due to drugs can be treated, if necessary, by reducing the dose of the drug or eliminating it altogether. The effects of folate antagonists which inhibit dihydrofolate reductase can be counteracted by folinic acid (citrovorum factor) in a dose of 100 to 200 mg per day. Since folinic acid is a derivative of tetrahydrofolate, it circumvents the block in folate metabolism imposed by dihydrofolate reductase inhibitors, replenishing the tissues with a form of folate which can directly enter the one-carbon donor pool. Certain of the congenital megaloblastic anemia–producing enzyme deficiencies can be treated by appropriate specific therapeutic regimens. For the megaloblastic forms of sideroblastic anemia, pyridoxine in pharmacologic doses (as high as 300 mg per day) should be tried. A few patients will respond to this therapy. Simple supportive measures are all that appear to be in order for treatment of refractory megaloblastic anemia. Acute erythroleukemia (di Guglielmo's disease) is usually treated like other types of acute nonlymphocytic leukemia (see Chap. 296).

REFERENCES

ALLEN RH: The plasma transport of vitamin B₁₂. Br J Haematol 36:153, 1976

BABIOR BM: The megaloblastic anemias, in *Hematology*, 4th ed, WJ Williams et al (eds). New York, McGraw-Hill, 1990

BORCH K: Epidemiologic, clinicopathologic, and economic aspects of gastroscopic screening of patients with pernicious anemia. Scand J Gastroenterol 21.21, 1986

COOPER BA, ROSENBLATT DS: Inherited defects of vitamin B₁₂ metabolism. Annu Rev Nutr 7:291, 1987

ERIKSSON S et al: Pernicious anemia as a risk factor in gastric cancer: The extent of the problem. Acta Med Scand 210:481, 1981

HERBERT V: Megaloblastic anemias. Lab Invest 52:3, 1985

———: Don't ignore low serum cobalamin (vitamin B₁₂) levels. Arch Intern Med 148:1705, 1988

KAPADIA CR, DONALDSON RM: Disorders of cobalamin (vitamin B₁₂) absorption and transport. Ann Rev Med 36:93, 1985

LAWSON DH et al: Early mortality in the megaloblastic anemias. Q J Med 41:1, 1972

LINDENBAUM J: Status of laboratory testing in the diagnosis of megaloblastic anemia. Blood 61:624, 1983

——— et al: Neuropsychiatric disorders caused by cobalamin deficiency in the absence of anemia or macrocytosis. N Engl J Med 318:1720, 1988

SAVAGE D, LINDENBAUM J: Anemia in alcoholics. Medicine 65:322, 1986

SHANE B, STOKSTAD EL: Vitamin B₁₂–folate interrelationships. Annu Rev Nutr 5:115, 1985

SCOTT JM, WEIR DG: Drug induced megaloblastic change. Clin Haematol 9:587, 1980

293 ANEMIA ASSOCIATED WITH CHRONIC DISORDERS

H. FRANKLIN BUNN

Among the most commonly encountered anemias are those that accompany a variety of chronic underlying diseases. They can be corrected only if the primary condition is reversible. As shown in Table 293-1, these anemias can be subdivided into several groups.

ANEMIA OF CHRONIC INFLAMMATION

CLINICAL FEATURES Patients who have a chronic systemic inflammatory disorder persisting more than a month usually develop a mild or moderate anemia. The extent of the anemia is roughly proportional to the duration and severity of the inflammatory process. These disorders include chronic infections such as subacute infective endocarditis, osteomyelitis, lung abscess, tuberculosis, and pyelonephritis. Among noninfectious causes of anemia of chronic inflammation, the most common is rheumatoid arthritis. Other noninfectious inflammatory disorders often associated with chronic anemia include systemic lupus erythematosus, vasculitides (such as temporal arteritis), sarcoidosis, regional enteritis, and tissue injury such as fracture.

This kind of anemia is also commonly encountered in neoplastic disorders, including Hodgkin's disease and a variety of solid tumors such as carcinoma of the lung and breast. Other factors may contribute to the development of more severe anemia in cancer patients. In those with gastrointestinal or uterine cancer, blood loss can be the predominant factor. Chronic bleeding will lead to iron deficiency. Furthermore, cancer patients may develop progressive anemia if the bone marrow is invaded with tumor cells. Myelophthisic anemia is discussed in Chap. 298. Cancer patients are often malnourished and may develop folate deficiency. Rarely, patients with disseminated malignancy develop severe traumatic hemolytic anemia (Chap. 294). Finally, suppression of hematopoiesis by chemotherapeutic agents or radiation therapy may aggravate anemia.

HEMATOLOGIC FEATURES Hemoglobin values generally range between 90 and 110 g/L. A hemoglobin level less than 80 g/L indicates the presence of one or more of the aggravating factors mentioned above. Although this group of anemias is generally classified as normocytic-normochromic, red blood cells are often slightly microcytic. The mean corpuscular hemoglobin concentration is about 320 g/L (normal ≅ 340 g/L). Examination of the bone marrow reveals normal erythroid maturation. However, the red blood cell precursors have less stainable iron than normal (i.e., fewer sideroblasts), while the macrophages in the marrow usually contain increased amounts of iron. Myeloid hyperplasia and an increase in plasma cells are often seen in chronic infections.

The corrected reticulocyte count is low. Careful measurement of red blood cell survival generally reveals moderately shortened erythrocyte life span. Cross-transfusion studies point to an extracorpuscular mechanism, probably hyperplasia of the mononuclear-phagocyte system. There is seldom any other evidence of significant hemolysis. However, in certain chronic infections such as subacute infective

TABLE 293-1 Anemias secondary to chronic systemic diseases

1 Anemia of chronic inflammation
  a Infection
  b Connective tissue disorders, etc.
  c Malignancy
2 Anemia of uremia
3 Anemia due to endocrine failure
4 Anemia of liver disease

endocarditis and miliary tuberculosis, splenomegaly can contribute to further shortening of the red blood cell life span, thereby increasing the severity of the anemia. In this setting spherocytes are often seen on the blood smear.

Serum iron is characteristically subnormal in this group of anemias, but in contrast to iron deficiency, the total transferrin level is also reduced (see Fig. 291-2). The fractional saturation of transferrin is lower than normal. The serum iron falls within hours or days following the onset of the inflammation, whereas several weeks elapse before the transferrin level falls. Serum ferritin is increased in patients with inflammatory disorders. Certain other plasma proteins are characteristically elevated in chronic inflammation, probably under the stimulus of interleukin 1, a protein hormone released by activated macrophages. These "phase reactants" include gamma globulin, the third component of complement, haptoglobin, alpha$_1$ antitrypsin, orosomucoid, and fibrinogen. The latter is usually not measured since protein electrophoresis is routinely done on serum rather than plasma. Elevation of these proteins is responsible for the increased rate of red blood cell sedimentation which is so commonly observed.

It is often difficult to detect iron deficiency in a patient with chronic inflammation. The serum iron is low, and red blood cell protoporphyrin is increased in both conditions. When iron deficiency is superimposed on a chronic inflammatory state, the serum ferritin falls and transferrin level rises, usually to within normal limits. Under such circumstances, the amount of storage iron in the bone marrow is unpredictable. This problem is commonly encountered in patients with rheumatoid arthritis who may have developed iron deficiency owing to gastrointestinal blood loss. Because of this diagnostic uncertainty, it is often prudent to give such a patient a trial of iron and ascertain whether the hemoglobin level increases. However, it is important to avoid prolonged administration of iron unless a true deficiency state persists.

PATHOGENESIS   The anemia of chronic inflammation is primarily due to defective red blood cell production and failure to compensate for the slightly decreased red blood cell life span. The subnormal amounts of iron in erythroblasts, in spite of an abundance of storage iron, suggest a defect in the transfer of iron to the developing erythroid cells. The cells that are formed are somewhat "iron deficient," and therefore tend to be small and pale. As in true iron deficiency, increased red blood cell protoporphyrin reflects the reduced availability of iron for heme synthesis. This defect can be quantitated by iron kinetic studies. If radioactive iron bound to transferrin is administered, there is normal uptake into erythroblasts and incorporation into circulating red cells. In contrast, if hemoglobin labeled with radioactive iron is injected, the incorporation of label into circulating red cells is only half normal. The hyperplastic mononuclear phagocyte system which is responsible for decreased survival of circulating red cells probably traps the hemoglobin iron and prevents its transfer to the bone marrow. The macrophages' increased avidity for iron may be due to one of the actions of interleukin 1, i.e., release of lactoferrin from neutrophils. The iron-binding protein lactoferrin captures free iron and rapidly transfers it to macrophages.

The modest suppression of red blood cell production is caused in part by decreased availability of iron. In addition, erythropoietin levels tend to be lower than expected for the degree of anemia. However, erythropoietin levels are not as low as in the anemia of renal failure (see below) and probably do not play a significant role in the pathogenesis of the anemia.

MANAGEMENT   The anemia of chronic inflammation is not responsive to hematinic agents such as iron, folic acid, or vitamin B$_{12}$. Since the anemia is seldom severe, blood transfusion is rarely indicated. Efforts should be directed toward correcting the underlying disorder. In addition, if the anemia is more severe than expected, it is essential to search for other factors such as blood loss or drug-induced myelosuppression that could contribute to the reduction of red blood cell mass.

ANEMIA OF UREMIA

Anemia almost always accompanies the uremic syndrome (Chap. 224). Although the hemoglobin level is highly variable among uremic patients, the severity of the anemia is roughly proportional to the degree of azotemia. The etiology of the renal failure usually has little bearing on the extent of anemia. However, for any level of serum creatinine patients with polycystic disease tend to be less anemic than those with other types of renal disease. In contrast to anemias associated with other chronic disorders discussed in this chapter, the anemia of uremia can be very severe, with hemoglobin levels as low as 40 g/L. However, patients often tolerate such marked anemia fairly well. This is largely due to compensatory adjustments such as redistribution of blood flow and a decrease in the oxygen affinity of the blood (see Chap. 61).

The anemia of uremia is normochromic and normocytic. Examination of the bone marrow seldom reveals any abnormalities. Red blood cell morphology is usually normal. In about one-third of patients, so-called burr cells are seen in the peripheral blood smear. These red blood cells have a characteristic evenly scalloped border (see Fig. A5-9). Neither the degree of anemia nor the red blood cell life span is influenced by the presence of burr cells. In most patients the corrected reticulocyte count is low and the red blood cell survival is only modestly decreased. Thus the low red blood cell mass is due to decreased red blood cell production. The primary basis for this defect is that the diseased kidneys are unable to secrete adequate amounts of erythropoietin. Plasma erythropoietin levels are lower than those of nonuremic patients with a comparable degree of anemia. Erythropoiesis is further impaired but not abolished in patients who have undergone bilateral nephrectomy. In addition, red blood cell production may be suppressed by the accumulation of substances that are normally cleared by the kidneys. Iron kinetic measurements reveal impaired incorporation of iron into circulating red blood cells. Thus, it is likely that the anemia is due in part to ineffective erythropoiesis (see Chap. 290). Improvement in the rate of utilization of iron by the bone marrow has been noted following hemodialysis.

A small minority of uremic patients, particularly those with advanced disease, have brisk hemolysis. Red blood cell survival studies indicate that the hemolysis is due to extracorpuscular factors. Either metabolic or mechanical factors may contribute to the hemolysis. Some patients may acquire a defect in the hexose monophosphate shunt which renders the red blood cell vulnerable to the formation of Heinz bodies (see Chap. 294). The hemolysis can be aggravated by oxidant drugs or oxidant compounds such as chloramine in the dialysis bath. If the renal failure is due to thrombotic thrombocytopenic purpura or hemolytic-uremic syndrome, patients will have a severe form of microangiopathic hemolytic anemia, with characteristic abnormalities of red blood cell morphology (see Chap. 294).

In some patients aluminum salts that contaminate the tap water used in hemodialysis cause a worsening of anemia and the emergence of microcytosis and hypochromia.

Treatment of the anemia of uremia should focus on an attempt to reverse the renal failure. The anemia may be modestly improved following hemodialysis. A prompt and dramatic correction of the anemia follows successful renal transplantation. Occasionally, polycythemia may be encountered following the renal engraftment, and may be a harbinger of impending rejection. In those patients who are not candidates for renal transplantation the administration of androgens provides a modest stimulation of erythropoiesis, particularly in patients who have not undergone bilateral nephrectomy.

The treatment of the anemia of uremia has been revolutionized by the development of recombinant human erythropoietin. Administration of this genetically engineered product thrice weekly by intravenous infusion results in correction of anemia and gratifying symptomatic improvement. The agent is identical in structure to native erythropoietin and therefore safe and virtually free of side effects. However, overtreatment should be avoided since it can aggravate hypertension and increase the likelihood of thromboses. Accordingly, sufficient recombinant erythropoietin should be given to maintain the patient's hematocrit between 0.33 and 0.38.

It is important to be aware of other factors that may aggravate the anemia of renal disease. Uremic patients have a propensity to hemorrhage, owing to a qualitative defect in platelet function. Thus, gastrointestinal blood loss is commonly encountered. Furthermore a small but significant amount of blood loss occurs during hemodialysis. For these reasons some uremic patients become iron deficient. Folic acid deficiency may also occur, owing to the poor nutrition of many patients or to the loss of this vitamin during dialysis.

ANEMIA SECONDARY TO ENDOCRINE FAILURE

A number of hormones, including thyroxine, glucocorticoids, testosterone, and growth hormone are known to affect proliferation of human erythroid cells in vitro. Therefore it is not surprising that a mild to moderate normochromic-normocytic anemia generally accompanies a number of endocrine deficiency states, including hypothyroidism, Addison's disease, hypogonadism, and panhypopituitarism. It is possible that the anemias associated with hypothyroidism and hypopituitarism are related to the decreased need for oxygen transport, since oxygen consumption is reduced when thyroid hormone or growth hormone is lacking.

The anemia of *myxedema* is usually normocytic. Red blood cell life span is normal and erythropoiesis is effective. A minority of patients have macrocytic red blood cells which can usually be attributed to either folic acid or B_{12} deficiency. Patients with myxedema have an increased incidence of pernicious anemia. Hypothyroid patients, particularly females with menorrhagia, often develop iron deficiency and a microcytic anemia. Because the plasma volume may be reduced along with the red blood cell mass, the anemia of hypothyroidism may be masked. Since the signs and symptoms of myxedema are sometimes elusive, this diagnosis should be considered in the evaluation of any patient with unexplained anemia.

The anemia of *Addison's disease* is also masked by a decrease in plasma volume. Untreated patients have an average hemoglobin level of about 130 g/L. Upon hormone replacement, the plasma volume is rapidly reconstituted and the hemoglobin level falls to 80 percent of its pretreatment value. With continued therapy, the red blood cell mass returns to normal.

Testosterone has a physiologic influence on red blood cell mass. During passage through adolescence the mean hemoglobin level of males increases from 130 to 150 g/L. Eunuchoid males generally have a mean hemoglobin level averaging 130 g/L. Pituitary dysfunction or ablation is associated with a mild normochromic normocytic anemia as well as occasional leukopenia.

The anemias secondary to endocrine failure are all readily corrected when adequate hormone replacement is given.

ANEMIA OF LIVER DISEASE

Patients with chronic liver disease, regardless of etiology, usually have a mild to moderate anemia which is normocytic or slightly macrocytic. An increased plasma volume may artificially lower the hematocrit and make the anemia seem worse than it is. Red blood cell morphology is normal, except for the presence of target cells (see Fig. A5-3) and occasional stomatocytes, which have increased membrane surface area owing to increased deposits of cholesterol and phospholipid. The bone marrow is usually normal. Erythropoiesis fails to compensate for a moderate shortening of red blood cell life span. The anemia persists as long as hepatic function is defective, but it may be corrected if normal hepatic function can be restored.

The situation is much more complex in patients with *alcoholic*

liver disease. Many factors can contribute to the development of anemia. Alcohol is a direct suppressor of erythropoiesis. In alcoholics who have continued to drink up to the time of clinical evaluation, the bone marrow often reveals vacuoles in the cytoplasm of red and white blood cell precursors. In addition, ringed sideroblasts may be observed, particularly in patients who are malnourished. In alcoholics there is often suboptimal intake of dietary folic acid and impairment of folate utilization. Furthermore, alcoholics commonly develop significant hemorrhage from gastritis, esophageal varices, or duodenal ulcer, which contributes to the anemia. The risk of gastrointestinal blood loss is further increased by the presence of thrombocytopenia or deficiencies in soluble clotting factors. Although alcoholics usually have increased iron stores, they may become iron-deficient after prolonged gastrointestinal bleeding. Rarely patients with alcoholic cirrhosis develop a severe hemolytic anemia accompanied by the appearance of rigid red blood cells with irregular borders called acanthocytes or "spur" cells (see Fig. A5-8). This entity is discussed in detail in Chap. 294. In addition, alcoholics may acquire a defect in the erythrocyte hexose monophosphate shunt, similar to that encountered in patients with uremia.

REFERENCES

BUDMAN DR, STEINBERG AD: Hematologic aspects of systemic lupus erythematosus. Ann Intern Med 86:220, 1977
ESCHBACH JW, ADAMSON J: Anemia of end-stage renal disease. Kideny Int 28:1, 1985
——— et al: Correction of the anemia of end-stage renal disease with recombinant human erythropoietin. N Engl J Med 316:73, 1987
LEE GR: The anemia of chronic disease. Semin Hematol 20:61, 1983
MOWAT AG: Hematologic abnormalities in rheumatoid arthritis. Semin Arthritis Rheum 1:195, 1972
NEFF MS et al: Anemia in chronic renal failure. Acta Endocrinol 271(Suppl):80, 1985
SAVAGE D, LINDENBAUM J: Anemia in alcoholics. Medicine 65:322, 1986

294 HEMOLYTIC ANEMIAS

RICHARD A. COOPER / H. FRANKLIN BUNN

Red blood cells undergo premature destruction by two general mechanisms. First, red blood cells may lyse in the circulation and release their contents directly into the plasma. Intravascular hemolysis may be caused by trauma to the red blood cell, by fixation of complement to the red blood cell, or by exogenous toxins. Second, and more commonly, red blood cells are taken up by macrophages in the spleen and liver (mononuclear-phagocyte system), where they are destroyed and digested (extravascular lysis). The mononuclear-phagocyte system clears the cells from the circulation under two general conditions: first, the presence of surface abnormalities such as bound immunoglobulin for which macrophages have specific receptors; second, the presence of physical characteristics that limit the deformability of red blood cells, thereby impeding their ability to traverse the fine filtering system of the spleen.

The discoid shape of red blood cells favors deformability, providing a surface area that is 60 to 70 percent in excess of the minimum that is necessary to encompass the content of the cell. Deformability is determined by three independent variables: (1) the viscoelastic properties of the red blood cell membrane, (2) the ratio of surface area to volume, and (3) the intracellular concentration of hemoglobin or the aggregation of hemoglobin into polymers or precipitates.

One or more of these factors play a role in the pathogenesis of the various hemolytic anemias that are described in this chapter. A classification of these anemias is shown in Table 294-1. A number of clinical and laboratory features are shared by various types of hemolytic anemia. Patients with congenital hemolysis often have

TABLE 294-1   Hemolytic anemias: Classification based on mechanism of hemolysis

Extracorpuscular
1 Extrinsic factors
  a Splenomegaly
  b Antibody: immunohemolytic anemias
  c Mechanical trauma: microangiopathic hemolytic anemia
  d Direct toxic effect: malaria, clostridial infection, etc.

Intracorpuscular
2 Membrane abnormalities
  a Spur cell anemia
  b Paroxysmal nocturnal hemoglobinuria
  c Hereditary spherocytosis (rare: elliptocytosis, stomatocytosis)
3 Abnormalities of red blood cell interior
  a Enzyme defects
  b Defects in the hexose monophosphate shunt
  c Hemoglobinopathies
  d Thalassemias

Acquired (1)

Hereditary (2, 3)

lifelong anemia and may have a positive family history. Splenomegaly is seen in most chronic hemolytic anemias, both congenital and acquired. Patients with significant red blood cell turnover may be icteric, owing to an increase in unconjugated bilirubin.

LABORATORY EVALUATION OF HEMOLYSIS

The reticulocyte count is the single most useful test in the initial evaluation (Table 294-2). Patients with hemolytic anemia generally have a brisk reticulocytosis. The bone marrow predictably reveals erythroid hyperplasia. Since it seldom provides useful additional information, a bone marrow examination is generally not indicated in the evaluation of a patient with hemolytic anemia, unless an associated disorder such as lymphoma is suspected.

A number of serum tests are useful in establishing the presence of hemolysis (see Table 294-2), most importantly, the measurement of bilirubin, a tetrapyrrole formed from the oxidative catabolism of heme. Unconjugated or "indirect" bilirubin circulates in the plasma in transit from the mononuclear-phagocyte system to the liver where it is conjugated. When measured accurately, unconjugated bilirubin is a reliable guide to the presence of increased heme catabolism and is usually elevated in patients with hemolysis. The serum level of conjugated or "direct" bilirubin is normal unless the patient has

TABLE 294-2   Laboratory evaluation of hemolysis

	Moderate hemolysis (RBC life span 20–40 days)	Severe hemolysis (RBC life span 5–20 days)
HEMATOLOGIC		
Routine blood film	Polychromatophilia	Polychromatophilia
Reticulocyte count	↑	↑ ↑
Bone marrow examination	Erythroid hyperplasia	Erythroid hyperplasia
PLASMA OR SERUM		
Bilirubin	↑ Unconjugated	↑ Unconjugated
Haptoglobin	↓ , absent	Absent
Hemopexin	Normal, ↓	↓ , absent
Plasma hemoglobin		
Lactate dehydrogenase	↑ (variable)	↑ ↑ (variable)
Methemalbumin	0	+ *
URINE		
Bilirubin	0	0
Urobilinogen	Variable	Variable
Hemosiderin	0, +	+
Hemoglobin	0	+ *

* Intravascular hemolysis.

associated hepatic or biliary dysfunction. Unconjugated bilirubin is also increased in patients with ineffective erythropoiesis, a condition in which there is enhanced destruction of red cell precursors within the bone marrow. Since circulating unconjugated bilirubin is tightly bound to albumin, it does not pass through renal glomeruli. Thus, patients with hemolytic anemia have acholuric jaundice, whereas the hyperbilirubinemia of liver disease is associated with bilirubin in the urine.

Other serum tests are also useful in the assessment of hemolysis. Haptoglobin is an alpha globulin which is present in high concentration (~ 1.0 g/L) in the plasma (and serum). It binds specifically and tightly to the protein (globin) in hemoglobin. The hemoglobin-haptoglobin complex is cleared within minutes by the mononuclear-phagocyte system, while free haptoglobin has a long circulation time ($t_{1/2} = 4$ days). Thus, patients with significant hemolysis, either intravascular or extravascular, have low or absent levels of serum haptoglobin. Haptoglobin synthesis is decreased in patients with hepatocellular disease. Conversely, synthesis is enhanced in inflammatory states. Haptoglobin, like alpha$_1$ antitrypsin, orosomucoid, and the third component of complement are acute phase reactants. These facts must be considered in the interpretation of serum haptoglobin. Hemopexin is a plasma beta globulin which binds specifically to heme. It becomes depleted in patients with moderate and severe hemolysis. In addition to that bound by hemopexin, some of the heme from circulating free hemoglobin is transferred to albumin, resulting in the formation of methemalbumin. This complex is encountered only in severe intravascular hemolysis. Plasma hemoglobin is increased in proportion to the degree of hemolysis, but may be falsely elevated owing to lysis of red cells in vitro.

Once the haptoglobin binding capacity of the plasma is exceeded, free hemoglobin permeates renal glomeruli, primarily as $\alpha\beta$ dimers with a molecular weight of 32,000. This filtered hemoglobin is reabsorbed by the proximal tubule, where it is catabolized in situ, and the heme iron is incorporated into storage proteins (ferritin and hemosiderin). The presence of hemosiderin in the urine, detected by staining the sediment with Prussian blue, indicates that a significant amount of circulating free hemoglobin has been filtered by the kidneys. When the absorptive capacity of the tubular cells is exceeded, hemoglobinuria ensues. The presence of hemoglobinuria indicates severe intravascular hemolysis. Sometimes the clinician is faced with the dilemma of whether benzidine-positive heme pigment in the urine is hemoglobin or myoglobin. The easiest way to distinguish between these alternatives is to examine an anticoagulated blood specimen after centrifugation. The plasma of patients with hemoglobinuria has a reddish-brown color. Conversely, patients with myoglobinuria have normal-appearing plasma. Because of its higher molecular weight, hemoglobin has lower glomerular permeability than myoglobin and is less rapidly cleared by the kidneys.

Tagging red cells with an appropriate isotopic label provides the most direct and precise measure of cell survival. The most commonly used label is sodium [^{51}Cr]chromate. Since it does not bind irreversibly to red cells, the measured survival of normal red cells ($t_{1/2} = 26$ to 32 days) is shorter than the true red cell survival ($t_{1/2} \simeq 60$ days). Such studies are not necessary or indicated in the diagnostic workup of the majority of patients with hemolytic anemia. However, scanning with a collimated detector can be employed to monitor the sequestration of ^{51}Cr-tagged red cells in the liver and spleen. This approach is sometimes useful in evaluating patients for possible splenectomy.

RED CELL MORPHOLOGY AS A CLUE TO DIAGNOSIS   Most hemolytic disorders are associated with a change in the morphologic appearance of red blood cells. Some of these are depicted in Atlas 5. Spherocytes are the most common morphologic abnormality in hemolytic diseases. Small numbers occur in many disorders. They are most striking in patients with hereditary spherocytosis and in patients with warm antibody-induced immunohemolytic disease (Figs. A5-10 and A5-11). Spherocytes are the hallmark of splenic conditioning. Fragmented red blood cells suggest traumatic injury of the red cell including valve hemolysis, one of the microangiopathic hemolytic anemias [thrombotic thrombocytopenic purpura (Fig. A5-7), hemolytic uremic syndrome], or disseminated intravascular coagulation. Target-shaped red blood cells which are well filled with hemoglobin occur in patients with hemoglobin C. They are prevalent in sickle cell anemia, where they were first described, and they are found in patients with the underhydrated form of hereditary stomatocytosis. The most common cause of target cells is liver disease (Fig. A5-3). Target cells which are deficient in hemoglobin (hypochromic) are the hallmark of the thalassemia syndromes (Fig. A5-5).

Spiculated red blood cells often cause confusion because of the frequency with which they are induced as an artifact during the preparation of a blood smear. Under these conditions, they are particularly frequent at the edges of the smear. When surrounded by otherwise normal-appearing red blood cells, spiculated red blood cells can be a clue to diagnosis. They occur, usually in small numbers, in conjunction with uremia or following splenectomy even in the absence of an underlying red blood cell disorder. Bizarrely spiculated red blood cells (acanthocytes) occur in the rare condition abetalipoproteinemia (Chap. 326) and in anorexia nervosa; however, in each of these instances minimal hemolysis is present. As discussed below, acanthocytes are a striking feature of spur cell anemia (Fig. A5-8).

Permanently sickled, crescent-shaped red blood cells (Fig. A5-6) are the hallmark of sickle cell anemia. Boat-shaped red cells are a clue to the double heterozygous state, hemoglobin SC disease. The presence of both crescent-shaped cells and hypochromic target cells on the same smear is suggestive of the doubly heterozygous state, sickle cell–β thalassemia (see Chap. 295).

While in no case can the peripheral blood smear be totally diagnostic, in many it is a low-cost, important clue to the diagnosis. In addition to red blood cell morphology, a large battery of specific diagnostic tests are available for determining the etiology of the various hemolytic anemias. These are discussed in broad outline in Chap. 61 (Table 61-1) and in detail in this chapter.

EXTRINSIC CAUSES OF HEMOLYSIS

SPLENOMEGALY The spleen is particularly efficient in trapping and destroying red blood cells which have minimal defects, often so mild as to be undetectable by in vitro techniques. This unique ability of the spleen to filter mildly damaged red blood cells results from its unusual vascular anatomy. Almost all the blood circulating through the spleen flows rapidly from arterioles in the white pulp to sinuses in the spleen's red pulp, and then on into the venous system. In contrast, a small portion of splenic blood flow (normally 1 to 2 percent) leaves the arterioles of the white pulp to enter a nonendothelialized portion of the spleen. In this sense, it is extravascular, although the entire spleen may be considered as a specialized part of the vascular system. This blood passes into the "marginal zone" of the lymphatic white pulp. Although the cells which occupy this zone are not phagocytic, they serve as a mechanical filter hindering the progress of severely damaged red blood cells. As red blood cells leave this zone and enter the red pulp, they flow into narrow cords which end blindly but which communicate with sinuses through small openings between the lining cells of the sinuses. These openings, averaging 3 μm in diameter, test the ability of red blood cells to undergo a deformation of shape. Red blood cells which do not pass the stringent test imposed upon them by the spleen filter are engulfed by phagocytic cells and destroyed.

The normal spleen poses no threat to normal red blood cells. However, splenomegaly exaggerates the adverse conditions to which red blood cells are exposed. Splenic enlargement may be considered in three broad categories. In the first are infiltrative disease (such as myeloproliferative disorders, Chap. 297), lymphomas (Chap. 302), and storage diseases (such as Gaucher's disease, Chap. 331). In the second are systemic inflammatory diseases leading to splenic hypertrophy. In the third are diseases which cause congestive splenomegaly. Hemolysis may occur whenever the spleen is enlarged. Its occurrence

TABLE 294-3 Hemolysis due to antibodies

I Warm-antibody immunohemolytic anemia
  A Idiopathic
  B Lymphomas: Chronic lymphocytic leukemia, non-Hodgkin's lymphomas, Hodgkin's disease (infrequent)
  C Systemic lupus erythematosus
  D Tumors (rare)
  E Drugs
    1 α-Methyldopa type
    2 Penicillin type (hapten)
    3 Quinidine type (innocent bystander)
II Cold-antibody immunohemolytic anemia
  A Cold agglutinin disease
    1 Acute: Mycoplasma infection, infectious mononucleosis
    2 Chronic: Idiopathic, lymphoma
  B Paroxysmal cold hemoglobinuria

is least predictable in infiltrative diseases of the spleen where substantial splenomegaly may exist with no apparent hemolysis. Inflammatory and congestive splenomegaly are commonly associated with mild to moderate shortening of red blood cell survival.

RED CELL ANTIBODIES Immune hemolysis in the adult may be induced by three general types of antibodies:

1 Alloantibodies acquired by blood transfusions or pregnancies and directed against transfused red blood cells (Chap. 286).
2 Antibodies reactive at body temperature and directed against the patient's own red blood cells (Table 294-3).
3 Antibodies reactive in the cold and directed against the patient's own red blood cells (Table 294-3).

Coombs' antiglobulin test is the major tool for diagnosing these disorders. This test relies on the ability of antibodies prepared in animals and directed against specific human serum proteins to agglutinate red blood cells if these human serum proteins are present on the red blood cell surface. The serum proteins of particular interest are IgG and C3. The ability of anti-IgG or anti-C3 antiserums to agglutinate the patient's red blood cells is referred to as the *direct Coombs test*. At times it is advantageous to know whether there is antibody in the serum of patients which is reactive against other human red blood cells, e.g., in cross matching prior to blood transfusion (Chap. 286). To determine this, an *indirect Coombs test* is performed by incubating normal ABO- and Rh-compatible red blood cells with the patient's serum and subsequently performing a direct Coombs test on these incubated red cells.

"Warm" antibodies Antibodies which react at body temperature are usually of the IgG class, although occasionally they are IgA. They induce a pattern of hemolysis which affects both the patient's own cells and normal transfused cells. This acquired syndrome is frequently designated *autoimmune hemolytic anemia*. In recent years, as a number of drugs which induce this clinical syndrome have become recognized, attention has focused on the exogenous factors which may underlie the formation of these red blood cell antibodies, and the expression *immunohemolytic anemia* is preferred.

CLINICAL MANIFESTATIONS Warm-antibody immunohemolytic anemia occurs at all ages but is more common in adults, particularly women and older individuals. In approximately one-fourth of patients this disorder occurs as a complication of an underlying disease affecting the immune system, especially chronic lymphocytic leukemia, non-Hodgkin's lymphoma, and systemic lupus erythematosus (SLE). Occasionally, immunohemolytic anemia is seen in patients with advanced, active Hodgkin's disease. Case reports link it to a variety of nonlymphoid neoplasms.

The presentation and course of immunohemolytic anemia are quite variable. In its mildest form, the only manifestation is a positive direct Coombs test. In this instance, insufficient antibody is present on the red blood cell surface to permit the reticuloendothelial system to recognize the cell as abnormal. This is particularly common in SLE. A large fraction of patients with immunohemolytic anemia have a chronic mild anemia and splenomegaly. The direct Coombs test is positive for IgG but seldom for C3, and the indirect Coombs test is negative. In other cases this disorder may be more severe, with hemoglobin levels less than 70 g/L and reticulocyte counts of 30 percent and higher. Spherocytosis is usually marked (Fig. A5-11). Coombs' test is positive for IgG and frequently for C3 as well. Large quantities of antibody are present not only on the patient's red blood cells but also in the patient's serum as demonstrated by the indirect Coombs test. Thrombocytopenia may also be present. The coexistence of immune destruction of red blood cells and platelets is referred to as *Evans' syndrome*, a disorder in which separate antibodies are directed against platelets and red blood cells. In its most severe form, immunohemolytic anemia presents with fulminant, overwhelming hemolysis associated with hemoglobinemia, hemoglobinuria, and shock, a syndrome which may be fatal.

Associated findings include hyperbilirubinemia, decreased or absent haptoglobin levels, and occasionally hepatomegaly. Fever and abdominal pain occur in some patients. Venous thrombosis occurs occasionally, the most frequent site being the deep veins of the legs, but thrombosis of mesenteric and portal veins has also been reported. Arterial thromboses occur as well.

PATHOGENESIS   Little is known about the origin of red blood cell antibodies in the immunohemolytic anemias. Much more information exists concerning the mechanism of destruction of red blood cells coated with IgG antibodies. Although spherocytosis is often a prominent feature of hemolysis in vivo, the simple exposure of normal red blood cells to IgG antibodies does not lead to spherocytosis in vitro. However, human red blood cells coated with IgG antibodies are bound to the surface of monocytes or splenic macrophages and undergo a spherical transformation. The ability to cause this red blood cell–leukocyte interaction is greatest with IgG of subclasses 1 and 3 (the most common subclasses). It is not shared by IgM or IgA. However, C3 on the red blood cell surface also promotes this cell-cell interaction, but binding may be more transient because of the ability of the plasma C3 inactivator to release bound cells. Indeed, IgG and C3 behave in a synergistic fashion in this regard, accounting for the more severe hemolytic disease in patients in whom both IgG and C3 are present on the red blood cell surface. Since the slow flow compartment of the spleen is particularly efficient in trapping red blood cells which are coated with IgG antibodies, the spleen is the major site of red blood cell destruction in this disorder.

THERAPY AND PROGNOSIS   In the initial evaluation of the patient, it is important to rule out drugs which are known to cause immunohemolytic anemia. This topic is discussed below.

Patients having a mild degree of hemolysis usually do not require therapy. In those with clinically significant hemolysis, initial therapy consists of glucocorticoids (e.g., prednisone, 1.0 mg/kg per day). A rise in hemoglobin is frequently noted within 3 or 4 days and occurs in most patients within 1 week. Prednisone is continued until the hemoglobin level has risen to normal values, and thereafter it is tapered slowly over the course of several months. More than 75 percent of patients will achieve a significant and sustained reduction in hemolysis; however, in half of these patients the disease will relapse either during the period of steroid tapering or following the cessation of steroid therapy. Steroids appear to have two modes of action: an immediate effect due to inhibition of the clearance of IgG-coated red blood cells by the mononuclear phagocyte system, and a later effect due to steroid-induced inhibition of antibody synthesis.

Patients with severe anemia may require blood transfusions. Because the antibody in this disease is a "panagglutinin," reacting with all normal donor cells, the usual cross matching is impossible. The goal in selecting blood for transfusion is to avoid administering red cells with antigens to which patients have previously been sensitized and which are known to be associated with complement lysis and intravascular hemolysis. In addition to A and B, Kell, Kidd (Jkᵃ), and Duffy (Fy) account for almost all examples of this type of hemolysis. A common procedure is to adsorb the panagglutinin present in patient's serum using the patient's own red cells from which antibody has previously been eluted. Serum freed of autoan-

tibody in this way can then be tested for the presence of alloantibody to specific donor blood groups. ABO-compatible red cells matched in this fashion are administered slowly with attention paid to the possibility of an immediate-type transfusion reaction.

Splenectomy is the second line of therapy in this disorder. It is recommended for patients who cannot tolerate steroid therapy, in whom steroid therapy has been insufficient to control the disease process, or in whom a normal hematologic status can be maintained only with excessive doses of steroids. To provide prophylaxis against pneumococcal infection, a risk in splenectomized individuals, patients should be immunized with polyvalent pneumococcal antiserum.

Patients who have been refractory to steroid therapy and to splenectomy have been treated with immunosuppressive drugs. The greatest experience is with azathioprine and cyclophosphamide. A variable success rate has been reported with each. Recently, intravenous gamma globulin has been administered to rare patients who have failed to respond to the therapies mentioned above. There is insufficient experience to date to assess its efficacy.

In the majority of patients, this disease is controlled by steroid therapy alone, by splenectomy, or by a combination. In most of the remaining patients, a partial degree of control is achieved. Fatalities occur among three categories: first, rare patients with overwhelming hemolysis in whom death is directly attributable to anemia; second, those with major thrombotic events coincident with active hemolysis; third, those whose host defenses are impaired by glucocorticoids, splenectomy, and/or immunosuppressives. In patients in whom immunohemolysis develops as a complication of an underlying disorder, the prognosis is dominated by that of the primary disease.

Immunohemolytic anemia secondary to drugs   Drugs which have been directly related to immunohemolytic anemia are of three kinds, as distinguished by their three mechanisms of actions: (1) Drugs, such as α-methyldopa (Chap. 196), which induce a disorder identical almost in every respect to the warm-antibody immunohemolytic anemia described above. (2) Drugs of the penicillin type which can become associated with the red blood cell surface and induce the formation of an antibody directed against the red blood cell–drug complex. (3) Drugs, such as quinidine, that form a complex with plasma proteins to which an antibody forms; this drug–plasma protein–antibody complex settles out on red blood cells or platelets, inducing destruction on an "innocent bystander" basis.

α-METHYLDOPA-TYPE ANTIBODIES   A positive direct Coombs test is observed in up to 10 percent of patients receiving α-methyldopa therapy in a dose of 2.0 g daily. A small minority of these patients develop spherocytosis and hemolysis, often of severe degree. This "autoimmune" disorder may be triggered by a deficiency of suppressor T lymphocytes. Two distinctive features are that the indirect Coombs test is positive in almost all patients with hemolysis and that the red cells are coated with IgG but not C3. The IgG antibody is directed against the Rh complex as it is in most patients with idiopathic immunohemolytic anemia due to IgG. Hemolysis decreases over the course of several weeks after cessation of drug therapy, although the direct Coombs test may remain positive for more than 1 year.

PENICILLIN (HAPTEN)-INDUCED IMMUNOHEMOLYSIS   An antibody directed against "penicillinized" red blood cells induces hemolysis in patients receiving large, intravenous doses of penicillin and penicillin-type antibiotics (e.g., 15 to 20 million units of penicillin per day, or 12 to 15 g oxacillin per day). Hemolysis usually begins 7 to 14 days after the start of penicillin therapy and is associated with spherocytosis and hyperbilirubinemia. The patient's red blood cells are Coombs-positive for IgG during the period of penicillin therapy. An indirect Coombs test can be demonstrated with the patient's serum using normal red blood cells "penicillinized" in vitro. Hemolysis ceases abruptly when penicillin therapy is stopped, although the serum antibody can be demonstrated for many weeks.

INNOCENT BYSTANDER IMMUNOHEMOLYSIS   Innocent bystander antibodies may be of either the IgG or IgM class, and the antigen-antibody complexes which adhere to the red blood cell surface are capable of fixing complement. The drug-antibody complex dissociates from the red blood cell, leaving only C3 to be detected by Coombs' test. The pattern of hemolysis may be primarily extravascular red blood cell destruction, or it may be intravascular hemolysis due to complement lysis with hemoglobinemia, hemoglobinuria, and acute renal failure. This is an uncommon form of hemolysis despite the fact that the drugs associated with it are in very common usage. They include quinine and quinidine, isoniazid, sulfonamides, phenacetin, stibophen, p-aminosalicylic acid, dipyrone, and various insecticides.

Immune hemolysis due to cold-reactive antibodies Antibodies which are reactive in the cold induce hemolysis under two general conditions. First, in cold agglutinin disease IgM antibodies, usually reactive with the I antigen, occur spontaneously, in the course of a lymphoproliferative disease or as a complication of infectious mononucleosis or mycoplasma pneumonia. Second, in paroxysmal cold hemoglobinuria, antibodies of the IgG class (Donath-Landsteiner) occur spontaneously or as a complication of certain viral diseases or of syphilis.

COLD AGGLUTININ DISEASE *Clinical manifestations* Agglutination of red blood cells by IgM cold agglutinins is most profound at very low temperatures, and disagglutination occurs quickly upon warming. In most patients agglutination ceases at 32°C. The fixation of complement is a warm-reactive process. Therefore, patients may have very high titers of cold agglutinins as measured at low temperatures, but these antibodies may be inefficient in fixing complement to the cell surface and totally unable to induce agglutination at temperatures achieved in the bloodstream. Most cold agglutinins cause little or no shortening of red blood cell survival.

In mycoplasma pneumonia, cold agglutinins are very common, whereas only the occasional patient will have significant hemolysis about 5 to 10 days after recovery from the infection. Spherocytes may be seen occasionally, but the red blood cell morphology is usually normal. The antibody is directed against the I antigen, and the entire process is self-limited.

The cold agglutinin in infectious mononucleosis is most frequently directed against the i antigen, an antigen accessible on the surface of fetal red blood cells but not adult red blood cells. Therefore, this cold agglutinin is of serologic interest, but rarely induces hemolysis in humans. Antibody directed against the I antigen and complex antibodies involving both antigens have also been reported, with hemolysis.

A chronic form of cold-induced hemolysis occurs in patients de novo or in association with lymphoid neoplasms. It most commonly affects individuals in their seventh or eighth decades. The clinical manifestations relate to hemolysis and less commonly to agglutination of red blood cells in capillaries in those portions of the body exposed to low temperature, causing acrocyanosis. Gangrene is uncommon. Hemoglobin levels are usually above 100 g/L and rarely below 70 g/L. Reticulocytes are fewer in number than might be anticipated, presumably because of the selective destruction of young cells (including reticulocytes) in this disorder.

In most patients with cold agglutinin disease, the antibody titer is very high (e.g., 1:10,000) at 4°C and very low (e.g., 1:16) at 37°C. In some patients the antibody shows a flatter thermal spectrum with a moderately high titer at 4°C (e.g., 1:320) and a readily demonstrable titer at 37°C (e.g., 1:64). Hemolysis tends to be more severe in this latter group. The Coombs test demonstrates the presence of C3 on the red blood cell surface, but IgM (which is responsible for the C3 coating of red cells) is not found.

Pathogenesis The etiology of the antibody is unknown. It appears to exert its hemolytic effect not through agglutination per se but rather by the fixation of C3 to the red blood cell surface. The liver is particularly efficient at detecting red blood cells coated with C3 in the form of C3b and clearing them from the circulation. A plasma enzyme, C3 inactivator, is capable of cleaving C3b into a small fragment (C3c) which leaves the cell surface and reenters the plasma, and C3d, which adheres to the red blood cell surface where it is recognized as C3 in Coombs' test but not as C3 by the mononuclear phagocyte system. The presence of C3d on the red blood cell surface

decreases the ability of IgM anti-I to begin anew the complement sequence and thereby reestablish C3b on the red cell surface. Because of this, red blood cells that have survived in the circulation for a period of time have become "protected," while the younger red blood cells are in greater jeopardy.

Therapy The cutaneous manifestations of this disorder are best treated by maintaining the patient in a warm environment. Because transfusion of normal blood presents to the patient a large number of red blood cells which have not previously been exposed to the cold agglutinin and are therefore not "protected," transfusion may be associated with an acceleration of the hemolytic process. Splenectomy is usually not of value in this disorder. Glucocorticoids are of limited value, although patients with the panthermal variety of cold agglutinin disease may respond favorably to this therapy. Chlorambucil and cyclophosphamide are the most commonly employed agents in those patients in whom therapy is indicated. Although some patients have experienced a dramatic improvement, the effectiveness of this therapy is usually marginal.

Cold agglutinin disease tends to be chronic and unremitting. The overall prognosis is dominated by the underlying lymphoproliferative disease, if present. In those patients in whom cold agglutinin disease appears to arise spontaneously, lymphoproliferative disease may become apparent after several years.

PAROXYSMAL COLD HEMOGLOBINURIA (PCH) Now a rare disorder, PCH was more frequent at a time when tertiary syphilis was more prevalent. It results from the formation of the Donath-Landsteiner antibody, an IgG antibody which is directed against the P antigen complex and which can induce complement-mediated lysis. Attacks are precipitated by exposure to cold and are associated with hemoglobinemia and hemoglobinuria, chills and fever, back, leg, and abdominal pain, headache, and malaise. Recovery from the acute episode is prompt, and between episodes patients are asymptomatic. When this syndrome accompanies acute viral infections (e.g., measles and mumps), it is self-limited. When secondary to syphilis, it responds favorably to specific therapy for this disorder. No specific therapy exists for idiopathic cases. Despite the severity of individual episodes, the natural history of this disease extends over many years.

TRAUMA IN THE CIRCULATION Mechanical trauma can cause hemolysis in three ways: (1) when red blood cells flow through small vessels over the surface of bony prominences and are subject to external impact during various physical activities; (2) when they flow across a pressure gradient created by an abnormal heart valve or valve prosthesis and are disrupted by a shear stress; and (3) when the deposition of fibrin in the microvasculature exposes them to a physical impediment that fragments them (Table 294-4).

External impact Hemoglobinemia and hemoglobinuria have been observed in individuals who have undergone a prolonged march or a

TABLE 294-4 Disturbances of the formed elements of blood secondary to intravascular trauma

Etiology	Fragments	Hemolysis	Thrombo-cytopenia
Impact: march hemoglobinuria, etc.	0	+	0
Cardiac (turbulence):			
Aortic valve prosthesis	+ + +	+ + + +	0
Mitral valve prosthesis	+ +	+ +	0
Calcific aortic stenoses	+	±	0
Vessel disease:			
Malignant hypertension			
Eclampsia			
Renal graft rejection	+ + +	+	+
Hemangiomas			
Immune disease (scleroderma)			
Thrombotic thrombocytopenic purpura	+ + + +	+ + + +	+ + + +
Hemolytic uremic syndrome	+ + + +	+ + + +	+ + + +
Disseminated intravascular coagulation	+ +	±	+ + + +

prolonged jog, most typically on a hard surface and while wearing thin-soled shoes. The role of direct external trauma in this process has been demonstrated by the fact that hemolysis can be prevented by the insertion of a soft inner sole in the runner's shoes. Similar types of hemolysis have been described following karate and the playing of bongo drums. No abnormality of red blood cell morphology has been demonstrated, even during the acute episode, and no underlying red blood cell abnormality has been uncovered. A large percentage of individuals will develop hemoglobinemia and hemoglobinuria when exposed to the conditions described above. As a result of muscle damage during some of these activities, myoglobinuria may also occur, but renal function is preserved. No specific therapy is required.

Cardiac hemolysis Hemolysis associated with fragmented red blood cells (Fig. A5-7) occurs in approximately 10 percent of patients with artificial aortic valve prostheses. This incidence is somewhat greater with valves having stellite rather than silastic occluders, greater with small valves as compared with larger valves, and greater when valves are cloth-covered or when there is a paravalvular leak. Traumatic hemolysis is much less common in recipients of porcine valves. Severe hemolysis may occur after repair of ostium primum or endocardial cushion defects with a prosthetic patch. Mitral valve prostheses have also been associated with hemolysis, but since the pressure gradient across these is lower than across aortic prostheses, the incidence is lower. A moderately shortened red blood cell survival with little or no anemia occurs in some patients with severe calcific aortic stenosis. Indeed, almost any intracardiac lesion which alters hemodynamics may lead to some shortening of red blood cell survival. In addition, traumatic hemolysis has been observed in patients who have undergone aortofemoral bypass.

CLINICAL MANIFESTATIONS In severe cases hemoglobin levels fall to 50 to 70 g/L with reticulocytosis, fragmented red blood cells in the peripheral blood, depressed haptoglobin, elevated serum lactic dehydrogenase, and hemoglobinemia and hemoglobinuria. Iron loss (as hemoglobin or hemosiderin) in the urine may lead to iron deficiency. Direct Coombs test may rarely become positive.

PATHOGENESIS A number of factors combine to cause the fragmentation and destruction of red blood cells in this disorder. Direct mechanical trauma of red blood cells at the time of seating of the occluder of the prosthetic valve, the deposition of fibrin across disrupted attachment points, but probably most important, the shear stress resulting from turbulent blood flow may all result in the fragmentation of red blood cells. The last explains the higher incidence of hemolysis in patients who have a paravalvular leak and therefore greater velocity of blood flow across the aortic orifice during systole.

THERAPY AND PROGNOSIS Iron deficiency should be corrected by the administration of oral iron. The elevated hemoglobin which results may permit a decrease in the cardiac output and a slowing of the hemolytic rate. Limitation in physical activity also lessens the hemolytic rate. When these measures fail, any paravalvular leak must be repaired or the prosthetic valve replaced.

Deposition of fibrin in the microvasculature Fibrin deposition in the microvasculature fragments red blood cells and traps platelets under three general conditions: (1) abnormalities of the vessel wall in recognized disorders, such as malignant hypertension, eclampsia, rejection of a renal allograft, disseminated cancer, and hemangiomas; (2) two potentially fatal syndromes of unknown etiology, thrombotic thrombocytopenic purpura and the hemolytic uremic syndrome; and (3) disseminated intravascular coagulation.

ABNORMALITIES OF THE VESSEL WALL The degree of hemolysis induced by this family of disorders is usually quite mild, although the number of fragments in the peripheral blood may be striking. In occasional patients, thrombocytopenia may be severe. In each case, therapy is best directed at the primary disease. Thus, reversal of renal graft rejection, treatment of malignant hypertension and eclampsia, control of cancer, etc., lead to a cessation of the hemolytic process. The relative importance of the primary vascular abnormality and of the deposition of fibrin in causing hemolysis is unclear.

Thrombotic thrombocytopenic purpura (TTP) This disease of unknown etiology affects individuals of all ages but primarily young adults, more often women.

CLINICAL MANIFESTATIONS Hemolysis is a striking feature of this disease. Anemia occurs in association with fragmented red blood cells, nucleated red cells in the peripheral blood, an elevated reticulocyte count, and thrombocytopenia of varying degree. Platelet counts range from 5000 to 100,000 per cubic millimeter. Jaundice is common, and petechiae may be present, although usually to a less striking degree than in idiopathic thrombocytopenic purpura (ITP). Tests of coagulation, such as the prothrombin time, partial thromboplastin time, fibrinogen concentration, and the level of fibrinogen split products, are usually normal or only mildly abnormal. If the coagulation tests indicate disseminated intravascular coagulation, the diagnosis of TTP is doubtful. Erythroid hyperplasia and an increased number of megakaryocytes are present in the bone marrow. The life span of platelets is decreased to hours, and no site of organ localization of destroyed platelets is observed. A positive antinuclear antibody (ANA) is obtained in approximately 20 percent of patients. Some patients experience significant, although not severe, bleeding of uterine, gastrointestinal, or other origin. Fever is present in almost all patients, and many experience nonspecific constitutional symptoms such as nausea, abdominal pain, and arthralgias. The spleen and liver may be palpable.

The course of TTP spans days to weeks in most patients, but occasionally continues for months. As the disease progresses, the brain and kidneys become progressively involved, and their dysfunction is the ultimate cause of death in the majority of patients. Proteinuria and a moderate elevation of blood urea nitrogen may be found on initial presentation, and there is a continued rise in blood urea nitrogen and a fall in urine output as the disease progresses. Neurologic symptoms evolve in more than 90 percent of patients whose disease terminates in death. Initially, there may be changes in mental status such as confusion, delirium, or altered states of consciousness. Focal findings include seizures, hemiparesis, aphasia, and visual field defects. These neurologic symptoms may fluctuate and terminate in coma. Involvement of myocardial blood vessels may be a cause of sudden death in some patients.

PATHOGENESIS The etiology of TTP is unknown. Arterioles are filled with hyalin material, presumably fibrin and platelets, and similar material may be seen beneath the endothelium of otherwise uninvolved vessels. Immunofluorescence studies have shown the presence of immunoglobulin and complement in arterioles. Microaneurysms of arterioles are often present. Controversy exists concerning the specificity of these changes, some authorities noting them in the hemolytic uremic syndrome (particularly in the kidney) and in disseminated intravascular coagulation. An association with systemic lupus erythematosus (SLE), scleroderma, and Sjögren's syndrome suggests an immunologic etiology. A high-molecular-weight form of von Willebrand's protein, as well as a platelet-aggregating protein, have been identified in the plasma of TTP patients and may contribute significantly to the pathogenesis of the microvascular defect.

DIAGNOSIS The combination of hemolytic anemia with fragmented and nucleated red blood cells, thrombocytopenia, fever, neurologic disorders, and renal dysfunction is virtually pathognomonic of TTP. The diagnosis is further supported by the finding of normal coagulation tests, although occasional patients have an isolated abnormality of coagulation. Although they are not usually required for diagnosis, biopsies of skin and muscle, gingiva, lymph node, or bone marrow will frequently reveal the pathologic abnormalities described above. TTP should be considered in every patient in whom the diagnosis of ITP or Evans' syndrome (ITP plus immunohemolytic anemia) is made. The finding of fragmented red blood cells in the peripheral blood is particularly helpful in this regard. Because the clinical course can fluctuate widely, therapy is difficult to evaluate.

THERAPY AND PROGNOSIS Until recently, this disease was almost universally fatal. A large number of therapeutic modalities have been attempted with variable success. These include glucocorticoids, plasma exchange, splenectomy, and antiplatelet drugs. Patients are initially treated with high doses of glucocorticoids (100 to 1000 mg prednisone per day). However, additional therapy is indicated. The most consistent improvement (60 to 75 percent) has been noted with exchange transfusion or plasmapheresis. In most patients plasmapheresis is as effective as exchange transfusion. In others the response may depend upon the infusion of plasma. Splenectomy is also effective, but with a lower frequency of response and with additional risk in these critically ill patients. The benefit of antiplatelet drugs (dipyridamole, sulfinpyrazone, dextran, aspirin) is unclear, but they are commonly used together with the therapeutic measures described above. Aspirin may increase the risk of bleeding and should be employed with caution. Vincristine may be effective in otherwise refractory patients. Because of the ever-present risk of sudden death, therapy should be instituted promptly. Even deep coma is not a contraindication to therapy since full neurologic recovery is the rule in patients responding to therapy. If treatment is instituted early in the disease, remission occurs in approximately two-thirds of patients. Relapses have been noted in approximately 10 percent of patients but are usually responsive to therapeutic intervention.

Hemolytic uremic syndrome The hemolytic uremic syndrome is a disorder usually encountered in young children and has laboratory features similar to those of TTP. Often the patient has a prodrome of a viral-like illness. Less commonly, the disorder appears to be familial. Patients present with acute hemolytic anemia, thrombocytopenic purpura, and acute oliguric renal failure. Most patients have either hemoglobinuria or anuria. Unlike TTP, neurologic manifestations are uncommon. The peripheral blood findings and coagulation tests are usually indistinguishable from those of TTP. Pathologic changes are similar but restricted to the kidney. Patients are treated with dialysis and transfusions. The efficacy of glucocorticoids, dextran, and heparin is uncertain. The mortality in children ranges from 5 to 20 percent, but is considerably higher in adults. A disorder resembling the hemolytic-uremic syndrome has recently been described in adults treated with the antineoplastic drug mitomycin C, usually in combination with other drugs.

Disseminated intravascular coagulation (DIC) Red blood cell fragmentation in the microvasculature (microangiopathic hemolytic anemia) is seen in about one-fourth of patients with DIC (Chap. 289). The degree of hemolysis is much less in DIC than in either TTP or the hemolytic uremic syndrome, and anemia with reticulocytosis and nucleated red blood cells is distinctly rare.

DIRECT TOXIC EFFECTS A variety of infections may be associated with severe hemolysis. The microorganisms in bartonellosis (Chap. 123) and malaria (Chap. 159) directly parasitize red blood cells. Babesiosis (Chap. 164) also may cause a mild to moderate hemolytic anemia by direct parasitization of red blood cells.

Other infectious organisms exert their damaging effects on red blood cells indirectly. The most striking is that resulting from septicemia with *Clostridium welchii* (Chap. 107). The phospholipase produced by this organism is capable of cleaving the phosphoryl bond of lecithin thereby lysing human red blood cells. A mild, transient hemolysis frequently accompanies bacteremia with diverse organisms such as pneumococci, staphylococci, and *Escherichia coli*.

Hemolysis may result from the direct action of snake and spider venoms on the red blood cell. Although cobra venom is directly lytic in vitro, the clinical disease induced by the bite of the cobra is one of moderate hemolysis associated with spherocytosis. Spider bites are known to induce acute intravascular hemolysis associated with spherocytosis. It is thought that the brown recluse spider which inhabits the central and southern portions of the United States and portions of South America is responsible. The hemolytic disease continues for several days up to 1 week.

Copper has a direct hemolytic effect on red blood cells. Hemolysis has been observed following exposure of individuals to copper salts (such as during hemodialysis). In addition, the transient episodes of hemolysis observed in patients with Wilson's disease are probably due to copper toxicity.

The red blood cell membrane is unstable at temperatures above 49°C due to denaturation of the cytoskeletal protein, spectrin. When studied in vitro, the red blood cell undergoes a process of budding, cleavage, and resealing above this temperature. The same process is observed in individuals who have suffered extensive burns. These patients have prominent spherocytosis as well as hemoglobinemia and sometimes hemoglobinuria.

MEMBRANE ABNORMALITIES

ACQUIRED DISORDERS OF THE MEMBRANE There are two well-defined acquired disorders of the red blood cell membrane: spur cell anemia and paroxysmal nocturnal hemoglobinuria (PNH).

Spur cell anemia Hemolytic anemia with bizarre-shaped red blood cells occurs in some patients with severe hepatocellular disease. Most patients with spur cell anemia have advanced Laennec's cirrhosis. This hemolytic disorder is observed in approximately 5 percent of patients with manifestations of severe cirrhosis, such as ascites, jaundice, and hepatic encephalopathy. Spur cell anemia has also been reported in neonatal hepatitis.

CLINICAL MANIFESTATIONS Anemia is moderate to severe, with hematocrit levels ranging from 0.16 to 0.30. Thus, the anemia is more severe than is observed in otherwise uncomplicated cirrhosis, in which hematocrit levels are rarely below 0.28, unless there is accompanying folic acid deficiency, blood loss, iron deficiency, etc. (Chap. 293). Splenomegaly is a constant feature, and the spleen is generally more prominent than in patients who have cirrhosis but who do not have spur cell anemia. Jaundice is also a constant feature, and hepatic encephalopathy is common. Other tests of liver function are similar to values obtained in most patients with severe cirrhosis, although there is a tendency to longer prothrombin times. Chromium half-survival times of red blood cells are decreased to as short as 6 days (normal being 26 to 32 days), and red cell destruction is localized to the spleen. Normal transfused red blood cells have a survival similar to that of the patient's own red blood cells. Red blood cells are irregularly shaped with multiple spicules, and a small number of bizarre-shaped fragments are commonly seen on peripheral blood smears (see Fig. A5-8). Reticulocytes range from 5 to 15 percent.

PATHOGENESIS The surface membrane of spur cells contains 50 to 70 percent excess cholesterol, but its total phospholipid content is normal. In this way, spur cells are distinct from the more usual target red blood cells in liver disease, which possess an excess of both cholesterol and phospholipid. Cholesterol out of proportion to phospholipid decreases the fluidity of the spur cell membrane, and cell deformability is also decreased. Normal red blood cells acquire the spur abnormality when incubated in serum from affected patients. This results from the presence in serum of an abnormal low-density lipoprotein with an increased mole ratio of free (unesterified) cholesterol to phospholipid. Thus, red blood cells in spur cell anemia may be considered to be "innocent bystanders." These rigid, cholesterol-laden red blood cells are detected by the filtering system of the spleen, aided by congestive splenomegaly in cirrhosis. In contrast to circulating spur cells, normal red blood cells which have acquired cholesterol in vitro have an increased surface area and a decreased osmotic fragility, and they have a regular pattern of spicule deformity. This is also true in vivo for normal red blood cells during their initial 24 h in the patient's circulation. However, during continued circulation in vivo in the presence of the spleen, cholesterol-rich spur cells lose surface area and transform to the irregular pattern of spiculation associated with acanthocytes (see "Red Blood Cell Morphology" above). This process of membrane "conditioning" by the spleen continues, and the cell is destroyed in the spleen.

DIAGNOSIS Increasing anemia in a patient with chronic cirrhosis most commonly results from blood loss, folic acid deficiency, or iron deficiency. The hemolytic rate may increase transiently during periods of acute fatty liver. The combination of an elevated reticulocyte count and elevated bilirubin in the presence of the characteristic morphologic abnormality on peripheral blood smear is diagnostic. Red blood cells of similar morphologic appearance are seen in patients with abeta-lipoproteinemia. However, these individuals have a minimal amount of hemolysis.

Spur cells and acanthocytes must be distinguished from regularly scalloped, crenated red blood cells (echinocytes). These are a frequent artifact on blood smears, and they are present in some patients with uremia ("burr cells") (Fig. A5-9). Small, dense crenated spheres (spheroechinocytes) are sometimes seen in congenital nonspherocytic hemolytic anemia due to enzyme deficiencies in the Embden-Meyerhof pathway (see below).

TREATMENT Since normal red blood cells acquire the spur abnormality when transfused into patients with this form of anemia, transfusion therapy is of limited benefit. Attempts to influence red blood cell cholesterol by the use of various lipid-lowering agents have been unsuccessful. Splenectomy has been reported to prevent both the conditioning of red blood cells in the spleen and their premature destruction. However, splenectomy carries a high risk in patients with severe liver disease complicated by portal hypertension and coagulation defects, and it must be reserved for selected patients in whom hemolysis is a major clinical problem and who appear to be relatively good surgical risks.

PROGNOSIS In most patients spur cell anemia occurs during the late stages of cirrhosis, and more than 90 percent of patients succumb to their underlying liver disease within 1 year of the diagnosis of spur cell anemia.

Paroxysmal nocturnal hemoglobinuria (PNH) This condition is distinctive among hemolytic disorders in humans because it is an intracorpuscular defect acquired at the stem cell level. It occurs primarily in young adults.

CLINICAL MANIFESTATIONS Anemia is of exceedingly variable degree with hematocrit values of 0.20 and lower in occasional patients and normal values in others. Mild granulocytopenia and thrombocytopenia are commonly present. Although regarded as a classic feature of this disease, gross hemoglobinuria is present only intermittently in most patients, and never occurs in some. Hemosiderinuria is usually present. Other features of diagnostic significance are a low leukocyte alkaline phosphatase and a low red blood cell acetylcholinesterase. Red blood cells are normochromic and normocytic unless iron deficiency has occurred from the chronic loss of iron in the urine. The diagnosis is established by a positive acid hemolysis test or sucrose lysis test, both of which demonstrate the enhanced sensitivity of PNH red blood cells to complement (see below). Venous thrombosis is a common complication of this disorder, and has been reported in peripheral veins as well as in mesenteric, hepatic, portal, and cerebral veins. Thrombosis is a common cause of death in patients severely affected with PNH. A second manifestation, possibly related to thromboses in small veins, is the occurrence of back and abdominal pain similar in character to that which occurs in sickle cell anemia. Headache has also been reported. Since the widespread use of the sucrose lysis test, many patients have been discovered with mild, chronic disease.

PATHOGENESIS The underlying abnormality which affects red blood cells, granulocytes, and platelets in PNH is an inordinate sensitivity to complement. This may be demonstrated in vitro using a complement-fixing antibody. PNH red blood cells fix more C1 than normal red cells per unit of antibody present, and this C1 promotes more C3 fixation per molecule of C1 than is seen with normal red cells. However, antibody is not necessary for the lysis of red blood cells in PNH. Rather, C3 is readily fixed to the red blood cell surface by means of the alternate (properdin) pathway. Careful analytic procedures have demonstrated two and in some cases three separate populations of red blood cells [type 1 (normal), type 2, type 3] with varying sensitivities to complement in patients with PNH. The clinical manifestations relate directly to the proportion of the red blood cells produced that are most sensitive to complement. Although platelets share with red blood cells this sensitivity to complement, platelet survival is normal in PNH. However, a functional modification of

platelets induced by complement may underlie the thrombotic complications of this disease. The increased sensitivity of red blood cells to complement has been demonstrated to result from the lack of a red cell membrane regulatory protein, decay-accelerating factor (DAF), which inhibits activation of C3 at the membrane and, in type 3 PNH cells, a deficiency of C8 binding protein which inhibits activation of C8 and C9. It is surely of pathophysiologic relevance that these two proteins, along with leukocyte alkaline phosphatase and erythrocyte acetylcholinesterase, share a common glycan-phosphatidyl membrane anchor.

Since it affects granulocytes, platelets, and red blood cells but not lymphocytes, this defect is thought to occur because of an acquired change in the pluripotent stem cell which generates these cells. In this respect it is similar to both acute myelogenous leukemia and the myeloproliferative syndromes, disorders which appear to affect the stem cells responsible for platelet, granulocyte, and red blood cell production. A number of patients with PNH have subsequently developed acute myelogenous leukemia. The red blood cell abnormality characteristic of PNH (complement sensitivity) occurs to a mild degree in some patients with aplastic anemia and in some with myelofibrosis, further linking this series of bone marrow disorders. It appears likely that PNH results from a somatic mutation in the marrow stem cell pool.

DIAGNOSIS As indicated above, PNH is commonly undiagnosed for a period of months to years. The classic manifestation of gross hemoglobinuria may be present only intermittently, and an awareness of its presence may be obtained only by repeated questioning of the patient. In some patients, a chronic hemolytic process occurs without gross hemoglobinuria. Therefore, diagnoses such as refractory anemia, hemolytic anemia of unknown etiology, and pancytopenia are common in patients subsequently proven to have PNH. A decreased leukocyte alkaline phosphatase is a clue to the diagnosis, and the presence of hemosiderin in the urine sediment is strongly suggestive. Hemosiderinuria may occur with intravascular hemolysis of any etiology. However, only a few disorders in humans result in intravascular hemolysis. These are PNH, paroxysmal cold hemoglobinuria, hemolytic transfusion reaction, traumatic hemolysis, and hemolysis due to lysins (snake venom, C. welchii bacteremia) or to extensive acute burns. The acid hemolysis test is also positive in the rare congenital disorder hereditary erythrocytic multinuclearity with positive acidified-serum test (HEMPAS). In this latter disorder, complement sensitivity results from an inordinate fixation of C4 molecules per molecule of C1. Since this sensitivity exists in the classic (antibody-mediated) pathway but not in the alternate (properdin) pathway, spontaneous fixation of complement with lysis in vivo is not a feature of the HEMPAS disorder.

It should be noted that in PNH chromium survival studies often produce confusing information. This results from the bi- or trimodal population of red blood cells. The cells most sensitive to complement have a very short survival, and they account for a minority of circulating red blood cells, whereas the cells less sensitive to complement have a more normal survival and account for the majority of circulating cells. Thus, the chromium survival is longer than might be anticipated from other measures of hemoglobin turnover.

TREATMENT Transfusion therapy is useful in PNH not only for raising the hemoglobin level but also for suppressing the marrow production of red blood cells during episodes of sustained hemoglobinuria or of sustained painful crisis. The transfusion of blood prior to surgery may reduce the incidence of postoperative thrombotic complications. For reasons that are still unclear, whole blood transfusions frequently cause an exacerbation of the hemolytic process. This can be prevented by using washed red blood cells rather than whole blood.

Therapy with androgens frequently results in a rise of hemoglobin level. Adrenocortical steroids may also be effective in reducing the rate of hemolysis.

Because of iron loss in the urine, iron deficiency is common. An exacerbation of hemolysis often follows the administration of iron because of the formation of a large number of young red blood cells, many of which are sensitive to complement. This may be minimized by suppressing the bone marrow with transfusions.

Splenectomy has been undertaken in some patients with the hope of decreasing the hemolytic rate and the transfusion requirement. However, because of the limited therapeutic benefit and the increased surgical risk in patients with PNH, splenectomy cannot be recommended.

Anticoagulation with coumarin-type drugs may have some benefit in preventing thromboses, particularly in the postsurgical patient. On the other hand, therapy with heparin has been noted to cause an increased amount of hemolysis in some patients with PNH, and caution must be exercised when using this drug.

PROGNOSIS   Most patients with classic PNH have a life expectancy of less than 10 years, although some survive for much longer. A series of 17 patients surviving more than 20 years has been compiled by questioning hematologists nationally. In more than one-third of these patients, there had been an amelioration of disease symptoms, and in two patients PNH was totally quiescent. The major morbidity relates to venous thromboses. Despite the marked degree of iron deposition in the kidney, death from renal failure is rare. The prognosis is uncertain in patients in whom the manifestations of PNH are more subtle and in whom the diagnosis was made because of the widespread use of the sucrose lysis test. Some patients may lead a normal life.

CONGENITAL ABNORMALITIES OF THE RED CELL MEMBRANE

There are four types of inherited abnormalities of the red cell membrane: hereditary spherocytosis, hereditary elliptocytosis, hereditary pyropoikilocytosis, and hereditary stomatocytosis. Each syndrome may represent a group of disorders with differing structural defects. The molecular pathogenesis of these disorders has not been completely defined.

Hereditary spherocytosis

This is a disease of autosomal dominant inheritance in which intrinsically abnormal red blood cells are destroyed in the presence of an otherwise normal spleen. Its incidence is approximately 1:4500. In 20 percent of patients the absence of hematologic abnormalities in family members suggests that a spontaneous mutation has occurred. The disorder is sometimes clinically apparent in early infancy, but often escapes detection until adult life.

CLINICAL MANIFESTATIONS   The major clinical features of hereditary spherocytosis are anemia, splenomegaly, and jaundice. The prominence of the latter finding accounts for its prior designation "congenital hemolytic jaundice" and is due to an increased concentration of unconjugated (indirect-reacting) bilirubin in plasma. Jaundice may be intermittent and tends to be less pronounced in early childhood. Because of the increased bile pigment production, gallstones of pigment type are common, even in childhood. Compensatory normoblastic hyperplasia of the bone marrow occurs with the extension of red marrow into the midshafts of long bones and occasionally with extramedullary erythropoiesis, at times leading to the formation of paravertebral masses visible on chest x-ray. Because the bone marrow's capacity to increase erythropoiesis by six- to tenfold exceeds the usual rate of hemolysis in this disease, anemia is usually mild or moderate and may even be absent in an otherwise healthy individual. Compensation may be temporarily interrupted by episodes of erythroid hypoplasia precipitated by infections, often of a minor nature. Splenomegaly is a constant feature of hereditary spherocytosis. The hemolytic rate may increase transiently during systemic infections which induce further splenic enlargement. Chronic leg ulcers, similar to those observed in sickle cell anemia, occasionally occur.

The characteristic erythrocyte abnormality is the spherocyte (Fig. A5-10). The mean corpuscular volume (MCV) is usually normal or slightly decreased, and the mean corpuscular hemoglobin concentration (MCHC) is increased to 350 to 380 g/L. Spheroidicity may be quantitatively assessed in terms of osmotic fragility (Fig. 294-1). Because spherocytes have a decreased surface area per unit volume, they lyse more readily when exposed to solutions of low salt concentration. On microscopic examination spherocytes are usually

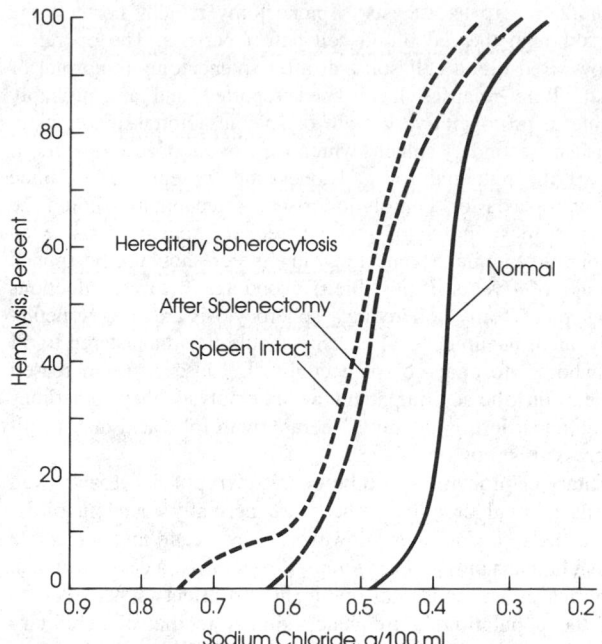

FIGURE 294-1   Osmotic fragility of red blood cells in hereditary spherocytosis. When the spleen is present, a small subpopulation of cells which are "conditioned" in the spleen form the fragile "tail" of the osmotic fragility curve. After splenectomy a single population exists which is more osmotically fragile than normal.

detected even when present in very small numbers. However, they will ordinarily not influence the osmotic fragility test unless they constitute more than 1 or 2 percent of the total cell population. A prominent increase in the osmotic fragility of red blood cells following sterile incubation of whole blood for 24 h at 37°C is also characteristic of hereditary spherocytosis. The autohemolysis test is an extension of this latter procedure and measures the amount of spontaneous hemolysis occurring after 48 h of sterile incubation. In hereditary spherocytosis about 10 to 50 percent of the red blood cells are lysed (versus less than 4 percent of normal red blood cells). Autohemolysis of these red blood cells is largely prevented by the addition of glucose prior to incubation.

PATHOGENESIS   The molecular abnormality in hereditary spherocytosis involves the proteins of the cytoskeleton. Nearly all patients have a significant deficiency of spectrin which correlates with the severity of the anemia. Some (perhaps most) patients have a decrease and/or a structural abnormality of ankyrin, the protein that links spectrin to protein 3 (see Fig. 290-6). The spheroidal contour and rigid structure of the red blood cells impede their passage through the spleen. There, the red blood cells are exposed to an environment in which their increased metabolic rate cannot be sustained. The first injury imposed upon them by the spleen is a further loss of surface membrane. This "conditioning" produces a subpopulation of hyperspheroidal red blood cells in the peripheral blood. These are subsequently destroyed in the spleen. The intracorpuscular nature of the red blood cell defect in hereditary spherocytosis is demonstrated by a diminished life span of the patient's red cells in normal subjects when the spleen is present and a normal survival of normal cells transfused into patients with hereditary spherocytosis.

DIAGNOSIS   Hereditary spherocytosis must be distinguished from the spherocytic hemolytic anemias associated with red blood cell antibodies. The family history is helpful, when present. The diagnosis of immune spherocytosis is usually readily established by a positive direct Coombs test. Spherocytes, often in considerable numbers, are seen in association with hemolysis induced by splenomegaly in patients with cirrhosis or chronic infections, and a few spherocytes are seen in the course of a wide variety of hemolytic disorders, particularly glucose-6-phosphate dehydrogenase (G6PD) deficiency.

TREATMENT AND PROGNOSIS   Splenectomy reliably corrects the anemia, although the red blood cell defect persists. The operative risk is low. Red blood cell survival after splenectomy is normal or nearly so. Rare relapses have been reported and are probably attributable to postoperative growth of splenic autotransplants or to hyperplasia of secondary spleens which were overlooked at operation. Because of the potential for gallstones and for episodes of bone marrow hypoplasia or hemolytic crises, splenectomy should be performed in most individuals with hereditary spherocytosis, even those with mild anemia. Splenectomy in children should be postponed until the age of 4 years, if possible. Beyond age 3, severe infections following splenectomy in hereditary spherocytosis are rare. Nonetheless, polyvalent pneumococcal vaccine should be administered to all patients who are to undergo splenectomy. Because of the increased requirement for folic acid in patients with hemolysis, they sometimes become deficient in this vitamin. Therapy with folic acid may result in an increased hemoglobin level.

Hereditary elliptocytosis and hereditary pyropoikilocytosis   Red blood cells of oval or elliptic shape are normally found in birds, reptiles, camels, and llamas; however, they occur in appreciable numbers in humans only in *hereditary elliptocytosis*, a disorder which is transmitted as an autosomal dominant and affects 1 per 4000 to 5000 of the population, a frequency similar to that of hereditary spherocytosis. It is also referred to as *hereditary ovalocytosis*. In most affected individuals, a structural abnormality of erythrocyte spectrin leads to impaired assembly. Others often have a deficiency of erythrocyte membrane protein 4.1, which is important in stabilizing the interaction of spectrin and actin in the cytoskeleton (see Fig. 290-6). Homozygotes with total absence of this protein have more marked hemolysis.

The great majority of patients manifest only mild hemolysis, with hemoglobin levels above 120 g/L, reticulocytes less than 4 percent, depressed haptoglobin levels, and red blood cell survivals within or just under the normal range. In 10 to 15 percent of patients the rate of hemolysis is substantially increased with chromium half-survival times of red blood cells as short as 5 days and reticulocytes ranging to 20 percent. Hemoglobin levels rarely fall below 90 to 100 g/L. Red blood cell destruction occurs predominantly in the spleen, which is enlarged in patients with overt hemolysis, and hemolysis is corrected by splenectomy.

In both the anemic and nonanemic varieties of this disorder the red blood cells are normochromic and normocytic. At least 25 percent and, more commonly, greater than 75 percent of red blood cells are elliptic, with an axial ratio (width/length) of less than 0.78. Patients with hemolysis frequently have microovalocytes, bizarre-shaped red blood cells, and red cell fragments, all of which increase in number following splenectomy. The degree of hemolysis does not correlate with the percentage of elliptocytes. Osmotic fragility is usually normal but may be increased in patients with overt hemolysis.

Hereditary pyropoikilocytosis (HPP) is thought to be related to hereditary elliptocytosis, since both have been reported in the same family. HPP is a rare disorder characterized by bizarre-shaped, microcytic red cells which undergo disruption at temperatures of 44 to 45°C (in contrast to the normal thermal instability at 49°C). This results from an abnormality of spectrin structure. Hemolysis, which is usually severe, is recognized in childhood and is partially responsive to splenectomy.

Hereditary stomatocytosis   Stomatocytes are red blood cells having a slit-like central zone of pallor on dried smears. The syndrome of hereditary hemolytic anemia and stomatocytic red blood cells is inherited in an autosomal dominant pattern. It may represent a number of discrete entities. Two major red blood cell defects have been delineated in this syndrome. First, the red blood cells have an increased permeability to sodium and potassium, which is compensated for by an increased active transport of these cations. Second, red cells have an increased surface area associated with an increase in membrane lipid content, particularly phosphatidylcholine. In some patients, the red blood cell is swollen with an excess of ions and

water and a decreased mean corpuscular hemoglobin concentration (overhydrated stomatocytes, "hydrocytosis"); in other patients the red cell is shrunken with a decreased ion and water content and an increased mean corpuscular hemoglobin concentration (dehydrated stomatocytes, "desiccytosis"). Those patients in whom the red blood cells are overhydrated have true stomatocytes on dried smears. Dehydrated stomatocytes assume the morphology of target cells on dried smears. In both instances, red blood cells are cup- or bowl-shaped when examined in wet preparation. Osmotic fragility is increased in overhydrated stomatocytes and decreased in underhydrated stomatocytes. Autohemolysis is increased and is corrected by glucose.

Most patients have splenomegaly and mild anemia. Splenectomy decreases but does not totally correct the hemolytic process. Its indications are similar to those for hereditary spherocytosis.

DISORDERS OF THE INTERIOR OF THE RED CELL

RED CELL ENZYME DEFECTS   During its maturation, the red blood cell loses its nucleus, ribosomes, and mitochondria and thus its capability for protein synthesis and oxidative phosphorylation. The mature circulating red blood cell has a relatively simple pattern of intermediary metabolism (Fig. 294-2) in keeping with its modest metabolic obligations. As discussed in Chap. 290, some ATP must be generated from the Embden-Meyerhof pathway to drive the cation pump which maintains the ionic milieu within the red blood cell. Smaller amounts of energy are needed for the preservation of hemoglobin iron in the ferrous (Fe^{2+}) state, and perhaps for the renewal of the lipids in the red blood cell membrane. About 10 percent of the glucose consumed by the red blood cell is metabolized via the hexose-monophosphate shunt (Fig. 294-2). This pathway protects both hemoglobin and the membrane from exogenous oxidants including certain drugs.

Studies of red blood cell enzyme defects have provided valuable information on the metabolic control of normal erythrocytes. Figure 294-2 shows a large number of recognized specific enzyme deficiency states affecting the glycolytic pathway or the hexose-monophosphate shunt. Many of these enzyme abnormalities appear to be restricted to red blood cells. The long life span of the red blood cell and its inability to synthesize proteins pose a challenge to the stability of its enzymes. Therefore, a mutation resulting in decreased stability will be expressed more readily in the red blood cell compared with other tissues.

Defects in the Embden-Meyerhof pathway   Deficiencies of most of the enzymes of the Embden-Meyerhof (or glycolytic) pathway have been reported. In general, all these enzymopathies have similar pathophysiologic and clinical features. Patients present with a congenital nonspherocytic hemolytic anemia of variable severity. The red blood cells are often relatively deficient in ATP, considering their young age. As a result, there is an increased leak of potassium ion from inside these cells. Abnormalities in red blood cell morphology (see below) indicate that the red cell membrane is secondarily affected by the enzyme defect. These red blood cells are apt to be rigid and thus more readily sequestered by the mononuclear-phagocyte system.

Some of these glycolytic enzyme deficiencies such as pyruvate kinase (PK) deficiency and hexokinase deficiency are localized to the red blood cell, with no apparent metabolic abnormality in leukocytes or other cells that have been studied. In other disorders, the enzyme deficiency is more widespread. Glucose phosphate isomerase deficiency and phosphoglycerate kinase deficiency also involve leukocytes, although affected individuals have no apparent abnormalities of white blood cell function. Individuals with deficiency of triose phosphate isomerase have decreased levels of enzyme in leukocytes, muscle cells, and central nervous system fluid. Furthermore, they have a progressive neurologic disorder. Some patients with phosphofructokinase deficiency have a myopathy.

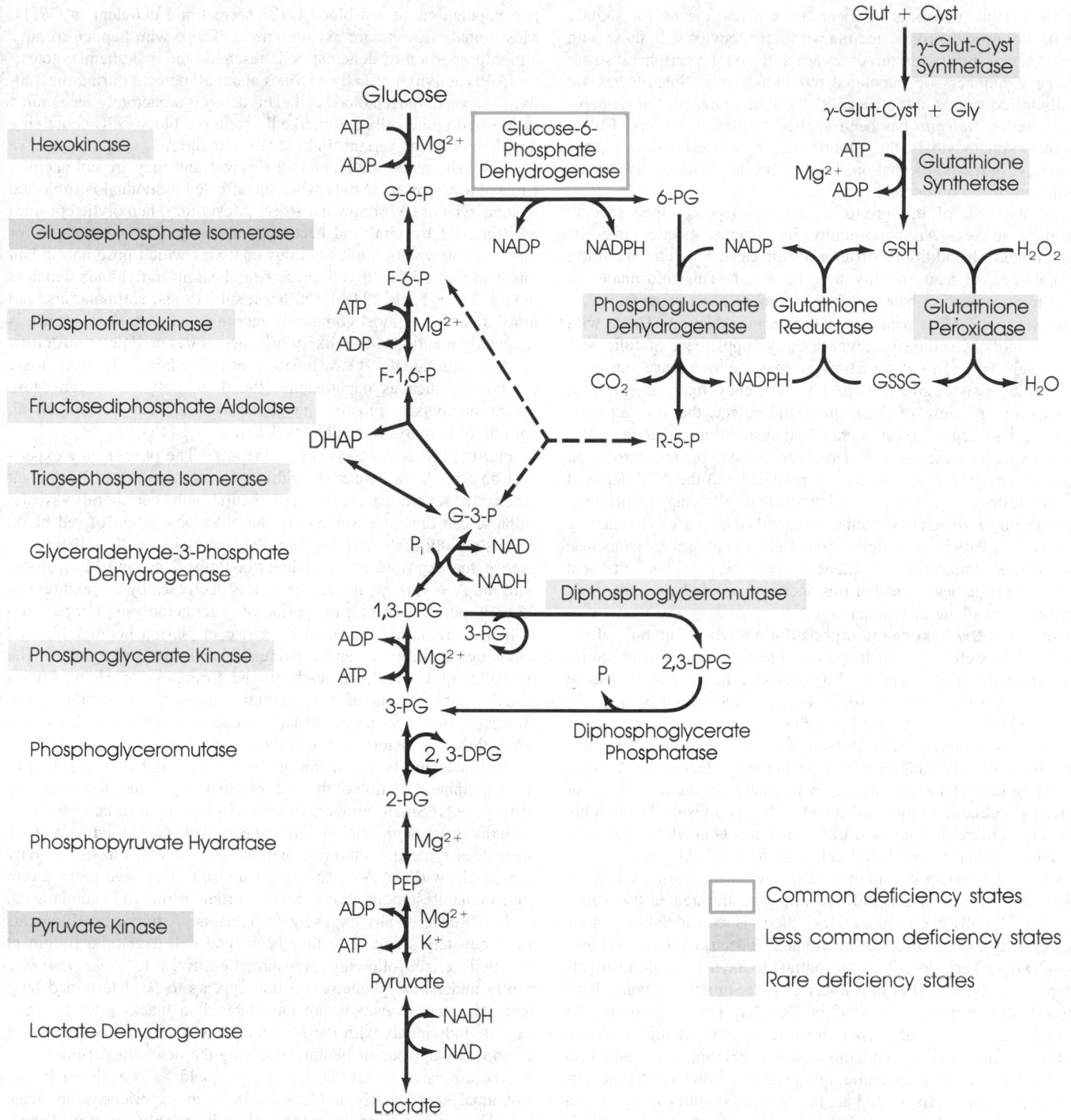

FIGURE 294-2   Metabolic pathways in the red blood cell. The glycolytic pathway is outlined vertically from glucose to lactate. The pentose phosphate pathway is shown on the right. Known enzyme deficiency states are shown. Bold solid lines denote common states, light solid lines less common ones, and dotted lines rare ones. (*From WN Valentine, Semin Hematol 8:309, 1971.*)

Among the reported defects of glycolytic enzymes, about 95 percent are due to PK deficiency and about 4 percent are due to glucose phosphate isomerase deficiency. The remainder shown in Fig. 294-2 are extremely rare. Most have been encountered in isolated families. There is considerable variability in the clinical manifestations and laboratory findings among reported cases of PK deficiency. This is probably due to the fact that a number of different PK variants have been reported. This heterogeneity probably also applies to the other less common glycolytic enzyme defects. Accordingly, the clinical manifestations of these disorders are quite variable.

GENETICS   Most of the glycolytic enzyme defects are inherited in an autosomal recessive pattern. Thus, the parents of affected patients are heterozygotes. Heterozygotes generally possess half-normal levels of enzyme activity which are more than adequate for normal metabolic function. Thus, these individuals are entirely asymptomatic. Since the gene frequency for this group of enzymopathies is low, it is not surprising that true homozygotes are often the offspring of a consanguineous mating. Alternatively, affected individuals may be double heterozygotes, inheriting an abnormal allele from each parent. Phosphoglycerate kinase deficiency is inherited as a sex-linked disorder. Affected males have a severe hemolytic anemia while female carriers may have a mild hemolytic process.

CLINICAL MANIFESTATIONS   Patients with severe hemolysis usually present during early childhood with anemia, icterus, and splenomegaly. Other stigmata of chronic hemolysis are occasionally seen. Occasionally, siblings are similarly affected.

LABORATORY FINDINGS Patients have a normocytic (or slightly macrocytic) normochromic anemia with reticulocytosis. In those with PK deficiency, bizarre erythrocytes are noted on the peripheral smear with large numbers of spiculated red blood cells. Spherocytes are usually infrequent or absent. Hence, the term *congenital nonspherocytic hemolytic anemia* has been applied to these disorders. Unlike hereditary spherocytosis, the osmotic fragility of freshly drawn blood is usually normal. Incubation brings out an osmotically fragile population of red blood cells.

The diagnosis of this group of anemias depends upon specific enzymatic assays. An abnormality in enzyme kinetics may be demonstrated. In addition, differences in electrophoretic mobility, pH optimum, or heat stability may be noted. This information is useful in documenting heterogeneity among enzyme variants.

TREATMENT Most patients do not require therapy. Those with severe hemolysis should be given a daily supplement of folic acid (1 mg per day). Blood transfusions may be necessary during a hypoplastic crisis. Patients with PK deficiency may benefit from splenectomy. Because of their enzymatic defect, the younger cells (reticulocytes) depend on mitochondrial respiration rather than glycolysis for maintenance of ATP. However, in the hypoxic environment of the spleen, aerobic metabolism is curtailed and the ATP-depleted cells are destroyed in situ. It is of interest that following splenectomy patients with PK deficiency often have a marked increase in circulating reticulocytes. Patients with deficiency of glucose phosphate isomerase may also be improved by splenectomy. There is not sufficient information to indicate whether this operation would help individuals with other glycolytic enzymopathies.

Defects in the hexose-monophosphate shunt The normal red blood cell is well endowed to protect itself against oxidant stress. Upon exposure to an offending drug or toxin, the amount of glucose that is metabolized via the hexose-monophosphate shunt is increased severalfold. In this way reduced glutathione is regenerated, protecting the sulfhydryl groups of hemoglobin and the red blood cell membrane from oxidation. Individuals with an inherited defect in the hexose-monophosphate shunt are unable to maintain an adequate level of reduced glutathione in their red blood cells. As a result, hemoglobin sulfhydryl groups become oxidized, and the hemoglobin tends to precipitate within the red blood cell forming Heinz bodies.

Among the congenital shunt defects, by far the most common is *G6PD deficiency*. It affects millions of people throughout the world. Like the glycolytic enzymopathies, there is considerable genetic heterogeneity among affected individuals. Indeed, over 250 variants of G6PD have been described. In contrast to the hemoglobin variants (Chap. 295) abnormalities in primary DNA or protein sequence have been established in only a few of the G6PD variants. The remainder are presumed to have abnormal structure because of differences in electrophoretic mobility, enzyme kinetics, pH optimum, and heat stability. Like many of the hemoglobin variants, some G6PD mutants were discovered by chance and are not associated with any significant functional abnormalities. The normal or "wild" form of G6PD is designated by type B. About 20 percent of blacks have a G6PD (designated A+) which differs electrophoretically but is functionally normal. Among the clinically significant G6PD variants, the most common is the so-called A− type encountered primarily in blacks who originated from central Africa. The A− G6PD has the same electrophoretic mobility as the A+ type, but it is unstable and has abnormal kinetic properties. Like the HbS gene, the A− type of G6PD may confer protection against malaria. This variant is found in about 15 percent of black males in the United States. A second relatively common G6PD variant is encountered among peoples of the eastern Mediterranean area, particularly Sephardic Jews. A third relatively common variant occurs in the Chinese.

The G6PD gene is located on the X chromosome. Thus the deficiency state is a sex-linked trait. Affected males (hemizygotes) inherit the abnormal gene from their mothers who are usually carriers (heterozygotes). Because of inactivation of one of the two X chromosomes (Lyon hypothesis, see Chap. 5), the heterozygote has

two populations of red blood cells: normal and deficient in G6PD. Most female carriers are asymptomatic. Those who happen to have a high proportion of deficient cells resemble the male hemizygotes.

G6PD activity normally declines about 50 percent during the 120-day life span of the red blood cell. This decay is moderately accelerated in A− red blood cells and markedly so in red blood cells containing the Mediterranean variant. Individuals with the A− variant may have a slightly shortened red blood cell survival, but they are not anemic. Clinical problems arise only when the affected individual is subjected to some type of environmental stress. Most often, hemolytic episodes are triggered by viral and bacterial infections. The mechanism for this is unknown. In addition drugs or toxins which pose an oxidant threat to the red blood cell cause hemolysis in individuals deficient in G6PD (see Table 294-5). Of these, sulfa drugs, antimalarials, and nitrofurantoin are most commonly incriminated. Although aspirin is frequently mentioned as a likely offender, it has no deleterious effect in A− individuals. Occasionally, accidental ingestion of toxic compounds such as naphthalene (found in moth balls) can cause severe hemolysis. Finally, metabolic acidosis can precipitate an episode of hemolysis in subjects deficient in G6PD.

CLINICAL AND LABORATORY FEATURES The patient may experience an acute hemolytic crisis within hours of exposure to the oxidant stress. In severe cases, hemoglobinuria and peripheral vascular collapse can develop. Since only the older population of red blood cells is rapidly destroyed, the hemolytic crisis is usually self-limited, even if the exposure to the oxidant continues. Among black males with the A− variant, the red cell mass decreases by a maximum of 25 to 30 percent. During the period of acute hemolysis, a rapid drop in hematocrit is accompanied by a rise in plasma hemoglobin and unconjugated bilirubin and a decrease in plasma haptoglobin. The oxidation of hemoglobin leads to the formation of Heinz bodies visualized by means of a supravital stain such as crystal violet. However, Heinz bodies are usually not seen after the first day or so, since these inclusions are readily removed by the spleen. Their removal leads to the formation of "bite cells," red cells which have lost a peripheral portion of the cell. Multiple bites cause the formation of fragments. Small numbers of spherocytes may also be present.

Individuals with the *Mediterranean type G6PD* have a more unstable enzyme and, therefore, a much lower overall enzyme activity than blacks with the A− variant. As a result, they have more severe clinical manifestations. Some have a chronic hemolytic anemia, even in the absence of any exposure to oxidants. A minority of patients are exquisitely sensitive to fava beans and will develop a fulminant hemolytic crisis following exposure. Sensitivity to *Vicia fava* is a poorly understood phenomenon that appears to be determined by a separate gene. Favism is not encountered in blacks with the A− variant. Individuals with the Mediterranean variant sometimes have a temporary episode of hemolysis during the newborn period.

The *diagnosis* of G6PD deficiency should be considered in any individual, particularly a black male, who experiences an acute hemolytic episode. The patient should be thoroughly questioned about possible exposure to oxidant agents. A number of screening tests are available to establish the diagnosis. However, since the deficiency occurs primarily in older red blood cells, a false-negative test may be seen during a hemolytic episode when there is a high proportion of young red blood cells. It may be necessary to repeat these diagnostic tests after the patient has recovered. Unusual features in

TABLE 294-5 Drugs causing hemolysis in subjects deficient in G6PD

Antimalarials: Primaquine, pamaquine, chloroquine, dapsone
Sulfonamides: Sulfanilamide, sulfasoxazole, etc.
Nitrofurantoin
Analgesics: Phenacetin, acetanilid
Miscellaneous: Vitamin K (water-soluble form), probenecid, methylene blue, p-aminosalicylic acid, nalidixic acid, quinine,* quinidine,* chloramphenicol*

* Not known to cause hemolysis in blacks with A− type G6PD.

the case should prompt further investigation including a more complete and specific characterization of the enzyme.

TREATMENT Since hemolysis in patients deficient in A − G6PD is usually self-limited, no specific treatment is necessary. Splenectomy does not appear to be of benefit to Mediterranean patients with chronic hemolysis. Blood transfusions are rarely indicated. If a patient develops a severe hemolytic episode with hemoglobinuria, maintaining adequate urine output is important.

Attention should be directed toward the *prevention* of hemolytic episodes. Infections ought to be treated promptly. Subjects deficient in G6PD should be warned about risks posed by oxidant drugs and fava beans. Any black patient about to be given an oxidant drug should be screened for G6PD deficiency.

OTHER DEFECTS OF THE HEXOSE-MONOPHOSPHATE SHUNT A few kindreds have been found to have congenital deficiency in red blood cell glutathione due to a defect in either of the two enzymes responsible for the synthesis of this tripeptide. Affected individuals have a hemolytic anemia with Heinz bodies that is aggravated by oxidant drugs. Deficiency of glutathione reductase has been reported, but its relationship to clinically significant hemolysis is not well established. Sometimes the deficiency state can be corrected by the administration of riboflavin (5 mg per day). There are also isolated reports of deficiencies of glutathione peroxidase and 6-phosphogluconate dehydrogenase, but, again, their association with hemolysis is uncertain.

Other enzyme defects Hemolytic anemia may sometimes be caused by abnormalities in enzymes of nucleotide metabolism. A growing number of individuals with pyrimidine 5′-nucleotidase deficiency have been encountered. Their red cells have marked basophilic stippling. Hemolytic anemia has also been noted in individuals whose red blood cells have supranormal levels of adenosine deaminase and relatively low levels of ATP.

HEMOGLOBINOPATHIES The sickling disorders constitute an important form of congenital hemolytic anemia. Less commonly, hemolysis may be due to the inheritance of an unstable hemoglobin variant. These disorders of hemoglobin are discussed in Chap. 295.

REFERENCES

ANTMAN KH et al: Microangiopathic hemolytic anemia and cancer: A review. Medicine 58:377, 1979
BYRNE JJ, MOAKE JL: Thrombotic thrombocytopenic purpura and haemolytic-uremic syndrome: Evolving concepts of pathogenesis and therapy. Clin Haematol 15:413, 1986
COOPER RA: Abnormalities of cell-membrane fluidity in the pathogenesis of disease. N Engl J Med 297:371, 1977
———: Hemolytic syndromes and red cell membrane abnormalities in liver disease. Semin Hematol 17:103, 1980
HIRONO A et al: Enzymatic diagnosis in non-spherocytic hemolytic anemia. Medicine 67:110, 1988
LUX SE: Disorders of the red cell membrane, in *Hematology of Infancy and Childhood*, DG Nathan, FA Oski (eds). Philadelphia, Saunders, 1987
PANGBURN et al: Paroxysmal nocturnal hemoglobinuria: Deficiency in factor H–like functions of the abnormal erythrocytes. J Exp Med 157:1971, 1983
PISCIOTTA AV: Thrombotic thrombocytopenic purpura. Ann Intern Med 92:249, 1980
ROSSE WF: Autoimmune hemolytic anemia. Hosp Prac 20:105, 1985
———: *Clinical Immunohematology*. Cambridge, Blackwell Scientific, 1989
———, PARKER CG: Paroxysmal nocturnal hemoglobinuria. Clin Haematol 14:105, 1985
SCHRIER SL (ed): The red blood cell membrane. Clin Haematol 14:1, 1985
VALENTINE WN et al: Hemolytic anemias and erythrocyte enzymopathies. Ann Intern Med 103:245, 1985

295 DISORDERS OF HEMOGLOBIN

H. FRANKLIN BUNN

In 1910, Herrick described a medical student from Jamaica who had a hemolytic anemia in conjunction with elongated "sickled" red blood cells. Subsequently, it was shown that all the red blood cells of such patients assume a classic holly leaf or sickle shape following deoxygenation of the blood. In 1949, Itano and Pauling discovered the association of sickle cell anemia with an electrophoretically abnormal hemoglobin. Eight years later, Ingram demonstrated that this hemoglobin (designated Hb S) differed from normal Hb A by the substitution of valine for glutamic acid at the sixth position of the β chain. Since then, over 400 structurally different human hemoglobin variants have been discovered in widely scattered parts of the world. Generally, a new hemoglobin is named after the place where it is first encountered. No more than a third of these mutant hemoglobins are associated with significant clinical manifestations. The remainder have been discovered by serendipity or as a result of large population surveys. All told, the hemoglobinopathies have taught us many valuable lessons in such diverse areas as the mechanisms of hemolysis, the pathophysiology of oxygen transport, the stereochemistry of hemoglobin function, and the genetic bases of protein synthesis.

This chapter focuses on the clinically significant variants. In addition, disorders of the biosynthesis of globin (the thalassemias) and methemoglobinemia are discussed.

GENETIC CONSIDERATIONS The synthesis of each of the subunits of hemoglobin (α, β, γ, δ, ϵ, ζ) is governed by separate genes. The ϵ and ζ subunits are found only in embryonic hemoglobin. Normal individuals inherit two β-chain genes (one from each parent), four α-chain genes, and four γ-chain genes. The ϵ-, γ-, δ-, and β-chain genes occupy adjacent loci on chromosome 11 (see Fig. 295-1). The ζ and α genes are located on chromosome 16. The structure and function of normal hemoglobin ($\alpha_2\beta_2$) are discussed in Chap. 290. The inheritance of abnormal hemoglobins follows classic mendelian genetics. If two parents are heterozygous for a hemoglobin variant such as Hb S, statistically one-quarter of the offspring will be SS homozygotes, another quarter will be normal (AA genotype), and half will have sickle trait (AS). The commonly encountered hemoglobinopathies such as S, C, and E are β-chain variants. Occasionally, an individual inherits two different β-chain variants, one from each parent. Hemoglobin SC disease is an example of such a double heterozygous state. Genes for β thalassemia are located on the β-chain structural gene. Accordingly, an individual can inherit from one parent (and pass on to a child) either β thalassemia or a β-chain variant, but not both. Among the hemoglobinopathies associated with sickling (described below), only the homozygous state (Hb SS) or double heterozygous state (Sβ thalassemia or SC) has important clinical manifestations. In contrast, the unstable variants and those having abnormal oxygen-binding properties are encountered only in heterozygotes. In some cases, the homozygous state would be incompatible with life.

About 90 percent of these abnormal hemoglobins are single amino acid replacements, due to a single base substitution in the corresponding triplet codon. The structural information accumulated on human mutant hemoglobins has provided ample verification of the fidelity of the genetic code. Other genetic mechanisms must be invoked to explain the structure of a few interesting hemoglobin variants. The Lepore hemoglobins have arisen because of nonhomologous crossover between the adjacent δ- and β-chain genes, giving rise to a fusion subunit in which the *N*-terminal end has the amino acid sequence of the δ chain and the *C*-terminal end has the sequence of the β chain (see Fig. 295-1). Some of the unstable hemoglobins have deletions of one or more residues in sequence within a subunit. Finally there are a few variants which have elongated subunits (e.g., Hb Constant

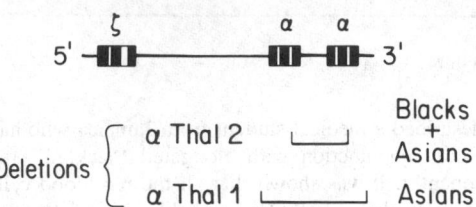

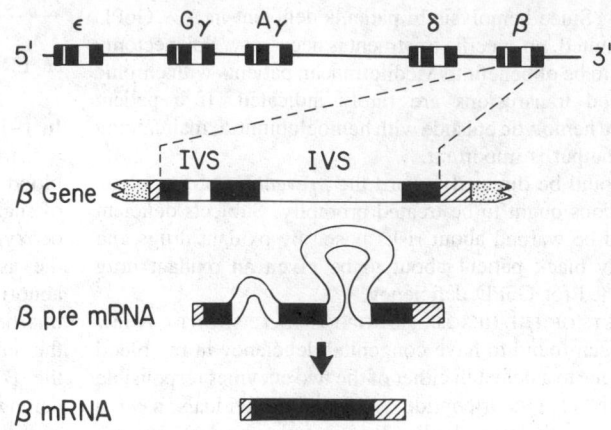

β^+ Thal: Impairment of IVS splicing

β^0 Thal: Nonsense mutation in coding region

FIGURE 295-1 Diagram of human globin genes. *Left:* The α-globin gene complex includes the embryonic ζ gene as well as two α genes. In the vast majority of individuals with α thalassemia 2 (α−) one α gene is deleted owing to a nonhomologous crossover between adjacent α genes. In α thalassemia 1 (− −) both α genes are deleted. *Right:* The β-globin gene complex includes the embryonic ε gene, two fetal genes ($^G\gamma$ and $^A\gamma$), the δ gene, and the β gene. Below is a diagram of the β gene showing the coding regions (■), the intervening segments (IVS) and the flanking regions (▨) that are transcribed into mRNA below. Most cases of β⁺ thalassemia in Mediterranean individuals involve a base substitution causing partial impairment of splicing of an IVS. Most cases of β⁰ thalassemia in Mediterraneans involve a base substitution that creates either a stop codon or a frame shift.

Spring). These have arisen either because of a base substitution in the termination codon or because of a frame shift which puts the termination codon out of phase.

CLINICAL CLASSIFICATION The clinically significant hemoglobin variants are classified in Table 295-1. By far the most important and prevalent type of hemoglobinopathy is due to the presence of sickle hemoglobin, either in the homozygous state or in conjunction with another type of hemoglobin abnormality. The inheritance of an unstable hemoglobin variant may give rise to congenital hemolytic anemia associated with the presence of inclusions of precipitated hemoglobin within the red blood cells (Heinz bodies). Finally, hemoglobin variants may have abnormal functional or spectral properties, resulting in familial erythrocytosis or familial cyanosis.

SICKLE SYNDROMES

SICKLE CELL TRAIT About 8 percent of black Americans are heterozygous for Hb S. The gene frequency is highest in central Africa, particularly in regions where malaria is endemic. In some parts of Nigeria, over 30 percent of the population has sickle trait. The gene has persisted because heterozygotes gain slight protection against falciparum malaria. This is an example of balanced polymorphism.

The diagnosis of sickle trait or any of the other sickle syndromes depends upon the demonstration of sickling under reduced oxygen tension. In the widely used sickle preparation, sickled cells can be visualized microscopically after the addition of an oxygen-consuming

TABLE 295-1   Clinically important hemoglobin variants

I Sickle syndromes
  A Sickle cell trait (AS)
  B Sickle cell anemia (SS)
  C Double heterozygous states: Sickle β thalassemia, sickle C disease (SC), sickle D disease (SD)
II Unstable hemoglobin variants: congenital Heinz body hemolytic anemia
III Variants with high oxygen affinity: familial erythrocytosis
IV M hemoglobins: familial cyanosis (see Table 295-3)

reagent such as metabisulfite. Many clinical laboratories prefer a solubility test which depends on the fact that deoxyhemoglobin S has a low solubility at high ionic strength. These tests are reasonably specific for Hb S although some of the unstable variants may give a false-positive solubility test. Therefore, if one of these screening tests is positive, hemoglobin electrophoresis should be performed. Individuals with sickle trait usually have about 35 to 40 percent Hb S and 55 to 60 percent Hb A.

Hemoglobin S heterozygotes have minimal clinical problems. Their overall life expectancy and frequency of hospitalization are no different from those of a comparable group of individuals with hemoglobin A. AS red blood cells require a much lower oxygen tension for sickling than SS red cells. Accordingly, individuals with sickle trait may develop sickle cell crises only if they become severely hypoxic. They may occasionally sustain a splenic infarct. As discussed below, the renal medulla is particularly susceptible to sickling. Many AS individuals have impaired ability to form concentrated urine, and a few have recurrent episodes of painless hematuria as a result of medullary infarction. Infarction due to sickling has been encountered in other organs in sickle trait but is extremely rare. For these reasons, AS individuals should not be placed in any high-risk group for employment or insurance considerations.

SICKLE CELL ANEMIA Sickle cell anemia is a significant cause of morbidity and mortality among black individuals. About 0.15 percent of black children in the United States have the disease. The prevalence is lower among adults because patients with sickle cell anemia have a decreased life expectancy. The protean clinical manifestations of this disorder can all be attributed to a specific molecular lesion: the substitution of valine for glutamic acid at the sixth residue of the β chain.

Molecular pathogenesis Upon deoxygenation, a red blood cell containing Hb S changes from a biconcave disk to an elongated crescent-shaped or ''sickle''-shaped cell (see Fig. 295-2). Electron micrographs reveal the presence of fibers having a diameter of about 20 nm. Each sickle fiber consists of a helical polymer with 14 strands. The polymer is stabilized by hydrophobic bonding between β6 valine and a complementary site on another portion of the β chain on an adjacent strand (Fig. 295-2). In addition, there are many other

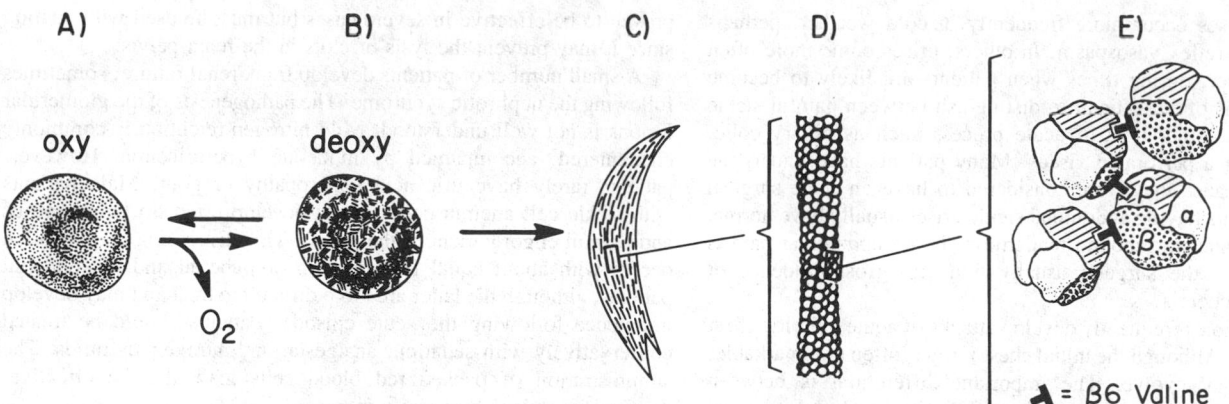

FIGURE 295-2 Polymerization of sickle hemoglobin. When the red cell (*A*) is deoxygenated, deoxyhemoglobin S aggregates to form domains of elongated rodlike polymers (*B*). In most cells these fibers align and distort the cell into the classic sickle shape (*C*). The individual Hb S molecules form a closely packed polymer consisting of 14 strands having a helical configuration (*D*). A close-up of the contacts between a pair of aligned strands (*E*) shows the abnormal β6 valine forming a hydrophobic contact with an acceptor site on the β chain of a molecule on the adjacent strand.

interactions between neighboring molecules. Sickling, both within the intact red blood cell and in free solution, is greatly affected by the presence of non-S hemoglobin. Hb A participates more readily than Hb F in copolymerization with Hb S.

Cellular pathogenesis As discussed in Chap. 290, the ability of red blood cells to traverse the microcirculation depends in large part on their pliability. As sickle polymers are formed during deoxygenation, the red blood cell becomes rigid, and, as a result, may obstruct capillary blood flow. The rate at which polymerization occurs depends primarily on the intracellular concentration of HbS and the extent of deoxygenation. If polymerization occurs before the red cell escapes the narrow-bore capillary, obstruction may occur, resulting in local tissue hypoxia, further deoxygenation, and further sickling. This vicious cycle may result in the amplification of microscopic obstruction into a larger area of infarction. The oxygen-dependent sickle cycle is ordinarily reversible. However, the membrane of SS red blood cells may become sufficiently damaged so that the cells lose potassium and water, leading to the formation of irreversibly sickled forms. In these cells, the characteristic sickle shape persists even after they are exposed to ambient oxygen tension at room temperature and can readily be seen on examination of Wright-stained blood films (see Fig. A5-6). The proportion of irreversibly sickled cells varies considerably among homozygous sicklers and is not correlated with clinical severity. Hemoglobin F is distributed unevenly among red blood cells of SS patients, and composes between 2 and 20 percent of the total hemoglobin (the remainder is almost entirely Hb S). Since Hb F inhibits the polymerization of Hb S, those cells that contain Hb F are protected from sickling, whereas those cells that lack Hb F are likely to become irreversibly sickled. It is not surprising that these rigid cells are readily culled from the circulation and destroyed. The continuous formation and destruction of irreversibly sickled cells contributes significantly to the severe hemolytic anemia shared by all patients with sickle cell anemia. Furthermore, these rigid cells may initiate small-vessel occlusions.

Factors such as acidosis or increased erythrocyte 2,3-diphosphoglycerate, which lower the oxygen affinity of red blood cells, will enhance the formation of deoxyhemoglobin and, therefore, promote intracellular polymerization and eventual sickling. In addition, sickling is highly dependent on hemoglobin concentration. Any pathophysiologic process which tends to pull water out of sickle red blood cells will greatly increase their tendency to sickle. Thus, the hypertonic environment of the renal medulla can cause local sickling and the formation of papillary infarcts, even in individuals with sickle trait.

Clinical manifestations Patients with homozygous sickle cell anemia have a variety of clinical problems broadly outlined in Table 295-2. Signs and symptoms usually do not appear until after the sixth month of life, at which time most of the Hb F has been replaced by Hb S. Among the *constitutional* manifestations of sickle cell anemia are delay of growth and development and a general failure to thrive. In addition, these patients have an increased tendency to develop serious infections, particularly due to pneumococcus. SS patients have marked impairment of splenic function, preventing effective clearance of circulating bacteria. With the passage of time, the organ sustains recurrent infarcts and eventually becomes a nubbin of fibrous tissue.

ANEMIA SS homozygotes have a severe hemolytic anemia with hematocrit values between 18 and 30 percent. The destruction of red blood cells is independent of cell age. The mean red blood cell survival is about 10 to 15 days. Those cells having relatively low levels of Hb F have a shorter life span, in part due to a greater chance of becoming irreversibly sickled. As a result of accelerated red blood cell breakdown, patients with sickle cell disease have characteristic clinical and laboratory findings discussed in Chap. 290. Even though hemolysis is primarily extravascular, plasma haptoglobin is generally low or absent, and plasma hemoglobin levels are moderately elevated.

The anemia becomes increasingly severe if erythropoiesis is suppressed. There are two main causes of "aplastic crises"—infection and folic acid deficiency. As discussed in Chap. 293, infection brings about a transient reduction in red blood cell production. In particular, parvovirus causes an abrupt suppression of erythropoiesis. In SS patients with severe ongoing hemolysis, this usually results in a rapid drop in hematocrit (Table 295-2).

VASOOCCLUSIVE PHENOMENA The morbidity and mortality of sickle cell disease are due primarily to recurrent vasoocclusive phenomena. As shown in Table 295-2, these can be divided into two groups. Throughout their lives, SS patients are plagued by recurrent *painful crises*. These episodes may appear with explosive suddenness and attack various parts of the body, particularly the abdomen, chest, back, and joints. About a third of painful crises are preceded by a viral or bacterial infection. The frequency of painful crises is highly variable. A given patient may have months or even years without a crisis and then have a cluster of frequent severe attacks. In some

TABLE 295-2 Clinical manifestations of sickle cell anemia

I Constitutional
  A Impaired growth and development
  B Increased susceptibility to infection

II Vasoocclusive
  A Microinfarcts → Painful crises
  B Macroinfarcts
       → Organ damage

III Anemia
  A Severe hemolysis
  B Aplastic crises

individuals, crises occur more frequently in cold weather, perhaps precipitated by reflex vasospasm. In others, crises come more often in warm weather, during times when patients are likely to become dehydrated. It is often difficult to distinguish between painful sickle crisis and some other type of acute process such as biliary colic, appendicitis, or a perforated viscus. Many patients have undergone exploration because they were considered to have an acute surgical problem. Patients having abdominal sickle crises usually have normal bowel sounds and no rebound tenderness. If the abdominal pain is due to sickling, the surgeon usually finds no gross evidence of infarction or ischemia.

SS homozygotes frequently develop attacks of acute pleuritic chest pain with fever. Although the initial chest x-ray is often unremarkable, an infiltrate may evolve. The important differential is between pneumonitis and pulmonary infarction. Culture and Gram's stain of the sputum will be helpful in establishing the presence of pneumonia. In these patients, pulmonary infarctions are much more likely due to thrombosis in situ than to emboli. Occasionally, pulmonary infarcts become secondarily infected.

When a sickle crisis is localized in the extremities, it may mimic osteomyelitis or an acute arthritis such as gout or rheumatoid arthritis. Patients commonly develop acute synovitis with joint effusion. Examination of the joint fluid is helpful in this differential diagnosis. If the effusion is due to sickling, the fluid will be clear and yellow, with a low white blood cell count (100 to 1000 mononuclear cells per cubic millimeter) and an absence of crystals or bacteria.

Sickle crises may occasionally involve the central nervous system. Patients can present with a seizure, stroke, or coma. Although such crises are frequently reversible, they may be fatal.

CHRONIC ORGAN DAMAGE By the time that patients reach adulthood, there is often objective evidence of anatomic or functional damage to various tissues, due to the cumulative effect of recurrent vasoocclusive episodes. Almost any organ may be involved, but the most common are the lungs, kidneys, liver, skeleton, and skin.

Cardiopulmonary Impairment of pulmonary function is a common complication of sickle cell disease. Resting arterial P_{O_2} is usually reduced in part because of intrapulmonary arterial-venous shunting. Since SS red blood cells have decreased oxygen affinity, arterial blood will be significantly undersaturated, leading to an increased tendency for red cells to sickle when they reach the peripheral circulation. SS homozygotes frequently develop congestive heart failure. The chronic severe anemia and hypoxemia impose a sustained burden on the heart. Most patients have a systolic ejection murmur as a result of their hyperdynamic circulation. Even though more oxygen is extracted by the myocardium than any other tissue, SS patients rarely develop myocardial infarction, probably because of rapid transit through the myocardial microcirculation.

Hepatobiliary Like other patients with congenital hemolytic anemia, those with sickle cell anemia have icterus and an increased tendency to form gallstones. It is often difficult to distinguish between the abdominal pain of acute cholecystitis and that due to a sickle crisis. Jaundice deepens markedly if a patient develops choledocholithiasis, and bilirubin levels as high as 855 μmol/L (50 mg/dL) have been reported. As a rule, cholecystectomy is not recommended unless gallstones cause symptoms. In addition, patients with sickle cell anemia may develop hepatic infarcts which occasionally become infected, resulting in abscess formation. If a significant portion of hepatic parenchyma becomes infarcted, fibrosis and deterioration of liver function may result, with deepening of jaundice.

Genitourinary (see also Chaps. 228 and 230) The hypertonic and acidic environment of the renal medulla promotes sickling, resulting in microinfarcts. Virtually all patients have isosthenuria. The inability to form concentrated urine increases the risk of significant dehydration. In addition, like those with sickle trait or SC disease, SS homozygotes may develop significant and prolonged painless hematuria as a result of papillary infarcts. Hematuria may be so extensive that iron deficiency develops. ε-Aminocaproic acid has proved to be effective in severe cases but must be used with caution since it may prevent the lysis of clots in the renal pelvis.

A small number of patients develop frank renal failure, sometimes following the nephrotic syndrome. The pathogenesis of the glomerular lesions is not well understood. Mild nitrogen retention is commonly encountered, accompanied by moderate hyperuricemia. However, patients rarely have uric acid nephropathy or gout. Male patients with sickle cell anemia occasionally develop priapism (spontaneous and painful engorgement of the penis). This distressing complication occurs with about equal frequency in prepubertal and postpubertal patients, although the latter are more difficult to treat and may develop impotence following the acute episode. Patients should be treated conservatively with sedation, analgesia, and intravenous fluids. The administration of packed red blood cells may also be effective. Surgical intervention is rarely indicated.

Skeletal Like other patients with congenital hemolytic anemia, patients with sickle cell anemia demonstrate radiologic abnormalities due to the expansion of red marrow. However, the development of bony infarcts results in more characteristic x-ray abnormalities. The biconcave or "fishmouth" vertebrae are pathognomonic of sickle cell disease. Skeletal infarction generally leads to increased bony trabeculation and sclerosis. Aseptic necrosis of the head of the femur is particularly common in patients with sickle cell disease and can lead to considerable disability. Like infarcts in other organs, bony infarctions are more likely to become infected. In patients who develop osteomyelitis, salmonella is a frequent pathogen.

Ocular A variety of ocular abnormalities are encountered in patients with SS and SC disease. These include retinal infarcts, peripheral vessel disease, arteriovenous anomalies, vitreous hemorrhage, retinitis proliferans, and retinal detachment. In addition, when viewed with a strong magnifying lens, angulated and "corkscrew" vessels can be seen in the bulbar conjunctiva. The major ocular complications are more commonly encountered in SC and sickle β thalassemia patients than in SS patients. The early diagnosis of retinal lesions in sickle disease is important since retinal detachment may be prevented by appropriate therapy.

Skin Chronic skin ulcers often occur in the distal lower extremities. The lesions appear to be commoner in patients with more severe anemia. Ankle ulcers have also been encountered in rare patients with other types of congenital hemolytic anemia. This complication is more commonly seen in tropical areas. Ankle ulcers generally respond to conservative management, such as elevation of the leg, maintenance of strict cleanliness, and application of a mild chemical debriding agent such as Dakin's solution. The weekly application of Unna boots has been effective. In patients with refractory ulcers, a hypertransfusion regimen is probably indicated. Skin grafting should be undertaken only after all other measures have failed.

Neurologic A variety of central nervous system manifestations may be encountered in sickle cell anemia. Although cerebral thrombosis is the principal neurologic complication, SS patients also have an increased incidence of subarachnoid hemorrhage. A patient has about a 25 percent chance of developing some type of neurologic complication during a lifetime. Hemiplegia is encountered more frequently than coma, convulsions, or visual disturbances. Patients generally make a full recovery, particularly from their first cerebral vascular accident. Preliminary studies in children indicate that a hypertransfusion program is beneficial to those who have sustained a major neurologic complication.

Diagnosis The diagnosis of sickle cell anemia should be considered in any black patient with a hemolytic anemia. The history of painful crises, arthropathy, ankle ulcers, etc., can be very helpful. If a patient has a relatively mild form of the disease, the diagnosis may not have been made during childhood. A number of laboratory tests are useful in distinguishing sickle cell anemia from other hemoglobinopathies. Examination of the peripheral blood smear reveals normochromic normocytic red blood cells, many of which appear as targets. The presence of irreversibly sickled forms is very helpful (see Fig. A5-6). In addition, the presence of Howell-Jolly bodies, siderocytes, and occasional normoblasts suggests the absence of effective splenic function. A positive test for sickling, such as the metabisulfite preparation or the solubility test, indicates the presence of Hb S but does not distinguish between SS, AS, and double heterozygotes (SβThal, SC). Hemoglobin electrophoresis is necessary to establish the diagnosis. Patients with homozygous sickle cell anemia have about 2 to 20 percent Hb F and 2 to 4 percent Hb A$_2$. The remainder is Hb S. No Hb A is detected unless the patient has been transfused within the past 4 months. Patients with sickle β thalassemia will have hypochromic microcytic red blood cells, fewer irreversibly sickled forms, and a variable proportion of Hb A (0 to 30 percent). SC diseases can be readily diagnosed by hemoglobin electrophoresis. In hemoglobin SD disease, the two hemoglobin variants comigrate during conventional electrophoresis at pH 8.6 but can be separated by agar gel electrophoresis at pH 6.0.

Treatment Understanding the molecular pathogenesis of sickling has not yet led to an effective form of therapy. A large array of antisickling regimens has been proposed, but thus far none has stood the test of time. Recent investigation has focused on stimulating the production of Hb F by agents such as hydroxyurea and perhaps recombinant erythropoietin. Currently accepted management of sickle cell anemia is primarily supportive and conservative. Since patients with sickle cell anemia are at increased risk of developing infections, many of which trigger painful and aplastic crises, it is very important to detect infection early and give appropriate antibiotics promptly. Malaria prophylaxis should be administered in endemic areas. The development of pneumococcal sepsis in children may be prevented by the administration of the polyvalent vaccine and prophylactic penicillin.

The anemia of sickle cell disease increases markedly if the patient becomes deficient in folic acid. Since these patients have a continuous increased requirement for folic acid, it is reasonable to maintain them on a daily oral supplement.

Painful crises should be treated promptly with adequate analgesia and hydration. Some patients feel that their crises can be aborted if treated early. Therefore, it is expedient to give these patients a supply of an analgesic such as codeine which can be taken at home. However, these patients are at risk of becoming addicted to opiates. Oxygen should be administered during acute pain crisis if the patient has arterial hypoxemia.

Blood transfusions play a limited role in the management of sickle cell anemia. Between crises, patients tolerate anemia quite well and do not derive much subjective benefit from transfusions. However, partial replacement of the patients' red blood cells by transfused red cells (hypertransfusion) may be an effective way of preventing vasoocclusive crises. In order to lower the viscosity of the patient's blood significantly, it is necessary that over 50 percent of the patient's red blood cells be of donor origin. Hypertransfusion is a reasonable approach to getting a patient through a limited period of risk such as surgery. However, the problems of isoimmunization, iron overload, and hepatitis dictate against its widespread use.

Prevention Genetic counseling can play an important role in the prevention of sickle cell anemia. Parents who are both AS heterozygotes should be informed that there is a 25 percent chance that their offspring will be homozygous. The antenatal diagnosis of sickle cell anemia can be made in the first trimester of pregnancy by obtaining fetal cells from a chorionic villus and analyzing the DNA following digestion with a restriction endonuclease that recognizes the codon involved in the β6 valine mutation. If it is established that the fetus is an SS homozygote, the parents may decide to terminate the pregnancy.

Prognosis The clinical course of patients with sickle cell anemia is highly variable. Many assessments of prognosis that have appeared in the literature have been unduly pessimistic. During the past 30 years there has been considerable improvement in the care of patients with sickle cell anemia. An increasing number of patients are surviving into adulthood and bearing offspring. There has also been a decline in the mortality of SS mothers during pregnancy and childbirth. However, in underdeveloped nations, the mortality in sickle cell anemia remains very high.

No single clinical or laboratory finding is a consistent predictor of prognosis in sickle cell disease. Although those patients who have relatively high amounts of Hb F tend to have milder clinical manifestations, this relationship is of no prognostic value in any given patient. Considerable variation in the severity of sickle cell disease has been reported among different ethnic and geographical groups. A group of Shi Arabs from Saudi Arabia has been found to have a benign form of sickle cell anemia with very high levels of Hb F (15 to 30 percent). A mild type of sickle cell anemia has also been encountered in central India. SS patients with coexisting α thalassemia have less severe hemolysis but do not have a significant reduction in vasoocclusive phenomena.

SICKLE β THALASSEMIA This disease is highly variable in its clinical severity and complications. It is commonly encountered in people from the Mediterranean countries as well as those from central Africa. Sickle β thalassemia tends to be milder in blacks, just as homozygous β thalassemia is much less severe in blacks than in the Mediterranean populations. Patients have a congenital hemolytic anemia of variable severity, accompanied by splenomegaly in about 70 percent of cases. Individuals who produce no normal β chains (sickle β^0 thalassemia) have vasoocclusive manifestations comparable to those encountered in homozygous SS disease. In contrast, patients who are able to produce some normal β chains (sickle β$^+$ thalassemia) have less severe anemia, fewer pain crises, and less organ damage.

Examination of the blood film reveals hypochromic microcytic red blood cells, with polychromatophilia, target cells, stippling, and rare fixed sickle forms. The electrophoretic pattern shows from 60 to 90 percent Hb S and 10 to 30 percent Hb F. Hemoglobin A will be about 10 to 30 percent if the β-thalassemia gene is capable of producing some β^A chains (β$^+$ thalassemia, see below). In patients who have sickle β^0 thalassemia, no Hb A will be present, and therefore the disorder may be difficult to distinguish from homozygous sickle cell anemia. Hemoglobin A$_2$ is moderately elevated in sickle β thalassemia, but it is difficult to measure this minor component accurately in the presence of Hb S. Occasional patients may derive benefit from splenectomy if the spleen is sequestering a significant amount of red blood cells.

SICKLE C DISEASE Although the gene frequency among blacks in the United States for Hb C (β6 Glu→Lys) is only one-fourth that for Hb S, the prevalence of SC disease among adults is almost as high as SS disease since the former group of patients has a nearly normal life expectancy. These individuals have a mild to moderate hemolytic anemia, usually accompanied by splenomegaly. On peripheral blood smears, target cells and occasional plump sickled forms are seen. Hemoglobin electrophoresis reveals 50 percent Hb S, 50 percent Hb C. Hemoglobin S copolymerizes with Hb C to the same extent as with Hb A. The increased tendency of SC red cells to sickle, compared with sickle trait cells, can be explained by two phenomena: increased intracellular hemoglobin concentration and significantly higher percent Hb S. Patients with SC disease may occasionally have painful crises or organ infarcts. They are at particular risk of developing ocular complications described above, including proliferative retinopathy and retinal detachment. In addition, patients with SC disease are at relatively high risk of developing hematuria from renal medullary infarcts and avascular necrosis of the femoral head. Pregnant women with SC disease have a high rate of complications during pregnancy. Individuals with an electrophoretic pattern suggestive of Hb SC disease but with more severe clinical manifestations may be double heterozygotes for Hb S and Hb O Arab (β121 Glu→Lys).

SICKLE D DISEASE A number of hemoglobins comigrate with Hb S on routine electrophoresis. The most commonly encountered variant is Hb D Los Angeles (β121 Glu→Gln). Hemoglobins S and

D can be separated by special electrophoretic methods. The diagnosis of Hb SD disease is suggested by the demonstration of a positive sickle cell preparation in only one of the patient's two parents. SD double heterozygotes have moderately severe anemia.

HOMOZYGOUS Hb C DISEASE Patients have a mild congenital hemolytic anemia accompanied by splenomegaly. Hemoglobin C has a tendency to form intracellular crystals, particularly if red blood cells are suspended in a hypertonic medium. The intracellular hemoglobin concentration is markedly increased owing to loss of potassium and water from the cytoplasm. As a result, the blood film reveals striking target cells. Red blood cell osmotic fragility is decreased. Patients rarely develop significant complications. No specific therapy is indicated.

UNSTABLE HEMOGLOBIN VARIANTS

In the early 1950s several patients in England were found to have congenital nonspherocytic hemolytic anemia associated with inclusions of precipitated hemoglobin (Heinz bodies) within red blood cells. The presence of an abnormal hemoglobin was suspected by the formation of a precipitate when the patients' hemolysates were gently heated. Currently, over 90 different unstable hemoglobin variants have been identified. The great majority are single amino acid substitutions in the β chain. A few are due to deletion of one or more amino acids within the β chain. Patients present with a hemolytic anemia of variable degree. Severe cases are usually detected in late infancy or early childhood and have jaundice, splenomegaly, and dark-colored urine. An autosomal dominant mode of inheritance can usually be established, although about a fifth of the cases appear to be spontaneous mutants.

Pathogenesis These hemoglobin variants have structural alterations at sites in the molecule that drastically affect its stability and solubility. Many involve an amino acid substitution in the portion of the subunit where heme is inserted. In such instances, the heme may be displaced from the heme pocket. As a result, the abnormal hemoglobin has decreased solubility and forms an intracellular precipitate (Heinz body). Red blood cells which contain this type of inclusion are recognized by the mononuclear phagocyte system and are either cleansed of their intracellular debris (pitting) or destroyed. The displaced heme moiety is aberrantly catabolized, forming dipyrroles, such as mesobilifuscin, instead of bilirubin. Pigmenturia is probably due to the excretion of these dipyrroles. The degree of instability of these hemoglobin variants and, therefore, the extent of hemolysis vary considerably. In some, such as Hb Zürich, an additional oxidant stress, such as the ingestion of certain drugs, is required for significant hemolysis. In contrast, patients with Hb Hammersmith have continuous and marked red blood cell breakdown. The degree of anemia is influenced not only by the severity of the hemolysis but also by the ability of the blood to unload oxygen. Thus, patients having unstable variants with increased oxygen affinity, such as Hb Köln, may have a near-normal hemoglobin level, i.e., compensated hemolysis.

Diagnosis The red blood cell morphology is somewhat variable. Often, patients with a functioning spleen have normal-appearing red blood cells. Slight hypochromia and basophilic stippling are not uncommon. The blood may have to be incubated in order to bring out Heinz bodies. In some cases, red blood cells appear as if a bite had been taken from a margin. It is tempting to speculate that at this site a Heinz body had been pitted. Following splenectomy, red blood cells appear much more abnormal, and Heinz bodies are larger and more numerous.

The diagnosis of a congenital Heinz body hemolytic anemia is established by the following laboratory tests and results:

1 *Hemoglobin electrophoresis* will often reveal an abnormal component, usually composing less than 30 percent of the total.
2 *Heinz bodies* can be demonstrated by incubating a freshly drawn sample of blood with a supravital stain.

3 A significant *precipitate* is formed when the hemolysate is incubated at 50°C, or in the presence of 17% isopropanol.
4 The unstable hemoglobins often have an abnormal *oxygen dissociation curve*.

If these tests are negative in a patient with congenital nonspherocytic hemolytic anemia, a defect of the membrane or one of the red blood cell enzymes is likely (Chap. 294).

Treatment The treatment of congenital Heinz body hemolytic anemia is primarily supportive. Anemia is rarely severe enough to warrant blood transfusion. Oxidant drugs should be avoided. Like others with chronic hemolysis, these patients have an increased requirement for folic acid. Those with severe hemolysis often benefit from prophylactic folate therapy. The red blood cell mass may fall during a period of bone marrow suppression, such as that resulting from folate deficiency or acute infection. Although patients with severe hemolysis may benefit from splenectomy, this operation is not curative. Because of the risk of bacterial sepsis in infants and young children who have been splenectomized, this treatment should be postponed until the child is over 4 years old. The diagnostic tests cited above become more abnormal following splenectomy. For this reason, in some cases the diagnosis may not be definitely established until after the operation.

STABLE VARIANTS HAVING ABNORMAL OXYGEN AFFINITY

In 1966 certain members of a large family were discovered to have erythrocytosis in association with an electrophoretically abnormal hemoglobin, Hb Chesapeake, which had a very high affinity for oxygen. Since then, more than 40 other stable high-affinity hemoglobin variants have been encountered in families with erythrocytosis. Their structural alterations tend to be at sites which influence hemoglobin's functional behavior. As a result of the hemoglobin's increased oxygen affinity, oxygen unloading to tissues is decreased, and there is an erythropoietin-mediated stimulus to erythropoiesis. This disorder is manifested in the heterozygous state and follows an autosomal codominant pattern of inheritance. Hematocrit levels are rarely high enough to cause a significant increase in blood viscosity. Thus, affected individuals are generally asymptomatic and lack any pertinent physical findings other than a ruddy complexion. The diagnosis should be suspected in all patients with unexplained erythrocytosis, particularly when other family members are similarly affected, and can be established by the demonstration of increased oxygen affinity of the whole blood. About two-thirds of the high-affinity variants can be readily separated from Hb A by electrophoresis. No treatment is indicated. The patient should be reassured that the disorder is benign.

Hemoglobin variants having a marked decrease in oxygen affinity cause one form of familial cyanosis (Table 295-3). Because of the abnormality of hemoglobin function, arterial blood is partially unsaturated despite normal oxygen tension. Thus, the cyanosis is due

---

TABLE 295-3 Differential diagnosis of cyanosis

I Decreased oxygenation of hemoglobin (↑ deoxyhemoglobin)
  A Reduced arterial oxygen tension (common)
    1 Pulmonary disease
    2 Cardiac right-to-left shunt
  B Hemoglobin variant having decreased oxygen affinity (rare)
II Methemoglobinemia (rare)
  A Hereditary
    1 M hemoglobins
    2 Cytochrome b_5 reductase deficiency
  B Acquired
    1 Nitrites and nitrates: sodium nitrite, amyl nitrite, nitroglycerin, nitroprusside, silver nitrate
    2 Aniline dyes
    3 Acetanilid and phenacetin
    4 Sulfonamides
    5 Other: lidocaine, chlorate, phenazopyridine

to increased levels of deoxyhemoglobin in the blood. Except for this cosmetic problem, affected individuals have no other clinical manifestations. Blood values are otherwise normal.

METHEMOGLOBINEMIA

Oxygen transport depends on the maintenance of intracellular hemoglobin in the reduced (Fe^{2+}) state. When hemoglobin is oxidized to methemoglobin, the heme iron becomes Fe^{3+} and is incapable of binding oxygen. Normal red cells contain less than 1 percent methemoglobin. A small amount of hemoglobin autooxidizes as red cells circulate. This process probably occurs by the dissociation of the superoxide anion from oxyhemoglobin:

$$Hb^{2+}O_2 \rightarrow Hb^{3+} + O_2^-$$

Normally, the methemoglobin that is formed is reduced by the following reaction:

$$Hb^{3+} + RedCyt\ b_5 \rightarrow Hb^{2+} + OxCyt\ b_5$$

Reduced cytochrome b_5 (RedCyt b_5) is regenerated by the enzyme cytochrome b_5 reductase (methemoglobin reductase):

$$OxCyt\ b_5 + NADH \xrightarrow[\text{reductase}]{\text{Cytochrome } b_5} RedCyt\ b_5 + NAD$$

Hereditary methemoglobinemia is due either to the presence of one of the M hemoglobins or to the deficiency of the enzyme cytochrome b_5 reductase (Table 295-3). These inherited disorders are clinically mild, while the induction of methemoglobinemia by drugs or toxins can be life-threatening.

If methemoglobin exceeds 15 g/L (1.5 g/dL) (10 percent of the total hemoglobin), affected individuals will have clinically obvious cyanosis. The color of the skin is indistinguishable from the much commoner cyanosis due to impairment of oxygen saturation that may occur in pulmonary and cardiac disorders (Table 295-3). With higher amounts of methemoglobin, patients become symptomatic. At a methemoglobin level of about 35 percent, the affected individual experiences headache, weakness, and breathlessness. Levels in excess of 80 percent are usually incompatible with life.

The toxicity of methemoglobinemia can be readily explained in terms of hemoglobin function. The fact that a certain proportion of the heme moieties is no longer able to bind oxygen is not a serious physiologic handicap per se. A proportion of 30 percent methemoglobin is much more deleterious than a 30 percent decrement in red cell mass, because the oxidized hemes have a profound effect on the remaining functional hemes in the hemoglobin tetramer. The conformation of methemoglobin (like that of carboxyhemoglobin) is very similar to that of oxyhemoglobin. Thus, a partially oxidized hemoglobin tetramer has the same tertiary and quaternary structure as a molecule which is comparably oxygenated. In each case, the affinity of the remaining hemes for oxygen is increased. For this reason, methemoglobinemia [as well as carbon monoxide (Chap. 374)] causes a "shift to the left" of the oxyhemoglobin dissociation curve and, consequently, impaired unloading of oxygen to tissues.

CYTOCHROME b_5 REDUCTASE (METHEMOGLOBIN REDUCTASE) DEFICIENCY This condition is inherited in an autosomal recessive pattern. The enzyme is a flavoprotein having properties similar to those of liver microsomal cytochrome b_5 reductase. The soluble erythrocyte enzyme is formed by cleavage of a hydrophobic tail from the microsomal enzyme.

Individuals with cytochrome b_5 reductase deficiency have lifelong cyanosis of variable degree, depending on the level of methemoglobin, but usually have no associated symptoms or other physical findings. Some may have mild polycythemia owing to increased oxygen affinity. Others have been noted to be mentally retarded. Untreated individuals usually have 15 to 30 percent methemoglobin. Methemoglobin levels are higher in the older population of red cells because the activity of the abnormal enzyme declines markedly with red cell age. There

appears to be considerable heterogeneity in the variant enzymes from different families, as shown by differences in their electrophoretic mobility and kinetic parameters. In these ways, cytochrome b_5 reductase deficiency resembles glucose-6-phosphate dehydrogenase deficiency (Chap. 294).

ACQUIRED METHEMOGLOBINEMIA This disorder is generally due to exposure to certain drugs or toxins. Compounds which can cause clinically significant methemoglobinemia are listed in Table 295-3. Some agents such as nitrite and chlorate oxidize the heme iron directly. Others such as sulfa drugs and aniline must undergo biochemical transformation before they cause methemoglobinemia. Few drugs currently in use cause significant methemoglobinemia, unless the individual is unusually susceptible. Exposure to local anesthetics such as procaine and to nitroprusside occasionally causes severe methemoglobinemia. As might be expected, individuals heterozygous for methemoglobin reductase deficiency are much more likely than normal individuals to develop clinically apparent methemoglobinemia after exposure to an oxidant stress. Thus, the extent of methemoglobinemia depends not only on the dose of the toxic agent but also on the susceptibility of the exposed individual.

M HEMOGLOBINS Five hemoglobin variants have abnormal absorbance spectra, owing to the oxidation of the heme iron in the affected subunit. They involve amino acid substitutions of residues responsible for the binding of the heme iron to the globin. These so-called M hemoglobins (Table 295-3) result in a rare form of congenital and familial cyanosis. Individuals with the α-chain variants Hb M Boston and Hb M Iwate are cyanotic at birth, while cyanosis does not appear in those with the β-chain variants (Hb M Saskatoon, Hb M Hyde Park, and Hb M Milwaukee) until about 4 to 6 months of age, when fetal hemoglobin has been replaced by adult hemoglobin. As with the unstable and high-affinity variants, an autosomal codominant inheritance pattern is found. Except for cyanosis, patients are asymptomatic.

DIAGNOSIS Methemoglobinemia should be considered in any cyanotic patient with no evidence of heart or lung disease. If the cyanosis is due to decreased oxygen saturation, a blood specimen will change from a purple to a red color upon mixing with air. In contrast, a blood specimen from a methemoglobinemic individual remains a chocolate brown color irrespective of exposure to air. Methemoglobinemia can be documented by spectroscopic examination of the hemolysate. Individuals with hereditary methemoglobinemia will have lower levels than patients symptomatic from acquired methemoglobinemia. Patients who have ingested an oxidant drug may have an additional hemoglobin derivative called sulfhemoglobin in which the protoporphyrin has been chemically modified. Sulfhemoglobinemia tends to cause cyanosis even more readily than methemoglobinemia. Unlike methemoglobin, the absorbance of sulfhemoglobin at 620 to 630 nm is not decreased by the addition of cyanide. The M hemoglobins have characteristic spectral abnormalities which differ from those obtained when normal Hb A is partially oxidized. Furthermore, these hemoglobin variants can be detected by hemoglobin electrophoresis.

Treatment In individuals with methemoglobin reductase deficiency, the oral administration of methylene blue (100 to 300 mg/d) or ascorbic acid (300 to 500 mg/d) will result in a marked reduction in the level of methemoglobin. The purpose of treatment is primarily cosmetic. Severe toxic methemoglobinemia is treated by the intravenous administration of methylene blue (2 mg/kg, repeat if needed). Within an hour, the methemoglobin level is usually reduced by at least 50 percent. Treatment is neither necessary nor possible in individuals having Hb M.

THALASSEMIAS

The thalassemias are a diverse group of congenital disorders in which there is a defect in the synthesis of one (or more) of the subunits of hemoglobin. As a result of decreased production of hemoglobin, the

TABLE 295-4   Classification of the thalassemias

Diagnosis	Globin chain synthesis in reticulocytes	RBC morphology	Hb electrophoresis	Clinical severity
α Thalassemia:	α/β*			
Silent carrier (α−/αα)	0.9	Normal	Normal, ↓ Hb A$_2$	0
α-thalassemia trait [(α−/α−) or (−−/αα)]	0.7	↓ MCV†	Normal, ↓ Hb A$_2$	0
Hb H disease (−−/α−)	0.3	↓ MCV Heinz bodies, targets	↑ Hb H (β$_4$) (10–15%)	2+
Hydrops fetalis (−−/−−)	0	↑↑ Nucleated RBC	↑↑ Hb Barts (γ$_4$)	4+
β Thalassemia:	β/α*			
Heterozygous	0.5	↓ MCV, stippling	↓ Hb A$_2$ (± ↑ Hb F)	0 to +
Homozygous (or double heterozygous)	0–0.3	↓ MCV, hypochromic Nucleated RBC, targets bizarre shapes	↑↑ Hb F	4+ (major) 2–3+ (intermedia)

* Normal = 1.
† MCV = mean corpuscular volume.

red blood cells are microcytic and hypochromic (Table 61-2). The thalassemias involve a spectrum ranging from subtle morphologic abnormalities to life-threatening disease. In contrast to the qualitative hemoglobin abnormalities listed in Table 295-1, the thalassemias are quantitative abnormalities of subunit synthesis. Thus, the β chains of patients with β thalassemia have normal structure but are produced in reduced and sometimes undetectable amounts. Conversely, patients with α thalassemia have impaired production of α chains. The reduction in globin chain synthesis can be demonstrated in vitro by incubating reticulocytes with labeled amino acids and determining the incorporation of radioactivity into globin subunits (Table 295-4). Most forms of thalassemia can be identified from the information summarized in Table 295-4. Occasionally, establishing a definitive diagnosis requires measurement of globin chain synthesis or analysis of globin gene structure.

α THALASSEMIA   As mentioned at the beginning of this chapter, normal individuals inherit two α-chain genes from each parent. The great majority of cases of α thalassemia can be explained by deletions of α-chain genes, owing to nonhomologous crossover (Fig. 295-1). Specific gene deletions can be identified by analysis of patients' DNA following digestion by restriction endonucleases. The clinical manifestations of α thalassemia depend upon the number of genes deleted (Table 295-4). In the silent carrier state, heterozygous α thalassemia 2 (α−/αα), one of the four genes is deleted. Affected individuals have no hematologic abnormalities. Individuals with deletion of two of the four α-chain genes (α-thalassemia trait) have either homozygous α thalassemia 2 (α−/α−) or heterozygous α thalassemia 1 (−−/αα). They have microcytic and slightly hypochromic red blood cells but no significant hemolysis or anemia. Hemoglobin electrophoresis is normal except for a decreased amount of Hb A$_2$. Deletion of three α-chain genes (−−/α−) produces a well-compensated hemolytic state with microcytic hypochromic red blood cells including many target cells. Intracellular inclusions or Heinz bodies are formed by the precipitation of Hb H, a tetramer composed of β chains which accumulates because of the marked impairment of α-chain synthesis. The most severe form of α thalassemia, hydrops fetalis, is usually due to deletion of all four α-chain genes. The affected fetus has red blood cells containing only Hb Barts, a tetramer composed of γ chains. This condition is incompatible with life, since oxygen transport depends upon the presence of heterotetramers such as α$_2$β$_2$ and α$_2$γ$_2$. In orientals both the α− and the −− haplotypes are relatively common; thus both Hb H disease and hydrops fetalis are frequently encountered. In contrast, blacks commonly have the α− haplotype (gene frequency ≅ 0.15) but rarely have the −− haploytpe. Therefore Hb H disease is very rare in blacks and hydrops fetalis has not been reported. Homozygous α thalassemia 2 is encountered in about 2 percent of blacks and is therefore a relatively common cause of microcytosis in an individual who is otherwise healthy and not iron-deficient.

The elongated α-chain variant Hb Constant Spring, commonly encountered among southeast Asians, also has an α-thalassemia phenotype, and when inherited with the −− haplotype can cause Hb H disease.

β THALASSEMIA   Since individuals inherit only one β-chain gene from each parent, affected individuals are either heterozygotes, homozygotes, or double heterozygotes. The gene frequency for β thalassemia approaches 0.1 in southern Italy and certain Mediterranean islands. β Thalassemia is also encountered quite commonly in central Africa, Asia, the south Pacific, and certain parts of India. Statistically, one-quarter of the offspring of two heterozygotes (β-thalassemia trait) will have the homozygous state: β thalassemia major or Cooley's anemia. An individual may inherit a β-thalassemia gene from one parent and a β-chain structural variant from the other Sickle β thalassemia (discussed above) is a commonly encountered example of such a double heterozygous state.

The molecular pathogenesis of the β thalassemias is more complex and heterogeneous than that of α thalassemia. In contrast to α thalassemia, gene deletion is an uncommon cause of β thalassemia. Among the recognized types of β-gene deletion, an entity known as "pancellular hereditary persistence of fetal hemoglobin" has minimal clinical manifestations owing to efficient synthesis of γ chains on the chromosome in which the β and δ genes are deleted. Hemoglobin Lepore is a fusion protein formed from a nonhomologous crossover between the δ and β genes resulting in the absence of normal β-chain synthesis and therefore a β-thalassemia phenotype (Fig. 295-1). In the great majority of cases of β thalassemia, restriction endonuclease maps reveal no gross abnormalities of the β-globin gene complex. Nevertheless, there are several steps in β-globin synthesis that could go awry and lead to a thalassemic phenotype. A number of cases involve mutations in or near one of the intervening sequences of the β-globin gene, leading to errors in the splicing of mRNA. Often β^A chains are made but in reduced amounts (β$^+$ thalassemia) (see Fig. 295-1). Other cases have nonsense mutations in the coding region, causing premature termination of β-globin chains. This is the most common cause of β^0 thalassemia (Fig. 295-1).

Cellular pathogenesis   As a result of imbalance in globin chain synthesis, the β thalassemias have varying degrees of ineffective erythropoiesis (Chap. 290) and hemolysis. In β thalassemia major there is a marked relative excess of α-chain production. Free α chains have decreased solubility and will form insoluble aggregates or inclusions within red blood cell precursors in the bone marrow. Like congenital Heinz body hemolytic anemia due to unstable hemoglobin variants, the inclusion bodies in thalassemia bring about abnormalities in membrane permeability as well as entrapment and destruction of red blood cells by the macrophages in the mononuclear phagoycte system. As a result, β thalassemia is characterized by both intramedullary erythroid destruction and also a shortening of the life span of circulating red blood cells that emerge from the bone marrow. Thus, these patients have the characteristic parameters of both ineffective erythropoiesis (increased plasma iron turnover, decreased incorporation of iron into red blood cells) and peripheral hemolysis. Because these red blood cells are under double jeopardy, there is an enormous compensatory stimulus to erythropoiesis, resulting both in expansion of the red marrow and in extramedullary hematopoiesis in the liver and spleen. Chain imbalance in β thalassemia is attenuated to a variable degree by the "compensatory" synthesis of γ chains which are able to combine with excess free α chains and form a stable tetramer (Hb F). Patients with Cooley's anemia who have a relatively high rate of γ-chain production have a less severe clinical course. Individuals with β thalassemia minor have absent or very mild ineffective erythropoiesis and hemolysis, detectable in some patients by a slight elevation in fecal urobilinogen and a modest shortening of the red blood cell life span.

In the α thalassemias a relative excess production of non-α chains can be detected, leading to the formation of Hb Barts (γ_4) in the newborn and young infant. Children and adults with deletion of 3 α-globin genes usually have Hb H (β_4). In contrast to the α-chain inclusions found in β thalassemia, the Heinz bodies due to Hb H are more stable and develop in mature circulating red blood cells. As a result, Hb H disease is primarily a hemolytic disorder without a significant amount of ineffective erythropoiesis.

β thalassemia minor This common entity, also referred to as β-*thalassemia trait*, is rarely associated with significant clinical manifestations. The diagnosis is generally made in patients being evaluated for mild anemia or in follow-up of abnormalities found on routine blood studies. Most individuals with β-thalassemia trait escape diagnosis. About one-fifth of affected individuals have splenomegaly. Icterus is occasionally noted, particularly in those individuals who also have Gilbert's disease, another common and benign congenital disorder (Chap. 251).

In otherwise healthy individuals with β-thalassemia trait, the mean hemoglobin level is about 15 percent lower than in normal persons of the same age and sex; the red blood cell count is usually elevated, and the cells are microcytic. Indeed, at any level of hematocrit, patients with β thalassemia minor have more marked microcytosis than those with iron deficiency. In contrast, the mean corpuscular hemoglobin concentration is normal. In addition to microcytosis, examination of the blood film reveals occasional target cells, cigar-shaped cells, and a moderate amount of basophilic stippling; the reticulocyte count is normal. Special isotope techniques are required to demonstrate a slightly reduced red blood cell life span. The red blood cells have decreased osmotic fragility. Serum iron is normal unless the patient also happens to be iron-deficient. Hemoglobin electrophoresis is very useful in establishing the diagnosis of β thalassemia minor. Most affected individuals will have a twofold increase in Hb A_2 (5 percent versus normal of 2.5 percent). In contrast, Hb A_2 is subnormal in α thalassemia, iron deficiency, and sideroblastic anemias. Patients with β-thalassemia trait who become iron-deficient usually have a "normal" level of Hb A_2 which increases to above normal after correction of the deficiency. Approximately half of individuals with β thalassemia minor also have a modest elevation of Hb F (2 to 3 percent). In the less common state, δβ thalassemia, in which there is a deletion of the adjacent δ and β chain genes, Hb A_2 levels will be normal or decreased, but Hb F is increased (5 to 15 percent).

No treatment is indicated for individuals with β-thalassemia trait. They should be reassured that they do not have a serious hematologic problem. The genetic implications of thalassemia should be explained, particularly to those of childbearing age. Many individuals have been given long-term iron treatment on the mistaken impression that they had iron-deficiency anemia. These patients may gradually develop clinically significant siderosis. Establishing the diagnosis of β thalassemia minor should prevent such inappropriate therapy.

β thalassemia major Also termed Cooley's anemia, this is probably the most severe form of congenital hemolytic anemia. Clinical manifestations generally appear after the first 4 to 6 months of life when the switch from γ-chain to β-chain production usually occurs. Patients develop a severe anemia with a hematocrit of less than 20 unless they are supported by transfusions. Accordingly, patients have all the signs and symptoms associated with severe anemia. In addition, they have findings related to severe intramedullary and peripheral hemolysis as well as to iron overload. Patients with β thalassemia major often have marked wasting and appear malnourished. Children have slow rates of growth and development. In adolescents, the onset and development of secondary sex characteristics are delayed. Patients have a peculiar skin color due to a combination of icterus, pallor, and increased melanin deposition. They usually have skeletal abnormalities, secondary to expansion of the erythroid marrow. Enlargement of the malar bones may give the characteristic "chipmunk" facies or cause malocclusion of the jaw. Patients invariably have cardiomegaly which may be accompanied by signs of congestive heart failure. Marked hepatomegaly and splenomegaly are always found in these patients.

The *diagnosis* of β thalassemia major should be considered in any patient with a severe hemolytic anemia and hypochromic microcytic red blood cells. Examination of the peripheral blood smear reveals marked variations in the size and shape of red blood cells, including many target and stippled cells as well as teardrop and cigar-shaped cells (see Fig. A5-5). Normoblasts are usually seen, particularly if the patient has undergone splenectomy. Hemoglobin electrophoresis shows the presence of increased amounts of Hb F and variable amounts of Hb A. In patients who are homozygous for β^0 thalassemia, no Hb A can be detected. Hemoglobin A_2 is usually increased about twofold, although it can be normal in β thalassemia major.

Patients with β thalassemia major have a short life expectancy. It is unusual for a patient with the most severe form of the disease to survive into adulthood. Most patients have such severe anemia that they are dependent upon transfusions. The chronic administration of large amounts of blood along with an inappropriate increase in iron absorption from the gastrointestinal tract inevitably leads to clinically significant hemosiderosis. As a result of iron overload, these patients develop abnormalities in cardiac, endocrine, and hepatic function. The combination of chronic hypoxia and myocardial siderosis leads to cardiac arrhythmias, congestive failure, and ultimately death.

Homozygotes who survive into adulthood are likely to have a less severe form of the disease, designated as β *thalassemia intermedia*. There are several genetic subtypes which are associated with less severe clinical manifestations: (1) β thalassemia with unusually high levels of Hb F synthesis, (2) δβ thalassemia in which there is absence of δ-chain as well as β-chain synthesis, and (3) the presence of α thalassemia in combination with homozygous β thalassemia, leading to more balanced subunit synthesis. A milder clinical course is also seen in individuals who are doubly heterozygous for β thalassemia and hereditary persistence of Hb F. Patients with the above genotypes usually have moderately severe anemia, but do not require transfusions.

Treatment of β thalassemia major is primarily supportive. The obvious benefits of transfusion therapy are partially offset by the risk of iron overload, hepatitis, and alloimmunization. Despite these problems, children with Cooley's anemia fare better if their hemoglobin is maintained at greater than 90 g/L (9 g/dL). In view of the increased demands of the hyperplastic marrow, it is reasonable to maintain these patients on a daily supplement of folic acid. Since splenic sequestration contributes to shortened red blood cell survival, many patients derive some benefit from splenectomy. The prevention and treatment of iron overload is a continuing concern in these patients. Continuous subcutaneous injection of desferrioxamine permits the mobilization and excretion of significant amounts of iron and, when administered over a prolonged period, can prevent or retard the development of chronic iron toxicity.

Considerations of genetic counseling and antenatal diagnosis are as relevant in the *prevention* of β thalassemia major as they are for sickle cell anemia (see above). Because of linkages between β thalassemias and restriction enzyme polymorphisms, prenatal diagnosis can often be made by DNA analysis of amniotic fluid cells.

However, in some cases it is necessary to take the risk of obtaining fetal red blood cells for globin chain synthesis measurements.

REFERENCES

Adams JG, Honig GR: *Human Hemoglobin Genetics.* New York, Springer Verlag, 1986
Bunn HF, Forget BG: *Hemoglobin: Molecular, Genetic and Clinical Aspects.* Philadelphia, Saunders, 1986
Castle WB: From man to molecule and back to mankind. Semin Hematol 13:159, 1976
Charache S: Advances in the understanding of sickle cell anemia. Hosp Pract 21:173, 182, 1986
Eaton WA, Hofrichter J: Hemoglobin S gelation and sickle cell disease. Blood 70:1245, 1987
Embury S: The clinical pathophysiology of sickle cell disease. Ann Rev Med 37:36, 1986
Kan YW: Thalassemia: Molecular mechanism and detection. Am J Hum Genet 38:4, 1986
Nienhuis AW et al: Advances in thalassemia research. Blood 63:738, 1984
Old JM et al: First trimester fetal diagnosis for haemoglobinopathies. Lancet 2:763, 1986
Schechter AN, Bunn HF: What determines severity in sickle cell disease. N Engl J Med 306:295, 1982
Serjeant GR: *The Clinical Features of Sickle Cell Disease.* New York, American Elsevier, 1986
Weatherall DJ, Clegg JB: *The Thalassemia Syndromes.* Oxford, Blackwell, 1982

296 THE LEUKEMIAS

RICHARD CHAMPLIN / DAVID W. GOLDE

The leukemias are a heterogeneous group of neoplasms arising from the malignant transformation of hematopoietic (blood-forming) cells. Leukemic cells proliferate primarily in the bone marrow and lymphoid tissues where they interfere with normal hematopoiesis and immunity. Ultimately they emigrate into the peripheral blood and infiltrate other tissues.

Leukemias are classified according to the cell types primarily involved (*myeloid* or *lymphoid*) and as *acute* or *chronic* based upon the natural history of the disease. Acute leukemias have a rapid clinical course, resulting in death within a matter of months without effective treatment, whereas chronic leukemias have a more prolonged natural history. This chapter will cover acute lymphocytic leukemia (ALL), acute myelogenous leukemia (AML), chronic lymphocytic leukemia (CLL), and hairy cell leukemia. Chronic myelogenous leukemia (CML) is discussed in Chap. 297.

ETIOLOGY   The cause of leukemia is not known in most patients, although both genetic and environmental factors may be important. There is a high concordance rate among identical twins if acute leukemia develops in the first year of life, and families with an excessive incidence of leukemia have been identified. Acute leukemia occurs with an increased frequency in a variety of congenital disorders, including Down's, Bloom's, Klinefelter's, Fanconi's, and the Wiskott-Aldrich syndromes.

Environmental factors are also known to play a role in the etiology of leukemia. Ionizing radiation causes leukemia in experimental animals, and there is a clear relationship between such exposure and the development of leukemia in humans. For example, individuals with occupational radiation exposure, patients receiving radiation therapy, or Japanese survivors of the atomic bomb explosions have a predictable and dose-related increased incidence of leukemia. Radiation exposure increases the risk of developing CML, AML, and possibly ALL, but there is no known relationship to CLL or to hairy cell leukemia. Chemicals such as benzene and other aromatic hydrocarbons have also been associated with the development of AML. Treatment with alkylating agents and other chemotherapeutic drugs also leads to an increased incidence of AML.

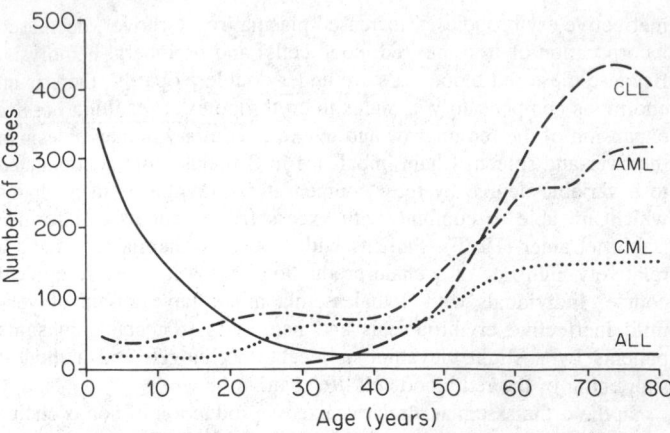

FIGURE 296-1   Age-related incidence of various forms of leukemia: ALL = acute lymphoblastic leukemia, AML = acute myelogenous leukemia, CLL = chronic lymphocytic leukemia, CML = chronic myelogenous leukemia. *(From Surveillance and Mortality Data 1973–1977, U.S. Department of Health and Human Resources.)*

While leukemias induced by retroviruses (RNA viruses) have been studied in laboratory animals for many years, it was not until recently that a viral etiology was established for a form of human leukemia. A unique human retrovirus, referred to as human T-cell leukemia virus I (HTLV-I) (see Chap. 134) has recently been identified as causing adult T-cell leukemia (ATL), an aggressive malignancy composed of mature T-lymphoid cells. A related virus, HTLV-II, has been isolated from cells of patients with rare and poorly defined chronic T-cell leukemias. Adult T-cell leukemia is endemic in southwestern Japan and parts of the Caribbean and central Africa. Except for the HTLV family, no virus has been causally associated with the more common human acute and chronic leukemias.

INCIDENCE AND PREVALENCE   The incidence of all leukemias is approximately 13 per 100,000 people per year, and the age-related incidence of the various forms of leukemia is shown in Fig. 296-1. The incidence of both acute and chronic leukemias is somewhat higher in men than in women. ALL is primarily a disease of children and young adults, whereas AML occurs at all ages. CLL and hairy cell leukemia tend to occur in the elderly.

There have been several epidemiologic reports of case clustering of leukemias within communities and even in successive occupants of the same house. The bulk of evidence, however, indicates that the common forms of acute and chronic leukemias are not contagious and the incidence of leukemia is not increased among close contacts, such as marital partners or in the offspring of women who develop leukemia during pregnancy. The clear exception is ATL caused by HTLV-I. The virus may be passed in blood products and from infected to uninfected individuals.

PATHOPHYSIOLOGY   Acute leukemia is characterized by proliferation of immature myeloid or lymphoid cells. The leukemia arises following malignant transformation of a single hematopoietic or lymphoid progenitor, followed by cellular replication and expansion of the transformed clone. The most prominent characteristic of the neoplastic cells in acute leukemia is a defect in maturation beyond the myeloblast or promyelocyte level in AML and the lymphoblast level in ALL. Leukemic cells accumulate in the bone marrow due both to excessive proliferation and to a defect in terminal maturation. The failure to mature to nonreplicating end cells is the major factor leading to the accumulation of leukemic cells in AML. The leukemic cells proliferate primarily in the bone marrow, circulate in the blood, and may infiltrate into other tissues such as lymph nodes, liver, spleen, skin, viscera, and the central nervous system.

The cellular blood elements are derived from pluripotent and committed hematopoietic stem cells which reside in the bone marrow.

Leukemic transformation may occur in cells at several levels of differentiation. In some patients with AML who are heterozygous for glucose-6-phosphate dehydrogenase (G6PD) isoenzymes, the granulocytes, macrophages, erythrocytes, and megakaryocytes all contain the single G6PD isoenzyme present in the leukemic cells, suggesting that these cells are derived from the malignant clone and that leukemic transformation involved a pluripotent stem cell. In other AML patients, only granulocytes and/or macrophages appear monoclonal, and in these patients, transformation may have occurred at the level of the committed granulocytic-macrophage progenitor.

The mechanism of neoplastic transformation producing leukemia is poorly understood but involves a fundamental alteration of DNA conferring hereditable malignant characteristics to the transformed cell and its progeny. A neoplastic phenotype can be induced in nonmalignant cells in vitro by transfer (transfection) of DNA from the leukemic cells. In animals, leukemias can be induced by retroviruses which either carry a transforming gene (viral oncogene) or integrate into specific sites in DNA causing activation of cellular proto-oncogenes (insertional mutagenesis). The role of oncogenes in the pathogenesis of neoplasia is discussed in Chap. 10. With sensitive techniques, clonal cytogenetic abnormalities can be detected in most patients with acute and chronic leukemias. A wide range of cytogenetic abnormalities is associated with the various forms of leukemias, and distinctive nonrandom chromosomal abnormalities are associated with AML, ALL, and CLL, as shown in Table 296-1. Chromosomal rearrangements in leukemic cells may alter the structure or regulation of cellular oncogenes, producing quantitative or qualitative changes in their gene products, which may play a role in initiating or maintaining the leukemic state. Most data suggest the development of leukemia is a multistep process. In many cases, acute leukemia develops in patients with a preexisting myelodysplastic or myeloproliferative disorder.

The pathophysiology of bone marrow failure in leukemia is complex. Pancytopenia is typically present and results at least in part from physical replacement of the normal precursor cells by leukemic cells. Some patients with acute leukemia and pancytopenia have a hypocellular bone marrow indicating that marrow failure is not simply due to overcrowding by leukemic cells. Leukemic cells may directly inhibit normal hematopoiesis via cell-mediated or humoral mechanisms. Alternatively, leukemic cells may occupy critical niches in the bone marrow (stromal) microenvironment and interfere with normal cellular interactions. Normal hematopoietic stem cells do remain in the bone marrow and are capable of proliferating and restoring hematopoiesis following effective antileukemic treatment.

Some patients develop AML after a preleukemic syndrome. The preleukemic and myelodysplastic syndromes are a heterogeneous group of disorders, and the nomenclature describing them is confusing. These syndromes generally occur in middle-aged or elderly patients. Included under the heading of myelodysplastic syndromes are refractory anemia with excess blasts, chronic myelomonocytic leukemia, and acquired idiopathic sideroblastic anemia. The term *preleukemia* should be reserved for a recognizable syndrome of hematopoietic dysfunction that typically precedes the classic findings of AML. This syndrome is usually characterized by a picture of ineffective hematopoiesis with anemia, thrombocytopenia, and sometimes granulocytopenia associated with a hypercellular, dysplastic bone marrow. In preleukemia, the leukemic clone is already established, and usually there is progressive impairment of hematopoiesis and accumulation of blasts. Megaloblastic hematopoiesis is common, and folate or vitamin B_{12} deficiency must be ruled out. Cytogenetic abnormalities are frequent; the most common chromosomal abnormalities are 5q−, −5, −7, and trisomy 8. When 5q− exists as the sole abnormality, the patient usually presents with refractory anemia associated with mild thrombocytosis. This disorder, referred to as the 5q− syndrome, usually does not progress to acute leukemia. Many patients with preleukemic or myelodysplastic syndromes never develop overt AML but die from complications of bone marrow failure. Smoldering AML refers to a syndrome in which the diagnostic features of acute leukemia are present, but the disease follows an indolent or subacute course. This disorder also tends to occur in elderly patients.

ACUTE LEUKEMIAS: ACUTE LYMPHOCYTIC LEUKEMIA (ALL) AND ACUTE MYELOGENOUS LEUKEMIA (AML)

PATHOLOGY AND CLASSIFICATION The diagnosis of acute leukemia requires the demonstration of leukemic cells in the bone marrow, peripheral blood, or extramedullary tissues. The bone marrow is typically hypercellular with a monomorphic infiltration of leukemic blasts and a marked reduction in normal bone marrow elements. It is critical to distinguish ALL from AML since these two diseases differ in natural history, prognosis, and response to various therapeutic agents.

Acute lymphocytic leukemia can be identified and classified on the basis of morphology and immunologic phenotype related to the stage of lymphoid differentiation. The leukemic lymphoblasts in ALL are generally smaller than myeloblasts (10 to 15 μm in diameter) and typically have only a thin rim of agranular cytoplasm. The nucleus may be round or convoluted (see Fig. A5-24). Three morphologic subtypes are included in the French-American-British classification: L1 cells are small and homogeneous with a regular nuclear membrane and a small nucleolus. L2 cells are larger and have a lower nuclear-cytoplasmic ratio with more pleomorphic size and shape; L2 cells typically have one or more prominent nucleoli. The L3 form of ALL is uncommon, occurring in less than 5 percent of cases; the leukemic cells in this variant contain large vesicular nuclei with basophilic, often vacuolated cytoplasm. L3 cells have a high mitotic index and represent the leukemic form of Burkitt's lymphoma.

Leukemic lymphoblasts in more than 90 percent of patients with

TABLE 296-1 Chromosomal abnormalities associated with acute leukemias

Abnormalities	Leukemia subtype	Relative prognosis
AML		
t(8;21)	M2 (myelocytic)	Good
+8	M1, M2, M4, M5	
t(15;17)	M3 (promyelocytic)	Good if remission is achieved
t(9;11)	M5 (monocytic)	Poor
inv 16	AML usually M4 with eosinophilia	Good
t(6;9)	AML with basophilia	—
5q−, −5, −7	AML following preleukemic syndrome or treatment-related leukemia	Poor
Ph¹, t(9;22)	Occasionally present in M1, M2, M4, M5, M6; must distinguish from CML blast crisis	Poor
ALL		
Hyperdiploidy	L1, L2	Good
6 q−	L1, L2	Good
14q+	L1, L2	—
t(8;14)	L3 (B-cell)	Poor
Ph¹, t(9;22)	L1, L2	Poor
t(4;11)	L2 (or M4 form AML)	Poor
CLL		
+12	B-cell type	Good
+12, 14 q+	B-cell type	Poor
+12, + other abnormalities	B-cell type	Poor
t(11;14)	B-cell type	Poor

1. RA + RARS
2. RA ē mild thrombocytosis (5q−)
3. RA ē Excess Blasts
4. Ch. Myelomonocytic leukemia

ALL contain a nuclear enzyme *terminal deoxynucleotidyl transferase* (Tdt) which is only rarely present in AML cells. An exception is the L3 subtype, which is Tdt-negative. The functional role of this enzyme is not known. Tdt is normally found in 1 percent of normal bone marrow cells and is present in immature T and B lymphocytes; it is absent in mature lymphocytes, hairy cell leukemia, and CLL. The leukemic cells from approximately half of patients with ALL react with the periodic acid Schiff stain showing blocklike inclusions of glycogen. Lymphoblasts do not contain granulocytic or monocytic lysosomal enzymes and therefore do not react with cytochemical stains for peroxidase, Sudan black, and nonspecific esterase.

Several forms of ALL can be defined based upon immunologic phenotype. Approximately 60 percent of cases are termed *common ALL;* the cells are Tdt-positive and have the common ALL antigen (CALLA) but do not express surface membrane immunoglobulin or T-cell antigens. These cells are usually derived from precursors of the B-cell lineage, as they may express immature B-cell antigens and have immunoglobulin gene rearrangements. CALLA is not a leukemia-specific antigen, since it is present on immature lymphoid cells including approximately 1 percent of cells in the normal bone marrow. About 20 percent of cases of ALL are of the *T-cell type,* where the T lymphoblasts express the E-rosette receptor or other T-lymphocyte-related antigens; these cells are Tdt-positive, usually CALLA-negative, and stain positively for acid phosphatase. T-cell ALL typically occurs in adolescent males and is frequently associated with a high leukocyte count and an anterior mediastinal mass. Less than 5 percent of cases of ALL are *B-cell type.* The cells in this variant produce a monoclonal immunoglobulin which is bound to the surface membrane and have L3 morphology. In B-cell ALL, the cells typically contain the t(8;14) chromosomal abnormality characteristic of Burkitt's lymphoma. Approximately 15 percent of cases of ALL are termed *null cell type* because the cells do not elaborate CALLA or T- or B-cell antigens.

The leukemic cells in AML are 12 to 20 μm in diameter, larger than lymphoblasts, and have a lower nuclear-cytoplasmic ratio. The leukemic myeloblasts usually have discrete nuclear chromatin and multiple nucleoli. The presence of Auer rods, abnormal primary granules, in the cytoplasm of leukemic cells is diagnostic of AML; these inclusions are present in 10 to 20 percent of patients with AML (see Fig. A5-22). Dysplastic morphologic abnormalities may be prominent in residual granulocytic, erythroid, and megakaryocytic cells. Cytochemical stains are often helpful in distinguishing AML from ALL and in classifying the pathologic subtypes of AML. Myeloperoxidase, α-naphthyl-AS-D-chloracetate esterase, and Sudan black are primarily present in cells undergoing granulocytic differentiation. Nonspecific esterase (α-naphthyl butyrate esterase) stains cells of the monocyte-macrophage lineage. A number of cell surface antigens present in AML cells have also been described. These stains and markers, however, may be negative in leukemias of undifferentiated cells.

A collaborative French-American-British group has divided AML into seven pathologic subtypes based upon the degree of differentiation and maturation of the predominant cells toward granulocytes, monocytes, erythrocytes, or megakaryocytes. The characteristics of each subtype are summarized in Table 296-2. There are only subtle differences in the clinical features of each subtype. The acute promyelocytic subtype (M3) is frequently associated with disseminated intravascular coagulation (DIC) induced by thromboplastic material released by the leukemic cells; DIC is usually present at the time of diagnosis and may be markedly exacerbated during chemotherapy. Acute myelomonocytic leukemia (M4) and acute monocytic leukemia (M5) are more likely than other subtypes to have extramedullary involvement of the skin, gingiva, central nervous system, and other tissues.

It is often difficult to distinguish the acute myelogenous leukemia without maturation (M1) from the L2 form of ALL by morphology alone. In these cases additional studies including cytochemical stains and analysis of myeloid and lymphoid antigens are required. Electron microscopy may be helpful in some cases to demonstrate small numbers of promyelocytic granules in cells that appear undifferentiated by light microscopy. Some patients appear to have a *biphenotypic acute leukemia.* In these patients, subpopulations of malignant cells contain both myeloid and lymphoid markers. These cells may represent leukemias of primitive pluripotent stem cells, or more likely they result from aberrant gene expression in a transformed myeloid or lymphoid progenitor.

CLINICAL AND LABORATORY FEATURES   ALL and AML share many clinical features. In the majority of patients, the initial symptoms of acute leukemia are present for less than 3 months. A preleukemic syndrome can be identified in approximately 25 percent

---

TABLE 296-2   Morphologic subtypes of AML

Subtype	% of AML	Morphology	Peroxidase Sudan black	Nonspecific esterase	Periodic acid Schiff
			Reactivity with special stains		
M1 AML without maturation	20	Few if any azurophilic granules	+/−	+/−	−
M2 AML with maturation	30	Blasts with promyelocytic granules, Auer rods may be present	+ + +	+/−	+
M3 Promyelocytic leukemia	5	Hypergranular promyelocytes often with multiple Auer rods per cell	+ + +	+	+
M4 Acute myelomonocytic leukemia	30	Monocytoid-appearing cells in peripheral blood associated with serum lysozyme	+ +	+ + +	+ +/+
M5 Acute monocytic leukemia	10	Two subtypes identified: (a) undifferentiated; (b) differentiated associated with serum lysozyme	+/−	+ + +	+ +/+
M6 Acute erythroleukemia	5	Predominance of erythroblasts and markedly dysplastic erythroid precursors	−	−	+ +
M7 Acute megakaryocytic leukemia	5	Undifferentiated blasts react with antiplatelet antibodies and contain platelet peroxidase	−	+/−	+

of patients with AML; in these patients, anemia and other cytopenias are usually present for months to years preceding the development of overt leukemia.

Patients with ALL and AML may present with pancytopenia without circulating blasts, with a normal leukocyte count, or with marked leukocytosis. Leukostasis due to occlusion of the microcirculation by leukemic blast cells can lead to hypoperfusion of vital tissues, most commonly lung and brain. Leukostasis becomes increasingly common when the number of circulating blasts exceeds 100×10^9 per liter and is seen more often with the larger blast cells in AML than in ALL. Patients may complain of manifestations of anemia such as pallor, easy fatigability, and dyspnea on mild exertion. The metabolic activity of large numbers of blasts can lead to artifactual results in laboratory tests, especially glucose and potassium concentrations and arterial blood gas analysis.

Bleeding is a major problem in patients with acute leukemia and is primarily related to thrombocytopenia. Coagulation defects may also be present. In some patients, megakaryocytes are derived from the leukemic clone and produce platelets with abnormal function. Petechiae and easy bruisability are common. Hemorrhage becomes increasingly common when the platelet count is less than 20×10^9 per liter, typically occurring from oral (particularly gingiva) and gastrointestinal mucous membranes. Spontaneous bleeding involving the central nervous system, lungs, or other viscera may also occur.

Infection is a frequent complication of acute leukemia. The incidence of infection is inversely related to the number of circulating neutrophils and becomes a major risk in patients with granulocyte counts less than 0.5×10^9 per liter. Neutrophils derived from leukemic progenitors may also function abnormally, further compromising host defenses. The leukemia and its treatment cause a breakdown of mucosal barriers, and systemic infections usually develop from organisms colonizing the skin, throat, and gastrointestinal tract. Common sites of infections in patients with acute leukemia include the skin, gingiva, perirectal tissues, lung, and urinary tract. Septicemia often occurs without an apparent source. Gram-negative bacteria, gram-positive cocci, and Candida species are frequent pathogens.

Hepatomegaly and splenomegaly due to leukemic infiltration are present in approximately one-half to three-fourths of patients with ALL and a minority of patients with AML. This visceral involvement can produce symptoms of nausea, abdominal fullness, or early satiety. Lymphadenopathy is more common in ALL than in AML. An anterior mediastinal mass is usually present in patients with the T-cell variant of ALL, and rarely occurs in other forms of ALL or in AML. Acute leukemia may infiltrate into extramedullary tissues such as the skin, lung, eye, nasopharynx, or kidneys. Testicular involvement is particularly common in males with ALL. Soft tissue masses of leukemic cells, "chloromas," can develop in any location. Occasionally, extramedullary leukemia can precede detectable involvement in the bone marrow.

Symptoms related to the expanding malignant cell mass, such as bone pain and sternal tenderness, occur in approximately half of patients with acute leukemia; osteolytic lesions are rare. Renal abnormalities can develop as a result of leukemic infiltration, ureteral obstruction by uric acid stones or enlarged lymph nodes, urate nephropathy, or from infectious or hemorrhagic complications. Gastrointestinal symptoms of early satiety, distention, and constipation may result from organomegaly or from leukemic infiltration or bleeding into the bowel and other viscera.

In acute leukemia, the neoplastic cells may infiltrate into the subarachnoid space, causing leukemic meningitis or direct involvement of the brain or spinal cord parenchyma. Neurologic involvement is unusual at the time of diagnosis, but the central nervous system is a frequent site of relapse, particularly in patients with ALL. The first symptoms of leukemic meningitis are usually headache and nausea. Papilledema, cranial nerve palsies, seizures, and altered mentation develop with disease progression. Cytocentrifuge preparations of cerebrospinal fluid (CSF) characteristically reveal leukemic

blast cells, an elevated CSF protein, and reduced glucose concentrations.

Patients with acute leukemia often develop metabolic abnormalities. Hyponatremia and hypokalemia are common due to renal tubular abnormalities induced by lysozyme or other products of the leukemic cells. The serum lactic acid dehydrogenase (LDH) level may be increased. Hyperuricemia may be present due to accelerated turnover of cells with increased purine release, and lactic acidosis rarely occurs in patients with a large burden of leukemic cells.

TREATMENT OF ACUTE LEUKEMIA: GENERAL CONSIDERATIONS The growth of leukemic cells follows a Gompertzian growth curve with near exponential growth at a lower cell mass and progressive slowing of the growth rate at higher leukemic cell burdens. The leukemic mass is usually between 10^{11} to 10^{12} cells at the time of diagnosis. Chemotherapeutic agents produce a fractional cell kill, that is, a percentage of tumor cells (not an absolute number) is killed with each course of treatment. Most chemotherapeutic regimens employed for acute leukemias are probably capable of a 3 to 5 log kill, resulting in the elimination of 99.9 to 99.999 percent of the leukemia cells. Another potential effect of some chemotherapeutic drugs is to induce maturation of the leukemic cells to mature nonproliferating cells. When the leukemia cell mass is reduced below approximately 10^9 cells, leukemia can no longer be detected in the blood or bone marrow, and the patient appears to be in complete remission. The clinical criteria for complete remission include (1) less than 5 percent blasts in the bone marrow and absence of leukemic cells in the peripheral blood, (2) the restoration of normal peripheral blood counts, and (3) the absence of physical findings attributable to extramedullary involvement of the leukemia. If no further treatment is given, however, the residual leukemic cells will proliferate, leading to relapse.

The treatment of acute leukemia is divided into distinct phases. Remission induction chemotherapy is the most critical phase. Intensive systemic chemotherapy is administered with the goal of reducing the leukemic cell mass below the level of detection. After remission is achieved, additional systemic chemotherapy must be given to further reduce the leukemic cell mass and, ideally, eradicate the leukemia. Intensive chemotherapy administered immediately following remission induction is referred to as consolidation or early intensification treatment. Lower dose chemotherapy that is generally continued over several years is referred to as maintenance treatment. Intensive chemotherapy administered more than 6 months after remission induction is termed late intensification. Another aspect of treatment involves local chemotherapy or radiation to frequent sites of relapse which are considered to be sanctuary sites, such as the central nervous system where systemic treatment may fail to eradicate the disease. The value of these forms of treatment for ALL and AML will be discussed separately.

Supportive care The supportive care of patients with pancytopenia is a critical aspect of the treatment of acute leukemia. This primarily involves the appropriate administration of blood products and management of infections.

Adequate levels of hemoglobin can usually be maintained with transfusions of packed red blood cells. An adequate number of circulating platelets can initially be attained by transfusions of platelets from unselected donors, but some transfused patients eventually develop antiplatelet antibodies which shorten platelet survival and render the patient unresponsive to further platelet transfusions. Patients who fail to respond to transfusions of platelets from unselected donors may respond to platelets from an HLA-identical donor. The risk of spontaneous hemorrhage is directly related to the degree of thrombocytopenia. It is generally advisable to transfuse platelets to maintain the platelet count above 20×10^9 per liter. Also, uterine bleeding should be minimized in menstruating women with thrombocytopenia by administering an anovulatory agent.

The potential therapeutic benefit of granulocyte transfusions has been extensively studied in patients receiving treatment for acute leukemia. Most data indicate that survival is not improved by granulocyte transfusions either to prevent infections or to treat documented infections, and that their routine use cannot be recommended. The major limitations in the use of granulocyte transfusions are the current technical difficulty in collecting sufficient numbers of granulocytes from normal donors and the adverse effects associated with their transfusion such as fever, leukoagglutination, pulmonary infiltrates, and transmission of cytomegalovirus (CMV) and other infections.

The prevention and treatment of infections is of critical importance in the management of patients with acute leukemia. Since most infections are caused by organisms colonizing the skin and gastrointestinal tract, a variety of approaches have been evaluated to suppress the endogenous flora in these sites. Most centers recommend the use of face masks, careful hand washing, oral nonabsorbable antibiotics, and reverse isolation for granulocytopenic patients. The development of bacterial and fungal infections may be delayed or avoided by these measures.

Granulocytopenic patients who develop fever or other signs of infection require prompt evaluation and treatment. Fever is usually due to a bacterial, fungal, or viral infection. Gram-negative sepsis is common in this setting and may be rapidly fatal. Granulocytopenic patients with unexplained fever or overt infections should be evaluated and receive empiric treatment for a presumed bacterial infection until a definitive diagnosis can be established. A combination of broad-spectrum antibiotics, such as an aminoglycoside or a third-generation cephalosporin in combination with a semisynthetic penicillin, should be employed and modified when the results of bacterial and fungal cultures are available. Systemic fungal infections are also common in granulocytopenic patients with leukemia and should be suspected in patients who fail to respond to antibiotic or who respond and develop recurrent fever. Definitive diagnosis of fungal infections may be difficult, and a therapeutic trial of amphotericin B is often indicated. The problem of infections in the immunocompromised host is discussed in Chap. 82.

TREATMENT OF ACUTE LYMPHOBLASTIC LEUKEMIA The treatment of ALL is one of the major successes in modern oncology. Forty years ago the disease was uniformly fatal and had a median survival of only 3 months. With current therapy, more than 50 percent of children with ALL achieve long-term remissions and probable cure. Adults and high-risk subgroups of children with ALL have a poorer prognosis, and long-term remissions are only achieved in a minority of patients. Therapy for ALL consists of three phases: (1) remission induction chemotherapy, (2) central nervous system prophylaxis, and (3) continuation (maintenance) chemotherapy.

The goal of remission induction chemotherapy is to eliminate all clinical signs and morphologic evidence of leukemia, as well as to restore normal bone marrow function. The intensity of treatment is important, because the duration of remission is prolonged by reducing the leukemic cell burden to the smallest possible fraction.

The combination of vincristine and prednisone plus either L-asparaginase or daunorubicin induces complete remissions in over 90 percent of children with ALL within 4 weeks. Some patients with persistent leukemia may achieve remission with 2 to 4 additional weeks of treatment with the same or alternate drugs. Failure to achieve remission can be attributed primarily to the development of drug resistance, severe infections, or central nervous system (CNS) leukemia.

In patients who achieve remission, prophylactic treatment to the CNS is required to prevent leukemic meningitis. The rationale for this treatment is based on the hypothesis that circulating leukemic cells infiltrate into the CNS and cerebrospinal fluid early in the course of the disease. Since the drugs used in remission induction in ALL generally penetrate poorly into the cerebrospinal fluid, these leukemic cells are sheltered from the effects of systemic chemotherapy. Over the ensuing months these cells may proliferate, producing overt leukemic meningitis. Leukemic meningitis is the initial site of relapse in up to two-thirds of patients with ALL who do not receive prophylactic therapy. Prophylactic treatment to the CNS,

instituted immediately after remission induction, has been successful in dramatically reducing the incidence of CNS relapse. Most centers employ 18- to 24-Gy whole-brain radiation in combination with intrathecal methotrexate. Cranial irradiation does produce subtle abnormalities in neurologic function, particularly in young children, and there is considerable interest in evaluating lower-dose radiotherapy regimens or alternative methods of CNS treatment. Preliminary data suggest that the combination of intrathecal and high-dose systemic methotrexate may provide adequate prophylactic treatment to the CNS.

Since patients in remission still harbor leukemia cells, further systemic treatment is required to prevent or delay leukemic relapse. The optimal approach to continuation therapy involves the administration of combination chemotherapy given in doses approaching maximal tolerance. As a rule, the drugs that are effective in inducing remission in ALL have not been useful in maintenance chemotherapy. The combination of 6-mercaptopurine and methotrexate is the most frequently employed maintenance regimen, but more intensive consolidation and maintenance regimens are required for adult patients and children with poor prognostic features.

The optimal duration of maintenance chemotherapy is unknown. Many patients can discontinue chemotherapy after 2 to 3 years and remain in long-term remission. Up to one-quarter of patients will relapse, however, after maintenance therapy is discontinued. It is not known whether maintenace therapy given for more than 3 years will further reduce the likelihood of relapse. Since there is currently no method to reliably detect small numbers of residual leukemic cells, there is no objective means to determine when therapy can be safely discontinued.

Complications of therapy for ALL Chemotherapy-induced myelosuppression and immunosuppression are inevitable side effects of the treatment for ALL. The chemotherapy directed toward the leukemic lymphoblasts also affects normal T and B lymphocytes, resulting in lymphocytopenia and immunodeficiency. Peripheral blood B cells generally recover to normal levels within several months after treatment is discontinued, but T-cell numbers and function may remain depressed for up to 1 year. *Pneumocystis carinii* pneumonia can occur while patients are in remission; trimethoprim-sulfamethoxazole prophylaxis is effective in preventing this complication. Growth in children is somewhat retarded during the administration of chemotherapy. Catch-up growth generally occurs once therapy is discontinued, and most children ultimately attain near normal height and weight. Sterility may result from treatment with most chemotherapeutic agents and irradiation. Gonadal function may recover after a prolonged interval. The gonads in prepubertal patients are relatively resistant to the effects of chemotherapy, and most patients undergo normal puberty after therapy is discontinued.

Prognosis in ALL The factors most affecting prognosis are age, the leukocyte count at the time of diagnosis, and cytogenetic abnormalities. Children between the ages of 3 and 9 years with white blood counts less than 10×10^9 per liter have the best prognosis; 50 to 70 percent achieve long-term survival and probable cure with current treatment. Older patients and those with higher leukocyte counts have a poorer prognosis. Fewer than 30 percent of adults with ALL are long-term survivors in most series, and it is uncertain whether the maintenance therapy which is effective in children is of benefit for adults. Males have a worse prognosis than females, due in part to the problem of testicular relapse. Children with the L1 morphologic subtype have a better prognosis than those with the L2 form, but this is probably not true in adults. Patients with T-cell ALL tend to have a poorer prognosis than the CALLA subgroup. These patients are generally older and present with a high white blood count, and it is uncertain if T-cell type, per se, is an independent poor prognostic factor. The B-cell (L3) variant of ALL has the worst prognosis.

Chromosomal abnormalities provide independent prognostic information. Approximately one-half of the patients with ALL have detectable cytogenetic abnormalities, including hypodiploidy, pseudodiploidy, or hyperdiploidy. A number of nonrandom chromosomal abnormalities are associated with ALL. Approximately 10 percent of patients with ALL have the Philadelphia (Ph¹) chromosome, an abnormality typical of chronic myelogenous leukemia. Associated with ALL, and possibly with hybrid (biphenotypic) leukemias, is t(4;11). Patients with pseudodiploidy, particularly t(4;11) and t(9;22), have a poor prognosis, while patients with hyperdiploidy have a better prognosis.

Remission and survival rates in adult patients with ALL (those over 15 years of age) are significantly lower than for children with the same disease. Remission induction rates in adults and high-risk children are generally between 50 to 70 percent following treatment with vincristine, prednisone, and daunorubicin; the median duration of remission is 10 to 12 months, and the 5-year survival rate is 10 to 30 percent with standard maintenance chemotherapy. Several centers have reported improved results in high-risk children and in adults with more intensive, multiple-drug consolidation and maintenance programs, but the optimal therapy for high-risk forms of ALL is uncertain.

Treatment of recurrent ALL Leukemia may recur either in the bone marrow or in extramedullary sites. Patients who relapse while receiving maintenance therapy have a very poor prognosis with little possibility of a long-term second remission. Combination chemotherapy with a three- or four-drug regimen including vincristine, prednisone, L-asparaginase, and/or daunorubicin results in a second remission in 50 to 70 percent of these patients. Remission duration, however, is usually brief, and subsequent relapse is inevitable. Patients who relapse after discontinuation of maintenance therapy have a better prognosis. Second remissions can be induced in about 90 percent of these patients. Although most will relapse again, some have achieved long-term survival. These patients should probably have CNS prophylaxis repeated to prevent recurrent disease in this extramedullary site.

Meningeal leukemia is the most common site of extramedullary relapse in patients with ALL. Cranial irradiation plus intrathecal methotrexate alone or in combination with cytarabine is the standard therapy for CNS leukemia. Testicular relapse is common in male patients with ALL and may occur during or after cessation of maintenance therapy. The treatment of choice is irradiation of the affected testicle. Patients with extramedullary relapse involving the CNS, testes, or other tissues are at very high risk for subsequent relapse in the bone marrow. Systemic reinduction therapy is indicated and may prevent generalized relapse of ALL.

TREATMENT OF ACUTE MYELOGENOUS LEUKEMIA The initial goal in the treatment of AML is to induce a complete hematologic remission. The drugs active in AML have little selectivity for leukemic cells over their normal bone marrow counterparts. Induction of severe myelosuppression is necessary in order to achieve a complete remission. The two most active drugs are cytarabine and daunorubicin. The combination of these agents with or without 6-thioguanine results in a complete remission rate of 60 to 80 percent. Mitoxantrone or amsacrine may be substituted for daunorubicin. If residual leukemia is present 2 to 4 weeks after chemotherapy, the treatment is repeated. Patients who fail to enter remission with this approach have a poor prognosis.

Patients with AML who achieve complete remission still have a substantial number of residual leukemic cells. Further therapy is required to reduce and hopefully to eradicate these occult leukemia cells. The benefits of available forms of consolidation and maintenance treatment are controversial. The best results have been achieved in patients receiving one to three intensive cycles of consolidation chemotherapy. Median remission duration varies from 9 months to 2 years in most series. Ten to thirty percent of patients survive over 5 years free of disease, and most of these patients are probably cured. Better results have been reported in preliminary studies using very intensive consolidation regimens, including high-dose cytarabine alone or in combination with other drugs. The results of these studies suggest a benefit for patients receiving consolidation treatment when

compared to historical controls, but these observations remain to be confirmed in prospectively controlled clinical trials.

Although some uncontrolled studies suggested that maintenance therapy with lower doses of these same agents or late intensification treatment improved remission duration, recent prospective controlled studies reported no benefit for patients receiving these forms of treatment. Current data suggest that the major benefit in therapy is achieved with intensive induction and consolidation treatment.

Most patients who achieve complete remission will ultimately relapse. At that point, the disease is usually much less responsive to therapy; only a minority of patients achieve a brief second remission, and median survival is 3 to 6 months.

Central nervous system leukemia in AML occurs in 10 to 20 percent of patients at some point in their disease, and most commonly develops in patients with monocytic (M5) or myelomonocytic (M4) subtypes. Unlike ALL, the CNS is rarely an isolated site of relapse in AML; CNS involvement usually occurs in the setting of systemic relapse. This may not be a biologically important leukemic sanctuary in patients with AML, and prophylactic treatment to the CNS has not improved remission duration or survival. Patients who develop meningeal leukemia are treated with cranial irradiation and intrathecal chemotherapy with cytarabine and/or methotrexate.

Prognostic factors in AML Chromosomal abnormalities in AML are of prognostic value; patients with abnormalities such as t(8;21), t(15;17), or inv 16 tend to have a relatively good prognosis, while -5, -7, t(9;22), and complex chromosomal abnormalities are associated with a poor prognosis.

Age is a major prognostic factor in many series; patients over 60 years of age are less likely to achieve complete remission. This group also tolerates intensive therapy poorly and is more difficult to support through the complications of pancytopenia. In addition, elderly patients are more likely to have leukemic cells with poor-risk chromosomal abnormalities such as -7, -5 and are more likely to have a defined preleukemic syndrome. However, elderly patients who do achieve remission have a similar remission duration and survival as younger patients. Since the major factor influencing survival is the achievement of complete remission, intensive chemotherapy should be administered to most elderly patients. Two controlled trials have shown that attenuated doses of daunorubicin in combination with full-dose cytarabine is less toxic and is as effective as higher dose regimens in elderly patients.

The leukemic subtype is of limited prognostic significance. Acute promyelocytic leukemia (M3) is typically associated with disseminated intravascular coagulation, and fatal CNS hemorrhage may complicate remission induction chemotherapy for this type of leukemia. Prophylactic heparin therapy is generally indicated during induction treatment to suppress DIC and prevent hemorrhagic complications. Heparin plus ε-aminocaproic acid is indicated in patients with excessive fibrinolysis. Patients with promyelocytic leukemia who do achieve remission appear to have a greater chance of long-term survival than other subgroups. Patients with monocytic or myelomonocytic leukemia may have a poorer prognosis than the M1 to M3 subgroups.

Patients with preleukemia evolving into AML or smoldering leukemia respond poorly to chemotherapy; less than half of these patients achieve complete remission. Such patients also tend to have prolonged bone marrow aplasia following treatment and often succumb to complications of pancytopenia. Patients who do achieve remission have a similar remission duration as patients with de novo AML, and intensive induction therapy is usually indicated. No treatment has been consistently effective during the preleukemic phase, and chemotherapy should be withheld until progressive overt leukemia develops. Low-dose cytarabine has been reported to be successful in occasional patients with preleukemia or smoldering AML; this therapy worsens cytopenias, and rare responses tend to be brief. An innovative approach to therapy for preleukemia involves agents such as retinoic acid which induce cellular maturation. A small number of patients with preleukemia (and progranulocytic leukemias) have had improvement in peripheral blood counts with retinoic acid therapy, but most patients fail to respond, and there is no evidence that survival is improved. Limited studies with hematopoietic hormones such as granulocyte-macrophage colony-stimulating factor (GM-CSF) suggest utility for this class of agents to improve hematopoiesis in preleukemia. Patients who develop acute leukemia after a preexisting myeloproliferative disorder or paroxysmal nocturnal hemoglobinuria usually have a poor prognosis.

Patients who receive cytotoxic chemotherapy with or without concomitant extensive radiation therapy have an increased risk of developing AML. Secondary or treatment-related leukemia is most commonly associated with prolonged therapy with alkylating agents, nitrosoureas, or procarbazine, and has been seen primarily in patients with Hodgkin's disease, multiple myeloma, and ovarian carcinoma. Almost all of the patients with treatment-related AML have chromosomal abnormalities, usually hypodiploidy with −5 and/or −7. These patients typically develop a preleukemic syndrome with pancytopenia several months before overt AML is recognized. They respond poorly to chemotherapy, and despite treatment, median survival is only 3 months after development of AML.

Other factors such as white blood and platelet counts, LDH level, and the presence of fever and hemorrhage have been reported to have prognostic importance. The impact of each of these variables is uncertain.

IMMUNOTHERAPY FOR ACUTE LEUKEMIAS Immunotherapy has been reported to be capable of suppressing small numbers of tumor cells in experimental animals. As such, immunotherapy has been evaluated to prevent leukemic relapse from the residual leukemic cells remaining after induction treatment in patients with ALL and AML. Unfortunately, clinical trials with nonspecific immune potentiating agents such as bacillus Calmette-Guérin (BCG), *Corynebacterium parvum*, or levamisole have not shown any benefit in prolonging the duration of remission. There are no convincing data to support the use of currently available immunotherapy in patients with either ALL or AML.

BONE MARROW TRANSPLANTATION FOR ACUTE LEUKEMIAS Bone marrow transplantation from an identical twin or an HLA-identical sibling donor is effective treatment for both ALL and AML. The objective of this approach is to administer very high doses of chemotherapy alone or with total-body irradiation, and then to rescue the patient from severe myelosuppression by the transplantation of bone marrow from a normal donor. In addition, the transplantation of allogeneic bone marrow may confer an immune-mediated graft-versus-leukemia effect. The current results with bone marrow transplantation are summarized in Table 296-3. Bone marrow transplantation is discussed in detail in Chap. 299.

Allogeneic bone marrow transplantation is associated with substantial risks. Approximately one-third of patients transplanted for leukemia will die from transplant-related complications including graft-versus-host disease, interstitial pneumonitis, and opportunistic infections. Most centers limit the use of bone marrow transplantation to patients under 45 years of age, since older patients generally have a poor outcome. Reports from several centers indicate that 10 to 15 percent of otherwise end-stage patients with refractory leukemia have achieved long-term disease-free survival and probable cure following bone marrow transplantation. Although only a small proportion of patients in this category benefit, the results compare favorably to those obtained with other forms of treatment.

These survival figures are substantially improved when bone marrow transplantation is performed during remission, the burden of leukemic cells is low, and the patients are in relatively good general condition. Because many children with ALL can achieve a prolonged initial remission with chemotherapy, bone marrow transplantation has generally been reserved for patients in second remission; in this group 30 to 60 percent have achieved prolonged survival with marrow transplantation. It is uncertain whether adults or children with high-risk forms of ALL should receive marrow transplants in first complete remission.

Approximately 30 percent of patients with AML transplanted in early relapse or second remission have achieved long-term survival. There is controversy as to whether patients with AML should receive allogeneic bone marrow transplantation or postremission chemotherapy while in first complete remission. Over 500 marrow transplants have been reported in this setting. It is clear that the risk of recurrent leukemia is lower following bone marrow transplantation than with postremission chemotherapy; however, bone marrow transplantation is more likely to be associated with fatal treatment complications. Overall 3- to 5-year survival is 40 to 60 percent with bone marrow transplantation compared with 10 to 50 percent survival achieved with optimal chemotherapy. Patient age is a major prognostic factor with bone marrow transplantation; the best results have been reported in children and young adults. Although young patients probably have better results with bone marrow transplantation than with chemotherapy, it is uncertain whether this is true for patients over 30 years of age. One major limitation of bone marrow transplantation as a general therapeutic approach is that only a minority of patients are currently eligible; most patients are either too old to be considered or lack an HLA-identical related donor. Recently several large registries of potential unrelated donors have been formed and bone marrow transplants from unrelated histocompatible donors are under active evaluation.

Autologous bone marrow transplantation has also been evaluated in patients with acute leukemia. With this approach, remission bone marrow is collected and cryopreserved. The patient may then receive intensive chemoradiotherapy followed by reinfusion of the cryopreserved bone marrow. Since remission bone marrow is likely to contain small numbers of residual leukemic cells, many centers have treated the collected marrow with antileukemic monoclonal antibodies or chemotherapy prior to cryopreservation. Selected patients with ALL and AML transplanted in first or second remission have achieved prolonged survival, but further studies are required to critically assess the efficacy of autologous marrow transplantation for acute leukemia. Furthermore the efficacy of ex vivo treatment of the collected bone marrow to eradicate contaminating malignant cells has not been conclusively demonstrated.

SUMMARY AND FUTURE DIRECTIONS IN ACUTE LEUKEMIA Effective induction chemotherapy capable of inducing remission in most patients with ALL and AML is now available, but long-term survival has been achieved in only a minority of patients. In the next decade, the focus of clinical research should be toward measures to prolong the duration of remission. Innovative methods of consolidation treatment with intensive chemotherapy or high-dose chemoradiotherapy and bone marrow transplantation must be evaluated for their effect on remission duration and survival. It will also be important to develop effective but less toxic approaches for favorable prognostic groups such as children with low-risk forms of ALL to improve the quality of life in long-term survivors. Innovative

TABLE 296-3   Representative results of bone marrow transplantation (BMT) compared with conventional chemotherapy for AML and ALL

	Survival >3 years, %	
	BMT	Chemotherapy
ALL		
First remission	30–60	20–70*
Second remission	30–50	<10
Third remission or relapse	10–20	0
AML		
First remission	40–60	10–50
Second remission or early relapse	30	<10
Third remission or relapse	10–20	0

* Best results in children with low white blood count.

new therapies are required for poor-risk groups, particularly the elderly and patients with preleukemic syndromes.

Sensitive techniques to detect residual leukemia during morphologic complete remission must also be developed to help guide the intensity and duration of treatment. Most importantly, new and effective drugs are required with selectivity toward leukemic cells which would spare the host from morbidity and mortality attendant to the currently available agents.

CHRONIC LYMPHOCYTIC LEUKEMIA

Chronic lymphocytic leukemia (CLL) is a hematologic neoplasm characterized by the accumulation of mature-appearing lymphocytes in the peripheral blood associated with infiltration of the bone marrow, spleen, and lymph nodes. The disease is uncommon before the fourth decade of life and is usually seen in patients over 50 years of age. It is the most common form of chronic leukemia in the United States but is rare in Orientals. CLL is more frequent in males than females.

CLL represents a clonal expansion of neoplastic B lymphocytes in more than 95 percent of cases. These cells commonly have trisomy 12 alone or with additional chromosomal abnormalities. Clonality has also been demonstrated by expression of a single light chain (κ or λ) or immunoglobulin idiotype specificity. In less than 5 percent of cases, CLL may be due to an expansion of T lymphocytes. An unusual type of T-cell CLL is seen in patients with ataxia-telangiectasia and is often associated with a translocation of genetic material between the number 14 chromosomes (t14;14). Other cytogenetic abnormalities occurring in CLL are listed in Table 296-1.

The diagnosis of CLL can usually be made on the basis of physical examination and a review of the peripheral blood smear. Leukocytosis is present, and the malignant cells characteristically appear as morphologically normal small lymphocytes (see Fig. A5-23). They have markers of B lymphocytes. In most cases a monoclonal immunoglobulin can be demonstrated on the cell surface, although immunofluorescent staining is usually weak. Monoclonal surface IgM with or without IgD is characteristically present, and a small amount of this IgM paraprotein can often be detected in the serum with sensitive techniques. The CLL cells also have receptors for the Fc portion of IgG, and complement receptors may or may not be present. Most patients develop some degree of hypogammaglobulinemia. Approximately 5 percent of patients have the T-cell form of CLL. The neoplastic cells form rosettes with sheep erythrocytes and contain other T-cell surface markers. T-cell CLL cannot usually be distinguished from B-cell CLL morphologically.

It is important to distinguish early CLL from reactive lymphocytosis in asymptomatic patients. In reactive lymphocytosis, the cells are polyclonal and predominantly T lymphocytes, whereas in CLL they are usually B cells. The demonstration of monoclonal surface membrane immunoglobulin unambiguously defines a B-cell lymphocytosis as neoplastic. T-cell CLL must be distinguished from Sézary syndrome where the cells have a characteristic lobulated nucleus and there is extensive skin involvement. T-cell CLL also must be distinguished from adult T-cell leukemia (ATL). Prolymphocytic leukemia is a CLL variant seen in older people and is characterized by massive splenomegaly, usually in the absence of lymphadenopathy. The neoplastic cell in prolymphocytic leukemia usually is of B-cell origin. It is larger than that seen in CLL and has a prominent nucleolus. Prolymphocytic leukemia is typically associated with very high white counts (in excess of 200×10^9 per liter) and a poor response to therapy. Lymphosarcoma cell leukemia represents a leukemic phase of lymphocytic lymphoma and is generally an aggressive disease (Chap. 302). The cellular morphology is suggestive of an acute rather than a chronic leukemia. Monoclonal immunoglobulin is usually easily detected on these cells, and the fluorescent staining is bright, often with spontaneous capping. Hairy cell leukemia is distinguished on the basis of the typical cellular morphology and the presence of tartrate-resistant acid phosphatase in the hairy cells.

Waldenström's macroglobulinemia is differentiated from CLL on the basis of bone marrow morphology and lower white blood cell counts, and the secretion of a large amount of a monoclonal IgM paraprotein.

CLINICAL FEATURES The clinical features of CLL are very different from acute leukemia. In more than 25 percent of patients with CLL, the disorder is discovered as an incidental finding. The common practice of ordering routine complete blood counts in adults has led to an earlier diagnosis of CLL in asymptomatic patients. The signs and symptoms of CLL usually relate to tissue infiltration, peripheral blood cytopenias, or immunosuppression. Patients may present with symptoms of anemia, lymph node enlargement, or intercurrent infection. Splenomegaly seldom leads to symptoms, and the liver is minimally enlarged in only about half of patients.

The white cell count ranges between 15×10^9 and 200×10^9 per liter, with a preponderance of mature-appearing lymphocytes. There is little correlation between the leukocyte count and symptomatology. Patients with advanced disease may present with anemia, granulocytopenia, and thrombocytopenia resulting from bone marrow infiltration by the leukemic cells. About 20 percent of patients develop a Coombs-positive autoimmune hemolytic anemia during the course of their disease. Occasionally, autoimmune thrombocytopenia may occur. Rarely, CLL evolves into an aggressive lymphocytic lymphoma referred to as *Richter's syndrome*, which is believed to be due to a clonal evolution of the original leukemia.

TREATMENT The therapeutic objectives in CLL differ sharply from those for the acute leukemias. The available drugs and radiation therapies are incapable of eradicating the leukemia and producing true complete remissions. Current therapy is effective to reduce the lymphocyte count and lymphadenopathy and to palliate symptoms produced by the leukemia. There is little evidence, however, that survival is substantially affected.

Although a number of prognostic classifications of CLL have been suggested, the new international classification appears most useful (Table 296-4). Prognosis correlates well with stage of disease; however, the rate of progression of patients from one stage to another is highly variable. Patients with stage A disease, in which the disease is limited to lymphocytosis alone or lymphocytosis plus limited lymphadenopathy, have a good prognosis. Median survival exceeds 7 years; these patients usually require no treatment. Patients with more substantial lymphadenopathy and hepatosplenomegaly (stage B) have an intermediate prognosis with a median survival of approximately 5 years. Patients with anemia or thrombocytopenia (stage C) have a worse prognosis with a median survival of less than 2 years.

The indications for therapy in CLL include hemolytic anemia, important cytopenias, disfiguring lymphadenopathy, symptomatic organomegaly, or marked systemic symptoms. When treatment is required, the cornerstone of therapy is usually an alkylating agent. Chlorambucil is the most frequently prescribed drug for CLL at a recommended daily dose of 0.1 to 0.2 mg/kg per day. The chlorambucil dose is generally reduced, and the drug is eventually stopped when the lymphocyte count falls below 20×10^9 per liter. The drug may also be given in pulses every 3 to 6 weeks, or continuously in low daily doses. Cyclophosphamide appears to be as effective as

TABLE 296-4 International workshop on CLL staging classification

Stage	Description	Median survival, years
A	Lymphocytosis with clinical involvement of fewer than 3 lymph node groups*; no anemia or thrombocytopenia	>10
B	More than 3 lymph node groups* involved	5
C	Anemia or thrombocytopenia regardless of number of lymph node groups involved	2

* Lymph node groups—cervical, axillary, inguinal, liver, spleen.

chlorambucil in the treatment of CLL. Maintenance therapy has no definite value, and continuing alkylating agent therapy may increase the risk of future development of AML.

Glucocorticosteroids are useful for CLL in special circumstances. These drugs do not have a prominent lympholytic effect in CLL and are therefore not effective as primary therapy. Glucocorticosteroids are useful, however, in the treatment of associated Coombs-positive hemolytic anemia or immune thrombocytopenia, and may be transiently effective in treating patients with pancytopenia and the "packed marrow" syndrome. Glucocorticosteroids have important side effects, including a predisposition to opportunistic infection. In more advanced CLL, combination chemotherapy may be useful. Regimens that include an alkylating agent, vincristine, and prednisone are often employed, and in advanced disease low-dose doxorubicin (Adriamycin) is often added. Pentostatin has been effective in selected patients. Splenectomy may be indicated in patients with hypersplenism, refractory hemolytic anemia, or thrombocytopenia. Radiation therapy may occasionally be useful for control of localized disease, and total-body radiation has rarely been useful in palliating end-stage disease. In preliminary trials, interferon does not appear to be effective in this disease, although agents such as deoxycoformycin, an adenosine deaminase inhibitor, are promising.

Hypogammaglobulinemia is common in patients with CLL, and life-threatening infectious complications may occur. Intramuscular injections of gamma globulin have not been effective, but recently developed intravenous immunoglobulin preparations may be useful in preventing infections in these patients.

HAIRY CELL LEUKEMIA

Hairy cell leukemia is a lymphoid neoplasm characterized by peripheral blood cytopenias, splenomegaly, and morphologically typical malignant cells in the blood and bone marrow. The disease superficially resembles CLL but has distinct clinical features and requires different therapy. Hairy cell leukemia is usually seen in patients over 40 years of age, and there is a very definite male preponderance. Originally, this disorder was thought to account for about 2 percent of all leukemias; however, the disease is now recognized with increased frequency, and many large series have been reported. Hairy cell leukemia has been reported to occur worldwide.

The disease was originally referred to as leukemic reticuloendotheliosis; however, the term *hairy cell leukemia* is now widely accepted because it is descriptive of the characteristic cytoplasmic projections seen on the leukemic cell. The disorder is due to expansion of neoplastic B lymphocytes which often produce monoclonal immunoglobulin; however, rare T-cell variants have been reported. The etiology of hairy cell leukemia is unknown; a single case of T-cell hairy cell leukemia has been reported, from which a unique species of human T-cell leukemia virus (HTLV-II) was recovered.

CLINICAL FEATURES AND PATHOLOGY Patients with hairy cell leukemia usually present with symptoms due to splenomegaly, infection caused by impaired host defense, or vasculitis. Many asymptomatic patients are detected on routine complete blood counts. More than three-quarters of patients will have palpable splenomegaly, and in some cases splenic involvement is massive. Lymphadenopathy is rare, and substantial hepatomegaly is uncommon at the time of diagnosis, although infiltration of the portal triads by hairy cells is often seen microscopically. Occasionally bone lesions may cause symptoms of hip pain. Approximately 30 percent of patients with hairy cell leukemia have an associated vasculitis-like disorder. Common manifestations include erythema nodosum and cutaneous nodules due to perivasculitis. Visceral involvement similar to polyarteritis nodosa may occur.

Moderate pancytopenia is usually present at diagnosis. The leukocyte count is normal or low, and characteristic hairy cells are seen in the peripheral blood. These cells are about 15 to 20 μm in diameter and have an eccentrically placed nucleus with characteristic foamy cytoplasm. Cytoplasmic projections may be seen on smear,

but they are best appreciated by phase microscopy. These cells stain positively for tartrate-resistant acid phosphatase (TRAP), which is a cytochemical stain for the isoenzyme 5 of acid phosphatase. Bone marrow aspiration is seldom successful because of reticulin fibrosis. The biopsy typically shows replacement of the normal architecture by mononuclear cells that are not packed together but maintain spaces between the intercellular contacts. Splenic histology is typical, consisting of mononuclear cell infiltration of the red pulp and engorgement of the sinuses.

Hairy cell leukemia must be distinguished from chronic lymphocytic leukemia, Waldenström's macroglobulinemia, and acute leukemia. Some patients with hairy cell leukemia present with a hypocellular bone marrow which may be misdiagnosed as aplastic anemia. The diagnosis depends on identifying the characteristic cells in the bone marrow and peripheral blood.

TREATMENT OF HAIRY CELL LEUKEMIA The course of hairy cell leukemia can be quite indolent; however, there is a wide spectrum of severity and rate of progression of the disease among patients. Approximately one-quarter of patients present without significant cytopenias and without other complications of the disease; these patients require no immediate treatment. They should be followed at intervals and closely observed for infections. Infection is the primary cause of death in patients with hairy cell leukemia. Common infections include *Legionella* pneumonitis, toxoplasmosis, tuberculosis, and atypical mycobacterial disease, nocardiosis, and pyogenic infections. Patients probably benefit from pneumococcal vaccination. Any significant fever should be thoroughly evaluated and aggressively treated with antibiotics. Since *Legionella* pneumonitis is relatively common in these patients, high-dose erythromycin should usually be administered to patients with pulmonary infiltrates.

Therapy directed at the leukemia is indicated in patients presenting with marked pancytopenia, a history of infections, massive splenomegaly, or a rapid rate of disease progression. The cornerstone of therapy has been splenectomy, which appears to ameliorate the disease in a majority of patients. The role of splenectomy, however, in patients with no splenic enlargement is uncertain. Patients with progressive disease following splenectomy or those who do not elect surgery should be treated with α-interferon. Interferon is now an approved drug highly effective in hairy cell leukemia. Virtually all treated patients respond to α-interferon with about 70 percent achieving major hematologic benefit. Complete remissions are rare, but retreatment of recurrent disease is often successful. Pentostatin is an experimental drug that is highly active in hairy cell leukemia and may become the treament of choice since it often induces complete remissions. Glucocorticosteroids are not effective in hairy cell leukemia, and they are potentially dangerous because they further predispose these patients to infections. Short courses of glucocorticosteroids may be useful, however, in controlling the vasculitis or autoimmune manifestations that are often associated with the disease. Chemotherapy with alkylating agents or other myelotoxic drugs is contraindicated in patients with hairy cell leukemia because of poor bone marrow reserve.

The prognosis in hairy cell leukemia is variable, and published series are outdated because of the recent improvements in diagnosis and treatment. At least 50 percent of patients survive more than 8 years from diagnosis, and this prognosis has improved considerably with the application of interferon, pentostatin, and better supportive care.

REFERENCES

General

GALE RP (ed): *Leukemia Treatment*. Boston, Blackwell, 1986
———, GOLDE DW (eds): *Recent Advances in Leukemia and Lymphoma*. New York, Alan R Liss Inc., 1987
GOLDE DW, TAKAKU E (eds): *Hematopoietic Stem Cells*. New York, Marcel Dekker Inc, 1985
GUNZ FW, HENDERSON ES (eds): *Leukemia*, 4th ed. New York, Grune & Stratton, 1983

ROWLEY JD: Biological implications of consistent chromosome rearrangements in leukemia and lymphoma. Cancer Res 44:3159, 1984

WONG-STAAL F, GALLO RC: The family of human T-lymphotropic leukemia viruses: HTLV-I as the cause of adult T cell leukemia and HTLV-III as the cause of acquired immunodeficiency syndrome. Blood 65:253, 1985

YUNIS JJ: The chromosomal basis of human neoplasia. Science 221:227, 1983

Acute leukemias

BENNETT JM et al: Criteria for the diagnosis of acute leukemia of megakaryocytic lineage. Ann Intern Med 103:460, 1985

CHAMPLIN R, GALE RP: Acute lymphoblastic leukemia: Recent advances in biology and therapy. Blood 73:2051, 1989

———: Bone marrow transplantation for leukemia: Recent advances and comparisons with alternative therapies. Semin Hematol 24:55, 1987

ALL

GAYNOR J et al: A cause-specific hazard rate analysis of prognostic factors among 199 adults with acute lymphoblastic leukemia: The Memorial Hospital experience. J Clin Oncol 6:1014, 1988

HOELZER D et al: Prognostic factors in a multicenter study for treatment of acute lymphoblastic leukemia in adults. Blood 71:123, 1988

JACOBS AD, GALE RP: Recent advances in the biology and treatment of acute lymphoblastic leukemia in adults. N Engl J Med 311:1219, 1984

JOHNSON FL et al: A comparison of marrow transplantation with chemotherapy for children with acute lymphoblastic leukemia in second or subsequent remission. N Engl J Med 305:846, 1981

MAUER AM: Therapy of acute lymphoblastic leukemia in childhood. Blood 56:1, 1980

RITZ J et al: Autologous bone marrow transplantation in CALLA-positive acute lymphoblastic leukemia after in vitro treatment with J5 monoclonal antibody and complement. Lancet 2:60, 1984

RIVERA GK, MAUER AM: Controversies in the management of childhood acute lymphoblastic leukemia: Treatment intensification, CNS leukaemia, and prognostic factors. Semin Hematol 24:12, 1987

AML

APPELBAUM FR et al: Bone marrow transplantation or chemotherapy after remission induction for adults with acute nonlymphoblastic leukemia. Ann Intern Med 101:581, 1984

BAGBY GC: The preleukemic syndrome (hematopoietic dysplasia). Blood Rev 2:194, 1988

CHAMPLIN RE et al: Treatment of acute myelogenous leukemia: A prospective controlled trial of bone marrow transplantation versus consolidation chemotherapy. Ann Intern Med 102:285, 1985

———, GALE RP: Acute myelogenous leukemia: Recent advances in therapy. Blood 69:1551, 1987

——— et al: Prolonged survival in acute myelogenous leukaemia without maintenance chemotherapy. Lancet 1:894, 1984

FIALKOW PJ et al: Acute nonlymphocytic leukemia: Heterogeneity of stem cell origin. Blood 57:1068, 1981

FOON KA et al: The role of immunotherapy in acute myelogenous leukemia. Arch Intern Med 143:1726, 1983

GALE RP, CHAMPLIN RE: How does bone marrow transplantation cure leukaemia? Lancet 2:28, 1984

GREENBERG PL: The smoldering myeloid leukemic states: Clinical and biologic features. Blood 61:1035, 1983

HERZIG RH et al: High-dose cytosine arabinoside therapy for refractory leukemia. Blood 62:361, 1983

KOEFFLER HP: Induction of differentiation of human acute myelogenous leukemia cells: Therapeutic implications. Blood 62:709, 1983

PREISLER HD: The treatment of acute nonlymphocytic leukemia. Blood Rev 1:97, 1987

WEINSTEIN HJ et al: Chemotherapy for acute myelogenous leukemia in children and adults: VAPA update. Blood 62:315, 1983

CLL

BINET J-L et al: Chronic lymphocytic leukaemia: Proposals for a revised prognostic staging system. Br J Haematol 48:365, 1981

CALIGARIS-CAPPIO F, JANOSSY G: Surface markers in chronic lymphoid leukemias of B cell type. Semin Hematol 22:1, 1985

FOON K, GALE RP: Staging and therapy of chronic lymphocytic leukemia. Semin Hematol 24:264, 1987

HAN T et al: Prognostic importance of cytogenetic abnormalities in patients with chronic lymphocytic leukemia. N Engl J Med 310:288, 1984

Hairy cell leukemia

CHESON BD, MARTIN A: Clinical trials in hairy cell leukemia. Current status and future directions. Ann Intern Med 106:871, 1987

GENOT E et al: Effect of interferon-alpha on the expression and release of the CD23 molecule in hairy cell leukemia. Blood 74:2455, 1989

GLASPY JA et al: Evolving therapy of hairy cell leukemia. Cancer 59:652, 1987

GOLOMB HM: The treatment of hairy cell leukemia. Blood 69:979, 1987

——— et al: Sequential evaluation of alpha-2b-interferon treatment in 128 patients with hairy cell leukemia. Semin Oncol 14(Suppl 2):13, 1987

JACOBS AD et al: Recombinant alpha-2 interferon for hairy cell leukemia. Blood 65:1017, 1985

SPIERS ASD et al: Remissions in hairy-cell leukemia with pentostatin (2'-deoxycoformycin). N Engl J Med 316:825, 1987

297 THE MYELOPROLIFERATIVE DISEASES

JOHN W. ADAMSON

DEFINITION The myeloproliferative diseases are neoplasms of the multipotent hematopoietic stem cell. They include chronic myelogenous leukemia (CML), polycythemia vera (PV), agnogenic myeloid metaplasia with myelofibrosis (AMM/MF), and essential thrombocytosis (ET). In addition to their common stem cell origin, other features are shared which occasionally lead to a blurring between the various disorders. However, apparent transitions from one disorder to another are uncommon. With the exception of CML, the diseases tend to run a chronic course over many years.

The stem cell origin and clonal nature of these diseases have been shown through cytogenetic analyses and through studies in female patients who are heterozygous for glucose-6-phosphate dehydrogenase (G6PD). Consistent with the stem cell origin and neoplastic nature of these diseases a single G6PD enzyme is found in peripheral blood granulocytes, platelets, red cells, and monocytes in patients who have been shown to be G6PD heterozygotes by analysis of skin fibroblasts. In at least some patients, the level of stem cell involvement includes a progenitor capable of giving rise to lymphocytes, as well. In patients with characteristic cytogenetic abnormalities, abnormal metaphases may be found in precursors of platelets, red cells, and granulocytes. These findings indicate that the diseases arise as clonal expansions of single transformed stem cells. At the time of diagnosis, virtually all of the myeloid cells of the blood are derived from the neoplastic clone.

CHRONIC MYELOGENOUS LEUKEMIA

DEFINITION AND ETIOLOGY CML is characterized by marked splenomegaly and the production of increased numbers of granulocytes, particularly neutrophils. The disorder is associated with a characteristic chromosomal abnormality (see below) and runs a generally mild course until it transforms to a frankly leukemic (blastic) phase. Usually no specific etiologic agent can be identified; however, an increased incidence of CML in atomic bomb survivors has been noted. CML occurs at any age, but the peak incidence occurs in the third and fourth decades. The sexes are affected equally.

PATHOPHYSIOLOGY AND SYMPTOMATOLOGY The natural course of CML can be divided into a chronic and a blastic or acute phase. The chronic phase of CML is characterized by an excessive proliferation and accumulation of granulocytes and their precursors in the marrow and blood. Typically, the white blood cell count is markedly elevated, often exceeding 200,000 per microliter. At this stage, myeloblasts are less than 5 percent of the cells in the marrow and blood. The diagnosis often is made because of incidental laboratory tests which reveal an elevated white blood count, or because a patient complains of left upper quadrant discomfort due to an enlarged spleen. About 20 percent of cases are diagnosed on the basis of an elevated blood count in the absence of symptoms. In the majority, however, the signs and symptoms of the disease are related to the expanded myeloid mass in the marrow and spleen. Presenting symptoms are related to splenomegaly, anemia, or hypermetabolism manifested by weight loss and fever. Arthralgias may be severe. Lymphadenopathy is rare in this phase. Thrombohemorrhagic complications such as excessive bleeding, either spontaneously or with surgical or dental procedures, are occasionally found. Ninety percent of patients have palpable splenomegaly.

During the course of the chronic phase of CML the disease transforms to the more malignant blastic phase. After the first 6 to 12 months following diagnosis, the rate of transformation to the blastic phase is about 25 percent of the remaining patients per year and over 85 percent of patients with CML will eventually die in this phase. Occasionally, patients may present in the blastic phase of the disease. The chronic phase may be restored if such patients respond successfully to chemotherapy. There is no single test which predicts precisely when a patient's disease will transform to the blastic phase, but certain features associated with early transformation include the degree of leukocytosis, the presence of an excessively large liver and spleen, the percentage of immature cells in the marrow, and the presence of large numbers of eosinophils or basophils. Overall survival for patients from the time of diagnosis averages $3\frac{1}{2}$ years.

The blastic phase of CML represents an evolution in the disease from hyperplasia of mature elements of the marrow to increased numbers of blasts and promyelocytes. Half of the patients progress to blast crisis through an "accelerated" phase characterized by progressively increasing leukocytosis, thrombocytosis or thrombocytopenia, and splenomegaly, which are refractory to previously effective drugs. In some patients, the transition to a state resembling acute myelogenous leukemia may take only a few weeks. A minority of patients will present with or develop extramedullary tumors, usually in lymph nodes or skin, or osteolytic bone lesions. Meningeal leukemia is rare.

The blastic phase may be lymphoid or myeloid in origin. One-third of cases have characteristics of lymphoblasts including the enzyme terminal deoxynucleotidyl transferase (Tdt), a DNA-synthesizing enzyme associated with acute lymphoblastic leukemia and normal thymic lymphocytes, as well as the common acute lymphoblastic leukemia antigen (CALLA). This is consistent with the known level of stem cell involvement in the original disease. Lymphoid blast crisis in some patients is associated with arrested rearrangements of the immunoglobulin genes, typical of pre-B cells. Myeloid blast crisis resembles acute myelogenous leukemia, but a few patients will have a basophilic or erythroleukemic conversion from the chronic phase of the disease. The latter, and the fact that the blasts may react positively with monoclonal antibodies to erythroid- or megakaryocyte-associated antigens, emphasize the diversity of this phase and the stem cell nature of the disease. Auer rods are virtually never seen in the myeloblasts of CML in blastic phase.

LABORATORY FINDINGS Table 297-1 summarizes the distinguishing laboratory features of the various myeloproliferative diseases. The most prominent laboratory finding in CML is the leukocytosis. Unlike the finding in leukemoid reactions, there is generally a bimodal distribution of neutrophils in the blood with a peak of mature polymorphonuclear neutrophils (PMNs) and a second peak of myelocytes or metamyelocytes. Platelet morphology is more normal than in the other myeloproliferative disorders, and in vitro platelet function, as marked by aggregation in the presence of agents such as epinephrine, is also generally normal. Basophilia, typical of all of the myeloproliferative disorders, may be prominent. A number of unique biochemical abnormalities are also found. Accompanying the leukocytosis of CML is a marked elevation of serum vitamin B_{12} levels, as well as an increased serum vitamin B_{12}-binding capacity. This is due to excessive serum levels of transcobalamin I, a glycoprotein of alpha globulin electrophoretic mobility. A vitamin B_{12}-binding protein with similar properties has been shown to be produced by mature normal and leukemic granulocytes in vitro. Elevated levels in the serum of patients with CML are probably derived from the turnover of the increased granulocytic mass. The high levels of vitamin B_{12}, as well as the increased serum binding capacity, return toward normal with

treatment of the disease. Leukocyte alkaline phosphatase, an enzyme in granulocytes, is markedly reduced in the granulocytes of nearly all patients with CML. However, with infection or glucocorticoid administration, the level of the enzyme in granulocytes may rise to the normal range. The levels of the enzyme may also return toward normal with successful therapy of the disease and reduction of the white cell count. The only other hematologic disorders with low or absent leukocyte alkaline phosphatase are paroxysmal nocturnal hemoglobinuria and occasional cases of myelodysplasia. The marrow as well as the spleen of patients with CML may contain glycolipid-laden phagocytes which resemble Gaucher cells. Hyperuricemia related to the increased cell turnover may occur in all the myeloproliferative diseases prior to therapy and can be exacerbated by treatment. The mature granulocyte in CML is a cell that is functionally normal with respect to phagocytosis and bactericidal activity. Granulocyte kinetics in CML have been studied with isotope-labeling techniques, and there is clear evidence for increased production of mature granulocytes. The numbers of primitive myeloid progenitors (colony-forming cells) in the marrow and blood of patients with CML are also increased. This includes both committed erythroid as well as granulocytic progenitors, and their numbers in the blood may be 10,000 times the normal number.

CYTOGENETICS More than 95 percent of patients with CML have a unique and characteristic chromosome marker in metaphases of marrow—the Philadelphia chromosome (Ph). This chromosomal abnormality represents a reciprocal translocation of genetic material between the long arms of chromosome 22 and chromosome 9. This particularly interesting chromosomal rearrangement involves break points near two cellular proto-oncogenes, c-abl on chromosome 9 and c-sis on chromosome 22. The proto-oncogene c-sis is the cellular homologue of the simian sarcoma virus oncogene and encodes sequences for platelet-derived growth factor (PDGF). The proto-oncogene c-abl is translocated to a specific region of chromosome 22, the breakpoint cluster region (bcr). As a result, a fusion gene product of bcr/abl is formed which has tyrosine kinase activity and may have a role in the development and persistence or progression of the disease. This chromosome abnormality persists throughout the course of the disease, in remission and relapse, and is unaffected by the usual therapies. It is present in virtually all metaphases of granulocytic, megakaryocytic, and erythroid precursors but not in traditionally prepared lymphocyte preparations or skin fibroblasts. Some patients with CML, who do not have the Ph chromosome abnormality by routine cytogenetic techniques, can be shown to have the bcr/abl rearrangement by molecular analysis. In addition to the Ph chromosome, the blastic phase of CML is often associated with the acquisition of other chromosomal abnormalities, such as aneuploidy, which reflect the more malignant character of this phase of the disease. Double Ph chromosomes also may be seen. Less than 5 percent of patients with clinically typical CML lack the Ph chromosome. These patients are generally younger and have a more rapidly progressive clinical course. Although considered with CML, this disease is probably a distinct myeloproliferative disorder.

While the Ph chromosome is a consistent feature of CML, there is evidence, using other cell markers such as G6PD, that the appearance of the chromosomal abnormality is not the primary event in the acquisition of the disease. Thus, some lymphocyte populations which appear by G6PD analysis to be clonally derived lack the Ph chromosome. These and other results suggest a multistep pathogenesis in

TABLE 297-1 The myeloproliferative diseases

Disease	Hematocrit	White blood cell count	Platelet count	Splenomegaly	Leukocyte alkaline phosphatase	Marrow fibrosis	Ph chromosome
CML	Normal or ↓	↑↑↑	↑ to ↓	+++	↓ to 0	±	+
PV	↑↑	↑	↑	+	↑↑	±	0
AMM/MF	↓	↑ to ↓	↑ to ↓	+++	↑ or normal	+++	0
ET	Normal	Normal	↑↑↑	+	↑ or normal	±	0

CML with the acquisition of the Ph chromosome as a secondary event.

DIAGNOSIS CML which presents with splenomegaly, a markedly elevated white cell count, a low leukocyte alkaline phosphatase, and the Ph chromosome is an easy diagnosis. Atypical presentations must be differentiated from leukemoid reactions associated with infections or neoplasms. In the latter, the leukocyte alkaline phosphatase is usually elevated and the Ph chromosome is absent. A closely related myeloproliferative disorder is agnogenic myeloid metaplasia (AMM/MF) (see below). This disease usually presents with marked myelofibrosis and splenomegaly. The white blood cell count and platelet count may be elevated, but leukocyte alkaline phosphatase is normal or increased and the Ph chromosome is absent. Among the myeloproliferative diseases, the serum vitamin B_{12} level cannot be used as a differential diagnostic test in patients with elevated white cell counts.

THERAPY Chronic phase CML can be controlled by a number of alkylating agents such as busulfan, cyclophosphamide, or melphalan, as well as hydroxyurea, a cell cycle–specific drug. Splenic irradiation is not as effective as chemotherapy for control of the disease. The most commonly used drug is busulfan. It may be administered on an intermittent schedule or on a continuous daily basis with approximately the same results. The most serious complication of busulfan therapy is prolonged myelosuppression. Occasionally, remission of the disease for periods in excess of 1 year may follow a single course of treatment. The principal side effects include increased skin pigmentation resembling that seen with adrenal insufficiency and, rarely, pulmonary or retroperitoneal fibrosis. An initial daily oral dose of 4 to 8 mg will reduce the white cell count to less than 20,000 per microliter in 2 to 3 weeks. The dose of busulfan should be reduced progressively, roughly in proportion to the reduction in white blood cell count. Patients achieve an excellent hematologic remission, with return of blood counts to normal and reduction in organomegaly. The Ph chromosome remains, however. A true remission of the disease does not occur; rather, the proliferating granulocyte mass is reduced to the point where immature cells disappear from the peripheral blood. Furthermore, neither conventional therapy nor high-dose combination chemotherapy designed to eradicate the Ph-positive clone significantly prolongs survival. Encouraging results with interferon, both in terms of reduction of the white cell count and the percent of Ph-positive metaphases in the marrow, have been reported, but the results of randomized trials with this or similar agents are not available.

Splenectomy has little place in the primary management of CML but may be reserved for those patients with evidence of hypersplenism or repeated painful splenic infarctions or for the rare instance in which prolonged thrombocytopenia follows busulfan therapy. Splenectomy in the chronic phase of CML does not prolong survival or delay the onset of blastic transformation.

Acceleration of the disease is reflected by progressive refractoriness to chemotherapy, increased leukocytosis with a larger proportion of immature forms, thrombocytosis, and increasing splenomegaly. Prior to blastic transformation, the drug hydroxyurea can effectively control the proliferative aspects of the disease. The dose ranges from 1 to 3 g/d by mouth. The blastic phase of CML is refractory to most drug regimens, but short-lived remissions in about 20 percent of cases have been obtained with the use of vincristine and prednisone or other intensive combination chemotherapy programs useful in the treatment of acute leukemia (see Chap. 296). There is a correlation between the appearance of Tdt in the blast cells and the response to vincristine and prednisone, drugs commonly used for acute lymphoblastic leukemia in childhood. However, the correlation is not perfect, and therapy for the blastic phase should begin with vincristine and prednisone, regardless of the presence or absence of Tdt or the morphology of the blasts. Hydroxyurea may be used here, as well, to suppress the proliferation of blasts; however, meaningful remissions are rarely, if ever, obtained and patients die of infection or bleeding. Symptomatic extramedullary myeloblastic tumors can be controlled with local radiation therapy.

It has been demonstrated that eradication of Ph-positive cells can be achieved in the majority of chronic phase patients treated with intensive chemotherapy and radiation and transplanted with bone marrow from an identical twin or sibling compatible for human histocompatibility leukocyte antigens (HLA). Analysis of patients receiving bone marrow transplantation suggests that the best results are obtained in patients transplanted in chronic phase within the first year of diagnosis. Busulfan or other alkylating agents should be avoided if marrow transplantation remains an option. Long-term disease-free survival in good-risk transplant patients is approximately 70 percent, although late relapses occur with reappearance of the Ph chromosome. Progressively poorer results with higher relapse rates are obtained if patients are transplanted in the accelerated or blastic phase of the disease.

POLYCYTHEMIA VERA

DEFINITION AND ETIOLOGY Polycythemia vera (PV) is characterized by splenomegaly and an increased production of all myeloid elements; however, the disease is generally dominated by an elevated hemoglobin concentration. PV is gradual in onset and runs a chronic but usually slowly progressive course.

The disease generally begins in late middle life and is slightly more common in males. Only rarely is PV found in children or multiple members of a single family. The disease is relatively uncommon in blacks and occurs with increased frequency in Jews of European ancestry.

PATHOPHYSIOLOGY AND SYMPTOMATOLOGY None of the recognized physiologic mechanisms of increased red blood cell production is present in PV. The disease must be distinguished from secondary forms of polycythemia, in which an elevated hemoglobin concentration results from increased erythropoietin production. Secondary polycythemia may arise through hypoxia or occasionally may be found with certain neoplasms. PV is also distinct from spurious (relative) polycythemia, which results from a decrease in the plasma volume rather than a true increase in red blood cell mass. Also, secondary causes of polycythemia are not associated with splenic enlargement or increased leukocytes and platelets, which are typical of PV.

In PV there is a unique relationship of erythropoietin to red blood cell production. As opposed to the findings in secondary forms of polycythemia, urine and serum levels of erythropoietin in patients with PV are reduced. Presumably, erythropoietin production is suppressed by the elevated hemoglobin concentration, since phlebotomy results in a rise in both erythropoietin levels and red blood cell production (provided that there is no deficiency in iron). This demonstrates the marrow's ability to respond to humoral regulation.

In cell culture, marrow from patients with PV forms colonies of hemoglobin-synthesizing cells in the absence of added erythropoietin. This is rarely the case with marrow cells from normal persons or from patients with secondary polycythemia. A reduced production of erythropoietin, the appearance of "endogenous" erythroid colonies in marrow cultures, and the clonal origin from the pluripotent hematopoietic stem cell indicate that hematopoiesis in PV is not regulated by the usual mechanisms.

PV produces symptoms associated with increased blood volume and blood viscosity. The hemoglobin concentration, hematocrit, and total blood volume may become markedly elevated, a consequence of the sharply increased red blood cell mass. The plasma volume is usually normal but may be increased. Associated with the expanded blood volume is a consistently elevated increase in cardiac output and a less uniform, but significant, increase in cardiac index. Reduction of the hematocrit and blood volume by phlebotomy leads to a reduction in the stroke volume and cardiac output in these patients and generally to an improvement in exercise tolerance. The increased cardiac output occurs in association with an increase in blood viscosity and, presumably, in vascular resistance associated with the elevated hematocrit.

Complaints related to the increased viscosity and/or decreased cerebral perfusion include headache, dizziness, vertigo, a sense of fullness of the head, rushing in the ears, visual alterations (scotomas, double vision, or blurred vision), tinnitus, syncope, and even chorea. Peripheral vascular symptoms of both arterial and venous insufficiency are common; in one large series, more than 35 percent of patients gave a history of some thrombotic or hemorrhagic event during the course of their disease. The risk of thrombosis may be increased by the accelerated atherosclerosis in this disease. Bleeding is common and comes most often from the nose or from peptic ulcer disease. Intramuscular hemorrhages and bruising also are seen. The tendency to increased bleeding may be due to the distended vasculature resulting from the increased blood volume. However, intrinsic platelet dysfunction also may contribute to bleeding, particularly from the gastrointestinal tract. The incidence of peptic ulcer disease is estimated to be four to five times higher in patients with PV than it is in the general population, although the reasons are unclear.

Late in the disease, the spleen may become greatly enlarged, producing symptoms of early satiety, a sense of abdominal fullness, and pleuritic chest or left upper quadrant pain secondary to capsular stretching or infarction. Pruritus, particularly after bathing, is reported frequently and may be disabling. Occasionally, urticaria is seen.

The increased cellular proliferation seen with PV results in hyperuricemia in 25 to 30 percent of patients and may be associated with formation of urate stones and uric acid nephropathy.

LABORATORY FINDINGS The most prominent laboratory feature is the elevated hemoglobin concentration. Unless altered by iron deficiency, the red blood cells are normochromic and normocytic. Polychromasia is frequently seen, and nucleated red blood cells may be found in the later stages of the disease. These findings represent cells released from extramedullary sites of hematopoiesis or reflect damage to marrow stroma due to fibrosis.

The white cell count is elevated in two-thirds of patients and is usually in the range of 15,000 to 25,000 per microliter but may be as high as 60,000 per microliter. An increase in the absolute basophil count (to more than 100 per microliter) is found in about 70 percent of patients. The leukocyte alkaline phosphatase is increased in more than 80 percent of cases. Serum vitamin B_{12} levels vary and are increased in about one-third of the patients; however, the binding capacity is increased in as many as 75 percent. In addition to increased transcobalamin I, transcobalamin III is also increased.

Thrombocytosis is seen in over half of all patients with PV. In vitro studies of platelet function demonstrate defective platelet adhesiveness and impaired secondary release of adenosine diphosphate (ADP) in response to epinephrine. These are poorly correlated with the bleeding time, and the contribution of these functional abnormalities to the thrombotic and hemorrhagic events in patients with PV is uncertain. Abnormal liver function studies, including an elevated alkaline phosphatase, may occur if there is massive hepatomegaly.

Splenomegaly occurs in 75 percent of patients but is usually not as marked as in CML or AMM/MF. Splenomegaly persists even when the elevated hemoglobin concentration has been reduced by repeated phlebotomies. Microscopic examination of the spleen reveals multiple foci of extramedullary hematopoiesis and fibrosis. The follicular pattern of the organ is retained, unlike the loss of normal architectural structure observed in CML. Foci of extramedullary hematopoiesis also may be found in the liver.

Bone marrow examination shows either erythroid hyperplasia or panhyperplasia without distinctive morphologic features. There is increased megakaryocyte nuclear ploidy in the face of thrombocytosis. This pattern of platelet regulation is different from that observed in the reactive thrombocytosis associated with inflammation or neoplasia, where megakaryocyte nuclear ploidy is inversely related to the peripheral platelet count. As PV progresses, fibrosis may appear in central areas of the marrow, and scanning techniques will demonstrate expansion of hematopoietic tissue to more peripheral skeletal sites.

Cytogenetic abnormalities, including trisomy 1, 8, or 9 and 20q−, have been reported in about 10 percent of untreated patients. Prior treatment with myelosuppressive agents or radioactive phosphorus (^{32}P) appears to increase the incidence of such abnormalities.

DIAGNOSIS The plethoric patient with pancytosis and splenomegaly, and without evidence of chronic cardiac or pulmonary disease, presents few diagnostic problems. However, it is more common to see patients with PV who have less than the full clinical disease or in whom an elevated hemoglobin or hematocrit has been discovered at the time of routine laboratory evaluation. Under these circumstances, it is important that the diagnosis of PV be made with certainty in order to direct therapeutic efforts appropriately.

First, there is little statistical likelihood that hematocrits consistently near or greater than 60 percent represent a simple decrease in plasma volume. When hematocrit levels are in the range of 50 to 55 percent, however, the likelihood of true erythrocytosis is reduced to about 50 percent and the red blood cell mass should be determined directly by isotope dilution using ^{51}Cr-labeled autologous red blood cells. While the plasma volume may be calculated indirectly from the red blood cell mass, it is preferable to measure this compartment independently using a second label. The results for red blood cell mass are best expressed as a function of the lean body mass, which may be estimated from the patient's height and weight. If the results of such a study are equivocal, the clinical findings must establish whether the patient has a true increase in red blood cell production or else the patient should be restudied at a later time.

The patient who presents with a hematocrit or hemoglobin in the high normal range, microcytosis, leukocytosis, and iron deficiency should be considered as possibly having PV. Evaluation of red and white blood cell morphology, basophil count, and platelet morphology should be carried out to make certain that this is not a patient with PV who has bled.

While measurements of red blood cell mass distinguish spurious from true erythrocytosis, the results do not distinguish between the various forms of polycythemia. If the diagnosis is uncertain, additional indexes which may be helpful include the absolute basophil count, the leukocyte alkaline phosphatase score, and results of radioisotope scanning to quantitate spleen size. This last is particularly useful in obese individuals or patients in whom the spleen is enlarged but not palpable.

If the diagnosis of PV remains obscure, an intravenous pyelogram or abdominal CT scan should be obtained to exclude hypernephroma or other renal pathology which might result in increased erythropoietin production. Arterial blood gas measurements should be obtained, including carboxyhemoglobin levels if the patient is a smoker. Perhaps 20 percent of patients with PV may have a hemoglobin oxygen saturation below 92 percent, but almost all will have a saturation equal to or greater than 88 percent. This modest impairment of oxygen loading may be due to decreased diffusing capacity of the lung, possibly triggered by repeated episodes of thromboembolism or thrombosis in situ.

When the diagnosis is not clear following routine investigation, measurement of serum erythropoietin levels by radioimmunoassay may be helpful. Patients with PV generally have lower plasma erythropoietin levels than do patients with secondary forms of polycythemia. In vitro growth characteristics of bone marrow cells from patients with PV also may be useful in diagnosis.

COURSE AND PROGNOSIS The course of PV has been a subject of disagreement, some observers believing that later complications are hastened by myelosuppressive therapy. About 15 to 20 percent of patients will progress to marrow fibrosis, marked splenomegaly, and anemia; one view holds that if patients live long enough, all will enter this so-called spent phase of the disease. However, the majority of patients die of vascular complications of their disease or of unrelated causes. Although the incidence is low, there is a statistically significant association of second hematologic neoplasms in patients with PV; these include non-Hodgkin's lymphomas and multiple myeloma. Of patients with PV, 1 to 2 percent experience transformation into acute leukemia even without prior radiation or chemotherapy.

THERAPY Optimal therapy of PV remains unsettled. The median survival has been extended to 10 to 12 years with phlebotomy alone, while patients receiving no therapy at all survive only 2 years. However, neither myelosuppressive therapy nor phlebotomy holds a clear advantage for survival. For many years after its introduction in 1940, ^{32}P was the therapy of choice. However, a retrospective analysis of a large number of cases suggested that ^{32}P increased the incidence of acute leukemia (to over 10 percent) while not clearly enhancing survival over other forms of therapy. In order to resolve the major questions regarding the most effective therapy, the incidence of complicating factors, and the prognostic implication of certain features such as thrombocytosis or cytogenetic abnormalities, the International Polycythemia Vera Study Group was established. This group prospectively assigned patients who met strict diagnostic criteria into three treatment programs at random: ^{32}P therapy augmented by phlebotomy, myelosuppressive therapy plus phlebotomy, and phlebotomy alone. Analysis of the survival curves demonstrated similar survivals for the various treatment groups until the seventh year after randomization. At that point, patients treated with alkylating agents had poorer survival. The findings indicated that those patients in the phlebotomy-only group suffered from increased risk of death due to hemorrhage or thrombosis within the first four years, while leukemia and other neoplasms were more prevalent later in the course of the patients treated with chemotherapy or ^{32}P. However, a simultaneous European cooperative therapy trial did not demonstrate increased leukemia in patients treated with chemotherapy, and the survival in those patients was superior to that of patients treated with phlebotomy alone.

Despite the controversy, certain therapeutic tenets meet with agreement. Phlebotomy is safe, can be done repeatedly, and is preferred in individuals with mild disease, young patients, or those with polycythemia of uncertain etiology. Myelosuppression is best in patients with extreme symptomatic thrombocytosis, rapidly enlarging spleen, or symptoms of hypermetabolism. It may also spare elderly patients the rigors of phlebotomy. Regardless of eventual decisions involving therapy, phlebotomy should be used initially to reduce the red blood cell mass and blood volume. The end point of phlebotomy therapy should be a hematocrit or hemoglobin value in the low-normal range. This form of treatment may lead to prolonged clinical remission. Iron should not be given if phlebotomy is the primary mode of therapy. Phlebotomy is especially important if a patient with PV must undergo emergency surgery, since intra- and postoperative morbidity and mortality are four to five times greater in uncontrolled as opposed to controlled (phlebotomized) patients. Under these circumstances, the red blood cell mass should be reduced acutely by exchange phlebotomies and the blood replaced with a suitable plasma expander. This will prevent the vascular instability associated with too rapid a reduction in total blood volume.

Marrow suppression may be achieved by radiation or chemotherapy. The administration of ^{32}P is easy, provides long, trouble-free remissions in most cases, and successfully reduces the morbidity associated with the disease. The regimen recommended by the International Polycythemia Vera Study Group consists of the intravenous administration initially of 85.2 MBq of ^{32}P/m^2 body surface area. The patient is then followed for a period of 3 months and retreated at that time, as needed, with a dose 25 percent greater than that given originally. This program may be repeated 3 months later but is rarely required. Remissions may last 6 to 24 months, during which time the patient is often symptom-free. This ^{32}P therapy may be repeated if relapse occurs. Exposure to ^{32}P increases the incidence of leukemia in patients with PV, and the risk of leukemic transformation may be related to the cumulative dose of isotope.

Suppression of marrow function with chemotherapy has been common during the last 15 years. Effective drugs include hydroxyurea, melphalan, busulfan, and chlorambucil. Busulfan, in doses of 4 to 6 mg/d orally, reduces the white blood cell and platelet counts, but suppression may be unpredictable and prolonged and the drug is relatively less effective in suppressing erythropoiesis. Moreover, continued use of this drug may lead to pulmonary fibrosis and a syndrome resembling adrenal insufficiency. Chlorambucil, originally employed in the prospective treatment trial by the International Polycythemia Vera Study Group, resulted in a high incidence (over 10 percent) of acute leukemia, and the study group has recommended against the routine use of this or other alkylating agents in this disease. Currently, no form of treatment is clearly better than any other in terms of patient survival, but management with ^{32}P may be simpler and particularly appropriate in elderly patients. Hydroxyurea, a drug active in the DNA synthetic phase of the cell cycle and not known to be leukemogenic, is effective. Hydroxyurea given orally in doses of 1 to 3 g/d may control symptoms of hypermetabolism and the elevated leukocyte and platelet counts, but phlebotomy is generally required for adequate control of the red cell mass. Small clinical trials of aspirin to control thrombotic complications have not shown benefit.

Other symptoms associated with PV may be managed conservatively. In the case of pruritus, cyproheptadine, 12 to 16 mg/d, may be effective. Allopurinol in doses of 300 mg/d will reduce serum uric acid. Symptomatic splenomegaly is usually improved with treatment, although splenectomy may be indicated in rare instances.

AGNOGENIC MYELOID METAPLASIA/MYELOFIBROSIS

DEFINITION AND ETIOLOGY AMM/MF is characterized by the tendency of the neoplastic stem cells to lodge and grow in multiple sites outside the marrow. Typically, there is progressive splenomegaly, the gradual replacement of marrow elements by fibrosis, progressive anemia, and variable changes in the number of granulocytes and platelets. The disease begins in late middle life and is gradual in onset, chronic, and progressive. Males and females are equally involved, and there is only rare familial occurrence.

While erythrocytes, granulocytes, and platelets are members of a single neoplastic clone, the fibrosis is reactive and not part of the abnormal clone. AMM is an integral part of the disease and is seen early in its course. There is no evidence that AMM arises in compensation for replacement of the marrow by fibrous tissue.

PATHOPHYSIOLOGY AND SYMPTOMATOLOGY AMM/MF presents most commonly with vague constitutional symptoms associated with anemia, such as fatigue, weakness, and anorexia, or with splenomegaly. An enlarged spleen is seen in virtually all patients; however, the disease progresses slowly and splenomegaly may be present for years prior to diagnosis. The enlargement may become so extensive as to produce symptoms of pain, abdominal fullness, and dyspnea. Hepatomegaly occurs in more than 50 percent of patients and also may become massive, but enlargement of the liver due to AMM does not occur in the absence of splenomegaly. Petechiae are found in 20 percent of patients as a result of thrombocytopenia, and a history of bleeding is obtained in 10 percent. Less common findings include lymphadenopathy, jaundice, ascites, and bone pain. Weight loss, fever, sweating, and extremity pain may occur occasionally and are associated with a hypermetabolic state. The increased cellular turnover results in hyperuricemia in 25 to 30 percent of patients.

LABORATORY FINDINGS The blood counts of patients with AMM/MF are variable. Mild anemia is observed in over one-half of the patients at the time of diagnosis and progresses during the course of the disease. Eventually, almost all patients become anemic. The recognized mechanisms leading to anemia include ineffective erythropoiesis, increased splenic pooling of red cells, and a decrease in red blood cell survival. Low serum folate and megaloblastic maturation may contribute. The peripheral blood smear usually shows dramatic changes in red cell and platelet morphology. Basophilic stippling is prominent and bizarre red cell shapes, including teardrop poikilocytes, fragmented cells, and nucleated red cells, are common, as are giant platelet forms.

An elevation in the white blood cell count is found in about 50 percent of patients, and values as high as 50,000 per microliter may be seen. However, 20 percent of patients are leukopenic, with white blood cell counts less than 4000 per microliter. Generally, there is a shift toward immature forms in granulocyte maturation, and circulating blast forms may be found. The appearance of these cells does not imply a bad prognosis. An increase in the absolute basophil count is observed in 25 percent of patients. The leukocyte alkaline phosphatase activity is elevated in about half the patients, the remainder being equally distributed between having normal or low values. Serum vitamin B_{12} levels are normal or slightly elevated, as are vitamin B_{12}-binding proteins. These values usually do not approach those seen with CML.

A normal or elevated platelet count is frequently found early in the course of the disease, but thrombocytopenia eventually develops in most patients, owing to ineffective production and splenic pooling. The circulating platelets vary considerably in size and shape, and megakaryocyte nuclei may be found on the peripheral blood smear. In vitro studies of platelet function reflect defective platelet adhesiveness and impaired secondary release of ADP in response to epinephrine. Abnormal liver function tests, including elevated bilirubin and alkaline phosphatase, may be associated with massive hepatomegaly.

The spleen may become massive. There are multiple foci of extramedullary hematopoiesis on pathologic examination, but the normal follicular architecture of the spleen is maintained. Other organs which may be involved include the kidneys, lymph nodes, adrenal glands, and lungs. Bone marrow examination early in the course of the disease reveals a hypercellular marrow in about 20 percent of patients and may be difficult to distinguish from PV. Special stains of the marrow reveal increased reticulin deposition. However, a minority of patients develops obvious patchy collagen fibrosis separating areas of hyperplastic marrow, or diffuse fibrosis with osteosclerosis. Megakaryocytes may be preserved remarkably well in the areas of fibrosis. One hypothesis to account for the marrow fibrosis is that neoplastic megakaryoblasts and megakaryocytes release growth factors, such as PDGF, which stimulate fibroblasts or other connective tissue cells to synthesize collagen or reticulin. This is also consistent with the fact that successful bone marrow transplantation leads to the reversal of established fibrosis.

The fibrosis and osteosclerosis of the marrow generally correlate with one another and also with the degree of splenomegaly. However, there is no clear relationship between the histopathology of the marrow and the peripheral blood counts. In 40 to 50 percent of patients, the appearance of marrow sclerosis is reflected on x-ray examination by increased bone density involving particularly the axial skeleton and proximal long bones. These x-ray changes result from thickened cortical bone and the loss of medullary spaces due to increased and thickened bony trabeculae.

No unique cytogenetic abnormalities have been described in AMM/MF; however, certain nonrandom abnormalities, including monosomy 7 and trisomy 9, have been found. Reports of the Ph chromosome in this disorder probably reflect examples of atypical CML.

DIAGNOSIS A bone marrow biopsy is essential to the evaluation of this disease, and without it the diagnosis cannot be made with certainty. This disorder may be difficult to distinguish from other myeloproliferative diseases.

In CML the white blood cell count is usually greater than 20,000 per microliter, while in AMM/MF it is generally 10,000 to 20,000 per microliter. Leukocyte alkaline phosphatase is usually lower in CML, and this determination may be useful in distinguishing between the two disorders. Fibrosis of the marrow is found in only 10 to 15 percent of patients with CML and is usually present only as a preterminal event; osteosclerosis is almost never seen. In the absence of the Ph chromosome, however, the distinction between these diseases is occasionally difficult.

The separation of PV and essential thrombocytosis (ET) from AMM/MF occasionally is troublesome because all may present with thrombocytosis, splenomegaly, leukocytosis, and anemia. However,

ET generally is not associated with advanced fibrosis. The most difficult distinction is between AMM/MF and the late stages of PV, and attempts to separate them are probably unwarranted. Approximately 15 to 25 percent of patients with PV progress to advanced marrow fibrosis and marked splenomegaly. It is impossible to be certain that a patient with typical AMM/MF did not initially have PV. Postpolycythemia myeloid metaplasia with myelofibrosis has a poorer prognosis.

Secondary causes of myelofibrosis include metastatic carcinoma, leukemia and lymphomas, tuberculosis, Gaucher's disease, Paget's disease, and exposure to toxins such as benzene or to x-rays. These associations are usually not difficult to distinguish from AMM/MF.

THERAPY There is no definitive therapy for this disorder, and no treatment has been shown to affect life span favorably. Anemia is treated with transfusions as required. Androgens may be administered to improve the anemia, although they are helpful in less than half of the cases. Oxymetholone (2 to 4 mg/kg per day) or fluoxymesterone may be given, particularly if there is marked ineffective erythropoiesis. Glucocorticoids may enhance the response to androgens but alone are not helpful. Myelosuppressive therapy is only occasionally indicated, but it may be used to control painful splenomegaly or marked thrombocytosis. Chlorambucil or melphalan may be employed, but other blood elements may be depressed and the period of remission is relatively short (4 to 5 months). External radiation to the spleen will reduce its size, but the effects are transient and therapy may lead to severe pancytopenia. Allopurinol may be given to reduce a high uric acid level.

The role of splenectomy in the treatment of AMM/MF is controversial. Late in the course of the disease the hazards of removing a massively enlarged organ are considerable, and intraoperative mortality and postoperative complications, particularly thrombosis and infection, are frequent. Early removal of the spleen, as soon as the diagnosis is made, does not clearly reduce later complications or make management easier. The only clear indications for splenectomy are hemolysis, severe thrombocytopenia, and intractable symptoms related to spleen size.

COURSE AND PROGNOSIS AMM/MF generally follows a prolonged course, with a median survival of 4 to 5 years from the time of diagnosis; 25 percent of patients may live 15 years. Anemia occurs eventually in most patients, and many will require transfusions. Complicating features of the disease include gout or other problems related to hyperuricemia and symptoms related to the enlarging spleen. Portal hypertension may be seen due to hepatic fibrosis, hepatic vein thrombosis, or the markedly increased blood flow through the spleen. Clinically evident bleeding occurs in about 25 percent, and it is important for thrombocytopenic patients to avoid drugs such as aspirin or nonsteroidal anti-inflammatory agents which further impair platelet function. While the degree of splenomegaly appears to be of no prognostic importance, a platelet count of less than 100,000 per microliter, hemoglobin of less than 100 g/L (10 g/dL), and hepatomegaly are associated with poorer survival.

The major causes of death include infection, congestive heart failure, renal failure, portal hypertension, and hemorrhage. Transformation to acute leukemia occurs in 5 to 10 percent of patients and may be related to radiation or chemotherapy. A particularly fulminant variant of AMM/MF, known as acute myelofibrosis, is characterized by rapid progression of fibrosis and pancytopenia without splenic enlargement. Death due to marrow failure usually occurs within 1 year of diagnosis. This disorder is now more correctly recognized as acute megakaryoblastic leukemia.

ESSENTIAL THROMBOCYTOSIS

DEFINITION AND ETIOLOGY Essential thrombocytosis (ET) is dominated clinically by a markedly elevated platelet count which is invariably above 400,000 per microliter and which may reach levels of 3 to 4 million per microliter. The disease closely resembles PV and AMM/MF. Although an elevated platelet count is the dominant laboratory feature, all cell lines are involved in the expansion of the neoplastic clone.

As opposed to secondary forms of thrombocytosis, which arise in response to inflammation, acute bleeding, iron deficiency, or neoplasms, ET represents the overproduction of platelets in the absence of a recognizable stimulus. In cultures of bone marrow cells from patients with ET, colonies of megakaryocytes from megakaryocytic progenitors often form in the absence of added stimulus. Endogenous erythroid colonies may also form. This does not happen with marrow cell cultures from normal individuals or patients with secondary thrombocytosis.

PATHOPHYSIOLOGY AND SYMPTOMATOLOGY Symptoms associated with ET are linked to the platelet dysfunction and perhaps to platelet aggregation in the microvasculature of the central nervous system. Patients with ET may present with erythromelalgia, venous or arterial thromboses, or spontaneous bleeding. This may be seen as easy bruisability, unusual bleeding following minor dental procedures or other surgery, or large-vessel bleeding into soft tissues or muscles in the absence of a history of trauma. The first clue may be such a hemorrhagic or thrombotic episode. Transient ischemic attacks or even frank strokes may occur in patients with markedly elevated platelet counts. In general, there is a correlation between symptomatology and platelet counts in patients with this disease. However, the correlation is imperfect and individual patients will manifest symptoms at different platelet levels. Young patients, particularly females, are generally asymptomatic, regardless of platelet count.

LABORATORY FINDINGS The most prominent laboratory feature is the elevated platelet count. Examination of the peripheral blood smear reveals platelets of markedly different morphology with many large forms and forms which appear hypogranular. In vitro platelet function tests typically reveal an abnormality in platelet aggregation in response to epinephrine, collagen, or ADP. The epinephrine defect is the most characteristic. These in vitro aggregation abnormalities do not correlate with the history of bleeding or thrombosis or with a prolonged bleeding time. Splenomegaly is seen in two-thirds of patients with this disease but is generally modest, and the spleen does not achieve the size observed in CML or AMM/MF. Bone marrow examination reveals large numbers of hyperploid megakaryocytes and, with disease progression, there may be evidence of fibrosis. This is rarely as marked as in AMM/MF.

DIAGNOSIS A markedly elevated platelet count with typical platelet morphology in the absence of a cause for secondary thrombocytosis is generally sufficient to make the diagnosis. Confirmation may be obtained by in vitro platelet function tests, measurement of bleeding time, or the association of splenomegaly. Cytogenetic abnormalities are uncommon with this disease. A useful feature is the matching of megakaryocyte size to platelet number on examination of a marrow aspirate and biopsy. Secondary thrombocytosis is associated with increased numbers of megakaryocytes which are of generally small diameter and lower ploidy. In ET, the elevated platelet number is associated with increased numbers of large, hyperploid megakaryocytes.

COURSE AND PROGNOSIS The median survival of patients with ET is not well-defined. A prospective study evaluating therapy in this disease is being conducted by the Polycythemia Vera Study Group. It is anticipated that survival will be at least as good as for those patients with PV. Complications of the disease, such as hemorrhage or fatal thrombosis, represent the terminal event in the majority of cases. In 1 or 2 percent of cases the disease transforms to a more aggressive or frankly leukemic phase. If this does occur, aggressive chemotherapy is rarely effective.

THERAPY The indications for therapy in ET are unsettled, particularly in young, asymptomatic patients, and the effect of therapy in prolonging survival has not been quantitated. However, there is agreement that patients with symptomatic thrombocytosis who have had bleeding or thrombotic episodes should be treated. Previous therapy has employed alkylating agents such as busulfan or chlor-

ambucil. However, because of the concern that these drugs may result in or enhance the likelihood of leukemic transformation, therapy with hydroxyurea is being evaluated. The available data suggest good control of the disease, but the overall effect on survival cannot be judged as yet. If patients are symptomatic at a particular platelet count, their counts should be maintained well below that level through the use of myelosuppression. Alkylating agents or ^{32}P may be used if hydroxyurea becomes ineffective. Treatment of acute events such as thrombosis or hemorrhage in an uncontrolled or previously undiagnosed patient with ET should be by emergent plateletpheresis. Aspirin and dipyridamole may prove useful in preventing thrombotic or ischemic symptoms in some patients with ET.

REFERENCES

Adamson JW, Fialkow PJ: Pathogenesis of the myeloproliferative syndromes. Br J Haematol 38:299, 1978

Allan HC: Therapeutic options in chronic myeloid leukemia. Blood Rev 3:45, 1989

Berk PD et al: Increased incidence of acute leukemia in polycythemia vera associated with chlorambucil therapy. N Engl J Med 304:441, 1981

Champlin RE, Golde DW: Chronic myelogenous leukemia (CML): Recent advances. Blood 65:1039, 1985

Hockin WG, Golde DW: Polycythemia: Evaluation and management. Blood Rev 3:57, 1989

Polycythemia vera: An update I and II. In *Seminars in Hematology,* vol 23, PA Miescher, ER Jaffe (eds). Orlando, Grune & Stratton, Nos 2 (April) and 3 (July), 1986

Silverstein MK: Primary thrombocythemia, in *Hematology,* WJ Williams et al (eds). New York, McGraw-Hill, 1983, pp 218–222

Stam K et al: Evidence of a new chimeric *bcr/abl* mRNA in patients with chronic myelocytic leukemia and the Philadelphia chromosome. N Engl J Med 313:1429, 1985

Talpaz M et al: Hematologic remission and cytogenetic improvement induced by recombinant human interferon alpha-a in chronic myelogenous leukemia. N Engl J Med 314:1065, 1986

Thomas ED et al: Marrow transplantation for the treatment of chronic myelogenous leukemia. Ann Intern Med 104:155, 1986

298 BONE MARROW FAILURE: APLASTIC ANEMIA AND OTHER PRIMARY BONE MARROW DISORDERS

JOEL M. RAPPEPORT / H. FRANKLIN BUNN

An important group of anemias is caused by primary disorders of the bone marrow which impair the formation of erythropoietic precursors. The term *aplastic anemia* should be restricted to conditions in which an acellular or markedly hypocellular bone marrow results in pancytopenia (anemia, neutropenia, and thrombocytopenia). Rare patients develop selective aplasia of only erythroid cells *(pure red blood cell aplasia)*. Alternatively, in *myelophthisic anemia*, erythropoiesis is suppressed because the marrow is infiltrated with tumor, granulomas, or fibrosis. The dysmyelopoietic or myelodysplastic anemias are associated with variable neutropenia and thrombocytopenia resulting from an acquired disorder of the hematopoietic pluripotent stem cell.

APLASTIC ANEMIA

ETIOLOGY Aplastic anemia is thought to be due to injury or destruction of a common pluripotential stem cell affecting all subsequent cell populations. The diverse factors associated with the development of aplastic anemia are listed in Table 298-1. In approximately half of the cases of aplastic anemia in the United States, no etiologic agent is identifiable. In areas of the world where a larger

TABLE 298-1   Causes of pancytopenia

I Aplastic anemia
   A Idiopathic anemias
   B Constitutional anemias (Fanconi's anemia)
   C Chemical and physical agents
      1 Dose-related: benzene, ionizing irradiation, alkylating agents, anti-metabolites (folic acid antagonists, purine and pyrimidine analogues), mitotic inhibitors, anthracyclines, inorganic arsenicals
      2 Idiosyncratic: chloramphenicol, phenylbutazone, sulfa drugs, methylphenylethylhydantoin, gold compounds, organic arsenicals, insecticides
   D Immunologically mediated aplasia
   E Other associations: hepatitis, other viral infections, systemic lupus erythematosus, diffuse eosinophilic faciitis
II Pancytopenia with normal or increased bone marrow cellularity
   A Myelodysplastic syndromes
   B Hypersplenism (Chap. 63)
   C Vitamin B_{12} and folate deficiencies (Chap. 292)
III Paroxysmal nocturnal hemoglobinuria (Chap. 294)
IV Bone marrow replacement
   A Hematologic malignancies (Chaps. 134, 296, 302)
   B Nonhematologic metastatic tumor
   C Storage cell disorders (Chap. 331)
   D Osteopetrosis (Chap. 345)
   E Myelofibrosis (Chap. 297)

percentage of the population may be exposed to toxins such as insecticides and benzenes in uncontrolled dose, the percentage of idiopathic cases is smaller. In some cases, a damaged marrow microenvironment may contribute to marrow failure. The role of lymphokines in aplasia is currently under intense study.

Congenital causes   Fanconi's anemia, the most common type of constitutional aplastic anemia, is an autosomal recessively inherited disease usually appearing in childhood. This disorder is often associated with multiple congenital somatic anomalies, including renal and cardiac malformations, hyperpigmentation of the skin, and bony abnormalities, particularly hypoplastic or absent thumbs or radii. Most patients have chromosomal abnormalities owing to a defect in DNA repair. Patients who survive the complications of progressive marrow failure are at high risk of developing leukemia or other malignancies. Other genetic syndromes have been associated with bone marrow failure including dyskeratosis congenita.

Immune causes   A number of clinical observations have led to the concept that a significant proportion of cases of aplastic anemia may be mediated by immunologic mechanisms. These include autologous recovery following immunosuppressive preparation for marrow grafting and failure of hematopoietic reconstitution in some patients following marrow transplantation from identical twin donors in the absence of immunosuppression. A variety of in vitro culture techniques have also supported the concept of an antibody or a cellular autoimmune process in some patients with aplasia. However, in any given case the identification of an immune process may be difficult.

Drugs and toxins   Multiple and seemingly unrelated drugs and chemical agents have been incriminated as etiologic agents in aplastic anemia. The association varies from a predictable dose-related aplasia to idiosyncratic reactions unrelated to dose.

The agents which in an adequate dose will predictably produce bone marrow depression are the antineoplastic and immunosuppressive drugs along with ionizing radiation. These drugs include folic acid antagonists, alkylating agents, the anthracyclines, and the nitrosoureas, as well as purine and pyrimidine analogues. The degree of aplasia is dose related but may vary from individual to individual. The effects of combination chemotherapy may be additive. Withdrawal of the drug usually permits recovery of the marrow elements, although irreversible aplasia is occasionally noted. Marrow aplasia may also be induced by therapeutic x-rays or, less commonly, by acute exposure from a laboratory or industrial accident. The severity of aplasia is dependent upon the dose and rate of the exposure as well as the extent of marrow irradiated.

Benzene derivatives have been associated with multiple hemato-

logic abnormalities including aplastic anemia. Benzene-induced aplasia may result from both industrial and domestic use of benzene-containing products. This aplasia may be reversible, although mild abnormalities such as macrocytosis may persist.

Chloramphenicol, a commonly used broad-spectrum antibiotic, is associated with two forms of bone marrow toxicity. The more common effect upon the bone marrow is a reversible dose-related suppression of erythroid and, on occasion, granulocytic and megakaryocytic precursors. This condition is characterized by a transient anemia, associated with a drop in reticulocytes and elevation of serum iron. This bone marrow suppression is related to the dose and duration of administration of chloramphenicol. The bone marrow reveals vacuoles in the cytoplasm of early erythroid and granulocytic precursors. Similar morphologic features are seen much more commonly in some patients who have ingested large amounts of alcohol.

The more serious form of bone marrow failure associated with chloramphenicol is an "idiosyncratic" reaction. This nitrobenzene compound has been the single most commonly incriminated drug in cases of aplastic anemia. These patients develop severe pancytopenia and often irreversible, fatal marrow aplasia. This complication occurs in approximately 1 in 50,000 patients who take the drug. The development of aplastic anemia seems to be unrelated to dose or duration of administration. Marrow aplasia cannot be anticipated or prevented by hematologic monitoring, since it may appear after cessation of the drug. Unfortunately, many cases of fatal aplastic anemia have occurred in patients who received chloramphenicol for trivial or dubious reasons. Therefore, this antibiotic should not be used when there are reasonable alternatives.

Other unrelated chemicals and drugs may be responsible for the development of aplastic anemia. These agents can be placed into two classes: those in which a number of associations have been reported and, therefore, a definite toxic potential has been established, and those in which only a few reported cases exist and, therefore, only a possibility of toxic potential exists at present. The establishment of these relationships is often further confused by the fact that many of the patients have taken multiple drugs. Agents in which a definite potential toxicity exists are shown in Table 298-1.

Infections   A number of cases of aplastic anemia have been reported following infectious hepatitis. The antecedent hepatitis is not distinguished by its severity, and the aplastic anemia commonly appears as the hepatitis resolves. Aplasia has usually followed non-A, non-B hepatitis but on occasion has been associated with types A and B. The aplasia tends to be severe and frequently has a fatal outcome. Other viruses, including Epstein-Barr virus, have been implicated in aplastic anemia. Many cases of so-called "idiopathic aplastic anemia" are preceded by a benign-appearing viral respiratory illness. Parvovirus selectively infects erythroblasts and therefore acutely aggravates anemia in patients with hemolysis (Chap. 294).

Some patients infected with human immunodeficiency virus will develop pancytopenia and a hypoplastic bone marrow. Contributing factors include direct suppression of hematopoietic cells by the virus, opportunistic infections such as cytomegalovirus or *Mycobacterium avium intracellulare,* and myelotoxic drugs such as trimethoprim-sulfamethoxazole and azidothymidine.

Aplastic anemia has also been reported in association with a number of other illnesses (Table 298-1). The clinical and laboratory findings associated with paroxysmal nocturnal hemoglobinuria may accompany or precede the development of aplasia. Aplastic anemia that develops during pregnancy may remit following delivery of the fetus.

CLINICAL MANIFESTATIONS   The onset of aplastic anemia is usually insidious. Initial presenting symptoms include mild progressive weakness and fatigue attributable to the anemia and/or hemorrhage from the skin, nose, gums, vagina, or gastrointestinal tract due to the thrombocytopenia. The bleeding is usually mild, but occasionally retinal or central nervous system hemorrhage may be the initial mode of presentation. Although the patient may be severely neutropenic, it is less common for the initial presentation to be a bacterial infection.

Physical examination generally reveals pallor. Petechiae or ecchymoses may be noted in the skin, mucous membranes, the conjunctivae, and fundi. Lymphadenopathy and hepatosplenomegaly are notably absent. Fever may be present, but despite the presence of an infection, the usual signs of inflammation may be absent because of neutropenia.

The *course* of the disease is generally determined by the severity of the aplasia, rather than by the etiology. Mild disease can progress to a more severe disorder. Conversely, complete recovery or partial recovery of one or more cell lines may develop. It is important to obtain an accurate assessment of the degree of aplasia. Severe aplasia is defined as marked pancytopenia with at least two of the following criteria: granulocytes fewer than 500 per microliter, platelets fewer than 20,000 per microliter, or anemia with corrected reticulocyte count less than 1 percent. The bone marrow is markedly hypoplastic and depleted of hematopoietic cells. Patients with severe disease have a high risk of dying from bleeding and/or infections in a matter of months, while patients with a milder form of the disease may live for years. The clinical course of the disease is affected primarily by infections and by the nature and location of bleeding. Although infections may not dominate the clinical picture initially, they assume greater importance with the passage of time. Because of the need for multiple red blood cell and platelet transfusions, over a period of time one may encounter the sequelae of hemosiderosis and/or hepatitis. Even those patients who recover may have mild thrombocytopenia and persistent macrocytosis for many years. Long-term survivors are at increased risk of developing either acute leukemia or the myelodysplastic syndrome.

LABORATORY DIAGNOSIS The diagnosis of aplastic anemia and the assessment of its relative severity depend upon a thorough laboratory evaluation. The peripheral blood usually shows pancytopenia. The absolute granulocyte count is low, or becomes progressively depressed during the illness. The red blood cells are normochromic and normocytic or mildly macrocytic reflecting stress erythropoiesis, and the corrected reticulocyte count is very low or zero. Since the incidence of serious bleeding and/or infection correlates with the degree of thrombocytopenia or neutropenia, these values must be determined initially and followed serially. A bone marrow aspirate may yield a "dry tap," but a bone marrow biopsy will reveal a severely hypocellular or aplastic marrow with replacement by fat. There is usually a severe depression of megakaryocytes and myeloid cells and a marked but relatively less severe depression of the erythroid precursors.

Elevated serum iron coupled with a normal level of transferrin results in elevated transferrin saturation. Because of the reduction in erythroid precursors, plasma iron clearance is prolonged, and incorporation of iron into red blood cells is markedly decreased. There is no evidence of increased red blood cell destruction.

DIFFERENTIAL DIAGNOSIS The diagnosis of aplastic anemia implies the exclusion of the other causes of pancytopenia that are listed in Table 298-1. Splenomegaly and/or lymphadenopathy argue strongly against aplastic anemia. Malignant and nonmalignant invasion of the bone marrow must be excluded by microscopic examination of the marrow. Paroxysmal nocturnal hemoglobinuria and systemic lupus erythematosus should be ruled out by appropriate tests including the sugar water and acid hemolysis tests. Vitamin B_{12} and folate deficiencies can be excluded by serum assays and morphologic changes. Pancytopenia rarely may be secondary to various infections. Before aplastic anemia can be classified as idiopathic, a careful history must exclude exposure to all known and suspected agents. In our complex society, all patients are exposed to potentially toxic agents in their environment. Nevertheless this difficulty should not discourage a careful and extensive search for a cause.

TREATMENT The management of aplastic anemia has become one of the most challenging aspects of modern medicine, requiring a diligent multidisciplinary team of care givers in a well-equipped tertiary care center. For patients with mild aplasia, every effort should be made to do as little as possible except to remove possible etiologic agents in expectation of spontaneous recovery. As noted below, androgens may be of value in mild aplasia. Patients with severe aplasia should be considered for a bone marrow transplantation, if a suitable donor is available. The efficacy of this treatment with complete correction of the hematopoietic defect has been most clearly demonstrated in younger patients (Chap. 299).

Supportive care Regardless of the therapy chosen, the mainstay of treatment is good supportive care. The first and most immediate step is the removal of any suspected etiologic agent. If the disease is mild at presentation, no further supportive care need be instituted, unless there is subsequent deterioration. If a severe neutropenia exists (polymorphonuclear leukocytes fewer than 500 per microliter), the patient should be shielded from potential infections. Prophylactic systemic antibiotics should not be utilized. Intramuscular injections should be minimized and, if necessary, should be administered with care. Established infections should be treated vigorously with specific antibiotics, and fever of undetermined etiology may, after appropriate evaluation, call for broad-spectrum antibiotic coverage until a specific diagnosis is established. Menstruating females should be placed on suppressive doses of birth control pills.

TRANSFUSIONS These should be used *judiciously* and restricted to appropriate component therapy, since future therapy and ultimate survival may be affected by transfusions. Red blood cells should be administered to maintain the well-being of the patient rather than to establish a certain hemoglobin level. Transfusions pose significant risks such as development of hepatitis or hemosiderosis, as well as sensitization to both red blood cell antigens and transplantation antigens. Platelet transfusions should be administered in the face of serious hemorrhage. Some groups employ prophylactic transfusions when the platelet count is lower than 20,000 per microliter. Others, fearful of the development of resistance to future transfusions, administer platelets only when faced with hemorrhage. Responses to platelet transfusions may be blunted by the presence of infection. If a patient develops immune resistance to platelet transfusions, HLA-compatible platelet transfusions may be useful (Chap. 286). Should a bone marrow transplant be considered, family members should be avoided as a source of blood products since the patient may develop antibodies to minor transplantation antigens. Leukocyte transfusions are not administered prophylactically. However, white blood cell infusions may be of value in patients with documented gram-negative infections and severe neutropenia who have failed to respond to antimicrobial therapy.

Marrow-stimulating agents Although patients with mild aplasia sometimes respond to androgens, and a few appear to be androgen-dependent, those with severe aplasia are usually unresponsive. Patients with mild aplasia should be treated with adequate doses of androgens as the initial mode of therapy. The most widely used drugs at present are oxymetholone, fluoxymesterone, and nandrolone decanoate. Responses may occur as long as 3 to 6 months after the initiation of therapy. The administration of recombinant granulocyte-macrophage colony stimulating factor is effective in treating pancytopenia associated with AIDS, myelodysplasia, or myelotoxic drugs. It is less effective in the treatment of aplastic anemia.

Immunosuppressive agents Increasing clinical and laboratory evidence suggests that 40 to 50 percent of patients will have a complete or, more likely, partial response to immunosuppressive therapy. The specificity and mechanism of this therapy is as yet undefined. The most commonly administered therapy is animal antisera directed against human lymphocytes and thymocytes. The effectiveness as well as the dose and duration of administration of these heterogeneous sera is variable from batch to batch. Serious side effects may accompany the administration of these heteroantisera. Very high doses of glucocorticoids or the immunosuppressive agent cyclosporine may yield similar responses.

In general, splenectomy has no role in the management of aplastic anemia.

Bone marrow transplantation (See Chap. 299)

OTHER PRIMARY BONE MARROW DISORDERS

PURE RED CELL APLASIA   Pure red cell aplasia involves a selective failure in the production of erythroid elements in the bone marrow. Granulopoiesis and megakaryocytopoiesis remain normal. Patients have a normochromic normocytic anemia with normal granulocyte count and platelet count. Severe reticulocytopenia exists, and the bone marrow is characterized by a virtual absence of any erythroid precursors in the face of otherwise normal cellular elements. An increase in lymphocytes may be seen in the marrow.

Constitutional red cell aplasia   Blackfan-Diamond syndrome, a rare chronic constitutional red blood cell aplasia, may appear in infants from the time of birth to the age of 2 years. Twenty-five percent of patients have minor congenital anomalies. The disorder is of unknown etiology, but has been corrected by both glucocorticoids and marrow transplantation.

Acquired red cell aplasia   The rare acquired form of pure red blood cell aplasia is seen predominantly in middle-aged adults. About one-third of patients have thymomas. Five percent of all patients with thymomas have pure red blood cell aplasia. The association between thymoma and myasthenia gravis is somewhat stronger. In many patients both with and without thymomas, erythropoiesis is inhibited by a complement-fixing IgG immunoglobulin which has selective cytotoxicity for marrow erythroblasts. A much smaller group of patients has been noted to have an inhibitor against erythropoietin. Occasionally, pure red cell aplasia is encountered in patients with T-cell chronic lymphatic leukemia. The circulating T cells are distinguished by the presence of receptors for the Fc portion of IgG.

TREATMENT   Since these patients have virtually no endogenous red blood cell production, they are totally dependent on red blood cell transfusion. If thymic enlargement is noted, a thymectomy may induce a remission in approximately 50 percent of patients. If the thymus is normal, thymectomy is of no benefit. Patients without thymoma or those with an unsuccessful thymectomy should receive glucocorticoids, alone or in combination with an immunosuppressive agent such as cyclophosphamide. Treatment often results in both prolonged clinical remission and disappearance of the inhibitor.

MYELODYSPLASTIC SYNDROMES   Also known as the refractory dysmyelopoietic anemias are a heterogeneous group of normocytic anemias often associated with neutropenia, thrombocytopenia, and/or monocytosis. The bone marrow varies in cellularity and usually reveals disordered maturation of erythroid, myeloid, and megakaryocytic cells. In some patients, erythroid cells accumulate large amounts of iron in mitochondria (ringed sideroblasts) (Chap. 291). The FAB (French, American, British) classification of the myelodysplastic syndrome includes five categories: refractory anemia (RA); refractory anemia with ringed sideroblasts (RARS); refractory anemia with excess of blasts (RAEB); chronic myelomonocytic leukemia (CMML); and refractory anemia with excess blasts in transformation (RAEB-T). This intrinsic disorder of the hematopoietic pluripotential stem cell is most frequently noted in older people. Although the etiology of these disorders is unclear, some patients appear to develop the syndrome secondary to chemotherapy, particularly alkylating agents with or without accompanying radiation therapy. The most common cytogenetic abnormalities noted include the deletion of the long arm of chromosome 5 (5q−), deletion of chromosome 7 or 5 (−7, −5), or trisomy 8. Over time, a variety of additional cytogenetic changes may be observed. Survival is variable among the subtypes with longer median survivals of 76 months noted in RARS and short median survivals of 3 to 6 months noted in RAEB-T. Patients may succumb to infections and hemorrhage because of the associated neutropenia and thrombocytopenia. These clonal disorders are frequently preleukemic with further evolution to a frank leukemic clone noted in 5 to 20 percent of patients with RARS and greater than 50 percent of patients with RAEB-T.

The mainstay of treatment is supportive: appropriate transfusion therapy and antibiotics for febrile episodes. Occasional long-term survivors may require therapy for iron overload. Rarely, patients with sideroblastic anemia will respond to pyridoxine or pyridoxal phosphate. Although differentiation agents such as vitamin D, retinoic acid, and low-dose cytosine arabinoside are effective in vitro, their therapeutic efficacy has been disappointing. Bone marrow transplantation in the appropriate setting has been curative for the myelodysplastic syndromes, as it has for de novo leukemias. Stimulation of the bone marrow by a variety of agents has been studied. Androgen therapy has in some cases resulted in moderate improvement. Hematopoietic growth factors, in particular recombinant granulocyte-macrophage colony stimulating factor (rGM-CSF), are currently under investigation and offer the potential for stimulating blood cell production. Both their long-term therapeutic effect and the possibility of accelerating the development of leukemia are still to be determined. The treatment of leukemia evolving from the myelodysplastic syndrome is discussed in Chap. 296.

MYELOPHTHISIC ANEMIA   Infiltration of the bone marrow with tumor, fibrosis, or granulomas can result in the development of a severe anemia. Tumor may be derived from cell lines indigenous to the bone marrow, as in leukemia, lymphoma, or myeloma, or the marrow may be invaded by metastatic deposits of solid tumor, usually carcinoma. Among the solid tumors most frequently associated with myelophthisic anemia are carcinoma of the breast, stomach, prostate, lung, and thyroid. Hepatomegaly and splenomegaly may develop in this setting, along with marrow fibrosis.

Fibrosis in the bone marrow, usually in association with myeloid metaplasia (see Chap. 297), can cause myelophthisic anemia. Granulomatous involvement of the bone marrow is usually due to advanced tuberculosis. Primary lipid storage disorders, such as Gaucher's disease and Niemann-Pick disease, occasionally produce a myelophthisic anemia, and the rare disorder osteopetrosis, or marble bone disease, may also give a similar hematologic picture.

The invasion of the bone marrow by tumor or granulomas impairs both erythropoiesis and thrombopoiesis. In contrast, neutrophil production is generally normal or increased. It is unlikely that the anemia and thrombocytopenia are due merely to "crowding" of the bone marrow space by extrinsic cells. Myelophthisis also causes a distortion of the microcirculation of the marrow, with premature release of immature cells.

Myelophthisis usually results in a severe normochromic normocytic anemia. A variety of misshapen erythrocytes are noted, particularly teardrop cells and fragmented cells with some basophilic stippling. In addition, normoblasts are usually seen in the peripheral blood. The reticulocyte percentage is often slightly increased (4 to 7 percent). However, when corrected for the anemia and the premature release from the bone marrow, the absolute reticulocyte count is actually reduced and reflects a decrease in red blood cell production. While thrombocytopenia is usually present, the white blood cell count is often elevated, with a marked shift to the left in the differential count. The combination of immature myeloid cells and normoblasts in the peripheral blood constitutes the "leukoerythroblastic" morphology so characteristic of myelophthisic anemia. Striking abnormalities are usually seen on examination of the bone marrow. Often an aspirate yields a "dry tap" owing to the infiltration of the marrow with abnormal tissue. Marrow biopsy is more likely to be diagnostic, revealing leukemia, lymphoma, or foci of metastatic tumors or granulomas. However, marrow involvement is often segmental, so that the primary pathologic process may be missed on a single biopsy.

Treatment   Treatment consists of attempts to reverse the primary pathologic process. It is particularly important to search for the presence of tuberculosis, since this disease is readily treatable. More often, however, the underlying disease is not amenable to therapy, and supportive measures, such as blood transfusions, must be employed.

REFERENCES

ANASETTI C et al: Marrow transplantation for severe aplastic anemia. Long-term outcome in fifty "untransfused" patients. Ann Intern Med 104:461, 1986

CAMITTA BM et al: Aplastic anemia: Pathogenesis, diagnosis, treatment and prognosis. N Engl J Med 306:645, 1982

CHIKKAPPA G et al: Pure red cell aplasia with chronic lymphatic leukemia. Medicine 65:339, 1986

CLARK DA et al: Studies on pure red cell aplasia. XI. Results of immunosuppressive treatment of 37 patients. Blood 63:277, 1984

GRIFFIN JD (ed): Myelodysplastic syndromes. Clin Haematol 15:909, 1986

HUMPHRIES RK, YOUNG N: Aplastic anemia and stem cell biology, in Aplastic Anemia. New York, AR Liss, 1984

KRANTZ SB, DESSYPRIS EN: Pure red cell aplasia, in Hematopoietic Stem Cells, DW Golde and F Takaka (eds). New York, Dekker, 1985

RAPPEPORT JM, NATHAN DG: Acquired aplastic anemia: Pathophysiology and treatment. Adv Intern Med 27:547, 1982

SPECK B et al: Treatment of severe aplastic anemia. Exp Hematol 14:126, 1986

VADHAN-RAJ S et al: Effects of recombinant human granulocyte-macrophage colony-stimulating factor in patients with myelodysplastic syndromes. N Engl J Med 317:1545, 1987

299 BONE MARROW TRANSPLANTATION

E. DONNALL THOMAS

SELECTION OF THE PATIENT Marrow transplantation is a rational therapeutic option only if the patient's disease involves the marrow or if hazard to the normal marrow is the limiting factor in aggressive treatment of a disease. A marrow transplant involves a transplant not only of the donor myeloid, erythroid, and megakaryocytic systems but also of the donor lymphoid and macrophage-monocyte systems. The rationale is illustrated by the three types of disease for which marrow transplantation has been widely utilized:

1 *Genetic disease.* For immunologic deficiency diseases, the objective is to replace the recipient's genetically defective lymphoid system with the normal lymphoid system of the donor. For genetic diseases such as thalassemia major, the abnormal marrow must be destroyed and replaced by normal marrow.
2 *Aplastic anemia.* Regardless of etiology, the disease process results in loss of the marrow, and the objective is to replace the defective organ with a normal functioning organ.
3 *Malignant disease.* For leukemia and other hematologic malignancies the objective is the complete destruction of the malignant cell population and, unavoidably, normal marrow cells by intensive chemoradiotherapy with restoration of normal marrow function by the transplanted marrow.

TYPES OF TRANSPLANTS A *syngeneic* graft describes a graft in which donor and recipient are genetically identical, i.e., identical twins. An *allogeneic* graft is one in which donor and recipient are of different genetic origins. A *chimera* is an individual whose body contains living, proliferating cells of different genetic origin. An *autologous* marrow graft refers to the removal of a patient's marrow, administration of chemo- and/or radiotherapy, and then return of the patient's own marrow.

SELECTION OF THE DONOR The donor must be in good health, and the donor, or an appropriate advocate, must be capable of giving informed consent. The principal risk is the anesthesia. Beyond these considerations, selection of the donor is largely determined by histocompatibility testing. Red blood cell incompatibility is not a barrier to marrow transplantation.

Histocompatibility typing (See Chap. 14) The HLA region is composed of a series of closely linked genes on chromosome 6. The array of genes encoded on a single chromosome is known as a *haplotype.* Each individual has two haplotypes, one inherited from each parent. The antigens encoded at HLA-A, -B, -C, -DR, and -DQ are detected on lymphocytes by serologic techniques in a microcytotoxicity assay and those of the D region are also detected by the mixed leukocyte culture reaction. Loci within the D region

can now be recognized serologically by typing of B lymphocytes. These closely linked genetic loci, each with a large number of known alleles, make the HLA region the most complex genetic polymorphism yet described. Despite this complexity, within a family there can be only four haplotypes. Therefore, for a given patient, each sibling has one chance in four of being HLA-identical with the patient. The most widely used transplants are those between HLA-identical siblings. There is now an increasing use of other family members and volunteer unrelated donors who match the patient or differ by only one HLA antigen.

PREPARATION OF THE PATIENT Infants with severe combined immunologic deficiency are conditioned to accept a transplant by the nature of their disease. All other patients are immunologically competent, to a greater or lesser degree, and are able to reject the marrow graft unless prepared with some form of immunosuppressive therapy. An immunosuppressive regimen commonly used for patients with aplastic anemia uses large doses of cyclophosphamide. Preparation of the patient with leukemia involves high-dose chemoradiotherapy for immunosuppression and to kill leukemic cells. A commonly used regimen involves cyclophosphamide followed by total-body irradiation (TBI). Approximately 10 gray (Gy) must be used for immunosuppression sufficient to permit consistent engraftment of marrow even though only 4 to 5 Gy will cause lethal marrow injury. Patients with genetic disease of the marrow may be prepared with busulfan or dimethyl busulfan to destroy the abnormal marrow along with cyclophosphamide for immunosuppression.

Marrow aspiration and infusion The pelvic bones are the most readily accessible sites for procurement, although marrow may be obtained from the sternum, ribs, or, in the case of children, the tibia. In the operating room and under general or spinal anesthesia multiple marrow aspirations are performed on the iliac crests. For adult donors, the volume of the mixture of blood and marrow cells is from 500 to 800 mL. As each aspiration is performed, the marrow is mixed with heparin and tissue culture medium. When the collection is completed, the marrow is passed through stainless steel screens to break up particles. It is then given to the recipient by intravenous infusion. The marrow stem cells pass through the lungs and subsequent growth and reconstitution of the marrow is confined almost exclusively to the medullary cavities.

Support for the patient without marrow function Usually 2 to 4 weeks are required before the transplanted marrow starts to produce the critical formed elements of the peripheral blood. Supportive care is crucial for survival. The patient should be cared for using the most effective available isolation facilities. Platelet transfusions are usually unnecessary at levels above 20,000 per microliter (see Chap. 287). Below that level, they should be used until values above 20,000 are sustained, especially if there is any evidence of bleeding. If the patient becomes refractory to random donor platelets, the use of platelets from HLA-matched family members or unrelated donors may be necessary. Aspirin and other drugs that depress platelet function should be avoided. Granulocyte transfusions (see Chaps. 81 and 82) may be indicated for therapy of refractory infection in a granulocytopenic patient. Packed red blood cells should be given as needed to control symptoms of anemia, usually to keep the hematocrit above 25 percent. All blood products should be irradiated with 1.5 Gy to inactivate lymphocytes that might cause a graft-versus-host reaction.

Since infection is an ever-present danger, bacteriologic cultures should be obtained frequently. Onset of significant fever (38.5°C) should arouse a strong suspicion of infection in the granulocytopenic patient. Fever with clinical signs of bacteremia or fever sustained more than 24 h is an indication for starting systemic antibacterial therapy even if cultures are negative. Initial therapy usually includes an aminoglycoside active against *Pseudomonas* (gentamicin, tobramycin, amikacin) and carbenicillin or ticarcillin with additional antibiotics added as indicated by culture results (see Chaps. 82 and 85). Subsequently, if cultures are negative but fever persists, therapy with a combination of trimethoprim and sulfamethoxazole or with amphotericin may be considered. Once broad-spectrum antibiotic therapy has been initiated, it should be continued until the granulocyte count rises above 200 per microliter even if clinical signs of infection disappear.

Many patients coming to marrow transplantation have had inadequate nutrition because of their disease or the efforts to treat it. The preparation for marrow grafting results in nausea, vomiting, and mucositis which results in poor oral intake for at least several weeks. A Hickman modification of the Broviac catheter is installed routinely. The catheter makes it possible to administer hyperalimentation, medications, and blood products and is also used for drawing blood samples. Although some catheters are removed because of infection or suspected infection, about 90 percent of the patients have the catheter in place for approximately 3 months, the period of time when it is needed.

ENGRAFTMENT AND PROOF OF ENGRAFTMENT Engraftment is signaled by a rise in granulocytes and platelets and the reappearance of reticulocytes. The median time required to reach a granulocyte count of 1000 per microliter is 26 days. The rise in platelet count usually occurs a week or two later.

Proof of engraftment depends upon use of cytogenetics, blood genetic markers, and/or restriction enzyme fragment length polymorphisms to distinguish donor from host cells. The regenerating marrow is usually entirely of donor type. Occasional patients show persistence of some host cells for a few weeks. Rare patients have an increasing number of host cells, and eventually the marrow is repopulated by host cells as the graft is lost.

COMPLICATIONS FOLLOWING ENGRAFTMENT The complications that may follow successful marrow engraftment are (1) graft rejection, a problem primarily occurring in patients with aplastic anemia; (2) infection, including early bacterial infections or later opportunistic infections such as cytomegalovirus interstitial pneumonia; (3) acute graft-versus-host disease (GVHD), the result of the immunologic reaction of the engrafted lymphoid elements against tissues of the recipient; (4) chronic GVHD; (5) recurrence of leukemia; and (6) miscellaneous complications such as hemorrhagic cystitis, cardiomyopathy, cataract formation, venocclusive liver disease, leukoencephalopathy, and sterility.

CLINICAL RESULTS OF MARROW TRANSPLANTATION Immunodeficiency diseases Despite the rarity of these disorders, these patients are unique in that immunosuppressive therapy is not necessary to condition the patient to accept a graft, and because some myeloid function is usually present, rapid marrow engraftment is not essential. One such patient was the first to be transplanted from an HLA-identical sibling, and more than 100 similar patients have been successfully reconstituted since then.

Genetically determined hematologic diseases Marrow grafts have now been reported for Kostmann's syndrome, chronic granulomatous disease, Chédiak-Higashi syndrome, Blackfan-Diamond syndrome, congenital aplastic anemia, and sickle cell disease (one patient, transplanted because of leukemia). Of particular interest is marrow transplantation for thalassemia major. Thalassemia major is a significant cause of death in children in many parts of the world. In developed countries, therapy with transfusions and chelating agents can prolong life for one to three decades but at great expense. In 1981, a patient with thalassemia major was prepared with dimethyl busulfan and cyclophosphamide and given a marrow graft from an HLA-identical older sister who did not have the thalassemia trait. There was prompt resolution of laboratory and clinical evidence of thalassemia, and the patient's growth and development are normal. Now more than 200 marrow transplants for thalassemia major have been done. Approximately 10 percent of the children died of complications of marrow grafting, and 10 percent have regenerated their own marrow and again have thalassemia major. Eighty percent of the patients appear to be cured of the disease although some 5 percent of the cured patients are under treatment for chronic GVHD. Results are better for patients less than 8 years of age, but good results are now being reported for older, multiply transfused patients.

Marrow grafting can cure genetically determined hematopoietic disorders which, at present, cannot be cured in any other way. Gene transfer for therapy of these diseases is an exciting possibility currently under investigation in many laboratories.

Transplantation for severe aplastic anemia (See Chap. 298) Because of the poor prognosis on conventional therapy, patients with severe aplastic anemia are logical candidates for marrow transplantation.

HLA-IDENTICAL SIBLING DONORS Patients with severe aplastic anemia must be prepared for engraftment with immunosuppressive therapy. The most widely used regimen is cyclophosphamide 50 mg/kg on each of 4 days followed 36 h later by donor marrow. The first two successful transplants were reported in 1972, and these recipients are alive and well.

For ethical reasons the initial marrow transplants were carried out in patients who had failed to benefit from conventional therapy. As a consequence these end-stage patients had already received multiple transfusions, and many were severely infected at the time of transplantation. One-third of the patients rejected the graft, and the long-term survival of these end-stage patients was 40 to 50 percent.

Since blood transfusions can sensitize an intended marrow transplant recipient, resulting in rejection of the marrow graft, patients with severe aplastic anemia were identified early in the course of the disease so that marrow transplantation could be carried out before blood transfusions were given. The long-term survival of these patients is more than 80 percent. Therefore, patients with severe aplastic anemia and their families should have tissue typing performed immediately upon diagnosis. If a suitable donor can be identified, marrow transplantation should be carried out promptly before transfusions become necessary.

However, many patients with severe aplastic anemia present to the physician with bleeding and/or infection, and transfusions must be given as an urgent medical necessity. Therefore, marrow transplant teams are investigating other preparative regimens designed to prevent graft rejection and to improve survival. These include regimens using various combinations of antithymocyte globulin, cyclophosphamide, and total-nodal irradiation. Another regimen is based on the fact that patients given a smaller number of marrow cells have had an increased probability of graft rejection. Since it was not practical to get more marrow cells from the donor, peripheral blood mononuclear cells have been used as an added source of donor cells. The standard cyclophosphamide regimen was administered followed by the marrow transplant. Then, on each of 3 to 5 days following marrow transplantation, buffy coat white blood cells were collected from 4 units of donor blood by a leukapheresis technique and administered intravenously to the recipient without in vitro irradiation. For patients who have been transfused, these modified regimens have largely solved the problem of graft rejection. Long-term survival is approximately 75 percent.

IDENTICAL TWIN DONORS Aplastic anemia is not a common disease, and to find a patient with it who has an identical twin is even more uncommon. Nevertheless, a number of transplants have been carried out for severe aplastic anemia using an identical twin as the marrow donor. In some patients the simple intravenous infusion of marrow without any immunosuppressive treatment resulted in recovery. These results reinforce the concept that aplastic anemia is due to an acquired abnormality of the stem cell which can be corrected by transplantation of normal syngeneic stem cells. However, some patients did not recover after simple intravenous marrow infusion. These patients were then treated with the cyclophosphamide regimen and given a second infusion of marrow from the twin which resulted in complete hematopoietic reconstitution. The results suggest that some cases may be due to an immune mechanism or abnormal regulators of cell growth. Whatever the mechanism, the rare patient with aplastic anemia who has a genetically identical twin has a 90 percent chance of being cured with marrow transplantation.

Transplantation for acute leukemia Acute leukemia (see Chap. 296) has served as a prototype malignant disease of the marrow for treatment by intensive chemoradiotherapy and marrow transplantation. Almost all regimens used for preparing leukemic patients for marrow transplantation have employed supralethal TBI. This has been done for several reasons: (1) irradiation is an effective means of eradicating leukemic cells; (2) irradiation penetrates to the so-called privileged sites where leukemic cells may be inaccessible to chemotherapeutic agents; and (3) irradiation is a powerful immunosuppressive agent. Cyclophosphamide or other antileukemic drugs are given with TBI. Regimens using busulfan and cyclophosphamide (without TBI) are also being explored.

ACUTE LEUKEMIA IN RELAPSE USING HLA-IDENTICAL SIBLING DONORS   For ethical reasons, marrow transplantation was initially attempted only in patients with acute leukemia in relapse after combination chemotherapy. These end-stage patients were poor candidates for any therapeutic procedure because they usually presented with a heavy body burden of leukemic cells, were usually granulocytopenic and thrombocytopenic, and often already infected with antibiotic-resistant bacteria and fungi. In early studies 10-Gy TBI was given in preparation for grafting. Then an attempt was made to kill more leukemic cells by giving cyclophosphamide a few days before administration of TBI and the marrow transplant. For these end-stage patients there were many deaths related to advanced illness at the time of transplantation, graft-versus-host disease, opportunistic infections, or recurrence of leukemia. An analysis of survival shows that 10 percent of these patients are long-term survivors with the leading patients now 18 years postgrafting. It appears that these patients, on no maintenance chemotherapy, are cured of their disease. Marrow transplant teams have utilized several different chemoradiotherapy preparative regimens for end-stage patients, but the long-term survival rate remains at 5 to 15 percent.

ACUTE LYMPHOBLASTIC LEUKEMIA (ALL) IN REMISSION USING HLA-IDENTICAL SIBLING DONORS   The fact that some patients in the end stages of acute leukemia could apparently be cured led to transplantation earlier in the course of disease. Many patients with ALL, particularly children in the "good-risk" category, can be cured by combination chemotherapy, but once marrow relapse has occurred, long-term survival is rare. Therefore, the decision was made to transplant patients in the second or subsequent remission. It was recognized that some of these patients would be lost early to transplant complications, but this risk seemed acceptable if some patients could, in fact, be cured. Most marrow transplant teams are reporting long-term survival and apparent cure of 25 to 50 percent of these patients. Recurrent leukemia is a major problem. These recurrences, in host-type cells, show that the preparative regimen was often ineffective in eradicating the residual leukemic cell population.

ACUTE NONLYMPHOBLASTIC LEUKEMIA (ANL) IN REMISSION USING HLA-IDENTICAL SIBLING DONORS   In contrast to patients with ALL, patients with ANL in first remission are known to have a poor prognosis. With combination chemotherapy the median duration of the first remission in most reported series is approximately 12 to 15 months, and only 20 to 25 percent of the patients are alive at 5 years after initial chemotherapy. Therefore, a study of marrow transplantation in these patients in first remission was considered to be ethically acceptable. Several hundred such transplants have now been carried out with various marrow transplant teams reporting 45 to 70 percent long-term disease-free survival.

PATIENTS WITH CHRONIC MYELOGENOUS LEUKEMIA (CML)   The term *chronic* is inappropriate in describing the clinical course of patients with CML. The conversion to blast crisis and death occurs at a fairly constant rate, and the median survival in most series of patients is approximately 30 to 40 months (see Chap. 297). Although a small fraction of patients may live for a long time in the chronic phase, in general, the outlook for most patients with CML is quite grim. When blast crisis appears, therapy is usually ineffective. A subset of patients whose blasts appear to be more like lymphoblasts (terminal transferase-positive) and with a hypodiploid number of chromosomes may respond for a period of a few months to treatment with vincristine and prednisone.

Marrow transplantation from HLA-identical donors has been carried out in patients with CML in blast crisis. As expected from the experience with acute leukemia in relapse, there were many deaths. However, 10 to 20 percent of these patients are long-term survivors without the Philadelphia (Ph) chromosome and appear to be cured.

A study of marrow transplantation during the chronic phase of the disease for patients with an identical twin to serve as marrow donor was initiated. The twin donors were clinically and hematologically normal. Preparation was with cyclophosphamide and TBI. Nine of 14 such patients are alive and well without the Ph chromosome 7 to 12 years later. These results of syngeneic marrow transplantation indicated that the Ph chromosome–positive leukemic cell clone can be eliminated and suggested that marrow transplantation could be carried out in the chronic phase of CML utilizing allogeneic donors. HLA-identical grafts have been performed for more than 600 patients in the chronic phase of CML. Long-term survival ranges from 50 to 80 percent and the absence of the Ph chromosome indicates cure for the majority of these patients.

PATIENTS WITH ACUTE LEUKEMIA USING DONORS OTHER THAN HLA-IDENTICAL SIBLINGS   The general experience in the United States has been that only one-third of the patients with acute leukemia will have an HLA-identical sibling. The majority of patients will not have an HLA-identical sibling. Marrow transplantation has been carried out in family member donor-recipient pairs in which one of the HLA haplotypes was genetically identical and the other haplotype phenotypically identical for one or more of the HLA loci. The results of these transplants when donor and recipient are phenotypically matched or mismatched at only one locus are quite similar to the results using an HLA-identical sibling donor. The outcome is largely a function of the stage of the disease in which the transplant was carried out. There are too few patients to permit an analysis according to the family relationship of the donor or according to the HLA locus involved in the mismatch.

Serologic HLA typing makes it technically possible to find a suitably matched unrelated donor, at least for patients with the more common HLA haplotypes, given a large panel of potential donors whose HLA types have been determined. The National Marrow Donor Program has recruited more than 20,000 HLA-typed donors, and more than 100 transplants from unrelated donors have been carried out.

Autologous marrow transplantation   The technique for procuring and cryopreserving marrow has been established for more than 20 years. The patient's own marrow can be cryopreserved during intensive chemoradiotherapy and then returned to the patient in order to avoid subsequent lethal marrow aplasia. The concept is attractive because use of the patient's own marrow avoids the risk of GVHD. The following points are pertinent in considering autologous marrow transplantation: (1) The patient's marrow should not be contaminated with malignant cells. (2) Autologous marrow is of value only in protecting the patient against lethal hematopoietic toxicity. If the regimen of chemoradiotherapy involves lethal toxicity to other organ systems, autologous marrow will not be of benefit. (3) The tumor being treated must show a dose-response curve such that supralethal chemoradiotherapy can be expected to result in a significantly enhanced antitumor response. Unfortunately, with currently available agents, only a few tumors appear to fall into this category. (4) The protocol must be designed so that the role of autologous marrow can be demonstrated. In animals it is feasible to administer "supralethal" therapy and to demonstrate that animals given syngeneic marrow will survive while those not given marrow will die. For obvious reasons, this kind of controlled experiment cannot be done in humans. Failure to recognize these four principles accounts for much of the current uncertainty about the value of autologous marrow transplantation in the treatment of patients with malignant disease.

Nevertheless, the potential use of autologous marrow is the subject of a new wave of interest, and some results are encouraging. The tumors that might be expected to show a significant improvement in response to high-dose chemoradiotherapy include the leukemias, Hodgkin's disease, non-Hodgkin's lymphoma, small cell cancer of the lung, breast cancer, testicular tumors, and ovarian tumors. Techniques being explored for removal of tumor cells from the marrow include physical separation, destruction by chemotherapeutic agents, and destruction by monoclonal antibodies. Several transplant centers are conducting studies of the utility of cryopreserved autologous marrow, and all have reported successful hematopoietic reconstitution in most patients. Most also describe the high complete remission rate and good disease-free survival over initial periods of 1 to 3 years. It is too early to evaluate fully the impact of these studies on the course of the several diseases.

IMMUNOLOGIC ASPECTS OF MARROW TRANSPLANTATION
Marrow graft rejection "Marrow graft rejection" describes a phenomenon in which the transplanted marrow graft begins to function, but after a few days or weeks, the peripheral blood counts suddenly drop and marrow biopsy shows the marrow to be devoid of myeloid elements. Immunologically mediated marrow graft rejection is usually a consequence of sensitization by transfusions. In addition, inadequate immunosuppressive therapy before grafting may facilitate marrow graft rejection. Marrow graft rejection is a common problem in patients with aplastic anemia, but is very uncommon in patients with leukemia, which may be due to several factors: (1) Transfusions are usually given to leukemic patients while they are receiving antileukemic chemotherapy which is also immunosuppressive. This chemotherapy may prevent sensitization to transplantation antigens contained in blood products. (2) Leukemia may damage the lymphoid system so that the disease process itself interferes with sensitization. (3) Leukemic patients receive a more intensive immunosuppressive regimen before grafting.

Marrow graft failure may be due to causes other than immunologic mechanisms. With a solid organ, such as the kidney, histologic proof of graft rejection is easily obtained, but such proof usually cannot be obtained with a marrow graft since the myeloid marrow simply disappears. Other possible mechanisms of graft failure include (1) defective or inadequate numbers of "stem cells" in the donor marrow; (2) defective microenvironment in the marrow recipient; (3) allogeneic resistance not associated with HLA; and (4) susceptibility of the donor marrow to the same etiologic mechanism(s) responsible for the original disease process.

Acute graft-versus-host disease (GVHD) A "wasting disease" or "runt disease" was described many years ago in newborn mice or in rodents exposed to lethal TBI and given infusions of allogeneic hematopoietic cells. These observations were later confirmed for other species, including humans, and were recognized to be due to an immunologic reaction of engrafted lymphoid cells, presumably T cells, against the tissues of the host. This graft-versus-host reaction is one of the major complications of marrow transplantation in humans. In patients given a marrow graft from an HLA-identical sibling and postgrafting immunosuppression, approximately one-half develop moderate to severe GVHD.

Acute GVHD in humans usually involves the skin, gastrointestinal tract, and/or the liver. A skin rash is usually the first sign of GVHD. Intestinal involvement results in diarrhea and may progress to abdominal pain and ileus. Liver disease is characterized by rises of bilirubin, serum glutamic oxaloacetic transaminase, and alkaline phosphatase. Severe immunologic deficiency accompanies GVHD, and death from infection is frequent.

Since GVHD is immunologically mediated, efforts to prevent its development have involved the use of immunosuppressive therapy. Of the many agents studied, methotrexate, glucocorticoids, and cyclosporine were found to be useful. One regimen consists of methotrexate, 15 mg/m^2 on day 1 postgrafting and 10 mg/m^2 on days 3, 6, 11, and 18, and weekly thereafter through day 102. Cyclosporine is a potent immunosuppressive agent. It is particularly valuable in organ grafts such as kidney, heart, and liver. Cyclosporine given after a marrow graft is useful because it does not cause mucositis as methotrexate does, and it does not suppress the marrow graft so that

effective marrow function is evident earlier. Cyclosporine is nephrotoxic, and marrow graft recipients often receive other nephrotoxic agents such as amphotericin for suspected fungal infection. Creatinine level and serum cyclosporine level must be monitored carefully with prompt reduction of dosage if renal function is threatened. A regimen using a short course of methotrexate along with cyclosporine has proved highly effective in reducing the incidence and severity of acute GVHD.

A number of studies have been carried out in an effort to treat acute GVHD once it becomes established. Recipients of HLA-identical marrow have been treated with rabbit, goat, or horse antithymocyte globulin, high-dose methyl prednisolone, cyclosporine, and/or anti-T-cell monoclonal antibodies. About two-thirds of patients will respond to one or another of these agents. However, about one-third of the patients who develop moderate to severe GVHD will die of it or its infectious complications. It is clear that the treatment of acute GVHD is unsatisfactory and that new approaches in preventing or treating GVHD must be found.

Experiments are underway designed to eliminate from the marrow inoculum the T cells believed to be responsible for GVHD while retaining hematopoietic stem cells. One approach involves treatment of the donor marrow with lectins for agglutination and separation of the T cells. Monoclonal antibodies that react with human T cells or subsets of T cells are being used in conjunction with complement, or are bound to toxins, such as the A chain of ricin, to create an immunotoxin. The preliminary results of these studies indicate a reduction in the incidence and severity of GVHD. However, the incidence of graft failure and of recurrence of leukemia is significantly increased. The explanation for these problems is unknown at present.

Chronic GVHD Chronic GVHD occurs in approximately one-fourth of those recipients of marrow from an HLA-identical sibling who survive beyond 100 days. The manifestations include skin disease, keratoconjunctivitis, buccal mucositis, esophageal strictures, small- and large-intestinal involvement, pulmonary insufficiency, chronic liver disease, and generalized wasting. Histologically, the disease resembles the systemic collagen vascular diseases, especially morphea and lupus erythematosus profundus. Chronic GVHD may be associated with recurrent and occasionally fatal bacterial infections.

Initial efforts to treat chronic GVHD with short courses of antithymocyte globulin or prolonged treatment with prednisone were ineffective. Recently, treatment with prednisone with or without azathioprine has resulted in recovery of about 80 percent of the patients, although treatment may be required for 1 or 2 years. Twenty percent continue to have problems which may be disabling, and cyclosporine, intermittent steroids, or monoclonal antibodies alone or bound to a toxin are being tried for the refractory patients.

Recovery of immunologic function Most patients given a marrow transplant from an HLA-identical sibling develop a functional graft with adequate levels of circulating granulocytes and platelets. Nevertheless, particularly in the first 3 months after grafting, these patients are susceptible to a wide variety of opportunistic infections. Approximately one-fifth of patients develop an interstitial pneumonia, and cytomegalovirus can be demonstrated in more than one-half of these pneumonias. The mortality rate is approximately 80 percent. Use of blood products from donors who are serologically negative for CMV for those donor-recipient pairs also serologically negative has almost eliminated CMV infection and pneumonia in this subset of patients. The high incidence of infection is the result of a very slow return of immunologic function, which may be made worse by GVHD and by efforts to prevent or treat GVHD. Fortunately, by the end of the first year after grafting, most patients have recovered immunologically and are able to lead normal lives without an increased incidence of infection.

Tolerance The long-term healthy human recipients of allogeneic marrow transplants are true chimeras. Their myeloid, lymphoid, and monocyte-macrophage systems are entirely made up of cells of donor origin. Clearly, these donor cells in the recipient are "tolerant" of the hosts' tissues. Studies of tolerance constitute a fascinating story in immunobiology, but a clear understanding of the state of tolerance has not emerged. At least three mechanisms may be operative, including classical central tolerance, tolerance maintained by ''blocking factors,'' and tolerance related to the presence of ''suppressor'' cells.

The effect of age The success of allogeneic marrow grafting is inversely proportional to the age of the recipient. For example, for patients transplanted in first remission of ANL, long-term survival for those under age 20 is approximately 75 percent and for patients aged 30 to 50, 40 percent. The most apparent explanation for this difference is the increased incidence and severity of GVHD in older patients. Most marrow transplant centers do not transplant patients over the age of 50. These age restrictions do not apply to syngeneic transplants since these patients do not have GVHD, although patients over the age of 50 do not tolerate intensive treatment as well as younger patients.

RECURRENT LEUKEMIA AFTER GRAFTING Frequency of recurrence of leukemia For patients with leukemia transplanted in relapse or in second remission, an actuarial analysis shows a rather constant rate of recurrence of leukemia in the first year, a decreasing rate in the second year, and few recurrences thereafter. If there were no other causes of death, approximately 35 percent of the patients would be cured, while 65 percent would be destined to relapse. However, the risk of relapse is only about 20 percent for patients with ANL transplanted in first remission or CML transplanted in chronic phase. It is evident that recurrent leukemia after grafting is a major problem for patients transplanted in relapse or in second or subsequent remission.

Nature of recurrent leukemia Blood genetic makers, cytogenetic techniques, and restriction enzyme fragment length polymorphisms can be used to identify the donor or host origin of the leukemic cells in patients who relapse after marrow transplantation. In the vast majority of patients the recurrent leukemia is in host-type cells, indicating that the preparative regimen and the graft did not eliminate all the leukemic cells. However, several cases have now been reported in which the recurrent leukemic cells were shown to be of donor origin. The mechanism of donor-cell transformation is unknown. In more than a dozen cases a lymphoblastic lymphoma associated with Epstein-Barr virus genomes has occurred in donor cells. These highly fatal lymphomas have usually occurred in patients undergoing intensive treatment for GVHD.

Graft-versus-leukemia In recipients of allogeneic marrow grafts, evidence supporting the existence of a graft-versus-leukemia effect has been difficult to obtain because of the large number of deaths from other causes among patients with severe GVHD. Statistical methods have shown that the relative relapse rate for patients transplanted in relapse or for ALL in second remission was 2.5 times greater in recipients without GVHD than in those with GVHD. Recipients of allogeneic marrow who did not develop GVHD had approximately the same relapse rate as recipients of syngeneic marrow, indicating that subclinical GVHD did not reduce the relapse rate.

GENERALIZATIONS ABOUT MARROW TRANSPLANTATION Because of the complexity of the marrow grafting regimens, transplantation should be undertaken only by teams with all of the resources

needed to ensure an optimal result. The number of such teams has increased rapidly over the past few years.

Marrow transplantation is obviously an expensive undertaking, primarily because of hospital costs, but cost has been reduced appreciably by transplantation earlier in the course of the disease when the patient is in relatively good condition. Cost analysis studies comparing marrow transplantation with combination therapy have found marrow transplantation to be more cost-effective.

The ethical problems of exposing a patient and donor to the marrow transplant regimen and the risk of death in the first 1 to 3 months after grafting have limited the use of marrow transplantation. However, the demonstration of better long-term survival rates with marrow transplantation compared to conventional therapy for several diseases and the cure of some diseases not cured by conventional therapy should alleviate the ethical concern. Extension of this form of therapy to other malignant diseases and to a variety of genetic disorders is being reported, and the current rapid rate of progress and the availability of unrelated volunteer donors may soon make a much broader application of marrow grafting a reality.

REFERENCES

APPELBAUM FR et al: Chemotherapy v. marrow transplantation for adults with acute nonlymphocytic leukemia: A five-year follow-up. Blood 72:179, 1988

BEATTY PG et al: Marrow transplantation from related donors other than HLA identical siblings. N Engl J Med 313:765, 1985

CLIFT RA et al: The treatment of acute non-lymphoblastic leukemia by allogeneic marrow transplantation. Bone Marrow Transplant 2:243, 1987

FEFER A et al: Treatment of chronic granulocytic leukemia with chemoradiotherapy and transplantation of marrow from identical twins. N Engl J Med 306:63, 1982

GOLDMAN JM et al: Bone marrow transplantation for chronic myelogenous leukemia in chronic phase. Ann Intern Med 108:806, 1988

MARTIN P et al: Effects of in vitro depletion of T cells in HLA-identical allogeneic marrow grafts. Blood 66:664, 1985

MEYERS JD, THOMAS ED: Infection complicating bone marrow transplantation, in *Clinical Approach to Infection in the Immunocompromised Host*, RH Rubin, LS Young (eds). New York, Plenum Press, 1981, p 507

O'REILLY RJ: Allogeneic bone marrow transplantation: Current status and future directions. Blood 62:941, 1983

PHILIP T et al: High-dose therapy and autologous bone marrow transplantation after failure of conventional chemotherapy in adults with intermediate-grade or high-grade non-Hodgkin's lymphoma. N Engl J Med 316:1493, 1987

RAPPEPORT JM et al: Application of bone marrow transplantation in genetic diseases. Clin Haematol 12:755, 1983

STORB R et al: Marrow transplantation for aplastic anemia. Semin Hematol 21:27, 1984

——— et al: Methotrexate and cyclosporine compared with cyclosporine alone for prophylaxis of acute graft versus host disease after marrow transplantation for leukemia. N Engl J Med 314:729, 1986

SULLIVAN KM et al: Chronic graft-versus-host disease in 52 patients: Adverse natural course and successful treatment with combination immunosuppression. Blood 57:267, 1981

THOMAS ED et al: Bone-marrow transplantation. N Engl J Med 292:832, 895, 1975

——— et al: Marrow transplantation for thalassemia. Lancet 2:227, 1982

——— et al: Marrow transplantation for the treatment of chronic myelogenous leukemia. Ann Intern Med 104:155, 1986

WEIDEN PL et al: Antileukemic effect of graft-versus-host disease in human recipients of allogeneic-marrow grafts. N Engl J Med 300:1068, 1979

YEAGER AM et al: Autologous bone marrow transplantation in patients with acute nonlymphocytic leukemia, using ex vivo marrow treatment with 4-hydroperoxycyclophosphamide. N Engl J Med 315:141, 1986

ZUTTER MM et al: Epstein-Barr virus lymphoproliferation after bone marrow transplantation. Blood 72:520, 1988

section 3 Neoplastic diseases

300 PRINCIPLES OF NEOPLASIA

JOHN MENDELSOHN

INTRODUCTION   The past few years have witnessed remarkable progress in understanding the biologic and biochemical bases for cancer. Gains in the treatment of nonresectable cancer in adults have been gradual and have focused upon those malignancies characterized by unusual sensitivity to radiation and chemotherapy. These include primarily acute leukemia, the lymphoproliferative malignancies, testicular cancer, and breast cancer. New treatment modalities involving immunotherapy and agents that promote normal cell maturation remain experimental and are under intensive investigation. Meanwhile, the search has begun for compounds which can interact with oncogene products, gene regulators, and growth factors and their receptors. Research employing modern technology in molecular genetics and immunology promises to provide a new array of anticancer agents which could move rapidly into clinical trials. This is possible because understanding cancer as a pathologic process is buttressed by new knowledge of cancer as an acquired genetic derangement.

This chapter provides an overview of the biology, etiology, and clinical sequelae of the neoplastic process, followed by a description of the general methods for diagnosing cancer and determining its stage, or extent of spread. Oncogenes and the molecular genetics of malignant transformation are discussed in Chap. 10. Cancer treatment is presented in the following chapter, and the details of managing patients with specific types of malignant disease will be found in the chapters devoted to disorders of various specific organs.

Definition   The terms cancer, neoplasia, and malignancy are usually used interchangeably in both the technical and popular literature. The disease called cancer is best defined by four characteristics which describe how cancer cells act differently from their normal counterparts.

1 *Clonality:* In most cases, cancer originates from a single stem cell which proliferates to form a clone of malignant cells.
2 *Autonomy:* Growth is not properly regulated by the normal biochemical and physical influences in the environment.
3 *Anaplasia:* There is a lack of normal, coordinated cell differentiation.
4 *Metastasis:* Cancer cells develop the capacity for discontinuous growth and dissemination to other parts of the body.

Properties similar to each of these characteristics *can* be expressed by normal, nonmalignant cells at certain appropriate times—for example, during embryogenesis and wound repair—but in cancer cells the characteristic is inappropriate or excessive. The process by which a normal cell is converted into one which exhibits these characteristic traits is termed *malignant transformation.*

THE CLINICAL PROBLEM   One-third of all individuals in the United States will develop cancer. The 5-year relative survival rate for these patients (the probability of escaping death from cancer for 5 years following diagnosis) has risen to nearly 50 percent as a result of progress in the early diagnosis and the therapy of this disease. However, cancer remains second only to cardiac disease as a cause

of death in this country. Twenty percent of Americans die from cancer; this amounted to 494,000 deaths in 1988. Half of the deaths were due to the three most common types of cancer: lung, breast, and colon-rectum. Lung cancer is more prevalent in males, while breast cancer is the commonest form of malignancy in females. Cancer of the colon and rectum is equally common in males and females.

Information is provided yearly by the American Cancer Society, summarizing the incidence and mortality rates for the common types of cancer. Table 300-1 and Fig. 300-1 present just a small portion of the extensive data available. Of particular importance is the clear documentation in Fig. 300-1 that deaths from lung cancer are increasing in the face of stable or falling rates for a number of other types of malignant disease.

Cancer typically presents to the physician as an abnormal growth, or tumor, which causes illness by production of biochemically active molecules, by local expansion, or by invasion into adjacent or distant tissue sites. The symptoms of the illness depend upon the specific molecular products and the location(s) of the tumor. Each type of cancer has a relatively distinctive natural history that describes the likely clinical course of the particular neoplastic process. Designing a proper treatment plan for an individual patient with malignant disease depends upon determining the extent of disease spread, together with a knowledge of the natural history and the available therapeutic alternatives for the particular type of cancer.

TUMOR CELL BIOLOGY AND BIOCHEMISTRY   Since all cells in an organism originate from a single fertilized egg (zygote), all carry the identical genetic information. The proliferation and differentiation of this cell into an embryo, and eventually into a mature organism, involve selective and coordinated expression of the genomic repertoire. Control of gene expression is accomplished through incompletely understood molecular interactions which can be modulated, in part, by chemical influences in the environment. The genomic repertoire includes information which permits cells to expand clonally, to function with varying degrees of autonomy, to differentiate and dedifferentiate, and to move from one part of the organism to another in a coordinated way. In the adult, the process of wound

TABLE 300-1   Estimated new cases and deaths for major sites of cancer—1988

Site or type	Number of cases	Deaths
Lung	152,000	139,000
Colon-rectum	147,000	62,000
Breast	136,000	42,000
Prostate	99,000	28,000
Urinary tract	69,000	20,000
Uterus	47,000*	10,000
Lymphoma	39,000	18,000
Oral	30,000	9,000
Pancreas	27,000	25,000
Leukemia	27,000	18,000
Melanoma	27,000†	6,000
Stomach	25,000	14,000
Ovary	19,000	12,000
All sites‡	985,000	494.000

* Includes cervix. If carcinoma in situ is included, cases total over 97,000.
† Estimated new cases of skin cancer (nonmelanoma) = about 500,000.
‡ Includes additional sites.
NOTE: Estimates are based on rates from the N.C.I. SEER program 1982–1984.

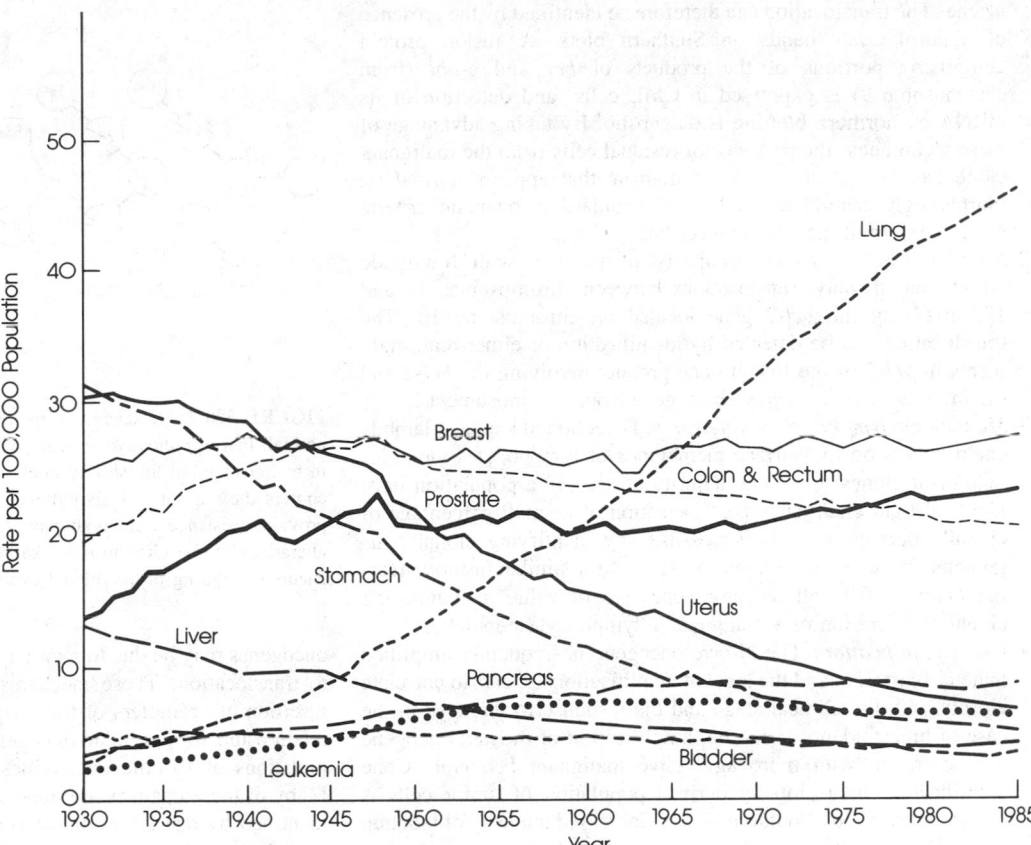

FIGURE 300-1 Cancer death rates by site in the United States, 1930 to 1985. *(Prepared by the American Cancer Society from data provided by the National Center for Health Statistics and the Bureau of the Census.)*

healing activates expression of these cellular characteristics in a more "embryo-like" fashion, but under well-coordinated control. In the case of malignancy, the normal control process is subverted or bypassed due to the anomalous activities of a select group of genes (oncogenes) which have central importance to the regulation of cellular activities. A detailed discussion of oncogenes is provided in Chap. 10.

Clonality Careful cytogenetic analysis of metaphase chromosome preparations from cancer cells has yielded a wealth of information about the neoplastic process. It has become clear that virtually all solid tumors and a majority of hematopoietic malignancies display abnormalities in the chromosomal karyotype which are inherited by the population of tumor cells. These may involve translocations of chromosomal fragments into new locations, as well as additions or deletions of parts of chromosomes or whole chromosomes. A particular karyotypic alteration often occurs in a substantial fraction of all patients with a form of cancer. The first and most well known example of this is the Philadelphia chromosome (Ph[1]) observed in 85 percent of patients with chronic myelogenous leukemia (CML), in which the long arm of chromosome 22 is translocated onto the long arm of chromosome 9. This alteration is so characteristic of CML that when analysis of some cases of acute lymphocytic leukemia demonstrated the identical translocation, it was inferred that the disease represented an unusual conversion from CML (which usually progresses to acute myelocytic leukemia). Characteristic chromosomal rearrangements have been described in a number of other human cancers.

The observation of uniform karyotypic abnormalities in all cells within a tumor provides strong evidence for the clonal origin of the tumor. In turn, the chromosomal abnormalities serve as markers of the presence of a common malignant state in the individual cells.

A remarkable concordance between the chromosome locations of a number of human cellular oncogenes and the break points involved in chromosome translocations in human malignancies has been demonstrated. Furthermore, in many cases, these locations correlate with "fragile" sites in the chromosome. Treatment of cultured cells

with agents that inhibit the DNA repair process induces chromosomal breaks far more frequently at many of these loci. A reasonable hypothesis, currently under investigation, links these phenomena and suggests that chromosome rearrangements may result in unregulated activation of cellular oncogenes. For example, in Burkitt's lymphoma, the typical translocation between chromosomes 8 and 14 places the cellular *myc* gene adjacent to the immunoglobulin heavy chain locus, a site of gene activation in the normal lymphocyte.

The new techniques of molecular genetics permit direct assessment of genetic alterations in DNA extracts from tissues suspected of harboring malignancy, using the method of *Southern blotting*. This involves restriction endonuclease digestion, agarose gel electrophoresis, and identification of specific DNA molecular species by hybridization with labeled specific probes. Changes in gene expression can be detected by a similar technique with RNA extracts known as *northern blotting*. The new technology of molecular genetics is more powerful than cytogenetics because (1) clonal genetic abnormalities can be identified in nondividing cells, (2) genetic rearrangements are detectable even when few tumor cells exist in a population of predominantly normal cells, and (3) the sensitivity of detection is greatly enhanced by obviating assays dependent on visual identification of altered staining patterns of chromosomes. The polymerase chain reaction takes advantage of the availability of appropriate primers for certain recombinant genes to amplify abnormal genetic material present in rare cells within a population, thereby enabling detection of genetic abnormalities in these cells by Southern blotting. These approaches to the diagnosis of genetic abnormalities are presented in detail in Chap. 6.

Clonal abnormalities in the genetic makeup of cells that can be detected with molecular techniques include gene mutation, rearrangement, translocation, deletion, and amplification. Some examples will serve to demonstrate the utility of these methods.

1 CML: The Ph[1] chromosome is formed by a translocation between chromosomes 9 and 22, with the break in chromosome 22 occurring in the break point cluster region (*bcr* region), which is the site of a gene. The translocation can therefore be identified by the presence of abnormal *bcr* bands on Southern blots. A fusion protein comprising portions of the products of *bcr* and c-*abl* (from chromosome 9) is expressed in CML cells, and detection of its mRNA by northern blotting is diagnostic. By taking advantage of these techniques, the presence of residual cells from the malignant clone can be detected in bone marrow that appears normal by morphologic criteria as well as by standard cytogenetic criteria (e.g., 30 normal metaphase spreads).

2 *Nodular lymphoma:* The majority of patients with low-grade lymphomas display translocations between chromosomes 14 and 18, involving the *bcl*-2 gene located on chromosome 18. The translocation can be detected by identification of either rearrangements in *bcl*-2 or the fusion gene product involving the *bcl*-2 and the immunoglobulin heavy chain gene from chromosome 14.

3 *Monoclonal lymphocyte proliferation:* Detection of kappa or lambda chain excess on the surface membranes of lymphocytes identifies malignant clones when the majority of cells in a population have identical light chain subtypes. Detection of a small percentage of clonally derived B cells is possible, by identifying clonal rearrangements of immunoglobulin genes. In a similar fashion, rearrangements of T-cell receptor genes are of value in diagnosing clonal proliferation of a malignant T-lymphocyte population.

4 *Gene amplification:* The N-*myc* oncogene is frequently amplified in neuroblastoma, and the level of amplification appears to correlate closely with the clinical stage and the response to therapy. In the case of breast adenocarcinoma, amplification of the *neu* oncogene may correlate with more aggressive malignant behavior. Gene amplification in a clonally derived population of tumor cells is detected directly on Southern blots as increased intensity of labeling of the DNA bands derived from the amplified gene.

Studies of the selective expression of the X-linked isoenzymes of glucose-6-phosphate dehydrogenase (G6PD) in heterozygotic patients have provided further evidence for the clonal origin of cancer from a single progenitor cell. Examination of both G6PD isoenzymes and chromosomal karyotypes in CML patients has demonstrated clonal abnormalities in erythroid, myeloid, and megakaryocytic cells, as well as B lymphocytes, suggesting that this malignancy originates in a precursor cell common to all of these cell lineages.

While there is convincing evidence for the origin of cancer from genetic alterations in a single cell, further heritable alterations commonly occur, resulting in the presence of a heterogeneous mixture of subclones in a mature tumor cell population which has proliferated enough to be clinically detectable. This heterogeneity can be demonstrated by assaying a variety of characteristics in the subpopulations within a tumor; for example, further abnormalities in the chromosomal karyotype, varied drug sensitivities and metastatic capacities, differences in growth rates, and the presence or absence of hormone receptors or particular cell surface glycoproteins. With time, therefore, the progressive accumulation of heritable abnormalities in tumor subpopulations typically results in highly significant phenotypic changes which have their clinical counterpart in development of resistance to previously effective therapy or in increased metastatic spread. The appearance of new chromosomal abnormalities in patients with Ph1-positive CML heralds the onset of a rapidly progressive, fatal phase of the disease. A schematic model of this process of clonal progression is shown in Fig. 300-2. It remains to be determined when in the life history of a typical malignancy the process of clonal progression occurs: the sequence of genetic alterations may occur early, with later expansion of selected subpopulations from a heterogeneous mixture of cells as circumstances change; alternatively the genetic alterations may occur close to the time when they are detected by changes in the behavior of the tumor cells.

Following the discovery of cellular oncogenes, evidence rapidly accumulated to show that unregulated activation of two or more of these genes may be the molecular genetic explanation for clonal progression in tumor cell subpopulations. Activation of cellular

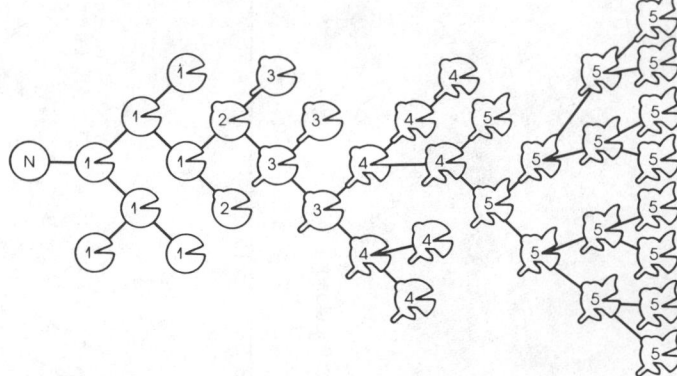

FIGURE 300-2   A schematic model of clonal progression. The N cell is normal. Five *hypothetical* genetic changes are noted. The first does not result in malignancy but the second does. The third adds invasiveness, the fourth confers the capacity to disseminate and produce metastases, and the fifth provides resistance to chemotherapy. Each may be accompanied by incremental alterations in the chromosomal karyotype, with an increasing tendency to aneuploidy during further clonal evolution.

oncogenes may be due to a variety of genetic mechanisms in addition to translocation. These mechanisms include gene amplification, or insertion of promoters of transcription adjacent to (*cis*) or in a *trans* relationship to a cellular oncogene, with or without accompanying mutations of specific nucleotides in the oncogene DNA sequence. Many of these changes are undetectable in the karyotype, but can be identified by restriction digest analysis of cellular DNA or by DNA sequencing.

Autonomy   Environmental influences which regulate the proliferation of normal cells are circumvented when the process of malignant transformation occurs. This is demonstrable by a variety of experimental assays which document, in different ways, the capacity of the malignant cells to continue to proliferate under normally nonconducive conditions. These assays are listed in Table 300-2.

At least initially, the autonomy of human malignancies is relative rather than absolute. The well-known experiments of Huggins and associates in the 1950s led to a new form of cancer therapy which took advantage of the initial dependence of certain tumors upon the normal influences of sex hormones. The conversion of many prostatic and breast cancers from sensitivity to resistance to hormone therapy vividly demonstrates the further development of autonomy through clonal progression.

Many tumor cell lines can proliferate in culture medium without the usual requirement for serum, provided that a "cocktail" containing three to five essential growth factors and other growth-promoting agents is added. Examples of such factors are epidermal growth

TABLE 300-2   Experimental detection of malignant transformation

Assay	Normal cell	Transformed cell
Capacity of single cells to form colonies in agar suspension	Unsuccessful	Successful
Density-dependent inhibition of cell proliferation in liquid culture	Yes	No
Generations obtained by continuous division in liquid culture	Limited to about 50	Unlimited
Requirements for serum or growth factors	Invariable	Reduced or absent
Capacity to grow as xenografts	Absent	Present

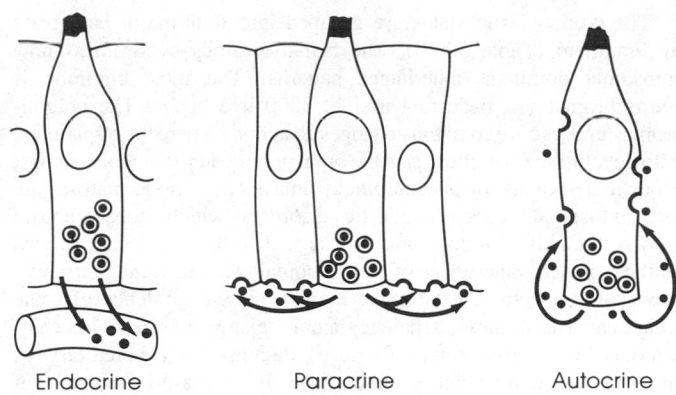

Endocrine   Paracrine   Autocrine

FIGURE 300-3   A diagrammatic representation of autocrine, paracrine, and endocrine secretion. Peptide growth factors are shown in latent form within the cell. The thickened, semicircular regions of the cell membrane represent receptor sites. *(From MB Sporn, GJ Todaro, N Engl J Med 303:878, 1980.)*

factor, platelet-derived growth factor, the carrier protein transferrin, and the hormone insulin. Malignant cells may obviate the requirements for even these essential factors. One mechanism, demonstrated experimentally and possibly of clinical significance, involves production of a growth factor (or its analogue) by the tumor cells themselves, a process called *autocrine secretion*. In this situation a polypeptide secreted by the tumor cells may have the capacity to bind to a receptor on the surface of the cells, resulting in autostimulation (Fig. 300-3). The first growth factor to be described with the potential for autocrine stimulation of tumor cells was transforming growth factor alpha, an analogue of epidermal growth factor (EGF), which also binds to the EGF receptor. Recent experiments have suggested that autocrine stimulation with platelet-derived growth factor (PDGF) may be accomplished by binding of ligand to the receptor intracellularly, prior to the expression of receptor on the cell surface. A second mechanism by which tumor cells can reduce dependence on growth factors involves expression of increased numbers of receptors on the cell surface. Increased expression of EGF receptors is a common event in epithelial tumors, occurring in all renal cell carcinomas and squamous lung carcinomas that have been examined, and in many other forms of malignancy. Tumor cells may develop a third mechanism for escaping regulation by a growth factor, by activating an internal biochemical process (e.g., a protein tyrosine kinase) ordinarily dependent upon binding of a specific growth factor to a cell surface receptor, thereby completely bypassing the need for exposure to the growth-promoting agent.

Anaplasia   Lack of normal differentiation is a most useful characteristic in the pathologic diagnosis of malignancy. While cancer cells usually bear some of the morphologic characteristics of their normal mature counterparts, they display cellular and histologic abnormalities readily detectable with the light microscope. The cells tend to have large nuclei, with more apparent chromatin and prominent nucleoli. There are increased mitoses, as well as abnormal mitoses and giant cells containing multiple nuclei, reflecting aneuploidy and/ or a failure of karyokinesis. The degree of morphologic derangement typically correlates with the extent of disease spread or the metastatic potential of the tumor. The histologic appearance of malignancy is one of disarray, with partial or complete loss of normal tissue architecture. Partial formation of structures such as glands or villi may be suggested, even in poorly differentiated malignancies.

Although the term is not used this way, the process of anaplasia may be expressed at a biochemical level as production of hormones or hormone-related peptides, which are either improperly regulated by normal feedback mechanisms (e.g., excessive corticosteroid production by an adrenal carcinoma), or are not appropriate for the particular cell type if it were normally differentiated (e.g., ACTH production by a carcinoma of the lung). In such cases, the genomic repertoire of the malignant cell is expressed inappropriately. Another

example is the unregulated production of immunoglobulin (partial or complete chains) by neoplastic derivatives of B lymphocytes.

Histologic features which are abnormal but do not meet the criteria of anaplasia (loss of differentiation) are designated *dysplastic*. Such changes may be seen in "premalignant" situations, for example, in the epithelial lining of the bronchi of cigarette smokers. These abnormalities are often reversible. Cessation of smoking can lead to normalization of the lung epithelium over a period of 5 years.

Metastasis   This term encompasses a number of phenotypic traits which together result in the clinical problem which most often leads to death from cancer. The cells lose their adherence and restrained position within an organized tissue, move into adjacent sites, develop the capacity both to invade and to egress from blood vessels, and become capable of proliferating in unnatural locations or environments. These changes in growth patterns are accompanied by biochemical alterations which have the capacity to promote the metastatic process. Invasive tumors may secrete, or may stimulate secretion of, a variety of tissue-degrading enzymes including collagenases and lysosomal hydrolases. Plasminogen activators which lead to promotion of fibrinolysis are also produced. Conversely, procoagulant compounds may be released into the environment of the tumor cells at stages when focal aggregation of cells might be of survival value. In experimental situations where tumor cells show a propensity to select a particular organ as a preferred site of metastasis, surface molecules on the metastatic cells appear to have a high affinity for endothelial cells in the vasculature of the specific target organ. The first step in tumor cell invasion probably involves attachment to the extracellular matrix, which is mediated by receptors on the cell plasma membrane that bind specifically to glycoproteins such as laminin and fibronectin. Additional biochemical steps are entailed in the progression of a tumor from a homogeneous proliferating clone to a group of heterogeneous subpopulations of cells, some of which have progressively accumulated the entire array of enzymes and surface molecules required for metastasis. It may be for this reason that the rate of metastasis is low during early tumor growth, in spite of the well-documented fact that malignant cells are often released from a tumor into the circulation continuously and in large numbers. Agents which could block critical steps in the metastatic process would be of great value in the armamentarium of antineoplastic agents.

It appears that clonal progression of a tumor generates biochemical or physiologic alterations which confer greater autonomy, greater degrees of anaplasia, and a greater capacity to metastasize. Because there is progressive selection for cells with increased tumorigenic capacity, the process has been called clonal evolution and has been compared to Darwinian evolution, in this case at a cellular level.

ETIOLOGY   Patterns of cancer incidence vary with sex, race, and geographic location. In addition, the types of tumors observed vary with age. Hereditary traits and variations in the internal environments around cells explain some of the differences in cancer incidence. It is clear from epidemiologic investigations that variations in diet and exposure to chemical and physical agents in the external environment contribute to the development of neoplasia. The environmental agents which have been linked to the incidence of cancer fall into three broad categories: radiation, a variety of chemicals, and viruses.

Genetic factors   Genetic alterations appear to play an essential role in oncogenesis. Several lines of evidence support this conclusion: (1) There are many examples of familial aggregation for specific histologic types of tumor (e.g., retinoblastoma). (2) Chromosomal abnormalities carried in the germ line confer increased risk of developing certain types of cancer (e.g., leukemia in trisomy 21). (3) Tumors often display specific somatic rearrangement of chromosomes or genes (e.g., CML). (4) Deficiency in the capacity to repair DNA damage by mutagens is accompanied by increased risk of malignancy (e.g., xeroderma pigmentosa). (5) The capacities for agents to mutate DNA and to elicit tumors are closely correlated, in studies of both bacteria and experimental animals (e.g., *Salmonella/* microsome test of Dr. Bruce Ames).

The molecular mechanisms explaining these genetic abnormalities are only beginning to be understood. They appear to fall into two categories: (1) genes which are deregulated and excessively expressed, displaying dominant genetic activity, such as the products of cellular proto-oncogenes; (2) genes which are suppressors of tumorigenic genetic activities and are recessive in that both alleles must be lacking for malignancy to occur, such as the retinoblastoma gene. The latter can appear to have a dominant inheritance pattern, because one of the alleles may be constitutionally deleted, so that a single genetic alteration (e.g., somatic mutation or loss) in the other allele results in neoplastic transformation. The retinoblastoma gene has been mapped to the q14 band of chromosome 13 and cloned. The cDNA has been used to demonstrate deletion of the retinoblastoma gene in some soft tissue sarcomas and other solid tumors.

There have been a number of reports of additional human malignancies which may be associated with chromosomal deletions and/or loss of restriction fragment length polymorphism (RFLP) alleles. These include Wilms's tumor (11p13), lung cancer (3p), renal cell carcinoma (3p), bladder cancer (11p), colorectal carcinoma (5q), and breast cancer (13). The nature of the information encoded by the genetic loci, in parentheses, is under intensive study. In the case of the retinoblastoma gene, the polypeptide product may bind to and inactivate a protein with enhancer-binding activity for DNA.

For many of the common malignancies, the incidence of cancer is higher among patients with positive family histories than among unselected patients, usually in the range of up to threefold. However, the risk can rise to as high as twenty-five- to thirtyfold in certain groups of patients with a familial history of breast cancer or bowel cancer. In addition, there are a number of uncommon inherited disorders involving either (1) a high risk for the occurrence of a particular neoplasm, or (2) the presence of multiple preneoplastic lesions that can progress to frank malignancy.

The hereditary neoplasms (Table 300-3) may occur as the only manifestation of a gene defect, or as part of a generalized syndrome involving multiple developmental abnormalities. The inheritance patterns in these disorders are generally autosomal dominant, with varying penetrance. Half of the children of patients with these disorders will inherit the gene defect.

TABLE 300-3 Hereditary cancer syndromes

I Hereditary neoplasms
  Retinoblastoma
  Nevoid basal cell carcinoma syndrome
  Multiple endocrine adenomatosis (Werner's syndrome)
  Pheochromocytoma and medullary thyroid carcinoma (Sipple's syndrome)
  Chemodectomas
  Polyposis coli
  Gardner's syndrome
  Tylosis with esophageal carcinoma
II Preneoplastic states
  A Hamartomatous syndromes
    Neurofibromatosis
    Tuberous sclerosis
    von Hippel–Lindau syndrome
    Multiple exostoses
    Peutz-Jeghers syndrome
    Cowden's multiple hamartoma syndrome
  B Genodermatoses
    Xeroderma pigmentosum
    Albinism
    Werner's syndrome
    Epidermodysplasia verruciformis
    Polydysplastic epidermolysis bullosa
    Dyskeratosis congenita
  C Chromosome breakage disorders
    Bloom's syndrome
    Fanconi's syndrome
  D Immune deficiency syndromes
    Ataxia-telangiectasia
    Wiskott-Aldrich syndrome
    Late-onset immunologic deficiency
    X-linked agammaglobulinemia

SOURCE: From JF Fraumeni, Jr, in JF Holland, E Frei.

The preneoplastic states are grouped into four major categories by Fraumeni (Table 300-3). The hamartomatous syndromes show autosomal dominant inheritance patterns. The most common is neurofibromatosis, occurring in 1 of 3000 live births. The neurofibromas undergo sarcomatous changes in about 10 percent of patients, with development of gliomas in the brain or optic nerve, meningiomas, acoustic neuromas, or pheochromocytomas. The genodermatoses are rare autosomal recessive genetic disorders which conspicuously involve the skin. Chromosome breakage disorders are characterized by the recessive inheritance of chromosomal instability and rearrangements of karyotypes; patients have an increased incidence of acute leukemia. The immune deficiency ataxic telangiectasia is also characterized by chromosomal fragility. Patients with hereditary or acquired immunodeficiency states have an increased incidence of neoplasia, most commonly the lymphoproliferative malignancies.

Race is a genetic factor in the incidence of cancer, but interpretation of epidemiologic data is made difficult by the concurrent effects of environmental and socioeconomic influences. Both the incidence and the death rate from cancer is higher in American blacks than in American whites, with all of the difference being accounted for by the higher cancer rate in black males. It is believed that later detection and less adequate treatment may account for part, but not all, of the difference in survival. The important effect of environmental factors is made clear by documented differences in cancer incidence for Asians living in Hawaii and in California.

Radiation It is estimated that less than 3 percent of cancers result from exposure to radiation. Radiation that can remove electrons from atoms is called ionizing radiation. It includes electromagnetic waves such as x-rays and gamma rays, as well as charged particles such as protons. The unit of radiation dose, the gray (Gy), measures the energy absorbed in matter as a result of exposure to radiation: 1 Gy = 100 rad.

Information on the capacity of radiation in relatively large doses to induce cancer in humans comes from studies on survivors of atomic bomb blasts, on individuals accidentally exposed to irradiation or radiative fallout, and on patients exposed to radiation for diagnostic purposes or for therapy. It has been learned that nearly all tissues are susceptible to tumor induction by radiation, but with variable sensitivity. The most sensitive tissues are the bone marrow, breast, and thyroid. The latent period is only 2 to 5 years for acute leukemia, and 5 to 10 years for most solid tumors. There is a higher incidence of leukemia in patients who have received radiation therapy for neoplastic diseases and for ankylosing spondylitis, and of thyroid cancer in children irradiated for thymic enlargement.

Solar radiation, resulting from exposure to electromagnetic radiation from the sun, is the primary risk factor in skin cancer. The evidence for this linkage comes from a variety of epidemiologic and experimental observations. Skin cancer is rare in blacks and the deeply pigmented racial groups, whereas it is especially common in fair-complexioned individuals. It occurs primarily on the parts of the body exposed to sunlight and has a higher incidence in outdoor workers. Patients with genetic diseases such as xeroderma pigmentosa and albinism, which are exacerbated by sunlight, have very high risks for the development of skin cancer.

The carcinogenic effect of solar irradiation is greatest in the spectral range of 290 to 320 nm (UV-B radiation), which produces delayed erythema in human skin (sunburn). This range of wavelengths correlates with the action spectrum for UV-induced damage to DNA.

Exposure to solar ultraviolet irradiation is also a risk factor in melanoma. As with skin cancer, there is a higher incidence of melanoma among populations living at a latitude nearer the equator, where exposure to UV irradiation is greatest.

Tobacco Numerous epidemiologic studies have demonstrated that the principal carcinogenic agent in our environment is inhaled tobacco smoke. The incidence of lung cancer is more than tenfold higher in male smokers than in nonsmokers. Furthermore, tobacco smoking is associated with increased rates of cancer of the oral cavity, esophagus, kidney, bladder, and pancreas. Particulate matter in

TABLE 300-4 Examples of occupational causes of cancer

Etiology	Site of malignancy
Arsenic (inorganic)	Lung, skin, liver
Asbestos	Mesothelium, lung
Benzene	Leukemia
Benzidine	Bladder
Chromium compounds	Lung
Radiation (mining, dial painting)	Numerous locations
Mustard gas	Lung
Polycyclic hydrocarbons (coal by-products)	Lung, skin
Vinyl chloride	Angiosarcoma of liver

tobacco smoke, known as "tar," contains a long list of chemicals, primarily polycyclic hydrocarbons, which have been shown experimentally to be contact carcinogens. In addition, the metabolic activation of tobacco components, for example, the cyclic *N*-nitrosamines, can produce carcinogens with the capacity to act upon the cells of internal organs. Tobacco-related malignancies account for one-third of all cancer deaths among men in the United States and for more than 10 percent of all female cancer deaths. Unfortunately, this figure is rising in females. As a result of increased use of tobacco by women in the period since World War II, the deaths from lung cancer in females exceeded deaths from breast cancer in 1988.

Clearly the single most effective action which could be taken against cancer at the present time involves not an application of molecular genetic research, but cessation of smoking. Fortunately, it appears that smoking cessation results in a gradual decrease in risk, so that after 10 to 15 years, exsmokers have nearly the same risk of lung cancer as nonsmokers. Because the habit of smoking is difficult to break, the physician's role in cessation of smoking is of critical importance. Doctors should deliver a *firm* antismoking message.

Occupational exposure The first report of cancer related to occupational hazards was Percival Pott's observation of an unusually high frequency of scrotal cancer among London chimney sweeps in 1775. It is now known that skin cancer (including scrotal) can be induced by a variety of coal tar products, such as the materials contacted in the London chimneys. Epidemiologic studies also have related lung cancer to exposure to coal by-products. Table 300-4 provides a partial listing of industrial agents which are known to cause cancer.

Air pollution It is clear that lung cancer incidence is increased by tobacco smoking and by certain industrial and occupational exposures (primarily related to coal tar and combustion by-products). Once the risks resulting from exposure to these factors are taken into account, the epidemiologic evidence that links ambient air pollution to lung cancer remains inconclusive. Studies correlating the incidence of lung cancer with increased levels of polycyclic hydrocarbons and benzo(a)pyrene in urban air are complicated by the difficulty of eliminating the contribution of exposure to these compounds through tobacco smoking as well as occupational exposure.

Medications Certain drugs and hormones have been shown to be carcinogenic. The synthetic nonsteroidal estrogen diethylstilbestrol (DES), which was used for a period of time to reduce fetal wastage in pregnant women, caused an increased incidence of vaginal and cervical cancer in daughters who were exposed in utero. Conjugated estrogens have been shown to increase the incidence of endometrial cancer in patients treated for menopausal symptoms. The use of progesterone concomitantly, together with decreased estrogen dose, may obviate this problem.

Alkylating agents have been shown to cause an increased incidence of acute myelocytic leukemia and probably other malignancies. They are used in therapeutic situations in which the poor prognosis of malignancy far outweighs the increased risk of an additional cancer in the future. However, because of this risk, new drug regimens which avoid the use of alkylating agents are being explored in situations where substantial long-term benefits from chemotherapy have been demonstrated, for example, in Hodgkin's disease.

The recipients of organ transplants who are treated with immunosuppressive agents, such as azathioprine and prednisone, have an increased incidence of histiocytic lymphoma as well as a variety of solid tumors. A similar increased incidence is observed in individuals with inherited and acquired immunodeficiency, for example, AIDS. This has been attributed to reduced immune surveillance, but a variety of other explanations are equally likely, such as activation of a latent oncogenic virus or chronic immunostimulation in conjunction with a compromised and malfunctioning immune system.

Diet The role of diet and nutrition in carcinogenesis has been the subject of intensive investigation and equally intensive controversy. There are numerous nutritional hypotheses of carcinogenesis. Some of these have led to unconventional forms of cancer therapy that are based upon no scientific evidence. Unfortunately, these putative dietary therapies are propagated upon a patient population for which proven treatment modalities are often unsuccessful in achieving cure, and at a time when there is a popular emphasis on healthful nutrition.

Epidemiologic analyses of international variations in cancer incidence and comparisons of the types and frequencies of cancer in populations with different dietary habits have yielded a great deal of evidence that cancers of most major sites are influenced by diet. These studies were reviewed in an authoritative publication, *Diet, Nutrition, and Cancer*. Interim dietary guidelines are suggested which are both consistent with good nutritional practices and likely to reduce the risk of cancer: (1) Reduce the intake of fat, saturated and unsaturated, from its present average level (40 percent) to 30 percent of total energy value in the diet. (2) Include fruits (especially citrus), vegetables (especially carotene-rich and cruciferous), and whole cereal grain (fiber) in the daily diet; these provide amounts of vitamins A and C as well as fiber adequate to obviate dietary supplements. (3) Minimize consumption of salt-cured or smoked food. (4) Use alcoholic beverages in moderation, since they increase the risk of certain cancers, especially when combined with cigarette smoking.

Experimental data lend support to the inferences from epidemiologic studies, but additional research is necessary to understand how dietary factors influence carcinogenesis. For example, epidemiologic evidence strongly correlates the intake of fat with the occurrence of cancer at several sites, especially the breast and colon. Possible explanations for this observation include increased adiposity, leading to greater conversion of androstenedione to estrone, which could influence carcinogenesis in the breast; and stimulation of increased bile salt excretion which could alter gut flora and thereby augment the production of carcinogenic substances by the bacteria in the colon. Vitamin C may act to prevent cancer by blocking endogenous formation of *N*-nitroso compounds in the gastrointestinal tract, but there are no data showing that taking vitamin C will prevent cancer in human beings. Dietary fiber enhances the rapid transit of potential carcinogens through the colon, which could explain the low incidence of bowel cancer and rectal cancer in tropical Africa.

It is important to stress that the accumulated scientific evidence does not support the anticarcinogenic value of particular vitamins, minerals, or nutritional supplements in amounts greater than provided by a prudent diet. Certainly their use in high doses in the therapy of established malignant disease is not indicated. The physician must be alert to the scientifically unproven dietary treatments which patients with cancer may be urged to undertake. Of course the greatest tragedy occurs when patients whose malignancy could be cured by proven therapeutic modalities are misled into depending upon such dietary manipulations.

Viruses Although there has been extensive research on viral oncogenesis with experimental murine tumors, viruses have been implicated as the direct cause of only one human cancer. Infection with human T-lymphotrophic virus I (HTLV-I) can lead to adult T-cell leukemia, an aggressive malignancy of T-lymphocytes, which has been reported in large series from Japan and the West Indies. The incidence of hepatocellular carcinoma in endemic regions of Asia and Africa is closely associated with previous infection with hepatitis B virus, followed by a carrier state, suggesting that a causal relationship is highly likely. Chronic hepatocyte infection by the virus might predispose to carcinogenesis in these cells. There may be a variety of contributing factors, including malaria, malnutrition, and exposure to aflatoxin. There also is a strong statistical correlation between herpes simplex 2 viral infection, which is sexually transmitted, and the incidence of cervical cancer. There are a number of situations in which viruses are linked to the occurrence of specific cancers with a high incidence in particular geographic locations, although a causative role has not been established. The Epstein-Barr virus is closely associated with African Burkitt's lymphoma as well as nasopharyngeal carcinoma in Asia. Cofactors in the development of these malignancies might be holoendemic malaria in African Burkitt's lymphoma, and a particular configuration of histocompatibility antigens in the case of nasopharyngeal carcinoma among Chinese. While the Epstein-Barr virus can infect human B lymphocytes (infectious mononucleosis) and transform them in cell culture, evidence is lacking that such a transformation is the cause of clinical malignancy.

Risk of cancer   Knowledge of genetic and environmental factors that may contribute to cancer incidence can be utilized by the conscientious physician to identify patients who have an increased risk of malignancy. The presence of certain hereditary diseases in a patient's family may suggest procedures that can lead to early detection and prevention, for example, early surveillance by colonoscopy and prevention by prophylactic colectomy in persons who have familial polyposis of the colon. Environmental factors that increase cancer risks should be identified and avoided. It is evident, however, that changing an individual's life-style in order to avoid exposure to a carcinogen can require an extraordinary level of effort on the part of both the patient and the physician.

CLINICAL SEQUELAE   The presence of a malignant lesion may not, in itself, cause symptoms in a patient with cancer. The primary lesion may, for a period of time, be unnoticed and unimportant for the normal maintenance of body functions, in which case its clinical significance is due to its potential for growth and spread. In addition, the presence of metastasis need not result in symptomatic illness. Patients with carcinoma of the bowel, whose disease may have spread beyond the limits of surgical curability, may live for many months or even years with easily detectable metastatic lesions in the lung or abdomen, yet remain free of symptoms until the function of a vital organ is compromised or obstructive problems appear.

Malignancies produce clinical symptoms in three general ways (Table 300-5): by direct effects resulting from invasion or compression of normal tissues; by release of cytokines, hormones, and other biologically active agents into the local and systemic environment; and by secondary psychological effects upon the patient. Each of these factors may contribute profoundly to the degree of illness experienced by the patient. Clinical symptoms resulting from released biologically active agents, as well as systemic problems caused by as yet undetermined mechanisms, are usually grouped under the category of "paraneoplastic syndromes."

Mass effects of malignancy   In most cases tumors produce clinical problems as a result of local expansion, with obliteration of normal tissues, as the malignant cells proliferate within the confines of the involved organ: marrow replacement by leukemia results in reduced production of the normal cellular elements of the blood; lung cancer compromises oxygen exchange in involved alveoli; primary or metastatic cancer in bone causes weakened trabecular architecture, resulting in pathologic fractures; hepatomas replace normal hepatocytes and interfere with liver function. A second result of local expansion is compression of normal structures, with partial or complete obstruction of tubular organs, blood vessels, and lymphatics: colonic cancer may obstruct the gastrointestinal tract; lung cancer blocks airflow through bronchi and can obstruct pulmonary venous return; hepatic and biliary malignancies produce obstructive jaundice; a variety of intraabdominal neoplasms can encase the ureters, causing renal failure; in the extreme case, penetration of blood vessels can

---

TABLE 300-5   Symptoms caused by malignant diseases

I Mass effects
  A Ablation by crowding or by invasion
  B Obstruction of vessels, tubes, and ducts
  C Rupture of blood vessels
II Remote effects (paraneoplastic syndromes)
  A Ectopic hormone production
  B Neuropathies and CNS abnormalities
  C Dermatologic abnormalities
  D Metabolic disorders
    1 Anorexia, weight loss
    2 Fever
    3 Chronic inflammation
  E Hematologic disorders
  F Immunosuppression
  G Collagen vascular disorders
III Psychosocial effects
  A Loss of control
  B Acceptance of personal finitude
  C Fear of pain and mutilation
  D Separation and loneliness

---

violate the integrity of the vasculature, resulting in hemorrhage. A third result of local expansion is pain, due to pressure on or stretching of nerve fibers. When neoplasia causes increased pressure on nervous tissue within the confines of the skull, the symptoms include headache and vomiting as well as seizure disorders and brain dysfunction.

Paraneoplastic syndromes   The malignant process is felt to develop as a result of the unregulated and/or inappropriate expression of certain genes crucial to cell proliferation and differentiation. The aggressiveness of the malignant process is increased by the subsequent uncovering of additional genetic information. In this evolutionary process, abnormal genetic information may be expressed which results in severe physiologic effects upon the patient. As noted above, there may be excessive synthesis of a gene product which is normally found in the particular cell type, or the malignant cell may produce a molecule which does not ordinarily originate from its normal counterpart.

A common type of molecule produced by malignant tumors falls into the category of polypeptide hormones. The synthesis of vasopressin or ACTH by small cell carcinoma of the lung or parathormone by some squamous cancers are examples. These can produce clinical illness by mediating normal physiologic functions to an excessive degree. Other active molecules have been detected which are homologous with or identical to known growth factors. The potential for autonomous stimulation of proliferation mediated by production of essential growth-promoting agents has been discussed.

From this brief introduction, it can be seen that biologically active agents produced by malignant cells can be clinically important for a number of reasons:

1 They may serve as markers for the presence of a type of tumor. Detection of such markers early in the course of the disease might increase chances for cure. They also may be used to follow the clinical progress of the disease and anticipate recurrence.
2 They may produce symptoms as a result of their intrinsic biologic activity. In some cases these can become the major clinical problems determining survival (e.g., hypercalcemia).
3 They may serve to promote the growth of the tumor directly. In turn, growth-promoting agents of this type may become the focus of new approaches to anticancer treatment.

The paraneoplastic sequelae of cancer which involve ectopic hormone production are described in Chap. 309, and the neurologic manifestations of neoplasia in Chap. 310. Cutaneous manifestations of internal malignancy are discussed in Chap. 59. The association of malignancy with certain metabolic disorders, hematologic abnormalities, and immunosuppression will be further described here.

Metabolic disorders   One of the major and most characteristic problems seen with cancer is weight loss, usually associated with anorexia. The extensive wasting which results is known as cachexia.

The cause for this commonly observed and often life-limiting disturbance remains to be determined in spite of the fact that many contributing factors have been identified. Abnormalities of taste and smell, physiologic malfunction of the gastrointestinal tract, excessive energy demands made by the tumor, and failure to adapt energy expenditure to the levels of nutrient intake have been implicated as causes of cachexia in patients with cancer. Biochemical abnormalities in energy metabolism have been well-characterized in these patients. Fatty acids are oxidized in preference to glucose, and anaerobic glucose metabolism is increased while oxidative phosphorylation is reduced. This results in an inefficient expenditure of ATP, which might lead to an energy deficit. However, none of these observations is felt to account for the magnitude of the problem.

Typically, the anorectic patient simply cannot ingest food, in spite of a clear understanding of the need for increased nourishment. The chief complaint is unpalatability. An aversion to meat has been clearly documented. While nausea may be a component of the syndrome, emesis occurs rarely. This may be because the patient feels so satiated that no food intake is tolerated.

Provision of alimentation through enteral tubes or by the intravenous route has the potential to provide total parenteral nutrition (TPN) to patients with cancer, and the techniques for performing these procedures have been well-described by investigators managing nonmalignant disease. At present there is no indication that the provision of nutritional support at this level can, by itself, affect the course of malignant disease. However, clinical trials have suggested a role for nutritional supplementation, including TPN, in preparing nutritionally deprived cancer patients for potentially beneficial surgical procedures or chemotherapy programs which otherwise might not have been tolerated due to the wasted state of the patient.

A polypeptide produced by macrophages has been isolated and named tumor necrosis factor (TNF), because of its capacity to cause lysis of certain types of tumor cells. Administration of TNF can mimic the syndrome of cachexia in experimental animals, and it is therefore also known as cachectin. Cytokines released by inflammatory cells and tumor cells are likely candidates as etiologic agents for the debilitation and wasting that accompany aggressive malignancy.

Fever is another sign associated with malignancy, and it is usually attributable to infection. Because of the debility which often accompanies cancer, and the depression in circulating granulocytes and mononuclear cells resulting from aggressive therapeutic measures, the types of infection seen may be unusual. Infection by endogenous bacteria, fungi, viruses, and protozoa must be considered when evaluating fever of unknown etiology in patients with malignancy (see Chap. 20). There remain unusual instances when fever cannot be explained by infection and must be attributed to a cause intrinsic to the neoplasm itself.

Hematologic abnormalities Anemia is found with increased incidence in advanced stages of malignant disease. The mechanisms accounting for anemia are, in nearly all cases, extrinsic to the tumor, and may be due to several mechanisms. Increased destruction of erythrocytes can result from hypersplenism, microangiopathic hemolysis, and autoantibodies, seen especially in the lymphoproliferative malignancies. Anemia due to occult bleeding is one of the cardinal signs of malignancy in the gastrointestinal tract. Decreased production of erythrocytes may result from iron deficiency related to bleeding, vitamin B_{12} or folate deficiency, erythron depletion due to tumor crowding in the marrow, toxicity secondary to chemotherapy or radiotherapy, and the anemia associated with chronic inflammatory disease.

Granulocytopenia is commonly associated with marrow infiltration by hematologic malignancies, and also results from chemotherapy. The etiologies of thrombocytopenia are comparable to those associated with anemia. Depression in one or all of the circulating hematopoietic elements may result from one of the various forms of marrow failure or aplastic anemia which are known to be preleukemic.

An increase in the formed elements of the blood may also occur. Erythrocytosis resulting from inappropriate production of erythropoietin is observed not only in polycythemia vera, but also in renal cell carcinoma, hepatoma, and cerebellar hemangioma. An elevated granulocyte count may result from marrow infiltration by tumor cells, or an inflammatory response to malignancy, and frank leukemoid reactions may be seen with nonhematopoietic tumors. Thrombocytosis unrelated to primary marrow disease is commonly associated with a systemic malignancy.

A hypercoagulable state is a rare clinical complication of malignancy, although it may be far more prevalent at a subclinical level. Mucin-producing tumors and adenocarcinomas, especially those of the pancreas and stomach, head the list of tumors reported to be associated with clinical disseminated coagulopathy (DIC). This may present as a migratory thrombophlebitis of unknown etiology, which can produce venous thrombosis as well as pulmonary embolism. Hypercoagulation also may be associated with marantic (nonbacterial) endocarditis and resultant thromboembolic episodes, which further complicate the clinical picture. The treatment of the primary malignancy is the only successful therapeutic attack on the problem. Anticoagulation, following the principles for treatment of DIC (Chaps. 62 and 289), may provide short-term benefits in acute situations, but with attendant risks.

Acute promyelocytic leukemia is often associated with abnormalities of hemostasis related to a hypercoagulable state. The malignant immature granulocytes can release procoagulant materials which initiate DIC. In this case, the addition of anticoagulation to the initial phase of antileukemia therapy results in an improved chance for a successful outcome.

Immunosuppression Advanced cancer is accompanied by abnormalities in immune function which can be demonstrated by skin testing against common antigens and by examination of lymphocyte responses to mitogenic stimulation in vitro. Moreover, in general, the extent of malignant disease correlates well with the degree of immune dysfunction. In spite of a vast experimental literature on this subject, the two significant questions concerning immunosuppression in cancer patients continue to be unanswered: (1) What is the mechanism(s) of inhibition? (2) Is the immunosuppression merely secondary to the malignant state, or could it play an etiologic role (failure of "immune surveillance")?

Experimental data have implicated defects in both T- and B-cell function, as well as abnormalities of macrophages, in the etiology of the reduced immune competence in cancer patients. Primary malignancies of lymphocytes are accompanied by abnormalities in the functioning of the particular cell type involved. Some of the lymphoproliferative malignancies are characterized by an increase in autoimmune reactions, most notably in 25 percent of patients with chronic lymphocytic leukemia. In addition, both chemotherapy and radiotherapy can produce long-standing suppression of immune function.

One approach to cancer treatment involves attempts to stimulate an effective immune response with the hope that immune antitumor activity can act alone or in concert with the standard therapeutic modalities to eliminate the malignant cell population. Monoclonal antibodies against antigens present in relatively increased quantities on tumor cells may provide ways to reconstitute or hyperconstitute immune responses to malignancy. Treatment with high concentrations of cytokines such as the interferons has produced responses in a number of types of malignancy, and this is especially effective in the therapy of hairy cell leukemia. Interleukin 2 (IL-2) is another cytokine which may produce antitumor responses in patients with melanoma and renal carcinoma, when administered in pharmacologic doses alone or in combination with lymphokine-activated killer (LAK) cells.

Psychosocial effects The diagnosis of cancer immediately raises in the mind of the patient and his or her family a host of questions and fears which require the undivided attention of an empathetic, considerate, and skilled physician. This is especially true when the particular form of cancer has a poor chance for cure, or when malignancy has recurred.

Of the variety of psychosocial problems experienced by patients, two which are particularly difficult to deal with are helplessness and loss of control. These involve both economic control and personal control of one's activity and one's future. Closely tied to these problems and adding to the feeling of helplessness is the difficulty of accepting personal finitude. A third major source of mental anguish is the fear of pain and mutilation. Finally, separation from loved ones, both anticipated and real, creates a void of loneliness and a fear of abandonment.

The reactions to the mental stresses which are produced by these problems can only be dealt with effectively by a professional who has become familiar with the patient's personality and his or her social and intellectual environment. Although one or another emotion may dominate at a particular time, the responses commonly observed include anger, denial, withdrawal, and depression. Added to these problems is the complexity resulting from the response of the patient's family to the illness and to the patient's own response to the illness. In spite of these stresses, some patients with incurable malignancies are able to adapt and reorient their lives in a creative and meaningful way. The intellectual and emotional challenge to the physician is obvious, and careful attention must be given to managing the patient's (and the family's) responses to malignancy in addition to providing specific treatment for the disease.

Does the patient's psychological attitude have a role in the cause or treatment of malignant disease? The question is a complex and controversial one. There is evidence, which is contested, that life stresses can predispose to systemic illness by producing anxiety or depression. One theory postulates that stress leads to a reduction in immunologic function, resulting in inadequate immune surveillance, but this explanation for the pathogenesis of cancer is not adequately supported by available clinical data. There are also claims that correction of emotional difficulties and development of positive attitudes can serve as effective anticancer therapy. In favor of psychological support and counseling is the clear benefit to the quality of life which can be achieved by helping patients with malignancy to develop positive attitudes and to gain some measure of control over *how* they are living. However, scientific evidence does not demonstrate that the patient's psyche can achieve regression or cure of the malignant process. Some of the strongest and most responsible advocates of counseling and attitudinal approaches to cancer patient management also stress the need for concurrent treatment with standard anticancer therapies.

DIAGNOSIS AND STAGING   There are five general goals in evaluating a patient for the presence of malignancy. First, information must be gathered leading to biopsy of a candidate lesion, which alone can establish the pathologic diagnosis of neoplasia. The second goal is to determine as precisely as possible the extent of tumor spread, both at the site of origin and as metastases. The process of obtaining this information is known as *staging*. The third goal is to determine the growth rate and time course of the neoplasm in the particular patient undergoing diagnostic evaluation. The dictum that "every person is different" holds for cancers as well. Each malignancy is different, although there is a natural history which broadly characterizes each type of neoplasm. The rate of tumor growth can be determined by sequential assessment, using physical examinations or radiologic techniques, occasionally aided by the measurement of serum markers of tumor activity. The physician's ingenuity and persistence often come into play; an example is determining the existence of past radiologic studies, locating them, and obtaining them for review. The fourth goal in the evaluation is to determine the effects of the malignancy upon the health and performance of the patient. The importance of this in the design of a management plan is obvious, since control of symptoms and proper modification of acitivity levels will improve the well-being of the patient. In addition, it has become increasingly evident that the patient's performance status provides important data in predicting prognosis as well as response to anticancer therapy. The final goal in the diagnostic evaluation is the selection of appropriate anticancer therapy. The

TABLE 300-6   Influence of pretreatment performance status on patients with inoperable lung cancer*

Performance status scale[†]			Median survival (weeks)	Patients in group (percent)
ECOG	Karnofsky	Definitions		
0	100	Asymptomatic, normal activity	34	2
1	80–90	Symptomatic, but ambulatory	24–27	32
2	60–70	Symptomatic, in bed less than 50% of day, needs minimal assistance	14–21	40
3	40–50	Symptomatic, in bed more than 50% of day, requires considerable assistance	7–9	22
4	20–30	100% bedridden, severely disabled	3–5	5

* N = 5022 males with inoperable lung cancer of all histologic types entered onto VA Lung Group protocols from 1968–1978.
† Eastern Cooperative Oncology Group (ECOG) performance status scale, and DA Karnofsky et al, Cancer 1:634, 1948.
SOURCE: Adapted from JD Minna et al, in VT DeVita, Jr et al.

choice will depend on the information gathered as outlined, plus a knowledge of the treatment regimens which have the highest likelihood of producing cure, durable remission, or palliation. The principles of cancer therapy are presented in Chap. 301.

There are two widely used clinical scales of performance status, the Karnofsky scale and a modification developed by the Eastern Cooperative Oncology Group. The influence of performance status upon prognosis is demonstrated by a report correlating performance and median survival in patients with inoperable lung cancer (Table 300-6).

Pathologic diagnosis   The diagnosis of cancer is made by pathologic examination. While there are definite limitations to histologic and cytologic examination of tumor specimens, this procedure is essential in order to exclude inflammatory processes as well as hyperplasia or benign tumors. In addition, the tissue of origin of a malignancy must be known in order to select the appropriate therapy. Specimens for pathologic examination are usually obtained by biopsy of a suspicious lesion. The procedure may involve a surgical operation under general anesthesia, but in many cases tissue specimens can be obtained through local incision (e.g., breast cancer) or by removal of a piece of tissue under direct visualization (bronchoscopy, colonoscopy). When direct visualization is not possible because of the internal location of a suspected lesion, it is often possible to obtain tissue fragments or clumps of cells by fine-needle biopsy aspiration, guided by computed tomography or fluoroscopy. In addition, suitable cytologic preparations can be obtained by washing or scraping surface lesions, as is commonly done to evaluate lesions on the cervix or in bronchi. Finally, in the case of malignancy involving the hematopoietic system or growing in body cavities (e.g., ascites), needle aspiration of tumor cells in suspension can be performed.

To make the diagnosis of cancer the pathologist looks for histologic and cytologic features characteristic of the disease. These include pleomorphism of cellular and nuclear structure, a high rate of mitosis and the presence of large or multiple nuclei, disordered tissue architecture, destruction or invasion of normal tissue boundaries, and the presence of cells in inappropriate locations (metastases). Special stains are useful for identifying chemical components characteristic of particular cell types and tissues. Additional evidence can be brought to bear upon the pathologic diagnosis, using the results of immunohistochemical studies, flow cytometry data on cellular DNA content, chromosomal karyotype analysis, Southern blotting for detection of diagnostic abnormalities in rearranged or amplified genes, and electron microscopy. However, in the overwhelming majority of cases, the diagnosis is made with the light microscope, on the basis of morphologic evaluation of the cells individually and as organized into tissue structures.

After the pathologic diagnosis of malignancy is established, the description usually includes three characteristics which classify the neoplasia:

1 The tissue of origin (e.g., adenocarcinoma, epidermoid carcinoma, sarcoma, leukemia)
2 Anatomic origin (e.g., colon, lung, breast)
3 Degree of differentiation (e.g., well-differentiated or poorly differentiated)

Each of these characteristics gives the therapist information relevant to the selection of treatment and to the prognosis. Although this terminology for classification is followed in general, there are many examples of exceptions based upon customary nomenclature involving particular tissues of origin or on the use of eponyms (e.g., Hodgkin's disease, glioblastoma multiforme).

Staging of cancer The staging of a cancer patient involves the detection of the anatomic extent of the tumor, both in its primary location and in metastatic sites. This process is of critical importance in the clinical management for a number of reasons:

1 The optimal treatment plan for an individual patient is selected on the basis of the stage of disease.
2 By determining the presence of early metastatic disease, treatment can often be designed which can increase the chance for cure, or delay the development of symptoms even if cure is not achievable.
3 Staging provides information from which the physician can better evaluate the prognosis.
4 Because half of the cases of cancer cannot be cured by the therapies available today and because rapid advances in the development of anticancer treatment are occurring, management of an individual patient often involves new drugs or experimental procedures which are in the process of being evaluated for toxicity and efficacy. Staging to determine the extent of disease accurately is essential for evaluating factors influencing the results of such new treatments.

The anatomic extent of disease is best described and communicated to other professionals by a standardized nomenclature known as the TNM system. The three elements characterized in this system are the primary *t*umor, the regional lymph *n*odes, and *m*etastases (Table 300-7). The details of classification were decided upon by the International Union against Cancer (UICC) and the American Joint Committee for Cancer Staging (AJCCS). There is a scale of subcategories with designations ranging from 0 to 4 for each of the three tumor characteristics listed in the table. These scales were chosen because they can provide useful predictions of the clinical course. The primary tumor is classified by its size and the extent of local involvement. The involvement of lymph nodes is typically stratified by the spread to locations at a varying distance from the primary lesion and by the number of involved nodes. The most relevant information regarding metastases is their presence or absence. The details of stratification within the TNM system vary for each type of malignancy and are highly individualized. They depend on the characteristic growth patterns and lymphatic drainage patterns of neoplasms of the various organs. There is not always agreement about the definitions of the TNM characteristics, which can create confusion.

The stage of the tumor is typically divided into three or four

TABLE 300-8 Stage Grouping of the New International Staging System for Lung Cancer*

Occult carcinoma	TX	N0	M0
Stage 0	TIS	Carcinoma in situ	
Stage I	T1	N0	M0
	T2	N0	M0
Stage II	T1	N1	M0
	T2	N1	M0
Stage IIIa	T3	N0	M0
	T3	N1	M0
	T1-3	N2	M0
Stage IIIb	Any T	N3	M0
	T4	Any N	M0
Stage IV	Any T	Any N	M1

* TX, positive cytology; TIS, carcinoma in situ; T1, less than or equal to 3 cm, no local invasion; T2, greater than 3 cm, more than 2 cm from carina; T3, direct extension to chest wall, diaphragm, pleura or pericardium; T4, invasion of mediastinum, intrathoracic organs, or vessels. N1, peribronchial or hilar nodes; N2, ipsilateral mediastinal nodes; N3, contralateral mediastinal nodes; M1, distant metastasis.
SOURCE: Mountain, CF: A new international staging system for lung cancer. Chest 89:225s–233s, 1986.

categories (e.g., I to IV). For each type of malignancy, the various T, N, and M designations are assigned to one of four stages, in order to develop separation into groupings which correlate with data on prognosis and clinical responses to therapy. This is best described by mentioning a specific example. For the neoplasm with the highest mortality rate, non-small cell carcinoma of the lung, the therapy which has the best chance for curing the patient is surgery. The staging system for lung cancer (Table 300-8) is designed in a way which stratifies patients into groups, for which different treatment protocols are indicated. For the stages I and II patients, surgery is the treatment of choice. The extent of the surgical procedure depends on the extent of disease designated by the T and N classification within these two stages. Total excision of all tumor is the therapeutic goal, with 5-year postresection survival rates of 50 percent for stage I, 30 percent for stage II, and 15 percent for stage IIIa.

Clinical evaluation How does the clinician proceed to evaluate a patient for the presence of malignant disease? Early detection depends primarily on awareness of the hereditary and environmental factors contributing to the incidence of cancer, combined with thorough exploration for symptoms and signs which could lead to further diagnostic workup. The seven warning signals widely publicized by the American Cancer Society are useful to remember (Table 300-9) and are usually covered in a review of systems. A careful physical examination is especially useful in detecting early breast cancer, cancer of the colon, skin cancer, and head-and-neck cancers. Three diagnostic screening tests have proved of value in early detection: (1) the exfoliative cytology ("Pap smear") screen for cervical cancer, (2) fecal occult blood testing, accompanied by periodic sigmoidoscopy, and (3) mammograms.

The prudent guidelines for early cancer detection provided by the American Cancer Society can be summarized as follows. A cancer-related checkup is recommended every 3 years for those 20 to 40 years of age. For breast cancer screening, an examination of patients in this age group by a physician is recommended every 3 years, a self-examination every month, and one baseline breast x-ray between the ages of 35 and 40. For detection of cervical and uterine cancer, an annual pelvic examination and Pap test are recommended, with a reduction in frequency after three normal examinations.

In the age group of 40 and over, a yearly cancer checkup is

TABLE 300-7 TNM system of anatomic staging

T: Primary tumor
  T0 No evidence of primary tumor
  T1–4 Ascending degrees of increase in tumor size and involvement
N: Regional lymph nodes
  N0 No evidence of disease in lymph nodes
  N1–4 Ascending degrees of nodal involvement
M: Distant metastasis
  M0 No evidence of metastasis
  M1–4 Ascending degrees of metastatic involvement

TABLE 300-9 Cancer's seven warning signals

Change in bowel or bladder habits
A sore that does not heal
Unusual bleeding or discharge
Thickening or lump in breast or elsewhere
Indigestion or difficulty in swallowing
Obvious change in wart or mole
Nagging cough or hoarseness

SOURCE: American Cancer Society.

TABLE 300-10   Methods for diagnosis and staging

I History
II Physical examination, including examination of oropharynx, Pap test, and proctoscopy
III Radiologic studies
  A Roentgenogram
  B Ultrasound
  C Computerized axial tomography
  D Angiography and lymphangiography
  E Nuclear medicine
  F Magnetic resonance imaging
IV Laboratory studies
  A Hematologic evaluation
  B Chemical tests of internal organ function
  C Tumor markers
V Pathologic examination of tissue
VI Cytogenetics and molecular genetics

recommended by the American Cancer Society. Women over 40 are advised to have a professional breast examination every year, a self-examination every month, and a breast x-ray every 1 to 2 years for those 40 to 49 years of age, and every year for those 50 and over. For screening of cervical and uterine cancer in this age group, an annual pelvic examination and Pap test are recommended, with a reduction in frequency after three normal examinations. An endometrial tissue sample is recommended at menopause if the patient has high-risk factors. For colon and rectal cancer, a digital rectal examination is suggested every year after 40, and a stool occult blood test every year after 50 as well as a sigmoidoscopic examination every 3 to 5 years after two initial negative tests 1 year apart. It is estimated by the American Cancer Society that the 5-year survival rate for colorectal cancer could be increased from the current level of 55 percent to as high as 85 percent, if these early detection techniques were generally applied.

The three most common malignancies involve bowel, lung, and breast, and it is significant that screening tests are suggested for only two of these. Unfortunately, trials of mass screening for lung cancer with chest x-rays and sputum cytology have not resulted in reduced mortality, even when subjects believed to be at high risk were followed. However, the physician who is evaluating a patient in order to attempt to detect cancer early must learn whether or not the patient smokes cigarettes and should attempt to intervene.

The approach to a patient who presents to the physician with a history of symptoms or with abnormal physical findings which could be attributed to cancer involves selection of appropriate diagnostic procedures from a wide variety of available radiologic tests and laboratory studies (Table 300-10). The choice of diagnostic procedures used in the staging of cancer patients is guided by the natural history of the various types of malignancy. For example, knowledge that distant spread of breast cancer most frequently occurs to the lung, liver, bone, brain, and contralateral breast leads to consideration of studies of each of these organs as part of the staging workup. In addition, the diagnostician must know the probability of spread to these various metastatic sites in the presence or absence of abnormal findings in the history, physical examination, and standard blood studies. For the asymptomatic patient with breast cancer who has no abnormal physical findings outside of a small palpable breast lesion, and normal hematologic and blood chemistry values, a chest x-ray and a mammogram are the tests typically performed to stage the patient prior to a decision for definitive therapy. Similar considerations go into planning the diagnostic workup for patients with each of the various forms of malignancy. It is for this reason that a thorough familiarity with the natural history of malignancies of the various organs, as well as the efficacy of a wide variety of diagnostic procedures in detecting these cancers, is essential.

Tumor markers   A tumor marker is an abnormality which is specific for a particular type of malignancy. For example, the Ph¹ chromosome abnormality in the karyotype is a marker for chronic myelogenous leukemia, and the exclusive presence of either κ or λ chains on the surface of a population of lymphocytes is a marker of the lymphoproliferative malignancies. Until recently there were no biochemical markers that were absolutely specific for and diagnostic of malignancy. However, utilization of molecular genetic technology has enabled detection of genetic alterations that are pathognomonic for particular malignancies (see discussion of "Clonality" above). In addition, recent reports demonstrate specific genetic abnormalities in a variety of types of cancer. Examples, some of which have been alluded to, include amplified *neu* or elevated *erb*B expression in breast cancer, elevated N-*myc* in neuroblastoma, overexpression of H-*ras* in bladder and prostate cancer, and amplified c-*myc* in small cell lung cancer. The term *marker* may also be used in a more restrictive sense, referring to molecules which are produced in abnormal amounts or under abnormal circumstances and are released into the circulation. The anaplasia and autonomy of the tumor cells permit production of molecules in greater than normal amounts or at inappropriate times in the life of the organism, and in this sense the abnormalities may become specific. Assays of such markers may be of great help to the clinician in a number of ways: (1) screening of high-risk individuals for the presence of malignancy, (2) diagnosis of malignancy, (3) monitoring of the effectiveness of therapy, (4) early detection of recurrence, and (5) immunodetection of metastatic sites, using radioactive-labeled antibodies against the markers.

The tumor marker of greatest use to the clinician is human chorionic gonadotropin (hCG), which has specificity because of its nearly exclusive production by the trophoblastic epithelium of the placenta under normal circumstances. The hCG levels rise during pregnancy. The hormone also may be secreted into the blood by trophoblastic tumors, as well as germ cell neoplasms of the testes and ovaries. Other neoplasms have been reported to be associated with elevated hCG levels, but the serum concentration rarely exceeds 10,000 ng/L (10 ng/mL) whereas trophoblastic tumors can produce concentrations over 100×10^6 ng/L (100,000 ng/mL). The usefulness of the assay for hCG is markedly enhanced by clinical data which show that changes in the serum hCG concentration in patients with secreting trophoblastic malignancies accurately reflect changes in the tumor burden. Therefore, decisions on the appropriate time to discontinue therapy can be based on the time course of serum levels, and decisions to reinstate therapy for recurrent disease are made on the basis of reappearance of hCG in the serum. The clinical test for hCG utilizes a radioimmunoassay for the beta subunit, to avoid cross reactivity with luteinizing hormone.

Two clinically useful tumor markers are products of genes which are expressed during the normal differentiation of fetal tissue but are partially or completely suppressed in the adult. These markers have been termed oncofetal antigens. Carcinoembryonic antigen (CEA) was originally thought to be specific for bowel cancer, but further studies have shown it to be a nonspecific tumor-associated antigen which also may be elevated in a variety of benign conditions. In the gastrointestinal tract, the molecule, a glycoprotein with a molecular weight of 180,000, is concentrated in the glycocalyx of epithelial cells, from which it is released into the lumen of the bowel. In the presence of malignancy, CEA concentrations may be elevated in the blood and other body fluids. Serum levels of CEA above the normal concentration of 2500 ng/L (2.5 ng/mL) are found in greater than 50 percent of neoplasms involving the colon, pancreas, stomach, lung, and breast. A variety of common nonmalignant conditions are associated with elevation of CEA, but typically not over 10,000 ng/L (10 ng/mL). These include cigarette smoking, chronic pulmonary disease, alcoholic cirrhosis, hepatitis, and inflammatory bowel disease. CEA is not selective for cancer, and measurements of its levels should not be used in screening for the presence of malignant disease. However, serial measurements of CEA levels in patients with secreting malignancies can provide valuable information on the efficacy of treatment and the recurrence of disease. The possibility that early elevation of serum CEA can predict recurrence of bowel cancer soon enough to allow further surgical resection for cure is under study.

The second clinically useful oncofetal antigen is alpha fetoprotein

(AFP), which is produced by the liver and gastrointestinal tract epithelium during gestation and which falls to levels less than 20,000 ng/L (20 ng/mL) after birth. Serum levels are elevated in 70 percent of patients with hepatocellular cancer, the majority of patients with nonseminomatous testicular cancer, and occasional patients with neoplasms of the gastrointestinal tract. As with CEA, the serum concentration of AFP may be elevated in benign conditions, especially in inflammatory disease of the liver. Its utility is in monitoring tumor activity, especially in the case of testicular tumors.

Elevation of either AFP or hCG is found in 80 to 90 percent of all nonseminomatous germ cell tumors of the testes. However, absence or normal levels of these biochemical markers of malignancy cannot be interpreted as proof that there is no tumor. Some tumors do not produce these marker molecules. Furthermore, because of tumor heterogeneity, it is possible for marker concentrations to fall in the presence of tumor, if a nonproducing subclone begins to grow preferentially. For this reason, recurrence of disease need not be accompanied by recurrence of elevated marker levels.

Other biochemical markers with clinical utility include calcitonin, with which familial medullary carcinoma of the thyroid can be detected in individuals who appear to be normal. Prostatic acid phosphatase levels are useful in determining the extent (stage) of prostatic cancer, and in monitoring the response to therapy.

There are many tumors which, because of increased cellular mass or loss of normal regulation, produce excessive quantities of polypeptides normally secreted into the circulation by the tissue of origin. Examples include the immunoglobulin molecules produced in multiple myeloma, and insulin or gastrin hypersecretion by islet cell tumors. In addition, tumors may secrete molecules which ordinarily are not produced in the tissue from which they are derived. This phenomenon has already been discussed in the description of the paraneoplastic syndromes, because in many cases these marker molecules have biologic activities which can produce clinical illness in the patient. In some cases of malignant disease, cultures of tumor cells have been found to secrete a variety of polypeptide hormones atypical of the tissue of origin. In addition, molecules related to normal hormones or to their precursor forms may be present in the patient's serum, in the absence of any demonstrable clinical effects. These observations provide evidence for the broad scope of genetic deregulation which may accompany the process of oncogene expression and carcinogenesis.

REFERENCES

CALABRESI P et al: *Medical Oncology: Basic Principles and Clinical Management of Cancer.* New York, Macmillan, 1985

CLINE MJ: Molecular diagnosis of human cancer. Lab Invest 61:368, 1989

DEVITA VT JR et al: *Cancer: Principles and Practices of Oncology.* Philadelphia, Lippincott, 1989

HOLLAND JF, FREI E: *Cancer Medicine.* Philadelphia, Lea & Febiger, 1982

MERKEL DE, MCGUIRE WL: Oncogenes and cancer prognosis, in *Important Advances in Oncology 1988,* VT DeVita Jr et al (eds). Philadelphia, Lippincott, 1988, chap 7

NORDENSKJOLD M, CAVENEE W: Genetics and the etiology of solid tumors, in *Important Advances in Oncology 1988,* VT DeVita Jr et al (eds). Philadelphia, Lippincott, 1988, chap 6

RUBIN P: *Clinical Oncology for Medical Students and Physicians.* New York, American Cancer Society, 1983

SCHOTTENFELD D, FRAUMENI JF JR: *Cancer Epidemiology and Prevention* Philadelphia, Saunders, 1982

301 CANCER CHEMOTHERAPY

EDWIN C. CADMAN / HENRY J. DURIVAGE

In the United States cancer is the second leading cause of death and in 1988 resulted in an estimated 480,000 deaths. This translates to 167 deaths per 100,000 population per year, or an estimated 21 percent of all deaths in the United States in 1988. Thus, someone born in the United States in 1990 has a greater than 1 in 3 chance of developing cancer in his or her lifetime. However, while a decade ago only 10,000 patients per year with metastatic cancer were cured by chemotherapy, at present this rate has increased to 30,000 patients per year.

There has been a systematic approach to the development of cancer chemotherapy in the United States. Since the creation of the National Cancer Chemotherapy Program in 1955, over 700,000 compounds and extracts have been screened for antineoplastic properties. In 1945 there was only one drug known to be effective—namely, nitrogen mustard. Today, there are nearly 50 chemotherapeutic agents used, singly or combined, in the treatment of malignancy.

The introduction of cancer chemotherapy followed closely on the wave of excitement concerning the antibiotic treatment of infectious diseases. In 1943, after it had been observed that World War II soldiers exposed to nitrogen mustard gases had a reduction in the size of their lymph nodes, mechlorethamine hydrochloride (chlormethine) was first used to treat Hodgkin's disease. A rapid decrease in these patients' lymph nodes was documented, but the remissions were very transient. At about the same time, based on knowledge regarding certain antimetabolite antibiotics, the antifolate agent aminopterin (methotrexate) was first used in 1947 to treat acute lymphocytic leukemia. The use of methotrexate as a single agent in gestational choriocarcinoma in 1955 resulted in the first cancer cures.

The lack of cure in other cancers similarly treated prompted investigators to examine combinations of chemotherapeutic agents based on the concept of "therapeutic synergism" developed for the treatment of infections using a combination of antibiotics. The first empirical trials using combinations of antineoplastic drugs were reported in 1957 and 1960 in patients with bronchogenic carcinoma and testicular carcinoma. In the latter up to 22 percent complete responses were recorded. However, substantial toxicity and drug-related deaths were major deterrents. In 1958 the first randomized study in children with acute lymphocytic leukemia was reported, and remarkable responses were observed.

In 1964 Skipper and his colleagues began the first studies in which the scientific knowledge of drug combinations was specifically evaluated. They utilized the murine leukemia L1210 cell line to examine the growth characteristics of tumors in a mouse model and to characterize the response of cancer cells to chemotherapy. Their study also provided an experimental model for "cure." Because of their laboratory success, other researchers were prompted to scientifically study cancer growth and chemotherapy with the goal of improving our ability to destroy cancer cells.

This early research also included attempts at biochemical modulation. Drug combinations were tested in various cancer cell lines using the in vivo mouse model. Combinations of drugs were tested which were predicted to cause sequential blockade (of two different sequential enzymes in a pathway) or concurrent blockade (of two different enzymes not in sequence which would both contribute to a reduction in a needed common end product) and result in therapeutic synergy. The results were disappointing, in part because the predictions were incorrect, but also because individually the drugs did not have dramatic cytotoxic effects. But a precedent for further research was established, and from this work the basic principles of cancer chemotherapy have evolved. In many cancers, chemotherapy can result in (1) significantly improved survival, (2) reproducible palliation without significantly improved survival, or (3) occasional responses at the expense of substantial toxicity. There are a few cancers that remain totally unresponsive to chemotherapy—namely, malignant melanoma with visceral metastases, hypernephroma, pancreatic carcinoma, and metastatic adenocarcinomas of unknown primary. The capacity to cure disseminated cancer is dependent on combination chemotherapy alone, or together with biologic therapy, surgery and/or radiotherapy. Further progress in deriving more effective combinations is dependent on a rational and scientific approach to developing and screening chemotherapeutic drug combinations.

As shown in Fig. 301-1, many cancers can be cured by surgical resection. Chemotherapy for cancer is used primarily in the treatment of nonoperable or metastatic malignancy or as an adjunct to primary surgical therapy. The most widespread use of adjuvant chemotherapy is for breast cancer. Modest estimates are that an additional 5 percent of patients who otherwise would have relapsed and died of breast cancer are now cured because they were given adjuvant chemotherapy.

Although the primary goal for chemotherapy is to cure, most patients are, in fact, not cured. Nearly all patients have some tumor response to their therapy, but only a small number have their lives substantially prolonged. Therefore, to improve our ability to treat cancer, patients should be offered the choice of participating in clinical trials. The standard use of the terms "complete response" or "partial response" is an important clinical determinant for assessing the results of therapy.

CELL KINETICS   Cancer is a clonal disease. A single cell becomes uninhibited in growth and continues to divide, leading to the formation of a tumor. The time for cellular division is generally quite long. The concept that all cancer cells multiply rapidly is incorrect. For example, breast cancer cells generally divide every 100 days. A simple series of mathematical evaluations yields compelling evidence that supports the contention that cancer has been present in any given individual for years prior to clinical detection. Given the average size of a cell of 1 μm, it will take 10^9 (1 billion) cells to form a 1-cm nodule, which is also equivalent to 1 g in weight. Assuming that all cells survived, it would take 30 cell doublings to achieve 1 billion cells from 1 cell; the first cancer cell divides to form two cancer cells; these two cells divide to form four cells, etc. This form of cell growth is exponential. If the time between doublings averages 100 days, then it will take almost 9 years for one cancer cell to result in a 1-cm nodule. A tumor which contains 10^{12} cells is equivalent to 1 kg. A cancer with this number of cells is a far-advanced malignancy which results in an extremely cachectic patient who is generally

FIGURE 301-1   Estimation of cancer patient results for the 1990s.

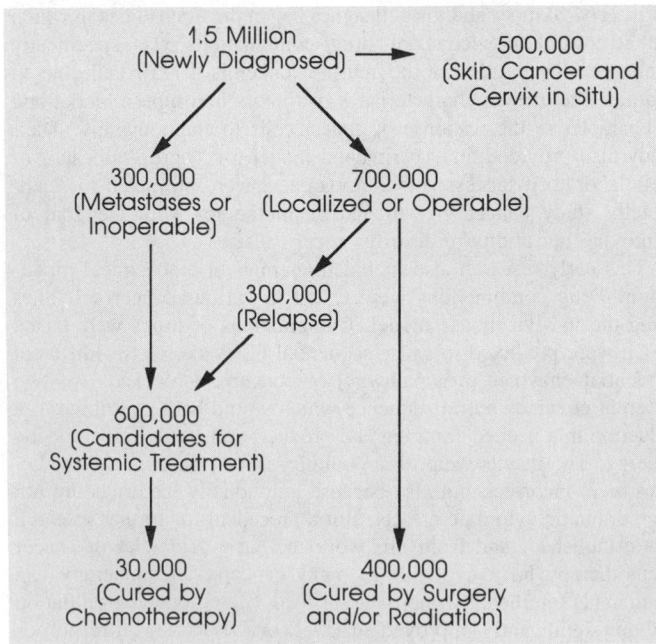

terminally ill. Only 10 more cell doublings are required to go from 10^9 cells to 10^{12} cells, which is approximately 3 years for a tumor whose cells divide every 100 days. Figure 301-2 describes tumor growth as a process that proceeds exponentially. Representative cancers and their doubling times, and the predicted time to form a 1-cm nodule, are presented in Table 301-1.

From this example, it is apparent that a small cancer is not a young tumor. Three-quarters of the cancer's "life" has been used to develop into a 1-cm lesion (30 doublings divided by 40 doublings). The actual growth kinetics of a cancer can vary considerably from this example, because this evaluation assumes linear growth and no natural cell loss. However, not all cells of a tumor divide simultaneously. The cell cycle (Fig. 301-3) consists of several phases, any of which contain various fractions of the cancer cell population.

Most chemotherapeutic agents affect cells during the synthesis of DNA. It is unclear if any of our current chemotherapeutic agents are effective in killing cells in G_0, or the resting phase. For example, methotrexate, which inhibits the formation of thymidylate (one of the four bases required for DNA synthesis), will not kill cells unless they are actively synthesizing this DNA precursor. Therefore, the success of chemotherapy is often highly dependent upon the cellular kinetics of the tumor at the time the drugs are administered.

The growth rate of malignant cells, which is exponential during the early phases of tumor growth, becomes less rapid in the later stages of tumor development. There are several reasons proposed for this reduction in the growth rate; these include (1) insufficient local nutrients (e.g., decreased blood supply) to support continued growth, (2) an increased rate of tumor cell death, and/or (3) fewer cells reentering the cell cycle. In general, the very small or undetected

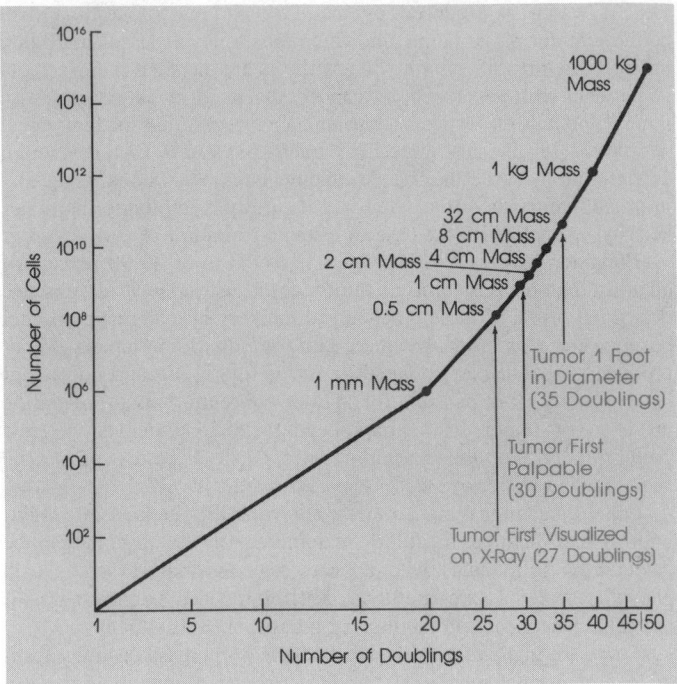

FIGURE 301-2   Schematic representation of the life cycle of a human tumor.

TABLE 301-1   Tumor doubling times and duration of growth

Tumor	Doubling, days	Time to a 1-cm tumor
Burkitt's lymphoma	1–5	30–150 days
Testicular cancer	20	1.6 years
Diffuse (high-grade) lymphoma	12–25	1–2.1 years
Lung cancer	100	8.2 years
Colon cancer	100	8.2 years
Breast cancer	100–130	8.2–10.6 years

SOURCE: Adapted from G Gordon Steel, *Growth Kinetics of Tumors*, Oxford, Clarendon Press, 1977.

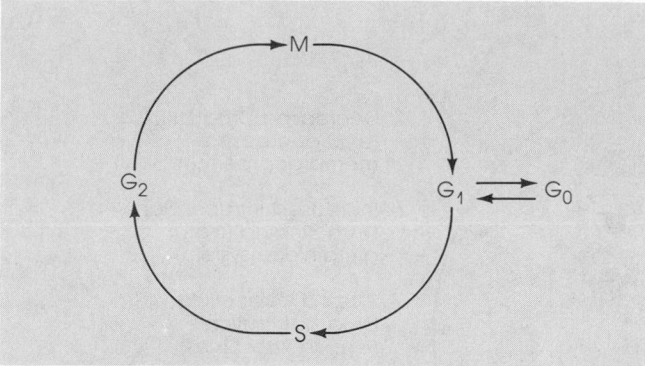

G_0 = resting phase (nonproliferation of cells)
G_1 = pre-DNA synthetic phase (12 h to a few days)
S = DNA synthesis (usually 2 to 4 h)
G_2 = post-DNA synthesis (2 to 4 h; cells are tetraploid in this stage)
M = mitosis (1 to 2 h)

FIGURE 301-3 The cell cycle.

TABLE 301-2 Some types of biologic and chemical agents used in the treatment of cancer

Hormones
Cytokines
   Interferons α, β, γ
   Interleukins, especially IL-2
   Tumor necrosis factor
Monoclonal antibodies coupled to tumoricidal agents
Cells
   Lymphokine activated killer (LAK) cells
   Tumor infiltrating lymphocytes (TIL)
Chemotherapeutic drugs

cancers undergo a more rapid proliferation than the larger clinically apparent tumors.

Adjuvant chemotherapy refers to the administration of drugs following primary surgical therapy when residual tumor is small and clinically undetectable and the cells are more likely to be actively dividing. It is self-evident that it is easier to kill 10^3 than 10^9 cells; therefore, assuming that drugs kill the same percentage of cells each time they are given, it will also take less time to get rid of 10^3 than 10^9 cells. These assumptions apply only if the drugs are toxic to the cancer cells. *Neoadjuvant therapy* refers to the use of chemotherapy prior to or immediately after a curative resection of a malignancy.

PRINCIPLES OF CHEMOTHERAPY To achieve a cure of a malignancy, presumably all of the cancer cells must be destroyed. For this to occur with chemotherapeutic drugs (1) the cancer cells must be sensitive to the agent; (2) the drug must reach the malignant cell; (3) if the drug is effective only in a phase of the cell cycle, it must be given frequently enough that all the cancer cells enter this phase of the cell cycle while the drug is present; and (4) the malignant cells must be destroyed before drug resistance emerges. There are obvious exceptions to the validity of these concepts. Thus, an innocuous dose of a drug over a long period of time will never be effective. It is assumed that high drug dose over a short time period is effective because sufficient amounts of the drug remain within the cells or the tumor environment to be lethal, even though the drug may not be detectable in the serum.

Experimental and clinical studies have demonstrated the importance of dose intensity for effective cancer treatment. Dose intensity is the amount of drug given per unit time. In general, more drug given over a short time period is superior to the same amount over a longer time period. The clinical implications of this principle are quite important—namely, patients who are treated with chemotherapy should be given the maximum tolerated dose frequently. Low, nontoxic, and nontumoricidal doses favor the emergence of drug-resistant cancer cells.

Table 301-2 lists some of the general types of biologic and chemical agents used in the treatment of cancer. The first tumor to be cured by chemotherapy was choriocarcinoma. Methotrexate was effective and continues to be the treatment of choice for this malignancy except in far-advanced stages. This tumor divides rapidly; presumably very few cells are in the resting phase (G_0). However, it is not surprising that very few malignancies have been cured by the administration of a single dose. The use of drug combinations has enhanced the possibility of cure or remission. The theoretical advantage of combination therapy is that several drugs can be given simultaneously or in close proximity to each other and thus lead to cell death by several mechanisms. This approach has been effective in the treatment of many cancers and reduces the emergence of drug-resistant cells. In general, if a cell is resistant to one drug, it is less likely also to be resistant to a second or third drug. However, certain caveats must be kept in mind. In selecting drug combinations, their site of action in the cell cycle is important. Thus, it makes little sense to use a drug that prevents DNA synthesis (viz., prevents cells from entering the S phase) together with an agent that is only effective on cells in the S phase. A negative aspect of combination therapy is that it is often associated with greater systemic toxicity.

Drug resistance The resistance of cancer cells to a cytotoxic drug is an inherent property of the cancer cell itself; it can be temporary or permanent. *Temporary resistance* can be due to environmental or local factors limiting cell killing as, for example, (1) by diminished blood supply to the tumor; (2) when cells are in "sanctuaries" such as the central nervous system and the drug does not cross the blood-brain barrier; or (3) when cells are in the wrong phase of the cell cycle.

The more significant problem, in general, is the development of genetic changes in the malignant cell leading to *permanent drug resistance*. Some of the major mechanisms include (1) increased intracellular inactivation of the drug; (2) increased efflux of the drug out of the cell by products of multidrug-resistant genes in the cell membrane (see below); (3) an increase in the number of target enzymes; (4) increased DNA repair, etc. (see Fig. 301-4).

Goldie and Coldman suggested in 1979 that just as bacteria mutate spontaneously to bacteriophage resistance, so cancer cells might develop resistance to drugs. They proposed that drug resistance was related to both *mutation rate* and *cell number* or size. Thus, if the intrinsic mutation rate is 10^{-6}, a tumor composed of 10^9 cells (approximately 1 cm in diameter) is very likely to develop a drug-resistant clone. Examples of this phenomenon probably occur in breast cancer, ovarian cancer, and acute leukemia with cancer cells responding initially but then becoming resistant with the emergence of resistant clones or cell lines.

A major clinical problem is that tumors of the visceral organs frequently are not responsive to chemotherapeutic agents. There may be several reasons for this. These tumors (e.g., colon, stomach, pancreas) may be inherently resistant due to the prior exposure of the normal tissue to the presence of these agents in the environment. Thus, they may have developed detoxification mechanisms to protect against the natural (? dietary) toxins from which many chemotherapeutic drugs have been developed. As shown in Fig. 301-2 the concept that a tumor 1 cm in size has gone through 30 doublings to reach 10^9 cells is based on exponential cell growth. This may not apply to all animal or human tumors. In fact, cell loss occurs in some tumors, and this may be as great as 90 percent. Thus, as many as 1200 doublings might be needed to reach 10^9 cells; this allows for an increased incidence of mutations to resistant cells, making it likely that the tumors are resistant to anticancer agents at the time of diagnosis.

A genetic mechanism leading to resistance of a wide range of drugs that have minimal, if any, relationship to each other involves pleiotropic or multidrug resistance (MDR). A single genetic step can

1. Increased Drug Efflux (e.g., p-glycoprotein in typical multidrug resistance)

2. Decreased Transformation from Inactive to Active Drug (e.g., mitomycin resistance)

3. Increased DNA Repair (e.g., increased O_6-methylguanine DNA methyltransferase in BCNU Resistance)

4. Increased Metabolism to Inactive Drug (e.g., increased aldehyde dehydrogenase in cyclophosphamide resistance)

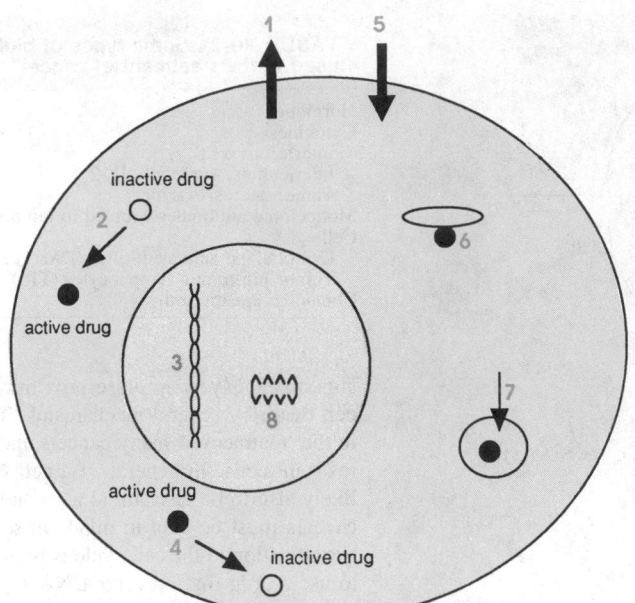

5. Decreased Drug Efflux (e.g., decreased membrane permeability)

6. Increased Intracellular Drug Binding (e.g., glutathione system)

7. Altered Intracellular Drug Distribution (e.g., to lysosomes)

8. Alteration of Specific Target Enzymes (e.g., altered topoisomerase II in etoposide resistance and increased dihydrofolate reductase in methotrexate resistance)

FIGURE 301-4 Potential sites for drug resistance at the cellular level.

make the cells resistant to the most effective and most used anticancer drugs. This genetic alteration leads to the expression on the cell surface of a 170-kDa glycoprotein (called P-glycoprotein, or P170). This protein leads to the increased drug efflux and, hence, reduced intracellular accumulation of the drug. However, a number of agents can reduce the actions of P170 and have been shown to potentiate the cytotoxic effects of certain drugs, at least in part by increasing their intracellular concentration. These agents include calcium channel antagonists, polyene antibiotics, and antiarrhythmic drugs (see Table 301-4).

Gene amplification can also be associated with drug resistance. This can occur as a result of gene reduplication if transcription is slowed down or stopped; it can also be induced by drugs that decrease DNA synthesis such as a low dose of alkylating agents or radiation. Therefore, giving a low dose or a weak antitumor agent or marginally effective x-radiation may induce resistance to drugs like methotrexate

without any prior exposure to the drug. This reduplication or amplification of DNA may result in as many as 100 copies of a given region on a chromosome. This amplification may take either of two forms: (1) the duplicated DNA may be tandemly organized at a single site leading to a *homogeneously staining region* (HSR) by microscopy; or (2) it may exist as small, chromosome-like structures referred to as *double minutes* on stained chromosome preparations.

CLINICAL TRIALS   The journey from basic research to clinically useful anticancer drugs takes many years. The time from a basic observation in the laboratory until sufficient information is obtained to support studies in human beings often ranges from 2 to 10 years. Once a drug has been proven safe and effective in rodents, it can enter clinical trials. The clinical trials program in this country is largely the result of coordinated efforts sponsored by the National Cancer Institute. There are three phases of clinical trials.

1 The purpose of phase 1 is primarily to determine the maximum tolerated dose and human pharmacology of the agent tested. Only patients with far-advanced cancer of any type for whom no further therapy is available or patients for whom no effective ("standard") therapy exists may be eligible to receive phase 1 drugs.

2 The purpose of phase 2 is to determine for which cancers the new drug is effective. Only patients with measurable tumors for whom either no further therapy is available or for whom no initial therapy is known to be effective can elect to participate in this phase. The patient must not be terminally ill. In general between 15 and 30 patients with specific types of cancer are entered into these studies. Ideally each drug should be tested in 7 and 10 different types of tumors.

3 As a result of phase 2 studies, the drug may have been shown to be effective against a specific type of cancer. In phase 3 studies, the new drug is given to a more uniform group of patients with the type of cancer for which the drug was determined to be effective in the phase 2 study. These patients have usually not been treated, and randomization between the new treatment and the nonstandard treatment is done or the new agent is added to a standard effective therapy and compared to the standard therapy alone. If there is no standard effective treatment, then randomization is not performed; for example, there is no effective standard treatment for squamous cell cancer of the lung. Therefore, patients with this cancer type should be entered into a phase 3 study.

To determine if a drug is effective against a given cancer in a phase 2 study, we must rely on statistical analysis to assist in the decision-making process. If we assume that we wish to find only

TABLE 301-3   Drugs that may modulate drug resistance

Drugs	Antineoplastic* drugs affected	Proposed mechanism of increased cytotoxicity
Calcium antagonists		
Verapamil	VCR, DNR, ADR	Increased accumulation by blocking efflux
Nifedipine		
Nitrendipine		
Caroverine		
Calmodulin inhibitors		
Prenylamine	VCR, DNR ADR	Same as above
Trifluoroperazine		
Clomipramine		
Amphotericin	ADR, ACT-D, BCNU	Alterations in lipid composition of plasma membrane leading to increased accumulation
Tween 80	ADR	
Perhexiline maleate	ADR	
Triparanol analogues		
Tamoxifen	ADR	Increased drug accumulation
Antiarrhythmic drugs		
Quinidine	ADR, VCR	Increased drug accumulation
Antihypertensive		
Reserpine	ADR	Increased drug accumulation
Thiol depleter		
Buthionine sulfoximine	L-PAM, PLAT, ADR	Drug inactivation, free radical metabolism, protection/repair of DNA

* ABBREVIATIONS: VCR, vincristine; DNR, daunorubicin; ADR, Adriamycin; L-PAM, melphalan; PLAT, cisplatin; BCNU, 1,3 bis(2 chloroethyl)1-nitrosourea; ACT-D, actinomycin D.

new drugs which have a minimum effectiveness of 20 percent, that is, that 20 percent of patients with cancer "X" will respond to the new drug, then projections to guide us can be made: Given this criterion, there is a 95 percent chance that in the first 14 patients with cancer "X" there will be at least 1 patient who responds to the new drug. If there is no response noted in the first 14 treated patients, then there is a 95 percent probability that the drug is not effective for the treatment of that type of cancer as defined by a minimum expected 20 percent response rate. The problem with this statistical reasoning is that it assumes that all 14 patients are similar. If a disparate group of patients (even if they have the same kind of cancer) is entered into the phase 2 study, the lack of response could be due to factors unrelated to the tumor type. Therefore, for a phase 2 study patients must be carefully selected.

Chemical and biologic agents in the treatment of cancer Many biologic and chemical agents can be given systemically to patients to produce destruction of cancer cells. These are shown in Table 301-4. As indicated above, in many instances these agents are used in combination rather than alone. Table 301-5 lists some drugs that are still investigational in the United States.

TABLE 301-4 Some commercially available anticancer drugs and hormones (dose-limiting effects are italicized)

Drug	Acute toxicity	Delayed toxicity*
Aminoglutethimide *Action:* Blocks steroidogenesis	Drowsiness; nausea; dizziness	Hypothyroidism (rare); bone marrow depression; fever; hypotension; masculinization
Asparaginase *Action:* Destroys essential amino acid (asparagine)	*Nausea and vomiting; fever;* chills; headache; hypersensitivity, anaphylaxis; abdominal pain; hyperglycemia leading to coma	CNS depression or hyperexcitability; acute hemorrhagic pancreatitis; coagulation defects; thrombosis; renal damage; hepatic damage
Bleomycin *Action:* Generates free radicals	*Nausea and vomiting; fever;* anaphylaxis and other allergic reactions	*Pneumonitis and pulmonary fibrosis; rash* and hyperpigmentation; stomatitis; alopecia; Raynaud's phenomenon; cavitating granulomas
Busulfan *Action:* Alkylates DNA	*Nausea and vomiting;* rare diarrhea	*Bone marrow depression;* pulmonary infiltrates and fibrosis; hyperpigmentation; alopecia; gynecomastia; ovarian failure; azoospermia; leukemia; chromosome aberrations; cataracts; hepatitis
Carboplatin *Action:* Cross-links DNA	*Nausea and vomiting*	*Bone marrow depression;* peripheral neuropathy (uncommon); hearing loss
Carmustine (BCNU) *Action:* Alkylates DNA	*Nausea and vomiting;* local phlebitis	*Delayed leukopenia and thrombocytopenia* (may be prolonged); pulmonary fibrosis (may be irreversible); delayed renal damage; gynecomastia; reversible liver damage; venoocclusive disease (hepatic or pulmonary) with high doses; leukemia
Chlorambucil *Action:* Alkylates DNA	Seizures; nausea and vomiting	*Bone marrow depression;* pulmonary infiltrates and fibrosis; leukemia; hepatic toxicity; sterility
Cisplatin (*cis*-DDP) *Action:* Cross-links DNA	*Nausea and vomiting;* anaphylactic reactions; fever; hemolytic-uremic syndrome	*Renal damage;* bone marrow depression; ototoxicity; hemolysis; hypomagnesemia; peripheral neuropathy; hypocalcemia; hypokalemia; Raynaud's disease; sterility; teratogenesis
Cyclophosphamide *Action:* Alkylates DNA	*Nausea and vomiting;* type 1 (anaphylactoid) hypersensitivity; facial burning with IV administration; visual blurring	*Bone marrow depression;* alopecia; hemorrhagic cystitis; sterility (may be temporary); pulmonary infiltrates and fibrosis; hyponatremia; leukemia; bladder cancer; teratogenesis; inappropriate ADH secretion
Cytarabine HCl *Action:* Inhibits DNA polymerase	*Nausea and vomiting;* diarrhea; anaphylaxis	*Bone marrow depression;* conjunctivitis; megaloblastosis; oral ulceration; hepatic damage; fever; pulmonary edema and central and peripheral neurotoxicity at high doses; rhabdomyolysis; pancreatitis when used with asparaginase
Dacarbazine *Action:* Alkylates DNA	*Nausea and vomiting;* diarrhea; anaphylaxis; pain on administration	*Bone marrow depression;* alopecia; flulike syndrome; renal impairment; hepatic necrosis; facial flushing; paresthesia; photosensitivity; urticarial rash
Dactinomycin *Action:* DNA intercalator	*Nausea and vomiting;* diarrhea; local reaction and phlebitis; anaphylactoid reaction	*Stomatitis; oral ulceration; bone marrow depression;* alopecia; folliculitis; dermatitis in previously irradiated areas
Daunorubicin HCl *Action:* DNA intercalator	*Nausea and vomiting;* diarrhea; red urine (not hematuria); severe local tissue damage and necrosis on extravasation; transient ECG changes; anaphylactoid reaction	*Bone marrow depression; cardiotoxicity;* alopecia; stomatitis; anorexia; diarrhea; fever and chills; dermatitis in previously irradiated areas
Doxorubicin HCl *Action:* DNA intercalator; generates free radicals	*Nausea and vomiting;* red urine (not hematuria); severe local tissue damage and necrosis on extravasation; diarrhea; fever; transient ECG changes; ventricular arrhythmia; anaphylactoid reaction	*Bone marrow depression; cardiotoxicity;* alopecia; stomatitis; anorexia; conjunctivitis; acral pigmentation; dermatitis in previously irradiated areas
Estramustine phosphate sodium *Action:* Combination of estrogen and nitrogen mustard	Nausea and vomiting; diarrhea	Mild gynecomastia; increased frequency of vascular accidents; myelosuppression (uncommon); edema; dyspnea; pulmonary infiltrates and fibrosis; leukemia

(continued)

TABLE 301-4 Some commercially available anticancer drugs and hormones (dose-limiting effects are italicized) (continued)

Drug	Acute toxicity	Delayed toxicity*
Etoposide (VP16-213) *Action:* Inhibits topoisomerase II	*Nausea and vomiting;* diarrhea; fever; hypotension; allergic reactions	*Bone marrow depression;* alopecia; peripheral neuropathy; mucositis and hepatic damage with high doses
Floxuridine *Action:* Inhibits thymidylate synthesis	*Nausea and vomiting;* diarrhea	*Oral and gastrointestinal ulceration; bone marrow depression;* alopecia; dermatitis; hepatic dysfunction with hepatic infusion
Fluorouracil (5-FU) *Action:* Inhibits thymidylate synthesis	*Nausea and vomiting;* diarrhea; hypersensitivity reaction	*Oral and GI ulcers; bone marrow depression;* diarrhea (especially with fluorouracilleucovorin); neurologic defects, usually cerebellar; cardiac arrhythmias; angina pectoris; alopecia; hyperpigmentation; palmar-plantar erythrodysesthesia; conjunctivitis; heart failure
Flutamide *Action:* Antiandrogen	Nausea; diarrhea	Gynecomastia; hepatotoxicity
Hydroxyurea (hydroxycarbamide) *Action:* Inhibits ribonucleotide reductase	Nausea and vomiting; allergic reactions to tartrazine dye	*Bone marrow depression;* stomatitis; dysuria; alopecia; rare neurologic disturbances
Ifosfamide *Action:* Alkylates DNA	Nausea and vomiting; confusion; nephrotoxicity; metabolic acidosis	*Bone marrow depression; hemorrhagic cystitis* (prevented by concurrent mesna); alopecia; inappropriate ADH secretion; neurotoxicity (somnolence, hallucinations, blurring of vision, coma); teratogenesis
Interferon Alfa-2a, Alfa-2b *Action:* Multifaceted, increases HLA expression	Fever; chills; myalgias; fatigue; headache; arthralgias; hypotension	Bone marrow depression; anorexia; renal damage; hepatic damage
Leuprolide acetate (LHRH-releasing factor analogue) *Action:* LHRH analogue	Transient increase in bone pain and ureteral obstruction; hot flashes	Impotence; amenorrhea; testicular atrophy
Lomustine (CCNU) *Action:* Alkylates DNA	*Nausea and vomiting*	*Delayed (4 to 6 weeks) leukopenia and thrombocytopenia* (may be prolonged); transient elevation of transaminase activity; neurologic reactions; pulmonary fibrosis; renal damage; leukemia
Mechlorethamine HCl (nitrogen mustard) *Action:* Alkylates DNA	*Nausea and vomiting;* local reaction and phlebitis	*Bone marrow depression;* alopecia; diarrhea; oral ulcers; leukemia; amenorrhea; sterility
Melphalan *Action:* Alkylates DNA	Mild nausea; hypersensitivity reactions	*Bone marrow depression* (especially platelets); pulmonary infiltrates and fibrosis; amenorrhea; sterility; leukemia; inappropriate ADH secretion
Mercaptopurine *Action:* Hypoxanthine analogue	Nausea and vomiting; diarrhea	*Bone marrow depression; cholestasis and rarely hepatic necrosis; oral and intestinal ulcers; pancreatitis;* allopurinol and azathioprine increase overall toxicity
Mesna *Action:* Used in conjunction with ifosfamide; inhibits hemorrhagic cystitis	Nausea and vomiting; diarrhea	
Methotrexate (MTX) *Action:* Inhibits dihydrofolate reductase (DHFR)	*Nausea and vomiting;* diarrhea; fever; anaphylaxis; hepatic necrosis	*Oral and gestrointestinal ulceration,* perforation may occur; *bone marrow depression;* hepatic toxicity including cirrhosis; renal toxicity; *pulmonary infiltrates and fibrosis;* osteoporosis; conjunctivitis; alopecia; depigmentation; menstrual dysfunction; encephalopathy and anaphylactoid reactions with high doses
Mitomycin *Action:* Cross-links DNA	*Nausea and vomiting;* local reaction; fever	*Bone marrow depression* (cumulative); stomatitis; alopecia; acute pulmonary toxicity; pulmonary fibrosis; hepatotoxicity; renal toxicity; amenorrhea; sterility; hemolytic-uremic syndrome; bladder calcification
Mitotane (o, p'-DDD) *Action:* Inhibits steroidogenesis	*Nausea and vomiting;* diarrhea	*CNS depression;* rash; visual disturbances; adrenal insufficiency; brain damage with long-term high dosage; hematuria; hemorrhagic cystitis; albuminuria; hypertension; orthostatic hypotension; cataracts
Mitoxantrone HCl *Action:* DNA intercalator	Blue-green pigment in urine; blue-green sclera; nausea and vomiting; stomatitis	Bone marrow depression; cardiotoxicity; alopecia; white hair; skin lesions; hepatic damage; renal failure
Octreotide *Action:* Somatostatin analogue	Nausea; diarrhea; abdominal pain	Steatorrhea
Plicamycin *Action:* DNA intercalator	*Nausea and vomiting; diarrhea; fever*	*Hemorrhagic diathesis; bone marrow depression* (thrombocytopenia); coagulation abnormalities; hepatic damage; hypocalcemia and hypokalemia; stomatitis; renal damage

TABLE 301-4 Some commercially available anticancer drugs and hormones (dose-limiting effects are italicized) (continued)

Drug	Acute toxicity	Delayed toxicity*
Procarbazine HCl Action: Alkylates DNA	*Nausea and vomiting;* CNS depression; disulfiram-like effect with alcohol	*Bone marrow depression;* stomatitis; peripheral neuropathy; pneumonitis; leukemia; interacts with tyramine in food to cause hypertensive crisis
Streptozocin Action: Alkylates DNA	*Nausea and vomiting;* local pain; chills and fever	*Renal damage;* hypoglycemia; hyperglycemia; liver damage; diarrhea; bone marrow depression (uncommon); fever; eosinophilia; nephrogenic diabetes insipidus
Tamoxifen citrate Action: Antiestrogen	Nausea and vomiting; hot flashes; transient increased bone or tumor pain; hypercalcemia	Vaginal bleeding and discharge; rash; thrombocytopenia; peripheral edema; depression; dizziness; headache; decreased visual acuity; corneal changes; retinopathy
Thioguanine Action: Purine analogue	Occasional nausea and vomiting	*Bone marrow depression;* hepatic damage; stomatitis
Thiotepa Action: Alkylates DNA	*Nausea and vomiting;* local pain	*Bone marrow depression;* menstrual dysfunction; interference with spermatogenesis; leukemia
Vinblastine sulfate Action: Inhibits tubulin function	*Nausea and vomiting;* local reaction and phlebitis with extravasation	*Bone marrow depression;* alopecia; stomatitis; loss of deep tendon reflexes; jaw pain; muscle pain; paralytic ileus; inappropriate ADH secretion
Vincristine sulfate Action: Mitotic arrest; inhibits tubulin function	Local reaction with extravasation	*Peripheral neuropathy;* alopecia; mild bone marrow depression; constipation; paralytic ileus; jaw pain; inappropriate ADH secretion

* Cutaneous reactions (sometimes severe), hyperpigmentation, and ocular toxicity have been reported with virtually all nonhormonal anticancer drugs.
SOURCE: Adapted from *The Medical Letter*, June 2, 1989, with permission.

Hormonal therapy The growth of many tissues is influenced by hormones, and some tumors continue to possess receptors for them. Lymphoid tumors have receptors for glucocorticoids, estrogen, and progesterone; receptors are present on some breast cancers and endometrial cancers, and prostate cancers have abundant androgen receptors. Hormones bind to receptors in the cytoplasm and nucleus; this is associated with a conformational change in the receptors that interact with the DNA in the nucleus leading to messenger RNA and protein synthesis.

Patients with breast cancer cells that have estrogen receptors have a greater than 50 percent chance of responding to hormonal agents such as tamoxifen, an antiestrogen (see Chap. 303). Endometrial

TABLE 301-5 Some investigational drugs (dose-limiting effects are in italics)

Drug	Acute toxicity	Delayed toxicity
Amsacrine (m-AMSA) Action: DNA intercalator	*Nausea and vomiting;* diarrhea; pain or phlebitis on infusion; anaphylaxis	*Bone marrow depression;* hepatic injury; convulsions; stomatitis; ventricular fibrillation; alopecia
Azacitidine Action: Inhibits DNA methylation	Nausea and vomiting; diarrhea; fever; drowsiness	Leukopenia (may be prolonged); thrombocytopenia; hepatic damage; muscle pain and weakness; bone marrow depression; possibly cardiotoxicity
Erythropoietin Action: Stimulates erythropoiesis	Fever; bone pain	Capillary leak; leukocytosis; local thrombosis
Hexamethylmelamine* (HMM) Action: Alkylates DNA	Nausea and vomiting	*Bone marrow depression;* visual disturbances (reversible); CNS depression; peripheral neuritis; visual hallucinations; ataxia
Interleukin 2 Action: Stimulates T-cell proliferation	*Fever; fluid retention;* rash; anemia; thrombocytopenia; nausea and vomiting; diarrhea; capillary leak syndrome; nephrotoxicity; myocardial toxicity; hepatotoxicity; erythema nodosum	Neuropsychiatric disorders; hypothyroidism
Mitoguazone (methyl-GAG; methyl glyoxal bis-guanylhydrazone; MGBG) Action: Alkylates DNA	*Nausea and vomiting;* fatigue	Myopathy; paresthesia; bone marrow depression; ventricular arrhythmias; stomatitis; gastrointestinal ulcerations
Pentostatin (2'-deoxycoformycin)	Nausea and vomiting; rash	Nephrotoxicity; CNS depression;
Semustine (methyl-CCNU) Action: Alkylates DNA	*Nausea and vomiting*	*Delayed leukopenia and thrombocytopenia* (may be prolonged); pulmonary fibrosis; renal failure; leukemia
Teniposide* (VM-26) Action: Multifactorial; mitotic arrest	Nausea and vomiting; diarrhea; phlebitis; anaphylactoid symptoms	Bone marrow depression; alopecia; peripheral neuropathy
Vindesine sulfate* Action: Inhibits tubulin function	Local reaction if extravasation; fever; nausea and vomiting; diarrhea	Bone marrow depression; alopecia; peripheral neuropathy; jaw pain

* Commercially available in Canada.
SOURCE: Adapted from *The Medical Letter*, June 2, 1989, with permission.

cancers may respond in one-third of patients to progestins; these hormones may also produce response in about 10 percent of patients with renal cancer, but the mechanism for this effect is not known.

Since prostate cancers grow under the influence of androgens, the hormonal treatment involves the use of agents with antiandrogen or estrogen properties. The development of nonsteroidal antiandrogens such as flutamide and antagonists of the hypothalamic releasing hormone LHRH such as leuprolide has produced promising clinical results in the treatment of prostatic cancer without the cardiovascular complications resulting from estrogen use.

Biologic agents   Biologic approaches to the treatment of cancer are varied but in general can be divided into three categories: (1) agents augmenting the defenses of the host, (2) agents that are directly tumoricidal, and (3) agents that modify the behavior of the tumor.

CYTOKINES   Agents that augment host defenses include the *cytokines* such as the interferons, interleukin 2, and tumor necrosis factor. *Interferons* (INF) are glycoproteins made by cells in response to viral infections. IFN-α is secreted by leukocytes, INF-β is secreted by fibroblasts, and IFN-γ is secreted by lymphocytes in response to mitogens. The mechanism by which IFNs are cytotoxic to cancer cells is not clear, but they inhibit cell proliferation and enhance T-cell cytotoxicity. IFN-α is the treatment of choice for hairy cell leukemia, producing a complete response in 50 percent of patients and a partial response in 90 percent. In addition, IFN-α has significant antitumor effects in renal cell carcinoma, ovarian cancer, melanoma, follicular lymphoma, and chronic myelogenous leukemia.

Interleukin 2 is a T-cell growth factor released by antigen-stimulated T cells. Purified IL-2 has been used to activate lymphocytes referred to as LAK cells (lymphokine activated killer cells) which differ from natural killer (NK) cells, to destroy tumor cells regardless of their immunogenicity. Clinical studies of so-called adoptive immunotherapy with concomitant administration of IL-2 and LAK cells have produced some complete and partial remissions in patients with advanced melanoma and renal cancers, with lesser responses in lung cancers. These studies suggest that tumor-infiltrating lymphocytes (TIL cells) plus IL-2 are somewhat more effective than LAK cells. However, there are significant systemic side effects associated with IL-2 administration, and this has limited its use.

Tumor necrosis factor (TNF) is produced and secreted by macrophages. It has been shown to have a direct cytotoxic effect against tumor cells, especially melanoma cells in culture. TNF has been cloned and produced in large quantities for clinical trials by recombinant techniques. However, in studies to date, TNF has not shown major cytotoxic activity in humans. Its toxicity is very similar to IL-2's.

Monoclonal antibodies   Since the development of the hybridoma technique in 1975, many monoclonal antibodies have been produced against tumor-associated antigens. The theoretical advantage of these antibodies is their selectivity and specificity for given antigens and, in general, in their not binding to normal cells. They are being evaluated to assess their use alone (as complement-fixing antibodies) or conjugated with toxins (e.g., ricin, *Pseudomonas* toxin) or coupled with radioisotopes (e.g., ^{131}I). Most experience has been with murine antibodies. Clinical efficacy to date has been limited for a number of reasons including tumor cell heterogeneity, lack of cytotoxicity, and development of human antimouse antibodies.

Antineoplastic drugs   One of the most important aspects of cancer chemotherapy trials in the 1960s and 1970s was the fact that drugs could *cure* some patients with cancer. Cancers can generally be grouped based on their response to antineoplastic drugs. Tables 301-6 to 301-8 list the tumors in which drugs have major, moderate, or minimal activity. In most cases maximum benefit is achieved by combination chemotherapy.

Antineoplastic drugs exert their cytotoxic effects by interfering with various cellular mechanisms involved in cell growth. The production of essential cellular components may be disrupted or damaged, or RNA and DNA synthesis and/or function may be altered. Figure 301-5 shows the major sites of action of most current antineoplastic drugs. The latter include alkylating agents, antineoplastic antibiotics, plant alkaloids, and antimetabolites.

Alkylating agents possess a characteristic alkyl moiety and exert their cytotoxic effects primarily by covalent bonding of the alkyl groups to cellular DNA or other molecules. Despite their apparent similarity, the alkylating agents exhibit a wide and varied spectrum of antitumor activity. Examples of alkylating agents are cyclophosphamide, the chlorethylnitrosoureas, and melphalan. *Antineoplastic antibiotics* have been isolated from microbial fermentation extracts. They also have a wide spectrum of antitumor activity and are largely responsible for the improved treatment of acute leukemias, lymphomas, and breast cancer. They include bleomycin, doxorubicin, mitomycin, and mitoxantrone. *Plant alkaloids* and other natural products have also yielded important antineoplastic drugs. The vinca alkaloids (e.g., vincristine, vinblastine) and podophyllotoxin derivatives (e.g., etoposide, teniposide) are examples of effective drugs derived from natural sources. *Antimetabolites* act by inhibiting crucial metabolic enzymes. Often prolonged exposure of these antimetabolites by continuous infusion is more effective than bolus administration. In general, antimetabolites such as 5-fluorouracil, methotrexate, and cytarabine are most effective on rapidly dividing cells.

SIDE EFFECTS OF CHEMOTHERAPEUTIC AGENTS AND THEIR MANAGEMENT   Antitumor agents exert their actions by interfering with cellular structures and function, and there is often a narrow "window" between therapeutic and adverse effects. Most acute toxicities are expressed in rapidly dividing tissues or organs such as the bone marrow, intestinal mucosa, and hair follicles. The important side effects are described below along with approaches to anticipate, prevent, or ameliorate them.

MYELOSUPPRESSION   Only a few anticancer agents directly suppress bone marrow stem cells. These include the alkylating drugs such as nitrogen mustard, cyclophosphamide, and the nitrosoureas. The reduction of the blood count for most other antineoplastic agents is the result of the inhibition of the proliferating committed cells in the marrow and not an effect on the nondividing stem cell. It is important to remember that a significant percentage of normal bone marrow cells are not actively dividing; this affords some selectivity in the choice of antitumor drugs.

In general, maximum bone marrow suppression occurs in the most actively dividing fractions such as platelets and granulocytes. Cell cycle–specific agents, such as the antimetabolites, seem to produce the most rapid granulocytopenic responses, but they are also associated with rapid recovery. For most anticancer drugs myelosuppression is the toxicity that determines the maximal dose that can be given. Only

TABLE 301-6   Diseases in which chemotherapy has major activity

Cancer	Drugs currently preferred	Alternative drugs
Acute lymphocytic leukemia (ALL)	Induction: vincristine + prednisone ± asparaginase ± doxorubicin or daunorubicin CNS prophylaxis: intrathecal methotrexate ± radiotherapy Maintenance: methotrexate + mercaptopurine Bone marrow transplant for chemotherapy failures	Etoposide + cytarabine, cyclophosphamide, cytarabine, thioguanine, teniposide,* mitoxantrone, etoposide, ifosfamide + mesna CNS prophylaxis: high-dose IV + intrathecal methotrexate, high-dose cytarabine, intrathecal cytarabine + methotrexate ± hydrocortisone Maintenance: doxorubicin and/or asparaginase in addition to methotrexate and mercaptopurine

TABLE 301-6 Diseases in which chemotherapy has major activity (*continued*)

Cancer	Drugs currently preferred	Alternative drugs
Acute myelogenous leukemia (AML)	Daunorubicin + cytarabine ± thioguanine Mitoxantrone + cytarabine ± daunorubicin Bone marrow transplant with cyclophosphamide plus either total-body irradiation or busulfan	High-dose cytarabine, mitoxantrone, amsacrine,* azacitidine,* etoposide, + eniposide,* ifosfamide + mesna
Breast cancer†,‡	Tamoxifen Cyclophosphamide + methotrexate + fluorouracil ± prednisone (CMF or CMFP) Cyclophosphamide + doxorubicin ± fluorouracil (AC or CAF)	Megestrol, leuprolide acetate, cisplatin ± vinblastine, ifosfamide + mesna, vincristine, mitomycin, mitoxantrone, etoposide, teniposide,* mitolactol,* estrogens, progestins, androgens, prednisone, aminoglutethimide
Choriocarcinoma	Methotrexate ± leucovorin ± dactinomycin	Vinblastine, chlorambucil, bleomycin, etoposide, cisplatin, methotrexate with leucovorin rescue
Embryonal rhabdomyosarcoma†	Vincristine + dactinomycin + cyclophosphamide (VAC) ± doxorubicin Vincristine + doxorubicin + cyclophosphamide	Methotrexate, cisplatin, ifosfamide + mesna
Ewing's sarcoma†	Cyclophosphamide + doxorubicin + vincristine (CAV)	Dactinomycin, etoposide ± ifosfamide with mesna
Hairy cell leukemia	Interferon or pentostatin*	Chlorambucil
Hodgkin's disease	Doxorubicin + bleomycin + vinblastine + dacarbazine (ABVD) ± cyclophosphamide ABVD alternated with MOPP Mechlorethamine + vincristine + procarbazine + prednisone (MOPP) Mechlorethamine + vincristine + procarbazine + doxorubicin + bleomycin + vinblastine (MOP/ABV) Chlorambucil + vinblastine + procarbazine + prednisone (CVPP) ± carmustine Marrow transplantation with lomustine, cyclophosphamide, etoposide	Lomustine, carmustine, etoposide, cisplatin + etoposide, teniposide,* streptozocin, methotrexate, ifosfamide + mesna, mitoguazone*
Lung, small cell (oat cell)	Cisplatin + etoposide (PE) Cyclophosphamide + doxorubicin + vincristine (CAV) PE alternated with CAV Cyclophosphamide + etoposide + cisplatin (CEP)	Methotrexate + doxorubicin + cyclophosphamide + lomustine (MACC) Ifosfamide + mesna, methotrexate,* cyclophosphamide, lomustine, carboplatin,* mechlorethamine
Non-Hodgkin's lymphoma, Burkitt's lymphoma	Cyclophosphamide Cyclophosphamide + vincristine + methotrexate Cyclophosphamide + high dose cytarabine ± methotrexate with leucovorin rescue	Carmustine, methotrexate, ifosfamide + mesna
Diffuse large cell lymphoma	Cyclophosphamide + doxorubicin + vincristine + prednisone (CHOP) Bleomycin + doxorubicin + cyclophosphamide + vincristine + prednisone (BACOP) Bleomycin + doxorubicin + cyclophosphamide + vincristine + prednisone + methotrexate with leucovorin rescue (M-BACOP) Prednisone + methotrexate-leucovorin + doxorubicin + cyclophosphamide + etoposide + mechlorethamine + vincristine + procarbazine + prednisone (ProMACE-MOPP) Bleomycin + doxorubicin + cyclophosphamide + vincristine + prednisone + procarbazine (COP-BLAM) Methotrexate with leucovorin + doxorubicin + cyclophosphamide + vincristine + prednisone + bleomycin (MACOP-B) Bone marrow transplantation with high-dose cyclophosphamide and total-body irradiation or with cyclophosphamide + carmustine + etoposide	Bleomycin, chlorambucil, lomustine, carmustine, cytarabine, etoposide, teniposide,* amsacrine,* methotrexate, high-dose cytarabine, ifosfamide + mesna, interferon (for follicular lymphomas), prednisone Cyclophosphamide + vincristine + methotrexate leucovorin + cytarabine (COMLA) Dexamethasone sometimes substituted for prednisone
Osteogenic sarcoma†	Doxorubicin and high-dose methotrexate + leucovorin rescue ± cisplatin ± bleomycin ± cyclophosphamide ± dactinomycin	Ifosfamide + mesna, etoposide
Testicular	Cisplatin + etoposide ± bleomycin (PEB) Cisplatin + vinblastine + bleomycin (PVB) Vinblastine + dactinomycin + bleomycin + cyclophosphamide + cisplatin (VAB-6) Autologous marrow transplantation with carboplatin + etoposide	Cisplatin + ifosfamide with mesna + vinblastine or etoposide Doxorubicin, vincristine, ifosfamide + mesna, carboplatin,* etoposide, cyclophosphamide, methotrexate, plicamycin, dactinomycin
Wilms' tumor†	Dactinomycin + vincristine ± doxorubicin ± cyclophosphamide	Doxorubicin, cyclophosphamide, cisplatin, ifosfamide + mesna, etoposide

* Available in the USA only for investigational use.
† Drugs have major activity only when combined with surgical resection, radiotherapy or both.
‡ For adjuvant treatment of breast cancer, tamoxifen is generally preferred for postmenopausal patients and combinations of other drugs for premenopausal node-positive patients.
SOURCE: Adapted from *The Medical Letter*, June 2, 1989, with permission.

TABLE 301-7   Diseases in which chemotherapy has moderate activity

Cancer	Drugs currently preferred	Alternative drugs
Adrenocortical carcinoma	Mitotane or cisplatin	Doxorubicin, aminoglutethimide
Bladder	Cisplatin and/or doxorubicin ± methotrexate ± vinblastine* Instillation of BCG or thiotepa or doxorubicin or mitomycin	Fluorouracil, vinblastine, methotrexate, instillation of interferon
Brain Glioblastoma	Carmustine or lomustine	Semustine,* procarbazine, cisplatin, cyclophosphamide, etoposide
Medulloblastoma	Vincristine + carmustine ± mechlorethamine ± methotrexate Mechlorethamine + vincristine + procarbazine + prednisone (MOPP) Vincristine + cisplatin ± cyclophosphamide	
Cervix	Cisplatin + bleomycin ± methotrexate Bleomycin + mitomycin + vincristine ± cisplatin	Cyclophosphamide, vincristine, methotrexate, mitomycin, fluorouracil, doxorubicin, vinblastine; ifosfamide + mesna
Chronic lymphocytic leukemia	Chlorambucil ± prednisone	Cyclophosphamide, vincristine, pentostatin*
Chronic myelogenous leukemia (CML) Chronic phase	Busulfan Hydroxyurea, interferon Bone marrow transplantation with cyclophosphamide and total-body irradiation	Mitobronitol,* mercaptopurine, thioguanine, melphalan
Acute phase	Daunorubicin + cytarabine + vincristine + prednisone ± thioguanine High-dose cytarabine ± daunorubicin Vincristine + prednisone for lymphoid variant	Amsacrine,* azacitidine,* vincristine ± plicamycin
Endometrial	Megestrol acetate or hydroxyprogesterone caproate or medroxyprogesterone acetate Doxorubicin ± cyclophosphamide ± cisplatin	Fluorouracil, tamoxifen, carboplatin
Gastric	Fluorouracil + doxorubicin + cisplatin, ± semustine or mitomycin	Cisplatin ± etoposide, fluorouracil
Head and neck, squamous cell	Cisplatin + fluorouracil Belomycin + cisplatin ± methotrexate	Methotrexate, mitomycin, doxorubicin
Islet cell carcinoma	Streptozocin ± fluorouracil ± doxorubicin	Doxorubicin, dacarbazine, octreotide
Kaposi's sarcoma (AIDS-related)	Etoposide or interferon or vinblastine	Cyclophosphamide, vincristine
Mycosis fungoides	Combination chemotherapy as in Hodgkin's disease or non-Hodgkin's lymphoma Mechlorethamine (topical)	Carmustine (topical), photopheresis (psoralen + extracorporeal ultraviolet light) Vinblastine, methotrexate, interferon, pentostatin,* etretinate
Myeloma	Melphalan (or cyclophosphamide) + prednisone Melphalan + carmustine + cyclophosphamide + prednisone Dexamethasone + doxorubicin + vincristine (VAD)	Carmustine, vincristine, lomustine, doxorubicin, interferon
Neuroblastoma	Doxorubicin + cyclophosphamide + cisplatin + teniposide* Doxorubicin + cyclophosphamide Cisplatin + cyclophosphamide	Mechlorethamine, daunorubicin, dacarbazine, vinblastine, prednisone, cisplatin, teniposide,* etoposide Bone marrow transplantation
Non-Hodgkin's lymphoma Follicular lymphoma	Cyclophosphamide or chlorambucil, ± vincristine and prednisone, ± etoposide (combinations not demonstrably superior to single agents)	Cytarabine, asparaginase, methotrexate, interferon

* Available in the United States only for investigational use.
SOURCE: Adapted from *The Medical Letter*, June 2, 1989, with permission.

recently, with the availability of colony stimulating factors has there been the opportunity to give these drugs beyond their previously defined maximal doses. The use of colony stimulating factors following chemotherapy results in a resurgence of proliferation of the dormant stem cells causing a rapid repopulation of normal functional cells.

With most agents, when given as a single therapeutic dose, the nadir of granulocyte and platelet counts occurs 7 to 14 days later, with recovery occurring by day 21 to 28. However, with mitomycin and most of the nitrosoureas (e.g., lomustine and carmustine) maximum myelosuppression occurs 4 to 5 weeks after the initial dose, with recovery 2 to 3 weeks later. Other drugs, such as bleomycin and vincristine, are less myelotoxic and are generally safe to administer when blood counts are low.

Antineoplastic drugs often lead to levels of myelosuppression without clinical complications at granulocyte levels of about 1500

cells per microliter and platelet counts 50,000 per microliter. Significant myelosuppression, leading to infectious or bleeding complications, generally occurs as a result of intentional high-dose chemotherapy (e.g., leukemia induction regimen) or in patients with tumors that involve the bone marrow. It is of critical importance to make certain that recent blood counts are available and that drug dosages are calculated accurately before the drugs are given. Preferably drug dosages should be calculated by two individuals before administration.

NAUSEA AND VOMITING Most but not all anticancer drugs cause nausea and vomiting, and despite substantial advances in antiemetic therapy, prevention of chemotherapy-induced nausea and vomiting continues to be a therapeutic challenge. At present, the treatment of choice involves metoclopramide plus dexamethasone-containing regimens. However, their use does not always prevent or relieve nausea and vomiting induced by highly emetogenic chemotherapy. Factors which influence whether or not nausea and vomiting

TABLE 301-8 Diseases in which chemotherapy has minor activity

Cancer	Drugs currently preferred	Alternative drugs
Colorectal	Fluorouracil + levamisole Intraarterial floxuridine (hepatic metastases)	Semustine,* mitomycin, leucovorin, + fluorouracil
Liver	Doxorubicin or fluorouracil	Floxuridine, intraarterial floxuridine
Lung (non-small cell)	Cyclophosphamide + doxorubicin + cisplatin (CAP) Vindesine† or vinblastine + cisplatin ± mitomycin Cisplatin + etoposide	Methotrexate + doxorubicin + cyclophosphamide + lomustine (MACC) Fluorouracil + doxorubicin + mitomycin (FAM) Methotrexate, mitomycin, carboplatin*
Melanoma	Interleukin 2* ± lymphokine activated killer (LAK) cells*; dacarbazine; semustine*	Dactinomycin, carmustine, interferon
Pancreatic	Fluorouracil Fluorouracil + doxorubicin + mitomycin (FAM) Streptozocin + mitomycin + fluorouracil (SMF)	Mitomycin, leuprolide acetate
Renal	Interleukin 2* or interferon	Vinblastine, lomustine, progestins

* Available in the USA only for investigational use.
† Not available in United States.
SOURCE: Adapted from *The Medical Letter*, June 2, 1989, with permission.

will occur or will be serious include: (1) the nature of the drug, (2) drug dosage, (3) schedule of administration (i.e., daily vs. repeated single doses), (4) time of day the drug is given, (5) the rate of administration (when given intravenously), and (6) combination drug therapy.

MECHANISMS OF NAUSEA AND VOMITING AND ANTIEMETIC PHARMACOLOGY The mechanisms by which antineoplastic drugs induce nausea and vomiting remain unclear, but the chemotrigger zone (CTZ) and emetic center of the brain appear to be involved. Emetogenic substances can reach the CTZ via the blood or cerebro-

FIGURE 301-5 Sites and mechanism of action of chemotherapeutic drugs.

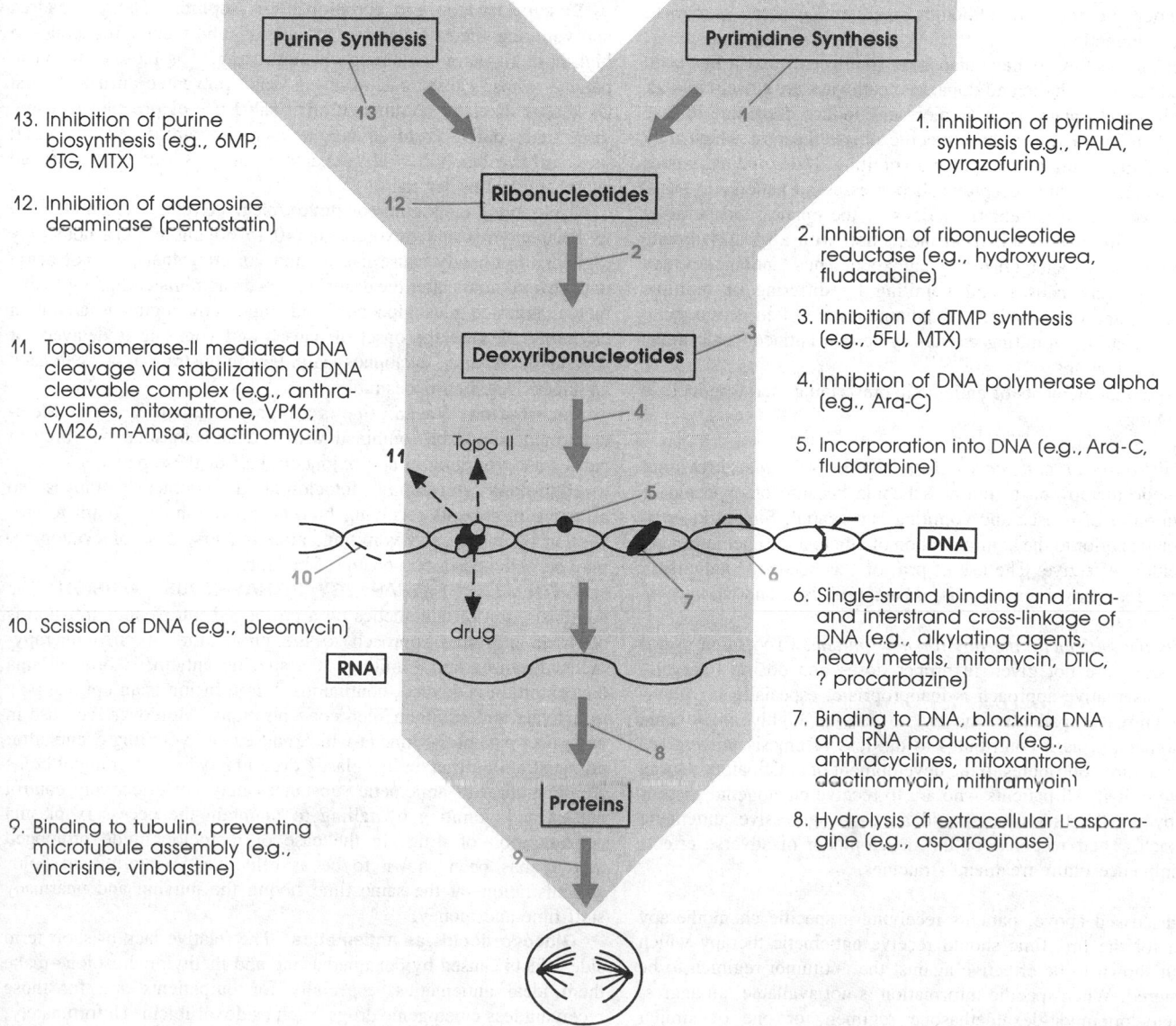

spinal fluid. Dopamine release induced by these drugs and subsequent dopamine binding to specific receptors in the emetic center may initiate nausea and vomiting. Many antineoplastic drugs are thought to cause nausea and vomiting through stimulation of the CTZ. However, there are many other neurotransmitters in this region, and a combination of neurotransmitters may be responsible for initiating nausea and vomiting.

Stimuli from outside the central nervous system (e.g., gastrointestinal tract) can induce nausea and vomiting. Peripheral stimuli travel via vagal and sympathetic afferents directly to the vomiting center. In cats with a surgically ablated CTZ, mechlorethamine and cisplatin can induce vomiting, presumably by stimulation of peripheral gastrointestinal pathways which may involve an interaction with peripheral serotonin receptors. In animals and in human beings, some antiserotonergic compounds have been shown to delay and, in some cases, to prevent the emetic actions of cisplatin, cyclophosphamide, and doxorubicin.

The response to sight and smell of higher centers in the brain can lead to nausea and vomiting. When anticipatory nausea and vomiting is present, stimulation of these centers may be involved. Vestibular pathways influenced by motion or movement may also contribute to nausea and vomiting after chemotherapy. This may in part explain why inpatients often experience better emesis control than outpatients receiving identical treatment. Further evidence that vestibular pathways may play a role in the causation of nausea and vomiting is provided by the fact that the anticholinergic drug scopolamine has been shown to be a useful addition to the metoclopramide-dexamethasone antiemetic regimen, although scopolamine alone is not an effective antiemetic.

Enkephalin pathways have also been implicated, and it has been suggested that enkephalin and dopamine pathways are closely linked. Enkephalins and opiates such as morphine induce dopamine release through their interaction with a specific opiate receptor which may be involved in stimulating nausea and vomiting. Naloxone has a poor binding affinity for this receptor and possesses no antiemetic properties. However, the antiemetic actions of the opiates and possibly the cannabinoids may result from interaction with a separate opiate receptor that can be antagonized by naloxone. Thus, antiemetics may reduce or prevent nausea and vomiting by differing or multiple mechanisms; and combinations of antiemetics are often necessary to prevent nausea and vomiting caused by certain antineoplastic drugs or drug combinations.

The essential elements of antiemetic prescribing therefore include the following:

1 *Administration of antiemetics on a routine schedule.* Providing antiemetic therapy on a routine schedule because of expected or known onset of nausea and vomiting is essential. Single doses of antiemetics prior to the administration of emetogenic chemotherapy are seldom effective. The use of prn, or "as needed," antiemetic therapy for known emetogens is inappropriate and should be discouraged.

2 *Aggressive antiemetic therapy for new patients.* Too often useful antiemetics are not given in proper doses and dosing intervals. This conservative approach is inappropriate, especially for previously untreated patients who are to receive highly emetogenic chemotherapy, as it contributes to the loss of emesis prevention, which in turn contributes to the development of anticipatory nausea and vomiting. All patients who are to receive emetogenic chemotherapy for the first time should have an aggressive antiemetic approach. Their response or the development of adverse effects will influence future treatment strategies.

As discussed above, patients receiving a specific chemotherapy regimen for the first time should receive antiemetic therapy which has been shown to be effective against the antitumor regimen to be administered. When specific information is not available, an aggressive metoclopramide-dexamethasone regimen, or one of similar

efficacy, should be described. The duration of antiemetic therapy will depend on the expected time course for the development of nausea and vomiting. Patients who previously experienced unsuccessful antiemetic therapy should have their previous regimen examined and optimized. If "optimal" antiemetic therapy was previously given and yet was unsuccessful, these patients should be considered for enrollment into clinical trials exploring new antiemetic treatments. Patients with refractory nausea and vomiting may benefit from heavy sedation and close inpatient monitoring during subsequent courses of chemotherapy.

ANTIEMETIC THERAPY FOR SPECIFIC ANTICANCER TREATMENTS Cisplatin, first 24 h Cisplatin is one of the most emetogenic antineoplastic drugs. Almost all patients receiving cisplatin will experience nausea and vomiting if no antiemetic protection is provided. However, metoclopramide plus dexamethasone regimens have been particularly effective. Major protection (fewer than two vomiting episodes) from cisplatin-induced nausea and vomiting occurs in 50 to 75 percent of the patients, but complete prevention rates are usually considerably lower.

Most commonly, metoclopramide, 2 mg/kg, is given intravenously every 2 h for four or five doses beginning 30 min prior to cisplatin administration. Dexamethasone, 10 to 20 mg intravenously, is also given 30 min before cisplatin and in many centers repeated with each metoclopramide dose. Alternatively, metoclopramide, 3 mg/kg, is given intravenously 30 min before and 1.5 h after cisplatin (with dexamethasone as above); this approach is as effective in a 2 mg/kg regimen and more suitable as an outpatient antiemetic regimen.

Delayed nausea and vomiting after cisplatin Delayed nausea and vomiting occurs frequently in patients who receive moderate- to high-dose cisplatin-containing chemotherapy; it is most common in patients whose nausea and vomiting is not prevented during the first 24 h after cisplatin administration. Oral doses of prochlorperazine, three times daily, 10 to 20 mg, or metoclopramide, 30 to 40 mg, used in combination with dexamethasone, 8 mg, have proved successful in this setting.

Cyclophosphamide and/or doxorubicin Cyclophosphamide (500 to 1000 mg/m^2) and doxorubicin (40 to 60 mg/m^2) chemotherapy regimens frequently cause nausea and vomiting that may not begin until several hours after the drugs have been administered. Aggressive metoclopramide plus glucocorticoid antiemetic regimens are often effective. Because the onset of nausea and vomiting is delayed for several hours after cyclophosphamide administration, an extended antiemetic regimen is desirable.

Dacarbazine Dacarbazine is a highly emetogenic agent. Metoclopramide alone or combined with a dexamethasone will prevent nausea and vomiting in approximately half of these patients.

High-dose cytarabine Metoclopramide antiemetic therapy is also effective in patients receiving high-dose cytarabine. Complete prevention of nausea and vomiting, after the first dose of cytarabine, may be obtained in 50 percent of patients.

ANTIEMETIC THERAPY BY INTRAVENOUS INFUSION The administration of antiemetics by a prolonged intravenous infusion is often an effective approach to the prevention of chemotherapy-induced nausea and vomiting. If a specific antiemetic drug plasma concentration is desired, continuous drug infusion is an optimal way to activate and maintain such concentrations. Moreover, because in any given patient the time at which nausea and vomiting occurs after administration of an antineoplastic drug may vary, intermittent bolus administration of antiemetic substances may not effectively control nausea and vomiting by failing to maintain the necessary plasma concentration of drug. In the case of metoclopramide prolonged therapy has been shown to be as effective as intermittent bolus administration, at the same time saving the nursing and pharmacy staff time and money.

Glucocorticoids as antiemetics The relative lack of short-term side effects caused by dexamethasone and methylprednisolone make them ideal antiemetics, especially for outpatients and for those receiving less emetogenic drugs, such as doxorubicin. Unfortunately, glucocorticoid antiemetic treatment alone is not optimal for patients receiving highly emetogenic drugs.

Benzodiazepines as adjuncts to antiemetic therapy The benzodiazepines have little, if any, antiemetic value by themselves. Their major effects are sedative, hypnotic, skeletal muscle relaxant, and amnesic; all of these may be desirable in some patients receiving emetogenic chemotherapy. Lorazepam is widely used as an adjunctive agent with metoclopramide-dexamethasone regimens; it lessens the anxiety associated with chemotherapy administration.

STOMATITIS AND MUCOSITIS Stomatitis is an inflammatory response of the oral mucosa and intraoral soft tissue structures that is not an uncommon response following the administration of cytotoxic drugs. Although there is much variability between individual patients, stomatitis is a complication of chemotherapy that is both drug- and dose-related. Almost all the anticancer drugs will cause stomatitis if a large enough dose is given. Patients undergoing induction chemotherapy for treatment of acute leukemia or as a preparative regimen before bone marrow transplantation are most likely to develop stomatitis. Some drugs, such as fluorouracil, cause stomatitis much more frequently than others. Stomatitis caused by methotrexate has been shown to be more a function of the duration of treatment rather than of peak drug plasma levels. The same is probably true for most, if not all, antitumor antimetabolites.

Early signs of stomatitis include mild erythema and edema of the buccal mucosa and/or tongue. This generalized inflammation may progress to painful ulcerations and secondary infections. Mouth sores usually occur 7 to 14 days after a dose of chemotherapy and take at least 7 days to heal after chemotherapy is discontinued. Stomatitis may lead to complications such as malnutrition (i.e., it may be too painful to eat), dehydration (i.e., pain on swallowing may prevent all oral intake), bleeding may be a sign of problems (such as thrombocytopenia), infection, and refusal of interruption of therapy.

The treatment of stomatitis includes good oral hygiene and providing pain relief. Topical anesthetics (e.g., viscous xylocaine) or mixtures containing a topical anesthetic may be needed, especially if the stomatitis interferes with eating. However, reducing subsequent doses of anticancer drugs may be necessary in patients with moderate to severe stomatitis.

ALOPECIA Antineoplastic drugs used singly or in combination often cause significant hair loss from the scalp. Although hair loss may seem relatively trivial compared to other side effects, it is often the most psychologically distressing complication of cancer chemotherapy. The hair loss produced by antineoplastic drugs is patchy and not similar to natural balding or thinning. It occurs over a few days, becoming maximal approximately 2 to 3 weeks after chemotherapy. The loss of hair is drug- and dose-dependent. The anthracyclines (doxorubicin and daunorubicin), cyclophosphamide, and vincristine commonly cause alopecia; but other drugs can also cause alopecia by themselves or in combination.

Scalp cooling undertaken for 30 to 60 min during and after treatment, can reduce hair loss. It is believed that when it works, it is due to decreased uptake of drugs by hair follicles.

REPRODUCTIVE EFFECTS Menstrual cycle changes (i.e., irregular periods, cessation of menses) in women and azoospermia in men, with elevation of serum follicle stimulating hormone (FSH), are relatively common side effects of chemotherapy. They occur more frequently with alkylating agents and patients receiving very intensive therapy. Men with Hodgkin's disease receiving 12 or more months of MOPP (mechlorethamine, oncovin, procarbazine, and prednisone) can all expect to become azoospermic. Sperm counts generally do not fully recover until 2 to 5 years after treatment has been discontinued. Ovarian dysfunction in women varies and appears to be related to age at the start of treatment, the specific drugs given, drug dose, and concomitant radiation therapy administered below the diaphragm. Almost all women with ovarian cancer receiving alkylating agents experience disruption of the menstrual cycle with a return to normal following completion of therapy.

In a retrospective study of over 2000 children who had received cancer chemotherapy during childhood or adolescence compared to a matched control group, fertility was not altered in the female group but was markedly decreased in males. Boys who received alkylating agents with or without radiation therapy below the diaphragm had a 60 percent decrease in fertility. This effect was greater if treatment was given after their fifteenth birthday than if given before.

Premenopausal women receiving adjuvant CMF (cyclophosphamide, methotrexate, fluorouracil) chemotherapy for breast cancer develop ovarian dysfunction that correlates with increasing age and duration of treatment. Nearly all women over 40 develop ovarian dysfunction after 4 to 6 months of treatment. Younger women may not have menstrual irregularities despite longer chemotherapy.

In men with testicular cancer, low sperm counts and/or abnormal sperm motility are often present before orchiectomy and may be accompanied by elevated levels of gonadotropins. Following aggressive cisplatin-etoposide (or vinblastine)-bleomycin chemotherapy, further impairment of spermatogenesis occurs, but is usually temporary. Full recovery of spermatogenesis is less likely in patients over age 30 receiving intensive chemotherapy and radiotherapy below the diaphragm.

REFERENCES

CUBEDDU LX et al: Efficacy of ondansetron (GR38032F) and the role of serotonin in cisplatin-induced nausea and vomiting. N Engl J Med 322:810, 1990

DEVITA VT JR: Principles of Chemotherapy, in *Cancer: Principles & Practice of Oncology,* 3d ed, VT DeVita Jr, S Hellman, SA Rosenberg (eds). Philadelphia, Lippincott, 1989, pp 276–300

DILLMAN RO: Monoclonal antibodies for treating cancer. Ann Intern Med 111:592, 1989

GOLDSTEIN LJ et al: Expression of a multidrug resistance gene in human cancers. J Natl Cancer Inst 81:116, 1989

GRECO FA, HAINSWORTH JD: The management of patients with adenocarcinoma and poorly differentiated carcinoma of unknown primary site. Semin Oncol 16:116, 1989

MUGGIA FM, NORRIS JR K: Future of cancer chemotherapy with cisplatin. Semin Oncol 16:123, 1989

302 THE MALIGNANT LYMPHOMAS

LEE M. NADLER

The malignant lymphomas, in contrast to leukemias, are neoplastic transformations of cells that reside predominantly in lymphoid tissues. The two major variants of malignant lymphoma are non-Hodgkin's lymphoma and Hodgkin's disease. Although both of these tumors infiltrate reticuloendothelial organs, their biologic and clinical behaviors suggest that they are probably not related. Table 302-1 compares non-Hodgkin's and Hodgkin's lymphomas with regard to cellular derivation, sites of disease, presence of systemic symptomatology, chromosomal translocations, and curability. This comparison supports the notion that they are fundamentally different diseases.

TABLE 302-1 The malignant lymphomas

	Non-Hodgkin's	Hodgkin's
Cellular derivation	90% B Cell 10% T Cell Rare monocytic	Unresolved
Sites of disease		
Localized	Uncommon	Common
Nodal spread	Discontiguous	Contiguous
Extranodal	Common	Uncommon
Mediastinal	Uncommon	Common
Abdominal	Common	Uncommon
Bone marrow	Common	Uncommon
B systemic symptoms*	Uncommon	Common
Chromosomal translocation	Common	Yet to be described
Curability	<25%	>75%

* Fever, night sweats, weight loss of greater than 10% of body weight.

CELLULAR AND DEVELOPMENTAL ASPECTS

To date, biologic studies have provided no clearcut explanations for the differences demonstrated in Table 302-1. It is important to examine the cellular origins of these tumors in an attempt to relate the neoplastic cell to its normal cellular counterpart. By understanding the lineage and corresponding normal stage of differentiation, it should be eventually possible to further group these tumors biologically according to cellular origin, ability to localize within specific microenvironments, propensity to further differentiate in vivo, production of cytokines, and response to therapy.

Non-Hodgkin's and Hodgkin's can be morphologically classified as shown in Tables 302-2 and 302-7. In order to understand the lineage derivation of these histologically defined subtypes, it is necessary to examine the normal populations of cells that reside in lymphoid tissues. To this end, B- and T-cell ontogeny will be reviewed and within this context the neoplastic lymphoma cell related to its normal cellular counterpart. Although histologic subtype is still the major basis for therapeutic decisions, the definition of immunologic phenotype is becoming more useful for classifying difficult cases.

Lymphocytes can be functionally subdivided into distinct populations by their expression of unique cell surface and molecular markers. In the past, human B cells were identified by their expression of cell surface or cytoplasmic immunoglobulin and their capacity to produce immunoglobulin. In contrast, human T lymphocytes were classically defined by the expression of sheep red blood cell receptors and their ability to regulate immune responses. During the past decade, the development of well-characterized monoclonal antibodies (MAbs) directed against T-cell surface molecules expressed on human lymphoid cells has led to very significant advances in both the phenotypic and functional characterization of these cells. MAbs have been useful in assigning cellular lineage and identifying normal stages of lymphoid differentiation. Similarly, molecular biologic techniques demonstrating gene rearrangements have been helpful in defining lineage, clonality, and, to a lesser extent, stage of differentiation.

NORMAL B-CELL ONTOGENY   Cell surface antigens   Normal B-cell ontogeny has been operationally divided into stages, namely pre-B cell, mature or resting B cell, activated/proliferating B cell, differentiating B cell, and plasma cell or secretory B cell (Fig. 302-1). These stages are delineated by the expression of unique cytoplasmic and cell surface antigens. Antigens can be clustered into pre-B, resting-B, activated-B, and plasma-cell subgroups. In addition, there are pan-B antigens. Several antigens have been useful in defining B-cell lineage since within the hematopoietic system they are uniquely expressed on B lymphocytes. Two of the most useful antigens are CD19 and CD20. Both are strongly expressed on the cell surface and, more importantly, their expression spans ontogeny from the early pre-B cells to the terminal stages of differentiation.

The most primitive pre-B cells have been defined by their coexpression of cell surface antigens, including Ia (of the major histocompatibility complex class II), CD19, and CD24. Stages of pre-B-cell ontogeny have been delineated by the sequential expression of CD10 (common acute lymphoblastic leukemia antigen, CALLA), CD20, and finally the appearance of cytoplasmic immunoglobulin mu (cμ) heavy chains without the expression of light chains. As pre-B cells mature, they are exported to the peripheral blood and lymphoid tissues where they reside until activated by antigen (mature B cell; Fig. 302-1).

Mature resting B cells continue to express cell surface Ia, CD antigens 19, 20, and 24, but no longer CD10. These cells also express cell surface immunoglobulins IgM and IgD (the B-cell antigen receptor); CD21, which is the receptor for the C3d cleavage fragment of complement and for Epstein-Barr virus (EBV); CD35, which is the C3b complement receptor; and CD22.

Following triggering by antigen or other signals of activation, mature resting B cells are activated and subsequently proliferate. In vitro, in vivo, and in situ studies show that the activation of resting B cells is accompanied by a sequence of cell surface antigenic changes. Resting B cells begin to lose cell surface IgD, CD21, and CD22. As these antigens are lost, a number of other antigens appear sequentially. These *activation antigens* are cell surface molecules involved in the regulation of cellular proliferation and/or differentiation or alternatively in the localization and binding of activated B cells. Activation antigens can be divided into those that are B-cell associated and those that are B-cell restricted. In the first group are CD71 (transferrin receptor), CD54 (ICAM-1, involved in homotypic aggregation), CD25 (low-affinity IL-2 receptor), CD5, and CD23 (low-affinity IgE receptor). Those that are B-cell restricted include B5, BB-1/B7, and Bac-1.

During differentiation there is a sequential loss of the B-cell activation antigens as well as pan-B-cell antigens, including Ia, CD19, -20, and -24. This stage is also characterized by the appearance of CD38 and PCA-1, which are expressed on plasma cells (secretory B cell).

Immunoglobulin gene rearrangements   A vast variety and number of possible immunoglobulin molecules exist, each corresponding to a unique antigenic epitope. This diversity is thought to result from genetic recombination within the DNA of B lymphocytes. The germline DNA contains segments coding for different subunits of the immunoglobulin molecule. For the immunoglobulin heavy chain, these consist of a very large number of different variable (V) segments, a smaller number of different diversity (D) segments, a few joining (J) segments, and a constant region for each subclass of immunoglobulin.

The usual mechanism for achieving recombination of the immunoglobulin heavy chain genes involves joining together single V, D, and J segments with the appropriate constant region segment and excising the unused segments. Therefore, the numbers of potential recombinants of V, D, and J segments are enormous. Light chain

TABLE 302-2   Histologic classification of non-Hodgkin's lymphoma

Working formulation, malignant lymphoma	Rappaport terminology	Cellular origin, % B	Cellular origin, % T	Chromosomal abnormalities
Low-grade				
A Small lymphocytic cell	Diffuse well-differentiated lymphocytic (DWDL)	98	2	Trisomy 12 t(11;14) t(14;19)
B Follicular, predominantly small cleaved cell	Nodular poorly differentiated lymphocytic (NPDL)	100		t(14;18)
C Follicular mixed, small cleaved and large cell	Nodular mixed lymphocytic histiocytic (NM)	100		t(14;18) Trisomy 8
Intermediate-grade				
D Follicular, predominantly large cell	Nodular histiocytic (NH)	100		Trisomy 7
E Diffuse small cleaved cell	Diffuse poorly differentiated lymphocytic (DPDL)	80	20	
F Diffuse mixed, small and large cell	Diffuse mixed lymphocytic-histiocytic (DM)	90	10	Trisomy 3
G Diffuse large cell	Diffuse histiocytic (DH)	80	20	Trisomy 7,18 t(14;18)
High-grade				
H Large cell immunoblastic	Diffuse histiocytic (DH)	80	20	
I Lymphoblastic	Diffuse lymphoblastic (LL)	10	90	
J Small noncleaved cell; Burkitt's	Diffuse undifferentiated (DUL)	95	5	t(8;14)

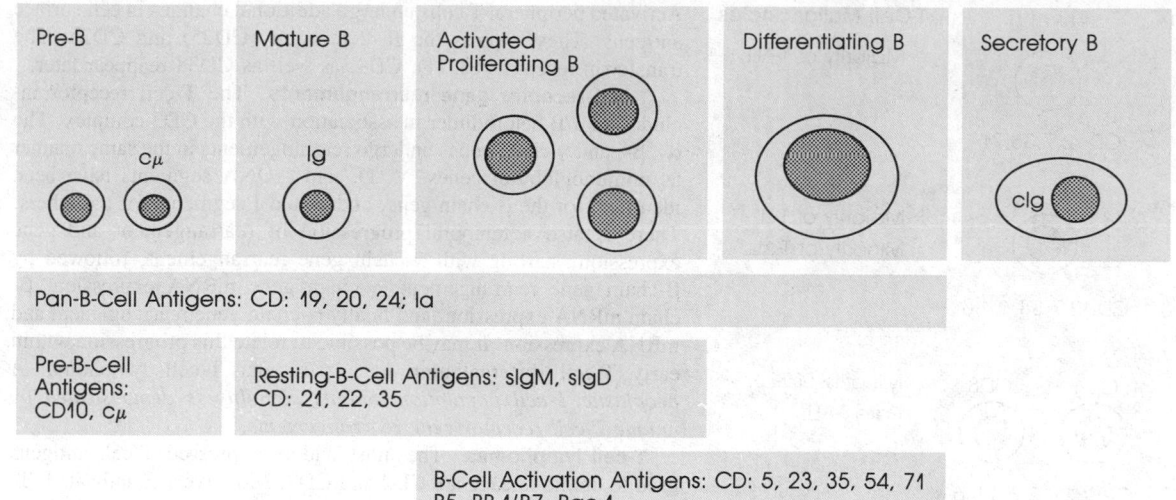

Pan-B-Cell Antigens: CD: 19, 20, 24; Ia

Pre-B-Cell Antigens: CD10, cμ

Resting-B-Cell Antigens: sIgM, sIgD CD: 21, 22, 35

B-Cell Activation Antigens: CD: 5, 23, 35, 54, 71 B5, BB-1/B7, Bac-1

Plasma Cell Antigens: CD38 PCA-1

FIGURE 302-1   Stages of normal B-cell ontogeny.

genes lack D segments but have a similar mechanism of rearrangement. A functional rearrangement of a heavy or light chain gene prevents rearrangements of another gene of the same chain type (allelic exclusion); however, an abnormal heavy or light chain rearrangement that cannot be transcribed will allow the other heavy chain allele or one of the other light chain alleles, respectively, to attempt rearrangement. This functional allelic exclusion insures that only one immunoglobulin is allowed for any one B cell. The heavy chain gene undergoes rearrangement first, followed by the kappa and then the lambda light chain genes. Clonal rearrangement of immunoglobulin genes is consistent with a B-cell lineage derivation of a lymphoma.

MALIGNANT LYMPHOMAS OF B-CELL ORIGIN   As seen in Table 302-2, more than 90 percent of all cases of non-Hodgkin's lymphomas are of B-cell derivation. This observation is based upon the expression of B-lineage–restricted antigens as well as clonal rearrangements of immunoglobulin heavy and light chain genes. Non-T-cell acute lymphoblastic leukemias antigenically correspond to discrete stages of pre-B-cell development. It is noteworthy that no B-cell neoplasm phenotypically corresponds to the resting B lymphocyte (mature B). Myelomas correspond to secretory B cells. Although most investigators have attempted to relate B-cell lymphomas to major steps of B-lymphocyte development (Fig. 302-1), it is becoming increasingly clear that these tumors correspond to major and minor subpopulations of activated/proliferating or differentiating B cells. All B-cell non-Hodgkin's lymphomas express the pan-B-cell antigens including Ia, CD19, and CD20. Moreover, virtually all B-

cell non-Hodgkin's lymphomas express one or more B-cell activation antigens. Although a common antigenic phenotype has been identified for each histologically defined subgroup, it should be stressed that significant antigenic heterogeneity exists within each subgroup. As indicated below, cell surface antigenic phenotype is considered within the context of the Working Formulation (Table 302-2). (MAbs commonly used in diagnosis of B-cell lymphomas are summarized in Table 302-3.)

Low-grade lymphoma   The commonest low-grade lymphomas are the small lymphocytic and follicular small cleaved cell lymphomas. Small lymphocytic lymphomas, like B-cell chronic lymphocytic leukemias, appear to correspond to a unique population of activated B cells that express pan-B-cell antigens as well as CD21, B5, and CD5. In contrast, follicular small cleaved cell lymphomas are thought to correspond to subpopulations of germinal center B cells. These lymphomas express pan-B-cell antigens and CD21, B5, and CD10. When small lymphocytic lymphomas or follicular small cleaved cell lymphomas "transform" and morphologically resemble diffuse large cell lymphoma cells, they retain their CD5 and CD10 positivity, respectively.

Intermediate-grade lymphoma   Within the intermediate-grade subgroup of B-cell lymphomas (Table 302-2), follicular large cell, diffuse large cell, and diffuse small cleaved cell lymphomas are immunologically distinct. Both subgroups of large cell lymphoma express pan-B-cell antigens and several B-cell activation antigens but less frequently express cell surface immunoglobulin or CD21. Follicular large cell, like follicular small cleaved cell lymphomas, express CD10, whereas B-cell diffuse large cell lymphomas are CD10 and CD5 negative. Diffuse small cleaved B-cell lymphomas morphologically and phenotypically resemble follicular small cleaved cell lymphomas. They both express pan-B-cell antigens and several of the B-cell activation antigens. Whereas follicular small cleaved cell lymphomas express CD10 and frequently demonstrate 14;18 translocations (see below), diffuse small cleaved cell lymphomas do not. A subgroup of diffuse small cleaved cell lymphomas, termed *mantle zone lymphomas*, are phenotypically identical to diffuse small cleaved cell lymphomas but also express CD5.

High-grade lymphoma   Large cell immunoblastic lymphomas are phenotypically identical to B-cell diffuse large cell lymphomas. In contrast, Burkitt's lymphomas are related to follicular lymphomas in that they express pan-B-cell antigens, B-cell activation antigens, and CD10. African Burkitt's cells express CD21 whereas the American variation does not.

TABLE 302-3   MAbs commonly used in diagnosis of B-cell lymphomas

CD	Common antibody terminology
5	Anti-T1, Leu 1, T101
10	J5, anti-CALLA, BA3
19	Anti-B4, anti-Leu 12
20	Anti-B1, anti-Leu 16, 1F5
21	Anti-B2
22	Anti-HD39 (anti-B3), SHCL-1
23	Anti-Blast-2 (anti-B5), MNM6
24	BA-1, J2
25	Anti-TAC, anti-IL-2R
38	Anti-T10
54	I-CAM-1
71	Anti-T9

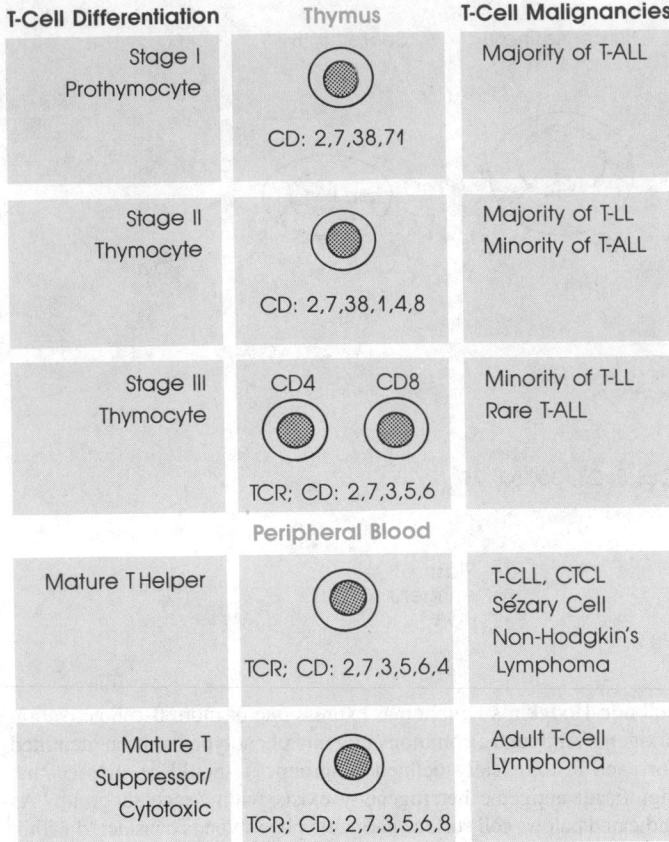

FIGURE 302-2   Correlation of T-cell differentiation and T-cell malignancies.

NORMAL T-CELL ONTOGENY   Cell surface antigens   A large number of MAbs have been developed that define cell surface antigens expressed on human T cells. These MAbs have been used to characterize the stages of T-cell ontogeny and differentiation, identify subsets of functionally distinct T cells, and elucidate the function of some of these cell surface antigens. Figure 302-2 summarizes the stages of normal T-cell ontogeny.

During embryonic and early postnatal development, bone marrow precursor cells migrate to the thymus. The thymic microenvironment provides a setting for the processing and eventual development of functionally competent T cells. These cells are subsequently exported into peripheral lymphoid tissues and the circulation. A sequence of changes in cell surface antigens identified by MAbs is observed to accompany intrathymic differentiation. The cells in the earliest stage (I) of intrathymic differentiation, which constitute 10 percent of the thymic lymphocytes, express CD2 (E-rosette receptor), CD71 (the transferrin receptor), CD38, and CD7.

Stage II thymocytes are characterized by the loss of CD71, the acquisition of CD1, and coexpression of CD4 and CD8. The population, coexpressing CD antigens 1, 2, 4, 7, 8, and 38, constitutes 70 percent of thymocytes.

With further maturation, cells lose CD1 and acquire mature T-cell antigens CD3, -5, and -6 (stage III). CD3 is a complex of chains that are noncovalently associated with the T-cell antigen receptor (TCR). In parallel with the expression of CD3, cells express TCR. It can exist as an α/β heterodimer and then recognizes antigen in the context of the major histocompatibility complex. A second T-cell receptor, also associated with CD3, is termed γ/δ. Cells that express the γ/δ TCR appear earlier in ontogeny than those expressing α/β. They are negative for CD4 and CD8 and are associated with natural killer cell (NK) activity.

When cells leave the thymus, they no longer express CD38 and are segregated into cells expressing either CD4 or CD8, constituting 60 to 70 percent and 30 to 40 percent of peripheral T cells, respectively.

Activated peripheral T cells undergo additional changes in cell surface antigens. They express the IL-2 receptor (CD25) and CD26. The transferrin receptor (CD71), CD9, as well as CD38 reappear later.

T-cell receptor gene rearrangements   The T-cell receptor includes an α/β heterodimer in association with the CD3 complex. The α-, β-, and γ-chain genes undergo rearrangements in the same manner as immunoglobulin genes. V, D, and J DNA segments have been identified for the β-chain gene, and V and J segments for the others. There is also a temporal progression of rearrangement and gene expression, starting with γ-chain gene rearrangement, followed by β-chain gene rearrangement, γ-chain gene mRNA expression, β-chain mRNA expression, and finally α-chain gene rearrangement and mRNA expression. It may be possible to relate this progression within early T-cell differentiation to a particular T-cell lymphoma. *A neoplastic T-cell population and its clonality is demonstrated by unique T-cell receptor gene rearrangements.*

T-cell lymphomas   The most widely expressed T-cell antigens used to define lineage are CD2 and CD7. Moreover, as indicated, T-cell neoplasms demonstrate rearrangement of TCR genes. As depicted in Fig. 302-2, T-cell malignancies clearly reflect distinct stages of T-cell ontogeny. Similar to B-cell neoplasms, the common antigenic phenotype for T-cell neoplasms will be presented; however, significant heterogeneity is observed within histologically defined subgroups.

Lymphoblastic lymphomas correspond to stage II thymocytes and the majority express CD1, -2, -4, -7, and -8. The remainder of the T-cell lymphomas correspond to mature T-cell populations (mature helper cells or mature cytotoxic/suppressor T cells). Although these tumors express the phenotype of mature functional T cells, few neoplasms retain function in vivo. Diffuse small cleaved cell and diffuse large cell lymphomas variably express the mature T-cell antigens CD2, -3, -5, -6, and -7. Most express CD4; a small fraction express CD8. Cutaneous T-cell lymphomas also express a mature phenotype: CD2, -3, -4, -5, and -7. Sézary cells generally lack CD7 and Ia antigens, whereas cells infiltrating the skin are CD7 positive and invariably express CD25 and CD71. Adult T-cell lymphomas are similar to the cutaneous T-cell lymphomas in that they express CD2, -3, -4, -5, and -7.

CELLULAR ORIGIN OF THE REED-STERNBERG CELL   Reed-Sternberg (RS) cells, in the appropriate cytoarchitectural milieu, are required for the diagnosis of Hodgkin's disease. The major obstacle to determining the cellular origin of Hodgkin's disease is the present inability to identify and isolate RS cells. Studies either have examined enriched populations of these cells or have examined them using immunologic staining techniques in tissue sections. As discussed below, evidence exists for both lymphoid and nonlymphoid origin. Unfortunately, these studies have been complicated by the contaminating effect of normal populations mixed with RS cells.

In Hodgkin's disease tissues the majority of cells are small lymphocytes with a "normal" T-cell phenotype (CD2, -3, -4 or -8, and -5) together with a variable number of presumably nonneoplastic B cells. Reed-Sternberg cells and their variants may be immunologically distinguished from the neoplastic cells of most non-Hodgkin's lymphomas by their lack of most T- and B-cell–associated antigens. Reed-Sternberg cells may contain intracellular immunoglobulin but this is polyclonal and is not thought to be produced by the RS cell. These cells express CD25 (low affinity IL-2 receptor) and the transferrin receptor (CD71), which are also expressed on activated B, activated T, and activated NK cells. They also express Ia antigens, certain antigens expressed on myeloid cells (e.g., CD13), receptors for peanut lectin, and the epithelial membrane antigen. Of great interest is the observation that RS cells of the lymphocyte-predominant form express the leukocyte common antigen (CD45R) whereas all other RS cells are negative.

Two unique antigens are expressed on the RS cell, and therefore MAbs directed against these antigens have proven to be diagnostically useful. The first is the Leu M1 antigen, which is expressed on RS cells in all subtypes of Hodgkin's disease except for the lymphocyte-predominant variant. The second antigen is the Ki-1 (CD30) antigen, which is expressed on virtually all RS cells. The Ki-1 antigen also is expressed on some activated B cells, activated T cells, EBV-transformed cell lines, and tumor cells isolated from some patients with immunoblastic lymphomas. Of great interest is the expression of CD30 on dendritic cells. Although these antigens are useful in the diagnosis of Hodgkin's disease, they have not been helpful in defining cellular lineage.

Recent molecular studies of RS-enriched populations have demonstrated immunoglobulin gene rearrangements in some specimens and T-cell β-chain rearrangements in others. Clonal rearrangements have not been seen in background lymphocytes. Although rearrangements of the T-cell γ-chain genes have been observed, they should not be misconstrued as evidence for a clonal T-cell origin since this gene may not provide evidence for clonality.

The lineage derivation of the RS cell is still unknown. Reed-Sternberg cells are not only observed in Hodgkin's disease but may be seen in small numbers in several variants of non-Hodgkin's lymphomas. Experts in the field believe that Hodgkin's disease is derived from subpopulations of activated B cells, activated T cells, or dendritic cells. The lack of expression of B- and T-lineage–restricted markers and lack of expression of the leukocyte common antigen suggest that they do not correspond to a known stage of B- or T-cell ontogeny. It is impossible to rigorously compare Hodgkin's to dendritic cells (either interdigitating or follicular) since these cells are also poorly characterized. Therefore, these studies support the notion that Hodgkin's and non-Hodgkin's lymphomas are derived from distinct cellular populations. Moreover, their distinct biologic and clinical behaviors (Table 302-1) are most probably a reflection of their divergent cellular origins.

NON-HODGKIN'S LYMPHOMA

EPIDEMIOLOGY About 30,000 new cases of non-Hodgkin's lymphoma occur each year in the United States and this number appears to be rising. Although the total number of patients is relatively small compared to some of the more common solid tumors, the malignant lymphomas are the commonest neoplasm of patients between the ages of 20 and 40. Moreover, they rank fourth in the total number of person-years of life lost each year from cancer. With the increasing incidence of acquired immunodeficiency syndrome (AIDS), the number of cases of non-Hodgkin's lymphoma has begun to increase sharply.

ETIOLOGY Animal studies suggest that lymphomas have a viral etiology. A herpesvirus has been isolated in avians, and C-type retroviruses have been identified in rodents, cows, and subhuman primates with lymphocytic lymphomas. In contrast, only endemic African Burkitt's lymphoma and adult T-cell lymphoma have been shown to have a viral etiology in humans. Thus, EBV has a strong association with the development of Burkitt's lymphoma, and the human T-cell leukemia virus appears to be the causative agent in adult T-cell lymphoma.

Although limited progress has been made in identifying agents that might be involved in inducing non-Hodgkin's lymphomas, exciting advances have been made in identifying those genes that appear to be involved in lymphomatous transformation. Cytogenetic abnormalities have been well documented in a number of non-Hodgkin's lymphomas (Table 302-2). DNA sequence analysis of several of these chromosomal translocations has demonstrated that genes that normally regulate heavy and light chain immunoglobulin synthesis have been juxtaposed to genes that regulate normal cellular activation and proliferation. It is postulated that these transforming genes or *oncogenes* have come under the control of those regulatory elements that normally control B-cell proliferation and differentiation. The best-studied example is the 14;8 translocation of Burkitt's lymphoma (see Chap. 7). In this disease, the c-*myc* oncogene on chromosome 8 is joined to the immunoglobulin heavy chain locus on chromosome 14. Another example is the 14;18 translocation

TABLE 302-4   Diseases or exposures associated with increased risk of development of malignant lymphoma

Inherited immunodeficiency diseases
  Klinefelter's syndrome
  Chédiak-Higashi syndrome
  Ataxia telangiectasia syndrome
  Wiscott-Aldrich syndrome
  Common variable immunodeficiency disease
Acquired immunodeficiency diseases
  Iatrogenic immunosuppression
  Acquired immunodeficiency syndrome
  Acquired hypogammaglobulinemia
Autoimmune diseases
  Sjögren's syndrome
  Nontropical sprue
  Rheumatoid arthritis and systemic lupus erythematosus
Chemical or drug exposures
  Phenytoin
  Radiation
  Prior combination chemotherapy and radiation therapy
Viral association (other than HIV)
  Epstein-Barr virus
  Human T-cell leukemia virus

commonly seen in follicular lymphomas where the oncogene termed *bcl*-2 (chromosome 18) is juxtaposed to the immunoglobulin heavy chain locus (chromosome 14). Table 302-2 summarizes the major chromosomal translocations associated with histologic subtypes of non-Hodgkin's lymphomas (see also Chap. 10).

In a number of primary diseases, increasingly often there is subsequent development of non-Hodgkin's lymphoma and, to a lesser extent, Hodgkin's disease. As seen in Table 302-4, diseases of inherited and acquired immunodeficiency as well as autoimmune diseases are associated with an increased incidence of lymphoma. Non-Hodgkin's lymphomas that occur in the context of drug-induced immunosuppression, acquired or congenital immunodeficiency, and AIDS are frequently associated with EBV. The association between immunosuppression and induction of non-Hodgkin's lymphomas appears to be compelling since, if the immunosuppression can be reversed (e.g., discontinuing immunosuppressive agents following organ transplantation), a percentage of these lymphomas regress spontaneously. The incidence of lymphoma in iatrogenic immuno-suppression, AIDS, and autoimmune disease argues strongly for immune dysregulation contributing to the development of lymphoma. Patients with certain environmental exposures have a higher incidence of lymphomas. Patients with Hodgkin's disease treated with radiation therapy and chemotherapy exhibit an increased risk of developing secondary large cell lymphomas. Lymphoma-like syndromes have also been found in patients treated with phenytoin. Although in most cases this disease regresses when the drug is stopped, a significant number of patients still develop true malignant lymphoma.

CLINICAL PRESENTATION AND DIFFERENTIAL DIAGNOSIS More than two-thirds of patients with non-Hodgkin's lymphoma present with persistent painless peripheral lymphadenopathy. At the time of presentation, differential diagnosis includes infections caused by bacteria, viruses (e.g., infectious mononucleosis, cytomegalovirus, and human immunodeficiency virus), and parasites (toxoplasmosis). In young patients, Hodgkin's lymphoma must be excluded. In older patients, other neoplasms must be considered. It is generally agreed that a firm spherical lymph node larger than 1 cm that is not associated with a documentable infection and that persists longer than 4 to 6 weeks should be biopsied. Certain clinical features suggest the diagnosis of non-Hodgkin's lymphoma. Involvement of Waldeyer's ring, epitrochlear, and mesenteric nodes are more suggestive of non-Hodgkin's than Hodgkin's. Unlike patients with Hodgkin's disease, who can present with weight loss, fever, or night sweats (so-called B symptoms), it is less common for patients with non-Hodgkin's lymphoma to present with systemic complaints.

Non-Hodgkin's lymphoma patients also present with chest, abdominal, or extranodal symptomatology. Although much less commonly than with Hodgkin's disease, approximately 20 percent of patients with non-Hodgkin's lymphoma have mediastinal adenopathy. These patients most frequently present with persistent cough, chest discomfort, or without symptoms but having an abnormal chest x-ray. Occasionally a superior vena cava syndrome accompanies presentation, especially in patients with T-cell lymphomas and, to a lesser extent, in those with B-cell diffuse large cell lymphoma. Differential diagnosis includes infections (e.g., histoplasmosis, tuberculosis, or infectious mononucleosis), sarcoidosis, Hodgkin's disease, as well as other neoplasms. Involvement of retroperitoneal, mesenteric, and pelvic nodes is common in most histologic subtypes of non-Hodgkin's lymphoma. Unless massive or leading to obstruction, these nodes usually produce no symptoms. In contrast, patients who come to medical attention because of an abdominal mass, massive splenomegaly, or primary gastrointestinal lymphoma present with complaints similar to those caused by other abdominal space-occupying lesions. These complaints include chronic pain, abdominal fullness, early satiety, symptoms associated with visceral obstruction, or even acute perforation and gastrointestinal hemorrhage. Symptoms due to extralymphatic disease are common in some subtypes of diffuse non-Hodgkin's lymphoma but are uncommon in follicular lymphomas. Rarely, some patients present with symptoms of unexplained anemia. Those with diffuse non-Hodgkin's lymphomas can present with primary cutaneous lesions, testicular masses, acute spinal cord compression, solitary bone lesions, and rarely lymphomatous meningitis. Historically, primary non-Hodgkin's lymphoma of the central nervous system was a very rare form of diffuse non-Hodgkin's lymphoma. However with AIDS and the increasing use of high dose immunosuppressive therapy, lymphoma may soon be one of the most common types of primary brain tumors.

PATHOLOGIC CLASSIFICATION   Rappaport and Working Formulation classification schemes   The pathologic classification of non-Hodgkin's lymphomas has been difficult for both pathologists and clinicians. In 1966, Henry Rappaport presented the first clinically relevant classification scheme for non-Hodgkin's lymphomas. This classification was based on assessment of the overall pattern of lymph node architecture (low-power microscopy) as well as the cytology of the neoplastic cell (high-power microscopy). The Rappaport classification subdivides the non-Hodgkin's lymphomas into two major subtypes, namely *diffuse* and *nodular* (follicular). Nodular lymphomas retain some features of normal lymph nodes in that the neoplastic cells appear to form "germinal centers" (nodules). In contrast, in diffuse lymphomas, the normal cortical and paracortical lymph node architecture is largely effaced. Rappaport also divided non-Hodgkin's lymphomas into subgroups according to whether the malignant cell was (1) well differentiated, (2) poorly differentiated, or (3) histiocytic. This suggested that these tumors corresponded morphologically to distinct stages of lymphoid and monocytic differentiation. The importance of the Rappaport classification (Table 302-2) was that each histologically defined subtype of non-Hodgkin's lymphoma exhibited a unique natural history and response to therapy.

With the advent of modern immunology, the Rappaport classification proved to have several biologic defects. First, the term *histiocytic* was incorrect since virtually all of these tumors were of lymphoid origin. Second, certain clinical entities were not accounted for by the scheme. Therefore, in 1974 the Lukes and Collins and Kiel classification schemes were proposed. The strength of these two was that they were "immunologically correct." However, by the late 1970s, six independent pathologic schemes were in use throughout the world and therefore therapeutic trials could not be compared. Because of this confusion, a classification scheme termed the *Working Formulation* was proposed (Table 302-2). It incorporates the best features of the various classification systems and, more importantly, retains clinical relevance. The Working Formulation subdivides non-Hodgkin's lymphomas into *low-*, *intermediate-*, and *high-grade* subgroups, depending on their natural history. Low-grade lymphomas are characterized by an indolent clinical course; their natural history is not significantly altered by therapy. Intermediate- and high-grade

TABLE 302-5   Ann Arbor staging system

Stage I	Involvement in single lymph node region or single extralymphatic site.
Stage II	Involvement of two or more lymph node regions on the same side of the diaphragm. Can also include localized involvement of extralymphatic site (stage IIE).
Stage III	Involvement of lymph node regions or extralymphatic sites on both sides of the diaphragm.
Stage IV	Disseminated involvement of one or more extralymphatic organs with or without lymph node involvement.

NOTE: Substage A = asymptomatic patients; substage B = Patients with history of fever, sweats, or weight loss of greater than 10% bodyweight.

lymphomas are associated with very short survivals. With the advent of aggressive combination chemotherapeutic regimens, some of these tumors demonstrate long-term disease-free survivals. Table 302-2 compares the Working Formulation and the Rappaport classifications. In clinical practice these classification schemes are frequently used interchangeably.

The histologic diagnosis of non-Hodgkin's lymphoma can only be reliably made on examination of lymph-node morphology. Since this is one of the most difficult areas of diagnosis, most cases should be reviewed by a hematopathologist. This is crucial, since therapeutic options are based on histologic subtype and only rarely by stage. The presence of follicular or diffuse patterns of the nodal architecture therefore predicts natural history and curability.

STAGING AND DISEASE DETECTION   Conventional staging   The Ann Arbor staging system developed for Hodgkin's disease has also been used in staging non-Hodgkin's lymphomas. This staging system focuses on the number of tumor sites (nodal and extranodal), location, and the presence or absence of systemic symptoms. Table 302-5 summarizes this staging system. In stages I and II sites of disease are on the same side of the diaphragm. Stage III disease involves both sides of the diaphragm, whereas stage IV is defined as extranodal lymphomatous involvement, most frequently of the bone marrow and liver. Systemic symptoms (fever, weight loss, and night sweats, i.e., B symptoms) are much less common in non-Hodgkin's lymphomas than in Hodgkins disease and therefore are not as useful in predicting prognosis. It must be emphasized that this classification scheme was specifically developed for Hodgkin's disease, which disseminates principally by contiguous lymphatic extension. Since non-Hodgkin's lymphomas most frequently disseminate hematogenously, for them this staging system has proven to be less useful.

The concept of staging is much less important in non-Hodgkin's lymphoma than in Hodgkin's disease. Since only 10 percent of patients with follicular lymphoma have localized disease, most advanced-stage patients are treated similarly. The majority of patients with diffuse lymphomas have advanced-stage disease and are therefore treated systemically. Thus, staging is undertaken in non-Hodgkin's lymphomas to identify the small number of patients who can be treated with local therapy and to stratify within histologic subtypes in order to prognosticate and to assess the impact of therapeutic regimens.

Staging procedures after biopsy diagnosis   Staging must be undertaken in the context of the Working Formulation histologic grade. A suggested staging workup for patients with non-Hodgkin's lymphoma is summarized in Table 302-6. An organized approach to staging a patient with non-Hodgkin's lymphoma is mandatory. After the initial excisional biopsy and documentation of the pathologic and, when possible, immunologic subtype of disease, blood tests should be obtained, including complete blood count, routine chemistry, liver function test, and serum protein electrophoresis to document the presence of circulating monoclonal paraprotein. Indirect laryngoscopy is highly recommended. Waldeyer's ring involvement is often associated with intestinal involvement, and gastrointestinal contrast studies or endoscopy are indicated if the patient appears to have localized disease. Chest x-ray is used to exclude mediastinal and hilar adenopathy, pleural effusions, and pulmonary parenchymal infiltration. Chest

TABLE 302-6 Staging tests for malignant lymphomas

Test	Non-Hodgkin's	Hodgkin's
Essential		
1 Pathologic documentation by hematopathologist	X	X
2 Physical examination detailing nodal sites	X	X
3 Documentation of B symptoms	X	X
4 Laboratory evaluation of:		
a Complete blood counts	X	X
b Liver function tests	X	X
c Renal function tests	X	X
d Alkaline phosphatase	X	X
5 Chest roentgenogram	X	X
6 CT scan of abdomen and pelvis	X	X
7 Bone marrow biopsy—bilateral	X	—
Essential under certain circumstances		
1 Bilateral lymphogram of lower extremities	—	X
2 Bone marrow biopsy—bilateral	—	X
3 Whole chest CT scan (if chest roentgenogram is abnormal)	X	X
4 Exploratory laparotomy	—	X
5 Liver biopsy	X	X
Useful tests under certain circumstances		
1 Bilateral lymphogram of lower extremities	X	—
2 Exploratory laparotomy	X	—
3 Abdominal ultrasonogram	X	—
4 Radionuclide scans		
a Bone	X	X
b Liver-spleen	X	X
c Gallium	X	X
5 Head CT scan	X	—
6 Magnetic resonance imaging	X	X
7 Immunologic markers	X	X
8 Gene rearrangement studies	X	X
9 Chromosomal analysis	X	—

computed tomographic scan is used to assess more precisely the extent of disease and is not a required screening test. However, abdominopelvic CT scan is essential for accurate staging to assess lymphadenopathy in retroperitoneal, mesenteric, and retrocrural areas. Lymphangiography is less useful than in Hodgkin's disease, since common sites of disease in non-Hodgkin's lymphoma include nodes in the mesentery, hilum of liver, spleen, or kidneys, as well as nodes in the deep bony pelvis, none of which can be visualized by this procedure. The lymphogram may be an accurate predictor of intra-abdominal lymphoma since the majority of patients with a positive lymphogram also have disease in the liver and in abdominal nodes. The major advantage of lymphangiography over abdominopelvic CT scan is its ability to detect infiltrated but normal-sized retroperitoneal nodes. Bilateral percutaneous bone marrow biopsies must be performed, since the likelihood of lymphomatous involvement of the marrow is relatively high, especially in low-grade lymphoma, where marrow involvement occurs in 60 to 80 percent of cases. If there is any indication of hepatic abnormalities on blood tests or on liver scan, a liver biopsy is highly recommended.

More invasive tests are reserved for the uncommon presentation with stage I or II non-Hodgkin's lymphoma. While staging laparotomy may be performed in Hodgkin's disease, this is not so in the non-Hodgkin's lymphomas. In the diffuse non-Hodgkin's lymphomas, stages II, III, and IV can all be considered as reflecting disseminated disease and are therefore usually treated with chemotherapy. In contrast, only true stage I disease or, depending on the histologic subtype, stage II disease will be considered as localized and treated with radiation alone. Therefore, for most patients with non-Hodgkin's lymphoma it is less critical to ascertain the precise pathologic stage of disease. Moreover, it is common for these patients to exhibit disseminated disease after routine staging tests (e.g., bone marrow or liver biopsy), thus obviating laparotomy to prove dissemination. For example, within follicular lymphomas the poorly differentiated and mixed subgroups comprise more than 80 percent of patients.

Following clinical staging and the minimally invasive techniques of bone marrow and liver biopsy, greater than 80 percent of these patients will have stage III or stage IV disease. Early in the staging process, only those diagnostic studies with low morbidity and a high probability of disclosing advanced disease should be employed. Bone marrow and liver biopsy, and, in selected patients, lymphangiography meet these requirements and usually obviate staging laparotomy. Thus, *surgical staging should never be considered a routine procedure in patients with non-Hodgkin's lymphoma.*

A number of other tests are becoming more important both in staging and in advancing our knowledge of the biology of non-Hodgkin's lymphoma. Radionuclide scans, especially with gallium, appear to have clinical utility. Gallium scans are commonly positive in intermediate- and high-grade lymphomas and in low-grade lymphomas that have converted to a higher histologic grade. Gallium, with high doses of isotope which permit delayed imaging, combined with single photon emission computed tomography (SPECT) are very sensitive in detecting tumor infiltration. These tests are also very useful in monitoring response to therapy and differentiating necrosis or fibrosis from active disease. The role of magnetic resonance (MR) imaging in detecting non-Hodgkin's lymphoma is under active investigation. Immunologic and molecular biologic studies are proving increasingly useful in confirming diagnosis. For example, in cases with difficult histopathologic patterns, cell surface markers can distinguish between non-Hodgkin's lymphoma and carcinoma (common leukocyte antigen, CD45-positive in lymphoma). Similarly, MAbs directed against lineage-restricted antigens and rearrangement of immunoglobulin or T-cell receptor genes are useful in identifying lymphoid tumors. Although therapeutic decisions are not currently made on the basis of lineage or state of differentiation of the neoplastic lymphocyte, these data may prove to be of prognostic importance. Moreover, delineation of the cell surface phenotype is becoming important because an increasing number of salvage treatment programs employ very high dose chemoradiotherapy and monoclonal-antibody–purged autologous bone marrow support (see below). Definition of a specific chromosomal abnormality may also have prognostic significance.

Sensitive techniques to detect minimal residual disease Monoclonal antibodies directed against cell surface antigens on lymphoid cells and molecular techniques to define immunoglobulin and T-cell-receptor gene rearrangements are very sensitive tools with which to assess tumor cell infiltration more accurately. Once the cell surface phenotype and genotype have been determined, one can examine other tissues for disease infiltration. The commonest and most accessible tissues to be tested include peripheral blood and bone marrow. Whereas conventional histologic analysis of the bone marrow can detect 1 lymphoma cell infiltrating 20 normal cells, immunologic flow cytometric and Southern blot analysis each improve this level of detection to approximately 1 lymphoma cell in approximately 100 normal cells. Similarly, flow cytometry has been used to detect "clonal excess" in the blood of patients with B-cell non-Hodgkin's lymphoma. More recently, newly developed molecular biologic techniques suggest that minimal disease detection can be markedly improved. For those non-Hodgkin's lymphomas with a known chromosomal translocation, it is now possible to identify a unique chromosomal "breakpoint." This has been most elegantly accomplished for the 14;18 translocation present in the majority of follicular lymphomas and in a smaller percentage of diffuse large cell lymphomas. This translocation, which occurs only in lymphoma cells, has been termed the *bcl*-2 breakpoint and its entire DNA sequence has been determined (see Chap. 10). Based on DNA sequence, it is possible to amplify this unique stretch of DNA using specific oligonucleotide primers and the polymerase chain reaction (PCR) (see Chap. 6). With this approach, 1 tumor cell in 100,000 cells can be detected. Thus, while other tests may be negative, PCR may demonstrate that the blood or bone marrow is contaminated by lymphoma cells. These biologic techniques are presently being compared to more conventional staging methods. Considering their sensitivity, they may be useful in more accurately assessing complete remission and, more importantly, determining whether treatment should be prolonged, altered, or intensified.

NATURAL HISTORY BY HISTOLOGIC SUBTYPE Considering the heterogeneity of non-Hodgkin's lymphoma and the unique clinical presentation and natural history within histologically defined subtypes, it is important to briefly review these subtypes.

Low grade SMALL LYMPHOCYTIC (DIFFUSE WELL-DIFFERENTIATED LYMPHOCYTIC) This disease is the lymphomatous presentation of chronic lymphocytic leukemia (CLL) and therefore occurs in middle- and older-aged patients. Patients usually present with generalized lymphadenopathy. Unlike CLL, the peripheral blood may be normal or reveal only a mild lymphocytosis (60 percent will have absolute lymphocytosis of >4000 per microliter at diagnosis). In contrast, the bone marrow is positive in 75 to 95 percent of cases. Serum paraprotein is found in about 20 percent of cases and hypogammaglobulinemia is common. Small lymphocytic lymphoma and CLL can convert to diffuse large cell lymphoma (Richter's syndrome, circulating large cell lymphoma). These patients usually present with abdominal masses and B symptoms and experience short survival.

FOLLICULAR, PREDOMINANTLY SMALL CLEAVED CELL (NODULAR POORLY DIFFERENTIATED LYMPHOCYTIC) Follicular lymphomas account for approximately 50 percent of the non-Hodgkin's lymphomas; the small cleaved cell variant is the most common subtype. Patients usually present with painless peripheral adenopathy in cervical, axillary, inguinal, and femoral regions. Patients frequently note that lymph node enlargement has been present for long periods of time and they have not sought medical attention because these nodes have "waxed and waned." Typically, there is enlargement of Waldeyer's ring, popliteal, and epitrochlear nodes. Some patients present with asymptomatic large abdominal masses with or without evidence of gastrointestinal and/or renal obstruction. Although patients may present with one or more sites of nodal disease, noninvasive workup usually demonstrates widely disseminated disease with involvement of spleen, liver, and bone marrow (80 to 90 percent with stage III or stage IV). Bone marrow involvement in follicular lymphoma reveals a unique pattern of paratrabecular infiltration. In contrast to diffuse lymphomas, very few patients present with extranodal disease and few present with B symptoms. The course of this disease is quite variable. Some patients can be observed with waxing and waning disease for 5 years without the need for therapy. Others demonstrate more disseminated and rapid growth and require treatment because massive nodal or organ enlargement leads to pain, lymphatic obstruction, organ obstruction, or, more rarely, neurologic symptoms. At the time of increasing generalized disease or rapid growth at a single site, involved nodes should be rebiopsied. At that time, a significant number of patients will demonstrate a "conversion" to a more aggressive histologic pattern, usually diffuse large cell. This conversion occurs in 60 percent of patients with follicular small cleaved cell lymphoma and is associated with infiltration of extranodal sites and, in some patients, with the development of systemic symptoms and a poorer prognosis, since the tumor is much less responsive to treatment. Late in the natural history of this disease, a number of patients circulate either small follicular cleaved cells or large cells as a leukemic phase. Historically, both disease-free and overall survivals of these patients have not changed in spite of many different therapeutic approaches. Few patients achieve complete remissions (noninvasively staged) with conventional single-agent or aggressive combination chemotherapy. However, these patients survive long periods of time with median survivals for patients with stages III and IV disease approaching 7 to 9 years.

FOLLICULAR, MIXED SMALL CLEAVED CELL AND LARGE CELL (NODULAR MIXED) This entity has similarities with both follicular small cleaved cell and follicular large cell lymphomas. Bone marrow infiltration at presentation is less common, but large abdominal masses are more commonly seen. It demonstrates a less favorable natural history with 35 percent disease-free survival at 2 years.

Intermediate grade FOLLICULAR, PREDOMINANTLY LARGE CELL (NODULAR HISTIOCYTIC) Although the follicular morphology is preserved, this disease behaves much more like diffuse large cell lymphoma. In contrast to other follicular lymphomas, this histologic variant has less infiltration of the marrow and liver and presents with larger masses. A finite cure rate has been reported. Most follicular large cell lymphomas that are not cured by treatment convert to diffuse large cell lymphomas.

DIFFUSE SMALL CLEAVED CELL (DIFFUSE POORLY DIFFERENTIATED LYMPHOCYTIC) This disease behaves like a follicular variant. Patients are middle-aged or older. At the time of presentation, most have stage IV disease with infiltration of the spleen, liver, and bone marrow. Marrow and hepatic infiltration occur in over 50 percent of patients. Later in the course of the disease, infiltration of other parenchymal organs (e.g., lung) is observed. Many patients present with massive splenomegaly and significant bone marrow infiltration. The overall survival is much shorter than observed in patients with low-grade lymphomas; however, like low-grade lymphoma, aggressive combination chemotherapy has not significantly changed the natural history of this disease.

DIFFUSE SMALL AND LARGE CELL (DIFFUSE MIXED) This tumor behaves most like diffuse large cell lymphoma. Some investigators consider these two tumors to be a spectrum of a single entity. Patients are usually older women with prominent extranodal disease, especially in the skin and gastrointestinal tract, and B symptoms are common. However, diffuse mixed lymphoma is a "wastebasket" of a number of pathologic entities and, therefore, it is difficult to compare clinical series with respect to disease presentation and response to treatment. In several clinical trials where patients with diffuse mixed and diffuse large cell lymphoma were treated identically, survival rates were comparable. However, in other series, a higher relapse rate was observed with diffuse mixed lymphoma.

DIFFUSE LARGE CELL (DIFFUSE HISTIOCYTIC) Patients present with either nodal enlargement (especially in the neck or abdomen) or extranodal disease (in the gastrointestinal tract, testes, bone, thyroid, salivary glands, skin, and brain). During the course of the disease, the liver, kidneys, and lung may be involved. Diffuse large cell lymphoma is highly invasive, with local compression of vessels or airways, involvement of peripheral nerves, and destruction of bone. Although bone marrow involvement initially is found in only 10 to 20 percent of patients, its detection is important because of its strong correlation with later spread to the central nervous system. Therefore, cytologic examination of spinal fluid is important in patients with bone marrow infiltration. Late in the disease, some patients demonstrate both extensive bone marrow infiltration and circulating large cell lymphoma cells. A number of clinical features reflect dissemination of disease and are considered to be associated with inability to achieve a complete remission and poor prognosis. These features include poor performance status, large tumor masses, bone marrow infiltration, multiple sites of extranodal disease, markedly elevated serum lactic dehydrogenase (LDH), and systemic B symptoms.

High grade LARGE CELL IMMUNOBLASTIC (DIFFUSE HISTIOCYTIC) This variant of diffuse large cell lymphoma demonstrates a unique pathologic appearance and the clinical course is usually fulminant. This disease usually occur in adults, commonly over age 50, and often in a setting of prior immune-mediated or lymphoproliferative disease (e.g., celiac disease, Hashimoto's thyroiditis, angioimmunoblastic lymphadenopathy, Sjögren's syndrome, Mediterranean lymphoma, cold aggulutinin disease, or Waldenström's macroglobulinemia). Anemia, lymphopenia, diffuse hypergammaglobulinemia, B symptoms, and advanced stage are common at presentation. Most patients present with extranodal disease and invasion of the bone marrow and central nervous system are common.

LYMPHOBLASTIC (DIFFUSE LYMPHOBLASTIC) Although lymphoblastic lymphomas represent a major subgroup of childhood non-Hodgkin's lymphomas, they are much less common in adults (less than 5 percent of adult non-Hodgkin's lymphomas). Patients are usually males in their twenties or thirties who present with lymphadenopathy in cervical, supraclavicular, and axillary regions (50 percent) or with a mediastinal mass (50 percent). In most patients the mediastinal mass is anterior, greater than 10 cm, and is associated with pleural effusions. Less commonly, patients present with extranodal disease (e.g., skin, testicular, or bony involvement). Greater than 90 percent of patients present with stage III or stage IV disease and half have B symptoms. Although the bone marrow is frequently normal at presentation, approximately 60 percent of patients develop bone marrow infiltration and a subsequent leukemic phase indistinguishable from T-cell acute lymphoblastic leukemia. Patients with bone marrow involvement have a very high incidence of CNS infiltration. Prior to current aggressive therapy, this disease was rapidly fatal.

SMALL NONCLEAVED CELL, BURKITT'S AND NON-BURKITT'S (DIFFUSE UNDIFFERENTIATED)   Burkitt's lymphoma is a childhood tumor that has two major clinical presentations. The *African* endemic form presents as a jaw tumor that spreads to extranodal sites, especially to the bone marrow and meninges. The *American* form has an abdominal presentation with massive disease and ascites and, like the African form, also spreads to the bone marrow and central nervous system. Prior to aggressive therapeutic programs, all children died rapidly. These tumors are now treated with very aggressive chemotherapeutic programs with more gratifying results. True Burkitt's lymphoma is uncommon in adults but is occasionally seen in patients up to age 35. In contrast, small noncleaved cell, non-Burkitt's lymphomas are observed and are very aggressive and frequently present in extranodal sites. Like Burkitt's, these tumors have a very high propensity to invade the bone marrow and central nervous system.

Other subtypes   AIDS-RELATED LYMPHOMAS   Non-Hodgkin's lymphoma occurs in 5 to 10 percent of patients with AIDS. Most cases are grouped with high-grade tumors including small noncleaved cell and large cell immunoblastic. In these cases extranodal involvement is common with central nervous system, bone marrow, and gastrointestinal tract the most frequent sites. Most patients present with rapid nodal enlargement, appearance of an extranodal mass, or severe B symptoms. Primary CNS lymphoma is common in AIDS patients, and it is predicted that within 5 or more years this will be one of the commonest presenting CNS malignancies. These lymphomas have been associated with chromosomal translocations (8;14 and 8;22) and with EBV, although a causal relationship has not been definitively demonstrated. Although treated with the most aggressive combinations of chemotherapy, results have been poor.

CUTANEOUS T-CELL LYMPHOMAS   Major variants include mycosis fungoides and Sézary syndrome. Both tumors are T-cell derived. Patients present with cutaneous manifestations, lymphadenopathy, and later with hepatic, splenic, and pulmonary infiltration. Infiltration of the bone marrow and circulating leukemia are also common late manifestations.

ADULT T-CELL LYMPHOMA   This entity has been observed in Japan, the Caribbean, and in blacks in the southeastern United States and is associated with the human T-cell leukemia virus (HTLV-I) C type retrovirus. Patients present with generalized adenopathy, hepatosplenomegaly, cutaneous infiltration, hypercalcemia, lytic bone lesions, and a profound leukemia characterized by pleomorphic CD4-positive T-cells. This disease has a fulminant course and its natural history has been little altered by aggressive combination chemotherapy.

ANGIOIMMUNOBLASTIC LYMPHADENOPATHY (CLASSIFIED WITH LARGE CELL IMMUNOBLASTIC)   This disease affects older adults who present with the acute onset of generalized lymphadenopathy, hepatosplenomegaly, and B symptoms. Immunologic abnormalities are common and include plasmacytosis, polyclonal hypergammaglobulinemia, and a positive Coombs test. Although this disease is progressive and frequently fatal, it is unresolved whether it is a hyperimmune disorder or a malignant lymphoma. Limited cytogenetic and clonal T-cell receptor β-chain rearrangements suggest a neoplasm akin to adult peripheral T-cell lymphoma.

TRUE HISTIOCYTIC LYMPHOMA   This is a rare entity that is the neoplastic counterpart of the true histiocyte (macrophage) and exhibits the curious phenomenon of erythrophagocytosis. This disease has an abrupt onset with fever, progressive pancytopenia, splenomegaly, and mild lymphadenopathy.

THERAPY   To decide the appropriate treatment regimen, the clinician must determine whether the histology is low-, intermediate-, or high-grade and whether the disease is localized or systemic. The next decision is whether or not to treat; if the treatment option is selected, whether the goal is to palliate symptoms or to cure. Although some general principles are agreed upon in the treatment of non-Hodgkin's lymphoma, therapeutic approaches for all histologic subtypes are actively being evaluated. Options to be chosen must consider age and the presence of comorbid diseases (cardiac, renal, pulmonary, etc.) that might significantly affect end-organ toxicity.

Radiotherapy   Radiation has a very limited role in the primary treatment of non-Hodgkin's lymphoma. It should only be considered as a potential curative modality in patients whose disease has been exhaustively staged and found to be true stage I intermediate- or high-grade or true stage I or II low-grade non-Hodgkin's lymphoma. Most of the radiotherapeutic principles developed for the treatment of Hodgkin's disease (see below) also apply to non-Hodgkin's lymphoma. For patients with stage I disease, involved-field radiotherapy is employed with the dose dependent upon the histologic subtype. Doses of less than 3000 cGy are usually sufficient for low-grade disease whereas high-grade disease is frequently treated with 5000 cGy or greater. For patients with true stage I non-Hodgkin's lymphoma, the long-term disease-free survival ranges from 60 to 80 percent. In addition to its curative potential in stage I patients, radiotherapy is frequently used in conjunction with systemic therapy to treat sites of bulk disease. Moreover, in low-grade lymphomas it has been commonly used to palliate sites of symptomatic disease. The use of local radiotherapy for patients not being treated for cure must be carefully evaluated in view of its potential later use as total-body irradiation in salvage therapy (i.e., bone marrow transplantation).

Chemotherapy   (See also Chap. 301 and Table 301-1 for abbreviations of standard regimens)   This modality is used for most patients with stage II and all patients with stages III and IV non-Hodgkin's lymphoma. Chemotherapeutic options are dictated by grade and histologic subtype and therefore treatment regimens depend upon the Working Formulation.

LOW-GRADE LYMPHOMA   For the most part, small lymphocytic (DWDL) and follicular small cleaved cell (NPDL) lymphomas are approached similarly. Traditionally, these tumors have not been treated until they produce symptoms. This was because single-agent chemotherapy or combinations of agents did not induce complete remissions and, more importantly, they did not change the overall survival of patients with these diseases. These regimens included the use of single alkylating agents like cyclophosphamide or chlorambucil or combinations like CVP (cyclophosphamide, vincristine, and prednisone) or CHOP (CVP plus adriamycin). More aggressive CHOP-like regimens (see intermediate-grade below) have produced more rapid and possibly higher percentages of complete remissions but unfortunately have not changed the overall survival rates for these diseases. In addition, attempts to treat patients for long periods of time with single-agent therapy or the addition of long-term "maintenance" treatment did not alter overall survival. If these diseases are to be cured, either more aggressive high-dose regimens must be evaluated or new therapeutic modalities must be employed. Recently, several institutions (e.g., National Cancer Institute, Dana Farber Cancer Institute, and St. Bartholomew's Hospital in London) have attempted to treat patients with advanced stage follicular lymphomas earlier in the course of their disease with aggressive chemotherapy combined with total nodal irradiation or with high-dose chemoradiotherapy and autologous bone marrow transplantation. These studies suggest that high complete-response rates in the range of 80 percent or greater are possible. However, the impact of these studies on long-term disease-free survival and possible cure is still uncertain.

INTERMEDIATE-GRADE LYMPHOMA   The regimen used to treat diffuse large cell lymphoma is now also employed to treat follicular mixed, follicular large cell, and diffuse small cleaved cell lymphomas. *The treatment of diffuse large cell lymphoma is one of the major successes of modern chemotherapy.* These tumors were initially treated with single agents and then CVP. This regimen induced disease regression in most patients, but few complete responses or improvement in disease-free survival were observed. The first successful regimen was CHOP, which induced complete remissions in approximately 50 percent of patients and with long-term disease-free survival for more than half of the complete responders. Success with this and subsequent regimens required attention to administering full doses and adhering to schedules as strictly as possible. Over the past 15 years, attempts have been made to improve the percentage of complete remissions and overall cure rate. Additional agents have been added to CHOP, including bleomycin, methotrexate, procarbazine, nitrogen mustard, cytarabine hydrochloride (cytosine arabinoside), and etoposide (e.g., BACOD, m-BACOD, ProMACE-MOPP, COP-BLAM, COMLA, ProMACE/CytaBOM, MACOP-B). In addition to the complexity of the regimen, the duration of treatment has been prolonged for up to 12 months. With these approaches, the complete-remission rate now approaches 80 percent for the most aggressive regimens. However, not surprisingly, toxicities have also increased (e.g., infections as well as cardiac and pulmonary complications.) Patients who survive 2 years disease-free have an excellent chance of being cured. Prolonged ''maintenance'' therapy has not improved overall survival. With the various treatment options, and until randomized studies are completed, the selection of a treatment regimen for diffuse large cell lymphoma should be based on the therapist's experience with a particular regimen and its toxicities.

Both nodular mixed and nodular large cell lymphomas have been treated with CHOP-like regimens with high complete-remission rates and good evidence for long-term disease-free survival. In contrast, diffuse small cleaved cell lymphoma has been treated with most of the above aggressive regimens but while complete-response rates are high, relapse is rapid and cure is rare.

HIGH-GRADE LYMPHOMA   These tumors have a very poor prognosis and need to be treated very aggressively. Lymphoblastic lymphoma and small noncleaved cell lymphomas have been treated with regimens even more aggressive than those used for diffuse large cell lymphoma. Although complete-remission rates are very high, the cure rate is still much less than is observed for diffuse large cell lymphoma. Groups with good prognostic features (bone marrow negative, low LDH) have better survival than those with poor prognostic characteristics. If there is CNS infiltration, intrathecal treatment or radiotherapy should be administered.

AIDS-RELATED LYMPHOMAS   These tumors are among the most aggressive of the non-Hodgkin's lymphomas. Most are intermediate-grade diffuse large cell with some high-grade B-cell lymphomas also observed. These tumors are becoming increasingly more common and their response to therapy and prognosis is radically different compared to non-AIDS-related intermediate- and high-grade lymphoma despite their histologic resemblance. Aggressive regimens have had limited impact with fewer than 25 percent achieving complete remissions and few, if any, cures. Salvage regimens have also been very disappointing, with patients dying of lymphoma as well as complications of aplasia. Bone marrow transplantation has not been attempted.

Salvage chemotherapy   Failure to achieve a complete remission or relapse following aggressive therapy is associated with short survival. Salvage chemotherapeutic regimens employing both higher doses and new drugs (e.g., ifosfamide, etoposide, and cisplatin) have therefore been used to induce remissions. Depending upon the histology and regimen, approximately one-third of patients attain a complete remission with partial remissions in another third. Unfortunately, these remissions tend to be short-lived with survival being less than 2 years.

Bone marrow transplantation (BMT)   Patients whose disease is resistant to conventional or salvage therapeutic regimens can still be induced into a complete remission with very high dosages of chemotherapy or chemoradiotherapy. This treatment approach is complicated by very significant and prolonged myelosuppression. To overcome the latter, bone marrow can be infused from an identical twin, an HLA-matched relative, or from the patient following the completion of therapy. Bone marrow transplantation has become widespread in the treatment of patients with refractory or relapsed non-Hodgkin's lymphoma, and retrospective analysis demonstrates that a subgroup of patients clearly benefits from this approach. Patients whose disease has never responded to therapy or, following relapse, is resistant to all forms of salvage therapy, have less than 20 percent long-term disease-free survival. In contrast, those patients whose disease is still responsive to therapy achieve approximately 40 percent long-term disease-free survival with BMT. Studies with BMT have reported treatment-related deaths in the range of 20 to 30 percent; however, as patients are treated earlier in the course of their disease this mortality has significantly decreased (10 percent or less). This lower mortality has led some to use BMT as consolidation therapy in patients with incurable non-Hodgkin's lymphomas. Although this modality is clearly capable of curing some patients with relapsed non-Hodgkin's lymphomas, many issues still remain. These include optimal therapeutic regimen, optimal time of transplantation, source of bone marrow, the question of purging autologous bone marrow, as well as methods to minimize morbidity and mortality.

Newer modalities   A variety of new therapeutic approaches have resulted from the advances in immunology and molecular biology. Over 10 years ago, MAbs directed against surface antigens expressed on non-Hodgkin's lymphoma cells were first used clinically in an attempt to specifically treat these tumors. The results of these studies suggest that MAbs by themselves do not induce significant tumor regressions. Although there was initial enthusiasm about using MAbs directed against unique idiotypes expressed on B-cell follicular lymphomas, many obstacles have been encountered. Some trials are evaluating MAbs coupled to radionuclides or toxins to specifically produce cytotoxic effects; other trials are using soluble factors (cytokines) that are potentially cytotoxic to tumor cells. The major cytokines being studied include the interferons, tumor necrosis factor, and interleukin 2 (IL-2). Recombinant hematopoietic growth factors that are responsible for growth of myeloid, lymphoid, and erythroid cells are also being tested. Conceptually, these growth factors will limit myelosuppression thereby permitting higher doses and more frequent administration of chemotherapeutic drugs. Early results are encouraging, and agents like granulocyte macrophage colony stimulating factor (GM-CSF) and G-CSF appear to hasten recovery of myeloid cells. The role of all of these agents in improving the treatment of lymphomas is being evaluated in many research centers.

HODGKIN'S DISEASE

EPIDEMIOLOGY AND ETIOLOGY   Approximately 7500 new cases of Hodgkin's disease are diagnosed annually in the United States. The epidemiology of this disease has provided important information regarding the possible role of age, genetic, and environmental factors associated with its development. While the interpretation of epidemiologic factors remains controversial, these data still provide a context within which to examine the population at risk for Hodgkin's disease. In non-Hodgkin's lymphomas there is a linear increase in incidence with age. In contrast, in Hodgkin's disease in the United States and developed western nations, the age-specific incidence curve is characteristically bimodal with an initial peak in young adults (15 to 35 years) and a second peak after age 50. However, in Japan, there is an absence of the early peak, and in underdeveloped, tropical countries there is a shift of the first peak into childhood. Hodgkin's disease is more prevalent in males, and when the age-specific incidence curve is compared to the sex distribution of the patients, the increased male prevalence is most prominent in young adults. A disproportionate number of patients in the first modal peak exhibit nodular sclerosis histology. In childhood Hodgkin's disease, this male predominance is even more striking with over 80 percent of patients being male. This has led some investigators to hypothesize a sex-linked genetic or hormonally related increase in susceptibility.

Although controversial, clusters of patients with Hodgkin's have been reported. Increased risk has been associated with decreased number of siblings, single family dwellings, decreased number of playmates, early birth order, sibling with Hodgkin's, tonsillectomy, and certain HLA antigens. These findings have been used to suggest that Hodgkin's disease is caused by a virus possessing an oncogenic potential that is low but that increases with age at the time of infection. These observations suggest that genetic and environmental factors may be associated with the development of this disease. As in non-Hodgkin's lymphomas, there is an increased risk of Hodgkin's in patients with immunodeficiencies and autoimmune diseases (Table 302-4). The major obstacle to examining the etiology of Hodgkin's disease is the inability to isolate and study the "real" neoplastic cell. Unlike non-Hodgkin's lymphomas, no chromosomal abnormalities have been consistently demonstrated.

CLINICAL FEATURES AND DIFFERENTIAL DIAGNOSIS Patients with Hodgkin's disease usually present with localized disease that subsequently spreads to contiguous lymphoid structures; it ultimately disseminates to nonlymphoid tissues with a potentially fatal outcome. Patients commonly present with a newly detected mass or group of lymph nodes that are firm, freely moveable, and usually nontender. Approximately half present with adenopathy in the neck or supraclavicular area, and over 70 percent present with superficial lymph node enlargement. Because these are frequently not painful, detection by the patient may be delayed until the lymph nodes are quite large. Approximately 50 to 60 percent of patients present with mediastinal adenopathy. This is sometimes first detected on a routine chest x-ray. Hodgkin's nodes tend to be centripetal or axial in contrast to non-Hodgkin's lymphomas, which have a tendency to be centrifugal involving epitrochlear, Waldeyer's ring, and abdominal nodes. In 2 to 5 percent of patients, lymph nodes or other tissues involved with Hodgkin's disease can become painful after the ingestion of alcohol. The growth of lymph nodes may be quite variable; some lesions can remain stable for long periods of time, while spontaneous and temporary regression of some nodes may also occur.

The majority of patients presenting with Hodgkin's disease have few or no symptoms related to their disease. However, 25 to 40 percent of patients have some constitutional symptoms; the most common is low-grade fever which can be associated with recurrent night sweats. For some patients, night sweats may be the sole complaint. A small number of patients may have high fluctuating fevers accompanied by drenching night sweats (Pel-Ebstein fevers). These fevers can persist for several weeks followed by afebrile intervals. Fevers and night sweats are more commonly seen in older patients and in those with more advanced-stage disease. Some patients with extensive abdominal but limited peripheral adenopathy are first evaluated for fever and night sweats. They undergo a workup for fever of unknown origin and usually are found to have lymphocyte-depleted Hodgkin's disease. Another important presenting symptom is weight loss of greater than 10 percent. *Fever, night sweats, and weight loss are referred to as B symptoms.* Other frequent symptoms include fatigue, malaise, and weakness. Pruritus occurs in approximately 10 percent of patients at initial diagnosis; it is usually generalized and may be associated with a skin rash. Rarely, pruritus may be the only disease manifestation. Site-specific symptoms are also rare. However, mediastinal, pulmonary, pleural, or pericardial involvement may be associated with cough, chest pain, shortness of breath, or hypertrophic osteoarthropathy; bone involvement may be associated with bone pain. Occasionally a patient will present with obstruction of the superior vena cava as the first symptom. Sudden

spinal cord compression can be a presenting complaint but is usually a complication of progressive disease. Headache or visual disturbances may be seen in the very rare patient with intracranial Hodgkin's disease, and abdominal involvement may result in abdominal pain, bowel disturbances, and even ascites.

Differential diagnosis is similar to that described for non-Hodgkin's lymphoma. Persistent lymph nodes larger than 1 cm present for 4 to 6 weeks should be biopsied. In patients with neck adenopathy, infections including bacterial or viral pharyngitis, infectious mononucleosis, and toxoplasmosis must be excluded. Other malignancies, such as non-Hodgkin's lymphomas, nasopharyngeal cancers, and thyroid cancers, can also present with localized neck adenopathy. Axillary adenopathy must be differentiated from non-Hodgkin's lymphoma and breast cancer. Since supraclavicular nodes drain both the thorax and the abdomen, regardless of infectious or neoplastic etiology, the left supraclavicular space is more commonly associated with lesions of the abdomen while the right side is more commonly associated with intrathoracic disease. Mediastinal adenopathy must be distinguished from infections, sarcoid, and other tumors. In older patients, the differential diagnosis includes tumors of the lung and mediastinum, specifically oat cell and epidermoid carcinomas. Reactive mediastinitis and hilar adenopathy from histoplasmosis can be confused with lymphoma since the former occurs in otherwise asymptomatic people. Primary abdominal disease with hepatomegaly, splenomegaly, and massive adenopathy is uncommon and may produce symptoms; other neoplastic diseases, especially non-Hodgkin's lymphoma, must be excluded under these circumstances.

DIAGNOSIS AND PATHOLOGIC CLASSIFICATION The diagnosis of Hodgkin's disease requires a biopsy that contains sufficient tissue to permit an accurate microscopic diagnosis. Biopsy specimens are usually from lymph nodes, but may occasionally be from other tissues. Needle aspirations or needle biopsies are not adequate for the histologic diagnosis of Hodgkin's disease.

The criteria for the diagnosis and classification of Hodgkin's disease have remained unchanged since 1966 when the Rye classification was adopted (Table 302-7). As indicated above, central to the diagnosis is the presence of the Reed-Sternberg cell, a large cell with a bilobed or multilobulated nucleus with prominent inclusion-like nucleoli. There are several morphologic variants of RS cells, and it is the frequency of these variants as well as the cellular and fibrous background of the proliferation that help to establish the histologic subtypes of Hodgkin's disease. It is important to note that RS cells may occasionally be found in other conditions such as infectious mononucleosis and non-Hodgkin's lymphoma. Thus, an accurate diagnosis of Hodgkin's disease depends on additional cellular and architectural features of the tissue and optimally also with supportive immunologic studies.

In the Rye classification, Hodgkin's disease is subdivided into four types: (1) lymphocyte-predominant, (2) nodular sclerosis, (3)

TABLE 302-7 Rye classification of Hodgkin's disease

Histologic subgroup	Incidence, %	Pathology RS*	Other	Prognosis
Lymphocyte-predominant	2–10	Rare	Predominance of normal-appearing lymphocytes	Excellent
Nodular sclerosis	40–80	Frequent "lacunae"	Lymphoid nodules, collagen bands	Very good
Mixed cellularity	20–40	Numerous	Pleomorphic infiltrate	Good
Lymphocyte-depleted	2–15	Numerous, often bizarre	Paucity of lymphocytes, pleomorphic, fibrosis	Poor

* RS = Reed-Sternberg cell.

mixed cellularity, and (4) lymphocyte-depleted. These variants define distinct entities with unique natural histories. Table 302-7 summarizes the major clinical characteristics of these types associated with the Rye classification. It is very important to stress that *treatment and prognosis in Hodgkin's disease are dependent on stage of disease whereas in non-Hodgkin's lymphoma, treatment and prognosis are largely based on histologic subtype.*

STAGING AND OTHER LABORATORY ABNORMALITIES   Ann Arbor classification   Following biopsy and histopathologic classification of Hodgkin's disease, one must define the extent of the disease (i.e., staging), which is essential for the selection of optimal therapy. In the Ann Arbor staging classification (Table 302-5), the patient receives both a clinical and a pathologic stage. The clinical stage is defined by the apparent extent of disease based on physical examination and other noninvasive studies. The pathologic stage is defined by data obtained from invasive tests including biopsy specimens obtained from different sites, usually during a staging laparotomy. The presence of localized extralymphatic disease is designated by the suffix E. Such extralymphatic involvement may include solitary involvement of lung, pericardium, or bone. Multifocal involvement in these organs usually is defined as disseminated disease. Bone involvement must be separated from bone marrow involvement, since bone marrow and liver involvement are always defined as stage IV disseminated disease.

The presence of systemic symptoms that are of prognostic importance is designated by the suffix B and their absence by the suffix A. B symptoms include loss of greater than 10 percent of body weight, fever, or night sweats. The presence of any of these symptoms results in a less favorable prognosis. As stated above, defining the pathologic stage is essential for determining optimal therapy. Patients with limited disease, such as pathologic stage IA or IIA, are effectively treated with radiotherapy alone, while patients with more disseminated disease, such as pathologic stage IIIB, IVA, or IVB, are most effectively treated with chemotherapy, alone or combined with radiotherapy.

Staging procedures after biopsy diagnosis   The diagnostic studies recommended for complete staging are outlined in Table 302-6. There is general agreement on the studies that are considered to be essential. Detailed physical examination with attention to documentation of all sites of nodal involvement and splenomegaly is essential. The chest radiograph is usually sufficient to exclude mediastinal, hilar, pleural, and parenchymal involvement. However, in patients with demonstrable thoracic disease, chest CT scan more accurately defines extent of disease. A CT scan of the abdomen and pelvis has a definite place in the staging of Hodgkin's disease for the assessment of nodal, splenic, and hepatic disease. It can detect the exact location and extent of all enlarged nodes including parailiac, mesenteric, and retrocrural nodal areas as compared to a lymphogram, which evaluates only the paraaortic and common internal and external iliac nodes. However, the abdominopelvic CT scan has several limitations; it requires nodal enlargement for detection and is less sensitive in detecting splenic involvement (50 to 60 percent) or hepatic infiltration (25 percent).

A number of more invasive diagnostic tests are required if patients are clinically stage I, II, or IIIA. Lymphograms of the lower extremities are very useful to demonstrate paraaortic and iliac nodal enlargement; they are more sensitive than abdominopelvic CT scans since they can detect disease in normal-sized nodes. Moreover, lymphograms are useful prior to staging laparotomy to direct the surgeon to the nodes to be biopsied. However, the safety and accuracy of this procedure is highly dependent on the experience of the radiologist. If a staging laparotomy is considered, patients should undergo *bilateral bone marrow biopsies* and percutaneous *liver biopsy* to exclude stage IV disease. The role of staging laparotomy is still controversial. Historically, staging laparotomy with splenectomy has played an important role in understanding the biology of Hodgkin's disease. Staging laparotomy includes biopsy of selected lymph nodes in the retroperitoneum, splenectomy, and several needle and wedge biopsies of the liver. Traditionally, all patients without obvious stage IV disease underwent laparotomy, and nearly one-third had their initial clinical stage changed as a result of the procedure. For example, one-third of patients with normal-sized spleens had demonstrable tumor infiltration at laparotomy, whereas 25 percent of patients with clinical splenomegaly had no histologic evidence of disease. Similarly, hepatic infiltration by Hodgkin's disease is associated with splenomegaly. The liver is rarely involved when splenic involvement is not associated with splenomegaly. Liver involvement is present in as many as 28 percent of patients with positive lymphograms and enlarged spleens. Although very important, the routine use of staging laparotomy in all patients may not be appropriate. Laparotomies should be utilized in patients whose clinical stages make them a candidate for treatment with radiation therapy alone and in whom evidence of unsuspected abdominal disease will significantly change treatment. A staging laparotomy should not be performed in patients who are to receive chemotherapy based upon their clinical stage since it is rare for the clinical stage to be lowered after a laparotomy. A staging laparotomy with splenectomy should be performed by a surgeon who is skilled in this procedure, after careful review of clinical, laboratory, pathologic, and radiologic studies. In selected patients, laparoscopy performed by a skilled practitioner may substitute for a laparotomy. Finally, a number of ancillary studies may be very useful in selected patients and are listed in Table 302-6. Gallium scintigraphy is useful in following response to treatment and in differentiating residual or recurrent disease from bulky nodal fibrosis, particularly in the abdomen and mediastinum. A scan is necessary at the time of initial staging to determine whether the lymphoma is gallium-avid.

Laboratory abnormalities   Routine blood counts, liver function tests, and renal function tests are all necessary parts of the medical workup, but do not provide information about the extent of Hodgkin's disease or of specific organ involvement. A moderate, normochromic, normocytic anemia associated with low serum iron and low iron-binding capacity, but with normal or increased iron stores in the bone marrow, may be present in patients with Hodgkin's disease as well as in those with other neoplastic and chronic diseases. A moderate to marked leukemoid reaction is common, particularly in symptomatic patients, and usually disappears with treatment. Mild peripheral absolute eosinophilia is not uncommon especially in patients with pruritus. Absolute monocytosis is also observed. Absolute lymphocytopenia (<1000 cells per cubic milliliter) usually occurs in patients with more advanced disease. Many tests have been evaluated as indicators of disease activity. To date, the erythrocyte sedimentation rate still is the best monitor but it suffers from its lack of specificity and can return to normal when residual disease is still demonstrable. Other abnormal tests include increased serum levels of copper, calcium, lactic acid, alkaline phosphatase, lysozyme, globulins, C-reactive protein, and other acute-phase reactants.

Immunologic abnormalities   Hodgkin's disease is associated with a well-described but poorly understood immunologic defect. Untreated patients, including those with limited disease, have defective cellular immunity characterized by anergy to routine skin tests. They also have a reversal of the CD4:CD8 ratio, suggesting that this anergy may be due to increased numbers of suppressor cells as well as decreased numbers of CD4-positive cells. In several studies, decreased immune reactivity correlates both with advanced stages of disease and the presence of systemic symptoms. However, anergy to recall and neoantigen appear to have no prognostic significance. Following successful therapy, anergy reverses to recall antigens but is still present to neoantigens in some patients. In addition to anergy, other tests of T-cell function, including response to mitogens and suppressor-cell function, suggest a defect in immune function prior to and following treatment. Humoral immunity with antibody production to soluble antigens is normal in untreated patients. Thus, patients who undergo staging laparotomy and splenectomy will develop humoral immunity to pneumococcal antigens if immunized with the pneumococcal vaccine prior to therapy. The clinical impact of these immune defects is limited. Except for a higher than normal incidence of herpes zoster, these patients are not plagued by opportunistic infections.

NATURAL HISTORY ACCORDING TO HISTOLOGIC SUBTYPE Patients with lymphocyte-predominant Hodgkin's disease are usually asymptomatic at presentation and tend to have localized disease. These patients are usually young, rarely have systemic symptoms or mediastinal mass, and are predominantly males. Nodular sclerosis Hodgkin's disease is found most frequently in adolescents and young adults who usually have localized disease; a preponderance are young women who present with a large mediastinal mass. Lymphocyte-depleted Hodgkin's disease is usually disseminated at the time of diagnosis and occurs in older patients who frequently have systemic symptoms. The mixed cellularity type occurs in all age groups and stages and is only slightly more common in males. There is a tendency toward an older age peak than with nodular sclerosis (30 to 40 years) and approximately half of these patients have advanced disease. Patients with lymphocyte-predominant and nodular sclerosis Hodgkin's disease, if untreated, have a more indolent disease associated with a longer survival and are more likely to be cured with radiotherapy. However, all Hodgkin's patients receiving chemotherapy have comparable long-term survivals irrespective of their histologic subtype.

There are several variables that adversely affect the prognosis of Hodgkin's disease. The number of involved sites and presence of bulky disease are the most important variables since extensive disease is often associated with high frequency of drug-resistant tumor cells. Large masses in the chest (greater than one-third the chest diameter) do poorly with radiotherapy or chemotherapy alone, but respond better to combined treatment. The prognosis is generally poor if a patient's disease is resistant to primary therapy or if relapse occurs within 12 months. Increased age and systemic B symptoms are poor prognostic signs regardless of stage. Systemic B symptoms forbode very poor prognosis, especially when all three symptoms are present. Lymphocyte-depleted histology, although very uncommon, is associated with a poor prognosis. Finally, males appear to have poorer prognosis than women when corrected for age, stage, and histology.

TREATMENT OF HODGKIN'S DISEASE Essentially all patients can and should be treated with curative intent. Radiotherapy may cure over 80 percent of patients with localized Hodgkin's disease, and chemotherapy over 50 percent of those with disseminated disease. *The choice of treatment regimen is totally dependent on stage of disease.* Thus, it is critical that pretreatment evaluation be precise and thorough with the objective of defining optimal therapy. This requires an integrated multidisciplinary effort at major oncology centers. As with all neoplasms, the therapy of Hodgkin's disease is constantly being reevaluated to improve disease-free survival and decrease toxicity.

Radiotherapy Radiation therapy alone has been evaluated in patients with pathologic stages IA, IIA, IB, IIB, and in some patients with stage IIIA. While lower doses of therapy will cause tumor regression, it was the recognition that 4000 cGy delivered at the rate of 1000 cGy per week could eradicate local Hodgkin's disease that revolutionized the treatment of this disease and led to substantial cure rates in patients with localized disease. With the knowledge that Hodgkin's disease spreads by lymphatic contiguity, three types of radiation fields were devised—namely, the mantle field, paraaortic field, and pelvic irradiation. The mantle field includes the submandibular, cervical, supraclavicular, infraclavicular, axillary, mediastinal, and hilar lymph nodes. The paraaortic field covers the transverse processes of the abdominal vertebral bodies and the spleen, if the spleen has not been removed. Pelvic irradiation includes the common iliac, hypogastric, external iliac, and inguinal nodes. When there is gross pelvic nodal involvement, the femoral nodes are also treated. Sometimes the pelvic and paraaortic fields are treated as one unit and it is commonly called the *inverted Y* field. The use of pelvic irradiation has been recently reduced since stages I and II supradiaphragmatic Hodgkin's disease can be treated without pelvic irradiation, and for stage III disease, total nodal irradiation has only a limited role.

Patients now receive mantle and paraaortic irradiation and only rarely total nodal irradiation. Patients receive doses of 3600 to 4000 cGy with an additional "cone down" dose for a total of 4000 to 4400 cGy to areas of bulk disease.

Patients with localized nodal Hodgkin's disease (pathologic stages IA and IIA) treated with mantle or paraaortic radiation therapy have a nearly 80 percent long-term disease-free survival. Patients with stages IB and IIB have reduced disease-free survival; however, most patients who relapse can be successfully treated with optimal combination chemotherapy. Early-stage patients with large mediastinal involvement appear to have a higher risk of relapse (disease-free survival of 40 to 55 percent) compared to patients with lesser or no mediastinal disease and should be managed with combined modality therapy.

Radiation therapy can lead to acute and late complications. Acute side effects of mantle irradiation include transient dry mouth, pharyngitis, fatigue, and weight loss; rarely, patients may develop transverse myelitis 9 months to several years later. Approximately 15 percent of patients within several months of mantle irradiation develop paresthesias in the lower extremities upon flexion of the neck or thighs (Lhermitte's syndrome). This syndrome usually resolves spontaneously; there is no correlation between this syndrome and irreversible spinal injury. With more recent techniques, including shielding and angling, this syndrome is rarely seen. Other long-term side effects include radiation pneumonitis (severe in less than 5 percent of patients) and subsequent pulmonary fibrosis. Late complications of mantle radiation include cardiac damage such as pericardial effusion with or without subsequent constrictive pericarditis and very rarely myocardial damage. Cardiac irradiation may also accelerate coronary artery disease and induce early myocardial infarctions. Chemical hypothyroidism may occur in up to 50 percent of patients with mantle irradiation. Paraaortic irradiation is rarely associated with significant side effects. Pelvic irradiation acutely induces transient diarrhea and bladder irradiation association with frequency. Chronic effects include potential long-term bone marrow suppression and sterility; therefore pelvic irradiation is less frequently employed. Moreover, increasing numbers of secondary tumors are being observed.

Chemotherapy By 1963 five agents had been identified as effective in the treatment of Hodgkin's disease, namely alkylating agents, vinca alkaloids, procarbazine, methotrexate, and prednisone. While disease regression occurred in 30 to 70 percent of patients, complete response occurred in only 10 percent. Based on the principles of dose, schedule, and combination chemotherapy, a four-drug combination regimen termed MOPP, meaning mechlorethamine (nitrogen mustard), Oncovin (vincristine), procarbazine, and prednisone, was introduced. In a "14 year median follow-up" of 188 patients, DeVita and his colleagues found that 84 percent had achieved a complete remission and 48 percent were alive. MOPP therapy has been associated with significant toxicity. Nearly all patients experience some degree of nausea and vomiting, which can be minimized by antiemetic therapy. Bone marrow suppression and associated leukopenia and occasional thrombocytopenia are frequently observed. Less commonly, absolute neutropenia occurs with increased susceptibility to infection. All males and nearly all older females become sterile following MOPP therapy, and all patients have a long-term risk of developing second malignancies.

Other multiple-drug regimens have been tested in the treatment of advanced Hodgkin's disease. However, none of the MOPP-derived combinations have been superior to the original MOPP administered at an optimal dose and schedule. Regimens have also been developed to treat MOPP-resistant patients. The best known of these is ABVD (adriamycin, bleomycin, vinblastine, and dacarbazine). A series of controlled clinical trials has demonstrated that ABVD is equivalent to MOPP in the successful treatment of primary advanced Hodgkin's disease. ABVD has also led to a significant number of prolonged complete remissions in MOPP treatment failures. Although most ABVD toxicities are identical to those from MOPP, the ABVD regimen produces only transient germ-cell toxicity in males, no drug-induced amenorrhea, and an apparent lower incidence of second tumors (although the data on this point are limited).

More recent studies have attempted to sequentially combine MOPP and ABVD to improve cure rate. The use of MOPP alternating with ABVD appears to produce higher complete remissions and disease-free survivals compared to MOPP alone, but longer periods of observations and more patients are necessary to confirm this observation.

Combined modality therapy In the past, combined modality therapy has been extensively employed in the treatment of intermediate- and advanced-stage Hodgkin's disease. Many patients received both MOPP and total nodal irradiation. Unfortunately, serious late consequences occurred. The most serious of these is the emergence of second malignancies, particularly acute nonlymphocytic leukemia and high-grade lymphomas. In patients treated with MOPP alone (or with one of its variants), the risk of leukemia within 10 years is 3 to 4 percent. The risk seems to be greater in patients over 40 years at the time of systemic treatment or when combined modality therapy is used (especially if salvage MOPP is administered after radiotherapy failure). The acute nonlymphocytic leukemia that occurs following MOPP differs from primary acute nonlymphocytic leukemia in that the former more commonly exhibits a preleukemia or myelodysplastic prodrome, a different cytogenetic profile with emphasis on partial or complete deletions of the 5th and 7th chromosomes, and a much lower response rate to antileukemia therapy. A recent study revealed an 18 percent cumulative actuarial risk of second tumors in 15-year survivors with Hodgkin's disease, and the risk of solid tumors appeared to continue to increase with time.

Salvage therapy After proper restaging, further radiotherapy can be delivered (if technically feasible) to patients who have shown relapse in areas outside a radiation port or following combination chemotherapy. In patients not achieving a complete remission or relapsing after MOPP, second line, non-cross-resistant regimens are available. If patients relapse more than 12 months after the completion of MOPP therapy, they should be retreated; if they relapse in less than 12 months, they should be treated with a salvage regimen. With ABVD as a salvage regimen, 50 percent of patients will achieve a complete remission and 20 percent will experience long-term disease-free survival. Selected chemotherapy patients who relapse after 12 months in limited nodal or pulmonary sites can be treated with salvage radiotherapy. Finally, as with non-Hodgkin's lymphoma, autologous or allogeneic bone marrow transplantation is an effective salvage treatment for some patients. Unlike in non-Hodgkin's lymphoma, total-body irradiation has minimal value and virtually all regimens include high-dose chemotherapy. Patients whose tumors are still sensitive to chemotherapeutic agents are more likely to experience long-term disease-free survival.

THERAPEUTIC RECOMMENDATION BY STAGE **Stages IA and IIA, nonbulky disease** Following staging laparotomy in patients with supradiaphragmatic disease, subtotal nodal irradiation is the treatment of choice. Rarely, in patients with subdiaphragmatic lymphoma, radiotherapy is delivered by an inverted Y field, including splenic pedicle in stage I disease and ranging through total nodal irradiation in stage II disease. Some suggest that treatment with involved-field radiotherapy combined with chemotherapy produces comparable results, but most do not consider this as an accepted treatment. For patients with subdiaphragmatic stage II disease of paraaortics, chemotherapy is recommended.

Stages IB and IIB, nonbulky disease The therapy is the same as for stages IA and IIA Hodgkin's disease; however, the relapse rate is higher. Relapse can usually be salvaged with chemotherapy. Previous studies have demonstrated that total nodal irradiation cures 80 percent and MOPP 60 percent of these patients. The combination of total nodal irradiation and MOPP is capable of producing a higher cure rate but also produces a significant incidence of second tumors and therefore is no longer recommended. If radiotherapy to the pelvis

is considered, bone marrow harvesting prior to treatment should be undertaken.

Stage II, bulky disease Stage II disease with bulky mediastinal or hilar adenopathy should be managed with combined modality therapy. This should include chemotherapy and radiotherapy to sites of bulk disease.

Stage IIIA Patients who present with minimal splenic disease respond equally well to subtotal lymphoid irradiation, combination chemotherapy with irradiation, or chemotherapy alone, with equivalent results. For patients with extensive splenic disease or enlarged paraaortic and pelvic nodes, the recommended treatment is combination chemotherapy with or without irradiation to involved sites. Alternative therapy includes either total nodal irradiation or combination chemotherapy, although these approaches are more controversial.

Stage IIIB, stage IV Combination chemotherapy is recommended, with alternatives including combination chemotherapy with irradiation to involved sites or alternating combination chemotherapy and irradiation.

REFERENCES

ANDERSON KC et al: Monoclonal antibodies: Their use in bone marrow transplantation. Prog Hematol XV: 137, 1987

ARMITAGE JO: Bone marrow transplantation in the treatment of patients with lymphoma. Blood 73(7):1749, 1989

CANELLOS GP (ed): Advances in chemotherapy for Hodgkin's and non-Hodgkins lymphomas. Semin Hematol, 25(2):1, 1988

COSSMAN J: T-cell neoplasms and Hodgkin's disease, in *Malignant Lymphoma*, CW Berard, RF Dorfman, N Kaufman (eds). Baltimore, Williams & Wilkins, 1987, pp 104–123

DEVITA VT JR et al: Lymphocytic lymphomas, in *Cancer: Principles and Practice of Oncology*, 3d ed, VT DeVita Jr, S Hellman, SA Rosenberg (eds). Philadelphia, Lippincott, 1989, pp 1741–1798

FREEDMAN AS, NADLER LM: Cell surface markers in hematologic malignancies. Semin Oncol 14(2):193, 1987

——— et al: Expression of B cell activation antigens on normal and malignant B cells. Leukemia 1:9, 1987

GRIBBEN JG et al: Successful treatment of refractory Hodgkin's disease by high-dose combination chemotherapy and autologous bone marrow transplantation. Blood 73(1):340, 1989

HELLMAN S et al: Hodgkin's disease, in *Cancer: Principles and Practice of Oncology*, 3d ed, VT DeVita Jr, S Hellman, SA Rosenberg (eds). Philadelphia, Lippincott, 1989, pp 1696–1740

KAPLAN HS: *Hodgkin's Disease*, 2d ed. Cambridge, Harvard University, 1980

KORSMEYER S: Immunoglobulin and T-cell receptor genes reveal the clonality, lineage, and translocations of lymphoid neoplasms, in *Important Advances in Oncology 1987*, VT DeVita Jr, S Hellman, SA Rosenberg (eds). Philadelphia, Lippincott, 1987, pp 3–26

SELTZER, SE, JOCHELSON MS (eds): Lymphoma, part I. Semin Ultrasound, CT, MR. 6(4):347, 1985

———, ———: Lymphoma, part II. Semin Ultrasound, CT, MR. 7(1):1, 1986

SHOWE LC, CROCE CM: Chromosomal translocations in B and T cell neoplasias. Semin Hematol 23(4):237, 1986

SKLAR JL et al: Diagnostic molecular biology of non-Hodgkin's lymphoma, in *Malignant Lymphoma*, CW Berard, RF Dorfman, N Kaufman (eds). Baltimore, Williams & Wilkins, 1987, pp 204–221

303 BREAST CANCER

CRAIG HENDERSON

Breast cancer is both one of the most common and one of the most treatable of all human malignancies. The incidence of this disease provides a poor estimate of the frequency with which breast problems are brought to the attention of physicians of all specialties. For each patient diagnosed with breast cancer, another 5 to 10 women are biopsied for suspicious symptoms, and for each patient biopsied, dozens seek consultation because of symptoms or concern. Breast cancer is one of the few tumors for which there is conclusive evidence that screening will substantially decrease mortality. In the treatment of breast cancer radical surgical procedures have been almost entirely replaced by more limited forms of surgery, such as the modified radical mastectomy, and most breast cancer patients now have the option of combining breast-sparing procedures (e.g., partial mastectomy or lumpectomy) with radiation therapy as an alternative to mastectomy. However, medical therapies are now an important component of the treatment of almost all stages of invasive breast cancer.

ETIOLOGY AND RISK FACTORS

Epidemiologic data suggest that genetic, endocrine, and environmental factors may be involved in the initiation and/or the promotion of breast cancer growth. Although the principal value of these studies is the identification of etiologic factors that may prove useful in primary prevention programs, epidemiologic data are often used to identify high-risk groups of women to be targeted for intensive surveillance or even prophylactic mastectomy. It has not been established, however, that these strategies will decrease breast cancer mortality in these high-risk groups, and an inappropriate emphasis on risk factors may obscure the fact that 70 to 80 percent of all breast cancers occur in patients without identifiable risk factors.

In the United States the cumulative lifetime probability of developing breast cancer is 10.2 percent and of dying from breast cancer, 3.6 percent. Most of the risk of developing breast cancer is expressed after age 50, and the highest risk is after age 75 (Table 303-1). In counseling women regarding their risk of developing breast cancer, the use of 20- to 40-year interval probabilities may be more meaningful than the lifetime probability. For example, the probability of a woman without defined risk factors developing breast cancer between the ages of 50 and 70 is 4.67 percent; that of dying from breast cancer is 1.04 percent. A patient with a relative risk of 3 (e.g., a woman whose mother and sister have been diagnosed with breast cancer) would then have a 14 percent probability of developing breast cancer and a 3.1 percent probability of dying from breast cancer during this interval. This likely explains why no risk group with an observed cumulative incidence of breast cancer in excess of 30 to 40 percent or cumulative mortality in excess of 10 to 20 percent has been identified.

Genetic factors Although all relatives of breast cancer patients are at some increased risk of developing breast cancer, first-degree relatives (siblings, parents, children) have a two- to threefold increase in risk compared to the general population. Thus, the cumulative probability that a 30-year-old woman whose sister or mother had breast cancer will herself develop breast cancer by age 70 is somewhere between 8 and 18 percent. Some investigators have observed an even higher risk when two or more relatives are affected, when the affected patient is premenopausal, or when the patient has bilateral breast cancer, but these observations have not been consistent among epidemiologic studies.

Endocrine factors Early age of menarche, late onset of menopause, nulliparity, and late age at first pregnancy appear to be independently associated with an increased incidence of breast cancer. Since both diet and exercise may affect both age of menarche and the regularity of menses, it has been suggested that this effect of diet and exercise may explain, at least in part, variations in breast cancer incidence among women with different lifestyles. Age at first full-term pregnancy is a more important determinant of risk than the number of pregnancies. Compared to women with a first pregnancy before age 18, the relative risk of breast cancer is doubled if the first pregnancy is delayed until after age 24 and about quadrupled after age 30. Several investigators have observed that the risk of breast cancer is actually higher among women with their first pregnancies after age 30 than among nulliparous women, and it has been suggested that early pregnancy is protective while late pregnancy may promote development of the disease. These observations are consistent with the hypothesis that events between menarche and the first pregnancy are critical in determining the lifetime probability of developing breast cancer.

The effect of exogenously administered hormones has been extensively studied with conflicting results. Although most studies on the effects of oral contraceptives have failed to establish a firm association with incidence of breast cancer, prolonged administration (e.g., 4 years or more), administration prior to the first pregnancy, and observation after a long latency period have been associated with a significantly increased risk in some studies. The reasons for the contradictory results are not readily apparent, and this is an issue about which physicians must suspend judgment until there are more definitive data. The results of studies on the use of estrogen replacement are also contradictory, but a review of all of the evidence suggests that there is a cumulative dose effect. A recently published prospective study of 23,244 Swedish women demonstrated that the relative risk of developing breast cancer was significantly increased to 1.7 after a little more than 9 years of therapy. The use of estrogens and progestins in sequence did not lessen the increased risk from estrogen use alone and may actually have augmented the risk and shortened the average latent interval. The use of conjugated estrogens, such as those most commonly used in the United States, may be associated with less risk than that following the use of estradiol, the major estrogen replacement therapy in the Swedish study. Although the effects of postmenopausal estrogen replacement on breast cancer incidence are substantially less than its effects on the incidence of endometrial cancer, moderate doses of conjugated estrogen for 15 to 20 years might increase the cumulative relative risk of breast cancer to 1.5 to 2.0.

Environmental factors Studies of atomic bomb blast victims in Hiroshima and Nagasaki demonstrate a radiation dose effect in the induction of breast cancer after a latent period of about 20 years. The highest incidence was observed among women who were aged 10 to 14 at the time of the explosion, and there was almost no increase in breast cancer incidence among women who were aged 30 to 49 at the time.

Breast cancer incidence varies widely around the world, and the highest rates occur in affluent and westernized countries. The lowest incidence is among Asians, but both immigrant and second-generation Japanese women migrating to Hawaii and southern California have an increasing risk of developing breast cancer with their greater longevity in the west. The search for environmental factors that might explain this phenomenon have centered on diet, and especially dietary fat. There is an excellent correlation between international variation in dietary fat intake and breast cancer incidence, and rats fed high-fat diets have a greater tendency to develop mammary tumors. However, epidemiologic studies have thus far failed to reproducibly

---

TABLE 303-1 Probability of a white female developing and dying of breast cancer

Age interval, years	Risk of developing breast cancer, %	Risk of dying of breast cancer, %
Birth to 110	10.20	3.60
20–30	0.04	0.00
20–40	0.49	0.09
35–45	0.88	0.14
35–55	2.53	0.56
50–60	1.95	0.33
50–70	4.67	1.04
65–75	3.17	0.43
65–85	5.48	1.01

SOURCE: From Seidman et al, CA 35:36, 1985.

demonstrate an association between dietary fat and the development of breast cancer. Postmenopausal women who are obese have an increased risk of breast cancer. Moderate alcohol intake has been repeatedly shown to be associated with an increased risk of 40 to 60 percent, but the explanation for this is not readily apparent. While points of circumstantial evidence linking environmental factors and breast cancer risk are numerous, none is sufficiently well-established to warrant strongly urging women to change their lifestyle in any particular way. Of course, recommendations to reduce dietary fat content and to maintain ideal body weight may be prudent because of their beneficial effects on other organ systems even if the benefits in reducing risk of breast cancer are minimal.

BENIGN BREAST DISEASE In general, a woman's risk of subsequently developing breast cancer after a biopsy that demonstrates benign disease is increased relative to the total population of women. The most common histologic diagnosis assigned to these biopsy specimens is "fibrocystic disease," a poorly defined term that implies the presence of macroscopic, fluid-filled cysts and a nonspecific proliferation of epithelial and mesenchymal tissue. This has led many physicians to equate all lumps and irregularities detected on physical examination or mammography with "fibrocystic disease," suggesting that the women examined are at increased risk of developing breast cancer. It has not been demonstrated that women with lumpy breasts who have *not* had a biopsy have an increased risk of breast cancer, and it is estimated that most women (probably more than 80 percent) have at least some irregular tissue densities on examination and/or mammography. For these reasons the diagnosis of "fibrocystic disease" should not be based on nonhistologic findings, and the term should probably be abandoned by pathologists as well because of its lack of specificity.

The increased risk of breast cancer among women with benign breast disease seems to be confined entirely to that group of women who have histologic evidence of ductal or lobular cell proliferation on biopsy (about 30 percent of all patients biopsied for benign conditions), and especially those who have atypical hyperplasia (about 3 percent of biopsied patients). The relative risk for developing breast cancer in this group is 4.4 times that of an age-matched population of unselected women. In women with both atypical hyperplasia and a first-degree relative with a history of breast cancer, the risk of subsequent breast cancer is increased about ninefold. Such patients are rare (representing about 1 percent of all biopsies for benign disease), and the *observed* cumulative risk of a patient in this very high risk group developing breast cancer over a 25-year period is about 40 percent; the cumulative risk of a woman in this group dying of breast cancer is less than 10 percent.

IN SITU BREAST CANCER There are two histologically and clinically distinct variants of carcinoma in situ (CIS): ductal and lobular. Traditionally, both were considered the earliest detectable form of malignant transformation in the breast, but increasingly lobular CIS (or lobular neoplasia) is viewed as a risk factor akin to atypical hyperplasia. Lobular CIS does not form a palpable tumor and is usually found as an incidental finding in a premenopausal woman biopsied for some other condition. Additional biopsies will usually demonstrate additional foci of lobular CIS in the same or even the contralateral breast, and any attempt to totally excise lobular CIS by any method other than mastectomy is likely to be ineffective. Patients who have no further treatment after a diagnosis of lobular CIS have an increased lifetime risk of subsequently developing an invasive breast cancer with either a ductal or a lobular histology. Without treatment, the cumulative incidence of a subsequent breast cancer of any type (invasive or ductal in situ) is about 25 percent and the cumulative mortality somewhat less than 10 percent. Most of these cancers occur after a latent period of 5 to 20 years and occur as often in the contralateral as in the biopsied breast. For this reason, most physicians now routinely offer these patients one of two treatment options: careful observation or bilateral simple mastectomies and breast reconstruction. A patient's choice between these two disparate

options is likely to depend on the anxiety generated by her perception of the risk associated with observation.

Ductal CIS (or intraductal carcinoma) may form palpable tumors. It occurs with almost equal frequency in premenopausal and postmenopausal women and is more often confined to one breast, even to one quadrant of the breast. Thus, it is possible to excise this type of cancer totally by more limited surgical procedures than mastectomy. Until recently, ductal CIS was uncommon, accounting for only about 1 percent of all cancers diagnosed in the United States. However, ductal CIS is often the cause of microcalcifications seen in mammograms, and it is estimated that ductal CIS constitutes almost 10 percent of all breast cancers now diagnosed in the United States due to the increased use of routine mammography. Because these changes in incidence and mode of diagnosis are recent, it is not certain that the natural history of the ductal CIS now being diagnosed is the same as that observed in earlier eras. The diagnosis of ductal CIS may be difficult. At one extreme, it may be mistaken for atypical hyperplasia, and at the other, microscopic foci of invasion may be overlooked. Electron microscopy will reveal additional areas of invasion, and this may account for the fact that axillary lymph node metastases are seen in 1 to 2 percent of patients with a diagnosis of ductal CIS.

The natural history of ductal CIS in patients treated with less than a mastectomy has been less extensively studied than that of lobular CIS. These patients, too, are at increased risk of developing a subsequent invasive cancer throughout life, but, unlike lobular CIS, this risk is more often expressed in the ipsilateral than in the contralateral breast. For this reason, a simple (or total) mastectomy *without node dissection* is still the standard treatment for this condition and is associated with a nearly 100 percent long-term survival. However, in recent years, wide excision alone, especially for very small tumors, or wide excision plus radiotherapy for larger tumors has been used in patients whose tumors can be totally excised. Although the initial results from these breast-conserving approaches are promising, more definite statements regarding the relative value of these treatments await longer follow-up and the completion of randomized trials in the United States and Europe.

Subsequent risk for invasive cancer in the contralateral breast after mastectomy The group of patients with the highest risk of developing breast cancer are those who have already had one breast cancer. The risk is lifelong and occurs at a rate of 0.5 to 1.0 percent per year of follow-up. Concurrent cancers in both breasts are diagnosed in about 4 percent of patients. However, the prognosis of a patient with two breast cancers, whether concurrent or sequential, is not measurably worse than that of a patient with only one breast cancer. Since the cancer with the worst clinical and pathologic stage determines the patient's overall prognosis, patients with a good prognosis after an initial diagnosis should be monitored carefully to detect a second cancer, should it occur, as early as possible.

SCREENING ASYMPTOMATIC PATIENTS

It has been firmly established by two randomized trials that periodic mammography performed in asymptomatic women will reduce breast cancer mortality by 20 to 30 percent. The only trial with follow-up in excess of 10 years was performed by the Health Insurance Plan (HIP) of New York. Patients in the study group of this trial were invited to undergo *both* mammography and physical examination at yearly intervals. Most of the benefits in the HIP trial derived from the physical examination, but this is likely due to the fact that the mammography equipment used was insensitive by modern standards. In the first reports from the HIP study, survival benefits were observed only for women in the study group over age 50. A more recent analysis has demonstrated a 24 percent reduction ($p < 0.05$) in mortality for all age groups at the end of 18 years of follow-up. The benefits of mammography in women 50 or over have been confirmed in almost all trials performed subsequent to the HIP study, and if the evidence from *all* of the available trials is considered together, there *may* be a much smaller but real benefit from screening women aged 40 to 49, as well. It is widely assumed that the benefits of screening are proportional to the patient's risk of developing breast cancer and that patients with a family history of breast cancer, benign breast disease, or those who are nulliparous should be screened at a younger age. These assumptions have not been prospectively or retrospectively evaluated in any study. Although yearly mammography and physical examination were used in the HIP trial, a Swedish trial demonstrated benefits of a similar magnitude in women over 50 years of age who received mammograms without physical examinations at 2- to 3-year intervals. No one has yet demonstrated that mortality is reduced by the use of a baseline mammography at age 35 or 40, even though many physicians employ this as a "halfway" measure.

Although there is an increasing tendency for professional societies in the United States to recommend yearly mammography for all women over the age of 40, some groups, such as the American College of Physicians and most European health services, have been more cautious in their interpretation of the available data. Large but still unpublished randomized trials from Great Britain and Canada may further alter the recommendations of these groups. However, based on the available evidence, the following guidelines appear reasonable:

1 Women age 50 and over should undergo an annual or biennial screening examination utilizing both mammography and physical examination.
2 Mammography should generally not be used in women under age 35.
3 Women between the ages of 40 and 49 may elect to undergo periodic screening examinations, but they should be informed about the controversies regarding the use of mammography in this age group.
4 Although not yet of proven value, it seems reasonable to recommend periodic screening mammography to high-risk patients over age 35. Mammography, with or without periodic physical examination, remains the only diagnostic tool of proven value in asymptomatic women. Although real, the risk of radiation-induced cancers is very small and is far outweighed by the benefits in women age 50 or over and probably in those age 40 to 49 as well. Ultrasound will not detect microcalcifications, often the only indication of tumor and especially of very small tumors. Thermography results in an unacceptably high false-positive and false-negative rate and has not even been shown to be helpful in identifying patients who should undergo mammography. Cancers appearing in patients who perform regular (e.g., monthly) breast self-examination (BSE) are, on average, smaller than those in patients who do not do BSE. The only known toxicity of BSE is the increased anxiety it causes some women. However, all published BSE studies have large length and lead-time biases. These biases occur because apparent survival advantages for patients whose cancers have been found by BSE may be due to a longer clinical observation period from diagnosis to death, or to the fact that slower growing tumors are more often detected by BSE, and not due to any improved efficacy of therapy, because the tumor was diagnosed before the onset of metastasis when it is theoretically more curable. It has not yet been shown in properly controlled trials that BSE will actually decrease breast cancer mortality.

DIAGNOSIS AND INITIAL EVALUATION

More than 80 percent of cancers are diagnosed because of a suspicious mass, usually a mass found by the patient. Pain without an immediately apparent mass is a less frequent presenting symptom, and increasingly breast cancer is being diagnosed on a routine mammogram in a totally asymptomatic patient. Nipple discharge is also an unusual presenting symptom. Most nipple discharges, whether serous or sanguineous, are caused by benign disorders, most commonly an intraductal papilloma. A nipple discharge with a negative test for hemoglobin is almost always benign, but breast cancer is the cause of a hemoglobin-positive discharge in less than 10 percent of such patients.

Physical examination should begin with a visual inspection of the breast while the patient is sitting. An underlying breast cancer may cause a protrusion, asymmetry in breast contour, or a subtle dimpling of the skin due to entrapment of Cooper's ligaments. Recent onset of nipple inversion may also be a sign of breast cancer, but both nipple inversion and asymmetry of breast size are common findings in the normal breast. Palpation of the breast is best performed when the patient is in a supine position. Breast cancers are most often described as irregularly shaped, firm or hard, painless nodules or masses, but in fact they may be of almost any shape or consistency. For this reason, any mass, lesion, or thickening that is distinctly different from the surrounding tissue (or "dominant") should be evaluated more carefully. The most common nonmalignant finding on breast examination is a diffuse, indistinct, and somewhat elastic amalgamation of lumps often mistakenly referred to as "fibrocystic disease" (see above). Well-defined cysts may be quite distinct but have a more elastic character than breast cancer. Benign fibroadenomas are often as firm as breast cancer but can be distinguished by their marblelike smoothness and slippery quality, their appearance in young women, and their recurrent nature. Fat necrosis and sclerosing adenosis, both benign conditions, can usually be distinguished from breast cancer only by biopsy. If there are signs of more locally advanced growth, mastectomy and/or radiotherapy are unlikely to substantially prolong a patient's life. These signs include fixation of the mass to the skin, the pectoralis muscle, or the chest wall, the presence of satellite skin nodules or ulcerations, the finding of matted axillary nodes, or the presence of any supraclavicular lymph nodes. Plugging of the dermal lymphatics will cause skin thickening and exaggeration of the usual skin markings, a process termed *peau d'orange*. When this is extensive and accompanied by inflammation, the patient usually has inflammatory breast cancer, a particularly virulent form of cancer best treated initially with chemotherapy and radiotherapy. Inflammatory breast cancer may be mistakenly diagnosed initially as mastitis, but infections or other inflammatory conditions of the breast are rare except in the first months postpartum or after trauma.

Further evaluation of a suspected cyst might include a repeat examination of the breast immediately following the next menstrual period in a premenopausal woman, the use of ultrasound to confirm the impression that the mass is fluid-filled, or removal of the cyst fluid with a fine-gauge needle *and reexamination of the breast to document that the cyst has disappeared.* The latter is the preferred approach in a symptomatic patient because it will usually relieve the pain and the patient will be reassured that this is not cancer, unless the cyst fluid is grossly bloody or reaccumulates rapidly.

Mammography   If breast examination leads to any suspicion that a mass is malignant, biopsy should be performed. Biopsy should be *preceded* by a mammogram, which may better define the extent of the lesion, demonstrate other suspicious masses, and serve as a baseline obtained before distortion of normal breast architecture by biopsy. Abnormalities on mammogram that suggest a breast cancer include: (1) distinct, irregular, often crablike densities (Fig. 303-1), (2) *clusters* of five or more microcalcifications, each less than 1 mm in diameter and all in an area of less than 1 cm (Fig. 303-2), or (3) architectural distortion without a benign explanation such as a scar from a prior biopsy. Although more than 80 percent of suspicious microcalcifications are benign, cancers associated with such microcalcifications are usually the most curable of all breast cancers. Diagnosis can be made by radiologic placement of needles under local anesthesia and subsequent biopsy of tissue surrounding the needle ends. The excised tissue should be x-rayed to ensure that the calcifications or other suspicious lesions have been removed, and/or

FIGURE 303-1   Focal compression mammogram shows a clinically occult 1-cm spiculated mass. Biopsy demonstrated infiltrating ductal breast cancer. *(Courtesy of Dr Paul Stomper.)*

the patient should have a repeat mammogram 4 to 6 weeks after biopsy when the breast is no longer tender.

In almost all instances, incisional or excisional biopsy of the breast may be performed under local anesthesia in a day surgery or an outpatient clinic, thus avoiding the additional risk of general anesthesia and permitting the patient to discuss and adjust to treatment options before undergoing definitive surgical treatment. Fine-needle aspiration and cytologic evaluation may also be diagnostic but is advisable *only* if an experienced cytologist is available and if all suspicious lesions read as negative are followed with a more definitive biopsy procedure. Tissue should be sent routinely for assay of estrogen and progesterone receptors. Additional staging procedures immediately following the diagnosis of breast cancer should include evaluation of those sites to which breast cancer most frequently metastasizes (see below).

NATURAL HISTORY AND PROGNOSTIC FACTORS

The natural history of breast cancer is characterized by long duration and marked heterogeneity. The median survival of patients who refuse all forms of treatment is between 2.5 and 3 years, but the

FIGURE 303-2   Mammogram shows a clinically occult 1-cm cluster of microcalcifications. Biopsy demonstrated infiltrating ductal breast cancer. *(Courtesy of Dr Paul Stomper.)*

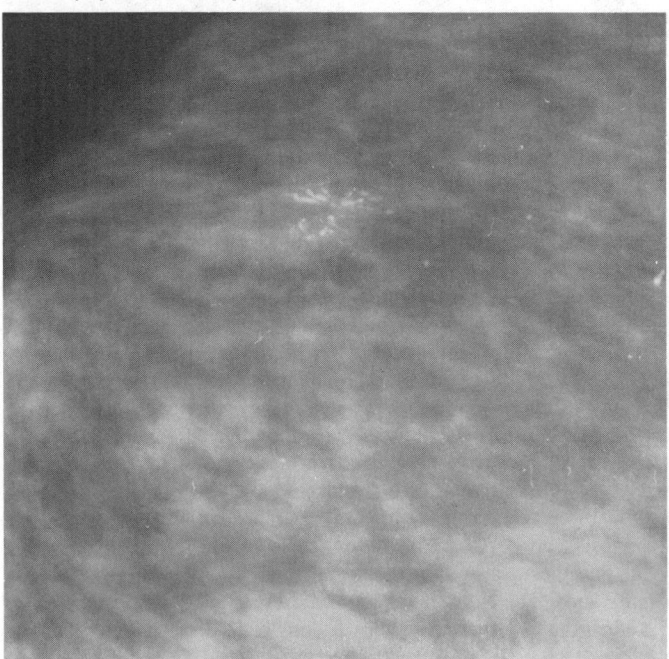

survival of an untreated patient may exceed 20 years. Breast cancer is certainly among the more slowly growing tumors, and it has been estimated that the average tumor doubles about three times per year. If this applies to the preclinical (or prediagnostic) period of tumor growth, then the average breast cancer requires 10 years or more to grow from a single cell to 1 cm, the size at which it can be readily detected by most patients or physicians. Presumably metastases may occur during much of this preclinical period but likely with greatest frequency during the last 3 to 4 years of preclinical growth, when the tumor mass increases from 10^6 cells to more than 10^9 cells. Because microscopic or clinically undetectable micrometastases are well-established by the time of diagnosis, most breast cancer patients treated with local therapy only (i.e., surgery and/or radiotherapy) eventually die in spite of excellent local control of their disease. Because many patients' tumors metastasize late in the preclinical course, early detection with mammography will increase the patient's survival. Because the growth rate of the disease is so variable, comparisons of treatment effects in even well-defined patient cohorts are often erroneous unless the treatment groups have been defined by large, randomized controlled trials.

Clinical pathologic staging   Clinical staging systems were developed by surgeons to identify *preoperatively* those patients unlikely to benefit from treatment with mastectomy. Although those with large tumor size and palpable axillary adenopathy were found to have a poorer long-term prognosis, the only patients categorically discouraged from undergoing mastectomy were those with signs of locally advanced disease (see above). About 25 to 35 percent of patients with axillary adenopathy will have no histologic evidence of tumor in lymph nodes, and the same percentage of patients without adenopathy *will* have histologic node involvement. Although information on histologic node involvement is of no value in deciding whether a patient should undergo mastectomy, this has proven to be the most accurate and reproducible prognostic factor worldwide. It is convenient to divide patients into three groups: those without node involvement, those with one to three positive nodes, or those with four or more positive nodes (Table 303-2). However, these divisions are arbitrary. A substantial number of node-negative patients will have recurrences and eventually die of breast cancer. Each additional positive node is associated with a worse prognosis, but some patients with more than 10 positive nodes will survive for 10 to 20 years or more. In general, the number of positive lymph nodes correlates with the time of recurrence as well as the probability of recurrence. For the data set shown in Table 303-2, the median time to recurrence was 2.1 years and the time to death 4 years for those patients with four or more positive nodes, compared to 4.1 years and >10 years, respectively, for those with one to three positive nodes. The hazard of recurrence decreased in all nodal subgroups after the first 3 years but remained fairly constant thereafter. This explains why the effects of therapy on recurrence rate, especially on recurrence in patients with many positive nodes, are apparent after a short follow-up, but the effects of therapy on survival may require much longer follow-up.

Patients with a larger breast mass or a higher clinical stage are more likely to have positive nodes, but within a single-node category the size of the breast cancer has independent prognostic value. This

TABLE 303-2   Ten-year survival and survival without recurrence relative to histologic node status at the time of radical mastectomy (no adjuvant systemic therapy given)

Node category	Survival, %	
	Overall	Without recurrence
All patients	60	47
Nodes negative	82	72
Nodes positive	40	25
1–3 nodes positive	54	34
4+ nodes positive	26	16

SOURCE: From Valagussa et al, CA 41:1170, 1978.

has led to the promulgation of staging systems that combine clinical and pathologic characteristics. However, these systems have changed so frequently and are used so differently by different specialists that the categorization of patients into one of four "stages" has lost all practical meaning. For example, a 3-cm tumor mass and no histologically involved lymph nodes is considered a stage II breast cancer, as is a 1-cm mass with eight positive nodes. Both the prognosis and the likely treatment of these two patients are substantially different. Therefore, a careful description of the patient's cancer, a precise measurement of tumor size, and a simple statement of the number of histologically positive lymph nodes will provide a more accurate description of "stage" than the use of stage numbers I to IV.

Histologic subtypes More than 80 percent of breast cancers are of the invasive ductal type. The next most common variety, infiltrating lobular, constitutes almost 10 percent of all cancers and has the same prognosis as infiltrating ductal carcinoma. Medullary carcinoma, representing about 5 percent of breast cancers, is less likely to metastasize to regional lymph nodes, but the prognosis of medullary cancers with nodal metastases is the same as that of the other major histologic groups with nodal metastases. The large number of histologic types that make up the remaining 5 percent of breast cancers are generally less malignant.

Tumor grade, defined by the degree of differentiation of cytoplasmic or nuclear features, has been shown repeatedly to correlate with the probability of recurrence or death from breast cancer. Other histologic characteristics that may be important include blood vessel or intramammary lymphatic vessel invasion, mitotic frequency, lymph node sinus histiocytosis, and tumor necrosis. However, the major limitation in the use of tumor histologic features is a lack of reproducibility from one pathologist to another, especially when the pathologist has not been specifically trained and is not very experienced in the use of these grading systems. For this reason, tumor grade is generally not used to make therapeutic decisions.

Estrogen receptors Tumors with an estrogen or progesterone receptor are more likely to respond to endocrine therapy used either as an adjuvant to mastectomy or radiotherapy soon after diagnosis or as a means of palliating metastatic disease symptoms later in a patient's course. In addition, most studies have demonstrated a significantly better disease-free survival and/or overall survival during the first 10 years of follow-up for patients who have one of these receptors. However, neither the estrogen nor the progesterone receptor identifies the 20 to 30 percent of node-negative patients likely to have recurrence, and at the end of 5 years, the difference in the recurrence rate among estrogen receptor–positive and –negative patients who are also node-negative is only about 5 percent.

Flow cytometry, ploidy, oncogenes The percentage of tumor cells undergoing mitosis has been shown in a number of experimental systems to be proportional to the growth fraction (i.e., the percentage of the tumor actually growing at any one point in time) and hence to the growth rate. This growth fraction can be estimated by thymidine labeling and autoradiography to obtain a thymidine labeling index (TLI) or by flow cytometry to estimate the fraction of cells in S phase (SPF). Clinical correlations have shown that a high TLI or high SPF is associated with early relapse and earlier breast cancer death, even after correction for other prognostic factors, such as lymph node and estrogen receptor status. However, as with other prognostic factors, these methods do not define distinct groups of patients, and, even though many clinical laboratories now routinely perform flow cytometry along with receptor determinations, there is still no standardization of methodology or established range of values associated with a particularly good or particularly poor prognosis. In general, patients with aneuploid tumors will have a worse prognosis than patients with predominantly diploid tumors, but early differences in relapse rate are not large, especially among node-negative patients.

Multiple genetic alterations have been described in breast cancers, including allelic deletions on chromosome 11 or 13 and amplification of the c-*myc* and *int*-2 genes. However, the most extensively studied is the amplification of the HER-2/*neu* (or c-*erb*B 2) gene. Some, but not all, studies have demonstrated a better survival among node-positive patients without amplification of this gene. The clinical importance of this relatively new area of study remains to be demonstrated, and the biologic importance of any of the known prognostic factors is still largely unexplored.

LOCAL THERAPY OF OPERABLE BREAST CANCER

Breast cancers are usually considered "operable" if it is technically possible to remove all cancerous tissue, if the tumor does not involve or has not become fixed to skin or structures deep to the breast, and if the tumor has not metastasized beyond the axillary or internal mammary lymph nodes. It has been demonstrated repeatedly in randomized clinical trials that more extensive surgical procedures will reduce the subsequent likelihood of tumor recurrence on the chest wall, in any remaining breast tissue, or in the nodal areas. However, these trials have failed to demonstrate that the type of surgery used will significantly affect patient survival. The evidence that local therapy has any effect on patient survival comes from the randomized trials of screening mammography (see above), in which it has demonstrated that early mastectomy results in a lower breast cancer mortality than late mastectomy.

The most extensive surgical procedure is the *radical mastectomy*, in which the breast is removed along with the pectoralis major and minor muscles and some overlying skin (at least 4 cm on each side of the tumor biopsy site), and there is an en bloc resection of all axillary contents, including lymph nodes beyond the subclavian vein. An *extended radical mastectomy* includes, as well, en bloc resection of the internal mammary nodes along with portions of the sternum and ribs. Because of the large cosmetic defect resulting from these procedures, neither is commonly used today, and it is doubtful whether their use is ever indicated, since the same or better local control of disease can be achieved with the use of radiotherapy added to less extensive surgical procedures. Most forms of the modified radical mastectomy leave the pectoralis major muscle intact, require the removal of less skin, and usually involve a less extensive node dissection. A *simple* or *total mastectomy* is the removal of the breast and a small amount of skin, but a simple mastectomy with node dissection approximates a modified radical mastectomy. Breast-conserving surgical procedures include wide excision, lumpectomy or tylectomy (Greek *tylos* = lump), segmental mastectomy, and quadrantectomy. These all require removal of the mass along with some normal surrounding tissue and differ only in the extent of the tissue excised. A separate excision for either a "sampling" of lymph nodes or a more complete lymph node dissection is possible with all of these procedures.

Radiotherapy When administered after a mastectomy, radiotherapy is usually referred to as "adjuvant," while radiotherapy given after breast-conserving surgery is often called "primary" radiotherapy. Adjuvant radiotherapy is less commonly used now than it once was because it was not possible to demonstrate in multiple randomized trials that its use prolonged survival. In addition, a small but statistically significant increase in mortality from second tumors and/or cardiovascular disease has been reported in patients who survived more than 10 to 15 years after receiving adjuvant radiotherapy. However, this finding was observed primarily in patients treated with now-outdated radiotherapy techniques.

When breast-conserving therapy is used, the resection margins ideally should be microscopically free of tumor before radiotherapy is given. Usually 4500 to 5000 cGy is administered in divided fractions over about 5 weeks. The same doses of radiotherapy may be administered to the axillary, supraclavicular, and internal mammary nodes, and a boost of 1600 to 1800 cGy may be added to the tumor bed. The treatment of axillary nodal areas and the use of a boost is variable and depends on the tumor characteristics of an individual patient and the treatment philosophy of the radiotherapist. When all areas are treated, "primary" radiotherapy is as extensive as the radical mastectomy, and local tumor control is as good or better.

The choice between breast-conserving surgery plus radiotherapy and mastectomy will depend on the patient's assessment of the relative benefits and side effects associated with each procedure. The only real advantage of breast-conserving procedures is the greater sense of body integrity and improved cosmesis that may result. This advantage may be lost if the tumor mass is large relative to the size of the breast, thus necessitating almost total removal of the breast to obtain tumor-free margins. Under the best of circumstances the cosmetic results of limited surgery plus radiotherapy are excellent, and the treated breast may feel entirely normal and appear indistinguishable from the contralateral breast. More often the treated breast will be somewhat smaller with limited induration around the biopsy site; uncommonly (in less than 5 percent of patients) there will be marked induration, breast shrinkage, and distortion of normal breast architecture. Other complications from radiotherapy, including broken bones, brachial plexopathy, and pneumonitis, are uncommon and rarely either cause symptoms or are the source of more than transient symptomatology. There may be a subgroup of patients who have a relatively high recurrence rate (23 percent by the end of 5 years) if treated with breast-conserving surgery and radiotherapy. The histologic appearance of the tumors in these patients is characterized by extensive intraductal carcinoma in *both* the area of invasive carcinoma and adjacent tissues ostensibly free of invasive carcinoma. Although a small intraductal component in an invasive carcinoma is normal, the intraductal component comprises more than 25 percent of all tumor tissue in these patients and appears to be a marker of a tumor likely to be multifocal throughout the breast. Very limited data suggest that patients who have recurrences some years after initial surgery and radiotherapy with tumor confined entirely to the breast or breast and regional lymph nodes may be successfully treated with a secondary mastectomy and that this type of recurrence may not compromise survival.

Breast-conserving surgery *without* radiotherapy is generally not used because of the very high likelihood of local recurrence. In the only randomized trial addressing this issue, patients with tumor-free resection margins who were treated with segmental mastectomy alone had a local recurrence rate of 28 percent at the end of 5 years, compared to 8 percent for patients treated with segmental mastectomy plus radiotherapy. At the end of nearly a decade of follow-up, the survival of patients in these three groups is not significantly different.

Breast reconstruction   Many patients will prefer mastectomy because it requires a shorter period of initial treatment and provides the patient with an added assurance that "all the tumor has been removed." Psychological studies demonstrate that most mastectomy patients have fully recovered from the initial emotional trauma of mastectomy by the end of 1 year. Many patients feel that their lives are simplified and their sense of body integrity restored by surgical reconstruction of the breast. This may be performed at the time of mastectomy or many years later. The procedures used include simple placement of a submuscular (or less commonly, subcutaneous) silicon implant, the use of a tissue expander followed by silicon implant, the transposition of muscle and blood supply from either the back of abdomen using the latissimus dorsi or the lower rectus abdominis muscle (TRAM flap), or the creation of a free tissue flap using the gluteus maximus muscle anastomosed to the internal mammary vessels. The choice among these procedures will depend on the extent of the patient's prior surgery and radiotherapy, the patient's willingness to undergo additional surgical procedures, and the experience and philosophy of the plastic surgeon. Under the best of circumstances the reconstructed breast will appear to be exactly the same size and shape as the contralateral breast, but, in addition to reconstruction of a nipple, this may require mammoplasty on the contralateral breast and several surgical procedures.

Node dissection   The main purpose of lymph node dissection is diagnostic, not therapeutic (see above). However, the morbidity associated with treatment of the lymph nodes is greater than with

any other aspect of local therapy. Even with a limited node sampling or node dissection limited to levels I and II (i.e., the areas medial and inferior to the subclavian muscle), the patient often will complain of lifelong discomfort, hyperesthesia or hypalgesia, and/or a sense of pulling and contraction. When more extensive surgery is used, when the radiotherapy field includes the upper axilla, and especially when both modalities are used, these symptoms increase in frequency and severity. Patients may experience edema of the arm and hand, and on rare occasions the patient may totally lose use of the involved extremity. For this reason a full node dissection, as employed in the radical mastectomy, followed by radiotherapy, is usually contraindicated, and whenever possible surgical excision should be limited to lower nodes and radiotherapy to this area avoided altogether.

Summary recommendations for local therapy   All patients with invasive operable breast cancer should receive some form of local therapy. In most cases this will be either a modified radical mastectomy (simple mastectomy plus node dissection) or breast-conserving surgery and limited node dissection followed by radiotherapy to the breast. Ideally, the patient will participate in the choice between these treatment alternatives and will see both a surgeon and a radiotherapist in the process of self-education regarding the benefits and limitations of these approaches.

ADJUVANT SYSTEMIC THERAPY

The use of systemic therapy, either chemotherapy or endocrine therapy, immediately after or as an "adjuvant" to local therapy will prolong the average time to recurrence of all patient groups. In addition, it has been reproducibly shown that the appropriate use of these therapies will significantly prolong the *survival* of some groups. Although theoretically possible, it has not yet been demonstrated that these therapies will "cure" any patient or group of patients not cured by local therapy alone.

An overview or meta-analysis of the large number of randomized adjuvant therapy trials has demonstrated that the use of adjuvant chemotherapy for some period in excess of 3 months will reduce a patient's odds of dying in the first 5 years after diagnosis by 14 ± 4 percent ($p = 0.003$). Although treatment prolongs the time to recurrence in women aged 50 and over as well as in those under age 50, adjuvant chemotherapy significantly improves survival only in those under 50 years of age. Among these younger women the odds of dying in the first 5 years may be reduced by 22 to 37 percent, and at the end of 5 years the survival of younger women given adjuvant chemotherapy was 7 to 9 percent higher than that of the control groups. The most commonly used and the most effective therapies in these studies were combinations that included cyclophosphamide, methotrexate, and 5-fluorouracil (CMF) (Table 303-3).

Adjuvant tamoxifen given for 1 year or more reduces the odds of death in the first 5 years after diagnosis by 16 ± 3 percent ($p <$

TABLE 303-3   Dose schedules of the drug regimens and endocrine therapies most frequently used to treat early and advanced breast cancer

Drug	Dose schedule
CMF(P) (28-day cycle)	
Cyclophosphamide	100 mg/m² PO days 1–14
Methotrexate	60 mg/m² IV days 1 and 8
5-Fluorouracil	600 mg/m² IV days 1 and 8
Prednisone (optional)	40 mg/m² PO days 1–14
CAF (21-day cycle)	
Cyclophosphamide	400–500 mg/m² IV day 1
Doxorubicin	40–50 mg/m² IV day 1
5-Fluorouracil	400–500 mg/m² IV days 1 and 8
Tamoxifen	10 mg PO bid
Megestrol acetate	40 mg PO qid
Aminoglutethimide	250 mg PO bid
+ hydrocortisone	10 mg PO qid

0.00001). However, when analyzed by age group, a significant survival benefit has been observed only in women aged 50 or more, where the reduction in the odds of death is 20 percent. At the end of 5 years the survival advantage for older, tamoxifen-treated women is about 6 percent. When tamoxifen was given from 2 to 5 years in these studies, it appeared to be more effective than when the duration of therapy was limited to 1 year.

Net benefit calculations There is no evidence that a patient who dies of breast cancer after mastectomy or radiotherapy has lived longer as a result of this local therapy. The patient is either cured or dies at about the same time she would have died without therapy. In contrast, systemic therapy may prolong life without curing the patient because systemic therapy causes a substantial but usually incomplete reduction in the size of tumor deposits at various metastatic sites. It is often erroneously assumed that a 10 percent survival advantage for the group of patients treated with adjuvant therapy means that *only* 10 percent of the patients have benefitted from therapy. In fact, the same survival difference between the treated and untreated patients can be obtained if *all* of the treated patients have a variable and transient prolongation of survival.

Calculation of the "average" size of this survival benefit requires long follow-up, and there is as yet no standard method for defining this average. However, it may be crudely estimated by subtracting the median survival of the patients randomized to the control group of a trial from the median survival of the treated group. When this is done for the premenopausal, node-positive patients randomized to receive 1 year of adjuvant CMF, the difference in median survivals exceeds 3 years, at least in one of the trials with the longest follow-up (the Milan trial). Of course, there is likely a wide range of effects around this average. Some patients may have had their lives shortened because of the toxicity of adjuvant chemotherapy. Some may have lived several decades longer as a result of treatment. The same calculations have been performed with data from a Scottish trial in which mostly postmenopausal, node-positive women were randomized to receive either 5 years of adjuvant tamoxifen or tamoxifen as first systemic therapy on relapse. The difference in median survival favored the treated patients and was just short of 2 years.

Most of these therapies, especially adjuvant chemotherapy, have well-known acute side effects and less well-defined delayed effects (see below). For this reason a real but small benefit may be outweighed by the toxicity of therapy. The expression of benefits as additional years of life eases this problem. For example, a premenopausal node-positive patient might subtract months during which CMF is administered (now usually about 6 months) and during which she experiences the toxicity of therapies from the 3 or more additional years of life gained from therapy to derive a "net" benefit of 2.5 or more years.

Node-negative patients Most of the early adjuvant trials included primarily or exclusively node-positive patients. However, since 20 to 30 percent of node-negative patients relapse and die of breast cancer in the first 10 years after diagnosis (Table 303-2), recent studies have included large numbers of node-negative patients, especially patients perceived as having the worst prognosis. Almost all of these trials demonstrate that adjuvant chemotherapy and adjuvant tamoxifen prolong the average time to recurrence of node-negative patients, but none of the large and more definitive trials has yet demonstrated a survival benefit. However, the interpretations of these trials are complicated by several additional considerations. Most node-positive patients eventually relapse and die of breast cancer, and therefore most node-positive patients will *potentially* benefit from adjuvant therapy. This is less true for node-negative patients, many of whom will be cured with local therapy and who will suffer the toxicities of therapy with no potential benefit. Further, the patients included in these trials had a higher relapse rate than that observed in previous studies of node-negative patients, suggesting that either previous studies have underestimated the virulence of breast cancer in node-negative patients or that the node-negative patients included in these adjuvant trials are not representative of all node-negative patients. The follow-up on these node-negative trials is still short,

and it will be several years before the size of a survival benefit, if any, can be estimated or a cost-benefit analysis performed. Since the risk of death is smaller and peaks later after diagnosis among node-negative than among node-positive patients, the size of the survival benefit may be smaller and the importance of delayed side effects proportionally greater. Conversely, if node-negative patients have smaller micrometastatic tumor deposits, adjuvant therapy, and especially adjuvant chemotherapy, may cure some portion of these patients. The precise role of adjuvant therapy in node-negative patients will be uncertain for some years yet, and its use now requires mature clinical judgment and a well-informed patient.

Principles for the selection of an adjuvant chemotherapy regimen Combinations of drugs, such as CMF, are somewhat more effective than single agents, such as melphalan. Short durations of therapy in the range of 4 to 6 months have been shown to be as effective as more prolonged durations, such as 12 to 24 months. The optimal drug combination, dose, and schedule of the commonly used cytotoxic agents are not well defined, and it has not been reproducibly demonstrated that the use of tamoxifen or oophorectomy with chemotherapy will provide a substantial or significant survival benefit for premenopausal women or that the addition of chemotherapy to tamoxifen will be more effective than tamoxifen alone for postmenopausal women. Adjuvant systemic therapy is usually initiated as soon as possible after the completion of local therapy, and it has been argued, largely on theoretical grounds and from uncontrolled clinical observations, that adjuvant chemotherapy should be given before definitive surgery ("neoadjuvant," "protoadjuvant," or "primary chemotherapy"). However, in a large, randomized study, chemotherapy begun 1 month after surgery was as effective as chemotherapy begun within 36 h.

Principles for the use of adjuvant endocrine therapy Although there are theoretical reasons why longer durations of tamoxifen therapy might be more effective, there are no published data from randomized trials evaluating different durations of tamoxifen therapy. The survival benefits were most certain in two studies, one utilizing a 2-year and the other a 5-year course of therapy. Two British studies have suggested that estrogen receptor measurements do not define a group of patients who derive no benefit at all from adjuvant therapy, but no one outside of Great Britain has systematically looked for or observed a benefit from adjuvant tamoxifen in patients with receptor-negative tumors. Since the British observations are inconsistent with the well-documented role of these receptors in mediating tamoxifen effects, they should probably be viewed skeptically until further clinical trial data are available.

A series of randomized ovarian ablation trials conducted between 1948 and 1970 were interpreted *at that time* as providing insufficient survival benefit to justify the routine use of this form of endocrine therapy. However, these studies were conducted prior to the discovery of the estrogen receptor, and new trials evaluating ovarian ablation with luteinizing hormone–releasing hormone agonists have been initiated. The use of ovarian ablation in place of or in addition to chemotherapy for premenopausal women should await the completion of these studies.

Summary recommendations for adjuvant systemic therapy Premenopausal, node-positive patients should routinely receive some form of adjuvant therapy after completion of local therapy. If a formal trial is unacceptable to the patient, 6 months of therapy with CMF might be considered standard. Postmenopausal, node-positive, receptor-positive patients should routinely receive tamoxifen for 2 to 5 years, either as part of a formal protocol or independent of any ongoing trial. There is at present no established role for adjuvant systemic therapy in patients with in situ breast cancer or those with very small, node-negative tumors, especially those that are impalpable (e.g., found only on mammography or diagnosed with needle localization) or those that are minimally invasive. The treatment of other groups of patients should be undertaken only after full consideration of the limitations in our knowledge regarding survival benefits and delayed toxicities.

TREATMENT OF DISTANT METASTASES

Breast cancer can and frequently does metastasize to almost every organ in the body, but most commonly to skin, lymph nodes, lungs, liver, and bones. More than 10 percent of patients with any metastases will have CNS metastases at some point in the course of the disease, and new onset of frequent headache, personality change, otherwise unexplained vomiting, or localized neurologic dysfunction should lead to a prompt evaluation that includes a head CT scan (or MRI) and cytocentrifuge examination of cerebrospinal fluid. Isolated metastases to the leptomeninges are not uncommon, and visual disturbances may be due to breast cancer metastatic to the choroid. Choroid metastases can usually be seen on funduscopic examination. Breast cancer not infrequently metastasizes to the ovary and adrenal gland, and metastases to the abdomen may mimic ovarian cancer with diffuse peritoneal studding and the development of ascites. Metastases to the skin may occur anywhere and commonly appear on the scalp. A standard evaluation for metastases might include a complete blood count, platelet count, liver function studies, chest x-ray, bone scan, and marker study such as the carcinoembryonic antigen (CEA) and CA15-3 in addition to the investigation of specific signs and symptoms.

CHOOSING AMONG THERAPIES Breast cancer recurrences, even recurrences in the skin or the chest wall or along the mastectomy scar, represent bloodborne metastases and are *never* truly isolated recurrences. Other organs will eventually manifest disease, and the time interval from the first recurrence to the second will be roughly *proportional* to the interval from primary diagnosis to the appearance of the first metastasis, usually referred to as the disease-free interval (DFI). Although the treatment of metastases may prolong median survival by some months and have a profound effect on the survival of a few patients, the major value of treatment for metastatic disease is palliation of symptoms. Surgery and radiotherapy are more certain to shrink disease and palliate symptoms in a given area than systemic therapies. Systemic therapies are more likely to achieve long-term control of the disease throughout the body. Metastases to the brain and the choroid of the eye are almost always treated with radiotherapy. A local recurrence to the chest wall without evidence of distant disease might reasonably be treated with radiotherapy if the DFI is long. Malignant pleural effusions are best treated with complete chest tube drainage followed by sclerosis because the effusion may not clear even in a patient whose disease is otherwise responding to chemotherapy or endocrine therapy. The pain from bone metastases may be relieved by either systemic therapy or radiotherapy, but in a patient with multiple lesions or a short DFI an initial course of systemic therapy is preferred, since all lesions will be affected by the systemic therapy. If the bone cortex is severely eroded, a surgical approach with placement of stabilizing rods may be preferred since there is a long period of decreased tensile strength in a bone even after a response to radiotherapy or systemic therapy.

The median survival of all patients with metastatic breast cancer exceeds 2.5 years, and most patients will reach several, and some patients more than a dozen, decision points when treatment should or could be offered. Patients given extensive radiotherapy to bone metastases may not tolerate chemotherapy because of the effect of the radiotherapy on the bone marrow. Patients given chemotherapy may not benefit from endocrine therapy administered secondarily. There is no evidence that the treatment of asymptomatic metastases significantly prolongs survival, and a physician or patient may decide to hold therapy for some period of time both to avoid the toxicity of therapy and to better assess the pace of disease. An asymptomatic but anxious patient who wishes to "do something" might explore the use of new or more experimental therapies first and hold therapies with known efficacy in reserve.

Endocrine therapy versus chemotherapy The patient most likely to respond to endocrine therapy is one with an estrogen and/or progesterone receptor, a long DFI, disease limited to soft tissues (e.g., lymph nodes, breast, skin) or bone as opposed to viscera, and

a prior documented response to endocrine therapy. The ideal patient for chemotherapy is anyone who is symptomatic and who is deemed a poor candidate for endocrine therapy. About two-thirds of all patients respond to chemotherapy. Although only one-third of unselected patients respond to endocrine therapy, two-thirds of patients with positive receptors and/or others of the characteristics listed above will respond to endocrine therapy. There is no evidence that a response to chemotherapy will occur more rapidly. The median duration of response to endocrine therapy, about 12 to 13 months, is somewhat longer than that to chemotherapy, about 9 to 12 months, but this likely reflects differences in the responding patient populations. Patients on either therapy may, on occasion, continue to respond for more than a decade. The choice between these two modalities will depend on the relative probability of benefit for an individual patient based on that patient's clinical characteristics.

ENDOCRINE THERAPY Patients who respond to one endocrine therapy frequently respond to a second, often to a third, and on occasion even to a fourth or fifth sequential endocrine manipulation. Patients who fail to respond at all are not likely to benefit from additional endocrine therapy. There is little difference in the efficacy of various forms of endocrine therapy, and for this reason, the least toxic therapy is usually used first. For postmenopausal women this is tamoxifen (Table 303-3); for premenopausal women it might be either tamoxifen or ovarian ablation by surgery or radiation. After response and progression of disease, a postmenopausal woman might be treated with either a progestin, such as megestrol acetate or medroxyprogesterone acetate, or aminoglutethimide plus hydrocortisone (Table 303-3).

Side effects of endocrine therapy More than 90 percent of patients treated with tamoxifen have no side effects at all. Others experience mild nausea that subsides after several weeks to a month, a flare reaction, menstrual disturbances if premenopausal, or hot flashes. The delayed side effects of tamoxifen, especially in patients receiving adjuvant tamoxifen, are still largely unknown. Preliminary evidence suggests that tamoxifen may decrease heart disease and osteoporosis while increasing the incidence of uterine cancer. Patients usually find weight gain due to increased appetite and fluid retention the most disturbing side effect of progestin therapies.

More than 10 percent of patients with metastatic breast cancer will experience hypercalcemia at some point in the course of their disease. Often this occurs soon after the initiation of endocrine therapy as part of a "flare." In addition to hypercalcemia, this syndrome is characterized by a sudden increase in bone pain, erythema around skin lesions, an increase in the number and intensity of lesions on bone scan, and an elevation of serum markers such as CEA and CA15-3. These signs and symptoms appear within hours to a few weeks after beginning endocrine therapy and subside by the end of a month. Unless hypercalcemia is life-threatening [calcium $\geq$ 3.5 mmol/L (14 mg/dL)], endocrine therapy should be continued and the underlying symptoms treated with pain medications, fluids, diuretics, and standard regimens for hypercalcemia (see Chap. 340).

CHEMOTHERAPY Although breast cancer responds to a long list of cytotoxic agents, three, and possibly four, appear to be especially effective and non-cross-resistant with each other: cyclophosphamide (C), doxorubicin (A, Adriamycin), mitomycin C, and vinblastine. Combinations of these drugs with each other and/or with methotrexate (M) and 5-fluorouracil (F) induce higher response rates and marginally improved survival compared to serial treatment with single agents. The most popular combinations are CMF, CMF plus prednisone, and CAF (Table 303-3). There is no evidence that survival is substantially improved by prolonged administration of these drugs, but the results of one randomized trial suggest that both response rate and quality of life are improved by some duration in excess of 3 months. A reduction of drug doses below those shown in Table 303-3 is likely to be associated with a lower response rate, but there is as yet no evidence of substantial benefit from exceeding these doses either. The use of very high dose therapy with autologous bone marrow support is an innovative therapy not yet proven to be beneficial in prolonging survival or improving quality of life.

Side effects of chemotherapy Although the acute side effects of chemotherapy often seem formidable, it has been repeatedly demonstrated in randomized trials that the efficacy of a regimen is a more important determinant of net quality of life than the side effects of treatment for patients with symptomatic, metastatic breast cancer. All of these drugs cause dose-related myelosuppression, thrombocytopenia, and, over some months, anemia. Gastrointestinal toxicity may include everything from mild nausea to protracted vomiting, severe mucositis, and diarrhea. Both myelosuppression and gastrointestinal toxicity are mitigated by the addition of prednisone to the regimen. Alopecia may be mild and gradual in onset with the use of CMF or abrupt and total with doxorubicin combinations. Doxorubicin cardiomyopathy occurs with increasing frequency after cumulative doses in excess of 450 mg/m³ body weight have been given. All of these agents, and especially the alkylating agents, such as cyclophosphamide, are potential carcinogens, but it is still too early to fully assess the incidence of second tumors in patients given adjuvant chemotherapy.

SPECIAL PROBLEMS

Male breast cancer occurs with less than 1 percent of the frequency of female breast cancer. Predisposing risk factors include states of hyperestrogenism, such as Klinefelter's syndrome, schistosomiasis, a family history of breast cancer, and radiation exposure. Gynecomastia, in itself, is not an established risk factor (see Chap. 323). In other respects male breast cancer is nearly identical to female breast cancer with a similar prognosis, stage per stage. The primary lesion is usually treated with mastectomy since most men are not concerned with saving the breast. There are no data from controlled trials regarding the use of adjuvant systemic therapy for men, but the treatment of metastatic disease is nearly identical.

Cystosarcoma phylloides is a rare tumor more closely related to either benign fibroadenoma, from which it apparently arises in most cases, or sarcoma. It metastasizes in less than 5 percent of cases, but the local recurrence rate may exceed 20 percent, especially if it is treated inadequately. Treatment of the benign variety of cystosarcoma phylloides consists of wide excision; for the malignant variety, wide excision or simple mastectomy. Node dissection is rarely indicated.

Paget's disease of the nipple is often mistaken initially for a simple eczema and treated with glucocorticoids. However, a crusting, eroding, or scaling nipple lesion that does not respond promptly to conservative therapy should be biopsied. Histologically, Paget's disease is characterized by noninvasive or minimally invasive tumor cells growing on the undersurface of the nipple. In some cases there will be no other tumor in the breast, and some physicians now treat apparently localized disease with wide excision. However, in over half of the cases a mass will be found deep within the breast, in which case the prognosis and treatment of Paget's disease will depend on the size of the mass and the presence of involvement. The majority of the patients with Paget's disease will be treated like any other breast cancer patient.

Breast cancer is particularly difficult to diagnose and treat when it occurs *during pregnancy,* but stage per stage the prognosis approximates that of patients diagnosed in a nonpregnant state. There is no evidence that therapeutic abortion improves the prognosis. Mastectomy can be performed in the second and third trimesters, and chemotherapy has been given in the third trimester without observed damage to the fetus. *Pregnancy 2 years or more after diagnosis of breast cancer* is not associated with a higher recurrence rate or shortened survival, and counselling women regarding the advisability of pregnancy depends more on the patient's feelings regarding the possibility of not being able to see her child reach adulthood than about any potential risk to the patient from the pregnancy.

REFERENCES

General, natural history, prognostic factors

HARRIS JR, HENDERSON IC: Natural history and staging of breast cancer, in *Breast Diseases,* JR Harris et al (eds). Philadelphia, Lippincott, 1987, pp 233–258

HENDERSON IC et al: Breast Cancer, in *Cancer: Principles and Practice of Oncology,* VT DeVita Jr et al (eds). Philadelphia, Lippincott, 1989, pp 1197–1268

Familial incidence

ANDERSON DE, BADZIOCH MD: Risk of familial breast cancer. Cancer 56:383, 1985

Endocrine factors

BERGKVIST L et al: The risk of breast cancer after estrogen and estrogen-progestin replacement. N Engl J Med 321:293, 1989

HENDERSON BE et al: Estrogens as a cause of human cancer: The Richard and Hinda Rosenthal Foundation Award Lecture. Cancer Res 48:246, 1988

Dietary factors

WILLETT WC et al: Dietary fat and risk of breast cancer. N Engl J Med 316:22, 1987

Benign breast disease, in situ carcinoma

DUPONT WD, PAGE DL: Risk factors for breast cancer in women with proliferative breast disease. N Engl J Med 312:146, 1985

SCHNITT SJ et al: Ductal carcinoma in situ (intraductal carcinoma) of the breast. N Engl J Med 318:898, 1988

Screening

CHU KC et al: Analysis of breast cancer mortality and stage distribution by age for the Health Insurance Plan clinical trial. J Natl Cancer Inst 80:1125, 1988

EDDY DM et al: The value of mammography screening in women under age 50 years. JAMA 259:1512, 1988

Biology

LIPPMAN ME et al: Autocrine and paracrine growth regulation of human breast cancer. Breast Cancer Res Treat 7:59, 1986

Local therapy

HARRIS JR, HELLMAN S: Conservative surgery and radiotherapy, in *Breast Diseases,* JR Harris et al (eds). Philadelphia, Lippincott, 1987, pp 299–324

Adjuvant therapy

EARLY BREAST CANCER TRIALISTS' COLLABORATIVE GROUP: The effects of adjuvant tamoxifen and of cytotoxic therapy on mortality in early breast cancer: An overview of 61 randomized trials among 28,896 women. N Engl J Med 319:1681, 1988

HENDERSON IC: Adjuvant systemic therapy for early breast cancer. Curr Probl Cancer 11:125, 1987

PRITCHARD KI: Systemic adjuvant therapy for node-negative breast cancer: Proven or premature. Ann Intern Med 111:1, 1989

Systemic therapy

HENDERSON IC: Chemotherapy for advanced disease, in *Breast Diseases,* JR Harris et al (eds). Philadelphia, Lippincott, 1987, pp 428–479

————: Endocrine therapy of metastatic breast cancer, in *Breast Diseases,* JR Harris et al (eds). Philadelphia, Lippincott, 1987, pp 398–428

304   CARCINOMA OF THE OVARY

FRED J. HENDLER

The occurrence rate of ovarian cancer is relatively low, only 1.5 percent, and it is only the seventh most common cause of cancer in women. However, cancer of the ovary is the leading cause of death from gynecologic malignancies and the fourth most common cause of cancer-related death among women. Survival is excellent with early stage disease and poor when extensive disease is present. The apparent discrepancy between incidence and survival reflects the fact that most women at diagnosis have extensive disease. The high death rate associated with advanced disease has led to the development of aggressive multimodal therapy encompassing surgery, radiation, and/or chemotherapy. As a result, survival in patients with advanced

TABLE 304-1   Incidence and death rate of invasive gynecologic cancer

Tissue	Incidence, per year	Deaths, per year
Ovarian	20,000	12,000
Cervix, invasive	13,000	7,000
Uterine corpus and endometrium	34,000	3,000
Others	4,900	1,100

SOURCE: Modified from the *National Cancer Institute's Surveillance, Epidemiology, and End Results Program (1983–1985).*

disease has improved, and some advanced ovarian carcinomas may be cured.

INCIDENCE AND EPIDEMIOLOGY

Each year 20,000 new cases are diagnosed, and about 12,000 women die in the United States from ovarian cancer (Table 304-1). The disease is responsible for a fifth of all pathologically documented ovarian masses and is the most frequent ovarian mass detected in postmenopausal women. The peak incidence is in the sixth and seventh decades, with the disease eventually affecting 1 in 70 women. The incidence and death rate have remained fairly constant during the past 20 years, namely 14 and 9, respectively, per 100,000 women per year.

The epidemiology varies with histologic cell type. In the United States ovarian germ cell tumors are more frequent in young nonwhite women, and epithelial tumors are more common among postmenopausal white women. The epidemiology of epithelial tumors is similar to that of breast cancer. The highest incidence of ovarian cancer is in the western industrialized countries, and the lowest incidence is in Japan and the Mediterranean countries. The rate of ovarian cancer is increased in Japanese immigrants to the United States and in their descendants, suggesting that environmental factors are important epidemiologic variables. Hormones may also influence the incidence. Risk is higher in nulliparous women, women who have difficulty conceiving, and women with fewer pregnancies. However, no conclusive data link exogenous estrogen administration with an increased incidence. In fact, birth control pills may reduce the risk of developing ovarian cancer. Familial ovarian cancer is not as common as familial breast cancer. Women with either breast or ovarian cancer have a two- to fourfold greater risk of developing the other malignancy as well. Genetic disorders that affect the intestinal epithelium, such as Peutz-Jeghers syndrome, are associated with a five- to tenfold increased risk. Some chromosomal abnormalities (pure gonadal dysgenesis of the 46,XY type and mixed gonadal dysgenesis of the 46,XY/45,X type) are associated with an increased incidence of gonadoblastomas, while others (gonadal dysgenesis of the 46,XX and 45,X types) are not associated with ovarian malignancies (see Chap. 324). Chromosomal changes have been described in ovarian cancer tissue, but these appear to be acquired defects.

HISTOLOGIC CLASSIFICATION

Tumors can arise from all of the component cells of the ovary—epithelial, germinal, and stromal (Table 304-2). They may be benign, have a borderline malignancy (i.e., have some but not all the features of malignancy), or be truly neoplastic. Even in the neoplastic category, many gradations exist. The histologic grade of the tumor is based on the most aggressive cytologic and histologic pattern that is identified. Approximately 85 percent of ovarian carcinomas are of epithelial origin, derived from the coelomic epithelium or mesothelium from the embryonal gonadal ridge. The remaining 15 percent encompass a wide variety of cell types. In most, the tissue of origin can be identified, and, when more than one cell type is present, tumors are classified by the predominant cell type.

TABLE 304-2   Primary ovarian neoplasms

Cell type	Incidence, %
I Epithelial cell	85
A Serous	
B Mucinous	
C Endometrioid	
D Mesonephroid (clear cell)	
E Brenner	
F Undifferentiated	
G Carcinosarcoma	
II Stromal cell	<10
A Granulosa	
B Thecoma	
C Arrhenoblastoma	
D Sertoli	
E Gynandroblastoma	
F Lipoid	
III Germ cell	<5
A Teratoma	
1 Not otherwise specified	
2 Dermoid cyst	
3 Struma ovarii	
B Teratocarcinoma	
C Dysgerminoma	
D Embryonal carcinoma	
E Endodermal sinus	
F Choriocarcinoma	
G Gonadoblastoma	
H Mixed tumors	
IV Mesenchymal cell	2

EPITHELIAL TUMORS

CLINICAL FEATURES AND DIAGNOSIS   Tumors derived from epithelial cells represent 85 percent of ovarian carcinomas. These malignancies most frequently occur in peri- or postmenopausal women. Frequently, the symptoms at presentation are nonspecific and usually include abdominal pain, increasing abdominal girth, and/or dysfunctional uterine bleeding. The symptoms have often been present for long periods and have been ignored. Thus, 75 percent of these tumors are widely disseminated at diagnosis. When the tumors are detected in premenopausal women, they may be more limited because menstrual abnormalities are associated with an earlier diagnosis.

Epithelial ovarian malignancies are rarely confined to one ovary and may be multifocal. Dissemination may occur early with small primary tumors. In limited disease, the tumors are confined to the ovaries and pelvic tissue. With extensive disease, the mode of spread is by diffuse peritoneal implantation of serosal surfaces and metastasis to regional lymphatics. The inferior surface of the right diaphragm is a frequent site for extrapelvic metastases. Hematogenous metastases are infrequent at the time of diagnosis. Careful examination of the entire abdominal cavity and retroperitoneal lymph nodes is required for accurate staging. Development of ascites with advanced disease is due to increased exudation and to blockage of diaphragmatic lymphatics.

PROGNOSTIC FACTORS   Tumor stage   A staging classification for all ovarian cancer was developed by the International Federation of Gynecology and Obstetrics (FIGO) in 1969 and revised in 1985. Tumor stage for epithelial carcinomas correlates the extent of disease with prognosis (Table 304-3). With a thorough and systematic diagnostic staging evaluation, many patients previously designated as stage I are now shown to have stage III disease. Similarly, malignant peritoneal washings in the presence of limited disease (stages Ic and IIc) probably indicate extensive disease outside the true pelvis, and such tumors should now be viewed as stage III. In short, many patients with apparent Ib, Ic, and IIc disease, when carefully staged, are at least stage III, and the prevalence of IIa and IIb disease has thereby been reduced. Apparently, only 20 to 30 percent of patients have limited ovarian cancer at presentation. By separating patients with previously unrecognized advanced disease, the prognosis in stages I and II has apparently improved to projected

TABLE 304-3 Pathologic staging of ovarian cancer

Stage	Extent of disease	Incidence, %	Projected 5-year survival, %
I	Involvement of ovaries only	15	80
a	Limited to one ovary, no ascites, external capsule intact		
b	Both ovaries involved, no ascites, external capsule intact		
c	Ia or Ib with tumor on surface of one or both ovaries or capsule ruptured or with malignant cells in peritoneal washings		
II	Ovarian involvement and extension into true pelvis	10	60
a	Extension or metastasis to uterus and/or tubes		
b	Extension to other pelvic tissues		
c	IIa or IIb with tumor on surface of one or both ovaries or capsule ruptured or with malignant ascites or with malignant cells in peritoneal washings		
III	Ovarian involvement with extension and/or metastasis into abdominal cavity including metastic implantation on the peritoneal surfaces of the liver and diaphragm and the serosal surface of the bowel	70	40
a	Tumor macroscopically limited to the true pelvis with negative nodes and with microscopic implantation on peritoneum		
b	Tumor limited to the true pelvis with negative nodes and with implantation on peritoneum none greater than 2 cm		
c	Retroperitoneal or inguinal node involvement or abdominal implants greater than 2 cm		
IV	Ovarian involvement with distant metastasis; pleural effusions must contain malignant cells; liver involvement must be parenchymal	5	0

TABLE 304-4 Five-year survival with respect to residual tumor size in stage III ovarian cancer

Tumor size, cm	Number of patients	Survival, %	
		Two years	Five years
0	31	80	63
0–1	84	70	41
1–2	46	49	15
3–6	144	28	8
7	309	16	3

SOURCE: Smith and Day, 1979.

invasion have the best prognosis. Well-differentiated tumors (lower histologic grades) have a better prognosis than do poorly differentiated tumors (higher histologic grades). The tumors with higher histologic grade are usually stages III and IV at presentation and respond poorly to radiation and/or chemotherapy.

The histologic cell type similarly appears to be an important prognostic factor (Fig. 304-1). Mucinous and endometrial tumors with good prognosis can be distinguished from those with moderately poor prognosis, such as serous tumors, and from those more-undifferentiated carcinomas with poor prognosis.

Biologic markers Alpha fetoprotein and human chorionic gonadotropin (hCG) are useful tumor markers in germ cell tumors but not in epithelial carcinoma of the ovary. Carcinoembryonic antigen is often detectable in patients with epithelial cell tumors who have ascites and/or liver involvement, but it does not fluctuate consistently with tumor burden. Using a monoclonal antibody (OC125), a mucin-like glycoprotein (CA125) can be detected in normal coelomic epithelium, in normal müllerian duct cells, and in serum in about 80 percent of patients with epithelial ovarian malignancies. CA125 is

FIGURE 304-1 Prognosis factors in carcinomas of the ovary. (*From K Sigurdsson et al. Reprinted with permission.*)

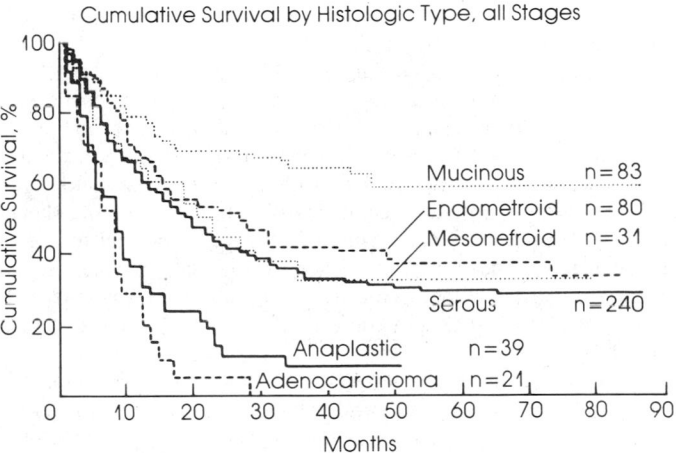

Cumulative Survival by Histologic Type, all Stages

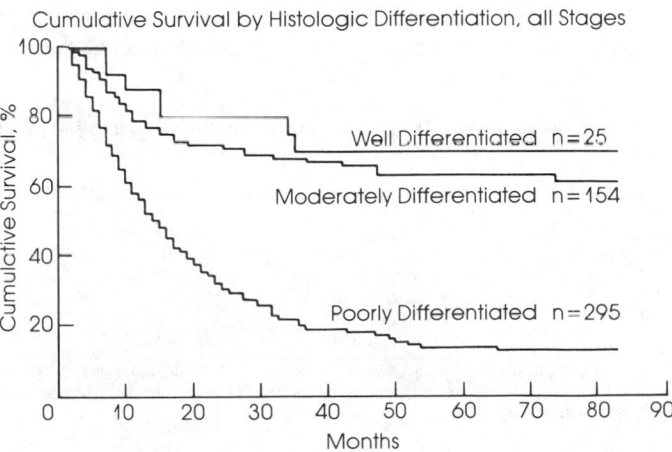

Cumulative Survival by Histologic Differentiation, all Stages

cure rates of approximately 80 percent and 60 percent, respectively. In addition, the prognosis of patients with stage II disease has improved because patients with less bulky disease have been added to this stage. These stage shifts have no effect on true prognosis. Nevertheless, the staging system has documented the importance of the tumor burden to the prognosis. Furthermore, modern chemotherapy has altered the natural history of ovarian cancer, prolonging the time to relapse. As a result, 5-year survival may no longer be synonymous with cure.

Tumor burden Confined disease, although bulky, has a better prognosis than does disease of similar total burden that is diffusely distributed. Survival is better for stage Ia than for Ic, and survival for stage IIa is better than for IIb or IIc. When extensive disease is present (stages III or IV), survival correlates with the tumor burden at presentation and with the minimal residual tumor burden following surgical debulking (Table 304-4).

Histologic grade and cell type The histologic grade of the tumor is an important prognostic factor. Histologic grading systems are applied to tumors with proliferative activity (not borderline malignancies) and are based on the ability of tumors to form papillary structures and glands and on the degree of cellular atypia (Broder's classification). The histologic grade correlates with survival (Fig. 304-1). Tumors of borderline malignancy which are characterized by the presence of malignant cells and mitosis without evidence of tumor

TABLE 304-5 Evaluation of epithelial ovarian carcinoma

I Staging evaluation
  A History and physical examination
  B Complete blood count, screening chemistries, CA125
  C Ultrasound, CT scan, or MRI of entire abdomen, including liver
  D Chest x-ray
  E Cystoscopy, intravenous pyelography, proctoscopy, and/or barium enema when indicated
  F Surgery
    1 Bilateral salpingo-oophorectomy
    2 Infracolic omentectomy, inspection of small bowel
    3 Periaortic node sampling
    4 Biopsy of liver, diaphragm, peritoneal gutters
    5 Peritoneal surface washing for cytologic examination
II Pathologic evaluation
  A Review of all tissue and peritoneal fluid blocks by at least two independent observers
  B Determination of histologic type
  C Determination of histologic grade
  D Review by ovarian cancer referral center

also present in serum from some patients with other adenocarcinomas, in some subjects with melanomas, and in some women who do not have carcinoma. The antigen level correlates with the extent of disease and fluctuates with therapy. However, the antigen level will often normalize while microscopic disease persists. In patients with known ovarian carcinoma an increase in the CA125 level in serum predicts recurrence.

STAGING EVALUATION A standard schema for evaluating suspected ovarian cancer is outlined in Table 304-5. Noninvasive diagnostic studies are of limited usefulness in detecting minimal abdominal involvement but are helpful in designing the surgical procedure.

The usual approach to staging an ovarian mass is to proceed directly to surgery once the diagnosis is suspected (Table 304-5). Paracentesis preoperatively is contraindicated in patients with ascites and a pelvic mass unless there is concern that the patient is infected. Once an epithelial cancer is diagnosed, the surgery should include (1) bilateral salpingo-oophorectomy, (2) hysterectomy, (3) omentectomy, (4) inspection and biopsy of the liver, diaphragmatic surfaces, and peritoneal gutters, and (5) cytologic examination of abdominal fluid and washings. Attempts should be made to remove all residual disease. When patients with bulk disease present following a diagnostic procedure, an aggressive surgical procedure should be undertaken. When patients present following an incomplete staging procedure with no clinical evidence of residual or bulk disease, peritoneoscopy should be performed; if disease is present, a second, more complete surgical procedure is indicated for complete staging and debulking.

THERAPEUTIC CONSIDERATIONS Stage I Stage I disease is adequately treated by a bilateral salpingo-oophorectomy and total abdominal hysterectomy done in the context of a staging procedure (Table 304-5). When the tumor is a borderline grade malignancy (approximately 25 percent of the stage I disease) and the patient is premenopausal and desires to have children, removal of the involved ovary and biopsy of the contralateral ovary may be adequate therapy.

However, if the lesion is frankly malignant, if tumor involves both ovaries (Ib), or if ascites is present (Ic) a complete staging procedure should be performed. The prognosis for stage I disease treated with surgery alone may be as high as 90 percent for 5-year survival. Postoperative therapy has not been shown to be beneficial.

Stage II With a careful staging procedure less than 10 percent of epithelial tumors are stage II. Patients with a good prognosis (low histologic grade) tend to be treated similarly to stage I poor prognosis patients. Poor prognosis stage II (aggressive histologic grade) are treated as having advanced disease. Clinical trials evaluating the benefits of postoperative therapy in stage II disease are ongoing. Preliminary results suggest that postoperative therapy prolongs relapse-free survival. Survival at 5 years in patients treated with postnecrotic therapy may approach 80 percent.

Stages III and IV At least 70 percent of patients with ovarian carcinoma present with advanced disease. Multiagent chemotherapy results in improved survival if the total measurable tumor mass is reduced to less than 2 cm in diameter prior to chemotherapy. Reduction of the tumor mass to a diameter between 0.5 and 1.5 cm may be associated with additional survival benefits. When the tumor bulk is reduced to microscopic disease, some patients may be cured. If a complete remission is not achieved, cytoreductive surgery may prolong survival but not alter the cure rate.

Chemotherapy in advanced ovarian cancer has improved the 5-year survival to between 20 and 30 percent and altered the natural history of the disease. It can palliate most patients and probably can cure some patients with advanced disease. The chemotherapeutic regimens induce approximately a 60 percent complete clinical response rate, and 30 percent of patients attain a pathologic complete remission. About 20 percent of tumors of stages III and IV, typically histologic grade IV, do not respond. The most effective drugs are cisplatin, carboplatin, doxorubicin, alkylating agents (cyclophosphamide, melphalan, and chlorambucil), and hexamethylmelamine. Polychemotherapy which includes a platin derivative appears to be most effective, but an ideal drug regimen has not yet been developed (Table 304-6). Thus, patients with stages III and IV disease should be entered into cooperative group clinical trials.

To achieve complete remissions in patients with residual disease following cytoreductive surgery and chemotherapy, many modes of therapy have been evaluated. Radiation therapy can reduce mass disease in stages III and IV patients and has a role in the treatment of advanced disease. Furthermore, radiation therapy following cytoreductive surgery and multiagent chemotherapy may increase the remission rate in patients with bulk residual disease but has not improved survival or cure rates. Intraperitoneal administration of chemotherapeutic or radioactive agents requires further evaluation but may be useful in patients with only residual microscopic disease. Selection of appropriate chemotherapeutic agents in an assay utilizing cloned tumor cells has not been shown to be useful in most patients who fail conventional treatment. High-dose chemotherapy with either autologous bone marrow support or with supplemental hematologic growth factors is under investigation as an alternative approach in patients who have not achieved a complete response to conventional therapy.

TABLE 304-6 Responses to combination chemotherapy in advanced ovarian carcinoma

Regimen*	Investigators	No. of patients	Overall responses, %	Complete responses, %	Pathologic complete responses, %
Hexa-CAF	Young, 1978	40	75	—	33
H-CAP	Greco, 1981	46	96	76	30
CHAD	Vogl, 1983	26	92	42	22
PAC	Ehrlich, 1983	56	79	41	18
CHAP-5	Neijt, 1984	84	79	—	30
CHEX-UP	Louie, 1986	62	69	47	19

* Hexa-CAF: altretamine, cyclophosphamide, methotrexate, 5-fluorouracil; H-CAP: altretamine, cyclophosphamide, doxorubicin, cisplatin; CHAD: cyclophosphamide, altretamine, doxorubicin, cisplatin; PAC: cisplatin, doxorubicin, cyclophosphamide; CHAP-5: cyclophosphamide, doxorubicin, altretamine, cisplatin; CHEX-UP: cyclophosphamide, altretamine, 5-fluorouracil, cisplatin.

STROMAL TUMORS

Stromal tumors constitute only a tenth of ovarian malignancies but account for most of the hormone-secreting tumors. The majority have either masculinizing or feminizing effects, and the severity of the clinical syndrome is dependent in part on the patient's age (see Chaps. 54 and 322). Tumors that secrete hormones have a better prognosis because the tumors are relatively well-differentiated and because of the earlier clinical awareness that is associated with the hormonal effects. Feminizing tumors of the granulosa-theca cell variety are readily detected in prepubescent children because of the resultant precocious puberty, with breast development and uterine bleeding, and in postmenopausal women as a result of dysfunctional uterine bleeding. However, in the reproductive years these tumors are usually insidious since menstrual irregularities are often disregarded. Androgen-secreting tumors, which include arrhenoblastoma, lipoid and hilar cell tumors, adrenal-rest tumors, and gynandroblastomas, are more readily diagnosed because of the hirsutism and virilization (see Chap. 54). The endocrine syndromes may be caused by secretions of a steroid hormone that acts directly as an estrogen or an androgen (e.g., estradiol synthesis by granulosa cell tumors, testosterone synthesis by arrhenoblastomas), by secretion of a hormone that must be converted peripherally to active androgens or estrogens (e.g., androstenedione by thecomas), or by secretion of a peptide hormone that induces the synthesis of steroid hormones by uninvolved ovarian tissue (e.g., hCG by germ cell tumors).

As a result of the endocrine abnormalities, stromal tumors are detected at earlier stages than are epithelial tumors. Prospective clinical studies on the response to therapy are not available, but the prognosis for a given tumor stage appears to be no different than that of epithelial tumors (Table 304-3). When stromal tumors are confined to one ovary in reproductive or prepubescent women, a conservative approach is warranted. Removal of the involved ovary with a biopsy of the contralateral ovary may be adequate and will maintain ovarian and reproductive function without jeopardizing survival. Platin-based polychemotherapy may have some efficacy in granulosa cell tumors. All other stromal tumors appear to be basically unresponsive to either chemotherapy or radiation therapy. Thus, extensive disease and late recurrences are often managed by surgical debulking.

GERM CELL TUMORS

Germ cell tumors comprise less than 5 percent of ovarian malignancies, occur in young women, and have a higher incidence in blacks than in whites. They are usually unilateral with metastases to regional lymph nodes, hematogenous spread to the lungs, and direct extension to other pelvic organs. Peritoneal implantation and ascites are rare. Tumors that contain yolk sac epithelium produce alpha fetoprotein, and those with syncytiotrophoblasts produce hCG. These tumor markers make it possible to monitor the disease status and response to therapy. High levels of hCG are associated with feminizing syndromes and with hyperthyroidism because of structural similarities of the hCG alpha chain with alpha chains of follicle-stimulating hormone and thyroid-stimulating hormone (see Chap. 309). Hyperthyroidism also occurs in struma ovarii which are derived from specialized thyroid tissue within teratomas. Struma carcinoid tumors can arise from argentaffin tissue in teratomas. However, carcinoid syndrome is more frequently associated with metatasis to the ovary from a primary intestinal tumor than from strumal carcinoid (see Chap. 262). Pure choriocarcinoma of the ovary is rare and is due to a primary ovarian gestation, to metastasis from a choriocarcinoma of the uterus, or to direct germ cell derivation. Most commonly, elements of choriocarcinoma are observed as a component of a mixed germ cell tumor.

When germ cell tumors are clinically stage I, surgical removal of the involved ovary, biopsy of the contralateral ovary, and a limited node dissection should be performed. However, these tumors tend to be disseminated at presentation. They are responsive to multiagent chemotherapy and poorly controlled by surgery and radiation therapy. Historically, most patients with disseminated germ cell tumors have been treated primarily with vincristine, actinomycin D, and cyclophosphamide. However, cisplatin-containing chemotherapeutic regimens that are effective in testicular cancer appear to be similarly effective in ovarian germ cell tumors and are becoming the therapy of choice (see Chap. 305).

REFERENCES

BAST RC et al: A radioimmunoassay using a monoclonal antibody to monitor the course of epithelial ovarian cancer. N Engl J Med 309:883, 1983

BEREK JS et al: CA 125 serum levels correlated with second-look operations among ovarian cancer patients. Obstet Gynecol 67:685, 1986

DEMBO AJ: Abdominopelvic radiotherapy in ovarian cancer: A 10-year experience. Cancer 55:2285, 1985

FUKS Z et al: Chemotherapeutic and surgical induction of pathologic complete remission and whole abdominal irradiation for consolidation does not enhance the cure of stage III ovarian carcinoma. J Clin Oncol 6:509, 1988

HEINTZ APM et al: Epidemiology and etiology of ovarian cancer: A review. Obstet Gynecol 66:127, 1985

——— et al: Cytoreductive surgery in ovarian carcinoma: Feasibility and morbidity. Obstet Gynecol 67:783, 1986

HOWELL SB et al: Long-term survival of patients with small-volume disease treated with intraperitoneal chemotherapy. J Clin Oncol 5:1607, 1987

INTERNATIONAL FEDERATION OF GYNECOLOGY AND OBSTETRICS: Changes in definitions of clinical staging for carcinoma of the cervix and ovary. Am J Obstet Gynecol 156:236, 1987

O'CONNELL GJ et al: Predictive value of CA 125 for ovarian carcinoma in patients presenting with pelvic masses. Obstet Gynecol 70:930, 1987

OZOLS RF, YOUNG RC: Ovarian cancer. Curr Probl Cancer 11:59, 1987

——— et al: Advanced ovarian cancer: Correlation of histologic grade with response to therapy. Cancer 45:572, 1980

RUBIN SC, LEWIS JL JR: Second-look surgery in ovarian carcinoma. CRC Crit Rev Oncol Hematol 8:75, 1988

——— et al: Peritoneal cytology as an indicator of disease in patients with residual ovarian carcinoma. Obstet Gynecol 71:851, 1988

SIGURDSSON K et al: Prognostic factors in malignant epithelial tumors. Gynecol Oncol 15:370, 1983

SMITH JP, DAY TG: Review of ovarian cancer at the University of Texas System Cancer Center, MD Anderson Hospital, and Tumor Institute. Am J Obstet Gynecol 135:984, 1979

YOUNG RC: Initial therapy for early ovarian cancer. Cancer 60:2049, 1987

——— et al: Staging laparotomy in early ovarian cancer. JAMA 250:3072, 1983

——— et al: Cancer of the ovary, in Cancer Principles and Pactice of Oncology, VT DeVita Jr, et al (eds). Philadelphia, Lippincott, 1989, pp 1162–1196

305 TESTICULAR CANCER AND OTHER TROPHOBLASTIC DISEASES

MARC B. GARNICK

TESTICULAR CANCER

Carcinoma of the testis is a disease that serves as a model of a curable, solid neoplasm. Patients with localized forms of germinal cell cancer have a high cure rate when treated either with surgery or radiation therapy, and the advanced, metastatic forms, which in the past were almost universally fatal, are now also potentially curable. In 1977 testicular cancer was the third leading cause of cancer death in men between the ages of 15 and 34, but by 1981 the disease was no longer among the top five causes of cancer death in the same age group. The multidisciplinary principles and strategies that evolved for the management of patients with advanced testicular cancer are now being applied to other cancers.

Approximately 5700 new cases are diagnosed annually. The incidence in blacks is substantially lower than in whites. There is a peak frequency in early childhood and a larger peak incidence between 20 and 35 years. The disease is uncommon after age 40. A lesion suggestive of testicular neoplasm in a patient over the age of 50 should suggest a lymphoma rather than primary germinal cell carcinoma. This is especially true if there is bilateral involvement of the testes.

Several factors are known to predispose to development of testicular tumor. Men with a history of cryptorchid (undescended) testes have a several-fold increased risk, intraabdominal testes being more at risk than high inguinal testes. Both the cryptorchid testis itself and the contralateral normally descended testis are at risk, suggesting that some underlying testicular defect may predispose both to maldescent and to tumor development. Although the effectiveness of orchiopexy in reducing risk is not established, it is generally agreed that a high inguinal testis should be brought into the scrotum so that it can be followed carefully. Abdominal testes that cannot be treated in this manner should probably be removed. Other predisposing factors include a history of mumps orchitis, inguinal hernia in childhood, and testicular cancer in the contralateral testis. In the majority of cases no predisposing factor can be identified.

CLINICAL FEATURES AND DIAGNOSIS The manifestations of testicular cancer range from an asymptomatic nodule or swelling detected while performing testicular self-examination to dyspnea secondary to massive pulmonary metastases. Most testicular cancers are diagnosed because of symptoms related to the testes, but significant delay in making a diagnosis is common and is the result of oversight by physicians and by patients. Thus, high school health programs that teach testicular self-examination should be encouraged. Such programs have allowed early diagnosis, leading to more successful treatment outcomes. Most testicular cancers occur in men under age 40, and the public should be educated to the need to seek prompt medical advice for any change in previously normal testes, including the presence of a mass, a feeling of heaviness, pain, hardness, and swelling. Other causes of testicular masses include hydrocele, epididymitis, spermatocele, and orchitis, but to reduce delay in reaching a diagnosis, physicians should consider any testicular mass to be malignant until proven otherwise. Patients with testicular tumors may have pain because of associated nonneoplastic lesions, such as epididymitis.

Back or abdominal pain secondary to retroperitoneal adenopathy, weight loss, dyspnea secondary to pulmonary metastases, gynecomastia, supraclavicular lymphadenopathy, and urinary obstruction may also be present at diagnosis.

A testicular sonogram can aid in establishing the presence of a testicular parenchymal abnormality. Once the diagnosis of a testicular neoplasm is suspected, a blood sample should be set aside, prior to orchiectomy, for subsequent determination of the tumor marker glycoproteins, alpha fetoprotein (AFP) and human chorionic gonadotropin (hCG). The correct operative approach is a high radical inguinal orchiectomy. A transscrotal biopsy of the testis or a transscrotal orchiectomy should never be performed if the diagnosis of testicular cancer is likely. Because the lymphatic drainage of the testis (to the retroperitoneal lymphatics between L1 and L3) differs from that of the scrotum (to superficial and deep inguinal groin nodes), a scrotal incision in the presence of a testicular cancer may predispose to the development of local recurrences and metastases to the inguinal lymphatics. This rarely happens if a radical, high inguinal orchiectomy is performed.

CLASSIFICATION AND PATHOLOGY The most widely used classification of testicular tumors is that of Mostofi and is based on the cell type from which the tumor is derived, namely germinal or stromal (Leydig and Sertoli) cells (Table 305-1). Germinal cell tumors, the most common of these tumors and the focus of this chapter, can be subdivided into seminomas and nonseminomas. Seminomas are characterized by large cells with clear cytoplasm in a delicate fibrovascular stroma infiltrated with lymphocytes. Indeed,

TABLE 305-1 Classification of testicular tumors

I Germinal cell tumors (95%)
  A Single cell tumors (60%)
    1 Seminomas
    2 Nonseminomas
      a Embryonal cell tumors (yolk sac tumors)
      b Teratomas
      c Choriocarcinomas
  B Combination tumors (40%)
II Tumors of gonadal stroma (1–2%)
  A Leydig cell
  B Sertoli cell
  C Primitive gonadal structures
III Gonadoblastoma: germinal cell + stomal cell

SOURCE: After FK Mostofi, Cancer 45:1735, 1980.

the granulomatous reaction around the tumor can be so intense as to suggest a graft-versus-host reaction. These tumors account for about half of all testicular neoplasms and can be divided into typical, spermatocytic, and anaplastic varieties. Germinal cell tumors of the nonseminoma type can be divided into embryonal cell tumors (yolk sac tumors), teratomas, and choriocarcinomas. Embryonal carcinomas are common in children and resemble embryonal carcinomas of the ovary. Choriocarcinomas contain syncytiotrophoblastic cells. Teratomas contain at least two types of germinal cell layers and in childhood are second in frequency to embryonal tumor. Mixed tumors that contain combinations of germinal cell types account for 40 percent of germinal cell tumors; the biology of such tumors is usually determined by the least differentiated (most malignant) elements. All four types of germinal cell tumors can also originate in extragonadal sites, most commonly the mediastinum or brain. Such extragonadal tumors are presumed to arise either from aberrant migration of germinal cells during embryogenesis or, alternatively, from some common precursor stem cell line that gives rise to the germinal cells, the thymus, and the pineal.

From the clinical standpoint, the critical distinction is between *seminomas* and *nonseminomas*, based upon the histopathology of the orchiectomy specimen. The former must be in pure form; the latter may either be a mixed cancer with both seminomatous and nonseminomatous components or a pure form of a nonseminoma, such as embryonal cell carcinoma, teratoma, or choriocarcinoma. The term *teratocarcinoma* generally refers to a mixed nonseminomatous cancer consisting of teratoma and embryonal cell cancer.

The distinction between seminoma and nonseminoma is important because the staging evaluation and subsequent management in the two differ as a consequence of the relative radioresponsiveness of seminomas compared to the radioresistance of nonseminomas. Radiation therapy to the lymphatics of the abdomen and/or chest is the mainstay of therapy in patients with pure seminoma but is rarely utilized in patients with nonseminoma. In addition, seminomas usually spread via the regional lymphatics to the retroperitoneal nodes of the abdomen and/or to the mediastinal and supraclavicular lymph nodes before gaining access to other visceral structures. Pulmonary and other hematogenous metastases (e.g., hepatic, CNS, osseous) are more common in patients with nonseminomas than in patients with seminomas.

BIOLOGIC TUMOR MARKERS Germinal cell cancers of the testis often secrete biologic tumor markers that can be detected in the peripheral blood (see Chap. 309). Following orchiectomy, the presence of such markers in blood reflects the presence of metastatic disease. Such assays can also be valuable in monitoring therapy (marker levels fall with disease regression and increase with disease progression), and elevated levels in blood may predate the detection of new clinical or radiologic metastatic disease by weeks to months. The two most common markers are AFP and hCG. AFP is commonly secreted by embryonal cell cancer: its biologic half-life is approximately 6 days. AFP is not produced by pure seminoma, and its detection implies the presence of nonseminomatous elements, either in the primary lesion itself or in the metastatic site, even when the primary orchiectomy specimen is thought to be a pure seminoma. hCG is secreted by syncytiotrophoblastic giant cells, present most commonly in choriocarcinomas; such giant cells may be present in embryonal cell components and occasionally in so-called pure seminomas. The biologic half-life of hCG is approximately 24 h. hCG may be biologically active, and hCG-enhanced secretion of estrogen by the testis is the cause of gynecomastia in such patients (see Chap. 323).

STAGING EVALUATION The function of staging is to determine whether the cancer is localized to the testis or to regional lymphatics or is widely disseminated. Such information is necessary to determine if disease is amenable to local or regional therapy. If the disease is disseminated at presentation, the initial staging evaluation serves as a baseline in assessing subsequent response. Since the approach to staging and management is dictated by the pathologic diagnosis of the orchiectomy specimen, the appropriate evaluation will be outlined for each.

Pure seminoma The routine workup involves careful physical examination, an abdominal-pelvic computed tomographic (CT) scan to determine the presence of retroperitoneal adenopathy or visceral involvement, a chest x-ray with or without lung tomography, measurement of routine chemistries, and assessment of the biologic markers (AFP and hCG). In most cases, the biologic markers are undetectable. If AFP is elevated, the patient should be treated as having a nonseminoma, even though the pathologic interpretation is pure seminoma.

The portals for radiation therapy for pure seminomas were traditionally determined on the basis of bipedal lymphangiography. However, the necessity of lymphangiography for such purposes is less imperative today because CT scanning may provide similar information.

If plasma hCG is elevated in a patient with a diagnosis of pure seminoma, a search should be made for syncytiotrophoblastic giant cells. Otherwise, there may be some uncertainty of whether occult foci of nonseminomatous components are responsible for the hCG production. Also, if the physical or radiographic examinations fail to reveal any evidence of metastatic disease and the hCG is elevated before orchiectomy, it is necessary to follow the level of hCG sequentially. If the marker does not decline as predicted by its biologic half-life, the presence of occult metastatic cancer should be considered.

Nonseminoma The staging evaluation outlined for the seminoma is employed for the patient with a nonseminomatous germinal cell tumor of the testis. On the basis of these noninvasive staging studies, patients can be categorized as having stage I, early stage II, advanced stage II, or stage III disease. Patients with stage I disease have no clinical, radiographic, or marker evidence of tumor presence beyond the confines of the testis. Patients with early stage II have nonpalpable, small, retroperitoneal adenopathy on CT scans, usually measuring <4 to 5 cm. Advanced stage II is defined as retroperitoneal lymphadenopathy measuring >5 cm on CT scan or palpable retroperitoneal adenopathy with disease limited to lymphatics below the diaphragm. Stage III disease includes visceral involvement below the diaphragm (e.g., liver or bowel) or above the diaphragm (e.g., lung or supraclavicular lymphadenopathy). Furthermore, patients with stage III disease can be further subdivided according to anatomic location and extent of disease. Treatment decisions are often based on volume of disease in stage III patients.

Conceptually, patients with testicular cancer can be categorized pathologically as having either *seminoma* or *nonseminoma* and staged as having either "early" or "advanced" disease. Patients with *early* disease would be considered to have stage I and early stage II disease, while patients with *advanced* disease have advanced stage II or any form of stage III disease. This formulation allows rational decision making for nearly all categories of disease.

TREATMENT MODALITIES ACCORDING TO HISTOLOGY AND STAGE (Table 305-2) **Early seminoma** These patients have either a normal abdominal CT scan or retroperitoneal lymphadenopathy measuring less than 5 cm in greatest diameter. Most such patients

TABLE 305-2 Testicular cancer: General approach to management and cure rates*

	Seminoma	% Cure	Nonseminoma	% Cure
Stage I	XRT	95–97	RPLND or orchiectomy alone/observation	97
Early stage II	XRT	85–90	RPLND ± chemo^a or Chemo^a	85–90
Advanced stage II Stage III	Chemo^a	80–85	Chemo^a ± TRS ± Chemo^b	80–85

* XRT = radiation therapy, delivered to subdiaphragmatic lymphatics; RPLND = retroperitoneal lymph node dissection; chemo^a = combination chemotherapy (see Table 305-3); TRS = tumor-reductive surgery; chemo^b = additional chemotherapy given if surgical specimen reveals viable cancer.

are treated with abdominal radiotherapy, delivering 30 Gy (3000 rad) to the subdiaphragmatic lymph nodes and ipsilateral groin and a 6-Gy (600-rad) boost in areas of known disease. Although prophylactic mediastinal and supraclavicular radiation therapy was used in the past, this practice is generally not employed today. When treated with radiation following orchiectomy, patients with clinical stage I have a 95 to 97 percent cure rate, and patients with early stage II disease have an 85 to 90 percent survival rate.

Advanced seminoma In the past, patients with large retroperitoneal masses or mediastinal involvement were often treated with radiation therapy to fields including the subdiaphragmatic lymph nodes, whole abdomen, mediastinum, and supraclavicular nodes; however, survival rates were only 40 to 70 percent. If these patients subsequently suffered a relapse in an area outside the radiation therapy field, the ability to administer myelosuppressive combination chemotherapy was diminished and was associated with drug-related morbidity. Today, most patients with advanced forms of seminoma are treated initially with combination chemotherapy that includes cisplatin. Substantial tumor shrinkage occurs in the majority of patients. However, the proper management for partially regressed retroperitoneal masses following chemotherapy is controversial. Patients are restaged following chemotherapy, and depending upon the individual treatment protocol, further treatment with chemotherapy, surgery, or radiation therapy is addressed.

Stage I nonseminoma Patients with stage I nonseminoma are routinely treated with a retroperitoneal lymph node dissection (RPLND), using either a transabdominal or a thoracoabdominal approach. The rationale for this operation is based upon the inexact data generated from the noninvasive staging evaluation of the retroperitoneal lymphatics. The false-negative rate of abdominal CT scans in patients with clinical stage I is 35 to 40 percent. Thus, surgical removal of the retroperitoneal lymph nodes not only serves as therapy but also determines the need for possible additional therapy. If microscopic disease is detected and surgically removed, an 85 to 90 percent cure rate can be expected following RPLND.

More recently, a policy of orchiectomy followed by surveillance has been used for selected stage I nonseminoma patients. This strategy avoids a retroperitoneal lymph node dissection in a large percentage of patients. If relapse occurs, chemotherapy can then be instituted with achievement of greater than 90 percent cure rates.

Stage II nonseminoma The optimal management of patients with retroperitoneal lymphadenopathy measuring between 2 and 5 cm on the CT scan is controversial. While RPLND may be curative, a relapse rate of 30 to 45 percent can be expected. If relapse occurs after RPLND, combination chemotherapy can be administered, or chemotherapy may sometimes be given as an adjuvant to RPLND. Alternatively, combination chemotherapy can be given prior to RPLND. If complete resolution of disease is achieved following chemotherapy, RPLND would not be performed, obviating the need for the operation in this subset of patients.

Advanced stage (bulky stage II or stage III) nonseminoma Cisplatin-containing programs are in nearly universal use today, either with vinblastine and bleomycin (PVB), the combination of cisplatin

TABLE 305-3 Commonly used chemotherapy programs for advanced testicular cancer

PVB	VAB-6	BEP
Vinblastine	Vinblastine	Etoposide
Bleomycin	Bleomycin	Bleomycin
Cisplatin	Cisplatin	Cisplatin
	Cyclophosphamide	
	Actinomycin D	

with vinblastine, actinomycin D, bleomycin, and cyclophosphamide (VAB program) or with etoposide and bleomycin (BEP) (Table 305-3). The use of these agents is associated with complete remission in as many as 80 to 85 percent of patients when administered cyclically over a 9- to 12-week period.

Following such therapy, patients are then restaged (with physical, radiographic, and biochemical examinations) to assess the response of areas which previously contained disease and to determine the need for additional therapy. Large abdominal masses may undergo astonishing regression. Pulmonary nodules often resolve completely, and biologic markers frequently return to normal after chemotherapy. If a residual abdominal or pulmonary mass persists despite normal levels of plasma markers, surgical removal of the mass(es) should be undertaken. Table 305-4 outlines current recommendations. Preoperatively, it is difficult to determine the nature of such residual masses. Approximately 20 percent contain residual, viable cancer; 40 percent contain fibrosis, necrosis, or hemorrhage, and an additional 40 percent demonstrate the phenomenon of "teratomatous transformation." The latter is thought to result either from chemotherapy-induced differentiation of the primary mass into a teratoma or from the selective elimination of the more malignant elements of the mass but persistence of residual teratomatous components. If either fibrosis, hemorrhage, or teratoma is found following chemotherapy, additional postsurgical chemotherapy is usually not indicated. If, however, residual cancer is demonstrated, additional cisplatin combination chemotherapy is required.

If biologic markers are persistently positive following remission induction chemotherapy, additional chemotherapy is also indicated. "Tumor-reductive" surgery should not be attempted until biologic markers return to normal. Some patients experience complete resolution of physical, radiographic, and biochemical marker abnormalities after cisplatin-containing chemotherapy and may require no additional chemotherapy or surgery following their program of chemotherapy.

Testicular cancer which is refractory of PVB, VAB-6, or BEP programs may sometimes respond to the addition of ifosfamide. Ifosfamide has been approved by the FDA for third-line treatment with other antineoplastics for patients with refractory germ cell tumors. The combination of cisplatin, etoposide, and ifosfamide will result in a second or third remission, which may be durable, in approximately 25 percent of patients. On occasion, bone marrow transplantation may be considered.

FOLLOW-UP OF PATIENTS WITH TESTICULAR CANCER All patients with testicular cancer, regardless of pathology or stage, require meticulous follow-up with monthly physical exams, chest x-

TABLE 305-4 Advanced testicular cancer, nonseminoma: Approach to management after initial chemotherapy

Biologic "markers"*	Radiographic abnormalities	Therapeutic choice
Positive	Present or absent	Additional chemotherapy†
Normal	Present	TRS‡ ± chemotherapy§
Normal	Absent	Observation

* Alpha fetoprotein and human chorionic gonadotropin.
† Chemotherapy with a "second-line" program, with attempts to "normalize" biologic markers.
‡ Tumor-reductive surgery.
§ Additional chemotherapy determined by presence of "viable" cancer in surgical specimen. Chemotherapy withheld if surgical specimen contains only fibrosis or teratoma.

rays, and assessment of markers for 18 to 24 months. Patients with stage I nonseminoma who are treated with a surveillance policy following orchiectomy will need frequent abdominal-pelvic CT scanning in addition to the other follow-up evaluations. The frequency of these tests can be decreased in the third or fourth year following diagnosis. The goal is to detect relapse when the tumor burden is minimal. Most relapses from testicular cancer occur within the first 2 years following diagnosis, but late relapses do occur.

SIDE EFFECTS OF THERAPY Radiation therapy and surgery Infertility can result both from radiation therapy and RPLND. Because these modalities are generally reserved for the management of early stage patients, a full discussion with patients about the potential loss of fertility is appropriate. Although of questionable benefit, the possibility of sperm banking should be considered prior to the initiation of either definitive radiation therapy for early stage seminomas or RPLND for early stage nonseminomas. Modifications in the surgical technique of RPLND (limited dissection) may decrease the incidence of fertility loss and ejaculatory disturbances.

Combination chemotherapy When standard cisplatin-vinblastine-bleomycin programs are employed, the major side effects are myelosuppression, potential for nephrotoxicity, nausea and vomiting, weight loss, anemia, ileus, pulmonary toxicity, ototoxicity, peripheral neuropathy, Raynaud's phenomenon, alopecia, hypomagnesemia, and stomatitis. Infertility is usual during therapy, although fertility may return years after completion of therapy. The use of the chemotherapy programs requires skill on the part of the treating physician and should not be attempted by the occasional user. With proper expertise these side effects can often be minimized. Hemorrhagic cystitis, which can occur with ifosfamide, can be minimized by concomitant use of the uroprotector mesna.

Bleomycin is known to cause pulmonary toxicity (see Chap. 205), and special precautions must be taken in patients who have received bleomycin and are scheduled for a surgical procedure. The acute respiratory distress syndrome has occurred in some and is thought to be related to excessive fluid overload and high inspired oxygen concentration (F_{IO_2}) during the operative procedure. Current recommendations now call for the F_{IO_2} to be maintained at ≤24 percent and for patients to be kept in a hypovolemic or euvolemic state in the perioperative period. Such measures seem to minimize the postoperative pulmonary complications.

THE EXTRAGONADAL GERMINAL CELL SYNDROME Patients with extragonadal germinal cell tumors may present with a large anterior mediastinal mass, central nervous system abnormalities, or retroperitoneal disease. The response to therapy is generally lower when compared to primary testicular cancer, justifying the need for more intensive therapy. Many patients relapse years after the original diagnosis, leading to a lower cure rate compared to patients with primary testicular cancer. However, a proportion of these patients may be cured when treated with chemotherapy and tumor-reductive surgery. In addition, patients with "undifferentiated" cancer of the mediastinum or retroperitoneum may have an unrecognized form of extragonadal germinal cell cancer. Biologic markers and immunohistochemical staining of the biopsy material for AFP or hCG may provide useful clues. If positive, these patients should be treated as if they have potentially curable advanced testicular cancer.

OTHER TROPHOBLASTIC DISEASES

Trophoblastic tumors of females encompass all proliferative trophoblastic growths that develop from pregnancy and are, hence, entitled *gestational trophoblastic neoplasms*. Gestational trophoblastic tumors arise most commonly from antecedent molar pregnancies, but may also follow term and ectopic pregnancy and spontaneous abortions. The incidence of choriocarcinoma occurring during a term pregnancy is approximately 1 in 150,000 and approximately 75 percent of these patients demonstrate metastatic disease, the lungs being the most frequent site of metastases. The incidence of choriocarcinoma occurring with an ectopic pregnancy is approximately 1 in 5000; the incidence with spontaneous abortion is approximately 1 in 15,000.

Pathologically, the morphology of gestational trophoblastic neoplasms includes the complete and partial hydatidiform mole, invasive mole, and choriocarcinoma. The distinction between complete and partial is based upon gross and microscopic appearance and karyotype. Complete moles usually demonstrate the absence of fetal or embryonic tissue; such tissue is present in a partial mole. Most complete moles have a 46,XX chromosome pattern; partial moles generally have a triploid karyotype, with the extra set of chromosomes of paternal derivation.

Based upon data generated by the New England Trophoblastic Disease Center, presenting signs of patients with complete hydatidiform mole are abnormal vaginal bleeding (>90 percent), anemia (>50 percent), enlargement of the uterus (>50 percent), toxemia of pregnancy (25 percent), hyperemesis gravidarum (25 percent), and infrequently, hyperthyroidism and trophoblastic emboli to the lung. Patients with trophoblastic moles often present with the signs and symptoms of a spontaneous abortion, with vaginal bleeding being the most common feature.

Following evacuation of the molar pregnancy, approximately 15 percent of patients demonstrate localized uterine invasion, and 4 percent demonstrate metastatic disease, most often associated with choriocarcinoma.

Gestational trophoblastic neoplasms can be staged according to the FIGO staging system. Stage I is tumor localized to the uterus; stage II is tumor involving the pelvis and/or vagina; stage III is tumor involving the lung; stage IV is tumor involving other organs. The stage of the patient is generally determined after an extensive diagnostic evaluation, including a history and physical examination, measurement of hCG levels, and routine biochemical and hematologic evaluation. The metastatic workup generally includes a chest x-ray, abdominal-pelvic ultrasonography, evaluation of the liver for hepatic metastases, and, on occasion, angiography of abdominal or pelvic organs. In individuals with choriocarcinoma and documented metastases, hCG values are often measured in the cerebral spinal fluid to detect asymptomatic central nervous system involvement. Likewise, stool guaiac tests are often done to rule out lesions to the gastrointestinal tract.

The most important aspect of gestational trophoblastic neoplasms is the fact that there is a 100 percent cure rate in patients with stages I to III and approximately an 85 percent cure rate in patients with stage IV. Depending upon the extent of disease and the level of hCG in the bloodstream, individuals are treated with evacuation of their pregnancy or chemotherapy. For patients having a good prognosis, single-agent methotrexate or actinomycin D are generally employed, while high-risk patients are generally treated with combination chemotherapy, including methotrexate, actinomycin D, and cyclophosphamide. More recently, for patients with evidence of metastatic disease, more intensive programs, including vinblastine, bleomycin, and cisplatin, have been used with excellent success. Treatment is continued until baselines of hCG have returned to normal.

Many patients can expect normal reproductive function following treatment. There is, however, an increased incidence of repeat episodes of moles or gestational trophoblastic neoplasms in subsequent pregnancies. The sequential determination of hCG has been extremely valuable in the monitoring of such patients.

REFERENCES

BERKOWITZ RS, GOLDSTEIN DP: Management of molar pregnancy and gestational trophoblastic disease, in *Gynecologic Oncology*, RC Knapp, RS Berkowitz (eds). New York, MacMillan, 1986
BOSL GJ: Treatment of germ cell tumors at Memorial Sloan-Kettering Cancer Center: 1960 to present, in *Genitourinary Cancer: Contemporary Issues in Clinical Oncology*, vol 5, MB Garnick (ed). New York, Churchill Livingstone, 1985
EINHORN EH (ed): *Testicular Tumors: Management and Treatment*. New York, Masson, 1980

————, DONOHUE JP: Cis-diamminedichloroplatinum, vinblastine, and bleomycin combination chemotherapy in disseminated testicular cancer. Ann Intern Med 87:293, 1977
FUNG CY, GARNICK MB: Clinical stage I carcinoma of the testis: A review. J Clin Oncol 6:734, 1988
GARNICK MB: Advanced testicular cancer: Treatment choices in the "land of plenty" (editorial). J Clin Oncol 3:294, 1985
———— (ed): Contemporary Issues in urologic cancer. Semin Oncol vol 4, August, 1988
———— et al: The treatment and surgical staging of testicular and primary extragonadal germ cell cancer. JAMA 250:1733, 1983
HAINSWORTH JD, GRECO FA: Testicular germ cell neoplasms. Am J Med 75:817, 1983
POTTERN LM et al: Testicular cancer risk among young men: Role of cryptorchidism and inguinal hernia. J Natl Cancer Inst 74:377, 1985
STEPHENS RL, WILLIAMSON SK: Clinical stage I testicular cancer: Orchiectomy without node dissection [Editorial]. Ann Intern Med 109:179, 1988
WILLIAMS SD et al: Treatment of disseminated germ-cell tumors with cisplatin, bleomycin, and either vinblastine or etoposide. N Engl J Med 316:1435, 1987
———— et al: Immediate adjuvant chemotherapy versus observation with treatment at relapse in pathological stage II testicular cancer. N Engl J Med 317:1433, 1987

306 HYPERPLASIA AND CARCINOMA OF THE PROSTATE

ARTHUR I. SAGALOWSKY / JEAN D. WILSON

PROSTATIC HYPERPLASIA

Development of prostatic hyperplasia is an almost universal phenomenon in aging men. The prostate weighs only a few grams at birth; at puberty it undergoes androgen-mediated growth and reaches the adult size of about 20 g by age 20. It remains stable in size for about 25 years, and during the fifth decade a second growth spurt commences in the majority of men. Consequently, the disease affects men over the age of 45 and increases in frequency with age so that by the eighth decade more than 90 percent of men have prostatic hyperplasia at autopsy. Because of refinements in prostatic surgery, the disorder is not a major cause of death, but it is a leading cause of morbidity in elderly men. The prostate surrounds the urethra, and any enlargement is a potential cause of urinary tract obstruction; indeed, prostatic hyperplasia is the most common cause of obstruction to urinary outflow in men. Overall, about 10 percent of men at some time require prostatic surgery to relieve urinary tract obstructions. The disorder occurs in all populations but is less common in the orient. The mean age for development of symptomatic disease is about 65 years for whites and about 60 years for blacks. It is probable that prostatic hyperplasia does not predispose to the development of prostatic cancer.

PATHOGENESIS Unlike the pubertal growth spurt which involves the gland diffusely, prostatic hyperplasia begins in the periurethral region as a localized proliferation and progresses to compress the remaining normal gland. Histologically, the hyperplastic tissue is nodular and composed of varying amounts of glandular epithelium, stroma, and smooth-muscle elements. The hyperplastic process can compress and obstruct the urethra; rarely, the hyperplastic gland grows posteriorly to obstruct the rectum and cause constipation.

The pathogenesis is not well-understood, but two necessary features for the process are aging and the presence of testes; whether the testes play a direct or permissive role is not known, but the active androgen that mediates prostatic growth at all ages is dihydrotestosterone, which is formed within the prostate from plasma testosterone (see Chap. 321). In the castrated dog, hormonal therapy that increases dihydrotestosterone levels in the prostate causes prostatic enlargement comparable to that seen in spontaneous canine prostatic hyperplasia. Estradiol levels in men increase with age (absolutely or relative to testosterone levels), and in dogs estrogen acts synergistically with dihydrotestosterone to induce prostatic growth by enhancing the amount of androgen receptor protein in the tissue. Consequently, the role of aging in the development of prostatic hyperplasia in men would be explained if dihydrotestosterone is the mediator of the hyperplasia and if estradiol augments dihydrotestosterone action.

DIAGNOSIS   Urethral obstruction results from the elongation, tortuosity, and compression of the posterior urethra, but there is no straightforward relationship between obstruction and prostatic size; indeed, severe obstruction can occur when the hyperplasia does not exceed the size of the normal gland. Early symptoms can be minimal because compensatory hypertrophy of the detrusor musculature of the bladder is capable of compensating for the increased resistance to urine flow. With increasing obstruction, diminution in the caliber and force of the urinary stream, hesitancy in initiating voiding, postvoiding dribbling, the sensation of incomplete emptying, and on occasion urinary retention supervene. These *obstructive* symptoms must be distinguished from *irritative* symptoms such as dysuria, frequency, and urgency that can result from inflammatory, infectious, or neoplastic causes. As the amount of residual urine increases, nocturia, overflow urinary incontinence, and a palpable bladder may be present. Eventually, the manifestations of chronic urinary retention and obstruction supervene, or acute urinary retention can be precipitated by infection, the ingestion of tranquilizing drugs, or alcohol. On occasion, profound obstruction can be compensated to the extent that symptoms are minimal or absent, and patients present with obstructive uropathy.

The prostate is palpated during digital rectal examination and should be characterized in regard to size, consistency, and shape. Hyperplasia commonly produces a smooth, firm, elastic enlargement, but it should be recognized that obstruction can occur in the absence of abnormalities on rectal examination. Ultrasonography with a rectal probe or magnetic resonance imaging allows a quantitative estimate of prostate size but ordinarily provides no information beyond that provided by rectal examination. An intravenous pyelogram with postvoiding film will document the degree of upper urinary tract obstruction and the extent of bladder emptying. To evaluate vesicle neck obstruction, cystourethroscopy is indicated. Measurement of urine flow rate and/or residual urine volume is recommended to document the degree of obstruction to outflow. More detailed urodynamic evaluation is occasionally required to rule out other causes of voiding dysfunction such as neurogenic bladder.

TREATMENT   The treatment is surgical, and when surgery is indicated, transurethral prostatectomy is the usual procedure of choice. In the case of massive glands, open prostatectomy may be employed using either retropubic, suprapubic, or perineal approaches. Because the majority of men above age 60 have some degree of prostatic hyperplasia, the presence of the disorder is not an indication for treatment. Indications for surgery include decrease in urine flow of sufficient magnitude to cause men to seek relief, persistent residual urine, acute urinary retention due to obstruction with no reversible precipitating cause, and hydronephrosis. In men who lack definite indications for prostatectomy, it is advisable that they be examined periodically to determine the natural history of the process; many patients who receive no therapy experience no progression in symptoms over many years.

PROSTATIC CARCINOMA

Cancer of the prostate is the second most common malignancy in men and is the third most common cause of cancer death in men older than age 55 (after carcinomas of the lung and colon). In 1987 there were some 96,000 newly diagnosed cases and over 26,000 deaths from the disorder in the United States. Only about a third of cases identified at autopsy are manifest clinically. The disease is rare before age 50, and the incidence increases with advancing age.

The frequency varies in different parts of the world. In terms of age-adjusted mortality rates, the United States has 14 deaths per 100,000 men per year compared to 22 for Sweden and 2 for Japan.

However, Japanese immigrants to the United States develop prostatic cancer at a frequency similar to other men in this country, suggesting that an environmental factor is the principal cause for population differences. The disease is more common among black men than white men in the United States; the reason for this difference is not known.

CLASSIFICATION   Some carcinomas of the prostate are slow-growing and may persist for long periods without causing significant symptoms, whereas others behave aggressively. It is not known whether tumors can become more malignant with time. Insight into the natural history of a given tumor is provided by careful histopathologic grading of the lesion combined with surgical evaluation of the pelvic lymph nodes.

Histologic grading   Over 95 percent of prostatic cancers are adenocarcinomas that arise in the prostatic acini. Adenocarcinoma may begin anywhere in the prostate but has a predilection for the periphery. The tumors are frequently multifocal. Variability in cellular size, nuclear and nucleolar shape, glandular differentiation, and the content of acid phosphatase and mucin may occur within a single specimen, but the most poorly differentiated area of tumor (i.e., the area with the highest histologic grade) appears to determine its biologic behavior. In the Gleason grading scheme the dominant and any other glandular histologic patterns are independently assigned numbers from 1 to 5 (best- to least-differentiated), and these numbers are summed to give a total score of 2 to 10 for each tumor. Such grading is reproducible and correlates with the course of the disease and with patient survival.

The remaining of prostatic cancers are divided among squamous-cell and transitional-cell carcinomas that arise in the prostatic ducts, carcinoma of the prostatic utricle (a müllerian duct remnant), carcinosarcomas that arise in the mesenchymal elements of the gland, and occasional metastatic tumors (usually carcinoma of the lung, melanoma, or lymphoma). These tumors will not be considered further.

Surgical staging   Adenocarcinoma of the prostate may spread by three routes: direct extension, the lymphatics, and the bloodstream. The prostatic capsule is a natural boundary against growth of tumor into adjacent structures, but direct extension occurs upward into the seminal vesicles and bladder floor. Lymphatic spread can best be assessed by surgical exploration; the frequency with which it occurs correlates with the size and the histologic grade of the tumor. Only about one-tenth of tumors with a grade of less than 5 have lymph node involvement, while more than 70 percent of tumors with a Gleason grade of 9 or 10 have coexisting lymphatic invasion at the time of diagnosis. The route of lymphatic spread (in decreasing order) is to obturator, internal iliac, common iliac, presacral, and paraaortic nodes. Hematogenous metastases occur to bone (pelvis > lumbar vertebrae > thoracic vertebrae > ribs) more frequently than to viscera (lung > liver > adrenal gland). Diffuse pulmonary involvement is infrequent.

The standard staging scheme is that of Whitmore. Stage A represents cancer not detectable by rectal examination but found in a surgical specimen obtained during operation for prostatic hyperplasia or at autopsy. Stage A is subdivided into two groups: stage A_1, in which well-differentiated tumor is present in only a few transurethral chips from one lobe; and stage A_2, in which involvement is more diffuse. Stage B disease is palpable but confined to the prostate. Stage B_1 disease is a single nodule involving only one lobe and surrounded by tissue that is normal to palpation; stage B_2 involves the gland more diffusely. In stage C, palpable tumor extends beyond the prostate, but there are no distant metastases. In stage D, metastatic disease is present. Stage D_1 refers to involvement of pelvic nodes only with no other metastases, whereas in the D_2 category metastatic disease is more widespread. Any of the lower stages (A, B, or C) may progress directly to stage D. Failure to include pelvic lymphadenectomy in the staging process results in marked underestimation of the frequency of lymph node metastases; for example, about one-fifth of tumors tentatively classified as A_2 solely on the basis of prostate pathology actually constitute stage D disease when appropriate surgical staging is performed. The frequency with which early hematogenous metastases are missed with the current staging procedures is uncertain.

DIAGNOSIS Symptoms and signs Both early and advanced carcinoma of the prostate may be asymptomatic at the time of diagnosis, and more than 80 percent of patients have stage C or D disease at the time of diagnosis. In symptomatic subjects common presenting complaints (in descending order) include dysuria, difficulty in voiding, increased urinary frequency, complete urinary retention, back or hip pain, and hematuria. A high index of suspicion should be entertained in all men over age 40 with dysuria, frequency, or difficulty in voiding in the absence of mechanical urethral obstruction. Additional complications of advanced disease may include spinal cord compression for dual metastases, deep venous thrombosis and pulmonary emboli, and myelophthisis.

Palpation of the prostate is the most appropriate test for detection of all stages of disease other than stage A. Indeed, the importance of the rectal examination in the routine physical examination of men cannot be stressed too strongly. The posterior surfaces of the lateral lobes, where carcinoma begins most often, are easily palpable on digital rectal examination. Carcinoma characteristically is hard, nodular, and irregular, but induration may also be due to fibrous areas in benign prostatic hyperplasia, to focal infarcts, or to calculi as well as to tumor. The midline furrow between the lateral lobes may be obscured by either benign or malignant enlargement. Local extraprostatic extension of tumor into the seminal vesicles can also be detected by rectal exam. Scrotal and/or lower extremity lymphedema secondary to infiltration of pelvic lymph nodes are manifestations of extensive disease.

With the use of transrectal prostatic sonography, carcinoma is revealed as hypoechoic densities within the peripheral zone. The procedure is a sensitive means of identifying prostate cancer but is not specific enough for use as a screening test. Ultrasonography is useful for directing needle biopsy and for documenting the degree of extension of the tumor into bladder and seminal vesicles. Magnetic resonance imaging (MRI) and to a lesser degree computed tomography (CT) of the prostate may also be helpful in defining the extent of tumor and locating nodes for aspiration needle biopsy.

Biopsy Biopsy of the prostate is essential for establishing the diagnosis and is indicated when an abnormality is detected by palpation and/or by imaging or when lower urinary tract symptoms occur in men who have no known cause of obstruction. Core-needle biopsy may be performed transperineally or transrectally with less risk of bacterial contamination with the former and more precise sampling with the latter. Fine-needle aspiration cytology offers immediate diagnosis with minimal patient discomfort and morbidity. Open perineal biopsy is performed infrequently because it carries risk of at least temporary impotence and is a more extensive surgical procedure. Transurethral biopsy is also used infrequently because most early lesions are in the peripheral regions of the gland.

Biochemical markers Several biochemical markers provide ancillary information in diagnosing prostatic cancer. Elevation of serum prostate specific antigen (PSA) or acid phosphatase is present in some localized disease, more commonly with bony metastases. PSA is more sensitive than acid phosphatase in the identification of prostate cancer. However, no technique of assay for either the enzyme (including counterimmune electrophoresis and radioimmunoassay) or the antigen is sufficiently specific or sensitive for use in screening, and the major application of the assays is in following the progress of the disease. Likewise, none of the other biochemical markers studied—bone marrow acid phosphatase, hydroxyproline, cholesterol, isoleucine, glycine, aspartic acid, glutamic acid, methionine, or spermidine—has sufficiently high specificity or sensitivity for routine screening.

Assessment of metastatic disease Bony metastases from prostatic carcinoma usually contain both osteoblastic and osteolytic components. The bony pelvis and lumbar vertebrae are involved most often, and metastases also occur in thoracic vertebrae, ribs, skull,

and long bones. Skeletal survey has a low sensitivity of detection because a significant portion of bone must be involved to permit detection on a routine x-ray. Bone scans using radionuclides such as technetium 99 are more sensitive, but the specificity is not high because positive scans may occur in any metabolically hyperactive bone; this includes sites of inflammation, healing fractures, osteoarthritis, and Paget's disease. Therefore, when a positive radionuclide scan is obtained during an initial survey for bone metastases, the presence of other lesions must be excluded by conventional radiography of the affected site. Radionuclide bone scans are also useful for monitoring progression and response to therapy.

Surgical staging is the common modality for assessing lymph node involvement and determining therapy. The procedure usually includes removal of the external iliac, internal iliac, and obturator lymph node chains and is either performed by itself or in conjunction with prostatic surgery or implantation of radioactive beads. In some centers the initial procedure is either lymphangiography or pelvic CT scan of the pelvis, followed when positive by confirmatory thin-needle biopsy of the affected lymph nodes. When the CT scan or the lymphangiogram is negative, however, operative staging is mandatory.

TREATMENT Surgery Total prostatoseminovesiculectomy is the oldest treatment for carcinoma of the prostate. Radical perineal prostatectomy allows an easier vesicourethral anastomosis and less bleeding, while radical retropubic prostatectomy affords access to the pelvic lymph nodes. In experienced hands both procedures have a low risk of urinary incontinence ($\sim$ 1 percent for radical perineal and 1 to 4 percent for radical retropubic prostatectomy). Formerly both operations caused impotence in most patients. Improvements in surgical technique for the retropubic procedure allow preservation of the neurovascular supply to the corpora cavernosa and preservation of potency in the majority of patients without compromising the thoroughness of the operation.

Radical prostatectomy is not indicated for most stage A_1 cancer, since this disease usually is cured definitively by the simple prostatectomy at which the diagnosis is made. The role of radical prostatectomy in stage A_2 is unsettled. However, true stage A_2 disease in which pelvic nodes show no evidence of metastases may behave aggressively and be benefited by radical surgery, particularly when the neoplasm is anaplastic. Indeed, 5- and 10-year survivals equivalent to those of age-matched controls have been reported following such treatment for stage A_2 disease.

Radical prostatectomy has its clearest indication in stage B disease. Nearly all of the apparent surgical cures in this stage are in men who have 1- to 2-cm nodules involving only one lobe of the prostate (e.g., stage B_1), a group comprising only 5 percent of prostatic carcinoma patients. In addition, subjects with true stage B_2 disease may also be appropriate candidates for radical prostatectomy.

The effectiveness of radical prostatectomy for stage C disease is less certain. Morbidity rates from local pelvic symptoms, bladder outlet obstruction, hematuria, and ureteral obstruction may be decreased by radical prostatectomy in stage C disease, but controlled studies comparing morbidity rates after surgery with those following other therapies are lacking. Radical prostatectomy has little if any place in the treatment of stage D disease, and lymph node removal has no therapeutic benefit. Therefore, other means of therapy should be tried.

Radiation Radiation therapy was developed as a primary treatment in prostatic carcinoma because of a desire to avoid the impotence and occasional incontinence that followed radical prostatectomy. In most series, approximately 60 to 70 Gy (6000 to 7000 rad) are administered to the prostate over 6 weeks by a variety of delivery patterns. Radiation to the pelvic nodes may or may not be performed. Acute proctitis and urethritis are common side effects but are usually controllable by local measures and adjustments in radiation therapy. Chronic complications after full courses of external beam radiation include impotence in 30 to 60 percent; chronic proctitis in 10 to 15 percent; and occasional rectal stricture, rectal fistula, or rectal bleeding. It is not clear whether external beam radiation actually eradicates prostatic carcinoma, because many patients in whom progression of the tumor is slowed or halted have persistent tumor on rebiopsy, and the biologic potential of these persistent tumors is not clear.

The largest series on external beam radiation for prostatic cancer is that of Bagshaw; a variety of delivery techniques and doses were utilized in nearly 1300 patients, many of whom had received prior hormone manipulation. There was about 50 percent 10-year survival in stages A and B and a mean 10-year survival of 30 percent in stage C. The 5-year survival in stage D patients who received radiation to the pelvis as well was 58 percent. Several smaller studies have reported responses that in the aggregate are similar. The best results are obtained when the tumors are less than 2 cm in size at the time of therapy. There appears to be no consistent correlation between tumor grade and radiosensitivity.

Focal external beam radiation may be palliative for bone pain due to metastases. The duration of relief is variable. Radiation is less effective for alleviating ureteral obstruction secondary to metastatic tumor because the time lag for a successful response may be 6 to 8 weeks.

Interstitial radiation involves retropubic or perineal implantation of seeds of ^{125}I or ^{198}Au. This treatment avoids major extirpative surgery and provides a concentrated delivery of radiation to the target tissue. Successful seed implantation requires a well-defined primary tumor with a diameter less than 5 cm, a tumor volume less than 30 to 40 mL, and uniform distribution of seeds throughout the prostate. In the initial reports, 5-year survival following staging pelvic lymphadenectomy and retropubic implantation of ^{125}I or ^{198}Au seeds was comparable to survival rates after other forms of treatment, but the incidence of tumor progression is higher. Potency is preserved in more than 90 percent, and early complications are fewer and less severe than those after external beam radiation.

In summary, except for impotence following external beam radiation, serious morbidity is infrequent following either form of radiation therapy. Practical considerations make ^{125}I or ^{198}Au seed implantation most suited to stage B$_1$ disease. The long-term efficacy of either form of radiation as compared to radical prostatectomy for treatment of localized carcinoma (stages A$_2$, B$_1$, and B$_2$) is not clear, but current data suggest that radiotherapy may be less curative than radical prostatectomy.

Androgen deprivation   Since growth of the normal prostate is dependent upon testicular androgens (see Chap. 321), it was logical to try androgen deprivation for treatment of prostatic cancer. Androgen deprivation can be achieved in four ways: (1) surgical extirpation of the glands that synthesize androgens (castration and adrenalectomy), (2) inhibition of pituitary gonadotropin (and/or adrenocorticotropic hormone, ACTH) production [estrogen therapy, hypophysectomy, or treatment with luteinizing hormone–releasing hormone (LHRH) analogues such as leuprolide or buserelin], (3) inhibition of androgen synthesis by the testes and adrenals (aminoglutethimide), and (4) inhibition of androgen binding to its receptor protein (cyproterone or flutamide).

The common means of achieving androgen deprivation at the clinical level are castration and estrogen therapy. Since testicular secretion accounts for more than 95 percent of testosterone production, bilateral orchiectomy results in a 90 percent decline of plasma levels. Estrogens such as diethylstilbestrol are potent inhibitors of the release from the pituitary gland of luteinizing hormone, the gonadotropin that regulates testosterone production, and consequently its administration also causes a fall in plasma testosterone to castration levels. Maximum depression of plasma testosterone is achieved with 3 mg of diethylstilbestrol per day. Other estrogens (conjugated estrogens, ethinyl estradiol, diethylstilbestrol diphosphate) are no more effective in lowering plasma testosterone than is diethylstilbestrol. Luteinizing hormone–releasing hormone analogues also inhibit luteinizing hormone secretion and lower plasma testosterone levels.

Androgen depletion beyond that achieved by surgical castration,

estrogen administration, or ACTH analogues can be accomplished by adrenalectomy. Since adrenal androgen production is under the control of ACTH, the adrenal sources of androgen can also be eliminated by hypophysectomy. The alternative to surgical ablation is the induction of a medical adrenalectomy and/or castration with drugs such as exogenous glucocorticoids that inhibit the synthesis of adrenal androgen or with agents such as flutamide that inhibit the binding of androgen to its cytoplasmic receptor protein. While these ancillary surgical and medical means have theoretical benefits for enhancing androgen deprivation, their usefulness in treating prostatic cancer is not established.

Androgen deprivation by means of bilateral orchiectomy, diethylstilbestrol therapy, or combined orchiectomy plus diethylstilbestrol was a standard form of treatment for carcinoma of the prostate for many years, based largely upon clinical reports comparing treatment groups with historical controls. Subsequently, in prospective control studies the effectiveness of high dose diethylstilbestrol or orchiectomy, alone or in combination, in enhancing survival in any stage of prostatic cancer was not clear cut. Furthermore, death from cardiovascular disease appeared to be more frequent in patients treated with large doses of diethylstilbestrol.

Even when there is no beneficial effect on survival, however, androgen deprivation decreases bone pain in two thirds of symptomatic stage D patients and hence constitutes a major therapy in the disease. Whether androgen deprivation therapy should be initiated early (asymptomatic phase) or late (symptomatic phase) in stage D disease is unsettled. Once the decision is made to institute such therapy, the choice must be made as to which form of androgen deprivation is appropriate. When acceptable to the patient, orchiectomy is safe and inexpensive and circumvents compliance problems. Diethylstilbestrol is also inexpensive and is usually safe in dosages of 3 mg per day or less in men who do not have preexisting cardiovascular disease. In men at risk for cardiovascular complications LHRH analogues appear to cause similar response rates and to have less cardiovascular complications than diethylstilbestrol. Hence, LHRH analogue treatment is an alternative to diethylstilbestrol and to orchiectomy.

Chemotherapy   The age group at greatest risk for prostatic cancer has poor tolerance for chemotherapy. This feature, coupled with the variable course of the disease, makes it difficult to determine the effectiveness of such therapy. However, several comprehensive trials utilizing chemotherapy have been undertaken in stage D disease following relapse after hormonal treatment, a situation in which mean survival time is only 7 to 8 months. The agents studied most extensively are estramustine phosphate, prednimustine, and cisplatin; more limited trials have been conducted with 5-fluorouracil, melphalan, and hydroxyurea. Complete response is rare, and only one-tenth of stage D patients have an objective partial response. In other trials combinations of chemotherapeutic agents have been tested in stage D disease, most commonly estramustine phosphate plus prednimustine or cyclophosphamide plus another agent. Complete response is again rare, and only one-fourth of patients or fewer show any objective improvement. For progressive, symptomatic stage D prostatic cancer, endocrine ablation therapy should be undertaken first, but chemotherapeutic agents may provide some benefit when such patients relapse.

REFERENCES

Benign prostatic hyperplasia

WALSH PC: Benign prostatic hyperplasia, in *Campbell's Urology*, PC Walsh et al (eds). Philadelphia, Saunders, 1986, p 1248–1267
WILSON JD: The pathogenesis of prostatic hyperplasia. Am J Med 68:745, 1980

Carcinoma of the prostate

BAGSHAW MA: External radiation therapy of carcinoma of the prostate. Cancer 45:1912, 1980
BYAR DP, CORLE DK: VACURG randomized trial of radical prostatectomy for Stages I and II prostate cancer. Urology 17(4) (Suppl):7, 1981

CATALONA WJ, SCOTT WW: Carcinoma of the prostate, in *Campbell's Urololgy*, PC Walsh et al (eds). Philadelphia, Saunders, 1986

EISENBERGER M et al: A reevaluation of nonhormonal cytotoxic chemotherapy for the treatment of prostatic carcinoma. J Clin Oncol 3:827, 1985

ERCOLE CJ et al: Prostatic specific antigen and prostatic acid phosphatase in the monitoring and staging of patients with prostatic cancer. J Urol 138:1181, 1987

GUINAN P et al: The accuracy of the rectal examination in the diagnosis of prostatic carcinoma. N Engl J Med 303:499, 1980

HENNRIKSSON P, JOHANSSON S-E: Prediction of cardiovascular complication in patients with prostatic cancer treated with estrogen. Am J Epidemiol 125:970, 1987

HERR HW: Iodine 125 implantation in the management of localized prostatic carcinoma. Urol Clin North Am 7:605, 1980

JEWETT HJ: Radical perineal prostatectomy for palpable clinically localized, non-obstructive cancer. Experience at the Johns Hopkins Hospital, 1909–1963. J Urol 124:492, 1980

KLEIN LA: Prostatic carcinoma. N Engl J Med 300:824, 1979

LEUPROLIDE STUDY GROUP: Leuprolide versus diethylstilbestrol for metastatic prostate cancer. N Engl J Med 311:1281, 1984

MURPHY GP et al: Current status of classification and staging of prostate cancer. Cancer 45:1889, 1980

NATIONAL INSTITUTES OF HEALTH CONSENSUS DEVELOPMENT CONFERENCE: The management of clinically localized prostate cancer. J Urol 138:1369, 1987

SCHMIDT JD: Chemotherapy of hormone-resistant stage D prostatic cancer. J Urol 123:797, 1980

SMITH JA JR: New methods of endocrine management of prostatic cancer. J Urol 137:1, 1987

STAMEY TA: Cancer of the prostate. An analysis of some important contributions and dilemmas. 1982 Monographs in Urology 3:67, 1983

WALSH PC: Physiologic basis for hormonal therapy in carcinoma of the prostate. Urol Clin N Am 2:125, 1975

——— et al: Radical surgery for prostatic cancer. Cancer 45:1906, 1980

307 SKIN CANCER

NEIL A. SWANSON

Cancer of the skin is the most common neoplasm among adults in the United States; more than 500,000 new cases of nonmelanoma skin cancer occur annually. The majority of nonmelanoma skin cancers are basal cell carcinomas (BCC). The second most common are squamous cell carcinomas (SCC). This chapter will concentrate on BCC, describing its etiology, clinical and histologic presentation, and treatment modalities. Once these are understood, a logical choice of treatment can be offered providing a success rate of greater than 95 percent.

ETIOLOGY Exposure to sunlight, principally ultraviolet (UV-B spectrum), is a primary etiologic factor for nonmelanoma skin cancer. These cancers occur principally on sun-exposed skin, commonly on the head and neck. There is abundant evidence to support the combined effects of UV light, immune system function (as affected by UV exposure), and the protection afforded by melanin in skin cancer. Individuals with outdoor occupations, for instance, sailors and farmers, have a higher incidence of cancer than persons with indoor occupations. The incidence of solar keratosis, sun damage, and skin cancers on the hand and forearm of automobile drivers correlates with local driving practices and occupations: in the United States, the left side of the body; in Australia, the right side of the body. Skin type also plays a role. Fair-skinned Caucasian persons of Scottish, English, or Irish descent with red or light blond hair, blue eyes, and freckles are particularly susceptible.

Other predisposing factors include exposure to carcinogens, trauma or scarring, chronic radiation damage, viral infection, and immunosuppression. Arsenic is the most common chemical carcinogen; exposure is through medicine (Fowler's solution) or well water, which induces nonmelanoma skin cancers with a latent period of decades. Both BCC and SCC may arise in areas of chronic scarring as well as in areas of chronic x-ray damage. In most instances the radiation damage occurs following x-ray therapy administered several decades before for the treatment of acne or as a depilatory. Viral oncogenesis in nonmelanoma skin cancer probably contributes as a cocarcinogen. Many subtypes of human papilloma virus (HPV) have

been found in verrucae, lesions of bowenoid papulosis, and genital neoplasms. HPV type 5 is most commonly found in benign lesions in patients with epidermal dysplasia verruciformis. HPV-5 has also been found in cancers developed from these lesions, and the papilloma virus, when combined with other oncogenic factors such as UV light and a decrease in cell-mediated immunity, can induce carcinomas. Defects in the immune system, seen most frequently with the use of immunosuppression in transplant patients, have produced a higher incidence of nonmelanoma skin cancers secondary to the immunosuppressive therapy. The behavior of these neoplasms is often aggressive. Lastly, genetic factors can play a role. The nevoid basal cell carcinoma syndrome is an autosomal dominant condition in which patients develop very large numbers of BCCs beginning in the second decade and eventually involving all parts of the skin. Xeroderma pigmentosum, an autosomal recessive disorder of defective DNA repair, is also associated with multiple cutaneous carcinomas.

CLINICAL PRESENTATION **Basal cell carcinoma** BCC usually occurs as a single lesion on hair-bearing and sun-exposed skin. There are five clinical types. The most common tumor is the *noduloulcerative* BCC. It usually presents as a raised, papular lesion that has translucent borders and exhibits telangiectasia and/or central ulceration. Histologic examination reveals circumscribed nests of tumor cells in the dermis with associated stromal retraction and palisading of the tumor cells at the periphery of the nests. Other clinical variants of BCC include *superficial* BCC, *pigmented* BCC, *morpheaform* BCC, and *keratotic* BCC. The superficial BCC can mimic chronic eczema in appearance, being red and scaly with a sharply marginated border. Pigmented BCC can have a smooth, somewhat translucent border with deep pigmentation, at times mimicking and being mistaken for malignant melanoma. More worrisome and difficult to treat, the morpheaform BCC often presents as a yellowish to white plaque-like lesion with telangiectasia, often mistaken clinically for morphea. It and the keratotic BCC (basosquamous carcinoma) are aggressive tumors with an infiltrative histology. BCC can recur within scar tissue, at the periphery of a scar or skin graft, or as a deep nodule. Care must be taken to examine any suspected recurrence and to biopsy and treat these lesions appropriately. BCC can recur up to 10 years after treatment, and there is a higher incidence of new primary nonmelanoma skin cancers in patients who have had a BCC than in individuals who have not. Therefore, long-term follow-up examination of the skin in these patients is important. The natural history of BCC is that of a slowly growing, locally invasive neoplasm. The degree of invasion depends on histologic subtype, with the morpheaform and keratotic BCCs as well as recurrent BCC being the most infiltrative and displaying more aggressive behavior. They also can be especially troublesome in immunosuppressed patients. Basal cell carcinoma rarely metastasizes; the incidence is less than 0.5 percent.

Squamous cell carcinoma SCC arises from epidermal keratinocytes. It commonly develops from sun-damaged skin or from a preexisting lesion such as chronic radiodermatitis, keratosis (solar or arsenical), chronic scar of any type (trauma), a lesion of lupus erythematosus, a chronic ulcer, a burn scar (Marjolin's ulcer), and other chronic inflammatory states. The red, scaly actinic keratosis can be premalignant, with SCC occasionally arising in a hypertrophic lesion.

SCC in situ occurs in the skin. It represents intraepidermal carcinoma consisting of atypical keratinocytes with pleomorphic nuclei confined to the epidermis. This clinically mimics chronic eczema but is more erythematous with a very sharply marginated border. Bowen's disease is the most common form of squamous cell carcinoma in situ. Erythroplasia of Queyrat is carcinoma in situ of the penis.

SCC can manifest as a noduloulcerative lesion with rolled margins. It can have satellite nodularity and can also be pigmented. Histologically the tumor has broad sheets and strands of atypical keratinocytes usually connected to the epidermis. These can infiltrate to the depths of the lower reticular dermis and subcutaneous tissue. Some pathologists grade SCC histologically as well, moderately, or poorly differentiated or as spindle cell tumor. This grading is not as critical as it is for other noncutaneous forms of SCC.

The natural history of SCC depends on its clinical nature, size, location, and depth of invasion. It has been stated that SCC arising in sun-exposed, actinically damaged skin has a lower metastatic rate than that arising on non-sun-exposed skin or in chronic scars and/or ulcers. This is probably true, but increasing evidence shows that this may be a result of the superficiality of actinically induced SCC. SCC that has infiltrated to the deep reticular dermis and fat, especially in the temple and periauricular areas, has a metastatic rate approaching that of de novo SCC, 10 to 30 percent. Mucocutaneous SCC, usually presenting on the lip, can metastasize in up to 12 percent of cases. Metastasis is usually angiolymphatic, presenting initially in local lymph nodes.

TREATMENT MODALITIES The treatment of BCC and SCC is similar, especially for small, histologically nonaggressive tumors. In order to determine the most appropriate type of treatment, a skin biopsy is necessary, not only to diagnose the tumor type, but also the histologic subtype. Incisional biopsies do not enhance metastasis, and a shave or punch biopsy can safely and adequately yield a diagnosis. In general, if the lesion is to be treated by a means other than excision, a shave biopsy is appropriate. A full-thickness biopsy, such as a punch, leaves a full-thickness scar that necessitates excision.

Treatment modalities used with basal cell carcinoma fall into the following groups: (1) excision, (2) electrodesiccation and curettage, (3) cryosurgery, (4) radiation therapy, and (5) Moh's surgery. A thorough discussion of these modalities is beyond the scope of this chapter. However, experience with all techniques, in conjunction with tumor type and clinical setting, is critical to ensure maximal therapeutic success while sparing as much normal tissue as possible. In most instances, SCCs are best treated with surgical excision or Moh's surgery. Actinic keratoses may be treated with topical liquid nitrogen.

REFERENCES

ALBRIGHT SD: Treatment of skin cancer using multiple modalities. J Am Acad Dermatol 7:143, 1982

FITZPATRICK TB et al (eds): Disorders of the dermis, in *Dermatology in General Medicine*, 3d ed. New York, McGraw-Hill, 1987, sect 16, pp 1033–1130

KOPF AW et al: Curettage-electrodesiccation treatment of basal cell carcinomas. Arch Dermatol 113:439, 1977

308 MELANOMA AND OTHER PIGMENTED SKIN LESIONS

ARTHUR J. SOBER / HOWARD K. KOH

Pigmented skin lesions are among the most common findings on physical examination. The challenge is to distinguish cutaneous melanoma, which may be lethal, from the remainder, which with rare exception are benign.

Melanoma originates from melanocytes, pigment cells present normally in epidermis and sometimes in dermis. This tumor affects approximately 28,000 individuals per year in the United States, resulting in 5800 deaths. The incidence has increased dramatically (700 percent increase in the past 40 years); it affects young individuals (onset from midteens); it has distinct clinical features which make it detectable at a time when cure by surgical excision is possible; and it is located on the skin surface, where it is visible. If the incidence continues to increase at the present rate, within a decade lifetime risk of melanoma will approximate 1 percent.

The reason for the increased incidence is uncertain, but may stem

TABLE 308-1   Risk factors for cutaneous melanoma

High risk (>50-fold increased risk)
  Persistently changing mole
  Dysplastic nevi in patient with two family members with melanoma
  Adulthood vs. childhood
  >50 nevi ≥2 mm
Intermediate risk (~10-fold)
  Family history of melanoma
  Sporadic dysplastic nevi
  Congenital nevi (?)
  Caucasians vs. blacks or Orientals
  Personal history of prior melanoma
Low risk (2- to 4-fold)
  Immunosuppression
  Sun sensitivity or excess exposure

SOURCE: Adapted from Rhodes et al.

from increased recreational sun exposure especially early in life. Individuals of similar ethnic background who emigrate after childhood to areas of high sun exposure (Israel, Australia) have lower melanoma rates than individuals of similar age either born in these countries or who emigrated before age 10. Individuals most susceptible to development of melanoma are those with fair complexions, red or blond hair, blue or gray eyes, and freckles, and who are poor tanners and easy sunburners. In one literature survey 9 of 11 studies linked increased melanoma risk to history of sunburn. Other factors associated with increased risk include family history of melanoma (approximately 1 in 10 melanoma patients have a family member with melanoma), presence of a dysplastic nevus (atypical mole), a giant congenital melanocytic nevus, a small to medium-sized congenital melanocytic nevus (see below), and immunosuppression (Table 308-1). The presence of a large number of normal nevi may also be a risk factor for melanoma. A 64-fold increased risk for individuals with 50 or more nevi ≥ 2 mm in size has been reported. Melanoma is relatively infrequent in heavily pigmented peoples. Dark-skinned populations (natives of India, Puerto Rico), blacks, and Orientals have rates one-seventh to one-tenth that noted for lighter skinned Caucasians.

CLINICAL CHARACTERISTICS There are four types of cutaneous melanoma (Table 308-2). Three of these—superficial spreading, lentigo maligna, and acral lentiginous melanoma have a period of superficial (radial) growth when the lesion increases in size but does not penetrate deeply. It is during the radial growth period that melanoma is most capable of cure by surgical excision. The fourth type, nodular melanoma, does not have a recognizable radial growth phase and usually presents as a deeply invasive lesion, fully capable of early metastasis. When tumors begin to penetrate deeply into the skin, they are in the vertical growth phase. Melanomas with radial growth phases are characterized by irregular and sometimes notched borders, variation in pigment pattern, and variation in color. Increase in size or change is noted by the patient in 70 percent of early lesions. Bleeding, ulceration, and pain are late signs and are of little help in early recognition. Nodular melanomas are dark brown–black to blue-black nodules. Melanoma may occasionally be amelanotic where the diagnosis of a new or changing skin nodule is established histologically as melanoma. Lentigo maligna melanoma confines itself to chronically sun-damaged, sun-exposed sites (face, neck, back of hands) in older individuals and appears to result from chronic solar damage similar to that seen with the nonmelanoma skin cancers (basal cell and squamous cell carcinomas). Acral lentiginous melanoma occurs on palms, soles, nail beds, and mucous membranes. While this type occurs in whites, it is most frequent (along with nodular melanoma) in blacks and Orientals. Superficial spreading melanoma (which in some cases may be deeply invasive) is most frequent in whites. Melanomas arising in dysplastic nevi (see below) are usually of this type. The back is the most common site for melanoma in men. In women the back and the lower leg from knee to ankle are frequent sites.

PROGNOSTIC FACTORS Prognostic factors are similar in white populations throughout the world (western Europe, United States,

TABLE 308-2 Clinical features of malignant melanoma

Type	Site	Average age at diagnosis, years	Duration of known existence, years	Color
Lentigo maligna melanoma	Sun-exposed surfaces, particularly malar region of cheek and temple	70	5–20* or longer	In flat portions, shades of brown and tan predominant, but whitish gray occasionally present; in nodules, shades of reddish brown, bluish gray, bluish black
Superficial spreading melanoma	Any site (more common on upper back and in women on lower legs)	40–50	1–7	Shades of brown mixed with bluish red (violaceous), bluish black, reddish brown, and often whitish pink, and the border of lesion is at least in part visibly and/or palpably elevated
Nodular melanoma	Any site	40–50	Months to less than 5 years	Reddish blue (purple) or bluish black; either uniform in color or mixed with brown or black
Acral lentiginous melanoma	Palm, sole, nail bed, mucous membrane	60	1–10	In flat portions, dark brown predominantly; in raised lesions (plaques) brown-black or blue-black predominantly

* During much of this time, the precursor stage, lentigo maligna, is actively confined to the epidermis.
SOURCE: Adapted from AJ Sober, in *Pathophysiology of Dermatologic Diseases*. NA Soter, HP Baden (eds), New York, McGraw-Hill, 1984.

Australia). The most important prognostic factor is stage at time of presentation. Five-year survival for clinical stage I (primary tumor; no clinical evidence of disease elsewhere) is about 85 percent. For clinical stage II (clinically palpable regional nodes that contain tumor), a 5-year survival of about 50 percent is noted when only one node is involved and about 15 to 20 percent when four or more nodes are involved. Five-year survival for clinical stage III (disseminated disease) is less than 5 percent. Fortunately, the majority of melanomas are diagnosed in clinical stage I. Within stage I, a gradient of prognosis can be delineated based on the thickness of the primary tumor (Table 308-3). This system is based on the rationale that the likelihood of metastasis should correlate with tumor volume. Thickness is the best single index of tumor volume. Melanomas less than 0.76 mm thick are usually cured by surgical removal (5-year survivals range from 96 to 99 percent). Approximately 40 percent of primary melanomas now fall into this low-risk category (thickness < 1 mm). When low-risk patients develop metastases, the primary tumors often exhibit either extensive microscopic features of regression or a small vertical growth phase. Approximately 60 percent of individuals with melanomas ≥ 3.65 mm thick will develop metastatic disease; most of these patients die from their melanoma. These thick tumors are almost always raised substantially above the plane of the skin. Two intermediate categories of thickness exist (Table 308-3). Certain anatomic sites appear to have more favorable prognoses, and some anatomic sites appear less favorable after adjusting for thickness. The favorable sites appear to be forearm and leg (excluding feet). Unfavorable sites include scalp, hands, feet, and mucous membranes. Survival for women in stage I is in general more favorable than for men, in part because of earlier diagnosis; women frequently have melanomas on the lower leg where self-recognition is more likely, and where prognosis is better. Older individuals, in general, have poorer prognoses. This has been explained, in part, on delayed diagnosis (thicker tumors) and a higher proportion of acral melanomas (palmar-plantar), which have relatively less favorable prognoses. As in breast cancer, recurrence of melanoma may occur after many years. About 10 to 15 percent of first time recurrences develop after 5 years so that prolonged follow-up (at least 10 years) is warranted. The time to recurrence varies inversely with tumor thickness. Other prognostic factors for stage I melanoma include presence of an ulcer in the primary tumor, mitotic rate, and the presence of microscopic tumor satellites (foci of tumor ≥0.05 mm in diameter) in the reticular dermis or subcutaneous fat distinct from the main body of the tumor. The presence of microscopic satellites is also predictive of microscopic metastases to the regional lymph nodes. An alternate prognostic scheme for clinical stage I melanoma is based on determination of anatomic level of invasion within the skin. Level I is intraepidermal (in situ), level II penetrates the papillary dermis, level III fills the papillary dermis, level IV penetrates the reticular dermis, and level V penetrates into the subcutaneous fat. Survival at 5 years by level of invasion averages 100, 95, 82, 71, and 49 percent, respectively.

NATURAL HISTORY As noted above, stage I melanoma usually behaves in a predictable manner. Melanomas may spread by the lymphatic channels or the bloodstream. Earliest metastases are to regional lymph nodes. Drainage pathways can be predicted based on anatomic charts (which are frequently wrong) or on lymphoscintigraphy using technetium 99m injected around the primary tumor site. Surgical lymphadenectomy usually controls regional disease.

Liver, lung, bone, and brain are common sites of hematogenous spread, but unusual sites such as the anterior chamber of the eye may also occur. Most deaths result from brain metastases. Once metastatic disease is established, likelihood of cure is negligible.

MANAGEMENT The entire cutaneous surface including scalp and mucous membranes should be examined in each patient. Bright room illumination is important, and a 7- to 10× hand lens is helpful for evaluating variation in pigment pattern. A history of relevant risk factors should be elicited. Any suspicious lesions should either be biopsied, referred to a specialist, or recorded by chart and/or photography for follow-up. Examination of the lymph nodes and palpation of the abdominal viscera is part of the staging examination for suspected melanoma. The patient should be advised to have other family members screened if either melanoma or dysplastic nevi are present. The detection of early melanoma in relatives upon screening has been reported. Until other causes of melanoma are more clearly understood, protection from the sun should be practiced by the patient. Routine use of a sunblock of SPF ≥ 15, use of protective clothing,

TABLE 308-3 Prognosis of stage I melanoma by thickness (Breslow): 5-year survival rates for stage I

Thickness, mm	Survival, %	
	Overall	MCCG*
<0.76	96	99
0.76–1.49	87	95
1.50–2.49	75	84
2.50–3.99	66	70
≥4.00	47	44

* MCCG = Melanoma Clinical Cooperative Group.
SOURCE: From Balch.

and avoiding intense midday ultraviolet exposure should be recommended. The patient should be educated in the clinical features of melanoma and advised to report any new growth or other change in a pigmented lesion. Patient education brochures are available from the American Cancer Society, the American Academy of Dermatology, and the Skin Cancer Foundation. Self-examination at 6- to 8-week intervals enhances the likelihood of detecting change between follow-up visits. The importance of routine follow-up visits for melanoma patients and patients with dysplastic nevi should be emphasized, since this facilitates early detection of new tumors.

PRECURSOR LESIONS A peculiar type of nevus termed the *dysplastic nevus* occurs in certain families affected by melanoma. In some families melanomas occur nearly exclusively in individuals with the dysplastic nevi. The nevi appear to be transmitted as an autosomal dominant trait. In other families the nevi may not be present in all individuals at risk of melanoma. The melanomas may arise within the dysplastic nevus (acting as a precursor) or in normal skin (the nevus acting as a marker of increased risk). An individual with dysplastic nevi and two family members with melanoma has a greater than 50 percent lifetime risk for developing melanoma. Table 308-4 lists the characteristic features of dysplastic nevi and their differentiation from benign acquired nevi. The number of dysplastic nevi may vary from one to several hundred. Dysplastic nevi usually look different one compared to another. The borders are often hazy and indistinct, and the pigment pattern is more highly variable than that in benign acquired nevi. Since the frequency of dysplastic nevi in melanoma-prone families is greater than 50 percent, some observers have suggested a polygenic inheritance rather than a single-gene pattern of inheritance. Of the 90 percent of melanoma patients regarded as sporadic (lacking a family history of melanoma), about 40 percent have dysplastic nevi, as compared to an estimated 5 percent of the population at large. Further studies to determine background frequency of dysplastic nevi are required once greater unanimity exists regarding the clinical and histopathologic features of dysplastic nevi. At present the diagnosis of dysplastic nevi is made microscopically. The fact that at least 20 percent of sporadic melanomas arise in association with a dysplastic nevus makes the dysplastic nevus the most important precursor for melanoma. Thus, recognition of the lesion is of paramount importance.

Less frequent precursors include the giant congenital melanocytic nevus and the small congenital melanocytic nevus. Congenital nevi are present at birth or appear in the neonatal period (tardive form). The giant melanocytic nevus, also called bathing trunk, cape, or garment nevus, is a rare malformation that affects perhaps 1 in 100,000 individuals. These nevi are usually greater than 20 cm in diameter and may cover more than half of the body surface. Giant nevi often occur in association with multiple small congenital nevi. The borders are sharp, and hair may be present. The lesions are usually dark brown and may have darker and lighter areas. Pigment is haphazardly displayed. The surface is smooth to rugose to cerebriform and may vary from one portion of the lesion to another. A lifetime risk of melanoma development of 6 percent has been estimated. The greatest risk is before age 5 and the next greatest period of risk is between ages 5 and 10. Early detection of melanoma is difficult in these lesions because of the deep dermal or subcutaneous origin of primary melanoma and because of the large and varied surface. Prophylactic excision early in life can be accomplished by staged removal with coverage by split-thickness skin grafts. The use of cultured keratinocytes for coverage appears promising.

The small to medium-sized congenital nevus, affecting approximately 1 percent of people, presents usually as a raised dark to medium brown lesion with a smooth or papillomatous surface. The border is sharp, and lesions may be oriented along lines of skin cleavage. Follicular hyper- and hypopigmentation may coexist in a salt-and-pepper configuration. The lesion may have an excess of thick coarse hairs. The risk of developing melanoma in these lesions is at present unknown; however, melanomas can arise in these lesions. From body surface area considerations, the coincidence of melanoma and small congenital nevi at the same site is probably higher than that calculated by chance. The remnants of a nevus with histopathologic features of a congenital nevus have been observed in 2 to 6 percent of melanomas. Management of small to medium-sized congenital nevi remains controversial, but at many medical centers consideration is given to prophylactic removal under local anesthesia in the early teen years. Melanomas in small congenital nevi appear to occur after this period of life.

DIFFERENTIAL DIAGNOSIS The aim of differential diagnosis is to separate benign pigmented lesions from melanoma and its precursors. If melanoma is a consideration, then biopsy or referral to a specialist is appropriate. It is appropriate to remove some benign look-alikes in order to decrease the chance of missing a melanoma. Table 308-5 summarizes the distinguishing features of benign lesions that may be confused with melanoma.

BIOPSY Any pigmented cutaneous lesion that has changed in size or shape or has other features suggestive of malignant melanoma should be biopsied. The recommended technique is a full-thickness excisional biopsy, as it facilitates pathologic assessment of the lesion, permits accurate measurement of thickness if the lesion is melanoma, and constitutes treatment if the lesion is benign. Shave biopsy or curettage of a suspected melanoma is contraindicated. For large lesions or lesions on anatomic sites where excisional biopsy may not be feasible (such as the face, hands, or feet), an incisional biopsy through the most nodular or darkest area of the lesion is acceptable; this should represent the vertical growth phase of the primary tumor. While there is a theoretical concern that an incisional biopsy might facilitate the spread of metastases, data from prospective studies do not support that concern.

STAGING Once the diagnosis of malignant melanoma has been confirmed, the tumor must be staged to determine prognosis and treatment. The history should probe for evidence of metastatic disease, such as malaise, weight loss, headaches, balance problem, visual difficulty, or bone pain. The physical examination should be especially directed to the skin, regional draining lymph nodes, central nervous system, liver, and spleen. In the absence of signs or symptoms of metastases, few laboratory or radiologic tests are indicated for staging purposes. Aside from a chest x-ray and, possibly, liver function tests, no other tests or scans are routinely indicated unless the history or physical examination suggests metastases to a specific organ. Specifically, liver-spleen scans and computed tomography have a low

---

TABLE 308-4 Clinical features distinguishing dysplastic nevi from benign acquired nevi

Clinical feature	Dysplastic nevi	Benign acquired nevi
Color	Variable mixtures of tan, brown, black, or red/pink within a single nevus; nevi may look very different from each other	Uniformly tan or brown.
Shape	Irregular borders; pigment may fade off into surrounding skin; macular portion at the edge of the nevus	Round; sharp, clear-cut borders between the nevus and the surrounding skin; may be flat or elevated.
Size	Usually more than 6 mm; may be more than 10 mm; occasionally smaller than 6 mm	Usually less than 6 mm in diameter.
Number	Often very many (more than 100), but occasionally may be only one	In a typical adult: 10 to 40 are scattered over the body; perhaps 15% of patients have no nevi.
Location	Sun-exposed areas; the back is the most common site, but dysplastic nevi may also be seen on the scalp, breasts, and buttocks	Generally on the sun-exposed surfaces of the skin above the waist; the scalp, breasts, and buttocks are rarely involved.

SOURCE: Modified from Friedman et al.

TABLE 308-5 Pigmented lesions that must be distinguished from cutaneous melanoma and its precursors

Lesion	Description
Blue nevus	Gun metal or cerulean blue, blue-gray. Stable over time. One-half occur on dorsa of hand and feet. Lesions are usually single, small, 3 mm to < 1 cm. Must be distinguished from nodular melanoma.
Compound nevus	Round or oval shape, well-demarcated, smooth-bordered. May be dome-shaped or papillomatous; colors range from flesh colored to very dark brown with individual nevi being relatively homogeneous in color.
Hemangioma	Dome-shaped reddish, purple, blue nodule. Compression with a glass microscope slide may result in blanching. Must be distinguished from nodular melanoma.
Junctional nevus	Flat to barely raised brown lesion. Sharp border. Fine pigmentary stippling noted especially upon magnification.

Lentigo
  Juvenile
  Solar
	Flat uniformly medium or dark brown lesion with sharp border. Solar lentigenes are acquired lesions on sites of chronic solar exposure (backs of hands/face). Lesions are 2 mm to ≥1 cm. Solar lentigenes have reticulate pigmentation upon magnification.

Pigmented basal cell carcinoma	Papular border. May have central ulceration. Usually solar exposed surface in older patient. Patient usually has dark brown eyes and dark brown or black hair.
Pigmented dermatofibroma	Lesion is not well demarcated visually, is firm, and dimples downward when compressed laterally. Usually on extremities. Usually < 6 mm.
Seborrheic keratosis	Rough, stuck on, waxy feeling lesions with sharp borders ranging in color from flesh to tan, to dark brown. Presence of keratin plugs in surface of help in discriminating especially dark lesions from melanoma.
Subungual hematoma	Maroon (red-brown) coloration. As lesion grows out from nailfold, a curving clear area seen.
Tattoo (medical or traumatic)	In medical tattoo lesions are small pigmentary dots often blue or green which make a regular pattern (rectangle). Traumatic tattoos are irregular, and pigmentation may appear black.

yield and are not cost-effective. However, if signs of metastases exist, favored sites of spread, such as the liver, lungs, bone, and brain, should be scanned.

Staging categories are stage I (confined to the skin), stage II disease (spread to regional lymph nodes), and stage III (distant metastases). It is important to indicate whether staging was clinically or pathologically determined, or both—for example, the disease in a patient without palpable adenopathy but with microscopic disease found on biopsy would be classified as clinical stage I and pathologic stage II and has a different prognosis from one that is stage I by both clinical and pathologic criteria.

SURGICAL MANAGEMENT For a newly diagnosed stage I cutaneous melanoma, wide surgical excision of the lesion with a margin of normal skin is necessary to remove all malignant cells and minimize local recurrence. The "5-cm rule" states that the normal skin within 5 cm of the edge of the primary cutaneous melanoma should be excised. Such margins often require split-thickness skin grafts and are cosmetically disfiguring. Narrower margins have been regarded as more appropriate by some, as they allow for primary closure and may obviate the need for grafts or flaps. The appropriate width of the narrow margin is a source of controversy. Some literature suggests that while narrower surgical margins increase rates of local tumor recurrence, they have little to no effect on overall survival. A World Health Organization trial prospectively randomized between 1-cm and 3-cm margins in 612 patients with thin malignant melanomas (≤ 2 mm in thickness) reported that the thinner surgical margin resulted in higher rates of local recurrence but no difference in nodal metastases, distant metastases, disease-free survival, or overall survival after 4½ years of follow-up. For thicker stage I lesions, definitive data are not available, but margins up to 3 cm appear to be reasonable. Once again, for lesions on the face, hands, and feet, strict adherence to margins must give way to individual considerations about the constraints of surgery and minimization of morbidity. In all instances, however, inclusion of subcutaneous fat in the surgical specimen allows for adequate thickness and assessment of surgical margins by the pathologist.

ELECTIVE REGIONAL NODE DISSECTION Elective regional node dissection in clinical stage I disease (without palpable adenopathy) has been advocated, based on the hypothesis that melanoma metastases disseminate in an orderly fashion from the skin to regional lymph nodes and finally to distant sites. Hence, surgical excision of nodal micrometastases could theoretically provide definitive treatment at a time of relatively low tumor burden and, hopefully, improve survival. The efficacy of this procedure remains unproven; while some retrospective series suggest a survival benefit, two randomized studies examining this question in patients with limb melanomas and clinical stage I disease showed no survival advantage between wide local excision followed by immediate elective regional node dissection and wide local excision followed by delayed dissection only if nodes became palpable. Furthermore, the procedure has associated morbidity and is complicated by the fact that many lesions, especially those on the trunk, have ambiguous nodal draining sites, making it difficult to decide which area to dissect. In situations of multiple draining sites, lymphoscintigraphy can be utilized to define the nodes that serve as the primary drainage area. Certainly, not all patients with clinical stage I disease require node dissections. Patients with lesions <0.75 mm thick have excellent prognoses and need no node dissection; at the other extreme, patients with lesions >3.50 mm have such a high risk for distant metastases that the possible benefit of an elective node dissection would be negated. A subset of patients with lesions of intermediate thickness may benefit the most from elective regional node dissection, but there is no consensus about which patients should undergo this procedure. Randomized studies may resolve this issue.

ADJUVANT THERAPY For patients free of disease but at high risk for metastases, adjuvant therapy that complements surgery is needed to destroy occult micrometastases, prolong disease-free survival, and improve cure rates. Many strategies have been tried, including chemotherapy, nonspecific immunotherapy such as immunization with bacillus Calmette-Guérin (BCG), chemoimmunotherapy, and radiation therapy. However, such studies have been hampered by improper stratification, lack of inclusion of those at high risk, lack of randomization, inadequate sample size, or inadequate length of follow-up. Hence, no consistent evidence documents adjuvant therapy as effective. Current trials are focused on specific active immunotherapy using viral antigens to induce tumor lysis. This is based on the hypothesis that the juxtaposition of strong viral antigens and putative weak tumor-associated or tumor-specific antigens can heighten a host immune response against micrometastases. Early studies are promising.

TREATMENT OF METASTATIC DISEASE Melanoma can metastasize to any organ, the brain being a particularly favored site. Metastatic melanoma is generally incurable, and survival is generally less than 1 year. Thus, the goal of treatment is usually palliative to improve the quality of life. Patients with soft-tissue and node metastases fare better than those with liver and brain metastases. If metastases are limited to regional nodes (stage II disease), a therapeutic lymph node dissection is indicated. Surgical excision of a single metastasis to the lung or surgically accessible brain site can also prolong survival. More often, however, patients have multiple brain metastases that require radiation and glucocorticoids. Radiation therapy is aimed at providing local palliation for recurrent tumors or metastatic sites. Chemotherapy has been generally disappointing, and the best single agent, imidazole carboximide (dacarbazine), has a response rate of only 20 to 25 percent and rarely induces complete remission. Combination chemotherapy does not result in consistent improvement in remission and survival rates compared to those of a single agent. Patients who have advanced regional disease isolated to a limb may benefit from hyperthermic limb perfusion with melphalan, which concentrates the chemotherapeutic agents and minimizes systemic leakage. In addition, in vitro and in vivo chemosensitivity tests may help select patients likely to benefit from chemotherapy. The lack of response to traditional treatments has spawned many trials using agents such as retinoids, high-dosage chemotherapy with autologous bone marrow transplantation, interferons, antipigmentary agents, and antibodies conjugated to isotopes, drugs, and toxins. Of all these investigational therapies, adoptive immunotherapy has the most promise; this treatment involves exposing lymphocytes from cancer patients to interleukin 2 (IL-2) to generate lymphokine-activated killer cells (LAK cells); the LAK cells are then reinfused in conjunction with IL-2 administration. This therapy may have particular relevance to melanoma because the immune system is suspected of having a critical role in the control of melanoma metastases. However, the early response rate appears to be only about 20 percent, most of these remissions are partial, are seen in patients with skin or lung metastases, and are of short duration. In addition, treatment with IL-2 has associated toxicities, especially related to increased capillary permeability. Research is now focusing on altering the administration of IL-2 to enhance the remission rate while minimizing the toxicity; trials include high-dose IL-2 either alone, with LAK cells, with even more potent tumor-infiltrating lymphocytes, or with other agents. The continued lack of curative treatment for metastatic disease underscores the importance of early detection and prevention of malignant melanoma to decrease avoidable mortality.

REFERENCES

ALBERT L et al: Dysplastic melanocytic nevi and cutaneous melanoma: Markers of increased melanoma risk for affected individuals and blood relatives. J Am Acad Dermatol (in press)

ARMSTRONG BK: Epidemiology of malignant melanoma: Intermittent or total accumulated exposure to the sun. J Dermatol Surg Oncol 14:835, 1988

BALCH CM et al (eds): Cutaneous Melanoma: Clinical Management and Treatment Results Worldwide. Philadelphia, Lippincott, 1985

CLARK WH JR et al: The histogenesis and biologic behavior of primary human malignant melanoma of the skin. Cancer Res 29:705, 1969

FRIEDMAN RJ et al: Early detection of malignant melanoma: The role of physical examination and self-examination of the skin. CA 35:130, 1985

GREENE MH et al: Acquired precursors of cutaneous malignant melanoma: The familial dysplastic nevus syndrome. N Engl J Med 312:91, 1985

ILLIG L et al: Congenital nevi ≤ 10 cm as precursors to melanoma: 52 cases, a review, and a new conception. Arch Dermatol 121:1274, 1985

KOH HK et al: Adjuvant therapy of cutaneous malignant melanoma: A critical review. Med Ped Oncol 13:244, 1985

KRAEMER KH et al: Risk of cutaneous melanoma in dysplastic nevus syndrome types A and B. N Engl J Med 315:1615, 1986

RHODES AR: Neoplasms: Benign neoplasias, hyperplasias, and dysplasias of melanocytes, in Dermatology in General Medicine, TB Fitzpatrick et al (eds). New York, McGraw-Hill, 1987, pp 877–946

——— et al: Risk factors for cutaneous melanoma. JAMA 258:3146, 1987

RIGEL DS et al: Dysplastic nevi. Markers for increased risk for melanoma. Cancer 63:386, 1989

ROSENBERG SA et al: New approaches to the immunotherapy of cancer using interleukin-2. Ann Intern Med 108:853, 1988

SOBER AJ et al: Early recognition of cutaneous melanoma. JAMA 242:2795, 1979

SWERDLOW AJ et al: Benign melanocytic nevi as a risk factor for malignant melanoma. Br Med J 292:1555, 1986

VERONESI U et al: Delayed regional lymph node dissection in stage 1 melanoma of the skin of the lower extremities. Cancer 49:2420, 1982

——— et al: Thin stage 1 primary cutaneous malignant melanoma: Comparison of excision with 1 or 3 centimeters. N Engl J Med 318:1159, 1988

309 ENDOCRINE MANIFESTATIONS OF NEOPLASIA

LAWRENCE A. FROHMAN

Hormone secretion by tumors derived from nonendocrine tissue has been recognized for more than 50 years. Initially, the majority of reported cases were associated with hypoglycemia and hypercalcemia, but the term *ectopic hormone secretion* was first used in relation to Cushing's syndrome caused by adrenocorticotropic hormone (ACTH) secretion from a variety of tumors. The spectrum of ectopic hormone secretion has expanded as a result of increased clinical awareness and the availability of more sophisticated and sensitive assay techniques. However, the use of the term *ectopic* in this regard has been questioned with the recognition that hormones once believed to be tissue-specific may have widespread sites of production, i.e., gonadotropins are produced by the normal gonad and intestine, thyrotropin-releasing hormone (TRH) and ACTH by the pancreas, and somatostatin by the kidney and thyroid C cells. Nevertheless, the original term serves to distinguish tumor-associated hormone production from syndromes due to excess secretion of the major and characteristic hormone of a specific endocrine gland.

THEORIES OF ECTOPIC HORMONE SECRETION   Several pathogenetic mechanisms have been proposed to explain ectopic hormone secretion. The "sponge" theory assumed a selective update of the circulating hormone by tumor tissue with subsequent release upon tumor cell death. This concept was abandoned, however, after the demonstration of arteriovenous differences of hormones across tumor vascular beds, of hormone mRNA in tumor tissue, and of hormone biosynthesis by tumors in vitro. The theory that random mutations resulted in altered DNA sequences and gene products was also discounted when it was established that the production of ectopic hormones by tumors is not random, i.e., that certain tumors commonly produce specific endocrinopathies. A third theory, that of gene derepression, proposed that regions of the genome not normally expressed become active and are transcribed in tumors, presumably as a result of loss of a normal suppressive mechanism during neoplastic transformation; in fact, however, there is no overall increase in gene transcription (derepression) in neoplastic cells. Two other explanations have also been proposed: *cellular dedifferentiation*, a theory that neoplastic cells revert to a more primitive level and again produce peptide hormones that were produced normally at an earlier developmental stage, and *arrested differentiation*, whereby hormone secretion is due to persistence of a function present during development because of a failure (arrest) of the developmental process. Arguments against these theories include an absence of evidence that cells can retrace their pathways of differentiation or that incompletely differentiated cells routinely secrete the hormone in question. Although the pathogenesis of ectopic hormone secretion is still unclear, the mechanism is likely the result of activation of selected gene expression by an oncogene.

CRITERIA FOR DIAGNOSIS   Criteria for the diagnosis of ectopic hormone secretion have changed as more precise laboratory methodology made it possible to recognize clinically inapparent cases (Table 309-1). Although many of these criteria cannot be satisfied in individual cases, the majority have been fulfilled in the commonly recognized syndromes.

TUMOR TYPES ASSOCIATED WITH ECTOPIC HORMONE SECRETION   Ectopic secretion of hormones is associated with a variety of tumors. Although original reports of these syndromes described primarily lung carcinomas, carcinoids, thymomas, and fibrosarcomas, virtually all tumors have the potential of hormone secretion. Nevertheless, the frequency of occurrence of ectopic hormone secretion among various tumor types is not random. The tumors most frequently associated with clinically recognized ectopic hormone production are small cell lung carcinomas, carcinoids, and pancreatic islet tumors.

TABLE 309-1 Criteria for establishing the diagnosis of ectopic hormone secretion

1 Association of a neoplasm with a syndrome attributable to excessive hormone secretion or with inappropriately elevated plasma and/or urine levels of a hormone not normally produced by the tissue from which the tumor is derived
2 Failure of plasma and/or urine hormone levels to respond to normal homeostatic suppression
3 Exclusion of other possible causal mechanisms for hormone hypersecretion
4 Reduction in hormone levels after tumor-specific therapy
5 Arteriovenous step-up gradients across tumor
6 Demonstration of hormone in tumor tissue
7 Biosynthesis and/or secretion of hormone by tumor tissue in vitro
8 Demonstration in the tumor of hormone-specific messenger RNA by cell-free translation or by hybridization with cDNA

Carcinoid tumors are generally found in the lung or the gastrointestinal tract. Gastrointestinal carcinoids may be present in either the foregut or the hindgut, though it is primarily foregut tumors that are hormonally active. In the lung these tumors are usually endobronchial and may remain undetected for long periods. There are many morphologic similarities between bronchial carcinoid tumors and small cell carcinoma of the lung. Indeed, the two types may have a common cell of origin, namely the Kulchitsky cell, a bronchial mucosal cell that has been called a neuroendocrine cell of the lung because of its peptide-containing granules observed on electron microscopy. A bombesin-like peptide (related to gastrin-releasing peptide) is present in Kulchitsky cells during fetal life and is the most frequent peptide produced by small cell carcinoma of the lung. Ectopic hormone secretion is also associated with other types of lung tumors, most commonly the squamous type of bronchogenic carcinomas.

In the 1960s Pearse proposed the theory that certain hormone-secreting cells are components of a "diffuse neuroendocrine system." Such cells were originally considered to be of neural crest or neuroectodermal origin and were designated APUD (amine precursor uptake and decarboxylation) cells on the basis of their ability to decarboxylate precursors of biogenic amines. Later it was discovered that many of these cells also produce the enzyme neuron-specific enolase and other neurosecretory cell markers. A corollary of the APUD theory was that tumors derived from APUD cells had the capability of hormone secretion. At present, there is doubt concerning the validity of the APUD theory on several grounds. First, all APUD cells are not of neuroectodermal origin. Second, the APUD function of these cells is not inherently linked with peptide hormone production, and third, some ectopic hormone-secreting tumors do not possess APUD characteristics. Nevertheless, the association of particular tumor types with the secretion of certain hormones is useful in evaluating these syndromes.

CHARACTERIZATION OF ECTOPIC HORMONES Type of hormone secreted Of the four classes of hormones—steroids, monoamines, substituted amino acids, and peptides/proteins—only the latter are secreted ectopically. Although the explanation is not known with certainty, the ectopic production of peptide/protein hormones may require less complicated derangements in cell metabolism. For example, an oncogene serving as an inducer or enhancer of gene transcription may be responsible for increasing the expression of a gene coding for a peptide hormone. In contrast, the synthesis of steroids, thyroid hormones, or monoamines requires multiple enzymatic steps and specifically targeted translocation of the precursor molecules through various cell compartments. The likelihood that this degree of cell specialization would occur as a consequence of neoplastic change is much less than the possibility that a process (protein synthesis) common to all cells might be initiated aberrantly. Ectopic secretion of nearly all peptide hormones has been reported. These hormones may be grouped according to their usual site of origin (Table 309-2). The first group of hormones, common to the central nervous system and gastrointestinal tract, are most frequently secreted by carcinoids, small cell lung carcinomas, and pancreatic islet tumors. The second group, normally produced by the fetoplacental

unit and/or the anterior pituitary, tends to be produced by gastrointestinal, hepatic, adrenal, and gonadal tumors. The third group, which includes insulin-like growth factors and parathyroid hormone–like factors, tends to be produced by mesenchymal, hepatic, genitourinary, and squamous cell lung tumors. In addition to the hormones listed, other humoral factors are believed responsible for tumor-associated syndromes such as hypertrophic osteoarthropathy, polyneuropathy, hypophosphatemic osteomalacia, and anorexia.

Relation to naturally secreted hormones The primary amino acid sequences of nearly all ectopically secreted hormones analyzed to date are identical to those of the native hormones. However, other differences in structure between ectopically secreted and native hormones can occur as a result of incomplete or abnormal processing of the precursor hormone. Several abnormal forms of ectopic hormones have been defined: (1) large-molecular-weight species due to incomplete enzymatic cleavage of the precursor (proopiomelanocortin); (2) small-molecular-weight fragments due to unregulated intracellular processing (fragments of growth hormone–releasing hormone); and (3) altered glycosylation species (microheterogeneity) due either to failed cleavage of carbohydrate residues during postribosomal hormone processing (glycosylated ACTH) or failure of normal glycosylation (the alpha subunit common to the gonadotropins and TSH). The usual consequence of such altered biosynthetic processing is a hormone variant with diminished biologic activity. If modification of hormone structure is sufficient to cause loss of all biologic activity, ectopic secretion is not accompanied by clinical manifestations. Even if a neoplastic cell can synthesize and store a biologically active hormone, a syndrome of hormone excess may not result if an intact secretory mechanism is absent. The frequency with which either an inactive hormone is synthesized or an active hormone is synthesized but not secreted is probably greater than that of classical ectopic hormone secretion since only a small percentage of tumors that contain ectopic hormones cause clinically recognizable syndromes attributable to hormone hypersecretion.

Other considerations Hormones may be secreted by both benign and malignant tumors. Although hormone secretion normally requires a high level of cellular differentiation, an incompletely differentiated tumor may still retain secretory capability. For example, the process of granule formation and hormone storage is not generally expressed by hormone-secreting tumors; consequently, the concentration of hormone in the tumor is usually low compared to that in endocrine glands. Overall hormone secretion per unit weight is also less and, as a result, considerable tumor mass is usually present before ectopic hormone secretion is clinically apparent. One notable exception is the relatively benign, highly differentiated neoplasm, usually a carcinoid or pancreatic islet tumor, that contains and secretes hormone at a level comparable to that of normal endocrine tissue and is sufficiently small to escape detection for long periods.

Many tumors produce multiple hormones. In some this is due to the existence of a common precursor for multiple hormones, e.g., ACTH, lipotropins, melanocyte-stimulating hormones (MSHs), and endorphins are all derived from a single precursor, proopiomelanocortin (POMC), and both vasoactive intestinal peptide (VIP) and peptide histidyl-methionine (PHM) are encoded in a single precursor. In other instances multiple hormones are produced in the absence of common precursors, e.g., production of ACTH, calcitonin, and somatostatin by medullary thyroid carcinoma and by small cell carcinoma of the lung. In some tumors separate cells secrete individual hormones, whereas in others multiple hormones are produced by the same cell. Furthermore, variation may occur in cell lines cloned from such tumors, suggesting that gene expression may be unstable in succeeding generations of tumor cells.

FREQUENCY The frequency of ectopic hormone secretion varies with the criteria used for its definition. The most frequently encountered syndromes are those of ACTH hypersecretion, hypercalcemia, and organic hypoglycemia. Ectopic ACTH secretion occurs in approximately 15 to 20 percent of patients with Cushing's syndrome. Thus, consideration of this diagnosis is of great importance. Similarly,

TABLE 309-2   Spectrum of ectopic hormone production

Group/hormone	Tumor type		Group/hormone	Tumor type	
	Common	Infrequent		Common	Infrequent
1 Neuroendocrine-gastrointestinal			j Glucagon		Lung carcinoma, Carcinoid, Renal carcinoma
a ACTH, β-lipotropin, endorphins, MSHs, enkephalins	Lung carcinoma (small cell), Thymoma, Pancreatic islet tumors, Carcinoid, Thyroid medullary carcinoma, Pheochromocytoma, Parotid tumor, Prostatic carcinoma, Renal carcinoma	Squamous cell, adenocarcinoma, and large cell carcinoma of the lung, Breast carcinoma, Colonic carcinoma, Gallbladder tumors, Testicular carcinoma, Uterine carcinoma, Laryngeal carcinoma, Plasmacytoma, Bladder small cell carcinoma	k Gastrin-releasing peptide (bombesin-like)	Lung carcinoma, Carcinoid	Medullary carcinoma of thyroid
			2 Fetoplacental and/or anterior pituitary		
			a Chorionic gonadotropin (and subunits)	Lung carcinoma, Gastric carcinoma, Ovarian carcinoma, Adeno- and islet cell carcinoma of the pancreas, Hepatoma, Genitourinary tract tumors	Testicular carcinoma, Ovarian carcinoma, Adrenocortical carcinoma, Breast carcinoma, Melanoma, Carcinoid
b Vasopressin, oxytocin, neurophysin	Lung carcinoma (small cell, anaplastic, adenocarcinoma), Carcinoid	Pancreatic carcinoma, Duodenal carcinoma	b Placental lactogen	Lung carcinoma (small cell)	Lymphoma, Pheochromocytoma, Hepatoma
c Corticotropin-releasing hormone	Lung carcinoma (small cell), Carcinoid	Pituitary gangliocytoma, Medullary carcinoma of thyroid	c Growth hormone		Lung carcinoma (large cell), Carcinoid, Pancreatic islet tumor
d Growth hormone–releasing hormone	Carcinoid, Pancreatic islet adenoma, Lung carcinoma (small cell)	Adrenocortical adenoma, Neurofibroma, Endometrial carcinoma, Pheochromocytoma, Pituitary gangliocytoma	d Prolactin		Lung carcinoma, Renal carcinoma, Gonadoblastoma
			3 Others		
			a Tissue growth factors (somatomedins)	Mesenchymal tumors (i.e., fibrosarcoma), Hepatoma, Adrenocortical carcinoma, Pancreatic/bile duct carcinoma	Lung carcinoma, Ovarian carcinoma, Neuroblastoma, Wilms's tumor
e Somatostatin	Lung carcinoma (small cell), Carcinoid, Pheochromocytoma		b Erythropoietin	Cerebellar hemangioblastoma, Uterine fibroma, Renal carcinoma	Adrenocortical carcinoma, Hepatoma, Pheochromocytoma
f Calcitonin	Lung carcinoma (small cell), Carcinoid	Breast carcinoma, Pheochromocytoma	c Humoral hypercalcemic factor of malignancy, osteoclast-activating factor	Renal carcinoma, Lung carcinoma (squamous), Hepatoma, Pancreatic islet tumors	GI tract tumors, Parotid tumors, Genitourinary tract tumors, Melanoma, Breast carcinoma
g Gastrin	Lung carcinoma (small cell)	Ovarian carcinoma			
h Vasoactive intestinal peptide	Lung carcinoma (small cell), Pancreatic islet tumors				
i Insulin		Gastric carcinoma, Lung carcinoma, Carcinoid	d 1,25-Dihydroxy vitamin D	Lymphoma	

nearly half of patients with hypercalcemia unrelated to volume depletion, excess ingestion of vitamin D, or sarcoidosis have a malignancy rather than hyperparathyroidism, and of these about 70 percent secrete a hypercalcemic peptide that has parathyroid hormone–like biologic activity and is structurally similar, though not identical, to parathyroid hormone. In contrast, hypoglycemia due to ectopic production of an insulin-like growth factor is infrequent in patients suspected of having an insulinoma, and ectopic growth hormone–releasing hormone (GRH) secretion is a rare (<1 percent) cause of acromegaly.

CONSEQUENCES OF ECTOPIC HORMONE SECRETION The consequences of ectopic hormone secretion may be of greater significance than the tumor itself. This is particularly true for patients with benign or slowly growing malignant ACTH- or gastrin-producing tumors in whom fulminant Cushing's syndrome or bleeding peptic ulceration may be life-threatening. In others, the hormone may cause medical problems that shorten the life span beyond that attributable to the tumor itself, i.e., severe hypercalcemia, hyponatremia, or hypoglycemia.

The symptoms of ectopic hormone secretion may be the presenting manifestations of the neoplasm or occur late in the course of the disease. The rapidity of onset of the clinical features of hormone hypersecretion affects the frequency with which the syndrome is recognized. For example, excessive secretion of ACTH or vasopressin is clinically evident within weeks or months; thus, a fully developed syndrome can be associated with rapidly growing malignant as well as benign tumors. In contrast, acromegaly due to ectopic GRH secretion typically requires years to become apparent and therefore is observed only when caused by benign or slowly growing malignant neoplasms. Ectopic hormone secretion, once established, does not necessarily persist for as long as the tumor is present. Hormone secretion may cease or decline to clinically insignificant levels either spontaneously or in response to radiation or chemotherapy. Hormone secretion usually, but not invariably, recurs with tumor relapse.

In addition to effects on the host, ectopic hormone secretion has numerous important biologic implications. Since tumor-secreted factors that exhibit biologic effects are unlikely to be unique substances, their identification and characterization can assist in the search for the naturally occurring (eutopic) peptide. For example, tumor-secreted GRH was the source for the purification, isolation, and structural characterization of hypothalamic GRH. Relatively little attention has been given to possible effects of ectopically secreted hormones on the growth or survival of the tumor.

DIAGNOSIS Occasionally, the clinical manifestations of ectopic hormone secretion are so distinctive that they suggest the diagnosis before any hormone measurements have been performed. The development of gynecomastia in the absence of associated diseases such as cirrhosis or testicular failure may suggest the presence of ectopic gonadotropin secretion, while Cushing's syndrome and increased pigmentation or severe muscle weakness (due to hypokalemia) point to ectopic ACTH secretion.

More commonly, however, clinical manifestations of hormone excess are subtle or absent. In such instances basal serum levels of hormones, e.g., ACTH, may be elevated out of proportion to the biologic effects observed. This may be the result of ACTH precursor molecules that have little or no biologic activity. Identification of these hormonal forms can be accomplished by molecular sieve chromatography or by multiple, site-specific radioimmunoassays of serum. Similarly, disproportionate elevations of hCG may reflect the presence of the glycoprotein alpha subunit, which is biologically inactive but exhibits cross-reactivity in some radioimmunoassays. A specific alpha-subunit assay is used to confirm the diagnosis.

In other instances the diagnosis of ectopic hormone secretion may be suggested by finding suppressed levels of hormones that are subject to feedback inhibition. Low or undetectable levels of insulin or parathyroid hormone in the presence of hypoglycemia or hypercalcemia are suggestive of tumors that secrete an insulin-like growth factor or a humoral hypercalcemic factor of malignancy, respectively.

Alterations in normal feedback regulation may also provide clues that elevated circulating hormone levels are derived from ectopic sources. Patients with ectopic ACTH production do not respond to suppression by glucocorticoids or to stimulation by corticotropin-releasing hormone (presumably because of the absence of appropriate receptors in the tumor tissue), an observation that helps distinguish them from patients with pituitary-dependent Cushing's disease. Apparent suppression of ACTH, which has been noted in several case reports, could be explained by intermittent secretion of ACTH by the tumor (an uncommon and poorly understood phenomenon of ectopic hormone secretion) or by the coproduction of corticotropin-releasing hormone.

If the diagnosis is still in doubt, or if the source of ectopic secretion is unknown, selective venous catheterization may be an effective means of locating the tumor. As long as the tumor is actually secreting hormone at the time of study, a step-up gradient in the concentration of the hormone is of value in tumor localization and/or a search for metastases.

THERAPY Primary treatment of ectopic hormone–secreting tumors should be directed, if possible, toward removal of the tumor. Measurement of circulating hormone levels can serve as a marker for completeness of tumor excision or of the effect of radiation and chemotherapy for tumors considered inoperable, i.e., small cell carcinoma of the lung. In addition, recurrence of tumor may be heralded by reappearance of elevated hormone levels prior to clinical evidence of the tumor mass. However, occasional tumors may not secrete hormones at the time of recurrence, so that one cannot rely entirely on hormone measurements as a marker of tumor activity.

Frequently, the tumor cannot be removed or is already metastatic at the time of diagnosis. In such cases, two other approaches are available for eliminating the effects of ectopic hormone secretion. Pharmacologic agents may be used to inhibit hormone release. Octreotide, a long-acting somatostatin analogue, has been used effectively in inhibiting growth hormone–releasing hormone secretion, VIP secretion, and the clinical symptoms of the carcinoid syndrome.

The other approach involves blocking the action of the hormone when its secretion cannot be altered. Pharmacologic agents may interfere with hormone effects on target tissues. Examples include (1) demeclocycline to inhibit vasopressin action on the renal tubule in the syndrome of inappropriate antidiuretic hormone (SIADH) associated with malignancy, and (2) ketoconazole and/or mitotane to inhibit adrenal steroidogenesis in the ectopic ACTH syndrome. Alternatively, surgical removal of the target tissue may avoid life-threatening complications and permit relatively symptom-free long-term survival if the tumor itself is benign or is slowly growing. Examples include adrenalectomy for the ectopic ACTH syndrome and gastrectomy for recurrent gastrointestinal bleeding caused by gastrin-producing tumors. This form of therapy will be used with

decreasing frequency as newer and more specific pharmacologic agents become available.

ECTOPIC HORMONES AS MARKERS FOR NEOPLASIA With the initial recognition of ectopic hormone secretion, it was hoped that by measuring these hormones a generally applicable means of screening for clinically silent tumors would become available. As knowledge of the spectrum of ectopic hormone secretion has increased, however, this hope has faded. The list of hormones that are secreted ectopically has lengthened to the point that cost considerations preclude the use of this form of screening. Even if the number of hormones were not as extensive, the limited correlation of tumor site and type with secretion of specific hormones necessitates an extensive workup to localize the tumor. Screening programs, when performed, have yielded relatively few positive results. Moreover evidence is lacking that earlier diagnosis, as a result of such procedures, reduces subsequent morbidity or mortality. Consequently, screening for ectopic hormone production is not justified as part of routine cancer detection programs.

REFERENCES

Bostwick DG et al: Expression of opioid peptides in tumors. N Engl J Med 17:1439, 1987

Broadus AE et al: Humoral hypercalcemia of cancer. Identification of a novel parathyroid hormone-like peptide. N Engl J Med 319:556, 1988

Frohman LA, Downs TR: Ectopic GRH syndrome, in *Acromegaly*, R Robbins et al (eds). New York, Plenum, 1987

Heitz PU et al: Ectopic hormone production by endocrine tumors: Localization of hormones at the cellular level by immunocytochemistry. Cancer 48:2029, 1981

Howlett TA, Rees LH: Ectopic hormones. Spec Top Endocrinol Metab 7:1, 1985

Insogna KL, Broadus AE: Hypercalcemia of malignancy. Annu Rev Med 38:241, 1987

Kohler PC, Trump DL: Ectopic hormones syndromes. Cancer Invest 4:543, 1986

Lokich JJ: The frequency and clinical biology of the ectopic hormone syndromes of small cell carcinoma. Cancer 50:2111, 1982

Melmed S et al: Acromegaly due to secretion of growth hormone by an ectopic pancreatic islet-cell tumor. N Engl J Med 312:9, 1985

———, Rushakoff RJ: Ectopic pituitary and hypothalamic hormone syndromes. Endocrinol Metab Clin North Am 16:805, 1987

Muddle AH et al: Ectopic production of 1,25-dihydroxyvitamin D by B-cell lymphoma as a cause of hypercalcemia. Cancer 59:1543, 1987

Orth D: Ectopic hormone production, in *Endocrinology and Metabolism*, 2d ed, P Felig et al (eds). New York, McGraw-Hill, 1987

Sano T et al: Growth hormone-releasing hormone-producing tumors: Clinical, biochemical, and morphological manifestations. Endocr Rev 9:357, 1988

Shah VM et al: Ectopic beta-human chorionic gonadotropin production by bladder urothelial neoplasia. Arch Pathol Lab Med 110:107, 1986

Wynick D et al: Symptomatic secondary hormone syndromes in patients with established malignant pancreatic endocrine tumors. N Engl J Med 319:605, 1988

310 PARANEOPLASTIC NEUROLOGIC SYNDROMES

ROBERT H. BROWN, JR.

Neoplasms can derange neurologic function in a number of ways (Table 310-1, see also Chap. 353). Paraneoplastic neurologic syndromes, which occur in the setting of a remotely located neoplasm, can present in several forms (Table 310-2). These paraneoplastic syndromes share several characteristics. They are clinically dramatic, arising subacutely in weeks or even days to produce neurologic symptoms that may be profoundly disabling. These syndromes may precede detection of the neoplasm by months or even years; their recognition should prompt a timely search for carcinoma. Although more than one syndrome may arise with a given neoplasm, certain clinical manifestations are often associated with particular types of tumors (Table 310-2).

The diagnosis of a paraneoplastic neurologic disorder depends primarily on (1) the presence of a recognized clinical syndrome; (2)

TABLE 310-1   Effects of malignancy on the nervous system

I Direct invasion
II Metastatic invasion
   A Parenchymatous
   B Vascular (neoplastic angioendotheliosis)
   C Meningeal (meningeal carcinomatosis)
III Opportunistic infections
   A Bacterial (e.g., *Listeria*)
   B Nonbacterial
     1 Typical and atypical viral (e.g., progressive multifocal leukoencephalopathy)
     2 Fungal (e.g., cryptococcus)
IV Complications of antineoplastic therapy
   A Radiation (e.g., radiation necrosis)
   B Chemotherapy (e.g., vincristine neuropathy)
V Metabolic complications
   A Nutritional deficiency
   B Ectopic hormone production
VI Paraneoplastic syndromes

careful exclusion of other cancer-related disorders listed in Table 310-1; and (3) in some instances, confirmatory laboratory studies such as an electromyogram typical of myasthenia gravis or the presence in serum of antibodies with specific patterns of reactivity. Cerebrospinal fluid (CSF) may show protein elevation and a mild lymphocytic pleocytosis.

INCIDENCE Studies of the incidence of these syndromes are problematic because the syndromes are rare and classifications vary somewhat among studies. In one series, these syndromes were detected in about 7 percent of nearly 1500 patients with tumors, although recent studies suggest the incidence is somewhat lower. Among malignant tumors with paraneoplastic neurologic syndromes, the most common are lung (47 percent), stomach (12 percent), breast (12 percent), ovary (9 percent), and colon (6 percent). These syndromes are encountered in one-sixth of all ovarian tumors, one-seventh of lung tumors, and less frequently in stomach, prostate, and breast cancers.

PATHOLOGIC CHANGES Pathologic features of these syndromes have been well defined. One of the most common findings is encephalomyelitis characterized by perivascular lymphocytosis, microglial proliferation, and loss of neurons. To emphasize involvement of neurons in gray matter, the process is sometimes described as *polioencephalomyelitis*. While these changes may be diffuse throughout the neuraxis, they often predominate in a specific anatomic location that dictates the resulting clinical abnormalities. Thus, as outlined below, the manifestations of limbic encephalitis may differ from those of brainstem encephalitis. Inflammation may be evident in dorsal root ganglia or in gray and white matter of the spinal cord, producing, respectively, ganglioradiculitis or subacute poliomyelitis. A second striking pathologic finding is severe, focal degeneration or loss of neurons without inflammation. This is exemplified by the selective but widespread loss of Purkinje neurons in the cerebellum in subacute cortical cerebellar degeneration. This may occur in isolation or concurrently with findings of encephalomyelitis; thus, in cortical cerebellar degeneration there may be some accompanying cerebellar inflammation. As outlined below, some paraneoplastic syndromes are associated with pathologic changes in the peripheral nervous system such as multifocal demyelination, myonecrosis, or ultrastructural changes in the neuromuscular junction.

Autoimmune mechanisms have been implicated in several instances. Some paraneoplastic disorders are characterized by serum and spinal fluid antibodies that have highly specific patterns of reactivity with neural tissue or muscle. These are exemplified by the Lambert-Eaton myasthenic syndrome and myasthenia gravis, in which affected individuals have circulating antibodies that react with pre- and postsynaptic proteins (see Chap. 366). Both syndromes have been reproduced in animals by passive administration of fractionated immunoglobulins. As another example, in some cases of cortical cerebellar degeneration serum and spinal fluid antibodies react specifically with cerebellar cytoplasmic antigens. By contrast, immu-

noglobulins from patients with different paraneoplastic neurologic syndromes may show similar patterns of reactivity with neural tissue. Thus, antibodies recognizing neuronal nuclear antigens are common in patients with small cell carcinoma of the lung and several paraneoplastic syndromes such as subacute sensory neuropathy. In this instance, it appears that one or more pathogenic antibodies, possibly cross-reacting with antigens on the tumor, may provoke autoimmune neural injury in more than one region of the neuraxis. Detection of such antibodies may confirm that an evolving neurologic disorder is of paraneoplastic origin even though the antibodies are not diagnostic of a specific neurologic syndrome.

TREATMENT Treatment of the paraneoplastic disorders is not uniformly successful. The most consistently beneficial treatments are anti-immune therapy such as plasma exchange or immunosuppression in those disorders that are clearly autoimmune. In some instances, the paraneoplastic syndromes have regressed after resection of the carcinoma. Otherwise, therapy is largely symptomatic.

The following is an outline of the salient features of the major paracarcinomatous neurologic syndromes.

BRAIN, CEREBELLUM, AND SPINAL CORD

VISUAL PARANEOPLASTIC SYNDROMES Patients with carcinoma of the lung or cervix may develop progressive, painless loss of vision because of degeneration of the rods and cones. The electroretinogram is abnormal, and cells may be present in the spinal fluid. Lymphocytic inflammation of the retina accompanies loss of rods and cones. Paraneoplastic visual loss may also occur because of antibody-mediated loss of retinal ganglion cells. Sera of affected patients contain antibodies that react with antigens shared by the retinal ganglion cell and the tumor (e.g., small cell lung carcinoma).

LIMBIC ENCEPHALITIS Encephalitis of limbic structures such as the hippocampus and amygdala produces affective changes in personality including anxiety and agitated depression in association with selective, early memory loss suggestive of Korsakoff's psychosis, and occasionally confusion and hallucinations. In some cases the initial presentation is an amnesic syndrome. The affective disorder often prompts psychiatric evaluation. Abnormalities of the electroencephalogram or overt seizures may be present early in the syndrome. While cognition may initially be spared, dementia is common. As the disorder progresses, symptoms referable to encephalitic involvement in other regions are often superimposed.

BRAINSTEM ENCEPHALITIS Symptoms of brainstem encephalitis relate directly to the distribution of the inflammation. Medullary involvement produces nausea, vomiting, nystagmus, possibly vertigo, and ataxia. A syndrome suggestive of progressive bulbar palsy with marked dysarthria and dysphagia is associated with pontine involvement. Mesencephalic inflammation and neuronal loss result in nuclear or internuclear eye movement abnormalities; diplopia and oscillopsia may be disabling. Rostral midbrain and nigral involvement may cause rigidity. Medullary symptoms typically predominate.

CEREBELLAR ENCEPHALITIS Inflammatory changes are rare in cerebellar cortex but may be severe in deep cerebellar nuclei such as the dentate nucleus. Inflammation within the dentate nucleus provokes myoclonus.

MYELITIS In paraneoplastic myelitis, the gray matter of the cord is diffusely inflamed with profound neuronal degeneration. This poliomyelitis may be widespread in the cord or restricted to a few segmental levels. Anterior horn cell destruction typically produces muscle weakness and neurogenic atrophy. Limb involvement is often asymmetric. There may be selective involvement of the neck and upper extremities or lower extremities alone. Corticospinal findings result from involvement of this tract in the cord or from brainstem disease. The corticospinal tract dysfunction and motor neuronopathy in these cases should not be confused with motor neuron disease; typical amyotrophic lateral sclerosis does not appear to arise on a paraneoplastic basis. The presence of sensory signs with cancer

TABLE 310-2 Paraneoplastic neurologic syndromes

Site	Evolution	Clinical features*	Cancer	Pathology
BRAIN AND CEREBELLUM				
Photoreceptor, retinal degeneration	Weeks to months	Painless visual loss progressing to blindness	Oat cell tumor; rarely cervical cancer	Loss of rods and cones; infiltration of retina with mononuclear cells
Limbic encephalitis	Weeks to months	Agitated, confusional state; memory loss followed by dementia[1]	Oat cell tumor of lung	Neuronal loss in medial temporal lobe and elsewhere in the limbic system; perivascular and meningeal lymphocytic infiltration
Brainstem encephalitis	Days to weeks	Nystagmus, diplopia, vertigo, ataxia, dysarthria, dysphagia[1]	Oat cell tumor	Neuronal loss in brainstem; inflammatory changes as above
Subacute cortical cerebellar degeneration	Weeks to months	Cerebellar ataxia, dysarthria[1,2]	Oat cell tumor; ovarian and breast cancer; Hodgkin's disease	Loss of Purkinje cells
Opsoclonus-myoclonus	Weeks	Dancing eyes and feet, cerebellar ataxia, and possibly encephalopathy	Neuroblastoma; bronchial carcinoma in adults	In adults, degeneration of dentate nuclei
SPINAL CORD				
Necrotizing myelopathy	Hours, days, or weeks	Para- or quadriplegia with areflexia; sensory loss and bladder dysfunction	Oat cell tumor, lymphoma	Severe necrosis of gray and white matter
Subacute motor neuronopathy	Weeks or months	Flaccid weakness and muscle atrophy; legs affected more than arms	Non-Hodgkin's lymphoma; loss of anterior horn cells	Inflammation of ventral horns
PERIPHERAL NERVE				
Acute demyelinating neuritis (Guillain-Barré, acute inflammatory demyelinating polyneuropathy, AIDP)	Hours to days	Ascending paralysis; areflexia; possibly ascending sensory loss; high CSF protein	Hodgkin's disease	Segmental demyelination; inflammation of peripheral nerves
Chronic inflammatory demyelinating polyneuropathy (CIDP)	Weeks to months	Chronic progressive or relapsing weakness with sensory loss; high CSF protein	Rarely lung, breast, and gastric cancer; lymphoma, myeloma	As in AIDP
Neuropathy with paraproteinemia	Weeks to months	Chronic; may be predominantly sensory[3] or motor[4]	Myeloma; osteosclerotic myeloma	As in CIDP
Subacute sensory neuronopathy	Weeks to months	Severe sensory loss with areflexia and ataxia; paresthesias, pain[1]	Oat cell and other lung tumors	Inflammation and neuronal degeneration in dorsal root ganglia; secondary axon loss
Sensorimotor neuropathy	Weeks to months	Distal motor and sensory loss[1]	Oat cell and other tumors	Axonopathy; some segmental loss of myelin
NEUROMUSCULAR JUNCTION				
Lambert-Eaton myasthenic syndrome	Weeks to months	Proximal weakness, fatigability; dry mouth; possibly ptosis[5]	Oat cell tumor, breast, prostate, stomach	Disruption of active zones on presynaptic terminals
Myasthenia gravis	Weeks to months	Weakness, fatigability, ptosis; diplopia[6]	Thymoma	Disruption of postsynaptic junctional membrane folds
MUSCLE				
Polymyositis	Months to years	Proximal weakness, myalgias, possibly cardiomyopathy; high creatine phosphokinase	Association with malignancy unclear; possibly breast, ovary, lung tumors; lymphoma	Lymphocytic inflammation of muscle interstitium; myofiber necrosis, phagocytosis
Necrotizing myopathy	Days to weeks	Rapidly progressive proximal weakness, possibly dysphagia, dyspnea	Bronchial carcinoma, Oat cell tumor	Severe myonecrosis with minimal inflammation or phagocytosis

* Superscript denotes possible immunoglobulin reactivity: (1) antineuronal nuclear antigen; (2) one or more cytoplasmic antigens expressed selectively in cerebellar Purkinje cells; (3) IgM M component reacting with myelin-associated glycoprotein; (4) IgG or IgA M component arising in association with osteosclerotic myeloma; (5) voltage-sensitive calcium channel at presynaptic terminal; (6) acetylcholine receptor on postsynaptic specialization.

denotes either dorsal root ganglioradiculitis or poliomyelitis involving the posterior horns.

NECROTIZING MYELOPATHY This syndrome, presenting clinically as a subacute transverse myelitis, often in a thoracic distribution, is distinguished from the less fulminant encephalomyelitis by the evolution of a densely necrotic, central thoracic cord lesion which tails off rostrally and caudally over several segmental levels. In some instances, there are multiple such lesions along the cord. Clinical findings include leg and possibly arm plegia, sensory loss, and loss of sphincter control. The lesion can initially be asymmetric, mimicking a Brown-Séquard syndrome. In severe cases, the spinal fluid protein and cell count are increased and myelography demonstrates focal cord swelling. Not all cases are associated with tumor; when present, the cancers are often lung, lymphoma, and leukemia.

OPSOCLONUS-MYOCLONUS   This syndrome of opsoclonus, myoclonus, and ataxia, or "dancing eyes–dancing feet," occurs in children and adults. About one-half of affected children are found to have differentiated neuroblastomas, usually in the thorax. In adults, the syndrome may be associated with solid tumors such as bronchial carcinoma. The onset is subacute, and in some instances the syndrome lasts for months to be followed by permanent encephalopathy or retardation. Pathologic findings in adults include prominent neuronal degeneration in the dentate nucleus of the cerebellum suggesting a relationship to cortical cerebellar degeneration. Occasionally there is lymphocytic cuffing diffusely in the central nervous system and cerebrospinal fluid pleocytosis. Some adults and children respond to treatment of the cancer or to glucocorticoids.

SUBACUTE CORTICAL CEREBELLAR DEGENERATION (SCCD)   This is a subacutely progressive cerebellar disorder characterized by profound truncal and appendicular ataxia arising within weeks in association with carcinoma, typically ovarian or oat cell of the lung. There often are superimposed symptoms potentially referable to the brainstem including vertigo, dysarthria, diplopia and nystagmus, or corticospinal signs. As a rule, any nonfamilial ataxia arising in patients over the age of 45 years should raise the suspicion of this entity. The predominant pathologic finding is widespread loss of cerebellar Purkinje cell neurons with some astrogliosis and secondary loss of Purkinje cell axons. Interestingly, in the purely degenerative disorder without inflammation elsewhere dentate neurons are largely spared, while they are often heavily damaged in encephalomyelitis. Many cases are associated with dementia for which an anatomic basis has not been established. The CSF commonly reveals a mild pleocytosis; cerebellar atrophy may be evident on neuroradiographic studies.

At least three types of anti-Purkinje cell antibodies have been detected in sera of patients with subacute cerebellar degeneration. Women with gynecologic cancer (breast, ovary) and SCCD have anti-Purkinje cell antibodies (APCA) recognizing cytoplasmic proteins of about 34 and 62 kDa. The former is a recently cloned, novel neuronal protein expressed selectively in cerebellar Purkinje cells. A different cytoplasmic antigen is recognized by immunoglobulins from patients with SCCD and adenocarcinoma of the lung; in this entity, the antibodies fail to recognize a specific protein on Western blots. In some patients with small cell carcinoma of the lung and SCCD, serum globulins ("anti-Hu" antibodies) stain nuclear antigens in many types of neurons. Anti-Hu antibodies are also detected in other paraneoplastic disorders (see below). APCA and anti-Hu antibody activities are of diagnostic significance as they help determine whether a neurologic syndrome is paraneoplastic. In addition, they underscore the likelihood that an antibody-mediated immunologic mechanism may underlie several of the paracarcinomatous syndromes.

PERIPHERAL NERVES

The diagnosis of peripheral neuropathy in association with cancer can be challenging. Paraneoplastic subacute sensory neuronopathy, arguably the most clinically distinctive, is a ganglioradiculitis which may arise with one or more other manifestations of encephalomyelitis. Other paraneoplastic neuropathies are difficult to distinguish from noncarcinomatous neuropathies. Their recognition is critical as they are relatively common and sometimes precede diagnosis of the underlying neoplasia. By electrodiagnostic criteria, neuropathy may be evident in as many as 50 percent of patients with lung cancer. In the evaluation of a possibly paracarcinomatous neuropathy, it is particularly helpful to ascertain whether the neuropathy (1) affects motor fibers, sensory fibers, or both; (2) predominantly involves axon or myelin; or (3) occurs with an abnormal serum paraprotein.

ACUTE INFLAMMATORY DEMYELINATING POLYNEURITIS (AIDP, GUILLAIN-BARRÉ)   This syndrome, discussed in detail elsewhere (Chap. 363), is characterized by subacutely ascending paralysis, sensory loss which is often mild by comparison with the motor deficits, areflexia, and a characteristic elevation of CSF protein without pleocytosis. Histopathology reveals lymphocytic infiltration of nerves, segmental demyelination, and relative axonal sparing. AIDP may be associated with Hodgkin's disease.

CHRONIC INFLAMMATORY DEMYELINATING POLYNEUROPATHY (CIDP)   This group of chronic progressive or relapsing, inflammatory demyelinative peripheral neuropathies is distinguished from acute polyneuritis by the time course, more prominent involvement of sensory nerves, lack of involvement of autonomic nerves, and responsiveness to immunotherapy. As in AIDP, the demyelinative nature of these neuropathies is defined physiologically by abnormalities such as slowed nerve conduction velocities or dispersion of compound muscle action potentials; as in AIDP, the pathologic hallmark is loss of myelin with relative preservation of axons or segmental demyelination. In some cases, physiologic studies may reveal only marginal slowing of conduction while the biopsy clearly demonstrates selective myelin loss. In other instances, a sural nerve biopsy may fail to reveal proximal demyelination detectable only with electrophysiologic methods. Elevation of the CSF protein helps confirm the diagnosis.

Rarely, CIDP occurs in association with solid tumors of lung, breast, and stomach. It also occurs with Waldenström's macroglobulinemia, gamma heavy chain disease, and lymphoma. In many instances, paraneoplastic CIDP is characterized by the presence of a serum paraprotein, typically a monoclonal immunoglobulin ("M component"). As many as 20 percent of patients with monoclonal gammopathies of undetermined significance develop significant hematologic disease, including malignancies.

Two chronic demyelinating neuropathies are particularly distinctive in this context. The first is associated with a monoclonal IgM that reacts with a myelin-associated glycoprotein (MAG) in peripheral nerve myelin. This pattern of reactivity occurs in about half of patients with an IgM gammopathy and neuropathy. This IgM anti-MAG neuropathy is more sensory than motor; it is only slowly progressive as compared to the subacute sensory neuronopathy (below). It remains to be established whether the anti-MAG antibody is a cause or consequence of the demyelination. The second distinctive subtype of CIDP occurs with osteosclerotic myeloma and monoclonal IgG or IgA antibodies that do not react with MAG. This polyneuropathy is predominantly motor and often quite indolent, although it may eventually produce severe limb wasting. Sensory and autonomic findings are unusual. A related group of CIDP patients develop polyneuropathy, organomegaly, endocrinopathy, the M protein, and skin changes (POEMS syndrome); one-half have osteosclerotic myeloma and IgG or IgA M proteins with lambda light chains. Some patients with demyelinative neuropathies and IgM M proteins respond well to immunosuppressive therapy. Those with osteosclerotic myeloma may improve after treatment of the underlying plasmacytoma, particularly if it is solitary.

SUBACUTE SENSORY NEURONOPATHY   By contrast with AIDP and CIDP, many paraneoplastic neuropathies primarily affect the axon with relative sparing of myelin. The best example is the paraneoplastic subacute sensory neuronopathy which, as noted above, is a ganglioradiculitis. Inflammatory destruction of the sensory neuronal cell bodies (hence the term *neuronopathy*) in the dorsal root ganglia results in wallerian degeneration of axons both in peripheral nerve and ascending sensory long tracts (posterior columns of the spinal cord). Clinically, this is heralded by the subacute appearance of paresthesias and pain in the distal limbs and truncal sensory ataxia. Limb pain may be severe, and sensory ataxia may be profoundly disabling. Although initially restricted only to arms or legs, the symptoms eventually affect all four limbs. In many cases, the underlying malignancy is oat cell cancer of the lung; the paraneoplastic neuropathy often precedes the diagnosis of the tumor by more than a year. Some patients' sera possess antibodies (anti-Hu) reactive with a 35- to 40-kDa protein present both in nuclei of neurons and in small cell lung cancers.

SENSORIMOTOR NEUROPATHY This category of mixed sensory and motor axonopathies is perhaps the most common paraneoplastic neuropathy. Symptoms depend in part upon the severity, but may include muscle wasting and weakness or distal limb paresthesias and even pain. Pathologically, there is noninflammatory degeneration of axons and mild myelin loss, presumably secondary to the axonopathy. Paraneoplastic sensorimotor neuropathy has been reported with several types of tumors (lung oat cell, breast, stomach) and hematologic malignancies (Hodgkin's disease, lymphoma, multiple myeloma). In amyloidosis, itself often associated with myeloma, there may be an axonal neuropathy with intraneural deposition of amyloid fibrils derived from immunoglobulin light chains. Axonal neuropathy has been reported as a manifestation of occult insulinoma, possibly as a consequence of hypoglycemia. Infrequently, these neuropathies remit spontaneously; often they progress even with aggressive treatment of the underlying malignancy.

SUBACUTE MOTOR NEURONOPATHY A subacute motor neuronopathy causes slowly progressive weakness in patients with lymphoma. Many patients seem to improve following immunosuppressive therapy for the malignancy. In others, progression of the weakness may cease after several months independently of the status of the lymphoma. Some myelomas are associated with subacute motor neuronopathy. Pathologic lesions include loss of motoneurons in the anterolateral gray matter of spinal cord, gliosis, loss of myelin in ventral roots, and some Schwann cell proliferation. There is no clearly effective treatment for this condition.

NEUROMUSCULAR JUNCTION

LAMBERT-EATON MYASTHENIC SYNDROME (LEMS) This syndrome afflicts men more than women, occurs in association with either malignancy or autoimmune diseases, and is characterized by weakness, myalgias, and fatigability, typically more severe in the lower extremities and proximal muscles. Ptosis may be seen. Dysautonomic features are common, including dryness of the mouth and eyes, impotence, diminished sweating, and orthostatic symptoms. The incidence of associated malignancy is 70 percent in men and 25 percent in women. In most cases the tumor is a small cell carcinoma of the lung. There is striking reduction in strength at rest with transient improvement in power on repetitive maximal exertion. Tensilon may marginally improve strength. Electromyography demonstrates motor unit potentials whose amplitude is low at rest but increases with exercise or tetanic stimulation; this contrasts with the electromyographic findings in myasthenia gravis. Electron microscopy of the presynaptic motor nerve terminals at the neuromuscular junction reveals a decrease in numbers of active zones believed to correspond to voltage-sensitive calcium channels. LEMS is believed to be an autoimmune disorder associated with diminished quantal release of acetylcholine. It is associated with other autoimmune disorders and appears to be HLA-linked (B8 and DRw3 antigens). Passive transfer of LEMS immunoglobulin in mice reproduces the ultrastructural findings. Electrophysiologic studies of affected mouse diaphragms suggest there is down-regulation of the voltage-sensitive calcium channels. Moreover, LEMS immunoglobulin also diminishes potassium-induced (voltage-dependent) influx of calcium into tumor cells cultured from small cell lung cancer. Treatment is directed toward the underlying neoplasm or autoimmune disease, or toward augmentation of acetylcholine release with drugs that prolong presynaptic depolarization and thereby enhance calcium influx. Guanidine hydrochloride and aminopyridine may be beneficial either in autoimmune or paraneoplastic LEMS; plasma exchange and immunosuppression may also be effective.

MYASTHENIA GRAVIS This disorder, discussed elsewhere in detail (Chap. 366), is characterized by exercise-induced muscle weakness caused by an antibody-mediated reduction in the numbers of acetylcholine receptors at the postsynaptic junction. About 15 percent of cases are associated with thymoma; many arise concurrently with other autoimmune or thyroid disorders.

MUSCLE

POLYMYOSITIS-DERMATOMYOSITIS This subject is reviewed fully elsewhere (Chap. 364). While an increased incidence of malignancy in elderly patients with dermatomyositis has long been suggested, this concept has recently been challenged by a retrospective analysis of experience with polymyositis at the Mayo Clinic.

NECROTIZING MYOPATHY Carcinoma of the bronchus may rarely be associated with a subacute, widespread, necrotizing myopathy that involves all muscles including bulbar and diaphragmatic muscles, weakness of which is often fatal. Intrafusal muscle fibers are also involved. Deep tendon reflexes are preserved. Muscle undergoes degeneration without phagocytosis or significant inflammatory response. The cause of the necrotizing process is unknown.

OTHER

Several other neurologic syndromes have been reported to be paraneoplastic but are less well characterized. *Stiff-man syndrome*, or diffuse hypertonia due to loss of inhibitory spinal interneurons, may arise in association with carcinoma of the pharynx. In this context, it is of interest that in nonneoplastic stiff-man syndrome autoantibodies have been detected that react with glutamic acid decarboxylase. This enzyme is essential for the synthesis of γ-aminobutyric acid, a central nervous system inhibitory neurotransmitter. Nonfamilial, subacute *chorea and dystonia* occur with oat cell carcinoma of the lung, and *optic neuritis* may develop as a paraneoplastic disorder. In the latter disorder, it is difficult to exclude direct involvement of the optic nerve or chiasm by cancer cells, or indirect effects of the underlying malignancy, as in Table 310-1.

REFERENCES

ANDERSON NE et al: Paraneoplastic degeneration: Clinical-immunological correlations. Ann Neurol 24:559, 1988

———— et al: Autoantibodies in paraneoplastic syndromes associated with small-cell lung carcinoma. Neurology 38:1391, 1988

FURNEAUX HM et al: Characterization of a cDNA encoding a 34-kDa Purkinje neuron protein recognized by sera from patients with paraneoplastic cerebellar degneration. Proc Natl Acad Sci USA 86:2873, 1989

GRAUS F et al: Sensory neuronopathy and small cell lung cancer. Am J Med 80:45, 1986

GRUNWALD GB et al: Autoimmune basis for visual paraneoplastic syndrome in patients with small cell lung carcinoma. Retinal immune deposits and ablation of retinal ganglion cells. Cancer 60:780, 1987

HENSON RA, URICH H: *Cancer and the Nervous System.* Oxford, Blackwell, 1982

KINSBOURNE M: Myoclonic encephalopathy of infants. J Neurol Neurosurg Psych 25.271, 1964

LAYZER RB: Stiff-man syndrome—an autoimmune disease? (editorial). N Engl J Med 318(16):1060, 1988

NAGEL A et al: Lambert-Eaton myasthenic syndrome IgG depletes presynaptic membrane active zone particles by antigenic modulation. Ann Neurol 24:552, 1988

POSNER JB: Paraneoplastic syndromes. Current Neurol 9:245, 1989

THIRKILL CE et al: Cancer-associated retinopathy (CAR syndrome) with antibodies reacting with retinal, optic-nerve, and cancer cells. N Engl J Med 321:1589, 1989

section 1 Endocrinology

311 HORMONES AND HORMONE ACTION

JEAN D. WILSON

Communication between cells is largely mediated by the endocrine and nervous systems. These two systems were originally considered distinct—information was thought to be carried either by neural impulses or by chemical mediators in the blood—but it is now clear that they constitute one coordinated network. Not only may neurotransmitters such as norepinephrine circulate in blood as hormones, but neural impulses have major effects on the release of chemical mediators such as testosterone and insulin. This interlocking relationship is most apparent in the hypothalamus, which serves as the highest integrative center for the two systems. Hence, one neuroendocrine system has evolved to integrate and coordinate the metabolic activities of the organism. Endocrinology deals largely with the chemical mediators in this system, but proper understanding of the role of hormones requires knowledge of the autonomic nervous system (Chap. 67) and of the metabolic capacities of cells.

The formulation of endocrinology has been blurred in additional ways. The term *hormone* originally referred to substances that are secreted into the circulation and act as chemical effectors in other tissues. However, the capacity to form such chemical mediators is not limited to so-called endocrine organs. Some hormones, such as angiotensins II and III, are formed in the bloodstream itself. Others, such as testosterone in women and dihydrotestosterone and estradiol in men, are in part secreted and in part formed in peripheral tissues from circulating precursors, so-called prohormones. Still other chemical mediators circulate only in restricted compartments such as the hypothalamic-pituitary portal system and do not reach the systemic circulation in appreciable quantities. Finally, certain hormones, such as insulin, dihydrotestosterone, and thyrotropin-releasing hormone (TRH), have paracrine actions in the same tissues in which they are formed and exert actions at distal sites, whereas other chemical mediators, such as müllerian-inhibiting substance, exert local actions exclusively.

BIOCHEMISTRY

SYNTHESIS The approximately 100 known mammalian hormones fall into three major categories—peptides or peptide derivatives, steroids, and amines. In the case of peptide hormones, genes code for messenger RNA, which is then translated into protein precursors. These proteins undergo posttranslational cleavage (pre-proparathyroid hormone → proparathyroid hormone → parathyroid hormone) and/or processing (thyroglobulin → thyroxine → triiodothyronine) to form the active hormone recognized by the target tissues. The distinct feature of peptide hormones is that one or a few structural genes code for the amino acid sequence of the peptide, and other genes are responsible for the alteration of the peptide to its final form. In the case of peptide hormones with subunits, the different subunits may be derived either from a single precursor (insulin) or from separate precursors [luteinizing hormone (LH)]. Furthermore, the same peptide hormone (somatostatin) can be formed from different prohormones encoded by distinct genes, individual prohormones such as proopiomelanocortin can be metabolized to different hormones in different cells, depending on the complement of processing enzymes in the cell in question, and the primary transcripts of genes such as that of the calcitonin gene can be alternatively spliced in different tissues to form messenger RNA for either calcitonin or calcitonin-related peptide. Peptide hormones may also be formed ectopically in malignancies of nonendocrine origin such as carcinoma of the lung and may be formed in small amounts in normal nonendocrine tissues (see Chap. 309).

In the case of steroid hormones the fundamental precursor—cholesterol (for most steroid hormones) or 7-dehydrocholesterol (for vitamin D metabolites)—undergoes a series of enzymatic transformations to form the final products. At least six enzymes and consequently a minimum of six genes are required to transform cholesterol to estradiol. Because of the number of enzymes required, the synthesis of steroids from cholesterol is unusual in malignancies of nonendocrine tissues. However, many tissues—malignant and nonmalignant—that cannot form steroid hormones de novo from cholesterol contain enzymes that convert circulating steroids to other hormones; examples are the conversion of androgens to estrogens by trophoblastic tumors and by normal adipocytes and the conversion of progesterone to deoxycorticosterone by the kidney.

Amine hormones are synthesized by a series of reactions similar to those involved in steroid hormone synthesis except that the precursors are amino acids. For example, tyrosine is the precursor for epinephrine and norepinephrine (see Chap. 67).

STORAGE Most tissues that synthesize hormones have a limited capacity to store the completed product. For example, the normal adult testes contain only about one-sixth of the quantity of testosterone needed for daily production, and consequently the testicular pool turns over several times to provide the normal daily output of hormone. Even when tissues have special storage organelles for hormone, the amount of hormone stored is usually limited: the insulin granules in the pancreatic beta cell ordinarily contain amounts of insulin sufficient only for short-term, reserve needs. (In contrast, nerve endings may contain a several-day supply of norepinephrine.) The limited capacity to store hormones in tissues is a chemical consequence of their unsuitability for incorporation into any of the three main storage compartments of the body (lipids, glycogen, or protein). For example, most steroid hormones are too polar to be stored in large quantities in lipid compartments, and peptide and amine hormones are unsuitable for incorporation into proteins. As a consequence of these factors the body pools of most hormones tend to be small. The major exceptions to this rule are those instances in which the precursor forms of hormone can be stored either as protein or in neutral lipid compartments; the normal thyroid gland contains the equivalent of a 2-week supply of thyroid hormones in the form of the protein thyroglobulin, and the precursor and intermediate forms of vitamin D can be stored in considerable quantity in hepatic lipid.

RELEASE The biochemical mechanisms involved in the release process are incompletely understood. In some instances they involve conversion of insoluble to soluble derivatives (proteolysis of thyroglobulin to thyroid hormones). In others, release is due to exocytosis of storage granules (insulin, glucagon, prolactin, growth hormone). Finally, release may involve passive diffusion of newly synthesized molecules such as steroid hormones down activity gradients into plasma; under this circumstance the rate of hormone release may be determined either by the rate of hormone synthesis or by the rate of blood flow to the tissue.

Because of the limited capacity for storage, most hormones are released into plasma at a pace reflecting the rates of formation. The pituitary trophic hormones [LH, adrenocorticotropin (ACTH), thyrotropin (TSH)] act in their target tissues to influence rates of both hormone synthesis and release. Even when peptide hormones are stored in granules, initial release of the stored material is followed by an enhanced rate of synthesis (as, for instance, the two-phase release of insulin induced by glucose infusion). For some hormones, major diurnal, sleep-related, developmental, and neural factors influence hormone release; again, it is assumed that in most of these instances synthesis and release are tightly linked.

The rate of hormone release in many instances is periodic or rhythmic, the cycle varying in frequency from minutes to hours (ultradian), to daily (circadian), to months or years (infradian). Hormones such as LH and follicle-stimulating hormone (FSH) are released in a pulsatile fashion with bursts of secretion occurring in a repetitive pattern: ACTH (and cortisol) release varies during a 24-h cycle, and thyroid hormone release can vary on longer cycles. Whether this intermittent release is a function of alterations in synthetic rates, changes in blood flow, or other mechanisms is uncertain, but most such cycles are under neurogenic control. In many instances the physiologic significance of pulsatile release is not fully understood, but in other instances changes in frequency or amplitude of the release pattern can have profound effects on hormone function; i.e., the pulsatile administration of luteinizing hormone–releasing hormone (LHRH) stimulates the release of LH by the pituitary, whereas the constant infusion of the same amount of hormone per unit time has the opposite effect. Furthermore, changes in frequency or amplitude of hormone release may characterize specific disease states; loss of the diurnal rhythm of cortisol release is characteristic of the early phase of Cushing's disease, and pulsatile release of LHRH is blunted in anorexia nervosa. Finally, understanding of the rhythms by which hormones are released is essential for interpreting plasma hormone levels.

TRANSPORT Hormones are transported via lymph, blood, and extracellular fluids from sites of synthesis to sites of cellular action and ultimately of metabolic inactivation and degradation. The plasma is probably a passive diluent for most peptide and amine hormones, and this feature explains the short half-lives (3 to 7 min) for most nonglycosylated peptide hormones. [Glycoprotein hormones such as human chorionic gonadotropin (hCG) have longer half-lives.] The more insoluble a hormone in water, the more important the role of transport proteins, and thyroid and steroid hormones are largely transported in protein-bound form. No transport protein yet characterized is exclusive; for example, testosterone can be transported both by a specific binding protein [testosterone-binding globulin (TeBG)]

and by albumin; thyroxine can be transported both by prealbumin and by thyroxine-binding globulin (TBG). Protein-bound hormone (HP) cannot enter most cellular compartments and serves as a reservoir from which free hormone (H) is liberated for diffusion into intracellular compartments:

$$H + P \rightleftharpoons HP$$

Distribution of bound and free hormone in plasma is determined by the amount of hormone, the amount of binding protein, and the binding affinity of hormone for the protein. However, in the intact organism the effective level of free hormone is influenced by additional factors. When the rate of dissociation of a hormone from a binding protein is rapid (more rapid than the capillary transit time for a specific organ), the functional free fraction in vivo is also influenced by capillary transit time and membrane permeability.

Understanding the relation between free and bound hormone is essential for assessment of endocrine function. First, the free (dialyzable) fraction in vitro is generally less than the actual free fraction available in vivo because the portion of hormone bound to weak binding proteins such as albumin (in contrast to that protein bound to specific, high-affinity binding proteins) rapidly dissociates from the albumin as the free fraction diffuses from the capillary; consequently the albumin-bound hormone can function in vivo as a free fraction. Under some conditions, measurement of the dialyzable fraction does provide a useful index of the in vivo apparent free fraction. However, in hypoalbuminemic states, the in vitro free (dialyzable) fraction may increase when the in vivo free hormone level is actually diminished. In addition, in those tissue compartments such as liver in which proteins including hormone-transport protein complexes are cleared (in contrast to peripheral tissues in which only the free hormone enters the cell) free hormone levels have lesser effects on hormone uptake by the tissue.

Second, the distribution of hormones between plasma and tissue is a function of the balance between tissue binding proteins and plasma binding proteins. Therefore, levels of true or apparent free hormone may not reflect the amounts of hormone within cells.

Third, only the free hormone interacts with receptors in target cells and participates in the regulatory feedback mechanisms that control the rates of hormone synthesis. As a consequence, changes in the amount of transport protein alone cannot cause endocrine pathology in the steady state, provided the remainder of the endocrine feedback loop is intact. For example, profound elevations or decreases in TBG (either because of genetic or other factors) are both compatible with a euthyroid state. To illustrate, an increase in TBG would lower the level of free (dialyzable) hormone and lower the amount bound to albumin; as a consequence TSH secretion would increase, and the output of thyroxine by the thyroid would increase *until* TBG is again saturated so that the level of free hormone returns to the normal range, at which time TSH levels and thyroid hormone secretion also return to normal. Likewise, a decrease in TBG would temporarily increase the level of free hormone, and TSH secretion and thyroxine output would fall until the free level returns to normal.

To summarize, a change in the amount of a specific, high-affinity binding protein can cause profound alterations in hormone levels but by itself does not cause either a steady state hormone excess or deficiency, provided the regulatory feedback mechanisms that control hormone synthesis are intact. In contrast, alteration of the amount of a binding protein may cause endocrine pathology when hormone formation is not regulated by ordinary feedback control mechanisms or when feedback control mechanisms are deranged. For example, testosterone production in women is not regulated directly by testosterone levels, and alterations in TeBG levels in women may alter the steady state levels of free testosterone. Likewise, changes in TBG levels in a hypothyroid patient receiving a fixed dose of levothyroxine can cause alterations in free thyroxine levels.

DEGRADATION AND TURNOVER The plasma level (PL) of any hormone is dependent on two factors—the secretion rate (SR) of the hormone and the rates of metabolism and excretion, the so-called metabolic clearance rate (MCR):

$$PL = SR/MCR \quad \text{or} \quad SR = MCR \times PL$$

Metabolic clearance of hormones is accomplished by several mechanisms. Only small fractions of hormones are excreted intact in urine or bile. Degradation and inactivation of the hormone can take place in target tissues, in nontarget tissues such as liver and kidneys, or in both target and nontarget tissues. Peptide hormones are in general inactivated by proteases, largely in target tissues. Hormone metabolism frequently facilitates excretion of steroid and thyroid hormone by rendering them soluble in urine or bile. Thyroid hormones are deiodinated, deaminated, and deconjugated primarily by the liver. Steroid hormones are reduced, hydroxylated, and converted into glucuronide and sulfate conjugates. Biliary conjugates may be hydrolyzed in the gastrointestinal tract and reabsorbed into the circulation. The degradative mechanisms for different hormones have one common feature, namely, that alternative pathways exist for the catabolism of all hormones described to date.

Because of the nature of feedback control of hormone secretion, changes in rates of hormone degradation alone, like changes in plasma protein binding, do not cause endocrine pathology, provided the feedback loops that regulate synthesis are intact. For example, in severe liver disease and in myxedema, the degradation of glucocorticoids by the liver is impaired; as a consequence the turnover of cortisol slows, but the plasma level does not rise because secretion of ACTH is inhibited. Thus, a normal level of free hormone is maintained by decreasing the rate of cortisol secretion. The opposite is the case when glucocorticoid degradation is enhanced (as in thyrotoxicosis); in this situation cortisol secretion rises to keep the level of the hormone normal.

Although changes in rates of hormone degradation alone do not result in hormone deficit or excess, such changes may cause profound alterations in endocrine pharmacology. Thus, ordinary doses of glucocorticoids may cause the Cushing syndrome in patients with myxedema or liver disease, and consequently glucocorticoid dosage must be reduced in both conditions. Likewise, doses of glucocorticoids may have to be increased in the presence of hyperthyroidism. In addition, the development of hyperthyroidism in a patient with inadequate adrenal reserve can precipitate adrenal crisis by accelerating the rate of glucocorticoid catabolism. Thus, in circumstances in which the normal control mechanisms that regulate hormone synthesis are either circumvented or inoperative, changes in rates of hormone degradation may aggravate or cause pathology.

REGULATION OF HORMONE PRODUCTION

As stated above, fluctuations of hormone levels in the normal person are determined primarily by changes in rates of production. A unifying feature of all endocrine systems is the fact that the production of most hormones is regulated directly or indirectly by the metabolic activity of the hormone itself. This regulation is accomplished through a series of negative (and positive) feedback loops (Fig. 311-1). In some cases a fairly constant blood level of hormone is required, and some sensing device must exist to monitor either the hormone level itself or some related function such as plasma osmolality, blood glucose, plasma calcium, or body sodium content. For example, hormones produced in response to pituitary trophic hormones (cortisol, thyroxine, gonadal steroids) feed back on the hypothalamic-pituitary system to regulate their own rates of secretion. Similarly, parathyroid hormone and insulin are secreted in response to feedback signals from serum calcium and glucose levels, respectively. Feedback systems are generally more complex than this description indicates, sometimes operating indirectly by several steps; when the hormone itself acts as the direct regulator of feedback (testosterone on the hypothalamic-pituitary axis), the effect is mediated by the same

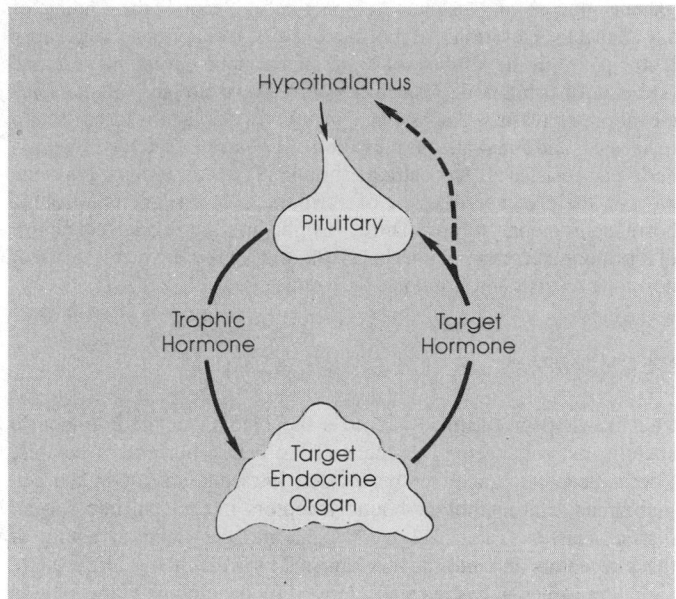

FIGURE 311-1 Feedback control of an endocrine organ such as the adrenal, thyroid, or gonads by the pituitary.

receptor-effector system by which the action of the hormone is accomplished in other target tissues. An example of positive feedback is the stimulation of LH release by estradiol prior to ovulation. Nonhormonal and environmental factors may alter both positive and negative feedback control mechanisms or the response to such control.

A usual feature of the feedback systems is rapidity of action; indeed, most respond within minutes or hours to varying metabolic demands to maintain homeostatic control within a narrow range. The main exceptions relate to gametogenesis in the ovary and testis (see Chaps. 321 and 322). In both instances, a complex differentiative process is involved. The steady state operation of these systems is such that sperm production tends to be relatively constant from day to day whereas ovulation is cyclic. However, spermatogenesis and export require approximately 2 months to complete so that changes in FSH levels may not result in altered levels of sperm in the ejaculate for long periods.

The fact that the secretion of hormones is under regulatory control has several important clinical implications. First, the significance of plasma levels of hormones may be interpretable only if the appropriate regulatory factors are taken into account (Fig. 311-2). The meaning of a borderline low plasma thyroxine may become clear only when thyroid-stimulating hormone (TSH) is measured simultaneously; likewise, plasma insulin and parathyroid hormone levels may be interpretable only in conjunction with simultaneous measurements of

FIGURE 311-2 Relation between target hormone level and trophic hormone level in normal and disease states (e.g., TSH and thyroid hormones, ACTH and cortisol, LH and testosterone).

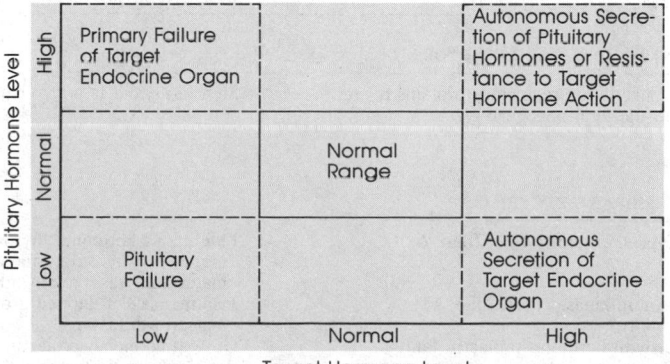

plasma glucose and calcium, respectively. Second, the finding of simultaneous elevations of hormone pairs (or hormone regulatory factor pairs) in the absence of signs of hormone excess suggests the presence of a hormone-resistance state. For example, simultaneous elevation of plasma glucose and insulin is characteristic of insulin resistance, and simultaneous elevation of LH and testosterone suggests androgen resistance. In contrast, simultaneous elevation of hormone pairs in the presence of signs of hormone excess suggests a trophic hormone–secreting tumor. Third, insight into the regulatory control of hormone secretion is the basis for the various dynamic tests of hormone reserve and hormone secretion.

MECHANISMS OF HORMONE ACTION

The first step in hormone action is the binding of the hormone to specific macromolecules in the cell, so-called hormone receptors. These receptors can either be located intracellularly or in the cell membrane, and membrane-bound receptors in turn fall into several distinct classes (Table 311-1). Insight into the chemical nature of these receptors and into the mechanisms by which they participate in signal transduction has been accelerated by the cloning of the cDNAs and the genes that encode these proteins (see Chap. 6).

INTRACELLULAR RECEPTORS   Most steroid and thyroid hormones are transported in plasma bound to carrier proteins (Fig. 311-3). The protein-bound hormones (HP) are in dynamic equilibrium with small amounts of free hormones (H) that diffuse by a passive mechanism into cells. In most instances the principal form of the hormone secreted into plasma (cortisol, progesterone, aldosterone, estradiol) undergoes no further metabolism within the cell and is responsible for hormone action within the target cell. Other hormones (thyroxine, testosterone) undergo chemical conversion to more active forms (triiodothyronine and dihydrotestosterone).

H binds to specific receptor proteins (R) in the cytoplasm or nucleus to form a hormone-receptor complex (HR). The hormone-receptor complex has the capacity to bind to specific regulatory sequences in DNA (so-called hormone regulatory elements) and thus acts as a regulator of transcription. As the result of this interaction with DNA new messenger RNAs (mRNAs) are formed, and the synthesis of cytoplasmic proteins is enhanced. The cytoplasmic proteins, in turn, mediate the effects of the hormone.

The cloning of the cDNAs for the various receptors revealed that receptors of this class bear a striking homology to the viral oncogene *erb*A and to each other. The fact that members of this family of hormone-dependent transcription factors are similar in structure suggests that these receptors have evolved from a common ancestral transcription factor. Each contains a hormone-binding domain, a DNA-binding domain, and an *N*-terminal variable or immunodominant domain (Fig. 311-4). An interesting feature of this class of receptors

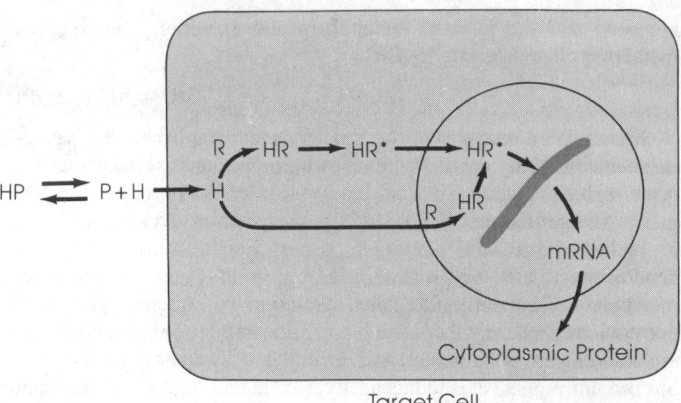

FIGURE 311-3   Mechanism of action of hormones with intracellular receptors. H = hormone; P = plasma transport protein; R = receptor; R* = activated receptor; mRNA = messenger RNA.

is that more than one receptor exists for certain hormones (thyroid hormones) and that candidate receptors have been identified for which no ligand is known. Elucidation of the structures of these receptors made it possible to analyze the mutations that impair hormone action and cause several hormone-resistance syndromes (see below).

MEMBRANE-BOUND RECEPTORS   G protein family   Receptors that bind GTP (G proteins) all work by similar mechanisms but are capable of mediating a complex range of actions. In every case, binding of ligand to the receptor produces a conformational change that causes GTP to bind to the protein at a special site. The active G protein then binds to a target protein and initiates a regulatory cascade involving one (or more) intracellular mediators including adenylate cyclase, phospholipase C, and arachidonic acid. The receptors of this class are monomeric proteins with an extracellular domain that binds ligand, an intracellular G protein–binding domain, and seven transmembrane-spanning regions. Elucidation of the molecular biology of the G protein has provided insight into the actions of drugs and signaling mechanisms in addition to hormones and into the pathophysiology of pseudohypoparathyroidism (see Chaps. 68 and 340 and below).

Protein kinases   Receptors of this class are glycoproteins typically composed of two alpha subunits and two beta subunits which are linked by sulfhydryl bonds (Fig. 311-5). The alpha subunits are extracellular and contain the hormone binding site, and the beta subunits are transmembrane proteins. The beta subunit of the receptor is a hormone-regulated protein kinase capable of phosphorylating itself and other substrates on tyrosine residues using ATP as the phosphate source. In the case of insulin the tyrosine activity of the receptor is essential for hormone action. Point mutations in the coding sequence of receptor genes that prevent the protein kinase activity

TABLE 311-1   Classification of hormone receptors

Type	Characteristic hormones	Disease states due to mutant receptor components
INTRACELLULAR RECEPTORS		
Transcription regulatory proteins related to the viral oncogene *erb*A	Steroid-thyroid family, vitamin A	Testicular feminization and related syndromes; cortisol resistance; vitamin D–dependent rickets, type II; thyroid hormone resistance; pseudohypoaldosteronism
MEMBRANE RECEPTORS		
G-protein family (see Chap. 68)	Luteinizing hormone, thyroid-stimulating hormone, parathyroid hormone, epinephrine, somatostatin, vasopressin, glucagon	Pseudohypoparathyroidism, nephrogenic diabetes insipidus
Protein kinases (see Chap. 11)	Insulin, platelet-derived growth factor, epidermal growth factor	Diabetes mellitus with profound insulin resistance
Growth hormone–prolactin family	Growth hormone, prolactin	Laron dwarfism
Guanylate cyclase	Atrial natriuretic factor	
Ion channels (see Chap. 11)	Acetylcholine (nicotinic)	Myasthenia gravis

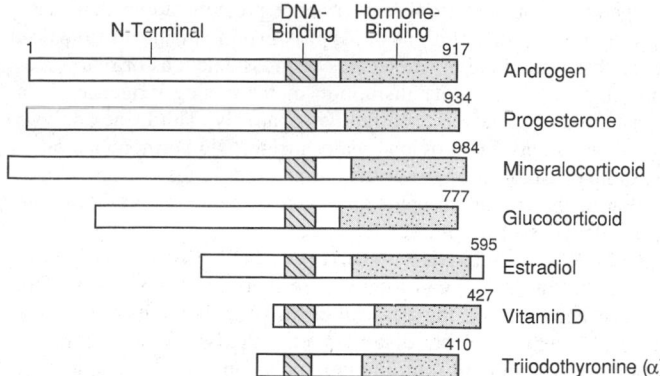

FIGURE 311-4 Intracellular receptors of the thyroid-steroid class. The areas of greatest homology (DNA-binding domain) are shown by the slanted bars, the areas of intermediate homology (hormone-binding domain) are shown by the stippled areas, and the areas with the least homology are shown by the open regions.

can cause profound resistance to insulin action (see below). Exactly how receptor kinase activity is transmitted into hormone action is not entirely clear. Several endogenous substrates of the enzyme have been identified, and physiologic effects of the hormone may either be indirect or direct consequences of the phosphorylation of the substrates or of the receptor itself.

Receptors of the growth hormone/prolactin class The growth hormone receptor is a protein of approximately 600 amino acids that contains a single, centrally located transmembrane domain. Interestingly, a high-affinity growth hormone–binding protein is present in the plasma; this protein corresponds to the extracellular hormone-binding domain of the growth hormone receptor and is believed to be cleaved from the receptor, but the role of the plasma protein in the regulation of growth is undefined. The growth hormone receptor shares approximately a 25 percent homology with the prolactin receptor (which may exist in more than one size) suggesting that the two receptors have evolved from a common ancestral gene. The mechanism(s) by which these receptors mediate hormone action is

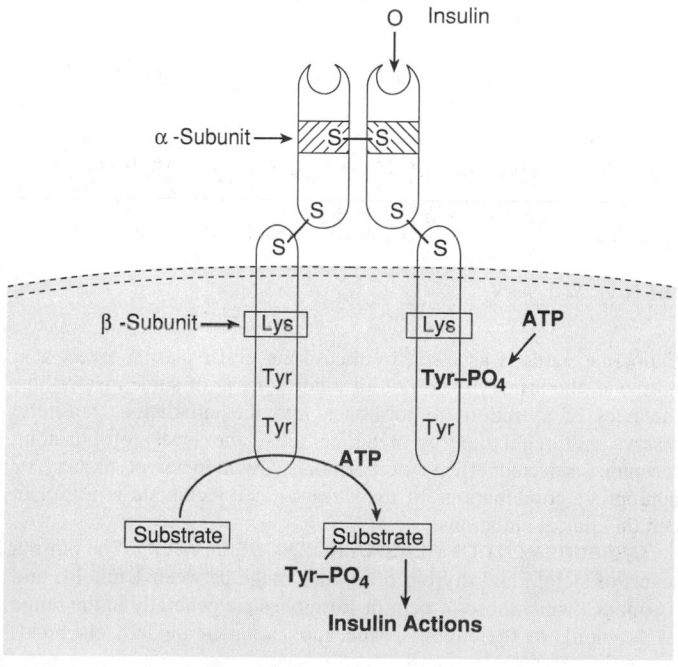

FIGURE 311-5 Schematic representation of the insulin receptor. As the result of the binding of insulin to the alpha subunit the protein kinase function of the beta receptor is activated, and both exogenous protein substrates and the beta subunit itself are phosphorylated.

unclear. Mutations that impair the function of the growth hormone receptor are responsible for Laron dwarfism (see below).

Other membrane-bound receptors The receptor for atrial natriuretic factor is a guanylate cyclase that spans the plasma membrane; the extracellular portion of the receptor binds the hormone, and the intracellular portion of the protein synthesizes guanosine-3′,5′-monophosphate (cyclic GMP) which serves as the second messenger for the hormone (see Chap. 68). The nicotinic acetylcholine receptor channel is a membrane-spanning complex of proteins that forms a true ion channel containing a central pore that can be opened and closed by ligand-binding-induced conformational change to allow sodium and potassium ions to cross the membrane and hence cause depolarization of cells that contain the receptors (see Chap. 11). Autoantibodies that block the function of this receptor cause myasthenia gravis (see Chap. 366).

ENDOCRINE DISORDERS

Endocrinopathy can result from hormone deficiency, hormone excess, or resistance to hormone action, and abnormalities in more than one endocrine system may coexist in the same individual.

DEFICIENCY STATES With few exceptions (calcitonin) hormone deficiency results in pathologic manifestations. The study of clinical disorders that result from hormone deficiency or absence played an important role in the evolution of endocrinology as a discipline. Such studies were followed by attempts to extract the responsible hormone from normal endocrine tissues, characterize the chemical nature (and ultimately synthesize the molecule), and administer the hormone to replace the deficit. The treatment of hypothyroidism by the administration of thyroid hormone is probably as successful as any therapeutic measure in medicine. Because clinical deficiency states can be induced in experimental animals by destruction or removal of the endocrine organ, an enormous amount is known about the pathophysiology of the deficiency states (diabetes mellitus, pituitary and adrenal insufficiency, hypothyroidism, and hypogonadism).

The nature of the destructive processes that cause failure of the endocrine organs is also understood in many instances; these include infections (adrenal insufficiency due to tuberculosis), infarction (postpartum pituitary failure) and tissue death of other causes (diabetes mellitus secondary to pancreatitis), tumors (chromophobe adenomas of the pituitary), autoimmune processes (Hashimoto's thyroiditis), dietary inadequacy (hypothyroidism due to iodine deficiency), and hereditary defects in hormone synthesis (pituitary dwarfism). In certain forms of diabetes mellitus, the cause may be a hereditary predisposition that renders the pancreas subject to destruction by several mechanisms (see Chap. 319). In other endocrine-deficiency diseases the etiology of the defect is unidentified (congenital anorchism).

HORMONE EXCESS With few exceptions (testosterone in men, progesterone in men and women) hormone excess causes pathologic effects. Four general types of hormone excess are recognized. In one, the hormone is overproduced by the gland that is the usual site of its production (hyperthyroidism, acromegaly, Cushing's disease); such excess production results from failure of circumvention of the feedback control mechanisms that regulate production of the hormone in the normal state, but the underlying mechanism is often obscure because animal models for the diseases are rare. The second type of hormone excess results when a hormone is produced by a tissue (usually malignant) that ordinarily is not a major endocrine organ (for example, ACTH production in oat cell carcinoma of the lung, thyroid hormone secretion by struma ovarii). Such hormone-excess states have been described for many hormones (see Chap. 309). A third type of hormone-excess state involves the overproduction of hormones in peripheral tissues from circulating precursors; for example, overproduction of estrogen in liver disease because of diversion of the precursor androstenedione from its usual sites of catabolism in the liver to sites of extraglandular estrogen formation. Finally, hormone excess all too commonly results from iatrogenic causes; for example, the complications resulting from glucocorticoid therapy (see Chap. 317).

Excess of a given hormone may result from more than one cause. Thyrotoxicosis can result from overproduction of hormone by the thyroid as a result of overproduction of TSH (rare); from stimulation by extrapituitary thyroid-stimulating factors; from autonomous thyroid hyperfunction; from leakage of preformed hormone from the thyroid due to an inflammatory injury; or from excess hormone from sources other than the thyroid itself, as in thyroid hormone overdosage, accidental ingestion of meats contaminated with thyroid tissue, or secretion by struma ovarii (see Chap. 316). The unraveling of the cause of specific hormone-excess states can be one of the most challenging problems of clinical endocrinology.

PRODUCTION OF ABNORMAL HORMONES In some instances abnormal hormones can cause endocrine disease. One form of diabetes mellitus is the result of a single-gene mutation that results in the production of an abnormal insulin molecule that is ineffective because of defective binding to the insulin receptor. In other cases, hormone precursors, hormone subunits, or incompletely processed peptide hormones may be released into the circulation, as is common in so-called ectopic hormone production of neoplasia (see Chap. 309). Alternatively, immunoglobulins may bind to hormone receptors and thus exert hormonal actions, for example, the thyroid-stimulating immunoglobulins that exert TSH-like actions in hyperthyroidism (see Chap. 316) or the antibodies to the insulin receptor that have insulin-like actions (see Chap. 319).

HORMONE RESISTANCE The concept that an endocrinopathy can result because the tissues cannot respond to normal (or increased) levels of a hormone evolved from the deduction that pseudohermaphroditism is due to peripheral resistance to the action of parathyroid hormone (see Chaps. 68 and 340). This concept has had far-reaching implications. First, the concept of hormone resistance served as a major stimulus for the study of how hormones act within cells. Second, more and more forms of hormone resistance have been identified, so that diseases are now recognized to result from resistance to most hormones. Such hormone resistance is frequently due to hereditary causes. Third, hormone resistance can be due to a variety of molecular abnormalities, including defects in receptors and in postreceptor effector mechanisms for hormones, development of antibodies to hormones or hormone receptors, and the absence of target cells. Fourth, abnormalities of receptors are now implicated in the pathogenesis of diseases outside the endocrine domain, such as familial hypercholesterolemia. Hormone resistance does not necessarily involve equally all target tissues for the hormone. For example, selective resistance to thyroid hormone can be restricted to the pituitary itself, and in one form of androgen resistance androgen action is more severely impaired in the testis than in other target tissues.

A common feature of hormone-resistance states is the coexistence of a normal or *elevated* level of the hormone in the circulation despite deficient hormone action. This feature is a consequence of the fact that most hormones are under regulatory feedback control and failure of hormone action usually leads to increased hormone production.

The elucidation of the structures of the various receptors and the cloning of the cDNAs for these proteins has made it possible to define the molecular defects in a number of hormone-resistance states (Table 311-1). Mutations of almost every class of receptor have now been identified, and several clinical implications are now apparent. First, in the past it was only possible to identify receptor defects that caused profound hormone resistance. Now that subtle defects in receptor function can be identified, hormone resistance may prove to be a common cause of human endocrinopathy. Second, when individual disorders are analyzed at the molecular level, it is apparent that the disorders are genetically heterogeneous. No two unrelated families with mutations of the insulin receptor, the growth hormone receptor, or the androgen receptor have proved to have identical disorders. Furthermore, in regard to individual receptors such as the

androgen receptor, mutations may either be point mutations that cause single amino acid substitutions in the protein or premature termination codons that result in short molecules or gross deletions or rearrangements that cause complete disruption of the coding sequence. It is thus necessary to analyze each family separately. Third, the analysis of these mutations has provided major insight into hormone action—for example, establishing the critical importance of the tyrosine kinase function of the insulin receptor and making it possible to define the various domains of the intracellular receptors.

DISEASES AFFECTING MULTIPLE ENDOCRINE SYSTEMS The fact that disorders can affect more than one endocrine system has been known since the description of panhypopituitarism in the nineteenth century. Such disorders encompass diverse etiologies including autoimmunity (autoimmune polyglandular dysfunction, or Schmidt's syndrome), receptor abnormalities (gonadotropin and thyrotropin resistance in pseudohypoparathyroidism), tumors (multiple endocrine neoplasia, or MEN) and hereditary disorders of unknown etiology (lipodystrophies) (see Chap. 325). They may include both hypo- and hyperfunctioning states, and some clinical syndromes may occur in the context of more than one polyendocrine state (pheochromocytoma in MEN II, MEN III, and von Hippel–Lindau disease; diabetes mellitus in Schmidt's syndrome and lipodystrophy).

Because each endocrinopathy in such a constellation can also occur alone, all endocrine patients must be approached with a high index of suspicion for abnormalities of multiple systems. This is of particular importance because treatment of one condition may cause worsening of another (surgical procedures such as thyroidectomy can cause worsening of unrecognized pheochromocytoma) and because in certain of the familial syndromes it is mandatory to make systematic searches for the disease in potentially affected family members.

REFERENCES

Evans RM: The steroid and thyroid hormone receptor superfamily. Science 240:889, 1988

Godowski PG et al: Characterization of the human growth hormone receptor gene and demonstration of a partial gene deletion in two patients with Laron-type dwarfism. Proc Natl Acad Sci USA 86:8083, 1989

Habener JF: Genetic control of hormone formation, in *Williams' Textbook of Endocrinology*, 7th ed, JD Wilson, DW Foster (eds). Philadelphia, Saunders, 1985, pp 9–32

Kahn CR, Goldstein BJ: Molecular defects in insulin action. Science 245:13, 1989

——, White MF: The insulin receptor and the molecular mechanism of insulin action. J Clin Invest 82:1151, 1988

Marcelli M et al: A single nucleotide substitution introduces a premature termination codon into the androgen receptor gene of a patient with receptor-negative androgen resistance. J Clin Invest Vol 85, 1990 In Press.

Pardridge WM: Serum bioavailability of sex steroid hormones. Clin Endocrinol Metab 15:259, 1986

312 ASSESSMENT OF ENDOCRINE FUNCTION

JEAN D. WILSON

Endocrine status is assessed by measuring either plasma levels of a hormone, the urinary excretion of a hormone or of some metabolite, the rates of secretion of hormones into the circulation, hormone reserve and regulation by dynamic tests, the levels of hormone receptors, selected effects of hormone action in target tissues, or appropriate combinations of these tests. Each technique is useful in certain clinical situations.

MEASUREMENT OF PLASMA HORMONE LEVELS The plasma levels of steroid and thyroid hormones range between 1 nmol/L and 1 μmol/L, while those of peptide hormones are generally in the range of 1 pmol/L to 0.1 nmol/L. The application of modern chemical, chromatographic, radioreceptor, and radioimmunoassay techniques for the assessment of plasma constituents in low concentrations constitutes one of the significant advances of modern medicine and has made clinical endocrinology a more quantitative discipline. In the case of hormones whose plasma levels are relatively constant from moment to moment and day to day (thyroxine and triiodothyronine), the measurement of isolated plasma levels alone provides a reliable assessment of the hormone status in most clinical situations.

For several reasons, however, care must be exercised in assessing isolated plasma levels. First, for hormones with relatively simple structures (steroid and thyroid hormones) chemical and radioimmunoassay techniques are reliable so that measured values usually reflect the plasma levels as of a given moment. In the case of the more complex peptide hormones, however, considerable variability may exist in the structure of physiologically active hormone molecules in the circulation, some of which may be measured poorly in specific radioimmunoassay procedures; for example, standard radioimmunoassays for luteinizing hormone (LH) and for parathyroid hormone may on occasion either underestimate or overestimate the amount of biologically active hormone in plasma. In such situations, radioreceptor assays or in vitro bioassays may provide a better assessment of endocrine status.

Second, in the case of hormones that undergo pulsatile secretion (LH, testosterone) a single value is usually not representative of mean plasma levels. In these instances it is necessary either to measure levels in several samples drawn at random or to pool aliquots of three or more samples of plasma drawn at 20- to 30-min intervals for a single determination.

Third, when plasma levels exhibit a characteristic, predictable fluctuation such as the diurnal variation of plasma cortisol, the timing of plasma sampling can be designed to provide a useful index of the hormone status. Even here, however, it is important to recognize that plasma levels may exhibit diurnal variation only during certain phases of life (plasma LH levels in early puberty). In women appropriate interpretation of plasma gonadotropins, progesterone, and estradiol during the reproductive years requires reference to the corresponding phase of the ovulatory and menstrual cycles, and it may be necessary to obtain sequential studies over many days to provide interpretable data. Seasonal variations also occur in the levels of certain hormones (such as thyroxine and testosterone), but these changes are generally so small that they do not affect the interpretation of individual values. In some situations variation in hormone levels is not the result of any obvious rhythmicity but rather the consequence of waxing and waning of disease processes; repeated measurements of cortisol or of calcium and parathyroid hormone levels over many months may be necessary to establish a diagnosis of Cushing's syndrome or of hyperparathyroidism.

Fourth, in the case of steroids, thyroid hormones, and some peptide hormones such as growth hormone that are transported in plasma largely bound to proteins, measurement of total hormone concentration provides an index of endocrine status *only* to the extent that it allows a deduction of the level of the free or unbound hormone. Indeed, direct measurements of the free levels of these hormones (usually 1 percent or less of the total) can be done only in a few laboratories. Since the amount of free hormone is a function of the amount and the affinity of binding of transport proteins and the amount of hormone, the total hormone level reflects the amount of free hormone only as long as the amount of binding protein(s) remains constant or fluctuates only within narrow limits. In those instances in which the level of binding protein is increased [e.g., thyroid-binding globulin (TBG) and testosterone-binding globulin (TeBG, or sex steroid–binding globulin, SHBG) in pregnancy] or decreased [hereditary decreases in TBG and cortisol-binding globulin (CBG)] it is essential to utilize some other assessment of the amount of binding protein to allow estimation of the free hormone level (T_3 resin uptake for TBG or direct measurement of TBG, TeBG, or CBG).

Fifth, the range of plasma levels of most hormones within the normal population is broad. As a consequence, the level of a hormone in an individual may be halved or doubled (and thus be grossly abnormal for that person) but still be within the so-called normal range. For this reason it is frequently useful to assess appropriate hormone pairs simultaneously (LH and testosterone, thyroxine and thyroid-stimulating hormone); a borderline low testosterone level in the presence of elevated plasma LH is indicative of testicular failure, whereas the same level of testosterone in the presence of a normal LH implies that the endocrine status is normal (Fig. 311-2). Likewise, in women with increased testosterone production and secondary decrease in TeBG, plasma testosterone concentration may be normal despite increased production of the hormone.

URINARY EXCRETION The measurement of urinary excretion of a hormone or a hormone metabolite that reflects plasma levels or secretory rates offers certain advantages over the measurement of isolated plasma levels, e.g., the urinary excretion reflects average plasma levels over the time of collection. Thus, a 24-h urine free cortisol value may provide a better estimate of the function of the adrenal cortex than isolated measurements of plasma cortisol. Again, however, certain limitations of the use of urinary measurements must be kept in mind. (1) Urinary creatinine should be measured routinely to document the adequacy of the urine collection. Women excrete on average about 1 g, and men excrete about 1.8 g/d. Day-to-day variation should not exceed 20 percent. (2) The excretion of individual metabolites may not reflect changes in hormone secretion under all conditions. For example, the formation of the 18-oxo derivative of aldosterone may be influenced by drugs that do not alter secretion or plasma levels of the hormone. (3) Urine values are obviously meaningless for those hormones (thyroxine, triiodothyronine) excreted into bile. Of more importance is the fact that peptide hormones such as gonadotropins may be metabolized differently in different individuals prior to excretion into the urine so that establishment of the range of normal is difficult. (4) Hormones from more than one source may be excreted as common metabolites; urinary 17-ketosteroids are derived from both adrenal and gonadal androgens, and consequently the measurement is of little value in assessing testicular androgen production in men. (5) Changes in renal function may influence rates of hormone excretion into urine. Such changes can in part be corrected by measurement of urine creatinine, but in the case of metabolites or conjugates formed in the kidney itself excretion patterns may be distorted out of proportion to the decrease in creatinine clearance.

SECRETION AND PRODUCTION RATES The measurement of the actual secretion rate of a hormone circumvents most problems inherent in measurement of plasma levels and urinary excretion. Such measurements involve the administration of radioactive hormone and measuring the dilution that such a hormone undergoes as a consequence of mixture with endogenously secreted, nonradioactive hormone over a given period of time. In practice the plasma hormone itself or a unique metabolite of the hormone from urine is isolated, purified to radiochemical homogeneity, and used to calculate the amount of the hormone secreted during the time of study. In the case of hormones formed principally in peripheral tissues (estradiol and dihydrotestosterone in men, triiodothyronine in both sexes) radioactive precursors can be administered, and the rates of conversion to the metabolites in question can be measured for assessment of overall production rates. Alternatively, as described above, clearance rates of hormones can be measured and, together with mean plasma levels, used to estimate secretion rates. Unfortunately, these various techniques are complex and expensive to perform, require use of radioactive isotopes, and can be done in only a few centers.

DYNAMIC TESTS OF HORMONE RESERVE AND REGULATION When hypo- or hyperfunction is severe, measurement of the level of hormone in blood or urine may be satisfactory for making a diagnosis, particularly when the tests demonstrate appropriate feedback relationships; e.g., low plasma testosterone coupled with high plasma LH indicates primary testicular failure. In less clear-cut instances, however, stimulation tests are useful in establishing the significance of borderline low values. Likewise, suppression tests are used to document the presence of hyperfunction of endocrine systems. All such dynamic tests are designed to take advantage of the known feedback control mechanisms for various hormones (Fig. 311-1).

Two types of stimulation tests are in common use. In one, endogenous hormone production or action is blocked (cortisol production by metyrapone, estradiol action by clomiphene), and the capacity of the pituitary to respond by increasing endogenous production of the trophic hormone and/or the capacity of the target tissue to respond are then assessed; ideally such tests measure the integrity of an entire hypothalamic–pituitary–target tissue loop. In the other type of stimulation test, the trophic hormone itself is administered under some standardized regimen, and the capacity of the target tissue to respond is determined (cortisol levels before and after ACTH administration). Stimulation tests are particularly useful in four situations: (1) assessing hormone status when precise quantification of plasma levels is difficult or imperfect (ACTH), (2) assessing endocrine status when static tests are borderline low, (3) distinguishing primary from secondary (pituitary) causes of endocrine failure, and (4) assessing gonadal reserve in prepubertal patients in whom plasma gonadotropins and gonadal steroids are difficult to interpret.

Suppression tests are useful for the diagnosis of hyperfunction because the hyperfunctioning gland by definition does not operate under normal control mechanisms. Suppression can either be quantitatively or qualitatively abnormal. For example, the feedback control of the pituitary may be reset to respond to high levels of the suppressing hormone (pituitary ACTH secretion in Cushing's disease), or secretion can be autonomous (ACTH secretion by carcinoma of the lung). In principle, the feedback regulator is administered, and the degree of inhibition of hormone secretion is assessed for the endocrine system in question (change in ^{131}I uptake after administration of thyroid hormones, change in cortisol secretion after the administration of potent exogenous glucocorticoids, suppressibility of plasma growth hormone by glucose).

The clinical usefulness of dynamic tests of endocrine function is limited by the fact that they are altered by a multitude of secondary factors. Age, coexisting disease states, and concurrent drug regimens all interact to influence responsiveness and hence to limit the specificity of such tests. In particular, psychiatric disorders such as endogenous depression may impair endocrine dynamic tests in the absence of specific endocrine pathology.

HORMONE RECEPTORS AND ANTIBODIES   The measurement of hormone receptors in biopsy material from target tissues or in fibroblasts propagated from biopsy material is useful—for example, in the diagnosis of partial hormone-resistance states such as rickets due to vitamin D resistance, hyperglycemia and hyperinsulinemia associated with insulin resistance, and male pseudohermaphroditism due to androgen resistance (see Chap. 311). In selected laboratories the cDNAs for some receptors can be sequenced to provide specific information about the structure of mutant proteins. Likewise, under selected conditions measurement of antibodies to hormones (such as antibodies to thyroid hormones that can cause hypothyroidism) or antibodies to target tissues (adrenal gland, gonads, thyroid) may be essential for the assessment of endocrine status. With certain exceptions (antibodies to thyroid tissue) these tests are not widely available.

TISSUE EFFECTS   Perhaps the ideal hormone test is the measurement of the peripheral end result of hormone action in the target tissues for the hormone. For example, demonstration of the capacity to concentrate urine maximally following water restriction indicates that the hypothalamic control mechanisms are intact, that the posterior pituitary has a normal capacity to secrete vasopressin, that the vasopressin receptor is intact, and that the postreceptor effector mechanisms for the hormone are operative. Optimally such a test assesses the function of the entire pathway of hormone secretion and action. In practice, many such tests are imperfect. For example, even though vasopressin secretion is normal, intrinsic renal disease can result in a fixed low urine osmolality and thus distort the interpretation of the functional test of vasopressin action. In other instances the tests are difficult to perform and subject both to artifact and to

influences from diverse parameters (for example, the metabolic rate is increased by fever even when thyroid function is normal). For these reasons, the identification of additional specific tissue markers for hormone action would be very useful.

IMAGING PROCEDURES   Developments in imaging have had a profound impact in endocrinology and provide better means of identifying abnormalities in almost every endocrine system, from delineating small lesions of the pituitary and hypothalamus, to using bone densitometry for assessing metabolic bone disease, to the noninvasive localization of functioning parathyroid tissue in patients with persistent or recurrent hyperparathyroidism. Because the rate of technologic advance in the field is so rapid, the literature evaluating the effectiveness (and limitations) of up-to-date processes inevitably lags.

A major problem in the interpretation of imaging procedures stems from the fact that small nodules of no functional significance are known from autopsy studies to occur in the pituitary, the adrenal, and, less commonly, the testes. The natural history of these nonfunctioning adenomas is not well understood; the vast majority appear to remain limited in size and nonfunctional for life, but in rare instances they may evolve into autonomous and/or hyperfunctioning tumors. In addition, malignancies—both metastatic and primary—can occur in these tissues. Now such lesions can be recognized in life, and the incidental discovery of adrenal and pituitary masses is a common result of CT scans performed for other reasons. Several types of criteria have been proposed for deciding which of these masses are likely to be benign and which should be removed. For example, by one guideline solid, endocrinologically silent lesions of the adrenal smaller than 3.5 cm may be followed safely with serial CT scans whereas larger lesions deserve further workup such as sonographically guided percutaneous needle biopsy or exploratory surgery. Additional experience will be required to establish the validity of these and other criteria for the assessment of such masses.

Another unresolved issue stems from the fact that it is not always clear which imaging procedure is best in a given clinical situation. In some instances evidence will be accrued that will make clear the indications for one or another procedure. In other instances definite guidelines may be harder to develop, as in the choice of MRI versus CT scans for delineation of the anatomy of the hypothalamic-pituitary system. In some patients small lesions are best seen with MRI whereas in others lesions in the same areas—equally small and with similar histologic features—are better delineated with CT scans. As a consequence, there is a tendency in the workup of complicated cases to order both procedures routinely. Although this practice is justified in some cases, the costs of diagnostic workups are thereby inflated.

An unexpected dividend of the developments in imaging is that it is now possible to chart the natural history of endocrine disease in a different way, as in the occasional documentation of hemorrhage into a pituitary tumor that eventuates in development of the empty sella syndrome or the uncovering of a functioning adrenal adenoma in the absence of biochemical or clinical evidence of Cushing's disease.

REFERENCES

BELLDEGRUN A et al: Incidentally discovered mass of the adrenal gland. Surg Gynecol Obstet 163:203, 1986

GORDEN P, WEINTRAUB BD: Radioreceptor and other functional hormone assays, in *Williams Textbook of Endocrinology*, 7th ed, JD Wilson, DW Foster (eds). Philadelphia, Saunders, 1985, pp 133–146

GRIFFIN JE: Assessment of endocrine function, in *Textbook of Endocrine Physiology*, JE Griffin, SR Ojeda (eds). New York, Oxford University Press, 1988, p 56

HAMPER UM et al: Primary adrenocortical carcinoma: Sonographic evaluation with clinical and pathologic correlation in 26 patients. Am J Roentgenog 148:915, 1987

VAITUKAITIS JL: Hormone assays, in *Endocrinology and Metabolism*, P Felig et al (eds). New York, McGraw-Hill, 1987, p 165

YALOW RS: Radioimmunoassay of hormones, in *Williams Textbook of Endocrinology*, 7th ed, JD Wilson, DW Foster (eds). Philadelphia, Saunders, 1985, pp 123–132

313 NEUROENDOCRINE REGULATION AND DISEASES OF THE ANTERIOR PITUITARY AND HYPOTHALAMUS

GILBERT H. DANIELS / JOSEPH B. MARTIN

The pituitary, appropriately titled the master gland, produces six major hormones and stores an additional two hormones (Fig. 313-1). Growth hormone (GH) regulates growth and has important influences on intermediary metabolism (see Chap. 314). Prolactin (PRL) is necessary for lactation. Luteinizing hormone (LH) and follicle-stimulating hormone (FSH) control the gonads in men and women. Thyroid-stimulating hormone (TSH, thyrotropin) regulates thyroid function. Adrenocorticotropin (ACTH) controls glucocorticoid function of the adrenal cortex. These hormones are all synthesized in the anterior pituitary. Vasopressin (AVP; antidiuretic hormone, ADH) and oxytocin are produced in neurons of the hypothalamus and stored in the posterior lobe of the pituitary (see Chap. 315). Vasopressin (AVP) controls water conservation by the kidneys; oxytocin is necessary for milk let-down during lactation.

A feedback relationship exists between the anterior pituitary and its three target endocrine glands—the gonads, the adrenal cortex, and the thyroid. When the gonads fail or are removed, the concentrations of LH and FSH rise, a condition known as primary hypogonadism. When the adrenal cortex is removed or destroyed, primary adrenal insufficiency (or Addison's disease) results, and the serum ACTH concentration increases. Thyroid failure results in the characteristic rise in TSH of primary hypothyroidism.

When the pituitary gland is removed or destroyed, loss of the trophic hormones results in secondary hypogonadism, adrenal insufficiency, or hypothyroidism. Growth hormone and prolactin function are also lost. AVP and oxytocin function are not affected by destruction of the pituitary provided their site of origin in the hypothalamus is intact.

FIGURE 313-1 The relationship between the hypothalamus and pituitary. See text for details.

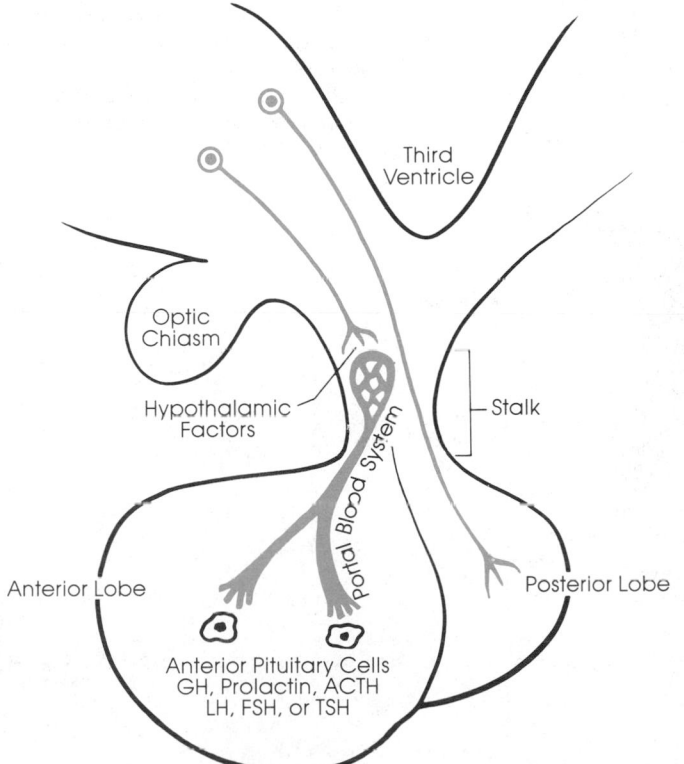

Third Ventricle

Optic Chiasm

Hypothalamic Factors

Stalk

Portal Blood System

Anterior Lobe

Posterior Lobe

Anterior Pituitary Cells
GH, Prolactin, ACTH
LH, FSH, or TSH

The pituitary is in turn under the control of the hypothalamus, which produces a number of chemical mediators. These hormones are synthesized in the hypothalamus and enter the portal vascular system which carries them through the pituitary stalk to the anterior lobe (Fig. 313-1). Interruption of the pituitary stalk is followed by reduction in the release of GH, LH, FSH, TSH, and ACTH from the anterior pituitary. This implies that stimulatory influences from the hypothalamus are necessary for release of these hormones. In contrast, the level of prolactin rises after interruption of the stalk, implying a normal tonic inhibitory hypothalamic influence on prolactin secretion. The rise in prolactin secretion indicates that stalk section does not lead to pituitary destruction. If the stalk section is not at too high a level, AVP and oxytocin release continue principally from axons that terminate in the median eminence of the hypothalamus. With hypothalamic ablation, the levels of GH, LH, FSH, TSH, ACTH, AVP, and oxytocin fall, whereas prolactin levels increase (Fig. 313-1).

Most hypothalamic factors that control secretion of the pituitary hormones are peptides (Table 313-1). Growth hormone–releasing hormone (GRH) is the dominant influence on GH release, and somatostatin acts as an inhibitory hormone for GH release. Although LH and FSH levels vary independently in physiologic states, one releasing hormone [luteinizing hormone–releasing hormone, LHRH, also called gonadotropin-releasing hormone (GnRH)] plays a major role in controlling their release. Thyrotropin-releasing hormone (TRH) controls TSH release and may also influence prolactin release. Corticotropin-releasing hormone (CRH) and other factors control ACTH release. In addition, dopamine acts as a prolactin inhibitory factor (PIF).

Pituitary tumors may lead to hormonal over- or underproduction or may cause mechanical problems by impinging on neighboring structures. The most common hormones produced by pituitary tumors are prolactin and GH. Prolactin excess leads to galactorrhea and/or hypogonadism; GH excess leads to gigantism and acromegaly. ACTH-secreting tumors produce Cushing's disease or Nelson's syndrome. TSH-secreting tumors are rare causes of hyperthyroidism. Gonadotropin-secreting tumors are paradoxically most often associated with hypogonadism. Large pituitary tumors may cause partial or complete hypopituitarism by compression of the adjacent normal gland or pituitary stalk and are associated with visual field disturbances due to compression of the optic chiasm with other neurologic disturbances caused by invasion of cavernous sinuses or cranial fossae.

TABLE 313-1   Anterior pituitary and hypophysiotropic hormones

Pituitary hormone	Hypophysiotropic hormones	
	Name	Structure
Thyrotropin (TSH)	Thyrotropin-releasing hormone (TRH)	Tripeptide
Adrenocorticotropin (ACTH)	Corticotropin-releasing hormone (CRH)	41 Amino acids
Luteinizing hormone (LH)	Luteinizing hormone releasing hormone (LHRH)	Decapeptide
Follicle-stimulating hormone (FSH)	LHRH	Decapeptide
Growth hormone (GH)	Growth hormone–releasing hormone (GRH)	44 Amino acids
	Growth hormone release–inhibiting hormone* (somatostatin, GIH)	14 Amino acids
Prolactin	Prolactin release–inhibiting factor (PIF)	Dopamine
	Prolactin-releasing factor (PRF)†	Peptide ? Vasoactive intestinal polypeptide (VIP)

* Somatostatin also inhibits TRH-stimulated TSH release.
† TRH stimulates prolactin release.

Hypothalamic disease may cause hypopituitarism with the exception that secretion of prolactin may be increased. Diabetes insipidus due to AVP deficiency is virtually diagnostic of hypothalamic disease or of high interruption of the pituitary stalk. Disturbances of thirst, temperature regulation, appetite, and blood pressure may occur with hypothalamic disorders as well. Large hypothalamic masses may lead to visual field disturbances, obstruction of the third ventricle, and invasion of surrounding brain tissue.

ANATOMY AND EMBRYOLOGY

The pituitary gland (hypophysis) sits within the sella turcica ("Turkish saddle") of the sphenoid bone at the base of the skull and is composed principally of the anterior (adenohypophysis) and posterior lobes (neurohypophysis). The intermediate lobe is rudimentary in humans. The normal pituitary gland weighs between 0.5 and 0.9 g.

The pituitary is separated from the brain by the diaphragma sella, an extension of the dura mater, and from the sphenoid sinus anteriorly and inferiorly by a thin layer of bone. The lateral walls of the sella abut on the cavernous sinuses, which contain the internal carotid arteries and cranial nerves III, IV, V, and VI. The optic chiasm is slightly anterior to the pituitary stalk, just above the diaphragma sella. Thus, tumors of the pituitary may lead to visual field defects, to cranial nerve palsies, or to invasion of the sphenoid sinus (Fig. 313-2).

The hypothalamus extends anteriorly to the margin of the optic chiasm and posteriorly to include the mammillary bodies. Superiorly, the hypothalamic sulcus of the third ventricle separates the thalamus from the hypothalamus. The rounded inferior base of the hypothalamus forms the tuber cinereum. The central portion of the base (termed the infundibulum or median eminence) is formed by the floor of the third ventricle and continues inferiorly to form the pituitary stalk. The releasing factors are synthesized in neurons that are along the margins of the third ventricle and that project fibers which terminate in the median eminence adjacent to the portal capillaries.

The cell bodies of the supraoptic and paraventricular nuclei of the hypothalamus produce vasopressin and oxytocin, which travel down nerve axons in the supraopticohypophysial and paraventriculohypophysial nerve tracts to reach the posterior lobe.

The communication between the hypothalamus and the anterior pituitary is chemical rather than physical. Releasing factors produced by hypothalamic neurons reach the anterior pituitary via the portal system to stimulate or inhibit hormone production. Some of the vasopressin-containing neurons also terminate in the median eminence, and vasopressin can stimulate release of ACTH and GH.

The anterior pituitary has the highest blood flow of any tissue in the body [0.8 (mL/g)/min]. The blood supply reaches the anterior pituitary by a circuitous route through the hypothalamus. Two derivatives of the internal carotid arteries, the superior hypophysial arteries (SHA), branch in the subarachnoid space around the pituitary stalk and terminate in the capillary network of the median eminence. These capillaries have a fenestrated endothelium which allows easy access to the hypothalamic releasing hormones. Transport of substances from the capillaries to the median eminence is also facilitated because the median eminence lies outside the blood-brain barrier. The capillaries then coalesce to form 6 to 10 straight veins known as the hypothalamic-pituitary portal circulation. These veins constitute the main blood supply to the anterior lobe and supply it with nutrients as well as information from the hypothalamus. A direct arterial blood supply to the anterior lobe is also present, but the magnitude and importance of that circulation are uncertain. The posterior pituitary is supplied entirely by blood from the inferior hypophysial arteries.

The anterior lobe is formed from the lateral proliferation of Rathke's pouch, an outpouching from the floor of the embryonic oral cavity. Rathke's pouch is met by a diverticulum from the floor of the third ventricle, which forms the posterior lobe.

Rathke's pouch is closed off by proliferation of the anterior and posterior lobe and forms a thin residual cleft in the gland (Rathke's cleft). This cleft may persist as a cyst lined with cuboidal or columnar epithelium. Since the pituitary rotates as it grows, these cysts usually lie in a position superior to the pituitary gland. The further growth and proliferation of these cysts can give rise to craniopharyngiomas, tumors that generally occupy a suprasellar position. Development of the sphenoid bone separates the pituitary from the oral cavity. Remnants of the pituitary, known as pharyngeal pituitaries, occa-

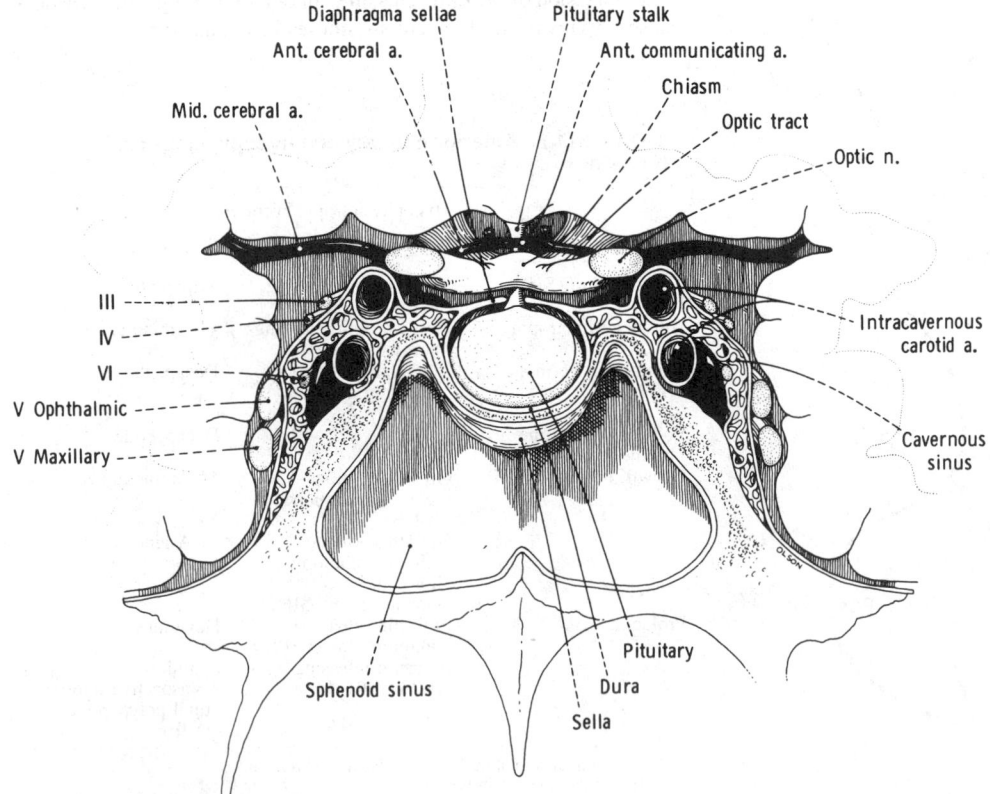

FIGURE 313-2 The relationship between the pituitary, cranial nerves, and the cavernous sinus as viewed in a coronal section through the sella. *(From JA Taren in RC Schneider et al (eds), Correlative Neurosurgery, 3d ed, Springfield, Ill., Charles C Thomas, 1982.)*

sionally persist within or below the sphenoid bone. These remnants may produce pituitary hormones and occasionally develop into pituitary tumors.

Five distinct cell types in the anterior pituitary secrete six different hormones: lactotrophs (prolactin), somatotrophs (GH), gonadotrophs (LH and FSH), thyrotrophs (TSH), and corticotrophs (ACTH).

PROLACTIN

PHYSIOLOGY   The lactotrophs constitute 10 to 25 percent of the normal pituitary and increase to 70 percent during pregnancy. The prolactin gene on chromosome 6 codes for a precursor molecule that is larger than the circulating hormone. The predominant form of the processed hormone contains 198 amino acids (23,000 mol wt) in a single polypeptide chain containing three intrachain disulfide bonds. Higher-molecular-weight forms of prolactin, up to 100,000 mol wt (''big'' and ''big-big'' prolactin), may be present in small amounts in the circulation of normal persons and in larger amounts in patients with pituitary adenomas; these molecules react in prolactin radioimmunoassays but do not have normal biologic potency.

Prolactin is essential for lactation. Receptors for the hormone are present in human breast and gonads, whereas in other animals they are found in additional tissues. Prolactin promotes breast cancer in rodents; a similar connection has not been established in human breast cancer (see Chap. 303).

During pregnancy increasing estrogen production stimulates the growth and replication of the pituitary lactotrophs and causes increased prolactin secretion. The pituitary doubles in size during pregnancy and returns to normal after delivery. Prolactin during pregnancy prepares the breast for postpartum lactation. High estrogen levels inhibit prolactin action at the breast, so that lactation does not commence until estrogen levels decline post partum. Prolactin levels rise in the fetus beginning at about 25 weeks, probably owing to maternal estrogen transfer and stimulation of the fetal pituitary. The level falls rapidly after delivery, reaching a nadir by 2 to 4 weeks post partum. High concentrations of prolactin are present in amniotic fluid, although the origin and functional significance are unknown.

Under normal circumstances, prolactin secretion by the anterior pituitary is restrained by the hypothalamus. With hypothalamic destruction or pituitary stalk section, prolactin secretion increases, and serum concentrations rise. The hypothalamic inhibitory factor for prolactin appears to be dopamine, although peptide inhibitory factors have been described. The arcuate nucleus is the primary hypothalamic site of dopamine synthesis; dopamine travels down axons to nerve terminals in the median eminence where it is released (tuberoinfundibular dopamine system) into the portal circulation and reaches the anterior pituitary to inhibit prolactin release. The intravenous administration of dopamine (2 μg/min per kilogram of body weight) or the oral administration of dopamine precursors (e.g., levodopa) or dopamine agonists (e.g., bromocriptine) inhibits prolactin release. Increased blood prolactin appears to increase hypothalamic dopamine production, which in turn partially inhibits prolactin release via a ''short'' feedback loop.

The prolactin rise during suckling appears to require a prolactin-releasing factor, which has not yet been conclusively identified. Vasoactive intestinal peptide (VIP) may be responsible, as it is a potent stimulator of prolactin release. Suckling-induced prolactin rise is blocked by serotonin antagonists, such as methysergide, which suggests an influence of serotonin on prolactin release. TRH is also a potent stimulator of prolactin release; indeed, the lowest dose of TRH capable of stimulating TSH stimulates prolactin release as well. However, TSH and prolactin release are under independent control in most physiologic states; lactation does not lead to TSH elevation, and primary hypothyroidism is rarely associated with prolactin excess.

Prolactin concentrations rise during sleep, a phenomenon that requires the input of higher centers into the hypothalamus. Stress-related prolactin release can be blocked by opiate antagonists such as naloxone and is probably mediated by endogenous opioids. Morphine can stimulate prolactin release, which may contribute to the amenorrhea of narcotic addiction, but basal prolactin secretion is not influenced by opiate antagonists.

HYPERPROLACTINEMIA   Clinical features   Prolactin excess (hyperprolactinemia) has many causes, is associated with hypogonadism and/or galactorrhea, and may indicate the presence of a pituitary adenoma or hypothalamic disease. Of women with amenorrhea, 10 to 40 percent have hyperprolactinemia, and about 30 percent of women with amenorrhea and galactorrhea have prolactin-secreting pituitary tumors.

The hypogonadism associated with hyperprolactinemia appears to be due to inhibition of hypothalamic release of LHRH, resulting in a decrease in LH and FSH secretion. This functional hypogonadism can be regarded, in part, as a physiologic mechanism since breast feeding causes decreased fertility and delayed resumption of menses. In general, the higher the plasma prolactin, the greater the likelihood of amenorrhea. Milder degrees of hyperprolactinemia in women cause irregular menses or infertility due to a shortened luteal phase. Prolactin excess in men can cause impotence and infertility. In some series 8 percent of men with impotence and 5 percent of men with infertility have hyperprolactinemia. With prolactin elevation, FSH and LH levels in men decline, and serum testosterone is often low.

Galactorrhea, defined as milk production in a patient who is not post partum, is present in 30 to 90 percent of hyperprolactinemic women (see Chap. 323). The variation in incidence reflects, in part, variation in the intensity with which clinicians search for this finding. Galactorrhea may occur without hyperprolactinemia, particularly in parous women. However, galactorrhea is often a clue to prolactin excess; when galactorrhea is coupled with amenorrhea, hyperprolactinemia is present in 75 percent of patients. Hyperprolactinemia in men rarely causes gynecomastia or galactorrhea (see Chap. 323).

Differential diagnosis   Prolactin excess has several mechanisms: (1) autonomous production (pituitary adenomas), (2) decreased dopamine or dopamine inhibitory action (e.g., due to hypothalamic disease or drugs that block dopamine synthesis, dopamine release, or dopamine action), (3) stimuli that overcome the normal dopaminergic inhibition (e.g., estrogens, possibly hypothyroidism), and (4) decreased clearance of prolactin (renal failure). No single suppression test can separate physiologic from pharmacologic or pathologic causes of hyperprolactinemia (Table 313-2).

Prolactin concentrations are slightly higher (<20 μg/L) in women than in men (<15 μg/L). During pregnancy, prolactin concentrations begin to increase during the second trimester and peak at term; maximal values are 100 to 300 μg/L, usually less than 200 μg/L. A pregnancy test is mandatory in all patients with hyperprolactinemic amenorrhea, as it is with amenorrhea alone. The mean prolactin level declines post partum but rises with each suckling episode. Over several months basal and suckling-stimulated prolactin concentrations diminish; by 4 to 6 months post partum, basal prolactin levels are normal, and the suckling-induced rise is absent despite continued nursing.

A careful drug history should be obtained in hyperprolactinemic patients. Dopamine-blocking drugs (e.g., phenothiazines, butyrophenones, metoclopramide) and dopamine-depleting drugs (e.g., methyldopa and reserpine) are important causes of hyperprolactinemia. Prolactin concentrations are rarely greater than 100 μg/L with these agents, provided renal failure is not present. Although high-dose estrogens cause hyperprolactinemia, oral contraceptives containing low doses of estrogen do not.

End-stage renal failure is associated with elevated serum prolactin in 70 to 90 percent of women and 25 to 60 percent of men. This contributes to hypogonadism in some patients with renal failure. Both decreased prolactin clearance and increased prolactin secretion may contribute to this elevation. The increased prolactin in cirrhosis of the liver has not been adequately explained.

Severe primary hypothyroidism may cause a mildly elevated serum prolactin, either due to elevated TRH or decreased dopaminergic

TABLE 313-2   Causes of hyperprolactinemia

I Physiologic states
  A Pregnancy
  B Nursing (early)
  C "Stress"
  D Sleep
  E Nipple stimulation
II Drugs
  A Dopamine receptor antagonists
    1 Phenothiazines
    2 Butyrophenones
    3 Thioxanthenes
    4 Metoclopramide
  B Dopamine-depleting agents
    1 Methyldopa
    2 Reserpine
  C Estrogens
  D Opiates
III Disease states
  A Pituitary tumors
    1 Prolactinomas
    2 Adenomas secreting GH and prolactin
    3 Adenomas secreting ACTH and prolactin (Nelson's syndrome and Cushing's disease)
    4 Nonfunctioning chromophobe adenomas with pituitary stalk compression
  B Hypothalamic and pituitary stalk disease
    1 Granulomatous diseases especially sarcoidosis
    2 Craniopharyngiomas and other tumors
    3 Cranial irradiation
    4 Stalk section
    5 Empty sella
    6 Vascular abnormalities including aneurysm
    7 Lymphocytic hypophysitis
  C Primary hypothyroidism
  D Chronic renal failure
  E Cirrhosis
  F Chest wall trauma (including surgery, *herpes zoster*)
  G Seizures

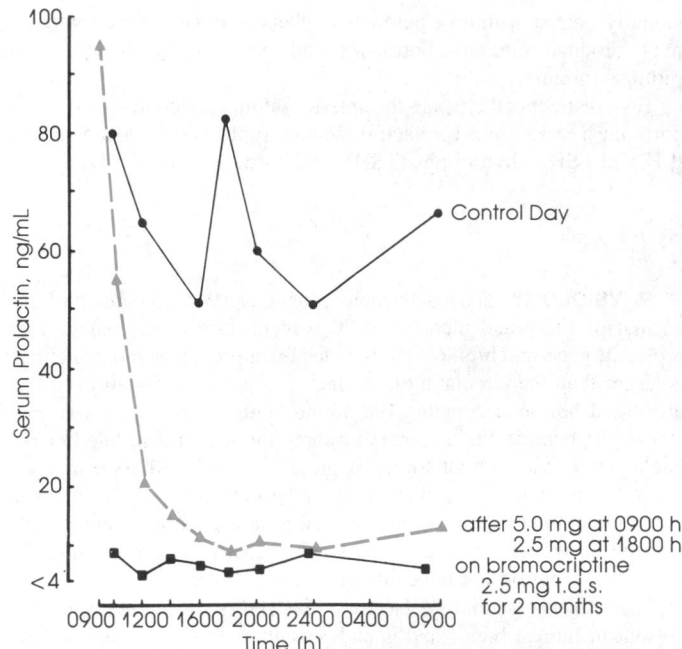

FIGURE 313-3 Changes in serum prolactin concentration in a woman with "idiopathic" hyperprolactinemia after an initial 5-mg dose of bromocriptine and when maintained on 7.5 mg daily. *(From GH Besser and MO Thorner, Postgrad Med J 52:66, 1976.)*

tone. Since primary hypothyroidism may also cause enlargement of the sella turcica, mimicking a pituitary adenoma, thyroid function tests are essential in all patients with elevated serum prolactin. Rarely, primary adrenal insufficiency causes reversible serum prolactin elevation.

If a hyperprolactinemic subject is not pregnant, post partum, cirrhotic, postictal, on medications, hypothyroid, or in renal failure, disease of the pituitary or hypothalamus is likely. Ectopic production of prolactin by nonpituitary tumors occurs rarely if at all. Diseases of the hypothalamus or pituitary stalk cause moderate prolactin elevation (usually less than 150 μg/L). Hyperprolactinemia occurs in 20 to 50 percent of patients with hypothalamic tumors.

Prolactin-secreting pituitary adenomas (prolactinomas) may either be small tumors in the parenchyma (so-called microadenomas) or cause enlargement of the pituitary (macroadenomas). Large, nonfunctioning pituitary adenomas may also cause modest prolactin elevation as a result of stalk compression and impedance of dopamine delivery to the gland. Acromegalics (25 to 45 percent) and patients with Nelson's syndrome (postadrenalectomy pituitary tumors in Cushing's disease) have elevated serum prolactin. Hyperprolactinemia is less common in untreated Cushing's disease.

Laboratory evaluation Serum prolactin levels should be measured in all patients with hypogonadism or galactorrhea. If basal prolactin concentration is elevated, further evaluation is warranted after establishing that minimal prolactin elevations (e.g., less than 30 μg/L) are not stress-related. Blood sampling from an indwelling catheter after a 90-min rest period will exclude "needle stick" hyperprolactinemia. Although there is no simple test to distinguish the various causes of hyperprolactinemia, a serum prolactin level of over 300 μg/L is diagnostic of a pituitary adenoma; a serum prolactin of over 100 μg/L in a nonpregnant patient is usually caused by a pituitary adenoma. Administration of dopamine agonists, such as bromocriptine, lowers prolactin regardless of the etiology and, therefore, is not useful as a differential test (Fig. 313-3). The majority of patients with prolactinomas have only a minimal or no rise in

prolactin in response to TRH, as compared to the normal rise of 200 percent or more and the intermediate response (usually a doubling at serum prolactin) in patients with hypothalamic disease and those on dopamine-blocking agents. Unfortunately, the response to TRH is too variable to be of diagnostic value in individual patients.

In general, patients with unexplained hyperprolactinemia require contrast-enhanced computed tomography (CT) scanning of the hypothalamus and pituitary or magnetic resonance imaging (MRI) of this area. Pituitary macroadenomas are easily visualized on these scans, but microadenomas (<10 mm) may be more difficult to delineate. Patients with amenorrhea and minimal prolactin elevations may also have hypothalamic lesions (e.g., craniopharyngiomas) or large "nonfunctioning" pituitary adenomas. When no radiologic abnormalities are found the disorder is designated "idiopathic hyperprolactinemia," although a microadenoma may still be present. Sella tomography is not a useful screening test for small pituitary adenomas because of the high frequency of false-positive and false-negative results.

Microprolactinomas do not cause hypopituitarism (except for hypogonadism). If a small pituitary lesion is seen in a patient with hypopituitarism and hyperprolactinemia, sarcoidosis or other lesions involving the pituitary stalk should be suspected, rather than a microprolactinoma. In patients with macroprolactinomas or hypothalamic lesions, evaluation of pituitary function and formal visual field examinations are essential.

Prolactinomas PATHOLOGY Prolactinomas are the most common functional pituitary adenomas. Small unsuspected microadenomas are found in 5 to 20 percent of unselected autopsies; 40 percent of these small tumors contain prolactin by immunologic staining techniques, but the fraction that actually secrete prolactin is unknown. About 70 percent of macroadenomas previously thought to be nonfunctioning are, in fact, prolactinomas. Prolactin-secreting pituitary carcinomas are rare.

Prolactinoma size correlates with hormonal output; in general, the larger the tumor, the higher the prolactin levels. Large pituitary tumors with modest prolactin elevation (50 to 100 μg/L) are not true prolactinomas and differ in their biologic behavior. Microprolactinomas cause only hyperprolactinemia and hypogonadotropism, whereas macroprolactinomas may influence other pituitary hormones and cause headaches, visual field disturbances, and other structural problems.

CLINICAL PRESENTATION   Microprolactinomas are more common than macroprolactinomas, and 90 percent of patients with microprolactinomas are women. In contrast, 60 percent of patients with macroprolactinomas are men. Irregular menses, amenorrhea, and galactorrhea are likely to result in early diagnosis, and this may explain the preponderance of microadenomas in women. Sexual dysfunction occurs in most men with prolactinomas, but this is the presenting complaint in 15 percent or less. Although delay in seeking medical help probably explains the larger tumors in men, more aggressive tumor behavior in men has not been excluded.

Estrogens promote the growth of lactotrophs, but an etiologic role has not been established for oral contraceptives in the pathogenesis of prolactinomas. Many women with prolactinomas first develop galactorrhea while on oral contraceptives or develop amenorrhea when the drug is discontinued. Some of these women may have been started on oral contraceptives for irregular menses that were the consequence of a prolactinoma. Although amenorrhea after discontinuing oral contraceptives is rare (about 2 percent), about a third of patients with postpill amenorrhea have prolactinomas. Development of galactorrhea in a woman on oral contraceptives mandates a prolactin determination. About 5 to 7 percent of prolactinoma patients have never menstruated (primary amenorrhea), making this an important treatable cause of primary amenorrhea. Prolactinomas may grow during pregnancy, and 15 percent of prolactinoma patients are first diagnosed in the postpartum period.

Women with prolactinomas who desire pregnancy need special consideration. Medical treatment of patients with microprolactinomas results in uneventful pregnancies 95 to 98 percent of the time; the remainder may develop headaches or visual field disturbances due to tumor enlargement that rarely requires therapy. Asymptomatic enlargement of microprolactinomas, as ascertained by radiologic studies, occurs in about 5 percent. With macroprolactinomas, the complications of tumor growth during pregnancy are more common. Symptomatic tumor enlargement occurs in about 15 percent of these patients, although individual series report complications in up to 35 percent. The majority of patients who develop symptoms do so during the first trimester.

In prolactinoma patients, the effect of pregnancy on prolactin secretion is variable. A further rise in prolactin during pregnancy may not occur even in patients in whom tumor growth occurs. Prolactin concentrations should be measured periodically throughout pregnancy in women with prolactinomas. If marked prolactin rise occurs (greater than 300 to 400 µg/L), then postpartum prolactin is usually greater than the prepartum level, and tumor growth is likely to have occurred. Patients with stable or declining prolactin concentrations during pregnancy may have lower prolactin concentrations after pregnancy than before. In such patients infarction or involution of the adenomas may have occurred during pregnancy. Rarely, macroprolactinomas in men grow as a consequence of replacement testosterone therapy, presumably as a result of extraglandular conversion of testosterone to estrogen.

THERAPY   The therapy of prolactinomas is influenced by the natural history of the disorder. Although large pituitary adenomas must begin as small tumors, most microadenomas do not progress to macroadenomas. Knowledge of the natural history of untreated microprolactinomas is incomplete; 90 to 95 percent may remain stable or demonstrate decreased serum prolactin concentrations after 7 years of follow-up. Many patients with ''idiopathic hyperprolactinemia'' are presumed to harbor small microadenomas. Serum prolactin returns to normal in a third of patients with idiopathic hyperprolactinemia followed for 5 years without therapy; in two-thirds of such patients in whom the basal prolactin is less than 40 µg/L serum prolactin levels return to normal over this time span.

Not all patients with microprolactinomas need therapy. Women with microprolactinomas require therapy when they desire pregnancy, have decreased libido or troublesome galactorrhea, desire regular

menses, or are at risk for osteoporosis. Men with microadenomas should be treated for decreased potency or libido or when infertility is a problem. Most patients with macroprolactinomas require therapy.

Dopamine agonist drugs lower prolactin concentrations in virtually all hyperprolactinemic patients (Fig. 313-3). Ovulatory menses and fertility are restored in 90 percent of premenopausal women, underscoring the direct relationship between hyperprolactinemia and amenorrhea. Bromocriptine, an ergot derivative with dopamine agonist actions, is the only effective prolactin-lowering agent licensed in the United States at this time. Bromocriptine should be given twice daily with food or a snack to prevent gastrointestinal irritation. Therapy should begin with 1.25 mg at bedtime to minimize the side effects of nausea, vomiting, fatigue, nasal stuffiness, and postural hypotension. The dosage is gradually increased to an average of 2.5 mg twice daily, although some patients can be treated with single daily doses. However, doses up to 15 mg/d may be required to return the prolactin concentration to normal in some patients with macroprolactinomas. Although the drug is expensive, it is effective in all forms of hyperprolactinemia and often abolishes nonhyperprolactinemic galactorrhea as well. Long-lasting (40-day) parenteral bromocriptine and long-lasting oral dopamine agonists are not licensed in the United States. Although these agents all have similar side effects, individuals may tolerate one but not the other.

Bromocriptine is the therapy of choice for patients with microprolactinomas who have one of the indications for treatment discussed above. Prolactin concentrations return to normal in almost all who tolerate the medication, usually within days of achieving full therapeutic dosages (Fig. 313-3). Menses usually resume within 2 months but may be delayed up to a year. Since pregnancy may occur without resumption of menses, a barrier contraceptive is recommended until menses become regular. In this way, bromocriptine can be stopped with the first missed period when pregnancy has occurred. Bromocriptine use during pregnancy is not, however, associated with an increased risk of congenital anomalies or fetal wastage. The effects of bromocriptine are usually not permanent, but a sixth of microprolactinoma patients maintain normal prolactin concentrations after stopping the drug.

In patients with macroprolactinomas, bromocriptine usually lowers the serum prolactin and may cause the tumor mass to shrink. In men testosterone concentrations usually begin to increase after 3 months of therapy and may reach normal levels by 6 to 8 months. Normal sperm counts are achieved in some.

One series of patients with large prolactinomas and suprasellar extension (mean prolactin of 1441 µg/L in women, 3451 µg/L in men) is of particular interest. Although prolactin levels fell to 10 percent of baseline in 96 percent of patients, most did not return to the normal range despite bromocriptine dosages of 7.5 to 20 mg/d. Visual field defects improved in 90 percent of those with field cuts. Tumor mass decreased by half or more in 60 percent of patients (see Fig. 313-4). When successful, bromocriptine alone is the therapy of choice in most patients with macroprolactinomas. With long-term (>2 years) therapy, the dosage of bromocriptine can often be reduced but rarely eliminated. In those patients in whom persistent hyperprolactinemia causes symptoms despite partial response to bromocriptine, radiation therapy and on occasion surgical debulking may be appropriate. In those women with large tumors who desire pregnancy, bromocriptine therapy during pregnancy should be considered, along with the alternatives of surgery or radiation therapy. Large nonfunctioning pituitary adenomas associated with hyperprolactinemia due to stalk compression usually do not shrink with bromocriptine therapy, although prolactin concentrations may on occasion return to normal. Patients with large prolactinomas, refractory to bromocriptine and other modalities of therapy, may partially respond to tamoxifen, an estrogen antagonist.

Following transsphenoidal resection of microprolactinomas, serum prolactin concentration returns to normal in up to 80 to 90 percent of patients, usually within 24 h. This procedure has low morbidity and mortality. Unfortunately, recurrence rates average 17 percent

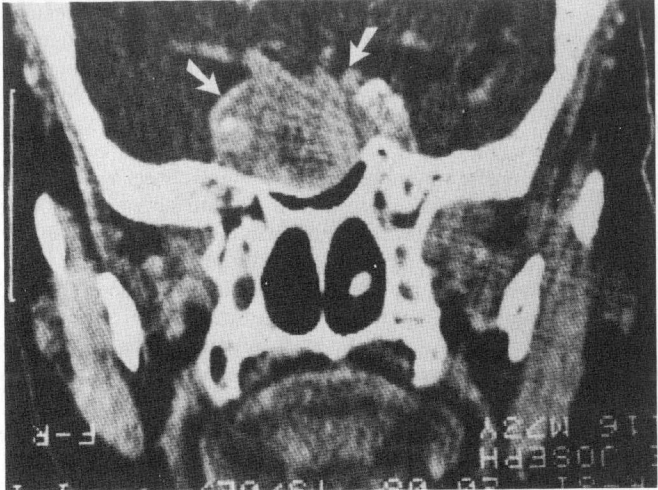

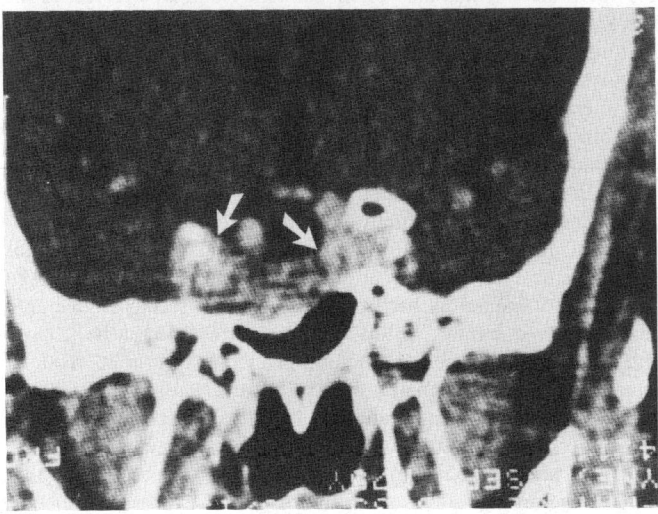

FIGURE 313-4 Frontal CT scan of a man with a large prolactin-secreting macroadenoma. *Top,* pretreatment scan. *Bottom,* scan after 1 year of treatment with bromocriptine. The upper border of the tumor is shown by arrows. *(From Molitch et al.)*

after "successful" surgery and may be as high as 40 percent after 6 years of follow-up. Surgery is appropriate for women with microprolactinomas who desire pregnancy and who cannot tolerate or do not wish to take dopamine agonist drugs.

Surgery, combined with bromocriptine and/or radiation therapy, is indicated for macroprolactinomas with suprasellar extension and persistent visual field defects and particularly in such patients desiring pregnancy. However, surgical resection, whether by transsphenoidal or transcranial approach, is rarely curative in patients with macroprolactinomas. Prolactin concentrations return to normal in about 30 percent, but even when they do, recurrence rates of up to 80 percent have been reported. In all patients in whom prolactin levels do not return to normal following surgery and in all with evidence of residual tumors after resection, long-term bromocriptine therapy and/or radiation should be given.

Conventional radiation therapy [4500 cGy (4500 rad) over 25 days] for prolactinomas causes a slow decline in serum prolactin concentration. Prolactin concentration returns to normal in about 30 percent of microprolactinoma patients 2 to 10 years after therapy. We do not favor this approach in patients with microprolactinomas because of the risk of their developing hypopituitarism. Radiation therapy is a useful adjunct to surgical or medical therapy in patients with macroprolactinomas; further growth is usually prevented, and shrinkage occurs in about half the patients. This therapy usually prevents tumor growth during subsequent pregnancies, but exceptions have been noted.

Heavy particle therapy with protons may be useful in treatment of macroprolactinomas without suprasellar extension or after surgical debulking of larger tumors. Occasional patients with microprolactinomas opt for this form of therapy. Long-term studies in prolactinoma patients are not available.

PROLACTIN DEFICIENCY Prolactin deficiency is manifested as an inability to lactate. Failure of lactation is often the earliest clue to panhypopituitarism resulting from pituitary infarction during the peripartum period. The lateral wings of the pituitary have a precarious blood supply; most lactotrophs reside in this area. During pregnancy, the hypertrophied and hyperplastic lactotrophs are at risk for necrosis. If systemic hypotension develops, as with postpartum hemorrhage, the hypertrophic and hyperplastic lactotrophs may infarct (Sheehan's syndrome). Patients with diabetes mellitus are susceptible to peripartum pituitary infarction even in the absence of significant hemorrhage. Autoimmune pituitary destruction (lymphocytic hypophysitis) may also occur during late pregnancy but often is associated with elevated prolactin levels.

Most prolactin radioimmunoassays cannot distinguish normal from low concentrations; hence, prolactin stimulation tests are needed to diagnose prolactin insufficiency. After administration of TRH or chlorpromazine, a rise in serum prolactin of less than 200 percent suggests prolactin deficiency. If prolactin deficiency is present, evaluation of other pituitary hormones is necessary as well to define other manifestations of hypopituitarism.

GROWTH HORMONE

PHYSIOLOGY Growth hormone (GH, somatotropin) is secreted by somatotrophs which make up about 50 percent of the anterior pituitary cells. The normal pituitary contains 3 to 5 mg of GH and secretes 500 to 875 μg of GH per day. The gene coding for GH is on chromosome 17; additional GH-related genes are of uncertain significance. Human growth hormone is a single polypeptide chain of 191 amino acids (22,000 mol wt) and contains two intrachain disulfide bonds. A larger (28,000 mol wt) precursor molecule is cleaved to yield GH. GH is stored in cytoplasmic granules in a high-molecular-weight polymeric form.

GH shares a 92 percent structural homology with human placental lactogen (hPL, chorionic somatomammotropin). GH and hPL genes are on the same chromosome and appear to have originated by gene duplication.

In the circulation, monomeric GH (22,000 mol wt) predominates. Larger molecular weight forms may represent dimers (i.e., "big" GH, 44,000 mol wt) that appear to be secreted by the pituitary gland into the circulation. Although "big" GH is measured by the GH radioimmunoassay, its biologic activity is reduced. Pulsatile release is characteristic. Circulating levels are immeasurably low for much of the day, punctuated by four to eight bursts after meals or exercise, during slow-wave sleep, or without obvious cause. The half-life of the hormone in plasma is 20 to 30 min.

GH is necessary for normal linear growth. Growth hormone deficiency causes short stature; growth hormone excess (prior to epiphyseal closure) leads to gigantism. GH does not appear to be the principal direct stimulator of growth but acts indirectly by stimulating the formation of other hormones. These factors, known as somatomedins (SM, somatotropin-mediating hormones) or insulin-like growth factors (IGF) are growth hormone–dependent and are responsible for growth stimulation (also see Chap. 314). Somatomedin C (insulin-like growth factor 1, IGF-1/SM-C), the most important somatomedin for postnatal growth, is produced in the liver and by other tissues as well. IGF-1/SM-C is a basic protein (7600 mol wt) that circulates bound to a large carrier molecule (140,000 mol wt). The complex has a half-life of 3 to 18 h, as compared to the half-life of 20 to 30 min for unbound hormone. As a consequence, the concentration of IGF-1/SM-C remains relatively constant throughout the 24 h period, in contrast to the fluctuating levels of GH itself. How the liver integrates GH pulses into somatomedin production is not known. Furthermore, local tissue generation of IGF-1/SM-C, particularly in bone, may play an important role in mediating growth through paracrine effects.

IGF-1 is structurally similar to proinsulin and exerts some insulin-like actions. Furthermore, GH is a trophic factor for insulin release, facilitating its release in response to various secretagogues, and GH-deficient individuals have impaired insulin release to glucose challenge. Technically, one might consider insulin a somatomedin.

During the prenatal and neonatal period growth is independent of GH, as shown by the normal birth length of GH-deficient children born to GH-deficient mothers. Nevertheless IGF-1/SM-C levels rise during pregnancy, and its concentration correlates with that of hPL, which may regulate somatomedin production. IGF-1/SM-C levels at birth are lower than those of adults and rise gradually during childhood to reach the adult range by age 8 to 10 years. IGF-1/SM-C levels are dependent upon nutritional status, declining in states of malnourishment. Elevated serum IGF-1/SM-C concentrations are present during the pubertal growth spurt, presumably accounting for the pubertal growth acceleration.

Although IGF-1/SM-C concentrations correlate with linear growth, the correlation is inexact, and therefore GH may have some direct influence on growth or cause somatomedin generation in target cells.

GH exerts additional metabolic effects, including stimulation of the incorporation of amino acids into protein. Although most of this action is somatomedin-mediated, GH can directly stimulate amino acid uptake in certain systems. Some amino acids, such as arginine, are potent stimuli for GH release.

GH may have a direct effect as an insulin antagonist. Patients with GH deficiency are prone to insulin-induced hypoglycemia; patients with GH excess develop insulin resistance. GH is one of the counterregulatory hormones that help restore a low blood sugar to normal (see Chap. 320). Hypoglycemia is a potent GH stimulus, and an acute rise in blood sugar inhibits GH release. GH increases free fatty acid release from adipocytes. The absence of this effect may be responsible for the pudgy appearance of children with GH deficiency. Increased serum free fatty acid concentrations tend to blunt GH release. GH opposes the action of insulin on sugar uptake and fatty acid release and complements the anabolic action of insulin on amino acid uptake.

GH is controlled by a dual hypothalamic regulation (Table 313-3). Secretion is stimulated by growth hormone–releasing hormone (GRH, somatocrinin) and inhibited by growth hormone release–inhibitory hormone (somatostatin, somatotropin release–inhibitory factor, SRIF). GRH appears to play the more important role, as stalk section leads to failure of GH release. In animals treated with anti-GRH antibodies the GH peaks disappear, and growth ceases; following treatment with antisomatostatin antibodies, the peaks remain, but the baseline values rise. After treatment with both anti-GRH and anti-somatostatin antibodies, the peaks disappear but the baseline rises. Although GRH- and somatostatin-containing neurons are separate, they have reciprocal interconnections.

Growth hormone–releasing hormone GRH has 44 amino acids, 29 of which are necessary for full potency. GRH belongs to a family of molecules that includes secretin, glucagon, vasoactive intestinal peptide (VIP), and gastric inhibitory peptide (GIP). The arcuate nucleus of the hypothalamus is the major site of GRH production, although a few such neurons are in the ventromedial nucleus as well. Axons containing the peptide project to the median eminence and terminate on the portal vessels. Whether GRH is also present in extracranial tissues is uncertain.

GRH stimulates GH release in vitro and in vivo, an effect that is calcium-dependent and appears to be mediated by cyclic adenosine monophosphate (cyclic AMP). Intravenous injection of GRH (0.1 to 3.3 μg/kg body weight) produces a peak GH response at 30 to 60 min with a return to baseline by 2 to 3 h postinjection (Fig. 313-5).

Somatostatin Somatostatin, a cyclic tetradecapeptide, is the most widely distributed of the hypothalamic releasing hormones.

TABLE 313-3 Growth hormone regulation

Class of agent	Stimulation	Inhibition
Hypothalamic factors	GRH	Somatostatin
Amines	Alpha-adrenergic stimuli (norepinephrine, clonidine)	Beta-adrenergic stimuli
	Beta-adrenergic blockers (propranolol)	Alpha-adrenergic blockers (phentolamine, dibenzyline)
	Dopaminergic stimuli (levodopa, bromocriptine, apomorphine)	Dopamine blockers (chlorpromazine)
	Serotonergic stimuli (L-tryptophan)	Serotonin blockers (methysergide, cyproheptadine)
Hormones	Decreased IGF-1/SM-C	Increased IGF-1/SM-C (obesity)
	Estrogen	Progestogens
	Vasopressin	Glucocorticoids
	Glucagon	
Fuels	Hypoglycemia*	Increased blood sugar
	Decreased free fatty acids	Increased free fatty acids
	Amino acids (arginine)*	
Others	Exercise*	
	Stress*	
	Sleep	

* Probably mediated through alpha-adrenergic stimulation.

The primary hypothalamic sources are the periventricular and medial preoptic areas of the anterior hypothalamus. Somatostatin is found in neurosecretory granules of axons that terminate in the median eminence. In addition to its function as a hormone, somatostatin is synthesized and distributed throughout the brain and serves as a neurotransmitter in many areas including the spinal cord, brainstem, and cerebral cortex. Somatostatin is also present in the gastrointestinal tract. Specific somatostatin-secreting cells (D cells) of the pancreatic islets participate in the regulation of insulin and glucagon secretion, an example of paracrine regulation by this hormone (see Chap. 319).

Somatostatin is produced by processing of a larger precursor molecule and exists in both 28– and 14–amino acid forms. The 28–amino acid somatostatin has a longer half-life and is a more potent inhibitor of GH and insulin secretion. Somatostatin 14 has a greater affinity for hypothalamic and cortical receptors and is more potent in inhibition of glucagon release. Somatostatin analogues are effective in the therapy of acromegaly, secretory pancreatic tumors, carcinoid syndrome, and other conditions.

Somatostatin inhibits GH secretion and decreases the GH response to secretagogues. Somatostatin also lowers serum TSH in normal and hypothyroid individuals and blunts TSH release in response to TRH. Somatostatin probably mediates the secondary hypothyroidism that may develop in GH-deficient children treated with GH. Somatostatin has no significant effect on the release of prolactin, gonadotropins, or ACTH in normal subjects but may lower ACTH concentrations in patients with Nelson's syndrome. Somatostatinomas are rare pancreatic islet cell or duodenal tumors that secrete somatostatin (see Chap. 262).

Growth hormone release is under complex physiologic control (Table 313-3). The various mediators appear to act through GRH and somatostatin. IGF-1/SM-C has an important feedback effect on GH secretion. An increased IGF-1/SM-C concentration inhibits GH release both through increased somatostatin production and by a direct action on the pituitary. A decrease in IGF-1/SM-C, as induced by starvation, leads to a compensatory increase in GH release.

A number of neurotransmitters influence GH release:

1 Hypothalamic dopamine, the important prolactin inhibitory factor, stimulates GH through an effect on GRH. Dopamine has a direct

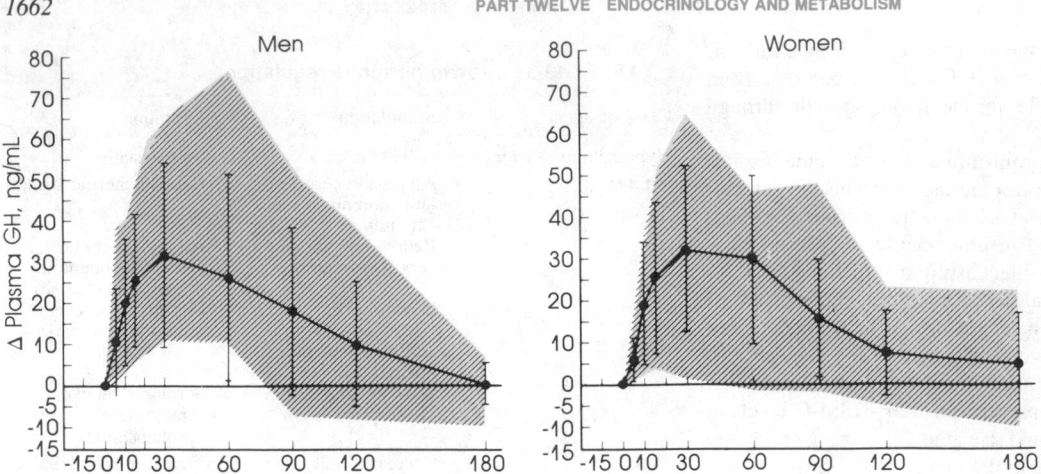

FIGURE 313-5 Response to GRH-44 (1 μg/kg) in eight men and eight women. The shaded area shows the full range of responses at each time point and the error bars indicate the mean ± 1 SD. *(From MC Gelato et al, J Clin Endocrinol Metab 59:200, 1984.)*

but weak inhibitory effect on GH release; this effect is overwhelmed by its hypothalamic stimulation of GRH secretion. Oral administration of dopamine precursors or agonists that cross the blood-brain barrier, such as levodopa, apomorphine, or bromocriptine, causes an increase in serum GH concentration. The effects of these stimuli can be utilized to test the adequacy of GH secretion (GH reserve).

2 Alpha-adrenergic agonists, such as clonidine, stimulate GRH and GH release whereas phentolamine, an alpha blocker, prevents the GH rise. A number of GH stimulators, including insulin hypoglycemia, arginine, and exercise, act through alpha-adrenergic mechanisms. Beta-adrenergic blockers potentiate the GH-stimulatory effect of clonidine (and of some other agents including levodopa), possibly by inhibiting somatostatin secretion.

3 Serotonin agonists stimulate GH release, and the nocturnal surge in GH secretion may be mediated by serotonin, as cyproheptadine (a serotonin antagonist) blocks the sleep-induced GH rise.

Obesity blunts GH release in response to many stimuli, including GRH itself. Weight reduction restores normal GH dynamics. In contrast, malnourished individuals, including women with anorexia nervosa, often have an increased GH concentration, probably as a result of decreased serum IGF-1/SM-C levels. Oral glucose administration decreases serum GH and the GH response to GRH.

A number of hormones influence GH release. Most factors that stimulate GH release are more potent in women than in men, an effect mediated by estrogen. In testing GH reserve in children, estrogen priming may be necessary before adequate GH release can be demonstrated. Although estrogen increases GH concentration, it decreases its biologic effect by blocking somatomedin production. This is similar to the estrogen effect on prolactin in which secretion is stimulated, but its action in promoting lactation is inhibited. Glucocorticoids inhibit GH release and may blunt somatomedin action as well, explaining the potent growth-inhibiting effects of these agents in children.

GROWTH HORMONE EXCESS: ACROMEGALY AND GIGANTISM   Clinical features   GH excess results in acromegaly, an insidious, chronic debilitating disease associated with bony and soft tissue overgrowth (Table 313-4). Acromegaly occurs most frequently in middle age. It is uncommon with a prevalence of 40 cases per million and an incidence of 3 cases per million per year. When GH excess develops prior to epiphyseal closure in children, increased linear growth and gigantism develop.

Most patients have soft tissue and bone enlargement which results in increased hand, foot, and hat size, prognathism, enlargement of the tongue, wide spacing of the teeth, and coarsening of facial features. Acromegalics are said to look more like each other than like their own family members (Fig. 313-6). Laryngeal hypertrophy and sinus enlargement lead to a hollow-sounding voice. A moist, doughy handshake, increased skin tags, acanthosis nigricans, and oily skin are common.

Acromegaly is more than a cosmetically disfiguring disease. Patients feel weak and tired. The basal metabolic rate increases, which in turn causes increased sweating. Obstructive sleep apnea may be an important cause of hypersomnolence. The majority have

TABLE 313-4   Acromegaly—manifestations

Location	Symptoms	Signs
General	Fatigue Increased sweating Heat intolerance Weight gain	
Skin and subcutaneous tissue	Enlarging hands, feet Coarsening facial features Oily skin Hypertrichosis	Moist, warm, fleshy, doughy handshake Skin tags Acanthosis nigricans Increased heel pad
Head	Headaches	Parotid enlargement, frontal bossing
Eyes	Decreased vision	Visual field defects
Ears		Otoscope speculum cannot be inserted
Nose-throat–paranasal sinuses	Sinus congestion	Enlarged furrowed tongue
	Increased tongue size	Tooth marks on tongue
	Malocclusion Voice change	Widely spaced teeth Prognathism
Neck		Goiter Obstructive sleep apnea Enlarged sinuses
Cardiorespiratory system	Congestive heart failure	Hypertension Cardiomegaly Left ventricular hypertrophy
Genitourinary system	Decreased libido Impotence Oligomenorrhea Infertility Kidney stones	
Neurologic system	Paresthesias Hypersomnolence	Carpal tunnel syndrome
Muscles	Weakness	Proximal myopathy
Skeletal system	Joint pains (shoulders, back, knees)	Osteoarthritis

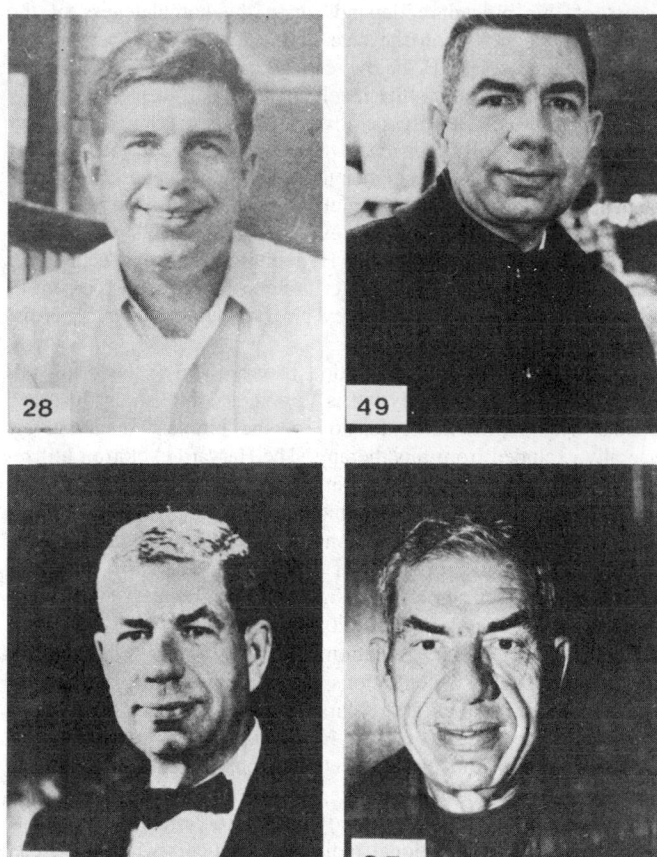

FIGURE 313-6 Serial photographs of a patient with acromegaly taken at ages 28, 49, 55, and 65 years, 6 months after removal of a GH-secreting adenoma. Note the gradual increase in the size of the nose, lips, and skin folds, particularly the nasolabial skin fold and forehead. *(From Reichlin, 1982.)*

neurologic and musculoskeletal symptoms including headaches, paresthesias (often due to carpal tunnel syndrome), muscle weakness, and arthralgias (particularly involving the shoulders, back, and knees). The cartilage hypertrophy and osseous overgrowth often lead to degenerative arthritis, and kyphoscoliosis may occur. Hypertension occurs in about one-third and is characterized by suppressed renin and aldosterone secretion associated with expansion of plasma volume and total body sodium. Almost all hypertensive acromegalics and about half of nonhypertensive acromegalics have increased left ventricular mass or left ventricular wall thickness. Although it is not established whether a specific cardiomyopathy occurs, acromegalics may develop congestive heart failure in the absence of other known underlying heart disease. Amenorrhea may occur with or without hyperprolactinemia, and hirsutism is often noted. Depression may persist after successful therapy for acromegaly. Many organs, including the liver and kidneys, increase in size with no evidence of functional impairment. Goiter is common, and 3 to 7 percent are hyperthyroid. Some series report abdominal pain and inguinal hernias each in about one-third of patients and nasal polyps in as many as 15 percent. Intracranial aneurysms coexist in 10 percent or less.

Patients with acromegaly probably have a shortened life expectancy with increased cardiovascular, cerebrovascular, and respiratory deaths. In studies in which modern therapy was available, effects on life expectancy are less striking. Patients with coexisting diabetes mellitus have increased mortality. Although increased prevalence of carcinoma has been reported in some series (including breast carcinoma in one series), the overall differences are not statistically significant. Skin tags appear to correlate with increased prevalence of colonic polyps and possibly with carcinoma of the colon.

Laboratory investigation   Insulin resistance occurs in 80 percent, although abnormal glucose tolerance (20 to 40 percent) and clinical diabetes mellitus (13 to 20 percent) are less common. Hypercalciuria is frequent, apparently due to increased levels of circulating 1,25-dihydroxyvitamin D; renal stones occur in about one-fifth of patients. Hypercalcemia, when it occurs, is not due to acromegaly per se but suggests primary hyperparathyroidism as part of the multiple endocrine neoplasia I (MEN I) syndrome (see Chap. 325). GH causes increased renal tubular reabsorption of phosphate by an undefined mechanism. Elevation of serum phosphate occurs in about one-half. Hyperprolactinemia occurs in up to one-half of patients and is responsible for much of the associated galactorrhea, amenorrhea, and decreased libido.

Pathophysiology   Well-defined pituitary adenomas are found in almost all patients with acromegaly and gigantism. The tumors tend to occur in the lateral wings of the sella where normal somatotrophs are found in abundance. Occasionally, tumors are found in ectopic locations along the lines of migration of Rathke's pouch, such as the sphenoid sinus or parapharyngeal regions.

GH levels correlate on average with tumor size. Tumors tend to be larger and may be more aggressive in younger patients. At the time of diagnosis 75 percent of somatotroph adenomas are macroadenomas, whereas two-thirds or more of prolactinomas are microadenomas at the time of diagnosis. Aggressive screening for acromegaly on the basis of subtle clinical clues might lead to early diagnosis while tumors are still small.

Immunohistochemical staining and electron microscopy of somatotroph tumors help to predict their behavior. Growth hormone–secreting carcinomas are rare and should be diagnosed only in the presence of distant metastases. Tumors that cause local invasion are called invasive adenomas.

Although hypothalamic GRH excess or somatostatin deficiency has been postulated to be the underlying abnormality leading to acromegaly, most acromegalics in fact have primary disease of the pituitary. Evidence for a pituitary etiology includes (1) low serum GRH in patients with acromegaly, (2) absence of somatotroph hyperplasia in the cells outside the adenomas, and (3) return of GH dynamics to normal upon successful removal of the somatotroph adenomas.

GRH-induced acromegaly is rare (less than 1 percent in a recent series). This diagnosis should be considered when pituitary somatotroph hyperplasia, rather than an adenoma, is diagnosed histologically. Bronchial carcinoids and pancreatic islet cell tumors are the most likely to secrete GRH, and certain of these tumors may cosecrete GH and/or IGF-1/SM-C as well. Hypothalamic gangliocytomas also produce GRH (as well as somatostatin) and may cause somatotroph hyperplasia and acromegaly. A number of other tumors (including small cell carcinoma of the lung, medullary carcinoma of the thyroid, and thymic carcinoid) contain GRH, but the amount of secretion from these tumors is unknown. These tumors also may be associated with ectopic ACTH production.

Isolated ectopic production of GH is rare but has been described in a patient with a pancreatic islet cell tumor; the tumor size in this instance (420 g) suggests inefficient GH production since GH-secreting pituitary tumors that cause acromegaly are usually much smaller.

Diagnosis   Patients with acromegaly have symptoms for an average of 9 years and often see several doctors before the diagnosis is made. Newly consulted physicians are more likely to suspect the diagnosis than is a physician or family member who has watched the insidious progress of the disease. When suggestive facial features are noted, a comparison with old pictures may be helpful (Fig. 313-6).

Basal or random GH determinations may be elevated in normal persons, particularly in women, and should not be used to screen for acromegaly. A physiologic test of the capacity to inhibit GH release must be utilized. The standard screening test is the measurement of serum GH concentrations 60 to 120 min after the oral administration of 100 g glucose. A serum GH concentration of less than 5 μg/L is usually taken as a normal response, although a postsuppression value of less than 2 μg/L is a more rigorous criterion. Acromegalics usually have a GH concentration after glucose administration of greater than 10 μg/L; however, some suppress to values below 5 but rarely below 2 μg/L.

GH concentrations in acromegaly may vary during the day, although they are never undetectable as in normal persons. After glucose administration to acromegalics the GH concentrations usually are unchanged or increase, but some GH lowering may occur. GH levels increase in response to insulin-induced hypoglycemia and arginine infusion, and the response to GRH is enhanced in most acromegalics. Somatostatin infusion lowers GH concentration but usually not to normal values. In addition, GH-secreting pituitary tumors respond to stimuli that do not affect normal somatotrophs: TRH increases GH in the majority (80 percent), and LHRH increases GH in about 10 to 15 percent. Dopamine agonists stimulate GH release in normal persons but inhibit GH release in 75 percent of acromegalics. Somatotroph tumors that cosecrete prolactin are most likely to show GH stimulation with TRH and GH inhibition with dopamine agonists.

Measurements of serum IGF-1/SM-C concentrations correlate with disease activity even in patients with basal GH concentrations below 10 μg/L. IGF-1/SM-C values vary considerably between laboratories. The levels do not correlate well with basal GH concentrations but do correlate with mean 24-h GH levels.

All patients with large pituitary adenomas should be screened with GH measurements, preferably after glucose ingestion. In rare cases patients with elevated serum GH and IGF-1/SM-C concentrations may have large pituitary tumors, without clinical evidence of acromegaly. This syndrome is unexplained.

Radiologic investigation is necessary once the laboratory tests confirm the clinical suspicion of acromegaly. Conventional skull x-rays or coned-down views of the sella turcica are abnormal in 90 percent of patients with acromegaly. CT scanning or MRI provides better definition of tumor size and is necessary for appropriate therapeutic planning. Additional clues to the diagnosis of acromegaly can be found on conventional skull x-rays and include thickening of the skull with increased bone density, enlargement of the paranasal sinuses and proliferation of the mastoid air cells, and prognathism if the jaw is included. On bone x-rays one may see enlarged vertebral bodies with anterior lipping, tufting of the distal phalanges of the hands and feet, increased thickness and lengthening of the ribs and clavicles, and bowing of the femur, tibia, and fibula. Soft tissue x-rays demonstrate increased thickness of the heel pad (greater than 18 mm in women and 21 mm in men).

Testing of anterior pituitary function for hypopituitarism and for increased prolactin should be performed. Large somatotrope adenomas commonly cause neurologic abnormalities. In addition, acromegaly may be associated with hyperparathyroidism and pancreatic islet cell tumors in the MEN I syndrome and rarely with pheochromocytomas or hyperaldosteronism. The alpha subunit of the glycoprotein hormones may be oversecreted in acromegaly and may serve as an additional marker of tumor regrowth.

Therapy The objectives of therapy are (1) return of GH levels to normal, (2) stabilization or decrease in tumor size, and (3) preservation of normal pituitary function. The available modalities are variably successful in achieving these goals, and none is perfect. Although GH values of less than 5 μg/L are frequently interpreted as representing cures, a value of less than 2 μg/L is a better criterion; patients with GH values between 2 and 5 μg/L may have persistent symptoms and increased IGF-1/SM-C concentrations.

Transsphenoidal surgery has the advantage of producing a rapid therapeutic response; it is potentially curative and is the procedure of choice. Anesthesiologists should be alerted to the potential of a difficult intubation due to anatomic changes in the jaw, tongue, epiglottis, and larynx. GH concentrations may fall to normal within hours, and soft tissue (but not bony) enlargement may melt away, even before the patient has been discharged from the hospital. The

success of this procedure depends upon the completeness of the resection and hence upon the size of the tumor. In expert hands, apparent cure rates (GH below 5 μg/L) average 75 percent in patients with preoperative GH levels of less than 40 μg/L but only 35 percent in those with preoperative GH levels greater than 40 μg/L. The occurrence of tumor regrowth and recurrent acromegaly after successful surgery may be higher than previously appreciated. Persistent GH response to TRH stimulation appears to have predictive value in assessing risk of relapse, even in those patients with normal postoperative GH concentrations. Hypopituitarism may occur in 10 to 20 percent of patients with larger tumors, but up to 10 percent of patients with pituitary insufficiency prior to surgery regain normal function.

Heavy particle pituitary radiation is successful in lowering GH concentrations in acromegaly but is slow in accomplishing this goal. Patients with suprasellar extension of the pituitary adenoma are generally excluded from this therapy. The Harvard cyclotron utilizes the Bragg peak with proton irradiation, achieving up to 12,000 cGy (12,000 rad) to the center of the pituitary adenoma. In patients with mean pretherapy GH concentration of 60 μg/L, GH concentrations are below 5 μg/L in 29 percent of patients at 2 years, 40 percent at 4 years, 75 percent at 10 years, and 92 percent by 20 years. Hypopituitarism occurs in about 20 percent.

Conventional pituitary radiation [4500 cGy (4500 rad)] also has its proponents. GH concentrations of less than 5 μg/L occur in 50 percent of acromegalics at 5 years and in 70 percent at 10 years (mean pretherapy GH 60 μg/L). Hypopituitarism is a sequela, and up to 50 percent of patients require replacement therapy. The hypopituitarism is most likely due to hypothalamic damage, which is less likely to occur with focused heavy particle radiation. We use heavy particle or conventional radiation in patients who have failed surgery or when surgery is contraindicated or is refused by the patient.

Bromocriptine is a useful adjunct to other modalities of therapy but rarely is successful alone. Clinical improvement is reported in up to 90 percent of patients with dosages of 20 to 60 mg/d. Objective decrease in hand and ring size as well as improvement in diabetes mellitus may occur in the absence of decreasing GH values. However, GH concentrations fall to less than 10 μg/L in only 35 percent, and values of less than 5 μg/L are achieved in only 15 percent. A decrease in tumor size occurs in a minority of patients.

A long-acting analogue of somatostatin (octreotide) lowers growth hormone to normal values in at least two-thirds of acromegalics and causes partial tumor regression (20 to 50 percent) in most. The drug must be administered subcutaneously (50 to 250 μg every 6 to 8 h). Side effects are minimal and include local pain, abdominal cramps, cholelithiasis, and temporary steatorrhea. This analogue is 40 to 50 times more potent in inhibiting GH secretion than in inhibiting insulin secretion, but abnormal glucose tolerance or worsening of diabetes mellitus occurs in some patients. Inhibition of TSH secretion does not appear to be a problem. It seems likely that this drug will be most useful as adjunctive therapy after external radiation or unsuccessful surgery. Indeed the success rate of surgery in acromegalic patients with invasive macroadenomas may be improved after octreotide pretreatment. The role of this agent as a primary treatment for acromegaly remains to be defined, but some patients have been treated successfully for as long as 2 years.

GH DEFICIENCY AND PITUITARY DWARFISM GH is often the first hormone to be lost in pituitary and hypothalamic disorders. In adults, GH deficiency is often cryptic and can only be diagnosed on the basis of stimulation tests for GH release. The consequences of GH deficiency in adults are still being explored. GH deficiency is probably responsible for the fine wrinkling of facial skin in patients with hypopituitarism. Diabetics with GH deficiency show a reduction in insulin requirements and may develop hypoglycemia. In children, GH deficiency leads to impaired growth and short stature and is often a consequence of hypothalamic GRH deficiency (see Chap. 314).

GONADOTROPINS

PHYSIOLOGY The gonadotropins, LH and FSH, are secreted by the gonadotrophs (also see Chaps. 321 and 322). These cells, which make up about 10 percent of the anterior pituitary, are dispersed throughout the anterior lobe, often situated close to the lactotrophs. Most gonadotrophs produce both LH and FSH, although a few cells produce only one hormone.

LH and FSH are glycoproteins of similar size (about 30,000 mol wt), which share a common alpha subunit [also present in TSH and human chorionic gonadotropin (hCG)] but have unique beta subunits. The alpha and beta chains are encoded in separate genes on separate chromosomes, and alpha chains are often produced in excess. The carbohydrate content of the molecules influences the biologic behavior and duration of action and may vary throughout the menstrual cycle. Although both FSH and LH are secreted in pulsatile fashion, the longer FSH half-life means that FSH concentrations fluctuate less throughout the day. FSH and LH regulate ovarian and testicular function.

FSH stimulates the growth of the granulosa cells of the ovarian follicle and controls the aromatase responsible for estradiol formation within these cells. LH stimulates the ovarian theca cells to produce androgens, which diffuse to the granulosa cells where they are converted to estrogens. Estradiol, the principal estrogen, peaks about 1 day prior to the LH surge, which in turn triggers ovulation. Postovulation, LH contributes to corpus luteum formation. Once conception has occurred, pituitary gonadotropin function is no longer necessary to sustain pregnancy.

In the testis LH is primarily responsible for controlling testosterone production in the Leydig cells. FSH, in conjunction with intratesticular testosterone, stimulates the seminiferous tubules to produce sperm. Thus LH and FSH are necessary for normal spermatogenesis, whereas testosterone production requires only LH.

Luteinizing hormone–releasing hormone [LHRH, also known as gonadotropin-releasing hormone (GnRH)], a decapeptide produced by the arcuate nuclei of the hypothalamus, is responsible for the release of both LH and FSH. Extrahypothalamic LHRH is present in other areas of the brain as well. Noradrenergic agonists appear to facilitate, whereas endogenous opioids inhibit, LHRH release.

LHRH stimulates and induces high-affinity pituitary receptors to stimulate LH and FSH production and release. The pituitary response to LHRH varies greatly throughout life. LHRH and the gonadotropins first appear in the fetus at about 10 weeks of gestation. During the first 3 months after birth, LHRH elicits a brisk gonadotropin rise. The sensitivity to LHRH then declines until the onset of puberty. Before puberty, the FSH response to LHRH is greater than that of LH. With the onset of puberty sensitivity to LHRH increases, and pulsatile LH secretion, first noted during sleep, ensues. Later in puberty and during the reproductive years, pulsations are present throughout the day, with LH responsiveness being greater than that of FSH. After the menopause FSH and LH concentrations rise, and postmenopausal FSH levels are higher than those of LH.

Pulsatile LHRH release results in pulsatile LH and FSH release. However, sustained infusion of LHRH and its analogues results in inhibition of LH and FSH release. This phenomenon has been utilized in the successful treatment of gonadotropin-mediated precocious puberty by the sustained administration of LHRH or its analogues. Conversely, in people with LHRH deficiency, the pulsatile administration of LHRH can restore a normal menstrual cycle or normal sperm and testosterone production.

The feedback relationship between the gonadal steroids and the hypothalamus and pituitary is detailed in Chaps. 321 and 322. Low doses of estrogens decrease the frequency of LHRH pulses and, more importantly, decrease the pituitary response to LHRH; this phenomenon is seen most clearly in postmenopausal women with elevated gonadotropins. However, sustained elevation of estrogens results in a positive feedback signal that stimulates LHRH and LH release; this phenomenon is responsible, in part, for the LH surge prior to ovulation. The sensitivity of LHRH to this positive feedback by estrogen increases during mid- to late puberty. Although progesterone decreases LHRH pulse frequency, the progesterone rise in the late follicular phase augments the pituitary LH response to LHRH and contributes to the LH surge. In castrated men, testosterone administration usually suppresses LH to undetectable levels and less often lowers FSH to normal (but not undetectable) concentrations. Inhibin, a peptide hormone produced by the testicular Sertoli cell and ovarian granulosa cell, is a potent inhibitor of FSH (but not LH) release. Its physiologic role is undefined. Testosterone decreases the frequency of LH pulsations, probably by a direct effect on LHRH release, and is converted in many tissues, including the brain, to estradiol, which inhibits the pituitary response to LHRH.

Gonadotropin measurements In postmenopausal women and men with primary hypogonadism, gonadal failure results in a marked increase in FSH and LH concentrations, providing an endogenous stimulation test. Such elevated gonadotropin concentrations ensure the adequacy of pituitary gonadotroph function. On the other hand, gonadotropin measurements are rarely indicated in a woman with ovulatory menses and in men with normal sperm counts. In evaluating gonadal failure associated with low testosterone concentrations in men or low estradiol levels in women, gonadotropin measurements help separate primary from central (secondary, hypogonadotropic) hypogonadism: high gonadotropin concentrations are indicative of primary gonadal failure; low or normal gonadotropin concentrations suggest hypothalamic or pituitary disease (see Chap. 312).

HYPOGONADOTROPIC (CENTRAL, SECONDARY) HYPOGONADISM Isolated gonadotropin deficiency may be present at birth as a congenital or hereditary disorder. Kallmann's syndrome is inherited as a single gene trait, afflicts men more severely than women, and is characterized by gonadotropin deficiency frequently associated with anosmia and midline anatomic defects. Kallmann's syndrome appears to be due to LHRH deficiency, as most patients secrete gonadotropins in response to LHRH administration after suitable priming. Acquired defects of LHRH production are common: hyperprolactinemia causes amenorrhea due to inhibition of LHRH release, possibly mediated by increased hypothalamic dopamine. Amenorrhea in anorexia nervosa, starvation, long-distance runners, and "stress" appears to be due to inhibition of LHRH release as well. Gonadotropin deficiency may be a relatively early defect in patients with large pituitary adenomas. Gonadotropin deficiency also occurs in patients with polyglandular endocrine deficiencies, presumably on an autoimmune basis (see Chap. 325) and in patients with hemochromatosis.

Patients with LHRH deficiency who desire fertility may respond to pulsatile therapy with LHRH or its agonists. When gonadotropin deficiency is due to pituitary disease, injections of FSH (menotropin) and chorionic gonadotropin (a hormone with LH-like activity) are necessary to achieve fertility.

ECTOPIC GONADOTROPIN SECRETION AND GONADOTROPIN-SECRETING TUMORS Ectopic gonadotropin production (usually hCG) can be associated with germinomas of the nonseminoma type (see Chap. 305), lung carcinomas, hepatomas, and other tumors. Children may develop precocious puberty, and men may develop gynecomastia. No distinct clinical syndrome occurs in women. Pituitary gonadotropin-secreting tumors are relatively common. Approximately 4 percent of all pituitary adenomas demonstrate gonadotropins or their subunits on immunologic staining; how often these tumors secrete gonadotropins is not clear.

FSH-secreting pituitary adenomas are large tumors, most commonly diagnosed in men with decreased libido, decreased serum testosterone, and normal prolactin levels. The finding of an increased FSH concentration may be misinterpreted as indicating primary hypogonadism if a pituitary adenoma is not suspected. The majority of these tumors overproduce intact FSH, but increased FSH beta and alpha subunits are common as well. About 40 percent demonstrate enhanced FSH secretion after TRH administration. Normal subjects and patients with primary hypogonadism do not have increased FSH secretion after TRH. Despite the normal or elevated LH concentrations in these patients, testosterone concentrations are low and respond normally to hCG administration. This suggests that the LH measured by radioimmunoassay is biologically inactive or that it represents immunologic cross-reactivity due to LH subunit overproduction.

LH-secreting pituitary adenomas are usually large tumors and are characterized by increased serum testosterone, elevated LH levels, and normal or low FSH concentrations, often with partial hypopituitarism. It is often difficult to diagnose gonadotropin-secreting pituitary adenomas in postmenopausal women because of the elevated gonadotropins associated with menopause. When faced with a large pituitary tumor and elevated plasma gonadotropin levels, with or without testosterone deficiency, the diagnosis is straightforward. However, differentiating primary hypogonadism (low testosterone with elevated FSH and LH) from the rare gonadotropin-secreting tumor of the pituitary with similar biochemistry presents a clinical dilemma. The preserved testicular response to exogenous hCG points toward a gonadotroph adenoma.

THYROTROPIN

PHYSIOLOGY TSH is a glycoprotein hormone (28,000 mol wt) composed of an alpha subunit which it shares with LH, FSH, and hCG and a unique beta subunit that confers specificity (also see Chap. 316). The genes coding for the alpha and beta subunits are on different chromosomes. TSH is produced by thyrotrophs which constitute about 10 percent of the cells of the anterior pituitary. TSH regulates the biosynthesis, storage, and release of thyroid hormones and determines thyroid gland size. TSH first appears in the fetal pituitary at about 10 weeks of gestation. TSH levels in normal subjects average 0.5 to 5.0 mU/L, with a slight increase in the nocturnal hours.

Thyrotropin-releasing hormone (TRH), the major hypothalamic mediator of TSH release, is a tripeptide found in highest concentrations in the medial division of the hypothalamic paraventricular nuclei and in the median eminence. Extrahypothalamic TRH is found in the posterior pituitary, in other parts of the brain and spinal cord, and in the gastrointestinal tract. TRH stimulates TSH secretion by increasing cytoplasmic free calcium; phosphatidylinositol and membrane phospholipids probably participate in TRH-stimulated TSH secretion. TRH stimulates the release of prolactin as well as that of TSH. The prolactin response is enhanced in hypothyroidism and diminished in hyperthyroidism. TRH-induced GH stimulation may occur in acromegaly, renal failure, depression, in many normal children, and in occasional normal adults.

The thyroid hormones thyroxine (T_4) and triiodothyronine (T_3) inhibit TSH production directly at the pituitary level. Both T_3 and T_4 bind to receptors on pituitary nuclei, but T_3 has a 40-fold greater affinity for these receptors than does T_4. Nevertheless, exogenous T_4 is more potent than T_3 in inhibiting TSH release because circulating T_4 is a more effective means of delivering T_3 to the pituitary than is T_3 itself. Half of intrapituitary T_3 is derived from T_4 conversion within the pituitary. The effects of T_4 and T_3 on hypothalamic TRH release in humans are unknown, but in animals they cause inhibition of TRH release. In hyperthyroidism TSH is suppressed, and the TSH response to TRH is absent; in primary hypothyroidism the basal TSH concentration is elevated, and the response to TRH is exaggerated.

Somatostatin decreases basal TSH release, the TSH response to TRH, and the nocturnal TSH peak. Dopamine and glucocorticoids decrease basal TSH concentration and the TSH response to TRH. Patients with untreated primary adrenal insufficiency may have slightly elevated TSH levels.

TSH concentrations can be interpreted only when serum thyroid hormone concentrations are known (see Chap. 312). In hyperthyroidism, thyroid hormone levels are elevated and TSH release is inhibited. Only sensitive TSH assays can differentiate between low and normal concentrations. A detectable serum TSH concentration by an ultrasensitive assay excludes conventional hyperthyroidism. Low thyroid hormone and elevated serum TSH concentrations are characteristic of primary hypothyroidism. Low thyroid hormone concentrations with a "normal" or "low" TSH concentration are found in central (secondary) hypothyroidism. The TRH stimulation test (no TSH response in hyperthyroidism, exaggerated TSH response in primary hypothyroidism) has largely been supplanted by sensitive TSH measurements. The TRH stimulation test is also not useful in the diagnosis of secondary hypothyroidism or in differentiating pituitary from hypothalamic disease.

PRIMARY HYPOTHYROIDISM Thyroid gland failure (primary hypothyroidism) leads to compensatory hypertrophy of the thyrotrophs. With thyroid failure of long duration, the pituitary gland and the sella turcica may enlarge. Although TSH-secreting tumors may develop in animals after thyroid gland removal, the increased TSH and pituitary size in human hypothyroidism is not autonomous and decreases with thyroid hormone replacement. Since hyperprolactinemia may also occur in patients with primary hypothyroidism, pituitary enlargement (hyperplasia) may be incorrectly diagnosed as a prolactinoma; however, the return to normal of prolactin concentrations with thyroid hormone therapy excludes that diagnosis. Severe primary hypothyroidism may occasionally cause impaired release of GH and ACTH after appropriate stimuli (so-called pituitary myxedema), and hypothyroid children may develop precocious puberty. These abnormalities are all corrected with thyroid hormone therapy.

SECONDARY HYPOTHYROIDISM Hypothyroidism due to pituitary or hypothalamic disease may be difficult to diagnose. With primary hypothyroidism serum TSH commonly rises before thyroid hormone concentrations decline below the normal range. No similar early laboratory clue exists in secondary hypothyroidism. Patients with central hypothyroidism usually do not have goiter, and many have deficiencies of other pituitary trophic hormones.

Some patients with hypothalamic hypothyroidism have mild TSH elevations, rather than normal or low concentrations as expected. Although the TSH elevations rarely exceed 10 mU/L, they are above the expected range for hypothyroidism due to TSH deficiency. Biologically inactive but immunologically active thyrotropin is present in such cases. After TRH injection, TSH concentration rises, and the biologic potency of the TSH is increased. This suggests an additional role for TRH in controlling the biologic activity of the TSH molecule by controlling its rate of glycosylation.

PITUITARY (TSH-INDUCED) HYPERTHYROIDISM Hyperthyroidism is not usually a disease of TSH overproduction. However, two types of TSH-mediated hyperthyroidism are recognized:

1 Pituitary tumors. These are usually macroadenomas with autonomous TSH secretion, unresponsive to thyroid hormone suppression or TRH stimulation. A hallmark of such tumors is overproduction of the glycoprotein hormone alpha subunit (TSH alpha), with a serum molar ratio of alpha to intact TSH of greater than 1:1. The free alpha subunit may be an important tumor marker and differs from the native alpha subunit in that one of its amino acids is carbohydrate-blocked and hence cannot combine with beta subunits. These tumors may produce other pituitary hormones in addition to TSH, most commonly GH. TSH and TSH alpha subunit secretion decrease with octreotide therapy.

2 Pituitary resistance to thyroid hormone. In this situation thyroid hormone fails to inhibit TSH secretion appropriately in the absence of a pituitary adenoma. Since TSH secretion is not inhibited, TSH rises and stimulates thyroid hormone overproduction. The peripheral tissues are not resistant to thyroid hormone, and clinical hyperthyroidism results. The pituitary resistance to thyroid hormone is incomplete since TSH can be suppressed with supraphysiologic levels of thyroid hormone and stimulated further with TRH; bromocriptine or octreotide may lower TSH as well. Pituitary resistance is usually diagnosed after thyroid gland ablation, when

TSH cannot be lowered to normal values with the usual therapeutic doses of thyroid hormone. However, once the hyperthyroidism has been treated, pituitary resistance is of no clinical consequence.

ADRENOCORTICOTROPIC HORMONE

PHYSIOLOGY ACTH is produced by corticotrophs which comprise about 15 percent of anterior pituitary cells, located principally in the central portion. ACTH is synthesized as part of a large precursor molecule termed pro-opiomelanocortin (POMC, 265 amino acids) (see Chap. 317). ACTH contains 39 amino acids, with near complete biologic activity residing in the N-terminal 26 amino acids. In the anterior pituitary POMC is cleaved to yield ACTH, β-lipotropin, and an N-terminal precursor.

ACTH controls the release of cortisol from the adrenal cortex. Although aldosterone is primarily controlled by the renin-angiotensin system, ACTH also stimulates aldosterone release acutely. Other derivatives of the POMC molecule, such as γ-melanocyte-stimulating hormone (γ-MSH), also influence aldosterone production and are found in increased concentrations in the plasma of patients with idiopathic hyperaldosteronism. Patients with ACTH deficiency have near-normal aldosterone production and do not require mineralocorticoid replacement therapy.

Corticotropin-releasing hormone (CRH) is the major but not exclusive regulator of ACTH release. CRH contains 41 amino acids on a single polypeptide chain. CRH is produced primarily by neurons of the paraventricular nuclei of the hypothalamus but is also present in other areas of the brain, including the limbic system and cortex, as well as in the pancreas, gut, and adrenal medulla. The placenta has the highest concentration outside the nervous system. CRH stimulates cyclic AMP production and regulates intracellular calcium and increases the concentration of POMC messenger RNA. Vasopressin potentiates the ACTH-releasing properties of CRH through a cyclic AMP–independent mechanism and may play a physiologic role in ACTH release. Beta-adrenergic stimuli and oxytocin cause ACTH release as well. Somatostatin blocks CRH-induced ACTH release.

ACTH is released in pulses with an overriding circadian rhythm. With a normal sleeping pattern, ACTH concentration is highest in the early morning (around 4 A.M.) and lowest in late evening. The characteristic diurnal rhythm of plasma cortisol occurs in response to these ACTH changes. In primary adrenal insufficiency (Addison's disease), cortisol concentrations fall and ACTH concentrations rise. This results in hyperpigmentation owing to the melanocyte-stimulating properties of ACTH. Cortisol administration inhibits ACTH release, a phenomenon dependent upon both the rate of rise of cortisol and its absolute concentration. Increased plasma cortisol inhibits CRH-induced ACTH release and may also inhibit CRH release. When supraphysiologic doses of glucocorticoids are given for prolonged periods, the hypothalamic-pituitary–adrenal cortex axis may remain suppressed for months after the drugs have been stopped, probably as the result of prolonged hypothalamic CRH suppression (see Chap. 317).

Stress, including hypoglycemia, surgery, and psychic distress, stimulates ACTH release, in part via increased CRH release. However, the magnitude of the ACTH release is greater than can be achieved during maximal stimulation with CRH. With severe illness, the requirements for cortisol may increase tenfold; failure to achieve these levels of cortisol during such periods may result in clinical adrenal insufficiency when adrenal reserve is impaired.

In normal persons ACTH circulates in low concentrations [2 to 18 pmol/L (10 to 80 pg/mL)]. It is difficult to measure ACTH in plasma and often not possible to separate low from normal values using commercial assays. Random ACTH measurements have little clinical significance. Tests for adrenal insufficiency and excess rely primarily on measurements of cortisol and its metabolites rather than on measurement of ACTH.

ACTH EXCESS (CUSHING'S DISEASE AND NELSON'S SYNDROME) Clinical features Cortisol excess is characterized by a central distribution of adipose tissue, muscle weakness, purplish striae, hypertension, amenorrhea, osteoporosis, fatigue, and psychiatric abnormalities. This syndrome may be caused by pituitary or ectopic ACTH overproduction, adrenal tumors, or exogenous glucocorticoid administration.

The presence of cortisol excess is established by the finding of increased excretion of urine free cortisol and/or 17-hydroxycorticosteroids that fails to decrease appropriately after either overnight (1 mg at midnight) or 2-day low-dose dexamethasone administration (0.5 mg every 6 h for eight doses). Additional suppression (and occasionally stimulation) tests are required to determine whether the Cushing's syndrome is due to a pituitary lesion. In patients with pituitary ACTH hypersecretion, either high-dose overnight (8 mg at midnight) or 2-day dexamethasone administration (2 mg every 6 h for 8 doses) results in suppression of urine 17-hydroxycorticosteroids and free cortisol and plasma cortisol, usually by greater than 50 percent. Urine 17-hydroxycorticosteroids increase after metyrapone administration in Cushing's disease. Plasma ACTH levels are normal or high-normal and show an exaggerated increase after CRH administration. Pituitary ACTH hypersecretion (Cushing's disease) is caused by a corticotroph microadenoma in 90 percent of patients and by a macroadenoma in most of the rest. Corticotroph hyperplasia has been documented in a few cases. The microadenomas are often small (3 mm or less) and may be difficult to find on CT or conventional MRI scanning. High-resolution MRI scanning with gadolinium may improve the localization of these tumors. Previously pituitary surgery was often recommended on the basis of dynamic testing alone. However, bilateral inferior petrosal sinus catheterization to localize the site of ACTH production can be used to confirm the pituitary source of ACTH production and to localize functioning adenomas when all imaging studies are negative.

Treatment Transsphenoidal microsurgery is successful in treating microadenomas in about 75 percent of patients. When surgery is successful, plasma cortisol concentrations fall almost to zero and often remain low for many months owing to delayed recovery of CRH and ACTH secretion by the hypothalamus and normal remaining pituitary. However, adrenal function eventually returns to normal in most patients. Cushing's syndrome may recur, however, even after apparently curative surgery. Previously, bilateral adrenalectomy was the therapy of choice for patients with pituitary Cushing's disease. Unfortunately, after this procedure enlarging pituitary adenomas with increased skin pigmentation (Nelson's syndrome) develop in 10 to 30 percent of patients.

Ectopic ACTH production is a relatively common disorder and can cause great difficulty in diagnosis (see Chaps. 309 and 317). When ACTH production is caused by rapidly growing tumors such as oat cell carcinoma of the lung, symptoms of Cushing's syndrome are blunted. Rather, patients have hypokalemia, muscle weakness, weight loss, and hyperpigmentation. ACTH concentrations often exceed 66 pmol/L (300 pg/mL) and do not change with dexamethasone administration. When slow-growing tumors such as thymic carcinoids, bronchial carcinoids, medullary carcinoma of the thyroid, and pancreatic islet cell tumors produce ACTH the typical features of Cushing's syndrome are common. In the latter group ACTH measurements and cortisol response to dexamethasone administration may mimic those found in patients with pituitary adenomas. However, with ectopic ACTH production ACTH concentrations generally do not change after CRH administration. When differentiation between pituitary and ectopic ACTH production is uncertain, bilateral inferior petrosal sinus catheterization is necessary. Cushing's syndrome can rarely be caused by ectopic production of CRH itself.

ACTH DEFICIENCY (SECONDARY ADRENAL INSUFFICIENCY) ACTH deficiency may be isolated or occur in association with other anterior pituitary hormone deficiencies. Reversible isolated ACTH deficiency is common after long-term glucocorticoid administration. If glucocorticoids are withdrawn suddenly in this situation or continued in physiologic doses when severe illness is present, adrenal insufficiency may occur (see Chap. 317). Symptoms include nausea, vomiting, fatigue, joint discomfort, and dizziness, and there may be fever, hypotension, hyponatremia, and hypoglycemia. Although cortisol is necessary for free water excretion, it is not needed for potassium excretion. Hence patients with ACTH deficiency are not hyperkalemic as are patients with primary adrenal insufficiency. Hyperpigmentation does not occur. These factors make diagnosis of secondary adrenal insufficiency more difficult than that of primary adrenal insufficiency. Isolated ACTH deficiency may occur without prior glucocorticoid therapy.

In general, patients undergoing pituitary surgery need to be treated with ''stress'' doses of glucocorticoids until normal adrenal function can be demonstrated postoperatively. All patients with pituitary macroadenomas or hypothalamic disease require testing of the pituitary-adrenal axis, but when pituitary surgery is planned testing can be limited in focus until after surgery is completed.

THE ENDOGENOUS OPIOID PEPTIDES

The endogenous opioid peptides, the enkephalins and endorphins, constitute approximately 10 to 15 substances that range in length from 5 to 31 amino acids (Fig. 313-7). Although these peptides are chemically unrelated to morphine, they bind to and act via the same opioid receptor. Although the opioid peptides have common chemical features, they arise via different biosynthetic pathways. In the pituitary β-endorphin, the most abundant endorphin, is synthesized as part of a larger precursor molecule (pro-opiomelanocortin, POMC) that also contains the full sequence of ACTH, α-melanocyte-stimulating hormone (α-MSH), β-MSH, and β-lipotropin (β-LPH) (Fig. 313-8). This precursor molecule also has the potential to generate other forms of endorphin, fragments termed α-endorphin and γ-endorphin. Cleavage sites within POMC allow the generation of each of the above-mentioned peptides in some anatomic sites. The biosynthetic pathway represents the only means by which the pituitary gland produces ACTH. Therefore, the biosyntheses of ACTH and β-endorphin are inextricably linked in the corticotroph cells of the pituitary by derivation from a single gene that encodes both hormones.

Different processing of POMC occurs within other tissues, depending on the enzymatic machinery within the tissues. For instance,

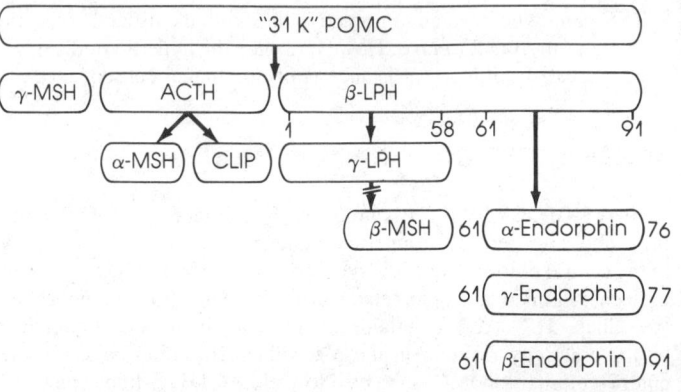

FIGURE 313-8 Biosynthetic pathway for β-endorphin in the pituitary gland. A single precursor protein, pro-opiomelanocortin (POMC) (molecular weight of approximately 31,000), is initially synthesized from translation of a gene that encodes the structure of adrenocorticotropin (ACTH), β-lipotropin (β-LPH), and β-endorphin. Prohormone-type cleavages can generate other hormones from the same precursor, although this occurs in tissues other than the pituitary. Abbreviations: MSH = melanocyte-stimulating hormone; LPH = lipotropin; CLIP = corticotropin-like intermediate peptide; ACTH = adrenocorticotropin.

although the pituitary does not metabolize ACTH to smaller fragments, the hypothalamus converts the precursor molecule to α-MSH. β-MSH is generated in the intermediate lobe of lower species. Humans lack an intermediate lobe and produce β-MSH in scattered cells within the pituitary. Although different cell types may synthesize the same primary gene product, the final profile of hormone secretion can differ completely.

The enkephalins are derived from different precursors. The adrenal glands synthesize enkephalins as part of a large protein, proenkephalin A, that contains six repeats of the Met-enkephalin sequence and one Leu-enkephalin structure. Dynorphins and enoendorphins are derived from a third distinct precursor molecule, proenkephalin B. Additional (''cryptic'') peptides are encoded within the structures of these precursor proteins and have the potential to be released by ''prohormone-type'' cleavages. It is not known whether these peptides are secreted into the blood in vivo.

ACTH, β-endorphin, and β-LPH synthesis and secretion by the

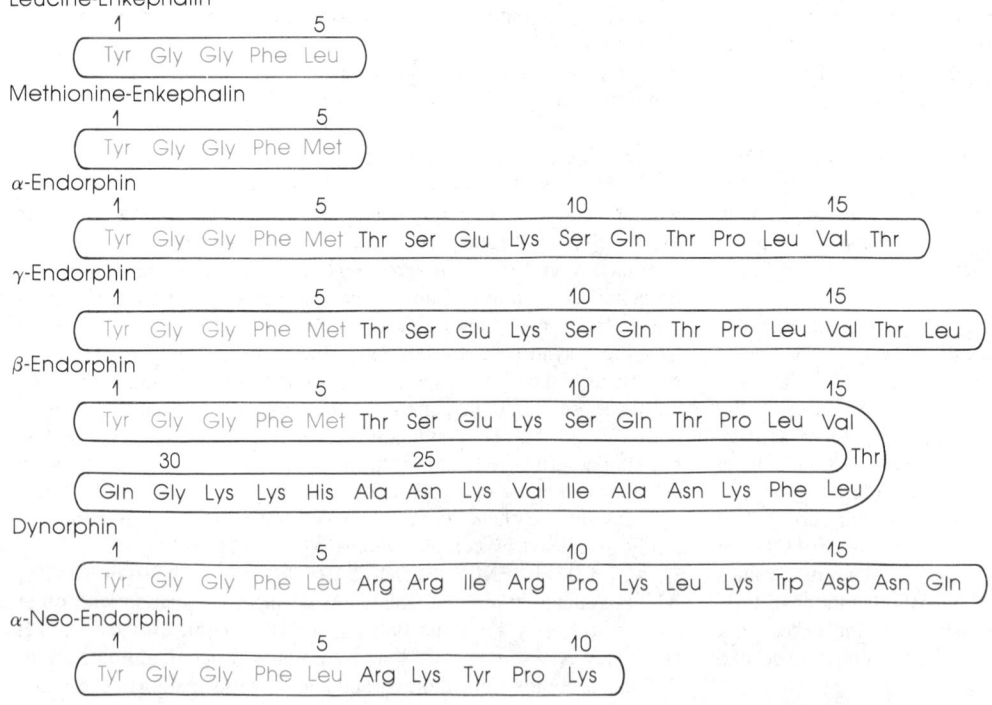

FIGURE 313-7 Structure of several endogenous opiate peptides. The amino-terminal (leftmost) four amino acids are identical in each peptide. At position 5, a methionine or leucine is found.

pituitary are linked both in normal and in abnormal states. Under normal conditions, β-LPH circulates in higher molar concentration than does β-endorphin, but the usual radioimmunoassays recognize both entities. Hence, levels of immunoreactive β-endorphin reflect the combined levels of β-endorphin and β-LPH. In adrenal insufficiency the plasma levels of both ACTH and β-endorphin are elevated; likewise, glucocorticoid replacement decreases the levels of both. Administration of corticotropin-releasing hormone (CRH) stimulates release of both ACTH and β-endorphin in a parallel manner, and in Nelson's syndrome the plasma levels of both ACTH and β-endorphin are elevated. Ectopic production of ACTH by tumors is also accompanied by β-endorphin excess. In the latter case, measurement of β-endorphin levels can be useful as a tumor marker and in some patients serves to monitor treatment. β-Endorphin and β-LPH have a longer half-life in blood than does ACTH, and measurement of plasma β-endorphin may be useful for the diagnosis of Cushing's disease.

The pituitary is the richest site of endorphin in the body. In the pituitary, ACTH and endorphin-containing cells are found in the anteromedial region of the anterior lobe, at the posterior boundary of the anterior lobe, and in nerve fibers of the posterior lobe. The hypothalamus also contains neurons that synthesize endorphin. These neurons have long projections to other regions of the brain. For example, regions of the brain associated with the limbic system contain substantial quantities of immunoreactive β-endorphin, suggesting a role in memory, learning, and emotions.

Neurons containing the enkephalins are even more widely distributed in the central nervous sytem. Levels are particularly high in the dorsal horn of the spinal cord, a region that contains opiate receptors and that is involved in the transmission of pain (see Chap. 15). Enkephalins are also present in the gastrointestinal tract. Concentrations in the myenteric plexus of the longitudinal muscles of the gut are higher than in the brain. Enkephalins are synthesized in the chromaffin cells of the adrenal medulla and packaged together with the catecholamines in the same secretory granules. Enkephalin is released as part of the sympathetic response to stress together with epinephrine and norepinephrine. Similarly, plasma enkephalin levels are high in pheochromocytoma.

Two general approaches have been employed to define the physiologic role of endorphins. One is to determine the effects of administration of endogenous opiate peptides to animals or humans. For example, the administration of β-endorphin produces an increase in the secretion of GH, prolactin, and vasopressin and a decrease in the secretion of ACTH, cortisol, LH, and FSH. The second approach is to assess the effects of antagonists of the opiates, such as naloxone. Such agents block the effects of endogenously secreted opiates, revealing the tonic or physiologic role of opiate peptides. Naloxone administration causes elevations in LH, FSH, and ACTH levels and prevents the stress-mediated rise in prolactin levels.

A variety of physiologic actions have been postulated for these hormones including: (1) morphine-like analgesic properties; (2) behavioral effects; and (3) neurotransmitter and neuromodulator functions. Indeed, these peptides may play a role in memory, learning, response to stress, reproduction, pain transmission, and regulation of appetite, temperature, and respiration. In addition, the placebo response, acupuncture-mediated analgesia, stress-induced amenorrhea, and the pathogenesis of shock may be mediated in part by enkephalins and the endorphins. Tranquilization, irritability, agitation, violent behavior, catalepsy, narcolepsy, catatonia, the smoking habit, alcoholism, and drug addiction may reflect biochemical abnormalities of the system.

DISEASES OF THE HYPOTHALAMUS AND PITUITARY

Diseases that affect the hypothalamus and pituitary can have both endocrine and nonendocrine manifestations.

HYPOTHALAMUS   The human hypothalamus weighs about 4 g; hypothalamic dysfunction occurs only when disease is bilateral.

Tumors in this region are often slow-growing and may achieve large size before symptoms appear. Signs of hydrocephalus or focal cerebral dysfunction may coexist with hypopituitarism and hypothalamic dysfunction. The hypothalamus exerts both endocrine and nonendocrine functions. Hypothalamic control of the pituitary gland has been discussed above. Nonendocrine functions are also influenced by the hypothalamus:

1 Food intake and feeding behavior. The basal hypothalamus controls maintenance of a stable weight. Several regions of the hypothalamus are implicated in hunger and satiety. The ventromedial nucleus is known to be involved in satiety, but it now appears that anterior hypothalamic regions are also concerned. Stimulation and termination of food ingestion appear to be affected by several neuropeptides, including the opioid peptides and neuropeptide Y. Hypothalamic obesity in humans is usually associated with lesions of the ventromedial nucleus; this obesity appears to involve a resetting of the weight set point. Marked hyperphagia, possibly related to rapid gastric emptying, occurs until the new weight set point is reached. Patients often demonstrate decreased activity and finicky eating once the new set point is reached. Other factors including thyroid and adrenal hormones also influence feeding behavior.

2 Temperature regulation. The anterior hypothalamus contains warm- and cold-sensitive neurons that respond to local and environmental thermal gradients. The posterior hypothalamus generates the signals necessary for heat dissipation. The temperature increase associated with infections is generated by the hypothalamus. Phagocytic cells throughout the body produce interleukin 1 (endogenous pyrogen) which stimulates the anterior hypothalamus to produce prostaglandin E_2. Prostaglandin E_2 raises the thermostat set point, leading to heat conservation (e.g., vasoconstriction) and increased heat production (e.g., muscle shivering) until blood and core temperatures match the new hypothalamic set point.

Abnormalities of temperature regulation may occur with hypothalamic disease. Hypothermia is a rare consequence of diffuse hypothalamic disease. Paroxysmal hypothermia with sweating, flushing, and a fall in body temperatures may occur, and sustained hyperthermia without tachycardia is reported with acute pathologic processes such as hemorrhage into the third ventricle. Poikilothermia (a change in body temperature of greater than 1°C with change in environmental temperature) is usually a consequence of posterior hypothalamic disease. Paroxysmal hyperthermia with episodic shaking chills, spiking fevers, and autonomic phenomena is a rare manifestation. It is important to remember that adrenal insufficiency can cause fever or hypothermia and that hypothyroidism may cause hypothermia.

3 Sleep-wake cycle. Lesions in the sleep center of the anterior hypothalamus result in insomnia. The posterior hypothalamus is important for arousal and maintenance of the waking state; posterior hypothalamic destruction due to ischemia, encephalitis, or trauma can result in a hypersomnolent state from which arousal is possible. Larger lesions extending to the reticular formation of the rostral midbrain cause coma (see Chap. 31).

4 Memory and behavior. Lesions of the ventromedial hypothalamus and premammillary region result in loss of short-term memory, often with Korsakoff's syndrome. Longer-term memory is often intact. Hypothalamic lesions may also cause a more typical picture of dementia. Rage reactions may result with ventromedial lesions, and lateral hypothalamic destruction may cause an apathetic state.

5 Thirst. The hypothalamus is the center for vasopressin production and for the control of thirst by serum osmolality. Impaired thirst may occur with hypothalamic lesions; rarely primary polydipsia without diabetes insipidus is a consequence of hypothalamic lesions.

6 Autonomic nervous system function. Parasympathetic pathways are stimulated by the anterior hypothalamus; sympathetic pathways are stimulated by the posterior hypothalamus. Diencephalic epilepsy is a rare syndrome associated with paroxysms of autonomic hyperactivity.

A diencephalic syndrome in children, characterized by emaciation, hyperkinesis and inappropriate affect, often with a cheerful disposition, can be caused by invasive tumors of the anterior and basal hypothalamus. Most of these children die by the age of 2 years, but in those who survive the clinical picture changes to one of increased appetite with obesity, irritability, and rage reactions.

In general, slow-growing tumors produce dementia, disturbances of food intake (obesity or emaciation), and endocrine dysfunction. Acute destructive processes are more likely to cause coma or disturbances of the autonomic nervous system.

Diseases of the anterior hypothalamus include craniopharyngiomas, gliomas of the optic nerve, sphenoid ridge meningiomas, granulomatous disease (including sarcoidosis), germinomas, and aneurysms of the internal carotid artery. Suprasellar pituitary adenomas and tuberculum sella meningiomas may grow into the hypothalamus as well. Lesions of the posterior hypothalamus include gliomas, hamartomas, ependymomas, germinomas, and teratomas.

Precocious puberty, particularly in males, can be associated with "pinealomas." However, these pinealomas actually are germinomas, and the precocious puberty appears to result from the ectopic production of chorionic gonadotropin by these tumors rather than from an effect on pituitary gonadotropins.

Craniopharyngiomas   Craniopharyngiomas arise from remnants of Rathke's pouch. Most of these tumors are suprasellar, but about 15 percent are intrasellar. The tumors are usually cystic or partially cystic, often contain calcium, and are lined with stratified squamous epithelium. Although craniopharyngiomas are usually manifested in childhood, 45 percent of patients are over the age of 20, and 20 percent are over the age of 40 at the time of diagnosis.

Children usually present with signs of increased intracranial pressure due to hydrocephalus (80 percent) including headache, vomiting, and papilledema. Visual abnormalities such as loss of vision and field cuts are found in 60 percent. Short stature is sometimes found (7 to 40 percent), but retarded bone age is more common. Delayed sexual development occurs in about 20 percent, and diabetes insipidus may be present.

About 80 percent of adults present with visual complaints, and an additional 10 percent have visual abnormalities on careful testing. Papilledema is present in about 15 percent of adults. Headaches (40 percent), mental deterioration or personality change (26 percent), and hypogonadism (35 percent) are relatively common in adults. Hyperprolactinemia is present in one-third to one-half of patients, but prolactin levels rarely exceed 100 to 150 µg/L. Diabetes insipidus (15 percent), weight gain (15 percent), and panhypopituitarism (7 percent) may occur as well. Rarely, the cyst contents spill into the cerebrospinal fluid, causing a picture of aseptic meningitis.

Suprasellar calcification (see Fig. 313-13) in a flocculent, granular, or curvilinear pattern is present on skull x-rays in most children and in some adults with craniopharyngioma. Calcification is evident on CT scan in most of these adults, however. Hypothalamic germinomas may calcify as well. Skull x-ray abnormalities include calcification, sellar enlargement, and signs of increased intracranial pressure in 90 percent of children and 60 percent of adults.

Therapy of craniopharyngiomas is often unsatisfactory. Total removal often results in major functional deficits. We generally favor biopsy and partial resection followed by conventional radiation as a more conservative approach. Tumors less than 3 cm in diameter have a better prognosis.

Germ cell tumors   Germinomas originate in the posterior third ventricle, anterior third ventricle (supra- or intrasellar), or in both locations (also see Chap. 305). Germinomas (also known as atypical teratomas) were previously confused with parenchymal tumors of the pineal (pinealomas); when located in the anterior third ventricle they were known as "ectopic pinealomas." Germinomas often infiltrate the hypothalamus and occasionally metastasize to the cerebrospinal fluid or distant sites.

The majority of patients have diabetes insipidus in association with variable anterior pituitary insufficiency. Precocious puberty may occur in boys, probably due to hCG production by these tumors. Diplopia, headache, vomiting, lethargy, weight loss, and hydrocephalus are common. The tumors usually begin in childhood but may be diagnosed in young adults. Because germinomas are radiosensitive, early recognition is important. When the tumor is located in the anterior third ventricle, biopsy by the transsphenoidal route is often possible. Tumors in the pineal region are more difficult to biopsy, leading some authors to recommend empirical radiation therapy or chemotherapy, whereas others prefer surgical biopsy or debulking followed by radiation and chemotherapy. Germinomas of the nonseminoma type may produce hCG and/or α-fetoprotein, whereas pure seminomas rarely produce tumor markers (see Chap. 305).

PITUITARY ADENOMAS   Pituitary adenomas account for about 10 to 15 percent of intracranial neoplasms. They can cause anterior pituitary hormonal imbalance, structural problems related to invasion of surrounding structures, or syndromes of hormone excess. Occasionally, the diagnosis is the result of incidental findings during skull x-ray examinations. Small pituitary tumors are present in 6 to 20 percent of adults at autopsy.

Pathology   Pituitary tumors were previously classified as basophilic, acidophilic, or chromophobic on the basis of hematoxylin and eosin staining. Corticotroph adenomas are generally basophilic; the more densely granulated prolactin-secreting tumors are acidophilic; the majority of prolactinomas, sparsely granulated GH-secreting tumors, TSH-secreting and gonadotropin-secreting tumors, and nonsecreting tumors are all chromophobic. Because this classification provides little insight into hormone production, it has been abandoned. Many nonfunctioning pituitary tumors are, however, still referred to as "chromophobes." Classification can also be based upon immunohistochemical staining or according to hormonal secretion, based upon hormone measurements in serum.

Furthermore, pituitary tumors have been classified by Hardy according to size and invasive characteristics. Stage I tumors are microadenomas (less than 10 mm in diameter) that may cause hormonal oversecretion but do not cause hypopituitarism and are not associated with structural problems. Stage II tumors are macroadenomas (greater than 10 mm) with or without suprasellar extension. Stage III tumors are macroadenomas that locally invade the floor of the sella and may cause sellar enlargement and suprasellar extension. Stage IV tumors are invasive macroadenomas with diffuse destruction of the sella, with or without suprasellar extension. The difficulty with this system of classification is that not all pituitary tumors fall neatly into one of these categories. For example, it may be difficult to separate thinning of the sellar floor (stage II) from erosion through the floor (stage III).

Endocrine manifestations   Anterior pituitary hormone overproduction is suspected on clinical grounds and confirmed by appropriate laboratory evaluation (see Table 313-5). The most common secretory pituitary tumors are prolactinomas. They cause galactorrhea and hypogonadism, including amenorrhea, infertility, and impotence. GH-secreting tumors are the next most common secretory pituitary tumors and cause acromegaly or gigantism. Next in frequency are corticotroph (ACTH-secreting) adenomas which cause cortisol excess (Cushing's disease). Glycoprotein hormone–secreting pituitary adenomas (secreting TSH, LH, or FSH) are the least common. TSH-secreting adenomas are a rare cause of hyperthyroidism. Paradoxically, most patients with gonadotropin-secreting adenomas have hypogonadism.

About 15 percent of patients with tumors that come to surgery have adenomas that secrete more than one pituitary hormone. The most common combination is GH and prolactin, and other common patterns are GH-TSH, GH-prolactin-TSH, and ACTH-prolactin. Most of these tumors have one cell secreting two hormones (unimorphous), but some tumors have two or more cell types, each of which produces a single hormone (polymorphous).

Prolactinomas in women and corticotroph adenomas in both sexes are usually diagnosed while still microadenomas. In contrast, the

TABLE 313-5 Pituitary hormone evaluation

Hormone	Excess	Deficiency
Growth hormone	*1* Measurement of plasma growth hormone 1 h following glucose PO	*1* Measurement of plasma growth hormone 30, 60, and 120 min after one of the following: *a* Regular insulin 0.1 to 0.15 unit/kg IV *b* Levodopa 10 mg/kg PO *c* L-Arginine 0.5 mg/kg intravenously over 30 min
	2 Measurement of IGF-1/SM-C	*2* ?Measurement of IGF-1/SM-C
Prolactin	*1* Measurement of basal serum prolactin	*1* Measurement of serum prolactin 10 to 20 min after one of the following: *a* TRH 200 to 500 μg IV *b* Chlorpromazine 25 mg IM
TSH	*1* Measurement of T₄, free T₄ index, T₃, TSH	*1* Measurement of T₄, free T₄, free T₄ index, TSH
Gonadotropins	*1* Measurement of FSH, LH, testosterone, FSH beta, FSH response to TRH	*1* Measurement of basal LH, FSH in postmenopausal women; no measurements in menstruating, ovulating women *2* Testosterone, FSH, and LH in men
ACTH	*1* Measurement of urine free cortisol*	*1* Measurement of serum cortisol at 30 and 60 min following regular insulin 0.05 to 0.15 units per kilogram IV
	2 Dexamethasone suppression by one of the following: *a* Measurement of 8 A.M. plasma cortisol after administration of 1 mg dexamethasone at midnight *b* Measurement of 8 A.M. plasma cortisol or 24-h urine 17-hydroxysteroids or free cortisol after 0.5 mg dexamethasone PO q 6 h for 8 doses	*2* Metyrapone response by one of the following: *a* Measurement of plasma 11-deoxycortisol at 8 A.M. after 30 mg/kg body wt metyrapone at midnight (maximal dose 2 g) *b* Measurement of 24-h urinary 17-hydroxycorticoids or plasma 11-deoxycortisol day of and day after 750 mg metyrapone q 4 h for 6 doses *c* Measurement of 24-h urinary 17-hydroxycorticoids day of and day after 500 mg metyrapone q 2 h for 12 doses
	3 High-dose dexamethasone suppression by one of the following: *a* Measurement of plasma cortisol after 8 mg dexamethasone PO at midnight *b* Measurement of 8 A.M. plasma cortisol or 24 h urine 17-hydroxysteroids or free cortisol after 2 mg dexamethasone q 6 h for 8 doses *4* Metyrapone response (same protocol as for deficiency testing) *5* Response of plasma ACTH to ovine corticotropin releasing hormone (1 μg/kg body wt)	*3* ACTH stimulation test: Measurement of plasma cortisol and aldosterone at 0 and 60 min after IM or IV administration of 0.25 mg cosyntropin
Arginine vasopressin (AVP)	*1* Measurement of serum sodium and osmolality, urine osmolality in presence of normal renal, adrenal, thyroid function *2* Simultaneous measurement of serum osmolality and ADH levels	*1* Comparison of urine osmolality and serum osmolality under conditions of increased AVP secretion† *2* Simultaneous measurement of serum osmolality and AVP levels

* Tests 1 and 2 establish the diagnosis of Cushing's syndrome. Tests 3, 4, and 5 localize the Cushing's disease to the pituitary gland. Occasionally bilateral inferior petrosal sinus catheterization will be necessary.
† May be achieved by water deprivation or saline administration.

majority of patients with acromegaly and most men with prolactinomas have macroadenomas at the time of diagnosis. Glycoprotein hormone–secreting tumors are also usually quite large at the time of diagnosis.

About 25 percent of pituitary adenomas that come to surgery are apparently nonsecretory, although some stain immunologically for pituitary hormones. In some cases, particularly in the case of gonadotropin-secreting tumors, hormonal secretion is overlooked. Some of the "nonfunctioning" pituitary tumors, as well as some functional ones, secrete part of the glycoprotein hormone molecule, most commonly the alpha subunit. In general tumors without endocrine-related symptoms are large at the time of diagnosis and often cause structural problems. Alpha subunit excess is a frequent finding in patients with TSH-secreting adenomas, and FSH beta may be hypersecreted in patients with gonadotropin-secreting tumors.

Null cell tumors (no specific hormones identified by immunostaining) also are generally large when diagnosed, since no hormonal overproduction is present to provide early clues to diagnosis. Oncocytomas are nonsecretory pituitary adenomas with abundant mitochondria, commonly found in older men.

Pituitary adenomas are occasionally part of the multiple endocrine neoplasia (MEN I) syndrome (see Chap. 325). This dominantly inherited disease causes adenomas of the pituitary gland, secretory tumors of the endocrine pancreas, and hyperparathyroidism due to generalized parathyroid hyperplasia. Pituitary adenomas may secrete GH or prolactin or may be nonfunctioning. Insulinomas and gastrinomas are the most common tumors in MEN I. Pancreatic GRH-secreting tumors can cause acromegaly and pituitary hyperplasia.

Mass effects of pituitary tumors   VISUAL FIELD DEFECTS   The optic chiasm lies anterior and superior to the pituitary gland and in 80 percent of normal persons overlies the pituitary fossa; in about 15 percent the chiasm is anterior to the tuberculum sella (prefixed), and in 5 percent it overlaps the dorsum sella posteriorly (postfixed). The chiasm is found at a variable distance above the diaphragma sella, with up to 1 cm of separation in some patients. Since 90 percent of the chiasmal axons originate in the macula, loss of central vision is an early finding. Foggy or dim vision is also described by many patients.

The most common visual field defect in patients with pituitary adenomas is a bitemporal hemianopsia, and about 8 percent of patients develop complete loss of vision in one eye with a temporal defect in the opposite eye. Alternatively, patients may demonstrate bitemporal scotomas rather than hemianopsia, particularly with a rapidly growing lesion in association with a prefixed chiasm (see Chap. 23). For this reason visual field examinations must assess more than the lateral fields of vision. Of those patients with field defects about 9 percent have a single eye defect, most commonly a superior temporal defect. Occasionally, there is a monocular field loss such as a central scotoma that mimics nonpituitary lesions. When pituitary adenomas cause visual field defects, sellar enlargement is the rule.

OCULOMOTOR PALSIES   Pituitary adenomas may extend laterally, invade the cavernous sinuses, and cause oculomotor palsies. When this occurs, visual field defects are usually not present. Involvement of the third cranial nerve is most common and may mimic diabetic third nerve neuropathy in that pupillary reactivity is usually preserved.

Additional findings associated with lateral extension of the adenoma may include involvement of the fourth and sixth cranial nerves, pain or numbness in the distribution of the fifth cranial nerve, and compression or obstruction of the carotid artery.

Headaches are common in patients with larger tumors and are also present in the majority of patients with acromegaly. Headaches may be exacerbated by coughing. Headaches are thought to be due to stretching of the diaphragma sella and may be referred to several locations, including the vertex of skull and to retroorbital, frontooccipital, frontotemporal, or occipital-cervical areas.

Very large pituitary tumors may invade the hypothalamus and cause hyperphagia, abnormal temperature regulation, loss of consciousness, and loss of hormonal input from the hypothalamus. Obstructive hydrocephalus involving the third ventricle is less common with pituitary adenomas than with craniopharyngiomas. Tumor invasion of the temporal lobe may cause complex partial seizures; invasion of the posterior fossa may be associated with brainstem dysfunction, and invasion into the frontal lobes causes alterations in mental state and frontal release signs.

PITUITARY APOPLEXY   Acute hemorrhagic infarction of a pituitary adenoma may cause a dramatic syndrome including severe headache, nausea, vomiting, and depression of consciousness. Ophthalmoplegia, visual and pupillary disturbances, and meningismus may be present. Most of these symptoms are caused by direct pressure from the tumor, whereas meningismus results from blood in the CSF. The syndrome may either evolve slowly over a period of 24 to 48 h or may lead to sudden death.

Pituitary apoplexy is most commonly found in patients with somatotroph or corticotroph adenomas, but it may be the first clinical manifestation of a pituitary tumor. Both anticoagulation and radiotherapy predispose to hemorrhagic infarction. Rarely, pituitary apoplexy produces "autohypophysectomy" with "cure" of acromegaly, Cushing's disease, or hyperprolactinemia. Hypopituitarism is a common sequela; although hormonal measurements may be normal during the acute phase, cortisol and gonadal steroid concentrations decline over the ensuing days, and thyroxine concentrations decline over weeks. Diabetes insipidus is rare.

It is important to differentiate between pituitary apoplexy and a leaking aneurysm; angiography is often required in this situation. Acute pituitary apoplexy is generally considered a neurosurgical emergency and may require acute decompression of the pituitary, generally via the transsphenoidal route.

Therapy of pituitary adenomas   Ideal therapy for pituitary adenomas would permanently correct hormonal hypersecretion without causing hypopituitarism and would shrink or remove the tumor mass without additional morbidity or mortality. Therapy for microadenomas may achieve both of these goals, whereas therapy for macroadenomas is usually less successful. In considering therapy it is critical to weigh the disability due to the tumor against any disability that may arise from the treatment. Regardless of tumor size the therapy should not be worse than the disease. Potentially serious diseases such as Cushing's disease or acromegaly may require more aggressive treatment than do prolactinomas.

MEDICAL THERAPY   Bromocriptine, a dopamine agonist, is currently the therapy of choice for patients with microprolactinomas who require therapy. Bromocriptine corrects hyperprolactinemia in almost all patients with microprolactinomas; however, when the drug is stopped, prolactin levels often return to pretreatment levels.

Bromocriptine side effects of nausea, gastric irritation, and postural hypotension can be minimized by initially giving a low dose (1.25 mg) at bedtime with a snack. Other side effects include headache, fatigue, abdominal cramps, nasal congestion, and constipation. The dosage is gradually increased to a twice-daily schedule (most commonly 2.5 mg bid).

Bromocriptine is also effective in larger prolactin-secreting macroadenomas. Bromocriptine lowers prolactin levels by about 90 percent in most patients with large tumors but usually not to normal. Tumor shrinkage of 50 percent or greater occurs in about half the patients, and visual field defects may return to normal. Tumor shrinkage is occasionally accompanied by reversal of hypopituitarism. With giant adenomas, bromocriptine-induced tumor shrinkage may rarely cause a devastating intracranial hemorrhage. Unfortunately macroadenomas usually regrow when bromocriptine is stopped.

If visual field defects are not rapidly (within 1 month) returned to normal with bromocriptine, we usually recommend surgery. Symptomatic hyperprolactinemia with inadequate response to bromocriptine also requires surgery or radiation therapy. When pregnancy is desired, the decision whether to continue bromocriptine through pregnancy needs to be weighed against the consequences of additional therapy (radiation or surgery).

The somatostatin analogue octreotide (see p. 1664) is probably the adjunctive therapy of choice in acromegaly and may be appropriate for primary therapy in some patients. Bromocriptine is a useful therapeutic adjunct in some patients with acromegaly, particularly in those with coexistent hyperprolactinemia. GH concentrations rarely return to normal, but symptomatic improvement is common and tumor shrinkage may occur. Bromocriptine should be considered in acromegalic subjects whose GH levels remain elevated following surgery or who are waiting for radiation therapy to take effect. Nonfunctioning chromophobe adenomas usually do not shrink in response to bromocriptine, even when high doses are used.

Tamoxifen is occasionally useful as an adjunct in the therapy of large prolactinomas refractory to therapy with dopamine antagonists. Cyproheptadine, a serotonin antagonist, has been reported to induce remissions in occasional patients with corticotroph adenomas. Octreotide may also be useful adjunctive therapy in patients with TSH-secreting adenomas.

SURGERY   Transsphenoidal surgery of pituitary microadenomas is safe and frequently corrects hormonal oversecretion. Hormonal overproduction is corrected within 24 h in 75 percent of patients with Cushing's disease due to corticotroph microadenomas, acromegaly with GH concentration less than 40 μg/L, and microprolactinomas associated with serum prolactin concentrations less than 200 μg/L. The initial success rate varies among institutions, with reported figures ranging from 50 to 95 percent. Unfortunately, after initially successful surgery hyperprolactinemia recurs in about 17 percent of patients followed for 3 to 5 years and possibly in 50 percent after 5 to 10 years. The recurrence rates after initially successful surgery in acromegaly and Cushing's disease are not established.

The mortality rate for transsphenoidal surgery of microadenomas is 0.27 percent with a morbidity rate of about 1.7 percent based on 2600 surgical procedures. Major complications include cerebrospinal fluid rhinorrhea, oculomotor palsy, and visual loss.

Pituitary surgery is less successful with larger secretory tumors. In patients with serum prolactin greater than 200 μg/L or GH greater than 40 μg/L, hormone concentrations return to normal in only 30 percent following surgery. Surgery is successful in about 60 percent of patients with Cushing's disease due to corticotroph macroadenomas. Recurrence rates with these secretory macroadenomas after a surgery-induced remission are uncertain; in the case of prolactin-secreting tumors, hyperprolactinemia recurs in 10 to 80 percent of patients. Pretreatment with octreotide in acromegalic patients with invasive macroadenomas may improve the surgical success rate.

Mass effects of large tumors are also rarely cured with surgery alone; in cases where surgery is the exclusive therapy, the 10-year recurrence of symptoms is 85 percent in patients not treated with radiation and/or bromocriptine. When radiation therapy is used in combination with surgery, the 10-year recurrence is 15 percent.

Surgery for macroadenomas has a mortality rate of around 0.86 percent and a morbidity rate of about 6.3 percent. Hypopituitarism occurs in an additional 10 percent of patients. Transient diabetes insipidus occurs in about 5 percent, and permanent diabetes insipidus occurs in 1 percent. Major complications of surgery for macroadenoma include cerebrospinal rhinorrhea (3.3 percent), permanent visual loss (1.5 percent), permanent oculomotor palsy (0.6 percent), and meningitis (0.5 percent).

RADIATION THERAPY   Conventional radiation therapy is effective in preventing tumor growth (70 to 100 percent) but is unsatisfactory in the acute management of pituitary hyperfunction. Therapy consists of delivery of 4500 cGy (4500 rad) over 4.5 to 5 weeks, using rotational techniques. GH values of less than 5 μg/L can be achieved in half of acromegalics after 5 years and in 70 percent after 10 years. Conventional radiation alone is rarely successful in treating corticotroph adenomas in adults. Long-term efficacy of radiation in patients with prolactinoma is currently being studied. Complications of conventional radiation therapy include hypopituitarism in up to 50 percent of patients. This may be used as primary therapy for nonfunctioning tumors without structural problems or as an adjunct to surgery for functioning and nonfunctioning tumors.

Heavy particle therapy with proton beam or alpha particles is effective in treating secretory adenomas, but response is slow. Tumors with suprasellar extension or tissue invasion are generally excluded from such series. With proton beam therapy at the Harvard cyclotron, radiation doses of up to 14,000 cGy (14,000 rad) can be given safely without damage to surrounding structures. At 2 years, 28 percent of acromegalics achieve GH values of less than 5 μg/L; the cure rate increases to 56 percent at 5 years and 75 percent by 10 years. With Cushing's disease proton beam corrects the hypercortisolism in 55 percent at 2 years and in 80 percent by 5 years. Proton beam therapy effectively lowers ACTH and stops growth of most corticotroph adenomas in patients with Nelson's syndrome with the exception of adenomas that are invasive at the time of therapy. Long-term results for treatment of prolactinomas with proton beam therapy are not available.

Complications of heavy particle therapy include hypopituitarism in at least 10 percent of patients, although the exact long-term prevalence of this complication is uncertain. Visual field defects and oculomotor dysfunction, usually temporary, have been reported in about 1.5 percent of patients. The major draw-back of this form of therapy and of conventional radiotherapy is the length of time that must elapse before hormonal hypersecretion is corrected.

We generally treat microprolactinomas with bromocriptine. However, we recommend surgery for those patients with microprolactinoma who require therapy and are intolerant of dopamine agonists. Surgery generally does not result in hypopituitarism in this relatively benign disease. Surgery is usually our treatment of choice in patients with acromegaly or Cushing's disease because in most instances rapid reversal of hormonal hypersecretion is essential, and cure can often be achieved. Since Cushing's disease and acromegaly are serious diseases, more extensive surgery that results in hypopituitarism may be required.

Many patients with macroprolactinomas are treated with bromocriptine alone, and a trial of this agent should be given. We recommend transsphenoidal surgery and/or radiation therapy for patients with large prolactinomas who desire pregnancy, show persistent structural abnormalities or symptomatic hyperprolactinemia despite dopamine agonists, and who are intolerant of dopaminergic agents and as an alternative to continued bromocriptine in those who desire pregnancy. Patients with nonfunctioning pituitary adenomas with structural abnormalities require transsphenoidal surgery, generally followed by conventional radiation therapy. Heavy particle therapy is an effective alternative to surgery in patients with acromegaly or Cushing's disease who have contraindications to or refuse surgery. Heavy particle or conventional radiation therapy is effective in treating patients with persistent GH elevation after transsphenoidal surgery, as is octreotide. Heavy particle therapy is effective in persistent Cushing's disease as well. Proton beam therapy is effective in most patients with Nelson's syndrome and may be a desirable alternative to conventional radiation therapy in patients with macroprolactinomas and nonsecretory macroadenomas. Transfrontal surgery is occasionally required, particularly in patients with giant adenomas.

HYPOPITUITARISM   *Hypopituitarism* refers to deficiency of one or more pituitary hormones and has many etiologies (see Table 313-6). Pituitary hormone deficiency may be congenital or acquired.

TABLE 313-6   Causes of hypopituitarism

A Isolated hormone deficiencies
  1 Congenital or acquired deficiencies
B Tumors
  1 Large pituitary adenomas
  2 Pituitary apoplexy
  3 Hypothalamic tumors, e.g., craniopharyngiomas, germinomas, chordomas, meningiomas, gliomas, and others
C Inflammatory diseases
  1 Granulomatous disease, e.g., sarcoidosis, tuberculosis, syphilis, granulomatous hypophysitis
  2 Eosinophilic granuloma
  3 Lymphocytic hypophysitis (autoimmune)
D Vascular diseases
  1 Sheehan's postpartum necrosis
  2 ? Diabetic peripartum necrosis
  3 Carotid aneurysm
E Destructive-traumatic events
  1 Surgery
  2 Stalk section
  3 Radiation (conventional—hypothalamus; heavy-particle—pituitary)
  4 Trauma
F Developmental anomalies
  1 Pituitary aplasia
  2 Basal encephalocoele
G Infiltration
  1 Hemochromatosis
  2 Amyloidosis
H "Idiopathic" causes
  1 ?Autoimmune disease

Isolated GH or gonadotropin deficiency is common. Temporary ACTH deficiency as a consequence of long-term glucocorticoid therapy is also common, but permanent isolated deficiency of ACTH or TSH is rare. Deficiency of any of the anterior pituitary hormones may occur at the level of the pituitary gland or the hypothalamus. When diabetes insipidus is present, the primary defect is almost invariably in the hypothalamus or high pituitary stalk, often in conjunction with mild hyperprolactinemia and anterior pituitary hypofunction.

Manifestations of hypopituitarism depend upon the specific pituitary hormones that are lacking. Growth failure due to GH deficiency is a common presenting complaint in children. GH deficiency in adults causes more subtle manifestations such as fine wrinkling around the eyes and mouth and in subjects with diabetes mellitus increased sensitivity to insulin. Complaints related to gonadotropin deficiency include amenorrhea and infertility in women and testosterone deficiency and decreased libido, decreased beard and body hair, and preservation of a youthful scalp hairline in men. TSH deficiency causes hypothyroidism with fatigue, cold intolerance, and puffy skin in the absence of goiter. ACTH deficiency results in cortisol deficiency, manifested by fatigue; decreased appetite; weight loss; decreased skin and nipple pigmentation; abnormal response to stress characterized by fever, hypotension, and hyponatremia; and a high mortality rate. Unlike primary adrenal insufficiency (Addison's disease) ACTH deficiency does not cause hyperpigmentation, hyperkalemia, or salt loss. With combined ACTH and gonadotropin deficiency, axillary and pubic hair may be lost. Children with combined GH and cortisol deficiency often develop hypoglycemia. AVP deficiency causes diabetes insipidus with polyuria and increased thirst. When pituitary adenomas impair anterior pituitary function, GH is often the first hormone to be compromised, followed by deficiencies of gonadotropins, TSH, and ACTH.

Etiology   Damage to the anterior pituitary is commonly due to a pituitary adenoma (with or without infarction), pituitary surgery, heavy particle pituitary irradiation, closed head trauma, or infarction during the postpartum period (Sheehan's syndrome). Postpartum pituitary infarction occurs because the enlarged pituitary gland of pregnancy becomes vulnerable to ischemia; postpartum hemorrhage with systemic hypotension can destroy the pituitary gland. Inability to lactate is the most common initial clinical clue, and other symptoms of hypopituitarism may unfold over months or years. The condition is sometimes diagnosed years after the primary event. Although clinical diabetes insipidus is rare in this setting, a decreased vasopressin response to appropriate stimuli is common. Patients with diabetes mellitus are also prone to develop hypopituitarism late in pregnancy.

Another cause of hypopituitarism in women is lymphocytic hypophysitis, a syndrome that usually occurs during pregnancy or in the postpartum period. In this syndrome, a mass lesion is often seen on CT scanning which, when biopsied, consists of lymphocytic infiltration. Lymphocytic hypophysitis is due to autoimmune pituitary destruction and often occurs with other autoimmune diseases such as Hashimoto's (autoimmune) thyroiditis and gastric atrophy (see Chap. 325). Circulating antibodies to prolactin cells have been identified in some patients. Although only 30 cases of lymphocytic hypophysitis have been reported, about 7 percent of patients with other autoimmune diseases have prolactin antibodies in serum. It is not clear whether autoimmune hypophysitis is a common cause of "idiopathic" hypopituitarism in adults.

Hypothalamic or pituitary stalk damage has many causes (see Table 313-6). Certain lesions in this region, such as sarcoidosis, metastatic carcinoma, germinomas, histiocytosis, and craniopharyngiomas, commonly cause diabetes insipidus along with hypofunction of the anterior pituitary. Pituitary insufficiency, resulting from conventional radiation to the brain or the pituitary, is thought to be largely hypothalamic in origin, although diabetes insipidus generally does not occur.

Diagnosis (See Table 313-5) To diagnose GH deficiency, the most reliable GH stimulus is insulin-induced hypoglycemia in which the blood sugar declines to less than 2.2 pmol/L (40 mg/dL) (Fig. 313-9). A GH concentration of greater than 10 μg/L after hypoglycemia, levodopa, or arginine effectively excludes GH deficiency.

FIGURE 313-9 The insulin tolerance test. After an intravenous injection of regular insulin (0.1 unit/kg body weight) a fall in blood sugar and rise in plasma GH and cortisol is expected. This test permits evaluation of both GH and ACTH in patients with pituitary disease. *(After KJ Catt, Lancet 1:933, 1970.)*

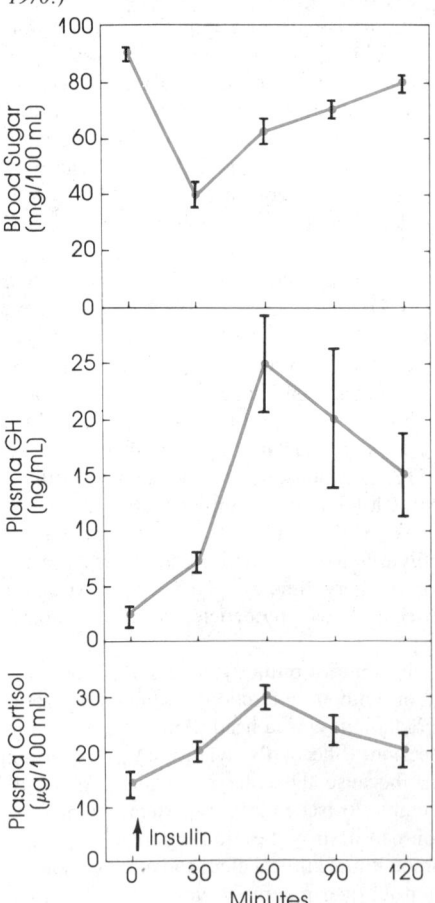

Measuring the basal GH or serum IGF-1/SM-C concentration is less reliable, because GH levels are undetectable in normal persons for much of the day and because IGF-1/SM-C concentrations in patients with GH deficiency may overlap the normal range.

Cortisol deficiency is potentially life-threatening. Basal cortisol function may be preserved in the face of extensive pituitary destruction; consequently, the ability of pituitary ACTH secretion to increase in response to "stress" must be assessed. Either the insulin tolerance test or the metyrapone test can be used to determine the adequacy of ACTH reserve; the ACTH stimulation test is a safer but less sensitive alternative.

The insulin tolerance test is safely performed on an outpatient basis in younger patients without heart disease or diseases predisposing to seizures (Fig. 313-9 and Table 313-5). Both cortisol and GH responses are measured. If hypopituitarism is strongly suspected, a lower dose of regular insulin (0.05 to 0.1 units per kilogram of body weight) should be employed. After adequate hypoglycemia, the peak plasma cortisol should be greater than 500 nmol/L (19 μg/dL), although other criteria have been suggested. Since the metyrapone test can precipitate acute adrenal insufficiency in patients with low basal cortisol secretory rates, it should always be performed in the hospital setting when the 8 A.M. basal plasma cortisol is less than 230 nmol/L (9 μg/dL). Furthermore, metyrapone administration in most patients should be preceded by a rapid ACTH stimulation test to ensure that the adrenals can respond to ACTH. A normal response to metyrapone administration (see Table 313-5) has been variably defined, but one criterion is an increase of plasma 11-deoxycortisol to greater than 200 nmol/L (7.5 μg/dL) and of the urinary 17-hydroxysteroids to at least twofold over baseline, usually to a value greater than 60 μmol/d (22 mg/d). The plasma cortisol must concomitantly fall to less than 110 nmol/L (4 μg/dL) to ensure that there has been an adequate stimulus for ACTH release if these criteria have not been met. Although ACTH responses to insulin-hypoglycemia and metyrapone have not been well-standardized, a peak ACTH concentration of greater than 40 pmol/L (200 pg/mL) is considered normal.

The rapid ACTH stimulation test (see Table 313-5) may be the safest and most convenient screening test for determining the adequacy of the pituitary-adrenal axis. Since the response of the adrenal gland to exogenous ACTH is dependent upon prior endogenous ACTH exposure, it follows that patients with profound ACTH deficiency will have a deficient adrenal response to exogenous ACTH stimulation. However, the rapid ACTH stimulation test may be normal in some patients with abnormal insulin tolerance tests and therefore may not detect all who are at risk for stress-induced adrenal insufficiency. Thus, whereas an abnormal ACTH stimulation test is indicative of an abnormal pituitary-adrenal axis, a normal response in the rapid ACTH stimulation test [cortisol greater than 500 nmol/L (19 μg/dL)] does not always establish that the pituitary-adrenal axis is normal.

Gonadotropin function is easier to evaluate. In women with regular menses gonadotropin secretion is normal, and gonadotropin measurements are superfluous. Likewise, a man with a normal serum testosterone and normal spermatogenesis need not have gonadotropins measured. In postmenopausal women gonadotropin levels are elevated (an endogenous stimulation test); "normal" levels suggest gonadotropin deficiency. Estrogen deficiency in women and testosterone deficiency in men in the absence of elevated gonadotropins imply gonadotropin deficiency.

To diagnose central hypothyroidism (thyrotropin deficiency), the serum T_4 and free T_4 (or T_3 resin uptake and free T_4 index) should first be measured. If these are in the midnormal range, TSH function is likely to be normal. If T_4 and free T_4 are low and the serum TSH is not elevated, central hypothyroidism is present. Minimal TSH elevation (with bioinactive TSH) can occur in hypothalamic hypothyroidism. Mild central hypothyroidism, a consideration in patients with known pituitary disease who have low-normal T_4 and free T_4 concentrations, remains a clinical diagnosis. Before considering the diagnosis of isolated TSH deficiency in patients with the biochemical features of central hypothyroidism without evidence of other pituitary hormone deficiency, it is important to exclude the thyroxine-binding globulin (TBG) deficiency syndrome (low T_4, increased T_3 resin uptake, low to low-normal free T_4 index, normal TSH) and the "sick euthyroid" syndrome (low T_4, low free T_4 or free T_4 index, normal TSH) (see Chap. 316).

Several diagnostic tests utilize hypothalamic-releasing hormones to assess pituitary reserve. While these tests are not helpful in assessing the adequacy of anterior pituitary function, they can be useful in certain situations. In patients with isolated gonadotropin deficiency, the gonadotropin response to gonadorelin (synthetic LHRH) may be useful in predicting which patients will respond to therapy with gonadorelin. CRH testing may be useful in the differential diagnosis of Cushing's syndrome but does not indicate whether the pituitary-adrenal axis will respond appropriately to stress. TRH stimulation testing is useful in some patients in supporting the diagnosis of hyperthyroidism or of acromegaly and in those cases in which documentation of prolactin deficiency is necessary to support a diagnosis of more generalized anterior pituitary hormone deficiency (e.g., mild central hypothyroidism). TRH testing is not necessary in the evaluation for central hypothyroidism and is not reliable in separating pituitary from hypothalamic hypothyroidism.

Therapy Multiple hormones must be replaced in patients with panhypopituitarism, but cortisol replacement is most important. We prefer prednisone for matters of convenience and cost, but many physicians use cortisone acetate. Prednisone (5 to 7.5 mg) or cortisone acetate (20 to 37.5 mg) can be given to some patients as a single morning dosage, whereas others require divided doses (two-thirds at 8 A.M., one-third at 3 A.M.). Hypopituitary patients may require lower daily glucocorticoid dosages than do patients with Addison's disease and do not require mineralocorticoid replacement. In stress situations or when preparing these patients for pituitary or other surgery, higher doses of glucocorticoids should be administered (e.g., for major surgery, hydrocortisone hemisuccinate 75 mg IM/IV every 6 h or methyl prednisolone sodium succinate 15 mg IM/IV every 6 h). Levothyroxine is the therapy of choice in central hypothyroidism (0.1 to 0.2 mg/d). Since thyroxine accelerates the degradation of cortisol and can precipitate adrenal crisis in patients with limited pituitary reserve, glucocorticoid replacement should always precede levothyroxine therapy in panhypopituitarism. Hypogonadism in women is treated with estrogen-progestogen combinations and in men with testosterone esters by injection. To achieve fertility gonadotropins must be administered by injection in patients with pituitary disease, whereas gonadorelin may be successful in those with hypothalamic disease. GH deficiency is not treated in adults; in children GH administration usually is required, but GRH injections may be effective in those with hypothalamic disease (see Chap. 314). Diabetes insipidus is treated with nasal desmopressin (usually 0.05 to 0.1 mL twice a day) (see Chap. 315).

RADIOLOGY OF THE PITUITARY Conventional posteroanterior and lateral skull x-rays define the contours of the sella turcica (Fig. 313-10). Abnormalities that may be identified on these films include enlargement, erosions, and calcifications in the region of the sella. CT scanning or magnetic resonance imaging (MRI) is necessary to define further intrapituitary and suprasellar lesions (Fig. 313-11). Angiography is routinely used when an aneurysm or vascular malformation is suspected as the cause of an enlarged sella and is occasionally necessary in patients with large pituitary or hypothalamic tumors. Intrasellar lesions can be visualized with direct coronal CT scanning, often with the aid of intravenous contrast material. High-resolution MRI scanning (sagittal and coronal views) using gadolinium (a paramagnetic MR contrast agent) provides comparable and in some cases superior information and avoids radiation exposure. The suprasellar region can be best visualized on axial CT views; however, the anatomic details of the optic chiasm obtained with MRI scanning make this the procedure of choice for imaging suprasellar pituitary tumors. Pneumoencephalography and metrizamide cisternography have been largely replaced by the newer modalities of CT and MR

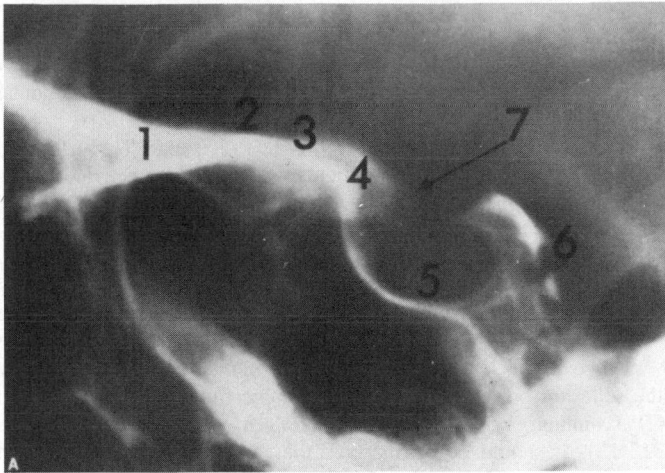

FIGURE 313-10 X-ray of the sella, lateral view. Note (1) planum sphenoidal, (2) limbus sphenoidal, (3) sulcus chiasmaticus, (4) tuberculum sellae, (5) sella floor with distinct lamina dura, (6) dorsum sellae, (7) anterior clinoid, and (8) sphenoid sinus. *(From SM Wolpert in Post et al.)*

FIGURE 313-11 Magnetic resonance imaging (MRI) in patient with a large pituitary adenoma. The arrow points to the adenoma which is seen on axial *(A)*, sagittal *(B)*, and coronal *(C)* views. *(From G Gerard et al, Hosp Pract 19:151, 1984.)*

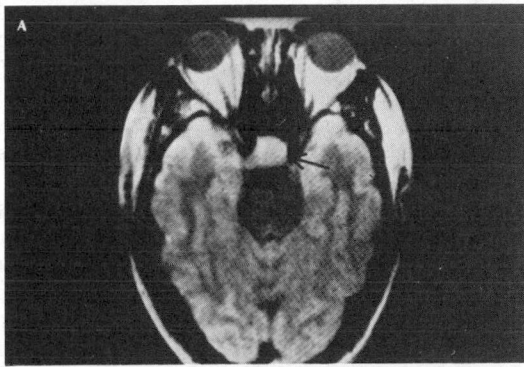

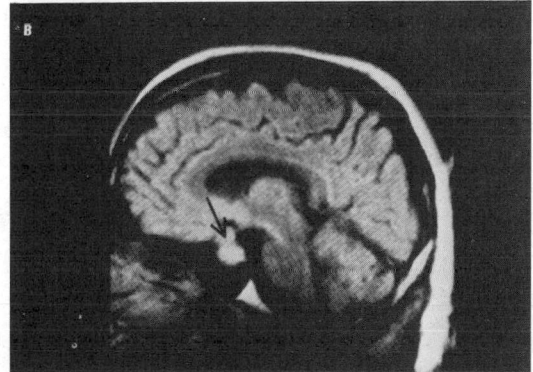

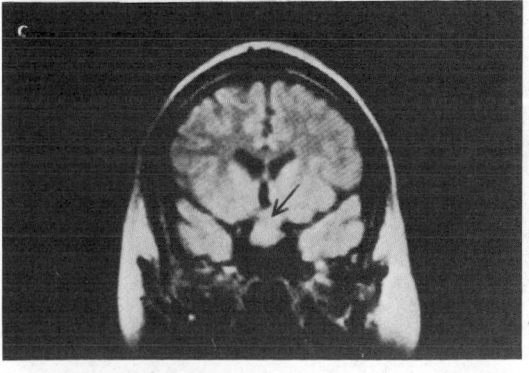

imaging. Sella tomography is not recommended, as it has a high frequency of false-positive and false-negative findings and exposes the lens of the eye to excessive radiation. Frontal tomography may be necessary for details of bony anatomy prior to transsphenoidal surgery.

The volume of the normal sella turcica (233 to 1092 mm³, mean 594 mm³) does not change in patients with pituitary microadenomas. With conventional radiography, pituitary microadenomas may be suspected on the basis of focal erosions or blistering of the floor of the sella, but these findings may also be present in normal individuals. Larger microadenomas may cause the floor of the sella to "tilt" when viewed in the frontal projection and may create the appearance of a double floor on lateral view (Fig. 313-12).

However, since most microadenomas neither affect the volume of the sella nor produce specific radiographic findings, high-resolution CT scanning or MR imaging is necessary for visualization (Fig. 313-13). It should be emphasized that localization of corticotroph adenomas in patients with Cushing's disease may be helpful in directing the surgical approach. In patients with modest prolactin elevations, however, the purpose of sella imaging is to exclude larger pathologic entities. Whether a microprolactinoma is actually visualized is less important, as this disorder is generally treated medically. On CT or MR images the normal pituitary gland has a height of 3 to 7 mm, although values up to 9 mm can be found in adolescents. The upper aspect is flat, concave, or, in younger patients, convex. The stalk is midline with a maximum diameter of 4 mm in axial sections. After intravenous contrast administration, the normal pituitary shows homogeneous enhancement on CT in 60 percent of patients and heterogeneous enhancement in 40 percent. Up to one-fifth of normal persons show discrete low-density areas on contrast-enhanced CT scanning. In random autopsies, one-fourth of individuals have small pituitary abnormalities (e.g., microadenomas, cysts, metastatic tumors, pituitary infarcts), but it is unclear whether such abnormalities correspond to the focal abnormal areas on CT scanning.

Microadenomas are best demonstrated on direct coronal CT scans taken in 1-mm sections after rapid infusion of contrast material or on sagittal or coronal MR images after intravenous gadolinium. On CT the normal pituitary enhances with contrast, as do the cavernous sinuses. Microadenomas, particularly microprolactinomas, usually appear hypodense with this technique (Fig. 313-13). T1-weighted coronal and sagittal views (MRI) and T2-weighted coronal views show the normal pituitary to be isointense with respect to cerebral

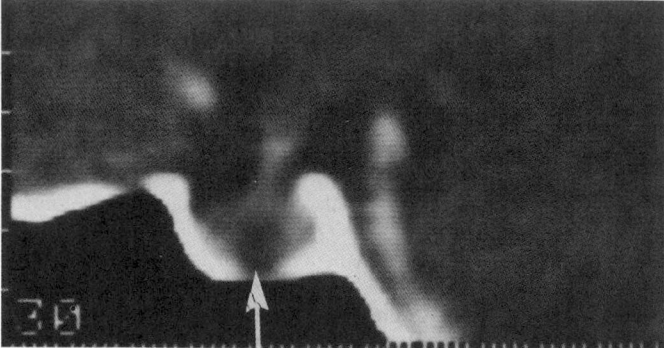

FIGURE 313-13 Sagittal CT scan of sella in patient with small microprolactinoma. The tumor has decreased density, and minimal erosion of the sella floor is demonstrated. Arrow points to tumor.

white matter. A small, bright, high-intensity area is seen in the posterior sella on T1 images, corresponding to the posterior pituitary. Microadenomas appear as low-intensity focal areas on T1- and high-intensity focal areas on T2-weighted images. Small corticotroph adenomas are particularly difficult to visualize; however, even these can often be seen on MRI if a high-field-strength magnet (1.5 T) and gadolinium are used. The specificity of CT and MR diagnosis of microadenomas is enhanced when upward convexity of the diaphragma sellae, contralateral deviation of the pituitary stalk (Fig. 313-14), and/or bony erosion (CT scan) are also found.

Pituitary macroadenomas generally cause sella enlargement on conventional radiography, with or without bony erosion. However, an enlarged sella is not sufficient to diagnose a pituitary adenoma (see below). Additional findings in plain skull x-rays in patients with acromegaly may include prognathism, enlarged paranasal sinuses, hyperostosis of the external occipital protuberance, increased density of the central bone of the sella, and an enlarged square sella with tapered tuberculum. GH-secreting adenomas may calcify and regress to leave a pituitary calculus or stone. Larger corticotroph adenomas may cause depression of the central floor of the sella.

CT scanning of macroadenomas may reveal enlargement of the sella, a mass in the sella with contrast enhancement of the tumor or its capsule, and obliteration of the suprasellar cistern. An area of decreased density within an enhancing mass is present in about 20 percent of patients (CT) and suggests cystic degeneration of an adenoma. An additional one-fifth of patients with macroadenomas have a partially empty sella with CSF density within the sella (see below). Axial views are preferred if suprasellar extension is clinically

FIGURE 313-12 Lateral view of the sella turcica demonstrating a "double floor" due to downward displacement by a pituitary adenoma. Top arrow points to normal floor; bottom arrow points to floor displaced by tumor.

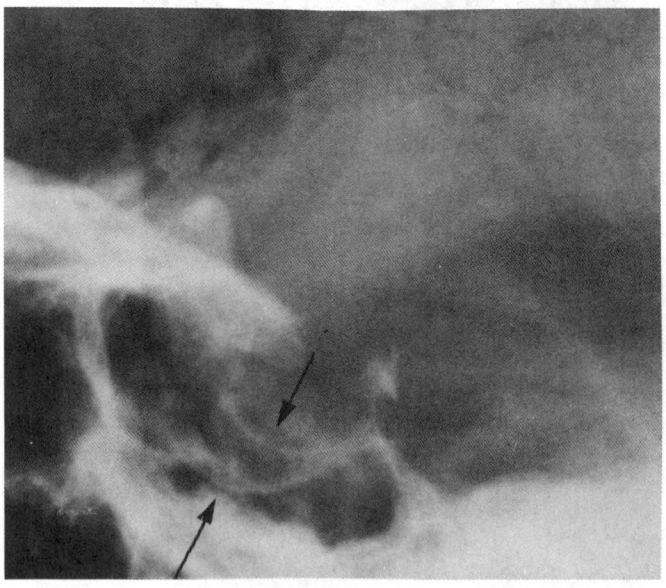

FIGURE 313-14 Coronal CT scan demonstrating 1.3-cm macroprolactinoma in a 30-year-old woman. Note decreased density of the tumor (arrow). The pituitary stalk is displaced to the left, and the floor of the sella slopes to the left as well.

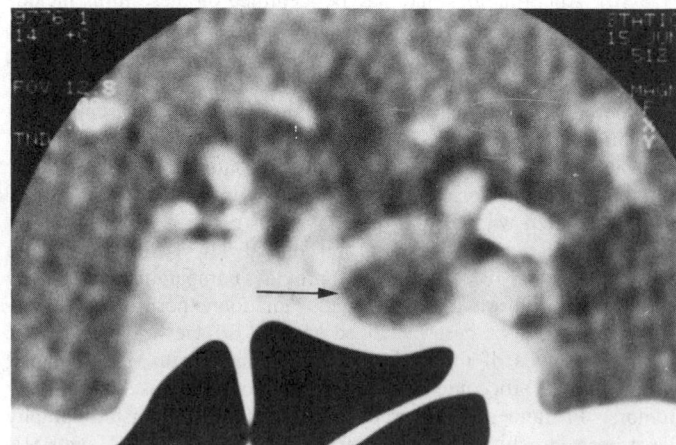

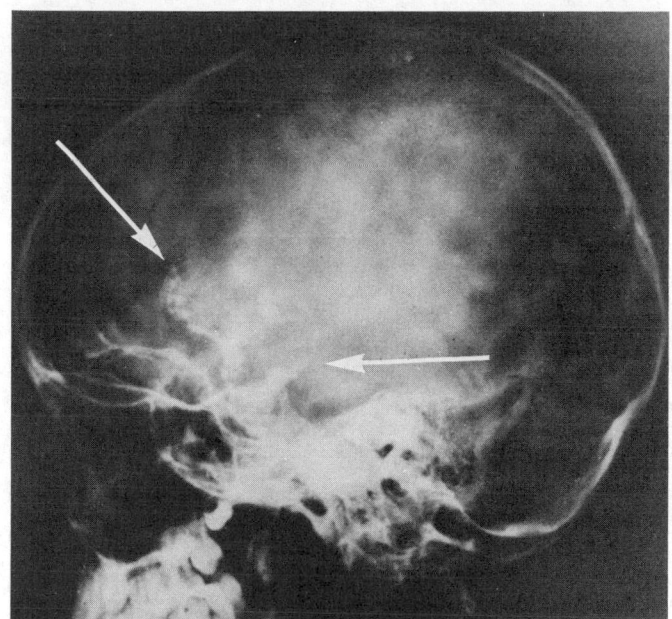

FIGURE 313-15 Lateral skull x-ray in a patient with a craniopharyngioma. Note dense calcification in suprasellar region (arrow).

suspected. On MRI, the adenomas are generally isointense on T1-weighted images and moderately hyperintense on T2-weighted images. Larger invasive tumors may extend into the cavernous sinus, sphenoid sinus, or any of the cranial fossae. Cavernous sinus invasion may be difficult to diagnose on CT and MRI; however, the flow void of the carotid artery on MRI does delineate tumors that surround the artery. Pituitary hyperplasia (e.g., thyrotroph hyperplasia in primary hypothyroidism or lactotroph hyperplasia during pregnancy) appears on CT as a full, enlarged sella that does not enhance after contrast administration.

Pituitary apoplexy is caused by a sudden increase in the size of a pituitary macroadenoma due to hemorrhage or infarction. Enlargement of the sella is almost always evident on plain films. In the case of hemorrhage, CT scanning reveals a high-density area within the adenoma during the acute phase and a decreased density, with or without marginal enhancement, as the hematoma is resorbed. With infarction, low-density areas are seen with or without enhancement. Two days after hemorrhage, MR scanning shows a high-intensity signal on T1 and T2 (due to methemoglobin) with some low-intensity signals intermixed (due to hemosiderin).

Craniopharyngiomas can often be suspected on plain skull x-rays on the basis of nodular or curvilinear calcification in the suprasellar region (Fig. 313-15). This calcification is visible in 80 to 90 percent

of children but in less than one-half of adults. Although the sella may be enlarged and ballooned, the cortical bone is usually preserved. With intrasellar craniopharyngiomas, the dorsum sella is often displaced backwards. On CT scanning cystic components are present with ring or nodular calcification in most children and 80 percent of adults. The noncystic areas show variable enhancement in children. On MRI craniopharyngiomas may be either slightly hyper- or hypointense on T1 images and markedly hypointense on T2 images. Unfortunately calcification is usually not seen on MRI unless large amounts are present.

Most meningiomas of the sellar region cause abnormalities on routine skull films that include calcifications of the tumor and hyperostosis of the planum sphenoidale or of the chiasmatic sulcus. Meningiomas may also cause sella enlargement and thereby mimic pituitary adenomas. On CT scanning, meningiomas may give the appearance of an aneurysm because of their dense homogeneous enhancement. Angiography may be required to exclude an aneurysm and to delineate the feeding vessels. On MRI, meningiomas have the same intensity as brain on both T1- and T2-weighted images, but the mass effect usually allows the lesion to be seen. While this pattern may allow distinction between a meningioma and an aneurysm, angiography is diagnostic.

Aneurysms in the region of the sella contain concentric calcifications demonstrable on plain skull films in about 30 percent of patients. Aneurysms may cause sella enlargement, usually with lateral depression and erosion of the sella floor; a "double floor" is therefore seen on lateral films. On CT scanning the aneurysm is hyperdense with homogeneous contrast enhancement. Most patients with hyperdense lesions that enlarge the sella need to be studied with digital subtraction or conventional angiography. When aneurysms clot the CT appearance may change: new clots show no enhancement whereas old clots enhance like adenomas. Complete thrombosis of an aneurysm is sometimes indistinguishable by CT criteria from a pituitary adenoma. On MRI, a decreased signal due to flowing blood appears and can often demonstrate an aneurysm. Thrombus in the aneurysm has an MRI appearance similar to that of hemorrhage (see above).

On CT scans enhancing masses of the suprasellar region include optic chiasm or hypothalamic gliomas, metastases to the hypothalamus or pituitary stalk, germinomas, sarcoid granulomas, histiocytosis, aneurysms, and craniopharyngiomas. Nonenhancing suprasellar masses include dermoid tumors, epidermoid tumors, and arachnoid cysts.

THE ENLARGED SELLA–EMPTY SELLA SYNDROME Enlargement of the sella can be caused by pituitary adenomas, hypothalamic masses and cysts, aneurysms, primary hypothyroidism or hypogonadism, and increased intracranial pressure. It can also occur in patients with the primary empty sella syndrome (Fig. 313-16). In this situation the sella tends to be symmetrically ballooned without bony erosion. The suprasellar subarachnoid space herniates through an incomplete diaphragma sella (Fig. 313-16) so that the sella is filled

FIGURE 313-16 The findings in patients with the empty sella syndrome. *Left panel* shows the normal anatomic relationships. With the empty sella syndrome (*right panel*) ballooning of the sella results when an arachnoid diverticulum herniates through an incompetent diaphragma sellae. (*After Jordan et al.*)

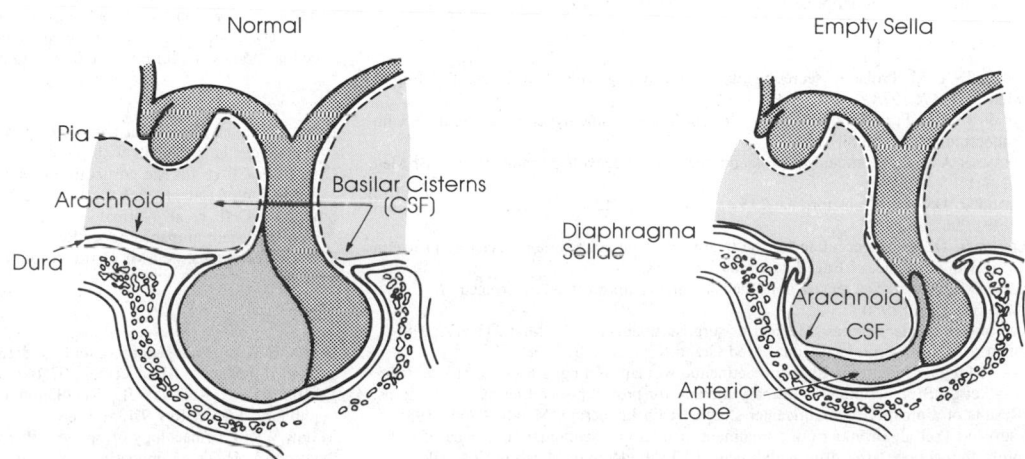

with CSF within an arachnoid-lined sac. An incomplete diaphragma sella is thought to be a prerequisite. It is not clear whether transient or persistent increased CSF pressure is necessary to produce sella enlargement in these patients, but CSF pressure is generally normal when measured. The pituitary is flattened and pushed to one side but tends to function normally. The fact that the CSF fills the sella can be demonstrated with high-resolution CT scanning, MRI, or metrizamide cisternography.

It is important to differentiate the primary empty sella from the enlarged partially empty sella due to a degenerated pituitary adenoma. In the former the pituitary volume is usually normal, in the latter the pituitary volume is generally increased.

Most patients with the primary empty sella syndrome are obese, multiparous women with headaches; about 30 percent have hypertension. It is of interest that multiparity, obesity, and hypertension are associated with increases in CSF pressure. Selection bias cannot be excluded in case reports since skull x-rays may be obtained in patients with headaches, which in turn uncovers the enlarged sella. Endocrine symptoms are uncommon. Hyperprolactinemia occurs on occasion, possibly due to stalk stretching or coincidental microprolactinomas. GH secretory reserve is often abnormal in these patients, probably the result of obesity. Spontaneous CSF rhinorrhea and pseudotumor cerebri have each been reported in about 10 percent of the cases, but this may represent a bias of ascertainment. CSF rhinorrhea often requires surgical correction. Visual field defects have been reported and are thought to be caused by herniation of the optic chiasm into the sella turcica. Once the diagnosis of the empty sella syndrome has been established by CT scan, MRI, or metrizamide cisternography, further diagnostic studies are superfluous, and the therapy is reassurance.

REFERENCES

General

ABBOUND CF, LAWS ER (JR): Diagnosis of pituitary tumors. Endocrinol Metab Clin North Am 17:241, 1988

BESSER GM: The hypothalamus and pituitary. Clin Endocrinol Metab 6:1, 1977

BLACK PMcL et al: *Secretory Tumors of the Pituitary Gland.* New York, Raven Press, 1984

BURROW GN et al: Microadenomas of the pituitary and abnormal sellar tomograms in an unselected autopsy series. N Engl J Med 304:156, 1981

DANIEL PM, PRICHARD MML: The human hypothalamus and pituitary stalk after hypophysectomy or pituitary stalk section. Brain 59:813, 1972

HOLLENHORST RW, YOUNGE BR: Ocular manifestations produced by adenoma of the pituitary gland. Analysis of 1000 cases, in *Diagnosis and Treatment of Pituitary Tumors,* PO Kohler, GT Ross (eds). Amsterdam, Excerpta Medica, 1973, p 53

IMURA H (ed): *The Pituitary Gland.* New York, Raven Press, 1985

KRIEGER DT, MARTIN JB: Brain peptides. N Engl J Med 304:876, 1981

MARTIN JB, REICHLIN S: *Clinical Neuroendocrinology,* 2d ed. Philadelphia, Davis, 1987

MOLITCH ME (ed): Pituitary tumors: Diagnosis and management. Endocrinol Metab Clin North Am 16:3, 1987

POST KD et al (eds): *The Pituitary Adenoma.* New York, Plenum, 1980

SCANLON ME: Neuroendocrinology. Clin Endocrinol Metab 12:467, 1983

VANCE ML et al: Bromocriptine. Ann Intern Med 100:78, 1984

Prolactin

CARTER JN et al: Prolactin secreting tumors and hypogonadism in 22 men. N Engl J Med 299:847, 1978

FERRARI C et al: Functional characterization of hypothalamic hyperprolactinemia. J Clin Endocrinol Metab 55:897, 1982

GROSSMAN A et al: Treatment of prolactinomas with megavoltage radiotherapy. Br Med J 288:1105, 1984

KLEINBERG DS et al: Galactorrhea: 235 cases including 48 with pituitary tumor. N Engl J Med 296:589, 1977

KLEINBERG DL et al: Pergolide for the treatment of pituitary tumors secreting prolactin or growth hormone. N Engl J Med 309:704, 1983

KLIBANSKI A et al: Decreased bone density in hyperprolactinemic women. N Engl J Med 303:1511, 1980

LAWTON NF: Prolactinomas: Medical or surgical treatment? Q J Med 243:577, 1987

MOLITCH ME: Hyperprolactinemia. Med Grand Rounds 1:307, 1982

———: Pregnancy and the hyperprolactinemic woman. N Engl J Med 321:1364, 1985

——— et al: Bromocriptine as primary therapy for prolactin-secreting macroadenomas: Results of a prospective multicenter study. J Clin Endocrinol Metab 60:698, 1985

MORIONDO P et al: Bromocriptine treatment of microprolactinomas: Evidence of stable prolactin decrease after drug withdrawal. J Clin Endocrinol Metab 60:764, 1985

SCHLECTE J et al: Prolactin-secreting pituitary tumors in ammenorrheic women: A comprehensive study. Endocr Rev 1:294, 1980

Growth hormone

ASA SL et al: A case for hypothalamic acromegaly: A clinicopathological study of six patients with hypothalamic gangliocytomas producing growth hormone–releasing factor. J Clin Endocrinol Metab 58:796, 1984

BARKAN AL et al: Treatment of acromegaly with the long-acting somatostatin analog SMS 201-995. J Clin Endocrinol Metab 66:16, 1988

——— et al: Preoperative treatment of acromegaly with long-acting somatostatin analog SMS 201-959: Shrinkage of invasive pituitary macroadenomas and improved surgical remission rate. J Clin Endocrinol Metab 67:1040, 1988

CLEMMONS DR et al: Evaluation of acromegaly by radioimmunoassay of somatomedin-C. N Engl J Med 301:1138, 1979

EASTMAN RC et al: Conventional supervoltage irradiation is an effective treatment for acromegaly. J Clin Endocrinol Metab 48:931, 1979

EDDY RL et al: Human growth hormone release: Comparison of provocative test procedures. Am J Med 56:179, 1974

FROHMAN LA, JANSSON J-O: Growth hormone–releasing hormone. Endocrinol Rev 7:223, 1986

GELATO MC et al: Effects of a growth hormone releasing factor in man. J Clin Endocrinol Metab 57:674, 1983

——— et al: Effects of growth hormone-releasing factor on growth hormone secretion in acromegaly. J Clin Endocrinol Metab 60:251, 1985

GROSSMAN A et al: Growth hormone releasing factor: Comparison of two analogues and demonstration of hypothalamic defect in growth hormone release after radiotherapy. Br Med J 288:1785, 1984

LAMBERTS SWJ: The role of somastostatin in the regulation of anterior pituitary hormone secretion and the use of its analogs in the treatment of human pituitary tumors. Endocr Rev 9:417, 1988

LAWRENCE JH et al: Successful treatment of acromegaly. Metabolic and clinical studies in 145 patients. J Clin Endocrinol Metab 31:180, 1970

MARTIN JB: Neural regulation of growth hormone secretion. N Engl J Med 288:1384, 1973

MELMED S et al: Pathophysiology of acromegaly. Endocr Rev 4:271, 1983

——— et al: Acromegaly due to secretion of growth hormone by an ectopic pancreatic islet-cell tumor. N Engl J. Med 312:9, 1985

MOSES AC et al: Bromocriptine therapy in acromegaly. Use in patients resistant to conventional therapy and effect on serum levels of somatomedin C. J Clin Endocrinol Metab 53:752, 1981

NABARRO JDN: Acromegaly. Clin Endocrinol 26:481, 1987

PHILLIPS LS, VASILOPOULOU-SELLIN R: Somatomedins. N Engl J Med 302:371, 1980

REICHLIN S: Acromegaly. Med Grand Rounds 1:9, 1982

———: Somatostatin. N Engl J Med 309:1495, 1983

SANO T et al: Growth hormone–releasing hormone-producing tumors: Clinical, biochemical and morphological manifestations. Endocr Rev 9:357, 1988

THORNER MO et al: Somatotroph hyperplasia: Successful treatment of acromegaly by removal of a pancreatic islet tumor secreting a growth hormone releasing factor. J Clin Invest 70:965, 1982

——— et al: Extrahypothalamic growth-hormone-releasing factor (GRF) secretion is a rare cause of acromegaly: Plasma GRF levels in 177 acromegalic patients. J Clin Endocrinol Metab 59:846, 1984

WRIGHT AD et al: Mortality in acromegaly. Q J Med 39:1, 1970

TSH

BECK-PECCOZ P et al: Decreased receptor binding of biologically inactive thyrotropin in central hypothyroidism. Effect of treatment with thyrotropin-releasing hormone. N Engl J Med 312:1085, 1985

BIGOS ST et al: Spectrum of pituitary alterations with mild and severe thyroid impairment. J Clin Endocrinol Metab 46:317, 1978

Gonadotropins

CUTLER GB JR: Therapeutic applications of luteinizing-hormone-releasing hormone and its analogs. Ann Intern Med 102:643, 1985

MARSHALL JC, KELCH RP: Gonadotropin-releasing hormone: Role of pulsatile secretion in the regulation of reproduction. N Engl J Med 313:1459, 1986

SNYDER PJ: Gonadotroph cell adenomas of the pituitary. Endocr Rev 6:552, 1985

——— et al: Secretion of uncombined subunits of luteinizing hormone by gonadotroph cell adenomas. J Clin Endocrinol Metab 59:1169, 1984

ACTH

BORST GC et al: Discordant cortisol response to exogenous ACTH and insulin-induced hypoglycemia in patients with pituitary disease. N Engl J Med 306:1462, 1982

CHROUSOS GP et al: The corticotropin-releasing factor stimulation test: An aid in the evaluation of patients with Cushing's syndrome. N Engl J Med 310:622, 1984

STREETEN DHP et al: Normal and abnormal function of the hypothalamic-pituitary-adrenal system in man. Endocr Rev 5:371, 1984

TAYLOR AL, FISHMAN LM: Corticotropin-releasing hormone. N Engl J Med 319:213, 1988

Endorphins

IMURA H et al: Endogenous opioids and related peptides: From molecular biology to clinical medicine. J Endocrinol 107:147, 1985

LUNDBLAD JR, ROBERTS JL: Regulation of proopiomelanocortin gene expression in pituitary. Endocr Rev 9:135, 1988

MARIN WR: Pharmacology of opioids. Pharmacol Rev 35:283, 1984

PFEIFFER A, HERZ A: Endocrine actions of opioids. Horm Metabol Res 16:386, 1984

Alpha Subunits

KLIBANSKI A et al: Pure alpha subunit-secreting pituitary tumors. J Neurosurg 59:585, 1983

Hypothalamus

BRAY GA, GALLAGHER TFJ: Manifestations of hypothalamic obesity in man: A comprehensive investigation of eight patients and a review of the literature. Medicine 54:301, 1974

DINARELLO CA: Interleukin-1 and the pathogenesis of the acute phase response. N Engl J Med 54:301, 1984

———, WOLFF SM: Molecular basis of fever in humans. Am J Med 72:799, 1982

PLUM F, VAN UITERT R: Nonendocrine diseases and disorders of the hypothalamus, in *The Hypothalamus*, S Reichlin et al (eds). New York, Raven Press, 1978, pp 415–473

Craniopharyngiomas

BANNA M: Craniopharyngiomas in adults. Surg Neurol 1:202, 1973

———: Craniopharyngioma: Based on 160 cases. Br J Radiol 49:206, 1976

Hypopituitarism

ABBOUD CF: Laboratory diagnosis of hypopituitarism. Mayo Clin Proc 61:35, 1986

ARAFAH BM: Reversible hypopituitarism in patients with large nonfunctioning pituitary adenomas. J Clin Endocrinol Metab 62:1173, 1986

ASA SL et al: Lymphocytic hypophysitis of pregnancy resulting in hypopituitarism: A distinct clinicopathologic entity. Ann Intern Med 95:166, 1981

EDWARDS OM, CLARK JDA: Post-traumatic hypopituitarism. Medicine 65:281, 1986

VELDHUIS JD, HAMMOND JM: Endocrine function after spontaneous infarction of the human pituitary: Report, review, and reappraisal. Endocr Rev 1:100, 1980

Radiology

BRUNETON JN et al: Normal variants of the sella turcica. Radiology 131:99, 1979

HEMINGHY S et al: Computed tomographic study of hormone-secreting microadenomas. Radiology 146:65, 1983

JORDAN RM et al: The primary empty sella syndrome. Analysis of the clinical characteristics, radiographic features, pituitary function, and cerebrospinal fluid adenohypophysial hormone concentrations. Am J Med 62:569, 1977

KUCHARCZYK W et al: Pituitary adenomas: High-resolution MR imaging at 1.5 T. Radiology 161:761, 1986

WOLPERT SM: The radiology of pituitary adenomas. Endocrinol Metab Clin North Am 16:553, 1987

314 DISORDERS OF GROWTH

RAYMOND L. HINTZ

NORMAL GROWTH   Children may grow rapidly over relatively short periods of time, and the physician must be aware of normal standards for growth and development as a function of age. A record of these changes can be utilized as a sensitive indicator of general health. Minimal aberrations in health may initially be reflected in a deviation from the normal growth rate; conversely, an actively growing child seldom has a serious systemic disease. Thus, height and growth rate provide important information.

Both longitudinal and cross-sectional studies indicate that differences exist in growth among different ethnic groups. However, normal well-nourished children have remarkably similar growth patterns. For example, the average length of children, which at birth is about 50 cm, increases by about 25 cm in the first year of life, 12.5 cm in the second year, and 6.2 cm per year thereafter until puberty. This formula can be used to estimate average height up to about 10 years of age. Nomograms have been constructed to give a more accurate picture of average growth and the range of normal deviations from the mean (Figs. 314-1 and 314-2).

CONTROL OF GROWTH   Growth involves both an increase in the total number of cells and the synthesis of macromolecules by individual cells. The relative importance of these processes varies from organ to organ and with age. The control and integration of growth also vary among tissues and with the stage of development.

Prenatal growth   Prenatal development exemplifies the complexities of the integration and control of growth. During this time, a

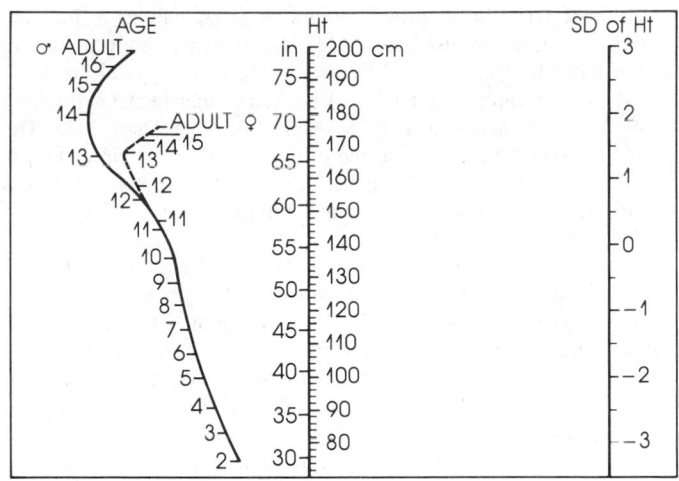

FIGURE 314-1   Nomogram for height of boys and girls.

single cell becomes a complex organism with billions of cells working in harmonious concert. The growth rate is astounding; the most rapid growth rate occurs during the second trimester. Prenatal growth may have different control mechanisms from those in the postnatal period. Growth hormone and thyroid hormone have relatively minor effects on growth during prenatal life. Prenatal growth rates are dependent on uterine blood flow and other maternal influences and are less dependent on the factors that determine ultimate stature. At birth the correlation between body length and adult height is weak ($r = 0.3$); by 2 years of age the correlation between body length and adult height is stronger ($r = 0.7$), indicating that the factors influencing adult stature begin operating early in postnatal life.

Genetic factors   Stature is a polygenic trait (see Chap. 5), so that there is no simple method of predicting on the basis of genetic factors the adult height of any given child. However, on average there is a correlation between the mean height of parents and the mean height attained by their children.

Nutrition   The next most important factor affecting growth is nutrition. Severe nutritional deprivation, as in marasmus or kwashiorkor (see Chap. 71), impairs growth. Selective deficiencies of vitamins and minerals, such as vitamin D, and subclinical deficiencies of nutrients may also retard growth. The trend toward increased adult stature in several countries over the last century may be due to improvement in diet, especially to an increase in protein intake during the growth period.

Hormones   GROWTH HORMONE   Growth hormone (GH, or somatotropin) plays the central role in the modulation of growth of children from birth until the completion of puberty. In the total

FIGURE 314-2   Nomogram for growth rate in boys and girls.

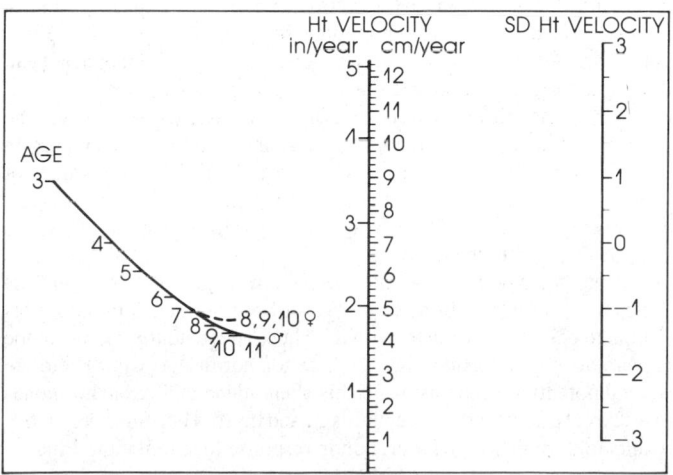

absence of GH, linear growth occurs at about half to a third the normal rate. GH may also play a role in the control of body anabolism throughout life.

GH is a member of a family of hormones that includes pituitary prolactin and human placental lactogen (hPL) (see Chap. 313). The most common form of GH in the pituitary and in the circulation is the 22,000-dalton (''22K'') form. This is the hormone that was purified and sequenced from human pituitary glands. The second most common form is a 20,000-dalton (''20K'') form. This variant is coded by the same gene sequence as the 22K growth hormone, but a segment of an exon (expressed part of the gene) in the growth hormone gene is not transcribed, thus resulting in a shorter hormone. Whether this variant fulfills some important metabolic function is not clear; the 20K form seems to have equivalent growth-promoting activity but may have a lesser effect on carbohydrate function than the 22K form.

GH secretion is under both positive and negative hypothalamic control (see Chap. 313). The somatotropin release–inhibiting factor (somatostatin, SRIF) is a 14-amino-acid peptide that is widely distributed in tissues outside the hypothalamus and is a potent inhibitor of the secretion of other hormones including insulin, glucagon, and gastrin.

The biologic action of GH-releasing hormone (GRH, somatocrinin) is contained in the first 29 amino acids of the 44-amino-acid peptide, and the aminoterminal amino acid is crucial for its biologic action. Patients with idiopathic GH deficiency may have a deficiency of GRH rather than an inability to make GH in the pituitary. Indeed, half or more of subjects with GH deficiency respond to prolonged pulsatile administration of GRH with an increase in plasma GH and with an accelerated growth rate.

The secretion of somatostatin and GRH, and hence the release of GH, is under the influence of several factors (Fig. 314-3). Higher centers in the central nervous system have synapses that terminate on hypothalamic cells that secrete somatostatin and GRH and exert both positive and negative influences. In addition, both GH and the GH-controlled somatomedin peptides influence the secretion or action of GRH and somatostatin. The secretion of GH is episodic with a relatively short (10- to 15-min) half-life in plasma. A significant proportion of GH in serum is bound to a binding protein that is structurally related to the GH receptor. Although small amounts of GH are secreted during waking periods, the major secretion of GH occurs during sleep, especially in association with third- and fourth-stage sleep.

THE SOMATOMEDINS   Although GH may exert some direct effects on growth, the majority of its growth-promoting actions are mediated by the insulin-like growth factor or somatomedin peptides. Two IGF peptides from human plasma, IGF-I and IGF-II, have about 50 percent homology to the structure of human insulin and 70 percent homology to each other. Somatomedin C (SM-C) and IGF-I are structurally and functionally equivalent. The IGF peptides are bound tightly to specific plasma proteins and have half-lives of hours rather than minutes. IGF levels are dependent on GH secretion and are consequently high in acromegaly and low in hypopituitarism. In addition, the normal values are age-dependent, with low levels in early childhood, a peak during adolescence, and a decline in average values after the age of 50 years. The plasma levels of IGF-II are also dependent on the presence of a minimal amount of GH, but pathologic increases in GH do not result in a further increase in IGF-II. Thus, the values of IGF-II are low in hypopituitarism but are not elevated in acromegaly. The average levels of IGF-II are constant from 1 year of age to beyond the eighth decade of life.

THYROID HORMONE   Unlike the pattern of growth seen with GH deficiency, the total absence of thyroid hormone leads to an almost complete cessation of linear growth. Thus, adequate thyroid hormone appears to be an absolute prerequisite for normal growth. There are several potential mechanisms for this phenomenon. Thyroid hormones exert direct effects on cell metabolism, and thyroid hormone deficiency results in diminished GH secretion in response to stimulation. Finally,

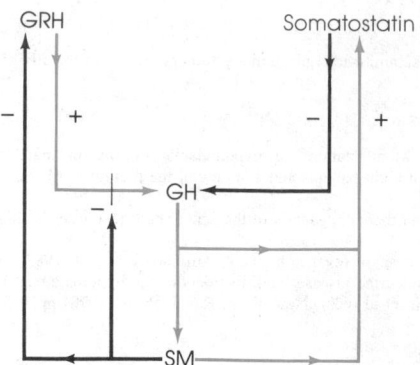

FIGURE 314-3 Feedback control of growth hormone secretion. GH = growth hormone; GRH = growth hormone–releasing hormone; SM = somatomedin. Stimulating influences are shown by arrows in color. Inhibitory influences are shown in black.

the action of IGF-I on cartilage cells may be dependent on thyroid hormone.

GONADAL STEROIDS   Androgens and estrogens exert their major role in the stimulation of growth at the time of puberty. Much of the pubertal growth spurt is due to these hormones. Androgens have a direct stimulatory effect on the growth and maturation of bone, cartilage, and muscle. Estrogens appear to have a biphasic action, stimulating growth at low levels and inhibiting growth at high levels.

INSULIN   Insulin has strong anabolic actions separate from its effects on carbohydrate metabolism. These actions include stimulation of protein synthesis and cell division. The excessive growth of some infants of diabetic mothers may be the consequence of high levels of plasma insulin in the fetus. The close structural relationship of insulin to the IGF group of growth factors and the ability of insulin to bind to the IGF-I receptor may explain some of these actions of insulin at high levels. However, insulin may also have growth-stimulating actions of its own at low levels in some cell types. The role of insulin in the control of normal growth is still unclear.

OTHER FACTORS   Nerve growth factor which is structurally related to the insulin-IGF-I/SM-C family of peptides has actions on the development of sympathetic neurons and possibly on the maintenance and repair of other neurons. Epidermal growth factor has potent actions on the maturation of epidermal features but also acts on other cell types. Platelet-derived growth factor is released from platelets upon clotting and is also a potent mitogen in many cell culture systems. The plasma levels, control mechanisms, interactions with other growth-stimulating hormones, and physiologic roles of these growth factors remain to be elucidated.

DIAGNOSIS OF GROWTH DISORDERS   Most individuals with short stature do not have a disease in the usual sense but exhibit some variation from the normal growth pattern (Table 314-1). Thus, the first step in dealing with growth disorders is to identify those individuals who have a normal variation in stature and who presumably do not require treatment.

Height and growth rate   One of the most important factors in the differential diagnosis of short stature is the determination of the height percentile of the patient, derived by a comparison to others of

TABLE 314-1   Causes of short stature

Diagnosis	Usual practice, %	Referral center, %
Constitutional growth delay	98	80
GH deficiency	0.1	10
Hypothyroidism	0.2	4
Systemic disease	0.3	3
Chromosomal disorders	0.1	1
Bone-cartilage dysplasia	0.3	1
Psychosocial disorders	1	1

SOURCE: Modified from Horner et al, 1978.

his or her age (Fig. 314-1). A straightedge is placed on the patient's age and present height. The intercept on the right-hand scale estimates the number of standard deviations (SD) from the mean height for age. In general, the further away the patient is from the mean height for age, the more likely a disease is present. A height above the -2-SD level indicates that the patient is likely normal. The patient's growth rate also should be determined, if possible, either from existing growth data or by observation (Fig. 314-2).

Because of the large number of normal children with short stature, clinical judgment plays a large role in the approach to this problem. Individuals with severe short stature (> -3 SD for age) should undergo immediate evaluation, while those with less severe short stature may be serially observed so that the growth rate can be assessed. A consistently low growth rate should lead to further investigation. The diagnosis of constitutional delay is one of exclusion. In general, if the physician has excluded hypothyroidism, GH deficiency, and the more common systemic diseases, it is reasonable to observe the patient. However, the boundaries between "normal" and "disease" may be blurred, and the indications for treatment may change. Furthermore, continued failure to maintain a normal growth rate is an indication for reinvestigation.

History Important features in the history include the weight and gestational age at birth, growth and development in early infancy, and presence of systemic disease. It is also crucial to assess the stature of the parents and first- and second-degree relatives and to review the growth and pubertal development patterns of parents, siblings, and other relatives. A family history of late pubertal development may be helpful diagnostically.

Physical examination The body proportions must be evaluated. Relatively short limbs compared to the trunk suggest either long-standing hypothyroidism or one of the chondrodystrophies. Achondroplastic dwarfism is an extreme example of this, but more subtle forms of chondrodystrophy may elude the casual examination. It is also important to note the height-to-weight ratio. A short child who is underweight for height may have malnutrition or systemic disease. On the other hand, a child who is short but overweight is more likely to have endocrine disease. Patients with Cushing's syndrome, GH deficiency, or hypothyroidism are frequently relatively overweight for their height. Specific physical findings may suggest hypothyroidism, GH deficiency, or other specific syndromes (Table 314-2).

Laboratory evaluation Laboratory tests may either confirm the clinical impression or reveal unsuspected pathology. Assessment of bone age is useful to indicate possible pathology and to estimate final adult height. Because the manifestations of hypothyroidism may be minimal, a serum thyroxine should be obtained routinely. IGF-I measurements are also useful screening procedures, since most patients with GH deficiency have low values. There are also syndromes of GH resistance, such as Laron dwarfism, that are characterized by low IGF-I levels and high GH levels. Specific chemistries may be ordered to screen for other disease states. Any girl with unexplained short stature should have a chromosomal karyotype. Useful laboratory studies for the evaluation of short stature are summarized in Table 314-3. Abnormalities of these tests should lead to more specific investigations.

TESTING OF GH SECRETION Because GH secretion is episodic and therefore variable, random measurements of plasma GH are not adequate tests of GH deficiency. Some GH stimulation tests for outpatient screening for GH deficiency are summarized in Table 314-4 (also see Chap. 313). Because of the long half-life of IGF-I, a random measurement of this hormone during the day is an accurate reflection of the mean plasma concentration. If care is taken to use age-related standards, measurement of IGF-I provides a reasonable screen for GH deficiency. Low levels of IGF-I should lead to more extensive evaluation. The other tests listed are indirect and largely nonphysiologic ways of provoking the release of GH. In our clinic, a GH level of 10 μg/L (10 ng/mL) after an exercise or clonidine test is interpreted as a normal response. If that level is not achieved, more definitive testing of GH reserve should be carried out as described in Chap. 313.

TREATMENT WITH GH GH deficiency The only established use of human GH is in the treatment of children who are GH-

TABLE 314-3 Screening laboratory investigations in short stature

Test or x-ray	Disorder
Serum thyroxine	Hypothyroidism
IGF-I	GH deficiency
Bone age	Constitutional delay, hypothyroidism, GH deficiency
Lateral skull film	Craniopharyngioma or other central nervous system lesion
Serum calcium	Pseudohypoparathyroidism
Serum phosphate	Vitamin D–resistant rickets
Serum bicarbonate	Renal tubular acidosis
Blood urea nitrogen	Renal failure
Complete blood count	Anemia, nutritional disorder
Sedimentation rate	Inflammatory disease of bowel
Chromosomal karyotype	Gonadal dysgenesis or other abnormality

TABLE 314-2 Physical findings in syndromes of short stature

Syndrome	Specific physical findings
GH deficiency	Frontal bossing, central obesity, high-pitched voice
Hypothyroidism	Dry skin, coarse hair, immature facies
Cushing's syndrome	Central obesity, striae, hypertension
Gonadal dysgenesis	Webbed neck, multiple pigmented nevi, shield chest, delayed sexual development
Pseudohypoparathyroidism	Moon facies and obesity, short metacarpals, mental retardation
Bone-cartilage dysplasia	Abnormal proportions, macrocephaly
Russell-Silver dwarfism	Small at birth, "pointed" facies, asymmetry

TABLE 314-4 Screening tests for assessing GH secretion

1 IGF-I radioimmunoassay
Age-related normals (may vary with method):

Age, years	Range, units/mL
<1	0.17–0.62
1–5	0.14–1.44
6–11	0.50–2.06
12–17	0.78–3.73
18–25	0.92–2.06
26–40	0.70–2.04

2 Exercise test:
Vigorous exercise (running or stairsteps) for 20 min
20-min rest
Samples for measurement of GH by radioimmunoassay at 0, 20, and 40 min from beginning
Normal response: GH greater than or equal to 10 μg/L (10 ng/mL) on any sample

3 Clonidine test:
NPO after midnight
Administration of clonidine by mouth

Body weight, kg	Dose, mg
5 to 15	0.05
15 to 25	0.1
25 to 35	0.15
35 to 50	0.2
>50	0.25

Samples for measurement of GH by radioimmunoassay at 0, 60, and 90 min
Side effects: Postural hypotension and somnolence
Keep patient supine until after postural hypotension is gone
Normal response: Greater than or equal to 10 μg/L (10 ng/mL) on any sample

deficient. Only between 1 in 4000 and 1 in 20,000 children have a GH deficiency. About half of these cases are due to idiopathic GH deficiency, and the other half are secondary to tumor and/or radiation therapy. In approximately one-third of the latter cases, only GH is deficient, and in the other two-thirds, there are multiple pituitary hormone deficiencies. If short stature is due to a systemic disease such as renal failure, treatment is directed toward the underlying disease state. Similarly, short stature due to hypothyroidism or cortisol excess is managed by treatment of the primary endocrine disorder. In general, the earlier the disorder is diagnosed and treated, the more successful the growth response will be; if treatment of the underlying disease is delayed until after puberty, little or no improvement in stature can be expected.

Unlike the broad species specificity of peptide hormones such as insulin, GH exhibits limited species specificity. Human GH stimulates linear growth in children with GH deficiency, whereas the bovine hormone is ineffective in humans. The collection of pituitary glands from autopsy material for the preparation of human GH did not supply adequate amounts of hormone for the treatment of all children who had GH deficiency, let alone provide sufficient material for the study of GH as a therapeutic agent for other conditions. Furthermore, the distribution of human pituitary GH in the United States and several other countries was discontinued in 1984 because of the development of Creutzfeldt-Jakob disease in four subjects who had been treated with human GH. The availability since 1985 of synthetic GH produced by recombinant DNA in bacteria has relieved the supply problem. Hormone is again available for patients with GH deficiency, and its relatively unlimited supply has allowed exploration of other therapeutic uses of GH, including the treatment of gonadal dysgenesis.

Most children with GH deficiency respond to GH treatment with an acceleration of growth rate to normal or even above normal rates. As with other peptide hormones, there is a dose-response curve to GH. The doses that have been tested range from 0.02 to 0.2 units (0.01 to 0.1 mg) per kilogram of body weight administered as an intramuscular injection three times a week. There is a wide variation in response, but the higher dosages in general result in higher average growth rates. It is possible that in selected clinical circumstances dosages of GH higher than those currently recommended should be administered. Treatment may be started at 0.06 or 0.1 units/kg body weight dosage. The majority of GH-deficient patients have a good growth response to this amount of GH. Daily subcutaneous injection of GH may be preferable; a starting dose of 0.025 or 0.05 units/kg body weight is used for daily therapy. If the patient fails to show an adequate growth rate, the dose can be increased until an adequate growth response is obtained or until the upper limit of 0.75 units/kg body weight per week is achieved. As doses of GH are increased above this level, the risk of glucose intolerance increases, particularly in children who are prediabetic.

An alternative method under study for the treatment of GH deficiency is the use of long-term, subcutaneous infusion of GH-releasing hormone (GRH). Since at least half of children with GH deficiency are able to secrete GH in response to GRH, this approach may ultimately be useful for those patients.

Short stature of other causes IDIOPATHIC SEVERE SHORT STATURE   Growth hormone has been used for some patients with growth failure not due to GH deficiency. Many children with severe short stature (more than 2.5 SD below the mean for age) do not have GH deficiency. Some workers propose that a subgroup of children without GH deficiency but with low IGF-I levels are responsive to GH treatment. These patients are believed to have a relatively inactive GH or to have a partial defect in the control of GH secretion. For example, although they do not fulfill the usual criteria for GH deficiency, they may not have normal bursts of GH secretion during certain physiologic circumstances such as sleep. Whatever the etiology, some of these children have a short-term increase in growth rate in response to GH therapy; whether the final height of these children after GH treatment is greater than their predicted height is not established. Furthermore, it is not known whether there are serious

side effects associated with the rise of GH levels to the supraphysiologic range.

GONADAL DYSGENESIS   GH may also have a therapeutic role in the treatment of gonadal dysgenesis (see Chap. 7). The majority of women with gonadal dysgenesis have an average adult height between 135 and 142 cm. Androgens can cause a short-term increase in the rate of growth of girls with the disorder but do not result in an increase in final adult stature. The use of GH at modest doses is also associated with a small increase in the rate of growth. Results of a multicenter group study utilizing synthetic GH either alone or in combination with androgens are encouraging in terms of initial growth response. It is not known whether GH therapy results in an increase in adult stature, although predicted heights do increase.

SKELETAL DISORDERS   Growth hormone has also been used to treat small numbers of subjects with a wide variety of other growth disorders including bone-cartilage dysplasias and other genetic syndromes associated with short stature. It is not clear whether GH is of use in any of these disorders.

REFERENCES

BROWN P: Potential epidemic of Creutzfeldt-Jacob disease from human growth hormone therapy. N Engl J Med 313:728, 1985

FRASIER SD: A review of growth hormone stimulation tests in children. Pediatrics 53:929, 1974

—— et al: A dose response curve for human growth hormone. J Clin Endocrinol Metab 53:1213, 1981

FURLANETTO R et al: Estimation of somatomedin-C levels in normals and patients with pituitary disease by radioimmunoassay. J Clin Invest 60:648, 1977

GERTNER J et al: Prospective clinical trial of human growth hormone in short children without growth hormone deficiency. J Pediatr 104:172, 1984

GRUMBACH M: Growth hormone therapy and the short end of the stick. N Engl J Med 319:238, 1988

HINDMARSH PC, BROOK CGD: Effect of growth hormone in normal short children. Br Med J 295:573, 1987

HINTZ RL: The somatomedins. Adv Pediatr 28:293, 1980

—— et al: Biosynthetic methionyl-human growth hormone is biologically active in adult man. Lancet 1:1276, 1982

HORNER JM et al: Growth deceleration patterns in children with constitutional short stature: An aid to diagnosis. Pediatrics 62:529, 1978

KASTRUP KW et al: Increased growth rate following transfer to daily sc administration from three weekly im injections of hGH. Acta Endocrinol (Copenh) 104:148, 1983

LANTOS J et al: Ethical issues on growth hormone therapy. JAMA 261:1020, 1989

LEWIS UJ et al: Human growth hormone: A complex of proteins. Recent Prog Horm Res 36: 477, 1980

RINDERKNECHT R, HUMBEL RE: Primary structure of human IGF-II. FEBS Lett 89:283, 1978

ROSENFELD RG et al: Three-year results of a randomized prospective trial of methionyl human growth hormone and oxandrolone in Turner's syndrome. J Pediatr 113:393, 1988

TANNER JM, ISREALSOHN WJ: Parent-child correlations for body measurements of children between the ages of one month and 7 years. Ann Hum Genet 26:245, 1963

—— et al: Effect of human growth hormone treatment for 1 to 7 years on growth of 100 children with growth hormone deficiency, inherited smallness, Turner's syndrome, and other complaints. Arch Dis Child 46:745, 1971

——, DAVIS PSW: Clinical longitudinal standards for height and height velocity for North American children. J Pediatr 107:317, 1985

THORNER MO et al: Acceleration of growth in two children treated with human growth hormone releasing factor. N Engl J Med 312:4, 1985

VIMPANI OV et al: Prevalence of severe growth hormone deficiency. Br Med J 2:427, 1977

WILSON DM et al: Subcutaneous versus intramuscular growth hormone therapy: Growth and acute somatomedin response. J Pediatr 76:361, 1985

315   DISORDERS OF THE NEUROHYPOPHYSIS

ARNOLD M. MOSES / DAVID H. P. STREETEN

There are two largely independent hypothalamic-neurohypophyseal systems composed of neurons in the supraoptic and paraventricular nuclei, from which axons extend through the pituitary stalk to the posterior pituitary. Hormones (vasopressin and oxytocin), formed within separate ganglion cells, migrate down the axons as part of precursor proteins. They are stored in secretory granules within the nerve terminals in the neurohypophysis and are released by exocytosis into the bloodstream in response to appropriate stimuli. Vasopressin or antidiuretic hormone (AVP or ADH) is predominantly concerned with the control of water conservation, and its release is coordinated with the activity of the thirst center that regulates fluid intake. Oxytocin stimulates uterine contractions and milk ejection.

VASOPRESSIN SYNTHESIS, RELEASE, AND ACTION

SYNTHESIS Vasopressin is synthesized in the magnocellular neurons of the anterior hypothalamus. It is translated as a prepro-hormone which is altered in the Golgi apparatus to form a prohormone. The prohormone is packaged into neurosecretory vesicles. While the prohormone is being transported to axonal terminals, enzymes generate the active nonapeptide (AVP), a 10,000 molecular weight protein called neurophysin, and a 39-amino acid glycopeptide. All three products are released into the peripheral circulation.

ACTIONS AVP conserves water by concentrating the urine. It binds to its V_2 receptor on the contraluminal surface of the distal tubular epithelium, mainly of the collecting ducts. At this site AVP enhances the hydrosmotic flow of water from the luminal fluid to the medullary interstitium and assists in maintaining constancy of the osmolality and volume of body fluids. High concentrations of AVP acting on V_1 receptors can cause vasoconstriction, as may occur in response to severe hypotension or to infusion of vasopressin for treatment of bleeding esophageal varices.

AVP, perhaps from axons that terminate in the cerebrum, may play a role in learning and memory, and AVP from fibers in the median eminence may influence corticotropin secretion.

NORMAL HORMONE LEVELS AVP concentrations in plasma and urine can be measured by radioimmunoassay. The results may be expressed either as units based on pressor activity in the rat or in terms of weight of purified vasopressin. Arginine vasopressin has a biologic activity of approximately 400 units per milligram (1 mU = 2.5 ng = 2.3 pmol). The neurohypophysis under conditions of random fluid intake contains approximately 8 units or 18 nmol (20 μg) of AVP. Under the same conditions peripheral plasma AVP concentration in ranges from 2.3 to 7.4 pmol/L (2.5 to 8 ng/L). At the latter level and above, urine osmolality is maximal. The AVP concentration of blood fluctuates, with a maximum late at night and in the early morning and a minimum in the early afternoon. Under conditions of normal hydration, healthy subjects release approximately 370 to 1400 pmol (400 to 1500 ng) from the pituitary and excrete 23 to 80 pmol (25 to 90 ng) AVP in urine in 24 h. During 24 to 28 h of dehydration the amount released increases three to five times with consequent increases in plasma and urinary levels.

METABOLISM Inactivation of AVP occurs largely in liver and kidneys, a major mechanism being the cleavage of the terminal glycinamide to produce a biologically inactive substance. Approximately 7 to 10 percent of secreted AVP is excreted in the urine as active hormone.

CONTROL OF AVP RELEASE The release of AVP is influenced by a number of stimuli.

Osmoregulation Under normal conditions AVP release is primarily regulated by osmoreceptors in the hypothalamus. Changes in the concentrations of plasma solutes to which the cellular membrane is impermeable cause alterations in the volume of the osmoreceptor cells, which in turn alter the electric activity of the neurons and control AVP release. Osmotic changes that stimulate release also enhance production of AVP. The servomechanism between effective plasma osmolality and AVP release normally maintains plasma osmolality within a very narrow range. The mean plasma osmolality of normal subjects following a water load of 20 mL per kilogram of body weight is 281.7 mosmol/kg, and the osmolality that initiates AVP release following infusion of hypertonic saline solution into water-loaded subjects is 287.3 mosmol/kg. Thus, the increase in plasma osmolality from full diuresis to the initiation of antidiuresis by hypertonic saline solution is only 5.6 mosmol/kg, or 2 percent.

The infusion of hypertonic saline solution at a constant rate into water-loaded subjects causes a linear rise in plasma osmolality with time. After an interval that depends on the infusion rate and the concentration of the saline solution, there is an abrupt, progressive fall in free water clearance without a significant change in solute or creatinine excretion. We have defined the osmotic threshold for AVP release as the plasma osmolality at the onset of antidiuresis under these conditions. In 73 normal subjects, this occurred at a mean plasma osmolality of 287 mosmol/kg. The osmotic threshold for AVP release may also be determined, with very similar results, by constructing a linear regression line between simultaneously obtained plasma osmolality and either plasma or urine AVP concentration during hypertonic saline infusion and extrapolating the regression line to the x-axis intercept (plasma osmolality).

Volume regulation Decreases in plasma volume, through effects on stretch receptors in the left atrium and perhaps in the pulmonary veins, stimulate the release of AVP by reducing the tonic inhibitory impulses from the left atrium to the hypothalamus. The neural impulses travel via the vagi to the reticular formation of the midbrain and diencephalon and thence to the supraoptic and paraventricular nuclei, where they are integrated with the other stimuli that affect AVP release. Positive pressure breathing, quiet standing, and vasodilatation due to a warm environment may activate this mechanism, which serves to restore plasma volume, even at times overriding osmotic inhibition of AVP release. Following volume contraction, circulating AVP concentrations may reach 10 times the levels induced by hypertonicity. Increased plasma volume inhibits AVP release by the reverse mechanisms, leading to a diuresis and correction of the hypervolemia. Negative pressure breathing, recumbency, lack of gravitational force (as occurs in space travel), submersion in water, and exposure to cold may activate this mechanism.

Baroreceptor regulation Activation of carotid and aortic baroreceptors in response to hypotension causes release of AVP. Hypotension due to blood loss is the most potent stimulus and may at times raise plasma levels of AVP to 2.3 nmol/L (2.5 μg/L). These concentrations of AVP may cause marked vasoconstriction, which probably plays a role in the restoration of blood pressure.

Neural regulation Many neurotransmitters and neuropeptides in the hypothalamus play a role in regulating and modulating the release of AVP. Acetylcholine stimulates AVP release by its nicotinic action on supraoptic neurons. Angiotensin II, histamine, bradykinin, and neuropeptide Y probably stimulate AVP release. Norepinephrine, prostaglandins, and dopamine stimulate or inhibit AVP release, depending on the experimental conditions. Gamma aminobutyric acid appears to act as an inhibitory neurotransmitter; serotonin and substance P are also present in the supraoptic nucleus, but their influence on magnocellular neuron activity is not clear. The regulatory action of opioid peptides on AVP release is unclear with reports indicating stimulation, inhibition, or no effect. Though the roles of these and other transmitters and peptides are still poorly defined, the antidiuretic actions of stress, emesis, and pain, and the diuretic actions of hypnosis, psychological conditioning, and inhalation of carbon dioxide certainly suggest an important influence of higher centers on the release of AVP.

Aging The aging process is associated with enhanced AVP release in response to a rising plasma osmolality and a progressive increase in plasma AVP concentration. These physiologic changes appear to place the older individual under greater risk of developing water retention and hyponatremia, despite a concomitant decline in maximal renal concentrating capacity in response to AVP, which is usually evident and progressive beyond 60 years of age.

Pharmacologic influences Pharmacologic agents that can stimulate AVP release include nicotine, morphine, vincristine, vinblastine, cyclophosphamide, clofibrate, chlorpropamide, and some of the tricyclic anticonvulsants and antidepressants. Ethanol has diuretic properties by inhibiting neurohypophyseal function under a variety of conditions. Some narcotic antagonists also inhibit AVP release. Experimentally chlorpromazine, reserpine, and phenytoin all diminish the loss of AVP from the pituitary and the rise in urinary excretion of AVP that result from water deprivation. In humans, phenytoin and chlorpromazine may inhibit AVP release and produce diuresis.

AVP RESPONSE TO WATER DEPRIVATION AND TO WATER LOAD Water deprivation provides both an osmotic and a volume stimulus to vasopressin release by increasing plasma osmolality and decreasing plasma volume. The maximum urinary osmolality after water deprivation varies, depending on renal medullary osmolality and other intrarenal factors. In response to fluid deprivation for 18 to 24 h, in normal individuals, plasma osmolality rarely rises above 292 mosmol/kg. The resultant stimulation of AVP release increases plasma AVP concentration to 14 to 23 pmol/L (15 to 25 ng/L).

The administration of water lowers plasma osmolality and expands blood volume, inhibiting the release of AVP via both the osmoreceptor and the atrial volume receptor mechanisms. An oral water load of 20 mL/kg in normal adults results in a fall in plasma osmolality to a mean of 281.7 mosmol/kg and causes a maximum diuresis in 1 to $1\frac{1}{2}$ h with free water clearance rising to approximately 12 mL/min and urine osmolality falling to 40 to 60 mosmol/kg. The delay in reaching maximal diuresis is accounted for by the time involved in absorption of water from the gut, in metabolizing previously secreted vasopressin, and in renal recovery from the action of vasopressin.

INTERACTION OF OSMOTIC AND VOLUME INFLUENCES Under conditions of water deprivation and of water loading, volume and osmotic influences act in parallel to influence AVP release. In other circumstances volume and osmotic influences may be competitive, and changes in plasma volume can modify the effects of hypertonic stimuli on AVP release. Osmotic factors ordinarily predominate to maintain plasma osmolality within a narrow range. Larger changes in blood volume, such as those induced by hemorrhage, may blunt and eventually overcome the osmotic influences, and hypotension can activate arterial baroreceptors and exert a powerful stimulus to the elaboration of AVP and override simultaneous inhibiting influences.

RELATION BETWEEN AVP RELEASE AND THIRST-INDUCED WATER INTAKE Under normal conditions there is close coordination between AVP release and thirst, both of which are regulated by small increases and decreases in plasma osmolality. The perception of thirst generally becomes apparent when plasma osmolality rises to values greater than 292 mosmol/kg. Thus, water intake is not stimulated until the urine is maximally concentrated. Angiotensin II increases thirst and AVP release under conditions of extracellular volume depletion. Normally, therefore, water losses lead to slight hypernatremia which increases thirst and fluid intake to an extent sufficient to restore and maintain normal plasma osmolality. In contrast, when there is loss of thirst perception (adipsia) fluid losses are uncorrected and hypernatremia occurs even though AVP release is adequate to concentrate the urine maximally.

EFFECTS OF GLUCOCORTICOIDS Hormones of the adrenal cortex and the posterior pituitary have antagonistic effects on water excretion. Cortisol elevates the osmotic threshold for AVP release elicited by hypertonic saline infusion in water-loaded normal subjects, and glucocorticoids protect against water intoxication and overcome the impaired response to water loading in adrenal insufficiency.

Although the subnormal ability to dilute the urine in adrenal insufficiency may in part be due to excessive circulating AVP, glucocorticoids can also act directly on the renal tubules to decrease water permeability and increase solute-free water in the absence of AVP.

CELLULAR MECHANISM OF AVP ACTIVITY The biochemical basis for the action of AVP on the renal tubule is shown in Fig. 315-1: (1) AVP binds to specific contraluminal V_2 receptor sites; (2) the receptor-hormone complex is coupled to and activates adenylate cyclase in the same contraluminal membrane via a guanine nucleotide binding stimulatory protein (see Chap. 68); (3) the production of

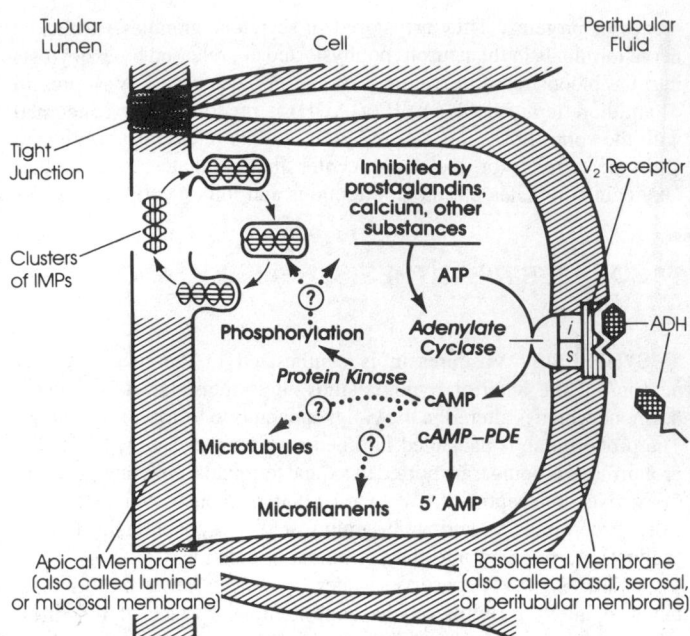

FIGURE 315-1 Schematic representation of the cellular action of vasopressin. The increased water permeability of responsive cells involves the V_2 receptor for vasopressin. Uninterrupted arrows denote steps that have been defined, interrupted arrows with question marks, postulated steps. ADH = antidiuretic hormone or vasopressin; i and s = inhibitory and stimulatory guanine nucleotide regulatory proteins; cAMP-PDE = phosphodiesterase; IMPs = intramembranous particles. [*From H Valtin, in Handbook of Physiology, Renal, Washington, DC, American Physiological Society (in press)*]

cyclic AMP is increased; (4) the cyclic AMP is translocated to the luminal cell membrane where it causes the activation of membrane-bound protein kinase; (5) the activated protein kinase causes the phosphorylation of membrane proteins; and (6) permeability of the luminal membrane to water is increased. The AVP-generated cyclic AMP may be inactivated by a phosphodiesterase that converts cyclic AMP to 5'-AMP. AVP also stimulates prostaglandin E_2 production which, in turn, acts as a feedback inhibitor of adenylate cyclase activation.

The final event in the transtubular movement of water is the appearance of particle aggregates in the luminal membrane of the cell (Fig. 315-2). These particles relieve the rate-limiting barrier to water flow. In the presence of the aggregates water molecules are able to move passively along an osmotic gradient. The transtubular movement of water depends also on the integrity of the microtubular system.

Various cations and drugs can influence the action of AVP. Calcium and lithium inhibit the adenylate cyclase response to vasopressin. Lithium also interferes with a subsequent biochemical action, as does potassium deficiency. Demeclocycline inhibits adenylate cyclase stimulation by AVP and also inhibits the cyclic AMP-dependent protein kinase. In contrast, chlorpropamide increases AVP-induced activation of adenylate cyclase.

DEFICIENCY OF VASOPRESSIN: DIABETES INSIPIDUS

Diabetes insipidus is a term which refers to the passage through the body of a large quantity of dilute fluid. This state of excessive water intake and hypotonic polyuria may be due to failure of AVP release in response to normal physiologic stimuli (central or neurogenic diabetes insipidus) or failure of the kidney to respond to AVP (nephrogenic diabetes insipidus).

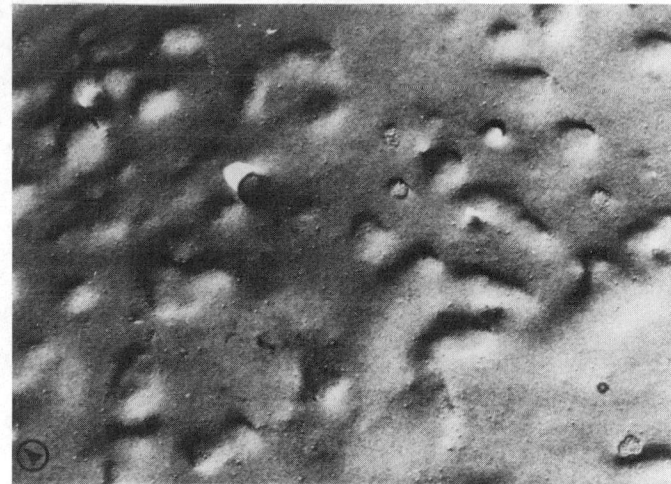

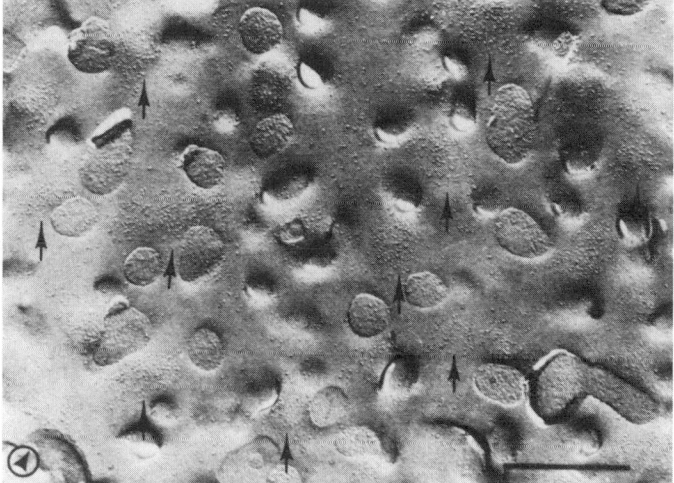

FIGURE 315-2 Virtual absence of particle clusters in renal collecting duct luminal membrane obtained from untreated Brattleboro (congenital diabetes insipidus) rat (*top*). Appearance of particle clusters (arrows) after treatment with AVP (*bottom*). *(From MC Harmanci et al, Am J Physiol 235:F440, 1978.)*

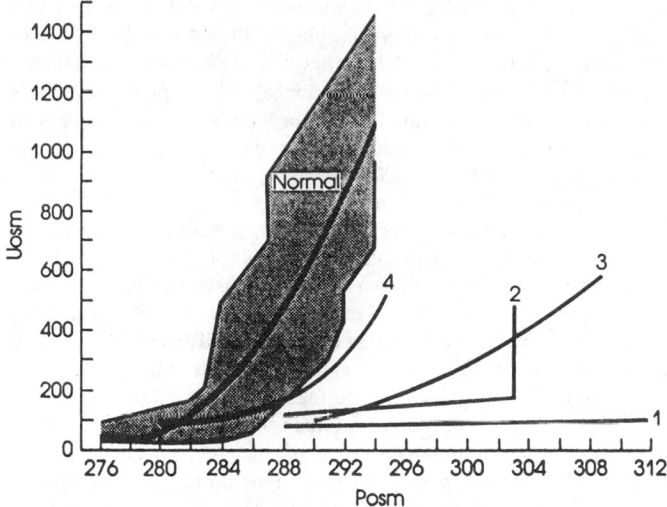

FIGURE 315-3 Relation of plasma and urinary osmolality during hydration and dehydration in normal adult subjects (shaded area) and in four types of patients with diabetes insipidus.

pamide, or clofibrate, indicating that the synthesis and storage of AVP are sufficient to allow for adequate urinary concentrating ability in the presence of an appropriate stimulus to release. In rare instances patients of the second to fourth types may present with asymptomatic hypernatremia associated with mild or absent evidence of diabetes insipidus.

ETIOLOGY The causes of central diabetes insipidus in 135 patients who satisfied the criteria described under ''Diagnostic Tests'' (below) and who had had diabetes insipidus for at least 6 months are shown in Table 315-1. Diabetes insipidus frequently starts in childhood or early adult life (median age of onset 21 years) and is more common in males than females. The major causes are as follows: (1) *Neoplastic or infiltrative lesions* of the hypothalamus or pituitary, including chromophobe adenomas, craniopharyngiomas, germinomas, pinealomas, metastatic tumors, leukemia, histiocytosis X, and sarcoidosis, caused diabetes insipidus in 37 patients. In approximately 60 percent of these patients evidence of partial or complete loss of anterior pituitary function was present. (2) *Pituitary or hypothalamic surgery or isotopic ablative therapy* caused diabetes insipidus in 32 patients and almost invariably was associated with anterior hypopituitarism.

PATHOPHYSIOLOGY Deficiency of vasopressin release in response to the appropriate stimuli may result from lesions at several functional sites in the physiologic chain of events which regulates discharge of the hormone into the bloodstream. For conceptual purposes four types of central diabetes insipidus can be defined. Patients of the first type show very little rise in urine osmolality, even with a marked increase in plasma osmolality (1, Fig. 315-3) and no evidence of AVP release during hypertonic saline infusion. They are essentially devoid of releasable AVP. In the second type there is an abrupt increase in urine osmolality during dehydration (2, Fig. 315-3), but there is no evidence of an osmotic threshold during saline infusion. These patients have a defective osmoreceptor mechanism but are capable of releasing AVP in response to the hypovolemia of severe dehydration. The third type of patient has some rise in urine osmolality with increasing plasma osmolality (3, Fig. 315-3) and has an elevated osmotic threshold for AVP release. These patients have a sluggish release mechanism and may be said to have a high-set osmoreceptor. In the fourth type of patient, urine and plasma osmolality coordinates are shifted to the right of normal (4, Fig. 315-3). AVP release in these patients is initiated at a normal plasma osmolality but is subnormal in amount.

The second to fourth types of patients may develop a good antidiuresis in response to nausea, nicotine, methacholine, chlorpro-

TABLE 315-1 Characteristics of 135 cases of longstanding* central diabetes insipidus diagnosed by the authors at SUNY Health Science Center, Syracuse. Categories are arranged in order of increasing median age of onset.

| Cause | Age of onset, years | | | | Percent of cases |
	Median†	Range	Males	Females	
Histiocytosis	2	1–30	3	2	4
Primary brain tumor —postoperative‡	15	6–50	9	11	15
Primary brain tumor —preoperative§	18	7–58	17	3	15
Idiopathic	20	<1–66	20	14	25
Head trauma	22	5–48	15	9	18
Nontraumatic encephalomalacia	43	15–73	3	4	5
Ruptured cerebral aneurysm	39		1	0	1
Post-hypophysectomy	42	24–68	4	8	9
Sarcoidosis	42		0	1	1
Metastatic cancer	56	32–72	6	5	8
			(58%)	(42%)	

* Longer than 6 months or until death.
† Median age of entire group = 24 years.
‡ 16 cases were of craniopharyngioma.
§ 5 cases were glioma, 7 germinoma, and 4 craniopharyngioma.

Surgically induced diabetes insipidus usually develops between 1 and 6 days after surgery and often disappears after a few days. It may remain absent or may recur and become chronic after an "interphase" of 1 to 5 days. Removal of the posterior lobe of the pituitary induces permanent diabetes insipidus only if the pituitary stalk is sectioned high enough to induce retrograde degeneration of most of the neurons of the supraoptic nucleus. (3) *Severe head injuries*, usually associated with fractures of the skull, caused diabetes insipidus in 24 patients and were associated with anterior hypopituitarism in only about one-sixth of patients. Spontaneous remissions of traumatic diabetes insipidus occasionally occur even after 6 months, presumably because of regeneration of disrupted axons within the pituitary stalk. (4) *Idiopathic diabetes insipidus* (in 34 patients) usually starts in childhood and is seldom (<20 percent) associated with anterior pituitary dysfunction. This diagnosis can be made only after a careful search has failed to reveal evidence of a tumor, infiltrative lesion, vascular lesion, or other presumptive cause of the AVP deficiency. The presence of anterior hypopituitarism or hyperprolactinemia or radiologic evidence of lesions within or above the sella should stimulate a continuing search for a causative lesion at 3- to 12-month intervals. The diagnosis of idiopathic diabetes insipidus is made with increasing confidence as the duration of negative findings on follow-up increases. A decrease in the number of neurons in the supraoptic and paraventricular nuclei has been reported in idiopathic diabetes insipidus, and circulating antibodies to hypothalamic nuclei may be present. In rare instances, dominant inheritance has been documented. (5) Seven patients had nontraumatic encephalomalacia from a variety of severe cerebral insults including shock, cardiopulmonary arrest, hypertensive encephalopathy, poisoning, and meningitis. All the patients were brain dead and had to be maintained on total life support systems.

CLINICAL MANIFESTATIONS *Polyuria, excessive thirst,* and *polydipsia* are almost invariably present in diabetes insipidus. Characteristically, these symptoms are sudden in onset, both when the disorder first presents itself and whenever the effects of administered vasopressin disappear during long-term therapy. In severe cases the urine is pale in color, and its volume may be immense (up to 16 to 24 L per day), requiring micturition every 30 to 60 min throughout the day and night. More frequently, however, the urine volume is only moderately increased (2.5 to 6 L per day), and occasionally it may be less than 2 liters per day, causing no complaints on the part of the patient. Urinary concentration (less than 290 mosmol/kg, specific gravity less than 1.010) is below that of the serum in severe cases but may be higher than that of serum (290 to 600 mosmol/kg) in patients with mild diabetes insipidus.

The slight rise in serum osmolality resulting from hypotonic polyuria stimulates thirst. Large volumes of fluid are imbibed, and cold drinks are preferred, patients often going to great trouble to secure cold fluids. Although thirst is probably secondary to loss of water, the administration of vasopressin often relieves or reduces thirst, even in the absence of fluid intake.

Normal function of the thirst center ensures that polydipsia closely matches polyuria, so that dehydration is seldom detectable except in the mild elevation of serum sodium concentration. However, when adequate replenishment of excreted water is interfered with, dehydration may become severe, causing weakness, fever, psychic disturbances, prostration, and death. These features are associated with a rising serum osmolality and serum sodium concentration, the latter sometimes exceeding 175 mmol/L. Adipsia is not found in idiopathic diabetes insipidus, but it may result from impaired function of the hypothalamic thirst center because of extension of the same abnormality that caused the diabetes insipidus. More frequently, dehydration occurs during unconsciousness produced by surgical anesthesia, head trauma, or other causes. It is particularly hazardous to administer large volumes of isotonic saline solution intravenously or of hyperosmolar protein by nasogastric tube unless adequate amounts of water are administered simultaneously in unconscious patients with untreated diabetes insipidus.

Hydronephrosis is a rare complication of the polyuria, especially in patients who fail to empty their bladders adequately because of bladder atony, uretheral strictures, or other causes.

DIAGNOSTIC TESTS The diagnostic procedures to establish the cause of hypotonic polyuria represent a pragmatic clinical approach in contrast to investigational studies on the pathophysiology of AVP release. Even though stimuli such as nausea, nicotine administration, hypoglycemia, and hypotension may release AVP, the results are clinically irrelevant. It is of little consequence to the patient with symptomatic diabetes insipidus that one or more of these nonosmotic stimuli retains its capacity to release AVP. The following procedures which utilize plasma and urine osmolality determinations are readily available, reliable, and safe and they allow the physician to establish the diagnosis rapidly and to initiate therapy. Measurement of plasma or urine AVP which are expensive and time-consuming are only occasionally needed, when osmolality measurements are inconclusive (Fig. 315-4). The tests should not be conducted in the presence of untreated thyroid or adrenocortical deficiency or in the presence of an osmotic diuresis (e.g., uncontrolled diabetes mellitus).

Assessment of the relation of plasma to urine osmolality The normal relationship between plasma osmolality (assuming no increase in blood urea or glucose) and urine osmolality is indicated in Fig. 315-3. If several simultaneously determined plasma and urine osmolalities in a patient with polyuria fall substantially to the right of the shaded area, the patient has central or nephrogenic diabetes insipidus. The latter diagnosis can be made if the response to injected vasopressin is subnormal (see "Dehydration Test" below) or if plasma or urinary AVP concentration is increased. The practice of relating plasma to urine osmolality is useful, particularly in postoperative neurosurgical cases or after head trauma, where its use can lead quickly to the differentiation of diabetes insipidus from parenteral fluid excess. In such patients, intravenous hydration can be slowed temporarily, and repeated plasma and urine osmolalities can be obtained and plotted as in Fig. 315-3, to determine whether the relationship is normal.

Dehydration test Comparison of the urinary osmolality after dehydration with that after vasopressin administration is a simple and reliable way of diagnosing diabetes insipidus and of differentiating vasopressin deficiency from other causes of polyuria. This test can and should be combined with the assessment of the relationship between plasma and urine osmolality.

FIGURE 315-4 Relationship between plasma osmolality (Posm) and urinary AVP excretion (U_{AVP}) in normal subjects (shaded area on left), patients with central diabetes insipidus (shaded area on right), and patients with nephrogenic diabetes insipidus (individual data points). Correlates in patients with SIADH fall to the left of the normal range. [*From AM Moses, in P Czernichow and AG Robinson (eds), Frontiers of Hormone Research, vol 13: Diabetes Insipidus in Man, Basel, Karger, 1985.*]

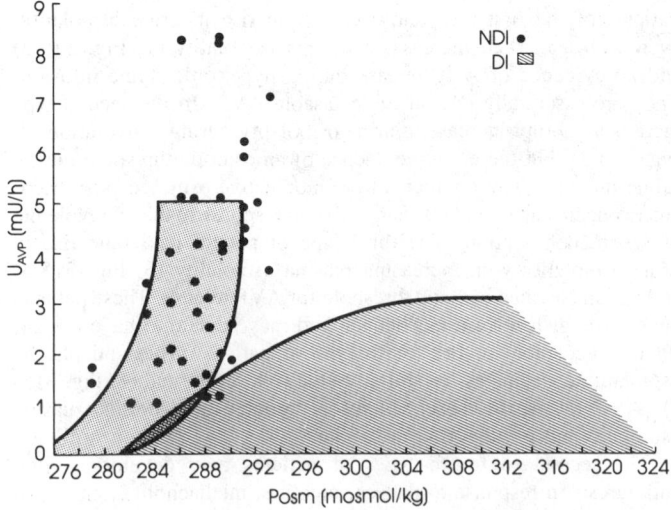

The maximal urinary concentrating capacity varies widely between individuals, and no absolute lower limits of "normal" can be defined in patients with nonspecific illnesses in whom AVP is produced in adequate amounts. It is impossible to distinguish between deficiency and sufficiency of AVP release solely by the level of the urinary osmolality attained after specified periods of water deprivation. On the other hand, if after prolonged dehydration vasopressin administration induces a further rise in urinary osmolality, there is a strong implication that vasopressin deficiency exists.

PROCEDURE

1 Fluids are withheld long enough to result in stable hourly urinary osmolalities (an hourly increase of <30 mosmol/kg for at least three successive hours). This is usually associated with a loss in body weight of at least 1 kg. In patients whose daily urinary volumes exceed 10 liters, the fluid deprivation should begin between 4 A.M. and 6 A.M. so that the patient can be carefully watched and the test terminated if weight loss exceeds 2 kg or the clinical condition deteriorates. In patients whose urinary volumes are only mildly increased or who are hyponatremic, water deprivation may be started about midnight.

2 Urine specimens are collected hourly for osmolality measurements from 6 A.M. at least until noon and preferably until the osmolality has been stable for three consecutive hours.

3 After the third hour of stable urinary osmolalities, the patient is given vasopressin as 5 units aqueous vasopressin or 1 μg desmopressin by subcutaneous injection or 10 μg desmopressin by nasal spray.

4 Plasma osmolality is determined immediately before the injection of vasopressin, and urinary osmolality is measured on the specimen collected between 30 and 60 min after the injection.

Vital signs should be monitored during the dehydration procedure, but when the test has been performed as described, adverse effects are rare.

INTERPRETATION In subjects with normal pituitary function, urinary osmolality does not rise by more than 9 percent after the injection of vasopressin, whatever the maximal urinary osmolality might be after dehydration alone. In central diabetes insipidus, the rise in urinary osmolality after vasopressin exceeds 9 percent. To ensure adequacy of dehydration, plasma osmolality before the vasopressin injection should be above 288 mosmol/kg. Patients who have polyuria from renal diseases, potassium depletion, or nephrogenic diabetes insipidus (see below) usually show little rise in urinary osmolality with dehydration and no further rise after vasopressin injection. Patients with compulsive water drinking (primary polydipsia) often require prolonged water deprivation before plasma osmolality reaches 288 mosmol/kg and before a plateau in urinary osmolality is reached; urinary osmolality rises by <9 percent after the administration of exogenous vasopressin.

Hypertonic saline infusions These tests are seldom necessary for the diagnosis of diabetes insipidus but are useful in the documentation of alterations in the osmotic threshold for AVP release; such changes may be of value in characterizing some cases of hypo- or hypernatremia. See references for details.

DIFFERENTIAL DIAGNOSIS Diabetes insipidus must be distinguished from other types of polyuria (Table 315-2). Several are recognizable by the history (e.g., recent lithium or mannitol administration, recent surgery under methoxyflurane anesthesia, or recent renal transplantation). In others the physical examination or simple laboratory procedures will indicate the diagnosis (evidence of glycosuria, renal disease, sickle cell anemia, hypercalcemia, or potassium depletion, including primary aldosteronism).

Congenital nephrogenic diabetes insipidus is a rare, usually familial, form of polyuria resulting from unresponsiveness to AVP. Females may have a less severe form of the disease than males, may concentrate urine reasonably well with water deprivation, and may be treatable with large amounts of desmopressin. One family with this disease has an abnormal gene located on the short arm of the X

TABLE 315-2 Major polyuric syndromes

I Primary disorders of water intake or output
  A Excessive water intake
    1 Psychogenic polydipsia
    2 Hypothalamic disease: histiocytosis X, sarcoidosis
    3 Drug-induced polydipsia
      a Thioridazine
      b Chlorpromazine
      c Anticholinergic drugs (dry mouth)
  B Inadequate tubular reabsorption of filtered water
    1 Vasopressin deficiency
      a Central diabetes insipidus
      b Drug-induced inhibition of AVP release
        (1) Narcotic antagonists
    2 Renal tubular unresponsiveness to AVP
      a Nephrogenic diabetes insipidus (congenital and familial)
      b Nephrogenic diabetes insipidus (acquired)
        (1) Several chronic renal diseases, after obstructive uropathy, unilateral renal arterial stenosis, after renal transplantation, after acute tubular necrosis
        (2) Potassium deficiencies, including primary aldosteronism
        (3) Chronic hypercalcemias, including hyperparathyroidism
        (4) Drug-induced: lithium, methoxyflurane anesthesia, demeclocycline
        (5) Various systemic disorders: multiple myeloma, amyloidosis, sickle cell anemia, Sjögren's syndrome
II Primary disorders of renal absorption of solutes (osmotic diuresis)
  A Glucose: diabetes mellitus
  B Salts, especially sodium chloride
    1 Various chronic renal diseases, especially chronic pyelonephritis
    2 After various diuretics, including mannitol

chromosome. Most patients studied appear to have a V_2-receptor abnormality, while some patients appear to have a postreceptor defect. All have normal V_1-receptor functions. Patients with congenital nephrogenic diabetes insipidus can be distinguished from those with vasopressin-deficient diabetes insipidus by the familial nature of the disorder (rare in central diabetes insipidus) and by lack of a dramatic reduction in daily urine volume when vasopressin or desmopressin is administered. When patients with nephrogenic and central diabetes insipidus cannot be differentiated with certainty by osmolality determinations alone, either elevated plasma, or urinary AVP concentration in relation to plasma osmolality (Fig. 315-4), or a high AVP concentration in relation to urine osmolality will allow the diagnosis of nephrogenic diabetes insipidus to be established.

Primary polydipsia Primary or psychogenic polydipsia is occasionally difficult to differentiate from diabetes insipidus and may occur in two forms. Chronic overingestion of water results in hypotonic polyuria and is often confused with diabetes insipidus. The intermittent ingestion of large quantities of fluid may also lead to water intoxication and dilutional hyponatremia even though there is normal urinary diluting capacity. This phenomenon is rare because normal adults can excrete between 10 and 14 mL/min of solute-free water, and it is an unusual circumstance which results in the ingestion of sufficiently more water than this to cause dilutional hyponatremia. The tendency to develop dilutional hyponatremia in these patients is increased because the chronic overingestion of fluids may limit their ability to excrete free water.

Polydipsia and polyuria are usually somewhat erratic, even in the chronic form of primary polydipsia. This is in contrast to the sustained polydipsia and polyuria of diabetes insipidus. These patients often have no nocturnal polyuria. Of 17 patients who were diagnosed as having sustained primary polydipsia, 10 were female and 7 were male with a median age of onset of 34 years (range 14 to 48). In three patients the onset of primary polydipsia followed head trauma, two had hypothalamic sarcoidosis, one was the sister of a patient with congenital nephrogenic diabetes insipidus, one was severely mentally retarded, and one had a hypothalamic lesion of unknown cause. The remaining nine patients had moderate to severe psychiatric disturbances and were frequently taking psychoactive drugs with anticholinergic properties. The syndrome has also been described in patients with anorexia nervosa who may drink huge quantities of

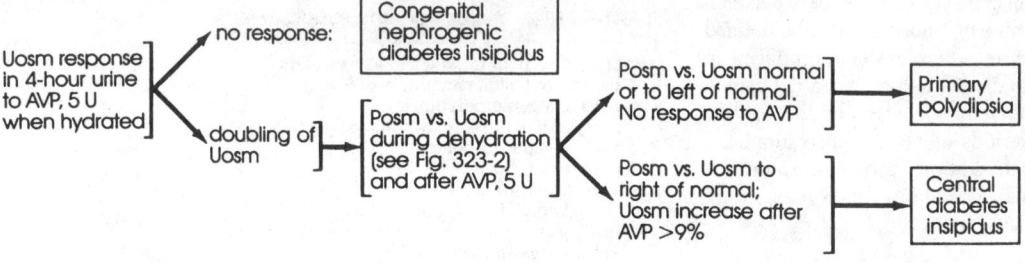

FIGURE 315-5 Approach to hypotonic polyurias

water; this consumption may markedly decrease when food intake increases. There is a predisposition toward dilutional hyponatremia in patients who ingest excessive fluids when urinary diluting capacity is impaired by therapeutic agents such as nonsteroidal anti-inflammatory drugs.

The diagnosis is usually evident from the combination of low plasma and urinary osmolalities. The relationship between urine and plasma osmolality during water deprivation is typically normal or supranormal (to left of normal in Fig. 315-3). There is an absent or minimal rise in urine osmolality after injection of vasopressin at the plateau of urine osmolality during the dehydration test. Because chronic overingestion of water may suppress release of AVP, and because chronic polyuria may cause a wash-out of the medullary osmotic gradient, urine osmolality may be subnormal in relation to plasma osmolality (to right of normal in Fig. 315-3). Therefore, it may be difficult, if not impossible, to differentiate patients with primary polydipsia from those with partial central diabetes insipidus. Indeed, there are probably patients with both problems. Attempts to treat these patients with vasopressin, even under close supervision, usually results in water intoxication.

A simple diagnostic approach to patients with hypotonic polyuria is shown in Fig. 315-5.

TREATMENT (See Table 315-3)   Diabetes insipidus can be treated by hormone replacement. As is true of most peptides, oral administration of vasopressin is ineffective. Aqueous vasopressin may be administered subcutaneously in doses of 5 to 10 units and usually has a duration of action of 3 to 6 h. The main use of this preparation is in initial management of unconscious patients with acute onset of diabetes insipidus following head trauma or a neurosurgical procedure. Its short duration of action allows recognition of the recovery of neurohypophyseal function and prevents the development of water intoxication in patients receiving intravenous fluids.

Desmopressin has prolonged antidiuretic activity and is almost completely devoid of pressor effects. When used intranasally in amounts between 10 and 20 μg (0.1 to 0.2 mL) or by subcutaneous injection (1 to 4 μg), it has an antidiuretic action for 12 to 24 h in most patients. This analogue is the drug of choice in the treatment

of most patients with diabetes insipidus. Lypressin is a nasal spray; a single application may result in an antidiuresis lasting approximately 4 to 6 h. Nasal absorption of both analogues may be decreased in the presence of an upper respiratory infection or allergic rhinitis with edema of the nasal mucosa. In such circumstances and in the unconscious patient with diabetes insipidus, desmopressin should be given by subcutaneous injection.

In the past, patients with an established diagnosis of diabetes insipidus were usually treated with intramuscular injections of vasopressin tannate in oil (2.5 or 5 units), which has an antidiuretic effect for 24 to 72 h. Since this material is a suspension of vasopressin tannate in peanut oil, it is essential that the ampul be warmed and then thoroughly shaken or inverted repeatedly until the brownish deposit of pituitary powder in the ampul is evenly distributed as a slightly cloudy suspension in the oil. A dry syringe should be used.

Patients with diabetes insipidus who have some residual releasable AVP (types 2 to 4) may respond to oral treatment with several nonhormonal agents. Chlorpropamide stimulates AVP release from the neurohypophysis and potentiates the action of submaximal amounts of AVP on the renal tubule, properties that make it of use in many patients with diabetes insipidus. Doses of 200 to 500 mg, usually taken once daily, are sufficient for an antidiuretic response. Its action starts within several hours of administration and usually lasts for 24 h. Chlorpropamide may also restore thirst perception and thus be useful in patients with thirst center defects. Hypoglycemia may occur but can usually be avoided by adherence to a regular schedule of meals. Clofibrate is capable of stimulating AVP release and has also been used in the treatment of diabetes insipidus. Doses of 500 mg four times a day often result in a prompt and sustained antidiuresis. In some patients, combined treatment with chlorpropamide and clofibrate results in complete restoration of water regulation to normal. Carbamazepine has also been observed to produce antidiuresis in patients with diabetes insipidus by stimulation of AVP release. Doses of 400 to 600 mg daily are effective, but the drug is not widely used owing to toxic side effects.

These therapeutic agents are effective only in central diabetes insipidus. In males with nephrogenic diabetes insipidus the only

TABLE 315-3 Agents used in treatment of diabetes insipidus

	Dose form	Usual dose	Duration of action, h
CENTRAL DIABETES INSIPIDUS			
Hormone replacement:			
Aqueous vasopressin	10 or 20 units/ampul	5–10 units subcutaneously	3–6
Desmopressin	2.5-mL intranasal preparation, 100 μg/mL; 1- or 10-mL ampul, for injection, 4 μg/mL	10–20 μg intranasally or 1–4 μg subcutaneously	12–24
Lypressin	5-mL bottle, 50 units/mL	2–4 units intranasally	4–6
Vasopressin tannate in oil	5 units/ampul	5 units intramuscularly	24–72
Nonhormonal agents:			
Chlorpropamide	100- and 250-mg tablets	200–500 mg daily	
Clofibrate	500-mg capsules	500 mg four times daily	
Carbamazepine	200-mg tablets	400–600 mg daily	
NEPHROGENIC DIABETES INSIPIDUS			
Hydrochlorothiazide	50-mg tablets	50–100 mg daily	
Chlorthalidone	50-mg tablets	50 mg daily	

agents of clinical value are thiazides and other diuretics. By producing sodium depletion, the diuretics cause a fall in glomerular filtration rate with enhanced reabsorption of fluid in the proximal portion of the nephron and decreased delivery of sodium to the ascending limb of the loop of Henle and consequently reduced capacity to dilute the urine. The therapeutic effect of diuretics in patients with nephrogenic diabetes insipidus is lost unless sodium intake is restricted. Some female patients with congenital nephrogenic diabetes insipidus and some patients with lithium-induced polyuria have been treated effectively with large doses of desmopressin.

PROGNOSIS The long-term prospects of a patient with diabetes insipidus are dependent primarily upon the underlying cause. In the absence of brain tumor or systemic disease, ready access to water and proper treatment of the polyuria usually lead to a normal life and life expectancy. Early recognition and treatment are important to prevent bladder distention, hydroureter, and hydronephrosis which may develop in patients with long-standing polyuria, particularly in patients with nephrogenic diabetes insipidus. The rare patient with adipsia or hypodipsia in association with diabetes insipidus is in danger of developing severe dehydration, which may lead to vascular collapse or central nervous system damage. Similarly severe complications may occur in patients with diabetes insipidus who develop impairment of consciousness. For this reason, all patients with diabetes insipidus should carry identification indicating the presence of the disorder and the necessity for treatment and fluid administration.

SYNDROMES ASSOCIATED WITH VASOPRESSIN EXCESS

Excessive blood levels or actions of vasopressin are associated with and probably cause water retention in several circumstances:

1 As a mechanism for *prevention of a rising plasma osmolality* which would otherwise result from sodium retention in edema, associated with congestive heart failure; cirrhosis with ascites; nephrosis; orthostatic edema; myxedema; and treatment with sodium-retaining drugs (fludrocortisone, nonsteroidal anti-inflammatory agents, and others)

2 As a mechanism of *defense against hypovolemia and/or hypotension* in adrenal insufficiency, excessive fluid losses (from vomiting, diarrhea, drug-induced diuresis, and excessive sweating), fluid deprivation, and probably positive pressure respiration

3 As a consequence of *drug- or disease-induced release of vasopressin from the neurohypophysis* caused by:

  a Central nervous system disorders: head trauma, subdural hematoma, subarachnoid hemorrhage, cerebral vascular thrombosis, brain tumor, cerebral atrophy, acute encephalitis, acute psychosis, tuberculous and other meningitides

  b Drugs that release or potentiate the action of AVP: chlorpropamide, vincristine, vinblastine, cyclophosphamide, carbamazepine, general anesthetics, tricyclic antidepressants

4 In ectopic AVP production and release:

  a From neoplastic tissue: oat cell carcinoma of lung, pancreatic carcinoma, lymphosarcoma, Hodgkin's disease, reticulum cell sarcoma, thymoma, carcinoma of duodenum or bladder

  b From inflammatory lung diseases: tuberculosis, lung abscess, pneumonias, empyema

5 Other conditions: Guillain-Barré syndrome, lupus erythematosus, acute intermittent porphyria, severe renovascular hypertension, and old age

SYNDROME OF INAPPROPRIATE AVP SECRETION OR SIADH SIADH is the term applied to vasopressin excess of types 3 to 5 above, associated with hyponatremia without edema (Table 315-4). In these patients the AVP excess is considered to be inappropriate since it occurs in the presence of plasma hypoosmolality. SIADH is analogous to abnormalities produced by administration of vasopressin and water to normal subjects. Although it might be

TABLE 315-4 Causes of SIADH

I Malignant neoplasms with autonomous AVP release
  A Oat cell carcinoma of lung
  B Carcinoma of pancreas
  C Lymphosarcoma, reticulum cell sarcoma, Hodgkin's disease
  D Carcinoma of duodenum
  E Thymoma
II Nonmalignant pulmonary diseases
  A Tuberculosis
  B Lung abscess
  C Pneumonia
  D Viral pneumonitis
  E Empyema
  F Chronic obstructive airways disease
III Central nervous system disorders
  A Skull fracture
  B Subdural hematoma
  C Subarachnoid hemorrhage
  D Cerebral vascular thrombosis
  E Cerebral atrophy
  F Acute encephalitis
  G Tuberculous meningitis
  H Purulent meningitis
  I Guillain-Barré syndrome
  J Lupus erythematosus
  K Acute intermittent porphyria
IV Drugs
  A Chlorpropamide
  B Vincristine
  C Vinblastine
  D Cyclophosphamide
  E Carbamazepine
  F Oxytocin
  G General anesthesia
  H Narcotics
  I Tricyclic antidepressants
V Miscellaneous causes
  A Hypothyroidism
  B Positive pressure respiration

conceptually valid to consider the AVP excess to be inappropriate in adrenal insufficiency and the edematous, hypovolemic, and hypotensive disorders listed in 1 and 2 above, their different pathogenic mechanisms and treatments make it clinically advisable not to consider these disorders as variants of the SIADH.

Pathogenesis of SIADH The ectopic origin of authentic AVP from neoplasms and pulmonary tissue of the types listed above has been documented by tissue analysis. Neoplastic cells obtained from the lungs of patients with SIADH can synthesize, store, and release AVP, and in some patients AVP release is not entirely autonomous, being partially suppressible by water loading of the patient. Both AVP and its associated neurophysin are elevated in the plasma of over 60 percent of patients with small cell carcinoma of the lung. There is excellent correlation between the increases in plasma AVP and neurophysin concentrations on the one hand and the clinical responses to treatment or the recurrences of disease on the other. Vasopressin has also been demonstrated in tuberculous lung tissue. It seems likely, but has not been established, that intracranial lesions (meningitis, encephalitis, trauma, vascular accidents) may cause nonspecific irritative stimulation of AVP release from the neurohypophysis. Some drugs, such as vincristine, chlorpropamide, and carbamazepine, stimulate excessive release of AVP from the neurohypophyseal system and others (e.g., chlorpropamide and nonsteroidal anti-inflammatory agents) potentiate the antidiuretic action of secreted AVP on the renal tubular concentrating mechanism.

Excessive release or excessive renal tubular activity of vasopressin results in the excretion of a concentrated urine (with a urinary osmolality usually over 300 mosmol/kg) despite a subnormal plasma osmolality and serum sodium concentration. Sodium excretion in the urine is maintained (usually above 20 mmol/L) by hypervolemia, suppression of the renin-angiotensin-aldosterone system, and increased plasma concentration of atrial natriuretic peptide; and reduction in sodium concentration may be low if sodium intake is low, and urinary sodium concentration is higher if sodium intake is high.

Blood urea nitrogen and uric acid concentrations tend to fall because of plasma dilution and increased excretion of nitrogenous compounds. Because of the hypervolemia, blood pressure shows no orthostatic fall, but in spite of hypervolemia there is no recumbent hypertension (except when plasma angiotensin II is simultaneously elevated in angiotensinogenic hypertension) and no edema (for an unknown reason). The extracellular hypotonicity leads to intracellular edema, and severe symptoms may result from the consequent cerebral edema.

Clinical manifestations of SIADH In general, the rate of fall in serum sodium concentration is more important in producing the neurologic features of SIADH than the absolute magnitude of the fall. When SIADH is mild, with serum Na concentrations of 130 to 135 mmol/L, or developing gradually over several weeks, symptoms are often absent or may be limited to anorexia, nausea, and vomiting, such as occurs in other forms of hyponatremia. When hyponatremia is severe or acute in onset, body weight increases, and the symptoms of cerebral edema become predominant, including restlessness, irritability, confusion, coma, and convulsions associated with nonspecific EEG changes. Edema is almost always absent.

Diagnosis SIADH may be strongly suspected in patients who have hyponatremia and a concentrated urine (osmolality >300 mosmol/kg) associated with lethargy and in the absence of edema, orthostatic hypotension, and features of dehydration. The diagnosis of SIADH is made when other causes known to stimulate AVP release are excluded. The diagnosis is supported by the finding of blood urea nitrogen, serum uric acid, creatinine, and albumin concentrations in the low-normal or subnormal range. However, it is essential in making the diagnosis of SIADH to differentiate the condition from (a) the *dilutional hyponatremias* listed in 2 above, particularly adrenocortical insufficiency, in which orthostatic hypotension with tachycardia and an elevated or high-normal BUN are characteristic; (b) the *edematous states* listed in 1 above, particularly congestive heart failure with hyponatremia, and hypothyroidism; (c) *hypertensive states* associated with hyponatremia caused by renovascular stenosis or by diuretic therapy; (d) *primary polydipsia* which is always associated with a dilute urine (osmolality <150 mosmol/kg); (e) *pseudohyponatremia* associated with excessive plasma glucose, triglyceride, or protein concentrations [conditions (a) through (e) are easily recognizable by the associated plasma abnormalities]; and (f) the *"sick-cell" syndrome* in which hyponatremia is due to a subnormal setting of the hypothalamic osmoreceptors, associated usually with a chronic, debilitating disease and polyuria.

When the diagnosis of SIADH is not obvious after excluding other causes of hyponatremia, a positive diagnosis can usually be made with a *water-load test*. The water-load test is particularly useful in differentiating patients with a low-set osmoreceptor (who excrete the water normally) from all other hyponatremic states associated with a concentrated urine. This test should not be performed unless or until the serum sodium concentration has been elevated to a safe level (above 125 mmol/L) by restriction of water intake, and/or if

necessary, saline administration. The patient is asked to drink the water load (20 mL per kilogram of body weight up to 1500 mL) in 10 to 20 min and urine is collected in hourly samples, with the patient recumbent between voidings, for 4 to 5 h in the morning. At least 65 percent of the water load should be excreted in 4 h or 80 percent in 5 h and the lowest urinary osmolality, usually reached in the second hour, should normally be below 100 mosmol/kg. It is essential, to prevent water intoxication in patients who have failed to excrete the water load normally, to allow no further water intake for the rest of that day. Failure to excrete the water load often occurs in adrenal insufficiency, or renal insufficiency, as well as in SIADH. It is important to appreciate, too, that SIADH cannot be diagnosed in the presence of severe pain, nausea, "stress," hypovolemia, hypotension, or other conditions that may stimulate AVP release even in the presence of plasma hypotonicity.

Measurements of plasma or urinary AVP (P_{AVP}, U_{AVP}) are useful adjuvants in establishing the diagnosis of SIADH. Plasma AVP is normally immeasurable in hyponatremic states but is detectable, even after a water load, in SIADH. The correlates of plasma osmolality (Posm) versus P_{AVP} or U_{AVP} concentration fall to the left of the normal values in SIADH (Fig. 315-4) and in any of the other hyponatremic states associated with a concentrated urine. Thus, in most patients with SIADH, P_{AVP} and U_{AVP} concentrations, which may fluctuate widely, are unrelated to concomitant changes in Posm. Occasionally, this lack of correlation between Posm and P_{AVP} or U_{AVP} may be inconsistent. Rarely, for instance, the baseline, unstimulated AVP level may be inappropriately elevated and may fail to change as Posm is raised until the Posm reaches the normal range. Further increases in Posm induced by hypertonic saline infusion or water deprivation may then result in normal or subnormal increases in P_{AVP} or U_{AVP}. This unusual phenomenon may reflect uncontrolled "leakage" of AVP from the neurohypophysis.

The diagnostic approach to SIADH is depicted in Fig. 315-6.

Treatment Restriction of fluid intake to 800 to 1000 mL daily is essential treatment. Since this intake will almost always be exceeded by urinary output plus insensible fluid loss, a negative water balance ensues that will result in gradual, daily reduction in weight, a progressive rise in serum Na concentration and osmolality, and symptomatic improvement. It is useful to verify the occurrence of these effects of fluid loss by documenting the changes in weight and serum Na concentration daily, until serum Na rises above 135 mmol/L.

Unless and until the underlying cause of the SIADH can be corrected, fluid intake should be appropriately restricted continuously, to maintain normonatremia. In addition to restriction of fluid intake, 5% sodium chloride solution, 200 to 300 mL, should be infused intravenously over 3 to 4 h in patients with severe confusion, convulsions, or coma. It is important to avoid the risk of inducing pontine myelinosis by not raising the serum Na concentration too rapidly. The possibility of causing congestive heart failure is remote

FIGURE 315-6 Approach to diagnosis of SIADH in patients with hyponatremia.

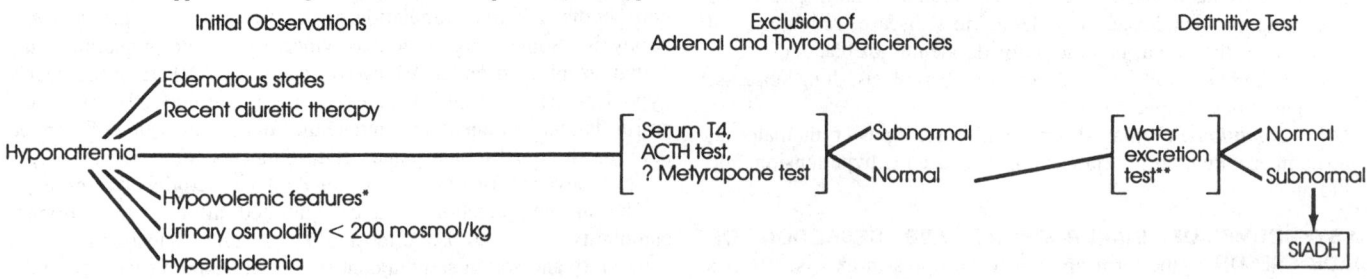

*Orthostatic hypotension and tachycardia, prerenal azotemia, etc.

**Water excretion test should only be performed when serum Na concentration has risen above 125 mEq/L, after water deprivation for as long as may be necessary.

as long as fluid is restricted, but this possibility may be further reduced by the simultaneous administration of furosemide, 40 mg intravenously.

Attempts should be made to identify and correct the cause of the SIADH as soon as possible. The administration of water-retaining drugs should be stopped. Treatment of hypothyroidism with thyroxine should be initiated. Pulmonary tuberculosis and other pulmonary infections should be appropriately treated, and meningitis or other CNS disorders should be sought and treated, if present. When a malignant tumor is the source of autonomous AVP release and SIADH, surgery, irradiation, and/or chemotherapy is often symptomatically beneficial even if the underlying neoplasm cannot be cured.

Antagonism of the release or actions of excessive AVP release is not often necessary and seldom successful. Although phenytoin inhibits AVP release, it is seldom effective in SIADH. Drugs that block the effect of AVP on the renal tubule may occasionally be useful in this syndrome. Demeclocycline is the most potent inhibitor of AVP action that is available for chronic administration, in doses of 900 to 1200 mg per day. Patients receiving demeclocycline should be carefully followed to detect any evidence of renal failure, bacterial superinfection, or excessive drug-induced water loss. Lithium salts interfere with AVP action on tubular water reabsorption and can cause polyuria by this mechanism. Unfortunately, lithium may have serious side effects in hyponatremic patients, and for this reason lithium salts are not recommended for treatment of SIADH.

Prognosis The prognosis of SIADH depends on the cause of the disorder. Drug-induced SIADH is rapidly and completely corrected by withdrawal of the causative agent. Similarly, the effective treatment of pulmonary or CNS infections results in improvement and eventual cure of SIADH caused by such lesions. Although SIADH resulting from oat cell carcinoma of the lung or other malignancies can often be controlled with vigorous restriction of fluid intake, the underlying malignancy determines the prognosis in these patients.

PARAVENTRICULAR-NEUROHYPOPHYSEAL SYSTEM AND OXYTOCIN

CHEMISTRY AND PHYSIOLOGY Oxytocin, a nonapeptide that differs by two amino acids from vasopressin, is produced predominantly in the cell bodies of the paraventricular nuclei and to a lesser extent in those of the supraoptic nuclei. It is synthesized and transported in neurosecretory granules by way of neuronal axons to the neurohypophysis, where it is stored or released, in conjunction with an oxytocin-specific neurophysin. Oxytocin release is stimulated by nerve impulses originating in the hypothalamus, which cause depolarization of the neurosecretory terminals of the posterior pituitary and subsequent release of oxytocin through a calcium-dependent process, similar to the mechanism for vasopressin. Estrogen stimulates release of oxytocin and its neurophysin. The secretion of oxytocin, as well as of vasopressin, is inhibited by ethanol. Some stimuli such as pain apparently release oxytocin and vasopressin simultaneously, but most stimuli release the two hormones independently. Oxytocin is primarily liberated during suckling, whereas vasopressin is released in much greater quantities than is oxytocin after an osmotic stimulus or hemorrhage. Manipulation or distention of the female genital tract, artificially or during parturition, is a more effective stimulus to oxytocin release than suckling.

Oxytocin acts on the membranes of myometrial and myoepithelial cells and results in an increased force of contraction. Sensitivity of the myometrium to oxytocin increases with the duration of pregnancy, but a role for oxytocin in the initiation and maintenance of labor is not established. Oxytocin may have survival value to the offspring since it may hasten the final stages of birth and lessen the chances of anoxia. Oxytocin also exerts a contractile action on the myometrium post partum and contracts the myoepithelial cells of the mammary alveoli, causing them to expel milk from the secretory tissue to the nipple. Oxytocin is 100 times more potent than vasopressin in its milk-ejecting activity in the human. In contrast, the antidiuretic potency of oxytocin relative to vasopressin is about 1:200. It is unlikely that oxytocin exerts any significant physiologic effect other than on the uterus and breast.

One milligram of purified preparation of oxytocin contains 450 IU of hormone, and the amount of oxytocin in the posterior pituitary ranges from 20 to 30 nmol (25 to 40 ng). In spite of the fact that there is no known role of oxytocin in the male, the male neural lobe stores oxytocin in amounts similar to those in the female. Plasma oxytocin concentration in both men and women exhibits episodic increases, with values ranging from a low of approximately 1 to 4 pmol/L (1.25 to 5 ng/L) but with no diurnal variation. In normal women there is a midcycle increase in plasma oxytocin concentration from a preovulatory value of approximately 2 pmol/L (2.5 ng/L) to a peak value of 4 to 8 pmol/L (5 to 10 ng/L) at the time of ovulation. During labor, plasma oxytocin concentrations may reach several hundred microunits per milliliter, with a rapid fall to prepartum levels after delivery. During suckling, plasma oxytocin levels of the mother vary but are usually about 10 to 20 pmol/L (12 to 25 ng/L). The half-life of oxytocin in plasma is about 3 to 5 min. Removal of oxytocin from the circulation is mainly by the kidneys and liver, although the uterus and mammary gland may remove some.

CLINICAL USE OF OXYTOCIN The clinical use of oxytocin is limited to the induction of labor, control of hemorrhage following incomplete abortion and curettage, and treatment of impaired milk ejection. For discussion of the obstetric uses of oxytocin, the reader is referred to textbooks on obstetrics. Care must be taken because oxytocin may cause uterine rupture and fetal death. The antidiuretic action of oxytocin can be elicited with single intravenous doses of as little as 100 mU. Maximal antidiuresis is reached with 40 to 50 mU/min. Since 10 to 40 units of oxytocin per liter of dextrose is often used in obstetric practice, water intoxication may result. The vasodilatory action of oxytocin may cause sudden death of obstetric patients with heart disease because of hypotension, tachycardia, and arrhythmias. Anesthetics may modify the cardiovascular responses to oxytocin. For instance, in patients under cyclopropane anesthesia, oxytocin produces more hypotension but less tachycardia than in unanesthetized subjects. The vasodilatory effect of oxytocin can be blocked by vasopressin.

REFERENCES

BARTTER FC, SCHWARTZ WB: The syndrome of inappropriate secretion of antidiuretic hormone. Am J Med 42:790, 1967

CROSS BA, LENG G: *Progress in Brain Research*, vol 60: *The Neurohypophysis: Structure, Function and Control*. Amsterdam, Elsevier, 1983

CZERNICHOW P, ROBINSON AG: *Frontiers of Hormone Research*, vol 13: *Diabetes Insipidus in Man*. Basel, Karger, 1985

GASH DM, BOER GJ (eds): *Vasopressin: Principles and Properties*. New York, Plenum, 1987

KNOBIL E, SAWYER WH (eds): *Handbook of Physiology*, sec 7, *Endocrinology*, vol IV: *The Pituitary Gland—Its Neuroendocrine Control*, part I. Washington, DC, American Physiological Society, 1974

MILLER M et al: Recognition of partial defects in antidiuretic hormone secretion. Ann Intern Med 73:721, 1970

MOSES AM: Osmotic thresholds for AVP release using plasma and urine AVP and free water clearance. Am J Physiol 256:R892, 1989

———— et al: Pathophysiologic and pharmacologic alterations in the release and action of ADH. Metabolism 25:697, 1976

———— et al: Marked hypotonic polyuria resulting from nephrogenic diabetes insipidus with partial sensitivity to vasopressin. J Clin Endocrinol Metab 59:1044, 1984

———— et al: Two distinct pathophysiological mechanisms in congenital nephrogenic diabetes insipidus. J Clin Endocrinol Metab 66:1259, 1988

REICHLIN S: *The Neurohypophysis. Physiological and Clinical Aspects*. New York, Plenum, 1984

ROBERTSON GL: The regulation of vasopressin function in health and disease. Rec Progr Hormone Res 33:333, 1977

316 DISEASES OF THE THYROID

LEONARD WARTOFSKY / SIDNEY H. INGBAR

Normal function of the thyroid gland is directed to the secretion of L-thyroxine (T_4) and 3,5,3'-triiodo-L-thyronine (T_3), iodinated amino acids that are the active thyroid hormones and that influence a diversity of metabolic processes (Fig. 316-1). Diseases of the thyroid are manifested by qualitative or quantitative alterations in hormone secretion, enlargement of the thyroid (goiter), or both. Insufficient hormone secretion results in *hypothyroidism* or *myxedema,* in which decreased caloric expenditure (hypometabolism) is a principal feature. Conversely, excessive secretion of hormone results in hypermetabolism and other features of a syndrome termed *hyperthyroidism* or *thyrotoxicosis.* Enlargement of the thyroid gland (normally 15 to 20 g in adults) may be generalized or focal. Generalized enlargements may not be symmetric, however, the right lobe tending to enlarge more than the left. They are associated with increased, normal, or decreased hormone secretion, depending upon the underlying disturbance. Focal enlargement usually reflects neoplastic disease, either benign or malignant, the former sometimes responsible for hypersecretion of hormone and hyperthyroidism, the latter rarely so. Any goiter may compress adjacent structures in the neck or mediastinum.

EMBRYOLOGY, ANATOMY, AND HISTOLOGY

The human thyroid originates embryologically from an evagination of the pharyngeal epithelium with some cellular contributions from the lateral pharyngeal pouches. Progressive descent of the midline thyroid anlage gives rise to the thyroglossal duct, which extends from the foramen cecum near the base of the tongue to the isthmus of the thyroid. Remnants of tissue may persist along the course of this tract as "lingual thyroid," as thyroglossal cysts or nodules, or as a structure contiguous with the thyroid isthmus called the *pyramidal lobe.* The latter is usually not discernible, except when the remainder of the gland is enlarged. Rarely, lingual thyroid may be the sole functioning thyroid tissue. In such cases, its secretion may or may not be sufficient to maintain a normal metabolic (euthyroid) state. Thyroid aplasia and functional failure of ectopic thyroid tissue are causes of sporadic neonatal hypo-

thyroidism (1 in every 4000 or 5000 newborns), which responds to early treatment.

The fetal thyroid acquires the capacity to collect and organify iodine at about 10 weeks' gestation. Both T_4 and thyroid-stimulating hormone (thyrotropin, TSH) are detectable in the blood soon thereafter and increase in concentration during the second trimester. The increase in serum T_4 is due both to increasing thyroid secretion and to the appearance in plasma of thyroxine-binding globulin (TBG), and the increase in TSH is a reflection of the maturation of the fetal hypothalamus with resulting secretion of thyrotropin-releasing hormone (TRH). Maternal TRH readily crosses the placenta and could play a role in the development of the fetal pituitary-thyroid axis. Maternal TSH, by contrast, does not cross the placenta. T_3 is detectable in the blood later during the second trimester, but its concentration in blood and amniotic fluid remains low until shortly after parturition. By contrast, the concentration of its analogue, 3,3',5'-triiodo-L-thyronine (reverse T_3, rT_3), is increased in fetal blood and amniotic fluid relative to that in maternal blood (Fig. 316-1). These differences are due to qualitative alterations in T_4 metabolism in the fetus. The low T_3 in fetal blood and amniotic fluid in the face of a high maternal concentration indicates that maternal-fetal transfer of T_3 is minimal, and the same is true of T_4. Hence, T_4 from the fetal thyroid is the major thyroid hormone available to the fetus. Except for the possible effect of maternal TRH, therefore, the fetal pituitary-thyroid axis is a functional unit distinct from that of the mother.

The normal adult thyroid contains two lobes joined by an isthmus and lies just anterior and caudad to the cartilages of the larynx. Fibrous septa divide the gland into pseudolobules which, in turn, are composed of vesicles, called *follicles* or *acini,* surrounded by a capillary network. Normally, the follicle walls are composed of cuboidal epithelium. The lumen is filled with a proteinaceous *colloid,* which contains a protein peculiar to the thyroid, *thyroglobulin,* within the peptide sequence of which T_4 and T_3 are synthesized and stored. The thyroid contains a smaller second population of cells, the C cells. They are the source of calcitonin and give rise to medullary thyroid carcinoma when they undergo malignant transformation.

THYROID HORMONE ECONOMY: NORMAL PHYSIOLOGY

The term *thyroid hormone economy* denotes the processes involved in the synthesis of hormones within the thyroid gland; their transport

FIGURE 316-1   Structural formulas of thyroxine, its precursors, and certain of its metabolites.

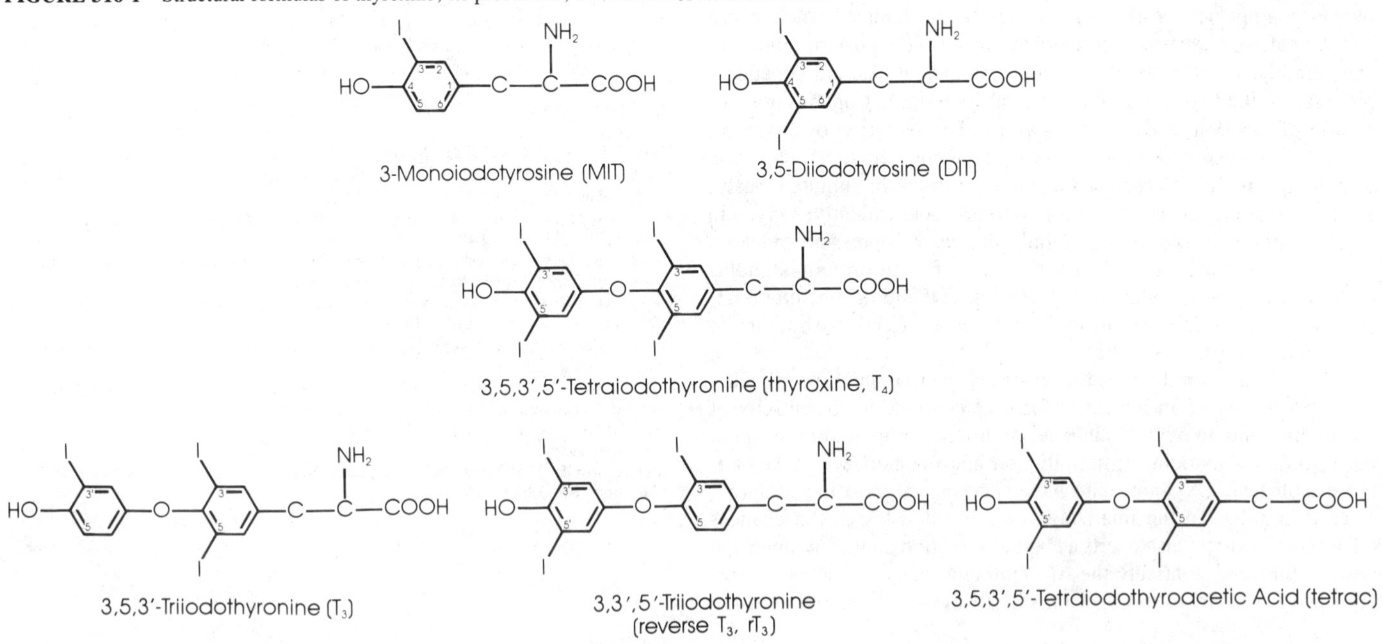

3-Monoiodotyrosine (MIT)

3,5-Diiodotyrosine (DIT)

3,5,3',5'-Tetraiodothyronine (thyroxine, T_4)

3,5,3'-Triiodothyronine (T_3)

3,3',5'-Triiodothyronine (reverse T_3, rT_3)

3,5,3',5'-Tetraiodothyroacetic Acid (tetrac)

in the circulation; their action and metabolism within the peripheral tissues; and the regulatory mechanisms that maintain a normal supply of thyroid hormones. This section describes the normal physiology and biochemistry of the thyroid hormone economy. Abnormalities in transport, action, and metabolism are described in the sections dealing with laboratory tests or specific disorders.

HORMONE SYNTHESIS AND SECRETION Thyroid hormone synthesis depends on entry into the thyroid of adequate quantities of iodine, a constituent of T_4 and T_3; normality of iodine metabolism within the gland; and concurrent synthesis of a receptor protein for iodine, thyroglobulin. The structure of thyroglobulin favors iodinations and particularly formation of T_4 and T_3. Secretion of normal quantities of hormone, in turn, requires both a normal rate of hormone synthesis and the integrity of processes within the gland by which thyroglobulin is hydrolyzed and the active hormones liberated. Iodine enters the thyroid from the bloodstream in the form of inorganic or ionic iodide whose source is twofold: iodide derived either from the deiodination of thyroid hormones, from iodinated agents that the patient may have received, or from iodide ingested in food, water, or medication. Formerly, a dietary iodine intake of approximately 200 μg was considered normal in the United States, and this was sufficient to sustain a plasma iodide concentration of approximately 40 nmol/L (0.5 μg/dL). However, owing to iodine contamination of some foods, and to the widespread use of iodine in drugs, vitamin preparations, and antiseptic agents, the average iodine intake has increased to about 500 μg/d, and in some areas may be as high as 1000 μg daily, with corresponding increases in plasma iodide concentration. Iodide is removed from the plasma by the thyroid, kidneys, and salivary and gastrointestinal glands, but since iodide that enters gastrointestinal secretions is reabsorbed, net clearance is effected only by the thyroid and kidneys. In effect, the thyroid and kidneys compete for plasma iodide. Renal clearance is largely a function of glomerular filtration rate and is not influenced by humoral factors or plasma iodide concentration; the kidney is normally a passive participant in this competition. Hence, adjustments in the rate of entry of iodide into the thyroid relative to the rate of urinary excretion are mediated by changes in thyroid rather than renal avidity.

The synthesis and secretion of the active thyroid hormones can be divided into four sequential steps (Fig. 316-2). The first involves active transport of iodide from the plasma into the thyroid cell and follicular lumen. This occurs at a rate that exceeds passive diffusion of iodide out of the gland, with the result that the thyroid maintains concentration gradients for iodide (thyroid/plasma concentration ratios) of substantial magnitude (usually of 25 but up to 500 or more under certain conditions). Energy for iodide transport depends upon oxidative metabolism within the gland. The second step in hormone biosynthesis involves oxidation of iodide to a higher valence form that is capable of iodinating tyrosyl residues in thyroglobulin, a glycoprotein of approximately 660,000 mol wt that is synthesized within the follicular cell. Oxidation of iodide is effected by a peroxidase, which utilizes hydrogen peroxide generated during the course of oxidative metabolism within the gland. Organic iodinations occur at the cell-colloid interface, where they take place to a large extent in newly synthesized thyroglobulin undergoing exocytosis into the follicular lumen. The consequence is the formation of the peptide-bound, hormonally inactive precursors, monoiodotyrosine (MIT) and diiodotyrosine (DIT). Subsequently, these iodotyrosines undergo oxidative condensation, again through the mediation of peroxidase. This coupling reaction occurs within the thyroglobulin molecule and yields a variety of iodothyronines, including T_4 and T_3. Although minute quantities of thyroglobulin are detectable in the blood, most thyroglobulin is retained for a time within the gland, serving as a storage form of thyroid hormone, or "prohormone." Liberation of the active hormones into the blood involves pinocytosis of follicular colloid at the apical margin of the cells to form colloid droplets. The colloid droplets fuse with thyroid lysosomes to form "phagolyso-somes," in which thyroglobulin is hydrolyzed by proteases and peptidases. The final step is release of the free iodothyronines, T_4

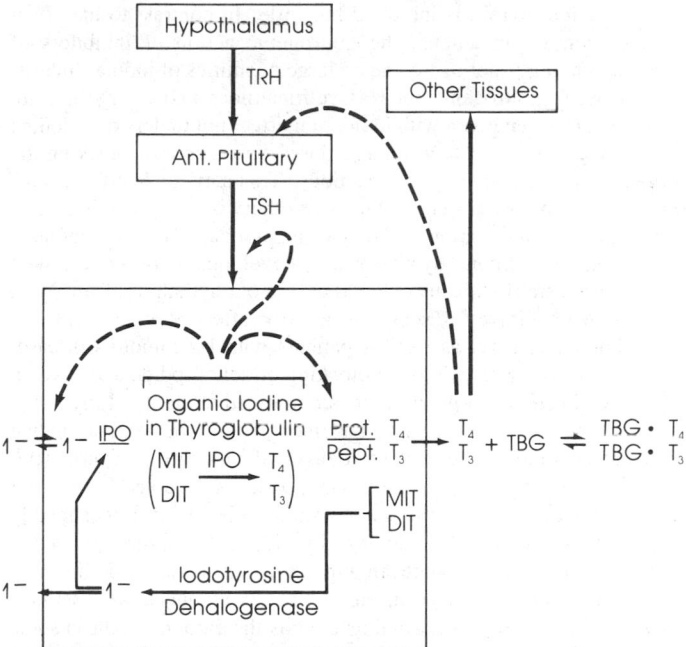

FIGURE 316-2 Schema depicting pathways in the synthesis and secretion of thyroid hormones and mechanisms for the suprathyroidal and intrathyroidal regulation of thyroid function. Small, solid arrows indicate pathways of iodine metabolism; open arrows indicate stimulation; cross-hatched arrows indicate inhibitory influences. TRH, thyrotropin-releasing hormone; TSH, thyroid-stimulating hormone; IPO, iodide peroxidase; prot., thyroid protease; peptid., thyroid peptidase; MIT, monoiodotyrosine; DIT, diiodotyrosine; T_4, thyroxine; T_3, 3,5,3'-triiodothyronine.

and T_3, into the blood. The thyroid gland is the only source of endogenous T_4; in contrast, thyroid secretion normally accounts for only about 20 percent of the T_3 produced, the remainder being generated in extraglandular tissues by the enzymatic removal of the 5'-iodine from the outer ring of T_4. Inactive iodotyrosines liberated by the hydrolysis of thyroglobulin are stripped of their iodine by an intrathyroid enzyme, iodotyrosine dehalogenase. Normally, iodide so liberated is reutilized in the synthesis of hormone, but a small proportion is lost into the blood (iodide leak); this proportion may become large under certain circumstances.

The thyroid is also capable of concentrating other monovalent anions such as pertechnetate, which is available as the radioactive isotope, sodium [⁹⁹ᵐTc]pertechnetate. Unlike iodide, little pertech-netate is organically bound; hence, its duration of stay within the thyroid is short. This property, together with its short physical half-life, makes pertechnetate a valuable radionuclide for imaging the thyroid by scintillation scanning.

The foregoing reactions are subject to inhibition by a variety of agents termed *goitrogens*, since, by virtue of their ability to inhibit hormone synthesis and indirectly stimulate TSH secretion, they induce goiter formation. Certain inorganic anions, notably perchlorate and thiocyanate, inhibit the iodide transport mechanism and thereby reduce substrate availability for hormone formation. The goiter and hypothyroidism that follow, however, can be prevented or relieved by doses of iodide sufficiently large to enable adequate quantities to enter the gland by passive diffusion. The commonly employed antithyroid agents, such as the derivatives of thiourea and mercap-toimidazole, exert more complex actions upon hormone biosynthesis. These agents, as well as certain aniline derivatives, inhibit the initial oxidation (organic binding) of iodide, decrease the proportion of DIT relative to MIT, and block coupling of iodotyrosines to form the hormonally active iodothyronines. The latter reaction is the most sensitive. Thus, it is possible for the synthesis of hormonally active iodothyronines to be decreased, although the total incorporation of iodine by the thyroid is inhibited but little. In contrast to the effect of the monovalent anions, the goitrogenic action of inhibitors of organic binding is not overcome by large quantities of iodine. Indeed, certain weak goitrogens, such as sulfonamides and antipyrine, are more potent when given with iodide, an effect not understood. Iodine itself, when given acutely in large doses, is capable of blocking the organic-binding and coupling reactions. This action (Wolff-Chaikoff effect) is normally transient, but in some otherwise normal individuals, prolonged administration of iodide is associated with continued inhibition of hormone synthesis and development of goiter, with hypothyroidism (iodide myxedema) or without hypothyroidism. Most patients with Graves' disease, especially after treatment with radioiodine or surgery, as well as patients with Hashimoto's disease, are inordinately sensitive to the blocking effect of iodide and develop hypothyroidism when given iodides chronically. The fetal thyroid is similarly sensitive, and pregnant women should not be given iodide in large amounts because of the danger of inducing goitrous hypothyroidism in the fetus. Iodide in large doses is capable of inhibiting proteolysis of thyroglobulin and hormone release, an effect readily demonstrable in hyperfunctioning thyroids and responsible for the ameliorative action of iodides in hyperthyroidism. Excess iodide may also induce thyrotoxicosis in susceptible individuals, as discussed below. Lithium, which is administered as the carbonate salt in some patients with depressive states, has several effects on intrathyroidal iodine metabolism, one of which is to inhibit hormone release. Dexamethasone in large doses also inhibits hormone release and, in conjunction with iodide, can effect a rapid reduction in the degree of thyrotoxicosis.

HORMONE TRANSPORT AND METABOLISM

HORMONE TRANSPORT   In the blood, T_4 and T_3 are almost entirely bound to plasma proteins. T_4 is bound, in decreasing order of intensity, to a globulin, termed thyroxine-binding globulin (TBG), to a T_4-binding prealbumin (TBPA), and to albumin. By virtue of its intense affinity for T_4, TBG is the major determinant of normal binding. The interaction between T_4 and its binding proteins conforms to a reversible binding equilibrium in which the majority of the hormone is bound and a small proportion (normally about 0.03 percent) is free. T_3 is not significantly bound by TBPA and is bound less firmly than T_4 by TBG. As a consequence, the normal proportion of free T_3 (approximately 0.3 percent) is 8 to 10 times greater than that of T_4. Only the free or unbound hormone is available to tissues; therefore, the metabolic state correlates more closely with the concentration of free than with the concentration of total hormone in plasma, and homeostatic regulation of thyroid function is directed toward maintenance of a normal concentration of free rather than total hormone. Moreover, the relatively weak binding of T_3 accounts for its more rapid onset and offset of action. Disturbances of the thyroid hormone–plasma protein interaction are of two general types (see Table 316-1). In the first, the thyroid-pituitary axis is intrinsically normal, and the homeostatic control of thyroid hormone secretion is intact. Under these circumstances, disordered binding interactions result from alterations in thyroid hormone binding. For example, an increase in TBG initially lowers the concentration of free hormone and thus diminishes the quantity of hormone available to tissues. Total hormone concentration in serum then increases until the concentration of free hormone is restored to normal. At this time, the proportions of free T_4 and T_3 are decreased. The increase in total hormone concentration counterbalances the decrease in the free proportion; as a result, the absolute concentration of free hormone is normal, and the metabolic state of the patient is normal. Opposite changes occur when the concentration of TBG declines. Table 316-2 summarizes those states associated with primary alterations in the concentration of TBG. Primary disturbances in thyroid hormone binding also occur when other binding proteins in blood are increased,

TABLE 316-1   Classification of the varieties of disordered thyroid hormone–plasma protein interactions

Type of abnormality	Serum T_4 and T_3	Percent FT_4 and FT_3 or RT_3U	FT_4 and FT_3 or FT_4I and FT_3I
I Primary abnormality in TBG			
A Increased concentration	↑	↓	N
B Decreased concentration	↓	↑	N
II Primary disorder of thyroid function			
A Hypothyroidism	↓	↓	↓
B Hyperthyroidism	↑	↑	↑

NOTE: FT_4 = free T_4; FT_3 = free T_3; FT_4I = free T_4 index; FT_3I = free T_3 index; RT_3U = resin-T_3 uptake; TBG = thyroid-binding globulin.

or when abnormal binding proteins appear. These are discussed below.

The second type of disturbance of thyroid hormone–binding interactions results from a primary alteration in the concentration of thyroid hormones in the blood, as in hypothyroidism or thyrotoxicosis. Here, normal homeostatic control of thyroid hormone secretion is lost, either because of disease within the control mechanism itself or because an intact control mechanism is incapable of overcoming the effects of disease elsewhere. Under these circumstances, the concentration of TBG is changed little, if at all, and the concentration of free hormone varies directly with the total concentration of hormone. Since homeostatic mechanisms cannot restore the concentration of free hormone to normal, primary changes in thyroid function are associated with persistent changes in the concentration of total and free hormone, and, consequently, with alterations in the metabolic state. In these disorders, the proportion of free hormone changes in a direction similar to that of the change in hormone supply.

HORMONE METABOLISM   Following penetration into the cell, T_4 and T_3 undergo a variety of reactions that lead ultimately to their excretion or inactivation. Thyroid hormones undergo metabolism mainly through the sequential removal of single iodine atoms (monodeiodinations) that ultimately yields the thyronine nucleus stripped of iodine. Deiodinative pathways account for approximately 70 percent of T_4 and T_3 disposal. In the case of T_4, the most important of these is the 5'-monodeiodination that leads to the generation of T_3. Since approximately 30 percent of T_4 is converted to T_3 and since T_3 has approximately three times the metabolic potency of T_4, virtually all of the metabolic action of T_4 can be ascribed to the action of the T_3 that it gives rise to. Normally, extraglandular formation accounts for about 80 percent of the T_3 in the blood and of overall T_3 production, the remainder coming from thyroid secretion. As a consequence, abnormal states and pharmacologic agents that impair T_3 formation lower the serum T_3 concentration (Table 316-3). When patients with thyroid hypofunction are treated with synthetic T_4 (levothyroxine) to sustain serum T_4 concentrations within or somewhat above the normal

TABLE 316-2   Circumstances associated with altered concentration of TBG

Increased TBG	Decreased TBG
Pregnancy	Androgens
Newborn state	Large doses of glucocorticoid
Oral contraceptives and other sources of estrogen	Chronic liver disease
	Severe systemic illness
Tamoxifen	Active acromegaly
Infectious and chronic active hepatitis	Nephrosis
	Genetically determined
Biliary cirrhosis	Asparaginase
Acute intermittent porphyria	
Perphenazine	
Genetically determined	

I Physiologic
   A Fetal and early neonatal life
   B ? Old age
II Pathologic
   A Fasting
   B Malnutrition
   C Systemic illness
   D Physical trauma
   E Postoperative state
   F Drugs (propylthiouracil, dexamethasone, propranolol, amiodarone)
   G Radiographic contrast agents (ipodate; iopanoic acid)

range, normal or nearly normal serum T$_3$ concentrations are maintained. The generalization that the thyroid secretes relatively little T$_3$ does not apply to states in which the thyroid is hyperfunctioning or under increased stimulation by TSH or when thyroid iodine content is reduced. Under these conditions, the T$_3$/T$_4$ ratio of the secretory product and the serum concentration of T$_3$ relative to that of T$_4$ are increased. In addition, when T$_4$ production is decreased, as in early thyroid failure or iodine deficiency, the T$_3$/T$_4$ concentration ratio in blood is increased still further by an autoregulatory mechanism that leads to an increase in the efficiency of T$_3$ formation.

Approximately 40 percent of T$_4$ disposal is accounted for by monodeiodination at the 5 position of its inner ring to yield rT$_3$; this process accounts for nearly all rT$_3$ produced. rT$_3$ has little if any metabolic potency; therefore, the relative rates of outer- and inner-ring monodeiodination of T$_4$ determine the quantity of metabolically active hormone available. Factors that impair T$_3$ formation almost invariably increase serum rT$_3$ concentrations. This increase is not due to an increase in the production of rT$_3$ from T$_4$, but rather to a decrease in the 5'-monodeiodination of rT$_3$ to yield 3,3'-diiodothyronine (3,3'T$_2$), i.e., both the decreased conversion of T$_4$ to T$_3$ and the decreased degradation of rT$_3$ are due to a selective impairment of 5'-monodeiodination.

A second major pathway of metabolism of T$_4$ and T$_3$ and of their metabolites is conjugation in the liver, principally with glucuronate and sulfate. Conjugates either undergo deiodination locally or are secreted into the bile, but the magnitude of the enterohepatic circulation in humans is unknown. Reabsorption is incomplete at best, since the fecal excretion of T$_4$, T$_3$, and their iodine-containing metabolites accounts for approximately 20 percent of overall T$_4$ disposal. About 20 percent of T$_4$ and T$_3$ undergoes oxidative deamination and decarboxylation of the alanine side chain to yield tetraiodo- and triiodothyroacetic acid (tetrac and triac, respectively).

Under certain circumstances, changes in hormone accumulation and metabolism are the major determinant of changes in the rates of metabolic clearance of T$_4$ and T$_3$. Both phenobarbital and phenytoin increase the metabolic clearance of thyroid hormones without increasing the proportion of free hormone in the blood. Indeed, in the case of phenytoin, both total and free T$_4$ concentrations are diminished. Nevertheless, a normal metabolic state is maintained possibly because of an increase in T$_3$ formation.

HORMONE ACTION   The thyroid hormones influence the growth and maturation of tissues, total energy expenditure, and the turnover of essentially all substrates, vitamins, and hormones, including the thyroid hormones themselves. The primary action of the hormone is exerted via binding to one or more intracellular receptor complexes which in turn bind to specific regulatory sites in the chromosomes to influence genomic expression (see Chap. 311). Other hormone actions may be mediated at the level of the mitochondrion to influence oxidative metabolism and at the level of the plasma membrane to influence the transcellular flux of substrates and cations.

REGULATION OF THYROID FUNCTION   Regulation of thyroid function is effected by two general mechanisms, one suprathyroid and one intrathyroid in locus (Fig. 316-2). The proximate mediator of suprathyroid regulation is thyrotropin (thyroid-stimulating hor-

mone, TSH), a glycoprotein secreted by basophilic (thyrotropic) cells in the anterior pituitary. TSH stimulates thyroid hypertrophy and hyperplasia; accelerates most aspects of intermediary metabolism in the thyroid; enhances synthesis of nucleic acid and protein, including thyroglobulin; and stimulates the synthesis and secretion of thyroid hormones. These actions of TSH result from binding of the hormone to specific receptors in the surface of the follicular cell and subsequent activation of the plasma membrane enzyme adenylate cyclase. The resulting increase in the cellular cyclic 3',5'-adenosine monophosphate (cyclic AMP) concentration initiates most or all of the responses that characterize the action of TSH.

Regulation of TSH secretion, in turn, is effected by two opposing influences at the level of the thyrotropic cell. Thyrotropin-releasing hormone (TRH), a tripeptide of hypothalamic origin, stimulates the secretion and synthesis of TSH, whereas thyroid hormones both inhibit the TSH secretory mechanism directly and antagonize the action of TRH. Thus, homeostatic control of TSH secretion is exerted in a negative-feedback manner by thyroid hormones, and the threshold for feedback inhibition is apparently set by TRH. TRH is synthesized in the hypothalamus, reaches the pituitary via the hypophyseal portal blood system, and binds to specific receptors on the plasma membrane of the thyrotropic cell. Either activation of the adenylate cyclase system or a concomitant translocation of extracellular calcium into the cell initiates release of TSH. To what extent, if any, suprahypothalamic centers influence the secretion of TRH is uncertain. The negative-feedback effect of the thyroid hormones appears to take place entirely at the level of the thyrotropic cell. Thyroid hormones do not directly affect the hypothalamic secretion of TRH but reduce the number of TRH receptors on the thyrotropic cell, thus impairing its responsiveness to TRH. The negative-feedback action of the thyroid hormones is apparently mediated by a protein whose synthesis is induced by binding of the hormones to specific receptors in the nucleus of the thyrotropic cell. The principal arbiter of thyroid hormone action within the pituitary is T$_3$, both that generated locally from intrapituitary T$_4$ and that derived from the pool of free T$_3$ in the plasma. To what extent T$_4$ itself is effective within the pituitary is uncertain, but other factors modify the secretion of TSH and its response to TRH. Both somatostatin and dopamine appear to be physiologic inhibitors of TRH secretion. Estrogens enhance responsiveness to TRH, whereas glucocorticoids inhibit this function.

Intrathyroid regulation of thyroid function is also important. In some manner, changes in glandular organic iodine content cause reciprocal changes in thyroid iodide transport activity and regulate growth, amino acid uptake, glucose metabolism, and nucleic acid synthesis. These influences are evident in the absence of TSH stimulation and hence may be termed *autoregulatory*, but their most important role is to modify (iodine-enrichment inhibiting and iodine-depletion enhancing) the response to TSH, probably by modifying the generation of cyclic AMP consequent to TSH stimulation.

LABORATORY TESTS

Laboratory tests of thyroid hormone economy can be divided into five general categories: direct tests of thyroid function, tests related to the concentration and binding of thyroid hormones in blood, metabolic indexes, tests of the homeostatic control of thyroid function, and various tests that do not fit into other categories.

DIRECT TESTS OF THYROID FUNCTION   Among all tests designed to assess thyroid status, only those that involve in vivo administration of radioactive iodine test glandular function per se, and measurement of the *thyroid radioactive iodine uptake* (RAIU) is the most common. ^{131}I has been used for this purpose, but ^{123}I is preferable because of the lower radiation dose that it delivers. The administered radioiodine mixes uniformly with the endogenous iodide in the extracellular fluid and, in the steady state, can be used to assess what percentage of the iodide entering and leaving the extracellular space per unit time is accumulated by the thyroid. The

RAIU is usually measured 24 h after administration of the isotope since it usually reaches a plateau value at this time, but in severe thyroid hyperfunction it may peak early. The RAIU varies inversely with the plasma iodide concentration and directly with the functional state of the thyroid. At usual levels of iodine intake in the United States (up to 1000 μg/d), the normal 24-h RAIU is approximately 5 to 30 percent of the administered dose. Consequently, this test discriminates poorly between normal and hypothyroid states. Values above the normal range, however, usually indicate thyroid hyperfunction and are useful in the diagnosis of hyperthyroidism. The RAIU is also a part of the thyroid suppression test (see below).

One valuable application of the RAIU is in the diagnosis of disorders in which thyrotoxicosis is associated with a low value of the RAIU. These include iodine-induced hyperthyroidism, thyrotoxicosis factitia, and the spontaneously resolving thyrotoxicosis that is associated with painless chronic thyroiditis or subacute thyroiditis.

TESTS RELATED TO HORMONE CONCENTRATION AND BINDING IN BLOOD Measurement of the concentration of T_4 and/or T_3 in serum, in conjunction with some assessment of hormone binding, is generally the means of confirming a diagnosis of hyperthyroidism or hypothyroidism. Highly specific and sensitive radioimmunoassays are used to measure *serum T_4* and T_3 concentrations and when indicated for measuring *serum rT_3* concentration. The approximate normal ranges are 60 to 150 nmol/L (5 to 12 μg/dL) for T_4, 1 to 3 nmol/L (70 to 190 ng/dL) for T_3, and 0.2 to 0.6 nmol/L (10 to 40 ng/dL) for rT_3.

As mentioned above, alterations in the intensity of hormone binding by plasma proteins, as well as alterations in the rate of hormone secretion, influence the concentration of hormone in the blood. However, only alterations in hormone secretion lead to steady state alterations in the concentration of free hormone. Because they most consistently reflect the rate of hormone production, free hormone concentrations usually correlate better with the metabolic state than do total hormone concentrations. The free T_4 concentration (FT_4) can be measured by equilibrium dialysis of serum enriched with a tracer quantity of labeled T_4. The percent of T_4 that is dialyzable or free is thereby determined, and the product of this value and the total T_4 is the FT_4. However, since the dialysis technique is cumbersome, an indirect assessment of hormone binding, the *in vitro uptake test*, is simple to perform and usually provides the same information. Here, the serum is enriched with labeled T_4 or labeled T_3 and is then incubated with an insoluble, particulate matter, such as resin or charcoal, that binds free hormone. The percent of labeled hormone taken up by the particulate material varies inversely with both the concentration of unoccupied sites among the serum proteins and their affinity for the particular hormone being used. Labeled T_3 is usually used in preference to labeled T_4, since it is less strongly bound in the serum and hence yields higher, and therefore more nearly accurate, uptake values (resin T_3 uptake, RT_3U). In most clinical conditions, values of the RT_3U are proportionate to those of the percent of FT_4 and percent of FT_3. This proportionality reflects the fact that in normal serum T_4 and T_3 are mainly bound by a common binding site on TBG. Therefore, alterations in binding produced by an excess or deficiency of TBG or by an excessive or insufficient supply of T_4 do not seriously disturb the relationship between the intensity of T_4 binding and that of T_3. Under these conditions, therefore, one may calculate a *free T_4 index* (FT_4I) and a *free T_3 index* (FT_3I) as the product of the RT_3U and the total T_4 and T_3 concentrations, respectively, and these are proportional to the actual FT_4 and FT_3. (In practice, values of the FT_3 and FT_3I are rarely determined.)

Primary alterations in plasma TBG concentration (Table 316-2) produce changes in the RT_3U that are inverse and approximately proportionate to those in the serum T_4 and serum T_3; as a result, the FT_4I and FT_3I remain normal. By contrast, alterations in T_4 secretion cause changes in the percent FT_4 and RT_3U that are in the same direction as those in serum T_4. As a result, the FT_4 and FT_4I deviate from normal values more markedly than do the percent FT_4 and RT_3U alone. Immunoradiometric (IRMA) and chemiluminescent assay

methods for the direct measurement of FT_4 have been developed; some provide reliable results in a wide range of disorders and may replace measurement of total T_4, RT_3U, and FT_4I in the diagnosis of thyrotoxicosis and hypothyroidism.

As noted earlier, several disorders are characterized by increased plasma binding of T_4 in which, because the protein involved is not TBG, the intensity of T_4 binding relative to that of T_3 is abnormal. Most commonly, binding of T_4 is enhanced, while that of T_3 is increased little, if at all. Included among these disorders is *familial dysalbuminemic hyperthyroxinemia (FDH)*, transmitted by autosomal dominant inheritance, in which the plasma concentration of an albumin variant with an unusually high affinity for T_4 is increased. As a result, the serum T_4 is markedly elevated, but, in keeping with the euthyroid state, FT_4 is normal. Because the RT_3U does not reflect the increase in the intensity of T_4 binding, calculated values of the FT_4I are greatly increased, often leading to a mistaken diagnosis of thyrotoxicosis. Similar findings occur when there is *increased T_4 binding by TBPA* or when the patient, usually one with autoimmune thyroid disease, develops *circulating antibodies* against T_4 itself.

In the foregoing disorders, in which the serum T_4 is increased owing to an increase in T_4 binding, the FT_4 and the metabolic state are normal. They are therefore classified among the disorders that lead to a state of *euthyroid hyperthyroxinemia*, a term that implies the presence of hyperthyroxinemia not caused by intrinsic thyroid disease (Table 316-4). The mechanism responsible for these findings is variable and in some cases uncertain. The increases in total T_4 do not appear to have any impact on the metabolic state, but the clinician should be aware of the causes of euthyroid hyperthyroxinemia lest hyperthyroidism be mistakenly diagnosed.

Some states are associated with an increased thyroid secretion of T_3, at least relative to the secretion of T_4. As a result, the serum T_3 concentration is disproportionately high relative to the prevailing serum T_4 concentration. This is apparently a consequence of hyperfunction of the follicular cell, since it is seen in all varieties of hyperthyroidism and in early thyroid failure, in which the gland is exposed to enhanced stimulation by TSH. Accordingly, the serum T_3 concentration and the derived FT_3I are generally superior to the corresponding values for T_4 in the diagnosis of hyperthyroidism. In *early* hypothyroidism, by contrast, the serum T_3 concentration and FT_3I may be normal despite subnormal values for the serum T_4 concentration and FT_4I. Consequently, the serum T_3 concentration is not reliable for the diagnosis of hypothyroidism.

Measurement of the serum rT_3 concentration is valuable in differentiating the "low T_3 syndrome" (see below) from intrinsic hypothyroidism; in the former the serum rT_3 concentration is increased, whereas in the latter it is usually subnormal.

METABOLIC INDEXES Tests in this category assess the metabolic impact of thyroid hormone in the peripheral tissues. Though tests of this type have value in the investigative setting, none of sufficient sensitivity, specificity, and ease of performance is available for routine use. Measurements of oxygen consumption in the basal state (basal metabolic rate, BMR) were once a mainstay in the diagnosis of thyroid disease but are now of historic interest. Several blood tests may be abnormal in patients with thyroid disease; their sensitivity may substantiate the diagnosis of thyroid dysfunction, but lack of specificity limits their utility. For example, serum concentrations of creatine phosphokinase and, less frequently, lactic dehydrogenase and aspartate aminotransferase are increased in hypothyroidism and may be slightly decreased in hyperthyroidism. The changes are nonspecific, and appreciation of them is important only in avoiding the inference that other diseases that produce similar changes are present. The concentrations in serum of testosterone-binding globulin (TeBG) and of angiotensin-converting enzyme are thyroid hormone–dependent and are, therefore, increased in thyrotoxicosis, but they are of no value in the diagnosis of thyroid disease. Increases in the *serum cholesterol concentration* are common in hypothyroidism of thyroid origin, and decreases in serum cholesterol are common in thyrotoxicosis. *Systolic time indexes,* such as the preejection period

TABLE 316-4 States associated with euthyroid hyperthyroxinemia

Disorder	FT₄	FT₄I	T₃	TSH	Comments
I Increased T₄ binding					
A Increased TBG	N	N	↑	N	See Tables 316-1 and 316-2
B FDH	N	↑	N,Sl↑	N	Autosomal dominant inheritance
C Increased TBPA binding	N	↑	N	N	Increased concentration (islet-cell tumor) or affinity
D Anti-T₄ antibody	N	↑	N	N	Anti-T₃ antibody may be present
II Pituitary and peripheral thyroid hormone resistance	↑	↑	↑	↑	If only pituitary resistant, patient thyrotoxic
III Various disorders					
A Sick euthyroid syndrome	↑ , N	↑	↓	N, ↓	Uncommon; poorly understood
B Acute psychiatric illness	↑ , N	↑	N, ↑	N, ↑	Remits without treatment in several weeks
C Hyperemesis gravidarum	↑	↑	N	↓	Remits in several weeks
IV Drugs					
A Inhibitors of T₃-formation					
1 Radiographic contrast agents	↑	↑	↓	↑	Particularly ipodate and iopanoate
2 Propranolol	↑	↑	↓	N, ↑	Especially with large doses
3 Amiodarone	↑	↑	↓	↑	Increased TSH during first several months
B Heparin	↑	↑	N	—	Requires only small intravenous doses
C Levothyroxine therapy	↑	↑	N	↓	Hyperthyroxinemia in about 50% of cases

NOTE: FT₄ = free T₄ concentration; FT₄I = free T₄ index calculated from an in vitro T₃ uptake test; TSH = basal serum TSH concentration and response to TRH; N = normal; Sl = slightly.

and pulse-wave arrival time, are prolonged in hypothyroidism and shortened in hyperthyroidism. They are of value in monitoring thyroid replacement therapy in elderly patients or in patients with coexisting heart disease.

TESTS OF HOMEOSTATIC CONTROL Measurement of the basal *serum TSH concentration* is useful in the diagnosis of both advanced and subclinical hypothyroidism. The latter state represents a stage in the evolution of hypothyroidism, in which a structural or functional abnormality that impairs hormone synthesis is compensated for by hypersecretion of TSH. The normal TSH level is less than 5 mU/L. In thyrotoxic states, serum TSH concentration is almost always low or undetectable. While the conventional radioimmunoassays cannot distinguish between normal and subnormal values, immunoradiometric or chemiluminescent techniques employing monoclonal antibodies provide exquisite sensitivity. Thyrotoxic patients tend to have undetectable levels (<0.1 mU/L) while values in most normal subjects range between 0.3 and 3.0 mU/L in these assays (Fig. 316-3). Serum TSH concentrations are absolutely or inappropriately elevated, relative to serum FT₄ and FT₃ values, in patients with TSH-induced hyperthyroidism. This rare syndrome results either from a TSH-secreting pituitary adenoma or resistance of the TSH secretory mechanism to feedback inhibition by T₄ and T₃. Measurement of serum TSH is the best means of distinguishing between untreated hypothyroidism of thyroid origin, in which the values are invariably increased, and pituitary or hypothalamic hypothyroidism, in which the values are usually undetectable or within the normal range. Occasional patients with hypothyroidism of hypothalamic or pituitary origin secrete a form of TSH that is immunoactive but not bioactive. Here, serum TSH concentrations may be elevated rather than depressed.

The *thyrotropin-releasing hormone (TRH) stimulation test* assesses the functional state of the TSH-secretory mechanism, and has diagnostic value in diverse circumstances. Following the intravenous injection of TRH in normal subjects, the serum TSH begins to increase within minutes, reaches a maximum between 20 and 45 min, and then rapidly declines. The nature of the pituitary feedback mechanism is such that when hypothalamic-pituitary function is normal, one would expect an increased response to TRH when the thyrotropic cell senses a deficiency of thyroid hormone, particularly T₃, and a decreased or absent response when there is thyroid hormone excess. Thus, except in the rare instances of pituitary resistance to thyroid hormone, in which responses are usually normal, thyrotoxicosis is invariably accompanied by a blunted or absent TSH response to TRH. Owing to extreme sensitivity of the TSH-secretory mechanism to feedback inhibition, diminished responses to TRH commonly occur in apparently euthyroid patients with serum T₄ or T₃ levels within the normal range but with marginally increased T₄ or T₃ output from autonomously functioning toxic adenomas or toxic multinodular goiters. Blunted TRH responses may be also seen in some patients with euthyroid Graves' disease. In addition, responses to TRH are often decreased in elderly individuals, especially men. Despite these exceptions, a subnormal or absent response to TRH is an excellent confirmatory test for thyrotoxicosis. TRH tests are of less value in the diagnosis of hypothyroidism. Responses are increased in patients with primary hypothyroidism, but the magnitude of increase is generally proportional to the extent of increase in basal serum TSH. Some patients with pituitary hypothyroidism have subnormal responses, and some with TRH deficiency owing to hypothalamic disease have a near-normal response, but these expected responses are not seen consistently. Further, in as many as one-fourth of patients with hypothyroidism due to hypothalamic-pituitary disease, basal serum TSH concentrations are normal or slightly elevated, and the response to TRH is exaggerated, although some of this TSH may not be bioactive.

The *thyroid suppression test* is used to assess whether thyroid

FIGURE 316-3 Utility of sensitive TSH assay in evaluation of suspected thyroid dysfunction in ambulatory patients.

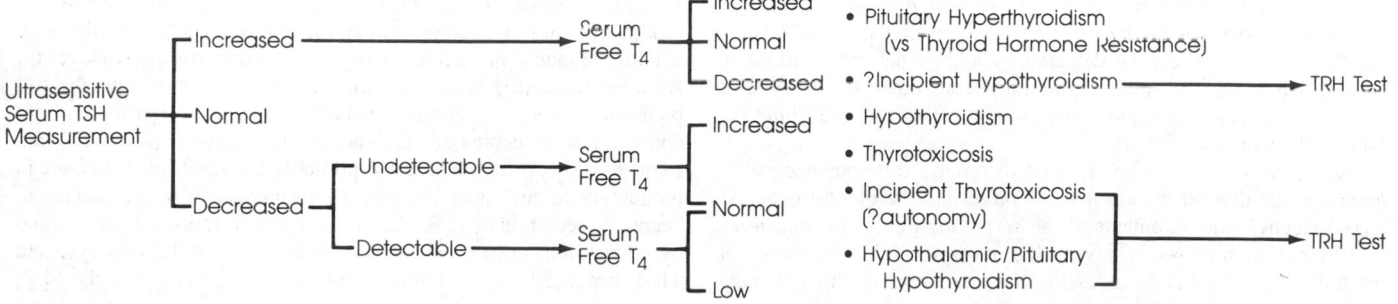

function is controlled by normal homeostatic mechanisms. Normally, exogenous thyroid hormone suppresses pituitary TSH secretion, resulting in a decrease in the RAIU. Since liothyronine is usually employed for the test (100 μg daily for 7 to 10 days), the resulting decline in serum T_4, as well as in the RAIU, can serve as an index of suppression. A normal suppressive response is a decrease of the RAIU to less than half of the control value and a decline of the serum T_4 to low normal or subnormal values. An abnormal suppression test is always present in hyperthyroidism, irrespective of the underlying cause; this indicates either autonomy of thyroid function, the presence of an abnormal (non-TSH) thyroid stimulator, or unremitting hypersecretion of TSH. A normal suppression test, on the other hand, is incompatible with and excludes a diagnosis of hyperthyroidism. An abnormal suppression test is not pathognomonic of hyperthyroidism, however, since it may persist after treatment of hyperthyroidism in Graves' disease and is seen in about half of the euthyroid patients with the ophthalmopathy of Graves' disease.

Because of the risk of adverse effects of exogenous thyroid hormone especially liothyronine in elderly patients and in those with cardiovascular disease, and since the TRH test is almost entirely devoid of undesirable side effects, the latter test has almost entirely supplanted the thyroid suppression test in the diagnosis of hyperthyroidism.

MISCELLANEOUS TESTS   Various tests that do not assess thyroid function are of value in defining the nature of the thyroid disorder or in planning therapy. For example, high titers of *antimicrosomal antibodies* or *antithyroglobulin antibodies* are found in the serum of most adults with Hashimoto's disease and in many patients with primary thyroprivic hypothyroidism or Graves' disease. In the latter, the serum also contains antibodies against the TSH receptor on thyroid plasma membranes. In general, these are capable of inhibiting the receptor binding of TSH (TSH-binding inhibitory immunoglobulins, TBII) and of stimulating the production of cyclic AMP therein (thyroid-stimulating immunoglobulins, TSI). The clinical utility of tests for TBII and TSI stems from the fact that the disappearance of the factors from the serum during a course of antithyroid therapy implies the likelihood of a long-term remission of hyperthyroidism when therapy is withdrawn. In some patients, analogous antibodies have no intrinsic stimulatory effect but block the response to endogenous TSH and produce nongoitrous hypothyroidism. Both stimulatory and blocking anti-TSH receptor antibodies have the ability to cross the placenta and, as a consequence, to produce transient hyperthyroidism (neonatal Graves' disease) or hypothyroidism, respectively, in the newborn. Measurement of these antibodies during the last months of pregnancy makes it possible to assess the likelihood of the disorders developing in the neonate.

Some patients, most commonly those with autoimmune thyroid disease, develop *circulating antibodies against T_3 or T_4*, or both. In radioimmunoassays for these hormones, because the endogenous antibody competes with the exogenous antibody for binding of the added labeled ligand, spurious values for the concentration of the hormone are obtained. These may be grossly elevated or greatly depressed, depending on the technique of radioimmunoassay used. The true concentration of the hormone, as determined in extracts of the serum, is increased owing to the additional binding sites provided by the antibody, but antibody-bound hormone is unavailable for metabolic action. In the case of anti-T_3 antibodies, which are the more common, values of the RT_3U are low because endogenous antibody competes with the resin for binding of the added labeled T_3. Such antibodies can be detected by adding labeled hormone to serum, separating the immunoglobulins from other serum proteins by any of several techniques, and demonstrating that they bind the labeled hormone.

Along with several other thyroid disorders, differentiated carcinomas of the thyroid release thyroglobulin into the bloodstream. As a consequence, measurements of the *serum thyroglobulin concentration* by radioimmunoassay have value not in the initial diagnosis of thyroid carcinoma but in assessing the adequacy of initial therapy

and in monitoring for recurrence or dissemination of the disease. In patients with thyrotoxicosis, subnormal serum thyroglobulin concentrations together with decreased values of the RAIU suggest the presence of thyrotoxicosis factitia.

Imaging by *scintiscanning* permits localization of sites of accumulation of radioiodine or sodium [^{99m}Tc]pertechnetate. This technique is useful for defining areas of increased or decreased function within the thyroid and for detecting retrosternal goiter, ectopic thyroid tissue, hemiagenesis of the thyroid, and functioning metastases of thyroid carcinoma. Ultrasonic examination of the thyroid is also a valuable technique for differentiating cystic nodules from those that are solid. Since ultrasonic scans provide an accurate indication of size, are noninvasive, and apparently have no injurious effects, sequential scans can be employed to assess changes in the size of the thyroid as a whole or of discrete nodules over time or in response to treatment.

SICK EUTHYROID SYNDROME

Severe illness, physical trauma, or physiologic stress can induce changes in one or more aspects of thyroid hormone economy, leading to findings referred to as the sick euthyroid syndrome (SES). Abnormalities in SES include alterations in the peripheral transport and metabolism of the thyroid hormones; the regulation of TSH secretion; and in some cases changes in thyroid function itself. Acting alone or together, these lead to changes in the concentrations of the circulating thyroid hormones, both total and free, that serve to define the several variants of the SES. Because of the frequency of illness in the general population and the nonspecificity of the disorders that cause it, SES is probably a more common cause of abnormalities in the concentration of thyroid hormones in the blood than intrinsic thyroid disease.

NORMAL-T_4 VARIANT OF SES   Decreased production of T_3 owing to inhibition of the peripheral 5'-monodeiodination of T_4 is a consistent feature of the SES. This is reflected in a decrease in the serum total T_3 concentration that varies in severity with that of the illness. In moderately ill patients, serum total T_4 concentration is within the normal range. A decrease in the intensity of protein binding, greater for T_4 than T_3, is an additional accompaniment. As a result, values of the RT_3U are moderately increased, and the percent FT_4 is increased to a proportionately greater extent. As a consequence, values of the free T_4 index (FT_4I) and those of the free T_4 concentrations (FT_4) are often increased. Serum rT_3 concentrations are increased, owing to a decrease in the plasma clearance of rT_3 secondary to inhibition of its 5'-monodeiodination. The plasma clearance rate of T_4 is increased, probably as a result of decreased T_4 binding, and this, in the face of normal T_4 concentrations, indicates that the overall rate of T_4 degradation and production is increased. Production rates for T_3 are decreased, and those for rT_3 are normal. Serum TSH concentration and the response of serum TSH to TRH are generally normal, though they may increase to supranormal values and then return to normal as recovery from the illness takes place. Despite the reduction in the serum T_3 concentration, this variant of the SES can be separated from intrinsic thyroid disease because the serum T_4 and TSH are normal and because the serum T_3 is not useful for diagnosing hypothyroidism in any event.

LOW-T_4 VARIANT OF SES   In more seriously ill patients, T_3 production rates and serum total and free T_3 concentrations decrease still further, and abnormalities in hormone binding increase in severity. As a consequence, serum T_4 concentrations decrease into the hypothyroid range, sometimes markedly so. This is partly but not entirely due to decreased T_4 binding since values of the FT_4 are frequently subnormal. These are probably the result of decreased T_4 production in the most severely ill patients and are secondary to decreased secretion of TSH. Serum TSH concentrations appear normal by conventional assay but are low with sensitive TSH assays, and TRH responses may be blunted. Hence, in this variant of the SES, there is an inappropriate hyposecretion of TSH, considering the low serum total and free T_4 and T_3 concentrations; its cause is unknown, but a diagnosis of pituitary hypothyroidism may be suggested. Production rates for rT_3 are diminished, owing to the decreased availability of its precursor T_4; nonetheless, serum rT_3 concentrations are increased, owing to retardation of its degradation, and this provides an important means of differentiating the SES from pituitary hypothyroidism, in which serum rT_3 concentrations are low. In patients with primary hypothyroidism who have associated illness, serum TSH concentrations remain elevated, though their concentrations are generally lower than they otherwise would be.

HIGH-T_4 VARIANT OF SES An unusual variant of the SES (approximately 1 percent of sick patients) is associated with increased serum total and free T_4 concentrations during acute illness and return to normal thereafter. This variant is most often seen in elderly women, many of whom have received medications that contain iodine. The principal source of diagnostic confusion is with the syndrome of "T_4 toxicosis," i.e., true thyrotoxicosis upon which illness has been superimposed, so that serum T_4 concentrations are increased and serum T_3 concentrations are normal. In the latter, however, serum rT_3 concentrations are higher, values of the serum total T_3 and FT_3I are higher, and TRH responses are blunted.

ABNORMALITIES IN HORMONE BINDING IN SES Multiple factors are responsible for the decreased binding of T_4 and, to a lesser extent, T_3 in the SES. Illness is associated with decreased synthesis of TBPA and a decrease in its serum concentration, but the extent to which this contributes to decreased T_4 binding is uncertain. In chronically ill patients, serum TBG concentration is subnormal. Most often, however, the extent of decreased T_4 binding cannot be explained by decreases in serum TBPA and TBG, and an inhibitor of hormone binding may be responsible. Its nature is uncertain, but it may be one or more fatty acids, which may also be responsible for diminished conversion of T_4 to T_3.

The importance of the SES is that the changes in circulating thyroid hormone concentrations that result should not be confused with those due to intrinsic thyroid or pituitary disease. Unresolved questions are whether the metabolic impact of thyroid hormone in peripheral tissues is decreased in the SES, whether the syndrome is a beneficial or adverse response to illness, and whether some patients would benefit from treatment with thyroid hormones.

SIMPLE (NONTOXIC) GOITER

Endemic goiter implies an etiologic factor or factors common to a particular geographic region. The term has been defined as the presence of generalized or localized thyroid enlargement in more than 10 percent of the population. *Sporadic* goiter arises in nonendemic areas as a result of factors that do not affect the population generally. Since these terms fail to define or distinguish the causes of such goiters and since thyroid enlargement of diverse etiology may exist in both endemic and nonendemic regions, it is prudent to employ a general term such as *simple* or *nontoxic goiter*. This all-inclusive category can be further subdivided into specific etiologic groups. Simple or nontoxic goiter can be defined as any enlargement of the thyroid gland that does not result from an inflammatory or neoplastic process and that is not initially associated with thyrotoxicosis or myxedema.

ETIOLOGY AND PATHOGENESIS Simple goiter is sometimes due to a definable cause of impaired thyroid hormone synthesis, such as iodine deficiency, ingestion of a goitrogen, or a demonstrable defect in a hormone biosynthetic pathway, but in most instances its cause is unknown. Whatever the cause, the clinical manifestations reflect the operation of a common pathophysiologic mechanism. Simple goiter occurs when one or more factors impair the capacity of the thyroid to secrete active hormones sufficient to meet the needs of the peripheral tissues. Although this has been presumed to lead to increased secretion of TSH, concentrations of TSH in the serum of

patients with established simple goiter are usually normal. Hence, some other mechanism of goitrogenesis may be operative. A likely possibility is that depletion of glandular organic iodine accompanying impaired hormone synthesis increases the responsiveness of thyroid structure and function to levels of TSH that remain within the normal range. The resulting increases in both functioning thyroid mass and cellular activity overcome mild impairment of hormone synthesis; thus, the patient is metabolically normal, though goitrous. When the underlying disorder is severe, compensatory responses, now including hypersecretion of TSH, are inadequate to overcome the impairment, and the patient is both goitrous and hypothyroid. Thus, simple goiter cannot be clearly separated in the pathogenetic sense from goitrous hypothyroidism. Specific causes of simple goiter may exist with or without hypothyroidism (Table 316-5). Defective iodination of thyroglobulin may be an important cause in many patients. The possibility that goiter can be due to antibodies that stimulate thyroid growth but not function remains to be substantiated.

PATHOLOGY The histopathology of the thyroid in simple goiter varies with the severity of the etiologic factor and the stage at which the examination is made. In its initial stages, the gland exhibits a uniform hypertrophy, hyperplasia, and hypervascularity. As the disorder persists or undergoes repeated exacerbations and remissions, uniformity of thyroidal architecture is lost. Occasionally, the greater part of the gland may display a uniform involution or hyperinvolution with colloid accumulation. More often such areas are interspersed with patchy areas of focal hyperplasia. Fibrosis may demarcate hyperplastic or involuted nodules. These may resemble true neoplasms (adenomas). Areas of hemorrhage and irregular calcification may be present. The evolution of the multinodular stage is almost always accompanied by the development of functional autonomy. Indeed, heterogeneity of structure and function and a greater or lesser degree of functional autonomy are the hallmarks of the mature stage of this disorder.

CLINICAL MANIFESTATIONS In simple goiter the clinical manifestations arise solely from enlargement of the thyroid since the metabolic state is normal. In goitrous hypothyroidism, symptoms caused by thyromegaly are accompanied by signs and symptoms of hormonal insufficiency. Mechanical sequelae include compression and displacement of the trachea or esophagus, occasionally with obstructive symptoms if the goiter becomes sufficiently large. Superior mediastinal obstruction may occur with large retrosternal goiters. Signs of compression can be induced in the case of large retrosternal goiters when the patient's arms are raised above the head (Pemberton's sign); suffusion of the face, giddiness, or syncope may result from this maneuver. Hoarseness due to compression of the recurrent laryngeal nerve is rare in simple goiter and suggests neoplasm. Sudden hemorrhage into a nodule may lead to an acute, painful swelling in the neck and may produce or enhance compressive symptoms.

TABLE 316-5 Classification of the causes of hypothyroidism

I Thyroid
  A Thyroprivic
    1 Congenital development defect
    2 Primary idiopathic
    3 Postablative (radioiodine, surgery)
    4 Postradiation (lymphoma)
  B Goitrous
    1 Heritable biosynthetic defects
    2 Maternally transmitted (iodides, antithyroid agents)
    3 Iodine deficiency
    4 Drug-elicited (aminosalicylic acid, iodides, phenylbutazone, iodoantipyrine, lithium)
    5 Chronic thyroiditis (Hashimoto's disease)
II Suprathyroid (trophoprivic)
  A Pituitary
  B Hypothalamic
III Self-limited
  A Following withdrawal of suppressive thyroid therapy
  B Subacute thyroiditis and chronic thyroiditis with transient hypothyroidism (usually after a phase of thyrotoxicosis)

Hyperthyroidism may supervene in long-standing multinodular goiter (toxic multinodular goiter). In both endemic and sporadic multinodular goiter, the ingestion of excess iodide may result in the development of thyrotoxicosis (jod-Basedow phenomenon).

In regions where iodine deficiency is severe, goitrous enlargement may also be associated with varying degrees of hypothyroidism. Cretinism, both goitrous and nongoitrous, occurs with increased frequency in the children of goitrous parents in many countries where goiter is common. Although iodine deficiency is doubtless a factor in the etiology of endemic goiter, the frequency of goiter differs greatly among areas of equally severe iodine deficiency. In such instances, dietary or waterborne goitrogens appear to be important conditioning factors. In some areas, these goitrogens may be sufficient to cause goiter in the absence of iodine deficiency.

DIAGNOSIS   The diagnosis of simple goiter requires, first, demonstration of a euthyroid state and, second, demonstration of normal serum T_4 and T_3 concentrations. The former may be difficult because manifestations of thyrotoxicosis may be subtle or atypical, especially among the elderly (see section on "Toxic Multinodular Goiter"). The latter may be problematic, since serum T_4 and especially T_3 concentrations may be near the upper limit of the normal range. In addition, the fact that serum T_3 concentrations decrease in the euthyroid elderly complicates interpretation of this test. The RAIU is usually normal but may be increased in the presence of iodine deficiency or a biosynthetic defect. Indeed, subclinical thyrotoxicosis may be present secondary to the significant functional autonomy of the goiter and consequently cause a decrease in both basal TSH and TSH response to TRH. Differentiation of nontoxic goiter from Hashimoto's disease is facilitated by the greater frequency of multinodularity in the former and by the presence of high titers of circulating antimicrosomal or antithyroglobulin antibodies in the latter. In some instances, emergence of a strongly dominant nodule may suggest the presence of a carcinoma. This is especially true if bleeding has caused it to increase in size rapidly and to lose the ability to accumulate iodine or pertechnetate.

TREATMENT   The object of treatment is to reduce the size of the goiter, either by relieving external encumbrances to hormone formation or by providing sufficient quantities of exogenous hormone to inhibit TSH secretion and thereby put the thyroid gland almost completely at rest. In disorders characterized by decreased thyroid iodide stores, such as iodine deficiency or impairment of the thyroid iodide-concentrating mechanism, small doses of iodide may prove effective. Occasionally, a known extrinsic goitrogen can be withdrawn. Most commonly, however, no specific etiologic factor can be detected, and thyroid hormone therapy is required. For this purpose, levothyroxine (L-thyroxine) is the agent of choice. In the younger patient with the early diffuse stage of simple goiter, treatment can be instituted with 100 μg of levothyroxine daily, and the dose is increased over the next month or so to a maximum of 150 or 200 μg daily (average dose of 1.8 μg/kg body weight per day). Complete suppression would imply reduction of serum TSH to levels less than 0.1 mU/L by an ultrasensitive assay. Until uncertainties about the association of long-term excess thyroid hormone therapy and loss of bone mineral (osteopenia) are resolved, patients should be titrated to slightly less than a fully suppressive dose. Adequacy of suppression also may be assessed by measuring the RAIU, which should decrease to less than 5 percent of the administered dose at 24 h. Lesser decreases indicate only partial suppression, which may reflect the presence of autonomous foci demonstrable by scanning techniques. In the elderly or the patient with long-standing multinodular goiter, an ultrasensitive TSH measurement or a TRH stimulation test should be undertaken before initiating treatment with levothyroxine to determine whether significant functional autonomy is present. If such is indicated by an undetectable basal TSH or a diminished or absent TSH responsiveness to TRH, suppressive therapy with levothyroxine is contraindicated since such patients are or will eventually become thyrotoxic. Rather, consideration should be given to radioiodine ablation of the autonomous foci (see later section on "Toxic Multi-

nodular Goiter"). On the other hand, if the TSH response to TRH is normal, excluding significant functional autonomy, treatment with levothyroxine can be initiated. In the elderly patient, the initial dose should not exceed 50 μg daily, and the dosage should be gradually increased, partial rather than complete suppression of the value for basal TSH and/or the RAIU being the end point. It is the practice to obtain a thyroid scan as part of the initial evaluation of all patients with multinodular goiter and to repeat the RAIU and scan (suppression scan), when practical, in patients receiving suppressive thyroid hormone therapy.

Results of therapy vary widely. The early diffuse, hyperplastic goiter responds well, with regression or disappearance in 3 to 6 months. In the authors' experience, the later, nodular stage responds less favorably, and significant reduction in gland size is achieved only in about one-third of the cases; however, in the remainder, suppressive treatment may forestall further glandular growth. Internodular tissue regresses more often than do nodules themselves. The latter may therefore appear to become more prominent during treatment. After maximum regression of the goiter, suppressive medication may be maintained for prolonged periods, reduced to minimal levels, or at times withdrawn. In an unpredictable manner, goiter may remain relieved or recur. In the latter instances, suppressive therapy should be reinstituted and continued indefinitely. In areas of endemic iodine deficiency, the size and prevalence of goiter and the frequency of cretinism can be reduced by the provision of iodized salt or water or the periodic injection of iodized oil.

Surgical therapy of simple goiter is physiologically unsound, but it may occasionally be necessary to relieve obstructive symptoms, especially those that persist after a trial of medical therapy. Surgical exploration of nodular goiter may be indicated in some individuals when evidence suggests carcinoma. However, the concept that subtotal resection of multinodular nontoxic goiter affords effective prophylaxis against the development of thyroid carcinoma is unsound. If for some reason subtotal thyroidectomy has been performed, levothyroxine in a usual dose of about 1.8 μg/kg body weight daily is recommended to inhibit regenerative hyperplasia and further goitrogenesis.

HYPOTHYROIDISM

Hypothyroidism can result from any of a variety of abnormalities that lead to insufficient synthesis of thyroid hormone. Hypothyroidism dating from birth and resulting in developmental abnormalities is termed *cretinism*. The term *myxedema* connotes severe hypothyroidism in which there is accumulation of hydrophilic mucopolysaccharides in the ground substance of the dermis and other tissues, leading to thickening of the facial features and doughy induration of the skin.

ETIOLOGY AND PATHOGENESIS   A classification of hypothyroidism is presented in Table 316-5. Overall, the thyroid varieties account for approximately 95 percent of cases, only 5 percent or less being suprathyroid in origin. In thyroprivic hypothyroidism, loss of thyroid tissue leads to inadequate synthesis of thyroid hormone, despite maximum stimulation of any thyroid remnant by TSH. The most common cause of thyroprivic hypothyroidism is surgical or radioiodine ablation of the thyroid gland in the treatment of Graves' disease. Thyroprivic hypothyroidism may also occur as a primary idiopathic disorder. Primary hypothyroidism is frequently associated with circulating antithyroid antibodies and in some cases may result from the action of antibodies that block the TSH receptor. It may coexist with diabetes mellitus and other diseases in which circulating autoantibodies are found, such as pernicious anemia, systemic lupus erythematosus, rheumatoid arthritis, Sjögren's syndrome, and chronic hepatitis. In addition, hypothyroidism can be one manifestation of a polyglandular endocrine deficiency state in which autoantibodies cause variable insufficiency of thyroid, adrenal, parathyroid, and gonadal function (see Chap. 325). All these diseases, including isolated primary hypothyroidism, are associated with an increased frequency of specific HLA haplotypes and may be diverse reflections of disordered immune regulation. Finally, a developmental defect may result in failure of the gland to function adequately, leading to sporadic nongoitrous cretinism or juvenile hypothyroidism. A self-limited period of hypothyroidism is common in the course of subacute thyroiditis and in the syndrome of "painless thyroiditis," including the postpartum variant and usually after a temporary period of thyrotoxicosis. Owing to a persisting lack of TSH stimulation, intrinsically euthyroid subjects from whom chronic suppressive therapy is abruptly withdrawn experience a several-week period of thyroid hypofunction.

Impairment in the ability to synthesize adequate quantities of thyroid hormone leads to hypersecretion of TSH and hence goiter. If this compensatory response is inadequate, goitrous hypothyroidism ensues. The commonest cause of goitrous hypothyroidism in North America is Hashimoto's disease, in which defective organic binding of iodide and abnormal secretion of iodoproteins are frequent abnormalities. Iodide-induced goiter with or without hypothyroidism appears to arise from an intrinsic defect in the organic binding mechanism, which permits a persistent Wolff-Chaikoff effect. Euthyroid patients with Graves' disease, especially after surgery or radioiodine treatment, those with Hashimoto's disease, and the normal fetus are particularly susceptible to iodide-induced goiter. In view of the susceptibility of the fetal thyroid to iodide, with resulting goiter and hypothyroidism, iodine in large doses should not be given during pregnancy. Less common causes of goitrous hypothyroidism are hereditary defects in hormone biosynthesis and ingestion of drugs that induce defects in hormone biosynthesis, such as aminosalicylic acid and lithium. Finally, in areas of environmental iodine deficiency, goitrous cretinism and hypothyroidism can occur on an endemic basis. Diminished thyroid reserve occurs as a stage in the evolution of both thyroprivic and goitrous hypothyroidism.

In hypothyroidism of suprathyroid origin, the thyroid is intrinsically normal but is deprived of stimulation by TSH. Deprivation of TSH, most commonly the result of postpartum pituitary necrosis or a tumor of the pituitary or adjacent regions, results in pituitary hypothyroidism. Hypothalamic hypothyroidism is less common and results from inadequate secretion of TRH.

CLINICAL PICTURE The appearance of children with hypothyroidism depends on the age at which the deficiency began and the promptness with which replacement therapy was instituted. Cretinism may be manifested at birth but usually becomes evident within the first several months, depending upon the extent of thyroid failure. Hypothyroidism is present in approximately 1 of every 5000 neonates and manifests itself in persistence of physiologic jaundice, hoarse cry, constipation, somnolence, and feeding problems; since clinical diagnosis is difficult and early treatment is crucial for normal intellectual development, all neonates should be screened for hypothyroidism with measurements of the serum T_4 or TSH. In later months, delay in reaching the normal milestones of development becomes evident, and the physical characteristics of the cretin appear. These include short stature, coarse features with protruding tongue, broad flat nose, widely set eyes, sparse hair, dry skin, protuberant abdomen with an umbilical hernia, and impaired mental development. X-ray examination reveals retarded bone age, epiphyseal dysgenesis, and delayed dentition.

In the older child, the clinical manifestations of hypothyroidism are intermediate between those of infantile and adult hypothyroidism. Retardation of linear growth is manifested by shortness of stature, and retardation of sexual maturation results in delay in the onset of puberty. Poor performance at school may call attention to the diagnosis. The manifestations of adult hypothyroidism are present to a variable degree. X-ray examination reveals delayed union of the epiphyses.

In the adult, early symptoms of hypothyroidism are nonspecific and of insidious onset. They may include lethargy, constipation, cold intolerance, stiffness and cramping of the muscles, the carpal tunnel syndrome, and menorrhagia. Over the succeeding months, intellectual and motor activity slows, appetite declines, and weight increases.

The hair becomes dry and tends to fall out, and the skin becomes dry. The voice becomes deeper and hoarse, and auditory acuity may deteriorate. Obstructive sleep apnea may occur. Ultimately, the clinical picture of florid myxedema appears, with dull expressionless face, sparse hair, periorbital puffiness, large tongue, and pale, cool skin that feels rough and doughy. Thyroid tissue is not readily palpable, except in the goitrous variety of hypothyroidism. The heart is enlarged owing to both dilation and pericardial effusion; if the heart is small, pituitary hypothyroidism (with adrenal insufficiency) should be considered. Adynamic ileus may result in megacolon or intestinal obstruction. Rarely, psychiatric symptoms or cerebellar ataxia may dominate the clinical picture. The relaxation phase of the deep tendon reflexes is characteristically prolonged, the so-called hung-up reflex. If left untreated, the patient with severe long-standing hypothyroidism may pass into a hypothermic, stuporous state (*myxedema coma*) that is frequently fatal. Respiratory depression is an important component of this state, and hence arterial P_{CO_2} may be increased. Factors that predispose to myxedema coma include cold exposure, trauma, infection, and administration of central nervous system depressants. Dilutional hyponatremia is common and results from impaired water excretion and from disordered regulation of vasopressin secretion.

LABORATORY TESTS The single most useful measurement is the serum TSH, which is invariably increased in the thyroprivic and goitrous varieties and is usually normal or undetectable in pituitary or hypothalamic hypothyroidism (Fig. 316-3). In the latter instances, hyposecretion of TSH is usually accompanied by hyposecretion of other pituitary hormones (see Chap. 313). A decrease in serum T_4 and in the FT_4I is common to all varieties of hypothyroidism. In the thyroid varieties, the serum T_3 may be decreased to a lesser extent than the serum T_4, the presumption being that the compensatory hypersecretion of TSH leads to a relative preponderance of T_3 secretion. In thyroprivic hypothyroidism the decreased RAIU is of limited diagnostic utility because of the low value for the lower limit of the normal range. In goitrous hypothyroidism, the RAIU may be increased or display an abnormal pattern of accumulation or retention.

Frequent manifestations of the hypothyroid state include an increased serum cholesterol in hypothyroidism of thyroid (but not pituitary) origin and increased concentrations in serum of creatine phosphokinase, aspartate transaminase, and lactic dehydrogenase. Systolic time intervals are altered in that the preejection period is prolonged, and the ratio of the preejection period to left ventricular ejection time is increased. Electrocardiographic changes include bradycardia, low-amplitude QRS complexes, and flattened or inverted T waves. In primary thyroprivic hypothyroidism, overt pernicious anemia occurs in about 12 percent of patients; histamine-fast achlorhydria and circulating antigastric parietal cell antibodies are more common.

Some patients who appear clinically euthyroid display laboratory evidence of early thyroid failure (subclinical hypothyroidism). In mild cases serum TSH and its response to TRH administration are increased while serum T_4 and T_3 concentrations are normal. When there is a greater degree of thyroid failure, serum T_4 concentration is decreased, but the serum T_3 concentration is normal or nearly so owing to TSH-induced hypersecretion of T_3 relative to T_4, and perhaps to more efficient conversion of T_4 to T_3. Subclinical hypothyroidism is most often seen in patients with Hashimoto's disease or those with Graves' disease who have been treated with ^{131}I or surgery and are usually stages in the evolution of frank hypothyroidism.

DIFFERENTIAL DIAGNOSIS Little difficulty will be experienced in diagnosing the classic picture of cretinism or juvenile and adult hypothyroidism. Occasionally, an infant with Down's syndrome may be confused with a cretin. However, the characteristic eye changes, Brushfield's spots in the iris, hyperextensibility of the joints, and normal skin and hair texture distinguish Down's syndrome from cretinism. Chronic nephritis and the nephrotic syndrome may simulate myxedema, particularly because of the facial puffiness and pallor. The nephrotic patient may have anemia, hypercholesterolemia, and anasarca, and the serum T_4 concentration may be decreased if there is significant loss of TBG into the urine. However, the FT_4I is normal or increased, the serum T_3 concentration is often subnormal, as in any severe systemic illness owing to impaired peripheral generation from T_4, and the serum TSH concentration is normal.

TREATMENT Two types of hormone are available for the treatment of hypothyroidism, synthetic hormone and thyroprotein derived from animal thyroids (Table 316-6). Synthetic hormones include levothyroxine (L-thyroxine), liothyronine (L-triiodothyronine), and liotrix (a combination of the two). The preparation of natural origin most commonly used is thyroid extract, USP. Because of their uniform potency, the authors prefer the synthetic preparations and specifically levothyroxine. Unlike liothyronine, liotrix, and even thyroid extract, ingestion of levothyroxine does not lead to abrupt increases in serum T_3 concentration, which can be dangerous in the older patient or in the patient with coexisting heart disease. Rather, a stable T_3 concentration is attained through continuous generation from administered levothyroxine.

In most instances, a normal metabolic state should be restored gradually, especially in the elderly or the patient with heart disease, since sudden increases in metabolic rate may tax cardiac or coronary reserve. In adults, an initial daily dose of 25 μg levothyroxine can be increased by 25- to 50-μg increments at 2- to 3-week intervals, until a normal metabolic state is attained. The dose necessary to sustain a normal metabolic state is usually about 1.8 μg/kg body weight per day, and this usually results in a serum T_4 at or somewhat above the upper limit of the normal range. The serum T_3 is superior to the serum T_4 as an indicator of the metabolic state in the patient receiving levothyroxine. Because of its long half-life, levothyroxine is administered as a single daily dose. The optimum dose for an individual should be based on clinical criteria and on measurements of serum TSH by an ultrasensitive assay or T_3. Elevations of the former indicate that treatment is insufficient and of the latter that it is excessive.

In neonatal, infantile, and juvenile hypothyroidism it is essential that full replacement therapy be begun as soon as possible; otherwise the chances of normal intellectual development and growth are poor. Infants and children require doses of levothyroxine that are disproportionately large in relation to body size. *In known or strongly suspected pituitary and hypothalamic hypothyroidism, thyroid replacement should not be instituted until treatment with hydrocortisone has been initiated*, since acute adrenocortical insufficiency may be precipitated by an increase in metabolic rate.

In some patients, hypothyroidism should be treated rapidly. This includes patients with myxedema coma and, because of the extreme sensitivity to central nervous system depressants, hypothyroid patients being prepared for emergency surgery. Here, intravenous administration of levothyroxine, in conjunction with the use of hydrocortisone, is indicated.

THYROTOXICOSIS

The term *thyrotoxicosis* denotes the clinical, physiologic, and biochemical findings that result when the tissues are exposed to, and

TABLE 316-6 Approximate therapeutic equivalence of various thyroid hormone preparations

Preparation	Average daily oral maintenance dose	Serum T_4
Thyroid extract, USP	120–180 mg	Normal
Levothyroxine	125 μg	Slightly increased
Liothyronine	50 μg	Decreased
Liotrix ($T_4/T_3 = 4{:}1$)	2 units	Normal

TABLE 316-7 Varieties of thyrotoxicosis

I Disorders associated with thyroid hyperfunction*
  A Excess production of TSH (rare)
  B Abnormal thyroid stimulator
    1 Graves' disease
    2 Trophoblastic tumor
  C Intrinsic thyroid autonomy
    1 Hyperfunctioning adenoma
    2 Toxic multinodular goiter
II Disorders not associated with thyroid hyperfunction†
  A Disorders of hormone storage
    1 Subacute thyroiditis
    2 Chronic thyroiditis with transient thyrotoxicosis
  B Extrathyroid source of hormone
    1 Thyrotoxicosis factitia
    2 Ectopic thyroid tissue
      a Struma ovarii
      b Functioning follicular cacinoma

* Associated with increased RAIU unless body iodine burden is excessive.
† Associated with decreased RAIU.

respond to, an excess supply of thyroid hormone. Rather than a specific disease, thyrotoxicosis is a syndrome that can originate in a variety of ways (Table 316-7). The first, and most important, encompasses those diseases that lead to sustained overproduction of hormone by the thyroid gland itself. Here, hyperfunction of the gland variously results from excessive secretion of TSH, a rare cause associated with pituitary tumor or with resistance to thyroid hormone in the pituitary but not in peripheral tissues; the action of an abnormal, homeostatically unregulated thyroid stimulator of extrapituitary origin, as in Graves' disease, hyperthyroidism in association with Hashimoto's disease, or trophoblastic tumors; or the development of one or more areas of autonomous hyperfunction within the gland itself. The second category encompasses the thyrotoxic states associated with subacute thyroiditis and the syndrome termed *chronic thyroiditis with spontaneously resolving thyrotoxicosis;* an excess of preformed hormone leaks from the gland owing to the presence of inflammatory disease. New hormone formation is decreased, however, owing to the suppression of TSH secretion by the hormone excess, and in some cases to the inflammatory injury itself. Since the inflammatory disorders are transitory and since stores of preformed hormone are ultimately depleted, the thyrotoxicosis in these disorders is self-limited and is often followed by a transient period of thyroid hormone insufficiency. The third category of thyrotoxic state is one in which the source of excess hormone is outside of the thyroid gland itself, as in thyrotoxicosis factitia, the rare functioning metastatic thyroid carcinoma, or struma ovarii.

Although all of the foregoing disorders are associated with thyrotoxicosis, not all are associated with hyperthyroidism, a term which should be used to denote only those conditions in which sustained hyperfunction of the thyroid leads to thyrotoxicosis. Thus, thyrotoxic states can be classified according to whether or not they are associated with hyperthyroidism. This distinction has implications for diagnosis and for treatment. In hyperthyroidism, hyperfunction of the thyroid is reflected in an increased RAIU, whereas in the nonhyperthyroid thyrotoxic states, thyroid function (as reflected in the RAIU) is subnormal. Further, treatment of thyrotoxicosis by means intended to decrease hormone synthesis (antithyroid agents, surgery, or radioiodine) is appropriate in hyperthyroidism but is inappropriate and ineffective in other forms of thyrotoxicosis.

Though the specific diseases that cause thyrotoxicosis each make their own imprint on the clinical picture, the manifestations of the thyrotoxic state are largely the same. In the discussion that ensues, the major diseases that lead to a thyrotoxic state are individually described. Since the first considered and most important is Graves' disease, the common manifestations of thyrotoxicosis are described in relation to Graves' disease.

GRAVES' DISEASE

Graves' disease, also known as Parry's or Basedow's disease, is a disorder with a triad of major manifestations: hyperthyroidism with diffuse goiter, ophthalmopathy, and dermopathy. Although part of the same disease complex, the three major manifestations need not appear together. Indeed, one or two need never appear, and, moreover, the three tend to run courses that are largely independent of one another.

PREVALENCE Graves' disease is a relatively common disorder that occurs at any age but is especially common in the third and fourth decades. The disease is more frequent in women than in men. In nongoitrous areas the ratio of predominance in women may be as high as 7:1. In areas of endemic goiter the ratio is lower. Genetic factors play an important role; there is an increased frequency of haplotypes HLA-B8 and -DRw3 in Caucasian, HLA-Bw36 in Japanese, and HLA-Bw46 in Chinese patients with the disease. Not surprisingly, there is a distinct familial predisposition to Graves' disease. In addition, among family members of patients with Graves' disease, a clinical and immunologic overlap exists with respect to Hashimoto's disease, primary thyroprivic hypothyroidism, and pernicious anemia and probably with respect to other diseases in which autoimmune features are prominent. In occasional patients, the disease picture may change from Graves' disease to Hashimoto's disease, or vice versa, and rarely patients with primary myxedema later become hyperthyroid. Thus, it is proper to consider Graves' disease, Hashimoto's disease, and primary myxedema as closely related autoimmune thyroid diseases.

ETIOLOGY AND PATHOGENESIS The cause is unknown. In view of the varied manifestations of Graves' disease and their differing courses, it is possible that no single factor is responsible for the entire syndrome. With respect to hyperthyroidism, the central disorder is a disruption of homeostatic mechanisms that normally adjust hormone secretion to meet the needs of peripheral tissues; if such were able to operate, hyperthyroidism could not be sustained. This homeostatic disruption results from the presence in plasma of an abnormal thyroid stimulator, first recognized when it was shown that the serum of patients with Graves' disease releases radioiodine from the prelabeled guinea pig or mouse thyroid. In view of its prolonged duration of action relative to that of TSH in this bioassay system, this material was designated the long-acting thyroid stimulator (LATS). LATS activity is present in one or more immunoglobulins of the IgG class elaborated by lymphocytes of patients with Graves' disease. LATS can be detected only in about half of patients with this disorder, and consequently its pathogenetic role was questioned. This failure to detect LATS in all patients with Graves' disease is due to the fact that the stimulator has variable actions in other species and is not uniformly detectable, therefore, in the conventional bioassay. When human thyroid tissue is used as the assay system, LATS-like responses can be demonstrated in the plasma of most patients. These responses and the corresponding names given to the responsible factors are as follows: prevention of the adsorption of LATS activity by human thyroid particulate fractions (LATS-protector, LATS-p), stimulation of colloid droplet or cyclic AMP generation in thyroid cells, slices, or membranes (thyroid-stimulating immunoglobulins, TSI), and inhibition of the binding of TSH to its receptors in human thyroid tissue (TSH-binding inhibitory immunoglobulins, TBII). These factors are probably antibodies against the thyroid TSH receptor. Activities of this type are also found in serum of some patients with euthyroid ophthalmic Graves' disease, an occasional patient with Hashimoto's disease, and some euthyroid relatives of patients with Graves' disease, though the reason for the absence of thyrotoxicosis in such instances is uncertain. Disappearance of these stimulatory factors from the serum during antithyroid treatment augurs well for long-term remission after treatment is withdrawn. Thus, while the basic cause of Graves' disease is not understood, an immunoglobulin or family of immunoglobulins directed against the TSH receptor mediates the thyroid stimulation of Graves' disease. A heritable abnormality in immune surveillance may permit particular lymphocytes to survive, proliferate, and secrete the stimulatory immunoglobulins in response to precipitating factors.

The pathogenesis of the ophthalmic component of Graves' disease is more enigmatic. One proposed mechanism is the development of antibodies against specific antigens in the extraocular muscles. Nothing is known of the pathogenesis of the dermopathy of Graves' disease.

PATHOLOGY In Graves' disease, the *thyroid gland* is diffusely enlarged, soft, and vascular. The essential pathology is that of parenchymatous hypertrophy and hyperplasia, characterized by increased height of the epithelium and redundancy of the follicular wall, giving the picture of papillary infoldings and cytologic evidence of increased activity. Such hyperplasia is usually accompanied by lymphocytic infiltration that reflects the immune aspect of the disease and that correlates in severity with levels of antithyroid antibodies in the blood. Following iodine medication, there is colloid storage, which sometimes causes enlargement and increased firmness of the gland. Graves' disease is associated with generalized lymphoid hyperplasia and infiltration and occasionally with enlargement of the spleen or thymus. Thyrotoxicosis may lead to degeneration of skeletal muscle fibers, enlargement of the heart, fatty infiltration or diffuse fibrosis of the liver, decalcification of the skeleton, and loss of body tissue (including fat deposits, osteoid, and muscle).

The *ophthalmopathy* is characterized by an inflammatory infiltrate of the orbital contents, exclusive of the globe, with lymphocytes, mast cells, and plasma cells. The orbital musculature is often enlarged, largely accounting for the increased volume of the orbital contents that causes the globe to protrude. Muscle fibers show degeneration and loss of striations, with ultimate fibrosis.

The *dermopathy* of Graves' disease is characterized by thickening of the dermis, which is infiltrated with lymphocytes and with hydrophilic, metachromatically staining mucopolysaccharides.

CLINICAL MANIFESTATIONS The manifestations comprise those that reflect the associated thyrotoxicosis and those specifically related to Graves' disease. The former vary in intensity with the severity of the thyrotoxicosis, the age of the patient, duration of the illness, and the presence of disease in other organs, such as the heart.

Manifestations of thyrotoxicosis Common manifestations include nervousness, emotional lability, inability to sleep, tremors, frequent bowel movements, excessive sweating, and heat intolerance. Weight loss is usual despite a well-maintained or increased appetite. Proximal muscle weakness is present with loss of strength often manifested by difficulty in climbing stairs. In premenopausal women, oligomenorrhea and amenorrhea tend to occur. Dyspnea, palpitations, and in older patients, enhancement of angina pectoris or cardiac failure may occur. In general, nervous symptoms dominate the clinical picture in younger individuals, whereas cardiovascular and myopathic symptoms predominate in older subjects.

Usually, the patient appears anxious, restless, and fidgety. The skin is warm and moist with a velvety texture, and palmar erythema is present. Separation of the fingernail from the nailbed (Plummer's nail) is common, especially on the ring finger. The hair is fine and silky. A fine tremor of the fingers and tongue, together with hyperreflexia, is characteristic. *Ocular signs* include a characteristic stare with widened palpebral fissures, infrequent blinking, lid lag, and failure to wrinkle the brow on upward gaze. These signs result from sympathetic overstimulation and usually subside when the thyrotoxicosis is corrected. They are to be distinguished from the *infiltrative ophthalmopathy* characteristic of Graves' disease, discussed below.

Cardiovascular findings include a wide pulse pressure, sinus tachycardia, atrial arrhythmias (especially atrial fibrillation), systolic murmurs, increased intensity of the apical first sound, cardiac enlargement, and, at times, overt heart failure. A to-and-fro, high-pitched sound may be audible in the pulmonic area and may simulate a pericardial friction rub (Means-Lerman scratch).

Manifestations of Graves' disease   The distinctive manifestations of Graves' disease, diffuse hyperfunctioning goiter, ophthalmopathy, and dermopathy, appear in varying combinations and in varying frequency, goiter being the most common. Premature graying of the hair and patchy vitiligo are not specific to Graves' disease but are also common in other autoimmune disorders.

The *diffuse toxic goiter* may be asymmetric and lobular. The presence of a bruit over the gland usually signifies that the patient is thyrotoxic, but it may rarely be present in other disorders in which the thyroid is hyperplastic. Venous hums and carotid souffles should be distinguished from true thyroid bruits. An enlarged pyramidal lobe of the thyroid may be palpable.

The clinical signs associated with the *ophthalmopathy* of Graves' disease may be divided into two components: the spastic and the mechanical. The former includes the stare, lid lag, and lid retraction that accompany thyrotoxicosis and account for the "frightened" facies and classic eye signs previously described. These findings need not be associated with proptosis and usually return to normal after correction of thyrotoxicosis. The mechanical component includes proptosis of varying degrees with ophthalmoplegia and congestive oculopathy characterized by chemosis, conjunctivitis, periorbital swelling, and the potential complications of corneal ulceration, optic neuritis, and optic atrophy. When exophthalmos progresses rapidly and becomes the major concern in Graves' disease, it is termed *progressive* and, if severe, *malignant exophthalmos*. The term *exophthalmic ophthalmoplegia* refers to the ocular muscle weakness that commonly accompanies this disorder and results in impaired upward gaze and convergence and strabismus with varying degrees of diplopia. Exophthalmos may be unilateral early in the course of the disorder but usually progresses to bilateral involvement.

The *dermopathy* of Graves' disease usually occurs over the dorsum of the legs or feet and is termed *localized* or *pretibial myxedema*. It occurs in patients with past or present Graves' disease and is not a manifestation of hypothyroidism. About half of cases occur during the active stage of thyrotoxicosis. The affected area is usually well demarcated from normal skin by the fact that it is raised, thickened, has a *peau d'orange* appearance, and may be pruritic and hyperpigmented. The lesions are usually discrete, assuming a plaquelike or nodular configuration but in some instances becoming confluent. Clubbing of the fingers and toes with characteristic bony changes that differ from those of hypertrophic pulmonary osteoarthropathy may accompany the dermal changes (*thyroid acropachy*). This disorder is usually self-limited.

DIAGNOSIS   When severe, Graves' disease presents little difficulty in diagnosis. Florid thyrotoxicosis is manifested by weakness, weight loss despite good appetite, nervous instability, tremor, intolerance to heat, sweating, palpitations, and hyperdefecation. When associated with diffuse thyroid enlargement, often accompanied by a bruit, and particularly when associated with ophthalmopathy, the clinical picture of Graves' disease is virtually unique. In such instances, laboratory tests documenting increased RAIU, serum T_4 and T_3, RT_3U, and FT_4I serve as baselines for evaluation of therapy, rather than necessary diagnostic aids. Occasionally, laboratory tests reveal a normal RAIU, normal serum T_4 and RT_3U, and elevated serum T_3 and FT_3I (T_3 toxicosis).

In less severe cases, particularly when ophthalmopathy is lacking, the diagnosis may be more difficult, since the symptoms of mild thyrotoxicosis are similar to those of other disorders (see "Differential Diagnosis" below). Presence of a goiter makes the diagnosis of hyperthyroidism likely, but careful palpation is necessary to determine whether toxic multinodular goiter, toxic adenoma, or subacute thyroiditis is present, since treatment of these disorders may differ from that of diffuse toxic goiter. Absence of thyroid enlargement makes the diagnosis of Graves' disease less likely but does not exclude it. In mild cases, confirmatory laboratory tests assume great importance. Unfortunately, mild thyrotoxicosis is often associated with marginal abnormalities in laboratory tests or values within the upper limit of the normal range. In such instances, an ultrasensitive TSH assay or the TRH stimulation test assumes crucial importance.

In a few (usually older) patients, the clinical picture may be one of apathy rather than hyperactivity, and evidence of hypermetabolism may be slight (*apathetic thyrotoxicosis*). In such patients, myopathic features may be pronounced. More often, cardiovascular manifestations predominate since mild hyperthyroidism may produce severe disability in patients with underlying heart disease. Hence, *all patients with unexplained cardiac failure or irregularities in rhythm, especially if atrial in origin, should be examined for thyrotoxicosis.* Clues to the diagnosis include a relatively rapid circulation time and resistance to the usual doses of digitalis, but laboratory confirmation is required.

DIFFERENTIAL DIAGNOSIS   Signs and symptoms in a number of nonthyroid disorders may simulate certain aspects of the thyrotoxic syndrome. Anxiety is a prominent feature of thyrotoxicosis, and there is thus some overlap in the symptomatology of thyrotoxicosis with that of anxiety states of emotional origin. Tachycardia, tremulousness, irritability, weakness, and fatigue are common to both disorders. In anxiety of emotional origin, however, the peripheral manifestations of excessive thyroid hormones are absent; the skin is usually cold and clammy rather than warm and moist. Weight loss, when present in emotional anxiety, is characteristically accompanied by anorexia, whereas in thyrotoxicosis the appetite is generally increased. Thyrotoxicosis can occasionally be confused with such disorders as metastatic carcinoma, cirrhosis of the liver, hyperparathyroidism, sprue, myasthenia gravis, and muscular dystrophy. Hypokalemic periodic paralysis is more common in thyrotoxic patients, especially in Oriental and Latin American men. Signs and symptoms of thyrotoxicosis may overlap with those of pheochromocytoma, which can cause heat intolerance, excessive perspiration, tachycardia with palpitations, and a hypermetabolic state. In the above disorders and in other conditions considered in the differential diagnosis, the judicious application of laboratory tests usually makes it possible to differentiate them from thyrotoxicosis.

When bilateral ophthalmopathy is accompanied by goiter and thyrotoxicosis, the origin of the ophthalmopathy in Graves' disease is virtually certain. The presence of unilateral ophthalmopathy, even when associated with thyrotoxicosis, raises the possibility of some other intraorbital or intracranial disease. In the euthyroid patient with either unilateral or bilateral ophthalmopathy other causes must be excluded. These include cavernous sinus thrombosis, sphenoidal ridge meningioma, retrobulbar tumors, including leukemic deposits, and the rare granulomatous disorder pseudotumor oculi. Exophthalmos may also be seen in certain systemic disorders, such as uremia, accelerated hypertension, chronic alcoholism, chronic obstructive pulmonary disease, superior mediastinal obstruction, and Cushing's syndrome. Ophthalmoplegia in the absence of overt infiltrative manifestations can be confused with that which occurs in diabetes mellitus, myasthenia gravis, and myopathies. When doubt exists about the cause of ophthalmopathy, the demonstration of significant titers of TSI or TBII or of an abnormal TRH stimulation or thyroid suppression test suggests that the cause is Graves' disease, though not all patients with "euthyroid Graves' disease" demonstrate abnormal responses. In such cases, ultrasonography or computed tomography of the orbits is valuable in demonstrating characteristic thickening of the extraocular muscles.

When a thyrotoxic state occurs in a patient lacking the characteristic ophthalmopathy of Graves' disease, other causes of thyrotoxicosis must be considered. Careful palpation of the thyroid and studies with radioactive iodine are important in this regard. A symmetric, diffuse goiter of moderate or large size suggests the diagnosis of Graves' disease, especially if a bruit is present. However, the uncommon patient whose hyperthyroidism is secondary to an excess of TSH (associated with a *pituitary tumor* or resistance to feedback suppression of TSH secretion) or an abnormal stimulator of trophoblastic origin (*hydatidiform mole* or *choriocarcinoma of uterus* or *testis;* see Chap. 309) may present in this way. A single, prominent thyroid nodule or multiple nodules suggest *toxic adenoma* or *toxic multinodular goiter*, respectively. Tenderness of the thyroid associated with firm nodularity strongly suggests *subacute thyroiditis*, while a small, firm, nontender goiter is consistent with the syndrome of chronic thyroiditis with spontaneously resolving thyrotoxicosis. The foregoing disorders are discussed more fully in later sections. Absence of a palpable thyroid gland suggests an extrathyroid source of hormone, such as ectopic thyroid tissue *(struma ovarii)* or, more commonly, self-administration of hormone *(thyrotoxicosis factitia)*. Studies with radioactive iodine are also helpful. Except when hormone overproduction is secondary to increased iodine intake, values of the RAIU are increased in all disorders producing hyperthyroidism, and scintillation scanning may aid in differentiating among them. Conversely, thyrotoxicosis that is not the result of hyperthyroidism is characterized by subnormal values of the RAIU. Subacute thyroiditis and chronic thyroiditis with spontaneously resolving thyrotoxicosis are the most common. Ectopic thyroid tissue producing thyrotoxicosis is rare. Here, the RAIU, as measured over the thyroid, is low since TSH secretion is suppressed, but despite this, urinary excretion of the dose of ^{131}I is slowed, owing to accumulation of ^{131}I by the ectopic tissue. Functioning ectopic tissue can be located by direct counting or scintillation scanning. Thyrotoxicosis factitia most frequently occurs in medical or para-medical personnel or in those who have easy access to thyroid hormone preparations. The disorder resembles thyrotoxicosis caused by ectopic thyroid tissue in that the patient's thyroid gland is suppressed. Consequently, the RAIU is very low, and most of an administered dose of ^{131}I is excreted promptly in the urine. When the disorder is caused by ingestion of preparations containing T_4, such as levothyroxine or thyroid extract, the serum T_4 is increased. On the other hand, when caused by liothyronine, the serum T_4 is subnormal. Irrespective of the preparation, the serum T_3 is increased but more so when liothyronine is the offending agent. Measurement of serum thyroglobulin is useful to confirm thyrotoxicosis factitia. Levels are elevated in Graves' disease and thyroiditis but are subnormal with exogenous thyroid hormone suppression.

The demonstration of elevated titers of antithyroid antibodies or of TSI or TBII activity in the blood also provides strong evidence that Graves' disease is the cause of thyrotoxicosis.

TREATMENT **Hyperthyroidism** The hyperthyroidism in Graves' disease is often characterized by cyclic phases of exacerbation and remission, each of unpredictable onset and duration. Moreover, long-standing disease may be associated with progressive thyroid failure, probably consequent to chronic thyroiditis, with the result that hypothyroidism or decreased thyroid reserve supervenes. These characteristics of Graves' disease have important implications in the choice of and response to therapy.

The major approaches to the treatment are directed to limiting the quantity of thyroid hormones the gland can produce. The use of antithyroid agents interposes a chemical blockade to hormone syn-thesis, the effect of which is operative only as long as the drug is administered. Thus, the agents can control a given phase of active thyrotoxicity but probably do not prevent exacerbation at some subsequent period. The second major approach is ablation of thyroid tissue, thereby limiting hormone production. This may be achieved either by surgery or by means of radioactive iodine. Since these procedures induce permanent anatomic alterations of the thyroid, they can control the individual active phase and are more likely to prevent a later exacerbation or recurrence. On the other hand, surgery or radiation is more likely to lead to hypothyroidism, either shortly after treatment or with the passage of years.

Each therapy has advantages and disadvantages, indications and contraindications. The latter are more often relative than absolute. In general, a trial of long-term antithyroid therapy is desirable in children, adolescents, young adults, and pregnant women but may also be employed in older patients. Indications for ablative procedures include relapse or recurrence following drug therapy, a large goiter, drug toxicity, failure to follow a medical regimen, or failure to return for periodic examinations. Subtotal thyroidectomy may be elected for patients under the age of 40 in whom ablative therapy is required; however, opinions differ, and some authorities employ radioactive iodine in the treatment of patients in the second or third decades. Surgery is also preferable in patients with very large goiters or with a coincident nonfunctioning nodule, especially if there is a history of radiation to the head and neck. Radioactive iodine is the ablative procedure of choice in older patients, in patients who have had previous thyroid surgery, and in those in whom systemic disease contraindicates elective surgery.

In patients selected for *long-term antithyroid therapy*, satisfactory control can almost always be achieved if sufficient drug is adminis-tered. Most patients can be managed with propylthiouracil, 100 to 150 mg every 6 or 8 h. In occasional patients with severe disease, larger doses are required for initial control. Methimazole is at least as effective as propylthiouracil when administered in one-tenth the dosage. However, propylthiouracil has the advantage of inhibiting the peripheral conversion of T_4 to T_3, thereby bringing about more rapid symptomatic improvement. Once euthyroidism is achieved, the daily dosage may be reduced to the smallest doses that control the thyrotoxicosis. In some clinics the initial dose is continued and is supplemented with levothyroxine. By this latter regimen, hypothy-roidism from overdosage of antithyroid drugs can be prevented. The undesirable consequences of hypothyroidism, such as enhancement of ophthalmopathy and enlargement of the goiter, may thereby be forestalled. The duration of therapy is difficult to predict in the individual patient and may be a function of the spontaneous course of the disease. The longer the course of therapy, the more likely it is that the patient will remain well when the drug is discontinued. In general a 12- to 24-month course is employed, following which one-third or one-half of patients remain well for a prolonged period or indefinitely. The likelihood of a prolonged remission is increased by a decrease in goiter size, reversion of the thyroid suppression test to normal, or disappearance of Graves' disease–related immunoglobulins (TSI and TBII) from the serum during treatment.

Leukopenia is the principal undesirable side effect of antithyroid drugs. A complete blood count should be obtained prior to initiating therapy to identify those patients with leukopenia related to Graves' disease. Mild transient leukopenia with antithyroid drugs may occur in approximately an additional 10 percent of patients and is not necessarily an indication for discontinuing therapy. When the absolute number of polymorphonuclear leukocytes reaches 1500 or less, antithyroid medication should be discontinued. Allergic rashes and drug sensitivity occur in a small percentage of patients. These may disappear with antihistamine therapy at the same or reduced dosage of antithyroid agent, but it is probably preferable when sensitivity reactions occur to change to another drug. On rare occasions (in less than 0.2 percent) agranulocytosis occurs. This may be sudden in onset. Hepatitis, drug fever, and arthralgias occur on occasion. In the authors' view, severe sensitivity reactions, including agranulo-cytosis, dictate the abandonment of antithyroid therapy, rather than recourse to an alternate drug.

Iodide inhibits the release of hormones from the hyperfunctioning thyroid gland, and its ameliorative effects occur more rapidly than those of agents that inhibit hormone synthesis. Hence, its main use is in patients with actual or impending thyrotoxic crisis and in patients with severe thyrocardiac disease. The response to iodide alone is often incomplete and transient. Furthermore, by expanding the thyroid store of hormone, iodide may prolong the latency of response to antithyroid therapy. Therefore, iodide is safely used only in con-junction with the antithyroid agents. If the clinical course is sufficiently severe to require iodide administration, antithyroid drugs are usually the primary therapeutic agents and should be given in large doses prior to iodide. Iodide is also useful in controlling thyrotoxicosis following ^{131}I administration, during the period in which the thera-peutic effect of radioiodine has not yet taken place. Large doses of *glucocorticoids* (2 mg of dexamethasone every 6 h) reduce the serum

T_4 concentration and should be added to the regimen when relief of thyrotoxicosis is urgent. The iodinated x-ray contrast agent sodium ipodate has a similar effect. Iodine liberated from this agent inhibits thyroid secretion of T_4 and T_3, and serum T_3 is further reduced by the inhibition by ipodate of peripheral T_3 formation. Daily doses of 1 g orally are effective, but the same precautions concerning the use of iodine therapy are applicable to ipodate as well.

Owing to the pronounced adrenergic component in thyrotoxicosis, various *adrenergic antagonists* have been employed in its management. Of these, propranolol is the agent of choice because of its relative freedom from side effects. In doses of 40 to 120 mg daily, propranolol alleviates such adrenergic manifestations as sweating, tremor, and tachycardia and may reduce to some extent the conversion of T_4 to T_3. However, propranolol should be used only as adjunctive therapy rather than sole therapy, as some have suggested, since the underlying metabolic abnormalities are not affected. Moreover, although the diminution in heart rate and cardiac work may be beneficial, the blocking of adrenergic support of myocardial contractility requires caution in its use in the patient with coexisting heart failure, unless rate- or rhythm-related. As adjunctive therapy, the major usefulness of propranolol is during the period when the response to conventional antithyroid agents or to radioiodine therapy is being awaited and in the management of thyrotoxic crisis. It has been employed as the sole agent in preparation for thyroidectomy, but its use in this setting is not recommended since it does not render the patient euthyroid, with a likely greater risk of surgically induced crisis.

Radioactive iodine (*^{131}I*) affords a relatively simple, effective, and economical means of treating thyrotoxicosis. It can produce the ablative effects of surgery without the immediate operative and postoperative complications. The principal disadvantage of ^{131}I therapy, in the dosage usually employed, is its tendency to produce hypothyroidism with a frequency that increases with time. As many as 40 to 70 percent of patients may develop this complication within 10 years after treatment. Although hypothyroidism is treatable, once diagnosed, the insidious onset may obscure the diagnosis until serious complications have developed. Hence, some recommend that all patients be treated with large doses of ^{131}I to ensure relief of thyrotoxicosis and then placed on permanent physiologic replacement doses of thyroid hormone.

There is no evidence of carcinogenic or leukemogenic effects of radioiodine when it is given to adults in the doses commonly used in treating hyperthyroidism. However, the susceptibility to carcinogenesis may be increased in the thyroids of children. Mutagenic effects have not been reported and would be difficult to document. For these reasons, many physicians prefer to reserve radioiodine therapy for patients over 30 years of age or those unlikely to have children subsequently. Moreover, the longer the life expectancy after ^{131}I therapy, the greater the likelihood that hypothyroidism will develop. Among younger patients, therefore, only those with recurrent thyrotoxicosis following surgery, those who refuse surgery, and those with complicating illness that contraindicates surgery are candidates for radioiodine therapy. In elderly patients, treatment with large doses of radioiodine is the general method of choice, so that the undesirable effects of incomplete treatment or recurrence can be avoided.

The usual therapeutic dose of ^{131}I [approximately 5.9 MBq (160 μCi) per gram of estimated gland weight] has led to the disturbingly high frequency of hypothyroidism. As a result, though continuing to use this dose, some authorities regularly administer prophylactic replacement doses of thyroid hormone. On the other hand, others have administered smaller doses [approximately 3.0 MBq/g (80 μCi/g)]. However, this does not diminish the frequency of late hypothyroidism but merely delays its onset. Moreover, the smaller dose is less likely to relieve thyrotoxicosis within a relatively short period. Antithyroid agents can be employed, however, to speed the attainment of a eumetabolic state, and propranolol can be given to relieve symptoms, while the effect of the ^{131}I is taking hold. There is general agreement that patients with coexisting cardiac disease should receive ^{131}I in large doses in view of the hazard of recurrent thyrotoxicosis.

Radiation thyroiditis is an occasional immediate complication of ^{131}I therapy. When present, it commonly appears within 7 to 10 days and is associated with excessive release of hormone into the blood. Rarely, radiation thyroiditis may be so severe as to cause thyrotoxic crisis (see below); this complication is most likely in the elderly thyrotoxic patient with other systemic illness. For these reasons, patients with severe hyperthyroidism or underlying heart disease should be rendered eumetabolic with antithyroid agents before ^{131}I is administered. Interruption of antithyroid therapy for 3 to 4 days before and after ^{131}I treatment suffices to permit adequate accumulation and retention of administered ^{131}I. Propranolol may be used as an adjunct both before and after ^{131}I administration but should not be relied upon to provide adequate prophylaxis if given alone. The swelling that accompanies radiation thyroiditis may contraindicate the use of large doses of ^{131}I in patients with large retrosternal goiters.

Before radioactive iodine was introduced, *subtotal thyroidectomy* was the standard form of ablative therapy, and it is still employed in younger patients in whom antithyroid therapy is unsuccessful. Although precise preoperative programs differ, several general principles should be emphasized. Patients should first be rendered euthyroid by means of antithyroid agents. Only then should iodide (five drops of Lugol's solution a day for approximately 10 days) be administered concomitantly to effect an involutional response in the gland. Antithyroid drugs should not be discontinued merely because treatment with iodide is instituted. The response of the patient, and not the calendar, should dictate when surgery is performed.

Hazards of subtotal thyroidectomy include immediate complications, such as anesthetic accidents, hemorrhage sometimes leading to respiratory obstruction, and damage to the recurrent laryngeal nerve leading to vocal cord paralysis. Later complications include wound infection, hemorrhage, hypoparathyroidism, or hypothyroidism. Subtotal thyroidectomy should be performed by a surgeon experienced in this procedure; under this condition surgery is effective and relatively safe. Postoperative recurrences are uncommon. However, carefully conducted follow-up studies reveal that hypothyroidism follows surgery more frequently than previously suspected, although not as commonly as following treatment with conventional doses of ^{131}I.

The *treatment of hyperthyroidism during pregnancy* is a subject of some disagreement. Most physicians believe that antithyroid therapy is preferable to surgery, which should not be performed in any event during the first and third trimesters. Antithyroid agents carry less risk to the patient and the pregnancy. Further, since they traverse the placental barrier, they have the theoretical advantage of preventing fetal and neonatal hyperthyroidism when maternal titers of thyroid-stimulating IgG are high. As a clue to the risk of fetal hyperthyroidism, assays of such stimulators should be conducted in pregnant women with a history of Graves' disease, whether treated or not. On the other hand, the major disadvantage of antithyroid therapy is the possibility of inducing hypothyroidism in the fetus. T_4 and T_3 traverse the human placenta from mother to fetus only slowly, if at all, and simultaneous administration of thyroid hormone and antithyroid drugs to the mother will not protect the fetus from developing hypothyroidism. Hence, the cardinal rule in using the antithyroid agents in pregnancy is that the dosage should be the smallest necessary to control hyperthyroidism in the mother. From the laboratory standpoint, the physician should aim to keep the serum FT_4 concentration or the FT_4I within the normal limits, remembering that pregnancy is normally associated with some elevation of the serum total T_4, owing to an increase in serum TBG concentration. Since pregnancy appears to attenuate the severity of hyperthyroidism, control can often be achieved with maintenance doses of 200 mg propylthiouracil daily or less. At this dose level, fetal goiter or hypothyroidism has not been a problem. Patients who require doses of 300 mg daily or more during the first trimester should probably be treated by subtotal thyroidectomy during the middle trimester. The authors believe that patients carried through pregnancy on antithyroid agents should not be given propranolol as adjunctive treatment, in view of reports that the agent may cause fetal growth retardation and neonatal respiratory depression. Radioiodine should never be administered to a pregnant woman, and all women of childbearing age who are about to receive ^{131}I should have a pregnancy test performed first.

Ophthalmopathy, dermopathy When severe and progressive, ophthalmopathy is the most difficult component of Graves' disease to treat satisfactorily. Fortunately, in most patients the disorder runs a benign course that is largely independent of the course of the hyperthyroidism. In most instances, the activity of even moderately severe disease declines and disappears with time, although some exophthalmos and ophthalmoplegia may persist. In mild disease, considerable benefit may be obtained from simple measures, such as elevating the head at night, administering diuretics to reduce edema, and providing tinted glasses for protection from sun, wind, and foreign bodies. A 1% solution of methylcellulose or plastic shields may prevent corneal drying in patients unable to oppose the lids during sleep. In more severe cases, as evidenced by progressive exophthalmos, chemosis, ophthalmoplegia, or loss of vision, large doses of prednisone (120 to 140 mg daily) should be administered, since this is usually effective in reducing the edematous and infiltrative components. With improvement, the dosage is reduced to the lowest effective level, to minimize the effects of glucocorticoid excess. Orbital radiation may be helpful in some patients with acute, severe infiltrative manifestations. In cases that progress despite these measures, orbital decompression, i.e., removal of part of the bony orbit, is required to relieve intraorbital pressure. The management must always be conducted in concert with an ophthalmologist.

In general, treatment of associated hyperthyroidism should be carried out much as would be the case were ophthalmopathy not present, since the mode of treatment of the hyperthyroidism does not influence the course of the ocular disease. The suggestion that total thyroid ablation by surgery and large doses of ^{131}I is beneficial to the ophthalmic disease has not been borne out. It is agreed, however, that hypothyroidism be avoided.

Severe dermopathy can be alleviated by the topical application of glucocorticoids.

TOXIC MULTINODULAR GOITER

Toxic multinodular goiter is an occasional consequence of long-standing simple goiter, although the proportion of cases in which this complication arises is uncertain. In areas of nonendemicity, the etiology of nontoxic multinodular goiter is usually indeterminate. Hence, it is unclear whether a specific etiologic factor underlies those cases of nontoxic multinodular goiter that progress to thyrotoxic phase. Common to many nontoxic multinodular goiters, even in areas of iodine sufficiency, is a decrease in the iodine content of thyroglobulin, suggesting either a conditioned deficiency of iodine or an impairment of its normal incorporation into iodinated amino acids. There is no pathologic feature to distinguish the nontoxic from the toxic multinodular goiter. However, the transition from nontoxic to toxic nodular goiter involves the development of functional autonomy, i.e., independence from TSH stimulation in one or more areas of the gland. Scattered foci of functional autonomy are present, even early in the disease process. These increase in size and number as time passes so that even among seemingly euthyroid patients with nontoxic nodular goiter, approximately a fourth display, as evidence of functional autonomy, subnormal or absent responses to TRH administration. As judged from scintillation scanning, functional patterns may be of two types. In the first and more common, iodine accumulation occurs diffusely but in patchy foci throughout the gland. The second, less common, pattern is that of iodine accumulation in one or more discrete nodules within the gland, the remainder appearing to be essentially nonfunctional. Histologic and autoradiographic

studies reveal marked heterogeneity of structure and function, the two being poorly correlated. In both endemic and sporadic nontoxic multinodular goiter, administration of iodides may lead to the development of thyrotoxicosis (jod-Basedow), a complication that is consonant with the functional autonomy that characterizes this disorder.

Because it arises in long-standing simple goiter, toxic multinodular goiter is a disease of the aging or elderly. For this reason and because of the nature of the underlying disease, the clinical presentation differs from that in Graves' disease. Ophthalmopathy is rare and would signal the emergence of Graves' disease superimposed on simple goiter. Some patients have typical thyrotoxicosis. Often, however, the degree of thyrotoxicosis is less severe than that in Graves' disease, although its physiologic impact upon specific organ systems may be great. Notable among these is the cardiovascular system, in which arrhythmias or congestive failure may be precipitated or accentuated by thyrotoxicosis that may be manifested only by subtle findings in other areas (apathetic hyperthyroidism). Weakness and wasting may predominate, frequently with loss of appetite rather than hyperphagia, suggesting the presence of a carcinoma.

In some patients, a definitive diagnosis of toxic nodular goiter is difficult to establish. On the one hand, enlargement or nodularity of the gland may escape detection because the patient has a short neck or is kyphotic or because the thyroid is substernal. When this is the case and when the clinical findings suggest thyrotoxicosis, RAIU and scintiscan may prove illuminating. On the other hand, even when a nodular goiter is palpable, the presence of mild but clinically significant thyrotoxicosis may be difficult to confirm, since values of the serum total T_4 and T_3, FT_4, and FT_4I, as well as the serum T_3, are often only near or slightly above the upper limit of the normal range. For example, a value for the serum T_3 that would be normal for a young adult may represent an increase in the elderly patient, since serum T_3 usually declines with age. Despite their value in situations such as this, thyroid suppression tests should not be undertaken in the elderly patient because of the hazard of adverse cardiovascular responses. Unfortunately, although a normal response to TRH would exclude a diagnosis of thyrotoxicosis in a patient with a nodular goiter, subnormal responses do not establish the diagnosis. Responses to TRH decline in the elderly, especially in men, and patients with nodular goiter who otherwise seem euthyroid may respond subnormally to TRH as a reflection of at least partial functional autonomy of the thyroid gland. An undetectable basal TSH and absent response to TRH by an ultrasensitive assay imply thyrotoxicosis (Fig. 316-3). When laboratory findings do not permit a clear diagnosis of thyrotoxicosis but suggestive clinical findings are present, a therapeutic trial of antithyroid drugs is indicated.

Radioactive iodine is the treatment of choice for toxic multinodular goiter. Large doses [740 to 1110 MBq (20 to 30 mCi)] are usually required, owing to the generally lower RAIU and to the variable degree of function throughout the gland. Moreover, the physiologic instability of the elderly patient makes definitive treatment desirable. For the same reason, it is usually wise to initiate therapy with antithyroid agents, withholding radioiodine until a euthyroid state is achieved, thereby forestalling an exacerbation of thyrotoxicosis should radiation thyroiditis occur. Unless contraindicated, propranolol is often useful in controlling manifestations of thyrotoxicosis both before and after radioiodine therapy, while its therapeutic effect is awaited. Hypothyroidism is an uncommon consequence of radioiodine treatment of toxic multinodular goiter, owing to the variable activity of differing portions of the gland, which permits previously quiescent areas to replace functionally those that have been destroyed by [131]I.

UNUSUAL VARIETIES OF THYROTOXICOSIS

In addition to Graves' disease and toxic multinodular goiter, thyrotoxicosis is seen in other disorders, including follicular adenoma of the thyroid and various forms of thyroiditis, which are discussed in later sections. This section will consider still other infrequent causes of thyrotoxicosis and unusual ways in which thyrotoxicosis may present from the laboratory standpoint.

UNUSUAL CAUSES OF THYROTOXICOSIS Rarely, hyperthyroidism and thyrotoxicosis are the result of sustained hypersecretion of TSH from either a *TSH-secreting pituitary adenoma* or a *selective resistance of the TSH-secretory mechanism* to feedback inhibition by thyroid hormones. The resistance syndrome may be a variant of a disorder in which both the pituitary and peripheral tissues are relatively resistant to thyroid hormones. TSH-secreting pituitary adenomas can be distinguished, in many cases, by radiologic evidence of pituitary tumor, by the fact that the concentration of free alpha subunits of TSH in serum is elevated, and by the fact that the response of the serum TSH to TRH is negligible. In the variant caused by pituitary resistance, subunit concentrations are not grossly elevated, and the TSH response to TRH is usually normal.

Patients with *trophoblastic tumor*, either choriocarcinoma or hydatidiform mole, frequently display elevations, sometimes marked, of serum total and free T_4 and T_3 concentrations. Clinical evidence of thyrotoxicosis may be lacking. Thyroid hyperfunction is caused by a circulating thyroid stimulator of trophoblastic origin, which is probably a variant of human chorionic gonadotropin (hCG), and abnormal thyroid function tests remit promptly after removal of the tumor.

Thyrotoxicosis factitia is a form of thyrotoxicosis without hyperthyroidism and results from purposeful or inadvertent ingestion of supraphysiologic quantities of thyroid hormone. The syndrome is usually a form of malingering and occurs most commonly in women with an underlying psychiatric disorder, usually paramedical personnel, or in patients who have taken thyroid hormones in the past or who have relatives that take thyroid hormones. In such patients, endogenous thyroid function is suppressed, as evidenced by subnormal values of the RAIU and serum thyroglobulin concentration. Both serum T_4 and T_3 concentrations are increased if the patient is taking a preparation that contains T_4, whereas the serum T_3 concentration is elevated and the serum T_4 depressed in patients taking T_3 alone. Factitious hyperthyroidism has also been described in people who ingest large quantities of ground meats contaminated with thyroid tissue.

Very rarely, thyrotoxicosis with a low RAIU is the result of excess hormone secretion by *ectopic thyroid tissue*, either widespread functioning metastases of thyroid carcinoma or struma ovarii.

The *jod-Basedow phenomenon* refers to the induction of thyrotoxicosis in a previously euthyroid patient as a result of exposure to increased quantities of iodine. It typically occurs in areas of endemic iodine deficiency when measures to increase iodine intake or body iodine stores are implemented. The presumption is that the supplemental iodine permits functionally autonomous thyroid tissue to produce and secrete excessive hormone. A similar phenomenon can occur in patients with nontoxic multinodular goiter who have received large doses of iodide. Since such patients tend to be elderly with the danger of serious cardiovascular manifestations should thyrotoxicosis ensue, large doses of iodine should not be given to those with multinodular goiter. Similarly, in such patients, pharmaceuticals containing iodine, most often x-ray contrast media, should be used only when indicated and with consideration of the possible hazard of inducing the jod-Basedow phenomenon. When a contrast study is indicated under these conditions, it may be judicious to administer large doses of propylthiouracil (450 to 600 mg/d) prior to and for a week after the procedure. Some patients may develop hyperthyroidism following exposure to large quantities of iodine despite the fact that after iodine is withdrawn, they recover, their thyroid function appears to be entirely normal, and evidence of functional autonomy is lacking.

UNUSUAL PRESENTATIONS OF THYROTOXICOSIS T₃ toxicosis Thyrotoxicosis in which serum T_4 is normal or low in the absence of a deficiency of TBG, while the serum T_3 is increased, is termed T_3 toxicosis. Although the production rate of T_3 is dispropor-

tionately increased relative to that of T_4 in patients with hyperthyroidism, in some this discrepancy is exaggerated. This may occur in association with Graves' disease, multinodular goiter, or hyperfunctioning adenoma. The diagnosis should be suspected in a patient with clinical manifestations of thyrotoxicosis in whom the serum T_4 and FT_4 are normal or low and the RAIU is normal or increased. This, together with the frequently palpable goiter, serves to differentiate this disorder from liothyronine-induced thyrotoxicosis factitia. In contrast to patients with nonthyroidal disorders that mimic thyrotoxicosis, patients with this disorder, as would be expected, demonstrate both nonsuppressibility of thyroid function in response to exogenous T_3 and blunted or absent responses to TRH. In many patients, thyrotoxicosis with increased serum T_3 and normal serum T_4 precedes emergence of typical increases in both, either during an initial episode of hyperthyroidism or more commonly during recurrence after previous treatment. In some patients in whom symptoms of thyrotoxicosis fail to regress completely during antithyroid therapy despite return of the serum T_4 concentration to normal, the serum T_3 concentration is persistently elevated. Such patients are prone to experience a recurrence of thyrotoxicosis when antithyroid therapy is withdrawn.

T₄ toxicosis In most patients with hyperthyroidism, the serum T_3 is increased to a relatively greater extent than is the serum T_4. This reflects the fact that in hyperthyroidism T_3 generated from T_4 peripherally is supplemented by release of substantial quantities of T_3 from the thyroid. However, thyrotoxicosis may sometimes be associated with a clear elevation of serum T_4 and a seemingly normal serum T_3 concentration. This syndrome of *T_4 toxicosis* occurs most commonly in patients who are elderly, ill, or both, and is, therefore, usually seen in a hospital setting. Presumably, the combination of high serum T_4 and normal serum T_3 concentration reflects inhibition of peripheral T_3 generation from T_4, with persistence of T_3 secretion along with T_4 from the thyroid.

MAJOR COMPLICATIONS OF THYROTOXICOSIS

CARDIAC DISEASE Thyrotoxicosis imposes a variety of burdens upon the heart. Hypermetabolism of the peripheral tissues increases both the metabolic and nonmetabolic (heat-loss) circulatory load, while direct effects of thyroid hormone on the myocardium increase the force, velocity, and rate of ventricular contraction. As a result, cardiac work and cardiac output are increased. Moreover, atrial irritability is enhanced, leading to arrhythmias, most importantly atrial fibrillation. In the patient with a normal heart, these burdens are usually tolerated. In the patient with underlying heart disease, however, cardiac insufficiency may be precipitated or aggravated. As would be expected, this complication is more common in the elderly patient and is common in the patient with toxic multinodular goiter, sometimes as the most prominent manifestation of the thyrotoxic state. In patients with cardiac insufficiency, clues to the presence of thyrotoxicosis include atrial fibrillation, relatively rapid circulation time, increased cardiac output (high-output failure), and resistance to the usual therapeutic doses of digitalis.

Treatment is directed at rapid alleviation of thyrotoxicosis and restoration of cardiac compensation. The former objective is best met by initiation of treatment with large doses of an antithyroid agent, followed by iodine if the clinical situation is urgent. In less severe cases, radioiodine treatment is preceded by antithyroid drug treatment alone. Management of the cardiac decompensation is carried out in the usual manner, employing larger than usual doses of digitalis but with care to avoid digitalis intoxication as thyrotoxicosis is alleviated. Adrenergic antagonists should not be employed in the presence of cardiac failure, unless failure is the consequence primarily of disturbance of cardiac rate or rhythm.

THYROTOXIC CRISIS Thyrotoxic crisis or storm causes a fulminating increase in the signs and symptoms of thyrotoxicosis. In the past, this disturbance was most often observed postoperatively in patients poorly prepared for surgery. However, with the preoperative use of antithyroid drugs and iodide and with appropriate measures directed to control of metabolic factors, weight, and nutritional status, postoperative thyrotoxic crisis should not occur. At present, so-called medical storm is more common and occurs in untreated or inadequately treated patients. It is precipitated by surgical emergency or complicating illness, usually sepsis. The syndrome is characterized by extreme irritability, delirium or coma, fever to 41°C or more, tachycardia, restlessness, hypotension, vomiting, and diarrhea. Rarely, the picture may be more subtle, with apathy, prostration, and coma, but with only slight elevation of temperature. Such postoperative complications as sepsis, septicemia, hemorrhage, and transfusion or drug reactions may mimic thyrotoxic crisis. The physiologic factor(s) that initiates thyrotoxic crisis is unknown. It does not appear to be an acute increase in the severity of thyroid hyperfunction. Rather, it may represent a shift from protein-bound to free hormone, secondary to circulating inhibitors to binding in systemic illness.

Treatment consists in providing general supportive therapy while undertaking measures for alleviating thyrotoxicosis as rapidly as possible. Supportive therapy includes treatment of dehydration and the intravenous administration of glucose and saline, vitamin B complex, and glucocorticoids. The latter are indicated because of the increased glucocorticoid requirements in thyrotoxicosis and because adrenal reserve may be reduced in this disorder. Patients should be placed in a cooled, humidified oxygen tent, and, if hyperpyrexia is present, a cooling blanket should be used. Digitalization is required to control ventricular rate in those with atrial fibrillation. If shock exists, intravenous pressor agents should be employed. Therapy of the hyperthyroidism consists of blockade of hormone synthesis by the immediate and continued administration of large doses of an antithyroid agent (e.g., 100 mg propylthiouracil every 2 h). If the patient is unable to swallow the medication, the tablets should be triturated and given by nasogastric tube, as parenteral preparations are unavailable. Following initiation of antithyroid therapy, inhibition of hormone release is sought through the administration of large doses of iodine intravenously or by mouth. The iodinated x-ray contrast agent sodium ipodate can be administered instead of iodine and has the added action of also inhibiting the peripheral conversion of T_4 to T_3. Doses of 1 g daily are effective. Adrenergic antagonists are an important, and perhaps critical, part of the therapeutic regimen, in the absence of cardiac failure. The beta-adrenergic blocking agent propranolol can be administered in doses of 40 to 80 mg every 6 h. If medications cannot be taken orally, 2 mg of propranolol may be given intravenously, with careful electrocardiographic monitoring. Large doses of dexamethasone (e.g., 2 mg every 6 h) should also be administered, since they inhibit hormone release, impair the peripheral generation of T_3 from T_4, and provide adrenal support. Indeed, with the combined use of propylthiouracil, iodine, and dexamethasone, the serum T_3 concentration generally returns to normal within 24 to 48 h. Antithyroid therapy, iodine, and dexamethasone must be continued until a normal metabolic state is approached, at which time iodine is progressively withdrawn and plans are made for definitive treatment.

NEOPLASMS

THYROID ADENOMAS True adenomas, as contrasted with localized adenomatous areas, are encapsulated and compress contiguous tissue. Adenomas vary in size and histologic characteristics and are classified into three major types: papillary, follicular, and Hürthle cell. The follicular adenomas can be subdivided according to the size of the follicles into colloid or macrofollicular, fetal or microfollicular, and embryonal varieties. There is variation in physiologic differentiation, as judged by the ability to concentrate radioiodine. The more highly differentiated adenomas (follicular) are the most common and are the most likely to mimic the function of normal thyroid tissue. Though their function may be responsive to TSH stimulation, usually it differs from that of normal thyroid tissue in being autonomous,

i.e., the basal activity is independent of TSH stimulation. Adenomas of this type are usually unifocal, presenting as a single nodule. Often the patient reports that the nodule has grown slowly over many years. Initially, its function is insufficient to disturb hormonal equilibrium though its capacity to accumulate radioiodine is evident in scintiscans as an area of increased density within the still-functioning extranodular tissue ("*warm*" *nodule*). At this stage, demonstration of the inherent autonomy of the nodule's function requires scintiscanning while the patient is receiving suppressive doses of exogenous thyroid hormone (suppression scan). With time the nodule grows larger, its function increasing until it is sufficient to suppress TSH secretion. Consequently, the remainder of the gland undergoes atrophy and loss of function, and the scintiscan reveals radioiodine accumulation only in the region of the nodule ("*hot*" *nodule*). At this time, the patient may or may not be overtly thyrotoxic, but frank thyrotoxicosis usually supervenes eventually (*toxic adenoma*), particularly after iodine exposure. Relative to its overall rate of occurrence, hyperfunctioning adenoma is a frequent cause of T_3 toxicosis. Hyperfunctioning adenomas are amenable to ablation by surgery or ^{131}I. Large doses of the latter are usually required to bring about prompt cure. Before such treatment it is desirable to administer TSH and demonstrate by scintiscan the latent functional capacity of the extranodular tissue. Although it has been thought that radiation damage would be confined solely to the hyperfunctioning nodule being treated with ^{131}I, the remaining tissue being spared, this may not always be the case, since some patients with hyperfunctioning adenoma become euthyroid after treatment with ^{131}I only to become hypothyroid years later.

Hyperfunctioning nodules are rarely the seat of carcinoma. However, hyperfunctioning adenomas not infrequently undergo hemorrhagic necrosis. The resulting pain and nodularity may suggest subacute thyroiditis. Subsequently, there is loss of function and the appearance of a "*cold*" *nodule* on scintiscanning, since the remainder of the thyroid will have resumed function. When this happens, the nodule is likely to be mistaken for a carcinoma. Indeed, hypofunctioning, hemorrhagic adenomas and thyroid cysts account for the majority of cold nodules initially suspected of being carcinomas.

THYROID CARCINOMAS Thyroid carcinoma may be classified into two varieties, depending upon whether the lesion arises in thyroid follicular epithelium or from the parafollicular or C cells. The latter disorder, medullary thyroid carcinoma, has distinctive physiologic and clinical characteristics and is discussed separately (see Chap. 325). The thyroid may also be the site of lymphoproliferative disease or of carcinoma metastatic from a diagnosed or undiagnosed primary tumor elsewhere.

Carcinomas of follicular epithelium The three general histologic types differ in their clinical course. The least common, *anaplastic carcinoma,* is histologically undifferentiated, usually afflicts the elderly, and is highly malignant. The lesion is rapidly fatal, owing to extensive local invasion which is refractory to radiation. The second type of tumor, *follicular carcinoma,* histologically mimics normal thyroid tissue. This lesion usually undergoes early hematogenous spread, and the patient may present with a distant metastasis, usually in lung or bone. Follicular carcinoma or follicular elements in papillary carcinoma are responsible for those instances in which thyroid carcinoma, in situ or in metastases, accumulates significant quantities of ^{131}I. The third and most common type of tumor, *papillary carcinoma,* has a bimodal frequency, peaks occurring in the second or third decades and again in later life. This lesion is slowly growing and typically spreads to the regional lymph nodes, where it may remain indolent for many years. Acceleration of the disease may take place at any time. Follicular elements are usually present in both the primary lesion and its metastases.

DIAGNOSIS AND MANAGEMENT The diagnosis and management of thyroid carcinoma are interwoven with the management of the nodular goiter. In the past, this subject has evoked a wide disparity of views among authorities, stemming from seemingly contradictory data. On the one hand, surgically excised specimens of thyroid nodules, particularly solitary nodules, revealed a high frequency of carcinoma (as much as 20 percent in some series). On the other hand, despite the frequency of nodular goiter in the general population (approximately 4 percent), the frequency of thyroid carcinoma, either newly diagnosed or as a cause of death, is low. These respective data led either to vigorous or to conservative approaches to the management of nodular goiter. This discordance can be explained by the ability of the physician to select for surgery those patients who are at high risk of harboring thyroid carcinoma, with consequent weighting of statistics from surgical series. This capability has increased, the as yet unrealized aim being to operate on only those patients whose thyroids harbor carcinoma and to avoid surgery in patients whose thyroids do not.

Several features suggest the presence of carcinoma. Recent growth of a thyroid nodule or mass, especially if rapid and unaccompanied by tenderness and hoarseness, is a source of suspicion. Of particular importance is a history of x-ray to the head or neck or upper mediastinum in infancy or childhood, since this is associated with a high incidence of thyroid disease, including carcinoma, later in life. Nodular disease develops in approximately 20 percent of patients so exposed and may not be apparent until 30 years or more after the radiation exposure. Among patients in this group who have palpable nodules, approximately a third have thyroid carcinoma at surgery, often multicentric and sometimes metastatic.

Skillful palpation of the thyroid provides important information. A nodule in an otherwise normal gland (solitary nodule) creates more suspicion of thyroid tumor than does one nodule among many, since the latter is more likely to be part of a diffuse process, such as simple goiter. In addition, carcinomas are usually firm or hard in consistency and nontender. Fixation to surrounding structures and lymphadenopathy are late features. Since purely cystic lesions, especially those that are less than a few centimeters in diameter, are less likely to reflect malignancy than solid lesions, transillumination is sometimes helpful, and ultrasonograms (see below) are particularly so. Age and sex of the patient also influence the clinical decision. Benign nodular lesions are more common in women than in men, malignant nodular lesions less so. Hence, nodular lesions in men create more suspicion of carcinoma than in women.

Laboratory tests are of little assistance in differentiating between malignant and nonmalignant thyroid nodules. Overall thyroid function is usually normal. Except in patients with medullary thyroid carcinoma, in whom serum calcitonin concentrations may be elevated, tumor markers are of little value. Elevations of serum thyroglobulin are present in many patients with differentiated thyroid carcinoma but are not useful in the initial diagnosis, since they may be elevated in patients with benign adenoma, simple goiter, or Graves' disease. Soft-tissue x-rays of the neck may be of assistance, since finely stippled calcification within the thyroid suggests the presence of psammoma bodies within a papillary carcinoma and more dense calcifications may signify medullary carcinoma.

Fine-needle aspiration for cytology is the initial procedure of choice in the evaluation of most patients (Fig. 316-4). The technique is simple to learn, free of complications, and applicable to most nodules. Optimal application of that technique rests upon the availability of experienced histopathologic interpretation of the specimen obtained. When such is available, aspiration biopsy provides a reliable means of differentiating between benign and malignant nodules in all except highly cellular lesions or follicular lesions, where evidence of vascular invasion may be required to differentiate benign from malignant forms. Despite the occasional occurrence of false-positives and -negatives, the procedure can reduce the number of operations performed for nodules that prove to be benign. Further, a diagnosis of carcinoma permits planning of the surgery to be undertaken preoperatively and is often useful in providing an impetus to surgery when the patient or physician is uncertain if surgery should be performed.

While fine-needle aspiration for cytology is the keystone in the approach to the management of the patient with nodular goiter, scintillation scanning may be also useful. Although only approximately 20 percent of nonfunctioning thyroid nodules prove to be malignant, demonstration that a nodule is cold adds substantial weight to the other factors suggesting carcinoma. Nodules that are hyperfunctioning are rarely malignant. Ultrasonograms of the thyroid have value in demonstrating whether nodules are cystic, solid, or a mixture of the two. Cystic nodules can be aspirated, a procedure that is often curative, and their contents should be subjected to cytopathologic examination. Solid or mixed lesions are consistent with tumor but may be either benign or malignant.

When the cytologic results are equivocal, the physician must decide whether to continue to observe the patient; to administer suppressive doses of thyroid hormone in the hope that the suspect nodule will shrink or disappear—a hope that in the authors' experience is usually unrealized; or to proceed to excisional biopsy and thyroidectomy. There are some patients in whom the authors choose the latter course. In general, these include patients with a history of radiation to the thyroid and one or more clearly palpable nodules, as well as young men and women with solitary cold nodules, particularly if hard, nontender, and changing rapidly in size. In the remainder,

FIGURE 316-4

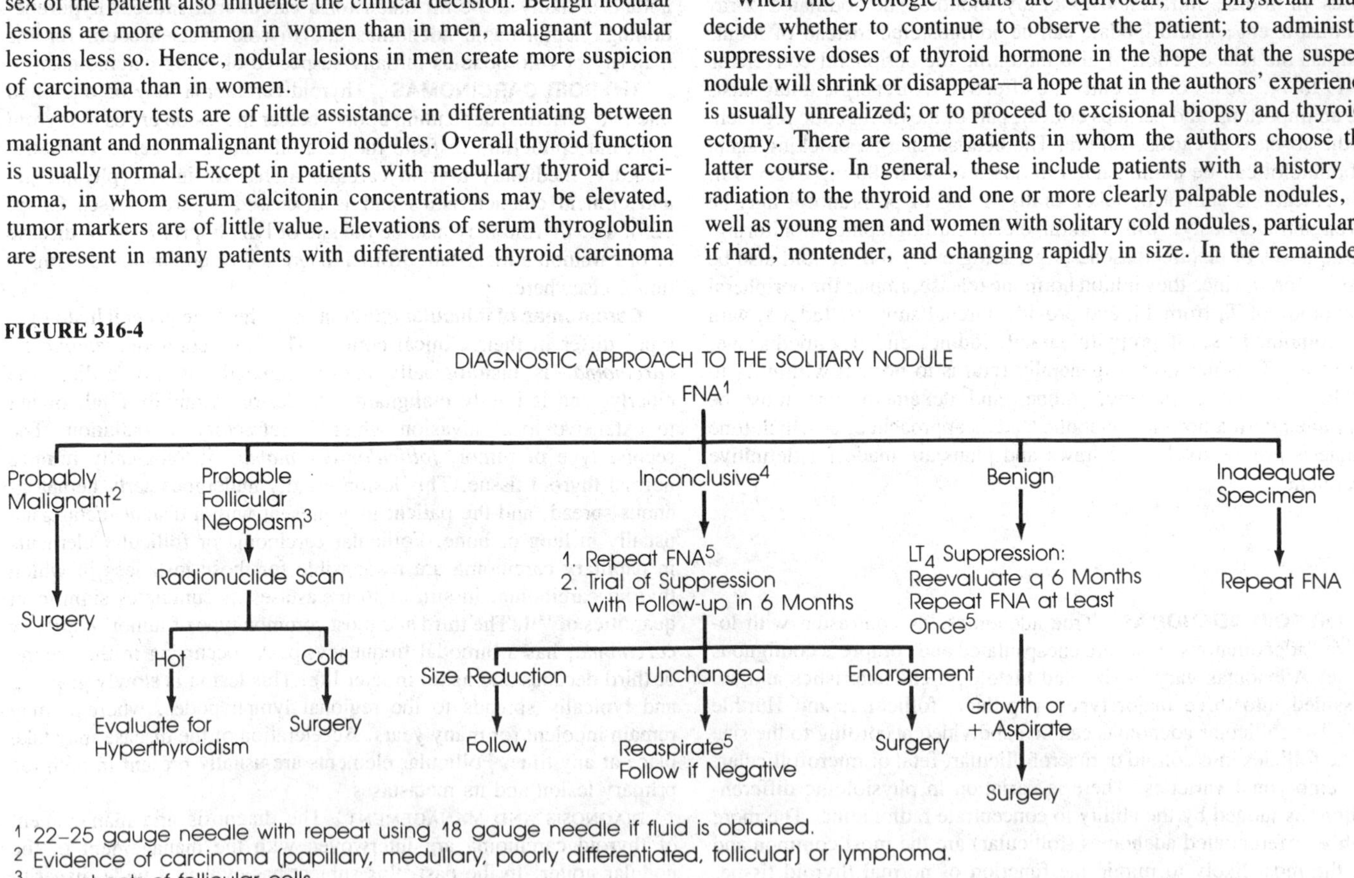

DIAGNOSTIC APPROACH TO THE SOLITARY NODULE

FNA[1]

| Probably Malignant[2] | Probable Follicular Neoplasm[3] | Inconclusive[4] | Benign | Inadequate Specimen |

Probably Malignant[2] → Surgery

Probable Follicular Neoplasm[3] → Radionuclide Scan → Hot → Evaluate for Hyperthyroidism; Cold → Surgery

Inconclusive[4] →
1. Repeat FNA[5]
2. Trial of Suppression with Follow-up in 6 Months
→ Size Reduction → Follow; Unchanged → Reaspirate[5] Follow if Negative; Enlargement → Surgery

Benign → LT₄ Suppression: Reevaluate q 6 Months Repeat FNA at Least Once[5] → Growth or + Aspirate → Surgery

Inadequate Specimen → Repeat FNA

[1] 22–25 gauge needle with repeat using 18 gauge needle if fluid is obtained.
[2] Evidence of carcinoma (papillary, medullary, poorly differentiated, follicular) or lymphoma.
[3] e.g., sheets of follicular cells.
[4] e.g., small groups of uniform follicular cells with little colloid.
[5] Changes in cytologic findings redirect clinician to the appropriate arm of the algorithm.

the authors recommend thyroid hormone therapy with repeat aspiration cytology in 3 to 6 months.

Regardless of the operative procedure planned, surgery for thyroid carcinoma should be performed by a surgeon experienced in the procedure. Should surgery be delayed, suppressive therapy with levothyroxine is often recommended preoperatively to facilitate the operative procedure and perhaps to decrease the likelihood of tumor dissemination. In patients in whom a definitive preoperative diagnosis, such as by biopsy, has not been made, the suspected lesion is removed en bloc with a wide margin of surrounding tissue and is examined by frozen section. Opinions vary as to the type of procedure that is preferable when carcinoma is found. For lesions of 2 cm or less that are not multicentric and that have not metastasized, some recommend ipsilateral lobectomy, isthmectomy, and possibly contralateral partial lobectomy. Despite its higher rate of morbidity, the authors prefer that a near-total thyroidectomy be performed, especially for lesions >2 cm, in view of the frequency of seeding of tumor throughout the gland by transglandular lymphatic spread and of evidence that both recurrence rates and subsequent mortality are lower after the more extensive operation. Regional lymph nodes should be explored and removed if there is evidence of involvement, but radical neck dissection is not justified. If permanent sections reveal carcinoma when frozen sections had failed to do so and the initial procedure was limited, secondary surgery should be undertaken to remove residual thyroid tissue.

Approximately 3 weeks after surgery, liothyronine (50 to 75 μg daily) is substituted for levothyroxine, since it permits a more rapid return of TSH secretion when withdrawn some 3 weeks later. After an additional 2 or 3 weeks, when the serum TSH concentration has risen to the range of 50 mU/L, a large scanning dose of ^{131}I [185 to 370 MBq (5 to 10 mCi)] is administered and whole-body scans are obtained at 72 h. If residual thyroid tissue is found, as is usually the case, a thyroid ablating dose of 1850 MBq (50 mCi) of ^{131}I is administered, and if functioning metastases are present, the dose is doubled. Suppressive therapy with levothyroxine is reinstituted 24 to 48 h later. Approximately 1 week after administration of the second dose of ^{131}I, whole-body scans are repeated, as the larger dose of radioiodine may permit demonstration of functioning metastases not seen after the smaller initial dose. When this proves to be the case, some clinics withdraw suppressive therapy, administer an additional 3700 MBq (100 mCi) of ^{131}I, and then reinstitute suppressive therapy with levothyroxine.

Patients are reexamined approximately 6 months after the initial operation and at least every 6 months for several years thereafter. At these examinations, the neck is palpated for evidence of recurrence of metastases, which often can be treated with selective surgical removal. Blood is drawn for a serum thyroglobulin measurement, since elevated values in patients receiving suppressive therapy signal the presence of metastatic disease. At the initial 6-month examination, patients in whom metastases had previously been found are prepared for a whole-body scan as described above. Those in whom no metastases had been demonstrated by earlier scans are not rescanned unless the serum thyroglobulin is elevated but are rescanned approximately 1 year after the initial surgery. Patients in whom whole-body scans are positive are reentered into the therapeutic algorithm, as described above. Those in whom scans are negative continue to be reexamined and have measurements of serum thyroglobulin concentrations at regular intervals. If both serum thyroglobulin concentrations and scans are unrevealing, patients are scanned for the last time after approximately 3 years, unless serum thyroglobulin concentrations rise. In some patients, serum thyroglobulin may be elevated despite the absence of demonstrable functioning metastases. Such patients obviously cannot be treated with ^{131}I but should be studied with x-rays and bone scans to ascertain the site of the thyroglobulin-secreting metastases.

A program of this nature, involving near-total thyroidectomy, long-term suppressive therapy, and treatment of functioning metastases with radioiodine reduces the recurrence rate and prolongs survival in patients with papillary carcinoma of the thyroid. Follicular carcinoma should be treated with even greater vigor, since the results are generally less favorable. Because follicular carcinoma metastasizes to lung and bone, appropriate follow-up x-rays in addition to serum thyroglobulin are warranted. Treatment of anaplastic carcinoma is largely palliative; most patients die within 6 months of diagnosis.

THYROIDITIS

Thyroiditis embraces disorders of differing etiology. Two are exceedingly uncommon, *pyogenic thyroiditis* and *chronic fibrosing (Riedel's) thyroiditis*. Pyogenic thyroiditis is usually anteceded by a pyogenic infection elsewhere and is characterized by tenderness and swelling of the thyroid, redness and warmth of the overlying skin, and constitutional signs of infection. Treatment consists of antibiotic therapy and incisional drainage if a fluctuant area within the thyroid should occur. Riedel's thyroiditis is a disorder in which intense fibrosis of the thyroid and surrounding structures, leading to induration of the tissues of the neck, may be associated with mediastinal and retroperitoneal fibrosis. The principal importance of this disorder is that it requires differentiation from thyroid neoplasia. The other forms of thyroiditis, comprising subacute thyroiditis, chronic thyroiditis with transient thyrotoxicosis (CT/TT), and Hashimoto's thyroiditis, are more common. They are notable for their different clinical courses and for the fact that each can be associated, at one time or another, with a euthyroid, thyrotoxic, or hypothyroid state.

SUBACUTE THYROIDITIS This disorder, also termed *granulomatous, giant cell,* or *de Quervain's thyroiditis*, is viral in origin. Symptoms of thyroiditis usually follow those of an upper respiratory infection and include pronounced asthenia, malaise, and symptoms referable to stretching of the thyroid capsule, principally pain over the thyroid or pain referred to the lower jaw, ear, or occiput. Referred pain may predominate. These symptoms may smolder for weeks before the diagnosis is suspected. Less commonly, the onset is acute, with severe pain over the thyroid, accompanied by fever and occasionally symptoms of thyrotoxicosis. Physical findings include exquisite tenderness and nodularity over the thyroid, which may be unilateral but which usually involves other areas of the gland. Although local or referred pain is the commonest symptom, occasional patients have other features typical of the disease but have no pain.

Two laboratory findings are characteristic: a high erythrocyte sedimentation rate (ESR) and a depressed RAIU. Values for the remaining tests depend upon the stage of the disease in which they are obtained. Early, many patients are mildly thyrotoxic owing to leakage of hormone from the gland. The serum T_4 and T_3 are high. Later, as glandular hormone is depleted, the patient may pass through a hypothyroid phase, in which serum T_4 and T_3 are low and TSH increased. Diagnosis of the thyrotoxic phase is especially troublesome in the painless variant since the patient may be thought to have Graves' disease or toxic nodular goiter and therapy inappropriate for subacute thyroiditis may be instituted. Demonstration of a low RAIU usually serves to differentiate subacute thyroiditis from these other causes of hyperthyroidism. Differentiation of painless subacute thyroiditis from chronic thyroiditis with transient thyrotoxicosis is discussed below.

The disorder may smolder for months but eventually subsides with a return of normal thyroid function. In mild cases, aspirin suffices to control the symptoms. In more severe cases, glucocorticoid (prednisone, 20 to 40 mg daily) is generally effective. Propranolol can be used to control associated thyrotoxicosis. When the RAIU and serum T_4 return to normal, therapy can be withdrawn without recurrence of symptoms.

CHRONIC THYROIDITIS WITH TRANSIENT THYROTOXICOSIS This term denotes a disorder in which a self-limited episode of thyrotoxicosis is associated with a histologic picture of chronic lymphocytic thyroiditis that differs from that of Hashimoto's disease. This syndrome has been variously designated as painless thyroiditis, silent thyroiditis, hyperthyroiditis, chronic thyroiditis with spontaneously resolving hyperthyroidism, or, as the author prefers, chronic thyroiditis with transient thyrotoxicosis (CT/TT). Designations that imply the existence of hyperthyroidism are inappropriate, since ongoing production of thyroid hormone is negligible and the RAIU is decreased.

The syndrome occurs in patients of any age, and although it occurs mainly in women the female/male ratio is not as high as in Graves' disease. Manifestations of thyrotoxicosis are usually mild but may be severe. The thyroid is nontender, firm, symmetrical, and enlarged only slightly or moderately. Laboratory features include elevations of the serum T_4 and T_3 concentrations consonant with the thyrotoxicosis and a markedly depressed RAIU. The ESR is normal or only slightly elevated, rarely exceeding 50 mm/h, and antithyroid antibodies, when present, are present in low titer.

The etiology, pathogenesis, and pathophysiology of this disorder are unclear. Viral antibody titers show no characteristic patterns. It is presumed that thyrotoxicosis results from leakage of hormone from the gland, as in subacute thyroiditis. Low values for the RAIU, in turn, reflect suppression of TSH secretion, since urinary iodine excretion is not greatly elevated. Some degree of thyroid malfunction is indicated by failure of the RAIU to respond briskly to exogenous TSH stimulation.

Thyrotoxicosis in CT/TT usually abates within 2 to 5 months. Many patients have recurrent episodes of thyrotoxicosis of similar nature, sometimes following pregnancy (postpartum thyroiditis). The thyrotoxic phase may be followed in several months by a phase of self-limited hypothyroidism. The latter, which has been noted particularly in the postpartum period, may be the only component of the disease that is diagnosed because the thyrotoxic phase may be very brief. In Japan, as many as 5 percent of pregnant women may experience the syndrome post partum.

This disorder, in the thyrotoxic phase, needs differentiation, first, from Graves' disease; this can be accomplished by demonstration of a depressed RAIU and absence of increased urinary iodine excretion. The latter serves also to exclude the jod-Basedow syndrome. When these data are available, the disorder must be differentiated from other causes of thyrotoxicosis with a low RAIU, principally subacute thyroiditis. Lack of tenderness or nodularity of the thyroid and absence of marked elevation of the ESR tend to exclude the latter diagnosis. Patients with functioning ectopic thyroid tissue and thyrotoxicosis factitia characteristically respond to exogenous TSH stimulation with a brisk increase in RAIU. Definitive diagnosis of CT/TT can be made by thyroid biopsy.

Since the thyroid is not hyperfunctioning in this disorder, measures used in the treatment of hyperthyroidism are useless. Symptomatic treatment with propranolol or mild sedatives is administered until the thyrotoxicosis abates.

HASHIMOTO'S THYROIDITIS   This disorder, also termed *lymphadenoid goiter*, is a common chronic inflammatory disease of the thyroid in which autoimmune factors play a prominent role. It occurs most frequently in women of middle age and is also the most common cause of sporadic goiter in children. Evidence of the participation of autoimmune factors includes the lymphocytic infiltration of the gland and the presence in the serum of increased concentrations of immunoglobulins and of antibodies against several components of thyroid tissue. Of these, the most important from the clinical standpoint are the antithyroglobulin antibody detected by the tanned red cell agglutination and the antimicrosomal antibody detected by immunofluorescence or complement fixation. This disorder also coexists with some frequency with other diseases of an autoimmune nature, including pernicious anemia, Sjögren's syndrome, chronic active hepatitis, systemic lupus erythematosus, rheumatoid arthritis, adrenal insufficiency, diabetes mellitus, and Graves' disease itself (see Chap. 325). These disorders, as well as Hashimoto's disease itself, also occur frequently in family members of patients with Hashimoto's disease.

Goiter is the outstanding feature. The enlargement involves the entire gland but not necessarily symmetrically. Typically, the consistency is rubbery, the margins are scalloped, and the general outline of the gland is preserved. The pyramidal lobe may be prominent. Early in the disease the patient is metabolically normal; however, even then decreased thyroid reserve is often manifest in an increase in serum TSH. The RAIU may be elevated early in the disease, reflecting the secretion of physiologically inactive iodoproteins, but the serum T_4 and T_3 are normal and the patient is euthyroid. As the disease progresses, thyroid failure, at first subclinical, may supervene owing to progressive replacement of thyroid parenchyma by lymphocytes or fibrous tissue. The thyroid failure is evident first in a rise in serum TSH concentration. With time, the serum T_4 concentration declines though the serum T_3 remains normal. Eventually, the serum T_3 concentration falls below normal, and frank hypothyroidism supervenes. High titers of antimicrosomal antibody are almost always present. High titers may also occur in other thyroid disorders, particularly primary thyroprivic hypothyroidism and Graves' disease but with lesser frequency. Although the foregoing findings usually suffice to permit a diagnosis, histologic confirmation by needle biopsy may be required. In view of the frequency with which hypothyroidism is either present or eventually develops, treatment with replacement doses of levothyroxine is indicated. In some patients, such therapy is associated with regression of goiter.

Occasional patients present with hyperthyroidism in association with a thyroid gland that is unusually firm and with high titers of circulating antithyroid antibodies, a combination which suggests, probably correctly, the concurrence of Graves' disease and Hashimoto's thyroiditis ("Hashitoxicosis"). In others, hyperthyroidism may supervene in a patient known to have Hashimoto's thyroiditis, presumably due to the emergence of clones of lymphocytes that produce stimulatory anti-TSH receptor antibodies. Hyperthyroidism in association with Hashimoto's thyroiditis is treated in a conventional manner, but ablative therapy is less commonly employed, since the associated chronic thyroiditis tends to limit the duration of thyroid hyperfunction and also predisposes the patient to the development of hypothyroidism after surgical or radioiodine treatment.

REFERENCES

BURMAN KD, BAKER JR JR: Immune mechanisms in Graves' disease. Endocr Rev 6:183, 1985

BURROW GN: The management of thyrotoxicosis in pregnancy. N Engl J Med 313:562, 1985

FRADKIN JE, WOLFF J: Iodide-induced thyrotoxicosis. Medicine 62:1, 1983

HAMBURGER JI: The autonomously functioning thyroid nodule: Goetsch's disease. Endocr Rev 8:439, 1987

HAY ID: Thyroiditis: A clinical update. Mayo Clin Proc 60:836, 1985

HENNESSEY JV et al: L-Thyroxine dosage: A re-evaluation of therapy with contemporary preparations. Ann Intern Med 105:11, 1986

INGBAR SH, BORGES M: Peripheral metabolism of the thyroid hormones, in *Free Thyroid Hormones*, R Ekins et al (eds). Amsterdam, Excerpta Medica, 1979, p 17

JACOBSON DH, GORMAN CA: Endocrine ophthalmopathy: Current ideas concerning etiology, pathogenesis, and treatment. Endocr Rev 5:200, 1984

OPPENHEIMER JH et al: Advances in our understanding of thyroid hormone action at the cellular level. Endocr Rev 8:288, 1987

ROJESKI MT, GHARIB H: Nodular thyroid disease. N Engl J Med 313:428, 1985

SCHNEIDER AB et al: Sequential serum thyroglobulin determinations, ^{131}I scans, and ^{131}I uptakes after triiodothyronine withdrawal in patients with thyroid cancer. J Clin Endocrinol Metab 53:1199, 1981

—— et al: Radiation-induced thyroid carcinoma, clinical course, and results of therapy in 296 patients. Ann Intern Med 105:405, 1986

SMALLRIDGE RC: Thyrotropin-secreting pituitary tumors. Endocrin Metab Clin 16:765, 1987

SPENCER CA: Clinical utility and cost effectiveness of sensitive thyrotropin assays in ambulatory and hospitalized patients. Mayo Clin Proc 63:1214, 1988

STOCKIGT JR, BARLOW JW: The diagnostic challenge of euthyroid hyperthyroxinemia. Aust NZ J Med 15:277, 1985

STUDER H, RAMELLI F: Simple goiter and its variants: Euthyroid and hyperthyroid multinodular goiters. Endocr Rev 3:40, 1982

WARTOFSKY L, OERTEL YC: Fine needle aspiration of thyroid nodules, in *Atlas of Nuclear Medicine*, D Van Nostrand, S Baum (eds). Philadelphia, Lippincott, 1988, p 193

——, BURMAN KD: Alterations in thyroid function in patients with systemic illness: The "euthyroid sick syndrome." Endocr Rev 3:164, 1982

317 DISEASES OF THE ADRENAL CORTEX

GORDON H. WILLIAMS / ROBERT G. DLUHY

BIOCHEMISTRY AND PHYSIOLOGY

STEROID NOMENCLATURE Steroids contain as their basic structure a cyclopentenoperhydrophenanthrane nucleus consisting of three 6-carbon hexane rings and a single 5-carbon pentane ring (Fig. 317-1). The carbon atoms are numbered in a sequence beginning with ring A. Adrenal steroids contain either 19 or 21 carbon atoms. The C_{19} steroids have methyl groups at positions C-18 and C-19. C_{19} steroids that have a ketone group at C-17 are termed *17-ketosteroids*. The C_{19} steroids have predominant androgenic activity. The C_{21} steroids have a 2-carbon side chain (C-20 and C-21) attached at position 17 and methyl groups at C-18 and C-19. C_{21} steroids that also possess a hydroxyl group at position 17 are termed *17-hydroxycorticosteroids*. The C_{21} steroids have either glucocorticoid or mineralocorticoid properties. *Glucocorticoid* signifies a C_{21} steroid with predominant action on intermediary metabolism; *mineralocorticoid* indicates a C_{21} steroid with predominant action on the metabolism of sodium and potassium.

BIOSYNTHESIS OF ADRENAL STEROIDS Cholesterol, derived from the diet and from endogenous synthesis, is the starting compound in steroidogenesis. The three major adrenal biosynthetic pathways lead to the production of glucocorticoids (cortisol), mineralocorticoids (aldosterone), and adrenal androgens (dehydroepiandrosterone). Separate zones of the adrenal cortex synthesize specific hormones; this reflects the enzymatic capacity of each zone to carry out certain transformations and hydroxylations (Fig. 317-2). The outer (glomerulosa) zone is mainly involved in aldosterone biosynthesis, and the inner (fasciculata-reticularis) zone is the site of cortisol and androgen biosynthesis.

STEROID TRANSPORT Some steroid hormones, e.g., testosterone and cortisol, circulate to a considerable extent bound to plasma proteins. Cortisol occurs in the plasma in three forms: free cortisol,

FIGURE 317-1 Basic steroid structure and nomenclature.

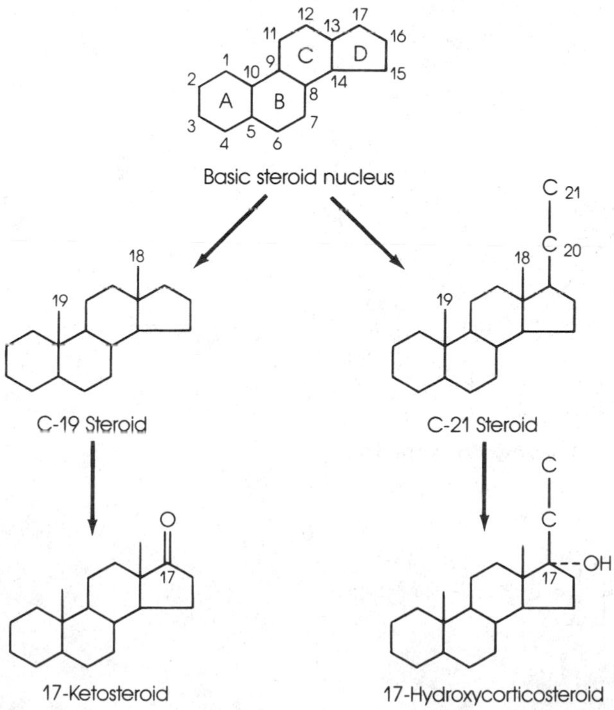

Basic steroid nucleus

C-19 Steroid

C-21 Steroid

17-Ketosteroid

17-Hydroxycorticosteroid

protein-bound cortisol, and cortisol metabolites. *Free cortisol* refers to that quantity which is physiologically active but not protein-bound and, therefore, represents a form of cortisol acting directly on tissue sites. Normally, less than 5 percent of circulating cortisol is free. Only the unbound cortisol and its metabolites are filtrable at the glomerulus. Increased quantities of free steroid are excreted in the urine in states characterized by hypersecretion of cortisol, as the unbound fraction of plasma cortisol rises. *Protein-bound cortisol* is that reversibly bound to circulating plasma proteins. There are two cortisol-binding systems of plasma. One is a high-affinity, low-capacity alpha₂ globulin termed *transcortin* or *cortisol-binding globulin* (CBG), and the other is a low-affinity, high-capacity protein, *albumin*. The binding affinity of CBG for cortisol is reduced in areas of inflammation, thus increasing the local concentration of free cortisol. This phenomenon may be important in the glucocorticoid response to stress. Cortisol-binding globulin in normal humans can bind approximately 700 nmol of cortisol per liter of plasma (25 μg/dL). When the concentration of cortisol exceeds this level, the excess becomes bound in part to albumin, and a greater proportion circulates unbound. The CBG level is increased in high-estrogen states (e.g., pregnancy, oral contraceptive administration). The rise in CBG is accompanied by a parallel rise in protein-bound cortisol, with the result that the plasma cortisol concentration is elevated. However, the free cortisol levels probably remain normal, and signs and symptoms of glucocorticoid excess are absent. Most synthetic glucocorticoid analogues bind less efficiently to CBG (approximately 70 percent binding). This may explain the propensity of some synthetic analogues to produce cushingoid side effects at low dosage. *Cortisol metabolites* are biologically inactive and bind only weakly to circulating plasma proteins.

Aldosterone is bound to proteins to a smaller extent than either testosterone or cortisol, and an ultrafiltrate of plasma contains as much as 50 percent of the circulating aldosterone. The limited binding of aldosterone by plasma protein is significant in the metabolism of this hormone.

STEROID METABOLISM AND EXCRETION Glucocorticoids The daily secretion of cortisol ranges between 40 and 80 μmol (15 and 30 mg), with a pronounced diurnal cycle. Cortisol is distributed in a volume of body fluids approximating the total extracellular fluid space, with more than 90 percent in the protein-bound fraction. The plasma concentration of cortisol is determined by the rate of secretion, the rate of inactivation, and the rate of excretion of free cortisol. The liver is the major organ responsible for steroid inactivation, by reduction of ring A and conjugation of the reduced products with glucuronic acid at position C-3 to form water-soluble compounds. The 11-dehydrogenase system converts cortisol to the inactive cortisone and is influenced by the level of circulating thyroid hormone, the oxidative reaction being increased in hyperthyroidism.

Mineralocorticoids In normal subjects on a normal salt intake, the average daily secretion of aldosterone ranges between 0.1 and 0.7 μmol (50 and 250 μg). Since aldosterone is only weakly bound to proteins, its volume of distribution is larger than that of cortisol and approximates 35 liters. During a single passage through the liver, more than 75 percent of circulating aldosterone is normally inactivated by ring A reduction and conjugation with glucuronic acid. However, under certain conditions, such as congestive failure, this inactivation is reduced.

From 7 to 15 percent of aldosterone is excreted in the urine as a glucuronide conjugate, from which free aldosterone is released on standing at pH 1. This *acid-labile conjugate* is formed in the liver and in the kidney. For average salt intake, the 24-h urine excretion of the acid-labile conjugate ranges from 15 to 50 nmol (5 to 19 μg), that of the reduced derivative from 70 to 100 nmol (25 to 35 μg), and that of the nonconjugated, nonreduced free aldosterone from 0.5 to 2 nmol (0.2 to 0.6 μg).

Adrenal androgens The major androgen secreted by the adrenal is dehydroepiandrosterone (DHEA) and its C-3 sulfuric acid ester. From 15 to 30 mg of these compounds are secreted daily. Smaller amounts of Δ^4-androstenedione, 11β-hydroxyandrostenedione, and testosterone are secreted. DHEA is the major precursor of the urinary 17-ketosteroids. Two-thirds of the urine 17-ketosteroids in the male is derived from adrenal metabolites, and the remaining one-third comes from testicular androgens. In the female, almost all urine 17-ketosteroids are derived from the adrenal.

ACTH PHYSIOLOGY   Corticotropin (ACTH) (see Chap. 313) is an unbranched polypeptide containing 39 amino acids. ACTH and a number of other peptides (lipotropins, endorphins, and melanocyte-

stimulating hormones) are processed from a larger precursor molecule of 31,000 mol wt—pro-opiomelanocortin (POMC) (see Chap. 313 and Fig. 317-3). ACTH is synthesized and stored in basophilic cells of the anterior pituitary gland. The basophilic staining of the corticotrophs is the result of the glycosylation of ACTH and related peptides. Much of the potential for the corticotropic actions of ACTH is present in smaller polypeptide fragments; the *N*-terminal 18-amino-acid structure retains full biologic potency, and shorter *N*-terminal fragments exhibit partial biologic activity. Release of ACTH and

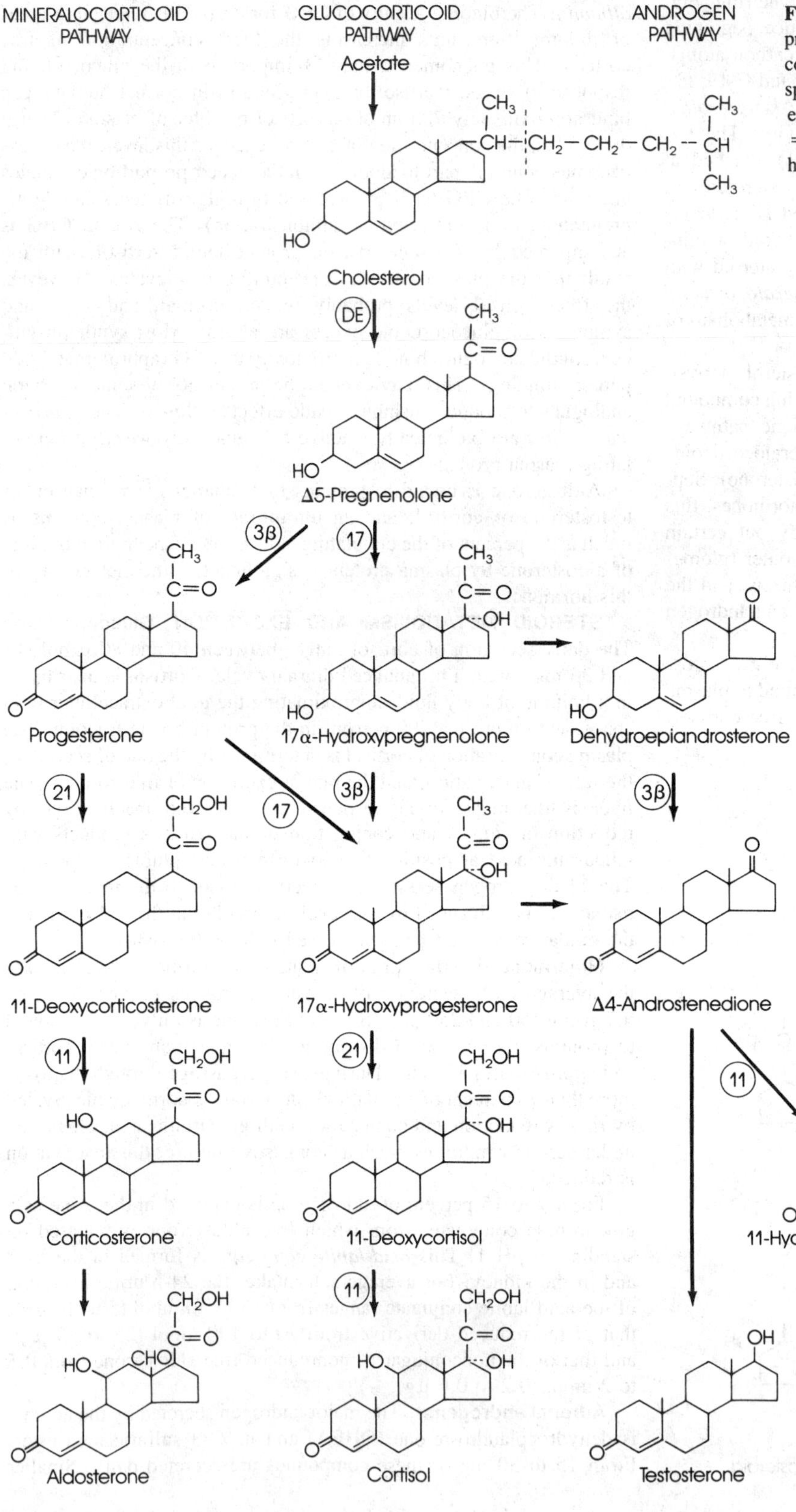

FIGURE 317-2 Biosynthetic pathways for adrenal steroid production; major pathways to mineralocorticoids, glucocorticoids, and androgens. Circled letters and numbers denote specific enzymes: DE = cholesterol side chain cleavage enzyme; 3β = 3β-ol-dehydrogenase with $\Delta^{4,5}$-isomerase; 11 = C-11 hydroxylase; 17 = C-17 hydroxylase; 21 = C-21 hydroxylase.

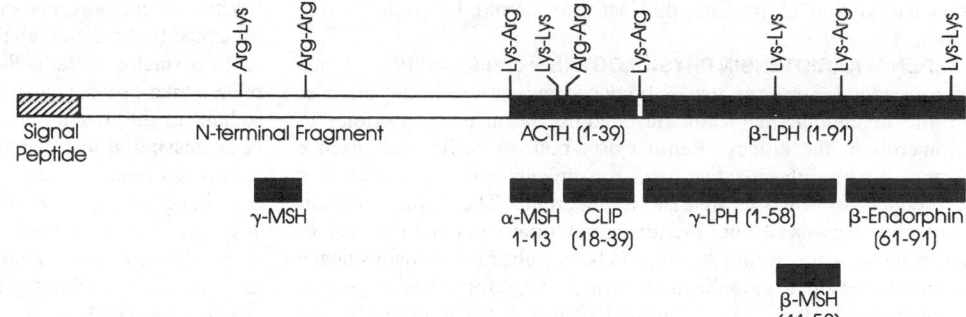

FIGURE 317-3 Schematic representation of the probable structure of the 31,000–mol wt pro-opiomelanocortin molecule. (*From DT Krieger, JB Martin, N Engl J Med 304:880, 1981. By permission of the New England Journal of Medicine.*)

related peptides from the anterior pituitary gland is governed by a "corticotropin-releasing center" in the median eminence of the hypothalamus, which upon stimulation releases a peptide with a chain of 41 amino acids (corticotropin-releasing hormone, CRH) that travels via the pituitary-stalk portal bloodstream to the anterior pituitary, where it effects the release of ACTH (Fig. 317-4). Some related peptides such as β-lipotropin (β-LPH) are released in equimolar concentrations with ACTH, suggesting enzymatic cleavage from the parent POMC prior to or concomitant with the secretory process. However, beta endorphin levels may vary disparately with circulating levels of ACTH depending on the nature of the stimulus. The functions and regulation of secretion of the related peptides derived from POMC are not understood.

The major factors controlling ACTH release include CRH, free cortisol concentration in plasma, stress, and the sleep-wake cycle (Fig. 317-4). The plasma level of ACTH varies during the day as a result of its pulsatile secretion but roughly follows a diurnal pattern, with a peak just prior to waking and a nadir before retiring. After several days on a new sleep-wake cycle, the pattern is altered to conform to the new cycle. ACTH and cortisol levels also increase in response to eating. Stress (e.g., pyrogens, surgery, hypoglycemia, exercise, and severe emotional trauma) can also enhance ACTH release. Stress-related secretion of ACTH abolishes circadian periodicity but is in turn suppressed by prior high-dose glucocorticoid administration. The secretion of ACTH following stress and the normal pulsatile, diurnal ACTH release are regulated by CRH; this is the so-called open feedback loop. CRH secretion, in turn, is influenced by hypothalamic neurotransmitters. For example, serotoninergic and cholinergic systems stimulate the secretion of CRH and ACTH; there is contradictory evidence regarding the inhibitory effects of α-adrenergic agonists and gamma-aminobutyric acid (GABA) on CRH release. In addition, there may be direct pituitary effects of these neurotransmitters. There is also evidence for peptidergic regulation of ACTH release. For example, beta endorphin and enkephalin inhibit and vasopressin and angiotensin II augment the secretion of ACTH. Finally, ACTH release is regulated by the free cortisol level in plasma. Cortisol decreases the responsiveness of adrenal corticotropic cells to CRH; i.e., in the presence of cortisol more CRH is required to produce a given increment of ACTH. The response of the POMC mRNA to CRH is also inhibited by glucocorticoids. In addition, glucocorticoids inhibit CRH release. This servomechanism establishes the primacy of blood cortisol concentration in the control of ACTH secretion. The inhibition of ACTH occurs in two phases: (1) an early fast feedback, possibly a membrane effect, lasting less than 10 min and dependent on the rate of increase of glucocorticoid levels; and (2) a time-dependent delayed feedback response, probably due to inhibition of synthesis of the precursor protein. The suppression of ACTH secretion that results in adrenal atrophy following *prolonged* glucocorticoid therapy may be primarily related to suppression of hypothalamic CRH release, since exogenous CRH administration in this circumstance produces a rise in plasma ACTH. Cortisol also exerts feedback on higher brain centers (hippocampus, reticular system, and septum) and perhaps on the adrenal cortex as well (Fig. 317-4).

The biologic half-life of ACTH in the circulation is less than 10 min. The action of ACTH is also rapid; within minutes of its release, the concentration of steroids in the adrenal venous blood increases. ACTH stimulates steroidogenesis via activation of the membrane-bound adenyl cyclase. Adenosine-3',5'-monophosphate (cyclic AMP) in turn activates protein kinase enzymes, thereby resulting in the

FIGURE 317-4 The hypothalamic-pituitary-adrenal axis. The dominant feedback control of plasma cortisol is on the pituitary gland (1) and on the hypothalamic corticotropin-releasing center (2). Feedback of plasma cortisol may also act on higher nerve centers (3) and/or on the adrenal gland itself (4). There also may be a short feedback inhibition of CRH by ACTH (5). Hypothalamic neurotransmitters influence CRH release; serotoninergic and cholinergic systems stimulate the secretion of CRH and ACTH; alpha-adrenergic agonists and gamma-aminobutyric acid (GABA) probably inhibit CRH release. The opioid peptides, beta endorphin and enkephalin, inhibit and vasopressin and angiotensin II augment the secretion of CRH and ACTH. CRH = corticotropin-releasing hormone; β-LPH = beta lipotropin; POMC = pro-opiomelanocortin.

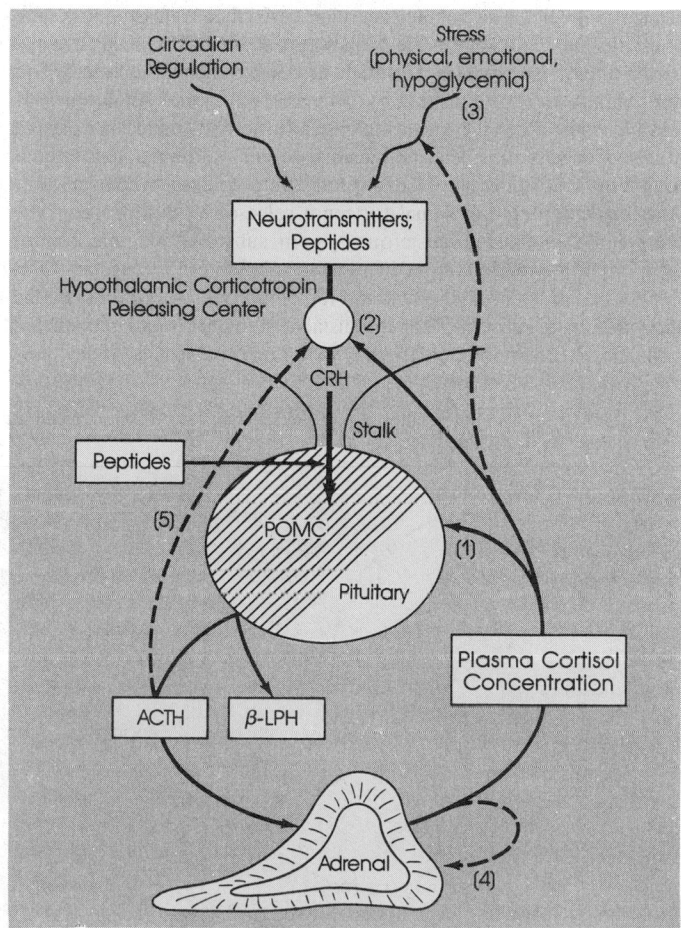

phosphorylation of proteins that activate steroid biosynthesis (see Chap. 68).

RENIN-ANGIOTENSIN PHYSIOLOGY (See also Chap. 196)   Renin is a proteolytic enzyme that is produced and stored in the granules of the juxtaglomerular cells surrounding the afferent arterioles of glomeruli in the kidney. Renin exists both in active and inactive forms. Whether the inactive form is a precursor (''prorenin'') or is a product formed after release is uncertain. The juxtaglomerular apparatus consists of both the juxtaglomerular cells and the cells of the macula densa. Renin acts on the basic substrate angiotensinogen (a circulating alpha$_2$ globulin made in the liver) to form the decapeptide angiotensin I (Fig. 317-5). Angiotensin I is then enzymatically transformed by converting enzyme, present in many tissues particularly in the pulmonary vascular endothelium, to the octapeptide angiotensin II by splitting off the two C-terminal amino acids. Angiotensin II is a potent pressor compound and exerts its pressor action by a direct effect on arteriolar smooth muscle. In addition, angiotensin II is a potent stimulus to the production of aldosterone by the zona glomerulosa of the adrenal cortex; the nonapeptide, angiotensin III, may also stimulate aldosterone production. Angiotensinases rapidly destroy angiotensin II (half-life approximately 1 min), while the half-life of renin is more prolonged (10 to 20 min). Other tissues, such as uterus, placenta, vascular tissue, brain, salivary glands, and adrenal cortex also produce renin-like substances, but the significance of these so-called tissue renins is not known.

Renal renin release is controlled by four interdependent factors, and the amount of renin released is a composite of the effects of all four. The *juxtaglomerular cells,* which are specialized myoepithelial cells cuffing the afferent arterioles, act as miniature pressure transducers, sensing renal perfusion pressure and corresponding changes in afferent arteriolar perfusion pressures. For example, under conditions of a reduction in circulating blood volume, there is a corresponding reduction in renal perfusion pressure and, therefore, in afferent arteriolar pressure (Fig. 317-5). This is perceived by the juxtaglomerular cells as a decreased stretch exerted on the afferent arteriolar walls. The juxtaglomerular cells then release increasing quantities of renin within the kidney circulation. This results in the formation of angiotensin I, which is converted in the kidney and peripherally to angiotensin II by converting enzyme. Angiotensin II stimulates the adrenal cortex to release aldosterone. Increasing plasma levels of aldosterone lead to increasing renal sodium retention and thus result in expansion of extracellular fluid volume, which, in turn, dampens the initiating signal for renin release. Within this context, the renin-angiotensin-aldosterone system subserves volume control by appropriate modifications of renal tubular sodium transport.

A second control mechanism for renin release centers in the *macula densa* cells, a group of distal convoluted tubular epithelial cells in direct apposition to the juxtaglomerular cells. They may function as chemoreceptors, monitoring the sodium (or chloride) load presented to the distal tubule, and such information may be conveyed to the juxtaglomerular cells, where appropriate modifications in renin release take place. Under conditions of increased delivery of filtered sodium to the macula densa, increasing release of renin is capable of decreasing glomerular filtration rate, thereby reducing the filtered load of sodium.

The *sympathetic nervous system* regulates release of renin in response to assuming the upright posture. The mechanism is either a direct effect on the juxtaglomerular cell to increase adenyl cyclase activity or an indirect effect on either the juxtaglomerular or the macula densa cells by way of a vasoconstrictive action on the afferent arteriole.

Finally, circulating factors may alter renin release. Increasing dietary *potassium* directly decreases renin release; decreasing potassium intake increases renin release. The significance of this potassium effect is unclear. *Angiotensin II* itself can exert a negative feedback control on renin release independent of alterations in renal blood flow, pressure, or aldosterone secretion. *Atrial natriuretic peptides* also may inhibit renin release. Thus, the control of renin release is complex, consisting of both *intrarenal* (pressor receptor and macula densa) and *extrarenal* (sympathetic nervous system, potassium, angiotensin, etc.) mechanisms. A given level of renin secretion probably reflects all these factors, with the intrarenal mechanism predominating.

GLUCOCORTICOID PHYSIOLOGY   The division of adrenal steroids into glucocorticoids and mineralocorticoids is arbitrary in that most glucocorticoids have some mineralocorticoid-like properties, and vice versa (see Chap. 311). The descriptive term *glucocorticoid* is applied to those adrenal steroids with a predominant action on intermediary metabolism. The principal glucocorticoid is cortisol (hydrocortisone). Cortisol enters the target cell by diffusion, combines with high-affinity cytoplasmic receptor proteins, and is transferred to acceptor sites on the chromosomes, which then results in an increase in RNA synthesis and later in protein synthesis. One way of defining glucocorticoid effects is as those mediated by one class of high-affinity cytoplasmic receptors (so called type II or glucorticoid receptors) (see Chap. 311). The physiologic actions of the glucocorticoids on intermediary metabolism include the regulation of protein, carbohydrate, lipid, and nucleic acid metabolism. Glucocorticoids raise blood glucose by acting as an insulin antagonist and by suppressing the secretion of insulin, thereby inhibiting glucose uptake in peripheral tissues and promoting hepatic synthesis of glucose (gluconeogenesis). The actions on protein metabolism appear to be mainly catabolic in effect, with an increased protein breakdown and nitrogen excretion. Glucocorticoids increase hepatic glycogen content and promote the hepatic synthesis of gluconeogenesis. These actions are in large part explained by the mobilization of glycogenic amino

FIGURE 317-5   The interrelationship of the volume and potassium feedback loops on aldosterone secretion. Integration of signals from each loop determines the level of aldosterone secretion.

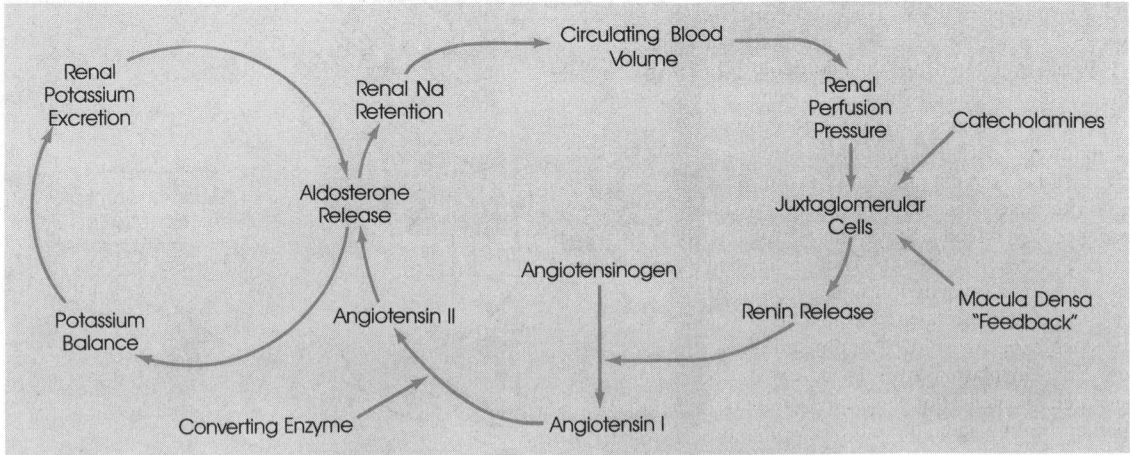

acid precursors from peripheral supporting structures, such as bone, skin, muscle, and connective tissue, due to protein breakdown and inhibition of protein synthesis and amino acid uptake. Glucocorticoid-induced hyperaminoacidemia also facilitates gluconeogenesis by stimulating glucagon secretion. Glucocorticoids act directly on the liver to stimulate the synthesis of certain enzymes, such as tyrosine amino transferase and tryptophan pyrrolase. Glucocorticoids inhibit the synthesis of nucleic acids in most body tissues, but in the liver RNA synthesis is stimulated. Glucocorticoids regulate fatty acid mobilization by enhancing activation of cellular lipase by lipid-mobilizing hormones (e.g., catecholamines and pituitary peptides).

The actions of cortisol on structural protein and on adipose tissue vary in different parts of the body. For example, pharmacologic doses of cortisol can deplete the protein matrix of the vertebral column (trabecular bone), but long bones (primarily compact bone) are affected only minimally; peripheral adipose tissue may diminish, whereas abdominal and interscapular fat may accumulate.

Glucocorticoids have anti-inflammatory properties, which are probably related to their actions on the microvasculature as well as to cellular effects. Cortisol maintains normal vascular responsiveness to circulating vasoconstrictor factors and opposes the increase in capillary permeability characteristic of acute inflammation. Glucocorticoids cause a polymorphonuclear leukocytosis; the circulating leukocyte mass is increased due to release from the bone marrow of mature cells as well as to inhibition of their egress through the capillary wall. Glucocorticoids produce a depletion of circulating eosinophils and of lymphoid tissue, specifically T cells (thymus-derived lymphocytes). The mechanism is by redistribution from the circulation into other compartments. Thus, cortisol impairs cellular-mediated immunity. Glucocorticoids also inhibit the production or action of the local mediators of inflammation such as the lymphokines and prostaglandins. These actions occur via the glucocorticoid receptors, and the effects are blocked by inhibitors of RNA and protein synthesis. Glucocorticoids inhibit actions and production of immune interferon by T lymphocytes, and the production of lymphocyte-activating factor (also known as interleukin 1) by macrophages. The action of glucocorticoids in suppressing fever may be explained by the latter effect since interleukin 1 appears to be identical to endogenous pyrogen, which can activate the hypothalamic fever center. Glucocorticoids also inhibit the production of T-cell growth factor (interleukin 2) by T lymphocytes. Glucocorticoids reverse macrophage activation and antagonize the action of migration-inhibiting factor (MIF), leading to reduced adherence of macrophages to vascular endothelium. Glucocorticoids inhibit prostaglandin and leukotriene production by inhibiting the activity of phospholipase A_2, thus blocking release of arachidonic acid from phospholipids. Finally, glucocorticoids inhibit the inflammatory actions induced by bradykinin and serotonin, such as increased vascular permeability. It is probably only at pharmacologic dosages that antibody production is reduced and lysosomal membranes stabilized, thereby suppressing the release of proteolytic acid hydrolases stored in these cytoplasmic organelles.

Cortisol levels are responsive within minutes to a variety of physical stresses (trauma, surgery, exercise) and psychological stresses (anxiety, depression). Hypoglycemia and fever are also potent stimuli of ACTH and cortisol secretion. The reasons why elevated glucocorticoid levels protect the organism under stress are not understood, but this action may be linked to the anti-inflammatory actions of cortisol in suppressing normal defense reactions, thus regulating the control of the inflammatory response in uninvolved tissues. In the absence of glucocorticoids, such stresses may cause hypotension, shock, and death. For these reasons, glucocorticoid administration should always be increased in individuals with hypofunction of the pituitary-adrenal axis during stress.

Cortisol has a major action on the distribution and excretion of body water. It subserves the extracellular fluid volume by retarding the migration of water into cells. It promotes renal water excretion by suppressing the secretion of vasopressin, increasing the rate of glomerular filtration, and acting directly on the renal tubule, the

consequence being to guard against water intoxication by increasing solute-free water clearance. Glucocorticoids also have weak mineralocorticoid-like properties, and increasing doses produce renal tubular sodium reabsorption and increased urine potassium excretion. Glucocorticoids can also influence behavior; emotional disorders may occur with either excesses or deficits of cortisol. Lastly, cortisol suppresses the secretion of pituitary POMC and peptides derived from this precursor molecule (ACTH, beta-endorphin, and beta-lipotropin) as well as the secretion of hypothalamic CRH and vasopressin.

MINERALOCORTICOID PHYSIOLOGY The major mineralocorticoid, aldosterone, has two important activities: (1) It is a major regulator of extracellular fluid volume, and (2) it is a major determinant of potassium metabolism. These effects are mediated by binding of aldosterone to high-affinity type I or mineralocorticoid receptor proteins in target tissues (see Chap. 311). Volume is regulated through a direct effect on the renal tubular transport of sodium. Aldosterone acts predominantly at the distal convoluted tubule, where it causes a decrease in the excretion of sodium and an increase in excretion of potassium. The reabsorption of sodium ions causes a fall in the transmembrane potential, thus enhancing the flow of positive ions out of the cell into the lumen. The major intracellular singly charged positive ion is potassium. Since its concentration in the cell is forty- to eightyfold greater than in the lumen, potassium passively follows this relative electric gradient to restore the normal positive charge to the lumen. The reabsorbed sodium ions are then transported out of the tubular epithelial cells into the interstitial fluid of the kidney and from there into the renal capillary circulation. Water passively follows the transported sodium.

Hydrogen ion is also abundant in the tubular epithelial cell. Since its concentration is greater in the lumen than in the cell, it is actively secreted, but the reduced intraluminal positivity allows more hydrogen to be secreted with the same amount of energy. Aldosterone and other mineralocorticoids also act on the epithelium of the salivary ducts, sweat glands, and gastrointestinal tract to cause reabsorption of sodium in "exchange" for potassium ions.

When normal individuals are given aldosterone (or deoxycorticosterone), an initial period of sodium retention is followed by a natriuresis, and sodium balance is reestablished after 3 to 5 days. As a result, edema does not develop. This phenomenon is referred to as the "escape phenomenon," signifying an "escape" by the renal tubules from the sodium-retaining action of chronically administered aldosterone.

Three primary mechanisms control aldosterone release—the renin-angiotensin system, potassium, and ACTH (Table 317-1). The renin-angiotensin system is the major system for control of extracellular fluid volume, via regulation of aldosterone secretion (Fig. 317-5). In effect, the renin-angiotensin system maintains the circulating blood volume constant by causing aldosterone-induced sodium retention

TABLE 317-1 Factors regulating aldosterone biosynthesis

Factors	Effects
I Renin-angiotensin system	Stimulate
II Sodium ion	Inhibit (?physiologic)
III Potassium ion	Stimulate
IV Neurotransmitters	
A Dopamine	Inhibit
B Serotonin	Stimulate
V Pituitary hormones	
A ACTH	Stimulate
B Non-ACTH pituitary hormones (e.g., growth hormone)	Permissive (for optimal response to sodium restriction)
C Unidentified pituitary factors	Stimulate
D Beta endorphin	Stimulate
E γ-MSH	Permissive
VI Natriuretic factors	
A Atrial peptide	Inhibit
B Ouabain-like factors	Inhibit

during periods registered as volume deficiencies and by decreasing aldosterone-dependent sodium retention under conditions in which volume is registered as being ample.

Potassium ions directly regulate aldosterone secretion independently of the renin-angiotensin system (Fig. 317-5). In normal humans, oral potassium loading increases aldosterone secretion, excretion, and plasma levels. In addition, an increase in serum potassium of as little as 0.1 mmol/L increases plasma aldosterone levels under certain circumstances.

Physiologic amounts of ACTH acutely stimulate aldosterone secretion, but this action is not sustained if ACTH is infused for periods greater than 10 to 12 h. Most studies relegate ACTH to a minor role in the control of aldosterone. For example, subjects on high-dose steroid therapy for several years and with presumably complete suppression of ACTH have normal aldosterone-secretory responses to sodium restriction. Therefore, chronic ACTH deficiency per se does not alter glomerulosa cell responsiveness.

The prior dietary intake of both potassium and sodium can alter the magnitude of the aldosterone response to acute stimulation. Increasing potassium intake or decreasing sodium intake sensitizes the response of the glomerulosa cells to acute stimulation by ACTH, angiotensin II, and/or potassium.

Neurotransmitters (dopamine and serotonin) and some peptides, such as atrial natriuretic factor, γ-melanocyte-stimulating hormone (γ-MSH), beta endorphin, and an unidentified pituitary aldosterone-stimulating factor, also participate in the regulation of aldosterone secretion (Table 317-1). Thus, the control of aldosterone secretion involves both stimulatory and inhibitory factors.

ANDROGEN PHYSIOLOGY   Androgens regulate male secondary sexual characteristics and can cause virilizing symptoms in women. They produce these actions by binding to high-affinity cytoplasmic receptors.

Steroids with predominant androgenic activity have 19 carbon atoms (Fig. 317-1). The principal adrenal androgens are dehydroepiandrosterone (DHEA), androstenedione, and 11-hydroxyandrostenedione. DHEA and its sulfate are *quantitatively* the major androgens secreted by the adrenal; DHEA and androstenedione are weak androgens, and they exert their effects via conversion in extraglandular tissues to the potent androgen, testosterone. The release of adrenal androgens is stimulated by ACTH, not by gonadotropins. With ACTH stimulation, 17-ketosteroids increase but to a lesser extent than do urine 17-hydroxycorticosteroids. It follows that adrenal androgens are suppressed by exogenous glucocorticoid administration.

LABORATORY EVALUATION OF ADRENOCORTICAL FUNCTION

The basic assumption in the measurement of plasma or urinary steroids is that they accurately reflect adrenal *secretory* rates of that steroid. A disadvantage of urine *excretion* values is that they may not truly reflect the secretion rate because of improper collection or altered metabolism. Measurement of the actual adrenal secretory rate of a given steroid would be preferable but is more difficult, involving isotope dilution techniques following administration of a radioactive steroid. Plasma levels reflect the level of secretion only at the time of measurement. The plasma level (PL) is dependent on two factors: the secretion rate (SR) of the hormone and the rate at which it is metabolized, i.e., its metabolic clearance rate (MCR). These three factors can be related mathematically as follows:

$$PL = \frac{SR}{MCR} \quad \text{or} \quad SR = MCR \times PL$$

BLOOD LEVELS (See Table 317-2)   **Peptides**   ACTH and angiotensin II can be measured by radioimmunoassay, but the measurements are technically difficult because of their low concentrations and their instability in human plasma. In addition, ACTH

TABLE 317-2   Range of normal values for tests of adrenal function

Test	Normal value, range
Plasma cortisol, nmol/L (μg/dL):	
8 A.M.	140–690 (5–24)
4 P.M.	80–330 (3–12)
Cortisol secretory rate, nmol/d (mg/d)	14–69 (5–25)
Urinary free cortisol, nmol/d (μg/d)	55–275 (20–100)
17-Hydroxycorticosteroids, μmol/d (mg/d)	5.5–28 (2–10)
Plasma testosterone, nmol/L (ng/mL):	
Men	10–35 (3–10)
Women	<3.5 (<1)
Plasma dehydroepiandrosterone (DHEA) nmol/L (μg/L)	7–31 (2–9)
Plasma DHEA sulfate, μmol/L (μg/L)	1.3–6.7 (500–2500)
Plasma 11-deoxycortisol (S), nmol/L (μg/dL)	<30 (<1)
Plasma 17OH progesterone, nmol/L (μg/L):	
Women	
Follicular phase	0.6–3 (0.2–1)
Luteal phase	1.5–10.6 (0.5–3.5)
Men	0.2–9 (0.06–3)
Plasma aldosterone, pmol/L (ng/dL) (100 mmol Na, 60–100 mmol K, supine, 8 A.M.)	<240 (<8)
Aldosterone secretion nmol/d (μg/d) (100 mmol Na, 600–100 mmol K)	140–690 (50–250)
Aldosterone excretion, nmol/d (μg/d) (100 mmol Na, 60–100 mmol K)	14–53 (5–19)
Plasma renin activity (μg/L)/h [(ng/mL)/h] (100 mmol Na, 60–100 mmol K, supine, 8 A.M.)	1–2.5 (1–2.5)
Plasma angiotensin II ng/L (pg/mL) (100 mmol Na, 60–100 mmol K, supine, 8 A.M.)	10–30 (10–30)
Plasma ACTH, pmol/L (pg/mL) (8 A.M.)	<18 (<80)

levels fluctuate from moment to moment, and a circadian rhythm is superimposed on basal ACTH secretion, with lower levels in the early evening than in the morning. Angiotensin II levels also vary diurnally but more importantly are influenced by dietary sodium intake and posture. Both upright posture and sodium restriction elevate angiotensin II levels.

Most clinical determinations of the renin-angiotensin system, however, involve measurements of peripheral "plasma renin activity" (PRA) in which the renin activity is gauged by the generation of angiotensin I during a standardized incubation period. This method depends on the presence of sufficient angiotensinogen in the patient's plasma as substrate. The generated angiotensin I is then measured by radioimmunoassay. Plasma renin activity depends on dietary sodium intake and whether the patient is ambulatory. In normal humans a diurnal rhythm for PRA is characterized by peak values in the morning with decreases in activity in the afternoon.

Steroids   Cortisol and aldosterone are both secreted episodically, and levels generally decline during the day with peak values in the morning and low levels in the evening. In addition, the plasma level of aldosterone, but not of cortisol, is increased by dietary potassium loading, sodium restriction, or assuming the upright posture. Measurement of the sulfate conjugate of DHEA is a useful index of adrenal androgen secretion since little is formed in the gonads and the half-life is 7 to 9 h.

URINE LEVELS   The urine *17-hydroxycorticosteroid* assay measures steroids with a "dihydroxyacetone" C-17 side chain, i.e., with hydroxyl groups on C-17 and C-21 and a ketone group on C-20. Therefore, this determination includes cortisol, cortisone, tetrahydrocortisol, tetrahydrocortisone, and 11-deoxycortisol (Fig. 317-2). Normally, daytime (7 A.M. to 7 P.M.) excretion exceeds night values (7 P.M. to 7 A.M.).

The urine *17-ketosteroids* are those containing a ketone group at C-17 (Fig. 317-1). They originate either in the adrenal gland or the gonad. In normal women, 90 percent or more of total urinary 17-ketosteroids is derived from the adrenal gland, while in men only 60 to 70 percent is of adrenal origin. Urine 17-ketosteroid values are highest in young adults and decline with age.

The determination of urinary free cortisol is perhaps more useful than 17-hydroxysteroid measurements since elevated excretion values correlate with states of hypercortisolism, reflecting changes in the unbound, physiologically active, circulating levels of cortisol.

A carefully timed urine collection is a prerequisite for all excretory determinations. Urinary creatinine should be measured simultaneously to demonstrate the accuracy and adequacy of the collection procedure. Adjustments for body size can be made; e.g., normal subjects excrete 8 to 20 μmol (3 to 7 mg) of 17-hydroxycorticosteroids per gram of creatinine.

STIMULATION TESTS Stimulation tests are useful in documenting the existence of a hormonal deficiency state. A standardized and specific stimulus for the production and release of a given hormone is applied, and the quantity of the released hormone can then be measured.

Tests of glucocorticoid reserve Within minutes after initiation of an infusion of ACTH, cortisol levels increase in adrenal venous blood. This responsiveness of the adrenal gland to ACTH is utilized as an index of the "functional reserve" of the gland for production of cortisol. Under maximal ACTH stimulation the cortisol secretion increases tenfold to 800 μmol/d (300 mg/d). Such maximal stimulation can be obtained only with prolonged ACTH infusions. For clinical purposes, the functional adrenal reserve for cortisol production is standardized with a 24-h ACTH infusion. Synthetic α^{1-24}-ACTH (cosyntropin) is usually given in 500 to 1000 mL normal saline at a rate of 2 units per hour for 24 h. Normal subjects increase 17-hydroxysteroid excretion rates to at least 70 μmol/d (25 mg/d), and plasma cortisol levels exceed 1100 nmol/L (40 μg/dL). In patients with secondary adrenal insufficiency, the maximal 17-hydroxysteroid excretion rate is 8 to 55 μmol/d (3 to 20 mg/d), and the plasma cortisol value at 24 h ranges between 280 and 1100 nmol/L (10 and 40 μg/dL). Patients with primary adrenal insufficiency have smaller responses.

A screening test (the so-called rapid ACTH stimulation test) involves the administration of 25 units (0.25 mg) cosyntropin intravenously or intramuscularly and measurement of plasma cortisol levels before and 30 and 60 min later; the test can be performed at any time of the day. The most clearcut criterion for a normal response is a stimulated cortisol level >500 nmol/L (18 μg/dL), and the minimal stimulated normal increment of cortisol is >200 nmol/L (7 mg/dL) above baseline. However, ill patients with elevated basal cortisol levels may show no further increases following acute ACTH administration.

Tests of mineralocorticoid reserve and stimulation of the renin-angiotensin system Stimulation tests utilize protocols of programmed volume depletion, such as sodium restriction, diuretic administration, or upright posture. A simple potent test consists of severe sodium restriction and upright posture. After 3 to 5 days of a 10-mmol sodium intake, aldosterone secretion or excretion rates should increase two- to threefold over control. Supine morning plasma aldosterone levels usually increase three- to sixfold. In addition, plasma levels increase two- to fourfold in response to 2 to 3 h of upright posture.

Stimulation tests on normal dietary sodium intake may be carried out by the administration of a potent diuretic, such as 40 to 80 mg furosemide, followed by 2 to 3 h of upright posture. The normal response is a two- to fourfold rise in plasma aldosterone levels.

SUPPRESSION TESTS Suppression tests to document hypersecretion of adrenocortical hormones are based on the demonstration of a decrease in the target hormone following standardized suppression of its tropic hormone.

Tests of pituitary-adrenal suppressibility The ACTH release mechanism is sensitive to the circulating blood level of glucocorticoids. When such blood levels are increased in the normal individual, less ACTH is released from the anterior pituitary and less steroid is produced by the adrenal gland. The integrity of this feedback mechanism can be tested clinically by giving a potent glucocorticoid and judging suppression of ACTH secretion by analysis of urine steroid excretory values and/or plasma cortisol and ACTH levels. A potent glucocorticoid such as dexamethasone is utilized in order that the administered compound can be given in such small amounts that it does not contribute significantly to the steroids to be analyzed.

The best *screening* procedure is the overnight dexamethasone suppression test. This involves the measurement of plasma cortisol levels at 8 A.M. following the oral administration of 1 mg dexamethasone the previous midnight. The 8 A.M. value for plasma cortisol in normal subjects should be less than 140 nmol/L (5 μg/dL).

The definitive test of adrenal suppressibility is to administer 0.5 mg dexamethasone every 6 h for two successive days while collecting urine over a 24-h period for determination of creatinine, 17-hydroxysteroids, and/or free cortisol and/or measuring plasma cortisol levels. In a patient with a normal hypothalamic pituitary ACTH release mechanism, a fall in the urine 17-hydroxycorticosteroids to less than 8 μmol/d (3 mg/d) on the second day of dexamethasone administration, urinary free cortisol to less than 80 nmol/d (30 μg/d), or plasma cortisol to less than 140 nmol/L (5 μg/dL) is seen.

Normal responses to either of the suppression tests implies that the ACTH control of the adrenal glands is physiologically normal. However, an isolated abnormal result, particularly when the overnight suppression test is being used, does not in itself imply pituitary and/or adrenal disease.

Tests of mineralocorticoid suppressibility Mineralocorticoid suppression procedures have been devised using saline infusions, oral salt loading, or deoxycorticosterone administration for expansion of the extracellular fluid volume. With expansion of extracellular fluid volume, there is a decrease in renal renin release, a decrease in circulating plasma renin activity, and a decrease in aldosterone secretion and/or excretion. Various tests differ in the rate at which extracellular fluid volume is expanded. One convenient suppression test is the intravenous infusion of 500 mL normal saline solution per hour for 4 h, which normally suppresses plasma aldosterone levels to <220 pmol/L (<8 ng/dL) on a sodium-restricted diet or to 140 pmol/L (<5 ng/dL) on a normal sodium intake. This test should not be performed in potassium-depleted subjects.

TESTS OF PITUITARY-ADRENAL RESPONSIVENESS Stimuli such as insulin hypoglycemia, arginine vasopressin, and pyrogen, cause release of ACTH from the pituitary by an action on higher nerve centers, the hypothalamus, or the pituitary itself. By measuring plasma ACTH or plasma glucocorticoids the status of pituitary ACTH can be evaluated. Insulin-induced hypoglycemia is particularly useful, since the release of growth hormone and of ACTH is stimulated. In this test 0.05 to 0.1 unit of regular insulin per kilogram of body weight is administered intravenously as a bolus to reduce fasting glucose levels at least 50 percent below basal. The normal cortisol response is a rise to more than 500 nmol/L (18 μg/dL).

One of the best ways to test integrity of the pituitary-adrenal axis is the metyrapone test. Metyrapone is a drug that inhibits 11β-hydroxylase in the adrenal gland. As a result, the conversion of 11-deoxycortisol (compound S) to cortisol is interfered with, and increased amounts of 11-deoxycortisol accumulate while blood levels of cortisol decrease (Fig. 317-2). The hypothalamic-pituitary axis responds to the declining cortisol blood levels by releasing more ACTH. The metabolites of 11-deoxycortisol are excreted in increasing amounts in the urine, where they are measured as 17 hydroxycorticosteroids. Alternatively, changes in plasma 11-deoxycortisol levels can be measured. *Note that the adrenal glands must be capable of being stimulated by ACTH, since assessment of the response depends both on an intact hypothalamic-pituitary axis and on adrenal steroid production.*

While a number of modifications of the original metyrapone test have been described, we believe the best involves administering orally 750 mg of the drug every 4 h over a 24-h period and comparing the control and the post-metyrapone 17-hydroxysteroid excretion rates and/or plasma 11-deoxycortisol, cortisol, and ACTH levels. Normal individuals respond with at least a doubling of their basal 17-

hydroxysteroid excretion; 11-deoxycortisol levels in the blood should exceed 290 nmol/L (10 μg/dL) following metyrapone administration. The metyrapone test does not accurately reflect ACTH reserve if subjects are ingesting exogenous glucocorticoids or drugs that accelerate the metabolism of metyrapone (e.g., phenytoin).

A direct and selective test of the pituitary corticotrophs can be achieved with the investigational agent corticotropin-releasing hormone (CRH). The bolus injection of 1 μg per kilogram of body weight of ovine CRH stimulates ACTH and beta lipotropin secretion in normal human subjects within 60 to 180 min. However, the magnitude of the ACTH response is less than that produced by the insulin tolerance test, which implies that additional factors (such as vasopressin) augment stress-induced increases in ACTH secretion.

Although the rapid ACTH stimulation test reliably diagnoses primary adrenal insufficiency, normal cortisol responsiveness may be seen in a subset of patients with secondary adrenocortical insufficiency where there is a partial ACTH deficit and absence of adrenal atrophy. These patients have inadequate pituitary ACTH reserve and fail to increase ACTH secretion in response to stress such as surgery or hypoglycemia. Since a bolus of exogenous ACTH does not invariably exclude a diagnosis of secondary adrenocortical insufficiency, direct tests of pituitary ACTH reserve (metyrapone, insulin tolerance testing) should be used in the appropriate clinical setting. On the other hand, the rapid ACTH test can distinguish between primary and secondary adrenal insufficiency since aldosterone secretion is preserved in secondary adrenal failure by the renin-angiotensin system and potassium. Twenty-five units of cosyntropin is given intravenously or intramuscularly, and plasma cortisol and aldosterone levels are obtained before and 30 and 60 min later. Although the cortisol response is abnormal in both groups, patients with secondary insufficiency increase aldosterone levels above control by at least 140 pmol/L (5 ng/dL). No aldosterone response is seen in patients with primary adrenocortical insufficiency in whom the adrenal cortex is destroyed.

HYPERFUNCTION OF THE ADRENAL CORTEX

Distinct clinical syndromes are produced when excess adrenocortical hormones are secreted. Thus, excess production of cortisol is associated with Cushing's syndrome, excess production of aldosterone causes aldosteronism, and excess production of adrenal androgens causes adrenal virilism. These syndromes do not always occur in the "pure" form but may have overlapping features.

CUSHING'S SYNDROME Etiology Cushing described a syndrome characterized by truncal obesity, hypertension, fatigability and weakness, amenorrhea, hirsutism, purplish abdominal striae, edema, glucosuria, osteoporosis, and a basophilic tumor of the pituitary. As awareness of this syndrome increased, the diagnosis of Cushing's syndrome has been broadened into the classification shown in Table 317-3. Regardless of etiology, all cases of endogenous Cushing's syndrome are due to increased production of cortisol by the adrenal

TABLE 317-3 Causes of Cushing's syndrome

I Adrenal hyperplasia
  A Secondary to pituitary ACTH overproduction
    1 Pituitary-hypothalamic dysfunction
    2 Pituitary ACTH-producing micro- or macroadenomas
  B Secondary to ACTH or CRH-producing nonendocrine tumors (bronchogenic carcinoma, carcinoid of the thymus, pancreatic carcinoma, bronchial adenoma)
II Adrenal nodular hyperplasia
III Adrenal neoplasia
  A Adenoma
  B Carcinoma
IV Exogenous, iatrogenic causes
  A Prolonged use of glucocorticoids
  B Prolonged use of ACTH

gland. Most are due to *bilateral adrenal hyperplasia*; the cause may be adrenocortical stimulation due to hypersecretion of pituitary ACTH or the production of ACTH by nonendocrine tumors. The incidence of pituitary-dependent adrenal hyperplasia in women is three times that in men, with the most frequent age of onset being the third or fourth decade. The cause of the hypersecretion of pituitary ACTH is still debated. Some speculate that the primary defect is the de novo development of a pituitary adenoma since in some reports tumors are found in over 90 percent of patients with pituitary-dependent adrenal hyperplasia. Alternatively, the defect may reside in the hypothalamus or in higher nerve centers, leading to release of CRH inappropriate to the level of circulating cortisol. The consequence would be that a higher level of cortisol is required to reduce ACTH secretion to normal. This primary defect would lead to hyperstimulation of the pituitary resulting in hyperplasia or tumor formation. As the pituitary tumor grows, it may become independent of the regulating influence of central nervous system factors and/or circulating cortisol levels. In surgical series most individuals with hypersecretion of pituitary ACTH have a microadenoma (<10 mm) (50 percent are 5 mm or less in diameter), but a macroadenoma (>10 mm) of the pituitary or diffuse hyperplasia of the corticotropic cells (hypothalamic-pituitary dysfunction) may also be found. The common finding of a microadenoma in pituitary-dependent adrenal hyperplasia does not rule out dysregulation of hypothalamic CRH as the defect in Cushing's disease. Long-term follow-up to determine the rate of recurrence following successful surgical resection is necessary to answer this issue. Traditionally, only an individual who has an ACTH-producing pituitary tumor has been defined as having *Cushing's disease*. However, in many centers, anyone who has hypersecretion of pituitary ACTH regardless of whether a tumor is identified by radiographic procedures is classified as having Cushing's disease. In this chapter we will use the traditional definition, although these definitions may become less distinct as small tumors are more easily diagnosed by high resolution scanning.

Nonendocrine tumors may secrete polypeptides that are biologically, chemically, and immunologically indistinguishable from either ACTH or CRH and that cause bilateral adrenal hyperplasia (see also Chap. 309). The ectopic production of CRH results in clinical, biochemical, and radiologic features indistinguishable from those caused by hypersecretion of pituitary ACTH. Often, but not invariably, the typical signs and symptoms of Cushing's syndrome are absent with ectopic ACTH production, and hypokalemic alkalosis and glucose intolerance are the prominent manifestations. The majority of these cases are associated with the primitive small-cell (oat cell) type of bronchogenic carcinoma or with tumors of the thymus, pancreas, or ovary, medullary carcinoma of the thyroid, or bronchial adenomas. The onset of Cushing's syndrome may be sudden, particularly in patients with oat cell carcinoma of the lung, and this feature accounts in part for the failure of these patients to exhibit the classic physical findings. On the other hand, patients with carcinoid tumors or pheochromocytomas have longer clinical courses and usually exhibit the typical cushingoid features. The secretion of ACTH by nonendocrine tumors is also accompanied by the accumulation of ACTH fragments in plasma and by elevated plasma levels of ACTH precursor molecules. Since such tumors may produce large amounts of ACTH, baseline steroid values are usually markedly elevated, and increased skin pigmentation is usually present. Indeed, hyperpigmentation in patients with Cushing's syndrome almost always points to an extraadrenal tumor, either in an extracranial location or within the cranium.

Approximately 20 to 25 percent of patients with Cushing's syndrome have primary overproduction of cortisol and other adrenal steroids due to an adrenal neoplasm. These tumors are usually unilateral, and about half are malignant. Occasionally, patients have biochemical features both of hypersecretion of pituitary ACTH and of an adrenal adenoma. These individuals usually have micro- or macro-nodularity of both adrenal glands resulting in *nodular hyperplasia*. In some this may be a familial autoimmune disorder often seen in children and young adults (so-called pigmented multinodular cortical dysplasia).

The most common cause of Cushing's syndrome is *iatrogenic* administration of steroids for other reasons. While the clinical features bear some resemblance to those of individuals with an adrenal adenoma, these patients are usually readily distinguishable on the basis of history and initial laboratory studies.

Clinical signs, symptoms, and laboratory findings Many of the signs and symptoms of Cushing's syndrome logically follow from the known action of glucocorticoids (Table 317-4). As a result of mobilization of peripheral supportive tissue, muscle weakness and fatigability, osteoporosis, cutaneous striae, and easy bruisability result. The latter two signs are secondary to weakening and rupture of collagen fibers in the dermis. The osteoporosis may be so severe that collapse of vertebral bodies and pathologic fractures of other bones occur. Increased hepatic gluconeogenesis and insulin resistance can cause impaired glucose tolerance. Overt diabetes occurs in less than 20 percent of patients, probably in individuals with a familial predisposition to this disorder. Hypercortisolism promotes the deposition of adipose tissue in characteristic sites, notably in the upper part of the face, the typical "moon" facies; in the interscapular area, the "buffalo" hump; and in the mesenteric bed, where it produces the classic "truncal" obesity (Fig. 317-6). Rarely, there may be episternal fatty tumors and mediastinal widening secondary to fat accumulation. The reason for this peculiar distribution of adipose tissue is not known. The face appears plethoric, even in the absence of any increase in red blood cell concentration. Hypertension is common, and frequently there are profound emotional changes, ranging from irritability or emotional lability to severe depression, confusion, or even frank psychosis. In women, increased adrenal androgen secretion can cause acne, hirsutism, and oligomenorrhea or amenorrhea. The most common signs and symptoms in patients with hypercortisolism, i.e., obesity, hypertension, osteoporosis, and diabetes, are nonspecific and therefore less helpful in diagnosing this condition. On the other hand, easy bruising, typical striae, myopathy, and androgen effects (although less frequent) are, if present, more suggestive of Cushing's syndrome.

Except in iatrogenic Cushing's syndrome, plasma and urine cortisol and urinary 17-hydroxycorticosteroid levels are variably elevated. Occasionally, hypokalemia, hypochloremia, and metabolic alkalosis are present, particularly in individuals who have ectopic production of ACTH.

Diagnosis The diagnosis of Cushing's syndrome depends on the demonstration of increased cortisol production and the failure to suppress endogenous cortisol secretion normally when dexamethasone is administered. Once the diagnosis is established, further testing is designed to determine the etiology of the hypercortisolism (see Fig. 317-7 and Table 317-5).

For initial screening, the overnight dexamethasone suppression test is recommended (see above). In difficult cases (e.g., in obesity) measurement of a 24-h free cortisol excretion rate can also be used as a screening test. A level greater than 275 nmol/d (100 μg/d) is suggestive of Cushing's syndrome. The definitive diagnosis is then established by failure to suppress urinary cortisol to less than 80 nmol/d (30 μg/d), plasma cortisol to less than 140 nmol/L (5μg/dL), or 17 hydroxysteroid excretion to less than 8 μmol/d (3 mg/d) after a standard low-dose dexamethasone suppression test (0.5 mg every

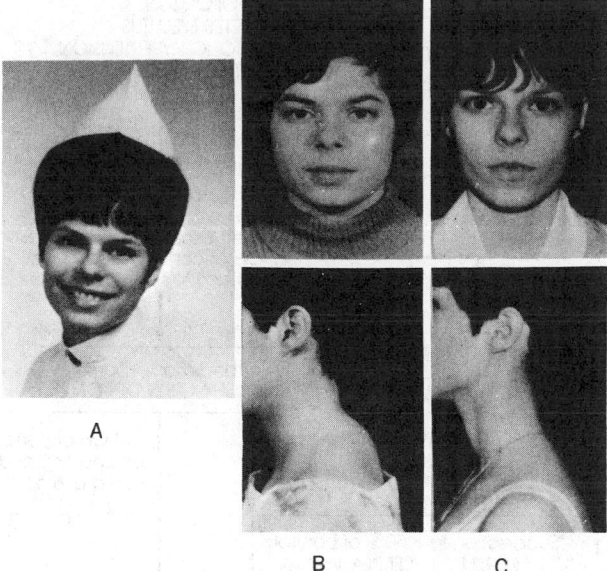

FIGURE 317-6 A 20-year-old woman with Cushing's syndrome due to a right adrenal cortical adenoma. *A.* Two years prior to surgery, age 18. *B.* One month prior to surgery, age 20. *C.* One year after surgery, age 21.

6 h for 48 h). Owing to diurnal variability, plasma cortisol and, to a certain extent, ACTH determinations are not meaningful when performed in isolation, but demonstration that the normal fall in P.M. levels of plasma corticoid does not occur may be useful.

Determining the etiology of Cushing's syndrome is complicated by the lack of specificity of all tests available and the spontaneous, sometimes clinical, changes in hormonal secretion, often dramatic, that may occur in the tumors producing this syndrome (periodic hormonogenesis). No test has a specificity greater than 95 percent, and it may be necessary to use a combination of tests to arrive at the correct diagnosis. A particularly useful first step is to determine the response of cortisol output to high-dose dexamethasone administration (2 mg every 6 h for 2 days). In most series, more than half of the patients so tested have a suppression of urine cortisol and/or 17-hydroxysteroid levels to less than 50 percent of basal values. These individuals usually have either an ACTH-secreting pituitary microadenoma or hypothalamic-pituitary dysfunction. Occasionally, in individuals with bilateral nodular hyperplasia and/or ectopic CRH production steroid output is also suppressed. Failure to suppress cortisol production after low- and high-dose dexamethasone administration (see Table 317-5) is usual in patients with adrenal hyperplasia secondary to an ACTH-secreting pituitary macroadenoma or ACTH-producing tumors of nonendocrine origin, and in adrenal neoplasms.

Theoretically, plasma ACTH levels should be useful in distinguishing the various causes of Cushing's syndrome, particularly in separating the ACTH-dependent from the ACTH-independent etiologies of the syndrome. In general, this is true for the ACTH-independent etiologies of the syndrome since most adrenal tumors have low or undetectable ACTH levels. Furthermore, ACTH-secreting pituitary macroadenomas and ACTH-producing nonendocrine tumors usually have elevated ACTH levels. In the ectopic ACTH syndrome, ACTH levels may be elevated above 110 pmol/L (500 pg/mL), with the majority above 40 pmol/L (200 pg/mL). In Cushing's syndrome, as the result of a microadenoma or pituitary hypothalamic dysfunction, ACTH levels range from 10 to 30 pmol/L (50 to 150 pg/mL) [normal <18 pmol/L (<80 pg/mL)], with half of values within the normal range. However, at least two problems hinder the utilization of ACTH levels in the differential diagnosis of Cushing's syndrome. First, reliable ACTH assays are still not widely available, and second, ACTH levels may be similar in individuals with hypothalamic-pituitary dysfunction, pituitary microadenomas, ectopic CRH pro-

TABLE 317-4 Incidence of signs and symptoms in Cushing's syndrome, percent			
Typical habitus	97	Amenorrhea	77
Increased body weight	94	Cutaneous striae	67
Fatigability and weakness	87	Personality changes	66
Hypertension		Ecchymoses	65
(>150/90)	82	Edema	62
		Polyuria, polydipsia	23
Hirsutism	80	Hypertrophy of clitoris	19

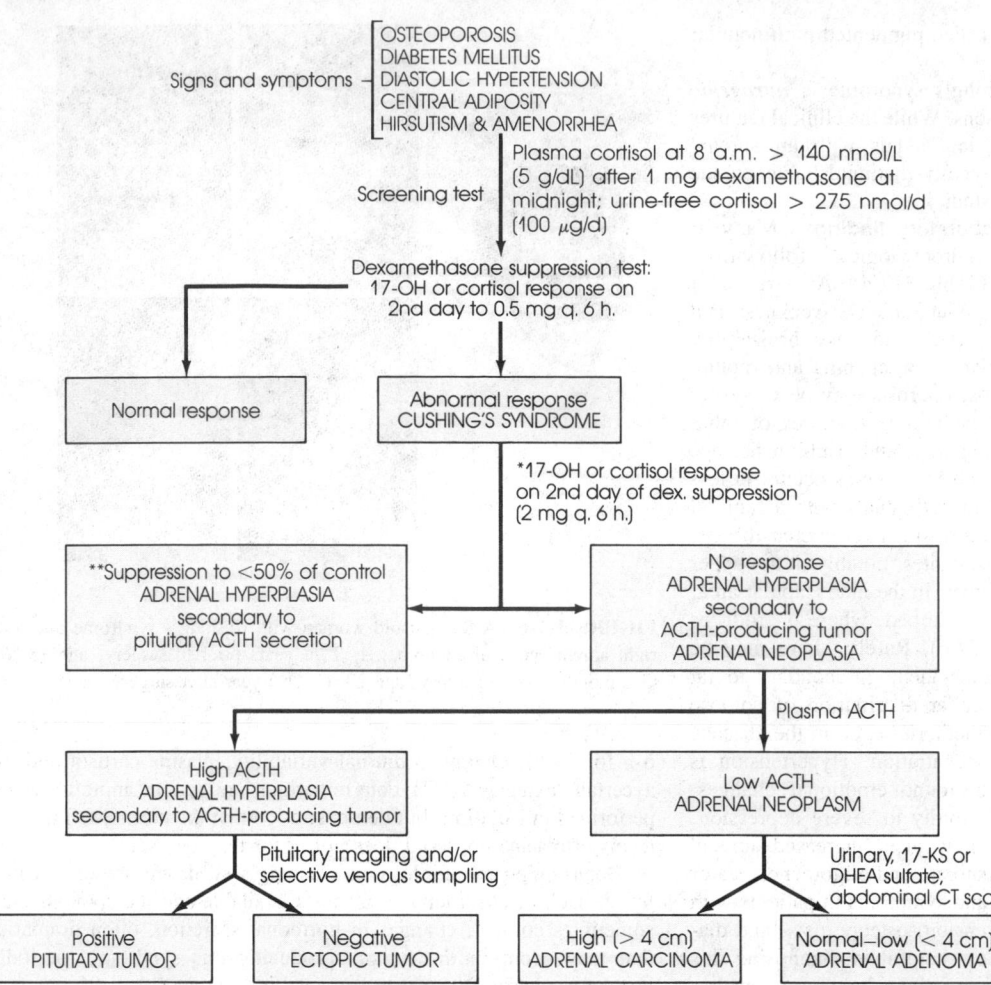

FIGURE 317-7 Diagnostic flow-chart for evaluating patients suspected of having Cushing's syndrome.

*The 17-hydroxycorticosteroid response to metyrapone (750 mg given orally every 4 h for six doses) may be used as an alternative test to the high-dose dexamethasone test (2 mg given orally every 6 h). Increased urinary 17-hydroxycorticosteroid excretion following metyrapone occurs in the majority of patients with adrenal hyperplasia secondary to pituitary ACTH secretion; no response suggests an adrenal neoplasm or adrenal hyperplasia secondary to a nonendocrine ACTH-producing tumor.

**This group of patients probably contains subjects with both pituitary-hypothalamic dysfunction and pituitary microadenomas. In some instances, a pituitary microadenoma may be visualized by CT scanning of the sella turcica.

duction, and ACTH production from some nonendocrine tumors (especially carcinoid tumors) (Table 317-5).

Because of these difficulties, several additional tests have been advocated, e.g., the metyrapone and the CRH infusion tests. The rationales underlying these tests are similar: Steroid hypersecretion secondary to an adrenal tumor or the ectopic production of ACTH will suppress the hypothalamic-pituitary axis so that inhibition of pituitary ACTH release can be demonstrated by either test. Thus, most patients with pituitary-hypothalamic dysfunction and/or a microadenoma have an increase in steroid or ACTH secretion in response to metyrapone and CRH administration while most ectopic ACTH-producing tumors and adrenal tumors will not. Most pituitary macroadenomas also respond to CRH, while their response to metyrapone

is variable. The utility of the CRH infusion test, however, is uncertain since only a limited number of studies have been performed and since CRH is not commonly available for testing. In addition, false-positive and -negative CRH tests in patients with nonendocrine and pituitary tumors have been reported.

The major diagnostic dilemma in Cushing's syndrome is to distinguish between those individuals with microadenoma of the pituitary and/or pituitary hypothalamic dysfunction from some paraendocrine tumors (e.g., carcinoids or pheochromocytoma) that ectopically produced CRH and/or ACTH. Clinical manifestations are similar unless the ectopic tumor produces other symptoms, such as diarrhea and flushing from a carcinoid tumor or episodic hypertension from a pheochromocytoma. Sometimes one can distinguish between ectopic and pituitary ACTH production by using metyrapone or CRH tests as noted above. In these situations computed tomography (CT) scan of the pituitary gland is usually within normal limits. Magnetic resonance imaging (MRI) with the enhancing agent gadolinium may be superior to CT scanning in demonstrating a pituitary microadenoma in some patients with Cushing's disease. However, finding a structural feature consistent with an adenoma does not prove that the lesion is secreting ACTH. In fact, as the resolution of scanners becomes greater more variations of the normal pituitary anatomy will be imaged. For this reason selective venous sampling for ACTH is employed in some centers. Demonstration of a gradient between ACTH level in the petrosal sinus and in peripheral blood localizes the source of ACTH overproduction to the pituitary gland but does not distinguish pituitary dependent adrenal hyperplasia from pituitary hyperplasia secondary to a tumor producing CRH. No reliable test is available to make this distinction if the ectopic tumor is not seen or if it produces no other hormones.

The diagnosis of *cortisol-producing adrenal adenoma* is suggested by disproprotionate elevations in baseline urine 17-hydroxycortico-

TABLE 317-5 **Diagnostic tests to determine the type of Cushing's syndrome**

Test	Pituitary macroadenoma	Pituitary-hypothalamic dysfunction or microadenoma	Ectopic ACTH or CRH production	Adrenal tumor
Measurement of plasma ACTH	↑ to ↑↑	N to ↑	↑ to ↑↑↑	↓
Response to high-dose dexamethasone, %	<10	>80	<10	<10
Response to metyrapone, %	>80	>90	<10	<10
Response to CRH, %	>90	>90	<10	<10

NOTE: N, normal; ↑, elevated; ↓, decreased.

steroid or free-cortisol levels with only modest rises or suppression of urinary 17-ketosteroids or plasma DHEA sulfate. Adrenal androgen secretion is usually reduced in these patients owing to the cortisol-induced suppression of ACTH and subsequent involution of the androgen-producing zona reticularis.

The diagnosis of *adrenal carcinoma* is suggested by a palpable abdominal mass and by *markedly* elevated baseline values *both* of urine 17-hydroxysteroids and of plasma DHEA sulfate. Plasma and urine cortisol levels are variably elevated. Adrenal carcinoma is usually resistant to both ACTH stimulation and dexamethasone suppression. Markedly elevated adrenal androgen secretion often leads to virilization in the female. Feminizing estrogen-producing adrenocortical carcinoma in the male usually presents with gynecomastia. These adrenal tumors secrete increased amounts of androstenedione which is peripherally converted to the estrogens, estrone and estradiol (see Chap. 323). Functioning adrenal carcinoma that produce Cushing's syndrome are most often associated with elevated values for the intermediates of steroid biosynthesis (especially 11-deoxycortisol), suggesting inefficient conversion of the intermediates to the final product. Approximately 20 percent of adrenal carcinomas are not associated with endocrine syndromes and are presumed to be nonfunctioning or to produce biologically inactive steroid precursors. In addition, the excessive production of gonadal steroids is not detectable in certain situations (e.g., androgens in adult men).

Differential diagnosis PSEUDOCUSHING'S SYNDROME A variety of groups may present problems in diagnosis; these are patients with obesity, chronic alcoholism, depression, and acute illness of any type. Extreme *obesity* is uncommon in Cushing's syndrome; furthermore, with exogenous obesity, the adiposity is generalized, not truncal. On adrenocortical testing, abnormalities in patients with exogenous obesity are usually modest. Basal urine steroid excretion levels in obese patients are either normal or slightly elevated, a finding similar to their cortisol secretory values. Some patients have elevated conversion of secreted cortisol into excreted metabolites. *Urinary* and *blood cortisol* levels are normal, and the diurnal pattern in blood and urine levels is normal. Patients with *chronic alcoholism* and *depression* share similar abnormalities in steroid output: elevated urinary 17-hydroxysteroids, absent diurnal rhythm of cortisol levels, and resistance to suppression with dexamethasone (particularly overnight and low dose). In contrast to alcoholic subjects, depressed patients do not have clinical signs and symptoms of Cushing's syndrome. Following discontinuation of alcohol and/or improvement of the emotional status, steroid testing usually returns to normal. A normal cortisol response to insulin-induced hypoglycemia may distinguish these patients from subjects with Cushing's syndrome. *Acutely ill* subjects often have abnormal laboratory tests and fail to suppress with dexamethasone since major stress (such as pain or fever) interrupts the normal regulation of ACTH secretion. *Iatrogenic Cushing's syndrome*, induced by the administration of potent synthetic glucocorticoids, is indistinguishable by physical findings from endogenous adrenocortical hyperfunction. This situation can be distinguished by measuring blood or urine cortisol levels or urinary 17-hydroxysteroid excretion in a basal state where the levels are low secondary to suppression of the pituitary-adrenal axis. The severity of iatrogenic Cushing's syndrome is related to the total steroid dose, to the biologic half-life of the steroid preparation, and to the duration of therapy. Also, individuals on afternoon and evening doses of steroid develop Cushing's syndrome more readily and on smaller total daily steroid doses than do patients on a steroid program limited to morning doses only. The enzymatic disposition and binding of administered steroids also differ among patients.

Radiologic evaluation for Cushing's syndrome The preferred radiologic study to visualize the adrenals is CT scan of the abdomen (Fig. 317-8). This procedure has largely replaced previous invasive procedures (such as selective adrenal arteriography and venography) and 19-[131I]iodocholesterol scanning; the CT scan is of value both in localizing adrenal tumors and in differentiating them from bilateral hyperplasia. All patients believed to have hypersecretion of pituitary

ACTH should have a pituitary MRI scan with the contrast agent gadolinium (if available) to establish whether a pituitary tumor is present. Even with this technique small microadenomas may be undetectable; alternatively, false-positive masses due to nonsecretory, variations of the normal pituitary anatomy may be imaged.

Evaluation of asymptomatic adrenal masses With abdominal CT scanning, many incidental adrenal masses are discovered. This is not surprising, since 10 to 20 percent of subjects at autopsy have adrenal cortical adenomas. The first step in evaluating such patients is to determine if the tumor is functioning by appropriate screening tests. However, in 90 percent of the cases tumors detected incidentally at the time of abdominal CT scanning are nonfunctioning. Fortunately, they also are seldom malignant. Yet, nonfunctioning tumors raise difficult therapeutic questions. Since 20 percent of adrenal carcinomas are nonfunctioning, one could argue that all such lesions should be removed. However, the frequency of adrenal carcinomas is low compared with the frequency of benign cortical adenomas (less than 1 percent), and surgery is not indicated in most cases. The size of the tumor sometimes is of value: Adrenal carcinomas are rarely smaller than 3 cm in diameter, and adrenal adenomas are usually smaller than 6 cm (Fig. 317-8). If surgery is not performed, a repeat CT scan in 3 to 6 months is usually required for followup.

Therapy ADRENAL NEOPLASMS When an adenoma or carcinoma is diagnosed, adrenal exploration is performed with excision of the tumor. Because of the possible atrophy of the contralateral adrenal, the patient is treated pre- and postoperatively as if for total adrenalectomy even when a unilateral lesion is suspected, the routine being similar to that for an Addisonian patient undergoing elective surgery (Table 317-11).

Despite operative intervention, most patients with adrenal carcinoma die within 3 years of diagnosis. Metastases occur most often to liver and lung. The principal antitumor drug used to treat metastatic adrenocortical carcinoma is mitotane (*o,p'*-DDD), an isomer of the insecticide DDT. This drug suppresses cortisol production and decreases plasma and urine steroid levels. Although its cytotoxic action is relatively selective for the glucocorticoid-secreting zone of the adrenal cortex, the zona glomerulosa may also be inhibited. Because mitotane also alters the extraadrenal metabolism of cortisol, plasma and urinary cortisol levels must be assessed to titrate the effect. The drug is usually given in divided doses three to four times a day, with the dose increased gradually to 8 to 10 g daily. Almost all patients experience gastrointestinal side effects (anorexia, diarrhea, or vomiting) or neuromuscular side effects (lethargy, somnolence, or dizziness). All patients treated with mitotane should be placed on long-term maintenance glucocorticoid therapy, and in some mineralocorticoid replacement is appropriate. In approximately one-third of patients regression of both tumor and metastases occurs, but long-term survival is limited. In many patients, mitotane only inhibits steroidogenesis and does not cause regression of tumor metastases. Osseous metastases are usually refractory to the drug and should be treated with radiation therapy. Mitotane can also be given as adjunctive therapy after surgical resection of an adrenal carcinoma.

BILATERAL HYPERPLASIA Patients with hyperplasia have a relative or absolute increase in ACTH levels. Since therapy would logically be directed at reducing ACTH levels, the ideal primary treatment for ACTH- or CRH-producing tumors, whether in the pituitary or ectopic, is surgical removal. Occasionally, this is not possible because the disease, particularly with ectopic ACTH production, is often far advanced. In this situation "medical" or surgical adrenalectomy may be indicated to correct the hypercortisolism.

Controversy exists as to the proper treatment for bilateral adrenal hyperplasia when the source of the ACTH overproduction is not apparent. In some centers, these patients (especially patients with a positive high-dose dexamethasone suppression test) have surgical exploration of the pituitary via a transsphenoidal approach in anticipation of a microadenoma being found. These explorations prove fruitful in between 20 and 70 percent of the cases, depending on the skill of the surgeon and the ability of the radiologist to localize the

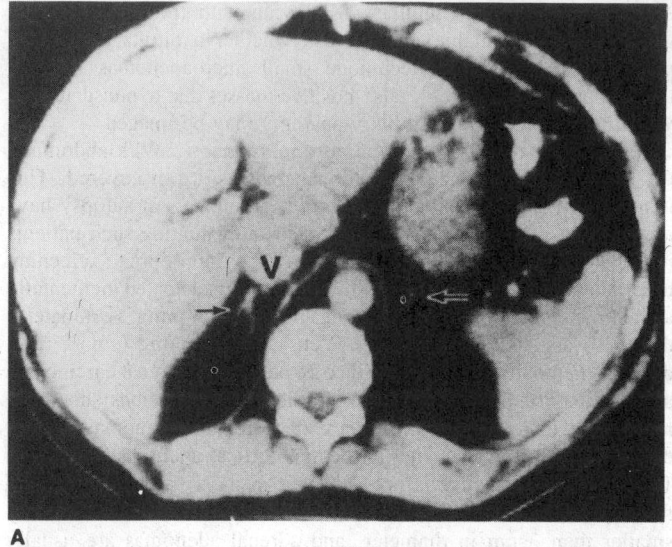

A

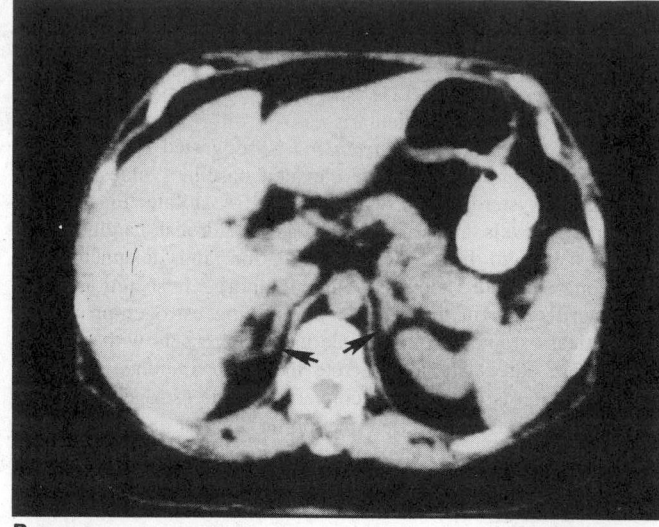

B

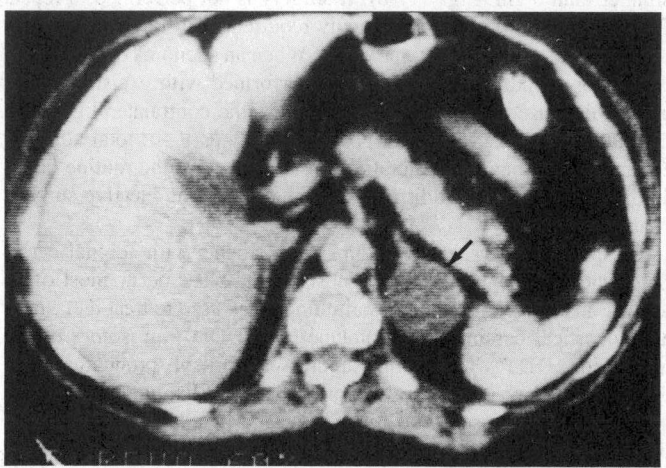

C

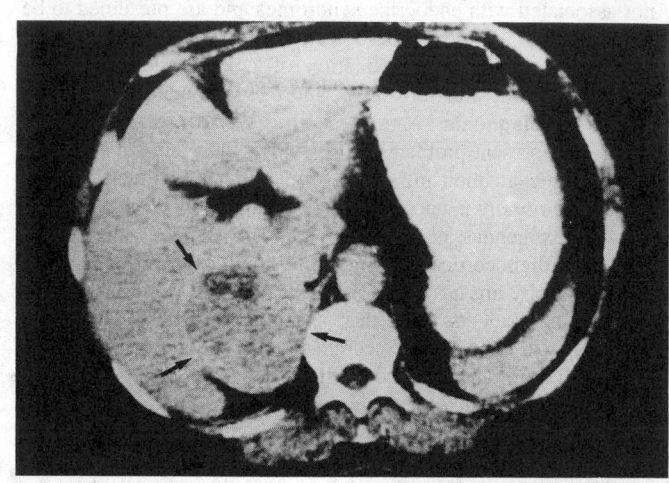

D

FIGURE 317-8 Computed tomography is the preferred method for visualizing the adrenal glands. The adrenal glands are indicated by arrows. *A.* The normal right adrenal gland is adjacent to the inferior vena cava (V) as it emerges from the liver. Approximately 90 percent of the right adrenal glands appear as linear structures extending posteriorly from the inferior vena cava into the space between the right lobe of the liver and the crus of the diaphragm. The normal left adrenal gland is lateral to the left crus of the diaphragm and below the stomach. The majority of left adrenal glands are shaped like an inverted "V" or "Y." *B.* Adrenal CT scan of a patient with ectopic ACTH production. Both adrenal glands (arrows) are enlarged (compare with A). In contrast, only 50 percent of patients with bilateral adrenal hyperplasia secondary to pituitary ACTH hypersecretion show enlargement of the adrenals when imaged by CT scan. *C.* CT scan of a patient with Cushing's syndrome with biochemical evidence only of cortisol overproduction. The left adrenal has been replaced by a racquet-shaped 2-cm tumor (arrow). Attenuation of the tumor is low because of its high lipid content. *D.* CT scan in a patient with Cushing's syndrome and biochemical evidence of an adrenal carcinoma. In contrast to *C*, the right-sided mass has a heterogeneous appearance and is larger in size—usual characteristics of an adrenal carcinoma.

microadenoma preoperatively. In equivocal circumstances selective venous sampling may be performed, or the patient may be referred to an appropriate center if the procedure is not locally available. In the event that a microadenoma is not found at the time of exploration, total hypophysectomy may be needed. Complications of transsphenoidal surgery include cerebrospinal fluid rhinorrhea, diabetes insipidus, panhypopituitarism, and optic or cranial nerve injuries. Furthermore, these pituitary neoplasms may recur if the primary abnormality actually resides in the hypothalamus.

In other centers, total adrenalectomy is the treatment of choice. Cure with this procedure is close to 100 percent. The adverse effects include the certain need for lifelong mineralocorticoid and glucocorticoid replacement therapy and a 10 to 20 percent probability of a pituitary tumor developing over the next 10 years, many requiring surgical therapy (Nelson's syndrome). It is uncertain whether in these individuals (see Chap. 313) the tumor develops de novo or is present prior to bilateral adrenalectomy but is so small that it is not detected by radiologic procedures. Periodic radiologic evaluation of the pituitary gland by CT scanning and serial ACTH levels should be obtained in any individual who has undergone bilateral adrenalectomy for Cushing's syndrome. Often, such pituitary tumors become locally invasive and impinge on the optic chiasm or extend into the cavernous or sphenoid sinuses. Thus, an aggressive surgical approach is often followed by postoperative irradiation.

In a few centers, pituitary irradiation is the primary treatment for pituitary ACTH overproduction, with the use of either conventional external or alpha (proton beam) radiation. The latter, while more effective, has a greater incidence of ocular motor palsy and hypopituitarism than does conventional radiation therapy. The long lag time between treatment and remission and the fact that the remission rate is less than 50 percent often contraindicate the use of external pituitary radiation in the presence of rapidly progressive or severe Cushing's syndrome.

Finally, in occasional patients in whom a surgical approach is not feasible, medical therapy directed at reducing hypothalamic CRH release either by administering the serotonin antagonist cyproheptadine or by administering an inhibitor of GABA transaminase, sodium valproate, has been successful in reducing cortisol secretion. Bromocriptine, a dopaminergic agonist, also suppresses ACTH output in occasional patients.

If ACTH levels cannot be successfully lowered by any of the above treatment modalities, then medical or surgical adrenalectomy may be indicated (Table 317-6). Inhibition of steroidogenesis may also be indicated in severely cushingoid subjects prior to surgical intervention. Chemical adrenalectomy may be accomplished by the administration of the inhibitor of steroidogenesis, ketoconazole (600 to 1200 mg/d). In addition, mitotane (2 or 3 g/d) and/or the blockers of steroid synthesis aminoglutethimide (1 g/d) and metyrapone (2 or 3 g/d) have been effective either singularly or in combination. Mitotane is slow in onset of action (over weeks). Hypoadrenalism is a risk with all these agents, and replacement steroids may be required.

ALDOSTERONISM Aldosteronism is a syndrome associated with hypersecretion of the major adrenal mineralocorticoid, aldosterone. *Primary* aldosteronism signifies that the stimulus for the excessive aldosterone production resides within the adrenal gland; in *secondary* aldosteronism the stimulus is extraadrenal.

Primary aldosteronism In the original case of excessive and inappropriate aldosterone production, the disease was the result of an *aldosterone-producing adrenal adenoma* (Conn's syndrome). The majority of cases involved a unilateral adenoma, usually small and occurring with equal frequency on either side. Rarely, primary aldosteronism occurs in association with adrenal carcinoma. It is twice as common in women as in men, occurs between the ages of 30 and 50, and is present in approximately 1 percent of unselected hypertensive patients. Many cases have clinical and biochemical features characteristic of primary aldosteronism, but a solitary adenoma is not found at surgery. Instead, these patients have *bilateral cortical nodular hyperplasia*. In the literature this disease has been alternatively termed "pseudo" primary aldosteronism, idiopathic hyperaldosteronism, or nodular hyperplasia. The cause is unknown.

SIGNS AND SYMPTOMS The continual hypersecretion of aldosterone increases the renal distal tubular exchange of intratubular sodium for secreted potassium and hydrogen ions, with progressive depletion of body potassium and development of hypokalemia. Most patients have diastolic hypertension, usually not of marked severity, and complain of headaches. The hypertension is probably due to the increased sodium reabsorption and extracellular volume expansion. Potassium depletion is responsible for the muscle weakness and fatigue and is related to the effect of potassium depletion on muscle membrane. The polyuria results from impairment of concentrating ability and is often associated with polydipsia. Electrocardiographic and roentgenographic signs of left ventricular enlargement are secondary to the hypertension. Electrocardiographic signs of potassium depletion, such as prominent U waves, cardiac arrhythmias, and premature contractions, are common. In the absence of associated congestive heart failure, renal disease, or preexisting abnormalities (such as thrombophlebitis), edema is characteristically absent. In cases of long duration, nephropathy with azotemia may be associated with congestive heart failure and edema.

LABORATORY FINDINGS Laboratory findings are dependent on both the duration and the severity of the potassium depletion. An

TABLE 317-6 Treatment modalities for patients with adrenal hyperplasia secondary to pituitary ACTH hypersecretion

I Reduce pituitary ACTH production
  A Transsphenoidal resection of microadenoma
  B Radiation
  C Treatment with hypothalamic serotonin antagonist (cyproheptadine) or GABA-transaminase inhibitor (sodium valproate)*
II Reduce or eliminate adrenocortical cortisol secretion
  A Bilateral adrenalectomy
  B Medical adrenalectomy (metyrapone, mitotane, aminoglutethimide, ketoconazole)*

* Not curative but effective as long as chronically administered in selected patients.

overnight concentration test often reveals impaired ability to concentrate the urine, probably secondary to the hypokalemia. Urine pH is neutral to alkaline, because of excessive secretion of ammonium and bicarbonate ions to compensate for a metabolic alkalosis. Tests of glucocorticoid and androgen secretion are within the normal range.

Hypokalemia may be severe (less than 3 mmol/L) and reflects significant body potassium depletion, usually in excess of 300 mmol. *Hypernatremia* is due to both sodium retention and a concomitant water loss from polyuria. Metabolic alkalosis and elevation of serum bicarbonate are a result of hydrogen ion loss into the urine and migration into potassium-depleted cells. The alkalosis is perpetuated by potassium deficiency, which increases the capacity of the proximal convoluted tubule to reabsorb filtered bicarbonate. If hypokalemia is severe, serum magnesium levels are also reduced. In the absence of azotemia, serum uric acid is normal.

Total body sodium content and total exchangeable sodium are increased, while total exchangeable body potassium is usually reduced. The expanded extracellular fluid volume may be responsible for the reversed diurnal excretory pattern for salt and water, with predominant salt and water excretion occurring during the night.

DIAGNOSIS The diagnosis is suggested by persistent hypokalemia in a nonedematous patient on a normal sodium intake who is not receiving potassium-wasting diuretics (furosemide, ethacrynic acid, thiazides). If hypokalemia occurs in a hypertensive patient on a potassium-wasting diuretic, the diuretic should be discontinued and the patient should be given potassium supplements. After 1 to 2 weeks the potassium level should be remeasured, and if hypokalemia persists, the patient should be evaluated for a mineralocorticoid excess syndrome (Fig. 317-9).

The criteria for the diagnosis of primary aldosteronism are (1) diastolic hypertension without edema, (2) hyposecretion of renin (as judged by low plasma renin activity levels) that fails to increase appropriately during volume depletion (upright posture, sodium depletion), and (3) hypersecretion of aldosterone that fails to suppress appropriately during volume expansion (salt loading).

Patients with primary aldosteronism characteristically *do not have edema,* since they exhibit an "escape" phenomenon from the sodium-retaining aspects of mineralocorticoids. Rarely, pretibial edema may be present in patients with associated nephropathy and azotemia.

The estimation of plasma renin activity is of limited value in separating patients with primary aldosteronism from those with other causes of hypertension. While the failure of plasma renin activity to rise normally during volume-depletion maneuvers is a criterion for primary aldosteronism, suppressed renin activity also occurs in about 25 percent of patients with essential hypertension.

Since the determination of plasma renin responsiveness is not sufficient, the demonstration of lack of suppression of aldosterone secretion is necessary to diagnose primary aldosteronism (Fig. 317-9). The autonomy exhibited by aldosterone tumors in these patients refers only to the resistance to suppression of secretion during volume expansion; such tumors can and do respond in normal or above normal fashion to the stimuli of potassium loading or ACTH infusion.

Once hyposecretion of renin and failure to suppress aldosterone secretion are demonstrated, localization of aldosterone-producing adenomas should be determined preoperatively by abdominal CT scan or by percutaneous transfemoral bilateral adrenal vein catheterization with simultaneous adrenal venography. The latter technique permits radiologic localization, and, in addition, the adrenal vein sampling may demonstrate a two- to threefold increase in plasma aldosterone concentration on the involved side compared with the uninvolved side. In cases of hyperaldosteronism secondary to cortical nodular hyperplasia, no localization is found. It is important for samples to be obtained simultaneously if possible and for cortisol levels to be measured to ensure that false localization does not reflect an ACTH- or stress-induced rise in aldosterone levels.

DIFFERENTIAL DIAGNOSIS Patients with hypertension and hypokalemia may have primary or secondary hyperaldosteronism (see Fig. 317-10). A useful maneuver to distinguish between them is the

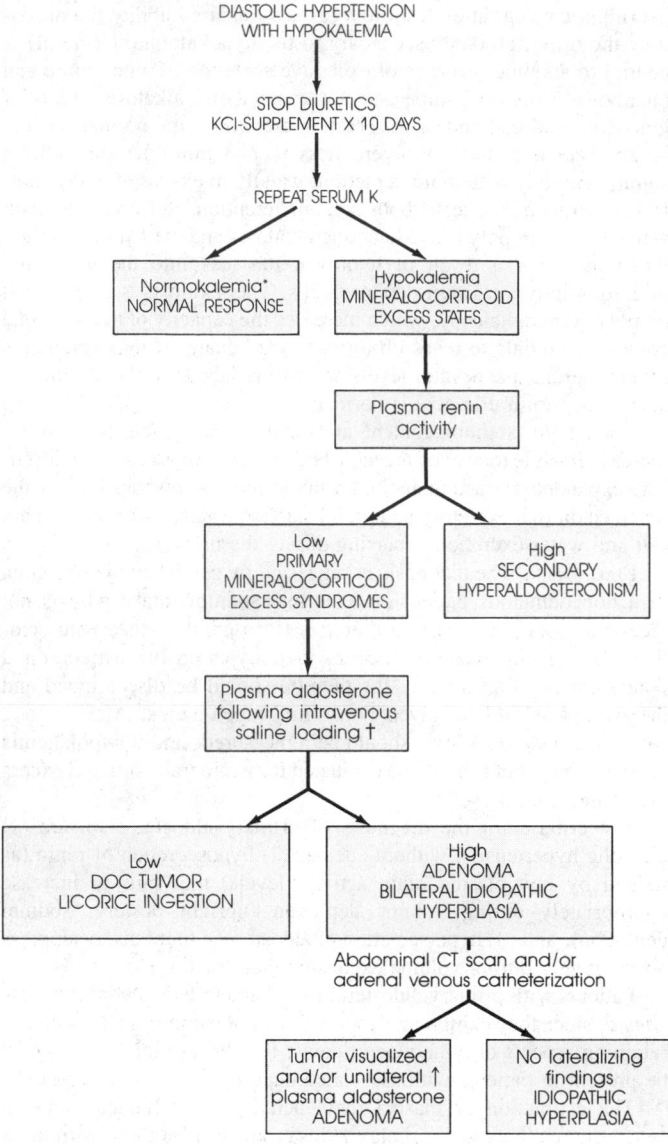

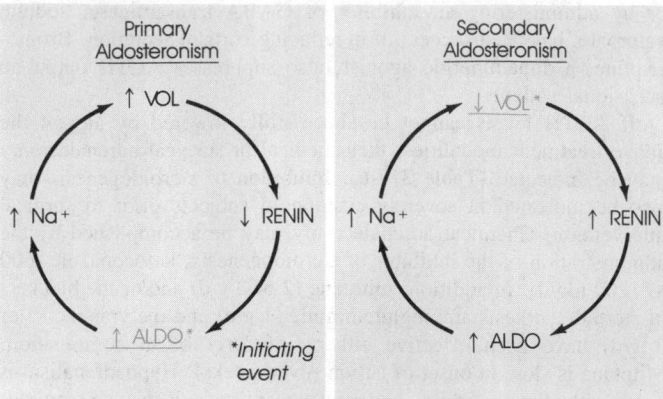

FIGURE 317-10 Responses of the renin-aldosterone volume control loop in primary versus secondary aldosteronism.

FIGURE 317-9 Diagnostic flowchart for evaluating patients with suspected primary aldosteronism.

*Serum K⁺ may be normal in some patients with hyperaldosteronism who are taking potassium-sparing diuretics (spironolactone, triamterene) or ingesting low sodium–high potassium intakes.

†This step should not be taken if hypertension is severe (diastolic pressure >115 mmHg) or if cardiac failure is present. Also, serum potassium levels should be corrected before the infusion of saline solution. Alternative methods producing comparable suppression of aldosterone secretion include oral sodium loading (200 mmol/d for 3 days) or 10 mg deoxycorticosterone acetate (DOCA) intramuscularly every 12 h for 3 days.

measurement of plasma renin activity. Secondary hyperaldosteronism in patients with accelerated hypertension is due to elevated plasma renin levels; in contrast, patients with primary aldosteronism have suppressed plasma renin levels.

Primary aldosteronism must also be distinguished from other *hypermineralocorticoid states.* The common problem is to distinguish between hyperaldosteronism due to an adenoma and that due to idiopathic bilateral nodular hyperplasia. This is of importance, since hypertension associated with idiopathic hyperplasia is usually not benefited by bilateral adrenalectomy, whereas hypertension associated with aldosterone-producing tumors is usually improved or cured following removal of the adenoma. Although patients with idiopathic bilateral nodular hyperplasia tend to have less severe hypokalemia, lower aldosterone secretion, and higher plasma renin activity than do

patients with primary aldosteronism, differentiation is impossible solely on clinical and/or biochemical grounds. An anomalous postural decrease in plasma aldosterone and elevated plasma 18-hydroxycorticosterone levels are present in the majority of patients with a unilateral lesion, but these tests are also of limited diagnostic value in the individual patient. A definitive diagnosis is best made by radiographic studies as noted above.

In a few instances, hypertensive patients with hypokalemic alkalosis have been found to have deoxycorticosterone (DOC)-secreting adenomas. Such patients have reduced plasma renin activity levels, but aldosterone measurements are either normal or reduced, suggesting the diagnosis of mineralocorticoid excess due to a hormone other than aldosterone. Rarely, hypermineralocorticoidism is due to a defect in cortisol biosynthesis, specifically 11- or 17-hydroxylation. ACTH levels are increased, with a resultant increase in the production of the mineralocorticoid 11-deoxycorticosterone. *Hypertension and hypokalemia can be corrected by glucocorticoid administration.* The definitive diagnosis is made by demonstrating an elevation of precursors of cortisol biosynthesis in the blood or urine. Occasionally, glucocorticoid administration produces normotension and normokalemia although a hydroxylase deficiency cannot be identified (Fig. 317-9). These patients have normal to slightly elevated aldosterone levels that do not fully suppress with saline but suppress after 2 to 8 weeks of dexamethasone (1 to 2 mg/d). The condition is familial and is termed *glucocorticoid suppressible hyperaldosteronism.*

Another rare cause of hyperkalemia and hypertension is 11 β-hydroxysteroid dehydrogenase deficiency in which cortisol cannot be converted to cortisone and hence binds to the mineralocorticoid type I receptor and acts as a mineralocorticoid (see Chap. 311). The ingestion of candies or chewing tobacco containing certain forms of licorice produces a syndrome mimicking primary aldosteronism. The sodium-retaining principle in such agent is glycyrrhizinic acid, which inhibits the 11 β-hydroxysteroid dehydrogenase and hence allows cortisol to act as a mineralocorticoid and causes sodium retention, expansion of the extracellular fluid volume, hypertension, depressed plasma renin levels, and suppressed aldosterone levels. The diagnosis is established or excluded by a careful history.

TREATMENT Primary aldosteronism due to an adenoma is usually treated by surgical excision. However, dietary sodium restriction and the administration of an aldosterone antagonist, spironolactone, are effective in many cases. Hypertension and hypokalemia are usually controlled by doses of 25 to 100 mg spironolactone every 8 h. Some patients have been successfully managed medically for years, but chronic therapy in men is usually limited by the development of gynecomastia, decreased libido, and impotence.

When bilateral hyperplasia is suspected, surgery is indicated only when significant, symptomatic hypokalemia cannot be controlled with medical therapy, e.g., by spironolactone, triamterene, or amiloride.

Dexamethasone, 1 mg every 12 h, may be tried for 4 to 6 weeks before surgery to rule out glucocorticoid-suppressible hyperaldosteronism. Hypertension associated with idiopathic hyperplasia is usually not benefited by bilateral adrenalectomy.

Secondary aldosteronism Secondary aldosteronism refers to an appropriately increased production of aldosterone in response to activation of the renin-angiotensin system (Fig. 317-10). The production rates of aldosterone are often higher in patients with secondary aldosteronism than in those with primary aldosteronism. Secondary aldosteronism usually occurs in association with the accelerated phase of hypertension or on the basis of an underlying edema disorder. Secondary aldosteronism in pregnancy is a normal physiologic response to estrogen-induced increases in circulating levels of renin substrate and plasma renin activity and to the antialdosterone actions of progestogens.

Secondary aldosteronism in hypertensive states either is secondary to a primary overproduction of renin (primary reninism) or is caused by an overproduction of renin which is secondary to a decrease in renal blood flow and/or perfusion pressure (Fig. 317-5). Secondary hypersecretion of renin can be due to a narrowing of one or both of the major renal arteries either by an atherosclerotic plaque or by fibromuscular hyperplasia. Overproduction of renin from both kidneys also occurs in association with severe arteriolar nephrosclerosis (malignant hypertension) or secondary to profound renal vasoconstriction (accelerated phase of hypertensive disease). The secondary aldosteronism is characterized by hypokalemic alkalosis, moderate to severe increases in plasma renin activity, and moderate to marked increases in aldosterone levels (see Chap. 196).

Secondary aldosteronism with hypertension can also be caused by a rare renin-producing tumor, in so-called primary reninism. These patients have the biochemical characteristics of renal vascular hypertension; however, the primary defect is renin secretion by a juxtaglomerular-cell tumor. The diagnosis can be made by the absence of changes in renal vasculature and/or demonstration of a space-occupying lesion in the kidney by radiographic techniques and documentation of unilateral increases in renal vein renin activity.

Secondary aldosteronism is present in many forms of *edema*. Increased aldosterone secretion rates are usual in patients with edema as a result of either cirrhosis or the nephrotic syndrome. In congestive heart failure, elevated aldosterone secretion varies depending on the severity of cardiac decompensation. The stimulus for aldosterone release in these conditions appears to be *arterial hypovolemia* and/or hypotension. Diuretic therapy often exaggerates the secondary aldosteronism via volume depletion; when this happens hypokalemia and on occasion alkalosis can become prominent features.

Secondary hyperaldosteronism rarely occurs without edema or hypertension (Bartter's syndrome). This syndrome is characterized by the signs of severe hyperaldosteronism (hypokalemic alkalosis) with moderate to marked increases in renin activity but normal blood pressure and absence of edema. Renal biopsy shows juxtaglomerular hyperplasia. The pathogenesis may be a defect in the renal conservation of sodium or chloride and/or an increased production of prostaglandins. The renal loss of sodium is thought to stimulate renin secretion and subsequent aldosterone production. Hyperaldosteronism produces potassium depletion, with the hypokalemia further elevating plasma renin activity. In some cases, the hypokalemia may be potentiated by a defect in renal conservation of potassium. Increased production of prostaglandins is present but is probably not a primary abnormality as administration of inhibitors of prostaglandin synthesis only temporarily reverses the features of this syndrome (see Chap. 231).

SYNDROMES OF ADRENAL ANDROGEN EXCESS The syndromes of adrenal androgen excess result from excess production of dehydroepiandrosterone and androstenedione, which are converted to testosterone in extraglandular tissues; the elevated testosterone levels account for most of the androgenic effects. Adrenal androgen excess may be associated with the secretion of greater or smaller amounts of other adrenal hormones and may, therefore, present as "pure"

syndromes of virilization or as "mixed" syndromes associated with excessive production of glucocorticoids and some characteristics of Cushing's syndrome.

Clinical signs and symptoms The signs and symptoms of androgen excess can be divided into four areas: hirsutism, oligomenorrhea, acne, and virilization. Clinically, it is important to distinguish between simple hirsutism and hirsutism associated with virilization. In most cases of simple hirsutism, there is no known cause for the increased hair growth. On the other hand, if the patient is virilized as well as hirsute, increased levels of androgens are usually present (see Chap. 54). In general, the degree of virilization reflects both the duration and the degree of excess androgen secretion, although significant virilization can result from minimal changes in testosterone production, and a significant increase in testosterone production may be associated with minimal signs of virilization. The occurrence of oligomenorrhea in a hirsute patient increases the probability that an excess secretion of androgens will be found. Thus, the evaluation of the hirsute patient should include a careful history of the onset of menarche, past and present menstrual history, and reproductive capacity and a careful physical examination for signs and symptoms of androgen excess.

Etiology As in other states of adrenocortical hyperfunction, the syndromes associated with androgen excess may result from hyperplasia, adenoma, or carcinoma (the latter two having been discussed above). Adrenal androgen overproduction may also arise from *congenital adrenal hyperplasia*, owing to enzymatic defects. In these patients, increased adrenal androgen production is associated either with excess or decreased secretion of mineralocorticoids or decreased production of glucocorticoids. Since, in humans, cortisol is the principal adrenal steroid regulating ACTH elaboration, and since the ACTH stimulates both cortisol and adrenal androgen production, an enzymatic interference with cortisol synthesis may result in the enhanced secretion of adrenal androgens. In severe congenital virilizing hyperplasia, the adrenal output of cortisol may be so compromised as to cause glucocorticoid deficiency despite anatomic adrenal hyperplasia.

Congenital adrenal hyperplasia is the most common adrenal disorder of infancy and childhood. These children usually have severe enzyme deficiencies (see Chap. 324). The deficiency of enzymes is the result of autosomal recessive mutations. Partial adrenal enzyme deficiencies can be expressed after adolescence, predominantly in women with hirsutism and oligomenorrhea but minimal virilization. Late onset adrenal hyperplasia may account for 5 to 25 percent of women with hirsutism and oligomenorrhea, depending on the patient population.

Congenital adrenal hyperplasia is secondary to one of several defects in steroid synthesis. To date, defects have been described in the C-21, C-18, C-17, and C-11 hydroxylase enzymes, as well as in the 3β-ol-dehydrogenase enzyme (see Fig. 317-2). These enzyme deficits usually occur singly. C-21 hydroxylase deficiency is closely linked to the histocompatibility leukocyte antigen (HLA-B) locus of chromosome 6 so that HLA typing can be used to detect the heterozygous carriers in some affected families (see Chap. 14). The clinical expression in the different disorders is variable, ranging from virilization of the female (C-21 deficiency) to feminization of the male (3β-ol-dehydrogenase deficiency). (See also Chap. 324.)

Adrenal virilization in the female at birth is associated with ambiguous external genitalia (*female pseudohermaphroditism*). The onset of virilization is most probably after the fifth month of embryonic development. At birth there may be enlarged genitalia in the male infant and enlargement of the clitoris, partial or complete fusion of the labia, and sometimes a urogenital sinus in the female. If the labial fusion is nearly complete, the female infant has external genitalia resembling a penis with hypospadias. In the *postnatal* period, congenital adrenal hyperplasia is associated with virilization in the female and isosexual precocity in the male. The excessive androgens result in accelerated growth, with bone age exceeding chronologic age. Since epiphyseal closure is hastened by excessive androgens, growth stops, but truncal development continues, giving the characteristic appearance of a child of short stature with well-developed trunk.

The most common form of congenital adrenal hyperplasia (95 percent of cases) is a result of impairment of *C-21 hydroxylation*. In addition to cortisol deficiency, there is an associated reduction in aldosterone secretion in approximately one-third of the patients. Thus, with C-21 hydroxylase deficiency, adrenal virilization occurs with or without an associated salt-losing tendency due to aldosterone deficiency (see Fig. 317-2).

C-11 hydroxylase deficiency causes a "hypertensive" variant of congenital adrenal hyperplasia. Hypertension and hypokalemia occur because of the impaired conversion of 11-deoxycorticosterone to corticosterone, resulting in the accumulation of 11-deoxycorticosterone, a potent mineralocorticoid. Increased shunting again occurs into the androgen pathway.

The *C-17 hydroxylase* deficiency is characterized by hypogonadism, hypokalemia, and hypertension. This rare deficiency causes decreased production of cortisol and shunting of precursors into the mineralocorticoid pathway with hypokalemic alkalosis, hypertension, and suppressed plasma renin activity. Usually, 11-deoxycorticosterone production is elevated. Because C-17 hydroxylation is required for biosynthesis of adrenal androgens as well as for biosynthesis of gonadal testosterone and estrogen, this defect is associated with sexual immaturity, high urinary gonadotropin levels, and low urinary 17-ketosteroid excretion. Female patients have primary amenorrhea and lack of development of secondary sexual characteristics. Because of deficient androgen production, male patients either have ambiguous external genitalia or a female phenotype (male pseudohermaphroditism). Exogenous glucocorticoids can correct the hypertensive syndrome, and treatment with appropriate gonadal steroids results in sexual maturation.

With 3β-ol-dehydrogenase deficiency, conversion of pregnenolone to progesterone is impaired, with the result that pathways to both cortisol and aldosterone are "blocked," with shunting then occurring into the adrenal androgen pathway via 17α-hydroxypregnenolone to dehydroepiandrosterone. Since dehydroepiandrosterone is a weak androgen and because this enzyme deficiency is also present in the gonad, the genitalia of the male fetus may be incompletely virilized or feminized. Conversely, in the female, overproduction of dehydroepiandrosterone may produce partial virilization.

Diagnosis The diagnosis of *congenital adrenal hyperplasia* should be considered in all infants exhibiting "failure to thrive," particularly those having episodes of acute adrenal insufficiency or salt wasting or showing sustained hypertension. The diagnosis is further suggested by the finding of hypertrophy of the clitoris, fused labia, or urogenital sinus in the female and isosexual precocity in the male. In infants and children with a *C-21 hydroxylation block*, increased urine 17-ketosteroid excretion and increased plasma DHEA sulfate are typically associated with an increase in the blood levels of 17-hydroxyprogesterone and the urinary excretion of the metabolite of this steroid, pregnanetriol.

The diagnosis of a *salt-losing form of congenital adrenal hyperplasia* due to defects in C-21 hydroxylase enzyme is suggested by episodes of acute adrenal insufficiency with hyponatremia, hyperkalemia, dehydration, and vomiting. These infants and children often crave salt and exhibit laboratory signs of concomitant deficits in both cortisol and aldosterone secretion.

With the *hypertensive form of congenital adrenal hyperplasia* due to impaired C-11 hydroxylation, 11-deoxycorticosterone and 11-deoxycortisol accumulate. Both urine 17-ketosteroid and 17-hydroxycorticosteroid excretion may be elevated, since 11-deoxycortisol is included in the analysis. The diagnosis is secured by demonstrating increased levels of 11-deoxycortisol in the blood or increased amounts of tetrahydro-11-deoxycortisol in the urine.

The finding of very high levels of urine dehydroepiandrosterone

with low levels of pregnanetriol and of cortisol metabolites in urine is characteristic of patients with 3β-ol-dehydrogenase deficiency. Marked salt wasting may also occur.

Patients with *late onset adrenal hyperplasia* (partial deficiency of C-21 hydroxylase) are characterized by normal or moderately elevated urinary 17-ketosteroids and plasma DHEA sulfate. A high basal level of a precursor of cortisol biosynthesis (such as 17-hydroxyprogesterone) or elevation of the precursor after ACTH stimulation confirms the diagnosis of a partial hydroxylase deficiency. It is uncertain how long the ACTH needs to be infused to unmask the enzyme deficiency, but it is likely that a 1-h infusion will pick up more than 75 percent and a 4-h infusion will detect more than 95 percent of those who have an enzyme deficiency documented with a 24-h ACTH infusion. Adrenal androgen output is easily suppressed by the standard low-dose (2 mg) dexamethasone test.

Differential diagnosis The causes of hirsutism can be divided into four broad categories: familial, idiopathic, androgen excess, and drugs. In general, the first two conditions are not associated with other signs of androgen excess, i.e., oligomenorrhea, significant acne, or virilization. Likewise, drug-induced hirsutism is usually not associated with other signs and symptoms of androgen excess, unless the drug is an androgen. The drugs that produce an increase in body hair include phenothiazines, minoxidil, and phenytoin. Each of these drugs, particularly minoxidil, produces a generalized increase in hair growth, not just an increase in hair growth in androgen target areas. The mechanism may be related to the ability of these drugs to convert vellus into terminal hair follicles.

If drugs are excluded, the only known causes of hirsutism amenable to treatment are those secondary to excess production of androgens by either the adrenal or the ovary.

In the female, the differential diagnosis of hirsutism and virilization is between adrenal and ovarian etiologies (Table 317-7). *Sudden onset of progressive hirsutism and virilization* suggests an adrenal or ovarian neoplasm. *Adrenal adenomas and carcinomas* may cause a pure or mixed virilizing syndrome. Since adrenal androgens are weak compared with gonadal androgens, adrenal virilization is characterized by *large increments in urine 17-ketosteroid excretion*. Virilizing adrenal adenomas are rare. *Virilizing adrenal carcinomas*, the most common adrenal tumors causing virilization, are associated with high plasma DHEA sulfate levels and high urinary 17-ketosteroid excretion rates; cortisol levels and 17-hydroxycorticosteroid excretion are normal or moderately elevated. Clinical differentiation between virilizing adrenal adenoma and carcinoma can usually be made preoperatively by CT scanning since carcinomas as a rule exceed 6 cm in size. Failure to reduce 17-ketosteroid levels and plasma DHEA sulfate levels to normal following dexamethasone suppression (0.5 mg given orally every 6 h for 2 days) further supports a diagnosis of virilizing adrenal tumor and excludes congenital adrenal hyperplasia. The most common virilizing *ovarian tumor* is the arrhenoblastoma, but other ovarian tumors, such as adrenal rest tumor, granulosa-cell tumor, hilar-cell tumor, and Brenner tumor, have been associated with virilization. Virilization due to ovarian tumors is usually characterized by normal levels of urinary 17-ketosteroids and DHEA sulfate, since the neoplasm usually secretes the potent androgen testosterone. Occasionally increases in 17-ketosteroid excretion occur

---

TABLE 317-7 Causes of hirsutism in women

I Familial
II Idiopathic
III Ovarian
   A Polycystic ovaries; hilus-cell hyperplasia
   B Tumor: arrhenoblastoma, hilus cell, adrenal rest
IV Adrenal
   A Congenital adrenal hyperplasia
   B Noncongenital adrenal hyperplasia (Cushing's)
   C Tumor: virilizing carcinoma or adenoma

in some patients with ovarian neoplasms, but baseline 17-ketosteroid excretion in excess of 100 μmol/d (30 mg/d) is rare with the exception of adrenal rest tumors. Like adrenal neoplasms, ovarian tumors are not suppressed by dexamethasone. With the exception of adrenal rest tumors, these tumors are largely independent of ACTH stimulation. Elevations of plasma testosterone or urinary testosterone excretion do not localize the neoplasm to the ovary, since testosterone can be elevated subsequent to peripheral conversion of adrenal precursors, such as DHEA (see Chap. 322).

The most common ovarian cause of excess androgen production is ovarian hyperthecosis or polycystic ovaries (see Chap. 322). As opposed to ovarian or adrenal tumors, virilization is less common with polycystic ovaries, whereas hirsutism is quite frequent. In most cases, the 17-ketosteroid excretion rate is greater than normal. Although the 17-ketosteroid excretion is partially reduced by dexamethasone, the residual level is often greater than in normal subjects. Plasma levels and production rates of androstenedione and to a lesser extent testosterone are usually increased. Follicle-stimulating hormone (FSH) levels tend to be lower than normal, and luteinizing hormone (LH) levels are tonically elevated, leading to the characteristic increased LH/FSH ratio. The laboratory findings in patients with hirsutism-virilizing syndromes are summarized in Table 317-8.

Treatment Treatment of adrenal virilism is dictated by the type of lesion. Patients with *congenital adrenal hyperplasia* have a fundamental defect of cortisol deficiency with resultant excessive ACTH stimulation, producing hyperplasia of the adrenal glands and causing additional "shunting" into the adrenal androgen pathway. Therapy in these patients consists of daily administration of glucocorticoids to suppress pituitary ACTH secretion. Because of its cost and intermediate half-life, prednisone is the drug of choice except in infants, when hydrocortisone is usually used. In adult patients with late-onset adrenal hyperplasia, a single bedtime dose of an intermediate-acting glucocorticoid, such as 2.5 or 5 mg of prednisone, suppresses pituitary ACTH secretion. The amount of steroid required by children with congenital adrenal hyperplasia is approximately 1 to 1.5 times the normal cortisol production rate of 33 to 35 μmol (12 to 13 mg) cortisol per square meter of body surface area per day and is given in divided doses two or three times per day. The dosage schedule is governed by repetitive analysis of the urinary 17-ketosteroids, plasma DHEA sulfate, and/or precursors of cortisol biosynthesis. Skeletal growth and maturation must also be closely monitored since overtreatment with glucocorticoid replacement therapy retards linear growth.

HYPOFUNCTION OF ADRENAL CORTEX

Adrenocortical hypofunction includes all conditions in which the secretion of adrenal steroid hormones falls below the requirements of the body. Adrenal insufficiency may be divided into two general categories: (1) those associated with primary inability of the adrenal to elaborate sufficient quantities of hormone and (2) those associated with a secondary failure due to a primary failure in the elaboration of ACTH (Table 317-9).

PRIMARY ADRENOCORTICAL DEFICIENCY (ADDISON'S DISEASE) Addison's description of "general languor and debility, remarkable feebleness of the heart's action, irritability of the stomach, and a peculiar change of the color of the skin," summarizes the dominant clinical features of the disease. Advanced cases are usually easy to diagnose, but recognition of the disease in its earlier phases may present a real challenge.

Incidence Primary adrenocortical insufficiency is relatively rare. It may occur at any age and affects both sexes with equal frequency. Because of increasing therapeutic use of exogenous steroids, secondary adrenal insufficiency is relatively common.

Etiology and pathogenesis Addison's disease results from progressive adrenocortical destruction, which must involve more than 90 percent of the glands before signs of adrenal insufficiency appear. The adrenal is a frequent site for chronic granulomatous diseases, predominantly tuberculosis but also histoplasmosis, coccidioidomycosis, and cryptococcosis. In previous years, tuberculosis was found at postmortem examination in 70 to 90 percent of cases; however, the most frequent finding at present is *idiopathic* atrophy, and an autoimmune mechanism is probably responsible. Rarely, other lesions are encountered, such as bilateral hemorrhage, tumor metastases, amyloidosis, or sarcoidosis.

Half of patients have circulating adrenal antibodies. Some patients also have antibodies to thyroid, parathyroid, and/or gonadal tissue (see also Chap. 325). There is also an increased incidence of chronic lymphocytic thyroiditis (Hashimoto's disease) and an increased incidence of premature ovarian failure, type I diabetes mellitus, and Graves' disease in patients with idiopathic adrenal insufficiency. The occurrence of two or more of these autoimmune endocrine disorders in the same individual defines the polyglandular autoimmune syndrome

TABLE 317-9 Classification of adrenal insufficiency

I Primary adrenal insufficiency
  A Anatomic destruction of gland (chronic and acute)
    1 "Idiopathic" atrophy (autoimmune)
    2 Surgical removal
    3 Infection (tuberculous, fungus, viral—especially in AIDS patients)
    4 Hemorrhage
    5 Invasion: metastatic
  B Metabolic failure in hormone production
    1 Congenital adrenal hyperplasia
    2 Enzyme inhibitors (metyrapone, ketoconazole, aminoglutethimide)
    3 Cytotoxic agents (mitotane)
II Secondary adrenal insufficiency
  A Hypopituitarism due to hypothalamic-pituitary disease
  B Suppression of hypothalamic-pituitary axis
    1 Exogenous steroid
    2 Endogenous steroid from tumor

TABLE 317-8 Laboratory evaluation of hirsutism-virilizing syndromes

	Ovarian		Adrenal			
	PCO	Ovarian tumor	CAH	Adrenal neoplasm	Cushing's syndrome	Idiopathic
Urinary 17-ketosteroids, plasma DHEA sulfate	N↑	N	N↑	↑↑↑	N↑	N
Plasma testosterone	N↑	↑↑	N↑	N↑	N↑	N
LH/FSH ratio	N↑	N	N	N	N	N
Precursors of cortisol biosynthesis:						
Basal	N	N	N↑	N↑	N	N
Following ACTH infusion	N	N	↑↑	N↑	N	N
Cortisol following overnight dexamethasone suppression test	N	N	N	↑	↑	N

NOTE: CAH, congenital adrenal hyperplasia; PCO, polycystic ovary syndrome; N, normal; ↑, elevated.

type II. Additional disorders in these patients include pernicious anemia, vitiligo, alopecia, nontropical sprue, and myasthenia gravis. Within families, multiple generations are affected by one or more of the above diseases. Type II polyglandular syndrome is the result of a mutant gene on the sixth chromosome and is associated with the HLA alleles B8 and DR3.

The combination of parathyroid and adrenal insufficiency and chronic mucocutaneous moniliasis constitutes a distinct familial syndrome (type I polyglandular autoimmune syndrome). Other autoimmune diseases also occur in higher frequency in these patients (e.g., pernicious anemia, chronic active hepatitis, alopecia, primary hypothyroidism, and premature gonadal failure). There is no HLA association; this syndrome is inherited in an autosomal recessive pattern, often with multiple affected siblings within a family. The type I syndrome usually presents during childhood, whereas the peak incidence of expression of the type II syndrome is in adulthood. The mechanisms by which genetic predisposition and/or autoimmunity interact in the pathogenesis of these disease states are unknown.

Clinical suspicion of adrenal insufficiency should be high in patients with acquired immunodeficiency syndrome (AIDS). Cytomegalovirus regularly involves the adrenal glands (so-called CMV necrotizing adrenalitis), and *mycobacterium avium-intracellulare, Cryptococcus,* and Kaposi's sarcoma involvement of the adrenals have also been reported. Clinical manifestations of adrenal insufficiency in AIDS patients may be uncommon, but tests of adrenal reserve are frequently abnormal. When interpreting tests of adrenocortical function, it is important to consider medications commonly used to treat AIDS patients that might potentiate or cause adrenal failure (rifampin, phenytoin, ketoconazole, and opiates).

Clinical signs and symptoms   Adrenocortical insufficiency caused by gradual adrenal destruction is characterized by an insidious onset of slowly progressive fatigability, weakness, anorexia, nausea and vomiting, weight loss, cutaneous and mucosal pigmentation, hypotension, and occasionally hypoglycemia (Table 317-10). However, the spectrum may vary, depending on the duration and degree of adrenal hypofunction, from a complaint of mild chronic fatigue to the fulminating shock associated with acute massive destruction of the glands in the syndrome described by Waterhouse and Friderichsen.

Asthenia is the cardinal symptom. Early it may be sporadic, usually most evident at times of stress; as adrenal function becomes more impaired, weakness progresses until the patient is continuously fatigued, necessitating bed rest.

Hyperpigmentation may be a striking sign, but its absence does not exclude this diagnosis. It commonly appears as a diffuse brown, tan, or bronze darkening of both exposed and unexposed parts such as elbows or creases of the hand and of areas normally pigmented such as the areolas about the nipples. Bluish-black patches may appear on the mucous membranes. Some patients develop dark freckles, and occasionally irregular areas of vitiligo may appear paradoxically. As an early sign, patients may notice an unusually persistent tanning following exposure to the sun.

Arterial hypotension is frequent, and in severe cases blood pressures may be in the range of 80/50 or less. Postural accentuation of hypotension is common.

Abnormalities of gastrointestinal function often are the presenting complaint. Symptoms may vary from mild anorexia with weight

loss to fulminating nausea, vomiting, diarrhea, and ill-defined abdominal pain, which at times may be so severe as to be confused with an acute abdomen. In addition, patients with adrenal insufficiency frequently have marked personality changes, usually in the form of excessive irritability and restlessness. Enhancement of the sensory modalities of taste, olfaction, and hearing is often present and is reversible with therapy. A decrease in axillary and pubic hair is common in women due to loss of adrenal androgen production.

Laboratory findings   In the early phase of gradual adrenal destruction, there may be no demonstrable abnormalities in the routine laboratory parameters, but adrenal reserve is decreased, that is, basal steroid output is normal but an increase does not occur in response to stress. Adrenal stimulation with ACTH uncovers abnormalities in this stage of the disease with a subnormal response and/or failure of cortisol levels to rise over basal. In more advanced stages of adrenal destruction, serum sodium, chloride, and bicarbonate are reduced while serum potassium is elevated. The hyponatremia is due to both loss of sodium into the urine (due to aldosterone deficiency) and movement into the intracellular compartment. This extravascular sodium loss depletes extracellular fluid volume and accentuates hypotension. Elevated plasma vasopressin and angiotensin II levels may be contributing factors to the hyponatremia through impairment of free water clearance. The hyperkalemia is due to a combination of aldosterone deficiency, impaired glomerular filtration, and acidosis. Basal levels of cortisol and aldosterone are subnormal and fail to increase following ACTH administration. Mild to moderate hypercalcemia occurs in 10 to 20 percent of patients; the reason for this is not understood. The electrocardiogram may show nonspecific changes, and the electroencephalogram exhibits a generalized reduction and slowing. There may be a normocytic anemia, a relative lymphocytosis, and usually a moderate eosinophilia.

Diagnosis   The diagnosis of adrenal insufficiency should be made only with ACTH stimulation testing to assay the adrenal reserve capacity for steroid production (see above for ACTH test protocols). In *severe adrenal insufficiency* the cortisol secretory rate is markedly decreased, and this may be ascertained indirectly by the finding of low to absent 24-h urine cortisol, 17-hydroxycorticosteroids, and 17-ketosteroids. With *mild adrenal insufficiency* (decreased adrenal reserve), urine and blood steroid values overlap the normal range; thus, a diagnosis of adrenal insufficiency should never be excluded solely on the basis of normal basal urine steroid determinations. Plasma cortisol values vary from zero to the lower range of normal. Aldosterone secretion is usually low, resulting in salt wasting and secondary rises in plasma renin levels. In primary adrenal insufficiency, plasma ACTH and associated peptides (β-lipotropin) are elevated because of loss of the usual cortisol-hypothalamic-pituitary feedback relationship, whereas in secondary adrenal insufficiency, plasma ACTH values are low, or "inappropriately" normal (Fig. 317-11).

Differential diagnosis   Since weakness and fatigue are common complaints, clinical diagnosis of early adrenocortical insufficiency is frequently difficult. However, mild gastrointestinal distress with weight loss, anorexia, and a suggestion of increased pigmentation make mandatory ACTH stimulation testing to rule out adrenal insufficiency, particularly before steroid treatment is begun. Weight loss is useful in evaluating the significance of weakness and malaise. Weight gain associated with lassitude is more characteristic of depressive syndromes. Racial pigmentation in many individuals may be a problem, but a *recent* and progressive *increase* is usually reported by the Addisonian patient with gradual adrenal destruction. However, hyperpigmentation is usually absent when adrenal destruction is rapid, as in bilateral adrenal hemorrhage. Hyperpigmentation in other diseases may also present a problem, but the appearance and distribution of pigment in Addison's disease are usually characteristic. When doubt exists, measurement of ACTH levels and testing of adrenal reserve with the infusion of ACTH provide clear-cut differentiation.

TABLE 317-10   Incidence of symptoms and signs in Addison's disease, percent

Weakness	99	Hypotension	
Pigmentation of skin	98	(<110/70)	87
Pigmentation of		Abdominal pain	34
mucous membranes	82	Salt craving	22
Weight loss	97	Diarrhea	20
Anorexia, nausea, and		Constipation	19
vomiting	90	Syncope	16
		Vitiligo	9

FIGURE 317-11 Diagnostic flowchart for evaluating patients with suspected adrenal insufficiency. Plasma ACTH levels are low in secondary adrenal insufficiency. In adrenal insufficiency secondary to pituitary tumors or idiopathic panhypopituitarism, other pituitary hormone deficiencies are present. On the other hand, ACTH deficiency may be isolated, as seen following prolonged use of exogenous glucocorticoids.

Since the isolated blood levels obtained in these screening tests may not be definitive, the diagnosis should always be confirmed by a continuous 24-h ACTH infusion. Normal subjects and patients with secondary adrenal insufficiency may be distinguished by insulin tolerance or metyrapone testing.

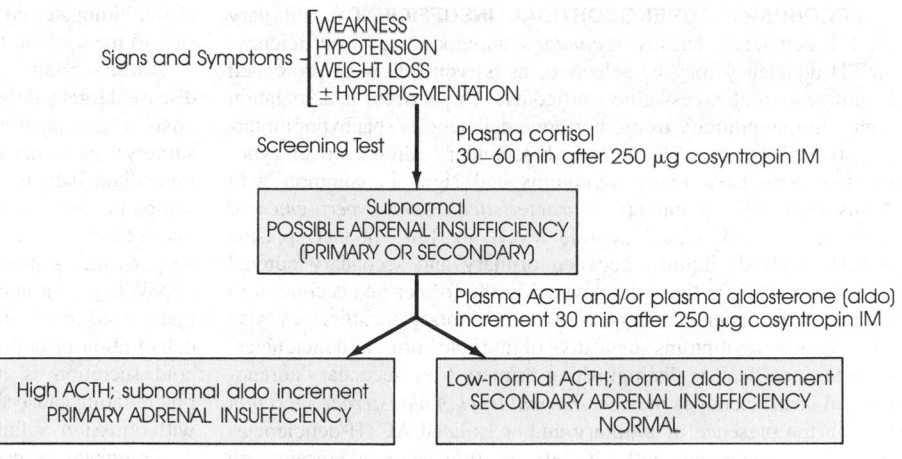

Treatment All patients with Addison's disease should receive specific hormone replacement. Like diabetics, these patients require careful and persistent education in regard to their disease. Since the adrenal gland elaborates three general classes of hormone, of which two, glucocorticoids and mineralocorticoids, are of primary clinical importance, replacement therapy should correct both deficiencies. Cortisone (or cortisol) is the mainstay of treatment. Cortisone dosage varies from 12.5 to 50 mg daily, with the majority of patients taking 25 to 37.5 mg in divided doses. Cortisol (30 mg daily) or prednisone (7.5 mg daily) in divided doses may also be given for substitution therapy. Patients are advised to take their glucocorticoid replacement medication with meals or, if this is impractical, with milk or an antacid because the drugs may increase gastric acidity. This is particularly important because if the steroid is biologically active, e.g., cortisol, prednisolone, and dexamethasone, it may exert local effects on the gastric mucosa. In addition, the larger proportion of the dose (e.g., 25 mg of cortisone) is taken in the morning, and the remainder (12.5 mg of cortisone) is taken in the late afternoon to simulate the normal diurnal adrenal rhythm. Some patients exhibit insomnia, irritability, and mental excitement after initiation of therapy; in these, the dosage should be reduced. Other indications for smaller amounts of glucocorticoids are hypertension, diabetes mellitus, or active tuberculosis.

Since this amount of cortisone or cortisol fails to replace the mineralocorticoid component of the adrenal gland, supplementary hormone is usually needed. This is accomplished by the daily oral administration of 0.05 to 0.1 mg fludrocortisone. Of course, patients should be instructed to ingest an ample intake of sodium (3 to 4 g/d). Adequacy of mineralocorticoid therapy can be assessed by measurement of blood pressure and serum electrolytes. Blood pressure should be normal and without postural change; serum sodium,

potassium, creatinine, and urea nitrogen should also be within the normal range.

Complications of glucocorticoid therapy, with the exception of gastritis, are *rare* in the dosage used in the treatment of Addison's disease. Complications of mineralocorticoid therapy occur more frequently and include hypokalemia, edema, hypertension, cardiac enlargement, or even congestive failure due to sodium retention. In the management of patients with Addison's disease, periodic measurements of body weight, serum potassium, and blood pressure are useful. All patients with adrenal insufficiency, including bilaterally adrenalectomized patients, should carry medical identification, should be instructed in the parenteral self-administration of steroids, and should be registered with a national medical alerting system.

Special therapeutic problems During periods of intercurrent illness, the dose of cortisone or cortisol should be increased to 75 to 150 mg/d. When oral administration is not possible, parenteral routes should be employed. Likewise, before surgery or dental extractions, supplemental glucocorticoids should be administered. Patients should also be advised to increase the dose of fludrocortisone and to add excess salt to their otherwise normal diet during periods of excessive exercise with sweating, during extremely hot weather, and with gastrointestinal upsets. For a representative program of steroid therapy for the patient with adrenal insufficiency who is undergoing a major operation, see Table 317-11. This schedule is designed to mimic on the day of surgery the output of cortisol in normal individuals undergoing prolonged major stress (10 mg/h, 250 to 300 mg/d). Thereafter, if the patient is progressing well and is afebrile, the dose of cortisol is tapered by 20 to 30 percent daily. Parenteral mineralocorticoid administration is unnecessary at cortisol doses greater than 100 mg/d because of the mineralocorticoid effects of cortisol at such dosages.

TABLE 317-11 Steroid therapy schedule for Addisonian patient undergoing a major operation*

	Cortisol phosphate (intramuscularly)		Cortisol infusion, continuous, mg/h	Cortisol (orally)		Fludro-cortisone (orally), 8 A.M.
	7 A.M.	7 P.M.		8 A.M.	4 P.M.	
Routine daily medication				20	10	0.1
Day before operation	50			20	10	0.1
Day of operation			10			
Postoperative:						
Day 1			5–7.5			
Day 2			2.5–5			
Day 3	50	50				
Day 4	50				20	0.1
Day 5				40	20	0.1
Day 6				20	20	0.1
Day 7				20	10	0.1

* All steroid doses are given in milligrams.

SECONDARY ADRENOCORTICAL INSUFFICIENCY Pituitary ACTH deficiency causes *secondary* adrenocortical insufficiency. ACTH deficiency may be selective, as is seen following prolonged administration of excess glucocorticoids, or may occur in association with multiple pituitary tropic hormone deficiencies (panhypopituitarism) (see Chap. 313). Patients with secondary adrenocortical hypofunction may have many symptoms and signs in common with Addisonian patients but are *characteristically not hyperpigmented* since ACTH and related peptide levels are low. In fact, plasma ACTH levels distinguish between primary and secondary adrenal insufficiency, since they are elevated in the former and decreased to absent in the latter. Patients with total pituitary insufficiency also have signs and symptoms suggestive of multiple hormone deficiencies. An additional feature distinguishing primary from secondary adrenocortical insufficiency is the *near-normal level of aldosterone secretion* seen in the presence of pituitary and/or isolated ACTH deficiencies (Fig. 317-11). Patients with pituitary insufficiency may present with hyponatremia, which may be dilutional or secondary to subnormal increments in aldosterone secretion in response to severe sodium restriction. However, the findings of severe *dehydration, hyponatremia,* and *hyperkalemia* are characteristic of severe mineralocorticoid insufficiency and favor a diagnosis of primary adrenocortical insufficiency.

Patients receiving long-term steroid therapy, despite physical findings of Cushing's syndrome, develop adrenal insufficiency because of prolonged pituitary-hypothalamic suppression and adrenal atrophy secondary to the loss of endogenous ACTH. Thus, these patients have two deficits, a loss of adrenal responsiveness to ACTH and a failure of pituitary ACTH release. These patients are characterized by low blood cortisol and ACTH levels, low baseline steroid excretion, and abnormal ACTH and metyrapone test results. Most patients with steroid-induced adrenal insufficiency eventually recover normal hypothalamic-pituitary-adrenal responsiveness, but individual response time varies from days to months. The rapid ACTH test can be used as a convenient assessment of recovery of hypothalamic-pituitary-adrenal function. Since the plasma cortisol concentrations after injection of cosyntropin and during insulin-induced hypoglycemia usually correlate closely, the rapid ACTH test assesses the integrated hypothalamic-pituitary-adrenal function (see ''Tests of Pituitary-Adrenal Responsiveness,'' above). Additional testing to assess endogenous pituitary ACTH reserve includes the standard metyrapone and the insulin tolerance tests.

Substitution glucocorticoid therapy in patients with secondary adrenocortical insufficiency does not differ from that for Addisonian patients. Mineralocorticoid replacement therapy is usually not necessary, since aldosterone secretion is preserved. Otherwise, the same basic principles should be applied to patients with secondary adrenocortical insufficiency.

ACUTE ADRENOCORTICAL INSUFFICIENCY Acute adrenocortical insufficiency may result from several processes. One of these, termed *adrenal crisis*, is a rapid and overwhelming intensification of chronic adrenal insufficiency, usually precipitated by sepsis or surgical stress. Another involves an acute hemorrhagic destruction of both adrenal glands. In children this is usually associated with septicemia with *Pseudomonas* or meningococcemia (Waterhouse-Friderichsen syndrome). In adults, anticoagulant therapy or a coagulation disorder may result in bilateral adrenal hemorrhage in patients undergoing major stress where there is increased adrenocortical activity. Occasionally, bilateral adrenal hemorrhage in the newborn results from birth trauma. Hemorrhage also has been observed during pregnancy, following idiopathic adrenal vein thrombosis, and as a complication of venography (e.g., infarction of an adenoma). A third, and probably the most frequent, cause of acute insufficiency results from the rapid withdrawal of steroids from patients with adrenal atrophy secondary to chronic steroid administration. In the presence of severe stress, acute adrenocortical insufficiency may also occur in patients with congenital adrenal hyperplasia or those with decreased adrenocortical reserve when they are given pharmacologic agents that are capable of inhibiting steroid synthesis (mitotane, ketoconazole) or increasing steroid metabolism (phenytoin, rifampin).

Adrenal crisis The long-term survival of patients with Addison's disease largely depends upon prevention and treatment of adrenal crisis. Consequently, the occurrence of infection, trauma (including surgery), gastrointestinal upsets, or other forms of stress requires an immediate increase in hormone. In untreated patients, preexisting symptoms are intensified. Nausea, vomiting, and abdominal pain may become intractable. Fever may be severe or absent. Lethargy deepens into somnolence, and the blood pressure and pulse fail as hypovolemic vascular shock ensues. In contrast, patients previously maintained on chronic glucocorticoid therapy may not exhibit severe dehydration or hypotension until preterminally, since mineralocorticoid secretion is usually preserved. In all patients in crisis, a precipitating cause should be sought. Intercurrent infection associated with omission or failure to increase maintenance therapy is common.

Treatment is primarily directed toward the rapid elevation of circulating glucocorticoid and the replacement of the sodium and water deficits. Hence, an intravenous infusion of 5% glucose in normal saline solution should be immediately started with a bolus intravenous infusion of 100 mg cortisol followed by a continuous infusion of cortisol at a rate of 10 mg/h. Effective treatment of hypotension consists of aggressive repletion of sodium and water deficits. If the crisis was preceded by prolonged nausea, vomiting, and dehydration, several liters of saline solution may be required within the first few hours. Vasoconstrictive agents (such as dopamine) may be indicated in extreme conditions as adjuncts to volume replacement. With large doses of steroid, as for example 100 to 200 mg cortisol, the patient receives a maximal mineralocorticoid effect, and supplementary mineralocorticoid is superfluous. Following improvement, the patient can be offered oral fluids and the steroid dosage is tapered over the next few days to maintenance levels, with reinstitution of supplementary mineralocorticoid if needed (Table 317-11).

HYPOALDOSTERONISM

Isolated aldosterone deficiency accompanied by normal cortisol production occurs in association with hyporeninism, as an inherited biosynthetic defect, postoperatively following removal of aldosterone-secreting adenomas, during protracted heparin or heparinoid administration, in pretectal disease of the nervous system, and in severe postural hypotension.

The feature common to all patients with hypoaldosteronism is the inability to increase aldosterone secretion appropriately during salt restriction. Most patients present with unexplained hyperkalemia often exacerbated by restriction of dietary sodium intake. In severe cases urine sodium wastage occurs on a normal salt intake, whereas in milder forms excessive losses of urine sodium occur only during salt restriction.

Most cases of isolated hypoaldosteronism occur in patients with a deficiency in renin production (so-called hyporeninemic hypoaldosteronism). This syndrome is most commonly seen in adults with mild renal failure and diabetes mellitus in association with hyperkalemia and metabolic acidosis out of proportion to the state of renal impairment. Plasma renin levels fail to rise normally following sodium restriction and postural changes. The pathogenesis is uncertain. Possibilities include renal disease (most likely), autonomic neuropathy, extracellular fluid volume expansion, and a defect in conversion of presumed renin precursors into active renin. Aldosterone levels also fail to rise normally following salt restriction and volume contraction; this is probably related to the hyporeninism since biosynthetic defects in aldosterone secretion cannot usually be demonstrated. In these patients, aldosterone secretion increases promptly following ACTH stimulation, but it is uncertain whether the magnitude of the response is normal. On the other hand, the level of aldosterone appears to be subnormal in relationship to the hyperkalemia.

Hypoaldosteronism can also be associated with high renin levels. In many of these subjects, a biosynthetic defect has been noted where there is an inability to transform the C-18 methyl group of corticosterone to the C-18 aldehyde of aldosterone due to a deficiency of the enzyme 18-hydroxysteroid dehydrogenase. These patients manifest not only low to absent aldosterone secretion and elevated plasma renin levels but also elevated values for the intermediates of aldosterone biosynthesis (corticosterone and 18-hydroxycorticosterone). Severely ill patients may also exhibit the syndrome of hyperreninemic hypoaldosteronism. This selective hypoaldosteronism is seen in hypotensive critically ill patients. Patients with this syndrome have a high mortality rate (80 percent). Hyperkalemia is not part of this syndrome. Possible explanations for the hypoaldosteronism include adrenal necrosis (uncommon) or an adaptation to severe illness by a shift in steroidogenesis from mineralocorticoids to glucocorticoids, possibly related to prolonged ACTH stimulation.

Before considering the diagnosis of isolated hypoaldosteronism in a patient with hyperkalemia, "pseudohyperkalemia" (e.g., hemolysis, thrombocytosis) should be excluded by measuring plasma potassium. The next step is to demonstrate a normal cortisol response to ACTH stimulation. Then stimulated (upright posture, sodium restriction) renin and aldosterone levels are obtained. Low renin–low aldosterone levels establish a diagnosis of hyporeninemic hypoaldosteronism. High renin–low aldosterone levels are consistent with an aldosterone biosynthetic defect or a selective unresponsiveness of the glomerulosa to angiotensin II. Finally, elevated renin and aldosterone levels suggest primary renal unresponsiveness to aldosterone, so-called pseudohypoaldosteronism.

The aim of treatment of isolated hypoaldosteronism is to replace the mineralocorticoid deficiency. For practical purposes, the oral administration of fludrocortisone in a dose of 0.1 to 0.2 mg daily should restore electrolyte balance, if salt intake is adequate (e.g., 150 to 200 mmol/d). However, patients with hyporeninemic hypoaldosteronism usually require higher doses of mineralocorticoid to correct the hyperkalemia. This poses a risk in those patients who also may have hypertension and mild renal insufficiency and/or congestive heart failure. Therefore, an alternative approach is to administer furosemide, which can ameliorate the acidosis and the hyperkalemia, and reduce the salt intake. Occasionally a combination of these two approaches is efficacious.

NONSPECIFIC CLINICAL USE OF ADRENAL STEROIDS AND ACTH

The widespread utilization of glucocorticoids and ACTH emphasizes the need for a thorough understanding of the metabolic effects of these agents when used nonspecifically, if optimum effectiveness is to be obtained and if undesirable side reactions are to be minimized. Before instituting adrenal hormone therapy, the gains that can reasonably be expected should be weighed against the potentially undesirable metabolic actions of pharmacologic doses of hormone.

HOW SERIOUS IS THE DISORDER? In a patient whose life is threatened by unexplained shock or in whom other measures have failed, the physician need not hesitate to employ large-dosage steroid therapy. On the other hand, one should exercise restraint in administering steroids to a patient with early rheumatoid arthritis who as yet has not been exposed to the possible benefits of physiotherapy, analgesics, and a well-organized program of general medical care.

HOW LONG WILL GLUCOCORTICOID THERAPY BE REQUIRED? The use of intravenously administered steroids for a period of 24 to 48 h in the treatment of such life-threatening situations as status asthmaticus or pseudotumor cerebri has little or no contraindication, in contrast to the initiation of a program of chronic steroid therapy for asthma, arthritis, or psoriasis. In the latter instances, the almost certain complication of a Cushing's syndrome of some degree must be weighed against the potential benefit. These side effects should be minimized by a careful choice of steroid preparations,

alternate-day or interrupted therapy programs, and the judicious use of supplementary adjuvants.

WHICH PREPARATION IS PREFERABLE? At least five considerations need to be taken into account in deciding which steroid preparation to use:

1 The biologic half-life of the compound. The rationale behind every-other-day therapy is to decrease the metabolic effects of the steroids for a significant amount of time over the 2-day period, yet at the same time to produce pharmacologic suppression of sufficient duration to maintain the disease in remission. Too long a half-life would defeat the first purpose, and too short a half-life would defeat the second. In general, the more potent the steroid, the longer its biologic half-life.

2 The importance of the mineralocorticoid effects of the steroid. Synthetic steroids have less mineralocorticoid effect relative to their glucocorticoid effect than do cortisol or cortisone (Table 317-12). This may be an important consideration in certain disease states.

3 The biologically active form of the steroid. Cortisone and prednisone, in contrast to the other glucocorticoids, have to be converted to biologically active equivalents before anti-inflammatory effects can occur. Because of this, in a condition in which steroids are known to be effective and when an adequate dose has been given without response, one should consider substituting cortisol or prednisolone for cortisone or prednisone.

4 The cost of the medication. This is a serious consideration if chronic administration is to be undertaken. Prednisone is the least expensive of available steroid preparations.

5 The variation in the manner in which preparations of glucosteroids are formulated. This factor may modify absorption. Thus, it is advisable for a patient whose steroid dosage has been standardized to continue to utilize the same pharmaceutical preparation to avoid relapse or overdosage.

ACTH VERSUS STEROIDS In general, adrenal steroid therapy is effective by mouth and can be regulated more accurately than ACTH therapy. The amount of steroid produced in response to ACTH varies from day to day, depending on the rate and extent of absorption of ACTH and on the state of the adrenal cortex. ACTH therapy stimulates the secretion of adrenal androgens as well as of hydroxysteroids. Sodium retention with ACTH is often more marked than with cortisone or prednisone therapy.

TABLE 317-12   Glucocorticoid preparations

Commonly used name*	Estimated potency†	
	Glucocorticoid	Mineralocorticoid
SHORT-ACTING		
Cortisol	1	1
Cortisone	0.8	0.8
INTERMEDIATE-ACTING		
Prednisone	4	0.25
Prednisolone	4	0.25
Methylprednisolone	5	<0.01
Triamcinolone	5	<0.01
LONG-ACTING		
Paramethasone	10	<0.01
Betamethasone	25	<0.01
Dexamethasone	30–40	<0.01

* The steroids are divided into three groups according to the duration of biologic activity. Short-acting preparations have a biologic half-life of less than 12 h; long-acting, greater than 48 h; and intermediate, between 12 and 36 h. Triamcinolone has the longest half-life of the intermediate-acting preparations.
† Relative milligram comparisons with cortisol, setting the glucocorticoid and mineralocorticoid properties of cortisol as 1. Sodium retention is insignificant in usual doses employed of methylprednisolone, triamcinolone, paramethasone, betamethasone, and dexamethasone.

TABLE 317-13   A "checklist" for use prior to the administration of glucocorticoids in pharmacologic dosages

1 Presence of tuberculosis or other chronic infection (chest x-ray, tuberculin test)
2 Evidence of glucose intolerance or history of gestational diabetes mellitus
3 Evidence of preexisting osteoporosis (spine x-ray or bone density assessment, if available, in postmenopausal patients)
4 History of peptic ulcer, gastritis, or esophagitis (stool guaiac test)
5 Evidence of hypertension or cardiovascular disease
6 History of psychological disorders

While some studies imply that ACTH may be superior to oral steroid therapy in the treatment of certain disorders such as dermatomyositis and multiple sclerosis, it is generally believed that the two agents are equally effective (or ineffective). Both ACTH and steroid therapy induce hypothalamopituitary suppression; however, in ACTH therapy adrenal gland size and activity are maintained, in contrast to the adrenal atrophy usually associated with steroid therapy.

EVALUATION OF PATIENT PRIOR TO INITIATING STEROID THERAPY (See Table 317-13)   **Chronic infection**   Three problems demand attention: (1) Any active infection, particularly tuberculosis, should be identified. If tuberculosis is present, steroid therapy can be employed, if indicated, in conjunction with antituberculous chemotherapy. (2) The chest film and tuberculin test provide baseline information for future comparison. Since high-dosage steroids minimize the tuberculin reaction, serial chest roentgenograms may be indicated. (3) Infection due to "opportunistic" low-virulence pathogens should be constantly considered in patients on high steroid dosage, especially when steroid therapy is combined with other immunosuppressive agents.

Diabetes mellitus   Prolonged glucocorticoid therapy may unmask latent diabetes mellitus or aggravate preexisting disease. The presence of diabetes mellitus or the demonstration of impaired glucose tolerance may affect the decision to institute adrenal hormone therapy.

Osteoporosis   All patients receiving long-continued steroid therapy are likely to develop some degree of osteoporosis. Indeed osteoporosis, with vertebral fractures or compression, is one of the most serious potential hazards of long-term steroid therapy. For patients at high risk (postmenopausal women, elderly men, and patients with restricted physical activity) initial films of the thoracolumbar segment of the spine are mandatory. Alternate-day or interrupted steroid therapy minimizes this complication (Table 317-14), and adjunctive therapies may be effective in the therapy of steroid osteoporosis (see Chap. 345).

Peptic ulcer, gastric hypersecretion, or esophagitis   In conventional therapeutic doses (equivalent to 15 mg prednisone per day or less) glucocorticoids probably do not cause peptic ulceration; whether higher doses are associated with increased incidence of peptic ulcer disease is not established and probably depends on duration of treatment (as well as dose) and the presence of predisposing factors

---

TABLE 317-14   Supplementary measures to minimize undesirable metabolic effects of glucocorticoids

I Monitor caloric intake to prevent weight gain.
II Restrict sodium intake to prevent edema and minimize hypertension and potassium loss.
III Supplement potassium if necessary.
IV Give antacid therapy and/or histamine receptor antagonist therapy.
V Institute alternate-day steroid schedule if possible. Patients on steroid therapy over a prolonged period should be protected by an appropriate increase in hormone level during periods of acute stress. A rule of thumb is to *double* the maintenance dose.
VI Minimize osteopenia by (not proved effective):
  A Estrogen therapy for postmenopausal women; 0.625–1.25 mg conjugated estrogens, may be given "cyclically." Regular Papanicolaou smear and breast examination and mammography mandatory (see Chap. 322).
  B Consider supplementary vitamin D and calcium.

---

such as hypoalbuminemia or cirrhosis. However, even in conventional doses patients with a history of ulcer may experience aggravation of symptoms while receiving glucocorticoids. Consequently, all individuals with a positive history or with known risk factors should be given a vigorous "ulcer combating" program (antacids, cimetidine) along with glucocorticoids. *The development of anemia in a patient receiving glucocorticoids should suggest gastrointestinal bleeding as a cause, and patients should be cautioned to note black stools.*

Hypertension or cardiovascular disease   In general, the sodium-retaining propensity of many adrenal steroid preparations requires that caution be used when they are given to patients with preexisting hypertension or cardiovascular or renal disease. Use of preparations in which sodium-retaining activity is minimal, restriction of dietary sodium intake, and the use of diuretic agents and supplementary potassium salts will minimize the mineralocorticoid actions of steroid therapy. However, hypertension may still be exacerbated by several mechanisms, including steroid-induced increases in renin substrate and consequently in angiotensin II levels, and reduction in vasodilator prostaglandin production. Additionally, steroids accelerate atherogenesis by induction of hypertension, glucose intolerance, and unfavorable lipid profiles. Glucocorticoid-associated lipid abnormalities include hypertriglyceridemia and hypercholesterolemia, particularly increased LDL cholesterol levels.

Psychological difficulties   Steroid therapy may be complicated by minor or severe psychological disturbances. In general, serious psychological disturbances are more closely related to the patient's personality structure than to the actual dose of hormone, although, as might be anticipated, larger doses of hormone are associated with more frequent serious reactions. At present there is no reliable method of determining beforehand a patient's psychological reaction to steroid therapy; moreover, previous tolerance of steroids does not necessarily ensure immunity to subsequent courses of therapy. Likewise, untoward psychological reactions on one occasion do not invariably mean that the patient will respond unfavorably to a second course of treatment; however, prophylactic treatment with lithium may be indicated.

Sleeplessness is a common complication and can be minimized by using the shorter-acting steroids and by prescribing the total dose as a single early-morning medication.

ALTERNATE-DAY STEROID THERAPY   The single most effective measure in minimizing the cushingoid effects of glucocorticoid therapy is to administer the total 48-h dose as a *single* dose of *intermediate-acting steroid* in the morning, *every other day*. If symptoms of the underlying disorder can be controlled by this technique, the therapeutic program offers a distinct advantage. Three special considerations deserve mention: (1) The alternate-day schedule may be approached through a series of transition dose schedules that permit the patient an opportunity to adjust to the ultimate program. (2) The physician should provide the patient with supplementary nonsteroid medications, if required, on the "off day" to minimize symptoms of the underlying disorder. (3) The physician and the patient should recognize that many symptoms noted during the off day (e.g., fatigue, joint pain, muscle stiffness or tenderness, and fever) are those of relative adrenal insufficiency, rather than an exacerbation of the underlying disease. Knowing this is of vital importance, since the physician can reassure the patient and avoid giving up the program on the basis of a misconception.

The alternate-day concept capitalizes on the fact that cortisol secretion and plasma levels normally are highest in the early morning and lowest in the evening. The normal pattern is mimicked by administering an intermediate-acting steroid in the morning (7 to 8 A.M.) (Table 317-12).

Initially the steroid program often requires daily or more frequent doses of steroid to accomplish the desired anti-inflammatory or immunity-suppressing action. *Only after this desired effect has been achieved is an attempt made to switch over to an alternate-day program.* A number of programs may be employed for transferring a patient from a daily to an alternate-day program. The key points to be considered are flexibility in arranging a program and the use of supportive measures on the off day. One may attempt a transition by a series of gradations rather than by an abrupt complete changeover. One approach is to keep the steroid dose constant on one day and gradually reduce the level on the alternate day. Alternatively, the steroid dose can be increased on one day while being reduced on the alternate day. In any case it is important to anticipate that the patient will experience some increase in pain or discomfort between the 36 to 48 h following the last dose of steroid.

The general principles advocated in the long-term use of steroids and in implementing an alternate-day schedule are as follows:

1 Utilize intermediate-acting steroids such as prednisone or prednisolone.
2 Give the total daily steroid as a single morning dose.
3 Begin a transition program as soon as the manifestations of the diseases are under reasonable control.
4 If possible, eliminate steroid medication on the alternate day.

WITHDRAWAL OF GLUCOCORTICOIDS FOLLOWING THEIR LONG-TERM USE AS PHARMACOLOGIC AGENTS Complete withdrawal of steroids should be initiated by implementing an alternate-day schedule. Patients on an alternate-day program for a month or more experience less difficulty during a subsequent termination regimen as far as pituitary-adrenal function is concerned. The dosage is gradually reduced and finally discontinued after a normal replacement dosage has been reached (e.g., 5 to 7.5 mg prednisone). Complications rarely ensue unless undue stress is experienced, and patients should understand that for 1 year or longer after the complete withdrawal from long-term high-dosage steroid therapy, they should receive supplementary hormone in the presence of serious infection, operation, or injury.

In patients on high-dose daily steroid therapy, it is frequently advised to reduce total steroid dosage to approximately 20 mg prednisone daily before beginning the transition to every-other-day therapy. If a patient cannot tolerate an alternate-day program, it is debatable as to whether complete discontinuance should be considered. Under these circumstances a daily replacement dose of steroid should be continued, and at some future date another trial of gradual transition to the alternate-day schedule should be attempted. These patients will not require mineralocorticoid therapy, as aldosterone secretion is usually adequate.

REFERENCES

BECKER DM et al: Relationship between corticosteroid exposure and plasma lipid levels in heart transplant recipients. Am J Med 85:632, 1988
CHROUSOS GP et al: Late onset of 21-hydroxylase deficiency mimicking idiopathic hirsutism or polycystic ovary disease. Ann Intern Med 96:143, 1982
CROCK PA et al: Multiple pituitary hormone gradients from inferior petrosal sinus sampling in Cushing's disease. Acta Endocrinologica 119:75, 1988
HOLLENBERG SM et al: Primary structure and expression of a functional human glucocorticoid receptor cDNA. Nature 318:635, 1985
MAMPALAM TJ et al: Transsphenoidal microsurgery for Cushing disease: A report of 216 cases. Ann Intern Med 109:487, 1988
METZLER CH et al: Increased synthesis and release of atrial peptide during mineralocorticoid escape in conscious dogs. Am J Physiol 252:R188, 1987
MUJAIS SK et al: Modulation of renal sodium-potassium-adenosine triphosphatase by aldosterone. J Clin Invest 76:170, 1985
MUNCK et al: Physiological functions of glucocorticoids in stress and their relation to pharmacological actions. Endocr Rev 5:25, 1984
NEW MI, LEVINE LS: Recent advances in 21-hydroxylase deficiency. Ann Rev Med 35:649, 1984
NOLAN PM et al: Therapeutic problems with transsphenoidal pituitary surgery for Cushing's disease. Clev Clin Q 49:199, 1982
ORTH DN: The old and the new in Cushing's syndrome. N Engl J Med 310:649, 1984
OLDFIELD EH et al: Preoperative lateralization of ACTH-secreting pituitary microadenomas by bilateral and simultaneous inferior petrosal venous sinus sampling. N Engl J Med 312:100, 1985
PEDERSEN RC et al: Pro-adrenocorticotropin/endorphin-derived peptides: Coordinated action on adrenal steroidogenesis. Science 208:1044, 1980
PEMBERTON et al: Hormone binding globulins undergo serpin conformational change in inflammation. Nature 336:257, 1988
RABINOWE SL et al: Ia-Positive T lymphocytes in recently diagnosed idiopathic Addison's disease. Am J Med 77:597, 1984
ROSS EJ, LYNCH DC: Cushing's syndrome—killing disease: Discriminatory value of signs and symptoms aiding early diagnosis. Lancet 2:646, 1982
SCHAMBELAN M et al: Prevalence, pathogenesis and functional significance of aldosterone deficiency in hyperkalemic patients with chronic renal insufficiency. Kidney Int 17:89, 1980
SCHULTE HM et al: Continuous administration of synthetic ovine corticotropin-releasing factor in man: Physiological and pathophysiological implications. J Clin Invest 75:1781, 1985
STEWART PM et al: Mineralocorticoid activity of liquorice: 11-Beta-hydroxysteroid dehydrogenase deficiency comes of age. Lancet 2:821, 1987
STEWART PM et al: Syndrome of apparent mineralocorticoid excess. A defect in the cortisol-cortisone shuttle. J Clin Invest 82:340, 1988
SUDA T et al: Effects of corticotropin-releasing hormone and dexamethasone on proopiomelanocortin messenger RNA level in human corticotroph adenoma cells in vitro. J Clin Invest 82:110, 1988
TYRRELL JB et al: An overnight high-dose dexamethasone suppression test: Rapid differential diagnosis of Cushing's syndrome. Ann Intern Med 104:180, 1986
WEINBERGER MH: Primary aldosteronism: Diagnosis and differentiation of subtypes. Ann Intern Med 100:300, 1984
WILLIAMS GH, DLUHY RG: Control of aldosterone secretion, in Hypertension, 2d ed, J Genest et al (eds). New York, McGraw-Hill, 1983, p 320
WILLIAMS GH, DLUHY RG: Diagnostic imaging of the adrenal gland, in Endocrinology, 2d ed, LG DeGroot et al (eds). Orlando, FL, Grune and Stratton 1989, p 1633
WULFRATT NM et al: Immunoglobulins of patients with Cushing's syndrome due to pigmented adrenocortical micronodular dysplasia stimulate in vitro steroidogenesis. J Clin Endocrinol Metab 66:301, 1988

318 PHEOCHROMOCYTOMA

LEWIS LANDSBERG / JAMES B. YOUNG

Pheochromocytomas, also known as chromaffin tumors, produce, store, and secrete catecholamines. They are derived most often from the adrenal medulla but may develop from chromaffin cells in or about sympathetic ganglia (extraadrenal pheochromocytomas or paragangliomas). Related tumors that secrete catecholamines and produce similar clinical syndromes include chemodectomas derived from the carotid body and ganglioneuromas derived from the postganglionic sympathetic neurons.

The clinical features and morbidity of these tumors are due predominantly to the release of catecholamines. Hypertension is the most common manifestation, and hypertensive paroxysms or crises, often spectacular and alarming, occur in over half the cases.

Pheochromocytoma occurs only in approximately 0.1 percent of the hypertensive population, but it is, nevertheless, an important correctable cause of high blood pressure. Indeed, it is usually curable if properly diagnosed and treated, but may be fatal if undiagnosed or mistreated. Postmortem series indicate that the majority of pheochromocytomas are unsuspected clinically and that in many of these cases the tumor is related to the fatal outcome.

PATHOLOGY Location and morphology In adults approximately 80 percent occur as a unilateral solitary lesion, 10 percent are bilateral, and 10 percent are extraadrenal. In children a fourth of tumors are bilateral, and an additional fourth are extraadrenal. Solitary lesions inexplicably favor the right side. Although pheochromocytomas may grow to large size (over 3 kg), most weigh less than 100 g and are less than 10 cm in diameter. The tumors are highly vascular with an arterial supply derived from any of the three arteries that normally supply the adrenal.

The tumors are made up of large, polyhedral, pleomorphic chromaffin cells. Less than 10 percent are malignant. As with other endocrine tumors malignancy cannot be determined by the histologic appearance; local invasion of surrounding tissues or distant metastases indicate malignancy.

FAMILIAL PHEOCHROMOCYTOMA In approximately 5 percent of cases pheochromocytoma is inherited as an autosomal dominant trait either alone or in combination with other abnormalities such as multiple endocrine neoplasia (MEN) type IIa (Sipple's syndrome) or type IIb (mucosal neuroma syndrome) (see Chap. 325), von Recklinghausen's neurofibromatosis, or von Hippel–Lindau's retinal cerebellar hemangioblastomatosis. Bilateral adrenal pheochromocytomas are common in the familial syndromes; within MEN kindreds over half with pheochromocytomas have bilateral lesions. A familial syndrome should be suspected in any patient presenting with bilateral pheochromocytomas.

EXTRAADRENAL PHEOCHROMOCYTOMAS Extraadrenal pheochromocytomas have an average weight of 20 to 40 g and are usually less than 5 cm in diameter. Most are located within the abdomen in association with the celiac, superior mesenteric, and inferior mesenteric ganglia. Approximately 1 percent are in the thorax in relation to the paravertebral sympathetic ganglia, 1 percent are within the urinary bladder, and less than 1 percent are in the neck, usually in association with the sympathetic ganglia or the extracranial branches of the ninth or tenth cranial nerves.

Catecholamine synthesis, storage, and release Pheochromocytomas synthesize and store catecholamines by processes resembling those of the normal adrenal medulla (Chap. 67). Little is known about the mechanisms of catecholamine release from pheochromocytomas, but changes in blood flow and necrosis within the tumor may be the cause in some instances. These tumors are not innervated, and catecholamine release does not result from neural stimulation. Pheochromocytomas also store and secrete a variety of peptides including endogenous opioids, neuropeptide Y, and chromagranin A (see Chap. 67). The functional and clinical significance of these peptides is uncertain.

EPINEPHRINE, NOREPINEPHRINE, AND DOPAMINE Most pheochromocytomas contain and secrete both norepinephrine and epinephrine, and the percentage of norepinephrine is usually greater than in the normal adrenal. Most extraadrenal pheochromocytomas secrete norepinephrine exclusively. Rarely, pheochromocytomas produce epinephrine alone, particularly in association with MEN. Although epinephrine-producing tumors may be associated with a preponderance of metabolic and beta-receptor effects, in general the predominant catecholamine secreted cannot be predicted from the clinical presentation. Increased production of dopamine and homovanillic acid (HVA) is uncommon with benign lesions; the excretion of these precursors is, however, increased in some patients with malignant pheochromocytoma.

CLINICAL FEATURES Pheochromocytoma occurs at all ages but is most common in young to midadult life. Some series show a slight female preponderance. Although the presentation is characteristically unpredictable, most patients come to medical attention as a result of hypertensive crisis, paroxysmal symptoms suggestive of seizure disorder or anxiety attacks, or hypertension that responds poorly to conventional treatment. Less commonly, unexplained hypotension or shock in association with surgery or trauma will suggest the diagnosis.

Hypertension Hypertension is the most common manifestation. In approximately 60 percent of cases the hypertension is sustained, although significant blood pressure lability is usually present and half of patients with sustained hypertension have distinct crises or paroxysms. The other 40 percent have blood pressure elevations only during an attack. The hypertension is often severe, occasionally malignant, and usually resistant to treatment with standard drugs used for therapy of essential hypertension.

Paroxysms or crises The paroxysm or crisis is a typical manifestation, occurring in over half of patients. In an individual patient the symptoms are often similar with each attack. The paroxysms are commonly frequent but may be sporadic at intervals as long as weeks or months. With time the paroxysms usually increase in frequency, duration, and severity.

The attack usually has a sudden onset. It may last from a few minutes to several hours or longer. Headache, profuse sweating, palpitations, and apprehension, often with a sense of impending doom, are common. Pain in the chest or abdomen may be associated with nausea and vomiting. Either pallor or flushing may occur during the attack. The blood pressure is elevated, often to alarming levels, and is usually accompanied by tachycardia.

The paroxysm may be precipitated by any activity that displaces the abdominal contents. In some cases a particular stimulus may reproduce an attack in a characteristic fashion, but no clearly defined precipitating event may be found. Although anxiety may accompany the attacks, mental stress or psychological tension does not usually provoke a crisis.

Other distinctive clinical features Symptoms and signs of an increased metabolic rate, such as profuse sweating and mild to moderate weight loss, are common. Orthostatic hypotension is a consequence of diminished plasma volume and blunted sympathetic reflexes. Both of these factors predispose the patient with unsuspected pheochromocytoma to hypotension or shock during surgery or major trauma.

CARDIAC MANIFESTATIONS Sinus tachycardia, sinus bradycardia, supraventricular arrhythmias, and ventricular premature contractions have all been noted. Angina and acute myocardial infarction may occur even in the absence of coronary artery disease. Catecholamine-induced increase in myocardial oxygen consumption and, perhaps, coronary spasm may be involved in the pathogenesis of these ischemic events. Electrocardiographic changes, including nonspecific ST-T wave changes, prominent U waves, left ventricular strain patterns, and right and left bundle branch blocks may be present in the absence of demonstrable ischemia or infarction. Cardiomyopathy, either congestive with myocarditis and myocardial fibrosis or hypertrophic with concentric or asymmetric hypertrophy, may be associated with heart failure and cardiac arrhythmias. Noncardiogenic pulmonary edema may also occur in patients with pheochromocytoma, secondary to either shifts in extracellular fluid, altered pulmonary capillary permeability, or increased pulmonary venous tone.

CARBOHYDRATE INTOLERANCE Over half of patients have impaired carbohydrate tolerance due to suppression of insulin and stimulation of hepatic glucose output. The impaired glucose tolerance rarely requires specific treatment with insulin and disappears after removal of the tumor.

HEMATOCRIT Patients may have an elevated hematocrit secondary to diminished plasma volume. Rarely production of erythropoietin by the pheochromocytoma may cause a true erythrocytosis.

PHEOCHROMOCYTOMA OF THE URINARY BLADDER Pheochromocytoma within the wall of the urinary bladder may result in typical paroxysms in relation to micturition. The unique location of these tumors within the bladder wall is responsible for the production of symptoms while the tumors are quite small, and consequently, urinary catecholamine excretion may be normal or only minimally elevated. Hematuria is present in over half, and the tumor can often be visualized at cystoscopy.

Adverse drug interactions Severe and occasionally fatal paroxysms have been induced by opiates, histamine, ACTH, saralasin, and glucagon. These agents appear to release catecholamines directly from the tumor. Indirect-acting sympathomimetic amines, including methyldopa (when administered intravenously), may cause an increase in blood pressure by releasing catecholamines from the augmented stores within nerve endings. Drugs that block neuronal uptake of catecholamines, such as tricyclic antidepressants or guanethidine, may enhance the physiologic effects of circulating catecholamines. These drugs should be avoided in patients with known or suspected pheochromocytoma; indeed all medications should be carefully considered and cautiously administered in such patients.

Associated diseases Pheochromocytoma is associated with medullary carcinoma of the thyroid in the familial MEN syndrome types IIa and IIb and with hyperparathyroidism in MEN IIa (see Chap. 325). Hypercalcemia, resolving after tumor resection, has also been described in patients with pheochromocytoma in the absence of parathyroid disease, reflecting, in some cases, secretion of a non-PTH humoral factor by the tumor. Every member of MEN IIa and IIb kindreds should be screened periodically for pheochromocytoma by assay of a 24-h urine sample for catecholamines, including measurement of epinephrine. Pheochromocytoma should be excluded or removed before thyroid or parathyroid surgery.

The association of pheochromocytoma and neurofibromatosis is well recognized but not common. Nevertheless, since incomplete forms of neurofibromatosis may be associated with pheochromocytoma, minor manifestations such as five to six café au lait spots, vertebral abnormalities, or kyphoscoliosis should increase the suspicion of pheochromocytoma in a patient with hypertension. The incidence of pheochromocytoma in some kindreds with von Hippel–Lindau disease may be as high as 10 to 25 percent. Many of these are unsuspected clinically and diagnosed postmortem.

The incidence of cholelithiasis is about 15 to 20 percent in patients with pheochromocytoma. Cushing's syndrome is rarely associated with pheochromocytoma, usually a consequence of ectopic secretion of ACTH either by the pheochromocytoma or, less commonly, by a coexistent medullary carcinoma of the thyroid.

DIAGNOSIS The diagnosis is established by the demonstration of increased amounts of catecholamines or catecholamine metabolites in a 24-h urine collection. The diagnosis can usually be made by the analysis of a single 24-h urine sample, provided the patient is hypertensive or symptomatic at the time of collection.

Biochemical tests The determinations employed in the diagnosis include vanillylmandelic acid (VMA), the metanephrines, and unconjugated or "free" catecholamines (Chap. 67). Although much has been written about the relative specificity and sensitivity of the different measurements, they are probably equivalent provided the assays are properly performed. Accuracy of diagnosis is improved when two of the three determinations are employed, although this is not essential as a screening procedure. The following considerations apply to all the urinary tests: (1) Despite claims for the adequacy of determinations made on random urine samples and expressed per milligram of creatinine, analysis of a full 24-h urine sample is preferable. Creatinine should be determined as well to assess the adequacy of collection. (2) Where possible the collection should be obtained when the patient is at rest, on no medication, and without recent exposure to radiographic contrast media. Where it is not practical to discontinue all medications, those drugs known specifically to interfere in the assays (as noted above) should be avoided. (3) The urine collection should be properly acidified and kept cold during and after collection. (4) With specific high-quality assays dietary restrictions are minimal and should be specified by the laboratory performing the analyses. (5) Although most patients with pheochromocytoma excrete increased quantities of catecholamines and catecholamine metabolites, the yield is increased in patients with paroxysmal hypertension if a 24-h urine collection is initiated during a crisis.

FREE CATECHOLAMINES The upper limit of normal for total catecholamines is between 590 and 885 nmol (100 and 150 μg) per 24 h. In most patients with pheochromocytoma values in excess of 1480 nmol (250 μg) per day are obtained. Specific measurement of epinephrine is often of value since increased epinephrine excretion [over 275 nmol (50 μg) per 24 h] is usually due to an adrenal lesion and may be the only abnormality in cases associated with MEN. False-positive increases in catecholamine excretion result from exogenous catecholamines and related drugs such as methyldopa, levodopa, labetalol, and sympathomimetic amines, which may elevate catecholamine excretion for up to 2 weeks. Endogenous catecholamines from stimulation of the sympathoadrenal system may also increase urinary catecholamine excretion and result in a false-positive test. The relevant clinical situations include hypoglycemia, strenuous exertion, central nervous system disease with increased intracranial pressure, and clonidine withdrawal.

METANEPHRINES AND VMA In most laboratories the upper limit of normal is 7 μmol (1.3 mg) of total metanephrine and 35 μmol (7.0 mg) of VMA excretion per 24 h. In most patients with pheochromocytoma the increase in excretion of these metabolites is

considerable, often more than three times the normal range. Metanephrine excretion is increased by exogenous and endogenous catecholamines and by treatment with monoamine oxidase inhibitors; propranolol may cause a spurious increase in metanephrine excretion, since a propranolol metabolite interferes in the commonly utilized spectrophotometric assay. VMA is less affected by endogenous and exogenous catecholamines but is spuriously increased by a variety of drugs, including carbidopa. VMA excretion is decreased by monoamine oxidase inhibitors.

PLASMA CATECHOLAMINES Measurement of plasma catecholamines has a limited application in the diagnosis. The care required in obtaining basal catecholamine levels (Chap. 67), the lack of readily available, reliable plasma catecholamine assays, and the satisfactory results obtained with urinary determinations make measurement of plasma catecholamines unnecessary in most cases. Plasma catecholamine levels are affected by the same drugs and physiologic perturbations that increase urinary catecholamine excretion. In addition, alpha- and beta-adrenergic receptor blocking agents may elevate plasma catecholamines by impairing catecholamine clearance.

In occasional patients, when the clinical features suggest pheochromocytoma and the urinary assays are borderline, measurement of plasma catecholamines may be worthwhile. Markedly elevated basal levels of total catecholamines support the diagnosis, although approximately one-third of patients with pheochromocytoma have normal or slightly elevated basal values. The usefulness of plasma catecholamine determinations may be increased by agents that suppress sympathetic nervous system activity. Clonidine and ganglionic blocking agents (Chap. 67) both markedly reduce plasma catecholamine levels in normal subjects and in patients with essential hypertension. These drugs have little effect on catecholamine levels in patients with pheochromocytoma. In patients with elevated or borderline basal catecholamine values, failure to suppress plasma or urinary levels with clonidine supports the diagnosis of pheochromocytoma.

Pharmacologic tests Reliable methods for the measurement of catecholamines and catecholamine metabolites in urine have rendered obsolete both the provocative and adrenolytic tests, which are nonspecific and entail considerable risk. A modified version of the adrenolytic test may be of some use, however, as a therapeutic trial in a patient in hypertensive crisis with features suggestive of pheochromocytoma. A positive response to phentolamine (5-mg bolus following a 0.5-mg test dose) is a reduction in blood pressure of at least 35/25 mmHg that becomes maximal after 2 min and persists for 10 to 15 min. The response to a pharmacologic agent is never diagnostic, and biochemical confirmation must always be obtained. Provocative tests in normotensive patients are potentially dangerous and rarely indicated. However, a glucagon provocative test may be of use in patients with paroxysmal hypertension and basal catecholamine levels below those usually found in patients with pheochromocytoma. Glucagon has a negligible effect on blood pressure or on plasma catecholamine levels in normal or hypertensive subjects. In patients with pheochromocytoma, on the other hand, glucagon may substantially increase both blood pressure and circulating catecholamine levels. The elevation in plasma catecholamine concentration, moreover, may occur in patients without a blood pressure response. It must be emphasized, however, that life-threatening pressor crises have occurred after administration of glucagon to patients with pheochromocytoma so that the test should never be performed casually. Careful continuous monitoring of the blood pressure is required, intravenous access must be adequate, and phentolamine must be at hand to terminate the test if a significant pressor reaction ensues.

Differential diagnosis Since the manifestations may be protean, the diagnosis must be considered and excluded in many patients with suggestive clinical features. In patients with essential hypertension and "hyperadrenergic" features such as tachycardia, sweating, and increased cardiac output, and in patients with anxiety attacks associated with blood pressure elevations, analysis of a 24-h urine collection is usually decisive in excluding the diagnosis. Repeated determinations on urine collected during attacks may be necessary, however, before the diagnosis can be excluded with certainty. The clonidine suppression and glucagon stimulation tests may occasionally be helpful in excluding the diagnosis in difficult cases. Pressor crises associated with clonidine withdrawal or the use of monoamine oxidase inhibitors (Chap. 67) may mimic the paroxysms of pheochromocytoma. Factitious crises may be produced by self-administration of sympathomimetic amines in psychiatrically disturbed patients, particularly among those employed in the health care professions.

Intracranial lesions, particularly posterior fossa tumors or subarachnoid hemorrhage, may be associated with hypertension and increased excretion of catecholamines or catecholamine metabolites. While this is most common in patients who have suffered an obvious neurologic catastrophe, the possibility of subarachnoid or intracranial hemorrhage secondary to pheochromocytoma should be considered. Diencephalic or autonomic epilepsy may be associated with paroxysmal spells, hypertension, and increased plasma catecholamine levels. This rare entity may be difficult to distinguish from pheochromocytoma, but an aura, an abnormal electroencephalogram, and a beneficial response to anticonvulsant medications will often suggest the proper diagnosis.

MANAGEMENT Preoperative management The induction of stable alpha-adrenergic blockade is the basis of preoperative management and provides the foundation for successful surgical treatment. Once the diagnosis is established, the patient should be placed on phenoxybenzamine to induce a long-lived, noncompetitive alpha-receptor blockade. The usual initial dose is 10 mg every 12 h with increments of 10 to 20 mg added every few days until the blood pressure is controlled and the paroxysms disappear. Because of the long duration of action the therapeutic effects are cumulative, and the optimal dose must be achieved gradually with careful monitoring of supine and upright blood pressures. Most patients require between 40 and 80 mg of phenoxybenzamine per day although in some cases 200 mg or more may be necessary. Phenoxybenzamine should be administered for at least 10 to 14 days prior to surgery. Over this time the combination of alpha-receptor blockade and a liberal salt intake will restore the contracted plasma volume to normal. Before adequate alpha-adrenergic blockade with phenoxybenzamine is achieved, paroxysms may be treated with intravenous phentolamine. Prazosin, the selective alpha₁ antagonist, has been employed in the preoperative management of a small number of patients. Doses in the range of 1.5 to 2.5 mg every 6 h have effectively controlled blood pressure and paroxysms. The role of this agent in the management of pheochromocytoma has not been established; the relatively short duration of action may be a disadvantage compared with phenoxybenzamine. Prazosin may be useful as an antihypertensive agent in patients with suspected pheochromocytoma while workup is in progress, since it is usually better tolerated than phenoxybenzamine and prevents serious pressor crises if pheochromocytoma is present. Nitroprusside is the only other antihypertensive agent that reliably reduces blood pressure in patients with pheochromocytoma and may be useful on occasion.

Beta-adrenergic receptor-blocking agents should be given only after alpha blockade has been established, since administration of such agents by themselves may cause a paradoxic increase in blood pressure by antagonizing beta-mediated vasodilatation in skeletal muscle. Beta blockade is usually initiated when tachycardia develops during the induction of alpha-adrenergic blockade. Low doses often suffice, and a reasonable starting dose is 10 mg propranolol 3 to 4 times per day, increased as needed to control the pulse rate. Beta blockade is effective treatment for catecholamine-induced arrhythmias, particularly those potentiated by anesthetic agents.

Preoperative localization of the tumor Surgical removal of pheochromocytoma is facilitated if the location of the tumor, or tumors, can be established preoperatively. Once pheochromocytoma is diagnosed, localization should be undertaken while the patient is being prepared for surgery by the administration of alpha-receptor

blocking agents. Computed tomography or magnetic resonance imaging of the adrenals is usually successful in identifying the intraadrenal lesions. Conventional chest roentgenograms and computed tomography of the chest usually suffice to identify intrathoracic lesions. If these studies are negative, abdominal aortography (once alpha-adrenergic blockade is complete) may be useful in identifying extraadrenal pheochromocytomas within the abdomen, since these lesions are often supplied by a large aberrant artery. If aortography and computed tomography fail to localize the lesion, venous sampling at different levels of the inferior and superior vena cava may reveal a step-up in catecholamine concentration in the region drained by the tumor; this area may then be restudied by selective angiography or directed scanning by computed tomography. An additional localization technique involves a radionuclide scintiscan after administration of an investigational radiopharmaceutical ¹³¹I-metaiodobenzylguanidine (MIBG). This agent is concentrated by the amine uptake process and produces an external scintigraphic image at the site of the tumor. This type of scanning may be useful in characterizing lesions discovered by computed tomography when biochemical confirmation is indeterminate, as well as in localizing extraadrenal pheochromocytomas. Percutaneous fine-needle aspiration of chromaffin tumors is contraindicated; pheochromocytoma should be considered before adrenal lesions discovered by scanning techniques are aspirated.

Surgery Surgery is best performed in centers with experience in the preoperative, anesthetic, and intraoperative management of pheochromocytoma patients. In experienced hands surgical mortality is below 2 or 3 percent.

Adequate monitoring during the surgical procedure should include continuous recording of arterial pressure, central venous pressure, and electrocardiogram; in the presence of cardiac disease or if congestive failure has been present, pulmonary capillary wedge pressure should be monitored as well. Adequate fluid replacement is crucial. Intraoperative hypotension responds better to volume replacement than to the administration of vasoconstrictors. Hypertension and cardiac arrhythmias are most likely to occur during induction of anesthesia, intubation, and manipulation of the tumor. Intravenous phentolamine is usually sufficient to control the blood pressure, but nitroprusside may be required. Propranolol may be given in the treatment of tachycardia or ventricular ectopy.

PHEOCHROMOCYTOMA IN PREGNANCY Spontaneous labor and vaginal delivery in unprepared patients are usually disastrous for mother and fetus. In early pregnancy it seems reasonable to prepare the patient with phenoxybenzamine and remove the tumor as soon as the diagnosis is confirmed. The pregnancy need not be terminated, but the operative procedure itself may result in spontaneous abortion. In the third trimester, treatment with adrenergic blocking agents should be undertaken; when the fetus is of sufficient size cesarean section followed by extirpation of the tumor may be undertaken. Although the safety of adrenergic blocking drugs in pregnancy has not been established, these agents have been administered in several cases without obvious adverse effect.

UNRESECTABLE AND MALIGNANT TUMORS In cases of metastatic or locally invasive tumor or in patients with intercurrent illness that precludes surgery, long-term medical management is required. When the manifestations of pheochromocytoma cannot be adequately controlled by the chronic administration of adrenergic blocking agents, the concomitant administration of metyrosine may be required. This agent inhibits tyrosine hydroxylase, diminishes catecholamine production by the tumor, and often simplifies chronic management. Malignant pheochromocytoma frequently recurs in the retroperitoneum and metastasizes most commonly to bone and lung. Although these are resistant to radiotherapy, combination chemotherapy has had limited success in the treatment of the malignant tumors.

PROGNOSIS AND FOLLOW-UP The 5-year survival after surgery is usually over 95 percent, and the recurrence rate is less than 10 percent. After successful surgery catecholamine excretion returns to normal in about 1 week and should be measured to ensure complete tumor removal. Catecholamine excretion should be assessed at the reappearance of suggestive symptoms or yearly for several years, if the patient remains asymptomatic. In malignant pheochromocytoma the 5-year survival is less than 50 percent.

Complete removal of the pheochromocytoma cures the hypertension in approximately three-fourths. In the remainder hypertension recurs but is usually well controlled by standard antihypertensive agents. In this group either underlying essential hypertension or irreversible vascular damage induced by catecholamines may cause the persistence of the hypertension.

REFERENCES

AVERBUCH SD et al: Malignant pheochromocytoma: Effective treatment with a combination of cyclophosphamide, vincristine, and dacarbazine. Ann Intern Med 109:267, 1988

BRAVO EL, GIFFORD RW: Pheochromocytoma: Diagnosis, localization, and management. N Engl J Med 311:1298, 1984

BROWN MJ et al: Increased sensitivity and accuracy of phaeochromocytoma diagnosis achieved by use of plasma-adrenaline estimations and a pentolinium-suppression test. Lancet 1:174, 1981

DUNCAN MW et al: Measurement of norepinephrine and 3,4-dihydroxyphenylglycol in urine and plasma for the diagnosis of pheochromocytoma. N Engl J Med 319:136, 1988

ENGELMAN K: Phaeochromocytoma. Clin Endocrinol Metab 6:769, 1977

FUDGE TL et al: Current surgical management of pheochromocytoma during pregnancy. Arch Surg 115:1224, 1980

GLUSHIEN AS et al: Pheochromocytoma: Its relationship to the neurocutaneous syndromes. Am J Med 14:318, 1953

HAMILTON BP et al: Measurement of urinary epinephrine in screening for pheochromocytoma in multiple endocrine neoplasia type II. Am J Med 65:1027, 1978

HORTON WA et al: Von Hippel–Lindau disease: Clinical and pathological manifestations in nine families with 50 affected members. Arch Intern Med 136:769, 1976

JONES DH et al: The biochemical diagnosis, localization and followup of phaeochromocytoma: The role of plasma and urinary catecholamine measurements. Q J Med 49:431, 1980

KHAIRI MRA et al: Mucosal neuroma, pheochromocytoma and medullary thyroid carcinoma: Multiple endocrine neoplasia type 3. Medicine 54:89, 1975

LAURSEN K, DAMGAARD-PEDERSON K: CT for pheochromocytoma diagnosis. AJR 134:277, 1980

MACDOUGALL IC et al: Overnight clonidine suppression test in the diagnosis and exclusion of pheochromocytoma. Am J Med 84:993, 1988

MANGER WM, GIFFORD RW JR: *Pheochromocytoma.* New York, Springer-Verlag, 1977

McCORKELL SJ, NILES NL: Fine-needle aspiration of catecholamine-producing adrenal masses: A possibly fatal mistake. Am J Roentgenol 145:113, 1985

PALUBINSKAS AJ et al: Localization of functioning pheochromocytomas by venous sampling and radioenzymatic analysis. Radiology 136:495, 1980

REINIG JW, DOPPMAN JL: Magnetic resonance imaging of the adrenal. Radiologe 26:186, 1986

REMINE WH et al: Current management of pheochromocytoma. Ann Surg 179:740, 1974

ROSS EJ et al: Preoperative and operative management of patients with pheochromocytoma. Br Med J 1:191, 1971

ST JOHN WM, GIFFORD RW JR: Prevalence of clinically unsuspected pheochromocytoma. Mayo Clin Proc 56:354, 1981

SISSON JC et al: Scintigraphic localization of pheochromocytoma. N Engl J Med 305:12, 1981

SJOERDSMA A et al: Pheochromocytoma: Current concepts of diagnosis and treatment. Ann Intern Med 65:1302, 1966

STEINER AL et al: Study of a kindred with pheochromocytoma, medullary thyroid carcinoma, hyperparathyroidism and Cushing's disease: Multiple endocrine neoplasia, type 2. Medicine 47:371, 1968

STEWART AF et al: Hypercalcemia in pheochromocytoma. Ann Intern Med 102:776, 1985

319 DIABETES MELLITUS

DANIEL W. FOSTER

Diabetes mellitus is the most common endocrine disease. The true frequency is difficult to ascertain because of differing standards of diagnosis but probably is between 1 and 2 percent. The disease is characterized by metabolic abnormalities; by long-term complications involving the eyes, kidneys, nerves, and blood vessels; and by a lesion of the basement membranes demonstrable by electron micros-

TABLE 319-1 Classification of diabetes

A Primary
  1 Insulin-dependent diabetes mellitus (IDDM, type 1)
  2 Non-insulin-dependent diabetes mellitus (NIDDM, type 2)
    a Nonobese NIDDM (type 1 IDDM in evolution?)
    b Obese NIDDM
    c Maturity-onset diabetes of the young (MODY)
B Secondary
  1 Pancreatic disease
  2 Hormonal abnormalities
  3 Drug or chemical induced
  4 Insulin receptor abnormalities
  5 Genetic syndromes
  6 Other

copy. Patients fulfilling these criteria are not homogeneous, and several distinct diabetic syndromes have been delineated.

DIAGNOSIS The diagnosis of symptomatic diabetes is not difficult. When a patient presents with signs and symptoms attributable to an osmotic diuresis and is found to have hyperglycemia, essentially all physicians agree that diabetes is present. There is likewise little disagreement about an asymptomatic patient with persistently elevated fasting plasma glucose concentrations. The problem arises with the asymptomatic patient who for one reason or another is considered to be a potential diabetic but has a normal fasting glucose concentration in plasma. Such patients are often given an oral glucose tolerance test, and, if abnormal values are found, diagnosed as having "chemical" diabetes. There seems to be little question that normal glucose tolerance is strong evidence against the presence of diabetes; the predictive value of a positive test is less certain. Much evidence suggests that the standard oral glucose tolerance test overdiagnoses diabetes to a remarkable degree, probably because a variety of stresses can produce an abnormal response. The operative mechanism is thought to be epinephrine discharge. Epinephrine blocks insulin secretion, stimulates glucagon release, activates glycogen breakdown, and impairs insulin action in target tissues such that hepatic glucose production is increased and the capacity to dispose of an exogenous glucose load is impaired. Even anxiety over venipunctures may generate sufficient epinephrine to produce an abnormal test. Concomitant illness, inadequate diet, and lack of physical exercise also contribute to false-positive examinations.

In an attempt to deal with these problems, the National Diabetes Data Group of the National Institutes of Health in 1979 provided revised criteria for the diagnosis of diabetes following a challenge with oral glucose:

1 Fasting (overnight): Venous plasma glucose concentration ≥7.8 mmol/L (140 mg/dL) on at least two separate occasions.[1]
2 Following ingestion of 75 g of glucose: Venous plasma glucose concentration ≥11.1 mmol/L (200 mg/dL) at 2 h and on at least one other occasion during the 2-h test; i.e., *two* values ≥11.1 mmol/L (≥200 mg/dL) must be obtained for diagnosis.

If the 2-h value is between 7.8 and 11.1 mmol/L (140 and 200 mg/dL) and one other value during the 2-h test period is equal to or greater than 11.1 mmol/L (200 mg/dL), a diagnosis of "impaired glucose tolerance" is suggested. The interpretation would be that persons in this category are at increased risk for the development of fasting hyperglycemia or symptomatic diabetes but that such progression is not predictable in an individual patient. Most patients (~75 percent) with impaired glucose tolerance never develop diabetes, and many subjects diagnosed as having diabetes by the second criterion may never manifest fasting hyperglycemia or symptomatic deterioration. Consequently, the oral glucose tolerance test is rarely indicated in clinical practice although it is useful as a research tool.

CLASSIFICATION A classification of diabetes is given in Table 319-1. The basic categories are those recommended by the National

[1] Venous whole blood concentrations are 15 percent lower than plasma values. Capillary whole blood, utilized in patient self-monitoring, is equivalent to venous plasma.

Diabetes Data Group except for division into primary and secondary types. Primary implies that no associated disease is present while in the secondary category some other identifiable condition causes or allows a diabetic syndrome to develop. Insulin dependence in this classification is not equivalent to insulin therapy. Rather, the term means that the patient is at risk for ketoacidosis in the absence of insulin. Many patients classified as non-insulin-dependent require insulin for control of hyperglycemia although they do not become ketoacidotic if insulin is withdrawn.

The term *type 1* is often used as a synonym for insulin-dependent diabetes (IDDM), and *type 2* diabetes has been considered equivalent to non-insulin-dependent disease (NIDDM). This probably is not ideal since some patients with apparent non-insulin-dependent diabetes may in fact be destined to become fully insulin-dependent and prone to ketoacidosis. The subset of patients in this category are nonobese subjects who usually express HLA antigens associated with susceptibility to insulin-dependent diabetes and exhibit islet cell antibodies in the blood (see "Pathogenesis" below). For this reason it has been suggested that the classification shown in Table 319-1 be modified such that the terms *insulin-dependent* and *non-insulin-dependent* describe physiologic states (ketoacidosis-prone and ketoacidosis-resistant, respectively) while the terms *type 1* and *type 2* refer to pathogenetic mechanisms (immune-mediated and non-immune-mediated, respectively). Using such a classification three major forms of primary diabetes would be recognized: (1) type 1 insulin-dependent diabetes, (2) type 1 non-insulin-dependent diabetes, and (3) type 2 non-insulin-dependent diabetes. Category 2 can be considered as type 1 insulin-dependent diabetes in evolution; i.e., autoimmune beta-cell destruction occurs slowly rather than rapidly with the result that there is a delay in reaching the ketoacidotic threshold of insulin deficiency.

Secondary forms of diabetes encompass a host of conditions. *Pancreatic disease*, particularly chronic pancreatitis in alcoholics, is a common cause. Destruction of the beta-cell mass is the etiologic mechanism. *Hormonal causes* include pheochromocytoma, acromegaly, Cushing's syndrome, and therapeutic administration of steroid hormones. "Stress hyperglycemia," associated with severe burns, acute myocardial infarctions, and other life-threatening illnesses, is due to endogenous release of glucagon and catecholamines. Mechanisms of hormonal hyperglycemia include varying combinations of impairment of insulin release and induction of insulin resistance. A large number of *drugs* can lead to hyperglycemia, but most simply produce impaired glucose tolerance. Hyperglycemia and even ketoacidosis may occur as a result of abnormalities at the level of the *insulin receptor*. The dysfunction may be due to quantitative or qualitative defects in the receptor itself or to antibodies directed against it (see "Insulin Resistance," below). The mechanism is essentially pure insulin resistance. A number of *genetic syndromes* are associated with impaired glucose tolerance or hyperglycemia. The three most common are the lipodystrophies, myotonic dystrophy, and ataxia-telangiectasia. The final category, *other*, is poorly defined and is meant to include any condition which does not fit elsewhere in the etiologic scheme. The appearance of abnormal carbohydrate metabolism in association with any of the secondary causes does not necessarily indicate the presence of underlying diabetes although in some cases a mild, asymptomatic primary diabetes may be made overt by the secondary illness.

PREVALENCE Prevalence of diabetes is difficult to determine because various standards, many no longer acceptable, have been used in diagnosis. The National Diabetes Data Group, utilizing the 75-g oral glucose tolerance test as the diagnostic criterion, has estimated the prevalence of diabetes at 6.6 percent, with 11.2 percent of the population having impaired glucose tolerance. These figures are almost certainly too high. The estimate of 1 to 2 percent prevalence given at the beginning of this chapter is based on actual experience in long-term follow-up of patients who had a single abnormal glucose tolerance test suggestive of diabetes. Over a 5-year period less than a third of patients developed overt diabetes. Similar conclusions have been reached in Sweden where a prevalence of 1.5 percent has been

estimated. Estimates for insulin-dependent diabetes are more reliable than for the non-insulin-dependent form since most patients are diagnosed after the abrupt appearance of symptoms. In England prevalence of the type 1 illness has been estimated to be 0.22 percent by age 16, and a study in the United States suggested a prevalence of 0.26 percent by age 20. If the prevalence of diabetes is about 1 percent, it follows that about one-fourth of cases have insulin-dependent disease while three-fourths are non-insulin-dependent. The relative frequency of insulin-dependent to non-insulin-dependent diabetes varies with age, being higher if a young population is studied and lower in the older age range. The cited prevalences are for the population as a whole. Certain subsets have different rates. For example, more than 40 percent of Pima Indians in the United States have type 2 NIDDM.

PATHOGENESIS OF TYPE 1 DIABETES MELLITUS By the time insulin-dependent diabetes mellitus appears, most of the beta cells in the pancreas have been destroyed. The destructive process is almost certainly autoimmune in nature, although details remain obscure. A tentative overview of the pathogenetic sequence is given in Table 319-2. *First*, genetic susceptibility to the disease must be present. *Second*, an environmental event ordinarily initiates the process in genetically susceptible individuals. Viral infection is believed to be a common triggering mechanism. The best evidence that an environmental insult is required comes from studies in monozygotic twins, in whom the concordance rate for diabetes is no more than 50 percent. If diabetes were a purely genetic illness, concordance rates would be approximately 100 percent. The *third* step in the sequence is an inflammatory response in the pancreas called "insulitis." The cells that infiltrate the islets are activated T lymphocytes. The *fourth* step is an alteration or transformation of the surface of the beta cell such that it is no longer recognized as "self" but is seen by the immune system as a foreign cell or "nonself." The *fifth* step is the development of an immune response. Because the islets are now considered "nonself," cytotoxic antibodies develop and act in concert with cell-mediated immune mechanisms. The end result is the destruction of the beta cell and the appearance of diabetes. Rarely, type 1 diabetes may develop from an exclusive environmental insult. An example is the ingestion of Vacor, a rat poison. It is also possible that in some cases autoimmune diabetes develops in the absence of an environmental trigger; i.e., it is purely genetic. Usually, however, the pathogenetic sequence is genetic predisposition → environmental insult → insulitis → conversion of beta cell from "self" to "nonself" → activation of the immune system → destruction of the beta cell → diabetes mellitus.

Genetics Although insulin-dependent diabetes aggregates in families, the mechanism of inheritance is unclear in mendelian terms. Transmission has been postulated to be autosomal dominant, recessive, and mixed, but none has been proven. The genetic predisposition is probably permissive and not causal.

Analysis of pedigrees shows a low prevalence of direct vertical

TABLE 319-2   The pathogenesis of type 1 diabetes mellitus

Step	Event	Agent or response
1	Genetic susceptibility	HLAD region genes (T-cell receptor?)
2	Environmental event	Virus (?)
3	Insulitis	Infiltration of activated T lymphocytes
4	Activation of autoimmunity	Self → nonself transition
5	Immune attack on beta cells	Islet cell antibodies, cell-mediated immunity
6	Diabetes mellitus	>90 percent beta cells destroyed (alpha cells unopposed)

transmission. In one series of 35 families in which there was a child with classic insulin-dependent diabetes only four of the index cases had a parent with diabetes and two had a diabetic grandparent. Of the 99 siblings of these diabetic children only 6 had overt disease. Overall the chance of a child developing type 1 diabetes when another first-degree relative has the disease is only 5 to 10 percent. HLA identity of siblings (see below) increases the risk while nonidentity decreases it. Haploidentity (sharing of one HLA genotype) is an intermediate risk. The presence of non-insulin-dependent disease in a parent increases the risk for insulin-dependent diabetes in the offspring. It is not known whether the intermixing of IDDM and NIDDM in the same family represents a single genetic trait (i.e., the apparent NIDDM is really type 1 NIDDM) or whether two common genetic predispositions coexist in the same family by chance, each perhaps influencing the expression of the other. Low rates of transmission of IDDM make it difficult to discern mechanisms of inheritance through study of families but are reassuring to diabetic parents who may wish to have children.

One of the susceptibility genes in IDDM likely resides on the sixth chromosome in view of strong associations between diabetes and certain HLAs coded by the major histocompatibility region on this chromosome (see Chap. 14). Four loci designated by the letters A, B, C, and D (Fig. 319-1) are recognized with alleles at each site identified by numbers (e.g., DR3). A lower case w indicates that identification is provisional (e.g., DQw8). Gene products of the A, B, and C regions are called class I molecules while D-region products are called class II molecules. The D region is subdivided into DR, DP, and DQ and also contains several less well understood regions (DO, DX, DZ). HLA gene products are located in the plasma membranes of cells and are best considered as recognition and/or programming signals for initiation and amplification of immune responses in the body. Class I molecules are present on all nucleated cells and function primarily in defense against infections (especially viruses). They may also be involved in immune surveillance against malignancy. Class II molecules (also called Ia) are normally present on circulating and tissue macrophages, endothelial cells, B lymphocytes, and activated T lymphocytes. They function in the regulatory (helper-suppressor) T-cell system. They also are important in autoimmune diseases such as type 1 diabetes. Activation of the immune system is "MHC restricted." This means that antigens are recognized only if they reach the cell surface in association with a "self" HLA allele which "fits" the receptor on the responding T cell. Thus activation of cytotoxic T lymphocytes to fight a viral infection requires that a neoantigen be formed by the "self" class I molecule and the viral antigen. Similar restriction applies to antigen presentation by macrophages and B lymphocytes to helper T cells.

While definite associations exist between class I alleles and type 1 diabetes (B8, B15), the D locus is considered of primary importance with the class I loci involved through nonrandom associations with D (linkage disequilibrium). Because about 95 percent of white, type 1 IDDM patients express either DR3 or DR4 or the heterozygous DR3/DR4 configuration, it was initially thought that a susceptibility gene might be located nearby. Focus has now shifted to the DQ locus

and to single amino acid changes in the gene product. Persons with alleles coding for aspartic acid in position 57 of the DQ_β chain have low susceptibility to type 1 diabetes, and persons who are homozygous $Asp_\beta57$-negative are at increased risk. A single $Asp_\beta57$ appears to exert intermediate protection in some populations but not in others. It is likely that other amino acids are also important because $Asp_\beta57$ does not appear to be protective in DR4/DR4 homozygotes. In these individuals the amino acid at position 45 appears crucial. At the time of this writing an extended allele designated DQw7 (previously DQw3.1) appears to confer protection while DQw8 (previously DQw3.2) confers maximum risk. DQw7 includes the code for $Asp_\beta57$. Interestingly, DR2/DR2 homozygotes also appear to be protected unless the DR2 clusters with a DQ_β susceptibility gene.

There seems to be little doubt that the HLA-D region is somehow involved in susceptibility to type 1 diabetes. The findings described above have narrowed the search, but other amino acid configurations may alter the function of class II molecules in such a way as to favor development of autoimmune diabetes. It is likely that allelic variation in the T-cell receptor is also involved in susceptibility to autoimmune disease, but understanding of these variations is less well developed than with the HLA side of the equation. How susceptibility or resistance is conferred remains unknown, although one theory proposes that induction of class II molecules on the surface of the beta cell (where they are normally not present) is important in initiating the destruction that leads to type 1 diabetes (see below).

Environmental event As noted earlier, the fact that a significant proportion of monozygotic twins remain discordant for diabetes (one twin with, the other without) has suggested that nongenetic factors are required for expression of diabetes in humans. Similar arguments derive from the fact that HLA identity or haploidentity does not ensure concordance.

The environmental factor in most cases is believed to be a virus capable of infecting the beta cell. A viral etiology was originally suggested by seasonal variations in the onset of the disease and what appeared to be more than a chance relationship between appearance of diabetes and preceding episodes of mumps, hepatitis, infectious mononucleosis, congenital rubella, and coxsackievirus infections. The viral hypothesis gained support from studies showing that certain strains of encephalomyocarditis virus cause diabetes in genetically susceptible mice. The isolation of a coxsackievirus B4 from the pancreas of a previously healthy boy who died following an episode of ketoacidosis and the induction of diabetes in experimental animals inoculated with the isolated virus also suggest that viruses can cause diabetes in humans. A rise in titer of neutralizing antibody to coxsackievirus over the weeks prior to death of the patient indicated that the virus was recently acquired. Further support for the viral theory comes from the observation that congenital rubella is associated with subsequent development of IDDM in about 20 percent of affected individuals in the United States. Cytomegalovirus genes have been found in the genome of a fifth of patients with type 1 diabetes. Presumably viral infections of the pancreas could induce diabetes by two mechanisms: direct inflammatory disruption of islets or induction of an immune response.

Despite its attractiveness, considerable caution should be reserved for the viral theory. Serologic studies seeking evidence of recent viral infection in patients with new-onset insulin-dependent diabetes are inconclusive at best.

Insulitis In animals activated T lymphocytes infiltrate the pancreatic islets prior to or simultaneous with development of diabetes. Lymphocytes are also found in the islets of young persons dying from new-onset diabetes, and radioactively labeled lymphocytes localize in the pancreas in humans with IDDM. These findings are in accord with the observation that immune endocrinopathies in general are associated with lymphocytic infiltration of the affected tissue. However, the insulitis might be an epiphenomenon not causally related to the pathogenetic sequence. This follows from the fact that in the low-dose streptozocin model of diabetes in rodents, which is immunologically mediated, loss of beta-cell mass occurs prior to

FIGURE 319-1 A schematic representation of the major histocompatibility complex on chromosome 6. (*Courtesy of Dr. J. Harold Helderman.*)

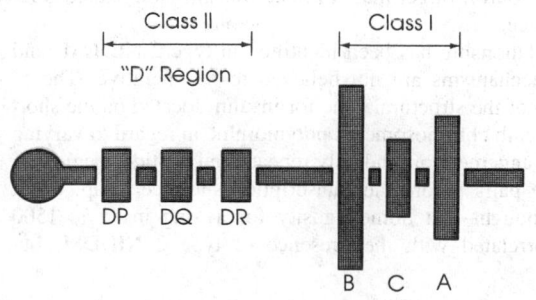

development of insulitis. Moreover, experiments in mice with immune deficiency indicate that T lymphocytes are not necessary for the beta-cell destruction induced by low-dose streptozocin.

Conversion of the beta cell from "self" to "nonself" and activation of the immune system HLA-DR3 and -B15, known to be associated with immune endocrinopathy, are found with increased frequency in insulin-dependent diabetic subjects. There is a frequent coexistence of IDDM and other forms of autoimmune endocrinopathy such as adrenal insufficiency, Hashimoto's thyroiditis, hyperthyroidism, pernicious anemia, vitiligo, myasthenia gravis, and collagen-vascular disease (see Chap. 325). All of these conditions tend to run in families. In addition, islet cell antibodies are found in a high percentage of patients with insulin-dependent diabetes who are examined during the first year after diagnosis. These antibodies are also present in the blood of nonconcordant monozygotic twins or triplets destined to become concordant in the future. The same is true for siblings of patients with insulin-dependent diabetes mellitus. Killer T cells are present in 50 to 60 percent of recently diagnosed diabetic children, a value higher than in control populations. It is noteworthy that diabetes similar to human type 1 disease develops spontaneously in the BB rat. Affected animals exhibit insulitis, thyroiditis, and autoantibodies to pancreatic islets, smooth muscle, thyroid colloid, and gastric parietal cells. Diabetes in these animals can be prevented or reversed by immune modulation. The same is true for the NOD mouse.

What causes the autoimmune process? Early studies reported an increase in the ratio of helper to suppressor T cells in the circulation. The increase in this ratio was due to a deficiency of suppressor T cells. An unbalanced helper-T-cell population would predispose to exuberant antibody formation on exposure to antigen. Subsequent studies failed to confirm an increase in the ratio and noted lymphopenia with a greater diminution in CD4 (largely helper) than CD8 (largely suppressor) T lymphocytes. It is conceivable that early in the disease the CD4/CD8 ratio is high, changing as islet cell destruction proceeds, but this is not established.

The nature of the "self" to "nonself" transition that activates the autoimmune process remains a mystery. One theory is that the key event is an appearance of class II molecules on the surface of the insulin-producing beta cells. The idea is that these cells do not normally express D-region products but that in response to a virus (probably through production of γ-interferon) expression is induced. This would presumably allow the cell to function in antigen presentation utilizing either "self" or foreign antigens. Such antigen presentation would cause the cell to be recognized as "nonself." Whether this actually occurred would depend on the genetic makeup. Thus, if DQw7 were induced, autoimmunity and diabetes would not result, while a person bearing DQw8 would be vulnerable. Susceptibility is probably linked to the fit between newly appearing class II molecules, the requisite membrane antigen (foreign or autologous), and a particular form of the T-cell receptor on the helper T cell. This may account for the appearance of IDDM in the absence of high-risk HLA genes; i.e., in certain cases the class II molecule–T-cell receptor fit occurs even with an ordinarily low-risk allele. As attractive as the formulation is, it has been questioned because of discordant experiments that cannot be reviewed here. However, in the author's opinion it should not be dismissed, especially since alternative explanations have even more problems.

As is true in other immune-mediated endocrinopathies, evidence of an activated immune system may disappear with time. Thus, the islet cell antibodies present in newly diagnosed patients with type 1 IDDM disappear within a year or so. The presence of islet cell antibodies correlates with residual beta-cell mass as assessed in vivo by the capacity to release endogenous insulin in response to a fuel stimulus. As the capacity for endogenous insulin secretion disappears, so do islet cell antibodies. The implication is that as beta cells die, the stimulus to the immune response disappears.

Destruction of beta cells and development of IDDM Because

persons developing insulin-dependent diabetes often have a rather abrupt onset of symptomatic hyperglycemia with polyuria and/or ketoacidosis, it was long assumed that beta-cell damage occurred rapidly. It is now believed that in most cases there is a slow loss of insulin reserve over a few to many years. This insight came from studies of discordant monozygotic diabetic twins and triplets where one twin or triplet developed diabetes long after the index case. In the slow course the earliest sign of abnormality is the development of islet cell antibodies at a time when there is no elevation of the blood sugar and glucose tolerance is normal. Insulin responses to a glucose load are intact. A phase then ensues in which the only metabolic abnormality is decreased glucose tolerance. Fasting blood sugar remains normal. In the third stage fasting hyperglycemia develops, but ketosis does not occur even when the diabetes is poorly controlled. The clinical appearance is that of non-insulin-dependent diabetes mellitus. With time, however, insulin dependence and ketoacidosis may develop, especially with stress. Many nonobese patients with non-insulin-dependent diabetes mellitus may have a slow autoimmune form of the disease as mentioned earlier.

The immune-directed destruction of beta cells probably involves both humoral and cell-mediated mechanisms, the latter being more important. Two types of antibodies have been identified: cytoplasmic and surface. Usually both are present simultaneously in a given patient, but either can occur alone. Islet cell surface antibodies have the capacity to fix complement and lyse beta cells. Surface antibodies appear to impair insulin release even before the beta cell is physically damaged. They interact with a membrane antigen that has not been precisely characterized. A 64,000-mol-wt peptide has received most attention, but other candidate antigens exist. One attractive target is the islet-specific glucose transport protein, since in all forms of diabetes loss of glucose-stimulated insulin secretion is the initial lesion. The fact that antibodies against insulin and proinsulin are often recognized early in the course has led some authors to feel that all such antibodies are secondary to leakage from damaged endocrine cells in the pancreas rather than a primary attack mechanism. At some point in the course cytotoxic T lymphocytes and antibody-dependent killer T cells participate in and complete the destructive process. Cytokines such as interleukin 1 (IL-1) and tumor necrosis factor (TNF-α) are likely also important. By the time overt diabetes appears, most insulin-producing cells have disappeared. In one study pancreatic mass at autopsy averaged 40 g in type 1 diabetes versus 82 g in controls. Endocrine cell mass in subjects with IDDM decreased from 1395 to 413 mg, and beta cells, which averaged 850 mg in normals, were unmeasurable. Since alpha cells remained essentially intact, the ratio of glucagon- to insulin-producing cells approached infinity.

PATHOGENESIS OF TYPE 2 NON-INSULIN-DEPENDENT DIABETES Little progress has been made in understanding the pathogenesis of non-insulin-dependent diabetes mellitus. Although the disease runs in families, modes of inheritance are not known except for the variant known as *maturity-onset diabetes of the young* (MODY). This disease is manifested by mild hyperglycemia in young persons who are resistant to ketosis. Four lines of evidence suggest transmission as an autosomal dominant trait. First, three-generation direct transmission has been demonstrated in over 20 families. Second, a 1:1 ratio of diabetic to nondiabetic children is found when one parent has the disease. Third, about 90 percent of obligate carriers have diabetes. Fourth, direct male-to-male transmission excludes X-linked inheritance.

No HLA relationship has been identified in type 2 NIDDM, and autoimmune mechanisms are not believed to be operative. The 5' flanking region of the structural gene for insulin, located on the short arm of the eleventh chromosome, is polymorphic in regard to varying number and arrangement of tandemly repeated nucleotides beginning some 363 base pairs before the transcription site (see Chap. 6). It was initially thought that homozygosity for a long insert (>1500 base pairs) correlated with the presence of type 2 NIDDM, but subsequent studies failed to confirm a unique relationship. Alcohol-induced flushing after priming with chlorpropamide has also been suggested as a genetic marker for certain forms of the type 2 illness. The fact that patients with IDDM given chlorpropamide also flush after alcohol ingestion has cast doubt on this assumption. Whatever its nature, the genetic influence is powerful, since the concordance rate for diabetes in monozygotic twins with type 2 disease approaches 100 percent. Risk to offspring and siblings of patients with NIDDM is higher than in type 1 diabetes. Nearly four-tenths of siblings and one-third of offspring eventually develop abnormal glucose tolerance or frank diabetes.

Patients with type 2 NIDDM have two physiologic defects: abnormal insulin secretion and resistance to insulin action in target tissues. The primacy of the secretory defect versus the insulin resistance is not established. Most patients with type 2 diabetes are obese, often massively so, and it has been speculated that obesity-induced insulin resistance leads to exhaustion of the beta cell; i.e., the secretory defect is secondary. On the other hand, many massively obese patients do not have diabetes or glucose intolerance, suggesting that obesity does not lead to diabetes in the presence of normal beta-cell responsiveness. The picture is further complicated by the observations that hyperglycemia per se may induce a beta-cell secretory defect and that relative insulin deficiency can cause insulin resistance. A period of aggressive dietary or insulin therapy leading to return of the blood sugar to normal may partially restore insulin secretory capacity as well as sensitivity to insulin action. Unfortunately this does not help in deciding primacy between a secretory defect and insulin resistance. The author favors the view that an islet cell abnormality is primary and necessary for development of diabetes but that acquired insulin resistance, usually obesity-related, is required for overt hyperglycemia to develop. Beta-cell mass is intact in type 2 NIDDM, in contrast to the situation with type 1 IDDM. The alpha-cell population is increased, resulting in an elevated alpha- to beta-cell ratio. This accounts for the excess of glucagon relative to insulin that characterizes NIDDM and that is a feature of all hyperglycemic states.

Although insulin resistance in type 2 NIDDM is associated with decreased numbers of insulin receptors, the bulk of the resistance is postreceptor in type (see below). Insulin resistance in NIDDM may exist independent of obesity. It has long been known that deposits of amyloid are found in the pancreas of patients with type 2 diabetes. This material is a 37-amino acid peptide termed *amylin*. Amylin is normally copackaged with insulin in secretory granules and is released simultaneously in response to insulin secretagogues. In animals amylin appears to induce insulin resistance. Its deposition in the islets may be the consequence of overproduction secondary to the insulin resistance to which it contributes. Alternatively, accumulation of amylin in the islets may contribute to the late failure of insulin production with longstanding NIDDM. The exact role of amylin is not defined.

A rare form of type 2 NIDDM, clinically mild, is due to production of an abnormal insulin that does not bind well to insulin receptors. Such persons respond normally to exogenous insulin.

CLINICAL FEATURES The manifestations of symptomatic diabetes mellitus vary from patient to patient. Most often medical help is sought because of symptoms related to hyperglycemia (polyuria, polydipsia, polyphagia), but the first event may be an acute metabolic decompensation resulting in diabetic coma. Occasionally, the initial expression is a degenerative complication such as neuropathy in the absence of symptomatic hyperglycemia. The metabolic derangements of diabetes are due to relative or absolute deficiency of insulin and relative or absolute excess of glucagon. Normally it is a rise in the molar ratio of glucagon to insulin that leads to metabolic decompensation. Changes in this ratio can be caused by a fall in insulin or a rise in glucagon concentration, separately or together. Conceptually alteration in biologic response to either hormone would have the same effect. Thus insulin resistance could cause metabolic effects

TABLE 319-3 General characteristics of IDDM and NIDDM diabetes

	IDDM	NIDDM
Genetic locus	Chromosome 6	Chromosome 11 (?)
Age of onset	<40	>40
Body habitus	Normal to wasted	Obese
Plasma insulin	Low to absent	Normal to high
Plasma glucagon	High, suppressible	High, resistant
Acute complication	Ketoacidosis	Hyperosmolar coma
Insulin therapy	Responsive	Responsive to resistant
Sulfonylurea therapy	Unresponsive	Responsive

expected of an elevated glucagon:insulin ratio even though the ratio assessed by immunoassay of the two hormones in plasma was not markedly abnormal or even decreased (the glucagon being biologically active, the insulin relatively inactive). The relationship between metabolic abnormalities and degenerative complications will be discussed subsequently. Typically, the clinical features of IDDM and NIDDM are distinctive.

Insulin-dependent diabetes Insulin-dependent diabetes usually begins before the age of 40; in the United States peak incidence is around age 14. Some patients develop type 1 diabetes late in life, with the first episode of ketoacidosis occurring at age 50 or even later in rare instances. These patients, who on the basis of age should have type 2 NIDDM, are usually not obese. Onset of symptoms may be abrupt, with thirst, excessive urination, increased appetite, and weight loss developing over a several-day period. In some cases the disease is heralded by the appearance of ketoacidosis during an intercurrent illness or following surgery. As outlined in Table 319-3, type 1 patients vary from normal weight to wasted, depending on the length of time between onset of symptoms and start of treatment. Characteristically the plasma insulin is low or immeasurable. Glucagon levels are elevated but suppressible with insulin. Once symptoms have developed, insulin therapy is required. Occasionally an initial episode of ketoacidosis is followed by a symptom-free interval (the "honeymoon" period) during which no treatment is required. The likely explanation for this phenomenon is shown in Fig. 319-2.

FIGURE 319-2 Schematic representation of the "honeymoon" period. In this graph insulin secretory capacity is shown gradually decreasing in a patient destined to develop diabetes. At approximately $13\frac{1}{2}$ years insulin would become insufficient to maintain plasma glucose in the normal range. An initial episode of ketoacidosis, for example, in association with acute appendicitis, is shown occurring in the twelfth year. Presumably stress-induced epinephrine release blocks insulin secretion and causes the syndrome. In normal subjects insulin reserve is such that hormone release is adequate, even in the face of stress. Following recovery from the stressful episode insulin secretory capacity returns to the previous level and remains sufficient for an additional year as indicated by the shaded area—the "honeymoon" period.

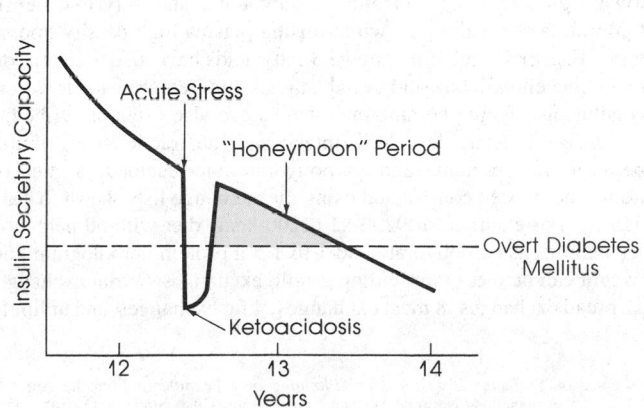

Non-insulin-dependent diabetes This disorder usually begins in middle life or beyond. The typical patient is overweight. Symptoms begin more gradually than in IDDM, and the diagnosis is frequently made when an asymptomatic person is found to have an elevated plasma glucose on routine laboratory examination. In contrast to insulin-dependent disease, plasma insulin levels are normal to high in absolute terms, although they are lower than predicted for the level of the plasma glucose; i.e., relative insulin deficiency is present. Stated in another way, if plasma glucose concentrations in nondiabetic subjects were raised to levels equivalent to those found in diabetic patients, insulin values would be higher in the normal group. This reflects the previously mentioned insulin secretory defect in NIDDM. Glucagon metabolism in non-insulin-dependent diabetes is complex. While the elevated fasting plasma concentrations can be lowered by large amounts of insulin, the exaggerated glucagon response to ingested nutrients cannot be suppressed; i.e., alpha-cell function remains abnormal. For unknown reasons non-insulin-dependent diabetics do not develop ketoacidosis. In the decompensated state they are susceptible to the syndrome of hyperosmolar, nonketotic coma. One hypothesis to explain the absence of ketoacidosis during stress is that the liver is resistant to glucagon so that malonyl-CoA levels remain high, inhibiting the fatty acid oxidation–ketogenic pathway (see below). If weight loss can be induced, patients may be managed by diet alone. The majority of patients failing dietary therapy respond to sulfonylureas, but improvement of hyperglycemia in many is not sufficient for control of diabetes. For this reason a high percentage of patients with NIDDM are treated with insulin.

TREATMENT Diet An estimate is made of the total energy intake needed per day based on ideal body weight (determined from life insurance tables). A decision is then made regarding carbohydrate, fat, and protein content, and an appropriate diet is constructed from the exchange system provided by the American Diabetes Association. Caloric recommendations from the Food and Nutrition Board for adults carrying out "average" activity decrease with age and range from 175 kJ per kilogram body weight (42 kcal/kg) in 18-year-old men to 140 kJ/kg (33 kcal/kg) for 75-year-old women. Intakes slightly less than official recommendations are usually preferable; 150 kJ/kg (36 kcal/kg) for men and 140 kJ/kg (34 kcal/kg) for women are reasonable initial values in most patients, but upward or downward adjustments may be necessary to achieve desired weight.

The minimal protein requirement for good nutrition is about 0.9 g per kilogram body weight per day. Recommended carbohydrate content is 40 to 60 percent of total energy intake, although fractional intakes as high as 85 percent have been prescribed. Protein and carbohydrate calories are supplemented with sufficient fat to bring energy intake to the desired level. Although sucrose is ordinarily not allowed in diabetic diets, a number of reports indicate that in moderation ordinary sugar does not exaggerate postprandial hyperglycemia. Currently most diabetic diets emphasize polyunsaturated fats as an antiatherogenic measure. Alternatively, monounsaturated fats can be used. A 50 percent fat diet containing 33 percent monounsaturated fatty acids and 35 percent carbohydrate reportedly lowers glucose levels, insulin requirements, and very low density lipoprotein concentrations while raising plasma high density lipoproteins. Fish oils containing omega 3 fatty acids have also been reported to be beneficial, but additional studies are required to draw firm conclusions. Increased amounts of fiber are also often prescribed.

Once the desirable caloric intake and the fractional distribution between fat, protein, and carbohydrate are decided, a diet has traditionally been constructed using the exchange lists shown in Table 319-4.[2] For example, a 9200-kJ (2200-kcal) diet with 50 percent of the calories as carbohydrate and 1 to 1.5 g protein per kilogram body weight can be met by providing 2 milk exchanges, 7 fruit exchanges, 12 bread exchanges, 8 meat exchanges, 4 fat exchanges, and unlimited

² Copies of *Exchange Lists for Meal Planning* may be ordered from the American Diabetes Association, National Service Center, 1660 Duke Street, P.O. Box 25757, Alexandria, VA 22313, or from any local affiliate of the association.

TABLE 319-4 Composition of food exchanges*

Exchange	kJ (kcal)	Carbohydrate, g	Fat, g	Protein, g
Milk	711 (170)	12	10	8
Vegetable†	146 (35)	7	—	2
Fruit	167 (40)	10	—	—
Bread	293 (70)‡	15	—	2
Meat	314 (75)‡	—	5	7
Fat	188 (45)	—	5	—

* Composition listed for one exchange.
† Type A vegetables contain little carbohydrate, fat, or protein and can be eaten in any amount. Exchange values are for type B vegetables.
‡ Calculated value for bread exchange is 285 kJ (68 kcal) and for meat exchange is 306 kJ (73 kcal) using 17 kJ/g (4 kcal/g) for carbohydrate and protein and 38 kJ/g (9 kcal/g) for fat.

type A vegetables (Table 319-5). In practice, precalculated diets of given caloric content prepared by the American Diabetes Association are usually used. Care must be taken to emphasize foods the patient likes and can obtain. As in any dietary regimen it is important to emphasize that it is the long-term, overall dietary pattern which counts. Deviation for one meal or two meals does not matter much. Thus a teenage diabetic may be allowed to eat a dessert, ordinarily forbidden, as a special treat with the understanding that resumption of the diet will be necessary the next day. Even in adults the "treat" technique often ensures better dietary cooperation than more rigid demands. Ideally patients should be trained by dieticians in a formal teaching program. Such classes are available in most large hospitals. If a patient is from a smaller community, it will probably be helpful to refer to a larger center for initial training.

In insulin-requiring diabetics the distribution of calories is also important if hypoglycemia is to be avoided. A typical pattern might include 20 percent of the total for breakfast, 35 percent for lunch, 30 percent for dinner, and 15 percent as a late-evening feeding. Occasionally a midafternoon snack is necessary. Different distributions may be required for different lifestyles; i.e., a person employed on a late-evening or night shift would not eat the major meal at noon. When regimens of meticulous control are attempted using multiple injections of insulin or insulin pumps, more frequent feedings are often prescribed. Thus one might recommend 20 percent of energy intake at both breakfast and lunch, 30 percent at dinner, and the remaining 30 percent as midmorning, midafternoon, and late-evening snacks depending on the pattern of plasma glucose during the day.

The traditional approach to dietary therapy has come under question as a result of experiments designed to measure actual blood sugar responses to ingested foods. It is now clear that the exchanges are not necessarily equivalent; i.e., foods of the same weight and similar fat, carbohydrate, or protein content may result in different postprandial increases in the plasma glucose. The term *glycemic index* has been coined to express these differences. In calculating a glycemic index the mean plasma glucose is measured over a 2- to 3-h period after ingestion of a test food and compared to the response with a reference standard of defined composition such as bread. Although

TABLE 319-5 9400-KJ (2200 kcal) diabetic diet (50 percent carbohydrate)

Exchange	No.	kJ (kcal)	Carbohydrate, g	Fat, g	Protein, g
Milk	2	1420 (340)	24	20	16
Vegetable*					
Fruit	7	1170 (280)	70	—	—
Bread	12	3520 (840)	180	—	24
Meat	8	2510 (600)	—	40	56
Fat	4	750 (180)	—	20	—
Total		9370 (2240)	274 (50%)	80 (33%)	96 (17%)

* Type B vegetables include beets, carrots, onions, green peas, pumpkin, rutabagas, winter squash, and turnips. If these are desired, ½ to 1 cup can be substituted for one fruit exchange. All other common vegetables can be eaten as desired.

in principle the approach is attractive because it measures actual glycemic response to foods, its applicability to the general diabetic population is not established. One of the problems is that a glycemic index determined for a food ingested by itself may not apply in a normal mixed meal.

The importance of diet in the management of diabetes varies with type of disease. In insulin-dependent patients, particularly those on intensive insulin regimens, the composition of the diet is not of critical importance since adjustment of insulin can cover wide variations in food ingestion. In non-insulin-dependent patients not treated with exogenous insulin more rigorous adherence to a fixed diet is required since endogenous insulin reserve is limited. Such patients cannot respond to increased demand produced by excess calories or increased intake of rapidly absorbed carbohydrate.

Insulin   Insulin is required for treatment of all patients with IDDM and many patients with non-insulin-dependent disease. If the physician does not use oral agents (see below), all diet-unresponsive NIDDM subjects must be given the hormone. It is fairly easy to control the symptoms of diabetes with insulin, but it is difficult to maintain a normal blood sugar throughout 24 h even if one utilizes multiple injections of regular insulin or infusion pumps. It is even more difficult to maintain normal blood sugars utilizing traditional insulin therapy given as one or two injections a day. Nondiabetic subjects maintain the plasma glucose concentration within a narrow range at all times despite episodic food intake. When a meal is eaten, a prompt rise in insulin release occurs such that absorbed carbohydrate is rapidly transported into the liver and other tissues. Even after meals, therefore, the plasma glucose in normal subjects does not rise into the hyperglycemic or glycosuric range. As the plasma glucose falls under the influence of insulin, release of the hormone is damped, and counterregulatory hormones enter the circulation to prevent hypoglycemia, ensuring smooth control of plasma glucose throughout the absorptive process. The diabetic treated with insulin by injection cannot reproduce these physiologic responses. If enough insulin is given to keep the postprandial glucose normal, inevitably too much insulin will be present during the postabsorptive phase and hypoglycemia will result. The same problem exists when insulin infusion pumps or multiple injections of insulin are utilized in an attempt to control diabetes tightly.

Because evidence suggests that some of the complications of diabetes may be prevented or partially reversed by maintenance of normal or near normal plasma glucose concentrations throughout the day, aggressive insulin therapy is frequently prescribed despite these difficulties. Three treatment regimens will be described: conventional, multiple subcutaneous injections (MSI), and continuous subcutaneous insulin infusion (CSII). *Conventional insulin therapy* involves the administration of one or two injections a day of intermediate acting insulin such as zinc insulin (lente insulin) or isophane insulin (NPH insulin) with or without the addition of small amounts of regular insulin. If the newly diagnosed diabetic is not in acute distress, therapy can be started as an outpatient, provided instruction in diet, insulin use, and monitoring are adequate and the physician can be reached by telephone for consultation. Adults of normal weight may be started on 15 to 20 units a day (the estimated daily insulin production rate in nondiabetic subjects of normal size is about 25 units a day). Obese patients, because of insulin resistance, may be started on 25 to 30 units a day. It is preferable to use the same quantity of insulin for several days before changing, the one exception being the hypoglycemic patient, for whom the dose should be immediately decreased unless a nonrecurrent cause of hypoglycemia (such as excessive exercise) is present. Generally changes should be no more than 5 or 10 units per step. It is probable that a single injection of insulin provides adequate control only in patients who have some residual capacity for insulin secretion. Poorly controlled patients should be placed on split therapy with about two-thirds of the total insulin given before breakfast and the remainder before supper. Two injections are almost always used when the total dose reaches 50 or 60 units a day but may be helpful at smaller doses as

well since the peak action of intermediate insulins appears to be dose-related; i.e., a low dose may exhibit maximal activity earlier and disappear sooner than a large dose. Many physicians routinely add regular insulin to the intermediate dose even at initiation of therapy. Thus in a single-dose schedule one might begin with 20 units of intermediate and 5 units of regular insulin rather than 25 units of intermediate alone. This practice is based upon the concept that the regular insulin lowers the plasma glucose rapidly after which the more slowly absorbed insulin maintains the lowered level. Most patients on twice-daily insulin injections are also treated with a mixture of intermediate and regular insulin; e.g., 25 units NPH plus 10 units of regular before breakfast and 10 units of NPH plus 5 units of regular before supper. All patients should be taught to decrease insulin when significant extra activity or exercise is anticipated. The proper decrement must be determined by trial and error, although a reduction of 5 to 10 units is a reasonable first step. The blood glucose–lowering effect of exercise is primarily due to increased energy demands in previously non-contracting muscle; enhanced absorption of insulin from depot sites secondary to increased blood flow plays a minor role. Conversely a small amount of extra regular insulin can be taken before a meal that contains extra calories or food ordinarily not allowed (e.g., when the diabetic must eat out at a banquet or the teenager goes out on a date). For patients willing to self-monitor plasma glucose an algorithm for adjusting insulin can be provided. A typical protocol is shown in Table 319-6. Patients with complicated control problems may require hospitalization, where frequent plasma glucose determinations can guide therapy.

The *multiple subcutaneous insulin injection technique* most commonly involves administration of intermediate or long-acting insulin in the evening as a single dose together with regular insulin prior to each meal. Home glucose monitoring by the patient is necessary if the goal is the return of the plasma glucose to normal. One approach to initiation of therapy involves administration of 25 percent of the previous daily insulin dose in the patient's conventional regimen at bedtime as intermediate insulin [NPH or zinc (lente) insulin] with the other 75 percent given as regular insulin divided such that 40, 30, and 30 percent is given 30 min before breakfast, lunch, and supper, respectively. Alternatively, a three-injection schedule can be designated by omitting the night intermediate insulin and giving a long-acting insulin, such as insulin zinc extended (ultralente insulin) or protamine zinc insulin (PZI insulin), before the evening meal. Adjustments of dosage depend on response of the plasma glucose. A number of different protocols have been utilized, all of which represent sliding scales of insulin based on the plasma glucose. A typical schedule based on home monitoring of plasma glucose is shown in Table 319-7. Individual patients may require different dosages. For specific details the reader should consult one of the published papers utilizing the technique (e.g., Schriffrin and Belmonte). MSI can be effective in controlling the plasma glucose and in some studies appears to match goals achieved with CSII.

TABLE 319-6   Adjusting insulin dosage in conventional insulin therapy*

Blood glucose		Regular insulin, units	
mmol/L	mg/dL	Breakfast (to be mixed with intermediate dosage)	Supper
2.8–5.5	51–100	8	4
5.6–8.3	101–150	10	5
8.4–11.1	151–200	12	6
11.2–13.9	201–250	14	7
14.0–16.6	251–300	16	8
>16.6	>300	20	10

* Once the patient has most blood sugars in the reasonable range, a prescription can be written for varying the regular insulin dosage as illustrated. The prescription in this case was for a patient in reasonable control on 25 units of NPH plus 10 units of regular before breakfast and 10 units of NPH plus 5 units of regular before supper. Change in metabolic status may require adjustments in both intermediate insulin and the sliding scale of regular insulin.

TABLE 319-7 Adjusting insulin dosage in a multiple-injection schedule*

I Initiation of therapy
  A 0.6 to 0.7 units insulin per kilogram body weight
  B 25% NPH at 9 P.M.; 75% regular in divided doses
    (40% before breakfast, 30% before lunch, 30% before supper)
  C Adjust NPH every 48 h based on fasting blood glucose
      <3.3 mmol/L (<60 mg/dL)   − 2 units
      >5.0 mmol/L (>90 mg/dL)   + 2 units
  D Adjust regular insulin every 48 h based on 1-h postprandial glucose
      <3.3 mmol/L (<60 mg/dL)   − 2 units
      >7.8 mmol/L (>140 mg/dL)   + 2 units
II Daily therapy

Preprandial glucose		Regular insulin, units
mmol/L	mg/dL	
<33	<60	− 2
3.4–5.0	61– 90	No change
5.1–6.7	91–120	+ 1
6.8–8.3	121–150	+ 2
8.4–11.0	151–200	+ 3
11.1–13.9	201–250	+ 4
>13.9	>250	+ 6

* With initiation of therapy insulin dosage is changed until target range is reached (see Table 319-8). After initial stabilization a variable insulin schedule is prescribed to maintain tight control. For example, if the patient after initiation is found to generally require 12 units of regular insulin before breakfast but has a prebreakfast blood sugar of 8.9 mmol/L (160 mg/dL), 15 units of regular insulin instead of the usual 12 would be taken.
SOURCE: Adapted from Schiffrin and Belmonte.

Continuous subcutaneous insulin infusion involves use of a small battery-driven pump that delivers insulin subcutaneously into the abdominal wall, usually through a 27-gauge butterfly needle. With CSII insulin is delivered at a basal rate continuously throughout the day with increased rates programmed prior to meals. Adjustments in dosage are made in response to measured capillary glucose values in a fashion similar to that used in MSI. Ordinarily about 40 percent of the total daily dose is given at the basal rate, the remainder being administered as preprandial boluses. There is little question that CSII can improve diabetic control relative to conventional therapy. Most patients report positive feelings of well-being as control improves. Nevertheless, although insulin infusion pumps have caught the attention of the public and many physicians, they should not be used indiscriminately. The danger of hypoglycemia is real, especially during the night in patients who maintain the plasma glucose consistently below 5.5 mmol/L (100 mg/dL). A fall in plasma glucose of 2.7 mmol/L (50 mg/dL) may not be important if the starting value is 8.3 mmol/L (150 mg/dL) but may be fatal if it occurs against a steady-state level of 3.3 mmol/L (60 mg/dL). Several deaths from hypoglycemia have occurred in pump users. Pumps should be prescribed only in disciplined and motivated patients who are followed by physicians with extensive experience in their use. Apart from problems of hypoglycemia, local insulin reactions and abscess formation may occur.

In some centers catheters for the insulin infusion pumps have been placed intravenously rather than subcutaneously. While few difficulties have been reported, this procedure appears unwise for routine use. Intraabdominal insulin pumps with reservoirs refillable from outside the body have been tried on experimental protocols. At present no advantage is apparent except that a pump does not have to be worn externally.

Alternative methods of insulin delivery are under study. One approach involves intranasal administration in a detergent carrier analogous to desmopressin for the treatment of diabetes insipidus. In animals insulin-secreting cells have been implanted in semipermeable membranes. The cells function for prolonged periods and respond in physiologic fashion to changing concentrations of plasma glucose. No similar human experiments have been reported.

Who should be recommended for meticulous control utilizing either MSI or CSII? There are only two absolute indications: pregnancy and renal transplantation. Maintenance of a normal plasma glucose during pregnancy prevents fetal macrosomy and respiratory distress and lowers perinatal mortality. Unfortunately, congenital malformations due to diabetes cannot be prevented by control of the blood sugar after conception occurs. This means that maximal safety for the fetus can only be provided by meticulous treatment of diabetes *prior* to impregnation. While a multicenter trial concluded that no relationship existed between degree of diabetic control and malformed fetuses, the author believes that routine treatment of diabetes in pregnancy is not an option; aggressive therapy should be initiated at the time pregnancy is planned. Inclusion of patients with renal transplants in the nonoptional category follows from the fact that diabetic nephropathy develops early in normal transplanted kidneys. The hope is that with improved metabolic control the acquired lesions can be slowed or prevented.

Meticulous control is an option for most other patients with insulin-dependent diabetes. Since the treatment schedules require much effort on the part of the patient, reliability and willingness to accept responsibility for self-care must be assessed ahead of time. Glucose monitoring is not inexpensive, and the financial status of the patient also has to be considered. Even if meticulous control does not achieve the goal of preventing late complications, in properly chosen patients it seems worthwhile in and of itself both because patients generally feel better when metabolically normal and because attention to clinical detail provides a sense of self-sufficiency and independence that is otherwise easily lost in diabetes. Meticulous control is rarely appropriate for patients whose life expectancy is shortened because of age, cardiovascular, cerebrovascular, or diabetic complications.

For surgical procedures in diabetic patients, intermediate insulin is omitted, and treatment is carried out with regular insulin alone. An effective method is to add 10 to 20 units of insulin to a liter of 5% glucose in water with infusion at a rate of 100 to 150 mL/h. Measurement of plasma glucose in capillary blood allows change of rate to avoid significant hypo- or hyperglycemia. It is also possible to administer 10 units of regular insulin subcutaneously and infuse 5 or 10% glucose at rates sufficient to avoid major changes in glucose concentration. Following surgery a sliding scale can be constructed for use in postoperative management.

Types of insulin A variety of insulins are available for use in the treatment of diabetes. Rapidly acting preparations are used in diabetic emergencies and in CSII and MSI programs. Intermediate preparations are used in conventional and MSI regimens. As noted, long-acting formulations are used in three-injection MSI schedules. Peak effects and duration vary from patient to patient and depend not only on route of administration but on dose. Hypoglycemic effects in insulin-treated diabetics appear to be delayed relative to normal subjects, probably because of the presence of anti-insulin antibodies in plasma. In one study in diabetics, regular insulin given subcutaneously had its onset of action at about 1 h, reached a peak at 6 h, and had measurable effects on average for 16 h, whereas in normal persons onset is within minutes, maximal action is around 2 h, and duration is only 6 to 8 h. With NPH insulin, diabetics exhibited an onset of action at 2.5 h, a peak at 11 h, and a total period of action of 25 h, more closely approximating values in normal subjects.

Commercial insulins are prepared in concentrations of 100 units per milliliter (U100) although higher concentrations can be obtained (e.g., U500). All commercial insulins are now "purified," meaning that they have a contamination with proinsulin <10 parts per million. Some preparations contain as little as 1 part per million. Animal insulins (beef, pork) are still in use, but insulin identical to the human molecule is now available. The advantages of purified animal insulins and "human" insulin are that insulin allergy, fat atrophy, and fat hypertrophy occur less frequently than with the previous preparations. It is possible that anti-insulin antibody (IgG) formation is slightly less with the "human" hormone. Given equivalent price structure it is appropriate to prescribe "human" insulin routinely. As stated above, the various insulins are available as rapid, intermediate, and long-acting preparations, although not all manufacturers offer all varieties. Lente and NPH insulin are used in most conventional therapy and are roughly equivalent in biologic effects, although lente appears to be slightly more immunogenic and to mix less well with regular insulin than does NPH.

Self-glucose monitoring   For many years effectiveness of treatment for diabetes was followed by reviewing symptoms (such as frequency of nocturia) and measurement of glucose in the urine by semiquantitative techniques. Since the renal threshold for glucose in normal persons is in the range of 10 to 11 mmol/L (180 to 200 mg/dL) plasma glucose and may increase with the appearance of renal disease, assessment of glycosuria is of little value if the goal of therapy is to maintain the plasma glucose near normal. In consequence most insulin-requiring patients now monitor control and alter therapy based on self-measurement of the capillary blood sugar. In addition to the fact that such measurements are necessary in all treatment schedules utilizing variable insulin dosage the ability to assess the blood glucose as needed has other positive benefits. It bestows a sense of confidence and independence in the patient, has a reinforcing effect on therapeutic goals (for example, the effect of dietary indiscretion can be immediately seen), serves to give early warning of incipient hypoglycemia, and allows documentation of hypoglycemia when suggestive symptoms are present.

Although blood glucose can be estimated visually utilizing reagent strips, it is generally preferable to use an instrument for readings. This is because it is difficult for many patients to extrapolate accurately between the color changes and because subjective wishes may influence the extrapolation. It is harder to ignore a number appearing in a machine. A variety of glucose analyzers are available. The system chosen should be "dry" (i.e., not require washing of the reagent strip). In general, the cost of a machine, spring-driven lancet holder, and lancets is around $200, and many insurance carriers reimburse for the purchase. The patient needs to have supervised training in the technique, and simultaneous checks of the blood sugar in a laboratory should be done periodically to test accuracy of the self-analysis. Repeated studies show that patients can measure blood glucose accurately using these techniques.

Although urine testing for glucose is now rarely used to follow diabetes, the measurement of ketones in the urine remains important.

Goals of therapy   Target levels for glucose control vary amongst diabetologists. The schedule shown in Table 319-8 lists the ranges considered acceptable and ideal by the author. The "acceptable" category would apply in conventional therapy utilizing a two-dose schedule of intermediate and regular insulin. The upper limit of 11.1 mmol/L (200 mg/dL) postprandially is arbitrary but is based on the finding in the Pima Indian population that complications of diabetes are rare if the 2-h value in the oral glucose tolerance test is less than 11.1 mmol/L. The "ideal" column represents values targeted in meticulous control regimens. Although some authors are more stringent and prefer the 1-h postprandial value to be no more than 7.8 mmol/L (140 mg/dL), the risk of hypoglycemia is greater under these circumstances. In general avoidance of serious hypoglycemia is more important than avoidance of hyperglycemia because the former has immediate consequences that may threaten the life of the patient or others (e.g., through an automobile accident) while the detrimental effects of hyperglycemia are long-term and less certain.

Hypoglycemia, the Somogyi effect, and the dawn phenomenon (See also Chap. 320)   The problem of hypoglycemia is common in insulin-dependent diabetics, particularly when aggressive efforts are made to keep both the fasting plasma glucose and postprandial hyperglycemia within the normal range. Hypoglycemia may be caused by missing a meal or doing unexpected exercise but can occur in the absence of known precipitating events. Daytime episodes of hypoglycemia are usually recognized by autonomic symptoms, such as sweating, nervousness, tremor, and hunger. Hypoglycemia during sleep may produce no symptoms or cause night sweats, unpleasant dreams, and early-morning headache. In one study of insulin-dependent diabetic children monitored throughout 24 h, 18 percent had asymptomatic nocturnal hypoglycemia. If hypoglycemia is not aborted by the countercurrent regulatory mechanisms or by ingestion of carbohydrate, central nervous system symptoms ensue: confusion, abnormal behavior, loss of consciousness, or convulsions. As diabetes progresses, particularly with the development of neuropathy, epinephrine-induced symptoms may become blunted and lose their effectiveness as warning signals, with the consequence that central nervous system signs predominate. This syndrome has been dubbed *hypoglycemia unawareness.* Some authors have suggested that "human" insulin is more likely to cause unrecognized hypoglycemia than animal insulins, but this has not been observed in the United States. Up to 7 percent of deaths in insulin-dependent diabetic subjects are attributed to hypoglycemia.

Protection against hypoglycemia is normally provided by two mechanisms as plasma glucose concentrations fall: cessation of insulin release and mobilization of counterregulatory hormones. The latter act to increase hepatic glucose production and decrease glucose utilization in nonhepatic tissues. Glucagon is the primary counterregulatory hormone, while epinephrine and norepinephrine released from the sympathetic nervous system serve as the major backup. Epinephrine is not required for maintenance of the plasma glucose provided glucagon is available but becomes critical in its absence. Cortisol and growth hormone do not function acutely but come into play with prolonged fasting or sustained hypoglycemia. Diabetic patients are vulnerable to hypoglycemia because of both insulin excess and counterregulatory failure. Since insulin is given by injection or infusion, the capacity to decrease plasma concentrations of the hormone as glucose levels fall is not available. Very early on the diabetic subject with type 1 insulin-dependent disease loses the capacity to increase glucagon release in response to hypoglycemia. Protection is thus dependent on epinephrine. Unfortunately, many patients subsequently also lose the capacity to release epinephrine and norepinephrine in response to hypoglycemia. In most circumstances catecholamine deficiency is probably due to diabetic autonomic neuropathy, but the defect may occur in the absence of clinically demonstrable nerve dysfunction. While failure of catecholamine release is usually a late event in diabetes, it can occur early. It is thought that beta-adrenergic blocking agents have the same effects as deficiencies of epinephrine, although a prospective clinical trial on the dangers of such agents in producing hypoglycemia under real life circumstances has not been carried out.

Counterregulatory hormone failure is especially dangerous when intensive insulin therapy is prescribed. The incidence of hypoglycemia is inversely related to the mean level of plasma glucose. Unfortunately there is no easy way to predict the occurrence of clinically significant counterregulatory failure. Experimentally an insulin infusion test can be used for this purpose but is probably not practical for routine use. In this test neuroglycopenic symptoms in the absence of autonomic signs or delay in return of plasma glucose from nadir after infusion of a standard amount of insulin are utilized to identify defects in the response system. Perhaps the best clinical clue to counterregulatory failure is the presence of frequent hypoglycemia not explicable by change in diet or exercise. Of additional concern are reports that intensive insulin therapy (meticulous control) may itself produce abnormal glucose counterregulation.

An important question is whether hypoglycemic symptoms can occur in the absence of low plasma glucose levels, for example, in response to a rapid fall in glucose concentrations. This question

TABLE 319-8   Goals for blood glucose in the control of diabetes*

Goal	Acceptable		Ideal	
	mmol/L	mg/dL	mmol/L	mg/dL
Fasting	3.3–7.2	60–130	3.9–5.6	70–100
Preprandial	3.3–7.2	60–130	3.9–5.6	70–100
Postprandial (1 h)	<11.1	<200	<8.9	<160
3 A.M.	>3.6	>65	>3.6	>65

* Values for healthy patients below the age of 65. Goals my be shifted upward in older patients.

cannot be answered with certainty, but most evidence suggests that neither rate nor magnitude of the fall signals counterregulatory release, only a low plasma glucose. It has been traditionally believed that counterregulatory hormone release and autonomic symptoms are not triggered until the plasma glucose approaches 3 mmol/L (50 to 55 mg/dL). Careful studies in humans utilizing auditory or visual evoked potentials as a measure of cortical function in the brain have shown abnormalities at a level of 4 mmol/L glucose (70 to 72 mg/dL). A monitored drop of glucose of only 0.5 mmol/L (10 mg/dL) resulted in delay of the evoked potential and, with time, release of counterregulatory hormones. Whether the cumulative effect of mild, asymptomatic falls in plasma glucose could permanently damage the brain is unknown.

From time to time patients with diabetes report symptoms suggestive of catecholamine release in the presence of documented hyperglycemia. The cause of these episodes is unknown, but theories include simple anxiety, insulin-induced vascular permeability with hypotensive response, and sympathetic nervous system activation by insulin-enhanced carbohydrate utilization. Some authors have suggested that the threshold for CNS-stimulated autonomic activation is changed in subjects with chronic hyperglycemia, but no experimental support for this view is available.

Hypoglycemia can occur in diabetic patients consequent to other mechanisms. Diabetic renal disease is not infrequently accompanied by diminished insulin requirements and may lead to frank hypoglycemia if adjustments in dosage are not made. The mechanism is not known. Although half-times for insulin in plasma are increased in diabetic nephropathy, other factors doubtless play a role.

Hypoglycemia may be due to the development of autoimmune adrenal insufficiency as part of polyglandular autoimmune deficiency (see Chap. 325), which is more frequent in diabetics than in the population as a whole. Some patients develop hypoglycemia in association with high levels of circulating insulin antibodies. The exact mechanism has not been established. Occasionally an insulinoma may develop in a diabetic patient. Very rarely, permanent remission of apparently typical diabetes occurs. The reason is not known, but the initial sign may be frequent hypoglycemia in a previously well-controlled patient.

It must be emphasized that hypoglycemic attacks are dangerous and if frequent portend a serious or even fatal outcome. If the patient is conscious, sugar, candy, or a sugar-containing beverage can be given. If the patient is unarousable or unconscious, intravenous glucose is required. Patients should have a vial of glucagon available as well. If access to medical care is delayed, administration of 1 mg glucagon intramuscularly frequently aborts the attack.

The *Somogyi phenomenon* refers to rebound hyperglycemia following an episode of hypoglycemia due to counterregulatory hormone release. It should be suspected whenever wide swings in the plasma glucose occur over short time intervals even if symptoms are not reported. Such rapid changes contrast with the alterations seen following insulin withdrawal in previously well-controlled diabetic patients in whom hyperglycemia and ketosis develop gradually and smoothly over a 12- to 24-h period. Excessive hunger and weight gain occurring in the context of worsening hyperglycemia are clues that the insulin dosage may be too high, since poor control due to underinsulinization usually results in weight loss (because of osmotic diuresis and glucose wastage). If the Somogyi phenomenon is suspected, the insulin dose should be decreased as a trial, even when specific symptoms of overinsulinization are absent. The Somogyi phenomenon is probably rare in adults but may be more frequent in children.

The *dawn phenomenon* refers to an early morning rise in plasma glucose requiring increased amounts of insulin to maintain euglycemia. Although similar early morning hyperglycemia may result from hypoglycemia, as just described, the dawn phenomenon itself is thought to be independent of the Somogyi mechanism. The nocturnal surge of growth hormone release may be a factor. Increased clearance of insulin also occurs in the early morning hours, but the changes are probably not of major importance. Differentiation between the dawn phenomenon and posthypoglycemic hyperglycemia can usually be accomplished by measuring the blood glucose at 3 A.M. This is important since the Somogyi phenomenon is avoided by decreasing insulin dosages for the critical time period while the dawn phenomenon usually requires increased insulin to maintain glucose in the normal range.

Oral agents   Non-insulin-dependent diabetes that cannot be controlled by dietary management often responds to sulfonylureas. The drugs are easy to use and appear to be safe. Fear that sulfonylureas might increase deaths from heart attacks, prompted by reports of the University Group Diabetes Program (UGDP), has largely dissipated because of questions about the design of that study and failure of other studies to confirm risks. On the other hand use of the oral drugs has decreased concomitant with the emphasis on better control as a possible means of slowing the development of late complications. While some patients with relatively mild disease have return of plasma glucose to normal on oral drugs, those with significant hyperglycemia tend to improve but do not approach the normal range. Thus a high percentage of non-insulin-dependent diabetics are now treated with insulin.

Sulfonylureas act primarily by stimulating release of insulin from the beta cell. They have the capacity to increase the number of insulin receptors in target tissues and also enhance insulin-mediated glucose disposal independent of an increase in insulin binding, but these effects are physiologically unimportant. Mean levels of plasma insulin do not increase following treatment with sulfonylureas despite significantly improved mean plasma glucose concentrations. The paradox of improved glucose metabolism in the absence of higher steady-state levels of insulin has been resolved by studies which show that elevation of plasma glucose to pretreatment values results in a rise of plasma insulin to levels higher than those seen pretreatment. Thus, the initial action of the drugs is to increase insulin release with lowering of the plasma glucose. As glucose concentrations fall, insulin levels also decrease since plasma glucose is the major stimulus to insulin release, thereby masking the initial stimulation of insulin secretion. The insulinogenic effect can then be unmasked by raising the plasma glucose to the previous elevated levels. The fact that sulfonylureas are ineffective in IDDM, where beta-cell mass is diminished, supports the pancreatic effect as primary, although as noted extrapancreatic mechanisms may play a minor role.

The characteristics of the sulfonylureas are summarized in Table 319-9. The newer drugs such as glipizide and glyburide are effective in smaller doses but otherwise differ little from agents in long use such as chlorpropamide and tolbutamide. In patients who have significant renal disease it is preferable to treat with tolbutamide or tolazamide since these agents are exclusively metabolized and inactivated by the liver. Chlorpropamide has the capacity to sensitize the renal tubule to antidiuretic hormone. It thus is helpful in some patients with partial diabetes insipidus but may cause water retention in patients with diabetes mellitus. Hypoglycemia is less common with oral agents than with insulin, but when it occurs it tends to be severe and prolonged. Some patients have required massive glucose infusions for days following the last dose of sulfonylurea. For this reason hospitalization is mandatory in patients with sulfonylurea-induced hypoglycemia.

The only other oral agents effective in the treatment of maturity-onset diabetes are the biguanides. They presumably lower plasma glucose by inhibiting gluconeogenesis in the liver although phenformin may increase the number of insulin receptors in some tissues. The drugs are ordinarily used only in combination with sulfonylureas under circumstances in which control is inadequate with sulfonylurea alone. Because of many reports linking phenformin to the appearance of lactic acidosis, the Food and Drug Administration removed the agent from routine clinical use in the United States. Phenformin and other biguanides are still used elsewhere in the world. Biguanides

TABLE 319-9 The sulfonylureas

Agent	Daily dose, mg	Doses per day	Duration of hyperglycemic action, h	Metabolism/excretion
Acetohexamide	250–1500	1–2	12–18	Liver/kidney
Chlorpropamide	100–500	1	60	Kidney
Tolazamide	100–1000	1–2	12–14	Liver
Tolbutamide	500–3000	2–3	6–12	Liver
Glyburide	1.25–20	1–2	Up to 24	Liver/kidney
Glipizide	2.5–40	1–2	Up to 24	Liver/kidney
Glibornuride	12.5–100	1–2	Up to 24	Liver/kidney

SOURCE: RH Unger, DW Foster.

should not be given to patients with renal disease and should be stopped if nausea, vomiting, diarrhea, or any intercurrent illness appears.

Two naturally occurring peptides are currently under investigation as adjuncts to treatment in NIDDM. Both insulin-like growth factor 1 (IGF-1, somatomedin C) and a product of the glucagon precursor gene called GLP-1 (glucagon-like peptide 1) or insulinotropin lower plasma glucose in normal subjects and in patients with type 2 diabetes. Their ultimate usefulness is not established.

Monitoring control of diabetes For those patients who measure blood glucose frequently for adjustment of insulin dosage an estimate of mean ambient glucose concentrations is readily available. For other patients, and as a check on accuracy of the self measurements, most diabetologists now measure hemoglobin A_{1c} to assess long-term control. Hemoglobin A_{1c}, a fast-moving minor hemoglobin component, is present in normal persons but increases in the presence of hyperglycemia. Its enhanced electrophoretic mobility is due to nonenzymatic glycation of the amino acids valine and lysine. The reaction is as follows:

$$
\begin{array}{ccc}
\text{HC}{=}\text{O} & \text{HC}{=}\text{N}{-}\beta\text{A} & \text{CH}_2{-}\text{N}^+\text{H}_2{-}\beta\text{A} \\
| & | & | \\
\text{HCOH} & \text{HCOH} & \text{C}{=}\text{O} \\
| & | & | \\
\text{HOCH} & \text{HOCH} & \text{HOCH} \\
\beta\text{-NH}_2 + \quad | \rightleftharpoons | \longrightarrow | \\
\text{HCOH} & \text{HCOH} & \text{HCOH} \\
| & | & | \\
\text{HCOH} & \text{HCOH} & \text{HCOH} \\
| & | & | \\
\text{CH}_2\text{OH} & \text{CH}_2\text{OH} & \text{CH}_2\text{OH} \\
\text{Glucose} & \text{Aldimine} & \text{Ketoamine} \\
& \text{(Schiff base)} & \\
\end{array}
$$

$$\text{Hb A} \xrightarrow[\text{Rapid}]{\rightleftharpoons} \text{pre A}_{1c} \xrightarrow{\text{Slow}} \text{Hb A}_{1c}$$

In this scheme β-NH$_2$ stands for the terminal valine of the β chain of hemoglobin. Aldimine formation is reversible so that pre-A$_{1c}$ is labile while ketoamine formation is irreversible and thus stable. Pre-A$_{1c}$ levels depend on the ambient glucose concentrations and do not reflect long-term control although they are measured in chromatographic methods for determining hemoglobin A$_{1c}$. Pre-A$_{1c}$ must thus be removed to assess true Hb A$_{1c}$ values accurately. Many laboratories employ high-performance liquid chromatography (HPLC) to make the measurement. A colorimetric method utilizing thiobarbituric acid also does not measure the labile pre-A$_{1c}$ fraction. When properly assayed, the percent of glycated hemoglobin gives an estimate of diabetic control for the preceding 3-month period. Normal values must be obtained for each lab; on average nondiabetic subjects have Hb A$_{1c}$ values of around 6 percent, and levels in poorly controlled diabetics may reach 10 to 12 percent. Measurement of glycated hemoglobin gives an objective assessment of metabolic control. Discrepancies between reported plasma glucose values and hemoglobin A$_{1c}$ concentrations suggest either that measurement or reporting of the former is not accurate. Measurement of glycated albumin,

because of its short half-life, can be used to monitor diabetic control over a 1- to 2-week period but clinically is rarely used.

ACUTE METABOLIC COMPLICATIONS In addition to hypoglycemia, diabetics are susceptible to two major acute metabolic complications: diabetic ketoacidosis and hyperosmolar, nonketotic coma. The former is a complication of insulin-dependent diabetes, while the latter usually occurs in the setting of non-insulin-dependent disease. Ketoacidosis rarely, if ever, develops in true type 2 diabetes.

Diabetic ketoacidosis Diabetic ketoacidosis appears to require insulin deficiency coupled with a relative or absolute increase in glucagon concentration. It is often caused by cessation of insulin intake but may result from physical (e.g., infection, surgery) or emotional stress despite continued insulin therapy. In the former case the concentration of glucagon rises secondary to insulin withdrawal, while in stress the operative stimulus is probably epinephrine and/or norepinephrine. In addition to stimulating glucagon secretion epinephrine presumably blocks release of the small amount of residual insulin found in some subjects with IDDM and inhibits insulin-induced glucose transport in peripheral tissues. These hormonal changes have multiple effects, but two are critical: (1) They induce maximal gluconeogenesis and impair peripheral utilization of glucose, causing severe hyperglycemia. Glucagon facilitates gluconeogenesis by inducing a fall in fructose-2,6-bisphosphate, an intermediate that stimulates glycolysis through activation of phosphofructokinase and blocks gluconeogenesis by inhibiting fructose bisphosphatase. When fructose-2,6-bisphosphate concentrations fall, glycolysis is inhibited, and gluconeogenesis is enhanced. The resultant hyperglycemia induces an osmotic diuresis that leads to the volume depletion and dehydration that characterize the ketoacidotic state. (2) They activate the ketogenic process and thus initiate development of metabolic acidosis. For ketosis to occur, changes must be produced in both adipose tissue and the liver. Free fatty acids from adipose stores represent the primary substrate for ketone body formation, and plasma levels of free fatty acids must rise if high rates of ketogenesis are to develop. However, fatty acids delivered to the liver are simply reesterified and stored as hepatic triglyceride or converted into very low density lipoproteins and transported back into the circulation unless the hepatic oxidative machinery for fatty acids is activated. While free fatty acid release is enhanced directly by insulin deficiency, accelerated fatty acid oxidation in the liver is primarily induced by glucagon, via action on the carnitine palmitoyltransferase system of enzymes responsible for the transport of fatty acids into the mitochondria following their esterification to coenzyme A. As shown in Fig. 319-3 carnitine palmitoyltransferase I transesterifies fatty acyl-CoA to fatty acylcarnitine, which then traverses the inner mitochondrial membrane via translocase. Reversal of the reaction occurs internally under the influence of carnitine palmitoyltransferase II. In the fed state carnitine palmitoyltransferase I is inactive, and, as a consequence, long-chain fatty acids cannot reach the β-oxidative enzymes for ketone body production. During starvation or uncontrolled diabetes the system is activated; under these circumstances the rate of ketogenesis is a first-order function of the concentration of fatty acids reaching transferase I.

Glucagon (or a change in the glucagon/insulin ratio) activates the

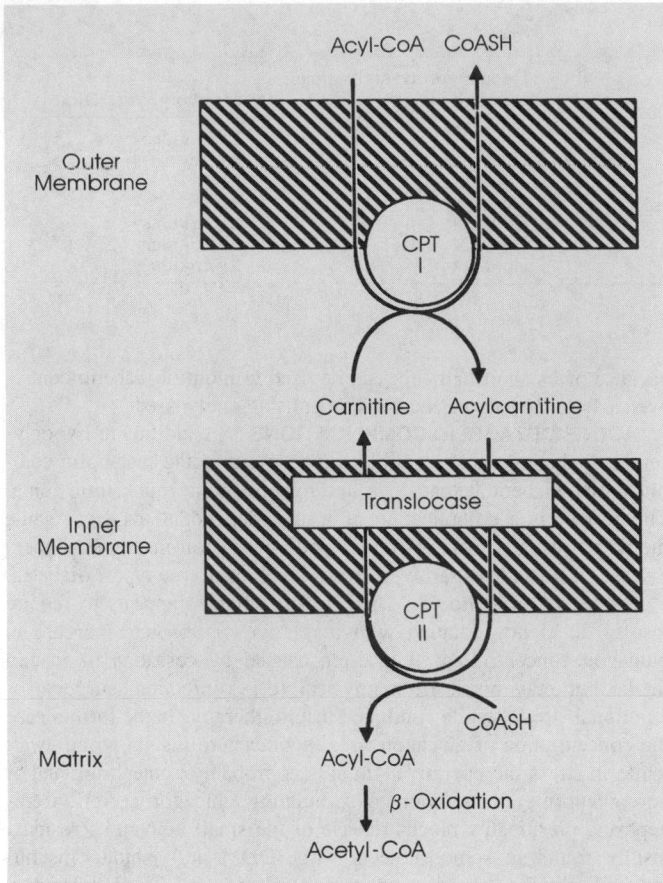

FIGURE 319-3 The carnitine palmitoyltransferase system. Long-chain fatty acyl-CoA molecules require transesterification to carnitine to traverse the inner mitochondrial membrane. Once across, the transesterification is reversed, and the fatty acyl-CoA is oxidized to either ketone bodies (liver) or CO_2 and water with the generation of ATP (nonhepatic tissues). CPT I is the rate-limiting step, controlled by malonyl-CoA levels in tissue. CPT I, carnitine palmitoyltransferase I; CPT II, palmitoyltransferase II.

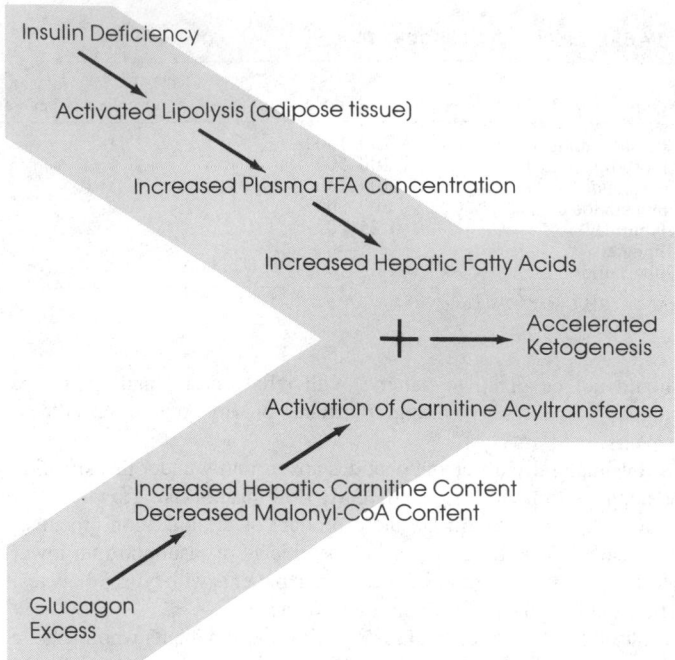

FIGURE 319-4 The regulation of ketogenesis. Significant production of acetoacetate and β-hydroxybutyrate by the liver requires provision of adequate free fatty acid substrate and activation of fatty acid oxidation. Lipolysis is primarily increased by insulin deficiency while the fatty acid oxidative sequence is activated primarily by glucagon. The immediate signal for oxidation is a fall in malonyl CoA content. (*After JD McGarry, DW Foster, Am J Med 61:9, 1976.*)

transport system in two ways. First, glucagon causes a rapid fall in hepatic malonyl-CoA content. It does so by interrupting the sequence glucose-6-phosphate → pyruvate → citrate → acetyl CoA → malonyl CoA via the previously mentioned decrease in fructose-2,6-bisphosphate. Malonyl-CoA, the first committed intermediate in the synthesis of fatty acids from glucose, is a competitive inhibitor of carnitine palmitoyltransferase I, and a fall in its concentration activates the enzyme. Second, glucagon causes a rise in hepatic carnitine concentration, which then drives the reaction toward fatty acylcarnitine formation by mass action. These events are summarized schematically in Fig. 319-4. At high plasma fatty acid concentrations hepatic uptake of fatty acids is sufficient to saturate both oxidative and esterifying pathways, resulting in fatty liver, hypertriglyceridemia, and ketoacidosis. Overproduction of ketones by the liver is the primary event in ketotic states, but limitation of peripheral utilization also plays a role at high concentrations of acetoacetate and β-hydroxybutyrate.

Clinically ketoacidosis begins with anorexia, nausea, and vomiting, coupled with an increased rate of urine formation. Abdominal pain may be present. If untreated, altered consciousness or frank coma may occur. Initial examination usually shows Kussmaul respiration, together with signs of volume depletion. Rarely the latter is sufficient to cause vascular collapse and renal shutdown. Body temperature is normal or below normal in uncomplicated ketoacidosis, and fever suggests the presence of infection. Leukocytosis, frequently very marked, is a feature of diabetic acidosis per se and may not indicate infection.

The characteristic metabolic abnormalities of diabetic coma are shown in Table 319-10. Several features deserve comment. The metabolic acidosis and anion gap are almost totally accounted for by the elevated plasma levels of acetoacetate and β-hydroxybutyrate, although other acids (e.g., lactate, free fatty acids, phosphates) contribute. Despite initial potassium concentrations that are normal to high, there is a total body potassium deficit of several hundred millimoles. Similarly, initial serum phosphorus may be high despite depletion of body stores. Magnesium deficiency may also be present. The serum sodium concentration tends to be low in the face of modest osmolar concentration because of the hyperglycemia that draws intracellular water into the plasma space. A very low serum sodium (e.g., 110 mmol/L) suggests an artifact due to severe hypertriglyceridemia. The latter is common in ketoacidosis and is the consequence of both impaired activity of lipoprotein lipase (a disposal defect) and the hepatic overproduction of very low density lipoproteins. If a fat meal has been ingested prior to the onset of ketoacidosis, chylomicrons

TABLE 319-10 Initial laboratory findings in diabetic ketoacidosis

Series		Dallas*	Los Angeles†	Washington‡
Age, y	HL	38	36	43
Glucose, mmol/L (mg/dL)		26(475)	37(675)	41(733)
Sodium, mmol/L		132	131	132
Potassium, mmol/L		4.8	5.3	6.0
Bicarbonate, mmol/L		<10	6	10
BUN, mmol/L (mg/dL)		9(25)	11(32)	15(42)
Acetoacetate, mmol/L		4.8	—	—
β-Hydroxybutyrate, mmol/L		137	—	—
Free fatty acids, mmol/L		2.1	—	2.3
Lactate, mmol/L		4.6	—	—
Osmolarity, mosmol/liter		310	323	331

* Eighty-eight consecutive episodes of ketoacidosis at Parkland Memorial Hospital (DW Foster, unpublished observations).
† Mean data from 308 episodes of nonfatal ketoacidosis (PM Beigelman, Diabetes 20:490, 1971).
‡ Mean data from 10 episodes of ketoacidosis (JE Gerich et al, Diabetes 20:228, 1971).

may make up a major portion of the circulating fat. Lipemia is usually visible if triglyceride concentration is above 4.5 mmol/L (400 mg/dL). True hyponatremia may occur if the patient has vomited repeatedly and continued to drink water. Prerenal azotemia, reflecting volume depletion, is usually modest in degree and reversible with treatment. The serum amylase may be elevated, and frank pancreatitis can occur.

The diagnosis of ketoacidosis in a known diabetic is not difficult. Its appearance in a patient not previously known to have diabetes requires differentiation from the other common causes of metabolic acidosis with an anion gap: lactic acidosis, uremia, alcoholic ketoacidosis, and certain poisonings. The first step is to test the urine for glucose and ketones. If urine ketones are negative, another cause for the acidosis is likely. If positive, plasma examination is required to be certain that something more than starvation ketosis is present. Since quantitative determinations of acetoacetate and β-hydroxybutyrate are not routinely available, semiquantitative tests must be done using ketone reagent strips. Serial dilutions of plasma can be made and tested. A strong test may occur in undiluted plasma owing to starvation alone; a strong reaction beyond 1:1 dilution is presumptive evidence for ketoacidosis. Apart from diabetes the only other common ketoacidotic state is alcoholic ketoacidosis. This syndrome, which by definition occurs in chronic alcoholics, usually follows a debauch, but the patient may not have had alcohol for 24 h or longer. It never occurs in the absence of starvation and frequently is associated with severe vomiting and abdominal pain. Pancreatitis is present in up to 75 percent of patients. A plasma glucose of less than 8.3 mmol/L (150 mg/dL) was found in three-fourths of cases and in 15 percent was less than 2.8 mmol/L (50 mg/dL) on arrival at the hospital. Hyperglycemia may occur but is usually mild and rarely, if ever, above 17 mmol/L (300 mg/dL). Plasma free fatty acid concentrations are higher (mean 2.9 mmol/L) than in normal starvation (range 0.7 to 1.0 mmol/L), reaching levels seen in diabetic ketoacidosis. Presumably the liver is activated for ketogenesis by starvation in these patients and driven to maximal rates of ketone formation by the high fatty acid levels. Why some alcoholics mobilize fatty acids excessively is not known. In contrast to diabetic acidosis, the syndrome is rapidly reversible by the intravenous administration of glucose. As in all alcoholics given glucose, thiamine should be supplied to avoid precipitation of acute beriberi. (Other water-soluble vitamins, though not as critical, should also be infused.) Insulin is required only if hyperglycemia persists during therapy.

Diabetic ketoacidosis cannot be reversed without insulin. For decades 50 or more units of insulin were given per hour until ketosis was reversed, but now most patients are treated by "low-dose" insulin schedules in which 8 to 10 units of insulin are infused intravenously each hour. Most diabetic acidosis can be reversed adequately with low-dose treatment, but some patients do not respond. Presumably the insulin resistance that is characteristic of diabetic ketoacidosis is more pronounced in these patients than in responsive subjects. The problem is that resistant subjects cannot be identified prospectively. For this reason it is probably preferable to treat ketoacidosis with 25 to 50 units of regular insulin intravenously hourly until the acidosis is reversed. It can be given as a bolus or by constant infusion. There are no known toxic effects of larger insulin doses, since maximal physiologic response is obtained once insulin receptors are saturated regardless of how much insulin is given. The advantage of the higher dosage schedule is that it ensures saturation of the receptors in the face of competing antibodies or other resistance factors. High concentrations of insulin probably accelerate the reversal of ketoacidosis by acting via the IgF-1 receptor. Hormonal interaction with this receptor can lower plasma glucose by a mechanism independent of the insulin receptor. If physicians choose to use the low-dose insulin schedule, they should be alert to the possibility of resistance. Should acidosis persist unabated after several hours of treatment, larger amounts of insulin are clearly indicated. Ketoacidosis can also be adequately treated with intramuscular (but not subcutaneous) insulin.

Therapy of ketoacidosis also requires intravenous fluids. The usual fluid deficit is 3 to 5 liters, and both salt solutions and free water are needed. One to two liters of isotonic saline or Ringer's lactate should be given rapidly intravenously on arrival, with additional amounts determined by urine output and clinical assessment of the fluid state. When the plasma glucose falls to about 17 mmol/L (300 mg/dL), 5% glucose solutions should be given, both as a source of free water and as a prophylactic measure to prevent the late cerebral edema syndrome. The latter is a rare complication of ketoacidosis occurring most often in children. It is suspected when the patient remains comatose or lapses into coma following reversal of acidosis.

Potassium replacement is always necessary, but the time of administration will vary. The initial potassium is often high despite a total body deficit because of the severe acidosis. In this case the cation will ordinarily not be needed until 3 to 4 h after initiation of therapy, when reversal of acidosis and the action of insulin cause a shift of K^+ into intracellular water. On the other hand if the admission value is normal or low, potassium should be given early, since plasma concentrations fall rapidly during therapy, predisposing the patient to cardiac arrhythmias. In view of the phosphate depletion of ketoacidosis, potassium should be administered initially as the phosphate salt rather than as potassium chloride.

Bicarbonate therapy is indicated in severely acidotic patients (pH 7.0 or below), especially if hypotension is present (acidosis itself can cause vascular collapse). It is not used routinely in less acutely ill subjects since rapid alkalinization may have detrimental effects on oxygen delivery to tissues. The hemoglobin-oxygen dissociation curve is normal in diabetic ketoacidosis because of the opposing effects of acidosis and deficiency of red blood cell 2,3-diphosphoglycerate (2,3-DPG). If the acidosis is rapidly reversed, the deficiency of 2,3-DPG becomes manifest, increasing the avidity with which hemoglobin binds oxygen and impairing the release of oxygen in peripheral tissues. In a volume-depleted patient with poor tissue perfusion such a change theoretically could predispose to the development of lactic acidosis. It is also thought that bicarbonate may impair left ventricular function through paradoxical acidification due to more rapid entry of CO_2 than bicarbonate into intracellular water. If bicarbonate is given, the infusion should be stopped when the pH reaches 7.2 to minimize possible detrimental side effects and to prevent metabolic alkalosis as circulating ketones are metabolized to bicarbonate with reversal of ketoacidosis.

In following the response to treatment, two points should be emphasized. (1) Plasma glucose invariably falls more rapidly than plasma ketones. Insulin should not be stopped because glucose concentrations approach normal; rather, as mentioned, glucose should be infused and insulin continued until the ketosis has cleared. (2) Plasma ketone values are not very helpful. The testing materials measure acetoacetate and acetone but not β-hydroxybutyrate. Since β-hydroxybutyrate must be oxidized to acetoacetate prior to utilization, it is characteristic for the plasma ketones measured by reagent strip to remain stable or even rise early in therapy at a time when total ketone concentration (acetoacetate plus β-hydroxybutyrate) is steadily falling. Because β-hydroxybutyrate and acetoacetate represent a redox couple in equilibrium with mitochondrial NADH/NAD concentrations, vascular collapse or severe hypoxia may mask the presence of ketoacidosis as acetoacetate is reduced to β-hydroxybutyrate. Under these circumstances the β-hydroxybutyrate/acetoacetate ratio, normally about 3:1, may reach 7:1 or 8:1. Paradoxically, in such a situation, ketosis may seem to worsen as the patient gets better because of conversion of β-hydroxybutyrate to acetoacetate when the circulation is reestablished and tissue oxygenation is restored. The key parameters to follow are the pH and the calculated anion gap since these give a more accurate assessment of therapeutic progress. The usual picture is for the pH to rise and the anion gap to narrow even though the plasma bicarbonate remains low. The persistently low bicarbonate is the consequence of hyperchloremia that develops because of rapid infusion of sodium chloride, the loss of potential bicarbonate from the body in urine as ketones, and exchanges with intracellular buffers. Some patients demonstrate a persistent anion gap despite clinical improvement and a rising pH. Presumably, the unmeasured anion derives from tissue buffers. If the anion gap remains elevated and pH is persistently low, this indicates insulin resistance and requires aggressive increase in the amount of insulin administered. On the other hand, persistence of the anion gap does not indicate resistance when present in the face of clinical improvement and a rising pH.

All patients should be followed with a flow sheet outlining amounts and timing of insulin and fluids together with a record of vital signs, urine volume, and blood chemistries. Without such a record therapy tends to become chaotic.

Most patients with diabetic ketoacidosis recover when properly treated. While mortality in large series is reported to be around 10 percent, the majority of deaths result from late complications rather than from ketoacidosis itself. The major causes are myocardial infarction and infection, particularly pneumonia. Poor prognostic signs on admission include hypotension, azotemia, deep coma, and associated illness. In children, cerebral edema is a common cause of death (less frequent in adults). The cause of the brain swelling is not known. Theories include osmotic disequilibrium between brain and plasma as glucose is rapidly lowered, decreased plasma oncotic pressure due to infusion of large amounts of saline, and insulin-induced ion flux across the blood-brain barrier. Whatever the mechanism, mortality rates are high. Diagnosis is usually made by CT scan. Treatment involves the bolus infusion of 1 g mannitol per kilogram body weight in the form of a 20% solution. Although of questionable benefit, dexamethasone is also usually given: 12 mg initially then 4 mg every 6 h. If there is no response, hyperventilation to an arterial P_{CO_2} of about 28 mmHg should be carried out by an anesthesiologist or pulmonary specialist.

Other acute complications of ketoacidosis include vascular thrombosis and the adult respiratory distress syndrome. The former is induced by volume depletion, hyperosmolarity, increased viscosity of blood, and changes in clotting factors favoring thrombosis. The cause of the pulmonary lesion is not known; it is probably not related to the metabolic acidosis since respiratory distress syndrome occurs in hyperosmolar coma as well. Acute gastric dilatation is another rare complication. A rare infection associated with ketoacidosis is mucormycosis (see below). Table 319-11 summarizes the complications of diabetic ketoacidosis and its treatment.

Hyperosmolar coma Hyperosmolar nonketotic diabetic coma is usually a complication of non-insulin-dependent diabetes. It is a syndrome of profound dehydration resulting from a sustained hyperglycemic diuresis under circumstances in which the patient is unable to drink sufficient water to keep up with urinary fluid losses. Commonly an elderly diabetic—often living alone or in a nursing home—develops a stroke or infection, which worsens hyperglycemia and prevents adequate water intake. The full-blown syndrome probably does not occur until volume depletion has become severe enough to decrease urine output. Hyperosmolar coma has also been precipitated by therapeutic procedures such as peritoneal dialysis or hemodialysis, tube feeding of high-protein formulas, high-carbohydrate infusion loads, and the use of osmotic agents such as mannitol and urea. Phenytoin, steroids, immunosuppressive agents, and diuretics have also been reported to initiate the disorder.

The absence of ketoacidosis is important in the pathophysiology. When ketoacidosis occurs in an insulin-dependent diabetic, nausea, vomiting, and air hunger bring the patient to the physician before extreme dehydration can occur. Such a protective mechanism is not operative in the ketoacidosis-resistant, maturity-onset diabetic. Interestingly, hyperosmolar coma can occur in insulin-dependent diabetic patients given sufficient insulin to prevent ketosis but insufficient to control hyperglycemia. Although unusual, the same patient may present on one occasion with ketoacidosis and on the next with hyperosmolar coma.

The reason for the absence of ketoacidosis in maturity-onset diabetics is not known. The hepatic ketogenic machinery is not impaired since the patients frequently have ketone concentrations in the starvation range (2 to 4 mmol/L). Free fatty acid levels are lower in hyperosmolar coma than in ketoacidosis, and substrate deficiency may limit ketone formation. That this is the sole mechanism seems unlikely since some patients with hyperosmolar coma have high levels of free fatty acids in plasma. A more likely explanation is that insulin concentrations in the portal vein of type 2 diabetics are higher than those of insulin-dependent subjects and prevent full activation of the hepatic carnitine palmitoyltransferase system. Other possibilities include glucagon resistance, previously mentioned, and maintenance of high malonyl-CoA levels via increased Cori cycle activity. The Cori cycle refers to conversion of circulating glucose to lactate in peripheral tissues with return of lactate to the liver for gluconeogenesis. Lactate is also a precursor of malonyl-CoA.

Clinically patients present with extreme hyperglycemia, hyperosmolality, and volume depletion, coupled with central nervous system signs ranging from clouded sensorium to coma. Seizure activity—sometimes Jacksonian in type—is not unusual, and transient hemiplegia may be seen. Infections, particularly pneumonia and gram-negative sepsis, are common and indicate a grave prognosis. Pneumonia is often due to gram-negative organisms. A high index of suspicion for infection should be maintained, and routine culture of the blood and spinal fluid is indicated. Because of the extreme dehydration plasma viscosity is high, and widespread in situ thrombosis has been found at post mortem. Bleeding, probably the consequence of disseminated intravascular coagulation and acute pancreatitis, may accompany the illness.

The laboratory findings in two large series are shown in Table 319-12. Plasma glucose is generally around 55 mmol/L (1000 mg/dL), about twice the value seen in ketoacidosis. The serum osmolality is extremely high, but because of the hyperglycemia the absolute serum sodium concentration is often not elevated.[3] Prerenal azotemia with marked elevation of BUN and creatinine is characteristic. A mild metabolic acidosis is present, plasma bicarbonate on the average being about 20 mmol/L. The acidosis is due to a combination of

TABLE 319-11 Clues to complications in diabetic ketoacidosis

Complication	Clues
Acute gastric dilatation or erosive gastritis	Vomiting of blood or coffee-ground material
Cerebral edema	Obtundation or coma with or without neurologic signs, especially if occurring after initial improvement
Hyperkalemia	Cardiac arrest
Hypoglycemia	Adrenergic or neurologic signs; rebound ketosis
Hypokalemia	Cardiac arrhythmias
Infection	Fever
Insulin resistance	Unremitting acidosis after 4–6 h of adequate therapy
Myocardial infarction	Chest pain, appearance of heart failure; appearance of hypotension despite adequate fluids
Mucormycosis	Facial pain, bloody nasal discharge, blackened nasal turbinates, blurred vision, proptosis
Respiratory distress syndrome	Hypoxemia in the absence of pneumonia, chronic pulmonary disease, or heart failure
Vascular thrombosis	Strokelike picture or signs of ischemia in nonnervous tissue

SOURCE: Adapted from DW Foster, in *Current Therapy in Endocrinology and Metabolism 1985–1986*, DT Krieger, CW Bardin (eds), Toronto/Philadelphia, Decker, 1985.

---

[3] Serum osmolality can be estimated from the formula

Serum osmolality (mosmol/L)
$$= 2\,([Na^+] + [K^+])(mmol/L) + glucose(mmol/L) + BUN(mmol/L)$$

In practice the contribution of the BUN is often ignored since it contributes to total osmolality but does not reflect the free water deficit. There are situations in which an increased osmolality is not equivalent to dehydration. Severe alcohol intoxication is one example, the ethanol itself providing the measured milliosmoles.

TABLE 319-12 Initial laboratory findings in hyperosmolar coma

Series		Brooklyn*	Washington†
Age, y	HL	60	57
Glucose, mmol/L (mg/dL)		65(1166)	54(976)
Sodium, mmol/L		144	142
Potassium, mmol/L		5	5
Chloride, mmol/L		99	98
Bicarbonate, mmol/L		17	22
BUN, mmol/L (mg/dL)		31(87)	23(65)
Creatinine, mmol/L (mg/dL)		490(5.5)	—
Free fatty acids, mmol/L		0.73	0.96
Osmolarity, mosmol/L		384	374

* Mean data from 33 episodes of hyperosmolar coma (AA Arieff, HJ Carroll, Medicine 51:73, 1972).
† Mean data from 20 episodes of hyperosmolar coma (JE Gerich et al, Diabetes 20:228, 1971).

starvation ketosis, retention of inorganic acids secondary to the azotemia, and modest elevation of plasma lactate, the latter the consequence of volume depletion. If the bicarbonate is less than 10 mmol/L and plasma ketones are not elevated, it can be assumed that lactic acidosis is present.

The mortality rate in hyperosmolar coma is high (>50 percent). As a consequence immediate treatment is urgent. The most important measure is rapid administration of large amounts of intravenous fluids to reestablish the circulation and urine flow. The average fluid deficit is 10 liters. While free water will ultimately be needed, initial therapy should be with isotonic salt solutions, and 2 to 3 liters should be given over the first 1 to 2 h. Subsequently half-strength saline can be used. As the plasma glucose approaches normal levels, 5% dextrose can be given as a vehicle for free water. While hyperosmolar coma may be reversed by fluids alone, insulin should be given to control the hyperglycemia more rapidly. Many authors recommend small doses of insulin, but larger amounts may be necessary, particularly in the obese patient. Potassium salts are usually required earlier in the treatment of hyperosmolar coma than in ketoacidosis because the intracellular shift of plasma K^+ during therapy is accelerated in the absence of acidosis. If lactic acidosis is present, sodium bicarbonate should be given until tissue perfusion can be reestablished. Antibiotics are required if infection complicates the picture.

LATE COMPLICATIONS OF DIABETES The diabetic patient is susceptible to a series of complications that cause morbidity and premature mortality. While some patients may never develop these problems and others note their onset early, on average symptoms develop 15 to 20 years following the appearance of overt hyperglycemia. A given patient may experience several complications simultaneously, or a single problem may dominate the picture.

Circulatory abnormalities Arteriosclerosis of the type seen in nondiabetics occurs more extensively and earlier than in the general population. The cause for this accelerated atherosclerosis is not known, although, as discussed below, nonenzymatic glycation of lipoproteins may be important. Oxidized low density lipoproteins (LDL) are important in the generation of atherosclerosis. They bind not to the normal LDL receptor but to an alternative receptor (the acetyl LDL receptor). It is not known if diabetes enhances oxidation of LDL, although the ratio of high density lipoprotein (HDL) to LDL is altered (see below). Other factors of potential importance are increased platelet adhesiveness, possibly due to enhanced thromboxane A_2 synthesis, and decreased prostacyclin synthesis. Atherosclerotic lesions produce symptoms in a variety of sites. Peripheral deposits may cause intermittent claudication, gangrene, and, in men, organic impotence on a vascular basis. Surgical repair of large vessel lesions may be unsuccessful because of the simultaneous presence of widespread disease of the small vessels. Coronary artery disease and stroke are common. Silent myocardial infarction is thought to occur with increased frequency in diabetics and should be suspected whenever symptoms of left ventricular failure appear suddenly.

Diabetes may also be associated with the clinical picture of cardiomyopathy, in which heart failure occurs in the face of angiographically normal coronary arteries and the absence of other identifiable causes of heart disease. As in nondiabetic subjects, smoking is a major risk factor for both coronary and peripheral vascular disease and should be avoided.

Retinopathy Diabetic retinopathy is a leading cause of blindness in the United States. On the other hand, most diabetics never become blind. Retinopathic lesions are divided into two large categories, *simple* (background) and *proliferative* (Table 319-13). The earliest sign of retinal change is an increased capillary permeability that is evidenced by leakage of dye into the vitreous humor after fluorescein injection. Occlusion of retinal capillaries follows, with subsequent formation of saccular and fusiform aneurysms. Arteriovenous shunts also occur. The vascular lesions are accompanied by proliferation of lining endothelial cells and a loss of the pericytes that surround and support the vessels. Hemorrhages into the inner retinal areas are dot-shaped, while bleeding into the more superficial nerve fiber layer causes flame-shaped, blot, or linear lesions. Preretinal hemorrhages characteristically have a boat-shaped appearance. Exudates are of two types. Cotton-wool spots can be shown by angiography to be microinfarcts—nonperfused areas surrounded by a ring of dilated capillaries. A sudden increase in the number of cotton-wool spots represents an ominous prognostic sign and may herald the appearance of rapidly advancing retinopathy. Hard exudates are more common than cotton-wool spots and probably represent leakage of protein and lipids from damaged capillaries.

The fundamental characteristics of proliferative retinopathy are new vessel formation and scarring. The stimulus for neovascularization may be hypoxia secondary to capillary or arteriolar occlusion. Two serious complications of proliferative retinopathy are vitreal hemorrhage and retinal detachment. Either may cause a sudden loss of vision in one eye.

The frequency of diabetic retinopathy appears to vary with the age of onset as well as the duration of the disease. Approximately 85 percent of patients eventually develop the complication, but some never develop lesions even after 30 years of disease. Retinopathy appears to develop earlier in older patients, but proliferative retinopathy is less common. Some 10 to 18 percent of patients with simple retinopathy progress to proliferative disease in a 10-year period. About half of patients with proliferative disease progress to blindness within 5 years.

Treatment for diabetic retinopathy is photocoagulation. Such treatment decreases the incidence of hemorrhage and scarring and is always indicated when new vessel formation occurs. Photocoagulation is also useful in treatment of microaneurysms, hemorrhages, and edema even if the proliferative stage has not begun. Panretinal photocoagulation is sometimes used to diminish retinal demands for oxygen in the hope that the stimulus for neovascularization will be decreased. In this technique several thousand lesions are produced

TABLE 319-13 Lesions of diabetic retinopathy

BACKGROUND

Increased capillary permeability
Capillary closure and dilatation
Microaneurysms
Arteriovenous shunts
Dilated veins
Hemorrhages (dot and blot)
Cotton-wool spots
Hard exudates

PROLIFERATIVE

New vessels
Scar (retinitis proliferans)
Vitreal hemorrhage
Retinal detachment

over a 2-week period. Complications of photocoagulation are within the acceptable range. Some loss of peripheral vision is inevitable with extensive burns. Another surgical technique, pars plana vitrectomy, is utilized for treatment of nonresolving vitreal hemorrhage and retinal detachment. Postoperative complications are more frequent than with photocoagulation and include retinal tears, retinal detachment, cataracts, recurrent vitreal hemorrhage, glaucoma, infection, and loss of the eye. Hypophysectomy, once widely performed for diabetic retinopathy, is no longer recommended. There is hope that inhibition of angiogenesis by drugs such as the experimental heparin analogue, beta-cyclodextrin tetradecasulfate, may prevent proliferative retinopathy. All patients with diabetic retinopathy should be followed by retinal specialists.

Diabetic nephropathy   Renal disease is a leading cause of death and disability in diabetes. About half of end-stage renal disease in the United States is now due to diabetic nephropathy. Approximately 40 to 50 percent of patients with insulin-dependent diabetes develop this complication. Prevalence may be somewhat less with the non-insulin-dependent form of the disease, possibly because duration of illness tends to be shorter. However, two-thirds of diabetic Pima Indians (who have non-insulin-dependent diabetes) have diabetic glomerulosclerosis at autopsy. It is probable that nephropathy, like other complications, is influenced by the genetic background of the patient (it is rare in Japanese Americans with diabetes). Some families with multiple diabetic members rarely have renal disease while in others more than 80 percent of persons at risk have nephropathy.

Diabetic nephropathy involves two distinct pathologic patterns that may or may not coexist: diffuse and nodular. The former, which is more common, consists of widening of the glomerular basement membrane together with generalized mesangial thickening. In the nodular form large accumulations of PAS-positive material are deposited at the periphery of the glomerular tufts, the Kimmelstiel-Wilson lesion. In addition, there may be hyalinization of afferent and efferent arterioles, "drops" in Bowman's capsule, fibrin caps, and occlusion of glomeruli. Deposition of albumin and other proteins occurs in both glomeruli and tubules. The most specific lesions of diabetic glomerulosclerosis are hyalinization of afferent glomerular arterioles and the Kimmelstiel-Wilson nodules. Clinical renal dysfunction in diabetes does not correlate well with the histologic abnormalities.

Diabetic nephropathy may be functionally silent for long periods (~10 to 15 years). At onset of diabetes the kidneys are usually enlarged with "superfunction," i.e., glomerular filtration rates may be 40 percent above normal. The next stage is the appearance of *microproteinuria* (microalbuminuria), the excretion of albumin in the range of 30 to 550 mg/d. Normal persons excrete less than 30 mg/d. Microalbuminuria is not detected by reagent sticks for urinary protein, which generally become positive only when proteinuria is greater than 550 mg/d, a degree of leakage termed *macroproteinuria*. Since microalbuminuria is initially transient and can be induced by mechanisms other than diabetes, diagnosis requires an excretion rate of albumin greater than 15 µg/h (~30 mg/d) in two of three samples collected in a 6-month period. Persistent leakage of protein >50 mg/d is predictive of subsequent macroproteinuria. Once the macroproteinuric phase begins, there is a steady decline in renal function with glomerular filtration rate falling, on average, about 1 mL/min per month. A plot of the reciprocal of the serum creatinine against time usually results in a straight line and allows prediction of the rate of deterioration. Ordinarily azotemia begins about 12 years after diagnosis of diabetes. The nephrotic syndrome may occur prior to azotemia. Progression of renal disease is accelerated by hypertension.

There is no specific treatment for diabetic nephropathy. Meticulous control of diabetes can reverse microalbuminuria in some patients, but there is no evidence that diabetic nephropathy can be prevented by intensive insulin therapy. Hypertension must be treated aggressively whenever present. Low-protein diets may be useful, based on experimental studies in animals. A prospective study testing protein restriction in humans is underway. Once the azotemic phase is reached, treatment does not differ from other forms of renal failure. Chronic dialysis and renal transplantation are routine in patients with renal failure due to diabetes. Hyporeninemic hypoaldosteronism, which is associated with renal tubular acidosis, may require alkalinizing solutions (Shohl's solution) and avoidance of external potassium loads. Rarely, fludrocortisone may be required to control hyperkalemia.

Diabetic neuropathy   Diabetic neuropathy may affect every part of the nervous system with the possible exception of the brain. While it is rarely a direct cause of death, it is a major cause of morbidity. Distinct syndromes can be recognized, and several different types of neuropathy may be present in the same patient. The most common picture is that of *peripheral polyneuropathy*. Usually bilateral, the symptoms include numbness, paresthesias, severe hyperesthesias, and pain. The pain, which may be deep-seated and severe, is often worse at night. It is occasionally lancinating or lightning in type, resembling tabes dorsalis (pseudotabes). Fortunately extreme pain syndromes are usually self-limited, lasting from a few months to a few years. Involvement of proprioceptive fibers leads to abnormalities of gait and development of typical Charcot joints, particularly in the feet. Loss of arch with multiple fractures of tarsal bones is a common finding by x-ray. On physical examination absent stretch reflexes and loss of vibratory sense are early signs. Diabetic neuropathy may also cause delay in return of the ankle reflex identical to that seen in hypothyroidism. *Mononeuropathy*, though less common than polyneuropathy, may also occur. Characteristically there is a sudden wrist drop, foot drop, or paralysis of the third, fourth, or sixth cranial nerves. Other single nerves, including the recurrent laryngeal, have been reported to be involved. Mononeuropathy is characterized by a high degree of spontaneous reversibility, usually over a several-week period. *Radiculopathy* is a sensory syndrome in which pain occurs over the distribution of one or more spinal nerves, usually in the chest wall or abdomen. The severe pain may mimic herpes zoster or an acute surgical abdomen. Like mononeuropathy, the lesion is usually self-limited. *Autonomic neuropathy* may present in a variety of ways. The gastrointestinal tract is a prime target, and there may be esophageal dysfunction with difficulty in swallowing, delayed gastric emptying, constipation, or diarrhea. The last is often nocturnal. Incompetence of the internal anal sphincter may mimic diabetic diarrhea. Orthostatic hypotension and frank syncope may occur. Cardiorespiratory arrest and sudden death, thought to be due solely to autonomic neuropathy, have been reported. Bladder dysfunction or paralysis is particularly distressing and often leads to the necessity of chronic catheter drainage. Impotence and retrograde ejaculation are additional manifestations in the male. Clues to autonomic neuropathy can be obtained by clinical tests such as measuring response of the heart rate to the Valsalva maneuver or standing. In both tests the subject has an electrocardiograph running for assessment of heart rate. In the former the subject blows against an anaeroid or mercury manometer to 40 mmHg pressure for 15 s. The test is performed three times with a rest period of 1 min in between. Normally the heart rate speeds during Valsalva such that the ratio of the longest interval between beats after release to the shortest interval during the test is >1.2. In autonomic neuropathy involving the parasympathetic system the ratio is <1:1. Similarly the ratio at the thirtieth beat after standing relative to that at the fifteenth beat should be >1.0. It is <1 in autonomic neuropathy. Diabetic *amyotrophy* is likely a form of neuropathy, although atrophy and weakness of the large muscles in the upper leg and pelvic girdle resemble primary muscle disease. Anorexia and depression may accompany amyotrophy. Because of the weight loss, such patients are often thought to have a paraneoplastic neuropathy.

Treatment of diabetic neuropathy is unsatisfactory in most respects. When pain is severe, it is easy for the patient to become habituated or addicted to narcotics or powerful nonnarcotic analgesics such as pentazocine. If the pain requires something stronger than aspirin, acetaminophen, or other nonsteroidal anti-inflammatory agents, codeine is the drug of choice. Phenytoin is used by some physicians, but others have not found it helpful. Combination therapy with amitriptyline and fluphenazine causes relief of pain in some patients and should always be tried. The recommended dosage is 75 mg amitriptyline at bedtime and 1 mg fluphenazine three times a day. Mononeuropathies and radiculopathies usually require no specific therapy since they are self-limited. Diabetic diarrhea often responds to treatment with diphenoxylate and atropine or loperamide. Orthostatic hypotension is best treated by having the patient sleep with the head of the bed elevated, avoidance of sudden assumption of the upright position, and the use of full-length elastic stockings. Occasionally volume expansion with fludrocortisone is required as in other forms of orthostatic hypotension.

Experimental therapy with aldose reductase inhibitors and myoinositol have failed to provide significant clinical benefit although enhanced regeneration of nerves has been reported in humans treated with an aldose reductase antagonist.

Diabetic foot ulcers A special problem in the diabetic patient is the development of ulcers of the feet and lower extremities. The ulcers appear to be primarily due to abnormal pressure distribution secondary to diabetic neuropathy. The problem is accentuated when there is bony distortion in the feet. Callus formation is usually the initial abnormality. Alternatively the ulcer may be initiated by ill-fitting shoes which cause blister formation in patients whose sensory deficits preclude recognition of pain. Cuts and punctures from foreign bodies such as needles, tacks, and glass are common, and a foreign body of which the patient is unaware may be found in the soft tissue. For this reason all patients with ulcers should have x-rays made of the feet. Vascular disease with diminished blood supply contributes to development of the lesion, and infection is common, often with multiple organisms. While no specific therapy is available for diabetic ulcers, aggressive supportive treatment can often lead to salvation of the leg without amputation. One approach is to simply put the patient to bed using hydrotherapy and debridement to remove nonviable tissue. Others recommend casting the leg with plaster to redistribute weight bearing and protect the lesion.

All diabetics should be instructed about proper foot care in an attempt to prevent ulcers. Feet should be kept clean and dry at all times. Patients with neuropathy should not be allowed to walk barefoot, even in the home. Properly fitted shoes are essential. This is a particular problem with women, since an adequate shoe for the diabetic is not often stylish. The feet should be carefully inspected daily for callus, infection, abrasions, or blisters and the physician consulted for any potentially troublesome lesion. Treatment with growth factors (e.g., fibroblast growth factor) may prove useful in the future.

What causes the complications of diabetes? The cause of diabetic complications is not known and may be multifactorial. Major emphasis has been placed on the polyol pathway wherein glucose is reduced to sorbitol by the enzyme aldol reductase. Sorbitol, which appears to function as a tissue toxin, has been implicated in the pathogenesis of retinopathy, neuropathy, cataracts, nephropathy, and aortic disease. The mechanism is perhaps best worked out in experimental diabetic neuropathy where sorbitol accumulation is associated with a decrease in myoinositol content, abnormal phosphoinositide metabolism, and a decrease in Na^+,K^+-ATPase activity. In experimental models primacy of the polyol pathway in initiating neuropathy was proven by showing that inhibition of aldol reductase prevented the fall in tissue myoinositol content and the decrease in ATPase activity. Myoinositol deficiency was not found in sural nerve biopsies from humans with diabetic neuropathy, in contrast to animals. Aldol reductase inhibition has also been shown to prevent experimental cataracts and retinopathy. It thus seems possible that neuropathy and retinopathy are primarily due to activation of the polyol pathway. It may also play a role in diabetic nephropathy.

A second mechanism of potential pathogenetic importance is glycation of proteins. (Current terminology uses *glycation* for nonenzymatic addition of hexoses to proteins and *glycosylation* for enzymatic addition.) The effect of such glycation on hemoglobin has been mentioned, but multiple proteins in the body are altered in the same way, often with disturbed functions. Examples include plasma albumin, lens protein, fibrin, collagen, lipoproteins, and the glycoprotein recognition system of hepatic endothelial cells. Particularly intriguing is the effect of glycation on lipoproteins. Glycated LDL is not recognized by the normal LDL receptor, and its plasma half-life is increased. Conversely, glycated HDL turns over more rapidly than native HDL. It has also been reported that glycated collagen traps LDL at rates two to three times greater than normal collagen. Conceivably the accelerated atherosclerosis of diabetes might be related to the combined effect of a glycated LDL that did not bind normally to LDL receptors but would be trapped to a greater than normal extent by macrophages and glycated collagen of blood vessels and other tissues. Dysfunctional HDL could contribute by diminishing cholesterol transport out of affected sites.

Glycated collagen is less soluble and more resistant to degradation by collagenase than native collagen. However, it is not clear that this is related either to the basement membrane thickening or the tight, waxy skin syndrome with limited joint mobility (scleroderma-like) seen in some patients with insulin-dependent diabetes (see "Miscellaneous Abnormalities," below). Although it is attractive to presume that nonenzymatic glycation of proteins plays a role in some degenerative complications, the evidence is less direct than with the polyol pathway. Linkage between the polyol pathway and the glycation sequence occurs as a result of the glycation of collagen and other proteins by fructose generated from sorbitol.

Increased blood flow has been postulated to play an initiating role in diabetic complications, possibly by increasing filtration of macromolecules that function as tissue toxins. There is supportive evidence for a role of hyperperfusion in diabetic nephropathy, but the hemodynamic hypothesis does not appear as attractive as the first two.

Can diabetic complications be prevented by meticulous control of diabetes? The critical question in diabetic therapy is whether hyperglycemia or some associated metabolic disorder causes or accelerates the development of the long-term complications just discussed. The alternative possibility is that complications are primarily determined by genetic factors independent of hyperglycemia. Perhaps the strongest evidence that the metabolic environment per se causes complications comes from the observation that kidneys from donors who have neither diabetes nor a family history of diabetes develop characteristic lesions of diabetic nephropathy within 3 to 5 years after transplantation into a diabetic recipient. Diabetic nephropathy did not develop when a kidney was transplanted into a diabetic subject whose disease had been reversed by pancreatic transplantation prior to renal transplantation. It has also been reported that kidneys with the lesions of diabetic nephropathy demonstrated reversal of the lesion when transplanted into normal recipients. All of these findings suggest that hyperglycemia or some other aspect of the abnormal metabolism of diabetes causes or influences the development of complications. On the other hand additional factors, probably genetic, must play a role. This follows from the fact that diabetic subjects with decades of poor control may escape the ravages of the late complications and from the fact that typical diabetic complications may be found in patients at the time of diagnosis of diabetes or even in the absence of hyperglycemia.

Meticulous control with insulin infusion pumps has been reported to decrease microalbuminuria, alter motor nerve conduction velocity, lower plasma lipoproteins, and decrease capillary leakage of fluorescein in the retina. Width of the capillary basement membrane in skeletal muscle has also been decreased. The changes are small in general, however, and of questionable biologic significance. Firm evidence does not exist to show that late complications can be either prevented or reversed by long-term near-normalization of the plasma glucose. Progression of retinopathy has been reported despite successful reversal of diabetes by pancreatic transplantation. Hopefully, definitive answers to this question may be forthcoming from a large multicenter trial now underway under the sponsorship of the National Institutes of Health.

Until the issue is clarified it is prudent to maintain the plasma glucose as near normal as possible in all diabetic patients. About this there appears to be no disagreement. The only question is whether insulin therapy should be routinely aggressive to the point where recurrent hypoglycemia occurs. A mild insulin reaction consisting of nervousness, tremor, hunger, and sweating that is rapidly interrupted by carbohydrate intake is probably not harmful except for the possibility of worsening diabetic control via the Somogyi reaction. Unfortunately, as stated earlier, many diabetics, particularly those with long-standing disease and autonomic neuropathy, do not have or do not recognize the usual warning signals and progress to altered central nervous system function with abnormal behavior, loss of consciousness, or even convulsions. The latter reactions are dangerous for both patient and society. Every effort should be made to control hyperglycemia, but the limit of therapy should be the appearance of hypoglycemic reactions. It does not seem wise to induce a condition that can cause immediate and irreversible damage to a patient in the unproven hope that late complications might be prevented.

Miscellaneous abnormalities of diabetes   Diabetes affects almost every system in the body. Space limitations preclude discussion of all associated features, but several deserve comment. *Infections* in diabetics may not occur more frequently than in normal subjects, but they tend to be more severe. This may be due to impaired leukocyte function, a frequent accompaniment of poor control. In addition to common infections of the skin, urinary tract, lungs, and bloodstream, four unusual conditions appear to have specific relationship with diabetes. *Malignant external otitis,* usually due to *Pseudomonas aeruginosa,* tends to occur in older patients and is characterized by severe pain in the ear, drainage, fever, and leukocytosis. Soft tissues around the ear are swollen and tender. A mound of granulation tissue is characteristically present internally at the junction of the osseous and cartilaginous portions of the ear. The facial nerve becomes paralyzed in half the cases, and other cranial nerves may also be involved. Facial nerve paralysis is a poor prognostic sign, and mortality approximates 50 percent in this subset of patients. A 6-week course of ticarcillin or carbenicillin together with tobramycin is the treatment of choice. Surgical debridement is often necessary. *Rhinocerebral mucormycosis* is a rare fungal infection which usually develops in patients during or following an episode of diabetic ketoacidosis. Organisms are from the genera *Mucor, Rhizopus,* and *Absidia.* Onset is sudden with periorbital and perinasal swelling, pain, bloody nasal discharge, and increased lacrimation. The nasal mucosa and underlying tissues become black and necrotic. Cranial nerve palsies are not uncommon. There may be thrombosis of the internal jugular vein or sinuses of the brain. Proptosis, chemosis, and retinal vein engorgement indicate cavernous sinus thrombosis. Untreated, death usually occurs in a week to 10 days. Amphotericin B and aggressive debridement are the indicated therapies. *Emphysematous cholecystitis* tends to affect diabetic men (in contrast to ordinary cholecystitis, a disease predominantly present in women). Gangrene of the gallbladder is 30 times more frequent than in the usual forms, accounting for high rates of perforation and a mortality rate 3 to 10 times higher than in ordinary cholecystitis. Diagnosis is made when gas is seen in the gallbladder wall on plain films of the abdomen. Clostridial species are frequently cultured from bile, but other organisms may be present. Treatment is cholecystectomy coupled with broad-spectrum antibiotics. Clindamycin and an aminoglycoside are adequate coverage until cultures are returned. *Emphysematous pyelonephritis* is signalled by the presence of gas in the kidney or perirenal space. Antibiotic therapy is usually ineffective, and nephrectomy may be required. Mortality rates of 80 percent have been reported.

Hypertriglyceridemia is common in diabetes and is usually due to insulin deficiency. Both overproduction of very low density

lipoproteins in the liver and a disposal defect in the periphery appear to be operative. The latter is a consequence of lipoprotein lipase deficiency, an insulin-dependent enzyme. Some diabetics exhibit hyperlipemia even when diabetic control is adequate, and these patients may have a primary familial hyperlipoproteinemia that is independent of diabetes. Patients who do not respond to dietary therapy should be treated for hypertriglyceridemia and hypercholesterolemia with drugs, as in nondiabetic subjects (see Chap. 326).

Some diabetics have *recurrent hyperkalemia* in association with hyperglycemia. Traditionally these patients have been considered to have hyporeninemic hypoaldosteronism although basal renin and aldosterone concentrations may be normal. Since the capacity to increase aldosterone production in response to stimulatory signals is impaired even when basal levels are normal, functional hypoaldosteronism probably plays a central role in the syndrome. With a deficiency of aldosterone, renal secretion of potassium is impaired and disposal of a potassium load is dependent on insulin-mediated transport of the cation into the intracellular space. Administration of potassium salts or triamterene to such patients may be dangerous. Whether potassium transport is directly regulated by insulin or is secondary to glucose movement is not clear. Affected subjects almost always have a hyperchloremic renal tubular acidosis.

A variety of skin lesions occur in diabetes. *Necrobiosis lipoidica diabeticorum* is a plaque-like lesion with a central yellowish area surrounded by a brownish border. It is usually found over the anterior surfaces of the legs. Ulceration may occur (see Fig. A1-28). *Diabetic dermopathy* (''shin spots'') is also usually located over the anterior tibial surface. The lesions are small rounded plaques with a raised border which may crust at the edges and ulcerate centrally. Several plaques may be arranged in linear fashion. Pigmentation is not prominent early, but as the lesion heals a depressed scar occurs with diffuse brown discoloration. A rarer abnormality is *bullosis diabeticorum.* The bullae may be superficial with clear serum or may be mildly hemorrhagic. The cause is unknown. *Infestations of the skin* with *Candida* and dermatophytes are common, and bacterial infections of a variety of types occur. In women *vaginal moniliasis* may be troublesome during hyperglycemic-glycosuric periods. While the symptoms respond to nystatin or gentian violet, recurrence is inevitable unless glycosuria is reversed. *Atrophy of adipose tissue* may occur at the site of insulin injections. The lipoatrophy is said to respond to injection of purified insulin into the atrophic area. Hypertrophy of fat may also occur, producing a lipoma-like lesion visible on physical examination.

Hyperviscosity occurs in diabetes, and *platelets aggregate abnormally.* The latter may be caused by increased prostaglandin synthesis. *Wound healing* is impaired in experimental diabetes but probably is not a major factor clinically. An interesting accompaniment of insulin-dependent diabetes is the presence of *joint contractures* (Dupuytren's contracture) coupled with *tight, waxy skin* over the dorsum of the hands. The hands resemble those in patients with scleroderma. The cause of the tendon contractures is unknown although alterations of cross-linking in collagen has been proposed. Patients with the joint contracture–waxy skin syndrome appear to have accelerated development of other diabetic complications. *Scleredema* is a common finding in diabetes. The lesion is a thickening of the skin over the shoulders and upper back that resembles scleroderma. The condition is benign.

NONROUTINE THERAPY   Transplantation with whole pancreas or segments has cured diabetes in a number of patients but is usually performed only when kidney transplantation is required. Half the grafts have failed at 1 year. Islet cell transplantation has not been successful in humans. Prevention of type 1 diabetes by suppression of the immune system remains a hoped-for goal. Cyclosporine given within a 6-week period after the appearance of hyperglycemia may reverse the metabolic abnormalities and allow discontinuation of insulin therapy in a significant number of patients. However, its long-term use is too dangerous to be recommended. New immunosuppressive agents have considerable promise, however.

INSULIN RESISTANCE Insulin resistance in diabetic subjects is arbitrarily defined as the requirement of 200 or more units of insulin per day to control hyperglycemia and prevent ketosis. Relative insulin resistance is present in essentially all persons with diabetes when carefully looked for using the glucose clamp technique. It is the consequence of near complete insulin deficiency in IDDM, whereas in NIDDM the major problem is obesity.

Normal anabolic metabolism, mediated by insulin, requires the secretion of adequate amounts of normal hormone in response to meals. Insulin must then bind to a specific insulin receptor in target tissues (see Chap. 320). The insulin receptor is a tetrameric glycoprotein consisting of two alpha subunits and two beta subunits linked by disulfide bonds. The beta subunit is a tyrosine kinase that is activated when insulin binds to the alpha subunit. The tyrosine kinase autophosphorylates the insulin receptor and initiates subsequent intracellular phosphorylations that mediate the multiple actions of insulin. The only such action which is reasonably understood is glucose transport. Glucose enters the cell by facilitated diffusion utilizing "glucose transporter" molecules. While some of these are always present in the plasma membrane, insulin binding to the receptor initiates a rapid mobilization of intracellular stores of the transporter to the plasma membrane while simultaneously activating units already in place. In poorly controlled diabetes the number of stored transporters appears to be deficient.

Insulin resistance is characterized as *prereceptor* (abnormal insulin or insulin antibodies), *receptor* (decreased receptor number or diminished binding of insulin), or *postreceptor* (abnormal signal transduction, especially failure to activate the receptor tyrosine kinase). Combinations may exist. The nature of the molecular defect is known in some syndromes of insulin resistance but in many the defect has not been pinpointed.

In diabetic subjects with fullblown insulin resistance (>200 units of insulin per day) the problem is usually prereceptor resistance due to insulin antibodies. Insulin antibodies of IgG type are present in essentially all diabetics within 60 days of the initiation of insulin therapy. The titer of these antibodies fluctuates for reasons that are not clear. Although the correlation between antibody titer and functional resistance is not close, insulin binding by high levels of antibody is presumed to be the primary mechanism in most cases. Probably less than 0.1 percent of insulin-treated diabetics ever have significant resistance. The problem may appear within a few weeks of the start of therapy or many years later. The onset may be abrupt, resulting in ketoacidosis, but usually is gradual, with uncontrollable hyperglycemia being the major problem. About 20 to 30 percent of patients have concomitant insulin allergy. Therapy of the syndrome requires prednisone in large amounts—80 to 100 mg/d initially. Response often occurs in 48 to 72 h but may take longer. If no improvement has resulted after 3 to 4 weeks, it can be assumed that steroids will not be effective. Once insulin requirements begin to fall, prednisone dosage can be rapidly decreased by 10 to 20 mg every 3 to 7 days until a maintenance level of 5 to 10 mg/d is reached. These levels may be required for many months. Whether remission has occurred, allowing cessation of therapy, can only be determined by trial. Sulfated insulin may also be of benefit. On rare occasions insulin resistance in diabetics appears to be due to enhanced destruction of the hormone at the subcutaneous injection site. Such patients tend to respond normally to insulin given intravenously or intraperitoneally. In some patients addition of a protease inhibitor (aprotinin) to the insulin mixture has been helpful. When resistance is extreme, U500 regular insulin should be used in order to control the volume of the injection.

Insulin resistance occurs in diseases other than diabetes. In such disorders *acanthosis nigricans* is a physical sign of its presence. Acanthosis nigricans is a brown to black, velvety hyperpigmentation of the skin, most often present in the posterior and lateral folds of the neck. It is also found in the axilla, groin, umbilicus, and other areas. Acanthosis nigricans is common, occurring in 7 percent of 1412 children who made up the 6th and 8th grade populations of the public schools in one study. Higher prevalence was found in Hispanics and blacks than in whites. Although acanthosis nigricans may be a sign of occult malignancy, it is not associated with neoplasia in the insulin-resistant states. A list of the major syndromes of insulin resistance is given in Table 319-14.

Obesity is the most common cause of insulin resistance. It is associated with decreased receptor number, but the major problem is at the postreceptor level, where there is apparently a failure to activate the tyrosine kinase. *Werner's syndrome* is an autosomal recessive illness with a high incidence of hyperglycemia despite elevated concentrations of plasma insulin (see Chap. 325). There is little response to exogenous hormone. Other features include growth retardation, alopecia or premature graying of the hair, cataracts, hypogonadism, leg ulcers, atrophy of muscle, fat, and bone, soft-tissue calcification, and a high frequency of sarcomas and meningiomas.

Of the rare conditions associated with acanthosis nigricans, women with *insulin receptor abnormalities* have attracted the greatest interest. Type A patients are tall young women with a tendency to hirsutism and abnormalities of the reproductive tract who most probably have polycystic ovaries. However, other causes of androgen excess are associated with the syndrome. Most patients have an absolute decrease in the number of insulin receptors, but in some receptor function is qualitatively abnormal. At the molecular level defects range from a decrease in mRNA for the receptor to mutations that alter receptor processing or insertion into the membrane. Type B subjects are older women with evidence of immunologic disease. The clinical picture includes arthralgias, alopecia, enlarged salivary glands, proteinuria, leukopenia, and antinuclear and anti-DNA antibodies. Insulin resistance in these patients is due to blocking antibodies to the insulin receptor (not to insulin itself). Interestingly, antireceptor antibodies may also cause hypoglycemia. The determinant of agonist (hypoglycemia) or antagonist (insulin resistance) activity presumably depends on the site of binding to the insulin receptor. Both A and B patients have high plasma insulin concentrations.

Generalized and *partial lipodystrophies* are fat depletion syndromes differing primarily in the extent of fat atrophy (see Chap. 338). In the generalized form essentially all body fat is missing, while the more common partial type exhibits atrophy of fat in the face and trunk with normal or increased adiposity in the lower half of the body. The disease can be either congenital or acquired. Typically the patients develop hyperglycemia at puberty, but ketoacidosis never occurs. Marked hypertriglyceridemia with eruptive xanthoma is a frequent feature. Characteristic features are hepatomegaly, splenomegaly, cardiomegaly, hirsutism, lymphadenopathy, hypertrophy of the external genitalia, varicose veins, and (in the congenital forms) muscle hypertrophy. Mental retardation is common, and renal disease may develop. The term *lipoatrophic diabetes* is synonymous with total lipodystrophy. All patients have elevated plasma insulin levels. Resistance may be due to decreased number of receptors, diminished affinity of the receptor for insulin, or a postreceptor defect.

The *pineal hypertrophy syndrome* is characterized by insulin

---

TABLE 319-14 Insulin-resistant states

I Prereceptor resistance
   A Mutated insulins
   B Anti-insulin antibodies
II Receptor and postreceptor resistance
   A Obesity
   B Type A syndrome (absent or dysfunctional receptor)
   C Type B syndrome (antibody to insulin receptor)
   D Lipodystrophic states (partial or generalized)
   E Leprechaunism
   F Ataxia-telangiectasia
   G Rabson-Mendenhall syndrome
   H Werner syndrome
   I Alström syndrome
   J Pineal hyperplasia syndrome

resistance, early dentition with malformed teeth, dry skin, thick nails, hirsutism, and a peculiar sexual precocity with enlargement of the external genitalia. The latter may reach near adult size by age 3 or 4. The insulin resistance is severe, and ketoacidosis may occur despite high endogenous insulin levels. The *Alström syndrome* is a rare autosomal recessive disease characterized by childhood blindness due to retinal degeneration, nerve deafness, vasopressin-resistant diabetes insipidus, and, in males, hypogonadism with high plasma gonadotropin levels. The patients thus appear to have end organ resistance to multiple hormones. Other features include baldness, hyperuricemia, hypertriglyceridemia, and aminoaciduria. Superficially the patients may resemble subjects with the Lawrence-Moon-Biedl syndrome but can be differentiated on initial exam by the absence of polydactyly and mental deficiency. Insulin resistance in the Alström syndrome is mild. *Ataxia-telangiectasia* is characterized by cerebellar ataxia, telangiectasia, and a variety of abnormalities in the immune system in addition to insulin resistance. The *Rabson-Mendenhall syndrome* consists of dental dysplasia, dystrophic nails, premature puberty, and acanthosis nigricans. The insulin resistance is probably due to an insulin receptor abnormality. *Leprechaunism* is characterized by an elfin appearance of the face, hirsutism, absence of subcutaneous fat, thickened skin, and insulin resistance. The latter is probably due to abnormal receptor function. Not listed in Table 319-14 is insulin resistance due to hormone excess (acromegaly, Cushing's syndrome), myotonic dystrophy, and thalassemia major. The insulin resistance in these conditions is usually not clinically significant.

INSULIN ALLERGY Insulin allergy is due to IgE antibodies to insulin. Manifestations include immediate reactions with local stinging or itching, delayed local reactions with brawny swelling lasting up to 30 h, and generalized urticaria or frank anaphylaxis. Systemic reactions are usually seen in patients who have stopped insulin therapy for one reason or another and have then resumed treatment. The allergic reaction may occur as early as the second injection on resumption of therapy. Mild reactions can be treated with antihistamines. If the problem is severe, desensitization procedures are required. A 1-day insulin desensitization procedure is shown in Table 319-15. Once the patient is desensitized, insulin therapy should not be interrupted.

THE EMOTIONAL RESPONSE TO DIABETES Acceptance of the fact that a person has a chronic disease that requires a change in lifestyle is always difficult. This is particularly true in the case of diabetes since patients generally are aware that they are vulnerable to late complications and that life expectancy is shortened. It is not surprising that the emotional response to diabetes often hampers treatment. On the one hand, the primary reaction may be denial with an accompanying refusal to cooperate. At the other extreme is excessive preoccupation with the illness. The physician should make every effort to define a middle ground wherein the patient acknowl-

edges his or her disease and responds prudently without becoming obsessed. The goal is to live with diabetes not for it. Diabetics are no different from other patients in that they may attempt to use their disease manipulatively with both family and physician. The problems are particularly acute with children and adolescents. While the psychiatric aspects of diabetes are not discussed here, most problems can be anticipated and handled if common sense is coupled with sympathy and firmness. It is also appropriate to offer cautious hope that the disease will be handled better in the future than is possible now.

REFERENCES

General review

UNGER RH, FOSTER DW: Diabetes mellitus, in *Williams' Textbook of Endocrinology*, 8th ed, JD Wilson, DW Foster (eds). Philadelphia, Saunders, 1990, in press

Pathophysiology

BANERJI MA, LEBOVITZ HE: Insulin-sensitive and insulin-resistant variants in NIDDM. Diabetes 38:784, 1989

BOTTAZZO GF et al: In situ characterization of autoimmune phenomena and expression of HLA molecules in the pancreas in diabetic insulitis. N Engl J Med 313:353, 1985

EISENBARTH GS et al: The "natural" history of type 1 diabetes. Diabetes Metab Rev 3:873, 1987

HARRISON LC et al: MHC molecules and β-cell destructive immune and nonimmune mechanisms. Diabetes 38:815, 1989

KWOK WW et al: Mutational analysis of the HLA-DQ 3.2 insulin-dependent diabetes susceptibility gene. Proc Natl Acad Sci (USA) 86:1027, 1989

LEIGHTON B, COOPER GJS: Pancreatic amylin and calcitonin gene-related peptide cause resistance to insulin in skeletal muscle *in vitro*. Nature 335:632, 1988

REAVEN GM: Banting Lecture 1988. Role of insulin resistance in human disease. Diabetes 37:1595, 1988

SHEEHY MJ et al: Diabetes-susceptible HLA haplotype is best defined by a combination of HLA-DR and -DQ alleles. J Clin Invest 83:830, 1989

TODD JA et al: HLA-DQβ gene contributes to susceptibility and resistance to insulin-dependent diabetes mellitus. Nature 329:599, 1987

Acute complications

CARROLL P, MATZ R: Uncontrolled diabetes mellitus in adults: Experience in treating diabetic ketoacidosis and hyperosmolar nonketotic coma with low-dose insulin and a uniform treatment regimen. Diabetes Care 6:579, 1983

FOSTER DW, McGARRY JD: The metabolic derangements and treatment of diabetic ketoacidosis. N Engl J Med 309:159, 1983

FRANKLIN B et al: Cerebral edema and ophthalmoplegia reversed by mannitol in a new case of insulin-dependent diabetes mellitus. Pediatrics 69:87, 1982

KITABCHI AE: Low-dose insulin therapy in diabetic ketoacidosis: Fact or fiction? Diabetes Metab Rev 5:337, 1989

Late complications

BROWNLEE M et al: Advanced products of nonenzymatic glycosylation and the pathogenesis of diabetic vascular disease. Diabetes Metab Rev 5:437, 1988

LoGERFO FW, COFFMAN JD: Vascular and microvascular disease of the foot in diabetes. N Engl J Med 311:1615, 1984

MOGENSEN CE, CHRISTENSEN CK: Predicting diabetic nephropathy in insulin-dependent patients. N Engl J Med 311:89, 1984

PARVING HH et al: Hemodynamic factors in the genesis of diabetic microangiopathy. Metabolism 32:943, 1983

RAMSAY RC et al: Progression of diabetic retinopathy after pancreas transplantation for insulin-dependent diabetes mellitus. N Engl J Med 318:208, 1988

ROSENSTOCK J, RASKIN P: Diabetes and its complications: Blood glucose control versus genetic susceptibility. Diabetes Metab Rev 4:417, 1988

SEQUIST ER et al: Familial clustering of diabetic renal disease. Evidence for genetic susceptibility and diabetic nephropathy. N Engl J Med 320:1161, 1989

WINEGRAD AI: Banting Lecture 1986. Does a common mechanism induce the diverse complications of diabetes? Diabetes 36:396, 1986

Treatment

COUSTAN DR: Pregnancy in diabetic women. N Engl J Med 319:1663, 1988

CRYER PE et al: Hypoglycemia in IDDM. Diabetes 38:1193, 1989

LEBOVITZ HE, FEINGLOS MN: The oral hypoglycemic agents, in *Diabetes Mellitus: Theory and Practice*, 3d ed, M Ellenberg, H Rifkin (eds). New Hyde Park, Medical Examination Publishing, 1983, pp 591–610

MECKENBURG RS et al: Long-term metabolic control with insulin pump therapy. N Engl J Med 313:464, 1985

SCHADE DS: Surgery and diabetes. Med Clin North Am 72:1531, 1988

SCHIFFRIN A, BELMONTE MM: Comparison between subcutaneous insulin infusion and multiple injections of insulin: A one year prospective study. Diabetes 31:255, 1982

SKYLER JS: Insulin pharmacology. Med Clin North Am 72:1337, 1988

SUTHERLAND DER: Who should get a pancreas transplant? Diabetes Care 11:681, 1988

ZINMAN B: The physiologic replacement of insulin. An elusive goal. N Engl J Med 321:363, 1989

TABLE 319-15 Insulin desensitization*

Time, h	Dose, units	Route
0	0.001	Intradermal
0.5	0.002	Intradermal
1	0.004	Subcutaneous
1.5	0.01	Subcutaneous
2	0.02	Subcutaneous
2.5	0.04	Subcutaneous
3	0.1	Subcutaneous
3.5	0.2	Subcutaneous
4	0.5	Subcutaneous
4.5	1	Subcutaneous
5	2	Subcutaneous
5.5	4	Subcutaneous
6	8	Subcutaneous

* Following desensitization, use 2 to 10 units of regular insulin every 4 to 6 h for 24 to 36 h after the 6-h injection before switching to intermediate-acting insulin.
SOURCE: *Schedule of JA Galloway*. For detailed information see JA Galloway, R Bressler, Med Clin North Am 62:663, 1978.

Insulin resistance

FLIER JS et al: Acanthosis nigricans in obese women with hyperandrogenism. Characterization of an insulin-resistance state distinct from the type A and B syndromes. Diabetes 34:101, 1985

KAHN CR, WHITE MF: The insulin receptor and the molecular mechanisms of insulin action. J Clin Invest 82:1151, 1988

———, GOLDSTEIN BJ: Molecular defects in insulin action. Science 245:13, 1989

KURTZ AB, NABARRO JDN: Circulating insulin-binding antibodies. Diabetologia 19:329, 1980

STUART CA et al: Prevalence of acanthosis nigricans in an unselected population. Am J Med 87:269, 1989

320   HYPOGLYCEMIA

DANIEL W. FOSTER / ARTHUR H. RUBENSTEIN

Maintenance of the plasma glucose concentration within narrow bounds is essential for health. Hypoglycemia is dangerous (in the short run more serious than hyperglycemia) because glucose is the primary energy substrate of the brain. Its absence, like that of oxygen, produces deranged function, tissue damage, or even death if the deficit is prolonged. The vulnerability of the brain to hypoglycemia is due to the fact that it cannot utilize circulating free fatty acids as an energy source in contrast to other tissues of the body. Short-chain metabolites of the free fatty acids, acetoacetic and β-hydroxybutyric acids ("ketone bodies," "ketoacids"), are efficiently oxidized by brain and can protect the central nervous system from damage by hypoglycemia when present at moderate concentrations in plasma. However, development of ketosis requires a number of hours in humans. Ketogenesis is not, therefore, an effective protective mechanism against acute hypoglycemia. Preservation of central nervous system function in the early phases of fasting or during hypoglycemia thus requires a prompt increase in the production of glucose by the liver. At the same time glucose utilization in other tissues is diminished by provision of free fatty acids as alternative substrate. These adaptive mechanisms are hormonally controlled and, under ordinary circumstances, are extremely effective. Occasionally, however, the system breaks down or is overwhelmed, resulting in the clinical syndrome hypoglycemia.

DEFENSE AGAINST HYPOGLYCEMIA   The hypoglycemic states can best be understood as derangements of normal fuel metabolism. Under ordinary circumstances energy needs are met by exogenous substrate derived from food. Oxidation of the constituent molecules of food to carbon dioxide and water is accompanied by the generation of adenosine triphosphate (ATP), the principal high-energy compound of the body. In one sense, life can be defined as the continued ability to generate ATP (and related high-energy nucleotides) for the preservation of cellular integrity in all its manifestations. When caloric intake is greater than immediate oxidative needs, as after the usual meal, excess substrate is stored as fat, structural protein, and glycogen. Substrate flux in this phase of metabolism, called *anabolic*, proceeds from intestine to liver to utilization and storage sites. Insulin is the primary hormone mediating the anabolic phase, and counterregulatory hormone levels are suppressed.

The *catabolic* phase of metabolism begins about 5 to 6 h after a meal. Normally the only significant period of catabolism is during the overnight fast, but under some circumstances, particularly serious illness, it may be prolonged. During fasting/catabolism a series of metabolic adjustments maintain the plasma glucose in a safe range for central nervous system metabolism while at the same time providing energy for other tissues in the body. First, the liver is activated for glucose production, and second, a lipid economy is established for most other tissues of the body. Initially glucose from the liver is derived almost exclusively from hepatic glycogen. Because there is only about 70 g of glycogen available in the average human liver, glycogenolysis can only sustain the plasma glucose for a short time, ordinarily 8 to 10 h. Exercise may shorten the protective period, as may the stress of severe illness. To compensate for glycogen depletion gluconeogenesis begins early, with flux of substrate from muscle and adipose tissue stores to liver and then to utilization sites.

The precursors for hepatic glucose synthesis are lactate/pyruvate and amino acids (primarily alanine) derived from muscle and glycerol released from adipose tissue consequent to lipolysis. Amino acids constitute the primary substrate for gluconeogenesis. Most of the lactate is recycled from preformed glucose (*Cori cycle*), the only net contribution coming from the breakdown of muscle glycogen. Glycerol is initially a minor substrate but increases in importance with time. With prolonged fasting the kidney also becomes a gluconeogenic organ and contributes to total glucose production. The primary renal substrate is glutamine, not alanine. Proteolysis required to provide amino acids for gluconeogenesis accounts for the negative nitrogen balance of starvation. The same mechanism is operative in the stress of trauma, surgery, and severe infection. In quantitative terms the liver produces about 11 μmol/kg per min (2 mg/kg per min) of glucose in the initial phases of fasting. Higher glucose turnover indicates increased utilization of glucose, an important consideration in the differential diagnosis of hypoglycemia.

The switch to fat metabolism is accomplished by activation of the hormone-sensitive lipase in adipose tissue, which hydrolyzes stored triglycerides to long-chain fatty acids and glycerol. The long-chain fatty acids have two fates. The bulk (normally about 120 g/d) is utilized directly, and the remainder (about 40 g/d) is oxidized in the liver to acetoacetic and β-hydroxybutyric acids. Ketoacids can be utilized efficiently as an energy source by most tissues (liver only minimally), but their primary importance is as backup substrate for the brain, as noted above. The shift of most tissues to lipid metabolism is important since the preferential oxidation of free fatty acids and ketones in place of glucose spares the latter for utilization by the central nervous system.

Catabolic metabolism is initiated by a fall in insulin concentration in plasma coupled with secretion of the four counterregulatory hormones glucagon, epinephrine, cortisol, and growth hormone. In addition norepinephrine is released directly in tissues from sympathetic neurons. Glucagon is the primary hormone of glucose maintenance with epinephrine playing a backup or secondary role. The latter is particularly important in the defense against hypoglycemia in diabetes mellitus where the glucagon response is lost early (see Chap. 319). Cortisol and growth hormone function by antagonizing insulin action and act synergistically ("permissively") with other hormones to promote mobilization of substrate and activation of gluconeogenesis.

The anabolic and catabolic phases of metabolism are summarized in Table 320-1. Breakdown in any of the adaptive mechanisms can lead to hypoglycemia.

SYMPTOMATOLOGY   Symptoms of hypoglycemia fall into two main categories: those induced by an *excessive secretion of epinephrine* and those due to *dysfunction of the central nervous system*. Rapid epinephrine release causes sweating, tremor, tachycardia, anxiety, and hunger. Central nervous system symptoms include dizziness, headache, clouding of vision, blunted mental acuity, loss of fine motor skill, confusion, abnormal behavior, convulsions, and loss of consciousness. When the onset of hypoglycemia is gradual central nervous system symptoms predominate, and the epinephrine phase may not be recognizable. With more rapid drops in plasma glucose (as in insulin reactions), adrenergic symptoms are prominent. In the diabetic subject adrenergic symptoms may not be manifest if severe neuropathy is present.

The level of plasma glucose required to impair metabolism is not uniform. In nondiabetic persons acute lowering of the plasma glucose to around 2.8 mmol/L (50 mg/dL) produces autonomic nervous system symptoms and induces release of counterregulatory hormones.

TABLE 320-1   The feeding-fasting cycle

Phase	Primary hormone	Plasma substrates	Substrate flux	Active process
Anabolic*	Insulin	↑ Glucose ↑ Triglycerides ↑ Branched-chain amino acids ↓ Free fatty acids ↓ Ketones	Splanchnic bed → storage and utilization sites	Glycogen storage Protein synthesis Triglyceride formation
Catabolic†	Glucagon	↓ Glucose ↓ Triglycerides ↑ Alanine and glutamine‡ ↑ Free fatty acids ↑ Ketones	Storage sites → liver and utilization sites	Glycogenolysis Gluconeogenesis Proteolysis Lipolysis Ketogenesis

* Expected findings during the first several hours after ingestion of a mixed meal of fat, carbohydrate, and protein.
† The major catabolic phase occurs during the overnight fast, although partial catabolic cycles occur between meals.
‡ Arrows indicate plasma concentrations except for alanine and glutamine. While arterial concentrations of these amino acids are relatively constant, uptake by the liver and intestine is increased in the catabolic phase.

However, utilizing auditory evoked potentials as a sensitive indicator of central nervous system function, abnormalities can be seen in normal persons with a drop in glucose from 4.8 to 4.0 mmol/L (87 to 72 mg/dL). When blood glucose is sustained at 4.0 mmol/L (72 mg/dL) counterregulatory release eventually occurs (2 to 3 h) despite the fact that no symptoms are produced. Major symptoms of nervous system dysfunction may not occur until plasma glucose concentrations approximate 1 mmol/L (20 mg/dL). This is because normal persons have the capacity to increase cerebral blood flow sufficiently to deliver adequate glucose to the brain even with low concentrations. Cerebral atherosclerosis, with its nonelastic blood vessels, compromises this protective mechanism and allows symptomatic distress at higher glucose levels. Symptoms (adrenergic or CNS) due to hypoglycemia are unlikely with a plasma glucose above 3.0 mmol/L (60 mg/dL) in nondiabetic persons, recognizing that the physiologic sequence induced by hypoglycemia is subliminal CNS dysfunction, adrenergic symptoms, and then overt CNS dysfunction. Poorly controlled patients with diabetes mellitus appear to develop symptoms at higher glucose concentrations [4.3 mmol/L (80 mg/dL) in one report] while meticulously controlled diabetic patients have a lowering of the symptomatic threshold.

CLASSIFICATION It is traditional to classify hypoglycemia as either *postprandial* (reactive) or *fasting*. Pathologically low plasma glucose concentrations occur in the former only in response to meals, while in the latter only after fasting for a few to many hours. Patients with fasting hypoglycemia (particularly those with insulinomas) may exhibit a reactive component, but reactive patients do not have symptoms when food is withdrawn. Fasting hypoglycemia usually means that a disease process is associated with the lowered plasma glucose, but symptoms suggestive of postprandial hypoglycemia are often found in the absence of recognizable disease.

CAUSES OF HYPOGLYCEMIA   Postprandial hypoglycemia The most common cause of postprandial hypoglycemia is alimentary hyperinsulinism (Table 320-2). Patients who have undergone gastrectomy, gastrojejunostomy, pyloroplasty, or vagotomy are subject to hypoglycemia following meals, presumably because of rapid gastric emptying with brisk absorption of glucose and excessive insulin release. Glucose concentrations fall more rapidly than insulin under these circumstances, and the resulting insulin-glucose imbalance leads to hypoglycemia. Ingestion of fructose or galactose induces hypoglycemia in children with fructose intolerance and galactosemia (Chap. 337), respectively. Leucine intake can rarely cause the syndrome in

TABLE 320-2   Causes of postprandial (reactive) hypoglycemia

Alimentary hyperinsulinism
Hereditary fructose intolerance
Galactosemia
Leucine sensitivity
Idiopathic

susceptible infants. Diabetes mellitus in its early phase is usually listed as a cause of reactive hypoglycemia, but in our experience symptomatic hypoglycemia as a premonitory symptom of diabetes is uncommon. Prediabetics, who by definition are normoglycemic, may have a late fall in plasma glucose after oral glucose tolerance testing, but this does not mean hypoglycemia. In fact, this pattern is similar to that frequently present in asymptomatic, healthy individuals (see below).

Idiopathic alimentary hypoglycemia consists of two syndromes: *true hypoglycemia* and *pseudohypoglycemia*. In the former, adrenergic symptoms appear postprandially and are accompanied by a low plasma glucose at the time the symptoms appear spontaneously during everyday life. The symptoms are relieved by ingestion of carbohydrate, which raises the plasma glucose. Such patients are rare. The mechanism is unknown, although subtle (nonanatomic) dysfunction of the gastrointestinal tract might be operative. Some patients with true postprandial hypoglycemia turn out to have insulinomas (see below). *Pseudohypoglycemia* describes the condition of patients who reproducibly develop adrenergic symptoms suggestive of hypoglycemia 2 to 5 h after a meal but who do not have low plasma glucose concentrations when symptoms appear spontaneously in everyday life. The condition is often self-diagnosed with "confirmation" coming from a 5-h glucose tolerance test that reveals a lower than "normal" plasma glucose between 2 and 5 h.

Two questions have to be asked about pseudohypoglycemia. First, what are the symptoms (which may be incapacitating) due to? Second, can a valid diagnosis of hypoglycemia be made by a glucose tolerance test? The symptoms of nervousness, weakness, tremor, tachycardia, dizziness, and sweating reported by these patients are probably due to epinephrine release. Many otherwise normal persons experience similar symptoms at some time in their lives and may even have gained relief by eating. Patients with pseudohypoglycemia, on the other hand, develop the symptoms regularly and repetitively. In one study 80 consecutive subjects with reproducible postprandial symptoms by history were studied by 5-h glucose tolerance testing. Hypoglycemia was considered to be present if (1) the plasma glucose fell below 3.3 mmol/L (60 mg/dL) during the test, (2) symptoms or signs compatible with hypoglycemia were present, and (3) at least a doubling of plasma cortisol occurred 39 to 90 min after the nadir of plasma glucose (suggesting hypoglycemia sufficient to activate the hypothalamic-pituitary-adrenal axis). Only 18 of the 80 (23 percent) who by history were candidates for postprandial hypoglycemia fulfilled these criteria. Twenty-five percent of asymptomatic matched normal controls also met all three criteria. When the patients and controls were tested after a mixed meal, no subject in either group had a plasma glucose below 3.3 mmol/L (60 mg/dL), yet 14 of the 18 patients (78 percent) had symptoms typical of those occurring spontaneously and after glucose tolerance testing. The absence of hypoglycemia after mixed meals despite the presence of typical symptoms has been confirmed in other studies. *Pseudohypoglycemia* appears to be an accurate descriptive term for the syndrome and is preferable to "idiopathic postprandial syndrome" which has also been used. Many such patients are thought to have stress or anxiety as a predisposing factor. Presumably they have enhanced catecholamine release following a meal, although they might be abnormally sensitive to normal postprandial norepinephrine/epinephrine release.

Fasting hypoglycemia The causes of fasting hypoglycemia are many, but in all there is an imbalance between the production of glucose by the liver and its utilization in peripheral tissues. In some, hypoglycemia is due primarily to a defect in glucose production, while in others the problem is excess glucose utilization. Both defects may be present. For example, with insulin excess there is driven glucose utilization coupled with blunted hepatic glucose production. The latter is caused by insulin's capacity to block the glycogenolytic/gluconeogenic effects of the counterregulatory hormones. Dual defects are probably operative in disorders of fat oxidation and non-insulin-producing tumors as well.

Supply-side hypoglycemia (impaired production of glucose) characteristically requires much less glucose during therapy than does *demand-side hypoglycemia* (overutilization of glucose) (Table 320-3). As noted above, glucose production during a fast approximates 11 μmol/kg per min (2 mg/kg per min) in normal persons, but with insulin stimulation this increases to about 67 μmol/kg per min (12 mg/kg per min). Thus if more than 56 mmol (10 g) of glucose per hour is required to prevent or reverse hypoglycemia it can be assumed that overutilization is present.

UNDERPRODUCTION OF GLUCOSE As discussed earlier, the production of glucose by the liver initially involves the breakdown of stored glycogen and subsequently depends on gluconeogenesis, the synthesis of glucose from precursors delivered to the liver from peripheral tissues. The causes of inadequate production of glucose during fasting can be grouped into five categories: (1) hormone

TABLE 320-3 Major causes of fasting hypoglycemia

I Conditions primarily due to underproduction of glucose
  A Hormone deficiencies
    1 Hypopituitarism
    2 Adrenal insufficiency
    3 Catecholamine deficiency
    4 Glucagon deficiency
  B Enzyme defects
    1 Glucose-6-phosphatase
    2 Liver phosphorylase
    3 Pyruvate carboxylase
    4 Phosphoenolpyruvate carboxykinase
    5 Fructose-1,6-diphosphatase
    6 Glycogen synthetase
  C Substrate deficiency
    1 Ketotic hypoglycemia of infancy
    2 Severe malnutrition, muscle wasting
    3 Late pregnancy
  D Acquired liver disease
    1 Hepatic congestion
    2 Severe hepatitis
    3 Cirrhosis
    4 Uremia (probably multiple mechanisms)
    5 Hypothermia
  E Drugs
    1 Alcohol
    2 Propranolol
    3 Salicylates
II Conditions primarily due to overutilization of glucose
  A Hyperinsulinism
    1 Insulinoma
    2 Exogenous insulin
    3 Sulfonylureas
    4 Immune disease with insulin or insulin receptor antibodies
    5 Drugs: quinine in falciparum malaria, disopyramide, pentamidine
    6 Endotoxic shock
  B Appropriate insulin levels
    1 Extrapancreatic tumors
    2 Systemic carnitine deficiency
    3 Deficiency in enzymes of fat oxidation
    4 3-Hydroxy-3-methylglutaryl-CoA lyase deficiency
    5 Cachexia with fat depletion

deficiencies, (2) defects in glycogenolytic or gluconeogenic enzymes, (3) inadequate substrate delivery, (4) liver disease, and (5) drugs. Hypopituitarism and adrenal insufficiency are the most common of the hormone deficiency states causing hypoglycemia. Defects in catecholamine or glucagon release are rare. Enzymic abnormalities causing hypoglycemia are generally seen in children and not adults. Glucose-6-phosphatase deficiency is the classic example of a defect in glycogen breakdown, but hypoglycemia may occur in young children with deficiencies of hepatic glycogen phosphorylase and in other forms of glycogen storage disease (Chap. 332). The inability to make glycogen because of inadequate glycogen synthetase activity also renders the infant susceptible to fasting hypoglycemia. In addition to glucose-6-phosphatase, three other enzymes are necessary for gluconeogenesis: pyruvate carboxylase, phosphoenolpyruvate carboxykinase, and fructose-1,6-bisphosphatase (fructose-1,6-diphosphatase) (Fig. 320-1). Hypoglycemia can occur with decreased activities of any of these enzymes, often in association with lactic acidosis. The cause of lactic acidosis in these disorders is not known, although impaired hepatic lactate uptake due to the gluconeogenic defect probably plays a role. Substrate deficiency appears to be one of the mechanisms operative in ketotic hypoglycemia of infancy, since alanine turnover in such patients is low. Inadequate substrate supply may also contribute to hypoglycemia in malnutrition, muscle-wasting states, chronic renal failure, and late pregnancy. Acquired liver disease can cause serious hypoglycemia. Hepatic congestion due to right-sided heart failure is particularly troublesome, but severe viral hepatitis or cirrhosis may also cause symptomatic hypoglycemia. Hypothermia, especially in association with alcohol, may cause very low levels of plasma glucose. Slowed enzymatic activity of the liver is the likely mechanism. The hypoglycemia of renal failure probably has multiple causes. In addition to impairing substrate delivery, uremic toxins may suppress hepatic gluconeogenesis. Decreased renal clearance of insulin and impairment of renal gluconeogenesis may contribute to the problem.

A number of drugs cause hypoglycemia. The most common, apart from insulin and sulfonylureas, is alcohol. Alcohol induces hypoglycemia only after a period of fasting sufficient to deplete liver glycogen stores. In this circumstance hepatic glucose production is dependent on gluconeogenesis. The oxidation of ethanol in the liver is accompanied by generation of high concentrations of NADH, the reduced form of nicotinamide adenine dinucleotide (NAD), in the cytosol of the cell. The increased NADH/NAD ratio diverts oxaloacetate into malate formation, diminishing its availability to the gluconeogenic sequence via the action of phosphoenolpyruvate carboxykinase (Fig. 320-1). The normal pathway of gluconeogenesis from pyruvate is thus blocked, leading to a drop in hepatic glucose output and hypoglycemia. Large amounts of ethanol are not required to produce this syndrome, and plasma alcohol concentrations may be as low as 5.4 mmol/L (25 mg/dL) at the time symptoms occur. Ethanol-induced hypoglycemia usually occurs in adults but can be seen in children who drink alcohol unknowingly. Salicylates (in children) and propranolol are the next most frequently involved drugs. Propranolol presumably causes difficulty in fasting patients or insulin-requiring diabetics by impairing the glycogenolytic response. In diabetes the drug may also prevent recognition of impending hypoglycemia by blunting the symptomatic response to epinephrine release. Other drugs have been reported to cause hypoglycemia in isolated cases, but the relationship is often unproved. Some drugs enhance glucose utilization. Pentamidine and disopyramide cause hyperinsulinism, the former by beta cell cytolysis ("insulin leak") and the latter by an unknown mechanism, perhaps as a direct insulin secretagogue. Quinine given in falciparum malaria has been reported to cause hyperinsulinemic hypoglycemia, but the issue is clouded because hypoglycemia occurs in untreated malaria as well, possibly secondary to malnutrition or liver involvement.

OVERUTILIZATION OF GLUCOSE Overutilization of glucose occurs in two settings. In the first, hyperinsulinism is present, and in the second, plasma insulin concentrations are low. There are basically

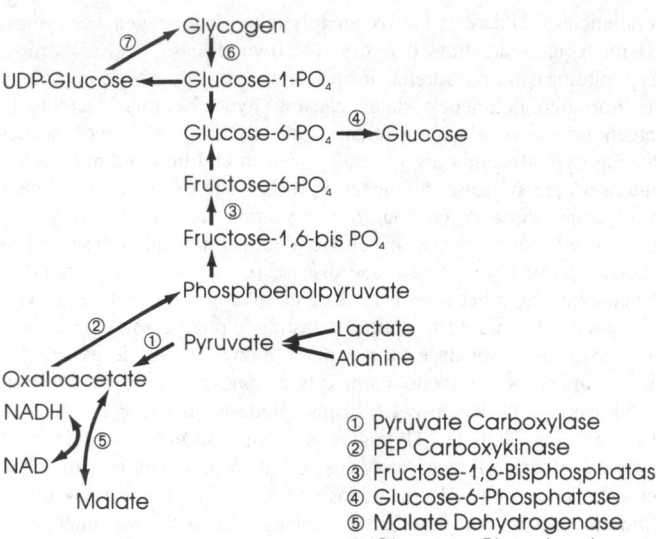

FIGURE 320-1 Scheme of hepatic carbohydrate metabolism. Only the sequence for gluconeogenesis, glycogen synthesis, and glycogenolysis is shown.

① Pyruvate Carboxylase
② PEP Carboxykinase
③ Fructose-1,6-Bisphosphatase
④ Glucose-6-Phosphatase
⑤ Malate Dehydrogenase
⑥ Glycogen Phosphorylase
⑦ Glycogen Synthetase

four causes of hyperinsulinemic hypoglycemia: insulinoma, exogenous insulin administration, sulfonylureas, and a peculiar form of insulin autoimmunity. Insulinoma is used generically here to include single solid tumors, microadenomatosis, and islet cell hyperplasia (nesidioblastosis), a rare syndrome in adults. Hypoglycemia in a diabetic taking prescribed insulin or oral agents is not a diagnostic problem. The difficulty comes when a nondiabetic subject induces hypoglycemia deliberately and surreptitiously because of psychiatric disturbance, raising the possibility of an insulin-producing tumor. The differential diagnosis between insulinoma and factitious hypoglycemia is considered below. Rarely hypoglycemia with hyperinsulinism occurs in autoimmune disease associated with antibodies to endogenous insulin. Mechanisms are not well understood, although dissociation of free insulin from hormone-antibody complexes at inappropriate times is probably most important. Idiotypic antibodies (antibodies against the anti-insulin antibodies) might also develop, functioning as insulin agonists with the insulin receptor. By binding insulin the antibodies may also induce excessive insulin release from the pancreas. Some patients have alternating insulin resistance/hyperglycemia and hypoglycemia. Insulin autoantibodies have been seen most frequently in subjects with hyperthyroidism treated with methimazole (thiamazole) but presumably they might arise in any autoimmune syndrome. Antibodies directed against the insulin receptor, usually a cause of insulin resistance, may also induce hypoglycemia with high plasma insulin levels. Under these circumstances conformational configuration of the antibody is thought to allow it to activate the insulin receptor, simultaneously blocking access of native insulin and impairing its clearance.

Sepsis with endotoxinemia causes hyperglycemia followed by hypoglycemia in experimental animals. Plasma insulin levels increase. Since hypoglycemia accompanying gram-negative sepsis has not been well studied in humans, its inclusion as a hyperinsulinemic state is tentative.

Hypoglycemia in the context of glucose overutilization and appropriately low plasma insulin concentrations occurs in two situations. The first is in association with solid extrapancreatic tumors, usually of large size. The most common are of mesothelial origin and include fibromas and sarcomas. The syndrome can also be seen with hepatomas, carcinomas of the gastrointestinal tract, and adrenal cancers. The mechanism of the hypoglycemia is not clear, although high levels of insulin-like growth factors may play a role. Indeed, in some studies insulin-like growth factors are present in essentially all

such tumors. Presumably such factors, if present, act via the insulin receptor rather than by binding to their own receptors. One patient with tumor-associated hypoglycemia was reported to have an increased number of insulin receptors in liver, muscle, and circulating mononuclear cells, but the significance of the finding is not clear.

Symptomatic hypoglycemia due to overutilization may also occur in situations where free fatty acids and ketones are not available for oxidation in muscle and other tissues. Patients with *systemic carnitine deficiency* may have severe hypoglycemia. In this condition carnitine, which is necessary to transport fatty acids into mitochondria for oxidation, is low in plasma, muscle, liver, and other tissues. As a consequence, peripheral tissues cannot utilize fatty acids for energy production, and the liver cannot make ketone bodies as alternative substrate. The result is that all tissues become glucose-dependent, exceeding the capacity of the liver to meet the demand. Other features of systemic carnitine deficiency include nausea, vomiting, elevated blood ammonia levels, and hepatic encephalopathy. The illness thus constitutes one form of the Reye's syndrome. (In *myopathic carnitine deficiency* only muscle is involved, and a polymyositis-like syndrome without hypoglycemia is produced.) Nonketotic (or hypoketotic) hypoglycemia with secondary systemic carnitine deficiency and the Reye syndrome also accompany *deficiencies of medium- and long-chain acyl-CoA dehydrogenases and 3-hydroxy-3-methylglutaryl-CoA lyase (HMG-CoA lyase)*. The first two enzymes operate in the fatty acid oxidative sequence while HMG-CoA lyase catalyzes the conversion HMG-CoA to acetoacetate and acetyl-CoA in the ketogenic cycle. Any time there is a block in fatty acid oxidation or ketone formation a secondary carnitine deficiency may develop. Accumulated acyl-CoA is transesterified to form acyl carnitine, which is then lost in the urine. Systemic carnitine deficiency in the absence of enzymic defect probably is due to a primary renal leak. It is not known whether the block in ketone production per se leads to hypoglycemia or whether secondary carnitine deficiency is required. If the former, ketones must become a primary (necessary) substrate during an extended fast. Hypoglycemia is less common with deficiency of *carnitine palmitoyltransferase*, the enzyme that transesterifies fatty acyl coenzyme A (CoA) to carnitine for oxidation. Presumably the defect is not complete in most patients, allowing some fatty acid oxidation to occur so that the tendency to hypoglycemia is minimized. The clinical picture is that of an exercise-induced myopathy with myoglobinuria. Hypoglycemia also occurs in patients with cachexia due to advanced cancer. At autopsy no recognizable triglyceride stores are present in adipose tissue, suggesting free fatty acid deficiency as the primary mechanism.

Causes of hypoglycemia in hospitalized patients Frequencies of diagnoses vary in unselected series. Drugs constitute the most common cause, the three most common agents being insulin, sulfonylureas, and alcohol. It has been estimated that 60 percent of the time one of these three agents is involved when hypoglycemia is diagnosed. Renal failure was present in nearly 30 percent of hypoglycemic episodes in hospitalized patients in one series but overall makes up about 15 percent of cases. Liver disease (about 15 percent), malnutrition (about 10 percent), and sepsis (about 5 percent) are the other common causes. A high index of suspicion for insulinoma, solid tumors, enzymatic defects, or hormonal deficiencies should be engendered by the finding of hypoglycemia in nondiabetic persons without uremia, liver disease, cachexia, or history of alcohol intake.

DIAGNOSIS Fasting hypoglycemia If a person with diabetes mellitus presents with symptoms of hypoglycemia, it is usually safe to conclude that no special diagnostic tests are needed since the hypoglycemia is almost always related to therapy. If a nondiabetic appears with similar symptoms—particularly if confusion, loss of consciousness, or convulsions are present—it is critical to draw blood for assay before intravenous glucose is administered. *The best time to obtain diagnostic laboratory tests with spontaneous hypoglycemia is at presentation.* The goal is to assess plasma insulin level and counterregulatory hormone response while the plasma glucose is low.

Assays should be carried out for glucose, insulin, insulin connecting peptide (C peptide), cortisol, drugs, and toxins, especially sulfonylureas and alcohol. It is often wise to freeze a separate sample of plasma for subsequent tests (e.g., proinsulin, carnitine, insulin antibodies, lactate) should the diagnosis not be clear from initial evaluation. Demonstration that hypoglycemia is accompanied by inappropriate insulin levels sharply narrows the clinical possibilities. Routine laboratory exams may also be helpful. For example, the absence of ketones or the presence of a metabolic acidosis may be clues to the primary problem.

Once the patient has become alert (assuming altered mental status is present on arrival), it is important to take a detailed history and carry out a physical examination. Special emphasis should be placed on food intake in the preceding 24 h and the possibility of drug ingestion. Signs of heart failure and hepatic congestion should be sought, and the presence and thickness of the adipose tissue mass should be noted. Pigmentation of the skin may suggest Addison's disease. Workup includes liver function studies and computed tomography (CT) scanning or abdominal sonography (to look for solid tumors in the retroperitoneal space or abdominal cavity). Patients with enzyme defects and rare hormonal deficiencies (epinephrine, glucagon) usually require evaluation in referral centers, since definitive assays for these hormones and enzymes are not routinely available. For reasons cited above it is important to quantitate the amount of glucose required to prevent recurrent hypoglycemia during acute phase therapy; i.e., if 8 to 10 g of glucose per hour is sufficient to prevent hypoglycemia, diminished glucose production is probably operative. A requirement for higher infusion rates suggests enhanced glucose utilization.

If the patient has a history compatible with hypoglycemia but does not have symptoms at the time of examination, hospitalization for fasting is generally required. The fast should be carried out for at least 72 h unless symptoms develop. Plasma glucose, insulin, C peptide, and cortisol should be measured every 6 h. Occasionally quantitation of plasma free fatty acids, glucagon, and total ketones is helpful. (For glucagon, a protease inhibitor such as aprotinin must be added.) Two points are at issue. First, does the patient have fasting hypoglycemia? Second, is the hypoglycemia associated with hyperinsulinism? Neither question is easy to answer. There is no definitive lower limit of plasma glucose that unequivocally defines pathologic hypoglycemia during a 72-h fast. Values of the nadir in one study are shown in Table 320-4. Women usually develop lower levels than men. Another series reported mean minimal levels of 3.4 mmol/L (62 mg/dL) in men and 2.9 mmol/L (52 mg/dL) in women during a 72-h fast. However, values as low as 1.2 mmol/L (22 mg/dL) may occur in normal women without symptoms. On balance, a presumptive diagnosis of hypoglycemia is probably justified if the plasma glucose falls below 2.8 mmol/L (50 mg/dL) in men and 2.5 mmol/L (45 mg/dL) in women at any time during the fast, provided typical symptoms are induced. The diagnosis of hypoglycemia is strengthened if symptoms are rapidly relieved by administration of carbohydrate. If symptoms are not produced, the diagnosis of hypoglycemia should be made with caution.

Absolute insulin values are not always helpful in diagnosing hyperinsulinism. In normal subjects when glucose concentrations rise insulin levels also increase, and when plasma glucose concentrations fall insulin release is inhibited. This means that plasma insulin concentrations must be interpreted in the light of the simultaneously determined glucose value. Thus, a "normal" absolute insulin level may be abnormal in the face of hypoglycemia, while high absolute levels may be appropriate if the glucose concentration is elevated. In an attempt to relate the two parameters the concept of the insulin/glucose ratio

$$\frac{\text{Plasma insulin } (\mu U/mL)}{\text{Plasma glucose } (mg/dL)}$$

was developed utilizing conventional laboratory units. In normal persons the ratio is always less than 0.4, while most (but not all) patients with insulinoma have ratios greater than 0.4—often above 1.0. When the ratio is calculated in SI units [plasma insulin (pmol/L)/plasma glucose (mmol/L)] the normal value is less than 50. Patients with insulinoma may secrete insulin episodically; the ratio may, therefore, be normal on one occasion and abnormal on another. The insulin/glucose ratio tends to fall during fasting in normal individuals but increases in patients with insulinoma.

Plasma insulin concentration generally reaches background levels for the assay when the plasma glucose falls below about 4.4 mmol/L (80 mg/dL). While some studies have shown lower cutoff points, it is probable that any measurable insulin concentration should be considered suspicious if the plasma glucose is below 2.8 mmol/L (50 mg/dL) in men or 2.5 mmol/L (45 mg/dL) in women, regardless of the value of the insulin/glucose ratio. If hyperinsulinism is not demonstrated, one of the other causes of fasting hypoglycemia must be sought.

Should hypoglycemia not develop during fasting, insulinoma or other hypoglycemia-producing organic disease is unlikely, although insulinomas may rarely present solely as postprandial hypoglycemia with no depression of the plasma glucose even during a prolonged fast. Diagnosis usually is suspected in such cases because inappropriate insulin levels are shown during the postmeal episodes. Some authors recommend provocative tests with calcium, tolbutamide, glucagon, or leucine in suspected islet cell tumors, but overlap between normal subjects and patients with insulinoma is so great as to render the tests of little value in a given individual.

Postprandial hypoglycemia In patients presumed to have postprandial hypoglycemia the most widely used test has been a 5-h oral glucose tolerance examination. Since normal persons may have chemical hypoglycemia without symptoms in the glucose tolerance test while subjects with pseudohypoglycemia have symptoms in the absence of hypoglycemia following meal testing, the 5-h glucose tolerance test should be abandoned as a tool for diagnosis. The only unequivocal diagnostic test for true pseudohypoglycemia is the demonstration of a low plasma glucose concentration (less than 2.8 mmol/L or 50 mg/dL) during spontaneously developed symptoms. Some physicians utilize a home glucose analyzer in diagnosis. If no hypoglycemia is demonstrated during one week of testing (on arising,

TABLE 320-4 Mean plasma glucose and insulin during fasting

| Assay | Subjects | Hours of fast | | | | |
		0*	24	36	48	72
Glucose mmol/L (mg/dL)	Men	4.7 (85)	4.6 (83)	4.3 (78)	4.3 (78)	3.9 (71)
	Women	4.6 (83)	3.5 (63)	2.8 (50)	2.6 (46)	2.7 (48)
Insulin pmol/L (µU/mL)	Men	100 (14)	64 (9)	57 (8)	57 (8)	43 (6)
	Women	86 (12)	43 (6)	29 (4)	21 (3)	29 (4)

* Zero values were obtained after overnight fast. Results are mean values for 20 normal men and 60 normal women.
SOURCE: TJ Merimee, JE Tyson, Diabetes 26:161, 1977.

TABLE 320-5   Differential diagnosis of insulinoma and factitious hyperinsulinism

Test	Insulinoma	Exogenous insulin	Sulfonylurea
Plasma insulin	High	Very high*	High
Insulin/glucose ratio	High	Very high	High
Proinsulin	Increased	Normal or low	Normal
C peptide	Increased	Normal or low†	Increased
Insulin antibodies	Absent	± Present‡	Absent
Plasma or urine sulfonylurea	Absent	Absent	Present

* Total plasma insulin in patients with insulinoma is rarely above 1435 pmol/L (200 μU/mL) in the basal state and often much lower. Values greater than 7175 pmol/L (1000 μU/mL) are highly suggestive of exogenous insulin injection.

† C peptide may be normal in absolute terms, but low in relation to the increased insulin value. See text for C-peptide suppression test.

‡ Insulin antibodies may not be present if only a few injections have been given, especially with purified insulins.

2 h after each meal, at bedtime, and during symptoms) the diagnosis of true postprandial hypoglycemia is rejected. Patients with pseudohypoglycemia usually have slightly elevated glucose concentrations during spontaneous attacks because of the hyperglycemic action of epinephrine, the stress hormone that induces the symptoms.

Insulinoma versus factitious hypoglycemia   The self-induction of hypoglycemia by the injection of insulin or the ingestion of sulfonylureas is so common as to equal or exceed the incidence of insulinoma. The demonstration of hyperinsulinism during hypoglycemia cannot, therefore, be taken as definitive evidence of the presence of an islet cell tumor. Factitious disease should always be suspected when hypoglycemic symptoms appear in medical personnel or families of diabetic patients. Several tests are helpful in distinguishing insulinoma from factitious disease once hyperinsulinism has been established. Patients with insulinoma tend to have high concentrations of proinsulin in plasma (>20 percent of total insulin). Plasma proinsulin is not elevated by the administration of commercial insulin preparations or sulfonylureas. Measurement of the insulin connecting peptide (C peptide) will indicate whether the insulin circulating in plasma is of endogenous or exogenous origin. When insulin is cleaved from its precursor proinsulin molecule, C peptide is released into the portal vein in a 1:1 ratio with insulin. Thus, patients with insulinoma should have C-peptide concentrations that parallel the plasma insulin values. The characteristic pattern in factitious hypoglycemia due to

insulin injection is a high circulating level of insulin with relatively suppressed C-peptide values because exogenous insulin suppresses endogenous insulin release in normal persons. Suppression does not usually occur in insulinoma. Some investigators recommend a C-peptide suppression test in equivocal situations. In this test 0.1 unit of insulin per kilogram of body weight is infused intravenously over 60 min. C-peptide concentration should be less than 1.2 ng/mL at the end of the test, provided the plasma glucose has dropped to 2.2 mmol/L (40 mg/dL) or less. Antibodies to insulin are helpful if present since they usually indicate chronic insulin injection. However, as noted earlier, autoantibodies directed against insulin may develop in hyperthyroidism and other autoimmune diseases. Anti-insulin antibodies cannot be taken as evidence of insulin injection under these circumstances. Sulfonylureas elevate both the C-peptide and insulin concentrations in plasma. Therefore, factitious hypoglycemia due to oral agents can only be diagnosed by a high index of suspicion coupled with assay of the drug in plasma or urine. The differential characteristics of insulinoma and the two types of factitious hypoglycemia are shown in Table 320-5.

TREATMENT   The initial treatment of serious hypoglycemia (producing confusion or coma) is the intravenous administration of a bolus of 25 or 50 g glucose as a 50% solution followed by constant infusion of glucose until the patient is able to eat a meal. The importance of the meal resides in the fact that hepatic glycogen repletion is not effective with small quantities of intravenous glucose. Patients in the overutilization category may require large amounts of intravenous glucose to maintain consciousness. It is not enough to infuse 5% dextrose at a rate of 1 to 2 mL/min and assume the patient is protected (20 to 30% dextrose solutions may be required in some cases). Frequent measurement of capillary glucose concentrations should be carried out using glucose-sensitive reagent strips to assess effectiveness of glucose infusion rates. Intravenous glucose can usually be stopped once the patient has eaten, but this can only be determined by trial. Adrenergic reactions without central nervous system abnormalities can be treated with oral carbohydrate and do not require parenteral therapy.

Hypoglycemia from sulfonylureas may last for prolonged periods (days) (Fig. 320-2). It is common for patients to lapse back into coma if glucose infusions are stopped too soon. The reason for the prolonged effect is not always clear, though drug interactions, hepatic disease, and renal failure may play a role in some cases.

Surgery is the treatment of choice for insulinoma. Localization

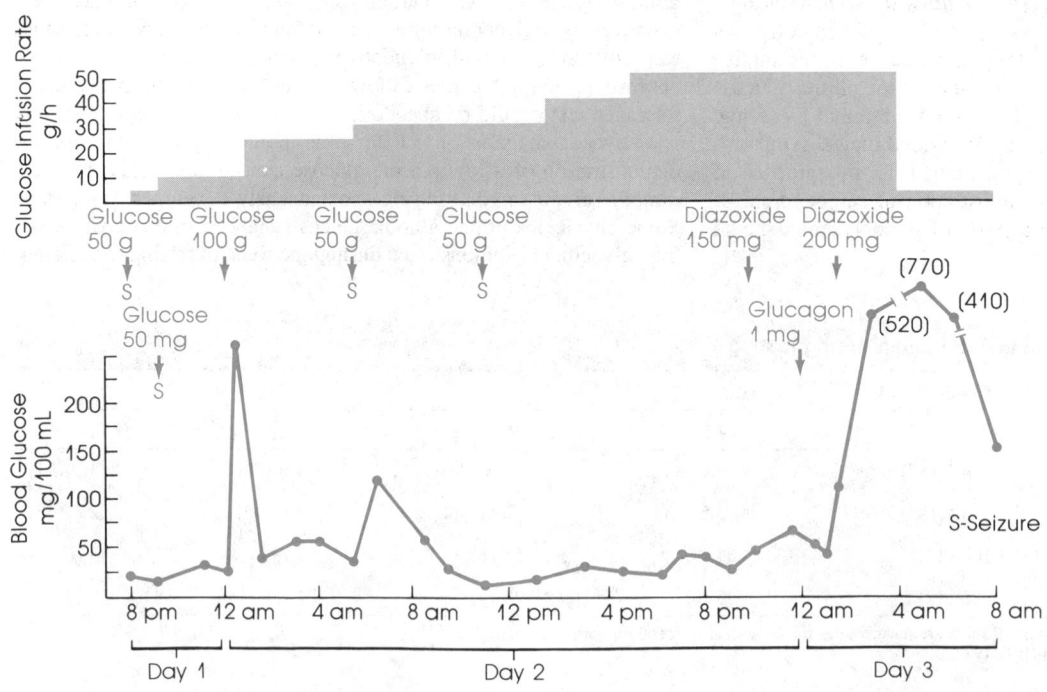

FIGURE 320-2 Prolonged and refractory hypoglycemia in factitious hypoglycemia due to chlorpropamide in an alcoholic. Note continued hypoglycemia despite the infusion of glucose at rates up to 50 g/h. *(From RM Jordan et al, Arch Intern Med 137:390, 1977. Copyright 1977, American Medical Association. Used by permission.)*

should be attempted with CT scan or sonography prior to exploration. Arteriography (celiac or superior mesenteric) is less effective. In some centers preoperative or operative sampling of insulin concentrations by selective pancreatic vein catheterization has been performed but appears to be of minimal benefit even if a rapid insulin assay is available. If the tumor cannot be palpated in the pancreas or located in an extrapancreatic site at the time of surgery, stepwise pancreatectomy (from tail to head) should be carried out with frozen sections made of sequential slices. Capillary glucose should be measured frequently (at each stage of the resection if the tumor is not obvious). A rise in plasma glucose may indicate removal of a small, nonpalpable lesion. In general, resection is stopped with an 85 percent pancreatectomy, even if the tumor is not found, to avoid malabsorptive complications. While a majority of patients are cured by surgery, as many as 15 percent have persistent hypoglycemia. Postoperative complications included acute pancreatitis, peritonitis, fistulas, pseudocyst formation, and chronic hyperglycemia (acquired diabetes).

Medical treatment is indicated in insulinoma only in preparation for surgery or after failure to find the tumor at operation. Two drugs are available, diazoxide and octreotide, a long-acting octapeptide analogue of somatostatin. Diazoxide can be given intravenously or orally in doses of 300 to 1200 mg/d and because of its salt-retaining properties must be accompanied by a diuretic. Octreotide is given subcutaneously in divided doses of 150 to 450 μg/d and may cause nausea and diarrhea and predispose to cholelithiasis. Treatment of metastatic insulin-producing carcinomas is unsatisfactory. Streptozocin, plicamycin, and doxorubicin have been tried in these malignancies, but the results are dismal. One multicenter trial reported improved results when streptozocin was combined with fluorouracil. Despite the generally poor prognosis, occasional patients with insulin-producing islet cell carcinomas survive for long periods.

Therapy of other forms of recurrent hypoglycemia, apart from hormone replacement in pituitary or adrenal insufficiency, is dietary. In most cases avoidance of fasting is all that is required. This is critical in diseases of fat oxidation or ketone synthesis. If intercurrent illness prevents eating, hospitalization for intravenous glucose is absolutely required. A high-protein, low-carbohydrate diet is frequently prescribed for patients with pseudohypoglycemia and often relieves symptoms. With true alimentary hypoglycemia it is probably important to keep the size of the individual meals small. The practice of giving massive amounts of vitamin E, crude adrenocortical extract, and trace metals to patients with pseudohypoglycemia is useless even if harmless (which has not been proved).

REFERENCES

AVRAM MM et al: Uremic hypoglycemia. A preventable life-threatening complication. NY State J Med 84:593, 1984

BERNSTEIN RK: Meaningful screening test for reactive hypoglycemia. Diabetes Care 10:792, 1987

BOYLE PJ et al: Plasma glucose concentrations at the onset of hypoglycemic symptoms in patients with poorly controlled diabetes and in nondiabetics. N Engl J Med 318:1487, 1988

CHARLES MA et al: Comparison of oral glucose tolerance tests and mixed meals in patients with apparent idiopathic postabsorptive hypoglycemia. Absence of hypoglycemia after meals. Diabetes 30:465, 1981

CLUTTER WE et al: Regulation of glucose metabolism by sympathochromaffin catecholamines. Diabetes/Metabolism Rev 4:1, 1988

COHEN RM et al: Proinsulin radioimmunoassay in the evaluation of insulinomas and familial hyperproinsulinemia. Metabolism 35:1137, 1986

DE FEO P et al: Modest decrements in plasma glucose concentration cause early impairment in cognitive function and later activation of glucose counterregulation in the absence of hypoglycemic symptoms in normal man. J Clin Invest 82:436, 1988

FERNER RE, NEIL HAW: Sulphonylureas and hypoglycaemia. Br Med J 296:949, 1988

FISCHER KF et al: Hypoglycemia in hospitalized patients. Causes and outcomes. N Engl J Med 315:1245, 1986

FOSTER DW, MCGARRY JD: Glucose, lipid and protein metabolism, in *Textbook of Endocrine Physiology*, JE Griffin, SR Ojeda (eds). New York, Oxford, 1988, pp 302–326

GERICH JE, CAMPBELL PJ: Overview of counterregulation and its abnormalities in diabetes mellitus and other conditions. Diabetes/Metabolism Rev 4:93, 1988

GIBSON KM et al: 3-Hydroxy-3-methylglutaryl-coenzyme A lyase deficiency: Report of five new patients. J Inher Metab Dis 11:76, 1988

GRUNBERGER G et al: Factitious hypoglycemia due to surreptitious administration of insulin. Diagnosis, treatment, and long-term follow-up. Ann Intern Med 108:252, 1988

HALE DE et al: Long-chain acyl coenzyme A dehydrogenase deficiency: An inherited cause of nonketotic hypoglycemia. Pediatr Res 19:666, 1985

MALOUF R, BRUST JCM: Hypoglycemia: Causes, neurological manifestations, and outcome. Ann Neurol 17:421, 1985

MERIMEE TJ: Insulin-like growth factors in patients with nonislet cell tumors and hypoglycemia. Metabolism 35:360, 1986

NAYLOR JM, KRONFELD DS: In vivo studies of hypoglycemia and lactic acidosis in endotoxic shock. Am J Physiol 248:E309, 1985

SERVICE FJ et al: Insulinoma. Clinical and diagnostic features of 60 consecutive cases. Mayo Clin Proc 51:417, 1976

TAYLOR TE et al: Blood glucose levels in Malawian children before and during the administration of intravenous quinine for severe falciparum malaria. N Engl J Med 319:1040, 1988

WASKIN H et al: Risk factors for hypoglycemia associated with pentamidine therapy for *Pneumocystis* pneumonia. JAMA 260:345, 1988

WEINSTOCK G et al: Islet cell hyperplasia: An unusual cause of hypoglycemia in an adult. Metabolism 35:110, 1986

321 DISORDERS OF THE TESTIS

JAMES E. GRIFFIN / JEAN D. WILSON

The testis produces sperm and the steroid hormones that regulate male sexual life. Both functions are under complex feedback control by the hypothalamic-pituitary system so that the testis has biosynthetic and regulatory features similar to those of the ovary and the adrenal. Testicular hormones are also responsible for the formation of the basic male phenotype during embryogenesis. The function of the embryonic testis and the disorders of sexual differentiation are described in Chap. 324.

PHYSIOLOGY AND REGULATION OF TESTICULAR FUNCTION

The testis consists of two components—a system of spermatogenic tubules for the production and transport of sperm and clusters of interstitial or Leydig cells that produce androgenic steroids.

THE LEYDIG CELL   Testosterone synthesis   The biochemical pathway by which the 27-carbon sterol cholesterol is converted to androgens and estrogens is depicted in Fig. 321-1. Cholesterol can either be synthesized de novo in the Leydig cell or derived from plasma lipoproteins. Five enzymatic transformations are required for the conversion of cholesterol to testosterone. In this process the side chain of cholesterol is cleaved in two steps to reduce the size from 27 to 19 carbons, and the A ring of the steroid is converted to the Δ^4-3-keto configuration. The five transformations are the 20,22-desmolase, the 3β-hydroxysteroid dehydrogenase-$\Delta^{4,5}$-isomerase-complex, 17α-hydroxylase, 17,20-desmolase, and 17β-hydroxysteroid dehydrogenase reactions. The first four reactions also take place in the adrenal.

The rate-limiting process in testosterone synthesis is the conversion of cholesterol to pregnenolone by the 20,22-desmolase reaction; luteinizing hormone (LH) from the pituitary regulates the activity of this enzyme and of other enzymes in the pathway. Other steroids including estradiol are synthesized in small amounts in the Leydig cell.

Testosterone secretion and transport   Only about 70 nmol (20 μg) of testosterone is stored in the normal testes, so that the total hormone content turns over about 200 times each day to provide the average of 17 to 20 μmol (5 to 6 mg) that is secreted into plasma in normal young men (Fig. 321-2). Testosterone is transported in plasma bound to protein, largely to albumin and to a specific transport protein, testosterone-binding globulin (TeBG, also called sex hormone–binding globulin, SHBG). The bound and unbound fractions

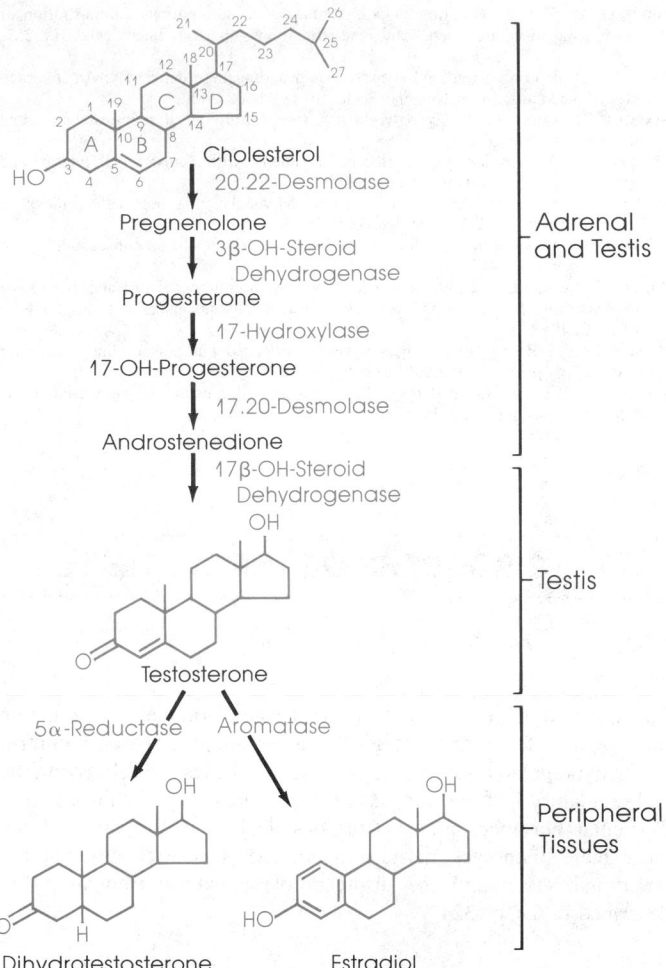

FIGURE 321-1 Pathways of androgen formation in the testis and the conversion of androgens to other active hormones in peripheral tissues.

from circulating testosterone, 50 percent is derived from the weak estrogen estrone, and 15 percent is secreted directly into the circulation by the testes. When gonadotropin levels are elevated, the amount of estradiol secretion by the testis is increased.

The 5α-reduced and estrogenic metabolites can exert local (paracrine) actions in the tissues in which they are formed or enter the circulation and act as hormones at other sites. Circulating dihydrotestosterone is formed principally in the androgen target tissues, and estrogen formation takes place in many tissues, the most significant being adipose tissue. The overall rate of extraglandular estrogen formation increases with increasing amounts of adipose tissue and with age.

Plasma testosterone and its active metabolites are converted to inactive metabolites in the liver and excreted predominantly in the urine; approximately half of the daily turnover is excreted in the form of urinary 17-ketosteroids (primarily androsterone and etiocholanolone), and the remainder is excreted as a series of polar compounds (diols, triols, and conjugates).

Gonadotropin regulation and testosterone secretion Testosterone secretion is regulated by pituitary LH (Fig. 321-3). (For the details of pituitary function, see Chap. 313.) Follicle-stimulating hormone (FSH) may also augment testosterone secretion, possibly by inducing maturation of the Leydig cell. Testosterone also regulates the sensitivity of the pituitary to the hypothalamic-releasing factor luteinizing hormone–releasing hormone (LHRH, also called gonadotropin-releasing hormone, GnRH). Although the pituitary can convert testosterone to dihydrotestosterone and to estrogens, testosterone itself is the primary regulator of gonadotropin secretion. Testosterone also acts in the central nervous system to slow the rate of LHRH formation or secretion and consequently to decrease the frequency of pulsatile LH release. Under ordinary circumstances, LH secretion is exquisitely sensitive to the feedback effects of testosterone, with complete suppression following the administration of amounts of exogenous androgen that approximate the normal daily secretory rate of testosterone (about 20 μmol or 6 mg). However, prolonged elevation of plasma LH (as in testicular deficiency) renders the pituitary less sensitive to negative feedback control by exogenous androgen.

Neither the plasma concentration of testosterone nor that of LH is constant, each showing fluctuations of a pulsatile nature that reflect changes in secretory rates (Fig. 321-4). Major sleep-related surges in the pulsatile secretion of both LH and testosterone signal the initiation of male puberty. In the adult the diurnal variation in the magnitude of this episodic secretion of LH and testosterone is minor

in plasma are in dynamic equilibrium, only about 1 to 3 percent being present in the free fraction. The fraction of circulating testosterone available for entry into tissues approximates the sum of the free and albumin-bound fractions or about 40 to 50 percent of the total plasma testosterone.

Peripheral metabolism of androgens Testosterone serves as a circulating precursor (or prohormone) for the formation of two other types of active metabolites that mediate many of the physiologic processes involved in androgen action (Fig. 321-1). Testosterone can be 5α-reduced to dihydrotestosterone, which performs many of the differentiative, growth-promoting, and functional actions involved in male sexual differentiation and virilization. Circulating androgens in both sexes can also be converted to estrogens in extraglandular tissues. In men estrogens act in some instances in concert with androgens but can also have effects independent of or opposite to those of androgens. Thus, the physiologic effects of testosterone are the result of the combined effects of testosterone itself plus those of the active androgen and estrogen metabolites of the parent molecule. (In normal men small amounts of estradiol and dihydrotestosterone are also derived by direct secretion from the testis and indirectly from the weak adrenal androgen androstenedione.)

The quantitative relation between circulating androgens and the formation of estrogen in normal young men is illustrated diagrammatically in Fig. 321-2. The production rates of testosterone and androstenedione average about 20 and 10 μmol (6 and 3 mg), respectively, per day. All of estrone production [averaging about 240 nmol (66 μg) per day] can be accounted for by formation from circulating precursors. The mean estradiol production rate is about 170 nmol (45 μg) per day; about 35 percent of this amount is derived

FIGURE 321-2 Androgen and estrogen production in normal young men. Average production of androstenedione and testosterone are shown in the top boxes, and mean daily production of estrone and estradiol is shown in the lower boxes. Estrogen is formed by extraglandular aromatization (braces) or by direct secretion from the testes. Vertical arrows indicate the rates of extraglandular aromatization of androgens, and the horizontal arrows indicate the interconversion of androgen and estrogens by 17β-hydroxysteroid dehydrogenase. Thus estradiol arises from plasma testosterone, from estrone, and from direct secretion by the testes. *(Adapted from PC MacDonald et al.)*

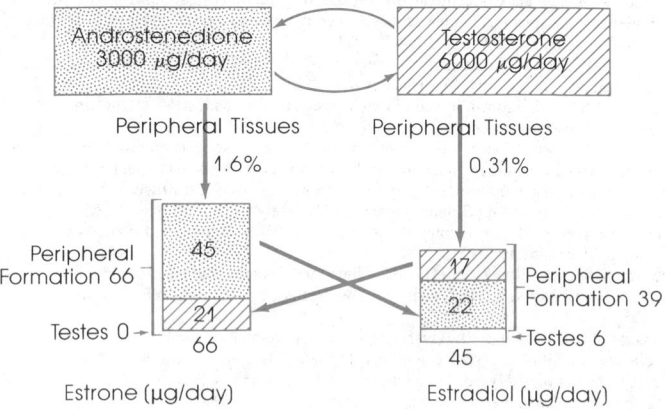

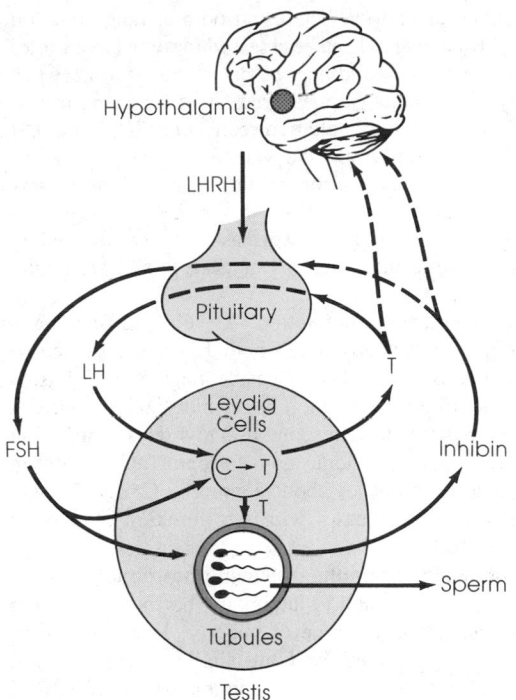

FIGURE 321-3   Regulation of testosterone and sperm production by LH and FSH. (C, cholesterol; T, testosterone.)

with peak morning levels only about 10 to 15 percent higher than during the rest of the day.

Androgen action   The major functions of androgen are the regulation of gonadotropin secretion, the formation of the male phenotype during sexual differentiation, and the induction of sexual maturation and function following puberty. The cellular mechanisms by which androgens perform these functions are summarized schematically in Fig. 321-5. Testosterone (T) enters the cell by passive diffusion. Inside the cell T can be converted to dihydrotestosterone (D) by the 5α-reductase enzyme. T or D is then bound to the androgen-receptor protein in the cytosol (R). The hormone-receptor complex (TR or DR) is transformed to the DNA-binding state (TR* or DR*) and translocated to the nucleus, where it attaches to specific chromosomal sites; as a result, new messenger RNA is transcribed, and new protein appears within the cytoplasm of the cell. The androgen receptor protein is coded by a gene on the long arm of the X chromosome; it contains 917 amino acids and has a molecular mass of about 100 kDa. It is similar in structure to other steroid hormone receptors and has distinct hormone-binding, DNA-binding, and functional domains.

FIGURE 321-4   Twenty-four-hour pattern of plasma LH and testosterone in a normal man sampled every 20 min. (*Reprinted from Griffin and Wilson, 1985.*)

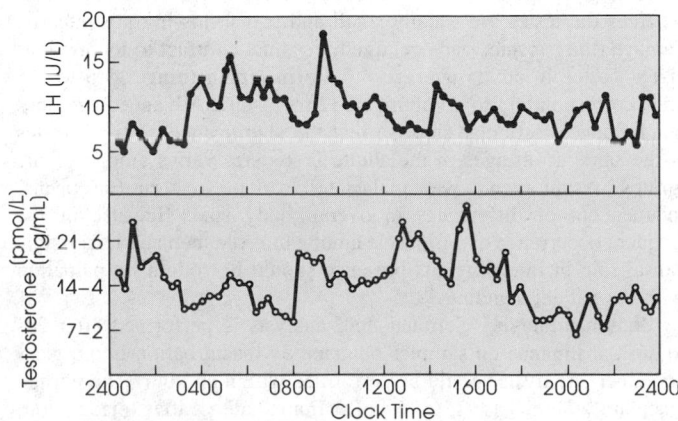

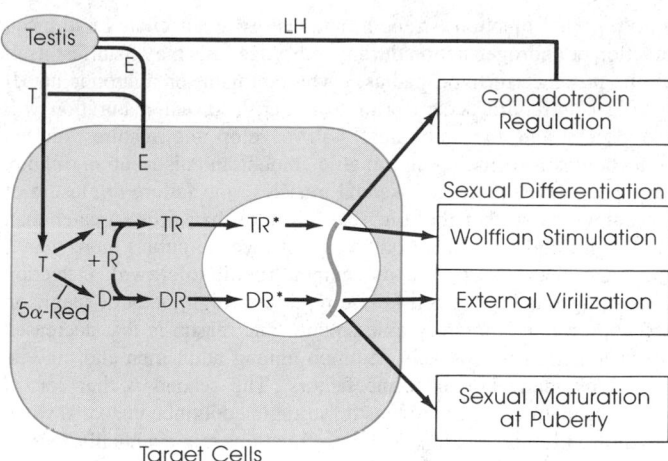

FIGURE 321-5   Current concepts of androgen action. (T, testosterone; D, dihydrotestosterone; E, estradiol; R, receptor protein; R*, transformed receptor protein; LH, luteinizing hormone; 5α-Red, 5α-reductase.)

Although testosterone and dihydrotestosterone bind to the same receptor, their physiologic roles differ. The testosterone-receptor complex regulates gonadotropin secretion and is responsible for the Wolffian stimulation phase of sexual differentiation (see Chap. 324), whereas the dihydrotestosterone-receptor complex is responsible for external virilization during embryogenesis and the major portion of androgen action during sexual maturation and adult sexual life, including the initiation and maintenance of spermatogenesis. The mechanism by which testosterone and dihydrotestosterone mediate these different functions is not known. The mechanisms by which estrogens act to augment or block androgen effects are also not known. It is presumed that estradiol acts by a mechanism similar to that of androgens but involving its own receptor protein (see Chap. 322).

THE SEMINIFEROUS TUBULE AND SPERMATOGENESIS
Normal function of the seminiferous tubule is dependent on the pituitary and on the adjacent Leydig cells, both FSH and androgen being essential for initiating and maintaining normal spermatogenesis (Fig. 321-3). The major site of FSH action is the Sertoli cell in the seminiferous tubules. The seminiferous tubule also contains androgen receptors. Androgen appears to be essential for the initial phase of spermatogenesis, whereas FSH is required for the terminal phases of spermatid development. In the normal adult male this machinery produces more than 200 million sperm per day.

The Sertoli cell cannot synthesize steroid hormones de novo and is dependent on testosterone that diffuses in from adjacent Leydig cells. Sertoli cells can convert testosterone to estradiol and to dihydrotestosterone. The seminiferous tubules also produce the peptide hormone inhibin that regulates the secretion of FSH by the hypothalamic-pituitary axis (Fig. 321-3). Inhibin, a peptide hormone produced by Sertoli cells, is the primary physiologic regulator of FSH, but testosterone and estradiol also can inhibit FSH secretion.

The interlocking system in which two pituitary hormones regulate testicular function provides a precise dual-control mechanism by which Leydig cells and the spermatogenic tubules produce factors that feed back upon the hypothalamic-pituitary system to regulate their own function (Fig. 321-3).

ASSESSMENT OF TESTICULAR FUNCTION

LEYDIG CELL FUNCTION   **History and physical examination**
The assessment of Leydig cell function and androgen status should include inquiry about the presence at birth of developmental abnormalities of the urogenital tract, the timing and extent of sexual maturation at puberty, the rate of beard growth, and the current

libido, sexual function, strength, and energy. Inadequate Leydig cell function or androgen action during embryogenesis may manifest itself by the presence of hypospadias, cryptorchidism, or microphallus. If Leydig cell failure occurs prior to puberty, sexual maturation will not occur, and the individual will develop the features termed eunuchoidism, including an infantile amount and distribution of body hair, poor development of skeletal muscles, and failure of closure of the epiphyses so that the arm span is more than 5 cm greater than the height, and the lower body segment (heel to pubic) more than 5 cm longer than the upper body segment (pubic to crown). Detection of postpubertal Leydig cell failure requires a high index of suspicion and appropriate laboratory assessment. One reason is that decreased sexual function is relatively common among adult men and may be caused by many nonendocrine factors. The second is that certain functions that require androgens for initiation continue unabated when Leydig cell failure occurs, and those functions that eventually regress may do so very slowly. For example, the frequency of shaving may not decrease for many months or even years because of the slow decline in rate of beard growth once established.

Plasma testosterone and dihydrotestosterone levels   Plasma testosterone is measured by a specific radioimmunoassay. Testosterone is secreted into plasma in a pulsatile fashion every 60 to 90 min (Fig. 321-4); a single random sample provides a result within ±20 percent of the true mean value only two-thirds of the time while three equally spaced samples 15 to 20 min apart provide a more accurate assessment. The samples do not need to be assayed separately, and aliquots of the three samples can be pooled for a single determination. The range of plasma testosterone in normal adult men is 10 to 35 nmol/L (3 to 10 ng/mL). In adult men the plasma values vary slightly throughout the day and at different times of the year, but these variations are not as great as those for plasma cortisol and are not significant in routine clinical assessment. Plasma levels of testosterone correlate in general with testosterone secretory rates as measured by isotope infusion. Estimation of TeBG concentration is sometimes useful in the interpretation of total plasma testosterone levels. Such assays can be done either by measuring the binding capacity of radioactive androgen or with a specific radioimmunoassay. Estimates of bio-available testosterone in plasma can be made by measuring the non-TeBG-bound fraction of testosterone.

The plasma testosterone value in prepubertal children is statistically higher in boys than girls, the range in both being 0.2 to 0.7 nmol/L (0.05 to 0.2 ng/mL). The rise in plasma testosterone at the start of puberty begins as a result of sleep-related nocturnal gonadotropin surges, so that during the initial phases plasma testosterone and LH are higher at night than during the day. The random daytime levels of plasma testosterone increase gradually as puberty progresses and reach adult levels at about age 17.

Dihydrotestosterone is also measured by radioimmunoassay. In normal young men the plasma dihydrotestosterone level is about one-tenth that of the testosterone value and averages around 2 nmol/L (0.5 ng/mL). In older men with benign prostatic hyperplasia, plasma dihydrotestosterone levels are higher and average about 3 nmol/L (0.9 ng/mL).

Urinary 17-ketosteroids   The measurement of urinary 17-ketosteroids is not a valid way to assess testicular function. Urinary 17-ketosteroids are mainly weak adrenal androgens or their metabolites, and testosterone contributes only about 40 percent of daily 17-ketosteroid production in men.

Plasma LH   Plasma LH is measured by specific radioimmunoassay. LH is also secreted in a pulsatile fashion and fluctuates more widely than does plasma testosterone so that in adult men an isolated random plasma LH is likely to be within ±20 percent of true mean value only a third of the time. Again, assay of a pool of plasma comprised of equal portions of three samples drawn 6 to 18 min apart as described above provides a value approaching the true mean. In early puberty plasma LH secretion increases only during sleep, but the pulsatile secretion in the adult is of similar magnitude during sleep and waking periods. The normal plasma LH values should be established for a given laboratory. The usual normal range in adult men is 5 to 20 IU/L. Bioactive LH can be assessed in some laboratories by the rat interstitial cell assay and may be detectable at times when the immunoreactive LH cannot be measured. A low plasma testosterone concentration can be interpreted correctly only if plasma LH is also measured simultaneously, and likewise the "appropriateness" of a given plasma LH must be interpreted in relation to the plasma testosterone. For example, a low plasma testosterone coupled with a low LH implies hypothalamic or pituitary disease, whereas the finding of a low plasma testosterone and a high LH suggests primary testicular insufficiency (see Chap. 312).

Response to gonadotropin stimulation   Leydig cell function is difficult to assess prior to puberty when both LH and testosterone levels are low, and it is common to measure response of plasma testosterone to gonadotropin stimulation as an index of Leydig cell capacity. Normal prepubertal boys respond to 3 to 5 days of injection of 1000 to 2000 IU human chorionic gonadotropin (hCG) with an increase in plasma testosterone to about 7 nmol/L (2 ng/mL); the magnitude of the response increases with the initiation of puberty and peaks in early puberty.

Response to luteinizing hormone–releasing hormone   The responsiveness of the pituitary gland to luteinizing hormone–releasing hormone (LHRH) changes at the time of puberty. Prior to puberty quantitative responses to LH and FSH are similar. With pubertal development the LH response to acute administration of LHRH increases while the FSH response remains the same. The amount of LH released following acute administration of LHRH probably reflects the amount of stored hormone in the pituitary. When 100 μg of LHRH is given subcutaneously or intravenously to normal men, there is, on average, a four- to fivefold increase in LH with the peak level at 30 min. However, the range of response is broad, with some normal men having less than a doubling of LH levels. In general, the peak LH following a single LHRH injection correlates with the basal levels. In patients with primary testicular failure measurement of basal LH is usually sufficient, and measurement of LHRH response adds little to aid the diagnosis. Men with either pituitary disease or hypothalamic disease may have a normal or an abnormal LH response to an acute dose of LHRH. Therefore, a normal response is of no diagnostic value, either in determining the presence or absence of disease or in distinguishing hypothalamic from pituitary disease. A subnormal response is of value in determining that an abnormality exists, even though the site is not determined. The LHRH test is most useful in the evaluation of men with secondary hypogonadism and subnormal LH response to an acute dose of LHRH. If daily infusions of LHRH for a week lead to the development of a normal LH response to an acute dose, a hypothalamic etiology is likely.

SEMINIFEROUS TUBULE FUNCTION   Examination of the testes Evaluation of the testes is an essential portion of the physical examination. The seminiferous tubules account for about 60 percent of testicular volume. The prepubertal testis measures about 2 cm in length and 2 mL in volume and increases in size during puberty to reach the adult proportions by age 16. When damage to the seminiferous tubules occurs prior to puberty the testes are small and firm, whereas the testes are usually small and soft following postpubertal damage (the capsule, once enlarged, does not contract to its previous size). Testes in adults average 4.6 cm in length (range, 3.5 to 5.5 cm), corresponding to a volume of 12 to 25 mL. Advanced age does not influence testicular size, so that the significance of small testes is the same at all ages in the adult. Testis size varies among ethnic groups. Asian men have smaller testes than western Europeans, independent of differences in overall body size. Because of the frequent occurrence of varicocele among infertile men and its possible causal role in infertility, its presence should be sought by palpation with the patient standing.

Semen analysis   Seminal fluid analysis is performed after 24- to 36-h abstinence on samples obtained by masturbation into a glass container. Analysis should be performed within an hour. The normal ejaculate volume is 2 to 6 mL. Immediately after ejaculation, coagulation of the seminal fluid occurs, followed within 15 to 30 min by liquefaction. Estimation of motility should be made on undiluted seminal fluid; more than 60 percent of the sperm should be motile and of normal morphology. The normal range for sperm density is generally considered to be greater than 20 million per milliliter with a total count per ejaculate of more than 60 million, but the definition of a minimally adequate ejaculate is not clear. Some men with low sperm counts are nevertheless fertile. This uncertainty as to the lower level of sperm density, percent motility, and percent normal forms in fertile semen stems from two issues. First, many factors produce temporary aberrations in sperm count, and in men who present with semen of equivocal quality it is necessary to examine three or more ejaculates to determine whether abnormal findings are permanent or temporary. Second, routine evaluation of the seminal fluid is dependent on tests that do not assess the functional capacity of the sperm. Although methods to measure sperm penetration of bovine cervical mucus and zona-free hamster ova have been developed, they are not sufficiently standardized to permit general use.

Plasma FSH Plasma FSH as measured by specific radioimmunoassay usually correlates inversely with spermatogenesis. In normal adult men, the range of plasma FSH is 5 to 20 IU/L. Men with intact hypothalamic-pituitary axes have elevations of FSH when damage to the germinal epithelium is severe.

Testicular biopsy Testicular biospy is useful in some patients with oligospermia and azoospermia both as an aid in diagnosis and as an indication of feasibility of treatment. For example, a normal testicular biopsy and a normal FSH in an azoospermic man suggest obstruction of the vas deferens, which may be surgically correctible. Tissue culture of the biopsy material with subsequent karyotypic analysis is necessary to identify those instances of Klinefelter syndrome secondary to chromosomal mosaicism in which the abnormality is limited to the testes. Testicular biopsy is often followed by a transient decrease in sperm counts, but there are no permanent adverse effects.

ESTROGENIC FUNCTION Examination of the breasts Breast enlargement (gynecomastia) is the most consistent feature of feminizing states in men (see Chap. 323). Gynecomastia is due to the proliferation of both glandular and adipose tissue. The presence of gynecomastia should be sought by examining the patient while he is in the sitting position using the fingers to grasp glandular tissue. Palpation with the flat of the hand while the patient is supine may result in failure to detect early or minimal breast enlargement. In obese men it is important to try to define the edge of the rim of glandular tissue that separates it from adipose tissue of the chest wall.

Plasma estrogen As discussed above, most of the estradiol and all of the estrone produced in normal men is formed by extraglandular aromatization of circulating androgens. Plasma estradiol is usually less than 180 pmol/L (50 pg/mL) in normal men; plasma estrone is somewhat higher but usually less than 300 pmol/L (80 pg/mL). Elevated estrogen production and elevated plasma levels can be due to elevations in plasma precursors (liver or adrenal disease), to increases in extraglandular aromatization (obesity), or to increased production by the testes (testicular tumors or androgen resistance).

PHASES OF NORMAL TESTICULAR FUNCTION

The phases of male sexual life can be defined in terms of the plasma testosterone value (Fig. 321-6). In the male embryo the production of testosterone by the testis commences at about 7 weeks of gestation. Shortly thereafter plasma testosterone attains a high value that is maintained until it falls late in gestation so that at the time of birth plasma testosterone is only slightly higher in males than in females. Shortly after birth, plasma testosterone in the male infant again begins to rise and remains elevated for approximately 3 months, falling to low levels by age 6 months to 1 year. The concentration then remains low (but slightly higher in boys than girls) until the onset of puberty,

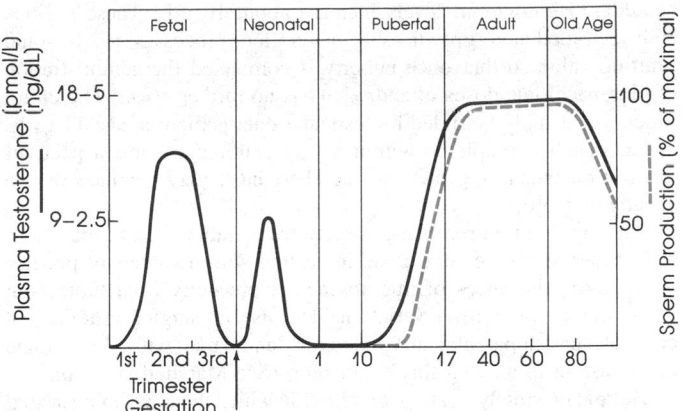

FIGURE 321-6 Phases of male sexual life. *(Reprinted from Griffin and Wilson, 1985.)*

when it begins to rise in boys, reaching adult levels by about age 17. The mean plasma level remains more or less constant in the adult until late middle age and then declines slowly during the later decades of life. During the third or adult phase of male sexual life sperm production becomes sufficient to allow reproduction to take place. The physiologic events that take place during these various phases differ, as do the pathologic consequences of derangements in testicular function at different stages of life. Male sexual differentiation during embryogenesis is considered in Chap. 324. The role of the surge of testosterone formation during the first year of life is unknown. The focus of this chapter is on testicular pathophysiology during puberty, mature sexual life, and old age.

ABNORMALITIES OF TESTICULAR FUNCTION

PUBERTY The factors that ultimately determine the onset of puberty are poorly understood and may reside in the hypothalamic-pituitary system, the testis, or the adrenal. Prior to the onset of puberty, gonadotropin secretion by the pituitary is low but appears to be under regulatory control by the testis, as prepubertal castration results in a rise in plasma gonadotropin levels. This suggests that prior to puberty the negative feedback control of gonadotropin secretion is exquisitely sensitive to the small amount of circulating testosterone. The onset of puberty is heralded by sleep-associated surges in gonadotropin secretion. Later in puberty the rises in LH and FSH persist throughout the day. Thus, with maturation the hypothalamic-pituitary system becomes less sensitive to negative feedback control, and the consequences are a higher mean plasma testosterone, maturation of the testes, and the onset of spermatogenesis. The rise in gonadotropin secretion is the consequence both of an increase in LHRH secretion and an increased sensitivity of the pituitary to LHRH. Plasma levels of bioactive LH increase even more than those of the immunoreactive hormone. The anatomic and developmental changes at the time of puberty are secondary to the rise in plasma testosterone. Maturation of the accessory organs of male reproduction (the penis, the prostate, the seminal vesicles, and the epididymides) accounts for about one-fourth of androgen-mediated nitrogen retention during puberty. The characteristic hair growth of male puberty involves development of mustache and beard, regression of the scalp line, appearance of body, extremity, and perianal hair, and extension of the pubic hair upward into a diamond-shaped pattern. Growth of axillary and pubic hair is initiated under the control of adrenal androgens and is promoted by testicular androgens. The larynx enlarges, and the vocal cords become thickened, resulting in a lowering of the pitch of the voice. Accelerated linear growth is accompanied by growth of muscle and connective tissue, accounting for the major portion of nitrogen retention at puberty. The principal androgen-sensitive muscles are those of the pectoral region and the shoulder. Hemoglobin levels increase about 10 g/L. These various androgen-mediated growth and maturation processes reach some limiting value so that once puberty is completed the administration of pharmacologic doses of androgen has no further effect. The entire process is usually heralded by testicular enlargement at age 11 to 12 and is usually completed within 5 years, although some aspects of virilization, such as growth of the chest hair, may continue over a decade or more.

The events of normal male puberty are variable in onset, duration, and sequence. The central issue in dealing with disorders of puberty is separating instances of true absence or precocity from subjects at the extremes of normal variation. The use of staging criteria that correlate developmental and anatomic landmarks with chronologic age is useful in making this distinction. (See Marshall and Tanner.)

Sexual precocity   Those disorders in which the developing sexual characteristics are appropriate for the phenotype, i.e., virilization in boys, are termed *isosexual precocity*. *Heterosexual precocity* refers to feminizing syndromes in boys.

ISOSEXUAL PRECOCITY   Sexual development prior to age 9 in boys is generally considered abnormal. *True precocious puberty* or *complete isosexual precocity* occurs when both premature virilization and spermatogenesis take place, and *precocious pseudopuberty* or *incomplete isosexual precocity* refers to virilization unaccompanied by spermatogenesis, indicating that androgen formation is not the result of premature activation of the hypothalamic-pituitary system. This distinction is blurred in practice because pure virilizing syndromes may cause activation of gonadotropin secretion secondarily and thus be followed by development of spermatogenesis. Furthermore, local androgen production in the testis, as in Leydig cell tumors, can cause local areas of spermatogenesis around the tumor and thus cause limited sperm production. We therefore prefer a simple two-part classification: virilizing syndromes (in which hypothalamic-pituitary activity is appropriate for age) and premature activation of the hypothalamic-pituitary system.

Virilizing syndromes can result from Leydig cell tumors, human chorionic gonadotropin (hCG)–secreting tumors, adrenal tumors, congenital adrenal hyperplasia (most commonly 21-hydroxylase deficiency), androgen administration, or Leydig cell hyperplasia. In all these situations plasma testosterone is inappropriately elevated for the age. Leydig cell tumors are rare in children but should be suspected when the testes are asymmetric in size (see Chap. 305). Virilizing adrenal tumors secrete large amounts of adrenal androgen (mainly androstenedione and dehydroepiandrosterone, some of which is converted to testosterone) and consequently cause elevated 17-ketosteroid secretion. Glucocorticoid administration does not suppress 17-ketosteroid excretion to normal in patients with testicular or adrenal tumors, in contrast to the prompt decrease that occurs following such treatment in congenital adrenal hyperplasia. Congenital adrenal hyperplasia leads to elevated 17-hydroxyprogesterone levels and as a consequence elevated androgen levels (see Chaps. 317 and 324). When this disorder is treated with glucocorticoids, true precocious puberty can then result if sufficient hypothalamic maturation has been produced by the increased androgen levels.

Gonadotropin-independent sexual precocity in boys may occur as a result of autonomous Leydig cell hyperplasia in the absence of Leydig cell tumor formation. The disorder is inherited as a male-limited autosomal disorder either from father to son or from mothers who are unaffected carriers. Virilization begins usually by age 2. Testosterone levels are elevated, often to the adult male range; however, immunoreactive and bioactive LH levels and the response to LHRH are prepubertal. Many of these boys were mistakenly thought to have true precocious puberty in the past because of the presence of spermatogenesis.

Premature activation of the hypothalamic-pituitary system may be "idiopathic" or due to central nervous system tumors, infections, or injuries. Such early hypothalamic-pituitary activation typically is associated with characteristics of normal puberty, i.e., sleep-related

gonadotropin secretion, elevated plasma bioactive LH, and enhanced gonadotropin response to LHRH. Since the diagnosis of idiopathic true precocious puberty is one of exclusion, rare patients later prove to have been misclassified and to have an identifiable central nervous system abnormality. With improved means of diagnosis, such as computed tomographic scans and magnetic resonance imaging, delays in diagnosis will probably be less frequent.

Management of sexual precocity due to steroid- or gonadotropin-producing tumors, congenital adrenal hyperplasia, or an identified CNS abnormality is directed toward the primary disease. In boys with Leydig cell hyperplasia attempts have been made to lower plasma testosterone with medroxyprogesterone acetate or ketoconazole, but the long-term efficacy and safety of these agents is unknown. Idiopathic true precocious puberty and true precocious puberty due to inoperable CNS lesions are treated with LHRH analogue therapy, resulting in reversal of the pubertal maturation including decreased rate of skeletal development.

HETEROSEXUAL PRECOCITY   Feminization in prepubertal boys can result from absolute or relative increases in estrogen due to a variety of causes (see Chap. 323).

Delayed or incomplete puberty   The separation of failure of puberty from variants of normal is one of the most difficult problems in endocrinology. Some patients fail to show the normal spurt of growth and sexual development at the usual time but eventually commence puberty by age 16 or older. Adolescence may then either progress rapidly, or there may be a slow development and growth that continues until age 20 to 22. Many men with delayed onset of puberty attain heights within the normal adult range. At times the history reveals that a parent or sibling has shown a similar pattern of development. The major problem is to separate this group of patients with delayed puberty from patients with organic disorders that impair puberty. Panhypopituitarism and hypothyroidism can cause pubertal failure in males (see Chaps. 313 and 316). Absent puberty can also result from primary disease of the testis including defects in testicular development; this diagnosis is suspected on the basis of low plasma testosterone and elevated FSH and LH. Hereditary androgen resistance (in which plasma testosterone and LH are both high) usually results in hereditary male pseudohermaphroditism but in milder cases may be manifested by absent or incomplete puberty (see Chap. 324).

The most frequent finding in boys with absent puberty is both low plasma testosterone and low gonadotropin levels; in these patients it is necessary to distinguish those with delayed puberty from those with isolated gonadotropin deficiency or idiopathic *hypogonadotropic hypogonadism* (*the Kallman syndrome*). The manifestations of isolated gonadotropin deficiency vary from boys with eunuchoidal features and testes of prepubertal size to those with partial manifestations of LH and FSH deficiency and partial degrees of testicular enlargement and pubertal development. One less severe form of this disorder in which plasma FSH levels and spermatogenesis appear to be normal is termed the *fertile eunuch syndrome.*. Anosmia or hyposmia and cryptorchidism are common. Histologic examination of the testis reveals undifferentiated Leydig cells and immature germinal epithelium similar to a normal prepubertal testis. The disorder is inherited as an X-linked recessive trait or an autosomal dominant trait with variable expressivity. Serum FSH and LH levels are usually below the normal male range, and plasma testosterone levels are low for the age. The secretion of other pituitary hormones is usually normal. The defect appears to be in the synthesis or release of LHRH with the resultant gonadotropin pattern ranging from absence of pulsatile LH secretion to defects in amplitude and frequency of LH secretion; the administration of synthetic LHRH for a sufficient period corrects the endocrine abnormalities and initiates spermatogenesis. If untreated, these patients usually remain in the prepubertal state indefinitely. A prepubertal manifestation is microphallus, in which the size of the penis is below the fifth percentile for the age. Indeed, a fourth or more of isolated prepubertal microphallus is due to hypogonadotropic hypogonadism. Distinction between this disorder and delayed puberty is particularly difficult in patients of early or midpubertal age; the presence of microphallus, anosmia, or a family history of hypogonadotropic hypogonadism may help to establish the diagnosis. In the absence of such evidence, differentiation of the two states may become clear only after several years of observation. In some cases the response of plasma LH to LHRH stimulation may be helpful in suggesting that puberty is imminent.

ADULT ABNORMALITIES OF TESTICULAR FUNCTION   At the completion of puberty, plasma testosterone levels reach the adult level of 10 to 35 nmol/L (3 to 10 ng/mL) throughout the day, plasma gonadotropins are 5 to 20 IU/L each for LH and FSH, and sperm production is sufficient to allow reproduction. The adult set of the complex regulatory system (Fig. 321-3) is sustained in the normal man for more than 40 years. However, the system is subject to a variety of influences, both at the level of the testis and of the hypothalamic-pituitary system. Spermatogenesis is exquisitely sensitive to alterations in temperature, and brief increases either in systemic or local temperature (as in a hot bath) can be followed by temporary decreases in sperm production. The system is likewise subject to influence by diet, drugs, alcohol, environmental agents, and psychological stress, all of which may cause temporary decreases in sperm count.

Persistent abnormalities of testicular function after the time of normal puberty can be due to hypothalamic-pituitary abnormalities (see Chap. 313), testicular defects, or to abnormalities of sperm transport. Certain of these conditions tend to affect Leydig cell function or spermatogenesis selectively, but most influence both aspects of testicular function and cause both underandrogenization and infertility (Table 321-1). The interlocking of defective Leydig cell function and infertility is a consequence of the dependence of spermatogenesis on androgen formation. Even partial decreases in testosterone production can cause infertility. Certain disorders (hyperprolactinemia, radiation, cyclophosphamide therapy, autoimmunity, paraplegia, androgen resistance) can cause either isolated infertility or a combined defect in testicular function in different subjects.

Hypothalamic-pituitary disorders   Disorders of the hypothalamus and pituitary can impair secretion of gonadotropins (and cause as a consequence decreased androgen production and defective spermatogenesis) either as a portion of generalized disease of the anterior pituitary (see Chap. 313) or as an isolated defect, usually hypogonadotropic hypogonadism, in which secretion of both LH and FSH are impaired; hypogonadotropic hypogonadism can either be congenital or, rarely, an acquired idiopathic defect. Alternatively, gonadotropin secretion can be altered by factors other than hypothalamic pituitary pathology. For example, elevation of plasma cortisol in the *Cushing syndrome* can depress LH secretion independent of a space-occupying lesion of the pituitary. Some patients with *congenital adrenal hyperplasia* have suppressed gonadotropin secretion and consequent infertility. *Hyperprolactinemia* (either as the consequence of pituitary adenomas or of drugs such as phenothiazines) has been associated with combined Leydig cell and seminiferous tubule dysfunction, presumably the consequence of inhibition of LH and FSH secretion by prolactin. Occasionally, impaired fertility in hyperprolactinemia is associated with normal gonadotropin and androgen levels and is presumed to result from direct inhibition of sexual function or spermatogenesis by prolactin. *Hemochromatosis* impairs testicular function most commonly as the result of effects on the pituitary; less often it affects the testis directly (see Chap. 327). The use of *androgens* for purposes other than replacement therapy is often associated with impaired sperm production (see below). In several other conditions testosterone levels may be decreased in association with normal LH levels, and the mechanism is less clear. Men with massive obesity have decreased TeBG and decreased levels of total and bioavailable testosterone that return toward normal with weight loss. Obesity may be part of the mechanism for decreased testosterone levels in the subset of such men with Pickwickian syndrome (see Chap. 217). Some men with seizures of temporal lobe origin also

TABLE 321-1   Classification of abnormalities of testicular function in the adult

Site of defect	Presentation	
	Infertility with underandrogenization	Infertility with normal virilization
Hypothalamic-pituitary	Panhypopituitarism	
	Hypogonadotropic hypogonadism	Isolated FSH deficiency
	Cushing's syndrome	Congenital adrenal hyperplasia
	Hyperprolactinemia	Hyperprolactinemia
	Hemochromatosis	Androgen use
Testicular	Developmental and structural defects:	
	Klinefelter's syndrome*	Germinal cell aplasia
	XX male	Cryptorchidism
		Varicocele
		Immotile cilia syndrome
	Acquired defects:	
	Viral orchitis*	*Mycoplasma* infection
	Trauma	
	Radiation	Radiation
	Drugs (spironolactone, alcohol, ketoconazole, cyclophosphamide)	Drugs (cyclophosphamide) Environmental toxins
	Autoimmunity	Autoimmunity
	Granulomatous disease	
	Associated with systemic diseases:	
	Liver disease	Febrile illness
	Renal failure	Celiac disease
	Sickle cell disease	
	Neurologic diseases (myotonic dystrophy and paraplegia)	Neurologic disease (paraplegia)
	Androgen resistance	Androgen resistance
Sperm transport		Obstruction of the epididymis or vas deferens (cystic fibrosis, diethylstilbesterol exposure, congenital absence)

* The common testicular causes of underandrogenization and infertility in adults—Klinefelter's syndrome and viral orchitis—are associated with small testes.

have a hormonal pattern consistent with hypogonadotropic hypogonadism.

Testicular defects   Abnormalities of testicular function in the adult can be grouped into several categories: developmental and structural defects of the testes, acquired testicular defects, and disorders secondary to systemic and/or neurologic disease.

DEVELOPMENTAL ABNORMALITIES   The *Klinefelter syndrome* (both the classic and mosaic forms) and the *XX male syndrome* are usually not recognized until after the time of expected puberty (see Chap. 324). Some developmental defects cause infertility in the presence of normal androgen production. These include varicocele, germinal cell aplasia, and cryptorchidism. *Varicocele* may be of etiologic importance in as much as one-third of all male infertility. It is caused by retrograde flow of blood into the internal spermatic vein that eventuates in progressive, often palpable dilatation of the peritesticular pampiniform plexus of veins. Varicocele occurs in about 10 to 15 percent in the general population and 20 to 40 percent in men with infertility and is thought to result from incompetence of the valve between the internal spermatic vein and the renal vein. It is more common on the left (85 percent). Unilateral varicocele increases the blood flow and the temperature of both testes as a result of the extensive anastomoses of the venous systems. The increased scrotal (and testicular) temperature is believed to be the cause of the poor-quality semen and infertility (the testes do not have the usual 2°C lower temperature than that of the abdominal cavity). The findings on semen analysis are usually nonspecific with all parameters showing some abnormality. In some studies, surgical resection results in improved fertility, with the best results (70 percent pregnancy rate) obtained in men whose preoperative sperm counts are over 10 million per milliliter.

Some patients with *germinal cell aplasia* (the Sertoli cell–only syndrome) have a positive family history and may constitute a specific entity in which the germinal epithelium is missing with resulting azoospermia; plasma testosterone and LH values are normal, and plasma FSH levels are elevated. Other patients with identical histologic and clinical findings have androgen resistance or a history of viral orchitis or cryptorchidism. Consequently a variety of conditions are commonly lumped under this term. The syndrome accounts for less than 10 percent of patients with azoospermia.

Unilateral *cryptorchidism,* even when corrected prior to puberty, is associated with abnormal semen in many individuals. This suggests that even in unilateral cryptorchidism the testicular abnormality is usually bilateral.

The *immotile cilia syndrome* is an autosomal recessive defect characterized by immotility or poor motility of the cilia of the airways and of the sperm. Kartagener's syndrome is a subgroup of the immotile cilia syndrome associated with situs inversus, chronic sinusitis, and bronchiectasis (see Chap. 208). The immotile sperm cannot fertilize. The structural abnormality leading to impaired motility of cilia can usually be defined by the electron-microscopic appearance. The specific defects that are known to cause the syndrome include defects in the dynein arms, spokes, or microtubule doublets. Cilia from epithelia and sperm tails from the same individual exhibit the same defects, but the pulmonary manifestations may be minor. *Other structural defects of sperm* that are less well understood can apparently lead to immotile sperm without involvement of cilia in the lung.

ACQUIRED TESTICULAR DEFECTS   The most common cause of acquired testicular failure in the adult is *viral orchitis*. The responsible viruses include mumps virus, echovirus, lymphocytic choriomeningitis virus, and group B arboviruses. The orchitis is due to actual infection of the tissue by virus rather than indirect effects of the infection. Orchitis is the most common complication of mumps in adult men, occurring in as many as one-fourth of men who have the disease. In about two-thirds of the cases orchitis is unilateral, and in the remainder it is bilateral. It usually develops within a few days after the onset of parotitis but may precede it. The testis may return to normal size and function or undergo atrophy. Atrophy is believed to be due both to direct effects of the virus on the seminiferous tubules and to ischemia secondary to pressure and edema within the taut tunica albuginea. Semen analysis returns to normal in three-fourths of men with unilateral involvement and in only one-third of men with bilateral orchitis. Atrophy is usually perceptible within 1 to 6 months after the orchitis subsides, and the degree of atrophy is not necessarily proportional to the severity of the acute orchitis or the development of infertility. Unilateral atrophy occurs in approximately one-third of cases of mumps orchitis, and bilateral atrophy occurs in about one-tenth.

Trauma is the second most common cause of secondary atrophy of the testes. The exposed position of the testis in the scrotum renders it susceptible to both thermal and physical trauma—particularly in individuals with hazardous occupations.

Both the seminiferous tubules and the Leydig cells are sensitive to *radiation damage;* decreased secretion of testosterone appears to be a consequence of diminished testicular blood flow. Doses higher than 200 mGy (20 rad) cause increases in plasma FSH and LH levels and damage to the spermatogonia. After doses of about 800 mGy (80 rad) oligospermia or azoospermia develops. Higher doses may obliterate the germinal epithelium except for occasional stem and Sertoli cells. Fractionated radiation may have a more profound effect than single-dose radiation. Recovery of sperm density occurs in a dose-related fashion, and complete recovery of sperm density to preradiation levels may require as long as 5 years. Permanent infertility can occur after radiation therapy of malignant lymphoma in spite of shielding the testes. Permanent androgen deficiency in adult men is uncommon after doses of radiation in the therapeutic range; however, most boys receiving direct testicular radiation for acute lymphoblastic leukemia have permanently low plasma testosterone levels.

In general, *drugs* interfere with testicular function in one of four ways—inhibition of testosterone synthesis, blockade of the peripheral action of androgen, enhancement of estrogen levels, or direct inhibition of spermatogenesis. Certain drugs have multiple effects, and agents such as guanethidine that block the sympathetic nervous system can impair sexual function in men whose pituitary-testicular axis is normal.

Spironolactone and ketoconazole block the synthesis of androgen by interfering with the late reactions in androgen biosynthesis. Spironolactone and cimetidine compete with androgen for the cytoplasmic receptor protein and thus interfere with androgen action in the target cell. Testosterone levels may be low and estradiol levels may be elevated in patients taking large amounts of marijuana, heroin, or methadone, although the exact reasons are unclear. Alcohol, when consumed in excess for prolonged periods, causes decreased plasma testosterone, independent of liver disease or malnutrition. Elevated plasma estradiol and decreased plasma testosterone have been reported in men taking digitalis.

Antineoplastic and chemotherapeutic agents commonly interfere with spermatogenesis. Cyclophosphamide causes azoospermia or extreme oligospermia within a few weeks after the initiation of therapy. Cessation of therapy is followed by a return of spermatogenesis within 3 years in about half of patients. Combination chemotherapy for acute leukemia, Hodgkin's disease, and other malignancies may also impair Leydig cell function. In pubertal boys this is manifested by decreased serum testosterone and elevated LH levels while in adult men testosterone levels do not decline and the impaired Leydig cell function may only be detected as exaggeration of LH response to LHRH. The alkylating agents in the chemotherapeutic regimens seem to be responsible for the toxic effects on the Leydig cell.

Because of the potentially toxic effects of many physical and chemical agents on spermatogenesis, the occupational and recreational history should be carefully evaluated in all men with infertility. Known environmental hazards include chemicals, such as the nematocide dibromochloropropane, cadmium, and lead, microwaves, and ultrasound.

Testicular failure also occurs as a part of a generalized disorder of *autoimmunity* in which multiple primary endocrine deficiencies coexist (Schmidt's syndrome) and in which circulating antibodies to the basement membrane of the testes are present (see Chap. 325). Sperm antibodies are also a cause of isolated male infertility. In some instances such antibodies may be secondary phenomena resulting from duct obstruction or vasectomy. *Granulomatous diseases* can also destroy the testes, the most common such disorder being leprosy. Testicular atrophy occurs in 10 to 20 percent of men with lepromatous leprosy, the result of direct invasion of the tissue by the mycobacteria. The tubules are involved initially, followed by endarteritis and destruction of Leydig cells.

TESTICULAR ABNORMALITIES ASSOCIATED WITH SYSTEMIC DISEASE   The common systemic diseases that cause underandrogenization and infertility are liver disease and renal failure. In *cirrhosis of the liver* a combined testicular and pituitary abnormality leads to decreased testosterone production independent of the direct toxic effects of ethanol. Although plasma LH is elevated, the level may be below the expected range given the degree of androgen deficiency. This is most likely the result of inhibition of LH secretion by the higher estrogen concentrations in patients with chronic liver disease. Increased estrogen production results from impaired hepatic extraction of adrenal androstenedione and subsequent increased peripheral conversion to estrone and estradiol. In effect there is shunting of estrogen precursors to sites of extraglandular aromatization. Testicular atrophy and gynecomastia are present in about half of men with cirrhosis, and many such men are impotent.

In chronic *renal failure* decreased androgen synthesis and diminution of sperm production develop in the setting of elevated plasma gonadotropins. The elevated LH is due to increased production as well as reduced clearance but is incapable of effecting normal testosterone production. In addition, about one-fourth of men with chronic renal failure have hyperprolactinemia. Low testosterone coupled with normal or increased plasma estrogen levels probably account for the presence of gynecomastia in about half of men on chronic hemodialysis. The role of the hyperprolactinemia in decreasing testosterone production is unclear. About half of men with renal failure on dialysis experience decreased libido and impotence. The etiology of the testicular abnormalities in renal failure is not well understood. Improvement in testosterone production with hemodialysis is incomplete, but successful transplantation may lead to return of testicular function to normal.

Men with *sickle cell anemia* usually have impaired secondary sexual development, and testicular atrophy is present in one-third. The defect may be either at the testicular or hypothalamic-pituitary level. Abnormalities in Leydig cell function, frequently accompanied by decreased sperm density, have been noted in a variety of chronic systemic diseases including protein-energy *malnutrition*, advanced *Hodgkin's disease* and *cancer* prior to chemotherapy, and *amyloidosis*. Most of these disorders cause a lowered plasma testosterone coupled with a normal to increased plasma LH, suggesting combined hypothalamic-pituitary and testicular defects. The low plasma testosterone is not the result of inhibitors that interfere with the binding to TeBG and hence is not analogous to the euthyroid sick syndrome. Similar hormone changes occur following *surgery*, *myocardial infarction*, and severe *burns*, and thus may be a nonspecific effect of illness.

The temporary decrease in sperm density after *acute febrile illness* usually occurs in the absence of any changes in testosterone production. Infertility in men with *celiac disease* is associated with a hormonal pattern typical of androgen resistance, namely elevated testosterone and LH levels. *Neurologic diseases* associated with altered testicular function include myotonic dystrophy and paraplegia. In myotonic dystrophy small testes may be associated with abnormalities of both spermatogenesis and Leydig cell function. Spinal cord lesions resulting in paraplegia lead to a temporary decrease in testosterone levels that tend to return to normal but persistent defects in spermatogenesis; some patients retain the capacity to obtain erection and to ejaculate.

ANDROGEN RESISTANCE Defects of the androgen receptor cause resistance to the action of androgen usually associated with defective male phenotypic development as well as infertility and underandrogenization (see Chap. 324). A less severe form of androgen resistance is associated with infertility due to oligo- or azoospermia in otherwise phenotypically normal men; this form of androgen resistance may cause a significant fraction of infertility previously classified as idiopathic azoospermia.

Impairment of sperm transport Disorders of sperm transport may lead to infertility in as many as 6 percent of infertile men with normal virilization. The obstruction may be unilateral or bilateral, congenital or acquired. In men with unilateral obstruction of sperm transport the infertility may result from antisperm antibodies. Obstructive azoospermia at the level of the epididymis also occurs in association with chronic infections of the paranasal sinuses and lungs. Tuberculosis, leprosy, and gonorrhea are rare causes of acquired obstruction of ejaculatory structures. Congenital defects of the vas deferens can occur as an isolated abnormality associated with absence of the seminal vesicles (and consequently absence of fructose in the ejaculate), in patients with *cystic fibrosis*, or in men whose mothers received *diethylstilbestrol* during pregnancy.

At least 40 percent of infertile men have infertility of unknown etiology; none of the above conditions is found on careful search.

The therapy in all forms of male infertility except surgically correctable varicocele, vas deferens obstruction or treatable endocrinopathy, is unsatisfactory. Empirical therapy with androgens or gonadotropins has no significant effect on fertility. Although the semen quality may improve with such treatment, the pregnancy rate is usually no greater than in infertile men given no therapy (25 percent fertility in patients followed for a year). This latter fact should be kept in mind, namely that spontaneous resolution may occur in up to one-fourth of patients with idiopathic infertility followed with no treatment. Many forms of male infertility associated with some motile sperm in the semen can be treated by in vitro fertilization.

Fertility control in the male Although a variety of approaches to fertility control in men have been tried, including the condom as a safe barrier method that also prevents sexually transmitted disease, the most practical means is ligation of the vas deferens, a procedure that has been successful in large numbers of men and can be performed on an outpatient basis. The time required for azoospermia to occur following the operation depends upon the number of sperm in the terminal vas deferens and ejaculatory ducts at the time of surgery but is usually less than 40 days. Azoospermia should be documented in each case to prove effectiveness. No deleterious effects on either testosterone production or the hypothalamic-pituitary axis have been documented. Despite reports of immune-complex-associated accelerated atherosclerosis in vasectomized nonhuman primates, there does not appear to be any association between vasectomy and atherosclerosis in men. Vasectomy should only be recommended for men requesting permanent sterilization. Vasovasostomy for reanastomosis of the vas has a success rate of about 80 to 90 percent as judged by return of sperm to the ejaculate, but only about 30 to 40 percent subsequently achieve fertility. This discrepancy is possibly due to the development of antisperm antibodies as a consequence of the vasectomy.

OLD AGE Beginning at about age 60 mean plasma total and bioavailable testosterone concentrations decline. Nevertheless, though statistically lower than levels in young men, the concentrations of testosterone in elderly men usually remain within the normal range. The cause of the decreased testosterone level is likely decreased Leydig cell numbers in the testes. There is also a decline in seminiferous tubule function and decreased sperm production in older men. Plasma LH and FSH levels are usually increased in elderly men, and an increase in the rate of conversion of androgen to estrogen in peripheral tissues results in a decrease in the effective ratio of androgen to estrogen. These latter endocrine changes may play a role in the development of prostatic hyperplasia and possibly in development of gynecomastia in aging men (see Chap. 323). Male sexual function gradually declines after early adulthood, but there is no convincing evidence that hormonal changes have any direct bearing on changes in sexual function with age.

Prostatic hyperplasia See Chap. 306.

Cancer of the prostate See Chap. 306.

DISORDERS OF ALL AGES **Testicular tumors** (See Chap. 305) Chorionic gonadotropin is present in normal testes, and it is therefore not surprising that plasma gonadotropins are elevated in testicular tumors. Indeed, an elevated plasma level of the beta subunit of human chorionic gonadotropins (hCG-β) serves as a sensitive and specific marker of tumor activity in some men with germ cell tumors. Plasma levels of the beta subunit are elevated in all patients with choriocarcinoma, in one-third of embryonal carcinomas and teratocarcinomas, and rarely in seminomas. There is a good correlation between change in hCG-β levels and response to therapy.

Elevated estradiol and testosterone production in patients with testicular tumors can arise by at least two mechanisms. In trophoblastic tumors and in tumors of Leydig and Sertoli cells production of both hormones occurs autonomously in the tumor tissue itself; in these instances plasma gonadotropin levels and hormone production by the uninvolved portions of the testes are depressed, and azoospermia is common. However, when gonadotropins are secreted by the tumor, the gonadotropin acts to increase estradiol and testosterone production in the unaffected areas of the testes, and azoospermia is uncommon. When estrogens and androgens are formed (directly or indirectly) by the tumors, feminization, virilization, or no obvious change may result, depending on the pattern of hormones produced and the age of the patients. Other cellular markers of testicular tumor activity have been described in individual cases, including alpha fetoprotein.

Gynecomastia See Chap. 323.

HORMONAL THERAPY

ANDROGENS Pharmacologic preparations Effective androgen therapy requires the use of chemically modified analogues of testosterone. When testosterone itself is administered by mouth, it is absorbed into the portal blood and degraded promptly by the liver so that insignificant amounts reach the systemic circulation; when injected parenterally testosterone is rapidly absorbed from the injection vehicle so that it is difficult to sustain effective levels in the plasma. As a consequence, effective androgen therapy requires either the administration in a slowly absorbed form of testosterone (dermal patches or micronized oral preparation) or the administration of chemically modified analogues. Such chemical modifications either retard the rate of absorption or catabolism, so as to sustain effective blood levels, or enhance the androgenic potency of each molecule, so that full androgenic effects can be achieved at a lower blood level of the drug. Three types of modification of the molecule have received widespread clinical application (Fig. 321-7), namely esterification of the 17β-hydroxyl group, alkylation at the 17α position, and modification of the ring structure, particularly substitutions at the 2, 9, and 11 positions. Most agents actually contain combinations of ring structure alterations and either 17α-alkylation or esterification of the 17-hydroxyl. Esterification serves to decrease the polarity of the

FIGURE 321-7 Some of the androgen preparations available for pharmacologic use.

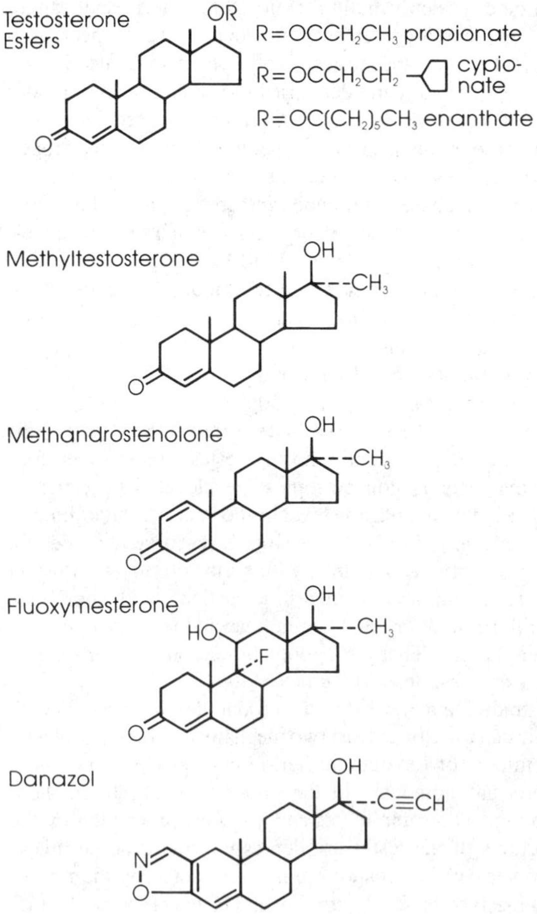

Testosterone Esters

R = OCCH₂CH₃ propionate
R = OCCH₂CH₂ cypionate
R = OC(CH₂)₅CH₃ enanthate

Methyltestosterone

Methandrostenolone

Fluoxymesterone

Danazol

molecule. Consequently, the steroid is more soluble in the fat vehicles used for injection, and release of the steroid into the circulation is slowed. Most esters must be injected parenterally. The more carbon molecules in the acid esterified, the more prolonged the action. Currently available esters such as testosterone cypionate and testosterone enanthate can be injected every 1 to 3 weeks. Because the esters are hydrolyzed before the hormones act, the effectiveness of therapy can be monitored by assaying the plasma level of testosterone with time following administration.

The effectiveness of 17α-alkylated androgens (such as methyltestosterone and methandrostenolone) when given by mouth is due to slower hepatic catabolism than occurs with testosterone itself so that the alkylated derivatives escape degradation by the liver and reach the systemic circulation. For this reason 17α-methyl or -ethyl substitution is a common feature of most orally active androgens. Unfortunately, all 17α-alkylated steroids may cause abnormalities of liver function, and for this reason they have a limited role in medicine.

Other alterations of the ring structure of the androgen molecule have been adopted empirically; in some instances the modification slows the rate of inactivation, in others it enhances the potency of a given molecule, and in still others it alters the conversion to other active metabolites. For example, the potency of fluoxymesterone may be due to the fact that, unlike most androgens, it is a poor precursor for conversion to estrogens in peripheral tissues. A transdermal therapeutic preparation of testosterone in which a testosterone-loaded film is applied each day to scrotal skin in the form of a patch makes it possible to sustain serum levels in the normal male range throughout the day. This therapy avoids the wide swings in serum testosterone values that occur between injections of testosterone esters.

Side effects of androgens All androgens carry the risk of inducing virilization in women. Among the early manifestations are acne, coarsening of the voice, and development of hirsutism. Menstrual irregularities are common. If treatment is discontinued as soon as these effects develop, the manifestations may slowly subside. With prolonged treatment, male-pattern baldness, worsening of the hirsutism and voice changes, and hypertrophy of the clitoris develop and are largely irreversible. There is considerable variation in the frequency and the degree to which these signs develop in women, probably because of individual differences in susceptibility, in steady-state blood levels among individuals, and in duration of therapy. In general, the younger the patient, the more striking the virilizing signs; nevertheless, florid virilization can also occur in adult women. At physiologic replacement doses testosterone esters have no known side effects in mature men. At supraphysiologic doses, however, gonadotropin secretion is inhibited, the testes decrease in volume, and the sperm count falls (indeed, low sperm counts may persist for as long as 9 months after such agents are discontinued). The so-called toxic side effects differ among the different agents and depending on the clinical setting in which they are used.

Retention of a limited amount of sodium is an inevitable consequence of androgen therapy, but in patients with underlying heart disease or renal failure or when androgens are administered in enormous amounts, as in some patients with carcinoma of the breast, the degree of sodium retention may lead to edema. Although androgens do not cause malignancy, they may promote growth of and intensify pain from carcinoma of the prostate and from breast carcinoma in men.

Feminizing side effects of androgen therapy in men are poorly understood. Testosterone itself can be converted (aromatized) in extraglandular tissues to estradiol. In contrast, 5α-reduction of the molecule precludes estrogen formation. The commonest manifestation of feminization is development of gynecomastia. Such breast enlargement is common in children given androgens and correlates with an increase in urinary estrogens, possibly because of a greater capacity to convert androgens to estrogens in childhood. The administration of testosterone esters to men results in an increase in plasma estrogen levels. In men with normal liver function, gynecomastia usually develops only after high doses of androgens.

All 17α-alkylated androgens can produce liver function abnormalities such as elevation of plasma alkaline phosphatase and conjugated bilirubin. The incidence of clinical liver disease probably depends upon the previous integrity of the liver, but jaundice may occur in the absence of preexisting liver disease. 17α-Alkylated drugs also cause an increase in a variety of plasma proteins that are synthesized in the liver. The most serious complications of oral androgen therapy are the development of peliosis hepatis (blood-filled cysts in the liver) and hepatoma. These disorders were initially described in patients with aplastic anemia, many of whom have Fanconi anemia, itself a predisposing factor for the development of malignancy. However, both lesions have also been reported in patients who received oral androgens for a variety of other causes, including use by athletes. There may be a similar increased incidence of hepatocellular neoplasms in women taking oral contraceptives. In some individuals these tumors regress and follow a benign course after discontinuation of the drugs, and in others the course is rapidly fatal.

One indication for the use of 17α-alkylated androgens is in hereditary angioedema; in this disorder the desired therapeutic benefit (increase in the level of the inhibitor of the first component of complement) may actually be a side effect of the 17-alkylated steroid rather than an effect of the parent androgen itself. As a consequence, weak androgens such as danazol are effective in this disorder (Fig. 321-7). Another indication for danazol is in the management of endometriosis (see Chap. 53).

Replacement therapy   The aim of androgen therapy in hypogonadal men is to restore or bring to normal male secondary sexual characteristics (beard, body hair, external genitalia) and male sexual behavior and to mimic the hormonal effects on somatic development (hemoglobin, muscle mass, nitrogen balance, and epiphyseal closure). Since an assay for plasma testosterone is available for monitoring therapy, the treatment of androgen deficiency is almost universally successful. The parenteral administration of a long-acting testosterone ester such as 100 to 200 mg testosterone enanthate at 1- to 3-week intervals results in a sustained increase in plasma testosterone to the normal male range. Such esters act only through the release of testosterone itself into the circulation. If the hypogonadism is primary and of long duration (as in the Klinefelter syndrome) suppression of plasma LH to the normal range may not occur for many weeks, if at all. Considerable variability exists in the relation between plasma testosterone and male sexual behavior, but in postpubertal testicular failure (even of many years duration) resumption of normal sexual activity is usual following adequate replacement. Androgen does not restore spermatogenesis in hypogonadal states, but the volume of the ejaculate (derived largely from the prostate and seminal vesicles) and male secondary sex characteristics return to normal. The effects of endogenous androgen on hemoglobin, nitrogen retention, and skeletal development are also reproduced.

In patients of all ages in whom hypogonadism developed prior to expected puberty (such as patients with hypogonadotropic hypogonadism), it is appropriate to bring plasma testosterone slowly into the adult range. When therapy is commenced at the time of expected puberty in such patients, the normal events of puberty proceed in the usual fashion. If therapy is delayed until after the time of usual puberty, the degree to which normal virilization will occur is variable, but many patients undergo a relatively complete anatomic and functional maturation. Intermittent low-dose androgen therapy is indicated in prepubertal hypogonadal boys with microphallus to bring the external genitalia into the normal range. If such patients are monitored closely and given androgens only for short periods, such therapy usually has no adverse effects on somatic growth.

In boys of pubertal age with either isolated hypogonadotropic hypogonadism or primary testicular deficiency, the usual practice is to institute androgen therapy between the ages of 12 and 14 years, depending on the subjective need for sexual development. The initial administration of small doses of testosterone esters followed by a gradual increase to 100 to 150 mg/m² of body surface area every 1

to 3 weeks should result in a normal pubertal growth spurt. The time from the start of treatment to the appearance of secondary sex characteristics is variable. Penile development, deepening of the voice, and other secondary sexual characteristics usually commence during the first year of treatment. In normal boys puberty extends over several years, and treatment designed to replicate normal development does not shorten the process greatly.

Testosterone exerts its full action only in the presence of a balanced hormonal environment and, particularly, in the presence of adequate levels of growth hormone. Consequently, prepubertal boys who have coexisting growth hormone deficiency exhibit a diminished response to androgens both in regard to growth and to the development of secondary sex characteristics unless sufficient growth hormone is given simultaneously.

Pharmacologic uses   Androgens have been used for a variety of disorders unassociated with hypogonadism, in the hope that potential benefits from the nonvirilizing actions of the agents (such as increase in nitrogen retention and muscle mass, increased hemoglobin, etc.) would outweigh any deleterious actions of the drugs. The most common nonreplacement uses of androgen have been attempts to improve nitrogen balance in catabolic states, self-administration by athletes in the belief that muscle mass and/or athletic performance will be improved, attempts to enhance erythropoiesis in refractory anemias including the anemia of renal failure, adjuvant therapy in carcinoma of the breast, treatment of hereditary angioedema and endometriosis, and management of growth retardation of various etiologies. Most expectations of beneficial effects in these disorders have been illusory for two reasons. First, pharmacologic doses of androgens do little if anything in men beyond the normal testicular androgen, and in women the virilizing side effects of androgens are formidable. Second, no androgen has been devised that exhibits only the nonvirilizing effects of the hormone. This is not surprising in view of the fact that all actions of androgens are mediated by a single high-affinity receptor protein in the cytoplasm (Fig. 321-5).

The most pervasive form of androgen abuse is by male athletes in the expectation that muscle development and athletic performance will be improved. In fact, however, in adequately controlled studies such therapy does not improve performance consistently, and in those rare instances in which it does, such improvement may be the consequence of sodium retention and expansion of the blood volume rather than of an effect on muscle development or strength. However, published trials of efficacy involve the administration of drugs at smaller doses than are usually taken by athletes; since the drugs at high dosage have multiple side effects, some of which preclude studies of efficacy in a double-blind fashion, it is not clear whether the question of efficacy can ever be resolved scientifically. Under no circumstances do putative benefits outweigh the risks associated with the use of oral androgens, a practice that cannot be condemned too harshly. At present, the only established indications for androgen therapy outside of male hypogonadism are in selected patients with anemia due to bone marrow failure, hereditary angioedema, or endometriosis.

Parenteral administration of testosterone esters to normal men results in little effects of any kind, except for the suppression of gonadotropin secretion by the hypothalamic-pituitary system and a consequent decrease in the production of sperm. There is no established contraindication to their administration to men with those disorders (such as short stature) where their use has been advocated, but the efficacy is not yet established. However, the virilizing side effects in women of androgens in usual dosages preclude their use in all except life-threatening situations. Even in potentially fatal diseases in women such as bone marrow failure and carcinoma of the breast great care must be exercised in androgen use.

GONADOTROPINS   Treatment with gonadotropins is utilized to establish or restore fertility in patients with gonadotropin deficiency of all causes. Two gonadotropin preparations are available: human menopausal gonadotropins (hMG) (purified from the urine of postmenopausal women) and human chorionic gonadotropin (hCG) (purified from the urine of pregnant women). hMG contains 75 IU FSH and 75 IU LH per vial. hCG has little FSH activity and resembles LH in its ability to stimulate testosterone production by Leydig cells. Because of the expense of hMG, treatment is usually begun with hCG alone, and hMG is added later to stimulate the FSH-dependent stages of spermatid development. A high ratio of LH to FSH activity and a long duration of treatment (3 to 6 months) are necessary to bring about the maturation of the prepubertal testis. Once spermatogenesis is restored in hypophysectomized patients or initiated in hypogonadotropic hypogonadal men by combined therapy, it can usually be maintained with hCG alone.

Men with oligospermia of unknown etiology have also been treated with gonadotropins; the incidence of fertility in such patients is probably no greater than in similar groups of untreated controls.

The dosage of hCG required to maintain a normal testosterone level varies from 1000 to 5000 IU weekly. A variety of regimens have been utilized to induce maturation of spermatogenesis. Most involve starting with 2000 IU hCG three or more times a week until most of the clinical parameters, including plasma testosterone, indicate normal adult male development. hMG (usually one ampul) is then added three times a week to complete the development of spermatogenesis. After regression of spermatogenesis has occurred, the length of therapy required to restore spermatogenesis may be as long as 12 months.

LUTEINIZING HORMONE–RELEASING HORMONE LHRH (gonadorelin) is now available for endocrine testing. LHRH therapy is now used by some physicians for chronic therapy of the infertility of hypogonadotropic hypogonadism. It is necessary to administer LHRH in frequent boluses (25 to 200 ng/kg of body weight every 2 h), requiring the use of portable infusion pumps or periodic nasal application. In general, LHRH does not appear to be more efficacious than gonadotropin in returning sperm counts to normal.

REFERENCES

CARR BR, GRIFFIN JE: Fertility control and its complications, in *Williams' Textbook of Endocrinology*, 7th ed, JD Wilson, DW Foster (eds). Philadelphia, Saunders, 1985, pp 452–475

DAVIS JE: Male sterilization. Clin Obstet Gynaecol 6:97, 1979

DE KRETSER DM: The effects of systemic disease on the function of the testis. Clin Endocrinol Metabol 8:487, 1979

———, ROBERTSON DM: The isolation and physiology of inhibin and related proteins. Biol Reprod 40:33, 1989

GOLDZIEHER JW et al:Improving the diagnostic reliability of rapidly fluctuating plasma hormone levels by optimized multiple-sampling techniques. J Clin Endocrinol Metab 43:824, 1976

GRIFFIN JE, WILSON JD: Disorders of the testes and male reproductive tract, in *Williams' Textbook of Endocrinology*, 7th ed, JD Wilson, DW Foster (eds). Philadelphia, Saunders, 1985, pp 259–312

LAUE L et al: Treatment of familial male precocious puberty with spironolactone and testolactone. N Engl J Med 320:496, 1989

MacDONALD PC et al: Origin of estrogen in normal men and in women with testicular feminization. J Clin Endocrinol Metab 49:905, 1979

MARSHALL WA, TANNER JM: Variation in the pattern of pubertal changes in boys. Arch Dis Child 45:13, 1970

MASSEY FJ et al: Vasectomy and health: Results from a large cohort study. JAMA 252:1023, 1984

SANTORO N et al: Hypogonadotropic disorders in men and women: Diagnosis and therapy with pulsatile gonadotropin-releasing hormone. Endocr Rev 7:11, 1986

SHERINS RH et al: Male infertility, in *Campbell's Urology*, 5th ed, PC Walsh et al (eds). Philadelphia, Saunders, 1985, pp 640–699

SNYDER PF, LAWRENCE DA: Treatment of male hypogonadism with testosterone enanthate. J Clin Endocrinol Metab 51:1335, 1980

SPRATT DI, CROWLEY WF: Hypogonadotropic hypogonadism: GnRH therapy, in *Current Therapy in Endocrinology and Metabolism*, 3d ed, CW Bardin (ed). Toronto, Decker, 1988, pp 221–225

STYNE DM, GRUMBACH MM: Puberty in the male and female: Its physiology and disorders, in *Reproductive Endocrinology: Physiology, Pathophysiology and Clinical Management*, 2d ed, SSC Yen, RB Jaffe (eds). Philadelphia, Saunders, 1986, pp 313–384

WILSON JD: Androgen abuse by athletes. Endocr Rev 9:181, 1988

———, GRIFFIN JE: The use and misuse of androgens. Metabolism 29:1278, 1980

322 DISORDERS OF THE OVARY AND FEMALE REPRODUCTIVE TRACT

BRUCE R. CARR / JEAN D. WILSON

The ovary is the source of ova for reproduction and of the hormones that regulate female sexual life. The anatomic structure, response to hormonal stimuli, and secretory capacity of the ovary are different at different periods of life. This chapter will review normal ovarian physiology as a background for understanding the abnormalities of the ovary and other tissues of the female reproductive tract.

DEVELOPMENT, STRUCTURE, AND FUNCTION OF THE OVARY

EMBRYOLOGY During the third week of gestation the primordial germ cells arise from the endoderm lining the yolk sac at the caudal end of the embryo. The germ cells migrate to the genital ridge adjacent to the mesonephric kidney by the fifth week of gestation and undergo mitotic divisions. The gonads exist in an undifferentiated state until the seventh week of fetal life, at which time the primitive ovary can be differentiated from the testis (see Chap. 324). Estrogen formation in the ovary commences between weeks 8 and 10, and by 10 to 11 weeks of gestation some oogonia in the developing ovarian cortex begin developing into primary oocytes. The ovary contains a finite number of germ cells, the maximal number of about 7 million oogonia being reached by the fifth to sixth month of gestation. Afterward, the germ cells begin to decrease in number through a process of atresia such that only 1 million remain at birth, 400,000 are present at the time of menarche, and only a few remain at menopause. Two X chromosomes are required for normal development of the ovary; in individuals with a 45,X karyotype ovarian development occurs, but the rate of atresia is accelerated so that only a fibrous streak remains at the time of birth (see Chap. 324).

After the oogonia cease to proliferate, meiosis commences, proceeds until the diplotene stage of the first meiotic division is completed, and then remains stationary until the time of onset of ovulation at puberty. During the fifth month of fetal life, the primordial follicle consists of the primary oocyte arrested in meiosis, a single surrounding layer of granulosa cells, and a basement membrane that separates the primordial follicle from surrounding stromal (interstitial) tissues.

PUBERTAL MATURATION Final maturation of ovarian follicles commences during puberty. The two major hormones that regulate follicular development are the pituitary gonadotropins—follicle-stimulating hormone (FSH) and luteinizing hormone (LH) (Fig. 322-1). During the second trimester of fetal development the plasma gonadotropins rise to levels equivalent to those at menopause. This peak in gonadotropin levels may be causally related to the simultaneous peak in replication of oocytes. The hypothalamic-pituitary axis (the so-called gonadostat) undergoes maturation and becomes sensitive after the second trimester to negative feedback by circulating steroid hormones, particularly estrogen and progesterone produced in the placenta. The circulating gonadotropins decrease thereafter and are almost undetectable at the time of birth. In the neonate, concomitant with the decrease in estrogen and progesterone levels due to separation from the placenta at birth, there is a rebound increase in gonadotropin secretion that persists for the first few months of life. With continued maturation of the hypothalamic-pituitary system the gonadostat becomes sensitive to negative feedback control by the low levels of circulating steroid hormones, and plasma gonadotropins again decrease.

As the time of puberty nears, a decrease in the sensitivity of the gonadostat allows for increased secretion of FSH and LH, possibly

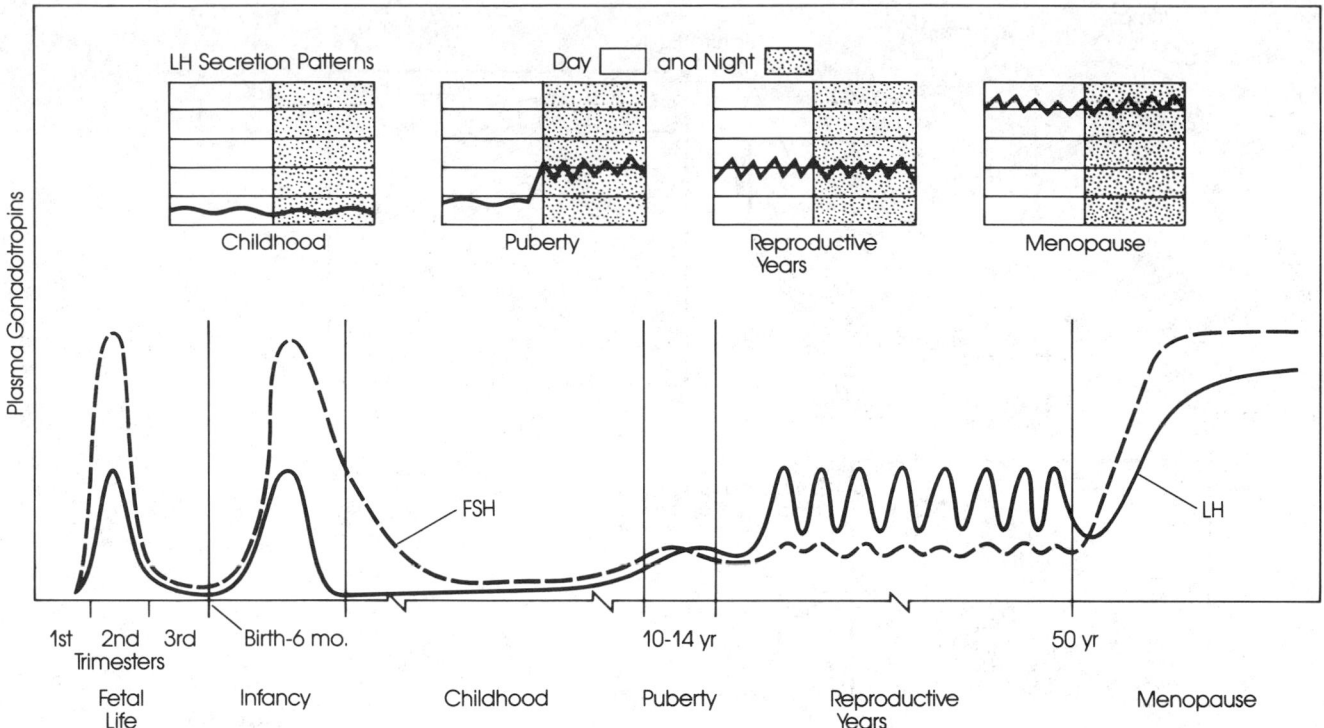

FIGURE 322-1 Pattern of gonadotropin secretion during different stages of life in women. FSH (follicle-stimulating hormone), LH (luteinizing hormone). The secretory patterns of LH during the waking hours (clear area) and night (stippled area) for each stage are indicated in the upper insets. (*After C Faiman et al.*)

secondary to increased episodic or pulsatile secretion of luteinizing hormone–releasing hormone (LHRH) by the hypothalamus (see Chap. 313). A sleep-induced, pulsatile pattern of LH secretion then ensues, the first step in the development of a cyclic pattern of gonadotropin secretion (Fig. 322-1). The increase in estrogen secretion subsequently exerts a positive feedback which leads to an exaggeration of the pulsatile release of LH and eventually to ovulation and the menarche, after which mean plasma gonadotropin concentrations reach adult values in which day and night levels are similar. After the menopause plasma gonadotropin levels rise, plateau 5 to 10 years later, and remain fairly constant until the eighth to ninth decade of life when the plasma levels may fall. Although ovarian function is regulated primarily by LH and FSH, the ovary is a source of several peptide and protein hormones and growth factors, raising the possibility that they play a role in ovarian pathophysiology.

With the development at puberty of decreased sensitivity of the hypothalamic-pituitary centers to circulating steroid hormones, LHRH release by the hypothalamus increases, gonadotropin secretion by the pituitary is enhanced, ovarian estrogen secretion increases, and the anatomic changes of puberty ensue. At age 10 to 11 the first secondary sexual characteristics begin to appear in girls, namely, development of the breast buds (thelarche), followed by the development of pubic hair (pubarche), and later by the development of axillary hair (adrenarche). The appearance of pubic and axillary hair is believed to be the result of an increase in adrenal androgens, commencing at approximately 6 to 8 years of age. A growth spurt ensues, and peak growth rate is attained at a mean age of 12 years.

The culmination of puberty is the onset of predictable, cyclic menses. The average time between the beginning of breast development and the onset of menses (menarche) is 2 years. During the first few years after menarche, menstrual cycles are often irregular and unpredictable due to anovulation. The age of menarche is variable and is determined in part by socioeconomic as well as by genetic factors and general health. In the United States the mean age of menarche is believed to have decreased at a rate of 3 to 4 months per decade over the last 100 years and is now around 13 years, a

decrease believed to be due to an improvement in nutrition in the population at large. A critical body weight of around 48 kg or a critical combination of weight, body water, and body fat is associated with development of hypothalamic insensitivity to circulating steroids that leads to increased secretion of gonadotropins and finally to menarche. Obese girls with a body weight 20 to 30 percent above ideal have earlier menarche than do girls with normal weights. In contrast, participation in certain sports or ballet, malnutrition, and chronic debilitating disease commonly cause delayed menarche.

MATURE OVARY Morphology The anatomic components and function of the adult ovary are illustrated schematically in Fig. 322-2. Under the influence of gonadotropins, a group of primary follicles is recruited, and by day 6 to 8 of the menstrual cycle one follicle becomes mature or "dominant," a process characterized by accelerated growth of granulosa cells and enlargement of the fluid-filled antrum. The recruited follicles not destined to ovulate begin to undergo degeneration, similar to the atresia observed in other follicles during embryogenesis. Just prior to ovulation, meiosis resumes in the ova of the dominant follicle, and the first meiotic division is completed with formation of the first polar body. Rapid enlargement of the antrum (up to 10 to 25 mm in size) occurs with an associated increase in follicular fluid, followed by a thinning of the follicular surface and formation of a conical stigma. Ovulation from the dominant follicle occurs some 16 to 23 h after the LH peak or 24 to 38 h after the onset of the LH surge as the result of rupture of the follicular wall at the area of the stigma, followed by expulsion of the ovum together with a mass of surrounding granulosa cells called cumulus cells. The rupture is believed to result from the action of hydrolyzing enzymes on the surface of the follicle, possibly under the control of prostaglandins. The second meiotic division begins after the egg is fertilized by a sperm, and a second polar body is then extruded. Following ovulation, the formation of the corpus luteum begins in the retained remnant of the ovulated follicle; the remaining granulosa and theca cells increase in size and accumulate lipids and a yellow pigment, lutein, to become "luteinized." The basement membrane that separated the granulosa cells from the stroma

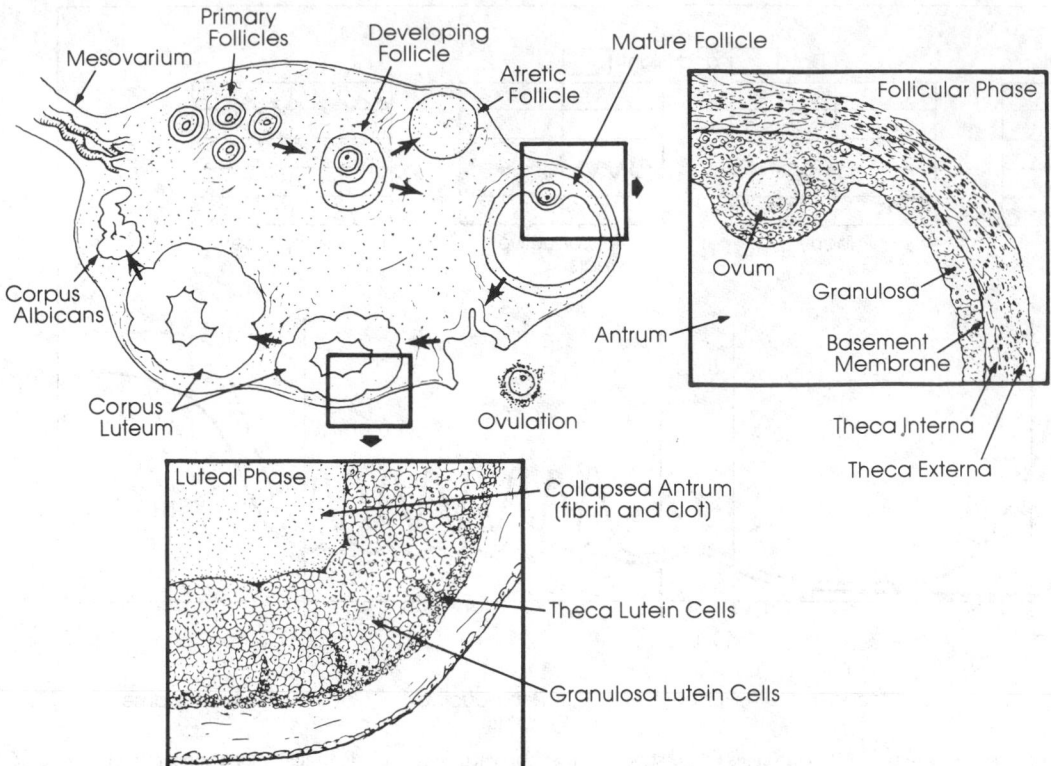

FIGURE 322-2 Developmental changes in the adult ovary during a complete 28-day cycle.

and blood vessels breaks, and capillaries, fibroblasts, and lymphatics from the theca invade the granulosa cells and reach the central cavity, thereby filling it with blood. After a period of 14 ± 2 days (the functional life of the corpus luteum) regression of vessels and atrophy of the corpus luteum commence and eventuate in replacement of the corpus luteum by a fibrous scar, the corpus albicans. The factors that limit the life span of the human corpus luteum are not known. However, if pregnancy occurs, the corpus luteum persists under the influence of placental or chorionic gonadotropins, and progesterone is produced by the corpus luteum for the support of early pregnancy.

Hormone formation STEROID HORMONES Like other steroid hormones, ovarian steroids are derived from cholesterol (Fig. 322-3). The ovary can synthesize cholesterol de novo from 2-carbon precursors and can also utilize cholesterol from circulating low-density lipoproteins (LDL) as substrate for steroid hormone formation (Fig. 322-4). Virtually all ovarian cells are believed to possess the complete enzymatic complement required for the conversion of cholesterol to estradiol (Fig. 322-3); however, different cell types within the ovary contain different amounts of these enzymes so that the predominant steroids produced differ in the various compartments. For example, the corpus luteum forms progesterone and 17-hydroxyprogesterone predominantly, whereas theca and stromal cells convert cholesterol to the androgens androstenedione and testosterone. Granulosa cells are particularly rich in the aromatase activity responsible for conversion of androgens to estrogen and utilize as substrates for this process androgens synthesized within the granulosa cells and in the adjacent theca cells.

The principal sites of action of LH and FSH are also illustrated in Figs. 322-3 and 322-4. LH acts primarily to regulate the first step in steroid hormone biosynthesis, namely the conversion of cholesterol to pregnenolone, and also induces subsequent enzymes in the pathway. FSH acts to regulate the final process by which androgens are aromatized to estrogens. As a consequence, in the absence of FSH, LH enhances substrate flow and the formation of androgens and/or progesterone, whereas FSH action is impeded in the absence of LH because of diminished substrate for aromatization.

Estrogens. Naturally occurring estrogens are 18-carbon steroids characterized by an aromatic A ring, a phenolic hydroxyl group at C-3, and either a hydroxyl group (estradiol) or a ketone (estrone) at C-17 (Fig. 322-3). (For the numbering of the steroid ring see Fig. 321-1.) The principal estrogen secreted by the ovary and the most potent naturally occurring estrogen is estradiol. Estrone is also secreted by the ovary, but the principal source of estrone is from extraglandular conversion of androstenedione in peripheral tissues. Estriol (16-hydroxyestradiol), the most abundant estrogen in urine, arises from the 16-hydroxylation of estrone and estradiol. Catechol estrogens are formed by hydroxylation of estrogens at the C-2 or C-4 position and may act as the intracellular mediators of some estrogen action. Estrogens promote development of the secondary sexual characteristics in women and cause uterine growth, thickening of the vaginal mucosa, thinning of the cervical mucus, and development of the ductular system of the breasts. The mechanism of estrogen action in target tissues is similar to that for other steroid hormones and involves the binding to a specific receptor protein, subsequent conformational change of the hormone-receptor complex, attachment of the complex to DNA, and initiation of the transcription of messenger RNA, which in turn causes increased protein synthesis in the cell cytoplasm (see Chap. 311).

Progesterone. Progesterone, a 21-carbon steroid (Fig. 322-3), is the principal hormone secreted by the corpus luteum and is responsible for progestational effects, namely induction of secretory activity in the endometrium of the estrogen-primed uterus in preparation for implantation of the fertilized egg. Progesterone also induces a decidual reaction in endometrium. Other effects include inhibition of uterine contractions, increased viscosity of cervical mucus, glandular development of the breasts, and increase in basal body temperature (thermogenic effect).

Androgens. The ovary synthesizes a variety of 19-carbon steroids including dehydroepiandrosterone, androstenedione, testosterone, and dihydrotestosterone, principally in stromal and thecal cells. The major ovarian 19-carbon steroid is androstenedione (Fig. 322-3), part of which is secreted into plasma and the remainder of which is converted to estrogen in granulosa cells or to testosterone in the interstitium.

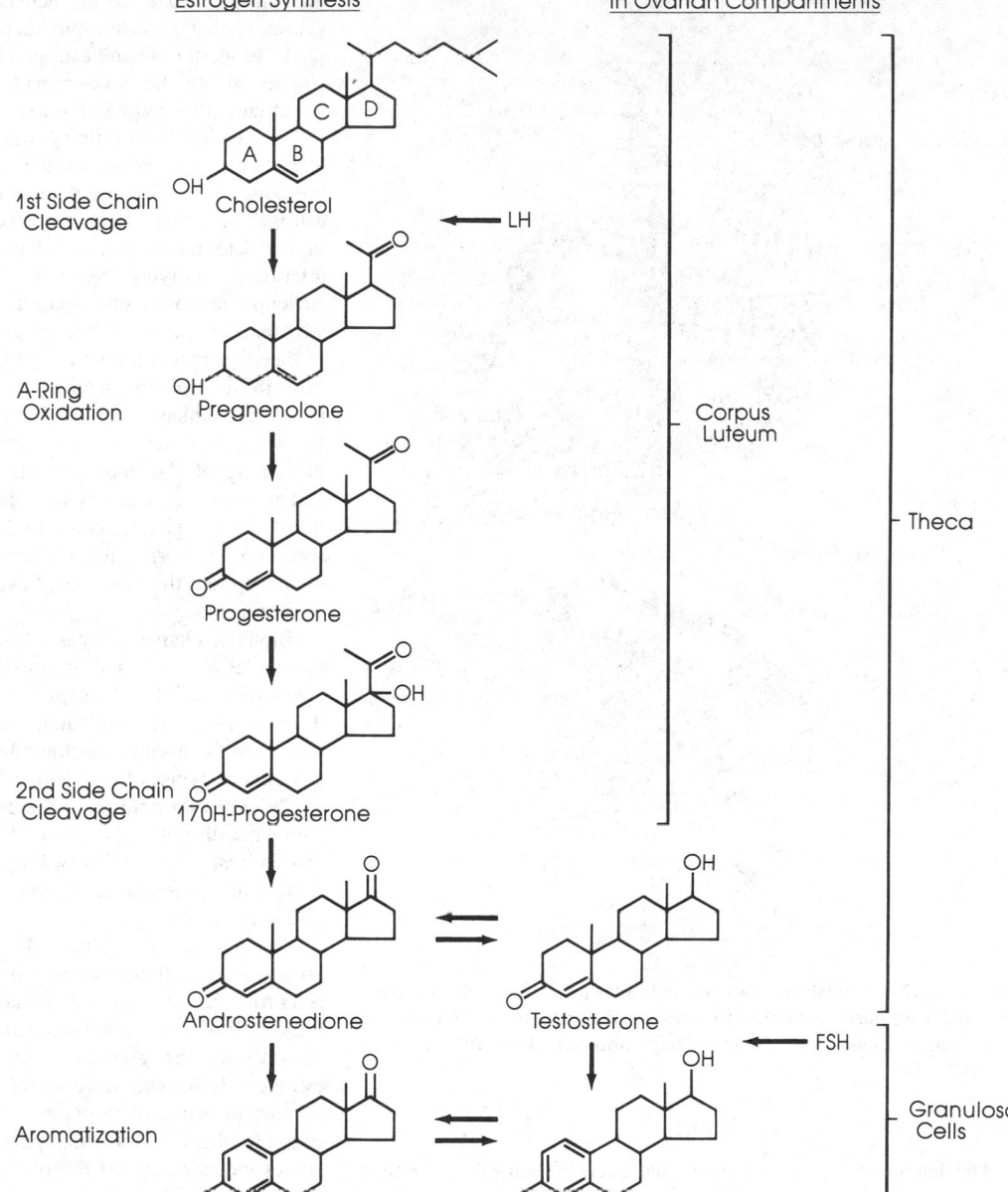

FIGURE 322-3 The principal pathway of steroid hormone biosynthesis in the ovary. Although every ovarian cell probably contains the complete enzyme complement required for the formation of estradiol from cholesterol, the amounts of the various enzymes and consequently the predominant hormones formed differ among the various cell types. The major enzyme complements for the corpus luteum, stroma, and granulosa cells are shown by the brackets; as a consequence these cells produce predominantly progesterone and 17-OH progesterone, androgen, and estrogen, respectively. The major sites of action of LH and FSH in mediating this pathway are shown in the horizontal arrows.

In peripheral tissues androstenedione can also be converted to testosterone and to estrogens. Only testosterone and dihydrotestosterone are true androgens with the capacity of interacting with the androgen receptor and thus inducing virilizing signs in women (see Chaps. 54 and 321).

OTHER HORMONES Other ovarian hormones play an uncertain role in human physiology. *Relaxin,* a polypeptide hormone produced by the human corpus luteum as well as by the decidua, causes softening of the cervix and loosening of the symphysis pubis in preparation for parturition in animals. *Oxytocin, vasopressin,* and other hypothalamic and pituitary hormones have also been found in granulosa and/or luteal cells, but their function in these cells is unknown. *Follicular inhibin* or *folliculostatin* (the equivalent of testicular inhibin) is secreted by the follicle and is believed to regulate the release of FSH by the hypothalamic-pituitary unit. *Follicle regulatory protein* (FRP) of human follicular fluid inhibits granulosa secretion and growth. *Gonadocrinins,* peptides purified from rat follicular fluid, stimulate the release of both FSH and LH from the pituitary in vitro and in vivo. Granulosa cells secrete *oocyte maturation*

inhibitor (OMI), a factor that prevents premature ovulation. In addition, in the gonads of both sexes a *meiosis-inducing substance* (MIS) triggers the onset of meiosis, an event that occurs earlier in ovarian than in testicular development. A variety of growth factors produced locally (including IGF) have been shown to influence steroid secretion by the ovary.

The normal menstrual cycle The menstrual cycle is usually divided into a follicular or proliferative phase and a luteal or secretory phase (Fig. 322-5). The secretion of FSH and LH is fundamentally under negative feedback control by ovarian steroids (particularly estradiol) and probably by inhibin, but the response of gonadotropins to different levels of estradiol varies. FSH secretion is inhibited progressively as estrogen levels increase—typical negative feedback. In contrast, LH secretion is suppressed maximally by estrogen in low amounts and is enhanced in response to a rising and sustained elevation of estradiol—so-called positive feedback control. Negative feedback of estrogen involves both the hypothalamus and pituitary, whereas positive feedback operates primarily at the level of the pituitary.

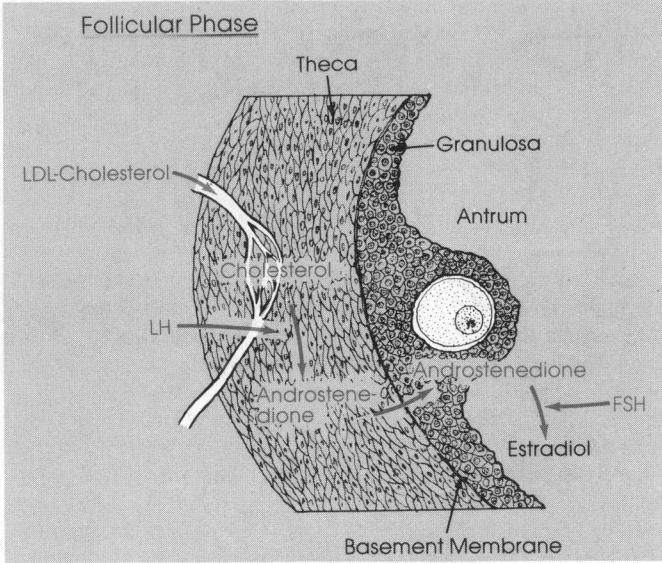

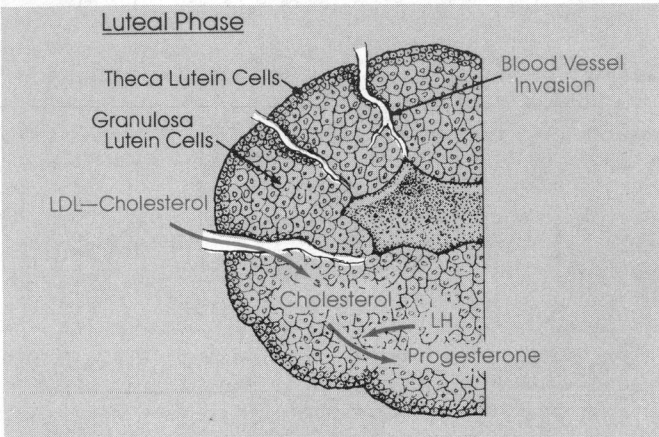

FIGURE 322-4 Cellular interactions in the ovary during the follicular phase (top) and luteal phase (bottom); LDL (low-density lipoprotein), FSH (follicle-stimulating hormone), and LH (luteinizing hormone). (*From BR Carr et al, 1982.*)

The length of the normal menstrual cycle is defined as the time from the onset of one menstrual bleeding episode to the onset of the next. In women of reproductive age the menstrual cycle averages 28 ± 3 days, and the mean duration of flow is 4 ± 2 days. Longer menstrual cycles (usually characterized by anovulation) occur at menarche and prior to menopause. At the end of one menstrual cycle and in the face of a waning corpus luteum, plasma levels of estrogen and progesterone fall, and circulating levels of FSH increase concomitantly. Under the influence of increasing levels of FSH, follicular recruitment is initiated to effect development of the follicle that will be dominant during the next cycle.

After the onset of menses, follicular development continues, but FSH levels decrease. Approximately 8 to 10 days prior to the midcycle LH surge, plasma estradiol levels begin to rise as the result of secretion of estradiol by the granulosa cells of the enlarging dominant follicle. During the second half of the follicular phase, LH levels also begin to rise (positive feedback). Just prior to ovulation, estradiol secretion reaches a peak and then falls. Immediately thereafter, a further rise in the plasma level of LH mediates the final maturation of the follicle, followed by follicular rupture and ovulation 16 to 23 h after the LH peak. Concomitant with the rise in LH is a smaller increase in the level of plasma FSH, the physiologic significance of which is unclear. Plasma progesterone also begins to rise just prior to midcycle and facilitates the positive feedback action of estradiol on LH secretion.

At the onset of the luteal phase plasma gonadotropins decrease, and plasma progesterone increases. A secondary rise in estrogens causes further gonadotropin suppression. Near the end of the luteal phase progesterone and estrogen levels fall, and FSH levels begin to rise to initiate the development of the next follicle (usually in the contralateral ovary) and the next menstrual cycle.

The endometrium lining the uterine cavity undergoes marked alterations in response to the changing plasma levels of ovarian hormones (Fig. 322-5). Concomitant with the decrease in plasma estrogen and progesterone and the decline of corpus luteum function in the late luteal phase, intense vasospasm occurs in the spiral arterioles supplying blood to the endometrium, followed by an ischemic necrosis, endometrial desquamation, and bleeding. This vasospasm is caused by locally synthesized prostaglandins. The onset of bleeding marks the first day of the menstrual cycle. By the fourth to fifth day of the cycle the endometrium is thin. During the proliferative phase glandular growth of the endometrium is mediated by estrogen. After ovulation increased progesterone leads to further thickening of the endometrium, but the rapid growth slows. The endometrium then enters the secretory phase characterized by tortuosity of the glands, curling of the spiral arterioles, and glandular secretion. As corpus luteum function begins to wane in the absence of conception, the sequence of events leading to menstruation is again set into action.

Biphasic changes in basal body temperature are characteristic of the ovulatory cycle and are mediated by alterations in progesterone levels (Fig. 322-5). An increase in basal body temperature of 0.3 to 0.5°C begins after ovulation, persists during the luteal phase, and returns to the normal baseline (36.2 to 36.4°C) after the onset of the subsequent menses (see Chap. 20).

Cellular interactions in the ovary during the normal cycle LH stimulates thecal cells surrounding the follicle to form androgens, and androstenedione diffuses across the basement membrane of the follicle into granulosa cells where it is aromatized to estrogen (Figs. 322-3 and 322-4).

The increase of FSH late in the preceding menstrual cycle stimulates growth and recruitment of the primary follicles by enhancing granulosa cell proliferation, resulting ultimately in the formation of the dominant follicle. FSH also stimulates activity and the amount of aromatizing enzymes in the granulosa cells that convert androstenedione to estrogen. Enhanced secretion of estradiol causes an increase in the number of estradiol receptors and further proliferation of granulosa cells. In the late follicular phase FSH, in concert with estradiol, causes induction of LH receptors on the granulosa cells. LH acts via these receptors to increase progesterone secretion at midcycle. The amount of progesterone formed by the follicle is believed to be limited by the availability of LDL-cholesterol to serve as substrate for steroidogenesis and by the fact that most of the progesterone formed is further metabolized to androstenedione by thecal cells. Prior to ovulation the granulosa cells of the follicle are bathed in follicular fluid but have limited access to circulating blood and consequently to plasma LDL. As depicted in Fig. 322-4, the granulosa cells become vascularized after ovulation, and plasma LDL-cholesterol becomes available to serve as the major substrate for progesterone synthesis by the corpus luteum. Thus, increased progesterone synthesis by the corpus luteum is the consequence of increased substrate availability. The peak in progesterone secretion by the corpus luteum is attained 8 days after ovulation at the time of maximal vascularization of the granulosa cells.

MENOPAUSE The menopause is defined as the final episode of menstrual bleeding in women. However, the term is used commonly to refer to the period of the female climacteric that encompasses the transitional period between the reproductive years up to and beyond the last episode of menstrual bleeding. During this period there is a gradual but progressive loss of ovarian function and a variety of endocrine, somatic, and psychological changes.

The median age of women at the time of cessation of menstrual bleeding is 50 to 51 years. Since the life expectancy in women is now close to 80 years, approximately one-third of life occurs after cessation of reproductive function. Preceding the menopause, the pattern of menstrual cycles is variable, but the interval between menses usually becomes longer. In addition, there is an increase in the mean levels of plasma FSH and LH, despite the continuation of ovulatory cycles. Thus, the ovary appears to become less responsive to gonadotropins prior to the menopause.

The menopause is the consequence of the exhaustion of ovarian follicles. The decrease in the number of ova begins in intrauterine life; by the time of the menopause few ova remain, and these appear to be nonfunctional. Only a small number of ova are lost as the result of ovulation during reproductive life, the majority of follicles and associated ova being lost by atresia. The cessation of follicular development results in a drop in the production of estradiol and other hormones, which in turn causes a loss of negative feedback on the hypothalamic-pituitary centers. In turn, the levels of plasma gonadotropins increase with FSH levels rising earlier and to a greater extent than those of LH (Figs. 322-1 and 322-6). The higher concentration of FSH than LH in postmenopausal women may result from the decrease in inhibin secretion by the ovary, from the fact that FSH is cleared from plasma less rapidly than LH due to its higher sialic acid content, and possibly from the loss of positive feedback on LH production by estradiol. Intravenous administration of LHRH to menopausal women results in a pronounced increase in the secretion of both FSH and LH, consistent with the enhanced hypothalamic-pituitary secretory activity in other forms of primary ovarian failure.

The ovaries of postmenopausal women are small, and the residual cells are predominantly stromal in type. Estrogen and androgen levels in plasma are reduced but not absent from the circulation (Fig. 322-6). Prior to the menopause, plasma androstenedione is derived almost equally from the adrenals and the ovaries; after menopause the ovarian contribution ceases so that the plasma levels of androstenedione fall by 50 percent (Fig. 322-6). However, the menopausal ovary continues to secrete testosterone, presumably formed in stromal cells.

Circulating estrogens in the ovulating woman are derived from two sources. Sixty percent of mean estrogen formation during the menstrual cycle is in the form of estradiol formed primarily by ovaries, and the remainder is estrone formed mainly in extraglandular tissues from androstenedione. After menopause, extraglandular estrogen formation becomes the major pathway for estrogen synthesis. Estrogen production by the menopausal ovary is minimal, and subsequent oophorectomy is not followed by any further decrease in estrogen levels. Plasma levels of estradiol, the principal estrogen secreted by the follicle, are lower in postmenopausal women than are the levels of estrone. The rate of peripheral formation of estrone increases somewhat in menopausal women so that estrone production is usually only slightly less than prior to the menopause, despite the fall in plasma androstenedione. Because a major site of extraglandular estrogen production is adipose tissue, peripheral estrogen formation may actually be enhanced in obese postmenopausal women, so that total estrogen production rates may be as great or greater than in premenopausal women. The predominant estrogen formed is estrone rather than estradiol.

The most common menopausal symptoms are those of vasomotor instability (hot flash), atrophy of the urogenital epithelium and skin, decreased size of the breasts, and osteoporosis. Approximately 40 percent of women in the postmenopausal period develop symptoms serious enough to seek medical assistance.

The pathogenesis of the hot flash is uncertain. There is a close temporal relationship between the onset of the hot flash and pulses of LH secretion; however, hot flashes occur in women with absence of pituitary function and following treatment with LHRH analogues where LH levels are absent or low. Alterations in catecholamine, prostaglandin, endorphin, or neurotensin metabolism in conjunction

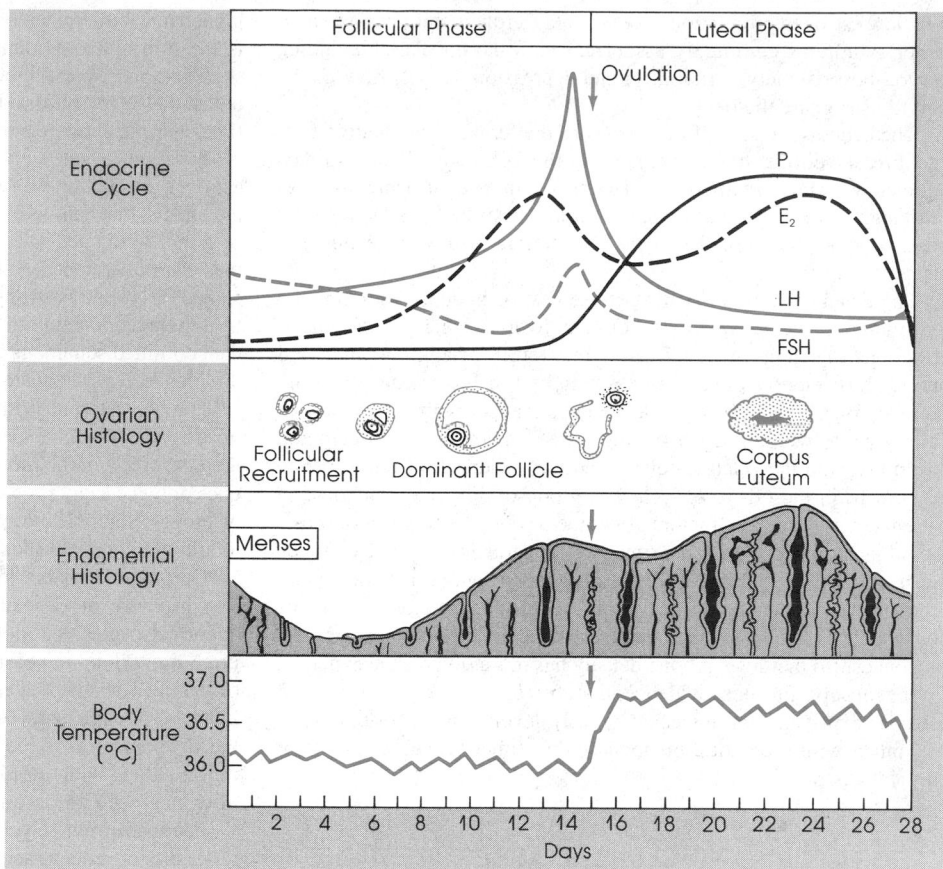

FIGURE 322-5 The hormonal, ovarian, endometrial, and basal body temperature changes and relationship throughout the normal menstrual cycle.

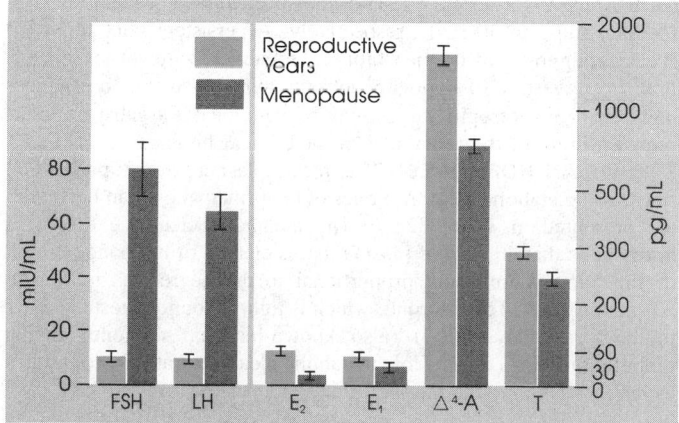

FIGURE 322-6 Differences in hormone concentration in women during the reproductive years and in women during the menopause. FSH (follicle-stimulating hormone), LH (luteinizing hormone), E_2 (estradiol-17β), E_1 (estrone), Δ^4-A (androstenedione), T (testosterone). (*From SSC Yen and RB Jaffe, 1986, and from DR Mishell, Jr, and V Davajan.*)

with low estrogen production may also play a role in this phenomenon. Other symptoms commonly associated with the hot flash, including nervousness, anxiety, irritability, and depression, may or may not be due to estrogen deficiency.

The decrease in size of the organs of the female reproductive tract and breasts during the menopause is the consequence of estrogen deficiency. The endometrium becomes thin and atrophic in most (although cystic hyperplasia may occur in one-fifth of postmenopausal women), and the vaginal mucosa and urethra also become thin and atrophic.

There is a close relationship between estrogen deprivation and the development of osteoporosis. Osteoporosis is one of the dread afflictions of aging. Approximately one-fourth of aging women and one-tenth of elderly men sustain a vertebral or hip fracture between the ages of 60 and 90, and the incidence appears to be greatest in elderly white women. Such fractures are a major cause of death and morbidity, and the fracture-related mortality increases from less than 10 percent in the 60- to 64-year age group to 30 percent or more in patients over 80. Many factors affect the development of osteoporosis including diet, activity, smoking, and general health, and estrogen deprivation is of particular importance in this regard. White postmenopausal women are more predisposed to osteoporosis and its consequences because bone density in such subjects is lower prior to menopause so that loss in bone density has more severe consequences in the group. Further evidence that osteoporosis is a disease of estrogen deprivation is suggested by early development of osteoporosis in women with premature menopause due either to natural causes or surgical castration.

LABORATORY AND CLINICAL ASSESSMENT OF HORMONAL STATUS

Assessment of the hormonal status of women can usually be made by obtaining a thorough history and physical examination. In general, presence of secondary sexual characteristics such as normal female breast development indicates adequate estrogen secretion in the past, and the presence of regular, predictable, cyclic menses implies that ovulation and the production of gonadotropins, estrogen, progesterone, and androgens are adequate and that the outflow tract is intact. Such a history may be more valuable than laboratory tests in evaluating ovarian hormone status. However, laboratory tests provide valuable ancillary information in the workup of women with endocrine dysfunction or infertility.

PITUITARY GONADOTROPINS Plasma gonadotropins are assessed by radioimmunoassay. Because both FSH and LH are secreted in pulsatile manner, the results obtained from a single serum sample may be difficult to interpret. Consequently, multiple samples at 20-min intervals for 2 h may be pooled to obtain a mean value. Serum gonadotropin measurements are of most use in evaluating women with suspected ovarian failure and in supporting the diagnosis of polycystic ovarian disease and hypogonadotropic hypogonadism. The normal ranges for serum LH and FSH in ovulating women are 5 to 25 IU/L and 5 to 30 IU/L, respectively. A persistent FSH above 40 IU/L is diagnostic of ovarian failure, and an LH value of less than 5 IU/L is suggestive of hypogonadotropic hypogonadism. In practice, however, gonadotropin values may be equivocal and must be interpreted in light of the remainder of the clinical findings.

OVARIAN HORMONES The mean plasma levels, production rates, and metabolic clearance rates of the principal ovarian hormones are presented in Table 322-1. The metabolic clearance rate of a hormone is that amount of plasma that is cleared of hormone per unit of time and is inversely proportional to the degree of binding to plasma proteins. Testosterone, which is tightly bound to testosterone-binding globulin (TeBG) (also known as sex hormone–binding globulin or SHBG), has a low metabolic clearance rate. Steroids such as androstenedione that are not tightly bound to carrier proteins have

higher metabolic clearance rates. The production rate of a hormone is the sum of the amount of hormone produced by direct glandular secretion and by extraglandular conversion of prohormones and can be estimated by multiplying the concentration of hormone in plasma times the metabolic clearance rate of that hormone.

Estrogen Normal secondary sexual characteristics imply that estrogen production was adequate in the past. Indication of the current estrogen status can be obtained by pelvic examination. The presence of a moist, rugated vagina with copious, clear, thin cervical mucus that can be stretched and that exhibits arborization or ferning when spread on a slide is strong evidence of adequate estrogen production. Cytologic demonstration of mature vaginal epithelial cells and abundant cornified squamous epithelial cells with pyknotic nuclei confirms the presence of adequate estrogen levels.

The progesterone-withdrawal test provides a functional assessment of estrogen status. If menses appear within a week to 10 days after the end of a trial of medroxyprogesterone acetate (10 mg by mouth once or twice a day for 5 days) or after a single intramuscular injection of progesterone (100 mg), then prior estrogen priming was adequate to allow withdrawal bleeding.

Due to its variable level in plasma during the normal cycle and the difficulty of estimating the day of the cycle in women with abnormal cycles, the determination of estrogen levels in plasma or urine by radioimmunoassay is of little use in the routine assessment of estrogen status. Plasma estradiol is measured during attempts to induce ovulation with human menopausal gonadotropins to prevent the development of the ovarian hyperstimulation syndrome and is utilized along with ultrasound assessment to monitor follicular growth in women who are to undergo in vitro fertilization.

Progesterone Cyclic, predictable menses also imply that adequate progesterone is secreted during the luteal phase of the menstrual cycle. The indications for specific assay of progesterone are to document ovulation or evaluate the adequacy of the luteal phase in the evaluation of infertile women and to separate subjects with müllerian agenesis from those with the testicular feminization syndrome. Several functional assays of progesterone secretion can be utilized. The least expensive and most useful is the daily measurement of basal body temperature throughout a cycle. Due to the thermogenic properties of progesterone, documentation of the monthly biphasic curve with an elevated temperature for approximately 2 weeks after ovulation is a valid indication of progesterone secretion during the luteal phase (Fig. 322-5). Presence of viscous cervical mucus that does not stretch or fern and the presence of predominant intermediate cells on vaginal cytology or demonstration of a secretory epithelium in an endometrial biopsy during the luteal phase on day 20 to 22 of the cycle provide additional evidence of progesterone secretion. In

TABLE 322-1 Concentrations, metabolic clearance rates, and production rates of the major ovarian steroid hormones in blood of ovulatory women

Steroid	Binding	Phase of menstrual cycle	Plasma concentration nmol/L (ng/ml)	Production rate, μmol/d (mg/d)
Estradiol	TeBG and albumin	Follicular	0.07–2.6 (0.02–0.7)	0.3–3.6 (0.08–1.0)
		Luteal	0.7 (0.2)	0.9 (0.25)
Estrone	Albumin	Follicular	0.2–1.1 (0.05–0.3)	0.4–2.6 (0.1–0.7)
		Luteal	0.4 (0.1)	0.9 (0.24)
Progesterone	CBG and albumin	Follicular	3 (1)	6.4 (2)
		Luteal	16–80 (5–25)	80 (25)
Androstenedione	Albumin	—	5.6 (1.6)	10 (3)
Testosterone	TeBG and albumin	—	1.4 (0.4)	0.9 (0.25)

NOTE: TeBG, testosterone-binding globulin; CBG, cortisol-binding globulin; MCR, metabolic clearance rate.
SOURCE: Derived in part from MB Lipsett, in *Reproductive Endocrinology*, SSC Yen, RB Jaffe (eds). Philadelphia, Saunders, 1986.

addition measurement of serum progesterone by radioimmunoassay can be used to estimate progesterone secretion by the corpus luteum.

Androgen Under normal conditions the ovary secretes androstenedione, testosterone, and dehydroepiandrosterone. In conditions of androgen excess, hirsutism and/or virilization are common. The evaluation of androgen excess is discussed in Chap. 54.

DIAGNOSIS OF PREGNANCY Pregnancy is usually suspected and diagnosed on the basis of the history and findings on physical examination. Namely, a woman with previous cyclic, predictable menses develops amenorrhea accompanied by breast tenderness, malaise, lassitude, and nausea, and on physical examination a softening and enlargement of the uterus is found.

Laboratory assays of placental products excreted in urine facilitate the diagnosis of pregnancy. Human chorionic gonadotropin (hCG) is secreted by the trophoblastic cells of the placenta into the maternal plasma and excreted in the urine. Assays of urinary hCG make it feasible to detect the presence of functioning trophoblasts earlier than can be recognized by clinical assessments. Assays for measurement of hCG content of serum or urine utilize either antibody against hCG or receptor for hCG. With radioimmunoassays and simplified immunoassay kits it is possible to detect pregnancies 8 to 10 days after ovulation and before the first missed menstrual period. Radioimmunoassay of the β subunit of hCG in serum or urine makes it possible to differentiate between excess LH and hCG, an important distinction in evaluating women with trophoblastic disease such as hydatidiform mole or choriocarcinoma.

DISORDERS OF OVARIAN FUNCTION

PREPUBERTAL YEARS Puberty is said to be precocious if the onset of breast budding occurs before age 8 or if menarche commences before age 9. Those disorders in which the developing sexual characteristics are appropriate for the genetic and gonadal sex, i.e., feminization in girls or virilization in boys, are termed *isosexual precocity*, whereas *heterosexual precocity* occurs when sexual characteristics are not in accord with the genetic sex, namely virilization in girls or feminization in boys. Pubertal disorders of boys are described in Chap. 321.

Isosexual precocious puberty Isosexual precocious puberty in girls can be divided into three major categories (Table 322-2).

TRUE PRECOCIOUS PUBERTY True precocious puberty is characterized by an early but otherwise normal sequence of pubertal development, including increased secretion of gonadotropins and ovulatory menstrual cycles. Constitutional or idiopathic precocious puberty comprises 90 percent of cases. In these individuals no cause for the premature maturation of the central nervous system–hypothalamic-pituitary axis can be identified, and the diagnosis is one of exclusion. As many as half of these individuals have abnormal electroencephalograms. Premature appearance of secondary sexual characteristics and of ovulatory cycles with the accompanying risk of fertility may result in significant emotional disturbances. Therefore, prompt initiation of therapy is imperative. The usual treatment is medroxyprogesterone acetate in doses of 100 to 200 mg given intramuscularly every 2 to 4 weeks to suppress gonadotropin secretion. Such a regimen is usually effective in inhibiting ovarian estrogen production and ovulation but does not consistently control bone growth or prevent premature epiphyseal closure and the resultant short stature. LHRH analogues have been utilized to inhibit estrogen synthesis and thus inhibit precocious puberty, and there is evidence to suggest that they also prevent premature closure of the epiphyses.

About 10 percent of cases are due to organic brain diseases, including brain tumors (hypothalamic gliomas, astrocytomas, ependymomas, germinomas, and hamartomas), encephalitis, meningitis, hydrocephalus, head injury, tuberous sclerosis, and neurofibromatosis. It is essential to separate this group of patients from those with the idiopathic disorder, and patients designated as idiopathic occasionally

---

TABLE 322-2 Differential diagnosis of sexual precocity

I Isosexual precocity
  A True precocious puberty
    1 Constitutional
    2 Organic brain disease
    3 Congenital adrenal hyperplasia
  B Precocious pseudopuberty
    1 Ovarian tumors
    2 Adrenal tumors
    3 McCune-Albright syndrome
    4 Hypothyroidism
    5 Silver syndrome
    6 Estrogen-containing medications
  C Incomplete sexual precocity
    1 Premature thelarche
    2 Premature adrenarche
    3 Premature pubarche
II Heterosexual precocity
  A Ovarian tumors
  B Adrenal tumors
  C Congenital adrenal hyperplasia

---

prove to have such tumors. Fortunately, most patients with organic lesions serious enough to cause precocious puberty have obvious neurologic signs and symptoms. Evaluation of all patients with precocious puberty should include, at a minimum, skull films and computed tomography scans of the brain. The success of treatment depends upon the nature of the lesion, but surgical and radiation treatment of well-localized tumors is occasionally successful.

A rare cause of isosexual precocity is virilizing congenital adrenal hyperplasia due to 21-hydroxylase deficiency in girls in whom treatment is delayed until 4 to 8 years of age. After initiation of glucocorticoid replacement, such individuals may undergo true isosexual precocious puberty (see Chap. 317).

PRECOCIOUS PSEUDOPUBERTY Precocious pseudopuberty occurs when girls feminize as a consequence of enhanced estrogen formation but do not ovulate or develop cyclic menses. Ovarian cysts or tumors that secrete estrogen (granulosa-theca cell tumors) are the most frequent cause of precocious pseudopuberty. Granulosa-theca-cell tumors associated with intestinal polyps and pigmentation of the mucous membranes occur in the Peutz-Jeghers syndrome. Other ovarian tumors that secrete estrogens (or androgens that can be converted to estrogens at extraglandular sites) include dysgerminomas, teratomas, cystadenomas, and ovarian carcinomas (also see Chap. 304). Ovarian tumors can usually be detected by rectoabdominal examination, and sonography, computed tomography, and/or laparoscopy may also be of help. Ovarian teratomas and choriocarcinomas and other carcinomas that secrete hCG do not cause precocious puberty in girls unless there is concomitant secretion of estrogen by the tumor (hCG or LH in the absence of FSH does not induce ovarian estrogen production). Rarely, feminizing tumors of the adrenal cause isosexual precocious puberty, either by formation of estrogens directly or by secretion of weak androgens to serve as estrogenic precursors in extraglandular tissues.

Other causes of precocious pseudopuberty include the following: (1) The McCune-Albright syndrome (polyostotic fibrous dysplasia), characterized by café au lait spots, cystic fibrous dysplasia of bones, and sexual precocity. Some of these individuals have increased gonadotropin secretion, whereas others have functional ovarian cysts in the presence of low gonadotropins, which represents a form of gonadotropin-independent sexual precocity. Occasionally, this disorder leads to true precocious puberty (see Chap. 325). (2) Primary hypothyroidism in which secretion of thyrotropin-releasing hormone (TRH) as well as the secretion of other hypothalamic hormones is enhanced, leading to increased FSH levels and ovarian estrogen secretion, frequently with galactorrhea. (3) The Silver syndrome, or congenital asymmetry associated with short stature and precocious feminization. (4) Estrogen-containing medications including use of estrogen-containing creams for diaper rash or the ingestion of meat from estrogen-treated animals or poultry or any estrogen by mouth.

INCOMPLETE ISOSEXUAL PRECOCITY   This term is used to describe the premature development of a single pubertal event and encompasses several entities. The appearance of breast budding prior to the age of 8 (premature thelarche) without other evidence of estrogen secretion and without premature bone maturation is believed to be due to a transient increase in estrogen secretion or a temporary increase in sensitivity to the small amounts of circulating estrogens formed prior to puberty. Usually the disorder is self-limited and resolves spontaneously. Occasionally axillary hair and/or pubic hair (so-called *premature adrenarche* and *pubarche*) appear without any other secondary sexual development. The phenomenon is associated with adrenal androgen secretion in the range of normal puberty and can be distinguished from syndromes of virilization by the absence of clitoromegaly. It requires no treatment, and patients enter puberty at about the average time.

Heterosexual precocity   Virilization in a prepubertal female is usually due to congenital adrenal hyperplasia or to androgen secretion by an ovarian or adrenal tumor. The manifestations of virilization are described in Chap. 54. Virilization in girls with congenital adrenal hyperplasia usually takes place in a background of variable sexual ambiguity (see Chap. 324).

Evaluation of sexual precocity   The evaluation of sexual precocity involves a careful history and physical examination including rectoabdominal examination, abdominal sonography, determination of bone age, and measurement of gonadotropins (and androgen or estrogen levels when appropriate). Skull films and further diagnostic tests are indicated if a neurologic disorder is suspected and no evidence of ovarian or adrenal tumor is found.

REPRODUCTIVE YEARS Disorders of the menstrual cycle   ABNORMAL UTERINE BLEEDING   Between menarche and the menopause, almost every woman experiences one or more episodes of abnormal uterine bleeding, here defined as any bleeding pattern that differs in frequency, duration, or amount from the pattern observed during a normal menstrual cycle. A variety of descriptive terms (such as *menorrhagia, metrorrhagia,* and *menometrorrhagia*) have been used to characterize patterns of abnormal uterine bleeding. A more logical approach is to divide abnormal uterine bleeding into those patterns associated with ovulatory cycles and those associated with anovulatory cycles.

OVULATORY CYCLES   Normal menstrual bleeding with ovulatory cycles is spontaneous, regular, cyclic, and predictable and frequently associated with discomfort (dysmenorrhea). Deviations from this pattern associated with cycles that are still regular and predictable are most often due to organic disease of the outflow tract. For example, regular but prolonged and excessive bleeding episodes unassociated with bleeding dyscrasias (hypermenorrhea or menorrhagia) can result from abnormalities of the uterus such as submucous leiomyomas, adenomyosis, or endometrial polyps. Regular, cyclical, predictable menstruation characterized by spotting or light bleeding is termed *hypomenorrhea* and is due to obstruction of the outflow tract as from intrauterine synechiae or scarring of the cervix. Intermenstrual bleeding between episodes of regular, ovulatory menstruation is also often due to cervical or endometrial lesions. An exception to the association between organic disease of the uterus and abnormal uterine bleeding is the occurrence of episodes of regular bleeding more frequently than 21 days apart (polymenorrhea). These cycles may be a normal variant.

ANOVULATORY CYCLES   Uterine bleeding that is unpredictable with respect to amount, onset, and duration and is usually painless is described as *dysfunctional uterine bleeding*. This disorder is not due to abnormalities of the uterus but rather to chronic anovulation and occurs when there is interruption of the normal progressive sequence of follicular and luteal phases under the influence of a dominant follicle and its resulting corpus luteum. As discussed above normal uterine bleeding in ovulatory cycles is due to progesterone

withdrawal and requires that the endometrium first be primed with estrogen (when castrates or postmenopausal women are given progesterone withdrawal bleeding usually does not occur).

Dysfunctional uterine bleeding can occur in women who have a transient disruption of the synchronous hypothalamic-pituitary-ovarian patterns necessary for regular ovulatory cycles, most often at the extremes of the reproductive life, namely in the early menarche and in the perimenopausal period, but also as the secondary consequence of temporary stresses or intercurrent illnesses.

On the other hand, primary *dysfunctional uterine bleeding* can result from at least three pathophysiologic mechanisms.

1 *Estrogen withdrawal bleeding* occurs when estrogen is given to a castrate or postmenopausal woman and then withdrawn. As in other types of dysfunctional uterine bleeding, this form of menstrual bleeding is usually painless.
2 *Estrogen breakthrough bleeding* occurs when there is prolonged continuous estrogen stimulation of the endometrium not interrupted by cyclic progesterone secretion and withdrawal. This is the most common type of dysfunctional uterine bleeding and is usually due to anovulation associated with chronic acyclic estrogen production as in women with polycystic ovarian disease. Such women may have histories of irregular, unpredictable menses, oligomenorrhea, or amenorrhea (see below). Alternatively, estrogen breakthrough bleeding can occur in hypogonadal women given estrogens chronically rather than intermittently or in women with estrogen-secreting tumors of the ovary. Estrogen breakthrough bleeding may be profuse and is unpredictable with respect to duration, amount of flow, and time of occurrence. The endometrium is typically thin because its repair between episodes of bleeding is incomplete.
3 *Progesterone breakthrough bleeding* occurs in the presence of abnormally high ratios of progesterone to estrogen, for example, in women on continuous low-dose oral contraceptives.

The approach to a patient with dysfunctional uterine bleeding in the reproductive years begins with a careful history of menstrual patterns and prior hormonal therapy. Since not all bleeding from the urogenital tract is from the uterus, rectal, bladder, and vaginal or cervical sources must be excluded by physical examination. If the bleeding is from the uterus a pregnancy-related disorder such as abortion or ectopic pregnancy must also be excluded. Once the diagnosis of dysfunctional uterine bleeding is established a rational approach to management is as follows. During a first episode of dysfunctional bleeding the patient can simply be observed, provided the bleeding is not copious and no evidence of bleeding dyscrasia is present. If bleeding is moderately severe, control can be achieved with relatively high dose estrogen oral contraceptives for 3 weeks. Alternatively, a regimen of three or four low-dose oral contraceptive pills per day for 1 week followed by tapering to the usual dosage for up to 3 weeks is also effective. If uterine bleeding is more severe, hospitalization, bed rest, and intramuscular injections of estradiol valerate (10 mg) and 17α-hydroxyprogesterone caproate (500 mg) or intravenous or intramuscular conjugated estrogens (25 mg) usually control the bleeding. After initial treatment iron replacement should be instituted, and recurrence can be prevented by cyclic oral contraceptives for 2 to 3 months (or more if pregnancy is not desired). Alternatively, menses should be induced every 2 to 3 months with medroxyprogesterone acetate 10 mg by mouth once or twice a day for 10 days. If hormone therapy fails to control uterine bleeding, an endometrial biopsy or dilatation and curettage may be required for diagnosis and therapy. Indeed, uterine sampling may be indicated prior to hormone therapy in women at risk for endometrial cancer (i.e., in women approaching the age of menopause or in the massively obese); endometrial cancer is rare in ovulatory women of reproductive age.

AMENORRHEA   An acceptable definition of amenorrhea is failure of menarche by age 16, irrespective of the presence or absence of secondary sexual characteristics, or the absence of menstruation for 6 months in a woman with previous periodic menses. However, women who do not fulfill these criteria should be evaluated if (1) the subject and/or her family are greatly concerned, (2) no breast development has occurred by age 14, or (3) any sexual ambiguity or virilization is present (Chap. 324). Amenorrhea is usually categorized as either primary (in a woman who has never menstruated) or secondary (in a woman in whom menstruation is present for a variable time and then ceases); some disorders can cause either primary or secondary amenorrhea. For example, most women with gonadal dysgenesis have primary amenorrhea, but occasional such patients have some follicles and ovulate for short periods so that pregnancies may rarely occur. Furthermore, patients with chronic anovulation (polycystic ovarian disease) most often have secondary amenorrhea but occasionally present with primary amenorrhea. For these reasons, categorization of amenorrhea into primary and secondary types is less helpful in the differential diagnosis than a classification based upon the major underlying physiologic derangements: (1) anatomic defects, (2) ovarian failure, and (3) chronic anovulation with or without estrogen present.

Anatomic defects. A variety of anatomic or structural defects of the female genital tract can preclude menstrual bleeding. Starting from the caudal end of the female genital tract, labial agglutination or fusion is often associated with disorders of sexual development, particularly female pseudohermaphroditism (congenital adrenal hyperplasia or exposure to maternal androgens in utero). (See Chap. 324.) Congenital defects of the vagina, imperforate hymen, and transverse vaginal septae can also cause amenorrhea. These women frequently have accumulation of menstrual blood behind the obstruction and may have cyclic, predictable episodes of abdominal pain.

More severe müllerian anomalies include müllerian agenesis (the Mayer-Rokitansky-Küster-Hauser syndrome) (see Chap. 324), second in frequency only to gonadal dysgenesis as a cause of primary amenorrhea. Women with this syndrome have a 46,XX karyotype, female secondary sex characteristics, and normal ovarian function, including cyclical ovulation, but have absence or severe hypoplasia of the vagina. The uterus usually consists of only rudimentary bicornuate cords, but if the uterus contains endometrium, cyclic abdominal pain and accumulation of blood may occur as in other forms of outlet obstruction. One-third of patients have abnormalities of the urogenital tract, and one-tenth have skeletal anomalies, usually involving the spine. The major diagnostic problem is separating müllerian agenesis from complete testicular feminization in which 46,XY genetic males with testes differentiate as phenotypic women with a blind vaginal pouch and an absent uterus. Women with testicular feminization have feminized breasts but a paucity of pubic and axillary hair. The disorder is due to a defect in the androgen-receptor protein that causes profound resistance to the action of testosterone (see Chap. 324). Testicular feminization can be diagnosed by demonstrating a male level of serum testosterone or a 46,XY karyotype, whereas the diagnosis of müllerian agenesis is established by demonstrating a 46,XX karyotype, biphasic basal body temperatures characteristic of ovulating women, and elevated levels of progesterone during the luteal phase.

A rare cause of absence of uterus in 46,XY phenotypic women who are sexually infantile is the so-called testicular regression syndrome or testicular agenesis (see Chap. 324).

Other abnormalities of the uterus that cause amenorrhea include obstruction due to scarring or stenosis of the cervix, often resulting from surgery, electrocautery, laser therapy, or cryosurgery. Destruction of the endometrium (Asherman's syndrome) may follow vigorous curettage, usually in association with postpartum hemorrhage or therapeutic abortion complicated by infection. This diagnosis is confirmed by hysterosalpingography or by direct vision of the endometrial scarring or synechiae using a hysteroscope.

Treatment of disorders of the outflow tract is surgical. Repair of vaginal agenesis results in normal menstruation and potential fertility only if an intact uterus is present.

Ovarian failure. Primary ovarian failure is associated with elevated plasma gonadotropins and can result from several causes. The most frequent cause is *gonadal dysgenesis*, in which the germ cells are lacking and the ovary is replaced by a fibrous streak. (Also see Chaps. 7 and 324.) Women with gonadal dysgenesis can be divided into two broad groups on the basis of chromosomal karyotype. The most common is due to deletion of genetic material in the X chromosomes and accounts for about two-thirds of gonadal dysgenesis. A 45,X karyotype is found in about half, and most have somatic defects including short stature, webbed neck, shield chest, and cardiovascular defects, collectively termed the Turner phenotype. The remainder of patients with identifiable abnormalities of the X chromosome have chromosomal mosaicism with or without associated structural abnormalities of the X chromosome. The most common form of mosaicism is 45,X/46,XX. Gonadal tumors are rare in 45,X patients, but gonadal malignancies have been reported in women with chromosomal mosaicism involving the Y chromosome. Therefore, a chromosomal analysis should be obtained in all cases of amenorrhea associated with ovarian failure, and the streak gonad should be removed if a Y chromosome is present. Approximately 90 percent of individuals with gonadal dysgenesis associated with deletion of genetic material in the X chromosome never have menstrual bleeding, and the remaining 10 percent have sufficient residual follicles to experience menses and, rarely, fertility; the menstrual and reproductive lives of such individuals are invariably brief.

A tenth of subjects with bilateral streak gonads have a normal 46,XX or 46,XY karyotype and are said to have *pure gonadal dysgenesis*. These individuals have either normal or above-average stature due to failure of estrogen-mediated epiphyseal closure in the presence of a normal chromosomal constitution. Pure gonadal dysgenesis does not constitute a phenotypic or chromosomally homogeneous disorder. Some are the result of X-linked or autosomal gene defects. Other possible causes include chromosomal mosaicism limited to gonadal tissue and destruction of germinal tissue in utero by environmental or infectious processes. Approximately one-tenth of such individuals with a 46,XY karyotype develop signs of virilization including clitoromegaly and have an increased incidence of tumors in the gonadal streaks; as a consequence gonadal streaks should be removed prophylactically as previously discussed when a Y chromosome is present. Approximately two-thirds of individuals with 46,XX karyotype experience no menses while the remainder have one or more menstrual episodes and are occasionally fertile.

Other causes of ovarian failure and amenorrhea include 17α-hydroxylase or 17,20-desmolase deficiency, premature ovarian failure, the resistant-ovary syndrome, and ovarian failure secondary to chemotherapy or radiation therapy for malignancy. *17α-Hydroxylase deficiency* is characterized by primary amenorrhea, sexual infantilism, and hypertension that is due to increased production of desoxycorticosterone (DOC), whereas women with 17,20-desmolase deficiency have primary amenorrhea and sexual infantilism with normal blood pressure (see Chaps. 317 and 324). The diagnosis of *premature ovarian failure* or *premature menopause* is applied to women who cease menstruating prior to the age of 40. The ovaries are similar to the ovaries of postmenopausal women, namely, paucity or absence of follicles as the result of accelerated follicular atresia. Premature ovarian failure due to ovarian antibodies may be one component of polyglandular failure together with adrenal insufficiency, hypothyroidism, and other autoimmune disorders (see Chap. 325). A rare form of ovarian failure is the *resistant-ovary syndrome* in which the ovaries contain many follicles arrested in development prior to the antral stage, possibly because of resistance to the action of FSH in the ovary. To differentiate this disorder from the 46,XX variety of pure gonadal dysgenesis, both of which are associated with sexual immaturity, it is necessary to perform ovarian biopsy. However, such a distinction is not clinically useful since the treatment of infertility in both conditions is usually unsuccessful.

CHRONIC ANOVULATION   At least 80 percent or more of gynecologic endocrine problems result from chronic anovulation. Women with chronic anovulation fail to ovulate spontaneously but may ovulate with appropriate therapy. The ovaries of such women do not secrete estrogen in a normal cyclic pattern; it is clinically useful to differentiate those women who produce sufficient estrogen to have withdrawal bleeding after progesterone therapy from those who fail to produce enough estrogen to have progesterone withdrawal bleeding and who often have hypothalamic-pituitary dysfunction.

Chronic anovulation with estrogen present.   Women with chronic anovulation who experience withdrawal bleeding after progesterone administration are said to be in a state of "estrus" due to the acyclic production of estrogen, largely estrone, by extraglandular aromatization of circulating androstenedione. The most common term for this disorder is *polycystic ovarian disease* (PCOD), a syndrome characterized by infertility, hirsutism, obesity, and amenorrhea or oligomenorrhea. When spontaneous uterine bleeding occurs in subjects with PCOD, it is unpredictable with respect to time of onset, duration, and amount, and on occasion the bleeding can be severe. The dysfunctional uterine bleeding is usually due to estrogen breakthrough (see above).

The disorder, which may be transmitted as an autosomal dominant or X-linked trait, was originally described by Stein and Leventhal as characterized by enlarged, polycystic ovaries, but the syndrome and its accompanying endocrine abnormalities are now known to be associated with a variety of pathologic findings in the ovaries, only some of which result in enlargement of the ovaries and none of which are pathognomonic. The most common finding is a white, smooth, sclerotic ovary with a thickened capsule, multiple follicular cysts in various stages of atresia, a hyperplastic theca and stroma, and rare or absent corpora albicans. Other ovaries have hyperthecosis in which the ovarian stroma is hyperplastic and may contain lipid-laden luteal cells. Thus, the diagnosis of PCOD is a clinical one, based upon the coexistence of chronic anovulation and varying degrees of androgen excess.

In most women with PCOD menarche occurs at the expected time, but uterine bleeding is unpredictable in onset, duration, and amount. Amenorrhea ensues after a variable time, although primary amenorrhea occurs in some women. Signs of androgen excess (hirsutism) usually become evident around the time of menarche. One formulation suggests that this disorder originates as an exaggerated adrenarche in obese girls (Fig. 322-7). The combination of elevated adrenal androgens and obesity would result in increased formation of extraglandular estrogen and lead to an acyclic positive feedback on LH secretion and negative feedback on FSH secretion so that the characteristic LH/FSH ratios in plasma would be greater than 2. The increased LH levels could then lead to hyperplasia of the ovarian stroma and theca cells and increased androgen production, which in turn would provide more substrate for peripheral aromatization and perpetuate the chronic anovulation. In the advanced state the ovary is the major site of androgen production, but the adrenal may continue to secrete excess androgen as well. The greater the obesity, the more this sequence would be perpetuated because adipose tissue stromal cells aromatize androgens to estrogens, which in turn exaggerates inappropriate LH release by positive feedback.

Thus, the fundamental defect in PCOD is viewed as one of inappropriate signals to the hypothalamus and pituitary. In fact, the hypothalamic-pituitary axis responds appropriately to high levels of estrogen, and ovulation can be induced with antiestrogens such as clomiphene citrate. Increased levels of plasma endorphins and inhibin may contribute to the perpetuation of the defect. The concept that the fundamental defect is one of inappropriate signals is supported by the findings in the ovary itself. Ovarian follicles from women with PCOD have low aromatase activity, but normal aromatase can be induced when the follicles are treated with FSH. In short, the anovulation is not due to an intrinsic abnormality in the ovary itself but rather the result of FSH deficiency and LH excess. An association exists between PCOD or hyperthecosis, acanthosis nigricans, and insulin resistance. The meaning of this association is not clear.

Treatment of PCOD is directed toward interrupting this self-perpetuating cycle and can be accomplished in several ways, including decreasing ovarian androgen secretion (wedge resection or oral contraceptive agents), decreasing peripheral estrogen formation (weight reduction), enhancing FSH secretion [administration of clomiphene, human menopausal gonadotropin (hMG), LHRH (gonadorelin) by portable infusion pump, or purified FSH (urofollitropin)]. The choice

FIGURE 322-7 Proposed mechanism for the initiation and perpetuation of chronic anovulation in polycystic ovarian disease (PCOD). This cycle may be entered or initiated via adrenal androgen excess or obesity, both of which result in enhanced extraglandular formation of estrogens. The therapy of PCOD involves interruption of the cycle at various sites. (*From SSC Yen and RB Jaffe, 1986, and from U Goebelsmann in DR Mishell, Jr, and V Davajan.*)

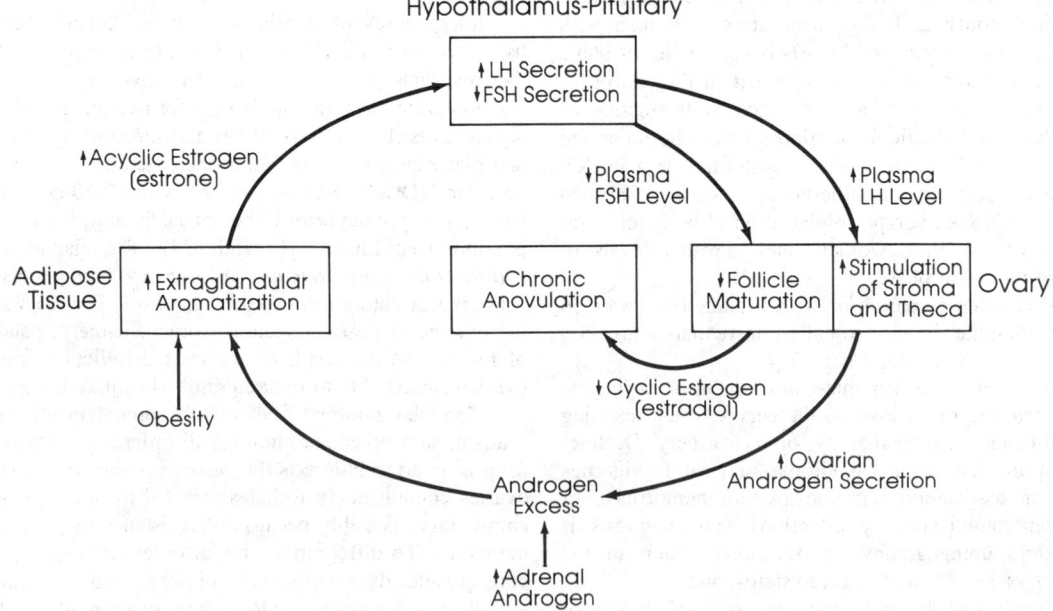

of therapy depends on the clinical findings and the needs of the patient. Attempt at weight reduction is appropriate in all who are obese. If the woman is not hirsute and does not desire pregnancy, periodic withdrawal menses can be induced with medroxyprogesterone acetate 10 days per month; such treatment prevents development of endometrial hyperplasia. If the woman is hirsute but does not desire pregnancy, the ovarian (and possibly the adrenal) component of androgen production can be suppressed with combined estrogen-progestogen oral contraceptive agents. Combined oral contraceptives are also indicated if prolonged or excessive menstrual bleeding is present. Once androgen excess is controlled, treatment of previously existing hair growth by shaving, depilatories, or electrolysis may be indicated (see Chap. 54). If the woman wants to become pregnant, induction of ovulation is necessary. The drug of choice for this purpose is clomiphene, which promotes ovulation in three-fourths of cases, or treatment with hMG, urofollitropin, or gonadorelin. Pretreatment with LHRH analogues prior to hMG, urofollitropin, or gonadorelin has been utilized to improve ovulation and pregnancy rates. Wedge resection of the ovaries is rarely indicated today because of the development of adhesions but may be successful on occasion.

Chronic anovulation with estrogen present may also occur with tumors of the ovary. These include granulosa-theca cell tumors, Brenner tumors, cystic teratomas, mucous cystadenomas, and Krukenberg tumors (also see Chap. 304). These tumors can either secrete excess estrogen themselves or produce androgens that can then be aromatized in extraglandular sites. As a result, chronic anovulation and the clinical features of PCOD are produced. Occasionally areas of the ovary not involved with tumors show the characteristic histologic changes of PCOD. Other causes of chronic anovulation with estrogen present include adrenal production of excess androgen (usually adult onset adrenal hyperplasia due to partial 21-hydroxylase deficiency) and various thyroid disorders.

Chronic anovulation with estrogen absent. Women with chronic anovulation who have low or absent estrogen production and do not experience withdrawal bleeding after progestogen treatment usually have hypogonadotropic hypogonadism due either to pituitary disease or to any of several organic or functional disorders of the central nervous system.

Isolated hypogonadotropic hypogonadism associated with defects of smell (olfactory bulb defects) is known as the Kallman syndrome (see Chaps. 313 and 321). Affected women are sexually infantile with a eunuchoid habitus and appear to have a defect in either the synthesis or release of LHRH. A variety of rare hypothalamic lesions can also impair LHRH production and cause hypogonadotropic hypogonadism; these include craniopharyngioma, germinoma (pinealoma), glioma, Hand-Schüller-Christian disease, teratomas, endodermal-sinus tumors, tuberculosis, sarcoidosis, and metastatic tumors that cause suppression or destruction of the hypothalamus. Central nervous system trauma and radiation can also cause hypothalamic amenorrhea and deficiencies in secretion of growth hormone, ACTH, vasopressin, and thyroid hormone.

More commonly, gonadotropin deficiency leading to chronic anovulation is believed to arise from functional disorders of the hypothalamus or higher centers. A history of a stressful event in a young woman is frequent. For example, chronic anovulation can begin suddenly in a woman who leaves home for the first time or experiences the death of a loved one. Gonadotropin and estrogen levels are in the low to low-normal range as compared to normal women in the early follicular phase of the cycle. In addition, rigorous exercise such as jogging or ballet and diets that result in excessive weight loss may lead to the development of chronic anovulation particularly in girls with a history of prior menstrual irregularity. The amenorrhea in these women does not appear to be due to weight loss alone but to a combination of a decrease in the percentage of body fat and chronic stress. An extreme form of weight loss with chronic anovulation is seen in anorexia nervosa. Anorexia nervosa is char-

acterized by the development in a young woman of amenorrhea with associated severe weight loss, distorted attitudes toward eating and weight gain, self-induced vomiting, extreme emaciation, and distorted body image. Amenorrhea in anorexia nervosa can precede, follow, or appear coincidentally with the loss in body weight (see Chap. 73). During successful therapy gonadotropin changes recapitulate those observed during normal puberty (Fig. 322-1).

In addition, chronic debilitating diseases such as end-stage kidney disease, malignancy, or the malabsorption syndrome are believed to lead to development of hypogonadotropic hypogonadism via a hypothalamic mechanism.

Treatment of chronic anovulation due to hypothalamic disorders includes reversal of the stressful situation, reducing exercise, or correction of weight loss if appropriate. These women appear to be susceptible to the development of osteoporosis, and estrogen replacement therapy to induce and maintain normal secondary sexual characteristics and prevent bone loss is recommended in those who do not desire pregnancy, and gonadotropin or gonadorelin therapy is indicated when pregnancy is desired (see therapy section). When appropriate, therapy is directed at the primary disease of the hypothalamus.

Disorders of the pituitary can lead to the estrogen-deficient form of chronic anovulation by at least two mechanisms—direct interference with gonadotropin secretion by lesions that either obliterate or interfere with the gonadotropic cells (chromophobe adenomas, Sheehan's syndrome) or inhibition of gonadotropin secretion in association with excess prolactin (prolactinoma). *Pituitary tumors* make up approximately 10 percent of all intracranial tumors and may secrete no hormone, one hormone, or more than one hormone (see Chap. 313). In the past most pituitary tumors were assumed to be nonfunctional chromophobe adenomas, but prolactin levels are elevated in 50 to 70 percent of cases, either because of prolactin secretion by the tumor (prolactinomas) or interference by tumor mass with the normal inhibitory influence of the hypothalamus on prolactin secretion.

Prolactinomas can be divided into microadenomas (less than 10 mm in diameter) and macroadenomas (greater than 10 mm). Prolactin excess associated with low levels of LH and FSH constitutes a specific subgroup of hypogonadotropic hypogonadism. One-tenth or more of amenorrheic women have increased levels of serum prolactin, and more than half of women with both galactorrhea and amenorrhea have elevated prolactin levels. The amenorrhea in this disorder is most often associated with decreased or absent estrogen production, but prolactin-secreting tumors may on occasion be associated with normal ovulatory menses or chronic anovulation with estrogen present. Most prolactin-secreting adenomas grow slowly, and some cease growth after attainment of a certain size. The increased frequency of diagnosis of prolactin-secreting adenomas is probably due to several factors, including increased awareness, improved radiographic detection methods, and availability of radioimmunoassays for prolactin. However, since in older autopsy series a 9 to 23 percent prevalence of pituitary adenomas was observed in asymptomatic women, the clinical and prognostic significance of small microadenomas remains to be established. When tumors of any size are associated with symptoms of amenorrhea or galactorrhea, however, therapy should be considered, and when visual field defects or severe headaches are present bromocriptine therapy or neurosurgical evaluation is mandatory. The evaluation, differential diagnosis, and management of hyperprolactinemia is described in Chap. 313. In the latter half of pregnancy, prolactin-secreting pituitary tumors may expand, leading to headaches, compression of the optic chiasm, and blindness. Therefore, prior to induction of ovulation for the purposes of achieving pregnancy, it is mandatory to exclude the presence of a pituitary tumor.

Large pituitary tumors such as chromophobe adenomas—whether or not hyperprolactinemia is present—are likely to be associated with deficiency of hormones in addition to gonadotropins (Chap. 313).

Craniopharyngiomas, thought to arise from remnants of Rathke's pouch, account for 3 percent of intracranial neoplasms, occur most frequently in the second decade of life, and may extend into the suprasellar region. A large percentage of these tumors calcify and can be diagnosed by conventional skull films. Patients often present with sexual infantilism, delayed puberty, and amenorrhea due to gonadotropin deficiency. Craniopharyngioma may also result in impaired secretion of TSH, ACTH, growth hormone, and vasopressin.

Panhypopituitarism may occur spontaneously, result from surgical or radiation treatment of pituitary adenomas, or develop after postpartum hemorrhage (Sheehan's syndrome). The latter patients exhibit characteristic clinical manifestations including failure to lactate or ovulate, loss of genital and axillary hair, hypothyroidism, and adrenal insufficiency (see Chap. 313).

Evaluation of amenorrhea. A general schema for the evaluation of women with amenorrhea is given in Fig. 322-8. In the initial physical examination, special attention should be given to three features: (1) degree of maturation of the breasts, the pubic and axillary hair, and the external genitalia; (2) the current estrogen status; and (3) the presence or absence of a uterus. All women with amenorrhea should be assumed to be pregnant until proven otherwise. Even when history and physical examination are not suggestive, it is prudent to exclude pregnancy by a suitable screening test. Once this is done, the cause of amenorrhea can frequently be diagnosed by history and physical examination. For example, Asherman's syndrome is suggested by a history of curettage in a woman who previously menstruated; in women with primary amenorrhea and sexual infantilism the essential differential diagnosis is between gonadal dysgenesis and hypopituitarism, and, in addition, the diagnosis of gonadal dysgenesis (Turner's syndrome) or of anatomic defects of the outflow tract (müllerian agenesis, testicular feminization, and cervical stenosis) is frequently suggested on the basis of physical findings. When a specific cause is suspected, it is appropriate to proceed directly to confirm the diagnosis (such as obtaining a chromosomal karyotype or measurement of plasma gonadotropins). It is also useful to measure serum prolactin level during the initial evaluation.

Estrogen status is evaluated by determining if the vaginal mucosa is moist and rugated and if the cervical mucus can be stretched and shown to fern upon drying. If these criteria are indeterminate a progestational challenge is indicated, most often administration of 10 mg of medroxyprogesterone acetate by mouth once or twice daily for 5 days or 100 mg of progesterone in oil intramuscularly. (It should be emphasized that progestogen should never be administered until pregnancy is excluded.) If estrogen levels are adequate (and the outflow tract is intact) menstrual bleeding should occur within 1 week of ending the progestogen treatment. If withdrawal bleeding occurs, the diagnosis is chronic anovulation with estrogen present, usually polycystic ovarian disease.

If no withdrawal bleeding or only minimal vaginal spotting occurs, the nature of the subsequent workup is dependent on the results of the initial prolactin assay. If plasma prolactin is elevated or if galactorrhea is present, radiography of the pituitary should be undertaken. When the plasma prolactin is normal in the anovulatory woman with estrogen absent, plasma gonadotropins should be measured. If the gonadotropin levels are elevated, the diagnosis is ovarian failure. If the gonadotropins are in the low or normal range, the diagnosis is either hypothalamic-pituitary disorder or anatomic defect of the outflow tract. As indicated previously, the diagnosis of outflow tract disorder is usually suspected or established on the basis of history and physical findings. When the physical findings are not clear-cut, it is useful to administer cyclic estrogen plus progestogen (1.25 mg of oral conjugated estrogens per day for 3 weeks with 10 mg of medroxyprogesterone acetate added for the last 7 to 10 days of estrogen treatment) followed by 10 days of observation. If no bleeding occurs, the diagnosis of Asherman's syndrome or other anatomic defect of the outflow tract is confirmed by hysterosalpingography or hysteroscopy. If withdrawal bleeding occurs following the estrogen-progestogen combination, the diagnosis of chronic anovulation with estrogen absent (functional hypothalamic amenorrhea) is suggested. Radiologic evaluations of the pituitary-hypothalamic areas may be indicated in the latter cases—irrespective of the prolactin level—because of the danger of overlooking a pituitary-hypothalamic tumor and because the diagnosis of functional hypothalamic amenorrhea is one of exclusion (see Chap. 313).

Infertility Infertility, the failure to become pregnant after 1 year of unprotected intercourse, affects approximately 10 to 15 percent of couples and is one of the common complaints for which women seek gynecologic assistance. Male factors account for 40 percent of infertility problems (see Chaps. 52 and 321). In women, failure of ovulation accounts for 30 percent, pelvic factors such as tubal disease and endometriosis account for half, and a cervical factor is implicated in about one-tenth of infertility evaluations. In 10 to 20 percent of infertile women no etiology is found. An immunologic cause may explain a portion of infertility in these couples. Finally, infertility in women may be due to *luteal phase dysfunction* in which ovulation is assumed to occur but progesterone formation is insufficient to allow preparation of the endometrium for implantation; the disorder

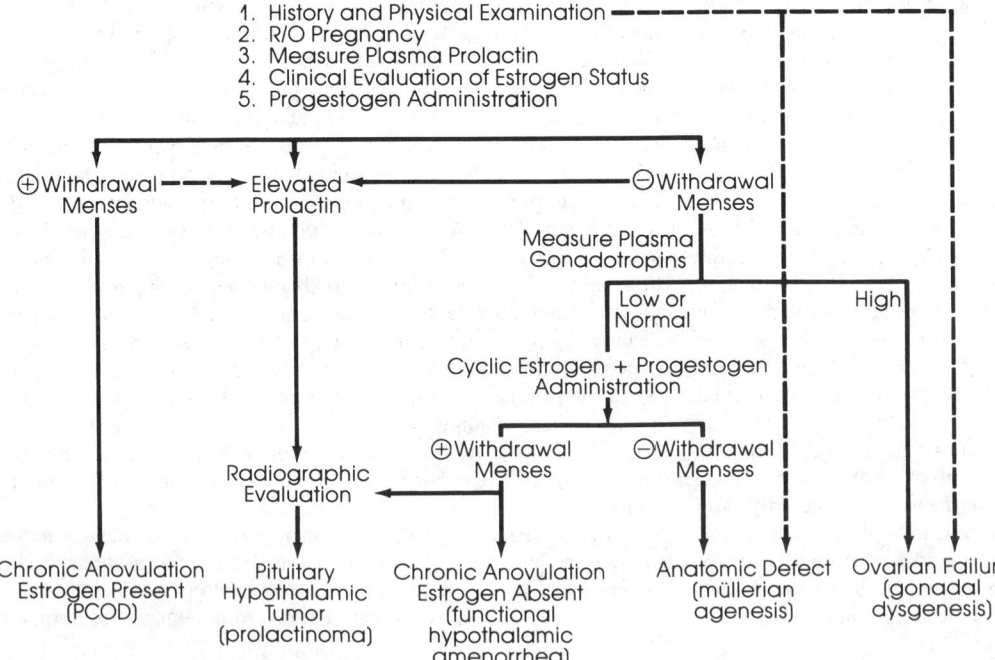

1. History and Physical Examination
2. R/O Pregnancy
3. Measure Plasma Prolactin
4. Clinical Evaluation of Estrogen Status
5. Progestogen Administration

⊕Withdrawal Menses — Elevated Prolactin ← ⊖Withdrawal Menses

Measure Plasma Gonadotropins

Low or Normal — High

Cyclic Estrogen + Progestogen Administration

Radiographic Evaluation — ⊕Withdrawal Menses — ⊖Withdrawal Menses

Chronic Anovulation Estrogen Present (PCOD)

Pituitary Hypothalamic Tumor (prolactinoma)

Chronic Anovulation Estrogen Absent (functional hypothalamic amenorrhea)

Anatomic Defect (müllerian agenesis)

Ovarian Failure (gonadal dysgenesis)

FIGURE 322-8 Flow diagram for the evaluation of women with amenorrhea. The most common diagnosis for each category is shown in parentheses. The dotted lines indicate that in some instances a correct diagnosis can be reached on the basis of history and physical exam alone.

is believed to be due to inadequate FSH secretion or action and consequent inadequate estrogen formation by the dominant follicle during the follicular phase.

The first diagnostic step in evaluation of the infertile couple is to determine whether the man or woman is the infertile partner, ordinarily by first obtaining a semen analysis in the man (see Chap. 321) and demonstration of presumed ovulation in the woman. Documentation of ovulatory cycles is obtained by daily measurement of basal body temperatures throughout the month. Occasionally, accurate basal body temperature records are not obtained, and demonstration of elevated serum progesterone levels during the luteal phase may be used as evidence of ovulation. Dating of endometrium by histologic examination of a biopsy sample is also useful for establishing ovulation or luteal phase dysfunction.

If the infertility is associated with amenorrhea, then the workup is that described in Fig. 322-8. If anovulation due to polycystic ovarian disease is the basis for infertility, ovulation can be induced utilizing clomiphene, gonadotropins, gonadorelin, or, on occasion, wedge resection of the ovaries. Bromocriptine is used to induce ovulation in cases of hyperprolactinemia. In the presence of prolactinomas the appropriate therapy prior to induction of ovulation remains controversial. Recommended therapies in this situation include observation, reinstitution of bromocriptine therapy, radiation therapy, or surgical resection of the tumor (see Chap. 313).

Hysterosalpingograms may be obtained to evaluate the fallopian tubes and uterine cavity. Further evaluation of tubal and ovarian disease is obtained by diagnostic laparoscopy and the demonstration of dye spillage from the fimbria after transcervical injection of dye during laparoscopy. Microsurgical repair of damaged or previously ligated fallopian tubes has resulted in an apparent increase in pregnancy rates. Removal of peritubular and fimbrial adhesions utilizing laser beam surgery is another treatment mode. Endometriosis can be diagnosed by laparoscopy, and treatment of endometriosis associated with infertility includes surgical resection of the endometrial implants or temporary gonadotropin suppression utilizing danazol (400 to 800 mg orally in divided doses for 4 to 6 months), LHRH analogues given by nasal spray or subcutaneous injection, or continuous low-dose oral contraceptive agents to promote regression of the implants.

The cervical factor in infertility is evaluated by study of cervical mucus at an appropriate time after coitus. The test is preferably performed just prior to ovulation (day 12 to 13) when cervical mucus is thin and stretches and provides information as to the penetration and survival of the sperm in the female genital tract. Preferred treatment of infertility due to such abnormality is intrauterine insemination with washed sperm.

When other treatment modalities are unsuccessful, in vitro fertilization and embryo transfer (IVF-ET) may be tried. Indications for the use of IVF-ET in infertile couples include tubal obstructive disease, cervical factors, endometriosis, oligospermia, and unexplained infertility. Multiple follicles are induced with clomiphene and/or gonadotropins, and follicles are obtained by laparoscopy or transabdominal or transvaginal aspiration with ultrasound monitoring. After fertilization and cleavage, embryos are transferred to the uterine cavity. Although pregnancy rates vary, successful pregnancy has been reported in as high as 30 percent of cases after IVF-ET. Other techniques that have been successful include a modification of IVF-ET, known as gamete-intrafallopian transfer (GIFT) in which a mixture of sperm and ova are introduced into the end of the fallopian tube at laparoscopy, and intrauterine insemination after gonadotropin stimulation.

Medical aspects of pregnancy The possibility of pregnancy should be considered in all women of reproductive age who are evaluated for medical illness or considered for surgery. Procedures such as x-ray exposure, drugs, and anesthetics may be harmful to the developing fetus, and a variety of medical problems may worsen during pregnancy, including hypertension; diseases of the heart, lungs, kidney, and liver; and metabolic and endocrine disorders. Indeed, all women who present with abnormal vaginal bleeding or amenorrhea during the reproductive years should be assumed to have a complication of pregnancy, such as incomplete abortion, ectopic pregnancy, or trophoblastic disease (hydatidiform mole or choriocarcinoma). Women who present with these complications of pregnancy often have histories of abdominal pain and vaginal bleeding and may have evidence of intraabdominal hemorrhage.

Choriocarcinoma is a particular problem because of its protean manifestations. Half of these malignancies follow pregnancies complicated by hydatidiform mole, and the remainder occur after spontaneous abortion, ectopic pregnancy, or normal deliveries. Patients may present with intraabdominal bleeding due to rupture of the uterus, liver, or ovary, with pulmonary manifestations (cough, hemoptysis, pleuritic pain, dyspnea, and respiratory failure), or with gastrointestinal symptoms, usually chronic blood loss or melena. In addition, patients can present with cerebral metastases or renal involvement. The diagnosis can be established by demonstrating an elevated level of the β subunit of hCG in plasma. Treatment and cure are possible with chemotherapeutic agents (dactinomycin and/or methotrexate). (For manifestations of choriocarcinoma in men see Chap. 305.)

Ovarian tumors See Chap. 304.

TREATMENT

PROGESTOGENS The major use of progestogen is in conjunction with estrogen to ensure the full maturation of the endometrium, both in combination birth control pills and in the therapy of hypogonadal states. In certain circumstances, however, progestogen therapy is appropriate by itself—to induce a progestational effect on the estrogen-primed endometrium (diagnostic tests for the evaluation of amenorrhea), to inhibit pituitary gonadotropins (precocious puberty in girls, and the progestogen-only birth control pill), for prophylaxis to prevent hyperplasia in PCOD, and for palliation in endometrial and breast carcinoma or treatment of endometriosis. Even when a direct progestational effect is desired, the available oral drugs substitute a synthetic derivative for the naturally occurring hormone. Oral progestogens include medroxyprogesterone acetate, megestrol acetate, norethindrone, norgestrel, and micronized progesterone. Parenteral agents include progesterone in oil, medroxyprogesterone acetate suspension, and 17-hydroxyprogesterone caproate. Vaginal progesterone suppositories are used for treatment of luteal phase defects.

The most common undesirable side effect is breakthrough bleeding, which occurs when progestogens are used continuously. Other complications include nausea, vomiting, and hirsutism. Abnormal liver function is a side effect of those derivatives with alkyl substitution in the 17α position. Progestogens are contraindicated if pregnancy is known or suspected because of the risk of birth defects.

ESTROGENS Estrogenic drugs are used for three purposes—the treatment of gonadal failure, control of fertility, and in the management of dysfunctional uterine bleeding and carcinoma of the breast. (The use of estrogens in management of carcinoma of the breast is discussed in Chap. 303.) However, none of the presently available orally active or parenteral hormones replaces the pattern of concentration of estradiol characteristic of the normally cycling, premenopausal woman (Fig. 322-5). Estrogens that can be given by mouth are either nonsteroidal agents (such as diethylstilbestrol) that mimic the action of estradiol, estrogen conjugates that must be hydrolyzed before they become active (estrogen sulfates, predominantly estrone sulfate from pregnant mare's urine), or estrogen analogues that cannot be metabolized to estradiol (mestranol, quinestrol) (Fig. 322-9). Even when micronized estradiol is given orally, it is rapidly converted in the body to estrone. Because oral therapy neither replaces nor mimics the daily secretory pattern of the lost hormone, such therapy must be viewed as a pharmacologic substitution rather than a physiologic replacement. Likewise, the use of parenteral estrogens rarely mimics the physiologic situation. Parenteral preparations of conjugated es-

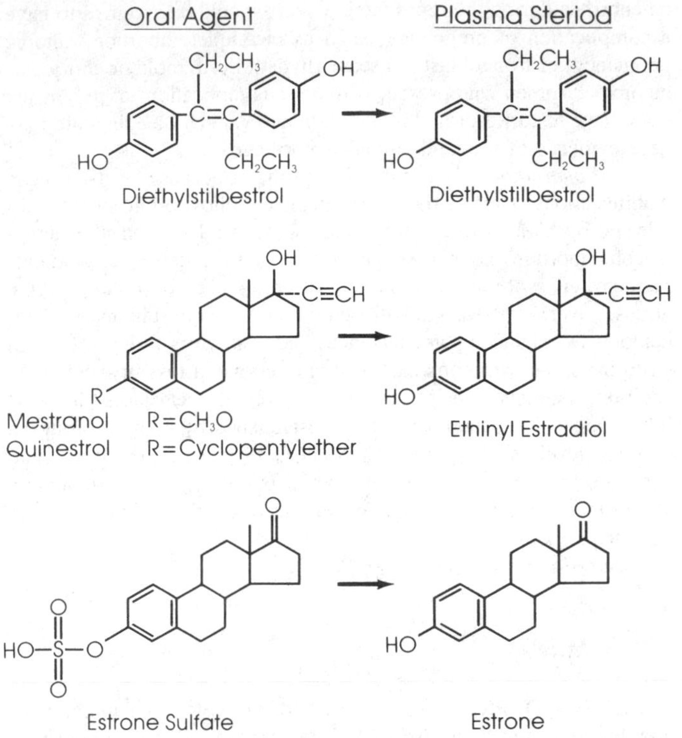

Oral Agent

Plasma Steriod

Diethylstilbestrol

Diethylstilbestrol

Mestranol   R=CH₃O
Quinestrol   R=Cyclopentylether

Ethinyl Estradiol

Estrone Sulfate

Estrone

FIGURE 322-9 The circulating forms of administered estrogenic drugs.

trogens, like the oral derivatives, are poor precursors of estradiol, and estradiol esters (estradiol benzoate and valerate) rarely cause plasma estradiol levels that mimic the normal monthly secretory pattern of the hormone. Transdermal estrogen results in constant levels of blood estrogen and is effective in the treatment of menopausal symptoms. The side effects of estrogen substitution differ at various times of life.

Hypoestrogenism In women with decreased estrogen production, whether due to disease of the ovaries (gonadal dysgenesis) or to hypogonadotropic hypogonadism, treatment with cyclic estrogens should be instituted at the time of expected puberty for development and maintenance of female secondary sexual characteristics and prevention of osteoporosis. The most commonly used medications are conjugated estrogens (0.625 to 1.25 mg per day by mouth) or ethinyl estradiol or its precursors (0.02 to 0.05 mg by mouth). The addition of medroxyprogesterone acetate (5 to 10 mg daily) is recommended by most physicians during the last several days of monthly estrogen treatment to prevent development of endometrial hyperplasia during long-term estrogen treatment. Abnormal bleeding in women receiving estrogen replacement requires histologic evaluation of the endometrium. Such substitution therapy or the use of oral contraceptives (see below) may also be used for the purpose of suppressing pituitary gonadotropins, as in women with PCOD in whom the major therapeutic aim is suppression of ovarian androgen production prior to the time when fertility is desired.

Temporary administration of estrogens in larger quantities (up to two times the usual adult maintenance dose) may be necessary to induce full development of secondary sexual characteristics in girls and for the control of menopausal symptoms. Even larger doses of parenteral estrogens (10 mg of estradiol valerate or 25 mg of conjugated estrogen) in conjunction with progestogen may be required in some instances of dysfunctional uterine bleeding. Estrogen replacement (100 ng/kg) stimulates growth in women with gonadal dysgenesis, but at high doses (400 ng/kg) has no effect on growth. In addition to the potential long-term side effects of all estrogens (see below), these dosages may cause specific problems including nausea, vomiting, and edema.

Fertility control Since the use of all contraceptive methods is associated with diverse side effects, an understanding of the use, methods of actions, and consequences of these agents is important to all physicians. Furthermore, since pregnancy may aggravate a variety of chronic illnesses, fertility control should be recommended in many patients.

To be effective, fertility control requires patient acceptance and compliance. The most widely utilized methods include (1) rhythm and withdrawal techniques; (2) barrier methods including the condom, jellies, foam, suppositories, and diaphragms; (3) intrauterine devices (IUD); (4) hormonal contraceptives; (5) sterilization; and (6) abortion.

The rhythm and withdrawal technique and the barrier methods are effective if used correctly and consistently but in actual practice result in high failure rates because of imperfect compliance. Nevertheless, these methods carry the lowest incidence of side effects, and the side effects, when produced, are minor except for local allergic reactions. Their use should be recommended when there is a relative or absolute contraindication to other therapy.

The most widely utilized nonsurgical methods of contraception, the IUD and birth control pills, are effective but may be associated with significant side effects.

IUD The success rates of most IUDs are 95 to 98 percent. Only two devices are marketed in the United States. Both are T-shaped, cause minimal pain at insertion, and are associated with low expulsion rates. One of these IUDs contains copper, which enhances effectiveness, and is replaced at 4-year intervals. The other contains slow-release progesterone, which makes annual replacement necessary. The IUD is believed to prevent pregnancy by the induction of a chronic inflammatory reaction in the endometrium, resulting in an unfavorable environment for the implantation of the blastocyst.

Once the IUD is inserted, it is necessary to check periodically to be certain that the device is in place. Both minor and serious side effects can occur. Intermenstrual spotting and increased bleeding and pain or cramps at the time of menses are frequent causes of discontinuation of the IUD. In addition, the device may be expelled spontaneously during a menstrual period without the subject being aware of its loss. The most serious side effect is pelvic infection, occasionally leading to the development of tuboovarian abscess and subsequent infertility. The incidence of pelvic infection is more frequent than in users of oral or barrier contraceptives but no greater than in women using no contraception. Women with multiple sex partners are at greatest risk for pelvic infection. For this reason, use in nulligravida women is not advocated by many gynecologists. In addition, pregnancy with an IUD in place is more likely to be ectopic since intrauterine but not extrauterine pregnancies are inhibited. Because of the increased incidence of spontaneous and septic abortions when IUDs are in place, the device should be removed if pregnancy is detected. Any user who develops persistent, severe bleeding, lower abdominal pain, fever, or discharge should have the IUD removed.

ORAL CONTRACEPTIVES Oral contraceptive agents have been used by over 200 million women worldwide and by 1 out of 4 women in the United States under the age of 45. These agents are popular because of ease of administration, low pregnancy rate (less than 1 percent), and a relatively low incidence of side effects.

The most widely utilized oral contraceptive pills are either combination tablets or biphasic or triphasic formulations. A list of oral contraceptives marketed in the United States is given in Table 322-3. Combination oral contraceptive tablets contain one of two synthetic estrogens (mestranol or ethinyl estradiol) and one of five synthetic progestogens (norethindrone, norethindrone acetate, norethynodrel, norgestrel, or ethynodiol diacetate). The agents now available all contain no more than 50 μg ethinyl estradiol or its equivalent. The combination or biphasic or triphasic tablets are taken for 21 consecutive days followed by 7 days' rest. Progestogen-only tablets are taken continuously on a daily basis. Presumably, the ideal contraceptive contains the lowest amount of steroid to minimize side effects but an amount that is at the same time sufficient to prevent

TABLE 322-3   Composition of currently marketed oral contraceptives

Name	Estrogen	μg	Progestogen	mg
COMBINATION-TYPE				
Fixed type				
Estrogen content = 50 μg:				
Ortho-Novum 1/50	Mestranol	50	Norethindrone	1.0
Norinyl 1/50	Mestranol	50	Norethindrone	1.0
Ovcon 50	Ethinyl estradiol	50	Norethindrone	1.0
Ovral	Ethinyl estradiol	50	Norgestrel	0.5
Demulen	Ethinyl estradiol	50	Ethynodiol diacetate	1.0
Norlestrin 2.5/50	Ethinyl estradiol	50	Norethindrone acetate	2.5
Norlestrin 1/50	Ethinyl estradiol	50	Norethindrone acetate	1.0
Estrogen content <50 μg:				
Ortho-Novum 1/35	Ethinyl estradiol	35	Norethindrone	1.0
Norinyl 1+35	Ethinyl estradiol	35	Norethindrone	1.0
Modicon	Ethinyl estradiol	35	Norethindrone	0.5
Brevicon	Ethinyl estradiol	35	Norethindrone	0.5
Ovcon 35	Ethinyl estradiol	35	Norethindrone	0.4
Demulen 1/35	Ethinyl estradiol	35	Ethynodiol diacetate	1.0
Loestrin 1.5/30	Ethinyl estradiol	30	Norethindrone acetate	1.5
Loestrin 1/20	Ethinyl estradiol	20	Norethindrone acetate	1.0
Nordette	Ethinyl estradiol	30	Levonorgestrel	0.15
Lo-Ovral	Ethinyl estradiol	30	Norgestrel	0.3
Biphasic type				
Ortho-Novum 10/11				
First 10 days	Ethinyl estradiol	35	Norethindrone	0.5
Next 11 days	Ethinyl estradiol	35	Norethindrone	1.0
Triphasic type				
Ortho-Novum 7/7/7				
First 7 days	Ethinyl estradiol	35	Norethindrone	0.5
Second 7 days	Ethinyl estradiol	35	Norethindrone	0.75
Third 7 days	Ethinyl estradiol	35	Norethindrone	1.0
Tri-Norinyl				
First 7 days	Ethinyl estradiol	35	Norethindrone	0.5
Next 9 days	Ethinyl estradiol	35	Norethindrone	1.0
Next 5 days	Ethinyl estradiol	35	Norethindrone	0.5
Triphasil				
First 6 days	Ethinyl estradiol	30	Levonorgestrel	0.05
Second 5 days	Ethinyl estradiol	40	Levonorgestrel	0.075
Third 10 days	Ethinyl estradiol	30	Levonorgestrel	0.125
Tri-Levein				
First 6 days	Ethinyl estradiol	30	Levonorgestrel	0.05
Second 5 days	Ethinyl estradiol	40	Levonorgestrel	0.075
Third 10 days	Ethinyl estradiol	30	Levonorgestrel	0.125
PROGESTOGEN ONLY				
Micronor	None		Norethindrone	0.35
Nor Q.D.	None		Norethindrone	0.35
Ovrette	None		Norgestrel	0.075

pregnancy or breakthrough bleeding. The triphasic tablets containing 35 μg or less of estrogen and less than 1 mg of progestogen come closest to this goal.

Oral contraceptives inhibit ovulation by suppressing FSH and LH secretion. As a consequence, the secretion of all ovarian steroids is also suppressed, including estrogen, progesterone, and androgen (Fig. 322-10). These agents also exert minor direct inhibitory effects on the reproductive tract, altering the cervical mucus and thereby decreasing sperm penetration and decreasing the motility and secretions of the fallopian tubes and uterus.

The death rates associated with oral contraceptives and other forms of birth control are summarized in Table 322-4. Up to age 40 the mortality rates in women using oral contraceptives and IUDs are lower than in women using no form of contraception (this difference is because of the increased risk of death associated with pregnancy). The decrease in death rate below age 40 is even more striking in nonsmokers than in smokers using contraceptives. In fact, the death rates in nonsmoking women age 15 to 24 who use oral agents are lower than those with other forms of fertility control. The increased death rates in women using rhythm or barrier techniques probably results from the higher failure rate and the consequent risk of pregnancy in such women. Oral contraceptive agents are not recommended for smoking women after age 35, rarely in women after age 40, and women of all ages who are at increased risk for myocardial infarction.

Despite the overall safety of these agents, users are at risk for several serious side effects. In most retrospective and prospective studies an increased incidence has been found for *deep vein thrombosis* and *pulmonary embolism*. The relative increased risk varies from two- to twelvefold and is greater for women taking tablets containing more than 50 μg estrogen. The use of oral contraceptives is also associated with an increased risk of thromboembolism after surgery, and for this reason these agents should be discontinued at least 1 month prior to elective surgery. In retrospective studies there is a 3- to 9-times increased risk for *thromboembolic stroke* and a twofold greater risk for *hemorrhagic stroke* in users of oral contraceptives. However, three large prospective studies have demonstrated only a slight increase in hemorrhagic stroke in oral contraceptive users. Therefore, the drugs should be discontinued in women who experience visual complaints or severe headaches. Smoking and age increase the risk for stroke as well as the frequency of death from complications of deep venous thrombosis, pulmonary emboli, and myocardial infarction.

A small rise in blood pressure while taking oral contraceptives is common, and 5 percent of women develop significant *hypertension*

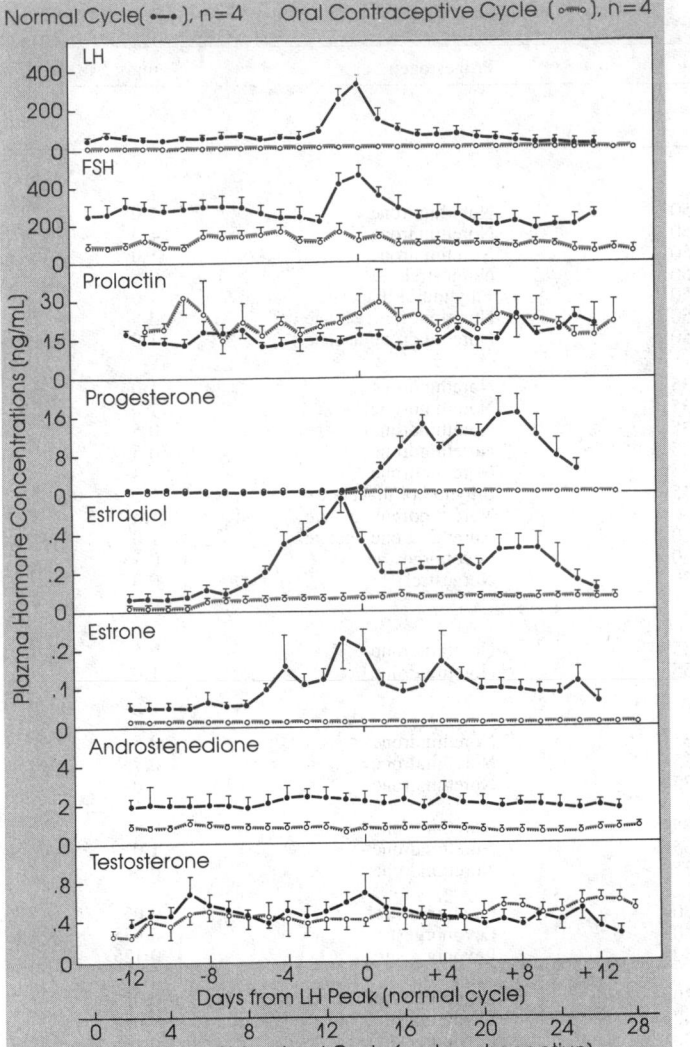

Normal Cycle(●–●), n=4   Oral Contraceptive Cycle (○–○), n=4

FIGURE 322-10 The mechanism of action of the birth control tablet. Mean daily plasma hormone concentrations during the ovarian cycle are shown for four ovulating women and four women treated with combination-type oral contraceptives. Data for the normal ovarian cycle are presented in relationship to the day of the LH peak; day 1 of the contraceptive cycle corresponds to the first day of uterine bleeding. The values are the mean ± SE obtained from four women. (*From BR Carr et al, 1979.*)

In most cases, blood pressure returns to normal when oral contraceptives are discontinued.

Serum lipids and lipoproteins are altered in women on oral contraceptives, the nature of the change depending on the specific components of the oral contraceptives. In general, estrogens increase serum high-density (HDL) and very low density lipoproteins (VLDL). Progestogens depress the concentration of HDL.

A few women taking oral contraceptives develop *impairment of glucose tolerance* as manifested by abnormal glucose levels and elevated plasma insulin after an oral glucose load, both of which usually return to normal after discontinuing the agents. Because juvenile-onset and adult-onset diabetes may be associated with increased incidence of cardiovascular disease, it is also preferable to utilize other forms of contraception in these individuals.

Oral contraceptives should not be used by women with abnormal liver function tests or in women with acute or chronic liver disease. A rare complication linked to the long-term use of oral contraceptives is the development of peliosis hepatis, which can cause death due to sudden rupture and hemorrhage of the liver. Cholestatic jaundice may occur in those women predisposed to the development of the syndrome of recurrent jaundice of pregnancy.

Oral contraceptives cause an increased concentration of cholesterol in the bile, which is probably the cause for the twofold increase in *cholelithiasis* and cholecystitis in women on oral contraceptives.

Estrogens induce elevation of a variety of proteins secreted by the liver including cortisol-binding globulin (CBG), testosterone-binding globulin (TeBG), and thyroxine-binding globulin (TBG). Consequently, various laboratory tests of adrenal and thyroid function may be altered and must be interpreted with caution (see Chaps. 312 and 316). Oral contraceptives also slightly lower plasma ACTH levels, possibly due to an inhibitory effect on ACTH secretion or cortisol catabolism. Finally, serum prolactin levels are slightly elevated in women on oral contraceptives, but such treatment is not believed to play a role in the development of pituitary prolactinomas.

Other effects of oral contraceptive pills include minor dyspepsia, breast discomfort, weight gain, development of pigmentation of the face (chloasma), which is augmented by exposure to the sun, and a variety of psychological effects, such as depression and changes in libido. There is no convincing evidence that oral contraceptives are associated with an increased incidence of cancer of the uterus, cervix, or breast. In fact, oral contraceptives have many beneficial effects including control of dysmenorrhea and anovulatory bleeding, prevention of sexually transmitted diseases, and decreased incidence of endometrial and ovarian cancer.

The absolute contraindications to the use of oral contraceptives include previous thromboembolic disorders, cerebral vascular or coronary artery disease, known or suspected carcinoma of the breast or estrogen-dependent neoplasia, undiagnosed abnormal genital bleeding, or known or suspected pregnancy. Relative contraindications must be weighed against the risk-benefit ratio of the oral contraceptive pills and include hypertension, migraine headaches, diabetes mellitus, uterine leiomyomas, sickle cell anemia, hyperlipemia, and elective surgery.

OTHER STEROID CONTRACEPTIVES   Types of steroid contraception

(blood pressure greater than 140/90) after 5 years of continuous use. Estrogens induce the synthesis of a variety of proteins by the liver including the renin substrate angiotensinogen. The resulting increased formation of angiotensin is believed to be involved in the development of hypertension. Alternatively, the progestogen component of oral contraceptives may be associated with increased risk of hypertension.

TABLE 322-4   Annual death rates associated with fertility control per 100,000 women

Contraceptive techniques	Age group					
	15–19	20–24	25–29	30–34	35–39	40–44
None (birth-related)	7.0	7.4	9.1	14.8	25.7	28.2
Oral contraceptives						
Smokers	2.4	3.6	6.8	13.7	51.4	117.6
Nonsmokers	0.5	0.7	1.1	2.1	14.1	32.0
IUD	1.3	1.1	1.3	1.3	1.9	2.1
Abortion	0.5	1.1	1.3	1.9	1.8	1.1
Barrier methods (birth-related)	1.5	1.4	1.0	0.8	1.3	7.6

SOURCE: Adapted from Ory.

other than the conventional oral contraceptives include (1) postcoital contraception and (2) injectable steroids. Use of high-dose estrogen for 5 days during the fertile part of the cycle (the morning-after pill) is an effective method of contraception, but is associated with significant side effects, particularly nausea. Administration of progestogens by injection, implants, or vaginal rings is used infrequently in the United States.

Estrogen treatment of the menopause   The use of estrogens in postmenopausal women with osteoporosis is based on the belief that such therapy may relieve many of the disorders of the menopause and indeed of aging itself. In some parts of the United States by the mid-1970s as many as half of women in the menopausal age group used one or more forms of estrogen replacement for a median period of 5 years, accounting for more than 30 million prescriptions per year.

The menopause is not associated with a simple state of estrogen deprivation since some estrogens continue to be produced but is instead a state of altered estrogen metabolism; the predominant estrogen becomes estrone formed by extraglandular conversion of prehormone rather than estradiol secretion by the ovary. As is true for all estrogen therapy, the estrogen treatment of the menopause is actually a pharmacologic substitution of one or another estrogen analogue for the physiologic estradiol rather than a physiologic replacement of the missing steroid. Estrogens available for replacement therapy include conjugated estrogens, estrogen substitutes (diethylstilbestrol), synthetic estrogen (ethinyl estradiol or derivatives), micronized estradiol, estrogen-containing vaginal creams, and estrogen-containing dermal patches. Regimens associated with low risk of complications include (1) cyclic estrogen therapy in the lowest effective dose for 21 to 25 days per month, and (2) cyclic estrogens plus the addition of progestogen during the last 10 to 13 days of estrogen therapy.

The most clear-cut benefit of estrogen therapy in the menopause is the relief of vasomotor instability (hot flashes) and of atrophy of the urogenital epithelium and skin. Estrogen therapy ameliorates these symptoms in the majority of cases. When estrogen therapy is designed to treat hot flashes alone, such therapy should be continued for only a few years since hot flashes tend to diminish after 3 to 4 years in untreated women.

Several lines of evidence indicate that routine estrogen therapy is beneficial in preventing the complications of menopausal osteoporosis, especially in high-risk women (i.e., thin white women). First, in women undergoing premature menopause the incidence and complication rates of osteoporosis are increased, and long-term estrogen replacement appears to be beneficial. Second, estrogen therapy has short-term positive effects on calcium balance and long-term beneficial effects on bone density. Third, in women given estrogen therapy, the incidence of fractures is decreased.

Of the potential side effects, the possibility of an increased risk of endometrial carcinoma is perhaps most worrisome. The relative risk of developing endometrial adenocarcinoma in estrogen users is between 6 and 8. The risk is increased with duration and dosage of estrogen but is decreased in women given combination estrogen-progestogen therapy.

Despite the large body of evidence linking endometrial carcinoma and estrogen use, two types of doubt have been raised about the clinical significance of the association. First, some epidemiologists have argued that the increased risk associated with estrogens has been exaggerated because of problems inherent in obtaining adequate controls in retrospective analyses. Second, in spite of an increased incidence of endometrial carcinoma in the United States, there was no concomitant increased mortality from this disease. Indeed the increased incidence apparently involves low-grade malignancies which may be difficult to distinguish histologically from various forms of hyperplasia. These forms of malignancy have little effect on life expectancy.

Apprehension concerning worsening of hypertension and thromboembolic disease appears to be due to reports of the effects of estrogen-progesterone oral contraceptive pills during the reproductive years and not to estrogen use in menopausal women. There is no documented evidence that low-dose estrogen therapy in the menopause enhances the development or the severity of thromboembolic disease, breast cancer, or hypertension. Low-dose estrogen treatment in the menopause does not appear to influence the development of atherosclerosis, myocardial infarction, or stroke. Some evidence suggests that in fact estrogens may decrease the incidence of death from myocardial infarction. There is a slightly increased risk for the development of gallbladder disease with estrogen use in the menopause.

A reasonable approach to the use of estrogens in the menopause is as follows: (1) For long-term use, estrogens should be given in the minimal effective doses (0.625 mg conjugated estrogen or 0.01 to 0.02 mg ethinyl estradiol per day). Except when hot flashes preclude intermittent use, the agents are often prescribed for 25 days each month followed by a rest period. (For women with an intact uterus it is the practice in some clinics to give estrogens alone for 15 days, estrogen plus a daily progestogen for an additional 10 to 13 days, and nothing for a week.) (2) Such replacement therapy is indicated routinely in women undergoing premature menopause (surgically induced or spontaneous) at least until the age of normal menopause. (3) Estrogen therapy is also indicated routinely in women of all ages who have severe hot flashes or symptomatic atrophy of the urogenital epithelium. Hot flashes rarely persist for longer than 4 years, so that if given for this purpose the duration of therapy can be limited. (4) In women who have had prior hysterectomy potential benefits of treatment appear to outweigh the dangers. Whether estrogens should be given routinely to all women with intact uteri is unsettled, but the authors prescribe it routinely in the absence of contraindications in hopes of ameliorating osteoporosis (in combination with calcium). (5) Each woman receiving estrogens must be monitored indefinitely and frequently.

DRUGS TO INDUCE OVULATION   The most common treatment for ovulation induction in women with PCOD is *clomiphene*. This antiestrogen is believed to act by binding to estrogen receptors in the hypothalamus and allowing FSH to rise to stimulate follicular development and ultimately result in ovulation. Clomiphene therapy is usually begun in a dose of 50 mg by mouth daily for 5 days commencing on the fifth day of progestin-induced uterine bleeding. If ovulation does not occur, the dose may be increased to 100 or 150 mg per day. Such treatment results in ovulatory cycles in 60 percent of women with PCOD. Additional regimens include clomiphene in combination with human menopausal gonadotropins (hMG), estrogen, glucocorticoids, or human chorionic gonadotropin (hCG).

The most commonly used gonadotropins for induction of ovulation are hMG, urofollitropin, and hCG. These agents are indicated in women who fail to ovulate on clomiphene. (For women with hypogonadotropic hypogonadism urofollitropin is not recommended.) The usual treatment regimen requires 1 to 3 ampuls of hMG or urofollitropin per day over an 8- to 12-day period to achieve adequate follicular stimulation and growth, followed by a single injection of 10,000 units of hCG 12 to 24 h after the last injection of hMG. For women with PCOD, pretreatment with LHRH analogues prior to hMG or urofollitropin appears to improve ovulation and pregnancy rates. Ovulation is successful in 90 percent of women, and pregnancy rates exceed 50 to 60 percent. Measurement of daily estrogen levels and frequent evaluation of ovarian size by ultrasound are indicated to prevent ovarian hyperstimulation. Ovarian hyperstimulation syndrome results from excessive stimulation of ovarian follicles with resultant enlargement of the ovaries and may progress to the development of ascites, hypotension, and shock. Therapy using hMG, urofollitropin, and hCG also carries a 20 percent risk of multiple pregnancies.

Bromocriptine is a dopamine agonist that is effective in inducing ovulation in women with elevated prolactin levels. Treatment is instituted at a usual dosage of 2.5 mg by mouth two or three times a day. Treatment should be discontinued as soon as pregnancy is diagnosed. The management of prolactin-secreting pituitary tumors is discussed in Chap. 313.

Luteinizing hormone–releasing hormone (LHRH, gonadorelin) and analogues Gonadorelin has been used successfully to induce ovulation in infertile women. The agent is infused subcutaneously or intravenously by a portable infusion pump which administers pulses at 90- to 120-min intervals for 10 to 20 days. After ovulation has occurred hCG is given to maintain corpus luteum function.

LHRH analogues that block ovulation have been used to treat a variety of gynecologic disorders; ovulation and ovarian steroidogenesis are inhibited due to down-regulation of LHRH receptors with a resultant decreased release of gonadotropins. Conditions in which these agents are under trial include fertility control, true precocious puberty, endometriosis, uterine leiomyomas, hirsutism, and, in combination with gonadotropins, ovulation induction and in vitro fertilization.

OTHER DISORDERS OF THE FEMALE REPRODUCTIVE TRACT

VULVA Most disorders of the vulva are due to venereal disease, most commonly syphilis (painless chancre), condyloma acuminata (venereal warts), and herpes vulvitis (painful ulcers) (see Chap. 93). All other lesions of the vulva, particularly in older women, must be biopsied. Early biopsy of cancer of the vulva is mandatory, because when it becomes symptomatic (pruritus and bleeding), it has often progressed to an advanced stage.

VAGINA Infections of the vagina usually present as vaginal discharge and pruritus. The most frequent organisms are *Trichomonas*, *Candida albicans*, and *Gardnerella vaginalis* (also see Chap. 93). The diagnosis is made by microscopic examination of the discharge, and appropriate therapy can be instituted utilizing vaginal or oral antibiotics.

Abnormalities of the vagina and cervix in female offsprings of women given diethylstilbestrol during pregnancy include adenosis of the vagina as well as structural abnormalities of the vagina, cervix, and uterus; the risk of developing a rare form of vaginal cancer (adenocarcinoma, clear cell type) is increased (2 per 10,000 exposed women). Periodic examination of women at risk should commence at age 12 to 14, and reevaluation should be undertaken after any episode of abnormal bleeding.

CERVIX Preinvasive lesions of the cervix (also known as cervical intraepithelial neoplasia) as well as invasive carcinoma of the cervix can be detected reliably by obtaining a Papanicolaou smear (Pap smear). Current recommendations by the American Cancer Society are that a Pap smear be obtained every 3 years after 2 negative Pap smears were obtained at yearly intervals. However, many gynecologists recommend yearly Pap smears especially in patients with more than one sexual partner.

UTERUS Only 40 percent of endometrial adenocarcinoma is detected by Pap smears. In women at high risk for endometrial carcinoma (obesity, history of chronic anovulatory cycles, diabetes, hypertension, estrogen treatment), yearly endometrial sampling should be performed. Low-dose oral estrogen therapy rarely causes breakthrough or withdrawal bleeding in menopausal women. Therefore, irrespective of whether the patient is on estrogen therapy, occurrence of postmenopausal bleeding makes it mandatory to obtain a tissue diagnosis to exclude endometrial cancer either by endometrial sampling or by curettage.

One of the most common disorders of the uterus and the most frequent tumor of women (1 of 4 women affected) is the uterine leiomyoma, or fibroid tumor. Three-fourths of women with leiomyoma are asymptomatic, and the diagnosis is made on routine pelvic examination. When associated with excessive menstrual blood loss, excessive size or rapid growth, or significant pelvic pain (see Chap. 53), the preferred treatment is surgical removal by hysterectomy if there is no desire for further childbearing. In young women myo-

mectomy may on occasion be indicated when infertility or repeated fetal wastage is a manifestation or where future childbearing is desired.

FALLOPIAN TUBES AND OVARIES Infectious pelvic inflammatory disease is a common disorder of the fallopian tubes and usually becomes symptomatic after a menstrual period; the symptoms include fever, chills, abdominal pain, and vaginal discharge, and pelvic tenderness on physical examination is common. The initiating organism most often is *chlamydia trachomatis* or *Neisseria gonorrhoeae*, but tuboovarian abscess and sterility are probably caused by mixed aerobic and anaerobic superinfections and require widespectrum antibiotic treatment (see Chap. 94).

Endometriosis is a benign disorder characterized by the presence and proliferation of endometrial tissue (stroma and glands) outside the endometrial cavity. The clinical manifestations are variable. Endometriosis occurs most commonly between the ages of 30 to 40 and is found incidentally at the time of surgery in approximately onefifth of all gynecologic operations. The fertility rate is significantly reduced in affected women. The disorder usually involves the posterior cul-de-sac or the ovaries and can give rise to ovarian enlargement (endometriomas), although it may also involve sites distant to the pelvis (lung, umbilicus). The most significant symptom is pelvic pain, characteristically dysmenorrhea (see Chap. 53). However, the frequency and degree of pelvic symptomatology correlate poorly with the extent of disease. Other symptoms include dyspareunia, pain with defecation, and infertility. The characteristic physical findings are multiple tender nodules palpable along the uterosacral ligament at the time of rectal-vaginal examination, a posteriorly fixed uterus, or enlarged cystic ovaries. The diagnosis can only be confirmed by direct visualization, usually at diagnostic laparoscopy. Treatment depends on the degree of involvement and the desires of the patient and includes observation for mild disease with no associated infertility or pain, hormonal suppressive therapy (see infertility), conservative surgery if fertility is desired, or removal of the uterus, tubes, and ovaries in severe disease. Endometriosis is rarely found after the menopause.

Any adnexal mass that persists for more than 6 weeks or is larger than 6 cm must be evaluated. Although ovarian cysts and neoplasms compose the largest group of pelvic adnexal masses (see above), tumors of the fallopian tubes, uterus, gastrointestinal tract, or urinary tract should also be considered. Sonography or radiographic evaluation is often helpful in identifying the nature of the adnexal mass prior to surgical exploration.

REFERENCES

CARR BR, GRIFFIN JD: Fertility control and its complications, in *Williams' Textbook of Endocrinology*, 7th ed, JD Wilson, DW Foster (eds). Philadelphia, Saunders, 1985, pp 452–475
———— et al: Plasma levels of adrenocorticotropin and cortisol in women receiving oral contraceptive steroid treatment. J Clin Endocrinol Metab 49:346, 1979
———— et al: Plasma lipoprotein regulation or progesterone biosynthesis by human corpus luteum tissue in organ culture. J Clin Endocrinol Metab 52:875, 1981
———— et al: The role of lipoproteins in the regulation of progesterone secretion by human corpus luteum. Fertil Steril 38:303, 1982
CUNNINGHAM FG et al: *Williams' Obstetrics*, 18th ed. Norwalk, Appleton-Lange, 1989
D'ARMIENTO M et al: McCune-Albright syndrome: Evidence for autonomous multiendocrine hyperfunction. J Pediatr 102:584, 1983
DIZEREGA GS, HODGEN GD: Folliculogenesis in the primate ovarian cycle. Endocrinol Rev 2:27, 1981
———— et al: The possible role for a follicular protein in the intraovarian regulation of steroidogenesis. Semin Reprod Endocrinol 1:309, 1983
DMOWSKI WP: Endocrine properties and clinical applications of danazol. Fertil Steril 31:237, 1979
DROEGEMULLER W et al: *Comprehensive Gynecology*. St. Louis, Mosby, 1987
ERICKSON GF et al: Functional studies of aromatase activity in human granulosa cells from normal and polycystic ovaries. J Clin Endocrinol Metab 49:514, 1979
FAIMAN C et al: Patterns of gonadotropins and gonadal steroids throughout life. Clin Obstet Gynaecol 3:467, 1976
FRASIER SD: *Pediatric Endocrinology*. New York, Grune & Stratton, 1980
FUTTERWEIT W: *Polycystic Ovarian Disease*. New York, Springer-Verlag, 1984
GEMZELL C, WANG CF: Outcome of pregnancy in women with pituitary adenoma. Fertil Steril 31:363, 1979

GLUCKMAN PD et al: The human fetal hypothalamus and pituitary gland, in *Maternal-Fetal Endocrinology*, D Tulchinsky, KJ Ryan (eds). Philadelphia, Saunders, 1980

GOLDZIEHER JW: Polycystic ovarian disease. Fertil Steril 35:371, 1981

HATCHER RA et al: *Contraceptive Technology 1986–1987*. New York, Irvington, 1986

HSUEH AJW et al: Hormonal regulation of the differentiation of cultured ovarian granulosa cells. Endocr Rev 5:76, 1984

JONES HW JR et al (eds): *In Vitro Fertilization*. Baltimore, Williams & Wilkins, 1986

JUDD HL et al: Estrogen replacement therapy: Indications and complications. Ann Intern Med 98:195, 1983

KASE N, WEINGOLD A: *Principles and Practice of Clinical Gynecology*. New York, Wiley, 1983

KELCH RP: Management of precocious puberty. N Engl J Med 312:1057, 1985

KNOBIL E, NEILL JD (eds): *The Physiology of Reproduction*. New York, Raven , 1988

MATTINGLY RF, THOMPSON JD: *Operative Gynecology*. Philadelphia, Lippincott, 1985

MISHELL DR JR, DAVAJAN V (eds): *Reproductive Endocrinology, Infertility, and Contraception*, 2d ed. Philadelphia, Davis, 1986

PIEPER DR et al: Ovarian gonadatropin-releasing hormone (GnRH) receptors: Characterization, distribution, and induction by GnRH. Endocrinology 108:1148, 1981

RIGGS BL et al: Effect of the fluoride/calcium regimen on vertebral fracture occurrence in postmenopausal osteoporosis. N Engl J Med 306:446, 1982

ROSS GT: Disorders of the ovary and female reproductive tract, in *Williams' Textbook of Endocrinology*, 7th ed, JD Wilson, DW Foster (eds). Philadelphia, Saunders, 1985, pp 206–258

ROSS JL et al: A preliminary study of the effect of estrogen dose on growth in Turner's syndrome. N Engl J Med 309:1104, 1983

SCULLY RE: Ovarian tumors: A review. Am J Pathol 87:686, 1977

SEIBEL MM: A new era in reproductive technology. N Engl J Med 318:828, 1988

SHEARMAN RP (ed): *Clinical Reproductive Endocrinology*, Edinburgh, Churchill Livingston, 1985

SITTERI PK, MacDONALD PC: Role of extraglandular estrogen in human endocrinology, in *Handbook of Physiology*, sec 7, *Endocrinology*, SR Geiger et al (eds). Washington, DC, American Physiological Society, 1973, p 615

SPEROFF L: Menopause. Semin Reprod Endocrinol 1:1, 1983

———— et al: The ovary, in *Endocrinology and Metabolism*, P Felig et al (eds). New York, McGraw-Hill, 1981, p 669

———— et al: *Clinical Gynecologic Endocrinology and Infertility*, 4th ed. Baltimore, Williams & Wilkins, 1989

STEINGOLD KA et al: Treatment of hot flashes with transdermal estradiol administration. J Clin Endocrinol Metab 61:627, 1985

STUDD JWW, WHITEHEAD MI (eds): *The Menopause*. Oxford, Blackwell, 1988

STYNE DM, GRUMBACH MM: Puberty in the male and female: Its physiology and disorders, in *Reproductive Endocrinology*, SSC Yen, RB Jaffe (eds). Philadelphia, Saunders, 1986, pp 331–384

WALLACH EE, KEMPERS RD: *Modern Trends in Infertility and Contraception Control*, vol 3. Baltimore, Williams & Wilkins, 1985

WENTZ AC et al: *Gynecologic Endocrinology and Infertility*, Baltimore, Williams & Wilkins, 1988

YEN SSC: Neuroendocrine regulation of the menstrual cycle. Hosp Prac 14.84, 1979

————: Clinical application of gonadotropin-releasing hormone and gonadotropin-releasing hormone analogs. Fertil Steril 39:257, 1983

————, JAFFE RB (eds): *Reproductive Endocrinology*, 2d ed. Philadelphia, Saunders, 1986

YING SY et al: Gonadocrinins: Peptides in ovarian follicular fluid stimulating the secretion of pituitary gonadotropins. Endocrinology 108:1206, 1981

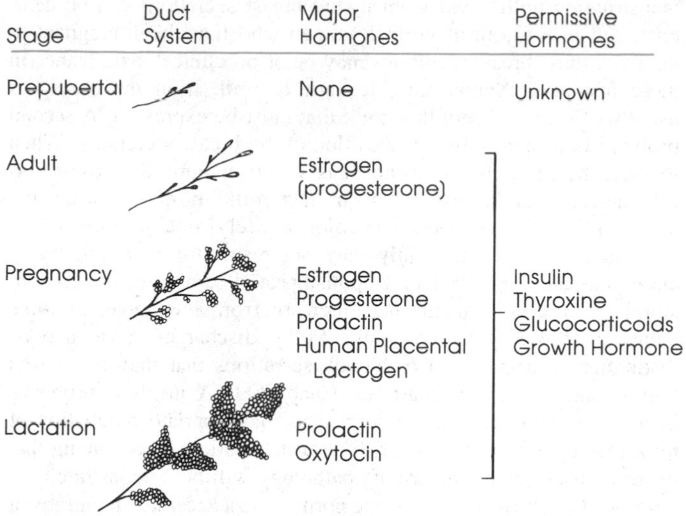

FIGURE 323-1   Endocrine control of female breast development and function at various stages of life.

323   ENDOCRINE DISORDERS OF THE BREAST

JEAN D. WILSON

Examination of the breasts is an important part of the physical examination. The breasts are the site of fatal and preventable disease in women and frequently provide clues to underlying systemic illness in both men and women. The internist frequently does not examine the male breast and is apt to refer the evaluation of the female breast to a gynecologist. It is the duty of every physician to distinguish the abnormal from the normal at the earliest possible stage and to call for assistance if there is any doubt. (For cancer of the breast see Chap. 303.)

ENDOCRINE CONTROL OF THE BREAST   There is no histologic or functional difference in the breasts of boys and girls prior to the onset of puberty, but a profound sexual dimorphism in breast development ensues at the time of puberty. The endocrine control of female breast development is illustrated in Fig. 323-1. The pubertal growth of the female breast is dependent primarily upon the action

of estradiol, which induces the growth, division, and elongation of the tubular duct system and maturation of the nipples. In men the administration of estrogen is equally effective in this regard. To produce true alveolar development at the ends of the ducts, however, the synergistic action of progesterone is required, a ratio of estrogen to progesterone of 1:20 to 1:100 being optimal. Once the anatomic development of the ducts and alveoli is complete, the continued action of estrogen and progesterone does not appear to be required for lactation itself.

The endocrine control of milk formation by the differentiated breast is complex, requiring, in addition to appropriate priming by estrogen and progesterone, specific lactogenic hormone and the permissive action of glucocorticoid, insulin, thyroxine, and in some species growth hormone. There are two lactogenic hormones. Human placental lactogen (hPL or chorionic somatomammotropin) is secreted in large amounts by the placenta during the latter phases of gestation and prepares the breast for milk production. It disappears from the fetal (and maternal) circulation shortly after termination of pregnancy. The pituitary hormone prolactin (see Chap. 313) plays the critical role in the initiation and maintenance of normal as well as inappropriate lactation. The plasma level of prolactin rises during pregnancy; during late pregnancy and lactation 60 to 80 percent of the anterior pituitary may consist of prolactin-secreting cells.

Unlike most pituitary hormones, the predominant regulation of prolactin secretion is negative, i.e., under ordinary basal conditions the hypothalamus secretes one or more inhibitory hormones, the most important being dopamine, which are delivered to the pituitary via the hypothalamic portal system and inhibit the release of prolactin into the blood (see Chap. 313). Most factors that influence prolactin secretion do so by affecting the synthesis or release of the inhibiting factors. Basal prolactin levels fall following delivery, but prolactin secretion is enhanced by stimulation of the breasts such as the act of nursing (the so-called sucking reflex), a phenomenon that is probably mediated by the reflex release of oxytocin. In the postgestational state the normal woman is capable of forming about a liter of milk per day containing 38 g fat, 70 g lactose, and 12 g protein. Normal lactation can be suppressed by the administration of estrogens or diethylstilbestrol, which inhibit milk production by direct effects on the breast, or bromocriptine, which inhibits prolactin secretion by the pituitary. Alternatively, if a woman does not nurse or empty her breasts post partum, lactation usually ceases of its own accord in 1 to 2 weeks.

GALACTORRHEA   Exactly what constitutes nonpuerperal or inappropriate lactation is not always clearly defined in the literature. According to the studies of Friedman and Goldfein, it is not possible to demonstrate any breast secretion whatsoever in normal, regularly menstruating nulligravid women, but breast secretions can be demonstrated in a fourth of normal women who have been pregnant in the past; thus, breast secretions may be of no clinical significance in these instances. Spontaneous leakage of milk from the breasts is usually of more concern than milk that must be expressed. A second problem is related to the composition of the breast secretions. When the secretion is milky or white, it is safe to assume that it contains fat, casein, and lactose and is in fact milk; however, when the secretion is brown or greenish in color, it rarely contains normal milk constituents and consequently may not result from an underlying endocrinopathy. Furthermore, upon repeated sampling, the composition of milk constituents may increase from low, colostrum-like values to those typical of milk. Milky discharges must also be distinguished from blood or bloody secretions that may be present with neoplasms of the breast (see Chap. 303). With these problems in mind galactorrhea can be defined as inappropriate production of milk that is persistent or worrisome to the patient, recognizing that in some instances no underlying pathology will be demonstrated.

Since the action of a lactogenic hormone is a necessary requirement for the initiation of milk production, it is logical to consider galactorrhea as a manifestation of deranged prolactin physiology. However, as indicated above, a complex endocrinologic milieu is necessary for lactation, and in many instances in which prolactin is elevated, both in women who have not been appropriately primed and in men, no production of milk takes place. As a consequence, hyperprolactinemia is more common than galactorrhea. Furthermore, although enhanced prolactin secretion is necessary for the initiation of lactation, production can be maintained in the presence of minimally elevated or intermittently elevated prolactin levels so that basal plasma prolactin levels are not always elevated in patients with galactorrhea. For example, repeated stimulation of the nipples of women who have previously been pregnant can cause galactorrhea with minimal elevations of basal prolactin (the wet nurse phenomenon) similar to those in normal nursing mothers. Perhaps the strongest evidence that prolactin is always involved in galactorrhea is the fact that administration of bromocriptine, which suppresses plasma prolactin levels, causes a disappearance of galactorrhea even when the basal plasma prolactin levels are normal.

Differential diagnosis It is thus appropriate to consider galactorrhea as the result of a failure of the normal hypothalamic inhibition of prolactin release, of enhanced prolactin-releasing factor, or of autonomous prolactin secretion by tumors (Table 323-1). Pituitary stalk section in humans results in a striking increase in prolactin secretion, as the result of the inhibition of the delivery of prolactin inhibitory factors to the pituitary. Likewise, many drugs that influence the central nervous system (including virtually all psychotropic agents, methyldopa, reserpine, and antiemetics) cause enhanced prolactin release, presumably by inhibiting synthesis or release of dopamine or other prolactin inhibitory factors. Estrogens enhance prolactin levels by an uncertain mechanism. Extrapituitary central nervous system diseases can cause galactorrhea, presumably by interfering with delivery of the inhibitory factors to the pituitary (central nervous system sarcoidosis, craniopharyngioma, pinealoma, encephalitis, meningitis, hydrocephalus, hypothalamic tumors).

In one pathologic state, primary hypothyroidism, galactorrhea results from enhanced prolactin-releasing activity. Thyrotropin-releasing hormone (TRH) stimulates prolactin release, and thyroid hormone replacement cures the galactorrhea. A similar mechanism, namely, enhanced secretion of oxytocin, may be involved in the galactorrhea of breast trauma.

Enhanced prolactin release can also occur from pituitary or nonpituitary tumors. Three types of pituitary tumors (see Chap. 313) may be associated with galactorrhea: pure prolactin-secreting tumors (micro- or macroadenomas), mixed tumors that secrete both growth hormone and prolactin and result in acromegaly with galactorrhea, and some chromophobe adenomas. The latter may either secrete prolactin or interfere with the delivery of inhibitory factors to the pituitary. Prolactin can also be secreted on occasion by other malignancies such as bronchogenic carcinoma, and hydatidiform moles and choriocarcinomas may secrete placental lactogen.

The known etiologies account for only a part of the cases of galactorrhea. In four published series totaling more than 500 carefully studied patients, a pituitary tumor was identified in about one-fourth of the patients, other known causes could be identified in another fourth or fifth, and the remaining half fall into the unknown category. Many patients may prove ultimately to have prolactin-secreting pituitary tumors, some probably have subtle disorders of hypothalamic function, and in others a drug-related cause may have been missed, but the fact remains that no satisfactory diagnosis is reached in many patients. When normal menses and galactorrhea coexist, the likelihood of establishing a diagnosis is poor.

Galactorrhea is unusual in men, even in the presence of profound elevations of plasma prolactin; when it does occur, it is usually upon the background of a feminizing state (see below).

Diagnostic evaluation If hyperprolactinemia is present, the workup is fundamentally that of a pituitary tumor once drug causes and hypothyroidism are excluded (see Chap. 313). Even when a specific cause cannot be identified and a diagnosis of idiopathic galactorrhea is made by exclusion, it is necessary to remember that pituitary tumors may subsequently become manifest. The higher the prolactin values and the more persistent the galactorrhea, the greater the likelihood of such a development.

Treatment The aim of treatment is to remove the source of the elevated prolactin, and resection of pituitary tumor, cessation of causative drugs, or correction of hypothyroidism is often followed by the disappearance of galactorrhea. Two other forms of therapy may have some usefulness. Breast binders can be effective in patients with mild galactorrhea of unknown etiology, presumably by preventing stimulation of the nipple and the consequent perpetuation of lactation. Bromocriptine, which suppresses plasma prolactin, has been used to treat patients with idiopathic hyperprolactinemia as well as patients with prolactin-secreting tumors of the pituitary. This drug not only suppresses lactation but may also cause resumption of normal menstrual cycles (and even fertility) in patients in whom amenorrhea accompanies galactorrhea.

GYNECOMASTIA A central issue in the evaluation of breast tissue in adult men is the separation of the normal from the abnormal. Whereas in autopsy data the incidence of active gynecomastia is between 5 and 9 percent, Nuttall and his colleagues have reported that approximately 40 percent of normal men and up to 70 percent of hospitalized men have palpable breast tissue. The reason for this discrepancy is not clear. On the one hand, it may be difficult to distinguish true breast tissue from masses of adipose tissue without true breast enlargement (lipomastia); in such cases true gynecomastia can be separated from lipomastia by mammography or by sonography. Alternatively, a true increase in the incidence of gynecomastia may have taken place, or the autopsy data may underestimate the frequency of palpable breast tissue. Regardless, we are left with major uncertainties; the finding of gynecomastia (distinct from lipomastia) could

---

TABLE 323-1 A physiologic classification of galactorrhea

I Failure of normal hypothalamic inhibition of prolactin release
  A Pituitary stalk section
  B Drugs (phenothiazines, butyrophenones, methyldopa, tricyclic antidepressants, opiates, reserpine, verapamil)
  C Central nervous system disease, including extrapituitary tumors
II Enhanced prolactin-releasing factor
  Hypothyroidism
  Sucking reflex and breast trauma
III Autonomous prolactin release
  A Pituitary tumors
    1 Prolactin-secreting tumors
    2 Mixed growth hormone and prolactin-secreting tumors
    3 Chromophobe adenomas
  B Ectopic production of human placental lactogen and/or prolactin
    1 Hydatidiform moles and choriocarcinomas
    2 Bronchogenic carcinoma and hypernephroma
IV Idiopathic

indicate underlying pathology or a normal variant. For the purposes of this discussion, we shall assume that any palpable breast tissue in men (except for the three so-called physiologic states) may reflect an underlying endocrinopathy and deserves a limited evaluation.

Early gynecomastia is characterized by proliferation in the breast of both the fibroblastic stroma and the duct system, which elongates, buds, and duplicates. As gynecomastia persists, progressive fibrosis and hyalinization are associated with regression of epithelial proliferation. Eventually the number of ducts decreases. Resolution occurs by reduction in size and epithelial content with gradual disappearance of the ducts, leaving hyaline bands that eventually disappear.

Growth of the breast in men, as in women, is mediated by estrogen and results from disturbances of the normal ratio of active androgen to estrogen in plasma or within the breast itself. As described in Chap. 321 estradiol formation in the normal man occurs principally by the conversion of circulating androgens to estrogens in peripheral tissues; the normal ratio of production of testosterone to estradiol in adult men is approximately 100:1 (6 mg versus 45 μg), and the normal ratio of the two hormones in plasma is about 300:1. Feminization results when there is a significant decrease in this effective ratio, as the result of diminished testosterone production or action, enhanced estrogen formation, or both processes occurring simultaneously. The predominant manifestation of feminization in men is enlargement of the breasts.

Enlargement of the male breast can occur as a normal physiologic phenomenon at certain stages of life or as the result of a variety of pathologic conditions (Table 323-2).

Physiologic gynecomastia In the *newborn* transient enlargement of the breast results from the action of maternal and/or placental estrogens. The enlargement ordinarily disappears in a few weeks but may persist longer. *Adolescent* gynecomastia occurs in many boys at some time during puberty. The median age of onset is 14; it is often

---

TABLE 323-2 Differential diagnosis of gynecomastia

PHYSIOLOGIC GYNECOMASTIA

Newborn
Adolescence
Aging

PATHOLOGIC GYNECOMASTIA

Deficient production or action of testosterone:
  Congenital defects:
    Congenital anorchia
    Klinefelter syndrome
    Androgen resistance (testicular feminization and Reifenstein syndrome)
    Defects of testosterone synthesis
  Secondary testicular failure:
    Viral orchitis
    Trauma
    Castration
    Neurologic and granulomatous diseases
    Renal failure
Increased estrogen production:
  Estrogen secretion:
    True hermaphroditism
    Testicular tumors
    Carcinoma of the lung and other tumors producing hCG
  Increased substrate for extraglandular aromatase:
    Adrenal disease
    Liver disease
    Starvation
    Thyrotoxicosis
  Increase in extraglandular aromatase
Drugs:
  Estrogens (diethylstilbestrol, birth control pills, digitalis, estrogen-containing cosmetics, estrogen-contaminated foods)
  Drugs that enhance endogenous estrogen secretion (gonadotropins, clomiphene)
  Inhibitors of testosterone synthesis and/or action (ketoconazole, metronidazole, alkylating agents, cisplatin, spironolactone, cimetidine)
  Unknown mechanisms (busulfan, isoniazid, methyldopa, tricyclic antidepressants, penicillamine, diazepam, marijuana, heroin)
Idiopathic

---

asymmetric, occasionally unilateral for a portion of its course, and frequently tender, and it regresses so that by age 20 only a small number of men have palpable vestiges of gynecomastia in one or both breasts. Although the origin of the excess estrogen has not been identified, the onset of gynecomastia correlates with transient elevations of plasma estradiol prior to the completion of puberty so that the androgen/estrogen ratio is altered. *Gynecomastia of aging* also occurs in otherwise healthy men. Forty percent or more of aged men have gynecomastia. A likely explanation is the increase with age in the conversion of androgens to estrogens in extraglandular tissues. Abnormal liver function or drug therapy may be contributing causes to gynecomastia in such men.

Pathologic gynecomastia Pathologic gynecomastia can result from one of three basic mechanisms: deficiency in testosterone production or action (with or without a secondary increase in estrogen production), increase in estrogen production, or drugs (Table 323-2). Most of the individual disorders that cause primary and secondary testicular failure have been discussed in Chap. 321. The fact that a deficiency in testosterone production per se can cause gynecomastia is illustrated by the syndrome of congenital anorchia in which normal (or slightly low) estradiol production in the presence of profoundly decreased testosterone production results in florid gynecomastia. Such is the case in some patients with Klinefelter syndrome. In the inherited syndromes of androgen resistance, such as testicular feminization, deficient androgen action and increased testicular estrogen production are both present, although diminished androgen action is the more critical in inducing gynecomastia.

A primary increase in estrogen production can result from a variety of causes. Increased testicular estrogen secretion may result from elevations in plasma gonadotropins, for example, in cases of aberrant production of chorionic gonadotropin by testicular tumors or by bronchogenic carcinoma, from the ovarian elements in the gonads of men with true hermaphroditism, or as the result of direct secretion by testicular tumors (particularly Leydig cell and Sertoli cell tumors). Increased conversion of androgen to estrogens in peripheral tissues can either be due to increased availability of substrate for extraglandular estrogen formation or to increased amount of the enzymes of estrogen formation in peripheral tissues. Increased substrate availability for extraglandular conversion can result from increased production of androgens such as androstenedione (congenital adrenal hyperplasia, hyperthyroidism, and most feminizing adrenal tumors) or because of diminished catabolism of androstenedione by the usual pathways (liver disease). Increased amount of extraglandular aromatase can be caused by a rare hereditary abnormality or by tumors of the liver or adrenal gland.

Drugs can cause gynecomastia by several mechanisms. Many drugs either act directly as estrogens or cause an increase in plasma estrogen activity, for example, in men receiving diethylstilbestrol for prostatic carcinoma and in transsexuals in preparation for sex-change operations. Boys and young men are particularly sensitive to estrogen and can develop gynecomastia after the use of dermal ointments containing estrogen or after the ingestion of milk or meat from estrogen treated animals. The gynecomastia of digitalis ingestion is usually attributed to an estrogen-like side effect of the drug, but in the experience of the author it is usually associated with abnormal liver function tests. A second mechanism by which drugs can induce gynecomastia is illustrated by gonadotropin, such as from human chorionic gonadotropin (hCG)–secreting tumors, which causes enhanced testicular secretion of estrogen. Other drugs cause gynecomastia by interfering with testosterone synthesis (ketoconazole and alkylating agents) and/or testosterone action, for instance by blocking the binding of androgen to its cytosol receptor protein in target tissues (spironolactone and cimetidine). Finally, drugs that cause gynecomastia by mechanisms which have not been defined include busulfan, ethionamide, isoniazid, methyldopa, tricyclic antidepressants, penicillamine, and diazepam, marijuana, and heroin. In some instances the feminization is due to effects of drugs on liver function.

Diagnostic evaluation The evaluation of patients with gynecomastia should include the following procedures: (1) a careful drug history; (2) measurement and examination of the testes (if both are small, a chromosomal karyotype should be obtained; if they are asymmetric, an evaluation for testicular tumor should be instituted); (3) an evaluation of liver function; (4) an endocrine evaluation to include measurement of serum androstenedione or 24-h urinary 17-ketosteroids (usually elevated in feminizing adrenal states), measurement of plasma estradiol and hCG (helpful if elevated but usually normal), and measurement of plasma luteinizing hormone (LH) and testosterone. If LH is high and testosterone is low, the diagnosis is usually testicular failure; if LH and testosterone are both low, the diagnosis is most likely increased primary estrogen production (for example, a Sertoli cell tumor of the testis); and if both LH and testosterone are elevated, the diagnosis is either an androgen-resistance state or a gonadotropin-secreting tumor.

A satisfactory diagnosis can be made in only half or fewer of the patients referred for gynecomastia by using these various tests. This implies either that the diagnostic techniques are not sufficiently refined to recognize mild disturbances, that many causes of gynecomastia are as yet undefined, that the causes may be transient and difficult to diagnose, or, as suggested by Nuttall, that gynecomastia may in some instances be normal rather than due to a pathologic state. Because of the problem of separating the normal from the pathologic, gynecomastia should probably be routinely worked up only if the drug history is negative, if the breast is tender (indicating rapid growth), or if the breast mass is larger than 4 cm in diameter. In other instances a decision to perform an endocrine evaluation depends on the clinical context. For example, gynecomastia associated with signs of under-androgenization should be evaluated.

Treatment   When the primary cause of the overestrogenization can be identified and corrected, the breast enlargement usually subsides promptly and eventually disappears. However, if the gynecomastia is of long duration (and fibrosis has replaced the original ductal hyperplasia), correction of the primary defect may not be followed by resolution. In such instances and when the primary cause cannot be corrected, surgery is the only effective therapy. Indications for surgery include several psychologic and/or cosmetic problems, continued growth, or a suspected malignancy. Although the relative risk of carcinoma of the breast is increased in men with gynecomastia, it is rare nevertheless. Prophylactic radiation of the breasts prior to the institution of diethylstilbestrol therapy is effective in preventing gynecomastia and has a low complication rate in elderly men. In rare patients who have painful gynecomastia and who are not candidates for other therapy, treatment with antiestrogens such as tamoxifen may be indicated.

REFERENCES

Galactorrhea

CHOTINER HC et al: Lactose and casein content of nonpuerperal breast secretion. J Reprod Med 22:267, 1979

DAVAJAN V: The significance of galactorrhea in patients with normal menses, oligomenorrhea, and secondary amenorrhea. Am J Obstet Gynecol 130:894, 1978

FRANTZ AG, WILSON JD: Endocrine disorders of the breast, in Williams' Textbook of Endocrinology, 8th ed, JD Wilson, DW Foster (eds). Philadelphia, Saunders, 1990, In press

FRIEDMAN S, GOLDFEIN A: Breast secretions in normal women. Am J Obstet Gynecol 104:846, 1969

JOHNSON DG et al: Prolactin secretion and biological activity in females with galactorrhoea and normal circulating prolactin concentrations at rest. Clin Endocrinol 22:661, 1985

KLEINBERG DL et al: Galactorrhea: A study of 235 cases, including 48 with pituitary tumors. N Engl J Med 296:589, 1977

KOPPELMAN MCS et al: Hyperprolactinemia, amenorrhea, and galactorrhea. A retrospective assessment of twenty-five cases. Ann Intern Med 100:115, 1984

KULSKI JK et al: Changes in the milk composition of nonpuerperal women. Am J Obstet Gynecol 139:597, 1981

RUIZ-VELASCO V: Hyperprolactinemia and mammary prostheses. A report of eight cases. J Reprod Med 31:267, 1986

SAUER HJ: Physiology of lactation and factors affecting lactation. Obstet Gynecol Clin North Am 14:615, 1987

TOLTS G: Prolactin: Physiology and pathology. Hosp Prac February 1980, p 85

TURKSOY RN et al: Diagnostic and therapeutic modalities in women with galactorrhea. Obstet Gynecol 56:323, 1980

Gynecomastia

ANDERSON JA, GROOM JB: Male breast at autopsy. Acta Pathol Microbiol Immunol Scand 90:191, 1982

CARLSON HE: Gynecomastia. N Engl J Med 303:795, 1980

CIMORA GA et al: Percutaneous oestrogen-induced gynecomastia: A case report. Br J Plast Surg 35:209, 1982

FASS D et al: Radiotherapeutic prophylaxis of estrogen-induced gynecomastia: A study of late sequela. Int J Radiation Oncology Bio Phys 12:407, 1986

FELDMAN D: Ketoconazole and other imidazole derivatives as inhibitors of steroidogenesis. Endocr Rev 7:409, 1986

FRANTZ AG, WILSON JD: Endocrine disorders of the breast, in Williams' Textbook of Endocrinology, 8th ed, JD Wilson, DW Foster (eds). Philadelphia, Saunders, 1990, In press

KORENMAN SG: The endocrinology of the abnormal male breast. Ann NY Acad Sci 464:400, 1986

MABUCHI K et al: Risk factors for male breast cancer. J Natl Cancer Inst 74:371, 1985

NIEWOEHNER CV, NUTTALL FQ: Gynecomastia in a hospitalized male population. Am J Med 77:633, 1984

NUTTALL FQ: Gynecomastia as a physical finding in normal men. J Clin Endocrinol Metab 48:338, 1979

PARKER LN et al: Treatment of gynecomastia with tamoxifen: A double-blind crossover study. Metabolism 8:705, 1986

---

324   DISORDERS OF SEXUAL DIFFERENTIATION

JEAN D. WILSON / JAMES E. GRIFFIN

Sexual differentiation is a sequential and ordered process. *Chromosomal sex*, established at the moment of fertilization, determines *gonadal sex*, and *gonadal sex* in turn causes the development of *phenotypic sex* in which the male or female urogenital tract is formed (Table 324-1). A disturbance of any step in this developmental process during embryogenesis may result in a disorder of sexual differentiation. Known causes of abnormalities in sexual development include environmental insults as in the ingestion of a virilizing drug during pregnancy, nonfamilial aberrations of the sex chromosomes as in 45,X gonadal dysgenesis, developmental birth defects of multifactorial etiology as in most cases of hypospadias, and hereditary disorders resulting from single gene mutations as in the testicular feminization syndrome.

Limitations of knowledge make it necessary to make empiric assignments as to the nature of the derangement in certain disorders. Nevertheless, a specific diagnosis can usually be made as the result of genetic, endocrine, phenotypic, and chromosomal assessment. As a consequence, appropriate gender assignment can be made, even in extreme instances of ambiguous genitalia, and tailoring of the phenotype can be undertaken when appropriate.

TABLE 324-1   Classification of disorders of sexual development

Disorders of chromosomal sex:
    Klinefelter syndrome
    XX male
    Gonadal dysgenesis
    Mixed gonadal dysgenesis
    True hermaphroditism
Disorders of gonadal sex:
    Pure gonadal dysgenesis
    Absent testis syndrome
Disorders of phenotypic sex:
    Female pseudohermaphroditism:
        Congenital adrenal hyperplasia
        Nonadrenal female pseudohermaphroditism
        Developmental disorders of müllerian ducts
    Male pseudohermaphroditism:
        Abnormalities in androgen synthesis
        Abnormalities in androgen action
        Persistent müllerian duct syndrome
        Development defects of male genitalia

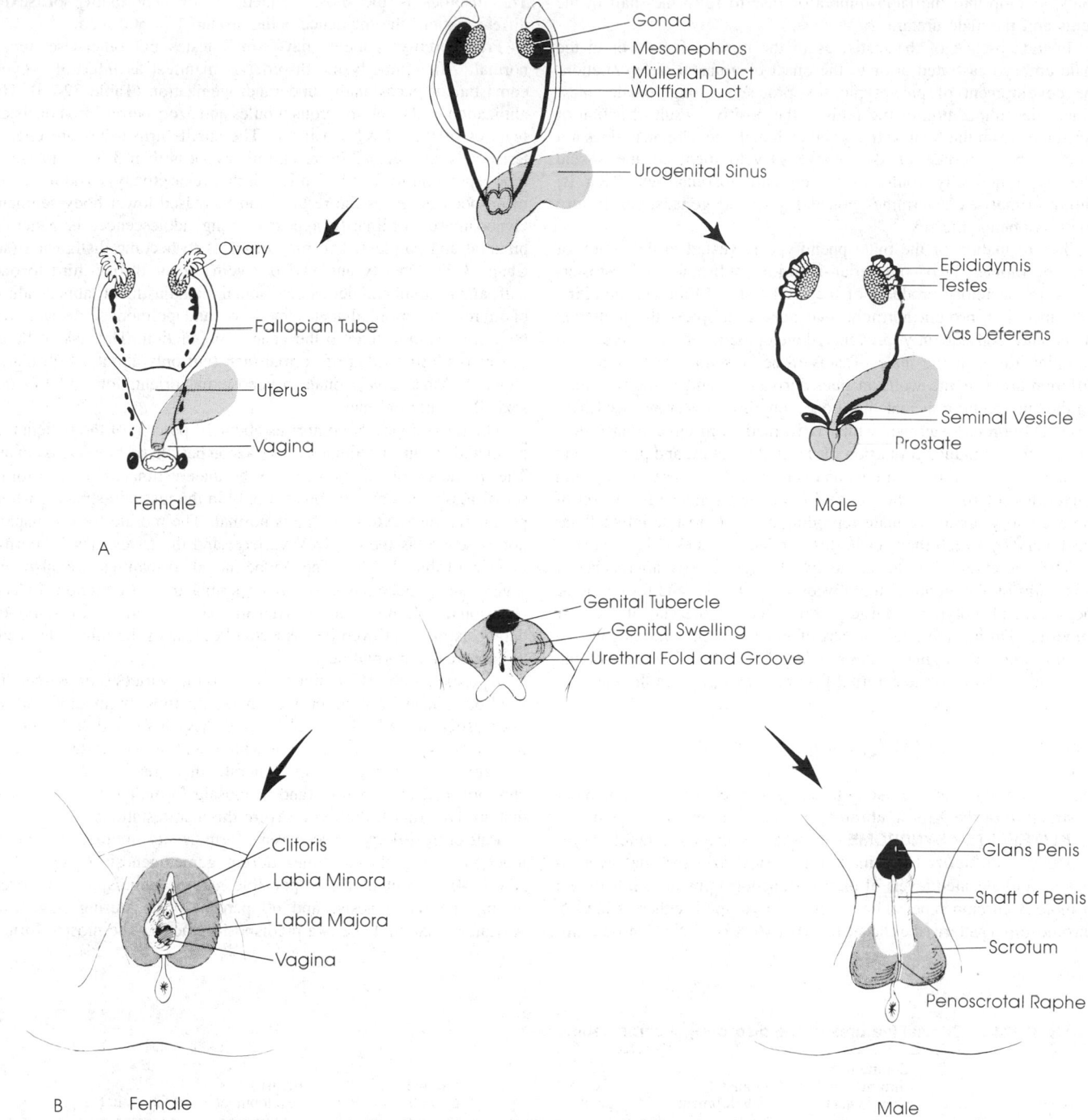

FIGURE 324-1 Normal sexual differentiation. *A*. Internal genitalia. *B*. External genitalia.

NORMAL SEXUAL DIFFERENTIATION

The first process in sexual differentiation is the establishment of chromosomal sex, the heterogametic sex (XY) being male and the homogametic sex (XX) female. The embryos of both sexes then develop in an identical fashion until approximately 40 days of gestation. The second phase of sexual differentiation is the conversion of the indifferent gonad into a testis or an ovary. The differentiation of the indifferent gonad into a testis is mediated by one or more testis determining factor (TDF) genes on the short arm of the Y chromosome; indeed, no matter how many X chromosomes are present (as in XXY, XXXY, etc.), a testis will develop as long as a Y chromosome is present. The final process, the translation of gonadal sex into phenotypic sex, is the direct consequence of the type of gonad formed and the endocrine secretions of the fetal gonads. The development

of phenotypic sex results in the formation of the male and female urogenital tracts.

The internal genitalia are derived from the wolffian and müllerian ducts that exist side by side in early embryos of both sexes (Fig. 324-1*A*). In the male the wolffian ducts give rise to the epididymides, vasa deferentia, and seminal vesicles, and the müllerian ducts disappear. In the female the fallopian tubes, uterus, and upper vagina are derived from the müllerian ducts, and the wolffian ducts regress. The external genitalia and urethra in the two sexes develop from common anlage—the urogenital sinus and the genital tubercle, folds, and swellings (Fig. 324-1*B*). The urogenital sinus gives rise to the prostate and prostatic urethra in the male and to the urethra and lower portion of the vagina in the female. The genital tubercle is the origin of the glans penis in the male and clitoris in the female. The urogenital swellings become the scrotum or the labia majora, and the urethral folds develop into the labia minora or fuse to form the shaft of the penis and the male urethra.

In the absence of the testis, as in the normal female or in the male embryo castrated prior to the onset of gonadal differentiation, the development of phenotypic sex proceeds along female lines. Thus, masculinization of the fetus is the positive result of action of hormones from the fetal testis, whereas female development does not require the presence of the ovary. Development of the sexual phenotype normally conforms to the chromosomal sex. That is, chromosomal sex determines gonadal sex, and gonadal sex in turn controls phenotypic sex.

The formation of the male phenotype is vested in the action of three hormones. Two—müllerian-inhibiting substance and testosterone—are secretory products of the fetal testis. Müllerian-inhibiting substance is a protein hormone that acts to suppress the müllerian ducts and consequently prevents development of the uterus and fallopian tubes in the male. Testosterone acts directly to stimulate differentiation of the wolffian duct derivatives and is the precursor for the third embryonic male hormone, dihydrotestosterone (see Chap. 321). Dihydrotestosterone, which is formed from circulating testosterone, acts to induce formation of the male urethra and prostate and to cause formation of the penis and scrotum. Thus, testosterone and dihydrotestosterone function during fetal life to induce formation of the accessory organs of male reproduction by the same intracellular machinery by which they act in differentiated tissues (Chap. 321).

The secretion of testosterone by the fetal testis approaches a maximum by the eighth to tenth week of gestation, and formation of the sexual phenotypes is largely completed by the end of the first trimester. During the latter phases of gestation the ovarian follicles develop and the vagina matures in the female, and descent of the testes and growth of the external genitalia take place in the male.

DISORDERS OF CHROMOSOMAL SEX

Disorders of chromosomal sex (Table 324-2) occur when the number or structure of the X or Y chromosomes is abnormal (see Chap. 7).

KLINEFELTER SYNDROME   Clinical features   Klinefelter syndrome is characterized by small, firm testes, azoospermia, gynecomastia, and elevated levels of plasma gonadotropins in men with two or more X chromosomes. The common karyotype is either a 47,XXY chromosomal pattern (the classic form) or 46,XY/47,XXY mosaicism.

The disorder is the most frequent major abnormality of sexual differentiation, the incidence being around 1 in 500 men.

Prepubertally, patients have small testes but otherwise appear normal. After puberty the disorder is manifest as infertility, gynecomastia, or occasionally underandrogenization (Table 324-3). Hyalinization of the seminiferous tubules and azoospermia are consistent features of the 47,XXY variety. The small, firm testes are characteristically less than 2.0 cm and always less than 3.5 cm in length (corresponding to 2 and 12 mL volume, respectively). The increased mean body height is the result of an increased lower body segment. Gynecomastia ordinarily appears during adolescence, is generally bilateral and painless, and may progress to become disfiguring (see Chap. 323). Obesity and varicose veins occur in one-third to one-half, and mild mental deficiency, social maladjustment, abnormalities of thyroid function, diabetes mellitus, and pulmonary disease may be more common than in the general population. The risk of breast cancer is 20 times that of normal men (but only about a fifth that in women). Most have a male psychosexual orientation and function sexually as normal men.

The mosaic variant comprises about 10 percent of the patients, as estimated by chromosomal karyotypes on peripheral blood leukocytes. The frequency of this variant may be underestimated since chromosomal mosaicism may be present only in the testes in subjects whose peripheral leukocyte karotype is normal. The mosaic form is usually not as severe as the 47,XXY variety, and the testes may be normal in size (Table 324-3). The endocrine abnormalities are also less severe, and gynecomastia and azoospermia are less common. Indeed, occasional patients with mosaicism may be fertile. In some the diagnosis may not even be suspected because of the minor degree of the physical abnormalities.

Approximately 30 additional karyotypic varieties of Klinefelter syndrome have been described, including those with uniform cell lines (such as XXYY, XXXY, and XXXXY) and a variety of mosaicisms of the X chromosome with or without associated structural abnormalities of the X. In general, the greater the degree of chromosomal abnormality (and in mosaic forms the more cell lines that are abnormal), the more severe the manifestations.

Pathophysiology   The classic form is due to meiotic nondisjunction of the chromosomes during gametogenesis (Fig. 324-2). About 40 percent of the responsible meiotic nondisjunctions occur during spermatogenesis, and 60 percent occur during oogenesis. Advanced maternal age is a predisposing factor. The mosaic form is

TABLE 324-2   Clinical features of the disorders of chromosomal sex

Disorder	Common chromosomal complement	Gonadal development	External genitalia	Internal genitalia	Breast development	Comment
Klinefelter syndrome	47,XXY or 46,XY/47,XXY	Hyalinized testes	Normal male	Normal male	Gynecomastia	Most common disorder of sexual differentiation; tall stature.
XX male	46,XX	Hyalinized testes	Normal male	Normal male	Gynecomastia	Shorter than normal men; increased incidence of hypospadias. Similar to Klinefelter syndrome. May be familial.
Gonadal dysgenesis (Turner syndrome)	45,X or 46,XX/45,X	Streak gonads	Immature female	Hypoplastic female	Immature female	Short stature and multiple somatic abnormalities. May be 46,XX with structurally abnormal X chromosome.
Mixed gonadal dysgenesis	46,XY/45,X or 46,XY	Testis and streak gonad	Variable but almost always ambiguous; 60% reared as female	Uterus, vagina, and one fallopian tube	Usually male	Second most common cause of ambiguous genitalia in the newborn; tumors common.
True hermaphroditism	46,XX or 46,XY or mosaics	Testis and ovary or ovotestis	Variable but usually ambiguous; 60% reared as males	Usually a uterus and urogenital sinus; ducts correspond to gonad	Gynecomastia in 75%	May be familial.

TABLE 324-3 Characteristics of patients with classic versus mosaic Klinefelter syndrome*

	47,XXY, %	46,XY/47,XXY, %
Abnormal testicular histology	100	94†
Decreased length of testis	99	73†
Azoospermia	93	50†
Decreased testosterone	79	33
Decreased facial hair	77	64
Increased gonadotropins	75	33†
Decreased sexual function	68	56
Gynecomastia	55	33†
Decreased axillary hair	49	46
Decreased length of penis	41	21

* Table based on 519 XXY patients and 51 XY/XXY patients.
† Significantly different at $p < .05$ or better.
SOURCE: After Gordon et al.

thought to result from chromosomal mitotic nondisjunction after fertilization of the zygote and can take place either in a 46,XY zygote (Fig. 324-2) or a 47,XXY zygote. The latter defect or double nondisjunction (meiotic and mitotic) may be the usual cause and thus explain why the mosaic form is less frequent than the classic disorder.

Plasma follicle-stimulating hormone (FSH) and luteinizing hormone (LH) are usually high; FSH shows the best discrimination, and little overlap occurs with normals, a consequence of the consistent damage to the seminiferous tubules. The plasma testosterone averages half normal, but the range of values overlaps the normal range. Mean plasma estradiol levels are elevated, the cause of which is not entirely clear. Early in the course, the testes may secrete increased amounts of estradiol in response to the elevated plasma LH, but the testicular secretion of estradiol (and testosterone) eventually declines. Elevated plasma estradiol late in the course is probably due to a combination of a decreased metabolic clearance rate and an increased rate of conversion of testosterone to estradiol in extragonadal tissues. The net result both early and late is a variable degree of insufficient androgenization and enhanced feminization. The feminization, including gynecomastia, depends on the ratio of circulating estrogen to androgen (relative or absolute), and subjects with lower plasma testosterone and higher plasma estradiol levels are more likely to develop gynecomastia (see Chap. 323). The increase in plasma gonadotropins following the administration of luteinizing hormone–releasing hormone (LHRH) is exaggerated after the age of expected puberty, and the normal feedback inhibition of testosterone on pituitary LH secretion is diminished. Subjects with untreated Klinefelter syndrome may have "reactive pituitary abnormalities" in the form of enlarged or abnormal sella turcicas, presumably secondary to the

persistent lack of gonadal feedback and hypertrophy of the gonadotrophs in response to stimulation by LHRH. It is not known whether actual adenoma formation occurs.

Management   No method is available for reversing the infertility, and surgical removal is the only means for effective treatment of the gynecomastia. Some underandrogenized patients benefit from supplemental androgen, but such treatment may paradoxically worsen the gynecomastia, presumably by providing increased androgen substrate for the conversion to estrogens in the peripheral tissues. Androgen should be administered in the form of testosterone cypionate or testosterone enanthate. Following the administration of testosterone, plasma LH returns to normal only after several months, if at all.

XX MALE SYNDROME   The incidence of a 46,XX karyotype in phenotypic males is approximately 1 in 20,000 to 24,000 male births. Affected individuals have absence of all female internal genitalia and male psychosexual identification. Indeed, the findings resemble those in the Klinefelter syndrome: the testes are small and firm (generally less than 2 cm), gynecomastia is frequent, the penis is normal to small in size, azoospermia and hyalinization of the seminiferous tubules are usual, mean plasma testosterone is low, plasma estradiol is elevated, and plasma gonadotropin levels are high. Affected individuals differ from typical Klinefelter patients only in that average height is less than in normal men, the incidence of mental deficiency is not increased, and the incidence of hypospadias is increased.

Four theories have been proposed to explain the pathogenesis of this disorder: (1) translocation of a portion of a Y chromosome to the X chromosome, (2) mosaicism for a Y chromosome in some cell lines or early loss of a Y chromosome, (3) mutation of an autosomal gene, or (4) deletion of genetic material on the X chromosome that normally has a negative regulatory effect on testis development. Mosaicism has not been documented, and no clearcut evidence has been adduced for an autosomal gene mutation. The majority of XX males whose DNA is probed with Y-chromosome DNA fragments containing the TDF gene are positive for Y-related DNA; thus, an X-Y interchange appears to be the common cause of the disorder. The management is similar to that of Klinefelter syndrome.

GONADAL DYSGENESIS (TURNER SYNDROME)   Clinical features   Gonadal dysgenesis is characterized by primary amenorrhea, sexual infantilism, short stature, multiple congenital anomalies, and bilateral streak gonads in phenotypic women with any of several defects of the X chromosome. This condition should be distinguished from (1) mixed gonadal dysgenesis in which a unilateral testis and a contralateral streak gonad are present; (2) pure gonadal dysgenesis in which bilateral streak gonads are associated with a normal 46,XX or 46,XY karyotype, normal stature, and primary amenorrhea; and (3) the Noonan syndrome, an autosomal dominant disorder of males and females characterized by webbed neck, short stature, congenital

FIGURE 324-2   Schema for normal spermatogenesis and fertilization showing effects of meiotic and mitotic nondisjunction leading to classic Klinefelter syndrome, Turner syndrome, and mosaic Klinefelter syndrome. The schema would be similar if the abnormal events took place during oogenesis.

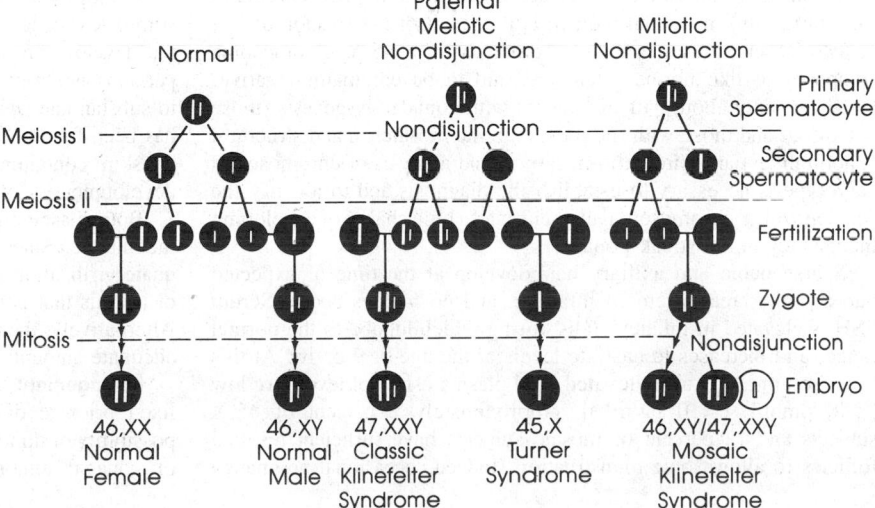

heart disease, cubitus valgus, and other congenital defects despite normal karyotypes and normal gonads.

The incidence is estimated at 1 in 2500 newborn females. The diagnosis is either made at birth because of the associated anomalies or more frequently at puberty when amenorrhea and failure of sexual development are noted in conjunction with the associated anomalies. Gonadal dysgenesis is the most common cause of primary amenorrhea, accounting for a third of such patients. The external genitalia are unambiguously female but remain immature, and there is no breast development unless the patient is treated with exogenous estrogen. The internal genitalia consist of infantile fallopian tubes and uterus and bilateral streak gonads located in the broad ligaments. Primordial germ cells are present transiently during embryogenesis but disappear as the result of an accelerated rate of atresia (see Chap. 322). After the age of expected puberty these streaks lack identifiable follicles and ova but contain fibrous tissue that is indistinguishable from normal ovarian stroma.

The associated somatic anomalies primarily involve the skeleton and connective tissue. Lymphedema of the hands and feet, webbing of the neck, low hair line, redundant skin folds on the back of the neck, a shield-like chest with widely spaced nipples, and a low birth weight are features that suggest the diagnosis in infancy. In addition, the facies may be characterized by micrognathia, epicanthal folds, prominent low-set or deformed ears, a fishlike mouth, and ptosis. Short fourth metacarpals are present in half, and 10 to 20 percent have coarctation of the aorta. In adults the average height rarely exceeds 150 cm. Associated conditions include renal malformations, pigmented nevi, hypoplastic nails, tendency to keloid formation, perceptive hearing loss, unexplained hypertension, and autoimmune disorders. Frank hypothyroidism is present in 20 percent.

Pathophysiology   About half have a 45,X karyotype, approximately one-fourth have mosaicism with no structural abnormality (46,XX/45,X), and the remainder have a structurally abnormal X chromosome with or without mosaicism (see Chap. 7). The 45,X variety may result from chromosome loss during gametogenesis in either parent or a mitotic error during one of the early cleavage divisions of the fertilized zygote (Fig. 324-2). Short stature and other somatic features result from loss of genetic material on the short arm of the X chromosome. Streak gonads result when genetic material is missing from either the long or short arm of the X. In individuals with mosaicism or structural abnormalities of the X, phenotypes on average are intermediate in severity between that seen in the 45,X variety and the normal. In some patients with hypertrophy of the clitoris, there is an unidentified fragment of a chromosome present in addition to the X chromosome, assumed to be an abnormal Y; malignancy may develop in the streak gonads in this subset of patients. Rarely, familial transmission of gonadal dysgenesis can be the result of a balanced X-autosome translocation (see Chap. 7).

Assessment of sex chromatin was previously utilized as a means of screening for abnormalities of the X chromosome. Sex chromatin (the Barr body) in normal women is the result of inactivation of one of two X chromosomes, and women with a 45,X chromosome composition, like normal men, are said to be chromatin-negative. However, only about half of patients with gonadal dysgenesis (those with 45,X and those with the most extreme mosaicism and structural abnormalities) are chromatin-negative, and analysis of chromosomal karyotype is necessary to establish the diagnosis and to identify the fraction with Y chromosomal elements and a high chance of developing malignancy in the streak gonads.

Sparse pubic and axillary hair develop at the time of expected puberty, the breasts remain infantile, and no menses occur. Serum FSH is elevated in infancy, falls during midchildhood to the normal range, and increases to castrate levels at the age of 9 or 10. At this time, serum LH is also elevated, and plasma estradiol levels are low [<40 pmol/L (<10 pg/mL)]. Approximately 2 percent of 45,X subjects and 12 percent of mosaic subjects have sufficient residual follicles to allow some menstruation. Indeed, occasional pregnancy has been reported in minimally affected individuals; the reproductive life in such individuals is brief.

Management   At the anticipated time of puberty replacement therapy with estrogen should be instituted to induce maturation of the breasts, labia, vagina, uterus, and fallopian tubes (see Chap. 322). Linear growth and bone maturation rates are approximately doubled during the first year of treatment with estradiol, but the eventual height of patients rarely approaches the predicted height. Treatment with growth hormone accelerates growth, but it is not established whether such therapy has an effect on final height (see Chap. 314).

Gonadal tumors are rare in 45,X patients but have occurred in several patients with mosaicism involving the Y chromosome; consequently, streak gonads should be removed in any patient with evidence of virilization or a Y-containing cell line.

MIXED GONADAL DYSGENESIS   Clinical features   Mixed gonadal dysgenesis is an entity in which phenotypic males or females have a testis on one side and streak gonad on the other. Most have 45,X/46,XY mosaicism, but the clinical entity is not confined to that chromosomal pattern. The incidence is unknown, but in most hospitals it is the second most common cause of ambiguous genitalia in the neonate after congenital adrenal hyperplasia.

About two-thirds are reared as females, and most phenotypic males are incompletely virilized at birth. The majority have ambiguous genitalia, including some degree of phallic enlargement, a urogenital sinus, and varying degrees of labioscrotal fusion. In most the testis is located intraabdominally; individuals with a testis in the inguinal or scrotal position are usually reared as males. A uterus, vagina, and at least one fallopian tube are almost invariably present.

The prepubertal testis appears relatively normal. The postpubertal testis contains abundant mature Leydig cells, but the seminiferous tubules lack germinal elements and contain only Sertoli cells. The streak gonad, a thin, pale, elongated structure located either in the broad ligament or along the pelvic wall, is composed of ovarian stroma. At puberty the testis secretes androgen, and virilization and phallic enlargement both occur. Feminization is rare; when it occurs, estrogen secretion from a gonadal tumor should be suspected.

Approximately a third exhibit the somatic features of 45,X gonadal dysgenesis, i.e., low posterior hairline, shield chest, multiple pigmented nevi, cubitus valgus, webbing of the neck, and short stature (height less than 150 cm).

Virtually all are chromatin-negative. In one series, two-thirds had the 45,X/46,XY karyotype, and in the remainder a 46,XY karyotype was present but mosaicism might have gone undetected or been limited to certain cell lines. The origin of 45,X/46,XY mosaicism is best explained by the loss of a Y chromosome during an early mitotic division of an XY zygote similar to the postulated loss of the X chromosome in the 46,XY/47,XXY mosaicism shown in Fig. 324-2.

Pathophysiology   It has been assumed that the 46,XY cell line stimulates testicular differentiation whereas the 45,X stem leads to the development of the contralateral streak gonad, but actual comparisons between karyotype and phenotypic expression have failed to substantiate such a relationship. Furthermore, no clear correlation has been found between the percentage of cells cultured from blood or skin containing 45,X or 46,XY and the degree of gonadal development or of somatic anomalies.

Both masculinization and müllerian duct regression in utero are incomplete. Since Leydig cell function is normal at puberty, inadequate virilization in utero may be the result of delayed development of a testis that is ultimately capable of normal Leydig cell function. Alternatively, the fetal testis may simply be incapable of synthesizing adequate amounts of müllerian-inhibiting substance and androgen.

Management   For the older child or adult in whom gender is fixed prior to diagnosis, the central issue in management is the possibility of tumor development in the gonads. The overall incidence of gonadal tumors is about 25 percent. Seminomas occur more frequently than gonadoblastomas, and the tumors may occur prior to puberty. The tumors occur most frequently in patients with a female phenotype who lack the somatic features typical of 45,X gonadal dysgenesis and are more common in intraabdominal testes than in the streak gonad. When the diagnosis is established in phenotypic females, early exploratory laparotomy and prophylactic gonadectomy should be undertaken both because gonadal tumors may occur in childhood and because the testis secretes androgen at puberty and thus causes virilization. Such subjects, like those with gonadal dysgenesis, are then given estrogen to induce and maintain feminization.

When the diagnosis is established in phenotypic males during late childhood or in adults the management is more complicated. Phenotypic males with mixed gonadal dysgenesis are infertile (no germinal elements are present in the testes) and have a high risk of developing gonadal tumors. Which testes can be safely conserved? In general the following observations apply: (1) tumors develop in scrotal streak gonads but not in scrotal testes, (2) tumors that develop in intraabdominal testes are always associated with ipsilateral müllerian duct structures, and (3) tumors in streak gonads are always associated with tumors in the contralateral abdominal testis. Based on these observations, it is recommended that (1) all streak gonads should be removed, (2) scrotal testes should be preserved, and (3) intraabdominal testes should be excised unless they can be relocated in the scrotum and are not associated with ipsilateral müllerian duct structures. Decisions as to reconstructive surgery of the phallus depend upon the nature of the defect.

When the diagnosis is established in early infancy and the genitalia are ambiguous, gender assignment is usually female. Resection of the enlarged phallus and gonadectomy can then be accomplished in infancy, sometimes in one procedure. If the decision is for male gender assignment, the same criteria apply as to which testes should be removed in infants as in older males.

TRUE HERMAPHRODITISM   Clinical features   True hermaphroditism is a condition in which both an ovary and a testis or a gonad with histologic features of both (ovotestis) is present. To justify the diagnosis there must be histologic documentation of both types of gonadal epithelium, the presence of ovarian stroma without oocytes not being sufficient. The incidence is unknown, but more than 400 cases have been reported. Three categories are recognized: (1) one-fifth are bilateral—testicular and ovarian tissue (ovotestes) on each side, (2) two-fifths are unilateral—an ovotestis on one side and an ovary or a testis on the other, and (3) the remainder are lateral—a testis on one side and an ovary on the other.

The external genitalia display all gradations of the male-to-female spectrum. Two-thirds are sufficiently masculinized to be reared as males. However, less than one-tenth have normal male external genitalia; most have hypospadias, and more than half have incomplete labioscrotal fusion. Two-thirds of phenotypic females have an enlarged clitoris, and most have a urogenital sinus. Differentiation of the internal ducts usually corresponds to the adjacent gonad. Although an epididymis usually develops adjacent to a testis, development of the vas deferens is complete in only one-third. Of the patients with an ovotestis, three-fourths have an epididymis, two-thirds have a fallopian tube, one-tenth have a vas deferens, and one-tenth have both a vas deferens and a fallopian tube. A uterus is usually present although it may be hypoplastic or unicornuate. The ovary usually occupies the normal position, but the testis or ovotestis may be found at any level along the route of embryonic testicular descent, frequently associated with an inguinal hernia. Testicular tissue is present in the scrotum or the labioscrotal fold in one-third, in the inguinal canal in one-third, and in the abdominal area in one-third.

Variable feminization and virilization ensue at puberty, three-fourths develop gynecomastia, and about half menstruate. In phenotypic men menstruation presents as cyclic hematuria. Ovulation occurs in approximately one-fourth and is more common than spermatogenesis. In men ovulation may present as testicular pain.

Fertility has been reported in women following removal of an ovotestis and in a man who fathered two children. Congenital malformations of other systems are rare.

Pathophysiology   About two-thirds of subjects have a 46,XX karyotype, a tenth have a 46,XY karyotype, and the remainder are chromosomal mosaics in which a Y cell line is present. The mechanism responsible for the gonadal development is unknown. Even though not demonstrable with conventional karyotyping methods, it was assumed that sufficient genetic material from the Y chromosome was present (as the result of translocation, nondisjunction, or mutation) to induce the development of testicular tissue. However, hybridization studies with Y chromosome–specific probes in the 46,XX disorder have failed to demonstrate the presence of DNA from the short arm of the Y. In rare instances multiple sibs with a 46,XX karyotype are affected, possibly the result of an autosomal or X-linked mutation.

Because corpora lutea are present in the ovaries of more than one-fourth of subjects, it can be deduced that a female neuroendocrine axis is present and functions normally in such individuals. Feminization (gynecomastia and menstruation) is the result of secretion of estradiol by the ovarian tissue present. In masculinized patients secretion of androgen predominates over secretion of estrogen, and some produce sperm.

Management   When the diagnosis is made in a newborn or early infant, gender assignment depends upon the anatomic features. In older children and adults gonads and internal duct structures that are contradictory to the predominant phenotype (and the gender of rearing) should be removed, and when necessary the external genitalia should be modified appropriately. Although gonadal tumors are rare in true hermaphroditism, a gonadoblastoma has been reported in an individual with an XY cell line. Consequently, the possibility of future tumor development must be taken into account when the decision regarding conservation of gonadal tissue is made.

DISORDERS OF GONADAL SEX

Disorders of gonadal sex result when chromosomal sex is normal, but for one of several reasons differentiation of the gonads is abnormal. Thus, gonadal and phenotypic sex do not correspond to chromosomal sex.

PURE GONADAL DYSGENESIS   Clinical features   Pure gonadal dysgenesis is a disorder in which phenotypic females with gonads and genitalia identical to those with gonadal dysgenesis (bilateral streaks, infantile uterus and fallopian tubes, and sexual infantilism) have normal height, few if any congenital anomalies, and either a normal 46,XX or 46,XY karyotype. This disorder is only about one-tenth as common as gonadal dysgenesis. On genetic grounds this can be considered a separate disorder from gonadal dysgenesis, but it cannot be distinguished clinically from those instances of gonadal dysgenesis associated with minimal somatic abnormalities. The height is normal or greater than normal, some subjects being over 170 cm. Estrogen levels vary from profound deficiency typical of 45,X gonadal dysgenesis to some breast development and appearance of menses that terminate in an early menopause. About 40 percent have some feminization. Axillary and pubic hair are scanty, and the internal genitalia consist of müllerian derivatives only.

Tumors may develop in the streak gonads, particularly dysgerminoma or gonadoblastoma in the 46,XY disorder. Such tumors are frequently heralded by the development of virilizing signs or a pelvic mass.

Pathophysiology   Although chromosomal mosaicisms have been described under this nosology, the designation here is restricted to subjects with uniform 46,XX or 46,XY karyotypes. (Those with mosaicism are variants of gonadal dysgenesis or mixed gonadal dysgenesis as described above.) The rationale for this restricted definition is based upon the fact that both the XX and XY varieties can result from single gene mutations. Several sibships have been reported in which more than one individual is affected with the 46,XX type of the disorder, frequently the result of consanguineous matings, suggesting an autosomal recessive pattern of inheritance. Familial occurrence of the 46,XY variety has also been described; in some the mutation appears to be inherited in an X-linked recessive pattern, while in other families the occurrence is compatible with a male-limited autosomal recessive inheritance. In some patients with the 46,XY form of the disorder, the TDF region of the Y chromosome is deleted. In both the 46,XX and the 46,XY forms the disorder prevents differentiation of ovary or testis, respectively; the development of the female phenotype is the consequence of the failure of gonadal development. As in all individuals with nonfunctional gonads, gonadotropin secretion is elevated, and estrogen secretion is low.

Management   The management of the estrogen deficiency is identical to that in gonadal dysgenesis, namely, appropriate estrogen replacement therapy is initiated at the time of expected puberty and maintained in adult life (see Chap. 322). Because of the high frequency of gonadal tumors in the 46,XY variety, the streak gonads should be removed once the diagnosis is made. The development of virilizing signs is indication for immediate surgery. The natural history of the gonadal tumors in this disorder is uncertain, but the prognosis after surgical removal is usually good.

THE ABSENT TESTES SYNDROME (ANORCHIA, TESTICULAR REGRESSION, GONADAL AGENESIS, AGONADISM)   Clinical features   A spectrum of phenotypes has been described in 46,XY males with absent or rudimentary testes but in whom unequivocal evidence exists that endocrine function of the testis (e.g., invariable müllerian duct regression and variable testosterone synthesis) was present at some time during embryonic life. This rare disorder can be distinguished from pure gonadal dysgenesis in which no evidence can be inferred for gonadal function during embryonic development. The disorder varies in its manifestations from complete failure of virilization through varying degrees of incomplete virilization of the external genitalia to otherwise normal males with bilateral anorchia.

The purest form is represented by 46,XY phenotypic females with absent testes, sexual infantilism, and absence of both müllerian duct derivatives and accessory organs of male reproduction. Such individuals differ from 46,XY pure gonadal dysgenesis in that no gonadal remnant can be identified, including no streak gonad, and in the absence of müllerian derivatives. Testicular failure must have occurred between the onset of formation of müllerian-inhibiting substance and the secretion of testosterone, that is, after development of the seminiferous tubules but before the onset of Leydig cell function.

In others the testicular failure must have occurred later in gestation, and these individuals may constitute problems in gender assignment. In some, failure of müllerian regression is more pronounced than failure of testosterone secretion, but none exhibit normal müllerian development. In those with more extensive virilization the external genitalia are phenotypically male, but rudimentary oviducts and vasa deferentia may coexist internally.

At the final extreme is the syndrome of bilateral anorchia in which phenotypic men have absence of müllerian structures and gonads but male development of the wolffian system and external genitalia. Microphallus implies that failure of androgen-mediated growth occurred late in embryogenesis after anatomic development of the male urethra is complete. Persistent gynecomastia may or may not develop.

Pathophysiology   The pathogenesis is not understood. The testicular regression could be the result of mutant genes, teratogen, or trauma. Multiple instances of agonadism in the same family have been reported, some of whom have unilateral and others bilateral defects.

The quantitative dynamics of gonadal steroid production have been studied in only a few patients. In two phenotypic women with primary amenorrhea, sexual infantilism, and no internal genital structures, androgen and estrogen kinetics were similar to those in gonadal dysgenesis; production rates of estrogen were low, and no glandular secretion of testosterone was found, confirming the func-

tional as well as anatomic absence of the testes. In one phenotypic male with bilateral anorchia, testosterone and estrogen production was accounted for by peripheral conversion from plasma androstenedione. However, some subjects in whom no testes can be identified at laparotomy have blood testosterone values clearly above the castrate range, presumably derived from remnant testes.

Management   The management of the two extremes is clearcut. Sexually infantile, phenotypic females should be treated like patients with gonadal dysgenesis, namely, given adequate estrogen to ensure appropriate breast and female somatic development, and any coexisting vaginal agenesis should be treated by surgical or medical means. Likewise, phenotypic males with anorchia should be given adequate androgen replacement to allow normal male secondary sexual development. The cases with incomplete virilization or ambiguous development of the external genitalia are more complex and require hormonal therapy at the time of expected puberty and individual assessment as to whether surgical therapy is appropriate.

DISORDERS OF PHENOTYPIC SEX

FEMALE PSEUDOHERMAPHRODITISM   Congenital adrenal hyperplasia   CLINICAL FEATURES   The pathways by which glucocorticoids are synthesized in the adrenal gland and androgens are formed in the testis and adrenal are summarized in Fig. 324-3. Three reactions are common to the formation of glucocorticoids and androgens (20,22-desmolase, 3β-hydroxysteroid dehydrogenase, and 17α-hydroxylase); impairment of any of these reactions results in deficiency of glucocorticoid and androgen synthesis and consequently in both congenital adrenal hyperplasia (due to enhanced ACTH levels) and defective virilization of the male embryo (male pseudohermaphroditism). Two enzyme reactions are involved exclusively in androgen synthesis (17,20-desmolase and 17β-hydroxysteroid dehydrogenase); deficiency in either results in pure male pseudohermaphroditism with normal glucocorticoid synthesis. Deficiency of either of the terminal two enzymes of glucocorticoid synthesis (21-hydroxylase and 11β-hydroxylase) results in defective formation of hydrocortisone; the compensatory increase in ACTH secretion causes adrenal hyperplasia and a secondary increase in androgen formation that results in virilization in the female or precocious masculinization in the male.

The *adrenal insufficiency* in these disorders may produce equally severe and life-threatening problems in both sexes and is described in detail in Chap. 317. The major features of congenital adrenal hyperplasia are listed in Table 324-4. From the standpoint of *abnormal sexual development,* some defects in steroidogenesis result in female pseudohermaphroditism and some cause male pseudohermaphroditism. (One disorder, 3β-hydroxysteroid dehydrogenase deficiency, can cause either male or female pseudohermaphroditism, but since the more common genital defect is incomplete virilization of the male, it will be discussed as an abnormality of male phenotypic differentiation.)

Congenital adrenal hyperplasia due to 21-hydroxylase deficiency is the most common cause of ambiguous genitalia in the newborn, with an incidence of between 1:5000 and 1:15,000 in Europe and the United States. Virilization is usually apparent at birth in the female and within the first 2 to 3 years of life in the male. Manifestations in females include hypertrophy of the clitoris with ventral binding (chordee), partial fusion of the labioscrotal folds, and variable virilization of the urethra. The internal female structures and ovaries remain unaltered, and the wolffian ducts regress normally, probably because adrenal function begins relatively late in embryogenesis. The external appearance of affected females is similar to that of a male with bilateral cryptorchidism and hypospadias. The labioscrotal folds are bulbous and rugated and resemble a scrotum. Rarely the virilization is so severe that development of a complete male penile urethra and prostate results in errors in sex assignment at birth. Radiography following the injection of radiopaque dye into the external genital orifice is helpful in demonstrating the presence of a vagina, uterus,

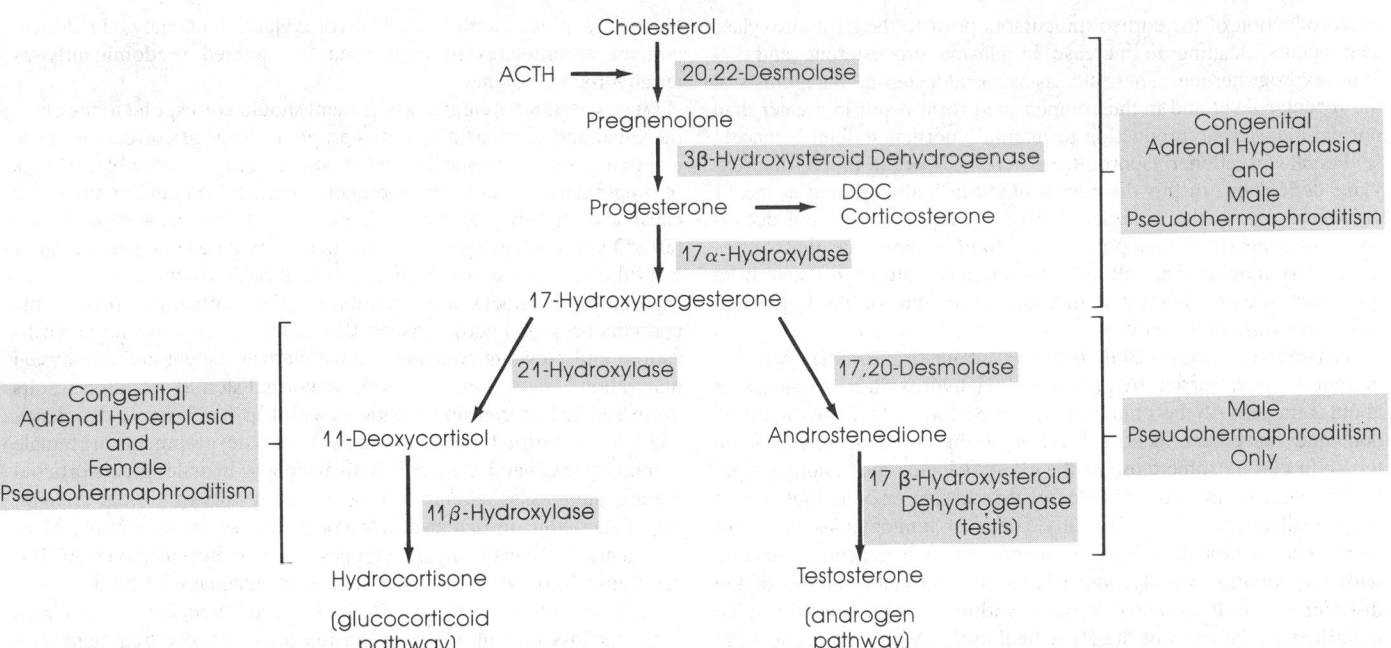

FIGURE 324-3 Pathways of glucocorticoid and androgen synthesis. Note abnormal conditions corresponding to impaired enzyme reactions.

and sometimes even fallopian tubes. In a few cases virilization of the female is slight or absent at birth and becomes evident in later infancy, adolescence, or adulthood, presumably as the result of allelic variation of the mutant genes (the so-called late-onset or adult form of the disorder). The untreated female with the congenital form of the disorder grows rapidly during the first year of life and has progressive virilization. At the time of expected puberty there is a failure of normal female sexual development and absence of menstruation. In both sexes rapid somatic maturation results in premature epiphyseal closure and a short adult height.

Since male phenotypic differentiation is normal, the condition is usually not recognized in the male at birth in the absence of overt adrenal insufficiency. However, early growth and maturation of the external genitalia, appearance of secondary sex characteristics, coarsening of the voice, frequent erections, and excessive muscular development are noticeable in the first few years of life. Virilization in the male can follow either of two patterns. Excessive adrenal androgens can inhibit gonadotropin production so that the testes remain infantile in size despite the acceleration of masculinization.

Such untreated adult men are capable of erection and ejaculation but have no spermatogenesis. Alternatively, adrenal androgen secretion can activate a premature maturation of the hypothalamic-pituitary axis and initiate a true precocious puberty including early maturation of spermatogenesis (see Chap. 321). The untreated male is also subject to the development of ACTH-dependent "tumors" of the testis composed of adrenal rest cells.

In 21-hydroxylase deficiency, which accounts for about 95 percent of congenital adrenal hyperplasia, decreased production of hydrocortisone leads to increased release of ACTH, enlargement of the adrenal glands, and partial or complete compensation of the defect in the secretion of hydrocortisone. In about half the enzyme defect appears to be partial, and cortisol secretion is normal. This form is termed "simple virilizing" or "compensated." In the remainder there seems to be a more complete deficiency of the enzyme; the enlarged adrenal fails to produce adequate amounts of cortisol and aldosterone leading to severe salt wastage with anorexia, vomiting, volume depletion, and collapse within the first few weeks of life, the so-called salt-losing form of 21-hydroxylase deficiency. In all untreated patients

TABLE 324-4 Forms of congenital adrenal hyperplasia

Deficiency	Cortisol	Aldosterone	Degree of virilization of females	Failure of virilization in males	Dominant steroid secreted	Comment
21-Hydroxylase, partial (simple virilizing or compensated)	Normal	↑	+ + + +	0	17-Hydroxy-progesterone	Most common type (~95% of total); from one- to two-thirds salt losers
Severe (salt-losing)	↓	↓	+ + + +	0	17-Hydroxy-progesterone	
11β-Hydroxylase (hypertension)	↓	↓	+ + + +	0	11-Deoxycortisol and 11-deoxy-corticosterone	Hypertension
3β-Hydroxysteroid dehydrogenase	0	0	+	+ + + +	Δ⁵-3β-OH compounds (dehydroepiandrosterone)	Probably second most common, usually salt loss
17α-Hydroxylase	↓	↓	0	+ + + +	Corticosterone and 11-deoxy-corticosterone	No feminization of female, hypertension
20,22-Desmolase (lipoid adrenal hyperplasia)	0	0	0	+ + + +	Cholesterol(?)	Rare, usually salt loss

overproduction of the cortisol precursors prior to the 21-hydroxylase step occurs, leading to increase in plasma progesterone and 17-hydroxyprogesterone. These act as weak aldosterone antagonists at the receptor level and in the compensated form result in greater than normal aldosterone production to maintain normal sodium balance.

Female pseudohermaphroditism may also occur in 11β-hydroxylase deficiency. In this disorder a block in hydroxylation at the 11 carbon results in the accumulation of 11-deoxycortisol and deoxycorticosterone (DOC), a potent salt-retaining hormone that causes hypertension rather than salt loss. The clinical features that stem from glucocorticoid deficiency and androgen excess are similar to those in 21-hydroxylase deficiency.

PATHOPHYSIOLOGY   Both disorders are due to autosomal recessive mutations. The carrier frequency for 21-hydroxylase deficiency is about 1 in 50. At the clinical level three forms of 21-hydroxylase deficiency have been identified, all involving mutations of a gene on the sixth chromosome close to the HLA-B locus: the common type, which acts like an ordinary autosomal recessive enzyme mutation; a cryptic allele, which is clinically silent in homozygous form but which causes typical disease when present as a genetic compound with the common variety; and a late-onset variant. Carriers of the disorder (as well as homozygotes) within a given family can be identified on the basis of the HLA haplotype. At the molecular level the mutations that give rise to 21-hydroxylase deficiency are even more polymorphic; indeed, deletions of portions of the gene, conversion of the gene from a functional state to a form that is not transcribed normally, and point mutations have been characterized in different families with the disorder. 11β-Hydroxylase deficiency is due to mutation of the normal gene for the enzyme on chromosome 8.

For discussion of the endocrine pathology see Chap. 317. In brief, urinary excretion of ketosteroids is elevated, as is the excretion of the major metabolites that accumulate proximal to the enzymatic blocks. Plasma ACTH is elevated. In 21-hydroxylase deficiency, 17-hydroxyprogesterone accumulates in blood and is excreted predominantly as pregnanetriol. In 11-hydroxylase deficiency, 11-deoxycortisol accumulates in blood and is excreted predominantly as tetrahydrocortexolone.

MANAGEMENT   Gender assignment should correspond to the chromosomal and gonadal sex, and appropriate surgical correction of the external genitalia should be undertaken as early as possible. This is of importance because appropriately treated men and women are capable of fertility. However, if the correct diagnosis is made late (after 3 years of age) gender assignment should be changed only after careful consideration of the psychosexual background.

Medical treatment with appropriate glucocorticoids prevents the consequences of hydrocortisone deficiency, arrests the rapid virilization, and prevents premature somatic advancement and epiphyseal maturation. The suppression of the abnormal steroid secretion results in cure of the hypertension in patients with 11β-hydroxylase deficiency and allows normal onset of menses and development of female secondary sex characteristics in both disorders. In males glucocorticoid therapy suppresses adrenal androgens and results in normal gonadotropin secretion, testicular development, and spermatogenesis. Measurements of plasma 17-hydroxyprogesterone, androstenedione, ACTH, and renin have all been used to assess adequacy of replacement therapy. In severe forms of 21-hydroxylase deficiency associated with salt loss or with elevated plasma renin activity treatment with mineralocorticoids is also indicated. In such patients the monitoring of plasma renin is useful for determining the adequacy of mineralocorticoid replacement.

Other causes of female pseudohermaphroditism   Female pseudohermaphroditism may also occur in babies born to mothers who have virilizing tumors of the ovary (e.g., arrhenoblastomas or luteomas of pregnancy) and, rarely, to mothers with virilizing adrenal tumors. In the past, the administration to pregnant women of progestational agents with androgenic side effects (such as 17α-ethinyl-19-nor-testosterone) to prevent abortion resulted in masculinization of female fetuses.

TABLE 324-5   Anatomic, genetic, and endocrine profile of hereditary male pseudohermaphroditism

| Disorder | Inheritance | Phenotype | | | | |
		Müllerian ducts	Wolffian ducts	Spermatogenesis	Urogenital sinus	External genitalia
DEFECTS IN TESTOSTERONE SYNTHESIS						
Five enzyme deficiencies	Autosomal or X-linked recessive	Absent	Variable development	Normal or decreased	Variable from male to female	Generally female
DEFECTS IN ANDROGEN ACTION						
5α-Reductase deficiency	Autosomal recessive	Absent	Male	Normal or decreased	Female	Clitoromegaly
Receptor disorders:						
Complete testicular feminization	X-linked recessive	Absent	Absent	Absent	Female	Female
Incomplete testicular feminization	X-linked recessive	Absent	Male	Absent	Female	Clitoromegaly and posterior fusion
Reifenstein syndrome	X-linked recessive	Absent	Variable development	Absent	Variable from male to female	Incomplete male development
Infertile male syndrome	X-linked recessive	Absent	Male	Absent or decreased	Male	Male
Undervirilized fertile male	X-linked recessive	Absent	Male	Normal or decreased	Male	Male
Receptor-positive resistance	Uncertain	Absent	Variable	Absent or decreased	Variable	Female to male
DEFECTS IN MÜLLERIAN REGRESSION						
Persistent müllerian duct syndrome	Autosomal or X-linked recessive	Rudimentary uterus and fallopian tubes	Male	Normal	Male	Male

CHAPTER 324 DISORDERS OF SEXUAL DIFFERENTIATION

Developmental disorders of müllerian ducts (congenital absence of the vagina, müllerian agenesis) CLINICAL FEATURES Congenital hypoplasia or absence of the vagina in combination with abnormal or absent uterus (the Mayer-Rokitansky-Kuster-Hauser syndrome) is second to gonadal dysgenesis as a cause of primary amenorrhea. Most patients are ascertained after the time of expected puberty because of failure to menstruate. The height and intelligence are normal, and the breasts, axillary and pubic hair, and habitus are feminine in character. The uterus can vary from almost normal, lacking only a conduit to the introitus, to the characteristic rudimentary bicornuate cords with or without a lumen. In some patients cyclical abdominal pain indicates that sufficient functional endometrium is present to result in retrograde menstruation and/or hematometra.

About one-third have abnormal kidneys, most commonly agenesis or ectopy. Fused kidneys of the horseshoe type and solitary ectopic kidneys located in the pelvis also occur. Skeletal abnormalities are present in one-tenth; two-thirds involve the spine, and limb and rib abnormalities account for the remainder. Specific bone abnormalities include wedge vertebrae, fused rudimentary or asymmetric vertebral bodies, and supernumerary vertebrae. The Klippel-Feil syndrome (congenital fusion of the cervical spine, short neck, low posterior hairline, and painless limitation of cervical movement) is a frequent association.

PATHOPHYSIOLOGY The karyotype is 46,XX. Most are believed to be sporadic in nature, but familial occurrence has been described. The pattern of inheritance in most familial cases is consistent with a sex-limited autosomal dominant mutation. Sporadic cases may represent new mutations of the type responsible for the familial disorder or be multifactorial in etiology. In the familial cases expressivity is variable; some affected family members have skeletal or renal abnormalities only, and some have other abnormalities of müllerian derivatives such as a double uterus. Bilateral renal aplasia in stillborn infants is commonly associated with absence of the uterus and vagina. Thus, the family history should be probed for isolated skeletal and renal abnormalities and for stillbirths that might result from congenital absence of both kidneys.

Documentation of ovulatory peaks of plasma LH and biphasic temperature curves during the cycle suggest that ovarian function is normal, and successful pregnancies have occurred after corrective vaginal surgery in patients with normal uteri.

MANAGEMENT Vaginal agenesis can be treated by surgical or nonsurgical means. Surgical repair generally utilizes a split-thickness skin graft around a solid rubber mold for the creation of an artificial vagina. Medical treatment consists of the repeated application of pressure against the vaginal dimple with a simple dilator to cause development of adequate vaginal depth. In view of complication rates of 5 to 10 percent in surgical series, medical treatment should be tried in most, and surgery should be reserved for patients in whom a well-formed uterus is present and the possibility of fertility exists. Frequent coitus or instrumental dilatation is essential for maintaining the neovagina formed by either technique.

MALE PSEUDOHERMAPHRODITISM Defective virilization of the male embryo (male pseudohermaphroditism) can result from defects in androgen synthesis, defects in androgen action, defects in müllerian duct regression, and uncertain causes. Four-fifths of male pseudohermaphrodites have normal androgen synthesis.

Abnormalities in androgen synthesis CLINICAL FEATURES- Enzymatic defects that result in defective testosterone synthesis (Fig. 324-3) can cause incomplete virilization of the male embryo during embryogenesis (Tables 324-4 and 324-5). Each of the defects blocks a step in the conversion of cholesterol to testosterone. Three (20,22-desmolase, 3β-hydroxysteroid dehydrogenase, and 17α-hydroxylase) are common to the synthesis of other adrenal hormones as well; consequently, their deficiency results in congenital adrenal hyperplasia (Table 324-4) as well as male pseudohermaphroditism. Two others (17,20-desmolase, and 17β-hydroxysteroid dehydrogenase) are unique to the pathway of androgen synthesis, and their deficiency results only in male pseudohermaphroditism. Since androgens are obligatory precursors of estrogens, synthesis of estrogen is also low in affected men and women in all but the terminal defect (17β-hydroxysteroid dehydrogenase deficiency).

The adrenal dysfunction is described in Chap. 317, and the present discussion concerns the abnormal sexual development. In 46,XY subjects there is usually no trace of uterus or fallopian tubes, indicating that the müllerian-inhibiting function of the testis during embryogenesis was normal. The masculinization of the wolffian ducts, urogenital sinus, and urogenital tubercle and the degree of virilization at puberty vary from almost normal to absent, and therefore, the clinical picture spans the range from phenotypic men with mild hypospadias to phenotypic women who prior to puberty resemble patients with complete testicular feminization. This variability is the consequence of varying severity of the enzymatic defects in different patients and of varying effects of the steroids that accumulate proximal to the metabolic blocks in the different disorders. In patients with partial defects and in whom plasma testosterone is normal the diagnosis can only be made by measuring the steroids that accumulate proximal to the metabolic block.

20,22-Desmolase deficiency (lipoid adrenal hyperplasia) is a form of congenital adrenal hyperplasia in which virtually no urinary steroids (either 17-ketosteroids or 17-hydroxycorticoids) can be detected. The defect is prior to the formation of pregnenolone and is assumed to involve the 20,22-desmolase (side-chain cleavage) enzyme responsible for the conversion of cholesterol to pregnenolone. The syndrome is associated with salt wasting and profound adrenal insufficiency, and most affected individuals die during infancy. At autopsy the adrenals and testes are enlarged and infiltrated with lipid. Affected males are incompletely masculinized whereas affected female infants have normal genital development. The gene for the human enzyme is located on chromosome 15.

3β-Hydroxysteroid dehydrogenase deficiency causes varying failure of masculinization and development of a vagina in male infants. Female infants may be modestly virilized at birth due to the weak

| | Endocrine profile relative to normal male | | |
Breast	Testosterone production	Estrogen production	LH
Usually male	Normal to decreased	Variable	High
Male	Normal	Normal	Normal or increased
Female	High	High	High
Female	High	High	High
Female	High	High	High
Usually male	Normal or high	Normal or high	Normal or high
Female	Normal or high	Normal or high	Normal or high
Variable	Normal or high	Normal or high	Normal or high
Male	Normal	Normal	Normal

androgenic potency of dehydroepiandrosterone, the major steroid secreted. If the enzyme is absent in both the adrenal and testis, no urinary steroids contain a Δ^4-3-keto configuration, whereas in patients in whom the defect is partial or affects only the testis, the urine may contain normal or elevated levels of Δ^4-3-ketosteroids. Most patients have marked salt wasting and profound adrenal insufficiency, and long-term survival in untreated cases occurs only in states of partial deficiency. Affected males may experience an otherwise normal male puberty except for profound gynecomastia. In these individuals a low-normal blood testosterone level is accompanied by elevated Δ^5 precursors. The enzyme in different tissues must be under complex control since deficiency of the enzyme in the testis may be less severe than in the adrenal and since enzyme activity in the liver may be normal in the face of profound deficiency in the adrenal and testis. Individuals with normal liver enzymes can be mistakenly identified as having 21-hydroxylase deficiency if urinary Δ^5-pregnenetriol is not documented to be greater than urinary pregnanetriol.

17α-Hydroxylase–17,20-desmolase deficiency impairs the introduction of the 17 hydroxyl and the scission of the C-17,20 carbon bond that convert pregnenolone and progesterone to dehydroepiandrosterone and androstenedione, respectively. These reactions are mediated by a single cytochrome P_{450} enzyme encoded on chromosome 10, and it is unclear why both reactions occur in the ovary and testis whereas in the adrenal 17-hydroxy progesterone is largely converted to glucocorticoids and mineralocorticoids rather than the 19 carbon steroids. Likewise, it is unclear why some patients have selective impairment of either 17α-hydroxylase or 17,20-desmolase activity; the distinction between these activities must be functional and may involve the relative concentration of steroid substrates and competing enzymes. Whatever the explanation, the clinical consequences of 17α-hydroxylase and 17,20-desmolase deficiencies are different.

17α-Hydroxylase deficiency characteristically results in hypogonadism, absence of secondary sex characteristics, hypokalemic alkalosis, hypertension, and virtually undetectable hydrocortisone secretion in phenotypic women. The secretion of both corticosterone and desoxycorticosterone (DOC) by the adrenal is elevated, and urinary 17-ketosteroids are low. Aldosterone secretion is low due to high plasma DOC and depressed angiotensin levels and returns to normal after suppressive doses of hydrocortisone are administered. In 46,XX subjects amenorrhea, absent sexual hair, and hypertension are common, but, since gonadal steroids are not required for female development during embryogenesis, the phenotype is that of a normal prepubertal woman. In males the deficiency results in defective virilization that varies from complete male pseudohermaphroditism to ambiguous genitalia with perineoscrotal hypospadias and, in some, gynecomastia. Adrenal insufficiency does not develop, since the secretion of both corticosterone (a weak glucocorticoid) and DOC (a mineralocorticoid) is elevated. Hypertension and hypokalemia are prominent features of the disorder (even in the neonatal period) and remit after suppression of the DOC secretion by adequate glucocorticoid replacement.

17,20-Desmolase deficiency in males is associated with normal function of the adrenal cortex and a variable pattern of male pseudohermaphroditism. In the majority there is genital ambiguity at birth with some virilization at the time of expected puberty. Rare 46,XY patients have had a female phenotype and no virilization at the time of expected puberty. The disorder has been recognized in one 46,XX woman with sexual infantilism.

17β-Hydroxysteroid dehydrogenase deficiency involves the final step in testosterone biosynthesis, reduction of the 17-keto group of androstenedione. This is the most common of the enzymatic defects in testosterone synthesis. Affected 46,XY males usually have a female phenotype with a blind-ending vagina and absence of müllerian derivatives, but inguinal or abdominal testes and virilized wolffian duct structures are present. At the time of expected puberty, both virilization (with phallic enlargement and development of facial and body hair) and a variable degree of female breast development take place. In some untreated patients reversal of gender behavior from female to male occurs at puberty. Androgen and estrogen dynamics have not been elucidated in detail, but the 17-keto reduction of estrone to estradiol by the gonads is also low. 17β-Hydroxysteroid dehydrogenase is normally present in many tissues besides the gonads, and only the gonadal enzyme appears to be defective in this disorder. Plasma testosterone may be in the low-normal range, making it essential to document elevation in plasma androstenedione to make the diagnosis.

PATHOPHYSIOLOGY   The available data for these various disorders are compatible with autosomal recessive inheritance. The pattern of steroid secretion and excretion depends on the site of the various metabolic blocks (Fig. 324-3). In general, gonadotropin secretion is high, and as a consequence many individuals with incomplete defects are able to compensate so that the steady-state levels of end products such as testosterone may be normal or almost normal.

In some cases of male pseudohermaphroditism testosterone formation is deficient for reasons other than a single enzyme defect in androgen synthesis. These include disorders in which Leydig cell agenesis (possibly due to absence of the LH receptor) or the secretion of a biologically inactive LH molecule is thought to be the primary defect. In addition, as described above, in several disorders including familial XY gonadal dysgenesis, sporadic dysgenetic testes, and the absent testis syndrome, deficient testosterone production is secondary to abnormal gonadal development.

MANAGEMENT   Therapy with glucocorticoids and in some instances mineralocorticoids is indicated in those disorders causing adrenal hyperplasia. The decision as to the management of the genital abnormalities depends upon the individual case. Fertility has not been reported, and its consideration does not enter into sex assignment. In genetic females there is no problem (except in diagnosis) in that affected individuals are raised appropriately as females, and suitable estrogen replacement is administered at the time of expected puberty to promote development of normal secondary sex characteristics. The decision as to whether newborn males with ambiguous genitalia should be raised as males or females depends upon the anatomic defect; in general the more severely affected should be raised as females, and corrective surgery of the genitalia and removal of the testes should be undertaken as early as possible. In such subjects estrogen therapy is also indicated at the appropriate age to allow development of normal female secondary sex characteristics. In individuals raised as males, corrective surgery is indicated for any coexisting hypospadias, and monitoring of plasma androgens and estrogens should be undertaken at the time of expected puberty to determine whether supplemental testosterone therapy is appropriate.

Abnormalities in androgen action   Several disorders of male phenotypic development result from abnormalities of androgen action. The spectrum of phenotypes is described in Tables 324-4 and -5. In these disorders testosterone formation and müllerian regression are normal, but male development is impaired to a variable degree as a result of resistance to androgen action in the target cells.

5α-REDUCTASE DEFICIENCY   This autosomal recessive disorder is characterized by (1) severe perineoscrotal hypospadias; (2) a blind vaginal pouch of variable size opening either into the urogenital sinus or into the urethra; (3) testes with normal epididymides, vasa deferentia, and seminal vesicles, and termination of the ejaculatory ducts into the blind-ending vagina; (4) a female habitus without female breast development but with normal axillary and pubic hair; (5) the absence of female internal genitalia; (6) normal male plasma testosterone; and (7) masculinization to a variable degree at the time of puberty.

The fact that virilization during embryogenesis is defective only in the urogenital sinus and the external genitalia provided insight into the fundamental abnormality. Testosterone, the androgen secreted by the fetal testis, is responsible for differentiation of the wolffian duct into the epididymis, the vas deferens, and the seminal vesicle, whereas dihydrotestosterone mediates virilization of the urogenital sinus and the external genitalia. Consequently, a failure of dihydrotestosterone formation in a male embryo would be expected to cause the phenotype observed in this disorder, normal male wolffian duct derivatives with defective masculinization of the external genitalia and urogenital sinus. Since testosterone itself regulates LH secretion (see Chap. 321), plasma LH is usually normal or minimally elevated. As a result, testosterone and estrogen production rates are those of normal men, and gynecomastia does not develop.

The fact that the 5α-reductase enzyme is deficient in this disorder was established by assay of biopsied tissues and cultured fibroblasts from affected individuals. In most subjects the 5α-reductase is either profoundly deficient or functionally absent, and in others the enzyme protein is normal in amount but structurally abnormal.

RECEPTOR DISORDERS   The androgen receptor is a typical member of the steroid/thyroid family of receptors with steroid-binding, DNA-binding, and functional domains and is encoded by a gene on the long arm of the X-chromosome. A variety of mutations of this gene impair receptor function and hence impair male phenotypic differentiation and/or virilization.

Clinical features.   Complete testicular feminization is the most common form of male pseudohermaphroditism; estimates of frequency vary from 1 in 20,000 to 1 in 64,000 male births. It is the third most common cause of primary amenorrhea in phenotypic women after gonadal dysgenesis and congenital absence of the vagina. The features are characteristic. Namely, a woman is seen by the physician either because of inguinal hernia (prepubertal) or primary amenorrhea (postpubertal). The development of the breasts after puberty, the general habitus, and the distribution of body fat are female in character so that most patients have a truly feminine appearance. Axillary and pubic hair are absent or scanty, but some vulval hair is usually present. Scalp hair is that of a normal woman, and facial hair is absent. The external genitalia are unambiguously female, and the clitoris is normal. The vagina is short and blind-ending and may be absent or rudimentary. All internal genitalia are absent except for undescended testes that contain normal Leydig cells and seminiferous tubules without spermatogenesis.

The testes may be located in the abdomen, along the course of the inguinal canal, or in the labia majora. Occasionally, remnants of müllerian or wolffian duct origin are present in the paratesticular fascia or in fibrous bands extending from the testis. Patients tend to be rather tall and bone age is normal. Psychosexual development is unmistakably female in regard to behavior, outlook, and maternal instincts.

The major complication of undescended testes in this disorder as in all forms of cryptorchidism is the development of tumors (Chap. 305). Since affected individuals undergo a normal pubertal growth spurt and feminize successfully at the time of expected puberty and since testicular tumors rarely develop until after puberty, it is usual to delay castration until after the time of expected puberty. Prepubertal castration is indicated if the testes are present in the inguinal region or the labia majora and result in discomfort or hernia formation. (If hernia repair is indicated prepubertally, most physicians prefer to remove the testes at the same time to limit the number of operative procedures.) If the testes are removed prepubertally, estrogen therapy is required at the appropriate age to ensure normal growth and breast development. When castration is performed postpubertally, meno-pausal symptoms and other evidences of estrogen withdrawal supervene, and suitable estrogen replacement is indicated (see Chap. 322).

Incomplete testicular feminization is about one-tenth as frequent as the complete form. In the incomplete disorder there is a minor virilization of the external genitalia (partial fusion of the labioscrotal folds and some degree of clitoromegaly), normal pubic hair, and some virilization as well as feminization at the time of expected puberty. The vagina is short and blind-ending, but in contrast to the complete form, the wolffian duct derivatives are often partially developed. The management of patients with the complete and incomplete forms of testicular feminization differs. Since patients

with the incomplete disorder virilize at the time of expected puberty, gonadectomy should be performed before the expected time of puberty in all prepubertal patients with clitoromegaly or posterior labial fusion.

Reifenstein syndrome is the term applied to forms of incomplete male pseudohermaphroditism initially described by a number of eponyms (Reifenstein syndrome, Gilbert-Dreyfus syndrome, Lubs syndrome). Each of these phenotypes was originally assumed to be a distinct entity, but these syndromes are now known to constitute variable manifestations of a single mutation. The most common phenotype is a man with perineoscrotal hypospadias and gynecomastia, but the spectrum of defective virilization in affected families ranges from men with azoospermia to phenotypic women with pseudovaginas. Axillary and pubic hair are normal, but chest and facial hair are minimal. Cryptorchidism is common, the testes are small, and azoospermia is present. Some have defects in wolffian duct derivatives such as absence or hypoplasia of the vas deferens. Since the psychological development in most is unequivocally male, the hypospadias and cryptorchidism should be corrected surgically. The only successful form of treatment of the gynecomastia is surgical removal.

The *infertile male syndrome* is probably the most common disorder of the androgen receptor and is not actually a form of male pseudohermaphroditism. Some such individuals are minimally affected subjects in families with Reifenstein syndrome with azoospermia as the only manifestation of the receptor abnormality. More commonly, the individuals present with male infertility and have negative family histories; indeed a disorder of the androgen receptor may be present in a fifth or more of men with idiopathic azoospermia. The *undervirilized fertile male* is an even less severe manifestation of an androgen receptor defect. In these families affected men have gynecomastia and undervirilization, and some are fertile.

Pathophysiology.   The karyotype is 46,XY, and the mutant gene is X-linked. The frequency of a positive family history varies from about two-thirds of patients with testicular feminization and Reifenstein syndrome to only occasional patients with the infertile male syndrome. The patients with a negative family history are believed to be the result of new mutations.

Hormone dynamics are similar in all disorders of the androgen receptor. Plasma testosterone levels and rates of testosterone production by the testes are normal or higher than normal. The elevated testosterone production is caused by the high mean plasma level of LH, which in turn is due to defective feedback regulation caused by resistance to the action of androgen at the hypothalamic-pituitary level. Elevated LH concentration is responsible also for the increased estrogen production by the testes (see Chap. 321). (In normal men most estrogen is derived from peripheral formation from circulating androgens, but when plasma LH is elevated the testes secrete increased amounts of estrogen into the circulation.) Thus, resistance to the feedback regulation of LH secretion by circulating androgen results in elevated plasma LH levels, and this in turn results in the enhanced secretion of both testosterone and estradiol by the testes. Gonadotropin levels rise even higher (and menopausal symptoms may develop) when the testes are removed, indicating that gonadotropin secretion is under partial regulatory control. Presumably, in the steady state and in the absence of an androgen effect, estrogen alone regulates LH secretion, a control purchased at the expense of an elevated plasma estrogen concentration for a male. The hormonal changes in the infertile male syndrome are similar to those in the other receptor disorders but less marked. Some men with this syndrome do not have an elevation of plasma LH or plasma testosterone.

Feminization in these disorders is the result of two interlocking phenomena. First, androgens and estrogens have antagonistic effects, and virilization occurs in normal men when the ratio of androgen to estrogen is 100 to 1 or greater; in the absence of androgen action the cellular effect of estrogen is unopposed. Second, the testicular production of estradiol is greater than that of the normal male (although less than that of the normal female). Variable degrees of androgen resistance coupled with variably enhanced estradiol production result in different degrees of defective virilization and enhanced feminization in the four clinical syndromes.

Each of these syndromes is the result of an abnormality of the androgen receptor. Initially fibroblasts cultured from the skin of some subjects with complete testicular feminization were shown to have a near absence of high-affinity dihydrotestosterone binding. Subsequently, other individuals with complete testicular feminization as well as subjects with incomplete testicular feminization, Reifenstein syndrome, the infertile male syndrome, and undervirilization with fertility have been found to have either a decreased amount of an apparently normal receptor or a qualitatively abnormal androgen receptor. In some families, the fundamental defect is due to the deletion of a portion of the gene, in others the disorder is due to point mutations in the coding sequence, and in still others the defect appears to impair the transcription of the messenger RNA that encodes the receptor.

RECEPTOR-POSITIVE RESISTANCE   A category of androgen resistance that does not appear to involve either the 5α-reductase or the androgen receptor was first identified in a family with the syndrome of testicular feminization. Subsequent patients have been described with phenotypes ranging from incomplete testicular feminization to the Reifenstein syndrome. The hormonal profile is similar to that in the receptor disorders. The site of the molecular abnormality in these patients is unclear. It could be due to receptor defects too subtle to be detected by the usual assay. If the defect is truly distal to the receptor, there could be failure of generation of specific messenger RNA or an abnormality of RNA processing. Indeed, the disorder may represent a heterogeneous group of molecular abnormalities.

Persistent müllerian duct syndrome   Men with this disorder have testes and normal phenotypic development and in addition have bilateral fallopian tubes, a uterus, and an upper vagina, and variable development of the vas deferens. The subjects commonly present with inguinal hernias that contain the uterus, and cryptorchidism is common. Most have uninformative family histories, but in some families the condition is inherited either as an autosomal recessive or an X-linked recessive mutation. Because the external genitalia are well developed and the patients masculinize normally at puberty, it is assumed that during the critical stage of embryonic sexual differentiation the fetal testes produce a normal amount of androgen. However, müllerian regression does not occur for one of two reasons: some individuals fail to produce müllerian-inhibiting substance, and others produce normal amounts but do not respond to the hormone. To minimize the chance of tumor development and to maintain virilization, orchiopexy should be performed. Malignancy in the uterus or vagina has not been described, and because the vasa deferentia are closely associated with the broad ligaments, the uterus and vagina should be left in place to avoid disruption of the vasa deferentia during removal and consequently to preserve possible fertility.

Developmental defects of the male genitalia   HYPOSPADIAS Hypospadias is a congenital anomaly in which the urethra terminates in an abnormal position along the midline of the ventral surface of the penis at some site between the normal urethral meatus and the perineum. This malformation is often associated with ventral contraction and bowing of the penis (chordee) and occurs in 0.5 to 0.8 percent of male births in the United States. It is common to categorize hypospadias as glandular (involving the glans penis), penile, or perineoscrotal. Since penile development is mediated by androgens, it is assumed that hypospadias results from some defect in androgen formation or androgen action during embryogenesis. Indeed hypospadias occurs in most disorders of male sexual differentiation. A rare cause of hypospadias is maternal ingestion of progestational agents early in pregnancy. However, the known causes (single gene defects, chromosomal abnormalities, and maternal drug ingestion) at best can account for only about one-fourth of cases, and the etiology of most remains unknown. The management is surgical.

CRYPTORCHIDISM   The normal descent of the testis is perhaps the most poorly understood portion of male sexual differentiation, both in regard to the nature of the forces that result in the movement and to the hormonal factors that regulate the process. In anatomic terms testicular descent can be divided into three phases: (1) transabdominal movement of the testis from its site of origin above the kidney to the inguinal ring, (2) formation of the opening in the inguinal canal (processus vaginalis) through which the testis exits the abdominal cavity, and (3) actual movement of the testis through the inguinal canal to its permanent site in the scrotum. This entire process occurs over a 6- to 7-month period during gestation, beginning at about the sixth week and not completed in some normal individuals until after birth. Whatever its involvement, androgen is probably not the sole hormone responsible for normal descent. Failure of any of the above anatomic events can be responsible for the failure of descent of one or both testes. About 3 percent of full-term and 30 percent of premature male infants have at least one cryptorchid testis at birth but completion of descent can occur within the first few weeks of life so that the incidence of failure of descent by 6 to 9 months of age is only 0.6 to 0.7 percent. It is this latter category of maldescent that requires intervention.

Permanent cryptorchidism can be classified as intraabdominal (10 percent), canalicular (in the inguinal canal) (20 percent), high scrotal (40 percent), or obstructed (30 percent) in which maldescent is due to a physical barrier between the inguinal pouch and the inlet of the scrotum. These disorders must be distinguished from the temporarily retracted normal testis.

The cryptorchid testis functions poorly after puberty, but the extent to which maldescent is the result of an abnormality of the testis or the cause of abnormal function is unknown. Two general theories have been advanced as to the etiology—inadequate intraabdominal pressure and deficient endocrine function of the testis either because of deficient testosterone synthesis or inadequate formation of müllerian-inhibiting substance. Indeed, hereditary defects that result in inadequate development of intraabdominal pressure or inadequate development of the testes themselves can cause cryptorchidism. As is true for hypospadias, however, the known causes of cryptorchidism constitute only a small fraction of the cases, and the etiology in most remains to be identified. Two complications of cryptorchidism are important; spermatogenesis cannot occur at the temperature of the abdominal cavity, and it is therefore necessary to correct the process as early as possible to allow possible fertility. However, the fact that infertility is common in men who have been treated for unilateral as well as bilateral cryptorchidism suggests that maldescent is usually the consequence rather than the cause of the testicular malfunction. There is also a greater frequency of malignancy in undescended testis, and all should be surgically corrected for this reason (see Chap. 305).

REFERENCES

BROWN TR et al: Deletion of the steroid-binding domain of the human androgen receptor gene in one family with complete androgen insensitivity syndrome: Evidence for further genetic heterogeneity in this syndrome. Proc Natl Acad Sci USA 85:8151, 1988

DE LA CHAPELLE A: The etiology of maleness in XX men. Hum Genet 58:105, 1981

DONAHOE PK et al: Mixed gonadal dysgenesis, pathogenesis and management. J Pediatr Surg 14:287, 1979

EDMAN CD et al: Embryonic testicular regression: A clinical spectrum of XY agonadal individuals. Obstet Gynecol 49:208, 1977

GEORGE FW, WILSON JD: Sex determination and differentiation, in The Physiology of Reproduction, E Knobil, JD Neill (eds). New York, Raven, 1988, vol 1, pp 3–26

GORDON DL et al: Pathologic testicular findings in Klinefelter's syndrome. 47,XXY vs 46,XY/47,XXY. Arch Intern Med 130:726, 1972

GRIFFIN JE et al: Congenital absence of the vagina. The Mayer-Rokitansky-Kuster-Hauser syndrome. Ann Intern Med 85:224, 1976

———, WILSON JD: Disorder of sexual differentiation, in Campbell's Textbook of Urology, 5th ed, PC Walsh et al (eds). Philadelphia, Saunders, 1986, pp 1819–1855

———, The androgen resistance syndromes: 5α-Reductase deficiency, and related disorders, in The Metabolic Basis of Inherited Disease, 6th ed, CR Scriver et al (eds). New York, McGraw-Hill, 1989, pp 1919–1944

GRINO PB et al: A mutation of the androgen receptor associated with partial androgen resistance, familial gynecomastia, and fertility. J Clin Endocrinol Metab 66:754, 1988

GRUMBACH MM, CONTE FA: Disorders of sexual differentiation, in *Williams' Textbook of Endocrinology*, 7th ed, JD Wilson, DW Foster (eds). Philadelphia, Saunders, 1985, pp 312–401

GUERRIER D et al: The persistent müllerian duct syndrome: A molecular approach. J Clin Endocrinol Metab 68:46, 1989

LEONARD JM et al: The classification of Klinefelter's syndrome, in *Genetic Mechanism of Sexual Development*, HL Vallet, IH Porter (eds). New York, Academic, 1979

MILLER WL: Molecular biology of steroid hormone synthesis. Endocrinol Rev 9:295, 1988

NEW M et al: Congenital adrenal hyperplasia and related conditions, in *The Metabolic Basis of Inherited Disease*, 6th ed, CR Scriver et al (eds). New York, McGraw-Hill, 1989, pp 1881–1917

PAGE DC et al: The sex-determining region of the human Y chromosome encodes a finger protein. Cell 51:1091, 1987

RAMSAY M et al: XX True hermaphroditism in Southern African blacks: An enigma of primary sexual differentiation. Am J Hum Genet Vol 43:4, 1988

SIMPSON JL: Gonadal dysgenesis and sex chromosome abnormalities: Phenotypic-karyotypic correlations, in *Genetic Mechanisms of Sexual Development*, HL Vallet, IH Porter (eds). New York, Academic, 1979

——— et al: XY gonadal dysgenesis: Genetic heterogeneity based upon clinical observations, H-Y antigen status and segregation analysis. Hum Genet 58:91, 1981

ZAH W et al: Mixed gonadal dysgenesis. A case report and review of the world literature. Acta Endocrinol Suppl 197:3, 1975

325 DISORDERS AFFECTING MULTIPLE ENDOCRINE SYSTEMS

R. NEIL SCHIMKE

Multiple endocrine gland hyper- or hypofunction can result from mechanisms other than a primary abnormality in the hypothalamic-pituitary axis. While not common, certain of the conditions that affect multiple endocrine systems are inherited and thus have significance out of proportion to their frequency.

SYNDROMES WITH MULTISYSTEM HYPERFUNCTION

MULTIPLE ENDOCRINE NEOPLASIA, TYPE I (MEN I) This disorder, also termed the *Wermer syndrome*, comprises tumors or hyperplasia of the parathyroids, pancreatic islet cells, and pituitary. The clinical presentation is variable, depending on which of the potentially affected glands is hyperfunctioning at the time of diagnosis. About two-thirds of patients have adenomas of two or more endocrine systems, and one-fifth develop tumors of three or more systems.

The majority of affected subjects present with one of the following problems: (1) peptic ulcer and its complications, (2) hypoglycemia, (3) hypercalcemia and/or nephrocalcinosis, (4) complaints referable to pituitary dysfunction such as headaches, visual field defects, and secondary amenorrhea, and (5) multiple lipomas of the skin. A minority (probably <10 percent) come to medical attention with acromegaly, Cushing's syndrome, nonfunctional thyroid adenomas, hyperthyroidism, hepatomegaly (due to metastatic liver disease), or flushing (associated with the carcinoid syndrome).

Parathyroid involvement in MEN I may be asymptomatic for prolonged periods, although most patients eventually show signs of hyperparathyroidism. Tumors of the islet cells may elaborate excessive insulin or gastrin. Insulinomas cause hypoglycemia (Chap. 320), whereas excess gastrin secretion causes the Zollinger-Ellison syndrome with its multifocal or atypically located ulcers and massive hypersecretion of gastric acid. Symptoms may be identical with those of ordinary peptic ulcer, but there is a higher incidence of complications, including perforation, bleeding, and obstruction. Diarrhea is frequent, often with steatorrhea. Radiographic findings include giant gastric rugae, duodenal nodularity, ectopic ulcers in the esophagus, lower duodenum, and jejunum, and intestinal hyperperistalsis. Associated endocrine abnormalities consistent with the MEN syndrome are present in over one-quarter of patients with the Zollinger-Ellison syndrome and in half of the first-degree relatives of such patients. MEN I should be considered in a patient with the Zollinger-Ellison syndrome even when no other endocrine abnormalities are apparent.

Islet-cell tumors may also produce glucagon, vasoactive intestinal polypeptide (VIP), prostaglandins, adrenocorticotropic hormone (ACTH), parathyroid hormone, antidiuretic hormone (ADH), serotonin, somatostatin, calcitonin, and pancreatic polypeptide (also see Chap. 262). Glucagonomas cause hyperglycemia, weight loss, stomatitis, and a peculiar skin rash called *necrotizing migratory erythema*. VIP and prostaglandins have been implicated in the watery diarrhea (pancreatic cholera) syndrome sometimes seen in MEN I. Adrenal adenomas are common in MEN I but are rarely functional. Cushing's syndrome in patients with MEN I is usually of pituitary origin or due to ectopic ACTH or CRH secretion of an islet-cell or carcinoid tumor. Only a single aldosteronoma has been described in MEN I. Similarly, thyroid involvement is so variable and inconsistent that thyroid disease should not be considered intrinsic to MEN I. Other reported features of MEN I include small-intestinal and bronchial carcinoid tumors, schwannomas, thymomas, multiple lipomas, inclusion cysts, and cutaneous leiomyomas.

Patients with MEN I may develop symptoms at any age, but the condition presents rarely in childhood or after the age of 60. Affected individuals may demonstrate multiple endocrine system involvement simultaneously, or years may elapse between the discovery of one adenoma and the appearance of the next. Once the diagnosis is established, the patient must be surveyed periodically for appearance of new facets of the syndrome. By the same token, all first-degree relatives should be studied. A reasonable approach for screening relatives at risk is as follows: (1) review history for symptoms of peptic ulcer disease, hypoglycemia, renal calculi, lipomas, or hypopituitarism; (2) examine for multiple lipomas; (3) assay serum calcium, phosphorus, prolactin, and gastrin. Upper gastrointestinal series and sella turcica x-rays are of no proven value as screening tests. Serum pancreatic polypeptide determinations may be useful in centers where the assay is available.

The fundamental lesion in MEN I is unknown. Many classify MEN I as a neurocrestopathy thereby implicating faulty differentiation or regulation of the embryonic neural crest, which is the anlage of at least part of the endocrine system. The endocrine components of the neural crest have been classified into a subsystem of APUD cells, so named because of their capacity for amine precursor uptake and decarboxylation. The evidence supporting the contention that all APUD cells are derived from neural crest is not strong; instead, cells of diverse origin probably develop similar characteristics; i.e., they represent a structural-functional convergence. A circulating factor that has mitogenic factor for the parathyroid glands has been found in MEN I patients, suggesting a humoral cause for involvement of the parathyroids in the disorder. The MEN I gene has been tentatively mapped to chromosome 11.

The pituitary and parathyroid tumors in MEN I are usually benign, but pancreatic tumors are frequently malignant. Surgical removal of the affected gland is the usual therapy, although standard radiation techniques may be employed for the pituitary tumors, and bromocriptine is useful in prolactinomas. Hyperparathyroidism may be due to a single adenoma, but diffuse hyperplasia of more than one gland is more common. Since new adenomas may arise later, some have advocated removal of all the parathyroid glands with transplantation of extirpated fragments into the thigh or forearm, where they can be easily removed should hyperparathyroidism recur. Successful transplantation obviates the need for long-term therapy of hypoparathyroidism. In hypergastrinemia due to islet-cell lesions, total gastrectomy has been used to prevent recurrent peptic ulcers, and in rare cases distant metastases have regressed after this procedure. Histamine-2-receptor antagonists are efficacious in controlling the hyperacidity and diarrhea seen with hypergastrinemia.

MULTIPLE ENDOCRINE NEOPLASIA, TYPE IIa (MEN IIa OR MEN II)   MEN IIa, also known as the *Sipple syndrome*, consists of pheochromocytoma (frequently bilateral and occasionally extraadrenal), medullary thyroid carcinoma (MTC), and, in about half of cases, parathyroid hyperplasia. MEN IIa can be related more directly to abnormal neural crest development than can MEN I, since both the adrenal medulla and the parafollicular or C cells of the thyroid originate in neural crest. However, there is no evidence that the parenchymal component of the parathyroid glands are so derived. The parafollicular cell elaborates calcitonin, the primary marker of medullary carcinoma of the thyroid. MTC is not common, comprising less than 10 percent of thyroid malignancies. At least 10 percent of MTC cases are familial, usually appearing as a component of MEN IIa or MEN IIb (see below). Medullary carcinoma may also occur in families without other associated endocrine dysfunction; this form is also transmitted as an autosomal dominant trait. MTC may present as a thyroidal mass or be clinically silent and undetectable by palpation or radioiodine scanning. The diagnosis is usually established by immunoassay of serum calcitonin, provided ectopic sites of calcitonin production can be excluded, e.g., breast, lung, and pancreatic islet-cell tumors. Occasionally, basal serum calcitonin levels are borderline in at-risk individuals, and measurement of plasma levels after calcium-pentagastrin infusion can be used to establish the diagnosis. MTC may on occasion secrete substances other than calcitonin, including ACTH, prolactin, serotonin, VIP, histamine, and various prostaglandins, resulting in a confusing array of symptoms.

The pheochromocytoma of MEN IIa may produce the classic signs of catecholamine excess as described in Chap. 318 or be asymptomatic. Approximately 5 percent of patients who present with pheochromocytomas also have MTC. Symptoms of hyperparathyroidism rarely bring the patient with MEN IIa to initial clinical attention.

Examination of cells from both the MTC and the pheochromocytoma components of MEN IIa using X-linked gene markers has led to the conclusion that the inherited defect produces multiple clones of abnormal cells; tumors then develop from a second mutation in the abnormal clone, accounting for the appearance of varying clinical patterns. The MEN IIa gene has been mapped to chromosome 10. Other tumors in MEN IIa include gliomas, glioblastomas, and meningiomas, all of which may be derived from the neural crest.

The age of the patient at the time of diagnosis varies from 2 to 67 years. C-cell hyperplasia of the thyroid may precede development of malignancy by many years, making early screening studies for calcitonin elevation mandatory in all family members at risk. The only effective therapy for MTC is surgical removal of the entire thyroid, as the tumors are multifocal in origin. Limited node dissection is often indicated since the cancer may progress slowly despite an aggressive histologic appearance, and prolonged survival is seen in patients with known metastatic disease. Serum calcitonin levels can be used to assess completeness of surgical removal of the tumor and in concert with selective venous catheterization may be utilized to locate metastases that are surgically accessible. Neither standard radioiodine nor x-ray therapy is helpful in disseminated medullary thyroid cancer, and chemotherapy has been of limited value (see Chap. 316). The pheochromocytomas are usually benign and are also treated surgically. Unresectable malignant pheochromocytoma requires long-term sympathetic blockade. A new radiopharmaceutical, *meta*-iodobenzyl guanidine, shows promise as both a diagnostic and a therapeutic agent.

MULTIPLE ENDOCRINE NEOPLASIA, TYPE IIb (MEN IIb OR MEN III)   MEN IIb also consists of medullary thyroid carcinoma and pheochromocytoma, but affected individuals have striking dysmorphic features such as neuromas of the conjunctival, labial, and buccal mucosa, the tongue, the larynx, and the gastrointestinal tract; hence the alternate designation of the condition as the *mucosal neuroma syndrome*. Other physical findings include enlarged corneal nerves, "blubbery" lips, soft-tissue prognathism, and a habitus resembling that seen in the Marfan syndrome with hypotonia, lax joints, kyphoscoliosis, genu valgus, and pès cavus. The patients may have café au lait spots or a diffuse lentiginous type of skin pigmentation along with cutaneous neuromas or neurofibromas. Megacolon may occur.

MEN IIb and MEN IIa appear to be distinct syndromes. For example, both parathyroid hyperplasia and production of hormones other than calcitonin by MTC are rare in MEN IIb. The mean survival of patients with MEN IIb is around 30 years compared with 60 years for those with MEN IIa, suggesting a more malignant course in the former disorder, although histologically the thyroid tumors appear to be identical. As with MEN IIa treatment of the medullary carcinoma is surgical. The unusual physical features of MEN IIb should immediately suggest the diagnosis of underlying thyroid malignancy. MTC has been documented in asymptomatic children with MEN IIb, and C-cell hyperplasia has been found at operation as early as 15 months of age. Clinically, the associated pheochromocytomas behave as expected (Chap. 318). The MEN IIb gene has not been mapped.

McCUNE-ALBRIGHT SYNDROME   This condition is characterized by the triad of polyostotic fibrous dysplasia, café au lait spots, and isosexual precocity, the latter occurring predominantly but not exclusively in females. The isosexual precocity may be hypothalamic in origin, but gonadotropin-independent ovarian function has been implicated in some cases (see Chap. 322). Cushing's syndrome, gigantism or acromegaly, and hyperprolactinemia may also occur in affected patients. The Cushing's syndrome may result from abnormal ACTH production or adrenal adenomas. Nodular toxic goiter and pheochromocytoma have also been reported. The bone lesion resembles that seen in hyperparathyroidism, and parathyroid hyperplasia has been described histologically but not clinically. The condition is usually sporadic, but pedigrees compatible with autosomal dominant inheritance have been seen. The cause of the condition is unknown (see Chap. 345).

SYNDROMES WITH MULTISYSTEM HYPOFUNCTION

POLYGLANDULAR AUTOIMMUNE SYNDROME TYPE I (CANDIDIASIS-ENDOCRINOPATHY SYNDROME)   Features that differentiate this autoimmune condition from polyglandular autoimmune syndrome type II (see below) include childhood onset and extensive mucocutaneous monilial infection that becomes evident shortly after birth. Hypoparathyroidism is common, and adrenal insufficiency may develop acutely. Diabetes is rare. Organ-specific antibodies against a variety of endocrine glands may be detected early, and pernicious anemia, sprue, chronic active hepatitis, and membranoproliferative glomerulonephritis have been seen. Defective cellular immunity to *Candida albicans* is present; some have more generalized anergy. A cause-and-effect relationship between the monilial infection and the endocrinopathy has not been established. The disorder has occurred in sibs, occasionally from consanguineous unions, and the disease may be inherited as an autosomal recessive trait. No association with the HLA system has been demonstrated, but affected individuals may have a deficiency of immunoglobulin A and hypergammaglobulinemia. Suppressor T-cell function may be defective, but the immune profile can be variable even in sibs. The fungal infection is usually refractory to conventional chemotherapeutic drugs, although partial remission has been reported with a combination of ketoconazole and transfer factor. Amelioration of the candidiasis in no way affects the endocrinopathy, and conventional replacement therapy is required.

POLYGLANDULAR AUTOIMMUNE SYNDROME TYPE II (SCHMIDT SYNDROME)   (See also Chaps. 316 and 317)   This polyglandular deficiency state was first described by Schmidt in patients with both Addison's disease and lymphocytic thyroiditis. This syndrome has subsequently been expanded to include any combination of adrenal insufficiency, lymphocytic thyroiditis, hypoparathyroidism, and gonadal failure. Diabetes mellitus is frequent. The manifestations may be so extensive as to simulate panhypopituitarism; rarely, true pituitary deficiency has been described. The first evidence of endocrinopathy generally appears in adult life. The most significant laboratory feature, in addition to the low levels of circulating hormones, is the presence of antibodies to one or more endocrine glands. The antibodies may be directed against a clinically normal gland, but with time hypofunction usually supervenes. Additional evidence for an immune pathogenesis is provided by the increased frequency of antibodies to parietal cells of the stomach, with or without overt achlorhydria or pernicious anemia, and the presence of other disorders felt to have an autoimmune basis such as sprue, vitiligo, myasthenia gravis, pure red cell aplasia, and antibody-mediated immunoglobulin A deficiency. Hyperthyroidism may complicate the clinical picture.

The majority of affected individuals are female, and most cases are sporadic. A few reports have noted multiple affected family members, suggesting a genetic basis. Members of these families who show no endocrine disability frequently have serologic abnormalities indicative of a disturbance in immune function. Many of the component endocrine disorders in this syndrome are associated with the presence of certain HLA antigens, notably HLA-B8 and -Dw3 (in white populations). Other racial groups show different associations, e.g., hyperthyroidism with HLA-Bw35 in the Japanese. Because of this association it has been postulated that the basic lesion may reside in a mutation of an inherited immunologic mechanism. For example, a selective immunodeficient state might render an individual unduly susceptible to certain environmental antigens (e.g., viruses) that have a predilection for the endocrine system. Cell lysis or damage could result in release of intracellular contents and lead to development of autoantibodies. Such autoantibodies would not necessarily be pathogenic but could represent secondary phenomena, important as markers

of potential clinical disease. Alternatively, the defect could reside in a genetically determined defect in suppressor T cells with consequent inadequate suppression of antibody synthesis. The syndrome is probably etiologically heterogeneous, and several pathogenetic mechanisms may be operative. At present, treatment is confined to providing hormone replacement.

LIPODYSTROPHIC SYNDROMES   The lipodystrophic syndromes are described in Chap. 338. Insulin-resistant diabetes mellitus is common and may be associated with hyperlipoproteinemia, elevated growth hormone levels, and an increased incidence of polycystic ovarian disease.

DIABETES MELLITUS, DIABETES INSIPIDUS, AND OPTIC ATROPHY (WOLFRAM SYNDROME)   This clinical triad has been noted in sibs and likely constitutes a rare autosomal recessive defect. Nerve deafness, usually mild, may also occur. The diabetes mellitus is of the early-onset insulin-dependent type. The diabetes insipidus usually appears prior to age 20. The varying manifestations are difficult to reconcile, and treatment requires replacement of the missing hormones.

OBESITY-HYPOGONADISM SYNDROMES   A number of seemingly discrete entities share obesity, generally with frank diabetes mellitus, and hypogonadism that may be either primary or secondary. The *Laurence-Moon-Biedl syndrome* features retinitis pigmentosa, polydactyly, mental retardation, and renal anomalies along with obesity, hypogonadotropic hypogonadism, and in some patients, diabetes mellitus. There is sufficient resemblance between this syndrome and the *Alström syndrome* (retinitis pigmentosa, nerve deafness, diabetes mellitus, and primary gonadal failure) to cause

TABLE 325-1   Disorders with common polyglandular manifestations

| Condition | Clinical features | Type of endocrine involvement | | | | | | |
		Hypothalamic-pituitary	Thyroid	Parathyroid	Pancreas	Adrenal	Gonads	Inheritance
Ataxia-telangiectasia	Early ataxia Oculocutaneous telangiectasia Immunologic deficiency	?Variably decreased pituitary reserve			Diabetes mellitus	Cortical hypoplasia	Dysgenetic gonads; gonadoblastomas later in females	Autosomal recessive
Pseudohypoparathyroidism	Short stature Short metacarpals and metatarsals Round facies Ectopic calcification	Variable deficiency of all pituitary hormones, including prolactin	Hypo- or hyperthyroidism	Elevated parathyroid hormone levels with either normo- or hypocalcemia	Diabetes mellitus		Ovarian failure	Probable X-linked dominant; heterogeneous
Myotonic dystrophy	Muscular dystrophy Premature baldness Mental retardation	Gonadotropin, growth hormone abnormalities, related to central integrative defect (?)	Hypothyroidism		Diabetes mellitus		Primary failure	Autosomal dominant
Noonan syndrome	Short stature Ptosis Webbed neck Pulmonary stenosis	Gonadotropin deficiency	Thyroiditis				Primary failure	Autosomal dominant
Fanconi syndrome	Short stature Bone marrow hypoplasia Abnormal skin pigmentation Radius malformations	Panhypopituitarism			Diabetes mellitus	Adrenal atrophy	Gonadal atrophy	Autosomal recessive
Werner syndrome	Premature aging of all organ systems Atrophic skin Cataracts Early osteoporosis		Papillary carcinoma		Diabetes mellitus		Gonadal atrophy	Autosomal recessive

frequent diagnostic confusion. Both are autosomal recessive disorders. However, polydactyly and mental retardation do not occur in the Alström syndrome. A similar condition is the *Biemond syndrome* in which obesity, diabetes mellitus, secondary hypogonadism, and postaxial polydactyly are combined with iris colobomata rather than pigmentary retinopathy. Patients with the *Prader-Willi syndrome* (obesity, hypogonadism, hypotonia, mental retardation) also have diabetes mellitus of the maturity-onset type. A genetic basis has not been established for the Biemond or the Prader-Willi syndromes. A small deletion of chromosome 15 is present in some patients with the latter disorder.

CHROMOSOMAL DISORDERS WITH ENDOCRINE DEFICIENCY
(See also Chaps. 7 and 324)   Patients with gonadal dysgenesis have hypogonadism and an increased incidence of diabetes mellitus and thyroiditis, thought to be on an autoimmune basis. In the Klinefelter syndrome an increased frequency of diabetes mellitus may occur along with gonadal failure. In the Down syndrome hypogonadism is probably universal in males, and menstrual irregularities and early menopause are common in women; in addition, increased prevalences of lymphocytic thyroiditis and diabetes mellitus have been reported.

OTHER CONDITIONS WITH MULTISYSTEM MANIFESTATIONS
There are a number of other rare conditions in which involvement of more than one endocrine gland has been recorded often enough to constitute a significant facet of the syndrome. Some, like neurofibromatosis (von Recklinghausen's disease) and tuberous sclerosis, may show either hypo- or hyperfunction of endocrine glands because of interference with central regulatory mechanisms caused by the brain tumors characteristic of the diseases. By the same token, pheochromocytomas and carcinoid tumors may occur in neurofibromatosis because these tissues are ultimately derived from the same embryonic source.

Table 325-1 lists some additional conditions in which disorders of multiple endocrine systems have been seen. It is noteworthy that both primary and secondary failures have been reported within the diagnostic confines of the same syndrome. For example, both gonadotropin deficiency and primary testicular atrophy have been documented in patients with the Noonan syndrome and in unaffected members of the same families. Whenever a clinical condition like diabetes mellitus occurs in such distinct entities as myotonic dystrophy and ataxia-telangiectasia, the molecular mechanisms underlying the disease are probably heterogeneous. A better understanding of the genetic defect would provide insight into the function of the endocrine system.

REFERENCES

BRANDI ML et al: Parathyroid mitogenic activity in plasma from patients with familial multiple endocrine neoplasia type 1. N Engl J Med 314:1287, 1986

FARID NR (ed): *Immunogenetics of Endocrine Disorders*. New York, Liss, 1988

LEE PA et al: McCune-Albright syndrome. Long-term follow-up. JAMA 256:2980, 1986

LIPS CJM et al: Multiple endocrine neoplasia syndromes. CRC Crit Rev Oncol/Hematol 2:117, 1984

NEUFELD M et al: Two types of autoimmune Addison's disease associated with different polyglandular autoimmune syndromes. Medicine 60:355, 1981

RIMOIN DL, ROTTER JI: Genetic syndromes associated with diabetes mellitus and glucose intolerance, in *The Genetics of Diabetes Mellitus*, J Köbberling, R Tattersall (eds). New York, Academic, 1982, pp 149–181

section 2 Disorders of intermediary metabolism

326   THE HYPERLIPOPROTEINEMIAS AND OTHER DISORDERS OF LIPID METABOLISM

MICHAEL S. BROWN / JOSEPH L. GOLDSTEIN

The *hyperlipoproteinemias* are disturbances of lipid transport that result from accelerated synthesis or retarded degradation of lipoproteins that transport cholesterol and triglycerides through plasma. Elevated plasma lipoprotein levels are important clinically because they can cause two life-threatening diseases: atherosclerosis and pancreatitis. A reduction in cholesterol-carrying lipoproteins, achieved by diet and drugs, reduces the risk of myocardial infarction in subjects with hyperlipoproteinemia. Some hyperlipoproteinemias are the direct result of *primary* defects in the synthesis or degradation of lipoprotein particles. Other hyperlipoproteinemias are *secondary*, that is, the elevated plasma lipoprotein level occurs as part of a constellation of abnormalities caused by an underlying disorder in a related metabolic system, such as thyroid hormone deficiency or insulin deficiency. The primary hyperlipoproteinemias can be divided into two broad categories: (1) *single-gene disorders* that are transmitted by simple dominant or recessive mechanisms and (2) *multifactorial disorders* with complex inheritance patterns in which multiple variant genes, each having a subtle effect, interact with environmental factors to produce varying degrees of hyperlipoproteinemia in members of a family.

ROLE OF LIPOPROTEINS IN LIPID TRANSPORT   The lipoproteins are globular particles of high molecular weight that transport nonpolar lipids (primarily *triglycerides* and *cholesteryl esters*) through the plasma. A general model for the structure of a lipoprotein particle is shown in Fig. 326-1. Each lipoprotein particle contains a nonpolar *core*, in which many molecules of hydrophobic lipid are packed to form an oil droplet. This hydrophobic core, which accounts for most of the mass of the particle, consists of triglycerides and cholesteryl esters in varying proportions. Surrounding the core is a polar *surface coat* of phospholipids that stabilize the lipoprotein particle so that it can remain in solution in the plasma. In addition to phospholipids, the polar coat contains small amounts of unesterified cholesterol. Each lipoprotein particle also contains specific proteins (termed *apoproteins*) that are exposed at the surface. The apoproteins bind to specific enzymes or transport proteins on cell membranes, thus directing the lipoprotein to its sites of metabolism.

Table 326-1 describes the characteristics of the five major classes of lipoproteins that normally circulate in human plasma. These lipoprotein classes differ in the composition of the nonpolar lipids in the core; in the composition of the apoproteins; and in density, size, and electrophoretic mobility.

Lipid transport: The exogenous pathway   Figure 326-2 shows the pathways by which lipoproteins transport lipids in plasma. The largest amounts of lipoproteins are involved in the transport of dietary fat, which amounts to more than 100 g triglyceride and about 1 g

FIGURE 326-1   *A*. Diagrammatic representation of the structure of a typical plasma lipoprotein particle. The *core* of the spherical lipoprotein particle is composed of two nonpolar lipids, triglyceride and cholesteryl ester, which are present in different lipoproteins in varying amounts. The nonpolar core is surrounded by a *surface coat* composed primarily of phospholipids. Apoproteins are exposed at the surface and extend into the core. Variable amounts of unesterified cholesterol are interdigitated with the phospholipids of the surface coat. The qualitative composition of each of the five major classes of lipoprotein particles in human plasma is summarized in Table 326-1. *B*. Structures of the two nonpolar lipids, triglyceride and cholesteryl ester. In order for these nonpolar lipids to be assimilated into tissues, the ester bonds between the fatty acids and either glycerol (triglycerides) or cholesterol (cholesteryl esters) must be broken by lipoprotein lipase and the lysosomal cholesterol esterase, respectively.

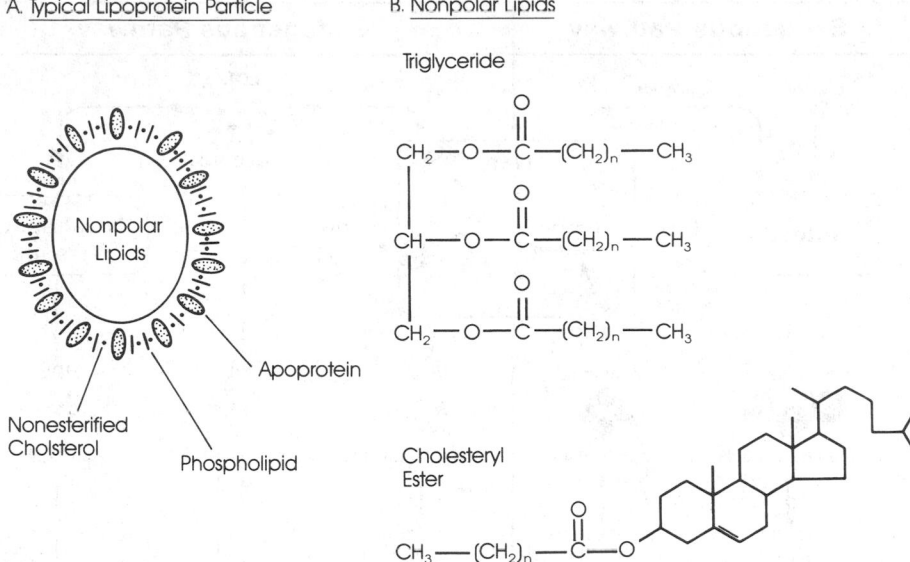

cholesterol per day. Within intestinal epithelial cells, dietary triglycerides and cholesterol are incorporated into large lipoprotein particles called *chylomicrons*. The chylomicrons are secreted into the intestinal lymph and pass into the general circulation for transport to the capillaries of adipose tissue and skeletal muscle, where they adhere to binding sites on the capillary walls. While bound to these endothelial surfaces, the chylomicrons are exposed to the enzyme *lipoprotein lipase*. The chylomicrons contain an apoprotein, apoprotein CII, that activates the lipase, liberating free fatty acids and monoglycerides (Fig. 326-3). The fatty acids pass through the endothelial cells and enter the underlying adipocytes or muscle cells, where they are either reesterified to triglycerides or oxidized.

After the core triglycerides have been removed, the remainder of the chylomicron dissociates from the capillary endothelium and reenters the circulation. It has now been transformed into a particle that is relatively poor in triglyceride and enriched in cholesteryl esters. It has also undergone an exchange of apoproteins with other plasma lipoproteins. The net result is the conversion of the chylomicron to a *chylomicron remnant particle,* enriched in cholesteryl esters and apoproteins B48 and E. This remnant travels to the liver, where it is taken up with great efficiency. This uptake is mediated by the binding of apoprotein E to specific receptors, called *chylomicron remnant receptors,* on the surface of the hepatocytes. The surface-bound remnants are taken into the cell and degraded within lysosomes by a process called receptor-mediated endocytosis (Fig. 326-3). The overall result of the chylomicron transport process is to deliver dietary triglyceride to adipose tissue and cholesterol to the liver.

Some of the cholesterol that reaches the liver is converted to bile acids, which are excreted into the intestine to act as detergents and facilitate the absorption of dietary fat. In addition, some cholesterol is excreted into the bile without metabolism to bile acids. The liver also distributes cholesterol to other tissues by the endogenous pathway, which is discussed below.

Lipid transport: The endogenous pathway   Triglyceride synthesis in the liver is enhanced when the diet contains excess carbohydrates. The liver converts the carbohydrate to fatty acids, esterifies the fatty acids with glycerol to form triglycerides, and secretes the triglyceride into the bloodstream in the core of *very low density lipoprotein (VLDL)*. The VLDL particles are relatively large, carry 5 to 10 times more triglycerides than cholesteryl esters, and contain a form of apoprotein B, designated B100, that differs from the apoprotein B48 of chylomicrons (Table 326-1).

The VLDL particles are transported to tissue capillaries, where they interact with the same lipoprotein lipase enzyme that catabolizes chylomicrons. The core triglycerides of the VLDL are hydrolyzed, and the fatty acids are used for triglyceride synthesis within adipose tissue. The remnants generated from the action of lipoprotein-lipase on VLDL are designated *intermediate-density lipoprotein (IDL)*. A portion of the IDL particles are catabolized by the liver through binding to receptors called *low-density lipoprotein (LDL) receptors,* which are distinct from the chylomicron remnant receptors. The remaining IDL remain in plasma, where they undergo a further transformation in which nearly all the residual triglycerides are removed. During this conversion, all the apoproteins are removed from the particle with the exception of apoprotein B100. The result is the transformation of the IDL particle into cholesterol-rich LDL. The core of LDL is composed almost entirely of cholesteryl esters, and the surface coat contains only one apoprotein, apoprotein B100. In humans a relatively high fraction of IDL escapes hepatic uptake, and consequently humans have relatively high circulating levels of LDL. Indeed, about three-fourths of the total cholesterol in normal human plasma is contained within LDL particles.

One function of LDL is to supply cholesterol to a variety of extrahepatic parenchymal cells, such as adrenal cortical cells, lymphocytes, and renal cells. These cells have *LDL receptors* localized on the cell surface. LDL that binds to this receptor is taken up by

TABLE 326-1   Characteristics of the major classes of lipoproteins in human plasma

Lipoprotein class	Major lipids	Apoproteins	Density, g/mL	Diameter, nm	Electrophoretic mobility
Chylomicrons and remnants	Dietary triglycerides	AI, AII, B48, CI, CII, CIII, E	<1.006	800–5000	Remains at origin
VLDL	Endogenous triglycerides	B48, CI, CII, CIII, E	<1.006	300–800	Pre-β
IDL	Cholesteryl esters, triglycerides	B100, CIII, E	<1.019	250–350	Slow pre-β
LDL	Cholesteryl esters	B100	1.019–1.063	180–280	β
HDL	Cholesteryl esters	AI, AII	1.063–1.210	50–120	α

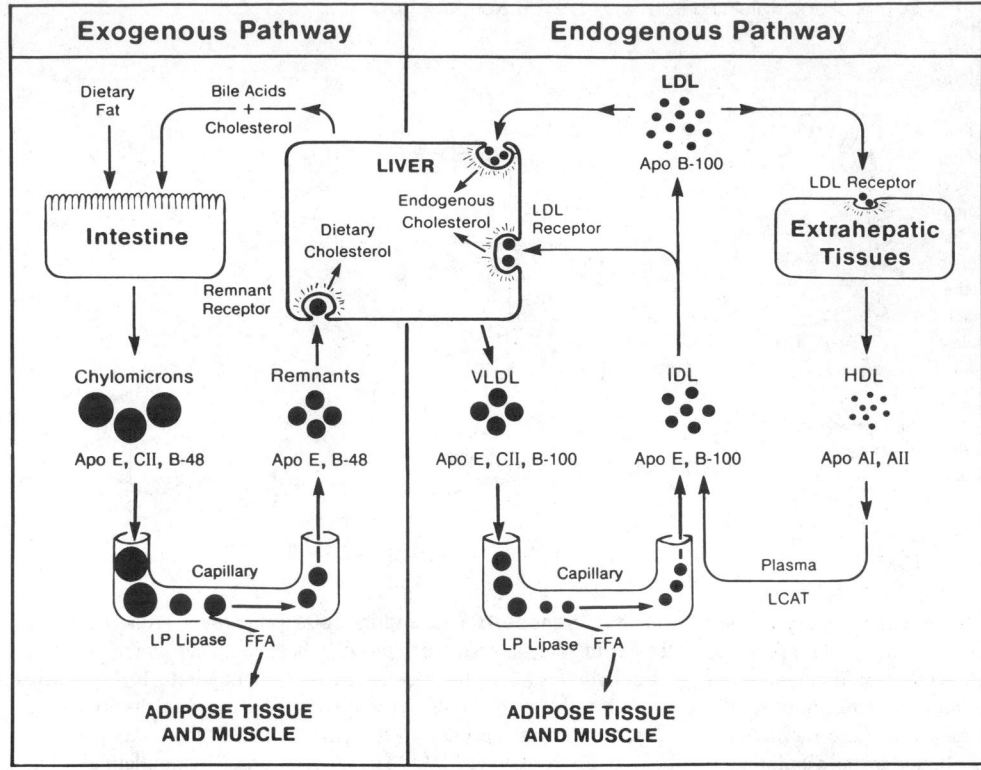

FIGURE 326-2 Model for plasma triglyceride and cholesterol transport in humans. The details of this model are described in the text. VLDL, very low density lipoprotein; IDL, intermediate-density lipoprotein; LDL, low-density lipoprotein; HDL, high-density lipoprotein; LCAT, lecithin:cholesterol acyltransferase; LP lipase, lipoprotein lipase; FFA, free fatty acids. The major apoprotein for each class of lipoproteins is shown. Other apoproteins are also present, and these are listed in Table 326-1.

receptor-mediated endocytosis and digested by lysosomes within the cells (Fig. 326-3). The cholesteryl esters of LDL are hydrolyzed by a lysosomal cholesteryl esterase (acid lipase), and the liberated cholesterol is used for membrane synthesis, as a precursor for steroid hormone synthesis, and as a regulatory molecule that suppresses the synthesis of new LDL receptors. Like extrahepatic tissues, the liver also has abundant LDL receptors; it uses the LDL-cholesterol for synthesis of bile acids and for generation of free cholesterol, which is secreted into the bile. In humans 70 to 80 percent of LDL is removed from the plasma each day by the LDL receptor pathway. Much of the remainder is degraded by a scavenger cell system in phagocytic cells in the reticuloendothelial system. In contrast to the receptor-mediated pathway for LDL degradation, the scavenger cell pathway is thought to function solely to degrade LDL when the lipoprotein reaches high concentrations in plasma rather than to supply cholesterol to cells.

As the membranes of parenchymal and scavenger cells undergo turnover and as cells die and are renewed, unesterified cholesterol is released into plasma, where it binds initially to *high-density lipoprotein* (*HDL*). This unesterified cholesterol is then coupled to a fatty acid in an esterification reaction catalyzed by the plasma enzyme *lecithin:cholesterol acyltransferase* (*LCAT*). The cholesteryl esters that are formed on the surface of HDL are transferred to VLDL and eventually appear in LDL. This establishes a cycle by which LDL delivers cholesterol to extrahepatic cells and by which cholesterol is returned to LDL from extrahepatic cells via HDL. Most of the cholesterol released from extrahepatic tissues is transported to the liver for excretion in the bile.

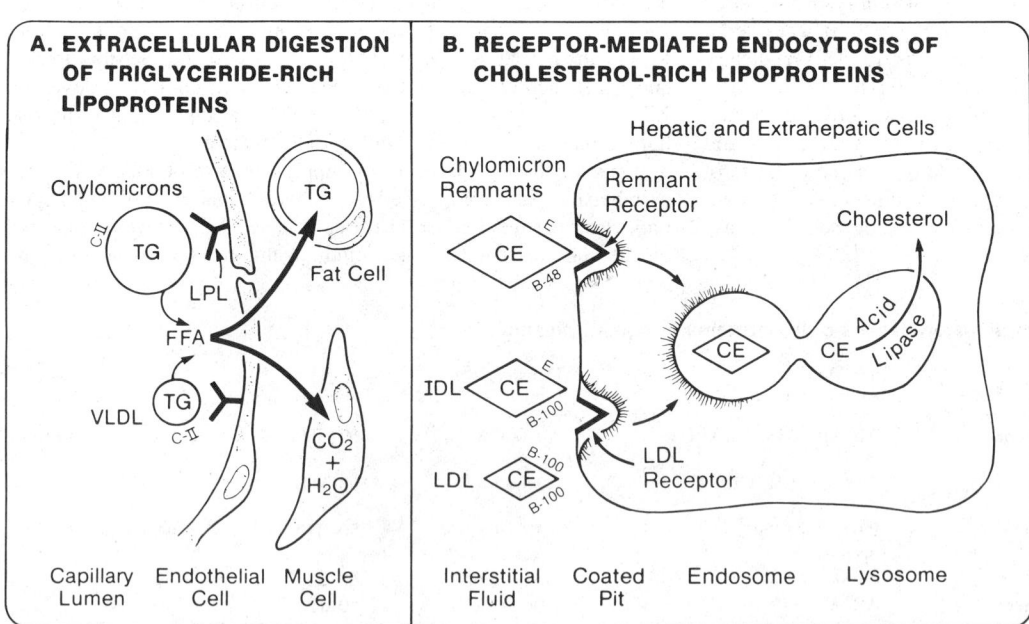

FIGURE 326-3 Comparison of the mechanisms by which triglyceride-rich lipoproteins and cholesterol-rich lipoproteins deliver their core lipids to target tissues. Triglycerides are hydrolyzed by an extracellular enzyme (LPL) that is attached to endothelial cells and operates at the endothelial surface. Cholesteryl esters are hydrolyzed by an intracellular enzyme, acid lipase, that is located in lysosomes and cleaves the esters that enter cells via receptor-mediated endocytosis. TG, triglycerides; LPL, lipoprotein lipase; VLDL, very low density lipoproteins; CE, cholesteryl esters; IDL, intermediate-density lipoproteins; LDL, low-density lipoproteins; FFA, free fatty acid. The apoproteins responsible for the interactions (CII, B, and E) are indicated.

TABLE 326-2 Patterns of lipoprotein elevation in plasma (lipoprotein types)

Lipoprotein pattern	Major elevation in plasma	
	Lipoprotein	Lipid
Type 1	Chylomicrons	Triglycerides
Type 2a	LDL	Cholesterol
Type 2b	LDL and VLDL	Cholesterol and triglycerides
Type 3	Chylomicron remnants and IDL	Triglycerides and cholesterol
Type 4	VLDL	Triglycerides
Type 5	VLDL and chylomicrons	Triglycerides and cholesterol

DIAGNOSIS OF HYPERLIPOPROTEINEMIA

A variety of diseases cause elevations in the concentrations of one or more lipoprotein classes in plasma. In general, these abnormalities are detected by the finding of an elevated concentration of triglycerides or cholesterol in fasting plasma, a condition called *hyperlipidemia*. The value for plasma cholesterol represents the total cholesterol, which includes both cholesteryl esters and unesterified cholesterol. The plasma cholesterol and triglyceride levels provide information regarding the nature of the lipoprotein particle that is increased. An isolated elevation in plasma triglycerides indicates that the concentrations of chylomicrons or VLDL are increased. On the other hand, an isolated elevation of plasma cholesterol nearly always indicates that the concentration of LDL is increased. Frequently, both triglycerides and cholesterol are elevated. Such a combined abnormality may be produced by a marked elevation in chylomicrons or VLDL, in which case the ratio of triglyceride to cholesterol in plasma will be greater than 5:1. Alternatively, there may be an elevation of both VLDL and LDL, in which case the triglyceride/cholesterol ratio in plasma is usually less than 5:1.

The definition of hyperlipoproteinemia is arbitrary because plasma lipid and lipoprotein levels exhibit a bell-shaped distribution in the population, without clear separation between normal and abnormal values. Since lipoprotein concentrations are influenced by diet and other environmental factors, standards must be established for the population under consideration. Usually, arbitrary statistical limits of normal concentrations are selected, based on the examination of a large number of healthy-appearing subjects of different ages. The usual cut-off limit is the upper 5 to 10 percent of values (i.e., the 90th to 95th percentile values). However, analysis of blood lipid levels in individuals from industrialized and more agrarian cultures

indicates that lipid and lipoprotein concentrations that are "normal" in a statistical sense are not necessarily healthy. As a working rule, hyperlipoproteinemia is considered to be present whenever the plasma cholesterol level exceeds 5.2 mmol/L (200 mg/dL) or the triglyceride level exceeds 2.2 mmol/L (200 mg/dL).

The various combinations of elevated lipoproteins that occur in disease states have been divided into six lipoprotein types or patterns (Table 326-2). Most of the lipoprotein types can be caused by several different genetic diseases (Table 326-3); conversely, some genetic diseases can produce more than one lipoprotein type. In addition, each of the abnormal lipoprotein types can occur as a secondary consequence of another metabolic disease (Table 326-4). Hence, the lipoprotein type must be considered a shorthand notation to describe an abnormal lipoprotein pattern in plasma and not a designation of a specific disease.

Ordinarily, the simple measurement of plasma lipid levels, coupled with a clinical assessment, is sufficient to classify the type of lipoprotein abnormality present (Table 326-2). Occasionally, electrophoresis of the plasma on agarose gels is useful either when an elevation in remnant particles is suspected (type 3 lipoprotein pattern giving a "broad beta" band on electrophoresis) or when chylomicronemia is a possibility (type 1 pattern). When the total cholesterol level exceeds 6.2 mmol/L (240 mg/dL), HDL levels should be measured, since low levels of this lipoprotein class are statistically associated with an increased risk of myocardial infarction (see Chap. 195). The level of HDL can be estimated in clinical laboratories using standardized lipoprotein separation techniques.

THERAPEUTIC APPROACHES

The first approach for treatment of all hyperlipoproteinemias is dietary. Individuals who are overweight should be placed on a weight-reducing regimen. Virtually all patients with hyperlipoproteinemia, either primary or secondary, can be treated with a single diet that is low in cholesterol and saturated animal fats and relatively (but not absolutely) high in polyunsaturated vegetable oils, which reduce concentrations of plasma LDL.

The second therapeutic aim is to eliminate aggravating factors, such as diabetes mellitus, alcoholism, or hypothyroidism. Patients with hyperlipoproteinemia should also be encouraged to reduce all other risk factors that predispose to atherosclerosis. These include cessation of smoking, treatment of hypertension, maintenance of a good exercise and physical fitness program, and control of blood glucose in subjects with diabetes mellitus (see Chap. 195).

The final aspect of therapy involves the use of drugs that lower plasma concentrations of lipoproteins, either by decreasing their production or by increasing their removal from plasma. The drugs available for this purpose are discussed below.

TABLE 326-3 Characteristics of the primary hyperlipoproteinemias resulting from single-gene mutations

Genetic disorder	Primary biochemical defect	Plasma lipoprotein elevation (pattern)	Typical clinical findings	Lipoprotein pattern in affected relatives	Drug therapy	
					First choice	Other
Familial lipoprotein lipase deficiency	Deficiency of lipoprotein lipase	Chylomicrons (1)	Eruptive xanthomas, pancreatitis	1	None	None
Familial apoprotein CII deficiency	Deficiency of apoprotein CII	Chylomicrons and VLDL (1 or 5)	Pancreatitis	1 or 5	None	None
Familial type 3 hyperlipoproteinemia	Abnormal apoprotein E of VLDL	Chylomicron remnants and IDL (3)		3, 2a, 2b, or 4	Gemfibrozil; clofibrate	Nicotinic acid
Familial hypercholesterolemia	Deficiency of LDL receptor	LDL (2a, rarely 2b)	Palmar and tuberous xanthomas; premature atherosclerosis	2a (rarely 2b)	Bile acid–binding resin plus lovastatin	Nicotinic acid; probucol
Familial hypertriglyceridemia	Unknown	VLDL (rarely chylomicrons) (4, rarely 5)	Tendon xanthomas; premature atherosclerosis	4 (rarely 5)	Gemfibrozil; nicotinic acid	Clofibrate
Multiple lipoprotein-type hyperlipidemia (familial combined hyperlipidemia)	Unknown	LDL and VLDL (2a, 2b, or 4, rarely 5)	(Eruptive xanthomas; premature atherosclerosis)	2a, 2b, or 4 (rarely 5)	Gemfibrozil; nicotinic acid	Lovastatin

TABLE 326-4 Clinical disorders associated with secondary hyperlipoproteinemia

Underlying disorder	Plasma lipoprotein elevation				Lipoprotein type	Proposed mechanism for hyperlipoproteinemia	Associated abnormality of carbohydrate metabolism
	Chylomicrons	IDL	VLDL	LDL			
ENDOCRINE AND METABOLIC							
Diabetes mellitus	+		+ + +		4 (rarely 5)	Increased secretion of VLDL. Decreased catabolism of VLDL and chylomicrons due to reduced lipoprotein lipase activity	Insulin deficiency or resistance
von Gierke's disease (glycogen storage disease, type I)	+		+ + +		4 (rarely 5)	Increased secretion of VLDL. Decreased catabolism of VLDL and chylomicrons due to reduced lipoprotein lipase activity	Hypoglycemia with decreased insulin secretion
Lipodystrophies (congenital and acquired forms)			+ +		4	Increased secretion of VLDL	Insulin resistance
Cushing's syndrome			+	+ +	2a or 2b	Increased secretion of VLDL with conversion to LDL	Insulin resistance
Sexual ateliotic dwarfism (isolated growth hormone deficiency)			+ +	+ +	2b	Increased secretion of VLDL with conversion to LDL	Insulin deficiency or resistance
Acromegaly			+		4	Increased secretion of VLDL	Insulin resistance
Hypothyroidism		+		+ + +	2a (rarely 3)	Decreased catabolism of VLDL and IDL	
Anorexia nervosa				+ +	2a	Reduced biliary excretion of cholesterol and bile acids	
Werner's syndrome				+ +	2a	Unknown	Insulin resistance
Acute intermittent porphyria				+ +	2a	Unknown	
DRUG-INDUCED							
Alcohol	+		+ + +		4 (rarely 5)	Increased secretion of VLDL in individuals genetically predisposed to hypertriglyceridemia	
Oral contraceptives	+		+ + +		4 (rarely 5)	Increased secretion of VLDL in individuals genetically predisposed to hypertriglyceridemia	Insulin resistance
Glucocorticoids			+	+ +	2a or 2b	Increased secretion of VLDL with conversion to LDL	Insulin resistance
RENAL							
Uremia			+ + +		4	Decreased catabolism of VLDL due to reduced lipoprotein lipase activity	Insulin resistance
Nephrotic syndrome			+ +	+ + +	2a or 2b	Increased secretion of VLDL. Direct secretion of LDL from liver. Decreased catabolism of VLDL and LDL	
HEPATIC							
Primary biliary cirrhosis and extrahepatic biliary obstruction					↑ Cholesterol ↑ Phospholipids ↑ Lipoprotein X	Diversion of biliary cholesterol and phospholipids into bloodstream	
Acute hepatitis (nonfulminant)			+ + +		4	Decreased hepatic secretion of lecithin: cholesterol acyltransferase (LCAT)	

TABLE 326-4 Clinical disorders associated with secondary hyperlipoproteinemia *(continued)*

Underlying disorder	Plasma lipoprotein elevation				Lipoprotein type	Proposed mechanism for hyperlipoproteinemia	Associated abnormality of carbohydrate metabolism
	Chylomi-crons	IDL	VLDL	LDL			
HEPATIC *(continued)*							
Hepatoma				+ +	2a	Lack of feedback inhibition of hepatic cholesterol synthesis by dietary cholesterol	
IMMUNOLOGIC							
Systemic lupus erythematosus	+ +				1	Presence of IgG or IgM that binds heparin, thereby decreasing activity of lipoprotein lipase	
Monoclonal gammopathies (myeloma, macroglobulinemia, lymphoma)	+ +	+ +	+ +		3 or 4	Presence of IgG or IgM that forms immune complex with chylomicron remnants and/or VLDL, thereby decreasing their catabolism	
STRESS-INDUCED							
Emotional stress, acute myocardial infarction, extensive burns, acute gram-negative sepsis			+ +		4	Increased secretion and decreased catabolism of VLDL	

PRIMARY HYPERLIPOPROTEINEMIAS RESULTING FROM SINGLE-GENE MUTATIONS

FAMILIAL LIPOPROTEIN LIPASE DEFICIENCY This rare autosomal recessive disorder is attributable to the absence or marked reduction in the activity of the enzyme lipoprotein lipase. This deficiency leads to a metabolic block in the metabolism of chylomicrons, causing these lipoproteins to accumulate to massive levels in plasma.

Clinical features The disease usually presents in infancy or childhood with recurrent attacks of abdominal pain. The pain is caused by pancreatitis occurring as a consequence of the massive elevation of chylomicrons in plasma. Affected individuals intermittently develop eruptive xanthomas, small yellowish papules, frequently surrounded by an erythematous base, that appear predominantly on the buttocks and other pressure-sensitive surfaces. The xanthomas are caused by the deposition of large amounts of chylomicron triglycerides in cutaneous histiocytes. Triglycerides are also deposited in phagocytes of the reticuloendothelial system, producing hepatomegaly, splenomegaly, and foam cell infiltration of the bone marrow. When the level of chylomicrons in the blood is massively elevated [(i.e., plasma triglyceride level greater than 22 mmol/L (2000 mg/dL)], the blood appears pale and creamy and is said to be *lipemic*. When viewed with the ophthalmoscope, the retina is pale, and the retinal vessels are white, producing the appearance of lipemia retinalis. Despite the massive elevation of plasma triglycerides, accelerated atherosclerosis does not occur.

Pathogenesis Affected individuals are homozygous for a mutation that prevents normal expression of lipoprotein lipase activity. The primary genetic defect appears to involve the structure of the enzyme itself; the activator of lipoprotein lipase, apoprotein CII, is present in normal amounts. The parents are obligate heterozygotes for the lipoprotein lipase defect, but they are clinically normal. As a result of the deficiency of lipoprotein lipase in homozygotes, chylomicrons cannot be metabolized normally, and the level of chylomicrons in the blood rises to high levels after a fat meal. In normal individuals chylomicrons disappear from the blood after a 12-h fast.

However, in affected patients high levels of chylomicrons are found in the plasma even after several days of fasting or ingestion of a fat-free diet.

The circulating chylomicrons inflame the pancreas when they pass through its capillaries. Within the capillary lumen in the pancreas, chylomicrons are exposed to small amounts of pancreatic lipase that leaks from the tissue. Partial hydrolysis of the triglycerides and phospholipids of the chylomicron produces toxic products, including fatty acids and lysolecithin, that break down tissue membranes, produce further leakage of lipase from the pancreatic acinar cells, and eventually cause fulminant pancreatitis.

Diagnosis The diagnosis of familial lipoprotein lipase deficiency is suggested by the finding of lipemic plasma in a young individual who has been fasting for at least 12 h. This lipemic plasma, when collected in the presence of EDTA, has a characteristic appearance after it has incubated overnight in a refrigerator at 4°C. A white layer of cream (which consists of chylomicrons) appears at the top of the tube. The layer beneath the cream is clear. The diagnosis of familial lipoprotein lipase deficiency is supported by the finding of a type 1 pattern on lipoprotein electrophoresis. It is confirmed by the demonstration that lipoprotein lipase levels in plasma fail to increase following the infusion of heparin. In normal individuals, intravenous heparin releases lipoprotein lipase from its binding sites within the capillary endothelium, and increased amounts of enzyme can then be assayed in the plasma. Gel electrophoresis of VLDL apoproteins in patients with lipoprotein lipase deficiency shows a normal amount of activator apoprotein CII, thus distinguishing these patients from those with the related disorder, familial apoprotein CII deficiency (see below).

Treatment The symptoms and signs of the disease recede when the patient is placed on a fat-free diet. Every attempt should be made to maintain the fasting plasma triglyceride level below 11 mmol/L (1000 mg/dL) to prevent pancreatitis. It has been found empirically that the chronic fat intake in affected adults must be less than 20 g/d to prevent symptomatic hyperlipemia. Since medium-chain triglycerides are not incorporated into chylomicrons, they have been employed to help achieve normal caloric intake. The diet should be supplemented with fat-soluble vitamins.

FAMILIAL APOPROTEIN CII DEFICIENCY This rare autosomal recessive disorder is due to the absence of apoprotein CII, an essential cofactor for lipoprotein lipase. Deficiency of this peptide creates a functional lipoprotein lipase deficiency, thus producing a syndrome that is similar but not identical to familial lipoprotein lipase deficiency (see above). Because of the apoprotein CII deficiency, lipoprotein lipase is not activated, and its two substrate lipoproteins, chylomicrons and VLDL, accumulate in the blood, thus causing hypertriglyceridemia (type 1 or type 5 lipoprotein pattern). The disorder is diagnosed in children or adults on the basis of recurrent attacks of pancreatitis or by milky plasma detected by chance. The diagnosis is made by showing an absence of apoprotein CII on gel electrophoresis of VLDL apoproteins. Transfusion of normal plasma (which contains abundant apoprotein CII) into the patient is followed by a dramatic fall in plasma triglyceride levels. Heterozygotes, who have 50 percent reduction in apoprotein CII levels, may exhibit slightly elevated triglyceride concentrations but do not have pancreatitis. Treatment involves use of a fat-restricted diet throughout life. In case of severe pancreatitis, transfusion of one or two units of normal plasma is helpful. As compared with patients with familial lipoprotein lipase deficiency, subjects with homozygous apoprotein CII deficiency are generally detected at a later age, accumulate more VLDL in their plasma, and rarely show cutaneous eruptive xanthomas. The reason for these clinical differences is not known.

FAMILIAL TYPE 3 HYPERLIPOPROTEINEMIA This is an inherited disorder in which the plasma concentrations of both cholesterol and triglycerides are elevated owing to the accumulation in plasma of remnant-like particles derived from the partial catabolism of VLDL. Also called familial dysbetalipoproteinemia, the disorder is transmitted by a single-gene mechanism, but its expression appears to require the presence of contributory environmental and/or genetic factors (discussed below).

Clinical features Affected individuals characteristically do not manifest hyperlipidemia or any clinical feature of the disease until after age 20. A unique clinical feature is the occurrence of two types of cutaneous xanthomas: xanthoma striata palmaris, which appear as orange or yellow discolorations of the palmar and digital creases, and tuberous or tuberoeruptive xanthomas, which are bulbous cutaneous xanthomas that may vary from pea to lemon size. The tuberous xanthomas are characteristically located over the elbows and knees. Xanthelasmas of the eyelids also occur but are not unique to this disorder (see ''Familial Hypercholesterolemia'' below).

Severe and fulminant atherosclerosis involves the coronary arteries, the internal carotids, and the abdominal aorta and its branches. The sequelae include premature myocardial infarctions, strokes, intermittent claudication, and gangrene of the lower extremities. Patients who develop clinical manifestations of this disorder often have hypothyroidism, obesity, or diabetes mellitus as aggravating factors.

Pathogenesis The hyperlipidemia is caused by the accumulation of large lipoprotein particles that contain both triglycerides and cholesteryl esters. These particles consist of chylomicron remnants produced from the catabolism of chylomicrons and IDL produced from the catabolism of VLDL through the action of lipoprotein lipase. In normal subjects, chylomicron remnant particles are rapidly taken up by the liver, and hence they are barely detectable in plasma. A portion of the IDL is also taken up by the liver while the rest is converted to LDL. In patients with type 3 hyperlipoproteinemia the uptake of IDL and chylomicron remnants by the liver is blocked, and these lipoproteins accumulate to high levels in plasma and tissues, producing xanthomas and atherosclerosis.

The mutation responsible for this disease involves the gene that encodes the structure of apoprotein E, a protein normally found in IDL and chylomicron remnants. This protein binds with very high affinity to both the chylomicron remnant receptor and the LDL receptor. Apoprotein E thus mediates the rapid uptake of chylomicron remnants and IDL by the liver. The gene for apoprotein E is polymorphic in the population. There are three common alleles, designated E^2, E^3, and E^4, with approximate frequencies of 0.12,

0.75, and 0.13 in the population. Each allele specifies a distinctive form of apoprotein E that differs from the others by a single amino acid substitution. This structural alteration allows each protein to be detected by isoelectric focusing. The three alleles create six genotypes: E^2/E^2, E^3/E^3, E^4/E^4, E^2/E^3, E^2/E^4, and E^3/E^4. Type 3 hyperlipoproteinemia occurs only in individuals who are homozygous for the E^2 allele (genotype, E^2/E^2). The protein produced by the E^2 allele is defective in its ability to bind to the liver receptors that mediate uptake of chylomicron remnants and IDL, as a result of which these particles accumulate in plasma.

The frequency of the E^2/E^2 genotype in the population is about 1 in 100. Yet the frequency of type 3 hyperlipoproteinemia is only about 1 in 10,000. Thus, only 1 percent of the individuals having genotype E^2/E^2 have symptomatic disease. It seems that most homozygotes for the E^2 allele are somehow able to compensate for the abnormal apoprotein E, because other apoproteins such as apoproteins B48 and B100 can also mediate binding to liver receptors, albeit less efficiently than apoprotein E. Familial type 3 hyperlipoproteinemia occurs only in those individuals who are homozygous for the E^2 allele and who are also unable to compensate for the abnormal function of the E protein. The inability to compensate may be caused by the independent inheritance of another defect in lipoprotein metabolism, such as familial hypercholesterolemia or multiple lipoprotein–type hyperlipoproteinemia (see below). When an individual is a heterozygote for one of these dominant diseases and is also homozygous for the E^2 allele, he or she expresses the syndrome of type 3 hyperlipoproteinemia. The expression of hyperlipoproteinemia is also brought out when an individual of genotype E^2/E^2 develops hypothyroidism, diabetes mellitus, or obesity. It should be emphasized that heterozygotes for the E^2 allele never show the clinical syndrome of familial type 3 hyperlipoproteinemia.

Diagnosis The diagnosis is suggested by the finding of palmar or tuberous xanthomas in a patient with elevated plasma levels of both cholesterol and triglyceride. Approximately 80 percent of symptomatic patients exhibit these xanthomas. The diagnosis is also suggested when a moderate elevation in the plasma concentration of both cholesterol and triglyceride occurs in such a way that the absolute concentrations of cholesterol and triglyceride are similar (e.g., the plasma cholesterol is about 7.8 mmol/L (300 mg/dL) and the triglyceride level is about 3.4 mmol/L (300 mg/dL). However, this finding does not always hold true and becomes especially unreliable when the disease is in severe exacerbation, in which case the plasma triglyceride tends to rise higher than the cholesterol.

The diagnosis is supported by the finding of a so-called broad beta band on lipoprotein electrophoresis (type 3 pattern). This appearance results from the presence of chylomicron remnants and IDL. The diagnosis can be established in specialized laboratories by two procedures. First, the plasma can be subjected to ultracentrifugation, and the chemical composition of the VLDL fraction can be measured. In affected patients, the VLDL fraction contains IDL and chylomicron remnants that have a relatively high ratio of cholesterol to triglyceride. Second, the diagnosis can be confirmed by the finding of homozygosity for the E^2 allele on isoelectric focusing of the proteins extracted from the remnant particles.

Treatment A vigorous search for occult hypothyroidism should be made, including measurement of plasma thyroid stimulating hormone (TSH) levels. If hypothyroidism exists, levothyroxine should be instituted. Patients who have hypothyroidism show a dramatic lowering of lipid levels with treatment. In addition, attempts should be made to control obesity and diabetes mellitus through diet and insulin treatment. If these measures are not successful, patients with type 3 hyperlipoproteinemia should be treated with a fibric acid, such as gemfibrozil or clofibrate. Affected patients usually show a dramatic and sustained reduction in plasma lipid levels when treated with these drugs. Nicotinic acid may be effective in the severely hyperlipidemic patient who does not respond to gemfibrozil or clofibrate.

FAMILIAL HYPERCHOLESTEROLEMIA This common autosomal dominant disorder affects approximately 1 in every 500 persons.

It is caused by a mutation in the gene for the LDL receptor. Heterozygotes manifest a two- to threefold elevation in the concentration of total plasma cholesterol which is attributable to an elevation in the level of LDL. Patients with two mutant LDL receptor genes (called familial hypercholesterolemia homozygotes) have six- to eightfold elevations in plasma LDL-cholesterol levels.

Clinical features   Heterozygotes with familial hypercholesterolemia can be diagnosed at birth because their umbilical cord blood contains a two- to threefold increase in the concentration of LDL and hence a similar increase in total cholesterol. The elevated levels of plasma LDL persist throughout life, but symptoms typically do not develop until the third or fourth decade. The most important feature is the occurrence of premature and accelerated coronary atherosclerosis. Myocardial infarctions begin to occur in affected men in the third decade and peak in the fourth and fifth decades. By age 60, approximately 85 percent have experienced a myocardial infarction. In women the incidence of myocardial infarction is also increased, but the mean age of onset is delayed 10 years as compared with men. Heterozygotes for this disorder constitute about 5 percent of all patients who have a myocardial infarction.

Xanthomas of the tendons constitute the second major clinical manifestation of the heterozygous state. These xanthomas are nodular swellings that typically involve the Achilles and other tendons about the knee, elbow, and dorsum of the hand. They are formed by the deposition of LDL-derived cholesteryl esters in tissue macrophages. The macrophages are swollen with lipid droplets and form foam cells. Cholesterol is also deposited in the soft tissue of the eyelid, producing xanthelasma, and within the cornea, producing arcus corneae. Whereas tendon xanthomas are essentially diagnostic of familial hypercholesterolemia, xanthelasma and arcus corneae also occur in many adults with normal plasma lipid levels. The incidence of tendon xanthomas in familial hypercholesterolemia increases with age, and up to 75 percent of heterozygotes display this sign. The absence of tendon xanthomas does not rule out familial hypercholesterolemia.

Approximately 1 in 1 million persons in the general population inherits two copies of the familial hypercholesterolemia gene and is a homozygote for the disorder. These individuals have marked elevations in the plasma level of LDL from birth. A unique type of planar cutaneous xanthoma is often present at birth and always develops within the first 6 years of life. These xanthomas are raised, yellow, plaque-like lesions at points of cutaneous trauma, such as the knees, elbows, and buttocks. Xanthomas are almost always present in the interdigital webs of the hands, particularly between the thumb and index finger. Tendon xanthomas, arcus corneae, and xanthelasma are also characteristic. Coronary artery atherosclerosis frequently has its clinical onset before age 10, and myocardial infarction has been reported as early as 18 months of age. In addition, cholesterol deposition in the aortic valve may produce symptomatic aortic stenosis. Homozygotes usually succumb to the complications of myocardial infarction before age 20.

Obesity and diabetes mellitus do not occur with increased frequency in familial hypercholesterolemia. A slender body habitus is the rule.

Pathogenesis   The primary defect resides in the gene for the LDL receptor. Studies of DNA from affected individuals suggest that at least 100 mutant alleles occur at this locus. These mutant alleles can be grouped into three classes. The most common, designated receptor-negative, specifies a gene product that is nonfunctional. The second most frequent mutant, designated receptor-defective, produces a receptor that has 1 to 10 percent of normal LDL binding activity. The third type, designated internalization-defective, produces a receptor that binds LDL normally but is unable to transport the receptor-bound lipoprotein into the cell. This rare allele produces the so-called internalization defect.

Phenotypic homozygotes possess two mutant alleles at the LDL receptor locus, and hence their cells show a total or near-total inability to bind or take up LDL. Heterozygotes have one normal allele and one mutant allele at the LDL receptor locus, and hence their cells are able to bind and take up LDL at approximately half the normal rate.

Because of the reduction in LDL receptor activity, LDL catabolism is blocked, and the level of LDL in plasma rises in a manner that is inversely proportional to the reduction in LDL receptors. In addition to the impaired catabolism of LDL, LDL production is increased. Enhanced production of LDL has been attributed to the lack of an LDL receptor on liver cells. The liver fails to remove IDL from the plasma normally, with the result that an increased amount of IDL is converted to LDL. This overproduction of LDL, together with its inefficient catabolism, accounts for the high concentrations in affected patients. The elevated LDL levels cause an increase in the uptake of LDL by scavenger cells, which accumulate at various sites in the body, producing xanthomas.

The accelerated coronary atherosclerosis in familial hypercholesterolemia results from the high LDL levels, which lead to an enhanced infiltration of LDL into the artery wall following episodes of endothelial damage. The large amounts of LDL that penetrate the artery wall cannot be cleared from the interstitial space by the scavenger cells, and atherosclerosis ultimately results. Some of the lipids in LDL may undergo oxidation when the lipoprotein enters the artery wall, and the resultant products may be toxic to endothelial cells, thereby accelerating the damage. High LDL levels may also act to accelerate platelet aggregation at sites of endothelial injury, thereby enhancing the growth of the atherosclerotic plaque (see Chap. 195).

Diagnosis   The diagnosis of heterozygous familial hypercholesterolemia is suggested by the finding of an isolated elevation of plasma cholesterol, with a normal concentration of plasma triglycerides. Such an isolated elevation in plasma cholesterol is usually due to an elevation in the plasma concentration of LDL alone (type 2a pattern). However, most individuals in the general population with type 2a hyperlipoproteinemia do not have familial hypercholesterolemia. Rather, they have a form of polygenic hypercholesterolemia that puts them on the upper end of the bell-shaped curve for the general population (see "Polygenic Hypercholesterolemia" below). Type 2a hyperlipoproteinemia is also caused by multiple lipoprotein-type hyperlipidemia (discussed below). In addition, a variety of metabolic disorders, including hypothyroidism and nephrotic syndrome, can cause type 2a hyperlipoproteinemia (Table 326-4).

Among individuals who have a type 2a lipoprotein pattern, those with heterozygous familial hypercholesterolemia can be distinguished from those with polygenic hypercholesterolemia and multiple lipoprotein-type hyperlipidemia on several grounds. (1) In familial hypercholesterolemia the plasma cholesterol level tends to be higher. A plasma cholesterol level in the range of 9 to 10 mmol/L (350 to 400 mg/dL) is highly suggestive of heterozygous familial hypercholesterolemia. However, many patients with heterozygous familial hypercholesterolemia have cholesterol levels of 7 to 9 mmol/L (285 to 350 mg/dL), a range in which the other disorders cannot be excluded. (2) The occurrence of tendon xanthomas virtually establishes the diagnosis of familial hypercholesterolemia, since such xanthomas usually do not occur in patients with other forms of hyperlipidemia. (3) In cases in which the diagnosis is in doubt, other family members should be surveyed. In familial hypercholesterolemia half of the first-degree relatives show an elevated plasma cholesterol level. Hypercholesterolemia in relatives is particularly informative when it occurs in children, since elevated levels of cholesterol in childhood are characteristic of familial hypercholesterolemia but not of the other disorders.

Approximately 10 percent of heterozygotes with familial hypercholesterolemia have a concomitant elevation in plasma triglyceride levels (type 2b pattern). In these cases, the disease is difficult to differentiate from multiple lipoprotein-type hyperlipidemia. The finding of a tendon xanthoma or a hypercholesterolemic child in the family establishes the diagnosis of familial hypercholesterolemia.

The diagnosis of homozygous familial hypercholesterolemia ordinarily affords no problem, providing the physician is familiar with the clinical picture. Most patients are first seen by dermatologists in childhood because of the cutaneous xanthomas. Occasionally, the presentation is delayed until the onset of angina pectoris or until the child suffers a syncopal episode owing to the xanthomatous aortic stenosis. The finding of a cholesterol level greater than 16 mmol/L (600 mg/dL) with normal triglyceride values in a nonjaundiced child is highly suggestive of the diagnosis. Both parents should have elevated cholesterol levels and other features of heterozygous familial hypercholesterolemia.

In specialized laboratories the diagnosis of both heterozygous and homozygous familial hypercholesterolemia can be made by direct measurement of the number of LDL receptors on cultured skin fibroblasts or freshly isolated blood lymphocytes. Homozygous familial hypercholesterolemia has been diagnosed in utero by the absence of LDL receptors on cultured amniotic fluid cells. The mutant genes for the LDL receptor can also be visualized directly in genomic DNA from affected individuals by using restriction enzyme digests and Southern blots (see Chap. 6).

Treatment   Inasmuch as the atherosclerosis in this disorder is a consequence of the long-standing elevation in plasma LDL levels, every effort should be made to lower the plasma LDL level into the normal range. Patients should be placed on a diet that is low in cholesterol, low in saturated fats, and high in polyunsaturated fats. This generally means the avoidance of milk, butter, cheese, chocolate, shellfish, and fatty meats and the addition of polyunsaturated cooking oils such as corn oil and safflower oil. With such a diet heterozygotes usually show a 10 to 15 percent drop in plasma cholesterol level.

Bile acid–binding resins, such as cholestyramine, should be added to the regimen when dietary therapy fails to lower the cholesterol levels to the normal range. These resins trap the bile acids excreted by the liver into the intestine and prevent their reabsorption. The liver responds to bile acid depletion by converting additional cholesterol into bile acids. This leads to an enhanced production of LDL receptors by the liver, which in turn lowers the plasma level of LDL. Unfortunately, affected subjects also respond to bile acid depletion by enhancing cholesterol synthesis in the liver, and this compensatory response ultimately limits the long-term success of bile acid sequestrant therapy. With the combination of diet and bile acid–binding resins, the extent of reduction in plasma cholesterol level usually is in the range of 15 to 20 percent in heterozygotes. The addition of nicotinic acid may help to block the compensatory increase in hepatic cholesterol synthesis, thus allowing a further lowering of the cholesterol. Major side effects of bile acid–binding resins include gastrointestinal bloating, cramps, and constipation. The major side effect of nicotinic acid is hepatotoxicity; it also produces flushing and headaches in most patients. Probucol has also been used for the treatment of familial hypercholesterolemia. Its mechanism of action is unknown.

A new class of drugs shows great promise for treatment of hypercholesterolemia. These drugs inhibit 3-hydroxy-3-methylglutaryl coenzyme A (HMG CoA) reductase, an enzyme in the cholesterol biosynthetic pathway. When cholesterol synthesis is inhibited, the production of LDL is diminished and the clearance of LDL by the liver is enhanced as a result of an increased production of LDL receptors. These two effects combine to lower plasma LDL levels by 30 to 50 percent. The HMG CoA reductase inhibitors are even more effective when given together with a bile acid–binding resin such as cholestyramine. One of the inhibitors, lovastatin, is available in the United States, and another inhibitor, simvastatin, is available in other countries. The major side effects of these drugs are myopathy (0.5 percent) and asymptomatic but persistent increases in plasma transaminases (1.9 percent). Both side effects are reversible on discontinuation of therapy. Myopathy is seen primarily in patients who are treated concomitantly with immunosuppressive drugs, gemfibrozil, or nicotinic acid.

Heterozygotes often show a moderate to marked lowering of plasma cholesterol level in response to the creation of an intestinal anastomosis that bypasses the ileum. This operation has the same functional effect as bile acid–binding resins, i.e., it accelerates the loss of bile acids in the stool. In certain patients in whom drug therapy is not tolerated, the creation of an ileal bypass may be indicated.

Homozygotes tend to be more resistant to treatment, probably because they are unable to increase production of LDL receptors. In general, combination therapy consisting of diet, a bile acid–binding resin, and nicotinic acid has little effect. Ileal bypass is uniformly ineffective. Several homozygous children have responded to surgical creation of a portacaval anastomosis. However, this procedure is still experimental. The use of a continuous-flow blood cell centrifuge to perform plasma exchanges at monthly intervals lowers the cholesterol in all homozygotes. After each plasma exchange, the plasma cholesterol level drops to about 8 mmol/L (300 mg/dL) and then gradually rises over the ensuing 4 weeks to the pretreatment level. If facilities are available, plasma exchange is the treatment of choice for homozygotes. One homozygous child has been treated with liver transplantation, which provided LDL receptors and lowered LDL levels by 80 percent.

FAMILIAL HYPERTRIGLYCERIDEMIA   This is a common autosomal dominant disorder in which the concentration of VLDL is elevated in the plasma, causing hypertriglyceridemia.

Clinical features   Affected individuals do not usually express hypertriglyceridemia until puberty or early adulthood. Thereafter, the fasting plasma triglyceride level tends to be moderately elevated in the range of 2 to 6 mmol/L (200 to 500 mg/dL) (type 4 lipoprotein pattern). The typical patient exhibits the clinical triad of obesity, hyperglycemia, and hyperinsulinemia. Hypertension and hyperuricemia are also frequent.

The incidence of atherosclerosis is increased. In one study affected patients constituted 6 percent of all individuals with myocardial infarction. However, it has not been established that the hypertriglyceridemia per se causes the increased atherosclerosis. As discussed above, many patients with this disease have diabetes, obesity, and hypertension. Each of these disorders by itself may predispose to atherosclerosis. Xanthomas are not a characteristic feature of familial hypertriglyceridemia.

Affected patients ordinarily have mild to moderate hypertriglyceridemia but may develop a severe exacerbation when exposed to a variety of precipitating factors. These include poorly controlled diabetes mellitus, excessive consumption of alcohol, ingestion of birth control pills containing estrogen, and the development of hypothyroidism. In response to any of these stimuli, the plasma triglyceride level can rise to more than 11 mmol/L (1000 mg/dL). During exacerbations such patients develop *mixed hyperlipidemia;* that is, they show an elevation in the concentration of both VLDL and chylomicrons (type 5 lipoprotein pattern). Whenever the concentration of chylomicrons rises to high levels, patients are predisposed to the formation of eruptive xanthomas and the development of pancreatitis. With treatment of the exacerbating condition, the chylomicron-like particles disappear from plasma, and the concentration of triglycerides returns to the moderately elevated basal condition.

In certain families some patients exhibit a severe mixed hyperlipidemia, even in the absence of known exacerbating factors. This is the so-called familial type 5 hyperlipidemia. Other individuals in the same family may have only the mild form of the disease with moderate hypertriglyceridemia and no hyperchylomicronemia (type 4 pattern).

Pathogenesis   Familial hypertriglyceridemia is transmitted as an autosomal dominant trait, implying a mutation in a single gene. However, the nature of the mutant gene and the mechanism by which it produces hypertriglyceridemia have not been identified. It is likely that the disorder is genetically heterogeneous; that is, the hypertriglyceridemia phenotype in different families may result from different mutations.

Some patients with familial hypertriglyceridemia seem to have an underlying defect in the ability to catabolize the triglycerides of VLDL. When VLDL production rates become elevated due to obesity or diabetes, they are unable to increase the catabolism of VLDL proportionately, and hypertriglyceridemia results. The reason for this defect in catabolism is not apparent. Lipoprotein lipase activity increases normally in plasma after the administration of heparin, and no abnormalities of lipoprotein structure have been identified.

The increased prevalence of diabetes and obesity in this syndrome is believed to be fortuitous, owing to the fact that both conditions tend to increase VLDL production and hence to exacerbate hypertriglyceridemia. In family studies, one can find relatives who have diabetes without hypertriglyceridemia and relatives who have hypertriglyceridemia without diabetes, indicating that the two are inherited by independent mechanisms. When an individual inherits the gene(s) for diabetes as well as the gene for hypertriglyceridemia, the hypertriglyceridemia is more severe, and such a person is more apt to come to medical attention. Similarly, an individual with familial hypertriglyceridemia who has a normal weight usually has mild hypertriglyceridemia and is less likely to come to medical attention. However, if obesity develops, the hypertriglyceridemia worsens, and a diagnosis is more likely to be made.

Diagnosis   A moderate elevation in the plasma triglyceride level, together with a normal cholesterol level, raises the possibility of familial hypertriglyceridemia. In most patients, the plasma is clear to somewhat cloudy on inspection. Chylomicrons typically are not found at the top of the plasma after overnight refrigeration. Electrophoresis of the plasma reveals an increase in the pre-β fraction (type 4 lipoprotein pattern). As mentioned above, an occasional patient exhibits severe hypertriglyceridemia with an elevation in both chylomicrons and VLDL. In this case, a cream layer develops on top (chylomicrons) and a cloudy infranatant (VLDL) is present after overnight storage of plasma in the refrigerator (type 5 lipoprotein pattern).

Given an individual who has an elevation in VLDL levels with or without an elevation in chylomicrons, there is no simple test to determine whether this subject has familial hypertriglyceridemia or hypertriglyceridemia due to some other genetic or acquired cause, such as multiple lipoprotein-type hyperlipidemia or sporadic hypertriglyceridemia. In a typical case of familial hypertriglyceridemia, half of the first-degree relatives have hypertriglyceridemia and no relatives have isolated hypercholesterolemia. Measurement of plasma lipid levels in children is not helpful inasmuch as the disease is typically not manifest until the time of puberty.

Treatment   Attempts should be made to control all the exacerbating conditions. Caloric restriction is required in the obese subject. The dietary content of saturated fat should also be limited. Alcohol and oral contraceptives should be avoided. Diabetes mellitus, if present, should be treated vigorously. Thyroid function should be checked, and hypothyroidism treated if found. If the above measures fail, some patients respond to the administration of gemfibrozil or nicotinic acid. Clofibrate may also be useful in certain patients. The mechanism of action of neither drug is well defined. Patients with severe hypertriglyceridemia frequently show a dramatic response to a fish oil diet.

MULTIPLE LIPOPROTEIN-TYPE HYPERLIPIDEMIA   This common disorder, which is also called familial combined hyperlipidemia, is inherited as an autosomal dominant trait. Affected individuals in a single family characteristically show one of three different lipoprotein patterns: hypercholesterolemia (type 2a), hypertriglyceridemia (type 4), or both hypercholesterolemia and hypertriglyceridemia (type 2b).

Clinical features   Hyperlipidemia is not present in childhood. Elevations in the plasma cholesterol and/or triglyceride level appear at puberty and continue throughout life. The lipid elevations tend to be mild and vary from time to time so that affected individuals may have a mildly elevated cholesterol level at one examination and/or a mildly elevated triglyceride level at another time. Xanthomas are not a feature. However, premature atherosclerosis occurs, and the incidence of myocardial infarction in middle age is elevated in affected women as well as men.

Patients usually have a strong family history of premature coronary artery disease. This disorder is found in about 10 percent of all patients who have a myocardial infarction. The frequency of obesity,

hyperuricemia, and glucose intolerance is increased in affected individuals, especially those with hypertriglyceridemia. However, this association is not as striking as in familial hypertriglyceridemia.

Pathogenesis   The disease is transmitted within families as an autosomal dominant trait, implying a mutation in a single gene. Family studies show that about half of the first-degree relatives of an affected individual have hyperlipidemia. However, blood lipid levels are variable among affected individuals in the same family as well as in the same individual at different times. About one-third of hyperlipidemic relatives have hypercholesterolemia (type 2a lipoprotein pattern), one-third hypertriglyceridemia (type 4), and one-third both hypercholesterolemia and hypertriglyceridemia (type 2b). In most affected relatives the plasma lipid levels tend to be just above the 95th percentile for the population and to dip into the normal range intermittently.

While the extent (if any) of the genetic heterogeneity and the nature of the underlying biochemical mechanisms are not known, affected individuals may have an elevated rate of secretion of VLDL by the liver. Depending on the interplay of factors governing the efficiency of conversion of VLDL to LDL and the efficiency of catabolism of LDL, this overproduction of VLDL may manifest itself alternatively as an elevation in plasma VLDL levels (hypertriglyceridemia), an elevation in LDL levels (hypercholesterolemia), or both. The hyperlipidemia is worsened by diabetes, alcoholism, and hypothyroidism.

Diagnosis   No clinical or laboratory methods exist by which to determine whether an individual with hyperlipidemia has the multiple lipoprotein-type disorder. The 2a, 2b, and 4 lipoprotein patterns can each occur in patients with several other diseases (see Tables 326-3 and 326-4). However, this disorder should be suspected in any individual whose hyperlipoproteinemia is mild and whose lipoprotein type changes with time. The diagnosis is supported by the finding of multiple abnormal lipoprotein types in relatives. The diagnosis can be ruled out by the finding of tendon xanthomas in the patient or the patient's relatives or by the finding of hypercholesterolemia in a relative under the age of 10 years.

Treatment   Therapy should be directed at the predominant lipid elevated at the time of examination. General measures such as weight reduction, restriction of dietary saturated fat and cholesterol, and avoidance of alcohol and oral contraceptives are useful. Triglyceride elevations may respond to nicotinic acid or gemfibrozil. When only the cholesterol level is elevated, a bile acid–binding resin or lovastatin should be given. However, in some individuals the lowering of cholesterol levels with such a drug is accompanied by an increase in triglyceride levels.

PRIMARY HYPERLIPOPROTEINEMIAS OF UNKNOWN ETIOLOGY

POLYGENIC HYPERCHOLESTEROLEMIA   By definition, 5 percent of individuals in the general population have LDL-cholesterol levels that exceed the 95th percentile and therefore have hypercholesterolemia (type 2a or type 2b lipoprotein patterns). On the average, among every 20 such hypercholesterolemic persons, 1 person has the heterozygous form of familial hypercholesterolemia, and 2 have multiple lipoprotein-type hyperlipidemia. The remaining 17 have a form of hypercholesterolemia, designated polygenic hypercholesterolemia, that owes its origin not to a single mutant gene but rather to a complex interaction of multiple genetic and environmental factors.

Most of the factors that place an individual in the upper part of the bell-shaped curve for cholesterol levels are not known. It is likely that subtle genetic differences exist among people with regard to many processes governing cholesterol metabolism. For example, among normal people there may be genetic polymorphisms in the proteins that govern the rates of intestinal cholesterol absorption, bile acid synthesis, cholesterol synthesis, and LDL synthesis or catabolism. Certain unfavorable combinations of these mildly altered proteins, coupled with an environmental challenge, such as a diet high in cholesterol or saturated fat, may raise the plasma cholesterol level.

Clinically, polygenic hypercholesterolemia can be distinguished from familial hypercholesterolemia and multiple lipoprotein-type hyperlipidemia in two ways: (1) family studies (hyperlipidemia is present in no more than 10 percent of first-degree relatives in polygenic hypercholesterolemia in contrast to 50 percent in the other two disorders) and (2) examination for tendon xanthomas (absent in both polygenic hypercholesterolemia and multiple lipoprotein-type hyperlipidemia but present in about 75 percent of adult heterozygotes with familial hypercholesterolemia).

Certain patients with polygenic hypercholesterolemia respond to dietary restriction of saturated fat and cholesterol. Other patients require drug therapy. A bile acid–binding resin with or without lovastatin or nicotinic acid may also be used.

SPORADIC HYPERTRIGLYCERIDEMIA   In addition to the forms of primary hypertriglyceridemia that show familial aggregation, endogenous hypertriglyceridemia with or without hyperchylomicronemia is sometimes seen in individuals whose relatives do not manifest hyperlipidemia. For purposes of classification, this disorder is called sporadic hypertriglyceridemia. Affected patients comprise a heterogeneous group. Some would undoubtedly be classified under one of the genetic disorders described above if a larger number of relatives were available for lipid measurements. Other than an absence of hyperlipidemic relatives, patients with sporadic hypertriglyceridemia cannot be distinguished clinically from patients with the single-gene forms of primary hypertriglyceridemia. Inasmuch as patients with sporadic hypertriglyceridemia may develop hyperchylomicronemia and pancreatitis, they should be treated with diet and drugs as in the familial disease.

FAMILIAL HYPERALPHALIPOPROTEINEMIA   This entity is characterized by elevated plasma levels of HDL, also called alpha lipoprotein. The plasma levels of LDL, VLDL, and triglycerides are normal. The elevated HDL causes a slight elevation in the total plasma cholesterol level. Although a selective elevation in plasma HDL cholesterol can be observed in individuals after exposure to chlorinated hydrocarbon pesticides, in alcoholism and after administration of estrogen, most cases of hyperalphalipoproteinemia have a genetic basis. In some families, hyperalphalipoproteinemia is inherited as an autosomal dominant trait, while in others a multifactorial or polygenic basis is suspected. Individual subjects with familial hyperalphalipoproteinemia show no distinctive clinical features.

Hyperalphalipoproteinemia is associated with a slightly increased longevity and an apparent protection against myocardial infarction. The mechanism for the increase in plasma HDL levels in this disorder has not been determined.

SECONDARY HYPERLIPOPROTEINEMIAS

A variety of clinical disorders produce secondary hyperlipoproteinemias. These are summarized in Table 326-4. The most frequently encountered forms of secondary hyperlipoproteinemia occur in association with diabetes mellitus, consumption of alcohol, and ingestion of oral contraceptives.

DIABETES MELLITUS   Three distinct patterns of hypertriglyceridemia occur in patients with diabetes mellitus. Classic "diabetic hyperlipemia" consists of a massive elevation in the plasma triglyceride level that occurs in patients who have suffered from insulin deficiency or insulin resistance for many weeks or months. Such insulin-deprived patients develop a progressive increase in concentration of plasma VLDL and eventually of chylomicrons as well. Triglyceride levels as high as 280 mmol/L (25,000 mg/dL) are seen. Eruptive xanthomas, lipemia retinalis, and hepatomegaly can occur. Ketosis is frequently present, but severe acidosis is not characteristic. This form of massive hyperlipoproteinemia is seen only in partial insulin deficiency. Patients with this form of diabetic hyperlipidemia

usually respond to a fat-free diet and to the administration of insulin, although triglyceride levels may not return entirely to normal.

The second type of hypertriglyceridemia in diabetics is associated with acute ketoacidosis. Such patients usually exhibit a mild hyperlipidemia with elevations of VLDL but not chylomicrons. On occasion, however, marked elevations of triglyceride are seen with lipemia retinalis. In this case both VLDL and chylomicrons are present.

The third type of hypertriglyceridemia is a mild to moderate elevation in plasma VLDL that persists even when patients appear to be adequately treated for their diabetes. This chronic triglyceride elevation generally occurs in patients who are obese. Inasmuch as most patients with well-controlled diabetes have normal plasma triglyceride levels, the occasional patient with persistent hypertriglyceridemia is likely to have an underlying familial hyperlipoproteinemic disorder. Indeed, family studies indicate that many of these patients have inherited the trait for familial hypertriglyceridemia in a pattern independent of the inheritance of diabetes mellitus.

The insulin deficiency or insulin resistance of diabetes produces a high VLDL level by two mechanisms. With acute insulin deprivation there is an increase in VLDL secretion from the liver as a secondary response to the increased mobilization of free fatty acids from adipose tissue. As the state of insulin deprivation becomes prolonged, the rate of removal of VLDL and chylomicrons from the circulation declines because lipoprotein lipase activity becomes diminished.

ALCOHOL CONSUMPTION   In any individual the daily consumption of large amounts of ethanol can produce a mild, asymptomatic elevation in the plasma triglyceride level due to an elevation of VLDL. However, in a subgroup ethanol ingestion regularly produces massive and clinically significant hyperlipidemia with elevations in both VLDL and chylomicrons (type 5 lipoprotein pattern). In most of this group, the VLDL level remains mildly elevated (type 4 lipoprotein pattern), even in the basal state after recovery from the severe alcoholic hyperlipidemia. This suggests that these individuals have a form of familial hypertriglyceridemia or multiple lipoprotein-type hyperlipidemia that is exacerbated and converted to a type 5 pattern by the ethanol ingestion.

Ethanol elevates the plasma triglyceride level primarily because it inhibits fatty acid oxidation and enhances fatty acid synthesis in the liver. The excess fatty acids are esterified to triglyceride. Some of this excess triglyceride accumulates in the liver, producing the characteristic enlarged fatty liver of alcoholics. The remainder of the newly formed triglyceride is secreted into plasma, resulting in an increased secretion of VLDL. In those who develop massive alcoholic hyperlipidemia, there appears to be a partial defect in the catabolism of these VLDL particles. As the concentration of VLDL increases, the lipoprotein begins to compete with chylomicrons for hydrolysis by lipoprotein lipase, and the plasma concentration of chylomicrons also rises.

In severe alcoholic hyperlipidemia, eruptive xanthomas and lipemia retinalis are frequent. The most serious complication, pancreatitis, may be difficult to diagnose, since elevated triglyceride levels can interfere with the estimation of serum amylase. There is no evidence to indicate that pancreatitis can cause hyperlipidemia; rather the hyperlipidemia is the cause of the pancreatitis.

Plasma from patients with alcoholic hyperlipidemia is creamy in appearance. If a blood sample is drawn in calcium edetate and the plasma placed in the refrigerator at 4°C overnight, the chylomicrons float to the top, and the infranatant layer is turbid, owing to the combined elevation of VLDL and chylomicrons (type 5 pattern).

ORAL CONTRACEPTIVES   The ingestion of estrogen-containing birth control pills causes an increase in the VLDL secretion rate from the liver. In most women the catabolism of VLDL also increases, so that the overall increase in plasma triglyceride level is modest. However, in women who have an underlying genetic disorder (such as familial hypertriglyceridemia or multiple lipoprotein-type hyperlipidemia) the plasma VLDL-triglyceride level can increase markedly, and hyperchylomicronemia can develop when estrogen-containing

TABLE 326-5 Rare autosomal recessive disorders of lipid metabolism

Disorder	Typical age of onset	Plasma lipid abnormality	Major clinical manifestations	Pathogenesis	Treatment
Abetalipoproteinemia	Early childhood	Very low cholesterol and triglyceride levels	Malabsorption of fat, ataxia, neuropathy, retinitis pigmentosa, acanthocytosis	Defective synthesis of apoprotein B leads to absence of chylomicrons, VLDL, and LDL in plasma	Vitamin E
Tangier disease	Childhood	Low cholesterol; triglycerides, normal to slightly elevated	Large orange tonsils, corneal opacities, relapsing polyneuropathy No premature atherosclerosis	Absence of HDL from plasma leads to generation of abnormal chylomicron remnants, which are taken up and stored as cholesteryl esters in phagocytic cells	None
Lecithin:cholesterol acyltransferase (LCAT) deficiency	Young adult	Total plasma cholesterol level variable with marked decrease in esterified cholesterol and increase in unesterified cholesterol; elevated VLDL level; structure of all lipoproteins is abnormal	Corneal opacities, hemolytic anemia, renal insufficiency, premature atherosclerosis	Decreased LCAT activity in plasma leads to accumulation of excess unesterified cholesterol in plasma and body tissues	Fat-restricted diet, kidney transplantation
Cerebrotendinous xanthomatosis	Young adult	None	Progressive cerebellar ataxia, dementia and spinal cord paresis, subnormal intelligence, tendon xanthomas, cataracts	Defective synthesis of primary bile acids in liver leads to increased hepatic synthesis of cholesterol and cholestanol, which accumulate in brain, tendons, and other tissues	None
Sitosterolemia	Childhood	Elevated levels of plant sterols in plasma, elevated or normal levels of cholesterol, normal triglyceride levels	Tendon xanthomas	Increased intestinal absorption of dietary cholesterol, sitosterol, and other plant sterols with accumulation in plasma and tendons	Diet low in plant sterols and cholesterol

medications are taken. These women generally have mild hypertriglyceridemia prior to the institution of oral contraceptive therapy, and they presumably are unable to increase VLDL catabolism in response to the stimulation of VLDL production. The elevated VLDL prevents the normal catabolism of chylomicrons by lipoprotein lipase, and secondary hyperchylomicronemia ensues. When the latter develops, severe pancreatitis can occur.

Ingestion of oral contraceptives may be a risk factor in promoting thromboembolic disease in young women, especially those with preexisting hypercholesterolemia. Thus, it is important to measure the plasma cholesterol and triglyceride levels prior to the institution of birth control therapy. The finding of hyperlipidemia is a contraindication to the use of these drugs.

RARE DISORDERS OF LIPID METABOLISM

Table 326-5 summarizes the clinical and pathophysiologic features of five rare autosomal recessive disorders of lipid metabolism. In two—abetalipoproteinemia and Tangier disease—the major effect of the abnormality is to cause a decrease in lipid levels in plasma. In two cerebrotendinous xanthomatosis and sitosterolemia—the major effect of the inborn error is to cause an accumulation of unusual sterols in tissues. In LCAT deficiency, the underlying mutation produces both an abnormal pattern of lipoproteins in plasma and an accumulation of unesterified cholesterol in tissues.

REFERENCES

BROWN MS, GOLDSTEIN JL: A receptor-mediated pathway for cholesterol homeostasis. Science 232:34, 1986

———, ———: Drugs used in the treatment of hyperlipoproteinemias, in *The Pharmacological Basis of Therapeutics*, 7th ed, AG Gilman et al (eds). New York, Macmillan, 1986, chap 34

BRUNZELL JD: Familial lipoprotein lipase deficiency and other causes of the chylomicronemia syndrome, in *The Metabolic Basis of Inherited Disease*, 6th ed, CR Scriver et al (eds). New York, McGraw-Hill, 1989, chap 45

CONNOR WE et al: Reduction of plasma lipids, lipoproteins and apoproteins by dietary fish oils in patients with hypertriglyceridemia. N Engl J Med 312:1210, 1985

GOLDSTEIN JL, BROWN MS: Familial hypercholesterolemia, in *The Metabolic Basis of Inherited Disease*, 6th ed, CR Scriver et al (eds). New York, McGraw-Hill, 1989, chap 48

HAVEL RJ: Lowering cholesterol, 1988: Rationale, mechanisms and means. J Clin Invest 81:1653, 1988

MAHLEY RW, RALL SC: Type III hyperlipoproteinemia (dysbetalipoproteinemia): The role of apolipoprotein E in normal and abnormal lipoprotein metabolism, in *The Metabolic Basis of Inherited Disease*, 6th ed, CR Scriver et al (eds). New York, McGraw-Hill, 1989, chap 47

SCRIVER CR et al: *The Metabolic Basis of Inherited Disease*, 6th ed. New York, McGraw-Hill, 1989, chaps 44, 46, 49, 50, and 51

327 HEMOCHROMATOSIS

LAWRIE W. POWELL / KURT J. ISSELBACHER

DEFINITION Hemochromatosis is an iron-storage disorder in which an inappropriate increase in intestinal iron absorption results in deposition of iron with eventual tissue damage and functional impairment of the organs involved, especially the liver, pancreas, heart, and pituitary. In 1889, von Recklinghausen named the disease *hemochromatosis* and the iron-storage pigment *hemosiderin* because he believed that the pigment was derived from the blood. The terms *hemosiderosis* and *siderosis* are often used to describe the presence of stainable iron in tissues, but quantitative measurement of tissue iron is necessary for accurate assessment of body iron status (see below and Chap. 291). *Hemochromatosis* implies progressive iron overload leading to fibrosis and organ failure. Although there is debate about definitions, it seems logical to use the following terminology: (1) *genetic hemochromatosis*—the inherited disease now known to be associated with an abnormal gene tightly linked to the A locus of the HLA complex on chromosome 6, (2) *acquired hemochromatosis*—iron overload with tissue injury arising secondarily to other disease, usually an iron-loading anemia such as thalassemia or sideroblastic anemia, in which increased erythropoiesis is present. It should be emphasized, however, that in these acquired iron-loading disorders massive iron deposits in parenchymal tissues can lead to the same clinical and pathologic features that are seen in genetic hemochromatosis.

The metabolic defect leading to increased iron absorption in hemochromatosis is unknown. The genetic disease can now be recognized during its early stages when the iron overload is of lesser degree and organ damage is minimal. At this stage the disease is best referred to as *early* or *precirrhotic hemochromatosis* (see Fig. 327-1).

PREVALENCE   Genetic hemochromatosis is now known to be one of the most common genetic diseases inherited as an autosomal recessive trait. In European Anglo-Saxon populations the gene frequency is approximately 5 percent, giving a disease (homozygote) frequency of approximately 0.3 percent, and a carrier (heterozygote) frequency of approximately 10 percent. However, expression of the disease is modified by several factors, especially blood loss associated with menstruation and pregnancies in women. The clinical expression of disease is 5 to 10 times more frequent in males than in females. Nearly 70 percent of patients develop their first symptoms between ages 40 and 60. The disease is rarely clinically evident below age 20, although with family screening (see below) asymptomatic subjects with iron overload can be identified, including young menstruating women.

PATHOGENESIS   Normally the body iron content of 3 to 4 g is maintained such that intestinal mucosal absorption of iron is equal to loss. This amount is approximately 1 mg per day in men and 1.5 mg per day in menstruating women. In hemochromatosis mucosal absorption is inappropriate to body needs, amounting to 4 mg per day or more. The resulting progressive accumulation of iron is reflected in an early elevation in the plasma iron and an increased saturation of transferrin. In advanced disease, the body may contain over 20 g iron. This excess iron is deposited mainly in parenchymal cells of the liver, pancreas, and heart. Iron in the liver and pancreas may increase 50 to 100 times; in the heart, 5 to 25 times; in the spleen, kidney, and skin, about 5 times. Tissue injury may result from disruption of iron-laden lysosomes and lipid peroxidation of subcellular organelles by excess iron. The demonstration of an association between hemochromatosis and the histocompatibility antigens HLA-A3, HLA-B14, and HLA-B7 has confirmed the genetic basis for the disease. The mode of inheritance is autosomal recessive, with homozygotes usually developing severe iron overload and symptomatic disease. In contrast, heterozygotes show no abnormalities or develop only minor derangements in iron metabolism without progressive iron overload or clinical evidence of the disease. In the absence of a genetic marker heterozygotes in the population cannot at this time be differentiated with certainty from normal subjects.

Gross parenchymal iron overload leading to *acquired* hemochromatosis occurs in association with chronic disorders of erythropoiesis, particularly in those with a defect in hemoglobin synthesis and ineffective erythropoiesis such as sideroblastic anemia and thalassemia. In this group of disorders the absorption of iron is increased, and these patients are also frequently treated with iron and blood transfusions. Porphyria cutanea tarda, a disorder characterized by a defect in porphyrin biosynthesis (Chap. 328), is also sometimes associated with excessive parenchymal iron deposits; however, the magnitude of the iron load is usually insufficient to produce tissue damage.

Alcoholic subjects with chronic liver disease may have increased tissue iron stores. They can be divided into two groups. The first group comprises patients who have a mild to moderate increase in stainable hepatic iron but relatively normal body iron stores. These patients have alcoholic liver disease (usually cirrhosis) but not hemochromatosis. The reason for the increased iron may be related in part to cell necrosis and uptake of iron released from adjacent Kupffer and parenchymal cells. The second (less common) group of alcoholic subjects with increased hepatic iron have gross iron deposition and increased body iron stores and are usually found to have genetic hemochromatosis with or without superimposed alcoholic liver disease. Hemochromatosis in a heavy drinker may be distinguished from alcoholic liver disease by two means: (1) measurement of hepatic iron concentration (see below and Table 327-1) and (2) studying relatives for evidence of the disease, including HLA typing of family members.

Excessive iron ingestion over many years has been reported to result in the clinical and pathologic features of hemochromatosis. This used to be common in certain South African blacks (Bantu) in whom the intake of excessive iron in an alcoholic beverage resulted from the practice of brewing fermented beverages in vessels made of iron. In other populations there are a few isolated reports of hemochromatosis developing in apparently normal subjects who have taken medicinal iron over many years, but it is probable that such individuals have the genetic trait. Family studies may be helpful.

The basic defect in hemochromatosis is not known but may involve the reciprocal relation between ferritin mRNA and transferrin receptor mRNA expression in the intestinal mucosa cell. Diagnosis is dependent

FIGURE 327-1 Sequence of events in genetic hemochromatosis and their correlation with the serum ferritin concentration. Increased iron absorption is present throughout life. Overt, symptomatic disease usually develops between ages 40 and 60, but latent precirrhotic disease can be detected long before this.

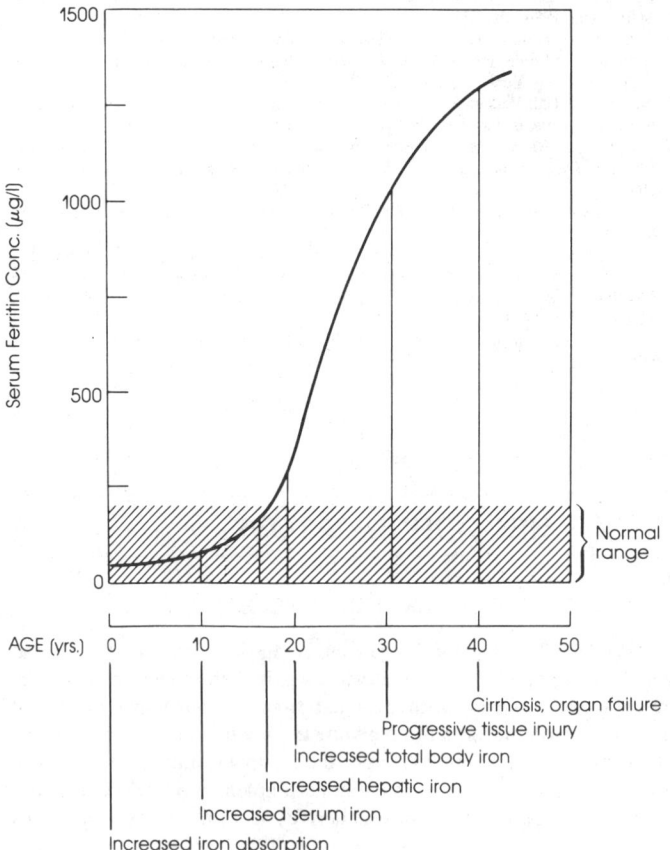

TABLE 327-1 Representative iron values in normal subjects, patients with hemochromatosis, and patients with alcoholic liver disease

Determination	Normal	Symptomatic hemochromatosis	Homozygotes with early, asymptomatic hemochromatosis	Alcoholic liver disease
Plasma iron, μmol/L (μg/dL)	9–27 (50–150)	32–54 (180–300)	Usually elevated	Often elevated
Total iron-binding capacity, μmol/L (μg/dL)	45–66 (250–370)	36–54 (200–300)	36–54 (200–300)	45–66 (250–370)
Transferrin saturation, percent	22–46	50–100	50–100	27–60
Serum ferritin, μg/L	10–200	900–6000	200–500	10–500
Urinary iron,* mg/24 h	0–2	9–23	2.5	Usually <5
Liver iron, μg/100 ng dry wt	30–140	600–1800	200–400	30–200

* After intramuscular administration of 0.5 g deferoxamine.

on the phenotypic expression of the disease (i.e., increased body iron stores), and the rate of iron accumulation may be modified by other factors such as blood loss and oral iron ingestion. The common denominator in all patients with hemochromatosis is the presence of *excessive amounts of iron in parenchymal tissues*. Parenteral administration of iron in the form of transfusions or iron preparations results in predominantly *reticuloendothelial cell* iron overload. This appears to lead to less tissue damage than iron loading of parenchymal cells.

PATHOLOGY At autopsy the enlarged, nodular liver and pancreas present a striking ochre color. Histologically iron is found in increased amounts in many organs, particularly in the liver and pancreas and to a lesser extent in the endocrine glands and the heart. A notable exception is the testis, the iron content of which is relatively low despite the fact that gonadal failure is a characteristic and early feature of the disease. In contrast, the pituitary gland is almost always involved. The epidermis of the skin is thin, and increased *melanin* is found in the cells of the basal layer. Deposits of iron are present around the synovial lining cells of the joints, and calcium pyrophosphate crystals may be seen to lie within deposits of calcium embedded in the synovial tissue.

The parenchymal deposits of iron in the liver of patients with genetic hemochromatosis are in the form of ferritin and hemosiderin. In the early stages, these deposits are found in the periportal parenchymal cells, especially within lysosomes in the pericanalicular cytoplasm of the hepatocytes. This stage progresses to perilobular fibrosis and deposition of iron in bile duct epithelium, Kupffer cells, and fibrous septa. Inflammatory cells are few in contrast to prominent proliferation of bile ductules. Wedge biopsy specimens show a characteristic pattern of fibrosis with dense fibrous septa surrounding groups of lobules somewhat analogous to the pattern in chronic biliary disease. In the advanced stage, a macronodular or mixed macro- and micronodular cirrhosis develops.

CLINICAL MANIFESTATIONS The symptoms and signs include skin pigmentation, diabetes mellitus, liver and cardiac impairment, arthropathy, and hypogonadism. The most frequently encountered initial symptoms are weakness, lassitude, weight loss, change in skin color, abdominal pain, loss of libido, and symptoms related to the onset of diabetes mellitus. Hepatomegaly, pigmentation, spider angiomas, splenomegaly, arthropathy, ascites, cardiac arrhythmias, congestive heart failure, loss of body hair, testicular atrophy, and jaundice are prominent physical signs in fully established disease.

The *liver* is usually the first organ to be affected, and hepatomegaly is present in more than 95 percent of symptomatic patients. Hepatic enlargement may exist in the absence of symptoms or in the presence of normal liver function tests. Indeed, over half the patients with symptomatic hemochromatosis have little or no laboratory evidence of functional impairment of the liver, in spite of hepatomegaly and fibrosis. Loss of body hair, palmar erythema, testicular atrophy, and gynecomastia are common. Manifestations of portal hypertension and esophageal varices occur less commonly than in Laennec's cirrhosis.

Splenomegaly is present in approximately half the symptomatic cases. Hepatocellular carcinoma develops in about 30 percent of patients with cirrhosis. The incidence of this complication increases with age and is now the most common cause of death in treated patients. However, it appears to occur only in cirrhotic patients; hence the importance of early diagnosis and therapy.

Excessive *skin pigmentation* is present in about 90 percent of symptomatic patients at the time of diagnosis. Melanin deposition in the skin usually gives rise to bronzing. The characteristic metallic gray hue is believed to result from the presence of increased melanin or both melanin and iron in the dermis. Pigmentation usually is diffuse and generalized, but frequently it is deeper on the face, neck, extensor aspects of the lower forearms, dorsa of the hands, lower legs, genital regions, and in scars. In only 10 to 15 percent of cases is there demonstrable pigmentation of the oral mucosa. Pigmentation of the hard palate and retina has been described.

Diabetes mellitus occurs in about 65 percent of patients and is more likely to develop in patients with a family history of diabetes mellitus. The presence of a genetic prediposition and direct damage to the pancreas by iron deposition both contribute to the development of diabetes mellitus. The management of the diabetes mellitus is similar to that of other forms of diabetes mellitus except for a higher incidence of insulin resistance. Late degenerative sequelae are the same as in diabetes mellitus.

Arthropathy develops in 25 to 50 percent of patients. It most commonly occurs after the age of 50 but may occur at any time in the course of the disease, even as a first manifestation or long after therapy. The small joints of the hands, especially the second and third metacarpophalangeal joints, are commonly the first joints to be involved. A progressive polyarthritis involving wrists, hips, ankles, and knees may ensue. Acute brief attacks of synovitis may occur, associated with deposition of calcium pyrophosphate (chondrocalcinosis or pseudogout), chiefly in the knees. Roentgenologic manifestations consist of cystic changes of sclerosis of the subchondral bones, loss of articular cartilage with narrowing of the joint space, diffuse demineralization, hypertrophic bone proliferation, and calcification of the synovium. The mechanism of these abnormalities and their relationship to iron metabolism are not known.

Cardiac involvement is the presenting manifestation in about 15 percent of patients. The most common cardiac manifestation, congestive heart failure, occurs in about 10 percent of young adults with the disease. Symptoms of congestive failure may develop suddenly, with rapid progression to death if untreated. The heart is diffusely enlarged, and such cases may be misdiagnosed as idiopathic cardiomyopathy if other overt manifestations are absent. A variety of cardiac arrhythmias may be present, particularly supraventricular beats and paroxysmal tachyarrhythmias. Atrial flutter, atrial fibrillation, and varying degrees of atrioventricular block have also been described.

Loss of libido and *testicular atrophy* are common. The former may antedate other clinical manifestations of the disease. Testicular atrophy is usually due to the decreased production of gonadotropins associated with impaired hypothalamic-pituitary function due to iron deposition. Adrenal insufficiency, hypothyroidism, and hypoparathyroidism have been described but are rare.

DIAGNOSIS   The association of (1) hepatomegaly, (2) skin pigmentation, (3) diabetes mellitus, (4) heart disease, (5) arthritis, and (6) evidence of hypogonadism should suggest the diagnosis of hemochromatosis. However, a parenchymal iron overload of comparatively short duration or modest degree may exist without any of these clinical manifestations, or with only some of them [e.g., in young subjects (see Fig. 327-1)]. Therefore, the diagnosis should be considered in any patient with unexplained hepatomegaly, idiopathic cardiomyopathy, abnormal skin pigmentation, loss of libido, diabetes mellitus, or arthritis.

The history should be particularly detailed in regard to disease in other family members, alcohol ingestion, iron intake, and the ingestion of large doses of ascorbic acid, which promotes iron absorption. The blood should be examined for evidence of anemia and abnormal erythropoiesis to rule out iron loading secondary to a hematologic disorder. Confirmation of the presence of liver, pancreatic, cardiac, and joint disease should be obtained by physical examination, roentgenography, and routine function tests of these organs. It then remains to be demonstrated that there is an increase in total-body iron stores and, in particular, an increased parenchymal iron concentration associated with tissue damage.

The methods available for the demonstration of excessive parenchymal iron stores include (1) measurement of serum iron and determination of percent saturation of transferrin, (2) estimation of chelatable iron stores using the agent deferoxamine, (3) measurement of serum ferritin concentration, (4) liver biopsy (Table 327-1), and (5) computed tomography and/or magnetic resonance imaging of the liver. Each has its inherent advantages and limitations. The serum iron level and percent saturation of transferrin are elevated early in the course of the disease, but their specificity is reduced by relatively high false-positive and false-negative rates. In particular, an increased serum iron concentration may be present in patients with alcoholic liver disease without iron overload; in this situation, however, the iron-binding capacity is usually not decreased as in hemochromatosis (Table 327-1). Population studies suggest that in otherwise healthy persons a fasting serum transferrin saturation greater than 62 percent strongly suggests homozygosity for hemochromatosis.

The serum ferritin concentration is usually a good index of body iron stores, whether they are decreased or increased. In most untreated patients with hemochromatosis, the serum ferritin level is greatly increased (Fig. 327-1 and Table 327-1). This test is also useful as a noninvasive screening test for the diagnosis of early disease, since it is usually abnormal before there is any morphologic evidence of liver damage and the ferritin concentration correlates with the magnitude of body iron stores.

These tests have, therefore, generally replaced the more cumbersome screening tests involving measurement of urinary iron excretion. However, in patients with inflammation and hepatocellular necrosis serum ferritin levels may be elevated out of proportion to body iron stores due to increased rate of release from tissues. A repeat determination of serum ferritin should therefore be carried out when any concurrent acute hepatocellular damage has subsided, e.g., in alcoholic liver disease. In some families serum ferritin levels in symptomatic relatives are normal despite increased iron stores; the reason for this finding is unclear, but it would appear to be unusual. In clinical practice, the *combined measurements* of the (1) percent transferrin saturation and (2) serum ferritin level provide the simplest and most reliable screening test for hemochromatosis, including the precirrhotic phase of the disease. If either of these tests is abnormal, liver biopsy should be performed since it is the *definitive* test for the diagnosis of hemochromatosis. It permits histochemical estimation of tissue iron, measurement of hepatic iron concentration, and assessment of the extent of tissue damage. Computed tomography

shows increased density of the liver due to iron deposition. However, dual-energy scanning and experienced personnel are required, and the lower limits for accurate detection of increased tissue iron are still unclear. Magnetic resonance imaging may also detect increased tissue iron, but the sensitivity requires further evaluation.

When the diagnosis of hemochromatosis is established, it is of particular importance to examine family members at risk. Asymptomatic as well as symptomatic family members with the disease usually have an increased saturation of transferrin and an increased or increasing serum ferritin concentration. These changes occur even before the iron stores are greatly increased (see Fig. 327-1). A liver biopsy should then be performed, since it is imperative to establish the diagnosis and begin therapy before tissue damage occurs. Since the hemochromatosis allele lies close to the HLA-A locus on chromosome 6, HLA typing is helpful in evaluating families with the disease. Affected siblings (putative homozygotes) usually have both HLA haplotypes identical with those of the proband, and where children of a proband are affected, a homozygous-heterozygous mating probably occurred. Siblings sharing only one HLA haplotype with a patient (putative heterozygotes) will probably not develop progressive iron overload. Thus, HLA typing helps greatly in determining the probability of a sibling later developing the disease and therefore the desirable frequency of screening.

The distinction between hemochromatosis and alcoholic cirrhosis associated with increased tissue iron is usually not difficult if measurement is made of liver iron concentration and hepatic iron index (concentration divided by age) (Table 327-1). Where biopsy is not possible the deferoxamine excretion test can provide diagnostic information.

TREATMENT   The therapy of genetic hemochromatosis involves the removal of the excess body iron and supportive treatment of damaged organs.

Iron is best removed from the body by weekly or twice weekly phlebotomy of 500 mL. Although there is an initial modest decline in the volume of packed red blood cells to about 35 mL/dL, the level stabilizes after several weeks. The plasma transferrin saturation remains increased until the available iron stores are depleted. In contrast, the plasma ferritin concentration falls progressively, reflecting the gradual decrease in body iron stores. Since one 500-mL unit of blood contains from 200 to 250 mg iron and about 25 g iron must be removed, weekly phlebotomy is usually required for 2 or 3 years. When the transferrin saturation and ferritin level become normal, phlebotomies are performed at such time intervals as are required to maintain these levels within the normal range. The measurements promptly become abnormal with iron reaccumulation. Usually one phlebotomy every 3 months will suffice.

Chelating agents such as deferoxamine, when given parenterally, remove 10 to 20 mg iron per day, less than half that mobilized by once weekly phlebotomy. Phlebotomy is also generally less expensive, more convenient, and safer for patients with genetic hemochromatosis, but chelating agents are indicated when anemia or hypoproteinemia is severe enough to preclude phlebotomy. Subcutaneous infusions of deferoxamine using a portable slow pump are the most effective means of administration.

The management of the hepatic failure, cardiac failure, and diabetes mellitus differs little from conventional management of these conditions. Loss of libido and change in secondary sex characteristics are partially relieved by parenteral testosterone or gonadotropin therapy (see Chap. 321).

PROGNOSIS   The principal causes of death in *untreated* patients are cardiac failure (30 percent), hepatocellular failure or portal hypertension (25 percent), and hepatocellular carcinoma (30 percent).

Life expectancy of symptomatic patients is extended considerably by removal of the excessive stores of iron and maintenance of these stores at near-normal levels. The 5-year survival rate with therapy increases from 33 to 89 percent. With removal of iron by repeated phlebotomy, the liver and spleen decrease in size, liver function studies return to normal, pigmentation of skin decreases, and cardiac failure is reversed. Carbohydrate tolerance improves in about 40 percent. Removal of excess iron has little or no effect on hypogonadism or arthropathy. The fibrosis in the liver may decrease, but cirrhosis is irreversible. Hepatocellular carcinoma occurs as a late sequela in about one-third of patients who are cirrhotic at presentation despite adequate iron removal. The apparent increase in its incidence in treated patients is probably related in part to their increased life span. This complication does not appear to develop if the disease is treated in the precirrhotic stage, and the life expectancy of homozygotes diagnosed and treated before the development of cirrhosis does not differ significantly from that of the normal population. Hence, the importance of family screening and early therapy cannot be emphasized too strongly. Asymptomatic subjects who are detected by family studies should have phlebotomy therapy if iron stores are moderately to severely increased. Screening for increasing iron stores at appropriate intervals is also important. With this approach most manifestations of the disease can be prevented.

REFERENCES

BASSETT ML et al: HLA typing in idiopathic hemochromatosis: Distinction between homozygotes and heterozygotes with biochemical expression. Hepatology 1:120, 1981
——— et al: Value of hepatic iron measurements in early hemochromatosis and determination of the critical iron levels associated with fibrosis. Hepatology 318:24, 1986
EDWARDS CQ et al: Prevalence of hemochromatosis among 11,065 presumably healthy blood donors. N Engl J Med 318:1355, 1988
KLAUSNER RD, HARFORD JB: Cis-trans models for post-transcriptional gene regulation. Science 246:870, 1989
NEIDERAU C et al: Survival and causes of death in cirrhotic and in noncirrhotic patients with primary hemochromatosis. N Engl J Med 313:1256, 1985
POWELL LW, KERR JFR: The pathology of liver in hemochromatosis, in Pathobiology Annual, H Joacim (ed). New York, Appleton-Century-Crofts, 1975
——— et al: Expression of hemochromatosis in homozygous subjects: Implications for early diagnosis and prevention. Gastroenterology (in press) 1990
STEVENS RG et al: Body iron stores and the risk of cancer. N Engl J Med 319:1047, 1988

328 PORPHYRIAS

URS A. MEYER

The porphyrias are inherited or acquired disturbances in heme biosynthesis. Porphyrins are tetrapyrrole intermediates in this pathway and are formed from the precursors δ-aminolevulinic acid (ALA) and porphobilinogen. Heme, the ferrous iron complex of protoporphyrin IX, functions as a prosthetic group for hemoproteins such as hemoglobin, cytochromes, catalase, and tryptophan oxygenase. Heme biosynthesis is essential to life and is operative in all aerobic cells.

Each of the porphyrias is characterized by a unique pattern of overproduction, accumulation, and excretion of intermediates of heme biosynthesis. These patterns are the metabolic expression of deficiencies of specific enzymes of the heme biosynthetic pathway (Table 328-1, Fig. 328-1).

The main clinical manifestations are intermittent attacks of nervous system dysfunction and/or sensitivity of the skin to sunlight. The *neurologic syndrome* is characteristically precipitated by drugs such as barbiturates and results in abdominal pain, peripheral neuropathy, and mental disturbance. The neuropsychiatric symptoms occur only in those porphyrias in which there is great overproduction of the porphyrin precursors ALA and porphobilinogen. The pathogenesis of the neurologic lesion is unclear. The *skin photosensitivity* is related to increased porphyrin accumulation, although the lesions differ among the different disorders. When radiated with ultraviolet light of wavelength ≈400 nm, the conjugated double-bond structure of the tetrapyrrole nucleus causes porphyrins to become unstable, highly reactive oxidizing agents that react with molecules in the upper dermis

and lower epidermis. The dominantly inherited human porphyrias exhibit variable expressivity. Only the biochemical or enzymatic abnormalities may be apparent. Such latent disease may occur as a phase or persist throughout life, or manifestations can be precipitated by factors such as drugs, hormones, or liver disease.

CLASSIFICATION The porphyrias are usually divided into two main groups, erythropoietic and hepatic, according to the two major sites of heme synthesis where the error of metabolism is predominantly expressed (Table 328-1). Erythropoietic forms of porphyria are the rare *congenital erythropoietic porphyria* (CEP) and *protoporphyria* (PP). But in some patients with PP, porphyrins accumulate both in erythropoietic and hepatic tissue. In *intermittent acute porphyria* (IAP), *hereditary coproporphyria* (HCP), and *variegate porphyria* (VP), heme biosynthesis is impaired predominantly in the liver, without affecting hemoglobin formation. *Porphyria cutanea tarda* (PCT) occurs both as a familial and as a sporadic disease. All patients with PCT have a deficiency of uroporphyrinogen decarboxylase in the liver. Acquired PCT occurs in individuals exposed to polyhalogenated hydrocarbons and in association with hepatic tumors. Poisoning with lead and hereditary tyrosinemia also produce abnormalities in porphyrin and heme synthesis (see Chap. 375). Small increases in urinary excretion of porphyrins or precursors and accumulation of porphyrins in erythrocytes may accompany numerous clinical conditions; these secondary phenomena do not produce symptoms or signs of porphyria.

BIOCHEMICAL CONSIDERATIONS The reactions that lead from the substrates glycine and succinyl coenzyme A to ALA, porphobilinogen (PBG), and finally heme are mediated by four mitochondrial and four cytosolic enzymes (Fig. 328-2). Differences exist in the regulation of heme biosynthesis among tissues.

In the liver ALA synthase catalyzes the rate-limiting reaction for heme formation under physiologic conditions. The enzymes subsequent to ALA synthase are present in excess. The principal regulation of ALA synthase is feedback repression by heme, the end product of the pathway. Increased demands for heme are met by the synthesis of ALA synthase. Hepatic ALA synthase can be induced by a large number of lipid-soluble drugs, steroids, and chemicals that are substrates and inducers of cytochrome P_{450} hemoproteins, the terminal oxidases in microsomal drug metabolism. This induction is modulated by genetic, metabolic, and environmental factors. The interdependence of heme synthesis and microsomal drug oxidation is important in several hepatic porphyrias where symptoms are precipitated by these drugs.

In the bone marrow ALA synthase is also rate-limiting in cells with fully expressed heme synthesis, but little is known of the role of the enzyme during division, differentiation, and maturation of erythroid cells. With maturation of erythroid cells the nuclei and mitochondria are extruded, and the mitochondrial enzymes of heme synthesis disappear, while the cytosolic enzymes catalyzing the reactions between ALA and coproporphyrinogen persist. Therefore, erythrocytes can be used for the diagnosis of porphyrias that are due to a defect in a cytosolic enzyme.

Control of heme synthesis differs in bone marrow and liver. The level of ALA synthase is the major determinant of heme formation in the liver, while heme synthesis in the bone marrow is triggered by the complex process of erythroid differentiation. These considerations probably explain the different manifestations of enzyme defects of heme synthesis in erythroid cells and liver.

The colorless and nonfluorescent porphyrinogens serve as intermediates between porphobilinogen and protoporphyrin. With the exception of protoporphyrin, porphyrins are by-products that have escaped from the biosynthetic path by irreversible oxidation of the corresponding porphyrinogen. Porphyrins do not possess physiologic function but are responsible, through their red-purple color and fluorescent properties, for the spectacular appearance of urine and erythrocytes in some patients.

The arrangement of two substituent side chains on the pyrrole ring of porphyrins determines the structural isomer types, numbered

TABLE 328-1　Characteristics of the porphyrias

	Erythropoietic porphyrias		Hepatic porphyrias				
	Congenital erythropoietic porphyria (CEP)	Protoporphyria (PP)	Intermittent acute porphyria (IAP)	Hereditary coproporphyria (HCP)	Variegate porphyria (VP)	Porphobilinogen synthase deficiency	Porphyria cutanea tarda (PCT)
Enzyme deficiency	Uroporphyrinogen III cosynthase (?)	Ferrochelatase	Porphobilinogen deaminase	Coproporphyrinogen oxidase	Protoporphyrinogen oxidase	Porphobilinogen synthase	Uroporphyrinogen decarboxylase
Inheritance	Autosomal recessive	Autosomal dominant	Autosomal dominant	Autosomal dominant	Autosomal dominant	Autosomal recessive	Autosomal dominant (familial form)
Metabolic expression	Erythroid cells	Erythroid cells and liver	Liver	Liver	Liver	Liver	Liver
Signs and symptoms:							
Photosensitive cutaneous lesions	Yes	Yes	No	Infrequent	Yes	No	Yes
Attacks of abdominal pain, neuropsychiatric syndrome	No	No	Yes	Yes	Yes	Yes	No
Laboratory abnormalities:							
Red blood cells:							
Uroporphyrin	+ + +	N	N	N	N		N
Coproporphyrin	+ +	+	N	N	N		N
Protoporphyrin	(+)	+ + +	N	N	N	+	N
Urine:							
δ-Aminolevulinic acid	N	N	(+ + +)	(+ + +)	(+ + +)	+ + +	N
Porphobilinogen	N	N	(+ + +)	(+ + +)	(+ + +)	+	N
Uroporphyrin	+ + +	N	+ +	+	+	+	+ + +
Coproporphyrin	+ +	(+)	N	+ +	+ +	+ + +	+
Feces:							
Coproporphyrin	+	(+)	N	+ + +	+	N	(+)
Protoporphyrin	+	+ +	N	+	+ + +	N	N

NOTE: N, normal; +, increased levels or excretion; + +, moderately increased; + + +, markedly increased; (+), increased in some patients only; (+ + +), frequently increased only during acute attacks.

I to IV. In nature only types I and III have been identified, and only type III is a substrate for the terminal steps of the pathway leading to protoporphyrin IX and heme. The catabolism of heme does not lead to porphyrins but to noncyclic tetrapyrroles referred to as *bile pigments*.

CONGENITAL ERYTHROPOIETIC PORPHYRIA

DEFINITION　Congenital erythropoietic porphyria (CEP; Günther's disease, congenital photosensitive porphyria, erythropoietic uroporphyria) is a rare, recessively inherited defect that causes chronic photosensitivity with severe, mutilating skin lesions and hemolytic anemia.

GENETICS, INCIDENCE, AND PATHOGENESIS　CEP is the rarest of the inherited porphyrias, less than 100 cases having been reported. Affected individuals are homozygous for an autosomal recessive gene; heterozygotes rarely have demonstrable abnormalities in porphyrin metabolism and appear normal. The underlying enzyme abnormality is a primary genetic deficiency of uroporphyrinogen III cosynthase with compensatory increases in the activities of ALA

synthase and PBG deaminase in erythroid tissue. The defect is expressed solely in maturing erythroid cells and results in massive overproduction of uroporphyrinogen I while the production of uroporphyrinogen III is normal or slightly increased. Uroporphyrinogen I cannot be used for heme synthesis but is converted to coproporphyrinogen I. Uroporphyrin I, coproporphyrinogen I, and coproporphyrin I accumulate in tissues and are excreted in excess amounts in urine and feces.

CLINICAL PRESENTATION AND DIAGNOSIS　Porphyrins accumulate in affected individuals during fetal development. Excretion of pink or red urine usually begins at or shortly after birth, whereas cutaneous photosensitivity, intermittent hemolysis, and splenomegaly may be manifested later. Hypertrichosis and red discoloration of the teeth (erythrodontia) and bones are common. Death may occur in childhood. With longer survival, severe scarring and mutilation occur, mostly affecting fingers, nose, and ears. The urine contains high concentrations of uroporphyrin I, coproporphyrin, and porphyrins with seven, six, five, and three carboxyl groups, whereas the excretion of ALA and PBG is normal. Large amounts of coproporphyrin I are found in the feces. Normoblasts, reticulocytes, and erythrocytes contain large quantities of uroporphyrin I and lower concentrations

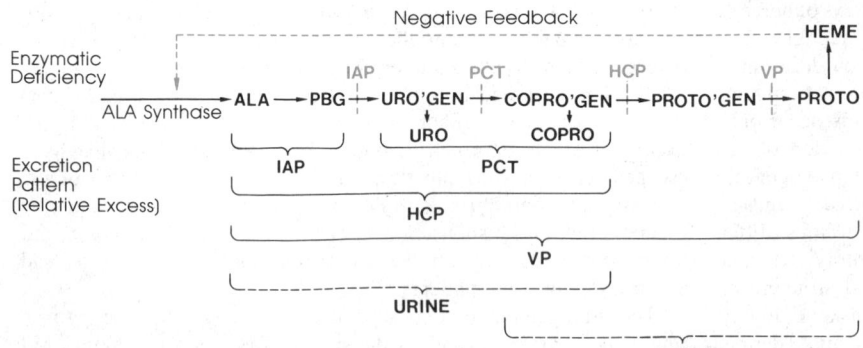

FIGURE 328-1　Patterns of urinary porphyrin and porphyrin precursor excretion in the hepatic porphyrias in relation to the enzymatic deficiency in the pathway of heme biosynthesis. Intermediates of the pathway excreted excessively during the acute phase of each of the hepatic porphyrias are within the respective brackets. (ALA, δ-aminolevulinic acid; PBG, porphobilinogen; URO'GEN, uroporphyrinogen; COPRO'GEN, coproporphyrinogen; PROTO'GEN, protoporphyrinogen; PROTO, protoporphyrin; IAP, intermittent acute porphyria; PCT, porphyria cutanea tarda; HCP, hereditary coproporphyria; VP, variegate porphyria.)

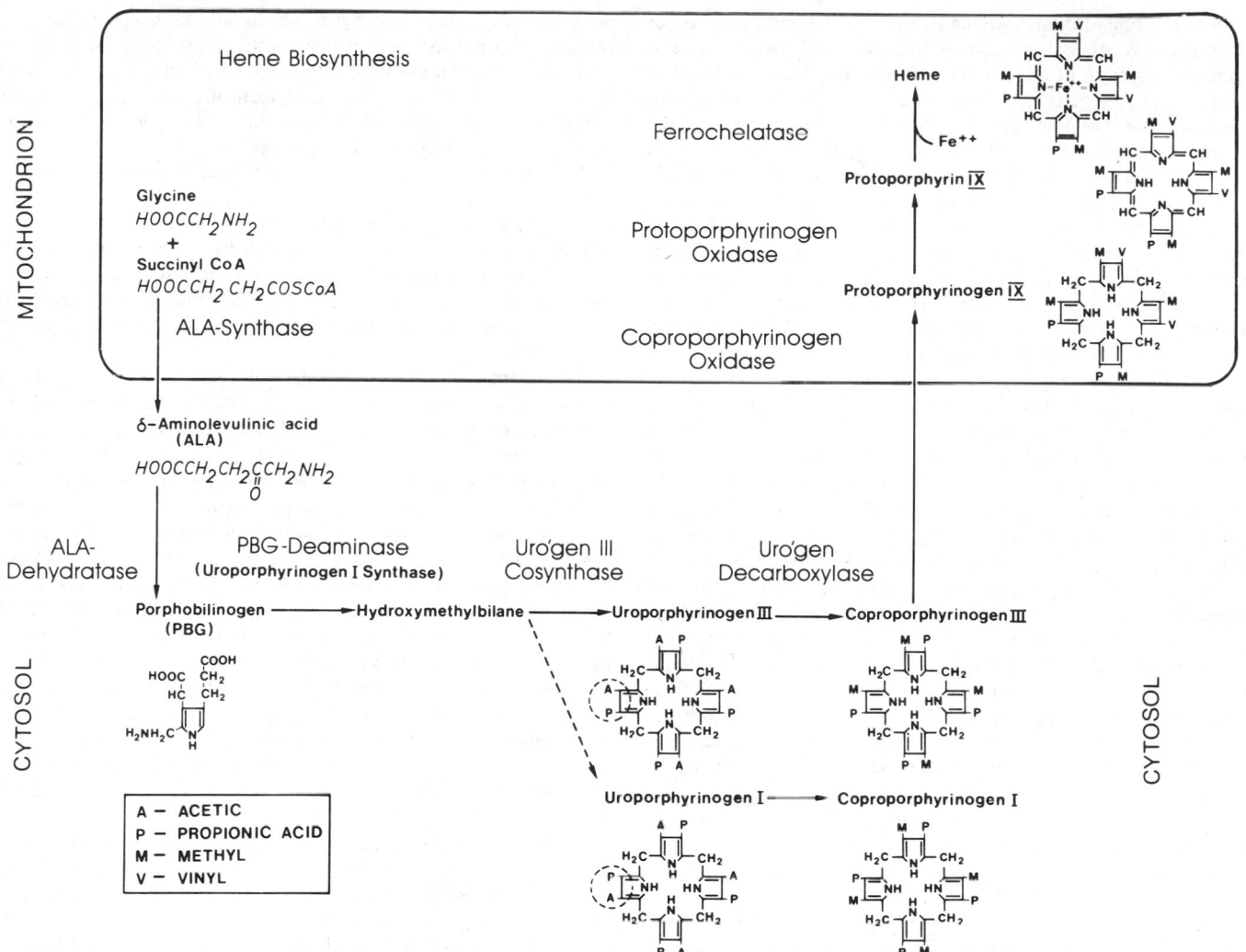

FIGURE 328-2 Outline of heme biosynthesis. (ALA, δ-aminolevulinic acid; PBG, porphobilinogen; URO'GEN, uroporphyrinogen.)

of coproporphyrinogen I. Normoblasts and reticulocytes exhibit intense red fluorescence. In accord with the normal excretion of ALA and PBG, neurologic disturbance does not occur.

TREATMENT Exposure to sunlight and trauma to the skin should be minimized. Oral carotenoids often decrease the photosensitivity (for details, see section on protoporphyria). In some cases, splenectomy has temporarily ameliorated hemolytic anemia, porphyrin excretion, and photosensitivity. The use of hematin infusions and packed erythrocyte transfusions to reduce hemolysis are other possibilities.

HEPATIC PORPHYRIAS

Three hepatic porphyrias, intermittent acute porphyria (IAP), hereditary coproporphyria (HCP), and variegate porphyria (VP), have many features in common. All are transmitted as autosomal dominants. Acute attacks of a life-threatening neurologic syndrome are precipitated by a variety of drugs, hormones, and other agents. During acute attacks increased urinary excretion of ALA and PBG occurs in all, but the patterns of porphyrins in urine and feces differ (Fig. 378-1). A recessively inherited deficiency of PBG synthase with extremely high urinary levels of ALA (but only slightly increased PBG) and a neurological syndrome identical to that of IAP, HCP, and VP has been described in a few homozygous patients (Table 328-1).

INTERMITTENT ACUTE PORPHYRIA Definition Intermittent acute porphyria [IAP, acute intermittent porphyria (AIP), pyrroloporphyria] is characterized by recurrent attacks of neurologic and psychiatric dysfunction. Photosensitivity does not occur. The primary defect is in porphobilinogen deaminase.

Genetics, incidence, and pathogenesis IAP is an autosomal dominant trait with variable expressivity. The frequency of the abnormal gene is estimated to be between 1 in 10,000 and 1 in 100,000, but in certain regions the incidence may be higher. Homozygous cases have not been observed. The defect consists of a partial (50 percent) deficiency of porphobilinogen deaminase, the enzyme that converts PBG to uroporphyrinogen I. Studies with antisera against human porphobilinogen deaminase suggest that at least four different classes of mutations can cause IAP. The most common mutation results in a decreased amount or absence of immunoreactive enzyme protein. The molecular defect at the gene level has not been defined. In the liver a partial deficiency of the enzyme leads to increased activity and/or inducibility of ALA synthase by drugs and other factors and, consequently, to increased formation and urinary excretion of ALA and PBG. Preformed porphyrins do not accumulate, and, therefore, cutaneous photosensitivity does not occur. Decreased porphobilinogen deaminase activity is observed in liver, erythrocytes, cultured skin fibroblasts, lymphocytes, and amniotic cells of patients with IAP. Thus, the enzymatic defect is present, albeit metabolically unexpressed, in tissues other than liver in most IAP patients examined. Deficiency of the enzyme does not necessarily result in clinical manifestations of acute porphyria without additional acquired factors, and only a third or less of individuals with the genetic defect ever experience an attack of porphyria. The relation between the genetic defect and the neurologic lesions is unknown.

Clinical presentation and diagnosis Symptoms rarely occur before puberty. Abdominal pain is frequently the initial and most prominent symptom of the porphyric attack. It may be moderate or severe, colicky, localized or generalized; radiation to the back or loins may occur. The pain probably results from autonomic neuropathy causing disturbed gastrointestinal motility with alternate areas of spasm and dilatation. The abdomen is usually soft, and tenderness is not marked. Because it is often accompanied by fever and leukocytosis, the acute porphyric attack can mimic any inflammatory abdominal disease. Severe vomiting and persistent constipation are common. Characteristically, the urine of patients with acute hepatic porphyria has a dark-red or "port-wine" appearance. Neurologic manifestations and mental disturbance are variable. Peripheral nerves, the autonomic nervous system, brainstem, cranial nerves, or cerebral function may be involved. Sinus tachycardia and labile hypertension with postural hypotension, urinary retention, and excessive sweating are frequent. Hypertension and tachycardia correlate with increased excretion of catecholamines. Peripheral neuropathy is predominantly motor, but sensory components may be present. Deep tendon reflexes are diminished or absent. Neuritic pain in the extremities, areas of hypesthesia and paresthesia, and foot and wrist drop are typical. Paraplegia or complete flaccid quadriplegia may ensue. Cranial nerve involvement may lead to optic nerve atrophy, ophthalmoplegia, and dysphagia. With more severe CNS involvement, delirium, coma, and seizures occur. Although the neuropathy is reversible to a surprising degree, residual paresis may last for years following an acute attack. Many patients have a long history of vague nervousness, emotional instability, and functional disturbances. Signs of mental disturbance occur in one-third, and an organic brain syndrome with restlessness, disorientation, and visual hallucinations may supervene. Hyponatremia can be severe. Multiple mechanisms (including gastrointestinal loss of sodium, imprudent fluid therapy, inappropriate secretion of antidiuretic hormone (vasopressin), and a sodium-losing nephropathy related to a toxic effect of ALA) have been implicated. Hypomagnesemia may cause tetany.

Acute attacks may last from days to months and vary in frequency and severity. In periods of remission symptoms may be slight or completely absent. Clinical (and biochemical) manifestations may be precipitated by usual therapeutic doses of barbiturates, anticonvulsants, estrogens, contraceptives, or alcohol. All these drugs are oxidized by hemoproteins of the cytochrome P$_{450}$ system. Impaired hepatic metabolism of some of these drugs can occur during acute attacks. In some women, exacerbations correlate with the menstrual cycle, and latent porphyria may become manifest late in pregnancy or shortly after delivery. Prolonged periods of decreased caloric intake (fasting) and infections may also provoke attacks.

Laboratory findings Excessive excretion of ALA and PBG in the urine is characteristic during acute attacks and does not differentiate IAP from HCP and VP. The levels in urine do not correlate with the severity of the symptoms. The qualitative determination of porphobilinogen in the urine by the Watson-Schwartz or the Hoesch test is a simple and valuable screening aid for the diagnosis of an acute attack in IAP, HCP, and VP. These tests are almost always positive during episodes of neuropsychiatric dysfunction but are positive only when the concentration of PBG in the urine is three to five times the upper limit of normal; as a consequence, both assays may be negative in latent cases and in patients in whom urinary excretion of PBG becomes normal following recovery from an acute attack. In these instances urinary ALA and PBG excretion should be quantified by chromatographic methods. In latent IAP with normal excretion of ALA and PBG, diagnosis is possible by measuring the activity of porphobilinogen deaminase in erythrocytes, lymphocytes, or cultured skin fibroblasts. However, there is an overlap between the activities of the enzyme in erythrocytes from normals and patients with IAP, and definite diagnosis is not always possible.

In IAP the porphyrin precursors ALA and PBG are excreted in increased amounts, consistent with the enzymatic defect. Freshly passed urine is, therefore, usually colorless and contains little preformed uro- or coproporphyrin. The urine may darken on standing because PBG polymerizes spontaneously to uroporphyrin and porphobilin, a dark-brown pigment of unknown structure. However, some patients have enough nonenzymatically formed pigments to impart a dark-red appearance to freshly voided urine. The fecal porphyrin concentration is usually normal.

Conventional liver function tests are normal. A moderate reduction in red blood cell mass and blood volume and a transient normochromic, normocytic anemia are the only hematologic disturbances. Metabolic abnormalities during acute attacks include hypercholesterolemia with increased low-density lipoprotein levels, increased serum thyroxine, impaired glucose tolerance, and defective 5α-reduction of testosterone in liver. The relationship of these abnormalities to the genetic defect is unknown.

Treatment The treatment of the acute attack is identical in IAP, HCP, and VP. Some acute attacks seemingly can be aborted by administration of large quantities (500 g/d) of carbohydrates (glucose effect), although no objective study of the efficacy of this therapy has been performed. Intravenous administration of glucose at a rate of 20 g/h is recommended. If the patient does not improve within 48 h of continued glucose infusion or if neuropsychiatric symptoms progress, intravenous infusion of hematin (4 mg per kilogram of body weight infused over 10 to 15 min every 12 h for 3 to 6 days) should be tried. Hematin is commercially available in the United States as lyophilized powder (Panhematin); solutions are prepared immediately before infusion. Complications of hematin treatment seem to be rare. Thrombophlebitis at the site of infusion, a coagulopathy (manifested by thrombocytopenia, prolonged prothrombin time, abnormal partial thromboplastin time, and hypofibrinogenemia), and hemolysis have been reported. These complications apparently are caused by degradation products of unstable heme solutions. They occur less frequently or not at all with freshly prepared hematin or with stable solutions of heme-arginate, available in Europe (Normosang). Both hematin and glucose prevent the induction of hepatic ALA-synthase in animals, and both may reverse the biochemical abnormalities and cause improvement within 48 h. Supportive treatment with careful monitoring of fluid and electrolytes is important to prevent and/or correct hyponatremia, hypomagnesemia, and azotemia. Tachycardia and hypertension should be treated with beta-adrenergic blocking drugs. A list of agents considered to be "safe" or "probably safe" in patients with latent and acute IAP, HCP, and VP is given in Table 328-2. Acute attacks carry a substantial risk of fatality if

---

TABLE 328-2 Drugs considered to be safe (or probably safe) in patients with intermittent acute porphyria, hereditary coproporphyria, and variegate porphyria

Analgesics:
　Acetaminophen, aspirin, ibuprofen
　Morphine and related opiates (meperidine, codeine)
Antibiotics:
　Penicillins, cephalosporins
　Methenamide, aminoglycosides
Psychoactive drugs:
　Phenothiazines (chlorpromazine), lithium, nortriptyline
Antihistamines:
　Diphenhydramine
Antihypertensives:
　Atenolol
　Propranolol
　Reserpine, thiazides
Miscellaneous:
　Atropine
　Cyclopropane, diethylether
　Neostigmine
　Propanidid
　Procaine
　Succinylcholine
　Nitrous oxide
　Glucocorticoids
　Oxazepam
　Chlordiazepoxide
　Insulin
　Heparin

the diagnosis is delayed and neurologic lesions progress, e.g., to respiratory paralysis. Complete recovery occurs in the majority, but neurologic deficits may require months or years to resolve. The most important measure in the management is prevention of acute attacks by instructing the patient to avoid provocative factors, such as drugs, steroids, alcohol excess, and deliberate fasting.

Some women with acute hepatic porphyria (IAP, HCP, or VP) have disabling premenstrual attacks with every cycle. These attacks can be prevented by daily intranasal or subcutaneous administration of a long-acting agonist of luteinizing hormone–releasing hormone (LHRH) such as leuprolide (leuproelin). The long-term effects of this treatment have not been evaluated.

HEREDITARY COPROPORPHYRIA **Definition and genetics** Hereditary coproporphyria (HCP) is a hepatic porphyria characterized by attacks of neuropsychiatric dysfunction identical with those of IAP and VP. Photosensitivity occurs in some. The primary genetic defect is a partial deficiency of coproporphyrinogen oxidase. The disease is inherited as an autosomal dominant trait. The incidence of HCP is uncertain since the majority of affected individuals remain asymptomatic.

Pathogenesis and clinical picture HCP is characterized by the excretion of large amounts of coproporphyrin III, mainly in feces but also in urine. Excretion of ALA and PBG is increased during acute attacks (positive Watson-Schwartz or Hoesch test) but usually returns to normal during remission. Acute attacks are indistinguishable from those of IAP and VP and are precipitated by the same factors. Skin photosensitivity occurs in approximately one-third of patients with overt disease. Its onset is frequently associated with intercurrent hepatic disease. A partial deficiency of coproporphyrinogen oxidase can be demonstrated in liver and other tissues.

Treatment Treatment is identical with that described for IAP.

VARIEGATE PORPHYRIA **Definition** Variegate porphyria (VP; South African genetic porphyria) is characterized both by acute attacks of neuropsychiatric dysfunction and by skin sensitivity to sunlight and to mechanical trauma. The primary enzymatic lesion in heme biosynthesis is a partial deficiency of protoporphyrinogen oxidase.

Genetics, incidence, and pathogenesis VP is inherited as an autosomal dominant trait. The disease is particularly common among the white population of South Africa, where its incidence is estimated at 1 in 400, and many cases have been identified as descendants of a woman who emigrated to Cape Town from the Netherlands in 1688. Elsewhere the disease is much less frequent, but VP has been recognized in many countries. The defect leads to the excretion of large amounts of protoporphyrin in bile and feces (with lesser increases in the fecal excretion of coproporphyrin) and to increased urinary excretion of ALA, PBG, and coproporphyrin during acute attacks.

Clinical presentation and diagnosis Overt cases with VP usually present in the second or third decade. The features include acute attacks of abdominal pain and neuropsychiatric symptoms, coupled with photocutaneous lesions. Neurologic and cutaneous manifestations may occur simultaneously or at different times. Most South African patients have cutaneous involvement, consisting of dermal abrasions, superficial erosions, and blister formation after trivial mechanical trauma. The mechanical fragility usually is limited to light-exposed parts of the skin. The lesions often leave depigmented or pigmented scars. Hyperpigmentation of the face and hands is common, and women often have hirsutism. The skin lesions are indistinguishable from those of porphyria cutanea tarda (PCT). Acute attacks of neuropsychiatric dysfunction are indistinguishable from those of IAP and HCP and are precipitated by the same factors. The characteristic chemical finding in VP is the continuous excretion of large amounts of proto- and coproporphyrin, even when clinical manifestations are minimal or absent. Urinary excretion of ALA, PBG, and porphyrins is either normal or moderately increased in asymptomatic patients or those who have only skin symptoms. During acute attacks the urinary excretion of ALA and PBG is increased (positive Watson-Schwartz or Hoesch test), and there also is increased urinary coproporphyrin

and uroporphyrin. Erythrocyte porphyrins are normal, allowing distinction from protoporphyria.

Treatment Prophylactic measures and treatment of the acute attack with glucose and possibly hematin infusions are the same as for IAP and HCP, although the experience with hematin in VP is limited. Avoidance of exposure to direct sunlight and use of protective clothing (gloves, hats) are advocated. The prognosis is similar to or better than that of patients with IAP.

PORPHYRIA CUTANEA TARDA **Definition** Porphyria cutanea tarda (PCT; symptomatic cutaneous hepatic porphyria, symptomatic porphyria) is characterized by chronic lesions on light-exposed areas of the skin and a distinct pattern of urinary excretion of porphyrins. The disorder is caused by an inherited or acquired deficiency of hepatic uroporphyrinogen decarboxylase. Neurologic manifestations are absent.

Genetics, incidence, and pathogenesis There are at least four distinct types of PCT: (1) *familial PCT*, inherited as an autosomal dominant trait, in which uroporphyrinogen decarboxylase is decreased ≈50 percent in liver, erythrocytes, and other tissues; (2) *sporadic PCT*, associated with the use of alcohol or contraceptive steroids, in which a partial deficiency of uroporphyrinogen decarboxylase is restricted to the liver; (3) *hepatoerythropoietic porphyria (HEP)*, which may represent a rare homozygous form of PCT, with a marked generalized decrease in uroporphyrinogen decarboxylase to <10 percent of normal and severe clinical manifestations beginning in infancy; (4) *toxic PCT*, occurring in individuals exposed to polyhalogenated hydrocarbons, notably hexachlorobenzene, and presumably also due to decreased hepatic uroporphyrinogen decarboxylase.

The incidence of the disease is not established, but sporadic PCT is the most commonly recognized type of human porphyria. It is unknown if decreased hepatic uroporphyrinogen decarboxylase in sporadic PCT is a consequence of a genetic or acquired (toxic) mechanism. Deficiency (of whatever etiology) in uroporphyrinogen decarboxylase, which catalyzes the conversion of uroporphyrinogen to coproporphyrinogen, may lead to a disturbance of hepatic heme synthesis and consequent skin photosensitivity only in the presence of additional factors such as iron overload, usually in association with alcoholic liver disease or the prolonged administration of estrogens. The mechanism by which iron overload and hormones cause clinical expression of latent PCT is unknown. In contrast to IAP, HCP, and VP, the enzymatic defect in PCT does not result in altered regulation of hepatic heme synthesis, and ALA synthase activity is normal or minimally increased even in overt cases. This probably accounts for the absence of acute neuropsychiatric attacks, the usually normal urinary ALA and PBG, and the lack of sensitivity to drugs such as barbiturates.

Clinical presentation and diagnosis Photosensitivity is the only major manifestation. The skin lesions are indistinguishable from those in VP. Skin symptoms usually begin insidiously, most often in men aged 40 to 60, and consist of enhanced facial pigmentation, increased fragility to trauma, erythema, and vesicular and ulcerative lesions. Sclerodermatous changes and increased hair on the forehead, malar region, or forearms are common.

Liver disease, frequently related to alcohol, is common, and hepatic siderosis is an almost constant finding, particularly in sporadic PCT, although the degree of iron deposition is variable and rarely severe. Spontaneous remission may occur. Estrogens (including contraceptive pills) or known hepatotoxic drugs may precipitate the clinical disease. The incidence of diabetes mellitus is increased in PCT, and association with systemic lupus erythematosus and other autoimmune syndromes has been noted.

The excretion in urine of uroporphyrin and, to a lesser extent, coproporphyrin is increased. The urine may be pink or brown. The excretion of ALA and PBG in urine is usually normal (negative Watson-Schwartz or Hoesch test). Although uroporphyrin is the major porphyrin in the urine, intermediary porphyrins (particularly heptacarboxylic porphyrin) are also found. Increases in fecal porphyrins are less marked and usually restricted to the coproporphyrin fraction.

The diagnosis is established by the combined presence of skin photosensitivity, increased urinary uroporphyrin excretion, the lack of an increase in porphyrin precursors (ALA, PBG), and absence of a history of neuropsychiatric attacks.

Toxic acquired porphyria resembling PCT can occur in individuals accidentally exposed to polyhalogenated hydrocarbons, best documented for hexachlorobenzene. Moreover, PCT may occur in association with benign or malignant primary tumors of the liver. A syndrome apparently analogous to PCT but with no abnormalities of porphyrin excretion (pseudoporphyria) has been described in patients with chronic renal failure on hemodialysis.

Treatment   Once the diagnosis of PCT is established, avoidance of alcohol, estrogens, and exposure to halogenated hydrocarbons often results in clinical and biochemical remission. Removal of hepatic iron by repeated phlebotomy may lead to long-lasting remissions within 6 to 9 months: 400 mL of blood (or the equivalent amount of erythrocytes) is removed weekly or less frequently with careful monitoring of the hemoglobin and plasma protein levels. For patients unable to tolerate phlebotomy, the administration of small doses of chloroquine (125 to 250 mg twice weekly) apparently removes uroporphyrins from the liver and has produced remissions. However, chloroquine carries the risk of hepatotoxicity. Chelation therapy with desferoxamine is another alternative to remove iron. Topical sunscreens and oral carotenoids are not effective in protecting against the skin lesions of PCT.

PROTOPORPHYRIA

DEFINITION   Protoporphyria (PP; erythropoietic protoporphyria, erythrohepatic protoporphyria), a disorder in which mild skin photosensitivity is associated with high concentrations of protoporphyrin in erythrocytes, is due to a deficiency of ferrochelatase. Protoporphyrin may also accumulate in the liver.

GENETICS, INCIDENCE, AND PATHOGENESIS   PP is inherited as an autosomal dominant trait with variable expressivity. The prevalence of PP is not established but seems to be similar to that of PCT. Activity of ferrochelatase, the mitochondrial enzyme that catalyzes the incorporation of ferrous iron into protoporphyrin, is deficient in bone marrow, peripheral blood, liver, and cultured skin fibroblasts. This deficiency results in the excessive accumulation of protoporphyrin in late normoblasts, reticulocytes, and young erythrocytes; protoporphyrin leaks into the plasma from erythrocytes as they age. Photosensitivity is mediated by protoporphyrin in plasma and skin and is evoked by visible light (380 to 560 nm). Skin photosensitivity shows seasonal variability. The liver participates in excess porphyrin production in some patients or, alternatively, may take up protoporphyrin from plasma. Many carriers of the defect remain clinically (and chemically) asymptomatic, and diagnosis may be possible only through enzymatic studies.

CLINICAL PRESENTATION AND DIAGNOSIS   Mild photosensitivity usually begins in childhood. Exposure to sunlight for minutes or hours is followed by painful burning or stinging sensations, pruritus, erythema, and occasional edema (solar urticaria). The lesions subside over hours or days without scarring; alternatively, the initial skin lesions may progress to a chronic eczematous phase (solar eczema). There is no abnormal mechanical fragility or blister formation in skin as is characteristic for VP and PCT. Erythrodontia, hypertrichosis, and hyperpigmentation are absent. Attacks of neuropsychiatric dysfunction do not occur.

PP is generally benign, but may be associated with abnormalities of liver, biliary tract, or blood. The incidence of cholelithiasis is increased, and the gallstones contain protoporphyrin. Liver disease due to massive deposition of protoporphyrin may rarely progress to fatal cirrhosis. All patients therefore should have routine evaluation of liver function. Mild anemia is common.

PP is diagnosed by the detection of high concentrations of protoporphyrin in erythrocytes. Large numbers of red-fluorescing erythrocytes are seen by fluorescent microscopy. Protoporphyrin may also be elevated in plasma and feces, while urinary porphyrins, ALA, and PBG are usually normal.

TREATMENT   Topical sunscreens usually are ineffective. Orally administered β-carotene (usually as a mixture of β-carotene and canthaxanthine) substantially improves the tolerance to sunlight. Serum β-carotene levels should be maintained between 10 and 15 μmol/L (600 and 800 μg/dL). The efficacy of carotenoid treatment is considered to be related to its ability to quench singlet oxygen and to act as free radical scavenger.

REFERENCES

BLOOMER JR: Protoporphyria, Semin Liver Dis: 2, 143, 1982

BONKOVSKY HL: Porphyria: Practical advice for the clinical gastroenterologist and hepatologist. Dig Dis 5, 179, 1987

KAPPAS A et al: The porphyrias, in *The Metabolic Basis of Inherited Disease*, 5th ed, JB Stanbury et al (eds). New York, McGraw-Hill, 1983

MASCARO JM (ed): The porphyrias. Semin Dermatol 5:69, 1986

MUSTAJOKI P, TENHUNEN R: Haem arginate in the treatment of hepatic porphyrias. Br Med J 293:538, 1986

PIERACH CA: Hematin therapy for the porphyric attack. Semin Liver Dis 2:125, 1982

PIMSTONE NR: Porphyria cutanea tarda. Semin Liver Dis 2:132, 1982

YEUNG LAIWAH AC, MCCOLL KEL: Management of attacks of acute porphyria. Drugs 34:604, 1987

329   GOUT AND OTHER DISORDERS OF PURINE METABOLISM

WILLIAM N. KELLEY / THOMAS D. PALELLA

GOUT

Gout is a term representing a heterogeneous group of diseases, which in their full development are manifested by (1) an increase in the serum urate concentration; (2) recurrent attacks of a characteristic acute arthritis, in which crystals of monosodium urate monohydrate are demonstrable in leukocytes of synovial fluid; (3) aggregated deposits of monosodium urate monohydrate (tophi) chiefly in and around the joints of the extremities and sometimes leading to severe crippling and deformity; (4) renal disease involving interstitial tissues and blood vessels; and (5) uric acid nephrolithiasis. These may occur singly or in combination.

PREVALENCE AND EPIDEMIOLOGY   The serum urate value is elevated in an absolute sense when it exceeds the limit of solubility of monosodium urate in serum. At 37°C the saturation value of urate in plasma is about 415 μmol/L (7.0 mg/dL); a value above this represents supersaturation in a physicochemical sense. The serum urate concentration is relatively elevated when it exceeds the upper limit of an arbitrary normal range, usually defined as the mean serum urate value plus 2 standard deviations in a healthy population matched for age and sex. In most studies the upper limit is about 415 μmol/L (7.0 mg/dL) in men and 360 μmol/L (6.0 mg/dL) in women. In epidemiologic terms a serum urate value in excess of 415 μmol/L (7.0 mg/dL) carries an increased risk of gouty arthritis or renal stones.

Sex and age influence urate levels. In both boys and girls the serum urate concentration before puberty averages approximately 200 μmol/L (3.6 mg/dL). After puberty, levels increase in boys more than in girls. Values in men reach a plateau in the early twenties and are essentially stable thereafter. Values in women are constant from age 20 through 40, but with menopause the values rise and approach or equal those in men. These age and sex differences are thought to be related to differences in the renal clearance of urate, perhaps influenced by the levels of estrogens and androgens. Certain physiologic variables such as height, body weight, creatinine, blood urea nitrogen, serum creatinine, and blood pressure correlate with serum urate concentration. Other factors, including warm ambient temperature, alcohol intake, high social status, and achievement or intelligence also appear to correlate with a higher serum urate concentration.

Hyperuricemia by one or more of the above definitions is present in 2 to 18 percent of the population. In one hospitalized group, 13 percent of adult men exhibited a serum urate concentration in excess of 415 μmol/L (7.0 mg/dL).

The incidence and prevalence of gout are less than those of hyperuricemia. In most of the western world the overall prevalence is 0.13 to 0.37 percent of the population. The prevalence relates both to the degree of elevation of the serum urate and to the duration over which this elevation is sustained. Gout is therefore primarily a disease of adult men, and only about 5 percent of cases occur in women; it occurs rarely in the prepubertal child of either sex. The usual form is uncommon before the third decade, and the peak incidence is in the fifth decade.

INHERITANCE   A family history of gout is obtained in 6 to 18 percent of gouty subjects, and figures as high as 75 percent are noted after persistent questioning. A precise definition of the inheritance of gout is complicated by the environmental factors that alter the serum urate concentration. In addition, the identification of several specific causes of gout indicates that the disorder is the common clinical manifestation of a heterogeneous group of diseases. Accordingly, analysis of the inheritance of hyperuricemia and gout in the population or even within families is difficult. Two specific enzymatic causes of gout, hypoxanthine-guanine phosphoribosyltransferase deficiency and 5-phosphoribosyl-1-pyrophosphate (PRPP) synthetase overactivity, are X-linked. In other families the inheritance is consistent with an autosomal dominant mode. More commonly, genetic studies suggest multifactorial inheritance.

CLINICAL FEATURES   The full natural history of gout comprises four stages: asymptomatic hyperuricemia, acute gouty arthritis, intercritical gout, and chronic tophaceous gout. Nephrolithiasis may occur in any stage but the first.

Asymptomatic hyperuricemia   Asymptomatic hyperuricemia is that stage in which the serum urate level is raised but arthritic symptoms, tophi, or uric acid stones have not yet appeared. In men vulnerable to classic gout, hyperuricemia begins at puberty, whereas in women at risk hyperuricemia is usually delayed until menopause. In contrast, patients with certain of the enzyme defects to be described later may be hyperuricemic from birth. While asymptomatic hyperuricemia may last throughout the lifetime with no recognizable consequences, the tendency toward acute gouty arthritis increases as a function of the level and the duration of hyperuricemia. The risk of nephrolithiasis also increases as serum urate values increase and correlates with the magnitude of uric acid excretion. While virtually all gouty subjects are hyperuricemic, only about 5 percent of hyperuricemics ever develop gout.

The phase of asymptomatic hyperuricemia ends with the first attack of gouty arthritis or nephrolithiasis. In most, gout comes before stone, usually after at least 20 to 30 years of sustained hyperuricemia. However, between 10 and 40 percent of gouty subjects have renal colic prior to the first episode of arthritis.

Acute gouty arthritis   The primary manifestation of acute gout is exquisitely painful arthritis, at first usually monoarticular and associated with few constitutional symptoms but later often polyarticular and accompanied by fever. Estimates vary as to the percentage of patients in whom the initial gouty episode is polyarticular. Some authors' estimates are as high as 40 percent, and the majority of reports range from 3 to 14 percent. Attacks last a variable but limited period of time and are separated by asymptomatic intervals. In at least half the initial attack occurs in the first metatarsal phalangeal joint. Ultimately, 90 percent of patients experience an acute attack in the great toe (podagra).

Acute gouty arthritis is predominantly a disease of the lower extremities. The more distal the site of involvement the more typical

are the attacks. Following the toe in order of frequency as sites of initial involvement are the insteps, ankles, heels, knees, wrists, fingers, and elbows. Acute attacks in the shoulder, hips, spine, sacroiliac, sternoclavicular, and mandibular joints are rare except in patients with established, severe disease. Gouty bursitis also occurs, the prepatellar and olecranon bursae being the most commonly involved sites. The patient may report trivial episodes of pain, often described as "twinges," preceding the first dramatic gouty attack. More commonly, the initial attack is unheralded and explosive. Often, the major attack begins at night, is exquisitely painful with inflamed joints, and may be triggered by a specific event such as trauma, alcohol ingestion, certain drugs, dietary excess, or surgery. The pain reaches peak intensity within several hours, and the associated signs of inflammation progress. The inflammatory response is typically so intense as to suggest pyogenic arthritis. Systemic signs may include fever, leukocytosis, and an elevated sedimentation rate. It is difficult to improve upon Sydenham's classic description:

The victim goes to bed and sleeps in good health. About two o'clock in the morning he is awakened by a severe pain in the great toe; more rarely in the heel, ankle, or instep. This pain is like that of a dislocation, and yet the parts feel as if cold water were poured over them. Then follow chills and shivers, and a little fever. The pain, which was at first moderate, becomes more intense. With its intensity the chills and shivers increase. After a time this comes to its height, accommodating itself to the bones and ligaments of the tarsus and metatarsus. Now it is a violent stretching and tearing of the ligaments—now it is a gnawing pain and now a pressure and tightening. So exquisite and lively meanwhile is the feeling of the part affected, that it cannot bear the weight of bedclothes nor the jar of a person walking in the room. The night is passed in torture, sleeplessness, turning of the part affected, and perpetual change of posture; the tossing about of the body being as incessant as the pain of the tortured joint, and being worse as the fit comes on. Hence the vain effort by change of posture, both in the body and the limb affected, to obtain an abatement of the pain.

The initial gouty episode indicates the serum urate concentration has been sufficiently elevated for a long enough period of time to result in tissue deposition of substantial amounts of urate.

Intercritical period   The attack of gout may last only a day or two or up to several weeks but characteristically subsides spontaneously. No sequelae ensue, and resolution is complete. An asymptomatic phase termed the *intercritical period* then commences. The patient is totally free of symptoms during this stage, a feature that is diagnostically important. While approximately 7 percent never have a second attack, approximately 60 percent experience a recurrence within 1 year. However, the intercritical period may last up to 10 years and is terminated by successive attacks each of which may last longer and resolve less completely than its predecessors. Later attacks tend to be polyarticular, more severe, more prolonged, and associated with fever. In this stage gout may be difficult to differentiate from other types of polyarticular arthritis such as rheumatoid arthritis. Rare patients progress directly from the initial acute attack to chronic polyarticular disease with no remissions.

Tophi and chronic gouty arthritis   In the untreated patient the rate of urate production exceeds the rate of urate disposition. As a result, the urate pool expands, and crystal deposits of monosodium urate eventually appear in cartilage, synovial membranes, tendons, and soft tissues. The rate of formation of these tophaceous deposits is a function of the degree and duration of hyperuricemia and of the severity of renal disease. The classic, but by no means the most common, location of a tophus is the helix or antihelix of the ear (Fig. 329-1). Tophi also commonly occur along the ulnar surface of the forearm, as saccular distensions of the olecranon bursae (Fig. 329-2), as enlargements of the Achilles tendon, or at other pressure points. Patients with the most severe tophi, interestingly, often have sparing of the helix and antihelix of the ear.

Tophi are difficult to differentiate from rheumatoid nodules and other types of subcutaneous nodules. They may ulcerate and exude chalky or pasty material rich in monosodium urate crystals. In contrast

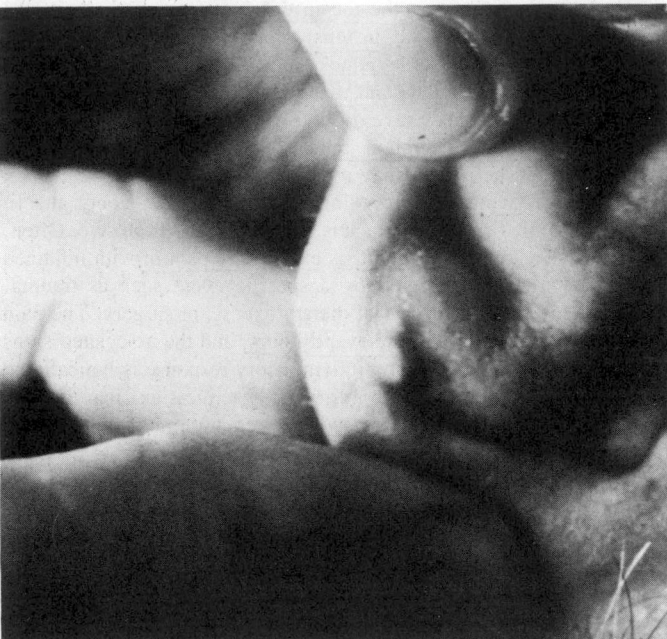

FIGURE 329-1 Tophus of the helix of the ear adjacent to the auricular tubercle.

to other subcutaneous nodules, tophi are rarely transient although they may resolve slowly in response to treatment of hyperuricemia. Documentation of monosodium urate crystals by polarizing microscopy of an aspirate establishes the nodule in question as a tophus. It is rare for a tophus to become infected. Patients with severe tophaceous disease appear to have milder and less frequent attacks of acute gouty arthritis than do nontophaceous subjects. Chronic tophaceous gout rarely occurs prior to the onset of gouty arthritis.

Effective therapy alters the natural history of the disease. Since the advent of effective antihyperuricemic therapy, only a minority of patients develop visible tophi, permanent joint changes, or chronic symptoms.

Nephropathy   Some renal dysfunction occurs in up to 90 percent of subjects with gouty arthritis. Prior to the advent of chronic hemodialysis, renal failure accounted for 17 to 25 percent of deaths in the gouty population. The initial manifestation of renal involvement may be albuminuria or isosthenuria. If the patient presents in an advanced stage of renal failure it may be difficult to determine whether renal failure is a consequence of hyperuricemia or hyperuricemia is the result of renal disease.

FIGURE 329-2 Effusions of olecranon bursae of patient with gout. Note also the cutaneous deposits of urate and the minimal inflammatory response.

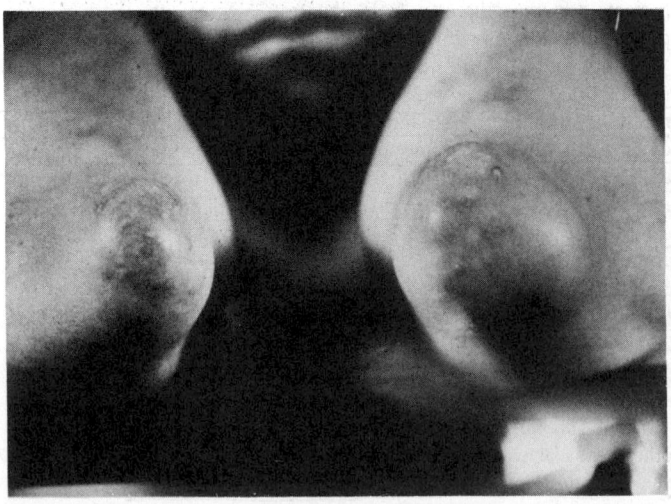

Two types of parenchymal renal damage have been described. The first, urate nephropathy, has been attributed to the deposition of monosodium urate crystals in the renal interstitial tissue. The second, obstructive uropathy, is due to the formation of uric acid crystals in the collecting tubules, renal pelvis, or ureter, with resulting blockage of urine flow.

There is considerable controversy over the pathogenesis of urate nephropathy. While crystals of monosodium urate have been demonstrated in the interstitium of kidneys from some gouty subjects, such crystals are not present in the kidneys of most people with gout. Conversely, renal interstitial urate deposition may occur in the absence of gout, although the clinical significance of such deposition is unclear. Unidentified factors may participate in the formation of urate deposits in the kidney. Further, there is a close correlation between the development of renal disease and the presence of hypertension in patients with gout. It is frequently not clear whether the hypertension causes the renal disease or the gouty renal disease is the cause of the hypertension.

Acute obstructive uropathy is a severe form of acute renal failure due to the precipitation of uric acid crystals in collecting ducts and ureters. Renal failure in this setting correlates more strongly with hyperuricaciduria than with hyperuricemia. This condition occurs most commonly in (1) patients with profound overproduction of uric acid, particularly subjects with leukemia or lymphoma who are subjected to aggressive chemotherapy, (2) patients with gout and marked hyperuricaciduria, and (3) (possibly) patients following severe exercise, rhabdomyolysis, or convulsions. Aciduria favors the formation of the relatively insoluble nonionized uric acid and, hence, may contribute to crystal precipitation in any of these conditions. Postmortem studies reveal intraluminal precipitates of uric acid with dilatation of proximal tubules. Therapy designed to decrease the formation of uric acid, accelerate urine flow, and increase the fraction of uric acid present as the more soluble ionized form, monosodium urate, is effective in the reversal of this process.

Nephrolithiasis   While the prevalence of subjects with uric acid stones in the United States is about 0.01 percent, the prevalence in gouty subjects ranges from 10 to 25 percent. The major factor favoring formation of uric acid stones is the increased urinary excretion of uric acid. Hyperuricaciduria may be due to primary gout, inborn errors of metabolism resulting in the overproduction of uric acid, myeloproliferative disease, and other neoplastic disorders. When the urinary uric acid exceeds 6.5 mmol/d (1100 mg/d), the incidence reaches 50 percent. There is also correlation with increasing serum urate concentrations, the prevalence reaching approximately 50 percent at a serum urate value of 770 μmol/L (13 mg/dL) or above. Other factors contributing to the formation of uric acid stones include (1) undue acidity of the urine, (2) increased urine concentration, and (3) (perhaps) abnormalities of urinary constituents that affect the solubility of uric acid itself.

Gouty subjects also have an increased frequency of calcium-containing stones; the occurrence in gout is 1 to 3 percent, while that in the general population is about 0.1 percent. While the mechanisms for this association are unclear, there is a high frequency of hyperuricemia and hyperuricaciduria in patients seen because of calcium stones. Uric acid crystals may serve as a nidus for calcium stone formation.

Associated conditions   Obesity, hypertriglyceridemia, and hypertension are common. The hypertriglyceridemia of primary gout is more closely associated with obesity or alcohol ingestion than with hyperuricemia itself. The incidence of hypertension in the nongouty population is correlated with age, sex, and obesity; when these factors are appropriately scored, there appears to be little or no direct relationship between hyperuricemia and hypertension. The increased frequency of diabetes is also probably related to factors such as age and obesity and not to hyperuricemia itself. In addition, the increased incidence of atherosclerosis has been attributed to the concomitant obesity, hypertension, diabetes, and hypertriglyceridemia. Independent analysis of these variables suggests that obesity is

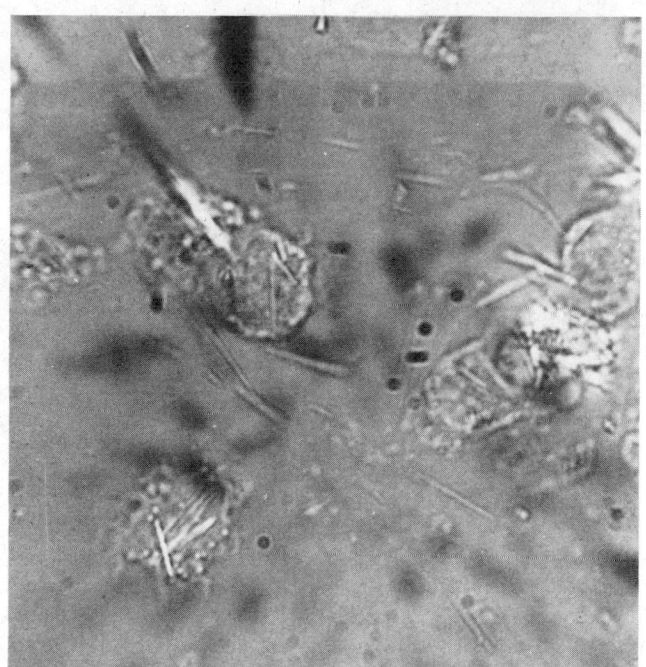

FIGURE 329-3   Crystals of monosodium urate monohydrate in joint aspirate.

most important. Hyperuricemia in the obese subject appears to be related to both increased production and reduced excretion of uric acid. Chronic alcohol ingestion also results in both overproduction and underexcretion of uric acid.

Rheumatoid arthritis, systemic lupus erythematosus, and amyloidosis rarely coexist with gout. The reasons for these negative associations are not known.

Acute gout should be suspected in any patient presenting with the sudden onset of monoarthritis, particularly in a distal joint of the lower extremity. Synovial aspiration should be performed in all such patients. The diagnosis of gout is established with certainty upon demonstration of monosodium urate crystals in leukocytes of synovial fluid from the involved joint by compensated polarized light microscopy (Fig. 329-3). The crystals are typically needle-shaped and negatively birefringent. Such crystals can be identified in synovial fluid of over 95 percent of patients with acute gouty arthritis. Failure to demonstrate urate crystals in synovial fluid after careful search under appropriate conditions makes the diagnosis unlikely. The presence of intracellular urate crystals establishes the diagnosis but does not exclude the possibility that another type of arthropathy is present concurrently.

Infection or pseudogout (calcium pyrophosphate dihydrate deposition) may coexist with gout. A Gram stain of the synovial fluid should be examined, and cultures should be obtained to exclude coexistent infection. Calcium pyrophosphate dihydrate is weakly positively birefringent and is more rectangular than monosodium urate. With polarized light microscopy, the crystals are easily differentiated. Synovial aspiration need not be repeated with subsequent episodes unless an alternative diagnosis is being considered.

During asymptomatic intercritical periods, synovial aspiration may still be helpful. Extracellular urate crystals can be found in more than two-thirds of aspirates from the first metatarsophalangeal joints of asymptomatic gouty patients Less than 5 percent of hyperuricemic patients without gout have such crystals.

Synovial fluid analysis may also be helpful in other ways. The total leukocyte count may be low or high. The predominant cell type is the polymorphonuclear leukocyte. As with other inflammatory fluids, the mucin clot is fair to poor. The concentrations of glucose and uric acid are the same as in serum.

In the patient in whom synovial fluid cannot be obtained or in whom intracellular crystals cannot be demonstrated, a presumptive

diagnosis of gout can be seriously entertained if the patient has (1) hyperuricemia, (2) the classic clinical features described above, and (3) a dramatic response to colchicine. In the absence of crystals or this highly suggestive triad, the diagnosis of gout should be considered tentative. A dramatic therapeutic response to colchicine is strongly suggestive of the diagnosis of gouty arthritis but is not pathognomonic by itself.

Acute gouty arthritis must be differentiated from other causes of monarticular and polyarticular arthritis. A common initial presentation in the gouty patient is podagra, but many conditions mimic the painful, swollen big toe characteristic of the disease. These include soft tissue infection, pyogenic arthritis, inflamed bunions, local trauma, rheumatoid arthritis, degenerative arthritis with acute inflammation, acute sarcoidosis, psoriatic arthritis, pseudogout, acute calcific tendonitis, palindromic rheumatism, Reiter's disease, and sporotrichosis. Rarely, confusion may be caused by cellulitis, gonorrhea, fibrosis of the sole and heel, hematoma, and subacute bacterial endocarditis with embolization or suppurative arthritis. Gouty involvement of other joints such as the knee must also be differentiated from acute rheumatic fever, serum sickness, hemarthrosis, and the peripheral joint involvement of ankylosing spondylitis or inflammatory bowel disease.

Chronic gouty arthritis must be differentiated from rheumatoid arthritis, inflammatory osteoarthritis, psoriatic arthritis, enteropathic arthritis, and the peripheral arthritis associated with the spondyloarthropathies. A history of antecedent, self-limited monarticular arthritis, the presence of tophi, typical radiographic changes, and the demonstration of hyperuricemia add support to the diagnosis of chronic gout. Chronic gout can be similar to other inflammatory arthropathies. The existence of effective therapy for gout justifies a vigorous workup to establish or exclude this diagnosis.

PATHOPHYSIOLOGY OF HYPERURICEMIA Classification The biochemical hallmark and prerequisite of gout is hyperuricemia. The concentration of uric acid in body fluids is determined by the balance between rates of production and elimination. Uric acid is formed by oxidation of purine bases, which may be exogenous or endogenous in origin. About two-thirds of uric acid is excreted into the urine [1.8 to 3.6 mmol/d (300 to 600 mg/d)], and approximately one-third is excreted into the gastrointestinal tract, where it is ultimately destroyed by bacteria. Hyperuricemia may be due to an excessive rate of uric acid production, a decrease in the renal excretion of uric acid, or a combination of both events.

Hyperuricemia and gout may be classified as metabolic or renal (Table 329-1). In those patients with hyperuricemia of metabolic origin, there is an increased production of uric acid, whereas in those with hyperuricemia of renal origin, decreased renal excretion of uric acid causes hyperuricemia. The distinction between metabolic and renal origins of hyperuricemia is not always clear-cut. A large number of gouty subjects have evidence of both mechanisms when thoroughly investigated. In such cases, the dominant component—renal or metabolic—directs classification. In the classification used here *primary* refers to those cases in which gout or hyperuricemia is the central manifestation of the disease, namely, gout that is neither secondary to another acquired disorder nor a subordinate manifestation of an inborn error that leads initially to a major disease unlike gout. While some cases of primary gout have a defined genetic basis, others do not. *Secondary* hyperuricemia or gout refers to those cases which develop in the course of another disease or as a consequence of drugs.

Overproduction of uric acid Overproducers of uric acid by definition excrete in excess of 3.6 mmol/d (600 mg/d) after a 5-day period of dietary purine restriction; such patients probably represent less than 10 percent of the gouty population. In these patients there is an acceleration in the rate of purine biosynthesis de novo or an increased turnover of purines. Understanding the basic mechanisms responsible for these abnormalities requires an understanding of purine metabolism (Fig. 329-4).

The purine nucleotides, adenylic acid (AMP), inosinic acid (IMP),

TABLE 329-1   Classification of hyperuricemia and gout

Type	Metabolic disturbance	Inheritance
Metabolic (10%):		
Primary		
Molecular defects undefined	Not established	Polygenic
Associated with specific enzyme defects		
PRPP synthetase variants, increased activity	Overproduction of PRPP and of uric acid	X-linked
Hypoxanthine-guanine phosphoribosyltransferase deficiency, partial	Overproduction of uric acid, increased purine biosynthesis de novo driven by surplus PRPP	X-linked
Secondary		
Associated with increased purine biosynthesis de novo		
Glucose-6-phosphatase deficiency or absence	Overproduction plus underexcretion of uric acid; glycogen storage disease, type I (von Gierke)	Autosomal recessive
Hypoxanthine-guanine phosphoribosyltransferase deficiency, "virtually complete"	Overproduction of uric acid; Lesch-Nyhan syndrome	X-linked
Associated with increased nucleic acid turnover	Overproduction of uric acid	
Renal (90%):		
Primary		
Secondary		

and guanylic acid (GMP), are the end products of purine biosynthesis. They can be synthesized in one of two ways: either directly from the purine bases, e.g., guanine to GMP, hypoxanthine to IMP, and adenine to AMP; or they may be synthesized de novo, beginning with nonpurine precursors and progressing through a series of steps to the formation of IMP, which is the common intermediate purine nucleotide. IMP can be converted either to AMP or to GMP. Once the purine nucleotides are formed, they are utilized for the synthesis of nucleic acids, adenosine triphosphate (ATP), cyclic AMP, cyclic GMP, and certain cofactors.

The various purine components are degraded to the purine nucleotide monophosphates. GMP is degraded via guanosine, guanine, and xanthine to uric acid. IMP is degraded through inosine, hypoxanthine, and xanthine to uric acid. AMP can be deaminated to IMP and further catabolized through inosine to uric acid, or it may be degraded to inosine by an alternate pathway with the intermediate formation of adenosine.

While the purine pathway is regulated in a complex manner, the intracellular concentration of 5-phosphoribosyl-1-pyrophosphate (PRPP) appears to be a major determinant of the rate of synthesis of uric acid in humans. Generally, when the concentration of PRPP in the cell is high, uric acid synthesis is elevated; when the concentration of PRPP is reduced, the synthesis of uric acid is also reduced.

Overproduction of uric acid in a small minority of adult gouty subjects occurs as either a primary or a secondary manifestation of an inborn error in metabolism. Hyperuricemia and gout occur as a primary manifestation of partial hypoxanthine-guanine phosphoribosyltransferase deficiency (reaction 2, Fig. 329-4) and of PRPP synthetase superactivity (reaction 3, Fig. 329-4). In the Lesch-Nyhan syndrome, the virtually complete deficiency of hypoxanthine-guanine phosphoribosyltransferase results in secondary hyperuricemia. These important inborn errors are discussed more fully below.

These two inborn errors of purine metabolism, hypoxanthine-guanine phosphoribosyltransferase deficiency and PRPP synthetase overactivity, account for less than 15 percent of all patients with primary hyperuricemia associated with an overproduction of uric acid. The cause of the overproduction in the majority of patients has not been defined.

There are numerous causes of secondary hyperuricemia associated with an increased production of uric acid. In some, the increased excretion of uric acid is related, as it is in primary gout, to an accelerated rate of purine biosynthesis de novo. Patients with glucose-

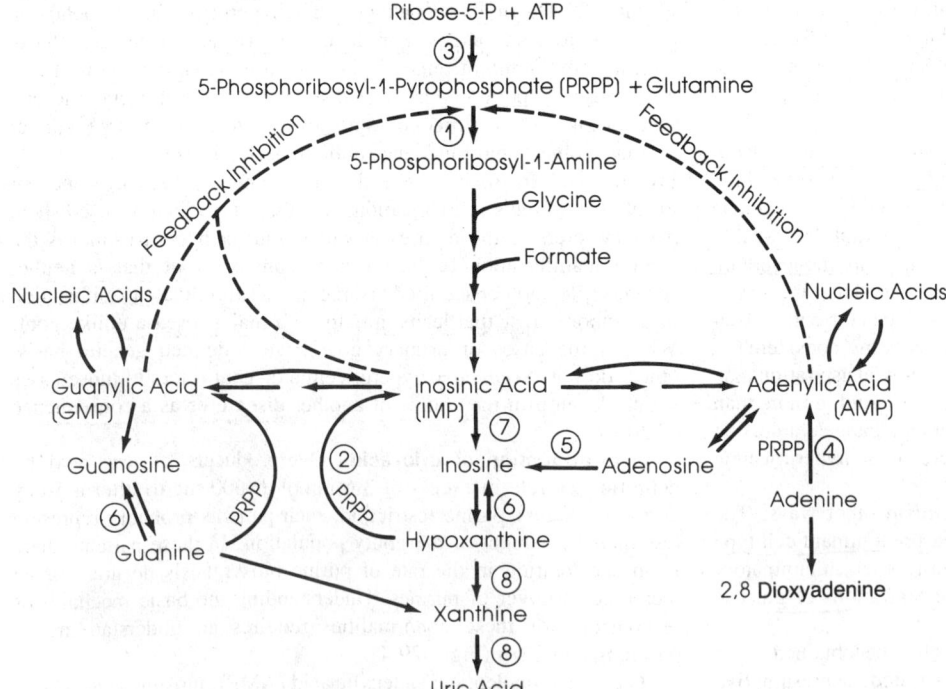

FIGURE 329-4 Outline of purine metabolism: (1) amidophosphoribosyltransferase; (2) hypoxanthine-guanine phosphoribosyltransferase; (3) PRPP synthetase; (4) adenine phosphoribosyltransferase; (5) adenosine deaminase; (6) purine nucleoside phosphorylase; (7) 5'-nucleotidase; (8) xanthine oxidase.

6-phosphatase deficiency (type I glycogen storage disease) uniformly exhibit an increased production of uric acid as well as an accelerated rate of purine biosynthesis de novo (see Chap. 332). Overproduction of uric acid in patients with this enzyme defect is multifactorial. An accelerated rate of de novo purine synthesis may be due in part to accelerated synthesis of PRPP. Additionally, accelerated degradation of purine nucleotides contributes to an increased rate of uric acid excretion. Both of these mechanisms are due to the deficiency of glucose as an energy source, and the production of uric acid can be decreased by the sustained correction of hypoglycemia in this disorder.

In the majority of patients with secondary hyperuricemia due to an overproduction of uric acid, the predominant abnormality appears to be an increased turnover of nucleic acids. A number of diseases, including the myeloproliferative and lymphoproliferative disorders, multiple myeloma, secondary polycythemia, pernicious anemia, certain hemoglobinopathies, thalassemia, other hemolytic anemias, infectious mononucleosis, and some carcinomas, may be associated with increased marrow activity or increased cell turnover in the marrow or at other sites and an associated increased turnover of nucleic acids. The increased turnover in nucleic acids leads in turn to hyperuricemia, hyperuricaciduria, and a compensatory increase in the rate of purine biosynthesis de novo.

Reduced excretion A large proportion of gouty subjects require a plasma urate value 60 to 120 μmol/L (1 to 2 mg/dL) higher than normal subjects to achieve a given rate of uric acid excretion (Fig. 329-5). This abnormality is most prominent in the gouty subject with a normal production of uric acid and is not present in most subjects with overproduction of uric acid.

The excretion of urate is dependent on glomerular filtration, tubular reabsorption, and tubular secretion. Uric acid appears to be completely filtered at the glomerulus and reabsorbed in the proximal tubule (i.e., presecretory reabsorption). Uric acid secretion then

occurs in a subsequent segment of the proximal tubule, and partial reabsorption takes place at a second reabsorptive site in the distal portion of the proximal tubule (i.e., postsecretory reabsorption). While some uric acid reabsorption may also occur in the ascending limb of the loop of Henle and in the collecting duct, these latter two sites are thought to be quantitatively less important. The nature of these latter sites and the magnitude of their contribution to uric acid transport is not known.

Theoretically, the altered renal excretion of uric acid exhibited by most patients with gout could be due to (1) reduced filtration of uric acid, (2) enhanced reabsorption, or (3) decreased secretion. No unequivocal data establish any one of these mechanisms as the basic defect, and it is likely that all three are operative within the gouty population.

Numerous secondary causes of hyperuricemia and gout can also be attributed to a decrease in the renal excretion of uric acid. A reduction in the glomerular filtration rate leads to a decrease in the filtered load of uric acid and thus to hyperuricemia; patients with renal disease are hyperuricemic on this basis. Other factors, such as decreased secretion of uric acid, have been postulated in patients with some types of renal disease (e.g., polycystic kidney disease and lead nephropathy). Gout is a rare complication of the secondary hyperuricemia due to renal disease.

Diuretic therapy is one of the most important causes of secondary hyperuricemia. Diuretic-induced volume depletion leads to enhanced tubular reabsorption of uric acid as well as decreased uric acid filtration. Decreased secretion of uric acid may also be a mechanism in diuretic-induced hyperuricemia. Other drugs lead to hyperuricemia by undefined renal mechanisms; these agents include low-dose aspirin, pyrazinamide, nicotinic acid, ethambutol, and ethanol.

Impaired renal excretion of uric acid is thought to be an important mechanism for the hyperuricemia associated with several disease states. Volume depletion may be important in patients with hyperuricemia associated with adrenal insufficiency and nephrogenic diabetes insipidus. In some situations hyperuricemia has been attributed to competitive inhibition of uric acid secretion by excess organic acids thought to be secreted by the same renal tubular mechanism responsible for uric acid secretion. Examples include starvation (ketosis and free fatty acids), alcoholic ketosis, diabetic ketoacidosis, maple syrup urine disease, and lactic acidosis of any cause. Hyperuricemia in conditions such as hyperparathyroidism, hypoparathyroidism, pseudohypoparathyroidism, and hypothyroidism may also have a renal basis, but the mechanism is unclear.

PATHOGENESIS OF ACUTE GOUTY ARTHRITIS The events leading to the initial crystallization of monosodium urate in a joint after an average of 30 years of asymptomatic hyperuricemia are not completely understood. Sustained hyperuricemia leads eventually to the development of microtophi in the synovial lining cells and perhaps to an accumulation in cartilage of monosodium urate on proteoglycans that have a high affinity for urate. By one of several mechanisms, probably including trauma with disruption of the microtophi and increased turnover of the cartilage proteoglycans, there is an episodic release of urate crystals into the synovial fluid. Other factors, such as a lower temperature in the joint space or an unequal reabsorption of water and urate from the synovial fluid, may accelerate urate precipitation.

A sufficient amount of crystals in the joint space triggers the acute attack by a process that appears to include (1) phagocytosis of the crystals by leukocytes with the rapid release of a chemotactic protein from the leukocytes, (2) activation of the kallikrein system, (3) activation of complement with the consequent formation of the chemotactic complement components, and (4) the ultimate urate-mediated disruption of lysosomes within the leukocytes, leading to destruction of white blood cells and release of lysosomal products into the synovial fluid. While progress in the understanding of acute gouty arthritis has occurred, questions about factors responsible for spontaneous resolution of the acute attack and the effect of colchicine remain to be answered.

FIGURE 329-5 Rate of uric acid excretion at various plasma urate levels in nongouty (solid symbols) and gouty (open symbols) subjects. Large symbols represent mean values; small symbols represent individual data of a few mean values selected to illustrate the degree of scatter within groups. Studies were conducted under basal conditions, after RNA feeding, and after infusions of lithium urate. (*From Wyngaarden. Reproduced by permission of Academic Press.*)

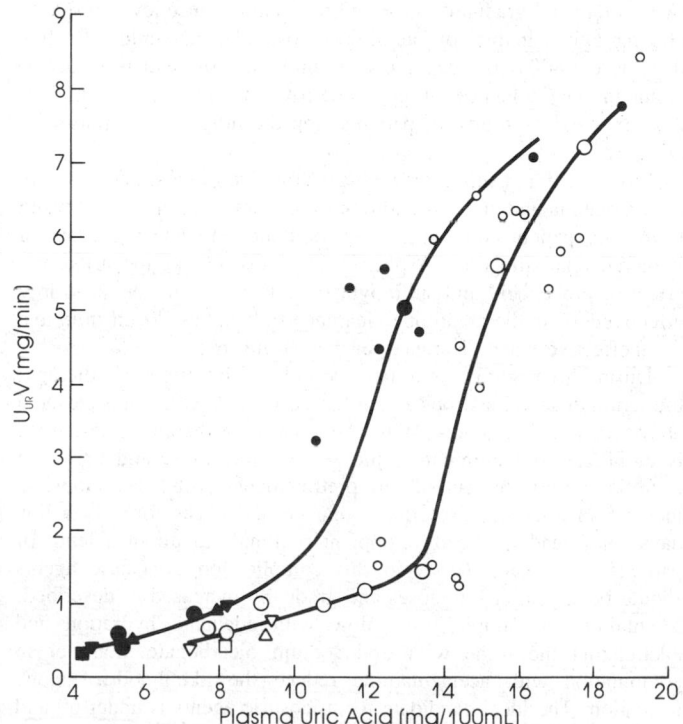

TREATMENT   The therapeutic aims in gout are (1) to terminate the acute attack as promptly and gently as possible; (2) to prevent recurrences of acute gouty arthritis; (3) to prevent or reverse complications of the disease resulting from deposition of monosodium urate crystals in joints, kidneys, and other sites; (4) to prevent or reverse associated features such as obesity, hypertriglyceridemia, or hypertension; and (5) to prevent formation of uric acid kidney stones.

Treatment of the acute gouty attack   Acute gouty arthritis is treated with an anti-inflammatory agent. Colchicine is the drug most frequently employed. Standard therapy involves administration of 0.5 mg each hour or 1.0 mg every 2 h by mouth until one of three things occurs: (1) the patient improves, (2) gastrointestinal side effects develop, or (3) a maximum of 6 mg is taken without relief. Colchicine is most effective if therapy is begun shortly after the onset of symptoms. Over 75 percent of patients with gout show major improvement in symptoms within the first 12 h of treatment. However, as many as 80 percent of patients are unable to tolerate an optimal dose because of gastrointestinal side effects, which may precede or coincide with clinical improvement. Orally administered colchicine results in peak plasma levels in approximately 2 h. Consequently, it has been suggested that 1.0 mg every 2 h is less likely to lead to the accumulation of toxic levels before the onset of therapeutic effect. However, since therapeutic benefit relates to colchicine levels within leukocytes rather than plasma levels, the efficacy of this regimen requires further evaluation.

Intravenous administration of colchicine eliminates gastrointestinal side effects and provides a more rapid response. Colchicine levels become high in leukocytes, remain constant for 24 h, and are detectable for over 10 days after a single intravenous infusion. As an initial dose 2 mg should be given intravenously, followed by two additional doses of 1 mg at 6-h intervals if needed. Special care must be taken in the intravenous administration of colchicine. The drug is irritative and can lead to severe pain and necrosis if allowed to extravasate to surrounding tissues. It is important to make certain that the intravenous route is secure and that the drug is diluted with 5 to 10 volumes of normal saline solution and infused over a period of no less than 5 min. Colchicine by either oral or parenteral route may cause bone marrow depression, alopecia, hepatocellular failure, mental depression, seizures, ascending paralysis, respiratory depression, and death. Toxic effects are more likely in patients with hepatic, bone marrow, or renal disease and in those subjects on maintenance colchicine. The dosage should be reduced for these individuals, and the drug should not be used in neutropenic patients.

Other anti-inflammatory agents, including indomethacin, phenylbutazone, naproxen, and fenoprofen, are also effective in the treatment of acute gouty arthritis. Indomethacin may be given at a dose of 75 mg orally, followed by 50 mg every 6 h and continued at that dose for 24 h after relief is obtained. The drug is then tapered to 50 mg every 8 h for three doses and then to 25 mg every 8 h for three doses. Side effects of indomethacin include gastrointestinal toxicity, sodium retention, and complaints referable to the central nervous system. While the incidence of side effects may be as high as 60 percent in patients taking the doses described above, the drug is generally better tolerated than colchicine and probably is the treatment of choice in the patient with a well-established diagnosis of acute gouty arthritis. To improve the therapeutic response and thus diminish morbidity of the disease, the patient may be instructed to begin therapy with an anti-inflammatory agent at the first twinge of an acute attack. Uricosuric drugs and allopurinol have no role in the treatment of the acute gouty attack.

Systemic or locally administered (i.e., intraarticular) glucocorticoids are useful in treating acute gout particularly when colchicine and nonsteroidal anti-inflammatory drugs are contraindicated or ineffective. When given systemically, moderate doses should be administered either by the oral or intravenous route for several days at most before the drug is rapidly tapered and discontinued. An isolated monarthritis or bursitis can be terminated within 24 or 36 h by the intraarticular instillation of a long-acting steroid preparation

(e.g., triamcinolone hexacetonide, 15 to 30 mg). This is particularly useful when standard drug regimens are not practical.

Prophylaxis   Once the acute episode has resolved, a number of measures can reduce the likelihood of recurrence: (1) the institution of prophylactic daily colchicine or indomethacin, (2) controlled weight reduction for the obese patient, (3) avoidance of known precipitating factors such as heavy alcohol consumption or a diet rich in purines, and (4) the institution of antihyperuricemic therapy.

The administration of small daily doses of colchicine is effective prophylaxis against further acute attacks. A program of 1 to 2 mg colchicine a day is successful in about three-fourths of patients with gout and fails completely in only about 5 percent. In addition, this program is safe and essentially free of side effects. However, unless serum urate is maintained at normal levels, the patient is spared only acute arthritis and may develop other manifestations of gout. Maintenance colchicine therapy is particularly helpful during the first year or two after institution of antihyperuricemic drugs.

Prevention or reversal of the deposition of monosodium urate in tissues   Antihyperuricemic agents are effective in reducing serum urate concentration and should be used in patients with (1) one or more attacks of acute gouty arthritis, (2) one or more tophi, and (3) uric acid nephrolithiasis. The aim of antihyperuricemic therapy is to maintain the serum urate below 415 μmol/L (7.0 mg/dL), the minimal concentration at which urate saturates the extracellular fluid. Reduction to these levels may be achieved by use of drugs that increase the renal excretion of uric acid or decrease uric acid production. Antihyperuricemic drugs generally do not have anti-inflammatory properties. Uricosuric agents reduce serum urate by enhancing the renal excretion. While a large number of drugs exhibit this property, the most effective agents available in the United States are probenecid and sulfinpyrazone. Probenecid is usually started in doses of 250 mg twice a day; it is increased over a period of several weeks to the dose necessary to achieve effective reversal of the hyperuricemia. A total dose of 1 g/d is appropriate for half of patients; the maximum dose should not exceed 3.0 g/d. Because the half-life is 6 to 12 h, it should be given in two to four evenly spaced doses per day. Hypersensitivity, skin rash, and gastrointestinal complaints are the major side effects. Although serious toxicity is rare, side effects may cause up to a third of the patients to discontinue probenecid.

Sulfinpyrazone is a metabolite of phenylbutazone with no anti-inflammatory activity. The drug is usually started at a dose of 50 mg twice a day and gradually increased to a maintenance level of 300 to 400 mg/d given in three or four divided doses. The maximum effective daily dose is 800 mg. Side effects are similar to those with probenecid, although the incidence of bone marrow toxicity may be higher. Approximately a fourth of patients stop the drug for one reason or another.

Probenecid and sulfinpyrazone are effective in most patients with hyperuricemia and gout. In addition to intolerance, failures can result from poor patient compliance, concomitant salicylate ingestion, or impaired renal function. Aspirin at any dose blocks the uricosuric effect of probenecid and sulfinpyrazone. These agents begin to lose effectiveness as the creatinine clearance falls below 80 mL/min and are ineffective when clearance reaches 30 mL/min.

During the negative urate balance induced by uricosuric therapy, the serum urate value drops and urinary uric acid excretion is elevated above pretreatment levels. With continuation of therapy excess urate is mobilized and eliminated, the serum urate falls, and uric acid excretion returns essentially to pretreatment levels. The transient increase in uric acid excretion, which usually lasts for only a few days, may lead to the development of renal calculi in a tenth of patients so treated. To avoid this complication uricosuric agents should be started at low doses and gradually increased as described. Maintaining an ample urine flow with adequate hydration and alkalinizing the urine with oral sodium bicarbonate alone or in combination with acetazolamide reduce the likelihood of stone formation. The ideal candidate for uricosuric agents is under 60 and has normal renal function, uric acid excretion of less than 700 mg/d on a general diet, and no history of renal stones.

Hyperuricemia may also be controlled by allopurinol, a drug that decreases uric acid synthesis. Allopurinol inhibits xanthine oxidase (reaction 8, Fig. 329-4), the enzyme that catalyzes the oxidation of hypoxanthine to xanthine and xanthine to uric acid. While allopurinol has a half-life in vivo of only 2 to 3 h, it is metabolized largely to oxipurinol, which also is an effective inhibitor of xanthine oxidase and has a half-life ranging from 18 to 30 h. In most patients 300 mg/d is an effective antihyperuricemic dose. Because of the long half-life of the major metabolite the drug may be administered once a day. Since oxipurinol is largely excreted in the urine, its half-life is prolonged in patients with renal insufficiency. The dose of allopurinol should, therefore, be reduced by half in patients with significant renal dysfunction.

Significant side effects of allopurinol include gastrointestinal distress, skin rashes, fever, toxic epidermal necrolysis, alopecia, bone marrow suppression, hepatitis, jaundice, and vasculitis. The overall incidence of side effects is about 20 percent; they are more common in the presence of renal insufficiency. In only 5 percent of patients the side effects are sufficient to force discontinuation of the drug. Important drug-drug interactions involving allopurinol include prolongation of the half-lives of mercaptopurine and azathioprine and enhancement of the toxicity of cyclophosphamide.

Specific indications for choosing allopurinol over a uricosuric drug include (1) an increased urinary uric acid excretion (greater than 700 mg/d on a general diet), (2) impairment of renal function with a creatinine clearance less than 80 mL/min, (3) tophaceous gout regardless of renal function, (4) uric acid nephrolithiasis, and (5) gout not controlled by uricosuric agents because of ineffectiveness or intolerance. Allopurinol and a uricosuric drug may be used simultaneously in the rare patient who cannot be controlled by a single medication. Such combination therapy requires no modification in the dosage of either agent and usually results in further lowering of the serum urate concentration.

Acute gouty arthritis may occur whenever there is a rapid and substantial change in the serum urate concentration. Thus, the initiation of antihyperuricemic therapy with any agent may precipitate acute gouty arthritis. In addition, recurrent attacks may occur for a year or longer when large tophaceous deposits are present, even if hyperuricemia is controlled. For these reasons, it is prudent to begin prophylactic therapy with colchicine prior to initiation of antihyperuricemic drugs and to continue it until the serum urate is controlled for at least a year or until all tophi have resolved. Patients should be warned of the possibility of flare-up during the early phase of therapy. While it is not necessary in most gouty patients, strict dietary purine restriction should be instituted in patients with severe tophaceous gout and/or renal failure.

Prevention and treatment of acute uric acid nephropathy Immediate and vigorous therapy is essential for acute uric acid nephropathy. The first step is to increase urine flow by vigorous hydration coupled with administration of a potent diuretic such as furosemide. The urine should be alkalinized to achieve conversion of uric acid to the more soluble monosodium urate. Alkalinization can be accomplished by the administration of sodium bicarbonate alone or in combination with acetazolamide. Allopurinol should also be administered to reduce uric acid formation. The initial dose in this setting should be 8 mg/kg body weight per day given as a single daily dose. The dose should be decreased after 3 or 4 days to 100 to 200 mg/d if renal insufficiency persists. Treatment for uric acid kidney stones is similar to that for acute uric acid nephropathy. In most cases allopurinol combined only with high fluid intake is effective.

WORKUP OF THE HYPERURICEMIC PATIENT Evaluation of the patient with hyperuricemia is directed toward (1) defining the cause of the hyperuricemia (which may disclose an important disease other than gout), (2) assessing the presence and extent of damage to tissues and organs, and (3) identifying associated abnormalities. From a practical standpoint these inquiries are pursued simultaneously,

since decisions about the significance of hyperuricemia and about therapy depend on the answers to all of these.

The most important single test in the hyperuricemic patient is analysis of the urine for uric acid. If a history of stone disease is present, a flat plate of the abdomen and intravenous pyelogram may be indicated. If a renal stone is recovered, analysis for uric acid and other constituents is useful. If joint disease is present, synovial fluid analysis and x-rays of the involved joints are helpful. If there is a history of exposure to lead, measurement of urinary lead excretion after an infusion of calcium edetate may be useful in documenting the presence of gout due to lead exposure. In cases where the patient appears to be an overproducer, measurement of erythrocyte hypoxanthine-guanine phosphoribosyltransferase and PRPP synthetase levels may be indicated.

Management of asymptomatic hyperuricemia There is considerable controversy about the indications for therapy of the patient with asymptomatic hyperuricemia. Generally, treatment should be withheld unless the patient (1) becomes symptomatic; (2) has a strong family history for gout, nephrolithiasis, or renal failure; or (3) excretes large quantities of uric acid (greater than 6.5 mmol/d (1100 mg/d).

OTHER DISORDERS OF PURINE METABOLISM ASSOCIATED WITH HYPERURICEMIA AND GOUT

HYPOXANTHINE-GUANINE PHOSPHORIBOSYLTRANSFERASE DEFICIENCY STATES Hypoxanthine-guanine phosphoribosyltransferase catalyzes the conversion of hypoxanthine to inosinic acid and guanine to guanosinic acid (reaction 2, Fig. 329-4). PRPP serves as the phosphoribosyl donor. The deficiency of hypoxanthine-guanine phosphoribosyltransferase leads to decreased consumption of PRPP, which accumulates to higher than normal levels. The excess PRPP accelerates de novo purine biosynthesis and consequently increases uric acid production.

The Lesch-Nyhan syndrome is an X-linked disorder. The characteristic biochemical abnormality is a profound deficiency of the enzyme hypoxanthine-guanine phosphoribosyltransferase (reaction 2, Fig. 329-4). Affected patients have hyperuricemia and a profound overproduction of uric acid. In addition, they have a bizarre neurologic disorder characterized by self-mutilation, choreoathetosis, spasticity, and retardation of growth and mental function. The incidence is estimated at 1:100,000 births.

From 0.5 to 1.0 percent of adult gouty subjects with overproduction of uric acid have a partial deficiency of hypoxanthine-guanine phosphoribosyltransferase. These patients typically have the onset of gouty arthritis at a young age (15 to 30 years), a high incidence of uric acid stones (75 percent), and the occasional occurrence of mild neurologic dysfunction characterized by dysarthria, hyperreflexia, incoordination, and/or mental retardation. This disease is inherited as an X-linked trait so that men are affected through carrier females.

The enzyme whose deficiency results in these disorders, hypoxanthine-guanine phosphoribosyltransferase, is of considerable interest in genetics. With the possible exception of the globin gene family, the hypoxanthine-guanine phosphoribosyltransferase locus is the single most studied human gene.

Human hypoxanthine-guanine phosphoribosyltransferase has been purified to homogeneity, and its amino acid sequence has been determined. The normal enzyme has a native subunit molecular weight of 24,470 and consists of 217 amino acid residues. The normal enzyme is a tetramer with four identical subunits. The DNA sequence complementary to messenger RNA encoding hypoxanthine-guanine phosphoribosyltransferase has been cloned and sequenced as well. As a molecular probe, this cDNA sequence has been used to identify carrier status in a female at risk for whom conventional carrier detection techniques were not successful. The mutations that cause hypoxanthine-guanine phosphoribosyltransferase deficiency are heterogeneous. Protein sequencing techniques have been used to identify the amino acid substitutions in four variant forms of hypoxanthine-

TABLE 329-2 Structural and functional abnormalities in mutant forms of hypoxanthine-guanine phosphoribosyltransferase (HPRT)

| | | Mutation | | Functional abnormalities | | | |
| | | | | Intracellular concentration, % normal | Maximal velocity | Michaelis constants | |
Mutant enzyme	Clinical presentation	Nucleotide substitution	Amino acid substitution			Hypoxanthine	PRPP
HPRT$_{Detroit}$	Lesch-Nyhan syndrome	T$_{122}$→C	Leu$_{41}$→Pro	ND	NM	NM	NM
HPRT$_{Toronto}$	Gout	ND	Arg$_{51}$→Gly	52	Normal	Normal	Normal
HPRT$_{New\ Haven}$	Lesch-Nyhan syndrome	G$_{209}$→A	Gly$_{70}$→Glu	50	NM	NM	NM
HPRT$_{Yale}$	Lesch-Nyhan syndrome	G$_{211}$→C	Gly$_{71}$→Arg	92	NM	NM	NM
HPRT$_{Flint}$	Lesch-Nyhan syndrome	C$_{222}$→A	Phe$_{74}$→Leu	<0.3	NM	NM	NM
HPRT$_{Arlington}$	Gout	A$_{239}$→T	Asp$_{80}$→Val	ND	NM	NM	NM
HPRT$_{Munich}$	Gout	C$_{397}$→A	Ser$_{104}$→Arg	79	↓	↑	Normal
HPRT$_{London}$	Gout	C$_{329}$→T	Ser$_{110}$→Leu	35–52	Normal	↑	Normal
HPRT$_{Midland}$	Lesch-Nyhan syndrome	T$_{389}$→A	Val$_{130}$→Asp	<0.3	NM	NM	NM
HPRT$_{Ann\ Arbor}$	Nephrolithiasis	T$_{396}$→G	Ile$_{132}$→Met	11	Normal	Normal	Normal
HPRT$_{Milwaukee}$	Gout	A$_{481}$→T	Ala$_{161}$→Ser	3	NM	NM	NM
HPRT$_{Kinston}$	Lesch-Nyhan syndrome	ND	Asp$_{194}$→Asn	72	Normal	↑	↑
HPRT$_{New\ Britain}$	Lesch-Nyhan syndrome	T$_{595}$→G	Phe$_{199}$→Val	<0.3	NM	NM	NM
HPRT$_{Ashville}$	Gout	A$_{602}$→G	Asp$_{201}$→Gly	4	NM	NM	NM

NOTES: PRPP denotes 5-phosphoribosyl-1-pyrophosphate; Ala, alanine; Arg, arginine; Asp, aspartic acid; Asn, asparagine; Glu, glutamic acid; Gly, glycine; Ile, isoleucine; Leu, leucine; Met, methionine; Phe, phenylalanine; Pro, proline; Ser, serine; Val, valine; ND, not determined; NM, not measured because of diminished catalytic activity; →, is replaced by; ↑, increased; ↓, decreased.
SOURCE: Wilson et al. and Davidson et al.

guanine phosphoribosyltransferase derived from deficient subjects: HPRT$_{Toronto}$, HPRT$_{Munich}$, HPRT$_{London}$, and HPRT$_{Kinston}$ (Table 329-2). More recently, recombinant techniques have been used to identify the actual mutation responsible for enzymic deficiency in more subjects. In each of the 14 examples in Table 329-2 a single amino acid substitution leads to either a catalytically incompetent protein or decreased steady-state concentration of hypoxanthine-guanine phosphoribosyltransferase as a result of diminished synthesis or accelerated degradation of the mutant protein. Although point mutations are the most common mechanism leading to hypoxanthine-guanine phosphoribosyltransferase deficiency, gene rearrangement, partial deletions, and insertions have also been described.

Human hypoxanthine-guanine phosphoribosyltransferase gene sequences have been transferred to mice via retroviral vector–infected bone marrow transplantation and by direct infection of brain tissue by recombinant herpes simplex virus type 1 vectors. A transgenic strain of mice that expresses the human enzyme has also been established. More recently, two strains of hypoxanthine-guanine phosphoribosyltransferase–deficient mice have been described. Neither strain displays the altered phenotype, and, therefore, these animals do not constitute an authentic model for the Lesch-Nyhan syndrome.

The associated biochemical abnormalities leading to the devastating neurologic consequences of the Lesch-Nyhan syndrome are incompletely understood. Evidence obtained from postmortem examination of brains from subjects with the Lesch-Nyhan syndrome indicates a specific defect in the central dopaminergic pathways, particularly those found in the basal ganglia and nucleus accumbens. Corroborating in vivo evidence is emerging from positron emission tomography studies of subjects deficient in hypoxanthine-guanine phosphoribosyltransferase. A defect in the metabolism of 2′-fluorodeoxyglucose in the caudate nuclei is present in the majority of subjects studied with this technique. The relationships between dopaminergic nervous system abnormalities and the aberrant metabolism of purines remain unknown.

The hyperuricemia resulting from partial or complete deficiency of hypoxanthine-guanine phosphoribosyltransferase can be successfully controlled with allopurinol, an inhibitor of xanthine oxidase. A few patients have developed xanthine stones with such therapy, but in the majority the renal stones and gout are effectively treated. No specific therapy exists for the neurologic abnormalities in the Lesch-Nyhan syndrome.

PRPP SYNTHETASE VARIANTS Several families are described in which there is increased activity of the enzyme PRPP synthetase (reaction 3, Fig. 329-4). The mutant enzymes, of which three different types are recognized, all exhibit increased activity, resulting in increased intracellular concentrations of PRPP, accelerated purine biosynthesis, and elevated excretion of uric acid. The inheritance pattern in this disease is also X-linked. These patients, like those with partial hypoxanthine-guanine phosphoribosyltransferase deficiency, generally develop gout in the second or third decade and have a high incidence of uric acid stones. Several kindred have been described in which nerve deafness is associated with PRPP synthetase overactivity groups.

OTHER DISORDERS OF PURINE METABOLISM Adenine phosphoribosyltransferase deficiency Adenine phosphoribosyltransferase catalyzes the conversion of adenine to AMP (reaction 4, Fig. 329-4). The first subjects described with a deficiency of this enzyme were heterozygous for deficiency of the enzyme and had no associated disease. It subsequently became apparent that heterozygosity for this deficiency is common, perhaps as frequent as 1:100. A homozygous deficiency of this enzyme has now been described in 11 patients with a history of renal stones composed of 2,8-dioxyadenine. Because of chemical similarity, 2,8-dioxyadenine may be confused with uric acid, and in each of these patients an incorrect diagnosis of uric acid nephrolithiasis was made initially.

Adenosine deaminase deficiency and purine nucleoside phosphorylase deficiency See Chap. 263.

Xanthine oxidase deficiency Xanthine oxidase catalyzes the oxidation of hypoxanthine to xanthine, xanthine to uric acid, and adenine to 2,8-dioxyadenine (reaction 8, Fig. 329-4). Xanthinuria, the first inborn error of purine metabolism to be defined at the enzyme level, is due to a deficiency of xanthine oxidase. As a result, affected patients with xanthinuria have hypouricemia and hypouricaciduria as well as an increased urinary excretion of the oxypurines, hypoxanthine, and xanthine. Half are asymptomatic, and a third have urinary xanthine stones. Several patients have been noted to have a myopathy. Three patients have been reported with polyarthritis, which may represent a crystal-induced synovitis. Precipitation of xanthine is thought to be the important factor in the development of each of these clinical manifestations.

Four patients have been described with combined congenital deficiencies of xanthine oxidase and sulfate oxidase. The clinical presentation is dominated by the serious neurologic abnormalities in the neonatal period seen in isolated sulfate oxidase deficiency. Although deficiency of a molybdate cofactor required by both enzymes has been postulated as the primary abnormality, therapy with ammonium molybdate has little effect on the neurologic manifestation. An acquired disorder mimicking combined xanthine oxidase and sulfate oxidase deficiency has been described in a patient on chronic total parenteral nutrition. Therapy with oral ammonium molybdate successfully restored enzymatic function and resulted in clinical resolution.

Myoadenylate deaminase deficiency Myoadenylate deaminase is an isozyme of adenylate deaminase found only in skeletal muscle. This enzyme catalyzes the conversion of adenylate (AMP) to inosinic acid (IMP). This reaction is a component of the purine nucleotide cycle and is probably important in the maintenance of energy production and utilization in skeletal muscle.

Deficiency of this enzyme is limited to skeletal muscle. The majority of deficient patients demonstrate exercise-induced myalgias, muscle cramps, and fatigue. Approximately one-third report weakness even in the absence of exercise. A few patients are apparently asymptomatic.

The disorder typically presents in childhood or adolescence. The clinical manifestations are those of a metabolic myopathy. Creatine kinase is elevated in less than half of subjects. Electromyograms and routine histology of muscle biopsies show nonspecific abnormalities. Presumptive evidence of adenylate deaminase deficiency can be obtained from performance of an ischemic forearm exercise test. Ammonia production is reduced in deficient patients since AMP deamination is blocked. The diagnosis must be confirmed by actual assay of AMP deaminase activity in a skeletal muscle biopsy since reduced ammonia production with exercise occurs in other myopathies. The disorder is slowly progressive, leading to mild disability in most cases. No specific therapy has been shown to be effective.

Adenylosuccinase deficiency Subjects deficient in adenylosuccinase are mentally retarded and often autistic. Additional neurologic abnormalities include seizures, psychomotor retardation, and other movement disorders. Urinary excretion of succinylamino-imidazole carboxamide riboside and succinyladenosine is elevated. Diagnosis depends upon demonstration of partial or complete absence of enzyme activity in liver, kidney, or skeletal muscle. Lymphocytes and fibroblasts show a partial deficiency. The prognosis is not known, and no specific therapy exists.

REFERENCES

DAVIDSON BL et al: The molecular basis of HPRT deficiency in ten subjects determined by direct sequencing of amplified transcripts. J Clin Invest, 84:342, 1989

KELLEY WN: Crystal-induced arthropathies, in *The Clinics in Rheumatic Diseases*. Philadelphia, Saunders, 1977, vol 3, pp 1–171

———, Fox IH: Antihyperuricemic drugs, in *Textbook of Rheumatology*, 3d ed, WN Kelley et al (eds). Philadelphia, Saunders, 1989, pp 884–899

——— et al: Gout and related disorders of purine metabolism, in *Textbook of Rheumatology*, 3d ed, WN Kelley et al (eds). Philadelphia, Saunders, 1989, pp 1395–1435

——— et al: Hypoxanthine-guanine phosphoribosyltransferase deficiency in gout. Ann Intern Med, 70:155, 1969

PALELLA TD, Fox IH: Hyperuricemia and gout, in *The Metabolic Basis of Inherited Disease*, 6th ed, CR Scriver et al (eds). New York, McGraw-Hill, 1989, chap 37

TALBOTT JH, YU TF: *Gout and Uric Acid Metabolism*. New York, Grune & Stratton, 1976

WILSON JM et al: Hypoxanthine-guanine phosphoribosyltransferase deficiency: The molecular basis of the clinical syndromes. N Engl J Med 309:900, 1983

——— et al: A molecular survey of hypoxanthine-guanine phosphoribosyltransferase deficiency in man. J Clin Invest 77:188, 1986

WYNGAARDEN JB: Gout, in *Advances in Metabolic Disorders*, R Levine and R Luft (eds). New York, Academic, 1965, vol 2, pp 2–78

———, KELLEY WN: *Gout and Hyperuricemia*. New York, Grune & Stratton, 1976

330 WILSON'S DISEASE

I. HERBERT SCHEINBERG

Wilson's disease is an autosomal recessive abnormality in the hepatic excretion of copper that results in toxic accumulations of the metal in liver, brain, and other organs. The disease occurs in populations of every ethnic and geographic origin and has a worldwide prevalence of about 1 in 30,000. Deficiency of the plasma copper protein ceruloplasmin is a characteristic feature.

NATURAL HISTORY Normal babies have low levels of plasma ceruloplasmin and high concentrations of hepatic copper. During the first year of life ceruloplasmin values rise and hepatic copper concentrations fall to normal adult levels. In contrast, serum ceruloplasmin changes very little in homozygotes for the Wilson's disease gene, and the concentration of hepatic copper remains elevated. However, clinical manifestations of copper excess are extremely rare before age 6, and about half of untreated patients remain asymptomatic through adolescence.

Wilson's disease presents with hepatic involvement in about half of patients. The toxic effects of copper in the liver may be manifest in four ways: as acute hepatitis, fulminant hepatitis, chronic active hepatitis, or cirrhosis. Acute hepatitis is often mistaken for viral hepatitis or infectious mononucleosis and is usually self-limited. Fulminant hepatitis, generally lethal, is characterized by progressive jaundice, malaise, ascites, hypoalbuminemia, and elevated plasma levels of liver enzymes. Sufficient copper may be released from necrosing hepatocytes to cause a hemolytic anemia. Parenchymal liver disease may persist following acute hepatitis or develop insidiously without prior acute disease into a clinical and histologic picture indistinguishable from chronic active hepatitis and always accompanied by cirrhosis. Finally, decades may elapse with no sign or symptom of liver disease but with the insidious development of cirrhosis. In all patients the past history of an episode of hepatitis can be overlooked unless they are questioned carefully.

In other patients the initial manifestations are extrahepatic. Neurologic or psychiatric disturbances are generally the first clinical signs in most of this group and are always accompanied by Kayser-Fleischer rings (Fig. A4-16). These green or golden deposits of copper in Descemet's membrane of the cornea do not interfere with vision but indicate that hepatic copper has been released and has caused brain damage. Rarely Kayser-Fleischer rings may be accompanied by sunflower cataracts. If a patient with frank neurologic or psychiatric disease does not have Kayser-Fleischer rings when examined by a trained observer using a slit lamp, the diagnosis of Wilson's disease can be excluded.

The primary neurologic manifestations are those of a movement disorder, particularly resting and intention tremors. Spasticity, rigidity, chorea, drooling, dysphagia, and dysarthria are common. Babinski responses and absent abdominal reflexes are occasionally noted; sensory changes, save for headache, never occur. Psychiatric disturbances, primarily due to the toxic effects of copper on the brain, but in some degree reactions to a life-threatening disease, are present in most patients with symptomatic disease. Syndromes indistinguishable from schizophrenia, manic-depressive psychoses, and classic neuroses may occur, and some bizarre behavioral disturbances defy classification. Improvement in the psychiatric state can occur with pharmacologic reduction of the copper excess, but psychotherapy is often also required.

In occasional patients the clinical onset reflects neither a hepatic nor a central nervous system disturbance. For example, primary or secondary amenorrhea may be the first evidence of disease in some young women; in others, repeated spontaneous abortions may be due to excess free copper in intrauterine secretions. Routine ophthalmo-

TABLE 330-1   Summary of analytic data in patients with Wilson's disease, heterozygous carriers, and control subjects

Group	Serum ceruloplasmin		Hepatic copper concentration	
	No. of patients	Mean ± SD, mg/L	No. of patients	Mean ± SD, μg/g dry weight
Wilson's disease:				
Asymptomatic	31	36 ± 53	36	983.5 ± 368
Symptomatic	84	59 ± 71	33	588.3 ± 304
Heterozygous carriers	95*	284 ± 85	14	117.0 ± 51
Normal subjects	180	307 ± 35	16	31.5 ± 6.8

* 71 parents of patients with Wilson's disease and 24 children, each of whom had one parent with Wilson's disease.
SOURCE: Sternlieb and Scheinberg, 1968.

logic examination in asymptomatic patients occasionally reveals Kayser-Fleischer rings, leading to the diagnosis.

PATHOGENESIS   The metabolic defect in Wilson's disease is an inability to maintain a near-zero balance of copper. Excess copper, small amounts of which are essential to life, accumulates possibly because hepatic lysosomes lack the normal mechanism to excrete into bile the copper that has been catabolically cleaved from ceruloplasmin. This may cause deficiency of ceruloplasmin since a stoichiometric excess of copper in vitro inhibits the formation of ceruloplasmin from apoceruloplasmin and copper. The capacity of hepatocytes to store copper is eventually exceeded, and release into blood and uptake in extrahepatic sites occurs accompanied by a decrease in the hepatic copper concentration (Table 330-1).

Under normal circumstances essentially all tissue copper is present as the prosthetic element of copper proteins including cytochrome oxidase, tyrosinase, superoxide dismutase, and ceruloplasmin. There is normally little or no free (non-protein-bound) copper. In Wilson's disease more copper is present than can be bound by specific copper proteins; such copper is as toxic as excess iron, zinc, mercury, or lead. Toxicity of these cations is probably effected in large degree by pathologic combinations with proteins that ordinarily do not contain metal.

The pathologic consequences of the accumulated copper occur first in the liver. Abnormal fat and glycogen deposits are the earliest findings by light microscopy (Fig. 330-1). With electron microscopy mitochondrial abnormalities are observed early and appear to be specific for Wilson's disease (Fig. 330-2). Later, necrosis, inflammation, fibrosis, bile duct proliferation, and cirrhosis occur. Abnormalities in liver chemistries may be seen in any of these stages.

Death can occur from the effects of copper toxicosis in the central nervous system. In the brain the excess copper is distributed ubiquitously. Necrosis of neurons with cavitation may be preceded by the appearance of Opalski and Alzheimer type II cells; however, neither is specific for Wilson's disease.

Increased copper in the kidney produces little if any structural change and commonly does not alter renal function. Hematuria, proteinuria, the Fanconi syndrome, and renal tubular acidosis, though commonly seen in untreated patients, almost never lead to clinical renal disease. Pathologic effects in other organs and tissues are minor.

DIAGNOSIS   The diagnosis is easy—*provided it is suspected.* Wilson's disease should be considered in any patient under the age of 40 with an unexplained disorder of the central nervous system, signs or symptoms of chronic active hepatitis, unexplained persistent elevations of serum transaminase, hemolytic anemia in the presence of hepatitis, unexplained cirrhosis, or in any patient who has a blood relative with Wilson's disease.

The diagnosis is confirmed in suspected cases by the demonstration either of (1) a serum concentration of ceruloplasmin less than 200 mg/L (20 mg/dL) and Kayser-Fleischer rings; or (2) a serum ceruloplasmin less than 200 mg/L (20 mg/dL) and a concentration of copper in a liver biopsy sample greater than 250 μg per gram of dry weight. Most symptomatic patients also excrete more than 100 μg copper per day in urine and exhibit histologic abnormalities on liver biopsy.

About 5 percent of patients have a serum concentration of ceruloplasmin greater than 200 mg/L (20 mg/dL), and some patients with other hepatic disorders, chiefly primary biliary cirrhosis, have elevated hepatic copper levels and, rarely, Kayser-Fleischer rings. In either circumstance measurement of the ability to incorporate radioactive copper into ceruloplasmin is useful as a discriminating test. Even in the presence of a normal concentration of ceruloplasmin, patients with Wilson's disease incorporate little or no isotope into the protein, while patients with other liver disorders and elevated hepatic copper incorporate the isotope normally.

TREATMENT   Treatment consists of removing and detoxifying the deposits of copper as rapidly as possible and should be instituted once the diagnosis is secure whether the patient is ill or asymptomatic. The drug of choice is penicillamine. It is administered orally in an initial dose of 1 g daily, usually in divided doses 30 min before meals and at bedtime. Since penicillamine has an antipyridoxine effect in animals, 25 mg/d of vitamin B_6 is also given. Effectiveness of therapy should be assayed chemically and clinically. Initially, the

FIGURE 330-1   Fatty changes, glycogen deposits, and cellular infiltrates in a hematoxylin and eosin–stained section of liver from an asymptomatic boy with Wilson's disease.

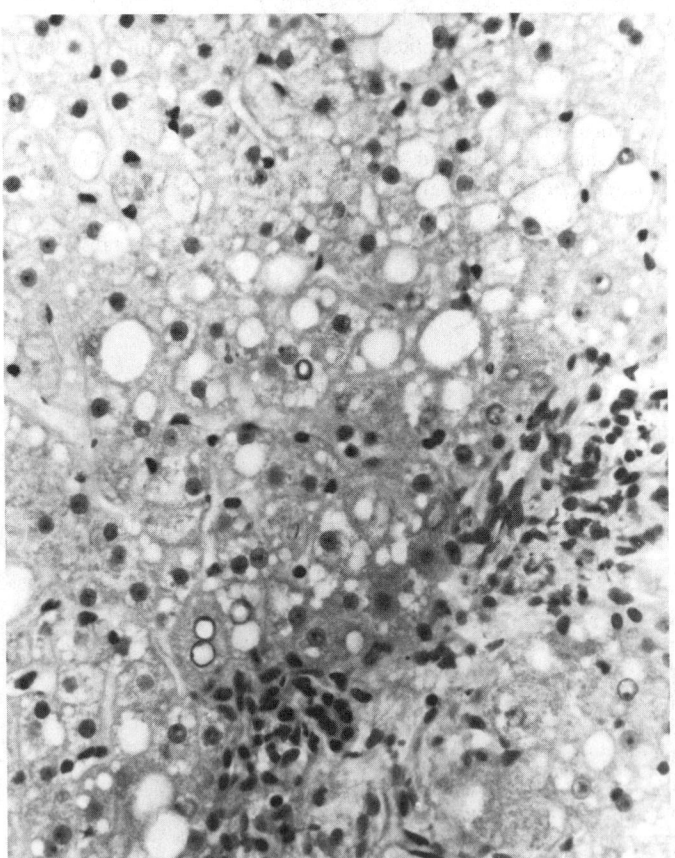

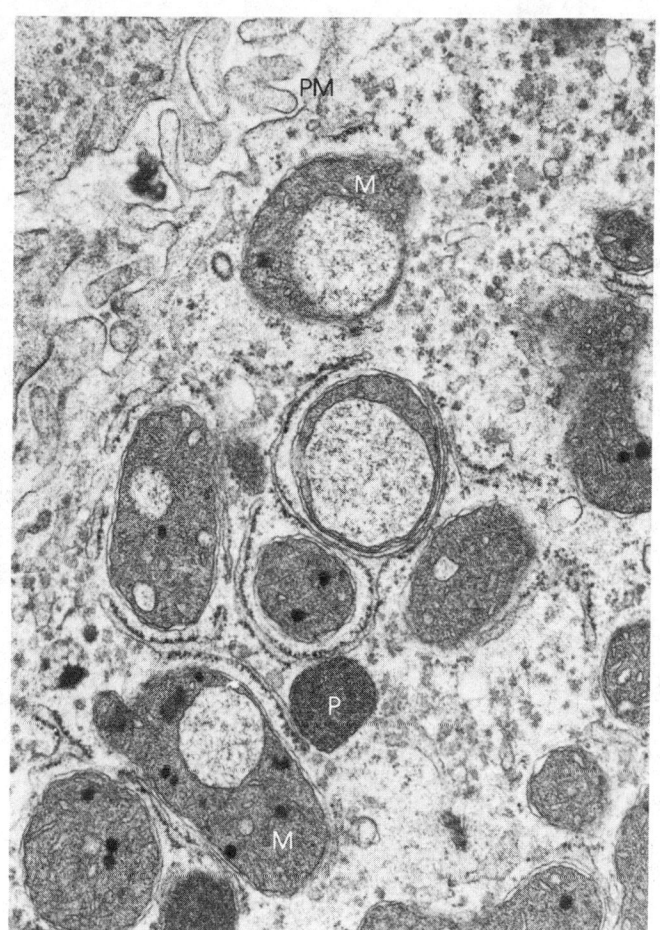

FIGURE 330-2 Electron micrograph of a liver biopsy sample from a 6-year-old asymptomatic boy. There are prominent vacuoles, containing granular material, in mitochondria (M). P, peroxisome; PM, plasma membrane.

24-h urinary excretion of copper should increase fivefold or more over the pretreatment level, and 1 to 3 mg copper per day may be excreted during the first months of therapy.

White blood cell and platelet counts, urinalysis, and body temperature should be monitored several times weekly for the first month of therapy and at intervals thereafter. Sensitivity to penicillamine usually appears within the first 14 days of treatment and may cause rash, fever, leukopenia, thrombocytopenia, lymphadenopathy, or proteinuria. Discontinuation of treatment is required if sensitivity develops. Therapy can often be resumed if the drug is reinstituted in small and gradually increasing dosage, although reactions are less likely to recur if 20 mg of prednisone is given daily for the first 2 weeks of penicillamine treatment and subsequently gradually discontinued. Reactions requiring a desensitizing regimen may recur several times before penicillamine can be administered without a steroid.

Lifelong and continual treatment is required. Inadequate treatment or interruption of therapy causes relapse that may be irreversible. Thus, of 11 patients who voluntarily discontinued penicillamine, after years of successful treatment, 8 died after an average survival of 2.6 years of noncompliance. Reinstitution of penicillamine after temporary interruption of therapy may be accompanied by the appearance or reappearance of sensitivity reactions. At any time—even after years of uneventful administration—granulocytopenia (or agranulocytosis), thrombocytopenia, the nephrotic syndrome, Goodpasture's syndrome, systemic lupus erythematosus, severe arthralgias, or myasthenia gravis may supervene. Toxicity is sometimes dose-related, and reduction of the dose to a level that is therapeutically effective but nontoxic may be possible. Continued low dosage of glucocorticoids may control penicillamine-associated lupus or arthralgias. After temporary interruption of the drug in patients with the nephrotic syndrome, it is sometimes possible to reinstitute therapy without recurrence of proteinuria. However, although irreversible intolerance to penicillamine is rare, the toxicity may be such that the drug must be withdrawn permanently and replaced by trientine, an orphan drug approved by the Food and Drug Administration in 1985.

After therapy with penicillamine has been successfully instituted, the patient should be seen indefinitely at 1- to 3-month intervals to detect drug toxicity and to manage the disease. Physical examination, including relevant neurologic assessment and inspection of the corneas with a slit lamp, and the patient's own evaluation provide the best indicators of the efficacy of treatment. Serial determinations of serum transaminase levels, albumin, and bilirubin are useful in following the course of liver function. Lack of clinical improvement or worsening of the disease may be due to irreversible damage present before therapy was begun, poor compliance, or inadequate dosage of penicillamine. Quantitative determinations of urinary copper excretion and of free copper in serum (total serum copper minus ceruloplasmin-bound copper) can help determine which is the case. After treatment for long periods, the level of urinary copper should be lower than at the onset of therapy, and rarely exceeds 1.5 mg/d. Even more helpful, the concentration of free serum copper is generally less than 2 μmol/L (10 μg/dL) in the adequately treated patient. After a patient has remained asymptomatic with no laboratory evidence of liver dysfunction for a year and in patients with minimal residual disease that has not changed, the dose of penicillamine may be reduced to 0.75 g/d.

Treatment of more than 100 asymptomatic patients with a confirmed diagnosis has established that continued administration of penicillamine can prevent virtually every manifestation of this disease.

REFERENCES

SCHEINBERG IH, STERNLIEB I: Wilson's disease, in *Major Problems in Internal Medicine.* Philadelphia, Saunders, 1984

—— et al: The use of trientine in preventing the effects of interrupting penicillamine therapy in Wilson's disease. N Engl J Med 317:209, 1987

—— et al: Penicillamine may detoxify copper in Wilson's disease. Lancet 2:95, 1987

STERNLIEB I: Evolution of the hepatic lesion in Wilson's disease (hepatolenticular degeneration), in *Progress in Liver Diseases*, H Popper et al (eds). New York, Grune & Stratton, 1972, vol IV, pp 511–526

——, SCHEINBERG IH: Prevention of Wilson's disease in asymptomatic patients. N Engl J Med 278:352, 1968

——, ——: Chronic hepatitis as a first manifestation of Wilson's disease. Ann Intern Med 76:59, 1972

WALSHE JM: Wilson's disease (hepatolenticular degeneration), in *Handbook of Clinical Neurology*, PJ Vinken et al (eds). New York, American Elsevier, 1976, vol 27

331 LYSOSOMAL STORAGE DISEASES

ARTHUR L. BEAUDET

GENERAL FEATURES

DEFINITION Lysosomes are cytoplasmic organelles that enclose an acidic environment and contain numerous enzymes capable of hydrolyzing most biologic macromolecules (Fig. 331-1). Primary lysosomes, the original bodies derived from the Golgi apparatus, may fuse with other membrane-bound vesicles to form secondary lysosomes. Secondary lysosomes contain material derived from outside the cell through endocytosis or material from within the cell through autophagy. A major function of the lysosome is degradation of used macromolecules related to normal turnover and tissue remodeling. Studies of the metabolism of vitamin B_{12}, lipoproteins, peptide hormones, and growth factors indicate that the lysosome is also important in the uptake of molecules through the process of adsorptive endocytosis. The initial cellular vacuole resulting from

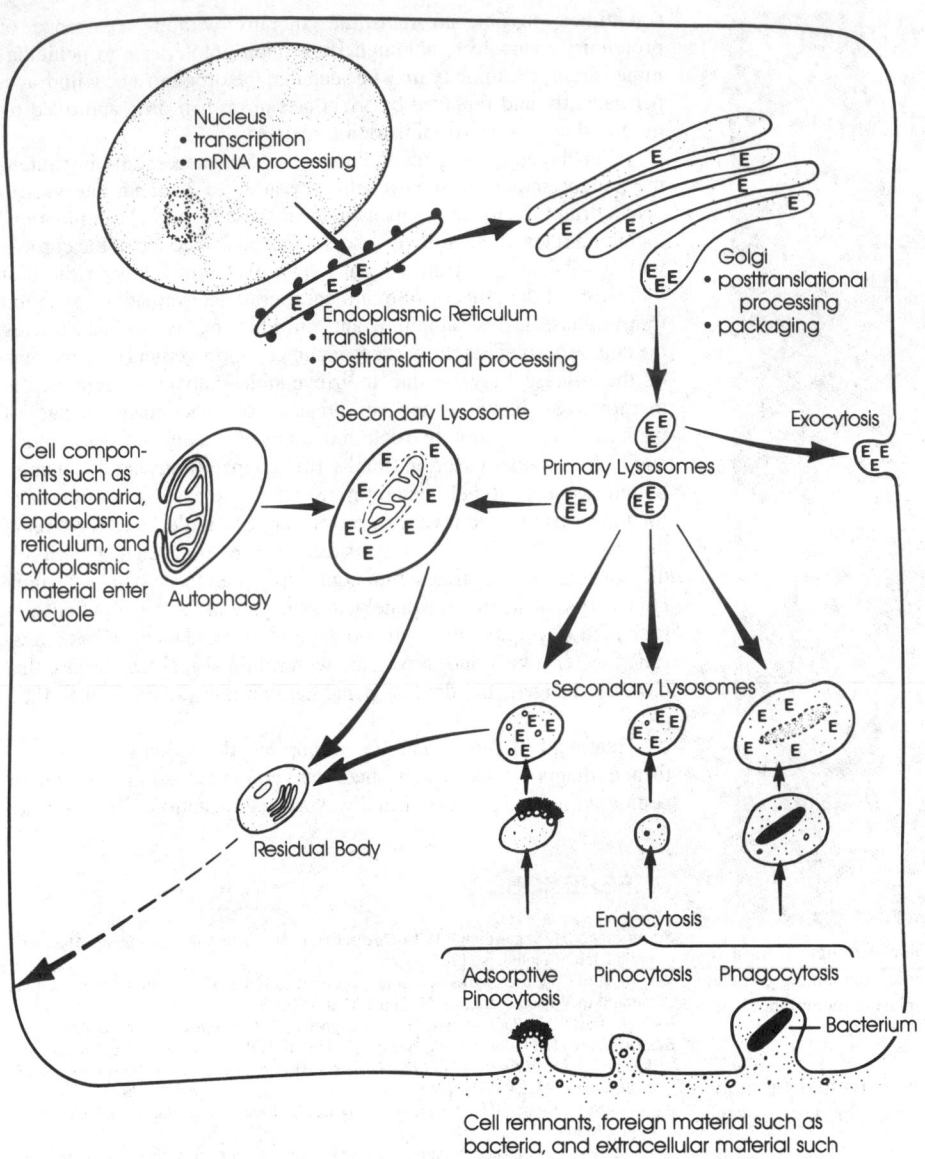

FIGURE 331-1 Biology of lysosomes. E represents lysosomal enzymes, including precursor forms. Lysosomal enzymes are synthesized in the endoplasmic reticulum and then undergo posttranslational processing that allows packaging into the primary lysosomes. The primary lysosomes can then undergo any of the several fates outlined.

In the figure: Nucleus • transcription • mRNA processing; Endoplasmic Reticulum • translation • posttranslational processing; Golgi • posttranslational processing • packaging; Secondary Lysosome; Primary Lysosomes; Exocytosis; Cell components such as mitochondria, endoplasmic reticulum, and cytoplasmic material enter vacuole; Autophagy; Residual Body; Secondary Lysosomes; Endocytosis; Adsorptive Pinocytosis; Pinocytosis; Phagocytosis; Bacterium; Cell remnants, foreign material such as bacteria, and extracellular material such as mucopolysaccharide and lipoprotein enter cell.

adsorptive endocytosis is the receptosome, or endosome, and this vacuole fuses with lysosomes. The lysosomal enzymes are glycoproteins which are synthesized within the endoplasmic reticulum. The initial products of protein synthesis undergo extensive modification including proteolytic cleavage, addition of complex oligosaccharides, synthesis of recognition markers (mannose-6-phosphate in some instances), and compartmentalization into primary lysosomes. These processes occur in the endoplasmic reticulum, in the Golgi apparatus, and probably in the primary, if not secondary, lysosomes as well. (See Chap. 3 in Scriver et al. for more details of lysosomal biology and biogenesis.)

The concept of lysosomal storage diseases arose from the studies of type II (Pompe) glycogen storage disease. The demonstration of lysosomal accumulation of glycogen as the result of α-glucosidase deficiency and data from other disorders led Hers to define an inborn lysosomal disease as one in which (1) a single lysosomal enzyme is deficient and (2) abnormal deposits (of substrate) are present within vacuoles related to lysosomes. This definition can be modified to include single-gene defects affecting one or more lysosomal enzymes and thus encompass disorders such as the mucolipidoses and multiple sulfatase deficiency. The concept also can be expanded to include the deficiency of other proteins necessary for lysosomal function, such as sphingolipid activator proteins. Biochemical and genetic

evidence indicates that these activator proteins are essential for hydrolysis of some substrates.

The lysosomal storage diseases include most of the lipid storage disorders, the mucopolysaccharidoses, the mucolipidoses, glycoprotein storage diseases, and others, as indicated in Table 331-1. The enzyme deficiencies have an autosomal recessive basis with the exception of Hunter's mucopolysaccharidosis II (MPS II), which is X-linked recessive, and Fabry's disease, which is X-linked with frequent manifestations in females. The target organs are determined by the usual sites of degradation for a macromolecule. For example, cerebral white matter is affected in patients with defects in degradation of myelin, hepatosplenomegaly develops in those with defects in degradation of glycolipids from red cell stroma, and generalized tissue involvement may occur in patients with defects in the degradation of ubiquitous mucopolysaccharides. The accumulated material often causes visceromegaly or macrocephaly, but secondary atrophy also can occur, particularly in brain or muscle. In simple terms, the symptoms appear to be due to damage from stored material, but exactly how this causes cell death or dysfunction often is unclear. All the disorders are progressive, and many are fatal in childhood or adolescence. Definitive diagnosis is accomplished best by specific enzyme assays on serum, leukocytes, or cultured skin fibroblasts, selecting the appropriate tests on clinical grounds. There is extensive phenotypic variation within disorders with infantile, juvenile, and adult forms of many entities. In addition, varying combinations of visceral, skeletal, and neurologic involvement can occur within a single enzyme disorder.

DIAGNOSIS A lysosomal storage disease is usually suspected on the basis of progressive neurologic dysfunction, visceromegaly, skeletal dysostosis, or some more specific finding, as outlined in Table 331-1. Progressive or degenerative disease is the hallmark of these disorders. The superimposition of degeneration upon normal childhood development results in a slowing of progress prior to loss of previously acquired abilities. The history should focus on the course of childhood development, neurologic symptoms, including seizures and visual or auditory impairment, the course of physical growth, and more specific findings such as coarsening facies, corneal clouding, exaggerated startle response, abdominal distention, joint pain, joint stiffness, hernias, and recurrent infection. The family history may reveal similarly affected siblings or consanguinity in autosomal recessive disease or other affected male family members in X-linked disorders. Ethnic background may be helpful because several lipid storage diseases are more frequent in Ashkenazi Jews, and mannosidosis and aspartylglucosaminuria may occur with increased frequency in Scandinavian populations. The juvenile form of sialidosis is frequent in the Japanese.

On physical examination the head circumference may be enlarged. Gigantism occurs early in the course of some mucopolysaccharidoses and glycoprotein storage diseases, while short stature is a later finding in many disorders. Ophthalmologic examination should include slit-lamp and careful funduscopic examination. Enlargement of the tongue, coarsening of the facies, and hepatosplenomegaly may occur. Skeletal findings may include gibbus deformity, broadening of the long bones, and joint stiffness. Cutaneous findings are rare except in fucosidosis, sialidosis, Fabry's disease, and Hunter's disease. Careful neurologic examination should attempt to distinguish the extent of involvement of gray matter, white matter, and peripheral nerves. Preliminary diagnostic studies should include examination of the peripheral blood smear for vacuolated or granulated leukocytes, urinary spot test for mucopolysaccharide, and radiologic bone survey. The preferred method of diagnosis is to use the above information to select specific enzyme assays in serum, leukocytes, or cultured skin fibroblasts. If a mucopolysaccharide screening test is positive or if clinical findings are suggestive, quantitative mucopolysaccharide analysis can be carried out. If a specific diagnosis is not readily established, biopsy of skin, bone marrow, rectal mucosa, liver, peripheral nerve, conjunctiva, or other tissue for light and electron microscopy can be helpful. Electron-microscopic findings can direct one toward or away from the general category of lysosomal storage diseases based on the presence or absence of engorged lysosomes. Again, enzyme assay is the proper method for diagnosis of the standard disorders. When significant evidence favors a lysosomal storage disease but no enzyme deficiency is demonstrable, chemical analysis of biopsy tissue from liver or brain may be an appropriate research starting point.

The diagnosis of lysosomal storage diseases in adults is often difficult, although studies such as bone marrow aspiration in Gaucher's disease and renal biopsy in Fabry's disease may be pathognomonic. The diagnosis is difficult in the face of insidious, slowly progressive neurologic and psychiatric symptoms as described below for deficiencies of aryl sulfatase A, hexosaminidase A, or β-galactosidase. Erroneous diagnoses are common in these disorders, and a high index of suspicion is required. Lysosomal α-glucosidase deficiency mimics muscular dystrophy (see Chap. 365).

HETEROGENEITY There is extensive clinical and biochemical heterogeneity within the lysosomal storage diseases. The biochemical genetic principles underlying this heterogeneity are reviewed in Chaps. 5 and 6. In general, a structural gene for lysosomal enzyme produces products that undergo posttranslational modification to become glycoproteins, often resulting in a series of electrophoretic variants, or isozymes. These isozymes may hydrolyze one or a variety of substrates, and the substrate specificity of particular isozymes may vary. Differences in substrate specificity also arise from the occurrence of similar but genetically distinct enzymes, for example, the β-galactosidases. Mutations within a gene may totally eliminate or reduce enzyme activity, alter posttranslational modification, or alter the activity of the enzyme for specific substrates.

In most instances different mutations within the structural genes for lysosomal enzymes account for varying degrees of severity from individual to individual as well as for the diverse combinations of visceral, skeletal, neurologic, ocular, and other manifestations. The heterogeneity is increased further by the recessive nature of most of the conditions in that each affected individual must have two mutant genes at the same locus. The exact mutation may vary in the two copies of the gene, making the patient a genetic compound heterozygote. In this instance either one or both genes may encode some form of residual enzyme activity for one or more substrates. Patients with intermediate clinical phenotypes with mucopolysaccharidosis type I (MPS I) have been cited as likely examples of compound heterozygotes. At a molecular level the majority of lysosomal storage disease patients might prove to be compound heterozygotes. Although it is useful to characterize clinical phenotypes as infantile, juvenile, adult, neuropathic, or nonneuropathic, the existence of different mutant alleles and of genetic compounds provides an explanation for those occasional patients who appear aberrant or intermediate as compared with the usual phenotype. Another type of heterogeneity is illustrated by MPS III A, B, C, and D, which are very similar disorders caused by different gene defects. Thus, biochemical heterogeneity can underlie apparent clinical homogeneity.

Further complexity results from the fact that certain enzyme activities are derived from complexes of nonidentical subunits. As a consequence, different mutations can cause deficiency of the same enzyme, for example, hexosaminidase A deficiency in Tay-Sachs and Sandhoff's diseases, and can explain multiple enzyme deficiencies due to a single-gene defect as in Sandhoff's disease. Genetic disorders that affect the posttranslational modification of lysosomal enzymes and defects in the lysosome itself may also cause lysosomal storage diseases. The mucolipidoses II and III are situations in which a single-gene defect alters the ability of a number of lysosomal enzymes to enter the lysosome. Thus, mutations outside the structural genes for the enzymes can account for further heterogeneity. Better understanding of the identity, subunit structure, posttranslational processing, and substrate specificities of lysosomal enzymes should provide further insight into phenotypic and genotypic heterogeneity.

Clinical diagnosis is facilitated but also somewhat complicated by the widespread use of synthetic substrates for measuring lysosomal enzyme activities. These substrates often measure a group of related activities attributable to different enzymes. Thus, the activity of β-galactosidase using an artificial substrate may represent the sum of various β-galactosidases encoded by different structural genes and having different substrate specificities. Clinical reliability generally is achieved by manipulating in vitro conditions to reflect that enzyme activity whose deficiency is characteristic of a clinical disorder. Genetic heterogeneity has, however, resulted in individuals with a mutant enzyme that either hydrolyzes the natural substrate and not the artificial substrate, or vice versa. This is exemplified by the normal individuals who have hexosaminidase A deficiency using artificial substrate and by patients with Tay-Sachs disease who have substantial levels of hexosaminidase A activity with artificial substrates. The presence or absence of disease correlates with ability to hydrolyze the natural G_{M2} ganglioside substrate. These phenomena have considerable significance for identification of affected patients, for heterozygote screening, and for prenatal diagnosis. They indicate the need to go beyond artificial substrate enzyme assays if normal results occur in the face of overwhelming clinical, electron-microscopic, or chemical evidence of a storage disease.

MANAGEMENT AND PREVENTION Specific therapy is not effective in lysosomal storage diseases at present, and care is largely symptomatic. The relentless, progressive course in many instances represents a tragic burden. Transplantation is effective in reversing

TABLE 331-1 Summary of lysosomal storage diseases

Disorder*	Heterogeneity (onset)	Enzyme deficiency	Stored material	Neurologic
G_{M1} gangliosidosis (71)	Infantile (birth) Juvenile (6–20 mo) Adult	β-Galactosidase	G_{M1} ganglioside Glycoproteins Keratan sulfate	Mental retardation, seizures, blindness; later in juvenile form, variable in adults
Tay-Sachs and variants, G_{M2} gangliosidosis (72)	Infantile (3–6 mo) Juvenile Adult forms	Hexosaminidase A	G_{M2} ganglioside	Mental retardation, seizures, blindness; later in juvenile form
Sandhoff, G_{M2} gangliosidosis (72)	Infantile (3–6 mo)	Hexosaminidase A and B	G_{M2} ganglioside Globoside	Mental retardation, seizures, blindness
G_{M2} gangliosidosis, AB variant (72)	Findings similar to Tay-Sachs except primary defect is a ganglioside activator protein.			
Krabbe, galactosylceramide lipidosis (68)	Infantile (2–6 mo) Late onset	Galactosylceramide β-Galactosidase	↑ Galactoscerebroside/ sulfatide ratio	Mental retardation, leukodystrophy; variable in late onset
Metachromatic leukodystrophy, sulfatide lipidosis (69)	Late infantile (1–4 yr) Juvenile (4–20 yr) Adult	Arylsulfatase A (cerebroside sulfatase)	Galactosyl sulfatides	Mental retardation, leukodystrophy, psychosis and dementia in adults
Sphingolipid activator protein 1 deficiency (69)	Findings similar to metachromatic leukodystrophy except primary defect is activator protein.			
Niemann-Pick, sphingomyelin lipidosis (66)	Infantile neuropathic (1–4 mo) Late onset neuropathic Visceral	Sphingomyelinase in types A and B but not type C	Sphingomyelin Cholesterol	Mental retardation, ataxia, and seizures in neuropathic forms
Gaucher, glucosylceramide lipidosis (67)	Infantile (1–12 mo) Juvenile (2–6 yr) Adult	β-Glucocerebrosidase	Glucosylceramide	Mental retardation; spastic, later flaccid, ataxia in juvenile; no neurologic symptoms in adult form
Fabry, trihexosyl ceramidosis (70)	Hemizygous males Heterozygous females	α-Galactosidase A	Trihexosylceramide	Painful neuropathy
Acid lipase deficiency (64)	Infantile Wolman's disease (0–3 mo) Late onset cholesteryl ester storage disease (CESD)	Acid lipase	Cholesteryl ester Triglyceride	Mental retardation but mild related to growth failure in Wolman; none in CESD
Farber, ceramide deficiency (65)	Infantile (0–4 mo) Rare juvenile	Ceramidase	Ceramide	Occasional mental retardation, but may be secondary to somatic features
Pompe, glycogen storage type II (12)	Infantile (0–6 mo) Juvenile Adult	Acid maltase (α-1,4- and 1,6-glucosidase)	Glycogen	Probably normal mentally
Fucosidosis (63)	Infantile (3–12 mo) Juvenile	α-Fucosidase	Glycopeptides Glycolipids Oligosaccharides	Mental retardation
Mannosidosis (63)	Infantile (6–18 mo) Milder form	α-Mannosidase	Oligosaccharides	Mental retardation
Aspartylglucosaminuria (63)	Young adult onset	Aspartylglucosamine amidase	Aspartylglucosamine Glycopeptides	Mental retardation
Mucopolysaccharidosis IH and IS (61)	Infantile Hurler (6–12 mo) Intermediate Adult Scheie	α-Iduronidase	Dermatan sulfate Heparan sulfate	Mental retardation, absent in Scheie
Hunter, mucopolysaccharidosis II (61)	Severe infantile (6–12 mo) Mild juvenile	Iduronosulfate sulfatase	Dermatan sulfate Heparan sulfate	Mental retardation, less in mild form

* Numbers in parentheses refer to the chapters in Scriver et al. in which the disorder is discussed in detail.

TABLE 331-1 Summary of lysosomal storage diseases *(continued)*

Liver and/or spleen enlargement	Skeletal dysplasia	Ophthalmic	Hematologic	Genetics	Unique manifestations
+ + + + Less in juvenile, variable in adult	+ + + + Variable in juvenile and adult forms	Cherry-red spot in 50% of infantile; corneal clouding variable but more in adults	Foam cells Vacuolated lymphocytes	AR†	Coarse facies, edema, macroglossia, mucopolysacchariduria; early blindness in infantile, milder in juvenile; in adults often spondyloepiphyseal dysplasia +/− mucopolysacchariduria
0	0	Cherry-red spot in infantile form, rare in juvenile	0	AR	Macrocephaly, hyperacusis in infantile; increased in Ashkenazi Jews
0	0	Cherry-red spot	0	AR	Macrocephaly, hyperacusis, visceral histiocytosis
0	0	Optic atrophy	0	AR	Extreme irritability, ↑ CSF protein, fever, globoid cell neuropathology
0	0	Optic atrophy, less in juvenile and adult forms	0	AR	↑ CSF protein and early gait abnormalities in late infantile; peripheral neuropathy
+ + + + Less prominent in late onset forms	0	Macular degeneration and cherry-red spot in neuropathic forms	Distinctive foam cell Vacuolated lymphocytes	AR	Pulmonary infiltrates, brownish skin, infantile neuronopathic form increased in Ashkenazi Jews, seablue histiocytes
+ + + + Hypersplenism common	+ +	Usually normal	Distinctive foam cell	AR	Adult form includes ↑ acid phosphatase, pathologic fractures; Ashkenazi Jewish predilection
0	0	Corneal dystrophy, vascular lesions, cataracts	0	X-linked dominant	Cutaneous angiokeratoma, vascular thromboses, hypohidrosis
+ + +	0	0	Foam cells Vacuolated lymphocytes	AR	Adrenal calcification, anemia, vomiting and poor growth in Wolman; hepatic fibrosis and ↑ blood cholesterol in CESD
+/−	?	Mild macular degeneration	0	AR	Arthropathy—subcutaneous, periarticular and visceral nodules (lipogranulomatosis); ↑ CSF protein
Mild hepatomegaly	0	0	0	AR	Lethal skeletal and cardiac myopathy in infantile; primarily skeletal myopathy in adults
+ +	+ +	0	Vacuolated lymphocytes Foam cells	AR	Coarse facies, increased sweat electrolytes, angiokeratoma in juvenile
+ + +	+ +	Cataracts, corneal clouding	Vacuolated lymphocytes Granulated neutrophils	AR	Coarse facies, enlarged tongue
0	+ +	Lens opacities	Vacuolated lymphocytes	AR	Coarse facies, detectable by urine amino acid analysis
+ + +	+ + + +	Corneal clouding	Granulated lymphocytes	AR	Coarse facies, cardiovascular involvement, joint stiffness
+ + +	+ + + +	Retinal degeneration, no significant corneal clouding	Granulated lymphocytes	X-linked	Coarse facies, cardiovascular involvement, joint stiffness

† AR = autosomal recective.

(Table continues next page)

TABLE 331-1   Summary of lysosomal storage diseases (*continued*)

Disorder*	Heterogeneity (onset)	Enzyme deficiency	Stored material	Neurologic
Sanfilippo A, muco-polysaccharidosis III A (61)	Late infantile (1–4 yr)	Heparan N-sulfatase (sulfamidase)	Heparan sulfate	Severe mental retardation
Sanfilippo B, muco-polysaccharidosis III B (61)		N-Acetyl-α-glucosaminidase		
Sanfilippo C, muco-polysaccharidosis III C (61)		Acetyl-CoA:α-glucosaminide N-acetyltransferase		
Sanfilippo D, mucopolysac-charidosis III D (61)		N-Acetylglucosamine-6-sulfate sulfatase		
Morquio, mucopolysaccha-ridosis IV (61)	Some variation	N-Acetylgalactosamine-6-sulfate sulfatase	Keratan sulfate	0
Maroteaux-Lamy, muco-polysaccharidosis VI (61)	Variation in severity and cardiovascular involvement	N-Acetylhexosamine-4-sulfate sulfatase (aryl-sulfatase B)	Dermatan sulfate	0
β-Glucuronidase deficiency, mucopolysaccharidosis VII (61)	Few patients; infantile to adult forms	β-Glucuronidase	Dermatan sulfate ? Heparan sulfate	Mental retardation ? absent in some adults
Multiple sulfatase deficiency (69)	Late infantile (1–4 yr)	Arylsulfatases A, B, and C Other sulfatases	Sulfatides Mucopolysaccharides	Mental retardation
Sialidosis (63)	Congenital, infantile, juvenile, cherry-red spot myoclonus	Glycoprotein neuraminidase (sialidase)	Sialyloligosaccharides	Mental retardation, myoclonus
Galactosialidosis (71)	Infantile Juvenile	Protective glycoprotein	Sialyloligosaccharides	Mental retardation
Mucolipidosis II, I cell disease (62)	Infantile (0–3 mo)	UDP-N-acetylglucosamine (GlcNAc):glycoprotein GlcNAc-1-phosphotransferase	Glycoproteins Glycolipids	Mental retardation
Mucolipidosis III, pseudo-Hurler polydystrophy (62)	Late infantile (>2 yr)		Glycoproteins Glycolipids	Mild mental retardation
Mucolipidosis IV (71)	Infantile	? Ganglioside neuraminidase	? Multiple	Mental retardation
Neuronal ceroid lipofusci-noses	Late infantile Juvenile Adult	Unknown	"Ceroid" "Lipofuscin"	Mental retardation, dementia variable in adults, seizures

* Numbers in parentheses refer to the chapters in Scriver et al. in which the disorder is discussed in detail.

the renal failure in Fabry's disease, and splenectomy may be helpful in adult Gaucher's disease. Considerable attention has been focused on enzyme replacement for lysosomal storage diseases using organ or fibroblast transplantation or the infusion of plasma, leukocytes, purified enzyme itself, or enzyme trapped in erythrocytes or liposomes. Although these approaches offer promise for treatment of manifestations outside the central nervous system, they are not of proven efficacy. The most distressing manifestations of lysosomal storage diseases involve the central nervous system, where the blood-brain barrier presents an additional obstacle to effective enzyme replacement therapy.

Genetic counseling is important in the management of these disorders. All the lysosomal storage diseases in which the specific enzyme deficiency is known either have been or presumably could be diagnosed in utero, since lysosomal enzyme activities are expressed in cultured amniotic fluid cells as well as in cultured skin fibroblasts. Prenatal diagnosis can also be made using chorionic villus biopsy. Although the incidence of miscarriage after this procedure may be slightly higher, the possibility of earlier diagnosis is attractive to families at risk. Heterozygote detection in close relatives is sometimes possible, although it can be difficult to achieve adequate statistical confidence for such determinations. Heterozygote detection is further complicated by random inactivation of X chromosomes in 46,XX carriers of X-linked diseases, but women at risk in such families should be counseled. More effective approaches to prevention require identification of heterozygous couples prior to the birth of an affected offspring. The feasibility of this approach has been demonstrated by heterozygote testing programs for Tay-Sachs disease. Such programs could result in a decreased frequency of these disorders through extensive testing and appropriate reproductive decisions by the rare couples at risk for affected offspring; the high frequency of the heterozygous state in Ashkenazi Jews and reliable methods for carrier detection for Tay-Sachs disease have facilitated this program. Efficient, accurate heterozygote detection methods would be needed to apply this approach to other diseases and to populations with lower heterozygote frequencies. Even under optimal conditions genetic variants may cause false-positive or false-negative results in any screening process.

TABLE 331-1 Summary of lysosomal storage diseases (continued)

Liver and/or spleen enlargement	Skeletal dysplasia	Ophthalmic	Hematologic	Genetics	Unique manifestations
+	+	0	Granulated lymphocytes	AR	Mild coarsening of facies
+	Severe, distinctive	Corneal clouding	Granulated neutrophils	AR	Severe deformity, odontoid hypoplasia, aortic regurgitation
+ +	+ + + +	Corneal clouding	Granulated neutrophils and lymphocytes	AR	Mild coarsening of facies, joint stiffness, valvular heart disease
+ + +	+ + +	Corneal clouding	Granulated neutrophils	AR	Coarse facies, ↑ vascular involvement
+	MPS features	Retinal degeneration	Vacuolated and granulated cells	AR	Icthyosis, combined MPS and metachromatic leukodystrophy phenotype
+ + Less in late form	+ + Less or absent in late form	Cherry-red spot	Vacuolated lymphocytes	AR	MPS phenotype in all but cherry-red spot myoclonus
+ + Less in juvenile	+ +	Cherry-red spot, corneal clouding	Vacuolated lymphocytes	AR	Angiokeratoma in juvenile; dysotosis multiplex
0/ +	+ + + +	Corneal clouding	Vacuolated and granulated neutrophils	AR	Coarse facies, inclusions in cultured fibroblasts, normal mucopolysacchariduria
0	+ + +	Corneal clouding	Vacuolated plasma cells	AR	Coarse facies, inclusions in cultured fibroblasts, joint contractures, valvular heart disease, normal mucopolysacchariduria
0	0	Corneal clouding, retinal degeneration	0	AR	Diagnosis based on electron microscopy; ? Ashkenazi Jewish predilection
0	0	Optic atrophy, macular degeneration, retinitis pigmentosa	Vacuolated lymphocytes Granulated neutrophils	AR	Electron microscopy helpful, degree of genetic heterogeneity unknown

MOLECULAR ANALYSIS Many of the lysosomal genes have been cloned. Specific mutations are being identified, and it may become possible to correlate severity of the phenotype with specific homozygous or compound heterozygous molecular genotypes. Molecular diagnosis is likely to supplement but not replace enzymatic diagnosis in most circumstances. It is also possible that availability of the cloned genes might allow for gene or enzyme replacement therapy.

SPECIFIC DISORDERS

SPHINGOLIPIDOSES G_{M1} gangliosidosis G_{M1} gangliosidosis is due to deficiency of β-galactosidase. The features of the infantile form are summarized in Table 331-1. The juvenile form is characterized by a later onset, survival to the latter half of the first decade of life, neurologic impairment and seizures, and milder skeletal and ocular findings. In adults, one phenotype (sometimes called Morquio B) includes corneal clouding, normal intelligence, and spondyloepi-

physeal dysplasia similar to that seen in MPS IV. Other adults have minimal bony abnormalities but exhibit spasticity, ataxia, or myoclonus. Patients with slowly progressive extrapyramidal signs with prominent dystonia, cerebral and caudate atrophy, and absence of visceral findings have been misdiagnosed as juvenile parkinsonism. A high index of suspicion is necessary to recognize the diverse phenotypes caused by β-galactosidase deficiency in juvenile and adult patients, since a wide range of skeletal, ocular, neurologic, and visceral findings can occur. Isozymes of β-galactosidase occur, but the diversity of phenotypes is believed to be due to different mutations in the same structural gene. All forms of G_{M1} gangliosidosis have an autosomal recessive inheritance. The frequency of the disease is low, with fewer than 50 patients reported for any given phenotype. Patients with isolated β-galactosidase deficiency must be distinguished from those with combined deficiency of neuraminidase and β-galactosidase.

G_{M2} gangliosidosis Tay-Sachs disease is a relatively common inborn error of metabolism with thousands of documented cases. Although it is clinically very similar to Sandhoff's disease, the two are genetically distinct with deficiency of hexosaminidase A in the former and hexosaminidase A and B in the latter. An additional disorder, called the AB variant of G_{M2} gangliosidosis, occurs with normal hexosaminidase A and B activity. This variant is due to a deficiency of a protein factor (activator) necessary for activity of the enzyme against natural substrate. The presenting features are similar in all of the infantile disorders and include a developmental delay beginning in the third to sixth month with subsequent, rapidly progressive neurologic deterioration. Macrocephaly, seizures, retinal cherry-red spot, and an augmented startle response to sound suggest the diagnosis. The diagnosis is confirmed by enzyme assay. Most juvenile-onset patients with hexosaminidase deficiency present with dementia, seizures, and ocular findings, and some have an atypical spinocerebellar degeneration.

The neurologic manifestations of hexosaminidase A deficiency in adults are variable. Ataxia, dysarthria, lower motor neuron disease, pyramidal signs, and recurrent psychosis are common. Misdiagnoses have included Kugelberg-Welander spinal muscular atrophy, amyotropic lateral sclerosis, cerebellar or spinocerebellar ataxia, atypical Friedreich's ataxia, muscular dystrophy, dementia, schizophrenia, and others. The manifestations are slowly progressive, and, if considered, the diagnosis is easily established by serum enzyme assay.

Sandhoff's disease is nonallelic with Tay-Sachs disease, whereas the juvenile forms of hexosaminidase deficiency are usually allelic with Tay-Sachs disease. Tay-Sachs disease is the most frequent form of hexosaminidase deficiency, the risk being about 100 times higher in Ashkenazi Jews than in other ethnic groups. All forms of G_{M2} gangliosidosis are autosomal recessive. Hexosaminidase B is composed of β subunits whose structural locus is on chromosome 5, while hexosaminidase A is composed of α and β subunits with the structural locus for the α subunit on chromosome 15. Thus there is a defect in the α subunit in Tay-Sachs disease and in the β subunit in Sandhoff's disease.

Although no specific therapy is available, extensive programs for heterozygote detection to prevent Tay-Sachs disease have been carried out throughout the world. As of 1985, more than 530,000 people had been tested, and more than 21,000 heterozygotes and 527 couples at risk for Tay-Sachs in their offspring had been identified. Over 800 pregnancies had been monitored by prenatal diagnosis because of a previous affected child, and 602 pregnancies had been monitored based on results of carrier screening by 1985. The incidence of the disease has been reduced by 80 to 90 percent in the Jewish population in the United States and Canada.

LEUKODYSTROPHIES Krabbe's galactosylceramide lipidosis or globoid cell leukodystrophy is an infantile disease due to deficiency of galactosylceramide β-galactosidase. The clinical features are summarized in Table 331-1. Rapid neurologic deterioration and death occur within 1 to 2 years of onset. Premortem diagnosis is accomplished by enzyme assay. The presence of globoid cells in the brain is a characteristic postmortem finding. Galactosylceramide β-galactosidase is different from the β-galactosidase that is deficient in G_{M1} gangliosidosis. Krabbe's disease is an autosomal recessive disorder, and diagnosis can be made prenatally. Juvenile or adult forms are rare.

Deficiency of arylsulfatase A (cerebroside sulfatase) is the basis of metachromatic leukodystrophy, a lipid storage disease with a frequency of 1 in 40,000. The age of onset is later than that in Tay-Sachs disease or Krabbe's disease. Patients usually attain the ability to walk and frequently present with gait abnormalities in the second to fourth year of life. Initially the patients may be hypotonic with decreased deep tendon reflexes, the latter reflecting peripheral nerve involvement. The disease progresses over the first decade to include ataxia, increased muscle tone, decorticate or decerebrate posturing, and eventual loss of all contact with surroundings. Rare patients with a juvenile form of metachromatic leukodystrophy have the clinical onset between 4 and 20 years of age and progress more slowly.

The adult form deserves special mention as an example of the difficulties presented by subtle, slowly progressive forms of lysosomal storage diseases. The onset is in the second to fifth decade with a slowly progressive dementia. Emotional difficulties, motor dysfunction, and indistinct speech are often present. Even though conduction velocity in peripheral nerves is usually diminished, the deep tendon reflexes are often increased. Typical misdiagnoses include organic dementia, multiple sclerosis, and schizophrenia; psychiatric hospitalization is common. Premortem diagnosis was rare in the past, but the presence of periventricular hypodensities of white matter on computed tomography (CT) scan or abnormalities of periventricular white matter on magnetic resonance imaging (MRI) of the brain may suggest the diagnosis which should be confirmed by enzyme assay.

Although some diagnostic studies have been performed on urine, leukocytes or fibroblasts are preferable for diagnostic enzyme assay. Changes demonstrable on metachromatic staining of nerve tissue are nonspecific and not an adequate substitute for enzyme assay.

Arylsulfatase A is routinely measured using artificial substrate, and complexities involving low levels of activity in normal individuals and moderate levels of residual activity in symptomatic patients have been described. Heterogeneity involving mutations in multiple components of the cerebroside sulfatase activity may exist, but the majority of patients probably have simple allelic disorders on an autosomal recessive basis. A few patients with a phenotype similar to metachromatic leukodystrophy have been shown to have deficiency of a sphingolipid activator protein. Arylsulfatase A deficiency also occurs in multiple sulfatase deficiency.

NIEMANN-PICK DISEASE Niemann-Pick disease is a sphingomyelin lipidosis. In type A and B disease, there is a clear deficiency of sphingomyelinase, an enzyme that hydrolyzes sphingomyelin to yield ceramide and phosphorylcholine. The most common disorder, Niemann-Pick A, begins shortly after birth with hepatosplenomegaly, failure to thrive, and neurologic impairment. Retinal cherry-red spots occur, but seizures and hypersplenism are rare. The diagnosis can be made by recognition of the distinctive Niemann-Pick cell in the bone marrow but should be confirmed by enzyme assay. Niemann-Pick B disease is a relatively benign disorder with hepatosplenomegaly, sphingomyelinase deficiency, and sometimes pulmonary infiltrates; but there is no neurologic involvement. Niemann-Pick C disease is characterized by sphingomyelin lipidosis and progressive neurologic deterioration in childhood. Niemann-Pick C disease is not due to sphingomyelinase deficiency but is associated with a massive lysosomal accumulation of cholesterol due to an incompletely characterized defect in intracellular utilization of cholesterol.

GAUCHER'S DISEASE Gaucher's disease is a glucosylceramide lipidosis caused by deficiency of glucosylceramidase. An infantile form is characterized by early onset, marked hepatosplenomegaly, and severe neurologic progression to early death. A juvenile form with milder neurologic involvement exists. The type 1 or nonneuronopathic form (commonly called adult Gaucher's) is the most common lysosomal storage disease. The diagnosis of Gaucher's disease should be established by enzyme analysis. All forms of Gaucher's disease have an autosomal recessive genetic basis and are allelic disorders. Type 1 is about 30 times more frequent in Ashkenazi Jews, with an incidence in this group of about 1 in 2500 births. Absence of neurologic involvement is the criterion for inclusion in the type 1 or adult category.

Clinical manifestations include incidental discovery of painless splenomegaly; thrombocytopenia, anemia, or leukopenia secondary to hypersplenism; and bone pain. The course is variable, ranging from confinement to a wheelchair early in life to asymptomatic diagnosis in the ninth decade. Most patients have a mild course with relatively normal life expectancy. Partial or total splenectomy may be required. Pneumococcal vaccine should be administered prior to splenectomy. Careful management of postsplenectomy infection risks are important, and prophylactic antibiotics are recommended. The extent of bone disease is variable and includes bone pain, pathologic fractures, vertebral collapse, and aseptic necrosis of the femoral head. Bone pain with fever is termed pseudoosteomyelitis. MRI is particularly effective in demonstrating and differentiating bony abnormalities in Gaucher's disease. Moderate hepatic dysfunction is common, and, rarely, severe hepatic failure, portal hypertension, pulmonary infiltrates, and pulmonary hypertension may develop. Serum acid phosphatase is characteristically elevated. A distinctive storage cell is present in the bone marrow in all forms of Gaucher's disease, but enzyme assay should be performed because the Gaucher cell may also be found in patients with granulocytic leukemia and myeloma. Bone marrow transplantation may be considered in the rare case of life-threatening complications from the disease.

FABRY'S DISEASE Fabry's disease involves the accumulation of a trihexoside, galactosylgalactosylglucosylceramide, due to deficiency of α-galactosidase A. The disorder is X-linked. The most severe symptoms occur in hemizygous males with an incidence of about 1 in 40,000; milder symptoms occur in heterozygous females. Painful neuropathy is the most prominent symptom in younger men. The pain may be constant or cause intermittent crises of burning pain particularly in the palms and soles. Painful crises may mimic appendicitis or renal colic, and associated low grade fever may lead to misdiagnoses of inflammatory processes.

The diagnosis can be suggested by the astute dermatologist or ophthalmologist. Cutaneous manifestations include angiokeratoma and decreased sweating. The angiokeratoma occur as clusters of red angiectases in the superficial skin. They do not blanch with pressure and are located on the trunk, perineal area, penis, and scrotum. The anhidrosis or hypohidrosis can predispose to heat stroke with vigorous exercise, as in military training. A characteristic corneal opacity occurs in males and in most heterozygous females. Lenticular opacities and tortuosity of the conjunctival and retinal vessels also occur.

Cardiovascular manifestations include direct involvement of the myocardium with lipid deposition, arrhythmias, valvular dysfunction, and myocardial infarction. Cerebral vascular manifestations secondary to involvement of small vessels are not rare, and frank cerebral hemorrhage can occur. Deposition of lipid in the kidney results in progressive renal impairment with renal failure in middle age (see also Chap. 228). The mean age at death of males not treated for renal failure was 41 years in one study. The diagnosis is often recognized at renal biopsy on the basis of lipid vacuoles in glomerular and tubular epithelial cells.

Heterozygous females are affected more mildly, but corneal dystrophy and cutaneous manifestations may be seen on careful examination. Life expectancy is near normal in women, although the more serious complications occur rarely.

Therapeutic intervention of several types may be helpful. Counseling regarding the risks of hypohidrosis is important. Painful neuropathy frequently responds to administration of phenytoin. Renal failure can be treated by chronic dialysis, and the patients are acceptable candidates for transplantation since the donor kidney will not be impaired by the disease. The disease in the future might be amenable to enzyme replacement therapy, since the central nervous system is spared.

ACID LIPASE DEFICIENCY The infantile form of acid lipase deficiency, Wolman's disease, is listed in Table 331-1. Cholesteryl ester storage disease in adulthood and adolescence is a rare disorder with mild phenotypic features by comparison. The usual features are hepatosplenomegaly, lipid deposition in the liver, and increased plasma cholesterol. Hepatic fibrosis, esophageal varices, and poor growth may occur.

GLYCOPROTEIN STORAGE DISORDERS Fucosidosis, mannosidosis, and aspartylglucosaminuria are rare, autosomal recessive disorders involving hydrolases that degrade polysaccharide linkages. Glycolipids as well as glycoproteins are accumulated in fucosidosis. All are characterized by neurologic impairment and varying somatic involvements, as outlined in Table 331-1. Fucosidosis and mannosidosis are most often lethal disorders in childhood, while aspartylglucosaminuria presents as a late-onset lysosomal storage disease with prominent mental retardation and a prolonged course. Abnormal sweat electrolytes and cutaneous angiokeratomas are distinctive in fucosidosis, and an unusual cartwheel-type cataract occurs in man-

nosidosis. Aspartylglucosaminuria is remarkable in that urinary amino acid analysis is diagnostic with an increase of aspartylglucosamine; it is more frequent in the Finnish population. Sialidosis encompasses a group of phenotypes associated with glycoprotein neuraminidase (sialidase) deficiency. The phenotypes include an adult cherry-red spot myoclonus syndrome, infantile and juvenile presentations with mucopolysaccharidosis-like phenotypes, and a congenital presentation with hydrops fetalis. Many patients previously classified as having mucolipidosis I have been proven to have mannosidosis or sialidosis. Some patients with sialidosis have β-galactosidase deficiency as well as neuraminidase deficiency. The combined β-galactosidase and neuraminidase deficiency is due to a defect in a "protective protein." Each of the glycoprotein storage diseases can be diagnosed by appropriate enzyme assay.

MUCOPOLYSACCHARIDOSIS (MPS) The mucopolysaccharidoses represent a broad spectrum of disorders due to deficiencies of one of a group of enzymes which degrade three classes of mucopolysaccharides: heparan sulfate, dermatan sulfate, and keratan sulfate. The general MPS phenotype includes coarse facies, corneal clouding, hepatosplenomegaly, joint stiffness, hernias, dysostosis multiplex, mucopolysaccharide excretion in the urine, and metachromatic staining in peripheral leukocytes and bone marrow. Various components of the MPS phenotype are also found in the mucolipidoses, glycoprotein storage disorders, and other lysosomal storage diseases. Detailed clinical and radiologic evaluation and identification of the type of MPS excreted in the urine help to narrow the diagnostic possibilities. Definitive diagnosis requires assay of specific enzymes in various tissues such as cultured skin fibroblasts.

Hurler's or MPS IH disorder is the prototype MPS. Virtually all the components of the phenotype mentioned above are present and expressed in a severe degree. Nasal congestion and grossly visible corneal clouding are early features. Excessive growth during the first year of life is followed by poor growth late in the course. Radiologic features include enlargement of the sella turcica with a distinctive "shoe-shaped" fossa, broadening and shortening of the long bones, and hypoplasia and beaking of the vertebrae in the lumbar area. The vertebral beaking gives rise to an accentuated kyphosis or gibbus deformity. Death occurs within the first decade; postmortem findings include hydrocephalus and cardiovascular disease with occlusion of the coronary arteries. The biochemical defect is α-iduronidase deficiency with accumulation of heparan sulfate and dermatan sulfate.

MPS IS, or Scheie's syndrome, a clinically distinct disorder with childhood onset but adult survival, is characterized by joint stiffness, corneal clouding, aortic regurgitation, and usually normal intelligence. Surprisingly, this much milder disorder is also the result of α-iduronidase deficiency; it is allelic with Hurler's syndrome, as shown by lack of cross-correction of enzyme activity in cocultures of skin fibroblasts. Phenotypes occur that are clearly intermediate between Hurler's and Scheie's syndromes. It is believed that patients with an intermediate phenotype represent genetic compounds with one Hurler's allele and one Scheie's allele. Although genetic compounds must occur, in any one case their existence is difficult to distinguish from still other mutations of intermediate severity.

Hunter's, or MPS II, syndrome is distinguishable from Hurler's phenotype by the absence of gross corneal clouding and the X-linked recessive inheritance. The infantile form resembles the Hurler's disease phenotype, and a milder form allows survival into adulthood. The severe and mild forms may be allelic, since both are X-linked and share the same enzyme deficiency (iduronosulfate sulfatase).

Sanfilippo's mucopolysaccharidoses (MPS IIIA, IIIB, IIIC, and IIID) are distinguished by the accumulation of heparan sulfate without dermatan or keratan sulfate and by the marked central nervous system involvement with milder somatic involvement. Sanfilippo's mucopolysaccharidosis usually is diagnosed in the evaluation of mental retardation in childhood. Because the somatic features of this MPS are mild, the condition can be overlooked in the evaluation of an apparently isolated central nervous system problem. Death usually occurs during the second or third decade. The MPS III disorders are approximate genocopies. That is, four different enzyme deficiencies give rise to relatively indistinguishable clinical phenotypes with the same storage product. The four MPS III disorders can be diagnosed and distinguished by enzyme assay (Table 331-1).

Morquio's or MPS IV syndrome is distinguished by the absence of mental retardation and the presence of a distinctive bony dystrophy which can be classified as a spondyloepiphyseal dysplasia. Marked hypoplasia of the odontoid process can cause cervical dislocation and usually leads to some degree of spinal cord compression. Aortic regurgitation is frequent. The deficiency of N-acetylgalactosamine-6-sulfate sulfatase is the basis for this condition. Bone changes somewhat suggestive of Morquio's syndrome may also occur in β-galactosidase deficiency and in other forms of spondyloepiphyseal dysplasia. Maroteaux-Lamy's or MPS VI disorder is characterized by prominent osseous involvement, corneal clouding, and normal intellect. Allelic forms with variable severity but the same deficiency of arylsulfatase B (N-acetylhexosamine-4-sulfate sulfatase) have been described. MPS VII, or β-glucuronidase deficiency, has been described in only a few patients with a rather complete MPS phenotype. Extreme variability from a lethal infantile form to a mild adult disease occurs.

MUCOLIPIDOSES Mucolipidosis is a general term for lysosomal storage diseases involving some combination of MPS, glycoprotein, oligosaccharide, and glycolipids. The category of mucolipidosis I probably can be abandoned since most or all of these patients actually have a specific glycoprotein storage disease.

Mucolipidosis II, or I-cell disease, is an early onset disorder with mental retardation and an MPS phenotype. The distinctive features are striking inclusions in cultured skin fibroblasts and markedly elevated serum levels of lysosomal enzymes. The disorder has an autosomal recessive basis and is now known to represent a defect in the posttranslational processing of lysosomal enzymes. Mucolipidosis III, or pseudo-Hurler's polydystrophy, is a milder disorder with many aspects of the MPS phenotype, particularly dysostosis multiplex. The disorder presents in the first decade with joint stiffness, the diagnosis of rheumatoid arthritis often being considered. The major handicaps are progressive physical disabilities, particularly claw hand deformity and hip dysplasia. Mild mental retardation is common. Aortic and/or mitral valvular disease is routinely present, although often not functionally significant. Survival into adult life with possible stabilization of the condition is characteristic, with greater disability in males than in females. Inclusions in cultured skin fibroblasts and elevation of serum lysosomal enzymes are essentially identical with the findings in mucolipidosis II, suggesting that these are allelic disorders. The primary defect in mucolipidosis II and III is deficiency of UDP-N-acetylglucosamine (GLcNAc):glycoprotein GLcNAc-1-phosphotransferase, an enzyme involved in posttranslational synthesis of the oligosaccharide portion of the lysosomal enzymes.

NEURONAL CEROID LIPOFUSCINOSES The neuronal ceroid lipofuscinosis disorders include a wide clinical spectrum with onset in childhood, juvenile, or adult periods. It is uncertain if these disorders are true lysosomal storage diseases, indeed whether single or multiple biochemical genetic disorders are present. The clinical features include central nervous system deterioration with cerebral atrophy, usually commensurate with degree of impairment. Seizures, particularly myoclonic jerks, are prominent. Ocular involvement with optic atrophy, retinitis pigmentosa, and macular degeneration is present in the infantile and juvenile disorders but often absent in adult forms. Autosomal recessive inheritance is likely in most instances. The neuropathologic findings form the basis of the descriptive term for the disease. Electron microscopy demonstrates abnormal inclusions within lysosomes throughout a wide variety of tissues, despite the rather isolated neurologic clinical involvement. The presence of curvilinear bodies, electron-dense material, and fingerprint profiles on electron microscopy of white blood cells, liver biopsy, or muscle biopsy can be helpful diagnostically.

OTHER LYSOSOMAL STORAGE DISEASES Glycogen storage disease type II (Pompe's disease) is the prototype lysosomal storage disease. The predominant clinical features of skeletal and cardiac

myopathy are described in Chap. 332. Some rarer disorders are included in Table 331-1. Multiple sulfatase deficiency is an autosomal recessive disorder characterized by a deficiency of five or more cellular sulfatases: aryl sulfatase A, aryl sulfatase B, other mucopolysaccharide sulfatases, and a nonlysosomal steroid sulfatase. The clinical picture combines features of metachromatic leukodystrophy, an MPS phenotype, and ichthyosis. Other neurodegenerative diseases may eventually be classifiable as lysosomal storage diseases. Disorders such as juvenile dystonic lipidosis, neuroaxonal dystrophy, Hallervorden-Spatz disease, Pelizaeus-Merzbacher disease, and other candidates exist. In addition, it is not unusual to identify patients with distinctive clinical features suggestive of lipidosis, mucolipidosis, or mucopolysaccharidosis, in which none of the present biochemically identifiable disorders can be identified. For these reasons, the number of distinct lysosomal storage diseases is likely to continue to increase.

REFERENCES

ARGOV Z, NAVON R: Clinical and genetic variations in the syndrome of adult GM$_2$ gangliosidosis resulting from hexosaminidase A deficiency. Ann Neurol 16:14, 1984

BEUTLER E: Gaucher disease. Blood Rev 2:59, 1988

DURAND P, O'BRIEN JS (eds): *Genetic Errors of Glycoprotein Metabolism*, Berlin, Springer-Verlag, 1982

LANIR A et al: Gaucher disease: Assessment with MR imaging. Radiology 161:239, 1986

SCRIVER CR et al (eds): *The Metabolic Basis of Inherited Disease*, 6th ed. New York, McGraw-Hill, 1989, chaps 12 and 61–72

TSUJI S et al: Genetic heterogeneity in type 1 Gaucher disease: Multiple genotypes in Ashkenazic and non-Ashkenazic individuals. Proc Natl Acad Sci USA 85:2349, 1988

WALTZ G et al: Adult metachromatic leukodystrophy. Arch Neurol 44:225, 1987

332 THE GLYCOGEN STORAGE DISEASES

ARTHUR L. BEAUDET

The glycogen storage diseases are a group of genetic disorders involving the pathways for storage of carbohydrate as glycogen and for its utilization to maintain blood sugar and to provide energy. Some forms are not associated with actual increases in glycogen content in tissues.

Glycogen is a highly branched polymer of glucose with the majority of residues in 1,4 linkage and with 7 to 10 percent of residues in 1,6 linkage. The treelike structure undergoes addition and removal of residues at its periphery. Glycogen molecules have molecular weights of many millions, and molecules may aggregate to form structures recognizable by electron microscopy. Liver generally contains less than 70 mg glycogen per gram of tissue, and muscle usually contains less than 15 mg/g, but these levels fluctuate as a consequence of feeding and hormonal stimuli. Abnormalities of glycogen structure can result either from decreased or increased branching.

The metabolic pathways involved in glycogen synthesis and breakdown are outlined in Fig. 332-1. These pathways differ among tissues; for example, certain reactions are active in liver but trivial or absent in muscle, and some enzyme functions are encoded by different genes in muscle and liver. Plasma glucose enters the cell and is phosphorylated by glucokinase or hexokinase. The former enzyme is found in liver where it accomplishes the majority of phosphorylation of glucose, while multiple hexokinases are distributed more widely in tissues. Glucose-6-phosphate (G6P) is converted to glucose-1-phosphate (G1P) in a reversible reaction catalyzed by phosphoglucomutase. Uridine diphosphate glucose (UDPG) is synthesized from G1P and UTP by UDPG pyrophosphorylase. Genetic

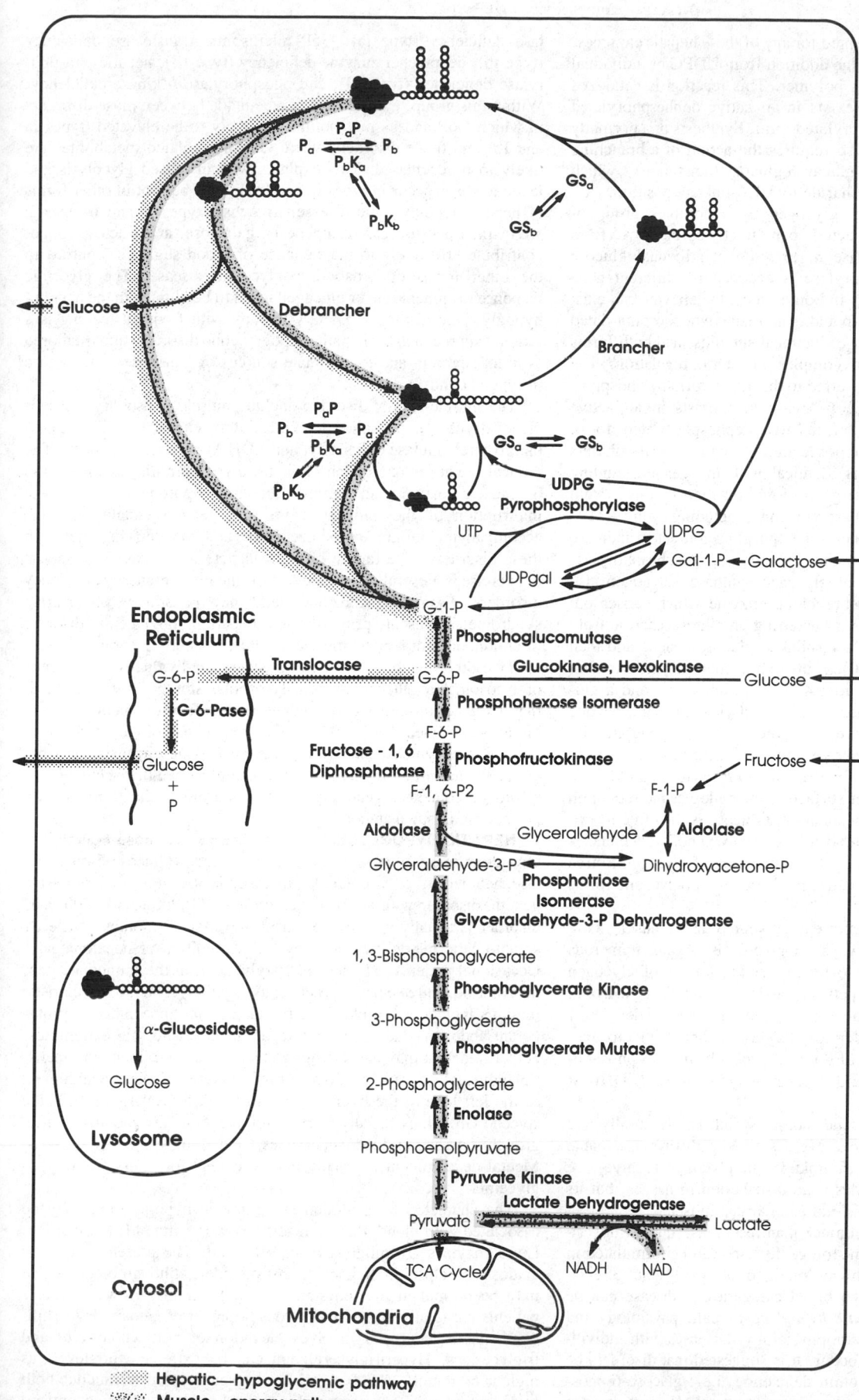

FIGURE 332-1 Metabolic pathways related to glycogen storage disease. A hypothetical composite cell is shown depicting both hepatic and muscle pathways. The shaded areas depict pathways that are blocked in the hepatic-hypoglycemic diseases or in the muscle-energy diseases. Nonstandard abbreviations are as follows: GS_a, active glycogen synthase; GS_b, inactive glycogen synthase; P_a, active phosphorylase; P_b, inactive phosphorylase; P_aP, phosphorylase a phosphatase; P_bK_a, active phosphorylase b kinase; P_bK_b, inactive phosphorylase b kinase.

deficiency has not been documented for any of these hepatic enzymes. Glycogen is then elongated by the addition from UDPG of individual glucose residues to an existing polymer. This reaction is catalyzed by glycogen synthase, which exists in an active dephosphorylated form and in an inactive phosphorylated form. Synthesis of a normally branched glycogen structure also requires the action of a branching enzyme (1,4-α-glucan:1,4-α-glucan-6-glucosyltransferase) which transfers a 1,4-linked oligosaccharide to a 1,6-linkage position.

Glucose is mobilized from glycogen by a complex group of enzyme reactions. Glycogen is acted upon directly by the active form of phosphorylase, phosphorylase a, to remove individual glucose units and yield G1P. Phosphorylase is encoded by different gene products in muscle and in liver. In both tissues, the enzyme can exist in an active phosphorylated form and in an inactive dephosphorylated form. Phosphorylase is a dimer of identical subunits, and both forms of the enzyme are subject to complex allosteric regulation. The inactive phosphorylase b is converted to the active form by phosphorylase b kinase. Phosphorylase b kinase also exists in an active phosphorylated form and in an inactive dephosphorylated form. Phosphorylase b kinase is composed of four nonidentical subunits $(\alpha,\beta,\gamma,\delta)_4$, and the δ chain is identical with the calcium-binding protein calmodulin. The rate of glucose mobilization by this system is regulated by a cascade of kinase reactions, including cyclic AMP–dependent protein kinase. Epinephrine and glucagon act to increase blood sugar via this cascade system by activation of phosphorylase and simultaneous inactivation of glycogen synthase. Glycogen also is acted upon directly by a debranching enzyme which carries out the debranching process by first transferring an oligosaccharide from a branch point to leave a single 1,6-linked glucose residue and then hydrolyzing the 1,6 linkage. Thus, the debrancher enzyme has both glucan transferase activity (oligo-1,4 → 1,4-transferase) and a glucosidase (amylo-1,6-glucosidase) activity and yields a single residue of glucose for each branch point removed. The G1P generated by phosphorylase, as mentioned above, must be further metabolized to G6P by phosphoglucomutase. In the liver G6P is transported by a specific translocase to the inner surface of the endoplasmic reticulum for hydrolysis by glucose-6-phosphatase. Glucose is then free to exit the hepatic cell to maintain blood levels. Many genetic deficiencies occur in the enzymes required for the conversion of glycogen to free glucose in the liver, and these cause the hepatic-hypoglycemic forms of glycogen storage disease.

If glycogen is used as a direct energy source, as in muscle, G6P and G1P must enter the pathways for glycolysis. Again, numerous enzymes are required in muscle for proper breakdown of glycogen and entry into the glycolytic pathway and tricarboxylic acid cycle. The enzymatic steps known to be associated with genetic deficiency states in muscle include muscle phosphorylase, debranching enzyme, muscle phosphofructokinase (PFK), and probably muscle phosphoglycerate mutase (PGAM) and lactate dehydrogenase (LDH) M subunit.

The lysosomal enzyme α-glucosidase, which is structurally and metabolically separate from the above-described pathways, is capable of degrading both 1,4 and 1,6 linkages in glycogen to give free glucose. This enzyme has widespread distribution in tissues, but its deficiency affects primarily skeletal and cardiac muscle.

CLASSIFICATION The clinical manifestations, diagnostic criteria, and therapy for glycogen storage diseases can be formulated in terms of the metabolic pathway outlined above (Table 332-1). According to this schema, two broad categories of disease can be delineated—those with a *hepatic-hypoglycemic* pathophysiology and those with a *muscle-energy* pathophysiology. Diseases with individualized pathophysiology also occur. It is suggested that disorders be designated by the specific protein deficiency, i.e., glucose-6-phosphatase deficiency. Although the roman numeral designations for types I through VII are in widespread use, numbering for higher types is confused and is to be avoided. Eponyms are of historical interest.

The hepatic-hypoglycemic disorders include glucose-6-phospha-tase deficiency (type Ia), G6P microsomal translocase deficiency (type Ib), debrancher enzyme deficiency (type III), hepatic phosphorylase deficiency (type VI), and phosphorylase b kinase deficiency. Within this group, a distinction can be made between those disorders in which G6P and its metabolites are likely to be elevated (types Ia and Ib) and those disorders where G6P and related metabolites are likely to be decreased. This explains why increased glycolysis and lactic acidosis occur in types Ia and Ib disease but not in other forms of hepatic-hypoglycemic disease. Likewise, types Ia and Ib disease are distinct because gluconeogenesis, galactose, and fructose cannot contribute effectively to maintenance of blood sugar, in contrast to the other forms of hepatic-hypoglycemic disease. The glycemic response to epinephrine or glucagon tends to be blunted in the hepatic-hypoglycemic disorders. Dietary therapy with frequent feeding is a rational approach to the hepatic-hypoglycemic disorders and is tailored to reduce protein and to eliminate sources of galactose and fructose in types Ia and Ib disease.

The muscle-energy disorders include muscle phosphorylase deficiency (type V), phosphofructokinase deficiency (type VII), phosphoglycerate mutase deficiency, and LDH M-subunit deficiency. The clinical picture is one of muscle pain, myoglobinuria, and elevation of muscle enzymes in serum following vigorous exercise. The interruption of the pathway from glycogen to lactate with the accompanying failure to oxidize NADH is the unifying theme in these disorders. The failure of blood lactate to increase in response to exercise is a useful diagnostic test for the muscle-energy deficiency disorders. Debrancher enzyme deficiency constitutes an overlap syndrome; it presents primarily as a hepatic-hypoglycemic disorder in childhood, but serious muscle weakness occurs in some adults.

Two other disorders are best considered individually. Deficiency of lysosomal α-glucosidase is a lysosomal storage disease without major impact on either carbohydrate metabolism or maintenance of blood sugar (see Chap. 331). The major pathologic process in branching enzyme deficiency is a severe hepatic cirrhosis, possibly due to the harmful effects of the abnormal glycogen that accumulates. Glycogen content is generally normal, and the ability to maintain a normal blood sugar is not impaired.

HEPATIC-HYPOGLYCEMIC   DISEASES   Glucose-6-phosphatase deficiency, type Ia CLINICAL FEATURES   Glucose-6-phosphatase deficiency, or von Gierke disease, is an autosomal recessive genetic disorder with an incidence of 1 in 100,000 to 400,000. The disorder is usually manifested during the first 12 months of life by symptomatic hypoglycemia or by the recognition of hepatomegaly. Occasional patients experience hypoglycemia in the immediate neonatal period, and rare patients never have hypoglycemia. Characteristic findings include a full-cheeked, rounded facial appearance; a protuberant abdomen due to marked hepatomegaly; and thin extremities. Hyperlipidemia may cause eruptive xanthomas and lipemia retinalis. Splenomegaly is usually mild or absent, although massive enlargement of the left lobe of the liver may be mistaken for enlargement of the spleen. Growth is usually normal for the first few months of life; growth retardation then supervenes, and adolescence is delayed. Mental development is usually normal except for injury from hypoglycemia.

The characteristic profound symptomatic hypoglycemia may be associated with blood glucose levels below 0.8 mmol/L (15 mg/dL). Liver enzymes are mildly elevated if at all. The presence of lactic acidosis is helpful in diagnosing this disorder, although blood lactate may be normal in the fed state in young infants. However, these patients are relatively resistant to development of ketosis. Hyperlipidemia is frequent and involves elevation of both cholesterol and triglycerides. Hypertriglyceridemia can be extreme with levels as high as 60 mmol/L (5000 mg/dL) or higher. Hyperuricemia due both to decreased renal excretion and increased production is frequent and often becomes more severe after adolescence. The rise in plasma glucose following administration of epinephrine or glucagon is impaired, as is the rise in blood glucose following administration of galactose by mouth. The pathogenesis of most of the metabolic

TABLE 332-1 Glycogen storage diseases

Type	Basic defect*	Clinical findings	Laboratory	Diagnosis	Treatment	Comments
DISORDERS WITH HEPATIC-HYPOGLYCEMIC PATHOPHYSIOLOGY						
Ia von Gierke	Glucose-6-phospha-tase deficiency	Hypoglycemia, hepatomegaly, bleeding diathesis, short stature, delayed adolescence, hepatic adenomas, enlarged kidneys	Increased lactate, cholesterol, tri-glyceride, and uric acid	Enzyme assay on liver or intestine, increased glycogen with normal structure in liver	Frequent feeding, nighttime tube feeding, 60–70% carbohydrate, restrict sucrose and lactose, bicarbonate and allopurinol as needed	Common, severe, autosomal recessive
Ib	G6P microsomal translocase deficiency	As for Ia with addition of neutropenia and recurrent infection	As for Ia	Enzyme assay on liver with and without detergent	As for Ia	Rare, severe, autosomal recessive
III Cori	Debrancher enzyme deficiency	Hypoglycemia, hepatomegaly, some short stature and delayed adolescence, mild myopathy worsening in some adults	Normal lactate and uric acid; increased cholesterol, triglyceride, and SGOT	Enzyme assay on liver, muscle, or fibroblasts; leukocytes variable; increased glycogen with abnormal structure in liver and muscle	Frequent feeding, nighttime tube feeding, 50% carbohydrate and 15–20% protein	Common, intermediate severity, some hepatic fibrosis
VI Hers	Hepatic phosphorylase deficiency	Hepatomegaly, variable hypoglycemia	Minimal changes, ? hyperlipidemia	Enzyme assay on liver, increased hepatic glycogen with normal structure	Dietary therapy as for type III, often little treatment required	Rare and poorly characterized; ? autosomal recessive
Formerly VIb, VIII, or IX	Hepatic phosphorylase b kinase deficiency	Hepatomegaly, variable hypoglycemia, occasional findings in heterozygous females	Minimal changes	Enzyme assay on leukocytes, fibroblasts, or liver; increased hepatic glycogen with normal structure	Dietary therapy as for type III, often little treatment required	Very mild but may be fairly common, X-linked
DISORDERS WITH MUSCLE-ENERGY PATHOPHYSIOLOGY						
V McArdle	Muscle phosphorylase deficiency	Pain, cramps, and myoglobinuria on strenuous exercise	Increased CPK with episodes, deficient lactate production with ischemic exercise test	Muscle enzyme assay, increased muscle glycogen with normal structure	Avoid exercise, glucose or fructose before exercise	Some clearly autosomal recessive, male preponderance
VII	Muscle phosphofructokinase deficiency	As for type V, mild hemolytic anemia	As for type V	Muscle enzyme assay, increased muscle glycogen with normal structure	As for type V	Rare, autosomal recessive
	Muscle phosphoglycerate mutase deficiency	As for type V	As for Type V	Muscle enzyme assay, normal glycogen content	? As for type V	Based on one affected male
	LDH M-subunit deficiency	As for type V	Increased CPK with episodes; pyruvate but not lactate rises with ischemic exercise test	LDH isozymes on serum, erythrocytes or leukocytes; enzyme assay on muscle; ? glycogen content normal	? As for type V	Based on sibship of 3 males and 1 female affected
DISORDERS WITH INDIVIDUAL PATHOPHYSIOLOGY						
II Pompe	Lysosomal α-glucosidase deficiency	*Infantile:* hypotonia, muscle weakness, cardiac enlargement and failure, enlarged tongue, fatal early; *juvenile:* progressive skeletal muscle weakness; *adult:* progressive skeletal muscle weakness, pulmonary insufficiency presentation	Increased CPK, no hypoglycemia	Enzymes assay on muscle or fibroblasts, enzyme assay on leukocytes possible but pitfalls are serious	No effective treatment	Common, autosomal recessive, prenatal diagnosis available and widely utilized in infantile
IV Andersen	Brancher enzyme deficiency	Infantile failure to thrive, cirrhosis and liver failure, extreme hypotonia and weakness in some, fatal early	No hypoglycemia, changes of liver disease	Enzyme assay on liver, muscle, leukocytes or fibroblasts; glycogen content not remarkable but structure abnormal	No effective treatment	Very rare, autosomal recessive

* These defects provide the preferred nomenclature for the diseases.

abnormalities is not well understood; lactic acidosis may be due to increased glycolysis, and other abnormalities including poor growth may be the result of chronically altered levels of insulin and glucagon. Renal enlargement can be demonstrated by radiologic or sonographic techniques. Mild renal tubular dysfunction or the Fanconi syndrome may occur. Moderate anemia is usually due to recurrent nosebleeds and chronic acidosis but may become severe after prolonged acidosis. A bleeding diathesis is due to a platelet dysfunction.

Once type Ia disease is suspected clinically, the diagnosis is established by liver biopsy. Type Ia disease is suggested by lactic acidosis, an abnormal galactose tolerance test, or renal enlargement. Proper handling of biopsy material should be arranged to distinguish types Ia and Ib. Sufficient material for enzyme assay may be obtained by needle biopsy provided the bleeding time is normal, or alternatively, open liver biopsy provides more tissue for analysis. Microscopic examination of liver reveals increased glycogen in cytoplasm and nuclei; lipid vacuoles in hepatocytes are prominent, and fibrosis is usually absent.

The hypoglycemia and lactic acid acidosis may be life-threatening. Other troublesome features include short stature, delayed adolescence, and hyperuricemia. During adult years uric acid nephropathy and glomerulosclerosis may lead to renal failure. Hepatic adenomata are common after adolescence. There is a significant risk of hepatic malignant degeneration, often during the third decade, and subjects who live long enough are probably at increased risk for atherosclerosis.

TREATMENT   The mainstay of management is frequent feeding. The most widely used approach in children has been the combination of frequent daytime feeding by mouth and continuous nighttime feeding by nasogastric tube (see Chap. 74). The regimen should include approximately 60 percent carbohydrate, and no significant portion of carbohydrate should come from sources containing galactose or fructose, which cannot be utilized effectively to maintain blood sugar. Raw cornstarch feeding provides a convenient, economical, and palatable source of slowly digested glucose polymer, and cornstarch therapy may become the primary dietary treatment for this disease. The ability of a family to carry out such a program is a significant variable, but in some instances the metabolic abnormalities and the rate of growth have improved substantially. Optimal management requires a team attentive to the dietary and psychosocial needs of patient and family. Control of elevated plasma urate may require the addition of allopurinol. This regimen provides a reasonably optimistic short-term prognosis, but it is not known whether the long-term risks of hepatic malignancy and atherosclerosis are ameliorated. Portacaval anastomosis is no longer used in the management of glycogen storage disease. Prenatal diagnosis is not possible at present.

G6P microsomal translocase deficiency, type Ib   G6P microsomal translocase deficiency, historically referred to as *pseudo type I,* has an incidence of one-fifth to one-tenth that of type Ia. The term *microsomal translocase* describes the capacity to transport G6P into the endoplasmic reticulum. The clinical features are similar to those in type Ia, but unique features include neutropenia, impaired neutrophil migration, and recurrent pyogenic infections; in general, type Ib is more severe than Ia. Laboratory findings, responses to tolerance tests, and management are similar in the two disorders.

Type Ib disease was initially distinguished from type Ia by the presence of normal glucose-6-phosphatase activity on assay of biopsy tissue in the presence of detergent. However, glucose-6-phosphatase activity is low in type Ib disease when fresh tissue is homogenized and assayed in the absence of detergent. These results have been interpreted to imply a genetic deficiency of a microsomal G6P transport system as a primary defect in type Ib glycogen storage disease. The cause for the neutropenia and abnormal neutrophil migration is unknown, although the disease suggests a role for G6P transport in these cells.

Debrancher deficiency, type III   CLINICAL FEATURES   Debrancher enzyme deficiency, also known historically as Cori disease, is an autosomal recessive disorder and is one of the more frequent forms of glycogen storage diseases, occurring with a particularly high

frequency in North African Jews. Symptomatic disease in the newborn period is unusual, and patients usually present with hypoglycemia or hepatomegaly during the first year of life. The physical findings are similar to those in type Ia, except that splenomegaly is more prominent, but the clinical course tends to be less severe. The skeletal or cardiac myopathy is usually mild or insignificant in childhood but may be disabling and progressive in adults. Some patients with myopathy are first diagnosed as adults because the features in childhood were mild and overlooked.

Fasting hypoglycemia occurs in about 80 percent of patients. The glucose response after glucagon or epinephrine is abnormal in the fasting state but may be normal shortly after eating since the terminal glucose residues in glycogen can be mobilized. The galactose tolerance test is usually normal. Ketosis is prominent, and blood lactate is normal. Serum transaminase is elevated, and further increases may occur with minor illnesses. Blood cholesterol and triglyceride are elevated in about two-thirds. Hyperuricemia is rare.

Two diagnostic modalities are used to establish the diagnosis—analysis of glycogen and measurement of debranching enzyme in tissue samples. The glycogen content of red blood cells and liver is increased in almost all, whereas glycogen content of muscle is increased only in some. Documentation of abnormal structure of glycogen with the use of spectrophotometric techniques is a more consistent finding than the increase in glycogen content. The establishment of the diagnosis by enzymatic assay is complicated both by methodologic problems and what is believed to be genetic heterogeneity. Both debrancher functions—the glucan transferase activity and glucosidase activity—are believed to reside in a single polypeptide, but as many as six subtypes of the disease may occur. While the diagnosis can be made in some patients using red cells, leukocytes, or fibroblasts, it is generally preferable to document the abnormal glycogen structure and the enzyme deficiency directly in biopsy material from liver or muscle. The pathologic findings in liver are similar to those in type Ia except for less lipid deposition and more prominent fibrous septae.

In regard to growth retardation and abdominal protuberance, the course is one of progressive improvement following adolescence, so that the adult appearance may be normal and hypoglycemia is less frequent. Liver tumors are not reported, and there is no information regarding the long-term risks of hyperlipidemia. The fraction of adult patients who develop a debilitating myopathy is probably low. Affected patients have had children.

TREATMENT   Frequent feeding is also the mainstay of therapy for type III in childhood. Gluconeogenesis is normal and, as described above, patients can ingest galactose, fructose, or protein to help maintain blood glucose. Thus, dietary therapy can include a larger percentage of calories as protein, but carbohydrate intake should be 40 to 50 percent of the total. An evening feeding is often sufficient to avoid hypoglycemia, but nighttime nasogastric tube feeding or cornstarch therapy may be required in severely affected children. Attempts to lower blood lipids using dietary means are desirable. Prenatal diagnosis is possible.

Hepatic phosphorylase deficiency, type VI   The diagnosis of hepatic phosphorylase deficiency, or Hers disease, was previously applied to a diverse group of patients with reduced hepatic phosphorylase levels due to a variety of causes but is now limited to patients in whom deficiency of hepatic phosphorylase is the primary defect. This nosologic difficulty is a consequence of the fact that phosphorylase exists in both active and inactive forms, and many factors may inhibit the activation of the enzyme secondarily. Consequently, diagnosis requires documentation that phosphorylase is absent and that the phosphorylase *b* kinase responsible for its activation is normal. The disorder is probably due to an autosomal recessive mutation.

Most patients have features similar to those in type III but in a milder form. The diagnosis is suspected because of hepatomegaly or hypoglycemia, and patients generally respond to dietary management similar to that employed in type III disease.

Phosphorylase *b* kinase deficiency Phosphorylase *b* kinase deficiency, now known to be a separate entity, was previously included in the type VI category. Various authors have designated this disorder as type VIa, type VIII, or type IX, but it is best termed *phosphorylase b kinase deficiency*. The best characterized form of the disorder is the X-linked variety, but there is potential for genetic heterogeneity, since the enzyme is composed of four nonidentical subunits. This disorder is relatively benign and is manifested in affected males by hepatomegaly, occasional fasting hypoglycemia, and some growth retardation, all of which tend to resolve spontaneously at the time of adolescence. Mild hepatomegaly may occur in female heterozygotes. The diagnosis can be established by specific enzyme assay of leukocytes or liver. Muscle phosphorylase *b* kinase is believed to be normal in this condition. Dietary management similar to that employed in type III can be employed for hypoglycemia or growth retardation. It is possible that this condition is relatively common and passes undiagnosed. Healthy adults with a history of abdominal protuberance in childhood are often identified during family studies of patients with this condition.

MUSCLE-ENERGY DISEASES (See also Chap. 365) In recognizing the various glycogen storage diseases that affect muscle, the *ischemic exercise test* is of particular use in the initial evaluation. A blood pressure cuff is inflated above arterial pressure, and the ischemic hand is exercised to maximum effort. The pressure cuff is released, and blood is drawn from the other arm at 2, 5, 10, 20, and 30 min for assay of lactate and pyruvate, muscle enzymes, and myoglobin.

Myophosphorylase deficiency, type V Myophosphorylase deficiency, or McArdle disease, is uncommon. Symptoms of pain and cramps after exercise usually develop during the second or third decade. A history of myoglobinuria is present in most, and on occasion myoglobinuria can cause renal failure. Affected individuals are otherwise healthy, without evidence of hepatic, cardiac, or metabolic disturbance. Performance of an ischemic exercise test usually causes painful cramping, which is helpful diagnostically. In addition, blood lactate does not rise whereas serum creatine phosphokinase is elevated after strenuous exercise.

The diagnosis is established by documentation of elevated glycogen content and reduced phosphorylase activity in biopsied muscle tissue. The glycogen is usually deposited in subsarcolemmal regions of the muscle. The gene for human myophosphorylase has been cloned and is located on chromosome 11, in keeping with the autosomal recessive nature of the disease. There is an excess of male patients, which may be due to better ascertainment in males, genetic heterogeneity, or other factors. A fatal infantile form of hypotonia in association with myophosphorylase deficiency also has been described.

Management of myophosphorylase deficiency requires the avoidance of strenuous exercise. Glucose or fructose ingestion prior to exercise can reduce symptoms.

Muscle phosphofructokinase deficiency, type VII There are two genetically distinct forms of phosphofructokinase. Activity in muscle is due to a distinct muscle isoenzyme, whereas activity in red cells is due both to a red cell isoenzyme and to the muscle form of the enzyme. A small number of families have been identified with deficiency of the muscle isoenzyme. Symptoms similar to those in myophosphorylase deficiency were present with pain and cramps, myoglobinuria, and elevated muscle enzymes in serum after strenuous exercise. Lactate production was impaired, and a mild nonspherocytic hemolytic anemia was present. Other patients have the anemia but no muscle symptoms; the latter phenomenon might be due to a qualitatively abnormal, unstable enzyme that rapidly disappears from the anucleate red cell but is replaced effectively in muscle cells and consequently prevents muscle symptoms.

Other muscle-energy diseases A group of even rarer familial metabolic disorders must be considered in the differential diagnosis of patients with myoglobinuria and elevated muscle enzymes in serum after exercise. These include phosphoglycerate mutase deficiency, LDH M-subunit deficiency, and carnitine palmityl transferase deficiency. (Older reports of phosphoglucomutase deficiency and phosphohexoseisomerase deficiency seem inconclusive by current standards.) When myophosphorylase, phosphofructokinase, or phosphoglycerate mutase are deficient, neither lactate nor pyruvate rises following exercise, whereas in deficiency of LDH M subunit there is a rise in pyruvate in the face of a failure of lactate production. Carnitine palmityl transferase deficiency is a disorder of lipid metabolism and is discussed in Chap. 320. Definitive diagnosis of these disorders must be established by enzyme assay of muscle tissue. Some patients with this clinical presentation have none of the above-mentioned enzyme deficiencies, and identification of other defects in muscle metabolism is likely in the future.

DISORDERS WITH INDIVIDUAL PATHOPHYSIOLOGY α-Glucosidase deficiency, type II Alpha-glucosidase deficiency, or Pompe disease, is a lysosomal storage disease, and the pathophysiology is discussed in Chap. 331. The incidence is not known but may exceed 1 in 100,000. The disorder is not associated with hypoglycemia, ketosis, or other abnormalities of intermediary metabolism.

The infantile form presents within the first 6 months of life and may be manifested at birth. Clinical features include skeletal muscle hypotonia and weakness, massive cardiac enlargement, enlargement of the tongue, and varying degrees of hepatomegaly. Muscle enzymes such as creatine phosphokinase and aldolase are usually elevated, and the ECG may show large QRS complexes and a shortened PR interval. Motor weakness and developmental delay may be present. Death occurs in the first 2 to 3 years in most cases due to the cardiac involvement.

The juvenile form has features suggestive of a progressive form of muscular dystrophy. These patients have gait abnormalities but no cardiac symptoms. Plasma creatine phosphokinase and aldolase are elevated, and the length of survival is variable. An even milder adult form presents as skeletal muscle weakness in the third to the fifth decade. Again, cardiac symptoms are absent, and serum muscle enzymes are elevated. Some patients have respiratory failure due to involvement of the muscles of respiration and are often misdiagnosed as having some form of muscular dystrophy.

Vacuolization of muscle and increased glycogen content are demonstrable on muscle biopsy. Electron-microscopic studies demonstrate membrane-bound vacuoles containing glycogen, a finding strongly suggestive of the disorder. Excessive glycogen is also found in other tissues including liver and central nervous system, particularly in the anterior horn cells of the spinal cord. Specific diagnosis is made by enzyme assay in biopsy material from muscle or liver or in cultured skin fibroblasts. In general, some residual enzyme activity is present in patients with the adult form of disease, but the exact level is not of prognostic significance. Prenatal diagnosis is reliable and has been used extensively for the infantile form. Various forms of enzyme infusion therapy have been tried but are ineffective.

Brancher deficiency, type IV Brancher enzyme deficiency, or Andersen disease, is a rare, autosomal recessive disorder. Features in infants include hepatomegaly, failure to thrive, and hypotonia in the first few months of life with subsequent development of progressive cirrhosis. In other patients the predominant feature is cardiac involvement and/or extreme hypotonia similar to that observed in spinal muscular atrophy and anterior horn cell degeneration. Death usually occurs within the first 2 or 3 years, although a more benign course is possible.

The symptoms are thought to be related primarily to the abnormal glycogen structure that results from a generalized deficiency of brancher enzyme. The presence of long outer chains on the glycogen molecules has led to the designation of the disease as amylopectinosis. The laboratory findings are generally those associated with severe liver disease except that hypoglycemia usually does not occur. The absence of hypoglycemia and the presence of normal glycogen content in the liver make the diagnosis difficult to establish. The diagnosis is suggested by finding abnormally structured glycogen in biopsy material and is established by direct assay of the enzyme in liver, leukocytes, or cultured skin fibroblasts. No effective treatment is known, but prenatal diagnosis is possible using cultured amniotic cells.

Other possible disorders of glycogen metabolism   Deficiency of glycogen synthase has been reported in a small number of families. Affected patients usually have fasting hypoglycemia, seizures, and some degree of mental impairment. The presence of some hepatic glycogen, the increase in plasma glucose in response to glucagon or galactose, and the known lability of the activation system for glycogen synthase have all led to skepticism as to whether such a disorder actually exists. This syndrome may be confused with ketotic hypoglycemia of childhood (see Chap. 320).

There are also reports of more than one enzyme defect in the same patient and of different enzyme defects among siblings. Many of these reports may be related to difficulties inherent in measuring enzymes of glycogen metabolism in human pathologic tissue. At present no specific syndrome of multiple primary enzyme deficiency is documented.

REFERENCES

CHEN Y-T et al: Renal disease in type I glycogen storage disease. N Engl J Med 318:7, 1988

FERNANDEZ J et al: Glycogen storage disease. Recommendations for treatment. Eur J Pediatr 147:226, 1988

HERS H-G et al: Glycogen storage diseases, in *The Metabolic Basis of Inherited Disease*, 6th ed, CR Scriver et al (eds). New York, McGraw-Hill, 1989, p 425

MOSES SW et al: Neuromuscular involvement in glycogen storage disease type III. Acta Paediatr Scand 75:289, 1986

333   HERITABLE DISORDERS OF CONNECTIVE TISSUE

DARWIN J. PROCKOP

Heritable disorders that involve the major connective tissues of the body such as bone, ligaments, blood vessels, and skin are among the most common genetic diseases in humans. The three major categories of the diseases are osteogenesis imperfecta (OI), Ehlers-Danlos syndrome (EDS), and the Marfan syndrome (MS). This system of classification is in part historical and is in part based on the clusters of signs and symptoms in patients and in affected members of their families. Some patients are readily classified as OI because their bones are so brittle they suffer multiple fractures from minor trauma, and they have characteristic features such as blue sclerae and opalescent teeth. Some patients are easily recognized as EDS because their skin is grossly hyperelastic and ligaments are so loose that permanent dislocations develop in major joints. Similarly, many patients can be unequivocally classified as MS because of the characteristic triad of long and thin extremities, dislocations of the lenses, and life-threatening aortic aneurysms. However, many patients are difficult to classify because they have one or two cardinal features of one of the diseases but lack the others, and some patients have signs and symptoms of more than one of these diseases, e.g., blue sclerae suggestive of OI and joint dislocations suggestive of EDS. Attempts have been made to overcome these problems of nosology by defining a series of subtypes of the three major disease categories. However, the value of the more elaborate classification schemes has not been fully established. Many patients still cannot be precisely categorized. Moreover, many of the clinically defined types and subtypes do not reflect the mutations that cause the diseases. For example, most patients with OI have mutations that change the primary structure of type I procollagen. However, similar mutations changing the structure of type I procollagen occur in some patients

with type VII EDS who have permanent joint dislocations but not fractures. At the same time, data on the molecular defects are not complete enough or readily enough available on individual patients to develop a new scheme of classification. Therefore, the current classification of OI, EDS, and MS based primarily on clinical criteria remains the best available system for diagnosis even though it will eventually be replaced by classifications based on the molecular defects that cause the diseases. Also, it is likely that additional information about the molecular defects will blur the distinction now made between OI, MS, and EDS and more common diseases of connective tissue such as familial forms of osteoporosis and aortic aneurysms.

DEFINITION AND CHEMICAL COMPOSITION OF CONNECTIVE TISSUES   Connective tissues are loosely defined as the extracellular compartments and components that provide the structural support of the body and bind together its cells, organs, and tissues. The major connective tissues are bone, skin, tendons, ligaments, and cartilage. The term is also applied to blood vessels and to synovial spaces and fluids. Indeed, all organs and tissues contain some connective tissue in the form of membranes and septa.

Connective tissues contain large amounts of water, salt, albumin, and other components of plasma. The distinguishing feature of connective tissues, however, is that they contain a series of specific macromolecules that are assembled into a large and insoluble extracellular matrix (Table 333-1). The macromolecules include at least 13 different types of collagens, the related fibrous protein known as elastin, a series of proteoglycans, and additional components whose structure and function have been only partially defined.

Connective tissues such as bone, skin, and cartilage obviously differ both in appearance and function. The differences are in part explained by differences in their content of specific macromolecules. For example, tendons and ligaments consist primarily of type I collagen fibrils associated with other types of collagen that bind to and probably help organize the fibrils of type I collagen into larger fibers. Cartilage consists primarily of fibrils of type II collagen in the form of arcade-like structures that are distended by the presence of highly charged proteoglycans. Large blood vessels such as the aorta contain several different kinds of collagens and large amounts of elastin. The differences between the different connective tissues, however, also depend on variations in the size, orientation, and packing of collagen fibrils. The type I collagen fibrils in tendon are packed into thick, parallel bundles of fibers. In skin, type I collagen fibrils are randomly oriented in the plane of the skin. In cortical bone, type I collagen fibrils are deposited in intricate helical arrays around haversian canals. Therefore, the morphology and function of connective tissues are in part based on their content of specific macromolecules and in part on the three-dimensional organization of the macromolecules.

BIOSYNTHESIS OF CONNECTIVE TISSUE   Assembly of the massive structures found in connective tissues is largely governed by the principle of *self-assembly,* whereby a molecular subunit of the correct size, shape, and surface properties binds to other molecules with the same structure, or with similar structures, in a spontaneous and highly ordered manner. Therefore, the molecular mechanisms and driving forces are similar to those involved in the formation of large inorganic crystals and organic polymers.

The principle of self-assembly of macromolecules in connective tissues is best illustrated by the assembly of collagen into fibrils. The collagen molecule is a long, thin rod consisting of three α-polypeptide chains wrapped into a rigid, ropelike triple helix not found in most other proteins (Fig. 333-1). Collagen has a triple-helical conformation, because each of the three α chains has a simple, repetitive amino acid sequence. Glycine (Gly) appears as every third amino acid. Therefore, the central sequence of 1,014 amino acids in each α chain can be designed as $(-Gly-X-Y-)_{338}$, where X and Y represent amino acids other than glycine. It is essential that every third amino acid be glycine, the smallest amino acid, since this residue must fit in a sterically restricted space where the three chains of the triple helix

TABLE 333-1   Constituents of connective tissue in various tissues

Connective tissue	Known constituents	Approximate amounts (% dry wt)	Characteristics
Skin (dermis), ligaments, tendons	Type I collagen	80	Bundles of fibers of high tensile strength
	Type III collagen	5 to 15	Thin fibrils
	Type IV collagen, laminin, entactin, nidogen	<5	In basal laminae under epithelium and in blood vessels
	Types V to VII	<5	Distributions and functions unclear
	Fibronectin	<5	Associated with collagen fibers and cell surfaces
	Proteoglycans*	0.5	Provides resiliency
	Hyaluronate	0.5	Provides resiliency
Bone (demineralized)	Type I collagen	90	Complex organization of fibrils
	Type V collagen	1 to 2	Function unclear
	Proteoglycans	1	Function unclear
	Sialoproteins	1	Function unclear
	Osteonectin	2 to 3	Role in ossification
	Osteocalcin	1	Probable role in ossification
	α_2-Glycoprotein	1	Possible role in ossification
Aorta	Type I collagen	20 to 40	
	Type III collagen	20 to 40	Thin fibrils
	Elastin, microfibrillar protein	20 to 40	Amorphous, elastic fibrils
	Type IV collagen, laminin, entactin, nidogen	<5	In basal lamina
	Types V and VI collagens	<2	Functions unclear
	Proteoglycans	<3	Mucopolysaccharides, mainly chondroitin sulfate and dermatan sulfate; heparan sulfate in basal lamina
Cartilage	Type II collagen	40 to 50	Thin fibrils
	Types IX and X collagen	5 to 25	Possible role in maturation
	Proteoglycans	15 to 50	Provides resiliency
	Hyaluronate	0.5 to 2	Provides resiliency

* Proteoglycan structures are incompletely defined. About five different protein cores have been identified, and each has one or more kind of mucopolysaccharides attached. Major mucopolysaccharides of skin and tendon are dermatan sulfate and chondroitin-4-sulfate; of aorta, chondroitin-4-sulfate and dermatan sulfate; of cartilage, chondroitin-4-sulfate, chondroitin-6-sulfate, and keratan sulfate. Basal lamina contains heparan sulfate.

come together. The X- and Y-position amino acids are frequently the ring amino acids proline and hydroxyproline, which give rigidity to the triple helical structure. The remaining X- and Y-position amino acids form clusters of hydrophobic and charged regions on the surface of the molecule that direct how one molecule spontaneously binds to other collagen molecules and thereby self-assembles into the large collagen fibrils found in tissues (Fig. 333-1).

About half of the 13 or so collagens in the body are called fibrillar because they form similar fibrils. Each contains three α chains that are folded into a triple helix. Type I collagen contains two identical

FIGURE 333-1 Schematic representation of synthesis of a type I collagen fibril by a fibroblast. *A.* Intracellular steps in the assembly of the procollagen molecule. Hydroxylations and glycosylations of the proα chains begin soon after the *N* termini pass into the cisternae of the rough endoplasmic reticulum and continue after the three chains associate through their *C*-propeptides and become disulfide-linked. *B.* Cleavage of procollagen to collagen, self-assembly of the collagen molecule into quarter-staggered fibrils, and cross-linking of the molecules in the fibrils. Cleavage of the propeptides may occur within crypts of the fibroblast, as shown here, or some distance from the cell. (*Reproduced with permission from Prockop and Kivirikko.*)

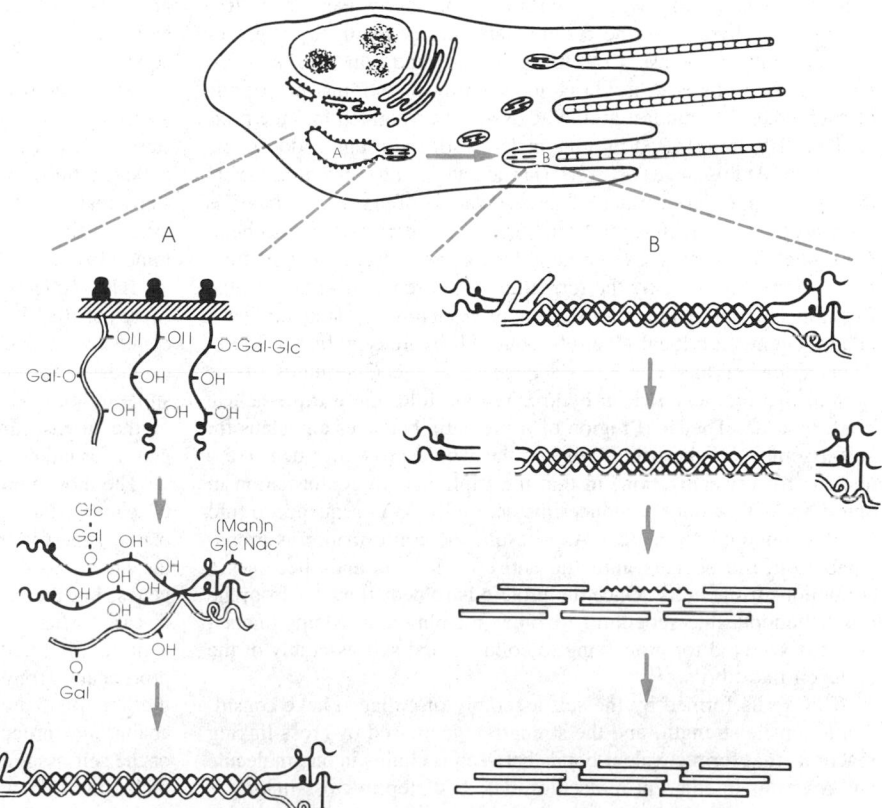

α chains called α1(I) and one slightly different chain called α2(I). Type II collagen and the type III collagen contain three identical chains called α1(II) and α1(III), respectively. About half of the known collagens are nonfibrillar. They are similar to the fibrillar collagens in that they contain -Gly-X-Y- sequences of amino acids that form triple-helical domains, but they also contain large globular domains. Self-assembly of most of the nonfibrillar collagens involves binding together of the globular domains to form networklike structures. For example, the type IV collagen found in basement membranes self-assembles into an amorphous network that provides a diffusion barrier and support for epithelial and endothelial cells in the renal glomerulus, skin, and most blood vessels.

Because fibrillar collagens spontaneously self-assemble into fibrils, they are first synthesized as larger and more soluble precursors called procollagens. The procollagen forms of type I, II, and III collagens are 1.5 times the mass of the corresponding collagens. The additional mass is in the form of amino acid sequences located at both the N-terminus and C-terminus of the molecule and called propeptides. To generate collagen fibrils, the N-terminal propeptides of procollagen must be cleaved by a specific procollagen N-proteinase, and the C-terminal propeptides must be cleaved by a specific procollagen C-proteinase. The cleavage of procollagens to collagens occurs after the molecules are secreted. The rates and order in which the propeptides are cleaved in different tissues probably influence the number of collagen fibrils formed and their morphology.

Assembly of the procollagens from the constitutive polypeptide chains, called proα chains, requires a large number of intracellular processing steps (Fig. 333-1). It also involves an unusual self-assembly step whereby the three chains fold into a triple-helical conformation. As the proα chains of procollagen are translated from mRNA on ribosomes, they pass into the cisternae of the rough endoplasmic reticulum. Hydrophobic "signal peptides" at the N-terminus are cleaved, and a series of additional posttranslational reactions begins. Proline residues in the Y position are converted to hydroxyproline by a specific prolylhydroxylase requiring ascorbic acid. Lysine residues in the Y position are similarly hydroxylated to hydroxylysine by a specific lysylhydroxylase also requiring ascorbic acid. The requirement for ascorbic acid by the two hydroxylases probably explains why wounds fail to heal in scurvy (see Chap. 76). Many of the hydroxylysine residues are further modified by glycosylation with galactose or with galactose and glucose. A large mannose-rich oligosaccharide is added to the C-terminal propeptide of each chain. As the last amino acids are incorporated into the proα chains, they are released into the cisternae of the rough endoplasmic reticulum. At this stage two proα1(I) and one proα2(I) chains associate through their C-propeptides. The association of the proα chains is directed by the structure and the surface properties of the globular C-propeptides. After the C-propeptides assemble correctly, the structure is locked in place by the formation of interchain disulfide bonds. Posttranslational modifications of the proα chains continue until each chain acquires a critical level of about 100 hydroxyproline residues. Then a few of the -Gly-X-Y- sequences at the C-terminus of the protein that are very rich in hydroxyproline fold into a triple-helical conformation. The short region of triple helix becomes a nucleus for self-assembly of the triple helix of the whole protein, much like a nucleus for crystallization, in that the triple-helical conformation in one -Gly-X-Y- sequence induces the next -Gly-X-Y- sequence to fold into the same conformation. As a result, the conformation is propagated from the nucleus until the entire α-chain domain becomes a continuous triple helix. Once the protein is folded, it passes from the rough endoplasmic reticulum to other membranous compartments, and it is secreted for processing to collagen and self-assembly of the collagen into fibrils.

The fibrils formed by the self-assembly of collagen have considerable tensile strength, and the strength is increased by cross-linking reactions that form covalent bonds between α chains in one molecule and α chains in adjacent molecules. The first step in cross-linking is oxidation by the enzyme lysyl oxidase of amino groups on lysine or hydroxylysine residues to form aldehydes. The aldehydes then interact to form stable covalent bonds.

The collagen fibrils and fibers in skin and tendon undergo repeated synthesis, degradation, and resynthesis during growth and development. They remain stable throughout most of adult life and turn over only with marked starvation or tissue destruction. The degradation of collagen fibers is initiated by specific collagenases found in fibroblasts, synovial cells, and other cell types. The collagenases cleave the collagen molecule at a point about three-quarters of the distance from its N-terminus. The cleavage triggers further degradation by other proteinases. In contrast to other connective tissue, collagen fibrils in bone undergo repeated degradation and synthesis throughout life as part of the continual remodeling of bone.

Essentially the same biosynthetic steps and the same posttranslational enzymes are involved in the biosynthesis of all collagens. Assembly of nonfibrillar collagens such as the type IV of basement membranes does not, however, involve cleavage of the globular domains at the ends of the protein since these are required for the self-assembly of the proteins into networklike structures. Elastin fibers are also assembled by a similar pathway. The elastin monomer, however, is a single polypeptide chain without a defined three-dimensional structure. It spontaneously self-assembles into amorphous elastic fibers, and the fibers then become tightly cross-linked through oxidation of lysine residues to aldehydes and complex interactions of the aldehydes.

Proteoglycan synthesis resembles collagen synthesis in that it involves a large number of posttranslational modifications. The synthesis begins with assembly of a core protein in the cisternae of the rough endoplasmic reticulum. The core protein then undergoes modifications by a series of sugar and sulfate transferases that generate large side chains of glycosaminoglycans. After secretion into the extracellular space, the core protein with its side chains binds to a smaller protein called a link protein. The complex of core protein and link protein then spontaneously binds to a long chain of hyaluronic acid to form a huge copolymer called a proteoglycan aggregate. Some of the four or more different kinds of proteoglycans in connective tissues bind to collagen fibrils and may thereby regulate the diameters of the fibrils. Others are closely associated with cell membranes and probably have an important role in the binding of cells to the extracellular matrix or in signal transduction from the matrix to the cell.

The assembly of bone follows much the same principles as the assembly of other connective tissues (see also Chap. 339). The first step is deposition of osteoid tissue that consists largely of type I collagen fibrils (Fig. 333-1). Mineralization of osteoid occurs by steps that are still incompletely defined; specific proteins probably bind to the collagen fibrils and then chelate calcium to initiate mineralization.

THE MUTATIONS THAT IMPAIR CONNECTIVE TISSUES Because of the large number of tissue-specific macromolecules in connective tissues, a large number of gene-protein systems are candidates for mutations that might cause disease. However, the situation may be simpler than originally assumed in that most forms of the disease appear to be caused by mutations in the structural genes for either type I or type III procollagens.

The most complete data are available on OI. About 90 percent of OI patients have mutations in either the gene for the proα1(I) chain or the gene for the proα2(I) chain of type I procollagen. A few of the mutations decrease expression of protein from one allele of the genes, but these are present in patients with the mildest form of the disease. Most of the mutations cause synthesis of a structurally abnormal but partially functional proα chain. Synthesis of abnormal proα chains from one mutant allele causes devastating effects because the abnormal proα chains interfere with assembly of normal proα chains into procollagen, the processing of procollagen to collagen, or the self-assembly of normal collagen into fibrils (Fig. 333-2). The mutations that underlie structurally abnormal proα chains include partial gene deletions, RNA splicing mutations, and a series of single

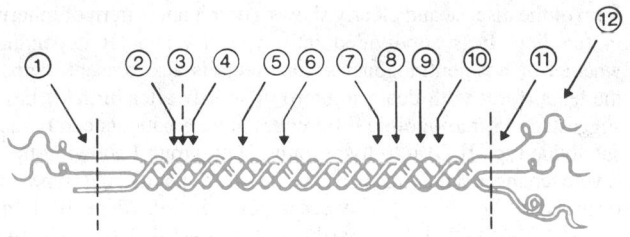

Pro α1

①	Splice Exon 6 (−24 aas)	EDS VII
②	$Gly^{175} \rightarrow Cys$	OI
③	Insertion 50-70 aas	Lethal OI
④	$Gly^{256} \rightarrow Val$	Lethal OI
⑤	$Gly^{391} \rightarrow Arg$	Lethal OI
⑥	Deletion Exons 24-26 (−84 aas)	Lethal OI
⑦	$Gly^{664} \rightarrow Arg$	Lethal OI
⑧	$Gly^{748} \rightarrow Cys$	Lethal OI
⑨	$Gly^{904} \rightarrow Cys$	Lethal OI
⑩	$Gly^{988} \rightarrow Cys$	Lethal OI
⑪	$Gly^{CT3} \rightarrow Cys$	OI
⑫	Frameshift Deletion of 5 bp	OI

FIGURE 333-2 Partial list of the mutations in the gene for the proα1(I) chain of type I procollagen that cause either OI or the type VII form of Ehlers-Danlos syndrome. Similar mutations have been found in the gene for the proα2(I) chains. (*Reproduced with permission from Prockop et al.*)

base mutations that substitute amino acids with bulkier side chains for glycines. The structurally abnormal proα chains exert their clinical effects through at least three molecular mechanisms (Fig. 333-3). First, the presence of an abnormal proα chain in a procollagen

FIGURE 333-3 Schematic summary of three mechanisms (see text) whereby mutations that cause biosynthesis of structurally abnormal proα1(I) or proα2(I) chains of type I procollagen interfere with either the assembly of the protein (*A*) or its processing to normal collagen fibrils (*B*). (*Reproduced with permission from Prockop et al.*)

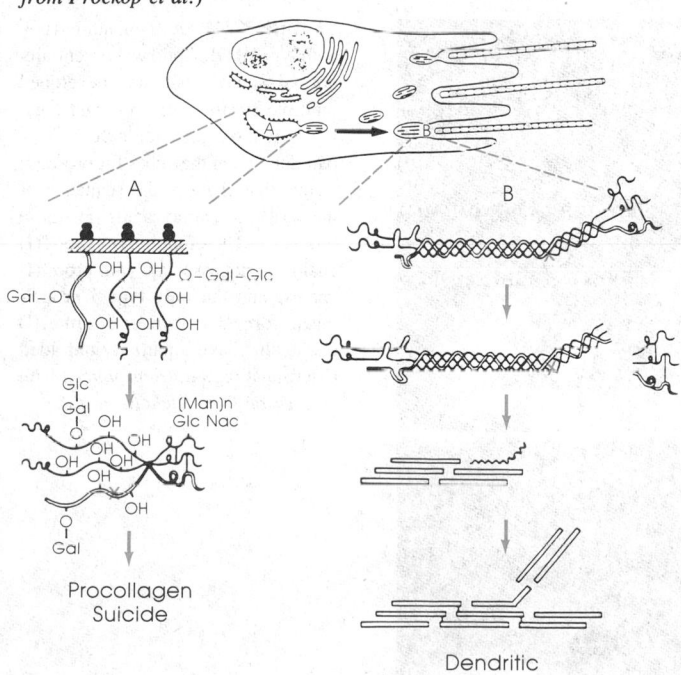

molecule containing two normal proα chains can prevent folding of the protein into a triple-helical conformation and lead to degradation of the whole molecule in a process called "procollagen suicide." Second, the presence of one abnormal proα chain in a procollagen molecule can interfere with cleavage of the N-propeptide from the protein by procollagen N-proteinase. The enzyme is unusual among proteinases in that it will not cleave procollagen substrate if the conformation of the cleavage site is disturbed. Therefore, mutations that change the amino acid sequence of a proα chain far from the cleavage site itself can markedly decrease or prevent cleavage of the N-propeptide from all three chains. The persistence of the N-propeptide on a fraction of the molecules produced by fibroblasts interferes with the self-assembly of normal collagen produced by the same cell so that abnormally thin and irregular collagen fibrils are formed. Third, the substitution of a bulkier amino acid for glycine can produce a kink in the triple-helical structure. A small amount of collagen containing such a kink can cause assembly of abnormally branched or dendritic collagen fibrils.

Type I procollagen genes harbor most of the mutations that cause OI for several reasons. One is that the collagen fibrils are a principal source of the structural strength of bone. Therefore, the whole structure is weakened by any mutation that drastically reduces the amount of collagen or distorts the normal geometry of collagen fibrils. A second reason derives from the extensive use of the principle of self-assembly in the synthesis of collagen fibrils. The advantage of the self-assembly principle is that highly ordered, large structures can be generated efficiently from small subunits with the correct properties. The disadvantage is that the presence of a few slightly flawed subunits can disrupt the process. In the assembly of procollagen, a flaw in one of 338 -Gly-X-Y- subunits in one proα chain can disrupt the triple-helix formed by all three proα chains and produce procollagen suicide. In the assembly of collagen into fibrils, the presence of a few incompletely processed or flawed collagen monomers can extensively distort the morphology of the fibrils formed. Hence, the two large genes for type I procollagen are highly vulnerable to disease-producing mutations in the sense that a mutation at any one of a large number of different sites can alter the assembly of collagen fibrils and produce an inherent weakness of bone and other connective tissues.

Over 30 mutations that cause synthesis of structurally abnormal type I procollagen and that produce OI have now been defined (Fig. 333-2). Similar mutations in the gene for type III procollagen are found in patients with the type IV variant of EDS, the most severe form of the disease that causes early death because of rupture of the aorta or other hollow organs. Data on one family indicate that some variants of the MS can also be produced by mutations in the type III procollagen gene that cause synthesis of structurally abnormal proα(III) chains. To date, the same mutation in a type I or type III procollagen gene has not been found in two unrelated people with OI, EDS, or MS. Similar mutations in the same genes and proteins can produce different disease syndromes, apparently because some features of the proteins are more important for the normal function of some connective tissues than others. There may, however, be more complex explanations for the marked differences among patients. Affected members of the same family tend to have the same manifestations and clinical course, but heterogeneity can be seen even within the same family. Because of the large size of the genes (20 to 40 kb), defining the mutation in a new patient or proband is a time-consuming process that can only be carried out in a research laboratory. Once the mutation in a family is found, however, it is relatively simple to use the polymerase chain reaction and appropriate primers together with allele-specific oligonucleotides to test other members of the same family.

Two forms of EDS are caused by mutations that are not in the structural genes for procollagen but instead are in the genes for two of the procollagen processing enzymes. Some variants of the ocular form of EDS (type VI) are caused by a deficiency of lysylhydroxylase, the enzyme that synthesizes the hydroxylysine in collagen. Some variants of type VII EDS are caused by deficiencies of procollagen N-proteinase. Such enzyme deficiencies appear to be rare causes of connective tissue diseases because, as with most enzyme deficiencies, a homozygous state in which the patient inherited two defective genes is necessary to reduce enzymic activity sufficiently to cause symptoms. To date, no mutations in genes for structural proteins other than collagens have been found to cause OI, EDS, or MS. This may in part be because detecting mutations in the genes is still technically difficult and in part because mutations in these genes may be so deleterious that they cause death at early stages of intrauterine development. Alternatively, mutations in the genes may be of less consequence than mutations in procollagen genes because less of the structure of the macromolecules they code for is essential for normal biologic function.

OSTEOGENESIS IMPERFECTA

General features   The term osteogenesis imperfecta (OI) is used for heritable defects that make bones brittle. The increased fragility of bone is frequently associated with blue sclerae, characteristic dental abnormalities (dentinogenesis imperfecta), progressive hearing loss, and a family history of the disease. The most severe forms of OI produce death in utero, at birth, or shortly thereafter. The clinical course of more moderate forms is variable. Some patients have fractures at birth and then improve so that they have little incapacity in childhood or adulthood. Some appear normal at birth (see Fig. 333-4) and then become progressively worse. Some patients suffer from multiple fractures in childhood, improve after puberty, and begin to fracture more frequently later in life with a marked increase in women during pregnancy and after menopause. Some individuals from families with OI do not develop fracture until after menopause and their disease is difficult to distinguish from postmenopausal osteoporosis. Also, some individuals with osteoporosis are heterozygous carriers for gene defects that produce OI in homozygotes. Therefore, some forms of postmenopausal osteoporosis are in the same spectrum of diseases as OI.

Classification into types   OI was initially classified as being either OI congenita or OI tarda, depending on whether fractures were present at birth or developed later. Currently, the most commonly used classification scheme for OI is the one developed by Sillence (Table 333-2). In the Sillence classification, type I is the mildest

form of the disease and clearly shows a dominant pattern of inheritance in families. It is subdivided into types IA and IB depending on whether or not dentinogenesis imperfecta is also present. Type II is the lethal form with death in utero or shortly after birth. It has been suggested that radiograpic differences among patients can be used to subdivide type II OI into five groups, with group I showing the most severe changes and group V the least. Type III and type IV are intermediate in severity between types I and II. Type III is distinguished from type IV primarily on the basis that type III tends to become progressively severe with age. Also, type III is recessively inherited whereas type IV is dominantly inherited. The mode of inheritance, however, is frequently difficult to establish because many patients have sporadic mutations and, therefore, are the first affected member of the family. Also, many couples with one OI child elect not to have additional children, and most patients with type III or type IV OI do not have children.

Incidence   Type I OI has both a birth incidence of 1:30,000 and a population frequency of 1:30,000. Type II OI has a birth incidence of about 1:60,000. Type III and type IV OI are less common.

Skeletal changes   In type I OI the fragility of bones may be severe enough to limit physical activity or so mild that individuals are unaware of any debility. Radiographs of the skull of some patients with relatively mild syndromes show a mottled or wormian appearance, apparently because of small islands of irregular ossification. In type II OI, bones and other connective tissues are extremely fragile so that massive injuries can occur in utero or during delivery. Ossification of many bones is frequently incomplete. Continuously beaded ribs and crumpled long bones (accordian femora) are frequently seen radiographically. For reasons that are not apparent, the long bones may be either unusually thick or thin. In types III and IV, multiple fractures from minor physical stress can cause stunting of growth and skeletal abnormalities. Severe kyphoscoliosis may cause respiratory impairment and predispose to pulmonary infections. The appearance on radiographs of "popcorn-like" deposits of mineral on the ends of long bones is usually an ominous sign.

In all forms of OI, bone mineral density in unfractured bone is decreased compared to age-matched controls. However, the degree of intrinsic osteopenia is frequently difficult to evaluate, because recurrent fractures limit exercise and thereby exacerbate the decrease in bone mass. The healing of fractures appears to be as normal.

Ocular changes   The sclerae can vary in color from normal to a slightly bluish or slate color to a bright blue. The blueness is probably

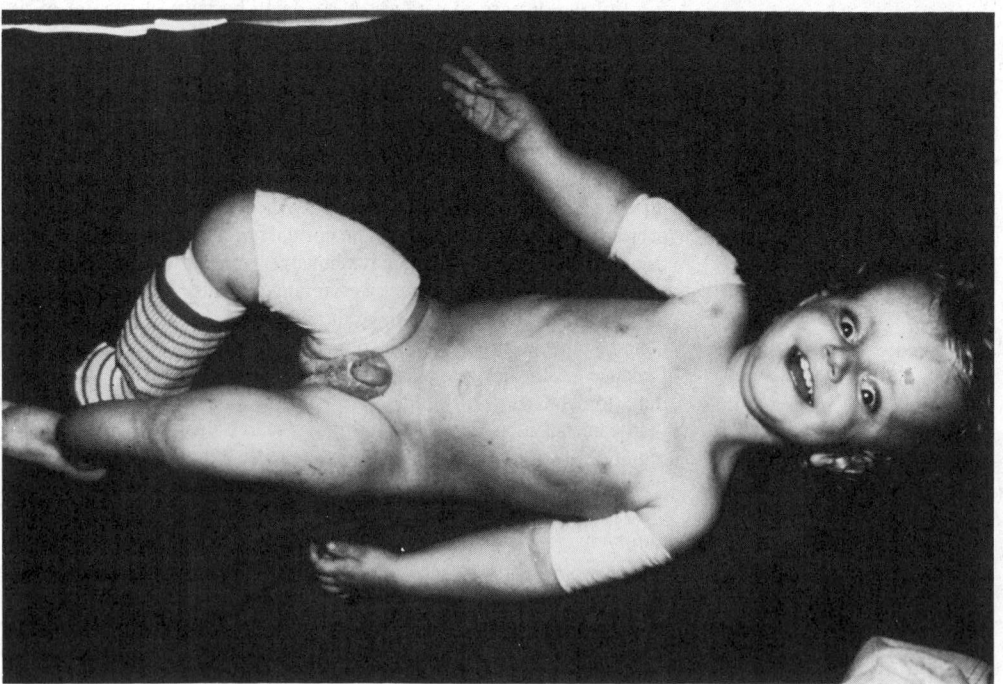

FIGURE 333-4 A 21-month-old boy with type III OI. Child was essentially normal at birth but then developed multiple fractures of arms and legs. He is homozygous for a four-base-pair deletion in the genes for proα2(I) chains that changes the sequence of the last 33 amino acids in these proteins. Therefore, the proα2(I) chains do not associate with proα1(I) chains, and the only type I procollagens formed are trimers of proα1(I) chains that have a partially unfolded C-terminal region. (*Reproduced with permission from Nicholls et al.*)

TABLE 333-2 Classification of osteogenesis imperfecta (OI) based on clinical manifestations and mode of inheritance as proposed by Sillence

Type	Bone fragility	Blue sclerae	Abnormal dentition	Hearing loss	Inheritance*
I	Mild	Present	Absent in IA, present in IB	Present in most	AD
II	Extreme	Present	Present in some	Unknown	AR or S
III	Severe	Bluish at birth	Present in some	High incidence	AR
IV	Variable	Absent	Absent in IVA, present in IVB	High incidence	AD

* AD, autosomal dominant; AR, autosomal recessive; S, sporadic.

caused by a thinness of the collagen layers of the sclerae that allows the choroid layers to be seen. Blue sclerae is an inherited trait in some families without evidence of increased bone fragility.

Dentinogenesis imperfecta The enamel of teeth is relatively normal, but the teeth frequently have a characteristic amber, yellowish-brown or translucent bluish-gray color because of improper deposition or deficiency of dentin. The deciduous teeth are usually smaller than normal, whereas permanent teeth are frequently bell-shaped and restricted at the base. The defect in dentin is directly attributable to the fact that the tissue is normally rich in type I collagen fibers. Some families show indistinguishable inherited teeth defects without any evidence of OI.

Hearing loss Deafness usually begins during the second decade of life, and hearing loss can be detected in 90 percent of patients over 30 years of age. The loss is primarily sensorineural, but the middle ear may also be involved. The histologic features include deficient ossification, persistence of cartilage in areas that are normally ossified, and abnormal calcium deposits.

Associated features Many patients and families show involvement of other connective tissues. Some patients have very thin skin and scar easily. Others have joint changes indistinguishable from those of EDS (see below). A few patients have cardiovascular manifestations such as aortic regurgitation, floppy mitral valves, mitral incompetence, and fragility of large blood vessels. For unknown reasons, some patients develop a hypermetabolic state with elevated serum thyroxine levels, hyperthermia, and excessive sweating.

Molecular defects Most patients with OI have mutations in one of the two genes for type I procollagen. In more severe forms of OI (types II, III, and IV), most of the mutations are dominant and cause synthesis of structurally abnormal proα chains whose effects are amplified by the three molecular mechanisms discussed above. The mutations that change the structure of the protein near the N-proteinase cleavage site tend to produce the extremely lax joints characteristic of type VII EDS rather than OI. Mutations that change the structure near the middle of the molecule or near the C-terminus tend to produce severe or lethal variants of OI. It has been difficult, however, to establish more extensive correlations between the site and nature of the mutation and the clinical phenotype. Also, a few patients with the mildest form of the disease (type I) have unidentified defects that decrease the rate of synthesis of proα1(I) chains. One patient was shown homozygous for a mutated allele for proα2(I) chains, and another patient was a compound heterozygote with independent mutations in two alleles for proα2(I) chains (Fig. 333-3). Such homozygous or compound heterozygous defects, however, tend to be rare. Data from one family suggest that heterozygous carriers for homozygous defects may be prone to osteopenia and perhaps osteoporosis.

Mosaicism in germline cells and in somatic cells The lethal variants of OI are, by definition, sporadic or new mutations. The frequency of a second child with lethal OI in the same family, however, is higher than the expected incidence of new mutations. Therefore, some parents of a child with type II OI apparently have mosaicism in their germline cells. Hence, they should be counseled that the chance of a recurrence is not negligible.

One asymptomatic woman was found to have mosaicism in her somatic cells for a mutation in a type I procollagen gene that produced lethal OI in one of her children. The woman subsequently had two normal children and had no evidence of any bone abnormalities at the age of 35. However, she was short compared to other members of her family, and she had temporal bossing and the triangular facies characteristic of many patients with OI. Such findings are frequently present in parents of children with OI and, therefore, somatic cell mosaicism may be more frequent than previously supposed.

Diagnosis The diagnosis is usually made on the basis of clinical criteria alone. The presence of fractures together with either blue sclerae, dentinogenesis imperfecta, or family history of the disease is usually sufficient to make the diagnosis. However, it is important to rule out other possible causes of fractures such as battered child syndrome, nutritional deficiencies, malignancies, and other heritable disorders including skeletal dysplasias and hypophosphatasia (Table 333-3). There is no consensus as to whether or not characteristic morphologic changes can be detected by electron microscopy of bone specimens. Procedures currently available in research laboratories can identify abnormal proα chains of type I procollagen by polyacrylamide gel electrophoresis of the protein synthesized by cultured fibroblasts in one-third or more of patients. Also, research procedures are available to identify mutations by analysis of mRNA or genomic DNA for type I procollagen; improvements in DNA technologies may make them generally available in the future. After a mutation in a type I procollagen gene has been definitively identified in a patient, a simple test based on polymerase chain reaction can be used to screen members of the same family and for prenatal diagnosis.

Treatment No convincing data have been presented that OI can be effectively treated. Many patients appear to be unusually intelligent and have successful careers in spite of severe deformities. Patients with mild forms may need little treatment after fractures decrease at the age of 15 to 20 years, but women may need special attention during pregnancy or after menopause when fractures again increase. More severely affected children require a comprehensive program of physical therapy, surgical management of fractures and skeletal deformities, and vocational education; emotional support for patients and parents is also necessary. Many of the fractures are only slightly displaced and have little soft tissue swelling. Therefore, they can be

TABLE 333-3 Partial differential diagnosis of OI

Age	Diagnosis	Distinguishing features
At birth	Hypophosphatasia	Unmineralized skull
	Achondrogenesis	Unmineralized vertebrae
	Thanatophoric dwarfism	H-shaped vertebrae
	Asphyxiating thoracic dystrophy	Cylindrical thorax
	Achondroplasia	Large head, short, tubular bones
Infancy	Battered child syndrome	Skull and rib fractures more common
	Immobilization osteogenesis	
	Scurvy	
	Congenital syphilis	
Childhood	Homocystinuria	Marfanoid appearance and mental deficiency
	Celiac disease	Steatorrhea, anemia
	Adrenal cortical tumor	
	Glucocorticoid therapy	

SOURCE: Modified from Smith et al., p. 126

treated with minimal support or traction for a week or two followed by a light cast. If fractures are relatively painless, physical therapy can be initiated early. A judicious amount of exercise is obviously important to prevent loss of bone mass secondary to physical inactivity. Some physicians advocate insertion of steel rods into long bones to correct limb deformities. The major rationale for the procedure is that correcting the deformities during childhood may make it possible to keep patients ambulatory. However, the risk-benefits and cost-benefits of the procedures are difficult to evaluate. A program for careful orthotic management developed by Bleck is a useful guide for the management of many patients.

EHLERS-DANLOS SYNDROME

General features The Ehlers-Danlos syndrome (EDS) describes a group of heritable disorders characterized by hypermobile joints and abnormalities of skin (Fig. 333-5). Beighton initially identified five types of EDS (Table 333-4). Type I is the classical, severe form of the disease with both joint hypermobility and characteristically velvety and hyperextensible skin. Type II is similar to type I but milder. In type III joint hypermobility is more prominent than the skin changes. Type IV is characterized by a striking thinness of skin and a predisposition to sudden death from rupture of large blood vessels or the large bowel. Type V is similar to type II but characterized by X-linked inheritance.

Types VI, VII, and IX were defined because of the presence of biochemical defects and phenotypes that did not fit into the types defined by Beighton. However, not all patients with these phenotypes have the molecular defect initially used to establish the classification. Type VIII was identified by the presence of generalized periodontitis together with moderate joint and skin changes. Because of overlapping signs and symptoms many patients and families cannot be assigned to any of the nine defined types of EDS.

Ligaments and joint changes Laxity and hypermobility of joints can vary from mild changes to changes severe enough to produce unreducible dislocations of hips and other joints. In milder forms, patients learn to reduce dislocations themselves or to avoid them by limiting physical activity. In more severe forms, surgical repair is required. Some patients have progressive difficulty with increasing age, but severe joint laxity can be compatible with a normal life span.

Skin The skin changes vary from a slight thinness and soft or velvety appearance to marked hyperextensibility or skin that is easily torn. Patients with several types of EDS also have easy bruisability. In patients with type IV EDS marked thinness of skin makes the subcutaneous blood vessels unusually prominent. Patients with type I EDS may have characteristic ''cigarette-paper'' scars of the skin from minor trauma. Similar but milder evidence of abnormal repair occurs in other forms, particularly type V. In type VIII, the skin is more fragile than hyperextensible, and it heals with atrophic, pigmented scars.

Associated changes Changes in connective tissues other than joints and skin include mitral valve prolapse, particularly in type I EDS. Pes planus and mild to moderate scoliosis are common. Extreme joint laxity and repeated dislocations may lead to early osteoarthritis. Hernias are frequent in those with types I and IX. Patients with type IV may have spontaneous rupture of the aorta or intestine. In type VI rupture of the eye with minimal trauma frequently occurs, and kyphoscoliosis can produce respiratory impairment. Also, sclerae are frequently blue in type VI. In type IX changes in joints and skin are minimal. This type is primarily defined by the presence of abnormalities in copper metabolism and includes diseases previously classified as X-linked cutis laxa, X-linked EDS, and Menkes's syndrome. Patients frequently have bladder diverticuli that can rupture, hernias, skeletal abnormalities that include characteristic occipital horns, and laxity of skin. In the variants formerly defined as cutis laxa, skin laxity is the most prominent finding and results in an

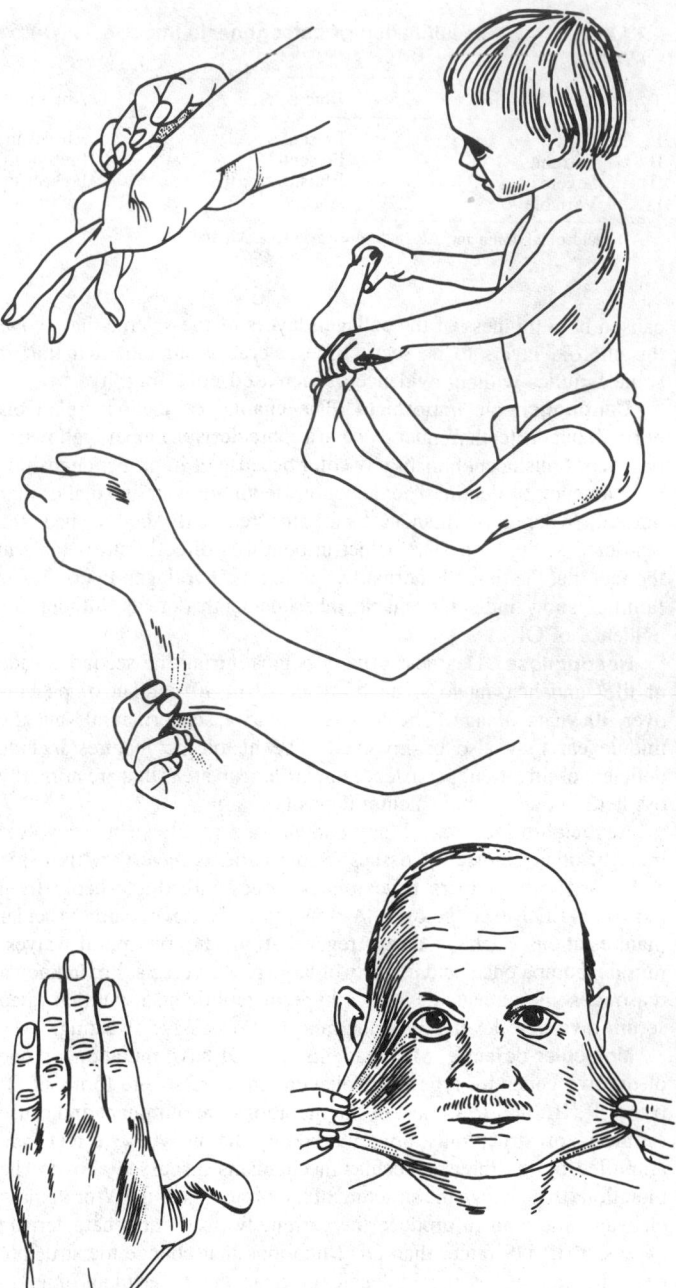

FIGURE 333-5 Schematic of the skin and joint changes in EDS. Girl in upper right has type VIIB EDS with dislocations of both hips that were not corrected by surgery. (*Reproduced with permission from Prockop and Guzman, Hosp Prac, 12(12):61, 1977.*)

appearance of premature senescence. These patients frequently develop pulmonary emphysema and pulmonary stenosis.

Molecular defects The molecular defects in the type I, type II, and type III variants of EDS are unknown. Electron microscopy of the skin from some patients has shown an unusual morphology of collagen fibers, but similar types of collagen fibrils are occasionally seen in normal skin.

Most patients with the type IV variant have a defect either in the synthesis or structure of type III procollagen. A defect in type III procollagen is consistent with the fact that these patients are prone to spontaneous rupture of the aorta and intestines, tissues that are rich in type III collagen. The mutations identified in the type III procollagen gene include partial gene deletions, RNA splicing mutations, and single-base mutations that convert codons for glycine to codons for amino acids with bulkier side chains. Therefore, most of

TABLE 333-4 Classification of EDS based on clinical manifestations and mode of inheritance

Type*	Joint hypermobility	Skin extensibility	Fragility	Bruisability	Other manifestations	Inheritance†
I	Marked	Marked	Marked	Marked	Skin characteristically soft, velvety; cigarette-paper scars; hernias; varicose veins; premature birth because rupture of fetal membranes	AD
II	Moderate	Moderate	Absent	Moderate	Milder than type I	AD
III	Marked	Minimal	Minimal	Minimal	Joint dislocations with minimal changes in skin	AD
IV	Small joints only	Minimal	Marked	Marked	Rupture of large arteries and bowel; thin skin with prominent venous network; characteristic facies in some	AD or AR
V	Moderate	Moderate	Absent	Moderate	Similar to type II	XL
VI	Minimal	Moderate	Moderate	Moderate	Similar to type II; intramuscular hemorrhage or keratoconus in some	XL
VII	Marked	Moderate	Moderate	Moderate	Multiple dislocations	AR or AD
VIII	Moderate	Moderate	Marked	Moderate	Advanced periodontitis; atrophic pigmented scars of skin	AD
IX	Mild	Mild	Absent	Absent	Bladder diverticuli with spontaneous rupture; hernias; skeletal abnormalities; skin laxity	XL

* Alternative designations; type I, gravis; type II, mitis; type III, benign familial hypermobility; type IV, ecchymotic or aortic; type V, X-linked; type VI, ocular; type VII, arthrochalosis multiplex congenita; type VIII, periodontal form; type IX, EDS with abnormal copper metabolism, Menkes's steely-hair syndrome (some variants) and cutis laxa (some variants).
† AD, autosomal dominant; AR, autosomal recessive; XL, X-linked.

the mutations lead to synthesis of abnormal but partially functional proα1(III) chains that produce "procollagen suicide," interfere with the processing of the N-propeptide, or alter fibril formation by the same mechanisms that amplify the effects of mutations in the genes for type I procollagen.

Type VI EDS was first characterized in two sisters by the fact that their collagen contained a decreased amount of hydroxylysine secondary to a deficiency of lysyl hydroxylase; a similar enzyme deficiency has been detected in other patients. Some patients with the clinical features of type VI EDS, however, do not have deficiency of lysyl hydroxylase.

Type VII EDS was first identified as a defect in the conversion of procollagen to collagen in patients with joint hypermobility and joint dislocations. At the molecular level, two kinds of genetic changes produce this disease. One, defined as type VIIA, is a deficiency of procollagen N-proteinase, the enzyme that removes the N-terminal peptide from type I procollagen. This form is inherited as an autosomal recessive trait. The second form, defined as type VIIB, involves a series of different mutations that make the type I procollagen resistant to cleavage by N-proteinase. The change in amino acid sequences of the proα chains of type I procollagen can be located as much as 90 amino acids away from the site at which the enzyme cleaves the protein. In both type VIIA and type VIIB variants, the persistence of the N-propeptide on the molecule causes the formation of fibrils that are unusually thin. Apparently, such thin fibrils can provide a scaffolding for bone but do not provide the necessary tensile strength for ligaments and joint capsules.

A defect in copper metabolism is present in most patients studied with type IX EDS (see Chap. 77). Low levels of serum copper and serum ceruloplasmin are accompanied by marked elevation of copper within cells. The molecular defects in some patients appear to be linked to synthesis of a diffusable factor involved either in regulation of the metallothionein gene or in some other aspect of copper metabolism.

Diagnosis Diagnosis is still based primarily on clinical evaluation of patients. Biochemical assays for known defects in EDS are still difficult and time-consuming. In type IV variants, incubation of cultured skin fibroblasts with radioactive proline or glycine followed

by gel electrophoresis of the newly synthesized proteins will usually demonstrate a defect in the synthesis or secretion of type III procollagen. A protocol for observing both the secretion and the rate of processing of type I procollagen in cultures of skin fibroblasts provides a simple method of identifying deficiencies of procollagen N-proteinase and structural mutations that prevent cleavage of the N-propeptide. It should therefore be useful in the diagnosis of both type VIIA and type VIIB EDS. However, some patients with OI are also positive by this assay. In patients suspected of having type IX EDS, the assignment to this general category can be confirmed by assays of copper and ceruloplasmin in serum and in fibroblast cultures. Specific DNA tests should be available in the future for families in which the exact mutations in type I and type III genes have been defined.

Treatment There are no specific treatments for the disease. Surgical repair and tightening of the joint ligament require careful evaluation of individual patients since the ligaments frequently will not hold sutures. The cardiovascular status should be evaluated in all patients, particularly those suspected of having type IV. Patients with bruisability should be evaluated for specific bleeding disorders, but such tests are usually negative.

THE MARFAN SYNDROME

Diagnosis The Marfan syndrome is defined on the basis of characteristic changes in three connective tissue systems: the skeleton, the eyes, and the cardiovascular system. The disease is inherited as an autosomal dominant trait, and 15 to 30 percent of cases may be due to new mutations. "Skipped generations" due to variable expressivity is relatively common. Also, the typical marfanoid habitus, lens dislocations, and cardiovascular abnormalities can each be inherited independently in some families. Therefore, the diagnosis is usually not made unless at least one member of a family has characteristic changes in at least two of the three connective tissue systems.

Skeletal changes Patients are unusually tall compared to other members of the same family and have unusually long limbs. The ratio of the upper segment (top of head to top of pubic ramus) to the lower segment (top of pubic ramus to floor) is usually 2 standard deviations below mean for age, race, and sex. The patients usually have long and slender fingers and toes (called arachnodactyly or dolichostenomelia), but these are difficult to evaluate objectively. Because of longitudinal overgrowth of the ribs, many patients have chest deformities, including depression (pectus excavatum), protrusion (pectus carinatum), or marked asymmetry. Scoliosis is usually present, often accompanied by kyphosis.

Patients fall into three categories in terms of joint mobility. Most have moderate hypermobility of most joints. Some have marked hypermobility similar to that in EDS, but a few have exceptionally tight joints with contractures of hands and fingers. The group with the latter disorder, which is known as contractural arachnodactyly, appears to be less prone to cardiovascular problems.

Cardiovascular changes Mitral valve prolapse and aortic dilatation are common. Dilatation of the aorta begins in the root and is usually progressive so that dissection and rupture are common. Echocardiography is particularly helpful in evaluation.

Ocular changes The characteristic finding is subluxation of the lens (ectopia lentis), usually in an upward direction. The lens dislocation, however, may be detectable only by slit lamp examination. Displacement of the lens into the anterior chamber may cause glaucoma, but glaucoma is more frequent after surgical removal of the lens. The axial length of the globe is greater than normal, predisposing to myopia and retinal detachment.

Associated changes Striae may occur over the shoulders and buttocks. Otherwise the skin is normal. A number of patients develop spontaneous pneumothorax. High-arched palate and high pedal arches are frequent.

Molecular defects In spite of intensive efforts by many investigators, the molecular defects in most variants of MS are still unknown. Family studies with restriction fragment length polymorphisms have tended to rule out mutations in the genes for type I and type III procollagen. However, a mutation in the gene for proα2(I) chain of type I procollagen was found in one patient with an atypical form of the disease. A single-base mutation that converted a codon for glycine to a codon for arginine in the type III procollagen gene was found in one family with a history of early deaths from ruptured aortic aneurysms, arachnodactyly, easy bruisability, and bleeding tendencies.

Diagnosis The diagnosis is easiest to establish if the patient or members of the family have objective evidence of subluxed lenses, aortic dilatation, and severe kyphoscoliosis or chest deformities. The diagnosis is frequently made if ectopia lentis and an aneurysm of the ascending aorta are present without evidence of a Marfan habitus or a positive family history. All patients in whom the diagnosis is suspected should have a slit lamp examination and an echocardiogram. Also, homocystinuria (Table 333-3) should be ruled out by a negative cyanide-nitroprusside test for disulfides in the urine. Patients with types I, II, and III EDS may have ectopia lentis but lack the Marfan habitus and have characteristic skin changes not present in the Marfan syndrome.

Treatment There is no established treatment. Several investigators have recommended use of propranolol to delay or prevent the severe aortic complications, but the therapy is unproven. Surgical replacement of the aorta, aortic valve, and mitral valve has been undertaken in a number of patients.

The scoliosis tends to be progressive and should be treated by mechanical bracing and physical therapy if greater than 20° or by surgery if it continues to progress and becomes greater than 45°. Estrogen to induce menarche has been tried in girls with progressive scoliosis, but the results are inconclusive. The subluxated lens rarely requires surgical removal, but patients should be followed closely for signs of retinal detachment.

Counseling is based on a 50 percent probability of passing on the defective gene. Because of the heterogeneity of the disease, offspring

may be more or less severely affected than the parents. Women should be advised that the cardiovascular risk of pregnancy is high.

REFERENCES

BLECK EE: Non-operative treatment of osteogenesis imperfecta: Orthotic and mobility management. Clin Orthop 159:115, 1981
BYERS PH et al: Ehlers-Danlos syndrome, in *Principles and Practice of Medical Genetics*, vol 2, AEH Emery, DL Rimoin (eds). New York, Churchill Livingston, 1983, p 36
MCKUSICK VA: *Heritable Disorders of Connective Tissue*, 4th ed. St. Louis, Mosby, 1972
NICHOLLS AC et al: The clinical features of homozygous α-2(I) collagen deficient osteogenesis imperfecta. J Med Genet 21:257, 1984
PROCKOP DJ, KIVIRIKKO KI: Heritable diseases of collagen. N Engl J Med 311:376, 1984
——— et al: Type I procollagen: The gene-protein system that harbors most of the mutations causing osteogenesis imperfecta and probably more common disorders of connective tissue. Am J Med Genet 34:60, 1989
PYERITZ RE: Marfan syndrome, in *Principles and Practice of Medical Genetics*, vol 2, AEH Emery, DL Rimoin (eds). New York, Churchill Livingston, 1983, p 57
SILLENCE DO: Osteogenesis imperfecta: An expanding panorama of variance. Clin Orthop 191:11, 1981
———: Disorders of bone density, volume and mineralization, in *Principles and Practice of Medical Genetics*, vol 2, AEH Emery, DL Rimoin (eds). New York, Churchill Livingston, 1983, p 736
SMITH R et al: *The Brittle Bone Syndrome: Osteogenesis Imperfecta*. London, Butterworths, 1983
UITTO J, BAUER AE: Diseases associated with collagen abnormalities, in *Collagen in Health and Disease*, JB Weiss, MID Jayson (eds). New York, Churchill Livingston, 1982, p 289

334 INHERITED DISORDERS OF AMINO ACID METABOLISM

LEON E. ROSENBERG

All polypeptides and proteins are polymers of 20 different amino acids. Eight of these, referred to as *essential,* cannot be synthesized by humans and must be obtained from dietary sources. The others are formed endogenously. Although most of the body's amino acids are "tied up" in proteins, small intracellular pools of *free* amino acids are in equilibrium with extracellular reservoirs in plasma, cerebrospinal fluid, and the lumina of the gut and kidney. Physiologically, amino acids are more than mere "building blocks." Some (glycine, γ-aminobutyric acid) are neurotransmitters. Others (phenylalanine, tyrosine, tryptophan, glycine) are precursors of hormones, coenzymes, pigments, purines, or pyrimidines. Each has a unique degradative pathway by which its nitrogen and carbon components are used for the synthesis of other amino acids, carbohydrates, and lipids.

Current concepts of inherited metabolic diseases are based to a considerable degree on investigations of amino acid disorders. More than 70 such disorders are now known, the catabolic defects (approximately 60) discussed in this and the following chapter far outnumbering the transport abnormalities (approximately 10) considered in Chap. 336. Each of these disorders is rare—the incidences range from 1 in 10,000 for cystinuria or phenylketonuria to 1 in 200,000 for homocystinuria or alkaptonuria. Collectively, however, they occur in perhaps 1 in 500 to 1 in 1000 live births.

The salient features of inherited disorders of amino acid catabolism are summarized in Table 334-1. In general, these disorders are named for the compound which accumulates to highest concentration in blood (*-emias*) or urine (*-urias*). For many conditions (often called aminoacidopathie), the parent amino acid is found in excess; for others, generally referred to as organic acidemias, products in the catabolic pathway accumulate. Which compound(s) accumulates depends, of course, on the site of the enzymatic block, the reversibility of the reactions proximal to the lesion, and the existence of alternate pathways of metabolic "run-off." For some amino acids, such as the sulfur-containing or branched-chain molecules, defects at nearly each step in the catabolic pathway have been described. For others numerous gaps in our knowledge of defective reactions remain. Biochemical and genetic heterogeneity are common among the aminoacidopathies and the organic acidemias. Five distinct forms of hyperphenylalaninemia, seven forms of homocystinuria, and seven types of methylmalonic acidemia are recognized. Such heterogeneity reflects the presence of many different molecular defects and is of clinical importance as well as scientific interest.

The manifestations of these conditions differ widely (Table 334-1). Some, such as sarcosinemia or hyperprolinemia, appear to produce no clinical consequences. At the other extreme, complete deficiency of ornithine transcarbamylase or of branched-chain keto acid dehydrogenase causes neonatal death in the untreated patient. Central nervous system dysfunction, in the form of developmental retardation, seizures, alterations in sensorium, or behavioral disturbances, occurs in more than half of the disorders. Protein-induced vomiting, neurologic dysfunction, and hyperammonemia occur in many disorders of urea cycle intermediates. Metabolic ketoacidosis often accompanied by hyperammonemia is a frequent presenting finding in the disorders of branched-chain amino acid metabolism. Occasional disorders produce focal tissue or organ involvement such as liver disease, renal failure, cutaneous abnormalities, or ocular lesions.

The clinical manifestations in many of these conditions can be prevented or mitigated if diagnosis is achieved early and appropriate treatment (i.e., dietary protein or amino acid restriction or vitamin supplementation) is instituted promptly. For this reason, a growing number of aminoacidopathies and organic acidemias are screened for in mass newborn surveys which analyze blood or urine with an array of chemical and microbiologic techniques. Once a presumptive diagnosis is made, confirmation can be provided by direct enzyme assay on extracts of leukocytes, erythrocytes, or cultured fibroblasts. DNA-based diagnostic capability is possible for several disorders. For example, substitutions, deletions, and insertions have been used to diagnose and characterize phenylketonuria, ornithine transcarbamylase deficiency, citrullinemia, gyrate atrophy of the retina, propionic acidemia, and methylmalonic acidemia (see also Chap. 6). As additional genes are cloned, DNA-based analysis will become more common.

Several of these disorders (including branched chain ketoaciduria, isovaleric acidemia, propionic acidemia, methylmalonic acidemia, homocystinuria, cystinosis, phenylketonuria, ornithine transcarbamylase deficiency, citrullinemia, argininosuccinic aciduria) can be diagnosed prenatally by chemical analysis of amniotic fluid or by chemical, enzymatic, or DNA-based studies of fresh or cultured amniotic fluid cells. In addition to permitting selective termination of at-risk pregnancies, such diagnosis has led to improved postnatal treatment.

The remainder of this and the subsequent chapter focus on selected disorders that illustrate the principles, properties, and problems presented by the disorders of amino acid metabolism.

THE HYPERPHENYLALANINEMIAS

DEFINITION The hyperphenylalaninemias (Table 334-1), result from impaired conversion of phenylalanine to tyrosine. The most common and clinically important is phenylketonuria, which is characterized by an increased concentration of phenylalanine in blood, increased concentrations of phenylalanine and its by-products (notably phenylpyruvate, phenylacetate, phenyllactate, and phenylacetylglutamine) in urine, and severe mental retardation.

ETIOLOGY AND PATHOGENESIS Each of the hyperphenylalaninemias results from reduced activity of the enzyme complex called *phenylalanine hydroxylase*. In humans this complete enzyme system is expressed only in liver. Phenylalanine and molecular oxygen are substrates for the enzyme which requires a reduced pteridine, tetrahydrobiopterin, as a cofactor (Fig. 334-1). Tyrosine and dihydrobiopterin are the products of this catalytic system, the latter being reconverted to tetrahydrobiopterin by a second enzyme, dihydropteridine reductase. In classic phenylketonuria, activity of the hydroxylase apoenzyme, whose gene locus has been mapped to the q22–q24.1 region of chromosome 12, is almost totally deficient. Six different mutations leading to such complete deficiency are recognized. These include missense changes, splicing defects, and partial deletions. Benign hyperphenylalaninemia results from a less complete deficiency, whereas transient hyperphenylalaninemia (sometimes called transient phenylketonuria) is caused by a delayed maturation of the hydroxylase apoenzyme. In "malignant" hyperphenylalaninemia, however, persistently impaired hydroxylating activity results not from abnormality in the apohydroxylase but from a lack of tetrahydrobiopterin. The tetrahydrobiopterin deficiency has three metabolic causes: two distinct blocks in the pathway by which tetrahydrobiopterin is synthesized from GTP, or deficiency of dihydropteridine reductase, the enzyme that regenerates tetrahydrobiopterin from dihydrobiopterin (see Fig. 334-1). This reductase system is also needed by tyrosine hydroxylase and tryptophan hydroxylase.

As a group the hyperphenylalaninemias occur in about 1 in 10,000 births. Classic phenylketonuria, which accounts for nearly two-thirds of these, is an autosomal recessive trait and is widely distributed among whites and Orientals. It is rare in blacks. Phenylalanine hydroxylase activity in obligate heterozygotes is less than normal but distinctly higher than in affected homozygotes. Heterozygous carriers are clinically well but may have slightly increased phenylalanine concentrations in plasma. The other hyperphenylalaninemias are also inherited as autosomal recessive traits.

Phenylalanine accumulation in blood and urine and reduced tyrosine formation are direct consequences of the impaired hydroxylation. In untreated phenylketonuria and in its tetrahydrobiopterin-deficient variants, plasma concentrations of phenylalanine become sufficiently high [greater than 1200 μmol/L (20 mg/dL)] to activate alternate pathways of metabolism and lead to formation of phenylpyruvate, phenylacetate, phenyllactate, and other derivatives that are rapidly cleared by the kidney and excreted in urine. Plasma concentrations of several other amino acids are moderately reduced, probably secondary to inhibition of gastrointestinal absorption or impairment of renal tubular reabsorption by the excess phenylalanine in body fluids. The severe brain damage appears to be related to several consequences of phenylalanine accumulation: competitive inhibition of transport of other amino acids required for protein synthesis, impaired polyribosome formation or stabilization, reduced myelin synthesis, and inadequate formation of norepinephrine and serotonin. Phenylalanine is a competitive inhibitor of tyrosinase, a key enzyme in the pathway of melanin synthesis. This block plus reduced availability of the melanin precursor, tyrosine, accounts for the hypopigmentation of hair and skin.

CLINICAL MANIFESTATIONS No abnormalities are apparent at birth. Untreated children with classic phenylketonuria fail to attain early developmental milestones and demonstrate progressive impairment of cerebral function. Most require chronic institutionalization within a few years of birth because of the hyperactivity and seizures that accompany the severe mental retardation. Electroencephalographic abnormalities, "mousy" odor of skin, hair, and urine (due to phenylacetate accumulation), and a tendency to hypopigmentation and eczema complete the devastating clinical picture. In contrast, affected children who are detected at birth and treated promptly show none of these abnormalities. Children with transient hyperphenylalaninemia or with the benign variant are not at risk for any of the clinical consequences seen in untreated classic phenylketonuria. Those children with tetrahydrobiopterin deficiency, however, are the most unfortunate. Seizures appear early, followed by progressive cerebral

TABLE 334-1 Inherited disorders of amino acid catabolism

Amino acid(s) affected	Disorder or condition	Enzyme defect	Clinical manifestations*			
			Mental retardation	Neuropsychiatric dysfunction	Protein intolerance	Metabolic ketoacidosis
AROMATIC—HETEROCYCLIC						
Phenylalanine	Classic phenylketonuria	Phenylalanine hydroxylase	+	+	−	−
	Benign hyperphenylala-ninemia	Phenylalanine hydroxylase	−	−	−	−
	Transient hyperphenylala-ninemia	Phenylalanine hydroxylase	−	−	−	−
	Malignant hyperphenyl-alaninemia	Dihydropteridine reductase	+	+	−	−
	Malignant hyperphenyl-alaninemia	GTP cyclohydrolase	+	+	−	−
	Malignant hyperphenyl-alaninemia	6-Pyruvoyltetrahydrobiop-terin synthase	+	+	−	−
Tyrosine	Hypertyrosinemia	Tyrosine aminotransferase (cytosol)	+	−	−	−
	Tyrosinosis	Tyrosine aminotransferase (?)	−	−	−	−
	Hereditary tyrosinemia	Fumarylacetoacetate hydro-lase	−	−	−	−
	Alkaptonuria	Homogentisic acid oxidase	−	−	−	−
	Albinism (oculocuta-neous)	Tyrosinase	−	−	−	−
	Albinism (ocular)	Unknown	−	−	−	−
Tryptophan	Tryptophanuria	Unknown	+	+	−	−
	Xanthurenic aciduria	Kynureninase	?	−	−	−
Histidine	Histidinemia	Histidine-ammonia lyase	±	±	−	−
	Urocanic aciduria	Urocanase	+	+	−	−
	Formiminoglutamic aciduria	Formiminotransferase	?	+	−	−
GLYCINE-IMINO ACIDS						
Glycine	Hyperglycinemia	Glycine cleavage	+	+	−	−
	Sarcosinemia	Sarcosine dehydrogenase	−	−	−	−
	Hyperoxaluria (type I)	Alanine: glyoxylate amino-transferase	−	−	−	−
	Hyperoxaluria (type II)	D-Glyceric acid dehydrogen-ase	−	−	−	−
Imino acids	Hyperprolinemia (type I)	Proline oxidase	−	−	−	−
	Hyperprolinemia (type II)	Δ′-Pyrroline dehydrogenase	−	−	−	−
	Hyperhydroxyprolinemia	Hydroxyproline reductase	−	−	−	−
	Iminopeptiduria	Prolidase	+	−	−	−
SULFUR-CONTAINING						
Methionine	Hypermethioninemia	Methionine adenosyltransfer-ase	−	−	−	−
Homocystine	Homocystinuria	Cystathionine β-synthase	±	±	−	−
	Homocystinuria	5,10-Methylenetetrahydro-folate reductase	±	±	−	−
	Homocystinuria and methylmalonic acidemia (cbl C, D)‡	Cobalamin (vitamin B_{12}) re-ductase (cytosol) (?)	±	±	−	−
	Homocystinuria and methylmalonic acidemia (cblF)	Lysosomal efflux	+	+	−	−
	Homocystinuria (cblE, G)	Methyltransferase-associated cobalamin reductase (?)	+	+	−	−
Cystathionine	Cystathioninuria	Cystathionase	±	−	−	−
Cystine	Cystinosis	Lysosomal efflux	−	−	−	−
S-Sulfo-L-cys-teine	S-Sulfo-L-cysteine, sul-fite, and thiosulfaturia	Sulfite oxidase	+	+	−	−
CATIONIC						
Lysine	Hyperlysinemia (type I)	Lysine dehydrogenase	−	+	+	−
	Hyperlysinemia (type II)	Lysine: α-ketoglutarate re-ductase	±	±	−	−
	Saccharopinuria	Saccharopine dehydrogenase	−	−	−	−
	Hydroxylysinemia	Unknown	+	−	−	−
	Pipecolic acidemia	Unknown	+	+	−	−
	α-Ketoadipic aciduria	α-Ketoadipic acid decarbox-ylase	±	±	−	−
	Glutaric aciduria (type I)	Glutaryl CoA dehydrogenase	−	+	−	−
	Glutaric aciduria (type II)	Medium-chain acyl CoA de-hydrogenase (?)	−	+	−	−

* +, Regularly present; ±, sometimes present; −, absent; ?, uncertain; all designations refer to manifestations in untreated disorder.
† AR, autosomal recessive; XL, X-linked; (AR), probably autosomal recessive.
‡ Designations in parentheses refer to complementation groups assigned by genetic analysis with cultured cells.

Ammonia intoxication	Other	Inheritance pattern†
–	Hypopigmented skin and hair, eczema	AR
–		AR
–		(AR)
–		(AR)
–		(AR)
–		AR
–	Palmar keratosis, corneal dystrophy	(AR)
–	Myasthenia gravis	?
–	Cirrhosis, hepatic failure, renal tubular dysfunction	AR
–	Ochronosis, arthritis	AR
–	Hypopigmentation of hair, skin, and optic fundus	AR
–	Hypopigmentation of optic fundus	XL
–	Photosensitive skin rash	AR
–		?
–	Hearing and speech deficit	AR
–		?
–		(AR)
–		AR
–		AR
–	Renal failure	AR
–	Calcium oxalate nephrolithiasis, renal failure	AR
–		AR
–		AR
–		AR
–	Crusting erythematous, ecchymotic dermatitis	AR
–		?
–	Dislocated lenses, osteoporosis, thrombotic vascular disease	AR
–		(AR)
–	Megaloblastic anemia	(AR)
–		(?)
–	Megaloblastic anemia	AR
–		AR
–	Fanconi syndrome, renal failure, photophobia	AR
–	Dislocated lenses	AR
+		?
–		AR
–		?
–		(AR)
–	Hepatomegaly, dysplastic optic disks	?
–		?
–		AR
–	Hypoglycemia	?

(Table continues next page)

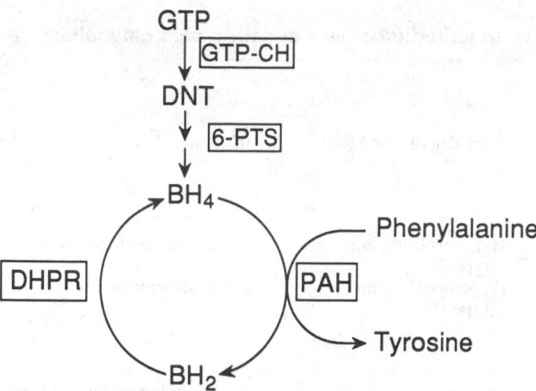

FIGURE 334-1 Pathways, enzymes, and coenzymes involved in the hyperphenylalaninemias. Blocked-in symbols highlight points of etiologic or therapeutic significance to the various genetic defects underlying these disorders. Abbreviations: GTP, guanosine triphosphate; GTP-CH, guanosine triphosphate cyclohydrolase; DNT, dihydroneopterin triphosphate; 6-PTS, 6-pyruvoyltetrahydropterin synthase; BH_4, tetrahydrobiopterin; BH_2, dihydrobiopterin; DHPR, dihydropteridine reductase; PAH, phenylalanine hydroxylase.

and basal ganglia dysfunction (rigidity, chorea, spasms, hypotonia). Most have succumbed to secondary infection within a few years despite early diagnosis and vigorous treatment.

A number of women with phenylketonuria who have been treated since infancy are now reaching adulthood and becoming pregnant. More than 90 percent of their offspring are markedly retarded, and many exhibit other congenital anomalies such as microcephaly, growth retardation, and congenital heart defects. Since these children are heterozygous, not homozygous for a phenylketonuria mutation, the clinical manifestations must be attributed to damage produced by the elevated maternal concentrations of phenylalanine to which they have been exposed in utero. This alarming syndrome is called maternal phenylketonuria.

DIAGNOSIS Plasma phenylalanine concentrations may be normal at birth in all the hyperphenylalaninemias but rise rapidly after institution of protein feedings and are usually abnormal by day 4. Since diagnosis and initiation of dietary treatment of classic phenylketonuria must be completed before the child is 30 days of age if developmental retardation is to be prevented, most newborns in North America and Europe are screened by determinations of blood phenylalanine concentration using the Guthrie bacterial inhibition assay. Infants with abnormal values are followed up with more quantitative fluorometric or chromatographic assays. In classic phenylketonuria and in tetrahydrobiopterin deficiency, values greater than 1200 μmol/L (20 mg/dL) are regularly observed. In transient or benign hyperphenylalaninemia concentrations are usually lower but above control values of less than 60 μmol/L (1 mg/dL). Distinction of classic phenylketonuria from its benign variants depends on following serial plasma phenylalanine concentrations as a function of age and dietary restriction. In transient hyperphenylalaninemia plasma values return to normal within 3 to 4 months. In benign hyperphenylalaninemia dietary restriction produces a more profound fall in plasma phenylalanine than that observed in classic phenylketonuria. Deficiency of tetrahydrobiopterin must be considered in any child with hyperphenylalaninemia who develops progressive neurologic impairment despite prompt diagnosis and dietary treatment. Diagnostic confirmation of these variants, which account for 1 to 5 percent of phenylketonuric children, can be achieved by enzyme assay on cultured fibroblasts. Of potentially greater therapeutic value, however, is the observation that administration of oral tetrahydrobiopterin loads can distinguish children with classic phenylketonuria (who show no chemical response) from those with tetrahydrobiopterin deficiency (who exhibit a sharp fall in plasma phenylalanine). Prenatal diagnosis of classic phenylketonuria is now feasible using DNA-based tests capable of detecting specific mutations or linked restriction fragment length

TABLE 334-1   Inherited disorders of amino acid catabolism (*continued*)

Amino acid(s) affected	Disorder or condition	Enzyme defect	Clinical manifestations*			
			Mental retardation	Neuropsychiatric dysfunction	Protein intolerance	Metabolic ketoacidosis
CATIONIC ()						
Ornithine	Hyperornithinemia (type I)	Ornithine decarboxylase	+	+	+	−
	Hyperornithinemia (type II)	Ornithine aminotransferase	−	−	−	−
UREA CYCLE						
Carbamyl-phosphate	Hyperammonemia (type I)	Carbamylphosphate synthetase I	+	+	+	−
N-acetylgluta-mate	Hyperammonemia (type IA)	N-acetylglutamate synthetase	?	+	+	−
Ornithine	Hyperammonemia (type II)	Ornithine transcarbamylase	±	+	+	−
Citrulline	Citrullinemia	Argininosuccinate synthetase	+	+	+	−
Argininosuc-cinic acid	Argininosuccinic aciduria	Argininosuccinase	+	+	+	−
Arginine	Argininemia	Arginase	+	+	+	−
BRANCHED-CHAIN						
Valine	Hypervalinemia	Valine aminotransferase	+	+	+	−
Leucine, isoleucine	Hyperleucine-isoleucinemia	Leucine-isoleucine aminotransferase	+	+	+	−
Valine, leucine, isoleucine	Classic branched-chain ketoaciduria	Branched-chain ketoacid dehydrogenase	+	+	+	
	Intermittent branched-chain ketoaciduria	Branched-chain ketoacid dehydrogenase	±	−	+	+
Leucine	Isovaleric acidemia	Isovaleryl CoA dehydrogenase	±	±	+	+
	β-Methylcrotonyl glycinuria	β-Methylcrotonyl CoA carboxylase	+	+	−	+
	β-Hydroxy-β-methylglutaric aciduria	β-Hydroxy-β-methylglutaryl CoA lyase	−	+	+	+
Isoleucine, valine	α-Methylacetoacetic aciduria	β-Ketothiolase	±	±	+	+
	Propionic acidemia (pcc A, B, C)‡	Propionyl CoA carboxylase	±	±	+	+
	Propionic acidemia (bio)‡	Holocarboxylase synthetase; biotinidase	+	±	+	+
	Methylmalonic acidemia (mut)‡	Methylmalonyl CoA mutase	±	±	+	+
	Methylmalonic acidemia (cbl A)‡	Cobalamin (vitamin B_{12}) reductase (mitochondrial) (?)	±	±	+	+
	Methylmalonic acidemia (cbl B)‡	Cobalamin (vitamin B_{12}): ATP adenosyltransferase	±	±	+	+
DICARBOXYLIC						
Glutamic acid	Glutathionemia	γ-Glutamyl-transpeptidase	+	−	−	−
5-Oxoprolinuria	Glutathione synthetase	±	±	±		

* +, Regularly present; ±, sometimes present; −, absent; ?, uncertain; all designations refer to manifestations in untreated disorder.
† AR, autosomal recessive; XL, X-linked; (AR), probably autosomal recessive.
‡ Designations in parentheses refer to complementation groups.

polymorphisms (RFLPs). Dihydropteridine reductase deficiency and the blocks in tetrahydrobiopterin synthesis can also be detected in utero using assays on cultured amniocytes.

TREATMENT   Classic phenylketonuria is the first inherited metabolic disease in which it was demonstrated that mitigating the accumulation of the offending metabolite prevented the dire clinical consequences. This is accomplished by a special diet in which the bulk of protein is replaced by an artificial amino acid mixture low in phenylalanine. By supplementing this formula with a small amount of natural foods, an amount of dietary phenylalanine is provided that is sufficient for normal growth but is insufficient to produce markedly increased quantities of phenylalanine in blood. Ordinarily, plasma phenylalanine concentrations are maintained between 180 and 700 μmol/L (3 and 12 mg/dL).

To be maximally effective, such diet therapy must be instituted during the first month of life. Even then, modest nervous system dysfunction is often seen. Because uncontrolled hyperphenylalaninemia results in brain damage throughout childhood (and perhaps in adults), dietary restriction in classic phenylketonuria should be continued indefinitely. The transient and benign forms of hyperphenylalaninemia do not require long-term dietary restriction. As mentioned earlier, children with tetrahydrobiopterin deficiency deteriorate despite dietary phenylalanine restriction; efficacy of pteridine cofactor replacement is under study. Such patients may be helped, however, by a regimen in which dietary phenylalanine restriction is combined with supplements of levodopa and 5-hydroxytryptophan. Finally, the deleterious consequences of maternal phenylketonuria can be minimized by instituting dietary phenylalanine restriction prior to con-

Ammonia intoxication	Other	Inheritance pattern†
+		(AR)
−	Gyrate atrophy of choroid and retina	AR
+		AR
+		XL
+		AR
+		AR
+		AR
+		
−		?
−		?
−	"Maple syrup" odor	AR
−		AR
±	"Sweaty feet" odor	AR
−	"Cat's urine" odor	AR
−		?
+		AR
+		AR
−		?
+		AR
+		AR
+		AR
−		?
−		AR

ception and continuing such treatment throughout gestation. This means that women with phenylketonuria should stay on a phenylalanine-restricted diet from birth through the child-bearing years.

THE HOMOCYSTINURIAS

The homocystinurias are seven biochemically and clinically distinct disorders (Table 334-1), each characterized by increased concentration of the sulfur-containing amino acid, homocystine, in blood and urine. The most common form results from reduced activity of cystathionine β-synthase, an enzyme in the transsulfuration pathway by which methionine is converted to cysteine. All the other forms are the result of impaired conversion of homocysteine to methionine, a reaction catalyzed by homocysteine:methyltetrahydrofolate methyltransferase and two essential cofactors methyltetrahydrofolate and methylcobalamine (methyl–vitamin B_{12}). Depending on the underlying disorder, some patients with each of the homocystinurias show chemical and, in some instances, clinical improvement following administration of specific vitamin supplements (pyridoxine, folate, or cobalamin).

CYSTATHIONINE β-SYNTHASE DEFICIENCY **Definition** Deficiency of this enzyme leads to increased concentrations of methionine and homocystine in body fluids and to decreased concentrations of cysteine and cystine. The clinical hallmark is dislocated optic lenses. Mental retardation, osteoporosis, and thrombotic vascular disease are frequent.

Etiology and pathogenesis The sulfur atom of the essential amino acid methionine is transferred ultimately to cysteine by a series of reactions designated as the transsulfuration pathway (Fig. 334-2). In one of these steps, homocysteine condenses with serine to form cystathionine. This reaction is catalyzed by the pyridoxal phosphate–dependent enzyme, cystathionine β-synthase. The locus for this homodimeric enzyme has been mapped to the q21 region of chromosome 21. More than 600 patients have been described with deficiency of this enzyme. The condition is common in Ireland (1 in 40,000 births) but rare elsewhere (less than 1 in 200,000 births).

Homocysteine and methionine accumulate in cells and body fluids; cysteine synthesis is impaired, resulting in reduced concentrations of this amino acid and its disulfide form, cystine. In approximately half of patients synthase activity in liver, brain, leukocytes, and cultured fibroblasts is undetectable. In the remaining patients, tissues retain 1 to 5 percent of normal activity, and this residual activity can often be stimulated by pyridoxine supplementation. Heterozygous carriers of this autosomal recessive trait show no reproducible chemical abnormalities in body fluids but have reduced tissue synthase activity.

Homocysteine interferes with the normal cross-linking of collagen, an effect that likely plays an important role in the ocular, skeletal, and vascular complications. Altered collagen in the suspensory ligament of the optic lens and in bone matrix may account for the dislocated lenses and osteoporosis. Similarly, interference with normal ground substance metabolism in vascular walls may predispose to the arterial and venous thrombotic diathesis. Increased platelet adhesiveness may result from homocysteine accumulation, thereby contributing to the thrombotic occlusive disease so often observed. Recurrent cerebrovascular accidents secondary to thrombotic disease may account for the mental retardation, but direct chemical effects on cerebral cell metabolism have not been excluded.

Clinical manifestations More than 80 percent of homozygotes for complete synthase deficiency have dislocated optic lenses. This abnormality usually appears by 3 to 4 years of age and often results in acute glaucoma as well as impaired visual acuity. Mental retardation occurs in about half of such patients, often accompanied by ill-defined behavioral disturbances. Osteoporosis is a common radiologic finding (seen in two-thirds of patients by age 15) but rarely causes clinical disease. Life-threatening vascular complications, probably initiated by damage to vascular endothelium, are the major cause of morbidity and mortality. Occlusion of coronary, renal, and cerebral arteries with attendant tissue infarction can occur during the first decade of life. Nearly one-quarter of patients die of vascular disease before age 30. These vascular complications seem to be exacerbated by angiographic procedures. Importantly, pyridoxine-responsive patients have milder clinical manifestations in all regards. Heterozygous carriers for synthase deficiency (about 1 in 70 in the population) may be at increased risk for premature peripheral and cerebral occlusive vascular disease.

Diagnosis The cyanide-nitroprusside test is a simple way of demonstrating increased excretion of sulfhydryl-containing compounds in urine. Since cystine and S-sulfocysteine also give a positive test, other disorders of sulfur metabolism must be excluded, but this is usually possible on clinical grounds. Distinction of cystathionine β-synthase deficiency from other causes of homocystinuria can usually be accomplished by measurements of plasma methionine, which tend

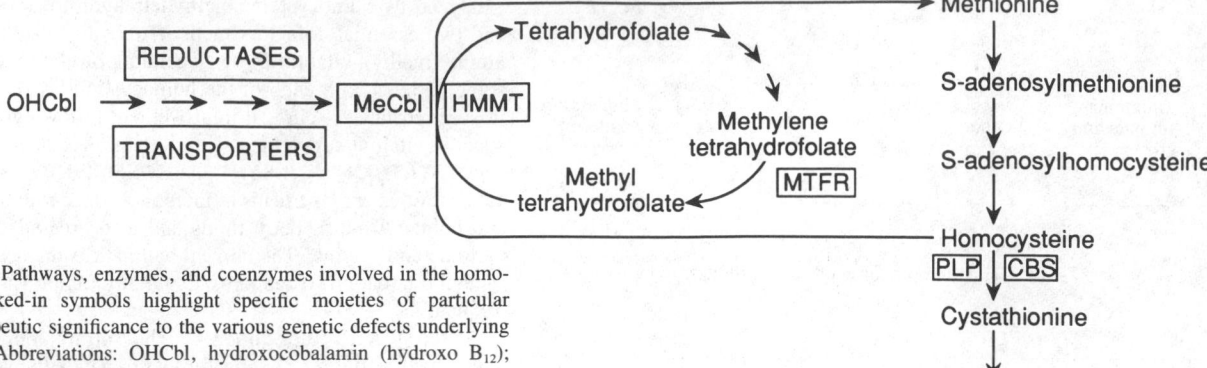

FIGURE 334-2 Pathways, enzymes, and coenzymes involved in the homocystinurias. Blocked-in symbols highlight specific moieties of particular etiologic or therapeutic significance to the various genetic defects underlying these disorders. Abbreviations: OHCbl, hydroxocobalamin (hydroxo B_{12}); MeCbl, methylcobalamin; MTFR, methylene tetrahydrofolate reductase; PLP, pyridoxal phosphate; CBS, cystathionine β-synthase.

to be increased in synthase-deficient patients and normal or low in those with impaired methionine formation (see below). Diagnostic confirmation depends on measurements of synthase activity in tissue extracts. Heterozygotes can be identified by measurement of peak serum homocystine after an oral methionine load and by measurement of tissue synthase activity.

Treatment As with classic phenylketonuria, effective treatment depends on early diagnosis. A number of infants diagnosed in the newborn period have been treated successfully with methionine-restricted, cystine-supplemented diets. Their clinical course has, thus far, been benign compared with that of untreated affected siblings. In approximately half of patients, oral supplements of pyridoxine (25 to 500 mg per day) produce a fall in plasma and urinary methionine and homocystine and an increase in cystine concentration in body fluids. This effect probably reflects a modest increase in synthase activity in cells of patients in whom the enzymatic defect is characterized by either reduced affinity for cofactor or accelerated degradation of mutant enzyme. Since such vitamin supplementation is simple and apparently harmless, it should be tried in all patients. There are no reports of the effect of pyridoxine supplementation therapy initiated soon after birth. Similarly, there are no data regarding pyridoxine supplements in heterozygous carriers.

5,10-METHYLENETETRAHYDROFOLATE REDUCTASE DEFICIENCY Definition In this form of homocystinuria, methionine concentrations in body fluids are normal or decreased because deficiency of 5,10-methylenetetrahydrofolate reductase leads to impaired synthesis of 5-methyltetrahydrofolate, a cofactor in the enzymatic formation of methionine from homocysteine (see Fig. 334-2). Central nervous system dysfunction occurs in most patients.

Etiology and pathogenesis 5-Methyltetrahydrofolate:homocysteine methyltransferase catalyzes the conversion of homocysteine to methionine. The methyl group transferred in this reaction comes from 5-methyltetrahydrofolate, which is converted to tetrahydrofolate in the process. 5-Methyltetrahydrofolate, in turn, is synthesized enzymatically from 5,10-methylenetetrahydrofolate by another enzyme, 5,10-methylenetetrahydrofolate reductase. Thus, reductase activity controls both methionine synthesis and tetrahydrofolate generation. This series of reactions is critical to normal DNA and RNA synthesis. A primary defect in the reductase activity results, secondarily, in deficient methyltransferase activity and impaired conversion of homocysteine to methionine. Methionine deficiency and impaired nucleic acid synthesis may contribute to the central nervous system dysfunction. The disorder appears to be inherited as an autosomal recessive trait.

Clinical manifestations More than 25 children with homocystinuria due to reductase deficiency have been reported. The most severely affected have presented with profound developmental retardation and cerebral atrophy early in life. Others manifested behavioral disturbances (catatonia) during the second decade or mild retardation. Presumably the severity of the clinical manifestations reflects the severity of the reductase deficiency.

Diagnosis and treatment The combination of increased concentrations of homocystine in body fluids with normal or decreased concentrations of methionine should suggest this entity. Serum folate concentrations are low in some patients. Confirmation requires direct reductase assays in tissue extracts (brain, liver, cultured fibroblasts). Although therapeutic experience is limited, one teenage girl with a catatonic psychosis responded dramatically, both chemically and clinically, to folate supplements (5 to 10 mg per day). When the folate was withdrawn, behavior worsened. This observation suggests that early diagnosis followed by folate supplementation may forestall neurologic or psychiatric disturbances.

DEFICIENCY OF COBALAMIN (VITAMIN B_{12}) COENZYME SYNTHESIS Definition Five other forms of homocystinuria also reflect impaired conversion of homocysteine to methionine. The primary defects in these entities, however, are in the synthesis of methylcobalamin, a cobalamin (vitamin B_{12}) coenzyme required by methyltetrahydrofolate:homocysteine methyltransferase (see Fig. 334-2). In some of these disorders methylmalonic acid accumulates in body fluids as well because synthesis of a second coenzyme, adenosylcobalamin, required for isomerization of methylmalonyl coenzyme A (CoA) to succinyl CoA is also impaired. These disorders are designated cblC, D, E, F, and G.

Etiology and pathogenesis As with 5,10-methylenetetrahydrofolate reductase deficiency, each disorder impairs remethylation of homocysteine. Since methylcobalamin is required for methyl-group transfer from methyltetrahydrofolate to homocysteine, impaired cobalamin metabolism leads to deficient methyltransferase activity. The defects responsible for impaired synthesis of methylcobalamin involve one of several steps in lysosomal or cytosolic activation of the vitamin precursor (see Fig. 334-2). In the cblF disorder, the transport of cobalamins out of lysosomes is impaired. In cblC and D, a reductase needed for formation of both methylcobalamin and adenosylcobalamin is deficient. In cblE and G, some component required to maintain a reduced form of cobalamin on the methyltransferase apoenzyme is impaired. Somatic cell genetic studies indicate that each of these abnormalities is distinct and imply that all are inherited as autosomal recessive traits.

Clinical manifestations The first reported patient with the cblC defect had profoundly arrested development and died of infection at age 6 weeks. More than 25 patients—mostly children—with these defects in cobalamin metabolism have been described subsequently. Although clinical manifestations vary considerably, neurologic and hematologic abnormalities include developmental delay, dementia, spasticity, megaloblastic anemia, and pancytopenia. It is not possible to define a specific clinical syndrome for each of the five defects in cobalamin metabolism.

Diagnosis and treatment Homocystinuria, homocysteinemia, and hypomethioninemia are the chemical hallmarks. Methylmalonic acidemia, too, has been noted in those defects resulting from defective synthesis of both cobalamin coenzymes. These findings may also be present in juvenile- or adult-onset pernicious anemia in which intestinal cobalamin absorption is impaired. Measurement of serum cobalamin concentrations, low in pernicious anemia and normal in patients with defective conversion of cobalamin vitamin to coenzymes, helps in the differential diagnosis. Definitive diagnosis depends on demonstrating impaired coenzyme synthesis in cultured cells. Treatment of affected children with cobalamin supplements (1 to 2 mg per day) shows promise: homocystine and methylmalonate excretion fall to near normal values; the hematologic and neurologic deficits have also lessened to a variable degree in several patients. Intervention early in life seems to offer the best long-term prognosis.

REFERENCES

BOERS GHJ et al: Heterozygosity for homocystinuria in premature peripheral and cerebral occlusive arterial disease. N Engl J Med 313:709, 1985

FENTON WA, ROSENBERG LE: Inherited disorders of cobalamin transport and metabolism, in *The Metabolic Basis of Inherited Disease*, 6th ed, CR Scriver et al (eds). New York, McGraw-Hill, 1989, pp 2065–2082

MUDD SH et al: Natural history of homocystinuria due to cystathionine β-synthase deficiency. Am J Hum Genet 37:709, 1985

———— et al: Disorders of transsulfuration, in *The Metabolic Basis of Inherited Disease*, 6th ed, CR Scriver et al (eds). New York, McGraw-Hill, 1989 pp 693–734

ROSENBERG LE, SCRIVER CR: Disorders of amino acid metabolism, in *Metabolic Control and Disease*, 8th ed, PK Bondy, LE Rosenberg (eds). Philadelphia, Saunders 1980, pp 583–776

SCRIVER CR et al: The hyperphenylalaninemias, in *The Metabolic Basis of Inherited Disease*, 6th ed, CR Scriver et al (eds). New York, McGraw-Hill, 1989, pp 495–546

335 STORAGE DISEASES OF AMINO ACID METABOLISM

LEON E. ROSENBERG

A number of inherited metabolic disorders are characterized by deposition or storage of particular metabolites in tissues. In most, storage reflects impaired degradation of the substance in question; in others, the mechanism is unknown. Many storage diseases involve large molecules such as glycogen, sphingolipids, mucolipids, cholesterol esters, and mucopolysaccharides (see Chaps. 332, 326, and 331); in others, metals such as iron and copper are deposited (see Chaps. 327 and 330). Finally, there is a group of storage diseases in which relatively small organic molecules are deposited. These include gout (see Chap. 329) and disorders of amino acid metabolism.

ALKAPTONURIA

DEFINITION Alkaptonuria is a rare disorder of tyrosine catabolism. Deficiency of the enzyme homogentisic acid oxidase leads to excretion of large amounts of homogentisic acid in urine and to accumulation of oxidized homogentisic acid pigment in connective tissues (ochronosis). After many years ochronosis produces a distinctive form of degenerative arthritis.

ETIOLOGY AND PATHOGENESIS Homogentisic acid is an intermediate in the catabolism of tyrosine to fumarate and acetoacetate. Activity of homogentisic acid oxidase, the enzyme that catalyzes the opening of the phenolic ring yielding maleylacetoacetic acid, is deficient in liver and kidney of patients with alkaptonuria, and homogentisic acid accumulates in cells and body fluids. Patients have minimally increased concentrations of homogentisic acid in blood because it is rapidly cleared by the kidney. As much as 3 to 7 g homogentisic acid may be excreted in the urine per day, but this is of little pathophysiologic significance. However, homogentisic acid and its oxidized polymers bind to collagen, leading to the progressive deposition of a gray to bluish-black pigment. The mechanism(s) by

which degenerative changes develop in cartilage, intervertebral disk, and other connective tissues is unknown but may involve direct chemical irritation, impaired collagen cross-linking, disturbed articular chondrocyte metabolism, or some combination of factors.

Alkaptonuria was the first human disease shown to be inherited as an autosomal recessive trait. Affected homozygotes occur with a frequency around 1 in 200,000. Heterozygous carriers are clinically well and excrete no homogentisic acid in urine, even after loading doses of tyrosine.

CLINICAL MANIFESTATIONS Alkaptonuria may go unrecognized until middle life when degenerative joint disease develops in the majority. Prior to this time the tendency of the patient's urine to darken on standing may go unnoticed, as may slight discoloration of the sclerae and ears. The latter manifestations are generally the earliest external evidence of the disorder and develop after age 20 to 30. Foci of gray-brown scleral pigment and generalized darkening of the concha, antihelix, and, finally, helix of the ear are typical. Ear cartilages may be irregular and thickened. *Ochronotic arthritis* is heralded by pain, stiffness, and some limitation of motion of the hips, knees, and shoulders. Intermittent periods of acute arthritis, which may resemble rheumatoid arthritis, occur, but small joints are usually spared. Limitation of motion and ankylosis of the lumbosacral spine are common late manifestations. Pigmentation of heart valves, larynx, tympanic membranes, and skin occurs, and occasional patients develop pigmented renal or prostatic calculi. An increased incidence of degenerative cardiovascular disease may occur in older patients.

DIAGNOSIS A patient whose urine darkens to blackness on standing must be suspected of having alkaptonuria, but because of modern plumbing conditions this finding is not often observed. The diagnosis is usually made from the triad of degenerative arthritis, ochronotic pigmentation, and urine which turns black upon alkalinization. Homogentisic acid in urine may be identified presumptively by other tests: upon addition of ferric chloride, a purple-black color is observed; treatment with Benedict's reagent yields a brown color; addition of a saturated silver nitrate solution produces an immediate black color. These screening tests can be confirmed by chromatographic, enzymatic, or spectrophotometric determinations of homogentisic acid. X-rays of the lumbar spine are virtually pathognomonic. They show degeneration and dense calcification of the intervertebral disks and narrowing of the intervertebral spaces.

TREATMENT There is no specific treatment for ochronotic arthritis. Joint manifestations might be mitigated if homogentisic acid accumulation and deposition could be curbed by dietary restriction of phenylalanine and tyrosine, but the long course of the disease has discouraged such therapeutic attempts. Since ascorbic acid impedes oxidation and polymerization of homogentisic acid in vitro, its use has been suggested as a possible means of decreasing pigment formation and deposition. The efficacy of this form of treatment has not been established. Symptomatic treatment is similar to that for osteoarthritis (Chap. 281).

CYSTINOSIS

DEFINITION Cystinosis is a rare disorder characterized by the intralysosomal accumulation of free cystine in body tissues. This results in the appearance of cystine crystals in the cornea, conjunctiva, bone marrow, lymph nodes, leukocytes, and internal organs. Three variants have been identified: an infantile (nephropathic) form leading to the Fanconi syndrome and renal insufficiency in the first decade; a juvenile (intermediate) form in which renal disease becomes manifest during the second decade; and an adult (benign) form characterized by deposition of cystine in the cornea but not in the kidney.

ETIOLOGY AND PATHOGENESIS The basic defect in cystinosis involves impaired efflux of cystine from lysosomes rather than an abnormality in cystine catabolism. Lysosomal cystine efflux is an active, ATP-dependent process. The cystine content of tissues may be more than 100 times normal in the infantile form, more than 30 times normal in the adult form. Intracellular cystine appears to be located in lysosomes and does not exchange with other intracellular or extracellular pools of this amino acid. Neither plasma nor urinary concentrations of cystine are particularly elevated.

The extent of cystine crystal deposition varies from patient to patient, depending on the form of the disease and on the methods used to prepare pathologic specimens. Cystine accumulation in the kidney causes renal insufficiency in the infantile and juvenile forms. The kidneys are pale and shrunken, the capsule is adherent, and the corticomedullary junction is obscured. Microscopically, nephron organization is interrupted, glomeruli are hyalinized, connective tissue is increased, and the normal epithelium of the tubules is replaced by cuboidal cells. Narrowing and shortening of the proximal tubule produces the swan neck deformity that is characteristic of but not specific for cystinosis. Patchy depigmentation and degeneration of the peripheral retina occurs in the infantile and juvenile forms. Cystine crystals may also be deposited in the cornea, ocular conjunctiva, or uvea.

Each form of cystinosis appears to be inherited as an autosomal recessive trait. Obligate heterozygotes have intracellular cystine contents intermediate between those of normal persons and affected patients but are free of clinical abnormalities.

CLINICAL MANIFESTATIONS   In the infantile form abnormalities are usually apparent by 4 to 6 months of age. Growth retardation, vomiting, fever, vitamin D–resistant rickets, polyuria, dehydration, and metabolic acidosis are prominent. Generalized proximal tubular dysfunction (the Fanconi syndrome) leads to hyperphosphaturia and hypophosphatemia, renal glycosuria, generalized aminoaciduria, hypouricemia, and often hypokalemia. Pyelonephritis may contribute, along with interstitial fibrosis, to progressive glomerular insufficiency. Death due to uremia or intercurrent infection usually occurs before age 10. Ocular manifestations are prominent. Photophobia is usually demonstrable within the first few years of life due to cystine deposits in the cornea, and retinal degeneration may appear even earlier.

In contrast, patients with the adult form manifest only ocular abnormalities. Photophobia, headache, and burning or itching of the eyes are major complaints. Glomerular and tubular function and the integrity of the retina are preserved. The findings in the juvenile variant fall between these extremes. These patients have both ocular and renal manifestations, but the latter do not become significant until the second decade. The renal lesion, albeit milder than that seen in the infantile form, eventually leads to renal insufficiency.

DIAGNOSIS   Cystinosis must be considered in any child with vitamin D–resistant rickets, the Fanconi syndrome, or glomerular insufficiency. Hexagonal or rectangular cystine crystals can be detected in the cornea (by slit-lamp examination), in leukocytes from peripheral blood or bone marrow, or in biopsies of rectal mucosa. Diagnosis can be confirmed by quantification of cystine in peripheral blood leukocytes or cultured fibroblasts. The infantile form has been diagnosed prenatally by the demonstration of increased cystine content in cultured amniotic fluid cells.

TREATMENT   The adult form is benign and requires no treatment. Symptomatic treatment of renal disease in the infantile or juvenile form of cystinosis does not differ from that of other forms of chronic renal insufficiency: maintenance of adequate fluid intake to prevent dehydration; correction of the metabolic acidosis; and ingestion of supplementary calcium, phosphate, and vitamin D to heal the rickets. Such measures are effective in maintaining growth, development, and well-being in affected children for a time. Two types of more specific therapy have been attempted. Cystine-restricted diets have not prevented progression of renal disease. This is not surprising given the nature of the primary defect and the large amount of cystine produced endogenously by cellular protein turnover. Whereas the early use of thiol reagents such as penicillamine and dimercaprol yielded no long-term benefits, administration of the free thiol, cysteamine, is helpful in slowing the progression of renal dysfunction, in improving growth, and in dissolving corneal cystine crystals. This compound acts in lysosomes by forming a mixed disulfide with

cysteine that can be transported out of the organelle efficiently by a different transporter from that deficient in the disease.

The most successful form of therapy for nephropathic cystinosis is renal transplantation. Hundreds of affected children with end-stage renal disease have been so treated. Those patients who tolerated the procedure and did not develop immunologic problems have shown return of kidney function toward normal. The transplanted kidneys have not developed the functional abnormalities typical of cystinosis (i.e., the Fanconi syndrome or glomerular insufficiency). They may, however, continue to accumulate cystine in the cornea and other ocular tissues. Because the usual life span of a transplanted kidney is generally 15 to 20 years, some patients with the infantile form of cystinosis have received two or more transplanted kidneys.

PRIMARY HYPEROXALURIA

DEFINITION   Primary hyperoxaluria is the designation for two rare disorders characterized by chronic excessive urinary excretion of oxalic acid and by calcium oxalate nephrolithiasis and nephrocalcinosis. Typically, patients with both forms develop renal insufficiency early in life and die of uremia. At postmortem examination, calcium oxalate deposits are widespread in renal and extrarenal tissues, a condition referred to as *oxalosis*.

ETIOLOGY AND PATHOGENESIS   The metabolic basis for the primary hyperoxalurias involves pathways of glyoxylate metabolism. In type I hyperoxaluria, urinary excretion of oxalate and of the oxidized and reduced forms of glyoxylate is increased. The excessive synthesis of these substances results from a block in glyoxylate metabolism. The primary defect is deficiency of the hepatic peroxisomal enzyme, alanine:glyoxylate amino transferase. The resulting expansion of the glyoxylate pool leads to enhanced oxidation of glyoxylate to oxalate and to enhanced reduction of glyoxylate to glycolate. Each of these 2-carbon acids is then excreted in excess in the urine. In type II hyperoxaluria, L-glyceric acid is excreted in excess along with oxalate. In this condition, activity of D-glyceric acid dehydrogenase, which catalyzes the reduction of hydroxypyruvate to D-glyceric acid in the catabolic pathway of serine metabolism, is absent in leukocytes (and presumably other tissues). The accumulated hydroxypyruvate is instead reduced by lactic dehydrogenase to the L-isomer of glycerate, which is excreted in the urine. The reduction of hydroxypyruvate is coupled in some way to the oxidation of glyoxylate to oxalate, thus causing the formation of increased oxalate. Both disorders appear to be inherited as autosomal recessive traits. Heterozygotes are asymptomatic.

The pathogenesis of stone formation, nephrocalcinosis, and oxalosis relates directly to the insolubility of calcium oxalate. Extrarenal deposits of oxalate are prominent in the heart, walls of arteries and veins, male urogenital tract, and bone.

CLINICAL MANIFESTATIONS   Nephrolithiasis and oxalosis may be manifest during the first year of life. Most patients experience renal colic or hematuria between ages 2 and 10 and succumb to uremia before age 20. With the onset of uremia, patients may develop severe peripheral arterial spasm and necrosis with resulting vascular insufficiency. Oxalate excretion falls as renal failure worsens. In patients with delayed onset of symptoms, survival to age 50 or 60 has been reported, despite recurrent nephrolithiasis.

DIAGNOSIS   Oxalate excretion in normal children or adults is less than 0.5 mmol (60 mg) per 1.73 m^2 surface area per day. Patients with type I or type II hyperoxaluria generally excrete two to four times this amount. Distinction between the two types of primary hyperoxaluria depends on measurements of the other organic acids that identify them: glycolic acid in type I and L-glyceric acid in type II. Since patients with pyridoxine deficiency or chronic ileal disease may excrete excessive amounts of oxalate, these conditions must be excluded.

TREATMENT   There is no satisfactory treatment. Urinary oxalate concentration can be transiently reduced by increasing the urinary flow rate. Large doses of pyridoxine (100 mg per day) may reduce urinary oxalate, but long-term effects are not dramatic. A diet high in phosphate content seems to reduce the frequency of attacks of renal colic, but oxalate excretion is unaffected. Finally, after renal transplantation renal function is lost because of calcium oxalate deposition in the transplanted kidney. The beneficial effects of combined liver-kidney transplantation observed in a single patient warrant additional study.

REFERENCES

GAHL WA et al: Lysosomal transport disorders, in *The Metabolic Basis of Inherited Disease*, 6th ed, CR Scriver et al (eds). New York, McGraw-Hill, 1989, pp 2619–2648

HILLMAN RE: Primary hyperoxalurias, in *The Metabolic Basis of Inherited Disease*, 6th ed, CR Scriver et al (eds). New York, McGraw-Hill, 1989, pp 933–944

LADU BN: Alcaptonuria, in *The Metabolic Basis of Inherited Disease*, 6th ed, CR Scriver et al (eds). New York, McGraw-Hill, 1989, pp 775–790

336 INHERITED DEFECTS OF MEMBRANE TRANSPORT

LEON E. ROSENBERG / ELIZABETH M. SHORT

The passage of certain molecules across plasma cell membranes depends on specific transport systems that owe their specificity to membrane receptor and "carrier" proteins. These membrane constituents recognize individual molecules or structurally related substances and catalyze their transmembrane movement by mechanisms poorly understood. The disorders considered in this chapter have three features in common: each is characterized by a specific defect in the transport of one or more compounds; each is inherited as a dominant or recessive trait, implying that a single genetic locus is involved; and each is presumed to reflect a primary alteration in a specific membrane protein. Many of these defects have been well characterized physiologically, but in none has the putative mutant transport protein been isolated. However, the cloning of the gene for the intestinal glucose transporter, whose deficiency underlies the glucose-galactose malabsorption syndrome, makes it possible to begin to characterize the molecular pathology in these syndromes.

More than 20 inherited disorders of membrane transport have been described in humans (Table 336-1). Most affect the gut and/or kidney only. Numerous classes of substrates are represented, including amino acids, sugars, cations, anions, vitamins, and water. Some are discussed elsewhere in this text. Those impairing the transport of amino acids, hexoses, urate, and chloride are discussed here as examples of the abnormalities encountered.

DISORDERS OF AMINO ACID TRANSPORT

As noted in Table 336-1, 10 disorders of amino acid transport have been described. Five of these (cystinuria, dibasicaminoaciduria, Hartnup disease, iminoglycinuria, and dicarboxylicaminoaciduria) show transport abnormalities for structurally related amino acids, thereby implying the existence of group-specific membrane receptors or carriers. With the exception of iminoglycinuria and dicarboxylic-aminoaciduria, these defects have important clinical consequences. The remaining five disorders affect the transport of only one amino acid, implying the existence of substrate-specific transport systems. Each of these conditions affects transport in the kidney, gut, or both; none has been shown to alter transport in other tissues.

CYSTINURIA Definition Cystinuria, the most common inborn error of amino acid transport, is characterized by excessive urinary excretion of the dibasic amino acids: lysine, arginine, ornithine, and cystine. This aminoaciduria results from impaired tubular reabsorption of these amino acids. A similar transport defect exists in the intestinal mucosa. Because cystine is the least soluble of the naturally occurring amino acids, its overexcretion predisposes to the formation of renal, ureteral, and bladder calculi. Such calculi are responsible for the signs and symptoms of the disorder.

Etiology and pathogenesis Massive excretion of cystine and the other dibasic amino acids occurs only in classic cystinuria. The disorder, inherited as an autosomal recessive trait, is believed to result from alterations in a membrane carrier protein essential for transport of this group of amino acids in the apical brush border of proximal renal tubule and small intestinal cells. The putative protein has a greater affinity for ornithine and arginine than for lysine and cystine. Although the renal clearance of all four amino acids is increased in homozygotes, the presence of some residual transport capacity for these compounds plus the existence of three other disorders marked by selective excretion of members of this group (dibasicaminoaciduria, hypercystinuria, lysinuria) argues for the existence of at least three discrete renal transport systems for these amino acids: one for each amino acid alone; one shared by lysine, arginine, and ornithine; and one for all four amino acids.

Whereas urinary excretion patterns and renal clearance abnormalities in all homozygotes are similar, evidence for three allelic variants has come from studies of intestinal transport in homozygotes and of urinary excretion in obligate heterozygotes. Type I homozygotes lack mediated intestinal transport of cystine, lysine, arginine, and ornithine; heterozygotes have normal urinary amino acid excretion patterns. Type II homozygotes lack mediated lysine transport in the gut but retain some capacity for cystine transport; heterozygotes have moderately increased urinary excretion of each of the four amino acids. Type III homozygotes retain some capacity for mediated intestinal transport of the four involved substrates; heterozygotes have modestly increased urinary lysine and cystine.

Clinical manifestations Cystinuria is among the most common inborn errors, homozygotes occurring with a frequency of 1 in 10,000 to 1 in 15,000 in many ethnic groups. Two-thirds of adults with cystinuria are type I homozygotes. Cystine stones account for 1 to 2 percent of all urinary tract calculi. The maximum solubility of cystine in the physiologic urinary pH range of 4.5 to 7.0 is about 1200 μmol/L (300 mg/L). Since affected homozygotes regularly excrete 2400 to 7200 μmol (600 to 1800 mg) per day, crystalluria and calculus formation are a constant threat. Cystine stone formation usually becomes manifest in the second or third decade but may occur in the first year of life. Symptoms and signs are those typical of urolithiasis: hematuria, flank pain, renal colic, obstructive uropathy, and infection. Recurrent urolithiasis may lead to progressive renal insufficiency.

Diagnosis The presence of cystine in a urinary tract stone is pathognomonic of cystinuria. However, since 50 percent of the stones excreted by cystinuric subjects are of mixed composition and since as many as 10 percent may contain *no* detectable cystine, a urinary nitroprusside test should be done on all patients with urolithiasis to exclude this diagnosis. The nitroprusside test is also positive (appearance of a cherry red color) in some heterozygotes for cystinuria, in patients with hypercystinuria, homocystinuria, and cysteine β-mercaptolactate disulfiduria, and in the presence of acetone in the urine. When cystine content exceeds 1000 μmol/L (250 mg/L), cystine crystals may be seen in the sediment of acidified, concentrated, chilled urine. These hexagonal crystals are pathognomonic of cystine overexcretion in patients not taking sulfonamides.

Diagnostic confirmation of cystinuria depends upon the demonstration of the characteristic amino acid excretion pattern in the urine. Selective excretion of cystine, lysine, arginine, and ornithine can be demonstrated by paper chromatography or electrophoresis, and quantitative determinations can be made by column chromatography.

TABLE 336-1   Genetic disorders of membrane transport

Class of substance and disorder	Individual substrates	Tissues manifesting transport defect	Proposed molecular basis of defect	Major clinical manifestations	Mode of inheritance	Location of discussion
AMINO ACIDS						
Classic cystinuria	Cystine, lysine, arginine, ornithine	Proximal renal tubule, jejunal mucosa	Mutation of shared dibasic-cystine transport protein	Cystine nephrolithiasis	Autosomal recessive	Chap. 336
Dibasicamino-aciduria	Lysine, arginine, ornithine	Proximal renal tubule, jejunal mucosa	Mutation of dibasic transport protein	Type I: Benign Type II: Protein intolerance, hyperammonemia, retardation	Autosomal recessive	Chap. 336
Hypercystinuria	Cystine	Proximal renal tubule	Mutation of cystine transport protein	Some risk of cystine nephrolithiasis	Autosomal recessive	Chap. 336
Lysinuria	Lysine	Proximal renal tubule, jejunal mucosa	Mutation of lysine transport protein	Seizures, physical and mental retardation	Possible autosomal recessive	Chap. 336
Hartnup disease	Neutral amino acids	Proximal renal tubule, jejunal mucosa	Mutation of shared neutral amino acid transport protein	Constant neutral aminoaciduria, intermittent symptoms of pellagra	Autosomal recessive	Chap. 336
Tryptophan malabsorption	Tryptophan	Jejunal mucosa	Mutation of tryptophan transport protein	Indoluria, ?hypercalcemia, ?nephrocalcinosis	Probable autosomal recessive	Chap. 336
Methionine malabsorption	Methionine	Jejunal mucosa	Mutation of methionine transport protein	α-Hydroxybutyric-aciduria, white hair, mental retardation, convulsions, hyperpneic attacks, edema	Probable autosomal recessive	Chap. 336
Histidinuria	Histidine	Proximal renal tubule, jejunal mucosa	Mutation of histidine transport protein	Mental retardation	Autosomal recessive	Chap. 336
Iminoglycinuria	Glycine, proline, hydroxyproline	Proximal renal tubule, jejunal mucosa	Mutation of shared glycine–imino acid transport protein	None	Autosomal recessive	Chap. 336
Dicarboxylic-aminoaciduria	Glutamic acid, aspartic acid	Proximal renal tubule, jejunal mucosa	Mutation of shared dicarboxylic amino acid transport protein	None	Probable autosomal recessive	Chap. 336
HEXOSES						
Renal glycosuria	D-Glucose	Proximal renal tubule	Mutation of D-glucose transport protein	Glycosuria with normal blood glucose	Autosomal recessive	Chap. 336
Glucose-galactose malabsorption	D-Glucose D-Galactose	Jejunal mucosa, proximal renal tubule	Mutation of shared Na^+-dependent glucose-galactose transport protein	Watery diarrhea on feeding glucose, lactose, sucrose, or galactose	Autosomal recessive	Chaps. 240, 336
LIPIDS						
Familial hypercholesterolemia	Cholesterol	Fibroblasts, lymphoid lines, leukocytes	Mutation of membrane LDL–cholesterol receptor protein	Hypercholesterolemia, tendon xanthomas, arcus corneae, coronary artery atherosclerosis	Autosomal dominant	Chap. 326
URATE						
Hypouricemia	Uric acid	Proximal renal tubule	Mutation of urate transport protein	Hypouricemia, hyperuricosuria, ?hypercalcinuria	Autosomal recessive	Chap. 336
ANIONS						
Familial hypophosphatemic rickets	Inorganic phosphate	Proximal renal tubule, jejunal mucosa	Mutation of inorganic phosphate transport protein	Hypophosphatemia, phosphaturia, phosphatopenic rickets/osteomalacia	X-linked dominant	Chap. 341

TABLE 336-1   Genetic disorders of membrane transport (*continued*)

Class of substance and disorder	Individual substrates	Tissues manifesting transport defect	Proposed molecular basis of defect	Major clinical manifestations	Mode of inheritance	Location of discussion
ANIONS (*continued*)						
Congenital chloridorrhea	Chloride	Ileal and colonic mucosa	Mutation of Cl^-/HCO_3^- exchange pump carrier protein	Hydramnios, watery diarrhea, elevated fecal chloride, achloriduria, metabolic alkalosis with volume depletion, hyperaldosteronism	Autosomal recessive	Chaps. 240, 336
Familial goiter	Inorganic iodide	Thyroid gland, salivary gland, gastric mucosa	Mutation of iodide transport protein	Congenital hypothyroidism (cretinism), goiter	Probable autosomal recessive	Chap. 316
CATIONS						
Distal renal tubular acidosis (type I—gradient)	Hydrogen ion	Distal renal tubule	Mutation of distal tubule H^+ pump carrier protein	Hyperchloremic acidosis, hypokalemia, acquired nephrocalcinosis, and hypercalcinuria	Autosomal dominant	Chap. 231
Proximal renal tubular acidosis (type II—HCO_3^- wasting)	Hydrogen ion	Proximal renal tubule	Mutation of proximal tubule H^+ pump carrier protein	Hyperchloremic acidosis, bicarbonate wasting	Probable autosomal recessive	Chap. 231
Menkes' disease	Copper	Duodenal and jejunal intestinal cells	Possible serosal transport protein or intracellular transport defect	Severe mental retardation, pili torti (kinky hair), typical facies, arterial tortuosity, excess Wormian bones, thermal instability	X-linked recessive	Chaps. 77
Hereditary Spherocytosis Elliptocytosis Ovalocytosis Stomatocytosis	Sodium	Red blood cell (RBC) membranes	Mutation of membrane structure (? lipid or protein) resulting in increased sodium permeability	Increased RBC fragility resulting in variable degrees of hemolytic anemia, splenomegaly, and jaundice; RBC shape respectively spherocytic, elliptocytic, ovalocytic, or stomatocytic (target-shaped)	Each of these diseases of RBC morphology is a separately inherited autosomal dominant	Chap. 294
WATER						
Nephrogenic diabetes insipidus (AVP-resistant)	Water	Distal renal tubule	Lack of activation of AVP-responsive luminal membrane adenylate cyclase, possible defect in receptor or enzyme protein	Polyuria, polydipsia, hyposthenuria	X-linked recessive	Chap. 231
VITAMINS						
Juvenile pernicious anemia	Cobalamin (vitamin B_{12})	Ileal mucosa	Mutation of receptor for intrinsic factor–cobalamin complex	Megaloblastic anemia	Autosomal recessive	Chap. 292
Folate malabsorption	Folic acid	Small bowel	Mutation of folate transport protein	Megaloblastic anemia	Autosomal recessive	Chap. 292

Quantitation is important for differentiating some heterozygotes from homozygotes and documenting the reduction of free cystine excretion during therapy.

Treatment   Medical management is aimed at reducing the concentration of cystine in urine. The most important treatment is maintenance of a large urine volume. Fluid ingestion in excess of 4 L/d is essential, and 5 to 7 L/d is optimal. Urinary cystine excretion should measure less than 1000 to 1200 μmol/L (250 to 300 mg/L). The daily fluid ingestion necessary to maintain this dilution of excreted cystine should be spaced over the waking hours, with one-quarter to one-third of the total volume ingested at bedtime. Stones can be prevented and even dissolved by such hydration. It must be made clear to the cystinuric subject that water is a drug. Solubility of cystine rises sharply in urine above pH 7.5, and urinary alkalinization can be therapeutic in some situations. Vigorous administration of sodium bicarbonate, acetazolamide, and polycitrates is required to maintain a persistently alkaline pH, but this measure introduces the danger of inducing formation of other "alkaline" stones (calcium oxalate, calcium phosphate, magnesium ammonium phosphate) and even of producing nephrocalcinosis.

Another treatment involves administration of penicillamine which undergoes sulfhydryl-disulfide exchange with cystine to form the mixed disulfide of penicillamine and cysteine. Since this disulfide is more than 50 times as soluble as cystine, penicillamine (in doses of 1 to 3 g per day) has the capacity to reduce free cystine excretion markedly, thereby preventing new stone formation and promoting dissolution of existing calculi. Unfortunately, allergic manifestations include acute serum sickness, agranulocytosis, pancytopenia, immune glomerulitis, and the Goodpasture syndrome. Thus, its use should be reserved for patients who fail to respond to hydration alone or who are in a high-risk category (one remaining kidney, renal insufficiency). Those patients unable to tolerate penicillamine may benefit from α-mercaptopropionylglycine, an experimental drug whose mechanism of action is similar to that of penicillamine but whose structure, and hence toxicity, is different. As many as two-thirds of patients unable to tolerate penicillamine may take α-mercaptopropionylglycine without ill effects. When medical management fails, urologic surgery is required. An occasional patient may require renal transplantation because of renal failure.

DIBASICAMINOACIDURIA Families have been described in which affected members have a defect in renal tubular reabsorption of lysine, arginine, and ornithine but *not* of cystine. The disorder almost surely reflects mutations in the genes coding for widely distributed transport protein used by the three dibasic amino acids only. Two variants have been observed, each apparently inherited as an autosomal recessive trait. Manifestations are related to the losses of ornithine, arginine, and perhaps lysine.

In the common form of dibasicaminoaciduria (type II), also known as lysinuric protein intolerance and much more common in Finland (1 in 60,000) than elsewhere in the world, homozygotes show defective intestinal transport of dibasic amino acids as well as exaggerated renal losses. The transport defect affects basolateral rather than luminal membrane transport. A defect in uptake of these substances by cultured fibroblasts and hepatocytes has also been reported. Affected patients present in childhood with hepatosplenomegaly, protein intolerance, and episodic ammonia intoxication. Plasma concentrations of lysine, arginine, and ornithine are reduced. The clinical findings have been attributed to hyperammonemia resulting from insufficient amounts of arginine and ornithine to maintain proper function of the urea cycle. Treatment includes dietary protein restriction and supplementation with citrulline, a neutral amino acid whose intestinal and hepatic transport are unimpaired, and which, when metabolized to arginine and ornithine, fuels the urea cycle. With 2.0 to 3.0 g of oral citrulline daily, dietary protein intake can be increased and growth improved in pediatric patients. Obligate heterozygotes are healthy and show no excess urinary loss of dibasic amino acids.

Type I dibasicaminoaciduria has been described in a large French-Canadian kindred. The female proband was moderately mentally retarded but had no clear history of protein intolerance or hyperammonemia. Her urinary losses of dibasic amino acids were not as great as those seen in type II homozygotes. The condition was distinguished from type II by the presence of modest excesses of dibasic amino acids in urine of both asymptomatic parents. A large number of chemically affected members of the family were also symptom-free. Other pedigrees containing asymptomatic heterozygotes have been identified by urinary screening programs. Type I disease may involve the same transport system as that impaired in the more common and severe type II disorder.

HARTNUP DISEASE Pellagra-like skin lesions, variable neurologic manifestations, and aminoaciduria for the monoaminomonocarboxylic amino acids with neutral or aromatic side chains characterize symptomatic Hartnup disease. Alanine, serine, threonine, valine, leucine, isoleucine, phenylalanine, tyrosine, tryptophan, glutamine, asparagine, and histidine are excreted in urine in quantities 5 to 10 times normal, and intestinal transport for these same amino acids is defective. The clinical manifestations result from nutritional deficiency of the essential amino acid tryptophan, caused by the combination of intestinal malabsorption and renal loss. Disease manifestations are episodic, related, at least in part, to metabolic demands for tryptophan. Only a small fraction of patients with the chemical findings typical of this disorder develop a pellagra-like syndrome, implying that onset of the clinical picture depends on factors over and above the transport defect.

The major pathway of tryptophan metabolism leads to the synthesis of niacin and nicotinamide-adenine dinucleotide (NAD). This pathway supplies about 50 percent of daily niacin needs. In patients with Hartnup disease, the renal and intestinal transport defect for tryptophan leads to niacin deficiency. The transport defect likely reflects abnormalities of a group-specific system for neutral amino acids. Some residual reabsorptive capacity persists for each involved amino acid. This suggests that they are transported by other carrier systems as well, a conclusion supported by the identification of patients with substrate-specific transport errors for tryptophan, methionine, and histidine.

Hartnup disease is inherited as an autosomal recessive trait. Homozygotes occur with a frequency of about 1 in 24,000 births. Heterozygotes exhibit no clinical or chemical abnormalities.

Pellagra is the clinical syndrome produced by dietary niacin deficiency, and its clinical features are those that characterize Hartnup disease (see Chap. 76). The diagnosis should be suspected in any patient with pellagra without a history of dietary niacin deficiency. The neurologic and psychiatric manifestations range from attacks of cerebellar ataxia to mild emotional lability to frank delirium and usually accompany exacerbations of the erythematous, eczematoid skin rash. Fever, sunlight, stress, and sulfonamide therapy provoke clinical relapses. Diagnosis is made by detection of the neutral aminoaciduria that does not occur in dietary niacin deficiency. Treatment is directed at niacin repletion and includes a high-protein diet and daily nicotinamide supplementation (50 to 250 mg).

IMINOGLYCINURIA This trait is characterized by excessive urinary excretion of glycine and the imino acids proline and hydroxyproline. Homozygotes for this autosomal recessive disorder occur with a frequency of about 1 in 16,000. The exaggerated renal clearance of glycine, proline, and hydroxyproline reflects a defect in the tubular transport system shared by these three compounds. An intestinal transport defect may also be present. This suggests that more than one mutation may lead to persistent iminoglycinuria, a thesis corroborated by the demonstration that obligate heterozygotes from some but not all families manifest glycinuria. No consistent clinical abnormalities have been reported in homozygotes, who are usually detected by urinary amino acid screening programs. Individuals with iminoglycinuria should be reassured as to the benign nature of the disturbance.

DICARBOXYLICAMINOACIDURIA Selective urinary loss and exaggerated endogenous renal clearance of glutamic and aspartic acids have been described in two unrelated children. Intestinal absorption of these dicarboxylic amino acids was impaired in one. This patient suffered from recurrent hypoglycemia; the other was asymptomatic.

SUBSTRATE-SPECIFIC DEFECTS IN AMINO ACID TRANSPORT
Rare pedigrees exist in which individuals have defective renal tubular reabsorption and/or impaired intestinal absorption of a single free amino acid. These disorders, each apparently inherited as an autosomal recessive trait, suggest that transport of amino acids is catalyzed by substrate-specific as well as group-specific transport mechanisms.

Hypercystinuria Two siblings exhibited modest cystinuria without excessive urinary excretion of lysine, arginine, or ornithine. Fractional tubular reabsorption of cystine was reduced to about 80 percent of the filtered load, and up to 250 mg per day was excreted in the urine. Neither sibling showed any abnormality in intestinal absorption of cystine. Both were clinically well, although the cystine excretion places them at risk for cystine urolithiasis. Urinary cystine excretion by the parents was normal.

Lysinuria A child with selective impairment of renal tubular reabsorption of lysine has been described. Endogenous lysine clearance was increased; intestinal transport was impaired; plasma lysine was reduced. Mental and growth retardation and seizures were present. A lysine-supplemented diet stimulated growth. Urinary lysine excretion was normal in the parents.

Histidinuria Two siblings, each with mental retardation, exhibited a renal transport defect for histidine only. Urinary loss of histidine approached 40 to 50 percent of the filtered load, and an intestinal transport defect for histidine was also present. The clinically normal parents had normal urinary excretion but a modest defect in intestinal absorption of histidine. In two additional cases of isolated histidinuria myoclonic seizures occurred.

Methionine malabsorption Single children from two pedigrees have shown an intestinal transport defect for methionine. One may have had a renal transport defect as well. This disorder was detected because of urinary excretion of α-hydroxybutyric acid, a by-product of the intestinal bacterial breakdown of the unabsorbed methionine. This compound, which gives an odor resembling malt or dried celery to the urine, appears to be responsible for the white hair, attacks of hyperpnea, convulsions, edema, and mental retardation. Treatment of one of these children with a methionine-restricted diet caused improvement in all clinical manifestations.

Tryptophan malabsorption An isolated defect in intestinal absorption of tryptophan has been described in two siblings. The renal tubular reabsorption of tryptophan was normal. A variety of indoles were excreted in stool and urine. These compounds result from chemical degradation of unabsorbed tryptophan by intestinal bacteria and may be present in patients with Hartnup disease as well. Because of concomitant renal disease, hydrolytic enzymes were released into the urine, acted upon the indoles found there, and led to the formation of a blue pigment, indigotin. This sequence of events earned this condition the sobriquet "blue-diaper syndrome." No pellagra-like symptoms were described. The mother also excreted indole compounds, suggesting that she is a carrier of this trait.

DISORDERS OF HEXOSE TRANSPORT

Nondiabetic melituria occurs in a number of conditions. Pentoses, hexoses, heptoses, and disaccharides have been identified in the urine; all except sucrose yield a positive test for reducing substances. Some meliturias result from diffuse renal injury, others from ingestion of nonmetabolizable sugars. In still others the sugars accumulate in blood owing to deficient activity of catabolizing enzyme systems and "spill" into the urine. Only among the hexoses have specific inherited disorders of sugar transport been identified. The existence of renal glycosuria and intestinal glucose-galactose malabsorption as heritable, autosomal recessive disorders points to the existence of at least two specific carrier proteins for hexoses in human jejunal and renal brush border membranes: one for glucose and one shared by glucose and galactose.

RENAL GLYCOSURIA To avoid confusion with diabetes mellitus, Marble's criteria for the diagnosis of renal glycosuria should be followed: (1) glycosuria in the absence of hyperglycemia, (2) constant glycosuria with little fluctuation related to diet, (3) normal (or slightly flat) oral glucose tolerance test, (4) identification of urinary reducing substance as glucose, and (5) normal storage and utilization of carbohydrates. The Fanconi syndrome, in which renal glycosuria occurs as part of generalized proximal tubular dysfunction, should also be excluded. The condition is benign, but occasionally glycosuria may be great enough to cause polyuria and polydipsia. Even more rarely, dehydration or ketosis may develop under conditions of stress such as pregnancy or starvation.

In normal persons glucose is present in the glomerular filtrate at a concentration equal to that in plasma water and is reabsorbed throughout the proximal renal tubule by a sodium-dependent, phlorizin-inhibitable transport process. Reabsorptive capacity exceeds normal plasma glucose concentration. Thus, glucose does not appear in the urine until the threshold for reabsorption is reached. The plasma concentration at which filtered glucose begins to escape proximal tubular reabsorption is usually around 10 mmol/L (200 mg/dL). Maximal renal reabsorptive capacity is exceeded at a filtered load of around 2 mmol (325 mg)/min per 1.73 m² body surface area, and this value is defined as the tubular maximum for glucose (TmG).

Two patterns of glycosuria are recognized: type A characterized by a reduced tubular maximum reabsorptive capacity and type B showing a reduced threshold for glycosuria, an increased "splay" in the titration curve, and a normal TmG. Marked renal glycosuria occurs in individuals homozygous for either of these recessively inherited mutations and in genetic compounds for these presumably allelic mutations. Modest reduction in renal threshold or TmG is present in obligate heterozygotes in some pedigrees; modest glycosuria occurs in such family members when plasma glucose is elevated. The gene responsible for renal glycosuria segregates with the human histocompatibility leukocyte antigen (HLA) haplotype suggesting its location on chromosome 6. No linkage disequilibrium was observed, and no specific HLA antigens have been associated with renal glycosuria.

GLUCOSE-GALACTOSE MALABSORPTION In this condition, infants develop a profuse, watery diarrhea when fed milk or foods containing lactose, sucrose, glucose, or galactose. Fructose or carbohydrate-free formulas are well tolerated. A specific defect in intestinal absorption of glucose and galactose can be demonstrated by oral tolerance tests that produce little or no increase in plasma glucose or galactose. The primary defect involves the sodium/hexose cotransporter found in the intestinal and renal brush border. Active D-glucose and D-galactose transport are absent in affected children, and intermediate transport capacity is present in their parents. These findings confirm the specificity and the autosomal recessive inheritance of the disorder. Treatment with a glucose- and galactose-free diet leads to resolution of symptoms in childhood. Although the basic transport defect is present throughout life, most patients show an improved tolerance for glucose and galactose with age.

A number of these patients have renal glycosuria at normal plasma glucose concentrations. Renal titration studies generally demonstrate a reduced threshold for glucose reabsorption (type B renal glycosuria) with a normal TmG. Urinary glucose loss is not as severe as in isolated renal glycosuria. This finding suggests the presence of multiple glucose transport proteins in the kidney. One, responsible for the bulk of glucose reabsorption and specific for glucose only, is affected in renal glycosuria; another, shared by glucose and galactose and responsible for transporting less of the filtered load of glucose, is affected in glucose-galactose malabsorption. Either the former is not present in intestinal mucosa, or the shared system is more important in that tissue. In both disorders transport of sugars in all other tested tissues is normal, reflecting the multiplicity and tissue specificity of membrane transport proteins.

DEFECTIVE URATE TRANSPORT: HYPOURICEMIA

Individuals with a selective defect in renal tubular reabsorption of sodium urate have marked hypouricemia. Since little serum urate is bound to plasma proteins, failure to reabsorb filtered urate results in a serum urate ranging from 12 to 110 μmol/L (0.2 to 1.8 mg/dL). Moderate uricosuria is present, and half of patients have renal calculi.

Renal urate clearance normally averages 15 percent of glomerular filtration rate, and the excreted urate is composed both of filtered urate that has escaped reabsorption and secreted urate. Subjects with isolated hypouricemia have urate clearances averaging from 33 to 85 percent of the filtration rate; in some, urate clearance exceeds the glomerular filtration rate. Studies with probenecid, which blocks tubular reabsorption of urate, and pyrazinamide, which blocks tubular secretion, reveal that six of the eight families described have a presecretory urate reabsorptive defect, and two have defective transport affecting the entire tubule. In four families hypercalciuria due to enhanced intestinal calcium absorption is also present, but in others only uricosuria has been demonstrated. The defect is inherited as an autosomal recessive trait. Urate transport has not been studied in nonrenal tissue or in obligate heterozygotes. The defect is presumed to reflect mutation of one or both of the proximal renal tubular membrane proteins that transport sodium urate. The findings in these families support the hypothesis that renal urate reabsorption is controlled by more than one transport protein.

DEFECTIVE ANION TRANSPORT: CHLORIDORRHEA

This rare, autosomal recessive disease results from impairment of active transport of chloride in the ileum and colon. Absence of the chloride-bicarbonate ion exchange "pump" causes profound symptoms even before birth (polyhydramnios and absence of meconium). Massive watery diarrhea is apparent from the first days of life. This fluid loss, with its attendant impairment of electrolyte homeostasis, is life-threatening. A hypokalemic, hypochloremic, hyponatremic metabolic alkalosis develops with dehydration and secondary hyperaldosteronism. Fecal fluid contains an excess of chloride ion over the sum of the accompanying cations, sodium and potassium. Fecal chloride concentration always exceeds 90 mmol/L when volume and serum electrolyte disturbances are corrected, and this chloridorrhea is diagnostic. Renal chloride transport is normal. Decreased urine chloride results from the kidney's attempts to conserve salt and water.

Treatment requires adequate, life-long repletion of electrolyte and fluid losses, since no way has yet been found to mitigate the transport disorder. Exact replacement of water, sodium chloride, and potassium chloride can prevent the growth and psychomotor retardation and the development of progressive renal damage. The renal lesion, with hyalinized glomeruli, juxtaglomerular hyperplasia, calcifications, and arteriolar changes, is probably a result of chronic volume depletion. Treatment of hyperreninemia and hypokalemia with prostaglandin inhibitors may reduce renal damage but does not alter intestinal symptoms or the need for chronic sodium chloride repletion.

REFERENCES

DESJEUX JF: Congenital selective Na$^+$ D-glucose cotransport defects leading to renal glycosuria and congenital selective intestinal malabsorption of glucose and galactose, in *The Metabolic Basis of Inherited Disease*, 6th ed, CR Scriver et al (eds). New York, McGraw-Hill, 1989, pp 2463–2478

ELSAS LJ, ROSENBERG LE: Renal glycosuria, in *Strauss and Welt's Diseases of the Kidney*, 3d ed, LE Earley, CW Gottschalk (eds). Boston, Little, Brown, 1979, pp 1021–1028

HOLMBERG C, PERHEENTUPA J: Congenital chloride diarrhoea (CCD), in *Population Structure and Genetic Disorders*, AW Erikson et al (eds). New York, Academic, 1980, pp 596–599

KAMOUN PP et al: Renal histidinuria. J Inherited Metab Dis 4:217, 1981

LEVY HL: Hartnup disorder, in *The Metabolic Basis of Inherited Disease*, 6th ed, CR Scriver et al (eds). New York, McGraw-Hill, 1989, pp 2515–2528

ROSENBERG LE: Intestinal hexose transport in familial glucose-galactose malabsorption, in *Membranes and Disease*, L Bolis et al (eds). New York, Raven Press, 1976, pp 253–262

———, SCRIVER CR: Disorders of amino acid metabolism, in *Metabolic Control and Disease*, 8th ed, PK Bondy, LE Rosenberg (eds). Philadelphia, Saunders, 1980, pp 616–645

SEGAL S, THIER SO: Cystinurias, in *The Metabolic Basis of Inherited Disease*, 6th ed, CR Scriver et al (eds). New York, McGraw-Hill, 1989, pp 2479–2496

SHORT EM, ROSENBERG LE: Renal aminoaciduria, in *Strauss and Welt's Diseases of the Kidney*, 3d ed, LE Earley, CW Gottschalk (eds). Boston, Little, Brown, 1979, pp 975–1020

SIMELL O: Lysinuric protein intolerance and other cationic aminoacidurias, in *The Metabolic Basis of Inherited Disease*, 6th ed, CR Scriver et al (eds). New York, McGraw-Hill, 1989, pp 2497–2514

WEITZ R, SPERLING O: Hereditary renal hypouricemia: Isolated tubular defect of urate reabsorption. J Pediatr 96:850, 1980

337   GALACTOSEMIA, GALACTOKINASE DEFICIENCY, AND OTHER RARE DISORDERS OF CARBOHYDRATE METABOLISM

KURT J. ISSELBACHER

DEFINITION   Galactosemia refers to any of three inborn errors of galactose metabolism. "*Classic*" galactosemia is due to the deficiency of galactose-1-phosphate uridyl transferase (GALT) and is typically associated with cataract formation, mental retardation, and cirrhosis. The second disorder, *galactokinase deficiency*, leads primarily to cataract formation. The third, *UDP-galactose-4-epimerase deficiency*, is the rarest of the group; few cases have been described, and the eventual outcome is uncertain.

PATHOGENESIS   Lactose, the main carbohydrate in milk, is a disaccharide containing galactose and glucose; when ingested it is hydrolyzed by intestinal lactase. Normally the absorbed galactose is converted to glucose in the liver. The first reaction in this pathway is the phosphorylation of galactose to galactose-1-phosphate by galactokinase (specified by a gene on chromosome 17):

$$\text{Galactose} + \text{ATP} \xrightarrow{\text{galactokinase}} \text{galactose-1-phosphate}$$

The next step involves the conversion of galactose-1-phosphate to glucose-1-phosphate by GALT, the gene for which is on chromosome 9:

$$\text{Galactose-1-phosphate} + \text{UDP-glucose} \xrightarrow{\text{GALT}}$$
$$\text{UDP-galactose} + \text{glucose-1-phosphate}$$

The uridine diphosphate (UDP) sugars can be reversibly interconverted by an epimerase reaction (UDP-galactose-4-epimerase):

$$\text{UDP-galactose} \longleftrightarrow \text{UDP-glucose}$$

Galactose can also be metabolized by alternative pathways. It can be converted (reduced) in the presence of NADPH (or NADH) to galactitol (dulcitol) by aldose reductase. It can also be oxidized to a limited extent by galactose dehydrogenase, leading to the formation of galactonic acid, xyulose, and CO_2. These pathways account for limited galactose metabolism in patients with galactosemia.

In galactokinase deficiency, galactose accumulates in the blood and tissues. In the lens galactose is converted by aldose reductase to galactitol, a sugar to which the lens is impermeable. As a consequence, excessive hydration occurs which, together with a decrease in glutathione in the lens, leads to cataract formation.

In classic galactosemia, GALT deficiency results in tissue accumulation of galactose-1-phosphate and galactose. As in galactokinase deficiency, cataracts develop secondary to galactitol accumulation in the lens. It is assumed that the cirrhosis and mental retardation of classic galactosemia are related to increased amounts of galactose-1-phosphate in these tissues. Elevated blood galactose levels may lead to a decreased hepatic output of glucose and hence to hypoglycemia. In the kidney and intestine accumulation of galactose and galactose-1-phosphate appears to lead to an inhibition of amino acid transport. In female homozygotes there is an increased incidence of hypergonadotrophic hypogonadism in which ovarian failure develops at an early age.

Both galactokinase and GALT deficiencies are transmitted as autosomal recessive traits. Heterozygotes for these disorders have half-normal enzyme levels but are asymptomatic. Maternal deficiency of galactokinase, together with lactose intake during pregnancy, may contribute to cataract formation during fetal development. However, not all persons with half-normal GALT enzymes in their cells are carriers of classic galactosemia. Some individuals homozygous for another gene, called the *Duarte variant*, normally have half-normal GALT levels and are asymptomatic. This group can be differentiated from classic galactosemia heterozygotes on the basis of the electrophoretic properties of the mutant enzyme. In both galactokinase deficiency and classic galactosemia there is a functional deficiency or absence of the involved enzyme. Classic galactosemia is due to a structural gene mutation, and the altered enzyme (GALT) protein does not function normally. Other clinical variants with altered enzyme electrophoretic mobility have been described.

The incidence of classic galactosemia is about 1 per 80,000 births in the white population. Approximately 0.8 to 1.3 percent of the population are heterozygotes for the galactosemia (GALT) gene, and about 10 percent carry the Duarte variant. During screening of newborns for galactosemia the most frequent cause of an abnormal result is compound heterozygosity for the Duarte variant and for classic galactosemia in which GALT levels are about 17 percent of normal. Such individuals are clinically asymptomatic.

CLINICAL FEATURES Symptoms of classic galactosemia usually begin within days to weeks after birth. The infant usually is reluctant to ingest breast milk or milk formulas, develops vomiting, shows poor nutrition, and fails to thrive. Jaundice, hepatomegaly, and evidence of liver disease may develop. Cataracts are usually not present at birth but develop gradually over weeks to months. Mental retardation becomes evident after 6 to 12 months and is usually not reversible. Infants with classic galactosemia are subject to bacterial sepsis (especially with *Escherichia coli*), and this may be the leading cause of death in the neonatal period. The only consistent feature of galactokinase deficiency is cataract formation.

DIAGNOSIS Galactokinase deficiency should be suspected in infants or children with cataract formation who have non-glucose-reducing substances in the urine. The diagnosis is made by demonstrating the deficiency of galactokinase in red blood cells.

Classic galactosemia must be considered when one or more of the clinical features described above are found. If the patient is ingesting milk, reducing sugar is present in the urine but gives a negative glucose oxidase reaction (i.e., is not glucose) and is identified as galactose by other techniques, such as chromatography. If the child is vomiting, has a poor food intake, or is on intravenous glucose feedings, galactose may not be present in the urine. The definitive diagnosis is made by demonstrating a lack or deficiency of red cell GALT by one of several techniques. The disease can also be diagnosed prenatally by enzyme studies on culture amniocentesis cells or by demonstrating increased galactitol in amniotic fluid. A nonenzymatic glycosylation of hemoglobin, analogous to that in diabetes mellitus, can be detected in patients with galactosemia as manifested by increased concentrations in the blood of Hb A_{lab} rather than Hb A_{1c}.

In the neonatal period galactosemia needs to be differentiated from primary liver disease. With liver damage, galactose removal from the blood is impaired, and elevated blood galactose levels and galactosuria may be present. However, GALT levels are normal in patients with liver damage.

TREATMENT The treatment of galactosemia consists of the removal of galactose-containing foods from the diet, especially milk. Milk substitutes such as Nutramigen are often used. Although soybean preparations contain polysaccharide-bound galactose, they appear to be well tolerated because the bound galactose is not readily liberated. In general, the red cell levels of galactose-1-phosphate are not increased in affected infants fed soybean formulas.

The institution of a galactose-free diet usually leads to a dramatic improvement in all clinical features except for mental retardation. Patients should be kept on galactose-free diets indefinitely or at least until they have attained adequate physical and neurologic development.

OTHER DISORDERS OF CARBOHYDRATE METABOLISM Features of hereditary fructose intolerance and fructose-1,6-diphosphatase deficiency, two autosomal recessive disorders of fructose metabolism that lead to hypoglycemia, are summarized in Table 337-1 (also see Chaps. 332 and 320).

REFERENCES

ALLEN TJ et al: Evidence of galactosemia in utero. Lancet 1:603, 1980

BURMAN D et al (eds): *Inborn Errors of Carbohydrate Metabolism.* Lancaster, MTP Press, 1979

GITZELMANN R et al: Essential fructosuria, heredity fructose intolerance, and fructose 1,6-diphosphatase deficiency, in *The Metabolic Basis of Inherited Disease,* 5th ed, JB Stanbury et al (eds). New York, McGraw-Hill, 1983, p 118

KAUFMAN FR et al: Correlation of ovarian function with galactose-1-phosphate uridyl transferase levels in galactosemia. J Pediatr 112:754, 1988

NG WG et al: Transferase-deficiency galactosemia and the Duarte variant. JAMA 257:187, 1987

SARDHARWALLA IB, WRAITH JE: Galactosemia. Nutr Health 5:175, 1987

SEGAL S: Disorders of galactose metabolism, in *The Metabolic Basis of Inherited Disease,* 5th ed, JB Stanbury et al (eds). New York, McGraw-Hill, 1983, p 167

338 THE LIPODYSTROPHIES AND OTHER RARE DISORDERS OF ADIPOSE TISSUE

DANIEL W. FOSTER

This chapter is concerned with abnormalities in adipose tissue. The disorders are rare, the pathophysiology is frequently not clear, and only clinical descriptions can be given.

THE LIPODYSTROPHIES

The lipodystrophies are characterized by generalized or partial loss of body fat and metabolic abnormalities, including insulin resistance, hyperglycemia, and hypertriglyceridemia. A classification is shown in Table 338-1. In *generalized lipodystrophy* essentially all body fat is lost, while in *partial lipodystrophy* fat atrophy is limited. The

TABLE 337-1 Some other disorders of carbohydrate metabolism

Disorder	Metabolic defect	Manifestations
Hereditary fructose intolerance	Deficiency of fructose-l-phosphate aldolase leads to accumulation of fructose-1-PO$_4$ in tissues.	Liver disease, renal tubular damage, and hypoglycemia.
Fructose-1,6-diphosphatase deficiency	Deficiency of the enzyme prevents gluconeogenesis from its normal precursors, lactate, glycerol, and alanine. Thus, maintenance of blood sugar is dependent upon exogenous glucose.	Lactic acidosis leads to hyperventilation, somnolence, and coma, usually with hypoglycemia and ketosis.

TABLE 338-1 The lipodystrophies

1 Generalized lipodystrophy
  a Congenital (familial or sporadic)
  b Acquired (sporadic)
2 Partial lipodystrophy
  a Common (sporadic)
  b Dominant (familial)
    (*1*) Limb and trunk
    (*2*) With Rieger anomaly
3 Localized lipodystrophy
  a Inflammatory
  b Noninflammatory

common acquired form of partial lipodystrophy ordinarily involves half the body, usually the upper segment. Dominantly transmitted partial lipodystrophy tends to spare the face. One variant is associated with eye and tooth malformations, the Rieger anomaly. *Localized lipodystrophy* may be either inflammatory or noninflammatory. The best-studied syndrome is *centrifugal lipodystrophy* in which fat atrophy begins in the groins or axillae of children under the age of 3 and spreads centrally to involve the entire abdomen. The edge of the lesion is red and scaly with an inflammatory infiltrate demonstrable on histologic examination. Fat atrophy usually disappears spontaneously when the patient is around 13 years of age.

GENERALIZED LIPODYSTROPHY   Generalized lipodystrophy (also called lipoatrophic diabetes) may be either congenital or acquired. The congenital form is transmitted as an autosomal recessive trait. Males and females are equally affected. Rates of parental consanguinity are high. Loss of fat is usually obvious at birth, but the rest of the clinical picture may not appear until later (up to 30 years). The acquired disease often develops after some other illness. Measles, chicken pox, whooping cough, or infectious mononucleosis are common precipitating events, but hypothyroidism, hyperthyroidism, and pregnancy have been implicated. Some cases begin with the appearance of painful nodular swellings of adipose tissue resembling acute panniculitis (see below). The congenital and acquired forms are similar in clinical manifestations (Table 338-2).

Fat atrophy   Loss of body fat is the characteristic feature. In congenital cases the skin of the face is tightly drawn over the bony structures, and the entire body is devoid of adipose tissue. Rarely, a small amount of breast fat remains. In the acquired form the face may be spared, but all other fat disappears. Adipose tissue cells can be identified microscopically, but they contain no triglyceride stores. Paradoxically the liver is engorged with fat, and the reticuloendothelial system contains lipid-laden macrophages (foam cells). The cause of the fat atrophy is not known. Fat-mobilizing polypeptides have been reported in the urine of patients with generalized lipodystrophy, but their role in the disease is uncertain.

A candidate molecule for the induction of lipodystrophy is a compound similar to cachectin (tumor necrosis factor), which is a potent inhibitor of lipoprotein lipase and causes fat depletion and hypertriglyceridemia when injected into animals. Lipoprotein lipase activity is low in generalized lipodystrophy, as would be predicted if a cachectin-like inducer were the cause. However, plasma levels of tumor necrosis factor were normal in two of the author's patients. Hepatic lipase is not impaired. Since triglyceride content of the adipocyte is the result of a balance between fat synthesis and fat breakdown, an alternative mechanism might involve activation of the hormone-sensitive lipase that catalyzes hydrolysis of triglycerides in the fat cell. For example, a defect in a natural inhibitor of the lipase, such as adenosine, could result in enhanced response to physiologic (nonelevated) concentrations of lipolytic hormones. Release of free fatty acids into plasma following norepinephrine infusion is impaired, but this may simply reflect the depleted triglyceride stores.

Although an inducing molecule could act as a circulating hormone in generalized lipodystrophy, such an etiology is unlikely in partial lipodystrophy where autotransplantation of adipocytes from an affected area to a nonaffected site resulted in reaccumulation of fat, and reverse transplantation from normal to affected site resulted in fat atrophy. An autocrine or paracrine function may be involved. In the former a cellular product would act on the cell of origin while in the latter a cellular product would act on adjacent cells, but in neither case would the putative inducer of lipodystrophy enter the circulation to act as a typical hormone.

Growth and maturation   Linear growth is accelerated in the first few years of life in the congenital disorder and in acquired disease that begins early in childhood. Epiphyses close early, however, so that the final height is usually normal. True muscular hypertrophy is present, and patients may have an acromegalic appearance with coarse facial features and large hands and feet. The ears tend to be prominent in the congenital form. Many viscera are enlarged, and generalized lymphadenopathy may be present. The cause of the growth disorder is not known. Levels of growth hormone and insulin-like growth factor I (IGF-I, somatomedin C) are normal or low. Insulin-like growth factor II has not been systematically assessed. One possibility is that abnormal growth and pseudoacromegaly are due to high concentrations of insulin in plasma secondary to insulin resistance (see below). The elevated insulin might cross-react with the IGF-I receptor in muscle and cartilage and promote growth via this mechanism.

Liver   Enlargement of the liver causes protuberance of the abdomen. Fatty liver may progress to cirrhosis, especially in the acquired disorder. Several patients have died from bleeding esophageal varices. Splenomegaly does not occur in the absence of portal hypertension.

Kidneys   The kidneys are usually enlarged. Subjects with the acquired disorder may have proteinuria and the nephrotic syndrome, although not as frequently as in partial lipodystrophy. Moderate hypertension is common.

Genitalia   The external genitalia (penis and testes in males, clitoris and labia majora in females) are usually hypertrophied in congenital disease. In women polycystic ovaries are common, resulting in the clinical picture of Stein-Leventhal syndrome. The cause of the genital abnormalities is not known. Systematic investigation of gonadotropin, estrogen, and androgen metabolism has not been carried out.

Skin   Acanthosis nigricans is present in most. Hypertrichosis of face, neck, trunk, and limbs is frequent. Scalp hair is usually thick and curly, particularly early in life.

Central nervous system   Mental retardation is present in about half the congenital cases. Dilatation of the third ventricle and basal cisterns has been demonstrated by pneumoencephalography. Central nervous system involvement appears to be less marked in the acquired disease, although two patients had astrocytomas arising in the floor of the third ventricle. Few patients have been examined with computed tomography or magnetic resonance imaging so that firm conclusions regarding CNS abnormalities cannot be drawn.

TABLE 338-2   Characteristics of the lipodystrophies

Finding	Congenital general	Acquired general	Acquired partial	Dominant partial
Inheritance	Autosomal recessive	Sporadic	Usually sporadic	Autosomal dominant
Age of onset	Infancy	Childhood to adult	Childhood to adult	Puberty
Sex incidence	Males and females equal	Female preponderance	Female preponderance	Female preponderance
Lipoatrophy	Face, trunk, limbs	Face, trunk, limbs	Face, upper trunk, upper limbs	Trunk and limbs
Liver involvement	+	+ +	Rare	0
Renal disease	+	+	+ +	0
Insulin resistance	+	+	+	+
Hyperglycemia	+	+	+	+
Hypertriglyceridemia	+	+	+	+
Acanthosis nigricans	+	+	Rare	+
Genital hypertrophy	+	+	Rare	+
Bone age	Accelerated	Normal to accelerated	Normal	Normal

Other abnormalities Bones tend to be sclerotic in generalized lipodystrophy, and cystic angiomatosis may be present. Cardiomegaly is common, but heart failure appears to be rare. Goiter is frequent. The associated abnormalities in generalized lipodystrophy are summarized in Table 338-3.

Metabolic and endocrine abnormalities Three major metabolic disturbances are characteristic.

1 Insulin resistance. Insulin resistance may be mild or severe. When severe the hyperglycemia may be difficult to control. Insulin and C-peptide concentrations are relatively or absolutely elevated, and response to exogenous insulin is impaired. Resistance is due to several causes, and affected siblings may exhibit different mechanisms. Increased insulin clearance, decreased number of insulin receptors, diminished affinity of the receptor for insulin, and postreceptor defects have all been reported. Insulin in the plasma of affected subjects is biologically active. Although glucagon levels are high (indicating insulin resistance in the alpha cell of the islets of Langerhans) and free fatty acid concentrations are elevated, ketoacidosis is unusual. One patient had recurrent epidoses of metabolic acidosis considered to be ketoacidosis, but concentrations of acetoacetate and β-hydroxybutyrate were characteristic of fasting ketosis, not ketoacidosis; presumably lactate or other organic acids were involved.

Ketoacidosis may be infrequent because insulin resistance spares liver and skeletal muscle (or is less severe); glycogen levels in the liver are high (insulin stimulates glycogen synthesis), and branched-chain amino acids fall normally in response to injected insulin. Elevated insulin levels in portal vein plasma would counteract the actions of glucagon in the insulin-responsive hepatocyte. This would prevent activation of the ketone body synthesis in liver and assure utilization of incoming fatty acids for triglyceride synthesis and production of very low density lipoproteins. The elevated long-chain fatty acids in the plasma are of dietary origin and fall toward normal with restriction of dietary fat. The diabetes mellitus accompanying lipodystrophy appears to be typical apart from insulin resistance, including the propensity to develop late degenerative complications. High levels of insulin in plasma and resistance to ketoacidosis distinguish this condition from type I (autoimmune) insulin-dependent diabetes mellitus, although both conditions begin in childhood or early adult life. Some subjects with insulin resistance and lipodystrophy have point mutations of the insulin receptor (see Chap. 311).

2 Hypertriglyceridemia with accumulation of both chylomicrons and very low density lipoproteins in the blood. Eruptive xanthomas, lipemia retinalis, and recurrent pancreatitis may be seen. Although lipoprotein lipase is low, as noted, and there is a defect in disposal of triglycerides in the atrophied fat tissue, the major cause for the hypertriglyceridemia is overproduction of very low density lipoproteins (VLDL) in the liver. This overproduction is probably driven by the elevated free fatty acids in blood since dietary fat restriction results in a fall of VLDL production rates toward normal. Hyperinsulinemia may contribute by enhancing hepatic fat synthesis.

3 A hypermetabolic state with normal thyroid function. Basal metabolic rates are usually elevated although thyroid hormone values (thyroxine, triiodothyronine, reverse triiodothyronine) are normal.

Patients do not gain weight with excessive caloric intake, indicating a facile capacity to waste calories as heat. Food intakes as high as 21,000 kJ (5000 kcal)/d are not unusual. One 16-month-old child ate 10,000 kJ (2400 kcal)/d. Following thyroidectomy in one patient, the basal metabolic rate decreased but did not return to normal; symptoms and signs of hypothyroidism supervened requiring treatment with thyroid hormone despite continued high metabolic rates. It thus seems clear that hypermetabolism is not due to hyperthyroidism. There is also no evidence of mitochondrial disease. Abnormal dietary thermogenesis, mediated by the sympathetic nervous system, is the likely cause of the increased metabolic rate. There is no evidence for adrenal medullary dysfunction.

Course and treatment Patients with generalized lipodystrophy may die at an early age. Hepatic failure, hemorrhage from esophageal varices, and renal failure are common causes of death. Despite the almost constant hypertriglyceridemia, symptomatic coronary artery disease is rare. There is no specific treatment for lipodystrophy, although dietary fat restriction is generally recommended. Medium-chain triglyceride supplementation has been reported to be of benefit. Pimozide therapy, hypophysectomy, and plasmapheresis are ineffective.

ACQUIRED PARTIAL LIPODYSTROPHY This is the most common of the lipodystrophies and usually affects women. Fat atrophy occurs in the upper half of the body, including the face, but spares the lower extremities. Rarely the lower half of the body is affected, leaving the upper torso intact. Occasionally the lesion affects only one side. The other anatomic features of generalized lipodystrophy are usually absent, and liver disease is unusual. Proteinuria, with or without the nephrotic syndrome, occurs more frequently than in other forms. The complement system is abnormal, and C3 levels tend to be low. C3 nephritic factor, a polyclonal IgG immunoglobulin that interacts with alternative pathway convertase to augment C3 activation, is present in serum. C3 levels may be low in unaffected first-degree relatives, but C3 nephritic factor is absent. Complement abnormalities disappeared after renal transplantation in one subject. Dermatomyositis and Sjögren's syndrome may occur. Rarely partial lipodystrophy progresses to the generalized form of the disease.

LIPODYSTROPHY WITH DOMINANT TRANSMISSION This variant is characterized by fat atrophy of the limbs and trunk with sparing of the face, which may actually be rounded. The neck may also be exempt. The disease usually begins at puberty but may not appear until middle age. Males are rarely affected. In families with the Rieger anomaly onset tends to be in infancy. Insulin resistance and hyperglycemia are usual, and severe hypertriglyceridemia with eruptive xanthoma may occur. The labia majora are hypertrophied, and polycystic ovaries may be seen. Acanthosis nigricans is usually present. Liver and renal disease do not occur.

LOCALIZED LIPODYSTROPHY Localized lipodystrophy takes several patterns. Centrifugal lipodystrophy (*lipodystrophia centrifugalis abdominalis infantilis*) has already been mentioned. Annular lipoatrophy is a bandlike ring of fat atrophy encircling a limb or the ankles. Occasionally only half the limb is involved, in which case the term often used is *lipoatrophia semicircularis*. On biopsy inflammatory infiltrates are usually present in the areas of fat atrophy. Localized lipodystrophy may also occur secondary to injection of insulin, iron dextrans, triamcinolone, and diphtheria/pertussis/tetanus vaccine.

TABLE 338-3 Accompanying abnormalities of lipodystrophy

Bone	Sclerosis, cystic angiomatosis
Brain	Mental retardation, third ventricle dilatation
Genitalia	Clitoromegaly, polycystic ovaries, penile hypertrophy
Heart	Cardiomegaly
Kidneys	Hypertrophy without renal failure
Liver	Hepatomegaly, fatty liver, cirrhosis, hepatic failure
Lymph nodes	Generalized lymphadenopathy
Skin	Acanthosis nigricans, hypertrichosis
Thyroid	Goiter, euthyroid state

MULTIPLE SYMMETRIC LIPOMATOSIS

Multiple symmetric lipomatosis, a disease found predominantly in men, is characterized by formation of multiple nonencapsulated lipomas in various areas. Two patterns of distribution are noted. In the *type I* variant, lipomas are primarily in the nape of the neck and in the supraclavicular and deltoid regions, resulting in an extraordinary bull-necked appearance (*Madelung collar*). Extension into the mediastinum may produce obstruction of the trachea or vena cava. Fat over the remainder of the body appears normal. In the *type II* pattern, lipomas are not localized to the neck but extend down over the body giving the appearance of simple obesity. Correct diagnosis requires recognition that the fat masses are symmetric and that the distal arms and legs are spared. Deep lipomatosis is absent in type II disease, and vena caval and tracheal compression do not occur.

Multiple symmetric lipomatosis may occur sporadically or in families. Autosomal dominant transmission has been postulated in the latter. Alcoholism is common. Coexisting folate deficiency, macrocytic anemia, and abnormal liver function may be due to alcohol and not lipomatosis. Neuropathy, which may be sensory, motor, or autonomic, is prominent, and neuropathic foot ulcers may be present. Histologic evidence from sural nerve biopsies suggests that the neuropathy is integral to the disease and not due to alcohol. The lesion is a chronic distal atrophy without the axonal degeneration and demyelination characteristic of alcohol injury.

Metabolic abnormalities include hyperuricemia, hypertriglyceridemia (VLDL, chylomicrons) and, paradoxically, an elevation of high-density lipoproteins (HDL) as well. Diabetes mellitus has not been reported, although hyperinsulinism may be present. A few patients have had renal tubular acidosis.

The cause of multiple symmetric lipomatosis is not known. The fat cells are slightly smaller than normal, suggesting hyperplasia. Isolated adipocytes appear to have a marked increase in lipoprotein lipase activity and a defect in adrenergic lipolysis. Lipolytic response to cyclic AMP is intact, suggesting an abnormality at the hormone receptor/adenylate cyclase unit. The biochemical abnormalities are not present in all cases.

There is no treatment except for surgical removal of lipomas that cause compression. They may also be removed for cosmetic reasons.

MEDIASTINO-ABDOMINAL LIPOMATOSIS

This syndrome may be a variant of multiple symmetric lipomatosis. The features include (1) exertional dyspnea due to compression of airways by lipomas of the mediastinum, (2) massive enlargement of the abdomen (pseudoascites) due to intraperitoneal and retroperitoneal fat, and (3) abnormal glucose tolerance or diabetes mellitus. The metabolic abnormalities and enzymic changes in adipocytes are identical with those in multiple symmetric lipomatosis except that HDL levels are not elevated.

ACUTE PANNICULITIS (NODULAR FAT NECROSIS)

The appearance of single or multiple crops of tender nodules in subcutaneous fat with a histologic picture of fat-cell necrosis, infiltration of inflammatory cells, and development of fat-filled macrophages (foam cells) is the hallmark of acute panniculitis. The nodules range in size from 0.5 to 10 cm and may be firm or fluctuant. They are usually, but not always, tender. On occasion they drain an oily solution, and suppuration may occur. Individual lesions last from 1 to 8 weeks before disappearing, and a pigmented depressed area may be left at the involved site. While some patients have only nodular panniculitis, which may or may not be relapsing, others develop fever, abnormal liver function, involvement of the bone marrow with leukemoid response, bleeding tendencies, nodular pulmonary lesions, and evidence of pancreatic disease with elevated plasma amylase and lipase levels. In the past this constellation of findings was called *Weber-Christian disease*. However, since painful or nonpainful panniculitis may result from a variety of conditions, Weber-Christian disease is not a specific entity, and the term should probably be abandoned.

It is not possible to develop a firm classification of acute panniculitis since the lesions may appear in sporadic fashion with many conditions. One classification system is given in Table 338-4.

TABLE 338-4   Causes of panniculitis

1 Panniculitis without systemic disease
   a Trauma
   b Cold
   c Subcutaneous fat necrosis of the newborn
2 Panniculitis with systemic disease
   a Connective tissue disorders (lupus erythematosus, scleroderma)
   b Lymphoproliferative disease (lymphoma, histiocytosis)
   c α_1-Antitrypsin deficiency
   d Pancreatic disease (cancer, pancreatitis)
   e Generalized lipodystrophy
   f Paraproteinemia with C_1 inhibition deficiency

Panniculitis without systemic disease is usually due to trauma (sometimes factitiously induced) or cold. For example, in equestrian cold panniculitis the lesions appear in the outer thighs of persons riding horseback for several hours in icy weather. One variant, subcutaneous fat necrosis of the newborn, may be due to a combination of obstetric trauma and hypothermia.

Panniculitis with systemic disease can be divided into several large categories. Collagen vascular disease is a frequent cause, although few patients with connective tissue disorders develop this complication. Lupus is probably most common, and scleroderma is second. About 2 to 3 percent of patients with lupus have nodular fat necrosis; it is more common in discoid lupus than in the systemic variant. Lymphomas and histiocytosis represent a second category. Histiocytic cytophagic panniculitis is a disease characterized by fever, serositis (pleural effusions), hepatosplenomegaly, panniculitis, anemia, leukopenia, thrombocytopenia, and coagulation defects. The characteristic lesion is the "beanbag" histiocyte containing ingested lymphocytes, red cells, and platelets. While some patients have a benign course, the majority have a fatal outcome due to hemorrhagic complications. Deficiencies of α_1-antitrypsin have been found in a number of patients with acute panniculitis and should be looked for in every suspected case. It is postulated that the α_1-antitrypsin deficiency predisposes to panniculitis secondary to trauma and induces a hyperactive immune response. Panniculitis with systemic symptoms, including fever and hepatitis, has also been seen with light-chain paraproteinemia and acquired deficiency of C_1 inhibitor in the classical complement-generating sequence. Severe pancreatic disease may also cause acute panniculitis. One distinct syndrome has been called *disseminated fat necrosis* and is described below. Finally, panniculitis may be associated with generalized lipodystrophy, especially the acquired type.

Acute panniculitis can be diagnosed only histologically. Once the lesion is identified a search for the cause must be made. If systemic symptoms are present and the course is rapidly downhill, the primary differential diagnosis is between collagen vascular disease, lymphoproliferative disorder, and pancreatitis or pancreatic cancer. Milder cases raise the possibility of α_1-antitrypsin deficiency.

Treatment is often unsatisfactory. Some patients with histiocytic cytophagic panniculitis respond to combined chemotherapy with cyclophosphamide, bleomycin, and prednisone. Patients with α_1-antitrypsin deficiency may respond to dapsone but should be given α_1-antiprotease concentrate (60 mg/kg body weight weekly) if this fails.

DISSEMINATED FAT NECROSIS

Disseminated fat necrosis (also called metastatic fat necrosis) is a syndrome in which patients with pancreatitis (two-thirds) or carcinoma of the pancreas (one-third) develop lesions that appear to be similar to or identical with nodular panniculitis. The fat necrosis has a predilection for periarticular sites. Fever is almost invariably present. Arthritis occurs in about 60 percent of cases and may be severe, resulting in destruction of the joint. Often there are sinus tracts running from the site of subcutaneous fat necrosis into the joint space, leading to deposition of necrotic material. Lytic bone lesions may underlie the site of fat necrosis. Polyserositis and vasculitis may be present. Since complement levels are low and immunofluorescent staining shows deposition of complement and IgG, the syndrome resembles, in some respects, lupus-associated panniculitis. Serologic studies for lupus have not been systematically carried out. Antinuclear antibody (ANA) and rheumatoid factor were negative in one patient.

Disseminated fat necrosis may be due to release of pancreatic enzymes into blood or lymph, and these enzymes may initiate fat necrosis at distal sites. Presumably free fatty acids released by pancreatic lipase and phospholipase A, both of which may be elevated in serum, induce tissue necrosis, with trypsin playing an ancillary role. Experimentally, necrosis can be induced in pericardial, subpleural, and subcutaneous fat by ligation of pancreatic ducts. Amylase and lipase levels may be elevated in pleural, pericardial, and ascitic fluid. These enzymes have also been found in fluid aspirated from subcutaneous nodules. A fistula developed between a pancreatic pseudocyst and the portal vein in one patient; shortly thereafter nodular fat necrosis appeared over most of the body. On the other hand an immune mechanism may be causal, given that polyserositis is common and that low complement levels and vasculitis may be present. The meaning of the eosinophilia that frequently accompanies disseminated fat necrosis is not known.

Mortality rates are high (even in the absence of pancreatic carcinoma), and death may occur in weeks to months. No treatment is known. Infusion of the protease inhibitor aprotinin appeared to have beneficial effects in one patient.

ADIPOSIS DOLOROSA

Adiposis dolorosa (Dercum's disease) is characterized by painful circumscribed adipose tissue deposits in subcutaneous tissues of the extremities and of other parts of the body. Juxtaarticular areas, particularly the knees, are the most common sites. Lesions vary from 0.5 to 5.0 cm. Pain and paresthesias may occur spontaneously or result from pressure. Affected subjects are frequently women (30:1). They are usually obese. The syndrome is associated with weakness, fatigue, emotional instability, and occasional dementia. The condition rarely begins until after menopause. Most cases are sporadic, but familial occurrence has been noted with a presumed dominant inheritance. Multiple associations have been reported, but they are probably chance phenomena. Autopsy reports from early in the century suggested abnormalities of the pituitary and other endocrine glands, but modern endocrinologic evaluations have not been undertaken.

Biopsy of affected sites may show no abnormalities, but granulomas with giant cell formations are usually seen. Fat necrosis is rare, thus separating the condition from acute panniculitis.

Treatment is unsatisfactory, although intravenous lidocaine has apparently provided relief in two cases.

REFERENCES

Lipodystrophy

BILLINGS JK et al: Lipoatrophic panniculitis: A possible autoimmune inflammatory disease of fat. Report of three cases. Arch Dermatol 123:1662, 1987

DUNNIGAN MG et al: Familial lipoatrophic diabetes with dominant transmission: A new syndrome. Q J Med 43:33, 1974

FRANKLIN B et al: Very low-density lipoprotein metabolism in an unusual case of lipoatrophic diabetes. Metabolism 33:814, 1984

LILLYSTONE D, WEST RJ: Lipodystrophy of limbs associated with insulin resistance Arch Dis Child 50:737, 1975

SEIP M: Generalized lipodystrophy, in *Ergebnisse der Inneren Medizin und Kinderheilkunde*, P Frick et al (eds). Berlin, Springer Verlag, 1971, pp 59–95

SOLER NG et al: Lipoatrophic diabetes: Endocrine dysfunction and the response to control of hypertriglyceridemia. Metabolism 31:19, 1982

WACHSLICHT-RODBARD H et al: Heterogeneity of the insulin-receptor interaction in lipoatrophic diabetes. J Clin Endocrinol Metab 52:416, 1981

WILSON DE et al: Eucaloric substitution of medium chain triglycerides for dietary long chain fatty acids in acquired total lipodystrophy: Effects on hyperlipoproteinemia and endogenous insulin resistance. J Clin Endocrinol Metab 57:517, 1983

Multiple symmetric lipomatosis

ENZI G: Multiple symmetric lipomatosis: An updated clinical report. Medicine 63:56, 1984

LEUNG NWY et al: Multiple symmetric lipomatosis (Launois-Bensaude syndrome): Effect of oral salbutamol. Clin Endocrinol 7:601, 1987

POLLOCK M et al: Neuropathy in multiple symmetric lipomatosis. Madelung's disease. Brain 111:1157, 1988

RUZICKA T et al: Benign symmetric lipomatosis Launois-Bensaude. Report of ten cases and review of the literature. J Am Acad Dermatol 17:663, 1987

Mediastino-abdominal lipomatosis

ENZI G et al: Mediastino-abdominal lipomatosis: Deep accumulation of fat mimicking a respiratory disease and ascites. Clinical aspects and metabolic studies *in vitro*. Q J Med 53:453, 1984

Acute panniculitis

ALEGRE VA, WINKELMANN RK: Histiocytic cytophagic panniculitis. J Am Acad Dermatol 20:177, 1989

ARONSON IK et al: Panniculitis associated with cutaneous T-cell lymphoma and cytophagocytic histiocytosis. Br J Dermatol 112:87, 1985

PASCUAL M et al: Recurrent febrile panniculitis and hepatitis in two patients with acquired complement deficiency and paraproteinemia. Am J Med 83:959, 1987

PATTERSON JW: Panniculitis. New findings in the "third compartment," editorial. Arch Dermatol 123:1615, 1987

SMITH KC et al: Panniculitis associated with severe α_1-antitrypsin deficiency. Treatment and review of the literature. Arch Dermatol 123:1655, 1987

WINKELMANN RK: Panniculitis in connective tissue disease. Arch Dermatol 119:336, 1983

Disseminated fat necrosis

PHILLIPS MR JR et al: Inflammatory arthritis and subcutaneous fat necrosis associated with acute and chronic pancreatitis. Arthritis Rheum 23:355, 1980

WILSON HA et al: Pancreatitis with arthropathy and subcutaneous fat necrosis. Evidence for the pathogenicity of lipolytic enzymes. Arthritis Rheum 26:121, 1983

Adiposis dolorosa

ATKINSON RL: Intravenous lidocaine for the treatment of intractable pain of adiposis dolorosa. Int J Obes 6:351, 1982

section 3 # Disorders of bone and mineral metabolism

339 CALCIUM, PHOSPHORUS, AND BONE METABOLISM: CALCIUM-REGULATING HORMONES

MICHAEL F. HOLICK / STEPHEN M. KRANE / JOHN T. POTTS, JR.

BONE STRUCTURE AND METABOLISM (See also Chap. 341) Bone is a dynamic tissue that is constantly remodeled throughout life. The arrangement of compact and cancellous bone provides a combination of strength and density suitable for mobility. In addition, bone provides calcium, magnesium, phosphorus, sodium, and other ions necessary for the support of homeostatic functions. The skeleton is highly vascular and receives about 10 percent of the cardiac output.

The properties of bone are a function of its extracellular components. The structure consists of a solid mineral phase in close association with an organic matrix of which 90 to 95 percent is type I collagen (see Chap. 333). The noncollagenous portion of the organic matrix contains proteins derived from serum (albumin and α_2-HS glycoproteins), α-carboxyglutamic acid (GLA)–containing proteins (*bone GLA protein*, or *BGP*, or *osteocalcin* and a matrix GLA protein), a glycoprotein called *osteonectin*, a phosphoprotein called *osteopontin*, sialoproteins, *thrombospondin*, and other less well characterized proteins. Some of these proteins may function in initiating mineralization and in binding of the mineral phase to the matrix. The mineral phase is made up of calcium and phosphate, best characterized as a poorly crystalline hydroxyapatite, although the calcium/phosphate molar ratio is less than the 1.67 of hydroxyapatite [empiric formula, $Ca_{10}(PO_4)_6(OH)_2$]. In addition, other ions are present, predominantly in the surface layers. The mineral phase of bone is deposited in intimate relation to the collagen fibrils and is found largely in specific locations within the "holes" of the collagen fibrils that result from the manner in which the collagen molecules are packed. This architectural organization of mineral and matrix results in a two-phase material uniquely suited to withstand mechanical stresses. The formation and the localization of the inorganic phase are probably determined in part by the organic matrix.

Bone is formed by cells of mesenchymal origin, *osteoblasts,* that synthesize and secrete the organic matrix. Mineralization of the matrix, particularly in *osteons* (haversian systems), begins soon after the matrix is secreted (primary mineralization) but is not completed until after several weeks (secondary mineralization). Osteoblasts are derived from mesenchymal stem cells and are characterized by their location and morphology, the presence of a specific skeletal form of alkaline phosphatase, receptors for parathyroid hormone (PTH) and 1,25-dihydroxyvitamin D [$1,25(OH)_2D$], and the ability to synthesize specific matrix proteins such as type I collagen, osteocalcin, and osteopontin. As an *osteoblast* secretes matrix which is then mineralized, the cell becomes surrounded by matrix and becomes an *osteocyte*, still connected with its blood supply through a series of canaliculi. Resorption of bone is carried out mainly by *osteoclasts*. Osteoclasts are multinucleated cells formed by fusion of precursor cells derived from a hematopoietic stem cell related to the mononuclear phagocyte series. Resorption of bone takes place in scalloped spaces (Howship's lacunae) where the osteoclasts are attached to the bone matrix through a ring of contractile proteins (clear zone) and form a specialized ruffled border. Mineral and matrix are removed in this space where the ruffled border is folded and is in contact with the bone. Proteins including a proton pump ATPase are found in the ruffled border membrane, which contributes to the production of a unique acid environment in the enclosed extracellular compartment and results in solubilization of the mineral phase. In addition to the proton pump, carbonic anhydrase (type II isoenzyme) is required to maintain the acid pH. Other features of osteoclasts include the presence of tartrate-resistant acid phosphatase, cell surface receptors for calcitonin, an integrin (vitronectin) receptor, and an ability to resorb mineralized bone. The bone matrix is resorbed in the acid environment adjacent to the ruffled border by acid hydrolyases following solubilization of the mineral phase. Several soluble ligands modulate the differentiation of osteoblasts or osteoclasts from precursor cells and modulate the function of the differentiated cells. Bone is a storehouse for growth regulatory factors. Some that affect osteoblast function include transforming growth factors (TGF-β I and II), acidic and basic fibroblast growth factors (FGF), platelet-derived growth factors (PDGF), and insulin-like growth factors (IGF-1 and -2). In addition, several proteins have the capacity to induce ectopic bone formation and may have a role in bone remodeling, e.g., osteoinductive factor, osteogenin, and bone morphogenic proteins. Other cytokines modulate resorption through effects on osteoclasts, e.g., interleukin 1 (IL-1), tumor necrosis factor (TNF), γ-interferon, and colony stimulating factors. Some of these effects on osteoclasts are mediated by osteoblasts and adjacent stromal fibroblasts in the marrow. For example, PTH receptors are not found on osteoclasts, and PTH increases osteoclastic bone resorption by first acting on osteoblasts or stromal fibroblasts. $1,25(OH)_2D$ receptors are found in precursor cells, which can differentiate into monocytes as well as osteoclasts, and $1,25(OH)_2D$ can induce differentiation along the osteoclast pathway. The effects of some cytokines such as IL-1 and TGF-α may be mediated by local production of prostaglandins. What had initially been termed *osteoclast-activity factor* is currently thought to reflect the presence of cytokines such as IL-1, TNF-α, TNF-β (lymphotoxin), and probably others as well.

In the embryo and in the growing child, bone develops either by remodeling and replacing previously calcified cartilage (endochondral bone formation), or it is formed without a cartilage matrix (intramembranous bone formation). New bone, whether in embryos or infants or that formed in adults during repair, has a relatively high ratio of cells to matrix and is characterized by coarse fiber bundles of collagen that are interlaced and randomly dispersed (woven bone). In adults, the more mature bone is organized with fiber bundles regularly arranged in parallel or concentric sheets (lamellar bone). In long bones, the lamellar bone is deposited in a concentric arrangement around blood vessels and forms the haversian systems. Growth in length of bones is dependent upon proliferation of cartilage cells and on the endochondral sequence at the growth plate. Growth in width and thickness is accomplished by formation of bone at the periosteal surface and by resorption at the endosteal surface with the rate of formation exceeding that of resorption. In adults, after the epiphyses close, growth in length and endochondral bone formation cease, except for some activity in the cartilage cells beneath the articular

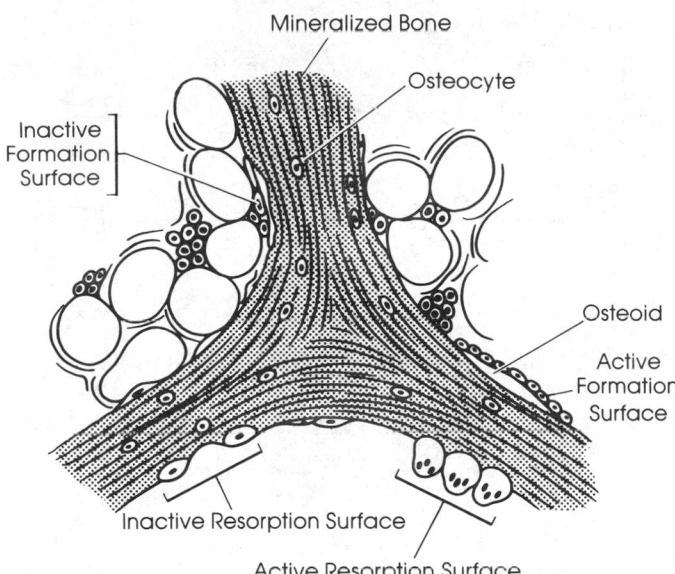

Mineralized Bone

Osteocyte

Inactive Formation Surface

Osteoid

Active Formation Surface

Inactive Resorption Surface

Active Resorption Surface

FIGURE 339-1 Schematic representation of bone remodeling surfaces in trabecular bone. Most bone surfaces in adults are involved in neither formation nor resorption. Such surfaces are usually smooth, have no osteoid seam, and are covered either by no visible cells or by flattened cells. Active formation surfaces are smooth and covered by osteoblasts which have an osteoid seam (clear), normally no thicker than 12 μm. The calcification front is located at the junction of the osteoid seam and mineralized bone (stippled). Inactive forming surfaces are not covered by osteoblasts but by only a few flattened cells. Active resorbing surfaces are irregular or scalloped and contain multinucleated osteoclasts. The latter are not seen on inactive resorbing surfaces.

surface. Even in adults, however, remodeling of bone (remodeling of haversian systems as well as trabecular bone) continues through life, as can be shown by microradiographic studies utilizing radioisotopes or fluorescence of tetracyclines fixed in bone in regions of new mineralization. Quantitative histomorphometric studies demonstrate that newly forming surfaces are characterized by smooth character, by uptake of tetracycline, and by relatively low mineral density. Actively forming surfaces are covered by active osteoblasts. The osteoid seam that results from the relative lag in mineralization of the newly formed organic matrix is normally no greater than about 12 μm. An index of the rate of bone formation can be obtained by examination of undemineralized sections of bone biopsies obtained from individuals who have received tetracycline for two periods separated by a drug-free interval. The distance between the fluorescent bands on the sections reflects the new bone formed. Resorption areas are characterized by their irregular configurations and the presence of osteoclasts (Fig. 339-1). Resorption precedes formation and is more intense, but it does not persist as long as formation. In adults, approximately 4 percent of the surface of trabecular bone (such as iliac crest) is involved in active resorption, whereas 10 to 15 percent of trabecular surfaces is covered with osteoid. Kinetic studies using isotopes such as radioactive calcium (^{47}Ca) provide estimates that as much as 18 percent of the total skeletal calcium may be deposited and removed each year. Thus, bone is an active metabolizing tissue that is dependent upon an intact blood supply. The remodeling of bone occurs in a manner somehow related to the continuous mechanical stresses to which it is subjected. Bone also serves as an important reservoir of mineral ions, particularly calcium, which are critical for a variety of processes.

The response of bone to injuries, such as fractures, infection, and interruption of blood supply, and to expanding lesions is relatively limited. Dead bone must be resorbed, and new bone must be formed, a process carried out in association with new blood vessels growing into the involved area. In injuries that disrupt the organization of the tissue, such as a fracture in which apposition of fragments is poor

and motion exists at the fracture site, the osteoprogenitor stromal cells differentiate into cells with functional capacities other than those of osteoblasts, and repair is accompanied by formation of varying amounts of fibrous tissue and cartilage. When there is good apposition with fixation and little motion at the fracture site, repair occurs predominantly by formation of new bone without other scar tissue. Remodeling of this bone occurs along lines of force determined by mechanical stresses that are somehow translated into biologic response.

Expanding lesions in bone, such as tumors, induce resorption at the surface in contact with the tumor. A bowing deformity causes increased new bone formation at the concave surface and resorption at the convex surface, all seemingly designed to produce the strongest mechanical structure. Even in a disorder as architecturally disruptive as Paget's disease, remodeling is dictated by mechanical forces. Thus, the plasticity of bone is due to the response of cells interacting with each other and with the environment.

Mechanisms of bone formation and resorption Bone formation is an orderly process in which inorganic mineral is deposited in relation to an organic matrix. The mineral phase is composed of calcium and phosphorus, and the concentration of these ions in the plasma and extracellular fluid influences the rate at which the mineral phase is formed. In vitro, mineralization can proceed, and crystals of hydroxyapatite can grow at concentrations of calcium and phosphorus similar to those in an ultrafiltrate of plasma. However, the concentration of these ions at the sites of mineralization is unknown, and the cells involved (osteoblasts, osteocytes) may somehow regulate the local concentration of calcium, phosphorus, and other ions. Collagens from a variety of sources can catalyze the nucleation of a mineral phase of calcium and phosphorus from solutions of these ions, and the initial mineral phase is deposited in specific locations in the holes produced by the particular packing arrangement of the collagen molecules. The organization of collagen probably influences the amount and type of mineral phase formed in bone. There is one gene for each of the two α1 chains and the single α2 chain that make up type I collagen. The primary structures of type I collagen in skin and bone tissues are similar. There are differences, however, in posttranslational modifications of type I collagen such as hydroxylation, glycosylation, and the type, number, and distribution of intermolecular cross-links. In addition, the "holes" in the packing structure of the collagen are larger in normally mineralized collagen of bone and dentin than in unmineralized collagens such as tendon. The fact that single amino acid substitutions in the helical portion of either the α1 or α2 chains of type I collagen that result from mutations in the col1A1 or col1A2 genes in osteogenesis imperfecta markedly disrupt the organization of bone indicates the importance of the fibrillar matrix in the structure of bone (see also Chap. 333). The noncollagenous organic components such as osteocalcin, osteonectin, or osteopontin may also play a role in the formation of the mineral phase of bone. Alkaline phosphatase is a marker for osteoblasts, and cellular levels of this enzyme correlate with mineralization potential of osteoblasts. Although mineralization defects occur in individuals with decreased levels of alkaline phosphatase (hypophosphatasia), the function of alkaline phosphatase in the mineralization process is not completely understood. To explain how collagens from tissues that are normally not mineralized can catalyze nucleation of an inorganic phase from solutions similar to normal extracellular fluid, regulation of mineralization by inhibitory substances has been suggested. Inorganic pyrophosphate is a potent inhibitor of mineralization at concentrations below those necessary to bind calcium ions. Since alkaline phosphatase, present in osteoblasts and other cells, can catalyze the hydrolysis of inorganic pyrophosphate at neutral pH, this enzyme could regulate mineralization by controlling the concentrations of pyrophosphate. In addition, macromolecular inhibitors such as the proteoglycan aggregates may also influence the rate and extent of mineralization. In cartilage undergoing calcification, membrane-bound vesicles containing mineral are present outside the cells, and it has been suggested that this is the initial mineral phase.

In bone, the calcium phosphate solid phase at the inception of mineralization is brushite ($CaHPO_4 \cdot 2H_2O$). As mineralization progresses, the solid phase is a poorly crystalline hydroxyapatite with a relatively low ($\sim$ 1.2) calcium/phosphate molar ratio. With age and maturation, the degree of crystal perfection increases as does the calcium/phosphate ratio. Fluoride ions, when incorporated into the mineral phase, decrease the proportion of amorphous calcium phosphate and increase crystallinity.

There is a limit for the concentration of calcium and phosphorus ions in the extracellular fluid below which mineralization will not occur. A "solubility product" for bone mineral is difficult to calculate since the mineral phase itself is of variable composition and the true nature of species in solution governing this solubility product is not known. Nevertheless, when the concentrations of calcium and phosphorus in extracellular fluid are excessive, a mineral phase may be formed in areas that are not normally mineralized.

When bone is resorbed, calcium and phosphorus ions from the solid phase are released into the extracellular space adjacent to the ruffled border of the osteoclast, and the organic matrix is then resorbed. The fact that bone resorption takes place in the region of the osteoclast adjacent to the bone surface, where the extracellular pH is low, lends support to the concept that this unique acid environment is required for solubilization of the bone mineral. The alkaline phosphatase of bone cells is an ectoenzyme that is released into the extracellular fluid. Increased circulating levels of the bone-derived enzyme are correlated with rates of bone formation. Other circulating markers of bone formation include osteocalcin and type I procollagen peptides. Markers for bone resorption are urinary excretion of hydroxyproline, hydroxylysine and its glycosides, and the bone-specific hydroxypyridinium collagen cross-links.

CALCIUM METABOLISM   There is about 1 to 2 kg calcium in the average adult human body, of which over 98 percent is in the skeleton. The calcium of the mineral phase at the surface of the crystals is in equilibrium with ions of the extracellular fluid, but only a minor proportion of the total calcium (about 0.5 percent) is exchangeable. The calcium in the extracellular fluid is critical for a variety of functions, and it is remarkably constant. In normal adults, the range of plasma concentration is 2.2 to 2.6 mmol/L (8.8 to 10.4 mg/dL). The calcium in plasma is in three forms: as free ions, bound to plasma proteins, and, to a small extent, as diffusible complexes. The concentration of free calcium ions, mean 1.2 mmol/L (4.8 mg/dL), influences neuromuscular irritability and other cellular functions and is subjected to tight hormonal control, especially through parathyroid hormone, as described below. The concentration of serum proteins is an important factor in determining the concentration of calcium ions; most of the protein binding is to albumin. One formula that approximates the amount of calcium bound to proteins is

$$\% \text{ protein-bound Ca} = 0.8 \times \text{albumin (g/L)} \\ + 0.2 \times \text{globulin (g/L)} + 3$$

Another correction is to subtract 0.25 mmol/L from the serum calcium concentration for every 10 g/L serum albumin lower than 40 g/L. Thus the concentration of ultrafiltrable calcium is usually about half the total calcium. In most laboratories only total calcium is determined, and knowledge of the concentration of proteins is essential to estimate concentration of calcium ions. Free ions can be measured directly with the use of calcium-specific electrodes.

Calcium ions inside the cell mediate a variety of cellular functions (see also Chap. 68). Most of the cellular calcium is in the form of insoluble complexes. The concentration of free calcium within the cell, which is critical for functional regulation, is low, approximately 0.1 μmol/L; thus, the gradient between plasma and intracellular free calcium is about 10,000 to 1. This gradient is tightly regulated. The concentration of calcium ions in the extracellular fluid is kept constant by the interaction of processes that constantly feed calcium into and withdraw calcium from the extracellular fluid. Calcium enters the plasma via absorption from the intestinal tract and by resorption of ions from the bone mineral. Calcium leaves the extracellular fluid

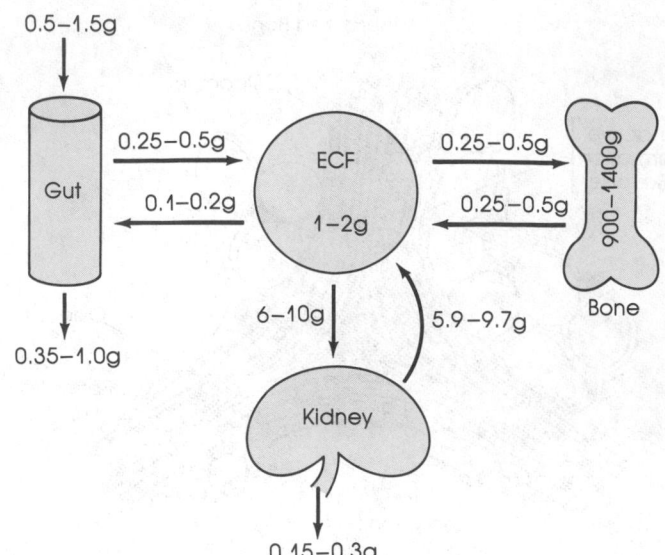

FIGURE 339-2 Calcium homeostasis. Schematic illustration of calcium content of extracellular fluid (ECF) and bone as well as of diet and feces; magnitude of calcium flux per day as calculated by various methods is shown at sites of transport in intestine, kidney, and bone. Ranges of values shown are approximate and chosen to illustrate certain points discussed in text. In intestine, absorption efficiency varies inversely with dietary calcium (chronic adaptation). This is reflected in typical quantities absorbed and excreted in feces; with 0.5-g intake, 50 percent absorption is depicted to occur (0.25 g), but at 1.5 g only 30 percent (0.5 g). Endogenous fecal calcium, the 0.1 to 0.2 g secreted into the intestinal lumen daily, is constant and does not vary with calcium intake or absorption. Quantities of calcium depicted as filtered, reabsorbed, and excreted at the kidney are chosen arbitrarily to indicate that at lower rates of filtration of calcium (expected at lower glomerular filtration rates), most is reabsorbed (e.g., 5.85 of 6 g), leading to urinary excretion of 150 mg; at higher rates of filtration (at high dietary calcium intake), slightly less is reabsorbed (e.g., 9.7 of 10 g), leading to a higher urinary excretion, 300 mg. In all situations, renal calcium reabsorption exceeds 95 percent of filtered load. Urinary calcium excretion is seen, therefore, to increase by only 150 mg despite a 1-g increase in dietary intake. In conditions of calcium balance, rates of calcium release from and uptake into bone are equal.

via secretion into the gastrointestinal tract, urinary excretion, deposition in bone mineral, and, to a minor extent, via losses in sweat. Resorption and formation are usually tightly coupled, approximately 12 mmol (500 mg) calcium entering and leaving the skeleton daily (Fig. 339-2).

The average dietary calcium intake for adults in the United States when surveyed has been found lower than expected [15 to 20 mmol/d (0.6 to 0.8 g/d)]. However, with the heightened awareness of the role of adequate calcium intake for the prevention of osteoporosis, those on some type of supplement have an average intake of 20 to 37 mmol/d (0.8 to 1.5 g/d). In adults less than half of the calcium in the diet is absorbed. Calcium absorption increases during periods of rapid growth in children, in pregnancy, and in lactation and decreases with advancing age. If adequate vitamin D is available and vitamin D metabolism is normal, more dietary calcium is absorbed (adaptation). Most of the calcium is absorbed in the proximal small intestine, and the efficiency of absorption decreases in the more distal intestinal segments. Both active transport and diffusion-limited absorption are involved; the former is more important in the upper, and the latter is more important in the lower, intestine. Both are influenced by vitamin D through the action of its metabolites. All forms of calcium in the diet may not be equally absorbed; even with defined salts, calcium as the chloride is probably absorbed more efficiently than that in other preparations.

Calcium is also secreted into the lumen of the gastrointestinal tract. When isotopes of radioactive calcium are administered intravenously, radioactivity appears in the feces, making possible calculations of *endogenous fecal calcium* (Fig. 339-2). Higher estimates of calcium losses in intestinal juices have been made by other approaches. Secretion of calcium into the intestinal lumen is constant and independent of absorption. If calcium availability in the diet is low [less than 12 mmol/d (500 mg/d)], positive calcium balance requires an efficiency of absorption greater than 30 to 40 percent if intestinal uptake is sufficient to exceed losses via intestinal secretion and to match calcium losses through renal calcium excretion.

The urinary calcium excretion of normal adults on average calcium intakes ranges between 2.5 and 10 mmol/d (100 and 400 mg/d). When the dietary calcium is below 5 mmol (200 mg) daily, urinary calcium excretion is usually less than 5 mmol (200 mg/d). However, in most normal individuals the level of dietary intake over a wide range has relatively little effect on the urinary excretion of calcium. Hence, in individuals on diets low in calcium, this relative inefficiency of renal calcium conservation leads to negative calcium balance unless calcium absorption is maximally efficient (Fig. 339-2).

The amount of calcium in the urine is minute compared with that filtered through the glomerulus [about 150 to 250 mmol/d (6 to 10 g/d)]. The rates of reabsorption of the filtered calcium are high compared to rates of excretion. Reabsorption takes place predominantly in the proximal tubule (~60 percent) and in Henle's loop (~25 percent). Relatively small amounts of filtered calcium are reabsorbed in the distal tubule. It is not certain whether non-protein-bound, nonionic forms of calcium (e.g., calcium citrate) are cleared at different rates. The excretion of other electrolytes affects the urinary excretion of calcium. For example, urinary calcium is usually proportional to urinary sodium; sulfate also increases calcium excretion.

Maintenance of calcium balance (Fig. 339-2) is dependent upon the efficiency of intestinal absorption. Deficiency of parathyroid hormone or vitamin D, intestinal disease, or severe dietary calcium deprivation may provide challenges to calcium homeostasis that cannot be compensated adequately by renal calcium conservation, resulting in negative calcium balance. Increased bone resorption may protect against extracellular fluid calcium depletion even in states of chronic negative calcium balance but only at the expense of progressive osteopenia.

Pathophysiology Decrease in the concentration of free calcium ions in plasma results in increased neuromuscular irritability and the syndrome of tetany. This syndrome is characterized, when fully expressed, by peripheral and perioral paresthesias, carpal spasm, pedal spasm, anxiety, seizures, bronchospasm, laryngospasm, Chvostek's, Trousseau's, and Erb's signs, and lengthening of the QT interval of the electrocardiogram. In infants tetany may be manifested only by irritability and lethargy. The level of calcium ions that determines which features of tetany will be manifested varies among individuals. Tetany is also influenced by the concentration of other components of the extracellular fluid. For example, hypomagnesemia and alkalosis lower the threshold for tetany, whereas hypokalemia and acidosis raise the threshold.

Increases in total serum calcium are usually accompanied by increases in calcium ions and may be associated with anorexia, nausea, vomiting, constipation, hypotonia, depression, and occasionally lethargy and coma. Persistent hypercalcemia, especially when accompanied by normal or elevated levels of serum phosphate, may result in ectopic deposition of a solid phase of calcium and phosphate in walls of blood vessels, connective tissue about the joints, gastric mucosa, cornea, and renal parenchyma. Hypercalcemia per se alters renal function in addition to the pathologic effects of calcium-phosphate deposits in the lumen of renal tubules and in the interstitial areas of the kidney.

PHOSPHORUS METABOLISM Phosphorus is a major component of bone and of all other tissues and in some form is involved in almost all metabolic processes. The total amount of phosphorus in the normal adult is about 32 mol (1 kg), of which about 85 percent is in the skeleton.

In fasting plasma most of the phosphorus is present as inorganic orthophosphate in concentrations of approximately 0.9 to 1.3 mmol/L (2.8 to 4 mg/dL). In contrast to calcium, where about 50 percent is bound, only about 12 percent of the phosphorus in plasma is bound to proteins. Free HPO_4^{2-} and $NaHPO_4^-$ normally are about 75 percent of the total plasma phosphorus, and free $H_2PO_4^-$ is 10 percent. Since so many species are present, depending upon pH and other factors, it has been the convention to express concentrations in terms of mass of elemental phosphorus, i.e., milligrams phosphorus per deciliter, or molarity. Total phosphorus levels are higher in children and tend to rise in women after the menopause. There is a circadian variation of phosphorus concentration even during a 24-h fast, mediated in part by the adrenal cortex. The nadir occurs at about 9 A.M., and the maximum is at about 2 P.M. The magnitudes of the peaks and troughs vary with phosphorus intake but occur regardless of whether the intake is high or low. Despite changes in serum phosphorus levels of nearly twofold, serum ionized calcium levels do not change significantly.

During phosphate depletion, phosphaturia decreases before phosphatemia. This adaptive response of increasing tubular transport when luminal concentrations are decreasing can be observed in the coupled sodium/phosphorus transport of isolated renal tubular cells and is thus an intrinsic property of these cells. There is also heterogeneity of phosphorus transport among different segments of proximal renal tubules. Tubular fluxes of phosphorus rather than hypophosphatemia per se may be critical in modulating effects of hypophosphatemia such as the stimulation of 25(OH)D-1α-hydroxylase. Conversely, increased phosphorus loads and increased renal tubular phosphorus fluxes result in decreased renal tubular reabsorption of phosphorus and increased clearance and suppress the activity of 25(OH)D-1α-hydroxylase (see below). Ingestion of carbohydrate depresses serum phosphorus acutely by 0.3 to 0.5 mmol/L (1 to 1.5 mg/dL), presumably as the result of cellular uptake and formation of phosphate esters. Ingestion of phosphorus per se increases serum levels. Therefore, it is essential for the interpretation of serum levels and urinary clearances that samples be obtained in the fasting state. Decreases in plasma phosphorus also occur during induction of alkalosis.

Whereas only a small proportion of dietary calcium is absorbed from the intestine, phosphorus absorption is remarkably efficient. At low levels of dietary intake (less than 2 mg/kg body weight per day) 80 to 90 percent of ingested phosphorus is absorbed. Even with the higher levels of intake (greater than 10 mg/kg body weight per day) in the form of dairy products, cereals, eggs, and meat, absorption is about 70 percent. Hypophosphatemia due to deficient intestinal absorption is unusual except when excessive quantities of nonabsorbable antacids are consumed; the antacids bind phosphorus and prevent absorption from the intestinal lumen.

The major control of phosphorus economy is exerted at the level of the kidney. Phosphorus filtered through the glomerulus is largely reabsorbed in the proximal tubule (there is homeostatically important distal reabsorption as well) so that normally only about 10 to 15 percent of the filtered load is excreted. When filtered loads of phosphorus decrease, proximal tubular reabsorption increases. Conversely, when phosphorus loads are increased, tubular reabsorption decreases, and clearance rises. Thus, the urinary excretion of phosphorus normally reflects dietary intake, and conservation or elimination of excessive amounts of the ion depends upon adequate renal handling (Fig. 339-3). There is no good evidence for renal tubular phosphate secretion. Proximal reabsorption of phosphorus is dependent upon parallel sodium reabsorption, but whereas the sodium rejected by the proximal tubule may be reabsorbed distally, the rejected phosphorus is not. Therefore, the effects of volume expansion and decreased sodium reabsorption are to increase phosphorus clearance; similarly, diuretics such as acetazolamide, which act proximally, are phosphaturic parallel to the degree to which they are natriuretic.

Pathophysiology No direct symptoms result from hyperphosphatemia. However, when high levels are maintained for long periods, the driving force for mineralization is increased, and calcium phosphate may be deposited in abnormal sites. Ectopic calcification of

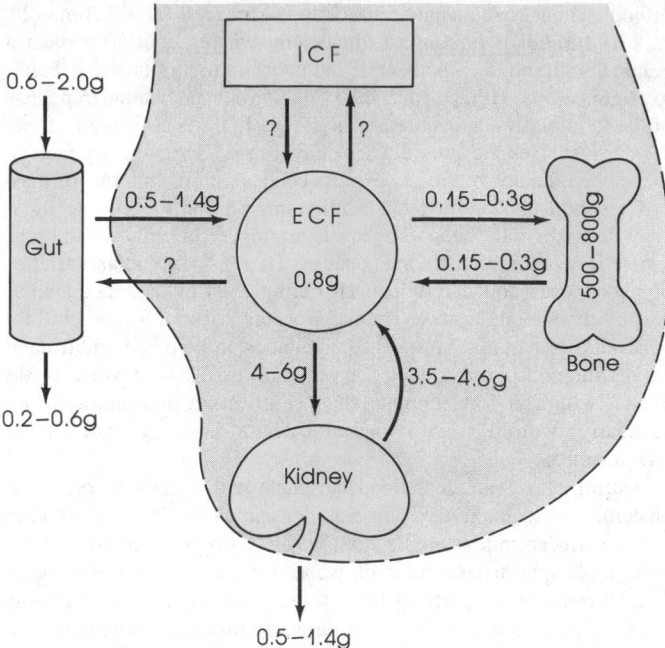

FIGURE 339-3 Phosphate homeostasis. Schematic illustration of inorganic phosphorus content (termed here phosphate) in extracellular fluid (ECF) and bone as well as diet and feces; magnitude of phosphorus flux per day as estimated by various methods is shown at transport sites in intestine, kidney, and bone. Range of values shown illustrates special features of phosphorus metabolism discussed in text. Intestinal phosphorus absorption is highly efficient, 85 percent at a lower intake (0.5 g of a 0.6-g intake) and 70 percent at a higher intake (1.4 g of a 2.0-g intake). Estimates of magnitude of endogenous fecal phosphate are less well established than for calcium. Contribution of at least 0.15 g is estimated to be added to the nonabsorbed phosphorus to provide a total of 0.2 g fecal phosphorus at the low intake level. At high phosphorus dietary intakes, no correction for endogenous fecal phosphate is calculated. Higher quantities of phosphorus are excreted in urine at all levels of dietary intake than for corresponding intakes of calcium; quantities excreted match closely the quantities absorbed, thereby maintaining phosphorus balance (no correction in this illustration is made for endogenous fecal phosphorus). Note that renal phosphorus reabsorption, in contrast to high and relatively invariant renal calcium reabsorption, varies from a low of 75 percent of filtered load to greater than 85 percent. The compartment labeled ICF refers to intracellular phosphorus, both organic and inorganic; rapid shifts of phosphorus into cells (and corresponding, possibly slower, efflux of phosphorus from cells) contribute to changes in ECF phosphorus. These shifts between ECF and ICF and phosphorus release from and uptake by bone are equal in conditions of phosphorus balance.

this type is thus encountered in untreated chronic renal failure with severe hypercalcemia and in vitamin D intoxication. *Tumoral calcinosis* is a rare heritable disorder in which ectopic calcification is associated with hyperphosphatemia and normal glomerular filtration rates (GFR). The disorder is characterized by high ratio of phosphorus tubule maximum (TmP) to GFR and increased serum levels of 1,25(OH)$_2$D. The latter is a paradoxical finding and presumably is related to the abnormal renal tubular phosphate fluxes. Severe, acute hypophosphatemia may or may not be accompanied by symptoms such as anorexia, dizziness, bone pain, proximal muscular weakness, and waddling gait. Significant hypophosphatemia is encountered in severe alcoholics and is aggravated after repletion of nutrients, in the course of therapy of diabetic ketoacidosis, and for various reasons in severely ill, hospitalized elderly patients (see also Chap. 342). Myopathy may be present when hypophosphatemia is severe and may be accompanied by elevations in levels of serum creatinine kinase and rhabdomyolysis. Severe congestive cardiomyopathy has also been noted with chronic hypophosphatemia; restoration of phosphorus deficits leads to prompt reversal of the abnormalities.

Respiratory muscle weakness is also common in the setting of severe hypophosphatemia and may improve with phosphate repletion. The bone pain and waddling gait are attributed to the osteomalacia which develops as a result of phosphate depletion. The muscular weakness may be due either to direct effects of hypophosphatemia on nerves and muscle or, in some instances, to the effects of hyperparathyroidism (either primary or secondary) which may have a role in the etiology of the hypophosphatemia. Defective growth in children may also be due to phosphate depletion. Hypophosphatemia results in decreased levels of 2,3-diphosphoglyceric acid and adenosine triphosphate (ATP) in erythrocytes which in turn alter the dissociation of oxyhemoglobin so that less oxygen is delivered in the periphery. Hemolytic anemia may be produced as the result of impairment of the ability of erythrocytes to deform in small vessels.

Negative phosphorus balance (Fig. 339-3) is rarely caused by inadequate phosphorus absorption in the intestine, and maintenance of normal phosphorus balance is dependent upon efficiency of renal excretion or conservation. In severe renal failure, hyperphosphatemia results from inadequate renal phosphorus clearance; heritable or acquired renal tubular defects may lead to hypophosphatemia due to inadequate renal conservation of phosphorus.

VITAMIN D

Vitamin D is a hormone, not a vitamin. With adequate exposure to sunlight, no dietary supplements are needed. The active principle of vitamin D is synthesized under metabolic control via successive hydroxylations in the liver and kidney and is transported through the blood to its target tissues (the small intestine and bone) to help maintain calcium homeostasis. Calcium and phosphate ions, parathyroid hormone, and possibly other peptide and steroid hormones play major roles directly or indirectly in the regulation of the renal metabolism of vitamin D. Analysis of hereditary and acquired defects in these metabolic processes have provided new insights into the pathophysiology of several disorders involving calcium, phosphorus, and bone metabolism. These discoveries have been the impetus for several advances, including the chemical synthesis of active vitamin D metabolites and analogues, the clinical use of 1α,25-dihydroxyvitamin D$_3$ [1,25(OH)$_2$D$_3$] (calcitriol) in many vitamin D–resistant disorders, the development and application of assays for measuring vitamin D metabolites in blood to define suspected abnormalities in vitamin D metabolism, and a growing interest in developing more potent vitamin D analogues for clinical use.

PHOTOBIOGENESIS OF VITAMIN D Vitamin D$_3$ is a derivative of 7-dehydrocholesterol (provitamin D$_3$), the immediate precursor of cholesterol. When skin is exposed to sunlight or certain artifical light sources, the ultraviolet radiation enters the epidermis and causes a variety of photobiochemical events. Among them is the transformation of 7-dehydrocholesterol to vitamin D$_3$. Wavelengths between 290 and 315 nm are absorbed by the conjugated double bonds at C$_5$ and C$_7$ of 7-dehydrocholesterol that result in the fragmentation of the B ring between C$_9$ and C$_{10}$ to yield a 9,10-secosterol (*seco* means "split"), previtamin D$_3$ (Fig. 339-4). Previtamin D$_3$ is biologically inert but is thermally labile and spontaneously undergoes a temperature-dependent molecular rearrangement of its conjugated triene system (three double bonds) to form the thermally stable 9,10-secosterol, vitamin D$_3$ (Fig. 339-4). At body temperature it takes approximately 3 days for previtamin D$_3$ to convert completely into vitamin D$_3$. Large changes in the temperature of the surface of the skin do not affect the rate of this conversion because the process occurs in the actively growing layers of the epidermis where the temperature is relatively constant; changes in the core body temperature also have little effect on this reaction. Once vitamin D$_3$ is synthesized, it is translocated from the epidermis into the circulation by the vitamin D–binding protein. Thus, vitamin D$_3$ is made in the skin from previtamin for days after a single sun exposure (Fig. 339-4). Although melanin in the skin competes with 7-dehydrocho-

FIGURE 339-4 Photobiogenesis and metabolic pathways for vitamin D production and metabolism. Circled letters and numbers denote specific enzymes: *7* = 7-dehydrocholesterol reductase; *25* = vitamin D-25-hydroxylase; *1α* = 25(OH)D-1α-hydroxylase; *24R* = 25(OH)D-24R-hydroxylase; *26* = 25(OH)D-26-hydroxylase. The insert denotes the basic $\Delta^{5,7}$-diene steroid structures for the precursors of vitamin D_2 (ergosterol) and vitamin D_3 (7-dehydrocholesterol) and the 9,10-secosteroid structures of vitamin D_2 (ergocalciferol) and vitamin D_3 (cholecalciferol). Historically, the subscripts for vitamin D are related to the order in which the compounds were isolated and characterized. What was originally called vitamin D_1 is a mixture of compounds, and the term is no longer used. The next two vitamin D compounds, vitamin D_2 and vitamin D_3, were isolated, respectively, from the irradiation products of ergosterol (a $\Delta^{5,7}$-diene steroid found primarily in plants) and 7-dehydrocholesterol (a $\Delta^{5,7}$-diene steroid precursor of cholesterol present in animal tissues, including humans). Vitamin D_2 and D_3 differ in their side chains; the side chain for vitamin D_2 contains a Δ^{22} and a C_{24}-methyl group. Even though vitamin D_3 is the only endogenous form of vitamin D in skin, both vitamins D_2 and D_3 are metabolized identically and have equivalent biologic potencies in most mammals; in the absence of subscript the term vitamin D may refer to either compound.

In steroid nomenclature, substituents on the steroid ring skeleton that are spatially oriented below the plane of the molecule (drawn as a broken line) are called α *substituents,* and those substituents spatially oriented above the plane of the molecule (drawn as a solid line) are called β *substituents.* Because vitamin D is a structural derivative of a $\Delta^{5,7}$-diene steroid, by convention the numbering of the carbon atoms and the stereochemical designation of the functional groups remain the same as for the parent steroid. During the transformation $\Delta^{5,7}$-diene→previtamin D→vitamin D, the geometric position of ring A is altered, thereby changing the stereochemical orientation of its substituents; nonetheless, the original designation(s) of the hydroxyl function(s) on ring A of the steroid precursor are retained. The R,S notation, as in 24R,25-dihydroxy-vitamin D_3, specifies the spatial configuration of a substituent at an asymmetric carbon center.

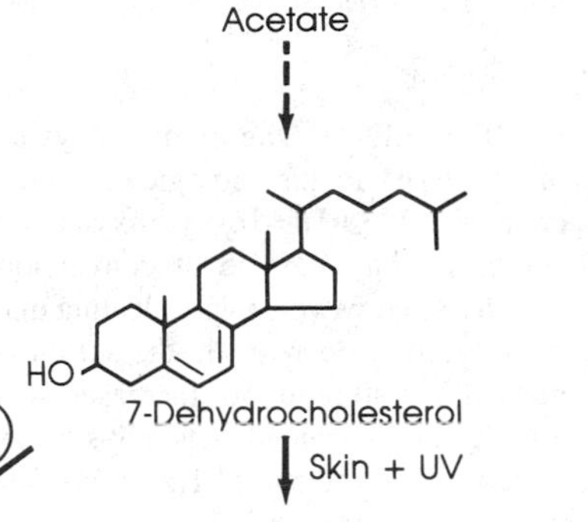

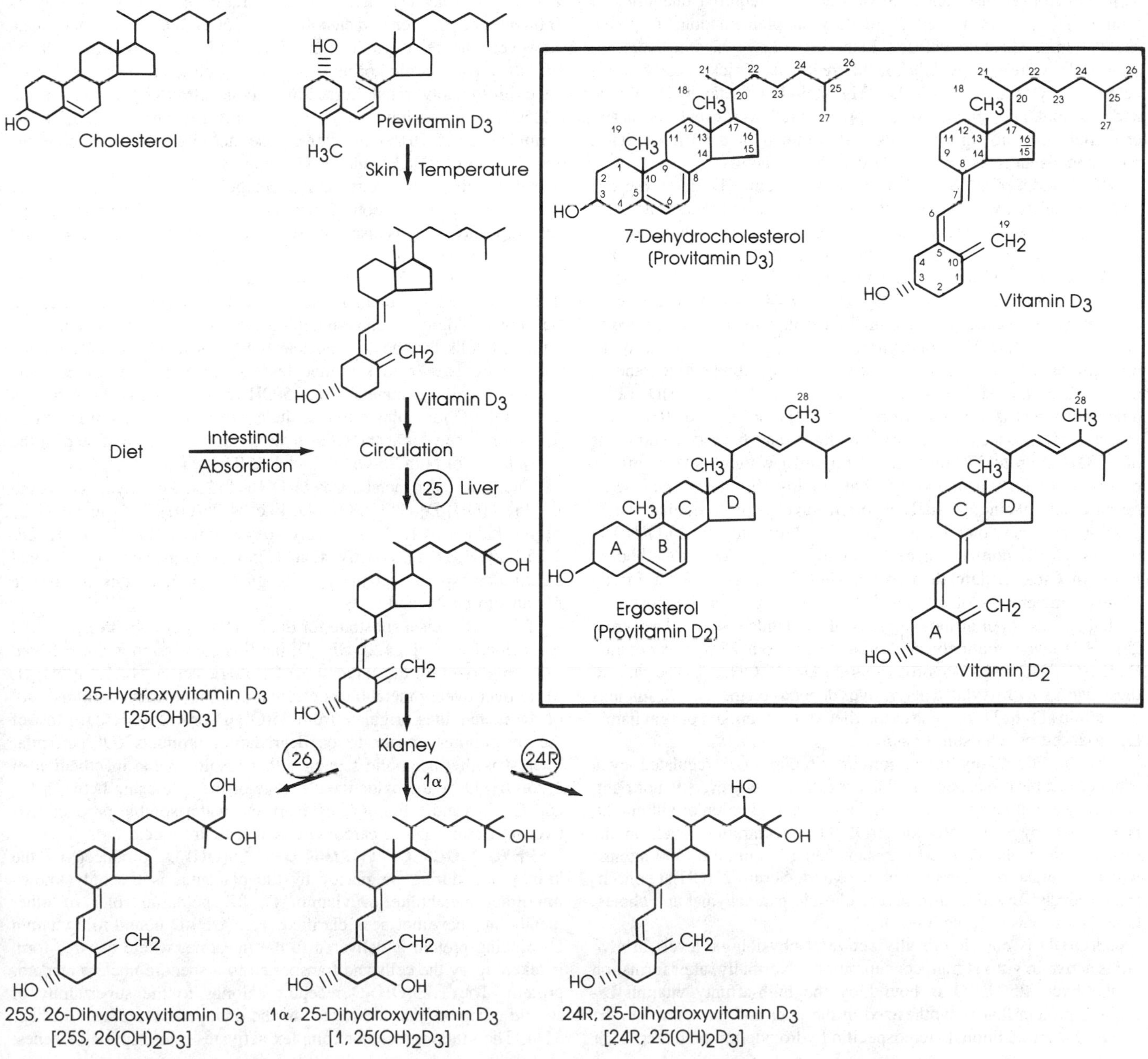

lesterol for ultraviolet photons and thus can limit the synthesis of previtamin D_3, the photochemical isomerization of previtamin D_3 to two biologically inert products (lumisterol$_3$ and tachysterol$_3$) appears to be more important in preventing excessive production of previtamin D_3 during prolonged exposure to the sun.

Aging decreases the capacity of the skin to produce vitamin D_3; greater than twofold reduction occurs after the age of 70 years. Topical sunscreens reduce cutaneous vitamin D_3 production by absorbing the solar radiation that is responsible for vitamin D_3 synthesis in the skin. Other factors that affect the cutaneous synthesis of vitamin D_3 include altitude, geographical location, time of day, and area of exposure. Latitude has profound effects on the cutaneous synthesis of vitamin D_3. As the zenith angle of the sun increases with approaching winter more of the high-energy ultraviolet photons responsible for previtamin D_3 synthesis are absorbed by the ozone layer. In Boston (42°N) and in Edmonton (52°N) the absorption of these photons is so complete that no vitamin D_3 is made in the skin between the months of November through February and October through March respectively. When the entire body is exposed to sufficient sunlight to cause mild erythema, the increase in the blood vitamin D is equivalent to consuming an oral dose of 10,000 international units (1 IU = 0.025 μg) of vitamin D_3. Only when skin radiation is insufficient to produce the required quantities of vitamin D_3 is there a need for dietary supplementation to prevent skeletal mineralization defects. Fish liver oils, a natural source of vitamin D, were used widely for the treatment of rickets early in this century. Crystalline vitamin D_2 (Fig. 339-4) or vitamin D_3 is now added to milk and cereals. Such supplementations prevent rickets and osteomalacia. The National Research Council of the United States recommends an intake of 200 IU per day for adults.

METABOLISM OF VITAMIN D   Once vitamin D enters the circulation, either by its absorption from the diet or through the skin, it is transported to the liver bound to a specific alpha$_1$ globulin (vitamin D–binding protein). In the liver, vitamin D is metabolized to 25-hydroxyvitamin D [25(OH)D] by hepatic mitochondrial and/or microsomal enzyme(s) (Fig. 339-4). 25(OH)D is one of the major circulating metabolites of vitamin D, and its half-life is estimated to be about 21 days. The concentration of 25(OH)D and some of its metabolites in the serum is measured using competitive binding assays. The normal circulating concentration of 25(OH)D varies among different laboratories from 12 to 200 nmol/L (5 to 80 ng/mL). Individuals exposed to excessive sunlight may have concentrations of 25(OH)D up to 370 nmol/L (150 ng/mL) without adverse effects on calcium metabolism. Assays that employ chromatographic separation prior to binding analysis often have a lower normal range, possibly because other vitamin D metabolites simulate 25(OH)D in this assay. The normal range, apparently independent of method, is lower in Great Britain than in the United States; in Great Britain dietary supplements of vitamin D are not routine, and exposure to sunlight is less than in most regions of the United States. The serum 25(OH)D levels routinely measured reflect both 25-hydroxyvitamin D_2 [25(OH)D_2] and 25-hydroxyvitamin D_3 [25(OH)D_3]. The ratio of these two 25-hydroxylated derivatives depends on the relative amounts of vitamins D_2 or D_3 present in the diet and the amount of previtamin D_3 produced by exposure to sunlight.

The hepatic 25-hydroxylation of vitamin D is regulated by a product feedback mechanism. This regulation, however, is not tight; an increase in dietary intake or endogenous production of vitamin D_3 is reflected by elevations in 25(OH)D concentration levels in the serum. The levels can rise to greater than 1200 nmol/L (500 ng/mL) when the intake of vitamin D is increased. Serum 25(OH)D concentration levels are reduced in severe chronic parenchymal and cholestatic liver disease (Table 339-1).

25(OH)D is not biologically active at physiologic levels in vivo but is active in vitro at high concentrations. Normally, after formation in the liver, 25(OH)D is bound by the high-affinity vitamin D–binding protein that is synthesized in the liver and transported to the kidney for an additional stereospecific hydroxylation on either C_1 or

TABLE 339-1   Serum concentrations of 25(OH)D in disorders of calcium, phosphorus, and bone metabolism

Disease states	Serum 25(OH)D
Vitamin D deficiency	↓
Intestinal malabsorption syndromes	↓
Liver disorders (chronic and severe)	↓
Nephrotic syndrome	↓
Osteopenia in the aged	N or ↓
Vitamin D intoxication	↑

NOTE: ↓ = decreased; N = normal; ↑ = increased.

C_{24} (Fig. 339-4). The kidney plays a pivotal role in the metabolism of 25(OH)D to the biologically active metabolite. The renal mitochondrial 25(OH)D-1α-hydroxylase activity is enhanced by hypocalcemia so that the rate of conversion of 25(OH)D to 1,25(OH)$_2$D increases. However, hypocalcemia may not control this hydroxylation directly. Any decrease in the serum concentration of calcium below normal is a stimulus for increased secretion of parathyroid hormone. Parathyroid hormone acts physiologically as a tropic hormone to increase the synthesis of 1,25(OH)$_2$D in the renal proximal convoluted tubule. The mechanism by which parathyroid hormone exerts its influence on the renal metabolism of 25(OH)D is not established; however, the renal production of 1,25(OH)$_2$D correlates with the effects of parathyroid hormone in lowering circulating concentrations (and presumably renal intracellular concentrations) of phosphate. 1,25(OH)$_2$D also influences the renal metabolism of 25(OH)D by diminishing 25(OH)D-1α-hydroxylase activity and enhancing the metabolism of 24R,25-dihydroxyvitamin D [24,25(OH)$_2$D].

24,25(OH)$_2$D is a circulating metabolite of 25(OH)D normally present in serum at a concentration of 1 to 10 nmol (0.5 to 5.0 ng/mL). 24,25(OH)$_2$D is also a substrate for renal 25(OH)D-1α-hydroxylase and is converted to 1α,24R,25-trihydroxyvitamin D [1,24,25(OH)$_3$D]. This trihydroxy metabolite is less potent than 1,25(OH)$_2$D in stimulating intestinal calcium transport; whether it has a physiologic role in maintaining calcium homeostasis is unclear. Cultured cells that possess nuclear receptors for 1,25(OH)$_2$D, such as chondrocytes, skin keratinocytes and fibroblasts, intestinal, and melanoma cells, also metabolize 25(OH)D to 24,25(OH)$_2$D. Although 24,25(OH)$_2$D may play a role in the expression of vitamin D action, it is more likely, that the C-24 hydroxylation is the first step in the degradation of both 25(OH)D and 1,25(OH)$_2$D.

The kidney also metabolizes 25(OH)D to 25S,26-dihydroxyvitamin D [25,26(OH)$_2$D]. 25,26(OH)$_2$D, like 24,25(OH)$_2$D, is metabolized by the kidney to 1α,25S,26-trihydroxyvitamin D [1,25,26(OH)$_3$D]. 1,25,26(OH)$_3$D is less active than 1,25(OH)$_2$D in inducing intestinal calcium transport, and the physiologic function of this metabolite remains to be defined.

1,25(OH)$_2$D is a substrate for the 25(OH)D–24R-hydroxylase and is metabolized to 1,24,25(OH)$_3$D, but this conversion is not believed to be important for the expression of biologic activity of 1,25(OH)$_2$D. More than twenty metabolites of vitamin D have been identified. All of the metabolites originate from 25(OH)D or 1,25(OH)$_2$D. Most of the metabolites appear to be degradation products. Of particular interest is the metabolic sequence that results in the inactivation of 1,25(OH)$_2$D by the oxidative cleavage of the side chain between C_{23} and C_{24} to yield a biologically inert and water-soluble product, 1α-hydroxyvitamin D–23-carboxylic acid (calcitroic acid).

PHYSIOLOGY OF VITAMIN D   1,25(OH)$_2$D, produced by the kidney and during pregnancy by the placenta, is the only known important metabolite of vitamin D; the potential roles of other metabolites have not been clarified. 1,25(OH)$_2$D bound to a vitamin D–binding protein is delivered to the intestine, where the free form is taken up by the cells and transported to a specific nuclear receptor protein. The 1,25(OH)$_2$D receptor belongs to the superfamily of steroid receptors that are related to the oncogene v-erbA (see Chap. 311). The vitamin-receptor complex activates transcription of genes;

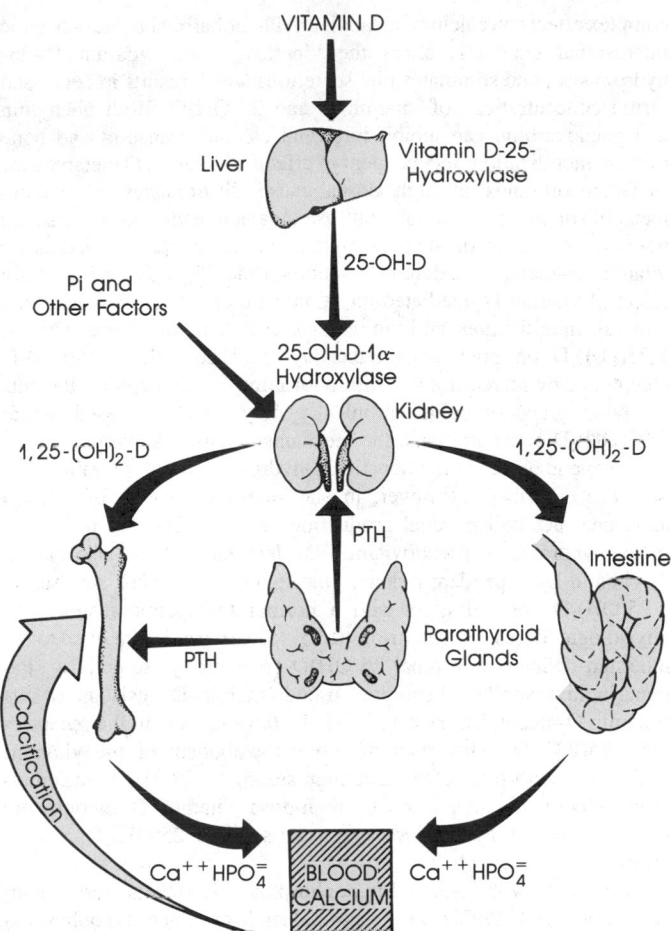

FIGURE 339-5 Schematic representation of the hormonal control loop for vitamin D metabolism and function. A reduction in the serum calcium below approximately 2.2 mmol/L (8.8 mg/dL) prompts a proportional secretion of parathyroid hormone that acts to mobilize calcium stores from the bone. Parathyroid hormone also promotes the synthesis of 1,25(OH)$_2$D in the kidney, which, in turn, stimulates the mobilization of calcium from bone and intestine. (*From MF Holick, Kidney Int 32:912, 1987.*)

eration of human keratinocytes and fibroblasts, stimulates terminal differentiation of human keratinocytes, induces monocytes to produce interleukin 1 and to mature into macrophages and osteoclast-like cells, and inhibits interleukin 2 and immunoglobulin production by activated T and B lymphocytes, respectively. In addition, a variety of tumor cell lines including breast carcinomas, melanomas, and promyeloblasts possess receptors for 1,25(OH)$_2$D.

Cultured tumor cell lines that possess receptors for this hormone respond to the hormone by decreasing the rate of proliferation and by enhancing differentiation. For example, when malignant, receptor-positive human promyelocytic cells (HL-60) are exposed to 1,25(OH)$_2$D, the cells mature into functioning macrophages within 1 week. Although the mechanism of 1,25(OH)$_2$D induction of maturation is unknown, 1,25(OH)$_2$D decreases the expression of c-*myc* oncogene coincident with decreasing replication. This effect, however, is not a lasting one; when the metabolite is removed from maturing HL-60 promyelocytes, the cells revert to their original malignant state, and expression of c-*myc* oncogene is no longer suppressed.

The importance of 1,25(OH)$_2$D in the regulation of differentiation and immunoregulation is unknown. Patients with vitamin D–dependent rickets type II who are unable to respond to physiologic concentrations of 1,25(OH)$_2$D (because of insufficient or defective receptors for this hormone) appear to have no demonstrable in vivo defects in the cellular immune response and in the growth of skin (with the exception of the associated alopecia) and other tissues. It is also interesting that when these patients receive infusions of calcium the metabolic bone disease is reversed. Although the use of 1,25(OH)$_2$D (calcitriol) for the treatment of leukemia is not efficacious, the antiproliferative activity of calcitriol has been used for the treatment of psoriasis.

Most measurements of circulating 1,25(OH)$_2$D in humans in various physiologic or pathologic states utilize a receptor/competitive binding assay (Table 339-2). Serum concentrations of vitamin D and 25(OH)D vary with the season and with vitamin D intake. Serum concentrations of 1,25(OH)$_2$D, however, appear to be unaltered by seasonal variation, by increases in dietary vitamin D, or by exposure to sunlight; as long as vitamin D supplies and circulating concentrations of 25(OH)D are sufficient, metabolic influences operate on the renal

in the intestine calcium-binding protein is synthesized, and in bone osteocalcin is produced. Some evidence suggests that 1,25(OH)$_2$D may also have nonnuclear effects on its target tissues; 1,25(OH)$_2$D increases the transport of calcium from the extracellular to intracellular space, and it can mobilize intracellular calcium concentrations from intracellular calcium pools. In the intestine the net effect of 1,25(OH)$_2$D is to stimulate calcium and phosphate transport from the small intestinal lumen into the circulation (Fig. 339-5). The effect of 1,25(OH)$_2$D on the enhancement of bone resorption is believed to be synergistic with parathyroid hormone. Mature osteoclasts do not possess receptors either for parathyroid hormone or 1,25(OH)$_2$D. Some evidence suggests that parathyroid hormone and 1,25(OH)$_2$D increase bone resorption activity by stimulating immature osteoclastic precursors that possess receptors for both parathyroid hormone and 1,25(OH)$_2$D to become mature osteoclasts and/or by interacting with osteoblasts to produce cytokines that enhance the activity of mature osteoclasts. The role of 1,25(OH)$_2$D on the renal handling of calcium and phosphorus remains uncertain.

Receptors for 1,25(OH)$_2$D are present in intestine, bone, and kidney and in tissues and cells that have not classically been recognized as target organs for this hormone, including skin, breast, pituitary gland, parathyroid glands, beta cells of the pancreatic islets, gonads, brain, skeletal muscle, circulating monocytes, and activated B and T lymphocytes. Although the physiologic role of 1,25(OH)$_2$D in these cells remains to be determined, 1,25(OH)$_2$D in vitro inhibits prolif-

TABLE 339-2 Serum concentrations of 1,25(OH)$_2$D in disorders of calcium, phosphorus, and bone metabolism

Disease states	Serum 1,25(OH)$_2$D
Vitamin D deficiency	↓ *
Renal failure:	
GFR > (30 mL/min)/1.7 m^2	↓ or N
GFR < (30 mL/min)/1.7 m^2	↓
Hypoparathyroidism	↓ or N
Pseudohypoparathyroidism	↓ or N
Vitamin D–dependent rickets:	
Type I	↓ or N
Type II	↑ or N
X-linked vitamin D–resistant rickets	↓ or N
Tumor-induced osteomalacia	↓
Oncogenic hypercalcemia	↓
Some lymphomas	↑
Hyperparathyroidism	↑
Sarcoidosis, tuberculosis, silicosis	↑
Idiopathic hypercalciuria	N or ↑
Williams' syndrome	↑
Vitamin D intoxication	↓ or N

* Serum 1,25(OH)$_2$D concentrations are normal or elevated in occasional patients with biopsy-proven osteomalacia and undetectable or low circulating concentrations of 25(OH)D. These patients also have secondary hyperparathyroidism, and they may represent a partially treated state; if a small amount of vitamin D is obtained from the diet or generated in the skin in these patients, the vitamin is efficiently converted to 1,25(OH)$_2$D. The net effect is low or undetectable circulating concentrations of 25(OH)D along with normal or elevated concentrations of 1,25(OH)$_2$D. However, in extreme vitamin D deficiency, circulating concentrations of 1,25(OH)$_2$D are low or undetectable.

NOTE: ↓ = decreased; N = normal; ↑ = increased; GFR = glomerular filtration rate.

25(OH)D-1α-hydroxylase to ensure a closely regulated circulating concentration of 1,25(OH)$_2$D. The serum concentration of 1,25(OH)$_2$D ranges from 40 to 160 pmol/L (16 to 65 pg/mL). The serum half-life of 1,25(OH)$_2$D is from 3 to 6 h.

When the serum calcium falls below normal, secretion of parathyroid hormone is enhanced, resulting in increased production of 1,25(OH)$_2$D. The principal physiologic regulation of the production of 1,25(OH)$_2$D appears to involve changes in serum calcium concentrations that result in reciprocal changes in secretion of parathyroid hormone, the latter controlling, possibly through actions on serum or tissue phosphorus concentrations, the rate of 1,25(OH)$_2$D production. Other factors that enhance 1,25(OH)$_2$D production in animals include estrogen, prolactin, and growth hormone. Humans adapt to increased calcium requirements during growth, pregnancy, and lactation by increasing the efficiency of intestinal calcium absorption, possibly by enhancing 25(OH)D-1α-hydroxylase activity. During the first two trimesters of pregnancy the concentrations of 1,25(OH)$_2$D increase proportional to increases in the concentrations of the vitamin D–binding protein; concentrations of free 1,25(OH)$_2$D do not change. During the last trimester when maximal mineralization of the fetal skeleton takes place, the increased demand for calcium is met by an increase in the free concentrations of 1,25(OH)$_2$D, which in turn enhance maternal intestinal calcium absorption.

PATHOPHYSIOLOGY OF DISORDERS OF VITAMIN D NUTRITION AND METABOLISM *Hypovitaminosis D* results from inadequate endogenous production of vitamin D$_3$ in the skin, insufficient dietary supplementation, and/or the inability of the small intestine to absorb adequate amounts of vitamin D from the diet. Disease states equivalent to hypovitaminosis D result from (1) effects of drugs that antagonize vitamin D action, (2) alterations in the metabolism of vitamin D, or (3) deficient or defective receptors for 1,25(OH)$_2$D. Hypovitaminosis D results in (1) disturbances of mineral ion metabolism and secretion of parathyroid hormone and (2) mineralization defects in the skeleton (e.g., rickets in children, osteomalacia in adults). The changes in the skeleton are described in Chap. 341. With regard to calcium metabolism, lack of vitamin D action leads to insufficient intestinal calcium absorption and to hypocalcemia. The latter stimulates the secretion of parathyroid hormone (secondary hyperparathyroidism), which enhances calcium release from bone and decreases calcium clearance by the kidney, and tends to blunt the hypocalcemia. (Late in the course of untreated hypovitaminosis D, severe hypocalcemia develops.) Hypophosphatemia is more marked than hypocalcemia, especially in early stages of vitamin D deficiency. The efficiency of intestinal phosphate absorption, similar to that of calcium absorption, is decreased. The increased secretion of parathyroid hormone, although partially effective in minimizing hypocalcemia, leads to urinary phosphate wasting through decreases in renal tubular reabsorption. This latter effect may be the most significant factor in causing hypophosphatemia. With an adequate glomerular filtration rate, the predominant changes in blood are severe hypophosphatemia, moderate or slightly low levels of calcium, and increased levels of parathyroid hormone. Blood levels of 25(OH)D are low (Table 339-1). As discussed in Chap. 341 defects in skeletal mineralization may accompany these disturbances in mineral ion metabolism.

Although the conversion of vitamin D to 25(OH)D is impaired in liver disease, there is no strong correlation between low serum 25(OH)D levels and osteopenia; multiple effects of the primary disease state seem to affect skeletal metabolism as well. Patients with nephrotic syndrome who excrete more than 4 g/d of protein in urine often have low 25(OH)D levels due to the loss in the urine of the vitamin D–binding protein with its associated tightly bound 25(OH)D. Circulating concentrations of 25(OH)D can also be decreased when 25(OH)D metabolism is increased, as in sarcoidosis and hyperparathyroidism. There is a relation between chronic anticonvulsant therapy and the development of osteomalacia or rickets; mineralization defects are worse in patients on multiple drug therapy and when vitamin D intake or exposure to sunlight is inadequate. Drugs have multiple and complex effects on calcium metabolism. Phenobarbital induces hepatic microsomal enzymes, alters the kinetics of the vitamin D–25-hydroxylase, and stimulates bile secretion, which results in decreased serum concentrations of vitamin D and 25(OH)D. Both phenytoin and phenobarbital can inhibit intestinal calcium transport and bone mineral mobilization, independent of effects of vitamin D metabolism.

Glucocorticoids in high doses cause disturbances in calcium metabolism and osteoporosis, but osteomalacia and rickets per se are not a consequence of such therapy. Actions of glucocorticoids on vitamin D–mediated calcium metabolism include a direct inhibitory effect of vitamin D–mediated intestinal calcium absorption and bone mineral mobilization and an enhancement of the sensitivity of 1,25(OH)$_2$D on bone cells either by stabilizing the 1,25(OH)$_2$D receptor or by increasing the affinity or number of receptors. Patients receiving glucocorticoids chronically may have depressed serum 1,25(OH)$_2$D concentrations; the mechanism(s) is unknown.

A genetic defect in the hepatic 25-hydroxylation of vitamin D has not been described. However, in one inherited disorder of calcium and bone metabolism renal production of 1,25(OH)$_2$D is defective. In the syndrome of pseudovitamin D–deficient rickets (also known as vitamin D–dependent rickets, type I; see Chap. 341), low serum 1,25(OH)$_2$D concentrations and a normal therapeutic response to physiologic doses of calcitriol (0.25 to 1.0 μg/d) are due to an inherited deficiency in renal 25(OH)D-1α-hydroxylase activity. Patients with a similar phenotype, pseudovitamin D–resistant rickets (vitamin D–dependent rickets, type II), have defects in the receptors for 1,25(OH)$_2$D rather than defective metabolism of the vitamin. Individuals with this defect have high serum 1,25(OH)$_2$D concentrations; therapeutic responses to high-dose vitamin D therapy are associated with a further increase in the serum 1,25(OH)$_2$D concentrations.

In patients with X-linked hypophosphatemic rickets, serum concentrations of 1,25(OH)$_2$D are normal or low. Since hypophosphatemia is a potent stimulus for the renal 25(OH)D-1α-hydroxylase, the serum 1,25(OH)$_2$D concentrations should be high. Thus, even a normal serum 1,25(OH)$_2$D concentration suggests a functional defect in the 25(OH)D-1α-hydroxylase system. In some cases, the combination of calcitriol and phosphate supplements offers a therapeutic advantage to phosphate therapy by itself (Chap. 341). In patients with mild to moderate chronic renal failure [glomerular filtration rate >0.5 mL/s (>30 mL/min)] and decreased phosphate clearance, hyperphosphatemia and acidosis play important roles in suppressing the renal production of 1,25(OH)$_2$D despite high circulating concentrations of parathyroid hormone. As the destruction of the renal cortex progresses, the reserves of the 25(OH)D-1α-hydroxylase are depleted to a point at which the kidney is unable to produce sufficient quantities of 1,25(OH)$_2$D to maintain calcium homeostasis, even when serum phosphorus concentrations are normal. Under these circumstances replacement therapy with calcitriol is most beneficial (Chap. 341). Aging decreases the responsiveness of the renal 25(OH)D-1α-hydroxylase to parathyroid hormone; this causes a slight lowering of 1,25(OH)$_2$D levels in the blood and may contribute to decreased calcium absorption in the elderly.

Patients with hypocalcemia due to hypoparathyroidism or pseudohypoparathyroidism have lower than normal mean serum concentrations of 1,25(OH)$_2$D although individual values may overlap with the normal range. In these patients favorable response to small replacement doses of calcitriol (0.25 to 1.0 μg/d; see Chap. 340) occurs even when the serum 25(OH)D concentrations are higher than normal. These observations are consistent with the concept that patients with absent or ineffective action of parathyroid hormone have defective function of renal 25(OH)D-1α-hydroxylase. It is not known to what extent serum 1,25(OH)$_2$D concentrations would be restored toward normal if the hyperphosphatemia were adequately controlled.

Patients with tumor-induced (oncogenic) osteomalacia have low serum phosphorus and 1,25(OH)$_2$D levels. These tumors presumably secrete a substance(s) that causes renal phosphorus wasting and inhibits the formation of $1,25(OH)_2D$; after removal of the tumor the serum phosphorus and $1,25(OH)_2D$ levels return to normal.

In disease states equivalent to hypervitaminosis D such as sarcoidosis (and other chronic granulomatous disorders), lymphomas, idiopathic hypercalciuria, and Williams' syndrome there is an abnormality in the metabolism of $25(OH)D$ to $1,25(OH)_2D$ (Table 339-2). Hypercalcemia and hypercalciuria in sarcoidosis are associated with elevated circulating concentrations of $1,25(OH)_2D$; sarcoid granulomas metabolize $25(OH)D$ to $1,25(OH)_2D$ in an unregulated manner, and pulmonary alveolar macrophages from patients with sarcoidosis synthesize $1,25(OH)_2D$. In addition, normal pulmonary macrophages can be induced to metabolize $25(OH)D$ to $1,25(OH)_2D$ in vitro when exposed either to lipopolysaccharides from the cell wall of gram-negative bacteria or to γ-interferon. Most patients with tumor-induced hypercalcemia have low circulating concentrations of $1,25(OH)_2D$ (Table 339-2). The exceptions are patients with several types of lymphoma (including T-cell, mixed histiocytic-lymphocytic, and B-cell immunoblastic lymphomas) whose hypercalcemia is associated with elevated concentrations of $1,25(OH)_2D$. In one report, surgical excision of a solitary splenic lymphoma resulted in rapid return of elevated serum $1,25(OH)_2D$ and calcium levels to normal suggesting that the lymphoma metabolized $25(OH)D$ to $1,25(OH)_2D$ in an unregulated manner. Hypercalcemic patients with elevated blood levels of $1,25(OH)_2D$ due to unregulated production of the hormone at an extrarenal site respond to glucocorticoid therapy with a decrease in the blood concentration of $1,25(OH)_2D$ and a return of the serum calcium level to normal. There is an association between elevated circulating concentrations of $1,25(OH)_2D$ in patients with primary hyperparathyrodisim, hypercalciuria, and renal stones. Similarly, in some instances of idiopathic hypercalciuria, intestinal calcium absorption is inappropriately increased. Approximately one-third of these patients have elevated circulating $1,25(OH)_2D$. These findings are consistent with the hypothesis that excessive $1,25(OH)_2D$ production is responsible for the hyperabsorption of calcium by the small intestine. Infants with hypercalcemia associated with supravalvular aortic stenosis, mental retardation, and elfin facies (*Williams' syndrome*) also have elevated serum $1,25(OH)_2D$ concentrations. It is not clear whether the increased levels result from abnormal synthesis or degradation of $1,25(OH)_2D$.

PHARMACOLOGY OF VITAMIN D AND ITS METABOLITES A variety of over-the-counter vitamin preparations contain 400 IU of either vitamin D_2 or vitamin D_3. More potent forms of vitamin D (calciferol) are available in capsule and tablet form (50,000 IU) as well as in oil (500,000 IU/mL) and in oral solution (8000 IU/mL). A single oral dose of 50,000 IU of vitamin D_2 increases the circulating concentrations of vitamin D from less than 25 nmol/L (10 ng/mL) to 130 to 260 nmol/L (50 to 100 ng/mL) within 12 to 24 h; the plasma half-life is about 2 days. Serum concentrations of $25(OH)D$ and $1,25(OH)_2D$ are not changed. For treatment of vitamin D deficiency, 50,000 IU of vitamin D twice a week for several weeks raises the circulating concentration of $25(OH)D$ into the normal range; in the presence of secondary hyperparathyroidism the circulating concentrations of $1,25(OH)_2D$ can increase to supranormal levels [(up to 600 pmol/L (250 pg/mL)]. $25(OH)D_3$ (calcifediol) is available in capsules containing either 20 or 50 μg. This drug may be useful in treating vitamin D deficiency [low $25(OH)D$ concentrations] in patients with severe liver dysfunction. Pharmacologic doses are used to treat disorders of $25(OH)D$ metabolism; in pharmacologic doses $25(OH)D_3$ is believed to be effective through its interaction with the receptor for $1,25(OH)_2D$. $1,25(OH)_2D$ (calcitriol) is available in capsules containing 0.25 or 0.5 μg and as a solution for intravenous use (1.0 and 2.0 μg/mL). Calcitriol is efficacious in a variety of calcium metabolic disorders (see Chap. 340). 1α-Hydroxyvitamin D_3 [$1(OH)D_3$] is also a potent $1,25(OH)_2D_3$ agonist. The structure of this analogue is identical to that of the natural renal hormone with the exception that it lacks a C_{25}-OH (Fig. 339-6). In humans, this analogue is rapidly metabolized by the liver to $1,25(OH)_2D_3$. This analogue is used in Europe and Japan.

When vitamin D is chemically manipulated to rotate the A ring through 180 degrees, the C_3-β-OH assumes a geometric position that mimics the C_1-α-OH (Fig. 339-6). These compounds, called pseudo-1α-hydroxyvitamin D analogues, include dihydrotachysterol and 5,6-*trans*-vitamin D. These analogues are less effective in stimulating intestinal calcium transport on a weight basis than either vitamin D or $1,25(OH)_2D$. However, because the pseudo-1α-hydroxyvitamin D analogues do not require a renal 1α-hydroxylation to be active on intestinal calcium transport, they are 3 to 10 times more potent than vitamin D in disease states that adversely affect the renal $25(OH)D$-1α-hydroxylase, such as hypoparathyroidism and chronic renal failure. These analogues are efficiently metabolized in the liver to the corresponding 25-hydroxy derivatives, which are the biologically active forms.

PARATHYROID HORMONE Physiology The function of parathyroid hormone is to maintain extracellular fluid calcium concentration. The hormone acts directly on bone and kidney and indirectly on intestine through its effects on synthesis of $1,25(OH)_2D$ to increase serum calcium; in turn, parathyroid hormone production is closely regulated by the concentration of serum ionized calcium. This feedback system is one of the most important homeostatic mechanisms. Any tendency toward hypocalcemia, as might be induced by calcium-deficient diets, is counteracted by an increased rate of secretion of parathyroid hormone. This in turn (1) acts to increase the rate of dissolution of bone mineral, thereby increasing the flow of calcium from bone into blood, (2) reduces the renal clearance of calcium, returning more of the calcium filtered at the glomerulus into extracellular fluid, and (3) increases the efficiency of calcium absorption in the intestine. The relative physiologic importance in minute-to-minute calcium homeostasis of these three actions of parathyroid hormone, stimulation of calcium transport in bone, kidney, and intestine, is not clear, but most evidence suggests that immediate control of blood calcium is due to effects of the hormone on bone and, to a lesser extent, on renal calcium clearance. Maintenance of calcium balance, on the other hand, is probably due to the effects of the hormone on $1,25(OH)_2D$ levels and hence on the efficiency of intestinal calcium absorption. As much as 12 mmol (500 mg) calcium is transferred between extracellular fluid and bone each day (a large amount in relation to the total extracellular fluid calcium pool), and parathyroid hormone has a major effect on this transfer. The action of the hormone tends to preserve calcium concentration in blood acutely at the cost of bone destruction and bone mineral release. The action of parathyroid hormone on kidney to increase the reabsorption of filtered calcium may also contribute to rapid regulation of blood calcium concentration.

Parathyroid hormone has a dual action on bone, the *calcium replacement* and the *bone remodeling* effects. There is an increased rate of release of calcium from bone into blood after administration of parathyroid hormone, the time period needed to observe the change varying with the dose of hormone and the overall metabolic status (influenced by age, diet, etc.). Usually 30 min to 1 h is required to detect a significant increase in blood calcium, but with the use of radioisotopes changes in bone calcium release can be seen within minutes. When studied carefully in animals a rapid efflux of calcium out of blood into bone, presumably into bone cells, precedes the release of calcium. On the other hand, the more chronic effects of parathyroid hormone, mainly increase in the number of osteoclasts and a general increase in the remodeling of bone, are apparent only hours after the hormone is given. These latter actions, which involve increased protein synthesis, persist for hours after parathyroid hormone has been given. It is not clear whether the two effects of parathyroid action on bone represent a continuous spectrum with a common initiating biochemical event or whether they are separate actions.

Osteoblastic cells but not osteoclasts have receptors for parathyroid hormone. The action of PTH on osteoclasts is indirect, through cytokines released from osteoblasts to activate osteoclasts, e.g., osteoblasts must be present along with osteoclasts for PTH to activate osteoclasts to resorb bone.

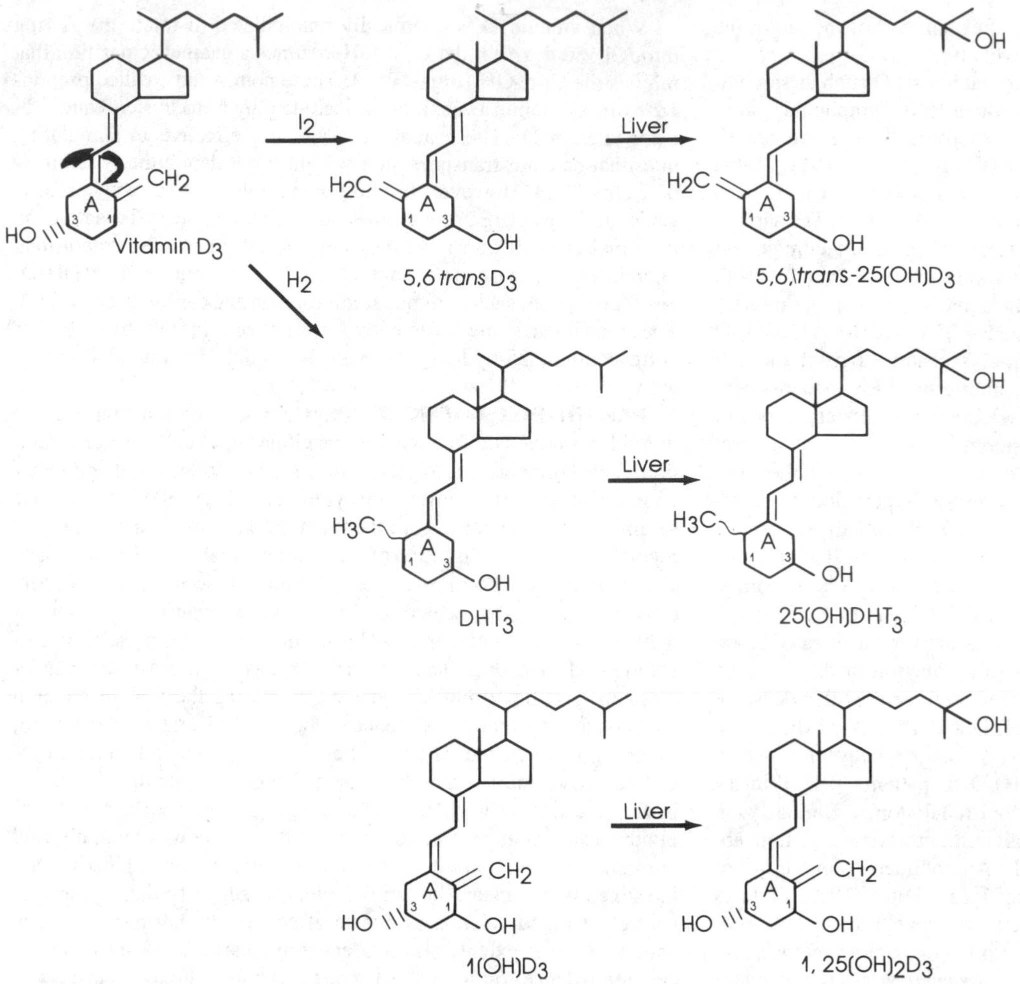

FIGURE 339-6 When vitamin D is treated with I_2 or reduced with H_2, ring A of the vitamin D molecule rotates 180° to reorient spatially the 3β-OH in a pseudo-1α-OH position. These analogues, 5,6-*trans*-vitamin D_3 and dihydrotachysterol, (DHT_3), are called pseudo-1α-hydroxy analogues. $1(OH)D_3$ is a synthetic analogue of $1,25(OH)_2D_3$ that lacks a C_{25}-OH. $1(OH)D_3$, 5,6-*trans*-vitamin D_3, and DHT_3 all undergo a hepatic C_{25}-hydroxylation before they are biologically active.

The nature of the cytokines that stimulate osteoclasts is a subject of major interest. IGF-1 and possibly other agents are candidates, but the definitive messenger(s) has not been determined.

Chemistry The complete amino acid sequences of the major forms of parathyroid hormone from cow, pig, rat, and human have been defined. The peptides consist of a single-chain structure composed of 84 amino acids. The molecules lack cysteine or cystine; the sequences of the four forms of the hormone are similar, as is illustrated in Fig. 339-7. The sequence of chicken parathyroid hormone has been deduced from the nucleotide sequence of the cloned cDNA. This molecule differs substantially from the mammalian hormones. One large sequence deletion in the middle of the molecule and a larger addition near the carboxy terminus result in a molecule of 88 rather than 84 amino acids. There is conservation in the amino-terminal portion needed for biologic actions of the molecule.

The structural requirements for the binding of the hormone to receptors and hence for its biologic activity have been defined. Synthetic fragments containing the amino-terminal sequence residues 1-34 or even shorter sequences, 2-26 being minimally active, exert the known biologic actions of the hormone on mineral ion transport in kidney and bone and by stimulating the renal 25-hydroxyvitamin D-1α-hydroxylase also exert the capacity of the hormone to stimulate intestinal calcium absorption. Since osteoblasts but not osteoclasts have receptors for parathyroid hormone, the effects of parathyroid hormone on stimulating osteoclastic bone resorption are indirect.

Fragments shortened at the amino terminus lose binding affinity more slowly than capacity to stimulate biologic response. The peptide 7-34 is a competitive inhibitor of the binding of active hormone to receptors in vitro and serves as a competitive inhibitor of the renal responses to the hormone, including the increased excretion of cyclic AMP and the enhanced clearance of phosphate. Rapid mobilization of calcium from bone is also blocked in certain test systems in vivo.

Biosynthesis, secretion, metabolism, and mode of action Several larger molecular forms have been identified in the biosynthetic sequence leading from gene transcription and translation to final packaging of the 84-amino acid peptide in secretory granules prior to secretion. The earliest detected precursor form, termed *preproparathyroid hormone,* consists of 115 amino acids; this molecular form is converted to an intermediate form of 90 amino acids termed *proparathyroid hormone,* then to the secreted product of 84 amino acids, parathyroid hormone. Parathyroid hormone shares, with other polypeptides and proteins destined for secretion from cells, this complex pattern of initial synthesis as a larger molecule which is then reduced in size by several cleavages prior to secretion. The regulation of these sequential steps in parathyroid hormone biosynthesis is unknown except by analogy with regulatory steps in biosynthesis, transport, and packaging of other proteins destined for secretion. The hydrophobic regions of the preproparathyroid hormone are similar to preprotein-specific regions of other cell-secreted proteins and serve a role in guiding transport of the polypeptide from sites of synthesis on polyribosomes through the endoplasmic reticulum to secretory granules. The genes for bovine, rat, and human parathyroid hormone have been cloned, and their structures have been determined. There are considerable homologies in the gene structures from these three species. Studies with cloned and expressed parathyroid hormone genes in vitro have demonstrated regions for control of gene expression at the transcriptional level, including sites for interaction and regulation by $1,25(OH)_2D$ and its receptor and "upstream" silencer elements as well as sites in which ambient calcium concentration regulates transcription. These in vitro observations are not well understood in terms of physiologic regulation of parathyroid hormone biosynthesis and secretion; the processing of hormone precursors (a posttranslational step of regulation of hormone production) may be more central to hormone availability than changes in transcription. It does not

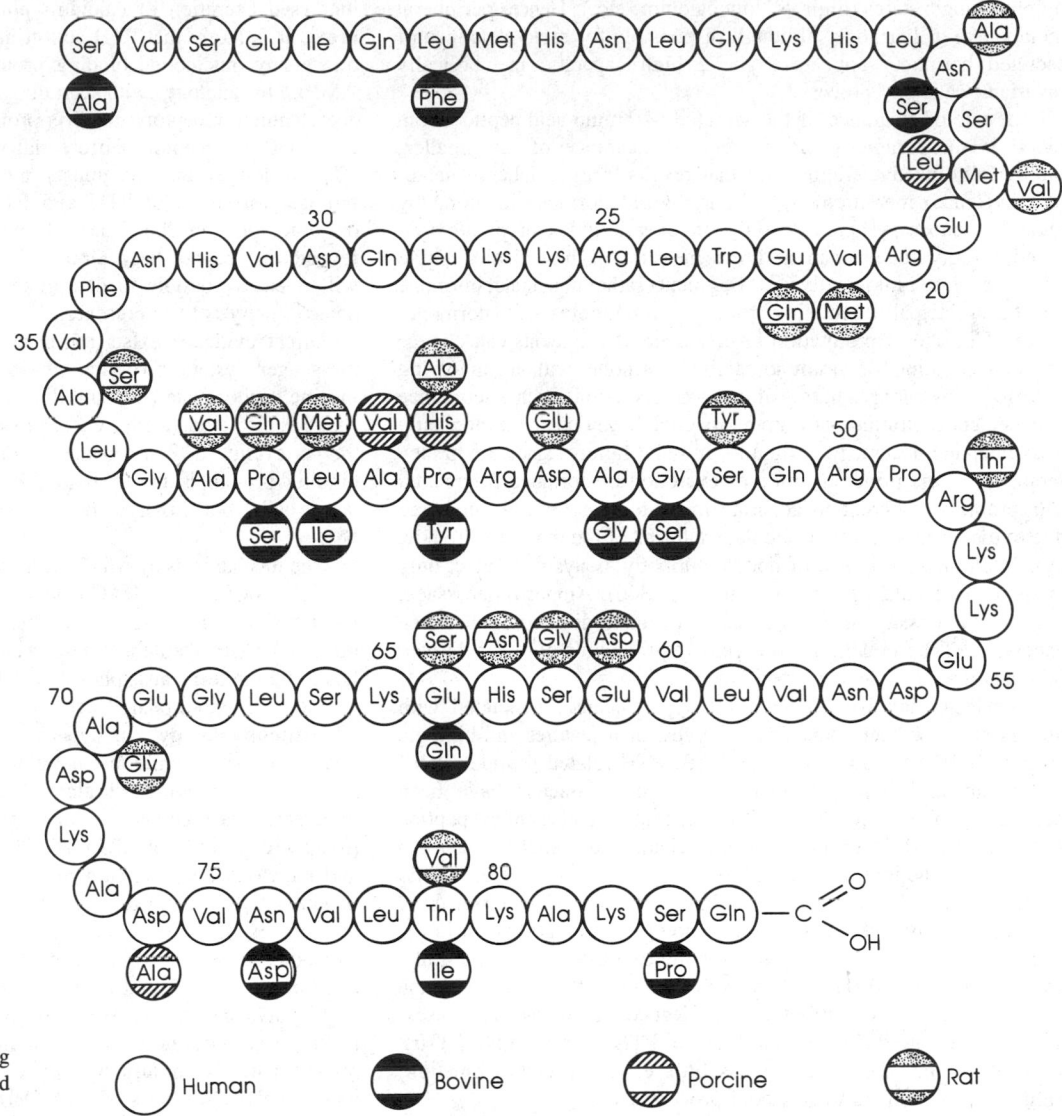

FIGURE 339-7 Model illustrating the sequence of human, cow, rat, and pig parathyroid hormone.

appear that changes in transcriptional activity of the parathyroid gene in the normal physiologic range of levels of blood calcium and 1,25(OH)$_2$D nor in short-term environmental stresses (e.g., fasting for 24 h) are important in control of blood levels of the hormone. Control is exerted by precise and rapid variation of rates of hormone secretion under the control of extracellular fluid calcium.

Blood calcium concentration over wide ranges controls the secretion of parathyroid hormone; the ionized fraction of blood calcium is the important determinant of hormone secretion. Hormone secretion increases steeply to a maximum value of fivefold above basal rates of secretion as calcium concentration falls from normal to the range of 1.9 to 2.0 mmol/L (7.5 to 8.0 mg/dL) (measured as total calcium). Beta-adrenergic agonists such as epinephrine and histamine-2 agonists may also increase hormone secretion, but the physiologic significance of these secretagogues is not established. Furthermore, drugs such as propranolol or cimetidine do not reproducibly decrease circulating parathyroid hormone levels.

Magnesium may influence hormone secretion in the same direction as calcium, but is a less potent secretagogue. It is unlikely that physiologic variations in magnesium concentration affect parathyroid secretion, but severe intracellular magnesium deficiency is associated with defective hormone secretion.

The hormone secreted in vivo from normal bovine and human parathyroid glands and from parathyroid adenomas is indistinguishable by immunologic criteria and by molecular size from the 84-amino acid peptide (molecular weight 9500) extracted from glands. However, much of the immunoreactive material found in the peripheral circu-

lation of humans and animals (cow, dog) is smaller than the extracted or secreted hormone. The principal circulating fragments of immunoreactive hormone (approximate molecular weight 7000) lack a portion of the critical amino-terminal sequence required for biologic activity and, hence, are biologically inactive hormonal fragments. The nature of the cleavage process suggests that an endopeptidase cuts the molecule into two pieces.

Cleavage of the native peptide by an endopeptidase would be expected to result in formation of a second fragment, molecular weight 2000 to 3000, representing the amino-terminal, biologically active, portion of the hormone. There has been uncertainty concerning the presence or absence of such a circulating amino-terminal fragment. It has been also unclear (1) as to what extent peripheral metabolism accounts for the circulating fragment(s) of hormone as contrasted with intraglandular cleavage and subsequent secretion of hormone fragments and (2) whether peripheral metabolism is a purely catabolic process concerned only with hormone destruction or whether the peripheral cleavage results in formation of a metabolically active amino-terminal fragment of parathyroid hormone. Present evidence suggests that the liver and kidney are the principal sites at which peripheral metabolism of hormone occurs. Cleavages in these organs could regulate the concentration of hormonally active polypeptides in the circulation. Peripheral metabolism, in turn, may be affected by pathologic processes, such as renal failure or severe hepatic dysfunction. Certain conclusions can be made. There is no convincing evidence that circulating biologically active fragments are produced by peripheral metabolism; the latter process does not seem regulated by physiologic states (high vs. low calcium, etc.). Hence, peripheral metabolism of hormone, although responsible for rapid clearance of secreted hormone, appears to be a high capacity, metabolically invariant, catabolic process.

The rate of clearance of the secreted 84-amino acid peptide from blood is more rapid than the rate of clearance of the smaller, biologically inactive fragment(s) that results from peripheral metabolism. Hence, measurements of parathyroid hormone in blood by most immunoassays provide only an overall index of parathyroid gland activity rather than a direct measure of biologically active hormone, since biologically inert fragments rather than intact hormone are the principal circulating form of immunoreactive hormone. Changes in rate of production or clearance of fragments can change the concentration of immunoreactive hormone without involving corresponding changes in rate of hormone secretion. Such discordance between concentrations of immunoreactive hormone and biologically active peptide occurs, for example, in renal failure, since the kidney seems to be the principal route of excretion of hormone fragments. The problems inherent in accurate measurements of PTH in blood due to the heterogeneity of circulating forms of the molecule are now largely eliminated by use of double-antibody assays that detect only the intact molecule (as discussed in Chap. 340). Among other issues, the improved assays make it possible to make distinctions between excessive PTH production and excessive production of tumor-derived products that also elevate blood calcium.

One factor involved in humoral hypercalcemia associated with tumors has now been identified. The chemical features and biologic properties of the tumor factor (PTHrP, PTH-related peptide; HHM factor, humoral hypercalcemia of malignancy factor) have been deduced by use of recombinant DNA techniques and chemical peptide synthesis. PTHrP is a product of normal squamous epithelial cells in skin and may be involved in milk production in mammary tissue and in placental calcium metabolism in sheep. PTHrP is a larger molecule, 144 amino acids, and shares little homology with PTH except in the amino-terminal region; the genes for the two molecules are located on different chromosomes. The two peptides both interact with the PTH receptor. The tumor factor does affect certain biologic responses, however, that are different from those of PTH. For example, PTHrP stimulates bone resorption but has little effect on bone formation, unlike PTH which stimulates both processes.

The action of parathyroid hormone at the biochemical level involves effects on receptor(s) and second messengers in target cells. Stimulation of enzyme activity (adenyl cyclase, phospholipase C) during specific hormone–target cell membrane interaction leads to an increase in second messengers, intracellular cyclic AMP, and products of polyphosphoinositol metabolism (see also Chap. 68). Parathyroid hormone interacts with a specific receptor/adenylate cyclase complex on plasma membranes of target cells consisting of hormone receptor, enzyme catalytic unit (adenylate cyclase), and a guanyl nucleotide (GTP or GDP)–binding regulatory protein (G unit or N protein). The latter protein consists of α subunits that bind GTP or GDP and β subunits that dissociate when the α subunits bind GTP and reassociate when the α subunits bind GDP. The α subunit with bound GTP complexes with adenylate cyclase, thereby activating the enzyme to increase the rate of cyclic AMP production from ATP. Hydrolysis of the GTP to GDP on the α subunit leads to reassociation of the G units and reduction in adenylate cyclase activity. In short, hormone binding to its receptor initiates a cycle of α subunit/GTP binding and enzyme activation.

Following the administration of parathyroid hormone a rise in urinary cyclic AMP precedes any observable increase in phosphate excretion. Likewise, the effects on bone adenylate cyclase activity can be detected within 1 min of the addition of parathyroid hormone to a suspension of bone cells. In addition, administration of dibutyryl cyclic AMP simulates many of the actions of parathyroid hormone in parathyroidectomized animals. Dibutyryl cyclic AMP leads to a rise in serum calcium, a lowering of serum phosphate, and an increased excretion of calcium, phosphate, and hydroxyproline in urine. It is likely that PTH action involves more than one receptor, one guanyl nucleotide binding protein, and one messenger (cyclic AMP). In analogy with certain other peptide, adrenergic, and acetylcholine receptors, there is probably more than one chemically distinct PTH receptor. Differential responses with certain synthetic PTH analogues and antagonists and some distinctions between the biologic responses of PTH and PTHrP are best explained by the existence of more than one PTH receptor. The cDNA for the PTH receptor(s) has not been cloned, however; only successful cloning will make it possible to determine whether the suspected receptor heterogeneity is truly present.

Direct evidence exists for participation of the alternate second messenger system involving phospholipase C/polyphosphoinositol/inosine triphosphate (IP$_3$) and diacyl glycerol (DAG) in PTH action. There is also evidence for a PTH-mediated calcium channel response that is cyclic AMP independent. Presumably, a distinctive guanyl binding protein is involved in PTH-mediated responses in certain target cells, but this hypothesis also awaits testing (see also Chap. 68).

The mechanisms by which an increased intracellular concentration of cyclic AMP, IP$_3$, or DAG lead to changes in calcium and phosphate ion translocation is unknown. There is evidence for stimulation of protein kinases (protein kinase A, cyclic AMP; protein kinase C, DAG) that in turn cause phosphorylation of proteins that are believed to initiate the hormonal effect.

Pathophysiology In hyperparathyroidism there is an overproduction of parathyroid hormone by tumors of the parathyroid or hyperplasia involving all glands. The excess hormone results in hypercalcemia secondary to increased intestinal calcium absorption [increased synthesis of 1,25(OH)$_2$D], reduced renal calcium clearance, and increased bone calcium release. Bone turnover increases in all patients, with resorption exceeding formation in many. Individual patients respond to the excess hormone variably at intestinal, renal, and bone target sites; the factors influencing the variable response from patient to patient are not known.

Hypophosphatemia results from the actions of the excessive parathyroid hormone on renal tubular phosphate reabsorption. Hypophosphatemia in turn aggravates the hypercalcemia in part by increasing the synthesis of 1,25(OH)$_2$D and by increasing the sensitivity of the bone to PTH action. The hypophosphatemia may also interfere with the normal mineralization of bone leading to a mixed picture of both increased resorption and deficient mineralization in adjacent skeletal sites.

Hypoparathyroidism causes hypocalcemia and hyperphosphatemia, a reversal of the response seen with hormone excess.

CALCITONIN (See also Chap. 325) Calcitonin is the potent hypocalcemic peptide hormone that, in many ways, acts as the physiologic antagonist to parathyroid hormone. Calcitonin reduces bone resorption and has opposing effects to parathyroid hormone on the kidney in that it increases renal calcium clearance. Calcitonin exerts at least some effects through stimulation of membrane-bound adenylate cyclase in receptor cells in kidney and bone. There is a variable hormonal responsiveness of renal tubular cells to calcitonin, parathyroid hormone, and vasopressin. In some portions of the nephron, there are cells that respond to all three hormones, whereas in other areas of the tubules the response is restricted to one or two of the hormones. In bone, osteoclasts possess calcitonin receptors, in contrast to the absence of receptors for PTH on osteoclasts. Indeed, direct effects of calcitonin on osteoclast morphology can be shown in vitro.

The thyroid gland is the major source of the hormone in mammalian species, and the cells involved in calcitonin synthesis arise from neural crest tissue. During embryogenesis these cells migrate into the ultimobranchial body. The latter body or gland arises from the last branchial pouch, hence the name *ultimobranchial body*. In submammalian vertebrates the ultimobranchial body remains as a discrete organ, anatomically separate from the thyroid gland. In mammals the ultimobranchial gland fuses with and is incorporated into the thyroid gland. Calcitonin is found in all vertebrate classes.

The naturally occurring calcitonins consist of a peptide chain of 32 amino acids. There is a considerable amount of variability in sequence among species. The entire chain of 32 amino acids appears to be required for biologic activity in the whole animal, although fragments function in in vitro systems. Calcitonin from salmon is 25 to 100 times more potent by weight in lowering serum calcium in animals than are mammalian forms of calcitonin; eel calcitonin is also highly potent. For example, the salmon hormone is at least 10 times more potent in humans than human calcitonin. Slow turnover may explain in part the greater biologic potency of salmon calcitonin, but the hormone binds more strongly to receptor sites as well. Calcitonin is synthesized as a precursor molecule, the parent molecule being four times larger than calcitonin itself. Analysis of the sequence of the coding portions of the gene for rat calcitonin indicates that at least two peptides flank calcitonin from which they are separated by basic residues. It is likely (in analogy with the common precursor for ACTH and endorphin) that these peptides are released along with calcitonin. Despite suggestions that one of the derivative peptides might have hypocalcemic action, there is, at present, no known biologic role for these noncalcitonin peptides.

There are two calcitonin genes, α and β, located on chromosome 11 in the general region of the beta globin and parathyroid hormone genes. The transcription of the calcitonin gene is complex. Two different messenger RNA molecules are transcribed from the α gene; one is translated into the precursor for calcitonin, and the other message is transcribed into an alternate product, calcitonin-gene-related peptide (CGRP). The two genes are sometimes called calcitonin/CGRP-1 and /CGRP-2 genes. CGRP is synthesized wherever the calcitonin message is expressed, for example, in medullary carcinoma of the thyroid. The β, or CGRP-2, gene is transcribed into the messenger RNA for CGRP in the central nervous system in animals; this gene is silent for calcitonin production. CGRP has cardiovascular actions and may serve a neurotransmitter or developmental role in CNS.

The secretion of calcitonin is under the direct control of blood calcium: an increase in calcium causes an increase and a decrease in calcium causes a decrease in calcitonin levels. Once secreted, calcitonin disappears rapidly from the circulation with a half-life of 2 to 15 min.

The concentration of calcitonin in the peripheral blood of normal humans is lower than in many other species. Basal and stimulated immunoreactive calcitonin levels are lower in women than in men and tend to decrease with age to a greater extent in women.

The physiologic role of calcitonin is incompletely understood. In animals calcitonin acts to lower both blood calcium and blood phosphate; the principal action is inhibition of bone resorption. The importance of calcitonin in increasing urinary calcium and phosphate clearance is synergistic with its effects on bone resorption. The actions of calcitonin on kidney and bone are in turn modulated by the regulation of calcitonin production by serum calcium. The view that calcitonin serves to protect against hypercalcemia is thus explained by the hypocalcemic effects of calcitonin triggered in response to hypercalcemia.

The role of calcitonin, if any, however, in normal adult humans is unknown. Changes in calcium and phosphate metabolism are not seen in humans despite extremes of variation in hormone production; there are no definite effects attributable to calcitonin deficiency (totally thyroidectomized patients receiving only replacement thyroxine) or excess (patients with the calcitonin-secreting tumor, medullary carcinoma of the thyroid). Patients with the latter disorder suffer multiple deleterious consequences of their malignancy (see Chap. 325), but no abnormalities in calcium or bone metabolism are recognized, perhaps because they become refractory to the skeletal effects of calcitonin.

Medical interest in calcitonin, therefore, at present is centered principally upon its use as a therapeutic agent and its usefulness, when deployed in radioimmunoassays, for detection of medullary carcinoma (Chap. 325). The use of calcitonin in the treatment of Paget's disease of bone is established (Chap. 344).

REFERENCES

Calcium, phosphorous, and bone metabolism

AVIOLI LV, KRANE SM (eds): *Metabolic Bone Disease and Clinically Related Disorders.* Philadelphia, Saunders, 1990

AZRIA M: The value of biomarkers in detecting alterations in bone metabolism. Calcif Tissue Int 45:7, 1989

BRINGHURST FR: Calcium and phosphate distribution, turnover, and metabolic actions, in *Endocrinology*, 2d ed, LJ DeGroot et al (eds). Philadelphia, Saunders, 1989, p 805

CANALIS E et al: Growth factors and the skeletal system. J Endocrinol Invest 12:577, 1989

COHN DV et al (eds): *Calcium Regulation and Bone Metabolism. Basic and Clinical Aspects.* Amsterdam, Excerpta-Medica, 1987

EPSTEIN S: Serum and urinary markers of bone remodeling: Assessment of bone turnover. Endocrine Rev 9:437, 1988

ERICKSEN EF: Normal and pathological remodeling of human trabecular bone: Three dimensional reconstruction of the remodeling sequence in normals and in metabolic bone disease. Endocrine Rev 7:379, 1986

EVERED D, HARNETT S (eds): *Cell and Molecular Biology of Vertebrate Hard Tissues.* Chichester, Wiley, 1988

GRAVELYN TR et al: Hypophosphatemia-associated respiratory muscle weakness in a general inpatient population. Am J Med 84:870, 1988

KANDERS B et al: Interaction of calcium nutrition and physical activity on bone mass in young women. J Bone Min Res 3:145, 1988

KLEEREKOPER M, KRANE SM (eds): *Clinical Disorders of Bone and Mineral Metabolism.* New York, Mary Ann Liebert, 1989

KRANE SM, SCHILLER AL: Metabolic bone disease. Introduction and Classification, in *Endocrinology*, 2d ed, LJ DeGroot et al (eds). Philadelphia, Saunders, 1989, vol 2, p 1151

LYLES KW et al: Correlations of serum concentrations of 1,25-dihydroxyvitamin D, phosphorus, and parathyroid hormone in tumoral calcinosis. J Clin Endocrinol Metab 67:88, 1988

MUNDY GR: Identifying mechanisms for increasing bone mass. J Natl Inst Health Res 1:65, 1989

O'GARA A: Peptide regulatory factors. Interleukins and the immune system 1. Lancet 1:943, 1989

PARFITT AM: The coupling of bone formation: A critical analysis of the concept and of its relevance to the pathogenesis of osteoporosis. Metab Bone Dis Relat Res 4:1, 1982

———: The cellular basis of bone remodeling: The quantum concept reexamined in light of recent advances in the cell biology of bone. Calcif Tissue Int 36:S37, 1984

PORTALE AA et al: Physiologic regulation of the serum concentration of 1,25-dihydroxyvitamin D by phosphorus in normal men. J Clin Invest 83:1494, 1989

POUILLES JM et al: Sensitivity of dual-photon absorptiometry in spinal osteoporosis. Calcif Tissue Int 43:329, 1988

RAISZ LG, KREAM BE: Regulation of bone formation. N Engl J Med 309:29, 1983

RECKER RR et al: Static and tetracycline-based bone histomorphometric data from 34 normal postmenopausal females. J Bone Min Res 3:133, 1988

RISTELI L et al: Radioimmunoassays for monitoring connective tissue metabolism. Rheumatology 10:216, 1986

TRACEY KJ et al: Peptide regulatory factors. Cachectin/tumour necrosis factor. Lancet 1:1122, 1989

URIST MR et al: Bone cell differentiation and growth factors. Science 220:680, 1983

Vitamin D

HOLICK MF: Vitamin D: Biosynthesis, metabolism, and mode of action, in *Endocrinology*, 2d ed, LJ DeGroot et al (eds). Philadelphia, Saunders, 1989, vol 2, chap 56

———: 1,25-Dihydroxyvitamin D_3 and the skin: A unique application for the treatment of psoriasis. Proc Soc Exper Biol Med 191:246, 1989

——— et al: Age, vitamin D, and solar ultraviolet. Lancet 2:1104, 1989

REICHEL H et al: The role of the vitamin D endocrine system in health and disease. N Engl J Med 320:981, 1989

WEBB AR et al: Influence of season and latitude on the cutaneous synthesis of vitamin D_3: Exposure to winter sunlight in Boston and Edmonton will not promote vitamin D_3 synthesis in human skin. J Clin Endocrinol Metab 67:373, 1988

Parathyroid hormone and calcitonin

ARNOLD A et al: Molecular cloning and chromosomal mapping of DNA rearranged with the parathyroid hormone gene in a parathyroid adenoma. J Clin Inv 83:2034, 1989

FRIEDMAN E et al: Clonality of parathyroid tumors in familial multiple endocrine neoplasia type 1. N Engl J Med 321:213, 1989

HOCK JM et al: Comparison of the anabolic effects of synthetic parathyroid hormone-related protein (PTHrP) 1-34 and PTH 1-34 on bone in rats. Endocrinology 25:2022, 1989

JUPPNER H et al: The parathyroid hormone-like peptide associated with humoral hypercalcemia of malignancy and parathyroid hormone bind to the same receptor on the plasma membrane of ROS 17/2.8 cells. J Biol Chem 263:8557, 1988

KHOSLA S et al: Nucleotide-sequence of cloned cDNAs encoding chicken preproparathyroid hormone. J Bone Min Res 3:689, 1988

MACINTYRE I: Calcitonin: Physiology, biosynthesis, secretion, metabolism, and mode of action, in Endocrinology, 2d ed, LJ DeGroot et al (eds). Philadelphia, Saunders, 1989, vol 2, chap 55

MANGIN M et al: Identification of a cDNA encoding a parathyroid hormone-like peptide from a human tumor associated with humoral hypercalcemia of malignancy. Proc Natl Acad Sci USA 85:597, 1988

NISHI M et al: Human islet amyloid polypeptide gene: Complete nucleotide sequence, chromosomal localization, and evolutionary history. Mol Endocrinol 3:11, 1775, 1989

NISSENSEN RA et al: Parathyroid hormone-like protein from human renal carcinoma cells: Structural and functional homology with parathyroid hormone. J Clin Invest 80:1803, 1987

RODDA CP et al: Regulation of fetal calcium metabolism: Evidence for a novel parathyroid hormone-related protein promoting placental calcium transport. J Bone Min Res 3 (Suppl):S213, 1988

ROSENBLATT M et al: Parathyroid hormone: Physiology, chemistry, biosynthesis, secretion, metabolism, and mode of action, in Endocrinology, 2d ed, LJ DeGroot et al (eds). Philadelphia, Saunders, 1989, vol 2, chap 54

RUSSELL J, SHERWOOD LM: Nucleotide sequence of the DNA complementary to avian (chicken) preproparathyroid hormone mRNA and the deduced sequence of the precursor. Mol Endocrinol 3:325, 1989

SUVA LJ et al: A parathyroid hormone-related protein implicated in malignancy hypercalcemia: Cloning and expression. Science 237:893, 1987

THAKKER RV et al: Association of parathyroid tumors in multiple endocrine neoplasia type 1 with loss of alleles on chromosome 11. N Engl J Med 321:218, 1989

THIEDE MA, RODAN GA: Expression of a calcium mobilizing parathyroid hormone-like peptide in lactating mammary tissue. Science 242:278, 1988

TRIMBLE ER et al: Secretin stimulates cyclic AMP and inositol trisphosphate production in rat pancreatic acinar tissue by two fully independent mechanisms. Proc Natl Acad Sci USA 84:3146, 1987

WAKELAM MJO et al: Activation of two signal-transduction systems in hepatocytes by glucagon. Nature 323:68, 1986

YAMADA H et al: Effects of human PTH-related peptide and human PTH on cyclic AMP production and cytosolic free calcium in an osteoblastic cell clone. Bone Min, 6:45, 1989

340 DISEASES OF THE PARATHYROID GLAND AND OTHER HYPER- AND HYPOCALCEMIC DISORDERS

JOHN T. POTTS, JR.

HYPERCALCEMIA

Hypercalcemia can be a manifestation of a serious illness such as malignancy or can be detected coincidentally by laboratory testing in a patient with no obvious illness. Management is a particular problem when the patient is asymptomatic. The number of patients recognized with asymptomatic hypercalcemia has increased severalfold in the last two decades. Does the hypercalcemia always require further evaluation? What are the most probable causes of hypercalcemia, and how can they be diagnosed? Can asymptomatic patients be followed, or is definitive therapy to eliminate the hypercalcemia the optimal medical management?

Whenever hypercalcemia is confirmed, a definitive diagnosis must be established. Although hyperparathyroidism, a frequent cause of asymptomatic hypercalcemia, is a chronic disorder in which manifestations, if any, may be expressed only over months or years, hypercalcemia can also be the earliest clue to the presence of malignancy, the second most common cause of hypercalcemia in the adult. The causes of hypercalcemia are numerous (Table 340-1), but hyperparathyroidism and cancer account for 90 percent of cases. Diagnosis can usually be established, but management of asymptomatic patients is still unsettled.

Before undertaking an evaluation of hypercalcemia, it is essential to be sure that true hypercalcemia, not a false-positive laboratory test, is present. Hypercalcemia is a chronic problem, and it is cost-effective to obtain several serum calcium measurements; these tests need not be in the fasting state. False-positive calcium tests are usually the result of inadvertent hemoconcentration during blood

TABLE 340-1   Classification of causes of hypercalcemia

Parathyroid-related:
1 Primary hyperparathyroidism
  a Solitary adenomas
  b Multiple endocrine neoplasia
2 Lithium therapy
3 Familial hypocalciuric hypercalcemia

Malignancy-related:
1 Solid tumor with metastases (breast)
2 Solid tumor with humoral mediation of hypercalcemia (lung, kidney)
3 Hematologic malignancies (multiple myeloma, lymphoma, leukemia)

Vitamin D–related:
1 Vitamin D intoxication
2 ↑ 1,25(OH)$_2$D; sarcoidosis and other granulomatous diseases
3 Idiopathic hypercalcemia of infancy

Associated with high bone turnover:
1 Hyperthyroidism
2 Immobilization
3 Thiazides
4 Vitamin A intoxication

Associated with renal failure:
1 Severe secondary hyperparathyrodism
2 Aluminum intoxication
3 Milk-alkali syndrome

collection or elevation in serum proteins, particularly albumin. Measurement of ionized calcium is technically feasible, but there is no advantage, except in research applications, to measurement of ionized rather than total calcium.

Clinical features alone are helpful in differential diagnosis. Hypercalcemia in an adult who is asymptomatic is usually due to primary hyperparathyroidism. In most cases of malignancy-associated hypercalcemia the disease is not occult; rather, symptoms of the underlying malignancy bring the patient to the physician, and hypercalcemia is discovered during the workup. In patients with malignancy the interval between detection of hypercalcemia and death is often less than 6 months. Accordingly, if an asymptomatic individual has had hypercalcemia or some manifestation of hypercalcemia, such as kidney stones, for more than 1 or 2 years, it is unlikely that malignancy is the cause. As discussed below, however, differentiating primary hyperparathyroidism from occult malignancy can occasionally be a problem, and careful evaluation of patients is required, particularly when the duration of the hypercalcemia is unknown.

Hypercalcemia not due to hyperparathyroidism or malignancy can result from excessive vitamin D action, high bone turnover from any of several causes, or from renal failure (Table 340-1). The sensitivity and specificity of various diagnostic tests for the differential diagnosis were previously not optimal, but newer parathyroid hormone (PTH) immunoassays based on double-antibody methods are more reliable. Dietary history and a history of ingestion of vitamins and drugs are often helpful in recognizing some of the less frequent causes. Except in malignancy-associated hypercalcemia, acute management of the hypercalcemia is usually successful prior to the institution of definitive therapy. The type of treatment is based on the severity of the hypercalcemia and the nature of associated symptoms.

Hypercalcemia from any cause can result in fatigue, depression, mental confusion, anorexia, nausea, vomiting, constipation, reversible renal tubular defects, increased urination, alteration in the electrocardiogram (a short QT interval), and, in some patients, cardiac arrhythmias. There is a variable relation between the severity of hypercalcemia and the presence or absence of symptoms from one patient to the next. Generally, symptoms are more common at calcium levels above 2.9 to 3 mmol/L (11.5 to 12.0 mg/dL), but some patients, even at this level, are asymptomatic. When calcium exceeds 3.2 mmol/L (13 mg/dL), renal insufficiency and calcification in kidneys, skin, vessels, lungs, heart, and stomach may occur, particularly if blood phosphate levels are normal or elevated due to impaired renal function. Severe hypercalcemia, usually defined as 3.7 mmol/L (15 mg/dL) or above, is a medical emergency. When serum calcium is 3.7 to 4.5 mmol/L (15 to 18 mg/dL) or higher, coma and cardiac arrest can occur.

PARATHYROID-RELATED HYPERCALCEMIA Primary hyperparathyroidism   NATURAL HISTORY AND INCIDENCE Primary hyperparathyroidism is a generalized disorder of calcium, phosphate, and bone metabolism that results from an increased secretion of parathyroid hormone. The excessive concentration of circulating hormone usually leads to hypercalcemia and hypophosphatemia. There is great variation in the clinical presentation. Patients may present with multiple signs and symptoms, including recurrent nephrolithiasis, peptic ulcers, mental changes, and, less frequently, extensive bone resorption. However, with greater awareness of the disease and wider use of multiphasic screening tests, including blood calcium determinations, the diagnosis is frequently made in patients who have no symptoms and minimal, if any, signs of the disease other than hypercalcemia and elevated levels of parathyroid hormone. If the frequency of diagnosis in referral centers reflects the incidence of the disease, hyperparathyroidism is more common than previously appreciated. In fact, the incidence of primary hyperparathyroidism may approximate *1 case per 1000 per year* in men over the age of 60 and *2 per 1000* in women 60 years of age or older. This incidence is greater than earlier estimates of *1 case per 10,000 persons per year* which were based on evaluation of patients with symptoms such as calcium-containing kidney stones. The clinical manifestations may be subtle, and the disease may have a benign course for many years or a full lifetime. Rarely, the disease seems to appear abruptly, and patients may exhibit severe complications, such as marked dehydration and coma, so-called hypercalcemic parathyroid crisis. The disease is most common in adults, with peak incidence between the third and fifth decades, but it occurs in young children and in the elderly.

ETIOLOGY AND PATHOLOGY   *Solitary adenomas*   The cause of hyperparathyroidism is one or more hyperfunctioning glands. The traditional view has been that a single abnormal gland is the cause in approximately 80 percent of patients; the abnormal gland is usually a benign neoplasm or adenoma and rarely a malignant tumor or parathyroid carcinoma. In a second group, approximately 15 percent, all glands are hyperfunctioning; this is termed *chief cell parathyroid hyperplasia*. The remaining few percent seem to have more than one abnormal gland but not necessarily all glands involved as in hyperplasia; this disorder is labeled *double or multiple adenoma*. There is considerable disagreement about this etiologic classification, particularly about the frequency of disorders involving single, several, and all-abnormal glands. This uncertainty has led to an associated disagreement about surgical management, in particular about how much tissue to remove to cure the disease and restore the euparathyroid state (discussed below).

Benign neoplasms are thought to be monoclonal, that is, one originally abnormal cell, losing growth control but not function, multiplies into an abnormal gland mass, or adenoma. In women, studies using X-linked markers that undergo random inactivation permit direct tests of monoclonality versus polyclonality of excised parathyroid tumors and indicate that adenomas are monoclonal; in turn a single abnormal gland is predicted in such patients. The tests have only been utilized in a few patients, however. In some series there are abnormalities in more than one but not all glands (*double adenoma*) in as many as 40 percent of patients or more. The functional significance of the enlarged glands is unknown—perhaps only one gland is truly hyperfunctioning. Tests of monoclonality versus polyclonality of the abnormal glands in this disorder have not been performed. The majority of evidence still favors a single, benign, monoclonal parathyroid adenoma as the cause of hyperparathyroidism in most patients because removal of a single gland usually restores the eucalcemic state.

Adenomas are most often located in the inferior parathyroid gland but are found in unusual locations in 6 to 10 percent of patients; such parathyroid adenomas may be located in the thymus, the thyroid, the pericardium, or behind the esophagus. Adenomas are usually 0.5 to 5 g in size but may be as large as 10 to 20 g (normal glands are 25 mg in weight on average). Chief cells are predominant in both hyperplasia and adenoma. The adenoma is sometimes encapsulated by a rim of normal tissue. Chief cell hyperplasia is especially common in familial cases of hyperparathyroidism and those that are part of the multiple endocrine neoplasia syndromes (see Chap. 325). With hyperplasia the enlargement may be so asymmetric that some involved glands appear grossly normal. In this case, histologic examination reveals a uniform pattern of chief cells and disappearance of fat even in the absence of an increase in gland weight. Thus, microscopic examination of biopsy specimens of several glands is essential to interpret findings at surgery. When an adenoma is present, the other glands are normal and contain a normal distribution of all cell types (rather than only chief cells) and normal amounts of fat.

Parathyroid carcinoma is usually not aggressive in character. Long-term survival without recurrence is common if at initial operation the entire gland is removed without rupture of the capsule. Even recurrent parathyroid carcinoma is usually slow-growing with local spread in the neck, and surgical correction of recurrent disease may be feasible. Occasionally, parathyroid carcinoma is more aggressive in character, with distant metastases (lung, liver, and bone) found at the time of initial operation. It may be difficult to appreciate initially that a primary tumor is carcinoma; increased numbers of mitotic figures and increased fibrosis of the gland stroma may precede invasive features. The diagnosis of carcinoma is often made in retrospect. Hyperparathyroidism from a parathyroid carcinoma may be clinically indistinguishable from other forms of primary hyperparathyroidism; a potential clue to the diagnosis, however, is provided by the degree of calcium elevation. Calcium values of 3.5 to 3.7 mmol/L (14 to 15 mg/dL) are frequent with carcinoma; this finding may alert the surgeon to remove the abnormal gland with care to avoid capsular rupture.

Multiple endocrine neoplasia   Hyperparathyroidism may occur in a familial pattern without other endocrinologic abnormality. More often, however, hereditary hyperparathyroidism is part of a multiglandular endocrinopathy (see Chap. 325). There are several distinct syndromes of multiple endocrine neoplasia (MEN). The type I disorder (MEN I, Wermer's syndrome) consists of hyperparathyroidism and tumors of the pituitary and pancreatic islet cells, often associated with peptic ulcer and gastric hypersecretion (the Zollinger-Ellison syndrome). A mitogenic factor for parathyroid tissue is present in the sera of patients with MEN I. Another distinct constellation of endocrinologic abnormalities consists of hyperparathyroidism associated with pheochromocytoma and medullary carcinoma of the thyroid (MEN IIa). The pattern of inheritance is autosomal dominant. Tumors of the thyroid and adrenal medulla are not found in patients with MEN I, and pancreatic and pituitary tumors do not occur in patients with MEN IIa. Since the different endocrine tumors can develop at widely separated intervals, hyperparathyroidism and the related endocrine disorders should be carefully and repeatedly searched for in kindreds afflicted with the MEN syndromes.

SIGNS AND SYMPTOMS   Half or more of patients with hyperparathyroidism are asymptomatic. These patients are either followed without therapy or are operated upon, eliminating the disease state. Manifestations of hyperparathyroidism involve primarily the kidneys and the skeletal system. Kidney involvement, due either to deposition of calcium in the renal parenchyma or to recurrent nephrolithiasis, was present in 60 to 70 percent of patients prior to 1970. With the increased frequency of detection of asymptomatic individuals, renal complications are less common.

Renal stones are usually composed of either calcium oxalate or calcium phosphate. Repeated episodes of nephrolithiasis or the formation of large calculi may lead to urinary tract obstruction and infection and may result in loss of renal function. Nephrocalcinosis may also cause decreased renal function and phosphate retention.

The unique bone involvement in hyperparathyroidism is osteitis fibrosa cystica. In the past osteitis fibrosa cystica occurred in 10 to 25 percent of patients with hyperparathyroidism. Histologically the pathognomonic features are a reduction in the number of trabeculae, an increase in the giant multinucleated osteoclasts in scalloped areas on the surface of the bone (Howship's lacunae), and a replacement of the normal cellular and marrow elements by fibrous tissues. Other bone changes include resorption of the phalangeal tufts and a replacement of the usually sharp cortical outline of the bone in the digits by an irregular outline (subperiosteal resorption). Loss of the lamina dura of the teeth is less specific. Tiny, "punched-out" lesions may be present in the skull, producing the so-called salt-and-pepper appearance.

Osteitis fibrosa cystica is now uncommon, even though the disease may be of long standing. The reduced frequency has not been explained. Other manifestations of bone disease, however, are frequent. Histomorphometric analyses of biopsied bone reveal an abnormality in bone turnover in most patients, even in those who do not evidence progressive loss of net bone mass; in such patients, rates of bone formation and bone restoration may be increased but balanced. In some patients, however, who do not have symptomatic bone disease or osteitis fibrosa cystica, rates of formation and resorption are not balanced so that a progressive loss of bone mineral mass causes osteopenia, indicating the need for surgery. There are no pathognomonic criteria to separate unequivocally parathyroid-dependent osteopenia from "high-turnover" osteoporosis as occurs in patients who are not hyperparathyroid.

Improved techniques are now available for monitoring bone mineral density. Computed tomography of the spine provides reproducible quantitative estimates (within a few percent) of spinal bone density. Similar, highly reproducible quantitation is also possible by photon densitometry for measurement of cortical bone density in the extremities, and dual-beam photometry can be used to estimate bone density in the spine or to measure total-body calcium. Serial measurements with these techniques can provide an early indication of whether or not progressive osteopenia is present. In some patients surgery is recommended because of progressive loss of bone, with the presumption that the progressive osteopenia is parathyroid hormone–dependent and hence treatable by correction of the hyperparathyroidism. Some patients have been followed for years, on the other hand, without evidence of loss of bone mass. Hence, bone disease with primary hyperparathyroidism can be quite variable.

Dysfunctions of the central nervous system, peripheral nerve and muscle, the gastrointestinal tract, and the joints also occur. An awareness of the signs and symptoms that may be seen in hyperparathyroidism may give the initial clue in the diagnosis. In some instances severe neuropsychiatric manifestations reverse after parathyroidectomy; in these patients there appears to be a cause and effect relationship. Generally, however, the fact that hyperparathyroidism is common in elderly patients, in whom there are often other problems, makes cause and effect of such problems as hypertension, renal deterioration, and depression uncertain and suggests caution in recommending surgery as a cure for hyperparathyroid patients. It is not apparent why some patients with hyperparathyroidism have no symptoms, while others with an equal degree of biochemical abnormality develop symptomatic disease.

Neuromuscular manifestations include proximal muscle weakness, easy fatigability, and atrophy of muscles. The clinical signs in these patients may be so striking as to suggest a primary neuromuscular disorder. The distinguishing feature is the complete regression of neuromuscular disease after surgical correction of the hyperparathyroidism.

Gastrointestinal manifestations of hyperparathyroidism are sometimes subtle and include vague abdominal complaints and disorders of the stomach and pancreas. Again, cause and effect are unclear, except in certain situations such as the multiple endocrine syndromes. In MEN I patients with hyperparathyroidism, duodenal ulcer is a result of the associated pancreatic tumors that secrete excessive quantities of gastrin (the Zollinger-Ellison syndrome). Pancreatitis has been reported in association with hyperparathyroidism, but the incidence and the mechanism are not established.

Chondrocalcinosis and pseudogout are said to be sufficiently frequent in hyperparathyroidism that screening of such patients is warranted. Occasionally, pseudogout is the initial manifestation.

DIAGNOSIS The diagnosis is made primarily on clinical grounds. ... immunoassay for PTH is of particular value as a diagnostic test.

Since hypercalcemia can be the presenting evidence for malignancy or other serious disease, a thorough evaluation of possible etiologies, including hyperparathyroidism, is indicated even in asymptomatic subjects. If the diagnosis of hyperparathyroidism is suspected after such an evaluation, a decision may be made to follow the patient for a time rather than to recommend surgery.

Hypercalcemia is the most common manifestation—either sustained or intermittent hypercalcemia. Careful consideration must be given to the justification for surgical exploration in the absence of hypercalcemia. So-called normocalcemic hyperparathyroidism, that is, surgically proven hyperparathyroidism accompanied by a normal calcium level but elevated values of immunoreactive PTH (iPTH), is rare in the absence of renal failure or gastrointestinal disease. If such patients have coexisting conditions that interfere with the calcium-elevating actions of PTH, such as chronic renal failure, severe malabsorption, or vitamin D deficiency, then the lack of calcium elevation need not argue against the presence of true hyperparathyroidism. Confusing situations can arise, however, in patients with recurrent kidney stones who are suspected of having hyperparathyroidism because of elevated iPTH levels but who have normal serum calcium. These patients may have true normocalcemic hyperparathyroidism. In situations in which the symptoms call for an early definitive diagnosis, it may be useful to search for postabsorptive hypercalcemia (detectable in certain patients when fasting hypercalcemia is absent) or to use a provocative test with benzothiadiazides (see below).

Hypercalciuria is common in hyperparathyroidism. However, PTH actually reduces calcium clearance, and the daily excretion of calcium in urine is lower than in patients with equivalent degrees of hypercalcemia from nonparathyroid causes.

Serum phosphate is usually low but may be normal, especially if renal failure has developed. Hypophosphatemia is a less useful diagnostic finding than hypercalcemia for two reasons. One, phosphate levels are influenced by dietary intake, diurnal variations, and other factors; to be useful, samples must be obtained in the morning under fasting conditions. Two, patients with severe hypercalcemia of all causes may have a low serum phosphate.

Many tests based on renal responses to excess parathyroid hormone (renal calcium and phosphate clearance; blood phosphate, chloride, magnesium; urinary or nephrogenous cyclic AMP) have been proposed and used in the past. These tests have low specificity for hyperparathyroidism and are not cost-effective; the improvement in the PTH immunoassay, long awaited, provide the more promising approach (as discussed below under differential diagnosis) in specificity and economy.

TREATMENT *Medical treatment* The medical treatment of hyperparathyroidism involves two separate issues. If hypercalcemia is severe and symptomatic, then the calcium must be lowered (the measures are described below. Hypercalcemia is not symptomatic in most patients with hyperparathyroidism, and it is usually not difficult to control the hypercalcemia. Simple hydration will often suffice to lower the calcium concentration to values below 2.9 mmol/L (11.5 mg/dL). There have been discussions in the past about whether chronic management of the hypercalcemia of hyperparathyroidism should be undertaken with oral phosphate therapy. Although the calcium concentration is lowered by phosphate in most patients, this is accompanied by an increase in iPTH levels in blood; it is unclear whether the increased PTH levels would cause more or less organ deterioration. There have been no systemic trials to evaluate effects of specific medical therapy for hypercalcemia.

Rather, the usual issue is to decide whether surgical intervention is required in a particular patient. If not, medical management consists of following the patient without specific therapy but monitoring bone and renal function periodically to ensure that silent osseous and renal deterioration does not occur. In postmenopausal women with hyperparathyroidism who are either unwilling or unable to undergo parathyroid surgery, estrogen therapy may retard demineralization of the skeleton and, in some, reduce blood and urinary calcium levels. If undesirable signs or symptoms occur, surgical intervention can then be recommended.

The natural history of the disease has been studied in several centers. Several hundred patients have been followed in attempts to afford a rational explanation for the benefits of surgery or the risks of medical observation. Large-scale randomized prospective clinical trials have not been undertaken, however. Rather, the long-term effects of hyperparathyroidism have been assessed in patients who do not have kidney stones, osteitis fibrosa cystica, or other clear-cut symptoms. Of principle concern is the possibility of progressive loss of bone density, a worrying problem in women who face the problem of age-dependent and estrogen-deficient bone loss in the absence of hyperparathyroidism. The concern is that such patients, even though asymptomatic, will suffer a degree of bone loss due to PTH excess that will leave them more vulnerable later in life to developing symptomatic osteoporosis. No generalization can be made in this regard other than that some patients, followed by noninvasive techniques for measuring bone density, show no evidence of substantial bone loss, while others show progressive bone loss. The reproducibility of the available noninvasive techniques for assessing bone density is 1 to 2 percent, and if progressive bone loss becomes significant, for example, in premenopausal women, surgery should be recommended to prevent further bone loss. Such decisions are more arbitrary in the elderly, in whom loss of bone may not be due to the hyperparathyroidism and bone loss may not cease once the patient is rendered euparathyroid. It is not that one can guarantee that parathyroidectomy will arrest progressive bone loss but rather that one cannot afford, except in a very elderly patient, to run the risk that persistent hyperparathyroidism may accelerate skeletal disease.

There are no indexes that help in predicting whether bone loss will be progressive or skeletal mass will remain stable. Hence, if patients wish to avoid surgery, bone mass must be monitored at intervals of 6 months to 1 year, then less frequently if bone mass is stable. Loss of renal function, on the other hand, occurs only rarely in the absence of kidney stones or infection.

No uniform recommendation can be made regarding medical (nonsurgical) management of patients with hyperparathyroidism. Decisions must be made in the light of the age of the patient and social and psychological factors. Most physicians believe it is appropriate to operate on young persons to avoid lifelong monitoring by time-consuming and expensive studies, particularly since surgical treatment is usually successful and does not carry a significant risk of mortality or morbidity. In patients over the age of 50, conservative evaluation without surgery is reasonable if the patient prefers and if progressive bone loss is not seen. The operation can be recommended for any patient in whom progressive bone loss is documented or in whom other symptoms of the disease appear, or for whom the stress of long-term follow-up is greater than the desire for surgical "cure." Estrogen therapy is appropriate for the management of postmenopausal women with hyperparathyroidism who are poor candidates for surgery; such therapy may not only protect the skeleton but also may reduce blood and urinary calcium levels.

Surgical treatment Parathyroid exploration is best undertaken by an experienced surgeon with the help of an experienced pathologist. Certain clinical features help in predicting the pathology; for example, in familial cases, multiple abnormal glands are likely. However, some critical decisions regarding management can be made only during the operation. The examination by frozen section of tissue removed at surgery helps direct the subsequent course of the operation.

As discussed under etiology there are many unresolved issues to consider in surgery for hyperparathyroidism. At the extreme of conservatism, the surgical approach is based on the view that typically only one gland (the adenoma) is abnormal. If an enlarged gland is found, a normal gland should be sought. If a biopsy of a normal-sized second gland confirms its histologic and therefore presumed

functional normality, no further exploration, biopsy, or excision is needed. At the other extreme is the minority viewpoint that not only should all four glands be sought but also most of the total parathyroid tissue mass should be removed.

The concern with the former approach is that the rate of recurrence of hyperparathyroidism will be unnecessarily high because a second abnormal gland will sometimes be missed; the latter approach could involve unnecessary surgery and an unacceptable rate of hypoparathyroidism.

The majority viewpoint, judged by surgical reviews, is that conservative surgery, i.e., removal of what is usually only one enlarged gland after four-gland exploration, leads to cure in most cases.

Known hyperplasia, as predicted in familial cases, poses more difficult questions of surgical management. Once a diagnosis of hyperplasia is established, it is necessary to identify all the glands. It is usually recommended that three glands be totally removed and the fourth gland be partially excised; care should be taken to leave a good blood supply for the remaining gland. Some surgeons advocate transplantation of a portion of the removed, minced parathyroid tissue into the muscles of the forearm. Cryopreservation is also being explored. When parathyroid carcinoma is encountered, the tissue should be widely excised; care must be taken to avoid rupture of the capsule to prevent local seeding of the tumor.

If no glandular abnormalities are found in the neck, the issue of further exploration must be decided. There are documented cases of five or six parathyroid glands and, therefore, of unusual locations for adenomas. A variety of techniques have been developed to aid in the preoperative localization of the abnormal parathyroid tissue; usually these techniques are used in patients with unsuccessful neck explorations before further surgery is undertaken. The early techniques featured either selective intraarterial angiography or selective venous catheterization of the thyroid venous plexus and adjacent areas coupled with radioimmunoassay for PTH. The techniques were often successful, but the frequency of detection was less than or at least not higher than the rate of success of an experienced parathyroid surgeon in finding the abnormal tissue at the first operation, so the morbidity and expense of the procedures are not warranted. Noninvasive techniques have also been utilized for preoperative localization, including ultrasound, computed tomography of the neck and mediastinum, differential scanning after simultaneous radiothallium and technetium administration, and intraarterial digital angiography.

Ultrasound is reported to detect abnormal parathyroid tissue in 60 to 70 percent of cases and is most useful for lesions in the vicinity of the thyroid and less successful for lesions in the anterior mediastinum. The technique may assist the surgeon even in the initial operation by directing the surgery to the side of the neck where the abnormal gland is located. Computed tomography has a similar success rate and is more helpful with mediastinal glands, although false-positives are noted. The subtraction of the technetium image, which targets the thyroid, from the radiothallium image, which targets both thyroid and parathyroid, has led to successful preoperative localization in approximately half of patients undergoing a second exploration.

Several generalizations seem warranted. Localization and removal of a single abnormal parathyroid gland at the first operation is usually successful, depending upon the experience of the surgeon (greater than 90 percent success for experienced surgeons). Preoperative localization techniques, therefore, which are less than 90 percent successful, should be reserved for patients in whom initial exploration is unsuccessful. When a second parathyroid exploration is indicated, ultrasound, computed tomography, and thallium-technetium scanning should probably be combined with selective digital arteriography in one of the centers specializing in these techniques. At one center, there has been experience with angiographic ablation of mediastinal adenomas with reports of long-term cure using selective embolization or deliberate excessive injection of contrast material into the endarterial circulation feeding the parathyroid tumor.

A decline in serum calcium occurs within 24 h after successful surgery; usually blood calcium falls to low normal values for 3 to 5 days until the remaining parathyroid tissue resumes hormone secretion. It may develop that intraoperative monitoring of parathyroid hormone levels by rapid PTH immunoassays will prove useful in guiding the surgery, as suggested by some studies (see below). Severe postoperative hypocalcemia is likely only if osteitis cystica is present or if injury to all the normal parathyroid glands occurs during surgery.

In general, patients with good renal and gastrointestinal function, who do not have symptomatic bone disease and a large deficit in bone mineral, have few problems with postoperative hypocalcemia. The extent of postoperative hypocalcemia varies with the surgical approach. If all glands are biopsied, hypocalcemia may be more prolonged and may be transiently symptomatic. Symptomatic hypocalcemia is more likely to occur after second parathyroid explorations, when normal parathyroid tissue may have been removed at the unsuccessful initial operation and when the manipulation and/or biopsy of the remaining normal gland has been more extensive in the search for the missing adenoma. Patients with hyperparathyroidism have efficient intestinal calcium absorption due to the increased levels of $1,25(OH)_2D$ stimulated by parathyroid excess. Once hypocalcemia signifies successful surgery, patients can be put on a high calcium intake or be given oral calcium supplements. Despite manifestations of mild hypocalcemia, most patients do not require parenteral therapy and do not experience severe symptoms. If the serum calcium falls below 2 mmol/L (8 mg/dL), *in particular if the phosphate level simultaneously rises,* the possibility of hypoparathyroidism must be considered. Coexistent hypomagnesemia should be checked for, as it interferes with PTH secretion and causes a relative hypoparathyroidism. Parenteral calcium replacement at a low level should be instituted if symptomatic hypocalcemia supervenes. Such symptoms include a general sense of anxiety and positive Chvostek and Trousseau signs coupled with serum calcium consistently below 2 mmol/L (8 mg/dL). For parenteral therapy, calcium (gluconate or chloride) solutions are prepared at a concentration of 1 mg/mL in 5% dextrose in water. The rate and duration of intravenous therapy are determined by the severity of the symptoms and the response of the serum calcium. A rate of infusion of 0.5 to 2 (mg/kg)/h or 30 to 100 mL/h of a 1 mg/mL solution usually suffices to relieve symptoms. Generally, parenteral therapy is required for only a few days. If symptoms become severe or if the need for parenteral calcium continues for more than 2 to 3 days, replacement therapy with vitamin D and/or oral calcium (2 to 4 g/d) should be started (see below). It is cost-effective to use calcitriol (doses of 0.5 to 1.0 μg per 24 h) because of the rapidity of onset and rapidity of cessation of action, in contrast to vitamin D per se (see below). A sudden rise in blood calcium after several months of vitamin D replacement may indicate restoration of parathyroid function to normal. This problem is minimized by use of calcitriol rather than vitamin D. It is also appropriate to monitor serum PTH serially to estimate gland function in such patients.

Magnesium deficiency may also complicate the postoperative course. Magnesium deficiency impairs the secretion of PTH, and, therefore, hypomagnesemia should be corrected whenever detected. Magnesium chloride is effective by mouth, but this compound is not widely available. Accordingly, repletion is usually parenteral. Only a fraction of body magnesium is present in extracellular fluid, but total-body magnesium deficiency is reflected by hypomagnesemia. Since the depressant effect of magnesium on central and peripheral nerve functions does not occur below 2 mmol/L (normal range, 0.8 to 1.2 mmol/L), parenteral replacement can be given rapidly. A cumulative dose as great as 0.5 to 1 mmol/kg body weight can be administered if severe hypomagnesemia is present; often, however, total doses of 12 to 15 mmol are sufficient. The magnesium is given either as an intravenous infusion over 8 to 12 h or in divided doses intramuscularly (magnesium sulfate, USP).

Lithium therapy Lithium, used in the management of bipolar depression and other psychiatric disorders, causes hypercalcemia in approximately 10 percent of patients. The parathyroids are involved in mediation of the hypercalcemia, and PTH levels may be elevated. The hypercalcemia is dependent on continued lithium treatment, remitting and recurring when lithium is stopped and restarted. In a few patients who were explored parathyroid adenomas were found. Histologic findings in the remaining parathyroid glands in these patients have not been described, but the implication is that there is a single abnormal gland.

The presence of hypercalcemia does not correlate with plasma lithium level, but the frequency with which hypercalcemia occurs is sufficiently high to support a causal relationship between lithium and the hypercalcemia, particularly the dependence of the hypercalcemia on the continuation of the lithium. It is presumed that in most cases an adenoma is not present, merely hyperfunctioning glands. Lithium, at the levels achieved in blood in treated patients, can be shown in vitro to shift the curve describing PTH secretion as a function of calcium level to the right, i.e., higher calcium levels are required to lower PTH secretion. It is logical to assume this effect can cause elevated PTH and consequent hypercalcemia in otherwise normal individuals. If careful studies were done, elevated PTH levels might be found in more patients treated with lithium than the 10 percent in whom frank hypercalcemia is detected. The adenomas reported in a few hypercalcemia patients with lithium therapy may reflect the presence of an independently occurring parathyroid tumor; an effect of lithium on parathyroid gland growth need not be implicated (although it is not excluded), since the majority of patients have complete reversal of hypercalcemia when lithium is stopped. Long-term follow-ups have not been reported; many patients are continued on lithium to treat psychiatric problems. These patients are presumably best managed according to the principles used in asymptomatic hypercalcemia independent of lithium administration. If troubling symptoms or unfavorable signs, such as rising blood calcium levels, progressive bone demineralization, or kidney stones, develop, it may be necessary to try alternate psychotropic medication. Since it is unclear how often parathyroid adenomas will be found, it does not seem wise to recommend parathyroid surgery unless the hypercalcemia and elevated PTH persist after lithium is discontinued.

Familial hypocalciuric hypercalcemia Familial hypocalciuric hypercalcemia (familial benign hypercalcemia; FHH) is transmitted as an autosomal dominant trait. Affected individuals are frequently discovered because of asymptomatic hypercalcemia; surgical exploration of the parathyroids is not indicated because parathyroidectomy does not cure the disorder. It is, therefore, important to separate such patients from those with primary hyperparathyroidism.

The pathophysiology is not understood, and there is no single biochemical marker to distinguish these patients from patients with primary hyperparathyroidism. Nonetheless, the aggregate evidence serves to separate FHH clearly from primary hyperparathyroidism. The majority of patients with primary hyperparathyroidism have less than 99 percent renal calcium reabsorption, and most patients with FHH exceed 99 percent reabsorption. The hypercalcemia may be detectable in affected members of the kindreds in the first decade of life, whereas hypercalcemia rarely occurs in primary hyperparathyroidism and the MEN syndromes under the age of 10 years. The iPTH values may be elevated in FHH, but the values are usually normal or lower than in patients with primary hyperparathyroidism. In patients who are inadvertently operated upon, hypercalcemia and hypocalciuria persist without elevated PTH; the hypercalcemia and hypocalciuria, therefore, do not seem PTH-dependent. Serum magnesium levels are, on average, higher in FHH than in primary hyperparathyroidism. The overall evidence favors some as yet uncharacterized non-parathyroid-dependent defect in calcium transport into or out of extracellular fluid.

Few clinical signs of symptoms are present in patients with FHH. Unlike the MEN syndromes, other endocrine abnormalities are not present. Most patients are detected as a result of family screening after the diagnosis has been made in one member of the kindred. All too commonly, the initial patient is operated upon without reversal of the hypercalcemia. At operation, the glands appear normal, or a moderate degree of hyperplasia of all parathyroid glands is seen. No patient has had reversal of hypercalcemia by surgery unless all of the parathyroid tissue has been inadvertently removed, rendering the patient hypoparathyroid, a most undesirable result. The high renal calcium reabsorption and the prompt recurrence of hypercalcemia as long as any parathyroid tissue remains establish that there is some abnormality in the regulation of the ratio of extracellular-to-intracellular calcium concentration or some abnormal mechanisms of calcium sensing in cell membranes in the kidney and/or elsewhere independent of parathyroid hormone excess. The exact nature of this disorder and its natural history are not clear yet, but since the parathyroid glands are permissive rather than responsible for the syndrome, parathyroid surgery is not to be advocated, nor, in view of the lack of symptoms, is medical treatment needed to lower the calcium.

Malignancy-related hypercalcemia CLINICAL SYNDROMES AND MECHANISMS OF HYPERCALCEMIA Hypercalcemia due to malignancy is common (occurring with 10 to 15 percent of certain types of tumor, such as lung carcinoma), often severe and difficult to manage, confusing as to etiology, and sometimes difficult to distinguish from primary hyperparathyroidism. Traditionally, hypercalcemia in malignancy was thought to be due to a local invasion and destruction of bone by tumor cells and, only in a minority of cases, to the elaboration by the malignant cells of humoral mediators of hypercalcemia.

Although the presence of malignancy is often clinically obvious, hypercalcemia can occasionally be due to an occult tumor. With occult malignancy, diagnosis and definitive treatment must be accomplished quickly if the patient is to be protected from the complications of the underlying malignancy.

Humoral hypercalcemia of malignancy occurs in patients with cancers of the lung and kidney in which bone metastases are absent, minimal, or not detectable clinically. The clinical picture resembles primary hyperparathyroidism (hypophosphatemia accompanies hypercalcemia), and elimination or regression of the primary tumor leads to disappearance of the hypercalcemia. Ectopic production of PTH by the tumor was initially felt to be the mechanism of the hypercalcemia, but the disease mechanisms are now appreciated to be due to humoral mechanisms unrelated to ectopic PTH production.

Many patients with the humoral hypercalcemia of malignancy have elevated urinary nephrogenous cyclic AMP excretion, hypophosphatemia, and increased urinary phosphate clearance, findings compatible with the actions of a humoral agent that emulates PTH action. On the other hand, these patients not only have lower iPTH levels generally than patients with hyperparathyroidism but also high, rather than low, renal calcium clearance (relative to serum calcium when compared to true hyperparathyroidism), and low to normal levels of 1,25-dihydroxyvitamin D [$1,25(OH)_2D$], all consistent with mediation by humoral factors distinct from PTH.

The histologic character of the tumor is more important than the extent of skeletal metastases in predicting hypercalcemia. Small cell carcinoma (oat cell) and adenocarcinoma of lung, although the most common lung tumors associated with skeletal metastases, rarely cause hypercalcemia. By contrast, as many as 10 percent of patients with squamous cell carcinoma of the lung develop hypercalcemia. Histologic studies of bone in patients with squamous cell or epidermoid carcinoma of the lung, in sites invaded by tumor as well as areas remote from tumor invasion, reveal bone remodeling, including osteoclastic and osteoblastic activity. In contrast, minimal evidence of skeletal metabolic activation is seen despite extensive skeletal metastases of small cell (oat cell) carcinoma.

The cumulative findings suggest that agents other than PTH must be responsible for hypercalcemia and that only certain tumor types produce these factors. At least two general mechanisms of hypercalcemia are suspected. Most solid tumors associated with hypercalcemia, particularly squamous cell and renal tumors, produce and secrete cellular factors that are believed to cause increased bone resorption and to mediate the hypercalcemia through systemic actions on the skeleton as a whole by stimulation of bone resorption. Substances produced by cells involved in the marrow response to hematologic malignancies or breast carcinoma resorb bone through local destruction and may be identical or analogous to some of the known lymphokines and cytokines.

Classification of the hypercalcemia of malignancy is arbitrary (Table 340-2). Multiple myeloma and other hematologic malignancies involving the bone marrow have been typically classified as one group; bone destruction and hypercalcemia are believed to be caused through local mechanisms of malignant cells spread widely throughout the marrow spaces. Breast carcinoma is typical of solid tumors that cause hypercalcemia through *localized osteolytic destruction*, probably mediated by locally secreted tumor products different from those involved in multiple myeloma or lymphoma. Finally, solid tumors can cause hypercalcemia from secretion of one or more distinctive mediators (Table 340-2).

In addition to the bone-resorbing factors elaborated by malignant cells in patients with hypercalcemia of malignancy, there may be variable synergism and antagonism between various bone-active agents secreted by the tumors. In the humoral hypercalcemia of malignancy, osteoclastic resorption is generalized, and there is an absence of an osteoblastic or bone-forming response to the surge of bone resorption, implying some inhibition of the normal coupling of formation and resorption. Cooperativity and antagonism in the skeletal actions of locally released cytokines may include blockade of cytokine-induced bone resorption by interferon or related cytokines, both the bone-resorbing and bone-resorbing-blocking cytokines being secreted in response to interactions among tumor cells and host inflammatory cells. Thus, the interaction of more than one substance may determine whether hypercalcemia develops with a particular tumor.

Several hormones, hormone analogues, specific cytokines, and/or growth factors have been implicated as the result of clinical assays, in vitro tests, or chemical isolation. In some lymphomas, typically B-cell lymphomas, there is an increased blood level of $1,25(OH)_2D$. It is not clear whether the increased $1,25(OH)_2D$ is produced by stimulation of the renal 1α-hydroxylase or whether the metabolite is produced ectopically by lymphocytes; the latter seems likely, based on studies with the malignant cells. The principal interest in etiologic mechanisms in hematologic malignancies has focused on the production of distinctive bone-resorbing factors by activated normal lymphocytes and by myeloma and lymphoma cells. This factor(s), termed *osteoclast activation factor* (OAF), now appears to represent the biologic action of several different cytokines, probably interleukin 1 and lymphotoxin or tumor necrosis factor, two closely related cytokines.

In most instances, breast carcinoma is believed to cause hypercalcemia by local stimulation of osteoclasts directly by products secreted by the metastatic breast carcinoma cells and associated inflammatory cells. Breast carcinoma cells produce and secrete prostaglandins of the E series, which are potent local stimulators of bone-resorbing cells.

More than one factor may be responsible for humorally mediated hypercalcemia in patients with solid tumors, but, as discussed in the

---

TABLE 340-2 Classification of tumor hypercalcemia

1 Hematologic malignancies
   a Local bone destruction (OAF, interleukin 1, tumor necrosis factor, lymphotoxin)
     Multiple myeloma
     Lymphomas
   b Humoral mediation [$1,25(OH)_2D$, ?PTH-rP]
     Lymphomas

2 Solid tumors
   a Local bone destruction (prostaglandin, E series)
     Breast carcinoma
   b Humoral mediation (PTH-rP, ?other agents)
     Lung (squamous cell)
     Kidney
     Urogenital tract
     Other squamous tumors

preceding chapter, work by several laboratories has resulted in identification of a hitherto unrecognized factor that resembles but is distinct from PTH and fulfills criteria of a humoral agent for the hypercalcemia syndrome. The factor, termed PTH-rP (parathyroid hormone–related protein), competes with PTH for PTH receptor occupancy in binding and receptor labeling assays, stimulates cyclic AMP production in in vitro assays, causes bone resorption in vitro, and induces hypercalcemia in test animals. These data indicate that PTH-rP acts through activation of the PTH receptor(s).

Other lines of investigation point to the possible role of other factors in the genesis of tumor hypercalcemia. Levels of urinary cyclic AMP rise in test animals treated with synthetic PTH-rP, but $1,25(OH)_2D$ levels also rise, which is at variance with the fact that patients with the humoral syndrome have normal or depressed levels of $1,25(OH)_2D$. Tumor-derived growth factors, believed to act as autocrine regulators to maintain the transformation and growth of tumor cells, and cellular growth factors produced by nonmalignant cells are also potent bone-resorbing agents in vitro. Still other factors potentially involved in tumor hypercalcemia are known only by their bone-resorbing properties and lack of stimulation of renal or bone cell cyclic AMP production. Several of these factors stimulate production of prostaglandins of the E_2 type.

Thus, although identification of PTH-rP represents a singular advance, it is not established to what extent the substance constitutes the sole pathophysiologic mechanism in the humoral hypercalcemia of malignancy. Immunoassays or bioassays of sufficient sensitivity and specificity to detect the presence of the PTH-rP in the circulation of hypercalcemic cancer patients or any human subject are needed.

Diagnostic issues and treatment Ordinarily, the diagnosis of hypercalcemia secondary to tumor is not difficult to make because the tumor symptoms are prominent at the time the hypercalcemia is detected. Indeed, the hypercalcemia may be noted incidentally during the workup of a patient with known or suspected malignancy. Patients with malignancy and hypercalcemia may have a coexistent parathyroid adenoma, some reports suggesting an incidence as high as 10 percent. Laboratory testing becomes critical when occult carcinoma is suspected. Levels of iPTH by the newer double-antibody technique are undetectable or extremely low in tumor hypercalcemia, as would be expected with the mediation of the hypercalcemia by a nonparathyroid agent (the hypercalcemia suppressing the normal parathyroid glands). This improvement in the usefulness of the PTH assay is a significant advance in laboratory diagnosis. (Earlier assays gave equivocal results.) An assay that could detect PTH-rP should be helpful; low or undetectable PTH and elevated PTH-rP would serve to focus attention on the presence of an occult malignancy [although reports that PTH-rP is produced in parathyroid adenomas and that there are multiple forms of the protein produced through alternate gene splicing and tissue metabolism (Chap. 339) may mean that the utility of the PTH-rP assay would be limited].

Hypercalcemia in association with truly occult malignancy, however, is rare. Clinical suspicion that malignancy is the cause of the hypercalcemia is heightened when symptoms associated with the paraneoplastic syndromes, such as weight loss, fatigue, muscle weakness, and unexplained skin rash, or symptoms specific for a particular tumor are present. Squamous cell tumors are most frequently associated with hypercalcemia, and the tumors most frequently arise in the lung, kidney, and urogenital tract. X-ray examinations can focus on these areas when clinical evidence is unclear. Bone scans with technetium-labeled diphosphonate are useful for detection of osteolytic metastases; the sensitivity is high, but specificity is low; results must be confirmed by conventional x-rays to be certain that areas of increased uptake are due to osteolytic metastases per se. Bone marrow biopsies are helpful in patients with anemia or abnormal peripheral blood smears.

Treatment of the hypercalcemia of malignancy must be considered in the perspective of the history and presumed course of the individual patient. Control of the tumor is the principal objective, and reduction of tumor mass is usually also the key to satisfactory control of

hypercalcemia. If a patient has severe hypercalcemia yet has an excellent chance for effective tumor therapy, treatment of the hypercalcemia should be vigorous. If hypercalcemia, on the other hand, is an accompaniment of the late stages of a tumor that is resistant to therapy, the treatment of the hypercalcemia should not be vigorous, as hypercalcemia can have a mild sedating effect. Standard therapies for hypercalcemia (discussed below) are applicable to patients with malignancy.

VITAMIN D–RELATED HYPERCALCEMIA Hypercalcemia related to abnormal vitamin D action can be due to *excessive ingestion* of vitamin D or *abnormal metabolism* of the vitamin. Abnormal metabolism of the vitamin is usually acquired in association with some widespread granulomatous disorder, but there is one, rare hereditary form of vitamin D sensitivity in infants associated with other developmental anomalies. As discussed in Chap. 339, vitamin D metabolism is carefully regulated, particularly the activity of the renal 1α-hydroxylase responsible for the production of $1,25(OH)_2D$. Many details of the regulation of 1α-hydroxylase remain unclarified, but the normal feedback suppression by $1,25(OH)_2D$ on the enzyme seems to work less well in infants than in adults and operates poorly, if at all, in ectopic sites, as distinct from the renal tubule; these facts explain the occurrence of hypercalcemia secondary to excessive $1,25(OH)_2D_3$ production in certain infants (Williams' syndrome) and in adults with granulomatous disease (sarcoidosis) or certain lymphomas.

Vitamin D intoxication The chronic ingestion of large doses of vitamin D, usually at least 50 to 100 times the normal physiologic requirement (doses in excess of 50,000 to 100,000 units per day), is required to produce hypercalcemia in normal individuals. In animals, vitamin D intoxication causes increased bone resorption as well as increased intestinal calcium absorption. In humans, excessive vitamin D action leads to an increase in intestinal calcium absorption, but it is not known whether increased bone resorption contributes to the hypercalcemia.

The immediate mechanism for the hypercalcemia is presumed to be an excessive production of $1,25(OH)_2D$ as a consequence of an increase in the substrate for the renal 1α-hydroxylase, namely, $25(OH)D$ production is less tightly regulated than is the production of $1,25(OH)_2D$. Hence, concentrations of $25(OH)D$ average 5 to 10 times above normal in patients on high-dose vitamin D, whether therapeutically, as in hypoparathyroidism, or accidentally, as in vitamin D intoxication. $25(OH)D$ has a definite, if low, biologic activity in intestine and bone. Hence, part of vitamin D intoxication may be attributable to the high levels of $25(OH)D$ itself, as well as supernormal levels of $1,25(OH)_2D$. Because of the infrequency of vitamin D intoxication, there have been few reports of the actual level of $1,25(OH)_2D$ in patients with vitamin D intoxication. Presumably, the presence of normal renal function and parathyroid reserve would lead to higher rates of formation of $1,25(OH)_2D$ than would occur in patients, for example, with impaired renal function or absence of PTH secretion in whom high doses of vitamins may be given to counter calcium deficiency.

The diagnosis is substantiated by documenting concentrations of $25(OH)D$ in excess of the upper limit of normal. Hypercalcemia is usually controlled by restriction of dietary calcium intake and appropriate attention to hydration. These measures, plus discontinuation of vitamin D, usually lead to satisfactory management, but vitamin D stores in fat may be substantial, and vitamin D intoxication may persist for weeks after vitamin D ingestion is terminated. Such patients are sensitive to glucocorticoids, which in doses of 100 mg of hydrocortisone per day, or its equivalent, return calcium levels to normal over several days.

Sarcoidosis and other granulomatous diseases Normal relations between $25(OH)D$ and the product, the active metabolite $1,25(OH)_2D$, are not maintained in patients with sarcoidosis and other granulomatous diseases. There is a positive correlation between $25(OH)D$ levels (reflecting vitamin D intake) and the circulating concentrations of $1,25(OH)_2D$; normally there is no increase in the active metabolite with increasing 25(OH)D levels. In patients with sarcoidosis, the site of synthesis of 1,25(OH)$_2$D is believed to be in macrophages or other cells associated with granulomatous deposits. Hypercalcemia has been reported in an anephric sarcoidosis patient in association with increased 1,25(OH)$_2$D levels. Macrophages obtained from granulomatous tissue form 1,25(OH)$_2$D at an increased rate when 25(OH)D is provided as substrate. Thus, the usual regulation of active metabolite production by calcium or PTH is circumvented in these patients, and hypercalcemia does not lead to a reduction in the blood levels of 1,25(OH)$_2$D in patients with sarcoidosis. PTH-independent production of 1,25(OH)$_2$D is suggested by normal 1,25(OH)$_2$D production in a patient with sarcoidosis and hypoparathyroidism. Clearance of 1,25(OH)$_2$D from blood may be decreased in sarcoidosis as well.

Even normocalcemic patients with sarcoidosis have unregulated production of 1,25(OH)$_2$D in response to vitamin D loading. Exposure to sunlight or administration of as little as 9000 units of vitamin D daily is followed by increased levels of the active metabolite. Treatment with moderate doses of steroids leads to a reversal of the hypercalcemia, as in other cases of excessive vitamin D action such as vitamin D intoxication, and reversal of the abnormal reponsiveness of 1,25(OH)$_2$D levels to vitamin D challenge. Presumably, steroid administration causes multiple effects in the disease, and both excessive production of the metabolite and the responsiveness to it in target organs are blocked.

Variation in reported frequency of hypercalcemia in sarcoidosis (10 percent or less in recent reports, 60 percent or more in older reports) is probably explained in part by the moderating influence of steroids used to control pulmonary complications and other manifestations of the granulomatous disease. Lytic lesions also occur in bone so that increased bone resorption could play a role in some cases. In most, however, hypercalcemia is directly related to an increased intestinal calcium absorption. Clinically, hypercalcemia is usually a manifestation of disseminated disease. Hence, pulmonary involvement is usual; chest x-ray may reveal a diffuse fibronodular infiltrate and/or prominent hilar adenopathy. Blood gamma globulin may also be elevated. The most useful diagnostic procedure is demonstration of noncaseating granulomas in liver or lymph node biopsy. The hypercalcemia of sarcoidosis can present a difficult problem in differential diagnosis, especially when many of the typical features of the disease are lacking (see Chap. 277).

Management of the hypercalcemia in these patients can be accomplished by avoiding excessive sunlight exposure and by limiting vitamin D and calcium intake; glucocorticoids in the equivalent of 100 mg hydrocortisone per day or less are sufficient to control hypercalcemia when it occurs. Presumably, however, the abnormal sensitivity to vitamin D and abnormal regulation of 1,25(OH)$_2$D synthesis will persist as long as the disease is active. PTH levels are usually suppressed and 1,25(OH)$_2$D levels are elevated, but primary hyperparathyroidism and sarcoidosis may occur in some patients.

Idiopathic hypercalcemia of infancy This unusual disorder, sometimes referred to as Williams' syndrome, consists of multiple congenital development defects, including supravalvular aortic stenosis, mental retardation, and an elfin facies, in association with hypercalcemia due to abnormal sensitivity to vitamin D. The syndrome was first recognized in England after the introduction of vitamin D fortification of milk. Hypercalcemia develops with vitamin D intakes as small as 2000 to 4000 units per day. Levels of 1,25(OH)$_2$D are elevated, ranging from 46 to 120 nmol/L (150 to 500 pg/mL). The mechanism of the abnormal sensitivity to vitamin D and of the increased circulating levels of 1,25(OH)$_2$D is unclear. The children become hypercalcemic because of excessive intestinal calcium absorption. The abnormality in vitamin D metabolism and the increased sensitivity to vitamin D intake are not seen after the first year of life. Treatment is restriction of calcium intake. Occasionally, the hypercalcemia can be severe, and calcium values above 4 mmol/L (16 mg/dL) are recorded. Treatment with glucocorticoids in the doses used

for vitamin D intoxication or sarcoidosis, adjusted for body weight, rapidly reverses the hypercalcemia.

HYPERCALCEMIA ASSOCIATED WITH HIGH BONE TURNOVER

Hyperthyroidism Mild elevation of serum calcium is common in patients with hyperthyroidism, and hypercalciuria is even more common. As many as 20 percent of patients show high normal or mildly elevated serum calcium concentrations. The hypercalcemia seems due to increased bone turnover with bone resorption exceeding bone formation; direct effects of thyroid hormone on the skeleton seems to be responsible. Severe calcium elevations are not typical, however, and the presence of such suggests a concomitant disease such as hyperparathyroidism. Indeed, patients with thyrotoxicosis are more sensitive to the hypercalcemic effects of PTH. Usually, the hyperthyroidism is obvious, and the hypercalcemia is managed by specific therapy of the hyperthyroidism. Signs of hyperthyroidism may occasionally be occult, particularly in the elderly.

Immobilization Immobilization in adults is rarely associated with hypercalcemia in the absence of an associated disease, but may cause hypercalcemia in children and adolescents, particularly after spinal cord injury and paraplegia or quadriplegia. With resumption of some ambulation, the hypercalcemia in children usually returns to normal spontaneously.

The mechanism appears to involve a disproportion between rates of bone formation and bone resorption that results from the sudden loss of weight bearing. Hypercalciuria and increased mobilization of skeletal calcium can be seen in normal volunteers subjected to extensive bed rest, although hypercalcemia does not usually occur. An underlying disease associated with high bone turnover, such as Paget's disease, may cause hypercalcemia with immobilization even in older adults.

Thiazides Administration of benzothiadiazines (thiazides) can cause hypercalcemia in patients with high rates of bone turnover, such as patients with hypoparathyroidism treated with high doses of vitamin D. Traditionally, thiazides are associated with aggravation of hypercalcemia in primary hyperparathyroidism and have been used as a provocative test to bring out hypercalcemia that is borderline in patients suspected of having hyperparathyroidism. However, this effect can be seen in other high-bone-turnover states as well. The mechanism of action of the drugs is complex, but the overall result seems to be to impose a challenge to calcium homeostasis by actions on renal calcium excretion, on bone-calcium turnover, and on the efficiency of parathyroid action per se. Thiazide administration in normal individuals causes a transient increase in blood calcium (but usually within the high normal range) which reverts to preexisting levels after a week or more of continued administration. If normal hormonal function and calcium and bone metabolism are present, homeostatic controls are reset to counteract the calcium-elevating effect of the thiazides. In the presence of hyperparathyroidism or increased bone turnover from another cause, homeostatic mechanisms cannot be reset. The abnormal effects of the thiazide on calcium metabolism disappear within days of cessation of the drug.

Many aspects of the action of the thiazides in normal subjects and in patients with hyperparathyroidism remain unclear. The drug clearly augments PTH responsiveness on target cells of bone and renal tubule. Chronic thiazide administration leads to reduction in urinary calcium excretion; the hypocalciuric effect of the drug appears to reflect the enhancement of proximal tubular resorption of sodium and calcium in response to sodium depletion. Some of this renal action reflects augmentation of PTH actions and is clearly more pronounced in subjects with intact parathyroid secretion than, for example, in a group of hypoparathyroid patients whose renal calcium clearance initially was reported to be unresponsive. However, a substantial hypocalciuric effect can be achieved in hypoparathyroid patients on high-dose vitamin D and oral calcium replacement if sodium intake is restricted. This finding is the rationale for the use of thiazides as an adjunct to therapy in hypoparathyroid patients as discussed below.

Vitamin A intoxication Vitamin A intoxication is a rare cause of hypercalcemia. Most vitamin A intoxication results inadvertently

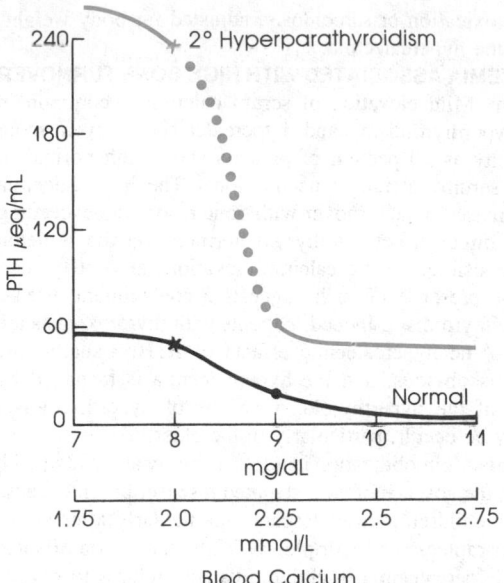

FIGURE 340-1 The relation between blood calcium and iPTH in normal subjects and subjects with secondary (2°) hyperparathyroidism. This model of secondary hyperparathyroidism assumes that there is an increased mass of parathyroid tissue. The lower line represents normal secretory patterns, and the upper line describes the exaggerated secretion (steeper slope) typical of secondary hyperparathyroidism. When calcium level in blood is raised by calcium infusion and multiple measurements of PTH and calcium are made, some portion of hormone secretion in normals is constant despite high calcium levels in blood (nonsuppressible secretion), and this secretion is higher in hyperparathyroidism. An elevation of blood calcium from low normal levels [(2 mmol/L (8 mg/dL)] to high normal levels [(2.2 mmol/L (9 mg/dL)] results in a reduction in PTH in both normal and hyperparathyroid individuals, but true involution of secondary hyperparathyroidism with treatment can be confirmed only by showing a return of the exaggerated response curve to normal.

from experiments with nutritional supplements. Calcium levels can be elevated into the 3 to 3.5 mmol/L (12 to 14 mg/dL) range after the ingestion of 50,000 to 100,000 units of vitamin A daily (10 to 20 times the minimum daily requirement). The patients have typical features of severe hypercalcemia that include fatigue and anorexia. They also have severe muscle pain and sometimes diffuse bone pain. The excess vitamin A intake is presumed to increase bone resorption.

Diagnosis can be established by history and by confirmatory measurements of vitamin A levels in serum, which may be increased severalfold above normal. Occasionally, skeletal x-rays reveal periosteal calcifications, particularly, in the hands. Withdrawal of the vitamin is usually associated with the prompt disappearance of the hypercalcemia and reversal of the skeletal changes. As in vitamin D intoxication, administration of 100 mg hydrocortisone or its equivalent per day leads to a rapid return of the serum calcium to normal.

HYPERCALCEMIA ASSOCIATED WITH RENAL FAILURE Severe secondary hyperparathyroidism Secondary hyperparathyroidism is the state in which excessive production of PTH is due to partial resistance to the metabolic actions of the hormone. Parathyroid gland hyperplasia with resultant increased secretion of PTH occurs because resistance to the normal level of the hormone leads to hypocalcemia which, in turn, is a stimulus to enlargement of the parathyroid glands by mechanisms direct or indirect, still not defined. This concept is based on animal and human studies, the former involving experimental renal failure with phosphatase retention and the latter involving treatment of patients with diphosphonates that block skeletal resorptive response. Figure 340-1 ilustrates the pathophysiology of hormone production in secondary hyperparathyroidism. When the parathyroid secretory reserve is tested by deliberately lowering blood calcium, the extent of rise in PTH for each milligram of decrement of plasma

calcium is greater with parathyroid hyperplasia than with normal glands. There is, therefore, a higher concentration of hormone at any given level of calcium concentration. Since a portion of PTH secretion by each individual parathyroid cell is not suppressible by any degree of elevation of blood calcium concentration, larger glands (more cells) have a higher concentration of hormone output at the hypercalcemic end of the dose-response curve.

Secondary hyperparathyroidism occurs in patients with renal failure, osteomalacia (vitamin D deficiency), and pseudohypoparathyroidism (deficient response to PTH at the level of the receptor). The clinical manifestations of secondary hyperparathyroidism vary in these states. Hypocalcemia seems to be the common denominator in secondary hyperparathyroidism. Primary and secondary hyperparathyroidism can be distinguished by the autonomous nature of the growth of the parathyroid glands in primary hyperparathyroidism (presumably irreversible) and the adaptive increase in parathyroid gland size in secondary hyperparathyroidism (presumably reversible). In fact, reversal from an abnormal pattern of secretion, presumably accompanied by an involution of parathyroid gland mass to a normal pattern of function, may occur in patients treated with diphosphonate after the drug is withdrawn (Fig. 340-1).

In progressive kidney disease, the initial tendency to hypocalcemia seems attributable to two causes: phosphate retention that develops because of the reduced excretion of phosphate and reduced concentrations of 1,25(OH)$_2$D associated with progressive renal damage. The two disturbances reduce skeletal responsiveness to PTH. The deficient 1,25(OH)$_2$D also interferes with the absorption of calcium from the intestine, already impaired in uremia. The ultimate pathophysiologic consequences in any given patient with chronic renal failure represent the outcome of competing physiologic adaptations, stimuli that cause parathyroid gland hyperplasia (tendency toward hypercalcemia and excessive bone resorption) versus those that modify the hormonal responsiveness of the end organs—bone, gut, and residual renal tubules (tendency toward hypocalcemia, hyperphosphatemia, and reduced bone resorption). Typically patients with renal failure exhibit hyperphosphatemia (renal retention and increased bone breakdown) and a low normal or moderately low blood calcium (calcium-lowering action of the phosphate elevation and reduced availability of calcium from bone and gut). In patients with severe secondary hyperparathyroidism, hypercalcemia and hyperphosphatemia both develop due to an increase in bone resorption; parathyroid hypersecretion "overshoots" the degree of resistance to hormone action.

In addition to hypercalcemia and hyperphosphatemia, patients with symptomatic or severe secondary hyperparathyroidism may develop bone pain, ectopic calcification, and pruritus. The bone disease in patients with secondary hyperparathyroidism and renal failure is usually termed *renal osteodystrophy*. Concomitant osteomalacia (vitamin D and calcium deficiency) and osteitis fibrosa cystica (excessive PTH action on bone) may be seen. In fact, osteitis fibrosa cystica is now more common in untreated renal failure than in primary hyperparathyroidism.

Judicious medical therapy, which includes reduction of excessive blood phosphate by dietary phosphate restriction plus the use of nonabsorbable antacids and careful, selective addition of calcitriol (0.25 to 2.0 μg/d), may reverse severe secondary hyperparathyroidism. As illustrated in Fig. 340-1, involution of the parathyroids then occurs; reduction of increased cellular mass causes the exaggerated secretory response to return to normal. The level of PTH at any given level of blood calcium is now more appropriate, and excessive parathyroid action is reversed. Somewhat paradoxically, during successful medical reversal of secondary hyperparathyroidism, elevated serum calcium and phosphate levels return to normal despite the administration of increased amounts of calcium and vitamin D metabolites.

Aluminum intoxication Aluminum intoxication occurs in patients on chronic dialysis; manifestations include acute dementia and unresponsive, severe osteomalacia. Bone pain, multiple nonhealing fractures, particularly of the ribs and pelvis, and a proximal myopathy may occur. Hypercalcemia develops when attempts are made to treat these patients as one treats those with renal osteodystrophy due to renal failure, namely, by administration of vitamin D or calcitriol. Acute hypercalcemia occurs after administration of vitamin D because of impaired skeletal responsiveness. Aluminum is present at the site of osteoid mineralization, and osteoblastic activity is minimal. Presumably, these patients are unable to incorporate the increased blood calcium into the skeleton. Prevention is accomplished by avoidance of aluminum excess in the dialysis regimen; treatment involves mobilizing aluminum through the use of the chelating agent deferoxamine. Aluminum is mobilized from bone and, being tightly bound to the chelating agent, can be removed via dialysis. After aluminum toxicity is reversed, patients may show typical features of renal osteodystrophy and secondary hyperparathyroidism. They can then be managed like other patients with secondary hyperparathyroidism with renal disease. A failure to recognize the syndrome is associated with persistence of the disabling bone disease and a fatal course due to progressive features or to hypercalcemia inadvertently induced by treatment with vitamin D.

Milk-alkali syndrome The milk-alkali syndrome can cause several clinical presentations—acute, subacute, and chronic—all of which feature hypercalcemia, alkalosis, and renal failure. The syndrome is due to an excessive ingestion of calcium and absorbable antacids such as milk or calcium carbonate. The disorder is less frequent since nonabsorbable antacids and H-2 receptor antagonists such as cimetidine and ranitidine became available for the treatment of peptic ulcer disease.

Individual susceptibility must be important in pathogenesis, since many patients are treated with calcium carbonate without developing the syndrome. One variable is the fractional calcium absorption as a function of calcium intake. Some individuals absorb a high fraction of calcium, even with intakes as high as 2 g and more of elemental calcium per day, instead of reducing calcium absorption with high intake, as occurs in most normal subjects. Resultant, mild hypercalcemia after meals in such patients is postulated to be the critical factor in the generation of alkalosis. With the development of hypercalcemia, increased sodium excretion and some depletion of total-body water occurs. This phenomenon and perhaps, additionally, some suppression of endogenous PTH secretion due to mild hypercalcemia would lead to increased bicarbonate resorption. This bicarbonate retention then would lead to alkalosis in the face of continued calcium carbonate ingestion. Alkalosis per se causes selective enhancement of calcium resorption in the distal nephron, thus aggravating the hypercalcemia. The cycle of mild hypercalcemia → bicarbonate retention → alkalosis → renal calcium retention → severe hypercalcemia perpetuates and aggravates hypercalcemia and alkalosis as long as calcium and absorbable alkali are ingested.

Acute hypercalcemia and alkalosis occurring within days of beginning calcium and alkali ingestion, *acute milk-alkali syndrome,* is manifested by weakness, myalgia, irritability, and apathy. The impairment of renal function, including reduced renal concentrating ability and tubular dysfunction as well as hypercalcemia and alkalosis, reverse rapidly upon stopping the intake of calcium and alkali.

The far-advanced milk-alkali syndrome, sometimes referred to as *Burnett's syndrome,* is due to long-standing calcium and alkali ingestion. Severe hypercalcemia, irreversible renal failure, and phosphate retention may be accompanied by ectopic calcification. Some improvement may result when calcium and alkali ingestion is reduced, but prior to the availability of renal dialysis, renal failure led to death. There is an intermediate or subacute form in which the renal failure is reversible over a period of weeks after withdrawal of excessive calcium and alkali intake.

DIFFERENTIAL DIAGNOSIS: SPECIAL TESTS Differential diagnosis of hypercalcemia is best achieved by using clinical criteria, but the radioimmunoassay for PTH, as now modified, is useful in distinguishing among major causes. The clinical points that deserve major emphasis in arriving at a correct diagnosis are the presence or

TABLE 340-3 Differential diagnosis of hypercalcemia: Laboratory criteria

	Blood*			
	Ca	P_i	1,25(OH)$_2$D	iPTH
Primary hyperparathyroidism	↑	↓	↑,↔	↑(↔)
Malignancy-associated hypercalcemia:				
Humorally mediated (HHM)	↑↑	↓	↓,↔	↓ ↔
Local destruction (osteolytic metastases)	↑	↔	↓,↔	↓ ↔

* Symbols in parentheses refer to values rarely seen in the particular disease.
NOTE: P_i = inorganic phosphate; iPTH = immunoreactive parathyroid hormone.

absence of symptoms or signs of disease and evidence of chronicity. If one discounts fatigue or depression, patients with *asymptomatic hypercalcemia* have primary hyperparathyroidism in well over 90 percent of instances; symptoms of malignancy are usually present when hypercalcemia is due to cancer. Disorders other than hyperparathyroidism and malignancy cause no more than 10 percent of hypercalcemia, and some of the nonparathyroid causes are associated with manifestations such as renal failure.

Chronicity is the second most important clinical criterion. If hypercalcemia has been manifest for more than 1 year, malignancy can usually (not always) be excluded as the cause of hypercalcemia. A striking feature of malignancy-associated hypercalcemia is the rapidity of the course, whereby signs and symptoms relatable to the underlying malignancy are evident within months of the first detection of hypercalcemia. Hyperparathyroidism is the likely diagnosis in patients with *chronic hypercalcemia.* Diseases such as sarcoidosis are rare, alternative causes of chronic hypercalcemia. A careful *history* of dietary supplements and drug use will often readily reveal intoxication with vitamin D or A or the use of thiazides.

Although clinical considerations are helpful in arriving at the correct diagnosis of the cause of hypercalcemia, appropriate laboratory testing is essential for definitive diagnosis (Table 340-3). Theoretically, the radioimmunoassay for PTH should separate hyperparathyroidism from all other causes of hypercalcemia, those with hyperparathyroidism having elevated levels of iPTH despite hypercalcemia and patients with malignancy and the other causes of hypercalcemia (except for other disorders mediated by parathyroid hormone such as lithium-induced hypercalcemia) having levels of hormone below normal or undetectable. Assays in use over the last two decades sometimes gave equivocal results, but assays based on the double-antibody method separate hypercalcemic patients with malignancy from those with primary hyperparathyroidism (Fig. 340-2), thus establishing the method as possessing the relevant specificity and sensitivity in the two disorders that account for more than 90 percent of all cases of hypercalcemia. 1,25(OH)$_2$D levels are elevated in many patients (but not all) with primary hyperparathyroidism and are also increased in states of vitamin D intoxication, particularly sarcoidosis. In other disorders associated with hypercalcemia, concentrations of 1,25(OH)$_2$D are low or, at the most, normal. Since not all patients with hyperparathyroidism, however, have elevated 1,25(OH)$_2$D levels and since not all nonparathyroid hypercalcemic patients have suppressed 1,25(OH)$_2$D, the test is of low specificity and not cost-effective in differential diagnosis per se.

PTH levels are elevated in chronic renal failure; the elevation in older assays reflects, in part, accumulation of fragments secondary to renal failure rather than true parathyroid oversecretion. In general with the older type, single-antibody assays, those based on middle or carboxyl-region epitopes, give higher values than those based on amino-terminal recognition sites. The latter assays seemed to correlate better with other evidence of parathyroid overactivity such as osteitis fibrosa. Results with the double-antibody assay are similar to those seen with amino-terminal assays. Patients with sarcoidosis have low or undetectable levels of iPTH. No systematic surveys have been reported concerning double-antibody PTH radioimmunoassay results

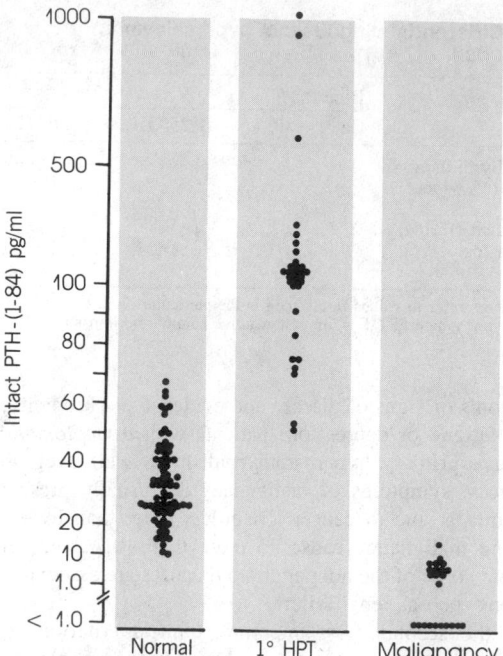

FIGURE 340-2 Levels of iPTH detected in normals, patients with primary hyperparathyroidism (1° HPT), and patients with hypercalcemia of malignancy by the double antibody assay. (*From SR Nussbaum et al: Highly sensitive two-site immunooradiometric assay of parathyrin and its clinical utility in evaluating patients with hypercalcemia. Clin Chem 33:1364, 1987.*)

in many of the other non-parathyroid-related causes of hypercalcemia shown in Table 340-1, largely because of the infrequency with which the disorders are encountered, but it is predicted they will be low or undetectable.

In summary, iPTH values are elevated in greater than 90 percent of parathyroid-related causes of hypercalcemia, undetectable or low in malignancy-related hypercalcemia, and undetectable or normal in vitamin D–related and high-bone-turnover-related causes of hypercalcemia (although there is a paucity of data for these latter categories; the same separation of groups is seen with measurements of 1,25(OH)$_2$D (Table 340-3).

Measurements of nephrogenous cyclic AMP are of limited value in distinguishing the two major causes of hypercalcemia: primary hyperparathyroidism and malignancy. Elevation of nephrogenous cyclic AMP occurs in some patients with malignancy and in essentially all patients with primary hyperparathyroidism. Specific laboratory tests are of utility in confirming the diagnosis of particular disorders (such as thyrotoxicosis); tests specific for tumor factors should be helpful when developed.

Some general recommendations can be made as to the differential diagnosis of hypercalcemia. Two independent causes of hypercalcemia in the same person, although reported, are rare. If a specific disease traditionally associated with hypercalcemia (Table 340-1) is clinically evident, it is reasonable to assume that the disease is responsible for the hypercalcemia. It is cost-effective in view of the specificity and speed of the PTH radioimmunoassay and the high frequency of hyperparathyroidism in hypercalcemic patients to measure the iPTH level in all hypercalcemic patients unless malignancy is clinically evident or a specific diagnosis of a nonparathyroid disease is obvious. If hypercalcemia disappears in response to control of hyperthyroidism, for example, or after reduction of excessive intake of fat-soluble vitamins or alkali and calcium, in the cases of vitamin D intoxication and milk-alkali syndrome, respectively, there is no need to search for a second cause of hypercalcemia. If specific treatment does not lead to a reversal of the hypercalcemia, a search for an additional cause, by detailed laboratory testing, must be undertaken. It also follows that if signs suggestive of malignancy are evident, the management of the patient focuses on management of the malignancy.

When no clues are evident as to the diagnosis, either because the patient is asymptomatic or because chronic illness obscures manifestations that might indicate the presence of malignancy, the following general approach can be used: If the patient is *asymptomatic* and if there is evidence by history of *chronicity* to the hypercalcemia, hyperparathyroidism is almost certainly the cause of the hypercalcemia. If iPTH levels (usually measured at least twice) are elevated, little additional evaluation is necessary. Hyperparathyroidism is never confirmed until abnormal parathyroid tissue is surgically removed and hypercalcemia is corrected, but patients with asymptomatic hypercalcemia who have the presumptive diagnosis on the basis of elevated concentration of iPTH can be followed without intervention but with careful monitoring or can be recommended for surgery with reasonable confidence of cure. If in such patients there is a family history suggestive of other endocrine abnormality, screening for multiple endocrine neoplasia should be undertaken in the patient and family.

If the patient does not have clear-cut symptoms and there is only a short history or no clue as to the duration of the hypercalcemia, *occult malignancy* must be considered with more care than if the hypercalcemia is known to be chronic. If the iPTH levels with the double-antibody technique are increased, the diagnosis of asymptomatic hyperparathyroidism is established.

If patients with a short history of hypercalcemia have clear-cut systemic symptoms and/or the iPTH levels are not elevated, then a thorough workup must be undertaken for malignancy, including chest x-ray, computed tomography of chest and abdomen, and bone scan. Attention should also be paid to clues for underlying hematologic disorders such as anemia, increased plasma globulin, and abnormal serum immunoelectrophoresis; bone scans can be negative in patients with multiple myeloma.

Finally, if a patient with *chronic hypercalcemia* is *asymptomatic* but iPTH values are not elevated and if malignancy seems unlikely on clinical grounds (*chronicity*), it is useful to search for other chronic illnesses that cause hypercalcemia, such as occult sarcoidosis.

MEDICAL TREATMENT OF HYPERCALCEMIA The acute treatment of hypercalcemia is usually successful. The serum calcium concentration can be decreased by 0.7 to 2.2 mmol/L (3 to 9 mg/dL) within 24 to 48 h in most patients, enough to relieve acute symptoms, prevent death from hypercalcemic crisis, and permit diagnostic evaluation. However, the chronic medical management of hypercalcemia is less satisfactory unless the underlying cause can be corrected because available therapies are inconvenient and may be toxic in chronic use.

Hypercalcemia develops because skeletal calcium release is excessive, intestinal calcium absorption is increased, or renal calcium excretion is inadequate. Understanding the particular pathogenesis helps guide therapy. For example, hypercalcemia in patients with osteolytic metastastes or acute immobilization is primarily due to excessive skeletal calcium release and is, therefore, minimally affected by restriction of dietary calcium. On the other hand, patients with vitamin D hypersensitivity or vitamin D intoxication have excessive intestinal calcium absorption, and restriction of dietary calcium is beneficial. Decreased renal function or extracellular fluid depletion decreases urinary calcium excretion. If additional abnormalities, such as increased bone breakdown, are present, hypercalcemia will develop. This may happen, for example, when patients with resorptive bone disease become dehydrated. In such situations, rehydration may rapidly reduce or reverse the hypercalcemia, even though excessive bone resorption and increased urinary calcium excretion continue.

Hydration, increased salt intake, mild and forced diuresis The first principle of treatment is to restore *normal hydration*. Many hypercalcemic patients are dehydrated because of vomiting, inanition, and/or hypercalcemia-induced defects in urinary concentrating ability. The resultant drop in glomerular filtration rate is accompanied by an additional decrease in renal tubular sodium and calcium clearance. Restoring a normal extracellular fluid volume corrects these abnormalities and increases urine calcium excretion by 2.5 to 7.5 mmol/d

(100 to 300 mg/d). Increased urinary sodium excretion to 400 to 500 mmol/d increases urinary calcium excretion even further than simple rehydration. Finally, after full benefits of simple rehydration have been achieved, saline can be administered or conventional doses of furosemide or ethacrynic acid can be given twice daily to depress the tubular reabsorptive mechanism for calcium (care must be taken to prevent the diuretic from provoking dehydration). The combined use of these therapies can increase urinary calcium excretion to 12.5 mmol/d (500 mg/d) or higher in most hypercalcemic patients. Since this is a substantial percentage of the exchangeable calcium pool, the serum calcium concentration usually falls 0.25 to 0.75 mmol/L (1 to 3 mg/dL) within 24 h. Precautions should be taken to prevent potassium and magnesium depletion during chronic therapy; calcium-containing renal calculi are a potential complication.

Under life-threatening circumstances, the above therapy can be pursued more aggressively, giving as much as 6 L isotonic saline (900 mmol sodium) daily plus furosemide or equivalent in doses up to 100 mg every 1 to 2 h or ethacrynic acid in doses to 40 mg every 1 to 2 h. Urinary calcium excretion may exceed 25 mmol/d (1000 mg/d), and the serum calcium may decrease by 1 mmol/L (4 mg/dL) or more within 24 h. Depletion of potassium and magnesium is inevitable unless replacements are given; pulmonary edema can be precipitated. The potential complications can be reduced by careful monitoring of central venous pressure and plasma or urine electrolytes; a bladder catheter may be necessary. The treatment approach should be immediately supplemented with agents to block bone resorption that become effective within a few days, since the forced diuresis therapy is difficult to sustain even in patients with good cardiopulmonary and renal function.

Plicamycin For the acute management of hypercalcemia, plicamycin (mithramycin), which inhibits bone resorption, is a useful therapeutic agent. Plicamycin must be given intravenously, either as a bolus injection or by slow infusion. The usual dose is 25 μg/kg body weight. In some patients, 10 μg/kg body weight can be given twice a week for chronic therapy. Treatment should not be repeated until hypercalcemia recurs, because the toxicity of the drug is dependent on the frequency of treatment and the total dosage. Careful monitoring is needed if repeated doses are used. The major side effects are thrombocytopenia, hepatocellular necrosis with increased lactic acid dehydrogenase (LDH) and aspartate aminotransferase (AST) levels, and decreased levels of clotting factors with resultant epistaxis, bruising, hemorrhage, and bleeding gums. Azotemia, proteinuria, and hypocalcemia may occur. Hypophosphatemia and hypokalemia may also develop, as may nausea, vomiting, stomatitis, and facial swelling. Toxicity is rare when only one or two doses are used and can be minimized by repeating single doses only when hypercalcemia recurs. Toxic effects other than hemorrhage can usually be reversed by stopping the drug.

Diphosphonates After an initial period of uncertainty relating to the divergent pharmacologic actions of this class of drugs (variable effects on bone formation vs. resorption and undesirable cellular effects—pyrexia, leukopenia), certain diphosphonates (bisphosphonates) are emerging as valuable, effective therapies with a favorable therapeutic/toxic ratio. Aminohydroxypropylidene diphosphonate (APD) is undergoing clinical trial. This drug acts primarily by blocking bone resorption without affecting bone formation. Diphosphonates, analogues of pyrophosphate, are "bone seeking" and have a long chemical half-life. The hypocalcemic action of APD lasts for weeks following intravenous administration to patients with hypercalcemia due to increased bone resorption such as in malignancy. If therapeutic actions are confirmed and toxicity remains minor, this drug class may be useful in the management of hypercalcemia; many new bisphosphonates are being evaluated.

Other therapies Glucocorticoids increase urinary calcium excretion and decrease intestinal calcium absorption when given in pharmacologic doses (e.g., 40 to 200 mg prednisone daily in divided doses), but they also cause negative skeletal calcium balance. In normal subjects and in patients with primary hyperparathyroidism,

glucocorticoids neither increase nor decrease the serum calcium concentration. In patients with hypercalcemia due to certain osteolytic malignancies, however, glucocorticoids may be effective as a result of antitumor effects. The malignancies in which hypercalcemia responds to glucocorticoids are usually hematologic malignancies such as multiple myeloma, leukemia, Hodgkin's disease, and other lymphomas; carcinoma of the breast may also respond, at least early in the course. Glucocorticoids are effective in treating hypercalcemia due to vitamin D intoxication and in the vitamin D hypersensitivity of sarcoidosis. In all the above situations, the hypocalcemic effect develops over several days, and the usual glucocorticoid dosage is 40 to 100 mg prednisone (or its equivalent) daily in four divided doses. The side effects of chronic glucocorticoid therapy may be acceptable in some circumstances.

Prostaglandins of the E series may play a role in the hypercalcemia of certain malignancies, especially those metastatic or primary in bone marrow. Prostaglandin synthesis can be blocked by indomethacin or aspirin; these drugs may correct the hypercalcemia in a subset of patients with osteolytic lesions or even humoral hypercalcemia of malignancy. The analytical methods necessary to define prostaglandin excess are not widely available, and correlations between prostaglandin levels and hypercalcemia are usually not available. In those cases when a therapeutic trial has been reported to be successful, indomethacin, 25 mg every 6 h, or aspirin in sufficient doses to produce a serum salicylate level of 1.4 to 1.8 mmol/L (20 to 25 mg/dL) have been used to lower the serum calcium concentrations over several days.

Hypercalcemia complicated by severe failure is difficult to manage; dialysis is often the treatment of choice. Peritoneal dialysis can remove 5 to 12.5 mmol (200 to 500 mg) of calcium in 24 to 48 h and lower the serum calcium concentration by 0.7 to 3 mmol/L (3 to 12 mg/dL) if calcium-free dialysis fluid is used. Large quantities of phosphate are lost during dialysis, and serum inorganic phosphate concentrations usually fall, thus aggravating hypercalcemia. Therefore, the serum inorganic phosphate concentration should be measured after dialysis, and phosphate supplements should be added to the diet or to dialysis fluids if necessary. APD may be helpful in such situations.

Calcitonin decreases the skeletal release of calcium, phosphorus, and hydroxyproline within minutes of its intravenous injection. The subsequent changes in serum calcium and phosphorus depend upon the initial magnitude of skeletal resorption; subjects with the most rapid bone turnover show the greatest reduction in serum calcium concentration. Calcitonin also increases the renal clearance of calcium and phosphorus (and sodium). Unfortunately, escape from drug action occurs in patients and animals invariably after 12 to 24 h of high-dose continuous therapy or after several days of repeated therapy with calcitonin. The mechanism of escape is unknown; coadministration of glucocorticoids and calcitonin may prevent escape. This promising lead deserves further clinical evaluation, since calcitonin causes minimal toxicity. Calcitonin is effective by intravenous, intramuscular, or subcutaneous injection; doses used are 25 to 50 units every 6 to 8 h, usually in the form of salmon calcitonin.

Phosphate Patients with primary hyperparathyroidism are frequently hypophosphatemic, and hypercalcemia of other causes may also be complicated by hypophosphatemia. Hypophosphatemia decreases the rate of calcium uptake into bone, increases intestinal calcium absorption, and directly and indirectly stimulates bone breakdown. These effects aggravate hypercalcemia, and correcting hypophosphatemia lowers the serum calcium concentration. The usual treatment is 1 to 1.5 g phosphorus per day for several days, given in four divided doses to minimize the chances of developing hyperphosphatemia. Such therapy has been administered for prolonged periods in selected patients. It is generally believed but not established that toxicity will not occur if the phosphate therapy is limited to restoring serum inorganic phosphate concentrations to normal rather than making them supranormal.

Raising the serum inorganic phosphate concentration above normal

TABLE 340-4 Commercially available phosphate preparations

	1000 mg P	mmol Na	mmol K
Oral phosphate preparations:			
Neutraphos (1250-mg capsule)	4 caps	28.5	28.5
Neutraphos-K (1450-mg capsule)	4 caps	—	57
Phos-Tabs (860-mg tablet)	6 tabs	—	51
Fleets Phospho-Soda (liquid)	6.7 mL	40	—
Intravenous phosphate preparations:			
In-Phos	40 mL	65	8
Hyper-Phos-K	15 mL	—	50

SOURCE: After Neer and Potts (with permission).

does decrease serum calcium levels, sometimes strikingly. Intravenous phosphate is one of the most dramatically effective treatments available for severe hypercalcemia but is toxic and even dangerous so that it is used rarely and *only* in severely hypercalcemic patients with cardiac or renal failure. A dose of 1500 mg phosphate phosphorus or more intravenously over 6 to 8 h leads to a prompt decrease in serum calcium of as much as 1.2 to 2.5 mmol/L (5 to 10 mg/dL) in patients with initially normal serum inorganic phosphate concentrations. This therapy should be employed only in extreme emergencies for two reasons. First, fatal hypocalcemia can be produced by excessive dosage; frequent serum calcium determinations are necessary if intravenous phosphate is administered. Second, unlike sodium chloride, sodium phosphate does not remove calcium from the body. In fact, urine calcium generally declines and fecal calcium declines or

remains the same. The decline in serum calcium reflects a redistribution of calcium within the body. There is a rapid efflux of calcium with no change in calcium influx to the circulation, findings indicative of precipitation of calcium phosphate salt. The calcium precipitates in bone, and metastatic calcification has also been reported in patients receiving oral or intravenous phosphate therapy for hypercalcemia. Indeed, hyperphosphatemia can cause metastatic calcification in normocalcemic animals. Thus, administration of intravenous phosphate in patients with compromised renal function who cannot have diuretic therapy is justifiable only as an emergency treatment.

Inorganic phosphate is commercially available for oral use in liquid, powder, and capsule form, and as a liquid for intravenous use. It is important to calculate doses in terms of phosphate phosphorus (see Table 340-4).

Anticancer drugs Several anticancer drugs have hypocalcemic effects independent of antitumor activity. Ethiofos (WR-2721), an organic thiophosphate, causes hypocalcemia in normocalcemic cancer patients; the action is attributed to inhibition of parathyroid hormone release. Extensive trials in vivo have not been reported.

Cisplatin has been tested in patients. The drug lowers serum calcium within days in the majority of treated patients with hypercalcemia and cancer; the beneficial effect lasts for weeks in most patients. The factors controlling responsiveness are unknown; the mode of action resembles that of mithramycin and diphosphonates: blockage of bone resorption. Similar effects and postulated mode of action have been reported with gallium nitrate, another experimental anticancer agent.

The ultimate utility of these agents is unclear, but their hypocalcemic effects represent a potentially useful therapy, especially in patients with malignancy.

Summary The various therapies for hypercalcemia are listed in Table 340-5. The choice depends upon the underlying disease, the

TABLE 340-5 Summary of treatments for hypercalcemia

Therapy	Therapeutic details	Indications	Complications	Precautions
MOST GENERALLY USEFUL THERAPIES				
Hydration	2 L or more	Universal	—	—
High salt intake	Achieve urine Na of 300 mmol/d or more	Universal	Edema	—
Furosemide or ethacrynic acid	40–160 mg/d 50–200 mg/d	Universal	↓ K and ↓ Mg	Measure serum K and Mg
Forced diuresis	4–6 L fluid IV/day containing 600–900 mmol Na plus furosemide every 1–2 h, plus at least 60 mmol K/day, plus at least 60 mmol Mg/day	Universal	Pulmonary edema; ↓ K and ↓ Mg	Intensive monitoring, including venous pressure and serum Mg and K
Oral phosphate	250 mg P every 6 h PO	Universal if serum P < 3 mg/dL	Ectopic calcification	Keep serum P below 5–6 mg/dL
Plicamycin	10–25 g/kg body weight IV, repeat PRN	Increased bone resorption	Liver; kidney; marrow toxicity	Monitor platelets, CBC, BUN, SCOT
Diphosphonate (aminohydroxypropylidene biphosphonate, APD)	15–30 mg IV every 2–6 h for 3–6 days or 1200 mg/d PO for 6 days	Increased bone resorption		
Prednisone or equivalent	5–15 mg every 6 h	Breast cancer, lymphomas, leukemias, multiple myeloma, vitamin D poisoning, sarcoidosis	Cushing's syndrome if chronic Rx	Alternate-day Rx for chronic use
SPECIAL THERAPIES FOR PARTICULAR USES				
IV phosphate	1500 mg P every 12 h until P is 2 mmol/L (6 mg/dL) or less	Severe hypercalcemia: diuresis or mithramycin contraindicated	Ectopic calcification: severe hypocalcemia	Monitor serum Ca and P closely
Calcitonin	2 units kg every 4 h subcutaneously	Adjunct in presence of bone reabsorption; paralysis; immobilization	—	—
Indomethacin	25 mg every 6 h PO	Certain types of pseudohyperparathyroidism	Na retention: GI bleeding; headache	Careful clinical monitoring
Dialysis	Lo-Ca bath	Acute renal failure	Multiple	Monitor serum P after dialysis

severity of the hypercalcemia, the serum inorganic phosphate level, and the renal, hepatic, and bone marrow function. Mild hypercalcemia [3 mmol/L (12 mg/dL) or less] can usually be managed by the sequence of hydration followed by intravenous sodium chloride and, if needed, small doses of furosemide or ethacrynic acid. Severe hypercalcemia [3.7 mmol/L (15 mg/dL)] requires rapid correction. Aggressive sodium-calcium diuresis with intravenous saline and large doses of furosemide and ethacrynic acid works but should be undertaken only if appropriate monitoring is available and cardiac function is adequate. Plicamycin has often been the drug of choice, but because of its potential toxicity plicamyin will probably be replaced by the diphosphonates, which also act by blocking bone resorption and, at present, seem safer and longer-acting.

There is a role for oral phosphate therapy in chronic management of hypercalcemia, unless its utility is superceded by the diphosphonates. Phosphate supplements should not be administered if hyperphosphatemia is present.

Severe dietary calcium restriction should be employed if intestinal absorption is enhanced (in sarcoidosis, vitamin D intoxication). Glucocorticoids and prostaglandin-synthesis inhibitors, even when effective in a particular disease, work slowly over several days and should not be relied upon as principal treatment for life-threatening hypercalcemia. Dialysis should be reserved for hypercalcemia complicating acute or chronic renal failure. There may be a role for calcitonin combined with glucocorticoids, but more experience is needed.

Chronic therapy of hypercalcemia poses greater problems of toxicity. One satisfactory regimen for chronic use is a combination of dietary calcium restriction, administration of sodium chloride with or without furosemide and ethacrynic acid, and moderate-dose oral phosphate (the patient is kept normophosphatemic). Some of the effective remedies (plicamycin, glucocorticoids, high-dose oral phosphate) may have significant toxicity when used chronically. Diphosphonates, if proven nontoxic, may become the chronic treatment of choice in cases of hypercalcemia where increased bone resorption is responsible for the disturbance in calcium metabolism.

HYPOCALCEMIA

PATHOPHYSIOLOGY OF HYPOCALCEMIA: CLASSIFICATION BASED ON MECHANISM *Chronic hypocalcemia* is less common than hypercalcemia; principal causes include chronic renal failure, hereditary and acquired hypoparathyroidism or vitamin D deficiency, and hypomagnesemia.

Critically ill patients may have *transient hypocalcemia* in association with severe sepsis, burns, acute renal failure, and extensive transfusions with citrated blood. In many instances, however, the hypocalcemia is more apparent than real. Although as many as half of patients in intensive care settings are reported to have calcium concentrations below 2.1 mmol/L (8.5 mg/dL), less than 10 percent have a reduction in ionized calcium. Patients with severe sepsis may have a decrease in ionized calcium (true hypocalcemia), but in other severely ill subjects hypoalbuminemia is the cause of the reduced total calcium concentration. Alkalosis, however, increases calcium binding to proteins, and in this setting direct measurements of ionized calcium should be made.

Medications such as protamine, heparin, and glucagon may cause transient hypocalcemia. These forms of hypocalcemia, apparent or real, are usually not associated with tetany and resolve with improvement in the overall medical condition. The transient hypocalcemia after repeated transfusions of citrated blood also usually resolves quickly.

Patients with acute *pancreatitis* have hypocalcemia that persists during the acute inflammation and varies in degree with the severity of the pancreatitis. The cause of hypocalcemia in pancreatitis remains unclear. Parathyroid hormone (PTH) values are variously reported to be low, normal, or elevated, and both resistance to PTH and impaired

TABLE 340-6   Functionally based classification of hypocalcemia (excluding neonatal conditions)

I PTH absent
  A Hereditary hypoparathyroidism
  B Acquired hypoparathyroidism
  C Hypomagnesemia
II PTH ineffective
  A Chronic renal failure
  B Active vitamin D lacking
    1 ↓ dietary intake or sunlight
    2 Defective metabolism:
      Anticonvulsant therapy
      Vitamin D–dependent rickets type I
  C Active vitamin D ineffective
    1 Intestinal malabsorption
    2 Vitamin D–dependent rickets type II
  D Pseudohypoparathyroidism
III PTH overwhelmed
  A Severe, acute hyperphosphatemia
    1 Tumor lysis
    2 Acute renal failure
    3 Rhabdomyolysis
  B Osteitis fibrosa after parathyroidectomy

PTH secretion have been postulated, leaving no clear view as to the principal mechanism. Occasionally a chronic low total-blood calcium is detected in an elderly patient, with documented reduction in ionized calcium concentration but without obvious cause and with a paucity of symptoms of hypocalcemia; the pathogenesis is unclear.

Neuromuscular and neurologic symptoms are the most common manifestations of chronic hypocalcemia and include muscle spasms, carpopedal spasm, facial grimacing, and, in extreme cases, laryngeal spasm and convulsions. Respiratory arrest may occur. Increased intracranial pressure occurs in some patients with long-standing hypocalcemia, often in association with papilledema. Chronic mental changes include irritability, depression, and psychosis. The QT interval on the electrocardiogram is prolonged, in contrast to its shortening with hypercalcemia. Arrhythmias are reported, and digitalis effectiveness may be reduced. Intestinal cramps and chronic malabsorption may occur. Chvostek's or Trousseau's signs can be used to confirm latent tetany.

The classification of hypocalcemia shown in Table 340-6 is based on the premise that PTH is responsible for minute-to-minute regulation of plasma calcium concentration within narrow limits and, therefore, that the occurrence of hypocalcemia must mean a failure of the homeostatic action of PTH. The classification is offered for simplicity of approach to diagnosis. Failure of the PTH response can occur if PTH is absent due to hereditary or acquired gland failure, if the hormone is rendered ineffective by mechanisms that interfere with its action at target organs, or if the action of the hormone to raise blood calcium is overwhelmed by the loss of calcium from the extracellular fluid at a rate faster than it can be replaced.

PTH ABSENT Hypoparathyroidism, whether hereditary or acquired, has a number of common components. Acute and chronic symptoms that result from untreated hypocalcemia are shared by both types of hypoparathyroidism, although typically the onset of hereditary hypoparathyroidism is more gradual and acquired hypoparathyroidism lacks associated developmental defects seen in hereditary hypoparathyroidism. In earlier decades, acquired hypoparathyroidism secondary to surgery in the neck was more common than hereditary hypoparathyroidism, but the frequency of surgically induced parathyroid failure has diminished with the recognition of the importance of parathyroid gland preservation and the use of nonsurgical approaches in treatment of hyperthyroidism. Basal ganglia calcification and extrapyramidal syndromes occur in both hereditary and acquired hypoparathyroidism but are more common and earlier in onset in hereditary hypoparathyroidism. Pseudohypoparathyroidism, an example of ineffective PTH action rather than a failure of parathyroid gland production, shares several features with hypoparathyroidism, including extraosseous calcification and extrapyramidal syndromes such as choreoathetotic movements and dystonia. Papilledema and raised intracranial pressure occur in both states, as do chronic changes in fingernails and hair and lenticular cataracts, the latter usually reversible with treatment of hypocalcemia. Certain skin manifestations, including alopecia and candidiasis, occur exclusively in hereditary hypoparathyroidism.

Hypocalcemia associated with hypomagnesemia is associated both with deficient PTH release and impaired responsiveness to the hormone (also see Chap. 343). Patients with hypocalcemia secondary to hypomagnesemia have absent or low levels of circulating iPTH, indicative of diminished hormone release despite maximum physiologic stimulus by hypocalcemia. Plasma PTH levels return to normal with correction of the hypomagnesemia. Thus, hypoparathyroidism associated with low levels of PTH in blood can be due to hereditary gland failure, acquired gland failure, or acute but reversible gland dysfunction (hypomagnesemia). Patients with acquired or hereditary hypoparathyroidism also have hyperphosphatemia and absent or low levels of $1,25(OH)_2D$.

Hereditary hypoparathyroidism Hypoparathyroidism can occur as an isolated entity without other endocrine or dermatologic manifestations or, more typically, in association with other abnormalities such as defective development of the thymus or failure of other endocrine organs such as the thyroid or ovary (see Chap. 325). Hereditary hypoparathyroidism is often manifest within the first decade but may appear later.

One rare form of hypoparathyroidism due to congenital aplasia of the parathyroid glands is manifested shortly after birth. A linkage between defective development of the thymus and the parathyroid glands is recognized in the *DiGeorge syndrome,* which is also associated with congenital cardiovascular and other developmental defects. Most patients die in early childhood.

Hypoparathyroidism can occur in association with other diverse developmental defects or as part of a complex autoimmune syndrome involving failure of the adrenals, the ovaries, and the parathyroids in association with recurrent mucocutaneous candidiasis, alopecia, vitiligo, and pernicious anemia (see Chap. 325). In many cases, antibodies to endocrine organs are present; there is, in addition, a failure of cell-mediated immunity. The inheritance of the autoimmune syndrome appears to be autosomal recessive, and some unaffected family members show antibodies to endocrine tissue without evidence of endocrine failure. The disorder is usually referred to as autoimmune polyglandular deficiency.

Hereditary hypoparathyroidism occurs also as an isolated entity without any other defects. The mechanism of inheritance varies from one kindred to another. Autosomal dominant, autosomal recessive, and X-linked inheritance patterns have all been identified. In one pedigree, a structural abnormality in the parathyroid hormone gene is suspected, but for most families the defect appears to involve some other gene(s) in control of parathyroid gland function.

Treatment of hereditary hypoparathyroidism is similar to that for acquired hypoparathyroidism and pseudohypoparathyroidism, although specific features of each disease lead to additional treatments. Replacement therapy with vitamin D or calcitriol combined with a high oral calcium intake usually suffices to regulate blood calcium and phosphate levels satisfactorily. Oral calcium and vitamin D restore the overall calcium-phosphate balance but do not reverse the lowered urinary calcium reabsorption typical of hypoparathyroidism. Therefore, care must be taken to avoid excessive urinary calcium excretion due to excessive vitamin D and calcium replacement therapy; otherwise kidney stones could develop. Thiazide diuretics lower urine calcium by as much as 100 mg/d in hypoparathyroid patients on vitamin D, provided patients are maintained on a low-sodium diet. Use of thiazides seems to be of benefit in preventing severe hypercalciuria and in improving the management of certain patients (see above).

Acquired hypoparathyroidism *Acquired chronic hypoparathyroidism* is usually the result of inadvertent surgical removal of all the parathyroid glands; in some instances, not all of the tissue is removed,

but the gland undergoes compromise of vascular supply secondary to fibrotic changes in the neck after surgery. In the past the most frequent cause of acquired hypoparathyroidism was surgery for hyperthyroidism. Chronic hypoparathyroidism now usually occurs after surgery for chief cell hyperplasia of the parathyroids where the surgeon, facing the dilemma of removing too little tissue and thus not curing the hyperparathyroidism, removes too much.

Parathyroid function is not totally absent in all patients with postsurgical hypoparathyroidism. Presumably, the persistence of some residual parathyroid activity reduces the amount of replacement therapy that is necessary, but suitable therapy varies greatly from patient to patient irrespective of the type of hypoparathyroidism or the question of residual parathyroid activity.

Other rare causes of acquired chronic hypoparathyroidism include radiation-induced damage subsequent to radioiodine therapy of hyperthyroidism or glandular damage in patients with hemochromatosis or with hemosiderosis after repeated blood transfusions. Although chronic infections may involve one or more of the parathyroids, they usually do not cause permanent hypoparathyroidism because all four glands are not usually involved.

Transient hypoparathyroidism is frequent following surgical exploration for hyperparathyroidism, particularly in patients in whom more than one exploration is required and in patients with multiple gland disease in which all glands must be identified and biopsied. Often, after a variable period of hypoparathyroidism, normal parathyroid function returns due to hyperplasia of remaining tissue. Occasionally, recovery occurs months after surgery. The management of transient, postoperative hypoparathyroidism is discussed under the surgical treatment of hyperparathyroidism. The treatment of chronic acquired hypoparathyroidism is similar to that used with idiopathic hypoparathyroidism: replacement with vitamin D and oral calcium.

Hypomagnesemia Hypomagnesemia of a severe degree is associated with severe hypocalcemia (also see Chap. 343). Restoration of the total-body magnesium deficits leads to rapid reversal of the hypocalcemia. There are at least two separate causes of the hypocalcemia—impaired secretion of PTH and reduced peripheral responsiveness to hormone action.

Hypomagnesemia is generally classified as primary or secondary; primary hypomagnesemia is due to hereditary defects in intestinal absorption or renal reabsorption of magnesium. Secondary hypomagnesemia, a more common condition, occurs on a nutritional basis or as a result of acquired intestinal or renal disorders. The most common causes of the secondary disorder are intestinal malabsorption syndromes, chronic alcoholism with poor nutritional intake, and parenteral nutrition in which magnesium replacement is omitted.

In experimental animals magnesium in extracellular fluid has effects similar to those of calcium on secretion of PTH; hypermagnesemia suppresses, and hypomagnesemia stimulates, PTH secretion. Effects of magnesium on hormone secretion are normally of little physiologic significance, however, because the effects of calcium dominate. Greater change in magnesium than in calcium is needed to influence hormone secretion. Nonetheless, hypomagnesemia, if it influences hormone secretion at all, might be expected to increase hormone secretion. It is, therefore, surprising to find that severe hypomagnesemia is associated with blunted secretion of PTH. The explanation for the paradox is that severe, chronic hypomagnesemia reflects intracellular magnesium deficiency; severe intracellular magnesium deficiency interferes with normal secretory mechanisms and normal peripheral responses to PTH. It is suspected that both effects involve function of adenyl cyclase in glandular and target tissues. Reduced intracellular stores of magnesium obscure any effects that might be brought about by acute changes in extracellular fluid magnesium in a magnesium-replete individual.

Severe hypocalcemia is often seen when serum magnesium is substantially below normal. Normal serum magnesium is 0.8 to 1.2 mmol/L (2 to 3 mg/dL). In most cases in which hypomagnesemia is associated with hypocalcemia, serum magnesium is below 0.4 mmol/L (1.0 mg/dL).

PTH levels are usually undetectable or inappropriately low despite the extreme stimulus of severe hypocalcemia. Even when iPTH levels are moderately elevated, acute repletion of magnesium leads to a further increase in iPTH concentration. The overall data indicate that PTH secretion is blunted in virtually all patients with severe hypomagnesemia; thus, absolute or relative hypoparathyroidism seems to be the rule in patients with hypocalcemia secondary to hypomagnesemia.

Diminished peripheral responsiveness to administered PTH can be shown in some patients with severe hypomagnesemia in addition. Some clinical reports document subnormal response in urinary phosphorus and urinary cyclic AMP excretion after administration of exogenous PTH to patients who are hypocalcemic and who have diminished PTH secretion. Both blunted PTH secretion and lack of renal response to administered PTH can occur in the same patient. Blunted skeletal responses have been claimed in many, but by no means all, patients studied with the hypomagnesemia-hypocalcemia syndrome. When acute magnesium repletion is undertaken, the restoration of PTH concentrations to normal or supranormal levels may precede by several days the restoration of normal serum calcium.

Overall, blunted PTH secretory response in hypomagnesemia seems the more important and invariant cause of hypocalcemia. The fact that impaired peripheral responsiveness, particularly renal response, is more variable from patient to patient may indicate that an even greater degree of magnesium deficiency is required to induce end organ resistance than to impair hormone secretion.

Several other features have been noted. The brisk response in hormone secretion following magnesium repletion, sometimes demonstrable within minutes of giving a large parenteral dose of magnesium, indicates that hormone biosynthesis is not impaired, only secretion. Serum phosphate levels are not elevated as they often are in patients with hypoparathyroidism, probably because phosphate deficiency is a frequent accompaniment of the nutritional deficiencies that cause hypomagnesemia. There have been a few reports of magnesium-wasting chronic renal disease; although magnesium is usually elevated in acute renal failure, increases in magnesium concentration are rare in chronic renal failure.

Repletion of magnesium is the cure of the condition, and attention must be given to restoring the intracellular deficiency, which may be considerable. After intravenous magnesium, serum magnesium may return to the normal range, but unless replacement therapy is continued, it will rapidly fall to subnormal levels again. If renal function is normal, a useful indicator of restoration of magnesium deficiency is the urinary magnesium excretion; magnesium is retained by the kidney until magnesium deficiencies are repleted. Intracellular deficits can be as great as 50 mmol or more, but in many cases parenteral administration of approximately 12 mmol magnesium reverses the signs of magnesium deficiency. Depending on the cause of the hypomagnesemia, treatment may have to be administered chronically to prevent recurrence.

PTH INEFFECTIVE PTH can be considered ineffective when the hormone's action to promote calcium absorption from the diet is interfered with because of a primary deficiency of vitamin D, because of conditions in which vitamin D is ineffective, or in chronic renal failure in which the calcium-elevating action of PTH is opposed by several different processes. Despite diverse pathophysiologic mechanisms, these conditions usually involve, but are not limited to, the unavailability of vitamin D as a cofactor for PTH. Hypocalcemia is usually mild rather than severe and is accompanied by hypophosphatemia. Typically, hypophosphatemia is more severe than hypocalcemia due to the increased secretion of PTH. Increased PTH is only partly effective in elevating blood calcium, yet it promotes renal phosphate excretion in a nearly unimpaired manner in vitamin D deficiency. Varying degrees of bone disease with impaired mineralization and/or frank osteomalacia are the more frequent and harmful consequences of chronic renal failure or inadequate or ineffective vitamin D action due to the hypophosphatemia.

Pseudohypoparathyroidism, on the other hand, is distinct in pathophysiology from the other disorders classified under ineffective PTH action. Pseudohypoparathyroidism resembles conditions in which there is an absence of PTH synthesis and secretion and is manifested, in the untreated state, by severe hypocalcemia and hyperphosphatemia. The cause of the disease, however, is inadequate peripheral response to PTH involving defective hormone binding to the receptor, deficient activation of guanyl nucleotide–binding proteins, and/or stimulation of adenyl cyclase to increase intracellular cyclic AMP (see Chap. 68).

Chronic renal failure Severe abnormalities in mineral ion and bone metabolism occur in chronic renal failure. Even prior to the initiation of extensive programs of dialysis, however, improved medical management of chronic renal failure and/or a more indolent course of the renal disease allowed many patients to survive for a sufficiently long period that renal osteodystrophy, the mixed bone disease associated with renal failure, became an important feature.

After the initiation of chronic dialysis programs, many of the impairments in mineral and bone metabolism became even more apparent. Now the roles of phosphate retention and impaired production of $1,24(OH)_2D$ are recognized as the principal factors responsible for inducing calcium deficiency, secondary hyperparathyroidism, and frequently a picture of severe bone disease. Less clearly, the uremic state appears to be associated with impairment of intestinal absorption by factors other than defects in vitamin D metabolism. Nonetheless, replacement of physiologic levels of $1,25(OH)_2$ usually leads to satisfactory calcium absorption, suggesting it is the lack of the vitamin D rather than intrinsic defects in intestinal cellular function that is the more important cause of the impaired mineral metabolism in chronic renal failure.

Hyperphosphatemia per se tends to lower blood calcium concentration by several actions; these include extraosseous deposition of calcium and phosphate, impaired sensitivity of the skeleton to the bone-resorbing action of PTH, reduced $1,25(OH)_2D$ production by surviving renal tissue, and reduction in calcium absorption due to trapping of calcium in insoluble form as calcium phosphate complexes. In animals, prevention of hyperphosphatemia by dietary means can block the development of secondary hyperparathyroidism, emphasizing the importance of phosphate retention in the pathogenesis of secondary hyperparathyroidism and the associated disorders of mineral and bone metabolism. Low levels of $1,25(OH)_2D$ are also critical in the hypocalcemia; the low levels of vitamin D metabolites are due to hyperphosphatemia and to destruction of renal tissue.

Therapy of chronic renal failure (see Chaps. 224 and 225) involves careful management of patients prior to dialysis as well as adjustment of dialysis regimens once this becomes necessary. Attention should be paid to restriction of phosphate in the diet, use of phosphate-binding antacids such as those based on aluminum hydroxide, provision of an adequate calcium intake by mouth, usually 1 to 2 g/d, and supplementation with calcitriol in doses of 0.25 to 1.0 μg/d. Each patient must be monitored closely. The aims of therapy are to restore normal calcium balance to prevent osteomalacia and secondary hyperparathyroidism. Renal osteodystrophy, as discussed above, is the principal disabling feature of chronic renal failure related to calcium metabolism. Reduction of hyperphosphatemia and restoration of normal intestinal calcium absorption by calcitriol can improve blood calcium concentration and reduce the manifestations of secondary hyperparathyroidism.

Vitamin D deficiency due to inadequate diet and/or sunlight Vitamin D deficiency is more common in the United States than previously recognized. Biopsies of bone in elderly patients with hip fracture (documenting osteomalacia) and abnormal concentrations of vitamin D metabolites, PTH, calcium, and phosphate have established that vitamin D deficiency may occur in as many as 25 percent of elderly patients, particularly in areas where there is little ambient sunlight. Concentrations of $25(OH)D$ are at the lower limits of normal or below normal in these patients. Quantitative histomorphometry of bone biopsy specimens reveals widened osteoid seams consistent with osteomalacia. PTH hypersecretion compensates for a tendency of the blood calcium level to fall, but with the consequence of inducing renal phosphate wasting and a combined mineral ion abnormality that results in osteomalacia.

The genesis of vitamin D deficiency is impaired intake of dairy products that are enriched with vitamin D, lack of vitamin supplementation, and reduced sunlight exposure in the elderly, particularly in winter in northern latitudes.

Treatment involves the administration of vitamin D and provision of 1 to 1.5 g calcium in the diet. Vitamin D supplementation should aim to provide several times the recommended daily requirement in younger people, which is probably a safe recommendation; a dosage of 1000 to 2000 units of vitamin D per day is satisfactory. Vitamin D is usually not available in multiple-dose forms. Hence, the administration of a capsule containing 50,000 units of vitamin D once-monthly is safe in elderly patients who have osteomalacia. The increased awareness of the importance of calcium supplementation, particularly in women, even without supplementation of vitamin D, may lessen the frequency of this problem. Severe hypocalcemia is rarely seen in the moderately severe vitamin D deficiency of the elderly, but vitamin D deficiency needs to be considered in the differential diagnosis of mild hypocalcemia.

Defective vitamin D metabolism   ANTICONVULSANT THERAPY Anticonvulsant therapy with any of several agents induces a state of acquired vitamin D deficiency by increasing the turnover of vitamin D into inactive compounds. The more marginal the degree of vitamin D intake in the diet, the more likely that anticonvulsant therapy will lead to abnormalities in mineral and bone metabolism. The syndrome at its extreme involves several rickets with bone fractures, hypocalcemia, and hypophosphatemia. Occasionally, a severe proximal myopathy is reported. More often, frank hypocalcemia is not detected, and mild osteomalacia is the only clinical symptom. In other patients on long-term anticonvulsant therapy, no symptoms or signs are present, but bone density is lower than normal and responds favorably to vitamin D supplementation.

Anticonvulsants stimulate the hepatic microsomal mixed-oxidase enzymes and hence increase the rate of clearance of vitamin D and its metabolites. Phenytoin also impairs intestinal calcium absorption independent of effects on vitamin D; the drug also has deleterious effects on bone cell function in vitro including inhibition of collagen synthesis. All manifestations of the syndrome can nevertheless be reversed with adequate vitamin D supplementation.

Although $1,25(OH)_2D$ levels are lower for the degree of vitamin D intake in patients treated with chronic anticonvulsants than in the normal population, there is a great deal of variation. The greater prevalence of the disorder in some European populations and in children in homes for the mentally retarded probably reflects the lower vitamin D intake of those groups. Restoration of bone mineral mass and reversal of hypocalcemia, when seen, can be accomplished with vitamin D replacement plus added oral calcium. Adjustments in dose are indicated depending on the age and body size of the patient, but approximately 50,000 units of vitamin D weekly plus 1 g elemental calcium per day for several months are usually sufficient. Alternatively, administration of one 50,000-unit capsule of vitamin D monthly may be preventative if the anticonvulsant therapy must be given chronically.

VITAMIN D-DEPENDENT RICKETS TYPE I   Rickets can be due to *resistance* to the *action* of vitamin D as well as to vitamin D deficiency. Vitamin D-dependent rickets type I, previously termed pseudo-vitamin D-dependent rickets, differs from vitamin D-resistant rickets in that it is less severe and in that the biochemical and radiographic abnormalities can be reversed with large doses of the vitamin.

Clinical features include hypocalcemia, often with tetany or convulsions, hypophosphatemia, secondary hyperparathyroidism, and osteomalacia, often associated with skeletal deformities and increased alkaline phosphatase. Doses of vitamin D or calcifediol, 100 to 1000 times above the usual amounts, are required to heal the bone disease, whereas physiologic amounts of calcitriol cure the disease. The

disorder, an autosomal recessive trait, is due to a defect in conversion of $25(OH)D$ to $1,25(OH)_2D$. Plasma levels of $1,25(OH)_2D$ are low or undetectable even after administration of large doses of vitamin D or calcifediol. Response to high doses of vitamin D or calcifediol is probably due to direct actions of high levels of $25(OH)D$. Treatment requires careful adjustment of calcitriol dose, particularly during growth periods.

Active vitamin D ineffective   INTESTINAL MALABSORPTION Mild hypocalcemia, secondary hyperparathyroidism, severe hypophosphatemia, and a variety of nutritional deficiencies occur with gastrointestinal diseases. Hepatocellular dysfunction can lead to reduction in $25(OH)D$ levels, as in portal or biliary cirrhosis of the liver. Malabsorption of vitamin D and its metabolites, including calcitriol, may occur in a variety of intestinal diseases, hereditary or acquired. Hypocalcemia itself can lead to steatorrhea, due to deficient production of pancreatic enzymes and bile salts. Depending on the disorder, vitamin D or its metabolites can be administered parenterally, thereby guaranteeing adequate blood levels of active metabolites.

VITAMIN D-DEPENDENT RICKETS TYPE II   Pseudo-vitamin D-dependent rickets can be due to defective response as well as to defective production of $1,25(OH)_2D$. This disorder, vitamin D-dependent rickets type II, results from any of several types of end organ resistance to the active metabolite, including absence or qualitative defects of the intracellular receptor protein for the hormone and postreceptor blocks in hormone action (see Chap. 311). The clinical features are similar to those with the type I disorder and include hypocalcemia, hypophosphatemia, secondary hyperparathyroidism, and rickets. Plasma levels of $1,25(OH)_2D$ are elevated at least three times above normal, in keeping with the refractoriness of the end organs. Severe alopecia totalis may commence early in life. Patients with this disorder usually require higher dose of vitamin D or vitamin D metabolites than with the type I disorder.

Pseudohypoparathyroidism   Pseudohypoparathyroidism (PHP) is a hereditary disorder characterized by symptoms and signs of hypoparathyroidism, typically in association with distinctive skeletal and developmental defects. The hypoparathyroidism is due to a deficient end organ response to PTH. Excessive secretion of PTH is the consequence of hyperplasia of the parathyroids, a response to the resistance to hormone action. The entity is actually a syndrome in which various individuals and kindreds exhibit different aberrancies in hormone receptor complex response.

A working classification of the various forms of pseudohypoparathyroidism is given in Table 340-7. The classification scheme is based on the signs of ineffective parathyroid hormone action (low calcium and high phosphate), urinary cyclic AMP response to exogenous PTH, the presence or absence of Albright's hereditary osteodystrophy (AHO), and assays of the concentration of the G_s subunits of the adenylate cyclase enzyme (see Chap. 68). Using these criteria there are four types: pseudohypoparathyroidism (PHP) type I, subdivided into a and b categories; PHP-II; and pseudopseudohypoparathyroidism (PPHP). Individuals with PHP-I, the most common of the disorders, show a deficient response in urinary cyclic AMP following administration of exogenous parathyroid hormone. Pseudohypoparathyroidism type II refers to patients with hypocalcemia and hyperphosphatemia who have a normal urinary cyclic AMP response to PTH. These patients are assumed to have a defect in the response to PTH at a locus beyond that of cyclic AMP production, although at least some patients reported to have PHP-II may instead have occult vitamin D deficiency. Patients with the PHP-I syndrome are divided into type a, with reduced activity of the stimulatory G protein subunit (G_s) in in vitro assays, and type b, with normal amounts of G_s in erythrocytes. Subjects with PHP-Ia also have shortened metacarpals and metatarsals and the other features of Albright's hereditary osteodystrophy syndrome and commonly show resistance to hormones in addition to PTH. Patients with PHP-Ib have a normal phenotype without the AHO syndrome and do not show resistance to any hormones other than parathyroid hormone. Fibroblasts cultured from the skin of some patients with PHP-Ib show

TABLE 340-7 Classification of pseudohypoparathyroidism (PHP) and pseudopseudohypoparathyroidism (PPHP)

Type	Hypocalcemia, hyperphosphatemia	Response of Urinary cAMP to PTH	Serum PTH	G_s subunit deficiency	AHO	Resistance to hormones in addition to PTH
PHP-Ia	Yes	↓	↑	Yes	Yes	Yes
PHP-Ib	Yes	↓	↑	No	No	No
PHP-II	Yes	Normal	↑	No	No	No
PPHP	No	Normal	Normal	Yes	Yes	±

NOTE: ↓ = decreased; ↑ = increased; AHO = Albright's hereditary osteodystrophy.

a much reduced response of cyclic AMP accumulation to PTH but not to other agents that stimulate adenylate cyclase such as prostaglandins and forskolin, consistent with the presence of a defective receptor. A subset of these patients, however, have a normal response to cyclic AMP production in fibroblasts in vitro.

Patients with PPHP have typical features of the hereditary osteodystrophy syndrome despite normal serum calciums and normal response of urinary cyclic AMP to exogenous PTH. These individuals are usually first-degree relatives of patients with PHP-Ia, and patients initially classified as having PPHP have subsequently developed mild hypocalcemia. Patients with PPHP on average have levels of G_s subunits that are half normal. These various features suggest that PPHP is a mild variant of PHP-Ia and illustrate the heterogeneity of the defect in PTH responsiveness. Further studies will be necessary to clarify the pathogenesis of these disorders.

Little is known about the pathophysiology of the skeletal defects. The AHO syndrome includes round facies, short stature, obesity, brachydactyly, and heterotopic calcification. Mental deficiency is frequent.

The mode of inheritance in these various disorders is uncertain and may itself be heterogeneous. In some families the disorder may be an X-linked dominant defect, whereas in others the disorder appears to result from an autosomal dominant mutation with variable expressivity.

The mineral deposits in ectopic sites may include true bone, whereas bone formation in ectopic sites never occurs in idiopathic hypoparathyroidism. Amorphous deposits of calcium and phosphate are found in the basal ganglia in about half of patients. The defects in metacarpal and metatarsal bones are sometimes accompanied by abnormal phalanges as well, possibly reflecting premature closing of the epiphyses. The typical findings are abnormally short fourth and fifth metacarpals and metatarsals. The defects are usually bilateral. Exostoses and radius curvus are frequent. Impairments in olfaction and taste and unusual dermatoglyphic abnormalities have been reported. There is little improvement in mental status even after adequate therapy with calcium and vitamin D.

The diagnosis can usually be made without difficulty. Positive family history for developmental defects and/or the presence of developmental defects characteristic of PHP-Ia, including brachydactyly, in association with the signs of hypoparathyroidism, low calcium, and high phosphate, essentially make the diagnosis on clinical grounds. On the other hand, patients with PHP-Ib or PHP-II do not have phenotypic abnormalities. In PHP-Ib, administration of exogenous parathyroid hormone can lead to detection of the blunted cyclic AMP response; such tests are usually used to confirm the diagnosis even in PHP-Ia. Low levels of G_s subunits in erythrocyte membranes can also distinguish patients with PHP-Ia from those with PHP-Ib. Patients in both categories have elevated serum PTH, particularly if they are hypocalcemic. The diagnosis of PHP-II is more complex, in that cyclic AMP responses in urine are, by definition, normal. Since vitamin D deficiency itself can result in dissociation between phosphaturic and urinary cyclic AMP responses to exogenous PTH, vitamin D deficiency must be excluded before diagnosis of PHP-II can be made. PHP-II is separated from hypoparathyroidism by finding of elevated PTH levels; this finding per se, however, does not distinguish between secretion of abnormal PTH and a post-cyclic AMP receptor defect. Some patients with the PHP-II phenotype may actually have hypoparathyroidism secondary to secretion of an abnormal, biologically inactive PTH.

Treatment of PHP and PPHP is similar to that of hypoparathyroidism, except that the dose of vitamin D and calcium is usually lower than that required in true hypoparathyroidism. Variations in individual responses make it necessary to establish the optimal therapeutic program for each patient, based on maintaining the appropriate blood calcium concentration and urinary calcium excretion.

PTH Overwhelmed Occasionally, loss of calcium from the extracellular fluid is so severe that PTH cannot compensate. Such situations include severe, acute hyperphosphatemia, often in association with renal failure, or acute pancreatitis, conditions in which there is rapid efflux of calcium from extracellular fluid. Severe hypocalcemia can occur quickly; PTH rises in response to hypocalcemia but does not return blood calcium to normal. The chance of hypocalcemia is enhanced when renal failure is present.

Severe, acute hyperphosphatemia Severe hyperphosphatemia occurs in situations associated with extensive tissue damage or cell destruction (also see Chap. 342). The combination of an increased release of phosphate from muscle and an impaired ability to excrete phosphorus secondary to the renal failure causes moderate to severe hyperphosphatemia, the latter causing calcium loss from the blood and hypocalcemia of mild to moderate severity. Hypocalcemia is usually reversed with tissue repair and restoration of renal function as phosphorus and creatinine values return to normal. There may even be a mild hypercalcemic period in the oliguric phase of recovery of renal function. This sequence, severe hypocalcemia followed by mild hypercalcemia, reflects widespread deposition of calcium in muscle with subsequent redistribution of some of the calcium to the extracellular fluid after restoration of phosphate levels to normal.

Other causes of hyperphosphatemia that lead to hypocalcemia include hypothermia, massive hepatic failure, and hematologic malignancies, either because of high cell turnover as part of the malignancy or because of cell destruction when chemotherapy is instituted.

Treatment is directed toward lowering of blood phosphate by the administration of phosphate-binding antacids or dialysis, often needed for the management of renal failure. Although calcium replacement may be necessary if hypocalcemia is severe and symptomatic, calcium administration during the hyperphosphatemic period may increase extraosseous cellular calcium deposition, thereby aggravating ultimate tissue damage. Although the levels of $1,25(OH)_2D$ may be low during the hyperphosphatemic phase and may return to normal during the oliguric phase of recovery, mineral ion imbalance per se seems to be the principal pathophysiologic mechanism.

Osteitis fibrosa after parathyroidectomy Severe hypocalcemia after parathyroid surgery is less common now that osteitis fibrosa cystica is an infrequent manifestation of hyperparathyroidism. When osteitis fibrosa cystica is severe, however, bone mineral deficits can be large, and after parathyroidectomy, blood calcium levels can fall to the hypocalcemic range and remain depressed for days if calcium replacement is inadequate. The mechanism of the hypocalcemia is complex. Increased cellularity of bone in severe osteitis fibrosa cystica involves both osteoblastic and osteoclastic cells. High levels of PTH enhance bone-blood exchange, with resorption favored over formation; an abrupt decrease in PTH levels with surgery leaves bone formation favored over resorption. Calcium loss from blood is increased, and temporary hyporesponsiveness of bone to the bone-resorbing actions of PTH (lowered hormone levels after parathyroid surgery in the presence of receptor down-regulation) may add to the imbalance between bone resorption and bone formation. Treatment may require parenteral administration of calcium; addition of calcitriol and oral calcium supplementation may hasten the ability to withdraw parenteral calcium supplementation and/or reduce the amount needed.

DIFFERENTIAL DIAGNOSIS Care must be taken to ensure that true hypocalcemia is present; in addition, acute transient hypocalcemia can be a manifestation of a variety of severe, acute illnesses as discussed above. *Chronic hypocalcemia,* however, can usually be ascribed to a few disorders associated with an absence of PTH or its ineffectiveness. Important clinical criteria include the duration of the illness, signs or symptoms of associated disorders, and the detection of features that suggest a hereditary abnormality in calcium and bone metabolism. A nutritional history can be helpful in detecting a low intake of vitamin D and calcium in the elderly, and a history of excessive alcohol intake can be the clue to magnesium deficiency.

Hypoparathyroidism and pseudohypoparathyroidism are typically lifelong illnesses; hence, a recent onset of hypocalcemia in an adult is usually due to nutritional deficiencies, renal failure, or intestinal disorders that result in vitamin D deficiency or ineffective vitamin D action. A history of seizure disorder raises the issue of anticonvulsive medication. Neck surgery, even long past, can be associated with a delayed onset of postsurgical hypoparathyroidism. Developmental defects, particularly in childhood and adolescence, may point to the diagnosis of pseudohypoparathyroidism. Rickets and a variety of neuromuscular syndromes and deformities may indicate ineffective vitamin D action, either due to hereditary defects in vitamin D metabolism or rarely to vitamin D deficiency.

A pattern of *low calcium* with *high phosphorus* in the absence of renal failure or massive tissue destruction almost invariably means hypoparathyroidism or pseudohypoparathyroidism. A *low calcium* with a *low phosphorus* points to absent or ineffective vitamin D, thereby rendering the action of PHT on calcium metabolism ineffective. The relative ineffectiveness of PTH in vitamin D deficiency, anticonvulsant therapy, gastrointestinal disorders, and hereditary defects in vitamin D metabolism leads to secondary hyperparathyroidism as a compensation. The relatively unopposed action of the excess PTH on renal tubule phosphate transport, less dependent on vitamin D sufficiency than calcium transport, accounts for renal phosphate wasting and hypophosphatemia.

Exceptions to these patterns may occur. Most forms of hypomagnesemia are due to long-standing nutritional deficiency, and, despite the fact that the hypocalcemia is due principally to an acute absence of PTH, phosphate levels are usually low rather than elevated as in hypoparathyroidism. Chronic renal failure is often associated with hypocalcemia and hyperphosphatemia, despite secondary hyperparathyroidism.

Diagnosis is usually established by application of the PTH radioimmunoassay, tests for vitamin D metabolites, and measurements of the urinary cyclic AMP response to exogenous PTH. In hereditary and acquired hypoparathyroidism and severe hypomagnesemia, PTH is either undetectable or in the normal range, especially with double-antibody assays; this result in a hypocalcemic patient is supportive of hypoparathyroidism, as distinct from ineffective PTH action, in which even mild hypocalcemia is associated with elevated PTH levels. Hence, a failure to detect elevated PTH levels establishes the diagnosis of hypoparathyroidism; elevated levels suggest the presence of secondary hyperparathyroidism as found in many of the situations in which the hormone is ineffective due to associated abnormalities in vitamin D action. Assays for 25(OH)D and 1,25(OH)$_2$D can be quite helpful. Low or low normal 25(OH)D indicates vitamin D deficiency due to lack of sunlight, inadequate vitamin D intake, or intestinal malabsorption. A low level of 1,25(OH)$_2$D in the presence of elevated concentrations of PTH suggests ineffective PTH action, including chronic renal failure, severe vitamin D deficiency, vitamin D-dependent rickets type I, and pseudohypoparathyroidism. Recognition that mild hypocalcemia, rickets, and hypophosphatemia are due to chronic anticonvulsant therapy is made by history.

TREATMENT OF HYPOCALCEMIA The chronic management of hypoparathyroidism or pseudohypoparathyroidism, chronic renal failure, and hereditary defects in vitamin D metabolism all feature the use of vitamin D or vitamin D metabolites and calcium supplementation. Vitamin D itself is the least expensive form of vitamin D replacement and is frequently used in the management of uncomplicated hypoparathyroidism and disorders associated with ineffective vitamin D action. When vitamin D is used prophylactically, as in the elderly or in those with chronic anticonvulsant therapy, there is a wider margin of safety than with the more potent metabolites. On the other hand, most of the conditions in which vitamin D is used for chronic management of hypocalcemia require the use of 50 to 100 times the daily replacement doses, because the formation of 1,25(OH)$_2$D is deficient. In such situations, vitamin D is no safer than the active metabolite because intoxication does occur with high-dose vitamin D therapy. Calcitriol is more rapid in onset of action and also has a short biologic half-life; in high doses vitamin D is stored in body tissues and is cleared slowly.

One to five micrograms per day of vitamin D or calcifediol and slightly lower doses of calcitriol (0.25 to 1.0 μg/d) are required to prevent rickets. In contrast, 500 to 3000 μg of vitamin D$_2$ or D$_3$ is typically required in hypoparathyroidism; doses of calcifediol are also high (several hundred micrograms per day) compared with doses required in euparathyroid individuals. The dose of calcitriol is unchanged in hypoparathyroidism since the defect is in hydroxylation by the 1α-hydroxylase.

The slightly greater therapeutic efficacy of calcifediol than vitamin D$_3$ in conditions in which the metabolism of the vitamin is impaired may be due to superior metabolic availability for the renal 1α-hydroxylase or to direct action directly by 25(OH)D at receptors in target tissues. Vitamin D is metabolized to a variety of compounds other than the principal product, 25(OH)D. Calcifediol bypasses these alternate pathways and is directly available for metabolism to 1,25(OH)$_2$D. In hypoparathyroidism and in hereditary defects in renal hydroxylase, the efficiency of formation of 1,25(OH)$_2$D from 25(OH)D is low, but some formation does occur with high substrate levels. Calcifediol has about 1 percent of the potency of calcitriol in in vivo and in vitro tests of vitamin D responsiveness.

Unless a loading dose is given, 2 to 4 weeks or even longer are required to achieve the maximum calcium replacement action of vitamin D or calcifediol; again, the onset of action of calcifediol is slightly more rapid. Calcitriol can be given for hypoparathyroidism at the same dose required for the prevention of rickets in euparathyroid individuals, 0.2 to 1.0 μg/d. Its onset of action is days rather than weeks. When vitamin D or calcifediol is withdrawn, weeks are required for the disappearance of the biologic effects, compared with a few days for calcitriol.

Patients with hypoparathyroidism should be given 2 to 3 g elemental calcium by mouth each day. The two agents, vitamin D (or vitamin D metabolites) and oral calcium, can be varied independently. Higher doses of vitamin D or its metabolites increase the efficiency of intestinal calcium absorption; higher intakes of oral calcium permit adequate calcium assimilation despite a lower efficiency of intestinal calcium absorption. In the event of hypercalcemia during the treatment of chronic hypocalcemia, the withdrawal of the supplemental oral calcium is effective in lowering calcium within 24 h, even more rapidly than withdrawal of calcitriol. Most patients with hypoparathyroidism can be managed with high-dose vitamin D therapy combined with 2 to 3 g oral calcium per day. If hypocalcemia alternates with episodes of hypercalcemia, then substitution of calcitriol will often make management easier.

The administration of thiazide diuretics in the usual antihypertensive doses and sodium restriction in patients with hypoparathyroidism lowers urinary calcium excretion. This hypocalciuric effect allows the calcium and vitamin D supplementation to be reduced. Patients will have a lower urinary calcium excretion at any given level of blood calcium on thiazides. The treatment also may protect against the development of kidney stones, a potential complication of the long-term management of hypoparathyroidism. If on dialysis, patients with chronic renal failure and hypocalcemia can have adjustments in dialysate calcium concentrations as an alternative to vitamin D and calcium supplementation. The doses of vitamin D and calcium required for the management of pseudohypoparathyroidism are usually lower than those required for hypoparathyroidism, reflecting incomplete resistance to the action of PTH in pseudohypoparathyroidism. The acute treatment of hypomagnesemia is discussed above; the use of magnesium chloride by mouth may be sufficient to restore blood magnesium.

REFERENCES

ADERKA D et al: Bacteremic hypocalcemia, a comparison between the calcium levels of bacteremic and nonbacteremic patients with infection. Arch Intern Med 147:232, 1987

AHN TG et al: Familial isolated hypoparathyroidism: A molecular genetic analysis of 8 families with 23 affected persons. Medicine 6502:73, 1986

AHONEN P : Autoimmune polyendocrinopathy–candidiasis–ectodermal dystrophy (APECED): Autosomal recessive inheritance. Clin Genet 27:535, 1985

BENSON L et al: Hyperparathyroidism presenting as the first lesion in multiple endocrine neoplasia type 1. Am J Med 82:731, 1987

BROADUS AE et al: Humoral hypercalcemia of cancer: Identification of a novel parathyroid hormone-like peptide. N Engl J Med 319:536, 1988

GARABEDIAN M et al: Elevated plasma 1,25-(OH)$_2$D concentrations in infants with hypercalcemia and elfin facies. N Engl J Med 312:948, 1985

KIYOKAWA T et al: Hypercalcemia and osteoclast proliferation in adult T-cell leukemia. Cancer 59:1187, 1987

LAD TE et al: Treatment of cancer-associated hypercalcemia with cisplatin. Arch Intern Med 147:329, 1987

LEVINE MA et al: Activity of the stimulatory guanine nucleotide–binding protein is reduced in erythrocytes from patients with pseudohypoparathyroidism and pseudo-pseudohypoparathyroidism: Biochemical, endocrine, and genetic analysis of Albright's hereditary osteodystrophy in six kindreds. J Clin Endocrinol Metab 62:497, 1986

———, AURBACH GD : Pseudohypoparathyroidism, in *Endocrinology*, LJ DeGroot et al (eds). Philadelphia, Saunders, 1989, vol 2, chap 65

LIBERMAN UA et al: Resistance to 1,25-(OH)$_2$ Association with heterogenous defects in cultured skin fibroblasts. J Clin Invest 7:192, 1983

MALLETTE LE, EICHORN E : Effects of lithium carbonate on human calcium metabolism. Arch Intern Med 146:770, 1986

MARTIN P et al: Partially reversible osteopenia after surgery for primary hyperparathyroidism. Arch Intern Med 146:689, 1986

MAYNARD FM : Immobilization hypercalcemia following spinal cord injury. Arch Phys Med Rehabil 67:41, 1986

MUDDE AH et al: Ectopic production of 1,25-dihydroxyvitamin D by B-cell lymphoma as a cause of hypercalcemia. Cancer 59:1543, 1987

MUNDY GR et al: Tumor products and the hypercalcemia of malignancy. J Clin Invest 76:391, 1985

NEER RM, POTTS JT JR : Medical management of hyperparathyroidism and hypercalcemia, in *Endocrinology*, 2d ed, LJ DeGroot et al (eds). Philadelphia, Saunders, 1989, vol 2, chap 61

NORTON JA et al: Effect of parathyroidectomy in patients with hyperparathyroidism, Zollinger-Ellison syndrome, and multiple endocrine neoplasia type I: A prospective study. Surgery 1026:958, 1987

NUSSBAUM SR et al: Highly sensitive two-site immunoradiometric assay of parathyrin and its clinical utility in evaluating patients with hypercalcemia. Clin Chem 33:1364, 1987

ORWOLL ES : The milk-alkali syndrome. Current concepts. Ann Intern Med 97:242, 1982

SALUSKY IB, COBURN JW: The renal osteodystrophies, in *Endocrinology*, 2d ed, LJ DeGroot et al (eds). Philadelphia, Saunders, 1989, vol 2, chap 63

STUCKEY BGA et al: Fasting calcium excretion and parathyroid hormone together distinguish familial hypocalciuric hypercalcaemia from primary hyperparathyroidism. Clin Endocrinol 27:525, 1987

THEIBAUD D et al: Oral versus intravenous AHP,BP (APD) in the treatment of hypercalcemia of malignancy. Bone 7:247, 1986

WARRELL RP JR et al: Metabolic effects of gallium nitrate administered by prolonged infusion. Cancer Treat Rep 69:653, 1985

341 METABOLIC BONE DISEASE

STEPHEN M. KRANE / MICHAEL F. HOLICK

OSTEOPOROSIS

GENERAL CONSIDERATIONS *Osteoporosis* is the term used for diseases of diverse etiology that cause a reduction in the mass of bone per unit volume. The reduction in mass is not accompanied by a significant reduction in the ratio of the mineral to the organic phase, nor by any known abnormality in bone mineral or organic matrix. Histologically, the disorder is characterized by a decrease in cortical thickness and in the number and size of the trabeculae of cancellous bone with normal width of the osteoid seams. Osteoporosis is the most common of the metabolic bone diseases (disorders in which all the skeleton is involved) and is an important cause of morbidity in the elderly.

The remodeling of bone (its formation and resorption) is a continuous process. Any changes in the rates of formation and resorption that result in bone resorption exceeding bone formation can cause a decrease in bone mass. In osteoporosis the bone mass *is* decreased, indicating that the rate of bone resorption must exceed that of bone formation. Bone formation is higher in cortical than in cancellous bone. This difference is exaggerated by the normal menopause and exaggerated even further in patients with osteoporosis because rates of formation of cancellous bone tend to be lower in patients with osteoporosis, particularly in women after the menopause. The fact that about a third of postmenopausal women have high skeletal turnover, assessed by whole-body retention of ^{99m}Tc-methylene diphosphonate and by other biochemical markers, could reflect the greater relative contribution of cortical remodeling in this group. After closure of epiphyses and cessation of longitudinal growth, there is a period of consolidation with a decrease in cortical porosity. When peak adult bone mass is reached at about age 30 to 35 for cortical bone and probably earlier for trabecular bone, rates of bone formation and resorption are relatively low (compared to the period of growth spurt) and approximately equal. The normal balance between bone formation and resorption results in maintenance of skeletal mass. The rates of remodeling are different, however, not only in cortical compared to trabecular bone but also in individual bones or portions of bones. Most of the bone surfaces are "inactive" and not involved at any given time either in formation or resorption. Active surfaces may be randomly distributed, but formation and resorption are locally coupled as units. Resorption areas are covered by osteoclasts if active; bone formation surfaces are characterized by the presence of osteoid seams and are covered by active osteoblasts. Resorption precedes formation and is probably more intense, but it does not last as long as formation. As a consequence, there are normally more sites of active formation than of resorption. Bone turnover is high when there are many units active and low when there are few. Unless formation compensates for resorption, bone mass decreases. In both sexes after age 40 to 50 there is a slow rate of loss of cortical bone, of about 0.3 to 0.5 percent per year. In women around the menopause an accelerated loss of cortical bone is superimposed upon the age-related loss. Loss of trabecular bone begins at an earlier age in both sexes but is probably greater in degree in women. The rate of bone loss in women may also be accelerated around the time of menopause. These losses of bone mass range from 20 to 30 percent in men and 40 to 50 percent for some women. In general, the pattern of bone loss involves predominantly trabecular bone in the spine and distal radius in women and the spine and hip in both women and men. The loss in selected regions has been documented using techniques such as single- and dual-photon absorptiometry, quantitative computed tomography, x-ray-based dual-energy densitometry, and neutron activation analysis of total-body calcium. For example, the rate of loss is greater in the metacarpals, the femoral neck, and the vertebral bodies than in the midshaft of the femur, the tibia, and the skull.

Although, as noted, skeletal turnover may be increased, turnover is usually normal or low. Bone formation is low in the majority, but the degree of reduction varies with the different bone surfaces. The major remodeling abnormalities in patients with vertebral crush fractures are a reduced frequency of activation of remodeling units and a decrease in the function of osteoblasts. Even in those individuals with increased bone resorption, however, bone formation does not compensate. At some critical point if the difference between rates of formation and resorption is maintained, loss of bone substance may become so marked that the bone can no longer resist the normal mechanical forces to which it is subjected, and fracture results. Osteoporosis then becomes a clinical problem. The level of reduction in bone mass sufficient to result in fractures after minimal trauma is variable. The strength of bones such as the vertebrae may depend upon additional factors such as adequacy of ligamentous support and the age-related changes in the intervertebral disks. The normal trabecular architecture is also disturbed. For example, the horizontal trabeculae of the vertebral bodies are preferentially lost in osteoporosis. Microfractures are also frequent. In elderly individuals with osteoporosis, age-related impairment of vision, hearing, and other neurologic and intellectual functions are additional contributions to the occurrence of fractures.

In the process of remodeling of lamellar bone in adults, most of the net resorption occurs at the corticoendosteal surface. The abnormal remodeling in osteoporosis follows the same pattern; the bone loss includes cancellous bone, cortical bone at the endosteal surface, and intracortical bone, resulting in enlargement of the medullary cavity and thinning of the cortex. Since bone formation at the periosteum continues at a slow rate, the diameter of the bone does not decrease, and the periosteal surface retains its smooth configuration. In addition, the cancellous bone also undergoes progressive resorption, with some trabeculae being resorbed at rates faster than others, particularly those vertebral trabeculae with horizontal orientation.

The loss of bone that accompanies advancing age begins earlier and proceeds more rapidly in women than in men, and there is a trend toward acceleration of bone loss in women before the menopause. All of the reasons for this age-associated bone loss are not known, although several risk factors have been identified. In general, white women have a greater risk than black women, and white men have a greater risk than black men. One explanation for these population differences is that the bone mass at skeletal maturity is one determinant of the bone mass at subsequent ages. The lower incidence of osteoporosis and hip fracture in black men and women has been attributed to a higher bone mineral content in blacks than in whites. Of interest is that bone formation is lower in blacks. Since formation and resorption are usually closely coupled and since bone mass is increased, bone resorption (and turnover) must also be reduced. Osteoporotic subjects are frequently less muscular and have lower average body weight. Exercise may have a beneficial effect in maintaining bone mass. The facts that accelerated bone loss accompanies the menopause in some women and that premature osteoporosis occurs when bilateral oophorectomy is performed prior to the age of normal menopause suggest that estrogens play a major role in preventing bone loss. Furthermore, osteoporotic women as a group may have an earlier menopause than age-matched nonosteoporotic women. Osteoporotic women also have a higher incidence of smoking; cigarette smoking might directly affect bone remodeling or have secondary effects on ovarian function. Excessive alcohol consumption, which can result in decreased bone formation, also is a risk factor for osteoporosis. Dietary calcium intake and the efficiency of intestinal calcium absorption may also influence bone mass. Inability to synthesize adequate amounts of $1\alpha,25$-dihydroxyvitamin D [$1,25(OH)_2D$] may play a role in the decreased calcium absorption, possibly because of decreased parathyroid hormone levels, impaired activity of the renal 25(OH)D-1α-hydroxylase, or altered responsiveness of the enzyme to parathyroid hormone.

Although increased production of interleukin 1 by blood mononuclear cells in patients with osteoporosis may be a consequence of estrogen deficiency, the contributing role of interleukin 1 and other cytokines that may modulate bone resorption or bone formation in the genesis of osteoporosis has yet to be established. Although osteoporosis occurs with Cushing's syndrome, there is no established role of adrenal steroids in the osteoporosis associated with the menopause or advancing age.

It is also possible that excessive acid intake, particularly in the form of high-protein diets, results in "dissolution" of bone in an attempt to buffer the extra acid. Acidosis may also directly increase osteoclast function. Prolonged use of heparin as an anticoagulant is also associated with osteoporosis, and heparin potentiates bone resorption in vitro. Patients with osteoporosis have increased numbers of mast cells, presumably capable of producing heparin and other substances that modulate bone cell function, in the bone marrow. Circumscribed and diffuse areas of osteoporosis occur in patients with systemic mastocytosis.

As mentioned earlier, the remodeling of bone is responsive to mechanical forces of many types. The early response to immobilization in the normal skeleton is an increase in bone resorption while bone formation remains normal or is decreased; later there is a compensatory increase in bone formation. In osteoporosis, immobilization tends to aggravate the defect by increasing the gap between formation and resorption. A sedentary life in an individual with poor musculature may reduce mechanical forces exerted on the skeleton and increase the tendency to bone loss.

CLASSIFICATION (See Table 341-1) In some instances osteoporosis is a feature of another disease such as Cushing's syndrome. Osteoporosis (decreased bone mass with normal mineralization) is characteristic of certain heritable diseases of connective tissue such as osteogenesis imperfecta (see Chap. 333). In most osteoporosis, however, no other disease is apparent. This category of osteoporosis can be conveniently considered to comprise several forms. One form occurs in children or young adults of both sexes and with normal gonadal function. This form is frequently termed *idiopathic osteoporosis*, although most of the other forms are in fact also of unknown pathogenesis. So-called *type I osteoporosis* occurs in a subset of postmenopausal women who are between 51 and 75 years of age and is characterized by an accelerated and disproportionate loss of trabecular bone as contrasted with cortical bone. Fractures of vertebral

---

TABLE 341-1 Classification of osteoporosis

I Common forms of osteoporosis unassociated with other disease
  A Idiopathic osteoporosis (juvenile and adult)
  B Type I osteoporosis
  C Type II osteoporosis
II Disorders or conditions in which osteoporosis is a common feature
  A Hypogonadism
  B Hyperadrenocorticism
  C Thyrotoxicosis
  D Malabsorption
  E Scurvy
  F Calcium deficiency
  G Immobilization
  H Chronic heparin administration
  I Systemic mastocytosis
  J Adult hypophosphatasia
  K Associated with other metabolic bone diseases
III Osteoporosis as a feature of heritable disorders of connective tissue
  A Osteogenesis imperfecta
  B Homocystinuria due to cystathionine synthase deficiency
  C Ehlers-Danlos syndrome
  D Marfan's syndrome
IV Disorders in which osteoporosis is associated but pathogenesis not understood
  A Rheumatoid arthritis
  B Malnutrition
  C Alcoholism
  D Epilepsy
  E Diabetes mellitus
  F Chronic obstructive pulmonary disease
  G Menkes' syndrome

bodies and the distal forearm are the most common complications. Decreased parathyroid gland function may be compensatory to increased bone resorption. So-called *type II osteoporosis* is found in a large proportion of women and men over the age of 70. Fractures of the femoral neck, proximal humerus, proximal tibia, and pelvis are most common in this group. These skeletal sites contain both cortical and trabecular bone. Circulating levels of parathyroid hormone tend to be higher than normal. Both groups have decreased mean circulating levels of $1,25(OH)_2D$.

GENERAL CLINICAL FEATURES Although osteoporosis is a generalized disorder of the skeleton, its major clinical sequelae result from fractures of the vertebrae, wrist, hip, humerus, and tibia, depending upon the pattern of the disease (type I or II osteoporosis). The most frequent symptoms from vertebral body fractures are pain in the back and deformity of the spine. Pain usually results from collapse of the vertebrae especially in the lower dorsal and upper lumbar regions, is typically acute in onset, and often radiates anteriorly around the flank into the abdomen. Such episodes may occur after sudden bending, lifting, or jumping movements that may seem to have been trivial; on some occasions they cannot be related to trauma. The pain may be increased even with slight movements such as turning in bed or by the Valsalva maneuver. Bed rest may relieve the pain temporarily, only for it to recur in spasms of variable duration. Radiation of pain down one leg is uncommon, and symptoms or signs of spinal cord compression are rare. The acute episodes of pain may also be accompanied by abdominal distention and ileus, thought to be due to retroperitoneal hemorrhage, but the use of narcotics at this stage also contributes to the ileus. Loss of appetite and apparent muscular weakness may also be present. Episodes of pain usually subside after several days to a week, and by 4 to 6 weeks patients may be fully ambulatory and able to resume normal activities. Although acute pain may be minimal, nagging, deep, dull, uncomfortable sensations may be localized to the area of fracture and brought about by straining or sudden changes in position. Patients may be unable to sit up in bed and have to arise by rolling over on the side and then propping themselves up. Most patients have disappearance or diminution of pain between episodes of vertebral body collapse. Others do not have acute episodes but complain of backache made worse by standing or moving suddenly. Tenderness is common over involved areas of the spinous processes or rib cage. The collapse fractures of the vertebral bodies are usually anterior, producing a wedge-shaped deformity and contributing to loss in height. This is particularly common in the middorsal region where collapse may be unassociated with pain but result in a dorsal kyphosis and exaggerated cervical lordosis described as a "dowager's" or "widow's" hump. Postural slumping with increase in existing curves also contributes to the loss of height. Scoliosis is also common in women with osteoporosis. Generalized skeletal pain is uncommon, and between fractures most patients are free of pain but may have other uncomfortable sensations in the back. Although recurrent episodes of collapse fractures of vertebral bodies, increasing spine deformity, and loss of height are common, the course in any one subject is not predictable, and there may be intervals of several years between fractures.

RADIOLOGIC FEATURES Prior to fracture and collapse the osteoporotic vertebral body shows a decrease in mineral density, increase in prominence of vertical striations due to a relatively greater loss of the horizontally oriented trabeculae, and prominence of the end plates. The bodies may become increasingly biconcave because of weakening of the subchondral plates and expansion of the intervertebral disks, resulting in the so-called codfish vertebrae. When collapse occurs it usually produces a decrease in the anterior height of the vertebral body and irregularity in the anterior cortex (Fig. 341-1). Older compression fractures may show reactive changes and osteophytes about the anterior margins. Most osteoporotic fractures occur in the middle and lower thoracic and upper lumbar vertebral bodies. Fractures of isolated vertebral bodies of T4 or higher should suggest malignancy. Although the cortices of long bones may be thin

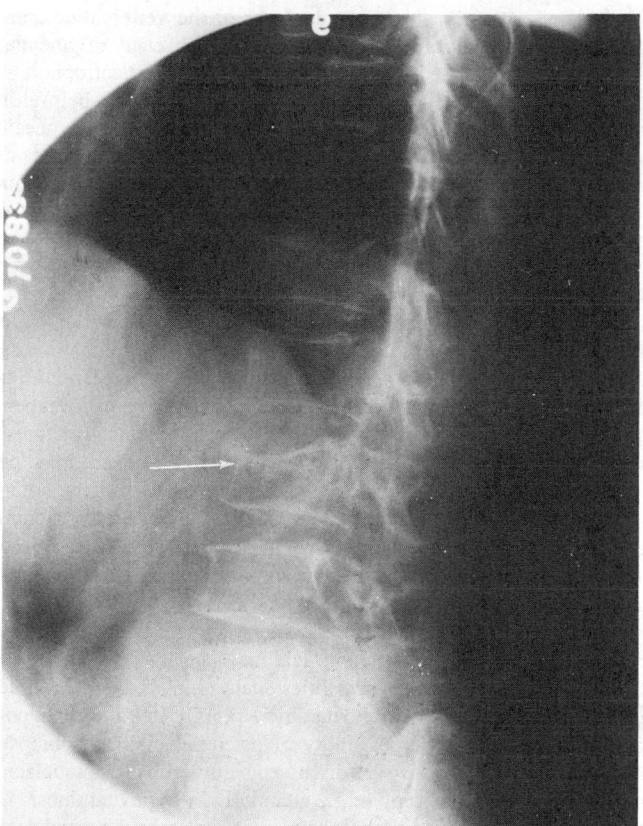

FIGURE 341-1 Lateral views of the lumbar spine of a 54-year-old man with idiopathic osteoporosis. A typical anterior compression fracture is indicated by the arrow.

because of excessive endosteal resorption, the outer margins are sharp in contrast to the typical effects of the subperiosteal resorption of hyperparathyroidism. Pseudofractures or Looser's zones are not present in osteoporosis in the absence of osteomalacia, but it may be impossible to distinguish osteoporosis from osteomalacia on radiologic grounds alone. In the absence of fractures standard roentgenograms are insensitive indicators of bone loss since as much as 30 percent decrease in bone mass may not be appreciated. Other procedures are required to establish whether a given individual has a sufficient decrease in bone mass to be at risk for fracture. These include single- and dual-photon absorptiometry, quantitative computed tomography, or neutron activation analysis of total-body calcium.

LABORATORY FINDINGS The concentrations of calcium and inorganic phosphorus in the blood are usually normal. Slight hyperphosphatemia is present in women who are past the menopause. The alkaline phosphatase in uncomplicated instances is normal, although slight increases may be seen after fractures. About 20 percent of postmenopausal women with osteoporosis have significant hypercalciuria. Urinary excretion of peptides containing hydroxyproline, an index of bone resorption, is usually normal or slightly increased in those with high-turnover osteoporosis. Serum levels of osteocalcin (bone GLA protein) and uptake of ^{99m}Tc-methylene diphosphonate also correlate with the rate of bone turnover.

DIFFERENTIAL DIAGNOSIS Since decrease in skeletal mass is a universal feature of aging, it is difficult to evaluate asymptomatic decreased bone density, determined radiographically, in older women, especially when unaccompanied by marked increase in biconcavity of vertebral bodies or fractures. Quantitative measurement of bone mass is, however, a predictor of future fractures. In the presence of bone pain with or without fracture or deformity, it is important to establish the presence or absence of known causes of osteoporosis as listed in Table 341-1 and to be certain that osteoporosis is the correct diagnosis. Malignancies of various types, particularly *multiple myeloma, lymphoma, leukemia,* and *carcinomatosis,* may result in diffuse loss of bone, especially the trabecular bone of the vertebral column, even in the absence of hypercalcemia. The absence of anemia, elevated erythrocyte sedimentation rate, abnormal electrophoretic patterns of serum proteins, and Bence Jones proteinuria is helpful in eliminating the possibility of multiple myeloma. However, needle bone biopsy or marrow aspiration may be appropriate in instances of severe osteoporosis with fractures. Quantitative histomorphometry on standard biopsy samples from the iliac crest is a research tool but is available in some referral laboratories. Bone biopsy samples must be properly fixed, not demineralized, and embedded in plastic to rule out osteomalacia, however.

Radiologic evidence of osteoporosis is common in patients with primary *hyperparathyroidism*, who may not have osteitis fibrosa (discrete lytic lesions of varying size and subperiosteal resorption) or elevation of serum alkaline phosphatase. Mild asymptomatic hyperparathyroidism is not a major risk factor for vertebral crush fractures, however. An element of secondary hyperparathyroidism may be present in some elderly patients with type II osteoporosis and in others with impairment of renal function, inadequate oral calcium intake, or decrease of intestinal calcium absorption. Increased numbers of osteoclasts may be present in bone biopsy specimens from such patients.

Osteomalacia may mimic osteoporosis or coexist with it, yet specific radiologic signs of osteomalacia may not always be present. Although the presence of abnormalities such as low or undetectable circulating levels of 25-hydroxyvitamin D [25(OH)D] and/or hypophosphatemia suggest the possibility of osteomalacia, bone biopsy may be essential for diagnosis, as discussed below. Since osteomalacia is more responsive to therapy (e.g., vitamin D in hypovitaminosis D or phosphate supplements in phosphate depletion) than the usual case of osteoporosis, such diagnostic procedures are often warranted.

In an occasional patient with *Paget's disease* the radiologic features may be almost purely lytic and be confused with osteoporosis. However, high alkaline phosphatase levels and moderately or markedly increased urinary excretion of hydroxyproline-containing peptides are clues to the presence of Paget's disease. Scanning procedures with bone-seeking isotopes are not helpful in differential diagnosis if fractures are present, because in any disease fractures demonstrate preferential uptake of isotope. However, in the absence of fracture, ''hot spots'' suggest tumor or early Paget's disease, particularly if present in the appendicular skeleton.

IDIOPATHIC OSTEOPOROSIS *Idiopathic osteoporosis* occurs in younger men and in premenopausal women in whom no other etiologic factor is detected. These patients probably have a number of different disorders with superficial resemblances. In some women the onset of the disease appears to be related to pregnancy and may represent a transient failure in homeostatic mechanisms such as failure to increase circulating levels of 1,25(OH)$_2$D and hence to protect the maternal skeleton from the stresses of childbirth (see Chap. 339). Some patients have low levels of serum alkaline phosphatase, though not low enough to fulfill diagnostic criteria for *hypophosphatasia*. Estrogens are ineffective in therapy. Losses of calcium and phosphorus are probably excessive, and it is unwise to permit women with osteoporosis to breast-feed since calcium losses via lactation are appreciable. Some patients have a disorder similar to mild forms of osteogenesis imperfecta, although such features as family history, blue scleras, and deafness are lacking. The course is variable; although recurrent episodes of fractures are characteristic, progressive deterioration does not occur in all patients, and in some the clinical problem is benign. Juvenile osteoporosis is a rare disorder with onset usually between the ages of 8 and 14 years and is characterized by the abrupt appearance of bone pain and fractures after minimal trauma. In many cases the disorder is self-limited, and recovery takes place spontaneously within 4 or 5 years.

GLUCOCORTICOID EXCESS Glucocorticoid excess does not appear to be involved in osteoporosis of the idiopathic variety or in the type I or II disorder. However, osteoporosis commonly accompanies Cushing's syndrome, both endogenous and exogenous, and in some instances is rapidly progressive, especially in children and in women over the age of 50. Bone loss of glucocorticoid excess is accounted for by a combination of low rates of bone formation (depressed osteoblastic oppositional rate) and high rates of bone resorption that accompany increased activation frequency of bone remodeling units. A part of the latter may be the result of glucocorticoid-induced secondary hyperparathyroidism, although increases in circulating parathyroid hormone have not been found consistently. Glucocorticoids, however, potentiate the effects of parathyroid hormone and 1,25(OH)$_2$D on bone cells in vitro. Glucocorticoids depress collagen synthesis in many tissues, as evidenced by delayed wound healing, thinning of the dermis, striae, and tendency to blue scleras. In some disorders in which glucocorticoids are administered in pharmacologic doses such as rheumatoid arthritis, a tendency to thin skin and osteoporosis is initially present, and the skeletal effects of the glucocorticoids may become particularly apparent. Even low dosages of glucocorticoids may accelerate bone loss in postmenopausal women as well as men with rheumatoid arthritis. Blood levels of 25(OH)D are normal or slightly decreased, and blood levels of 1,25(OH)$_2$D are usually normal. Glucocorticoids inhibit intestinal calcium absorption by a direct, vitamin D–independent action on the intestine. Osteomalacia is not observed histologically. Once osteoporosis develops in adults with Cushing's syndrome, the abnormality may persist indefinitely following alleviation of the glucocorticoid excess. In children, however, cure of the Cushing's syndrome may result in striking improvement in the appearance of the spine due to new endochondral bone formation around the less dense, older osteoporotic bone. Likewise, a striking increase in bone mass, increase in serum osteocalcin levels (indicative of increased osteoblastic function), and decrease in urinary hydroxyproline excretion may occur in young adults following therapy of Cushing's syndrome. Withdrawal of glucocorticoids or decrease of the dose by alternate-day schedule may thus be the only way to halt progression of the osteoporosis. Anabolic steroids are not effective in this regard. The defect in intestinal calcium absorption may be overcome by administering vitamin D in doses of 50,000 IU two times weekly plus supplemental oral calcium of 1 to 1.5 g per day. Vitamin D metabolites such as calcifediol [25(OH)D] may be more effective. When large doses of vitamin D are used, it is important to monitor serum and urinary calcium and serum 25(OH)D levels at intervals of 2 to 4 months, especially if glucocorticoid dosages are lowered. In Cushing's syndrome, spontaneous, symptomless fractures may occur in ribs and pubic and ischial rami even in the absence of marked osteoporosis of the spine. These fractures often heal partially with an exuberant calcified callus surrounding a radiolucent zone of nonunion, superficially resembling the pseudofractures of osteomalacia. If they appear in the thorax superimposed upon the lungs, they may be confused with nodules suggesting primary or metastatic tumor.

GONADAL DEFICIENCY Receptors for estrogens are in osteoblasts, and estrogens may function in these cells by stimulating production of substances that are anabolic for bone such as somatomedin C (insulin-like growth factor-1). Estrogen is deficient in the postmenopausal woman, and the administration of estrogen to such an individual reduces the negative calcium balance and decreases urinary hydroxyproline excretion. Estrogens are particularly useful in retarding the bone loss in women who have oophorectomy at an early age. Bone mass is also decreased in women athletes who are amenorrheic, such as marathon runners. Such women are particularly prone to tibial stress fractures. In patients of either sex castrated at an early age, the adult skeleton is smaller to begin with, and therefore age-related losses are more significant. Bone density is also decreased in women with hyperprolactinemia and in men with hypogonadism of all types.

THYROTOXICOSIS In many patients with hyperthyroidism, excessive bone resorption, occasionally marked in degree and far exceeding that in the usual patient with osteoporosis, can be associated with increased excretion of calcium and phosphorus in urine and feces. The excessive bone resorption is usually accompanied by a compensatory increase in bone formation. Parathyroid hormone secretion is decreased, and levels of $1,25(OH)_2D$ are normal or low. If the hyperthyroidism is of short duration, skeletal losses are inconsequential. However, in patients with chronic hyperthyroidism, especially in women after the menopause, this accelerated bone loss becomes clinically significant, and it is important to eliminate hyperthyroidism as a contributing cause of osteoporosis. Hypothyroid patients who are treated with excessive doses of levothyroxine may also have accelerated loss of bone mass. Although typical osteitis fibrosa (resorption lacunae containing osteoclasts and a fibrous stroma) may be seen on biopsy, the skeletal lesions have the radiologic appearance of osteoporosis.

ACROMEGALY Hypercalciuria and overall net negative calcium balance occur in acromegaly, and occasionally osteoporosis is an associated finding. The secondary panhypopituitarism and the associated gonadal insufficiency may be factors in production of the osteoporosis. In adult animals growth hormone decreases endosteal resorption and stimulates bone formation, and it is therefore unlikely that excessive secretion of growth hormone in itself produces osteoporosis.

DIABETES MELLITUS Individuals with juvenile or adult-onset diabetes mellitus have a decreased bone mass. In some series the incidence of hip fractures is increased, but studies of large groups of diabetic subjects have not revealed abnormal calcium metabolism or significant bone disease specifically attributable to the diabetes.

CALCIUM DEFICIENCY AND MALABSORPTION Although calcium deficiency may be a factor, it cannot be the sole or major cause in idiopathic, senile, or postmenopausal osteoporosis. Osteoporosis is an associated finding in a significant number of cases of steatorrhea, prolonged obstructive jaundice, and lactose intolerance and in patients following gastrectomy. Other patients may have a specific defect in calcium absorption or a failure to adapt adequately to a low-calcium diet either by increasing the percentage of dietary calcium absorbed or by decreasing urinary calcium excretion. Presumably, vitamin D is adequate in these instances to prevent osteomalacia.

HERITABLE DISORDERS OF CONNECTIVE TISSUE In the strict sense, the bone disease of osteogenesis imperfecta is osteoporosis (see Chap. 333). *Osteogenesis imperfecta* is clinically, genetically, and biochemically heterogeneous. Type I osteogenesis imperfecta is the autosomal dominant form characterized by mild to moderate bone fragility, blue sclerae, and premature deafness. The frequency of fractures tends to decrease around puberty, and another period of increased incidence occurs in women after the menopause. Type II is the lethal perinatal disorder. Type III is characterized by severe bone fragility, progressive bone deformity, and white sclerae. In type IV, sclerae are white, but other features are similar to those of type I disease. Many instances of osteogenesis imperfecta of all types have been linked to mutations in the *COL*1A1 and *COL*1A2 genes that encode type I collagen. Such linkage has been shown either by analysis of restriction fragment length polymorphisms (RFLPs) or by direct demonstration of mutations that produce amino acid substitutions or deletions. It is thought that the majority of patients with osteogenesis imperfecta will ultimately prove to have mutations in the type I collagen genes. In other individuals, defects in these genes may predispose to what is now diagnosed as idiopathic or postmenopausal osteoporosis, in the absence of other features of osteogenesis imperfecta. Osteoporosis also occurs in patients with *homocystinuria* due to cystathionine synthase deficiency, an autosomal recessive trait, associated with ectopia lentis, various deformities of the extremities, mental retardation, decreased pigmentation of hair and skin, and thromboembolism. The diagnosis is established by the finding of homocystine in urine. The osteoporosis may be due to the effect of homocysteine or other metabolites in interfering with the cross-linking of collagen.

THERAPY In considering treatment of osteoporosis, it should be emphasized that one is dealing with a group of disorders rather than a single entity. Even in patients within the same category, e.g., those with idiopathic osteoporosis, the etiologies may be different.

It is also difficult to predict the course, especially in patients seen because of pain and collapse-fracture. Many patients in the idiopathic, postmenopausal (type I), and senile (type II) groups have a few episodes of vertebral body collapse but then go for many years without symptoms or further loss in height. Furthermore, the acute pain associated with vertebral body fracture tends to subside in weeks, and *any* treatment administered at that time might be considered efficacious. Although accurate estimation of bone mass can help determine efficacy of therapy, clinical benefit (diminution of bone pain, decrease in incidence of fractures) is more difficult to assess in view of variability in disease progression. It is generally agreed, however, that estrogen replacement in women is effective in preventing bone loss after oophorectomy or early in the menopause.

General measures Patients with acute pain secondary to fracture of vertebral bodies frequently require rest in bed in a position of maximum comfort, local heat, adequate analgesics, and avoidance of constipation. Use of traction or plaster jacket splints is not indicated. As soon as pain permits, the patient should attempt to move out of bed, slowly at first, perhaps with support of a walker or crutches. Braces are commonly employed, but their efficacy in preventing progression of spinal deformity has not been established. A well-made corset may provide support and comfort. Exercises to correct postural deformity and increase muscle tone are useful. Patients should be taught to avoid sudden painful movements such as jumping and how to lift and carry objects with minimal back strain. After the fractures have healed, a supervised exercise program that includes daily walking may be helpful in preventing further skeletal losses.

Estrogens and androgens The use of estrogens in postmenopausal women causes a decrease in urinary calcium and hydroxyproline excretion, especially during the first few months of treatment (see Chap. 322). Estrogens may have direct effects on osteoblasts and also decrease the rate of bone resorption, but bone formation usually does not increase and eventually decreases. Nevertheless, estrogens produce significant calcium retention, decrease the difference between bone formation and resorption, and retard bone loss. Although any restoration of skeletal mass is minimal, the use of estrogens effectively prevents bone loss following castration and in the menopause and decreases the incidence of osteoporotic fracture in postmenopausal women. The major role of estrogens is in preventing osteoporosis in menopausal women rather than treating clinical disease already developed, although they may also be effective in the woman with mild or moderate disease during the first 10 years following cessation of ovarian function. The common dosage is 0.625 mg/d as conjugated estrogens, usually in a cyclic fashion for the first 25 days of each month. (Lower doses of estrogens are usually ineffective.) Estradiol can also be administered in a percutaneous patch or gel for transdermal absorption (see Chap. 322). In women after hysterectomy progestogens are not necessary, but in women with a uterus, a progestogen (e.g., medroxyprogesterone 5 or 10 mg/d) may be added for the last 10 days of estrogen administration (see Chap. 322). Testosterone preparations are useful in treatment of osteoporotic men with gonadal deficiency, but there are no convincing reports of their efficacy in men with normal gonadal function. There is also no proven advantage to combinations of estrogens and androgens.

Calcium supplements, vitamin D metabolites, and thiazide diuretics Women who are estrogen-deprived require an average oral intake of 1500 mg/d of elemental calcium to remain in calcium equilibrium. The recommendation of the National Institutes of Health of 1000 mg elemental calcium per day for women on estrogen replacement and for men is reasonable. In postmenopausal women unable to take estrogens, the use of 1500 mg/d of oral calcium may have minor benefit in preserving cortical bone mass but has no effects on trabecular bone mass. Adequate calcium intake before age 30 to 35 may have beneficial effects on the attainment of peak bone mass, however. The content of elemental calcium of available preparations varies, depending upon the accompanying anion and the composition (Table 341-2). Vitamin D preparations have been used in osteoporosis because calcium absorption is impaired and levels of the active

TABLE 341-2 Elemental calcium content of various oral calcium preparations

Calcium preparation	Elemental calcium content
Calcium citrate	40 mg/300 mg
Calcium carbonate	400 mg/g
Calcium lactate	80 mg/600 mg
Calcium gluconate	40 mg/500 mg
Calcium carbonate + 5 μg vitamin D_2 (Os – Cal 250)	250 mg/tablet

metabolite, $1,25(OH)_2D$, are marginally low in serum. The efficacy of vitamin D itself has never been established, although reports have appeared indicating that oral administration of calcitriol [$1,25(OH)_2D$] can improve intestinal calcium absorption, suppress bone resorption, and prevent bone loss in patients with postmenopausal osteoporosis. Bone formation is not increased, however, and at the dose used in one study (mean, 0.8 μg/d) hypercalcemia and hypercalciuria were complications. To establish whether beneficial effects would be achieved with lower doses of calcitriol would require additional study. Thiazide diuretics are useful in patients with high-turnover osteoporosis associated with hypercalciuria and secondary hyperparathyroidism. In the absence of secondary hyperparathyroidism the thiazide diuretics lower urinary calcium excretion, suppress parathyroid gland function, inhibit synthesis of $1,25(OH)_2D$, and reduce intestinal calcium absorption.

Calcitonin Calcitonin decreases bone resorption, and the use of salmon calcitonin in established osteoporosis has been recommended in doses of 50 units subcutaneously every other day. Only patients with high-turnover osteoporosis (elevated levels of serum osteocalcin, increased urinary hydroxyproline excretion, and increased total body retention of ^{99m}Tc-methylene diphosphonate) appear to respond with improvement in bone mass. Another approach involves the use of salmon calcitonin administered by nasal spray (200 units per day) to avoid injections.

Fluoride Fluoride ions are deposited in the skeleton where they become incorporated into the crystal lattice of hydroxyapatite, substituting for hydroxyl ions. This process results in a mineral phase of greater crystallinity. Sodium fluoride is also the only therapeutic agent that can stimulate osteoblastic proliferation and function and increase bone formation. Indeed, chronic ingestion of high amounts of fluoride ions, usually in endemic areas where fluoride content of drinking water is very high, produces a form of hyperostosis, with dense bones, exostoses, neurologic complications due to bony overgrowth, and ligament ossification. Increased amount of bone with excessive osteoid is evidence of stimulation of bone formation, and a decrease in the rate of new vertebral fractures suggests that the new bone is of reasonable structure. Not all patients respond and some develop side effects including knee, foot, and ankle pain attributed to microfractures; other patients cannot tolerate sodium fluoride because of nausea. An oral slow-release form is better tolerated with fewer gastrointestinal and rheumatologic complications. Sodium fluoride has been recommended only for treatment of established vertebral osteoporosis with symptomatic crush fracture syndrome that would not likely respond to other therapies. Caution about fluoride has been raised in view of increased incidence of hip fractures in some series.

RICKETS AND OSTEOMALACIA

Rickets and *osteomalacia* are disorders in which mineralization of the organic matrix of the skeleton is defective (Table 341-3). In *rickets* the growing skeleton is involved; defective mineralization occurs not only in bone but also in the cartilaginous matrix of the growth plate. The term *osteomalacia* is usually reserved for the disorder in the adult in whom the epiphyseal growth plates are closed.

A number of conditions result in rickets and/or osteomalacia such as inadequate dietary intake of vitamin D, inadequate exposure to solar ultraviolet radiation to form endogenous vitamin D, intestinal malabsorption of vitamin D, acquired and inherited disorders of vitamin D metabolism, inherited defects in the receptors for $1,25(OH)_2D$ in target tissues, chronic acidosis, renal tubular defects which produce hypophosphatemia or acidosis, aluminum intoxication, and chronic administration of anticonvulsants. In the renal tubular disorders rickets and osteomalacia develop in the presence of normal intestinal function and are not cured by treatment with doses of vitamin D adequate to cure deficiency rickets. Thus the term *vitamin D–resistant* (or

TABLE 341-3 Classification of rickets and osteomalacia

I Vitamin D deficiency
  A Dietary deficiency
  B Deficient endogenous synthesis
II Gastrointestinal
  A Small-intestinal diseases with malabsorption
  B Partial or total gastrectomy
  C Hepatobiliary disease
  D Chronic pancreatic insufficiency
III Disorders of vitamin D metabolism
  A Hereditary: pseudovitamin D deficiency or vitamin D dependency, types I and II
  B Acquired
    1 Anticonvulsants
    2 Chronic renal failure
IV Acidosis
  A Distal renal tubular acidosis (classic or type I)
  B Secondary forms of renal acidosis
  C Ureterosigmoidostomy
  D Drug-induced disease
    1 Chronic acetazolamide ingestion
    2 Chronic ammonium chloride ingestion
V Chronic renal failure
VI Phosphate depletion
  A Dietary: low phosphate intake plus ingestion of nonabsorbable antacids
  B Impaired renal tubular phosphate reabsorption
    1 Hereditary
      a X-linked hypophosphatemic rickets (vitamin D–resistant rickets)
      b Adult-onset vitamin D–resistant hypophosphatemic osteomalacia
    2 Acquired
      a Sporadic hypophosphatemic osteomalacia (phosphate diabetes)
      b Tumor-associated (oncogenous) rickets and osteomalacia
      c Neurofibromatosis
      d Fibrous dysplasia
VII Generalized renal tubular disorders (Fanconi's syndrome)
  A Primary renal
  B Associated with systemic metabolic abnormality
    1 Cystinosis
    2 Glycogenosis
    3 Lowe's syndrome
  C Systemic disorder with associated renal disease
    1 Hereditary
      a Inborn errors
        (1) Wilson's disease
        (2) Tyrosinemia
      b Neurofibromatosis
    2 Acquired
      a Multiple myeloma
      b Nephrotic syndrome
      c Transplanted kidney
    3 Intoxications
      a Cadmium
      b Lead
      c Outdated tetracycline
VIII Primary mineralization defects
  A Hereditary: hypophosphatasia
  B Acquired
    1 Diphosphonate (disodium etidronate) treatment
    2 Fluoride treatment
IX States of rapid bone formation with or without a relative defect in bone resorption
  A Postoperative hyperparathyroidism with osteitis fibrosa cystica
  B Osteopetrosis
X Defective matrix synthesis: fibrogenesis imperfecta ossium
XI Miscellaneous
  A Magnesium-dependent conditions
  B Axial osteomalacia
  C Parenteral alimentation
  D Aluminum intoxication

–refractory) *rickets* has been applied in these instances. Renal insufficiency, especially in children, and chronic hemodialysis per se are also associated with rickets or osteomalacia.

PATHOGENESIS AND HISTOPATHOLOGY For skeletal mineralization, sufficient calcium and phosphate must be present at the mineralization sites. Other conditions required for normal mineralization include intact metabolic and transport functions of osteoblasts and chondrocytes, adequate collagen matrix, possibly phosphorylation or other modifications of matrix components, and low concentrations of inhibitory substances such as proteoglycan aggregates or inorganic pyrophosphate. A specific function in the mineralization process for the γ-carboxyglutamic acid–containing proteins (e.g., osteocalcin, osteonectin, and phospho-sialoproteins) synthesized by bone cells has not been demonstrated, although they bind calcium ions. In cartilage the initial mineral phase is in membrane-bound extracellular vesicles. If the osteoblast continues to produce matrix components that cannot be adequately mineralized, rickets and osteomalacia result. If calcification continues to be inadequate, the production of organic matrix (osteoid) also gradually decreases. In bone there will be an increase in the fraction of the forming surface covered by incompletely mineralized osteoid, an increase in osteoid volume and thickness (the latter normally less than 12 to 14 μm), and a decrease in the calcification or mineralization front. The latter is detected in undemineralized sections by the fluorescence of previously ingested tetracycline or by special stains. There is a marked decrease in the rate of apposition of mineralized bone. A variety of methods are available to measure the thickness of the osteoid seams and the calcification front. In histologic sections stained with hematoxylin and eosin, the more heavily mineralized areas tend to appear violet or blue, whereas the osteoid seams appear pink. Subtle degrees of osteomalacia may not be appreciated with routine preparations, and undecalcified, thin sections (3 to 5 μm) stained, for example, with Goldner's trichrome method are necessary to establish its presence (Fig. 341-2). Rickets is also characterized by inadequate mineralization of the matrix of cartilage in the growing epiphyseal plate. Calcification in the interstitial regions of the hypertrophic zone is defective, the growth plate increases in thickness, the columns of cartilage cells (usually highly ordered) are disorganized, and there is

FIGURE 341-2 Photomicrograph of an undemineralized section stained with Goldner method of an iliac crest bone biopsy from a 45-year-old man with chronic renal failure maintained on hemodialysis. Almost the entire surface is covered by osteoid (O) readily distinguished from mineralized bone (MB). The thickness of the osteoid seams exceeds 100 μm in several areas.

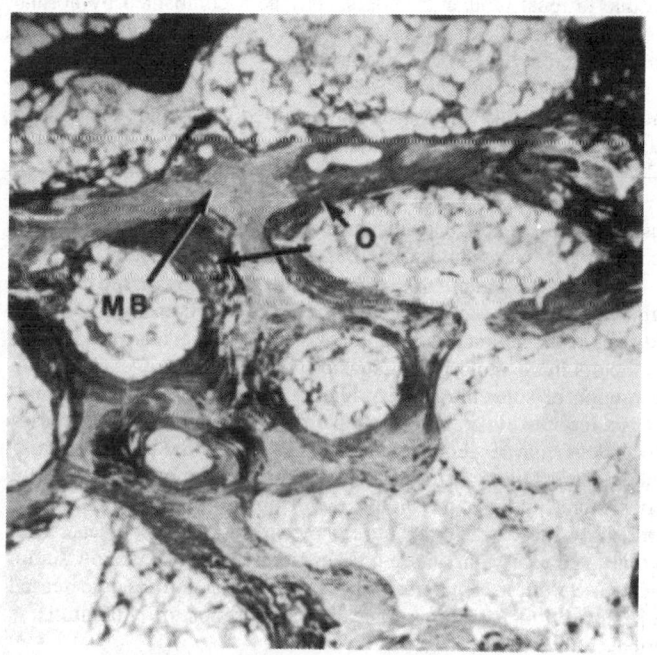

a variable cupping of the epiphyses. The rachitic bones are often incapable of withstanding usual mechanical stresses and tend to undergo bowing deformities. If rickets is untreated, growth at the epiphyseal plates is slowed, and the eventual length of the long bones is diminished.

It has not been established whether vitamin D, through one of its metabolites, has a major direct effect on mineralization. Its primary roles after metabolic conversion to 25(OH)D and 1,25(OH)$_2$D are to regulate and enhance absorption of calcium ions from the intestinal lumen and, possibly, to enhance differentiation of stem cells to form osteoclasts. Insufficiency of the active metabolites of vitamin D leads to decreased intestinal absorption of calcium and decreased mobilization of calcium from bone, resulting in hypocalcemia. This stimulates increased synthesis and secretion of parathyroid hormone (PTH) and hyperplasia of the parathyroid glands. The increased circulating concentration of PTH tends to increase plasma calcium and enhances renal phosphate clearance, which, in turn, produces hypophosphatemia. When the concentration of phosphorus in the extracellular fluid falls below a critical level, mineralization cannot proceed normally. In severe vitamin D deficiency, normal levels of serum calcium cannot be maintained, and the driving force for mineralization is further decreased. The absence of some critical metabolite of vitamin D that acts directly on the skeleton may also play a role in the defective mineralization of rickets and osteomalacia.

Phosphate depletion alone can produce osteomalacia as in patients consuming large amounts of nonabsorbable antacids and in patients with excessive renal loss of phosphate due to decreased tubular reabsorption. Secondary hyperparathyroidism is usually not present in these patients. Hypophosphatemia per se produces mineralization defects despite its effect on increasing the activity of the renal 25(OH)D-1α-hydroxylase, but it cannot account for the osteomalacia in all the disorders listed in Table 341-3. In chronic renal failure, for example, plasma phosphate levels are not decreased and usually are increased. Similarly, plasma phosphorus levels are not depressed in infants and children with osteomalacia secondary to hypophosphatasia, a hereditary deficiency in alkaline phosphatase. Osteomalacia in some patients with chronic renal failure is associated with accumulation of aluminum in bone, and the aluminum probably plays a role in production of the mineralization defect.

CLINICAL FINDINGS The clinical manifestations of rickets are the result of skeletal deformities, susceptibility to fractures, weakness and hypotonia, and disturbances in growth. In extreme instances of vitamin D–deficiency rickets, hypocalcemia may be sufficient to produce tetany which, when severe, may be accompanied by laryngeal spasm and convulsive seizures.

In infants and young children features include listlessness, irritability, and often profound hypotonia and muscular weakness. As the disorder progresses, children become unable to walk without support. Abnormal parietal flattening and frontal bossing develop in the skull. The calvaria are softened (craniotabes), and sutures may be widened. Prominence of the costochondral junctions is called the "rachitic rosary," and the indentation of the lower ribs at the site of attachment of the diaphragm is known as *Harrison's groove*. If untreated, progressive deformities of the pelvis and extremities result, with bowing particularly common in the tibia, femur, radius, and ulna. Fractures are frequent, dental eruption is often delayed, and enamel defects are common.

The presentation of osteomalacia in adults usually is not as dramatic as in infants and children. The skeletal deformities may be overlooked, and the features of the underlying disorder may dominate, as, for example, in the vitamin D deficiency of adult celiac disease. Symptoms, when they occur, include diffuse skeletal pain and bony tenderness. Pain may be prominent about the hips and result in an antalgic gait. Muscular weakness may be difficult to distinguish from hesitancy to move because of skeletal pain. Proximal weakness may mimic that of primary muscle disorders and contribute to the waddling gait. Pain and weakness may be sufficient to cause patients to be confined to bed and chair. Many factors, including the secondary hyperparathyroidism, contribute to the myopathy. Clinical improvement in the myopathy usually results from specific therapy such as vitamin D repletion in nutritional osteomalacia, phosphate replacement in renal hypophosphatemia, or correction of acidosis. Fractures of involved bones may occur with minimal trauma. When the ribs are involved, severe deformities may develop in the thoracic cage, and the collapse of vertebral bodies may produce loss of height.

RADIOLOGIC FEATURES   Radiologic changes reflect the pathologic changes. In rickets the alterations are most evident at the epiphyseal growth plate, which is increased in thickness, cupped, and hazy at the metaphyseal border due to decreased calcification of the hypertrophic zone and inadequate mineralization of the primary spongiosa. The trabecular pattern of the metaphyses is abnormal, the cortices of the diaphyses may be thinned, and the shafts may be bowed.

In osteomalacia decrease in bone density is usually associated with loss of trabeculae and variable thinning of the cortices. The radiologic changes may be indistinguishable from those in osteoporosis. Trabecular patterns may be blurred, producing a homogeneous ground glass appearance. The specific finding that suggests osteomalacia is the presence of radiolucent bands ranging from a few millimeters to several centimeters in length, usually perpendicular to the surface of the bones. They are particularly common at the inner aspects of the femur, especially near the femoral neck, in the pelvis, in the outer edge of the scapula, in the upper fibula, and in the metatarsals (Figs. 341-3 and 341-4). These radiolucent bands, called *pseudofractures* or *Looser's zones*, occur most often at sites where major arteries cross the bones and are thought to be due to the mechanical stress of the pulsation of these vessels. Subperiosteal

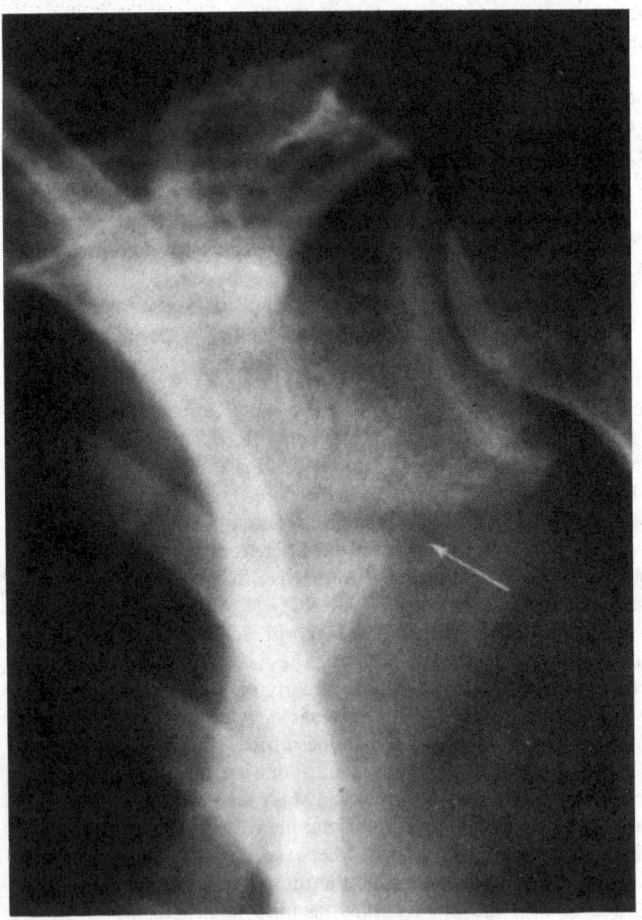

FIGURE 341-3   Radiographs of the scapula of a 58-year-old woman with phosphate diabetes. The presence of a pseudofracture or Looser's zone is indicated by the arrow.

erosions along the diaphyseal cortices are sometimes seen in secondary hyperparathyroidism.

Increased rather than decreased density of bones may be observed in patients with renal tubular disorders rather than with vitamin D deficiency and may produce a striking thickening of the cortices and trabeculae of spongy bone. Despite the increase in mass of bone per unit volume, the trabeculae are covered with thickened osteoid seams typical of osteomalacia. Similar findings may occur in patients with chronic renal failure. The reason for the hyperostosis is unknown; the bone is architecturally abnormal and subject to fracture with minimal trauma.

LABORATORY FINDINGS   Changes in serum concentrations of calcium, inorganic phosphorus, 25(OH)D, and 1,25(OH)$_2$D vary with the different disorders (see Chap. 339). In vitamin D deficiency, whether due to dietary lack, inadequate sunlight exposure, or intestinal malabsorption, serum calcium levels are normal or low, whereas phosphorus and 25(OH)D levels are characteristically low, the latter usually <12 nmol/L (<5 ng/mL) depending upon the assay. In contrast, levels of 1,25(OH)$_2$D may be normal or even elevated due to secondary hyperparathyroidism. Eventually, when levels of 25(OH)D become so low that there is inadequate substrate for the renal 25(OH)D-1α-hydroxylase, then the serum level of 1,25(OH)$_2$D will also decline. In adults the lower limit of serum phosphorus concentration is around 0.9 mmol/L (2.8 mg/dL); in children the lower limit of normal is closer to 1.3 to 1.5 mmol/L (4.0 to 4.5 mg/dL). In *severe* vitamin D depletion, hypocalcemia may be sufficient to produce tetany. Mild acidosis and generalized aminoaciduria also result from secondary hyperparathyroidism. As a rule, patients with renal tubular disorders maintain normal serum calcium levels, while hypophosphatemia is characteristic. Other laboratory findings such as glucosuria, aminoaciduria, acidosis, and hypouricemia reflect variable degrees of disturbance of proximal tubular function or features of the underlying disease (e.g., low plasma ceruloplasmin in Wilson's disease or abnormalities of immunoglobulins in multiple myeloma). In chronic renal failure hyperphosphatemia and some degree of hypocalcemia are usually accompanied by normal 25(OH)D and low 1,25(OH)$_2$D levels. In nephrotic syndrome serum 25(OH)D levels can be low due primarily to urinary losses of protein-bound 25(OH)D. Serum phosphorus levels are also normal or elevated in hypophosphatasia. Increased excretion of hydroxyproline-containing peptides occurs in those conditions in which secondary hyperparathyroidism and excessive bone resorption are associated with the defect in mineralization. Alkaline phosphatase levels in plasma are usually elevated in rickets or osteomalacia, but typical and even severe osteomalacia, especially that due to renal tubular disorders, may be accompanied by normal or only borderline elevations. Levels may increase during the early phases of therapy.

DIETARY VITAMIN D DEFICIENCY AND INADEQUATE ENDOGENOUS SYNTHESIS   Most foods unfortified with vitamin D contain insufficient amounts of the vitamin to prevent rickets in growing children or osteomalacia in adults living in temperate-zone cities. As discussed in Chap. 339, in the absence of supplements, vitamin D must be formed endogenously through the ultraviolet irradiation of precursor 7-dehydrocholesterol in the skin. Many factors decrease the formation of vitamin D$_3$ from its precursor: increased melanin pigmentation, hyperkeratosis, sunscreens, limited exposure of the body, short days of sunlight, oblique angle of ultraviolet irradiation, and factors in the atmosphere, such as smog, which prevent adequate penetration of solar ultraviolet radiation. Since fortification of milk and routine use of vitamin D supplements for infants have been in effect, deficiency rickets is unusual in the United States. Poor, dark-skinned infants living in crowded northern cities are most susceptible. Furthermore, elderly individuals with insufficient sun exposure, particularly those who are housebound or in nursing homes, drink no milk, and receive no vitamin D supplements, may have low serum levels of 25(OH)D, secondary hyperparathyroidism, and increased frequency of hip fractures. Intestinal absorption of vitamin D is normal in the elderly.

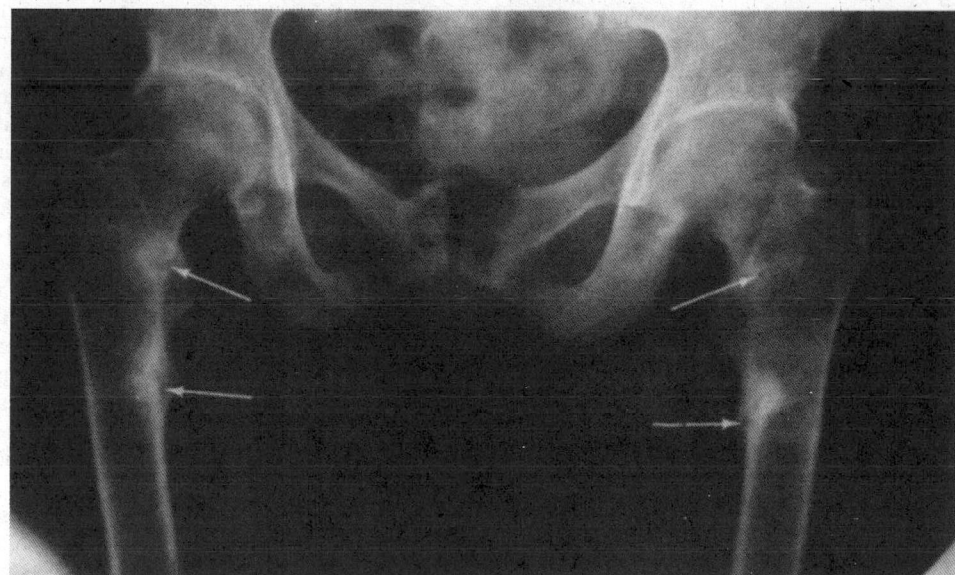

FIGURE 341-4 Radiograph of the femurs of a 47-year-old woman with Fanconi's syndrome of adult onset. The presence of multiple pseudofractures is indicated by the arrows.

VITAMIN D LOSS AND INTESTINAL MALABSORPTION Osteomalacia may be seen in patients with intestinal malabsorption such as in adult celiac disease and regional enteritis. Prior to the discovery of gluten sensitivity in some of these cases, celiac disease was among the more common disorders underlying osteomalacia. Vitamin D absorption, which normally occurs via chylomicrons, is impaired in diseases causing steatorrhea where emulsification of fat is disturbed, such as chronic biliary obstruction. Patients with cholestatic liver disease or extrahepatic biliary obstruction may have low serum levels of 25(OH)D and osteomalacia, due not only to poor vitamin D absorption but also to decreased hepatic production of 25(OH)D. Osteomalacia is less frequent in chronic pancreatic insufficiency. Patients who have had gastric surgery for peptic ulcer disease or gastric bypass for obesity may also develop osteomalacia, possibly due to malfunction of the proximal small bowel. Factors other than failure to absorb vitamin D may contribute to the osteomalacia in patients with small-bowel disease, such as inadequate absorbing surface and failure of intestinal cells to respond to the active metabolites of vitamin D. Secondary hyperparathyroidism is usually present in intestinal malabsorption, as it is in dietary lack of vitamin D, and may be particularly severe in patients who develop osteomalacia following intestinal bypass surgery. Some patients who lack vitamin D, usually associated with intestinal malabsorption, have normal circulating levels of $1,25(OH)_2D$, despite low or undetectable 25(OH)D. In these individuals the normal levels of $1,25(OH)_2D$ may be accounted for by ingestion of sufficient vitamin D in hospital diets to produce substrate 25(OH)D for 1α-hydroxylation by the renal enzyme that is increased in activity due to secondary hyperparathyroidism. In other patients, circulating $1,25(OH)_2D$ levels may not reflect levels at critical target cells.

ABNORMAL METABOLISM OF VITAMIN D Serum 25(OH)D levels are reduced in some instances of parenchymal and obstructive liver disease, but these findings have not yet been correlated with quantitative histologic studies of bone. Patients consuming anticonvulsant drugs such as phenobarbital, phenytoin, or carbamazepine may develop rickets or osteomalacia. For a given intake of vitamin D, patients receiving chronic anticonvulsant drugs have lower serum levels of calcium and 25(OH)D. Consumption of anticonvulsants may be especially important in individuals whose intake of vitamin D is marginal, who are nonambulatory and confined indoors, who have chronic recurrent infections, or in whom mild intestinal malfunction exists as in the postgastrectomy state. As discussed in Chap. 339 the anticonvulsant drugs have multiple actions on calcium homeostasis.

Two autosomal recessive syndromes associated with rickets have been termed *vitamin D–dependent rickets* (also see Chap. 311).

Features of *type I vitamin D–dependent rickets* include hypocalcemia, hypophosphatemia, short stature, skeletal deformities of rickets, dental enamel hypoplasia, frequently marked elevations of serum alkaline phosphatase activity, generalized aminoaciduria, and secondary hyperparathyroidism. Treatment with massive doses of vitamin D or small doses of calcitriol reverses the abnormal biochemical findings, induces healing of the rickets, and restores the rate of skeletal growth. The abnormalities are due to mutations that impair the renal 25(OH)D-1α-hydroxylase. *Type II vitamin D–dependent rickets*, also termed *hereditary resistance to $1,25(OH)_2D$*, has many clinical features of the type I syndrome. Rickets is usually of early onset but varies in severity in different kindreds. Distinguishing features include alopecia, which may develop during the first few months of age, and multiple milia and epidermal cysts. The type II disorder is due to mutations that impair the $1,25(OH)_2D$ receptor. Different molecular abnormalities have been demonstrated in different kindreds including mutations that impair binding of the receptor to DNA and mutations that cause the formation of incomplete receptor molecules.

Abnormalities in vitamin D metabolism, not on a genetic basis, as well as osteomalacia may be found in patients on long-term total parenteral nutrition. Some of these individuals have hypoparathyroidism but this cannot account for the osteomalacia. Serum levels of 25(OH)D are normal although levels of $1,25(OH)_2D$ may be low. Aluminum has been detected in increased amounts in plasma, urine, and bone and may play a role in genesis of the osteomalacia similar to that postulated in patients with renal failure on chronic hemodialysis.

RENAL TUBULAR DISORDERS Rickets and osteomalacia occur in association with a variety of disorders of proximal renal tubular function. These disorders have in common increased renal clearance of inorganic phosphorus and hypophosphatemia with normal or near normal glomerular filtration rate. Increased phosphate clearance with resultant hypophosphatemia is usually an isolated defect with no other abnormalities except for increase in urinary glycine excretion (hyperglycinuria). X-linked hypophosphatemia (*phosphate diabetes* and *vitamin D–resistant rickets* are terms applied to these cases especially when the disorder presents in early childhood) is characterized by rickets that develops in an otherwise well-nourished, healthy-appearing child. When the child begins to walk and bear weight, lower limb deformities appear and become progressively worse. The rate of linear growth is at first normal and then slowed. The inheritance pattern is X-linked dominant. Many of these individuals develop a unique disorder of tendons, ligaments, and joint capsules characterized by calcification or, more probably, ossification of insertions of tendons and ligaments and joint capsules (enthesopathy). In some patients spontaneous remissions may be followed by recurrences in adult life associated, for example, with pregnancy and lactation. Hypophosphatemia is due to defective renal conservation of phosphate, which in turn is due to defective phosphate transport across the luminal membrane of proximal renal tubular cells. [A model of the human disease has been found in a strain of hypophosphatemic (Hyp) mice.] On the basis of analysis of RFLP studies in several kindreds of X-linked hypophosphatemia, the gene has been mapped to the short arm of the X chromosome (Xp22.31-p21.3). The sequence of the normal gene and the nature of the defect that leads to altered phosphate transport have not been elucidated. In affected individuals, the serum levels of 25(OH)D are normal, and the levels of $1,25(OH)_2D$ are in the low-normal range. Since the induction of hypophosphatemia in normal individuals results in stimulation of the 25(OH)D-1α-hydroxylase and an increase in the levels of $1,25(OH)_2D$, it has been proposed that altered renal tubular cellular phosphate fluxes that result from the mutation in X-linked hypophosphatemia fail to stimulate the hydroxylase. Thus, levels of $1,25(OH)_2D$, although in the normal range, are inappropriately low relative to the phosphate depletion. The skeletal mineralization defect is ascribable not only to the low ambient phosphate levels but also to an intrinsic defect in osteoblast function possibly related to that in the renal tubular cells. Effective therapy therefore requires combination of phosphate repletion with large amounts of oral phosphate, combined with supplements of calcitriol (see below). Combined therapy with calcitriol and inorganic phosphorus reverses the osteomalacia of trabecular bone surfaces, corrects the microscopic periosteocytic mineralization defects, and results in improvement in longitudinal growth. After the rickets is healed, however, defects in phosphate clearance and hypophosphatemia persist and medical therapy is still required. The effects of excessive calcitriol administration, such as nephrocalcinosis and nephrolithiasis, must be avoided. Adults with X-linked hypophosphatemia frequently have pseudofractures; osteoarthritis in the sacroiliac joints, wrists, knees, hips, and feet; and marked enthesopathy. Another variant of hereditary rickets has been termed *hereditary hypophosphatemic rickets with hypercalciuria*. Muscular weakness, not a feature of X-linked hypophosphatemia, may be present. These individuals, whose disorder is probably inherited as an autosomal recessive trait, have normocalcemia, hypophosphatemia, and striking absorptive hypercalciuria; the latter disappears after fasting and returns after oral calcium loading. Levels of $1,25(OH)_2D$ in serum are elevated in contrast to low-normal levels in X-linked hypophosphatemia. These elevations of serum $1,25(OH)_2D$ are an appropriate response of the 25(OH)D-1α-hydroxylase to phosphate depletion. Phosphate replacement induces healing of the rachitic lesions.

Sporadic cases of hypophosphatemia have also been described in adults in whom family histories are negative and where proximal muscle weakness is a prominent feature (also see Chap. 342). These patients also are best treated with a combination of calcitriol and inorganic phosphorus. As mentioned above, in most untreated patients with renal tubular disorders associated with rickets and osteomalacia, secondary hyperparathyroidism is not present.

In other patients the disorder in tubular function may be more widespread, involving (besides phosphorus) glucose, potassium, amino acids, and uric acid; the various combinations are termed the de Toni-Debré-Fanconi syndrome. The more complete renal tubular defects may occur sporadically or in families. In some instances the lesion is part of a more widespread disorder as in Wilson's disease and cystinosis. The acidosis of proximal tubular defects also plays a role in development of osteomalacia, possibly by altering metabolism of vitamin D or the renal handling of calcium and phosphorus. In this regard osteomalacia has accompanied the hyperchloremic acidosis of ureterocolic anastomosis.

TUMOR-ASSOCIATED (ONCOGENOUS) OSTEOMALACIA Osteomalacia and hypophosphatemia with high renal phosphate clearance occur with a variety of mesenchymal tumors. The latter have included giant cell tumors (benign or malignant), reparative granulomas, hemangiomas, fibromas, and other mesenchymal neoplasms. A similar syndrome occurs in patients with prostatic carcinoma. In some instances, removal of the tumor resulted in return of renal phosphorus clearance to normal, rise in serum phosphorus levels, and healing of the osteomalacia (or rickets in children). Serum $1,25(OH)_2D$ levels are low or undetectable, although chronic administration of sufficient calcitriol to raise circulating levels of this metabolite to normal does not alter renal phosphorus clearance or serum phosphorus concentrations. Humoral factors released by these tumors may impair proximal tubular functions such as 1α-hydroxylation of 25(OH)D *and* phosphate transport; removal of the tumor results in a return of serum $1,25(OH)_2D$ and phosphorus levels to normal.

CHRONIC RENAL FAILURE Osteomalacia is common in patients with chronic renal failure; it often tends to be the predominant type of renal osteodystrophy in younger patients and is more frequent in those with the lower plasma levels of calcium and phosphorus. A component of secondary hyperparathyroidism and osteitis fibrosa almost always accompanies the defect in mineralization. The defect itself probably involves a decreased conversion of 25(OH)D to $1,25(OH)_2D$ either because of insufficient viable renal cortical tissue or the inhibitory effect of hyperphosphatemia on renal 25(OH)D-1α-hydroxylase activity. In addition, there may be a primary defect in intestinal calcium absorption. Part of the secondary hyperparathyroidism may also be due to decreased phosphate clearance and subsequent hyperphosphatemia. Under circumstances of hyperphosphatemia and near-normal plasma concentration of calcium, the presence of inhibitors probably accounts for the defective mineralization. In some patients the osteomalacia responds to large doses of vitamin D or dihydrotachysterol or to small doses of calcitriol or calcifediol. However, some patients with renal osteodystrophy do not respond to pharmacologic doses of vitamin D or improve when given calcitriol. In some of these subjects accumulation of aluminum in the bone accounts for the vitamin D–refractory osteomalacia. Aluminum deposits can be identified at the mineralization fronts, and bone apposition rates are low. These individuals have high levels of aluminum accumulation and uncoupling of matrix deposition and mineralization. Individuals with lower amounts of aluminum develop a form of "aplastic" bone disease where matrix deposition and mineralization are more closely coupled. Deferoxamine can mobilize aluminum from bone and other tissues and is effective therapy of the aluminum osteodystrophy. In some patients with renal osteodystrophy the total bone mass may be increased (osteosclerosis), resulting in increased density of bone. This is particularly evident in the spine, where a characteristic appearance is that of dense bone at the superior and inferior margins of the vertebral bodies with more radiolucent central portions ("rugger jersey sign"). Histologically, although there is more bone per unit area, each trabecula is covered by an abnormally wide osteoid seam.

HYPOPHOSPHATASIA Rickets is a feature of a deficiency of alkaline phosphatase in infants and children, termed *hypophosphatasia*. There are four forms of hypophosphatasia, i.e., lethal perinatal, infantile, childhood, and adult. Rickets occurs in the infantile and childhood forms. In adults, the disorder may not be recognized until middle age, but there is frequently a history of early loss of deciduous or permanent teeth. Osteomalacia and calcium pyrophosphate deposition disease occur in the adult form. The severe perinatal and infantile forms are inherited as autosomal recessive traits; the pattern of inheritance in the other forms is uncertain. The low levels of circulating alkaline phosphatase activity are explained by a deficiency of the liver-bone enzyme due to defects in the alkaline phosphatase gene.

Although alkaline phosphatase is abundant in osteoclasts, its function in mineralization is not established. In hypophosphatasia there is increased urinary excretion of phosphoethanolamine and increased circulating levels of pyridoxal-5'-phosphate. The metabolic origin of the phosphoethanolamine is not established. Concentrations of pyridoxal-5'-phosphate are not elevated intracellularly, and the extracellular increases are consistent with the function of alkaline phosphatase as an ectoenzyme; whether alterations of pyridoxal-5'-phosphate metabolism contribute to the clinical abnormalities in hypophosphatasia is not known. Inorganic pyrophosphate (PPi) is a substrate for alkaline phosphatase, which accounts for increased levels of PPi in urine and plasma and for the increased incidence of calcium pyrophosphate deposition disease in hypophosphatasia. Since PPi can also function to inhibit growth of the calcium-phosphate mineral phase, excessive concentrations of PPi may cause the rickets and osteomalacia. There is no effective therapy.

OTHER DISORDERS ASSOCIATED WITH DEFECTIVE MINERALIZATION Disturbances in mineralization may be seen in patients consuming high doses of fluoride ion and in patients with Paget's disease treated with diphosphonates such as etidronate. Some decrease in mineralization of newly forming matrix, increase in surface covered by osteoid, and increase in the width of the osteoid seams occur in conditions that are not usually considered as osteomalacia except by these criteria. Biopsies in some of these conditions show a normal calcification front. Examples include patients with the osteitis fibrosa of hyperparathyroidism following surgical cure. In these circumstances there is a temporary imbalance between the rate at which mineral is supplied to bone and the rate at which bone matrix is formed. Wide osteoid seams and hypophosphatemia are also seen in children with osteopetrosis in whom there is inadequate resorption of bone and calcified cartilage but active bone formation.

A condition that resembles osteomalacia and is associated with a coarsened, mottled bony trabecular pattern, pseudofractures, and bone pain but normal plasma levels of calcium and phosphorus is *fibrogenesis imperfecta ossium*. The bone has a distinctive histologic appearance, with wide osteoid seams, distortion of the birefringent pattern of normal bone, and abnormal collagen fibers by electron microscopy. The nature of the abnormality is not known.

TREATMENT OF RICKETS AND OSTEOMALACIA In rickets and osteomalacia due to dietary absence of vitamin D or inadequate exposure to sunlight, vitamin D_2 (cholecalciferol) or vitamin D_3 (ergocalciferol) is given orally in doses of 2000 to 4000 IU (0.05 to 0.1 mg) daily for 6 to 12 weeks, followed by daily supplements of 200 to 400 IU, which are adequate to prevent the development of the disorder in otherwise normal subjects. In infants and children such treatment causes improvement in muscle tone and strength, increase in serum calcium and phosphorus, and decrease in alkaline phosphatase levels after several weeks. Radiologic evidence of healing is first noted within weeks and may be complete by a few months. Calcium supplements and larger initial doses of vitamin D may be necessary in infants and children with tetany. In adults with nutritional osteomalacia healing of pseudofractures may be evident within 3 to 4 weeks after therapy with as little as 2000 IU (0.05 mg) vitamin D daily. Healing is complete usually by 6 months.

Patients with osteomalacia due to intestinal malabsorption do not respond to the relatively small doses of vitamin D that can cure osteomalacia due to dietary absence or inadequate sunlight. In the presence of active steatorrhea, daily oral doses of vitamin D of 50,000 to 100,000 IU (1.25 to 2.5 mg) and large doses of calcium (e.g., 15 g calcium lactate or 4 g calcium carbonate orally per day) may be required. In some instances oral vitamin D is ineffective, and the parenteral route is required (e.g., 10,000 IU intramuscularly per day). Another approach is the use of artificial ultraviolet B irradiation or exposure to sunlight in addition to supplemental calcium. Small doses of calcitriol (0.5 to 1.0 μg daily) are usually effective in this form of osteomalacia. Inorganic phosphate therapy is not indicated either in deficiency or in intestinal malabsorption of the vitamin, since hypocalcemia will develop and intestinal calcium absorption will remain inadequate. In all patients in whom large doses of vitamin D are used, periodic monitoring of serum calcium and 25(OH)D levels is essential. Semiquantitative urinary calcium measurements alone are inadequate.

In patients on anticonvulsants, it is usually necessary to continue the drugs while adding supplemental vitamin D and to monitor levels of serum calcium and serum 25(OH)D until a therapeutic response (evidence of radiologic healing, improvement in symptoms) is obtained. Doses varying from 4000 to 40,000 IU daily have been recommended.

Treatment of rickets and osteomalacia in the presence of renal tubular disorders is more difficult. In the past, the X-linked form of hypophosphatemic osteomalacia was treated with large doses of vitamin D (from 50,000 to several hundred thousand IU or more daily), but skeletal responses were rarely complete. The use of dihydrotachysterol, a pseudo-1α(OH)D analogue, 0.2 to 0.6 mg orally per day, in place of vitamin D had the advantage of shorter onset and duration of action and more consistent skeletal healing. With vitamin D therapy alone radiologic evidence of healing in many patients is incomplete; some hypophosphatemia persists, linear skeletal growth remains abnormally slow, and bony deformities continue to develop. In addition, hypercalcemia and its consequences are potential hazards. Currently oral supplements of inorganic phosphate in divided doses of phosphorus, 1.0 to 3.6 g/d, and calcitriol, 0.5 to 2.0 μg/d, constitute the best regimen. Restoration of skeletal growth and healing of the bone disease result. In some adults, therapy with inorganic phosphate alone abolishes muscle weakness and bone pain and produces radiologic and histologic healing. The addition of calcitriol improves calcium balance and helps decrease secondary hyperparathyroidism and maintain a sufficient level of serum phosphorus to permit complete healing. In some patients there may be temporary increase in bone pain and rise in serum alkaline phosphatase during the early phases of treatment. In the osteomalacia associated with the chronic acidosis of renal tubular disorders, the use of alkali may be of value in supplementing therapy with phosphate and calcitriol. In patients with ureterosigmoidostomy, oral sodium bicarbonate can reverse acidosis, improve serum phosphate level, and heal the bone disease; with maintenance doses of alkali, recurrence of symptoms can be prevented.

Patients with nephrotic syndrome and low serum 25(OH)D levels benefit from modest vitamin D supplementation. In chronic renal failure high doses of vitamin D, similar to those needed to treat osteomalacia of renal tubular disorders, are used. Dihydrotachysterol at doses of 0.2 to 1.0 mg daily is effective in treating hypocalcemia and osteodystrophy resulting from chronic renal failure. Calcitriol in small doses is equally effective in most cases of renal osteodystrophy. The recommended initial dose is 0.25 μg/d. If after 2 to 4 weeks on this dose the biochemical parameters are unaltered, the dose is increased by 0.25 μg/d every 2 to 4 weeks until a satisfactory clinical biochemical response (including elevation of serum calcium levels and decrease in PTH levels) is obtained. The usual dose is 0.5 to 1.0 μg/d. Calcitriol may also be administered intravenously (1.0 to 2.5 μg three times weekly) in patients on dialysis, particularly to treat refractory osteitis fibrosa. Because there are no regulatory mechanisms to control the biological responses to calcitriol, there is a high incidence of transient hypercalciuria and hypercalcemia, especially initially. Thus, serum calcium should be monitored frequently during the first 1 to 2 months of therapy and less frequently once a stable dose has been established. Since calcitriol has a short duration of action and is not stored in fat depots, hypercalcemia usually resolves in 2 to 7 days after the dose is discontinued or decreased. Phosphate supplements are, of course, contraindicated in the usual patient with chronic renal failure. Occasionally, however, hypophosphatemia may result from the excessive use of nonabsorbable antacids or from excessive removal of phosphate through hemodialysis.

In patients who have had rickets in childhood, the abnormal mechanical stress of severe deformities may contribute to the development of degenerative joint disease, particularly in hips and knees. Osteotomies at the proper time after healing may prevent this complication and more extensive arthroplasties later in life.

REFERENCES

Osteoporosis

ALOIA JF et al: Risk factors for postmenopausal osteoporosis. Am J Med 78:95, 1985

—— et al: Calcitriol in the treatment of postmenopausal osteoporosis. Am J Med 84:401, 1988

AVIOLI LV, KRANE SM (eds): *Metabolic Bone Disease and Clinically Related Disorders.* Philadelphia, Saunders, 1990

BARZEL US: Estrogens in the prevention and treatment of postmenopausal osteoporosis: A review. Am J Med 85:847, 1988

BERGKVIST L et al: The risk of breast cancer after estrogen and estrogen-progestin replacement. N Engl J Med 321:293, 1989

BILLER BMK et al: Mechanisms of osteoporosis in adult and adolescent women with anorexia nervosa. J Clin Endocrinol Metab 68:548, 1989

BOIVIN G et al: Fluoride content in human iliac bone: Results in controls, patients with fluorosis, and osteoporotic patients treated with fluoride. J Bone Min Res 3:497, 1988

BUCHANAN JR et al: Effect of excess endogenous androgens on bone density in young women. J Clin Endocrinol Metab 67:937, 1988

CHEEMA C et al: Effects of estrogen on circulating "free" and total 1,25-dihydroxyvitamin D and on the parathyroid-vitamin D axis in postmenopausal women. J Clin Invest 83:537, 1989

CIVITELLI R et al: Effects of one-year treatment with estrogens on bone mass, intestinal calcium absorption, and 25-hydroxyvitamin D-1α-hydroxylase reserve in postmenopausal osteoporosis. Calcif Tissue Int 42:77, 1988

—— et al: Bone turnover in postmenopausal osteoporosis. Effect of calcitonin treatment. J Clin Invest 82:1268, 1988

COLE WG et al: New insights into the molecular pathology of osteogenesis imperfecta. Q J Med 70:1, 1989

DEMPSTER DW: Bone histomorphometry in glucocorticoid-induced osteoporosis. J Bone Min Res 4:137, 1989

DIAMOND T et al: Ethanol reduces bone formation and may cause osteoporosis. Am J Med 86:282, 1989

DRINKWATER BL et al: Bone mineral content of amenorrheic and eumenorrheic athletes. N Engl J Med 311:277, 1984

EASTELL R et al: Colles' fracture and bone density of the ultradistal radius. J Bone Min Res 4:607, 1989

Editorial: Risk factors in postmenopausal osteoporosis. Lancet 1:1370, 1985

ETTINGER B et al: Postmenopausal bone loss is prevented by treatment with low-dosage estrogen with calcium. Ann Intern Med 106:40, 1987

EVANS RA et al: Bone mass is low in relatives of osteoporotic patients. Ann Intern Med 109:870, 1988

FINKELSTEIN JS et al: Osteoporosis in men with idiopathic hypogonadotropic hypogonadism. Ann Intern Med 106:354, 1987

GALLAGHER JC et al: Epidemiology of fractures of the proximal femur in Rochester, Minnesota. Clin Orthopaed Rel Res 150:163, 1980

HEDLUND LR, GALLAGHER JC: Increased incidence of hip fracture in osteoporotic women treated with sodium fluoride. J Bone Min Res 4:223, 1989

HODSMAN AB, DROST DJ: The response of vertebral bone mineral density during the treatment of osteoporosis with sodium fluoride. J Clin Endocrinol Metab 69:932, 1989

HOLBROOK TL et al: Dietary calcium and risk of hip fracture: 14-year prospective population study. Lancet 2:1046, 1988

HUPPERT LC: Hormonal replacement therapy. Benefits, risks, doses. Med Clin North Am 71:23, 1987

JENSEN J et al: Cigarette smoking, serum estrogens, and bone loss during hormone-replacement therapy early after menopause. N Engl J Med 313:973, 1985

KANIS JA: Treatment of osteoporotic fracture. Lancet 1:27, 1984

KELLY TL et al: Quantitative digital radiography versus dual photon absorptiometry of the lumbar spine. J Clin Endocrinol Metab 67:839, 1988

KRANE SM, SCHILLER AL: Metabolic bone disease, in *Endocrinology*, 2d ed, LJ DeGroot et al (eds). Philadelphia, Saunders, 1989, vol 2, p 1151

KRØLNER B et al: Physical exercise as prophylaxis against involutional vertebral bone loss: A controlled trial. Clin Sci Mol Med 64:541, 1983

LINDSAY R et al: Prevention of spinal osteoporosis in oophorectomised women. Lancet 2:1151, 1980

MAMELLE N et al: Risk-benefit ratio of sodium fluoride treatment in primary vertebral osteoporosis. Lancet 2:361, 1988

MARIE PJ et al: Osteocalcin and deoxyribonucleic acid synthesis *in vitro* and histomorphometric indices of bone formation in postmenopausal osteoporosis. J Clin Endocrinol Metab 69:272, 1989

MCDERMOTT MT, KIDD GS: The role of calcitonin in the development and treatment of osteoporosis. Endocrine Rev 8:377, 1987

MUNDY GR: Identifying mechanisms for increasing bone mass. J NIH Res 1:65, 1989

NAGANT DE DEUXCHAISNES C: Therapy for skeletal disorders. Curr Opin Rheumatol 1:98, 1989

PAK CYC et al: Safe and effective treatment of osteoporosis with intermittent slow release sodium fluoride: Augmentation of vertebral bone mass and inhibition of fractures. J Clin Endocrinol Metab 68:150, 1989

PARFITT AM: Dietary risk factors for age-related bone loss and fractures. Lancet 2:1181, 1983

—— et al: Relationships between surface, volume, and thickness of iliac trabecular bone in aging and in osteoporosis: Implications for the microanatomic and cellular mechanisms of bone loss. J Clin Invest 72:783, 1985

POCOCK NA et al: Recovery from steroid-induced osteoporosis. Ann Intern Med 107:319, 1987

PROCKOP DJ: Mutations in collagen genes: Consequences for rare and common diseases. J Clin Invest 75:783, 1985

REEVE J et al: The assessment of bone formation and bone resorption in osteoporosis: A comparison between tetracycline-based iliac histomorphometry and whole body ^{85}Sr kinetics. J Bone Min Res 2:479, 1987

REGINSTER JY et al: Relationship between whole plasma calcitonin levels, calcitonin secretory capacity, and plasma levels of estrone in healthy women and postmenopausal osteoporotics. J Clin Invest 83:1073, 1989

RIGGS BL: Osteoporosis, in *Endocrinology*, 2d ed, LJ DeGroot et al (eds). Philadelphia, Saunders, 1989, vol 2, p 1188

——, MELTON LJ III: Evidence for two distinct syndromes of involutional osteoporosis. Am J Med 75:899, 1983

——, ——: Involutional osteoporosis. N Engl J Med 314:1676, 1986

—— et al: Effect of the fluoride/calcium regimen on vertebral fracture occurrence in postmenopausal osteoporosis: Comparison with conventional therapy. N Engl J Med 306:446, 1982

—— et al: Changes in bone mineral density of the proximal femur and spine with aging: Differences between the postmenopausal and senile osteoporosis syndromes. J Clin Invest 70:716, 1982

—— et al: Incidence of hip fractures in osteoporotic women treated with sodium fluoride. J Bone Min Res 2:123, 1987

RIIS B et al: Does calcium supplementation prevent postmenopausal bone loss? N Engl J Med 316:173, 1987

SAKHAEE K et al: Postmenopausal osteoporosis as a manifestation of renal hypercalciuria with secondary hyperparathyroidism. J Clin Endocrinol Metab 61:368, 1985

SEEMAN E et al: Risk factors for spinal osteoporosis in men. Am J Med 75:977, 1983

—— et al: Effect of early menopause on bone mass in normal women and patients with osteoporosis. Am J Med 85:213, 1988

SILVERBERG SJ et al: Abnormalities in parathyroid hormone secretion and 1,25-dihydroxyvitamin D$_3$ formation in women with osteoporosis. N Engl J Med 320:277, 1989

SMITH R et al: Osteoporosis of pregnancy. Lancet 1:1178, 1985

SPENCER H et al: Chronic alcoholism: Frequently overlooked cause of osteoporosis in men. Am J Med 80:393, 1986

STEINBERG KK et al: Sex steroids and bone density in premenopausal and perimenopausal women. J Clin Endocrinol Metab 69:533, 1989

STEPAN JJ et al: Castrated men exhibit bone loss: Effect of calcitonin treatment on biochemical indices of bone remodeling. J Clin Endocrinol Metab 69:523, 1989

STEWART AF et al: Calcium homeostasis in immobilization: An example of resorptive hypercalciuria. N Engl J Med 306:1136, 1982

WEINSTEIN RS, BELL NH: Diminished rates of bone formation in normal black adults. N Engl J Med 319:1698, 1988

WHITEHEAD MI, FRASER D: Controversies concerning the safety of estrogen replacement therapy. Am J Obstet Gynecol 156:1313, 1987

WILSON RJ et al: Mild asymptomatic primary hyperparathyroidism is not a risk factor for vertebral fractures. Ann Intern Med 109:959, 1988

Osteomalacia

ANDRESS DL et al: Osteomalacia and aplastic bone disease in aluminum-related osteodystrophy. J Clin Endocrinol Metab 65:11, 1987

—— et al: Intravenous calcitriol in the treatment of refractory osteitis fibrosa of chronic renal failure. N Engl J Med 321:274, 1989

CHARHON SA et al: Effects of parathyroidectomy on bone formation and mineralization in hemodialyzed patients. Kidney Int 27:426, 1984

DELVIN EE et al: Vitamin D nutritional status and related biochemical indices in an autonomous elderly population. Am J Clin Nutr 48:373, 1988

FRASER D, SCRIVER CR: Hereditary rickets and osteomalacia associated with abnormalities in vitamin D metabolism (calcipenic rickets) or phosphate homeostasis (phosphopenic rickets), in *Endocrinology*, 2d ed, LJ DeGroot et al (eds). Philadelphia, Saunders, 1989, vol 2, p 1080

GLORIEUX FH: Disturbances of phosphate metabolism—effects on bone, in *Metabolic Bone Disease: Cellular and Tissue Mechanism*, CS Tam et al (eds). Boca Raton, Fla, CRC Press, 1988, p 215

GODSALL JW et al: Vitamin D metabolism and bone histomorphometry in patients with antacid-induced osteomalacia. Am J Med 77:747, 1984

GOLDRING SR, KRANE SM: Disorders of calcification: Osteomalacia and rickets, in *Endocrinology*, 2d ed, LJ DeGroot et al (eds). Philadelphia, Saunders, 1989, vol 2, p 1165

HARDY DC et al: X-linked hypophosphatemia in adults: Prevalence of skeletal radiographic and scintigraphic features. Radiology 171:403, 1989

HARRELL RM et al: Healing of bone disease in X-linked hypophosphatemic rickets/osteomalacia: Induction and maintenance with phosphorus and calcitriol. J Clin Invest 75:1858, 1985

HARVEY JA et al: Lack of effect of 24,25-dihydroxyvitamin D$_3$ administration on parameters of calcium metabolism. J Clin Endocrinol Metab 69:467, 1989

HOCHBERG Z et al: 1,25-dihydroxyvitamin D resistance, rickets, and alopecia. Am J Med 77:805, 1984

rickets, and alopecia. Am J Med 77:805, 1984

HODSMAN AB et al: Vitamin D–resistant osteomalacia in hemodialysis patients lacking secondary hyperparathyroidism. Ann Intern Med 94:629, 1981

—— et al: Bone aluminum and histomorphometric features of renal osteodystrophy. J Clin Endocrinol Metab 54:439, 1982

KLEEREKOPER M, KRANE SM (eds): *Clinical Disorders of Bone and Mineral Metabolism.* New York, Mary Ann Liebert, 1989

KLEIN GL, COBURN JW: Metabolic bone disease associated with total parenteral nutrition. Adv Nutr Res 6:67, 1984

KUMAR R: Hepatic and intestinal osteodystrophy and the hepatobiliary metabolism of vitamin D. Ann Intern Med 98:662, 1983

LIPS P et al: The effect of vitamin D supplementation on vitamin status and parathyroid function in elderly subjects. J Clin Endocrinol Metab 67:644, 1988

MALLOY PJ et al: Abnormal binding of vitamin D receptors to deoxyribonucleic acid in a kindred with vitamin D–dependent rickets, type II. J Clin Endocrinol Metab 68:263, 1989

MARIE PJ, GLORIEUX FH: Relation between hypomineralized periosteocytic lesions and bone mineralization in vitamin D–resistant rickets. Calcif Tissue Int 35:433, 1983

MCELDUFF A, POSEN S: Parathyroid hormone sensitivity in familial X-linked hypophosphatemic rickets. J Clin Endocrinol Metab 69:386, 1989

MIYAUCHI A et al: Hemangiopericytoma-induced osteomalacia: Tumor transplantation in nude mice causes hypophosphatemia and tumor extracts inhibit renal 25-hydroxy-vitamin-1-hydroxylase activity. J Clin Endocrinol Metab 67:46, 1988

NORDAL KP, DAHL E: Low dose calcitriol versus placebo in patients with predialysis chronic renal failure. J Clin Endocrinol Metab 67:929, 1988

PARFITT AM et al: Metabolic bone disease with and without osteomalacia after intestinal bypass surgery: A bone histomorphometric study. Bone 6:211, 1985

POLISSON RP et al: Calcification of entheses associated with X-linked hypophosphatemic osteomalacia. N Engl J Med 313:1, 1985

PORTALE AA et al: Physiologic regulation of the serum concentration of 1,25-dihydroxy-vitamin D by phosphorus in normal men. J Clin Invest 83:1494, 1989

RALPHS JR et al: Ultrastructural features of the osteoid of patients with fibrogenesis imperfecta ossium. Bone 10:243, 1989

REICHEL H et al: The role of the vitamin D endocrine system in health and disease. N Engl J Med 320:980, 1989

RYAN EA, REISS E: Oncogeneous osteomalacia: Review of the world literature of 42 cases and report of two new cases. Am J Med 77:501, 1984

WHYTE MP: Hypophosphatasia, in The Metabolic Basis of Inherited Disease, 6th ed, CR Scriver et al (eds). New York, McGraw-Hill, 1989, p 2843

342 DISORDERS OF PHOSPHORUS METABOLISM

JAMES P. KNOCHEL

Phosphorus is the most abundant intracellular anion and is critical for membrane structure, transport, and energy storage. The role of phosphate ions in tissues explains the systemic nature of cellular injury consequent to phosphorus deficiency.

At a plasma pH of 7.4, inorganic phosphate in plasma is a 4:1 mixture of HPO_4^{2-} and $H_2PO_4^-$. The sum of the products of the valences of these ions ($4 \times 2^- + 1 \times 1^-$) divided by the sum of the ions ($4 + 1$) is equal to 9/5 or an average valence of 1.8. Of the average 700 g of phosphorus in the body, 85 percent is in the skeleton, about 15 percent is in soft tissues, and 0.1 percent is in extracellular fluid. The phosphorus that is in extracellular fluid is in a freely diffusible form that (1) permits excretion of hydrogen ions as phosphate buffer into the urine and (2) is in diffusion equilibrium with cytosolic inorganic phosphate in cells.

A normal adult consumes approximately 1 g of phosphorus each day. Soluble phosphates in dairy products and meat are almost completely absorbed, predominantly in the midjejunum. Insoluble phosphates, in vegetables and seeds, are absorbable provided the phosphate can be digested from its ligand. For example, phosphorus in corn and oats is contained partly as phytic acid; these foods contain little phytase, which splits phytic acid into phosphate and inositol, and hence phosphorus from this source may be poorly absorbed. Thus, corn and oats may be rachitogenic in man if they comprise the major components of the diet.

Phosphorus absorption is under the influence of vitamin D, and phosphorus excretion is under the control of parathyroid hormone. Parathyroid hormone decreases tubular phosphate reabsorption and increases excretion into the urine. The effect of vitamin D on phosphate reabsorption by the kidney is relatively minor. The quantity of soluble phosphorus available for absorption from the diet varies, and excretion of phosphorus in the urine on a given day depends directly upon absorption. Accordingly, the range for phosphorus excretion in health is very broad.

HYPOPHOSPHATEMIA

CAUSES Hypophosphatemia has many causes (Table 342-1). The finding of hypophosphatemia is not always a reliable indicator of deficiency since a total-body deficiency of phosphorus may exist in the face of hyperphosphatemia as, for example, in diabetic ketoacidosis.

Hypophosphatemia can be moderate or severe. Decreased dietary intake is an unusual cause of hypophosphatemia because of the ubiquitous and abundant distribution of the mineral in foods. Decreased absorption of phosphorus from the small intestine occurs in a variety of malabsorptive states, but simple diarrhea is usually not a cause. One of the most common causes of hypophosphatemia is respiratory alkalosis. Indeed, discovery of hypophosphatemia should lead to a search for potentially serious causes of hyperventilation such as sepsis or otherwise unsuspected alcohol withdrawal. Reduction of intracellular P_{CO_2} and elevation of pH increase the activity of phosphofructokinase, the rate-limiting enzyme of glycolysis. Phosphorylation of glucose intermediates causes cellular uptake of phosphorus and hypophosphatemia. Administration of insulin or nutrients

TABLE 342-1 Causes of hypophosphatemia

I Decreased dietary intake
II Decreased intestinal absorption
  A Vitamin D deficiency
  B Malabsorption
  C Steatorrhea
  D Secretory diarrhea
  E Vomiting
  F PO₄-binding antacids
III Shifts from serum into cells
  A Respiratory alkalosis
    1 Sepsis
    2 Alcohol withdrawal
    3 Heat stroke
    4 Neuroleptic malignant syndrome
    5 Hepatic coma
    6 Salicylate poisoning
    7 Gout
    8 Panic attacks
    9 Psychiatric depression
  B Hormonal effects
    1 Insulin
    2 Glucagon
    3 Epinephrine
    4 Androgens
    5 Cortisol
    6 Anovulatory hormones
  C Nutrient effects
    1 Glucose
    2 Fructose
    3 Glycerol
    4 Lactate
    5 Amino acids
    6 Xylitol
  D Cellular uptake syndromes
    1 Recovery from hypothermia
    2 Burkitt's lymphoma
    3 Histiocytic lymphoma
    4 Acute myelomonocytic leukemia
    5 Acute myelogenous leukemia
    6 Treatment of pernicious anemia
    7 Hungry bone syndrome
      a Following parathyroidectomy
      b Acute leukemia
IV Increased excretion into the urine
  A Hyperparathyroidism
  B Renal tubular defects
    1 Renal rickets
    2 Polyostotic fibrous dysplasia
    3 Postrenal transplantation
    4 Oncogenic osteomalacia
  C Aldosteronism
  D Licorice ingestion
  E Volume expansion
  F Inappropriate secretion of vasopressin
  G Mineralocorticoid administration
  H Glucocorticoid therapy
  I Diuretics

TABLE 342-2 Causes of severe hypophosphatemia

Chronic alcoholism and alcohol withdrawal
Dietary deficiency and phosphate-binding antacids
Severe thermal burns
Recovery from diabetic ketoacidosis
Hyperalimentation
Nutritional recovery syndrome
Respiratory alkalosis
Therapeutic hyperthermia
Neuroleptic malignant syndrome
Recovery from exhaustive exercise
Renal transplantation
Acute renal failure

TABLE 342-3 Hypophosphatemic syndromes

Phosphate trapping
Rhabdomyolysis
Cardiomyopathy
Respiratory insufficiency
Erythrocyte dysfunction
Leukocyte dysfunction
Skeletal demineralization
Metabolic acidosis
Nervous system dysfunction

that stimulate insulin release is also a common cause of hypophosphatemia. Insulin stimulates phosphorus uptake by cells. Cellular phosphorus uptake also occurs in patients recovering from hypothermia as a result of reactivation of metabolism. Certain rapidly growing malignancies may take up enough phosphate to cause hypophosphatemia. Deposition of bone mineral following parathyroidectomy may also be a cause. Parathyroid hormone and volume expansion may independently reduce tubular reabsorption of phosphorus. A number of other conditions typified by chronic volume expansion may cause hypophosphatemia.

Severe hypophosphatemia is defined as phosphorus levels in serum below 0.3 mmol/L (1.0 mg/dL). Many of the conditions that result in such low levels are associated with prolonged hyperventilation with respiratory alkalosis or reflect rapid cellular uptake (see Table 342-2). Respiratory alkalosis does not cause phosphorus deficiency, but may reduce serum phosphorus values to 0.1 mmol/L (0.3 mg/dL) and urinary phosphorus excretion to virtually undetectable levels. Severe hypophosphatemia and severe total body deficiency of phosphorus occur in patients with poor dietary intake who consume phosphate-binding antacids. Similarly, treatment of diabetic ketoacidosis results in hypophosphatemia. Reduction of serum phosphorus below 0.3 mmol/L (1.0 mg/dL) suggests but does not prove the existence of serious phosphorus depletion. In chronic alcoholics, reduction of phosphorus content of skeletal muscle may be associated with reduction of muscle magnesium and potassium and accumulations of calcium, sodium, chloride, and water. These findings are not necessarily associated with elevations of creatine phosphokinase activity that would reflect acute muscle damage. However, during withdrawal from alcohol, phosphorus is often taken up rapidly into skeletal muscle or liver, resulting in severe hypophosphatemia, and in this instance hypophosphatemia may precipitate acute rhabdomyolysis.

Most patients with diabetic ketoacidosis are not severely depleted of phosphorus. Although, on the one hand, metabolic acidosis and insulin deficiency mobilize intracellular phosphate stores and lead to their excretion into the urine, most patients have not been sick long enough for severe phosphorus deficiency to occur. On the other hand, the existence of hypophosphatemia and hypokalemia, despite severe diabetic ketoacidosis, reflects severe body depletion of phosphorus and potassium that demands treatment. The history usually shows that this type of patient with diabetic ketoacidosis has been sick for many days, has not had significant vomiting, has been able to maintain a good intake of fluids, and has excreted phosphorus briskly for a period of many days, thus establishing severe deficiency. Such patients probably represent no more than 5 percent of all cases of diabetic ketoacidosis.

MANIFESTATIONS The major manifestations of phosphorus deficiency are listed in Table 342-3; it should be appreciated that many of these can occur simultaneously.

Phosphate trapping is an acute disorder resulting from reduction of intracellular inorganic phosphate concentration. The most common cause is administration of intravenous fructose. Fructose is metabolized by only three tissues in the body—the liver, the small bowel epithelium, and the proximal tubule of the kidney. When glucose is taken up into liver cells and phosphorylated by hexokinase, the

resulting glucose-6-phosphate inhibits hexokinase, producing a smoothly regulated uptake of glucose that does not deplete or trap stores of inorganic phosphate. When fructose is administered intravenously, it is taken up into liver cells where it is converted to fructose-1-phosphate by the enzyme fructokinase. Fructose-1-phosphate does not inhibit fructokinase, thus permitting rapid uptake of fructose into liver cells and trapping of available stores of inorganic phosphate. Reduced intracellular phosphate concentration activates AMP deaminase and nucleotidase. The consequent reduction of adenylate compounds is reflected by increased uric acid production and hyperuricemia. Acute liver cell damage may occur. Disturbances of renal function may also occur after intravenous fructose. Hepatic and renal metabolic disturbances that follow fructose administration are preventable by infusing inorganic phosphate. Whether large concentrations of oral fructose affect intestinal epithelium in a similar manner has not been examined.

Rhabdomyolysis predictably occurs in chronic alcoholics who become acutely hypophosphatemic during the course of alcohol withdrawal. Hypophosphatemic rhabdomyolysis occurs rarely during treatment for diabetic ketoacidosis, during the course of hyperalimentation, or while refeeding patients with malnutrition. In alcoholics, evidence of muscle cell injury has preceded the occurrence of hypophosphatemia. Presumably, severe hypophosphatemia triggers induction of acute rhabdomyolysis. This syndrome can be reproduced experimentally. It does not occur if hypophosphatemia is prevented during hyperalimentation.

Cardiomyopathy occurs in severe phosphorus depletion. The usual manifestations include reduction in cardiac output, hypotension, impaired pressor responsiveness to catecholamines, and a reduced threshold to ventricular arrhythmias.

Respiratory insufficiency is a hypophosphatemic syndrome in malnourished patients receiving intravenous nutrients with inadequate phosphorus who become progressively hypophosphatemic over 8 or 10 days. Profound weakness causes failure of diaphragm function, hypoxia, and respiratory acidosis. Despite severe hypophosphatemia, these patients rarely develop rhabdomyolysis, presumably because they had no preexistent muscle damage. The initial clue to this complication may be inability to extubate a patient from a ventilator at the anticipated time. This syndrome is seldom seen in chronic alcoholics because rhabdomyolysis in such patients may correct hypophosphatemia spontaneously. Rapid correction of chronic respiratory acidosis may also cause hypophosphatemia and diaphragm weakness. In these patients, administration of phosphorus rapidly corrects muscle weakness and respiratory insufficiency.

Erythrocyte dysfunction is due to a decrease in 2,3-diphosphoglycerate (2,3-DPG) content. The red cell is the only tissue in the body that produces this substance. Both 2,3-DPG and ATP facilitate dissociation of oxyhemoglobin and promote oxygen delivery to tissue. Reduced 2,3-DPG and ATP both enhance affinity of oxygen for hemoglobin and reduce tissue oxygenation. This mechanism may explain central nervous system dysfunction in hypophosphatemia. Hemolysis due to phosphorus deficiency probably does not occur.

Leukocyte dysfunction due to phosphorus deficiency results in impaired phagocytosis and opsonization. As a result, chronic hypophosphatemia increases susceptibility to bacterial fungal infections.

Skeletal demineralization is an important effect of phosphorus deficiency, especially in patients with a poor dietary intake who simultaneously ingest phosphate-binding antacids. Under conditions of increased bone turnover, in normal children or in adults with Paget's disease, hyperparathyroidism, or bony metastases, demineralization may occur at such a rate as to cause hypercalcemia. Osteopenia, bone pain, and a syndrome resembling osteomalacia occur in chronic phosphorus deficiency.

Metabolic acidosis may occur in children or adults with phosphorus deficiency due to vitamin D deficiency. Reduced phosphorus intake results in mobilization of hydroxyapatite from bone that serves to maintain normal levels of serum phosphorus. Hypercalciuria occurs normally as a result of phosphorus deprivation. Severe hypophosphatemia has two important metabolic effects on the kidney. First, inorganic phosphate excretion into the urine falls so that hydrogen excretion as NaH_2PO_4 into the urine is eliminated. Second, phosphorus deficiency also elevates renal intracellular pH, which results in a profound decrease in ammonia production. The reduction in ammonia production eliminates hydrogen excretion as ammonium ions (NH^{4+}). Since excretion of hydrogen as phosphate buffer or ammonium accounts for nearly all of the kidney's capacity to secrete acid, it is surprising that phosphorus deficiency is only rarely associated with metabolic acidosis. The explanation lies in the fact that mobilization of hydroxyapatite from bone provides carbonate ions; they in turn buffer the retained hydrogen ions that otherwise would be excreted in the urine. Under conditions in which hydroxyapatite cannot be mobilized during phosphorus deprivation (e.g., vitamin D deficiency, severe magnesium deficiency, and perhaps aluminum poisoning), buffer cannot be mobilized adequately, and metabolic acidosis ensues.

Nervous system dysfunction is one of the most distinctive and predictable abnormalities in severe hypophosphatemia and phosphorus deficiency. This syndrome usually occurs in the setting of refeeding or hyperalimentation-induced hypophosphatemia that develops over the course of 8 to 10 days. Such patients become irritable and apprehensive and hyperventilate sufficiently to cause paresthesias and numbness. Profound muscular weakness is followed by dysarthria, confusion, obtundation, convulsive seizures, coma, and death. Alternatively, ascending motor paralysis with or without sensory disturbances may resemble the Guillain-Barré syndrome. In such cases, the cerebrospinal fluid is normal. Ophthalmoplegia, diplopia, and dysphagia suggest botulism, and poorly defined defects in color perception (metachromatopsia) suggests cerebral cortical dysfunction. In these patients, as in those with respiratory failure, spontaneous rhabdomyolysis does not occur despite severe hypophosphatemia.

TREATMENT Before initiating treatment for hypophosphatemia, the cause should be ascertained. Measurement of arterial pH and blood gases and of phosphorus concentration in the urine are helpful.

Milk is an excellent source of phosphorus, containing 33 mmol/L (100 mg/dL). Phosphate salts are also available for oral use. They are less likely to cause diarrhea in a phosphorus-deficient patient than in a normal person. Phosphorus salts cannot be given by intramuscular or subcutaneous injection, but sodium phosphate and potassium phosphate are available for intravenous use. The potassium salt should be given when hypokalemia and hypophosphatemia coexist. A safe dosage regimen for treatment of alcoholics who are hypophosphatemic, hypokalemic, and hypomagnesemic is the infusion each 8 to 12 h of 1 L of 0.5 normal NaCl in 5% glucose containing 9 mmol of potassium phosphate and 4.2 mmol $MgSO_4$ (2.0 mL of 50% $MgSO_4$ solution). Serum concentrations of potassium, magnesium, and phosphate should be closely monitored. Such infusions should be stopped when oral intake becomes possible.

Hyperphosphatemia should be avoided since it can cause severe hypocalcemia and crystal deposition in important structures including blood vessels, the eye, lung, heart, and kidney. Fatal alveolar diffusion block has occurred, especially if the patient is alkalotic.

HYPERPHOSPHATEMIA

Causes of hyperphosphatemia include renal insufficiency, hypoparathyroidism, pseudohypoparathyroidism, active untreated acromegaly,

overmedication with phosphate salts, and acute tissue destruction. The latter instance occurs in rhabdomyolysis and during treatment for malignancy. Hyperphosphatemia in untreated diabetic ketoacidosis is best explained by cellular release of phosphorus because of acidosis and volume depletion.

Hyperphosphatemia is treated by dietary restriction, employment of phosphate-binding antacids, promotion of excretion by fluid administration, correction of acidosis, and administration of insulin.

REFERENCES

BLACHLEY JD et al: The harmful effects of ethanol on ion transport and cellular respiration. Am J Med Sci 289:22, 1985

BODE JC et al: Depletion of liver adenosine phosphates and metabolic effects of intravenous infusion of fructose or sorbitol in man and in the rat. Eur J Clin Invest 3:436, 1973

FULLER TJ et al: Reversible depression in myocardial performance in dogs with experimental phosphorus deficiency. J Clin Invest 62:1194, 1978

KNOCHEL JP : Hypophosphatemia in the alcoholic. Arch Intern Med 140:613, 1980

——— : The clinical status of hypophosphatemia. N Engl J Med 313:447, 1985

——— : Hypophosphatemia and phosphorus deficiency, in *The Kidney*, 4th ed, B Brenner, F Rector (eds). Philadelphia, Saunders, 1990

KONO N et al: Alteration of glycolytic intermediary metabolism in erythrocytes during diabetic ketoacidosis and its recovery phase. Diabetes 30:346, 1981

LOTZ M et al: Evidence for a phosphorus depletion syndrome in man. N Engl J Med 278:409, 1968

NEWMAN JH et al: Acute respiratory failure associated with hypophosphatemia. N Engl J Med 296:1101, 1977

VEECH RL et al: Cytosolic phosphorylation potential. J Biol Chem 254:6538, 1979

WEINSIER RL, KRUMDIECK CL : Death resulting from overzealous total parenteral nutrition: The refeeding syndrome revisited. Am J Clin Nutr 34:393, 1980

343 DISORDERS OF MAGNESIUM METABOLISM

JAMES P. KNOCHEL

Magnesium (Mg) is the most abundant intracellular divalent cation. The total magnesium content of a normal man is about 12.4 mmol (25 meq) per kilogram body weight. Of this, 1 percent is extracellular, 31 percent is in cells, and 67 percent is in bone. Serum magnesium ranges between 0.62 and 1 mmol/L (1.2 to 2.0 meq/L). Of this, the unbound diffusible concentration is about 0.6 mmol/L (1.2 meq/L). It exists in two forms in cells, one in solution which is in equilibrium with the diffusible form in plasma and a larger quantity bound to organic components. Since most magnesium inside cells is bound to ATP, in accordance with the principle of mass action, MgATP is in equilibrium with free magnesium ions. Thus, shifts in free magnesium concentration may help regulate stores of ATP. Since ATP is critical to nearly all metabolic transformations, a normal concentration of serum magnesium is essential for normal function. Magnesium ions may also act as cofactors that modify the activity of enzymes themselves.

The ideal intake of magnesium for an adult is 15 to 20 mmol (30 to 40 meq) per day. Foods rich in magnesium include seed grains, nuts, peas, and beans. Fresh meat, fish, and most fresh fruits contain relatively small amounts of magnesium. Magnesium is absorbed primarily in the jejunum and ileum, and healthy persons absorb about 30 to 40 percent of ingested magnesium. This may increase to 70 percent when intake is low or magnesium deficiency exists. The percentage of magnesium absorption is reduced by a high magnesium intake or, independently, by vitamin D deficiency. When magnesium intake is restricted, fecal excretion becomes neglible, and urinary excretion decreases to 0.5 to 1 mmol (1 to 2 meq) per day. Thus, magnesium retention by the kidney is very efficient. Magnesium excretion depends upon glomerular filtration of the unbound fraction, of which 25 percent is reabsorbed in the proximal tubule and 50 to 60 percent is reabsorbed in the loop of Henle. Loop diuretics, such as ethacrynic acid or furosemide, cause greater excretion of magnesium than do diuretics such as the thiazides that act on the distal tubule. Magnesium excretion is increased by expanding extracellular fluid volume by ingestion of water and salt, and aldosterone decreases reabsorption of magnesium by the renal tubule. Magnesium excretion increases sharply when the concentration in serum exceeds 0.85 mmol/L.

In health, slight hypomagnesemia occurs in highly trained individuals, hypermetabolic states such as cold acclimatization, or after experimental administration of thyroid hormone.

MAGNESIUM DEFICIENCY   When any of the three major intracellular elements—magnesium, potassium, and phosphorus—has been deprived or lost, losses of the others usually follow. For this reason, deficiency of a single intracellular component almost never occurs. A diet devoid of magnesium causes depletion of phosphorus and potassium in skeletal muscle. Selective potassium deficiency may cause reductions in magnesium and phosphorus. Phosphorus deficiency may cause reductions in potassium and magnesium contents of tissue. The usual somatic responses to selective deprivation of one major intracellular element are anorexia, cellular atrophy, a negative nitrogen balance, and net loss of the other two major intracellular elements. Shrinkage of the cell and expulsion of the elements not deprived help to maintain a normal intracellular composition.

During hyperalimentation a different situation prevails. Provision of a diet that is otherwise replete but deficient in one major intracellular element promotes an anabolic state, and protoplasm is synthesized that has a major deficit of the ion being withheld. In these situations, serious derangements of cellular composition include accumulations of sodium, chloride, calcium, and water, suggesting a major interference with cellular ion transport. Indeed, elevation of cellular calcium, by activating proteases and phospholipases, may be an important cause of cellular injury under these conditions.

As in deficiencies of other major intracellular elements, deficiency of body magnesium can exist even when serum values are normal. In addition, magnesium deficiency may be organ-selective, since certain tissues become deficient before others. The definition of a true deficit of an intracellular element is reduction of its ratio with nitrogen in tissue. In muscle, this ratio is about 0.3 mmol (0.6 meq) magnesium per gram nitrogen. Red cell magnesium content appears to decrease in all species during magnesium deficiency. In contrast, muscle magnesium content remains perfectly normal in some species. Because of the inconsistency of tissue levels and because measurement of tissue magnesium is difficult, the clinician must rely upon serum or plasma magnesium levels to detect magnesium deficiency or excess.

The clinical physiology of magnesium deficiency   Volunteers fed a diet deficient in magnesium eventually develop characteristic symptoms and findings. Within 3 to 7 days after reducing dietary magnesium intake to less than 0.5 mmol (1 meq) per day, renal excretion of magnesium declines to below 0.5 mmol (1 meq) per day. Anorexia, nausea, vomiting, lethargy, and weakness develop within weeks. Characteristic symptoms of magnesium deficiency consist of paresthesias, muscular cramps, irritability, decreased attention span, and mental confusion. These complaints may require months to appear.

The physical findings are manifestations of the associated hypocalcemia. These are a positive Trousseau test and a Chvostek's sign, peculiar movements of the fingers best described as athetoid tetany, and on occasion convulsive seizures. Muscle fasciculations may be precipitated by a sharp blow with a neurologic hammer to muscle. About half of patients with selective magnesium depletion become hypokalemic. In animals rhabdomyolysis may occur. Cardiac arrhythmias, disturbances of conduction, and even ventricular fibrillation and cardiac arrest can occur in patients with both hypokalemia and hypomagnesemia. In such instances, hypokalemia may be the cause of the associated ECG abnormalities. Digitalis potentiates the severity

TABLE 343-1   Causes of hypomagnesemia
I Primary nutritional disturbances
A Inadequate intake
B Total parenteral nutrition
C Refeeding syndrome
II Gastrointestinal disorders
A Specific absorptive defects
B Malabsorption syndromes
1 Enteric fistulas
2 Nontropical sprue
3 Whipples disease
4 Intestinal lymphoma
5 Chronic pancreatic insufficiency
6 Biliary diversion
7 Giardiasis
8 Short bowel syndrome
C Prolonged diarrhea
D Prolonged nasogastric suction
E Pancreatitis
III Endocrine disorders
A Hyperparathyroidism
B Hypoparathyroidism
C Hyperthyroidism
D Primary hyperaldosteronism
E Bartter's syndrome
F Diabetic ketoacidosis
G Alcoholic ketoacidosis
H Administration of epinephrine
I Syndrome of inappropriate secretion of antidiuretic hormone
J "Hungry bones" syndrome after parathyroidectomy
IV Chronic alcoholism; alcoholic withdrawal
V Increased renal excretion
A Idiopathic
B Following renal transplantation
C Cisplatin therapy
D Aminoglycoside therapy
E Amphotericin B therapy
F Diuretics
1 Furosemide
2 Ethacrynic acid
3 Acetazolamide
4 Thiazides
5 Chlorthalidone
6 Osmotic agents
G Recovery phase of acute tubular necrosis

and potential danger of arrhythmias. In the presence of QT prolongation, polymorphic ventricular tachycardia (torsade de pointes) may occur that responds to magnesium salts. The causes of magnesium deficiency are shown in Table 343-1.

Hypocalcemia usually does not develop until serum magnesium falls below 0.5 mmol/L (1.0 meq/L). Although mild magnesium deficiency may increase release of parathyroid hormone, severe hypomagnesemia [levels below 0.4 mmol/L (0.8 meq/L)] consistently blocks release of parathyroid hormone. The resulting hypocalcemia may be severe. In addition, magnesium deficiency impairs the normal calcemic response to parathyroid hormone at the level of the skeleton. Hypocalcemia can become sufficiently severe to cause tetany. Although tetany has been reported in patients with hypomagnesemia independently of hypocalcemia, both conditions usually exist in patients with this finding. The tetany does not respond to infusions of calcium but only to correction of magnesium levels. The hypocalcemia responds only to magnesium replacement therapy, usually requiring 2 to 7 days for correction. However, administration of magnesium salts intravenously to such a patient can cause prompt and sometimes explosive release of parathyroid hormone. In rare instances, acute hypercalcemia can occur.

Hypokalemia in patients with magnesium deficiency is less well understood. Aldosterone production may be enhanced, thus permitting loss of potassium into the urine. It is extremely difficult to correct the potassium deficiency with supplemental potassium salts. However, administration of magnesium salts sufficient to correct the hypomagnesemia promptly reduces potassium excretion and corrects the hypokalemia. For this reason, it should be kept in mind that hypokalemia refractory to KCl supplements may be due to magnesium deficiency. The causes of magnesium deficiency are shown in Table 343-1.

Gastrointestinal causes of magnesium deficiency Familial hypomagnesemia is manifested during childhood and is caused by reduced absorption of dietary magnesium. The most important cause of magnesium deficiency in adults is intestinal malabsorption and steatorrhea, as in nontropical sprue, the short bowel syndrome, chronic pancreatic insufficiency, or biliary diversion. Because of unabsorbed fat, complexes of nonabsorbable magnesium–fatty acid soaps are formed in the intestinal lumen. When long-standing, hypomagnesemia in such cases is often associated with hypocalcemia, hypokalemia, and hypophosphatemia. Because of steatorrhea, disorders related to malabsorption of fat-soluble vitamins, especially vitamins K, A, and D, may coexist. It is important to recognize that vitamin D deficiency associated with hypomagnesemia can cause severe weakness due to chronic proximal myopathy in association with pain in the lower back and hips reflecting osteomalacia. Such patients display multiple and complex nutritional deficiency.

Magnesium deficiency also occurs in patients undergoing prolonged nasogastric suction who have not received adequate supplies of magnesium salts. Acute hypomagnesemia, along with acute hypocalcemia, occurs in acute hemorrhagic pancreatitis because magnesium- and calcium-fatty acid soaps are formed in situ as a result of tissue necrosis.

Endocrine causes of hypomagnesemia Mild hypomagnesemia occurs in poorly controlled diabetes mellitus. Moderate hypomagnesemia may occur in hyperparathyroidism, hypoparathyroidism, hyperthyroidism, primary hyperaldosteronism, and during recovery from diabetic ketoacidosis. In primary hyperaldosteronism, aldosterone enhances magnesium excretion directly and acts via volume expansion to cause net losses of magnesium. These effects can be reversed by spironolactone. Hypomagnesemia may occur in hypokalemic and hyponatremic patients with the syndrome of inappropriate secretion of antidiuretic hormone (vasopressin). Presumably, this is the result of increased aldosterone production and overexpansion of the circulatory volume. Epinephrine and other potent beta agonists may cause transient hypomagnesemia. Experimentally, epinephrine administration causes uptake of magnesium ions into adipose tissue as fatty acids are released. Of interest, as catecholamines cause release of fatty acids into the blood, insoluble magnesium- and calcium-fatty acid complexes form. If serum is centrifuged, the precipitates settle to the bottom of the tube. As a result, spurious hypomagnesemia and hypocalcemia can be diagnosed. The latter event may explain the allegation that mild hypomagnesemia and hypocalcemia are common in seriously ill patients who have no predisposing cause for magnesium deficiency. Seriously ill patients often have elevated catecholamine levels in blood.

Hypomagnesemia associated with alcoholism Ethanol causes a transient loss of magnesium into the urine. Alcoholics with a reasonably normal nutrient intake and normal intestinal function usually have normal or only slightly depressed magnesium levels in blood. However, during alcoholic withdrawal, serum magnesium can decline in association with acute hypophosphatemia and acute hypokalemia. In animals, sustained ethanol administration in intoxicating doses causes severe depletion of phosphorus, moderate depletion of magnesium and potassium, and increases in intracellular sodium, chloride, water, and calcium. Selective depletion of phosphorus also causes magnesium wasting and muscle magnesium deficiency. Identical findings occur in muscles of severe alcoholic patients. In acute alcohol withdrawal, respiratory alkalosis and insulin release provoked by administration of nutrients act in concert to incorporate phosphate into cells. Increased ATP synthesis as a result of phosphate movement into cells may cause increased magnesium binding and coincident hypomagnesemia.

In alcoholics with intestinal malabsorption and steatorrhea, hypomagnesemia can be severe and is commonly associated with hypocalcemia, hypophosphatemia, and hypokalemia. Although a relationship has been claimed between hypomagnesemia and alcoholic

withdrawal seizures, essentially all alcoholics in a withdrawal state display prominent respiratory alkalosis. Alkalosis lowers the threshold for seizure activity. Thus, the relationship of hypomagnesemia to seizures in this setting is far from clear. Furthermore, correction of hypomagnesemia in a withdrawing alcoholic appears to have no favorable effect on the withdrawal syndrome.

Magnesium deficiency may play a role in the temporary hypertension during alcohol withdrawal. Magnesium deficiency is associated with accumulation of calcium in smooth muscle. Accumulation of calcium potentiates the pressor response to circulating catecholamines. Withdrawing alcoholics nearly always have elevations of circulating catecholamines. The combined effects of magnesium depletion, calcium accumulation in cells, and hyperresponsiveness to catecholamines may explain the common occurrence of hypertension in this setting.

Magnesium deficiency due to increased renal excretion Hypomagnesemia can also result from impaired renal tubular reabsorption. Most of these states are associated with renal potassium wasting and hypokalemia, and some patients are hypercalciuric. Transient hypomagnesemia due to reduced renal tubular reabsorption may follow renal transplantation.

Aminoglycoside antibiotics, cisplatin, diuretics, and cyclosporine can cause magnesium wasting in the urine. Gentamicin causes hypomagnesemia and hypokalemia as a result of impaired tubular reabsorption. Hypomagnesemia develops after prolonged treatment and usually in patients who have received more than 8.0 g. Total recovery is the rule after the drug has been stopped. The majority of patients treated with cisplatin develop hypomagnesemia that can be severe; hypokalemia is less common. Even after cisplatin is withdrawn, the absorptive defect in the nephron may persist for months or years. About one-fourth of patients treated with cyclosporine and prednisone after renal transplantation develop serum magnesium levels below 0.5 mmol/L (1 meq/L). As mentioned above, loop diuretics are potent magnesuric agents, but significant hypomagnesemia in patients medicated with diuretics is infrequent. Patients receiving large doses of these drugs or patients receiving two diuretics acting at different sites in the nephron are more likely to develop hypomagnesemia.

Treatment of hypomagnesemia and magnesium deficiency Treatment of hypomagnesemia and its associated disorders should be aimed at correcting the cause. Patients with inadequate dietary intake or with diseases that either reduce intestinal absorption or cause excessive losses into the urine can often be corrected by oral administration of magnesium salts. Patients with potentially serious cardiac arrhythmias or with nausea and vomiting should be given intravenous magnesium sulfate. Magnesium sulfate heptahydrate ($MgSO_4 \cdot 7 H_2O$) has a molecular weight of 234; thus, 1 mL of 50% solution contains 2.1 mmol (4.2 meq) magnesium. The usual adult dose of 50% magnesium sulfate is 2 mL every 6 h on the first day and half this quantity on each of the following 3 to 4 days. Magnesium sulfate may be given intramuscularly, but this is painful and may cause elevation of creatine phosphokinase levels reflecting muscle damage and thus blunting the value of measurements of the enzyme to detect rhabdomyolysis. It is preferable to infuse magnesium sulfate in a dose of 4.1 mmol (8.2 meq) each 6 h. Patients sufficiently ill to require intravenous magnesium sulfate are often hypokalemic and hypophosphatemic. Potassium phosphate and potassium chloride may be included with 50% magnesium sulfate in 0.5% saline containing 5% glucose. The total potassium content in each infusion bottle should represent one-fourth of the amount determined to be necessary each day. In patients who have an adequate urine flow, such solutions can be given in a quantity of 750 mL each 6 h until nausea and vomiting disappear and oral intake becomes possible. In patients with tetany due to magnesium deficiency, although hypocalcemia coexists, calcium is generally ineffective and infusions of magnesium salts usually require 2 h or more to relieve the tetany. Up to a full day may be required for all signs of latent tetany, such as Chvostek's or Trousseau's signs, to disappear completely. Several oral preparations of magnesium salts are available. Doses of 5 mL magnesium hydroxide containing antacids (Maalox, Gelusil, Mylanta) each contain 3.5 mmol (6.9 meq) magnesium. However, there are two theoretical objections to the use of these preparations. First, these compounds also contain aluminum salts that may be hazardous if the patient has renal impairment. Second, they bind phosphate in the gut, and it is known that phosphate deprivation by this method can itself promote loss of magnesium. Other preparations include magnesium chloride tablets, magnesium gluconate tablets, and commercially available magnesium oxide powder. Since both spironolactone and triamterene cause retention of magnesium and potassium, these drugs may be useful adjuncts to maintain normal serum magnesium levels in patients taking diuretics.

HYPERMAGNESEMIA Patients with end-stage renal disease frequently have modest hypermagnesemia and are at risk of developing significant hypermagnesemia in the event of the ingestion of magnesium-containing compounds such as antacids. Adrenal insufficiency may also cause modest hypermagnesemia. Symptomatic hypermagnesemia is uncommon and is usually precipitated by inadvertent overdose with magnesium salts or is deliberately induced to treat patients with eclampsia. Magnesium can reduce neuromuscular transmission and can act as a central nervous system depressant. Symptoms of hypermagnesemia usually correspond to serum levels. Nausea usually appears between 2 and 2.5 mmol/L (4 to 5 meq/L). Sedation, decreased deep tendon reflexes, and muscle weakness appear at levels of 2 to 3.5 mmol/L (4 to 7 meq/L). Hypotension, bradycardia, and diffuse vasodilatation appear between 2.5 to 5 mmol/L (5 to 10 meq/L). Areflexia, coma, and respiratory paralysis occur at levels between 5 and 7.5 mmol/L (10 and 15 meq/L). Patients treated for eclampsia must be observed very carefully for sequential signs of magnesium intoxication. If this occurs, symptoms and findings can be reversed very quickly by infusion of calcium salts since these ions electrically oppose one another at their sites of action.

REFERENCES

ALFREY AC et al: Evaluation of body magnesium stores. J Lab Clin Med 84:153, 1974

ANDERSON R et al: Skeletal muscle phosphorus and magnesium deficiency in alcoholic myopathy. Mineral Electrolyte Metab 4:106, 1980

CRONIN RE et al: Skeletal muscle injury after magnesium depletion in the dog. Am J Physiol 243:F113, 1982

———, KNOCHEL JP: Magnesium deficiency, in *Advances in Internal Medicine*, GH Stollerman (ed). Chicago, Yearbook Medical Publishers, 28:509, 1983

KNOCHEL JP: Hypophosphatemia in the alcoholic. Arch Intern Med 140:613, 1980

——— et al: The muscle cell in chronic alcoholism. The possible role of phosphate depletion in alcoholic myopathy. Ann N Y Acad Sci 252:274, 1975

KROENKE K et al: The value of serum magnesium determination in hypertensive patients receiving diuretics. Arch Intern Med 147:1553, 1987

QUAMME GA, DIRKS JH: Magnesium metabolism, in *Clinical Disorders of Fluid and Electrolyte Metabolism*, 4th ed, MH Maxwell, CR Kleeman, RG Narins (eds). New York, McGraw-Hill, 1987, chap 13, pp 297–316

RASMUSSEN HS et al: Magnesium and acute myocardial infarction. Arch Intern Med 146:872, 1986

SHILS ME: Experimental human magnesium depletion. Medicine 48:61, 1969

SHINE KI: Myocardial effects of magnesium. Am J Physiol 237:H413, 1979

TZIVONI D et al: Treatment of torsade de pointes with magnesium sulfate. Circulation 77:392, 1988

VELOSO D et al: The concentrations of free and bound magnesium in rat tissues. J Biol Chem 248:4811, 1973

VICTOR M: The role of hypomagnesemia and respiratory alkalosis in the genesis of alcohol withdrawal symptoms. Ann N Y Acad Sci 215:235, 1973

WHANG R et al: Frequency of hypomagnesemia in hospitalized patients receiving digitalis. Arch Intern Med 145:655, 1985

344   PAGET'S DISEASE OF BONE

STEPHEN M. KRANE

Paget's disease of bone (osteitis deformans) is usually focal but may be widespread. The initial event is excessive resorption of bone by cells such as osteoclasts, followed by the replacement of normal marrow by vascular, fibrous connective tissue. At some stage and to a variable degree, the resorbed bone is replaced by coarse-fibered, dense trabecular bone organized in haphazard fashion. The irregular and often rapid deposition of this new bone, to a great extent still lamellar, causes an increase in the number of prominent, irregular cement lines that give the bone its characteristic "mosaic" pattern. Most lesions show both excessive resorption and chaotic new bone formation.

INCIDENCE The prevalence is difficult to determine since it is often asymptomatic and is frequently detected when roentgenograms are obtained for other reasons or because of a high level of alkaline phosphatase on routine blood screening. On the basis of autopsy examination, the incidence is estimated to be about 3 percent in individuals over the age of 40; there is increased likelihood of occurrence with increasing age. The incidence varies in different parts of the world. Figures based on radiologic surveys indicate less than a 1 percent frequency in the adult populations in the United States, Great Britain, and Australia. In India, Japan, the Middle East, and Scandinavia, the disease is rare.

ETIOLOGY The etiology is unknown. No convincing evidence of endocrine abnormality has been produced. Likewise, although pagetic bone can be exceedingly vascular, it has not been established that the vascular abnormality is primary. Some of the manifestations can be suppressed with glucocorticoids, salicylates, and cytotoxic drugs, but there is no convincing evidence that the fundamental lesion is inflammatory. Intranuclear inclusions have been found by electron microscopy in osteoclasts in pagetic bone but not in osteoclasts or other bone cells in normal persons or patients with other bone diseases with the exception of pyknodysostosis. Some of the inclusions resemble nucleocapsids of viruses belonging to the measles group. Indirect immunofluorescence and immunoperoxidase studies using antibodies to measles virus support the suggestion that the inclusions are indeed measles virus nucleocapsids. Measles virus nucleocapsid mRNA has also been detected by in situ hybridization in bone cells from patients with Paget's disease. Other evidence suggests that the inclusions are due to respiratory syncytial virus. In one area of England ownership of dogs is more common in pagetic subjects than in controls, suggesting that a canine virus (for example, canine distemper) might be the infective agent. Thus, different viral agents might be responsible for Paget's disease in different patients.

PATHOPHYSIOLOGY The characteristic feature is increased resorption of bone accompanied by an increase in bone formation, which is usually adequate to compensate. In the early phase bone resorption predominates (for example, in the variant, *osteoporosis circumscripta*), and the bones are exceedingly vascular. This has been termed the *osteoporotic, osteolytic,* or *destructive phase* of disease in which the external calcium balance may be negative. Commonly the excessive resorption is followed closely by formation of new pagetic bone. In this so-called mixed phase of the disease, the rate of bone formation is so geared to that of bone resorption that the magnitude of the increase in bone turnover is not reflected in the overall calcium balance.

As the activity decreases, a progressive decrease in resorptive rate may occur, eventually leading to the occurrence of hard, dense, less vascular bone (the so-called *osteoplastic* or *sclerotic* phase) and a positive external calcium balance. The rates of bone turnover may be increased enormously in patients with active Paget's disease, occasionally more than 20 times normal. Quantitative histomorphometry of bone biopsies confirms the extent of remodeling with marked increase in resorption surfaces and deep scalloped lacunae containing giant osteoclasts with numerous nuclei and increased numbers of osteoblasts lining the edges. The calcification rate is also increased. The normal hematopoietic marrow is replaced by a loose stroma which may be highly vascular. The magnitude of the increase in turnover varies with the extent as well as the activity of the disease. The increase correlates with the increased plasma levels of bone alkaline phosphatase, which are higher in Paget's disease than in any other condition with the exception of hereditary hyperphosphatasia. Although increased bone resorption enhances release of calcium and phosphate ions from bone, utilization of these ions for new bone formation and, presumably, feedback control of parathyroid hormone secretion usually maintain the concentration of calcium ions in the plasma at normal levels. The concentration of phosphate in the plasma is normal or slightly elevated. When marked imbalance between bone formation and resorption occurs in favor of resorption, as after prolonged immobilization or fractures, urinary calcium excretion may be increased, and rarely hypercalcemia may occur. If, on the other hand, bone formation exceeds resorption (relatively uncommon), circulating levels of parathyroid hormone may be increased. Significant increases in trabecular bone resorption and osteoid surfaces in normal bone from patients with Paget's disease may be due to compensatory, secondary hyperparathyroidism. Resorption involves the organic phase of bone as well as the mineral phase. While the inorganic ions of the mineral phase are reutilized for bone formation, amino acids such as hydroxyproline and hydroxylysine are released during resorption of the collagen matrix of bone and are not reutilized for collagen biosynthesis. The urinary excretion of small peptides containing hydroxyproline is increased, reflecting the increased bone resorption. Peptides of about 1500 to 5000 mol wt containing hydroxyproline and other amino acids in proportions characteristic of collagen are also excreted in increased amounts in the urine and are correlated with increased bone formation. Other markers for increased matrix synthesis include elevated levels of osteocalcin (bone-GLA protein) (see Chap. 339) and procollagen extension fragments in plasma.

RADIOLOGIC CHANGES The radiologic findings reflect the underlying pathology and the phase of the disease that predominates at the time of the examination. The pelvic bones are most commonly involved, followed by the femur, skull, tibia, lumbosacral spine, dorsal spine, clavicles, and ribs; small bones are not as frequently diseased. The lytic phase of the disease may be overlooked except when it occurs in the skull as *osteoporosis circumscripta*, with areas of sharply demarcated radiolucency in the frontal, parietal, and occipital bones. In the long bones the lytic areas are usually first seen at one end, from which they progress toward the other end with a V-shaped advancing edge. The lesion may produce expansion of the cortex and exhibit features suggesting malignancy. Usually the lytic area is followed by a zone of increased density, representing the new bone formation of the mixed phase of the disease. In general, the bone shows enlargement with irregularly widened cortex in a coarse, striated pattern and increased density, occasionally focal in distribution. Perpendicular lines of radiolucency (cortical infractions) are frequent and occur on the convex side of bowed long bones, particularly the femur and tibia. Transverse fractures may also occur, some initiated at the sites of these cortical infractions. The remodeling of the pagetic bone usually follows the lines of stress produced by muscle pull or gravity, accounting for the characteristic lateral bowing of the femur or anterior bowing of the tibia and the tendency for most of the dense bone to be deposited on the concave side of the bowed bone. In the skull, in the mixed stage, there is enlargement and thickening, especially of the outer table, with irregular areas of increased density, often spotty (Fig. 344-1). Basilar invagination is common with involvement of the base of the skull. The changes in the pelvis also consist of bone resorption and new bone formation and are frequently accompanied by a characteristic thickening of the pelvic brim. In the sclerotic phase of the disease, the bone may show uniform increase in density, often in the absence of striations. This

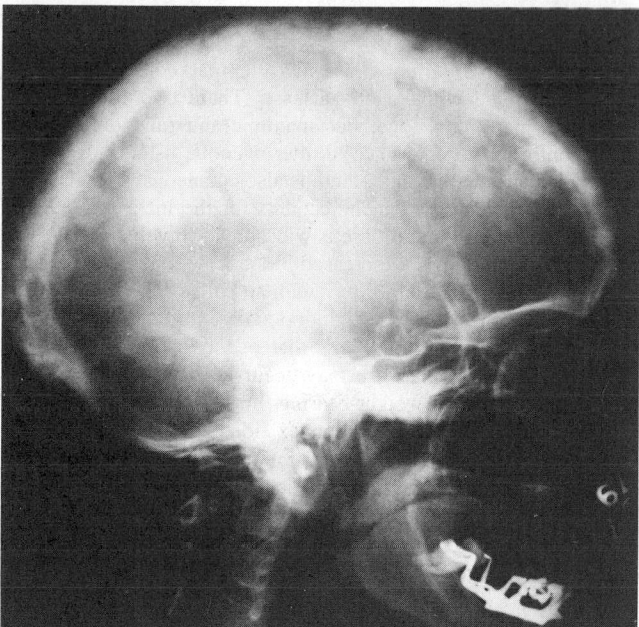

FIGURE 344-1 Lateral roentgenogram of the skull from a 58-year-old woman with Paget's disease of bone.

is common in the facial bones but is occasionally seen as well in the vertebrae where a homogeneous, dense pattern gives an "ivory" appearance similar to that typical of Hodgkin's disease, although the involved vertebrae are not enlarged in Hodgkin's disease. Computed tomography is useful in defining atypical lesions, particularly where neoplastic involvement is suspected. Technetium 99m diphosphonate bone scans are indicated to document the extent of disease when therapy is contemplated or to confirm the diagnosis when radiologic findings are inconclusive. Gallium 67 scans have also been used to define the extent of bone involvement.

CLINICAL PICTURE The clinical presentation is a function of the extent of the disease, the particular bones involved, and the presence of complications. Many patients are asymptomatic. In these individuals the disorder is discovered during radiologic examination of the pelvis or spine for an unrelated disease or complaint or because of the finding of an elevated level of plasma alkaline phosphatase. Other individuals may gradually become aware of a swelling or deformity of a long bone or develop a disturbance in gait due to unequal length of and change in the distribution of mechanical forces in the lower extremities. Enlargement of the skull is often not noticed by the patients, or they may be aware of increasing hat size. Pain in the face and headache are initial complaints in some; backache and pain in the lower extremities are common. The pain is usually dull but may be shooting or knifelike. Back pain is most common in the lumbar region and may radiate into the buttocks or lower extremities. This pain is probably due to the pagetic process itself, to distortion of articular facets, and to secondary osteoarthritis. Pain in the lower extremities may be associated with the transverse cortical infractions along the convex lateral surface of the femur or the anterior surface of the tibia. Often the new lytic lesions detected on bone scan are the most painful. Pain may also be due to involvement of the hip joint resembling degenerative joint disease and characterized by narrowing of the joint space, bony lipping at the margin of the acetabulum, and deepening of the acetabulum. Angioid streaks may be present in the retina. Hearing loss is due to direct involvement of the ossicles of the inner ear or of bone in the region of the cochlea or to impingement by bone on the eighth cranial nerve in the auditory foramen. More serious neurologic complications can result from overgrowth of bone at the base of the skull (platybasia) and compression of the brainstem. Compression of the spinal cord with paraplegia has been observed, particularly with involvement of the middorsal spine. Pathologic fractures of vertebrae may also produce spinal cord lesions.

COMPLICATIONS   Blood flow may be markedly increased in extremities involved with Paget's disease. There is proliferation of blood vessels in pagetic bone, but anatomic and functional studies have not confirmed the presence of arteriovenous fistulas. Although blood flow is increased in bone, there is also cutaneous vasodilatation in the pagetic extremities, which accounts for the increased warmth noted clinically. When the disease is widespread, involving one-third or more of the skeleton, the increased blood flow may be associated with *high cardiac output* and rarely with so-called high-output heart failure. However, heart disease in individuals with Paget's disease is usually due to the same conditions that occur in other patients of similar age. *Pathologic fracture* may occur in the destructive phase of the disease. In the weight-bearing bones fractures are often incomplete, multiple, and on the convex side of the bone. They may occur spontaneously or follow slight trauma; the lesions are painful but heal spontaneously with no major disability. More serious fractures may also occur. Complete fractures are often transverse as if the bone were snapped like a piece of chalk. Under these circumstances the fracture may upset the delicate balance between bone formation and resorption in favor of resorption. At this stage the imbalance may be reflected by increased urinary calcium excretion, and in rare instances the serum calcium level may rise to dangerous levels.

There is no characteristic level of urinary calcium excretion, although calcium excretion tends to be higher when the resorptive phase predominates. This may be a factor which accounts for the somewhat higher incidence of *urinary stone* in these patients. Secondary changes in the cartilage of the hip joints and knees may result in articular symptoms. Hyperuricemia and gout commonly occur in men with Paget's disease, and calcific periarthritis may occur.

Sarcoma is the dread complication. The incidence is probably no greater than 1 percent, although higher incidence has been noted in some series that include many patients with polyostotic involvement. The sarcomas most frequently arise in the femur, humerus, skull, facial bones, and pelvis, and rarely in the vertebrae. In about 20 percent the tumors are multicentric. Histologically, they are usually osteosarcomas, although fibrosarcomas and chondrosarcomas have also been found. Increase in pain and swelling are the common complaints that lead to recognition of the sarcomas. The extent and character of the neoplastic involvement are established by computed tomography and/or magnetic resonance imaging. The level of alkaline phosphatase in the serum of patients with sarcomas usually reflects the activity and extent of the Paget's disease. In occasional patients an "explosive rise" of the phosphatase level may accompany the growth of the sarcoma, whereas in patients with limited Paget's disease, phosphatase levels may be only slightly elevated and give no clue to the development of the malignant lesion. The prognosis is poor following the development of sarcomas, and ablative surgery is rarely successful. Although chemotherapy is successful for treatment of some osteosarcomas in children, such regimens have little effect on survival of patients in whom osteosarcomas develop on the background of Paget's disease. Reparative granulomas resembling giant cell tumors may be locally destructive, but they do not metastasize.

THERAPY   Most patients require no treatment, since the disease is localized and does not cause symptoms. Indications for therapy include persistent pain in involved bones, neural compression, rapidly progressive deformity resulting in disabling disturbance of posture and/or gait, high-output congestive heart failure, hypercalcemia, severe hypercalciuria with or without formation of renal stones, repeated fractures or nonunion, and preparation for major orthopedic surgery. *Aspirin* is an effective analgesic, and if it can be tolerated in large enough doses (3.6 to 4 g/d) for months or years, disease activity may be suppressed, as shown by decreases in the level of plasma alkaline phosphatase and urinary hydroxyproline excretion. Nonsteroidal anti-inflammatory drugs such as *indomethacin*, 25 mg

three or four times daily, may also relieve pain, especially in the presence of hip involvement. *Glucocorticoids* suppress the disease but only in large doses (greater than 60 mg prednisone per day) which are usually not tolerated and, therefore, are not recommended. It is of interest that the high cardiac output of some patients may be reduced significantly after only a few days of glucocorticoid treatment. Orthopedic procedures also have a role in the management of selected cases. Total hip replacement may be indicated, and osteotomy may correct marked bowing deformities, particularly of the tibia. In patients with fractures or orthopedic procedures or in patients immobilized for any reason, urinary and serum calcium levels should be measured at intervals to anticipate the development of hypercalciuria and hypercalcemia. Early ambulation and adequate fluid intake are essential. Preparations of inorganic phosphate may reduce hypercalciuria under these circumstances (5 to 6 g/d neutral sodium phosphate in divided doses for 1 to 2 weeks).

Several agents reduce the excessive bone resorption of Paget's disease and are of possible therapeutic value. The administration of porcine, salmon, and human *calcitonins* for prolonged periods to pagetic patients may cause a decrease in plasma alkaline phosphatase and in urinary hydroxyproline excretion. Treatment with calcitonin causes variable decrease in bone pain, improvement in neurologic symptoms, and decrease in elevated cardiac output. Some patients have not continued to respond to porcine and salmon calcitonins, possibly because of the development of neutralizing antibodies. These individuals usually continue to exhibit a satisfactory response to human calcitonin. In others the development of secondary hyperparathyroidism has been postulated as the cause for a diminished response, although this cannot account for resistance in all cases. The calcitonins are probably most useful in patients with pain in areas of pagetic involvement, not due to associated joint disease. The dose of salmon calcitonin (the form available in the United States) is 50 to 100 MRC units daily given subcutaneously. In some cases it may be possible to reduce the dose to three times weekly. In severe cases alkaline phosphatase levels decrease, but not to the normal range. The disorder relapses after weeks or months when the calcitonin is discontinued. Some patients develop a sensation of warmth and/or nausea 30 min to several hours after injection. This may occur after initiating treatment or after months or years of therapy. The etiology is unknown, but the symptoms may be severe enough to discontinue the medication. Nasal spray and suppository formulations of calcitonin are efficacious and in the future may replace subcutaneous injection.

Cytotoxic drugs such as plicamycin and dactinomycin are potent agents in the disorder. Parenteral administration of plicamycin, 10 to 25 μg/kg body weight per day for 10 to 14 days, has produced striking decrease in urinary hydroxyproline excretion with subsequent decreases in plasma alkaline phosphatase level and clinical improvement. The indexes of active disease again become abnormal within weeks to months following completion of plicamycin therapy. Maintenance therapy may be administered as a weekly intravenous bolus. With doses of less than 15 μg/kg per week toxicity is low despite potential risks. Although the risks of plicamycin therapy appear to be low, it is seldom used in Paget's disease because of the availability of other effective, and even safer, agents.

Etidronate, a diphosphonate compound, given orally in doses up to 20 mg/kg body weight per day is effective in reducing bone resorption in almost all and in producing clinical improvement in some. Biochemical indices may be brought to normal, but in most the responses are incomplete. Serum alkaline phosphatase and urinary hydroxyproline excretion remain decreased for several months after withdrawal of the drug and only gradually return to pretreatment levels. In doses of 20 mg/kg body weight per day for periods of 6 months or longer and even with lower doses, mineralization of new bone may be inhibited and predispose to fracture. Some patients develop disabling pain over pagetic lesions within weeks or months of starting treatment that may be severe enough to warrant discontinuing the drug. Radiographs in some instances show an increase in bone lysis that heals when the drug is stopped. It is therefore recommended that doses of 5 mg or occasionally 10 mg/kg body weight per day be used for 6-month periods. Treatment could be reinstituted within 3 to 12 months if biochemical relapse occurs.

Other diphosphonate compounds such as the dichloromethylidene, 3-amino-1-hydroxypropylidine, aminohexane, or aminobutane derivatives have been introduced for therapy in Europe. The daily administration of these agents intravenously for 1 to 2 weeks or orally for several months produces rapid decrease in urinary hydroxyproline excretion and the characteristic delayed fall in serum alkaline phosphatase levels which, in contrast to experience with calcitonin or etidronate, usually reach the normal range. There is no inhibition of mineralization, and remission usually persists for 1 to 2 years or longer. Several of these highly effective agents are under trial in the United States. Although the diphosphonates and calcitonins act primarily to decrease bone resorption, the rate of new bone formation subsequently falls. As a result, the state of high bone turnover is shifted to a state of lower turnover, where rates of formation and resorption are still apparently geared to each other. In this lower turnover state, collagen fibers of the bone matrix are deposited in a more orderly fashion similar to normal bone.

REFERENCES

ALTMAN R, SINGER FR (eds): Proceedings of the Kroc Foundation Conference on Paget's Disease of Bone. Arthritis Rheum 23:1073, 1980

BASLÉ MF et al: Measles virus RNA detected in Paget's disease bone tissue by *in situ* hybridization. J Gen Virol 67:907, 1986

BIJVOET OLM et al: Paget's disease of bones: Assessment, therapy, and secondary prevention, in *Clinical Disorders of Bone and Mineral Metabolism,* M Kleerekoper, SM Krane (eds). New York, Mary Ann Liebert, Inc., 1989

HARINCK HIJ et al: Relation between signs and symptoms in Paget's disease of bone. Q J Med 226:133, 1986

HUVOS AG: Osteogenic sarcoma of bones and soft tissues in older persons. Cancer 57:1442, 1986

———— et al: Osteogenic sarcoma associated with Paget's disease of bone. A clinico-pathologic study of 65 patients. Cancer 52:1489, 1983

KRANE SM: Etidronate disodium in the treatment of Paget's disease of bone. Ann Intern Med 96:619, 1982

McDONALD DJ, SIM FH: Total hip arthroplasty in Paget's disease. J Bone Joint Surg 69A:766, 1987

MILLS BG et al: Gallium-67 citrate localization in osteoclast nuclei of Paget's disease of bone. J Nucl Med 29:1083, 1988

NAGANT DE DEUXCHAISNES C, KRANE SM: Paget's disease of bone: Clinical and metabolic observations. Medicine 43:233, 1964

REBEL A (ed): Symposium on Paget's disease. Clin Orthop Rel Res 217:1, 1987

SERET P et al: Sarcomatous degeneration in Paget's bone disease. J Cancer Res Clin Oncol 113:392, 1987

SINGER FR, KRANE SM: Paget's disease of bone, in *Metabolic Bone Disease,* LV Avioli, SM Krane (eds). Philadelphia, Saunders, 1990

STRICKBERGER SA et al: Association of Paget's disease of bone with calcific aortic valve disease. Am J Med 82:953, 1987

UPCHURCH K et al: Giant cell reparative granuloma of Paget's disease of bone. A unique clinical entity. Ann Intern Med 98:35, 1983

345 HYPEROSTOSIS, NEOPLASMS, AND OTHER DISORDERS OF BONE AND CARTILAGE

STEPHEN M. KRANE / ALAN L. SCHILLER

HYPEROSTOSIS

A number of disease states have in common an increase in the mass of bone per unit volume (hyperostosis) (Table 345-1). Such increase in bone mass is detected radiologically as increased density of the bone, often associated with a variable disturbance in the architecture of the tissue. In the absence of quantitative histomorphometric data, it is usually not possible to distinguish between an increase in bone

TABLE 345-1 Causes of hyperostosis

1 Endocrine disorders
  a Primary hyperparathyroidism
  b Hypothyroidism
  c Acromegaly
2 Radiation osteitis
3 Chemical poisoning
  a Fluoride
  b Elemental phosphorus
  c Beryllium
  d Arsenic
  e Vitamin A intoxication
  f Lead
  g Bismuth
4 Osteomalacic disorders
  a Renal tubular osteomalacia (vitamin D resistance or phosphate diabetes)
  b Chronic renal glomerular failure
5 Osteosclerosis (localized) associated with chronic infection
6 Osteosclerotic phase of Paget's disease
7 Osteosclerosis associated with carcinomatous metastases, malignant lymphoma, and hematologic disorders (myeloproliferative disorders, sickle cell disease, leukemia, multiple myeloma, systemic mastocytosis)
8 Osteosclerosis of erythroblastosis fetalis
9 Osteopetrosis
  a Infantile (malignant, autosomal recessive form)
  b Adult (benign, dominant form)
  c Intermediate form with carbonic anhydrase II deficiency and renal tubular acidosis
10 Unclassified diseases
  a Pyknodysostosis
  b Osteomyelosclerosis
  c Hyperostosis corticalis generalisata
  d Hyperostosis generalisata with pachydermia
  e Hereditary hyperphosphatasia
  f Progressive diaphyseal dysplasia (osteopathia hyperostotica multiplex infantilis; Camurati-Engelmann disease)
  g Melorheostosis
  h Osteopoikilosis
  i Hyperostosis frontalis interna

mass due to excessive formation of new bone or to decreased resorption of bone already formed. When bone deposition is rapid, the new bone may be of the woven type, but if the process is more chronic, true lamellar bone is formed. The additional bone may be located at the periosteum, within the compact bone of the cortex, or in the trabeculae of the cancellous regions. In the medullary area, the new bone is deposited on and between the trabeculae and encroaches upon the medullary spaces. Typical examples of such responses are seen in areas adjacent to tumors or in association with infection. In some diseases, the increase in bone mass may be spotty, as in osteopoikilosis, whereas in others most of the skeleton may be involved, as in the malignant form of osteopetrosis in children. The increase in mass is usually not due to an excessive amount of mineral relative to matrix, except in disorders such as osteopetrosis where islands of calcified cartilage may persist. (The mineral density of calcified cartilage is greater than that of bone.) In some diseases, such as the osteosclerosis of renal insufficiency, the bone mass and radiodensity may be increased, even though the new bone formed is poorly mineralized and contains widened osteoid seams. Hyperostosis could be due to dysfunction of osteoblasts or osteoclasts. It is of interest, therefore, that infection of newborn mice produces an osteopetrosis-like phenotype in which osteoblast progenitors appear to induce increased bone formation. However, in human osteopetrosis of the relatively benign and sporadic type, viral nucleocapsid particles have been found in osteoclasts, and it is possible that viral infection causes disordered function in these cells to account for the excessive bone mass.

Several of these conditions are discussed in more detail in other chapters, although some generalizations are pertinent. Bone that is denser than normal may be seen occasionally in the osteitis fibrosa associated with hyperparathyroidism. When the hyperparathyroidism is successfully treated, the rate of bone resorption decreases abruptly out of proportion to the rate of bone formation; this imbalance may lead to the production of areas of bone density greater than in the surrounding skeleton, especially in the healing of brown tumors. In hypothyroidism, the rates of both bone formation and resorption may be decreased, but when the balance is in favor of formation bones are of increased density but normal architecture. Increased bone density also occurs in some instances of osteomalacia associated with disturbances in renal tubular function. The increased mass of bone occurs together with widened osteoid seams, as in chronic renal glomerular insufficiency. In the vertebral bodies the bone appears denser in transverse bands at the upper and lower margins, with a relatively radiolucent center. This "sandwich" appearance is similar to that seen in some patients with osteopetrosis and has been termed by the British the *rugger jersey sign*. Skeletal hyperostosis, including cortical hyperostoses, periostitis, and tendon and ligament ossification, is also a complication of long-term therapy with synthetic retinoids such as isotretinoin.

OSTEOPETROSIS Osteopetrosis (Albers-Schönberg or marble bone disease) is clinically, biochemically, and genetically heterogeneous. Although osteopetrosis has multiple causes, a defect in bone resorption is always the underlying mechanism. The most severe form in infants is due to defects in differentiation and/or function of osteoclasts. Several types of hereditary osteopetrosis which resemble the infantile human disease have been described in rodents, and in some the disorder can be cured by engraftment of hematopoietic cells from a normal donor. In humans infantile osteopetrosis is manifested in utero and progresses after birth with anemia, hepatosplenomegaly, hydrocephalus, cranial nerve involvement and death, often due to infections. In most of these instances the disorder is inherited as an autosomal recessive trait. Several attempts to transplant bone marrow from normal donors to provide normal osteoclast precursor cells have been successful, and osteopetrotic bone has been repopulated with functioning osteoclasts of donor origin that produce radiologic and/or bone biopsy evidence of bone resorption. One infant received a bone marrow transplant from a brother with successful response lasting more than 4 years, although vision was not restored. In other individuals with osteopetrosis, peripheral blood monocyte function is defective. In other cases of osteopetrosis, clinical improvement has been obtained using high doses of calcitriol.

Less fulminant forms of osteopetrosis are seen in older children and adults. In some of the latter the disorder is sporadic. In others the osteopetrosis is progressive with increasing age and is inherited as an autosomal dominant trait; anemia is not as severe, neurologic abnormalities are not as frequent, and recurrent pathologic fractures are the main feature. Although most cases are in infants and children, many are discovered first in adult life when roentgenograms are obtained because of fractures or unrelated diseases. There is no predilection for either sex. Even the inherited adult disorder is heterogeneous. Type I is characterized by increased thickness of the cranial vault, whereas rugger jersey sign and "endo bones" in the pelvis are features of type II. A defect in modeling of endosteal bone is present in both types, and there is an additional defect in the remodeling of trabecular bone in type II osteopetrosis.

In kindreds where it is associated with renal tubular acidosis and cerebral calcification, osteopetrosis is inherited as an autosomal recessive defect, is compatible with long survival, and is associated with a deficiency of one of the isoenzymes of carbonic anhydrase (carbonic anhydrase II). Carbonic anhydrase II is a major component of the enzyme system required for generation of the unique acid environment adjacent to the ruffled border of the osteoclast, and deficiency of carbonic anhydrase results in disordered bone resorption. Bone resorption is depressed. In some instances, islands of unresorbed calcified cartilage are encased in bone. The defect in remodeling results in disorganization of bone structure with thickened cortices and lack of funnelization of metaphyses. Despite increased density, the bone is abnormal mechanically and fractures readily. Osteomalacia or rickets is sometimes a component of the osteopetrosis in children (Fig. 345-1).

The histologic changes are reflected in the roentgenograms (Fig. 345-2), which reveal uniformly dense, sclerotic bone often without distinction between the cortical and cancellous regions. There is

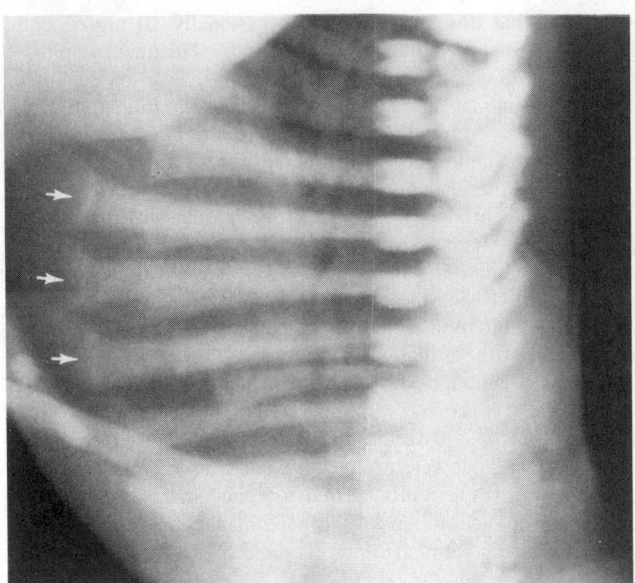

FIGURE 345-1 Lateral roentgenogram of the thorax of a 9-month-old boy with the "malignant" form of osteopetrosis. Note the uniform increase in mineral density of the vertebral bodies and the marked flaring of the ends of the ribs (arrows), indicative of rickets.

persistence of the primary spongiosa with central calcified cartilage cores surrounded by woven bone. Osteoclasts are often increased in number but apparently do not function properly. Osteoclasts may be morphologically normal or have loss of their ruffled borders suggesting that a spectrum of changes may occur. The variability may reflect heterogeneity in this syndrome, as in the osteopetrosis that occurs spontaneously in rodents. The long bones are usually involved, with increased density along the entire shaft. Foci of increased density

FIGURE 345-2 Roentgenogram of the spine and pelvis of a 55-year-old man with the more benign, dominant form of osteopetrosis.

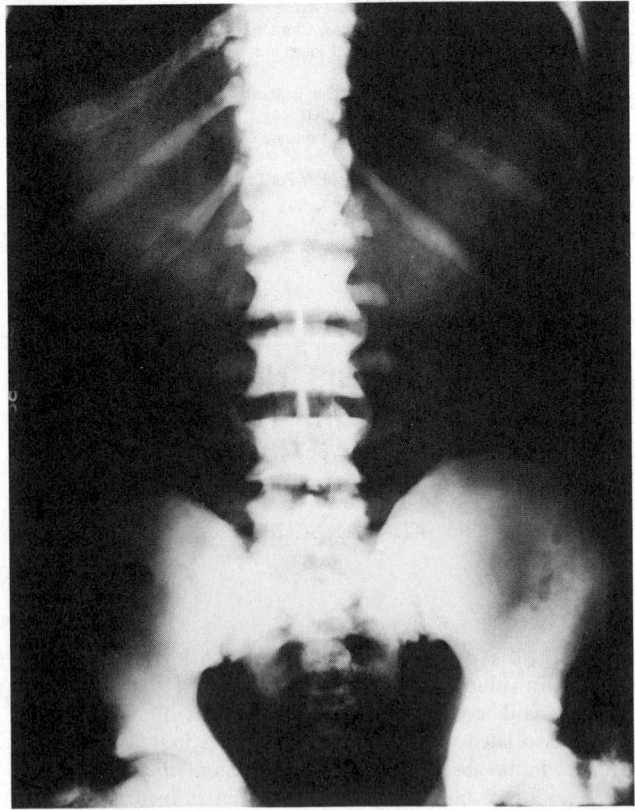

may be seen in the epiphyses corresponding to regions of unresorbed calcified cartilage. The metaphyses have a characteristic clubbed or splayed appearance. Horizontal bandings of increased density alternating with zones of decreased density in the long bones and vertebrae suggest that the defect is intermittent during periods of growth. The skull, pelvis, ribs, and other bones may be involved. The phalanges and the distal humerus may appear normal.

Encroachment of bone upon the marrow cavity, particularly in the malignant infantile disorder, is associated with anemia of the myelophthisic type with foci of extramedullary hematopoiesis in liver, spleen, and lymph nodes and enlargement of these organs. Neurologic abnormalities are associated with encroachment on cranial nerves and include optic atrophy, nystagmus, papilledema, exophthalmos, and impairment of extraocular motility. Facial paralysis and deafness are frequent; trigeminal lesions and anosmia are less common. In infants macrocephaly, hydrocephalus, and convulsions may occur, and infections such as osteomyelitis are frequent. Renal tubular acidosis is a feature of the form of osteopetrosis associated with a deficiency in carbonic anhydrase II.

In the milder dominant osteopetrosis, about half of the patients have no symptoms, and the disorder is discovered incidentally on roentgenograms. Other patients present because of fractures, bone pain, osteomyelitis, and cranial nerve palsies.

Fractures are a complication even with trivial trauma. Healing of such fractures is usually satisfactory, although delayed union may occur. When the disease is manifested first in adult life, fractures may be the only clinical problem. Levels of calcium and alkaline phosphatase in the plasma are usually normal in adults, although in children hypophosphatemia and, occasionally, moderate hypocalcemia have been noted. Serum acid phosphatase levels are usually increased.

The skeletal defect is not the same in all forms of osteopetrosis, and within a clinical subtype genetic and biochemical heterogeneity is common. As mentioned, several children with severe osteopetrosis have received bone marrow transplants from HLA-identical siblings which resulted in histologic and radiologic increases in bone resorption, accompanied by variable improvement in anemia, vision, hearing, and growth and development.

Unfortunately, it is not always possible to find appropriate donors for bone marrow transplantation, or patients may not be good candidates to receive transplants. Patients with the lethal forms have been treated with calcitriol. This therapy is associated with appearance of osteoclasts with normal ruffled borders and other evidence for increased bone resorption.

PYKNODYSOSTOSIS *Pyknodysostosis* resembles osteopetrosis but is a more benign condition not usually associated with hepatosplenomegaly, anemia, or cranial nerve involvement. In addition to a generalized increase in bone density, features include short stature, separated cranial sutures, hypoplasia of the mandible, kyphoscoliosis and deformities of the trunk, persistence of deciduous teeth, and progressive acroosteolysis of the terminal phalanges. Life span is usually unaffected, and the patient usually presents because of frequent fractures. Pyknodysostosis is inherited as an autosomal recessive trait. In one case levels of plasma calcitonin were intermittently elevated, and the response of the plasma calcitonin to infusions of calcium and glucagon was exaggerated. The gene that causes this disorder may be located on the short arm of a small acrocentric chromosome.

OSTEOMYELOSCLEROSIS *Osteomyelosclerosis* is a disorder in which the marrow cells are replaced by diffuse fibroplasia, occasionally accompanied by osseous metaplasia. When the latter is prominent, increased skeletal density is seen on roentgenograms. In early stages woven bone may be found in intratrabecular locations whereas in more advanced stages woven bone is observed in the medulla. The disorder is probably a phase in the course of the myeloproliferative disorders and is characteristically accompanied by extramedullary hematopoiesis.

Hyperostosis corticalis generalisata (van Buchem's disease) is characterized by osteosclerosis of the skull (base and calvaria), lower jaw, clavicles, and ribs, and thickening of the diaphyseal cortices of the long and short bones. Alkaline phosphatase levels in the serum are elevated, and the disorder may be due to increased formation of bone of normal structure. The major manifestations are due to neural compression and consist of optic atrophy, facial paralysis, and perception deafness. In *hyperostosis generalisata with pachydermia* (Uehlinger), the sclerosis is due to increased formation of subperiosteal spongy bone and involves the epiphyses, metaphyses, and diaphyses. Pain, swelling of joints, and thickening of the skin of the lower arms are common.

HEREDITARY HYPERPHOSPHATASIA This disorder is characterized by severe structural deformities of the skeleton with increase in thickness of the calvaria, large homogeneous areas of increased density at the base of the skull, and widening and loss of normal architecture of the shafts and the epiphyses of the long and short bones. There is a failure to deposit normal bone, with haphazard orientation of lamellae suggesting active remodeling that resembles Paget's disease of bone. Osteoclasts with multiple nuclei characteristic of Paget's disease and the typical "mosaic" pattern of faceted units of lamellar bone are not found, however. Levels of plasma alkaline phosphatase and urinary excretion of hydroxyproline peptides and other collagen degradation products are markedly increased. The disorder is apparently inherited as an autosomal recessive trait. Calcitonin therapy may be of value in some of these patients.

PROGRESSIVE DIAPHYSEAL DYSPLASIA A disorder in which a symmetric thickening and increased diameter of the diaphyses of long bones occurs, particularly in femurs, tibias, fibulas, radii, and ulnas, has been termed *progressive diaphyseal dysplasia* (Camurati-Engelmann disease). Pain over affected areas, fatigue, abnormal gait, and muscle wasting are the major manifestations. Serum alkaline phosphatase levels may be elevated and, on occasion, hypocalcemia and hyperphosphatemia may be found. Other abnormalities include anemia, leukopenia, and elevated erythrocyte sedimentation rate. Clinical and biochemical improvement may result from the use of glucocorticoids.

MELORHEOSTOSIS This rare condition usually begins in childhood and is characterized by a slowly progressive linear hyperostosis in one or more bones of one limb, usually in a lower extremity. All segments of the bone may be involved, with sclerotic areas that have a "flowing" distribution. The involved limb is often extremely painful.

OSTEOPOIKILOSIS This benign disorder is usually discovered by chance and is not associated with symptoms. It is characterized by dense spots of trabecular bone less than a centimeter in diameter, usually of uniform density, that are located in the epiphyses and adjacent parts of the metaphyses. All bones may be involved except the skull, ribs, and vertebrae.

HYPEROSTOSIS FRONTALIS INTERNA *Hyperostosis frontalis interna* is an abnormality of the inner table of the frontal bones of the skull consisting of smooth, rounded enostoses covered by dura and projecting into the cranial cavity. These enostoses are usually less than 1 cm at their greatest diameter and usually do not extend posteriorly beyond the coronal suture. The abnormality is found almost exclusively in women, who are frequently obese, hirsute, and who have a variety of neuropsychiatric complaints (Morgagni-Stewart-Morel syndrome). However, hyperostosis frontalis interna also occurs in women with no obvious illness or particular associated disease. The finding in the skull may be a manifestation of a generalized metabolic disorder.

NEOPLASMS OF BONE

Primary neoplasms of the skeletal system reflect in their histology the cellular and extracellular components of the skeleton. However, it is not always possible to prove that a tumor arises from the same type of tissue that it produces. The precursor cells of bone tissue are probably derived from distinct cell lines in which the osteoclasts arise from hematopoietic cells and the osteoblasts arise from the stromal cell system. The primitive stromal cell could differentiate into chondroblasts and fibroblasts as well as osteoblasts. Neoplasms can arise from all these cell types. Each of these cells can produce its characteristic extracellular matrix, and neoplasms arising from them may thus be recognized. Primary neoplasms of bone can arise also from other hematopoietic, vascular, and neural elements.

PATHOPHYSIOLOGY Neoplasms in bone induce resorption of skeletal tissue. This bone resorption results from production by the tumor cells of factors that stimulate osteoclast function and/or recruitment and differentiation of the osteoclast hematopoietic precursor cells. One of the factors produced by the tumor cells is the parathyroid hormone–related peptide (PTHrP) that interacts with the PTH receptor (see also Chap. 340). Other factors that induce bone resorption by modulating recruitment, differentiation, and/or activation of osteoclasts include cytokines such as transforming growth factor alpha, interleukins 1 and 6, tumor necrosis factor, and lymphotoxin derived from the tumor, resident bone cells, or infiltrating mononuclear inflammatory cells. What was initially termed "osteoclast activating factor" is now known to include cytokines such as interleukin 1 and lymphotoxin produced by monocytes and lymphocytes. Prostaglandin production by some tumors may also mediate bone resorption. T lymphocytes infected with some viruses can metabolize circulating $25(OH)D$ to $1,25(OH)_2D$, which may also stimulate bone resorption. Tumors may also alter blood supply to bone by obstructing vessels or inducing angiogenesis. Tumors may also produce reaction in surrounding bone and alter the normal contour. The epiphyseal plate, articular cartilage, cortex, and periosteum of bone often offer a barrier to the spread of neoplastic tissue. Alteration of the contour of the cortex is not due to "expansion" but to remodeling of the bone in the area and formation of new bone with the new contour. Some tumors induce primarily an osteoblastic or sclerotic reaction in surrounding bone, which results in increased radiodensity. Primary neoplasms may be less radiopaque than surrounding bone or more radiopaque, depending upon the degree of calcification or ossification of the matrix and the density of the tissue. Bone tumors may be recognized because of (1) the presence of a mass in the soft tissues, (2) deformity of a bone, (3) pain and tenderness, or (4) pathologic fractures. Tumors of bone may also be detected incidentally on roentgenograms obtained for other reasons. Although it is usually possible to classify bone tumors as benign or malignant, prediction of the clinical outcome on histologic and radiologic criteria is not always possible.

The extent of the lesions should be defined by standard and computed tomographic techniques and magnetic resonance imaging, if available. Lesions can also be assessed by bone scans utilizing ^{99m}Tc polyphosphonate. There are numerous pitfalls in the clinical diagnosis and interpretation of histologic features of tumors of bone. However, proper evaluation and selection of therapy require evaluation of both radiographic and histologic features. Management, therefore, requires cooperation of the orthopedist, oncologist, radiologist, radiotherapist, and pathologist.

BENIGN TUMORS The most common benign tumors are *osteochondromas* (exostoses) and *endochondromas* (which may be multiple in Ollier's disease), *benign giant cell tumors, unicameral bone cysts, osteoid osteomas*, and *nonossifying fibromas* (fibrous cortical defects). As a rule benign tumors are not painful except for osteoid osteomas, benign chondroblastomas, and benign chondromyxoidfibroma. The usual clinical problem is that of slowly progressing mass, pathologic fracture, or deformity. Treatment is usually accomplished by resection or curettage and bone grafting. When wide resection of tissue is necessary, insertion of metal and plastic prostheses or allograft transplantation may preserve limb function.

MALIGNANT TUMORS The most common malignant tumor of bone is multiple myeloma (see Chap. 265). Primary lymphoma may also arise locally in bone. Malignant tumors of nonhematopoietic origin include osteosarcomas, chondrosarcomas, fibrosarcomas, and Ewing's tumor. Giant cell tumors may be included here since they

may metastasize and are locally destructive. *Osteogenic sarcomas* are presumed to arise from osteoprogenitor cells and have a wide variation in histopathology, with at least six histologic types. These tumors always contain woven bone at least in small foci, and may contain in addition cartilaginous and fibrous elements. They are most common in the second and third decades and are less common under the age of 10 and over the age of 40. Genetic factors are important in the genesis of osteosarcomas particularly in children. Between 30 and 40 percent of patients with retinoblastoma have a hereditary predisposition to the tumor as well as to other cancers, particularly osteosarcomas. This predisposition is determined by a genetic locus within the q14 band of chromosome 13 that can be detected by analysis of restriction fragment length polymorphisms. Homozygosity for the mutant allele at the retinoblastoma locus in the osteoblast precursor could lead to osteosarcoma in the same way that homozygosity for the allele in a retinoblast could lead to retinoblastoma. In contrast, when osteosarcomas occur in older individuals, some predisposing cause is usually present such as Paget's disease, prior exposure to ionizing radiation, or a bone infarct. In primary osteogenic sarcomas the lesions usually arise in the metaphyseal region of long bones, especially in the distal femur, proximal tibia, and proximal humerus. The most common symptoms are pain and swelling which may be present for weeks or months. The roentgenographic features of osteosarcomas depend upon the degree of bone destruction, the extent to which mineralized bone is formed by and within the tumor, and the type of reaction in the surrounding bone. Thus, the lesions may vary from purely lytic lesions to dense areas containing radiopaque lumps, clouds, or spicules of tumor bone in varying patterns of organization. Discontinuities may occur in the cortex surrounding the lesion. In other cases, hyperostotic periosteal reactions may involve grossly layered bone. If the tumor grows rapidly, it may destroy the cortex and penetrate the soft tissue surrounding the bone; it leaves only a cuff of periosteal new bone at the peripheral margin of the tumor, just at the point of penetration (Codman's triangle). High plasma alkaline phosphatase levels in those sarcomas that are predominantly osteogenic parallel the course of the tumor. In general, high levels of serum alkaline phosphatase activity correlate with a poor prognosis. When lesions are adequately treated by amputation, chemotherapy, or radiation, the level of alkaline phosphatase falls, and when metastases appear, the level rises again, often reaching values higher than those present initially. When values are initially high, the course is often rapidly fatal. Metastases occur primarily by the hematogenous route especially to the lung.

The prognosis of osteosarcoma was very poor prior to development of effective chemotherapy, with radiologic evidence of pulmonary metastases usually occurring within a year following surgical amputation that was potentially curative. The course varies with the type of tumor; for example, a "telangiectatic" variant has a very poor prognosis, unless treated with aggressive chemotherapy, whereas the less common low-grade intramedullary type has a better prognosis. In the typical intramedullary type of osteosarcoma, death occurs within 6 months from the onset of detectable pulmonary metastases, suggesting that the lesions in the lungs were present at the time of amputation or that cells were shed from the tumor during the operation.

Several chemotherapeutic programs are efficacious. The disease-free and overall survival rates after 4 to 5 years in patients with no demonstrable metastases have increased from about 20 percent with ablative surgery alone to 80 percent or higher with current treatment programs. Since microscopic metastatic foci must be present when the bone tumors are first recognized, aggressive adjuvant chemotherapy is now routine. Chemotherapeutic programs include high-dose methotrexate with leucovorin rescue and various combinations of doxorubicin, cisplatin, bleomycin, cyclophosphamide, and dactinomycin. Amputation or surgical resection of the sarcoma leaving a wide margin of normal tissue is generally carried out. More frequently, a limb-sparing procedure is attempted, particularly in distal femoral osteosarcomas, with allograft bone and cartilage transplants and/or prosthetic devices used to preserve the joint. Resection of isolated pulmonary metastases combined with chemotherapy may also improve survival in younger individuals with primary osteosarcomas. The prognosis of osteosarcoma occurring on the background of Paget's disease in adults is still poor despite chemotherapy.

Chondrosarcomas are distinguishable from osteogenic sarcomas. In contrast to the latter, chondrosarcomas usually arise in adulthood and old age, with the peak incidence in the fourth, fifth, and sixth decades. Most are located in the pelvic girdle, ribs, and diaphyseal portions of the femur and humerus; distal portions of the extremities are involved rarely. Chondrosarcomas probably arise by malignant transformation in enchondromas and more rarely in the cartilaginous cap of osteochondromas. As a rule, chondrosarcomas are slow growing and slow to recur. Radiographically the lesions appear destructive, with mottled increases in radiodensity which reflect the variable degree of calcification of cartilaginous matrix and ossification. Radical excision is the treatment of choice. Histologic grading of the tumor can be valuable for predicting prognosis and determining appropriate surgical therapy.

Ewing's tumor   This is a malignant sarcoma composed of small, round cells that occurs most frequently in the first three decades of life. Most are located in the long bones, although any bone may be involved. Ewing's sarcoma is highly malignant with a low incidence of cure by ablative surgery with or without radiation. However, radiation therapy to the primary site and site(s) of metastases combined with chemotherapy with doxorubicin, cyclophosphamide, vincristine, and dactinomycin improves survival of patients with Ewing's sarcoma, including some with metastatic disease.

TUMORS METASTATIC TO BONE   The skeleton is a common site for metastases from carcinomas and occasionally even from sarcomas. Skeletal metastases may be silent or produce symptoms by the same mechanisms as primary tumors, i.e., pain, swelling, deformity, encroachment on hematopoietic tissue in the marrow, compression of spinal cord or nerve roots, and pathologic fractures. In addition, rapidly lytic skeletal metastases can result in hypercalcemia. The bones involved most commonly are the vertebrae, proximal femur, pelvis, ribs, sternum, and proximal humerus, in that order of frequency. The carcinomas that most frequently metastasize to bone arise in prostate, breast, lung, thyroid, kidney, and bladder. Malignant cells reach the skeleton via the bloodstream. Those that survive may proliferate and distort the normal architecture, probably by production of substances that cause dissolution of both mineral phase and organic matrix.

Osteolysis most often results from modulation of osteoprogenitor cells to osteoclasts in the surrounding bone. Some mediators involved in induction of osteoclasts were described earlier in this section. Some carcinoma cells may also act directly to resorb bone. Carcinomatous metastases (which are usually predominantly osteolytic) arise from thyroid, kidney, and lower bowel. Other tumors induce an *osteoblastic* response in which the new bone does not arise from the tumor itself, but is induced from normal skeletal cells by some product(s) of the tumor cells. The resulting lesion may be more dense than the surrounding tissue. Occasionally the increase in radiodensity is uniform, simulating osteosclerosis. Carcinoma of the prostate characteristically produces osteoblastic metastases. Carcinoma of the breast can cause both osteolytic and osteoblastic metastases. Malignant carcinoid tumors arising from the embryonic foregut and hindgut metastasize to bone with high frequency, producing an osteoblastic reaction. Hodgkin's disease in bone also produces an osteoblastic response both focal and diffuse. More malignant lymphomas in bone produce predominantly destructive lesions. As a rule, osteolytic metastases are the ones associated with hypercalcemia, hypercalciuria, and increased excretion of hydroxyproline-containing peptides (reflecting matrix destruction); they are usually associated with normal or only slightly increased levels of serum alkaline phosphatase. Osteoblastic metastases, on the other hand, may cause more marked elevations of serum alkaline phosphatase and may be associated with hypocalcemia. With some metastases (as in carcinoma of the breast) there may be phases in which osteolysis predominates (with hyper-calciuria, hypercalcemia, and normal alkaline phosphatase levels) alternating with phases in which alkaline phosphatase levels rise and the skeletal lesions become more sclerotic.

Treatment of skeletal metastases is usually palliative. In slowly growing localized lesions (as in some instances of carcinoma of the thyroid or occasionally in carcinoma of the kidney), local radiation is useful to relieve pain or reduce compression of surrounding structures. Many patients with carcinomas of breast or prostate survive for years even after extensive skeletal metastases are recognized. Castration and estrogen therapy or receptor antagonists may slow the progress of the lesions in patients with metastatic prostatic carcinoma (see Chap. 306). When patients with mammary cancer are treated with estrogens or androgens, the character of the reaction to the metastases may temporarily shift from a predominantly osteoblastic to a lytic phase with resultant hypercalcemia (see Chap. 303). Plicamycin, which inhibits osteoclast function and is effective in treating hypercalcemia associated with malignant disease, may also be useful in palliation of osteolytic metastases. The diphosphonates, which decrease bone resorption in Paget's disease, are useful in reducing bone metastases and the accompanying morbidity, such as bone pain, pathologic fractures, and hypercalcemia. The newer derivatives, such as the dichloromethylene and the aminohydroxy-propylidene analogues, as well as etidronate are effective, presumably by decreasing the ability of the tumor to establish itself in bone by blocking bone resorption. The bone pain in patients with metastatic carcinoma may also be relieved by the use of levodopa. Hypercalcemia in patients with malignant tumors is not due solely to skeletal metastases, although this is the most common cause. Production of circulating stimulators of osteoclast differentiation, such as PTHrP, is another cause of the humoral hypercalcemia of malignancy. Hypercalcemia per se, whether spontaneous or induced by therapy, may produce anorexia, polyuria, polydipsia, depression, and eventually coma. In addition, nephrocalcinosis can result from hypercalcemia, and death may result from renal insufficiency.

OTHER DISORDERS OF BONE AND CARTILAGE

FIBROUS DYSPLASIA (McCUNE-ALBRIGHT SYNDROME)   This syndrome is characterized by osteitis fibrosa disseminata, areas of pigmentation, and endocrine dysfunction, with precocious puberty in females. The bony lesions, called *fibrous dysplasia*, may occur in the absence of the other features. The fundamental nature of the disorder is unknown; the disease does not appear to be heritable, although it has been reported to affect monozygotic twins. The disease occurs with equal frequency in both sexes.

Incidence   The disease may be divided into three main categories: (1) monostotic, (2) polyostotic, and (3) McCune-Albright syndrome and its variants. The monostotic form is the most common. The lesions can be asymptomatic, associated with local pain, or predispose to pathologic fracture. The majority of the lesions are in the ribs or in the craniofacial bones, especially the maxillas. Many other bones may be affected, however, such as metaphyseal or diaphyseal portions of the proximal femurs or tibias. Monostotic fibrous dysplasia is most often diagnosed between 20 and 30 years of age. There are usually no associated skin lesions. Approximately a quarter of the individuals with the polyostotic form have more than half the skeleton involved by disease. One side of the body may be affected, and the lesions may be distributed segmentally in a limb, particularly in the lower extremities. Craniofacial lesions are present in approximately half of patients with the polyostotic form. Whereas the monostotic form is usually detected in young adults, fractures and skeletal deformities occur in childhood in the polyostotic form; the disease is generally more severe and deforming with early clinical onset. Lesions, especially monostotic lesions, may become quiescent around the time of puberty and may worsen during pregnancy. McCune-Albright syndrome is more common in females. Short stature is ascribed to premature closure of the epiphyses. The most frequent extraskeletal manifestations are the skin lesions.

Pathology All forms of fibrous dysplasia have an identical histologic appearance, although cartilage is more commonly involved in the polyostotic form. The marrow cavity is filled by gritty, gray-pink, rubbery tissue that replaces the normal cancellous bone. Often, the endosteal cortical surface is scalloped. Histologically, the lesions contain benign-appearing fibroblastic tissue arranged in a loose whorled pattern (Fig. 345-3). The grittiness is due to irregularly arranged woven bone spicules, most of which lack osteoblastic palisading or rimming, which are embedded in the fibrous tissue. These bone spicules may also have prominent cement lines. In approximately 10 percent of cases, islands of hyaline cartilage are present, and more rarely, myxoid tissue may predominate in young patients. Examination by polarized light and with the use of special stains indicates a contiguity of collagen fibers of the osseous and marrow tissue. In the polyostotic form cystic degeneration may be characterized by the presence of hemorrhage with hemosiderin-containing macrophages and osteoclast-type giant cells in the periphery of the cyst. Malignant transformation of either monostotic or polyostotic fibrous dysplasia occurs but with a frequency of less than 1 percent. The malignant change is usually detected in the third or fourth decades in individuals who have had lesions first identified in childhood. In about a third of the cases the neoplasms arise in previously radiated lesions. Ossifying fibroma of long bones is a peculiar fibroosseous cortical lesion which may be a variant of fibrous dysplasia. It is most common in the tibial shaft of teenagers. Although benign, the lesion has a tendency to recur if not adequately excised.

Radiologic changes The roentgenographic appearance of the lesions is that of a radiolucent area with a well-delineated, smooth or scalloped border, typically associated with focal thinning of the cortex of the bone (Fig. 345-4). Fibrous dysplasia and Paget's disease of bone are two disorders that can cause a bone to become larger than normal. The lesions of fibrous dysplasia are not usually cysts in the strict sense, since they are not fluid-filled cavities. They occasionally appear multiloculate. The so-called ground glass appearance reflects the content of the thin spicules of calcified, woven bone. Frequently, deformities are present such as coxa vara, shepherd's-crook deformity of the femur, bowing of the tibia, Harrison's grooves, and protrusio acetabuli. Involvement of facial bones, usually with lesions of increased radiodensity, may create a leonine appearance (leontiasis ossea) superficially resembling leprosy. Fibrous dysplasia of the temporal bones can cause progressive loss of hearing and obliteration of the external ear canal. Advanced skeletal age in females is correlated with sexual precocity but may also be seen in males without sexual precocity. The lesions tend to spare the epiphyseal regions before puberty, but in older individuals fibrous dysplasia may develop in the epiphyses. Occasionally, a focus of fibrous dysplasia

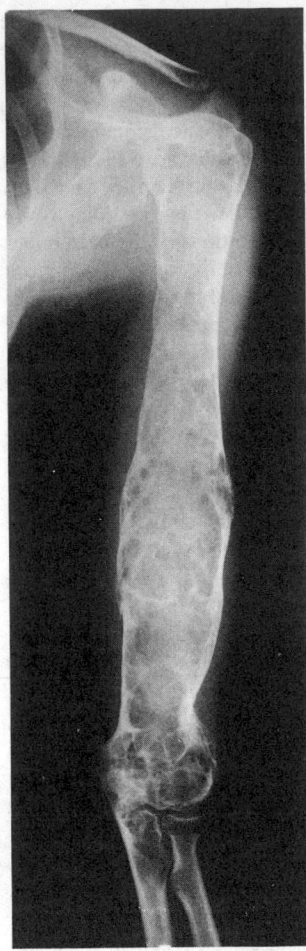

FIGURE 345-4 Roentgenogram of the upper extremity from a 33-year-old woman with fibrous dysplasia of bone. Typical lesions involve the entire humerus as well as the scapula and proximal ulna.

may undergo cystic degeneration with an enormous distortion of the shape of the bone, and mimic the so-called aneurysmal bone cyst.

Clinical picture The clinical course is variable. Skeletal lesions are usually detected because of localized pain, deformities, or fractures. Other symptoms ascribable to bone involvement are headache, seizures, cranial nerve abnormalities, hearing loss, narrowing of the external ear canal, or even spontaneous scalp hemorrhages if there is craniofacial bone disease. In some females and even less commonly in males, sexual precocity is the presenting complaint, occasionally before the appearance of skeletal symptoms. Serum calcium and phosphorus values are usually normal. In approximately one-third of patients, levels of serum alkaline phosphatase may be elevated to high values, and urinary hydroxyproline excretion is often increased. In some subjects, high cardiac output similar to that in extensive Paget's disease may be found. In general, patients with extensive involvement have widespread disease when symptoms first appear, whereas when disease is mild at the onset extensive disease does not usually develop.

The cutaneous pigmentation in most patients with McCune-Albright syndrome consists of isolated dark-brown to light-brown macules which tend to remain on one side of the midline (Fig. 345-5). The border is usually, although not always, irregular or jagged ("coast of Maine") in contrast to the smooth borders of the pigmented macules of neurofibromatosis ("coast of California"). As a rule there are fewer than six of the lesions, which range in size from 1 cm to those covering very large areas, particularly the back, buttocks, or sacral regions. When the lesions are present in the scalp, the overlying hair may be more deeply pigmented than that over the remainder of the scalp. Localized alopecia is associated with osteomas of the skin, and such lesions tend to have concordance with the skeletal lesions. The pigmentation tends to be on the same side as the skeletal lesions and actually overlie them.

FIGURE 345-3 Photomicrograph of the lesion of fibrous dysplasia. Note spicules of dark-staining woven bone (WB) surrounded by loose fibroblastic tissue.

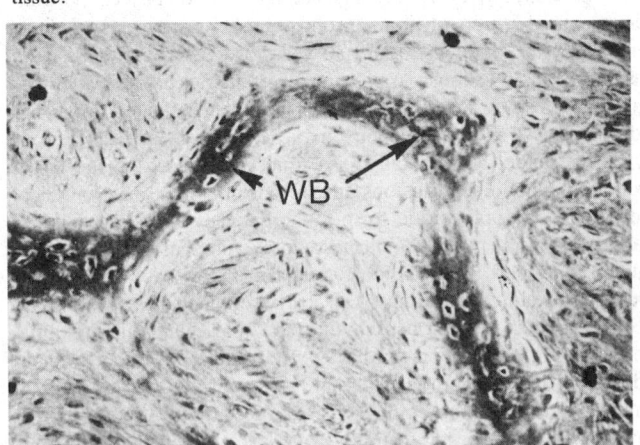

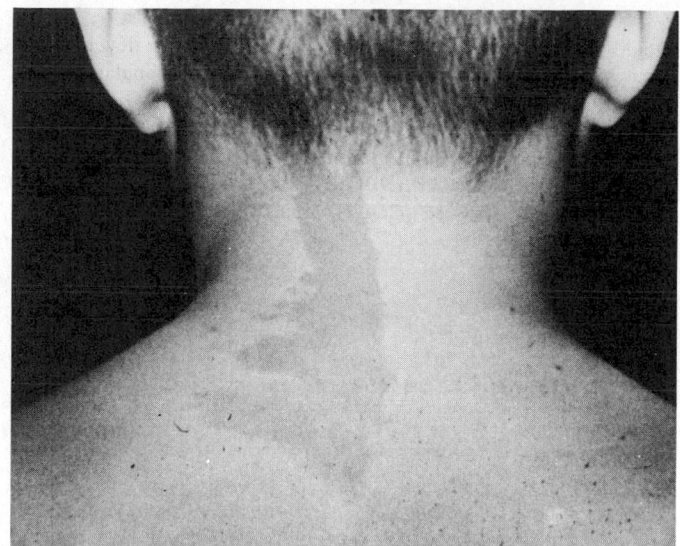

FIGURE 345-5 Typical pigmented café au lait lesion of the skin in an 11-year-old boy with polyostotic fibrous dysplasia. The border has the jagged "coast of Maine" appearance that is characteristic of McCune-Albright's syndrome. Note that the lesion is limited to one side (left) of the body.

The sexual precocity of unknown cause is found in females and rarely in males (see also Chaps. 321 and 322). Premature vaginal bleeding and development of axillary and pubic hair and of breasts are the main features. In the few ovaries that have been examined, no corpora lutea have been seen. The cause of the precocious sexuality is still not clear. In the few cases where measurements have been reported, the girls have high estrogen levels and low or undetectable gonadotropins. Autonomous hyperfunction of ovarian cysts may account for the high estrogen levels and sexual precocity. Estrogen receptors have been measured in the bone lesions. It is therefore not surprising that precocious sexuality is not limited to patients with cranial involvement. The characteristic pigmented macules are usual but not invariable. Another endocrine abnormality with increased frequency is hyperthyroidism. Rarer associations include Cushing's syndrome, acromegaly, possibly hypogonadotropic hypogonadism, and soft tissue myxomas. Hypophosphatemic osteomalacia may also accompany fibrous dysplasia and resembles the disorder associated with other skeletal and nonskeletal tumors. As mentioned, sarcomatous degeneration may rarely occur in fibrous dysplasia.

Although the lytic lesions of fibrous dysplasia resemble the brown tumors of hyperparathyroidism, the age of the patient, normal calcium levels, increased density of bone in the skull, and areas of cutaneous pigmentation identify the former condition. However, fibrous dysplasia and hyperparathyroidism may coexist. Neurofibromas may involve bone and produce cutaneous pigmentation as well as nodules in the skin. The pigmented macules of neurofibromatosis are more numerous and more widely distributed than in fibrous dysplasia, usually have smooth borders, and tend to involve areas such as the axillary folds. Other lesions that have roentgenographic features similar to those of isolated fibrous dysplasia are unicameral bone cysts, aneurysmal bone cysts, and nonossifying fibromas. Leontiasis ossea is most often due to fibrous dysplasia, although other disorders may also produce this appearance such as craniometaphyseal dysplasia, hyperphosphatasia, and, in adults, Paget's disease.

Treatment Fibrous dysplasia is not curable. The symptoms, however, can be managed using a variety of orthopedic procedures such as casting, osteotomy with internal fixation, curettage, and bone grafting depending upon the lesion and the age of the patient. Indications for such procedures include progressive deformity, nonunion of fractures, and pain unresponsive to conservative treatment. Calcitonin may be effective in treatment of widespread disease associated with bone pain and high serum alkaline phosphatase levels (see Chap. 344).

DYSPLASIAS AND CHONDRODYSTROPHIES A variety of diseases of bone and cartilage have been called *dystrophies* or *dysplasias*. The *osteochondrodysplasias* are heritable disorders of connective tissue that are characterized by primary abnormalities of cartilage that lead to disturbances in cartilage and bone growth and development. They comprise more than 100 distinct entities, which can be distinguished based on clinical, genetic, and radiologic features. The biochemical (and genetic) defects have been identified in few of these conditions. The greatest success has been in delineation of errors in metabolism of glycosaminoglycans (acid mucopolysaccharides) to explain the pathogenesis, for example, of Hunter's and Hurler's syndromes (see Chap. 331). Some reports suggest the presence of abnormalities in type II collagen in disorders such as Stickler's syndrome, Kniest dysplasia, and forms of achondrogenesis. In a related syndrome, spondyloepiphyseal dysplasia, a fragment of 36 amino acids in the helical region of type II collagen is deleted. A biochemical explanation for many of these conditions will permit more than a descriptive classification. At present, however, a useful scheme is that proposed by Rubin based on the consideration of errors in modeling of bone and cartilage (Table 345-2). Other clinical and genetic features form the basis of a classification by Rimoin. Pathologic processes in the skeletal dysplasias may be expressed as a deficiency (hypoplasia) or excess (hyperplasia) in relation to normal development.

Spondyloepiphyseal dysplasia The spondyloepiphyseal dysplasias are disorders in which abnormalities of growth occur in various bones including the vertebrae, pelvis, carpal and tarsal bones, and the epiphyses of tubular bones. On the basis of roentgenographic findings, this group can be divided into (1) those with generalized platyspondyly, (2) those with multiple epiphyseal dysplasias, and (3) those with epiphysometaphyseal dysplasias. *Morquio's syndrome*, in which there is a defect in degradation of glycosaminoglycans (therefore a "mucopolysaccharidosis") is inherited as an autosomal recessive trait and is associated with corneal opacities, dental defects, variable disturbances in intellect, and increased urinary excretion of keratosulfate, belongs in the first group. Other forms of spondyloepiphyseal dysplasia, some of which are accounted for by defects in type II collagen, may not be recognized until late in childhood or young

---

TABLE 345-2 Working classification of bone dysplasias

I Epiphyseal dysplasias
  A Epiphyseal hypoplasias
    1 Failure of articular cartilage: spondyloepiphyseal dysplasia, congenita and tarda
    2 Failure of ossification of center: multiple epiphyseal dysplasia, congenita and tarda
  B Epiphyseal hyperplasia
    1 Excess of articular cartilage: dysplasia epiphysialis hemimelica
II Physeal (growth plate) dysplasias
  A Cartilage hypoplasias
    1 Failure of proliferating cartilage: achondroplasia, congenita and tarda
    2 Failure of hypertrophic cartilage: metaphyseal dysostosis, congenita and tarda
  B Cartilage hyperplasias
    1 Excess of proliferating cartilage: hyperchondroplasia
    2 Excess of hypertrophic cartilage: enchondromatosis
III Metaphyseal dysplasias
  A Metaphyseal hypoplasias
    1 Failure to form primary spongiosa: hypophosphatasia, congenita and tarda
    2 Failure to absorb primary spongiosa: osteopetrosis, congenita and tarda
    3 Failure to absorb secondary spongiosa: craniometaphyseal dysplasia, congenita and tarda
  B Metaphyseal hyperplasia
    1 Excessive spongiosa: familial exostosis
IV Diaphyseal dysplasias
  A Diaphyseal hypoplasias
    1 Failure of periosteal bone formation: osteogenesis imperfecta, congenita and tarda
    2 Failure of endosteal bone formation: idiopathic osteoporosis
  B Diaphyseal hyperplasias
    1 Excessive periosteal bone formation: Engelmann's disease
    2 Excessive periosteal bone formation: hyperphosphatasia

adult life. Flat vertebral bodies are associated with other abnormalities in shape and alignment. The disordered development of the capital femoral epiphyses leads to irregularities in shape and flattening of the femoral heads and early onset of osteoarthritis of the hips.

Achondroplasia *Achondroplasia* is a physeal dysplasia in which dwarfism results from decrease in the proliferation of cartilage in the growth plate. This disorder is among the more common types of dwarfism and is inherited as an autosomal dominant trait. Histologic sections through the growth plate show a thin zone of cartilage cells with absence or abbreviation of the normal columnar arrangement and zone of provisional calcification, although endochondral ossification may not be completely disorganized. Formation of the primary spongiosa is reduced since there is often a transverse bar of bone sealing off the plate from further endochondral ossification. However, formation and maturation of the secondary ossification centers and articular cartilage are not disturbed. Appositional growth at the metaphysis continues, with resulting flare in this region of the bone; intramembranous bone formation at the periosteum is normal. The abnormal proliferation at the growth plate, leaving other areas relatively unaffected in the tubular bones, causes production of short bones that are proportionately thick. However, the length of the spine is almost always normal. The appearance of short limbs with a normal trunk is characteristically accompanied by a large head, saddlenose, and an exaggerated lumbar lordosis. The disease is usually recognized at birth. Those who survive the period of infancy usually have normal mental and sexual development, and life span may be normal. However, spinal deformity may lead to cord compression and nerve root encroachment, especially in those with kyphoscoliosis. Homozygous achondroplasia is a more serious disorder and a cause of neonatal death. In view of the observations in spondyloepiphyseal dysplasia, several of the achondroplasias may also eventually be explained on the basis of defects in genes encoding extracellular matrix components of cartilage such as proteoglycan core protein, types II or IX collagens, or link protein.

Enchondromatosis (dyschondroplasia, Ollier's disease)   This is also a disorder affecting the growth plate in which the hypertrophic cartilage is not resorbed and ossified in a normal fashion. It results in masses of cartilage with disorderly arrangement of the chondrocytes showing variable proliferative and hypertrophic changes. These masses are located in the metaphyses in close association with the growth plate in very young patients but often are diaphyseal in teenagers and young adults. The disorder is usually recognized in childhood by the appearance of deformities or retardation in growth. The most common sites of involvement are the ends of long bones, usually in the region where rate of growth is most marked. The pelvis is often involved, but ribs, sternum, and skull are seldom affected. There is also a tendency toward unilateral involvement. Chondrosarcoma develops occasionally in the enchondromata. The association of enchondromatosis and cavernous hemangiomata in the soft tissues including the skin is known as Maffucci's syndrome.

Multiple exostoses (diaphyseal aclasis or osteochondromatosis)   This is a disorder of the metaphysis, inherited as an autosomal dominant character, in which areas of the growth plate become displaced, presumably by growing through a defect in the perichondrium or so-called ring of Ranvier. The spongiosa forms within the mass as vessels invade the cartilage. Therefore, the diagnostic radiographic finding is the direct continuity of the mass to the marrow cavity of the parent bone with absence of underlying cortex. Usually the growth of these exostoses ceases when growth of the adjacent plate ceases. The lesions may be solitary or multiple and are usually located in the metaphyseal areas of long bones with the apex of the exostosis directed toward the diaphysis. Often the lesions produce no symptoms, but occasionally interference with the function of a joint or tendon or compression of nerves may result. Dwarfism may occur. The metacarpals may be shortened, resembling those seen in McCune-Albright's hereditary osteodystrophy. Multiple exostoses are sometimes seen in patients with pseudohypoparathyroidism.

An exostosis may suddenly begin to enlarge long after growth should have ceased, and rarely chondrosarcomas may develop from the cartilage cap of an exostosis. Pregnancy may stimulate growth of an exostosis that clinically may mimic malignancy. However, the lesion merely undergoes exuberant endochondral ossification and cartilage hyperplasia without malignant changes.

RELAPSING POLYCHONDRITIS   See Chap. 284.

TIETZE'S SYNDROME (COSTOCHONDRAL SYNDROME)   See Chap. 284.

REFERENCES

Hyperostosis

BOLLERSLEV J et al: Structural and histomorphometric studies of iliac crest trabecular and cortical bone in autosomal dominant osteopetrosis: A study of two radiological types. Bone 10:19, 1989

BOSTMAN OM et al: Osteosarcoma arising in a melorheostotic femur. J Bone Joint Surg 69A:1232, 1987

CANALIS E et al: Dynamic bone morphology and studies on the effects of serum on bone metabolism in vitro in a case of pycnodysostosis. Metab Bone Dis Rel Res 2:99, 1981

CAUDLE RJ et al: Melorheostosis of the hand. A case report with long-term follow-up. J Bone Joint Surg 69A:1229, 1987

CHAN Y-L et al: Dialysis osteodystrophy: A study involving 94 patients. Medicine 64:296, 1985

COCCIA PF et al: Successful bone-marrow transplantation for infantile malignant osteopetrosis. N Engl J Med 302:701, 1980

———— et al: Cells that resorb bone. N Engl J Med 310:456, 1984

COINDRE JM et al: Histomorphometric analysis of sclerotic bone from idiopathic myeloid metaplasia (nine cases). J Pathol 144:163, 1984

CRISP AJ, BRENTON DP: Engelmann's disease of bone—a systemic disorder? Ann Rheum Dis 41:183, 1982

DIGIOVANNA JJ et al: Extraspinal tendon and ligament calcification associated with long-term therapy with etretinate. N Engl J Med 315:1177, 1986

EINHORN TA et al: Hyperphosphatasemia in an adult. Clinical, roentgenographic, and histomorphometric findings and comparison to classical Paget's disease. Clin Orthop 204:253, 1986

GENNANT HK et al: Osteosclerosis in primary hyperparathyroidism. Am J Med 59:104, 1975

JACOBSON HG: Dense bone—too much bone: Radiological considerations and differential diagnosis. Part II. Skeletal Radiol 13:97, 1985

JOHNSON CC et al: Osteopetrosis: A clinical, genetic, metabolic and morphologic study of the dominantly inherited benign form. Medicine 47:149, 1968

KAPLAN FS et al: Successful treatment of infantile malignant osteopetrosis by bone-marrow transplantation. J Bone Joint Surg 70A:617, 1988

KEY L et al: Treatment of congenital osteopetrosis with high-dose calcitriol. N Engl J Med 310:409, 1984

KRAEMER KH et al: Prevention of skin cancer in xeroderma pigmentosum with the use of oral isotretinoin. N Engl J Med 318:1633, 1988

KUMAR R et al: An unusual case of pycnodysostosis. Arch Dis Child 63:558, 1988

MANZKE E et al: Skeletal remodeling and bone-related hormones in two adults with increased bone mass. Metabolism 31:25, 1982

MILLS BG et al: Osteoclasts in human osteopetrosis contain viral-nucleocapsid-like nuclear inclusions. J Bone Min Res 3:101, 1988

SCHMIDT J et al: Retrovirus-induced osteopetrosis in mice. Effects of viral infection on osteogenic differentiation in skeletoblast cell cultures. Am J Pathol 129:503, 1987

SHAPIRO F et al: Variable osteoclast appearance in human infantile osteopetrosis. Calcif Tissue Int 43:67, 1988

SHELDON J et al: Engelmann's disease (progressive diaphyseal dysplasia): A review and presentation of two cases with abnormal phosphate retention. Metab Bone Dis Rel Res 2:307, 1981

SLY WS et al: Carbonic anhydrase II deficiency in 12 families with the autosomal recessive syndrome of osteopetrosis with renal tubular acidosis and cerebral calcification. N Engl J Med 313:139, 1985

THOMPSON RC JR et al: Hereditary hyperphosphatasia. Am J Med 47:209, 1969

VAN BUCHEM FSP et al: Hyperostosis corticalis generalisata. Am J Med 33:387, 1962

Neoplasms of bone

BACCI G et al: Therapy for primary non-Hodgkin's lymphoma of bone and comparison of results with Ewing's sarcoma. Ten years' experience at the Istituto Ortopedico Rizzoli. Cancer 57:1468, 1986

———— et al: Neoadjuvant chemotherapy for osteosarcoma of the extremity. Clin Orthop 224:268, 1987

CHARHON SA et al: Parathyroid function and vitamin D status in patients with bone metastases of prostatic origin. Mineral Electrolyte Metab 11:117, 1985

DRYJA TP et al: Chromosome 13 homozygosity in osteosarcoma without retinoblastoma. Am J Hum Genet 38:59, 1986

ETTINGER LJ et al: Adjuvant adriamycin and cisplatin in newly diagnosed, nonmetastatic osteosarcoma of the extremity. J Clin Oncol 4:353, 1986

FECHNER RE et al: A symposium on the pathology of bone tumors. Pathol Ann 19(Part 1):125, 1984

GOORIN AM et al: Osteosarcoma: Fifteen years later. N Engl J Med 313:165, 1985

HAN M-T et al: Aggressive thoracotomy for pulmonary metastatic osteogenic sarcoma in children and young adolescents. J Pediatr Surg 16:928, 1981

HAYES FA et al: Metastatic Ewing's sarcoma: Remission induction and survival. J Clin Oncol 5:1199, 1987

VAN HOLTEN-VERZANTVOORT AT et al: Reduced morbidity from skeletal metastases in breast cancer patients during long-term bisphosphonate (APD) treatment. Lancet 2:983, 1987

HUVOS AG: Osteogenic sarcoma of bones and soft tissues in older persons. A clinicopathologic analysis of 117 patients older than 60 years. Cancer 57:1442, 1986

——— et al: Osteogenic sarcoma associated with Paget's disease of bone. A clinicopathologic study of 65 patients. Cancer 52:1489, 1983

KANIS JA (ed): Clodronate—a new perspective in the treatment of neoplastic bone disease. Bone 8(Suppl 1):S1, 1987

KLEEREKOPER M, KRANE SM (eds): Clinical Disorders of Bone and Mineral Metabolism. New York, Mary Ann Liebert, pp 1–649, 1989

MANKIN HJ, GEBHARDT MC: Advances in the management of bone tumors. Clin Orthop Rel Res 200:73, 1985

——— et al: The use of frozen cadaveric allografts in the management of patients with bone tumors of the extremities. Orthop Clin North Am 18:275, 1987

MISER JS et al: Preliminary results of treatment of Ewing's sarcoma of bone in children and young adults: Six months of intensive combined modality therapy without maintenance. J Clin Oncol 6:484, 1988

SCHILLER AL: Diagnosis of borderline cartilage lesions of bone. Semin Diag Pathol 2:42, 1985

SIMON MA, NACHMAN J: The clinical utility of preoperative therapy for sarcomas. J Bone Joint Surg 68A:1458, 1986

——— et al: Limb-salvage treatment versus amputation for osteosarcoma of the distal end of the femur. J Bone Joint Surg 68A:1331, 1986

SUIT HD et al: Treatment of the patient with stage M_0 soft tissue sarcoma. J Clin Oncol 6:854, 1988

SUTOW WW et al: Survival after metastasis in osteosarcoma. Natl Cancer Inst Monogr 56:227, 1981

UNNI KK et al: Conditions that simulate primary neoplasms of bone. Pathol Ann 15(Part 1):91, 1980

WIGGS J et al: Prediction of the risk of hereditary retinoblastoma, using DNA polymorphisms within the retinoblastoma gene. N Engl J Med 318:151, 1988

WINKLER K et al: Neoadjuvant chemotherapy of osteosarcoma: Results of a randomized cooperative trial (COSS-82) with salvage chemotherapy based on histological tumor response. J Clin Oncol 6:329, 1988

YUNIS EJ, BARNES L: The histologic diversity of osteosarcoma. Pathol Ann 21(Part 1):121, 1986

Other disorders of bone and cartilage

AKESON WH et al: Symposium on Heritable Disorders of Connective Tissue. St. Louis, Mosby, 1982

ALBRIGHT FA et al: Syndrome characterized by osteitis fibrosa disseminata, areas of pigmentation and endocrine dysfunction, with precocious puberty in females. Report of five cases. N Engl J Med 216:727, 1937

BENEDICT PH: Endocrine features in Albright's syndrome (fibrous dysplasia of bone). Metabolism 11:30, 1962

——— et al: Melanotic macules in Albright's syndrome and in neurofibromatosis. JAMA 205:618, 1968

GEFFNER ME et al: Treatment of acromegaly with a somatostatin analog in a patient with McCune-Albright syndrome. J Pediatr 111:740, 1987

GRABIAS SL, CAMPBELL CJ: Fibrous dysplasia. Orthop Clin North Am 8:771, 1977

HARRIS RI: Polyostotic fibrous dysplasia with acromegaly. Am J Med 78:539, 1985

HARRIS WH et al: The natural history of fibrous dysplasia: An orthopaedic, pathological and roentgenographic study. J Bone Joint Surg (Br) 44A:207, 1962

KAPLAN FS et al: Estrogen receptors in bone in a patient with polyostotic fibrous dysplasia (McCune-Albright syndrome). N Engl J Med 319:421, 1988

LEE B et al: Identification of the molecular defect in a family with spondyloepiphyseal dysplasia. Science 244:978, 1989

NAGER GT et al: Fibrous dysplasia: A review of the disease and its manifestations in the temporal bone. Ann Otol Rhinol Laryngol 91(suppl 92):1, 1982

PALOTIE A et al: Predisposition to familial osteoarthrosis linked to type II collagen gene. Lancet 1:924, 1989

RIMOIN DL: The chondrodystrophies. Adv Hum Genet 5:1, 1975

RUBIN P: Dynamic Classification of Bone Dysplasias. Chicago, Year Book, 1964

SAMBROOK PN et al: Synovial complications of spondylepiphyseal dysplasia of late onset. Arthritis Rheum 31:282, 1988

SILLENCE DO et al: Neonatal dwarfism. Pediatr Clin North Am 25:431, 1978

STEPHENSON RB et al: Fibrous dysplasia. An analysis of options for treatment. J Bone Joint Surg 69A:409, 1987

YABUL SM et al: Malignant transformation of fibrous dysplasia. A case report and review of the literature. Clin Orthop 281, 1988

346 IMPACT OF NEUROBIOLOGY ON NEUROLOGY AND PSYCHIATRY

JOSEPH B. MARTIN

Advances in molecular genetics, neurobiology, and brain imaging are having a major impact on neurology and psychiatry. These advances are changing our understanding of how the brain is constructed and of the way it functions. They are also expanding the repertoire of experimental approaches, some of which may be successful in solving both basic and clinical problems. The discoveries imply the possibility of defining a rational taxonomy for many of the inherited diseases affecting the nervous system, enable new approaches for understanding the molecular basis of development (and degeneration) of the nervous system, and permit analysis of cognitive brain function in ways not previously possible.

The advances have occurred on several fronts, which are now beginning to coalesce into a general move forward. The identification of genes responsible for several of the inherited neuropsychiatric diseases has provided insight into their pathogenesis. Research in molecular structure has disclosed several proteins that subserve receptor and membrane channel functions (see Chap. 11). Elucidation of neurotransmitter signal transduction has modified our perception of intercellular and intracellular communication. These discoveries have major implications for drug development by permitting identification of more selective receptor agonists and antagonists. There is also new insight into the mechanisms of cellular injury and neuronal death. The ability to analyze neuronal structure and function extends also to the intact brain. Positron emission tomography (PET) and in vivo magnetic resonance spectroscopy now provide means for analysis of the functional organization of the brain.

The impacts of some of these efforts are reviewed in this chapter.

MOLECULAR GENETICS Applications of molecular biology have already had a major effect on the clinical neurosciences. In the case of inherited neurologic diseases, there is the use of DNA probes that demonstrate restriction fragment length polymorphisms (RFLPs), which can be combined with linkage analysis in affected pedigrees (see Chap. 6). These tools have made possible the chromosomal localization of the mutant gene in Huntington's disease (see Chap. 359), some cases of familial Alzheimer's disease (see Chap. 359), neurofibromatosis (see Chap. 358), Friedreich's ataxia (see Chap. 359), spinal muscular atrophy, torsion dystonia, Wilson's disease, and several types of familial CNS tumors including retinoblastoma and von Hippel–Lindau disease (see Table 346-1). The use of linkage analysis with chromosome-specific RFLPs is the first step toward characterization of the abnormal gene product, a process referred to as "reverse genetics," i.e., analysis of gene structure makes possible studies of the abnormal cellular protein (see Chap. 285).

In two conditions this approach has already affected clinical practice. In Duchenne's dystrophy, an X-linked disorder, the muscle abnormality results from failure to encode for a membrane protein, *dystrophin*, which is absent from skeletal muscle in virtually all patients with the disorder (see Chap. 365). This discovery has proved of theoretical importance in a less severe allied condition, Becker's dystrophy, where dystrophin is present but in abnormal amounts or of abnormal size. Dystrophin is also present in smooth muscle, cardiac muscle, and brain. Its presence in the brain presumably accounts in some way yet to be defined for the frequent occurrence of mental retardation in individuals with Duchenne's dystrophy. The precise function of dystrophin remains to be elucidated, but it is now known to be a membrane-associated structural protein that appears to function as a strut to maintain membrane integrity during muscular contraction. The discovery of dystrophin demonstrates elegantly the power of reverse genetics. Decades of effort attempting to define the protein abnormality in Duchenne's dystrophy had been unsuccessful. The quantities of dystrophin present in muscle are so minute that it could not have been characterized by current biochemical approaches.

In retinoblastoma, identification of the protein encoded by the normal allele of the gene (a growth suppressor gene) that is absent from the tumor has provided insight into cellular growth. It is postulated that an inherited mutation affects one allele of the normal gene. If this is followed by a "second hit" mutation that eliminates the function of the second allele in one of the cells in the developing retina, the cell growth suppressor cannot be synthesized. The consequence is the abnormal division of cells in the retina and tumor formation (see also Chap. 10). Another tumor associated with hereditary retinoblastoma is osteosarcoma. A similar mechanism for tumor formation may be involved in Wilms' tumor (on chromosome 11) and in the von Hippel–Lindau syndrome, which leads to hemangioblastoma, pheochromocytoma, and renal cell carcinoma (shown by RFLPs to be located on chromosome 3) (see Table 346-1).

The application of RFLPs has provided new approaches to presymptomatic and prenatal diagnosis of Huntington's disease (Fig. 346-1), Duchenne's dystrophy, retinoblastoma, and von Hippel–Lindau disease (see also Chap. 353).

CHARACTERIZATION OF NEW NEUROTRANSMITTER CANDIDATES More than 60 neurotransmitter candidates have been identified in brain based upon localization within synaptic vesicles, release with depolarization, and interactions with postsynaptic receptors. The functions of these agents, many of which are small-molecular-weight peptides (neuropeptides), remain obscure in many cases. But some are known to modulate functions such as pain transmission (opioid peptides), satiety (cholecystokinin), and thirst (angiotensin).

The discovery of these molecules has made possible new approaches to defining neuronal populations in the human brain by immunohistochemical staining, autoradiography, and in situ messenger RNA hybridization. This information has made it possible to delineate the subclasses of cells affected in neurodegenerative diseases, such as Alzheimer's, Parkinson's, and Huntington's disease. Realization that dopamine cells are affected in Parkinson's disease led to the idea of therapy with levodopa. In Huntington's disease, it has been possible to define the subsets of neurons affected by the degenerative process in the striatum and to show selective sparing of other cell types (see Chap. 359). Although this has not led yet to specific theories about the mechanisms of cell death, it has resulted in speculations about potentially beneficial therapeutic strategies.

Many of these newly discovered neuropeptides appear to share

TABLE 346-1 Chromosomal localization and gene abnormalities in selected neurologic diseases

Genetic classification and disease	Chromosome	Gene defect	Comments on genetic heterogeneity
AUTOSOMAL DOMINANT			
Charcot-Marie-Tooth disease (type 1)	1p22–1q23	Unknown	Unknown
von Hippel–Lindau disease	3p	Unknown (possible deficiency in growth suppressor gene)	None demonstrated in over 10 pedigrees
Huntington's disease	4p16.3	Unknown	None demonstrated in over 100 pedigrees
Spinocerebellar ataxia (one form)	6p21.2–q12	Unknown	Unknown
Torsion dystonia	9q32–q34	Unknown	None demonstrated
Retinoblastoma	13q14	Absence of Rb protein	Allelic heterogeneity
von Recklinghausen's neurofibromatosis (NFl)	17q11.2	Unknown	None demonstrated in over 25 pedigrees
Familial amyloidotic polyneuropathy	18q11.2–q12.1	Single-base pair substitution in mRNA for transthyretin	Allelic heterogeneity
Myotonic dystrophy	19–centromere	Unknown	None demonstrated
Benign familial convulsions	20q13.2	Unknown	Unknown
Familial Alzheimer's disease	21q21	Unknown (not amyloid protein)	Probable heterogeneity
Bilateral acoustic neurofibromatosis (NF2)	22q11–q13	Unknown	Unknown
AUTOSOMAL RECESSIVE			
Gaucher's disease	1q21	Amino acid substitution in gluco-cerebrosidase	Allelic heterogeneity
Spinal muscular atrophy	5q11.2–q13.3		None demonstrated
Friedreich's ataxia	9p22–centromere	Unknown	None found in 23 pedigrees
Ataxia-telangiectasia	11q22–23	Unknown	None found in 31 families
Wilson's disease	13q14.11	Unknown (not ceruloplasmin)	Unknown
G_{M2} gangliosidosis			
Tay-Sachs disease (type 1)	15q22–q25	Mutation in gene encoding α chain of hexosaminidase	Allelic heterogeneity
Sandhoff's disease (type 2)	5q13	Mutation in gene encoding β chain of hexosaminidase	Allelic heterogeneity
X-LINKED RECESSIVE			
Duchenne's dystrophy	Xp21.21	Absence of dystrophin	Multiallelic heterogeneity
Becker's dystrophy	Xp21.21	Defect in dystrophin	Multiallelic heterogeneity
Pelizaeus-Merzbacher disease	Xq21–q22	Defect in myelin proteolipid protein	Unknown
Adrenoleukodystrophy	Xq27–q28	Unknown	Unknown
Lesch-Nyhan syndrome	Xq27	Hypoxanthine-guanine phosphoribo-syltransferase deficiency	Multiallelic heterogeneity
Emery-Dreifuss dystrophy	Xq28	Unknown	Unknown
MITOCHONDRIAL DISEASES WITH MATERNAL TRANSMISSION			
Mitochondrial myopathy		Deletion in mitochondrial DNA	
Leber's hereditary optic atrophy		Amino acid substitution in NADH dehydrogenase, subunit 4	

SOURCE: Modified from JB Martin, 1989. Reproduced with permission.

nerve terminals and often even secretory vesicles with conventional neurotransmitters. It appears likely that neuropeptides exert profound modulatory effects on the actions of the primary neurotransmitter. In other cases the peptide may influence neuronal plasticity, growth, or differentiation.

BIOCHEMICAL CLASSIFICATION OF RECEPTOR SUBTYPES Some of the most important insights from the new biology have resulted from the cloning of the genes of several neurotransmitter and hormone receptors that were identified originally by pharmacologic means. Based on pharmacologic analysis alone it was difficult to account for the diverse effects mediated by molecules of low molecular weight. For example, acetylcholine has many diverse effects that on pharmacologic analysis were divided into muscarinic and nicotinic effects. With the biochemical elucidation of acetylcholine receptor subtypes and through the use of molecular cloning techniques and molecular probes, it is now established that multiple forms of muscarinic (M1, M2, M3, M4, and M5) and nicotinic (N1 and N2) receptors exist in the brain and that their distribution varies from region to region. Thus, differences in receptor subtypes expressed in different regions of the brain can account for the complex multiple effects of the medications acting on cholinergic receptors. The molecular specificities of the various receptor subtypes provide sensitive systems with which to search for selective agonists and antagonists. For example, M1 agonists may facilitate memory. Regional differences in the distribution of the subtypes of the nicotinic

cholinergic receptor in the central nervous system make it possible to explore the neurologic basis of nicotine addiction.

Identification of the subclasses of the alpha- and beta-adrenergic receptors, of serotonin receptors, and of gamma-aminobutyric acid (GABA) receptors makes it possible to correlate structure and function and provide a rational basis for molecular classification of drug actions. In the case of the GABA receptor, structural features that account for the interaction of barbiturates and benzodiazepines can now be elucidated (see Snyder).

Subclasses of glutamate receptors that mediate excitatory amino acid neurotransmitter effects have also been defined. Glutamate, one of the most abundant of all neurotransmitters in the brain, functions to promote rapid neurotransmitter depolarization by opening membrane channels that permit diffusion of sodium and potassium ions. These rapid effects are mediated by two receptor subtypes, identified by ligand binding with kainate and quisqualate. The identification of an additional subtype of glutamate receptor which binds N-methyl-D-aspartate (the *NMDA receptor*) made possible identification of additional glutamate functions. The NMDA receptor appears to mediate other functions that heretofore were classed in the category of plasticity, a process considered important, for example, in memory and learning. The NMDA subtype of glutamate receptor is linked to a voltage-sensitive channel that responds to repetitive activation by the opening of an ion channel (Fig. 346-2; see also Chap. 11). The actions of calcium permit transduction of electrical events into

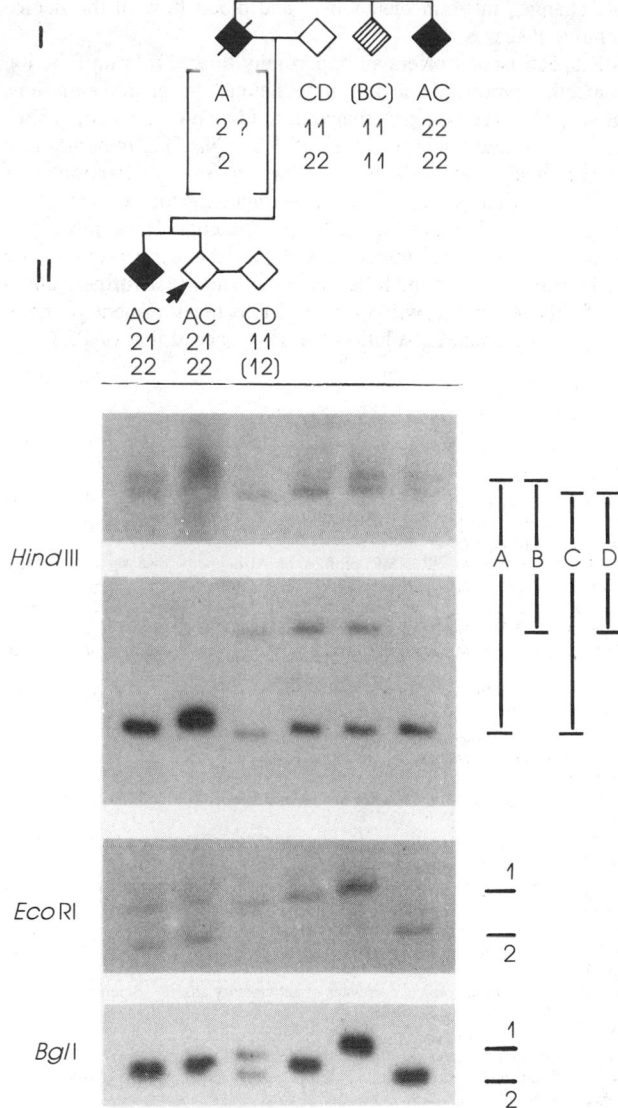

FIGURE 346-1 Sample family pedigree and Southern blot for a positive predictive test for Huntington's disease. Solid symbols denote a person with Huntington's disease; a diagonal line, a dead person; and crosshatched symbols, a person suspected to have Huntington's disease; the arrow indicates the family member who requested the predictive test. *Hind*III, *Eco*RI, and *Bgl*I were employed to detect alternate forms of RFLPs. *Hind*III recognized two different RFLPs, producing A, B, C, and D patterns, whereas *Eco*RI and *Bgl*I recognized only one RFLP (1 or 2). In cases in which the combination of alleles grouped together on a specific chromosome or phase could not be specified, alleles with alternative possible phases are depicted in parentheses (i.e., C11/D12 could be C12/D11 for subject II-3). Markers reconstructed for a deceased subject are enclosed in brackets. The affected sibling (I-4) of the affected parent (I-1) and the affected sibling (II-1) of the participant (II-2) had only the A22 haplotype (set of alleles located on same chromosome) in common; therefore, the Huntington's disease gene appeared to segregate with A22. A sibling (I-3) of the affected parent with neurologic symptoms that were suspected of indicating the presence of Huntington's disease did not have the A22 form of the marker. The participant inherited from the affected parent the A22 form of the marker allele apparently linked to the Huntington's disease gene, since the C12 was inherited from the unaffected parent. (*From GJ Meissen et al, with permission.*)

molecular changes that can alter neuronal function permanently, i.e., change cellular function to subserve a memory or learning response.

It now appears, on the basis of quite definitive experimentation, that activation of the NMDA receptor can also have deleterious effects on the cell, whereby calcium entry induces *neurotoxicity* that, if sufficiently severe, can lead to neuronal cell death. This mechanism

may explain some of the extensive neuronal cell damage that occurs in ischemia, hypoxia, epilepsy, and, perhaps, neurodegenerative diseases (see Choi).

These findings have resulted in great interest in the development of new drugs that might selectively block the NMDA receptor, thereby minimizing the effects of ischemia or hypoxia that occur in stroke or after cardiorespiratory arrest. The profound potential of this work is illustrated by the demonstration that NMDA receptor blockade induced even several hours after the neuronal insult may be "neuroprotective."

Cloning of cellular membrane channels (sodium, potassium, calcium) has also had a profound effect on defining mechanisms of neuronal excitability. It can be expected that these findings will also be translated into discovery of more effective neuroactive drugs.

BRAIN IMAGING The development of computed tomography and proton imaging by magnetic resonance has revolutionized our ability to define lesions in the brain and spinal cord (see Chap. 348). Other techniques have been developed to make it possible to study brain function as well as structure by the application of positron emission tomography (PET), single photon emission computed tomography (SPECT), and nuclear magnetic resonance spectroscopy (NMRS).

PET scanning involves the use of positron-emitting radionuclides with short half-lives in which particle disintegration is captured in a three-dimensional array by multiple sensors positioned about the head. With the use of radioisotopes for carbon (^{13}C), oxygen (^{15}O), and fluorine (^{18}F), it is possible to measure cerebral blood flow, cerebral oxygen metabolism, and cerebral glucose uptake (with ^{18}F-labeled deoxyglucose). The last technique uses the principles devel-

FIGURE 346-2 Model of proposed mechanisms of activation and deactivation of glutamate (GLU) *N*-methyl-D-aspartate (NMDA) receptor-channel complex. *A* and *B*. Glutamate attaches to receptor to cause opening of channel, first to Na⁺ and K⁺ and, after membrane depolarization, to Ca⁺⁺. Glycine (GLY) modulates effects of GLU. *C*. Competitive receptor antagonists, such as AP5 can prevent GLU activation. *D*. Other drugs and ions can block an opened channel by noncompetitive antagonism. These drugs include phencyclidine (PCP) and an experimental neuroprotective drug, MK801. Mg⁺⁺ can also block the channel.

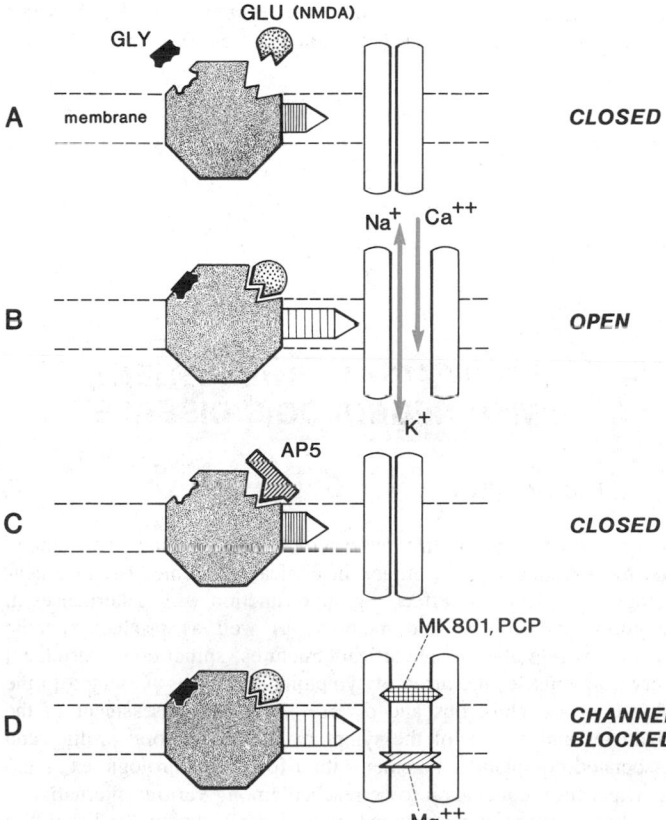

oped by Sokoloff and colleagues, who first used the technique of labeled deoxyglucose combined with tissue section autoradiography. PET scanning is also used to define regional changes in cerebral function associated with stroke, Alzheimer's disease, Huntington's disease, and schizophrenia, and it identifies foci of hyperactivity associated with seizures.

Perhaps the most creative use of PET techniques has been analysis of language function. Two theories of language had emerged from studies in neurology and linguistics. The first proposed that language function occurs serially, i.e., an object is first seen in the occipital lobes, its name is recalled by the temporal lobes, and the information is then sent to the frontal lobes, which direct formation of speech. PET studies have now confirmed the second of these hypotheses, which suggested from linguistic analysis that language occurs in a parallel array. Posner and colleagues, using subtraction techniques to isolate activity associated with a particular language task, have shown clearly that brain processing occurs simultaneously in several of the regions underlying a set of neurologic functions. These kinds of analyses now permit regionalized functional study of the brain in a manner not hitherto expected by the physical limits set by three-dimensional imaging using positron emitters. Regional studies of this kind have also shown that brain blood flow changes that occur in panic disorder and anticipatory anxiety correlate with anatomic loci in the temporal lobes.

There have also been important advances in the use of radioligands for neurotransmitter receptors. The imaging of dopamine and of dopamine receptors in the basal ganglia has been achieved in both normals and in patients with Parkinson's disease and with 1-methyl-4-phenyl-1,2,3,6-tetrahydropyridine (MPTP) poisoning. In the latter case deficits in basal ganglion function in asymptomatic subjects exposed to MPTP raise the possibility of identifying subclinical deficits and of following subjects over time to determine eventual outcome and prognosis.

SPECT imaging has been made possible by refinements in detection systems for single photon emitters. The resolution of SPECT does not yet reach the capacity of PET, but the longer half-lives of the isotopes and the simplicity of the detection systems make it less expensive and potentially more widely available. Its potential includes measurement of radioligand binding to receptors and determination of cerebral blood flow. Thus far, studies with SPECT have delineated regional changes in brain metabolism and blood flow in the neurodegenerative diseases.

NMR spectroscopy offers an opportunity to assess brain function at the subcellular molecular level. The technique uses natural emissions from atomic nuclei activated by magnetic fields to measure endogenous molecules. Potential nuclei include ^{31}P, ^{13}C, ^{23}Na, ^{7}Li, in addition to ^{1}H. The promise of analysis of ^{31}P is the closest to realization. It is possible to quantitate several phosphate-containing compounds (phosphocreatine, ATP, ADP, and inorganic phosphorus). The combination of spectral analysis with topical NMR permits localization within superficial regions of brain. It can be anticipated that further refinements of this technique will make possible measurement of brain metabolism with spatial resolution that may exceed that of PET.

REFERENCES

BREAKEFIELD XO, CAMBI F: Molecular genetic insights into neurologic diseases, in *Annual Review of Neuroscience*, vol 10, WM Cowan et al (eds). Palo Alto, Annual Reviews, 1987, pp 535–594

BROWN GG et al: In vivo ^{31}P NMR profiles of Alzheimer's disease and multiple subcortical infarct dementia. Neurology 39:1423, 1989

BUCKLEY NJ et al: Antagonist binding properties of five cloned muscarinic receptors expressed in CHO-K1 cells. Molec Pharmacol 35(4):469, 1989

CHOI D: Glutamate neurotoxicity and diseases of the nervous system. Neuron 1:623, 1989

COOPER JR et al: *The Biochemical Basis of Neuropharmacology*. New York, Oxford University Press, 1986

GUSELLA JF et al: DNA markers for nervous system diseases. Science 225:1320, 1984

MARTIN JB: Molecular genetics: Applications to the clinical neurosciences. Science 238:765, 1987

————: Molecular genetic studies in the neuropsychiatric disorders. Trends Neurosci 12:130, 1989

MEISSEN GJ et al: Predictive testing for Huntington's disease with use of a linked DNA marker. N Engl J Med 318:535, 1988

PETTEGREW JW et al: ^{31}P nuclear magnetic resonance studies of phosphoglyceride metabolism in developing and degenerating brain: Preliminary observations. J Neuropathol Exp Neurol 46:419, 1987

POSNER MI et al: Localization of cognitive operations in the human brain. Science 240:1627, 1988

REIMAN EM et al: Neuroanatomical correlates of anticipatory anxiety. Science 243:1071, 1989

ROWE CC et al: Localization of epileptic foci with postictal single photon emission computed tomography. Ann Neurol 26:660, 1989

SNYDER SH: Drug and neurotransmitter receptors: New perspectives with clinical relevance. JAMA 261:3126, 1989

section 1 The central nervous system

347 APPROACH TO THE PATIENT WITH NEUROLOGIC DISEASE

JOSEPH B. MARTIN

Symptoms and signs of disordered nervous system function are among the most frequent and complex in clinical medicine. Because neurologic disorders may affect cognitive function with disturbances in language, perception, and memory, as well as produce specific symptoms referable to subcortical structures, spinal cord, peripheral nerve, or muscle, the array of symptoms and signs presented to the physician are numerous and diverse. A careful assessment of the character and pattern of the symptoms, their temporal profile, and associated complaints, together with a focused neurologic examination, permit a conclusion to be reached among various alternatives.

These considerations are made more complicated by the difficulties that often arise in distinguishing so-called neurologic from psychiatric diseases. In general, the neurologist has defined disease of the nervous system as any condition that produces a visible anatomic or definable biochemical lesion. However, it is now recognized that many primary neurologic disorders, which present with severe clinical manifestations, fail to show any demonstrable neuropathologic or neurochemical abnormality, even when scrutinized by the most modern techniques of neurobiology. The conditions of dystonia musculorum deformans, spasmodic torticollis, tardive dyskinesia, and Gilles de la Tourette's syndrome, for example, are considered to be neurologic disorders, yet no defined structural abnormality has been reported. The possibility that such disorders are caused by abnormalities of neurotransmitter release or of receptor function is currently viewed as likely because of their partial response to various neuropharmacologic drugs. In other disorders traditionally treated by the psychiatrist, in particular the major psychoses of schizophrenia and of manic-depressive disease, accumulated evidence based on genetic analysis, responses to neuroactive agents, and documented neuroendocrine-biochemical abnormalities suggest that these, too, are primary disorders of nervous system function. This conclusion is supported further by observations that similar psychotic symptoms can be observed in patients with readily identifiable lesions of the nervous system (chronic temporal lobe seizures, brain tumor) or after the administration of certain drugs, such as lysergic acid or amphetamines.

Despite the importance of these areas of overlap between neurology and psychiatry, most neurologic conditions for which a patient seeks general medical care are due to readily demonstrated disease processes. It is the task of the clinician to develop a neurologic method of analysis that will result in accurate diagnosis of the site of the disorder and of its likely cause. Only then can effective approaches to management and treatment be developed.

In this and the subsequent sections, neurology and psychiatry are considered separately because many of the approaches to diagnosis and treatment remain distinct even today. In the chapters that follow, neurologic disorders and diseases are described as they present to the neurologist or general internist. Currently accepted explanations in terms of anatomy, physiology, pharmacology, and chemistry are offered. The section on psychiatric disorders is found in Chaps. 368 and 369. Dependency syndromes are described in Chaps. 370 to 373.

THE NEUROLOGIC METHOD OF CLINICAL EVALUATION   The strategy used in evaluating a patient with neurologic illness is to begin with the question, Where is the lesion that is causing the neurologic symptoms? The first clues to answering this question appear in the history, and the examination is then "tailor-made" to clarify uncertainties or to make distinctions suggested by the history. Thus, optokinetic nystagmus might be an important part of the examination in a patient with a left hemiparesis and dressing apraxia, but irrelevant to the examination of a patient complaining of burning feet. In a patient who presents with the history of ascending paresthesia and weakness, the examination must be *directed* to deciding, among other things, if the location of the lesion is the spinal cord or peripheral nerves. Notations regarding muscle stamina or endurance might be crucial to the examination of a patient with myasthenia gravis, as opposed to the usual tests of peak muscle power. What one does with the neurologic examination depends on what the questions are; the questions are formulated by a properly taken history.

Deciding "where the lesion is" accomplishes the task of delimiting the number of possible etiologies to a manageable, finite size. In addition, this strategy safeguards against making really tragic errors. Symptoms of recurrent vertigo, diplopia, and nystagmus should not trigger "multiple sclerosis" as an answer (etiology), but "brainstem" or "pons" (location); then a diagnosis of brainstem arteriovenous malformation will not be missed because it is not considered. The combination of optic neuritis and spastic, ataxic paraparesis should not be memorized as "multiple sclerosis"; then central nervous system syphilis and vitamin B_{12} deficiency (both treatable) will not be overlooked.

Only after the clinician decides "where the lesion is," should the question "what the lesion is" be asked.

The neurologic history   A bewildering array of clinical abnormalities require documentation and interpretation during the neurologic evaluation of a patient. The analysis becomes difficult because similar symptoms and signs may present in a patient with any of several disorders. A number of general principles relevant to obtaining a complete neurologic history are important for the physician, whether a generalist or a specialist. Careful attention to the description of the symptoms as experienced by the patient and substantiated by family members or friends permits, in many instances, an accurate localization and determination of the probable cause of the complaints even before an examination of the patient has been undertaken. Two principles should be followed. First, each complaint ought to be chased down as far as possible in an effort to delineate (before the examination) where the lesion might be or, more importantly, *to formulate a set of questions to be answered by the examination*. A patient complains of weakness of the right upper limb. What are the associated features? Is this weakness for brushing the hair or opening

a twist-top can? Second, in neurology—where many of the diseases are due to *anatomically restricted* lesions—*negative* associations may be crucial. A patient with a right hemiparesis without a language deficit likely has a different lesion (and likely etiology) than a patient with a right hemiparesis and aphasia. Several of the important factors that aid greatly in defining the nature of the neurologic disorder include:

1 *Temporal course of the illness*. It is particularly important to ascertain the precise rate of appearance and progression of the symptoms experienced by the patient. A paroxysmal onset of a neurologic complaint, occurring within seconds or minutes, usually indicates a cerebrovascular lesion or a seizure. Attention to the temporal march of symptoms may help define a focal seizure, a transient cerebral ischemic attack (TIA), or the onset of a migraine. For example, the onset of sensory symptoms located in one extremity that spreads over a few seconds to adjacent portions of that extremity and then to the other limb or to the face suggests a seizure. A more gradual onset involving less discrete regions of the extremities points to the possibility of a TIA. A similar, but slower progression of sensory change occurring in a young person together with other symptoms of headache, nausea, or visual disturbance suggest migraine. In general, the march of a migraine is slower than that of seizure, and a TIA tends to be more generalized in location on the side of the body or extremities. The presence of positive sensory symptoms or motor movements suggests a seizure; in contrast, transient loss of a function (negative symptom) suggests a TIA. A stuttering onset where symptoms appear, stabilize, regress, and then progress over hours or days also suggests the presence of impending vascular ischemia. In some cases, a demyelinating process may produce new symptoms over the course of a few hours. Progressing symptoms associated with the systemic manifestation of fever, stiff neck, and altered level of consciousness or awareness suggest the possibility of an infectious process. The course of the illness over years in terms of remissions and exacerbations offers additional clues to the nature of the process. Recurrent neurologic symptoms involving any level of the neuraxis with partial or complete recovery suggest the possibility of multiple sclerosis. Slowly progressive disorders without remissions tend to be characteristic of the neurodegenerative processes that affect the nervous system.

2 *Subjective descriptions of the complaint*. It is wise for the physician to recall that patient vocabularies are often limited and that symptoms are interpreted within the experience of the patient. Descriptions are highly introspective and subject to the patient's degree of intelligence and general familiarity with medical terminology. The same words often mean very different things to individual patients. For example, dizziness may be a description applied by the patient to impending syncope, to a sense of giddiness, or to true vertigo. Numbness may mean a complete loss of feeling, a positive sensation of tingling, or paralysis. Blurring of vision may be used to describe unilateral visual loss, as in amaurosis fugax, or diplopia. It is important to determine the level of understanding that the patient exhibits with respect to the complaint in order to assess accurately the precise significance of the symptom.

3 *Corroboration of the history by other close associates*. It is often useful to obtain additional information from family, friends, or observers to corroborate or expand the patient's description. Memory loss, personality change, drug abuse, excess alcohol intake, and other factors may severely impair the ability of patients to describe accurately their subjective experiences or prevent them from being completely open and forthright about the factors that have contributed to the illness. Complaints of loss of consciousness that may be due to syncope or seizures necessitate seeking details from patients and family to ascertain the exact circumstances. It is often important to recognize the major manifestations of depression and anxiety that may mask or color the presentation given by the patient. Failure to note these underlying factors which

interfere with the patient's performance may result in the incorrect interpretation that a variety of complaints are actually due to structural disease of the brain.

4 *Family history.* Many neurologic disorders, particularly those presenting in childhood or early adulthood, are familial or inherited conditions. It is important to ascertain the familial frequency of occurrence of systemic diseases such as hypertension, heart disease, or stroke, which may affect the nervous system. It is essential to inquire about the possibility of consanguinity of the parents or of the existence of similar symptoms in other members of the family. These may provide clues to a propensity toward a hereditary neurologic condition. It is critical to distinguish between a *negative* family history and an *incomplete* family history. It is insufficient to simply ask, Is there any similar illness in any member of your family? A negative response to such an inquiry may mean that there is, in fact, no such illness in the patient's family, but it may also mean that the patient is unfamiliar with relatives or their medical histories. It is wise to elicit specific positive or negative data about relatives as follows: Are your parents living? If so, are they well? If not, what illness did they have and how did they die? It should always be remembered that maternity is a fact, but paternity is only an assumption.

It is also important to elicit family history data regarding all illnesses rather than just neurologic and psychiatric disorders. Many familial neurologic illnesses are associated with signs and symptoms in other systems (e.g., the phakomatoses, hepatocerebral disorders, neuroophthalmic syndromes, etc.).

5 *Medical illnesses.* Many neurologic illnesses occur in the context of systemic disorders. A history of allergy and asthma may suggest the onset of polyarteritis, with mononeuritis multiplex. Previous or current medical illnesses such as diabetes mellitus, hypertension, and abnormalities of blood lipids may be relevant to evolving symptoms that affect the nervous system. Similarly, the presence of systemic diseases that have an increased association with peripheral neuropathy should be explored. Most patients with coma in a hospital setting can be shown to have a metabolic, toxic, or infectious process.

6 *The patient's perception of the disease.* It is frequently helpful to ask patients what they perceive to be wrong. Do they have a particular fear about a disease like Alzheimer's disease, a brain tumor, or multiple sclerosis? Increasingly, patients who complain of failing memory are concerned about early symptoms of Alzheimer's disease. Patients with headaches may fear that a tumor or an impending stroke is a possibility. Patients with sensory symptoms frequently are concerned about the possibility of multiple sclerosis. Or the patient may seek attention because a relative or friend has been diagnosed with a serious neurologic illness.

7 *Drug use and abuse and toxin exposure.* It is essential to inquire about the history of drug use, both prescribed and illicit. Complaints of yellow vision may occur with digitalis administration. Excessive vitamin administration may lead to peripheral neuropathy, as has been demonstrated in the case of pyridoxine. Aminoglycoside antibiotics may exacerbate symptoms of weakness in patients with disorders of neuromuscular transmission, such as myasthenia gravis. Dizziness may be secondary to ototoxicity caused by the aminoglycosides. In eliciting a history of drug use it is often necessary to be quite specific and to use lay terminology. Most patients are, for example, unaware that over-the-counter sleeping pills, cold preparations, and diet pills are actually drugs. Alcohol, the most prevalent neurotoxin, is often not recognized as such by patients. History of environmental or industrial exposure to neurotoxins may provide the essential clue; consultation with the patient's family or employer may be required.

8 *History of malignancy.* Because malignant tumors may present with nervous system metastases or occasionally with any of several paraneoplastic syndromes, it is important to determine whether any history of malignancy exists and whether chemotherapy or radio-

therapy was given. Patients with prior malignancy can present with unexpected and unusual neurologic complications.

9 *Formulating an impression of the patient.* Use the opportunity while taking the history to form an impression of the patient. Is there evidence of anxiety, depression, hypochondriasis? Are there any clues to defects of language, memory, inappropriate behavior, or secondary gain? The neurologic assessment begins as soon as the patient walks into the room and the first introduction is made.

The neurologic examination   After obtaining a complete medical and neurologic history, the physician should have reliable clues to the portions of the nervous system to be examined. By the elicitation of specific signs it is then determined whether the nervous system is affected, and, if so, to what degree and which part. The anatomic localization of the lesion assumes special significance in neurology, as certain diseases are known to affect certain regions of the nervous system and not to involve others. Recognition of a constellation of symptoms and signs (a syndrome) points to the possible existence of certain diseases and to the exclusion of others.

A systematic neurologic examination should encompass a survey of all functions from the cerebrum to peripheral nerve and muscle, i.e., from the mental status examination to the simplest reflexes. Such a detailed examination requires the performance of a series of physical tests aimed at eliciting the functional capacities of each part of the nervous system. The examiner must acquire skills that come only from the repeated use of the same techniques and instruments on a large number of normal and abnormal individuals. Errors and serious omissions are avoided if the examination procedure is orderly and systemic, beginning with mental (cerebral) functions and continuing with cranial nerves, then with motor, reflex, and sensory functions of the arms, trunk, and legs, and finishing with an analysis of posture and gait.

The mental status is already appreciated while the history is being taken. But rather profound disorders of recent memory or of spatial organization may be missed unless specifically tested for. Faults of memory, incoherence of thought, dominating ideas, peculiarities of mood and outlook, aphasic errors, problems of articulation, and loss of insight and judgment should be sought. If abnormalities are noted, a more formal analysis of these functions is undertaken along the lines suggested in Chaps. 29, 30, 32, and 33. The function of each cranial nerve is then examined in order, beginning with olfaction (see Chaps. 22, 23, 24, and 360). Examination of the motor system should include estimates of power of each of the major muscle groups, evidence of atrophy or fasciculation, and assessment of the tone of the musculature during passive manipulations, looking for signs of spasticity, rigidity, or hypotonia (as outlined in Chaps. 25 and 362). Speed and coordination of the limbs are assessed. Next, prevailing postures and the stance and gait are evaluated (Chap. 26). The tendon reflexes are examined for evidence of increased or decreased (or absent) response or of asymmetry between right and left sides or between arms and legs. The superficial cutaneous reflexes, abdominal and plantar, are then evaluated. Touch, pain, vibration, and joint-position sense are tested as the final part of the examination (see Chap. 28).

This detailed neurologic examination is undertaken only if there are symptoms of disturbed nervous system functioning. If none are present, it suffices to do an abbreviated examination which includes evaluation only of pupils, ocular movements, optic fundi, facial movements, speech, strength of arm and leg muscles, tendon and plantar reflexes, pain and vibratory sensation in hands and feet, and gait. All of this can be completed in 3 to 5 min. The findings, even in the short examination, should be recorded in the patient's record for future reference.

Two additional points about the examination are worth noting. First, in recording observations it is important for the physician to describe what is found, rather than to apply a poorly defined medical term (i.e., "patient groans to sternal rub" rather than "obtunded").

Second, if the patient's complaint is brought out by some activity, reproduce the activity in the office. If the complaint is of dizziness when raising the right arm and turning the head to the left, have the patient do it. If pain occurs after walking two blocks, have the patient demonstrate it and repeat the examination.

Experience teaches that the neurologic examination may be normal even in patients with a serious neurologic disease, such as one which causes seizures or syncope. Or the patient may arrive in a coma with no available history, and the examination proceeds along the lines described in Chap. 31. An inadequate history may to some extent be replaced by a succession of examinations from which the course of the illness may be plotted.

The formulation of the problem and establishment of an etiologic diagnosis The clinical data obtained from the history and the examination are assembled into one of the known syndromes and are interpreted and translated in terms of neuroanatomy and neurophysiology. From the syndrome the physician should be able to determine the anatomic localization(s) that best explains the clinical findings. The anatomic localization, mode of onset and course of illness, other medical data, and laboratory findings are then integrated. Finally, the etiologic diagnosis is reached, and therapy appropriate for the disorder is proposed.

The proper selection of laboratory tests which will assist in arriving at an anatomic, but more particularly at an etiologic, diagnosis poses another set of problems for the clinician. In Chaps. 348 and 362 are described the principal tests and when they should be used. Radiologic imaging techniques, utilizing computed tomography (CT) scanning, and magnetic resonance imaging (MRI) have had a major impact on the neurologic assessment. It cannot be overemphasized, however, that the anatomic method of physical diagnosis should proceed together with imaging studies for localization of the site of the disorder. There are commonly great discrepancies between the findings on examination and on brain imaging which are resolved only after continued careful assessment of the patient, together with further radiologic study. Assiduous attention to the clinical method in neurology remains as important today as it ever was.

REFERENCES

ADAMS RD, VICTOR M: *Principles of Neurology*, 4th ed. New York, McGraw-Hill, 1989

DEJONG RN: *The Neurologic Examination.* New York, Harper and Row, 1979

SWANSON PD: *Symptoms and Signs in Neurology.* Philadelphia, Lippincott, 1984

348 IMAGING OF THE NERVOUS SYSTEM

KENNETH R. DAVIS / JOSEPH B. MARTIN

Imaging of the brain and spinal cord has revolutionized the ability to visualize lesions that cause neurologic dysfunction. These developments have occurred as a result of the application to clinical problems of computed tomography (CT) scanning in the 1970s, magnetic resonance imaging (MRI) in the 1980s, and positron emission tomography (PET) and single-photon emission computed tomography (SPECT) in the past 5 years. Nuclear magnetic resonance spectroscopy (NMRS) has promise for the study of function in the central nervous system (CNS) to complement those currently available with PET and SPECT.

COMPUTED TOMOGRAPHY CT scanning provides a sensitive and reproducible method for evaluating suspected lesions in the CNS. It is often the procedure of choice whether or not MRI is available

and may also be complementary in circumstances where MRI is available. Its principal utility is when rapid information about the state of the CNS is desired, and it is particularly important for decisions related to emergent surgical versus medical management of patients with the sudden onset of a neurologic deficit. Such conditions include acute head or spinal trauma, stroke where a differentiation between hemorrhage and infarction is important, and other circumstances where a decision as to immediate operative intervention is important. CT continues to have an advantage over MRI in emergency settings in patients with acute neurologic deterioration. It has high specificity, particularly for the demonstration of acute hemorrhage, where its imaging capacity exceeds that of MRI.

The CT scan is also widely used for the evaluation of lesions that involve bone, such as metastatic disease at the base of the skull. However, the radionuclide bone scan provides a more sensitive and generalized evaluation for bone metastases than CT or MRI. Calcification within lesions of the brain is demonstrated best by CT rather than MRI. CT is also the better imaging method for fractures of the face, temporal bone, and base of the skull. It is also an important imaging technique for evaluating fractures of the spine, although soft tissue encroachment upon the spinal cord is better visualized by MRI.

MAGNETIC RESONANCE IMAGING MRI is useful in the following circumstances:

1 Screening for metastatic disease. With the administration of intravenous contrast material, such as gadolinium-DTPA, metastatic tumors can be visualized within the brain parenchyma, as well as primary tumors that cause a breakdown of the blood-brain barrier (Fig. 348-1). Imaging with gadolinium-DTPA may be more sensitive for these conditions than noncontrast MR or CT scanning with contrast. It is also the preferred method for visualization of pituitary tumors, acoustic neurinomas (Fig. 348-2), and other posterior fossa tumors, where CT artifacts from dental fillings on coronal scans of the sellar region and from nearby bony structures in the posterior fossa may prevent clear delineation of the lesion.

2 Imaging of demyelinating diseases such as multiple sclerosis (MS) and other white matter disorders of the brain and spinal cord (Fig. 348-3). It is possible to visualize small (2 to 5 mm) white matter lesions and to watch their progress over time. Contrast enhancement may make it possible to determine the acute perivascular involvement of new active lesions in MS. It is also the method of choice for evaluation of the leukodystrophies and for other white matter diseases such as Binswanger's disease (see Chap. 351).

3 Screening for the presence of arteriovenous malformation (AVM) and aneurysms, particularly when family members at risk require evaluation (Fig. 348-4). MRI is followed by angiography if more detailed visualization is necessary in preparation for surgical intervention, or if the findings are equivocal. Development of MRI methods for evaluation of blood flow (MRI angiography) promises to improve the ability to delineate blood flow and vascular lesions, including encroachment upon the lumen by atheromatous plaques in the carotid and vertebral basilar systems (Fig. 348-5).

4 Evaluation of congenital and developmental abnormalities of the CNS. These include the Chiari malformation, porencephalic cysts, as well as a variety of inherited abnormalities affecting the CNS (e.g., tuberous sclerosis).

5 Detection of posterior fossa vascular lesions. Small lacunes can be visualized within the brainstem that are not visible on CT scan (see Chap. 351). It is also the procedure of choice for the demonstration of small hemorrhages more than several days old in the posterior fossa. MRI angiography is capable of visualizing basilar and vertebral artery flow (Fig. 348-5).

6 Lesions intrinsic to the spinal cord. Particularly advantageous is the ability to examine the entire spinal cord and canal, a technique that has led to improved management, particularly of thoracic disc syndromes. Myelopathy should be evaluated first with an MRI to differentiate intramedullary from extramedullary lesions. Metastatic

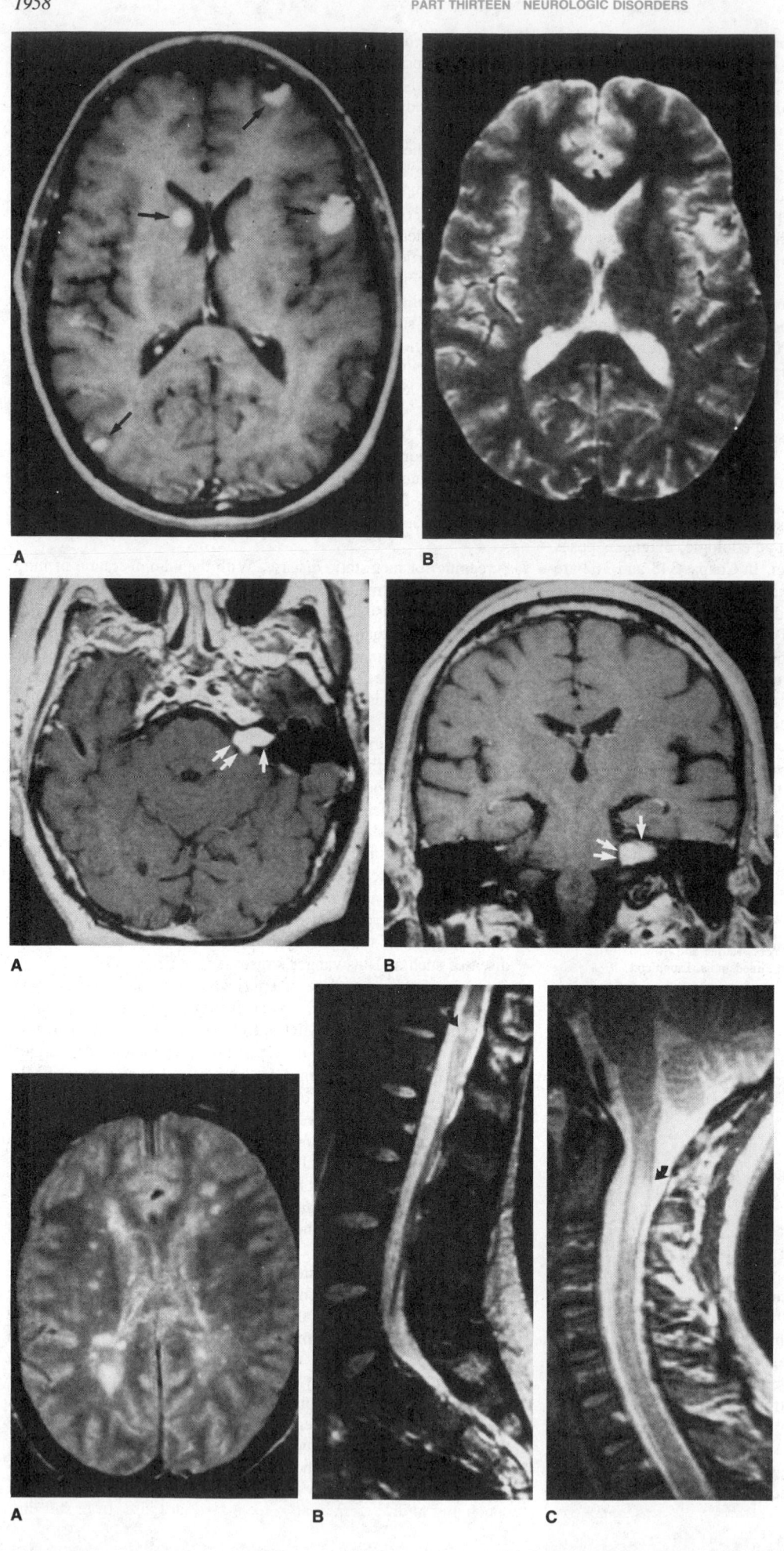

FIGURE 348-1 Cerebral metastases. Magnetic resonance scan of the brain showing many more obvious enhancing lung metastases on the T1-weighted image (*arrows*) with intravenous contrast material (*A*) than on the T2-weighted image prior to contrast injection (*B*).

FIGURE 348-2 Acoustic neurinoma. MRI with intravenous contrast material clearly depicts the intracanalicular (*arrow*) and cerebellopontine angle cistern (*double arrows*) components of an acoustic neurinoma on axial (*A*) and coronal (*B*) views. (*Courtesy of R.G. Gonzalez, M.D.*)

FIGURE 348-3 Multiple sclerosis. *A.* A proton-density MRI reveals multiple periventricular hyperintense multiple sclerosis plaques. The T2-weighted MRI of the spine shows a hyperintense plaque within the conus medullaris (*B*) and the upper cervical cord (*C*), respectively (*arrows*), in different patients. (*Courtesy of S. Sweriduk, M.D.*)

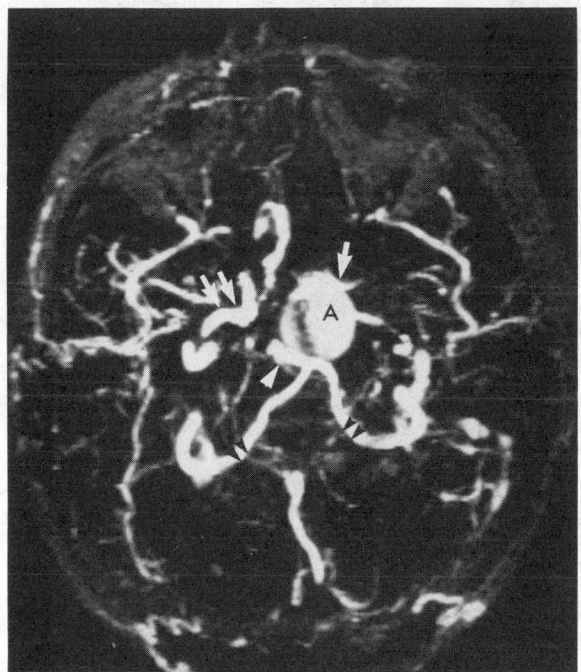

FIGURE 348-4 Cerebral aneurysm. MR angiography indicates the presence of a large aneurysm originating from the left internal carotid artery. A, aneurysm. Single arrow: left carotid artery. Double arrows: right carotid artery. Angle arrowhead: basilar artery. Double arrowheads: vertebral arteries. (*Courtesy of D. Mikulis, M.D.*)

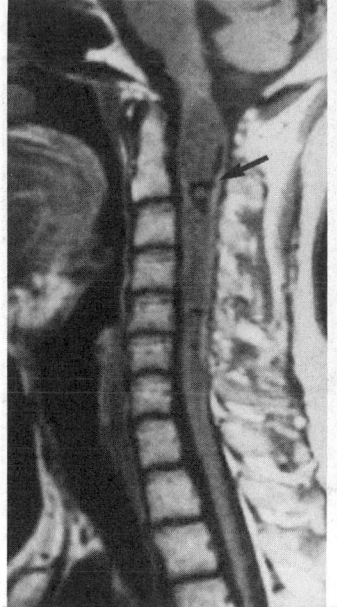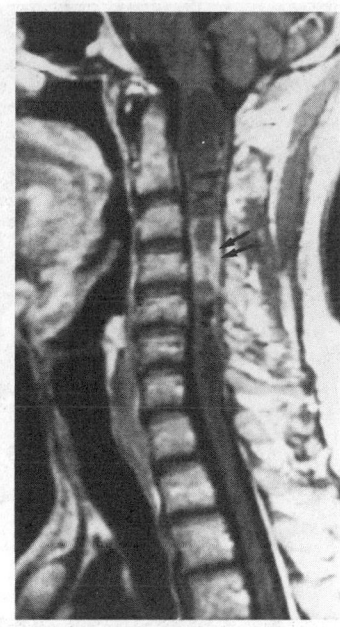

A   **B**

FIGURE 348-6 Ependymoma. *A.* A T1-weighted sagittal MRI of the cervical spine made without intravenous contrast shows expansion of the cervical cord by an ependymoma (*arrow*) with mixed hypointense signal intensities. *B.* Following intravenous injection of gadolinium DTPA contrast, the T1 image shows enhancement of a portion of the tumor (*double arrows*) that would be most likely to yield a positive biopsy.

disease affecting the spinal cord from an epidural location is easily visualized by MRI. It is also the best method for the demonstration of intrinsic spinal cord lesions including tumors (Fig. 348-6), syringomyelia, and areas of demyelination (Fig. 348-3). Use of intravenous contrast material may provide increased sensitivity or improved characterization of a lesion (Fig. 348-7). As compared to the myelogram, MRI allows visualization within and around the entire cord. The postmyelography CT scan is limited in the full evaluation of the spine because a large number of slices, and hence excessive time, are required. MRI is the choice for acute spinal cord syndromes caused by extramedullary lesions, including epidural abscess and metastases. Osteomyelitis of the spine and secondary abscess are readily visualized by MRI (Fig. 348-8).

FIGURE 348-5 Basilar artery stenosis. MR angiogram of the vertebral basilar circulation showing stenosis of the mid-basilar artery (*arrow*) with turbulent flow artifact above the stenosis. Double arrows: vertebral arteries. Arrowhead: normal lower basilar artery. (*Courtesy of Gilbert Vezina, M.D.*)

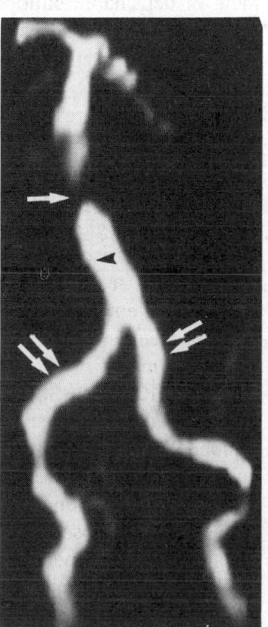

7 Although MRI is useful in the evaluation of all vertebral disc and spondylosis problems, it is particularly valuable for patients who have had previous back surgery. Following the administration of intravenous contrast material, it is possible to visualize extradural granulation tissue and to determine whether fibrosis (scarring) or recurrent disc protrusion is contributing to root symptoms. Fibrous granulation tissue usually shows early enhancement following intravenous contrast material, whereas a disc fragment may show delayed slight enhancement 15 to 20 min after injection.

8 Developmental lesions of the spinal cord such as syringomyelia, tethered cord, lipomas, and cavernous hemangiomas. MRI can demonstrate vascular lesions that subsequently may require angiography for definition, but may also demonstrate small intramedullary lesions that are not visible on the angiogram.

However, the problems of taking care of patients in the MRI scanner, particularly those who are unconscious on life support systems, who have gunshot wounds, or who are in MRI-incompatible tongs or halos for spinal traction or immobilization, limits the use of MRI. In these circumstances, it may be necessary to obtain a myelogram performed with a water-soluble, nonionic contrast material that permits a subsequent CT-myelogram.

MYELOGRAPHY If the MRI is insufficient to account for the clinical presentation, it may be necessary to perform a myelogram or CT-myelogram in which a water-soluble, nonionic contrast material is instilled into the subarachnoid space. Films are usually taken at the time of contrast injection and followed by a CT scan of the appropriate regions. The procedure is particularly useful in cervical spondylosis where an MRI may not demonstrate detail of a herniated disc or osteophyte. The safety of new nonionic, water-soluble contrast materials has made myelography a more feasible procedure associated with less risk. Iophendylate myelography, now rarely performed, does not permit subsequent CT evaluation. Furthermore, residual iophendylate after myelography may produce artifacts on subsequent MR scans. A CT-myelogram may be particularly useful in cervical disc disease and spondylosis to demonstrate narrowing of the neural foramen and to differentiate an osteophyte (hard disc) from soft disc

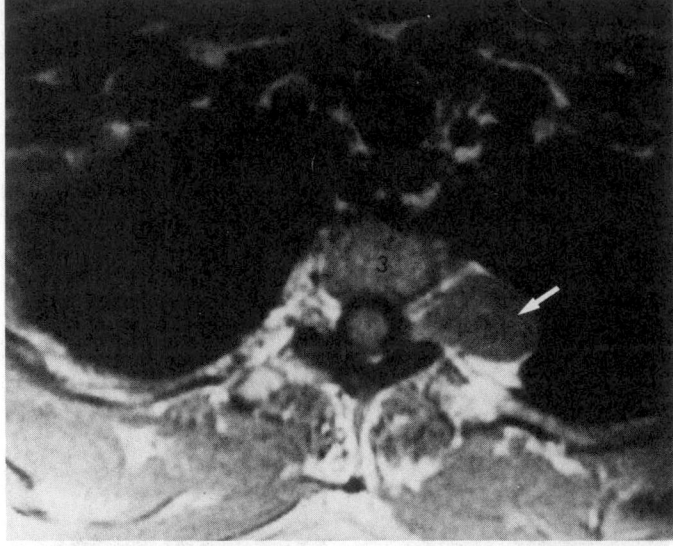

A

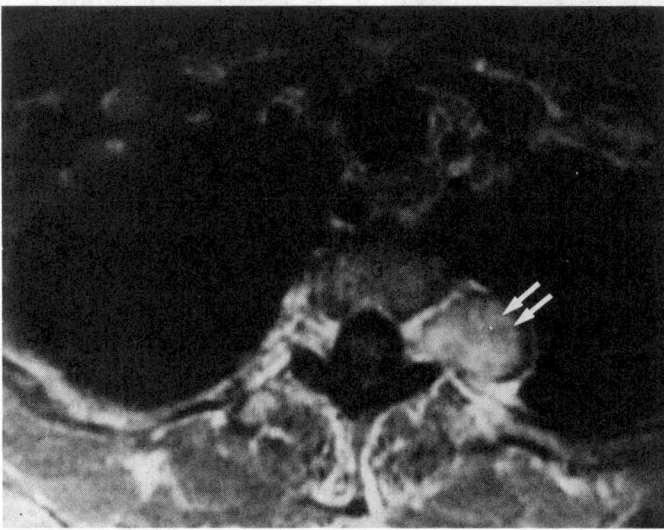

B

FIGURE 348-7   Neurofibroma. T1-weighted axial MRI of the spine through the D2-3 neural foramen reveals a hypointense foraminal and extraforaminal neurofibroma (*arrow*) extending into the left paraspinal region (*A*) that enhances (*double arrows*) with intravenous contrast (*B*).

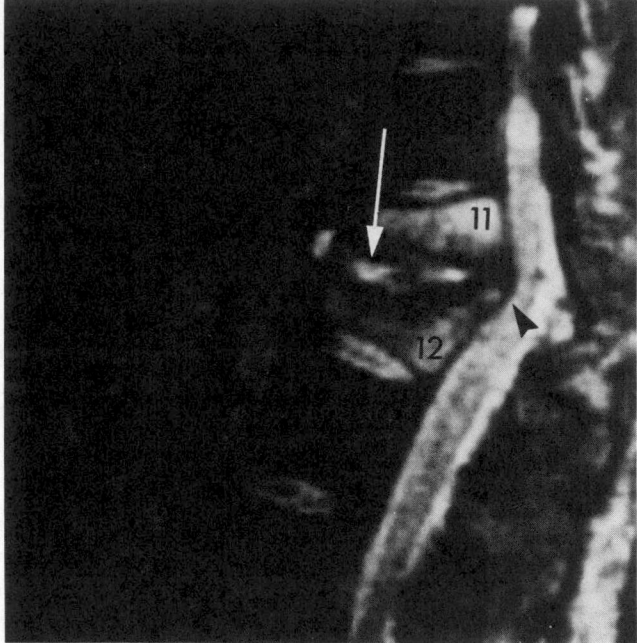

FIGURE 348-8   Osteomyelitis of the spine. A T2-weighted sagittal MRI indicates hyperintense signal of the remaining D11-12 disc space (*arrow*) between the collapsed, slightly hyperintense surrounding vertebral bodies. These findings are caused by disc space infection and surrounding osteomyelitis. Posterior extension of the epidural mass represents epidural abscess (*arrowhead*).

material. This may not always be optimally visualized on MRI. For tumors of the vertebral foramen, such as neurofibromas, a myelogram and CT-myelogram are not often necessary, given the availability of MRI and use of intravenous contrast material (see Fig. 348-9). Seeding of tumors along roots in the cauda equina is often visualized on MRI, but these may be too small to be identified or not enhance with intravenous contrast material. In this circumstance, a myelogram followed by a CT-myelogram may be the best choice. Herniated lumbar disc is usually detected by MRI (Fig. 348-9), but some physicians still prefer to have the anatomic details confirmed by CT and myelography prior to surgery. If the MRI is normal or equivocal, a myelogram may demonstrate enlarged veins in cases of suspected AVM of the cord, prior to deciding on spinal angiography. MRI may detect flow voids of the AVM and an abnormal signal within the cord. In such cases where AVM is suspected, a spinal angiogram rather than a myelogram will be the next step after an unremarkable MRI. Finally, a CT myelogram may be the examination of choice in spinal cord injury where ferromagnetic metal stabilization has been used and MRI-incompatible life-support systems are required. In these circumstances, it is difficult to perform an adequate MRI.

INTERVENTIONAL RADIOLOGY   It is now possible to navigate into small vessels using maneuverable microcatheters and to visualize the vasculature and microcatheter by high-resolution, digital fluoroscopic equipment with real-time roadmapping capabilities. The decrease in the time required for microcatheter entry and visualization of target vessels results in faster studies at lower risk. The studies are usually performed by transfemoral retrograde catheterization using specialized coaxial microcatheters that can enter small vessels in the distribution of the anterior, middle, and posterior cerebral, vertebral, basilar, external carotid, or spinal circulations. This technique, along with availability of polymerizing glues such as *n*-butyl-cyanoacrylate, microcoils, and various particulate agents, make endovascular embolization treatment of AVMs possible. Treatment may be partial, to facilitate surgical resection, or primary and definitive. The development of detachable balloons that are attached to microcatheters has made possible the endovascular treatment of fistulas, such as carotid-cavernous or vertebral-venous fistulas. Detachable balloons can also be used to occlude aneurysms or the parent feeding vessel. Nondetachable balloons are used to predict deficiencies of neurologic function that may follow permanent surgical or balloon occlusion of vessels. For example, selective microcatheterization of a vessel supplying an AVM followed by injection of amobarbital can be used to test for adverse neurologic effect prior to embolization. Nondetachable balloons may be used to dilate and treat certain cases of vasospasm secondary to subarachnoid hemorrhage from an aneurysm. Finally, preoperative embolization is often used to reduce vascularity in tumors such as meningiomas, glomus jugulare, and angiofibromas prior to surgical removal.

POSITRON EMISSION TOMOGRAPHY   PET is based upon three-dimensional reconstruction of brain sections using positron-emitting radionuclides. By utilization of a number of individual radionuclides and radiolabeled moieties, it provides an opportunity to measure quantitatively: regional cerebral blood flow, blood volume, oxygen metabolism, glucose transport and metabolism, and neurotransmitter metabolism; and it permits neurotransmitter receptor localization (see Table 348-1.) PET can provide spatial resolution, approaching 3 to 5 mm definition in sequential slices.

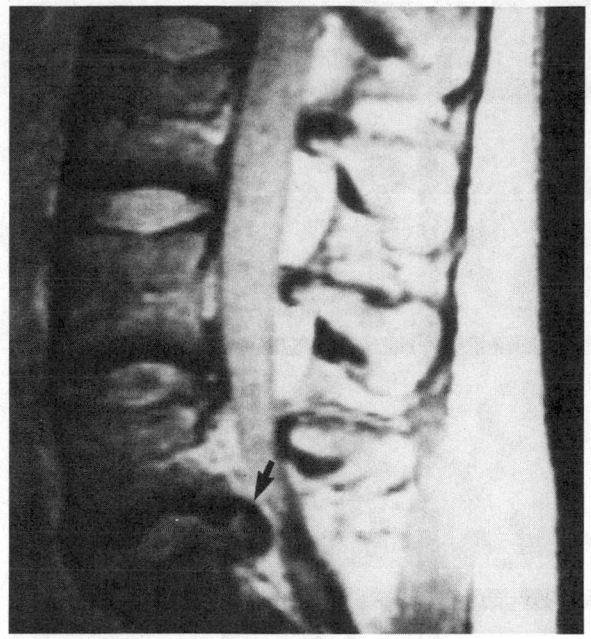
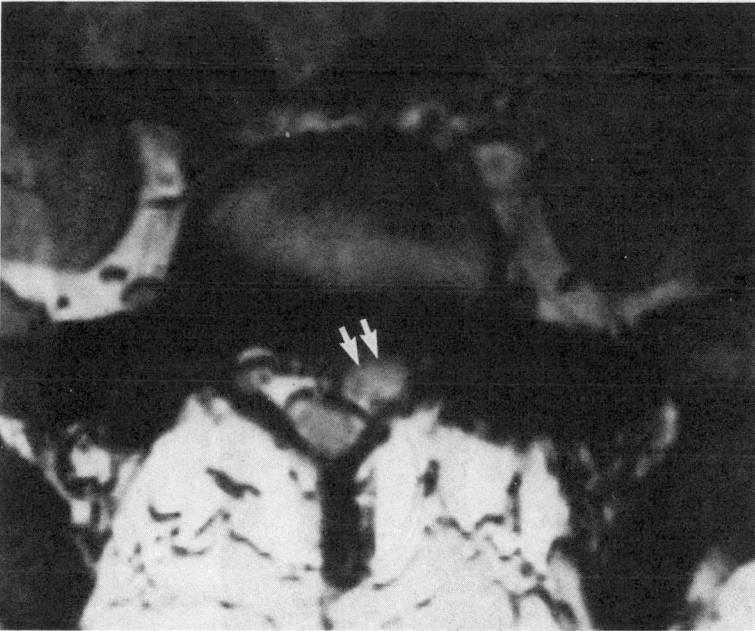

A   **B**

FIGURE 348-9 Herniated and extruded disc at L5-S1. *A*. The sagittal proton density MRI shows the abnormal hypointense disk (*arrow*) producing a large extradural defect. *B*. Using a 110-degree flip angle, the axial multiplanar gradient echo image shows the disc lateralized to the left (*double arrows*) compressing the S1 root sleeve and thecal sac as well as extruding caudally into the lateral recess of S1.

Cerebrovascular disease In acute ischemic injury to the brain, PET studies demonstrate functional alterations in blood flow and oxygen metabolism when the CT scan may be normal; however, the difficulty in obtaining emergency PET studies limits its usefulness in this setting. MRI scans do show acute changes in stroke more readily than CT and are now widely used. In the assessment of long-term neurologic dysfunction after a stroke, PET scanning with deoxyglucose may show focal abnormalities that extend well beyond the lesions seen on CT or MRI. Analysis in such circumstances may provide insight into neural connections important for cognition (Chap. 346).

Epilepsy The PET application most useful in epilepsy is assessment of glucose metabolism by measurement of brain uptake and phosphorylation of [^{18}F]fluorodeoxyglucose (FDG). The methods are based on those developed by Sokoloff and colleagues for 2-deoxy-glucose autoradiography in tissue sections. The PET scan summates approximately 40 min of local cerebral glucose metabolism and allows assessment of regional variations. PET studies have been most useful in patients with focal seizures. About 70 percent of patients with partial (focal) seizures that are refractory to medical treatment show zones of decreased glucose metabolism in the interictal state. The site of hypometabolism correlates with the epileptic focus in many patients. The same region often shows enhanced glucose metabolism if it is measured during a seizure discharge. In patients with temporal lobe seizures, it is common to find hypometabolism in one lobe.

The application of FDG-PET to evaluation of epilepsy patients undergoing consideration for surgical treatment is useful for confirming the unilaterality of sites producing electrical discharges and, in some cases, rendering intracerebral recordings unnecessary (Fig. 348-10).

Neurodegenerative diseases Parkinson's disease, caused by degeneration of the dopaminergic nigra-striatal pathway, can be demonstrated by [^{18}F]6-fluoro-L-dopa (^{18}F-FD) and PET. Decreased accumulation of ^{18}F-FD occurs in the striatum in Parkinson's disease and during normal aging. 6-Fluoro-L-dopa is decarboxylated to 6-fluoro-L-dopamine by the enzyme aromatic L-amino acid decarboxylase, and the product then enters nerve terminals. PET allows visualization of the entrapped labeled dopamine. Decreased dopamine levels have been demonstrated in patients with Parkinson's disease induced by 1-methyl-4-phenyl-1,2,3,6-tetrahydropyridine and in asymptomatic drug addicts exposed to the drug, who presumably have subclinical degeneration of the nigra-striatal pathway.

Abnormalities can also be detected by FDG-PET in the basal ganglia in Huntington's disease (decreased metabolism) and in the brainstem and cerebellum in degenerative diseases such as olivopontocerebellar degeneration and Friedreich's ataxia (decreased metabolism). Decreased oxygen extraction and metabolism in the cerebral

TABLE 348-1 Examples of tracers used in positron emission tomography of brain

Process	Tracer
Blood flow	$H_2^{15}O$, $C^{15}O_2$, ^{11}C-alcohols
Blood volume	$C^{15}O$-RBC, ^{11}CO-RBC, ^{68}Ga-labeled EDTA
Tissue pH	^{11}C-DMO, $^{11}CO_2$
Transport and metabolism	
Oxygen	^{15}O-O_2
Glucose, glucose analogues, carbohydrates	2-deoxy-2-^{18}F-fluoro-D-glucose, 2-^{11}C-deoxy-D-glucose, ^{11}C-D-glucose, ^{11}C-lactate, -pyruvate, -acetate, -succinate, -oxaloacetate
Amino acids: ^{13}N	L-^{13}N-glutamate, -glutamine, -alanine, -aspartate, -leucine, -valine, -isoleucine, -methionine
Amino acids: ^{11}C	L-^{11}C-aspartate, -glutamate, -valine, -leucine, -phenylalanine, -methionine
Molecular diffusion	^{68}Ga-EDTA
Protein synthesis	L-1-^{11}C-leucine, -methionine, -phenylalanine, L-^{11}C-methylmethionine
Receptor systems	
Dopaminergic	^{18}F-spiperone, ^{11}C-spiperone, ^{11}C-raclopride, ^{75}Br- and ^{76}Br-p-bromospiperone, ^{18}F-haloperidol, ^{11}C-pimozide, ^{11}C-methyl, -ethylspiperone, L-^{11}C-dopa, 6-^{18}F-fluoro-L-dopa, ^{18}F-ethylspiperone
Cholinergic	^{11}C-imipramine, ^{11}C-QNB
Benzodiazepine	^{11}C-flunitrazepam, -diazepam, -RO15-1788, ^{18}F-fluorovalium
Opiate	^{11}C-etorphine, N-methyl-^{11}C-morphine, ^{11}C-heroin, -carfentanil
Adrenergic	^{11}C-norepinephrine, -propranolol
Anticonvulsants	^{11}C-valproate, -phenytoin

SOURCE: Adapted from Phelps and Mazziotta, with permission.

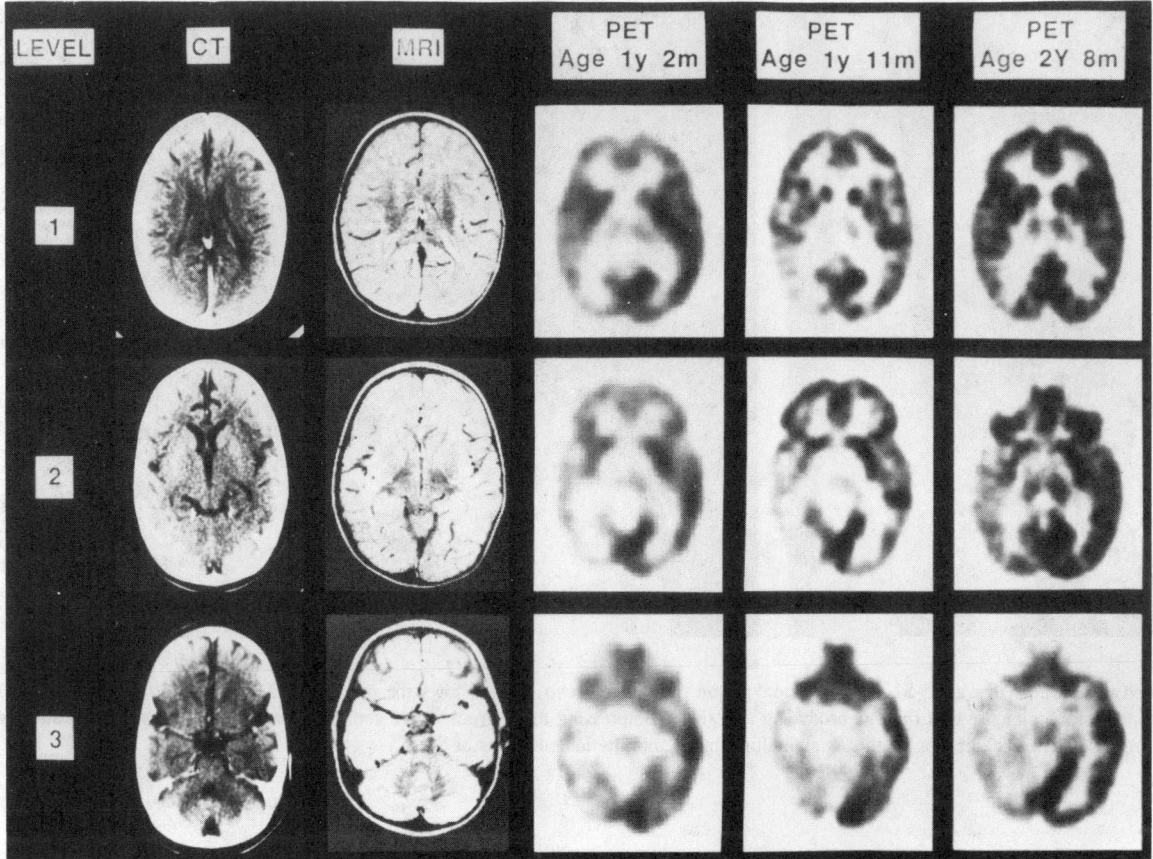

FIGURE 348-10   Preoperative CT, MRI, and FDG-PET images of a patient with infantile spasms (epilepsy). The right side of the brain is to the viewer's left. Both CT and MRI failed to show abnormalities. Interictal PET studies performed at ages 1 year 2 months, 1 year 11 months, and 2 years 8 months revealed right occipitotemporal hypometabolism, corresponding to the surface EEG localization of interictal discharges. (*Used with permission of Harry Chugani and Annals of Neurology.*)

cortex may be demonstrated in Alzheimer's disease and in schizophrenia. Abnormalities in dopamine receptors have also been documented in schizophrenia. PET studies are also valuable in neuropsychological studies (see Chap. 346).

Although PET is at present primarily a research tool, its increasing availability in medical centers for cardiac imaging (see Chap. 178) makes likely more widespread application to other neurologic and psychiatric diseases.

SINGLE-PHOTON EMISSION COMPUTED TOMOGRAPHY SPECT depends on gamma-emitting radionuclides attached to molecules that can readily cross the blood-brain barrier. SPECT allows for concurrent blood flow determination and visualization of neurotransmitter receptors (see also Chap. 346). For example, [^{123}I]isopropyl amphetamine (IMP) and [^{99}Tc]m-d, 1-hexamethyl-propylene-amine-oxime–labeled iodoamphetamine have been used to demonstrate abnormalities in epilepsy, Alzheimer's disease, and Parkinson's disease. However, present SPECT technology is relatively nonquantitative and insensitive in demonstrating changes, and its spatial resolution is considerably less than that of PET. On the other hand, SPECT is less expensive and more widely available. It is now widely acknowledged as a potentially important diagnostic tool for differentiation of dementia caused by Alzheimer's disease from that caused by vascular disease (multi-infarct dementia) (see Chap. 30).

NUCLEAR MAGNETIC RESONANCE SPECTROSCOPY NMRS offers the potential of assessing brain function at metabolic and molecular levels. NMRS uses naturally occurring nonradioactive measurements of ^{31}P, ^{13}C, ^{23}Na, ^{7}Li, and ^{1}H. The ^{31}P NMR spectrum can detect tissue concentrations of the phosphomonoesters phosphocholine and inorganic orthophosphate, the phosphodiesters glycerol-3-phospho-ethanolamine and glycerol-3-phosphocholine, the triphosphate ATP, and other phosphorus-containing molecules including phosphocreatinine. The ^{31}P NMR spectrum gives quantitative analysis of these compounds in vivo with the potential of three-dimensional resolution within the brain. At present, much of the work in this area is experimental (see also Chap. 346).

REFERENCES

BRANT-ZAWADSKI M, NORMAN D (eds): *Magnetic Resonance Imaging of the Central Nervous System*. New York, Raven, 1987

CHUGANI HT et al: Infantile spasms: I. PET identifies focal cortical dysgenesis in cryptogenic cases for surgical treatment. Ann Neurol (1990)

DUARA R et al: Positron emission tomography in Alzheimer's disease. Neurology 36:879, 1986

FELIX R et al: Brain tumors: MR imaging with gadolinium-DTPA. Radiology 156:681, 1985

JOHNSON KA et al: Single photon emission computed tomography in Alzheimer's disease: Abnormal iofetamine I 123 uptake reflects dementia severity. Arch Neurol 45:392, 1988

JUNCK L et al: PET imaging of human gliomas with ligands for the peripheral benzodiazepine binding site. Ann Neurol 26:752, 1989

LATCHAW RE (ed): *Computed Tomography of the Head, Neck and Spine*. Chicago. Year Book, 1985

LEE SH, RAO KCVG (eds): *Cranial Computed Tomography and MRI*, 2d ed. New York, McGraw-Hill, 1987

MCGEER PL et al: Positron emission tomography in patients with clinically diagnosed Alzheimer's disease. Can Med Assoc J 134:597, 1986

MODIC MT, MASARYK TJ, ROSS JS (eds): *Magnetic Resonance Imaging of the Spine*. Chicago, Year Book, 1989

PETTEGREW JW et al: ^{31}P nuclear magnetic resonance study of the brain in Alzheimer's disease. J Neuropath Exp Neurol 47:235, 1988

PHELPS ME, MAZZIOTTA JC: Positron emission tomography: Human brain function and biochemistry. Science 228:799, 1985

ROSS JS et al: Magnetic resonance angiography of the extracranial carotid arteries and intracranial vessels: A review. Neurology 39:1369, 1989

WILLIAMS AL, HAUGHTON VM (eds): *Cranial Computed Tomography. A Comprehensive Text*. St. Louis, Mosby, 1985

WONG DF et al: Positron emission tomography reveals elevated D_2 dopamine receptors in drug-naive schizophrenics. Science 234:1558, 1986

ZAWADZKI MB, NORMAN D: *Magnetic Resonance Imaging of the Central Nervous System*. New York, Raven, 1987

349 CLINICAL ELECTROPHYSIOLOGY AND OTHER DIAGNOSTIC METHODS

KEITH CHIAPPA / BHAGWAN SHAHANI / JOSEPH B. MARTIN

Clinical neurophysiologic techniques provide an objective, quantitative measure of function of the central and peripheral nervous systems (CNS and PNS), including the autonomic nervous system. These studies have proved useful in the investigation and understanding of a variety of neurologic disorders. Because many of the procedures are time-consuming and costly, they should be undertaken only when they can shed new light on the clinical problem by providing data that are otherwise unavailable. Clinical neurophysiologic studies are also useful for monitoring and following the progression or recovery of patients with certain neurologic disorders.

NEUROPHYSIOLOGIC STUDIES OF MUSCLE AND NERVE

ELECTROMYOGRAPHY Electromyography refers to several diagnostic procedures in which electrical activity of nerve and muscle is studied. Strictly speaking, the term *electromyography* (EMG) is used when a needle electrode is inserted into a skeletal muscle to study changes in electric potential (voltage) during a state of complete relaxation and with graded voluntary activity. There are no EMG wave forms that are diagnostic for a particular disease entity, and it is not possible to sample every muscle in the body. Electromyography is an extension of the clinical neurologic examination and, by itself, cannot be used to arrive at a specific clinical entity. Clinical applications of EMG and conventional nerve conduction studies for the diagnosis of disorders affecting skeletal muscles, peripheral nerves, and neuromuscular junctions are described in Chap. 362.

Newer EMG techniques for evaluation of nerve conduction Methods for study of electrical conduction in proximal nerve segments include measurements of latencies for F responses, H reflexes, and blink reflexes. These techniques determine conduction times in nerves from the periphery (of a limb or the face) to the central nervous system (spinal cord or brainstem) and back again.

The *F response* measures the time required for a stimulus applied to the axon of an alpha motor neuron to propagate antidromically to the anterior horn of the spinal cord and then to return orthodromically down the same axon. The *H reflex* measures the time required for orthodromic conduction up the nerve via group IA sensory fibers, through the spinal monosynaptic connection with the alpha motor neuron, and then orthodromically down the motor axon. Conduction along proximal sensory and motor nerves and spinal roots can be measured. The application of these techniques to the measurement of proximal nerve conduction has increased recognition of abnormal conduction velocity in patients with peripheral neuropathy to between 80 and 90 percent. These studies are also useful in documenting a *conduction block* in proximal segments of peripheral nerves and roots in patients with inflammatory and demyelinating neuropathies (e.g., Guillain-Barré syndrome).

The *blink reflexes* measure conduction in branches of the trigeminal and facial nerves. The blink reflex is evoked by electric stimulation of the supraorbital branches of the trigeminal nerve and measures latency to blink response. It permits localization of lesions in the distribution of the facial or trigeminal nerve.

Nerve conduction studies, both conventional (see Chap. 362) as well as the late-response studies described here, only give information regarding large-diameter fast-conducting axons and do not provide information regarding conduction in intermediate and small-diameter nerve fibers. By applying physiologic principles of collision of nerve impulses evoked by stimulation at two different sites (proximal and distal) in the same nerve, it is possible to measure conduction in motor axons with small diameters. Abnormal conduction velocities of intermediate size fibers can be demonstrated in some patients with metabolic and nutritional neuropathies in whom conventional methods and late-response studies are normal.

Single-fiber EMG and macro EMG In addition to conventional EMG with concentric needle electrodes, specialized techniques permit the recording of the EMG of single fibers or of the entire motor unit (macro EMG). Single-fiber techniques, by recording *jitter* (variations in potentials) in individual fibers, can measure accurately, within microseconds, the performance of individual neuromuscular junctions. Characteristic quantitative abnormalities are found in patients with myasthenia gravis, Lambert-Eaton syndrome, and other disorders of neuromuscular transmission. Single-fiber EMG studies are also used to calculate *fiber density,* the number of single muscle fiber action potentials belonging to one motor unit within the recording area of the single-fiber EMG electrode (approximately 200 μm). Fiber density values are increased after disorders that cause denervation followed by reinnervation.

Macro EMG techniques presumably measure summated electrical activity of all fibers belonging to a motor unit and allow estimation of true motor unit size. The amplitude and area of macro EMG motor unit potentials is increased in reinnervation and decreased in primary muscle diseases that cause reduction in the number of muscle fibers per motor unit.

EMG in disorders of the CNS The application of EMG and nerve conduction studies to evaluation of CNS function is termed *central EMG.* Since the motor unit is the final common path for all nerve impulses controlling skeletal muscles, disorders of motor control produced by lesions of the CNS may result in abnormal discharge patterns of motor neurons that can be documented by electrophysiologic techniques. For example, surface EMG recordings from pairs of agonist and antagonist muscles, analysis of single motor unit recruitment patterns, and microneurographic studies are useful in evaluating different types of tremor, including rest tremor of Parkinson's disease, familial essential tremor, and physiologic tremor (see Chap. 25). Cerebellar ataxia can usually be differentiated from other tremors and from sensory ataxia. Asterixis can be distinguished from tremor, and different types of myoclonus can be documented. Studies of proprioceptive and exteroceptive reflexes are helpful in the differential diagnosis of movement disorders and in differentiating spasticity from other types of disorders of tone, such as rigidity. Studies of the H reflex and F responses provide information regarding the excitability of the motor neuron pool. The effect of vibration on the H reflex has been used to evaluate *presynaptic inhibition* in different neurologic disorders. *Silent-period studies* have been used to evaluate function of proprioceptive input from muscle spindles. Mismatching of information from muscle spindles and joint receptors can result in an apparent "cerebellar" ataxia in patients with acute inflammatory polyneuropathy (Fisher syndrome) due to a lesion in the peripheral nervous system. EMG recordings and blink reflexes are useful in documenting clinically inapparent lesions of the brainstem in multiple sclerosis and in localizing early compressive lesions of trigeminal and facial nerves produced by small posterior fossa tumors.

QUANTITATIVE SENSORY TESTING Light touch and vibratory sensation are mediated by large-diameter myelinated nerve fibers (see Chaps. 28 and 363). Small myelinated nerve fibers convey messages encoded by cold receptors and some nociceptors, and unmyelinated sensory pathways transmit impulses generated by warmth receptors and polymodal nociceptors. A reproducible quantitative examination of several sensory modalities can be performed in approximately 1 h.

Vibratory perception can be determined by a hand-held vibrator equipped with an indicator for monitoring the pressure applied to the skin. The stimulus strength is measured by peak-to-peak displacement of the vibratory rod and the perception and disappearance thresholds for vibratory sensation are recorded at least three times. The technique of vibrametry is now used widely to assess and follow patients with peripheral neuropathies, including those in whom sensory nerve action potentials are absent.

Thermal threshold determination is performed with a special probe in which temperature varies at a constant rate. The probe is either warmed or cooled. The thermal stimulator is applied to the skin at different sites, and the temperature of the probe measured by a thermocouple is recorded. Thresholds for cold and warmth perception and for cold and heat pain are obtained by asking the subject to press a button when a given perception is felt. Using quantitative thermal testing in patients with Guillain-Barré syndrome, for example, it is possible to document impairment of cold perception thresholds (small myelinated fibers) and preservation of warmth perception thresholds (unmyelinated sensory fibers). Sensory pathways, which are inaccessible to conventional electrophysiologic testing, can be studied by this technique.

AUTONOMIC TESTING   Two simple electrophysiologic techniques are often used to evaluate function of the autonomic nervous system. The *sympathetic skin response* (SSR), which is a voltage change recorded from the skin, is evoked by a variety of stimuli, including an electrical stimulus, a loud noise, or deep inspiration. The SSR can be easily recorded from hands and feet of all normal subjects. Using a commercially available EMG machine provided with bandpass filters to include low frequencies (low-frequency cutoff of 0.16 Hz), SSR evaluates function of a subset of sympathetic nerve fibers that mediate sudomotor (sweating) function. SSR abnormalities are more commonly associated with axonal neuropathies than with demyelinating neuropathies. Quantitative in vitro studies of a group of patients with sural nerve biopsy has shown that absent SSR is due to loss of unmyelinated nerve fibers.

Using standard EMG equipment the QRS complex can be recorded through surface electrodes placed over the dorsum of each hand. By superimposing pairs of QRS complexes, it is possible to measure *RR-interval variation* at rest and during deep breathing. RR-interval variation is abnormal in many patients with Guillain-Barré syndrome who have involvement of small myelinated nerve fibers in the vagus nerve.

In most patients with clinical symptoms and signs of dysautonomia, one of these two electrophysiologic tests is abnormal. Both the SSR and RR-interval tests are simple and reproducible and they are useful to rule out involvement of the autonomic nervous system in patients referred to the laboratory for evaluation of peripheral neuropathy.

ELECTROENCEPHALOGRAPHY

The electroencephalographic (EEG) examination is part of the clinical study of many patients suspected of having disease of the CNS, either primary or secondary to a systemic medical illness. The conventional EEG recording should include the resting record and a number of *activating procedures* as follows: (1) The patient is requested to breathe deeply 20 times a minute for 3 min. The resulting alkalosis and cerebral vasoconstriction may activate characteristic seizure patterns or other abnormalities. (2) A powerful light (a stroboscope) is placed over the patient's face and flashed at frequencies from 1 to 20 per s with the patient's eyes open and closed. The EEG may then show abnormal discharges in photosensitive patients. (3) The EEG is recorded after the patient is allowed to fall asleep naturally or following sedative drugs given by mouth or by vein. Procedures 1 and 2 are routinely employed, but sleep may be extremely helpful in bringing out certain abnormalities, especially where temporal lobe epilepsy and other seizures are suspected. Sleep deprivation the night prior to the EEG study is useful when a sleeping record is desirable.

Certain preparations are necessary if EEG is to be most useful. The patient should not be sedated and should not have been for a long time without food, for both sedative drugs and relative hypoglycemia modify the normal EEG pattern. The same may be said of mental concentration, extreme nervousness, or drowsiness, all of which tend to suppress the normal alpha rhythm and increase muscle artifacts. When dealing with patients suspected of having epilepsy who are already being treated for it, most physicians prefer to record the first EEG while the patient continues to receive drugs.

TYPES OF NORMAL RECORDINGS   The normal EEG in adults shows somewhat asymmetric 8- to 12-Hz, 50-μV sinusoidal *alpha waves* in both occipital and parietal regions. These waves wax and wane spontaneously and usually disappear promptly when patients open their eyes or fix their attention on something. Waves faster than 13 Hz and of lower amplitude (10 to 20 μV), called *beta waves*, are also seen symmetrically in the frontal regions. Very slow waves *(delta waves)*, sharp waves, or other unusual patterns are absent in a normal record. When normal subjects fall asleep, the rhythm slows symmetrically, and characteristic waveforms *(vertex sharp waves* and *sleep spindles)* appear (see Chap. 34 for a more detailed description of polysomnography and the EEG in sleep); if the sleep is induced by barbiturates or benzodiazepines, an increase in the fast frequencies is seen and is considered to be normal. Excessive fast activity should raise the possibility that a patient is receiving one of these classes of compounds. In addition, there are many common and uncommon normal variants that should not be mistaken for abnormalities (e.g., drowsy hypersynchrony, 14 + 6 positive spikes, 6 per s spike-wave, rhythmic midtemporal discharge, and benign epileptiform transients of sleep).

The most pathologic finding of all is "electrocerebral inactivity," which means that the electrical activity of the cortical mantle, measured at the scalp, is below 2 μV and probably absent. Acute intoxication with anesthetic levels of drugs, such as barbiturates, and extreme hypothermia [<21°C(<70°F)] can also produce this sort of isoelectric EEG. However, in the absence of CNS depressants or extreme hypothermia, a record that is "flat" at highest recording sensitivity all over the head (except for artifacts such as EKG whose presence is a biologic calibration that indicates that the recording system is functioning properly) is the result of cerebral hypoxia, ischemia, or widespread cortical destruction. Such a patient, without EEG activity, reflexes (other than spinal), spontaneous respiration, or muscular activity of any kind for 6 h or more, is said to be in "irreversible coma." The brain of such patients is largely necrotic. There is no chance for neurologic recovery, and the patient may be considered dead, despite the preservation of vegetative (cardiovascular) functions supported by mechanical means, such as respirators (see also the discussion of brain death in Chap. 31). There has been no exception to this statement in over 1000 patients examined at the Massachusetts General Hospital in the past 20 years. Although the demonstration of electrocerebral silence by EEG should not be a legal requirement for the determination of brain death, it can be a very useful confirmation of the clinical conclusion.

Localized regions with absence of EEG activity may rarely be seen when there is a large area of infarction or an extensive surface tumor clot lying between the cerebral cortex and the electrodes. The localization of this abnormality is precise, but of course the nature of the lesion cannot be ascertained by EEG. Most such lesions, however, are too small, relative to the recording arrangement, to be visible, and the EEG may then record abnormal waves arising from functional, though ⌐ ¬anged, brain at the borders of the lesion. These abnormal waves are slower and of higher amplitude (50 to 350 μV) than normal. Those which are less than 4 Hz are called *delta waves;* those from 4 to 7 Hz are called *theta waves;* and the higher-voltage, faster waves are known as spikes or sharp waves. These fast and slow waves may be combined, and when a series of them suddenly interrupts relatively normal EEG patterns in a paroxysmal fashion, they are highly suggestive of epilepsy.

NEUROLOGIC CONDITIONS WITH ABNORMAL EEG   In the following groups of neurologic disorders, the EEG may be of considerable help in reaching the correct diagnosis.

Epilepsy   EEG correlates of the epilepsies are discussed in Chap. 350, and the review of this topic by Engel is highly recommended.

Brain tumor, abscess, and subdural hematoma Clinically significant intracranial space-occupying lesions are characteristically associated with abnormalities in the EEG, depending on their type and location, in some 90 percent of patients. In addition to diffuse changes, the classic abnormalities are focal or localized slow waves (usually delta), or, occasionally, seizure activity and decreased amplitude and synchronization of normal rhythms. As a rule, those lesions which expand more rapidly (abscess, some metastases, glioblastoma), especially when situated supratentorially, have the greatest frequency of EEG abnormalities (90 to 95 percent of the latter two and virtually 100 percent of abscesses). Slower growing tumors (astrocytomas) and particularly those outside the cerebral hemispheres (meningiomas, pituitary tumors) may produce no change in the EEG, though they may be very evident clinically or on imaging. The EEG abnormality has the correct lateralization in as many as 75 to 90 percent of patients with supratentorial tumors or abscesses. The EEG may be focally abnormal at a time when a cerebral metastasis is not yet visible on a computed tomography scan. A normal EEG and CT scan together almost exclude the presence of a supratentorial brain tumor or abscess. The EEG may be normal, however, in 20 to 25 percent of patients with infratentorial tumors.

Cerebrovascular disease Both the diffuse and localized EEG changes produced by vascular lesions such as cerebral infarcts and intracranial hemorrhages depend on their location and size rather than their type. The EEG has been shown to be useful in the differential diagnosis of vascular hemiplegia. If the lesion responsible is in the internal carotid or a major cerebral artery, an area of decreased normal activity and excessive slowing is practically always seen acutely in the appropriate region. If the hemiplegia is due to small vessel disease, i.e., a lacunar infarction deep in the cerebrum or brainstem (see Chap. 351), the EEG is usually normal. Large hemispheral lesions associated with acutely depressed levels of consciousness also produce widespread, diffuse, slow-wave activity of a nonspecific type as is seen with stupor or a coma from any cause. Resolution begins after a few days, cerebral edema subsides, and focal activity may then be seen (slow-wave activity or suppression of normal background rhythms). Smaller infarctions are associated with acute focal abnormalities that lateralize the lesion well but do not localize it precisely. In contrast with tumors, further resolution continues, and after 3 to 6 months roughly 50 percent of patients with cerebrovascular accidents have a normal EEG despite the persistence of clinical abnormalities. Under these circumstances the prognosis for further recovery is poor. Persistence of moderate- to high-voltage EEG abnormalities after this time period, particularly if spikes or sharp waves are present, suggests the presence of abnormally functioning tissue, which might be epileptogenic. The EEG may be of lateralizing value in acute subarachnoid hemorrhage, depending upon the extent to which the adjacent cerebrum is affected.

Brain injury Cerebral contusion or laceration produces EEG changes similar to those described for cerebrovascular disease. Diffuse changes often give way to focal ones, especially if the lesions are on the lateral or superior surface of the brain, and these in turn usually disappear over a period of weeks or months unless seizures supervene. Sharp waves or spikes sometimes emerge as the focal slow-wave abnormality resolves. These or failure of the EEG to "normalize" usually precede the occurrence of posttraumatic epilepsy. Following head injury, therefore, serial EEGs may be of prognostic value as regards the prospect of epilepsy.

Diseases that cause coma and states of impaired consciousness The EEG is abnormal in almost all conditions in which there is some impairment of consciousness. With hypothyroidism the rhythms are normal in configuration but are usually slow. In general, the more profound the change in consciousness, the more abnormal the EEG recording. In these latter situations slow waves (delta) are bilateral, are of high amplitude, and tend to predominate over the frontal regions. This pertains to such differing conditions as acute meningitis or encephalitis, severe disorders of blood gases, glucose, electrolyte and water balance, uremia, diabetic coma, liver coma, or impairment of consciousness accompanying the large cerebral lesions discussed above. In hepatic coma, the degree of abnormality in the EEG corresponds to the degree of confusion, stupor, or coma. Moreover, paroxysms of bilaterally synchronous large, sharp "triphasic waves" are characteristic, though they may also be seen with other metabolic encephalopathies associated with renal or pulmonary failure. Diffuse diseases (e.g., Alzheimer's disease) affecting the cerebral cortex are accompanied by a relatively slight degree of diffuse, slow-wave abnormality in the theta (4- to 7-Hz) range. Certain more rapidly progressive ones, such as subacute sclerosing panencephalitis (SSPE), Creutzfeldt-Jakob disease, and to a lesser extent the cerebral lipidoses, have, in addition, very characteristic, almost pathognomonic EEG changes consisting of recurring complex bursts of sharp and slow activity. A focal, temporal EEG abnormality in a patient suspected of having herpes simplex encephalitis may indicate the side for cerebral biopsy or may be sufficient confirmation to allow initiation of antiviral therapy. A normal EEG in a patient who is apathetic, slow, depressed, or forgetful is a point in favor of the diagnosis of an affective disorder or schizophrenia.

An EEG may also assist the physician in caring for a comatose patient when the pertinent history is unavailable. It may point to such otherwise unexpected causes as hepatic encephalopathy (bilaterally synchronous triphasic waves), intoxication with barbiturates or benzodiazepines [(excess fast activity), clinically inapparent continuous epileptic discharges (status epilepticus), a large space-occupying lesion, or diffuse anoxia-ischemia ("burst-suppression") pattern with repetitive generalized complexes separated by periods with very little EEG].

Other diseases of the cerebrum There are many disorders of nervous function that cause little or no alteration in the EEG. Multiple sclerosis and other demyelinating diseases are examples, though as many as 50 percent of advanced cases will have an abnormal record. Delirium tremens, Wernicke-Korsakoff disease, transient global amnesia, and withdrawal seizures, despite the dramatic nature of the clinical picture, cause little or no changes in the EEG. Some degree of slowing often accompanies confusional states. Interestingly, anxiety states and psychoses, such as manic-depressive disorders or schizophrenia, abnormal states due to hallucinogenic drugs such as LSD, and the majority of cases of mental retardation are associated with no important modification of the normal record or with nonspecific abnormalities.

SPECIAL APPLICATIONS OF THE EEG Because the EEG provides information about the status and function of the brain, it is useful as a monitor in the operating room to ensure the presence of a viable brain during the increasingly extensive procedures of modern cardiovascular surgery. The presence of EEG patterns appropriate to the depth of anesthesia and the agents in use is the final common denominator and confirms the adequacy of cerebral blood flow and oxygenation. It is routine practice now for the EEG to be monitored continuously during carotid endarterectomies in patients with stenotic or ulcerative carotid artery disease. Characteristic EEG changes (particularly marked voltage attenuation) signal the need for a temporary bypass shunt to maintain sufficient cerebral blood flow to preclude ischemic cerebral damage during surgery. Observing EEG changes may eventually be shown to be useful in monitoring the cerebral status of all patients during surgical anesthesia.

In the neurosurgical operating room the EEG can be recorded from exposed brain (electrocorticogram), and seizure patterns can be localized more precisely than from the scalp so that resection of such physiologically abnormal tissue may be undertaken (see Chap. 350).

The routine EEG can be of value in the diagnosis of hysterical blindness. Similarly, a response evoked by noise during light sleep can be helpful in confirming the presence of hearing in a patient who feigns total deafness. These responses may also be useful in evaluating hearing and vision in infants. Ambulatory EEG monitoring over a 24-h period, in which a miniature EEG recorder allows the patient to engage in normal daily activities at home or work, may assist in the evaluation of unexplained episodes of disturbed consciousness.

EVOKED RESPONSES

An evoked response (sometimes termed an evoked potential) is the record of electrical activity produced by groups of neurons within the cord, brainstem, thalamus, or cerebral hemispheres following stimulation of one or another sensory system by means of visual, auditory, or tactile input. The amplitude of these potentials, as recorded from the scalp using ordinary EEG electrodes, ranges from less than 0.5 to 20 μV. Because of their extremely small size, they can rarely be recognized on the ink-written EEG record with the background of ongoing EEG activity, which itself is usually 50 μV or more in amplitude. Therefore, special techniques, requiring simple computers, must be used to extract the evoked response waveform that one is interested in, from the continuous background EEG activity. These techniques are called "averaging" because the process involves repeating 100 to 1000 precisely timed stimuli and recording the electrical activity during a certain brief interval following each stimulus. The random ongoing EEG activity which, at any given point in time following the stimulus, is sometimes negative and at other times positive in polarity, tends to cancel out with sufficient repetition. The evoked response, however, is time-locked to the stimulus, and at a given time following the stimulus always has the same electrical sign as well as shape. The evoked response thus grows larger with repetition while the background averages out and becomes smaller. It is important to have special amplifiers, to apply the electrodes to the surface of the scalp with great care, and to time stimuli precisely with a minimum of accompanying electrical artifact. These evoked responses provide sensitive, objective extensions of the clinical neurologic examination of the related sensory system, but they are no more specific etiologically and must be carefully integrated into the clinical situation by a physician familiar with the clinical use of the test. The physician must decide if other procedures are indicated to differentiate the possible causes of the conduction abnormality.

VISUAL EVOKED RESPONSES Visual evoked responses produced by a pattern shift (PSVER) have the longest history of clinical usefulness. During this test, patients are asked to watch an alternating black and white checkerboard pattern which is projected on a screen. When patients watch this pattern shift, it produces a characteristic waveform which can be recorded from the scalp over the posterior portion of the head. Under normal circumstances, this triphasic wave has a distinctive positive peak at 95 to 115 ms latency (usually called P100) from the time of pattern reversal. This latency, the duration of the response, and the amplitude of the peak are measured; the latency is the most important parameter clinically. Each eye is tested independently. A purely monocular abnormality indicates that the conduction defect is anterior to the chiasm.

Many diseases processes affecting the optic nerve fibers in their intraocular, orbital, or cranial portions produce abnormalities of this potential. Glaucoma, compression of the optic nerve, chiasm, or tract by various space-occupying lesions, and degenerative disease of this system often produce a reduction in amplitude and/or prolonged latency of the PSVER. If the visual system is sufficiently affected, no response may be recorded by stimulation of one or both eyes. In a general hospital setting, however, the most common cause of abnormality in this response is optic neuritis, frequently associated with multiple sclerosis. Demyelination of the optic nerve fibers, as a primary demyelinating disease or due to one of the lesions listed above, slows conduction in the nerve fibers so that the latency of the positive peak of the PSVER is prolonged (115 to 200 ms). In fact, almost all patients with optic neuritis, even after the visual acuity has returned to normal, continue to show distinct abnormalities in this PSVER at a time when detailed ophthalmologic evaluations reveal no abnormality. In multiple sclerosis, if the PSVER is normal, the neuroophthalmologic examination is almost always normal (we have had no exceptions to this rule in more than 225 patients). Even when the PSVER is abnormal, the visual fields, visual acuity, pupillary

reactions, and optic fundus examination are normal in a considerable number of patients.

Approximately one-half of the patients with multiple sclerosis who have never had visual symptoms also show abnormalities, and this accounts for one of the most useful aspects of the test. If a patient presents with what appears to be the first episode of a neurologic illness in which the lesion is in the brainstem or spinal cord, a demonstration by means of an abnormal PSVER of another clinically unsuspected lesion in a different part of the central nervous system (the optic nerves) makes the diagnosis of multiple sclerosis more likely and may spare the patient certain neuroradiologic procedures.

Abnormalities in visual acuity have no effect on the PSVER unless the acuity is so poor that the patient cannot see the checkerboard pattern—patients with acuity of 20/200 or better are suitable for testing. The only other requirement is that the patient be cooperative enough to sit still for 20 min and watch the pattern. Infants and children can also be tested by using special techniques.

BRAINSTEM AUDITORY EVOKED RESPONSES Brainstem auditory evoked responses (BAERs) are more difficult to obtain than PSVERs because BAERs are much smaller, of the order of 0.5 μV. These are produced by clicks transmitted to one of a patient's ears through earphones. The patient may be alert or comatose and need not be particularly cooperative except that excess movement or muscle artifact makes the response even more difficult to obtain. BAERs of essentially normal appearance can be recorded from infants and children. BAERs consist of a series of seven waves which appear within the first 10 ms after the click. These (named I to VII) are considered to represent successive activation of the auditory nerve (I) and the brainstem auditory pathways (cochlear nucleus, II; superior olivary complex, III; lateral lemniscus, IV; inferior colliculus, V; and higher auditory centers, VI, VII). A lesion at or between any of these levels either obliterates or delays the appearance of waves from successively higher levels. The same is true of other lesions affecting the brainstem, such as small vascular lesions, central pontine myelinolysis or hypoxic damage. The waves that arise from structures caudal to the lesion are perfectly normal in latency, whereas those arising from structures cranial to the lesion are either obliterated or delayed. This allows one to pinpoint quite accurately the level of the lesion within the brainstem auditory pathways and provides a very neat opportunity for correlation of clinical observations with neurophysiologic and occasionally pathologic data. This test is useful as a screening test for patients with acoustic neuromas (who almost always show an abnormality), for patients suspected of having multiple sclerosis, for comatose patients in whom the level of lesion within the central nervous system is not clear, and for other patients in whom documentation of brainstem lesions is important. Hearing loss can often be recognized in this test, since changes in the latency of the first (and, therefore, subsequent) waves are produced, and these must be taken into consideration in the evaluation of the results obtained. Interwave latencies, which are the parameters used to measure central conduction, are not affected by hearing loss or stimulus intensity. The test is also useful in screening high-risk infants for hearing defects.

SOMATOSENSORY EVOKED RESPONSES Somatosensory evoked responses (SERs) are produced by small painless electrical stimuli administered to large sensory fibers in mixed nerves of the hand or leg. The afferent volley is recorded at many levels as it ascends the somatosensory pathways, and a series of waves can be recorded which reflect activity in peripheral nerve trunks, tracts in the spinal cord, gracile and cuneate nuclei, pontine and/or cerebellar structures, thalamus, thalamocortical radiations, and primary sensory fields of the cortex. Lesions of the pathways at any level affect the subsequent waves, thus providing localizing and confirmatory data in a similar fashion to the BAER.

Evoked responses can be used for a single evaluation of patients (looking for lesions in the various pathways discussed) or as a quantitative method for following a patient's course to document functional improvement or deterioration as time passes, following therapy, and so on. They also prove useful for on-line monitoring of function in optic nerve, brainstem, or spinal cord during neurosurgical procedures that involve manipulation of those structures. Since BAERs and SERs are unaffected by general anesthesia and high-dose barbiturates, they also can be used to follow CNS function in comatose patients. Longer latency auditory and somatosensory evoked responses have been studied for a number of years. These are largely cortically produced responses, dramatically affected by drowsiness, inattention, and other poorly controllable variables, and have not proven to be clinically useful. Neither have most visual evoked responses produced by stroboscopic flashes. They are very useful in evaluation of visual pathways in infants and young children who are not cooperative enough to watch the checkerboard pattern and in adults during surgery or when comatose. Under other circumstances, pattern-shift PSVERs afford a much more reliable and reproducible response.

MOTOR EVOKED RESPONSES In conventional motor nerve conduction studies, recordings are made from peripheral muscles and the nerve is stimulated at various sites between the muscle and the spinal cord. The rostral limit of such studies has been determined by the accessibility of the proximal parts of the peripheral nervous system to stimulation. Magnetic stimulators developed over the last few years induce sufficient current flow in conductive tissues to allow the motor cortex itself to be stimulated painlessly through the intact skull in humans. The resultant compound motor action potential, measured over peripheral muscles, has a very high amplitude (compared to SEP waveforms) and does not require signal averaging. Stimulation of the motor pathways at multiple sites allows the conduction properties of the intervening motor tracts, including central ones, to be studied in health and disease. This provides objective, numerical data relating to the functioning of central motor pathways, previously amenable only to peripheral tests usually dependent on patient cooperation (e.g., grip strength).

Clinical applications of these motor evoked responses have been reported and they show very good correlations with motor disabilities in multiple sclerosis and motor neuron diseases. In the latter disease, the motor cortex may be unexcitable by the transcranial magnetic stimulator, despite moderate preservation of voluntary strength.

LUMBAR PUNCTURE AND CEREBROSPINAL FLUID EXAMINATION

The information yielded by the examination of the cerebrospinal fluid (CSF) is often of crucial importance in diagnosis and treatment.

INDICATIONS FOR LUMBAR PUNCTURE Lumbar puncture is performed for the following reasons:

1 To obtain pressure measurements and to secure a sample of CSF for cellular, chemical, and bacteriologic examination.
2 To aid in therapy by the administration of spinal anesthetics and occasionally antibiotics or antitumor agents.
3 To inject air for air contrast myelography or, very rarely, for pneumoencephalography; a radiopaque substance or a water-soluble contrast medium for myelography; or a radioactive substance [e.g., indium or radioactive iodinated serum albumin (RISA)] for the study of CSF dynamics and to aid in the diagnosis of hydrocephalus or CSF leak.

Lumbar puncture carries a risk if the CSF pressure is high (evidenced by headache and papilledema), for it increases the possibility of fatal cerebellar or tentorial herniation. In doubtful cases, it is wise first to obtain a CT or magnetic resonance image (MRI) to exclude a mass lesion before proceeding to perform a lumbar puncture. However, if it seems important in a given case of suspected increased intracranial pressure to have the information yielded by CSF examination, the lumbar puncture may be performed with a fine-bore (no.

22 or 24 gauge) needle as the last part of the clinical study. (Note that if the pressure is over 400 mmHg, one should obtain the necessary sample of fluid, remove the needle, and then, according to the suspected clinical disease and patient's condition, administer mannitol in a dose of 0.75 to 1.0 mg/kg.) Dexamethasone should be started in a dose of 4 to 6 mg every 6 h in cases of tumor, cerebral trauma, hemorrhage, and certain types of encephalitis (acute hemorrhagic leukoencephalitis, herpes simplex encephalitis).

Cisternal puncture and lateral cervical puncture (C1–C2), although safe in the hands of the expert, are too hazardous to entrust to those without experience. The lumbar puncture is to be preferred except in obvious instances of spinal block requiring a sample of cisternal fluid or myelography above the lesions, or in rare instances where infection of the skin or subcutaneous tissue render needle penetration dangerous.

Experience teaches the importance of meticulous technique. Lumbar puncture should always be done under sterile conditions. If procaine is injected in and beneath the skin, the procedure should be painless. Failure to enter the lumbar subarachnoid space after two or three trials can usually be corrected by doing the puncture with patients in the sitting position and then assisting them to lie on their side for pressure measurements and fluid removal. The "dry tap" is more often due to an improperly placed needle than to a pathologic obliteration of subarachnoid space by compressive lesion of the spinal cord or chronic adhesive arachnoiditis. A bloody tap due to transfixation of a meningeal vessel may result in hopeless confusion of the diagnosis if it is falsely interpreted as indicating hemorrhage in the subarachnoid spaces and ventricles. Lumbar puncture should be undertaken with particular care in patients with thrombocytopenia or disorders of blood coagulation because serious hemorrhage into the extradural or intradural space may occur.

EXAMINATION PROCEDURES Once the lumbar puncture is successful, some or all of the following aspects of the CSF should be studied: (1) pressure and "dynamics"; (2) gross appearance of CSF including centrifugation, if blood is present, to examine the supernatant for xanthochromia; (3) number and type of cells and presence of microorganisms; (4) protein, sugar, and, in special instances, analysis of pigments; (5) exfoliative cytology using Millipore filters; (6) Wassermann reaction and appropriate serologic precipitation reactions (including cryptococcal antigen in patients with immunologic suppression, e.g., AIDS); (7) protein immunoelectrophoresis for determination of gamma globulin levels, and other special biochemical tests (for NH_3, pH, CO_2, enzymes, etc.); and (8) bacteriologic cultures and virus isolation. See the appendix for normal values of CSF constituents.

REFERENCES

CHIAPPA KH (ed.): *Evoked Potentials in Clinical Neurology*, 2nd ed. New York, Raven Press, 1989
EBERSOLE JS, BRIDGERS SL: Ambulatory EEG monitoring, in *Recent Advances in Epilepsy*, TA Pedley, BS Meldrum (eds). New York, Churchill Livingstone, 1986, pp 111–135
ENGEL J, JR: *Seizures and Epilepsy*. Philadelphia, F.A. Davis, 1989
ENGEL J JR: A practical guide for routine EEG studies in epilepsy. J Clin Neurophysiol 1(2):109, 1984
HESS CW et al: Magnetic brain stimulation: Central motor conduction studies in multiple sclerosis. Ann Neurol 22:744, 1987
KIMURA J: *Electrodiagnosis in Diseases of Nerve and Muscle*, 2d ed. Philadelphia, F.A. Davis, 1989
NIEDERMEYER E, LOPES DA SILVA F (eds): *Electroencephalography*, 2d ed. Baltimore, Urban & Schwarzenberg, 1987
OH SJ: *Electromyography, Neuromuscular Transmission Studies*. Baltimore, Williams & Wilkins, 1988
SHAHANI BT (ed): *Electromyography in CNS Disorders: Central EMG*. Boston, Butterworth, 1984
SPEHLMANN R: *EEG Primer*. New York, Elsevier Biomedical Press, 1981
STALBERG E, YOUNG RR (eds): *Clinical Neurophysiology*. London, Butterworth, 1981

350 THE EPILEPSIES AND CONVULSIVE DISORDERS

MARC A. DICHTER

The *epilepsies* are a group of disorders characterized by chronic, recurrent, paroxysmal changes in neurologic function caused by abnormalities in the electrical activity of the brain. They are estimated to affect between 0.5 and 2 percent of the population, and can occur at any age. Each episode of neurologic dysfunction is called a *seizure*. Seizures may be *convulsive* when they are accompanied by motor manifestations, or may be manifest by other changes in neurologic function (i.e., by sensory, cognitive, emotional events). Epilepsy can be acquired as a result of neurologic injury or a structural brain lesion and can also occur as a part of many systemic medical diseases. Epilepsy also occurs in an *idiopathic* form in an individual with neither a history of neurologic insult nor other apparent neurologic dysfunction. Isolated, nonrecurrent seizures may occur in otherwise healthy individuals for a variety of reasons, and under these circumstances, the individual is not said to have epilepsy.

CLASSIFICATION OF SEIZURES

The neurologic manifestations of epileptic seizures are varied, ranging from a brief lapse of attention to a prolonged loss of consciousness with abnormal motor activity. The proper classification of the kinds of seizures which an individual is experiencing is important for an appropriate diagnostic workup, prognostic evaluation, and selection of therapy. The classification of epileptic seizures provided in this chapter is based on the International Classification of Epileptic Seizures. It emphasizes the clinical seizure type and ictal (seizure-associated) and interictal (between seizure) electroencephalographic pattern (Table 350-1), whereas etiology, anatomic substrate, and pathways of spread are not major considerations. The older terminology of grand mal, petit mal, and psychomotor or temporal lobe epilepsy has been integrated into the current scheme. In addition to identifying the seizure types which an individual is experiencing, it is also useful to categorize the clinical context within which the seizures occur. Epilepsy syndromes that take into account the age of the patient, types of seizures, presence of underlying neurologic lesion, etc., help define groups of patients with relatively predictable prognoses and for whom specific therapies are indicated.

The major underlying premise of the seizure classification is that some seizures (partial or focal seizures) start in one area of the brain (cortex) and either remain localized or generalize (that is, spread throughout the brain), whereas other seizures appear to be general from their earliest manifestation.

PARTIAL OR FOCAL SEIZURES Partial or focal seizures begin with the activation of neurons in one area of the cortex. The specific clinical symptoms depend on the area of cortex involved and imply dysfunction in a limited area of the cortex. The lesion may be due to birth injury, postnatal trauma, tumor, abscess, infarction, vascular malformation, or some other structural abnormality. The abnormal area of the cortex underlying the seizure activity can be identified by the specific neurologic phenomena observed during the focal seizure. Partial seizures are classified as "simple" if there is no alteration of consciousness or awareness of the environment and "complex" if there is such a change.

Simple partial seizures Simple partial seizures can occur with motor, sensory, autonomic, or psychic symptoms. A simple partial seizure with motor signs consists of recurrent contractions of the muscles of one part of the body (finger, hand, arm, face, etc.) without loss of consciousness. Each muscular contraction is caused by the discharge of neurons in the corresponding area of the contralateral motor cortex.

TABLE 350-1 Classification of epileptic seizures

I Partial or focal seizures
  A Simple partial seizures (with motor, sensory, autonomic, or psychic signs)
  B Complex partial seizures (psychomotor or temporal lobe seizures)
  C Secondary generalized partial seizures
II Primary generalized seizures
  A Tonic-clonic (grand mal)
  B Tonic
  C Absence (petit mal)
  D Atypical absence
  E Myoclonic
  F Atonic
  G Infantile spasms
III Status epilepticus
  A Tonic-clonic status
  B Absence status
  C Epilepsia partialis continua
IV Recurrence patterns
  A Sporadic
  B Cyclic
  C Reflex (photomyoclonic, somatosensory, musicogenic, reading epilepsy)

The muscle activity of a partial seizure ("ictus") may remain confined to one area or may spread from the affected area to involve contiguous ipsilateral body parts (i.e., right thumb to right hand to right arm to right side of face). This "Jacksonian march," first described by Hughlings Jackson, is caused by a demonstrable progression of epileptiform discharges in the contralateral motor cortex and may occur over seconds or minutes. The EEG manifestations of this form of seizure are often very striking and consist of regularly occurring spike discharges in the appropriate area of the motor cortex. Between seizures (interictal period) this region may give rise to irregular spike discharges in the EEG.

Simple partial seizures may have other behavioral manifestations if the seizure discharges occur in other cortical regions. Thus, sensory symptoms (paresthesias, vertiginous feelings, simple auditory or visual hallucinations) occur with epileptiform discharges in the contralateral sensory cortex, and autonomic and psychic symptoms [i.e., the sensation of having experienced something before (déjà vu), unwarranted sense of fear or anger, illusions, and even complex hallucinations] occur with discharges in temporal and frontal lobes.

Complex partial seizures (temporal lobe or psychomotor seizures) Complex partial seizures are episodic changes in behavior in which an individual loses conscious contact with the environment. The onset of these seizures may consist of any of a variety of auras: an unusual smell (as of burning rubber), a feeling that the current experience has happened before (déjà vu), a sudden intense emotional feeling, a sensory illusion such as that of objects growing smaller (micropsia) or larger (macropsia), or a specific formed sensory hallucination. Patients may come to recognize these as heralding their seizures, or the memory of the aura may be lost in the postictal amnesia, which often occurs if the seizure becomes generalized. During complex partial seizures there may be a cessation of activity with some minor motor activity, such as lip smacking, swallowing, walking aimlessly, or picking at one's clothes (automatisms). Complex partial seizures may also be accompanied by the unconscious performance of highly skilled activities such as driving a car or playing complicated musical pieces. When the seizure ends, the individual is amnesic for events which took place during the seizure and may take minutes or hours to recover full consciousness.

Patients with complex partial seizures have EEGs that exhibit unilateral or bilateral spikes, sharp waves, or slow wave discharges over temporal or frontotemporal regions both interictally and during seizures. Most of these seizures originate from epileptiform activity in the temporal lobes—especially the hippocampus or amygdala—or other parts of the limbic system, but others have been shown to originate from mesial parasagittal or orbital frontal regions. Epilepsy manifest by these kinds of seizures is also referred to as "temporal lobe epilepsy'' and ''psychomotor epilepsy'' in older classification schemes.

Although often showing spike discharges or focal slowing during complex partial seizures, exceptionally the surface EEG may be normal. Sphenoidal electrodes may record the abnormal discharges, but in some cases only depth electrodes in the hippocampus or amygdala or other limbic structures will show seizure discharges. The occasional discrepancy between surface and depth electrophysiologic events is a particularly difficult problem when trying to use the surface EEG to determine the nature of an abnormal behavior in an individual susupected of having complex partial seizures. (See ''Differential Diagnosis of Seizures,'' below.)

Secondary generalization of partial seizures Simple or complex partial seizures can progress to generalized seizures with loss of consciousness and often with convulsive motor activity. This may occur immediately or after many seconds or a minute or two. In addition, many patients with focal seizures have generalized seizures without an obvious initial focal component which are difficult to distinguish from primary generalized seizures. The presence of an aura or the observation of any focal feature (twitching of one extremity, aphasia, tonic eye deviation) at the onset of the generalized seizure or the presence of a postictal focal neurologic deficit (Todd's paralysis) are important clues to a focal origin to the seizure.

PRIMARY GENERALIZED SEIZURES Tonic-clonic (grand mal) One of the most common kinds of epileptic paroxysms is the generalized tonic-clonic seizure. Some of these appear to be primary generalized seizures and others are the result of secondary generalization from partial seizures. In either case, the seizures follow a common pattern. The primary generalized seizures usually start without warning, although some individuals sense a vague, nonspecific sense of the impending event. The onset is heralded by a sudden loss of consciousness, a *tonic* contraction of the muscles, a loss of postural control, and a cry produced by a forced expiration caused by contraction of the respiratory muscles. The individual falls to the floor in an opisthotonic posture, often sustaining injury, and remains rigid for many seconds. There may be cyanosis as respiration is inhibited. Soon a series of rhythmic contractions of all four limbs occurs. This *clonic* phase can last for a variable period of time and ends when the muscles relax. The individual remains unconscious and unarousable for a period of minutes or longer. There is usually a gradual return to consciousness, and often a period of disorientation during recovery. The patient may even be combative if restrained. During the seizure, urinary or fecal incontinence and tongue biting may occur. Postictally there is amnesia for the seizure, and sometimes a retrograde amnesia as well. Headache and drowsiness are common sequelae, and the individual may not return to baseline functioning for days.

The EEG in patients with tonic-clonic seizures shows low-voltage fast (10-Hz or more) activity during the tonic phase, which converts gradually to slower, larger sharp waves throughout both hemispheres. During the clonic phase there are bursts of sharp waves associated with the rhythmic muscular contractions and slow waves coincident with the pauses. Often the excessive muscular activity of the seizure causes artifacts which interfere with ictal EEG recordings. Interictally, the EEG is often abnormal, with polyspike (or spike) and wave or occasionally sharp and slow wave discharges; interictal EEGs may also be normal.

Tonic seizures Tonic seizures are a less common form of primary generalized seizure which consist of the sudden occurrence of a rigid posturing of the limbs or torso, often with deviation of the head and eyes toward one side. They are not followed by a clonic phase, and are often of shorter duration than tonic-clonic seizures.

Absence seizures (petit mal) Pure absence seizures consist of the sudden cessation of ongoing conscious activity without convulsive muscular activity or loss of postural control. Such seizures may be so brief as to be inapparent. Usually they last for seconds and, occasionally, for as long as several minutes. The brief lapses of consciousness or awareness may be accompanied by minor motor manifestations such as eyelid fluttering, small chewing movements of the mouth, or mild shaking of the hands. During longer absences, automatisms may occur which may be difficult to distinguish from complex partial seizures. At the end of the absence seizure, the patient regains awareness of the environment very quickly, and there is usually no period of postictal confusion.

Absence seizures almost always begin in younger children (6 to 14 years of age) and rarely appear for the first time in adults. These brief seizures may occur hundreds or more times per day and go on for weeks or months before it is recognized that the child is having seizures. Absence seizures may first be recognized when the child begins having learning difficulties in school.

The EEG is pathognomonic in this form of seizure disorder. Brief 3-Hz spike and wave discharges, which appear synchronously throughout all the leads, occur interictally, but become clinically significant as absence seizures when they last more than several seconds. Interictal EEG background activity is otherwise normal. Often the EEG demonstrates that the child is having more seizures than was thought from clinical observation alone.

Absence seizures usually occur in otherwise neurologically normal children. These seizures are usually sensitive to antiepileptic drugs (see below). Children with this condition often do quite well once it is treated. Approximately one-third outgrow the seizure disorder, one-third continue to have only absence seizures, and one-third have concomitant generalized tonic-clonic seizures.

Absence seizures can be differentiated from absence-like attacks which occasionally occur in complex partial seizures by the lack of aura, immediate recovery from the absence, and typical 3-Hz spike and wave EEG pattern.

Atypical absence Atypical absence seizures are similar to absence seizures but coexist with other forms of generalized seizures, such as tonic seizures, myoclonic seizures, or atonic seizures (see below). The EEG is more heterogeneous, containing spike and wave discharges at 2 or 4 Hz during the absence attacks and poorly developed background with spike or polyspike activity during interictal periods.

Atypical absence seizures commonly occur in children with some other form of underlying neurologic dysfunction and tend to be resistant to medication. In the most severe form of this disorder, the Lennox-Gastaut syndrome, children have several kinds of generalized seizures and often have intellectual impairment.

Myoclonic seizures Myoclonic seizures are sudden, brief, single or repetitive muscle contractions involving one body part or the entire body. In the latter case, the seizure is accompanied by a violent fall, without a loss of consciousness. Myoclonic seizures often coexist with other seizure types but may occur alone. The EEG shows polyspike and wave discharges or sharp and slow waves, both ictally and interictally. Although often idiopathic, myoclonic seizures occur as a major neurologic symptom in a variety of medical conditions including uremia, hepatic failure, Creutzfeldt-Jakob disease, subacute leukoencephalopathies, and a hereditary degenerative condition, Lafora body disease.

Juvenile myoclonic epilepsy (of Janz) has been identified as a distinct syndrome which begins in adolescence and which has a genetic component. It often begins with postawakening myoclonic seizures, and later in its course, these may be followed by generalized tonic-clonic seizures.

Atonic seizures Atonic seizures are brief losses of consciousness and postural tone not associated with tonic muscular contractions. The individual may simply drop to the floor without apparent cause. Atonic seizures usually occur in children and are often accompanied by other forms of seizures. The EEG contains polyspikes and slow waves. The ''drop attacks'' of atonic seizures need to be distinguished from cataplexy seen in narcolepsy (where the patient remains conscious), transient brainstem ischemia, or sudden rises in intracranial pressure.

Infantile spasms or hypsarrhythmia These primary generalized seizures occur in infants between birth and approximately 12 months of age and consist of several types of brief synchronous contractions of the neck, torso, and both arms (usually in flexion). Infantile spasms often occur in children with underlying neurologic diseases, such as anoxic encephalopathy or tuberous sclerosis, but can rarely occur in an otherwise apparently normal infant. The prognosis for children with this form of seizure disorder is grave, and approximately 90 percent develop mental retardation in addition to their seizures. The EEG is characterized by a very disorganized background, random high-voltage slow waves, spikes, and burst suppression (hypsarrhythmia). The spasms and hypsarrhythmia tend to disappear over the first 3 to 5 years of life only to be replaced by other forms of generalized seizures. Infantile spasms sometimes respond to treatment with ACTH or valproic acid.

STATUS EPILEPTICUS   Prolonged or repetitive seizures without a period of recovery between attacks can occur with all forms of seizures and is defined as "status epilepticus." When tonic-clonic seizures are involved, this state can be life-threatening (see "Treatment of Seizures"). Absence status, on the other hand, may proceed for some time before it is recognized, because the patient does not lose consciousness or have convulsive movements. Status epilepticus of partial seizures is called *epilepsia partialis continua* and may occur with partial motor, sensory, or visceral seizures. Complex partial seizures may also present as status epilepticus.

RECURRENCE PATTERNS   All classes of recurrent seizures can occur sporadically or randomly, with no apparent triggering event, or can occur cyclically, i.e., in concert with the sleep-wake cycle or the menstrual cycle (catamenial epilepsy). Epileptic seizures can also occur as evoked reactions to a specific stimulus (reflex epilepsy), although this is relatively infrequent. Examples are seizures triggered by photic stimulation (photomyoclonic or photoconvulsive epilepsy), specific musical compositions (musicogenic epilepsy), tactile stimulation (somatosensory-induced epilepsy), or reading (reading or language epilepsy). The latter usually consists of brief myoclonic jerks of the jaw, cheek, and tongue which occur during silent or oral reading and may progress to generalized tonic-clonic seizures.

PATHOPHYSIOLOGY OF EPILEPSY

Epileptic seizures can be induced in any normal human (or vertebrate) brain with a variety of different electrical or chemical stimuli. The ease and rapidity with which these seizures can occur and the stereotyped nature of the seizures produced suggest that the normal brain, particularly the cerebral cortex, contains within its fine anatomic and physiologic structure a mechanism which is inherently unstable and which can be influenced in many different ways to produce a seizure. Thus, many different kinds of metabolic abnormalities and anatomic lesions of brain can produce seizures, and conversely, there is no pathognomonic lesion of the epileptic brain.

The hallmark of the altered physiologic state of epilepsy is a rhythmical and repetitive hypersynchronous discharge of many neurons in a localized area of the brain. A reflection of this hypersynchronous discharge can be observed in the electroencephalogram. The EEG records the integrated electrical activity generated by synaptic potentials in neurons in the superficial layers of a localized area of cortex. Normally, the EEG records unsynchronized activity during periods when the mind is actively working, or mildly synchronized activity when the mind is in a restful state (i.e., alpha waves during relaxation with closed eyes) or during various stages of sleep. In the epileptic focus, neurons in a small area of the cortex are activated for a brief period (50 to 100 ms) in an unusually synchronized manner, and this produces a larger, sharper waveform in the EEG—the spike discharge. If the synchronous neuronal discharge occurs over several seconds, a focal seizure follows; if it spreads through the brain and lasts for many seconds or minutes, a complex partial or generalized seizure (the ictus) will occur and the EEG can have a variety of appearances, depending on which areas of brain are involved and how the primary discharging areas project

to the superficial cortex. During the seizure the EEG may display low-voltage fast activity or high-voltage spikes or spike and wave discharges throughout both hemispheres.

During the interictal spike discharge, the neurons in the epileptic focus undergo a large membrane depolarization (the depolarizing shift, or DS) accompanied by action potential generation. After the DS, the neurons hyperpolarize and stop firing for several seconds. In areas around the discharging focus, the neurons are also inhibited. Thus, it appears as if the epileptic discharge is limited to a localized area of cortex by a ring of inhibition around the focus and slightly delayed inhibition within the focus. When the epileptic focus undergoes a transition from the isolated discharges to a seizure, the post-DS inhibition disappears and is replaced by a depolarizing potential. Neurons in contiguous areas and in synaptically connected distant areas are then recruited into the seizure and become activated. Local cortical circuits, long association pathways (including callosal), and subcortical pathways are all utilized for the spread of the discharges. Thus, a focal seizure can spread locally or generalize throughout the brain. Widely ramifying thalamocortical pathways are likely to be responsible for the rapid generalization of some forms of epilepsy, including absence seizures.

A number of metabolic events occur within the brain during the epileptic discharges which may contribute to the development of the focus, to the transition to seizures, or to postictal dysfunction. During the discharges, extracellular potassium concentration increases and extracellular calcium concentration decreases. Both of these changes have profound effects on neuronal excitability and neurotransmitter release and on neuronal metabolism. Neurotransmitters and neuropeptides are also released in unusually large amounts during seizure discharges. Some of these substances can have prolonged actions on central neurons and may be responsible for prolonged postictal phenomona such as Todd's paralysis. In addition to the ionic effects, seizures produce increases in cerebral blood flow to the primary involved areas, increases in glucose utilization, and alterations in oxidative metabolism and local pH. It is possible that these events are not just consequences of the seizures but actually contribute to the development of the seizure activity and that manipulation of such factors could become an effective means for controlling seizures.

There are many mechanisms by which seizures can develop in either normal or pathologic brains. Three common mechanisms include (1) diminution of inhibitory mechanisms, especially synaptic inhibition due to gamma-aminobutyric acid (GABA), (2) enhancement of excitatory synaptic mechanisms, especially those mediated by the N-methyl-D-aspartate (NMDA) component of glutamate responses, and (3) enhancement of endogenous neuronal burst firing (usually by enhancing voltage-dependent calcium currents). Different forms of human epilepsy may be caused by any one or combination of these mechanisms. For example, in some forms of chronic focal epilepsy, inhibitory interneurons appear to be preferentially lost; in other models, and possibly in cases of human hippocampal sclerosis, aberrant recurrent excitatory connections may form among surviving neurons. In primary generalized absence epilepsy, thalamic neurons with large, low-threshold, transient, voltage-dependent calcium currents may be responsible for generating the diffusely synchronous cortical spike and wave activity.

Currently available antiepileptic drugs appear to operate on several of these mechanisms. Phenytoin, carbamazepine, barbiturates, and valproic acid all appear able to block voltage-dependent sodium channels in a use-dependent manner, such that individual action potentials are relatively unaffected but high-frequency repetitive firing is reduced. The barbiturates and benzodiazepines can enhance GABA-mediated inhibition. Ethosuximide appears to block a low-threshold, transient calcium current in neurons. At present, no drugs are available for clinical use which specifically block excitatory synaptic systems, but much effort is being expended in this direction.

Electrical stimulation is another mechanism by which seizures can easily be produced in a normal brain. At certain current strengths and stimulus frequencies, seizure discharges are produced and become self-sustaining beyond the original stimulus. Generalized tonic-clonic seizures result. At lower stimulus parameters, seizure afterdischarges may not occur. However, if a stereotyped subthreshold stimulus is repeated at regular intervals (which may even be as infrequent as one stimulation per day), there is a gradual buildup of response until generalized seizures occur to the same stimulus which was originally subthreshold. Eventually spontaneous seizures may occur without any further electrical stimulation. This phenomenon has been called "kindling." Its relationship to the pathophysiology of posttraumatic epilepsy or to the issue of whether the occurrence of seizures themselves tends to foster the continued development of a seizure focus in human beings has not been resolved.

THE CAUSES OF EPILEPSY

The likely etiology of a given seizure depends on the age of the patient and the type of seizure (Table 350-2). In young infants, anoxia or ischemia before or during birth, intracranial birth injury, metabolic disturbances such as hypoglycemia, hypocalcemia, and hypomagnesemia, congenital malformations of the brain, and infections are the most common causes of seizures. In the young child, trauma and infections are common causes of epilepsy, although idiopathic seizures account for the majority of patients.

Genetic factors can influence the development of epilepsy and have also been shown to affect EEG patterns in general. Patients with primary generalized seizures, especially absence and myoclonic seizures, have a higher familial incidence of epilepsy than is found in the normal population, and relatives of such patients have higher incidences of dysrhythmic EEGs, even when they do not have seizures. The mode of inheritance of epilepsy susceptibility appears complicated and probably represents multiple genes with variable penetrance. Even in the highest risk group, however, the chance of a sibling or a child of an individual with generalized seizures also having epilepsy is below 10 percent.

Young children also frequently (approximately 2 to 5 percent of the population) develop seizures with febrile illnesses. These febrile convulsions are short generalized tonic-clonic convulsions which occur during the early phases of a febrile illness in children between the ages of 3 months and 5 years. Febrile seizures must be distinguished from seizures which are triggered by central nervous system infections which coincidentally produce fever (meningitis or encephalitis). There is minimal likelihood that the child will develop epilepsy or any neurologic impairment from the febrile convulsion if the seizure lasts less than 5 min, is generalized rather than focal, and is not associated with any interictal EEG abnormalities or abnormalities on neurologic examination. There may be a family history of this kind of febrile seizure. Febrile seizures of this kind are probably best treated with quick and relatively vigorous attempts to keep children from developing excessive fevers during various childhood illnesses but without specific antiepileptic medication. Some pediatricians prefer to maintain children susceptible to febrile convulsions on phenobarbital medication; others advocate administration of benzodiazepines at the first signs of illness. On the other hand, if the febrile convulsion is prolonged or focal or is associated with an abnormal EEG, or if the child has a neurologic abnormality, there is a significant risk of subsequent epilepsy. These children should be treated with chronic antiepileptic therapy.

In adolescents and young adults, head trauma is a major cause of focal epilepsy. Epilepsy can be caused by any kind of serious head injury, with the likelihood of developing recurrent seizures being proportional to the extent of the damage. Injuries which either cause dural penetration or produce posttraumatic amnesia of more than 24-h duration may result in a 40 to 50 percent incidence of later epilepsy, while the incidence with closed head injuries with cerebral contusion varies from 5 to 25 percent. Brief concussions or nonpenetrating head injuries without loss of consciousness are not usually epileptogenic. Seizures which occur immediately or within the first 24 h of injury are not associated with a poor prognosis, whereas seizures occurring after the first day and within the first 2 weeks indicate a high likelihood of posttraumatic epilepsy. Most recurring seizures develop by 2 years after the injury. Approximately 50 percent of patients with posttraumatic seizures spontaneously recover, 25 percent have medically controllable seizures, and 25 percent have seizures that are much more intractable to antiepileptic medication. The effectiveness of prophylactic anticonvulsant medication after head trauma still requires adequate documentation, although many physicians treat such patients (and other postoperative neurosurgical patients) with phenytoin or phenobarbital to attempt to prevent the development of posttraumatic seizures.

In the adolescent or young adult age group, generalized tonic-clonic seizures tend to be idiopathic or are associated with drug (especially barbiturate) or alcohol use or withdrawal. Arteriovenous malformations may present as focal seizures in this age group. Between ages 30 and 50, brain tumors become more common causes of seizures and may be present in 30 percent of patients with new focal seizures. In general, the incidence of seizures is higher with slowly growing brain tumors involving the cerebrum, such as meningiomas or low-grade gliomas, than with the more malignant types. However, seizures can occur in individuals with any kind of central nervous system mass lesion, including highly malignant metastatic tumors or completely benign vascular malformations.

Above age 50, cerebrovascular disease is the most common cause of focal or generalized seizures. Seizures can occur acutely in patients with an embolus, hemorrhage or, more rarely, a thrombosis but occur more often as a late sequel to these lesions. Seizures can also result from "silent" cerebral infarctions in patients with no known cerebrovascular disease. Brain tumors, either primary or metastatic, also present with seizures in the older age group.

At any age, a variety of medical diseases can produce metabolic disturbances which may present as seizures. Uremia, hepatic failure, hypo- or hypercalcemia, hypo- and hyperglycemia, or hypo- and hypernatremia may be associated with myoclonic seizures or generalized tonic-clonic seizures.

EVALUATION OF THE PATIENT WITH A SEIZURE

Individuals with seizures present to physicians either in an emergency room setting during the acute attack or in an office setting days after the epileptic event. In the former case, the seizure may be the presenting symptom of a serious central nervous system disorder

TABLE 350-2 The causes of seizures

Infant (0–2)	Paranatal hypoxia and ischemia Intracranial birth injury Acute infection Metabolic disturbances (hypoglycemia, hypocalcemia, hypomagnesemia, pyridoxine deficiency) Congenital malformation Genetic disorders
Child (2–12)	Idiopathic Acute infection Trauma Febrile convulsion
Adolescent (12–18)	Idiopathic Trauma Drug, alcohol withdrawal Arteriovenous malformations
Young adult (18–35)	Trauma Alcoholism Brain tumor
Older adult (>35)	Brain tumor Cerebrovascular disease Metabolic disorders (uremia, hepatic failure, electrolyte abnormality, hypoglycemia) Alcoholism

which requires immediate diagnosis and therapy. In the latter case, the seizure may be a symptom of a more chronic neurologic dysfunction and a different approach is warranted.

Initial emergency evaluation is directed toward ensuring adequate ventilation and perfusion and stopping the seizure (see "Treatment"). Once the patient is medically stable, the investigation is directed at determining the cause of the seizure. Often a careful history (either from the patient, if recovered, or from a friend or relative), a physical examination, and a few blood studies can provide the diagnosis.

A history suggesting a recent febrile illness accompanied by headaches, change in mental status, or confusion suggests an acute CNS infection (either meningitis or encephalitis) and indicates the need for urgent examination of the CSF. In this context, a complex partial seizure may be the presenting symptom of herpes simplex encephalitis. A history of headache and/or change in mental functioning preceding the seizure, coupled with either signs of increased intracranial pressure or a focal neurologic deficit, suggests an underlying mass lesion (tumor, abscess, arteriovenous malformation) or a chronic subdural hematoma. Seizures with a clear focal onset or aura are especially worrisome in this regard. An MRI or CT scan should be performed for a more definitive diagnosis.

The general physical examination may provide important etiologic information. Gum hyperplasia is usually the result of chronic phenytoin therapy. Exacerbation of a chronic seizure disorder due to intercurrent infection, alcohol, or cessation of therapy is a common cause of patients presenting to an emergency room. Skin examination may reveal the port wine facial stain of Sturge-Weber disease (with accompanying cerebral calcifications), the stigmata of tuberous sclerosis (adenoma sebaceum and shagreen patches), or neurofibromatosis (subcutaneous nodules, café au lait spots). Body or limb asymmetries may indicate hypotrophic somatic development contralateral to a congenital or infantile cerebral lesion.

The history or physical examination may also reveal evidence of chronic alcoholism. Heavy alcohol users commonly have seizures for any of several reasons—old cerebral contusion (from falls or fights), chronic subdural hematoma, metabolic derangements of undernutrition and liver disease, CNS infection, or alcohol withdrawal ("rum fits"). Seizures occurring during alcohol use or withdrawal, in the absence of other causes, are usually brief generalized tonic-clonic seizures which occur singly or in a flurry of two or three. Once the flurry is over, chronic antiepileptic treatment is unnecessary, since they are usually self-limiting. Seizures in alcoholics which occur at other times should be treated, but this group of patients presents a particular challenge because of lack of compliance and metabolic problems which complicate drug therapy.

Routine blood studies will indicate if the seizure was caused by hypoglycemia, hypo- or hypernatremia, or hypo- or hypercalcemia. These biochemical abnormalities should be corrected and the cause determined. In addition, other less common causes of seizures can be sought with appropriate tests: thyrotoxicosis, acute intermittent porphyria, and lead or arsenic intoxication.

In the older patient, a seizure may indicate an acute cerebrovascular accident or may be a delayed effect of an old cerebral infarct (even a silent one). The manner in which further evaluation proceeds is dictated by the patient's age, cardiovascular status, and accompanying symptoms.

Generalized tonic-clonic seizures can occur in neurologically normal individuals after moderate sleep deprivation. Such seizures can be seen in individuals working double shifts, in college students around examination time, and in soldiers returning from short leaves of absence. After the first seizure, if all investigations are normal, such individuals do not require further treatment.

If the patient's history, physical examination, and blood chemistries are all normal after a seizure, it is likely that the seizure was "idiopathic" and was not caused by a serious underlying CNS lesion. However, tumors or other mass lesions may be entirely asymptomatic, and every adult with an unexplained seizure should have an EEG

and an MRI or CT scan (both without and with contrast) and should be reexamined at regular intervals (3 to 6 months).

The EEG is important in relation to the differential diagnosis of the seizure, the determination of the cause of the seizure, and the proper classification of the seizure. When the diagnosis of a seizure is in doubt, as, for example, when trying to distinguish seizures from syncope, the presence of a paroxysmal EEG abnormality supports the diagnosis of epilepsy. For this purpose, special activation procedures (sleep recording, photic stimulation, or hyperventilation), special EEG leads (sphenoidal, nasopharyngeal, or nasoethmoidal) for recording from deep structures, or prolonged monitoring, even on an ambulatory basis, can be employed. The EEG can also reveal focal abnormalities (spikes, sharp waves, or focal slow waves) which would indicate the possibility of a focal neurologic lesion even if the seizure symptomatology appeared generalized from the outset.

The EEG is also used to help classify seizures. It can distinguish focal seizures with secondary generalization from primary generalized seizures and is especially useful in the differential diagnosis of brief lapses of consciousness. Absence seizures are always accompanied by bilateral spike and wave discharges, whereas complex partial seizures are accompanied by either focal paroxysmal spikes or slow waves or by a normal surface EEG. In cases of absence seizures, the EEG may reveal that the patient is having many more small seizures than was clinically apparent and may help in monitoring antiepileptic drug therapy.

In the past, lumbar puncture, skull x-rays, arteriography, and pneumoencephalography were important adjuncts to the evaluation of the seizure patient. Lumbar puncture is still employed in those situations where acute or chronic CNS infections or subarachnoid hemorrhage are suspected. MRI and CT scans can now provide more definitive information about anatomic lesions than the older, invasive techniques.

DIFFERENTIAL DIAGNOSIS OF SEIZURES

SYNCOPE VERSUS SEIZURE　Sudden loss of consciousness, usually without convulsive movements, presents a common diagnostic problem in both children and adults (see Chap. 21). Faints are often preceded by a feeling of light-headedness, of the room spinning, or of a flush, and are often, but not always, precipitated by an environmental stimulus such as prolonged standing in a hot, crowded area, the sight of blood, a fright, etc. In older people, pure syncope is most often secondary to cardiovascular problems, such as Stokes-Adams attacks, tachyarrhythmias, or orthostatic hypotension, and these may occur with or without a warning. A clear focal onset of the event (i.e., abnormal smell, head turning, staring, etc.) favors seizure as the cause. In addition, convulsive muscular contractions, tongue biting, or incontinence commonly accompany seizures but are much less common with fainting spells. Occasionally vasovagal or other types of fainting episodes can be accompanied by either clonic movements or brief generalized tonic-clonic seizures. If the original loss of consciousness can be ascribed to a clear nonepileptic cause (e.g., the patient was having blood drawn or a dental procedure at the time), it is not necessary to regard the episode as a manifestation of epilepsy, and antiepileptic drug therapy is not indicated.

When the origin of a syncopal episode is in doubt, the patient should undergo a complete cardiovascular evaluation, an EEG with sleep recording, and, if available, a prolonged ambulatory EEG monitoring. If the EEG shows paroxysmal activity (which is often brought out by drowsiness and sleep onset), and the patient has no signs of cardiac arrhythmia with ECG monitoring or of valvular disease on echocardiogram, it is likely that the syncopal episode represented a seizure and the patient should be evaluated and treated accordingly.

TRANSIENT ISCHEMIC ATTACKS AND MIGRAINE　Transient ischemic attacks (TIAs) and migraine episodes can present as a transient alteration in neurologic function (usually without loss of consciousness) which may be confused diagnostically with focal seizures. Neurologic dysfunction due to ischemia (TIA or migraine) is often a negative symptom (i.e., loss of feeling, numbness, visual field deficit, paralysis), whereas deficits due to focal seizure activity are often positive (twitching, paresthesias, visual distortion, or hallucination), although this distinction is not absolute. Brief stereotyped episodes which conform to dysfunction in a single vascular territory in an individual with either known vascular disease, heart disease, or with risk factors for vascular disease (diabetes, hypertension) are more likely TIAs. However, since cerebral infarcts are a common cause of subsequent seizures in older patients, a paroxysmal EEG focus should be sought.

Classic migraine headaches with a visual aura, unilateral headache, and gastrointestinal upset are usually easy to distinguish from seizures. However, some migraine patients have only "migraine equivalents" such as a hemiparesis, numbness, or aphasia and may not have subsequent headache. These episodes, especially when they occur in older individuals, are hard to distinguish from TIAs, but may also represent focal seizures. The presence of loss of consciousness after some forms of vertebrobasilar migraine and the common occurrence of headaches after seizures makes this differential diagnosis more difficult. The slower development of neurologic dysfunction in migraine (often occurring over minutes) is the most helpful point. Nevertheless, occasionally such patients need to be investigated for all three problems with an MRI or CT scan, carotid studies, and specialized EEG procedures before a diagnosis can be made. In some cases, a therapeutic trial with antiepileptic drugs (which, interestingly, can prevent migraines as well as seizures in some patients) will be necessary for the final diagnosis.

PSYCHOMOTOR VARIANTS AND "HYSTERICAL" SEIZURES As remarked above, patients with complex partial seizures often have bizarre behavioral manifestations of their seizures. These may consist of abrupt changes in personality, feelings of impending doom or of undirected fear, abnormal bodily sensations, episodic forgetfulness, or brief repetitive motor activities such as picking at one's clothes or stamping a foot. Many of these patients also have personality disorders and a significant proportion have had psychiatric intervention. It is common, especially if these patients do not have tonic-clonic seizures or loss of consciousness and when these patients appear emotionally disturbed, for these episodes of psychomotor seizures to be called "psychopathic fugues" or "hysterical seizures." This incorrect diagnosis is often reinforced by a "normal EEG" interictally, or even during one of these episodes. It must be emphasized that seizures can arise from foci deep in temporal lobe structures with *no* surface EEG manifestations. This has been repeatedly demonstrated with depth electrode recordings. Moreover, deep temporal seizures can be manifest only by the kinds of phenomena described above and may be free of the usual seizure phenomena of motor convulsions and loss of consciousness.

In a small number of cases, individuals present with seizure-like events which upon investigation turn out to be hysterical "pseudoseizures" or frank malingering. Often these individuals have had true seizures in the past or are acquainted with an individual with epilepsy. Such pseudoseizures can be quite difficult to distinguish from true seizures. Hysterical seizures are characterized by nonphysiologic events such as a progression of twitching from one hand to the other without spread to subjacent ipsilateral face or leg areas, twitching of all four extremities without loss of consciousness (or with surreptitious loss of consciousness), or careful attention to avoiding injury by moving away from a wall or bed edge while having motor convulsions. In addition, hysterical seizures, especially in adolescent girls, may have frankly sexual overtones, with pelvic thrusting or genital manipulation. While many forms of temporal lobe seizures can occur with normal surface EEGs, generalized tonic-clonic seizures always produce abnormal EEGs both during and after the seizure. Most generalized tonic-clonic seizures and many complex partial seizures

of moderate duration are accompanied by rises in serum prolactin (during the immediate 30-min postictal period), whereas "hysterical" seizures are not. Although not an absolute distinguishing point, such measurements, especially if positive, can be very helpful in characterizing the origin of a given "spell." After careful observation, especially with video-EEG monitoring, and after establishing a relationship with the patient, pseudoseizures can sometimes be elicited by suggestion. Frequently, when patients are appropriately confronted with this diagnosis, they respond well, and the pseudoseizures are eliminated or greatly reduced in frequency.

TREATMENT OF SEIZURES

Treatment of the patient with a seizure disorder is directed at eliminating the cause of the seizures, suppressing the expression of the seizures, and dealing with the psychosocial consequences which may occur as a result of the neurologic dysfunction underlying the seizure disorder or from the presence of a chronic disability.

If the seizure disorder is a result of a metabolic disturbance, such as hypoglycemia or hypocalcemia, restoration of normal metabolic function is usually accompanied by cessation of the seizures. If the seizures are caused by a structural brain lesion, such as a brain tumor, arteriovenous malformation, or cerebral cyst, removal of the offending lesion may eliminate the seizures. However, long-standing lesions, even nonprogressive ones, can result in gliosis and chronic denervation. These changes may lead to chronic epileptic foci which will not be eliminated by the subsequent removal of the original lesion. In such cases, surgical extirpation of the epileptic brain regions may be necessary for control of the epilepsy (see "Neurosurgical Approaches to Epilepsy," below).

There is complex interrelationship between the limbic system and neuroendocrine function which may have significant implications for patients with epilepsy. Normal hormonal fluctuations may influence the frequency of seizures, and epilepsy can cause changes in neuroendocrine function. For example, some women will have a marked change in the pattern of their seizures during particular parts of the menstrual cycle (catamenial epilepsy), while others may have changes in seizure frequency in response to oral contraceptives or pregnancy. In general, estrogens tend to exacerbate seizures, while progesterones tend to be more protective. On the other hand, some patients with epilepsy, especially complex partial seizures, may also have an associated reproductive endocrine dysfunction. Disorders in sexual interest, especially hyposexuality, are frequently observed. In addition, women may have polycystic ovary disease, and men may have disturbances in potency. Some patients with these endocrine disorders have not had clinical seizures but have significantly abnormal EEGs (often with temporal discharges). Whether the epilepsy causes the endocrine and/or behavioral dysfunction or whether the two conditions are separate manifestations of a common underlying neuropathologic process is not known. However, endocrine manipulation can sometimes be useful in controlling some forms of seizures, and antiepileptic medication may be a useful adjunct for treating some forms of endocrine dysfunction.

PHARMACOLOGIC CONTROL OF EPILEPSY The fundamental modality for the treatment of epilepsy is pharmacologic therapy. The goal is to protect the patient from having seizures without interfering with normal cognitive function (or, in the child, with development of normal intellectual function) and without producing harmful systemic side effects. If possible, the individual should be treated with the lowest possible dose of a single antiepileptic medication. Precise knowledge of the kind of seizure the patient is having, the spectrum of action of the available antiepileptic medications, and a few basic pharmacokinetic principles can result in the complete control of approximately 60 to 75 percent of patients with epilepsy. Many patients appear to be resistant to medications or develop unnecessary side effects because the medications chosen are not appropriate for the kind(s) of seizure or are not administered in the optimum doses.

The availability of serum levels of antiepileptic drugs makes it possible to optimize dosage regimens for individual patients and to monitor drug compliance. Thus, patients can be placed on a medication and after a suitable equilibration period (usually several weeks, but at least five "half-lives"), the amount of medication in the serum can be determined and compared to standard therapeutic ranges established for each drug. Utilizing blood levels to adjust doses can compensate for individual patient variability in absorption or metabolism of drugs.

Many antiepileptic drugs are bound by serum proteins, and it is the unbound, or "free," drug which is in equilibrium with extracellular spaces within the brain; this level correlates best with seizure control. However, "total" drug is measured in the serum by conventional assays. Under most circumstances, this is adequate for determining if the antiepileptic drug is in the therapeutic range. Occasionally, serum antiepileptic drug levels will be high, yet the patient continues to have seizures without any physiologic side effects of the drug. In these cases, it is possible that serum protein binding is higher than expected and that the patient is undermedicated in relation to the free drug available. Increase in dose may produce control without any untoward side effects (despite a blood level above the therapeutic range). Similarly, individuals with impaired liver or renal function may have low serum proteins or circulating "toxins," which reduces drug binding. In this case, toxicity may appear at unusually low serum levels because of a relatively higher free level of drug.

Intensive long-term EEG and video monitoring have demonstrated that careful characterization of seizures and selection of antiepileptic drugs can significantly increase seizure control in many patients whose seizures had previously been considered intractable to conventional antiepileptic drugs. In fact, often these patients can have one or more of their multiple drugs removed while still achieving better control.

INDICATIONS FOR USE OF SPECIFIC DRUGS Generalized tonic-clonic seizures (grand mal) There are four medications which are of proven value in this very common form of seizure—phenytoin (or diphenylhydantoin), carbamazepine, phenobarbital (and other long-acting barbiturates), and valproic acid (Table 350-3). Most patients will be controlled by adequate doses of any one of these, although individual patients may respond better to one or another. The choice among them often relates to minimizing undesirable side effects.

Phenytoin can often produce effective control with no sedation and very little, if any, intellectual impairment. However, phenytoin produces gum hyperplasia in some individuals, coarsening of facial features, and mild hirsutism, all of which can lead to long-term changes in appearance, which is especially unpleasant for young women. Phenytoin may produce lymphadenopathy and, in very high doses, may be toxic to the cerebellum.

Carbamazepine is equally effective and does not have many of the side effects seen with phenytoin. Cognitive function appears as well or even better preserved than with phenytoin. However, carbamazepine can cause gastrointestinal upset and may cause bone marrow depression with mild to moderate falls in peripheral white count (3.5 to 4 × 10^3 per microliter) which can occasionally become severe and which must be watched carefully. In addition, carbamazepine can produce hepatotoxicity. For these reasons, a complete blood count (CBC) and liver function tests should be performed before starting carbamazepine, and at 2-week intervals for a period after initiating therapy.

Phenobarbital is also effective against tonic-clonic seizures and has none of the side effects mentioned above. It commonly causes sedation and a dulling of intellect, however, especially early in its use, and this may lead to poor compliance. The sedation is dose-dependent and may limit the amount of drug which can be given to achieve complete control. However, if control can be achieved with nonsedative doses of phenobarbital, it may be the safest chronic

regimen. Primidone is a barbiturate which is metabolized to phenobarbital and phenylethylmalonamide (PEMA). In children, the barbiturates can produce a state of hyperactivity and hyperirritability which will limit their usefulness. Barbiturates may also exacerbate depression.

Valproic acid (sodium valproate) has also been shown to be effective for tonic-clonic seizures. It can cause gastrointestinal irritation, bone marrow suppression (especially thrombocytopenia), hyperammonemia, and hepatic dysfunction (including rare instances of fatal progressive hepatic failure which appear to be idiosyncratic rather than dose-related and are more common in children under 2 years of age). A CBC with platelet count and liver function tests should be performed before beginning therapy and at biweekly intervals after initiating therapy for a suitable period until the safety of the drug is established in the individual patient.

In addition to their systemic side effects, all four of these drugs have neurologic toxicities at higher doses. Nystagmus is common at therapeutic blood levels but ataxia, dizziness, tremor, intellectual dulling, forgetfulness, confusion, and even stupor may occur with increasing blood concentrations. These are reversible when blood levels fall back to therapeutic levels.

Partial seizures, including complex partial seizures (temporal lobe epilepsy) Three of the four groups of drugs which are useful for tonic-clonic seizures are also effective for partial seizures. Carbamazepine and phenytoin are the drugs of choice while the barbiturates may also be effective. In general, complex partial seizures are difficult to control, and patients with these seizures may require more than one medication (i.e., carbamazepine and a barbiturate, or phenytoin and a barbiturate, or any one of the primary drugs and high doses of methsuximide) and may become candidates for neurosurgical intervention. These are the kinds of seizures for which many epilepsy centers are conducting trials of new antiepileptic drugs.

Other primary generalized seizures [absence (petit mal), atypical absence, myoclonic] These seizures respond to different classes of medications than either tonic-clonic or focal seizures. For simple absence, ethosuximide and valproic acid are the drugs of choice. Side effects of ethosuximide include gastrointestinal upset, behavior changes, dizziness, and lethargy but are not often troublesome. For more difficult to control atypical absence seizures and for myoclonic seizures, valproic acid is the drug of choice. Clonazepam (a benzodiazepine) can also be used for atypical absence and myoclonic seizures. It can cause drowsiness and irritability, but usually does not cause other systemic side effects. Trimethadione was one of the first antiabsence drugs but is now rarely used because of its potential toxicity.

Approximately one-third of children who present with "pure" absence seizures also have tonic-clonic seizures at some later time. The question of whether these children should be treated prophylactically with an anti-tonic-clonic seizure medication has not been resolved. Since valproic acid has actions against both classes of seizures, its use has been increasing in children with absence. The concurrent use of phenobarbital with antiabsence drugs for this purpose should be avoided, as it may interfere with therapy for the absence.

Status epilepticus Generalized tonic-clonic status epilepticus is a life-threatening medical emergency, but overzealous and incautious treatment can produce more harm than good. Patients are in danger from hyperpyrexia and acidosis (from prolonged muscle activity) and less commonly, hypoxia or compromise of respiratory function. Immediate treatment for status is protection of the airway, protection of the tongue (with a soft object, large enough not to be swallowed, between the clenched teeth), protection of the head, and then establishment of a secure parenteral (intravenous) access. A bolus of 50% glucose in water (after blood is drawn for analysis), even if hypoglycemia is not expected, may stop the seizures. All further intravenous medication should be given after preparation for respiratory and circulatory support is available.

Phenytoin, 1000 to 1500 mg (18 to 20 mg/kg) in a slow intravenous

TABLE 350-3 Commonly used antiepileptic drugs

Generic name	Trade name	Principal uses	Dosage	Half-life	Therapeutic range	% Protein bound	Toxic effects Neurologic	Toxic effects Systemic	Drug interactions
Phenytoin (diphenylhydantoin)	Dilantin	Tonic-clonic (grand mal) Focal Complex partial	300–400 mg/d (3–5 mg/kg, adult) (4–7 mg/kg, child)	24 h (wide variation)	10–20 μg/mL	90	Ataxia Incoordination Confusion Cerebellar Skin rash	Gum hyperplasia Lymphadenopathy Hirsutism Osteomalacia Facial coarsening	Level increased by isoniazid, dicumarol, sulfonamides Level decreased by carbamazepine, phenobarbital Altered folate metabolism Folate interferes with effects
Carbamazepine	Tegretol	Tonic-clonic Focal Complex partial	600–1200 mg/d (20–30 mg/kg, child)	13–17 h	4–12 μg/mL	80	Ataxia Dizziness Diploplia Vertigo	Bone marrow suppression Gastrointestinal irritation Hepatotoxicity	Level decreased by phenobarbital, phenytoin
Phenobarbital	Luminol	Tonic-clonic Focal	60–120 mg/d (1–5 mg/kg, adult) (3–6 mg/kg, child)	90 h (shorter in children)	10–50 μg/mL	40–60	Sedation Ataxia Confusion Dizziness Decreased libido Depression	Skin rash	Level increased by valproic acid, phenytoin Enhances metabolism of other drugs via liver enzyme induction
Primidone	Mysoline	Tonic-clonic Focal	750–1000 mg/d (10–25 mg/kg)	Primidone, 8 h Phenylethylmalonomide, 24–48 h Phenobarbital, 90 h	Primidone, 2–10 μg/mL Phenobarbital, 10–50 μg/mL	Small for primidone or phenylethylmalonomide	Same as phenobarbital		
Sodium valproate (valproic acid)	Depakane Depakote	Absence Atypical absence Myoclonic Tonic-clonic	750–1250 mg/d (30–60 mg/kg)	15 h	50–100 μg/mL	80–94	Ataxia Sedation Tremor	Hepatotoxicity Bone marrow suppression Gastrointestinal irritation Weight gain Transient alopecia Hyperammonemia	May precipitate absence status if given with clonazepam Increases free phenytoin Decreases phenobarbital Increases active carbamazepine metabolites
Ethosuximide	Zarontin	Absence (petit mal)	750–1250 mg/d (20–40 mg/kg)	60 h, adult 30 h, child	40–100 μg/mL	Small	Ataxia Lethargy	Gastrointestinal irritation Skin rash Bone marrow suppression	
Methsuximide	Celontin	Absence (complex partial)	600–1200 mg/d	38–50 h	10–30 μg/mL (N-desmethyl methsuximide)	Small	Ataxia Lethargy	Same as ethosuximide	Increases phenytoin level Increases phenobarbital from primidone
Clonazepam	Clonopin	Absence Atypical absence Myoclonic	1–12 mg/d (0.1–0.2 mg/kg)	24–48 h	5–70 ng/mL	50	Ataxia Sedation Lethargy	Anorexia	May precipitate absence status if given with valproic acid
Trimethadione	Tridione	Absence Atypical absence (intractable seizures only)	900–2100 mg/d (20–60 mg/kg)	6–13 days (for dimethadione)	700 μg/mL (for dimethadione)	Small	Sedation Blurred vision	Skin rash Bone marrow suppression Nephrosis Hepatitis	

"push" (not in 5% dextrose in water—phenytoin precipitates in this low pH solution) no faster than 50 mg/min, is one of the drugs of choice. It does not depress respiration but may produce mild atrioventricular block and, if given too rapidly, can cause a serious fall in blood pressure. Blood pressure and EEG should be monitored.

The benzodiazepines, diazepam, 10 mg, or lorazepam, 4 mg (followed by another 4 mg if necessary), are also effective in stopping status epilepticus when administered intravenously. However, these drugs may depress respiratory function (or even cause respiratory arrest), and measures for respiratory support should be available before they are administered. The use of a benzodiazepine after phenobarbital administration carries a particular risk. The benzodiazepines are short-acting drugs in these circumstances, and after they are administered, a second, longer-acting antiepileptic such as phenytoin is usually required to prevent recurrence of seizures.

Phenobarbital, in a dose of 10 to 20 mg/kg (up to 1 g), divided into two to four doses at 30- to 60-minute intervals, can also be administered for status epilepticus. Phenobarbital also causes respiratory depression and should not be used immediately after treatment with intravenous diazepam.

If tonic-clonic seizures cannot be controlled within 30 to 60 min with the above sequence, the likelihood of serious neurologic sequelae or death becomes very high. Serious consideration needs to be given to anesthetizing the patient with barbiturates or inhalation anesthetics, with EEG monitoring to ensure that cessation of electrical seizure activity accompanies cessation of motor convulsions.

After stopping the seizures, it is imperative to determine the cause of the status epilepticus in order to prevent its recurrence. In most adults the cause can be determined and is usually tumor, vascular disease, infection, cerebral damage, or precipitous withdrawal from alcohol or antiepileptic medication. In children, the incidence of idiopathic status is higher (approximately 50 percent), and the remaining cases are divided between acute brain illnesses such as purulent meningitis, encephalitis and dehydration with electrolyte disturbances, and chronic encephalopathies. Tonic-clonic status epilepticus is a dangerous condition; the mortality may be over 10 percent with another 10 to 30 percent of patients being left with permanent neurologic sequelae.

NEUROSURGICAL TREATMENT OF EPILEPSY   If a structural lesion (i.e., tumor, cyst, abscess, etc.) is causing recurrent seizures, the removal of that lesion and nearby diseased brain will often eliminate the seizures or make them easier to control. Some patients, however, have uncontrollable seizures without a demonstrable structural lesion. These are often complex partial seizures with ictal and interictal EEG abnormalities emanating from one or both temporal lobes. Many surgical series have shown that if the epileptogenic lesion can be clearly localized to one temporal lobe, neurosurgical removal of that temporal lobe can result in significant improvement in 60 to 95 percent of the patients. Localization often depends on intensive EEG monitoring and may require intracranial recordings from the temporal or frontal lobes. In a high percentage of cases the removed temporal lobe can be shown to have microscopic pathology, such as hippocampal (or ''Ammon's horn'') sclerosis (loss of pyramidal cells in the hippocampus), a hamartoma, or cortical ectopia.

Some individuals with complex partial seizures also develop a psychiatric illness characterized most often as a borderline personality with certain specific behavioral manifestations including hypergraphia, hyperreligiosity, lack of sense of humor, and disordered sexuality. The psychiatric aspects of this illness may result from the epilepsy or may be independently produced by the same underlying brain lesion which produces the epilepsy. The personality disorder may not significantly change after epilepsy surgery, even if the seizures are controlled.

TREATMENT OF A SINGLE SEIZURE   Some individuals present with a single, brief, generalized tonic-clonic seizure and, after complete evaluation, are found to have a normal EEG and no underlying cause for the seizure. Some of these individuals (between 40 and 70 percent, depending on the series) go on to have recurrent seizures. The decision to treat such a patient with several years (at least) of antiepileptic medication must be made on an individual basis, considering the patient's lifestyle, risks from a sudden loss of consciousness, and feelings about medications.

CESSATION OF ANTIEPILEPTIC DRUG THERAPY   Many patients with epilepsy require antiepileptic drug therapy for life. However, a large proportion of epileptic patients become seizure-free on appropriate medication, and approximately half of such patients can eventually stop their medications and remain seizure-free. The patient who has had no seizures for 4 years, who had had relatively few seizures before control was attained, who only required a single medication, who has a normal neurologic exam and no structural lesion causing the seizures, and who has a normal EEG at the end of the therapeutic period has the best chance of remaining seizure-free if medication is slowly tapered (over 3 to 6 months). An abnormal EEG is not a contraindication to discontinuing medication. When considering the discontinuance of antiepileptic therapy, the consequences of the recurrence of seizures must be carefully considered. One inopportune seizure in a previously well-controlled patient who is not used to taking precautions may be a life-threatening event or lead to loss of a driver's license or loss of employment. Nevertheless, since all medications carry some risk of toxicity and since medication compliance in a healthy individual is often variable, it is worth a careful trial of medication tapering in individuals who meet the above criteria and are willing to accept the risk.

EPILEPSY AND PREGNANCY   Most women with epilepsy can undergo uneventful pregnancies and deliver healthy babies—even those taking antiepileptic medications. During the pregnant state, however, body metabolism changes, and close attention must be given to antiepileptic drug levels. Sometimes relatively high doses have to be given to ensure therapeutic levels. Most women who are well controlled before pregnancy will remain so during pregnancy and delivery. Women whose seizures are not under good control before becoming pregnant are at higher risk for having increased difficulties during the pregnancy.

One of the most serious complications of pregnancy, toxemia, often presents as a generalized tonic-clonic convulsion in the third trimester. This seizure is a symptom of a severe neurologic disturbance and is not a manifestation of epilepsy, nor is it more common in epileptic women. The toxemic state must be treated in order to control the seizures.

There is a two- to threefold higher incidence of significant fetal malformations in offspring of epileptic women, and this is likely due to a combination of a low incidence of medication-induced malformation and of genetic predisposition in this population. Among those malformations which do occur, a fetal-hydantoin (which is not unique to babies exposed to phenytoin) syndrome consisting of cleft lip and palate, heart defects, digital hypoplasia, and nail dysplasia has been identified.

Although it would be ideal for women contemplating pregnancy to have their antiepileptic drugs discontinued, it is likely that for a large number of women this would result in recurrence of seizures which would, in the long run, be more harmful for both mother and baby. If patients meet the criteria for discontinuance of medication, this should be done with a suitable interval before pregnancy is to occur. Other patients should be tapered to a minimal effective dosage and, if possible, maintained on only one medication. There are no clear data indicating differences in safety for phenobarbital, phenytoin, or carbamazepine when used alone. Less experience is available for valproate. Phenobarbital, primidone, or phenytoin can cause transient and reversible deficiency in vitamin K–dependent clotting factors in the neonate, and these should be promptly treated. Babies exposed to chronic barbiturates in utero are often transiently sluggish, hypotonic, jittery, and often show signs of barbiturate withdrawal. These babies should be considered at risk for neonatal problems and should be slowly withdrawn from barbiturates and closely observed in the nursery during the neonatal period.

DRIVING AND EPILEPSY   Each state has its own regulations for determining when an individual with epilepsy can obtain a driver's license, and several states have laws about the physician's obligations in either reporting epileptic patients to the registry or informing the patients of their responsibilities to do so. In general, patients can drive after a seizure-free interval (on or off medications) which ranges from 6 months to 2 years. In some states there is no fixed interval, but the individual is required to have a physician's letter attesting to seizure control. It is the physician's responsibility to warn the epileptic patient of the risks of driving when seizures are not under control.

SOCIAL AND EDUCATIONAL REHABILITATION Most people with epilepsy attain adequate control of their seizures and are able to attend school and obtain employment and live a relatively normal life. Children with epilepsy tend to have more problems in school than their peers, but every effort should be made to keep these children integrated into the mainstream of the educational process while supplying additional help in the form of academic tutoring or psychological counseling.

REFERENCES

AIRD R et al: *The Epilepsies: A Critical Review.* New York, Raven, 1984

CALLAGHAN N et al: Withdrawal of anticonvulsant drugs in patients free of seizures for two years. N Engl J Med 318:942, 1988

COMMISSION ON CLASSIFICATION AND TERMINOLOGY OF THE ILAE: Proposal for revised clinical classification of epileptic seizures. Epilepsia 22:489, 1981

DICHTER M, AYALA GF: Cellular mechanisms of epilepsy: A status report. Science 237:157, 1987

EMERSON R et al: Stopping medication in children with epilepsy. N Engl J Med 304:1125, 1981

ENGEL J JR: *Seizures and Epilepsy.* Philadelphia, Davis, 1989

——— (ed): *Surgical Treatment of the Epilepsies.* New York, Raven, 1987

LAIDLAW J, RICHENS A (eds): *A Textbook of Epilepsy,* 3d ed. London, Churchill Livingstone, 1988

LEVY R et al (eds): *Antiepileptic Drugs.* 3d ed. New York, Raven, 1989

MATTSON R et al: Comparison of carbamazepine, phenobarbital, phenytoin, and primidone in partial and secondarily generalized tonic-clonic seizures. N Engl J Med 313:145, 1985

351 CEREBROVASCULAR DISEASES

J. PHILIP KISTLER / ALLAN A. ROPPER / JOSEPH B. MARTIN

Cerebrovascular disease, the third leading cause of death after heart disease and cancer in developed countries, has an overall prevalence of 794 per 100,000. Five percent of the population over 65 are affected by a stroke, and, in the United States, it is estimated that more than 400,000 patients are discharged each year from hospitals after a stroke. The loss of these patients from the work force and the extended hospitalization they require during recovery make the economic impact of the disease one of the most devastating in medicine.

PATHOGENESIS AND PATHOLOGY OF STROKE Cerebrovascular disease is caused by one of several pathologic processes involving the blood vessels of the brain. The process may (1) be intrinsic to the vessel, as in atherosclerosis, lipohyalinosis, inflammation, amyloid deposition, arterial dissection, developmental malformation, aneurysmal dilation, or venous thrombosis; (2) originate remotely, as occurs when an embolus from the heart or extracranial circulation lodges in an intracranial vessel; (3) result from decreased perfusion pressure or increased blood viscosity with inadequate cerebral blood flow; or (4) result from rupture of a vessel in the subarachnoid space or intracerebral tissue.

A *stroke* is the acute neurologic injury occurring as a result of one of these pathologic processes. Other secondary symptoms may accompany stroke and vascular disease including pressure on cranial nerves from an aneurysm; vascular headache; or increased intracranial pressure with a venous thrombosis.

Normal brain function requires continuous supply of oxygenated blood. Cardiac arrest results in unconsciousness within 10 s; in animal experiments, total cessation of blood flow produces irreversible cerebral infarction within 3 min. Reduced blood flow may interfere with brain function, but the brain can remain viable for more prolonged periods. For example, patients who suffer cerebral embolism or cerebral vasospasm following subarachnoid hemorrhage often recover partially or completely, suggesting that focal areas of brain can remain functionless and ischemic for hours, even days, yet recover. This has led to the notion of an ischemic zone (penumbra or halo) that surrounds an infarct. There are also several secondary phenomena that may contribute to ongoing neuronal death. These include excitotoxins released by damaged neurons, cerebral edema, and alterations in local blood flow.

An infarcted brain is pale initially. Within hours to days, the gray matter becomes congested with engorged, dilated blood vessels and minute petechial hemorrhages. When an embolus blocking a major vessel migrates, lyses, or disperses within hours, recirculation into the ischemic area causes hemorrhagic infarction and may aggravate subsequent edema formation after the blood-brain barrier has been disrupted. A primary intracerebral hemorrhage, on the other hand, damages the brain by directly injuring tissue at the site of the hemorrhage and by compressing the surrounding tissue.

After an ischemic stroke, intracerebral hemorrhage, or transient episode of cerebral ischemia has occurred, the prelude to therapy is a precise diagnosis. The evaluation of a stroke must include clear definitions of the character and location of the lesion, the vascular pathologic process producing the symptoms, and the anatomy of spared collateral circulation to the ischemic area. The brain repairs itself only by forming fibrogliotic scar tissue at the site of an infarction or hemorrhage; therefore, therapeutic efforts after a stroke can only hope to minimize secondary loss. Such efforts should attempt to protect both the normal and ischemic brain from either initial or recurrent pathologic processes, as well as from the secondary effects of the stroke itself, e.g., brain compression from intracranial hemorrhage or edema. Such preventive therapy has three broad goals: (1) to reduce risk factors, thus attenuating the pathologic process; (2) to prevent recurrent stroke by removing the underlying pathologic process; and (3) to minimize secondary brain damage by maintaining adequate perfusion to marginally ischemic areas, and by reducing edema formation. Except for the elimination of risk factors, all aspects of therapy remain controversial. Because proof of efficacy is lacking for many therapies, current therapy is largely empirical and based on the physician's knowledge of the risks associated with various diagnostic procedures and therapeutic initiatives.

Strokes can be classified according to their pathophysiologic mechanism. The most important factor is an accurate assessment of the initial clinical presentation and temporal profile, which are determined by the pathologic process and the size and location of the diseased vessel and by the availability of collateral circulation (Figs. 351-1A–C and 351-2). The most important source of collateral flow for the internal carotid and vertebrobasilar arteries is the circle of Willis. When arteries distal to the circle of Willis, the middle, anterior, or posterior cerebral arteries are involved, collateral flow is limited to anastomoses over the cortical surface of the brain, the brainstem, or cerebellum. In these circumstances, or when the circle of Willis collateral is inadequate (Fig. 351-2, I–IV), factors that affect blood viscosity and clotting become increasingly important determinants of the extent of the stroke.

TIA syndrome The term *transient ischemic attack (TIA)* has usually been applied to any sudden focal neurologic deficit that clears completely in less than 24 h. This definition is probably too broad, because it includes other disease entities that are not necessarily caused by ischemia per se, e.g., a focal epileptic manifestation or a migraine attack with neurologic symptoms. Furthermore, ischemic symptoms that persist longer than an hour are usually accompanied by tissue injury, even though clinical recovery frequently occurs. Therefore, it is advisable to consider focal but totally reversible episodes lasting minutes to an hour as TIAs.

The specific symptoms of a TIA point to the particular arterial territory involved (carotid, middle cerebral, vertebrobasilar, or small penetrating artery). The duration, stereotypic nature, and frequency of repetitive spells suggest the underlying pathophysiologic mechanism. For example, repetitive (up to 5 to 10 per day), short-lived (15 min or less), stereotypic spells of hand and arm weakness suggest

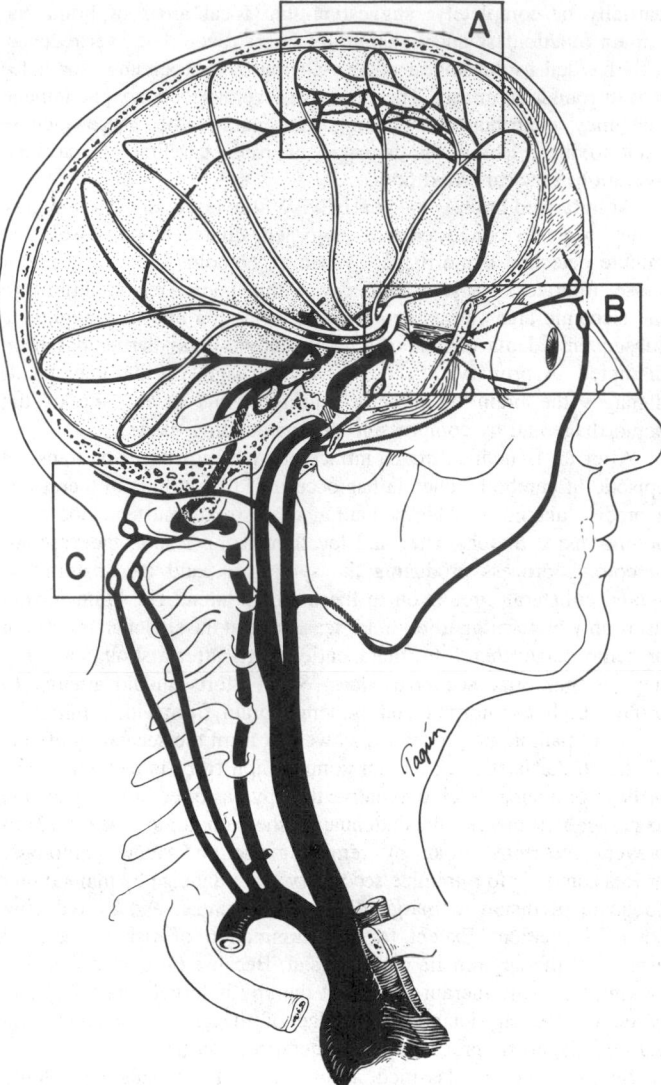

FIGURE 351-1   Arrangement of the major arteries of the right side carrying blood from the heart to the brain. Also shown are vessels of collateral circulation that may modify the effects of cerebral ischemia *(A,B,C)*. Not shown is the circle of Willis which also provides a source for collateral circulation. *A.* The anastomotic channels between the distal branches of the anterior and middle cerebral artery, termed borderzone or watershed anastomotic channels. Note that they also occur between the posterior and middle cerebral arteries and the anterior and posterior cerebral arteries. *B.* Anastomotic channels occurring through the orbit between branches of the external carotid artery and ophthalmic branch of the internal carotid artery. *C.* Wholly extracranial anastomotic channels between the muscular branches of the ascending cervical arteries and muscular branches of the occipital artery that anastomose with the distal vertebral artery. Note that the occipital artery arises from the external carotid artery, thereby allowing reconstitution of flow in the vertebral from the carotid circulation. *(Courtesy of C.M. Fisher, M.D.)*

that proximal arterial narrowing or occlusion have produced transient focal ischemia ("low flow") in the contralateral motor cortex. In contrast, a single episode of speech difficulty with or without hand, arm, or face weakness lasting 12 h suggests an embolic TIA in the contralateral frontal lobe. A transient short-lived episode (12 to 24 h) of pure motor hemiparesis—face, arm, leg, and foot—occurring *without* dysphasia or hemineglect suggests transient ischemia in the internal capsule or in the corticospinal tract of the ventral pons, territories supplied by penetrating arteries arising from larger parent vessels (a "lacunar TIA"). TIA in the vertebrobasilar system often presents with short-lived, repetitive episodes of dizziness, diplopia, and dysarthria. The repetitive, short-lived nature of these spells suggests transiently reduced blood flow rather than embolism.

The mechanism of embolic TIA is obvious, and only the source needs to be considered in deciding therapy. The mechanism of focal "low-flow" TIAs or lacunar TIAs, however, remains less certain. A critically stenotic or occluded artery can probably reduce flow to a focal region of brain. Poor collateral circulation contributes to the ischemia, but factors such as blood viscosity, vessel wall compliance, and other unknown factors may explain the transient reduction. Although TIAs resolve completely, they warn that a stroke may follow. Therefore, it becomes important to consider the pathophysiologic mechanisms of stroke and TIA together.

The terms *stroke in evolution* (also called *progressive stroke*) and *completed stroke* need special mention. Stroke in evolution refers to a neurologic deficit that progresses or fluctuates while the patient is under observation, whereas completed stroke implies that no further deterioration will occur. Several mechanisms have been proposed to explain stroke in evolution, among them progressive narrowing of an artery by thrombus, development of cerebral edema, thrombus propagation obliterating collateral branches to the ischemic brain, and systemic factors, e.g., arterial hypotension. Although these may have a role in some cases, it is more likely that fluctuating neurologic deficits are the result of emboli propagating, migrating, lysing, and dispersing, or are caused by recurrent artery-to-artery embolization, fluctuating collateral flow through the circle of Willis, through border zone anastomotic channels, or through orbital or cervicovertebral collaterals (Figs. 351-1*A–C* and 351-2). Fortunately, refinement in clinical diagnosis and new diagnostic techniques usually allow prediction of the type and location of strokes and their underlying vascular lesions, making a more focused approach to therapy both possible and mandatory.

Risk factors in stroke   Cerebral vascular disease is associated with several risk factors. An atherothrombotic stroke often indicates that the patient has cardiovascular or peripheral vascular disease. Atrial fibrillation, valvular heart disease, myocardial infarction, and bacterial endocarditis are sources of emboli, and their presence suggests embolism as the diagnosis. Severe hypertension is linked to small-vessel lipohyalinotic disease, lacunar strokes, and the formation of atherothrombotic lesions at the carotid bifurcation, in the middle cerebral artery stem, and in the vertebrobasilar system. Hypertension also predisposes to deep intracerebral hemorrhages. The advent of antihypertensive therapy is the principal factor accounting for the declining incidence of stroke. Smoking and familial hyperlipidemia, although less important than hypertension, are also associated with an increased risk of atherothrombotic disease and stroke. Racial differences predispose to specific types of stroke and may affect stroke incidence independently of other factors. Ischemic strokes occur more often in the early morning hours, whereas hemorrhages tend to occur during waking hours.

ISCHEMIC CEREBROVASCULAR DISEASE: GENERAL REMARKS

Ischemic cerebrovascular disease results from arterial narrowing or thrombosis or from arterial occlusion by embolism. Cerebral arterial thrombosis secondary to atherosclerosis and cerebral embolism cause similar symptoms and signs, but with different temporal profiles. Differences in symptomatology are discussed in the section on cerebral embolism.

Of the many causes of ischemic stroke listed in Table 351-1 and discussed elsewhere, thrombosis complicating atherosclerosis of intra- and extracranial vessels ultimately accounts for most cases. Atherosclerosis affects each artery at specific locations. In general, atheromatous plaques tend to form at branchings and curves of large vessels, and thrombosis is likely to occur at the site of maximal luminal narrowing.

The details of the process that superimposes thrombosis on artherosclerosis are discussed in Chap. 195. The damage that atherosclerotic thrombosis causes to the brain is determined by the

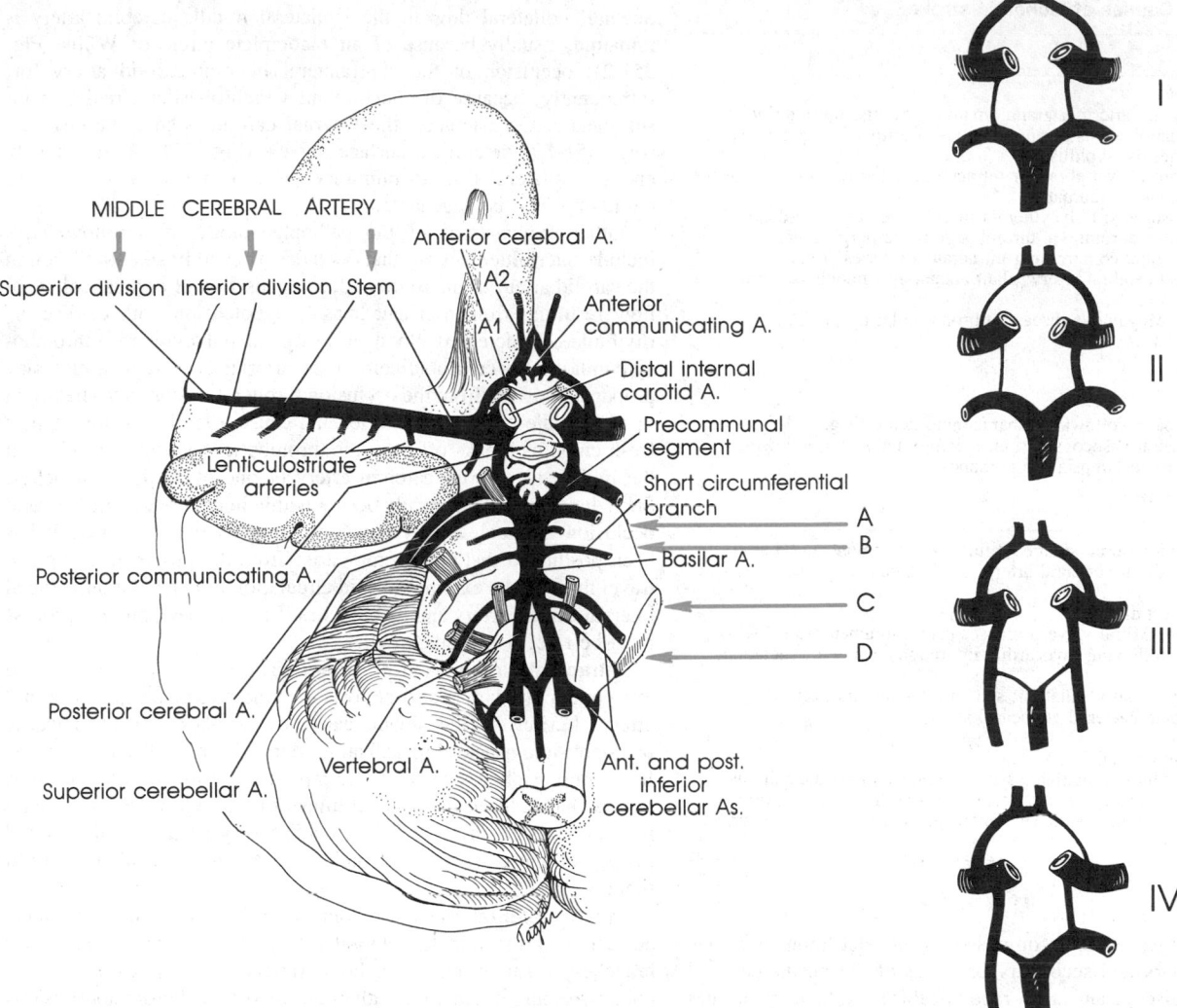

FIGURE 351-2 Diagram of the brainstem, cerebellum, inferior right frontal lobe, and temporal lobe transected. Principal branches of the vertebral basilar arterial system are pictured. Small branches of the vertebral and basilar artery that penetrate the medulla and pons are not pictured. The stem of the middle cerebral artery with its small, deep penetrating lenticulostriate arteries and the circle of Willis with its small, deep penetrating branches are shown. Roman numerals I, II, III, and IV represent some of the possible variations of the Circle of Willis due to atresia of one or more of its arterial components. *A, B, C,* and *D* arrows point to the four cross-sections of the brainstem diagrammed below (*D* = Fig. 351-7, *A* = Fig. 351-8, *B* = Fig. 351-9, *C* = Fig. 351-10). Although typical vascular syndromes of the pons and medulla have been designated by the shaded areas in Figs. 351-7 to 10, the shading is arbitrary. Great variability in infarct size and location occurs when the basilar or vertebral arteries, or one of their penetrating branches, becomes occluded. This variability is because of variation in arterial anatomic location and available collateral circulation. Thus the stroke syndromes produced are often atypical, incomplete, or merge with one another. *(Courtesy of C.M. Fisher, M.D.)*

available collateral flow, the speed of thrombotic occlusion, and by embolism distal to the thrombosis ("artery-to-artery" embolus). The clinical symptoms and signs resulting from occlusion of a particular artery differ from one patient to another, and many syndromes are partial representations of an idealized complete stroke in an arterial distribution. The following descriptions apply to infarction and ischemia in specific arteries due to thrombosis, recognizing that similar clinical pictures may occur after embolism. Occasionally, hemorrhage within these vascular territories also causes similar symptoms and signs.

ATHEROTHROMBOTIC DISEASE OF THE INTERNAL CAROTID ARTERY AND ITS BRANCHES

The origin of the carotid artery is the most common site of artherosclerosis and superimposed atherothrombosis that lead to TIA or stroke. Less often, disease at the siphon (S-shaped portion of the internal carotid artery in the cavernous sinus) or in the proximal segment (stem) of the middle or anterior cerebral arteries may be responsible for the symptom (rarely, the origin of the common carotid artery may be the site). The natural history of asymptomatic atherosclerotic stenosis or of ulcerated lesions at these locations is unknown. Presumably, in most instances the disease is progressive.

Internal carotid artery Atherosclerosis in the proximal internal carotid artery is usually most severe in the first 2 cm and arises from the posterior wall, often extending downward into the common carotid artery. Disease in this area is usually heralded by a minor stoke or TIA caused by embolism from the carotid artery to its intracranial branches or to a "low-flow" hemodynamic crisis. Emboli rather than low flow, however, probably cause most strokes or TIAs from carotid disease.

When *emboli* arise from a stenotic or ulcerated atherosclerotic lesion at the origin of the internal carotid artery, symptoms may result from occlusion of the ophthalmic artery, the middle cerebral artery stem or one or more of its branches, or, less often, the anterior cerebral artery. Small platelet emboli may occlude either only the ophthalmic artery or the very distal vessels of the middle cerebral artery, causing transient monocular blindness (*amaurosis fugax*) or small asymptomatic infarctions in the cerebral arterial watershed,

TABLE 351-1 Causes of ischemic stroke

THROMBOSIS

A Atherosclerosis
B* Arteritis: Temporal arteritis, granulomatous arteritis, polyarteritis, Wegener's granulomatosis, granulomatous arteritis of the great vessels (Takayasu's arteritis, syphilis)
C* Dissections: Carotid, vertebral, or intracranial arteries at the base of the brain (spontaneous or traumatic)
D* Hematologic disorders: Polycythemia first-degree or second-degree, sickle cell disease, thrombotic thrombocytopenic purpura, etc.
E* Cerebral mass effect compressing intracranial arteries: Tentorial herniation—post-cerebral artery; giant aneurysm—middle cerebral artery compression
F Miscellaneous: Moyamoya disease, fibromuscular dysplasia, Binswanger's disease

VASOCONSTRICTION

A* Cerebral vasospasm following subarachnoid hemorrhage
B* Reversible cerebral vasoconstriction: Etiology unknown, following migraine, trauma, eclampsia of pregnancy

EMBOLISM

A Atherothrombotic arterial source: Bifurcation common carotid artery, carotid siphon, distal vertebral artery, aortic arch
B* Cardiac source
  1 Structural heart disease
    a Congenital: Mitral valve prolapse, patent foramen ovale, etc.
    b Acquired: following myocardial infarction, marantic vegetation, etc.
  2 Dysrhythmia, atrial fibrillation, sick sinus syndrome, etc.
  3 Infection: acute bacterial endocarditis
C* Unknown source
  1 Healthy child or adult
  2 Associations: hypercoagulable state secondary to systemic disease, carcinoma (especially pancreatic), eclampsia of pregnancy, oral contraceptives, lupus, anticoagulants, factor C deficiency, factor S deficiency, etc.

* May occur in patients under 30.

respectively. Larger emboli composed of platelet-fibrin clot may occlude the primary and secondary branches of the middle cerebral artery leading to discrete and easily recognizable neurologic syndromes that suggest the area involved. Some emboli are large enough to occlude the proximal "stem" of the middle cerebral artery, leading to devastating ischemia of the entire middle cerebral territory (deep white matter, lenticular nuclei, and cortical surface). Other emboli large enough to occlude the middle cerebral stem may cause only deep infarction because collateral flow through the cortical surface is sufficient (Fig. 351-1A). Large emboli may not entirely occlude a major vessel or may migrate or lyse and disperse, causing a neurologic deficit that fluctuates (stroke in evolution) or resolves.

In a few symptomatic patients, an ulcerated plaque may be the only lesion in the carotid bifurcation, but far more often there is a stenotic lesion with a residual lumen diameter of less than 2 mm. The incidence of large embolic strokes resulting from an ulcerated lesion alone is undetermined, but it is probably low and mostly associated with large ulcers (4 mm or greater). *A nonstenotic or slightly stenotic carotid lesion in conjunction with a stroke or a single prolonged TIA suggests the heart as the source of the embolus.* Atheromatous lesions at the origin of the great vessels in the aortic arch can also produce cerebral emboli that cause transient ischemia or infarction, but the incidence of this mechanism, thought to be low, is also undetermined.

Internal carotid artery occlusion or severe stenosis (≤ 1 mm) may be entirely asymptomatic if collateral circulation through the circle of Willis is adequate. Inadequate collateral circulation may lead to a stroke or TIA. When *low arterial flow* results in cerebral infarction or transient ischemia, it does so in the border zone or "watershed" areas, approximately between the cortical surface branches of the middle cerebral and the anterior or posterior cerebral arteries (Fig. 351-1A). Two anatomic conditions contribute to this complication. First, the residual lumen diameter of carotid artery stenosis is typically less than 1.5 mm (80 to 90 percent occluded). Second, collateral flow to the ipsilateral middle cerebral artery is impaired, usually because of an incomplete circle of Willis (Fig. 351-2), occlusion of the contralateral internal carotid artery, or, infrequently, because of concomitant vertebrobasilar circulation insufficiency. Occasionally, the external carotid ophthalmic channels (Fig. 351-1B) or cortical surface vessels (Fig. 351-1A) can supply enough collateral flow to minimize the ischemic area, even if the circle of Willis is inadequate.

Other explanations of the pathophysiology of low-flow TIAs include intermittent spasm that occludes a severely stenotic lesion in the carotid artery or intermittent decompensation of cortical collateral flow resulting from transient spasm, hypotension with cardiac arrhythmia, or increased blood viscosity (in polycythemia, thrombocythemia, or macroglobulinemia). In arterial occlusion, a clot may propagate upward from the occlusion through the siphon to the origin of the middle or anterior arteries and cause a stroke. More often, a fresh embolus breaks off from the thrombotic material and lodges in the middle or anterior cerebral artery or one of its distal branches. Such distal embolism usually occurs within hours or days after carotid occlusion although it may develop 6 months or more later. It has been postulated that emboli may arise from the proximal stump and travel through the external carotid circulation to reach the intracranial internal carotid artery and its branches (Fig. 351-1B), but this process must be rare, if it occurs at all.

Intracranial internal carotid artery The carotid siphon is involved less commonly with atherosclerosis than the proximal internal carotid artery. Lesions in the siphon can cause strokes and TIAs whose pathophysiologic and clinical features duplicate those discussed above. In general, siphon stenosis is asymptomatic until the atheromatous process has reduced the residual lumen to 1.5 mm or less. Collateral flow around the circle of Willis undoubtedly influences the natural history of these lesions and their response to medical or surgical therapy.

Middle cerebral artery In contrast to the internal carotid artery, occlusion of the middle cerebral artery stem or one of its major branches is usually due to embolus (artery-to-artery, cardiac, or of unknown source) rather than atherothrombosis. Atheromatous lesions in the middle cerebral stem may cause ischemic symptoms either by narrowing the artery or by occluding the origin of one or more of the lenticulostriate arteries supplying the deep white matter and basal ganglia. Symptomatic atheroma rarely occurs distal to the first bifurcation of the middle cerebral artery. Because the circle of Willis is proximal to the origin of the middle cerebral artery, collateral blood flow to the middle cerebral artery territory must arise from small cortical-surface border zones and anastomotic vessels of the anterior and posterior cerebral arteries. Clinical evidence indicates that TIAs in the middle cerebral artery territory usually warn of vessel narrowing prior to thrombotic occlusion.

Anterior cerebral artery Atheromatous deposits in the proximal segment of the anterior cerebral artery rarely cause symptoms because the occlusion is circumvented by collateral circulation through the anterior communicating artery. However, if the anterior communicating artery is congenitally atretic or if the atheromatous lesion occurs distal in the anterior cerebral artery, TIAs and stroke may occur.

CLINICAL SYNDROMES Middle cerebral artery The cortical branches of the middle cerebral artery supply the lateral surface of the hemisphere except for (1) the frontal pole and a strip along the superomedial border of the frontal lobe supplied by the anterior cerebral artery, and (2) the lower temporal and occipital pole convolutions, which are in the territory of the posterior cerebral artery (Fig. 351-3).

The proximal middle cerebral artery gives rise to penetrating branches that supply the putamen, outer globus pallidus, posterior limb of the internal capsule above the plane of the upper border of the globus pallidus, the adjacent corona radiata, and the body, upper, and lateral head of the caudate nucleus. In the sylvian cistern, the

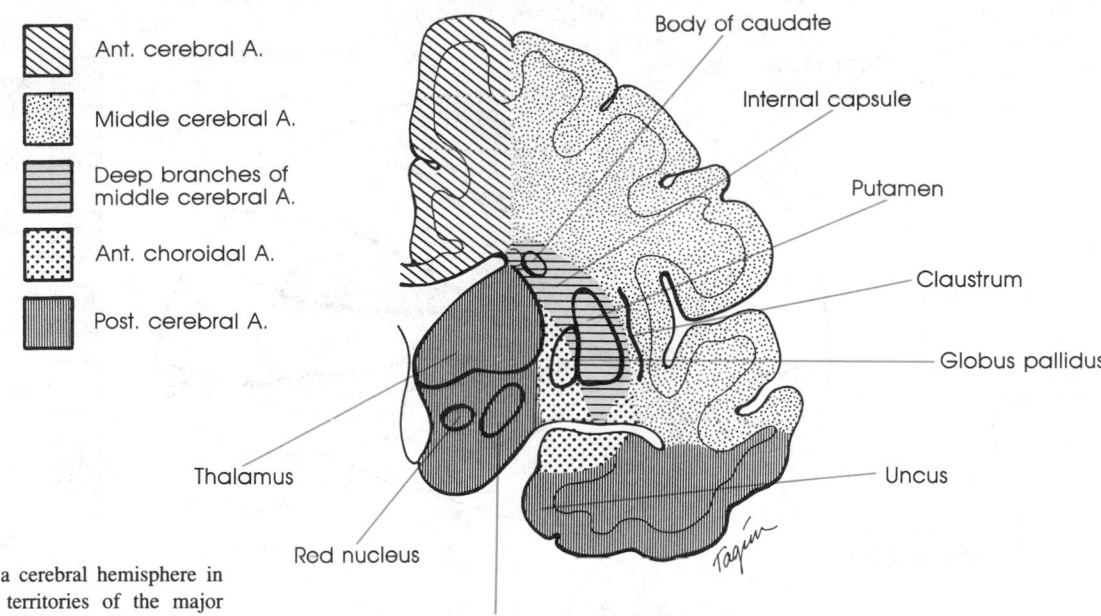

FIGURE 351-3 Diagram of a cerebral hemisphere in coronal section, showing the territories of the major cerebral vessels. *(Courtesy of C. M. Fisher, M.D.)*

middle cerebral artery stem in most patients divides into *superior* and *inferior divisions*. Branches of the inferior division supply the inferior parietal and temporal cortex, and those from the superior division supply the frontal and superior parietal cortex (Fig. 351-4). There is considerable variability in the parietal lobe supply between the two divisions, with about two-thirds of individuals having an inferior division that supplies regions above the angular gyrus.

If the entire middle cerebral artery is occluded at its stem, blocking both the penetrating and cortical branches, the clinical findings are contralateral hemiplegia and hemianesthesia. If the dominant hemisphere is involved, global aphasia is also present. If the nondominant hemisphere is affected, apractagnosia and anosognosia are found (Fig. 351-4). Dysarthria may also occur.

Complete middle cerebral territory syndromes occur most often when an embolus occludes the stem of the artery. Cortical collateral blood flow and differing arterial configurations are probably responsible for the development of partial middle cerebral artery syndromes. Partial middle cerebral territory syndromes may also be due to an embolus that enters the middle cerebral artery stem without complete occlusion or that lyses and moves distally. Symptoms and signs may fluctuate in such patients (stroke in evolution).

Partial syndromes resulting from embolic occlusion of a single branch include hand, or arm and hand, weakness alone (brachial syndrome), or facial weakness with motor aphasia, with or without arm weakness (frontal opercular syndrome). A combination of sensory disturbance, motor weakness, and motor aphasia suggests that an embolus has occluded the proximal superior division branch and infarcted large portions of the frontal and parietal cortices (Fig. 351-4). If Wernicke's aphasia occurs without weakness, the inferior division of the middle cerebral artery supplying the posterior part (temporal cortex) of the dominant hemisphere is probably involved (Fig. 351-4). Jargon speech and an inability to comprehend written and oral language are prominent features, often accompanied by a contralateral superior quadrantanopsia. Hemineglect or spatial agnosia without weakness indicates that the inferior division of the middle cerebral artery in the nondominant hemisphere is involved.

Anterior cerebral artery The anterior cerebral artery is divided into two segments: the precommunal (A1) circle of Willis, or stem, which connects the internal carotid artery to the anterior communicating artery, and the postcommunal (A2) segment distal to the anterior communicating artery (Fig. 351-2). The A1 segment of the anterior cerebral artery gives rise to several deep penetrating branches that supply the anterior limb of the internal capsule, the anterior

perforate substance, amygdala, anterior hypothalamus, and the inferior part of the head of the caudate nucleus (Fig. 351-3).

Infarction in the territory of the anterior cerebral artery is uncommon and most often due to embolism rather than artherothrombosis. Occlusion of the A1 segment of the anterior cerebral artery is usually well tolerated, because of collateral flow. If both A2 segments arise from a single anterior cerebral stem (contralateral A1 segment atresia), then the occlusion affects both hemispheres. Profound abulia (a delay in verbal and motor response) and bilateral pyramidal signs with paraplegia result. Occlusion of a single A2 segment of the anterior cerebral artery results in the contralateral symptoms noted in the legend of Fig. 351-5.

Anterior choroidal artery This artery arises from the internal carotid artery and supplies the posterior limb of the internal capsule and the white matter posterolateral to it, through which pass some of the geniculocalcarine fibers (Figs. 351-3 and 351-6). The complete clinical syndrome of anterior choroidal artery occlusion consists of contralateral hemiplegia, hemianesthesia (hypesthesia), and homonymous hemianopsia. However, because this territory is also supplied by penetrating vessels of the middle cerebral stem, the posterior communicating, and posterior choroidal arteries, syndromes with minimal deficits may occur and patients frequently recover partially or completely.

Internal carotid artery The clinical picture of internal carotid occlusion varies depending upon whether the cause of ischemia is propagated thrombus, embolism, or low flow. The cortex supplied by the middle cerebral territory is most often affected. With a competent circle of Willis, however, occlusion can be entirely asymptomatic. Less often, there is massive infarction of the deep white matter and cortical surface from propagation of a thrombus up the internal carotid artery, into the middle cerebral stem, or from embolization to the stem of the middle cerebral artery. Symptoms are identical to middle cerebral stem occlusion (see above). When the origins of both the anterior and middle cerebral arteries are occluded by embolus to the top of the carotid artery, abulia and/or stupor occurs with hemiplegia, hemianesthesia, and aphasia or anosognosia. When the posterior cerebral artery arises from the internal carotid artery (an unusual configuration called a fetal posterior cerebral artery), it also may become occluded and give rise to symptoms referable to its peripheral territory (Figs. 351-5 and 351-6).

Carotid occlusion may cause low-flow infarction if the circle of Willis is incomplete. The territory of the distal cortical branches of

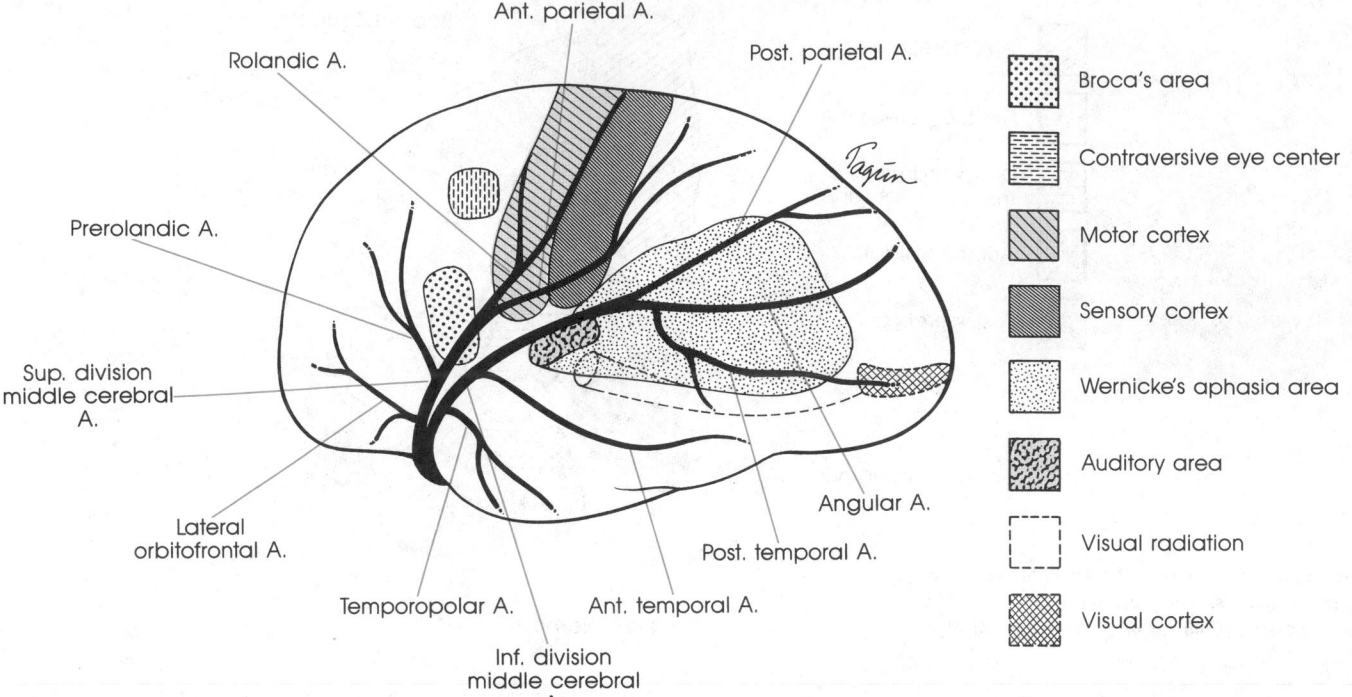

FIGURE 351-4 Diagram of a cerebral hemisphere, lateral aspect, showing the branches and distribution of the middle cerebral artery and the principal regions of cerebral localization. Note the bifurcation of the middle cerebral artery into a superior and inferior division (*Courtesy of C. M. Fisher, M.D.*)

Signs and symptoms	Structures involved
Paralysis of the contralateral face, arm, and leg; sensory impairment over the same area (pinprick, cotton touch, vibration, position, two-point discrimination, stereognosis, tactile localization, barognosis, cutaneographia)	Somatic motor area for face and arm and the fibers descending from the leg area to enter the corona radiata and corresponding somatic sensory system
Motor aphasia	Motor speech area of the dominant hemisphere
Central aphasia, word deafness, anomia, jargon speech, sensory agraphia, acalculia, alexia, finger agnosia, right-left confusion (the last four comprise the Gerstmann syndrome)	Central, suprasylvian speech area and parietooccipital cortex of the dominant hemisphere
Conduction aphasia	Central speech area (parietal operculum)
Apractognosia of the minor hemisphere (amorphosynthesis), anosognosia, hemiasomatognosia, unilateral neglect, agnosia for the left half of external space, dressing "apraxia," constructional "apraxia," distortion of visual coordinates, inaccurate localization in the half field, impaired ability to judge distance, upside-down reading, visual illusions (e.g., it may appear that another person walks through a table)	Nondominant parietal lobe (area corresponding to speech area in dominant hemisphere); loss of topographic memory is usually due to a nondominant lesion, occasionally to a dominant one
Homonymous hemianopsia (often homonymous inferior quadrantonopsia)	Optic radiation deep to second temporal convolution
Paralysis of conjugate gaze to the opposite side	Frontal contraversive field or fibers projecting therefrom

the middle cerebral artery tends to be involved, giving rise to transient or stepwise, progressive hip, shoulder, or arm weakness. Other TIAs suggestive of carotid insufficiency include recurrent unilateral tongue, lip, cheek, or hand numbness, with or without motor weakness.

In addition to supplying the ipsilateral brain, the internal carotid artery perfuses the optic nerve and retina via the ophthalmic artery (Fig. 351-1). In about 25 percent of symptomatic internal carotid disease, transient recurrent monocular blindness (TMB or amaurosis fugax) warns of the lesion. Patients may describe a shade that seems to sweep up, down, or across the field of vision or may say that the periphery of vision fades away. They may also complain that their vision was blurred in that eye or that the upper or lower half of vision disappeared. In most cases, these symptoms last only a few minutes. Rarely, ophthalmic or central retinal artery occlusion develops at the time of stroke.

Common carotid artery All the neurologic symptoms and signs of internal carotid occlusion may also be present with occlusion of the common carotid artery. Bilateral common carotid arterial occlusion at their origin may occur in "pulseless disease," or the aortic arch syndrome (see Chap. 197). Clues to this condition are absence of

pulsation in carotid and radial arteries, faintness on arising from the horizontal position, recurrent loss of consciousness, headache, neck pain, transient blindness (unilateral or bilateral), dim vision with exercise, premature cataracts, retinal atrophy and pigmentation, atrophy of the iris, leukomas, peripapillary arteriovenous anastomoses, optic atrophy, and/or claudication of the jaw muscles. An incomplete aortic arch syndrome has been reported consisting of various combinations of carotid, subclavian, or innominate stenosis or occlusion (see below).

LABORATORY INVESTIGATION Several diagnostic techniques are available for evaluating patients with a carotid bruit, carotid-territory stroke, or TIA.

Noninvasive carotid tests Noninvasive carotid tests reliably determine the severity and location of carotid atherothrombotic disease in over 90 percent of patients. Indirect assessment of pressure in the internal carotid artery is made by ophthalmodynamometry, oculoplethysmography, and directional supraorbital Doppler examination. Ultrasound techniques define directly the bifurcation of the common carotid artery by real-time B-mode imaging and analysis of the Doppler-shift signal of the returning echo of flowing blood. Ultrasound

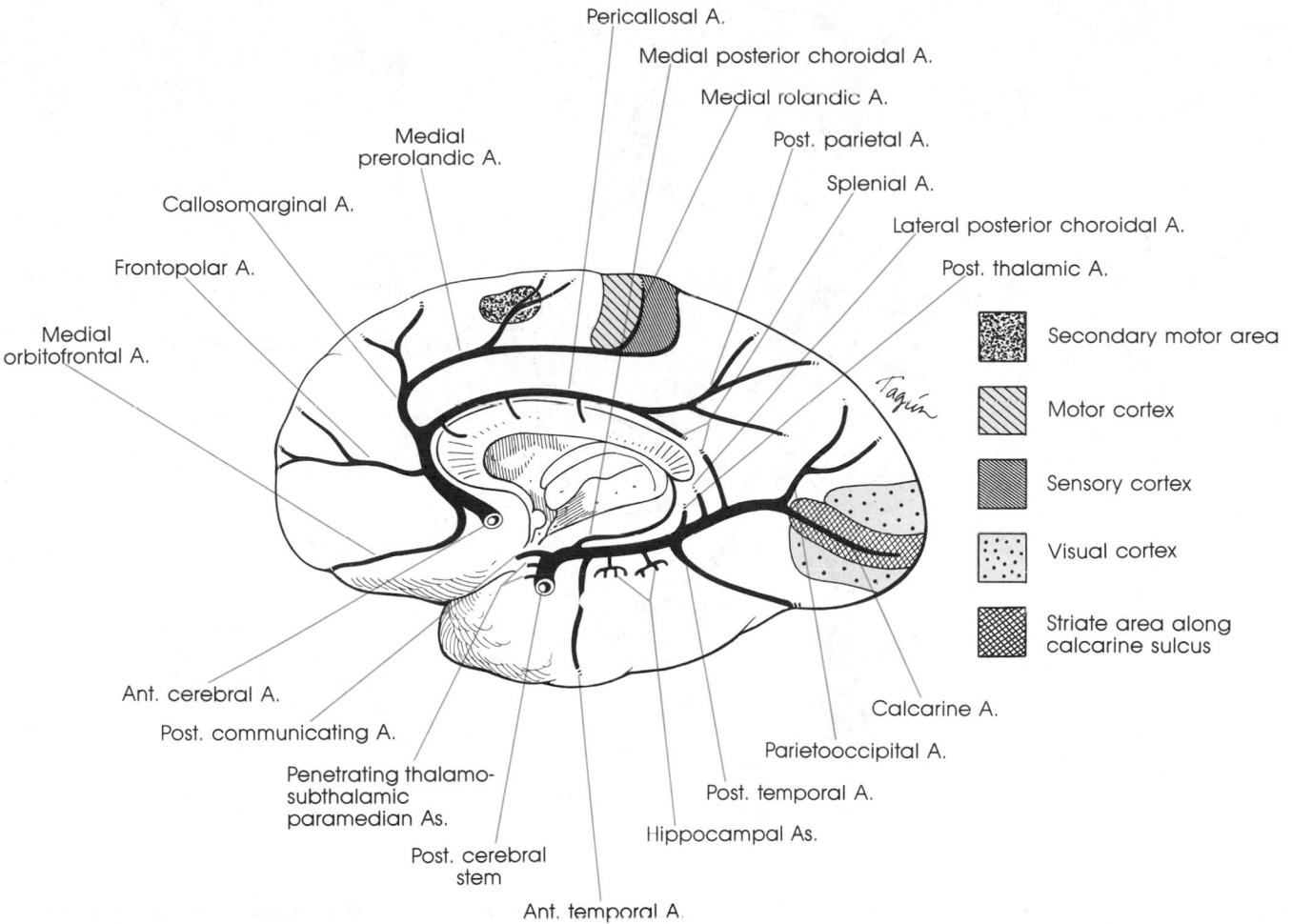

Pericallosal A.
Medial posterior choroidal A.
Medial rolandic A.
Post. parietal A.
Splenial A.
Lateral posterior choroidal A.
Post. thalamic A.
Medial prerolandic A.
Callosomarginal A.
Frontopolar A.
Medial orbitofrontal A.

Secondary motor area
Motor cortex
Sensory cortex
Visual cortex
Striate area along calcarine sulcus

Ant. cerebral A.
Post. communicating A.
Penetrating thalamo-subthalamic paramedian As.
Post. cerebral stem
Ant. temporal A.
Hippocampal As.
Post. temporal A.
Parietooccipital A.
Calcarine A.

FIGURE 351-5 Diagram of a cerebral hemisphere, medial aspect, showing the branches and distribution of the anterior cerebral artery and the principal regions of cerebral localization. (*Courtesy of C. M. Fisher, M.D.*)

Signs and symptoms	Structures involved
Paralysis of opposite foot and leg	Motor leg area
A lesser degree of paresis of opposite arm	Involvement of arm area of cortex or fibers descending to corona radiata therefrom
Cortical sensory loss over toes, foot, and leg	Sensory area for foot and leg
Urinary incontinence	Sensorimotor area in paracentral lobule
Contralateral grasp reflex, sucking reflex, gegenhalten (paratonic rigidity)	Medial surface of the posterior frontal lobe (?) supplemental motor area
Abulia (akinetic mutism), slowness, delay, intermittent interruption, lack of spontaneity, whispering, reflex distraction to sights and sounds	Uncertain localization—probably cingulate gyrus and medial inferior portion of frontal, parietal, and temporal lobes
Impairment of gait and stance (gait apraxia)	Frontal cortex near leg motor area
Dyspraxia of left limbs, tactile aphasia in left limbs	Corpus callosum

imaging can reliably identify most atheromatous lesions at the common carotid bifurcation. Atherosclerotic stenotic lesions alter normal laminar flow to rapid disturbed flow with a broad range of velocities immediately distal to the stenosis. These changes can be detected by continuous-wave or range-gated pulsed-Doppler techniques. Errors arise when calcification in a plaque prevents penetration of the ultrasound beam, and when a soft thrombus has the same density as flowing blood. Duplex ultrasound scanning combines B-mode images of the artery with range-gated pulsed-Doppler analysis of flowing blood at each point in the image. Recently, Doppler technology has been developed to allow analysis of intracranial blood flow in the middle and anterior cerebral artery stems, the distal internal carotid and ophthalmic arteries, and in the basilar and vertebral arteries (*transcranial Doppler*). Such studies of intracranial arterial flow are particularly helpful in assessing collateral flow in the circle of Willis, identifying middle cerebral artery stem stenosis or vasospasm, and

in documenting the direction and velocity of blood flow in the vertebral or basilar arteries.

Experience suggests that an optimal set of noninvasive tests includes (1) direct assessment of the bifurcation of the common carotid artery by B-mode ultrasound imaging and spectral analysis of the Doppler shift signal to give a semiquantitative assessment of the severity of the stenotic lesion (best expressed as residual lumen diameter) and (2) oculoplethysmography and transcranial Doppler analysis to provide an assessment of the hemodynamic significance of internal carotid origin or carotid siphon stenosis. Positive tests are more diagnostic than apparently normal patterns. However, none of these tests distinguishes reliably between a completely occluded internal carotid origin and one that is nearly completely occluded. Noninvasive testing is most helpful in assessing the carotid artery in patients with middle or anterior cerebral artery stroke or TIA of uncertain cause, in following the progress of a carotid stenosis

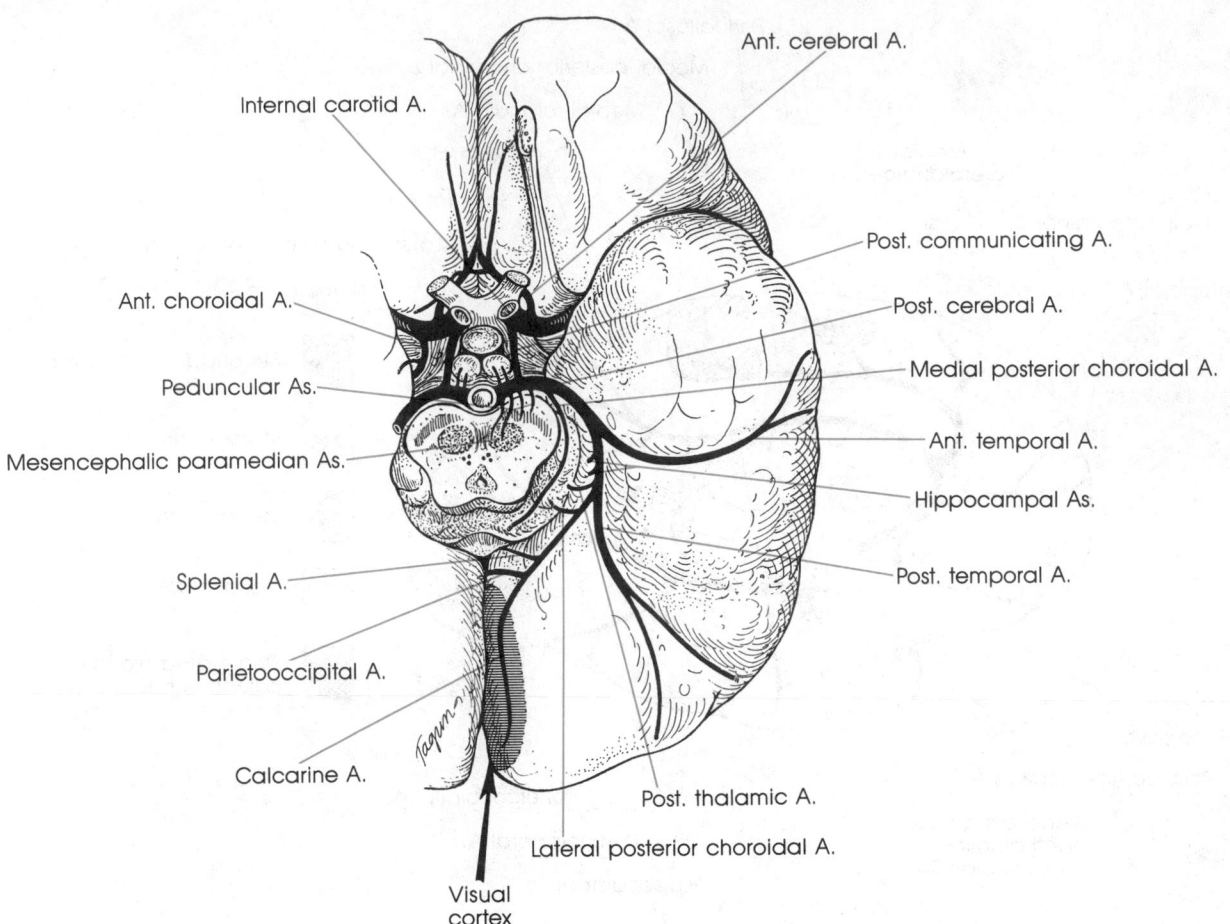

Internal carotid A.

Ant. choroidal A.

Peduncular As.

Mesencephalic paramedian As.

Splenial A.

Parietooccipital A.

Calcarine A.

Ant. cerebral A.

Post. communicating A.

Post. cerebral A.

Medial posterior choroidal A.

Ant. temporal A.

Hippocampal As.

Post. temporal A.

Post. thalamic A.

Lateral posterior choroidal A.

Visual cortex

FIGURE 351-6 Inferior aspect of the brain with the branches and distribution of the posterior cerebral artery and the principal anatomic structures shown. *(Courtesy of C. M. Fisher, M.D.)*

Signs and symptoms	Structures involved
Peripheral territory (see also Fig. 351-5)	
Homonymous hemianopsia (often upper quadrantic)	Calcarine cortex or optic radiation nearby
Bilateral homonymous hemianopsia, cortical blindness, awareness or denial of blindness; tactile naming, achromatopsia (color blindness), failure to see to-and-fro movements, inability to perceive objects not centrally located, apraxia of ocular movements, inability to count or enumerate objects, tendency to run into things which the patient sees and tries to avoid	Bilateral occipital lobe with possibly the parietal lobe involved.
Verbal dyslexia without agraphia, color anomia	Dominant calcarine lesion and posterior part of corpus callosum
Memory defect	Hippocampal lesion bilaterally or on the dominant side only
Topographic disorientation and prosopagnosia	Usually with lesions of nondominant, calcarine, and lingual gyrus
Simultagnosia, hemivisual neglect	Dominant visual cortex, contralateral hemisphere
Unformed visual hallucinations, peduncular hallucinosis, metamorphopsia, teleopsia, illusory visual spread, irreminiscence, paliopsia, distortion of outlines, central photophobia	Calcarine cortex
Complex hallucinations	Usually nondominant hemisphere
Central territory	
Thalamic syndrome: sensory loss (all modalities), spontaneous pain and dysesthesias, choreoathetosis, intention tremor, spasms of hand, mild hemiparesis	Posteroventral nucleus of thalamus; involvement of the adjacent subthalamus body or its afferent tracts
Thalamoperforate syndrome: crossed cerebellar ataxia with ipsilateral third nerve palsy (Claude's syndrome)	Dentatothalamic tract and issuing third nerve
Weber's syndrome: third nerve palsy and contralateral hemiplegia	Third nerve and cerebral peduncle
Contralateral hemiplegia	Cerebral peduncle
Paralysis or paresis of vertical eye movement, skew deviation, sluggish pupillary responses to light, slight miosis and ptosis (retraction nystagmus and "tucking" of the eyelids may be associated)	Supranuclear fibers to third nerve, interstitial nucleus of Cajal, nucleus of Darkschewitsch, and posterior commissure
Contralateral rhythmic, ataxic action tremor; rhythmic postural or "holding" tremor (rubral tremor)	Dentatothalamic tract (?)

detected by other means such as an asymptomatic bruit, or in assessing the patency of the middle cerebral stem or vertebrobasilar system in patients with appropriate symptoms.

Cerebral angiography Cerebral angiography performed by selective extracranial injection after transfemoral catheterization remains the most reliable method of assessing the cerebrovascular system. It can (1) detect ulcerative lesions, severe stenosis, and formation of a mural thrombus at the carotid bifurcation, (2) directly visualize atherothrombotic disease or dissection in the siphon and intracranial vessels, (3) demonstrate collateral circulation around the circle of Willis and on the cortical surface, and (4) show embolic occlusion of cerebral branch vessels. Although angiography cannot measure blood flow directly, it reflects relative pressures in major vessels and can suggest compromised flow in the internal carotid system. Computerized enhancement techniques have improved the resolution of angiography and reduced the amount of dye injections necessary.

However, the advantages of selective cerebral angiography must be assessed in the context of its risks. Complications range from 2 to 12 percent in various studies. The principal risks are aortic or carotid artery dissection and embolic stroke. Although rare, cholesterol microemboli from aortic arch atheroma can cause watershed cerebral infarction and renal failure. A skilled angiographer and careful attention to hydration can reduce these risks. Patients with recurrent headaches or a history of migrainous phenomena have been given glucocorticoids before angiography, but their value in preventing ischemic complications has not been established. In some patients the less risky technique of brachial artery injection offers as much relevant information as selective intracranial angiography from transfemoral catheterization.

Intravenous digital subtraction angiography is a computer-reconstruction method developed to circumvent problems inherent in arterial catheterization. However, its poor resolution and the need for large amounts of contrast material have made it virtually obsolete. Magnetic resonance techniques that image intracranial vessels are being developed (see below).

Cerebral imaging Brain imaging remains the most important acute test once a stroke has occurred. The extent and location of infarcted brain tissue can be assessed by CT scanning, which provides an estimate of extent and location of supratentorial cerebral infarction, including small 0.5- to 1.0-cm lacunar infarctions. In addition, CT scans immediately exclude hemorrhage as the cause of focal stroke and can detect surrounding edema, and less consistently, hemorrhagic infarction. *CT, however, cannot detect most cerebral infarctions for at least 48 h.* It does not reliably identify infarction of the cortical surface gray matter at any age. Furthermore, when infarction occurs in the brainstem—i.e., in the vertebral or basilar territories—CT is even less reliable because of bone and motion artifacts and the small size of many infarcts (see also Chap. 348).

Magnetic resonance imaging reveals more than CT scanning in patients with stroke. Within hours of onset, with MRI the extent and location of infarction on the cortical surface and small lacunar infarctions in the posterior fossa can be easily identified. The hemorrhagic components of infarction can be detected using high-field-strength magnets (1.5 to 4 tesla) and different pulse sequencing. Blood flow in many intracranial arteries can be detected by varying the image plane and using variable pulsing techniques. Future applications are likely to expand the angiographic capability. Tomographic assessment of cerebral blood flow and metabolism using nuclear magnetic spectroscopy may soon be possible (Chap. 348).

Xenon blood flow and positron emission tomography can assess cerebral blood flow and metabolism qualitatively and quantitatively. These methods remain time-consuming and expensive and are used largely to conduct research rather than to guide therapy (see Chap. 348).

THERAPY FOR CAROTID TERRITORY TIA
Anticoagulant therapy Heparin has been used when impending carotid or middle cerebral occlusion is suspected as the cause of TIA, but in the absence of established clinical proof of efficacy its use must be considered empirical. Heparin may be useful in the short term in stemming additional TIAs and in preventing complete occlusion of a tightly stenotic lesion while the patient is awaiting angiography, surgery, or oral anticoagulation. Heparin prevents clot formation and propagation by inhibiting the activation of prothrombin and by accelerating the rate of neutralization of several clotting factors and thrombin. However, in a few cases it has been thought to promote thrombosis, presumably by platelet activation and consumption in the clotting process. Thrombocytopenia may occur as a side effect.

The use of chronic anticoagulant therapy with sodium warfarin (coumadin) is even more controversial and problematic. Most studies of efficacy of chronic anticoagulant therapy to prevent stroke or to decrease TIAs are difficult to appraise for a number of reasons, e.g., lack of randomization, small number of patients, and lack of uniformity in the diagnosis of the cause of the TIA. In some studies, the inclusion of patients with other transient neurologic symptoms unrelated to ischemia have further complicated assessment of the results. Many believe that chronic anticoagulation therapy benefits patients with carotid-territory TIAs who are not candidates for surgery either because of medical conditions or because the lesion is surgically inaccessible (carotid siphon or middle cerebral stem). Because of the often devastating effect of middle cerebral artery occlusions, anticoagulation is similarly recommended when patients present with TIAs or minor strokes from a tightly stenotic lesion in the stem of the middle cerebral artery.

To minimize the bleeding complications of warfarin, it has been suggested that the prothrombin time should be maintained between 1.3 and 1.5 times control value (see "Embolism," below). Contraindications to anticoagulant therapy include an actively bleeding ulcer, malignant hypertension, uremia, hepatic failure, or poor patient compliance. Relative contraindications are old age, systolic blood pressure above 180 mmHg, or a history of bleeding ulcer, or bleeding diathesis.

Antiplatelet therapy Studies of the effect of antiplatelet agents on the natural history of TIAs and minor strokes can be criticized for the same reasons as the anticoagulation studies. Aspirin has been the agent most widely investigated in the prevention of stroke. Eight randomized trials have considered either aspirin alone or aspirin in combination with another antiplatelet agent. The two largest have suggested that aspirin alone may be beneficial in preventing further TIAs and strokes in symptomatic patients. Another study, in which angiography was performed routinely, suggested that aspirin benefitted patients who had TIAs associated with a lesion in the internal carotid artery, but not those who had a single TIA and no carotid lesion, i.e., those thought to have emboli from the heart. In these studies, aspirin has reduced the stroke risk over 3 years from approximately 19 to 12 percent. But endarterectomy, not aspirin, is the treatment of choice for most TIAs resulting from severe atherothrombotic disease of the internal carotid artery. Most physicians agree that aspirin may be used when TIAs are caused by inoperable carotid artery lesions or, perhaps, by ulcerative plaques.

There are theoretical reasons to avoid the excessive use of aspirin. Paradoxically, aspirin inhibits platelet formation of thromboxane A_2, a platelet-aggregating, vasoconstricting prostaglandin, but also inhibits the formation of prostacyclin, an antiaggregating vasodilating prostaglandin derived from endothelial cells. Aspirin in low doses predominantly inhibits the production of thromboxane A_2; therefore, many physicians recommend aspirin in doses of 300 mg or less per day.

Dipyridamole acts by inhibiting platelet phosphodiesterase, which is responsible for breakdown of cyclic adenosine monophosphate. The resulting elevation in platelet cyclic AMP level inhibits aggregation of platelets. Sulfinpyrazone inhibits the platelet-release reaction and interferes with platelet adhesion to subendothelial tissues. However, there is no compelling clinical evidence to suggest that dipyridamole, sulfinpyrazone, or other antiplatelet agents such as clofibrate or ibuprofen are better than aspirin in preventing recurrent TIAs or stroke in patients with symptomatic atherothrombotic cerebral vascular disease. Ticlopidine is thought to inhibit platelet binding to fibrinogen, and recent studies have compared its efficacy to aspirin's in preventing stroke in patients with TIAs or stroke. Unfortunately, these studies, like the aspirin studies, suffer from their failure to define precisely the cause of the cerebral symptoms. Ticlopidine has the disadvantage of producing a small risk of leukopenia, diarrhea, and rash.

Carotid endarterectomy Carotid endarterectomy remains the main therapy for TIAs caused by severe internal carotid stenosis, though its indications are being carefully scrutinized in several current studies. First introduced in 1954, the procedure has been associated with a morbidity ranging from 1 to 20 percent, depending on the patient population and the experience of surgeons and physicians. Although many studies suggest that this procedure is effective in preventing additional TIAs or strokes, its value has yet to be confirmed by a well-designed, controlled, randomized clinical trial. To make these surgical trials valid, the more threatening ($\leq$ 1.0-mm) lesions must be accurately identified. *Unless the acute combined complication rate of angiography and surgery is less than approximately 3 to 5 percent, carotid surgery is unlikely to be more effective than no treatment.*

Patients with a tightly stenotic lesion in one carotid artery and either an occlusion of the contralateral carotid artery or an inadequate circle of Willis are at somewhat higher risk of intraoperative stroke during endarterectomy. Intraoperative electroencephalographic or evoked potential monitoring can detect cerebral ischemia during the procedure and warn the surgeon to take steps to improve circulation.

Most patients who undergo endarterectomy have hypertensive arteriosclerotic cardiovascular disease and peripheral vascular disease. Active coronary diseases such as unstable angina, recent myocardial infarction (within 6 months), or congestive heart failure are contraindications to surgery. Severe hypertension is often corrected before surgery, but excessive lowering of the blood pressure should be avoided with tight carotid artery stenosis, because it can lead to vessel occlusion and stroke.

Stenosis can recur after surgery, although it seldom does. Poor surgical technique, excessive scar formation, and active arteriosclerotic disease have been implicated. Within the first year, the underlying pathologic process appears to be largely the proliferation of fibrous tissue; after the first year, of fibrous tissue and atherosclerosis. When stenosis recurs and gives rise to symptoms, surgery, although feasible, becomes more difficult technically.

Tandem stenotic lesions of the internal carotid artery—one at the carotid bifurcation and one at the carotid siphon—require special consideration. If the siphon stenosis has a residual lumen diameter of more than 2 mm and the lower carotid a diameter of less than 2 mm, then endarterectomy can generally be recommended. If the siphon narrowing is more severe, the value of endarterectomy is less certain. Anticoagulant or antiplatelet therapy may be preferable. But there is no consensus about the efficacy of either therapy in this setting.

Anastomosis of a superficial temporal branch of the external carotid artery to a cortical surface branch of the middle cerebral artery (EC/IC bypass) can provide collateral flow to the middle cerebral territory. Such surgery has been considered in patients with an occluded carotid artery or a tightly stenotic lesion of the carotid siphon or middle cerebral stem who present with recurrent TIAs or minor strokes. However, the results of a worldwide randomized study failed to prove greater benefit of surgical compared to anticoagulation or antiplatelet therapy in these conditions.

THERAPY FOR CAROTID TERRITORY STROKE The severity of a recent stroke in the territory of the internal carotid artery is an important factor in the decision about therapy. If there is a complete hemiplegia, severe aphasia, or anosognosia, indicating involvement of the major portions of the middle cerebral territory, the prevention of additional strokes in that arterial distribution becomes moot.

Instead, careful attention to maintenance of adequate blood pressure and prevention of delayed cerebral edema becomes important. There is little evidence to support the use of anticoagulant therapy once a "completed" or static major stroke deficit exists. However, if marked clinical improvement occurs during the first hours after onset or if the deficit is small, some anecdotal evidence suggests that short-term anticoagulation (heparin) prevents further damage, i.e., benefits "stroke in evolution." Given the pathophysiologic mechanisms of carotid stroke, many physicians use short-term anticoagulation in a patient with a slight stroke from a recently occluded or tightly stenotic internal carotid artery, hoping to prevent a second, possibly more devastating, event. In such patients, small ischemic infarcts may become hemorrhagic, but they rarely develop frank hemorrhages that act as a mass. Nonetheless, this possibility and the theoretical risk of thrombosis promotion make the timing and benefit of early heparinization controversial.

Even though no controlled studies exist, endarterectomy can tentatively be recommended for patients with tightly stenotic internal carotid lesions who present with a minor stroke in the territory distal to the lesion. The risk of surgery in experienced hands may be as low as 2 percent if the patient has no medical contraindications. When the contralateral carotid artery is tightly stenotic or occluded, endarterectomy of the ipsilateral carotid artery has a higher morbidity. Comparison of the natural history of cases of symptomatic tight carotid stenosis with surgical results has not been made, but some experience suggests that additional strokes develop in more than 3 percent of patients who are not treated surgically. Surgical trials will hopefully assess the degree of stenosis accurately enough to analyze separately the tightly stenotic ($\leq$ 1.0-mm) lesions.

Hemorrhage into a cerebral infarct is rare following internal carotid endarterectomy and probably occurs no more frequently than it would without surgery if postoperative hypertension is avoided. Nevertheless, most surgeons advise that carotid endarterectomy be delayed 2 to 6 weeks after a stroke. Earlier surgery, although controversial, may be preferable when the neurologic deficit is small or transient.

Surgery has also been performed in some cases of acute carotid artery occlusion, usually less than 8 h old, but the results are generally unsatisfactory once a major neurologic deficit is present. For most patients with a mild to moderate stroke and demonstrated occlusion of the internal carotid artery, alternative therapies include anticoagulants or antiplatelet agents, or neither. Some physicians prescribe warfarin for 6 months in hopes of preventing embolization of the propagated thrombus. In exceptional circumstances, endarterectomy of the external carotid artery or the contralateral stenotic internal carotid artery may be considered, depending on the findings at angiography and the nature of the recurrent clinical symptoms. An embolism from an occluded carotid artery suggests that the use of anticoagulation therapy may be helpful in preventing a second stroke, whereas recurrent symptoms suggestive of diminished blood flow in a hemisphere that is isolated from collateral sources of blood supply warrant consideration of surgery.

Therapy for stenosis of the carotid siphon or the middle cerebral stem associated with stroke or recurrent TIAs remains controversial. Because of the failure of external carotid–internal carotid (EC/IC) bypass surgery to reduce risks of ischemic stroke, antiplatelet therapy (aspirin) or anticoagulant therapy (warfarin) is recommended in most cases. In the absence of randomized studies to indicate which is more efficacious, antiplatelet therapy is usually recommended first for carotid siphon stenosis followed by anticoagulation if recurrent symptoms occur. Because of the potentially devastating effects of middle cerebral artery occlusion, anticoagulation with warfarin is recommended for symptomatic middle cerebral stem stenosis. In cases where recurrent symptoms occur in spite of this therapy, lowering of the blood viscosity may be helpful. Fortunately, with time, recurrent symptoms often diminish despite the treatment choice.

The unusual case of atherothrombotic stenosis or occlusion of the proximal anterior cerebral artery may cause intermittent symptoms involving the contralateral leg. Antiplatelet or anticoagulation therapy has been recommended, but no studies have documented the natural history of atherothrombotic disease at this location, and no surgical procedure protects the distal territory of the anterior cerebral artery from ischemia caused by proximal stenosis.

Experimental therapies Although much attention has been directed toward the investigation of the opioid-like substance naloxone in the treatment of acute ischemic infarction, it has yet to be shown to be efficacious. Several earlier studies suggested a beneficial effect on outcome with hemodilution, but randomized trials have given conflicting results. Reducing blood viscosity is a more promising innovative therapy for ischemic stroke. If the blood pressure remains constant, reduction of whole-blood viscosity (mainly by reduction in hematocrit and serum fibrinogen) results in increased flow through a stenotic lesion. In theory, this form of therapy increases flow to the ischemic zone (penumbra) that lies between infarcted and normal brain. This therapy has little risk. Preliminary work with drugs that block calcium influx into ischemic cells, either conventional calcium channel blockers or glutamate receptor blockers, has also had variable success in patients with stroke and in animal models.

ASYMPTOMATIC CAROTID BIFURCATION STENOSIS WITH BRUIT The natural history of an atherosclerotic lesion of the carotid bifurcation that causes a bruit but has not caused either a TIA or stroke is unknown. The available studies have examined small populations, and most failed to localize and quantitate the severity of the stenotic lesion. The studies of asymptomatic patients with cervical bruits who are about to undergo major surgical procedures have the same deficiencies. Although in some studies patients with cervical bruits were found to be at increased risk of heart disease, stroke, and death, the strokes did not necessarily occur in the vascular territory of the carotid giving rise to the bruit. At the present time, given these facts, there is little justification for operating on the carotid artery in such patients.

However, patients with tightly stenotic lesions at the origin of the internal carotid artery (1.5 mm or less) that reduces flow in the distal internal carotid artery may be at higher risk of thrombotic occlusion. Although such patients have reduced flow in the distal internal carotid artery, they may remain asymptomatic because of adequate collateral flow across the anterior circle of Willis. When stroke occurs, it is usually the result of ipsilateral artery-to-artery embolism. A high-pitched prolonged bruit fading into diastole is often associated with a tightly stenotic lesion at the origin of the internal carotid artery. It may become fainter as the stenosis progresses and flow is reduced and may disappear altogether when occlusion is imminent. Noninvasive carotid testing can often identify tightly stenotic lesions (see above). Two randomized trials are in progress to assess efficacy of surgery in patients with asymptomatic carotid stenosis. Surgery is considered only when hemodynamically significant stenotic lesions can be demonstrated. Antiplatelet therapy or observation is therefore recommended in most patients.

ATHEROTHROMBOTIC DISEASE OF THE VERTEBROBASILAR–POSTERIOR CEREBRAL ARTERY SYSTEM

The two vertebral arteries join to form the basilar artery at the pontomedullary junction. The basilar artery divides into two posterior cerebral arteries in the interpeduncular fossa (Fig. 351-2). Each of these major arteries gives rise to long and short circumferential branches and to smaller deep penetrating branches that supply the cerebellum, medulla, pons, midbrain, subthalamus, thalamus, hippocampus, and medial temporal and occipital lobes. Atherosclerosis has a predilection for the origin and the distal segments of the vertebral arteries, the proximal basilar artery, and the origin of the major and minor branches of the vertebral, basilar, and posterior cerebral arteries. Predictably, atheromatous disease at each site carries its own unique natural history, produces its own clinical syndromes, and has its own specific therapeutic implications.

POSTERIOR CEREBRAL ARTERY Pathophysiology In 70 percent of cases, both posterior cerebral arteries arise from the bifurcation of the basilar artery; in 22 percent, one or the other comes from the ipsilateral internal carotid artery; in 8 percent, both come from the ipsilateral internal carotid artery (Fig. 351-2) via the posterior communicating arteries. The precommunal segment (mesencephalic portion) of the true posterior cerebral artery is atretic in such cases (Fig. 351-2).

Atheroma formation at the top of the basilar artery or along the precommunal segment of the posterior cerebral artery may cause symptoms by narrowing one or more of the small brainstem-penetrating branches (Figs. 351-2 and 351-6) that supply the middle cerebral peduncles, the substantia nigra, red nucleus, oculomotor nuclei, midbrain reticular formation, subthalamic nucleus of Luys, decussation of superior cerebellar peduncles, the medial longitudinal fasciculus, and the medial lemniscus. The artery of Percheron (the posterior thalamosubthalamoparamedian artery), is a single artery that arises from either the right or the left precommunal segment of the posterior cerebral artery. It divides in the subthalamus to supply the inferior medial and the anterior portions of the thalamus and subthalamus bilaterally. The thalamogeniculate branches, which also originate from the precommunal portion of the posterior cerebral artery, supply the dorsal, dorsomedial, anterior, and inferior thalamus and the medial geniculate body. The medial posterior choroidal artery supplies the superior dorsomedial and dorsoanterior thalamus and the medial geniculate body in addition to the tela choroidea of the third ventricle. The lateral posterior choroidal artery supplies the choroid plexus of the lateral ventricle.

Atheroma in the posterior cerebral artery distal to the junction with the posterior communicating artery (Fig. 351-6) may occlude small circumferential branches that course around the midbrain to supply the lateral part of the cerebral peduncles, medial lemniscus, tegmentum of the midbrain, superior colliculi, lateral geniculate body, and posterior lateral nucleus of the thalamus, choroid plexus, and hippocampus. On the rare occasions when atheroma occur more distally in the posterior cerebral artery (Fig. 351-6), occlusion may produce ischemia and infarction in the medial inferior temporal lobe, parahippocampal and hippocampal gyri, and occipital lobe—including the calcarine cortex and the visual association areas 18 and 19.

Clinical manifestations The site of atheromas and the degree of narrowing determine the clinical syndrome. Although factors of collateral circulation or serum viscosity may play a role in some cases, embolic occlusion is the usual cause of stroke in this vascular territory. Two syndromes are commonly observed: (1) midbrain, subthalamic, and thalamic signs, which are due to disease of the precommunal segment of the posterior cerebral artery or of its penetrating branches; and (2) cortical temporal and occipital lobe syndromes, due to occlusion of the postcommunal segment.

PROXIMAL PRECOMMUNAL SYNDROMES (CENTRAL TERRITORY) If the proximal posterior cerebral artery is occluded, infarction usually occurs in the ipsilateral or bilateral subthalamus and medial thalamus and in the ipsilateral cerebral peduncle and midbrain, producing concomitant signs (Fig. 351-6). If the posterior communicating artery is atretic, the peripheral territory supplied by posterior cerebral artery is also affected (Fig. 351-6). If the posterior cerebral artery is completely occluded at its origin, hemiplegia secondary to infarction of the cerebral peduncle occurs. Involvement of the red nucleus and/or dentatorubrothalamic tract can produce contralateral ataxia. A third nerve palsy with contralateral ataxia (Claude's syndrome) or with contralateral hemiplegia (Weber's syndrome) may result. If the subthalamic nucleus of Luys is involved, contralateral hemiballismus may occur. Occlusion of the artery of Percheron produces paresis of upward gaze and drowsiness and is often associated with abulia. Extensive infarction in the midbrain of the subthalamus occurring with bilateral posterior cerebral stem occlusion is usually secondary to embolism. Coma, bilateral pyramidal signs, and ''decerebrate rigidity'' occur in this setting.

Atheromatous occlusion of the penetrating branches of the thalamic and thalamogeniculate arteries produces less extensive thalamic and thalamocapsular lacunar syndromes. The *thalamic syndrome of Dejerine and Roussy* is the best known. Its main feature is contralateral hemisensory loss of both superficial sensation (pain and temperature) and deep sensation (touch and proprioception). Occasionally, it may affect only pain and temperature or vibration and joint position sense. After a few weeks or months, an agonizing, searing pain may develop in the affected areas. Patients describe the pain as tight, drawing, icy, and knifelike. It is devastatingly persistent and responds poorly to analgesics. Occasionally, anticonvulsants are beneficial. If the posterior limb of the internal capsule is involved, hemiparesis or hemiplegia may accompany the hemisensory syndrome. Other associated motor signs include hemiballismus, choreoathetosis, intention tremor, incoordination, and posturing of the hand and arm, particularly while walking.

POSTCOMMUNAL SYNDROMES (PERIPHERAL OR CORTICAL TERRITORY) (Fig. 351-6) Occlusion of the posterior cerebral artery causes infarction of the cortical surface of the medial temporal and occipital lobes. Contralateral homonymous hemianopsia is the usual manifestation. Occasionally, only the upper quadrant of the visual field is involved. If the visual association areas are spared and only the calcarine cortex is involved, the patient is aware of visual defects. Central vision may be spared if middle cerebral artery branches supply the macular region of the occipital pole. Medial temporal lobe and hippocampal involvement may cause an acute disturbance in memory, particularly if it occurs in the dominant hemisphere, but the defect usually clears because memory has bilateral representation. If the dominant hemisphere is affected and the infarct extends to involve the splenium of the corpus callosum, the patient may demonstrate alexia without agraphia. Visual agnosia for faces, objects, mathematical symbols, and colors and anomia with paraphasic errors (amnestic aphasia) may also occur in this setting even without callosal involvement. Occlusion of the posterior cerebral artery can produce peduncular hallucinosis (visual hallucinations of brightly colored scenes and objects).

Bilateral infarction in the distal posterior cerebral arteries produces cortical blindness. The patient is often unaware of the blindness. The clinical clue to the site is a finding of normal pupillary reaction to light. Tiny islands of vision may persist; and the patient then reports that vision fluctuates as images are captured in the preserved portions. Rarely, only peripheral vision is lost and central vision is spared; resulting in "gun-barrel" vision. A constellation of symptoms termed *Balint's syndrome* can occur with unilateral or bilateral visual association area lesions. It includes optic ataxia (inability to visually guide limb movements), ocular ataxia (inability to direct eyes to a precise point in the visual field), inability to enumerate objects in a picture or extract meaning from a picture, and inability to avoid objects seen in one's path. Balint's syndrome is most often seen with bilateral infarctions, secondary to low flow in the distal posterior and or middle cerebral "watershed" territories as occurs after arrest. Embolic occlusion of the top of the basilar artery can produce a clinical picture that includes any or all of the central or peripheral territory symptoms. Its hallmark is suddenness of onset and bilaterality of symptoms including ptosis and somnolence (see above in the discussion of the artery of Percheron).

Laboratory evaluation   Infarction in the peripheral territory of the posterior cerebral artery can be easily documented by CT or MRI. Infarction in the central territory of the posterior cerebral artery, particularly in territories supplied by the penetrating branches of the posterior cerebral artery, is not reliably detected by CT scanning. MRI can detect infarctions greater than 0.5 cm in this area.

Therapy   Because infarction in the territory of the posterior cerebral artery is usually secondary to embolism from the vertebrobasilar system or from the heart, treatment with anticoagulants to prevent further embolic events is appropriate. Transient ischemic symptoms in the territory of the posterior cerebral artery may result from atherothrombotic stenosis of its proximal portion or one of its penetrating branches (lacunar TIA). The natural history of such atheromatous disease is unknown. Thus, the efficacy of anticoagulants vs. antiplatelet therapy vs. no medication is still uncertain. In general, antiplatelet therapy seems safest in this setting.

VERTEBRAL AND POSTERIOR INFERIOR CEREBELLAR ARTERIES   The *vertebral artery,* which arises from the innominate artery on the right and the subclavian artery on the left, divides into four anatomic segments. The first segment extends from its origin to its entrance into the sixth or fifth transverse vertebral foramen. The second segment traverses the vertebral foramina from C6 to C2. The third segment passes through the transverse foramen and circles around the arch of the atlas to pierce the dura at the foramen magnum. The fourth segment courses upward to join the other vertebral artery to form the basilar artery; only the fourth segment gives rise to branches that supply the brainstem and cerebellum. The *posterior inferior cerebellar artery* in its proximal segments supplies the lateral medulla and, in its distal branches, the inferior surface of the cerebellum. Anastomotic channels exist among the ascending cervical arteries, the thyrocervical arteries, the occipital artery (branch of the external carotid artery), and the second segment of the vertebral artery (Fig. 351-1). In 10 percent of patients, one vertebral artery is too small to contribute significant blood to the brainstem.

Atherothrombotic lesions have a predilection for the first and fourth segments of the vertebral artery. Although the atheromatous narrowing in the first segment (the origin) may be significant, it seldom produces brainstem ischemic strokes. Collateral flow from the contralateral vertebral artery or the ascending cervical and ascending thyrocervical or occipital arteries is usually sufficient to prevent ischemia (Fig. 351-1*D*). When one vertebral artery is atretic and an atherothrombotic lesion threatens the origin of the other, the only avenues for collateral circulation are through the ascending cervical artery, the thyrocervical artery, and the occipital artery, or by retrograde flow down the basilar artery via the posterior communicating artery (Fig. 351-2 and 351-6). In this setting, low flow in the vertebrobasilar system exists and TIAs may occur. In addition, incipient thrombosis in the proximal basilar or distal vertebral system may occur. If the subclavian is blocked proximal to the origin of the vertebral artery, exercise of the left arm may draw blood from the vertebrobasilar insufficiency (*subclavian steal*). It rarely leads to significant vertebrobasilar ischemia.

Atheroma in the fourth segment of the vertebral artery can occur proximal to or distal to the origin of the posterior inferior cerebral artery, as well as at the junction with the other vertebral artery to form the basilar artery. When it is proximal to the origin of the posterior inferior cerebral artery, a critical narrowing can threaten the lateral medulla and posterior inferior surface of the cerebellum.

Although atheromatous disease rarely narrows the second and third segments of the vertebral artery, this region is subject to dissection, fibromuscular dysplasia, and rarely to encroachment by osteophytic spurs within the vertebral foramina.

Clinical manifestations   *Transient cerebral ischemic attacks* resulting from vertebral artery insufficiency cause dizziness or vertigo, numbness of the ipsilateral face and contralateral limbs, diplopia, hoarseness, dysarthria, and dysphagia. Hemiparesis is rare. Such TIAs are usually short (up to 10 to 15 min) and repetitive.

When *infarction* ensues, it most often affects the lateral medulla with or without the posterior inferior cerebellum (Wallenberg's syndrome). Its features are listed in Fig. 351-7. In 70 to 80 percent of the cases, the syndrome occurs after ipsilateral vertebral artery occlusion; in the remainder it results from posterior inferior cerebellar artery occlusion. Atherothrombotic occlusion of the medullary penetrating branches of the vertebral or posterior inferior cerebellar artery results in partial syndromes of the ipsilateral, lateral, or medial medulla.

Rarely, a medial medullary syndrome occurs in which the pyramid becomes infarcted, causing a contralateral hemiparesis of the arm and leg, sparing the face. If the medial lemniscus and emerging hypoglossal nerve fibers are involved, contralateral loss of joint position sense and ipsilateral tongue weakness occur.

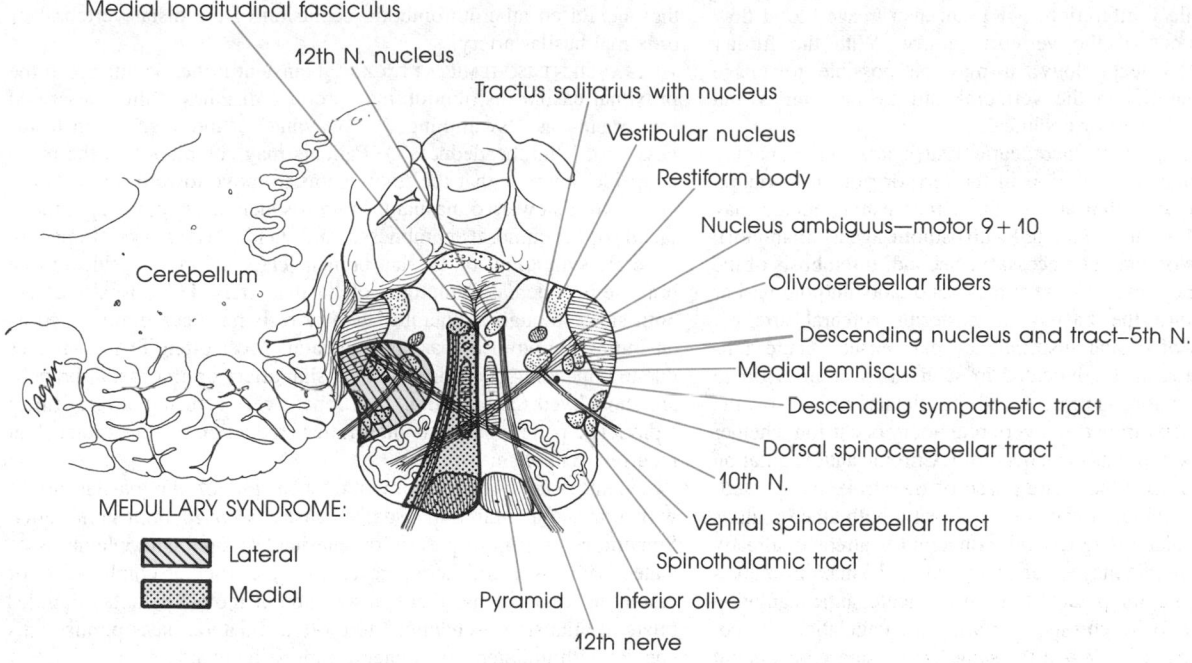

FIGURE 351-7 *(Courtesy of C. M. Fisher, M.D.)*

Signs and symptoms	Structures involved
1 Medial medullary syndrome (occlusion of vertebral artery or of branch of vertebral or lower basilar artery)	
On side of lesion:	
Paralysis with atrophy of half the tongue	Ipsilateral twelfth nerve
On side opposite lesion:	
Paralysis of arm and leg sparing face; impaired tactile and proprioceptive sense over half the body	Contralateral pyramidal tract and medial lemniscus
2 Lateral medullary syndrome (occlusion of any of five vessels may be responsible—vertebral, posterior inferior cerebellar, superior, middle, or inferior lateral medullary arteries)	
On side of lesion:	
Pain, numbness, impaired sensation over half the face	Descending tract and nucleus fifth nerve
Ataxia of limbs, falling to side of lesion	Uncertain—restiform body, cerebellar hemisphere, cerebellar fibers, spinocerebellar tract (?)
Nystagmus, diplopia, oscillopsia, vertigo, nausea, vomiting	Vestibular nucleus
Horner's syndrome (miosis, ptosis, decreased sweating)	Descending sympathetic tract
Dysphagia, hoarseness, paralysis of palate, paralysis of vocal cord, diminished gag reflex	Issuing fibers ninth and tenth nerves
Loss of taste	Nucleus and tractus solitarius
Numbness of ipsilateral arm, trunk, or leg	Cuneate and gracile nuclei
On side opposite lesion:	
Impaired pain and thermal sense over half the body, sometimes face	Spinothalamic tract
3 Total unilateral medullary syndrome (occlusion of vertebral artery): Combination of medial and lateral syndromes	
4 Lateral pontomedullary syndrome (occlusion of vertebral artery): Combination of lateral medullary and lateral inferior pontine syndromes	
5 Basilar artery syndrome (the syndrome of the lone vertebral artery is equivalent): A combination of the various brainstem syndromes plus those arising in the posterior cerebral artery distribution	
Bilateral long tract signs (sensory and motor; cerebellar and peripheral cranial nerve abnormalities)	Bilateral long tract; cerebellar and peripheral cranial nerves
Paralysis or weakness of all extremities, plus all bulbar musculature	Corticobulbar and corticospinal tracts bilaterally

Cerebellar infarction with edema formation can lead to *sudden respiratory arrest* due to raised intracranial pressure in the posterior fossa. Drowsiness, Babinski signs, dysarthria, and bifacial weakness may be absent or present only briefly before respiratory arrest ensues. Gait unsteadiness, dizziness, nausea, and vomiting may be the only early symptoms and signs and should arouse suspicion of this impending complication.

Laboratory evaluation When TIAs occur in the territory of the lateral medulla, it becomes important to determine the adequacy of blood flow in the distal vertebral artery and the posterior inferior cerebellar artery. Angiography is therefore considered if the diagnosis is unclear. CT scanning may detect a large cerebellar infarction in the territory of the posterior inferior cerebellar artery. MRI can detect cerebellar infarction earlier and, with high-resolution scanning, can detect lateral medullary infarction. MRI can also image blood flow in the fourth segment of the vertebral artery. With the further development of MRI technology, it may be possible to image atherothrombotic material in the vertebral and basilar arteries and determine if they are patent or occluded.

Therapy Four important therapeutic issues arise in managing patients with ischemia or infarction in the territory of the vertebral or posterior inferior cerebellar artery. First, the ensuing edema may be life-threatening. It should be treated with osmotic agents (mannitol); surgical decompression may be necessary. Second, thrombosis of the fourth segment of the vertebral artery may send clots into the basilar artery or emboli into the basilar or posterior cerebral arteries. Symptoms or signs of basilar insufficiency may ensue. Acute anticoagulation with heparin is advocated in such cases in an effort to prevent clot propagation. Third, some physicians argue for the prophylactic use of heparin in acute vertebral artery occlusion whether or not basilar artery symptoms have occurred. Chronic anticoagulation is not recommended after the acute phase of the stroke has passed. Fourth, when one vertebral artery is symptomatic with atheromatous disease and the contralateral vertebral is congenitally atretic or already occluded, basilar ischemia may ensue and proximal basilar thrombosis may develop. Despite its potential hazards, acute anticoagulation with heparin, followed by chronic warfarin anticoagulation, is recommended in such patients. When the same circumstance occurs but the symptomatic vertebral atherothrombotic lesion lies immediately proximal to the posterior inferior cerebellar artery, occipital-to–posterior inferior bypass grafting has been recommended. The efficacy of this surgery is unproven, and it should be considered only after anticoagulation therapy has failed.

BASILAR ARTERY Pathophysiology Branches of the basilar artery supply the base of the pontis and superior cerebellum and fall into three groups: (1) paramedian, seven to 10 in number, which supply a wedge of pons on either side of the midline; (2) short circumferential branches, five to seven in number, which supply the lateral two-thirds of the pons and middle and superior cerebellar peduncles; and (3) two bilateral long circumferential arteries (superior cerebellar and anterior inferior cerebellar arteries) which course around the pons to supply the cerebellar hemispheres.

Atheromatous lesions can occur anywhere along the basilar trunk, but are most often in the proximal basilar and distal vertebral segments. Typically, lesions occlude either the proximal basilar and one or both vertebral arteries. The clinical picture varies depending on the availability of retrograde collateral flow from the posterior communicating arteries.

Although atherothrombosis occasionally occludes the top of the basilar artery, emboli from the heart or proximal vertebral or basilar segments are more common.

Clinical manifestations Because the brainstem contains many structures in close approximation, a diversity of clinical syndromes may emerge with ischemia. Involvement of the corticospinal tracts, corticobulbar tracts, medial and superior cerebellar peduncles, spinothalamic tracts, and cranial nerve nuclei cause the common symptoms and signs (see Figs. 351-8 to 351-10).

Unfortunately, the symptoms of transient ischemia or infarction in the territory of the basilar artery often do not indicate whether the basilar artery itself or one of its branches is diseased, yet the distinction has important implications for therapy. The picture of complete basilar insufficiency, however, is easy to recognize. A combination of bilateral long tract signs (sensory and motor) with signs of cranial nerve and cerebellar dysfunction suggest this diagnosis. A ''locked-in'' state of quadriplegia occurs with bilateral basis pontis infarction. Coma due to dysfunction of the reticular activating system and quadriplegia with cranial nerve signs suggest complete and devastating pontine and upper midbrain infarction. The therapeutic goal, however, is to recognize impending basilar occlusion before such a devastating infarction occurs. A series of TIAs or a slowly progressive, fluctuating stroke become extremely significant when they herald an atherothrombotic occlusion of the distal vertebral or proximal basilar artery.

TRANSIENT ISCHEMIC ATTACKS Transient ischemic attacks in the proximal basilar distribution may produce dizziness (often described by patients as ''swimming,'' ''swaying,'' ''moving,'' ''unsteadiness,'' or ''lightheadedness''). Patients may complain that the room is upside down or that the floor seems to move toward them. Other symptoms that warn of basilar thrombosis include diplopia, dysarthria, facial or circumoral numbness, and hemisensory symptoms. In general, symptoms of basilar branch TIAs affect one side of the brainstem, whereas symptoms of basilar artery TIAs usually affect both sides, though a ''herald'' hemiparesis has been emphasized as an initial symptom of basilar occlusion. Most often TIAs, whether due to impending occlusion of the basilar artery or of a basilar branch, are short-lived (5 to 30 min) and repetitive, occurring several times a day. The pattern suggests intermittent reduction of flow rather than recurrent embolism.

INFARCTION Atherothrombotic occlusion of the basilar artery with brainstem infarction usually causes *bilateral* brainstem signs. Sometimes only gaze paresis or internuclear ophthalmoplegia associated with ipsilateral hemiparesis, i.e., a particular combination of cranial nerve and long tract (sensory and/or motor) deficits, signifies bilateral brainstem ischemia. More often, bilateral basis pontis signs coexist with unilateral or bilateral pontine tegmental signs.

Symptomatic atherothrombotic occlusion of a branch of the basilar artery usually causes *unilateral* symptoms and signs involving motor, sensory, and cranial nerves. Occlusions of the two long circumferential branches of the basilar artery produce specific clinical syndromes depending on the artery involved.

SUPERIOR CEREBELLAR ARTERY Occlusion of the superior cerebellar artery results in severe ipsilateral cerebellar ataxia (middle and/or superior cerebellar peduncles), nausea and vomiting, dysarthria, and contralateral loss of pain and temperature sensation over the extremities, body, and face (spino- and trigeminothalamic tract). Partial deafness, ataxic tremor of the ipsilateral upper extremity, Horner's syndrome, and palatal myoclonus may rarely occur. Partial syndromes occur frequently (see Fig. 351-8).

ANTERIOR INFERIOR CEREBELLAR ARTERY Occlusion of the anterior inferior cerebellar artery produces variable degrees of infarction because the size of this artery and the territory it supplies vary inversely with those of the posterior inferior cerebellar artery. The principal symptoms include ipsilateral deafness, facial weakness, true vertigo (whirling dizziness), nausea and vomiting, nystagmus, tinnitus and cerebellar ataxia, Horner's syndrome, and paresis of conjugate lateral gaze. The opposite side of the body loses pain and temperature sensation. An occlusion close to the origin of the artery may cause corticospinal tract signs (see Fig. 351-10).

Occlusion of one of the five to seven short circumferential branches of the basilar artery affects the lateral two-thirds of the pons and/or middle or superior cerebellar peduncle, whereas occlusion of one of the seven to ten paramedian branches of the basilar artery affects a wedge-shaped area on either side of the medial pons (Figs. 351-8 to 351-10). Many syndromes of brainstem syndromes with cranial nerve abnormalities and crossed hemiplegia have been given eponyms, e.g., Weber, Claude, Benedict, Foville, Raymong-Cestan, Millard-Gubler.

Laboratory evaluation MRI scanning can detect brainstem infarction due to either basilar artery or basilar branch occlusion. Application of defined pulse sequences can detect blood flow in the basilar artery. MRI scanning combined with transcranial Doppler analysis may eventually replace conventional angiography in documenting basilar artery potency. CT scanning is not reliable in detecting brainstem infarcts but can show hemorrhages and assess mass effect after large cerebellar infarctions.

Selective cerebral arteriography remains the best method to define atherothrombotic disease of the basilar artery. Since arteriography entails potential morbidity and may precipitate the very stroke one is seeking to prevent, it is recommended only when the information

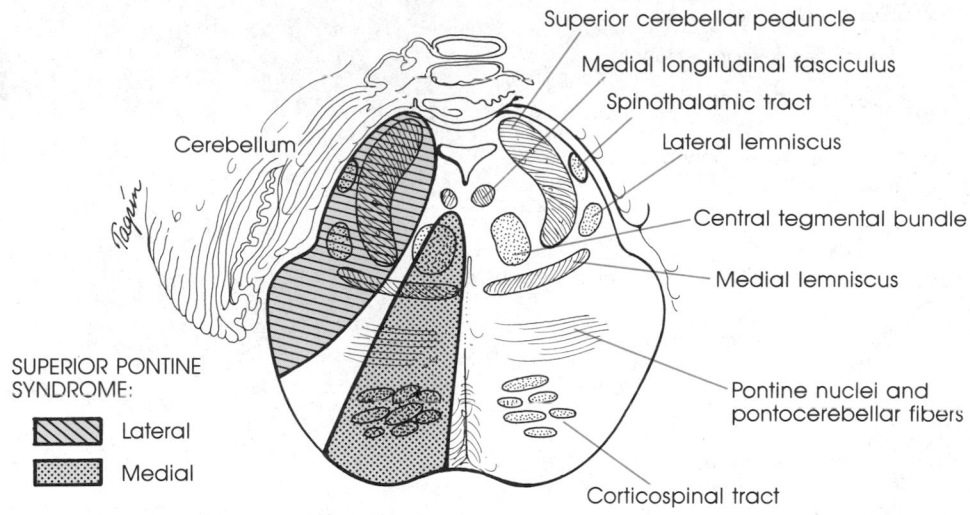

Superior cerebellar peduncle
Medial longitudinal fasciculus
Spinothalamic tract
Lateral lemniscus
Central tegmental bundle
Medial lemniscus
Pontine nuclei and pontocerebellar fibers
Corticospinal tract
Cerebellum

SUPERIOR PONTINE SYNDROME:

Lateral

Medial

FIGURE 351-8 *(Courtesy of C. M. Fisher, M.D.)*

Signs and symptoms	Structures involved
1 Medial superior pontine syndrome (paramedian branches of upper basilar artery)	
On side of lesion:	
Cerebellar ataxia (probably)	Superior and/or middle cerebellar peduncle
Internuclear ophthalmoplegia	Medial longitudinal fasciculus
Myoclonic syndrome, palate, pharnyx, vocal cords, respiratory apparatus, face, oculomotor apparatus, etc.	Localization uncertain—central tegmental bundle (?), dentate projection (?), inferior olivary nucleus (?)
On side opposite lesion:	
Paralysis of face, arm, and leg	Corticobulbar and corticospinal tract
Rarely touch, vibration, and position are affected	Medial lemniscus
2. Lateral superior pontine syndrome (syndrome of superior cerebellar artery)	
On side of lesion:	
Ataxia of limbs and gait, falling to side of lesion	Middle and superior cerebellar peduncles, superior surface of cerebellum, dentate nucleus
Dizziness, nausea, vomiting; horizontal nystagmus	Vestibular nucleus
Paresis of conjugate gaze (ipsilateral)	Pontine contralateral gaze
Skew deviation	Uncertain
Miosis, ptosis, decreased sweating over face (Horner's syndrome)	Descending sympathetic fibers
Static tremor reported in one case	Dentate nucleus (?), superior cerebellar peduncle (?)
On side opposite lesion:	
Impaired pain and thermal sense on face, limbs, and trunk	Spinothalamic tract
Impaired touch, vibration, and position sense, more in leg than arm (there is a tendency to incongruity of pain and touch deficits)	Medial lemniscus (lateral portion)

provided will assist in the management of the patient. Occasionally, injection of angiographic dye in the posterior circulation precipitates a delirious state sometimes associated with cortical blindness. This reversible state can last for 24 to 38 h or, rarely, several days.

Therapy Impending basilar occlusion causing transient or fluctuating symptoms should be treated with short-term anticoagulation with intravenous heparin, after MRI or CT scanning has excluded hemorrhage. When basilar artery stenosis or occlusion is associated with minor or improving stroke, long-term anticoagulation with warfarin is recommended. If, on the other hand, basilar branch disease is the cause, then the rationale for using warfarin is uncertain. While embolism from the heart or from atheroma in the distal vertebral system may occlude a penetrating basilar branch, this is unlikely. Therefore, long-term control of blood pressure and antiplatelet therapy are recommended as preventive measures in the management of small-vessel basilar branch disease. Because of the long-term accumulative risk of anticoagulation therapy, it is generally reserved for symptomatic large-vessel atherothrombotic disease.

LACUNAR DISEASE

The term *lacunar disease* refers to atherothrombotic and lipohyalinotic occlusive disease of the penetrating branches of the circle of Willis, middle cerebral artery stem, and vertebral and basilar arteries.

PATHOPHYSIOLOGY The middle cerebral artery stem, the arteries comprising the circle of Willis (A1 segment of the anterior cerebral artery, anterior and posterior communicating arteries, and precommunal segment of the posterior cerebral arteries), the basilar, and the vertebral arteries all give rise to 100- to 300-μm-diameter branches that penetrate the deep gray and white matter of the cerebrum or brainstem (Fig. 351-2). Each of these small branches can be thrombosed either by atherothrombotic disease at its origin or by the development of lipohyalinotic thickening. Thrombosis of these vessels causes small infarcts that are referred to as *lacunes*. They range in size from as small as 3 to 4 mm to 1 to 2 cm. Hypertension is the principal risk factor for such small-vessel disease. Lacunar infarcts represent approximately 10 percent of all strokes.

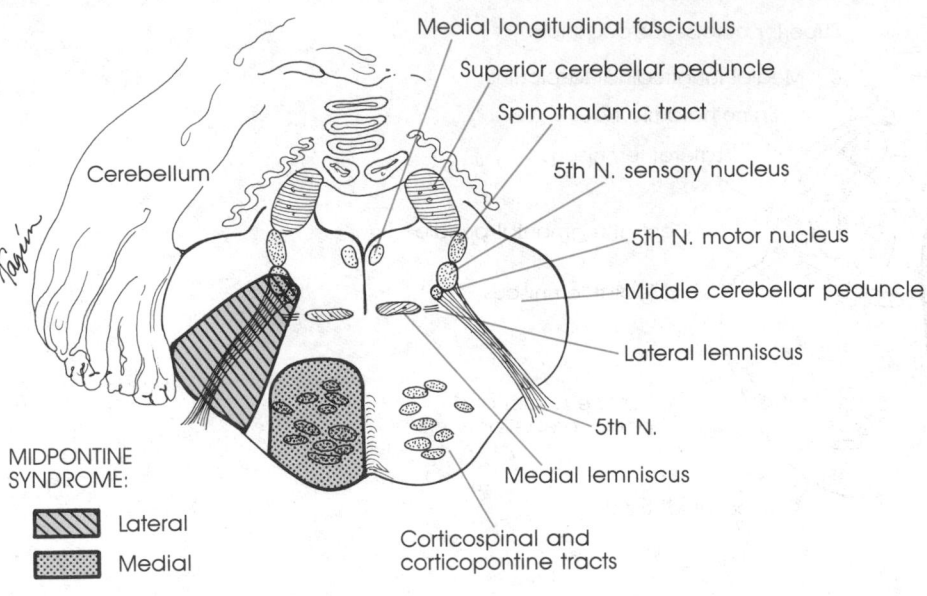

FIGURE 351-9 *(Courtesy of C. M. Fisher, M.D.)*

Signs and symptoms	Structures involved
1 Medial midpontine syndrome (paramedian branch of midbasilar artery)	
On side of lesion:	
Ataxia of limbs and gait (more prominent in bilateral involvement)	Pontine nuclei
On side opposite lesion:	
Paralysis of face, arm, and leg	Corticobulbar and corticospinal tract
Variable impaired touch and proprioception when lesion extends posteriorly	Medial lemniscus
2 Lateral midpontine syndrome (short circumferential artery)	
On side of lesion:	
Ataxia of limbs	Middle cerebellar peduncle
Paralysis of muscles of mastication	Motor fibers or nucleus of fifth nerve
Impaired sensation over side of face	Sensory fibers or nucleus of fifth nerve
On side opposite lesion:	
Impaired pain and thermal sense on limbs and trunk	Spinothalamic tract

CLINICAL MANIFESTATIONS Lacunar infarcts cause recognizable stroke syndromes that usually evolve over hours or longer. Transient symptoms (lacunar TIAs) may herald a lacunar infarct; they may occur several times a day, and last only a few minutes. When infarction occurs, it usually causes a sudden deficit, but may evolve in a progressive fashion over a few days. Recovery often begins within hours or days after the infarct, and over weeks or months may be complete or result in minimal residual deficit. In some cases significant disability persists.

The most common lacunar syndromes are the following:

1 *Pure motor hemiparesis* from an infarct in the posterior limb of the internal capsule or basis pontis. Here, the face, arm, leg, foot, and toes are almost always involved. The weakness may be intermittent (TIA), progress in a stepwise manner, or appear abruptly, and may progress to complete paralysis, but improvement occurs in many cases.
2 *Pure sensory stroke* from an infarct in the ventrolateral thalamus.
3 *Ataxic hemiparesis* from an infarct in the base of the pons or *dysarthria and a clumsy hand or arm* due to infarction in the base of the pons or in the genu of the internal capsule.
4 *Pure motor hemiparesis* with ''motor aphasia'' due to thrombotic occlusion of a lenticulostriate branch supplying the genu and anterior limb of the internal capsule and adjacent white matter of the corona radiata.

Before the advent of hypertensive therapy, multiple lacunes often caused *pseudobulbar palsy* with emotional instability, a slowed abulic state, and bilateral pyramidal signs. This syndrome is now uncommon.

Other lacunar syndromes have been described, some not correlated with arterial occlusion. An anarthric pseudobulbar syndrome due to bilateral infarctions in the internal capsule can occur from disease in the lenticulostriate arteries. Syndromes resulting from occlusion of the penetrating arteries of the proximal posterior cerebral artery were discussed above. Syndromes resulting from occlusion of the penetrating arteries of the basilar artery (Figs. 351-8 to 351-10) include ipsilateral ataxia and crural (leg) paresis, pure motor hemiparesis with horizontal gaze palsy, and hemiparesis with a crossed sixth nerve palsy. Lower basilar branch syndromes include sudden internuclear ophthalmoplegia, horizontal gaze palsy, and appendicular cerebellar ataxia.

Syndromes resulting from vertebral branch occlusions include pure motor hemiparesis sparing the face by involving the medullary pyramid, and syndromes that involve the lateral pontomedullary area, which may include vertigo, vomiting, facial weakness, Horner's syndrome, ipsilateral trigeminal numbness, and contralateral spinothalamic sensory loss.

LABORATORY EVALUATION The CT scan documents most supratentorial lacunar infarctions, and MRI successfully documents both supratentorial and infratentorial infarctions when the lacunes are 5 mm or greater. Lacunar infarction is diagnosed when the infarct size is less than 2 cm, and its location is attributable to occlusion of a small penetrating arterial branch of a major parent vessel. Larger

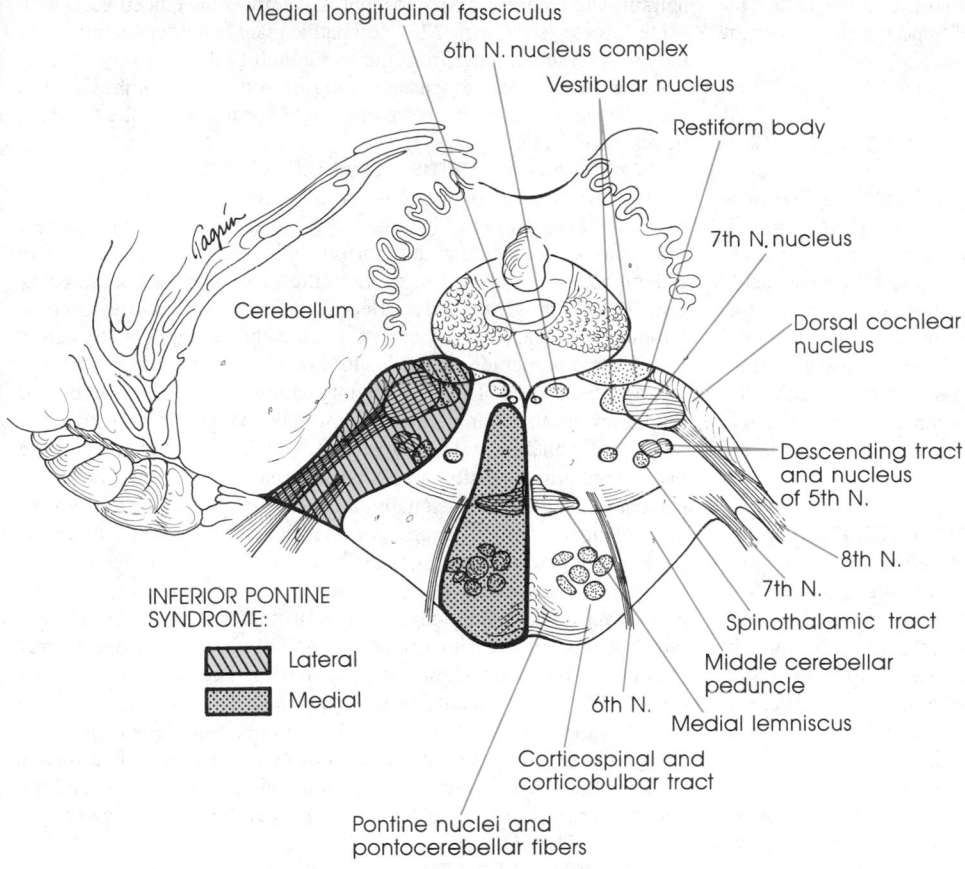

Medial longitudinal fasciculus
6th N. nucleus complex
Vestibular nucleus
Restiform body
Cerebellum
7th N. nucleus
Dorsal cochlear nucleus
Descending tract and nucleus of 5th N.
8th N.
7th N.
Spinothalamic tract
Middle cerebellar peduncle
Medial lemniscus
6th N.
Corticospinal and corticobulbar tract
Pontine nuclei and pontocerebellar fibers

INFERIOR PONTINE SYNDROME:
Lateral
Medial

FIGURE 351-10 *(Courtesy of C. M. Fisher, M.D.)*

Signs and symptoms	Structures involved
1 Medial inferior pontine syndrome (occlusion of paramedian branch of basilar artery)	
On side of lesion:	
Paralysis of conjugate gaze to side of lesion (preservation of convergence)	"Center" for conjugate lateral gaze
Nystagmus	Vestibular nucleus
Ataxia of limbs and gait	Middle cerebellar peduncle (?)
Diplopia on lateral gaze	Abducens nerve
On side opposite lesion:	
Paralysis of face, arm, and leg	Corticobulbar and corticospinal tract in lower pons
Impaired tactile and proprioceptive sense over half of the body	Medial lemniscus
2 Lateral inferior pontine syndrome (occlusion of anterior inferior cerebellar artery)	
On side of lesion:	
Horizontal and vertical nystagmus, vertigo, nausea, vomiting, oscillopsia	Vestibular nerve on nucleus
Facial paralysis	Seventh nerve
Paralysis of conjugate gaze to side of lesion	"Center" for conjugate lateral gaze
Deafness, tinnitus	Auditory nerve or cochlear nucleus
Ataxia	Middle cerebellar peduncle and cerebellar hemisphere
Impaired sensation over face	Descending tract and nucleus fifth nerve
On side opposite lesion:	
Impaired pain and thermal sense over half the body (may include face)	Spinothalamic tract

deep white matter infarcts in the territory of the middle cerebral artery (so-called giant lacunes) are probably due to embolism or large atherosclerotic plaques that occlude the mouths of several adjacent penetrating vessels. The electroencephalogram (EEG) is usually normal, or nearly so, in lacunar infarction but abnormal in cortical surface infarction.

THERAPY Lacunar strokes may present with a fluctuating progressive course, and acute reduction in blood pressure may worsen symptoms. Antihypertensive therapy is begun after the patient's symptoms become stable. Whether anticoagulant or antiplatelet agents benefit patients with lacunar TIAs and fluctuating stroke is unknown. Some studies suggest that thalamic lacunes may be associated with minor hemorrhage, since hemosiderin-laden macrophages are sometimes seen at autopsy. This circumstance increases the risk of using heparin. On the other hand, some patients with fluctuating hemiparesis from atherothrombotic disease of a basilar branch or of the middle cerebral stem lenticulostriate arteries may improve coincident with heparin administration. Most physicians, however, do not use anticoagulation in patients with typical lacunar strokes. Long-term therapy after lacunar stroke requires careful control of hypertension to prevent progression of vascular disease.

OTHER CAUSES OF CEREBRAL INFARCTION

VENOUS THROMBOSIS (Table 351-1) Lateral or sagittal sinus thrombosis or thrombosis of small cortical veins occurs as a complication of sepsis, intracranial infections (meningitis), conditions associated with hypercoagulable states such as polycythemia and sickle cell anemia, or during pregnancy or administration of oral contraceptives. Venous thromboses may cause an increase in intracranial pressure, headaches, focal seizures, and focal neurologic signs affecting the legs more than the arms. Massive venous infarction with secondary edema may be fatal. The CT scan shows hemorrhagic infarction underlying the occluded veins, and may show clot in the posterior sagittal sinus, but the definitive diagnosis is made with angiography.

DISSECTION OF THE CERVICOCEREBRAL ARTERIES Dissection of the large extracranial arteries may cause cerebral infarction, and is a frequent cause of stroke in children and young adults. The dissection divides the media of the vessel or separates the intima from the media. TIAs and infarction occur when the vessel is critically narrowed or occluded or when dissection causes emboli. Trauma, either severe or trivial, accounts for a substantial proportion of cases. Spontaneous dissection also occurs in atheromatous lesions and can occur in association with fibromuscular dysplasia, homocystinuria, or arteritis. The internal carotid artery is the most common site. An oculosympathetic palsy (Horner's syndrome) occurs in over half the cases. A self-audible bruit may appear, and tenderness over the carotid bulb may be present. In carotid dissection, transient monocular blindness or TIAs often precede embolic or "low-flow" watershed infarction, leaving time for therapeutic intervention. When the patient has only oculosympathetic palsy, TIAs, or a minor stroke, anticoagulation with heparin is recommended. Surgical exploration is only considered for patients with increasingly severe TIAs or a mild stroke that is worsening. After the patient's symptoms have stabilized, anticoagulation with warfarin is recommended for 6 months. Repeat angiography often demonstrates a reestablished lumen in the formerly occluded vessel.

Patients with symptomatic vertebral, middle cerebral, or posterior cerebral artery dissection may also be managed in the acute phase with heparin and later with warfarin.

FIBROMUSCULAR DYSPLASIA OF THE CERVICAL VESSELS Fibromuscular dysplasia of the cervical vessels occurs mainly in young women. The carotid or vertebral arteries show multiple rings of segmental narrowing alternating with dilatation. Occlusion is usually incomplete. The process is often asymptomatic, but occasionally is associated with an audible bruit, TIAs, or stroke. Hypertension, if present, may be the result of renal artery stenosis. The cause and natural history of fibromuscular dysplasia is unknown (see Chap. 230). Transient ischemic symptoms or embolic stroke generally occur only when the residual lumen diameter of the narrowed portion of the artery is less than 2 mm. Surgical dilatation of the cervical internal carotid artery is possible in symptomatic cases but is associated with considerable morbidity. Anticoagulation may be more successful than surgery in patients with TIAs of increasing severity.

ARTERITIS Arteritis due to bacterial or syphilitic infection is no longer a common cause of cerebral thrombosis. Other arteritides are rare but can cause cerebral thrombosis (see below and Chaps. 269 and 276). Necrotizing or granulomatous arteritis, occurring alone or in association with generalized polyarteritis nodosa or Wegener's granulomatosis, involves the distal small branches (less than 2-mm-diameter) of the main intracranial arteries and produces small ischemic infarcts in the brain, optic nerve, or spinal cord. The disease, although rare, is relentlessly progressive. The CSF often has cells. In some cases, glucocorticoid therapy (prednisone, 40 to 60 mg/d) has been helpful, and recently, immunosuppressive drugs have been used with some success (see Chap. 276). Idiopathic giant cell arteritis involving the great vessels arising from the aortic arch (Takayasu's syndrome) may, on rare occasions, cause carotid or vertebral thrombosis. It is an infrequent cause of the aortic arch syndrome in the western hemisphere (see Chap. 197).

TEMPORAL ARTERITIS (CRANIAL ARTERITIS) (See Chap. 276) This is a relatively common affliction of elderly persons in which the external carotid system, particularly the temporal arteries, is the site of a subacute granulomatous inflammation with an exudate of lymphocytes, monocytes, neutrophilic leukocytes, and giant cells. Usually the most severely affected parts of the artery become thrombosed. Headache or head pain is the chief complaint. Systemic manifestations include anorexia, loss of weight, malaise, and polymyalgia rheumatica. The inflammatory nature of the illness is indicated by one of the following: fever, slight leukocytosis, increased erythrocyte sedimentation rate, and anemia. Occlusion of branches of the ophthalmic artery results in blindness in one or both eyes in over 25 percent of patients. Occasionally, an ophthalmoplegia due to involvement of ocular nerves occurs. An arteritis of the aorta and its major branches, including carotid, subclavian, coronary, and femoral arteries, has been found at postmortem examination in some cases. Significant inflammatory involvement of intracranial arteries is rare, but strokes occur occasionally on the basis of occlusion of the internal carotid, middle cerebral, or vertebral arteries. The diagnosis depends on the finding of a tender thrombosed or thickened cranial artery and the demonstration of the lesion in a biopsy specimen. Glucocorticoids bring striking subjective relief and often prevent blindness. Prednisone is most often used, beginning with large daily doses of 80 to 120 mg and then tapering after 2 to 4 weeks using the erythrocyte sedimentation rate as a guide.

MOYAMOYA DISEASE Moyamoya disease is a poorly understood occlusive disease involving large intracranial arteries, especially the internal carotid artery and the stem of the middle and anterior cerebral artery. The lenticulostriate arteries develop a rich collateral flow circulation around the middle cerebral occlusive lesion that on cerebral angiography gives the impression of a puff of smoke (*moyamoya*). Other collaterals include transdural anastomoses between the cortical surface branches of the middle cerebral artery and the scalp arteries. The disease mainly occurs in the oriental population, but should be suspected when TIAs or stroke occur in children or young adults. Its etiology is unknown. Few pathologic studies have been made; they suggest that hyalinotic fibrous-type material is associated with the arterial narrowing. Because of the occurrence of subarachnoid hemorrhage from rupture of the transdural anastomotic channels, anticoagulation is not recommended in all symptomatic cases. Extracranial-intracranial (EC/IC) bypass grafting has been recommended in some cases, but its efficacy is not established.

ISCHEMIC DISEASES ASSOCIATED WITH HYPERCOAGULABLE STATE Certain diseases have been associated with ischemic infarction in special clinical circumstances through a mechanism of a hypercoagulable state (see Chaps. 287 and 288). They include polycythemia vera, thrombotic thrombocytopenic purpura, idiopathic thrombocytosis, hyperproteinemia, and sickle cell anemia. Furthermore, circulation of anticardiolipin antibodies ("lupus anticoagulant") has been associated with stroke in young adults, although its relative frequency is controversial. Some cases may be due to cerebral embolism (see below), but others seem to be caused by local arterial thrombosis.

REVERSIBLE CEREBRAL SEGMENTAL VASOCONSTRICTION Reversible, widespread cerebral segmental vasoconstriction has been noted in patients with severe headache and fluctuating neurologic symptoms and signs. Sometimes cerebral infarction has ensued. The cause is unknown. Eclampsia, the postpartum period, head injury, migraine, and sympathomimetic intoxication have all been associated with this entity. Angiography is the only means of establishing the diagnosis. The CSF is normal in most cases but an elevated protein and slight lymphocytic pleocytosis has been found in some cases.

No effective therapy is known. Maintenance of normal systemic arterial pressure or even increasing it modestly with adequate hydration seems important on empiric grounds. Glucocorticoids and vasodilators such as calcium channel blocking agents or intravenous nitroglycerin may be considered.

BINSWANGER'S DISEASE Binswanger's disease (chronic progressive subcortical encephalopathy) is a rare condition in which the subcortical white matter becomes subacutely infarcted. The CT or MRI scan detects periventricular areas of white matter disruption and gliosis. There is lipohyalinosis in the small arteries of the deep white matter, as in hypertension. There are usually associated lacunar or embolic strokes. Binswanger's disease may represent a type of border zone ischemic infarction in the deep white and gray matter between the penetrating arteries of the circle of Willis and of the cortex. Unfortunately, the pathophysiologic basis of the disease remains unknown, and the underlying microvascular pathology may be different in younger patients without hypertension and typical cases in older patients with severe long-standing hypertension. Binswanger's disease is one of the causes of gait disability and abulia in the elderly.

ORAL CONTRACEPTIVE AGENTS Oral contraceptive agents have been associated with an increased incidence of stroke in young women (13.2:100,000 among women who take oral contraceptives compared to 2.8:100,000 among those who do not). In most cases, there is no vascular occlusion on angiography; or if there is occlusion, it is found to have opened later, suggesting embolism as the cause of the stroke. The source of the embolus, however, is uncertain. Pathologic examination has shown that the affected arteries and the heart are normal. Migraine and cigarette smoking have been associated with increased frequency of strokes in young women on oral contraceptives and suggest that hypercoagulability may predispose to thrombosis formation and/or embolization.

CEREBRAL EMBOLISM

PATHOPHYSIOLOGY Cerebral embolism is the most common cause of ischemic stroke. The heart is the most common source of embolic material, with artery-to-artery embolism, usually arising from an atherothrombotic lesion in the carotid or vertebrobasilar system, a somewhat less frequent source (see above). Other causes, such as thrombus in the pulmonary vein, fat emboli, tumor emboli, marantic endocarditis, air emboli, paradoxical emboli, and complications of neck or thoracic surgery (Table 351-1), may occasionally be responsible. Frequently, however, embolic cerebral infarction occurs without an obvious source.

"Unknown source" cerebral embolism poses one of the most perplexing problems in cerebrovascular disease. Patients with hypercoagulability states due to oral contraceptive agents, anticardiolipin antibody, chronic illness, antithrombin 3 deficiency, or metastatic tumor may develop sudden cerebral embolism. In some patients, examination may fail to disclose potential sources of embolism such as the opening snap of mitral stenosis or intermittent atrial fibrillation. Many patients, especially those in the second to fifth decade, suffer sudden embolic strokes that leave no clue to their etiology.

The size, site, and to some extent the pathologic nature of the fragment determines the size, location, and character of the ensuing infarct. Emboli from the heart lodge in the middle cerebral artery or one of its branches 80 percent of the time, in the posterior cerebral artery or its branches 11 percent of the time, and in the vertebral or basilar arteries or the branches in the remainder. Cardiac emboli infrequently go to the anterior cerebral artery. Emboli large enough to occlude the stem of the middle cerebral artery (2 to 3 mm) lead to a large stroke, one that involves both deep gray and white matter as well as the cortical surface and its underlying white matter. A smaller embolus may occlude a small cortical or penetrating arterial branch. Characteristically embolic platelet fibrin clot has a tendency to migrate, lyse, and disperse, accounting for fluctuations in symptoms and, in some cases, complete recovery of the ischemic deficit. The location and size of an infarct also depends on the extent of spared collateral circulation.

Because emboli migrate and lyse, recirculation into the infarcted brain may cause petechial hemorrhages (*hemorrhagic infarction*). On rare occasions, petechial hemorrhages coalesce to form a significant hemorrhagic mass (*hemorrhage into infarction*). This is more likely to occur when the stem of the middle cerebral artery is occluded and large areas of infarction develop before recirculation occurs.

Many types of heart disease, including cardiac arrhythmias or diseases due to cardiac structural abnormalities, may produce cerebral emboli.

Cardiac arrhythmias of all types have been associated with cerebral and systemic embolism. Emboli associated with the sick sinus syndrome and atrial fibrillation are particularly common. There is a high incidence of cerebral embolism associated with atrial fibrillation in patients with rheumatic valvular disease. However, recent studies show that patients with atrial fibrillation from any cause are at risk of embolization. The incidence in patients with atrial fibrillation without valvular disease is estimated at 4 to 7 percent per year, and in most cases, the initial stroke causes severe disability.

Mural thrombus formation with embolism occurs relatively frequently in patients with arteriosclerotic cardiovascular disease and myocardial infarction.

Postsurgery embolization is a high risk in intracardiac surgery and prosthetic valve replacement (Starr-Edwards and Bjork-Shiley valves have been particularly implicated). Thoracic surgery (pulmonary vein embolism) and head-and-neck surgery (aortic or carotid artery-to-artery emboli) have an uncommon but definite association with cerebral embolism. Long bone fracture and thoracic surgery or angiography are associated with cerebral fat embolism and air embolism, both of which give rise to multiple areas of petechial hemorrhage. The principal complication of the use of artificial hearts is cerebral embolism. The overall risk of stroke after any type of general surgery is 0.2 to 1 percent.

Congenital septal defects may give rise to paradoxical embolism. Material (thrombus, tumor, infective or fibrous marantic vegetation) accumulating on a valve or the endocardial surface may become displaced. Vegetations on the aortic and mitral valves from rheumatic or marantic endocarditis are associated with systemic or cerebral emboli and can be diagnosed by a combination of history, physical examination, and laboratory tests. Typically flat vegetations under the mitral and, to a lesser extent, aortic valve leaflets have been noted in patients with systemic lupus erythematosus (Libman-Sacks vegetations). There may give rise to cerebral embolism but more often are a nidus for bacterial endocarditis.

The *vegetations of acute and subacute bacterial endocarditis* give rise to septic embolism (see Chap. 188) and can cause large areas of infarction similar to noninfective embolic infarction if they occlude a major intracranial artery. Alternatively, they may give rise to small septic infarcts with microscopic abscesses. Large brain abscesses, however, are not associated with embolization from subacute bacterial endocarditis. Mycotic aneurysms caused by septic embolism give rise to subarachnoid or intracerebral hemorrhage. Endocarditis should always be considered and ruled out when cerebral embolism is suspected.

Atrial myxoma results in tumor emboli arising from the endocardial surface. Physical signs of pulmonary hypertension or a high erythrocyte sedimentation rate together with signs of systemic illness (fever, malaise) may help in the differential diagnosis. *Mitral valve prolapse* with mural thrombus formation has been associated with cerebral embolism, but insufficient data exist based on the natural history of this abnormality to predict the incidence of recurrent embolism (presumably low). Echocardiography establishes this diagnosis.

CLINICAL MANIFESTATIONS The onset of the neurologic deficit from embolism is sudden and usually maximal. This temporal profile with a neurologic syndrome corresponding to the distribution of a major branch vessel points to cerebral embolism. Sometimes, however, the neurologic deficit may not be complete and after its sudden onset, may fluctuate. The neurologic signs may wax and wane, lasting only a few minutes or hours, then partially or completely disappear, suggesting an embolic TIA, or a mild deficit may progress to complete major infarction over hours. The neurologic deficit corresponds to the cerebral cortex supplied by the arterial territory affected. The resulting deficits resemble those caused by occlusive atheromatous lesions (see sections on atherothrombosis and lacunar stroke). Certain neurologic syndromes strongly suggest embolism as their cause. In the middle cerebral artery territory these include (1) the frontal opercular syndrome, in which there is facial weakness and severe aphasia or dysarthria; (2) the brachial or hand plegia syndrome, in which the arm and hand, or the hand is paralyzed with or without cortical sensory abnormalities; (3) the syndromes of Broca's or Wernicke's aphasia alone, when the dominant hemisphere is involved; or (4) the syndrome of left visual neglect, when the nondominant parietal lobe is involved; (5) a sudden hemianopic field defect, which suggests a posterior cerebral territory embolus; or (6) a sudden foot incoordination or weakness, suggesting an anterior cerebral territory embolus. Sudden gait unsteadiness may suggest a cerebellar embolus. Sudden sleepiness and an inability to look up associated with bilateral ptosis suggests an embolus to the top of the basilar artery, specifically to the artery of Percheron (the small vessel supplying both sides of the medial subthalamus and thalamus arising from the top of the basilar artery).

Seizures following cerebral infarction occur most often after embolic infarction and are not associated with deep white matter lacunar infarction. They are associated with supratentorial cortical surface infarction but are infrequent at the onset and are more often the result of gliotic scar that matures months or more after stroke. Seizures after infarction are rare before 6 months and peak in incidence at 12 to 18 months. Many cases of idiopathic epilepsy in the elderly are probably the result of silent cortical infarction.

LABORATORY EVALUATION Although early CT scanning is usually negative in embolic stroke, it serves to exclude hemorrhage. MRI scanning is better to document the extent and location of the embolic infarction, both supratentorially and infratentorially. Although endocarditis is rarely the cause of cerebral embolism, laboratory evaluation should include a sedimentation rate and blood cultures. Noninvasive carotid studies combined with transcranial Doppler analysis can exclude hemodynamically significant carotid stenosis as the source of emboli if there is any clinical or circumstantial reason to consider this source. Cerebral angiography is considered only when endarterectomy is considered and/or noninvasive tests for significant carotid stenosis have produced equivocal results. Twenty-four hours after cardiogenic cerebral embolism, angiography is often negative, indicating that the embolus has lysed and dispersed. An ECG may show an arrhythmia or myocardial infarction that may have contributed to the source of embolism. Echocardiography or more sophisticated techniques for imaging the ventricular chambers are often used to determine whether a cardiac thrombus was the source of embolism. These techniques are generally insensitive to small clots and are positive in less than 20 percent of patients who have had cerebral emboli. Even after extensive evaluation, including ECG, echocardiography, coagulation studies, etc., the majority of emboli have no evident source.

THERAPY Therapy of patients with embolic cerebral infarction consists of managing the stroke itself, in both the acute and chronic phases, and in preventing further embolic strokes. When cerebral embolism is suspected, the immediate goal is to keep cerebral perfusion in the ischemic area as adequate as possible. The blood pressure should not be lowered even if hypertension is found unless it is malignant hypertension (see Chap. 196). If the blood pressure is low, raising it is probably advisable in the hours after stroke. An excessive rise above normal may, however, aggravate edema formation. Approximately 5 percent or less of patients with middle cerebral artery strokes have enough *secondary cerebral edema* to cause clinical problems. These few patients who are at risk from edema have large regions of low density and slight mass effect on early CT scans, often involving both the middle and anterior cerebral artery territories. Once infarction becomes evident, edema seldom becomes problematic until the second or third day but can then cause mass effect for up to 10 days. Two observations governing the severity of the edema associated with cerebral embolism seem to apply. First, in instances of supratentorial embolic infarction, the larger the area of infarct, the more likely that edema formation will become a problem. Emboli that lodge in the middle cerebral artery stem are much more likely to cause symptomatic edema formation that leads, in a few patients, to coma and death than are emboli in a distal branch of the middle cerebral artery. Second, small amounts of edema formation in the cerebellum following embolic infarction, usually in the territory of the posterior inferior cerebellar artery (inferior cerebellum), can lead to an acute increase in intracranial pressure in the posterior fossa. The resulting compression of the brainstem may result in sudden coma and respiratory arrest requiring emergency surgical decompression. Water restriction and agents that raise the serum osmolarity should be considered early in both instances. Intravenous mannitol is most frequently used to raise the serum osmolality to approximately 300 mosmol/L; it is given as often as every 2 to 4 h. The acute management of artery-to-artery embolus, in either the carotid or vertebral territory, is discussed above (see "Ischemic Cerebrovascular Disease").

When the deficit is large enough to suggest that the embolus has lodged in the middle cerebral artery stem with corresponding infarction of the basal ganglion, deep white matter, and cortical surface, acute anticoagulation with heparin is generally avoided. On rare occasions symptomatic basal ganglion hemorrhage into infarcted tissue occurs. But when the stroke is smaller and involves the cortical surface or when the deficit fluctuates, suggesting partial arterial occlusion, then acute anticoagulation should be considered. For future stroke prevention, chronic anticoagulation with warfarin is general recommended beginning 2 to 5 days after the stroke. A second embolism is rare in the first 3 days. The usual duration of anticoagulation is 6 months or longer if chronic ventricular failure or ventricular aneurysms are present. Lifelong anticoagulation with warfarin may be legitimately instituted in patients who have evidence of recurrent embolism or embolism associated with chronic, intermittent, or sustained atrial fibrillation. Prophylactic anticoagulation for chronic atrial fibrillation without embolism remains controversial. It is the subject of several current randomized, controlled trials.

The appropriate dosage of warfarin has been debated. At the moment, the standard is "low-dose" warfarin (prothrombin time 1.3 to 1.5 times control), the exception being that prothrombin time in patients with prosthetic heart valves and high risk of embolism is often maintained at two times control. The minimal effective antithrombotic warfarin dose has yet to be determined. This determination may require newer, more sensitive methods for monitoring the hemostatic system or more sensitive, uniform thromboplastin reagents.

INTRACRANIAL HEMORRHAGE: GENERAL REMARKS

Of the many causes of nontraumatic intracranial hemorrhage, four are particularly common: deep hypertensive or spontaneous lobar intracerebral hemorrhage, ruptured saccular aneurysm, and bleeding from an arteriovenous malformation. Hemorrhage associated with a bleeding disorder and rupture of a mycotic aneurysm are less common. Rare causes include idiopathic brain purpura, brainstem (Duret) hemorrhages associated with brainstem compression during herniation, and small multifocal hemorrhages associated with hypertensive encephalopathy.

HYPERTENSIVE INTRACEREBRAL HEMORRHAGE

PATHOPHYSIOLOGY Hypertensive hemorrhages typically occur in one of four sites: (1) the putamen and adjacent internal capsule, (2) the thalamus, (3) the pons, and (4) the cerebellum. They rarely originate in the central white matter of the hemispheres. A penetrating artery arising from the middle cerebral artery stem, basilar artery, or circle of Willis is generally the source of hemorrhage, the same vessels that are known to be damaged by hypertension.

The hemorrhage begins as a small oval mass, then spreads by dissection, growing in volume, displacing and compressing adjacent brain tissue. Rupture or seepage into the ventricular system may occur. Primary intraventricular hemorrhage is rare.

Most hypertensive intracerebral hemorrhages develop over a few minutes, but some evolve over 30 to 60 min, and others, particularly those associated with anticoagulant therapy, may evolve for as long as 24 to 38 h. Once bleeding stops, it has generally been thought not to start again, but some larger clots have been shown by sequential CT scanning to have originated as smaller hemorrhages, and it is believed that the frequency of rebleeding or enlargement has been underestimated in the past. Edema in the compressed tissue around the hemorrhage often leads to increasing mass effect and, in some cases, worsening of the clinical state. Within 48 h, macrophages begin to phagocytize the hemorrhage at its outer surface. After 1 to 6 months, the hemorrhage mass is generally resolved to a slitlike orange cavity lined with glial scar tissue and hemosiderin-laden macrophages.

CLINICAL MANIFESTATIONS Hypertensive intracerebral hemorrhages are most common in patients with prolonged sustained hypertension. Although not particularly associated with exertion, intracerebral hemorrhages almost always occur while the patient is awake and sometimes when under stress. Unlike the sudden onset of embolism, these strokes usually evolve over a few minutes, with the neurologic signs and symptoms dependent on the site and size of the extravasation. Vomiting and headache are hallmarks of acute hemorrhages that distinguish them from other strokes. Seizures are uncommon but occur in a few instances.

Putamenal hemorrhage, the most common hypertensive hemorrhage, invariably disrupts the internal capsule adjacent to the basal ganglia. Contralateral hemiplegia is therefore the sentinel sign, but when these hemorrhages are large, the patient may become comatose within a few minutes. In milder cases, over 5 to 30 min, the face sags on one side, speech becomes slurred, the arm and leg gradually weaken, and *the eyes deviate away from the side of the hemiparesis.* The paralysis may worsen until the affected limbs become flaccid or extend rigidly with a Babinski sign on the same side. In the worst case, drowsiness gives way to stupor as signs of upper brainstem compression appear. Coma ensues, accompanied by deep, irregular, or intermittent respiration, a dilated and fixed ipsilateral pupil, bilateral Babinski signs, and decerebrate rigidity. Edema formation in the adjacent brain may cause progressive deterioration over 12 to 72 h.

Thalamic hemorrhages also produce a hemiplegia or hemiparesis from pressure on or dissection through the internal capsule adjacent to the thalamus. A prominent sensory deficit involving all modalities is usually present. Aphasia, often with preserved verbal repetition, may occur after hemorrhage into the dominant (left) thalamus, and apractagnosia or mutism occurs in some cases of nondominant hemorrhage. There also may be a transient homonymous visual field defect. Thalamic hemorrhages cause several typical ocular disturbances by virtue of extension medially into the upper midbrain. These include most characteristically: deviation of the eyes downward and inward, so they appear to be looking at the patient's nose; unequal pupils with absence of light reaction; skew deviation, with the eye opposite the hemorrhage displaced downward and medially; ipsilateral ptosis and miosis (Horner's syndrome); absence of convergence; paralysis of vertical gaze; an assortment of lateral gaze abnormalities (paresis or pseudoparesis of the sixth nerve), and retraction nystagmus.

In *pontine hemorrhages,* deep coma with quadriplegia usually occurs over a few minutes. There is often prominent decerebrate rigidity, and small (1-mm) pupils that react to light. There is impairment of reflex horizontal eye movements evoked by head turning (doll's-head or oculocephalic maneuver) or by irrigation of the ears with cold water (see Chap. 31). Hyperpnea, severe acute hypertension, and hyperhidrosis are common. Death usually occurs within a few hours, but there are exceptions where consciousness is retained because the hemorrhage is limited to the tegmentum.

Cerebellar hemorrhages usually develop over several hours with repeated vomiting and inability to walk or stand. In mild cases there may be no other neurologic signs; therefore it is imperative to test gait. Occipital headache and dizziness or vertigo may be prominent symptoms. There is often paresis of conjugate lateral gaze toward the side of the hemorrhage, forced deviation of the eyes to the opposite side, or an ipsilateral sixth nerve palsy. Other less frequent ocular signs include blepharospasm, involuntary closure of one eye, ocular bobbing, and skew deviation. There may be little or no evidence of the usual signs of cerebellar disease, and only a minority of cases show nystagmus or ataxia of the limbs. A mild ipsilateral facial weakness and a diminished corneal reflex are common. Dysarthria and dysphagia may occur. There are no Babinski signs until late in the evolution of the hemorrhage as it expands to brainstem. As the hours pass, and occasionally with unanticipated suddenness, the patient becomes stuporous, then comatose as a result of brainstem compression, at which point reversal of the syndrome by surgical removal of the clot is seldom successful.

In summary, ocular signs have been highlighted as a method of rapidly localizing hemorrhages. In putamenal hemorrhage, the eyes are deviated to the side opposite the paralysis; in thalamic hemorrhage, the eyes are deviated downward and the pupils may be 3 to 4 mm and unreactive; in pontine hemorrhage, the reflex lateral eye movements are impaired and the pupils are less than 1 mm yet reactive; and in cerebellar hemorrhage, the eyes may be deviated laterally (to the side opposite the lesion) in the absence of paralysis.

LABORATORY EVALUATION The CT scan reliably detects all acute hemorrhages of 1 cm or more in diameter in the cerebral or cerebellar hemispheres. After the first 2 weeks, x-ray attenuation values of clotted blood diminish until they become isodense with surrounding brain. Mass effect and edema may remain. In some cases, a surrounding rim of contrast enhancement appears after 2 to 4 weeks and may persist for months. Small pontine hemorrhages may not be identified because of motion and bone artifact that obscure structures in the posterior fossa. MRI, though more sensitive for delineating posterior fossa lesions, is not necessary in most instances. Proper pulse sequences on MRI can, however, differentiate a hematoma mass from edema. Images of flowing blood on MRI scan may identify arteriovenous malformations as the cause of the hemorrhage. Angiography is used when the etiology of intracranial hemorrhage is uncertain, particularly if the hematoma is not in one of the four usual sites for hypertensive hemorrhage. For example, hemorrhage into the temporal lobe suggests rupture of a middle cerebral artery berry aneurysm. Lumbar puncture carries considerable risk after intracerebral hemorrhage and should generally be avoided unless CT scanning is not available.

THERAPY The size and location of the hematoma determine the treatment and prognosis. Supratentorial hematomas greater than 5 cm in largest diameter generally have a poor prognosis, and infratentorial pontine hematomas greater than 3 cm in size are usually fatal. The occurrence of edema in the week after the intracerebral hemorrhage often worsens the prognosis. The tissue surrounding the hematoma is displaced and compressed but not necessarily infarcted. Hence, in survivors, improvement can result as the hematoma is reabsorbed and the tissue regains its function. Careful management of the patient during the critical acute phase of the cerebral hematoma can lead to considerable recovery.

Surgical removal of an acute supratentorial clot is controversial, but most surgeons have found it necessary on rare occasions. In stuporous patients who still have reflex eye movements and some pupillary reaction, surgery may prevent temporal lobe herniation and irreversible brainstem compression. One important randomized trial has shown a benefit of surgery, though marginal, only in patients in this state. Lifesaving surgery may nonetheless leave major neurologic residua. In contrast, surgical treatment of acute cerebellar hemorrhage is usually recommended because it prevents secondary brainstem compression that is the mechanism of death and it offers an excellent prognosis for recovery. If patients are alert without focal brainstem signs and if the cerebellar hematoma is small, acute surgical removal may not be necessary.

Mannitol and other osmotic agents reduce intracranial pressure that has been raised by the volume of the hematoma and edema (see Chap. 352). Steroids are of uncertain value in curtailing edema from intracerebral hematoma. Monitoring of the intracranial pressure may help to assess medical therapy. Both excessive hypo- and hypertension should be avoided. Toxemia of pregnancy and malignant hypertension associated with acute hemorrhage should be treated cautiously to avoid excessive or precipitous lowering of the blood pressure.

LOBAR INTRACEREBRAL HEMORRHAGE

As control of hypertension in the general population has improved, the relative proportion of hemorrhages outside the basal ganglia and thalamus has increased. These "lobar hemorrhages" appear on CT scan as oval or circular clots in the subcortical white matter. The role of chronic hypertension in their genesis is controversial, but many occur without a history of increased blood pressure. A number of other underlying conditions are found in almost half the cases, the most common being arteriovenous malformation. Others are due to bleeding diathesis, often associated with warfarin administration; hemorrhages into tumor, usually a melanoma or glioma; aneurysms of the circle of Willis that bleed into brain substance; and there are a large number whose causes remain undetermined even after extensive study including arteriography. Many of these are presumed to be from arteriovenous malformations that have become obliterated or are angiographically occult.

Amyloid angiopathy, a cause of both single and recurrent lobar hemorrhages in the elderly, can only be diagnosed by postmortem demonstration that cerebral vessels stain strongly with Congo red. Amyloid is deposited in the walls of the cerebral arteries, but not elsewhere in the body. Patients may have multiple hemorrhages, with months between occurrences.

CLINICAL MANIFESTATIONS The neurologic symptoms and signs of lobar hemorrhage appear suddenly, over one to several minutes. Most lobar hemorrhages are small enough to cause a restricted clinical syndrome that simulates an embolus to a vessel supplying one lobe. For example, the major neurologic deficit of occipital hemorrhage is hemianopsia; of left temporal hemorrhage, aphasia and delirium; of parietal hemorrhage, thalamic-like hemisensory loss; and of frontal hemorrhage, arm weakness. Large hemorrhages may be associated with stupor or coma if they secondarily compress the lower thalamus and midbrain, but the greater distance of lobar clots from these vital structures makes coma result less frequently than putamenal or thalamic hemorrhages.

Most patients with lobar hemorrhages have focal headaches that are attributable to the innervation of adjacent dural vessels: occipital hemorrhage causes pain over the ipsilateral eye; temporal hemorrhage, over the area around or anterior to the ipsilateral ear; frontal hemorrhage, over the forehead or diffusely in the frontal quadrant; and parietal hemorrhage, over the temple region. Stiff neck or seizures are uncommon, but more than half the patients vomit or are initially drowsy.

TREATMENT In awake or drowsy patients, surgical evacuation offers little benefit over medical management with fluid restriction, and osmotic agents. Stuporous or comatose patients who do not respond rapidly to medical therapy for raised intracranial pressure should generally have the clot evacuated.

SUBARACHNOID HEMORRHAGE—SACCULAR ANEURYSM

Rupture of an intracranial saccular aneurysm is the most common cause of subarachnoid hemorrhage, followed by arteriovenous malformation. Although autopsy studies have estimated that 5 percent of the population harbor aneurysms, the incidence of bleeding is about 4:100,000 per year. This devastating disease causes a greater than 10 percent mortality during the first day, and another 25 percent succumb in the first 3 months. Of those who survive, more than half are left with major neurologic deficits as a result of the initial hemorrhage or of a delayed complication, such as rehemorrhage, infarction from cerebral vasospasm, or hydrocephalus. Given these alarming figures, the major therapeutic emphasis should be on preventing the initial rupture and, if rupture occurs, preventing the predictable early complications.

PATHOPHYSIOLOGY Saccular aneurysms occur at the bifurcations of the large arteries at the base of the brain and rupture into the subarachnoid space of the basal cisterns. The common sites of saccular aneurysms include the junction of the anterior communicating artery with the anterior cerebral artery, the junction of the posterior communicating artery and the internal carotid artery, the bifurcation of the middle cerebral artery, the top of the basilar artery, the junction of the basilar artery and the superior cerebellar artery or the anterior inferior cerebellar artery, or the junction of the vertebral artery and the posterior inferior cerebellar artery. Approximately 85 percent of cases occur in the anterior circle of Willis; 10 to 30 percent of patients have multiple aneurysms; 10 to 20 percent occur in bilateral identical locations.

As an aneurysm develops, it often forms a neck with a dome. The length of the neck and the size of the dome, factors that are important in planning microsurgical obliteration, vary greatly. The arterial internal elastic lamina disappears at the base of the neck. The media thins, and connective tissue replaces smooth-muscle cells. At the site of rupture (most often the dome) the wall thins to less than 0.3 mm, and the tear that allows bleeding is often no more than 0.5 mm long.

It is not possible to determine which aneurysms are likely to rupture, but limited data suggest that those larger than 7 mm may warrant prophylactic surgical obliteration.

CLINICAL SYMPTOMS, EVOLUTION, AND MANAGEMENT Prodromal symptoms Prodromal symptoms may suggest the location of an unruptured aneurysm and suggest that it is progressively enlarging. A third nerve palsy, particularly when associated with pupillary dilatation, loss of light reflex, and focal pain above and behind the eye, indicates an expanding aneurysm at the junction of the posterior communicating artery and the internal carotid artery. Prompt surgery is indicated. A sixth nerve palsy may indicate an aneurysm in the cavernous sinus, and visual field defects can occur with an expanding supraclinoid carotid aneurysm. Occipital and posterior cervical pain may signal a posterior inferior cerebellar artery (PICA) or anterior inferior cerebellar artery (AICA) aneurysm. Pain in or behind the eye and in the low temple can occur with an expanding middle cerebral aneurysm.

It is not known for certain if an aneurysm can cause small intermittent bleeding into the subarachnoid space—so-called warning leaks. However, the importance of recognizing the smallest aneurysmal rupture or leak is undeniable. Sudden unexplained headache at any location should raise suspicion of subarachnoid hemorrhage and be investigated by a CT scan to look for blood in the basal cisterns. Often a small subarachnoid hemorrhage will not be seen by CT scan, necessitating a lumbar puncture to detect subarachnoid blood.

Initial clinical presentation: Acute major subarachnoid hemorrhage At the moment of aneurysmal rupture, with major subarachnoid hemorrhage, the intracranial pressure approaches the mean aterial pressure and cerebral perfusion pressure falls. This may account for the sudden transient loss of consciousness that occurs in up to 45 percent of cases. Sudden loss of consciousness may be preceded by a brief moment of excruciating headache, but most patients first complain of headache upon regaining consciousness. In 10 percent of cases, aneurysmal bleeding may be severe enough to cause loss of consciousness for several days. In about 45 percent of cases, severe headache, usually associated with exertion, is the presenting complaint. The headache is often called by the patient "the worst headache of my life." Words like "explode" or "burst" may be used. It may be "all over" or "in the back of the head and neck." Vomiting is a prominent symptom and when coupled with sudden headache should always raise the question of acute subarachnoid hemorrhage.

Although sudden headache in the absence of focal neurologic symptoms is the hallmark of aneurysmal rupture, focal neurologic deficits may occur (in addition to direct cranial nerve compression by the enlarging aneurysm as noted above). Anterior communicating artery aneurysms or middle cerebral bifurcation aneurysms may rupture into the subdural space, into the basal cisterns of the subarachnoid space, or directly into the underlying brain and form a clot large enough to produce a localized mass effect. The common deficits that result include hemiparesis, aphasia, anosognosia (hemineglect), memory loss, and abulia. An unusual acute unilateral hemispheric swelling with associated focal neurologic signs and stupor occurs rarely, immediately following aneurysmal rupture. Transient interruption of the cerebral circulation, possibly from acute vascular spasm, may underlie this complication.

Initial evaluation Over 75 percent of cases have evidence of a subarachnoid clot on a noncontrast CT scan obtained within 72 h of aneurysmal rupture. The extent and location of subarachnoid blood may help locate the underlying aneurysm and identify the cause of the initial neurologic deficit. The clot in the subarachnoid space may also help predict the delayed neurologic deficits due to cerebral vasospasm. *A noncontrast CT scan should be done first because arterial enhancement in the basal cisterns may be mistaken for clotted blood.* A later contrast CT scan may improve the definition of an aneurysm or demonstrate an unsuspected arteriovenous malformation. If the CT scan neither establishes the diagnosis of subarachnoid hemorrhage nor demonstrates a mass lesion or obstructive hydrocephalus, a lumbar puncture should be performed to establish the presence of subarachnoid blood. Lumbar puncture prior to scanning is indicated only if the CT scan is not available at the time of the suspected subarachnoid hemorrhage. MRI scanning may complement (or soon supplement) CT in the initial evaluation, but it is contraindicated postoperatively if metallic surgical clips were used.

Once the diagnosis of subarachnoid hemorrhage from ruptured saccular aneurysm has been established, angiography is generally delayed until just prior to surgery (though the time of surgery is becoming increasingly earlier). Angiography is performed to localize and define the anatomic details of the aneurysm and to determine if there is focal cerebral vasospasm. If an arteriovenous malformation or mycotic aneurysm is suspected because of the location of blood on CT, angiography should be done earlier.

The ECG frequently shows ST-segment and T-wave changes similar to those associated with ischemic coronary heart disease. Prolonged QRS complex, increased QT interval, and prominent "peaked" or deeply inverted symmetric T waves, although suggesting primary cardiac disease, are usually secondary to the intracranial hemorrhage. The cause of these changes is debated, but there is evidence that structural myocardial lesions may occur after acute hemorrhage.

Serum electrolyes are obtained because hyponatremia may develop from urinary sodium loss, possibly due to natriuretic peptides released by the brain or heart.

Initial management Following subarachnoid hemorrhage, a stuporous or comatose patient may have increased intracranial pressure.

Care is required to maintain adequate cerebral perfusion pressure while avoiding excessive elevation of mean arterial pressure. Frequent arterial blood-gas determinations are helpful to assess alveolar ventilation. If hypercapnia exists, mechanically assisted ventilation is necessary. If a subdural or intracerebral hematoma mass is causing neurologic deterioration, its surgical removal and, if feasible, obliteration of the aneurysm are undertaken.

Because rebleeding is possible all patients are put on bed rest in a quiet, preferably darkened room and are given adequate stool softeners to prevent constipation. If headache or neck pain is severe, mild sedation and analgesics are prescribed. Aspirin, an antiplatelet agent, is inappropriate, but acetaminophen, meperidine and phenobarbitol, or other sedatives may be used. Extreme sedation is generally avoided because it can obscure the assessment of initial or delayed neurologic deficits.

Seizures are uncommon at the onset of aneurysmal rupture. The quivering, jerking, and extensor posturing that usually accompany loss of consciousness are probably related to the sharp rise in intracranial pressure. However, phenytoin or phenobarbitol are sometimes given as prophylactic therapy, since a seizure may cause rebleeding.

Glucocorticoids may help reduce the head-and-neck ache caused by the irritative effect of blood in the subarachnoid space, but there is no evidence to suggest they help in treatment of the cerebral edema that is sometimes seen in patients immediately after a subarachnoid hemorrhage, and they are generally omitted.

DELAYED NEUROLOGIC DEFICITS There are three major causes of delayed neurologic deficits: *rerupture, hydrocephalus,* and *cerebral vasospasm.* Recognizing each of these depends upon knowing precisely the cause and character of the initial neurologic findings.

Rerupture The incidence of rerupture in the first 3 weeks following subarachnoid hemorrhage is 10 to 30 percent. Because rerupture is associated with death and poor outcome, numerous clinical investigations of the effects of antifibrinolytic agents have been undertaken. Most have demonstrated a reduced rebleeding rate but also an increased incidence of ischemic stroke, presumably from vasospasm.

In general, when a thick clot is seen in the basal cisterns on the CT scan 24 to 48 h after hemorrhage (see below), symptomatic vasospasm is likely to develop and the use of antifibrinolytic agents is probably inappropriate. On the other hand, minimal or no blood on the initial CT scan or on the 24- to 48-h scan suggests that the blood in the basal cisterns has washed out and that delayed vasospasm is unlikely. Antifibrinolytic therapy may then be considered in selected cases, particularly if surgery is delayed.

Hydrocephalus Acute hydrocephalus can cause stupor and coma and requires emergency ventricular drainage. More often, subacute hydrocephalus over a few days or a few weeks causes progressive drowsiness or abulia with incontinence. Differentiating hydrocephalus from symptomatic cerebral vasospasm in the anterior communicating arteries is often difficult. It may clear spontaneously or require temporary ventricular drainage. Permanent ventricular drainage, if necessary, is usually done at the time of aneurysmal surgery. A chronic hydrocephalus similar to normal-pressure hydrocephalus may appear a few weeks to months after subarachnoid hemorrhage. It may present with gait difficulty, incontinence, or slowed mentation (abulia). The clue to the diagnosis may be a lack of initiative in conversation or a failure to recover independence after the aneurysm has been surgically clipped. Ventricular shunting is the treatment of choice.

Cerebral vasospasm Narrowing of the arteries at the base of the brain following subarachnoid hemorrhage from ruptured saccular aneurysm (*cerebral vasospasm*) can lead to delayed cerebral ischemia and infarction. This *symptomatic cerebral vasospasm* after subarachnoid hemorrhage occurs in approximately 30 percent of patients and is the major cause of delayed morbidity or death. Signs of ischemia usually appear 4 to 14 days after the initial subarachnoid hemorrhage, most frequently at about 7 days. The new deficits may fluctuate and correspond to ischemia in specific arterial territories. The severity and distribution of vasospasm determines whether cerebral infarction will develop.

Clinical evidence suggests that the extent and location of clotted blood on CT scans can be used to predict the incidence, location, and severity of cerebral vasospasm in patients after subarachnoid hemorrhage. A high incidence of symptomatic cerebral vasospasm in the middle and anterior cerebral artery territories has been found in patients with early CT scans showing globular subarachnoid clots larger than 5×3 mm in the basal cisterns, or layers of blood 1 mm thick or greater in the cerebral fissures. CT scans less reliably predict vasospasm in the vertebral, basilar, or posterior cerebral arteries. The CT scan should be obtained between 24 and 96 h following subarachnoid hemorrhage since blood present initially can disappear or "wash out" on a scan obtained after 24 h. With the further passage of time, x-ray attenuation values of clotted blood diminish so that its full extent and location may not be reliably detected after 96 h.

Cerebral vasospasm is a local phenomenon related to the presence of blood in the cerebrospinal fluid, surrounding a basal vessel. Its cause is unknown. Laboratory studies have suggested that substances such as serotonin, prostaglandins, and catecholamines can produce arterial narrowing. However, all these compounds break down rapidly in vivo, and only large amounts produce spasm in vitro. More sustained arterial vasospasm has been produced by experiments with incubated whole blood and erythrocyte breakdown products. The best current hypothesis suggests that a clot encases the artery; then after a few days spasmogenic hemoglobin breakdown products induce spasm. Once the vessel is in spasm, high-energy phosphate metabolism becomes impaired, because the surrounding clot prevents cerebrospinal fluid from nourishing the vessels. Vasa vasorum are not present in the vessels at the base of the brain or over the cortical surface. The reduction in local ATP may prevent the artery from relaxing.

CLINICAL SYNDROMES   Symptomatic severe cerebral vasospasm presents with symptoms referable to the specific arterial territories involved. For example, spasm of the middle cerebral stem or its main branches causes contralateral hemiparesis, dysphasia (dominant hemisphere), anosognosia, or apractagnosia (nondominant hemisphere). Even severe vasospasm may not produce ischemic symptoms if sufficient collateral blood flow develops through border zone anastomotic channels (Fig. 351-1A). Proximal anterior cerebral artery vasospasm is associated with abulia and incontinence while severe vasospasm of the posterior cerebral artery is associated with hemianopic visual field defects. Severe spasm of the basilar or vertebral arteries occasionally produces focal brainstem ischemia. All of these focal neurologic symptoms may develop over a few days, fluctuate, or present abruptly.

TREATMENT   Therapeutic efforts to prevent or treat symptomatic cerebral vasospasm have been universally disappointing. The failure to find a satisfactory therapy for cerebral vasospasm has prompted a search for prophylactic measures to prevent or minimize its occurrence. Treatment with the calcium channel blocking agent nimodipine has been reported in several studies to have beneficial effects, but patients in both the treated and untreated groups developed symptomatic vasospasm.

The most commonly accepted form of therapy for symptomatic cerebral vasospasm is to increase the cerebral perfusion pressure by raising mean arterial pressure through plasma volume expansion and the judicious use of pressor agents, ordinarily phenylephrine or dopamine. Raised perfusion pressure has been associated with symptomatic improvement in some patients, but high arterial pressure may risk rebleeding. The therapies generally require monitoring the central venous pressure, arterial pressure, and, in severe cases, the intracranial and pulmonary artery wedge pressure. Angioplasty is currently under investigation.

Severe cerebral edema in patients with infarction from vasospasm may increase the intracranial pressure enough to reduce cerebral perfusion pressure. Treatment, as outlined in Chap. 352, is with mannitol and hyperventilation. Plasma osmolality is usually raised to approximately 300 mosmol/L. As a last resort, barbiturate-induced coma has been used to reduce intracranial pressure in some patients; it has not been proven to improve outcome.

Surgical treatment of saccular aneurysms   The advent of the operating microscope has made microsurgical obliteration of a ruptured aneurysm a safe and effective means of preventing disastrous rerupture. Some neurosurgeons delay surgery for at least 10 to 14 days, although the trend has been toward earlier surgery. Operation is undertaken when the patient is clinically stable. Delayed surgery allows cerebral swelling from the initial rupture time to resolve and minimizes the risk of symptomatic vasospasm in the postoperative period.

The wisdom of delaying surgery has been questioned, especially if the patient is neurologically intact. Surgery within the first 48 h eliminates the problem of rebleeding, can remove potentially spasmogenic clots from the basal cisterns, theoretically preventing vasospasm, and allows volume expansion or hypertensive therapy for vasospasm to be conducted without the risk of rebleeding. While it is technically possible to remove local clots and obliterate aneurysms early, some subarachnoid clots are too extensive for safe, complete removal. The timing of aneurysm surgery, still controversial, should therefore be tailored to the individual patient. Intravascular catheter techniques to obliterate aneurysms are investigational but may have a role in management of aneurysms considered to have a high surgical risk.

Giant aneurysms   Giant aneurysms larger than 2 cm in diameter occur at the same sites as small aneurysms. The three most common locations are the intracranial internal carotid, middle cerebral bifurcation, and top of the basilar arteries. Although they can bleed, they usually cause symptoms by compressing the adjacent brain or cranial nerves. Edema formation in the compressed brain can be relentless, compounding the mass effect. It is resistant to treatment and may be fatal. This progression is particularly likely if a giant aneurysm occurs at the bifurcation of the middle cerebral artery. Surgical decompression, until recently was the only adequate therapy. It is extremely difficult technically and carries a high morbidity in the presence of edema. Newer interventional neuroradiologic procedures may prove helpful (see Chap. 348).

Mycotic aneurysms   Mycotic aneurysms are located distal to the first bifurcation of major arteries of the circle of Willis. Emboli from bacterial endocarditis should be suspected and appropriate blood cultures taken. Because of their distal location in the arterial tree they rarely leave significant amounts of clotted blood in the basal cisterns, and severe cerebral vasospasm is infrequent. Mycotic aneurysms, however, are subject to rerupture. Although antibiotic therapy may reduce this risk, surgical obliteration remains the definitive treatment.

OTHER CAUSES OF INTRACRANIAL HEMORRHAGE

ARTERIOVENOUS MALFORMATION   An angioma, or hemangioma, consists of a tangle of abnormal vessels forming an abnormal communication between the arterial and venous systems. Most are developmental arteriovenous fistulas in which the constituent vessels enlarge and grow with the passage of time. Angiomas vary in size from a small blemish a few millimeters in diameter to a huge mass of tortuous channels composing an arteriovenous shunt of sufficient magnitude to raise the cardiac output. Hypertrophic dilated arterial "feeders" approach the main lesion, disappear below the cortex, and break up into a network of thin-walled blood vessels which connect directly with draining veins. These often form huge, dilated, pulsating channels, carrying away arterial blood. The blood vessels forming the tangle interposed between arteries and veins are usually abnormally thin and do not have a normal structure. Angiomas occur in all parts of the brain, brainstem, and spinal cord, but the larger ones are most frequently in the posterior half of the hemispheres, commonly forming a wedge-shaped lesion extending from the cortex to the ventricular lining.

Angiomas are more frequent in men and may occur in more than one member of a family in the same or successive generations. Although the lesion is present from birth, bleeding or other complaints are most common between the ages of 10 and 30, occasionally as late as the fifties.

The chief clinical symptoms and signs are headache, seizures, and those associated with rupture. When headache occurs (without bleeding), it may be hemicranial and throbbing, like migraine, or diffuse. There may be hemiplegia with headache, resembling hemiplegic migraines. Focal seizures that become generalized occur in about 30 percent of cases and are usually well managed with anticonvulsants. In half of cases, arteriovenous malformations become evident as intracerebral hemorrhages. In most of these cases, the hemorrhage is mainly intraparenchymal with a small amount of spillage into the subarachnoid space. Blood is usually not deposited in the basal cistern, and symptomatic cerebral vasospasm is therefore rare. The threat of rerupture in the first 3 weeks is low, so that there is no need to consider the use of antifibrinolytic agents. The hemorrhage may be massive, leading to death acutely, or may be as small as 1 cm in diameter, leading to minor focal symptoms or no deficit. In either case, the hemorrhagic mass may compress the arteriovenous malformation so completely that angiography cannot detect the malformation. Hence, when arteriovenous malformation (AVM) is suspected, angiography is best postponed until the hematoma has completely resolved, i.e., after 6 to 8 weeks. Rarely the angioma is large enough to steal blood away from adjacent normal brain tissue, rendering the surrounding brain ischemic. This deprivation is most often seen when large AVMs in the middle cerebral–posterior cerebral system or middle cerebral–anterior cerebral system extend from the cortical surface to the ventricular system. Hydrocephalus may result when the vein of Galen enlarges as a channel for drainage from the AVM.

Large AVMs of the carotid–middle cerebral system may be associated with a systolic and diastolic bruit (sometimes self-audible) over the eye, forehead, or neck where a bounding, forceful carotid pulse may be perceived. Headache at the onset of AVM rupture is not as prominent or as common as it is with a ruptured saccular aneurysm. Contrast CT scan can often detect the channels of an AVM prior to rupture; newer MRI techniques may prove more sensitive.

Although many AVMs eventually rupture, definitive surgical therapy is usually reserved until after the first episode of hemorrhage; the threat of rerupture is 3 percent per year thereafter. When surgery is not feasible because of the location and size of AVMs, other therapeutic options being evaluated include endovascular embolization and proton beam irradiation.

TRAUMA Head injury can result in intracerebral (especially temporal lobe and inferior frontal) hematoma and infratentorial hematomas, subarachnoid bleeding, acute and chronic subdural hematoma formation, and acute epidural hematoma formation. Trauma must be considered in any patient with an unexplained acute neurologic deficit (hemiparesis, stupor, or confusion), particularly if the deficit occurred in the context of a fall. These entities and their distinction from spontaneous hemorrhage are discussed more fully in Chap. 352.

HEMATOLOGIC DISORDERS Intracerebral hemorrhage associated with hematologic disorders (leukemia, aplastic anemia, thrombocytopenic purpura) can occur at any intracranial site and may present as multiple intracerebral hemorrhages. Skin and mucous membrane bleeding is usually evident and offers a diagnostic clue. Intracerebral hemorrhage associated with anticoagulant therapy can occur at any location, often lobar, and may evolve slowly over 24 to 48 h. Fresh frozen plasma and vitamin K are usually given immediately. When intracerebral hemorrhage is associated with aspirin, fresh platelet transfusions may be required.

BRAIN TUMORS Hemorrhage into a brain tumor may be the first manifestation of neoplasm. Choriocarcinoma, malignant melanoma, renal cell carcinoma, and bronchogenic carcinoma are among the most common metastatic tumors associated with intracerebral hemorrhage. Glioblastoma multiforme in adults and medulloblastoma in children may also have areas of intracerebral hemorrhage.

OTHER CAUSES Primary intraventricular hemorrhage is rare. It usually begins intraparenchymally and dissects into the ventricular system without leaving signs of intraparenchymal hemorrhage. Sepsis can cause small petechial hemorrhages through the cerebral white matter. There is no blood in the spinal fluid, and this condition should not be confused with a stroke. Inflammatory disease of the arteries and veins, especially polyarteritis nodosa and lupus erythematosus, can produce hemorrhage into the central nervous system. Most of the time it is associated with hypertension. An intensely inflammatory and hemorrhagic white matter process termed *Hurst's hemorrhagic leukoencephalitis* is probably a type of hyperacute multiple sclerosis. Moyamoya, mainly an obliterative disease that causes ischemic symptoms, may also have multiple small aneuysms that rupture in a small percentage of patients. Hemorrhages into the spinal cord are usually the result of an AVM or metastatic tumor. Epidural spinal hemorrhage usually compresses the cord rapidly and produces a transverse myelopathy (see Chap. 361).

HYPERTENSIVE ENCEPHALOPATHY (See Chap. 196)

In this acute syndrome, severe hypertension is associated with headache, nausea, vomiting, convulsions, confusion, stupor, and coma. Focal or lateralizing neurologic signs, either transitory or lasting, may occur but are infrequent and always suggest some other form of vascular disease (hemorrhage, embolism, or atherosclerotic thrombosis). By the time neurologic manifestations appear, the hypertension has usually reached the malignant state, with retinal hemorrhages, exudates, papilledema (hypertensive retinopathy grade IV), and evidence of renal and cardiac disease. In many, but not all, cases the cerebrospinal fluid pressure and the protein values are both elevated. The hypertension may be essential or due to chronic renal disease, acute glomerulonephritis, acute toxemia of pregnancy, pheochromocytoma, Cushing's syndrome, or ACTH toxicity. Lowering of the blood pressure with hypotensive drugs may reverse the process in several days if permanent damage is not severe. Neuropathologic examination may reveal a cerebral swelling or hemorrhages of various sizes from massive to petechial. A cerebellar pressure cone reflects increased pressure in the posterior fossa, and in some instances lumbar puncture has been fatal. Microscopically there are small hemorrhages, clusters of microglial cells, minute cerebral infarcts, and necrosis of arterioles.

The term *hypertensive encephalopathy* should be reserved for this syndrome and not for chronic recurrent headaches, dizziness, epileptic seizures, recurrent TIAs, or small strokes, which often occur in association with high blood pressure.

REFERENCES

AUSMAN JI et al: Vertebrobasilar insufficiency: A review. Arch Neurol 42:803, 1985

BAUER KA, ROSENBERG RD: The pathophysiology of the prethrombotic state in humans: Insights gained from studies using markers of hemostatic system activation. Blood 70:343, 1987

BOUGHNER DR, BARNETT HJM: The enigma of the risk of stroke in mitral valve prolapse. Stroke 16:175, 1985

BOUSSER MG et al: "AICLA" controlled trial of aspirin and dipyridamole in the secondary prevention of athero-thrombotic cerebral ischemia. Stroke 14:5, 1983

CALL G et al: Correlation of continuous-wave Doppler spectral flow analysis with gross pathology in carotid stenosis. Stroke 19:584, 1988

CANADIAN COOPERATIVE STUDY GROUP: A randomized trial of aspirin and sulfinpyrazone in threatened stroke. N Engl J Med 299:53, 1978

CAPLAN LR: "Top of the basilar" syndrome. Neurology 30:72, 1980

CEREBRAL EMBOLISM STUDY GROUP: Immediate anticoagulation of embolic stroke: Brain hemorrhage and management options. Stroke 15:779, 1984

CHAMBERS BR et al: Outcome in patients with asymptomatic neck bruits. N Engl J Med 315:860, 1986

EC/IC BYPASS STUDY GROUP: Failure of extracranial-intracranial arterial bypass to reduce the risk of ischemic stroke: Results of an international randomized trial. N Engl J Med 313:1191, 1985

FISHER CM: Occlusion of the internal carotid artery. Arch Neurol Psychiatry 65:346, 1951

——— et al: Lateral medullary infarction: The pattern of vascular occlusion. J Neuropathol Exp Neurol 20:323, 1961

——— et al: The arterial lesions underlying lacunes. Acta Neuropathol (Berl) 12:1, 1969

———: Clinical syndromes in cerebral thrombosis, hypertensive hemorrhage, and ruptured saccular aneurysm. Clin Neurosurg 22:117, 1975

——— et al: Atherosclerosis of the carotid and vertebral arteries—extracranial and intracranial. J Neuropathol Exp Neurol 24:455, 1965

——— et al: Cerebral vasospasm with ruptured saccular aneurysm: The clinical manifestations. Neurosurg 1:245, 1977

——— et al: Spontaneous dissection of cervico-cerebral arteries. Can J Neurol Sci 5:9, 1978

——— et al: The correlation of cerebral vasospasm and the amount of subarachnoid blood detected by computerized cranial tomography after ruptured aneurysm. Neurosurg 6:1, 1980

———: Late-life migraine accompaniments as a cause of unexplained transient ischemic attacks. Can J Neurol Sci 7:9, 1980

———: Lacunar strokes and infarcts: A review. Neurology 32:871, 1982

HINTON RC et al: Influence of etiology of atrial fibrillation on incidence of systemic embolism. Am J Cardiol 40:509, 1977

——— et al: Symptomatic middle artery stenosis. Ann Neurol 5:152, 1979

HIRSH J et al: Optimal therapeutic range for oral anticoagulants. Chest (Suppl) 95(2):5s, 1989

KISTLER JP: Cardiac embolic cerebrovascular disease. Primary Care 6:745, 1979

——— et al: Vertebral basilar territory stroke. Delineation by proton nuclear magnetic resonance imaging. Stroke 15:417, 1984

——— et al: Therapy of ischemic cerebral vascular disease due to atherothrombosis. N Engl J Med 311:27, 100, 1984

MOHR JP: Valvular disease, cardiac arrest, systemic hypotension, and cardiac surgery, in Handbook of Clinical Neurology, GW Bruyn, PJ Vinken (eds). Amsterdam, North-Holland, 1978

——— et al: The Harvard Cooperative Stroke Registry: A prospective registry. Neurology 28:754, 1978

———: Lacunes. Stroke 13:3, 1982

PHILLIPS SJ: An alternative view of heparin anticoagulation in acute focal brain ischemia. Stroke 20:295, 1989

ROPPER AH, DAVIS KR: Lobar cerebral hemorrhages: Acute clinical syndromes in 26 patients. Ann Neurol 8:141, 1980

WELIN L et al: Analysis of risk factors for stroke in a cohort of men born in 1913. N Engl J Med 317:521, 1987

WILKINS RH: Natural history of intracranial vascular malformation: A review. Neurosurg 16:421, 1985

WOLF PA et al: Atrial fibrillation, a major contributor to stroke in the elderly: The Framingham study. Arch Intern Med 147:1561, 1987

352   TRAUMA OF THE HEAD AND SPINAL CORD

ALLAN H. ROPPER

Head injuries are frequent in industrialized countries, affecting many patients in the prime of life. To appreciate the medical and social magnitude of this problem it needs only to be recognized that almost 10 million Americans have head injuries yearly, about 20 percent serious enough to cause brain damage. Among men under 35 years old, accidents, usually motor vehicle collisions, are the chief cause of death, and over 70 percent of these involve head injury. Minor head injuries are so common that almost all physicians encounter patients requiring immediate care or suffering from various sequelae. Traumatic spinal cord injuries often occur in conjunction with head injury. The two are best considered together in the context of trauma to the nervous system.

In the past two decades, declining mortality from head and spinal cord injuries can be attributed mainly to public health measures, such as use of seat belts and motorcycle helmets, and the development of ambulance systems with trained personnel. A systematic approach to the evaluation of patients with head and spine trauma, beginning at the scene of the accident, has improved outcome. An understanding of the pathologic lesions produced by trauma is essential for diagnosis and to provide a framework for management.

TYPES OF HEAD INJURIES

SKULL FRACTURES   A blow to the skull causes fractures if the elastic tolerance of the bone is exceeded. Significant intracranial lesions accompany two-thirds of skull fractures, and the presence of a skull fracture increases manyfold the chances of an underlying subdural or epidural hematoma. Consequently, fractures assume importance primarily as markers of the site and severity of injury. They also cause cranial nerve injuries and produce entry pathways to the cerebrospinal fluid (CSF) for bacteria (meningitis) and air (pneumocephalus), or for leakage of CSF. Fractures are classified as linear, basilar, compound, or depressed; linear fractures account for 80 percent of all skull fractures and are most often associated with subdural or epidural hematomas. Linear fractures usually extend from the point of impact toward the base of the skull.

Basilar skull fractures are often extensions of adjacent fractures over the convexity of the skull but may occur independently due to stresses on the floor of the middle cranial fossa or occiput. They are usually located parallel to the petrous bone or along the sphenoid bone toward the sella turcica and ethmoidal groove. Most are uncomplicated, but they may cause CSF leak, pneumocephalus, or cavernous-carotid fistula. Fractures of the basal skull bones are often accompanied by signs of hemotympanum (blood behind the tympanic membrane), delayed ecchymosis over the mastoid process (Battle's sign), or periorbital ecchymosis ("racoon sign"). Because routine x-ray examination can fail to disclose basilar fractures, they should be suspected in the presence of these clinical signs. Cerebrospinal fluid may also leak through the cribriform plate or the adjacent sinus and present as a watery discharge from the nose (CSF rhinorrhea). Persistence of rhinorrhea or recurrent meningitis is an indication for a surgical repair of torn dura underlying the fracture. The site of the leak is often difficult to determine, but useful diagnostic tests include metrizamide instillation into the CSF with subsequent computed tomography (CT) scans, or radionuclide or fluorescein injection into the CSF followed by assessment of uptake by absorptive nasal pledgets. The site of intermittent leaks is rarely delineated; most resolve spontaneously. Sellar fractures can also be radiologically occult, although they are sometimes associated with serious neuroendocrine dysfunction. Occasionally, fractures of the dorsum sella cause sixth or seventh nerve palsies or optic nerve damage. An air-fluid level in the sphenoid sinus suggests a fracture of the sellar floor.

About 20 percent of petrous bone fractures, usually along the long axis of the bone, are associated with facial palsy. Disruption of ear ossicles and CSF otorrhea are other complications. Transverse petrous fractures are less common, almost always damaging the cochlea or labyrinths and often the facial nerve. External bleeding from the ear can result from petrous bone fractures, though local laceration of the external canal from abrasions is more common. Frontal bone fractures are often depressed, involving the frontal and paranasal sinuses and the orbits; anosmia frequently follows if the olfactory filaments in the cribriform plate are disrupted.

Depressed skull fractures are often compound but are commonly asymptomatic, except for amnesia due to concussions, because the impact energy is dissipated in breaking the bone. Some cause brain contusions and focal neurologic signs appropriate to the underlying cortical area. Surgical repair and bone elevation with exploration of the dura is required in most cases. Delayed or incomplete debridement of the wound leads to a high incidence of infection. If the skin is lacerated over a skull fracture and the underlying meninges are torn, or if the fracture passes through the posterior wall of a nasal sinus, bacteria or air may enter the cranial cavity resulting in meningitis, abscess formation, or pneumocephalus.

CRANIAL NERVE INJURIES   Cranial nerves liable to injury with basilar skull fractures are the olfactory, optic, oculomotor, trochlear, first and second branches of the trigeminal, facial, and auditory. Anosmia and an apparent loss of taste (actually a loss of perception of aromatic flavors, with elementary tastes retained) occurs in approximately 10 percent of serious head injuries, particularly with falls on the back of the head. This results from displacement of the brain and shearing of the olfactory nerve filaments. Recovery usually occurs with residual hyposmia, but if bilateral anosmia persists for several months, the prognosis is poor. Fractures of the sphenoid bone may bruise or transect the optic nerve, resulting in unilateral partial or complete blindness, and an unreactive pupil usually equal in size to the other side, with a preserved consensual light response. Partial optic nerve injuries from closed trauma result in blurring of vision, central or paracentral scotomas, or sector defects. Prognosis for recovery of vision varies widely. Direct orbital injury may cause short-lived blurred vision for close objects because of reversible iridoplegia. Oculomotor nerve injury causes the globe to turn outward with loss of adduction and vertical movement and a fixed dilated pupil; vision is preserved. Diplopia only on looking down, which suggests trochlear nerve damage from fracture of the lesser sphenoid wing, is not uncommon as an isolated problem from minor injury and may be delayed in appearance for several days. Patients report correction of the diplopia by tilting the head away from the affected eye. Direct facial nerve injury by a basal fracture is present immediately in 3 percent of severe injuries or may also be delayed 5 to 7 days. Petrous fractures, particularly the less common transverse type, are liable to produce this injury. Delayed facial palsy has a good prognosis; its mechanism is not known. Injury to the eighth cranial nerve with fractures of the petrous bone causes loss of hearing, vertigo, and nystagmus immediately after injury; the nystagmus is frequently positional. Deafness due to nerve injury must be distinguished from rupture of the eardrum, blood in the middle ear, or disruption of the ossicles from fracture through the middle ear. A high-tone hearing loss occurs with direct cochlear concussion.

CONCUSSION Concussion refers to an immediate but transient loss of consciousness often described as dazed or "star-struck" and associated with a short period of amnesia. It typically occurs after blunt impact or deceleration of the frontal or occipital areas that creates sudden movement of the brain within the skull. In severe cases, a brief convulsion, or autonomic symptoms and signs such as facial pallor, bradycardia, faintness with mild hypotension, or sluggish pupillary reaction may occur, but most patients are neurologically normal. Higher primates are particularly susceptible to concussion; in contrast, billy goats, rams, and woodpeckers can tolerate impact velocity and deceleration a hundred times greater than that experienced by humans. The mechanism of loss of consciousness in concussion is believed to be transient electrophysiologic dysfunction of the reticular activating system in the upper midbrain caused by rotation of the cerebral hemispheres on the relatively fixed brainstem. The mechanism of the associated amnesia is not known. Gross and light microscopic changes in the brain are usually absent after concussion, but biochemical and ultrastructural changes such as mitochondrial ATP depletion and local disruption of the blood-brain barrier suggest that complex abnormalities occur. The CT and MRI scans are normal, and there are usually no red blood cells in the CSF as occurs with more severe injuries. Approximately 3 percent of patients who have sustained concussions will have an intracranial hemorrhage (subdural, epidural, or parenchymal), but the presence of a skull fracture increases the risk manyfold.

Amnesia after concussion typically follows a few moments of unresponsiveness after impact. Rarely there is no loss of consciousness. The memory loss spans the time of, and moments before, mild impact injuries but may encompass previous weeks (rarely months) in more severe trauma. Any anterograde amnesia is usually brief and disappears rapidly in alert patients. The extent of retrograde amnesia has been suggested as a coarse measure of the severity of injury. Improvement usually occurs in an orderly progression from most distant to recent memories, with islands of amnesia occasionally remaining in severe cases. Hysterical posttraumatic amnesia is not uncommon. It should be suspected when abnormalities of behavior occur, such as a tendency to recount events that cannot be recalled on later testing, bizarre affect, a person forgetting his or her own name, disproportionate or selective memory loss, or exaggerated anterograde deficit in comparison to the degree of injury.

A single uncomplicated head injury has not been shown to produce permanent neurobehavioral changes in most patients who are free of preexisting psychiatric problems and substance abuse. In some patients, however, there has been increasing attention to minor problems in memory and concentration that may have an anatomical correlate in small shearing lesions (see below).

CONTUSION, BRAIN HEMORRHAGES, AND SHEARING LESIONS Hemispheral lesions Contusions on the surface of the brain and deeper hemorrhages result from mechanical forces that move the hemispheres relative to the skull. Deceleration of the brain against the inner skull causes contusions, either under a point of impact (coup lesion) or in the antipolar area (contrecoup lesion). Trauma sufficient to cause prolonged unconsciousness beyond concussion usually produces contusions varying from small superficial cortical petechiae to hemorrhagic and necrotic destruction of large portions of a hemisphere. Because the motion of the hemispheres brings them into contact with the prominences of the sphenoid and other frontal basal bones, blunt impact, as from an automobile dashboard, typically causes contusions on the orbital surfaces of the frontal lobes and the anterior and basal portions of the temporal lobes. The anterior corpus callosum may also be bruised from striking the falx. With lateral forces, as from the doorframe of a car, contusions occur on the convexity of the hemispheres.

Contusions are visible on CT scan, appearing early as smudged hyperlucencies from scattered cortical and subcortical blood and a mass that distorts adjacent structures, most prominently the lateral ventricles. After several hours the surrounding edematous tissue appears as a ring of lower density. Confluent, roughly spherical contusions can be distinguished from spontaneous cerebral hemorrhages because the former characteristically extend to the cortical surface. After a week some contusions have a surrounding ringlike contrast-enhancing density that may be mistaken for tumor or abscess. Glial and macrophage reactions begin within 2 days, years later resulting in scarred hemosiderin-stained depressions on the surface (*plaques jaune*) that are one source of posttraumatic epilepsy. Large single hemorrhages after minor trauma are found in patients with a bleeding diathesis or in the elderly, sometimes related to cerebrovascular amyloidosis.

The clinical signs produced by contusions vary with their location and size; most often a hemiparesis or gaze preference is seen, similar to a middle cerebral artery stroke. Bilateral large contusions produce coma with extensor posturing; when contusions are limited to the frontal lobes, an abulic-taciturn state or inappropriate jocularity and indifference occur. Contusions of the temporal lobes cause an aggressive combative syndrome, described below. With large contusions the secondary effect of progressive edema is the most threatening aspect of the injury. Coma and signs of secondary brainstem compression (pupillary enlargement) then dominate the examination. Seizures soon after trauma are rare with contusions, as indeed they are for several weeks after most acute head injuries.

Deep hemorrhages in the central white matter may result from confluent contusions in the depths of a sulcus. However, ganglionic, diencephalic, and other deep hematomas due to torsion or shearing forces in the brain often occur independently of surface damage. The areas around these hematomas may become edematous, resulting in enlargement of the affected region and progressively raised intracranial pressure.

Another type of white matter, or "shearing," lesion consists pathologically of widespread acute disruption of axons. Axonal shearing occurs at, or soon after, impact. The affected areas of white matter are replaced with glial proliferation over a period of several months. There are characteristically small areas of tissue disruption in the corpus callosum and dorsolateral pons. Widespread axonal shearing lesions in the deep white matter of both hemispheres may explain persistent coma or vegetative state, but small hemorrhages in the midbrain and diencephalon are as often the cause. Shearing lesions are not usually visualized by CT scanning, but in severe cases small hemorrhages of the corpus callosum and centrum semiovale are seen.

On occasion, head trauma causes diffuse brain swelling within a few hours after injury. Most instances are due to widespread contusion though CT scanning fails to reveal significant focal lesions or hemorrhage. The edema creates a mass effect with disastrous consequences. This problem is encountered in children and young adults who may develop a virtually instantaneous generalized edema probably due to microvascular disruption, hypertension, and greatly increased cerebral blood flow.

Deep cerebral hemorrhages may occur several days after severe injury. Sudden neurologic deterioration, often in already comatose patients, or a sustained and unexplained rise in intracranial pressure should prompt a CT scan to detect delayed hemorrhage.

Brainstem hemorrhages   A syndrome with coma, midposition or larger pupils unreactive to light, and impaired or absent oculocephalic reflex eye movements results from small linear or oval-shaped hemorrhages in the high midbrain, visible on CT scan, though often delayed in appearance. Though extensor posturing occurs with stimulation, the limbs are otherwise flaccid. This clinical syndrome should be suspected even in the initial absence of a hemorrhage on CT scan. These acute midbrain hemorrhages may be the result of primary injury from rotational forces in the upper midbrain. They also occur from secondary compression of the brainstem by supratentorial hematomas and lateral tissue shifts or pressure from the adjacent temporal lobes. Magnetic resonance image (MRI) scanning shows many other small brainstem and hemispheric white matter lesions that are related to mechanical disruption of tissue, similar to shearing. In pathologic material from severe, acutely fatal injuries, small linear and oval hemorrhages are found in the low thalamic and subthalamic regions and throughout the midline of the brainstem (termed *Duret hemorrhages*).

Residual symptoms and signs of primary or secondary brainstem hemorrhages or ischemic lesions include tremor, pupillary enlargement, eye movement abnormalities, or the "locked-in" syndrome (see Chap. 31). Midbrain or diencephalic hemorrhages are the only well-defined traumatic brainstem lesions responsible for coma. Most other cases of coma without fixed pupils and unexplained by CT scan are probably due to diffuse axonal shearing injuries in the cerebral hemispheres.

SUBDURAL AND EPIDURAL HEMATOMAS   In severe head injury, hemorrhages beneath the dura (subdural) or between the dura and skull (epidural) may be combined with contusions and other injuries, making it difficult to determine their relative contribution to the clinical state. However, subdural and epidural hematomas often occur as the primary lesion, each with a characteristic clinical and radiologic appearance. Because the mass effect of the hemorrhage and rise in intracranial pressure may be life-threatening, it is important to make an immediate diagnosis by CT scanning and carry out surgical evacuation.

Acute subdural hematoma   Acute subdural hematomas become symptomatic in minutes to hours after injury. Up to one-third of patients have a lucid interval before coma supervenes, but the majority are drowsy or comatose from the moment of injury. Arousable patients complain of unilateral headache and frequently have a slightly enlarged pupil on that side. Stupor or coma with unilateral pupillary enlargement are the major signs in larger hematomas. Pupillary dilation is ipsilateral in most, but 5 to 10 percent are contralateral to the hematoma. Lateralizing signs such as a hemiparesis are helpful in only a few patients and may be ipsilateral to the clot. Acute seizures or isolated hemianopsias are uncommon. The CT scan shows the clot, allowing early evacuation. MRI scans may fail to demonstrate an acute collection of blood. Angiography with oblique projections can also outline subdural hematomas and has been used if CT scanning is unavailable. In an acutely deteriorating patient with rapidly diminishing alertness and pupillary enlargement, burr holes or an emergency

craniotomy are sometimes appropriate without prior radiographic confirmation of subdural hematoma. A subacute syndrome is seen in alcoholics and in the elderly, with drowsiness, headache, confusion, or mild hemiparesis occurring days to 2 weeks after injury.

Direct trauma or surface contusions are not required for the formation of acute subdural hemorrhage; acceleration forces alone, as from whiplash, are adequate, especially in the elderly. Most subdural hematomas are small crescentic collections over the hemispheral convexity, adjacent to variable degrees of surface hemorrhagic contusions. Larger clots are thought to be primarily venous in origin, though additional arterial bleeding sites are often found, and some, when explored surgically, appear to be exclusively arterial. Most are located over the frontotemporal region, less often in the inferior middle fossa or over the occipital poles. Less common instances of interhemispheric, posterior fossa, or bilateral convexity clots are difficult to diagnose clinically, although drowsiness and the signs expected for each region can be detected. Small subdural hematomas may be asymptomatic and usually do not require therapy.

Acute epidural hematoma   Epidural hematomas evolve more rapidly and therefore can be more treacherous. They occur in 1 to 3 percent of all head injuries and in up to 10 percent of severe ones. They are less often associated with underlying cortical damage than subdural hematomas. The majority of patients are unconscious when first seen, often with associated injuries of subdural clot and contusion. A "lucid interval" of several minutes to hours before coma supervenes is said to be most characteristic of epidural hemorrhage, though it is not common and by no means the only cause of this temporal profile. The findings of drowsiness progressing to coma, pupillary enlargement, and hemiplegia are similar in some respects to subdural hematoma, but occur more rapidly.

The location of epidural hematomas is explained by their origin from torn dural vessels, most commonly the middle meningeal artery. Epidural clots therefore overlie the lateral temporal convexity. The majority of patients have fractures of the squamous portion of the temporal bone, through the path of the torn vessel. Frontal, inferior temporal, or occipitoparietal epidural hematomas are less frequent, occurring when fractures disrupt branches of the middle meningeal artery. Dural laceration over the sagittal or lateral sinuses or rupture of small diploic veins can rarely cause venous epidural hemorrhages. Epidural hematomas strip the tightly attached dura from the inner table of the skull, producing a characteristic lenticular-shaped clot on CT scan. They may be relatively less frequent in the elderly because of the tighter attachment of dura to skull that occurs with aging. Posterior fossa epidural hematomas are rare and difficult to detect clinically (most result from surgery such as resection of an acoustic neuroma).

Chronic subdural hematoma   In chronic subdural hematoma, a preceding traumatic cause is less often clear; 20 to 30 percent of patients fail to give a history of injury. Elderly patients or those with a bleeding diathesis seemingly form clots spontaneously. The causative injury may be trivial (striking the head against the branch of a tree, a sudden stop in a car with lurching forward, or striking the head during a fall or faint) and is often forgotten because it was remote in time. A period of weeks, or even months, follows when headaches (common but not invariable), slowed thinking, confusion, changes in personality, seizures, or a mild hemiparesis are the main findings. Fluctuation in the severity of the headache is typical, often with positional changes. Many chronic subdural hematomas are bilateral and give particularly misleading clinical syndromes. The initial clinical impression is often a stroke, brain tumor, drug intoxication, or a depressive, senile, or other type of dementia, the latter because disturbances of consciousness (drowsiness, inattentiveness, incoherence of thought) are more prominent than focal or lateralizing signs such as hemiparesis. Hemianesthesia or hemianopsia are seldom observed, probably because the anatomic structures subserving these functions are deep and not easily compressed. The diagnosis should be considered in dementias of apparently rapid onset, particularly if headache is present. The condition does not usually progress. When it does, the patient may become comatose with fluctuations of alertness and pupillary dilation as occurs in acute subdural hematoma. Acute bleeding is superimposed on the chronic hematoma in these cases. Occasionally patients present with "spells" of hemiparesis or aphasia typically lasting more than 10 min, sometimes indistinguishable from a transient ischemic attack. Patients with undetected small bilateral subdural hematomas seem to tolerate surgery, anesthesia, and nervous system depressive drugs poorly, often remaining drowsy or confused for long periods postoperatively.

Skull x-rays are usually normal except for a shift of a calcified pineal body to one side or an occasional unexpected fracture. The CT scan without contrast infusion typically shows a low-density mass over the convexity of the hemisphere, but may show only a shift of the midline structures and compression of the lateral ventricles because the clot becomes isodense to adjacent brain after 2 to 6 weeks. Bilateral chronic hematomas are often missed because of the absence of lateral tissue shifts. A "hypernormal" CT scan with absent cortical sulci and small ventricles in an older patient should suggest the diagnosis of bilateral isodense hematomas. Contrast infusion demonstrates the chronic fibrous capsule in some cases. MRI scans are very reliable in identifying a clot. The CSF may be clear, bloody, or xanthochromic, depending on the presence or absence of recent or old contusion and subarachnoid hemorrhage, and the pressure is usually elevated. However, lumbar puncture is not recommended for diagnosis because of risk of worsening tissue shifts. Chronic subdural hematomas can gradually expand, and then behave clinically like a tumor. Treatment with glucocorticoids alone is sufficient in some cases, but surgical evacuation is most often successful. Fibrous membranes (pseudomembranes) grow from the dura and encapsulate the region. Craniotomy and removal of the membranes is required if there is recurrent fluid accumulation. Small hematomas are largely resorbed, and only the organizing membranes remain, becoming calcified after many years.

PENETRATING INJURIES, COMPRESSIONS, AND LACERATIONS Tangential scalp wounds from bullets can produce neurologic signs or delayed seizures due to small hemorrhages or contusions, even in the absence of missile penetration. Bullets entering the brain cause considerable damage because of tremendous kinetic energy. A cylindrical area of necrosis surrounds the bullet track. Injuries differ with varying projectiles; soft civilian bullets typically shatter on impact and leave a track of metallic fragments with disproportionately less parenchymal damage. Military bullets, because of high velocity and energy, disrupt tissue at great distances from the track and produce massive brain destruction.

Penetrating bullet injuries cause a rapid increase in intracranial pressure for several minutes followed by a drop depending on the volume of secondary hemorrhage and the degree of developing edema. Infection is a risk mainly from shell fragments, shrapnel, grenades, and mines, because such small projectiles carry surface bacteria and dirt into the brain. Nevertheless, most neurosurgeons administer systemic antibiotics prophylactically and perform local debridement in all types of penetrating injuries. Traumatic aneurysms can form due to disruption of vessel walls from the shock wave of the projectile; facial-orbital entrance wounds have the highest incidence. The aneurysms have an unpredictable course; most that rupture do so in the first month. The prognosis for survival after missile injuries is good if consciousness is preserved and poor if coma is present from the outset.

Other intracranial foreign bodies from knives, picks, studguns, or high-speed tool bits may be missed unless skull x-rays are taken after minor penetrating injuries. Surgical removal, debridement, and extensive exploration for hemorrhage and necrotic tissue is required. Simply removing a protruding object is not sufficient.

TRAUMATIC VASCULAR OCCLUSION AND DISSECTION Minor, sometimes unnoticed, neck trauma can produce dissection (stripping of the intima or the media) of the internal carotid or vertebral arteries. Chiropractic neck manipulation accounts for some cases. Severe blunt trauma to the neck can initiate a dissection several centimeters above the origin of the internal carotid artery. In awake patients there is usually local neck pain over the internal carotid artery, a Horner's syndrome, and headache over the ipsilateral anterior cranium. Some patients with carotid dissection subsequently have large middle cerebral artery strokes with hemiplegia, visual field and sensory deficits, and if the dominant hemisphere is affected, aphasia. In drowsy or comatose patients evidence of dissection or subsequent stroke is difficult to discern but is suggested by unexplained hemiplegia, unilateral miosis, or the appearance of cerebral infarction on CT scan. Angiography demonstrates either the typical "string sign" characterized by an elongated narrowed lumen extending over 5 to 10 cm, or complete occlusion of the carotid artery beginning several centimeters distal to the bifurcation, sometimes accompanied by a distal embolus in the middle cerebral artery. On rare occasion, basilar skull fractures cause carotid dissection beginning at the point of entry of the artery into the skull. Traumatic "false" aneurysms of the cervical carotid artery result from deep penetrating, and occasionally from nonpenetrating, blunt trauma of the neck. A pulsatile mass and bruit over the artery establish the diagnosis and mandate surgical repair. Traumatic vertebral artery dissection can produce vertigo, vomiting, suboccipital or supraorbital headache, and other signs of lateral medullary ischemia. These symptoms are frequently attributed to vestibular concussion. In drowsy or comatose patients the only indication of vertebral artery occlusion may be inferior cerebellar infarction on CT scan.

Intracranial vascular damage is rare except in penetrating injuries. High-velocity projectiles, as discussed above, disrupt vessel walls, leading to aneurysms of large vessels in the vicinity of the wound, usually a surface branch of the middle cerebral artery. Preexisting saccular aneurysms may rupture after basilar skull fractures, and this diagnosis should be considered if subarachnoid hemorrhage is profuse and inadequately explained by accompanying subdural blood on CT scan. Vasospasm from traumatic subarachnoid blood may be involved in the development of infarction after head injury.

Cavernous sinus arteriovenous fistulas are serious complications in patients surviving severe head injury. They are first evident as a self-audible bruit (many are also audible to the examiner), proptosis, conjunctival injection, or visual impairment. Angiography shows early filling of the cavernous sinus and its draining tributaries. The fistula generally enlarges, causing increasingly severe local changes around the eye and orbit and decreased chances of visual recovery. About 10 percent, mostly small fistulas, resolve spontaneously. Many surgical approaches have been tried including ligation of the carotid artery, direct obliteration of the fistula or cavernous sinus, and angiographic-guided balloon embolization. A detachable balloon technique has proved successful in many cases (see Chap. 348).

INTRACRANIAL PRESSURE AND CEREBRAL BLOOD FLOW

The pathophysiology of intracranial pressure (ICP) regulation and its relationship to cerebral blood flow (CBF), which is applicable to many pathologic processes including cerebral hemorrhage, encephalitis, and brain edema after stroke, is best understood in the context of head trauma. The components of the intracranial compartment are brain, CSF, and blood. Because the skull limits total intracranial content, the volume of these compartments is compromised by expanding lesions within the cranial cavity. The brain is virtually incompressible; therefore CSF and blood serve as the main buffers of increasing intracranial volume. The relationship between increments in intracranial volume and the associated rises in ICP, termed *compliance,* approximates an exponential function after the volume buffering capacity of CSF and blood are exceeded. ICP is normally between 2 and 12 mmHg. Raised ICP in the range 15 to 40 mmHg, while not harmful by itself, can rapidly result in secondary damage, either by precipitously decreasing global cerebral perfusion when ICP exceeds blood pressure in the cranium, or by associated shifts of brain tissue that damage the thalamus and brainstem. The global damage from increased ICP is therefore ischemic in nature and related to the arithmetic difference between ICP and blood pressure in the major cerebral arteries. This difference is termed *cerebral perfusion pressure*, or CPP. Cerebral perfusion pressure below 40 to 60 mmHg is considered detrimental to nerve cells; therapy is therefore directed toward maintaining perfusion above this range. The rationale for keeping CPP even higher (i.e., bringing ICP below 15 to 20 mmHg) is to afford a margin of safety should transient increases in ICP occur. Physiologic changes or medications that increase blood pressure do not necessarily improve CPP because increased vascular pressures exacerbate brain edema in damaged areas and induce plateau waves (see below), resulting in further increases in ICP that ultimately lower perfusion.

The most important secondary complication of head injury is raised intracranial pressure arising from the added volume of contusions, hematomas, and the progressive edema surrounding them. A close relationship exists between clinical outcome and ICP in patients with closed head injury. At least 50 percent of patients who die as a result of head injury do so solely because of uncontrolled rises in ICP, and outcome is inversely related to the level of ICP after acute injury. Aggressive treatment of raised ICP in modern intensive care units is believed to improve survival after severe head injury. The role of direct monitoring of ICP to guide therapy is controversial.

Resting ICP, CPP, and compliance are spontaneously interrupted by rises in ICP termed *plateau waves*. They often are precipitated by iatrogenic maneuvers such as suctioning, physical therapy, excess fluid administration, or pain. Such plateau waves (lasting 1 to 10 min, and ranging from 25 to 60 mmHg) are most pronounced in patients with diminished intracranial compliance. They are best observed on continuous recordings of ICP. Plateau waves are probably due to a loss of cerebrovascular tone with a resultant increase in cerebral blood volume. Signs of apparent transtentorial herniation such as pupillary enlargement may occur after plateau waves (they more often do not), and occasionally brain death ensues. The proximate cause of deterioration is probably a reflex rise in blood pressure, part of the Cushing reflex (hypertension and bradycardia), greatly increasing intracranial blood volume and cerebral edema.

There is little consensus about the importance of alterations in cerebral blood flow caused by head injury. For several minutes to an hour after acute head injury, cerebral blood flow may increase in some patients although metabolic demands and oxygen consumption are diminished. Autoregulation, the ability of the cerebral vasculature to keep blood flow constant in response to decreased or increased perfusion pressure, is also impaired in damaged regions. Vascular factors have been found to account for approximately two-thirds of the rise in ICP after severe head injury. The blood-brain barrier also becomes more permeable after head injury in badly damaged regions, making edema formation more likely.

There is a complex relationship between raised ICP and clinical signs such as coma and pupillary enlargement that accompany supratentorial masses. ICP represents the accommodation of intracranial contents to additional mass; clinical signs are a parallel barometer of tissue shifts, particularly affecting structures around the tentorial opening. Raised ICP per se does not cause signs (including coma) until it reaches levels that preclude cerebral perfusion; it then causes global ischemia in a fashion similar to acute hypotension. Coma and other secondary signs resulting from tissue shifts in the region of the tentorial opening are described in Chap. 31. Horizontal midline shift at the level of the pineal body is closely related to the level of consciousness with acute unilateral mass lesions.

Other secondary phenomena after severe head injury cause brain damage and alter outcome. Hypoxia, for example, is common from a number of causes, and when severe, is associated with a poorer outcome.

CLINICAL SYNDROMES AND TREATMENT OF HEAD INJURY

MINOR INJURY   A fully alert and attentive patient presenting after head injury with one or more symptoms of headache, faintness, nausea, a single episode of emesis, difficulty with concentration, or slight blurring of vision has a good prognosis with little risk of subsequent deterioration. Such patients have sustained a concussion or have been dazed, and have a brief amnestic epoch surrounding the moment of impact. Occasionally, vasovagal syncope occurs several minutes to an hour after the injury and causes concern. Constant generalized or frontal headache is common in the days following trauma; it is often throbbing or hemicranial in nature, like migraine. The majority of patients with a minor syndrome do not have a skull fracture on skull x-ray, or hemorrhage on CT scan. The decision to obtain these tests depends largely on the availability of CT or MRI scanning and clinical signs suggesting that the impact was severe (e.g., prolonged concussion, periorbital or mastoid hematoma, repeated vomiting, etc). Children and young adults are particularly prone to drowsiness, vomiting, and irritability, sometimes delayed for several hours after apparently minor injuries. After a period of observation for several hours, arrangements may be made for the patient to be accompanied home to be observed by family or friends.

Persistent severe headache and repeated vomiting in the context of normal alertness and no focal neurologic signs are usually benign, but CT or MRI scanning and/or skull x-rays should be obtained. Skull fractures increase the likelihood of a subdural or epidural hematoma. Patients with these exaggerated signs, even if they follow minor injury, deserve observation in the hospital for 24 h. Clinical judgment, the presence of associated noncranial injuries, the availability of others at home, and the examiner's certainty of a normal neurologic examination should guide the need for further surveillance.

INJURY OF INTERMEDIATE SEVERITY   Patients who are not comatose but who have persistent confusion, behavioral changes, less than normal alertness, extreme dizziness, or focal neurologic signs such as hemiparesis should be admitted to the hospital and have a CT scan. The clinical syndromes most common in this group, in addition to postconcussive headache and dizziness, unsteadiness, photophobia, and vomiting of minor injury, include (1) delirium with a disinclination to be examined or moved, expletive speech, and resistance if disturbed, most often associated with anterior temporal lobe contusions; (2) a quiet, disinterested, slowed mental state (abulia) with dull facial appearance and slight irascibility if bothered, the patient lying quietly with eyes closed when undisturbed, seen with inferior and frontopolar frontal contusions (usually without grasp responses); (3) severe memory loss with poor retrograde and anterograde performance, headache, and photophobia, with medial temporal lobe contusions or diffuse injury; (4) a focal deficit such as aphasia or mild hemiparesis (hemianopsia is rare as an isolated posttraumatic finding), suggesting subdural hematoma or convexity contusion; (5) global confusion with inattention, poor performance on simple mental tasks, fluctuating or slightly erroneous orientation, associated with several types of injuries including the first two described above as well as medial frontal contusions and interhemispheric subdural hematoma; (6) repetitive vomiting, nystagmus, drowsiness, and unsteadiness, usually from a labyrinthine concussion, but occasionally due to a posterior fossa subdural hematoma or vertebral artery dissection; (7) drowsiness alone or with muteness, often unassociated with significant CT scan abnormalities; and (8) diabetes insipidus with or without a frontal-temporal lobe syndrome, from damage to median eminence or pituitary stalk and adjacent medial cortex.

The syndromes of intermediate severity are usually preceded by brief loss of consciousness and many are associated with skull fractures. A CT scan is required to exclude surgically remediable subdural or epidural hematomas and to define areas of contusion that later enlarge with edema, or coalesce to form intraparenchymal hemorrhages. Paroxysmal or rhythmic EEG abnormalities, in contrast to acute convulsions, are common over the region of a large contusion. Many intermediate injuries are complicated by drug or alcohol intoxication, making toxic screening important.

Close clinical observation in a well-staffed setting is advisable in order to detect increasing drowsiness, change in respiratory pattern or pupillary enlargement, and to ensure fluid restriction. Fully awake or slightly drowsy patients with small subdural hematomas may be treated with glucocorticoids and fluid restriction; larger clots, especially with fluctuating or worsening alertness, require surgery. Epidural hematomas causing compression of adjacent brain should be evacuated in patients who have a good chance of recovery from other injuries. Free water intake should be limited, allowing serum osmolarity to rise spontaneously toward 290 mosmol/L. Fever must be treated assiduously with antipyretics or a cooling blanket, and its source must be identified (usually aspiration). So-called central fever is rare. The routine, acute administration of phenytoin is controversial. About half of neurosurgeons advocate its use, particularly in children and young adults, in the belief that it may reduce the incidence of posttraumatic epilepsy. Glucocorticoids may be useful if there is a contusion, hemorrhage, or edema on the CT scan; otherwise they complicate management and should be omitted. The possibility of associated cervical spine injuries should be considered in all patients with syndromes of intermediate severity. The neck should be immobilized, and adequate x-rays of the spine should be obtained.

The majority of patients with intermediate injury improve over 1 to 6 weeks. During the first week alertness, irascibility, memory, and mental performance fluctuate. Behavioral changes such as agitation are most evident at night and sometimes seem to be worsened by large doses of glucocorticoids or CNS-depressant drugs. Haloperidol is useful when used sparingly. Subtle abnormalities of intellectual function particularly attention, spontaneity, and memory, tend to return to normal later, and frequently do so abruptly.

SEVERE HEAD INJURY AND COMA Patients who are stuporous or comatose from the outset require immediate neurologic attention and often, resuscitation. There is often pupillary enlargement or asymmetry. Persistent unresponsiveness is a grave sign. After the patient is intubated and the blood pressure is stabilized, attention is given to life-threatening noncranial injuries, followed by a survey neurologic examination.

The possibility of cervical injuries should not be overlooked, and the cervical spine must be immobilized during the initial assessment. The depth of coma and the size of the pupils are most important. Most severely injured patients hyperventilate. Extensor limb posturing and bilateral Babinski signs, combined with apparently purposeful movements, are common. Asymmetry in limb posture, limb movement, or gaze perference suggest a subdural or epidural hematoma or a large contusion.

As soon as vital functions permit and cervical spine x-rays and a CT scan have been obtained, the patient should be taken to a critical care unit. The finding of an epidural or subdural hematoma or large intracerebral hemorrhage are usually indications for surgery and intracranial decompression. In one large series the time between injury and evacuation of acute subdural hematomas was the major determinant of outcome. If such lesions are not present and the patient is still comatose and critically ill, attention is directed toward treating raised ICP. Patients with abnormal CT scans showing contusions, hemorrhages, or tissue shifts are the best candidates for ICP monitoring. The lumbar CSF pressure does not accurately reflect the intracranial pressure and may increase the risk of brain herniation, therefore the practice in most head injury treatment centers is to use one of several devices that is inserted intracranially to measure ICP. The pressure can be monitored continuously, disturbances in compliance and falling CPP can be identified, and appearance of plateau waves can be noted.

The treatment of raised ICP is best guided by direct measurement but may proceed on a presumptive basis using clinical status and CT scan as guides. All potentially exacerbating factors must be eliminated.

Hypoxia, hyperthermia, hypercarbia, awkward head positions, and high mean airway pressures from mechanical ventilation all increase cerebral blood volume and ICP. Many, but not all, patients will have lower ICPs when the head and trunk are elevated. If raising the patient's head lowers blood pressure, then cerebral perfusion pressure may be optimal in the supine position. Active management of raised ICP includes induced hypocarbia to an initial level of 28 to 33 mmHg P_{CO_2} and hyperosmolar dehydration with 20% mannitol (0.25 to 1 g/kg every 3 to 6 h), preferably using directly measured ICP as a guide. Otherwise, a serum osmolality of 305 to 315 mosmol/L is desirable, as is ventricular or subarachnoid fluid drainage when it is possible.

Persistently raised ICP after inception of this conservative therapy generally indicates a poor outcome, but the addition of high-dose barbiturates may further lower ICP and salvage a small number of patients. In many instances barbiturates cause a parallel reduction in ICP and blood pressure without resulting in net improvement in cerebral perfusion. The beneficial effects of barbiturates, aside from their sedative and anticonvulsant activities, are not established, and they can cause disastrous hypotension so that their routine use in severe head injury remains controversial. Further details of treatment of raised ICP are given in Chap. 31. Systolic blood pressure should be maintained above 100 mmHg by vasopressor agents, if necessary, but when pressors are required to support barbiturate use, there is usually little improvement in CPP. Mean blood pressure levels above 110 to 120 mmHg may exaggerate brain edema and are associated with plateau waves; hypertension may be treated with diuretics and beta-adrenergic blocking agents, or intermittent doses of barbiturates. A number of other antihypertensive drugs, including some calcium-channel blockers, are relatively contraindicated because they may lower blood pressure while leaving ICP unchanged, or raising it. Fluid and electrolytes must be administered cautiously, and free water administration should be limited. Administration of phenytoin or phenobarbital to prevent seizures is recommended by many neurosurgeons. Hourly antacids by nasogastric tube to keep gastric pH above 3.5, and administration of sucralfate or cimetidine are used to prevent gastrointestinal bleeding. The use of large doses of glucocorticoids in severe head injury has not been shown to improve outcome. Several recent studies suggest that early nutritional support results in earlier neurologic recovery from head injury. If the patient remains comatose, it is worthwhile to repeat the CT scan to exclude a delayed surface or intracerebral hemorrhage. Intensive care salvages some critically ill head-injured patients by concentrating efforts on simple treatments that avoid medical complications, particularly pneumonia and sepsis, and preventable increases in ICP. Whether more assiduous control of ICP and CPP will produce better results remains to be proved.

ASSOCIATED DERANGEMENTS OCCURRING WITH SEVERE HEAD TRAUMA Injuries outside the cranium should be searched for at the outset, because they are likely to be forgotten if not initially noted. In particular, associated spinal, long bone, and abdominal injuries may cause delayed difficulties in management. However, secondary medical complications dominate the intermediate-term intensive care of head trauma patients.

Fluids and electrolytes Over half of patients who persist in coma for 24 h after head injury develop abnormalities of electrolytes or fluid balance. Frequently these are a consequence of therapy, but the metabolic responses to head trauma are similar to those produced by trauma elsewhere and are important in planning treatment. Daily input-output records and body weights, when possible, are important in management. Water restriction and osmotic agents render most patients hyperosmolar and hypovolemic, requiring monitoring of serum osmolality and sodium concentrations. Diabetes insipidus should be suspected if urine output increases and urine specific gravity is low. Replacement of water losses suffices for mild cases, but vasopressin may be required in persistent cases. Serum osmolality above approximately 325 mosmol/L should be avoided because of the associated decrease in cardiac output.

Aldosterone and antidiuretic hormone (ADH) secretion in response to stress favor sodium and free water retention, respectively. The latter usually predominates, leading to mild hypervolemic hyponatremia in untreated patients, but is obscured by concomitant administration of osmotic agents. Severe hyponatremia results from excessive ADH secretion, which may occur with raised ICP, basilar skull fractures, and after prolonged mechanical ventilation. Potassium is lost in head injury because of trauma-induced aldosterone hypersecretion, therapeutic osmotic diuresis, and glucocorticoids. Because potassium is predominantly an intracellular ion, hypokalemia is frequently manifested as a hypochloremic alkalosis with normal or minimally depressed serum potassium and requires adequate replacement therapy with KCl.

Respiratory complications   Some patients with head injuries have hypoxia acutely after injury without obvious pulmonary infiltrates. Aspiration pneumonia presents a great risk; acid burn injury from aspirated gastric contents, infection, and atelectasis may combine to produce the adult respiratory distress syndrome (ARDS) and severe arteriovenous shunting. Some evidence suggests that agents that coat the gastric lining without reducing pH, such as sucralfate, are associated with less aspiration pneumonia than are conventional prophylactic agents for gastric bleeding. ARDS can also occur due to disseminated intravascular coagulopathy, fat embolism, or rarely "neurogenic" pulmonary edema. Treatment is similar to other cases of ARDS with positive end-expiratory pressure (PEEP) to allow lowered inspired oxygen concentrations and to prevent further atelectasis. The effect of PEEP on ICP is complex, but PEEP should not be withheld if necessary for oxygenation.

Atelectasis is common in all poorly responsive patients and is treated with chest physical therapy and adequate ventilator tidal volumes. Pulmonary embolism is also a major threat to bedridden patients, and intermittent pneumatic calf compression or modest doses of subcutaneous heparin may be useful prophylaxis. The latter has not predisposed to intracerebral or gastrointestinal bleeding. Early recognition of deep leg vein thrombosis and aggressive treatment by occlusion of the inferior vena cava may prevent later emboli.

Gastrointestinal hemorrhage   The majority of patients with severe head injuries develop gastric erosions, but only a few have clinically significant hemorrhages. Gastrointestinal bleeding usually occurs in the first days to 1 week. Unlike most patients in shock or with stress ulceration, head-trauma patients often have elevated gastric acidity. The synergistic effect of glucocorticoids in causing upper tract hemorrhage has been questioned, but the incidence of viscus perforation, particularly of the cecum, is elevated. Prophylactic treatment with gastric coating agents, as discussed above, with cimetidine, or with frequent antacid administration to keep gastric pH high (above 3.5) reduces gastric hemorrhage in other stress states and is commonly used in head trauma.

Fat embolism   Patients with severe long bone injuries are subject to widespread cerebral fat embolism. This complication is seen less often than previously, perhaps due to better fluid replacement. In the typical case, head injury is a minor part of the overall trauma; in a few, severe cranial injury masks the syndrome. Several days after the bone fractures, restlessness, delirium, or drowsiness progressing to coma in severe cases, seizures, generalized brain edema, and hypoxia develop. About half have retinal and conjunctival punctate hemorrhages or visible fat in retinal vessels. A petechial rash, prominent in the anterior axillary folds and supraclavicular fossae, diffuse interstitial infiltrates on the chest x-ray, fat in the urine, or renal failure occur in some patients. Severe reduction in arterial oxygen content is common from widespread lung injury (ARDS). Cerebral fat embolism causes cerebral purpura, mainly in the white matter, due to capillary occlusion by fat globules. There is evidence that cases recognized and treated early have a better prognosis. Massive doses of glucocorticoids, reduction of ICP, and administration of positive-pressure ventilation with high end-expiratory pressures have been claimed to be useful. Heparin or intravenous alcohol are no longer recommended.

Cardiovascular changes   Acute head trauma may cause transient apnea and cardiac arrest. In the absence of overwhelming brain damage recovery from the arrest is the rule. Subsequently, raised ICP may cause systemic hypertension, either with the classically associated bradycardia (Cushing response) or, almost as frequently, with tachycardia. Cardiac arrhythmias are common, most notably sinus bradycardia, supraventricular tachycardias, nodal rhythm, and heart block. T-wave inversion and alterations in the ST segment may simulate subendocardial ischemia.

Neurogenic pulmonary edema is a form of ARDS in which the alveoli fill with fluid as they would in congestive heart failure but left ventricular end-diastolic pressure (measured by pulmonary capillary wedge pressure) is normal. A pulmonary vascular leak may be produced when a sudden shift of intravascular volume occurs from the systemic to pulmonary circulation, as occurs transiently with suddenly raised ICP. Once the pulmonary vasculature has been damaged, an alveolar capillary leak may continue despite return of blood pressure to normal. The result is pulmonary edema with normal central venous and wedge pressures after the initial injury.

Hematologic complications   A large number of patients demonstrate a mild coagulopathy, and 5 to 10 percent have various degrees of disseminated intravascular coagulation. A correlation may exist between the severity of injury and the level of increased fibrin degradation products in blood. The cause of the coagulopathy is thought to be the release of highly thromboplastic material into the systemic circulation from the damaged brain.

PROGNOSIS   Extensive work by Jennet's group in Glasgow and others has provided data on the outcome in severe head injury (Table 352-1). Verbal output, eye opening, and the best motor response are important predictors of ultimate outcome. Eighty-five percent of patients with aggregate Glasgow Coma Scale scores of 3 or 4 die 24 h after injury. Yet a number of patients with a poor initial prognosis, including absent pupillary light responses, survive, suggesting that aggressive management is justified in virtually all patients. Patients below approximately 20 years of age, particularly children, may make remarkable recoveries after grave early neurologic signs. In one large study of severe head injury, 55 percent of children had a good outcome at 1 year, compared to 21 percent of adults.

Evoked potentials have prognostic value in head injury, and their accuracy probably exceeds clinical observations and ICP measurements. Somatosensory evoked potentials are the most useful, with bilaterally absent cortical potentials (with more caudal potentials present) being predictive of death or a vegetative state in 85 to 95 percent of patients. Prediction of a good functional outcome in the presence of normal or mildly abnormal tests is less certain.

TABLE 352-1   Glasgow Coma Scale for head injury

Eye opening (E):	
Spontaneous	4
To loud voice	3
To pain	2
Nil	1
Best motor response (M):	
Obeys	6
Localizes	5
Withdraws (flexion)	4
Abnormal flexion posturing	3
Extension posturing	2
Nil	1
Verbal response (V):	
Oriented	5
Confused, disoriented	4
Inappropriate words	3
Incomprehensible sounds	2
Nil	1

NOTE: Coma score = E + M + V. Patients scoring 3 or 4 have an 85 percent chance of dying or remaining vegetative, while scores above 11 indicate 5 to 10 percent likelihood of death or vegetative state and 85 percent chance of moderate disability or good recovery. Intermediate scores correlate with proportional chances of patients recovering.

SPINAL CORD TRAUMA

Approximately 10,000 patients a year in the United States, mostly young and otherwise healthy, become paraplegic or quadriplegic because of spinal cord injuries. There are an estimated 200,000 quadriplegics in the country. The majority of cord injuries in civilian life result from damage to the surrounding vertebral column, from fracture, dislocation, or both. Vertical compression with flexion is the main mechanism of injury in the thoracic cord, and hyperextension or flexion is the main cause of injury in the cervical cord. Preexisting spondylosis, a congenitally narrowed spinal canal, hypertrophied ligamentum flavum (see Chap. 361), or instability of the apophyseal joints of adjacent vertebrae from diseases such as rheumatoid arthritis, predispose to severe spinal cord damage after minor degrees of injury.

PATHOPHYSIOLOGY AND PATHOLOGY OF CORD INJURY

Much damage to the spinal cord is due to secondary phenomena in the minutes and hours following injury. Even when a complete transverse myelopathy is evident immediately after impact, some secondary changes are avoidable, and the resultant damage may be reversible. The immediate injury causes pericapillary hemorrhages that coalesce and enlarge, particularly in the gray matter. Infarction of gray matter and early white matter edema are evident within 4 h of experimental blunt injury. Eight hours after injury there is global infarction at the injured level, and only at this point does necrosis of white matter and paralysis below the level of the lesion become irreversible. The necrosis and central hemorrhages enlarge to occupy one or two levels above, and below, the point of primary impact. Gliosis in these regions results in necrotic areas over several months and may cavitate causing a progressive syringomyelic syndrome.

The early phases of injury are associated with reduced regional blood flow from direct capillary damage and a more prolonged secondary ischemia. A number of interventions including opiate antagonists, thyrotropin-releasing hormone, local cord cooling, dextran infusion, adrenergic blockade, glucocorticoids, and hyperbaric oxygen are of uncertain clinical usefulness. More importantly, the critical factor for recoverable function is the time from injury to institution of therapy. Complete axonal disruption from the immediate trauma or secondary phenomena precludes recovery.

TYPES OF SPINAL CORD INJURY AND THEIR MANAGEMENT

Any patient with severe head injury potentially has an associated instability of the spinal column. The care of such patients begins at the scene of the accident. The neck should be immobilized to prevent cord damage, and care should be taken during transport and during the physical and radiologic examinations to avoid neck extension or rotation and to prevent torsion-rotation of the thoracic spine. Blood pressure, respiratory status, and systemic injuries are attended to rapidly. Most patients can be intubated, if necessary, by blind nasotracheal technique without neck extension. High thoracic or cervical cord trauma regularly cause mild hypotension and bradycardia because of functional sympathectomy (often corroborated by bilateral ptosis and miosis—Horner's syndrome) that responds to infusion of crystalloid or colloid.

The neurologic examination in the awake patient focuses on neck or back pain, diminished limb power, a sensory level on the trunk, and deep tendon reflexes, usually absent below the level of an acute cord injury. Injuries above C5 cause quadriplegia and respiratory failure. At C5 and C6 the biceps are also weak, and at C4 and C5 the deltoid and supra- and infraspinatus are weak. C7 injuries cause weakness of the triceps, wrist extensors, and forearm pronators. Injuries at T1 and below cause paraplegia; the precise level can be determined from the level of sensory loss. Compression in the low thoracic and lumbar region causes a conus medullaris or cauda equina syndrome (see Chap. 361). Cauda equina injuries are usually incomplete, involving peripheral nerves rather than spinal cord, and therefore are surgically remediable for longer periods after injury than spinal cord compression. In a comatose patient absent reflexes should be sought in the legs, or in all the extremities, associated in the latter case with small pupils or paradoxical breathing from high cervical cord injury.

The next priority is to exclude a surgically remediable and potentially reversible cord compression due to dislocation of a vertebral body. Many traumatic myelopathies have no clearly associated fracture or dislocation. If x-rays suggest any aberration in the position of vertebrae, then reduction should be quickly undertaken. The role of myelography is controversial, but many neurosurgeons instill a few drops of Pantopaque into the spinal subarachnoid space to demonstrate a block to the flow of CSF. At present, examination by CT and MRI are more useful. Decompression within 2 h of severe injury may lead to some recovery of cord function. With incomplete myelopathies, especially if the limbs are becoming progressively weaker, early decompression is strongly recommended, even many hours after injury. Surgical approaches to decompressing the spinal column depend upon the specific nature of the injury. In complete transverse myelopathies beyond 6 to 12 h in duration, decompressive laminectomies are usually unsuccessful in restoring function.

The concerns with spinal column fractures, with or without myelopathy, are threefold: (1) detection of vertebral dislocations causing cord compression, (2) instability caused by fractures that will lead to misalignment and cord compression in the future, and (3) the proper treatment of fractures through the pedicles, facets, or vertebral bodies. Some fractures heal with immobilizaton and time, usually 2 to 3 months; others require surgical fusion to ensure stability.

Atlantoaxial dislocations can cause immediate death from respiratory failure, an event that may occur with no neurologic signs. Rheumatoid arthritis predisposes to this injury. Atlantooccipital dislocations occur predominantly in children and are almost always fatal. "Jefferson's fractures" are burst fractures of the ring of the atlas resulting from a force descending on the vertex of the skull as in diving accidents; they are usually asymptomatic. "Hangman's fractures" are produced by hyperextension and longitudinal distraction of the upper cervical spine, as occurs with penal hanging or striking the chin on a steering wheel in head-on collisions. These are usually fractures through the pedicles of C2 with subluxation anteriorly of C2 on C3. Traction reduction and immobilization allow proper healing.

Hyperflexion dislocation of the cervical vertebrae commonly causes traumatic quadriplegia. Occasionally, a markedly displaced injury is unassociated with neurologic dysfunction, presenting only with neck pain. In most cases, however, minor subluxation is associated with a severe neurologic deficit. Ligamentous disruption presumably allows compression of the cord at the moment of impact, but the vertebral bodies return closer to their original stations afterward. Therefore, any degree of subluxation must be treated as potentially unstable.

Compression fractures of the cervical spine can cause neurologic damage if a bone fragment is driven backward (burst fracture) into the spinal cord. "Teardrop fractures" with crushing of a vertebral body, leaving a fragment of bone anteriorly, are usually associated with ligamentous disruption and spinal instability. Single compression fractures of the thoracic spine are usually stable because the thoracic cage provides support, but they may be associated with anterior cord compression and require decompression and stabilization with the insertion of metal rods.

Mild hyperextension injuries may cause only disruption of supporting ligamentous structures and be well tolerated. More severe injuries cause vertebral displacement and cord compression. The "central cord syndrome" is produced by brief compression of the cord and disruption of the central gray matter usually occurring in patients with an already narrow spinal canal, either congenitally or from cervical spondylosis. There is weakness of the arms, often with pinprick loss over the arms and shoulders, and relative sparing of leg power and sensation on the trunk and legs. Abnormality of bladder function is variable. The prognosis for recovery is good.

Thoracolumbar fractures are produced by impact in the high or midback, usually while the patient is bent over. Impingement on the spinal canal results in a complex combination of cauda equina and conus medullaris dysfunction. Pure lumbar fractures produce cauda equina compression. Myelography, MRI, or CT scan allows precise localization, and surgical decompression is usually recommended, even with complete deficits, because the potential for recovery of peripheral nerves is great.

The subsequent care of patients with spinal cord injury is best undertaken in specialized centers. General principles of medical and urologic management are discussed in Chap. 361.

REFERENCES

ADAMS JH et al: Diffuse brain damage of the immediate impact type. Brain 100:489, 1977

BAKAY L, GLASSAUER FE: *Head Injury*. Boston, Little, Brown, 1980

BECKER DP et al: Outcome from severe head injury with early diagnosis and intensive management. J Neurosurg 47:491, 1977

DACEY RG et al: Neurosurgical complications after apparently minor head injury. J Neurosurg 65:203, 1986

EISENBERG HM et al: High-dose barbiturate control of elevated intracranial pressure in patients with severe head injury. J Neurosurg 69:15, 1988

GOLDSTEIN M: Traumatic brain injury: A silent epidemic. Ann Neurol 27:327, 1990

JENNET B et al: Predicting outcome in individual patients after head injury. Lancet 1:1081, 1976

LANGFITT TW, GENARELLI TA: Can the outcome from head injury be improved? J Neurosurg 56:19, 1982

LEVIN HS et al: Neurobehavioral outcome following minor head injury: A three center study. J Neurosurg 66:234, 1987

MARSHALL LF et al: The outcome with aggressive treatment in severe head injury. I: The significance of intracranial pressure monitoring. II: Acute and chronic barbiturate administration in the management of head injury. J Neurosurg 50:20, 1979

ROPPER AH et al (eds): *Neurological and Neurosurgical Intensive Care*, 2d ed. Baltimore, Aspen, 1988

353   NEOPLASTIC DISEASES OF THE CENTRAL NERVOUS SYSTEM

FRED HOCHBERG / AMY PRUITT

Tumors of the brain, of its meningeal coverings, and of the spinal cord are estimated to cause the death of 90,000 patients in the United States each year. Of these tumors, more than three-quarters are *secondary* metastases arising in patients undergoing treatment for systemic cancer. *Primary* tumors arising within the meninges or the parenchyma of the brain or spinal cord are common at all ages of life. Brain neoplasms claim a disproportionate share of hospital beds, diagnostic tests, and other medical resources. One-fourth of the annual $4 billion cost for care of cancer patients in the United States is allocated to patients with neoplasms of the central nervous system.

Although the specialized care of such patients is usually delegated to the neurosurgeon, radiotherapist, or neurooncologist, with the advent of new imaging techniques the internist is increasingly involved in the initial diagnosis. Late in the course of the disease, such patients again may come under the care of a general physician. The proper care of patients with primary or metastatic tumors of the central nervous system requires a systematic approach that enables the physician to (1) distinguish tumor from other causes of neurologic dysfunction such as infection, metabolic derangement, pseudotumor cerebri, or subdural hematoma; (2) make proper use of sophisticated diagnostic techniques such as magnetic resonance imaging (MRI), computed tomography (CT), and of more invasive tests such as arteriography; (3) provide early therapy to control cerebral edema and avoid seizure activity; (4) exclude systemic malignancy prior to referring the patient for a biopsy; and (5) recognize the medical complications of the tumor and of its therapy.

APPROACH TO THE PATIENT WITH CENTRAL NERVOUS SYSTEM TUMORS

CLASSIFICATION OF TUMORS   Tumors of the CNS may originate in the brain or spinal cord (primary tumors) or may spread from systemic sites of cancer (metastatic tumors). Both benign and malignant primary CNS tumors are capable of producing neurologic impairment. Primary tumors arise from glial cells (astrocytoma, oligodendroglioma, glioblastoma), ependymal cells (ependymoma), or supporting tissue (meningioma, schwannoma, papilloma of the choroid plexus). In childhood, tumors arise from more primitive cells (medulloblastoma, neuroblastoma, chordoma). Malignant astrocytoma or glioblastoma is the most common type of primary tumor in adults over age 20. A classification of intracranial tumors is given in Table 353-1.

CLINICAL MANIFESTATIONS OF INTRACRANIAL TUMOR   Intracranial tumors may be located within the brain substance (intraaxial) or in close proximity to the brain (extraaxial). The latter produce symptoms by compression or infiltration of brain. Many of the symptoms caused by intracranial masses reflect tumor expansion within a fixed bony vault into space normally occupied by brain, blood, and cerebrospinal fluid (CSF). The nature and severity of these symptoms depend on the location of the tumor and the rate of its growth. Although brain tissue can accommodate the presence of slowly growing tumors, masses larger than 3 cm in diameter compress the brain, its blood supply, and CSF pathways. This compression is increased by peritumoral edema (vasogenic cerebral edema). Neurologic deterioration occurs as the tumor infiltrates or displaces normal brain structures; as the tumor develops areas of hemorrhage, necrosis, or cyst formation; or as the tumor obstructs the normal flow of CSF, producing hydrocephalus.

Papilledema, or choking of the optic nerve head, emerges in the setting of impaired retinal venous return or axoplasmic flow along the optic nerve. Increasing intracranial pressure caused by a mass in one hemisphere may displace the medial temporal lobe (uncus) through the tentorial notch. As the uncus is forced inferiorly (*uncal herniation*) the midbrain is displaced and the third cranial nerve is compressed. The clinical signs of a unilateral third-nerve palsy— fixed, dilated pupil followed shortly thereafter by depression of consciousness, dilation of the opposite pupil, and hemiparesis on the opposite side of the original pupillary abnormality—should alert the physician to uncal herniation. A mass located more centrally in the supratentorial region produces a less specific picture called *central herniation*. In this situation the patient develops depression of consciousness as supratentorial structures compress the diencephalon and upper midbrain. Cheyne-Stokes respiration develops, but there is preservation of pupillary activity until late in the course of the deterioration (see Chap. 31).

Cerebellar masses may cause the cerebellar tonsils to herniate into the foramen magnum. As the tonsils are pushed inferiorly, the medulla and portions of the cervical spinal cord are compressed or infarcted.

TABLE 353-1   Classification of intracranial tumors

Type of tumor	Percent of total	
Glioma:	40	
Glioblastoma		20
Astrocytoma grades I and II		10
Ependymoma		6
Medulloblastoma		2
Oligodendroglioma		1
Papilloma of choroid plexus		1
Metastases	23	
Meningioma	17	
Pituitary adenoma	5	
Schwannoma	5	
Lymphoma	3	
Miscellaneous (congenital tumors, PNETs*)	7	

* Primitive neuroectodermal tumors.

Abnormalities of cardiovascular regulation ensue. The resulting bradycardia and hypertension are followed by irregularity or cessation of respiration. Posterior fossa lesions of small size may produce early hydrocephalus by obstruction of CSF flow at the level of the fourth ventricle or aqueduct of Sylvius.

Symptoms of intracranial tumor may develop in patients with previously diagnosed systemic cancer or in those not known to harbor a malignancy. Patients with intracranial tumor usually present with one or more of the following groups of symptoms: (1) headache with or without evidence of increased intracranial pressure; (2) progressive generalized decline in cognitive abilities or impairment of specific neurologic functions affecting speech and language, gait, or memory; (3) adult-onset seizures or increased frequency or severity of previously documented seizure activity; or (4) focal neurologic symptoms reflecting the particular anatomic site of the tumor, such as those caused by acoustic schwannoma (neuroma) in the cerebellopontine angle or by meningioma of the olfactory groove, sella, or parasellar areas.

Headache is the initial symptom in half of patients with brain tumors. Traction on the dura, blood vessels, or cranial nerves results from local compression, elevation of intracranial pressure, edema, or hydrocephalus. In most patients with supratentorial tumor, pain radiates to the side of the tumor mass, whereas patients with posterior fossa masses describe retroorbital, retroauricular, or occipital pain. Emesis or hiccups, often without nausea, signals development of increased intracranial pressure and is especially common in patients with masses located beneath the tentorium.

Tumors of the frontal lobes may attain considerable size before symptoms develop, and then symptoms often are nonspecific. Subtle, progressive disturbances of mentation, slowness of comprehension, loss of acuity in business affairs, memory disorders, or apathy, lethargy, and drowsiness may be reported. Spontaneity of thought and activity is lost. Incontinence of urine and disordered gait may be seen by family members. The development of a true dysphasia and/or motor weakness signal progression of the tumor or its associated edema into motor cortex and speech areas of the frontoparietal region.

Masses in the temporal lobes are associated with personality changes that may resemble affective or psychotic thought disorders. Various combinations of auditory hallucinations, abrupt shifts in mood, and altered sleep, appetite, and sexual functions are soon interspersed with complex partial seizures possibly accompanied by visual field defects in the superior quadrants contralateral to the tumor.

Disorders of communication and vision characterize parietooccipital masses. Receptive aphasia with contralateral hemianopsia characterizes left parietal tumors, while a combination of spatial disorientation, constructional apraxia, and left homonymous hemianopsia bespeaks right parietal tumors.

Tumors of the diencephalon often present with a combination of failure of pupillary constriction to light, failure of upward gaze, and neuroendocrine abnormalities. Hydrocephalus due to obstruction to CSF flow at the level of the third ventricle leads to headache. Syndromes suggesting tumors of diencephalon or posterior fossa origin are more fully discussed in the section of this chapter devoted to neoplasms of these regions.

Cerebellar and brainstem lesions lead to a combination of cranial nerve palsies and incoordination of limbs or gait with or without accompanying signs of hydrocephalus. (See Chap. 360 for discussion of cranial nerve symptoms and signs.)

Seizures occur as the initial symptom in 20 percent of patients with brain tumors. Patients with new onset of epilepsy after the age of 35 must be evaluated for brain tumor. Similar high-risk groups of new seizure patients include those with previously diagnosed systemic cancer, longstanding neurologic diseases (including such neuroectodermal disorders as von Recklinghausen's disease and tuberous sclerosis), or acute or atypical psychiatric disorders. A carefully obtained history may uncover disordered time perceptions (déjà vu or déjà jamais), paroxysms of fear, and clinging "viscous" personality

changes in addition to obvious features such as "complex partial" (temporal lobe) seizures or personality changes that antedate the diagnosis by years. Occasionally, the first symptom simulates a transient ischemic attack with no residual deficit or discernible seizure, but more commonly the pattern of clinical seizures provides localizing information. Thus, the "Jacksonian march" of tonic-clonic seizure points to frontal tumors and a sensory march characterizes tumors of the sensory parietal cortex. Metastatic tumors, occupying the junction of gray and white matter, are more likely than are primary tumors to produce acute symptoms evolving in days to weeks. Even more rapid onset of symptoms reflects hemorrhage in tumors of lung, melanoma, renal cell, choriocarcinoma, or thyroid origins. In contrast, with the exception of oligodendroglioma and malignant astrocytoma, primary brain tumors are unlikely to hemorrhage.

PHYSICAL EXAMINATION OF THE PATIENT WITH SUSPECTED CNS TUMORS When the physician examines a brain tumor suspect who is not previously known to have a systemic cancer, the general examination should include (1) a survey of the skin for stigmata of neurocutaneous syndromes or melanoma, (2) a search for enlarged lymph nodes, (3) an examination of the abdomen for hepatic or splenic enlargement, (4) a rectal examination with stool guaiac test, (5) a breast and pelvic examination in female patients, and (6) a cardiopulmonary examination.

The neurologic examination of the patient with suspected brain tumor should focus first on an evaluation of the mental status. The examiner should look for evidence of specific localizing cognitive deficits, such as dysphasia, dyspraxia, or memory loss, in addition to gleaning a sense of any personality change which has occurred. The patient is examined for increased intracranial pressure (papilledema or sixth cranial nerve paresis) and for other cranial nerve abnormalities. Asymmetries of strength, sensation, visual fields, and reflex activity should be sought. Attention should be paid to the constellation of signs suggestive of tumors in specific supratentorial, diencephalic or posterior fossa sites (see above). Combinations of cranial nerve abnormalities and corticospinal or lumbosacral radicular signs raise suspicion of leptomeningeal metastases (see below).

INVESTIGATION OF THE PATIENT WITH INTRACRANIAL TUMOR Advances in neuroradiology have contributed greatly to the diagnosis and management of patients with suspected neoplastic disease of the CNS. A plan for appropriate diagnostic studies based on the initial MRI or CT scan results is outlined in Table 353-2. The language of neurooncology differs from that of medical oncology, familiar terms such as "benign," "malignant," and "metastasizing" taking on different connotations when the tumor involves the CNS. Benign and malignant tumors are not differentiated in the scheme of Table 353-2 because the initial clinical approach is identical. Although many primary CNS tumors exhibit microscopic characteristics classifiable as "benign" because they are well-differentiated histologically and grow slowly, they are, nevertheless, incurable. Tumors of identical histology may have very different prognoses, depending upon their location and amenability to resection. Secondary CNS tumors are malignant in the conventional sense, since they represent metastases and invade normal tissue. Both benign and malignant tumors may produce profound, irreversible neurologic impairment. Primary brain tumors, with rare exceptions, do not metastasize outside the CNS; however, virtually all primary brain tumors are capable of diffuse seeding to the leptomeninges. Thus, the approach to *all* intracranial tumors, summarized in Table 353-2, relies on the clinical history and physical examination and on information provided by MRI scan and CT.

The laboratory evaluation of intracranial tumors MRI and contrast-enhanced CT scanning have now largely replaced the combination of skull x-ray, electroencephalogram, radionuclide brain scan, and arteriography as the principal tests for the evaluation of patients with suspected brain tumor.

MAGNETIC RESONANCE IMAGING (MRI) MRI is the procedure of choice for the evaluation of neurologic dysfunction in a patient suspected of having cancer. MRI delineates most metastatic and

TABLE 353-2   Evaluation following MRI or CT scan of the patient with suspected neoplastic disease of the brain and spinal cord

CT/MRI result	Possible diagnosis	Pretreatment evaluation	Primary treatment	Secondary treatment
KNOWN SYSTEMIC CANCER: BRAIN				
Normal				
No focal deficits on examination	Infection, metabolic abnormality	Lumbar puncture, exclude infection or metabolic problem	See text	———
Focal deficits on examination	Vascular disease, carcinomatous meningitis, seizure, paraneoplastic syndrome, complications of therapy	Lumbar puncture, follow-up MRI 4–6 weeks, gadolinium MRI	See text	Glucocorticoids as needed
Solitary mass	Radioresistant or radiosensitive tumor, unrelated tumor	MRI (Gd-DTPA)*, metastatic evaluation, surgical opinion	Glucocorticoids, radiation if radiosensitive tumor or active systemic disease found	Glucocorticoids as needed
Multiple masses	Metastases	None	Glucocorticoids, radiation	Glucocorticoids as needed, radiation, chemotherapy as indicated
NO KNOWN SYSTEMIC CANCER: BRAIN				
Normal	No disease	Repeat MRI (Gd-DTPA) in 8–12 weeks if symptoms persist		———
Solitary mass	Neoplastic disease, primary or secondary tumor, benign or malignant tumor	Metastatic evaluation, surgical opinion, MRI (Gd-DTPA)	Glucocorticoids, biopsy, radiation	Glucocorticoids as needed
Multiple masses	Neoplastic disease, primary or secondary tumor	Metastatic evaluation	Glucocorticoids and radiation if systemic tumor identified Glucocorticoids, biopsy, and radiation if no systemic tumor is found	See text
KNOWN SYSTEMIC CANCER: SPINAL CORD				
Normal	Nonneoplastic disease Carcinomatous meningitis Paraneoplastic	CSF analysis CSF cytology CT/myelogram	See text	See text
Abnormal	Metastases vs. tumor vs. nonneoplastic	CSF cytology, CT/myelogram, metastatic evaluation, surgical opinion	Glucocorticoids, chemotherapy (meningeal disease), Radiation	See text
NO KNOWN SYSTEMIC CANCER: SPINAL CORD				
Normal	No disease	Further evaluation in 8–12 weeks if symptoms persist (EMG)	See text	See text
Abnormal	Metastases vs. primary tumor vs. nonneoplastic	Metastatic evaluation, CSF analysis and cytology, angiography, CT/myelogram, MRI (Gd-DTPA)	See text	———

* Gd-DTPA = gadolinium diethylenetriamine pentaacetic acid.

primary tumors of the nervous system (see also Chap. 348). Lesions of the skull base and those in the brainstem, cerebellum, and spinal cord are visualized with greater detail with MRI than with CT, myelographic, or radionuclide images (Fig. 353-1). In addition to great sensitivity and delineation of anatomic detail, MRI offers the advantages of requiring no radiation exposure or administration of contrast material. The "flow-void" characteristic of MRI images provides a measure of tumor vascularity and may be reconstructed to create an MRI angiogram that often removes the need for preoperative arteriography. Hemorrhage, seen in metastatic melanoma and glioblastoma, is easily identified as hemoglobin products or as ferritin. Tumors which contain fat (epidermoid, lipoma, craniopharyngioma) are recognized by their "bright" T2 signals as are those growths with cysts containing high concentrations of protein. The interpretation of MRI abnormalities can be very vexing, however. Many patients harbor unexplained white matter abnormalities ("unidentified bright objects," or UBOs) in close proximity to the ventricular system. Extensive areas of T2 signal abnormality on MRI are not clearly correlated with the extent of tumor on CT nor with the histologic tumor margin. These areas, reflecting cerebral edema, infarction, tumor necrosis, and the effects of prior irradiation and surgery, hinder the physician's attempt to use MRI for treatment planning.

Paramagnetic contrast with intravenous gadolinium diethylenetriamine pentaacetic acid (gadolinium DTPA) produces contrast changes in MRI similar to those observed following the use of organic iodides in CT. The combination of paramagnetic agents and higher energy MRI units may provide better separation of tumor from nontumor tissue and better resolution of the spinal cord and brachial plexus. Gadolinium DTPA administration occasionally produces hypotension and nausea or emesis. The agent is cleared through the kidneys and must be used with caution in hepatic failure because of altered iron metabolism. As red cell morphology may be altered, gadolinium DTPA should be used with caution in hemolytic anemia.

CT SCAN   Contrast-enhanced CT imaging delineates intracranial masses as small as 0.5 cm in diameter. Certain tumors whose density exceeds that of normal brain parenchyma, including meningioma, melanoma, and primary lymphoma, and tumors with spontaneous hemorrhage can be visualized without contrast enhancement. CT scanning may be better than MRI for definition of meningiomas and other calcium-containing tumors such as oligodendroglioma and pineal region tumors. Tumors commonly appear as homogeneous or ring-

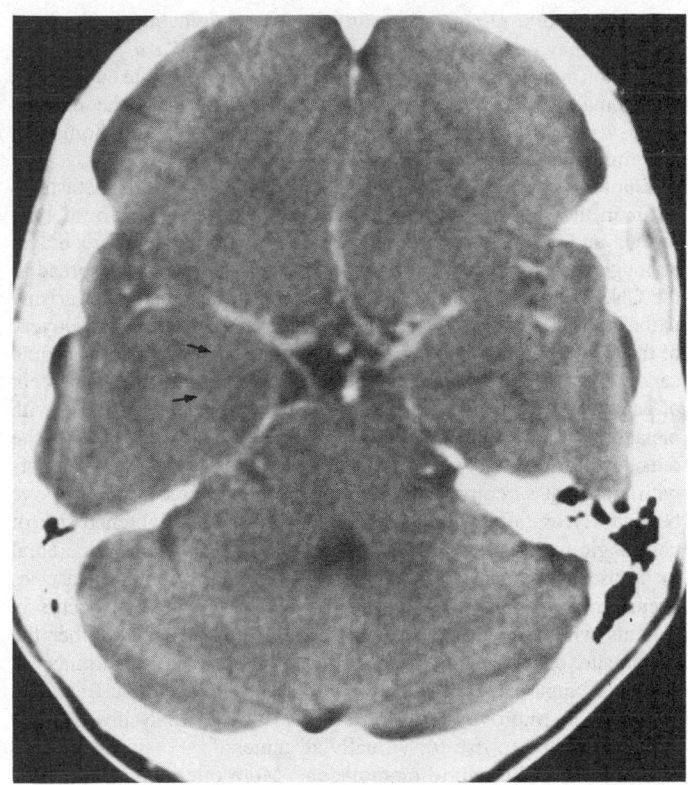

A

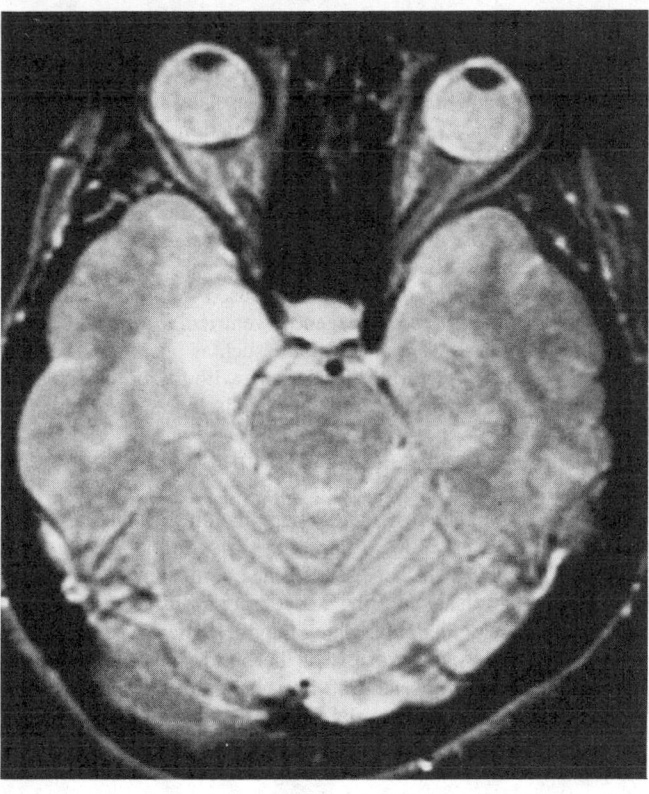

B

FIGURE 353-1 CT and MRI scans in a 57-year-old woman with a long history of temporal lobe epilepsy. *A*. Contrast-enhanced CT scan showed decreased absorption in the medial left temporal lobe (arrows) with no sign of contrast enhancement. Lesion was present on a CT scan taken 5 years earlier. *B*. Recent T2-weighted image shows a hyperintense circumscribed mass in the same lobe. Biopsy revealed a low-grade astrocytoma.

enhancing masses surrounded by variable amounts of edema. Reconstructions in coronal and sagittal planes and magnification of focal regions allow detection of 95 percent of intracranial masses and definition within 1 cm of the histologic border of the tumor. Although not a substitute for biopsy diagnosis, the CT often correctly predicts the histology of the tumor. Despite MRI advances CT remains the technique of choice for irradiation treatment planning and for the evaluation of the response of brain tumors to therapy.

Initial CT studies may show no abnormality in meningeal carcinomatosis, small metastases, primary brain lymphoma, or some glial tumors that emerge in the setting of chronic seizure activity. Repeat CT scanning, using single or double doses of contrast, 4 to 5 weeks later, usually provides tumor detection. However, if the initial CT scan of a patient with suspected CNS cancer is negative, MRI should be performed. The clinician should be wary of attributing all CT or MRI scan masses to tumor, as ringlike abnormalities may occur in abscesses, in recent cerebral infarction, in the plaques of multiple sclerosis, as a consequence of encephalitis, and in certain vascular malformations with or without hemorrhage. Asymptomatic meningioma and aneurysm are sometimes detected incidentally during evaluation for brain tumors.

Before MRI, brainstem, cerebellar, and spinal cord masses could be further defined by a combination of CT and subarachnoid administration of water-soluble contrast agents. MRI has largely supplanted this procedure except for the delineation of intradural lesions of the spinal cord.

ANGIOGRAPHY Transfemoral arteriography provides selective visualization of internal carotid and vertebral arteries and their branches. Vessels of malignant tumors are characterized by an angiographic "blush" with enlarged early draining veins, features not seen in association with an intracerebral hemorrhage, infarction, or abscess. The identification on MRI of "flow-voids" has diminished the requirement for arteriograms. Preoperative neurosurgical planning is often aided by knowledge of the vascular anatomy or by embolization of excessively vascularized tumors such as meningioma (see Chap. 348).

MANAGEMENT OF INTRACRANIAL TUMORS Surgery: Biopsy and resection Surgical exploration allows tumor identification in patients with either solitary or multiple intracranial masses. Surgical exploration may be necessary to obtain a diagnosis in patients with multiple CT masses in whom a thorough systemic evaluation, including hemogram, liver function studies, carcinoembryonic antigen, chest x-ray, sputum cytology, radionuclide bone and liver scans, and perhaps intravenous pyelography is unrewarding. Of patients with multiple CNS metastatic lesions, 20 percent have no evidence of systemic cancer.

Tumor biopsy is performed through an open craniotomy or with CT-guided stereotaxic techniques. The establishment of a diagnosis is important to determine prognosis and treatment. *Resection* is undertaken and may be curative for some primary tumors such as meningioma, ependymoma, oligodendroglioma, and low-grade astrocytoma (see below) in nondominant, frontal, anterior temporal, or occipital locations or in the ventricular system. *Partial resection* improves patient symptoms, often including better seizure control; by diminishing cerebral edema, it reduces dependence on glucocorticoids. Although resection offers little to patients with multiple intracranial lesions, such as those with brain lymphoma, it may be of value for solitary metastases. Resection of a *solitary tumor* in patients with known systemic cancer may be considered if (1) there is a greater than 2-year interval without known residual systemic malignancy, (2) relief of specific symptoms such as hydrocephalus is required, (3) the tumor is known to be radioresistant as in the case of melanoma, sarcoma, and renal or colonic carcinomas, (4) symptomatic tumor recurs after radiation and (5) the patient's systemic disease is under good control and the cerebral tumor is the limiting factor in quality of survival. For selected patients, this approach offers survival free of neurologic disease of more than 1 year.

Acute treatment of intracranial tumors   Clinical evidence of acute or subacute deterioration, such as stupor, focal neurologic signs, or evidence of transtentorial herniation, requires aggressive management. Treatment is directed to reducing cerebral edema, lowering intracranial pressure, and reducing the risk of seizures. Treatment with daily doses of dexamethasone 30 to 60 mg or methylprednisolone 120 to 200 mg in four to six divided doses reduces cerebral edema and associated surgical morbidity. Glucocorticoids may not control symptoms caused by obstruction of the ventricular system, and emergency ventricular drainage may be required. Anticonvulsant medications, such as phenytoin (300 to 400 mg/d), are usually prescribed for patients with seizures, though many physicians administer them prophylactically when intracranial tumor has been diagnosed.

PSEUDOTUMOR—BENIGN INTRACRANIAL HYPERTENSION
Symptoms of increased intracranial pressure may occur in the absence of demonstrable parenchymal or leptomeningeal tumor or hydrocephalus. However, little distinguishes the symptomatic presentation of true tumor from that of pseudotumor, which includes headache, neck stiffness, visual blurring and obscurations, diplopia, nausea, and vomiting. Papilledema, which may be unilateral or asymmetric, is accompanied by enlargement of the blind spot and altered visual acuity. Pseudotumor usually afflicts young, often obese women; it occurs most often in the absence of systemic cancer and focal neurologic difficulties. The marked increases in intracranial pressure may reflect impaired venous drainage within the brain or skull or may accompany the hormonal alterations of pregnancy, oral contraceptive use, or obesity. Less-common predisposing endocrinologic illnesses include both hypo- and hyperthyroidism, hypoparathyroidism, adrenal insufficiency, and both endogenous and exogenous excess of adrenocorticoids. Rare associations occur with sarcoidosis and lupus erythematosis. A variety of drugs have been implicated, including supplemental vitamin A, tetracycline, nalidixic acid, nitrofurantoin, sulfa preparations, lithium, indomethacin, phenytoin. The diagnosis is confirmed by the exclusion of an intracranial mass lesion or meningeal cancer. In the presence of a normal or small ventricular system on CT scan, lumbar puncture carries no risk for brain herniation. Cerebrospinal fluid is invariably under increased pressure but is otherwise unremarkable. Treatment is aimed at prevention of visual deficits and lasting symptoms by reducing the CSF volume by repetitive lumbar punctures. The removal of an offending drug or metabolic cause will reverse symptoms within 1 week's time. Patients refractory to this may benefit from acetazolamide, furosemide, or short-term glucocorticoid therapy. Lumboperitoneal shunting and surgical subtemporal decompression or optic nerve sheath fenestration are reserved for patients with progressive visual impairment who have failed medical therapy. The outlook for most patients is excellent—fully 80 percent respond to conservative therapy, but as many as 10 percent experience permanent or recurrent visual deficits.

SYSTEMIC CANCER AND THE CENTRAL NERVOUS SYSTEM

CEREBRAL METASTASES   The most common CNS tumors are metastatic. The following section discusses the approach to patients who present with a CNS tumor where systemic cancer must be considered.

Pathogenesis and pathology   Cerebral metastases occur in one-quarter of patients with systemic cancer. Spread to the calvarium, brain parenchyma, and subarachnoid space occurs through several mechanisms. *Hematogenous tumor embolism* from intermediate sites such as lung and liver is the most common mechanism in solid tumors of the breast and lung and in melanoma. Spread into the spinal canal via the *perivertebral venous system* occurs with uterine, colonic, and

prostatic tumors. *Direct extension* of tumors originating in the head and neck may occur through the base of the skull. *Paraspinal direct* infiltration may occur with lymphoma and with prostate and breast carcinomas. *Tumor passage from the eye* or through the choroid plexus to the brain and subarachnoid space occurs in lymphoma and leukemia.

Clinical manifestations   Sixty percent of cerebral metastases occur in the setting of diagnosed systemic cancer. Cancers of lung in men and of breast in women account for the largest percentage, although melanoma is the tumor with highest likelihood of spread to the CNS. Of patients with a cerebral metastasis (most often arising in the lung) 20 percent develop neurologic symptoms before discovery of the primary malignancy. At some point after diagnosis of systemic cancer, 25 percent of patients with lung carcinoma, 6 to 20 percent of patients with breast carcinoma, and about 50 percent of those with melanoma (when this last tumor has already metastasized to a site outside the CNS) develop tumors in brain or spinal cord. Patients with recurrent sarcoma or ovarian or colorectal cancer who survive beyond 3 years after the original diagnosis face a heightened risk of neurologic involvement. These tumors rarely accounted for cerebral metastases in the past. In the majority of patients, cerebral metastases occur with systemic relapse (Table 353-3). An exception occurs in patients with lung cancer, where the CNS is frequently either the initial site of presentation or of first demonstrated recurrence in otherwise apparently well-controlled disease. As systemic treatment continues to improve survival, the incidence of CNS involvement can be expected to rise for virtually all tumors.

Diagnosis of cerebral metastases   More often than is the case with primary brain tumors, those of metastatic origin occur in a setting of seizure activity, increasingly severe head pain, and motor weakness. These difficulties often evolve in days to weeks. MRI or contrast-enhanced CT scan is the procedure of choice for evaluating patients with known systemic cancer and new neurologic symptoms (Table 353-2). Tumors appear with equal frequency as multiple ring-shaped lesions or solitary masses. Three categories of patients without neurologic symptoms or signs are initially evaluated by MRI or CT scanning. First, patients with lung carcinoma for whom attempted cure with pulmonary lobectomy is planned should have a scan preoperatively, since 5 percent of such patients will have clinically unsuspected cerebral metastases. Second, prophylactic brain radiation for small cell carcinoma of the lung should be preceded by a scan. Third, patients with widely disseminated cancer due to breast or testicular tumors, sarcoma, or melanoma who are about to receive systemic chemotherapy should have a scan to stage the disease.

Ten percent of patients with cancer develop neurologic difficulties in the absence of an intracranial mass on CT scan. Most of these will be found to have an abnormality on MRI scan. Focal motor or cranial nerve symptoms, headache, or impaired intellectual performance may reflect cerebrovascular lesions known to be associated with systemic cancer, unwitnessed seizures, meningeal carcinomatosis, paraneoplastic syndromes, or complications of tumor therapy (Table 353-4).

Patients with systemic neoplasms can develop several types of cerebrovascular disease. Multiple cerebral infarctions are the most frequent in patients with solid tumors. Patients with lymphoma or leukemia may develop diffuse encephalopathic difficulties from infarcts due to disseminated intravascular coagulation; or may develop focal findings from emboli of nonbacterial thrombotic endocarditis, hemorrhage in the setting of clotting abnormalities, or thrombocytopenia. In the absence of an etiology, laboratory studies should be done to exclude a circulating anticoagulant.

Focal deficits in patients with negative MRI or CT scans may result from seizures due to undetectable metastatic disease or may be manifestations of meningeal carcinomatosis or paraneoplastic syndromes (see Chap. 310). Gadolinium DTPA MRI or repeat CT scan in 4 to 6 weeks often discloses the tumor if present. A lumbar puncture with cytologic examination is mandatory in such patients both to exclude infection and to search for leptomeningeal tumor (see

TABLE 353-3 Interval between diagnosis of cancer and occurrence of brain metastases

| Tumor | Patients with brain metastases, percent | | | Interval from diagnosis of primary tumor to diagnosis of brain metastasis, percent |
	At diagnosis of primary	Sometime during course of tumor growth	At autopsy	
Lung tumor	10–15	22–30	15–30	90 after 3 months
Breast tumor	1	6–20	15–30	90 after 1 year
Melanoma	6	50	40–80	80 after 1 year
Renal tumor	4	11–13	8–20	90 after 1 year
Colorectal tumor	1	—	1	75 after 2 years
Sarcoma	1	36	—	90 after 1 year

SOURCE: L Weiss et al, *Brain Metastases*, Boston, Hall, 1980; M Deutsch et al, Cancer 34:1607, 1974.

below). CSF pleocytosis with mild elevation of protein may be found with paraneoplastic disorders.

Treatment The common assumption that brain metastases represent a uniform disease has been proved invalid. Therapeutic decisions must be based on the type, extent, and radiosensitivity of the primary tumor, the morbidity produced, and the number and location of metastases.

Patients with solitary lesions and little or no active systemic disease may require surgery, whereas for those with advanced, widespread systemic cancer, comfort is the prime consideration. Steroids may be used in such patients to maximize neurologic function and to reduce headache (see "Acute Treatment of Intracranial Tumors").

RADIATION THERAPY After acute symptoms are treated, most patients with multiple cerebral metastases or unresectable solitary lesions receive radiation therapy. A common approach is palliative whole-brain radiation totaling about 30 Gy (3000 rad) given in 10 to 15 equal fractions. Three-quarters of patients improve clinically and by CT; over one-half are able to discontinue their steroid medication for a time. However, only 30 percent of patients who complete radiation therapy survive 6 months and fewer than 20 percent are alive at 1 year. Two-thirds of the latter patients die from recurrent systemic tumor and not from cerebral disease. Treatment is less effective in the elderly, in those with advanced systemic cancer, and in patients with radiation-resistant tumors such as melanoma and gastrointestinal and lung tumors. Reinstitution of glucocorticoids may be useful when progressive neurologic deterioration recurs.

TABLE 353-4 Complications of chemotherapy

Neurologic problem	Drug(s)	Route
Encephalopathy	Glucocorticoids	PO/IM/IV
	L-Asparaginase	IV
	Procarbazine	PO/IV
	Nitrosoureas	PO/IV/IA/HDIV
	Cytosine arabinoside	HDIV
	Cisplatin*	IV
Leucoencephalopathy	Methotrexate	HDIV/IT
Cerebral edema	Cisplatin	IA
	Nitrosoureas	IA/HDIV
Optic nerve damage	Nitrosoureas	IA/HDIV
Cerebellar ataxia	5-Fluorouracil	IV
	Cytosine arabinoside	IT
Cranial neuropathy	Vincristine	IV
	Cisplatin*	IV/IA
Myelopathy/radiculopathy	Thio-TEPA	IT
	Methotrexate	HDIV/IT
	Cytosine arabinoside	HDIV/IT
Peripheral neuropathy	Vincristine†	IV
	Cisplatin	IV
Myopathy	Glucocorticoids	PO/IM/IV
	Vincristine	IV

* Ototoxicity and vestibular toxicity.
† Autonomic neuropathy may be seen as well.
NOTES: IA = intraarterial; IM = intramuscular; IV = intravenous; PO = per os; IT = intrathecal; HDIV = high dose intravenous.
SOURCE: Modified from Young.

CHEMOTHERAPY Systemic (intravenous or intraarterial) chemotherapy has been used with some success to treat cerebral metastases of lung (small cell), breast, and testicular origin. Anecdotal reports of brain metastases of breast origin responding to tamoxifen or other systemic chemotherapy have appeared.

LEPTOMENINGEAL METASTASES Pathogenesis and pathology Eight percent of patients with cancer develop diffuse infiltration of the meninges. The cranial and spinal nerve roots are usually affected. Tumors that commonly invade the meninges include non-Hodgkin's lymphoma, leukemia, melanoma, and adenocarcinoma of breast, lung, or gastrointestinal origin.

Clinical manifestations The common symptoms are headache, alteration in mentation, cranial nerve abnormalities, and lumbosacral radiculopathies. Patients may also present with seizures. The MRI or CT scan usually is normal, but may reveal enlarged ventricles. With contrast injections, scans may reveal diffuse enhancement of the meninges over the cerebral hemispheres and at the base of the brain.

A lumbar puncture is required for diagnosis. Three-quarters of patients show a modest CSF mononuclear pleocytosis of 5 to 100 cells. Elevation of protein and lowered glucose content may occur, but demonstration of malignant cells is required to confirm the diagnosis. Repeat lumbar or cervical subarachnoid punctures may be necessary to obtain positive cytology. In the past, myelography was often done in such patients because of back pain and radicular symptoms; it often disclosed multiple small nodules on the nerve roots. MRI studies using surface coils provide equal sensitivity providing that arachnoiditis is not present. Larger lesions can be detected and treated with radiation.

Treatment Treatment of meningeal carcinomatosis usually requires a combination of cranial radiation and intrathecal administration of chemotherapeutic agents. Chemotherapy is given either into the lumbar subarachnoid space or (more effectively) into a reservoir connected to the lateral ventricle. Agents commonly used include methotrexate, triethylenethiophosphoramide (thio-TEPA), cytosine arabinoside, and methylprednisolone either alone or in combination.

About one-half of patients with breast carcinoma respond initially to these treatments, but the median survival is only 7 months. The prognosis is particularly grave for meningeal carcinomatosis of melanoma or lung tumor origin; few responses are seen. A much better prognosis is expected in patients with lymphoma or leukemia with control for 2 or more years being common. Treatment failures reflect tumor drug resistance, poor circulation of drug within the subarachnoid space, and complications arising from chemotherapy and radiation (see Table 353-4).

TOXIC EFFECTS OF CANCER TREATMENT Chemotherapy Chronic glucocorticoid therapy may induce insulin-dependent diabetes mellitus, myopathy, and aseptic necrosis of the hip and may predispose to thrombophlebitis. In the early stages the muscle changes reverse with steroid taper and intensive physical therapy. Administration of anticonvulsants is associated with cutaneous allergies. Anticonvulsant doses may need to be adjusted in patients receiving glucocorticoids. Allergy to an anticonvulsant may be masked while the patient receives glucocorticoids and revealed later when the steroid medication is tapered. Table 353-4 summarizes the neurologic toxicities of currently used *chemotherapeutic agents*.

Radiation therapy Radiation therapy may cause toxic effects on the CNS. Acute changes include lethargy, loss of appetite, alterations in mental status, or exacerbation of previous symptoms and signs. These develop within 1 to 2 weeks of its initiation. These effects are usually attributable to worsening cerebral edema and are best treated with increased doses of glucocorticoids. Subacute changes that develop between 3 and 18 months after treatment are ascribed to radiation-induced demyelination and are unresponsive to steroids. Reappearance of previous neurologic impairment and the appearance of a mass which is indistinguishable from recurrent tumor on MRI or CT scan may occur. These areas of radiation necrosis may be visualized by hypometabolism following the injection of positron-emitting ^{18}F-deoxyglucose (PET scan). Patients who have received spinal radiation may develop Lhermitte's phenomenon with tingling in the back and legs following flexion of the neck.

Between 18 and 60 months after radiation, still other less reversible changes occur. These include retarded growth rate and impaired intellectual development in children who have received more than 30 Gy (3000 rad) of whole-brain radiation. At doses above 50 Gy (5000 rad), adults may exhibit cortical atrophy, communicating hydrocephalus, and hypothalamic dysfunction with elevated prolactin levels and amenorrhea or impotence. Dementia resulting from these changes is irreversible and in the case of hydrocephalus is usually unimproved by ventricular shunting.

The peripheral nervous system can also be affected by radiation therapy. Localized dysfunction of the brachial or lumbosacral plexus may follow radiation in excess of 40 Gy (4000 rad), usually appearing more than 1 year after treatment (see Chap. 363). Unlike peripheral nerve problems due to tumor invasion, radiation plexopathy is commonly painless. Additional tests, including CT scan, may be necessary to distinguish tumor invasion from radiation toxicity. Glucocorticoids may afford some benefit.

PRIMARY BRAIN TUMORS

In the following section, the most common primary brain tumors in adults are discussed by histologic type. Other tumors which occur in characteristic locations and whose presenting symptoms therefore reflect site rather than specific histology are then discussed by location. These include tumors located in the diencephalon-third ventricle, the posterior fossa, and the skull base.

MALIGNANT ASTROCYTOMA (GLIOBLASTOMA) Definition Malignant astrocytoma or glioblastoma (also known as malignant glioma or grade 3 or 4 astrocytoma) and the less malignant anaplastic astrocytoma account for about one-quarter of the 5000 intracranial gliomas diagnosed yearly in the United States; 75 percent of gliomas in adults are of this category. Because of its profound and uniform morbidity, it contributes more to the cost of cancer on a per capita basis than does any other tumor. The patient, commonly stricken in the fifth decade of life, enters a cycle of repetitive hospitalizations and operations while experiencing the progressive complications associated with relatively ineffective treatments of radiation and chemotherapy.

Pathogenesis and pathology Epidemiologic studies offer few clues to the etiology of malignant astrocytoma. Some tumors arise in patients with longstanding seizure disorders or personality disorders resulting from temporal lobe dysfunction and in scars incurred from head trauma, suggesting that in certain instances the malignant cells emerge from a more benign glial proliferation. There are rare instances of malignant tumors occurring in families, suggesting a genetic propensity. At least four human oncogenes (*sis*, *myc*, *src*, n-*myc*) have been identified in cell lines derived from primary brain tumors, and there is overexpression for the receptors of both platelet-derived (PDGF) and epidermal (EGF) growth factors. Small clusters of tumors have appeared in certain occupational settings, notably in the petro-leum processing industry. The tumor has an appearance similar to that produced by a variety of viral agents inoculated into animals. On gross examination, the surrounding normal brain is distorted and infiltrated by yellow tumor tissue containing areas of necrosis, cysts, and hemorrhage. Microscopic examination reveals a highly cellular composite of heterogeneous glial cells with elongated or rounded astrocytes whose processes stain for glial fibrillary acidic protein. Giant cells may be seen along with mitotic figures and the proliferation of small capillaries.

Clinical manifestations Patients commonly present with a subacute progressive neurologic deficit exhibiting either focal signs or personality changes. Prior mental changes or seizures may antedate tumor diagnosis by months to years. Clinical symptoms may occur abruptly with seizures or with sudden deficits secondary to tumor hemorrhage. The CT scan reveals a heterogeneous pattern of tumor enhancement interspersed with hypodense foci presumably corresponding to tumor necrosis and edema. Multiple tumors can occur but are uncommon. MRI scans often define more extensive tumor involvement than is indicated on the CT scan.

Malignant astrocytoma can arise in the brainstem, cerebellum, or spinal cord in addition to the more common locations within the white matter of the cerebral hemispheres. The prognosis for any site, unfortunately, has not changed greatly in the last 20 years. Following treatment, less than 6 months of useful function can be expected for most patients before progression of symptoms signals recurrent tumor. Death results in 80 percent of patients from tumor recurrence within 6 to 12 months. Progressive neurologic deterioration is followed by stupor and coma. In patients who survive over 1 year, often young adults, CNS dissemination can occur to the meninges or the ventricular ependyma. Metastasis outside the CNS is extremely rare.

Treatment Confirmation of histology by biopsy should be performed in most patients; debulking of tumor is recommended if the tumor is located in an area that permits an extensive operation.

Therapeutic modalities are not highly effective. The average life expectancy of 17 weeks for untreated patients is improved by postoperative external beam radiation alone to 47 weeks and by radiation combined with chemotherapy to 62 weeks. A subgroup of young patients under age 50 obtains significant improvement in quality and duration of life. Such patients have a 20 percent 2-year survival after cranial radiation of 55 to 60 Gy (5500 to 6000 rad) combined with adjunctive chemotherapy with the nitrosoureas carmustine (BCNU) or lomustine (CCNU).

Efforts to improve prognosis for this malignancy include radiotherapy trials of implanted radiation sources of isotopic iodine (^{125}I brachytherapy). Current chemotherapeutic trials are based on the localized nature of the tumor and of its recurrence and involve local arterial infusions of cisplatin prior to radiation or at the time of tumor recurrence. Experimental approaches include the use of β-interferon, interleukin-stimulated lymphocyte killer cells (LAK) or monoclonal antibodies.

ASTROCYTOMA Definition Low-grade astrocytomas occur throughout the brain and spinal cord. The subcortical white matter is the most common site in adults. In children and young adults astrocytomas arise in the optic nerves, cerebellum (cystic, juvenile, pilocytic astrocytoma), and brainstem (pontine glioma). These tumors are also associated with neurofibromatosis and tuberous sclerosis and are found in 20 percent of patients undergoing temporal lobectomy for control of chronic seizure disorders.

Pathogenesis and pathology The tumors are avascular without necrosis and contain homogeneous populations of well-differentiated astrocytes. The astrocytomas are divided into those with good prognosis (80 percent survivorship at 5 years) (cystic cerebellar, "juvenile" pilocytic, giant cell subependymoma) and those with likely recurrence after surgery (infiltrating, gemistocytic, anaplastic).

Clinical manifestations The tumors evolve slowly over several years, producing symptoms by displacement of normal brain or by invasion of white matter tracts. Optic nerve gliomas cause progressive, monocular or bitemporal visual field defects leading eventually to

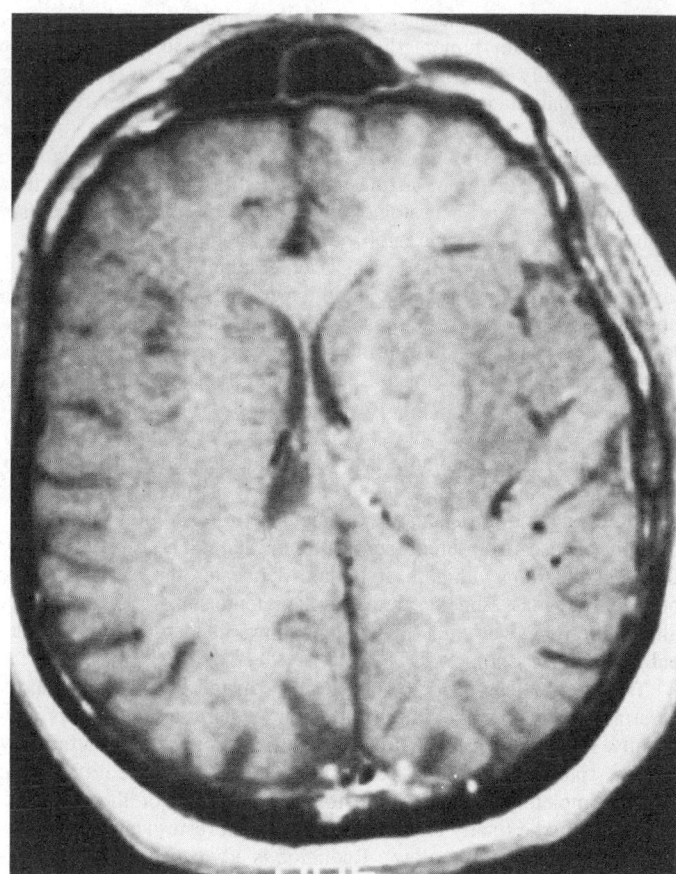

A

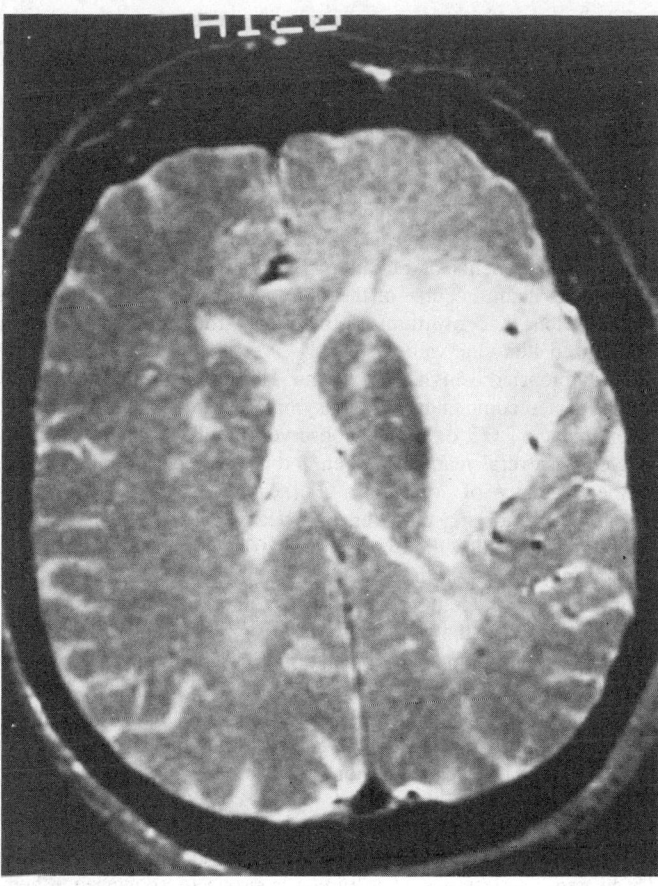

B

FIGURE 353-2 *A*. Gadolinium-DTPA-enhanced T1-weighted axial image demonstrating a decreased signal in the right temporoparietal region with no evidence of contrast enhancement. Mild effacement of the body of the left lateral ventricle without midline shift is present. Biopsy showed low-grade glioma. *B*. T2-weighted axial MRI of same tumor showed area of hyperintense signal corresponding to low signal area seen on T1 study.

blindness and sometimes proptosis. Hypothalamic compression may cause endocrine dysfunction. Hydrocephalus is rare. In the brainstem, such tumors typically involve several cranial nerves (often the abducens, facial, and trigeminal) and later impinge on corticospinal fibers and medial lemniscal and spinothalamic tracts. These symptoms must be distinguished from those caused by multiple sclerosis, arteriovenous malformations, cysts of cysticercosis and echinococcal origin, and extramedullary tumors such as schwannomas or meningiomas. Cerebellar astrocytomas cause progressive incoordination and gait ataxia combined with abnormalities of eye movements. In supratentorial locations, these tumors may produce seizures before any focal abnormality appears on clinical examination. In *gliomatosis cerebri,* slow infiltration of white matter occurs with atypical individual astrocytes without evidence of localized tumor.

Early use of MRI scanning may allow for earlier diagnosis and intervention (see Figs. 353-1, 353-2, and 353-3). MRI often demonstrates white matter abnormalities in patients with normal CT scans and is the preferred procedure for early diagnosis and follow-up. A stable clinical course is common with astrocytoma and repeat radiologic studies may show little change. The characteristic CT appearance is an indistinct mass that is hypodense with respect to surrounding brain and exhibits little or no contrast enhancement, calcification, or evidence of edema. Malignant degeneration of astrocytomas is heralded by rapid progression of symptoms and signs, evidence of expanded size or altered MRI T2 or CT signal, or the presence of new enhancement on MRI with gadolinium DTPA or CT with iodine contrast.

Treatment Because up to half of nonenhancing CT masses may be aggressive gliomas, many surgeons argue for early biopsy. This is especially true in the setting of seizure progression or increase in

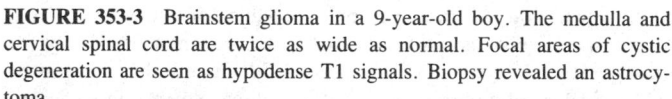

FIGURE 353-3 Brainstem glioma in a 9-year-old boy. The medulla and cervical spinal cord are twice as wide as normal. Focal areas of cystic degeneration are seen as hypodense T1 signals. Biopsy revealed an astrocytoma.

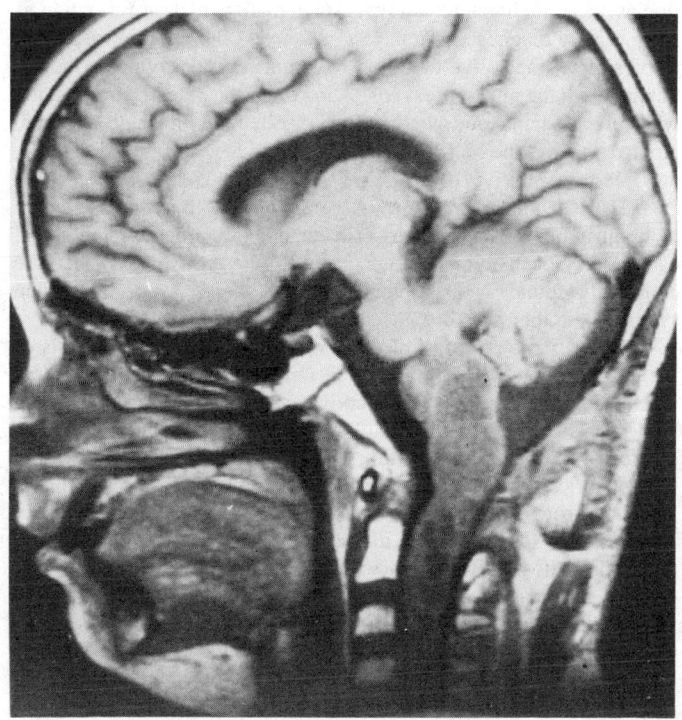

the size of the lesion. Surgical excision can be curative for some cerebellar, optic nerve, and lobar astrocytomas. Cyst drainage and partial resection are feasible for many. Biopsy should be obtained for supratentorial tumors but is less frequently considered for brainstem or spinal cord gliomas. Exceptions to the latter are tumors that have a cystic or extraaxial component. Postoperative radiation is recommended for incompletely resected tumors and for those involving the brainstem (for which multiple daily doses are often provided). Its role in the treatment of excised supratentorial tumors is less clear. The possible benefits of radiation therapy are weighed against the known long natural course of the astrocytoma and the complications of irradiation. A consortium of treatment groups has placed under randomized study the value of "early" versus "delayed" irradiation of newly biopsied benign astrocytoma. Until this study is completed, radiation is recommended when symptoms and signs progress or enlargement on CT or MRI is observed. Radiation may be safely delayed for several years in apparently totally resected tumors because of the accuracy of MRI and CT scans. The judicious use of glucocorticoids during radiation or when symptoms recur improves function. The median life expectancy is 67 months for supratentorial tumors and 89 months for cerebellar tumors. Average survivals of 15 months after radiation are reported for patients with brainstem tumors. However, the 5-year survival is only 30 percent. Chemotherapy, currently under investigation for brainstem tumors, may offer some improvement in survival.

OLIGODENDROGLIOMA   Definition   This tumor of oligodendroglial origin may develop in isolation or may be mixed with other glial cells. An uncommon tumor, it represents less then 10 percent of all gliomas.

Pathology   Microscopic examination discloses rounded cells containing darkly staining nuclei with poorly staining cytoplasm, the "fried egg" appearance. The tumor is prone to spontaneous hemorrhage. Both "benign" and "malignant" forms are seen.

Clinical manifestations   Presentation is most commonly in the third or fourth decade and tumors are most frequently in the frontal lobes or within the ventricles. CT reveals a well-defined, low-attenuation mass with fine speckled calcium deposits and small cysts.

Treatment   Although the oligodendroglioma is histologically benign, resection is curative in only one-third of patients. The role of postoperative radiation is uncertain; it is recommended only for incompletely resected tumors or those with mixed glial features or with evidence of progression after operation. Some oligodendrogliomas have malignant features. Such malignant transformation is more readily diagnosed if contrast-enhanced CT is used. Prospective studies of postoperative radiation have not been performed. Chemotherapy with the nitrosoureas lomustine or carmustine (in combination with procarbazine and vincristine) is effective in some patients. Approximately one-half of patients survive 5 years after diagnosis, and one-third survive 10 years.

MENINGIOMA   Definition   Meningiomas account for 20 percent of brain tumors. They can arise in either the cranium or the spinal canal. They occur more frequently at all sites in women. They are commonly found as asymptomatic tumors at postmortem. When symptomatic they usually present in the fifth or sixth decades.

Pathogenesis and pathology   Meningiomas arise from cells of the pia-arachnoid. Common sites include the midline along the falx cerebri and the lateral cerebral convexity, the olfactory groove and along the sphenoid ridge, the tuberculum sellae, foramen magnum, and tentorium of the cerebellum. They also arise on occasion within the ventricles, where on radiographic examination they are indistinguishable from a papilloma of the choroid plexus. Meningiomas may coexist with schwannomas in patients with the central form of neurofibromatosis. Both tumor types are related to the loss of a "tumor suppressor" gene on chromosome 22. They occur more frequently in women with breast cancer; some meningiomas contain estrogen and progesterone receptors.

On the basis of microscopic characteristics, meningiomas are divided into seven categories: syncytial, transitional, fibroblastic, microcystic, psammomatous, angioblastic, and malignant meningiomas. Malignant tumors display mitoses, invade normal brain, and occasionally develop CNS and extraneural metastases. Angioblastic and malignant forms are more likely than the other types to recur.

Clinical manifestations   The clinical presentation reflects the slow expansion of tumor in the characteristic locations within the skull and spine, with neurologic deficits evolving over many years. Tumors of the parasellar region produce a combination of second, third, fourth, fifth, and sixth cranial nerve deficits. Cerebellopontine tumors may produce a syndrome similar to that of acoustic schwannomas (see "Tumors of the Posterior Fossa" below). Early hearing loss is not a typical finding in meningioma. Parasagittal and frontal tumors may produce seizures or may be entirely asymptomatic, often growing to enormous size before they are discovered. Parasagittal lesions that attain sufficient size may cause spastic paraparesis and incontinence. Falx meningioma should be considered in the differential diagnosis of gait disorders in the middle-aged and elderly. In all locations, meningiomas must be distinguished from similar-appearing dural metastases from breast, prostate, and lung. The CT scan often discloses calcium within a tumor and delineates the close relation between the mass and the dura, falx, or tentorium, as well as the altered bony calvarium. MRI often shows isodense masses that enhance with gadolinium-DTPA.

Treatment   Tumor site, rather than histology, is the major determinant of outcome. Intraventricular or parasagittal tumors are usually resectable and recurrence is rare. Those in the olfactory groove, sphenoid ridge, and parasellar locations are more difficult to resect completely and are prone to recur. Tumors of the foramen magnum may be totally removed with microneurosurgical techniques (see "Spinal Tumors" below). Radiation is advocated for malignant meningiomas and for incompletely excised symptomatic tumors of other histologic subtypes. Chemotherapy is without apparent efficacy.

PAPILLOMA OF THE CHOROID PLEXUS   Definition   Neoplasms derived from choroid plexus epithelium are rare, representing only 0.5 percent of all intracranial tumors.

Pathogenesis and pathology   In children most such tumors occur in the lateral ventricles, whereas in adults the fourth ventricle is the most common site. The histologic structure resembles normal choroid plexus, with a connective tissue core covered by a single layer of cuboidal epithelium.

Clinical manifestations   Very rare examples of malignant transformation have been described. Metastases to the leptomeninges may occur. The tumor may secrete excessive CSF leading to communicating hydrocephalus.

Treatment   Surgery is the treatment of choice and is usually highly successful.

LIPOMA   Lipoma can develop anywhere within the brain or spinal cord, though the corpus callosum is the most common location. The association of lipomas with partial or complete agenesis of this structure and with other dysplastic or hamartomatous anomalies such as ectopias, colloid cysts, and epidermoids supports the theory that they are the result of disorders of development. Intraspinal lipomas are most common in the thoracic region and are associated with spina bifida in one-third of cases. All lipomas can be easily demonstrated by MRI. The treatment of symptomatic cranial and spinal lipomas is excision.

DERMOID AND EPIDERMOID TUMOR   Definition   The distinction between dermoid tumors and epidermoids (true cholesteatomas) is often difficult. Both result from inclusion of ectodermal tissue at the time of closure of the neural groove and soon thereafter.

Pathology and pathogenesis   Cholesteatomas are slowly growing tumors that most often afflict young adults, occurring commonly in lateral or midline locations within the skull, i.e., the cerebellopontine angle, the suprasellar region, the fourth ventricle, the pineal region, and over the hemispheres. No clear relationship has been established between cholesteatoma of the cerebellopontine angle and middle ear infection. Dermoid tumors, which are frequently cystic, occur largely in the posterior fossa or in the lumbosacral region. Rarely they are found in suprasellar or pineal regions.

Clinical manifestations Symptoms vary according to the location of these tumors, the general pattern being slow evolution of defects attributable to the specific area with seizures interspersed when the tumor occupies cortical regions. MRI provides excellent delineation.

Treatment Treatment of the cholesteatoma is total surgical removal of the tumor together with its capsule. Dermoid tumors similarly are curable if total surgical excision is possible.

PRIMARY LYMPHOMA OF THE CENTRAL NERVOUS SYSTEM

Definition Primary lymphomas are now recognized to be relatively common in the CNS. Before 1972, fewer than 25 cases had been identified at the Massachusetts General Hospital over a 50-year period. Since 1977, 10 cases per year have been diagnosed. Primary lymphoma is distinguished from the more frequent secondary involvement of the meninges that occurs in patients with poorly differentiated non-Hodgkin's lymphomas.

Pathogenesis and pathology The tumor is uncommon in patients without immunologic compromise. It is usually seen in patients with mixed humoral and cellular immune deficits. Three such disorders are recognized: inherited disorders of immunity such as combined immunodeficiency disease, selective IgM deficiency, or selective IgA abnormalities seen with combined immunodeficiency and Wiskott-Aldrich syndrome; acquired immunodeficiency syndrome (AIDS); and therapeutic immunosuppression following organ transplantation or treatment of autoimmune disorders. The demonstration of Epstein-Barr virus (EBV) DNA within primary lymphoma in some affected patients raises the possibility that this agent may play a role in the pathogenesis of this disease.

The tumor may be focal or multicentric in the subcortical white matter, the walls of the ventricles, or the subarachnoid space. Tumor cells are always found in a perivascular distribution. At biopsy, tumor cells are often indistinguishable from normal lymphocytes, leading to an erroneous early diagnosis of "encephalitis" or "nonspecific perivascular inflammation." The B-cell populations may be characterized as malignant by monoclonal antibodies to immunoglobulin surface proteins. The tumors contain cells defined histologically as diffuse histiocytic or poorly differentiated lymphocytes by the Rappaport system and as follicular center cells and small cleaved cells by the Lukes-Collins system (see Chap. 302). Burkitt-type lymphomas are rarely reported.

Clinical manifestations A history of personality change, focal deficits, or seizures evolving over several weeks in an immunosuppressed patient should raise the suspicion of cerebral lymphoma. Obviously, in these circumstances infection must be excluded. Patients with HIV infection are often treated presumptively for toxoplasmosis and brain lymphoma. The CT scan typically reveals multiple periventricular masses which enhance with contrast. Similar lesions are seen on T2-weighted MRI sections. These may persist when CT abnormalities have disappeared. A characteristic feature, rarely observed with other types of intracranial tumor, is the marked reduction or disappearance of lesions after a few weeks of high-dose glucocorticoid therapy (dexamethasone 6 to 10 mg four times daily). When both symptoms and CT abnormalities resolve after glucocorticoid therapy, remissions lasting several months are common, and steroids can be tapered. Spontaneous remissions without glucocorticoid therapy have been described. The usual clinical course is recurrence after 4 to 6 months, with resistance to steroid administration. The tumor may seed the meninges in one-quarter of patients. Systemic lymphoma is found in less than 10 percent of patients and occurs late in the course of the disease. However, uveitis or vitreitis may occur at the time of presentation or early in the evolution of the disease; when present, it is helpful in the initial diagnosis.

Treatment After biopsy or diagnosis by CSF cytology, the recommended treatment is chemotherapy consisting of high-dose methotrexate and glucocorticoids, alone or in combination with cyclophosphamide, doxorubicin, and vincristine, followed by radiation. Chemotherapy provides therapeutic drug levels in brain paren-

chyma and most importantly, in the CSF. Partial or complete remission occurs in over three-quarters of patients. When methotrexate is administered prior to radiation, there is a reduced risk of radiation or drug-induced white matter damage. The median survival following irradiation is 17 months. Radiation treatment is recommended for patients with brain lymphoma.

TUMORS OF THE THIRD VENTRICLE AND PINEAL REGION

Several categories of tumors occur in close proximity to the diencephalon, hypothalamus, and third ventricle; these are pituitary adenoma, craniopharyngioma, germ-cell neoplasms, pineal tumors, and glial, meningeal, or metastatic tumors.

Uncommon tumors of the pineal region include astrocytomas, glioblastomas, meningiomas, and metastases. Nonneoplastic masses occurring in this region include colloid cysts of the third ventricle (see "Colloid Cysts" below) and parasitic cysts (cysticercosis).

Pituitary adenomas These tumors are described in Chap. 313.

Craniopharyngiomas These tumors arise from remnants of Rathke's pouch, derived from the primitive stomatodeum. They are usually suprasellar in location and cause symptoms related to neuroendocrine dysfunction or visual compromise (see also Chap. 313). They are easily identified by a "bright" T2 signal on MRI (Fig. 353-4).

Germ-cell tumors DEFINITION Germ-cell tumors, which account for half of all pineal region neoplasms, arise primarily during childhood or early adolescence and include germinoma, teratoma, embryonal carcinoma, endodermal sinus tumor, and choriocarcinoma.

CLINICAL MANIFESTATIONS The most common of these germ-cell tumors is the germinoma. It may occur in the pineal region or at the base of the hypothalamus. It occurs more frequently in males,

FIGURE 353-4 This 39-year-old woman presented with headaches and gait disturbance (caused by a craniopharyngioma). On a T1-weighted coronal MRI, a large, lobulated hyperdense mass is visualized in the suprasellar cistern compressing the inferior third ventricle. There is enlargement of the frontal and temporal ventricles.

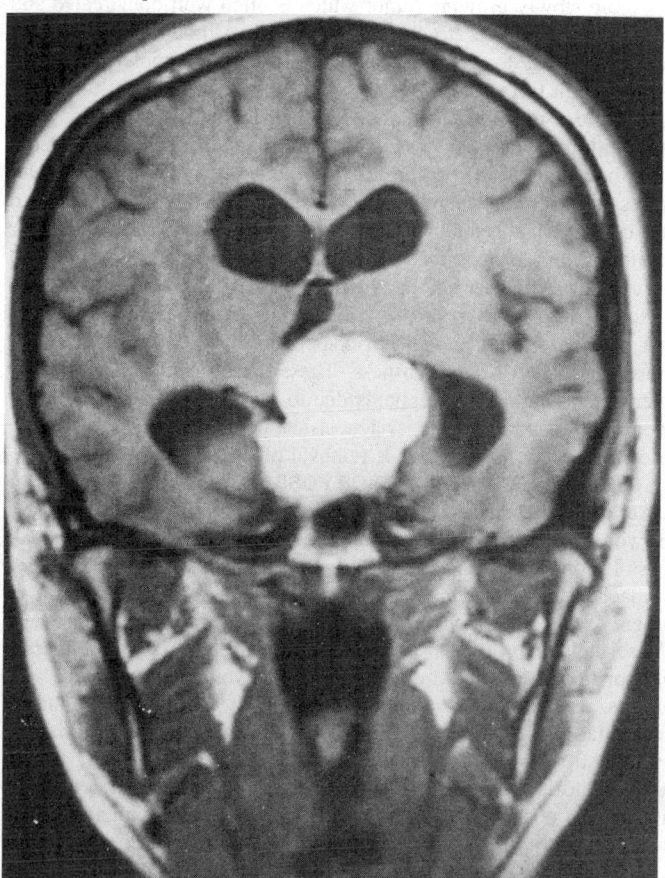

who present with findings of diabetes insipidus and other neuroendocrine deficiencies, bitemporal visual field defects, paralysis of upward gaze (see Chap. 23), and sometimes hydrocephalus. The typical features of pineal masses occur more commonly with nongerminomatous germ-cell tumors. Findings include Parinaud's syndrome—a failure of upward gaze and pupillary dilatation with deficiencies in response to light. Rarely, other signs such as nystagmus retractorius or brainstem signs due to compression may occur. Diagnosis may be assisted by the finding of elevated serum and CSF levels of alphafetoprotein (AFP) and of human chorionic gonadotropin (hCG) in germinomas. MRI and CT scans identify tumors of the pineal region *but offer no histologic differentiation.*

TREATMENT   Following biopsy by transcallosal or suboccipital route, radiation is given. Germinomas are radiosensitive; up to 80 percent are cured by well-tolerated doses of cranial radiation. Craniospinal irradiation is provided when tumor invades the ventricles or subarachnoid space, or is found outside the pineal region. Other histologic subtypes have poorer prognoses and recurrence is common, often with seeding of the cranial nerves and meninges. Recurrences sometimes respond to drug treatment with etoposide, cisplatin, and doxorubicin, which are beneficial in testicular tumors of similar histology.

Pineoblastoma and pineocytoma   These tumors account for 20 percent of growths in the pineal region.

PATHOGENESIS AND PATHOLOGY   Pineoblastoma and pineocytoma arise from pineal organ cells. The pineoblastoma is a primitive malignant tumor of childhood and early adult life and is indistinguishable both in appearance and natural history from primitive neuroectodermal tumors that arise elsewhere in the CNS. The tumor may contain astrocytic or neuronal elements. Recurrence is invariable and dissemination through the ventricular system and subarachnoid space is frequent.

TREATMENT   Brain and neuraxis radiation are recommended, and chemotherapy as outlined above for germ-cell tumors has been successful in producing remissions in a few patients. Chemotherapy prior to irradiation is reserved for pineoblastoma. The pineocytoma is a more slowly growing tumor which is often well-demarcated and resembles the normal structure of the pineal. Although histologically benign, it tends to recur, probably because of incomplete removal. It is resistant to radiation.

Colloid cysts   PATHOGENESIS AND PATHOLOGY   Colloid cysts arise within the anterior third ventricle and are considered to develop from the anlage of the paraphysis, a component of the third ventricle, or possibly from the ependyma itself. The cysts are well-encapsulated and consist of a layer of connective tissue covered with columnar ciliated cells. The cyst is filled with glycoproteinaceous material which stains with periodic acid Schiff (PAS).

CLINICAL MANIFESTATIONS   Symptoms occur usually in adults and may be dramatic, with episodes of headache, weakness of the limbs, and loss of consciousness. These symptoms are attributed to intermittent acute hydrocephalus due to blockage of the foramen of Monro by the mobile cyst. Diagnosis cannot be made with certainty prior to operation; treatment is removal of the cyst.

TUMORS OF THE POSTERIOR FOSSA   Tumors of the posterior fossa pose special problems in diagnosis and treatment. Rapidly growing tumors may cause obstructive hydrocephalus, and even small mass lesions in the posterior fossa may result in vomiting, lethargy, headache, and papilledema. Slowly growing tumors give rise to progressive signs which are recognized by rather specific syndromes. These include progressive unilateral hearing loss, facial weakness, pain or numbness, and a unilateral sixth nerve deficit occurring with tumors in the cerebellopontine angle. Gait ataxia and unilateral cerebellar signs occur with hemangioblastoma, medulloblastoma, or cystic astrocytoma of the cerebellum. Progressive diplopia, cranial nerve abnormalities, and crossed corticospinal tract and reflex abnormalities occur in brainstem glioma. Nuchal and occipital pain are common with all tumors of the posterior fossa. Corticospinal signs

develop with further tumor enlargement and encroachment on the brainstem.

Acoustic schwannoma   DEFINITION   The acoustic schwannoma (synonymous with acoustic neuroma) is composed of myelin-forming Schwann cells that cover the acoustic nerve fibers. Schwann cells normally replace oligodendroglia as the nerve leaves the brainstem to enter the internal auditory meatus.

PATHOGENESIS AND PATHOLOGY   Schwannomas are slow-growing masses that compress rather than invade normal tissue. When bilateral, they represent an inherited form of schwannoma which is diagnostic of ''central'' neurofibromatosis. Other CNS tumors associated with neurofibromatosis or von Recklinghausen's disease are schwannomas of spinal and other cranial nerves, intracranial and spinal meningiomas, gliomas, and ependymomas (see Chap. 358).

CLINICAL MANIFESTATIONS AND TREATMENT   Early detection of acoustic schwannomas at a time of minimal hearing deficit and minimal facial motor difficulty is essential, as hearing may be spared by microneurosurgical intervention while the tumor is still restricted to the canal. Brainstem auditory-evoked responses, CT and MRI studies, especially with contrast injection, have replaced metrizamide cisternography by enhancing the physician's ability to detect these tumors in their early stages.

Hemangioblastoma   DEFINITION   The cerebellar hemangioblastoma is an uncommon tumor that may be solitary but is frequently multiple. When the tumors are multiple, they are considered part of von Hippel-Lindau disease. This autosomal dominant disorder, linked to chromosome 3, typically consists of retinal, cerebellar, and spinal hemangioblastomas and visceral lesions, usually renal and/or pancreatic tumors or cysts. Polycythemia may be present.

PATHOGENESIS AND PATHOLOGY   Hemangioblastomas are well-circumscribed and often cystic. The tumor may consist solely of a small nodule attached to the wall of a large cyst. The lesion is usually highly vascular and may be mistaken for an arteriovenous malformation. The microscopic appearance is one of numerous capillary vessels separated by sheets of clear cells with an abundance of intracytoplasmic vacuoles. The tumors are probably derived from capillary endothelial cells.

CLINICAL MANIFESTATIONS   Dizziness, ataxia of gait or of the limbs, and symptoms of raised intracranial pressure are characteristic features of the cerebellar hemangioblastoma. The tumors may bleed spontaneously, resulting in a paroxysmal onset of headache and neurologic deficit. The MRI may show vascular ''flow voids'' or ferritin suggesting old hemorrhage.

TREATMENT   Craniotomy with opening of the cerebellar cyst and excision of the mural tumor may be curative. Though the tumor is histologically benign, postoperative recurrences and the appearance of less operable spinal lesions worsen the prognosis. Patients with the von Hippel-Lindau syndrome should have periodic ophthalmologic evaluation for the appearance of retinal angiomas and general medical follow-up for early detection of renal tumors.

Ependymoma   PATHOGENESIS AND PATHOLOGY   These are glial tumors that occur chiefly in childhood and young adulthood, with a typical cranial location in the fourth ventricle. The tumor is composed of uniform ependymal cells surrounding a central lumen. Spinal ependymomas, which are more common, arise within the dura of the lumbar spine and represent more than half of spinal intramedullary gliomas. In this location, the prognosis is excellent. Supratentorial tumors are often more aggressive in rate of growth.

TREATMENT   Resection and radiation to the tumor site results in 5-year survival in excess of 80 percent for spinal cord lesions and between 30 percent and 50 percent for posterior fossa tumors. The role of chemotherapy in the treatment of local recurrences and of seeding within the subarachnoid space is not established.

PRIMITIVE NEUROECTODERMAL TUMORS (PNET)   Several histologic varieties of tumor arise from primitive neuroectodermal tumors (PNET) which contain cells with a capacity to differentiate into medulloblasts, astrocytes, oligodendrocytes, ependyma, ganglion cells, or skeletal muscle. Some tumors have several cell types, but all PNETs share a propensity for local invasion, subarachnoid dissemination, and extraneural metastases. The initial evaluation should include CT scan and myelography with CSF cytology.

Medulloblastoma DEFINITION The *medulloblastoma* is the most common variety of PNET. It accounts for 25 percent of childhood brain tumors. However, one-fourth of medulloblastomas occur in patients over age 20.

PATHOGENESIS AND PATHOLOGY In children the tumor is usually located in the midline, in the inferior portion of the vermis of the cerebellum. In adults the cerebellar hemisphere is most often the site of occurrence. It is composed of small, densely staining cells which elicit a brisk glial response. Invasion of the meninges, ventricles, and subarachnoid space is common.

CLINICAL MANIFESTATIONS The common presentation is occipital headache, vomiting, and trunkal ataxia. Hydrocephalus is frequent. With enlargement of the tumor other signs of brainstem compression emerge. As spinal axis dissemination occurs in one-third of patients CSF cytologic examination and myelography are advocated during initial evaluation.

TREATMENT Resection of the tumor is usually attempted, followed by radiation in doses of 45 to 50 Gy (4500 to 5000 rad) to the posterior fossa, together with 40 Gy (4000 rad) to the whole brain and 35 to 40 Gy (3500 to 4000 rad) to the spinal cord. Chemotherapy prior to irradiation has not been shown to be effective, although it is used with some success in recurrent tumors. Nitrosourea, procarbazine, and vincristine combined with prednisone and intrathecal methotrexate are advocated. Five-year survival is nearly 75 percent. The posterior fossa remains the major site for recurrence. A pessimistic outlook exists for children under 3 years, those with large tumors, and those with subarachnoid spread. Metastases to lung, liver, vertebrae, and pelvis are reported. Some medulloblastomas may take on features reminiscent of neuroblastoma.

Neuroblastoma DEFINITION The neuroblastoma, a relatively common adrenal tumor, can rarely occur as a primary CNS tumor. Eighty percent of cases present during the first decade of life.

PATHOGENESIS AND PATHOLOGY Microscopically, neuroblastoma resembles medulloblastoma because of its small dense cells. Variations in pathology occur. Some tumors show differentiation to ganglion cells but do not have a better prognosis. These tumors appear to form a spectrum of tumors of embryonal origin, ranging from the aggressive, poorly differentiated PNETs to the very well differentiated and quite slow growing neurocytomas. The intraparenchymal tumors found in children resemble in clinical behavior the PNETs, with neuroaxis spread and occasional extraneural metastases. CT reveals a hypodense mass with dense uniform enhancement after contrast administration as well as variable hemorrhage and calcification. These tumors may present as slowly growing intraventricular masses in adults and may grow to large size before discovery.

TREATMENT The rarity of these tumors has prevented any randomized therapeutic trials. Optimal treatment may consist of radical excision with postoperative radiation, though definitive evidence that radiation increases survival is lacking. Because of the frequency of local recurrence and CSF metastases, prophylactic spinal irradiation may be justified. A trial of chemotherapy, either pre- or postirradiation may be worthwhile, especially in younger patients with more aggressive-appearing tumors. Long-term follow-up is complete but appears to have a greater than 30 percent 5-year survival. The survival of adults with intraventricular tumors may be better than that of other primitive CNS tumors.

TUMORS OF THE SKULL BASE Tumors in this region produce characteristic clinical presentations that pose unique diagnostic difficulties even with advanced neuroradiologic procedures. Meningiomas, tumors of bone (including epidermoid and dermoid tumors and osteomas), chordomas, schwannomas (neurofibromas) of the cranial nerves, nasopharyngeal carcinoma, and metastases may all present with pain localized to the lower face, ear, or occiput and

with involvement of one or more cranial nerves making exit from the skull. Metastases arise commonly from the lung, breast, nasopharynx, testicle, and prostate. Multiple myeloma and occasionally lymphoma may appear at this site. The mass may be palpable or may be visualized on polytomography, CT scan, or MRI; however, even a combination of all three studies may be negative. These studies usually differentiate successfully other erosive processes of the skull base, including fibrous dysplasia, Paget's disease, xanthomatosis, and osteitis fibrosa cystica. Enlargement of specific cranial nerve foramens may be the first evidence of schwannomas or of *glomus* tumors of the chromaffin cells in the jugular bulb. These last tumors invade temporal and occipital bone and produce hearing abnormalities and lower cranial nerve deficits.

Chordomas arise from remnants of the notochord. Of these, 60 percent are localized in the clivus, 30 percent in the sacral region, and the remaining 10 percent along the extent of the spine and skull base. The chordoma is not easily distinguished in appearance from radiation-sensitive chondrosarcomas and chondroid chordoma. They are highly invasive, expanding along the skull base and causing serial cranial nerve compression, sometimes with invasion of the nasopharynx. Up to one-third may metastasize via the subarachnoid space. A cauda equina syndrome (see "Spinal Tumors") results from sacral tumors. Clivus tumors may be difficult to visualize adequately on CT scan but are clearly delineated by MRI. Complete removal is rarely feasible and postoperative radiation therapy is recommended. Radiation with cyclotron-derived protons is followed by 80 percent survival at 5 years and 63 percent at 10 years with minimal complications.

Metastases to the skull base are treated with radiation therapy. In the presence of characteristic patterns of pain and cranial nerve deficit, radiation may be considered to treat presumptive metastases in patients with known systemic malignancy even when radiographic examinations are inconclusive.

SPINAL TUMORS Pathogenesis and pathology Tumors of the spinal canal and of the cord are only one-quarter as common as are intracranial tumors. Spinal neoplasms arise from the same types of cells as their counterparts in the cerebrum. They are classified according to location as intramedullary (within the substance of the spinal cord), extramedullary (or intradural), and extradural. Some tumors, such as schwannomas, may be both extradural and intradural. The most frequent location for all types of spinal neoplasms is in the thoracic cord, presumably reflecting its greater total length. These tumors arise from cells of the spinal cord, nerve roots, meninges, vascular structures, or the vertebral column. Tumors of the spinal cord parenchyma are relatively infrequent compared to lesions arising outside the substance of the cord. In one large series, nerve sheath tumors (schwannomas) accounted for 29 percent of all spinal tumors, meningiomas for 25.5 percent, gliomas for 22 percent, and sarcomas for 12 percent. Metastatic lesions represent about 13 percent of all spinal tumors, but as with intracranial tumors, these figures reflect neurosurgical service statistics and metastases are likely underrepresented.

Clinical manifestations Any lesion that narrows the spinal canal sufficiently to encroach on neural structures can give rise to neurologic symptoms. Dysfunction may arise from direct compression of the spinal cord and its nerve roots or from interference with blood supply. The rapid growth of metastatic lesions leads to motor and sensory symptoms over a period of days to weeks, whereas slowly growing astrocytomas and ependymomas produce symptoms over a period of months to years.

Extramedullary tumors (both intradural and epidural) cause symptoms by compressing the spinal cord or nerve roots. The initial symptoms are usually focal back pain and paresthesias followed by sensory loss below the level of the pain, weakness, and bladder and bowel dysfunction. Intramedullary lesions usually extend over several spinal cord segments, and their symptoms and signs are more varied than those of extramedullary tumors. A common pattern is dissociated sensory loss, with pain and temperature sensation impairment in the segments of tumor origin and with sparing of posterior column sensory function. Later, as the tumor grows peripherally, spinothalamic tracts may be involved. Since, in the thoracic and cervical regions, the sacral pain and temperature fibers lie superficial to those fibers representing more rostral regions, the sacral segments may be spared. Atrophy in the appropriate segments due to anterior horn cell involvement may combine with corticospinal tract signs.

These clinical presentations are not diagnostic of spinal cord neoplasm. Transverse myelitis from multiple sclerosis or other causes can lead to rapid onset of spinal cord dysfunction associated with pain, paresthesias, and weakness (see Chap. 361). A similar syndrome can occur as a paraneoplastic process, resulting from a necrotic myelopathy (see Chap. 310). Syringomyelia can produce a chronic syndrome indistinguishable from that produced by intramedullary neoplasms. Other diseases that can lead to a progressive spinal cord syndrome include combined system degeneration due to vitamin B_{12} deficiency, amyotrophic lateral sclerosis, cervical spondylosis, arachnoiditis, vascular anomalies, meningeal carcinomatosis, and spinal stenosis due to a combination of degenerative disk disease and hypertrophy of the ligamentum flavum (see Chap. 361).

Additional specific clinical syndromes occur in two other locations within the spinal canal. *Foramen magnum tumors* may extend into the cervical region or rostrally into the posterior fossa. A combination of signs and symptoms referrable to lower cranial nerves, sensory loss in the distribution of the second cervical segment, posterior headache, and asymmetric sensory and motor involvement of the limbs leads to the suspicion of such a tumor, most commonly a meningioma. *Tumors of the conus medullaris or cauda equina* produce pain in the back, rectum, and/or both legs and may mimic lumbosacral disk disease. With tumor growth, muscle atrophy in the legs associated with sphincter dysfunction and reflex changes usually point to the correct site of involvement.

Diagnosis of spinal cord tumors MRI has replaced all other modalities in the evaluation of the patient with cancer suspected to exist outside of or within the dura of the spinal canal (Fig. 353-5). In most centers MRI can be performed as an emergency procedure.

FIGURE 353-5 Sagittal T1-weighted MRI image of the conus medullaris (arrow) in a 26-year-old male with malignant primitive neuroectodermal tumor.

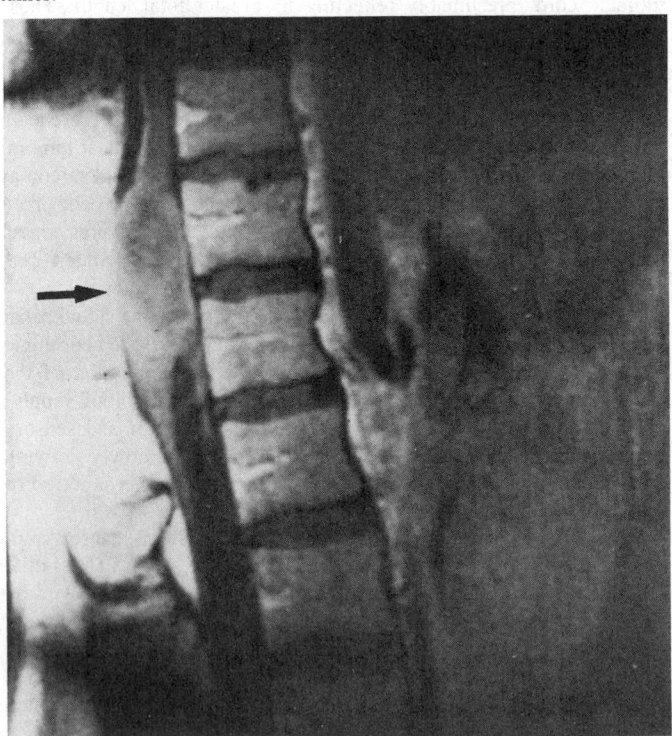

With or without gadolinium, these studies delineate the site, number, and extent of *extradural* deposits, while providing definitive information concerning the enlargement of neural foramens (which occur with schwannomas), distortion of paraspinal tissues with masses that have grown into the spinal canal from extraneural sites (as with lymphomatous spread), and the intricate anatomy of the cervicomedullary junction (as with meningioma or skull-base chordoma or nasopharyngeal metastases). MRI pictures have supplanted confusing arguments regarding "complete" or "incomplete" myelographic block. By identifying multiple extradural lesions needless surgery can be avoided and irradiation fields appropriately applied. Intradural, leptomeningeal metastases or tumors within the spinal cord or its roots are equally amenable to MRI visualization, especially when used following injection of gadolinium.

Myelography following the subarachnoid injection of nonionic contrast materials is often used to complement MRI studies or when they are unavailable. A small amount of contrast injected prior to CT evaluation of the spine is used to elucidate the coexistence of extradural tumor *and* calcified disk fragment, compression fracture of the bony vertebrae, osteomyelitis, or defects from prior surgery or irradiation. Similarly these CT studies identify intradural processes including arachnoiditis, lipomatous masses, and syrinx for which MRI experience remains scanty.

Cerebrospinal fluid removed at the time of myelography should be analyzed for cell count, protein content, and cytology. A specimen stained with Wright's stain should be analyzed and cells examined further after cytocentrifugation. The cell count is usually normal in spinal tumors unless there is meningeal tumor, but protein content is increased in virtually all cases of high-grade spinal cord block. The CSF glucose is usually normal unless there is meningeal tumor invasion.

Treatment Once the diagnosis of spinal cord tumor is established, rapid treatment is mandatory to maximize neurologic recovery. Extramedullary primary neoplasms are treated with microneurosurgery, and complete resection is usually possible. The most common intramedullary tumors, ependymomas and astrocytomas, usually can only be partially resected and are likely to recur. The role of radiation therapy for slowly growing tumors of this class is not well established; for high-grade astrocytomas a course of postoperative radiation is recommended. Glucocorticoids may improve function temporarily. There is no established role for chemotherapy of spinal neoplasms.

EPIDURAL CANCER: THE PATIENT WITH CANCER AND BACK PAIN Spinal epidural cancer should be suspected in patients with back pain and known systemic malignancy even in the absence of neurologic signs. Progressive paraparesis with bladder dysfunction and development of a sensory deficit may be avoided by early intervention. High doses of glucocorticoids (up to 100 mg dexamethasone per day) are administered immediately and radiation therapy is usually recommended. The results of treatment in the large series of patients with epidural cancer reported by Gilbert has led to the conclusion that radiation therapy is as effective as surgery in the relief of symptoms. The clinical condition of the patient at the time of diagnosis is the most important factor in prognosis; only 3 percent of patients paraplegic at the time of treatment, regardless of type of therapy, regain ambulation. Reconsideration is being given to surgical decompression as a primary mode of treatment in patients with radioresistant malignancies such as melanoma and lung, prostatic, and colonic cancers and in the setting of paraparesis of recent onset.

REFERENCES

BRANT-ZAWADZKI M: MR imaging of the brain. Radiology 166:1, 1988
BULLARD DE et al: Oligodendroglioma. An analysis of the value of radiation therapy. Cancer 60:2179, 1987
BYRNE TN, WAXSMAN SG: *Spinal Cord Compression; Diagnosis and Principles of Management*. Philadelphia, FA Davis 1990
CORBETT JJ et al: Visual loss in pseudotumor cerebri. Arch Neurol 39:461, 1982
GILBERT RW et al: Epidural spinal cord compression from metastatic tumor: Diagnosis and treatment. Ann Neurol 3:40, 1978

GUTIN PH: Recurrent malignant gliomas: Survival following interstitial brachytherapy with high activity iodine 125 sources. J Neurosurg 67:864, 1987

HART R et al: Acoustic tumors: Atypical features and recent diagnostic tests. Neurology 33:211, 1983.

HESSELINK JR, PRESS GA: MR contrast enhancement of intracranial lesions with Gd-DTPA. Radiol Clin North Am 26:873, 1988

HOCHBERG FH, MILLER DC: Primary central nervous system lymphoma. J Neurosurg 68:835, 1988

HUGHES EN et al: Medulloblastoma at the Joint Center for Radiation Therapy between 1968 and 1984. The influence of radiation dose on the patterns of failure and survival. Cancer 61:1992, 1988

JENNINGS MT et al: Intracranial germ cell tumors: Natural history and pathogenesis. J Neurosurg 63:155, 1985

LAWS ER et al: Neurosurgical management of low grade astrocytomas of the cerebral hemispheres. J Neurosurg 61:665, 1984

LINSTADT D et al: Radiotherapy of primary intracranial germinomas: The case against routine craniospinal irradiation. Int J Radiat Oncol Biol Phys 15:291, 1988

MIRA JG et al: Outcome of prophylactic and therapeutic cranial irradiation in disseminated small cell lung carcinoma. Int J Radiat Oncol Biol Phys 14:861, 1988

RECHT L et al: Central nervous system metastases from non-Hodgkin's lymphoma: Treatment and prophylaxis. Am J Med 84:425, 1988

SMOKER WR et al: The role of MR imaging in evaluating metastatic spinal disease. Am J Radiol 149:1241, 1987

SUNDAESAN N, GALICICH JH: Surgical treatment of brain metastases. Cancer 55:1382, 1985

WALKER MD (ed): Cancer Treatment and Research Series, Oncology of the Nervous System, WL McGuire (series ed). Boston, Martinus Nijhoff, 1983

————— et al: Randomized comparison of radiation therapy and nitrosoureas for the treatment of malignant glioma of the brain. N Engl J Med 303:1323, 1980

WASSERSTROM WR: Diagnosis and treatment of leptomeningeal metastases from solid tumors. Cancer 49:759, 1982

YOUNG DP: Neurology complications of chemotherapy, in Neurological Complications of Therapy, A Silverstein (ed). Mount Kisco, NY, Futura Publishing, 1982, p 57

354 BACTERIAL MENINGITIS AND BRAIN ABSCESS

DONALD H. HARTER / ROBERT G. PETERSDORF

Pyogenic infections of the cranial contents originate in one of two ways, by hematogenous spread or by extension from surface structures, paranasal sinuses, osteomyelitic foci in the skull, penetrating cranial injuries, congenital sinus tracts, or following neurosurgical procedures.

ACUTE BACTERIAL MENINGITIS

DEFINITION Bacterial meningitis may be defined as an inflammation in response to bacterial infection of the pia-arachnoid and the fluid residing in the space which it encloses and also of the fluid in the ventricles of the brain. Since the subarachnoid space is continuous around the brain, spinal cord, and the optic nerves, an infective agent (or tumor cells or blood) gaining entry to any one part of it may extend immediately to all of it, even its most remote recesses; therefore, meningitis is always *cerebrospinal*. It also reaches the ventricles, either directly from the choroid plexus or by reflux through the basal foramens of Magendie and Luschka.

PATHOLOGY The effect of bacteria or other organisms in the subarachnoid space is to cause an inflammatory reaction in the pia and arachnoid and in the cerebrospinal fluid (CSF); in pyogenic meningitis, pus accumulates in this space. The infective agent or its toxin (gram-negative endotoxins, pneumococcal cell wall fragments), if allowed sufficient time to act, injures those structures which lie within the subarachnoid space (cranial and spinal roots) or ventricles (choroid plexuses) and adjacent to it (pial arteries and veins, underlying cerebral and cerebellar cortices, subpial white matter of the spinal cord, peripheral fibers of optic nerves, ependymal and subependymal tissues). In addition, purulent material may interfere with the flow of CSF from the ventricles or along the subarachnoid space over the brainstem, with resulting obstructive hydrocephalus. Although the outer arachnoidal membrane proves to be a remarkably effective barrier to the extension of infection, some reaction in the cranial subdural space and even in the inner surface of the dura and the spinal epidural space may occur. This happens more often in infants, approximately 15 percent of whom develop subdural effusions in response to meningitis, than in adults.

ETIOLOGY The causes of bacterial meningitis vary with age as follows:

1 *Streptococcus pneumoniae* (see Chap. 99) causes 30 to 50 percent of cases in adults, 10 to 20 percent in children, and up to 5 percent of cases in infants.
2 *Neisseria meningitidis* (see Chap. 109) causes from 10 to 35 percent of cases in adults and from 25 to 40 percent in children up to age 15. It is a rare cause in infants.
3 *Haemophilus influenzae*, type B (see Chap. 115) is responsible for 40 to 60 percent of cases in children, but for only 1 to 3 percent in adults and for virtually none in infants.

Also important in the etiology of meningitis are *Staphylococcus aureus* and *Staph. epidermidis* (see Chap. 100); the latter accounts for 75 percent of infections associated with shunting procedures for hydrocephalus. *S. aureus* meningitis occurs largely in postoperative neurosurgical patients, in patients with vertebral infection, and as a complication of *S. aureus* endocarditis. Other causative organisms include group B streptococci, particularly in infants; anaerobic or microaerophilic streptococci and gram-negative bacilli, usually in association with brain abscess, epidural abscess, head trauma, neurosurgical procedures, or cranial thrombophlebitis; *Escherichia coli* and other Enterobacteriaceae such as *Klebsiella-Enterobacter, Proteus, Citrobacter, Pseudomonas,* and *Acinetobacter calcoaceticus* (see Chap. 111), usually as a consequence of head trauma, neurosurgical procedures, spinal anesthesia, lumbar puncture, or shunting procedures to relieve hydrocephalus. Heretofore, gram-negative bacilli were associated most often with neonatal meningitis, but the spectrum has shifted to adults with debilitating diseases and other predisposing causes. Almost one-fifth of bacterial meningitis cases occurring in persons 50 years of age or older are due to gram-negative enteric bacteria. The outcome in this group has been notoriously poor. Rare meningeal pathogens include *Salmonella, Shigella, Clostridium perfringens,* and *Neisseria gonorrhoeae*.

The changing etiology of bacterial meningitis is reflected by the appearance of *Listeria monocytogenes* as a major pathogen, particularly in infants or elderly, debilitated patients or in those with immunosuppression secondary to transplantation, those who are receiving therapy for cancer, or those with connective tissue diseases. Alcoholism and high-dose steroids also appear to be predisposing factors. *Listeria* meningitis accounts for approximately 2 percent of all reported cases of bacterial meningitis in the United States. The mortality rate in the adult group with severe underlying disease is 70 percent (see Chap. 103).

EPIDEMIOLOGY AND CLINICAL SETTING The incidence of bacterial meningitis is between 4.6 and 10 cases per 100,000 persons per year. More than 2000 deaths due to bacterial meningitis are reported in the United States every year. *H. influenzae* is the most frequent cause, followed by *N. meningitidis* and *S. pneumoniae*. About 70 percent of all cases occur in children under the age of 5. Pneumococcal, *H. influenzae*, and meningococcal infections have a worldwide distribution, tending to occur more often in males and during the fall, winter, and spring. *H. influenzae* meningitis is the most frequent meningeal infection in children between 2 months and 3 years of age. Meningococcal infections occur most often in children and adolescents, but they are also encountered throughout most of adult life with a sharp decline after age 50. Meningococcal meningitis differs from other forms of meningitis because it may occur in epidemics. Pneumococcal meningitis predominates in adults over 40 years of age.

A variety of factors apart from age predispose to the development of certain types of acute bacterial meningitis. Acute otitis media and mastoiditis occur in about 25 percent of patients with pneumococcal meningitis, and pneumonia occurs in another 25 percent. Recent head injury is recorded in 10 to 20 percent of patients with pneumococcal meningitis and may give rise to recurrent meningitis because of persistent cerebrospinal fluid rhinorrhea. Pneumococcal meningitis also occurs in patients with sickle cell disease, Hodgkin's disease, or multiple myeloma; in urban general hospitals many adults who develop pneumococcal infections suffer from chronic alcoholism. Immunoglobulin deficiency (whether congenital or acquired), splenectomy, and renal or bone marrow transplantation also predispose patients to pneumococcal infection. Adults who develop *H. influenzae* meningitis should be suspected of harboring an anatomic defect (dermal sinus tract, old skull fracture) or have abnormal immune defenses. Meningitis caused by *Staph. aureus* usually follows neurosurgical procedures, a penetrating cranial wound, vertebral osteomyelitis, epidural abscess, and bacterial endocarditis. This organism and *Staph. epidermidis* account for the majority of cerebral ventricular shunt infections and occasionally neonatal omphalitis and meningitis. Gram-negative bacillary infections also complicate neurosurgical operations and other nosocomial diseases; they are assuming progressively greater importance in meningitis in adults.

PATHOGENESIS The three most common meningeal pathogens are invasive and depend upon antiphagocytic capsular or surface antigens for survival in the tissues of the infected host; all express their pathogenicity largely in the form of extracellular proliferation. All three are inhabitants of the nasopharynx in a significant part of the population. It is evident from the frequency with which the carrier state is detected that nasal colonization is not a sufficient explanation for infection of the meninges. The factors which predispose the colonized patient to bloodstream invasion, which is the usual route by which bacteria reach the meninges, are obscure. They include (1) antecedent viral infections of the upper respiratory passages; (2) in the case of the pneumococcus, infections in the lung and the absence of bactericidal antibodies; and (3) deficiencies in the terminal components of complement in *H. influenzae* and meningococcal infection (see Chaps. 109 and 115). Once bloodborne, the factors that lead to meningeal localization of bacteria are unknown, but it has been postulated that pneumococci, *H. influenzae*, and meningococci possess a unique predilection for the meninges. Other possibilities are that the entry of bacteria into the subarachnoid space is facilitated by disruption of the blood-CSF barrier by trauma, circulating endotoxin, inflammatory cytokines (see Chap. 20), or an initial viral infection of the meninges. Once CSF entry occurs, bacterial replication proceeds readily because levels of immunoglobulins and complement are too low to permit opsonization and/or bacteriolysis and phagocytosis by neutrophils is impaired.

Avenues other than the bloodstream by which bacteria can gain access to the meninges include congenital neuroectodermal defects, craniotomy sites, diseases of the middle ear and paranasal sinuses, and cranial trauma, notably skull fractures. Occasionally brain abscesses may rupture into the subarachnoid space or ventricles, infecting the meninges. The isolation of anaerobic streptococci, *Bacteroides* spp., or *Actinomyces* or of a mixture of microorganisms in the CSF should suggest the possibility of a brain abscess occurring as an antecedent to meningitis.

Once developed, characteristic features of bacterial meningitis include an increase in intracranial pressure, disruption of the blood-brain barrier, cerebral edema, and alterations in cerebral blood flow.

SYMPTOMATOLOGY Fever, headache, photophobia, seizures, vomiting, impairment of consciousness, and stiff neck and back are common to bacterial meningitis irrespective of its etiology. When the initial symptoms are only pain in the neck or abdomen, a confusional state, or delirium, the diagnosis is difficult. Three patterns of onset have been documented. In approximately 25 percent of patients, meningitis has a fulminant onset and patients become seriously ill within 24 h, usually without antecedent respiratory tract infections. In over 50 percent, meningitis develops over 1 to 7 days and is associated with respiratory symptoms. Slightly less than 20 percent have meningeal symptoms after 1 to 3 weeks of respiratory symptoms.

In children, the onset is often nonspecific. Fever and vomiting are more frequent than headache. There is a higher incidence of seizures, and the error of misinterpreting seizures as febrile convulsions is greater. The classic signs of meningitis may be minimal in elderly, debilitated patients in whom low-grade fever and changes in mental status may occur without headache or nuchal rigidity.

There are certain special clinical features that correlate with particular types of meningitis. Meningococcal meningitis should always be suspected in epidemics of meningitis; when the evolution is extremely rapid; when the onset is attended by a morbilliform, petechial, or purpuric skin eruption, larger ecchymoses, and lividity of skin in the lower parts of the body; and when circulatory collapse has occurred. Since a rash accompanies approximately 50 percent of meningococcal infections, its presence should dictate immediate institution of therapy for a neisserial infection, even though similar rashes may be observed with echovirus type 9 meningitis and rarely with staphylococcal, *H. influenzae*, and streptococcal meningitis. Recurrent systemic infections with meningococcus or *Haemophilus* should lead to the suspicion of complement deficiency. A family history of fulminant meningococcal disease in males in skipped generations suggests properdin deficiency. Pneumococcal meningitis is usually preceded by an infection in the lungs, ears, and sinuses, and, rarely, endocarditis. In addition a pneumococcal etiology should be suspected in patients suffering from alcoholism, sickle cell disease, basal skull fracture, following splenectomy or organ transplantation, or when there are multiple recurrences of bacterial meningitis following head trauma. *H. influenzae* meningitis may follow upper respiratory and ear infections in young children.

The signs of meningeal irritation—stiff neck or positive Kernig's and Brudzinski's signs—may be absent in the very young, the very old, or the severely obtunded. Signs of focal cerebral disease, although seldom prominent, are more frequent in pneumococcal and *H. influenzae* meningitis and are associated with a comparatively poor prognosis. Seizures are encountered most often in children with *H. influenzae* meningitis. In some instances they are caused by hypoglycemia, hyponatremia, or penicillin neurotoxicity. Some of the more transitory focal cerebral signs may represent postictal phenomena (Todd's paralysis); stable, local, cerebral lesions are probably the result of vasculitis and occlusion of cerebral veins with infarction of cerebral tissue, or they may connote localization of pus as occurs in brain abscess or subdural empyema. Abnormalities involving the third, fourth, and sixth as well as other cranial nerves are particularly frequent with pneumococcal meningitis.

LABORATORY FINDINGS The alterations of the cerebrospinal fluid are diagnostic. The *number of leukocytes* in the CSF ranges between 1000 and 100,000 per milliliter but averages between 5000 and 20,000. Cell counts above 50,000 per milliliter raise suspicion of the possibility of a brain abscess having ruptured into the ventricle (ventricular empyema). Neutrophilic leukocytes generally predominate, but an increasing proportion of mononuclear cells are found in the exudate as the infection continues, especially in partially treated meningitis. CSF lymphocytosis occurs in about one-third of bacterial meningitis patients with CSF cell counts of 1000 per milliliter or less. In the early stages careful cytologic examination may reveal some of the mononuclear cells to be myelocytes or young neutrophils. Later, as treatment takes effect, the proportions of lymphocytes, plasma cells, and histiocytes steadily increase. Early in meningococcal meningitis with fulminant meningococcemia, or more rarely with pneumococcal meningitis, the cellular response may be minimal or absent despite the presence of bacteria.

The CSF *pressure* is so consistently elevated (above 180 mmH$_2$O) that a normal or low pressure on the initial lumbar puncture in a case of suspected bacterial meningitis should raise the possibility that the needle was partially occluded or that the spinal arachnoid space was blocked.

The *protein levels* of CSF are higher than 45 mg/dL in 90 percent of cases, and most determinations fall in the range of 150 to 500 mg/dL.

The *sugar concentration* of CSF is depressed, usually to a level lower than 40 mg/dL or less than 40 percent of the blood sugar concentration (measured concomitantly), provided the latter is less than 250 mg/dL. However in atypical or "culture-negative cases," other conditions associated with a depressed CSF glucose should be considered. These include hypoglycemia from any cause, sarcoidosis of the central nervous system, meningeal carcinomatosis or gliomatosis, fungal or tuberculous meningitis, and subarachnoid hemorrhage. In acute cases of pyogenic meningitis, the CSF glucose concentration often approaches zero.

Gram stain of sedimented CSF permits identification of the causative agent in most cases of bacterial meningitis; it will be positive in about three-fourths of patients with untreated bacterial meningitis. Pneumococci and *H. influenzae* are identified more readily than are meningococci. Small numbers of gram-negative diplococci present within leukocytes may be indistinguishable from nuclear material which may also be gram-negative and of the same shape. In such cases a thin film of uncentrifuged CSF may lend itself more readily to morphologic interpretation than will a smear of sedimented CSF. The commonest errors in reading Gram-stained smears of CSF are misinterpretation of precipitated dye or debris as gram-positive cocci and confusion of pneumococci with *H. influenzae*. *Haemophilus* organisms may stain heavily at the poles so that they resemble gram-positive diplococci, and older pneumococci often lose their capacity to take a gram-positive stain. *Listeria monocytogenes* may be misidentified as a "diphtheroid" or hemolytic streptococcus in the microbiology laboratory. Staining with acridine orange and examination under a fluorescence microscope may demonstrate bacteria not observed with the Gram stain.

Cerebrospinal fluid cultures are positive in 70 to 80 percent of cases. When brain abscess is suspected, anaerobic cultures should be made, and meningococci should be cultured under 10% CO_2 (see Chap. 80). Partially treated meningitis poses a most difficult problem in diagnosis because cultures are often negative. The measurement of bacterial antigen in the CSF by latex agglutination, countercurrent immune electrophoresis (CIE), radioimmunoassay, or enzyme-linked immunosorbent assay (ELISA) to determine the presence of a specific capsular polysaccharide associated with *H. influenzae* type B, *S. pneumoniae*, and meningococcal serogroups A, B, C, and Y has been helpful. It has limited value in *E. coli* and streptococcal group B infections. Latex agglutination tests typically have a sensitivity of 90 to 100 percent, compared to 65 to 75 percent for CIE. Detection of antigen in the serum or urine of bacterial meningitis patients is not a sensitive diagnostic method. The concentration of bacterial antigen diminishes as treatment progresses. Failure to detect antigen does not rule out bacterial meningitis.

In addition to CSF cultures, *blood cultures* should always be obtained because they are positive in 40 to 60 percent of patients with *H. influenzae* and with meningococcal and pneumococcal meningitis and may provide the only definitive clue to the causative agent (if CSF cultures are negative). Routine cultures of the pharynx or external ear are as often misleading as helpful because pneumococci, *H. influenzae*, and meningococci are such common inhabitants of these locations. However, culture of pus from the middle ear or sinuses is often helpful.

The *blood leukocyte count* is generally elevated, and usually there is a shift to the left. Most patients with meningitis are sufficiently ill to require determination of blood urea nitrogen and serum electrolytes. These may be abnormal because of severe dehydration and may reveal inappropriate secretion of antidiuretic hormone (AVP) with resultant hyponatremia.

ROENTGENOGRAPHIC STUDIES Patients with bacterial meningitis should have x-rays of the chest, skull, and sinuses as soon as possible after admission. Chest x-rays are particularly important because they may reveal a silent area of pneumonitis or abscess. Sinus and skull films may provide clues to the presence of cranial osteomyelitis, paranasal sinusitis, or skull fracture. Computed tomography (CT scan) is usually not necessary in bacterial meningitis and is normal early in most infections. It is indicated when there is a suspicion of purulent sinusitis, mastoiditis, or epidural and brain abscess and always in the presence of focal neurologic deficits. In severe cases it may show cerebritis, vascular occlusions, and encephalomalacia. Later in the course, CT will detect hydrocephalus, brain abscess, and subdural effusions or subdural empyema. If bacterial meningitis is suspected and the patient does not have papilledema or focal neurologic findings, lumbar puncture should not be delayed while waiting for a CT scan to be done. When, in the presence of suspected meningitis, a CT scan is indicated to exclude lesions that might cause herniation, antibiotics may be instituted after blood cultures have been obtained. Most of the time this preliminary antibiotic treatment will not interfere with isolation and identification of the organism from the CSF.

COMPLICATIONS OF BACTERIAL MENINGITIS The longer the duration of meningitis and the less effective the treatment, the greater the chances that complications and neurologic residua will develop. The cranial nerve palsies, usually third, sixth, seventh, and eighth nerves, which occur in some 10 to 20 percent of cases usually disappear within a few weeks. Approximately 10 percent of infants and children who have bacterial meningitis will be left with persistent unilateral or bilateral sensory hearing loss. Deafness is especially frequent with pneumococcal, *H. influenzae*, and meningococcal meningitis. If focal and lateralizing neurologic signs last for some days or occur late in the course of meningitis, they are usually indicative of a vasculitis and cerebral infarction. Such lesions are most extensive in children with *H. influenzae* meningitis who are inadequately treated. If these lesions are extensive, they may leave the child retarded and epileptic. Persistent coma is more common in pneumococcal meningitis in adults. In infants or very young children with bacterial meningitis (particularly due to *H. influenzae*), prolonged alteration in state of consciousness or increased intracranial pressure (ICP) should raise the suspicion of obstructive hydrocephalus and subdural effusions. Approximately 30 percent of children who have had bacterial meningitis later will turn out to have subtle learning deficits.

DIFFERENTIAL DIAGNOSIS The diagnosis of bacterial meningitis is not difficult, providing a high index of suspicion is maintained. All febrile patients with lethargy, headache, or confusion of sudden onset, even if only low-grade fever is present, should be subjected to lumbar puncture. It is particularly important to consider meningitis in febrile, confused alcoholic patients. Too often the symptoms are mistakenly ascribed to inebriation, delirium tremens, or hepatic encephalopathy until the CSF reveals a meningitis.

Bacterial meningitis can be diagnosed definitively only by examination of the CSF. Viral meningoencephalitis and tuberculous, leptospiral, and fungal meningitides often enter into the differential diagnosis. Also to be considered are Behçet's syndrome, a disease characterized by recurrent oral and genital ulcers along with meningitis, and Mollaret's meningitis, which consists of recurrent episodes of fever, headache, and meningeal irritation accompanied by a leukocytosis in the CSF.

Tuberculous meningitis is discussed in Chap. 125. The diagnosis of other intracranial suppurative diseases is detailed below.

PROGNOSIS The case fatality rate for bacterial meningitis in the United States approximates 14 percent; it is highest for gram-negative and miscellaneous causes of meningitis. Of the three common forms of meningitis, pneumococcal meningitis is the most lethal. The triad of pneumococcal meningitis, pneumonia, and endocarditis has a particularly high fatality rate. The case fatality rate of *H. influenzae* or meningococcal meningitis has remained fixed at 5 to 15 percent for many years. Also in meningococcal infection, because of the fulminating nature of the disease and the often complicating adrenocortical necrosis (Waterhouse-Friderichsen syndrome), the mortality rate remains significant. Old age, infancy, abrupt onset, bacteremia, coma, seizures, and a variety of concomitant diseases including alcoholism, diabetes mellitus, multiple myeloma, and head trauma all worsen the prognosis.

It is often impossible to explain the death of the patient or at least to trace it to a single specific mechanism. Bacteremia with hypotension or brain swelling and bilateral temporal and/or cerebellar herniation are clearly implicated in the deaths of some patients during the initial 48 h. These events may occur in bacterial meningitis of any etiology; however, some observations suggest that they are more important in meningococcal infection. There is experimental evidence that acute centrally mediated respiratory failure (rather than circulatory collapse) is the major mechanism of early death. Deaths occurring later during the course of illness may be due to necrosis of brain tissue and respiratory failure, often consequent to aspiration pneumonia.

TREATMENT **Antimicrobials** Bacterial meningitis is a medical emergency; the rapid destruction of bacteria in the meninges and in the CSF is essential to survival. For this reason, drugs and dosages which achieve bactericidal activity in the CSF should be used where possible. The following therapeutic regimens are recommended: [NOTE: Dosage reductions of the penicillins, cephalosporins, and trimethoprim-sulfamethoxazole are needed in patients with renal failure (see Chap. 85).]

1 For adults with pneumococcal, meningococcal, or *Listeria monocytogenes* meningitis, penicillin G, 18 to 24 million units intravenously each day in four to six divided doses, is recommended; for children the dose of penicillin G should be 300,000 to 400,000 units per kilogram per day in divided doses every 4 h. Ampicillin (12 to 18 g daily intravenously in divided doses) or chloramphenicol (4 to 6 g given intravenously in divided doses) are alternative treatment regimens in adults. Ampicillin can also be used in children at a dosage of 300 to 400 mg/kg per day. The third-generation cephalosporins, cefotaxime (2 g IV every 4 h), or ceftriaxone (2 g IV once daily) are effective in pneumococcal and meningococcal but *not* in *Listeria* meningitis. Trimethoprim-sulfamethoxazole (160 mg TMP/800 mg SMX intravenously every 6 h) or chloramphenicol should be used to treat *Listeria* meningitis in penicillin-allergic patients.

2 For children over 2 months of age with *H. influenzae* or uncomplicated meningitis of unknown etiology, cefotaxime, 200 mg/kg per day in divided doses every 4 to 6 h, or ceftriaxone, 100 mg/kg per day up to a maximum of 2 g/d as a once-daily dose, should be administered. The use of these cephalosporins has largely replaced, in the United States, the combination of ampicillin and chloramphenicol, although the two regimens are of equivalent efficacy. For the older regimen, ampicillin, 300 to 400 mg/kg per day intravenously in divided doses, plus chloramphenicol, 75 to 100 mg/kg per day intravenously, should be given. The reason for the use of two drugs is that 15 to 25 percent of *H. influenzae* isolates are resistant to ampicillin, and chloramphenicol-resistant *H. influenzae* have also been reported. In order to avoid interference between the two drugs, ampicillin should be given 30 min before chloramphenicol. Once the causative microorganism has been recovered and its sensitivity to antimicrobials has been determined, chloramphenicol can be discontinued if the organism is sensitive to ampicillin. If the isolate is resistant to both ampicillin and chloramphenicol or if the child is intolerant to chloramphenicol, cefotaxime or ceftriaxone should be used. In adults with *H. influenzae* meningitis, the doses of ampicillin (12 to 18 g/d) and chloramphenicol (4 to 6 g/d) are administered intravenously either as a constant infusion or in divided doses. Alternatively, therapy with cefotaxime or ceftriaxone as outlined for pneumococcal infections can be employed.

3 Adult patients with pneumococcal, meningococcal, or *H. influenzae* meningitis who may be allergic to the penicillins can be treated with chloramphenicol in dosage of 4 to 6 g/d, or with a third-generation cephalosporin as outlined above. If the history of penicillin allergy is one of acute anaphylaxis, chloramphenicol is the preferred choice.

4 In meningitis due to gram-negative enteric bacilli, the organism is usually susceptible to treatment with a third-generation cephalo-sporin or a combination of antibiotics. Therapy can be started with cefotaxime, 2 g intravenously every 4 h, ceftazidime, 2 g intravenously every 6 h, or ceftriaxone 2 g/d, and an aminoglycoside (gentamicin or tobramycin, 3 to 5 mg/kg per day). Intrathecal therapy with gentamicin (8 to 10 mg/d) should be considered. When the bacterial species has been identified and its sensitivity to antimicrobials determined, the antibiotic regimen can be modified. If *Pseudomonas aeruginosa* or *Acinetobacter calcoaceticus* is identified, parenteral and intrathecal gentamicin or tobramycin should be given in conjunction with ceftazidime. Trimethoprim-sulfamethoxazole may provide a useful alternative for gram-negative meningitis (except that caused by *P. aeruginosa*) when the causative agent is resistant to third-generation cephalosporins.

5 Meningitis due to *Staphylococcus aureus* should be treated with a penicillinase-resistant penicillin rather than penicillin G because over 80 percent of isolates are penicillin-resistant. Nafcillin or oxacillin in daily doses of 12 to 18 g can be used in adults. Patients with staphylococcal meningitis who are allergic to penicillin can be given vancomycin intravenously (1 g every 8 to 12 h to adults) and intrathecally 10 to 20 mg/d.

6 When the etiology of meningitis is unknown, the drugs of choice are as follows: in adults, ampicillin, 12 to 18 g/d, or penicillin, 18 to 24 million units per day in divided doses, plus cefotaxime or ceftriaxone. In the penicillin-allergic patient chloramphenicol, 75 to 100 mg/kg per day in divided doses, may be substituted. In children, a third-generation cephalosporin administered as outlined for treatment of *H. influenzae* is recommended; in neonates, ampicillin, 200 mg/kg per day, and an aminoglycoside, usually gentamicin (2.5 to 5.0 mg/kg per day), are recommended.

7 Foci of infection in the paranasal sinuses or mastoids, in an infected shunt, or in cranial osteomyelitis should be identified so that appropriate drainage may be carried out when the acute episode of meningitis has subsided. Removal of shunts or reservoirs should be considered and is often necessary.

8 In most patients bacterial meningitis need not be treated for longer than 10 days except when there is a persistent parameningeal focus of infection. Antibiotics should be administered in full doses parenterally (preferably intravenously) throughout the period of treatment to avoid treatment failures due to inadequate concentrations of antibiotic in the plasma and CSF. Meningitis caused by *P. aeruginosa* or *Listeria monocytogenes* is usually treated for 3 weeks to prevent relapse.

9 Repeated lumbar punctures are not necessary to follow the course of therapy as long as the patient is doing well and the pathogen has been identified. The CSF sugar may remain low for a number of days after cultures become negative and should cause concern only if bacteria are present. Likewise, persistent but steadily diminishing mononuclear pleocytosis following pyogenic meningitis is the rule. CSF examination at the end of treatment for bacterial meningitis in patients who have recovered clinically from pneumococcal, meningococcal, or *H. influenzae* meningitis is not useful because it may lead to unnecessarily prolonged hospitalization; relapse after recommended therapy is extremely unusual. In meningitis caused by enteric gram-negative bacilli, in particular, *P. aeruginosa*, periodic repeat CSF examinations are indicated to follow the therapeutic response and confirm culture negativity. Similarly, repeat CSF examination is indicated in patients with meningitis complicating shunt or reservoir insertion and can determine the need for removal of the foreign body.

Adrenocortical steroids The few controlled studies available have demonstrated that steroids exert no beneficial effects in pyogenic meningitis, except in children with meningitis caused by *H. influenzae*, in whom the incidence of postmeningeal nerve deafness is reduced by the administration of dexamethasone. For adults these drugs should not be used except as an adjunct to intravenous mannitol in severe cerebral edema.

Other forms of therapy Intrathecal administration of enzymes to lyse excessive subarachnoid cellular exudate which may be associated with spinal block or hydrocephalus in the subacute stages of bacterial meningitis is of no value. There is also no evidence to support the therapeutic efficacy of repeated drainage of CSF. In fact, increased CSF pressure in the acute phases of bacterial meningitis is largely a consequence of CSF outflow blockage, increased intracranial blood volume, and later cerebral edema. In this situation lumbar puncture may predispose to temporal lobe or cerebellar herniation and death. Mannitol and urea have been employed apparently successfully in some cases of severe brain swelling with unusually high initial CSF pressures (>400 mmH$_2$O). Either should be accompanied by dexamethasone in relatively high doses (4 to 10 mg intravenously every 6 h). An adequate but not excessive amount of parenteral fluids should be given, and phenytoin should be given to control seizures. In children care should be taken to avoid hyponatremia and water intoxication—a cause of brain swelling. Subdural effusions usually resolve spontaneously but must be followed by serial CT scans. Drainage is rarely necessary.

RECURRENT MENINGITIS

Recurrent attacks of bacterial meningitis usually follow in the wake of trauma. The interval between the traumatic episode and the initial bout of posttraumatic meningitis may be as long as several years. *S. pneumoniae* is the usual bacterial pathogen. Often it proves to be one of the higher serologic types, reflecting the predominance of such strains in nasal carriers. *CSF rhinorrhea* is present in most of these patients but may be transient. The patient with recurrent meningitis of inapparent origin should always be suspected of having a fistulous connection between the nasal sinuses and the subarachnoid space. The fistula is usually traumatic (old basal skull fracture), and the site is the frontal or ethmoid sinuses or the cribriform plate. The rhinorrhea may be difficult to demonstrate except by injecting a radioactive tracer into the CSF and watching for its appearance in nasal secretions. Cerebrospinal fluid rhinorrhea may also be detected by measuring the glucose concentration of nasal secretions. The usual mucous secretions contain little glucose, but in CSF rhinorrhea the amount approximates that in the CSF. The prognosis in recurrent meningitis is remarkably benign, and the mortality is much lower than in ordinary pneumococcal meningitis. Nevertheless, vaccination of these patients with pneumococcal vaccine is indicated, and long-term prophylactic chemotherapy with penicillin V should be considered. Treatment of recurrent meningitis is similar to that for first bouts. Attempts to demonstrate CSF rhinorrhea should be made only after the acute infection has subsided; if evidence of a fistula is found, surgical repair should be considered.

Other causes of recurrent meningitis include congenital bony abnormalities of the inner ear, congenital dermal sinus tract, and tumors at the base of the skull.

SUBDURAL EMPYEMA

DEFINITION Subdural empyema is a suppurative process in the cranial subdural space between the inner surface of the dura and the outer of the arachnoid. The proper term for this condition is not *abscess* but *empyema,* indicating suppuration in a preformed space. Subdural empyema accounts for approximately one-fifth of all localized intracranial infections. About three-fourths of cases are unilateral, and the remainder bilateral.

ETIOLOGY The infection usually gains entry to the subdural space from the frontal or ethmoid sinuses or, less often, from the mastoid cells. These cases are termed *primary* subdural empyema. The subdural space may also become infected by extension of bacteria from a contiguous site of osteomyelitis or from a brain abscess. Septic thrombophlebitis and venous drainage of bacteria to the subdural space may be important in its development. Rarely has it been observed with bloodstream infections. Secondary subdural empyema usually follows neurosurgical drainage of a chronic subdural hematoma.

The bacterial flora in subdural empyema closely resembles that seen in chronic sinusitis and brain abscess; it may be polymicrobial. Isolates in order of decreasing frequency include aerobic streptococci, staphylococci, microaerophilic and anaerobic streptococci, aerobic gram-negative rods, and other anaerobes.

PATHOLOGY A collection of subdural pus in quantities of a few milliliters to 100 to 200 mL lies over the cerebral hemisphere. It is often mistaken for meningitis. The arachnoid, when cleared of exudate, is cloudy, and thrombosis of meningeal veins may be seen. The underlying cerebral hemisphere is depressed, and in fatal cases there is often an ipsilateral temporal lobe pressure cone. Microscopic studies demonstrate various degrees of organization of the exudate on the inner surface of the dura and infiltration of the underlying pia with small numbers of neutrophilic leukocytes, lymphocytes, and mononuclear cells. There is superficial thrombophlebitis; the thrombi in cerebral veins appear to begin on the outer side (toward the empyema). The thrombosis extends to other dural sinuses, and the superficial layers of the cerebral cortex undergo ischemic necrosis, which probably accounts for the unilateral seizures and signs of disordered cerebral function.

SYMPTOMATOLOGY AND LABORATORY FINDINGS The usual history includes chronic sinusitis or otitis with a recent flare-up and evidence of local pain and increase in purulent nasal or aural discharge. The illness is severe and progressive. Generalized headache, fever, vomiting, and a depressed sensorium are the first indications of intracranial spread. They are followed within a few days by localizing signs including focal motor seizures, hemiplegia, hemianesthesia, and aphasia. Papilledema is present in one-half of the patients at the time of diagnosis. Stupor or coma develops rapidly as the cerebral symptoms progress. Fever is usually present, but the neck is not always stiff. There is a leukocytosis and increased erythrocyte sedimentation rate. Lumbar puncture poses a distinct risk because it may precipitate transtentorial herniation. It is generally contraindicated if the diagnosis of subdural empyema is suspected and certainly should not be performed in advance of a CT scan of the head. The CSF shows increased pressure, a raised white blood cell count in the range of 50 to 1000 per milliliter including both neutrophils and lymphocytes, elevated protein (75 to 300 mg/dL), and normal sugar values. Unless subdural empyema is complicated by bacterial meningitis, no bacteria can be recovered from the CSF. In the type of subdural empyema that follows drainage of a chronic subdural hematoma, the onset is more indolent, fever is lower, and there is usually a local wound infection.

DIAGNOSIS Skull films may show involvement of the sinus or mastoid. CT scanning is the method of choice for establishing the diagnosis and location of a subdural empyema. The usual CT scan appearance is a crescentic or elliptical hypodense area lying directly below the cranial vault or adjacent to the falx cerebri. After administration of contrast, the CT scan may demonstrate an intense line of enhancement between the subdural collection and cerebral cortex. False-negative CT scans have been reported. When there is question about the diagnosis after CT scanning, magnetic resonance imaging may be required to define the lesion; cerebral angiography is rarely necessary or useful. In secondary empyemas, CT scan is invariably positive. Several conditions need to be distinguished clinically from subdural empyema: cerebral thrombophlebitis, brain abscess, viral encephalitis, acute hemorrhagic encephalitis (see Chap. 355), and bacterial meningitis with localizing neurologic findings or seizures.

TREATMENT Drainage of pus is the single most important part of treatment. In particular, it is important to institute drainage early because delaying it sharply increases the mortality rate. Specimens of pus obtained at surgery should be transported to the laboratory in oxygen-free containers and cultured both aerobically and anaerobically. Initial treatment should be guided by the Gram stain of the pus. In the absence of an identifiable organism, appropriate empiric antibiotic therapy consists of 20 million units of penicillin per day plus chloramphenicol, 4 g/d, administered intravenously. If a foul odor is present suggesting anaerobic infection, metronidazole, 500 mg intravenously every 6 h, may be substituted for chloramphenicol. If staphylococcal infection is suspected, nafcillin should be substituted for penicillin G (12 to 18 g/d in divided doses for adults). In postoperative neurosurgical patients the possibility of methicillin-resistant *S. aureus* or *S. epidermidis* should be considered and vancomycin administered as described for meningitis. Without such massive antimicrobial therapy and surgery, most patients will die, usually within 7 to 14 days, often while the unsuspecting physician and surgeon are waiting for better localization of an assumed cerebral abscess, the most commonly mistaken diagnosis. Antibiotic therapy can be altered when final culture and sensitivity results are available. It should be continued for 3 to 6 weeks. Drugs to reduce cerebral edema and to prevent seizures should be given. Mortality in subdural empyema is now between 10 and 20 percent. Long-term sequelae include seizures, hemiparesis, and dysphasia.

CRANIAL EXTRADURAL ABSCESS

This condition is almost invariably associated with osteomyelitis in a cranial bone which originates from an infection in the ear or paranasal sinuses. Pus and granulation tissue accumulate on the outer surface of the dura, separating it from the cranial bone. Symptomatically, the effects are those of a local inflammatory process: frontal or auricular pain, purulent discharge from the sinuses or ear, and fever and local tenderness. Unrelenting headache is a frequent complaint. Focal neurologic signs are uncommon. A cranial epidural abscess characteristically enlarges too slowly to cause sudden neurologic abnormalities. The CSF is usually clear and under normal pressure but may contain a few lymphocytes and neutrophils (20 to 100 per milliliter) and slightly raised protein concentration. CT scan is the diagnostic procedure of choice. False-negative scans have been reported; the diagnosis can then be made by contrast-enhanced CT scan or magnetic resonance imaging (MRI). Treatment consists of prompt surgical drainage of the epidural space, debridement of infected bone, and appropriate systemic antibiotics. The primary sinusitis or mastoiditis, from which the extradural infection has arisen, may also require surgical drainage.

SPINAL EPIDURAL ABSCESS

This type of abscess possesses unique clinical features and constitutes an important neurologic and neurosurgical emergency. It is discussed in Chap. 361.

INTRACRANIAL THROMBOPHLEBITIS

The lateral, cavernous, and superior longitudinal sinuses are relatively uncommon sites of infection. Usually there is evidence that the intracranial process has extended from the middle ear and mastoid cells, the paranasal sinuses, and skin around the upper lip, nose, and eyes.

LATERAL SINUS THROMBOPHLEBITIS In lateral sinus thrombophlebitis, which usually follows otitis media and mastoiditis, the earache and mastoid tenderness are succeeded, after a period of days to a few weeks, by fever, headache, nausea, and vomiting due to increased ICP. There may be swelling over the mastoid region, distention of veins, and tenderness of the jugular vein in the neck. With jugular vein involvement, there may be neck pain and restriction of movement. Drowsiness and coma are common. Papilledema (unilateral in some patients) is seen in about one-half of cases. Convulsions occur, but focal neurologic findings are infrequent. Abducens nerve paralysis and trigeminal nerve involvement (Gradenigo's syndrome) are found when there is spread to the inferior petrosal sinus.

CAVERNOUS SINUS THROMBOPHLEBITIS In this condition, which is usually secondary to oculonasal infections, the clinical syndrome is one of orbital edema, chemosis, venous congestion, and evidence of palsy of the third, fourth, ophthalmic fifth, and sixth cranial nerves. Later spread through the circular sinus to the opposite cavernous sinus results in bilateral symptoms and signs. The posterior part of the cavernous sinus may be infected via the superior and inferior petrosal veins without the occurrence of orbital edema or ophthalmoplegia. The patient appears acutely ill with high fever, headache, nausea, and vomiting. There is eye pain and the orbits are tender to pressure. Chemosis, edema, and cyanosis of the upper face are present; the bulbs are proptosed. Sensorium may remain clear until late in the infection. Ophthalmoplegia, pupillary changes, retinal hemorrhages, papilledema, and sensory changes in the ophthalmic division of the trigeminal nerve may be present. The CSF is usually normal unless there is associated meningitis or subdural empyema. The only effective therapy in the fulminant variety, associated with thrombosis of the anterior portion of the sinus, has been antimicrobial therapy usually aimed at coagulase-positive staphylococci (see Chap. 100), anaerobic or microaerophilic streptococci (see Chap. 108), and occasionally gram-negative pathogens. Anticoagulants have been used occasionally, but their value has not been proven. Cavernous sinus thrombosis must be differentiated from mucormycosis, which may cause a similar clinical picture in uncontrolled diabetics or in immunosuppressed patients (see Chap. 151).

SUPERIOR LONGITUDINAL SINUS THROMBOPHLEBITIS The superior sagittal sinus may become infected by spread from the lateral or cavernous sinuses or by extension from the nasal cavities, from a focus of osteomyelitis, or from epidural or subdural infection. General signs include fever, headache, and papilledema. Edema of the forehead and anterior part of the scalp occur. The typical neurologic picture is one of unilateral convulsions and hemiplegia, first on one side of the body, then on the other, because of extension into the superior cerebral veins. The paralysis may be predominantly monoplegic and involve mainly the legs.

Cerebral angiography with particular attention to the late filling of venous sinuses is the most specific diagnostic test. Digital subtraction angiography has been useful in the diagnosis of sagittal sinus thrombosis. CT scans show normal or small ventricles, hemorrhages, low-density lesions, and a high-density lesion in the involved sinus. Postcontrast CT scan may demonstrate a filling defect in the involved sinus. Radionuclide dynamic and static scans may indicate termination of isotope activity in the midportion of the sinus. MRI may be the best and safest diagnostic approach.

All types of thrombophlebitis, especially those related to ear and paranasal sinus infection, may be complicated by other forms of intracranial suppuration including bacterial meningitis, subdural empyema, or brain abscess. The proper treatment of major sinus thrombosis due to infection is the systemic administration of antibiotics against organisms isolated from blood or pus or presumed to be present in the primary focus of infection. Antibiotics should be used in high dosage, and surgical drainage of infected bone and tissues should be carried out. The initiating focus should be brought under control by surgery if necessary. To operate on the primary focus before medical treatment is instituted is to court disaster. The better plan is to institute antibiotic therapy; surgery on the ears or sinuses should be decided upon only after the infection is controlled. In general, anticoagulants should be avoided because brain hemorrhage may result. Residual neurologic deficits are frequent, but the prognosis for recovery is good when optimal treatment is given early in the illness.

ASEPTIC THROMBOSIS OF INTRACRANIAL VENOUS SINUSES This may develop after sinus and ear infections and may lead to an obscure increase in intracranial pressure because of the occlusion of one lateral or superior sagittal sinus. The more common conditions which may be accompanied by aseptic thrombosis are postpartum and postoperative states, which are often characterized by thrombocytosis and hyperfibrinogenemia; use of oral contraceptive drugs;

congenital heart disease and marasmus in infants; systemic cancer; Behçet's disease; sickle cell disease; primary or secondary polycythemia; disseminated intravascular coagulation; and cryofibrinogenemia.

MALIGNANT EXTERNAL OTITIS

This paracranial infection is found in elderly patients with diabetes mellitus. Beginning in the external auditory canal, it spreads from the outer ear to the soft tissues below the temporal bone and invades the parotid gland, temporomandibular joint, masseter muscle, and temporal bone. *Pseudomonas aeruginosa* is responsible for the infection. The high mortality rate (initially reported at 40 percent) led to the term *malignant* for the condition; the adjective *necrotizing* or *invasive* may be preferable.

Symptoms and signs include pain in the ear with or without a purulent discharge, swelling of the parotid gland, trismus, and paralysis of the sixth to twelfth cranial nerves. Death is usually due to the development of meningitis. CT scan findings include obliteration of the normal fat planes in the subtemporal area and patchy destruction of the bony cortex of the mastoid. Radionuclide scans using Tc 99m or Ga 67 citrate are helpful in the initial identification of the disease and in following the course of the infection.

Prolonged intravenous administration of tobramycin, ticarcillin, ceftazidime, or imipenem is necessary to treat this condition. The choice of the β-lactam is determined by antimicrobial sensitivity testing. Antibiotics should be given for 6 weeks or for at least 2 weeks after all symptoms have resolved. Treatment for basal skull involvement may need to last at least 3 months, and, for prolonged treatment, oral ciprofloxacin may be a convenient and effective approach. Surgical debridement may be necessary.

BRAIN ABSCESS

PATHOGENESIS Most of the focal suppurative intracranial processes of this type are linked to chronic ear and sinus or pulmonary infections. About 25 percent of brain abscesses are due to disease of the middle ear, mastoids, or paranasal sinuses. Infection spreads to the brain directly across bone and dura mater or through vascular channels by septic thrombophlebitis or arteritis.

With frontal or ethmoid sinusitis, the abscess forms in the frontal lobe; with middle ear or mastoid infection, the abscess localizes to the temporal lobe or cerebellum. Of the remaining cases, about 25 percent are due to contaminated penetrating wounds or postoperative infections and about 25 percent are metastatic. Of these, about half are traceable to pleuropulmonary disease—usually bronchiectasis, empyema, lung abscess, or bronchopleural fistula. In the rest, the source of infection may be skin, bone, teeth, or heart. In about 20 percent of cases, the source cannot be ascertained. Brain abscess is seldom a consequence of bacterial meningitis. Brain abscess also occurs in patients whose immune systems are defective or suppressed. In these instances, *Nocardia* or nonbacterial causes such as fungi, protozoans, and helminths may be recovered from the abscess.

Brain abscess is particularly frequent in congenital heart disease with right-to-left shunts (e.g., tetralogy of Fallot) and may also complicate arteriovenous vascular abnormalities of the lung, as in cases of familial telangiectasia (Osler-Rendu-Weber syndrome). When brain abscess is associated with a right-to-left cardiac shunt, it is frequently single. With cranial trauma, the location of the abscess will depend on the site of the penetrating wound. In contrast to the otogenic and rhinogenic abscesses, abscesses of hematogenous origin are frequently multiple and may occur anywhere in the brain.

Bacterial endocarditis rarely gives rise to brain abscess. Instead, the picture is one of focal embolic encephalitis with or without signs of embolic vascular disease elsewhere (see Chap. 90). In subacute endocarditis the emboli are sterile and cause only infarction and

mycotic aneurysms. The CSF may contain a small number of neutrophilic leukocytes, lymphocytes, and red blood cells; the protein level may be elevated, but cultures are sterile and sugar values remain normal. In acute bacterial endocarditis caused by *S. aureus*, miliary abscesses and purulent meningitis may develop. There may be infarcts and subarachnoid or intracerebral hemorrhages secondary to rupture of a mycotic aneurysm. Rarely do the miliary abscesses progress to large ones. Rapidly evolving cerebral signs in endocarditis are nearly always caused by embolic infarction or hemorrhage.

ETIOLOGY Streptococci, including *S. milleri* (a member of the viridans group), other viridans and nonhemolytic streptococci, enterococci, β-hemolytic streptococci, and peptostreptococci, are the most commonly isolated group of microorganisms (see Chap. 108). Next in order of frequency are members of the *Bacteroides* group, Enterobacteriaceae (*Proteus, Escherichia coli, Klebsiella*), and *S. aureus*. Pneumococci, meningococci, and *H. influenzae* rarely cause brain abscess. In addition to *Bacteroides* and anaerobic streptococci, anaerobic actinomyces, veillonellae, and fusobacteria have been isolated. Bacterial species vary with the site of the abscess—staphylococcal abscesses are usually a consequence of penetrating head trauma or bacteremia; enteric organisms are almost always associated with ear infections; anaerobic streptococci are commonly metastatic from the lung. Two or more species of bacteria are identified in a single abscess in approximately 25 percent of cases, and mixtures of aerobes and anaerobes may be found. *Nocardia* species can cause brain abscesses. They often occur in association with pulmonary involvement and complicate immunosuppressive disease or therapy (see Chap. 152).

PATHOLOGY The location of brain abscess in decreasing order of frequency is in frontal, parietal, temporal, and occipital lobes, followed by cerebellum and basal ganglia. Abscesses rarely occur in the pituitary gland or brainstem. Localized inflammatory necrosis and edema, septic thrombosis of vessels, and aggregates of degenerating leukocytes (suppurative encephalitis) represent the early reaction of bacterial invasion of the brain. This is followed by encapsulation of the liquefied brain and of accumulated pus. The lesion becomes encapsulated by fibroblasts and newly formed vessels, and the capsule thickens over a period of weeks. The meninges adjacent to the abscess, especially near the point of entry of infection, are infiltrated by neutrophils, lymphocytes, and plasma cells. Cerebral edema associated with the abscess and products of bacterial metabolism (such as anaerobically produced gas) result in increased ICP. The evolution of cerebral abscess can be divided into four stages: early cerebritis (1 to 3 days), late cerebritis (4 to 9 days), early capsule formation (10 to 13 days), and late capsule formation (14 days and later).

CLINICAL MANIFESTATIONS Most patients have symptoms for less than 2 weeks. Characteristically the clinical presentation is more like that of an expanding intracranial mass lesion than an infectious process. In patients with chronic ear, sinus, or pulmonary infections, a recent reactivation of the infection usually precedes the onset of cerebral symptoms. In a number of patients, evidence of CNS invasion is acute, and headache, vomiting, increasing obtundation, seizures, and a variety of localizing neurologic signs appear within a few days. In other patients, bacterial invasion of the brain substance may be asymptomatic or may be attended only by a slowly developing focal neurologic disorder. Sometimes stiff neck accompanies generalized headache, suggesting the diagnosis of meningitis. Early symptoms may subside or appear to respond to antimicrobials. Within a week or two, recurrent headache, slowness in mentation, focal or generalized convulsions, progressive neurologic defects, and obvious signs of increased intracranial pressure provide evidence of a mass in the brain. At this stage, the symptoms of infection are not conspicuous. Fever is present in less than half of the patients. Symptoms are usually progressive in their intensity. On presentation less than half of patients will have altered consciousness with lethargy, irritability, confusion, or coma. Hemiplegia is the most common focal finding. Seizures, either focal or generalized, occur in about one-third of patients; papilledema and neck stiffness are present in about one-quarter of patients.

Patients demonstrate focal neurologic signs related to location of the abscess as described below.

Frontal lobe abscess   Headache, drowsiness, inattention, and general impairment of mental function are prominent. Hemiparesis with unilateral motor seizures and expressive aphasia are the most frequent neurologic signs.

Temporal lobe abscess   Headache is usually on the side of the abscess and is localized to the frontotemporal region. If the abscess lies in the dominant hemisphere, there is aphasia and anomia (inability to name objects). A homonymous upper quadrantic field defect may also be demonstrable owing to interruption of the inferior portion of the optic radiation. This may be the only sign in abscess of the right temporal lobe. Contralateral motor or sensory defects in the limbs tend to be minimal, though weakness of the lower face is often observed.

Cerebellar abscess   Headache in the postauricular or suboccipital region is usually the first symptom and may at first be ascribed to infection in the mastoid cells. Coarse nystagmus and gaze weakness to the side of the lesion and a cerebellar ataxia of the ipsilateral arm and leg are present in most patients. As a rule, the signs of increased ICP are more prominent than those of focal cerebral disease. Mild contralateral or bilateral pyramidal signs may provide evidence of ipsilateral brainstem compression.

DIAGNOSIS   The diagnosis of a brain abscess depends on (1) a demonstrated source of infection in the ears, sinuses, or lungs or the presence of a right-to-left cardiac shunt, (2) evidence of increased ICP, and (3) focal cerebral or cerebellar signs. Clues to the origin of the abscess are often present on initial evaluation. They include chronic ear disease with discharge, sinus infection, orbital cellulitis, pharyngitis, infected skin wound, and chest infection.

Lumbar puncture in suspected brain abscess is potentially dangerous, particularly when the ICP is obviously elevated, and the information to be derived is not specific enough to justify the risk. Routine x-rays of the skull may demonstrate gas in an abscess cavity. The electroencephalogram (EEG) is usually abnormal with focal changes.

The CT scan is the most valuable procedure for visualizing brain abscess(es). It also demonstrates ventricular distortion, surrounding edema of white matter, and the thickness of the capsule; it enables close follow-up of therapy. Injection of iodine-containing contrast material will enhance the selectivity of the CT scan and will permit the visualization of an abscess from the early stage of focal cerebritis to a densely encapsulated mass demonstrated as a "ring" that is sharply demarcated both internally and externally with a homogeneous central area of decreased attenuation. Generally only a CT scan is required to make the diagnosis. Peripheral ring enhancement may also be found in tumor, cerebral infarction, resolving hematoma, radiation necrosis, and recent surgery; these conditions may enter into the differential diagnosis of the CT scan findings. Although MRI is more sensitive than CT in the detection of changes produced by early cerebritis, the improved sensitivity of MRI is rarely clinically significant. If CT scanning is not available, radionuclide brain scan is a reliable method for localizing brain abscess. If both CT and radionuclide scans are negative, there is little likelihood of cerebral abscess. Scanning procedures have supplanted arteriography in nearly all instances.

When the typical clinical picture is present and CT scan corroborates the presence of a mass lesion, the diagnosis is easy. If there is no source of infection and there are only signs and symptoms of a mass lesion, the diagnosis may be difficult. Sometimes only surgical exploration will settle the issue.

TREATMENT   During the stage of acute suppurative cerebritis, intracranial operation accomplishes little and probably causes only additional trauma and swelling of brain tissue. If a predisposing factor is present and the presumed offending organism has been successfully cultured, there is good evidence that many brain abscesses

visible by CT scanning can be cured at this stage by the administration of adequate doses of antimicrobials. Since the bacteriologic diagnosis must be presumptive, the most widely used regimen for adults consists of 20 to 30 million units of penicillin G and 2 to 4 g of metronidazole, both drugs given intravenously in divided doses. Cefotaxime or ceftriaxone may be added empirically in dosages similar to those for meningitis. Chloramphenicol, 4 to 6 g/d in divided doses, may be substituted for penicillin in allergic patients. This choice of antimicrobial agents is based on the preponderance of anaerobic streptococci and *Bacteroides* that are usually isolated from brain abscess. Treatment should be continued for 6 to 8 weeks, and if there is clinical improvement and recovery during antibiotic treatment, surgical intervention can be withheld.

For well-defined brain abscesses, selection of specific antimicrobials requires recovery of the responsible microorganism(s). Pus from the abscess cavity can be obtained by needle puncture at the time of craniotomy or by CT-guided percutaneous stereotactic operation, a procedure that is performed under local anesthesia with a 1 percent mortality rate. The specimen should be sent to the laboratory for Gram stain and for routine and anaerobic bacteriologic and fungal cultures. Specimens must be handled in a way that will not kill fastidious bacteria. Once the infecting bacteria have been identified and their sensitivities determined, the appropriate antibiotic regimen can be chosen.

Serial CT scanning and prompt, aggressive antibiotic treatment have avoided surgical intervention in cases of well-formed, small (<3 cm) abscesses, particularly when an organism has been isolated elsewhere. The indications for medical management include presence of multiple abscesses after one has been aspirated for diagnosis and culture, small abscesses located in deep brain structures, concomitant meningitis or ependymitis, the presence of a ventricular shunt, and an uncorrectable bleeding diathesis. In many instances, surgery should be performed to confirm the diagnosis, culture the organism, and treat the condition. Since the advent of CT-directed stereotactic surgery entails minimal risk, the only absolute contraindication to surgery is a bleeding diathesis.

ICP monitoring may be useful in the management of some brain abscesses, but is not usually employed. Initial elevation of ICP and threatening temporal lobe or cerebellar herniation should be managed by the prompt intravenous injection of mannitol or dexamethasone. Persistence or progression of high ICP manifested by deepening coma requires operation, regardless of the stage of the abscess. Likewise, clear-cut evidence of a mass lesion that is not improving with antimicrobial therapy is an indication for surgery. Gas-containing abscesses should be aspirated surgically or excised. The usual methods of treatment of an abscess are total excision or drainage by aspiration. If the abscess is superficial and encapsulated, total excision is sometimes attempted; if it is deep, aspiration of the abscess is the least traumatic treatment but might have to be repeated.

PROGNOSIS   With the availability of CT scanning, more effective antimicrobials, and improved surgical techniques, abscesses have been treated earlier and more effectively. Mortality has fallen to approximately 10 percent. Neurologic abnormalities, particularly focal epilepsy, are rare, troublesome sequelae to brain abscess surgery. Following successful treatment of cerebral abscess in patients with congenital heart disease, correction of the cardiac anomaly is indicated to prevent recurrence.

REFERENCES

ANON JB, MILLER GW: Malignant external otitis. South Med J 77:1541, 1984

BLAQUIERE RM: The computed tomographic appearances of intra- and extracerebral abscesses. Br J Radiol 56:171, 1983

CHERUBIN CE, ENG RHK: Experience with the use of cefotaxime in the treatment of bacterial meningitis. Am J Med 80:398, 1986

DAGBJARTSSON A, LUDVIGSSON P: Bacterial meningitis: Diagnosis and initial antibiotic therapy. Pediatr Clin North Am 34:219, 1987

DURACK DT: Prevention of central nervous system infection in patients at risk. Am J Med 76(5A):231, 1984

GARVEY G: Current concepts of bacterial infections of the central nervous system: Bacterial meningitis and bacterial brain abscess. J Neurosurg 59:735, 1983

GORDON JJ et al: Meningitis due to *Staphylococcus aureus*. Am J Med 78:965, 1985

GORSE GJ et al: Bacterial meningitis in the elderly. Arch Intern Med 144:1603, 1984

HARRISON MJG: The clinical presentation of intracranial abscess. Q J Med 204:461, 1982

KAUFMAN DM et al: Subdural empyema: Analysis of 17 recent cases and review of the literature. Medicine 54:485, 1975

LEBEL MH et al: Dexamethasone therapy for bacterial meningitis. Results of two double-blind, placebo-controlled trials. N Engl J Med 319:964, 1988

LEFROCK JL et al: Gram-negative bacillary meningitis. Med Clin North Am 69:243, 1985

MANAPLANT TJ, ROSENBLUM MI: Trends in the management of bacterial brain abscesses: A review of 102 cases over 17 years. Neurosurgery 23:451, 1988

MARTON KI, GEAN AD: The spinal tap: A new look at an old test. Ann Intern Med 104:840, 1986

MAYHALL CG et al: Ventriculostomy-related infections: A prospective epidemiological study. N Engl J Med 310:553, 1984

POLLOCK SS et al: Infection of the central nervous system by *Listeria monocytogenes:* A review of 54 adult and juvenile cases. Q J Med 211:331, 1984

RAO KCVG et al: Computed tomographic findings in cerebral sinus and venous thrombosis. Radiology 140:391, 1981

ROSENBLUM ML et al: Controversies in the management of brain abscesses. Clin Neurosurg 33:603, 1986

SCHAAD UB et al: A comparison of ceftriaxone and cefuroxime for the treatment of bacterial meningitis in children. N Engl J Med 322:142, 1990

SZE G, ZIMMERMAN RD: The magnetic resonance imaging of infections and inflammatory diseases. Radiol Clin North Am 26:839, 1988

355 VIRAL DISEASES OF THE CENTRAL NERVOUS SYSTEM: ASEPTIC MENINGITIS AND ENCEPHALITIS

DONALD H. HARTER / ROBERT G. PETERSDORF

Viruses can affect the central nervous system in a variety of ways. Although much is known about the nature and replication of viruses, the correlation between viral properties and the type of the neurologic disease produced is inadequate or incomplete. Viruses that differ widely in their morphology, chemical composition, and replication can provoke identical clinical and pathologic changes in the CNS.

It is helpful to consider the time between the patient's first exposure to the viral agent and the appearance of disease, that is, to distinguish between CNS infections of a "fast" or "slow" nature. In fast or acute viral disease, neurologic changes occur very shortly after the patient first becomes infected by the virus. The illness follows a course of one to several weeks. In slow viral disease, the neurologic changes appear months to years after viral invasion, are insidious in development, and progress slowly.

ACUTE VIRAL CNS DISEASE

GENERAL CONSIDERATIONS Most viral CNS infections are the end result of preceding infection in other tissues and organs. There is usually a phase of extraneural viral replication before the nervous system becomes involved. Acute viral CNS infections are classified according to the clinical findings presented by the patient or, more indirectly, by the part of the nervous system involved by the disease process. In these terms, acute viral CNS disease is defined as meningitis, encephalitis, or myelitis, depending on the patient's symptoms and signs and the location of the infection. It is often difficult, however, to arrive at a single satisfactory localization on the basis of clinical findings alone. This leads to the use of compound terms such as meningoencephalitis or encephalomyelitis to describe the disease. This manner of classification is less than satisfactory because it gives no clear idea about the virus causing the condition.

Viruses vary in size, morphology, chemical composition, and effect on the host (see Chap. 133). Their common characteristics include a genome, which is either RNA or DNA surrounded by a protective protein shell; the fact that they multiply only inside the cell; and that the initial step in replication involves separation of the genome from its protective shell. They are divided into two broad categories on the basis of their nucleic acid content and then into major families and genera (Table 355-1). Certain common properties of viruses are important determinants of the disease they produce. Herpesviruses have a tendency to remain latent in cells. Togaviruses and bunyaviruses are transmitted by insect vectors. Enteroviruses replicate in the gastrointestinal tract and are transmitted by the oral-fecal route. Myxoviruses contain a segmented genome which is prone to genetic recombination. Selection of the most effective methods of virus isolation depends in great measure on the virus's properties. Knowledge of a virus's biochemical composition is of help in determining whether antiviral therapy can be used. Understanding the biologic features of viruses within the major families and genera permits associations which are impossible when the location of the disease process is considered alone (see Chap. 133).

ASEPTIC OR VIRAL MENINGITIS Etiology The term *aseptic meningitis* designates a disease characterized by an acute onset, meningeal symptoms, fever, cerebrospinal fluid (CSF) pleocytosis, and bacteriologically sterile cultures. The illness has a relatively benign clinical course of short duration, and recovery is the rule. With the introduction of more refined methods of viral isolation and the use of new culture techniques to define other microorganisms, it has become clear that aseptic meningitis is a syndrome of multiple etiologies. When viral infection produces the syndrome, the condition should be referred to as viral meningitis.

Epidemiology Aseptic meningitis affects between 9000 and 12,000 persons in the United States every year. Although all ages are involved, more than 90 percent of the patients are under age 30. The peak incidence of aseptic meningitis is in the late summer. The majority of cases seen in the summer are due to picornaviruses other than polioviruses, such as the coxsackie- and echoviruses. Mumps meningitis occurs more often in the winter and late spring. Both sexes are affected equally by enteroviruses, but there is a 2:1 or 3:1 male predominance in mumps meningitis. Acute aseptic meningitis may occur in the course of infection with Epstein-Barr virus (EBV) (see Chap. 137), cytomegalovirus (CMV) (see Chap. 138), herpes simplex virus type 2 (HSV-2) (see Chap. 135), varicella-zoster virus (VZV) (see Chap. 136), and human immunodeficiency virus (HIV) (see below and Chap. 264).

TABLE 355-1 Viruses of vertebrates

RNA-containing		DNA-containing
Picornavirus*	Paramyxovirus*	Hepadnavirus
Enterovirus*	Paramyxovirus*	
Cardiovirus	Morbillivirus*	Parvovirus
Rhinovirus	Pneumovirus	
Aphthovirus		Papovavirus*
Hepatitis A	Orthomyxovirus*	Papillomavirus
	Influenzavirus	Polyomavirus*
Calicivirus	Influenza C virus	Adenovirus
Togavirus*	Bunyavirus*	Herpesvirus*
Alphavirus*	Bunyavirus*	Alphaherpesvirus*
Rubivirus*	Phlebovirus	Betaherpesvirus*
Pestivirus	Nairovirus	Gammaherpesvirus*
Arterivirus	Uukuvirus	
	Hantavirus	Poxvirus
Flavivirus*		
	Arenavirus*	Iridovirus
Coronavirus		
	Reovirus	
Rhabdovirus*		
Vesiculovirus	Birnavirus	
Lyssavirus*		
	Retrovirus*	
Filovirus	Oncovirus	
	Spumavirus	
	Lentivirus*	

* Virus genera and families associated with neurologic illnesses.

Clinical picture   The symptoms and signs of viral meningitis are similar irrespective of the particular virus involved. The onset of illness is acute. There may be a prodromal "flulike" illness before the onset of meningitis, as in lymphocytic choriomeningitis. This biphasic pattern of illness also may be observed in young children with poliomyelitis or in illness due to other insect-borne viruses (see Chaps. 148 and 149). CNS involvement is manifested by an intense frontal or retroorbital headache. Malaise, nausea and vomiting, listlessness, and photophobia may be present. As a rule, there is little impairment of consciousness. The patient may be drowsy and slightly confused but is usually oriented and rational. Stupor and coma occur rarely. The temperature is usually elevated in the range of 38 to 40°C. There is neck stiffness on forward flexion. Kernig's and Brudzinski's signs are present in most cases but may be absent in patients with minimal meningeal irritation. Extension of the spine may be such that a child will sit with the head retracted and the arms extended posteriorly in the form of a tripod. Signs of focal damage to the central nervous system are rarely present. Occasionally, strabismus or diplopia, asymmetry of tendon reflexes, and an inconstant extensor plantar response may be found.

Clinical findings outside the nervous system may provide clues to the virus involved in the infection. Parotitis in association with viral meningitis suggests mumps. Skin rash has been a prominent feature of coxsackievirus or echovirus infections (see Chap. 144). Blotchy or punctate maculopapular rashes that involve the extremities and which occur chiefly in the summertime are commonly due to echovirus. Herpangina (large, painful vesicles in the posterior one-third of the oropharynx) are usually caused by coxsackieviruses. Sharp pains in the chest aggravated by deep respiration or coughing suggest the pleurodynia seen with Coxsackie B viruses. Infection with VZV, HSV, or EBV is usually dominated by nonneurologic manifestations.

Laboratory findings   The lumbar CSF is usually under increased pressure and clear or slightly turbid in appearance. Slight turbidity can be demonstrated by holding a tube containing CSF to the light and agitating the fluid with a gentle finger tap. CSF usually contains 10 to 100 cells per microliter. At times, the cell count rises to levels of 3000 per microliter or greater. The cells are usually more than three-fourths lymphocytes or mononuclear cells. Polymorphonuclear cells may predominate in the early phases of aseptic meningitis. The CSF protein and sugar concentrations are usually normal. Isolated instances of depressed CSF sugar in patients with infections due to mumps or HSV have been reported but are rare. If the patient presents with CSF that contains less sugar than expected, meningitis due to bacteria, mycobacteria, or fungi should receive first attention. Oligoclonal IgG bands may be found in the CSF of patients with viral meningitis. Gram stain and india ink preparations fail to identify an organism; bacterial and fungal cultures are negative. Although certain viruses (such as mumps, HSV, VZV, and CMV) can be recovered from CSF with relative ease, in most cases of viral meningitis, it is usually impossible to recover the responsible viral agent from the patient's CSF. The white cell count in the blood is usually normal, but leukopenia is present in about one-third of patients.

The specific viral diagnosis can usually be made by performing serologic tests on acute and convalescent sera and by attempting to isolate viruses from feces, urine, and throat washings. With the exception of CMV and HIV, performance of a Monospot test or specific measurement of antibodies to EBV can lead to the diagnosis of aseptic meningitis complicating infectious mononucleosis (see Chap. 137). Other useful tests can include CSF cytologies, a nontreponemal antibody test for syphilis (see Chap. 128) and serologies for *Borellia burgdorferi* (see Chap. 132). Attempts to isolate the agent from blood are usually unsuccessful.

Differential diagnosis   The syndrome of viral or aseptic meningitis can be caused by a number of different infectious and noninfectious agents. The majority of cases of viral origin are due to picornaviruses, togaviruses, herpesviruses, paramyxoviruses, and arenaviruses. The list of nonviral infectious causes of the aseptic meningitis syndrome is extensive. It includes intracranial infections located near the meninges (otitis, mastoiditis, vertebral osteomyelitis); brain abscess; partially treated bacterial meningitis; and mycobacterial, spirochetal, fungal, rickettsial, protozoan, or helminthic infections.

Noninfectious causes of the aseptic meningitis syndrome include the intrathecal introduction of drugs and agents for diagnostic tests and tumors in close proximity to the cerebral ventricles or that invade the subarachnoid space. Cytologic examination of cells in the CSF will distinguish neoplastic meningeal infiltration from viral meningitis. Systemic diseases such as sarcoidosis, disseminated lupus erythematosus, and infective endocarditis may be associated with aseptic meningitis.

Also, there are a number of infrequently encountered systemic diseases in which the CSF findings resemble viral meningitis. These include (1) Behçet's disease, characterized by uveitis, genital and oral ulcers, and focal neurologic abnormalities; (2) Vogt-Koyanagi and Harada's diseases, which combine uveitis, depigmentation of the hair and skin about the eyes, loss of eyelashes, and deafness; (3) Mollaret's meningitis; and (4) Lyme disease.

Treatment   The treatment of viral meningitis is symptomatic. Antiviral agents are not indicated in uncomplicated cases. Fever and other symptoms resolve in 3 to 5 days, and patients are usually entirely well within 2 weeks. CSF abnormalities are most pronounced from the fourth to sixth day, but the CSF white blood cell count may remain elevated for several weeks in patients who are otherwise asymptomatic. Initial therapy with antimicrobial agents may be appropriate if the initial elevation is not completely typical for viral infection. In most instances, patients recover from viral meningitis without sequelae. A limited number of patients may develop muscular weakness and other forms of motor disability. A very small number of patients may have recurrent attacks of viral meningitis; the multiple episodes are often due to different viruses. Acyclovir treatment can shorten the course of infection with HSV and VZV (see Chaps. 135 and 136).

Prognosis   It is important to recognize that viral meningitis is an acute and self-limited illness and to realize that it may mimic life-threatening CNS infections which are potentially treatable. Most important to appreciate is the similarity between viral meningitis and partially treated bacterial meningitis, tuberculous meningitis, or fungal meningitis. If the CSF changes are not completely characteristic of viral meningitis or if the patient's clinical response is atypical, it is important to perform repeated lumbar punctures and to reexamine the CSF within a relatively brief period of time, until the clinical picture becomes clear.

VIRAL ENCEPHALITIS   Definition   The term *encephalitis* is used when there is clinical and/or pathologic evidence of involvement of the cerebral hemispheres, brainstem, or cerebellum by the infectious process. It is customary to divide viral encephalitis into primary and postinfectious or parainfectious forms and to consider whether the disease is sporadic or epidemic. The *primary* form of the disease occurs when the encephalitis is the presenting form of the disease and is due to direct invasion and replication of virus within the CNS. The term *postinfectious* or *parainfectious* is used to describe an encephalitis that follows or occurs in combination with other viral illnesses or administration of certain vaccines (see Chap. 356). The cause of the encephalitis in such cases is believed to be a hypersensitivity reaction. The pathologic picture is typical of multifocal perivenous demyelination. The virus cannot be recovered from the CNS. If the inflammatory condition extends into the spinal cord, the term encephalomyelitis is used.

Clinical picture   When encephalitis is the primary illness, such as with togaviruses and herpesviruses, there may be a minor illness consisting of such systemic symptoms as headache, myalgia, malaise, and upper respiratory symptoms. These nonspecific symptoms may occur several days before neurologic complaints and signs are recognized.

The onset of neurologic symptoms is abrupt. There is alteration in the patient's state of consciousness with lethargy, drowsiness, or stupor. The patient's behavior may be abnormal as a consequence of confusion, disorientation, and hallucinations. A convulsion or series of convulsions may occur at the start of the illness, and seizures may be the sole presenting symptom. The patient usually complains of headache, nausea, and vomiting. Fever is usually present, and there may be stiffening of the neck on forward bending. Focal neurologic abnormalities are found, depending on the portion of the nervous system involved by the inflammatory process. Involvement of the cerebral hemispheres may result in aphasia, signs of corticospinal and corticobulbar tract lesions, involuntary movements, ataxia, sensory defects, and loss of retentive memory.

Laboratory examinations General laboratory tests are usually of little help in the diagnosis of encephalitis. They may provide evidence of systemic disease, such as abnormal lymphocytes in infectious mononucleosis and elevated amylase and transaminase levels in mumps and certain picornavirus infections.

Lumbar puncture, followed by examination of the CSF, is the most important diagnostic test. The CSF is usually under normal or slightly elevated pressure, clear or slightly turbid, and contains an increased number of white cells (in the range of 50 to 500 per microliter), a slight-to-moderate elevation of protein content, and a normal glucose level. There may be a predominance of polymorphonuclear leukocytes in the early phase of the illness. The protein content will often rise as the total cell count diminishes. In encephalitis caused by HSV-1, the CSF may be slightly bloody or xanthochromic and contain a significant number of red blood cells. This reflects the sometimes hemorrhagic nature of HSV encephalitis. Occasionally a viral encephalitis may exist without CSF abnormalities, which makes the diagnosis even more difficult.

The electroencephalogram may be of diagnostic help in suspected encephalitis. Diffuse or bilateral abnormalities can be defined by the EEG in patients who present with focal or unilateral neurologic deficits. A number of EEG changes may be seen, but the most common pattern is a diffuse slow wave activity with disruption of normal rhythms, punctuated at times with periodic high-amplitude bursts and spike-and-wave complexes. Computed tomography (CT), magnetic resonance imaging (MRI), and radionuclide scans may be helpful in demonstrating intracranial mass lesions or localized foci of infection about or within the brain. The cerebral cortex may be enhanced diffusely. Because of its sensitivity to altered water content, MRI detects changes of viral encephalitis before CT.

Diagnosis When presented with a patient with suspected viral encephalitis, it is important to exclude nonviral infections for which potential treatment is available. A number of conditions can mimic viral encephalitis (Table 355-2). It is imperative to consider these alternative causes when the patient is first evaluated. Once the

TABLE 355-2 Nonviral conditions mistaken for acute viral encephalitis

Infection:	
Bacterial	Early or imperfectly treated meningitis Brain abscess Parameningeal infections Illness due to mycobacteria, spirochetes, *Mycoplasma*
Fungi	*Cryptococcus, Coccidioides immitis, Histoplasma, Candida, Nocardia, Blastomyces*
Rickettsia	Rocky Mountain spotted fever
Protozoa	"Fresh water" amebiasis, malaria, toxoplasmosis
Metazoa	Cysticercosis, trichinosis, and others
Intoxication	Salicylates, barbiturates, heavy metals, tick paralysis
Endocrine and metabolic disorders	Acute sodium, calcium, or carbohydrate imbalance; porphyria, pheochromocytoma
Systemic diseases	Sarcoidosis, hyperglobulinemia, collagen disease, neoplasms, endocarditis with embolization
Acute psychotic disorders	

SOURCE: After Brown.

diagnosis of primary viral encephalitis is secure, it is important to determine if the illness is occurring as part of an epidemic or as an isolated sporadic event. Knowledge of the seasonal, geographic, and age group occurrence of the disease can often furnish enough information to make an informed guess about the correct viral etiology. During the summer and early fall, togaviruses, bunyaviruses, and picornaviruses may prevail. Some of these viruses may produce milder disease than others; some, such as western equine and California encephalitis viruses, affect a predominantly young age group. In the winter, epidemic encephalitis is more often associated with paramyxovirus, VZV, EBV, or rubella virus infection. HSV is responsible for more cases of nonepidemic sporadic encephalitis cases than any other virus.

The course of viral encephalitis is variable. It may be a short-lived, benign illness or a devastatingly severe one which leaves the patient with pronounced impairment of cerebral functions. Severe sequelae may be associated with certain viruses (HSV-1, eastern equine encephalitis, Japanese encephalitis, and St. Louis encephalitis). Other viruses cause milder disease (California encephalitis, western equine encephalitis). The acute phase of the disease usually lasts a few days to a week. Resolution can be abrupt or gradual. The disease may be complicated by a salt-wasting syndrome resulting from hypothalamic involvement and/or alterations in temperature or respiratory control centers owing to brainstem involvement. These events may occur rapidly and require prompt recognition and correction. Neurologic defects may continue to improve over a period of weeks to months.

In most instances of epidemic encephalitis, the viral diagnosis is made by serologic tests of acute and convalescent phase sera. Three major serologic tests are employed: complement-fixation, hemagglutination-inhibition, and neutralization. Because the serologic test is crucial for viral diagnosis, it is imperative to obtain an acute-phase serum as soon as the diagnosis of viral encephalitis is suspected. In vector-transmitted encephalitis which does not result in fatality, the blood is the most likely tissue source of viral isolation. Isolation of virus from blood is difficult, however, because viremia is usually brief and occurs before the onset of neurologic symptoms. In fatal cases, the virus can often be isolated from brain and spinal cord by inoculation of susceptible animals and tissue culture.

When HSV encephalitis is suspected, greater urgency is required in arriving at a viral diagnosis because there is a definite advantage in initiating antiviral therapy as quickly as possible (see Chap. 135). Serologic tests are not helpful. A number of patients with HSV encephalitis present with fever and neurologic findings compatible with a bilateral space-occupying lesion of the medial parts of the temporal and the orbital parts of the frontal lobes. A severe retentive memory defect is a frequent sequelum. HSV can be best demonstrated in brain tissue obtained by biopsy. Examination of the tissue by light, electron, and immunofluorescence microscopy and inoculation of a brain homogenate into cell cultures and animals permit a specific diagnosis of HSV early in the course of the patient's illness. However, many neurologists object to biopsy as a diagnostic procedure because the risks and sequelae outweigh the dangers of treatment. Moreover, enhanced CT scans, MRI, and radionuclide brain imaging often reveal the temporal lobe lesions which, when added to the clinical picture and a CSF pleocytosis, make the diagnosis fairly certain and permit treatment without brain biopsy. MRI may improve the sensitivity by detecting hemorrhage in certain HSV encephalitis patients.

Encephalitis may present as an infrequently encountered manifestation of a systemic disease such as measles, varicella, or neoplasia. When this is the case, the encephalitis occurs after the more characteristic features of the disease have become evident. Rarely, the systemic disease may appear after the diagnosis of encephalitis has been established.

UNUSUAL FORMS OF VIRAL ENCEPHALITIS *Acute cerebellar ataxia* may be associated with a number of different viruses (picornaviruses, VZV, and EBV). The illness usually afflicts children between the ages of 1 and 5 years. The majority of patients have had a preceding mild infectious illness a week or so before the onset of neurologic signs. The onset of the illness is characteristically abrupt with prominent ataxia of the trunk and limbs. Complete recovery is the rule, but a permanent cerebellar deficit may ensue in patients when ataxia is profound in the early stages of the illness. In some instances of VZV infection, the cerebellar lesions are of the parainfectious, demyelinating type (see Chap. 356).

Acute hemorrhagic leukoencephalitis is an infrequently encountered hyperacute disease of cerebral white matter which is often preceded by some form of systemic viral illness, most often an upper respiratory tract infection. The disease is marked by an acute onset, progressively deepening disturbance of consciousness, fever, seizures, and focal cortical abnormalities. Cerebral involvement is frequently unilateral. The course is rapid and usually fatal. There is a peripheral leukocytosis, and the CSF frequently contains mononuclear and polymorphonuclear leukocytes. The presence of mass effect or increased absorption coefficient on CT scan within the first 3 days of encephalitis should suggest this diagnosis. The cause of the disease is unknown. It has not been linked to infection by a specific virus or group of viruses and may well be allergic in nature. A virus has not been recovered from brain tissue. Treatment includes vigorous control of intracranial pressure and seizures and aggressive use of glucocorticoids in high dosage (see Chap. 356).

Limbic encephalitis is a form of encephalitis localized to the temporal and frontal lobes—the limbic part of the brain. It is encountered as a remote effect of malignancy—most commonly carcinoma of the lung. A viral etiology has been suspected but never proved. Patients with limbic encephalitis have marked impairment of recent memory manifested by a confabulatory-amnestic state, and generalized seizures. The patient's CSF often contains a limited number of lymphocytes and mononuclear cells. The EEG is characterized by paroxysmal and/or slow waves over one or both temporal lobes. Pathologic changes are most pronounced in the hippocampal formation and amygdaloid nuclei. Encephalitis with predilection for the brainstem has also been reported as a remote effect of tumor (see Chap. 310).

Encephalitis lethargica (von Economo's disease) first occurred during and for about 10 years after World War I. A causative viral agent was never identified, but the clinical and pathologic features were those of a viral infection of the thalamus and midbrain. The disease was characterized by pronounced somnolence and ophthalmoplegia. A high proportion of survivors developed a parkinsonian syndrome months or years after the encephalitis (see Chap. 359). Sporadic case reports of patients with the clinical features of encephalitis lethargica appear even to the present time.

MYELITIS Viral infection of the central nervous system may localize in the parenchyma of the spinal cord producing myelitis. Poliovirus infection with damage to spinal motor neurons is the prototype of a viral infection localized chiefly to the spinal cord. Vaccination has markedly reduced but not eliminated poliomyelitis because patients who have not been vaccinated remain susceptible. Progressive muscular weakness, fasciculations, and atrophy occur in some patients many years after an acute episode of poliomyelitis. The cause of this "postpolio" syndrome is still uncertain; it may be a recrudescence of viral activity (see Chap. 144).

Spinal paralytic disease has also been described with other enteroviruses (coxsackieviruses and echoviruses). The illness is characterized by an asymmetric flaccid paralysis of the limbs; it is usually less severe and has a higher rate of recovery from muscular weakness than poliomyelitis.

Other viruses have also been reported to affect the spinal cord directly. Herpesvirus type 2 infection in the genital and perineal region has been associated with paralysis of sphincter function, probably indicative of direct viral involvement of the sacral spinal cord. Myelitis due to VZV (aside from the ganglionitis and unilateral poliomyelitis) is another very rare cause of a leukomyelitis resulting in bilateral weakness of the legs with occasional ankle clonus or extensor plantar responses. Sphincter disturbances are present in two-thirds of patients and a sensory level in about one-half of patients. The CSF contains from 25 to 125 cells per microliter; the protein content may be normal or elevated. Recovery of function is the rule.

There may also be delayed involvement of the white matter of the spinal cord following viral infection. This is a parainfectious demyelinative process that interrupts sensory and motor tracts at one level and is termed an acute transverse myelitis. It begins with the abrupt onset of bilateral weakness of the legs and concomitant involvement of ascending sensory pathways. Urinary bladder and bowel functions are usually disturbed early in the course of the illness. An exanthem or respiratory infection not uncommonly precedes neurologic symptoms. Acute myelitis in the absence of encephalitis has been described in association with measles, VZV, echovirus, HSV, and infectious mononucleosis. It has also been observed after rabies and smallpox vaccination. Virus isolation from CSF has been unsuccessful. A small proportion of patients with acute transverse myelitis will later develop multiple sclerosis. Acute spinal epidural abscess should be considered and excluded in patients who present with an acute nontraumatic transverse spinal cord syndrome. Rarely schistosomiasis may present with transverse myelitis (see Chap. 170).

TREATMENT Of the various viruses that cause acute encephalitis, HSV is the most responsive to antiviral chemotherapy. The drug of choice is acyclovir, given intravenously. Details of therapy are given in Chap. 86.

CNS DISEASES DUE TO SLOW VIRUS INFECTION

In slow virus infections, a protracted period, often months or years, passes between the introduction of the infectious agent and the appearance of clinical illness. Once neurologic disease is established, it may progress slowly over many months or years. The reasons why a certain virus will cause acute illness in one patient and slow infection in another are still largely unknown. Viruses causing slow infections do not appear to share any common features. No single virus property can be correlated with the slow virus disease process. The factors invoked to explain slow virus infections include (1) a defect in the composition of the virus; (2) a change in the virus's antigenicity; (3) an altered or defective host immune response; (4) a special property of the virus which permits it to remain latent or to become integrated in the host cell's genome; or (5) a yet incompletely understood and possibly unique method of replication.

Slow virus CNS diseases affect the parenchyma of the cerebral hemispheres and, in some instances, the cerebellum, brainstem, and spinal cord. These infections are not grouped by their topography, i.e., the part of the nervous system that they damage, or by their clinical presentation. Some slow viruses provoke a mild conventional inflammatory response during the time they are clinically silent; others are able to reside within cells for long periods without causing detectable cytopathic changes. The role of immunity in slow virus infection is largely unknown. Some slow virus infections occur in the presence of elevated levels of circulating antibodies; in others, there may be no detectable immune response.

Because infective agents causing some human slow CNS diseases have not been demonstrated to contain nucleic acid, the slow viral CNS infections are divided into those due to conventional viruses and those due to unconventional agents whose viral nature has not been fully established (Table 355-3). There are currently nine well-defined neurologic diseases caused by slow viruses. No consistently effective therapy is now available for any of them. Conventional viruses have been recovered from the CNS of patients with subacute sclerosing panencephalitis (SSPE), progressive multifocal leukoencephalopathy (PML), progressive rubella encephalitis, tropical spastic paraparesis (TSP), and persistent viral infection in immunodeficient patients. Each of these is based on an inflammatory reaction in the CNS. Kuru, Creutzfeldt-Jakob disease (CJD), and Gerstmann-Sträussler-Scheinker (GSS) disease share common neuropathologic features

TABLE 355-3 Slow virus diseases of the CNS	
Conventional viruses	Subacute sclerosing panencephalitis (SSPE)
	Progressive multifocal leukoencephalopathy (PML)
	Progressive rubella encephalitis
	Tropical spastic parapheresis (TSP)
	Persistent infection in immunodeficiency:
	Congenital or primary
	Acquired or induced
Unconventional viruslike agents	Kuru
	Creutzfeldt-Jakob disease (CJD)
	Gerstmann-Sträussler-Scheinker disease (GSS)

which are noninflammatory. They produce fine vacuolation of nervous tissue and hence are referred to as the subacute spongiform virus encephalopathies. Although these diseases have been shown to be of infectious etiology by the transmission of neurologic illness to higher primates, their causative agents remain incompletely characterized. They are classified as the slow virus infections due to unconventional agents.

The best studied of the unconventional transmissible agents is scrapie, a neurologic disease of sheep. The true nature of the scrapie agent has not been defined. There is evidence that a surface membrane protease-resistant protein (PrP) is involved in the development of the disease. Concentrated and partially purified scrapie agent contains a sialoglycoprotein of approximately 27,000 to 30,000 mol wt, designated PrP 27-30, as a major component. PrP 27-30 is recovered from scrapie-infected brain; the protein is not found in normal brain. Because of this association, the term *prion* was introduced as an operational name for the putative infectious agent. Prion is defined as a small proteinaceous infectious particle that is resistant to inactivation by most procedures that modify nucleic acids.

PrP is a host-specified protein that is encoded by a single exon that can be expressed in both normal and diseased animals. Brains of scrapie-infected animals contain two isomorphs of PrP, a scrapie form (PrP^{Sc}) and cellular form (PrP^{C}). The two proteins have different physical differences that appear to be due to posttranslational modification. After proteolysis, PrP^{Sc} loses an amino-terminal peptide to become PrP 27-30. Homogenates of tissue culture cells expressing the cloned PrP gene fail to induce clinical signs of scrapie when inoculated into susceptible mice. PrPs have been recovered from the brains of patients with CJD and GSS disease and have been named PrP^{CJD} and PrP^{GSS}, respectively.

SUBACUTE SCLEROSING PANENCEPHALITIS (SSPE) This progressive and ultimately fatal disease of children and adolescents had been suspected to be of viral origin since its initial description as inclusion body encephalitis. Measles virus or a virus very closely related to measles virus has been recovered from the brains of patients with the disease. The disorder may be considered to be a slow form of measles encephalitis (see Chap. 141).

SSPE occurs in patients between the ages of 4 and 20; 80 percent are under 11. The disease affects boys 3 to 10 times as frequently as girls. Mean annual incidence rates have fallen rapidly in the last two decades; the drop in incidence roughly parallels the decline in the number of measles cases diagnosed since the introduction of live attenuated measles vaccine. Most patients are from rural areas or small towns. Characteristically, they are entirely well until the disease begins. The onset of usually insidious mental deterioration, often expressed by a decline in the patient's schoolwork, is the presenting symptom. Incoordination, ataxia, and myoclonic jerks develop within a few months along with abnormalities of the pyramidal and extrapyramidal motor systems. Cortical blindness, papilledema, and optic atrophy may be present; focal chorioretinitis has been described. A few cases have occurred in association with infectious mononucleosis.

The patient becomes bedridden within 6 to 9 months. Death results from superimposed pulmonary or urinary tract infections or from decubiti. Signs of meningeal irritation are absent. The differential diagnosis includes cerebral storage diseases, nonstorage poliodystrophies, leukodystrophies, and demyelinating diseases of childhood.

The CSF gamma-globulin level, as determined by electrophoresis, quantitative immunochemical assay, or colloidal gold curve, is elevated, but the fluid is otherwise normal. The EEG typically shows a "burst suppression" pattern characterized by synchronous and symmetrical spike and high-voltage slow wave activity followed by electrical inactivity. Elevated levels of measles antibody are found in the serum and CSF. CT scan abnormalities correlate with the stage and duration of the disease. They include lateral ventricular dilatation, cortical atrophy, low parenchymal attenuation, and brainstem and cerebellar atrophy.

Pathologic findings include lymphocyte and mononuclear infiltrations about small cerebral arteries and veins, intranuclear and intracytoplasmic inclusions in neurons and glial cells, and varying degrees of destruction of medullated nerve fibers. The lesions occur in the cerebral gray and white matter, brainstem, and cerebellum.

Measles virus is the etiologic agent. Electron-microscopic studies show that the intranuclear inclusions in brain cells are composed of hollow tubular filaments resembling the internal nucleocapsid component of a paramyxovirus. Staining of brain tissue from patients with the disease demonstrates measles virus antigen in the inclusions. An agent serologically identical with measles virus and having the properties of measles virus has been recovered from brain by cocultivating cell cultures originating from brain tissue with established laboratory cell lines.

Attempts to transmit the disease to animals have met with variable results. Ferrets inoculated with suspensions of brain from patients with the disease develop a nonfatal neurologic disorder with EEG changes.

There is evidence that SSPE patients have clinical measles at an unusually early age, but SSPE appears many years after the patient's initial rubeola infection. A few reported cases may have been related to measles vaccination. The risk of SSPE following measles vaccination is far less, however, than the risk of encephalitis or SSPE following natural measles.

SSPE patients lack antibody to one of the measles virus proteins (the M or matrix protein) despite high titers of antibodies to the other viral proteins. Extracts of SSPE-infected brain lack significant quantities of M antigen. The M protein is a nonglycosylated protein localized to the inner surface of the viral membrane; it is important in the assembly of the virus particle at the cell surface. SSPE brain cells do not appear capable of synthesizing the M protein even in normal amounts. The molecular reasons for the absence of M polypeptide in terminal SSPE may involve decreased transcription and translation of M messenger RNA.

Isoprinosine has been reported by some to affect the course of the disease favorably in an open therapeutic trial, but there is controversy about its effectiveness. The drug has not been approved by the Food and Drug Administration. Other forms of treatment (including interferon and plasmapheresis) have been ineffective.

PROGRESSIVE MULTIFOCAL LEUKOENCEPHALOPATHY (PML) This rare neurologic condition usually occurs in patients who have leukemia, malignant lymphoma, carcinomatosis, acquired immunodeficiency syndrome (AIDS), or a variety of other chronic disease processes, or who are involved with immunosuppressive therapy. The disease is consistently associated with disorders of cell-mediated immunity with which deficits in humoral antibody response may or may not coexist.

The disease affects adults of both sexes, and its duration from onset of symptoms to death is 1 to 6 or more months. The neurologic signs and symptoms reflect a diffuse, asymmetric involvement of the cerebral hemispheres. Hemiplegia, hemianopsia, aphasia or dysarthria, and organic mental changes are frequent; visual field abnormalities and complete or incomplete transverse myelitis may develop. Headache and convulsive seizures are rare, but EEG abnormalities consisting of diffuse or focal abnormalities are often present. Lesions in the white matter may be recognized on CT scans. MRI is helpful in demonstrating white matter destruction. CSF is normal. Specific diagnosis can be made by brain biopsy.

The pathologic changes consist of multiple areas of demyelination with little or no perivascular infiltration and abnormal mitotic figures in astrocytes. The presence of distinctive intranuclear inclusions in oligodendrocytes first suggested that the disease was of a viral etiology. Electron-microscopic observations show the intranuclear inclusion bodies to be composed of closely packed spheres, which have the physical dimensions and properties of the polyomavirus genus of the papovaviruses.

By employing tissue cultures derived from human fetal brain, it has been possible to recover a new human polyomavirus serotype (JC virus) from the brains of PML patients. Abundant virus particles are present in brain. Rapid identification of the virus in brain is possible using fluorescent antibody staining or electron-microscopic agglutination with monospecific hyperimmune rabbit serum. Serologic diagnosis using the patient's serum is unreliable. The virus has not been demonstrated in tissues other than brain; the disease has not been transmitted to animals. There are isolated reports of clinical remission with cytarabine hydrochloride, but no cures. Death usually occurs within 6 months of onset.

PML may result from the activation of a polyomavirus which has been latent in brain or other tissues since childhood infection. Alternatively, there may be certain individuals who fail to acquire immunity in childhood and have their first encounter with the virus when a disease that interferes with cell-mediated immunity develops.

PROGRESSIVE RUBELLA ENCEPHALITIS A chronic progressive encephalitis developing in boys with the typical stigmata of the congenital rubella syndrome (Chap. 142) and sharing some of the features of SSPE was first described in 1974. Fewer than 20 patients have been reported.

The illness begins in the second decade and is characterized by dementia, cerebellar ataxia, spasticity, and seizures. The CSF has an increased cell count, and the protein and IgG levels are elevated. High titers of antibody to rubella virus can be detected in both the serum and CSF. Rubella virus has been recovered from the brain by use of the cocultivation technique.

Unlike SSPE, patients with rubella panencephalitis have the stigmata of congenital rubella before the onset of progressive disease. Myoclonus is less constant, and the EEG does not show the burst suppression observed in SSPE. Histologic examination of the brain shows mineralization of old lesions and an inflammatory reaction, but not the inclusion bodies characteristically found in SSPE.

The clinical picture of progressive rubella encephalitis also resembles the rare case of juvenile paresis that may occur in patients with congenital syphilis. The immune status of patients with rubella encephalitis has not been fully defined, and the pathogenesis of the disease remains obscure.

TROPICAL SPASTIC PARAPARESIS (TSP) This slowly progressive disorder of the spinal cord has been described in patients living in circumscribed regions located in equatorial latitudes. It appears to be caused by infection with the human retrovirus, HTLV-I, an agent that is transmitted by sexual contact, from mother to fetus, by intravenous drug abuse, and by blood transfusion. HTLV-I virus is also the etiologic agent of adult T-cell leukemia. Foci of the disease have been encountered in the Caribbean, South India, South Africa, the Seychelles, and Colombia. A similar disease known as HTLV-I–associated myelopathy (HAM) has been reported in Japanese patients. The disease affects about 10 to 100 persons per 100,000 in a tropical HTLV-I endemic area. TSP afflicts both men and women in their middle age. The disease is slow in onset, chronically progressive, and characterized by a spastic weakness of both legs with pyramidal tract signs as well as bilateral symmetric loss of vibratory sensation distally in the feet. Achilles tendon reflexes are absent in about one-fourth of patients. There is no pleocytosis in the CSF, but the protein content is increased. Increased levels of CSF gamma globulin and oligoclonal bands are often detected.

Pathologic changes are observed in the lateral and anterior columns of the spinal cord where there is loss of myelin and axons. Perivascular and parenchymal infiltration with lymphocytes and macrophages, as well as astrocytosis, are found in the white and gray matter of the spinal cord. Lymphocytes also infiltrate the spinal cord's blood vessels and subarachnoid space.

Antibodies to HTLV-I have been demonstrated in sera and CSF from patients with TSP and HAM. Cultured peripheral blood lymphocytes from TSP patients form multinucleated giant cells and react with sera and monoclonal antibodies to HTLV-I. An HTLV-I-like virus has been isolated from T-cell lines derived from peripheral blood and CSF of TSP patients

PERSISTENT VIRAL DISEASE IN IMMUNODEFICIENT PATIENTS Persistent or chronic neurologic infections of the nervous system may occur in immunodeficient patients. The immunodeficiency state may be congenital (primary) or acquired. Enteroviruses may be recovered from the CSF of patients with primary agammaglobulinemia over a period of many years, during which time there is a persistent CSF pleocytosis. A chronic or subacute encephalitis has also been described in children with congenital hypogammaglobulinemia. A specific virus has not been associated with this disorder.

NEUROLOGIC CONDITIONS RELATED TO INFECTION WITH HUMAN IMMUNODEFICIENCY VIRUS (HIV-1) Involvement of the nervous system by HIV-1 produces complex clinical findings resulting from a primary neurotropic disorder as well as the immunologic compromise that permits other viruses to replicate in and damage nerve tissue.

The immunocompromised patient with AIDS is susceptible to a variety of infectious agents that can attack the CNS. The most common viral agents that assert themselves belong to the HSV and papovavirus groups, i.e., viruses that may remain latent until there is dysfunction of normal immunologic processes. The most commonly isolated viruses from these groups include HSV, CMV, and the PML agent (JC virus). Infection with these viruses in the patient with AIDS can produce a variety of neurologic conditions—most notably atypical aseptic meningitis, acute or subacute encephalitis, PML, and viral myelitis. In addition to viral encephalitis and PML, the patient with AIDS may also develop toxoplasma brain abscess and primary CNS lymphomas. Differentiation from PML is often difficult solely on the basis of CT, MRI, and other laboratory tests. Because treatment for these conditions varies, it may be necessary to perform a brain biopsy and obtain a specimen of the cerebral lesion to make the correct diagnosis.

Neurologic disease may be the only clinical manifestation of HIV infection. It can be expressed as subacute dementia, aseptic meningitis, peripheral neuropathy, or vacuolar myelopathy. Subacute encephalitis is the most frequent cause of neurologic abnormality in AIDS patients. Because of the terminal nature of overt CNS infection in patients with AIDS, brain biopsy is usually reserved for patients who have failed empiric treatment for toxoplasmosis and in whom the possibility of reversible disease exists.

There is evidence that HIV-1 replicates in brain, probably in macrophages. HIV-1 has been recovered from CSF, brain, spinal cord, and sural nerve, suggesting that the AIDS dementia, myelopathy, and peripheral neuropathy may be caused by infection with the retrovirus.

AIDS dementia is insidious in onset and progresses gradually. The early manifestations include an inability to recall, loss of capacity to concentrate, and difficulty in performing complex sequential tasks. There is slowing of verbal and motor responses; spontaneity and animation are reduced. The condition may be difficult to differentiate from depression. As the disease advances, there may be gait unsteadiness, leg weakness, impaired handwriting, and tremor. In the advanced stage, there is global cognitive impairment and pronounced psychomotor slowing. Initially, CT and MRI scans appear normal. As the disease progresses, cortical atrophy and enlargement of the ventricles may become prominent. The MRI scan may disclose only atrophy, but hyperintense abnormalities may be visualized in the central white matter of some patients with AIDS-associated dementia. The CSF may contain mononuclear cells and have mildly elevated protein content.

The brains of patients with AIDS demonstrate moderate to marked cerebral atrophy and histologic changes involving the white matter and subcortical structures; the cortical gray matter is largely spared. The microscopic findings include multifocal perivascular rarefaction and focal vacuolation of the white matter with perivascular and parenchymal collections of macrophages and multinucleated giant cells. Neuronal loss is present only in the most severe cases.

Clinical trials, some still in progress, suggest that zidovudine (formerly AZT) improves functional status in some patients with AIDS dementia.

KURU Kuru, or "trembling with fear," is a progressive and fatal neurologic disorder that occurs exclusively among natives of the New Guinea highland. The disease is rare and seems to be disappearing; its elucidation represented a major hallmark in microbiology.

Difficulty in walking is usually the first sign of kuru. This usually progresses from a minor disturbance in gait to marked ataxia with lurching and staggering. Eventually, ambulation becomes so incoordinated that patients are unable to walk independently or to use their limbs because of intention tremor. Patients display an inability to perform rapid alternating movements, hypotonia, and abnormal involuntary movements which take the form of myoclonus, athetosis, or chorea. Slurring of speech and convergent strabismus appear as the disease progresses. There are no abnormalities in the blood or CSF. Dementia develops in the later phases of the disease. The illness terminates fatally in 4 to 24 months, usually from decubitus ulcers or bronchopneumonia. Kuru was common in male and female children and in adult women, but rare in adult men. The incubation period may be longer than 20 years in older patients.

Pathologic changes are limited to the CNS and include widespread neuronal loss, intense astrocytosis and microglial proliferation, loss of myelinated fibers, and the presence of plaquelike bodies. Perivascular cuffing by lymphocytes and mononuclear cells is rarely present.

It was the close similarity between the neuropathologic and clinical findings found in kuru and in scrapie that suggested the possibility that kuru might be caused by a virus or some closely related infectious agent. The infectious origin of kuru was confirmed subsequently by the transfer of a kurulike syndrome in chimpanzees 10 to 82 months after intracerebral inoculation of suspensions of brain from human cases. Disease has also been produced in chimpanzees by inoculation of tissues other than brain. The clinical illness in chimpanzees appears 3 to 11 months after inoculation. The disease has also been successfully transmitted to a number of new world and old world monkeys as well as to other animals. The specific agent responsible for the disease has not been fully characterized.

Cannibalism is the probable mode of transmission of kuru. Native custom in New Guinea dictated that bone marrow, viscera, and brain be cooked and eaten. The agent may be introduced by conjunctival, nasal, or skin contamination during the practice of ritual cannibalism. The marked predilection of kuru for the adult female may be explained by the observation that cannibalism appears more prevalent among women and that males who practice cannibalism seldom eat the bodies of women. The recent influx of foreign settlers into the kuru area has led to increasing rejection of cannibalistic practices and this in turn may be responsible for the progressive decline in the number of cases of kuru since 1960.

CREUTZFELDT-JAKOB DISEASE (CJD) CJD is an invariably fatal degenerative disease of the CNS that usually afflicts persons between the ages of 50 to 75 years and presents as a rapidly evolving dementia with myoclonus. Unlike kuru, the disease is not geographically limited and has been reported from over 50 countries around the world. The annual incidence is about one case per million inhabitants in metropolitan areas. The majority of cases occur between the ages of 50 and 75, but patients as young as 16 and as old as 80 have been reported.

Although CJD may have diverse clinical presentations, it usually begins with gradually progressive mental deterioration in the form of memory loss, mood changes, and errors in judgment. Disturbances

of stance, gait, motor control, visual disturbances, and dizziness and vertigo may be prominent in the early stages of the disease. Some patients complain of headache. The patient may experience distortions in the shape and appearance of objects. Higher cortical function deficits, such as aphasia or apraxia, may occur. Hallucinations, delusional ideas, and confusion may appear as the disease progresses. In certain patients, cerebellar signs and visual abnormalities may predominate and may be confused initially with cerebrovascular insufficiency. As the condition worsens, the patient becomes mute, stuporous, spastic, and rigid. Myoclonic jerks and other abnormal movements become more prominent as the disease progresses. Visual deterioration may advance to cortical blindness. Disturbances of oculomotor control and of the autonomic nervous system have been noted.

The disease progresses rapidly. The majority of patients die within 6 months, most often 2 to 3 months after the onset of their disease. About 5 to 10 percent of cases will have an illness lasting 2 years or more.

Only rarely has a second member of a family been affected. Fifteen percent of CJD patients have a family history of the disease consistent with an autosomal dominant transmission; the onset of the illness in familial cases is earlier than in sporadic cases. A family history of presenile dementia can be obtained in about 10 percent of CJD patients.

The EEG is often helpful in making the correct diagnosis. During the early stages, it may only show mild, excessive generalized slowing more marked over one hemisphere or even focal. As the disease progresses, distinctive repetitive sharp waves with a characteristic interval of 0.5 to 1.0 s are seen. The sharp waves may first be unilateral, resembling periodic lateralized epileptiform discharges (PLEDS), but eventually they become bilateral and synchronous. In the final stages of the disease, all background EEG activity becomes progressively slower and of lower amplitude, sometimes with the persistence of periodic complexes. Repetitive sharp waves are also occasionally seen in the EEGs of patients with dementia due to other illnesses such as Alzheimer's disease or Binswanger's subcortical encephalopathy, but not with the regular rate found in CJD patients. Serial EEG tracings are helpful in questionable cases.

A CT scan of the brain is usually normal, but sulcal widening, ventricular enlargement, and moderate cortical atrophy may be visualized. Rapid progressive atrophic changes on serial CT scans may suggest the diagnosis. MRI scanning may demonstrate bilateral cortical atrophy without apparent white matter changes. Positron emission tomography (PET) has demonstrated temporal lobe hypometabolism with hemispheric asymmetry. The CSF is usually normal except for a slight elevation in the protein content. No immunologic response, either humoral or cellular, to the CJD agent has been demonstrated in the blood.

The cerebrum and cerebellum are affected predominantly. The brain may show cerebral atrophy. Microscopic examination demonstrates widespread status spongiosus, nerve cell loss, and intensive gliosis. Vacuoles are located within the neuropil, i.e., within axons, dendrites, and glial fibers. There is no inflammatory reaction.

Electron-microscopic observations in CJD have disclosed membrane fragments in vacuoles. Abnormal fibrils similar in appearance to the scrapie-associated fibrils (SAF) have been observed in CJD brain fractions. The exact composition of these fibrils is unclear. CJD brains have been shown to contain protease-resistant proteins (PrP^{CJD}) with molecular weights ranging from 10,000 to 50,000. These CJD proteins reacted with antibodies raised against the scrapie PrP 27-30. Immunologic identification by western blots provides a diagnostic adjunct to neuropathologic examination and animal transmission experiments. Protein polymers in CJD brain aggregate to form plaques with the staining properties of amyloid; these amyloid collections can be stained by antiserum to hamster scrapie PrP 27-30. The SAF and PrPs present in CJD brain resemble those observed in other naturally occurring and experimentally induced spongiform encephalopathies of humans and other animals. It is uncertain if they represent a form of the infectious agent or modified pathologic products.

Sixty percent of patients with kuru and CJD demonstrate an autoimmune antibody directed against 10-nm neurofilaments. The antibody usually appears late in the disease. It can occasionally be found in normal subjects. The significance of this antibody is unclear.

CJD may be mistaken for Alzheimer's disease with myoclonus. In this situation, the presence of cerebellar signs provides strong evidence against the possibility of Alzheimer's disease. At times, CJD can be confused with multi-infarct dementia, alcoholic or nutritional deficiency syndromes, or primary brain tumors. The hallmarks of the disorder (mental deterioration, multisystem neurologic signs, myoclonus, and typical EEG changes) evolving over a period of months in a middle-aged patient usually secures the diagnosis.

The CJD agent has been found in lymph nodes, liver, kidney, spleen, lung, cornea, and CSF of patients with the disorder. The way the disease is acquired naturally is unknown. Incubation periods as long as 20 years may occur in natural transmission. The higher incidence of CJD among Israelis of Libyan origin who eat sheep's eyeballs has led to speculation that the disease may be naturally transmitted by the ingestion of scrapie-infected meat. There is an unexpectedly high incidence of previous brain or eye operations among CJD patients. Human-to-human transmission has occurred by corneal transplantation, by the implantation of contaminated stereotactic electroencephalographic electrodes, by cadaveric dura mater graft, and by the parenteral administration of growth hormone prepared from cadaveric human pituitary glands. Transmission of CJD has not been linked to blood transfusion.

There is no evidence of an increased risk among spouses, friends, and medical or nursing personnel caring for CJD patients. The patient's CSF and blood should be considered, however, as potential sources of infection. Precautions should be taken to avoid autoinoculation with needles, scalpels, or other instruments that have been contaminated by the patient's tissues. Maximum care should be taken to avoid accidental percutaneous exposure to blood, CSF, or tissue. Contaminated skin can be disinfected by a 5- to 10-min exposure to 1 N sodium hydroxide followed by extensive washing with water. Contaminated material should be steam-autoclaved for 1 h at a temperature of at least 132°C or immersed for 1 h in 1 N sodium hydroxide or a 10% sodium hypochlorite solution. More detailed guidelines for the handling of materials from patients with these disorders have been developed by the Centers for Disease Control. These should be applied to all patients who have evidence of rapid intellectual deterioration, particularly when it is associated with myoclonus.

There is no effective treatment for CJD. Claims that amantadine hydrochloride is effective have not been substantiated.

GERSTMANN-STRÄUSSLER-SCHEINKER (GSS) DISEASE
GSS disease is an inherited autosomal dominant illness characterized by spinocerebellar ataxia with dementia and plaquelike deposits of amyloid in the brain. Inoculation of brain tissue from GSS disease produces spongiform encephalopathy in nonhuman primates. PrP and PrP-immunoreactive amyloid plaques accumulate in the brains of these patients. The putative gene for the syndrome is linked to the PrP gene, codon 102, on the short arm of chromosome 20. A substitution of leucine for proline at this codon may lead to the development of the GSS disease. The usual onset of the disease is in the fifth decade. GSS disease follows a lengthy course, usually on the order of 2 to 10 years. Ataxia is prominent in the early phase of the illness; dementia follows later. The patient's symptoms and signs are reminiscent of olivopontocerebellar atrophy. Pathologic changes include spinocerebellar and corticospinal tract degeneration, extensive amyloid deposits, and spongiform degeneration. Like other human spongiform encephalopathies, there is no effective treatment for GSS disease.

There have been isolated reports that brain tissues for a restricted number of patients with familial Alzheimer's disease induced neu-

rologic disease and spongiform changes in chimpanzees. Numerous other transmission attempts from patients with both familial and nonfamilial Alzheimer's disease have been negative. At present, there is no direct evidence to indicate that Alzheimer's disease is caused by a slow virus.

REFERENCES

BERGER JR et al: Progressive multifocal leukoencephalopathy associated with human immunodeficiency virus infection. A review of the literature with a report of sixteen cases. Ann Intern Med 107:78, 1987
BOCKMAN JM et al: Creutzfeldt-Jakob disease prion proteins in human brains. N Engl J Med 312:73, 1985
BROWN P: Acute viral encephalitis, in Current Diagnosis 7, RB Conn (ed). Philadelphia, Saunders, 1985, p 918
——— et al: The epidemiology of Creutzfeldt-Jakob disease: Conclusion of a 15-year investigation in France and review of the world literature. Neurology 37:895, 1987
DYKEN PR: Subacute sclerosing panencephalitis. Current status. Neurol Clin 3:179, 1985
GABUZDA DH, HIRSCH MS: Neurologic manifestations of infection with human immunodeficiency virus: Clinical features and pathogenesis. Ann Intern Med 107:383, 1987
GAJDUSEK DC: Unconventional viruses and the origin and disappearance of kuru. Science 197:943, 1977
GRIFFITH JF, CH'IEN LT: Herpes simplex virus encephalitis. Diagnostic and treatment considerations. Ann Neurol Med 67:991, 1983
HO DD, HIRSCH MS: Acute viral encephalitis. Med Clin North Am 69:415, 1985
HUDSON AJ et al: Gerstmann-Sträussler-Scheinker disease with coincidental familiar onset. Ann Neurol 14:670, 1983
JOHNSON RT: The pathogenesis of acute viral encephalitis and postinfectious encephalomyelitis. J Infect Dis 155:359, 1987
PRUSINER SB: Scrapie prions. Ann Rev Microbiol 43:345, 1989
RATZAN KR: Viral meningitis. Med Clin North Am 69:399, 1985
ROMAN GC, ROMAN LN: Tropical spastic paraparesis. A clinical study of 50 patients from Tumaco (Colombia) and review of the worldwide features of the syndrome. J Neurol Sci 87:121, 1988
ROSENBERG RN et al: Precautions in handling tissues, fluids, and other contaminated materials from patients with documented or suspected Creutzfeldt-Jakob disease. Ann Neurol 19:75, 1986
WALKER DL: Progressive multifocal leukoencephalopathy, in Handbook of Clinical Neurology, JC Koetsier (ed). Amsterdam, Elsevier Science Publishers 1985, vol 3(47), p 503
WEIL ML et al: Chronic progressive panencephalitis due to rubella virus simulating subacute sclerosing panencephalitis. N Engl J Med 292:994, 1975
WHITLEY RJ et al: Vidarabine versus acyclovir therapy in herpes simplex encephalitis. N Engl J Med 314:144, 1986

356 DEMYELINATING DISEASES

JACK P. ANTEL / BARRY G. W. ARNASON

The demyelinating diseases comprise a group of neurologic disorders important both because of the frequency with which they occur and the disability that they cause. Demyelinating diseases have in common the pathologic feature of focal or patchy destruction of myelin sheaths in the central nervous system accompanied by an inflammatory response. Some degree of axonal damage may occur as well, but demyelination always predominates. Multiple sclerosis is the most common of the demyelinating diseases. Its cause is not known. Current opinion holds that autoimmunity, perhaps induced by viral infection, is likely to be implicated in its pathogenesis. Acute disseminated encephalomyelitis and its hyperacute variant, acute hemorrhagic leukoencephalitis, are acute and monophasic immune-mediated demyelinating diseases. HTLV-I–associated myelopathy provides an example of a virus-initiated chronic demyelinating disease.

Myelin loss occurs in other conditions as well, but in these others an inflammatory response is lacking. Included are genetically determined defects in myelin metabolism, exposure to toxins such as carbon monoxide, and opportunistic viral infection of oligodendrocytes (e.g., progressive multifocal leukoencephalopathy) against a background of immune incompetence. These entities, which are usually not classified as demyelinating diseases, are discussed in Chaps. 355 and 359.

MULTIPLE SCLEROSIS

This disease usually presents in the form of recurrent attacks of focal or multifocal neurologic dysfunction, reflecting lesions within the central nervous system (CNS). Attacks occur, remit, and recur, seemingly randomly over many years. The disease begins most commonly in early adult life. The frequency of flare-ups is greatest during the first 3 to 4 years of disease, but a first attack, which may have been so mild as to escape medical attention and can barely be recalled, may not be followed by another attack for 10 to 20 years. During typical episodes, symptoms worsen over a period of a few days to 2 to 3 weeks and then remit. Recovery is usually rapid over a period of weeks, although at times it may extend over several months. The extent of recovery varies markedly between patients and from one attack to the next in the same person. Remission may be complete, particularly after early attacks; often, however, remission is incomplete and as one attack follows another, a stepwise downward progression ensues with increasing permanent deficit.

In perhaps as many as one-third of cases the disease declares itself as a slowly but inexorably progressive illness. This is particularly likely to be the case if onset is after age 40. Although occasional patients die within the first few years of disease onset, most do not, and the average survival from multiple sclerosis (MS) is better than 30 years after onset of disease.

Multiple sclerosis is pleomorphic in its presentations. The clinical picture is determined by the location of foci of demyelination within the CNS. Classic features include impaired vision, nystagmus, dysarthria, decreased perception of vibration and position sense, ataxia and intention tremor, weakness or paralysis of one or more limbs, spasticity, and bladder problems.

Criteria which must be satisfied to establish a diagnosis of clinically definite MS include a reliable history of at least two episodes of neurologic deficit and objective clinical signs of lesions at more than one site within the CNS. Demonstration of additional lesions by laboratory tests [e.g., evoked potentials, urologic studies, computed tomography, or, most sensitively, magnetic resonance imaging (MRI)], in concert with one objective clinical lesion, also fulfills the criteria. A finding of increased cerebrospinal fluid immunoglobulin with oligoclonal bands supports the diagnosis but will not substitute for the above criteria. Clinically probable MS is defined as either two attacks with clinical evidence of one lesion or one attack with clinical evidence of two lesions (or one clinical and one paraclinical lesion). Follow-up studies of probable MS patients indicate considerable diagnostic imprecision in this category. When signs pointing to damage of white matter tracts in optic nerves, brainstem, and spinal cord are present together and more than one attack is known to have occurred, a diagnosis of multiple sclerosis can be made with greater than 95 percent certainty. In the early years of the disease, when few relapses have occurred and fixed deficits are mild, the diagnosis may prove difficult, and single or multiple focal lesions due to other causes must be excluded.

PATHOLOGY Many scattered, discrete areas of demyelination, termed *plaques*, are the pathologic hallmark of multiple sclerosis. Macroscopically, plaques appear as gray-pink sharply defined areas which stand out against the surrounding white matter of the central nervous system. Lesions may extend into gray matter, although nerve cell bodies are seen to be preserved on microscopic examination. Plaques vary in size from a few millimeters to several centimeters; larger ones form by coalescence of smaller ones and by expansion of their margins. Plaques may be found anywhere in the white matter but typically occur in the paraventricular areas of the cerebrum and subpially, and within the brainstem and spinal cord. Their topography conforms to that of the venous drainage of the brain and spinal cord, and no particular anatomic structures are respected. The peripheral nervous system is not affected. The number of plaques found at autopsy invariably exceeds the number expected on the basis of physical signs. Many plaques, therefore, are clinically silent; this establishes that substantial impulse conduction occurs across regions of demyelination. In fact, autopsy studies indicate that 20 percent of multiple sclerosis cases are clinically silent during life.

The microscopic features of multiple sclerosis lesions depend on their age. Typically lesions of different ages and evidence of new activity about the margins of old lesions are encountered. Active multiple sclerosis lesions feature T-lymphocyte and monocyte-macrophage accumulations about venules and at plaque margins where myelin is being destroyed. The inflammatory cells that invade the white matter and the soluble mediators that they release (lymphokines and monokines) are held responsible for the myelin breakdown. Macrophages also function as scavengers of myelin debris; fat-laden macrophages may persist for months, perhaps for years, after the acute inflammatory response has subsided. Plasma cells accumulate within plaques and are usually found at or near their centers.

An astroglial response at or just beyond the margins of acutely demyelinating lesions is characteristic. In established, inactive plaques, a thick mat of fibrillary gliosis throughout the demyelinated regions is usual, and only a few residual perivascular macrophages are found. Oligodendrocyte number has been said to be normal or increased at the plaque margin. Yet, oligodendrocyte number is reduced within plaques, indicating that ultimately, this cell type is lost in multiple sclerosis. Indeed, damage to oligodendrocytes may be the primary event.

Only limited regeneration of myelin occurs in multiple sclerosis (shadow plaques). Absent remyelination, mechanisms responsible for recovery from an MS attack along segmentally demyelinated axons are likely multiple. Resolution of edema, as documented by MRI or CT scan, may permit return of saltatory conduction along segmentally demyelinated axons. Restoration of conduction may also relate, in part, to insertion of K^+ channels along the length of denuded axonal segments rather than exclusively at the nodes of Ranvier as is the situation in myelinated nerve.

Axons within plaques tend to be spared, although in acute lesions frank necrosis with loss of axons sometimes occurs. At least 10 percent of multiple sclerosis plaques show marked axonal loss, and ultrastructural studies indicate that loss of axons may be more general than can be appreciated by routine histology. All gradations of pathologic change between the extremes described above are encountered.

The pathologic features of MS fail to account for the hour-to-hour and day-to-day waxings and wanings in function so characteristic of the disease. Conduction of impulses through demyelinated nerve is compromised and is further altered by transient changes in the internal milieu such as alterations in temperature and in electrolyte balance or by stress. Fever, or even minor increases in body temperature, such as may follow a hot bath or exercise, may cause a failure of conduction through demyelinated regions and lead to evanescent symptoms and signs. The mechanism of this axonal fatigability is unknown, but some type of conduction block is assumed to occur. It is important to distinguish transient fluctuations in symptomatology of the type just described from attacks of disease.

ETIOLOGY The cause or causes of MS remain unknown. A role for immune-mediated or infectious factors has been proposed, but data to support these postulates are fragmentary and indirect. Isolation of HTLV-I–related viral components from CNS tissue in patients with MS is reported, but the etiologic significance of these findings remains uncertain (see Waksman).

Epidemiology Epidemiologic studies have established several facts which will ultimately have to be incorporated into any coherent theory of the disease. Average age of onset of the first clinical episode of MS falls within the third and fourth decades. Females account for 60 percent of cases. For disease to begin in childhood or beyond the sixth decade is uncommon but not unknown.

In general, incidence in temperate climatic zones exceeds that in tropical zones; but variations within regions with similar climates do exist; hence the effect is not simply one of latitude or temperature. The incidence of MS in northern Europe, Canada, and the northern United States is approximately 10 new cases each year per 100,000 persons between the ages of 20 and 50. The incidence in Australia, New Zealand, and the southern United States is one-third to one-half of that; in Japan, elsewhere in the Orient, and in Africa MS is rare. Some epidemiologic evidence also suggests that persons migrating from high- to low-risk regions as children may be partially protected from MS. The data are consistent with the existence of an environmental factor, possibly a virus, and perhaps geographically restricted, that influences development of MS.

Genetic factors   The incidence of MS among American Indians and blacks is lower than that among whites living in the same regions. This suggests that genetic factors also influence disease susceptibility. Blood relatives of MS patients (children, siblings) have an at least fifteenfold increased risk of developing MS. This could reflect an interplay of several genetic factors, shared exposure to an environmental factor, or a combination of the two. Concordance for MS between identical twins (25 percent) is markedly greater than for fraternal twins (2 to 3 percent). Family studies have failed to reveal any predictable genetic pattern but do argue persuasively for a genetically determined predisposition to disease.

Certain histocompatibility antigens (HLA) are overrepresented in patients with MS. Among whites with the disease the HLA-B7, -DR2, and -DQW1 alleles occur with increased frequency. Most illnesses with which an HLA association has been shown are autoimmune or infectious in nature, a finding in keeping with current thought about the etiology of MS. Many American blacks with MS express the DW2 allele; this allele is rare in blacks in Africa, among whom MS is virtually unknown. It follows that an HLA-linked genetic factor which predisposes to MS exists, but inasmuch as the vast majority of persons bearing DR2 or DQW1 do not develop the disease, additional genetic or environmental factors must play a role. Paradoxically, siblings concordant for MS have concordance rates for HLA haplotypes little above those expected by chance. The HLA-B12 allele is less frequent in MS than in the population at large. This finding suggests that genetically determined protective factors may operate in MS.

Autoimmune factors   The lesions of MS are mimicked by those of experimental allergic encephalomyelitis (EAE), an autoimmune disease induced in animals by immunization with myelin. Lesions of EAE are demyelinating, perivenular, plaque-like, occur in chronic and recrudescent forms, and have an inflammatory infiltrate composed of lymphocytes, macrophages, and plasma cells. T lymphocytes sensitized to specific myelin antigens (myelin basic protein or proteolipid protein) can adoptively transfer the disease. In MS, sensitivity to these myelin antigens cannot be demonstrated. Chronic demyelination can be a consequence of viral infection in animals. Demyelination follows infection of mice with Theiler's murine encephalomyelitis virus; infected animals do not exhibit sensitivity to myelin antigens. Attempts to find any antigen to which only MS patients react have failed.

Attacks of MS are associated with changes in peripheral blood monocyte and lymphocyte properties. Reported changes include heightened prostaglandin secretion by macrophages (which may in turn influence lymphocyte properties), reduced suppressor cell function, an increased number of activated T cells as evidenced by their expression of certain surface antigens, heightened T-cell–dependent in vitro immunoglobulin secretion, deficient interferon secretion, and possibly reduced natural killer (NK) cell function. Whether these changes relate to the etiology of MS is not known.

Within the cerebrospinal fluid (CSF), T-cell activation is apparent during active disease. Excessive IgG production within the CNS is characteristic of MS at all stages of disease; whether this reflects the presence of some stimulator of B cells in the brain in MS or is the result of a defect in immune regulation is not known. Viral infection of brain remains a possible cause of MS, despite the fact that all attempts to isolate, rescue, or "passage" a virus from MS brains or to visualize a virus within them have failed.

Precipitating factors   Most attacks of MS occur without any evident antecedent. There is a modestly increased risk for an attack following viral infections. Injury and even emotional upsets have been claimed to precipitate attacks of MS; evidence in support of these claims remains anecdotal and nonpersuasive. The probability that an attack of MS will occur during the first 6 months after pregnancy is greater than chance would predict, but this observation is counterbalanced by a decreased risk of an attack during the second and third trimesters of pregnancy. In established cases, trauma, including lumbar puncture, myelography, and surgery, has not been shown to relate to attacks or to progression of disability nor has emotional turmoil been shown to alter the tempo at which the disease evolves. Experience has also shown that vaccinations do not provoke attacks of MS.

CLINICAL MANIFESTATIONS   The first attack of MS may declare itself as a single symptom or sign (45 percent) or as more than one (55 percent). Approximately 40 percent of MS patients will have an episode of optic neuritis, either as their first difficulty or at some point along the course of their disease. Optic neuritis presents as loss of vision, partial or total, usually in one eye, seldom in both, and is often associated with pain on movement of the eye. Macular vision tends to be most affected (central scotoma), but a wide range of field defects may occur. Disturbances of color perception sometimes provide an early indication of mild disease. Fewer than half of optic neuritis patients will show evidence of an inflamed optic nerve head (papillitis); most show no changes in the optic disc at the outset, indicating that the demyelinating lesion is developing some distance behind the nerve head (retrobulbar neuritis). Both forms of optic neuritis will be followed by optic nerve atrophy, detected as pallor of the optic disc.

It is important to recognize that cases of optic neuritis occur as an isolated event. Nonetheless, 35 percent of men and 75 percent of women with optic neuritis go on to develop MS in the ensuing 15 years. Unfortunately, it is difficult to predict who will and who will not develop the disease, although presence of oligoclonal bands in the CSF and of multifocal cerebral lesions on MRI scanning are seemingly unfavorable findings. Whether optic neuritis occurring alone and for unknown reasons constitutes a *forme fruste* of MS with but a single attack is not known. Approximately one-third of patients with optic neuritis recover completely, one-third partially, and one-third little or not at all. Visual evoked response testing reveals prolonged latencies of the evoked potentials in more than 80 percent of established cases of MS; less than half of these can describe an antecedent optic neuritis. Clearly subclinical involvement of the optic pathways is common.

Symptoms and signs of neurologic dysfunction arising from brainstem, cerebellar, and spinal cord lesions are frequent in MS. Diplopia may occur either because the third, fourth, or sixth cranial nerve pathways are damaged along their course within the CNS or because an internuclear ophthalmoplegia (INO) has developed (see Chap. 23). An INO reflects involvement of the medial longitudinal fasciculus. The sign consists of an inability to adduct one eye on attempted lateral gaze together with full abduction of the other eye, which shows horizontal nystagmus. Bilateral INO in a young adult is virtually diagnostic of MS, although a few instances of bilateral INO in systemic lupus erythematosus are on record. Another clinical feature of brainstem involvement is either facial hypesthesia or tic douloureux (fifth cranial nerve). When tic douloureux occurs in a young adult, the possibility of underlying MS should be seriously entertained. Bell's palsy or hemifacial spasm (seventh cranial nerve), vertigo, vomiting, and nystagmus (vestibular connections of the eighth cranial nerve) are also frequent; less commonly there is complaint of deafness. Involvement of cerebellar connections results in ataxia which can affect speech (scanning), head or trunk (titubation), limbs (intention tremor), and stance and gait. Cerebellar ataxia may be combined with sensory ataxia due to involvement of the spinal cord.

Spinal cord lesions produce a myriad of motor and sensory problems. Corticospinal tract interruption results in the classical features of upper motor neuron dysfunction (weakness, spasticity, hyperreflexia, clonus, Babinski response, loss of abdominal skin reflexes). Posterior column lesions cause loss, or diminution, of joint-position and vibration senses as well as the frequently encountered complaints of tingling or tightness of the extremities and of bandlike sensations about the trunk. Less often pain and temperature sensations are lost or diminished, reflecting spinothalamic tract involvement. Partial lesions of sensory tracts or of the root entry zones of sensory nerves can produce painful dysesthesias as well as interruption of reflex arcs. On occasion, spinal cord lesions will result in paroxysmal symptoms including tonic spasms which can be painful.

Symptoms of bladder dysfunction, including hesitancy, urgency, frequency, and incontinence, are common features of spinal cord involvement. Equally common is bowel dysfunction, particularly constipation. Males with MS, if questioned, often complain of sexual impotence; methods exist to distinguish physical from psychogenic causes. Patients with MS may experience an electric shock-like sensation on flexion of the neck, called Lhermitte's sign.

Severe spinal cord lesions can result in loss of function, sometimes total, below the level of the lesion; less complete lesions can result in the hemicord syndrome of Brown-Séquard (see Chap. 361). When either of these events occurs, it is referred to as a transverse myelitis. A single episode of transverse myelitis not followed by subsequent progression of disease may, as with an isolated episode of optic neuritis, represent a *forme fruste* of MS, although less than 10 percent of acute transverse myelitis cases develop MS. Again as with optic neuritis, approximately one-third of patients with transverse myelitis recover completely, one-third partially, and one-third not at all. Spinal cord involvement is the predominating feature in most advanced cases of MS.

Cerebral symptoms may occur in MS due to extensive involvement of subcortical and central white matter. With extensive lesions of brain, intellect may suffer, sometimes disastrously. By far the most frequent emotional feature of MS is depression. Euphoria, when it occurs, indicates widespread cerebral disease and is often associated with dementia and pseudobulbar palsy. Three to five percent of patients (twice the expected rate) will have one or more epileptic seizures, presumably because of extension of plaques into gray matter. Focal neurologic signs of cerebral origin, such as hemiparesis, homonymous hemianopsia, and dysphasia, while seen in MS, are rare.

Neuromyelitis optica and MS   An ill-defined symptom complex known as Devic's syndrome, or neuromyelitis optica, is considered by some to be an entity distinguishable from MS. The complex is characterized by acute optic neuritis, usually bilateral, which is followed, or less frequently preceded, within hours to weeks by transverse myelitis. The cerebrospinal fluid (CSF) may show a pleocytosis with polymorphonuclear cells and a protein content that is higher than is usual for MS. Pathologic examination in fatal cases reveals more tissue destruction and cavitation than is expected in MS, although this may bespeak no more than the intensity of the process.

COURSE OF ILLNESS AND PROGNOSIS   The clinical course of MS is unpredictable. In general, symptoms which appear acutely and those referable to sensory paths and the cranial nerves have a more favorable prognosis than those developing insidiously or involving motor and especially cerebellar function. According to McAlpine, 80 percent of patients who have a purely exacerbating and remitting disease have unrestricted function after 10 years. Of cases in which exacerbations and remissions are superimposed on a progressive tempo of evolution, 50 percent are disabled after 10 years. In cases that have a purely progressive course from the outset (in these the brunt of the disease usually falls on the spinal cord) long-term prognosis for ambulation is poor.

Rarely MS may be fulminant and fatal within weeks to months. Such cases, which are referred to as acute MS, show intense inflammatory responses within the plaques. Onset in such patients may be with headache, vomiting, delirium, convulsions, even coma, plus an array of signs indicating severe compromise of cortical, brainstem, optic nerve, and spinal cord function. Distinction from acute disseminated encephalomyelitis may be difficult in life; at autopsy the lesions are larger and more like those of MS.

DIFFERENTIAL DIAGNOSIS   The diagnosis of MS becomes secure when signs referable to multiple lesions of CNS white matter have developed and remitted at different times. Particularly in the early phases of disease, the neurologic symptoms may suggest discrete dysfunction of the nervous system, and other causes of focal disease must be excluded. An excellent clinical rule is that MS should not be diagnosed when all the patient's symptoms and signs can be explained by a single lesion. A common aphorism is that MS presents with symptoms in one leg and signs in both.

Conditions to be excluded vary depending on the sites of the lesions. Abrupt monocular loss of vision may result from impaired vascular supply to the optic nerve, including embolic and thrombotic occlusion of the carotid, ophthalmic, or central retinal arteries, or as an accompaniment of migraine. When monocular visual loss is more gradual, compressive lesions affecting the optic nerve or an optic nerve glioma need to be considered.

In patients presenting with acute or progressive spinal cord disease, the presence of focal lesions affecting the cord and of degenerative-nutritional diseases which selectively affect spinal cord tracts should be considered (see Chaps. 357 and 361). Patients with progressive spastic paraplegia should be evaluated for the presence of intrathecal or extradural neoplasm, vascular malformations, and for cervical spondylosis. Such evaluation often requires a CT body scan, MRI, or myelography. Hereditary ataxias can present as degeneration of multiple CNS tracts, with or without involvement of the peripheral nervous system. Degeneration of posterior columns and corticospinal and spinocerebellar tracts is common in these disorders. Hereditary ataxias are slowly progressive and feature stereotyped symmetric involvement as well as a family history consistent with autosomal dominant, or recessive, inheritance. Amyotrophic lateral sclerosis (ALS) usually presents with prominent lower motor neuron signs (atrophy, weakness, and fasciculations) in addition to pyramidal signs (spasticity, hyperreflexia) and without sensory abnormalities. Subacute combined degeneration of the cord can be excluded by symmetry of spinal symptoms and by a normal serum vitamin B_{12} level, a normal bone marrow, and a normal Schilling test.

When progressive brainstem dysfunction occurs, posterior fossa tumor as well as brainstem encephalitis should be excluded. Single cranial nerve palsies, particularly Bell's palsy, trigeminal sensory neuropathy, or tic douloureux may occur as part of the MS picture, but evidence of multifocal disease must be present before they can be ascribed to MS. When vertigo is the complaint and nystagmus is detected, inner ear disease should be considered as well as the possibility that barbiturates or phenytoin have been taken.

There are several multifocal and recrudescent diseases of the central nervous system which may mimic MS. Systemic lupus erythematosus and other vasculitides may cause scattered and recurring lesions within brain, brainstem, and spinal cord, as can the mitochondrial encephalopathies (MELAS syndrome) (see Chap. 365). Behçet's disease is characterized by recurrent episodes of focal brain disease, CSF pleocytosis, oral and genital ulcers, and uveitis. Other disorders to be excluded include meningovascular syphilis, cryptococcosis, toxoplasmosis, other chronic nervous system infections, and sarcoidosis. Lyme disease can present with focal neurologic signs in the absence of antecedent skin lesions, arthralgias, or peripheral neuropathy (see Chap. 132). HTLV-I–induced disorders are described below. AIDS encephalopathy and myelopathy need also to be considered in progressive cases.

When complaints are vague and findings minimal, a diagnosis of conversion reaction (hysteria) may come to mind. This diagnosis should always be made on the basis of positive criteria for hysteria and never as a "diagnosis by exclusion." Early in its course, MS is mislabeled as hysteria with distressing frequency. Patients with MS may develop superimposed hysterical phenomena adding to the complexity of the clinical syndrome.

A few patients present with pain as their principal symptom. Awareness of its occurrence in MS and careful attention to a thorough examination will usually clarify the diagnosis.

A firm diagnosis of MS should only be made when the evidence is unequivocal. Aside from the distress that such a diagnosis causes, it will serve to explain almost any subsequent neurologic event and may divert attention away from other possibly treatable diseases.

LABORATORY TESTS   Although the diagnosis of MS continues to depend on its clinical features, laboratory aids have become increasingly useful as supports for the diagnosis. In the vast majority of patients with MS, one or more tests will be abnormal, although normal results do not rule out the diagnosis.

The CSF in MS patients typically reveals only a slight or no increase in cell number. Ninety percent of patients show fewer than 10 cells per microliter in their CSF; cell counts greater than 50 are rare. The cells in the CSF are predominantly T lymphocytes, although rare plasma cells may be found. Some correlation exists between the extent of pleocytosis and disease activity. Higher cell counts also are more typical in early stages of disease. Evidence that the lymphocytes in the CSF are activated not only during exacerbations of disease but also during seeming remission has been presented; this indicates that disease activity smolders at all times, even though neither the physician nor the patient may be able to detect changes. T-cell lines specifically reactive with various viral and nonviral antigens can be derived from the CSF of MS patients, again suggesting that a heterogeneous immune response is ongoing (see discussion of oligoclonal bands below). The CSF of 90 percent of patients contains less than 60 mg/dL of total protein; protein of greater than 100 mg/dL should raise questions about whether the diagnosis is correct.

The most characteristic CSF finding in MS is an increase in immunoglobulin G (IgG) which contrasts with relatively normal total protein and albumin concentrations. IgG levels are increased in 80 percent of MS patients; the increase is greatest in long-standing cases with severe neurologic deficits. Early in the disease, when the diagnosis is most in doubt, IgG values can be normal. IgG levels do not change in any meaningful way with relapses and remissions. Most of the IgG in the CSF is synthesized within the central nervous system. The increased IgG fraction in the CSF explains the first-zone abnormality of the colloidal gold curve, a test of historical interest.

When the CSF IgG from MS patients is subjected to electrophoresis or isoelectric focusing, it fractionates into a restricted number of bands (termed oligoclonal bands). Oligoclonal banding of IgG has also been found in the CSF in a number of acute and chronic central nervous system infections; in subacute sclerosing panencephalitis cases, these bands have been shown to be antibodies to the infective agent. In MS, the IgG bands have not been shown to be directed against any single viral or intrinsic brain antigen; more likely they represent a heterogeneous group of antibodies directed against many antigens. The number of bands in the CSF is greater in those with longer disease duration. It has also been suggested that high levels of IgG and many oligoclonal bands are associated with a severe course. The overall IgG shows further restrictions in its heterogeneity, with the IgG1 being mainly of the G1m$_1$ allotype. Rare cases of MS without increased CSF IgG synthesis or oligoclonal bands have been documented at autopsy.

Within CSF, myelin debris as well as myelin basic protein fragments appear during attacks of disease. Myelin basic protein levels can be measured by radioimmunoassay; the level seems to reflect the extent of myelin breakdown since levels also increase in other disorders associated with white matter breakdown such as stroke.

Conduction of nerve impulses along axons denuded of their myelin is slowed. Evoked response testing provides a sensitive means to detect slowed conduction of visual, auditory, or somatosensory impulses. Such tests employ repetitive sensory stimuli and utilize computer averaging techniques to record the electric responses evoked during the conduction of these stimuli along visual, auditory, or somatosensory afferent pathways. In normal subjects, the pattern of the evoked responses and time for conduction are highly predictable. One or more of the evoked response tests will reveal slowing of conduction in 80 percent of MS patients; in 30 to 40 percent of patients, abnormal evoked responses are detected without any clinical symptoms or signs in the involved pathway being apparent. Evoked response testing may confirm the presence of additional sites of disease in suspected cases with only a single clinically detectable lesion (see Chap. 349).

Computed tomography (CT) of the brain may reveal low-density lesions within white matter, usually in a paraventricular or subcortical distribution. Enhancement of lesions following intravenous infusion of iodine with delayed scanning indicates the presence of acute lesions with disruption of the blood-brain barrier. Enhancement may disappear as the clinical symptoms resolve. Cortical atrophy with enlarged ventricles is also found in some patients. The incidence of such abnormalities discovered by CT scanning is approximately 25 percent.

MRI is the most sensitive means of detecting lesions of MS. More than 90 percent of patients with clinically definite MS show multifocal cerebral white matter lesions on MRI, better seen with spin-echo (T2-weighted) than with inversion recovery (T1-weighted) images. Serial MRI studies of MS patients with relapsing disease indicate that the frequency of lesion formation, either arising de novo or as an expansion of a preexisting lesion, far exceeds clinical relapse rate. New lesion formation is also observed in progressive MS patients. Lesions typically develop over several weeks and resolve over 2 to 3 months; such resolving lesions likely reflect inflammation and edema rather than demyelination and gliosis. IV administration of gadolinium DTPA can enhance detection of "active" lesions on T1-weighted images (see Chap. 348). MRI lesions suggest that the MS disease process rarely "sleeps." Coalescence of MRI lesions appears to correlate with development of progressive disease. Multifocal cerebral white matter lesions are detected by MRI in 60 to 75 percent of cases of isolated optic neuritis and chronic progressive myelopathy. Technical advances now permit direct detection of inflammatory demyelinating lesions within the optic nerves and spinal cord.

Elevated CSF IgG, abnormal evoked responses, and lesions on CT scans and MRI provide useful adjuncts in evaluation of the patient with suspected MS; however, the clinical findings remain paramount in establishing the diagnosis.

TREATMENT OF MS   No effective treatment for MS is known. Therapeutic efforts are directed toward (1) amelioration of the acute episode, (2) prevention of relapses or progression of disease, and (3) relief of symptoms.

In acute flare-ups of disease, glucocorticoid treatment may lessen the severity of symptoms and speed recovery; however, ultimate recovery is not improved by this drug nor is the extent of permanent disability altered. Glucocorticoids likely act chiefly via mechanisms other than modulation of the immune response. They may improve the ability of demyelinated nerve to conduct and reduce edema and inflammation within plaques. Usual regimens utilize either ACTH, to stimulate endogenous glucocorticoid synthesis, or prednisone. ACTH is preferred by many clinicians since the only controlled trials that demonstrated the efficacy of glucocorticoid therapy in flare-ups of MS and in acute optic neuritis were performed with this drug. ACTH is commonly given in a dose of 80 units daily intravenously for 3 to 7 days, followed by intramuscular injections in periodically decreasing doses over the next 2 to 3 weeks. Prednisone, 15 mg qid, is sometimes given rather than ACTH, again, over 3 to 7 days with gradually tapering doses over the next 2 to 3 weeks. Since prednisone is taken by mouth, the treatment is simpler than with ACTH, and an admission to the hospital may sometimes be avoided. Use of long-term daily or alternate-day steroids is not advised.

Immunosuppressive agents such as azathioprine and cyclophosphamide have been claimed to reduce the number of relapses in several series, but there is no consensus about the efficacy of these drugs. Plasma exchange in combination with immunosuppression, total-lymphoid irradiation, cyclosporine A, α-interferon, β-interferon, or copolymer 1 remains under active investigation. γ-Interferon provokes exacerbations.

Symptomatic treatment should address both the physical and psychological needs of patients. Patients should avoid excess fatigue and extremes of temperature and eat a balanced diet. Diets containing low levels of saturated fats have been advocated. The use of belladonna alkaloids and bethanechol chloride can help bladder dysfunction. Periodic checks for urinary tract infection should be performed. Bowel training can alleviate disorders of bowel function. Drugs available for the treatment of spasticity include diazepam, baclofen, and dantrolene sodium. Painful dysesthesias, facial twitching, tic douloureux, and tonic spasms may respond to carbamazepine or phenytoin. Occasionally trigeminal root injection is required to relieve tic douloureux (see Chap. 360).

ACUTE DISSEMINATED ENCEPHALOMYELITIS

Acute disseminated encephalomyelitis (ADEM) may be defined as a monophasic encephalitis or myelitis of abrupt onset characterized by symptoms and signs indicative of damage chiefly of the white matter of the brain or spinal cord. The process may be severe, and even fatal, or mild and evanescent. Pathologic features are those of innumerable minute foci of perivenular lymphocyte and mononuclear cell infiltration with demyelination. The topography of the demyelination corresponds to that of the inflammatory infiltrates. The condition most commonly follows vaccinations against rabies or smallpox or acute infectious illnesses, especially measles, but may occur without any obvious antecedent. The cause is uncertain but is believed by some to represent a hypersensitivity, perhaps to myelin basic protein, and to be the human counterpart of experimentally induced EAE.

ETIOLOGY The entity has been described after two types of vaccination: after rabies vaccination with the Semple vaccine, which contains brain tissue, now seldom used, and after vaccination against smallpox, now seldom performed.

Shortly after introduction of rabies vaccination by Pasteur, it became evident that neuroparalytic accidents could follow this procedure. After a course of injections a sudden encephalitic or myelitic catastrophe might occur coincident with hypersensitivity-type reactions at the sites of vaccine injection. The process clearly involved hypersensitivity to nervous system antigens. The incidence was variously reported as between 1 in 1000 and 1 in 5000 persons vaccinated. An identical syndrome has followed inoculation with noninfected brain material, indicating that killed rabies virus was not the cause; with the introduction of duck embryo killed rabies virus vaccine (which is free of myelinated nervous tissue), the condition has markedly decreased in incidence, although cases continue to be reported from countries where Semple-type vaccines remain in use. Neuroparalytic accidents were most frequent in young adults, the peak age of occurrence corresponding to that of onset of MS. In some cases cellular immune sensitivity to myelin basic protein has been demonstrated.

Smallpox vaccination was also followed by an incidence of ADEM averaging perhaps 1 case per 5000 persons vaccinated but with marked differences between vaccination programs. The complication almost always occurred in conjunction with a primary take rather than a booster-type response. The encephalitis usually followed the peak of the vaccination response by a few days to a week or more but on occasion preceded it. The complication was unknown in children less than 2 years of age; in infants, smallpox vaccination was sometimes associated with an encephalopathy with brain swelling, i.e., toxic encephalopathy.

One case of measles in 1000 is followed by neurologic complications, which are often severe. The mortality rate averages 20 percent, and half the survivors are left with residual damage. The syndrome usually follows the rash by a few days. It bears no relationship to the severity of measles itself. Systemic lymphocyte sensitivity to myelin basic protein has been demonstrated in some

patients. All attempts to isolate a virus have failed. Abnormal CSF and changes in the electroencephalogram are observed in perhaps half the children who contract measles, suggesting that subclinical neurologic involvement may be much more widespread than is usually appreciated. A subtle decline in performance and changes in behavior following measles may reflect this inapparent nervous system involvement. Measles vaccination has drastically reduced the frequency of this complication.

An identical clinical picture was seen formerly as a complication of smallpox and is still encountered during or following chickenpox and extremely rarely as a complication of rubella. Demyelinating encephalomyelitis is very rare in mumps; instead there is often a true viral meningitis. A clinical picture identical to postinfectious encephalomyelitis has been described after mycoplasma infections. Despite its striking association with measles, the occurrence of the same clinical picture after several different infections fits better with the postulate that the basic process involves hypersensitivity rather than a direct viral infection of the brain and spinal cord.

CLINICAL MANIFESTATIONS The disease usually begins abruptly. Headache and delirium may give way to lethargy and coma. Coma has an ominous prognosis. Seizures at the onset or shortly thereafter are not infrequent. There may be stiffness of the neck, other signs of meningeal irritation, and fever. Focal signs may be engrafted on this picture, and spinal cord involvement with flaccid paralysis of all four limbs is particularly common. Monoparesis and hemiplegia are also seen. Tendon reflexes may be lost initially only to become hyperactive later; extensor plantar responses are the rule, and sphincter control is generally lost. Sensory loss is variable but may be extensive and severe. Brainstem involvement may be reflected by nystagmus, ocular palsies, and pupillary changes. Some cases may present as a purely spinal cord syndrome and in mild instances with minor signs such as a facial palsy. Chorea and athetosis are rare. Cerebellar signs may predominate, particularly in cases associated with chickenpox. Involvement of motor and sensory peripheral nerves can be documented clinically and electromyographically in some patients. The CSF almost always shows an increase in protein (50 to 100 mg/dL) and lymphocytes (10 to several hundred cells); rarely it is normal. The mortality is 20 percent, and perhaps half the survivors have residual deficits. Recurrences are almost unknown.

The diagnosis is not difficult if there is a history of rabies or smallpox vaccination or of measles. In cases without such a history, distinction from viral encephalitis may be difficult and at times not possible. Reye's syndrome may be difficult to distinguish from acute disseminated encephalomyelitis. Vomiting at onset, a normal CSF, hyperammonemia, and raised intracranial pressure should suggest Reye's syndrome; frequent convulsions and focal signs argue against it. A distinction from acute MS may not be possible.

PREVENTION AND TREATMENT Since smallpox has been eradicated, there is no longer reason to vaccinate against it. Use of duck embryo and human diploid vaccine in rabies prophylaxis has almost eliminated neuroparalytic accidents, and measles vaccination has drastically reduced what used to be the largest group of postinfectious encephalomyelitides.

Administration of high doses of glucocorticoids every 4 to 6 h is the treatment of choice though controlled trials have not been carried out.

ACUTE NECROTIZING HEMORRHAGIC ENCEPHALOMYELITIS

Acute necrotizing hemorrhagic encephalomyelitis is a rare tissue-destructive disease of the CNS which occurs with explosive suddenness within a few days of an upper respiratory infection. The pathologic findings are distinctive. On sectioning the brain, much of the white matter of one or both hemispheres is seen to be destroyed almost to the point of liquefaction. The involved tissue is pink or yellowish-gray and flecked with multiple small hemorrhages. Sometimes similar changes are localized to the brainstem or spinal cord. On histologic examination the core lesion resembles that of acute disseminated encephalomyelitis in showing perivenular foci of demyelination, all of like age. As in acute disseminated encephalomyelitis lymphocytes and macrophages are present in the regions of myelin loss, but superimposed on and dominating the picture is an intense polymorphonuclear infiltrate, in keeping with the necrotizing nature of the process. The vessels themselves are partially necrotic; they may contain platelet or fibrin thrombi within their lumens and fibrin deposits beyond their walls. Multiple small hemorrhages at sites of vessel damage are an invariable feature as is a violent inflammatory reaction in the meninges. Large necrotic foci form by coalescence of smaller lesions in the hemispheres, brainstem, or spinal cord.

The clinical course of the illness resembles that of acute disseminated encephalomyelitis save for its apoplectiform onset and rapidity of progress, sometimes leading to death within 48 h. Neurologic signs are frequently unilateral, reflecting disease in one cerebral hemisphere, but may be bilateral. It is probable that certain patients showing an explosive myelitic illness are suffering from a necrotizing myelitis of similar type, but pathologic evidence in support of this view has been difficult to obtain. The CSF examination discloses a more intense reaction than in other demyelinating diseases. Often a polymorphonuclear pleocytosis of up to 2000 cells and a considerable increase in amount of protein are detected. In cases of slower evolution the cell counts are lower and cells are mainly of the mononuclear type.

The etiology of this disease is not established; however, the entire clinical-pathologic entity bears a close resemblance to a hyperacute form of EAE that can be induced in animals by administration of endotoxin, pertussis vaccine, or the vaccine's histamine-sensitizing factor coincident with or shortly after injection of myelin in adjuvant. The lesions in this experimental disease can perhaps be considered as those of a Sanarelli-Shwartzman reaction within the brain superimposed on an acutely demyelinating process. Rarely a lesion like acute necrotizing hemorrhagic encephalomyelitis occurs in MS.

The differential diagnosis of this disorder includes acute encephalitis, particularly those types causing tissue necrosis (herpes simplex, arbovirus), acute bacterial cerebritis, septic embolic occlusion of an artery, thrombophlebitis, and suppurative brain abscess. The similarity of acute necrotizing hemorrhagic encephalomyelitis to acute disseminated encephaloymyelitis suggests that steroid therapy may be beneficial.

HTLV-I–ASSOCIATED MYELOPATHY (HAM)– TROPICAL SPASTIC PARAPARESIS (TSP)

HAM-TSP presents as a syndrome of progressive spasticity of the lower limbs associated with variable amounts of low back pain, bowel and bladder dysfunction, and disrupted superficial and proprioceptive sensations. The illness develops on a background of HTLV-I infection.

PATHOLOGY   The characteristic features are a chronic inflammatory response within the gray and white matter and the meninges, demyelination with relative axonal sparing, proliferation of small blood vessels with perivascular cuffing, and reactive astrocytosis; the above are more marked in the lateral columns of the spinal cord than in the spinothalamic and spinocerebellar tracts. In severe cases, focal spongiosus of tissue is found. Pathologic changes can extend into the brainstem, cerebellum, and cerebrum.

ETIOLOGY   Evidence that HTLV-I is the cause of this syndrome includes presence of serum and CSF anti-HTLV-I antibodies, isolation of HTLV-I from systemic and CSF white blood cells, and detection of viral particles within the CNS by electron microscopy. The fact that the immune response is activated coupled with the apparent response of HAM cases to glucocorticoid therapy argues for an immune component in the pathogenesis of tissue injury.

EPIDEMIOLOGY   HAM describes the progressive myelopathy syndrome endemic to southern Japan, a temperate climate zone; TSP

describes the same etiologic syndrome occurring in tropical regions of the Caribbean, South America, and Africa, affecting mainly, but not exclusively, individuals of black ethnic origin. Peak age of onset of clinical symptoms ranges from 30 to 60 years; childhood onset cases are rare but have been reported from Japan. Females are affected more frequently than males. In endemic areas, prevalence of serum HTLV-I antibodies in the population range from 5 to 20 percent, far exceeding the number of symptomatic individuals. Routes of disease transmission include sexual transmission from male to female, maternal-fetal passage, and blood transfusion. The latency period ranges from 2 years in transfusion cases to many years in maternal-fetal cases. Association of the neurologic syndrome with HTLV-I–induced adult T-cell leukemia is rare. HTLV-I–associated neurologic syndromes have begun to be reported in nonendemic areas.

GENETICS   In Japan, specific HLA-region haplotypes are associated with development of the neurologic syndrome; other haplotypes are associated with leukemia.

CLINICAL FEATURES   Initial symptoms are usually those of leg weakness with or without back pain. Less frequent complaints are leg paresthesias and bladder dysfunction. Clinical findings include spastic lower limbs with hyperreflexia and Babinski reflexes. In 10 to 60 percent of cases posterior column sensations (proprioception, vibration) are impaired, as are superficial sensations, sometimes with a sensory level that is less well defined than in spinal cord compression syndromes. Less frequent signs include upper limb weakness and spasticity, cerebellar dysfunction, and cranial nerve palsies.

CLINICAL COURSE   The progressive myelopathy typically evolves over many years; cases with a more rapid evolution and cases with apparent arrest are also observed.

DIFFERENTIAL DIAGNOSIS   Within endemic areas, other causes of myelopathy must be included. Epidemics of "TSP" are on record; such cases are often associated with optic neuropathy and deafness and may be attributable to toxin exposures, particularly with cyanide-containing cassava, malnutrition, or other infectious agents endemic to specific regions, such as treponema. The syndrome of tropical ataxic neuropathy (TAN), characterized by sensory ataxia and slowed peripheral nerve conduction velocities, is also induced by chronic cyanide intoxication (cassava) combined with dietary deficiency. Cases of MS within the endemic TSP-HAM regions do not demonstrate serologic evidence of HTLV-I infection. The severe HTLV-I cases associated with spongiosus of spinal cord need be distinguished from HIV-associated vacuolar myelopathy.

LABORATORY TESTS   Within the peripheral blood, T-cell ratios are usually normal, although occasional patients show inverted CD4/CD8 ratios. An increased proportion of T cells express activation antigens compared to controls. Some patients, particularly Japanese, have mild cellular responses within the CSF (up to 50 to 100 cells); in such cases, occasional leukemia-like cells may be found. CSF protein is modestly increased in about 50 percent of cases. Increased CSF immunoglobulin with oligoclonal banding is characteristic. In more than 80 percent of suspected cases, HTLV-I antibodies are detectable in serum and CSF. Virus can be isolated from peripheral blood and CSF. Cerebral lesions are observed on MRI in a minority of cases.

THERAPY   Beneficial response to glucocorticoid therapy is claimed in HAM cases; response is less in TSP cases. Viral-directed therapies are under study.

REFERENCES

GONZALEZ-SCARANO F et al: Multiple sclerosis disease activity correlates with gadolinium-enhanced magnetic resonance imaging. Ann Neurol 21:300, 1987

HEMACHUDHA T et al: Myelin basic protein as an encephalotigen in encephalomyelitis and polyneuritis following rabies vaccination. N Engl J Med 316:369, 1987

PATY DW et al: MRI in the diagnosis of MS: A prospective study with comparison of clinical evaluation, evoked potentials, oligoclonal banding, and CT. Neurology 38:180, 1988

POSER CM et al: New diagnostic criteria for multiple sclerosis: Guidelines for research protocols. Ann Neurol 13:227, 1983

RIZZO JF, LESSELL S: Risk of developing multiple sclerosis after uncomplicated optic neuritis: A long-term prospective study. Neurology 38:185, 1988

SEVER JL, GIBBS CJ (eds): *Retroviruses in the Nervous System, Proceedings of a Symposium Sponsored by the National Institutes of Health.* Ann Neurol (Suppl) 23, 1988

WAKSMAN BH: Multiple sclerosis—relationship to a retrovirus? Nature 337:599, 1989

WEINER HL, HAFLER DA: Immunotherapy of multiple sclerosis. Ann Neurol 23:211, 1988

357 NUTRITIONAL AND METABOLIC DISEASES OF THE NERVOUS SYSTEM

MAURICE VICTOR / JOSEPH B. MARTIN

Included under the title of this chapter is a large and diverse number of neurologic disorders that fall into two distinct types—acquired and inherited. In this chapter, emphasis will be on the *acquired* diseases, insofar as they are essentially disorders of adult life and a major source of concern to internist and neurologist alike. The *inherited* metabolic and nutritional diseases, on the other hand, are predominantly disorders of infancy and childhood and are more appropriately considered in a textbook of pediatrics (see also Chaps. 331 to 335). However, a small proportion of the inherited diseases permit survival to adolescence or early adult life or may even have their onset during these periods. These latter instances, which need to be differentiated from certain degenerative and acquired metabolic diseases, are discussed here briefly and in other chapters of this book to which the reader will be referred.

DISEASES DUE TO NUTRITIONAL DEFICIENCY

The general aspects of deficiency disease have been presented in Chap. 76, which should be reviewed as an introduction to the discussion of deficiency diseases of the nervous system. The term *deficiency* will be used here in its strictest sense, to designate those diseases or syndromes resulting from the *lack of an essential nutrient in the diet or from a conditioning factor that increases the need for that nutrient.* The neurologic diseases in this category are the following:

1 Wernicke's disease and Korsakoff's psychosis
2 "Alcoholic" cerebellar degeneration
3 Nutritional polyneuropathy
4 Pellagra
5 Deficiency amblyopia (nutritional optic neuropathy)
6 The syndrome of amblyopia, painful neuropathy, and orogenital dermatitis (Strachan's syndrome)
7 Subacute combined degeneration of the spinal cord (vitamin B_{12} deficiency)
8 Folic acid deficiency
9 Vitamin E deficiency

A number of general principles are applicable to all of the diseases under consideration. Of the known vitamin deficiencies, it is essentially the B deficiencies that are of importance in neurologic disease. Thiamine chloride, nicotinic acid, pyridoxine, pantothenic acid, and possibly folic acid and riboflavin each plays a role in carbohydrate metabolism, upon which the CNS depends for its principal source of energy. These vitamins function as coenzymes in the Krebs tricarboxylic acid cycle; in addition, thiamine is involved in the hexose-monophosphate shunt. Vitamin B_{12} is required for the conversion of methylmalonyl to succinyl coenzyme A and for the conversion of homocystine to methionine. Vitamin E deficiency is a rare cause of central nervous system disease.

Except for subacute combined degeneration of the spinal cord and other manifestations of vitamin B_{12} deficiency, it is not possible to relate the deficiency diseases in humans to the lack of one particular vitamin. For example, polyneuropathy may result from any one of several vitamin deficiencies [thiamine chloride (vitamin B_1), pyridoxine (vitamin B_6), pantothenic acid, and probably B_{12}]. Moreover, pellagra, beriberi, and Strachan's syndrome are probably related to a deficiency of several vitamins. These generalizations should not obscure the fact that certain manifestations of deficiency disease are related to the lack of a specific nutrient (e.g., the ocular signs of Wernicke's disease to a deficiency of thiamine).

In the western world, deficiency diseases of the nervous system occur most often in the alcoholic population of large urban centers. Alcohol acts mainly by displacing food in the diet, but it also increases the demand for B vitamins, which are necessary to metabolize the carbohydrate furnished by alcohol itself, and it may impair the gastrointestinal absorption of vitamins. Dietary faddism, impaired absorption of dietary nutrients (as occurs in sprue, after gastric plication for the treatment of obesity, or resection of stomach and small bowel), and the use of certain drugs (e.g., isoniazid and hydralazine, which interfere with the enzymatic function of pyridoxine) account for a small number of cases of deficiency disease.

Each of the deficiency diseases may occur in pure form and will be so described. More often they occur in various combinations. Stated in another way, deficiency diseases usually involve both the central and peripheral nervous systems, an attribute that they share with few other categories of disease. Also, the examination of patients with deficiency disease frequently discloses nonneurologic signs of malnutrition such as general wasting, lesions of the skin and mucous membranes, and circulatory abnormalities.

WERNICKE'S DISEASE OR ENCEPHALOPATHY Wernicke described an illness of acute onset characterized by mental disturbance, paralysis of eye movements, and ataxia of gait. Swelling of the optic discs and retinal hemorrhages were also present, and there was a progressive depression of the state of consciousness, leading to death, so that a fatal outcome was at one time considered a universal feature of this disease. Wernicke described focal vascular lesions in the gray matter around the third and fourth ventricles and aqueduct of Sylvius. He regarded the disease as inflammatory in nature and suggested the name *acute superior hemorrhagic polioencephalitis.* Since Wernicke's time, views regarding this disease have undergone considerable modification.

Symptoms and signs The most readily recognized abnormalities are the ocular motor signs, and it is difficult to make the clinical diagnosis without them. The usual ocular abnormality is a weakness or paralysis of abduction (sixth nerve palsy) which is invariably bilateral though rarely symmetric and is accompanied by horizontal diplopia, strabismus, and nystagmus. Three types of nystagmus may occur, conjugate horizontal or vertical gaze–evoked nystagmus being the most frequent. An asymmetric horizontal gaze–evoked nystagmus in the abducting eye is characteristic of internuclear ophthalmoplegia. Rarely, one sees a primary position upbeat or downbeat nystagmus with oscillopsia. Each of these abnormalities may be present alone, but far more often a constellation of signs of disordered motility is present, including supranuclear paralysis of gaze. Horizontal gaze palsy is more frequent than vertical gaze palsy. Rarely an isolated paralysis of downgaze or an isolated paralysis of convergence or divergence occurs. In advanced disease there may be complete loss of ocular movement, and the pupils, which ordinarily are spared, may become miotic and nonreacting. Ptosis is rare. The parenteral administration of thiamine in the early stages results in dramatic improvement of the eye movement disorders although horizontal nystagmus may persist.

The *ataxia* affects stance and gait predominantly. The patient may be unable to stand or walk without support. With specific treatment the disorder of equilibrium improves, and the patient is left with a wide-based, uncertain gait. The mildest degree of ataxia is brought out only by heel-to-toe walking. In contrast to the gross disorder of locomotion, an intention (cerebellar) tremor of the limbs is relatively infrequent. The latter abnormality, when present, affects the legs more than the arms. Scanning speech is present only in isolated cases.

A derangement of mental function is found in about 90 percent of patients and takes one of several forms: (1) The most common is a *global confusional-apathetic state*, characterized by profound listlessness, inattentiveness, indifference to the surroundings, and disorientation. Unconsciousness or deep stupor as the initial abnormality is distinctly rare, but drowsiness is common. Spontaneous speech is minimal. Many questions directed to the patient go unanswered, or the patient may fall asleep while being questioned, a state from which he or she can be readily aroused, however. Whatever questions the patient answers betray disorientation in time and place, misidentification of those nearby and an inability to grasp the meaning of the illness or immediate situation. Many of the patient's remarks are irrational and show no consistency from one moment to another. Under these circumstances a more extensive evaluation of intellectual function is seldom possible. (2) Some patients show a disproportionate disorder of retentive memory, i.e., the Korsakoff amnesic state (see Chap. 30 and later in this chapter). (3) A relatively small number of patients (less than 20 percent in our series) show the symptoms of alcohol withdrawal, either delirium tremens or a variant thereof.

The symptoms of Wernicke's disease may appear simultaneously and rather acutely, but more often ophthalmoplegia and/or ataxia precede the mental signs by days or weeks.

Wernicke's disease is usually associated with other nutritional disorders, both neurologic and nonneurologic. In more than 80 percent of patients, a *polyneuropathy* of varying degrees of severity is evident. Rarely, *amblyopia* or *spinal spastic ataxia* may be present. Many patients in the chronic stage demonstrate impaired olfactory discrimination, a defect that is most likely related to the diencephalic lesions (see below).

Full-blown beriberi heart disease occurs rarely in patients with Wernicke's disease, although indications of *disordered cardiovascular function* such as tachycardia, exertional dyspnea, postural hypotension, and minor ECG abnormalities are common. Occasionally patients die suddenly, the mode of death suggesting "cardiovascular collapse," and Wernicke's disease is characterized by a state of high cardiac output which is out of proportion to the oxygen consumption. This is probably due to an abnormal state of peripheral vasodilatation, which in turn may be related to thiamine deficiency. Postural hypotension and syncope are related to impaired function of the automatic nervous system, more specifically to a defect in sympathetic regulation.

Ancillary findings   Vestibular function, as measured by the response to standard caloric testing, is always impaired bilaterally and more or less symmetrically in the acute stages of Wernicke's disease (*vestibular paresis*). The cerebrospinal fluid (CSF) is normal or shows only a modest elevation of protein content; protein values above 1.0 g/L (100 mg/dL) or a pleocytosis should always suggest the presence of a complicating illness. In untreated cases of Wernicke's disease, there is invariably an elevation of the *blood pyruvate,* and a marked reduction in the *blood transketolase* (a thiamine-dependent enzyme of the hexose monophosphate shunt). Diffuse slowing of the EEG, mild to moderate in degree, occurs in about one-half of the patients. On the other hand, total cerebral blood flow and cerebral oxygen and glucose consumption may be greatly reduced in the acute stages and persist for several weeks after the institution of treatment.

Course of the illness   Death occurs in 15 to 20 percent of hospitalized patients and is usually due to a complicating infection (pneumonia, pulmonary tuberculosis, and septicemia being the most common) or to hepatic failure.

Patients who recover do so in a characteristic manner. Ocular palsies may *begin to improve* within hours after the administration of thiamine and practically always within several days. Failure to respond in this manner raises doubts about the diagnosis of Wernicke's disease. Sixth nerve palsies, ptosis, and vertical gaze palsies recover completely, within a week or two in most cases, but vertical gaze–evoked nystagmus may persist for months. Horizontal gaze palsies recover completely as a rule, but a fine horizontal gaze–evoked nystagmus usually remains as a permanent sequela of the disease.

Ataxia improves somewhat more slowly than the ocular motor abnormalities. Approximately half the patients recover incompletely and are left with a slow, shuffling, wide-based gait and inability to walk tandem. The residual gait disturbance and horizontal nystagmus provide a means of identifying obscure and chronic cases of dementia as alcoholic-nutritional in origin. Vestibular function, as measured by caloric testing, improves at about the same rate as the ataxia of stance and gait, i.e., over a period of weeks or months, and recovery is usually but not always complete.

The symptoms of apathy, drowsiness, and confusion recede gradually, and as they do, the *defect in retentive memory and learning (Korsakoff's psychosis;* see Chap. 30) stands out more clearly. It is important to emphasize that Wernicke's disease and Korsakoff's psychosis are not separate diseases, but that the changing ocular and ataxic signs and the transformation of the global confusion state into an amnesic syndrome are successive stages in the recovery of a single disease process. Stated in another way, Korsakoff's psychosis is the psychic component of Wernicke's disease. Hence the symptom complex should be called Wernicke's disease when the amnesic state is not evident and the Wernicke-Korsakoff syndrome when both the ocular-ataxic and amnesic symptoms can be recognized.

The outcome of Korsakoff's psychosis varies. Complete or almost complete recovery occurs in less than 20 percent of patients. In the remainder recovery is slow and incomplete. Depending on the severity of the residual symptoms, the patient may or may not be able to lead a supervised existence out of a hospital. The residual mental state is characterized by large gaps in memory, without confabulation, and an inability of the patient to sort out events in their proper temporal sequence. This late stage of the disease, when the ocular and ataxic signs have receded or are not recognized, is often loosely referred to as "alcoholic deteriorated state" or "alcoholic dementia."

Pathologic changes   Patients who die in the acute stages of Wernicke-Korsakoff disease have symmetrically placed lesions in the paraventricular regions of the thalamus and hypothalamus, the mamillary bodies, periaqueductal region of the midbrain, floor of the fourth ventricle, and anterior-superior folia of the cerebellum, particularly of the vermis. Lesions are invariably found in the mamillary bodies and less consistently in the other areas. Microscopically, the principal change consists of varying degrees of necrosis of parenchymal structures. Many nerve cells and fibers are destroyed; others remain intact and are seen against a background of reactive glial elements, both astrocytes and microgliocytes. The blood vessels are prominent, owing to adventitial and endothelial proliferation. Hemorrhagic lesions are present in a small proportion of cases and are usually of recent origin. The oculomotor and vestibular nuclei are regularly involved, but to a lesser degree.

Clinical-pathologic correlations   The ocular motor signs are attributable to lesions in the brainstem affecting the abducens nuclei and eye movement centers in the pons and rostral midbrain (see Chap. 23). The lesions of the vestibular nuclei are probably responsible for the loss of caloric responses and gross abnormality of equilibrium that characterize the initial stage of the disease. The lack of significant destruction of nerve cells in these lesions accounts for the rapid improvement in oculomotor and vestibular function.

The persistent ataxia of stance and gait is related to the loss of neurons in the superior vermis of the cerebellum; extension of the lesion into the anterior parts of the anterior lobes accounts for the ataxia of individual movements of the legs. These cerebellar lesions are indistinguishable from those of so-called *alcoholic cerebellar degeneration* (see below).

The amnesic defect is related to lesions in the diencephalon, more specifically to those in the medial dorsal nuclei of the thalami. Lesions in the mamillary bodies are probably not critical in respect to memory function since they are found in patients with Wernicke's disease who had shown no disorder of memory during life.

Etiology and pathogenesis Nutritional deficiency is the causal factor. Wernicke's disease has been encountered in prisoners-of-war and in patients with wasting diseases of varied origin, i.e., circumstances in which alcohol played no part. The specific factor responsible for most, if not all, of the symptoms of the Wernicke-Korsakoff syndrome is a deficiency of thiamine. The marked sensitivity of the ocular abnormalities to the administration of thiamine accounts for their rapid abatement after the ingestion of a meal or two. The quality of prompt reversibility indicates that the ocular signs are due to a biochemical abnormality and not to irreversible structural changes. On the other hand, the slow and incomplete recovery of the memory defect suggests that this symptom is due to irreversible structural changes, presumably in the medial dorsal nuclei.

The mechanism whereby thiamine deficiency causes brain lesions is not established. Thiamine is a cofactor for several enzymes including transketolase, pyruvate dehydrogenase, and α-ketoglutarate dehydrogenase. Thiamine deficiency produces a diffuse decrease in cerebral glucose utilization, and lesions in thiamine-deficient experimental animals are diminished by antagonists that block *N*-methyl-D-aspartate–preferring glutamic acid receptors. This latter finding suggests that the neurotoxicity of thiamine deficiency may be mediated by excitotoxicity evoked by glutamic acid release (see also Chaps. 346 and 359).

The selective vulnerability of certain periventricular regions to a deficiency of thiamine is not understood. McEntee and Mair have pointed out that the lesions lie in the monoamine-containing pathways and have presented evidence that 3-methoxy-4-hydroxyphenylglycol (MHPG), the primary brain metabolite of norepinephrine, is decreased in the CSF of alcoholic patients with Korsakoff's psychosis; moreover, the administration of clonidine, an alpha$_2$-adrenergic agonist, seemed to improve the memory disorder in these patients. These authors have theorized that damage to the ascending norepinephrine-containing neurons in the brainstem and diencephalon is the basis for the amnesia.

The topography of the lesions caused by thiamine deficiency has been studied in rhesus monkeys. Witt and Goldman-Rakic found that the severity and number of brain nuclei affected are related to the duration and number of bouts of thiamine deficiency.

Treatment of the Wernicke-Korsakoff syndrome Wernicke's disease represents a medical emergency, and its recognition demands the immediate administration of thiamine. A delay of a few hours may be crucial in determining whether the patient with ocular and ataxic signs will be prevented from developing Korsakoff's psychosis and whether the patient with early Korsakoff's changes will be restored to a state of mental competency. Although 2 to 3 mg of thiamine may modify the ocular signs, much larger doses are needed to replenish the thiamine stores—50 mg intravenously and 50 mg intramuscularly, the latter dose being repeated each day until the patient resumes a normal diet. The other B vitamins may be given by mouth in the dosages outlined in Chap. 76. If the patient cannot or will not eat, parenteral feeding and administration of B vitamins become necessary.

A particular danger attends the treatment of the severely depleted alcoholic patient with intravenous glucose solutions. Such infusions may exhaust the patient's reserve of B vitamins and either precipitate Wernicke's disease in a previously unaffected patient or cause a rapid worsening of an early form of the disease. For this reason, B vitamins must be administered to all alcoholic patients requiring parenteral glucose. The cardiovascular status of each patient should be monitored carefully. Since these patients are confused and forgetful, they must be supervised continually, preferably on a medical ward.

A special problem arises when the patient recovers from the acute phase of the illness and the amnesic psychosis becomes prominent. The disposition of the patient to family, nursing home, or mental institution should be made on the basis of the severity of the mental illness as well as the capacity of the family unit and social circumstances.

NUTRITIONAL POLYNEUROPATHY (See also Chaps. 76 and 363) Nutritional polyneuropathy is usually a disease of the alcoholic population. As mentioned above, it is present in most patients with the Wernicke-Korsakoff syndrome, but it may occur as the only manifestation of deficiency disease. The peripheral neuropathy of alcoholics ("alcoholic polyneuropathy") does not differ in any fundamental way from that of beriberi. The clinical features of nutritional polyneuropathy and its identity with beriberi are discussed in Chaps. 76 and 363. A deficiency of thiamine chloride, pyridoxine, pantothenic acid, vitamin B$_{12}$, and perhaps folic acid has been demonstrated in individual cases to cause nutritional polyneuropathy. In the alcoholic patient it is usually not possible to incriminate a particular vitamin.

"ALCOHOLIC" CEREBELLAR DEGENERATION This is the term applied to a common, stereotyped, nonfamilial form of cerebellar ataxia that occurs on a background of prolonged ingestion of alcohol. Usually the symptoms evolve in subacute fashion, i.e., over several weeks or months, sometimes more rapidly. In some patients the symptoms are present in mild but stable form and worsen after an attack of pneumonia or delirium tremens.

The signs are those of cerebellar dysfunction, affecting stance and gait predominantly. The legs are involved more severely than the arms, and nystagmus and speech disturbances occur relatively infrequently. Once established, the signs change very little, although some improvement of gait may follow the cessation of drinking, due probably to improvement in general nutrition and recovery from associated polyneuropathy.

The pathologic changes consist of degeneration of varying severity of all the neurocellular elements of the cerebellar cortex, particularly of the Purkinje cells, with a striking topographic restriction to the anterior and superior aspects of the vermis and adjacent parts of the anterior lobes of the cerebellum. The disorder of stance and gait is related to the lesion in the vermis, and the ataxia of the limbs is due to the involvement of the anterior lobes. A similar clinical-pathologic syndrome is observed occasionally in nutritionally depleted nonalcoholic patients.

Central nervous system disorders in alcoholism not associated with vitamin deficiency A number of alcohol-associated disorders are not attributable to nutritional deficiency or trauma. There appears to be an increased incidence of hypertension in alcoholics and probably of strokes, both ischemic infarction and spontaneous subarachnoid hemorrhage. Alcoholics as a group also show dilatation of the lateral ventricles and widening of sulci on CT or MRI scans. The nature of these changes is obscure. They do not correlate with any mental abnormality, nor do they represent cerebral atrophy insofar as partial and sometimes complete reversal occur with sustained abstinence. Some believe that alcohol can cause intellectual deterioration separate from effects due to nutritional deficiency, but an entity of "alcoholic dementia" has never been established on the basis of clinical and neuropathologic studies. A syndrome of progressive myelopathy occurring in alcoholics has also been described. Such patients are said to show no evidence of nutritional deficiency (B$_{12}$ or folic acid) or of liver disease. The nature of the spinal cord disease is unknown, and a causal relationship to the toxic effects of alcohol remains to be established.

PELLAGRA This disease is described in Chap. 76. Neurologic manifestations are quite diverse. Pellagra is essentially an encephalopathy, although involvement of the spinal cord and peripheral nerves may occur. The early mental symptoms—insomnia, fatigue, anxiety, nervousness, irritability, and depression—may be mistaken for a psychiatric disorder. However, as the disease advances, slowing and inefficiency of mental processes and impairment of memory become clear-cut. Pellagra may not only cause psychiatric manifestations but occasionally may result from them because certain mental illnesses, including alcoholism, cause anorexia and dietary deficiency.

The spinal cord involvement in pellagra has not been clearly delineated, perhaps because the mental state of the patients has precluded accurate testing. In general, there is both posterior and lateral column involvement, predominantly the former. Neuropathic signs are difficult to distinguish from other types of nutritional polyneuropathy. Other manifestations such as tremor, extrapyramidal rigidity, suck and grasp reflexes, and coma (referred to in the past as "nicotinic acid–deficiency encephalopathy") have indiscriminately been included in the pellagra syndrome, as have various disorders of the special senses.

A *spastic paretic syndrome,* apart from the other symptoms and signs of pellagra, may be a rare manifestation of nutritional deficiency. The chief signs are spastic weakness of the legs with absent abdominal and increased tendon reflexes, clonus, and extensor plantar responses. These signs are usually accompanied by other manifestations of nutritional deficiency, such as Wernicke's disease, amblyopia, and peripheral neuropathy.

Pathologic features   The distinctive neuropathologic changes in pellagra are most readily discerned in the large Betz cells of the motor cortex, although the same changes are seen to a lesser extent in the smaller pyramidal cells of the cerebral cortex and cells of the basal ganglia, cranial motor and dentate nuclei, and anterior horns of the spinal cord. The affected cells appear swollen and rounded with eccentric nuclei and loss of Nissl staining. This *central neuritis of pellagra,* as it is called, appears to represent a primary affection of the whole motor cell. The spinal cord lesions take the form of a symmetric degeneration of the dorsal columns, especially the fasciculus gracilis, and to a lesser extent of the corticospinal tracts. The posterior column degeneration is probably secondary to degeneration of specific dorsal root ganglion cells.

DEFICIENCY AMBLYOPIA (NUTRITIONAL OPTIC NEUROPATHY, TOBACCO-ALCOHOL AMBLYOPIA)   These terms refer to a characteristic form of visual impairment that complicates nutritional disease and is due to a lesion in the optic nerve, more or less confined to the zone of the papillomacular bundle. The cornea and other parts of the refractive mechanism are uninvolved, hence the term *amblyopia.*

The main symptoms are dimness or blurring of vision for near and distant objects and impairment of color vision, which worsens progressively and insidiously for several days or weeks. In addition to a reduction in visual acuity, examination discloses the presence of bilateral and roughly symmetric central or centrocecal scotomas, which are larger for colored than for white test objects. Pallor of the temporal portion of the optic disc is observed in some cases. Untreated, this condition progresses to irreversible optic atrophy.

Deficiency amblyopia was common in prisoners of war. Although this form of amblyopia had previously been described in association with beriberi (due to thiamine deficiency) and pellagra (due to niacin deficiency), the peak incidence among prisoners coincided with neither of these syndromes but with the syndrome of orogenital dermatitis and "burning feet" ("Strachan syndrome," see below).

In the United States, most, if not all, of the cases of retrobulbar neuropathy attributed to the toxic effects of alcohol or tobacco—so-called tobacco-alcohol amblyopia—are of nutritional origin. Optic neuropathy may occur as the only manifestation of vitamin deficiency, but more often it is combined with other evidence of nutritional deficiency, such as peripheral neuropathy and the Wernicke-Korsakoff syndrome.

Although the nutritional origin of this type of amblyopia has been established, the specific vitamin deficiency can rarely be determined. Observations in both humans and experimental animals indicate that a deficiency of thiamine (vitamin B_1), vitamin B_{12}, or perhaps riboflavin may cause lesions in the optic nerves. Two causative mechanisms for the pathogenesis of tobacco amblyopia have been proposed: (1) chronic cyanide (generated in tobacco smoke) poisoning; and (2) alterations of fatty acid metabolism resulting from derangement of proprionate metabolism in the central nervous system. The notion that cyanide or other substances in tobacco smoke have a toxic effect upon the optic nerves is not supported by experimental data. And, since fatty acids take part in the formation and preservation of myelin, the biochemical consequences of vitamin B_{12} deficiency may be sufficient to account for both ophthalmologic and other neurologic involvement. However, in only a small proportion of patients with this type of amblyopia can a vitamin B_{12} deficiency state be established.

Treatment consists of the administration of a balanced diet, supplemented with B vitamins, and the interdiction of alcohol where this is the cause of nutritional deficiency.

SYNDROME OF AMBLYOPIA, PAINFUL NEUROPATHY, AND OROGENITAL DERMATITIS (STRACHAN'S SYNDROME)   There have been many reports of a neurologic syndrome that is undoubtedly nutritional in origin but cannot be fitted into the boundaries of beriberi or pellagra. Strachan attributed the disorder to malaria. Originally known as "Jamaican neuritis," the syndrome occurs among the undernourished populations of many tropical countries. Large numbers of patients with this syndrome were observed also in the besieged population of Madrid during the Spanish Civil War and among prisoners of war during World War II in the Middle and Far East. In the United States, occasional alcoholic patients have this syndrome.

Strachan's syndrome is essentially a disorder of the peripheral and optic nerves. The peripheral nerve disorder is characterized mainly by sensory symptoms and signs (painful paresthesias of the feet, loss of superficial and deep sensation, and ataxia). On the other hand, foot drop and muscle weakness occur rarely. A frequently associated disorder is failing vision, which may go on to complete blindness and pallor of the optic discs. Deafness and vertigo are rare, but among some prisoners of war these symptoms were so prominent as to earn the epithet "camp dizziness." In these respects the syndrome differs from beriberi. Along with the neurologic signs there may be varying degrees of stomatoglossitis, corneal degeneration, and genital dermatitis. These mucocutaneous lesions are spoken of together as the *orogenital syndrome.* Because the genital dermatitis and stomatoglossitis are typical of pellagra and the ocular lesions, of vitamin A deficiency, it is possible Strachan's syndrome can be accounted for by multiple vitamin deficiencies.

There have been few pathologic studies of this syndrome. Aside from the damage to the papillomacular bundle in the optic nerve, the most consistent abnormality has been a loss of myelinated fibers in the posterior columns (fasciculus gracilis) of the spinal cord. This indicates a systematized degeneration of the central processes of the large bipolar sensory neurons of the lumbosacral spinal ganglia. Degeneration of the peripheral processes of these neurons probably accounts for the loss of pain and temperature sensation. There are no reliable data concerning the specific vitamin deficiencies that cause this disease.

SUBACUTE COMBINED DEGENERATION (SCD) OF THE SPINAL CORD (See also Chap. 76)   This term designates the spinal cord disease that is due to vitamin B_{12} deficiency. The brain, optic nerves, and peripheral nerves may also be affected but far less often than the spinal cord. The neurologic and hematologic manifestations (pernicious anemia) are distinctive insofar as they are caused not by a lack of vitamin B_{12} in the food but by an inability to transfer this nutrient across the intestinal mucosa. Such a nutritional disorder is referred to as a *conditioned deficiency,* since it depends upon the lack of an intrinsic factor in the gastric secretions (see Chap. 292). Rarely neurologic symptoms due to vitamin B_{12} deficiency occur in patients with disease of the distal small intestine (Crohn's disease, lymphoma) or after surgical resection.

Clinical manifestations   Neurologic symptoms are present in the majority of patients with vitamin B_{12} deficiency. The patient first notices general weakness and paresthesias, consisting of tingling, "pins-and-needles" feelings, or other vaguely described sensations in the distal parts of the limbs; the lower extremities may be involved before the upper ones or vice versa. The paresthesias tend to be constant, to progress steadily, and to be the source of much distress. As the illness progresses, the gait becomes unsteady, and movements of the limbs, especially the legs, become stiff and awkward.

Early in the course of the illness, when only paresthesias are present, there may be no objective signs. Later, the neurologic examination discloses a disorder of the posterior and lateral columns of the spinal cord, predominantly the former. Loss of vibration sense, the most consistent sign, is more pronounced in the legs than in the arms, and frequently it extends over the trunk. Position sense is involved to a somewhat lesser extent. The motor defects are usually limited to the legs and include loss of power, spasticity, changes in the tendon reflexes, clonus, and extensor plantar responses. At first the patellar and Achilles reflexes may be diminished, increased, or absent. With treatment, the reflexes may return to normal or become hyperactive. The gait at first is predominantly ataxic, later ataxic and spastic. If the disease remains untreated, an ataxic paraplegia with variable degrees of spasticity and contracture may develop.

A loss of superficial sensation below a segmental level on the trunk, implicating the spinothalamic tracts, occurs rarely, but such a finding should always suggest the possibility of some other disease of the spinal cord. More often the sensory defect takes the form of a blunting of tactile, painful, and thermal sensation over the distal segments of the lower limbs, implicating the peripheral nerves, but such findings are uncommon.

The nervous system involvement in vitamin B_{12} deficiency is characteristically, though not perfectly, symmetric. A definite asymmetry of motor or sensory findings, maintained over a period of weeks or months, should always cast doubt on the diagnosis.

Mental signs are frequent, ranging from irritability, apathy, somnolence, suspiciousness, and emotional instability to a marked confusional or depressive psychosis, or even to intellectual deterioration. Optic neuropathy with impaired acuity and cecocentral scotoma has been reported with virtually all forms of vitamin B_{12} deficiency. In all cases, variable improvement in acuity occurs once systemic vitamin B_{12} is administered. Although dementia and amblyopia are relatively uncommon manifestations of vitamin B_{12} deficiency, each may occasionally be the initial manifestation of the disease.

Pathology and pathogenesis The pathologic process takes the form of a diffuse, though uneven, degeneration of the white matter of the spinal cord and sometimes of the brain. At first there is swelling of myelin sheaths, characterized by separation of myelin lamellae and formation of intramyelinic vacuoles. This is followed by a coalescence of small foci of tissue destruction into larger ones, giving the tissue a vacuolated appearance. The myelin sheaths and the axis cylinders are both affected, the former perhaps earlier and to a greater extent than the latter. Astrocytic gliosis is minimal in the early lesions, but in the more chronic ones gliosis is pronounced. The changes begin in the posterior columns of the lower cervical and upper thoracic cord and spread from this region up and down the cord, as well as forward into the lateral columns. The lesions are not limited to specific systems of fibers within the posterior and lateral funiculi but are scattered irregularly through the white matter. The changes in the optic nerves are similar to those in other types of nutritional neuropathy, i.e., a degeneration of myelinated fibers in the territory of the papillomacular bundles.

The *pathogenesis* of the nervous system lesions in vitamin B_{12} deficiency is not well understood. Impairment of DNA synthesis probably accounts for the hematologic abnormalities and the production of megaloblasts; however, since neurons do not divide, this mechanism cannot be invoked to explain the central nervous system changes. One of the better-understood functions of vitamin B_{12} is its role as a coenzyme in the methylmalonyl CoA mutase reaction. Impairment of this metabolic step may lead to the production of abnormal fatty acids, which are important building blocks of cell membranes and of myelin. However, Carmel et al. have described a hereditary form of cobalamin deficiency, in which methylmalonyl CoA mutase activity was normal despite the presence of typical neurologic abnormalities. These authors attributed the neurologic abnormalities to an impairment of methionine synthase activity. These and other hypotheses have been reviewed by Beck.

Diagnosis and treatment The chief obstacle to early diagnosis is the lack of parallelism between the hematologic and neurologic signs. This is particularly true of patients who have received folic acid, which serves to maintain a hematologic remission for an indefinite period while the neurologic signs worsen, often to an

irreversible stage. Under these circumstances the most reliable diagnostic procedures are the measurement of the serum B_{12} concentration and the two-stage Schilling test (see Chap. 292). In rare instances, even these tests may be inconclusive, in which case the finding of high serum concentrations of cobalamin metabolites—methylmalonic acid and homocysteine—may be diagnostically useful.

The treatment of the neurologic manifestations of vitamin B_{12} deficiency differs in no way from the treatment of the hematologic ones. Patients whose vitamin B_{12} stores have been depleted require large doses of cobalamin—1000 μg intramuscularly each day during hospitalization, then weekly for a month, and then monthly for the remainder of the patient's life.

The most important factor influencing the *response to treatment* is the duration of the neurologic disease. Recovery may be complete if therapy is instituted within a few weeks of the onset of symptoms. For this reason SCD and the other neurologic complications of vitamin B_{12} deficiency represent medical emergencies. If symptoms have been present for longer than a month or two, only partial recovery can be expected, and in long-standing cases the best that can be expected is the arrest of progression of the symptoms.

FOLIC ACID DEFICIENCY Despite the frequent occurrence of folic acid deficiency, a role in the pathogenesis of nervous system disease has not been established beyond doubt. The polyneuropathies that occasionally complicate sprue and other malabsorption syndromes and the chronic administration of phenytoin have been attributed, on uncertain grounds, to folate deficiency. With respect to folate deficiency and spinal cord disease, the data are equally limited. Cases have been described (see Pincus) in which the neurologic signs of subacute combined degeneration were attributed to folic acid deficiency. In these cases there was no evidence of vitamin B_{12} deficiency but there was a resolution of both the hematologic and neurologic abnormalities after the institution of folate therapy.

VITAMIN E DEFICIENCY A rare neurologic disorder of childhood, consisting essentially of a spinocerebellar degeneration in association with a polyneuropathy and pigmentary retinopathy, has been related to a deficiency of vitamin E that develops after prolonged intestinal malabsorption (Satya-Murti et al.). The same mechanism has been proposed to explain the neurologic disorders that sometimes complicate abetalipoproteinemia, fibrocystic disease, and extensive intestinal resections (Harding et al.). Vitamin E deficiency also occurs in young children with chronic cholestatic hepatobiliary disease. Ataxia, loss of tendon reflexes, ophthalmoparesis, proximal muscle weakness with elevated serum creatine phosphokinase, and decreased sensation are the usual manifestations. These symptoms are referable to parts of the nervous system and musculature known to be involved in animals deprived of vitamin E—degeneration of Clarke's columns, spinocerebellar tracts, posterior columns, nuclei of Goll and Burdach, and sensory roots (Nelson et al.). In affected children neurologic function improves after the long-term correction of vitamin E deficiency.

NEUROLOGIC SYNDROMES CAUSED BY HYPERVITAMINOSIS Acute toxicity with vitamin A causes symptoms of headache, dizziness, irritability, and drowsiness. Chronic hypervitaminosis A can give rise to chronic increased intracranial pressure (pseudotumor cerebri) (see Chap. 76).

The ingestion of pyridoxine in excessive amounts (2 g or more daily) can cause a sensory neuropathy characterized clinically by progressive ataxia, impairment of position and vibration sense, and loss of deep tendon reflexes. Motor strength is preserved. The syndrome is reversible with discontinuation of pyridoxine.

ACQUIRED (SECONDARY) METABOLIC DISEASES OF THE NERVOUS SYSTEM

In this important category of neurologic disease, disturbance of cerebral function is due to disease in some other organ system—heart (and circulation), lungs (and respiration), kidneys, liver, endocrine glands, and possibly pancreas. Each of these diseases affects the nervous system in somewhat different ways.

ANOXIC-ISCHEMIC ENCEPHALOPATHY This common and often disastrous condition is caused by a lack of oxygen to the brain, resulting from hypotension or respiratory failure. Sometimes both are responsible, and one cannot say which predominates—hence, the ambiguous designation in clinical records, as "cardiorespiratory failure." The conditions that most often lead to anoxic-ischemic encephalopathy are (1) myocardial infarction; (2) cardiac arrest; (3) hemorrhage, with shock and circulatory collapse; in these situations vascular supply to the brain is compromised before respiration; (4) shock; (5) suffocation (from drowning, strangulation, aspiration of vomitus or blood, compression of the trachea by hemorrhage or a surgical pack, or a foreign body in the trachea); (6) diseases that paralyze the muscles of respiration or compromise the central nervous system respiratory drive (trauma, vascular disease of the brain, epilepsy), causing respiratory failure followed by cardiac failure; and (7) carbon monoxide (CO) poisoning, in which respiration fails first and then cardiovascular functions. Hypoxia alone may induce different clinicopathologic consequences than a combination of hypoxia and hypoperfusion (ischemia).

Clinical manifestations Mild degrees of hypoxia cause inattentiveness, impaired judgment, and motor incoordination but have no lasting effects. With severe hypoxia or anoxia, as occurs with cardiac arrest, consciousness is lost within seconds, but recovery will be complete if breathing, oxygenation of blood, and cardiac action are restored within 3 to 5 min. If anoxia persists beyond this time, there is serious and permanent injury to the brain, particularly to those parts in which the efficiency of circulation is marginal (globus pallidus, cerebellum, hippocampus, and the "borderzone regions" of the parietooccipital lobes). Clinically, it is difficult to judge the precise degree of hypoxia-ischemia since slight heart action or an imperceptible blood pressure may serve to maintain the circulation to some extent. Hence some individuals have made an excellent recovery after cerebral anoxia that allegedly lasted 8 to 10 min or longer. *An important clinical rule is that degrees of hypoxia which at no time abolish consciousness rarely if ever cause permanent damage to the nervous system.* P_{O_2} as low as 2.7 kPa (20 mmHg) is well tolerated if it develops gradually and blood pressure is normal. Also, subjects who demonstrate intact brainstem function (as indicated by normal ciliospinal, oculovestibular, and pupillary light responses, and intact doll's-head eye movements) usually have a better outlook for recovery of consciousness and perhaps all of their faculties. Conversely, absence of these reflexes and the presence of pupils that are persistently fixed to light indicate a grave prognosis.

Extreme or sustained global ischemia causes brain death (see Chap. 31). Immediately after resuscitation from cardiorespiratory arrest, the physical findings may suggest brain death (dilated, unresponsive pupils, absent brainstem reflexes and respiration, and isoelectric EEG), yet full recovery may occur. However, persistence of the unresponsive state for more than an hour or two invariably carries a poor prognosis. The diagnosis of brain death must be made with caution because anesthesia, drug intoxication, and hypothermia may also cause deep coma, absent brainstem reflexes, and an isoelectric EEG but permit recovery. The problem of brain death has been brought increasingly to public attention because of ethical and moral issues that surround the question of discontinuing supportive medical therapy. Issues of management are most difficult in the patient who has suffered severe but lesser degrees of cerebral anoxia.

Patients who suffer a severe anoxic encephalopathy, but one that falls short of causing "brain death," often stabilize breathing and heart action. Neurologic evaluation shows the patient to be profoundly comatose, with eyes slightly divergent and motionless but with reactive pupils, flaccid or intensely rigid limbs, and diminished tendon reflexes. Within a few minutes after cardiac action and breathing have been restored, generalized convulsions and isolated or grouped twitches of muscles (myoclonus) may supervene. Decerebrate or decorticate postures may be present or occur upon pinching the limbs,

and bilateral Babinski signs can be evoked. In the first 24 to 48 h death may occur in a setting of rising temperature, deepening coma, and circulatory collapse. Or, with somewhat lesser degrees of injury, where the cerebral and cerebellar cortices are partly or completely destroyed but brainstem-spinal structures remain intact, the individual may survive in a state referred to as "irreversible coma" or "persistent vegetative state" (see Chap. 31). The latter patients remain mute, unresponsive, and unaware of their environment for weeks, months, or years. Criteria to predict accurately the outcome of anoxic encephalopathy early in the comatose period have been developed (see Chap. 31). If intoxication can be excluded, the presence of fixed dilated pupils and paralysis of eye movement for 24 to 48 h, along with marked slowing of the EEG, usually signifies irreversible cerebral damage. Deep coma of this type, lasting more than a few days, is rarely attended by full recovery.

Patients with lesser degrees of injury improve after a period of coma. Consciousness is regained, and then various degrees of confusion, visual agnosia, extrapyramidal rigidity, or movement disorder (action or intention myoclonus, choreoathetosis, cerebellar ataxia) become manifest. Some of these patients quickly pass through this posthypoxic phase and proceed to make full recovery; others are left with permanent neurologic sequelae. The *posthypoxic syndromes* observed most frequently are (1) *persistent coma or stupor;* and, with lesser degrees of cerebral injury, (2) *dementia,* with or without extrapyramidal signs; (3) *visual agnosia;* (4) *parkinsonism;* (5) *choreoathetosis;* (6) *cerebellar ataxia;* (7) *intention or action myoclonus;* and (8) *Korsakoff's amnesic state. Seizures* may continue to be a problem but are uncommon.

A relatively uncommon and unexplained phenomenon is *delayed postanoxic encephalopathy.* Initial improvement, which appears to be complete, is followed after a variable period of time (several days to a week or longer) by a relapse, characterized by apathy, confusion, irritability, and occasionally agitation or mania. A few patients have recovered from this second episode, but in most the neurologic syndrome progresses, with shuffling gait, diffuse rigidity and spasticity, coma, and death after 1 to 2 weeks. Postmortem examination of these patients has shown the major abnormality to be widespread cerebral demyelination. Exceptionally, another delayed syndrome occurs, in which a period of hypoxia is followed by a slow, deteriorating state, affecting basal ganglia more than cerebral cortex and white matter and progressing for weeks to months until the patient is mute, rigid, and helpless.

The essential *mechanism* in hypoxic encephalopathy is a neuronal lack of oxygen and an arrest of all aerobic metabolic processes necessary to sustain the Krebs tricarboxylic cycle and the electron transport system. Lactic acid accumulates in the tissues. The pathophysiology of delayed progression is not understood. Experimental observations suggest that glutamate release from hypoxic-ischemic brain tissue can induce neurotoxicity by actions exerted through one subclass of glutamate receptor, the N-methyl-D-aspartate (NMDA) receptor.

Diagnosis This depends on (1) the history of a hypoxic-ischemic event and evidence of reduced oxygenation of arterial blood [$P_{O_2} < 5.3$ kPa (40 mmHg)], CO intoxication (indicated by its spectroscopic band or cherry-red color of the skin for a few minutes to hours after the episode), blood pressures below 9.3 kPa (70 mmHg) systolic, or cardiac arrest; and (2) as outlined above, the typical clinical sequence of events after a possible hypoxic-ischemic episode has terminated. Renal damage (anuria) and myocardial infarction may also have occurred and provide corroborative evidence of hypoxia.

Treatment The treatment of anoxic encephalopathy is directed mainly at the prevention of a critical degree of hypoxic injury. After a clear airway is secured, artificial respiration, external thoracic cardiac massage, the use of a cardiac defibrillator or pacemaker, and open chest surgery all have their place, and every second counts in their prompt utilization. Once cardiac and pulmonary function are restored, there is no evidence that any pharmacologic measure enhances recovery. Barbiturates, glucocorticoids, dimethyl sulfoxide, and benzodiazepines have been given without proof of benefit. A small proportion of patients develop secondary complications of diffuse brain swelling after cardiac arrest; this condition is more common in children. This is detected by compression of the lateral ventricles and cisterns on CT scan, or by very high lumbar CSF pressure. Seizures should be controlled by anticonvulsants. Posthypoxic myoclonus may respond to oral administration of clonazepam 8–12 mg/d. Other details of treatment are considered in Chap. 31.

HYPERCAPNIC ENCEPHALOPATHY Chronic emphysema and fibrosing lung disease and, in rare instances, an inadequacy of central respiratory drive lead to chronic respiratory acidosis, with an elevation of P_{CO_2} and a reduction in arterial P_{O_2}. Secondary polycythemia and cor pulmonale often accompany these pulmonary diseases.

Clinical Manifestations The clinical syndrome consequent upon hypercapnia (and hypoxia) consists of generalized or bilateral frontal or occipital headache, often intense and persistent for hours; papilledema; mental dullness, drowsiness, confusion, stupor, and coma; a fast-frequency action tremor and coarse twitching of all muscles, which are in a state of sustained contraction; and inability to maintain a fixed posture or interruption of a voluntary movement because of brief lapses of sustained muscle contraction (asterixis). Intermittent drowsiness, indifference and inattention to the environment, reduction of psychomotor activity, imperception of the sequence of events, and forgetfulness constitute the more subtle manifestations of this syndrome.

In fully developed cases, the cerebrospinal fluid (CSF) is under increased pressure, P_{CO_2} may exceed 10 kPa (75 mmHg), and oxygen saturation of the arterial blood ranges from 85 to 40 percent. The EEG reveals slow activity in the delta and theta range, sometimes bilaterally synchronous. The mechanism of the cerebral disorder is said to be CO_2 narcosis, but the biochemical mechanism is not known. The danger of administering morphine or sedatives, which blunt the respiratory drive (already depressed by the CO_2 retention), or inhaled O_2, which removes the sole stimulus (low P_{O_2}) to the respiratory center, is now widely recognized.

Treatment Forced ventilation with an intermittent positive-pressure respirator, treatment of heart failure with digitalis and diuretics, venesection to reduce the viscosity of the blood, and antibiotics to combat pulmonary infection are the most effective therapeutic measures. If stupor or coma persists, the arterial O_2 level should be rechecked; it may be critically reduced, and needs to be raised by controlled O_2 administration to a point [6.7 to 7.3 kPa (50 to 55 mmHg)] where consciousness is improved but the stimulus to respiratory drive is not removed. Also, the pH of the CSF may be very low, in the range of 7.15 to 7.25. In CO_2 narcosis, correction of the acidosis of blood is easier than that of CSF, which tends to lag. The management of respiratory failure is discussed in detail in Chap. 210.

Differential diagnosis Unlike pure hypoxic encephalopathy, hypercapnia rarely causes prolonged coma and is not a cause of irreversible brain damage. Papilledema and asterixis are important diagnostic features. (Asterixis is also characteristic of liver failure and uremia, and occasionally it is observed in other metabolic disorders.) The syndrome of hypercapnia is apt to be mistaken for brain tumor, a confusional psychosis of nondescript type, or a chronic extrapyramidal syndrome causing myoclonus or chorea.

HYPOGLYCEMIC ENCEPHALOPATHY (See also Chaps. 319 and 320) This condition is a frequent and important cause of episodic confusion, convulsions, coma, and sometimes of hemiparesis and other focal neurologic signs. The essential biochemical abnormality is a critical lowering of the blood glucose concentration to less than 1.4 mmol/L (25 mg/dL) (lower in infants), which, if it lasts for many minutes, leads to exhaustion of cerebral glucose reserve. As cerebral oxidation proceeds without exogenous glucose, the lipid and protein components of neurons are metabolized, and irreversible damage occurs. The severely hypoglycemic patient becomes deeply comatose before permanent damage occurs. Consequently prompt treatment is important.

Etiology The most common causes of hypoglycemic encephalopathy are (1) accidental or deliberate overdose of insulin or an oral antidiabetic agent, (2) islet cell, insulin-secreting tumor of the pancreas or retroperitoneal sarcoma, (3) ethanol ingestion, (4) acute, nonicteric hepatic encephalopathy of childhood (Reye's syndrome), and (5) an idiopathic syndrome occurring in the neonatal period. In the past, hypoglycemic encephalopathy was a frequent complication of "insulin shock" therapy of schizophrenia.

Clinical manifestations As the concentration of blood glucose decreases to about 1.7 mmol/L (30 mg/dL), the initial symptoms appear—nervousness, hunger, flushed facies, headache, palpitation, anxiety, sweating, and trembling—and these gradually give way to confusion, drowsiness, focal neurologic signs, and occasionally excitement or overactivity. In the next stage, forced sucking, grasping, motor restlessness, muscular spasms, and finally decerebrate rigidity occur, in that sequence. Myoclonic twitching and convulsions may develop in some patients. Blood levels of approximately 0.6 mmol/L (10 mg/dL) are associated with deep coma, dilatation of the pupils, pallor, shallow respirations, bradycardia, and hypotonicity of limb musculature—the so-called medullary phase of hypoglycemia. If glucose is administered before the medullary phase is reached, the patient is restored to normal within a few minutes, retracing the aforementioned steps in reverse order. Once the medullary phase appears, and particularly if it persists for a time before the hypoglycemia is corrected, neurologic recovery is delayed for a period of days or weeks and may be incomplete.

A huge dose of insulin that produces severe hypoglycemia, even of relatively brief duration (30 to 60 min), is more dangerous than a series of less severe hypoglycemic episodes from smaller doses of insulin, possibly because in the former the counterregulation mechanisms are likely to be less effective. In this situation massive amounts of glucose may have to be infused in order to maintain plasma glucose levels in the normal range (see Chap. 320).

Pathology The major *neuropathologic effect* is on the cerebral cortex; nerve cells degenerate and are replaced by microgliocytes and astrocytes. The distribution of lesions is similar though not identical to that in hypoxic encephalopathy (the cerebellar cortex is relatively spared in hypoglycemic encephalopathy). The sequelae of the two disorders are also much alike.

Episodes of chronic hypoglycemia may give rise to two other syndromes, both relatively uncommon. One, termed *subacute hypoglycemia,* is characterized by drowsiness and lethargy, diminution in psychomotor activity, deterioration of social behavior, and confusion. Oral or intravenous glucose immediately alleviates the symptoms. In the other, *more chronic syndrome,* there is gradual deterioration of intellectual function, raising the question of a presenile dementia, and in some reported instances there have been tremor, chorea, rigidity, cerebellar ataxia, and rarely signs of lower motor neuron involvement ("hypoglycemic amyotrophy"). These subacute and chronic forms of hypoglycemia have been observed with islet cell hyperplasia or tumor, carcinoma of the stomach, fibrous mesothelioma, carcinoma of the cecum, and hepatoma.

Differential diagnosis The major clinical differences between hypoglycemia and hypoxia are in the clinical setting and mode of evolution of the neurologic disorder. Hypoglycemia usually disturbs cerebral function more slowly than hypoxia, over a period of 30 to 60 min rather than in a few seconds or minutes. The recovery phase and sequelae of the two conditions are much the same. *Recurrent hypoglycemia,* as occurs with an islet cell tumor, may masquerade for some time as an episodic confusional psychosis or convulsive illness, and diagnosis awaits a period of demonstrably low blood glucose or hyperinsulinism (see Chap. 320).

Correction of the hypoglycemia at the earliest moment is the obvious therapy. It is not known whether hypothermia or other measures will increase the safety period in hypoglycemia or alter the outcome.

HYPERGLYCEMIC COMA Two hyperglycemic syndromes occur, mainly in the diabetic: (1) hyperglycemia with ketoacidosis and

(2) hyperosmolar nonketotic hyperglycemia. These are described in Chap. 319.

ACUTE HEPATIC ENCEPHALOPATHY Chronic hepatic insufficiency with portacaval shunting of blood is often punctuated by episodes of stupor, coma, and other neurologic symptoms, a state referred to as hepatic coma or portal-systemic encephalopathy. Also, hereditary hyperammonemic syndromes of infancy may lead to episodic coma with or without seizures. A special type of nonicteric hepatic encephalopathy (Reye's syndrome) occurs in children, presenting as acute brain swelling, in conjunction with rapid enlargement of the liver, fine droplets of fat in hepatocytes, high serum aspartate aminotransferase (AST, SGOT) and other liver enzymes, and very high levels of serum ammonia (see Chap. 256).

Clinical features The central feature of acute hepatic encephalopathy in the adult is a derangement of consciousness, presenting first as mental confusion with increased or decreased psychomotor activity, followed by progressive drowsiness, stupor, and coma. The confusional state that occurs before coma intervenes is frequently combined with characteristic lapses of sustained muscle contraction (asterixis). The EEG becomes abnormal during the earliest stages of the confusional state. Paroxysms of bilaterally synchronous delta waves, characteristically triphasic and prominent in the frontal regions, are at first interspersed with alpha activity and later, as the coma deepens, displace all normal activity. A variable, fluctuating rigidity of the trunk and limbs, grimacing, suck and grasp reflexes, exaggeration or asymmetry of tendon reflexes, Babinski signs, and focal or generalized seizures round out the clinical picture.

The syndrome usually evolves over a period of days to weeks and often terminates fatally. At times it does not advance beyond the stage of drowsiness and confusion with asterixis and EEG changes. This relatively mild form needs to be differentiated from other forms of acute confusional psychosis and delirium. If the metabolic disorder persists for months and years, a mild dementia and a disorder of posture and movement may gradually appear (grimacing, tremor, dysarthria, ataxia of gait, choreoathetosis), and the condition must then be distinguished from other dementing and extrapyramidal syndromes (see further on in this chapter).

Pathology and pathogenesis The striking *neuropathologic finding* in patients who die in a state of hepatic coma is a diffuse increase in the number and size of the protoplasmic astrocytes (Alzheimer type II astrocytes) in the deep layers of the cerebral cortex and in the lenticular nuclei, with little or no alteration in the nerve cells or other parenchymal elements.

The *pathogenesis* of hepatic encephalopathy is not fully understood. The most plausible theory relates it to an abnormality of nitrogen metabolism, wherein ammonia and/or other amines, which are formed in the bowel by the action of urease-containing organisms on dietary protein and are carried to the liver in the portal circulation, fail to be converted into urea, either because of hepatocellular disease or portal-systemic shunting of blood, or both. As a result, these substances reach the systemic circulation, where they interfere with cerebral metabolism in some obscure way. Other theories of causation have been discussed in Chap. 254 and have recently been reviewed by Zieve and by Cooper and Plum.

Treatment Despite an incomplete understanding of the genesis of hepatic coma, the most effective means of treating this disorder consists of restriction of dietary protein; mechanical cleansing of the colon; oral administration of antibiotics that suppress or eliminate urease-producing organisms in the bowel; and the use of lactulose, an inert sugar that acidifies the colonic contents. Additional methods of treatment, the practicality of which remain to be established, are discussed in Chap. 254.

In acute hepatitis, delirious, confusional, and comatose states also occur, but their mechanisms are not understood. Blood ammonia levels are usually elevated but of unclear significance, because of other associated metabolic abnormalities.

CHRONIC HEPATIC ENCEPHALOPATHY (ACQUIRED HEPATOCEREBRAL DEGENERATION) Clinical manifestations Patients who survive an episode or several episodes of hepatic coma are occasionally left with residual neurologic abnormalities, such as tremor of the head or arms, asterixis, grimacing, choreatic twitching of the limbs, dysarthria, ataxia of gait, or impairment of intellectual function, and these symptoms may worsen with repeated attacks of stupor and coma. In other patients with hepatic failure, these neurologic abnormalities become manifest in the absence of discrete episodes of hepatic coma. In either event, patients thus afflicted deteriorate neurologically over a period of months or years. As the condition evolves, a chronic characteristic dysarthria, mild ataxia, wide-based, unsteady gait, and choreoathetosis, mainly of the face, neck, and shoulders, are joined in a common syndrome. Mental function is slowly altered—a simple dementia with lack of concern and indifference to the illness evolves. A coarse rhythmic tremor of the arms, appearing with certain sustained postures, mild corticospinal tract signs, and diffuse EEG abnormalities complete the clinical picture. Other less frequent signs are muscular rigidity, grasp reflexes, tremor in repose, nystagmus, asterixis, and action or intention myoclonus. Many of the neurologic abnormalities that occur as part of acute hepatic encephalopathy may also be observed in patients with chronic hepatocerebral degeneration, the only difference being that the abnormalities are evanescent in the former and irreversible in the latter.

The chronic cerebral symptoms, like the transient ones, may occur with all varieties of chronic liver disease. Portacaval shunts are always present; jaundice, ascites, and esophageal varices are manifest in most of the cases.

Pathology Chronic hepatocerebral degeneration, like acute and subacute hepatic encephalopathy, is characterized by a widespread hyperplasia of protoplasmic astrocytes in the deep layers of the cerebral and cerebellar cortices as well as in the thalamic and lenticular nuclei and many other nuclear structures of the brainstem. In addition, in the chronic disease, medullated fibers and nerve cells are destroyed in the affected areas, and polymicrocavitation is prominent at the corticomedullary junction, in the striatum (particularly in the superior pole of the putamen), and in the cerebellar white matter. Protoplasmic astrocytic nuclei contain periodic acid Schiff (PAS)–positive glycogen granules. Nerve cells may appear swollen and chromatolyzed, accounting for the so-called Opalski cells. The similarity of these lesions to those observed in the familial form of hepatocerebral disease (Wilson's disease) suggests a common hepatogenesis.

UREMIC ENCEPHALOPATHY Episodic confusion and stupor and other neurologic symptoms may accompany any form of severe renal disease. In addition, a number of neurologic syndromes complicate chronic hemodialysis and kidney transplantation. Chronic polyneuropathy, the most common neurologic complication of renal failure, is discussed in Chap. 363.

Acute uremic encephalopathy The initial cerebral symptoms attributable to uremia consist of apathy, fatigue, inattentiveness, and irritability; later, confusion, disturbances of sensory perception, hallucinations, and stupor supervene. The later symptoms are practically always associated with twitching of the muscles and myoclonic jerks, and the patient may convulse.

Uremic encephalopathy, if associated with irreversible and progressive renal disease, can only be managed with dialysis or renal transplantation (see Chap. 225). Convulsions, which occur in about one-third of cases, often preterminally, respond to relatively low plasma concentrations of phenytoin and phenobarbital.

The brains of patients with uremic encephalopathy and the twitch-convulsive syndrome show hyperplasia of protoplasmic astrocytes in some cases but never to the degree observed in hepatic encephalopathy. Cerebral edema is notably absent. Restoration of renal function corrects the neurologic syndrome, attesting to a biochemical rather than a structural abnormality. Whether this is caused by the retention of organic acids, elevation of phosphate in the CSF, or by the action of other toxins has never been settled.

"Disequilibrium syndrome" and dialysis encephalopathy These terms refer to syndromes that commonly complicate hemodialysis or peritoneal dialysis. The *disequilibrium syndrome* is characterized by headaches, nausea, muscular cramps, nervous irritability, agitation, drowsiness, and convulsions. The headache develops in approximately 70 percent of patients, while the other symptoms are observed in 5 to 10 percent, usually in those undergoing rapid dialysis or in the early stages of a dialysis program. The symptoms tend to occur in the third to fourth hour of dialysis and last for several hours. Sometimes the symptoms appear 8 to 48 h after completing dialysis (see Chap. 225).

Dialysis encephalopathy or *dialysis dementia* is an uncommon complication of chronic hemodialysis. It begins with stuttering and dysarthria, coupled with a predominantly motor aphasia, to which are added facial and generalized myoclonus, focal and generalized seizures, personality changes and psychotic episodes, intellectual decline, progressive aphasic disorder, and EEG abnormalities. The latter consist of bisynchronous, predominantly frontal or multifocal bursts of slow wave discharges, associated with spikes and sharp waves. The CSF is usually normal. At first these symptoms are intermittent, occurring during or immediately after dialysis and lasting for only a few hours, but gradually they become more persistent and eventually permanent. Once established, the syndrome is usually steadily progressive over a 1- to 15-month period (average survival of 6 months in 42 cases analyzed by Lederman and Henry). A few patients have a waxing and waning course and survive for several years. In some patients the myoclonus and seizures subside for several months under the influence of clonazepam or diazepam.

The neuropathologic changes are subtle and consist of a mild microcavitation of the upper layers of the cerebral cortex. Although the changes are diffuse, the left (dominant) hemisphere is affected more than the right, and the left frontotemporal operculum more than other parts of the cortex (Winkelman). The predominant affection of the operculum would explain the striking disturbance of speech and language. Alfrey and his associates found that the cerebral gray matter of patients who died with dialysis encephalopathy contained a much greater amount of aluminum than analogous tissue from dialysis patients without encephalopathy. The aluminum was derived from both the dialysate and orally administered aluminum gels. The concept that dialysis encephalopathy represented a form of aluminum intoxication was supported by the observations that (1) the frequency of dialysis dementia was related to the concentrations of aluminum in the dialysate and (2) deionization of the water used in the dialysate prevented the occurrence of new cases. The possibility that other trace elements contribute to the syndrome has not been excluded.

Kidney transplantation is associated with an increased risk of developing primary cerebral lymphoma, Wernicke's encephalopathy, and central pontine myelinolysis. Systemic fungal infections are common at autopsy in patients who have had renal transplants and long periods of immunosuppressive treatment, and in some of these patients there is involvement of the central nervous system. *Cryptococcus, Listeria, Aspergillus, Candida, Nocardia,* and *Histoplasma* are the usual organisms. Other central nervous system infections that complicate transplantation are toxoplasmosis and cytomegalic inclusion disease.

ENCEPHALOPATHIES DUE TO ELECTROLYTE AND ENDOCRINE DISTURBANCES   Brief reference to these important groups of metabolic encephalopathies is given here. More detailed accounts are found in the cross-referenced chapters.

Metabolic acidosis [(arterial pH<7.30, P_{CO_2}<4.7 kPa (<35 mmHg), HCO_3<10 mmol/L)] due to diabetes mellitus, renal failure, lactic acidosis, or poisoning with an acid substance produces a syndrome characterized by drowsiness, stupor, and coma with dry skin and Kussmaul breathing, described in Chap. 51. Extreme degrees of *hyperosmolality* of the blood may develop in the course of diabetes mellitus [blood glucose>22 mmol/L (>400 μg/dL)] and in extreme hypernatremia, resulting in either case in tremulousness, convulsions, and coma. In some instances the movement disorder resembles chorea or the myoclonic twitching of uremia. *Hypokalemia* is characterized by extreme muscular weakness associated with a stuporous-confu-

sional state, and sometimes by striking changes in personality and behavior (see Chap. 51).

Hyponatremia, usually with water intoxication, is another cause of episodic coma, especially in infants. Among the many causes, the syndrome of inappropriate secretion of antidiuretic hormone (SIADH) is of special importance, since it commonly complicates neurologic diseases of many types—head trauma, bacterial meningitis and encephalitis, cerebral infarction and subarachnoid hemorrhage, neoplasm, and sometimes Guillain-Barré disease (see Chap. 315). The diagnosis of SIADH should be suspected in any critically ill neurologic or neurosurgical patient who excretes urine that is hypertonic relative to the plasma. As the hyponatremia develops, there is a decrease in alertness, which progresses through stages of confusion to coma, often with convulsions. Lack of recognition of this state may allow the serum Na^+ to fall to dangerously low levels, 100 mmol/L or lower. Treatment is described in Chap. 315. Replacement with intravenous NaCl in severe cases must be done cautiously because vigorous and rapid correction of severe hyponatremia has been incriminated in the pathogenesis of central pontine myelinolysis (CPM) and related brainstem, cerebellar, and cerebral lesions (Laureno). Ayus and colleagues emphasize the risks of persistent severe hyponatremia and suggest the following therapeutic guidelines: serum Na^+ above 120 mmol/L does not require immediate correction. If Na^+ is >105 mmol/L, it can be safely corrected to a level of 125 to 130 mmol/L at a rate of administration of Na^+ of 2 mmol/h. If serum Na^+ is less than 105 mmol/L, it is corrected by 20 mmol/L at a rate of 2 mmol/h and then permitted to return slowly to normal. More prospective studies are needed to determine the safest method of correcting severe hyponatremia.

In children more than adults, cholera being an exception, extremely *severe diarrhea* may be attended by an encephalopathy. Irritability, weakness, headache, seizures, stupor, and coma may develop over a period of 2 to 3 days and carry a grave prognosis unless promptly relieved. Presumably this is a metabolic encephalopathy due to loss of fluids and electrolytes and can be corrected by their replacement.

In the *endocrine encephalopathies* the clinical phenomena are even more abstruse. Confusional states may be combined with agitation, hallucinations, delusions, anxiety, and depression. And the duration of the illness may be measured in weeks and months, rather than days. Derangement of higher nervous function may follow the *administration of ACTH or glucocorticoids,* and the same symptoms have been reported in *Cushing's disease* (see Chap. 317). The neurologic manifestations of *thyrotoxicosis* are particularly elusive. Allusions to thyrotoxic psychosis are widely recorded in the medical literature; mental confusion, seizures, manic or depressive attacks, delusions, and chorea occur in various combinations with muscular weakness and atrophy, periodic paralysis, and myasthenia (see Chap. 316). Treatment of the hyperthyroidism gradually restores the patient to a normal mental state. *Myxedematous patients* may show slow mentation and depression, and in a small proportion there is a major change in cerebral function, taking the form of inattentiveness, apathy, and drowsiness or extreme somnolence. These symptoms can usually be reversed within weeks to months by thyroid medication. The association of myxedema and cerebellar ataxia is well documented, but the neuropathologic basis of this disorder remains unclear. In *hyperparathyroidism,* when the serum calcium levels reach 3.7 mmol/L (15 mg/dL) or higher, the patient sinks into a quiet state of inattentiveness, lethargy, and confusion. Stupor, coma, and death may be caused by extreme degrees of hypercalcemia such as occur occasionally in cases of hypervitaminosis D and metastatic tumors of the bones. Chronic *hypoparathyroidism,* either idiopathic or following thyroid or parathyroid resection may rarely give rise to intracranial calcifications and an extrapyramidal motor syndrome. Adrenal insufficiency may be attended by episodic confusion, stupor, or coma, without special identifying features (see Chap. 317).

The term *pancreatic encephalopathy* describes a syndrome of agitation and confusion, sometimes with hallucinations and clouding of consciousness, dysarthria, and changing rigidity of the limbs, in association with acute pancreatic disease. The status of this entity is uncertain. A uniform neuropathologic change has not been discerned. We agree with Pallis and Lewis who suggest that before such a diagnosis can be seriously entertained in a patient with acute pancreatitis, one should exclude delirium tremens, the cerebral effects of shock, renal or hepatic failure, hypoglycemia, diabetic acidosis, hyperosmolality, hypokalemia, hypo- or hypercalcemia, any one of which may complicate the underlying disease(s).

Lactic acidosis can cause encephalopathy in patients who undergo jejunoileostomy for treatment of morbid obesity. Such patients report episodes of confusion, ataxia, and slurred speech. D-Lactate, an isomer not normally found in the blood and a product of intestinal bacteria, is present in serum, urine, and stool in these patients. D-Lactate causes encephalopathy by interfering with pyruvate metabolism. Diagnosis is dependent upon recognition of metabolic acidosis associated with hyperchloremia and measurement of elevated D-lactate (see Dahlquist; Cross). A more common cause of encephalopathy in patients with jejunoileal shunting is hepatic (see Chap. 72).

HEREDITARY METABOLIC DISEASES OF LATE ONSET

Inherited metabolic disorders affecting amino acid metabolism (Chaps. 334 and 335), lysosomal enzyme functions (Chap. 331), and cerebral lipids (Chap. 331) are generally rare and first become manifest during infancy or childhood. In this chapter are described a small number of hereditary metabolic disorders that may have their onset in late adolescence and adulthood and may present diagnostic problems because of the similarity of clinical presentation to other more common acquired and degenerative diseases of the nervous system. Noteworthy attributes of these diseases are their chronicity and progressive nature.

METACHROMATIC LEUKODYSTROPHY (See Chap. 331)   Probably the most common member of this category is *adult metachromatic leukodystrophy (MLD)*. While the majority of cases appear in early childhood, approximately 25 percent manifest their first symptoms after age 21. Cases among men outnumber those in women 2:1. The mode of inheritance is autosomal recessive in almost all instances. The onset is insidious, and the course is protracted, over 20 or more years.

Mental symptoms tend to dominate the clinical picture. Failing scholastic performance, forgetfulness, and irrationality occur early in the illness but may be obscured by peculiarities of personality, such as suspiciousness, delusional thinking, and bizarre actions. These latter qualities may raise the question of schizophrenia or immature ("borderline") personality development. Sooner or later a mild cerebellar ataxia presenting as awkwardness and falling, mild pyramidal signs, masked facies, and bizarre postures stamp the illness as neurologic. Eventually mental processes deteriorate to the point where the patient is helpless, demented, mute, incontinent, and bedfast.

Specific diagnostic tests include (1) the demonstration of a diminished arylsulfatase A activity in white blood cells, serum, and urine, (2) increased excretion of sulfatides in the urine, (3) slowed conduction velocity in nerves, and (4) deposits of metachromatic material in nerve biopsies. No treatment is available.

ADRENOLEUKODYSTROPHY   In this X-linked metabolic disorder, either adrenal insufficiency or cerebral symptoms may be the initial manifestation. The cerebral lesions may present as a homonymous hemianopsia, cortical blindness, hemiparesis, aphasia, or dementia. Usually the signs are asymmetric at first and progress intermittently. Relatively pure polyneuropathic and myelopathic forms have also been described. The diagnosis is usually made by the finding of a low blood cortisol level in a man with cerebrospinal demyelinating disease, although a purely spinal type, taking the form of a progressive spastic paraparesis, has been described in the heterozygote (female carrier). Increased urinary concentration of C22-

C26 fatty acids is diagnostic. Glucocorticoid replacement therapy helps the symptoms of adrenal insufficiency but has no effect on the neurologic disorders. The latter progress intermittently over a few years, and usually the outcome is fatal.

ADULT LIPID STORAGE DISEASES G_{M2} *gangliosidosis* (hexosaminidase A deficiency) has been observed in young adults. Many are from non-Jewish families, and males and females in the same generation are equally affected. Generalized seizures may mark the beginning of a cerebral disorder that later is evidenced by alterations of behavior and intellectual decline. A progressive ataxia and mild signs of corticospinal disease, the combination of which interferes with independent locomotion, clarifies the diagnosis. The fundi and visual function are normal in most cases, but typical cherry-red macular spots are seen occasionally. The liver and spleen are normal or slightly enlarged. The CSF protein is normal. CT scans of the brain reveal a modest ventricular enlargement. A slowly developing dementia, cerebellar ataxia, polymyoclonus, and failing vision may characterize the clinical picture in some cases. In yet others, the presenting syndrome has consisted of prominent motor neuron involvement accompanied by muscle cramps, suggesting a diagnosis of spinal muscular atrophy or amyotrophic lateral sclerosis (see Chap. 359). G_{M2} ganglioside is increased in tissue obtained by cerebral biopsy. Membranous cytoplasmic bodies are visualized by electron microscopy of rectal, appendicular, and cortical neurons. *Gaucher's* and *Niemann-Pick* diseases are yet other storage diseases that may present in adult life. (See Chap. 331.)

Ceroid lipofuscinosis   The Kufs type of *ceroid lipofuscinosis* is a lipid storage disease that only becomes evident in adolescence or early adult life. Usually the disease begins with mental deterioration, followed by seizures, ataxia, increasing rigidity, athetotic posturing, and corticospinal signs. Skin and conjunctival biopsies, examined by electron microscopy, show lipofuscin storage material in fibroblasts and endothelial cells.

SUBACUTE NECROTIZING ENCEPHALOMYELOPATHY (LEIGH'S DISEASE)   Some cases of this disease begin in adolescence and take the form of a progressive polymyoclonus with seizures and cerebellar ataxia and relatively mild impairment of intellectual function.

SUMMARY   These rare forms of hereditary metabolic diseases should be considered whenever an adolescent or young adult becomes demented, shows a psychiatric syndrome with decline in cognitive functions, has seizures (especially with polymyoclonus), failing vision, and cerebellar ataxia in combination with corticospinal signs or a progressive polyneuropathy.

REFERENCES

ADAMS RD, FOLEY JM: The neurological disorder associated with liver disease of the nervous system. Proc Assoc Res Nerv Ment Dis 32:198, 1953

———, VICTOR M: *Principles of Neurology*, 4th ed. New York, McGraw-Hill, 1989

ALFREY AC et al: The dialysis encephalopathy syndrome: Possible aluminum intoxication. N Engl J Med 294:184, 1976

AYUS JC et al: Treatment of symptomatic hyponatremia and its relation to brain damage: A prospective study. N Engl J Med 317:1190, 1987

BECK WS: Cobalamin and the nervous system. N Engl J Med 318:1752, 1988

BLASS JP, GIBSON GE: Abnormality of a thiamine-requiring enzyme in patients with Wernicke-Korsakoff syndrome. N Engl J Med 297:1367, 1977

BRAIN RESUSCITATION CLINICAL TRIAL I STUDY GROUP: Randomized clinical study of thiopental loading in comatose survivors of cardiac arrest. N Engl J Med 314:397, 1986

CARDINALE GJ et al: Effect of methylmalonyl coenzyme A: A metabolite which accumulates in vitamin B_{12} deficiency on fatty acid synthesis. J Biol Chem 245:3771, 1970

CARMEL R et al: Hereditary defect of cobalamin metabolism (*cblG* mutation) presenting as a neurologic disorder in adulthood. N Engl J Med 318:1738, 1988

CHARNESS ME et al: Ethanol and the nervous system: Medical Progress. N Engl J Med 321:442, 1989

COOPER AJL, PLUM F: Biochemistry and physiology of brain ammonia. Physiol Rev 67:440, 1987

CREMER GM et al: Myxedema and ataxia. Neurology 19:37, 1969

CROSS SA, CALLOWAY WC: D-Lactic acidosis and selected cerebellar ataxias. Mayo Clin Proc 59:202, 1984

DAHLQUIST NR et al: D-Lactic acidosis and encephalopathy after jejunoileostomy: Response to overfeeding and to fasting in humans. Mayo Clin Proc 59:141, 1984

—— et al: D-Lactic acidosis and encephalopathy after jejunoileostomy: Response to overfeeding and to fasting in humans. Mayo Clinic Proc 59:141, 1984

HARDING AE et al: Spinocerebellar degeneration associated with a selective defect of vitamin E absorption. N Engl J Med 313:32, 1985

KLATSKY AL et al: Alcohol consumption and blood pressure. N Engl J Med 296:1194, 1977

KOLODNY EH, BOUSTANY RM: Storage diseases of the reticuloendothelial system, in *Hematology of Infancy and Childhood*, 3d ed, D Nathan, F Oski (eds). Philadelphia, Saunders, 1986

LAURENO R: Central pontine myelinolysis following rapid correction of hyponatremia. Ann Neurol 13:232, 1983

LEDERMAN RS, HENRY CE: Progressive dialysis encephalopathy. Ann Neurol 4:199, 1978

LINDENBAUM J et al: Neuropsychiatric disorders caused by cobalamin deficiency in the absence of anemia or macrocytosis. N Engl J Med 318:1720, 1988

MCENTEE WJ, MAIR RG: Memory enhancement in Korsakoff's phychosis by clonidine: Further evidence for a nonadrenergic deficit. Ann Neurol 7:466, 1980

MARKS R, ROSE FC: *Hypoglycemia*. Oxford, Blackwell, 1965

MOSER HW et al: Adrenoleukodystrophy: Studies of the phenotype, genetics and biochemistry. Johns Hopkins Med J 147:217, 1980

NELSON JS et al: Progressive neuropathic lesions in vitamin E–deficient rhesus monkeys. J Neuropathol Exp Neurol 40:166, 1981

PALLIS CA, LEWIS PD: *The Neurology of Gastrointestinal Disease*. Philadelphia, Saunders, 1974

PINCUS JH: Folic acid deficiency. A cause of subacute combined system degeneration, in *Folic Acid in Neurology, Psychiatry, and Internal Medicine*, MI Botez, EH Reynolds (eds). New York, Raven, 1979, pp 427–433

PLUM F, POSNER JB: *Diagnosis of Stupor and Coma*, 3d ed. Philadelphia, Davis, 1980

POTTS AM: Tobacco amblyopia. Surv Ophthalmol 17:313, 1973

RASKIN NH, FISHMAN RA: Neurologic disorders in renal failure. N Engl J Med 294:143, 204, 1976

SAGE JI et al: Alcoholic myelopathy without substantial liver disease. A syndrome of progressive dorsal and lateral column dysfunction. Arch Neurol 41:999, 1984

SATYA-MURTI S et al: The spectrum of neurologic disorders from vitamin E deficiency. Neurology 36:917, 1986

SCHAUMBURG HH et al: Sensory neuropathy from pyridoxine abuse. A new megavitamin syndrome. N Engl J Med 309:445, 1983

SERDARU M et al: The clinical spectrum of alcoholic pellagra encephalopathy. Brain 111:829, 1988

SHIMOJYO S et al: Cerebral blood flow and metabolism in the Wernicke-Korsakoff syndrome. J Clin Invest 46:849, 1967

VICTOR M: Polyneuropathy due to nutrional deficiency and alcoholism, in *Peripheral Neuropathy*, 2d ed, PJ Dyck et al (eds). Philadelphia, Saunders, 1984, pp 1899–1940

——, ADAMS RD: On the etiology of the alcoholic neurologic diseases: With special reference to the role of nutrition. Am J Clin Nutr 9:379, 1961

—— et al: A restricted form of cerebellar degeneration occurring in alcoholic patients. Arch Neurol 1:577, 1959

—— et al: Deficiency amblyopia in the alcoholic patient: A clinicopathologic study. Arch Ophthalmol 64:1, 1960

—— et al: The acquired (nonwilsonian) type of chronic hepatocerebral degeneration. Medicine 44:345, 1965

—— et al: *The Wernicke-Korsakoff Syndrome, and Related Neurologic Disorders Due to Alcoholism and Malnutrition*. Philadelphia, Davis, 1989

WILKINSON DS, PROCKOP LD: Hypoglycemia: Effects on the nervous system, in *Handbook of Clinical Neurology*, PJ Vinken, BW Bruyn (eds). Amsterdam, North-Holland, 1976, vol 27, pp 53–78

WINKELMAN MD, RICANATI ES: Dialysis encephalopathy: Neuropathologic aspects. Hum Pathol 17:823, 1986

WITT ED, GOLDMAN-RAKIC PS: Intermittent thiamine deficiency in the rhesus monkey. I. Progression of neurological signs and neuranatomical lesions. Ann Neurol 13:376, 1983

ZIEVE L: Pathogenesis of hepatic encephalopathy. Metab Brain Dis 2:147, 1987

and the skin, *developmental disorders principally affecting the nervous system*, and *neuroskeletal disorders*.

NEUROCUTANEOUS SYNDROMES

A large number of neurocutaneous disorders (also *phakomatoses* from Greek *phakos*, "lentil," "mole," or "freckle") are expressed in a patchy fashion in affected tissues. The most commonly encountered of these, reviewed below, are transmitted by autosomal dominant inheritance. The chromosomal linkage group has been (provisionally) identified for four of these dominantly transmitted forms (Table 358-1).

NEUROFIBROMATOSIS (VON RECKLINGHAUSEN'S DISEASE) The dominating feature of this disorder is the neurofibroma, a tumor that arises from the Schwann cells and fibroblasts of the neurilemmal sheath of the peripheral nerve. Two nonallelic heritable forms are now recognized. *Neurofibromatosis type 1*, carried on chromosome 17, is the classic autosomal dominant neurocutaneous disorder in which tumors involving the sheaths of peripheral nerves are associated with characteristic cream-brown cutaneous lesions (café-au-lait spots). The neurofibromas themselves are only occasionally symptomatic, as when they result in entrapment of a nerve root at the intervertebral foramina. The disorder may be associated with other tumors of the central nervous system including optic glioma, glioblastoma, and meningioma, and rarely with pheochromocytoma (see also Chap. 318). Other associated aberrations include hamartomas of the iris (Lisch nodules), freckling concentrated around the nipples and in the axillae, stenosis of the aqueduct of Sylvius, leading to obstructive hydrocephalus, and mild degrees of mental retardation, related presumably to developmental abnormalities of the cerebral cortex. *Neurofibromatosis type 2*, carried on chromosome 22, is also an autosomal dominant disorder in which neurofibromas involve the acoustic nerves exclusively and usually bilaterally. The acoustic neurinomas may produce deafness and other symptoms and signs of a cerebellopontine angle lesion (see Chap. 353). They may also be associated with meningiomas and astrocytomas.

TUBEROUS SCLEROSIS (BOURNEVILLE'S DISEASE) In this condition, cutaneous lesions of multiple types are associated with malformation and tumors of the central nervous system. Mental deficiency, though not invariable, may be profound and associated with a remarkably intractable seizure disorder. The earliest lesions to emerge are leaf-shaped hypopigmented spots ("white spots") scattered over the trunk and limbs. These are seen most clearly under ultraviolet light (Wood's lamp). The adenoma sebaceum, a hallmark of the disorder, is an angiofibroma, distributed in a butterfly pattern over the cheeks, chin, and forehead. The individual adenomas vary in size from 0.1 to 1.0 cm and are elevated and pinkish or pinkish-yellow in color. The skin over the lumbosacral region of the back

---

358 NEUROCUTANEOUS SYNDROMES AND OTHER DEVELOPMENTAL DISORDERS OF THE CENTRAL NERVOUS SYSTEM[1]

VERNE S. CAVINESS, JR.

Developmental disorders that involve the nervous system and are encountered in adult life are the emphasis of this chapter. The discussion is arranged according to broad phenotypic groupings, namely, *neurocutaneous syndromes* in which abnormalities of the nervous system are associated with abnormalities of osseous structures

[1] This is in part the revision of the chapter in the 11th edition by GR DeLong and RD Adams.

TABLE 358-1 Chromosomal locations of dominant mutant genes in the phakomatoses*

Disorder	Chromosome	Phenotypic signature	Mental retardation	Tumors
NF-1	17	Café-au-lait spots, neuro-fibromas	Occasionally	Multiple types: CNS, PNS, viscera
NF-2	22	Bilateral acoustic neuromas	No	Acoustic neuro-mas; other CNS
TS	9	White spots, adenoma sebacea	Frequent	CNS: tubers, gliomas; viscera
VH-L	3	Cerebral he-mangioblas-tomas, reti-nal angiomas	No	Angiomas of vis-cera; renal cell carcinomas

* NF-1 and NF-2 are neurofibromatosis types 1 and 2; TS, tuberosclerosis; VH-L, von Hippel-Lindau; CNS and PNS, central and peripheral nervous systems.

may be marked by a rough thickening which is yellowish in color like sharkskin or pigskin (shagreen patch). The cutaneous lesions may provide the earliest clue to the causation of mental retardation or infantile epilepsy. Rhabdomyoma of the heart and tumorous malformations (angiolciomyomas) of the kidney, liver, adrenal glands, and pancreas are also characteristic of this disorder. The disorder can be inherited as an autosomal dominant trait: linkage studies with restriction fragment length polymorphisms (RFLPs) in some pedigrees have located the mutant gene to chromosome 9.

In the brain multiple nodular tumors, composed of abnormal neurons and glial cells, often lie in the plane of the cerebral cortex itself. These can be diagnosed accurately in T2-weighted magnetic resonance scans. If calcified, they may also be visualized by CT scans or skull x-rays. Calcified nodules occur in brain subependymal regions adjacent to the ventricles. If large, they may obstruct the foramen of Monro, causing a unilateral or bilateral hydrocephalus. Masses of subependymal glial tissue forming nodules are likened to "candle gutterings" on the walls of the ventricles. The electroencephalogram is usually abnormal but without specific pattern. The only treatment is symptomatic. When severe epilepsy and mental retardation are present, prognosis for life beyond the third decade is poor. Death is usually due to seizures, associated tumors, or intercurrent diseases.

CEREBELLORETINAL HEMANGIOBLASTOMATOSIS (VON HIPPEL–LINDAU SYNDROME)

This syndrome of retinal and cerebellar hemangioblastoma is inherited as an autosomal dominant disorder (encoded on chromosome 3) (see Table 358-1). The retinal lesions are capillary angiomas, usually multiple, causing progressive loss of vision. The cerebellar hemangioblastomas, which may be multiple, are slowly growing cystic tumors. These may also occur in the medulla or in the spinal cord where they may be associated with a syrinx. Enlargement of cerebellar tumor may lead to obstructive hydrocephalus with headache, papilledema, and cerebellar ataxia. Only rarely do tumors become symptomatic before adolescence, but the diagnosis must be considered in all adults with a cerebellar tumor. Tumors of the central nervous system are a part of a constellation including agiomas and cysts of the liver, pancreas, and kidneys and tumors of the epididymis and kidney. The latter may be lethal. Pheochromocytomas may occur in this as in other kinds of phakomatoses (see Chap. 318). An association with renal cell carcinoma led to localization of the mutant gene on chromosome 3. Polycythemia, presumably the consequence of ectopic production of erythropoietin by the hemangioblastoma, may disappear after excision of the tumor.

ENCEPHALOTRIGEMINAL SYNDROME (STURGE-WEBER DISEASE)

Capillary or cavernous hemangiomas, within but not always limited to the cutaneous distribution of the trigeminal nerve, co-occur with a predominantly venous hemangioma that can spread through subjacent leptomeninges. The adjacent cerebral cortex is progressively destroyed, perhaps as a consequence of interruption of local blood flow. The first neurologic symptom is usually a focal seizure on the side opposite the skin lesion. Sensorimotor paralysis or permanent visual field defect, the most common sequelae, may be either of sudden or of insidious onset with progression. In time calcium is deposited within the area of involved cortex and may be visualized as a characteristic "railroad track" in conventional x-rays or CT scans. If the skin lesion is within the area of supply of the ophthalmic division of the trigeminal nerve, the occipital lobes are more commonly involved. A facial nevus is more often associated with involvement of the parietal and frontal lobes. The intracranial and cutaneous lesions may also occur separately. The disease is usually sporadic; a familial occurrence consistent with autosomal dominant inheritance is exceptional. Deeply situated arteriovenous malformations rarely coexist. Blindness in the eye on the side of the nevus is nearly always due to glaucoma. Most patients with this malformation survive for many years, often with mental defects and hemiparesis.

Hemangioma of the trunk or upper or lower extremity may be associated with a spinal cord vascular malformation (Klippel-Tren- aunay syndrome) and with hypertrophy of the involved extremity. The cord lesion may cause infarction in nervous tissue, producing a spinal sensorimotor paralysis. Surgical exploration and decompression are seldom beneficial.

DEVELOPMENTAL DISORDERS OF THE CENTRAL NERVOUS SYSTEM

Developmental disorders expressed largely or even exclusively as disturbance of neurologic functions afflict a substantial portion of the population. Certain of these, particularly when neurologic disability is severe, are complicated secondarily by restricted general somatic growth, articulatory contractures, and general medical disorders resulting from limited mobility and poor personal care. The discussion will be focused upon developmental disorders expressed predominantly as malfunction of the forebrain, particularly the cerebral hemispheres. Three general syndromes emerge: mental retardation, where the disability is predominantly in the domains of cognition, language, and memory; autism, where socialization is the prominently defective characteristic; and "cerebral palsy," where disability largely relates to motor function.

MENTAL RETARDATION Mental retardation specifies an IQ less than 70 resulting from a pathophysiologic process affecting the cerebrum during the developmental period. If IQ is normal, the diagnosis is not applied to more restricted learning disabilities including dyslexia, incompetence with mathematics, and a variety of developmental language disorders. Mental retardation, even if it is the predominant disability, is often conjoined with a complex of other disabilities which include disordered motor function, abnormalities of special senses, such as hearing and sight, and a variety of medical problems.

Etiology and pathogenesis The specific cause of abnormal cerebral development cannot be defined for as many as half of all mentally retarded persons. For many, the disorder is familial and may be due to either single-gene defects or polygenic inheritance. Among the remaining half in whom the cause can be identified, the recognized causes include the 21 trisomy and fragile X syndromes and intrauterine exposure to alcohol (see Chap. 7). Collectively these few disorders are responsible for a third of mental retardation in this country. Prevalence for each approximates 1:1000 live births. Other identifiable causes include encephaloclastic processes, such as infection, hypoxia-ischemia, trauma, and hydrocephalus, occurring either before or after birth. Intrauterine exposures to infectious and pharmacologic teratogenic agents are also common, including exposure to HIV infection or to cocaine and other "recreational" drugs. Malnutrition, hypothyroidism, and other metabolic disorders may also cause mental retardation if the conditions occur during intrauterine and postnatal life. Among the general medical conditions is a substantial list of heritable disorders of metabolism. The list is long and includes enzymopathies relating to amino acid, carbohydrate, organic acid, and lipid processing such as phenylketonuria (see Chap. 334), galactosemia (see Chap. 337), proprionic aciduria, and disorders of lysosomal enzyme function such as neuronal ceroid lipofuscinosis, the gangliosidoses, and the mucopolysaccharidoses (see also Chaps. 331 and 333).

Many chromosomal and single-gene disorders of metabolism may be diagnosed prenatally. Where diagnosis is made postnatally, it may be critical to do so expeditiously in the case of treatable CNS infections and correctable or manageable metabolic disorders, i.e., cretinism or phenylketonuria. During the first 2 years of life diagnosis and intervention are also critical for malnutrition, a state usually coupled to other socioeconomic deprivations. These deprivations may result in retarded brain growth and mental development that persist into adult life. If, however, such children are "rescued" by refeeding and placement in a stimulating and supportive environment, the effects of early malnutrition are largely reversible, and normal mental development can result.

Clinical manifestations The defining characteristic of this domain of cerebral disturbance, subnormal IQ, is an inexact but a meaningful predictor of behavioral capabilities. Severely retarded children, those with IQs of less than 20, are virtually unable to look after themselves. Often they never sit up, walk, or stand. Language is rudimentary; at most a few words are understood and uttered. They exhibit only primitive emotional reactions, and sphincteric control may never be achieved. Motor mannerisms such as rhythmic rocking, rolling, head banging, and bouncing movements are typical and often are accompanied by bleating sounds and squeals. Music may encourage rhythmic movements. The physical appearance may be unremarkable. However, if the insult to the brain occurs in utero or early in postnatal life, a variety of physical deformities, particularly microcephaly and variable degrees of joint contracture, are common in this group.

If the mental defect is less pronounced, that is, there is an IQ of 20 to 50, and if specific motor defects do not coexist, then sitting, walking, and speech are acquired, often after a delay. The existence of a cerebral defect may be noted for the first time when the child fails to speak normally during the second and third year of life and seems not to be able to learn the usual household tasks and play activities as well as other children. However, delay in speech development by itself is not a mark of mental retardation, for some children who are intelligent and show remarkable talent in communicating by gesture are slow in talking. Also the deaf child may be singled out by indifference to noise and reduced vocalization but otherwise normal development. Toilet training also may be difficult to accomplish in the retarded child, but again it may be delayed in an otherwise normal child.

The least severely retarded of these individuals (IQ of 50 to 70) grow and develop, in many ways not differently than the normal child during the early years of life. Their abilities and adaptations merge imperceptibly with those of the general population. Often there is neither somatic nor other specific neurologic abnormality. That such a child is handicapped may not be evident until it is apparent that scholastic pursuits are relatively unsuccessful. There may be manifest inability to learn with poor school progress, and the child with an IQ of 60 to 70 is generally unable to pass the sixth grade. Vocational training is of more value than other types of education. The mildly retarded child may be able to acquire useful occupational skills and to work under careful supervision.

Whereas IQ is a useful index of competence, the clinical and behavioral characteristics of individuals with retarded development cannot be adequately described by this single attribute. In particular, social competence, which may vary in ways that are not predicted by IQ, may largely determine the life expectations of retarded children. This aspect of behavior should be an organizing theme for education and training. Some mentally retarded persons are pleasant and amiable and achieve a satisfactory social adjustment. At the opposite extreme is the poorly understood syndrome of autism, associated with varying degrees of retardation, in which the child or older person fails to manifest any kind of interpersonal, social contact (see "Autism," below). Many retarded individuals are dull, apathetic, and underactive. Others display an incessant hyperactivity, characterized by a very short attention span, a restless inquisitive searching of the environment, and low frustration tolerance; they may be destructive or recklessly fearless and may seem strangely impervious to injury. As with the mentally normal but hyperactive, inattentive child, improvement in these children can often be achieved by using stimulants and desipramine.

Three specific disorders associated with mental retardation deserve separate description.

Fetal alcohol syndrome The fetal alcohol syndrome may be the most prevalent cause of defective cerebral development in industrialized nations. Its estimated frequency in the United States, 1:700 live births, is probably less than the actual occurrence and is even greater than the occurrences of trisomy 21 (Down's syndrome) and the fragile X syndrome. The fully developed disorder includes marked growth retardation, microcephaly, and cardiac valvular lesions. Characteristic facial features include hypotelorism, small palpebral fissures, small nasal bridge, and reduction of the vermillion border of the upper lip. Mental retardation may be profound. However, the less severely affected may have IQs in the normal range but be significantly disabled by attention deficit disorder with hyperactivity and learning disabilities. The severity of the disorder is related to alcohol dose, and the threshold for clinical expression appears to lie in the ingestion of 30 to 60 mL of absolute alcohol equivalent per day. Additional risk factors including exposure to multiple drugs or venereally transmitted infectious agents may interact with alcohol abuse. The potential risk to successive offspring is obvious.

Fragile X syndrome The fragile X chromosome anomaly is a phenotype that combines dysmorphic somatic characteristics with mental retardation. Cytogenetic analysis shows constriction of the terminal segment of the long arm of the affected X chromosome, and the fragile link is subject to breakage. Expression of the anomaly in standard tissue culture conditions is enhanced by folate deficiency and other modifications. The characteristic phenotype is expressed in approximately 80 percent of males and in 35 percent of females carrying a single affected X chromosome. It remains uncertain whether the chromosome anomaly is a determinant of, or simply marker for, the phenotypic anomalies. Stigmata include macroorchidism in males, possibly large ovaries in females, prognathism, and large everted ears. The skull is narrow and elongate. Mental retardation is usually mild to moderate and associated with dysphonic, sometimes echolalic speech. The association of the fragile X chromosome anomaly and autism in males (see below) has been estimated to be as high as 10 to 15 percent. A therapeutic response to treatment with folate has not been substantiated.

Down's syndrome (See Chap. 7) Down's syndrome accounts for about 1 percent of all mental retardation. Trisomy of chromosome 21 or translocation of parts of this chromosome is responsible for the disorder. Older mothers are more apt to have babies with Down's syndrome than are young mothers. The mean age of the mother is 37.

The degree of mental retardation in Down's syndrome varies from mild to severe and is associated with a characteristic facial appearance and small stature. Many stigmata can be recognized in the neonatal period. The head tends to be small and round, with sloping forehead. The ears are set low and are oval, with small lobules. The eyes slant slightly upward and outward owing to the presence of a medial epicanthal fold, which partly covers the angle of the palpebral fissure. The bridge of the nose is poorly developed. The mouth tends to hang open, and the tongue is usually enlarged, heavily fissured, and protruding. Gray-white specks of depigmentation are seen in the iris (Brushfield's spots). The little fingers are often short and curved inward (clinodactyly), owing to a hypoplastic middle phalanx. The hands are broad with a single transverse palmar crease. Lenticular opacities and congenital heart lesions (septal defects) are found in some cases. At birth these children are of average size, but at later periods of life they are characteristically small. The brain is of reduced weight with a relatively simple convolutional pattern. Of the patients who survive to puberty, many live to middle adult life and may develop a premature Alzheimer's type cerebral degeneration (onset in the majority by the age of 40) (see Chap. 359).

CRETINISM (See also Chap. 316) Cretinism and childhood hypothyroidism occur endemically in parts of the world where there is iodine deficiency and in infants everywhere with congenital disorders of thyroid function. The frequency is greater than that of phenylketonuria. For iodine deficiency to produce cretinism the mother must be lacking in iodine during the pregnancy, especially in the first trimester. Diagnosis rests with the clinical picture, for in the iodine-deficient state routine measures of thyroid function may be normal. Jaundice, umbilical hernia, noisy respirations, hypotonia, depression of reflexes, and lethargy are present at birth. Coarse facial features, large tongue, and constipation become manifest later. Among those with endemic cretinism, the neurologic abnormality consists of mental deficiency, deaf-mutism (or lesser degrees of hearing loss), and a combination of flexed posture with spasticity and rigidity of proximal limb musculature. These deficits persist throughout adult life.

AUTISM Autism is a mysterious and provocative condition. Long considered primarily psychiatric or a childhood form of schizophrenia, it is now generally thought to represent an organic defect in brain development characterized by failure to develop communicative language or other form of social communication. Some autistic persons often show motor and other skills far beyond that expected of a mentally retarded person. Often they are obsessively preoccupied with inanimate objects, such as lights, running water, or spinning objects. Most children with autism prove later to be retarded, and the ultimate level of disability depends largely on the IQ. Some gradually acquire language and may then exhibit certain exceptional talents, such as in mathematics (idiot savant). Upon reaching adult life they retain all the above characteristics. Not more than 1 in 20 improves significantly.

The etiology is unknown and there are likely to be multiple causes. A few detailed histopathologic studies identify abnormalities of forebrain limbic structures, and a reduction in volume of the midline region of the cerebellum is observed in CT and MR images. The abnormality of limbic structures is consistent with our understanding of the role of the medial temporal lobes in mediating language, affective, motivational, and social behavioral functions in human beings and also consistent with the finding that up to 30 percent of autistic children eventually manifest temporal lobe epilepsy. There is no specific therapy.

ABNORMALITIES OF MOTOR FUNCTION (CEREBRAL PALSY) *Cerebral palsy* refers to a developmental disorder of motor function that is present from infancy or early childhood and that is due to a nonprogressive cerebral disorder. The more commonly encountered conditions are spastic diplegia (affecting the legs), hemiplegia (affecting the arm and leg on the same side), and heterogeneous extrapyramidal syndromes. Cerebral infarction resulting from hypoxia and/or ischemia is one determinant of these disorders. For most the abnormal state has its origins before birth in events that go unrecognized. The insult may occur perinatally as a result of obstetrical mishap in 20 percent or less of cases. For some few an encephaloclastic event occurs in early childhood.

Spastic diplegia resulting from a prenatal or perinatal insult to the brain may not attract attention until several weeks or months after birth. There may be a delay in all normal developmental sequences, especially those that depend on the motor system. Once walking is attempted, usually much later than in the normal child, the characteristic stance and gait become manifest. The legs are advanced stiffly in short steps, each describing part of the arc of a circle: adduction is often so strong as to lead to actual crossing (scissors gait), with lower legs slightly splayed out and the feet flexed and turned in, the heels not touching the ground. Crural paraparesis is the rule, though in general it is associated with at least a mild affection of the arms as well. In the adolescent and adult, the legs tend to be short and small, but the muscles are not markedly atrophic, as in infantile muscular atrophy and dystrophy. Less commonly there may also be pseudobulbar dysarthria and athetosis.

Hemiplegia is a not uncommon condition of infancy and childhood, and a difference in function of the right and left extremities may be noticed soon after birth or during the first 6 to 12 months of life. The parents may be the first to notice that movements of prehension and exploration are carried out with only one arm. The affection of the leg is usually recognized later, i.e., during the first attempt to stand and walk. Mental defect is even less common than with cerebral diplegia and less common than in bilateral hemiplegia. Convulsions occur in 35 to 50 percent of children with congenital hemiplegia and may persist throughout life. If the hemiplegia is acquired during childhood, seizures often accompany the onset. They may be generalized but are frequently unilateral and limited to the hemiplegic side. Often, after a series of seizures, the affected side will be weak for several hours or longer (Todd's paralysis).

In *double hemiplegia,* a less frequent condition, the bilateral weakness of face, arms, and legs arises at any age under conditions of more severe acquired cerebral disease. The arms are severely affected, in contrast to their minimal involvement in cerebral diplegia. A quadriplegic state may occur without bulbar involvement. The condition is relatively rare and may result from a bilateral cerebral lesion or a high cervical cord lesion. Although this may occasionally result from cysts, tumors, and other malformations, it is usually produced in the infant by fracture-dislocation of the cervical spine, induced during a difficult breech delivery. Similarly, in paraplegia, with weakness or paralysis limited to the legs, the lesion may be either a cerebral form of diplegia or a spinal one. Sphincteric disturbances and a loss of sensation below a certain level on the trunk favor a spinal localization.

The spastic and rigid cerebral diplegias discussed above shade almost imperceptibly into the congenital extrapyramidal syndromes. Many such patients are found in every cerebral palsy clinic and ultimately reach adult medical clinics. Pyramidal tract signs may be absent. The nonprogressive extrapyramidal cases considered here are generally attributable to severe perinatal hypoxia; others represent separate diseases such as erythroblastosis fetalis with kernicterus. These are to be distinguished from the progressive acquired or hereditary postnatal syndromes such as familial athetosis, dystonia musculorum deformans, and cerebellar ataxia.

Congenital choreoathetosis (double athetosis) is probably the most frequent representative of this group. Like the spastic states, it may be recognized only after several months or a year have elapsed. Syndromes may be mixed, however. All combinations of chorea, athetosis, ballismus, myoclonus, and dystonia may be found in a single case, or one or another type of movement disorder may predominate. However, in all instances there is, in addition, a primary defect in voluntary movement. Choreoathetosis varies in severity. In some the disorder is so mild that the abnormal movements are misinterpreted as restlessness or "the fidgets"; in others, every voluntary act is marred by intense involuntary movements, leaving the patient nearly helpless. The severely handicapped patients, even with the help of rehabilitation clinics and corrective orthopedic operations, rarely achieve a degree of motor control that permits them to lead an independent life, and they need supportive treatment and help as adults. Intelligence may be preserved.

Kernicterus was a more common cause of abnormal cerebral development prior to the contemporary practice of restraining early postnatal serum bilirubin concentrations to levels below 250 μmol/L (15 mg/dL). The majority of infants with this disorder die within the first week of two of life, and those who survive are often mentally retarded, deaf, and totally unable to sit, stand, or walk. However, exceptional patients, obviously less damaged, are mentally normal or at most only slightly backward. Either athetosis or ataxia may be present. A few have rigid limbs and a picture not too different from that of cerebral spastic diplegia with involuntary movements. Kernicterus should always be suspected if an extrapyramidal syndrome is accompanied by bilateral deafness and palsy of upward gaze.

NEUROSKELETAL DISORDERS

The skull and vertebral column normally enlarge coordinately with growth of the central nervous system. Abnormalities in the size of the skull can occur secondary to underlying abnormalities of brain development. Abnormalities resulting primarily from derangements of osseous development may lead to aberrations in skull shape and to entrapment of the enclosed nervous system, as in the Chiari and related malformations.

SECONDARY MACROCRANIA AND MICROCRANIA Alterations in the circumference of the head greater than (macrocrania) or less than (microcrania) the 98th percentiles are considered abnormal. Macrocrania may result from potentially correctable hydrocephalus and is associated with headache, mental dullness, depression, visual blurring, difficulty walking, and urinary incontinence. Limited ability to elevate the eyes, ataxia of gait, hyperreflexia in the legs, and Babinski responses are common signs.

Developmental causes of *noncommunicating hydrocephalus* include aqueductal stenosis, the Dandy-Walker malformation in which the cerebrospinal fluid escape from the fourth ventricle is obstructed, and the Chiari malformations (see below). Neoplasms or cysts, particularly when located within the ventricular system or impinging upon structures of the posterior fossa, must be excluded. *Communicating hydrocephalus* may develop after recovery from disorders that cause scarring of the leptomeninges, such as intraventricular hemorrhage in the perinatal period, especially in premature infants, and meningitis. Localized head enlargement, associated with mental slowing and contralateral long tract signs, may complicate porencephalic cerebral defects resulting from a focal cerebral injury in the perinatal period or early childhood.

Macrocrania may also be the result of an abnormally large brain (macrocephaly). Benign, or asymptomatic, macrocephaly may be familial. Macrocephaly and a characteristic triangular face, moderate impairment of cognitive functions, and macrosomia constitute the syndrome of cerebral gigantism (Soto), which in some families appears to be transmitted by autosomal dominant inheritance. Symmetric or asymmetric macrocephaly, seizures, and cognitive impairment may occur with neurofibromatosis. Macrocephaly can also occur in certain lysosomal storage disorders that affect the brain, but such individuals rarely reach adulthood.

Microcrania is most commonly secondary to microcephaly. Typically this is a consequence of lack of brain growth and may result from virtually any heritable or acquired disorder that affects the developing brain. *Microcephaly vera* is a rare but distinctive disorder transmitted by autosomal recessive inheritance and associated mental retardation and brain weight less than 500 g. The face and facial features are distinctively prominent in relation to the small cranium.

PRIMARY DISORDERS OF SKELETAL DEVELOPMENT The Chiari malformations are among the most prevalent and complex neuroskeletal malformations. The characteristic feature is entrapment and compression of the rhombencephalon within an underdeveloped posterior cranial fossa (see Marin-Padilla). In the severest forms, typically apparent at birth, the cerebellar vermis, medulla, and fourth ventricle are herniated or extruded into the upper cervical canal (Chiari type II) or protrude exteriorly as an occipital encephalocele at the base of the skull (Chiari type III). Hydrocephalus and hydromyelia may be associated with meningomyelocele arising from the lumbosacral spinal cord. Milder degrees of herniation of the posteroinferior region of the cerebellum ("tonsils") into the cervical canal with little or no downward displacement of the fourth ventricle (Chiari type I) or milder degrees of the Chiari II deformity may become symptomatic only in adolescence or adult life. Symptoms typical of adult expression of the Chiari malformation include pain that is localized to the cranial-cervical junction, which is aggravated by head movement or Valsalva maneuver. There may be unsteadiness of gait, dysarthria, and dysphagia, corresponding to compromise of cerebellar-related connections and lower cranial nerve paresis. Downbeat nystagmus is characteristic.

Syringomyelia and *syringobulbia* occur in association with the Chiari malformations. Syringomyelia, a disorder of the cervical region of the spinal cord, can be viewed as a progressive destructive expansion of a central cavitation of the spinal cord. A variable number of segments of the upper cervical and thoracic cord, or of the medulla and pons in the case of syringobulbia, may be involved. Typically, the commissure and the posterior horns of the central gray and the axonal fascicles of the posterior and lateral columns of the cord are damaged. The neurologic manifestations include impairment of pain and temperature perception in a capelike distribution and impairment of perception of vibration and joint displacement and spasticity in the lower extremities. To the extent that anterior horn cells are destroyed at cervical segmental levels, muscle atrophy and weakness appear in the upper extremities (see Chap. 361). Extension of the

cystic cavity upwards into the brainstem can cause facial pain, nystagmus, and lower cranial nerve deficits.

Other disorders of the axial skeleton and the lower spinal cord and cauda equina are also characteristically associated with the Chiari malformation but may occur independently. The osseous anomalies include aberrations of the primary pattern of formation (absence or fusion) or the size of vertebrae, hemivertebrae, or fusion of vertebra and scapula (Sprengel's deformity). The Klippel-Feil deformity is a complex of osseous and visceral anomalies that include low hairline, platybasia, fusion of cervical vertebra with short neck, and deafness. These malformations may entrap and damage the brain and spinal cord. The disorders of the lower vertebral region may become symptomatic with rapid growth in adolescence or in adult life. Diastematomyelia, the protrusion of a bony spur into the vertebral canal, is of particular importance in adults because it represents a treatable form of deficit. Intermittent, generally progressive disturbances of somatic and visceral motor function, typically associated with pain, may be subtle clues to the diagnosis.

A cauda equina syndrome, that is, impairment of both somatic and visceral sensory and motor functions referable to the lower lumbar and sacral roots, may result from lipomas or dermoid cysts within the lower vertebral canal. A dimple or tuft of hair near the midline in the lumbar region or within the gluteal crease may suggest the persistence of a sinus tract or a deeper-lying anomaly affecting vertebral canal and spinal roots. Tethering of the cord to the lower end of the vertebral canal by fibrous bands may result in traction that becomes symptomatic with growth in adolescence. Stenosis of the lumbar vertebral elements may be associated with claudication, that is, symptoms of a cauda equina syndrome that develop with walking.

CT and MRI, particularly when utilized in conjunction with myelography for syrinx and other spinal disorders, are sensitive and efficient diagnostic procedures. Images obtained in the midsagittal plane are particularly appropriate for diagnosis of the Chiari malformation and syrinx and for abnormalities of the lumbosacral region. In principle, treatment is surgical. Decompression is appropriate for entrapment and compression; shunting is required for hydrocephalic (or syringomyelic) states. Mass lesions and bony spurs are excised.

SYNOSTOSES AND CRANIOFACIAL DEFORMITIES Cranial synostosis and some other craniofacial anomalies affect principally the rostral region and the vault of the skull. Premature closure of the sagittal suture results in an elongate (scaphocephalic) skull, and premature closure of the coronal sutures causes a broad and foreshortened (brachycephalic) skull. If all major sutures close prematurely, a tower (turricephalic) skull results, manifest by shallow orbits with bulging eyes. Other combinations may affect one or more sutures. Synostosis, particularly when generalized, may result in cerebral compression and hydrocephalus. Less extensive disorders are cosmetically disfiguring. Early surgical correction of the disorders is appropriate.

REFERENCES

ADAMS RD: Neurocutaneous disease, in *Dermatology in General Medicine*, 3d ed, TB Fitzpatrick et al (eds). New York, McGraw-Hill, 1986
——, Lyon G: *Neurology of Hereditary Metabolic Diseases of Children*. New York, McGraw-Hill, 1982
CAVINESS VS JR: The Chiari malformations of the posterior fossa and their relation to hydrocephalus. Dev Med Child Neurol 18:103, 1976
CHASNOFF IJ et al: Cocaine use in pregnancy. N Engl J Med 313:666, 1985
Ho HZ et al: The fragile-X syndrome. Dev Med Child Neurol 30:257, 1988
LAMIELL JM et al: Von Hippel-Lindau disease affecting 43 members of a single kindred. Medicine 68:1, 1989
MARIN-PADILLA M: Clinical and experimental rachischisis, in *Handbook of Clinical Neurology*, PJ Vinken, GW Bruyn (eds). Amsterdam, North Holland, 1978, pp 159–191
MARTUZA RL, ELDRIDGE R: Neurofibromatosis 2 (bilateral acoustic neurofibromatosis). N Engl J Med 318:684, 1988
RICCARDI VM: Von Recklinghausen neurofibromatosis. N Engl J Med 305:1617, 1981
SEIZINGER BR et al: Models for inherited susceptibility to cancer in the nervous system: A molecular-genetic approach to neurofibromatosis. Dev Neurosci 9:144, 1987

Smith DW: *Recognizable Patterns of Human Malformation*, 3d ed. Philadelphia, Saunders, 1982

Swaiman KF: *Pediatric Neurology: Principles and Practice*. St. Louis, Mosby, 1989

Volpe JJ: *Neurology of the Newborn*. Philadelphia, Saunders, 1987

359 DEGENERATIVE DISEASES OF THE NERVOUS SYSTEM

M. FLINT BEAL / EDWARD P. RICHARDSON, JR. / JOSEPH B. MARTIN

In classifying diseases of the nervous system, it is customary to designate a group of them as *degenerative*, indicating that they are characterized by gradually evolving, relentlessly progressive neuronal death occurring for reasons that are still largely unknown. The identification of these diseases depends upon exclusion of such possible causative factors as infections, metabolic derangements, and intoxications. A considerable proportion of the disorders classed as degenerative are genetic, with either dominant or recessive inheritance. Others, however, occur only sporadically—as isolated instances in a given family.

Classification of the degenerative diseases cannot be based upon any exact knowledge of cause or pathogenesis; their subdivision into individual syndromes rests on descriptive criteria based largely upon neuropathologic and clinical aspects. This group of diseases presents as several distinct clinical syndromes, the recognition of which can assist the clinician in arriving at a diagnosis.

GENERAL CONSIDERATIONS The degenerative disorders usually begin insidiously and run a gradually progressive course over many years. Their course is generally more protracted than that of the hereditary metabolic diseases of the nervous system (see Chap. 357). The earliest changes may be so subtle that it often is impossible to assign any precise time of onset. At times the history suggests an abrupt onset of disability—particularly when an injury or some other event in the patient's life has occurred to which illness might conceivably be related. By careful questioning, it is frequently evident that the patient or family has suddenly become aware of a condition that had, in fact, already been present but had passed unnoticed.

The family history is of great importance, and denial of familial occurrence cannot always be taken at face value. Some patients or their relatives are hesitant to disclose that a neurologic disease afflicts the family. In other cases, the extent of the disease affecting other family members may be so slight as to go unnoticed by the family—as may occur, for instance, in the group of the hereditary ataxias. Moreover, small sibships in a family may prevent well-established hereditary diseases from being recognized. Familial occurrence, of course, does not always mean that a disease is hereditary; it may indicate instead that there has been a common exposure to an infective or toxic agent.

Many of the degenerative nervous system diseases progress uninfluenced by therapeutic measures. Caring for such patients is often an anguishing experience for all concerned. In others, such as persons with Parkinson's disease, symptoms can often be alleviated by wise and skillful management. The physician's caring attention may be of great help even when curative measures cannot be offered.

The symptoms and signs of this group of diseases tend to have a bilaterally symmetric distribution. This aspect alone may help to distinguish the disorder from other varieties of neurologic disease. In some patients, in the early stages, one side of the body, or one limb, may become involved in the presence of normal findings elsewhere. Eventually, despite the asymmetric beginning, the inherently bilateral nature of the process generally asserts itself.

A striking characteristic of the degenerative disorders is that particular anatomic or physiologic systems of neurons may be selectively affected, leaving others entirely intact. This is exemplified in amyotrophic lateral sclerosis, in which the disease process is limited to cerebral and spinal motor neurons, and in some forms of progressive ataxia in which only the Purkinje cells of the cerebellum are affected. In Friedreich's ataxia and some other syndromes, the disease process affects multiple neuronal systems.

In this respect certain degenerative neuronal diseases resemble others of known cause, particularly intoxications, where similarly circumscribed effects occur. Diphtheria toxin, for example, produces selective breakdown of peripheral nerve myelin, triorthocresyl phosphate affects the corticospinal tracts in the spinal cord together with the peripheral nerves, and the neurotoxin 1-methyl-4-phenyl-1,2,3,6-tetrahydropyridine (MPTP) brings about death of dopamine-containing neurons in the substantia nigra. Selective involvement of particular neuronal systems is not, however, characteristic of all of the degenerative diseases; some are characterized by pathologic changes that are diffuse and unselective.

Typically, the pathologic process in the nervous system is one of slow involution of nerve cell bodies or their axonal extensions, unaccompanied by any intense tissue reaction or cellular response, although the loss of neurons and fibers is often accompanied by hyperplasia of fibrillary astrocytes (gliosis). The cerebrospinal fluid (CSF) shows little if any change—at most a slight elevation of protein, without abnormalities in specific proteins, cell count, or in other constituents. Moreover, since these diseases invariably result in tissue loss, rather than in new tissue formation, radiologic visualization of the brain, the ventricular system, or subarachnoid space shows either no change or an enlargement of the CSF compartments. These negative laboratory findings thus help to distinguish the degenerative disorders from the other large classes of progressive diseases of the nervous system—tumors and infections.

CLASSIFICATION Since etiologic classification is impossible, subdivision of the degenerative diseases into individual syndromes rests on descriptive criteria based largely on their clinical aspects and pathologic anatomy. Many of these syndromes are named after distinguished neurologists and neuropathologists. A useful classification is outlined in Table 359-1.

SYNDROMES IN WHICH PROGRESSIVE DEMENTIA PREDOMINATES

In the disease entities that follow, the clinical picture is dominated by gradual loss of intellectual capacities, i.e., by dementia. Other neurologic abnormalities, except in the terminal stages, are absent or relatively insignificant. (For further discussion of dementia, including its clinical evaluation, Chaps. 29, 30, and 32 should be consulted.)

ALZHEIMER'S DISEASE Alzheimer's disease is perhaps the most important of all the degenerative diseases because of its frequent occurrence and devastating nature. It is the commonest cause of dementia in the elderly, with all that this implies in the way of distress for patients and families, and economic loss in the form of the costs entailed in the long-term care of patients totally disabled by the disease. Historically, the term *Alzheimer's disease* was applied to progressive dementia coming on in late middle life but preceding the senile period, following the original description by Alois Alzheimer in 1907, in which the illness of a woman dying at the age of 55 was depicted clinically and pathologically. It became usual to classify cases of this kind under the heading of *presenile dementia*. Meanwhile, it became increasingly apparent that very old people dying with progressive mental deterioration, generally referred to as *senile dementia*, showed cerebral lesions that were identical to those found in cases of presenile dementia. Such cases are now designated as *senile dementia of the Alzheimer type*. Current evidence indicates that the disease process is the same, regardless of the age of onset. At the same time, Alzheimer's disease is clearly age-related. It is extremely uncommon in young people and rare in middle age; as age advances, however, it is increasingly frequent, such that its prevalence

TABLE 359-1   Clinical classification of the degenerative diseases of the nervous system

I Disorders characterized by progressive dementia in the absence of other prominent neurologic signs
  A Alzheimer's disease
  B Senile dementia of the Alzheimer type
  C Pick's disease (lobar atrophy)
II Syndromes combining progressive dementia with other prominent neurologic abnormalities
  A Mainly in adults
    1 Huntington's disease
    2 Multiple system atrophy combining dementia with ataxia and/or manifestations of Parkinson's disease
    3 Progressive supranuclear palsy (Steele-Richardson-Olszewski)
    4 Diffuse Lewy body disease
    5 Corticodentatonigral degeneration
  B Mainly in children or young adults
    1 Hallervorden-Spatz disease
    2 Progressive familial myoclonic epilepsy
III Syndromes of gradually developing abnormalities of posture and movement
  A Paralysis agitans (Parkinson's disease)
  B Striatonigral degeneration
  C Progressive supranuclear palsy (see *II, A, 3* above)
  D Torsion dystonia (torsion spasm; dystonia musculorum deformans)
  E Spasmodic torticollis and other restricted dyskinesias
  F Familial tremor
  G Gilles de la Tourette syndrome
IV Syndromes of progressive ataxia
  A Cerebellar degenerations
    1 Cerebellar cortical degeneration
    2 Olivopontocerebellar atrophy (OPCA)
  B Spinocerebellar degenerations (Friedreich's ataxia and related disorders)
V Syndrome of central autonomic nervous system failure (Shy-Drager syndrome)
VI Syndromes of muscular weakness and wasting without sensory changes (motor neuron disease)
  A Amyotrophic lateral sclerosis
  B Spinal muscular atrophy
    1 Infantile spinal muscular atrophy (Werdnig-Hoffmann)
    2 Juvenile spinal muscular atrophy (Wohlfart-Kugelberg-Welander)
    3 Other forms of familial spinal muscular atrophy
  C Primary lateral sclerosis
  D Hereditary spastic paraplegia
VII Syndromes combining muscular weakness and wasting with sensory changes (progressive neural muscular atrophy; chronic familial polyneuropathies)
  A Peroneal muscular atrophy (Charcot-Marie-Tooth)
  B Hypertrophic interstitial polyneuropathy (Dejerine-Sottas)
  C Miscellaneous forms of chronic progressive neuropathy
VIII Syndromes of progressive visual loss
  A Pigmentary degeneration of the retina (retinitis pigmentosa)
  B Hereditary optic atrophy (Leber's disease)

---

in persons over 80 years old is estimated at more than 20 percent. Advancing age is unmistakably a predisposing factor, but it is incorrect to consider Alzheimer's disease as the inevitable accompaniment of aging. Many elderly people remain mentally unimpaired into the ninth and tenth decades. Genetic predisposition to Alzheimer's disease emerges as a clear-cut pattern in some families, particularly in those with early age of onset. There are well-documented familial cases, some following an autosomal dominant pattern of inheritance. An exception to the statement that Alzheimer's disease is rare in young people occurs in the instance of Down's syndrome (trisomy 21), which leads to the development of the characteristic lesions of Alzheimer's disease in the majority of the patients after 40 years of age.

Pathology The outstanding pathologic feature is death and disappearance of nerve cells in the cerebral cortex. This leads ultimately to extensive convolutional atrophy, especially in the frontal, parietal, and medial temporal regions. There is a corresponding enlargement of the ventricular system, but this is usually not extreme.

Two kinds of microscopic lesions are distinctive for the disease. The first, originally described by Alzheimer, consists of intraneuronal accumulations of filamentous material in the form of loops, coils, or tangled masses—referred to as *Alzheimer neurofibrillary tangles*. Their nature is currently under active investigation. The neuropath-

ologic evidence strongly suggests that these fibrillar masses are of major importance in bringing about the death of neurons. Electron microscopy reveals accumulations of paired helical filaments that differ from normal neurofilaments and microtubules. Recent studies have shown that a major component is an abnormally phosphorylated form of the microtubule protein tau. Alzheimer neurofibrillary tangles also contain ubiquitin, a protein that marks cells for proteolysis.

Neurofibrillary tangles tend to be most abundant, together with the most extreme degrees of neuronal loss, in the hippocampus and adjacent parts of the temporal lobe—structures that have been found to be of greatest importance in memory function.

The other histopathologic change that characterizes Alzheimer's disease is the presence of intracortical clusters of thickened neuronal processes, both axons and dendrites (collectively referred to as *neurites*), generally in the form of an irregular ring surrounding a spherical deposit of amyloid fibrils. These lesions, which had been recognized before Alzheimer's description of the neurofibrillary change, were termed *senile plaques*. Recent elucidation of their structure has led to their current designation as *neuritic plaques*. They have been shown to contain paired helical filaments identical to those found in the perinuclear cytoplasm of the diseased neurons. One form of plaque, the *diffuse plaque*, consists of amorphous amyloid without neurites. The nature and origin of the amyloid component are being intensively studied. It is now evident that amyloid, identified by its staining reactions and ultrastructural features, is not a uniform substance; instead, its tinctorial and morphologic character depends upon a particular molecular spatial configuration (beta-pleated sheet fibrils) that can be brought about with various proteins, some of immunologic origin, some not.

There is another aspect to the problem of cerebral amyloidosis in Alzheimer's disease. In many, but not all, cases identical amyloid deposits may be found in the walls of small meningeal and intracortical arteries, and the question has arisen as to whether this cerebrovascular amyloidosis (often called *cerebral amyloid angiopathy* or *congophilic angiopathy* because of the characteristic staining of amyloid with the dye Congo red) has a close relationship, perhaps even causative, to plaque amyloidosis. The amyloid in the blood vessels in Alzheimer's disease, as well as that in the core of neuritic plaques, has been isolated and sequenced. The amyloid peptide (β- or A_4-peptide) gene is on chromosome 21, on which the familial Alzheimer's disease gene also has been localized in some families. However, the two loci are not identical. Antibodies against the cerebrovascular amyloid cross react with the amyloid in neuritic plaques. It is as yet unclear where the amyloid in plaques originates—whether from neurons or blood vessels; most investigators favor the former.

Biochemical studies show that choline acetyltransferase, the key enzyme required for the synthesis of acetylcholine, is decreased in the cerebral cortex in Alzheimer's disease. The major source of neocortical cholinergic innervation is a group of neurons situated in the basal part of the forebrain just beneath the corpus striatum—the nucleus basalis of Meynert. Careful neuropathologic investigations have shown that in Alzheimer's disease, this nucleus is a site of major neuronal loss and of frequent Alzheimer neurofibrillary tangles. These studies suggest that impairment of cholinergic transmission may play a part in the clinical expression of the disease. However, attempted therapy with cholinomimetic agents has been largely unsuccessful. Less consistent reductions in cortical norepinephrine and serotonin appear to be caused by neuronal loss in the locus coeruleus and raphé nucleus, respectively. Loss of peptidergic neurons in the cerebral cortex is associated with reduced cortical concentrations of somatostatin and corticotropin releasing factor. Reduction in CSF concentrations of somatostatin is also reported.

It is anticipated that investigations of the biochemistry of the cerebral lesions in Alzheimer's disease will lead ultimately to an understanding of their pathogenesis. The remarkable discovery that one form of progressive dementia, Creutzfeldt-Jakob disease, is the result of infection with a transmissible virus-like agent has led to the question as to whether Alzheimer's disease and other neuronal degenerations might be due to a similar form of infectious agent. All attempts to transmit Alzheimer's disease have failed, however, so that currently an infective basis is thought unlikely.

Clinical manifestations   The onset is insidious and subtle, with changes most noticeable first in memory for recent happenings and in other aspects of mental activity. Emotional disturbances such as depression, anxiety, or odd, unpredictable quirks of behavior, may be salient features in the early stages. Progression is usually slow and gradual, and unless other medical conditions supervene, it may smolder on for 10 or more years.

In the milder cases, including those of the senile period, the noteworthy features are those of simple dementia, as described in Chap. 32. More unusual disorders of thought and intellect, including aphasia, apraxic disturbances, and abnormalities of space perception, may be seen, especially in the presenile group. Exceptionally, and only in the advanced stages of the disease, extrapyramidal signs appear; the patient walks in a shuffling manner with short steps, and there is a generalized stiffness of the musculature with slowness and awkwardness of all movements. In some patients, sudden jerklike contractions of various muscles (myoclonus) may occur in the presence of otherwise typical Alzheimer's disease, but this is unusual and should immediately raise the suspicion of Creutzfeldt-Jakob disease (Chap. 355). Terminally the patient may become nearly decorticate, losing all ability to perceive, think, speak, or move.

Laboratory investigations, including blood and CSF determinations, do not yield any conclusive or pertinent data. There is a diffuse slowing in the electroencephalogram in the more advanced stages of the disease. Enlargement of the ventricular system and subarachnoid space resulting from brain atrophy can be demonstrated by computed tomography (CT) scan and by magnetic resonance imaging (MRI). These imaging procedures, however, are not decisive for making the diagnosis, especially in the earlier stages, because the degree of cerebral atrophy demonstrated may be no more than that seen in patients of a similar age group who are functioning normally. Recent studies with positron emission tomography have shown decreased glucose metabolism in the temporal and parietal lobes. During the course of the illness, occasional convulsive seizures may occur, but they are relatively rare and should raise suspicion of other diseases. Terminally, the patient dies from intercurrent disease, in a state of total helplessness. Institutional care is usually necessary long before the end.

Differential diagnosis   The physician should recognize that treatable conditions may at first appear to be dementia of the Alzheimer type. Space-occupying lesions, such as chronic subdural hematoma or slowly growing frontal neoplasms (meningioma or glioma) should be excluded. CT and MRI scanning usually demonstrate mass lesions of these kinds, as well as an unsuspected hydrocephalus, which, when treated by a shunt procedure for ventricular decompression, may lead to dramatic improvement in the patient's state. Other treatable conditions producing a dementia-like state include metabolic derangements (liver disease), vitamin B_{12} deficiency, and hypothyroidism. Elderly people may be unusually susceptible to the sedative effects of medications, so that chronic drug intoxication may need to be considered. Cerebrovascular disease is not ordinarily a cause of uncomplicated dementia, but finding multiple small infarcts on CT or MRI scanning raises the possibility of multi-infarct dementia. Depression can mimic dementia, particularly in the elderly, in whom it may be all too easy to attribute deficits in thinking, motivation, and memory to cerebral disease (see Chaps. 29 and 30). Depression may show a most gratifying response to appropriate treatment (see Chap. 368).

The evidence that cholinergic innervation may be impaired in Alzheimer's disease has led to attempts to correct the deficiency pharmacologically, but so far none of these has proved to be effective.

Practical measures that may help in the management of cases of Alzheimer's disease are suggested in Chaps. 29 and 30.

PICK'S DISEASE (LOBAR ATROPHY)   This remarkable form of cerebral disease, characterized by circumscribed cerebal atrophy (lobar

sclerosis), enters in the differential diagnosis of dementia in the presenile period. It is, however, an extremely rare condition as compared with diffuse cerebral atrophy of the Alzheimer type. Hereditary transmission (as a dominant trait) is frequent in Pick's disease, and women are more frequently affected than men. The age distribution is similar in both of these varieties of progressive dementia.

Pathology   So striking are the gross pathologic changes in the brain that in typical cases the diagnosis can be made at a glance. Severe atrophy of the anterior portions of the frontal and temporal lobes occurs, and there is a curiously sharp line of demarcation between the atrophied portions and the remainder of the brain, which appears normal or nearly so. In some cases, the frontal atrophy is more prominent; in others, the temporal lobes are more severely involved; in general, both regions are affected. Rarely, the disorder has a predominantly unilateral localization—as in cases described originally by Pick. Atrophic changes also occur in subcortical structures: caudate nucleus, putamen, thalamus, and substantia nigra, and in the descending frontopontine fiber system. There are striking changes in nerve cells in the affected regions in most cases. These consist of fibrillary deposits within the cytoplasm—masses of straight fibrils, differing from the paired helical filaments of Alzheimer's disease. In some neurons, densely packed spherical aggregates (Pick bodies) can be seen with silver-impregnation methods. In other affected neurons, the fibrils are more widely dispersed, and the neuronal cytoplasm takes on a rounded, distended appearance, forming ballooned cells. Recent evidence suggests that despite the morphologic differences, these neuronal changes are biochemically related to those in Alzheimer's disease, as indicated by common antigenic properties. In rare instances of Alzheimer's disease, disproportionate atrophy of the frontal and temporal lobes may suggest Pick's disease, but in such cases the distinguishing feature is the presence of the characteristic plaques and neurofibrillary tangles, which are not found in Pick's disease.

Clinical manifestations   If Pick's disease has any distinctive clinical features, they consist of unusually severe signs of frontal lobe or temporal lobe dysfunction (see Chap. 32). Typical early manifestations are a general impoverishment of mental function, changes in behavior patterns, and a striking lack of insight. The later phases of the disease are characterized by loss of retentive memory (with temporal lobe involvement), loss of all language functions, and, when the frontal lobes are mainly affected, prominent grasp and sucking reflexes. In CT and MRI scans the shrinkage of the cortex and the low density of the white matter in the affected lobes may be diagnostic. Progression, as in Alzheimer's disease, is slow and relentless, the average duration being about 7 years. In the late stages, rigidity, dystonic postures, and perhaps tremor may be prominent features; these can be ascribed to extension of the disease process into the basal ganglia.

Differential diagnosis   The considerations already noted with regard to Alzheimer's disease apply to Pick's disease as well.

SYNDROMES COMBINING DEMENTIA WITH OTHER NEUROLOGIC SIGNS

HUNTINGTON'S DISEASE   This disorder, characterized by a combination of choreoathetotic movements and progressive dementia usually beginning in midadult life, is transmitted as an autosomal dominant disease. Recent genetic studies have shown that the determining gene is located on the terminal segment of the short arm of chromosome 4. The classic description is that of George Huntington, who, together with his father and grandfather, all physicians, made clinical observations on familial cases living near their home on Long Island, New York. Huntington, writing in 1872, entitled his paper "On Chorea"; subsequently the disorder described by him came to be known as *Huntington's chorea*. The more general term used in this chapter—Huntington's disease—is preferable, since the disease state comprises more than abnormal movements, and the motor abnormalities often are more complex than would be implied by the unqualified term *chorea*.

Because of its distressing and incapacitating nature, and its implications for members of any family in which it appears (50 percent risk in all children of an affected parent), the disease has attracted attention in recent years and has been found to be considerably more frequent and widely distributed than once was thought. It is estimated that there are approximately 25,000 cases in the United States alone. In virtually all cases that come to the notice of a physician, there is a family history of the disease, although occasionally patients present with typical symptoms and no documentable family history; no proven case of a new mutation has occurred. Some of these cases are classified as senile chorea, where family members have died of other causes before the disease became manifest.

Pathology Distinctive for Huntington's disease is atrophy of the caudate nucleus and, to a lesser extent, other structures of the basal ganglia (putamen and globus pallidus), out of proportion to any other changes in the brain. The degree of atrophy is directly related to the severity and duration of the disease. In the late stages, the caudate nucleus, which normally forms a convexly rounded eminence in the lateral wall of the lateral ventricle, takes on instead a flattened or concave appearance. As the result of the tissue loss, the ventricular system becomes correspondingly widened, especially the frontal horns. Along with these changes in the basal ganglia, there characteristically is diffuse gyral atrophy, most severe over the convex aspect of the brain.

The atrophy of the caudate nucleus and putamen is seen microscopically to be due to extensive loss of neurons, which stands out in contrast to the intactness of adjacent structures such as the nucleus accumbens septi, the nucleus basalis of Meynert (so strikingly involved in Alzheimer's disease), and the thalamus.

There are no morphologically distinctive or characteristic cytopathologic alterations in the neurons in Huntington's disease such as occur in Alzheimer's and some other diseases. Neurochemical studies have shown a striking decrease of γ-aminobutyric acid (GABA) and of its synthesizing enzyme, glutamic acid decarboxylase, in the caudate nucleus, putamen, globus pallidus, and pars reticulata of the substantia nigra, and some decrease also in choline acetyltransferase in the caudate nucleus. The loss of GABA can be attributed to depletion of the abundant medium-sized *spiny* neurons within the striatum. Spiny neurons are characterized in Golgi studies by a large number of dendritic spines and have been shown to constitute the projection neurons of the striatum. They provide efferents to both the globus pallidus and substantia nigra. In contrast *aspiny* neurons, with few dendritic spines, are striatal interneurons with locally arborizing axons. In addition to GABA, other neurotransmitters contained within striatal spiny neurons, including substance P, enkephalins, and dynorphin, are similarly depleted in the striatum and its sites of projection.

Recent observations indicate that the peptide neurotransmitters somatostatin and neuropeptide y are relatively increased in the caudate nucleus and putamen in Huntington's disease, and cells identifiable as somatostatin–neuropeptide y neurons (*aspiny* neurons) are selectively preserved—in striking contrast to the loss of other neurons in the same regions. The large aspiny neurons containing acetylcholine are also preserved. The pathophysiologic meaning of this sparing is not clear as yet; its occurrence emphasizes the fact that in Huntington's disease, as in other neuronal-system degenerations, selective vulnerability of neurons occurs in a particular region with preservation of others. The pattern of resistance of certain neuronal groups has provided clues to a possible underlying pathogenesis of the disease. The susceptible spiny neurons have dense glutamate inputs from the cerebral cortex. The pattern of cell death can be reproduced experimentally by glutamate receptor agonists that act on the *N*-methyl-D-aspartate subclass of glutamate receptors (see Chaps. 11 and 346). These observations have led to the hypothesis that striatal neurons die as a result of glutamate-induced neurotoxicity.

The progressive dementia of Huntington's disease is still not well characterized neuropathologically. Pathologic examination reveals shrinkage of cortical volume, but it has been difficult to document cell loss. Biochemical studies, however, are consistent with a mild neuronal loss, particularly in the frontal cortex. Further correlative biochemical and neuropathologic studies, using careful quantitative methods, will be needed to resolve this issue.

Clinical aspects The disorder has a prevalence in Europe and North America of 7 to 10 per 100,000 population. The movement disorder generally makes its appearance in early to middle adult years (average age of onset about 35 to 40 years). It is characteristic of the disease that younger patients, with onset of symptoms in the age group of 15 to 40 years, suffer a more severe form of the disorder than older patients, with onset in the 50s and 60s, and the neuropathologic changes in the brain are correspondingly more extensive and severe in the younger as compared with the older patients. Huntington's disease is occasionally manifest in childhood (even before the age of 4); in such cases transmission usually occurs through the father. Such cases are rare and tend to be characterized more by rigidity than by chorea and by other atypical features such as convulsive seizures and cerebellar ataxia (Westphal's variant).

The involuntary movements (bizarre grimacing, respiratory irregularity, faulty articulation of speech, and irregular, arrhythmic, unpatterned movements of the limbs, imparting to the gait a peculiar dancing quality) tend to be less quick and more athetoid than in Sydenham's chorea (see Chap. 25). Some reported cases that on genealogic and pathologic grounds must be classified with Huntington's chorea have shown progressive rigidity rather than choreiform movements, even in the adult. As a general rule, dementia runs parallel with the motor disorder. Occasionally it may appear before or after chorea; very rarely it may be slight or lacking altogether. Neuropsychiatric manifestations of depression, erratic behavior, and emotional outbursts often seriously handicap the patient before dementia or the movement disorder are severe. The advance of the disease is slow, with death on average occurring 15 to 20 years after onset of symptoms. Increasing disability from involuntary movements and mental changes result in death from intercurrent infection or, not rarely, by suicide.

Differential diagnosis There is no difficulty in the recognition of typical cases. The relatively late onset, the slowly progressive course, the prominent dementia, and lack of association with rheumatic fever help to exclude Sydenham's chorea. Patients with Parkinson's disease when overdosed with levodopa may develop a widespread chorea or choreoathetosis, and this, combined with the early dementia that occurs in some patients, can reproduce the picture of Huntington's disease. Phenothiazine drugs may induce generalized chorea, unassociated with dementia, and the movement disorder may persist for months or years after the medication is discontinued (tardive dyskinesia). Typically, tardive dyskinesia spares the forehead and does not impair gait in contrast to the findings in Huntington's disease. Finally, there is a form of self-limited chorea, which, like other localized dyskinesias, may appear in older persons without identifiable cause. Hepatolenticular degeneration (Wilson's disease) and nonfamilial forms of hepatocerebral degeneration may display clinical abnormalities resembling those of Huntington's disease, but the specific changes characteristic of these disorders, including liver disease, corneal Kayser-Fleischer rings (in Wilson's disease), and the typical biochemical abnormalities, are absent in Huntington's disease (see Chap. 330). Choreoathetosis appearing during the second postnatal year and lasting throughout life is due to hypoxic birth injury or kernicterus. Sporadic cases of choreiform movements beginning in middle or late life may present a difficult problem in exact diagnosis. The occasional cases of violent choreiform movements produced by vascular lesions, classically in the subthalamic region, are characterized by sudden onset, unilateral distribution (hemiballismus), and a tendency to improve after a period of initial severity. A few cases of acute choreoathetosis have accompanied hyperthyroidism. Virus encephalitis may occasionally be associated with choreiform movements; acute development, fever, and pleocytosis in the CSF help in recognition of such cases. Hereditary acanthocytosis is a rare condition which can mimic Huntington's disease.

Treatment   No form of treatment has as yet been devised that halts the relentless progression of this disease, and therapeutic attempts to alleviate the abnormal movements have generally been unsatisfactory. Dopamine receptor antagonists (butyrophenones or phenothiazines) may partially ameliorate the chorea, but the side effects characteristic of this class of drugs limit their use. The depression, which is so common in many patients, usually responds to tricyclic antidepressants. The application of molecular genetic probes for presymptomatic and prenatal testing is available in several centers. However, until the gene itself is discovered, testing can only be performed in families by linkage analysis (see Chaps. 6 and 346).

MULTIPLE SYSTEM ATROPHY   General experience has indicated that cases of multiple affection of neuronal systems may occur in which progressive dementia is combined with varying degrees of ataxia, dysarthria, and parkinsonian dyskinesia, depending upon the pattern of anatomic distribution of the pathologic changes. For cases of this kind, the general term *multiple system atrophy* or *degeneration* has been applied. In some, loss of neurons in the cerebellar cortex and in the pontine nuclei and inferior olivary nuclei results in the predominating picture of *olivopontocerebellar degeneration,* to be discussed below as one of the syndromes of progressive ataxia. These changes may be combined with similar neuronal loss in the substantia nigra (and in the striatum in striatonigral degeneration), resulting in parkinsonian features (discussed below under ''Parkinson's Disease''). Pathologically, the disease process is characterized by death and disappearance of the affected cells and an accompanying reactive gliosis, without intracellular inclusions or other distinctive features. The cerebral cortex generally shows little discernible change, so that it may be difficult to ascribe a definite pathoanatomic basis for the dementia, which, for this reason, is sometimes designated as *subcortical.* Typically multiple system atrophy is a disorder of late adult life, occurring sporadically in some instances and genetically transmitted in others. Further details of individual syndromes are given in later sections.

PROGRESSIVE SUPRANUCLEAR PALSY (STEELE-RICHARDSON-OLSZEWSKI SYNDROME)   This disorder is discussed below among the syndromes characterized by gradually developing abnormalities of posture and movement. It is mentioned here because progressive dementia may accompany the other neurologic abnormalities, although it appears late in the course and generally is not severe.

DIFFUSE LEWY BODY DISEASE   Diffuse lewy body disease is a rare illness that presents with progressive dementia or psychosis. Parkinsonian signs, which may be absent or mild at the onset, eventually become common, and rigidity is usually severe. Tremor is often absent. Other features include involuntary movements, myoclonus, quadriparesis in flexion, orthostatic hypotension, and dysphagia in some cases. Lewy bodies are found profusely in the brainstem, basal forebrain, hypothalamic nuclei, and neocortex. The course of the illness is relentlessly progressive over several years.

CORTICODENTATONIGRAL DEGENERATION   Corticodentatonigral degeneration with neuronal achromasia is a rare illness which has also been termed cortical-basal ganglionic degeneration. Watts and colleagues have studied seven cases. The illness begins at age 55–75 and the initial symptoms are loss of dexterity in one limb (usually an arm) combined with rigidity and often a tremor in the limb. The illness then progresses steadily over several months to involve the other limbs with rigidity, postural imbalance, and masked facies. Dyspraxia is a prominent clinical feature but dementia is usually mild or absent until late in the clinical course. The findings at autopsy are severe neuronal loss and gliosis in cerebral cortex which is greatest in the perirolandic regions and mild neuronal loss and gliosis in the substantia nigra. In cortical areas many of the pyramidal neurons are swollen with indistinct nuclei and poorly stained pale cytoplasm (''achromasia'').

HALLERVORDEN-SPATZ DISEASE   This unusual disorder, often affecting several siblings in a family in a manner suggesting an autosomal recessive trait, is associated with a rather variable clinical picture in which abnormalities of posture and muscle tone, involuntary movements, and progressive dementia predominate. Pathologically, there are characteristic abnormalities in the basal ganglia, suggesting a localized disorder of metabolism. The features of the condition were classically described in an affected family by Hallervorden and Spatz (1922).

Pathology   Distinctive for this condition is the accumulation of large amounts of pigmented material in the globus pallidus and pars reticulata of the substantia nigra, resulting in grossly visible brownish discoloration of these regions. Microscopically, there are irregular pigmented, ferruginous concretions and granules of varying brownish or greenish hues, depending on the stains used. Although much of this pigment contains iron, serum iron and ferritin are normal, and there is no systemic disorder of iron metabolism. There also is loss of nerve cells. Another feature of the disease is the presence of focal swelling of axons, most probably in their terminal portions; this is especially pronounced in the regions affected by the pigmentary disorder, but typically can be found at all levels of the central nervous system, including the cerebral cortex. This neuroaxonal change may link the disease with childhood neuroaxonal dystrophy.

Clinical aspects   The disorder typically makes its appearance in childhood or adolescence, with abnormalities in muscle tone and movements, such as rigidity and choreoathetosis. Abnormal postures of the trunk characteristic of torsion spasm (dystonia) may be seen, or the clinical picture may be reminiscent of parkinsonism. Cerebellar ataxia is also present in some instances. Speech becomes indistinct, and there is progressive intellectual impairment. Eventually, the involuntary movements give way to increasing generalized rigidity, and death comes as a rule about 10 years after onset. A few cases of late onset have shown a parkinsonian syndrome.

Differential diagnosis   No feature of the clinical picture serves to distinguish this particular disorder from other conditions showing dementia with extrapyramidal motor abnormalities. Wilson's disease must be excluded by appropriate laboratory tests. The clearly progressive course sets this condition apart from clinically similar abnormalities resulting from accidents or illnesses at birth or in the neonatal period. It has lately been demonstrated that following intravenous injection of labeled ferrous citrate, there is a selective uptake of radioactive iron in the region of the basal ganglia; possibly a study of this kind would be helpful in diagnosis. In an advanced case, CT scanning may show extreme atrophy of the brain, especially including the structures of the basal ganglia, but the pigmented deposits do not show any increased radiographic density. In some cases there is lucency in the putamen and globus pallidus. MRI scans show a characteristic pattern of increased density in the globus pallidus surrounded by low density on T2-weighted images. This sign has been termed ''eye of the tiger.'' At present no effective treatment is known. Treatment with a chelating agent, deferoxamine mesylate, has not shown definite benefit, and levodopa and other antiparkinsonian medications, tryptophan, and megavitamin therapy have been of only temporary and questionable help.

PROGRESSIVE FAMILIAL MYOCLONIC EPILEPSY   There are several neurologic disorders that can result in a syndrome of convulsive seizures, myoclonic jerklike contractions of the musculature, and progressive dementia. Those most frequently encountered in practice are subacute sclerosing panencephalitis in children, adolescents, and young adults (Chap. 355), and subacute spongiform encephalopathy (Creutzfeldt-Jakob disease) in older adults (Chap. 355). The syndrome can also occur in some of the rare forms of metabolic familial disorders: neuraminidase deficiency associated with macular cherry-red spots (Chap. 331) and ceroid-lipofuscinosis (Chap. 338). When these and other disorders of known cause can be excluded from consideration, there remain some clinicopathologic entities which can appropriately be considered under the heading of the hereditary degenerative diseases. Several families presenting this syndrome have been carefully studied in northern Europe (Sweden and Finland), but there is no specific geographic distribution.

Lafora's disease This variety of recessively inherited progressive myoclonic epilepsy is characterized by distinctive intracytoplasmic inclusions in cerebral neurons, called Lafora bodies following their original description by Gonzalo Lafora (1911). These have been found to be composed of polymers of glucose (polyglucosans) and thus indicate a disorder of carbohydrate metabolism, but the biochemical defect that leads to their accumulation is unknown. The Lafora bodies are widely distributed, but most numerous in the thalamus, substantia nigra, and dentate nucleus of the cerebellum. Subsequent to Lafora's reports, similar polysaccharide deposits have been found in myocardial and skeletal muscle fibers, skin, and in the liver, and it is now possible to establish the diagnosis in the presymptomatic phase by skin or liver biopsy.

The disorder characteristically makes its appearance during childhood or adolescence in the form of recurrent seizures (generalized or restricted), or uncontrollable myoclonic jerks, or combinations of the two. With the passage of time, the myoclonic phenomena become increasingly severe, and there is deterioration of all intellectual functions. Death from intercurrent infection generally occurs before the age of 25. Anticonvulsive treatment may help in controlling the seizures, but there currently is no effective treatment for the underlying disease.

Unverricht-Lundborg disease This is a rare autosomal recessive illness with onset in adolescence of myoclonic and tonic-clonic seizures. Dementia is mild or absent at the outset, but eventually there is a gradual intellectual decline as well as dysarthria, ataxia, and intention tremor. Survival into adulthood is usual. Pathologic studies show widespread degenerative changes without evidence of storage material.

Other varieties of myoclonic epilepsy When Lafora's disease and the metabolic and infective disorders mentioned above have been excluded, there remains a rather heterogeneous group of progressive neurologic illnesses having in common autosomal recessive inheritance, myoclonic phenomena, convulsive seizures, and mild dementia. Ataxia of stance, gait, and limb movements is a prominent feature in most cases—so much so that the term introduced by Ramsay Hunt, *dyssynergia cerebellaris myoclonica*, is often applied. In a few cases, including some of those originally described by Hunt, there is an overlap with Friedreich's ataxia, or with chronic sensorimotor neuropathies (see Chaps. 361 and 363). The neuropathologic changes in the few cases that have come to postmortem examination have varied from case to case. In some, atrophy of the dentate nucleus and its fiber projections has been prominent; in others, there has been loss of neurons, especially Purkinje cells, in the cerebellar cortex; in still others, changes have been confined to long-tract degeneration (posterior columns and spinocerebellar tracts) in the spinal cord; a few patients have had cortical, basal-ganglionic, or retinal lesions. Variations also occur in the age of onset and the rate of progression. Until more is known about the biochemistry and genetics of this group of disorders, no satisfactory classification is possible. For further details of these syndromes, general reference works on neurology, such as that of Adams and Victor, should be consulted.

Treatment with appropriate anticonvulsant medications has been helpful in some mild cases, but phenytoin is contraindicated. L-Tryptophan and carbidopa or valproic acid have ameliorated myoclonus in a few cases.

SYNDROMES OF ABNORMAL POSTURE, TREMOR, AND INVOLUNTARY MOVEMENT

PARALYSIS AGITANS (PARKINSON'S DISEASE) This is a common condition first named and described by James Parkinson in 1817. His remarkably complete account gives this definition:

Involuntary tremulous motion, with lessened muscular power, in parts not in action and even when supported; with a propensity to bend the trunk forward, *and to pass from a walking to a running pace, the senses and intellects being uninjured.*

Typically, Parkinson's disease is a disorder of middle or late life, with very gradual progression and a prolonged course. Although it has been seen to occur in families (the estimated familial incidence is 1 to 2 percent), it usually is sporadic. It is well recognized, however, that the epidemic encephalitis of von Economo, which occurred in a worldwide distribution in the years following World War I, was followed by a syndrome clinically almost indistinguishable from paralysis agitans. It is usual in such instances to speak of postencephalitic parkinsonism, whereas the term *Parkinson's disease* should be reserved for true paralysis agitans of unknown cause. Parkinson's disease bears no consistent relation to any known disease process such as arteriosclerosis, trauma, or intoxication (except for MPTP, see below), although such conditions have often been invoked as etiologically significant and may at times produce somewhat similar clinical manifestations.

Pathology Despite the general medical familiarity with the condition and an extensive literature on the subject, it cannot be said that the pathologic changes of paralysis agitans are yet fully understood. The most regularly observed changes have been in the aggregates of melanin-containing nerve cells in the brainstem (substantia nigra, locus coeruleus), where there are varying degrees of nerve cell loss with reactive gliosis (most pronounced in the substantia nigra) along with distinctive eosinophilic intracytoplasmic inclusions (Lewy bodies). Similar changes are seen in the nucleus basalis of Meynert. Lesions in pigmented nuclei, but without Lewy bodies, characterize the pathologic findings in postencephalitic parkinsonism, in striatonigral degeneration, and in the Shy-Drager syndrome (discussed below).

Biochemical studies show a decrease of dopamine in the caudate nucleus and putamen, emphasizing the point that Parkinson's disease can be considered an example of neuronal system disease, involving mainly the nigrostriatal dopaminergic system. Confirmation of the importance of the nigrostriatal dopaminergic system arose from observations of the effects of accidental intoxication of drug users by self-injection with 1-methyl-4-phenyl-1,2,3,6-tetrahydropyridine (MPTP), which selectively destroys dopaminergic neurons of the substantia nigra. The typical clinical manifestations of this disease resemble closely those of Parkinson's disease. The pathologic features of MPTP-induced Parkinson's disease, however, differ from those of idiopathic cases in the absence of Lewy bodies and the lack of neuronal loss in the locus coeruleus, but the mechanism by which the drug kills substantia nigra neurons may provide new insights about the pathogenesis of the idiopathic illness.

Clinical aspects In its fully developed form, Parkinson's disease cannot be mistaken for any other. The stooped posture, the stiffness and slowness of movement, the fixity of facial expression, and the rhythmic tremor of the limbs, which subsides on active willed movement or complete relaxation, are familiar to every clinician. Although symmetric in the later stages, the disorder typically begins asymmetrically, e.g., as a slight tremor of the fingers of one hand or in one leg. Also typical are more or less general hypokinesia and stiffness of the musculature so that even where tremor is inapparent, the disease may betray itself by a somewhat staring and immobile facial expression, a monotonous voice, a general slowness and diminution of all motor activity, and a curious lack of the little spontaneous movements of postural adjustment that are so characteristic of the normal individual. When tremor is minimal, patients often are able to alleviate it by relaxation or by movement or to hide it by keeping their hands in their pockets. The tremor is generally most pronounced in the hands but may involve the legs (and thus secondarily the trunk), lips, tongue, and neck muscles, and is easily seen in the eyelids when they are lightly closed. Its frequency is 4 to 5 per second, but another faster (action) tremor (7 to 8 per second) predominates in some patients. There is never total paralysis, although this is implied by the name of the disease; nevertheless, general enfeeblement of voluntary movement is characteristic of the fully developed disorder. Generally accompanying the stooped attitude is the typical festinating gait, whereby the patient, prevented by the abnormality of postural tone from making the appropriate reflex adjustments required for effective walking, progresses with quick shuffling steps at an accelerating pace as if to catch up with the body's center of gravity. Clinical examination of the tendon and plantar reflexes discloses no abnormalities. There are no sensory changes, although deep aching in joints and muscles is common. Eventually, patients may become so incapacitated by rigidity and tremor as to be helpless in caring for themselves. It has often been observed, however, that even severely disabled patients may, when excited or under great emotional stress, perform complex motor acts quickly and efficiently. Although the temporary alleviation under extreme provocation can never be long maintained, it is nevertheless true that the severity of the symptoms is considerably influenced by emotional factors, being aggravated by anxiety, tension, and unhappiness, and minimal when the patient is in a contented frame of mind. Despite the inherently progressive nature of the condition, much can be achieved with good medical management, and patients may continue for years to live effective, happy lives.

Although intellectual deterioration is not a consistent feature of early Parkinson's disease, dementia has been increasingly recognized to be a feature of advanced Parkinson's disease. It eventually afflicts up to one-third of all cases. The dementia is typically insidious in onset and may be heralded by disorientation at night. In advanced cases patients may suffer from vivid auditory and visual hallucinations, often precipitated by levodopa therapy.

Differential diagnosis   In typical cases, this is not difficult. The extrapyramidal syndromes associated with most diseases of known cause or established nature, such as cerebrovascular disease, cerebral hypoxia (including carbon monoxide asphyxia), or metallic poisoning, differ from paralysis agitans in a number of respects, such as atypical behavior or tremor, presence of signs of corticospinal tract deficit, or early onset of dementia. The differentiation from postencephalitic parkinsonism may be impossible; a clear history of an attack of epidemic encephalitis (prolonged somnolence, disturbance of consciousness, diplopia) and relatively early age of onset of the disorder and the presence of tics, localized spasms, and oculogyric crises may be the only clues to this diagnosis. A neurologic disorder similar to some degree to Parkinson's disease occurs with the prolonged administration of large amounts of reserpine and phenothiazine drugs, as the result of their blocking action on dopaminergic transmission. This drug-induced syndrome usually subsides on discontinuation or decrease in the dosage of the drug, but it may continue indefinitely in the syndrome of *tardive dyskinesia*. MPTP-induced parkinsonism persists because of the destructive effects of the drug on the nigral dopaminergic neurons. Parkinsonism very rarely is produced by cerebral neoplasms or other focal lesions, but then only when the nigrostriatal system has been largely destroyed, with relative sparing of the corticospinal projections.

Some Parkinson-like postural and motor abnormalities may be seen following the repeated blows to the head sustained by boxers—in the "punch drunk" syndrome, in which lesions of the substantia nigra are one of the neuropathologic components. In this condition, dementia, ataxia, dysarthria, and inappropriate behavior are prominent, and neuronal cell loss with neurofibrillary tangles is evident in the cerebral cortex.

Multiple bilateral infarcts in the corticospinal pathways and central structures of the brain may induce a syndrome that in some ways resembles paralysis agitans (so-called arteriosclerotic parkinsonism), but careful clinical assessment of the history and findings, particularly the reflex status, serves to distinguish this disorder from true Parkinson's disease. Striatonigral degeneration is a rare syndrome which can be clinically indistinguishable from Parkinson's disease but which does not respond to dopaminergic agents (see below). Progressive supranuclear palsy may also present as a parkinsonian syndrome; however, eventually the characteristic abnormalities of eye movement become manifest.

Treatment   Although there is no treatment that is known to halt or reverse the neuronal degeneration that presumably underlies Parkinson's disease, methods are now available which can bring about a considerable degree of relief from symptoms in many patients. An important part of any therapeutic program is the maintenance of optimum general health and neuromuscular efficiency by planned programs of exercise, activity, and rest; expert physical therapy may be of great help in achieving these ends. In addition, the patient often needs much emotional support in meeting the stress of the illness, in comprehending its nature, and in carrying on courageously in spite of it. Along with these general supportive measures, which are applicable to many chronic illnesses, patients generally require a carefully thought-out program of treatment specifically aimed at counteracting the pathophysiologic disorder that produces their disabilities.

Drug therapy should be adapted to the patient's needs, which vary with the stage of the disease and the predominant manifestation(s). Usually anticholinergic drugs are most effective in suppressing tremor at rest, and propranolol or primidone is best for action tremor. Levodopa improves akinesia and postural imbalance; anticholinergic drugs have little effect on these two abnormalities.

The decision about whether to treat with a drug and the choice of drug(s) are influenced by the stage of the disease. The scale of Hoehn and Yahr is recommended:

Stage I: Unilateral involvement.
Stage II: Bilateral involvement but no postural abnormalities.
Stage III: Bilateral involvement with mild postural imbalance; the patient leads an independent life.
Stage IV: Bilateral involvement with postural instability; the patient requires substantial help.
Stage V: Severe, fully developed disease; the patient is restricted to bed and chair.

For patients with mild disease (stages I and II), no medication may be required, or only an anticholinergic drug, or amantadine (a dopamine agonist), or a combination of both. Levodopa is required for stages III, IV, and V. In each instance, one uses the lowest dose that gives satisfactory benefit; this decreases the chances of unwanted side effects such as dyskinesias, the on-off phenomenon, and mental confusion, as well as of loss of efficacy of the drug.

The anticholinergic drugs in use share the capacity to block muscarinic receptors and thereby to reduce cholinergic transmission. They are effective not only in relieving the rest tremor of mild Parkinson's disease but also may be combined with levodopa in the treatment of the severe forms of the disease. The anticholinergic drugs also reverse the dystonia and parkinsonian symptoms of neuroleptic drugs.

Currently available anticholinergic drugs are trihexyphenidyl, benztropine, biperiden, and procyclidine. The usual dose of trihexyphenidyl is 1 to 2 mg qid. Benztropine has both anticholinergic and antihistaminic properties; the usual dose is 0.5 to 1.0 mg tid. The optimal dose of all these medications varies for each patient and often needs adjusting. Low doses of these drugs cause dry mouth but few if any other side effects. Larger doses should be given with caution for in the elderly they may cause confusion, visual and tactile hallucinations, narrow-angle glaucoma, and urinary retention. Anticholinergic drugs may exacerbate dementia and should be withdrawn when dementia becomes clinically evident.

Propranolol, a beta-adrenergic antagonist, is helpful in suppressing the fast-frequency action tremor in Parkinson's disease and in the hereditary tremor syndrome. The usual dose is 40 to 80 mg tid. In large doses, it may slow the heart rate and lower blood pressure, which are disadvantages in patients with a tendency to orthostatic hypotension. Metoprolol, a specific beta-adrenergic antagonist, is also effective and is safer in patients with suspected asthma. Primidone in a dose of 50 mg at bedtime has also been shown to be effective. If the tremor is not improved after 1 week, the dose can be increased up to 250 mg daily. Many clinicians now initiate therapy with this regimen.

Amantadine was found by accident to be helpful in Parkinson's disease. Its effect is achieved by its capacity to release stored dopamine from presynaptic terminals; thus it is efficacious in the earlier stages of the disease, before the majority of the dopaminergic neurons in the midbrain have degenerated. It tends to be especially beneficial for tremor. The usual dosage is 100 mg bid; larger doses may produce side effects such as skin changes (livedo reticularis), ankle edema, and mental confusion. In some patients, the addition of amantadine to levodopa achieves better results than either medication alone.

Levodopa, which increases the dopamine levels in the striatum and restores neurotransmitter balance between dopamine and acetylcholine, improves akinesia and postural disorders (and sometimes rest tremor) in 75 percent of patients. Levodopa is now given in combination with a dopa-carboxylase inhibitor (carbidopa) which prevents destruction of levodopa in the bloodstream and peripheral tissues but does not pass the blood-brain barrier. This combination therefore makes it possible to achieve optimum effects with a smaller dosage of levodopa than would otherwise need to be used. In this way, some of the side effects of levodopa, particularly nausea and vomiting, can be greatly reduced. The combination (Sinemet) is available in ratios of 1:4 carbidopa to levodopa (25 mg/100 mg) or 1:10 (10/100, 25/250). A total dosage of levodopa from 300 to 2000 mg daily can be used; the relative amounts of carbidopa and levodopa, and the timing of the medications, should be adjusted according to the needs of the individual patient. Although levodopa now is the cornerstone of therapy, it can be combined with an anticholinergic drug, with amantadine, or with bromocriptine.

Bromocriptine is a dopamine agonist which acts directly upon dopamine receptors, unlike levodopa, which requires enzymatic transformation into dopamine within the brain. It has been found to be helpful in the treatment of Parkinson's disease, generally in combination with levodopa. When used alone, patients with mild early disease will often respond to doses of 15 to 30 mg daily. However, more advanced patients may need a dosage range of 50 to 100 mg daily. When given in combination with other drugs, smaller quantities should be used, beginning with 2.5 mg tid. Doses of bromocriptine ranging from 20 to 30 mg daily have been effective as an adjunct to levodopa therapy. Whether or not to use bromocriptine and the dosage are matters that must be decided on the basis of what seems best for an individual patient. The side effects are much the same as those with levodopa.

It must be said that although the modern treatment of Parkinson's disease is more successful than any that was available before the introduction of levodopa, including stereotactic surgery, there are still many problems. Underlying much of the difficulty undoubtedly is the fact that none of these therapeutic measures has an effect on the underlying disease process, which consists of neuronal degeneration. Ultimately a point seems to be reached where pharmacotherapy can no longer compensate for the loss. The major difficulties consist of fluctuations or sudden variations in the response to the drugs used (the on-off response), the development of weakness or immobility (akinesia), and dyskinesias, which increasingly become a problem as the years go by. The dyskinesias consist of choreiform or choreoathetotic movements, which in the late stages of the disease alternate with paralyzing akinesia depending upon a very narrow dosage variation (50 to 100 mg) of levodopa. Interference with absorption of levodopa may be partially responsible since continuous intravenous infusions of levodopa result in a stable clinical state. Loss of therapeutic efficacy also occurs: a single dose which at one time was effective for 5 to 6 h may last only an hour or so. Giving smaller amounts of medication more frequently is sometimes efficacious. In addition, agents acting directly on the postsynaptic receptor, such as

bromocriptine, are sometimes more effective. It has recently been shown that temporary levodopa withdrawal, advocated as a method of dealing with the long-term complications of Parkinson's disease, carries some risk and does not result in improved efficacy of levodopa.

Progressive dementia, which eventually overtakes one-third to one-half of the patients in later years, may render them less tolerant to medication. Visual and tactile hallucinations are especially prominent in this group of patients.

As many as one-half of patients with Parkinson's disease have depressive symptoms. They should be treated along the lines suggested in Chap. 369.

The introduction of stereotaxic surgery, with the placement of precisely localized focal lesions in central structures in the brain—mainly the ventrolateral thalamus, or globus pallidus contralateral to the side of the major symptoms—was an important advance in the attempt to relieve the symptoms of Parkinson's disease. The success that has been achieved with levodopa has largely supplanted these procedures, which, although very beneficial in well-chosen cases, were not without risk and at times were followed by severe disability. Neurosurgical treatment of this kind can still be recommended for patients who are relatively young and who have a severe unilateral disabling or disfiguring tremor. Recent interest has focused on adrenal medullary transplants to the striatum. Although initial reports indicated favorable responses, subsequent experience in many centers has failed to confirm the earlier report. Fetal tissue transplants containing substantia nigra neurons may be more effective. Clinical trials indicate that deprenyl (a monoamine oxidase B inhibitor) can retard clinical progression of the disease.

STRIATONIGRAL DEGENERATION   This rare syndrome closely resembles Parkinson's disease clinically, but clearly differs from it pathologically. The classic clinicopathologic description is that of Adams, van Bogaert, and Van der Eecken, who encountered the disorder in four middle-aged patients with no family history of similar disease. Three of the patients showed the typical clinical picture of Parkinson's disease; orthostatic hypotension was observed in one of them, and cerebellar ataxia in another.

The principal neuronal cell loss is in the striatum and substantia nigra. There is an association in some cases with a progressive ataxic disorder resembling olivopontocerebellar degeneration, and in others with degeneration of spinal cord neurons of the autonomic nervous system, similar to the Shy-Drager syndrome, in which postural hypotension is a major component (see below). The degree to which parkinsonian symptoms occur probably depends on the extent of the nigral lesions as balanced against those in the cerebellum and its connections. Cases of this kind represent examples of multiple system degeneration as described above.

The disorder characteristically occurs in late middle age. Treatment with anti-Parkinson's disease medications has usually not been successful. For measures which control hypotension see under "Shy-Drager Syndrome" (below and Chap. 21).

PROGRESSIVE SUPRANUCLEAR PALSY (STEELE-RICHARDSON-OLSZEWSKI SYNDROME)   This disorder, first clearly described in 1963 by Richardson, Steele, and Olszewski, occurs in elderly individuals in approximately the same age period as paralysis agitans. Moreover, it is among the group of parkinsonian patients that most of the examples of this disease are to be found.

Pathology   A loss of neurons and gliosis are found on postmortem examination in the tectum and tegmentum of the midbrain, the subthalamic nuclei of Luys, the vestibular nuclei, and to some extent the ocular nuclei. A characteristic finding is the presence of neurofibrillary tangles similar to those of Alzheimer's disease on light-microscopic examination, but differing from them on electron microscopy in that they are composed of straight rather than paired helical filaments. The cause of the disease is unknown. A slow virus has been suspected, but attempts to transfer it to monkeys by the intracerebral inoculation of brain tissue have failed.

Clinical manifestations The clinical features are quite distinctive: disturbances of balance and gait with unexpected falls; rigidity of the neck and other trunk muscles, resembling Parkinson's disease; "masking" of the face; reduction in the volume of the voice; extreme flexion or extension dystonia of the neck; and difficulty in looking down—all these are early symptoms and any one of them may first bring the patient to a physician. Ophthalmoplegia has been regarded as the cardinal clinical sign of the disease. Typically there is initial impairment of vertical saccadic movements and a loss of the fast component of optokinetic nystagmus usually affecting downward more than upward gaze. With progression of the disease horizontal eye movements are affected, with oculovestibular reflexes preserved. Symptoms progress over months and years, until the patient becomes virtually anarthric with total loss of voluntary control of eye movements, and severe cervical and truncal rigidity. Dementia is usually mild with forgetfulness, slowing of thought processes, apathy, and impaired ability to manipulate acquired knowledge. There are no impairments of vision, hearing, somatic sensation, or voluntary power, and signs of corticospinal involvement are minimal or absent. The diagnosis should be considered whenever an elderly patient begins to fall repeatedly and inexplicably and has extrapyramidal symptoms with a rigid neck and paralysis of conjugate or vertical gaze.

Treatment Treatment has been unsuccessful. Relatively little benefit comes from the administration of the antiparkinsonian group of drugs, although they should be tried. Occasionally levodopa, or a combination of levodopa with an anticholinergic drug, has helped to diminish some of the symptoms.

NORMAL-PRESSURE HYDROCEPHALUS Normal-pressure hydrocephalus (NPH) is a syndrome of communicating hydrocephalus in which intracranial hypertension is either absent or not recognized. It is discussed here because of the common association of the condition with dementia and abnormalities of gait.

Pathology and pathophysiology Although it is recognized that delayed hydrocephalus can occur after meningitis, head injury, or subarachnoid hemorrhage, the majority of patients presenting with NPH give no history of such an illness. Studies of isotope cisternography indicate that NPH is a communicating hydrocephalus presumed to be due to partial obliteration of the subarachnoid space with defective CSF reabsorption through the arachnoid villi. Whether episodes of increased intracranial pressure occur during the course of the illness is debated. Some patients monitored continuously show fluctuations in CSF pressure including so-called plateau waves.

Clinical manifestations Typically, the patient or family describe a subacute onset, over weeks, months, or sometimes years, of progressive intellectual deterioration accompanied by slowness and restriction of movements, particularly of gait. No single diagnostic gait disorder occurs (see description, Chap. 26). A broad-based stance with hesitant initiation of walking is common. In some patients ataxic features are present. Hyperreflexia in the legs and extensor plantar responses may be found. Urinary incontinence is noted in less than one-half of patients.

Differential diagnosis Parkinson's disease can be differentiated by its clinical features and the response to carbidopa-levodopa (Sinemet). Bifrontal disease due to tumor (butterfly glioma), metastases, or cerebral infarction can be identified by CT or MRI. Multi-infarct dementia with gait disorder can be recognized by focal, often asymmetric, neurologic signs and by CT changes. Aqueductal stenosis may present occasionally in late adulthood with hydrocephalus, headaches, dementia, and incontinence. The CT or MRI usually will demonstrate an enlarged third ventricle with normal fourth ventricle.

Treatment The diagnosis can be difficult because of the common association of ventricular enlargement and gait disorder in patients with degenerative brain conditions, particularly Alzheimer's disease. CSF pressure in NPH is usually in the normal range of 80 to 150 mmH$_2$O. Isotope cisternography demonstrating reflux into the ventricular system may be helpful in some cases. However, the finding of ventricular reflux has not proved to determine reliably which patients are likely to improve following a surgical shunt. Temporary benefit in the gait disorder after removal of 25 to 30 mL of CSF has been noted in some patients. When the history of dementia and gait disorder is subacute in onset and accompanied by considerable ventricular dilatation, surgical shunting is warranted. Ventricular-peritoneal shunting is the procedure most commonly performed. Between 40 and 70 percent of patients show benefit after surgery. The gait disorder tends to show a better response to shunting than the dementia (see Black et al. for review).

TORSION DYSTONIA (TORSION SPASM; DYSTONIA MUSCULORUM DEFORMANS) This is a syndrome of sustained muscular contraction frequently causing twisting and repetitive movements that result in abnormal, at times bizarre, postures of the limbs and trunk. Eventually these postures become more or less fixed. Underlying the clinical disorder may be any of several pathologic conditions, such as the lesions of neonatal hypoxia, Wilson's disease, the pigmented lesions of Hallervorden-Spatz disease (described above), GM$_1$ gangliosidosis, ataxia-telangiectasia, or kernicterus. There is, in addition, an important group of cases with a variable pattern of genetic transmission. Occasionally, a similar disorder occurs sporadically in late adult life. It is to these cases, both hereditary and sporadic, that the term *torsion dystonia* (torsion spasm, dystonia musculorum deformans) is correctly applied. In these conditions, the course tends to be progressive, and the cause and pathogenesis remain unknown. Genetic linkage studies have shown a positive correlation to markers on chromosome 9 and the mechanism is autosomal dominant inheritance.

Pathology Few cases of dystonia musculorum deformans not due to one of the definable disease processes indicated above have been adequately studied neuropathologically. Reported results from these cases has led to uncertainty as to what the pathologic-anatomic basis of the clinical state might be, although it was generally assumed that the basal ganglia were diseased. A careful study by Zeman and Dyken, which included comparison of the findings in patients with the disease with control material, failed to demonstrate any neuropathologic abnormality to which the clinical changes could reasonably be attributed. These negative findings, which are perhaps surprising, must not be interpreted as indicating that there is "no disease" in the brain, but rather that the pathologic state is not one that can be disclosed by the usual histopathologic techniques. It may well be that more careful quantitative assessments of certain populations of neurons and studies of the pathophysiology of neurotransmitters will result in further elucidation of this disease.

Clinical manifestations The motor abnormalities are described in Chap. 25. In the early stages, the involuntary muscular contractions are intermittent and variable in location and severity, but typically interfere with motor performance by superimposing an unwanted posture upon parts in use. One leg may briefly be pulled into a flexed or extended position or one shoulder elevated. Later the lingual, pharyngeal, neck, and thoracic muscles participate, and grimacing may occur. These latter may also be the first and only signs of disease for several years. Progression may be relatively rapid in cases with onset during early childhood, but is slow in those beginning in late childhood or adult life. The end result is extreme disability, with grossly distorted postures of the trunk and contractures of the limbs. Affection of face and tongue muscles results in faulty articulation of speech, which eventually becomes incomprehensible. The tendon and plantar reflexes are normal.

The most severe type, which occurs almost exclusively in Ashkenazi Jews, characteristically makes its appearance in childhood after a preceding period of normalcy. Typically it becomes first evident in the lower limbs and then evolves, sometimes relatively rapidly, into the generalized state of severe incapacity described above. The manner of genetic transmission—whether autosomal recessive or dominant with variable penetrance—is still not wholly settled. In the recognized autosomal dominant type, which occurs mainly in non-Jewish populations, the disorder comes on later (often in midadult life) and takes a milder form. It tends to appear first in the upper limbs and to remain more restricted in its extent than the early-onset variety, and progression is less relentless. The late-life sporadic cases are generally similar in character to those of the autosomal dominant form; here, the possibility of dominant transmission with incomplete penetrance cannot always be excluded.

FOCAL DYSTONIAS In addition to the generalized dystonias noted above, there is a group of focal or segmental dystonias which appear sporadically in adult life. Their clearly involuntary nature, and lack of susceptibility to willed control by the patient, distinguish them from the common tics, habit spasms, and mannerisms described in Chap. 25. They have often been erroneously interpreted as manifestations of hysteria. If the muscle contraction is frequent and prolonged, aching pain accompanies it—for which the spasm may mistakenly be blamed.

The most frequent and familiar type of focal dystonia is *spasmodic torticollis.* This is a disorder of adults that afflicts women somewhat more frequently than men. It consists of an involuntary turning of the head to one side—intermittent at first, then gradually worsening to the point of being more or less continuous. In some cases, torticollis is the first manifestation of a generalized dystonia, but more usually it remains focal and segmental.

Another frequent focal dystonia of adults is exemplified by *writer's cramp,* in which the dystonic postures and movements occur only during the performance of specific acts, to the extent that carrying out the act in the usual way, such as writing with a pen or pencil, becomes impossible, while other motor activities using the same musculature are unimpaired. An analogous disorder sometimes afflicts musicians.

The combination of blepharospasm and oromandibular dystonia—*cranial dystonia*—is sometimes referred to as Meige's syndrome. When the throat and respiratory muscles are involved, this interferes with speech production, resulting in spastic dysarthria. The muscles of the neck are variably affected. It should be recalled that similar dystonic states (facial-cervical and more extreme dyskinesias) can result from the use of phenothiazine and similar drugs. This sometimes persists after discontinuation of the medication as *tardive dyskinesia*—a troublesome condition that may resist all forms of treatment.

Differential diagnosis Hepatolenticular degeneration (Wilson's disease) should be seriously considered in any case presenting these motor symptoms and appropriate measures should be undertaken for its investigation (see Chap. 330). The progressive course, and possibly the family history, differentiate the degenerative group from the "symptomatic" dystonias resulting from infections or metabolic disorders occurring at birth or later. Hallervorden-Spatz disease, however, cannot be distinguished on clinical grounds alone. Rare instances of GM_1 gangliosidosis or other lipid storage diseases may begin in adult life with a dystonic syndrome, and drug-induced (tardive) dyskinesia must be considered in all cases of focal or generalized dystonia in adults, especially if they have or have had a psychiatric illness.

Treatment This is extremely difficult and often unsatisfactory. In the generalized dystonias, pharmacotherapy should certainly be attempted and, in most patients, needs to be individualized. Marsden and Fahn, whose experience with this disorder is extensive, suggest beginning with an anticholinergic agent such as trihexyphenidyl or ethopropazine and very gradually increasing the dosage until either benefit ensues or intolerable side effects appear. They found that the response in children (who may be able to take as much as 80 mg/d of trihexyphenidyl) was better than in adults, who tolerated the high doses less well, generally because of mental disturbances. In their experience, the next best group of drugs for ameliorating dystonic spasms are the benzodiazepines (such as diazepam) which likewise are used in high dosage after a very gradual introduction and increase (up to 80 mg of diazepam daily). Again, children are more tolerant of the side effects (mainly drowsiness). A combination of anticholinergics and benzodiazepines may work out best. Other drugs—both dopaminergic agonists and antagonists—have been used, occasionally with success.

Stereotaxic surgical operations have been used in the past to treat generalized dystonias, with insufficient benefit to counterbalance the risks. Cervical cord stimulation, a less hazardous procedure, has helped some patients; referral to a neurosurgeon with experience in the technique should be considered when medical treatment has failed.

The symptoms of the focal dystonias, if not severe, may be more acceptable to the patient than prolonged trials with various drugs or surgical intervention. Biofeedback techniques are sometimes helpful. Denervative surgical procedures may at times be beneficial if only a very restricted group of muscles is involved (as in torticollis). Blepharospasm has recently been successfully treated temporarily with local injection of botulinum toxin into the orbicularis oculi muscles. Beneficial effects last on average for 10 to 12 weeks. Neuroleptics (dopamine-antagonists) such as haloperidol or perphenazine may be useful in the treatment of focal dystonias. Here again, the program of management must be adapted to the individual patient's needs.

FAMILIAL TREMOR One of the commonest hereditary disorders of the human nervous system is that which gives rise to a fast-frequency (6 to 8 per second) action tremor. This may appear at any age but more often during adolescence and adult years; once started, it lasts throughout life. The heredity is dominant. Probably all cases are not the same, for some patients have tremors of slower frequency, looking more like those of Parkinson's disease, but lacking the slowness of movement, rigidity, and flexed postures of that disorder. In patients of advanced age it is called *senile tremor.* Consumption of alcohol suppresses the fast-frequency forms, as does a beta-adrenergic blocking agent (propranolol) in doses of 20 to 40 mg three times daily. The slightly slower rhythmic action tremors with frequencies of approximately 6 per second do not consistently respond to propranolol or alcohol. Primidone 50 mg at bedtime has recently been found to be effective and has been advocated for use as initial therapy. If there is no response after 1 week the dose should be increased gradually up to 250 mg at bedtime. Usually the tremor is the only abnormality, but in a few patients a cerebellar ataxia or an extrapyramidal syndrome may appear years later. The pathologic basis is unknown.

GILLES DE LA TOURETTE SYDROME This condition, of unknown cause and uncertain pathology, presents with multiple tics, associated with snorting, sniffing, and involuntary vocalizations. It begins in childhood, usually as isolated tics, which are at first difficult to distinguish from habit spasms. Progression occurs over years, and other behavioral findings appear; compulsive touching of others, repeating of words or phrases, and explosive utterance of obscenities (coprolalia). Careful attention to other members of the family has given evidence that the disease is hereditary, with an autosomal dominant pattern of transmission. Obsessive compulsive disorder appears to be an alternate phenotypic expression of the gene in these families.

The course of the illness is unpredictable. In some cases associated mild neurologic abnormalities are found with hyperactivity, disorders of attention, and abnormal psychologic tests. Dementia does not occur. In some patients the condition abates, in others it progresses, leading to serious disability. Treatment is only partially satisfactory. Haloperidol has received the most clinical attention, but should be used only in severe cases, and in the smallest effective dosage: 0.25 to 0.5 mg daily. Clonidine has proved effective in some cases.

SYNDROMES OF SLOWLY DEVELOPING ATAXIA

These conditions are distinguished clinically by progressive unsteadiness in standing and walking, along with impaired coordination of the limbs. Pathologically, they are characterized by degeneration of the cerebellum and/or its related fiber systems, and thus constitute classic examples of the system diseases. Although sporadic instances occur, hereditary transmission is an outstanding feature in most cases; as a result, this group of disorders is often referred to as the *hereditary ataxias.* Their subdivision into more or less separate entities is largely arbitrary, with pathologic changes of varying distribution underlying clinically indistinguishable symptom complexes. As yet, not enough is known about the underlying basis for the pathophysiologic alterations for a more satisfactory classification to be established.

Attempts to establish a classification on a genetic basis, on the presumption that a defective gene expressed as a progressive ataxia would produce a distinctive clinicopathologic picture, have not been successful. Instead, the phenotypic expression of the genetic abnormality commonly varies widely among affected members of an individual family. Because of these difficulties, the most that a clinician can do when confronted with a case is to exclude infective, toxic, metabolic, or neoplastic diseases for which there might be effective treatment, to search for evidence of genetic factors, and to assess the state of the patient as precisely as possible. There are now indications that some of the hereditary ataxic disorders may be associated with an identifiable biochemical abnormality though at present it is not possible to make use of this information in a way that would correct the abnormality and benefit the individual patient.

Nevertheless, if one takes a broad view of the whole group of hereditary ataxias, it turns out that there are certain clinicopathologic groupings that allow a very simplified descriptive classification. According to this principle, three main categories may be emphasized: (1) *cerebellar cortical degeneration*, (2) *olivopontocerebellar atrophy*, and (3) *spinocerebellar degenerations*, including *Friedreich's ataxia*.

CEREBELLAR CORTICAL DEGENERATION In this disorder, the principal neuropathologic feature is loss of neurons (mainly of Purkinje cells) in the cerebellar cortex. Cases of this kind characteristically occur in late adult life. Although the condition can occur sporadically, in the majority it is inherited as an autosomal dominant trait.

Pathology The loss of Purkinje cells tends to be most severe in the superior vermis and adjacent parts of the cerebellar cortex, but can be more extensive. The granule neurons are less affected. In long-standing cases, there is an associated atrophy of neurons in the olivary nuclei of the medulla, apparently representing a transsynaptic retrograde degeneration resulting from the loss of Purkinje cells, to which the olivocerebellar fibers project. In advanced cases atrophy of the cerebellar cortex can be readily demonstrated by CT scanning. In the purest forms of this disorder, as exemplified by the cases of late onset, slow progression, and dominant inheritance, other neuronal systems remain relatively intact.

Clinical manifestations Incoordination first appears in the legs, resulting in abnormal stance and an unsteadiness of gait of a wavering, lurching character typical of cerebellar ataxia (see Chap. 26). This gait disturbance is a consequence of degenerative changes in the superior vermis of the cerebellum and adjacent parts of the cerebellar cortex. With more extensive cerebellar involvement, a disturbance in articulation and rhythm of speech occurs and the arms become ataxic. There may be nystagmus. The illness progresses gradually, often extending over two or three decades, without appreciably curtailing the life span. Dementia tends to be mild or a late feature of this circumscribed cerebellar atrophy of late life. However, cerebellar cortical degeneration with very similar features may occur as a component in many of the ataxic disorders.

In addition to this slowly evolving, relatively circumscribed form of cerebellar cortical degeneration, there is a subacutely developing diffuse cerebellar cortical degeneration that affects all parts of the cerebellar cortex indiscriminately, often in association with some inflammatory changes. This disorder occurs in the presence of malignant neoplastic diseases of various kinds and is referred to as *carcinomatous cerebellar degeneration* (see Chap. 310). It is now apparent that this is one of a number of interrelated neurologic degenerative syndromes that occur on the background of malignant disease but do not result from any direct effect of the neoplasm on the nervous system such as invasion or metastasis. These so-called paraneoplastic disorders are etiologically unclarified; an immunologic or viral attack on neural structures has been postulated, but never proven. Paraneoplastic cerebellar degeneration produces a striking

clinicopathologic syndrome that tends to stand out as a particular entity (see Chap. 310).

OLIVOPONTOCEREBELLAR ATROPHY (OPCA) Grouped under this category are a number of similar disorders characterized by a combination of cerebellar cortical degeneration, atrophy of the inferior olivary nuclei secondary to this, and degeneration and disappearance of the neurons of the pontine nuclei and their fiber projections in the basis pontis and middle cerebellar peduncles. Konigsmark and Weiner distinguished five varieties on the basis of differences in the form of hereditary transmission and in the extent of other abnormalities both within and outside of the nervous system. Most instances of OPCA can now be considered to represent various forms of multiple system degeneration in which admixtures of parkinsonism, dementia, spasticity, choreoathetosis, retinal degeneration, myelopathy, and peripheral neuropathy may be encountered, sometimes obscuring the ataxic component. For present-day views of the classification of OPCA and the features of the various forms of disease brought under this heading, the monograph edited by Duvoisin and Plaitakis may be usefully consulted. The introduction of the new techniques of imaging—CT and MRI—now make it possible to visualize clearly the pontocerebellar lesions and some of the other atrophic changes in the central nervous system.

Autosomal dominant inheritance is characteristic in many families—most notably the Schut family, on which information extending over five generations has been obtained. Genetic linkage has shown localization to chromosome 6 in this family. Families of Portuguese ancestry, mainly from the Azores, who manifest the various syndromes that have been brought together under the heading of Joseph's disease have also been extensively studied. These families illustrate with striking clarity the varied phenotypic expression of what may turn out to be a single genetic abnormality.

Recessively transmitted OPCA has on the whole been less distinctly established than the dominant (or sporadic) forms, but of particular interest is a group of families with an autosomal recessive disorder and late-adult onset of neurologic symptoms, in whom the disease is characterized by multiple system degeneration, including a prominent OPCA component, and in which deficiency of glutamic acid dehydrogenase has been demonstrated in leukocytes and cultured fibroblasts from affected family members. Glutamate, among its other functions, acts as an excitatory neurotransmitter and is involved in the excitatory input to the Purkinje cells from the granule cells of the cerebellar cortex. In excess, this transmitter has neurotoxic effects, which might be the basis of the Purkinje cell degeneration that is so prominent in OPCA. These observations, and other biochemical leads that have opened up in connection with some of the dominant forms of OPCA, suggest a promising field of research that may give new etiologic and pathophysiologic insights into a wide group of neuronal degenerative diseases and may ultimately suggest avenues for therapeutic approach.

Pathology OPCA and the disorders related to it exemplify clearly the phenomenon of selective premature neuronal death, and of affection of particular, vulnerable neuronal systems with sparing of others. The distribution of neuronal lesions that characterizes OPCA as distinct from other neuronal system degenerations has already been indicated. The neuronal changes are in no way distinctive or specific in OPCA. Rather, it is the particular location of the neuronal loss that determines the clinicopathologic picture. Still not fully clarified in this group of disorders is what determines the dementia that so often accompanies them. It has been generally assumed that abnormalities occur in the cerebral cortex, but examination of the cortex in typical cases discloses insufficient abnormality to account for the cognitive and behavioral alterations. On the other hand, the lesions of the cerebellum and related systems provide a reasonable explanation for the incoordination (ataxia) that is observed; the lesions in the basal ganglia and substantia nigra (equivalent to striatonigral degeneration) underlie the features of parkinsonism and of other postural and movement disorders that are so frequently seen as manifestations of OPCA; and involvement of the peripheral motor neurons, similar to what occurs in the motor neuron disease group to be discussed later, produces the severe muscular weakness and atrophy that may be encountered. The disturbances of ocular motility that typify some cases still are in need of further anatomic elucidation.

Clinical manifestations There is great clinical variation among cases of OPCA. Some present a picture of a relatively pure cerebellar ataxia indistinguishable from that seen in cases with atrophy of the cerebellar cortex (and secondarily of the inferior olivary nuclei) alone. Others are characterized by parkinsonian features. Superimposed is an evolving dementia. For accounts of these varied forms of clinical expression, general neurologic reference works and specialized monographs (such as that edited by Duvoisin and Plaitakis) should be consulted.

SPINOCEREBELLAR DEGENERATIONS (FRIEDREICH'S ATAXIA)

This group of ataxic disorders is characterized by degeneration of long ascending and descending fiber systems in the spinal cord, including the spinocerebellar tracts, and concomitant degeneration of peripheral axons and myelin sheaths in the form of chronic peripheral neuronopathy.

The classic form of hereditary ataxia, first clearly depicted by Nikolaus Friedreich of Heidelberg in 1863, constitutes a relatively distinct symptom complex which generally runs true to form, although it overlaps other heredodegenerative syndromes, particularly other types of spinocerebellar atrophy. In some families, the disorder occurs with dominant inheritance; usually it is a recessive trait. Recent studies have linked the recessive form of the disease to chromosome 9.

Pathology The principal changes are cell loss in the dorsal root ganglia and secondary degeneration in the posterior columns and spinocerebellar tracts of the cord and in the peripheral nerves. Degeneration is also evident in the corticospinal tracts in most cases. The cerebellum is variably affected. In addition to these neuropathologic changes there is in some cases a peculiar form of myocardial degeneration resulting in fiber loss and fibrosis. There are no other associated visceral lesions.

Clinical manifestations As with other progressive ataxias, the disorder first appears in the legs, affecting the individual during late childhood. The patient, previously healthy, begins to stagger and lurch in walking and is unsteady on standing. Clumsiness and cerebellar tremor of the hands and arms appear later along with dysarthria and abnormal rhythm (scanning) of speech. These symptoms result from changes in the dorsal root ganglia, the spinocerebellar tracts, and cerebellum; it is not easy to ascertain the relative contribution of lesions in each structure to the ataxia. The limbs, in addition to being ataxic, generally show considerable weakness. Examination usually discloses nystagmus and skeletal deformities: kyphoscoliosis, the basis of which is not certain, and a peculiar foreshortening of the feet (pes cavus) with cocking of the toes, best ascribed to atrophy and contractures of the musculature of the feet at a time when the bones of the feet are malleable. Typically, there is the unusual combination of total absence of tendon reflexes with extensor plantar reflexes (Babinski sign). This results from the presence of degeneration of the corticospinal tracts together with the involvement of peripheral sensory neurons that relay afferent signals from muscle spindles. Impairment of position and vibration sense in the extremities is prominent and, in some patients, sensation of pain, temperature, and light touch is diminished in a distal and roughly symmetric distribution consistent with an axononeuropathy affecting small nerve fibers. Mentation is usually preserved, though a few of the patients have been of low intelligence or have become demented late in the course of the disease. Survival beyond early adult life is rare, with death frequently the result of associated cardiomyopathy.

Occasionally very mild or fragmentary forms of the disorder (such as pes cavus and absent or hyperactive tendon reflexes) may be encountered with little, if any, disability or progression. Such abnormalities are most likely to be seen in other members of the family of a patient afflicted with the fully developed form of the disease. A related syndrome, the Roussy-Lévy syndrome, shows similarities to Friedreich's ataxia and to peroneal muscular atrophy. Mild ataxia, pes cavus, absent ankle and knee tendon jerks, and atrophy of lower leg muscles occur. In some well-documented cases the peripheral nerves show hypertrophy due to proliferation of Schwann cells (see Chap. 363). Chronic familial polyneuropathies are particularly difficult to distinguish since they also give rise to sensory ataxia, but signs of pyramidal tract disease are absent (see Chap. 363). Hereditary forms of cerebellar ataxia with corticospinal signs (hyperactive tendon reflexes) and sensory disturbances are also known to occur in the adolescent or adult. Familial spastic paraplegia with or without optic atrophy (Behr's syndrome) is another closely related disease. In the absence of a family history, and with atypical clinical findings, further diagnostic studies to exclude congenital malformation, spinal cord compression, foramen magnum tumor, and multiple sclerosis will be necessary.

No treatment is of proven value. Earlier reports of disturbed pyruvate metabolism have not been confirmed.

DIFFERENTIAL DIAGNOSIS OF THE ATAXIAS The slow but relentless progression in the absence of abnormalities in other parts of the nervous system and in the CSF distinguishes the hereditary group from other diseases and other forms of cerebellar ataxia such as may occur with hereditary metabolic diseases, or with neoplastic, infectious, or demyelinative disease, or with drug intoxications (e.g., phenytoin) or with hyperpyrexia. The degenerative disorders under discussion tend to develop slowly over many years in a setting of otherwise good general health, and in the absence of other neurologic symptoms and signs; this, together with the other clinical differences, distinguishes them from such hereditary metabolic diseases as juvenile Gaucher's disease, juvenile Niemann-Pick disease, and juvenile hexosaminidase deficiency and from alcoholic cerebellar ataxia or nutritional deficiency disease, with or without Wernicke-Korsakoff syndrome. Alcoholic cerebellar degeneration usually develops over a few days to weeks, and then may remain more or less unchanged for the remainder of the patient's life (Chap. 357). A prolonged deficiency of vitamin E can result in progressive ataxia, incoordination of the limbs, areflexia, and distal loss of proprioception and vibratory sense, mimicking spinocerebellar degeneration. Most cases are associated with fat malabsorption

In the cases associated with carcinoma, the tempo of evolution of the process is relatively rapid, with severe disability coming on within a period of months. Vertigo, diplopia, and nausea may be prominent. In an occasional patient, the neurologic symptoms have appeared before there was any obvious evidence of carcinoma. Opsoclonus (rapid side-to-side jerking of the eyes) and oscillopsia (movement back and forth of objects seen) may be conjoined. In contrast to the consistently normal CSF findings in the forms of cerebellar degeneration noted above, the CSF in paraneoplastic degeneration may show increased lymphocytes and protein.

TREATMENT No specific treatment is available for any of the progressive ataxias, although encouragement to remain active is beneficial to health in general. Gait training is of relatively little value in enabling patients to compensate for their disability. In cases where parkinsonian features are prominent, antiparkinsonian medications should be tried (see above), but the response in the group of multiple system degenerations is generally unsatisfactory. Trauner has reported that baclofen in high dosage may help control involuntary movements in some cases of OPCA, but the ataxia is not benefited.

IDIOPATHIC AUTONOMIC FAILURE (IDIOPATHIC ORTHOSTATIC HYPOTENSION, SHY-DRAGER SYNDROME)

Abnormalities of central autonomic nervous system functions manifest principally by failure to maintain blood pressure and by urinary incontinence are now recognized to be caused in some cases by a progressive degenerative disorder of the CNS that affects several systems; in some patients the peripheral nervous system is also involved (postganglionic sympathetic neurons). Bradbury and Eggleston in 1925 called attention to the combination of postural hypotension, incontinence, impotence, and abnormality of sweating (anhidrosis). Symptoms of central neurologic origin develop later in many of these patients consisting predominantly of extrapyramidal or cerebellar dysfunction.

PATHOGENESIS AND PATHOLOGY The cause of the disorder is unknown. In 1960 Shy and Drager described neuropathologic changes in the brainstem and basal ganglia, and subsequently others showed a prominent loss of neurons in central regions of the autonomic nervous system, affecting in particular the cells of the intermediolateral column of the thoracic spinal cord. Abnormalities have also been found in peripheral autonomic ganglia (cell loss). In the brainstem and basal ganglia there is widespread symmetric neuronal degeneration affecting the caudate nucleus, substantia nigra, locus coeruleus, olivary nuclei, dorsal vagal nuclei, and in some cases affecting the cerebellum. Cell loss is accompanied by gliosis; Lewy bodies typical of Parkinson's disease are present in some cases. For these reasons many neurologists consider the Shy-Drager syndrome to be a unique form of multisystem degeneration resembling but distinct from either Parkinson's disease or OPCA.

Clinical manifestations The onset is insidious, usually in the sixth or seventh decade. Men are more frequently affected than women. Disturbances of urinary bladder function, including hesitancy and incontinence, postural dizziness and syncope, impotence, and decreased sweating are the presenting manifestations. Later symptoms of extrapyramidal dysfunction resembling parkinsonism or cerebellar findings may emerge. The condition becomes severely disabling over the course of 5 to 7 years in most patients. The hallmark of the condition is postural hypotension, defined as a fall in blood pressure greater than 30/20 mmHg on standing upright from a supine position (see Chap. 21). Despite this fall in blood pressure there is usually a total failure of compensatory tachycardia, the pulse rate remaining unchanged. Autonomic signs of pupillary asymmetry, partial Horner's syndrome, or partial parasympathetic denervation occur in some patients. Anhidrosis is common and can be demonstrated by placing the individual in a warm room after application of a starch-iodine mixture to the skin. The parkinsonian manifestations may be identical to those of idiopathic parkinsonism, although in many patients rigidity and bradykinesia are more prominent than tremor. Cerebellar gait ataxia and mild limb ataxia may be evident. Other findings include laryngeal paralysis and sleep apnea.

Treatment The treatment is symptomatic. The postural hypotension is usually the most disabling initial symptom. Antigravity stockings to minimize pooling of venous blood in the legs are recommended. A leotard that covers the lower abdomen may provide additional benefit. Pharmacologic agents are given to expand blood volume and to enhance vascular responsivity. Increased NaCl intake combined with fludrohydrocortisone 0.05 to 0.2 mg twice daily is usually beneficial (see Chap. 21). In severe cases, adrenergic drugs such as ephedrine, levodopa, or amphetamine may improve the disability. The parkinsonism symptoms often respond initially to Sinemet or bromocriptine, but later in the course most patients become refractory to these agents. Centrally acting alpha agonists (e.g., yohimbine or clonidine) may also be beneficial.

SYNDROMES OF MUSCULAR WEAKNESS AND WASTING WITHOUT SENSORY CHANGES: MOTOR NEURON DISEASE

AMYOTROPHIC LATERAL SCLEROSIS (ALS) ALS is the most frequently encountered form of progressive motor neuron disease, and it presents a clinical syndrome that is generally familiar to physicians who see patients with neurologic diseases. It is characteristically a disorder of late middle age. Most patients are older than 50 when symptoms begin. The disease rarely develops before the third decade, and patients whose symptoms begin in the late teenage

TABLE 359-2 Categories of degenerative motor neuron diseases

I Amyotrophic lateral sclerosis
  A Spinal muscular atrophy
  B Bulbar palsy
  C Primary lateral sclerosis
  D Pseudobulbar palsy
II Heritable motor neuron diseases
  A Autosomal recessive spinal muscular atrophy (SMA)
    1 Type I: Werdnig-Hoffmann, acute
    2 Type II: Werdnig-Hoffmann, chronic
    3 Type III: Kugelberg-Welander
    4 Type IV: Adult onset
  B Familial amyotrophic lateral sclerosis
  C Other
    1 Arthrogryposis multiplex congenita
    2 Progressive juvenile bulbar palsy (Fazio-Londe)
    3 Neuroaxonal dystrophy
III Associated with other degenerative disorders
  1 Olivopontocerebellar atrophies
  2 Peroneal muscular atrophy

years often seem to have an inherited variant of the disorder. Men are more frequently affected than women. Because of its restriction to motor neurons of the central nervous system, ALS represents another prime example of a neuronal system disease. It occurs sporadically in most instances. Familial occurrence, with transmission as an autosomal dominant trait, is observed in about 10 percent of cases and differs in some clinical and pathologic aspects (Table 359-2).

Pathology The disease is characterized by progressive loss of motor neurons, both in the cerebral cortex and in the anterior horns of the spinal cord, together with their homologues in some motor nuclei of the brainstem. It typically affects both upper and lower motor neurons, although variants may predominantly involve only particular subsets of motor neurons, particularly early in the course of the illness. Thus, in bulbar palsy and spinal muscular atrophy (or progressive muscular atrophy) the lower motor neurons of brainstem and spinal cord, respectively, are most severely involved while pseudobulbar palsy and primary lateral sclerosis affect upper motor neurons innervating the brainstem and spinal cord. The loss of motor neurons is not accompanied by any distinctive or unique cytopathologic features. The affected cells undergo shrinkage, often with some excessive accumulation of the pigmented lipid (lipofuscin) that normally develops in these cells with advancing age, and they eventually disappear. Focal enlargement of proximal motor axons is frequently seen; ultrastructurally, these "spheroids" are composed of accumulations of neurofilaments. Beyond some astroglial proliferation, which is the inevitable accompaniment of all disintegrative processes in the central nervous system, the interstitial and supportive tissues and the macrophage system remain largely inactive, and there is no inflammation. The death of the peripheral motor neurons in the brainstem and spinal cord leads to denervation and consequent atrophy of the corresponding muscle fibers. Histochemical and electrophysiologic evidence indicate that in the early phases of the illness denervated muscle can be reinnervated by sprouting of nearby distal motor nerve terminals, although reinnervation in this disease is considerably less extensive than in most other disorders affecting motor neurons (e.g., poliomyelitis, peripheral neuropathy). As denervation progresses, there is shrinkage of the musculature and a fiber atrophy that is readily recognized in muscle biopsies. It is this muscular atrophy that is designated by the term *amyotrophy*, which appears in the common name for the disease. The loss of motor neurons in the cortex results in disappearance of the long axons and their myelin sheaths that make up the corticospinal tracts, which travel via the internal capsule and extend through the brainstem, including the pyramids of the medulla oblongata, to the lateral (and a portion of the anterior) white matter columns of the spinal cord. The loss of fibers in the lateral columns, together with the fibrillary gliosis which imparts a particular firmness (sclerosis) to the affected tissues, makes up the lateral sclerosis component of the disease. The fact that the nerve fiber loss is more extensive in the distal parts of the affected tracts in the lower spinal cord rather than the more proximal parts, such as the internal capsule, suggests that the affected neurons first undergo disintegration at their distal terminals and the disease process proceeds in a centripetal direction until ultimately the parent cell body dies, a phenomenon referred to as "dying back." The disease clearly affects the large pyramidal neurons (Betz cells) of the motor cortex in the precentral gyrus, but in some cases the extent of degeneration in the long projection pathways provides evidence that many other neurons involved in voluntary movement, both in the cortex and in subcortical nuclei, are also affected.

A remarkable feature of the disease is the selectivity of neuronal cell death. The entire sensory apparatus, the regulatory mechanisms for the control and coordination of movement, and the components of the brain that are needed for intellect and thinking, remain intact. There is also some consistent selectivity in motor system involvement. The motor neurons required for ocular motility remain unaffected as do the parasympathetic neurons in the sacral spinal cord (the nucleus of Onufrowicz, or Onuf) which innervate the sphincters of the bowel and bladder.

Clinical manifestations The first evidence of the disease is manifest as insidiously developing asymmetric weakness, usually first apparent in one of the limbs. Fatigue and easy cramping of affected muscles can be prominent. The weakness is accompanied by visible wasting and atrophy of the muscles involved; particularly in the early stages of the disease, affected muscles may display focal twitchings—fasciculations—when not concealed by overlying adipose tissue. Virtually any muscle group may be the first to show signs of the disease, but as time passes, more and more muscles become involved until ultimately the disorder takes on a symmetric distribution in all regions, including the muscles of chewing, swallowing, and movements of the face and tongue. Early involvement of the muscles of respiration may lead to death before the disease is far advanced elsewhere; otherwise the disorder generally is terminated by pulmonary infection secondary to the profound generalized weakness.

The corticospinal component of the disease becomes apparent in the form of hyperactivity of the muscle-stretch reflexes (tendon jerks) and, often, spastic resistance to passive movements of the affected limbs. With corticospinal involvement the plantar reflex will be upgoing (the Babinski sign) until—as often occurs—lower motor neuron dysfunction in the legs advances sufficiently that extensor movement of the great toes is impossible. The disease process in the corticobulbar projections innervating the brainstem results in dysarthria and exaggeration of the motor expressions of emotion leading to involuntary weeping or laughter (so-called pseudobulbar affect), or strange admixtures of both. Ocular motility is spared, even when other brainstem functions are greatly impaired. Throughout the evolution of the disease, awareness and intellectual abilities typically remain intact. Dementia is not usually a component of ALS; when it occurs, it is due to the superimposition of another disease process.

The course is relentlessly progressive and leads ultimately to death, but the total duration of the illness is variable. In recent studies approximately 50 percent of patients can be expected to die within 3 to 5 years from the onset of the disease; some may live considerably longer. Very rarely, what seems to be ALS may become stabilized, or even regress to the point of recovery.

Differential diagnosis Because the underlying process in ALS is currently untreatable, it is imperative that potentially remediable causes of motor neuron dysfunction be excluded (see Table 359-3), particularly in atypical cases. Compression of the cervical cord or cervicomedullary junction from tumors in the cervical region or at the foramen magnum, or from cervical spondylosis with osteophytes projecting into the vertebral canal, can at times give rise to weakness, wasting, and fasciculations in the upper limbs and spasticity in the legs, thus closely resembling ALS. The absence of cranial nerve involvement may be helpful in differentiation, although some compressive lesions in the foramen magnum may implicate the twelfth

TABLE 359-3 Etiology and investigation of secondary motor neuron disorders

Diagnostic categories	Investigations
I Structural lesions	
A Parasagittal or foramen magnum tumors	MRI/CT scan—head, spine including foramen magnum
B Cervical spondylosis	MRI/CT scan or myelogram
C Chiari malformation or syrinx	
D Spinal cord arteriovenous malformation	
II Infections	
A Bacterial—tetanus	CSF exam
B Viral—poliomyelitis, herpes zoster	Antibody titers
III Intoxications, physical agents	
A Toxins—lead, aluminum, other metals	24-h urine for lead, mercury arsenic, thallium, aluminum
B Drugs—strychnine, phenytoin, dapsone	
C Electric shock	
D X-irradiation	Serum lead and aluminum
IV Immunologic mechanisms	
A Plasma cell dyscrasias	Complete blood count, sedimentation rate
B Autoimmune polyradiculoneuropathy	Immunoprotein electrophoresis, antinuclear antibody (ANA), cryoglobulins (+/−) bone marrow biopsy
V Paraneoplastic	
A Paracarcinomatous	
B Paralymphomatous; Hodgkin's disease	
VI Metabolic	
A Hypoglycemia	Fasting blood sugar (FBS)
B Hyperparathyroidism	Routine chemistries including calcium, magnesium, phosphate
C Hyperthroidism	Thyroid functions
D Vitamin B_{12}, Vitamin E deficiency	Vitamin B_{12}, folate, vitamin E levels
E Malabsorption	Stool fat (72-h; spot), carotene, prothrombin time (PT)
VII Hereditary biochemical disorders	
A Hexosaminidase A deficiency	Lysosomal enzyme screen
B α-Glucosidase deficiency (Pompe's)	
C Hyperlipidemia	Lipid electrophoresis
D Hyperglycinuria	Urine and serum amino acids
E Methylcrotonylglycinuria	CSF amino acids

cranial (hypoglossal) nerve, with resulting affection of the tongue. Absence of pain or of sensory changes, normal function of bowels and bladder, normal roentgenographic studies of the spine, and absence of changes in the composition or dynamics of the cerebrospinal fluid are all points in favor of ALS against spinal cord compression. Where doubt exists, MRI scans and contrast myelography should be performed in order to visualize the cervical spinal cord.

Other treatable disorders that occasionally can mimic ALS are chronic lead poisoning and thyrotoxicosis. These may be suggested by the patient's social or occupational history or by unusual clinical features. When the family history is positive, inherited enzyme disorders such as hexosaminidase A or α-glucosidase deficiency must be excluded (see Chap. 357). These can readily be identified by appropriate laboratory tests. Benign fasciculations are occasionally a source of concern because on inspection they resemble the fascicular twitchings that accompany motor neuron degeneration. The absence of weakness or atrophy, and of denervation phenomena on electrophysiologic examination, excludes ALS or other serious neurologic disease. Poliomyelitis is now recognized to result in a delayed progressive deterioration of motor neurons which presents clinically with progressive weakness, atrophy, and fasciculations. Its cause is unknown but is thought to reflect prior sublethal injury to motor neurons by the poliovirus.

Treatment There is no treatment that has influence on the underlying pathologic process in any form of motor neuron disease. Modern rehabilitative measures, including mechanical aids of various kinds, can do much in helping patients to overcome the effects of their disabilities and often, with respiratory support, to survive longer than would otherwise have been the case. Initial observations (reviewed by Tandan and Bradley) showed that intravenous (or intrathecal) infusions of thyrotropin releasing hormone (TRH) result in transitory improvement of motor functions in some patients with ALS. Unfortunately TRH has not shown any long-term benefits. A recent report showed beneficial effects of treatment with branched chain amino acids; this will require verification.

SPINAL MUSCULAR ATROPHY (SMA)   In the varieties of motor neuron disease that are grouped under this heading, the peripheral motor neurons are affected without evidence of involvement of the corticospinal motor system (Table 359-2). In comparison with ALS, SMA in general occurs in a younger age group, runs a slower, more protracted course (except in the infantile form), and tends to be hereditary (usually autosomal recessive) rather than sporadic. The SMA group undoubtedly includes several distinct disease processes that differ from one another genetically and phenotypically.

Infantile SMA (Werdnig-Hoffmann disease)   This rapidly fatal disorder is characterized by autosomal recessive transmission. Not infrequently, infantile SMA (sometimes also referred to as SMA type I) is apparent even before birth, as indicated by decreased fetal movements in comparison with what normally would be expected. The afflicted infants are weak and floppy (hypotonic), though alert, and muscle-stretch reflexes are absent. Weakness progresses relatively rapidly, and death ensues generally within the first year of life; rarely, the child survives to 3 years of age.

Neuropathologically, Werdnig-Hoffmann disease is characterized by extensive loss of the large motor neurons. Sections of the muscles show extreme degrees of denervation atrophy. During life, the diagnosis is made by electrophysiologic studies and by muscle biopsy, which shows the characteristic denervational pattern rather than an intrinsic myopathy or inflammatory disease of muscle. There is no effective treatment, but a family that has had an affected infant may be helped by genetic counseling.

There is another form of infantile muscular atrophy, also characterized by autosomal recessive inheritance, which appears to be distinct from Werdnig-Hoffmann disease in that the evolution is considerably slower, with survival into preadolescence or even into adult life. This disorder, which has been called *chronic childhood SMA*, or SMA type II, is considerably rarer than Werdnig-Hoffmann disease.

These motor neuron diseases can be distinguished from benign congenital hypotonia, which is a nonprogressive form of myopathy, by electrophysiologic assessment and by muscle biopsy.

Juvenile SMA (Wohlfart-Kugelberg-Welander disease)   This disorder, also referred to as SMA type III, manifests itself during late childhood and runs a slow, indolent course. Typically the muscles of the trunk and the proximal parts of the limb are earliest and most severely involved—a picture that closely resembles that of progressive muscular dystrophy, even to the presence of pseudohypertrophy of the calf muscles in some cases. Electrophysiologic and biopsy evidence of denervation in the affected muscles serves to distinguish this disease from any of the myopathic syndromes.

Other genetically determined varieties of SMA   In individual families, other syndromes characterized by SMA in varying patterns have been described. An infantile variety involving mainly the musculature innervated by the brainstem is referred to as the *Fazio-Londe syndrome*. In some juvenile cases, the distribution is distal, rather than proximal, as in the Wohlfart-Kugelberg-Welander variety. In addition, there is a slowly evolving adult form of SMA, sometimes called SMA type IV (Table 359-2). Depending upon the family, autosomal dominant, autosomal recessive, or X-linked recessive patterns of heredity may be discerned.

A component of SMA may also be found in some of the multiple system degenerations that have already been referred to, e.g., in Joseph's disease and in some of the syndromes characterized by olivopontocerebellar degeneration. Some of the recognized familial

metabolic disorders also present a striking picture of progressive symmetric muscular weakness and atrophy, for instance, adult hexosaminidase A deficiency (the enzymopathy that results in Tay-Sachs disease in infancy) and adrenomyeloneuropathy. For details and more extensive discussions of these disorders, specialized monographs (such as that edited by Rowland), reviews (Tandan and Bradley), and general reference works on neurology (Adams and Victor) should be consulted.

Primary lateral sclerosis (PLS)   It might be thought that this is a variant of ALS in which the amyotrophic component is lacking, but the few cases of this disorder that have been described have been encountered in remarkably pure form. It occurs as a sporadic disease of late life, affecting the same age group that is prone to develop ALS. The course may be similar to that of ALS with approximately 3 years from onset to death. Clinically, the illness is characterized by progressive spastic weakness of the limbs, preceded or followed by spastic dysarthria and dysphagia, indicative of corticobulbar tract involvement. Fasciculations, amyotrophy, and sensory changes are absent. On neuropathologic examination, there is selective loss of large pyramidal cells in the precentral gyrus and degeneration of the corticospinal and corticobulbar projections; the peripheral motor neurons and other neuronal systems are spared.

It may be necessary to consider PLS in the differential diagnosis of late-life progressive spastic paresis of the limbs, but obviously it is necessary, by appropriate studies of CSF and radiographic investigations, to exclude treatable disorders such as parasagittal intracranial tumors, neoplasms of the spinal cord, cervical spondylosis, or inflammatory diseases.

HEREDITARY SPASTIC PARAPLEGIA   This is a very rare disorder which differs from PLS in several respects. Instead of occurring sporadically, it is characterized by genetic transmission—as an autosomal dominant trait in the majority of cases. Several families are on record in which it has appeared in many successive generations. It appears at a younger age, usually in the fourth decade, and the course is very slowly progressive, to the extent that patients often live out a full life span. The condition is probably genetically heterogeneous; the group with onset in childhood or adolescence can be distinguished from those in whom the disease does not appear until the age of 35 years or older; as might be expected, there is considerable overlap between these groups. In a few families, a clinically indistinguishable disorder shows a pattern of autosomal recessive inheritance.

Pathology   Neuropathologically, there is degeneration of the corticospinal (pyramidal) tracts, which appear almost normal at brainstem levels but become increasingly atrophic as they descend through the spinal cord. In addition, the ascending tracts in the posterior columns and the spinocerebellar tracts show some loss of fibers so that the picture resembles to some degree the findings in Friedreich's ataxia. In fact, some individual cases of what seems to be a fairly pure spastic paraparesis may actually represent an incomplete form of Friedreich's ataxia. In such families spastic paraparesis is the outstanding phenotypic expression of Friedreich's ataxia.

Clinical manifestations   As the name implies, the lower limbs are affected earliest and most severely. The major cause of disability is spasticity rather than weakness. There is concomitant exaggeration of the muscle stretch reflexes. Late in the course, urinary urgency and incontinence, and sometimes fecal incontinence, may occur; sexual potency tends to be preserved. In pure forms of the disorder, ataxia and amyotrophy are absent or minimal. In some patients, minor sensory changes (in the form of impaired vibration and position sense) may be observed in the late stages.

It is important in cases of otherwise unexplained progressive spastic paraparesis, despite a negative family history, to examine as many family members as possible. Members of a family with minimal degrees of the disease may be asymptomatic and unaware of its presence, even though they can be shown on examination to have spasticity and hyperreflexia.

SYNDROMES COMBINING MUSCULAR WEAKNESS AND WASTING WITH SENSORY CHANGES

PROGRESSIVE NEURAL MUSCULAR ATROPHY The degenerative disorders characterized by progressive weakness and wasting of skeletal muscles combined with sensory changes are usually chronic diseases of peripheral nerves, often occurring as hereditary conditions. Although clinical and pathologic subvarieties exist, there is no sharp dividing line between them, and they are best considered together under the designation given above, in which the term *neural* emphasizes the peripheral nerve affection. Chronic peripheral neuropathy is an associated disorder in some of the hereditary ataxias and is regularly encountered in the classic form of Friedreich's ataxia. It is also a component of adrenomyeloneuropathy and other leukodystrophies (see Chap. 331). In some cases of progressive neural muscular atrophy, other genetically determined CNS diseases may occur such as progressive optic atrophy or pigmentary degeneration of the retina. The peripheral neuropathy begins distally and progresses in a centripetal fashion with the feet and legs first affected, and involvement of the hands and more proximal parts only after a considerable interval, usually several years.

The two most frequent forms of hereditary polyneuropathy, *peroneal muscular atrophy* (Charcot-Marie-Tooth disease) and *hypertrophic interstitial polyneuropathy* (Dejerine-Sottas disease), are described in Chap. 363. Brief reference is also made there to a rare condition known as *Refsum's disease*.

Although no specific treatment is available (except in Refsum's disease, as indicated in Chap. 363), patients whose disease is of slow progression and in whom conditions are otherwise favorable may be greatly helped by measures to ensure a stable walking surface, such as corrective shoes, braces to prevent foot drop, and even orthopedic procedures to stabilize the joints.

SYNDROMES OF PROGRESSIVE VISUAL LOSS Although the preceding discussion of the various hereditary progressive nervous system disorders categorized as degenerative has emphasized the intellectual, motor, and peripheral sensory derangements that result from these, many of these syndromes are accompanied by concomitant loss of the neural structures subserving vision. The hereditary ataxias, including Friedreich's, and hereditary spastic paraplegia stand out as examples. The pathologic changes, viewed broadly, take on two forms: selective degeneration of retinal ganglion cells with secondary optic atrophy, and a more diffuse degenerative process involving all retinal components, with subsequent migration of the melanin-containing cells of the pigment epithelium into the superficial retinal layers, resulting in the picture of *pigmentary degeneration of the retina* (formerly, but erroneously—since there is no inflammation—called retinitis pigmentosa). Occasionally, the peripheral visual system is the major, or only, site of disease resulting in progressive blindness without other neurologic defects. The major entities of this kind, including Leber's *hereditary optic atrophy*, are described in Chap. 360. A more complete review, with references to the pertinent literature, is given by Adams and Victor.

REFERENCES

General

ADAMS RD, VICTOR M: *Principles of Neurology*, 4th ed. New York, McGraw-Hill, 1989
——— et al: Striatonigral degeneration. J Neuropathol Exp Neurol 23:584, 1964
ASBURY AK et al: *Diseases of the Nervous System*, vols I and II. Philadelphia, Ardmore Medical Books, Saunders, 1986
GILMAN S et al: *Disorders of the Cerebellum*. Philadelphia, Davis, 1981
Greenfield's Neuropathology, 4th ed, JH Adams et al (eds). New York, Wiley, 1984
MARSDEN CD, FAHN S (eds): *Movement Disorders*. London, Butterworth, 1982
ROSENBERG RN: *Neurogenetics: Principles and Practice*. New York, Raven, 1986

Alzheimer's disease

BALL MJ: Alzheimer's disease: A challenging enigma. Arch Pathol Lab Med 106:157, 1982
FRIEDLAND RP et al: Alzheimer's disease: Clinical and biochemical heterogeneity. Ann Intern Med 109:298, 1988

GLENNER GG: On causative theories in Alzheimer's disease. Human Pathol 16:433, 1985
HAXBY JV et al: Heterogeneous anterior-posterior metabolic patterns on dementia of the Alzheimer type. Neurology 38:1853, 1988
HYMAN BT et al: Alzheimer's disease: Cell-specific pathology isolates the hippocampal formation. Science 225:1168, 1984
JOACHIM CL et al: Clinically diagnosed Alzheimer's disease: Autopsy results in 150 cases. Ann Neurol 24:50, 1988
KATZMAN R: Alzheimer's disease. N Engl J Med 314:964, 1986
PERL DP, BRODY AR: Alzheimer's disease: X-ray spectrometric evidence of aluminum accumulation in neurofibrillary tangle-bearing neurons. Science 208:297, 1980
PETRY S et al: Personality alterations in dementia of the Alzheimer type. Arch Neurol 45:1187, 1988
SCHEINBERG P: Dementia due to vascular disease—A multifactorial disorder. Stroke 19:1291, 1988
SELKOE DJ: Biochemistry of altered brain proteins in Alzheimer's disease. Ann Rev Neurosci 12:493, 1989
ST. GEORGE-HYSLOP PH et al: The genetic defect causing familial Alzheimer's disease maps on chromosome 21. Science 238:664, 1987
WHITEHOUSE PJ et al: Alzheimer's disease and senile dementia: Loss of neurons in the basal forebrain. Science 215:1237, 1982

Huntington's disease

FERRANTE RJ et al: Selective sparing of a class of striatal neurons in Huntington's disease. Science 230:561, 1985
HAYDEN MR: *Huntington's Chorea*. Berlin, Springer-Verlag, 1981
MARTIN JB, GUSELLA JF: Huntington's disease: Pathogenesis and management. N Engl J Med 315:1267, 1986
MEISSEN GJ et al: Predictive testing for Huntington's disease with use of a linked DNA marker. N Engl J Med 318:535, 1988
VONSATTEL JP et al: Neuropathological classification of Huntington's disease. J Neuropathol Exp Neurol 44:559, 1985

Parkinson's disease

FABBRINI G et al: Motor fluctuations in Parkinson's disease: Central pathophysiological mechanisms, part I. Ann Neurol 24:366, 1988
FAHN S et al (eds): *Recent Advances in Parkinson's Disease*. New York, Raven, 1986
GROWDON JH: Medical treatment of extrapyramidal diseases, in *Update III: Harrison's Principles of Internal Medicine*, KJ Isselbacher et al (eds). New York, McGraw-Hill, 1982
HOEHN MM, YAHR MD: Parkinsonism: Onset, progression and mortality. Neurology 17:427, 1967
LANGSTON JW et al: Chronic parkinsonism in humans due to a product of meperidine-analog synthesis. Science 219:979, 1983
MARTTILA RJ et al: Parkinson's disease in a nationwide twin cohort. Neurology 38:1217, 1988
MAYEUX R et al: Reappraisal of temporary levodopa withdrawal ("drug holiday") in Parkinson's disease. N Engl J Med 313:724, 1985
MOURADIAN MM et al: Motor fluctuations in Parkinson's disease: Central pathophysiological mechanisms, part II. Ann Neurol 24:372, 1988
NUTT JG et al: The "on-off" phenomenon in Parkinson's disease: Relation to levodopa absorption and transport. N Engl J Med 310:438, 1984
PARKINSON STUDY GROUP: Effect of deprenyl on the progression of disability in early Parkinson's disease. N Engl J Med 321:1364, 1989

Cerebellar degeneration

DUVOISIN RC, PLAITAKIS A (eds): *Advances in Neurology*, vol 41, *The Olivopontocerebellar Atrophies*. New York, Raven, 1984
KONIGSMARK BW, WEINER LP: The olivopontocerebellar atrophies: A review. Medicine 49:227, 1970
TRAUNER DA: Olivopontocerebellar atrophy with dementia, blindness, and chorea. Arch Neurol 42:757, 1985

Motor neuron disease

MITSUMOTO H et al: Amyotrophic lateral sclerosis: Recent advances in pathogenesis and therapeutic trials. Arch Neurol 45:189, 1988
PLAITAKIS A et al: Pilot trial of branched-chain amino acids in amyotrophic lateral sclerosis. Lancet 1:1015, 1988
ROWLAND LP (ed): *Advances in Neurology*, vol 36, *Human Motor Neuron Diseases*. New York, Raven, 1982
TANDAN R, BRADLEY WG: Amyotrophic lateral sclerosis: Part 1, Clinical features, pathology, and ethical issues in management. Ann Neurol 18:271, 1985
———, ———: Amyotrophic lateral sclerosis: Part 2, Etiopathogenesis. Ann Neurol 18:419, 1985

Miscellaneous

BAUMANN RJ et al: Lafora disease: Liver histopathology in presymptomatic children. Ann Neurol 14:86, 1983
BERKOVIC SF et al: Progressive myoclonic epilepsies: Specific causes and diagnosis. N Engl J Med 315:296, 1986
BLACK PM et al: CSF shunts for dementia, incontinence and gait disturbance. Clin Neurosurg 32:632, 1985
BURKHARDT CR et al: Diffuse Lewy body disease and progressive dementia. Neurology 38:1520, 1988
HARDING AE: Hereditary "pure" spastic paraplegia: A clinical and genetic study of 22 families. J Neurol Neurosurg Psychiatry 44:871, 1981

——— et al: Spinocerebellar degeneration associated with a selective deficit of vitamin E absorption. N Engl J Med 313:32, 1985

HENSON RA, URICH H: *Cancer and the Nervous System.* Blackwell Scientific, 1982

IIVANAINEN M, HIMBERG J-J: Valproate and clonazepam in the treatment of severe progressive myoclonus epilepsy. Arch Neurol 39:236, 1982

JANKOVIC J, ONMAN J: Botulinum A toxin for cranial-cervical dystonia: A double-blind, placebo-controlled study. Neurology 37:616, 1987

KRAMER PL et al: Dystonia gene in Ashkenazi Jewish population is located on chromosome 9q32–34. Ann Neurol 27:114, 1990

LOGIGIAN EL et al: Myoclonus epilepsy in two brothers: Clinical features and neuropathology of a unique syndrome. Brain 109:411, 1986

McGEER EG, McGEER PL: The dystonias. Can J Neurol Sci 15:447, 1988

McLEOD JG, TUCK RR: Disorders of the autonomic nervous system: Part 2. Investigation and treatment. Ann Neurol 21:519, 1987

MESULAM MM, PETERSEN RC: Treatment of Gilles de la Tourette syndrome: Eight-year, practice-based experience in a predominantly adult population. Neurology 37:1828, 1987

MUNOZ-GARCIA D, LUDWIN SK: Classic and generalized variants of Pick's disease: A clinicopathological, ultrastructural, and immunocytochemical study. Ann Neurol 16:467, 1984

PAULS OL, LECKMAN JF: The inheritance of Gilles de la Tourette syndrome and associated behaviors. N Engl J Med 315:993, 1986

SETHI KD et al: Hallervorden-Spatz syndrome: Clinical and magnetic resonance imaging correlations. Ann Neurol 24:692, 1988

STEELE JC: Progressive supranuclear palsy. Brain 95:693, 1972

TISSOT R et al: *La Maladie de Pick.* Paris, Masson et Cie, 1975

WATTS RL et al: Corticobasal ganglionic degeneration. Neurology 35:178, 1985

ZEMAN W, DYKEN P: Dystonia musculorum deformans: Clinical, genetic and pathoanatomical studies. Psychiatr Neurol Neurochir 70:77, 1967

360 DISORDERS OF THE CRANIAL NERVES

MAURICE VICTOR / JOSEPH B. MARTIN

The cranial nerves are susceptible to disorders that rarely affect the spinal peripheral nerves, and for this reason deserve to be considered separately. This chapter describes the principal syndromes of disordered function and the diseases that cause them. Cranial nerve disorders of taste and smell, vision and ocular movement, and vertigo and deafness are also discussed in Chaps. 22 to 24.

OLFACTORY NERVE (See Chap. 24)

OPTIC NERVE

TRANSIENT MONOCULAR BLINDNESS (AMAUROSIS FUGAX)
(See also Chap. 351) **Definition** Amaurosis fugax is the name applied to an attack of transient painless loss of vision in one eye. Frequently it is recurrent. (The term *amaurosis* refers to blindness from any cause, in distinction to *amblyopia*, which refers to a loss of vision from disease of structures other than the eye itself.)

Clinical manifestations Amaurosis fugax is a common clinical symptom indicative of transient retinal ischemia, usually associated with ipsilateral internal carotid artery stenosis or to embolism of the retinal arteries. In some cases the basis for the symptom cannot be discerned.

Typically, the episode of blindness evolves swiftly, in a matter of 10 to 15 s, and is described as a shade that falls smoothly and painlessly over the field until the eye is completely blind. Or, a similar obliteration of the visual field may occur from below. The blindness lasts for a few seconds or minutes, sometimes longer, then clears slowly and uniformly, the patient's vision returning in the reverse direction from that in which it was lost. Sometimes there is only a generalized dimness of vision, rather than a complete loss, or only a segment of the visual field may be involved. Many patients who experience amaurosis fugax on the basis of carotid stenosis also have transient attacks of contralateral hemiparesis, but it is uncommon for the two types of attack to occur simultaneously.

Diagnosis The transient visual loss that accompanies classic migraine is of a different type. Often it begins with unformed flashes of light (photopsia) or dazzling zigzag lines (fortification spectra or teichopsia), which move across the visual field for several minutes, leaving scotomatous or hemianopic defects. The patient with migraine may complain of blindness in one eye, but examination usually shows the defects to be bilateral and homonymous, i.e., they occupy corresponding halves of both visual fields. The latter symptoms point to an origin in the visual cortex of one occipital lobe. In so-called basilar migraine, in which the neurologic symptoms are referable to the territory of the basilar artery, the transient visual disturbances may occupy the whole of both visual fields.

Investigation and treatment Amaurosis fugax is most commonly a manifestation of ipsilateral internal carotid artery disease. Attention should be directed to carotid bruits, and noninvasive tests for carotid blood flow and lumen diameter should be carried out in every case. The decision of when to proceed to angiography is discussed in Chap. 351. Definitive treatment is dependent upon the results of these investigations. In the absence of carotid disease other possible sources of emboli (cardiac or aortic) should be sought. Amaurosis fugax may sometimes herald occlusion of the central retinal artery or anterior ischemic optic neuropathy due to giant cell arteritis or to nonarteritic (arteriosclerotic) disease. The sedimentation rate is usually elevated in giant cell arteritis (Chap. 276).

RETROBULBAR OPTIC NEUROPATHY OR NEURITIS **Definition** This syndrome is characterized by the rapid development (hours or days) of impaired vision in one or both eyes. In the latter case the eyes may be affected either simultaneously or sequentially. The visual loss in such cases is usually the result of acute demyelinative disease of optic nerves, although a number of other causes of unilateral or bilateral optic nerve disease must be sought (see below).

Clinical manifestations The most frequent setting is one in which a child, adolescent, or young adult notes a rapid diminution of vision in one eye (as though a veil or haze covered every object seen). The condition may progress to severe loss of vision (<20/100) within a few days, but complete blindness is rare. The optic disc and retina may appear normal, but in some patients the optic disc is hyperemic and elevated with blurring of the disc margins (papillitis). Peripapillary hemorrhages are seen infrequently, and the veins are not engorged. *Papillitis* is distinguished from *papilledema* due to increased intracranial pressure by the acute and often marked reduction of visual acuity that accompanies the former. Also, in retrobulbar neuropathy, there is often pain on movement of the eye or on pressure on the globe. After a few days or weeks the other eye may become similarly involved, with loss, typically, of central vision but with some preservation of peripheral vision. The pupillary light reflex is impaired. In a high percentage of patients, no cause can be found, and after days or weeks there is spontaneous recovery of vision. In the majority of patients the visual acuity returns to normal or near normal within months of the attack. Sometimes a small central scotoma persists. The optic disc later becomes slightly pale due to demyelination, often most prominent in the temporal region. The CSF may be normal or may contain from 10 to 20 lymphocytes, and the protein content, particularly the gamma globulin portion, may be increased. Oligoclonal bands are found in some patients.

About 50 percent of such patients will develop other symptoms and signs consistent with multiple sclerosis within 10 to 15 years, and even more will do so if the patients are observed for longer periods (see Chap. 356). Less is known about children with retrobulbar neuropathy, but the prognosis for them is considerably better than that for adults. Multiple sclerosis is the most common cause of a *unilateral retrobulbar neuritis.* Bilateral optic neuritis may occur a few days or weeks in advance of an attack of transverse myelitis. This combination is called neuromyelitis optica or Devic disease (Chap. 356).

Diagnosis Other causes of unilateral optic neuropathy, all of them rare, include postinfectious or disseminated encephalomyelitis, posterior uveitis, and, more commonly, vascular lesions of the optic nerve. *Anterior ischemic optic neuropathy (AION)* is a condition caused by interruption of blood supply to the optic nerve secondary to atherosclerotic or inflammatory disease of the ophthalmic artery or its branches (see Chap. 23). It presents clinically as acute, painless, visual loss in one eye, usually accompanied by an altitudinal visual field defect. In severe cases visual loss is complete and permanent. The fundus shows a pale swollen optic disc surrounded by splinter-shaped peripapillary hemorrhages. Occasionally only a section of the disc is pale and swollen. The macula and the retina are normal. Investigations are directed toward excluding temporal arteritis (see Chap. 276). Rarely, microemboli can cause occlusion of the posterior ciliary arteries and AION; for example, following open heart or coronary artery bypass surgery.

Central retinal artery occlusion (CRAO) also presents with sudden blindness. In this entity the optic disc initially appears normal. The retina is infarcted and appears pale with accentuation of the macular cherry-red spot. In all cases of unilateral involvement of the optic nerve, tumor (glioma, von Recklinghausen neurofibromatosis, meningioma) needs to be ruled out.

Treatment   Acute optic neuropathy due to demyelination usually resolves without specific treatment. Severe visual loss is commonly treated with prednisone 40 to 80 mg daily in divided doses for 7 to 10 days with gradual tapering over a few days. Some physicians recommend ACTH treatment. Both forms of treatment may hasten recovery from an individual attack, but do not prevent further attacks or modify their severity.

TOXIC-NUTRITIONAL OPTIC NEUROPATHY   Simultaneous impairment of vision in the two eyes, with central or centrocecal scotomas, occurring over a period of days or weeks, is usually due to a toxic or nutritional disorder rather than to a demyelinative process (see Chap. 357). Impairment of vision due to *methyl alcohol intoxication* is abrupt in onset and is characterized by large symmetric central scotomas, as well as by symptoms of systemic disease and acidosis (see Chap. 374). The lesion is in the retinal ganglion cells and their axons, which project into the optic nerve. The most important treatment is intravenous administration of sodium bicarbonate. Hemodialysis is a useful adjunct because of the slow rate of oxidation of methyl alcohol. Other drugs with proven but less devastating toxic effects on the optic nerve include chloramphenicol, ethambutol, isoniazid, streptomycin, sulfonamides, digitalis, ergot, disulfiram, and heavy metals.

Degenerative diseases may affect the retina or the optic nerves, taking the form of optic atrophy. There are several types of hereditary optic atrophy, the most frequent being the Leber type, which is sex-linked, occurring in males (see Chap. 23). An autosomal dominant form of congenital or early infantile optic atrophy and optic atrophy with diabetes mellitus and deafness are described. Senile macular degeneration and various forms of retinitis pigmentosa are important causes of visual loss (see Chap. 23).

BITEMPORAL HEMIANOPSIA   This type of visual disorder is usually related to suprasellar extension of a pituitary adenoma (often with an enlarged sella), but may also be due to a craniopharyngioma, saccular aneurysm of the circle of Willis, meningioma of the tuberculum sellae (normal sella or thickened tuberculum by radiography), and rarely sarcoidosis, metastatic carcinoma, and Hand-Schüller-Christian disease (see Chap. 313). The lesion involves the decussating nasal fibers from each retina.

OCULOMOTOR, TROCHLEAR, AND ABDUCENS NERVES (See Chap. 23)

TRIGEMINAL NERVE

The trigeminal nerve supplies sensation to the skin of the face and half of the vertex of the skull and motor innervation to the masseter and pterygoid masticatory muscles.

PAROXYSMAL FACIAL PAIN (TRIGEMINAL NEURALGIA, TIC DOULOUREUX)   Definition   The most striking disorder of trigeminal nerve function is tic douloureux, a condition characterized by excruciating paroxysms of pain in the lips, gums, cheek, or chin, and, very rarely, in the distribution of the ophthalmic division of the fifth nerve. The disorder occurs almost exclusively in middle-aged and elderly persons. The pain seldom lasts more than a few seconds or a minute or two but may be so intense that the patient winces, hence the term *tic*. The paroxysms recur frequently, both day and night, for several weeks at a time. Another characteristic feature is the initiation of pain by obvious stimuli applied to certain areas on the face, lips, or tongue (the so-called trigger zones) or by movement of these parts. Sensory loss cannot be demonstrated. In studying the relations between stimuli applied to the trigger zone and the paroxysm of pain, it is found that the adequate stimulus for precipitating an attack is a tactile one and possibly tickle, rather than a noxious or thermal stimulus. Usually a spatial and temporal summation of impulses is necessary to trigger an attack, which is followed by a refractory period of up to 2 or 3 min.

The diagnosis of this disorder rests upon these strict clinical criteria, and the condition must be distinguished from other forms of facial and cephalic neuralgia and pain arising from diseases of the jaw, teeth, or sinuses. Tic douloureux is usually without assignable cause; occasionally it is a manifestation of multiple sclerosis when it appears in younger adults and may be bilateral. Very rarely it may occur with herpes zoster or a tumor. To a degree that remains uncertain and controversial, pain of tic douloureux may be caused by a redundant or tortuous blood vessel in the posterior fossa, causing an irritative lesion of the nerve or its root. Usually, however, space-occupying lesions, such as aneurysms, neurofibromas, or meningiomas affecting the nerve, produce a loss of sensation (trigeminal neuropathy).

Treatment   The initial treatment of tic douloureux is pharmacologic. Carbamazepine is the drug of choice and is effective initially in 75 percent of patients. Unfortunately, up to one-third cannot tolerate the drug in the doses required to alleviate pain. Carbamazepine should be started gradually, 100 mg with food, as a single dose, and increased to 200 mg qid. Doses greater than 1200 to 1600 mg provide no additional benefit.

If drug treatment fails, surgical therapy should be offered. The most widely applied procedure is percutaneous retrogasserian rhizotomy accomplished by radiofrequency lesions. Relief is obtained by one to three procedures in more than 95 percent of patients. Later recurrences affect 7 to 31 percent of patients. Complications and morbidity are infrequent in experienced hands. The procedure results in partial numbness of the face and carries a risk of corneal denervation with secondary keratitis when used for first division trigeminal neuralgia.

A second treatment, microvascular dissection, requires a suboccipital craniectomy, a major procedure requiring about 1 week of hospitalization. It has an 80 percent efficacy but is accompanied by a 5 percent major complication rate. Not all patients operated upon have a demonstrated vascular or other compressive lesion of the trigeminal nerve. The most troublesome complication of all surgical treatments is the development of anesthesia dolorosa or denervation hypersensitivity. This condition responds poorly to treatment. Tricyclic antidepressants or phenothiazines are usually given with only partial success in alleviating the discomfort.

TRIGEMINAL NEUROPATHY   A variety of diseases may affect the trigeminal nerve in addition to those mentioned above. Most present with sensory loss on the face or with weakness of the jaw muscles. Deviation of the jaw on opening indicates weakness of the pterygoids of the side to which the jaw deviates. Tumors of the middle cranial fossa (meningiomas), of the trigeminal nerve (schwannomas), or of the base of the skull (metastatic) may cause a combination of motor and sensory signs. Lesions in the cavernous sinus can affect the first and second divisions of the trigeminal nerve, and lesions of the superior orbital fissure can affect the first (ophthalmic) division. The accompanying corneal anesthesia increases the risk of ulceration (neurokeratitis).

Anesthesia and analgesia of the face have been reported after treatment with stilbamidine (formerly used in the treatment of kala azar and multiple myeloma). Pain and itching may occur during recovery. Rarely, an idiopathic form of trigeminal neuropathy is observed. It is characterized by feelings of numbness and paresthesias, sometimes bilaterally, with loss of sensation in the territory of the trigeminal nerve but without weakness of the jaw. Recovery is the rule, but the symptoms may be troublesome for many months, or even years. Leprosy may involve the trigeminal nerves.

Tonic spasm of the masticatory muscles, known as *trismus*, is symptomatic of tetanus (see Chap. 105). It may also occur as an idiosyncratic reaction in patients treated with phenothiazine drugs; lesser degrees may be associated with disease of the pharynx, temporomaxillary joint, teeth, and gums.

FACIAL NERVE

FACIAL PALSY AND FACIAL SPASM   The seventh cranial nerve supplies all the muscles concerned with facial expression. The sensory component is small (the nervus intermedius of Wrisberg); it conveys taste sensation from the anterior two-thirds of the tongue and probably cutaneous impulses from the anterior wall of the external auditory canal. The motor nucleus of the seventh nerve lies anterior and lateral to the abducens nucleus. After leaving the pons the seventh nerve enters the internal auditory meatus with the acoustic nerve. The nerve continues its course through the middle ear to exit from the skull via the stylomastoid foramen. It then passes through the parotid gland and subdivides to supply the facial muscles.

A complete interruption of the facial nerve at the stylomastoid foramen paralyzes all muscles of facial expression. The corner of the mouth droops, the creases and skin folds are effaced, the forehead is unfurrowed, and the eyelids will not close. Upon attempted closure of the lids, the eye on the paralyzed side is seen to roll upward (Bell's phenomenon). The lower lid sags also, and the punctum falls away from the conjunctiva, permitting tears to spill over the cheek. Food collects between the teeth and lips, and saliva may dribble from the corner of the mouth. The patient complains of a heaviness or numbness in the face, but no sensory loss is demonstrable and taste is intact.

If the lesion is in the middle ear portion, taste is lost over the anterior two-thirds of the tongue on the same side. If the nerve to the stapedius is interrupted, there is hyperacusis (painful sensitivity to loud sounds). Lesions in the internal auditory meatus may also affect the adjacent auditory and vestibular nerves, causing deafness, tinnitus, or dizziness. Intrapontine lesions that paralyze the face usually affect the abducens nucleus and often the corticospinal and sensory tracts.

If the peripheral facial paralysis has existed for some time and recovery of motor function has begun but is incomplete, a kind of contracture (actually a continuous diffuse contraction) of facial muscles may appear. The palpebral fissure becomes narrowed and the nasolabial fold deepens. With the passage of time, the face and even the tip of the nose become pulled to the unaffected side. Attempts to move one group of facial muscles result in contraction of all of them (associated movements, or *synkinesis*). Facial spasms may develop and persist indefinitely, being initiated by every facial movement (hemifacial spasm). This condition may represent a transient or permanent sequela to a Bell's palsy but may also be due to an irritative lesion of the facial nerve (e.g., an acoustic neuroma, an aberrant artery which compresses the nerve and is relieved by surgery, or a basilar artery aneurysm). However, in the most common form of hemifacial spasm, the cause and pathology are unknown. Anomalous regeneration of the seventh nerve fibers may result in other curious disorders. If fibers originally connected with the orbicularis oculi come to innervate the orbicularis oris, closure of the lids may cause a retraction of the mouth; or if fibers originally connected with muscles of the face later innervate the lacrimal gland, anomalous tearing (crocodile tears) may occur with any activity of the facial muscles, such as eating. Yet another unusual facial synkinesia is one in which jaw opening causes a closure of the eyelids on the side of the facial palsy (jaw-winking).

BELL'S PALSY   Definition   The most common form of facial paralysis is idiopathic, i.e., *Bell's palsy*. The incidence rate of this disorder is about 23 per 100,000 annually, or about 1 in 60 or 70 persons in a lifetime. The pathogenesis of the paralysis is unknown. The few autopsied cases of this disease have shown only nondescript changes in the facial nerve and not inflammatory changes, as is commonly presumed.

Clinical manifestations   The onset of Bell's palsy is fairly abrupt, maximum weakness being attained by 48 h as a general rule. Pain behind the ear may precede the paralysis for a day or two. Taste sensation may be lost unilaterally, and hyperacusis may be present. In some cases there is mild CSF lymphocytosis. Fully 80 percent of patients recover within a few weeks or months. Electromyography may be of value in distinguishing a temporary conduction defect from a pathologic interruption in the continuity of nerve fibers. Evidence of denervation after 10 days indicates that there has been axonal degeneration and that there will be a long delay before regeneration occurs, and that it may be incomplete. The presence of incomplete paralysis in the first week is the most favorable prognostic sign.

Treatment   Protection of the eye during sleep, massage of the weakened muscles, and a splint to prevent drooping of the lower part of the face are the measures generally employed in the management of such cases. A course of prednisone beginning with 60 to 80 mg daily during the first 5 days and then tapered over the next 5 days may be beneficial. Unroofing of the facial nerve in the facial canal has been practiced, but there is no evidence that this measure is helpful, and it may be harmful.

Differential diagnosis   There are many other causes of facial palsy. Tumors that invade the temporal bone (carotid body, cholesteatoma, dermoid) may produce a facial palsy, but the onset is insidious and the course progressive. The *Ramsay Hunt syndrome*, presumably due to herpes zoster of the geniculate ganglion, consists of a severe facial palsy associated with a vesicular eruption in the pharynx, external auditory canal, and other parts of the cranial integument; often the eighth cranial nerve is affected as well. *Acoustic neuromas* frequently involve the facial nerve by local compression (see Chap. 353). Infarcts and tumors are the common pontine lesions which may interrupt the facial nerve fibers. Bilateral facial paralysis (facial diplegia) occurs in acute inflammatory polyradiculoneuritis (Guillain-Barré disease) and in a variety of sarcoidosis known as *uveoparotid fever* (*Heerfordt syndrome*). The *Melkersson-Rosenthal syndrome* consists of a rarely encountered triad of recurrent facial paralysis, recurrent—and eventually permanent—facial (particularly labial) edema, and less constantly, plication of the tongue; many causes of this rare syndrome have been suggested, but none has been established. Leprosy frequently involves the facial nerve.

A puzzling disorder is the *facial hemiatrophy of Romberg*. It occurs mainly in females and is characterized by a disappearance of fat in the dermal and subcutaneous tissues on one side of the face. It usually begins in adolescence or early adult years and is slowly progressive. In its advanced form the face is gaunt and the skin is thin, wrinkled, and rather brown. The facial hair may turn white and fall out, and the sebaceous glands become atrophic. The muscles and bones are not involved as a rule. Sometimes the atrophy becomes bilateral. The condition is a form of lipodystrophy, and the localization within a dermatome suggests a disorder of some neural trophic factor of unknown nature. The treatment is transplantation of skin and subcutaneous fat by a plastic surgeon.

Facial myokymia is a fine fibrillary activity of the facial muscles which may be caused by a plaque of multiple sclerosis. *Blepharospasm* is an involuntary recurrent spasm of both eyelids that occurs in elderly persons as an isolated phenomenon or with varying degrees of spasm of other facial muscles (see Chap. 25). Relaxant and sedative drugs are of little help, although in many patients this disorder subsides spontaneously. In severe persistent cases of blepharospasm or hemifacial spasm, an effective treatment has been differential facial nerve section of selected branches of the nerve or nerve decompression (from vessels) intracranially. Cases are now successfully treated by local injection of botulinus toxin into the orbicularis oculi; the spasms are relieved for 3 to 4 months, and the injections can be repeated without morbidity.

All these forms of nuclear or peripheral facial palsy must be distinguished from the supranuclear type. In the latter the frontalis and orbicularis oculi muscles are involved less than those of the lower part of the face, since the upper facial muscles are innervated by corticobulbar pathways from both motor cortices, whereas the lower facial muscles are innervated only by the opposite hemisphere. In supranuclear lesions there may be a dissociation of emotional and voluntary facial movements, and often some degree of paralysis of the arm and leg or an aphasia (in dominant hemisphere lesions) is conjoined.

VESTIBULAR NERVE

The eighth cranial nerve has two components, vestibular and auditory. Symptoms and signs of involvement of the vestibular portion are discussed in Chap. 22 and in this section. The auditory nerve and its disorders are discussed in Chap. 24.

MÉNIÈRE'S SYNDROME Definition and clinical manifestations Ménière's disease, or Ménière's syndrome, is the name applied to recurrent vertigo accompanied by tinnitus and deafness. The latter symptoms may be absent during the initial attack(s) of vertigo, but they invariably appear as the disease progresses and are increased in severity during an acute attack. With milder forms of the syndrome the patient may complain more of head discomfort, slight instability, and difficulty in concentration than of vertigo and may be considered to be anxious or depressed. Provided that deafness is not complete, the recruitment phenomenon can be demonstrated (see Chap. 24).

Ménière's disease has its onset most frequently in the fifth decade of life, though younger adults and the elderly are not spared. The pathologic changes are said to consist of a dilatation of the endolymphatic system which leads to a degeneration of the delicate vestibular and cochlear hair cells. The relation of these pathologic changes to the paroxysmal disorder of labyrinthine function is unknown.

Treatment During an acute attack, rest in bed is the most effective treatment, since the patient can usually find a position in which vertigo is minimal. Dimenhydrinate, cyclizine, or meclizine in doses of 25 to 50 mg tid is useful in the more protracted cases. A low-salt diet is still used in treatment, but its value is difficult to judge. Mild sedative drugs may help the anxious patient between attacks. Usually the deafness is unilateral and progressive, and when it is complete, the vertiginous attacks cease. However, the course is variable, and if the attacks persist in a severe manner, permanent relief can be obtained by surgical destruction of the labyrinth or section of the vestibular portion of the eighth nerve intracranially.

BENIGN POSITIONAL VERTIGO Another disorder of labyrinthine function is characterized by the occurrence of paroxysmal vertigo and nystagmus with the assumption of certain critical positions of the head. This is the positional vertigo of Bárány, of the so-called benign paroxysmal type (see Chap. 22). In refractory cases, in which attacks continue, vestibular exercises may be beneficial.

DIFFERENTIAL DIAGNOSIS OF VERTIGO There are many other causes of acute vertigo, such as purulent labyrinthitis complicating meningitis, serous labyrinthitis due to infection of the middle ear, "toxic labyrinthitis" due to drug intoxication (e.g., with alcohol, quinine, streptomycin, gentamicin, and other antibiotics), motion sickness, trauma, and hemorrhage into the internal ear. In these instances the attacks of vertigo tend to last longer than in the recurrent

form, but in other respects the symptoms are similar. Streptomycin or gentamicin may damage the fine hair cells of the vestibular end organs and cause a permanent disorder of equilibrium (as well as hearing), especially in older patients.

There has been described a dramatic clinical syndrome, characterized by the abrupt onset of severe vertigo, nausea, and vomiting, without tinnitus or hearing loss. The vertigo persists for several days or weeks, and labyrinthine function is permanently ablated on one side. Occlusion of the labyrinthine division of the internal auditory artery would logically explain this syndrome, but pathologic or angiographic confirmation of this hypothesis has so far not been obtained.

Vertigo of vestibular nerve origin may occur with diseases that involve the nerve in the petrous bone or the cerebellopontine angle. Except that it is less severe and is less frequently paroxysmal, it has many of the characteristics of labyrinthine vertigo. The adjacent auditory division of the eighth cranial nerve may also be affected, which explains the frequent association of vertigo with tinnitus and deafness. The function of the eighth cranial nerve may be disturbed by tumors of the lateral recess (especially acoustic neuroma), less frequently by meningeal inflammation in this region and rarely, by an abnormal vessel that compresses the nerve.

Vestibular neuronitis and *benign recurrent vertigo* are the names that have been applied to a clinical syndrome that occurs mainly in middle-aged and young adults (sometimes in children) and is characterized by the abrupt onset of vertigo, nausea, and vomiting, without impairment of hearing. The attacks are brief and leave the patient for some days with a mild positional vertigo. They may occur only once or recur in varying degrees of severity. The cause is unknown. The medical treatment is the same as for Ménière's disease.

A particular variety of paroxysmal vertigo affects children. The attacks occur in a setting of good health and are of sudden onset and brief duration. Pallor, sweating, and immobility are prominent manifestations, and occasionally vomiting and nystagmus occur. No relation to posture or movement of the head has been observed. The attacks are recurrent but tend to cease spontaneously after a period of several months or years. The outstanding abnormal finding is demonstrated by caloric testing, which shows impairment or loss of vestibular function, bilateral or unilateral, frequently persisting after the attacks have ceased; cochlear function is unimpaired, however. The pathologic basis of this disorder has not been determined.

GLOSSOPHARYNGEAL NERVE

GLOSSOPHARYNGEAL NEURALGIA Glossopharyngeal neuralgia resembles trigeminal neuralgia in many respects but is much less common. The pain is intense and paroxysmal; it originates in the throat, approximately in the tonsillar fossa. In some cases the pain is localized in the ear or may radiate from the throat to the ear, because of implication of the tympanic branch of the glossopharyngeal nerve (Jacobson's nerve). Spasms of pain may be initiated by swallowing. There is no demonstrable sensory or motor deficit. Cardiac symptoms of bradycardia with hypotension and fainting have been reported. A trial of carbamazepine or phenytoin is the recommended therapy, but if this is unsuccessful, division of the glossopharyngeal nerve near the medulla is the definitive treatment. Percutaneous rhizotomy of glossopharyngeal and vagal fibers in the jugular foramen alleviates pain in some patients.

Very rarely, herpes zoster may involve the glossopharyngeal nerve. Glossopharyngeal neuropathy in conjunction with vagus and accessory nerve palsies may occur due to a tumor or aneurysm in the posterior fossa or in the jugular foramen. Hoarseness due to vocal cord paralysis, some difficulty in swallowing, deviation of the soft palate to the intact side, anesthesia of the posterior wall of the pharynx, and weakness of the upper part of the trapezius and sternocleidomastoid muscles make up the syndrome (see Table 360-1, jugular foramen syndrome).

PART THIRTEEN NEUROLOGIC DISORDERS

TABLE 360-1 Cranial nerve syndromes

Site	Cranial nerves involved	Eponymic syndrome	Usual cause
Sphenoid fissure (superior orbital)	III, IV, first division V, VI	Foix	Invasive tumors of sphenoid bone; aneurysms
Lateral wall of cavernous sinus	III, IV, first division V, VI, often with proptosis	Foix Tolosa-Hunt	Aneurysms or thrombosis of cavernous sinus; invasive tumors from sinuses and sella turcica; benign granuloma responsive to steroids
Retrosphenoid space	II, III, IV, V, VI	Jacod	Large tumors of middle cranial fossa
Apex of petrous bone	V, VI	Gradenigo	Petrositis; tumors of petrous bone
Internal auditory meatus	VII, VIII		Tumors of petrous bone (dermoids, etc.); infectious processes; acoustic neuroma
Pontocerebellar angle	V, VII, VIII, and sometimes IX		Acoustic neuroma; meningioma
Jugular foramen	IX, X, XI	Vernet	Tumors and aneurysms
Posterior latero-condylar space	IX, X, XI, XII	Collet-Sicard	Tumors of parotid gland, carotid body, and metastatic tumor
Posterior retro-parotid space	IX, X, XI, XII and Horner syndrome	Villaret Mackenzie Tapia	Tumors of parotid gland, carotid body, lymph nodes; metastatic tumor; tuberculous adenitis

SPINAL ACCESSORY NERVE

Isolated involvement of the eleventh cranial nerve can occur anywhere along its route, resulting in partial or complete paralysis of the sternocleidomastoid and trapezius muscles. More commonly, involvement occurs in combination with deficits in the ninth and tenth cranial nerves in the jugular foramen or after exit from the skull (see Table 360-1).

VAGUS NERVE

DYSPHAGIA AND DYSPHONIA Complete interruption of the intracranial portion of one vagus nerve results in a characteristic paralysis. The soft palate droops ipsilaterally and does not rise in phonation. There is loss of the gag reflex on the affected side, as well as the "curtain movement" of the lateral wall of the pharynx, whereby the faucial pillars move medially as the palate rises in saying "ah." The voice is hoarse, slightly nasal, and the vocal cord lies immobile in the cadaveric position, i.e., midway between abduction and adduction. There may also be a loss of sensibility at the external auditory meatus and back of the pinna. Usually no change in visceral function can be demonstrated.

Complete interruption of both vagi is said to be incompatible with life, and this is probably true if the nuclei are involved in the medulla by poliomyelitis or some other disease. However, in the cervical region, both vagi have been blocked with procaine (Novocain) for the treatment of intractable asthma, without mishap. The pharyngeal branches of both vagi may be affected in diphtheria; the voice has a nasal quality, and regurgitation of liquids through the nose occurs during the act of swallowing.

The vagus nerve may be implicated at the meningeal level by neoplastic and infectious processes and within the medulla by tumors and vascular lesions, e.g., the lateral medullary syndrome of Wallenberg, and by motor neuron disease. This nerve may be involved by the inflammatory lesion of herpes zoster. Polymyositis and dermatomyositis, which cause hoarseness and dysphagia by direct involvement of laryngeal and pharyngeal muscles, may be confused with diseases of the vagus nerves. Also dysphagia is a symptom in some patients with myotonic dystrophy (see Chap. 42 for discussion of nonneurologic forms of dysphagia).

The recurrent laryngeal nerves, especially the left, are most often damaged as a result of intrathoracic disease. Aneurysm of the aortic arch, an enlarged left atrium, and tumors of the mediastinum and bronchi are much more frequent causes of an isolated vocal cord palsy than are intracranial disorders.

When confronted with a case of laryngeal palsy, the physician must attempt to determine the site of the lesion. If it is intramedullary, there are usually other signs, such as ipsilateral cerebellar dysfunction, loss of pain and temperature sensation over the ipsilateral face and contralateral arm and leg, and an ipsilateral Horner syndrome. If the lesion is extramedullary, the glossopharyngeal and spinal accessory nerves are frequently involved (see discussion of the jugular foramen syndrome above). If it is extracranial in the posterior laterocondylar or retroparotid space, there may be a combination of ninth, tenth, eleventh, and twelfth cranial nerve palsies and a Horner syndrome. Combinations of these lower cranial nerve palsies have a variety of eponymic designations, listed in Table 360-1. If there is no sensory loss over the palate and pharynx and no palatal weakness or dysphagia, the lesion is below the origin of the pharyngeal branches, which leave the vagus nerve high in the cervical region; the usual site of disease is then the mediastinum.

HYPOGLOSSAL NERVE

The twelfth cranial nerve supplies the ipsilateral muscles of the tongue. The nucleus of the nerve or its fibers of exit may be involved by intramedullary lesions (tumor, poliomyelitis, or motor neuron disease). Lesions of the basal meninges and the occipital bones (platybasia, Paget's disease) may compress the nerve in its extramedullary course or in the hypoglossal canal. Isolated lesions of unknown cause can occur. Atrophy and fasciculation of the tongue develop weeks to months after interruption of the nerve.

MULTIPLE CRANIAL NERVE PALSIES

Several cranial nerves may be affected by the same disease process. In this situation, the main clinical problem is to determine whether the lesion lies within the brainstem or outside of it. Lesions that lie on the surface of the brainstem are featured by involvement of adjacent cranial nerves (often occurring in succession) and late and rather slight involvement of the long sensory and motor pathways and segmental structures lying within the brainstem. The opposite is true of intramedullary, intrapontine, and intramesencephalic lesions. The extramedullary lesion is more likely to cause bone erosion or enlargement of the foramens of exit of cranial nerves. The intramedullary lesion involving cranial nerves often produces a crossed sensory or motor paralysis (cranial nerve signs on one side of the body and tract signs on the opposite side).

Involvement of multiple cranial nerves outside the brainstem is frequently the result of trauma (sudden onset), localized infections such as herpes zoster (acute onset), granulomatous disease such as Wegener's granulomatosis (subacute onset), Behçet's disease, or tumors and enlarging saccular aneurysms (chronic development). Of the tumors, neurofibromas, meningiomas, chordomas, cholesteatomas, carcinomas, and sarcomas have all been observed to implicate a succession of lower cranial nerves. Owing to their anatomic relationships, the multiple cranial nerve palsies form a number of distinctive syndromes, listed in Table 360-1. Sarcoidosis has been found to be the cause of some cases of multiple cranial neuropathy, and chronic glandular tuberculosis (scrofula) the cause of a few others. Malignant granuloma of the nasopharynx may also affect multiple cranial nerves, as do nasopharyngeal tumors, platybasia, and basilar invagination of the skull, and the Chiari malformation that becomes evident in adult life. A purely motor disorder without atrophy always raises the question of myasthenia gravis (see Chap. 366). Guillain-Barré syndrome commonly affects the facial nerves bilaterally (facial diplegia). In the Fisher variant of the Guillain-Barré syndrome oculomotor paresis occurs with ataxia and areflexia in the limbs. Wernicke encephalopathy can cause a severe ophthalmoplegia combined with other brainstem signs (see Chap. 357).

A benign idiopathic form of multiple cranial nerve involvement on one or both sides of the face is occasionally seen. The disease may recur over a period of years with variable degrees of recovery between attacks. The condition is called *polyneuritis cranialis multiplex.*

REFERENCES

ADAMS RD, VICTOR M: *Principles of Neurology*, 4th ed. New York, McGraw-Hill, 1989

BALOH RW: Vertigo, in *Current Therapy in Neurologic Disease* 2d ed, RT Johnson (ed). Philadelphia, Decker, 1987, pp 7–10

BRODAL A: The cranial nerves, in *Neurological Anatomy in Relation to Clinical Medicine*, 3d ed. New York, Oxford, 1980, chap 7, pp 448–577

BROWNSTONE PK et al: Bilateral superior laryngeal neuralgia. Arch Neurol 37:525, 1980

DALESSIO DJ: Trigeminal and glossopharyngeal neuralgia, in *Current Therapy in Neurologic Disease*, 2d ed, RT Johnson (ed). Philadelphia, Decker, 1987, pp 62–65

DURELLI L et al: The Melkersson-Rosenthal syndrome: A case with increased CNS IgG synthesis. Ann Neurol 18:623, 1985

EISEN A, BERTRAND G: Isolated accessory nerve palsy of spontaneous origin: A clinical and electromyographic study. Arch Neurol 27:496, 1972

ELSTON JS: Botulinum-toxin treatment of hemifacial spasm. J Neurol Neurosurg Psychiatr 49.824, 1986

GLASER JS: *Neuro-ophthalmology*. Hagerstown, Harper & Row, 1978

GROVES J: Bell's (idiopathic) facial palsy, in *Scientific Foundations of Otolaryngology*, R Hinchcliffe, D Harrison (eds). London, Heinemann, 1976, pp 446–459

HAUSER WA et al: Incidence and prognosis of Bell's palsy in the population of Rochester, Minnesota. Mayo Clin Proc 46:258, 1971

KARNES WE: Diseases of the seventh cranial nerve, in *Peripheral Neuropathy*, 2d ed, PJ Dyck et al (eds). Philadelphia, Saunders, 1984, chap 55, pp 1266–1299

KAYE AH, ADAMS CBT: Hemifacial spasm: A long-term follow-up of patients treated by posterior fossa surgery and nerve wrapping. J Neurol Neurosurg Psychiatry 44:1100, 1981

LECKY BRF et al: Trigeminal sensory neuropathy. Brain 110:1463, 1987

LIEBOLD JE: Drugs having a toxic effect on the optic nerve. Intern Ophthalmol Clin 11:137, 1970

SELBY G: Diseases of the fifth cranial nerve, in *Peripheral Neuropathy*, 2d ed, PJ Dyck et al (eds). Philadelphia, Saunders, 1984, chap 54, pp 1244–1265

SWEET WH: The treatment of trigeminal neuralgia (tic douloureux). N Engl J Med 315:174, 1986

————: Percutaneous methods for the treatment of trigeminal neuralgia and other faciocephalic pain; comparison with microvascular decompression. Semin Neurol 8:272, 1988

361 DISEASES OF THE SPINAL CORD

ALLAN H. ROPPER / JOSEPH B. MARTIN

Diseases of the spinal cord are frequently devastating, causing permanent and severe neurologic disability. Small lesions can produce quadriplegia, paraplegia, and sensory deficits far beyond the damage they would inflict elsewhere in the nervous system because the spinal cord contains, in a small cross-sectional area, almost the entire motor output and sensory input systems. Many spinal diseases are reversible, particularly extrinsic cord compression, making acute spinal cord lesions among the most critical of neurologic emergencies.

The stereotypic organization of the spinal cord, innervating the limbs and trunk segmentally through 31 pairs of spinal nerves, makes anatomic diagnosis relatively straightforward. A sensory level, par-

aplegia, or other typical syndromes usually permit recognition of a spinal cord process. Full assessment of cord disease requires a careful examination supplemented by laboratory tests, including magnetic resonance imaging (MRI), computed tomography (CT) scanning, myelography, analysis of cerebrospinal fluid (CSF), and somatosensory evoked responses. Most deficiencies in evaluating patients with signs of spinal cord disease result from cursory physical examination or inadequate x-rays. Computed tomography and MRI are replacing conventional myelography because of their ease of performance and better resolution; MRI gives particularly valuable information about intrinsic cord structure.

SPINAL COLUMN AND SPINAL CORD ANATOMY RELEVANT TO CLINICAL SIGNS The spinal cord is organized in a uniform somatotopic fashion throughout its length, giving rise to easily identifiable syndromes (see Chaps. 15, 25, and 28). The longitudinal location of lesions is established by the uppermost level of sensory and motor dysfunction. However, the relationship between the vertebral bodies of the spinal column (or their surface markers, the vertebral spines) and the cord segments that underlie them at times complicates the anatomic interpretation of signs of spinal cord diseases. Spinal cord syndromes are described according to the cord segment affected rather than by the surrounding vertebrae. During embryologic development the growth of the cord lags behind that of the spinal column, so that the cord ends behind the first lumbar vertebral body and the lower nerves must take an increasingly oblique downward course to exit near their targets in the limbs or viscera. The upper cervical cord segments lie behind the same numbered vertebral body, whereas the lower cervical segments are located one above each corresponding vertebral body, the upper thoracic cord two segments higher, and the lower thoracic cord, three segments higher. The lumbar and sacral cord segments, which form the conus medullaris, are located behind the ninth thoracic to first lumbar vertebrae. The cervical roots (except C8) exit from neural foramina above their respective vertebral bodies, while thoracic and lumbar roots exit below each body. In judging encroachment by various extrinsic masses, particularly spondylosis, careful radiographic measurement of the sagittal diameters of the spinal canal is often useful; they are normally 16 to 22 mm in the cervical and thoracic spine, 15 to 23 mm from L1 to L3, and 16 to 27 mm below.

CLINICAL SYNDROMES OF SPINAL CORD DISEASE The principal clinical signs of spinal cord damage are a "sensory level," i.e., loss of sensation below a circumferential horizontal line on the trunk, and weakness in the extremities innervated by the descending corticospinal fibers. Sensory symptoms, particularly paresthesias, may begin in the feet (or in one foot) and ascend, giving the impression early on of a polyneuropathy before a static sensory level is apparent. Lesions that disrupt descending corticospinal and bulbospinal tracts at a single cord level cause paraplegia or quadriplegia, with the characteristics of increased muscle tone, enhanced deep tendon reflexes, and Babinski signs. A careful examination often also elicits segmental signs that are approximate indicators of the location of a transverse lesion, such as a band of altered sensation at the rostral extent of the sensory level (hyperalgesia or hyperpathia), and isolated flaccidity, atrophy, or a single diminished deep tendon reflex. The sensory level to pinprick and temperature sensation is generally one or two segments below the level of an asymmetric lesion, but is at the level of the lesion in bilateral lesions. This is a result of the course of sensory fibers which ascend and cross to the opposite spinothalamic tract after synapsing in the dorsal horn. Midline back pain is also an accurate localizing sign, particularly in the thoracic region, where interscapular pain may be the first sign of cord compression. Radicular pain marks the primary site of a more laterally placed spinal lesion. Pain from lower cord (conus medullaris) lesions is often referred to the low back.

Early in the course of a severe and acute transverse lesion there may be flaccidity of the limbs rather than spasticity, due to so-called spinal shock. This state may last for several weeks and be mistaken for extensive segmental damage, but the reflexes later become increased. Brief clonic or myoclonic limb movements often precede paralysis in acute transverse lesions, particularly those due to infarction. Autonomic dysfunction, mainly urinary retention, is another prominent sign in transverse spinal lesions and should call attention to cord disease if it occurs in conjunction with spasticity or a sensory level.

Much is made of the clinical distinction between intramedullary (within the cord) and extramedullary compressive lesions, but most rules are approximations that do not distinguish one from the other dependably. Features that favor extramedullary lesions include radicular pain; a Brown-Séquard hemicord syndrome (see below); asymmetric lower motor neuron signs in one or two segments; early corticospinal signs; marked sacral sensory loss; and early, prominent CSF abnormalities. On the other hand, poorly localized burning pain, dissociated loss of pain sensation with sparing of joint position sensation, sparing of sensation in the perineal and sacral areas, late and less prominent corticospinal signs, and normal or minimally altered CSF generally favor an intramedullary lesion. "Sacral sparing" refers to the preservation of pinprick and temperature sensation in the sacral dermatomes, usually S3 to S5, with more rostral areas affected up to the sensory level. This is usually a dependable sign of intrinsic cord disease damaging the innermost fibers of the spinothalamic tracts while sparing those placed more laterally which subserve sacral sensation.

The *Brown-Séquard syndrome* is an eponym given to a hemicord syndrome consisting of ipsilateral mono- or hemiplegia, accompanied by ipsilateral loss of joint position and vibration sense, with contralateral loss of pain and temperature (spinothalamic) sensation. The segmental level for pain and temperature loss is sometimes one or two levels below the anatomic lesion. Segmental signs, such as radicular pain, muscle atrophy, or decreased tendon reflexes when they occur, are often unilateral.

Lesions limited to, or primarily within, the central portion of the cord preferentially damage gray matter neurons and segmental tracts crossing at that level. Traumatic contusion, developmental syringomyelia, tumors, and vascular lesions in the territory of the anterior spinal artery are the most common lesions localized to the central cord. Inflammatory diseases occur in this distribution less frequently. In the cervical cord, the central cord syndrome gives arm weakness out of proportion to leg weakness and a "dissociated" sensory loss signifying analgesia (loss of pin sensation), in a cape distribution over the shoulders, lower neck, and upper trunk without anesthesia (loss of touch sensation) or pallanesthesia (loss of vibration sense).

Lesions located in the region of the first lumbar vertebral body or below compress the spinal nerves of the cauda equina and cause a flaccid, areflexic, asymmetric paraparesis usually accompanied by bladder and bowel dysfunction. A sensory level is found in a saddle distribution up to L1, corresponding to the roots carried in the cauda equina. The Achilles and patellar reflexes are diminished or absent. Pain is common and projected to the perineum or thighs. With conus medullaris lesions pain is less prominent than in cauda equina lesions, and bladder and prominent bowel symptoms occur earlier. Compressive lesions may involve both the cauda and conus causing a combined syndrome of lower motor neuron signs and some hyperflexia or a Babinski sign.

The classic syndrome of the foramen magnum is weakness of the shoulder and arm followed by weakness of the ipsilateral leg, then contralateral leg, and finally, contralateral arm. Masses in this region sometimes produce suboccipital pain spreading to the neck and shoulders. A Horner's syndrome is another clue to a high cervical cord lesion; it does not occur with lesions below T2.

A few nontraumatic diseases are capable of producing sudden "strokelike" myelopathy without preceding symptoms. They include epidural hemorrhage, hematomyelia, cord infarction, nucleus pulposus embolism, and compression by spinal subluxation.

SPINAL CORD COMPRESSION   Tumors of the cord Tumors in the spinal canal may be primary or metastatic, and are classified as extradural ("epidural") or intradural, and the latter as intra- or

extramedullary (see Chap. 353). The majority of neoplastic lesions are epidural arising from metastases to the adjacent spinal column. Neoplasms originating in the prostate, breast, and lung, and lymphoma and plasma cell dyscrasias are particularly common, though virtually every malignant tumor has been reported to cause metastatic epidural cord compression. The initial symptom in epidural compression is usually local back pain, often worse in the recumbent position, and causing the patient to awaken at night. Radiating radicular pain exacerbated by coughing, sneezing, or straining may accompany the back pain. Pain and local tenderness often precede other symptoms by many weeks. Neurologic signs commonly evolve over several days to a few weeks. The cord syndrome begins with progressive weakness, eventually acquiring all the hallmarks of a transverse myelopathy with paraparesis and a sensory level. A plain radiograph may show lytic or blastic changes, or a compression fracture at the level appropriate to the cord syndrome; radionuclide bone scans are more frequently positive. CT scan, myelography, and particularly MRI remain the optimal way of demonstrating cord compression. A horizontally widened and flattened cord from extrinsic compression is seen at the margins of the subarachnoid block, and the adjacent vertebral body is usually abnormal (Fig. 361-1).

In the past, emergency laminectomies were considered necessary to treat epidural cord compression by tumor, but treatment with high-dose glucocorticoids and rapid, fractionated radiation therapy has been as successful. Outcome is most closely related to the tumor type and its radiosensitivity. Paraparesis frequently improves within 48 h of the administration of glucocorticoids. Some incomplete or early transverse cord syndromes may still be better treated surgically, but each case must be analyzed individually taking into account the radiosensitivity of the tumor, distribution of other metastases, and the patient's general medical condition. Whichever therapy is chosen, it is wise to proceed quickly and use glucocorticoids as soon as the diagnosis of cord compression is suspected.

Intradural, extramedullary tumors are a less frequent cause of spinal cord compression and evolve more slowly than extradural

FIGURE 361-1   Sagittal section MRI showing compression deformity of the T12 vertebral body from metastatic adenocarcinoma (below arrows), and compression and displacement of the spinal cord. *(Courtesy of Greg Shoukimas, M.D., Department of Radiology, Massachusetts General Hospital.)*

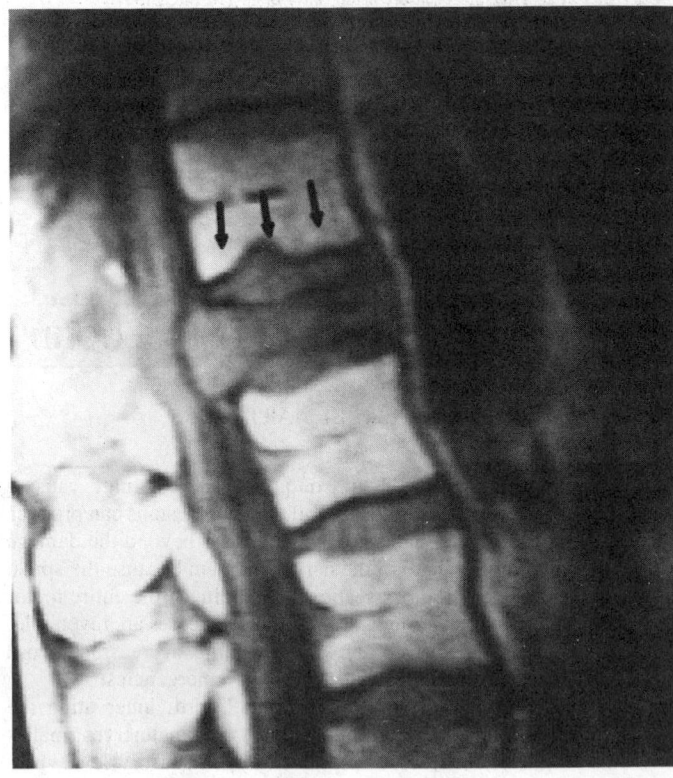

lesions. Meningiomas and neurofibromas are most common. Symptoms usually begin with radicular sensory changes and an asymmetric spinal cord syndrome. Radiologic studies show the typical appearance of dislocation of the cord to one side and an outline of the tumor within the subarachnoid space. Primary intramedullary tumors of the spinal cord are discussed in Chap. 353.

Neoplastic compressive myelopathies of all types initially cause minimal elevation of CSF protein, but with complete block of the subarachnoid space CSF protein concentration rises to the 1 to 10 g/L (100 to 1000 mg/dL) range due to impaired CSF circulation from the caudal sac to the intracranial subarachnoid space. There are usually few or no cells, cytology for malignant cells is often negative, and CSF glucose concentration remains normal unless there is accompanying widespread carcinomatous meningitis (see Chap. 353).

Epidural abscess This is a treacherous lesion, often misdiagnosed at first (see Chap. 354). The predisposing clinical settings are furunculosis of the back or scalp, bacteremia, or minor back injury. The condition can occur as a complication of local operation or very rarely after lumbar puncture. Spinal osteomyelitis acts as the nidus for the formation of an abscess that subsequently enlarges to compress the cord. The osteomyelitis is usually small and not often evident on plain radiographs. For several days to 2 weeks there may be only unexplained fever and mild spinal ache with local tenderness; later, radicular pain occurs. As the abscess expands, it rapidly causes cord compression with a transverse and usually complete transection syndrome. The proper treatment is rapid decompression by laminectomy and drainage, followed by appropriate antibiotics determined from culture of the purulent material. Incomplete drainage is not uncommon, resulting in a chronic granulomatous and fibrous reaction that may be sterilized with antibiotics but continues to act as a compressing mass. Tuberculous pyogenic abscess formation, more common in the past, is still a common cause of epidural abscess in developing countries.

Epidural hemorrhage and hematomyelia Hemorrhage into the spinal chord (hematomyelia) or epidural space produces an acute transverse myelopathy evolving over minutes or hours, accompanied by severe pain. Although these hemorrhages may originate from an arteriovenous malformation, or from hemorrhage into a tumor during anticoagulation with warfarin, they are more commonly spontaneous. Epidural hematoma may occur in the setting of minor trauma, lumbar puncture, warfarin anticoagulation, or secondary to coagulation disorders. Back and radicular pain can precede weakness by several minutes to hours, and be so severe that patients may be perceived to act in a peculiar, exaggerated fashion. Lumbar epidural hematoma results in loss of both knee and ankle reflexes, whereas retroperitoneal hematomas usually cause only absence of the knee reflexes. A myelogram or MRI defines the mass; CT scan is sometimes normal because the clot cannot be distinguished from adjacent bone. Subdural and subarachnoid clots are particularly painful and may occur spontaneously or under circumstances similar to those causing epidural hemorrhages. The CSF with epidural hemorrhage is usually clear or contains a few red blood cells; in subarachnoid or subdural hemorrhage the CSF is grossly bloody at first and later becomes discolored to a deep yellow-brown characteristic of blood pigments present in the CSF. There may be, in addition, a pleocytosis and lowered CSF glucose, giving the impression of bacterial meningitis.

Acute disk protrusion Lumbar disk herniation, a common disorder, is discussed in Chap. 19. Thoracic or cervical disk protrusion is less often a cause of spinal cord compression, usually occurring after direct trauma to the spinal column. Degeneration of cervical disk spaces with adjacent osteoarthritic hypertrophy causes a subacute spondylytic-compressive myelopathy in the cervical, and less often the thoracic region, discussed below. Embolism from nucleus pulposus material causing acute spinal cord infarction is also described below.

Other unusual compressive lesions Patients with iatrogenic or primary Cushing's syndrome have a tendency to form increased epidural fat tissue that rarely can reach a size large enough to compress the thoracic cord. Extramedullary hematopoiesis has caused cord

compression in a number of hematologic diseases. Eroding aortic aneurysms, echinococcal or other parasitic cysts, gummas, lymphomatoid-granulomatosis, mucopolysaccharidoses, and other rare lesions can also compress the cord.

Arthritic diseases of the spine occur in two clinical forms: a lumbar or cauda equina compression from ankylosing spondylitis, or cervical cord compression from destruction of the cervical apophyseal or atlantoaxial joints in rheumatoid arthritis. Spinal complications arising as one component of severe generalized joint disease in rheumatoid arthritis are often overlooked. Forward subluxation of cervical vertebral bodies, or of the atlas on the axis, can cause a devastating, even fatal, acute cord compression after minor trauma such as whiplash, or it may present as a chronic compressive myelopathy similar to cervical spondylosis. Separation of the odontoid process from the axis may narrow the upper spinal canal compressing the cervicomedullary junction, particularly in flexion movements.

NONCOMPRESSIVE NEOPLASTIC MYELOPATHIES Intramedullary metastasis, paracarcinomatous myelopathy, and radiation myelopathy In the context of known cancer most myelopathies are compressive. However, when radiologic studies fail to show compression, there is often difficulty distinguishing between several less common entities: intramedullary metastasis, paracarcinomatous myelopathy, and radiation myelopathy. In a patient with known metastatic cancer and a progressive myelopathy shown to be noncompressive, intramedullary metastasis is the most likely diagnosis since paraneoplastic myelopathy is rarer (see Chap. 310). Back pain is the most common initial symptom with intramedullary metastasis, though it is not invariable, followed by progressive spastic paraparesis and, less often, paresthesias. Dissociated sensory loss or sacral sparing, though characteristic of intrinsic compression, is uncommon, and asymmetric paraparesis with incomplete sensory loss is typical. Myelography, CT scan, or MRI may show a swollen cord without extrinsic compression; in almost half of patients CT or myelography are normal; MRI is more successful in outlining a metastatic mass or primary intramedullary tumor (Fig. 361-2). Intramedullary metastases usually

FIGURE 361-2 Sagittal MRI showing intrinsic fusiform enlargement of the cervical spinal cord from an intramedullary tumor. The tumor displays a low-density signal (arrows). (*Courtesy of Greg Shoukimas, M.D., Department of Radiology, Massachusetts General Hospital.*)

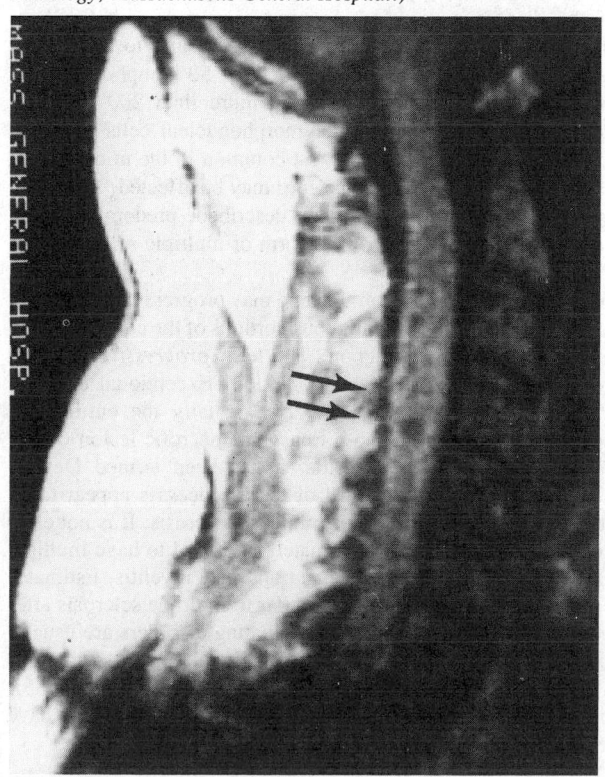

arise from bronchogenic carcinoma and less often from breast cancer and other solid tumors. Metastatic melanoma, an uncommon cause of extrinsic cord compression, more often presents as an intramedullary mass. The pathology of the metastasis is usually a single eccentrically placed nodule that presumably arrived hematogenously. Radiation therapy may be helpful in appropriate circumstances.

Carcinomatous meningitis, a common form of CNS invasion in malignancy, does not cause a myelopathy unless there is extensive subpial infiltration from adjacent roots causing nodules with secondary compression or infiltration of the cord. An incomplete, painless cauda equina syndrome can result from carcinomatous root infiltration (see Chap. 353). Headache is common, and repeated CSF examinations eventually reveal malignant cells, an elevated protein, and, in some cases, reduced CSF glucose concentration.

A progressive necrotic myelopathy associated with a paucity of inflammation can occur as a remote effect of cancer, usually with solid tumors. The radiologic studies and CSF are normal, or there may be slightly elevated protein. A subacute progressive spastic paraparesis evolves over days or weeks, usually asymmetrically, with distal paresthesias ascending to establish a sensory level, and late bladder dysfunction. Several adjacent segments of cord are involved.

Radiation may produce a delayed subacute progressive myelopathy due to microvascular hyalinization and vascular occlusion (see Chap. 353). It frequently presents a differential diagnostic problem when the cord lies within radiation portals used to treat other structures such as the mediastinal lymph nodes. Differentiation from paracarcinomatous myelopathy or intramedullary metastasis is difficult except by circumstantial history of prior radiation.

INFLAMMATORY MYELOPATHIES Acute myelitis, transverse myelitis, and necrotic myelopathy These are a group of related diseases marked by intrinsic inflammation of the cord and a clinical syndrome evolving over several days to 2 or 3 weeks. There may be a transverse or virtually complete spinal syndrome (transverse myelitis) or incomplete variants such as a posterior column myelopathy with ascending paresthesias and a sensory level for vibration; ascending, predominantly spinothalamic findings; or a Brown-Séquard syndrome with leg paresis and contralateral spinothalamic-type sensory changes. Many cases follow a viral illness. The most common presenting findings in transverse myelitis are back pain, progressive paraparesis, and asymmetric ascending paresthesias in the legs, later affecting the hands if the disease progresses, creating confusion with Guillain-Barré syndrome. Radiologic studies are necessary to exclude a compressive lesion. The CSF contains 5 to 50 lymphocytes per microliter in most patients; occasionally more than 200 cells per microliter are found, and rarely, polymorphonuclear cells predominate. The inflammatory process is most common in the mid and low thoracic regions, but any level of the cord may be affected. A chronic progressive cervical myelitis has been described, predominantly in older women, and is believed to be a form of multiple sclerosis (see Chap. 356).

In some cases necrosis is profound and may progress intermittently for several months to involve contiguous portions of the cord, reducing much of it to a thin gliotic ribbon. The term *progressive necrotic myelopathy* has been given to this condition. Exceptional cases of necrotic myelopathy progress to involve virtually the entire cord (necrotic panmyelopathy). When a transverse necrotic lesion occurs before or shortly after optic neuritis, it has been termed Devic's disease or neuromyelitis optica. All of these processes appear to be related to, and many are variants of, multiple sclerosis. It is not clear what proportion of patients will ultimately be found to have multiple sclerosis after a single episode of acute transverse myelitis. Estimates have been 15 to 80 percent, a range similar to multiple sclerosis after optic neuritis. The postinfectious demyelinating disorders are usually monophasic and only rarely recur, though fluctuation of symptoms related to a single level of the cord is common (see Chap. 355). Systemic lupus erythematosus and other autoimmune disorders have also been associated with myelitis.

Infectious myelopathy Direct viral infection of the cord produces specific types of myelitis. In the past, the most common form was poliomyelitis. Herpes zoster, preceded by radicular symptoms, is presently the most common cause of viral myelitis. The pathologic process is not restricted to the gray matter as is polio. Lymphocytes are always found in the CSF.

The human retroviruses HTLV-I and HIV may be associated with myelopathies (see Chap. 355). HTLV-I causes a chronic progressive, noninflammatory cord syndrome with symmetric spastic paraparesis and mild sensory and bladder disturbances. The disease is endemic in several areas where the virus is endemic, including areas of the Caribbean, South America, and southern Japan. It was identified as "tropical spastic paraparesis" before the virus was known. A myelopathy with vacuolar pathologic changes has been associated with HIV. There is generally no clear sensory level in the retroviral myelopathies.

Intramedullary cord abscesses caused by bacteria or mycobacteria arising in the context of systemic infection have been reported. Chronic meningitic lesions due to syphilis may produce a secondary subpial myelitis and radiculitis that evolve slowly (see below). An intense granulomatous, necrotic, and inflammatory myelitis is peculiar to infestation by *Schistosoma mansoni*, caused by a local response to tissue-digesting enzymes produced by ova from the parasite. Toxoplasmosis may also rarely cause a focal myelopathy.

Toxic myelopathy A toxic noninflammatory myelopathy, sometimes with optic atrophy, has been reported, mainly in Japan, and linked to ingestion of iodochlorhydroxyquinoline. Most patients have recovered, but many have persistent paresthesias.

Arachnoiditis This is a nonspecific term referring to inflammation, scarring, and fibrous thickening of the arachnoid membrane capable of compressing nerve roots or, rarely, the spinal cord. It is usually a postoperative complication or results from instillation of radiographic dye, antibiotics, or noxious chemicals into the subarachnoid space. The CSF contains many cells and an elevated protein concentration soon after the inciting event, but the inflammation then subsides. There may be slight fever in acute cases. Bilateral asymmetric radicular limb pain is the most prominent feature, with additional signs of root compression, such as reflex loss. Back pain and radicular symptoms are attributed to lumbar arachnoiditis, perhaps more often than justified. Arachnoiditis is not often responsible for cord compression (see Chap. 19). Treatment is controversial; laminectomy has led to improvement in some patients. Multiple meningeal cul-de-sacs, or arachnoid cysts, along nerve roots, occur as a congenital process that may produce severe radicular pain in midadulthood when the cysts enlarge and distort or exert traction on spinal nerve roots or ganglia. An unexplained delayed paraplegia has been reported after the use of chymopapain for the treatment of disk herniation.

SPINAL CORD INFARCTION Because the anterior or posterior spinal arteries are not usually involved by atherosclerosis, and only occasionally are affected by angiitis or emboli, most infarctions of the spinal cord are due to ischemia secondary to distant vascular occlusions. Aortic thrombosis or dissection causes cord infarction by interrupting the entire radicular and direct arterial supply to the anterior and posterior spinal arteries. The infarction typically occurs in a vascular watershed region of the thoracic cord between the large tributary to the spinal cord arising from the lower aorta, the artery of Adamkiewicz, and the anterior spinal artery arising from the vertebral arteries. The anterior spinal artery syndrome usually appears abruptly, like a stroke, or emerges postoperatively if the proximal aorta has been clamped. In some cases, however, symptoms progress over 24 to 72 h making diagnosis difficult. Spinal infarction has been reported rarely with systemic arteritis, immune reactions of serum sickness, and after intravascular contrast injection, heralded in the latter by severe back pain at the time of injection.

Cord infarction caused by microscopic fragments of herniated nucleus pulposus may occur after minor trauma, frequently during athletic activities. There is sharp local pain followed by a rapid paraplegia and a transverse cord syndrome evolving over several minutes to an hour. Pulposus tissue is found in small intramedullary vessels and often within the marrow of the adjacent vertebral body. The route from the disk space to marrow and thence to the cord is uncertain. This entity should be suspected in young adults with catastrophic transverse cord syndromes after back injury or exercise.

VASCULAR MALFORMATION OF THE SPINAL CORD Arteriovenous malformations (AVM) of the spinal cord are among the most difficult lesions to detect because of their great clinical variability. They may simulate multiple sclerosis, transverse myelitis, spinal cord stroke, or neoplastic compression. AVMs are most often found in the low thoracic or lumbar cord in middle-aged men. The majority begin with an incomplete progressive cord syndrome that may advance subacutely or episodically, like multiple sclerosis, producing bilateral corticospinal, spinothalamic, and posterior column symptoms and signs in any combination. Almost all patients are paraparetic and unable to walk within several years. About one-third have an abrupt syndrome with a single acute transverse myelopathy from bleeding, which simulates acute myelitis; others present with several acute exacerbations. About half have back or radicular pain, a few have a claudication syndrome similar to lumbar canal stenosis, and rare patients describe an acute onset with severe, localized back pain. Fluctuation of pain or neurologic signs with exercise, posture, or menses is helpful in suspecting the diagnosis. Bruits over the lesion are rare but should be sought at rest and after exercise. Most patients have mild elevation of CSF protein and a few show CSF pleocytosis. Bleeding into the cord or CSF may occur. Myelography, CT or MRI shows a lesion in 75 to 90 percent of cases. The anatomic details of most AVMs can be demonstrated with selective spinal angiography, a procedure requiring experience for safe and efficacious performance.

The pathogenesis of the myelopathy caused by AVMs (that have not bled) is incompletely understood, but appears to be a necrotic noninflammatory process consistent with ischemia. A dorsal AVM with a prominent progressive intramedullary syndrome (Foix-Alajouanine) has been reported with an adjacent necrotic myelopathy. The abnormal vessels have a characteristic thickened, hyalinized wall. Since any necrotic process within the cord may give rise to neovascularization and thick-walled vessels, the pathologic basis of

this vascular malformation remains controversial. Arteriovenous fistulas outside the spinal cord, including in visceral organs, have been associated with a vascular myelopathy due to large draining veins that traverse the spinal canal.

CHRONIC MYELOPATHIES Spondylosis This is a general term for several related degenerative changes of the spine giving rise to compression of the cervical cord and adjacent roots. Cervical spondylosis is primarily a disease of older patients, affecting men more often than women, and consisting of a combination of (1) narrowing of intervetebral disk spaces with nucleus pulposus herniation or annulus bulging, (2) osteophytic spur formation on the dorsal (posterior) aspect of the vertebral bodies, (3) partial subluxation of vertebrae, and (4) hypertrophy of the dorsal spinal ligament and dorsolateral facet articulations (see Chap. 19). The bony changes are reactive in nature, but there is no true arthritis. The most important feature causing spinal cord symptoms and signs is a "spondylitic bar" formed by osteophytes arising from the dorsal surfaces of adjacent vertebral bodies resulting in a horizontal compression of the ventral cord (Fig. 361-3A and B). Extension of the bar laterally, accompanied by articulatory hypertrophic changes or encroachment on the neural foramina, often causes additional radicular symptoms. The sagittal diameter of the spinal canal may be narrowed further by actual disk protrusion, or by hypertrophy or buckling of the dorsal spinal ligament, particularly during neck extension. Although the radiographic findings of spondylosis are common in the elderly, only a few patients develop myelopathy or radiculopathy, often dependent upon a congenitally narrow canal.

Neck and shoulder pain with stiffness are early symptoms; pressure on nerve roots is associated with radicular arm pain, most often in a C5 or C6 distribution. Compression of the cervical cord produces a slowly progressive spastic paraparesis, at times asymmetric, and often accompanied by paresthesias in the feet and hands. Vibratory sense is substantially diminished in the legs in most patients, and occasionally there is a sensory level for vibration on the upper thorax. Coughing or straining often produces leg weakness or radiating arm or shoulder pain. Dermatomal sensory loss in the arms, atrophy of intrinsic hand muscles, increased deep tendon reflexes in the legs, and asymmetric Babinski signs are common. Urinary urgency or incontinence do not occur unless the process is well-advanced. The reflexes in the arms are often diminished at some level, notably the biceps, corresponding to C5–C6 cord compression or root involvement. Either radicular, myelopathic, or combined signs may predominate. The diagnosis should be considered in cases of progressive cervical myelopathy, paresthesias of feet or hands, or wasting of the

FIGURE 361-3 *A.* Lateral x-ray of the cervical spine showing spondylitic "bar" formation from the junction of adjacent osteophytes at C6–C7 (arrow). *B.* Horizontal CT section at C6 from patient shown in *A*, after instillation of water-soluble dye into the subarachnoid space. A spur of the bony osteophyte compresses and distorts the spinal cord (arrows).

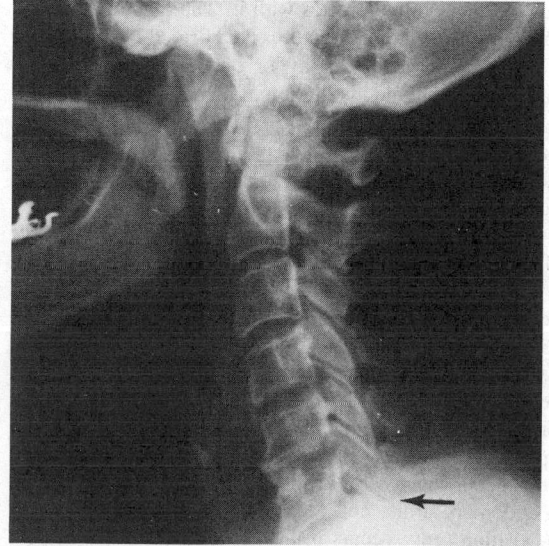

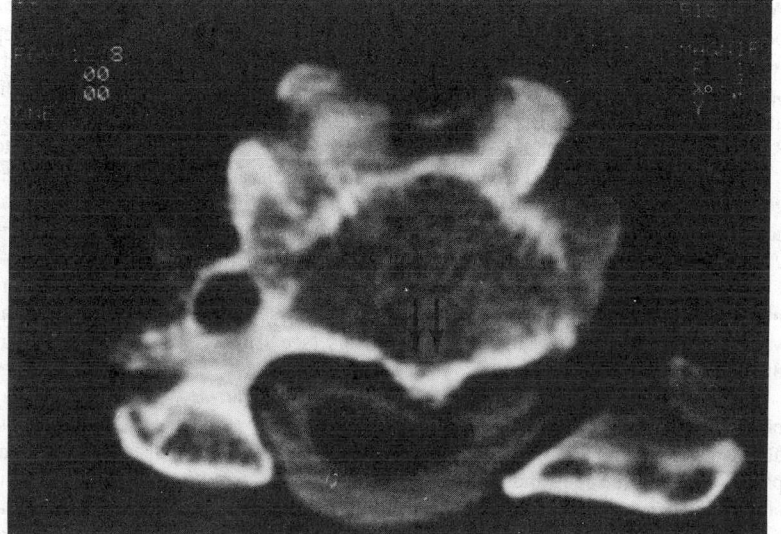

A   B

hands. Spondylosis is also one of the most common causes of gait difficulty in the elderly, often causing an otherwise unexplained increase in leg reflexes or Babinski signs.

Plain radiographs demonstrate spondylitic bars, intervertebral narrowing and subluxations, reversal of the normal cervical spine curvature, and reduction of the sagittal diameter of the canal to less than 11 mm, or to 7 mm with neck extension (Fig. 361-3A). The CSF is usually normal or shows a slightly elevated protein concentration. Somatosensory evoked potentials can be very helpful by demonstrating normal conduction in peripheral large sensory fibers and a delay in central conduction in the mid or high cervical cord. Electromyography may also be useful in demonstrating radicular compression.

Cervical spondylosis is both an under- and overdiagnosed disease. Many patient with intrinsic cord processes, particularly amyotrophic lateral sclerosis, multiple sclerosis, and subacute combined degeneration, have had cervical laminectomies in the belief that spondylosis was responsible. There may be temporary improvement suggesting that there was an element of spondylolytic compression, but the underlying intrinsic myelopathy soon progresses. A mild progressive gait disorder with sensory symptoms in the feet and hands caused by cervical spondylosis may also be incorrectly attributed to peripheral neuropathy.

Rest and cervical immobilization with a soft collar are helpful in minor cases, traction may be helpful in others, but an operation is advisable if there are advanced symptoms of gait difficulty, severe hand weakness, or bladder difficulty, particularly if there is a virtually complete block of the subarachnoid space on myelography or CT scan.

Lumbar stenosis (also discussed in Chap. 19) is an intermittent and chronic compression of the cauda equina usually based on congenital narrowing of the lumbar spinal canal, which is further compromised by disk protrusion or spondylitic changes. Exercise brings about an aching pain in the buttocks, thighs, and calves, frequently sciatic in distribution, ceasing with rest and thereby simulating vascular-induced claudication. During the peak of pain, deep tendon reflexes and sensation may be reduced as compared to the resting state; peripheral vascular studies are normal. Lumbar stenosis and cervical spondylosis commonly occur together, the former probably explaining occasional lower extremity fasciculations in cervical spondylosis.

Degenerative and inherited myelopathies   The prototype of the inherited disorders causing spinal cord syndromes is Friedreich's ataxia, a progressive, recessively inherited, leg and truncal ataxia of late childhood onset. Intention tremor, clumsiness of the arms, and, later, dysarthria occur. Kyphoscoliosis and pes cavus are common. Areflexia, Babinski signs, and severely impaired vibratory and joint position sense loss are found on examination. Fragmentary or milder forms of the illness occur and overlap with other syndromes including spastic paraparesis (Strümpell-Lorrain), cerebellar cortical degeneration with ataxia, and olivopontocerebellar atrophy (see also Chap. 359).

Amyotrophic lateral sclerosis (motor neuron disease) must be considered in patients with symmetric spastic paraparesis without sensory findings. It causes a pure motor syndrome with combined corticospinal, corticobulbar, and anterior horn cell involvement. Clinical or electromyographic evidence of widespread muscle fasciculations and denervation, in contrast to the limited segmental denervation of spondylosis, confirms the diagnosis (see Chaps. 359 and 362).

Subacute combined degeneration due to vitamin B$_{12}$ deficiency   This treatable myelopathy causes a progressive spastic and ataxic paraparesis and neuropathy, usually with prominent distal paresthesias of the feet and hands. It should be considered in cases simulating cervical spondylosis, late-onset degenerative myelopathies, and symmetric late-onset spinal multiple sclerosis. The disease can also involve the peripheral and optic nerves, and the brain. The diagnosis is confirmed by low B$_{12}$ serum concentration and a positive Schilling test. This entity and related nutritional degenerations are discussed in Chap. 357. Whether folate or vitamin E deficiencies can produce a similar syndrome is controversial. Rarely, multiple sclerosis and B$_{12}$ deficiency myelopathy are found in the same patient.

Syringomyelia   Syringomyelia is a progressive myelopathy characterized pathologically by cavitation of the central spinal cord. It is often idiopathic or developmental (see Chap. 358) but may result from trauma, primary intramedullary tumors, extrinsic compression with central cord necrosis, arachnoiditis, hematomyelia, or necrotic myelitis. The developmental type usually begins in the midcervical cord and extends upward to the medulla or downward as low as the lumbar cord. It commonly takes an eccentric position often causing unilateral long tract signs or reflex asymmetries. Many cases occur in association with craniovertebral abnormalities, most commonly the Arnold-Chiari malformation, but also including myelomeningocele, basilar skull impression (platybasia), atresia of the foramen of Magendie, or Dandy-Walker cysts (see Chap. 358).

The cardinal clinical signs of syringomyelia correspond to a central high cervical cord syndrome and depend on the extent of the syrinx and associated abnormalities such as the Arnold-Chiari malformation. The classic presentation is ① sensory loss, usually of a dissociated type (loss of pain and temperature and preservation of touch and vibration senses), which is "suspended" over the nape of the neck, shoulders, and upper arms (cape distribution), and eventually extends to the hands, ② wasting of muscles in the lower neck, shoulders, arms, and hands, with asymmetric or absent reflexes, and ③ high thoracic kyphoscoliosis. The majority begin asymmetrically with unilateral sensory loss. A number of patients develop loss of pin sensation on the face attributed to damage to the descending tract of the trigeminal nerve in the upper cervical cord. Cough-induced headache and neck pain are common with associated Arnold-Chiari malformations.

Symptoms in idiopathic cases begin in adolescence or early adulthood, progress irregularly, and frequently arrest for several years. A few patients escape major disability, but over half become wheelchair-bound. Analgesia leads to injuries, burns, and trophic ulcers in the fingertips. Charcot joints in the shoulders, elbows, or knees are common in advanced cases. Prominent lower extremity weakness or hyperreflexia suggest an associated abnormality at the craniovertebral junction. Syringobulbia results from extension of the cavity into the medulla, or rarely the pons, usually occupying the lateral medullary tegmentum. Palatal and vocal cord paralysis, dysarthria, nystagmus, episodic dizziness, tongue weakness, and Horner's syndrome may occur.

Slow enlargement of the cavity may create a narrowing or complete block of the subarachnoid space. The cavity is separate from the central canal but usually communicates with it. The diagnosis can be made dependably from the clinical features, confirmed by finding an enlarged cervical cord on myelography or on delayed CT images several hours after subarachnoid instillation of metrizamide or another water-soluble contrast material (Fig. 361-4A). Syrinx cavities are shown to greatest advantage by MRI (Fig. 361-4B). The cervicomedullary junction should be examined for associated developmental abnormalities.

Therapy is directed at decompressing the cavity to prevent progression of damage and decompressing the spinal canal if the cord is distended. Laminectomies and suboccipital decompression are sometimes recommended when an Arnold-Chiari malformation accompanies an enlarged cervical cord.

Tabes dorsalis   Tabes and meningovascular syphilis of the spinal cord are presently rare but at one time had to be considered in the differential diagnosis of most spinal cord syndromes. The most common symptoms of tabes are characteristic fleeting and repetitive, lancinating pains occurring mostly in the legs, less commonly in the back, thorax, abdomen, arms, and face. Severe gait and leg ataxia due to loss of position sense occurs in half of patients. Paresthesias, bladder disturbances, and acute abdominal pain with vomiting (visceral crisis) occur in 15 to 30 percent. The cardinal signs of tabes are loss

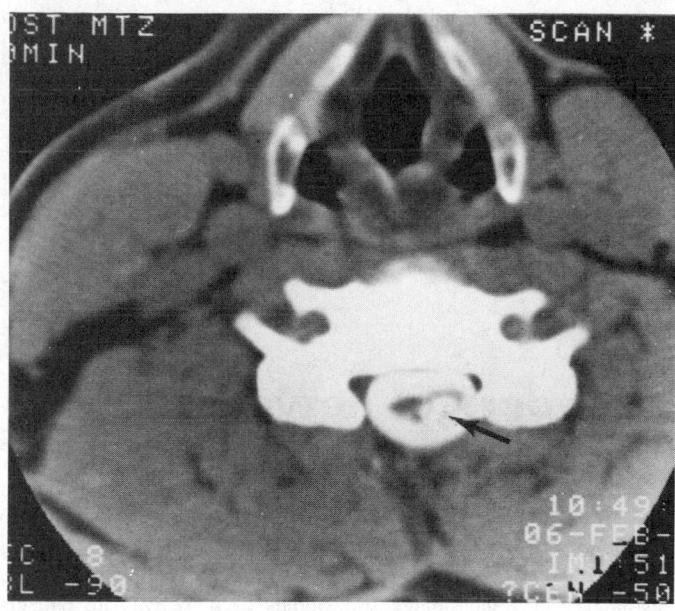

A

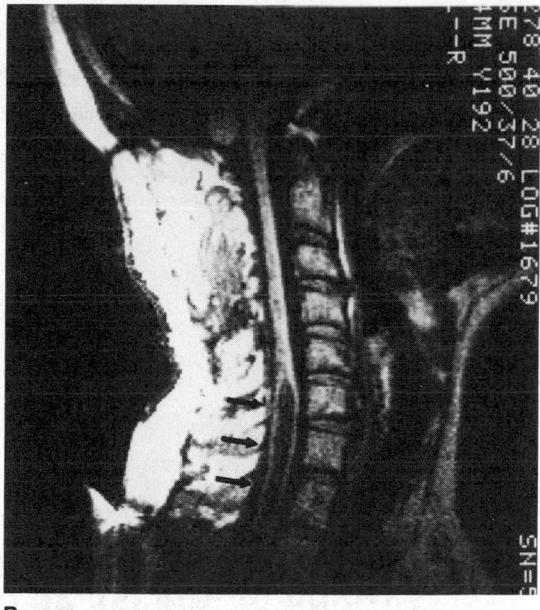

B

FIGURE 361-4 *A.* Horizontal CT section 1 h after subarachnoid instillation of water-soluble contrast medium showing the cervical spinal cord surrounded by contrast and dye in a large intramedullary syrinx cavity (arrow). *B.* Sagittal

MRI of same patient shown in *A* showing the syrinx cavity and enlargement of the spinal cord (arrows). *(Courtesy of Greg Shoukimas, M.D., Department of Radiology, Massachusetts General Hospital.)*

of reflexes in the legs, impaired position and vibratory sense, Romberg's sign, and bilateral, Argyll Robertson pupils, which fail to constrict to light but react with accommodation.

Traumatic spinal cord lesions and compression of the cord secondary to orthopedic disorders are discussed in the chapter on cranial and spinal injury (Chap. 352).

GENERAL CARE OF THE PATIENT WITH ACUTE PARAPLEGIA OR QUADRIPLEGIA Protection from secondary damage to the urinary tract is a high priority in the acute stages of paraplegia. The bladder is areflexic, retains urine, and the patient is unaware of bladder distention, making damage to the detrusor muscle from overdistention possible. Urologic rehabilitation requires bladder drainage and avoidance of urinary infection. This is best accomplished by intermittent catheterization by trained personnel. Continuous closed system urinary drainage, which is associated with a higher infection rate than intermittent catheterization, or suprapubic drainage are less desirable alternatives. Patients with acute lesions, especially those causing spinal shock, frequently need special cardiovascular care because of paroxysmal hypertension or hypotension. Ileus and gastric stress ulcers are other potential acute medical problems in patients with complete transverse cord lesions. Cimetidine, ranitidine, or sucralfate may be useful in these circumstances. Pulmonary embolism due to immobilization is a grave early risk occurring in approximately one-third of patients after acute cord trauma. Subcutaneous heparin may reduce the risk of early embolic complications. Rarely spinal injury patients have become hypercalcemic from immobilization.

High cervical cord lesions cause varying degrees of mechanical respiratory failure requiring artificial ventilation. In cases of incomplete respiratory failure with forced vital capacities of 10 to 20 mL/kg, chest physical therapy is useful, and a negative pressure cuirass may be used to alleviate atelectasis and fatigue, particularly if the major lesion is below C4. With severe respiratory failure, tracheal intubation (performed over an endoscope if the spine is unstable), followed by tracheostomy, provides tracheal access for ventilation and suctioning. A promising new technique is phrenic nerve pacing in patients with lesions at C5 or above.

As clinical signs stabilize, attention should be directed to the psychological state of the patient and the development of a rehabilitation plan framed by realistic expectations. An aggressive program

is often remarkably successful with younger and middle-aged patients allowing return to home and a productive lifestyle.

Chronic nursing care problems can be handled by patients with varying degrees of assistance. The major issues are related to immobilization: skin breakdown over pressure points, urinary sepsis, and autonomic instability, and the potential for pulmonary embolism. Early care includes frequent repositioning, application of skin emollients, and soft bed coverings. Specialized beds turn the patient or distribute body weight evenly rather than predominantly on bony prominences. If the sacral cord segments are undamaged, then a large degree of automatic voiding can be entrained. Patients initially void reflexly between catheterizations and later learn to induce voiding with various maneuvers. If residual urinary volumes lead to infection, surgical procedures or an indwelling catheter may be necessary. Bowel regimens and disimpaction are necessary in most patients to ensure at least biweekly evacuation and avoid colonic distention or obstruction.

Severe hypertension and bradycardia occur in response to noxious superficial stimuli, bladder or bowel distention, or surgery, particularly in patients with cervical and high thoracic cord lesions. Flushing and diaphoresis above the level of the lesion may accompany the hypertension. The mechanism of this dysautonomia is not well understood. A potent antihypertensive agent may be necessary, particularly during surgery, but beta-blocking drugs should probably be avoided. Some patients become severely bradycardic with tracheal suctioning; this can be prevented with small doses of atropine.

Detailed aspects of the physical therapy, rehabilitation, and orthotics related to severe spinal cord diseases may be found in specialized texts. The orthopedic stabilization of the spine in relation to cord trauma is discussed in Chap. 344.

REFERENCES

ADAMS CBT, LOGUE V: Studies in cervical spondylitic myelopathy. Brain 94:579, 1971

AMINOFF MJ, LOGUE V: Clinical features of spinal vascular malformations. Brain 97:197, 1974

AULD AW et al: Metastatic spinal epidural tumors: An analysis of 50 cases. Arch Neurol 15:100, 1966

BAKER AS et al: Spinal epidural abcess. N Engl J Med 293:463, 1975

BARNETT HJM et al: *Syringomyelia.* Philadelphia, Saunders, 1973

Byrne TN, Waxman SG: Spinal cord compression. Contemporary Neurology Series, vol 33. Philadelphia, Davis, 1990

Edelson R et al: Intramedullary spinal cord metastasis. Neurology 22:1222, 1972

Gilbert RW et al: Epidural cord compression from metastatic tumor: Diagnosis and treatment. Ann Neurol 3:40, 1978

Greenberg HS et al: Epidural spinal cord compression from metastatic tumor: Results with a new treatment protocol. Ann Neurol 8:361, 1980

Hardy AG, Rossier AB: *Spinal Cord Injuries: Orthopedic and Neurological Aspects.* Stuttgart, Thieme, 1975

Johnson RT, McArthur JC: Myelopathies and retroviral infections. Ann Neurol 21:113, 1987

Logue V: Angiomas of the spinal cord: Review of the pathogenesis, clinical features, and results of surgery. J Neurol Neurosurg Psychiatr 42:1, 1979

———, Edwards MR: Syringomyelia and its surgical treatment. J Neurol Neurosurg Psychiatr 44:273, 1981

McIlroy WJ, Richardson JC: Syringomyelia: A clinical review of 75 cases. J Can Med Assoc 93:731, 1965

Ropper AH, Poskanzer DC: Prognosis of acute and subacute transverse myelopathy based on early signs and symptoms. Ann Neurol 4:51, 1978

Rossier AB et al: Posttraumatic cervical syringomyelia. Brain 108:439, 1985

Srigley JR et al: Spinal cord infarction secondary to intervertebral disc embolism. Ann Neurol 9:296, 1981

section 2 Disorders of nerve and muscle

362 APPROACH TO THE PATIENT WITH NEUROMUSCULAR DISEASE

ROBERT C. GRIGGS / WALTER G. BRADLEY / BHAGWAN SHAHANI

The neuromuscular diseases are disorders of the *motor unit* and of the sensory and autonomic peripheral nerves. Each motor unit consists of: (1) the *motor neuron cell body*, located in either the spinal cord anterior horn (for muscles innervated by the spinal cord) or a cranial nerve nucleus (for ocular, facial, bulbar musculature); (2) the *axon* of the motor neuron in the peripheral (or cranial) nerve; (3) the *neuromuscular junction;* and, (4) the *muscle fibers* innervated by the motor neuron. The sensory peripheral nerves comprise (1) the *sensory neuron* cell body in the posterior root ganglion; (2) the *central axon* passing to the spinal cord in the posterior root; (3) the *distal axon* in the peripheral nerve; and (4) the *sensory nerve terminal* in skin, muscle, joint capsule, etc. The autonomic nerves are divided into *sympathetic* and *parasympathetic* fiber systems. The sympathetic preganglionic fibers arise from cell bodies in the intermediolateral column of the spinal cord and enter the sympathetic ganglia, where postganglionic fibers arise to innervate blood vessels or viscera. The parasympathetic preganglionic neurons lie in the brainstem and sacral spinal cord, and axons terminate in the viscera, special sensory organs, or skin, which contain the postganglionic neurons and their nerve terminals. Neuromuscular diseases are classified into four groups depending upon which portion of the motor unit is involved (see Table 362-1).

The major symptoms of diseases of the motor unit are muscle weakness, fatigue, cramps, pain, or stiffness. Symptoms of peripheral nerve disease include, in addition, decreased sensation (hypesthesia or hypalgesia), abnormal sensations (paresthesias), or painful sensations (dysesthesias) (see Chap. 28). Symptoms of autonomic nervous system disease include postural dizziness, and abnormal cardiac, visceral, and ocular function, and changes in sweating. The symptoms of neuromuscular disease, particularly those of weakness or sensory disturbance, do not necessarily distinguish disorders of the peripheral nervous system from those of the central nervous system. Most neuromuscular diseases are relatively symmetric in contrast to the asymmetry of many central nervous system diseases.

CLINICAL ASSESSMENT

History and physical examination will lead to a diagnosis in a majority of patients with neuromuscular disease. Failure to arrive at a diagnostic impression before routine and sophisticated laboratory studies often leads to diagnostic inaccuracy and confusion. Few of the biochemical, histologic, and electrodiagnostic studies used to evaluate patients with neuromuscular disease are pathognomonic since nerve and muscle can respond to disease processes in only a limited number of ways.

CLINICAL HISTORY Weakness and fatigue (See Chap. 25) The patient with weakness, particularly when of gradual onset, may not recognize it, emphasizing the useful axiom that "signs of muscle weakness precede symptoms of weakness." Words such as numbness, deadness, tiredness, or fatigue may be used by a patient unfamiliar with what is taking place. On the other hand, some complaints of "weakness" result from systemic rather than neuromuscular disease. In such patients, strength is often normal or only mildly reduced, since the complaint is usually loss of stamina and endurance. The patient with fatigue should be asked to distinguish between true weakness and the less specific symptoms of lassitude and asthenia. If the patient is unable to perform a normal activity, true weakness is suggested. Objective evidence of weakness is established if symptoms exceed the bounds of normal variation (e.g., double vision, drooping eye lids, difficulty in swallowing, aspiration of food or liquids into the airway) as opposed to the more subjective complaints of inability to lift, carry, or push an object.

The time-course and severity of weakness must be quantitated by questions concerning alterations in functional abilities: for the legs, difficulty in rising from a chair or commode, rising from a squatting position, or climbing up and down stairs, and a history of frequent tripping, stumbling, or falling; for the trunk, difficulty in sitting up from supine in bed; or for the arms, difficulty in washing the hair, opening jars, fastening buttons, or raising objects onto a shelf.

Abnormalities of sensation (See Chaps. 28 and 363) Sensory symptoms suggest peripheral nerve disease although, as with weakness, sensory abnormalities can occur with disease at any level of the nervous system. The characteristics and localization of sensory symptoms in the various peripheral nerve syndromes and diseases

TABLE 362-1 Classification of neuromuscular disease

Site of involvement	Typical example
Anterior horn cell	
Without upper motor neuron involvement	Spinal muscular atrophy
With upper motor neuron involvement	Amyotrophic lateral sclerosis
Peripheral nerve	
Unifocal	Carpal tunnel syndrome
Multifocal	Mononeuritis multiplex (e.g., polyarteritis nodosa)
Diffuse	Diabetic neuropathy
Neuromuscular junction	Myasthenia gravis
Muscle	Duchenne muscular dystrophy

are discussed in Chap. 28. In contradistinction to weakness, it is axiomatic that "sensory symptoms precede objective sensory signs."

Muscle pain (See Chap. 27) Muscle aches and pains may suggest inflammatory or metabolic muscle disease but are far commoner in bone, joint, and nerve disease. Persistent muscle pain in a patient with normal strength usually results from a cause other than myopathy. Intermittent muscle pain, however, particularly when precipitated by exercise, should raise a consideration of a substrate utilization defect such as a glycogen or lipid storage myopathy or the purine nucleotide cycle disorder, myoadenylate deaminase deficiency. It is important to determine if other factors, such as fasting, precipitate pain and then to inquire about associated findings such as dark urine which may be indicative of myoglobinuria.

Autonomic dysfunction The most common complaint is "dizziness," or "blackouts," which prove to be precipitated by the patient standing up from sitting or lying. Loss of potency in the male is frequent in autonomic neuropathies. Explosive diarrhea or cyclical diarrhea-constipation are sometimes present, as is partial urinary retention.

PHYSICAL EXAMINATION Strength testing Reliable testing of strength requires that the examiner have an adequate frame of reference for normal strength and that the patient be motivated and able to cooperate with testing. As with history taking, it is helpful to quantitate the ability to perform tasks required in daily living. The legs are particularly easy to test by observing: walking on heels and toes; rising from a chair, noting whether there is a need to use the arms; rising from a squat; and stepping up on to a chair. It is also important to examine the legs for a *knee extension lag,* the inability to fully extend the leg against gravity. The number of degrees of extension lag can be measured with a goniometer. Patients with even a minor extension lag almost invariably report frequent tripping and falling. The converse is also true: patients with muscle weakness who report frequent falls usually have quadriceps muscle weakness producing a knee extension lag. Trunk and neck muscles can be tested by having the patient sit up from supine; extending the head over the edge of an examining table is a sensitive method of detecting neck weakness. The arms are not as easily evaluated with function testing: inspection of shoulders for scapular winging as the arms are elevated and watching the patient lift the arms above the head test shoulder girdle function. Hand strength can be judged by determining the degree of difficulty in extracting two fingers from the grip of the patient and by noting the ability of the patient to blanch the knuckles when making a tight fist. When the lesion affects a specific region, e.g., the brachial plexus or the ulnar nerve, it is essential to test each individual muscle of the arm or hand.

Formal muscle testing, assigning a numerical grade to muscle strength, is usually based on the MRC (Medical Research Council of Great Britain) 0 to 5 scale:

5—normal
4—able to oppose gravity plus resistance
3—able to move fully against gravity but not resistance
2—able to move with gravity eliminated
1—trace movement
0—no movement

An important assessment is whether a muscle is indeed *weaker than one would expect,* after making allowances for age, male-female differences, inactivity, or generalized illness. If one has a limited time for the testing of muscle strength, the assessment of function is likely to be of more value than formal muscle testing.

Muscle bulk Muscle atrophy and hypertrophy are often difficult to recognize because of wide variation among normals. The problem is accentuated in young children and in obese patients because of overlying adipose tissue. Atrophy is easier to appreciate when asymmetric. Muscle enlargement or hypertrophy is a normal accompaniment of physical activity. It is occasionally a sign of disease in patients with long-standing spasticity or myotonic disorders. So-called pseudohypertrophy, in which the muscles become enlarged by

replacement with connective tissue or fat, may be prominent in certain of the muscular dystrophies but is also seen with spinal muscular atrophy and other denervating conditions. Actual hypertrophy of muscle fibers may also be present in these patients. Muscle enlargement may also be caused by infiltration with substances such as amyloid or by parasitic infestation (e.g., cysticercosis).

Focal muscle swelling may be due to inflammatory infiltrates, calcium deposits, or tendon rupture. Preservation of some parts of a muscle, while other parts atrophy, may occur in spinal muscular atrophy and some forms of muscular dystrophy, giving an appearance of a focal swelling during muscle contraction ("belly hypertrophy"). Single or multiple muscle masses in a patient without weakness may indicate a neoplastic process. Other causes of muscle enlargement include focal myositis, sarcoidosis, ectopic ossification, and tendon rupture.

Pathologic fatigue Patients with disorders of neuromuscular transmission such as myasthenia gravis can usually be shown to fatigue on examination. Sustained upward gaze produces gradual ptosis of the eyelids (curtain sign); eye movements become disconjugate on sustained horizontal gaze; the voice may become hoarse, slurred, or nasal with prolonged speech; or a smile may rapidly become a sneer when the patient cannot maintain facial muscle activity. Inability to sustain limb activity is less easily quantitated since patients who are weak from any cause may have decreased endurance.

Sensory testing Patients with peripheral neuropathy usually have sensory loss. The distribution of sensory disturbance as well as the modalities affected are often of diagnostic importance (see Chaps. 28 and 363).

Autonomic testing A fall of systolic blood pressure of more than 20 mmHg from lying to standing indicates impaired autonomic control of peripheral blood vessels. A greater fall often occurs with exercise in the erect position. The pulse rate does not increase normally in response to this hypotension if there is an autonomic neuropathy. Similarly, there is no slowing of the heart rate following a sustained Valsalva maneuver.

Other findings Myotonia, fasciculations, myokymia, and other spontaneous activity (Chap. 27) should be sought. Certain disorders such as myotonic dystrophy and facioscapulohumeral dystrophy have distinctive and virtually pathognomonic facial features. Less diagnostic but significant facial weakness is found in other myopathies and in myasthenia gravis. Contractures, particularly of the Achilles tendons, limitation of hip joint movement, and scoliosis may indicate that weakness is of long duration.

DIFFERENTIAL DIAGNOSIS Weaknesses produced by diseases of the motor unit are distinguishable from each other by their distribution, by the time-course of the illness, and by accompanying clinical findings such as muscle bulk and tone, reflexes, and sensory findings. The portion of the motor unit involved by a disease process is usually evident from clinical findings (Table 362-2). Motor neuron diseases (Chap. 359) are suggested in the patient whose weakness is accompanied by prominent atrophy, fasciculations, and lack of sensory involvement. The reflexes may be disproportionately depressed if anterior horn cell disease alone is present or pathologically increased if there is coexistent upper motor neuron disease, such as amyotrophic lateral sclerosis. Peripheral neuropathy (Chap. 363) is suggested by the presence of distal weakness associated with sensory involvement. In general, patients with peripheral neuropathy have depressed reflexes; preservation of reflexes in the presence of significant weakness suggests a cause other than neuropathy. Neuromuscular junction disorders (Chap. 366) are suggested if ocular and bulbar weakness is prominent, particularly if there is *diurnal variation,* with the patient becoming weaker as the day progresses. Pathologic fatigue can usually be demonstrated. Reflexes are preserved in most neuromuscular junction disorders, particularly myasthenia gravis.

Myopathy versus other neuromuscular disease Clinical features which suggest myopathy in contrast to other motor unit diseases include a proximal distribution of weakness, relative preservation or

TABLE 362-2   Presenting clinical features of the neuromuscular diseases

	Anterior horn cell	Peripheral nerve	Neuromuscular junction	Muscle
Distribution of weakness	Asymmetric limb or bulbar	Symmetric distal	Extraocular, bulbar, proximal limb	Symmetrical limb (bulbar in some)
Atrophy	Marked and early	Moderate	None	Slight early; marked later
Sensory involvement	None	Paresthesias, hypesthesia	None	None
Characteristic features	Fasciculations, cramps, tremor	Combined sensory and motor abnormality	Diurnal fluctuation	
Reflexes	Variable (depending on degree of upper motor neuronal involvement)	Decreased out of proportion to weakness	Normal	Decreased in proportion to weakness

increase of muscle bulk, and the preservation of reflexes. Table 362-3 presents a classification of primary muscle diseases. Many patients with muscle symptoms, however, have disorders that do not fit into this table because evaluation discloses disease in another portion of the motor unit or in another system (see Chap. 25). For example, a patient with a denervation produced by nerve root damage from a lumbar disc protrusion may have muscle cramps, pain, and weakness in muscles innervated by those nerve roots. Furthermore, fatigue, weakness, and pain are common accompaniments of derangements of cardiac, hematologic, gastrointestinal, pulmonary, renal, or hepatic function. Despite complaints of weakness and fatigue and the finding of atrophy, it is relatively infrequent for patients with pulmonary or cardiac disease to be mistaken for those with primary muscle disease.

Proximal weakness is so characteristic of myopathies that, by a somewhat circular argument, proximal weakness is usually attributed to "myopathy." In fact, neuropathies such as acute or chronic inflammatory polyneuropathy, the neuromuscular junction disorders, and many anterior horn cell diseases have predominantly proximal weakness. Proximal weakness, occurring in disorders such as hyperthyroidism and hyperparathyroidism and as a result of glucocorticoid administration, is often termed "myopathic," despite the fact that the underlying pathophysiology of the muscle disorders in these conditions has not been defined.

Acute generalized weakness   Weakness developing over the course of less than an hour is usually caused by a metabolic or toxic disorder affecting either the neuromuscular junction or muscle. A sudden alteration in circulating potassium, calcium, sodium, mag-

nesium, or phosphate may result in partial or complete paralysis of muscle. Acute failure of neuromuscular junction transmission may occur with botulism and other toxins, hypermagnesemia, aminoglycoside antibiotics, and other medications. Weakness developing over the course of 24 h may occur in electrolyte, metabolic, and toxic disorders; in periodic paralysis (Chap. 367); and in acute inflammatory myopathies, particularly those related to viral and parasitic infection (Chap. 364) and certain acute polyneuropathies (Chap. 363). Occasionally, patients with more chronic disorders first realize that they are weak when the insidious progression of their weakness produces an abrupt change in function.

Subacute weakness   Weakness developing over days is more common in peripheral nerve or neuromuscular junction diseases than in muscle or anterior horn cell disease. Acute inflammatory polyneuropathy (Guillain-Barré syndrome) and porphyric, diphtheritic, and toxic neuropathies are of subacute onset. Myasthenia gravis and other neuromuscular junction diseases must also be considered in the differential diagnosis. Subacute weakness can occur in severe polymyositis and dermatomyositis (see Chap. 364). Weakness from endocrine disorders and certain muscle toxins (Table 362-3) may also develop subacutely (Chap. 365). Of the anterior horn cell disorders only infections with poliomyelitis and other viruses commonly evolve subacutely. Amyotrophic lateral sclerosis occasionally pursues a subacute, severe course.

Slowly progressive weakness   *Slowly progressive proximal weakness* evolving over weeks to months may be caused by polymyositis or dermatomyositis or an unsuspected endocrinopathy. When the course has extended for a year or more, however, one of the muscular dystrophies, spinal muscular atrophy, or a neuromuscular junction defect such as myasthenia gravis may be present. Neuropathies are seldom proximal, the major exceptions being acute and chronic inflammatory polyneuropathy, porphyric neuropathy, and diabetic proximal mononeuropathy. *Slowly progressive distal weakness* is more characteristic of peripheral nerve or anterior horn cell disorders than of disorders of muscle or the neuromuscular junction. The only commonly encountered distal myopathy is myotonic dystrophy. Less common disorders such as distal muscular dystrophy, nemaline and centronuclear myopathies, and a variant of polymyositis known as inclusion body myositis may present with distal weakness. Prominent distal lower limb weakness is also present in the facioscapulohumeral and scapuloperoneal muscular dystrophies, but proximal involvement is invariably also present in such patients. *Slowly progressive bulbar weakness* is more typical of anterior horn cell or neuromuscular junction disorders than of myopathies. Bulbar weakness (difficulty in speaking, coughing, and swallowing) occurs commonly in motor neuron disease (especially amyotrophic lateral sclerosis) and neuromuscular junction disorders. It is also seen in oculopharyngeal dystrophy, myotonic dystrophy, and polymyositis or dermatomyositis. *Ocular muscle weakness and ptosis* do not occur in motor neuron disease and are uncommon in peripheral neuropathy. Ophthalmoparesis is typical of myasthenia gravis and may occur in myotonic and oculopharyngeal dystrophies. Weakness limited to or predominantly ocular in location (*progressive external ophthalmoplegia*) occurs in disorders such as the Kearns-Sayre syndrome (Chap. 365).

TABLE 362-3   Classification of primary muscle diseases

I   Hereditary
    A Muscular dystrophy (Chap. 365): Duchenne, myotonic, facioscapulohumeral, limb-girdle, oculopharyngeal, scapuloperoneal, congenital, distal, and ocular
    B Congenital myopathies (Chap. 365): Central core, nemaline, centronuclear, fiber-type disproportion
    C Metabolic myopathies (Chap. 365):
        1 Glycogen: Deficiencies of phosphorylase, phosphofructokinase, phosphoglyceromutase, acid maltase, others
        2 Lipid: Defective synthesis or transport of carnitine; deficiency of carnitine palmityl transferase
        3 Purine nucleotide cycle: Deficiency of myoadenylate deaminase
    D Myotonia (Chap. 365): Congenita, paramyotonia
    E Periodic paralysis (Chap. 27 and 367): Hypokalemic, hyperkalemic
II Inflammatory (Chap. 364)
    A Collagen disease: Systemic lupus erythematosus, rheumatoid arthritis, scleroderma, mixed-connective tissue
    B Sarcoidosis, carcinoid, neoplastic
    C Infections: Numerous, especially viral (influenza B), protozoal (toxoplasmosis), parasitic (trichinosis)
    D Idiopathic: Polymyositis, dermatomyositis
III Endocrine and metabolic (Chap. 365)
    A Electrolyte abnormalities: Calcium, phosphate, magnesium, sodium, potassium
    B Endocrine: Hypo- and hyperfunction of thyroid, adrenal, parathyroid, pituitary
IV Toxic (Chap. 365): Alcohol, opiates, pentazocine, clofibrate, others
V   Tumors and masses: Primary and metastatic neoplasms, infection, sarcoidosis, myositis ossificans, calcinosis, muscle rupture and hemorrhage

LABORATORY ASSESSMENT

Patients with significantly impaired strength and sensation merit thorough diagnostic study. The sequence of investigations should be based on the test's diagnostic specificity and sensitivity, level of patient discomfort, and cost. Hematologic, renal, and hepatic function and serum electrolytes should be evaluated. In many instances, thyroid, adrenal, and other endocrine studies may be indicated. Other useful diagnostic tests are the serum creatine kinase (CK) level, nerve conduction studies, electromyography, and in many instances muscle biopsy. Nerve biopsy is a more specialized technique with a relatively small number of specific indications (see Chap. 363). Repetitive stimulation of nerve with recording from muscle should be obtained when a neuromuscular junction defect is suspected. Since many diagnostic tests are uncomfortable and expensive, it is important to consider what information is being sought in requesting each test. Confounding features in the investigations must also be understood. For instance, muscle necrosis and inflammation and an elevated serum CK may occur after minor muscle trauma such as is caused by electromyography and intramuscular injection. Electromyography and muscle biopsy obtained from a muscle affected by past nerve root disease (e.g., from a herniated disk) may show neuropathic abnormalities unrelated to a new disease process. A patient complaining of weakness and fatigue who is found on examination to have no weakness should be examined during exercise. Some of these patients have a metabolic myopathy. Others may have a neuromuscular junction, central nervous system, or psychological problem requiring appropriate investigations.

BIOCHEMICAL EVALUATION OF NEUROMUSCULAR DISEASE Certain enzymes, especially CK, occur in high concentrations in the sarcoplasm of muscle, and may leak into blood to serve as an indicator of muscle damage. The serum CK, aldolase, lactic dehydrogenase (LDH), aspartate aminotransferase (AST, SGOT), and alanine aminotransferase (ALT, SGPT) may be elevated in the serum of a patient with active muscle destruction. Since several of these enzymes are used for screening for abnormalities of organs other than muscle, it is not uncommon for a patient with muscle disease to be first identified by an unexpected elevation in one of these enzymes. The clue to the muscle origin of the increased enzyme levels is that the degree of abnormality decreases in the order CK > aldolase > LDH > SGOT > SGPT. The serum CK level is the most sensitive test and may be very high (raised more than tenfold) in diseases with muscle fiber necrosis, such as the muscular dystrophies, polymyositis, and rhabdomyolysis. It is frequently slightly elevated in spinal muscular atrophy, amyotrophic lateral sclerosis, and other motor neuron disorders and is usually normal in peripheral neuropathies and neuromuscular junction disorders. Strenuous exercise in normal individuals can elevate the level of serum CK for 6 h or more. Three isoenzymes of CK occur: MM, MB, and BB. MM predominates in skeletal muscle, MB occurs mainly in cardiac muscle, and BB is mainly in brain. Elevations of CK-MB levels are used to indicate the presence of myocardial damage. CK elevation caused by acute muscle injury is usually due to the MM isoenzyme. However, in many patients with long-standing necrotizing muscular diseases and in athletes, the proportion of MB in skeletal muscle rises and in consequence the proportion of CK-MB in blood is elevated.

MUSCLE COMPOSITION AND MASS Computed tomography and magnetic resonance imaging can differentiate between muscle fibers, fat, and connective tissue and may show distinctive differences between muscular dystrophy and the other forms of muscle disease. The high cost and the nonspecificity of the findings limit the role of these techniques. Estimations of total muscle mass are of some importance in metabolic studies. A simple decline in muscle mass without weakness is indicative of a process other than a neuromuscular disease, for example, aging, neoplasm, impaired nutrition, renal or hepatic disease. The 24-h urinary creatinine excretion is the most widely available technique used to estimate muscle mass; it is decreased in patients with wasting from any cause.

METABOLIC, ENDOCRINE, AND OTHER STUDIES Hypo- and hyperkalemia, hypernatremia, hypo- and hypercalcemia, hypophosphatemia, and hypermagnesemia can all cause severe, usually acute, weakness. Serum potassium levels are labile and subject to rapid shifts induced by acidosis or alkalosis. The intracellular concentration of potassium is high, so that hemolysis during blood collection may spuriously elevate the potassium level. The extensive muscle damage in rhabdomyolysis may produce a true hyperkalemia. Such elevations in serum potassium are generally not greater than 0.1 meq/L, however, unless the serum is stained with hemoglobin, as occurs with hemolysis, or the urine with myoglobin, as occurs with rhabdomyolysis.

Chronic endocrine disorders, either hypo- or hyperfunction of thyroid, adrenal, or parathyroid glands, may cause weakness in the absence of other clinical evidence of endocrinopathy. Rheumatoid arthritis, systemic lupus erythematosus, scleroderma, and the polymyalgia rheumatica syndrome may be complicated by muscle weakness. Tests for these diseases are usually indicated in the evaluation of unexplained muscle pain and weakness. The weakness in most of these disorders is related to disuse atrophy and joint pain; muscle inflammation and evidence of muscle destruction are uncommon. Disorders of muscle mitochondrial function may cause a high plasma lactate level. Other laboratory investigations that may be indicated in patients with peripheral neuropathy include tests for diabetes mellitus; levels of serum vitamin B_{12}, folate, and lipids; serum protein electrophoresis; urinary and serum immunoelectrophoresis; lipoprotein electrophoresis; and urinary porphyrins and heavy metal levels. Diagnostic enzyme determinations are available in white blood cells in certain neuromuscular disorders, such as aryl sulfatase and acid maltase deficiencies.

MYOGLOBINURIA Acute muscle destruction, *rhabdomyolysis* associated with myoglobinuria, occurs with acute toxic, metabolic, inflammatory, infectious, and traumatic muscle damage (see Chap. 364). The molecular weight of myoglobin is lower than that of hemoglobin, so that the urine rather than the serum changes color in extensive rhabdomyolysis. Myoglobinuria causes a positive urine test for blood in the absence of urinary erythrocytes. Confirmatory testing for myoglobin uses a specific immunoassay.

EXERCISE TESTING (See Chap. 365) Patients with substrate utilization defects characteristically have decreased exercise tolerance and muscle pain and weakness during or following exercise. Most defects in the enzymatic pathways of glycolysis result in the failure of muscle to generate adenosine triphosphate (ATP) from glycogen and a diminished or absent production of lactic acid. Patients with these disorders can be evaluated with a forearm exercise test to evaluate the level of venous lactic acid. Patients with disturbance of fatty acid metabolism (such as carnitine palmityl transferase deficiency, in which long-chain fatty acids cannot be transferred into mitochondria for beta oxidation) generate lactic acid normally. Patients with myoadenylate deaminase deficiency generate lactate in normal or increased amounts but fail to produce ammonia in the exercise test (Chap. 365). Measurement of specific muscle enzymes can define the cause of the disorder.

ELECTROPHYSIOLOGIC STUDIES OF NEUROMUSCULAR DISEASE

NORMAL MOTOR UNIT PHYSIOLOGY The motor unit is the final common pathway for motor activity of the nervous system, and muscle is the final effector of the motor unit. All movement, posture, and reflex activity result from integrated discharge of large numbers of motor units by spinal and supraspinal mechanisms. The strength of a muscle contraction depends upon the number of motor units recruited, the frequency of motor unit discharge, the speed of contraction of muscle fibers in the motor unit, and the nature of the motor unit (whether fatigue-resistant or fatigue-prone). The number of motor units varies greatly among muscles, ranging from as few as 10 in the extraocular muscles, to approximately 100 in the intrinsic muscles of the hands, to nearly 2000 in leg muscles such as the gastrocnemius. The number of muscle fibers per muscle varies up to a thousandfold, from 1000 in extraocular muscles to over 1 million in large leg muscles. The muscle fibers of the motor unit are dispersed randomly within a muscle, and fibers innervated by the same anterior horn cell are generally not contiguous. An understanding of the organization of motor units and their patterns of firing is important in the interpretation of clinical and laboratory findings in normal and diseased muscle.

The physiologic characterization of the muscle fibers relate importantly to the exercise capacity of muscle. Motor units that innervate type 1, slow-twitch muscle fibers are designed for continuous and prolonged activity, since their energy supply is derived from the oxidative metabolism of mitochondria. These motor units are smaller and are activated (*recruited*) by low-intensity efforts. High-intensity effort or rapid muscle contraction, such as lifting of a heavy weight or sprinting, recruits larger motor units that innervate rapid-twitch type 2 muscle fibers, which derive their energy supply from anaerobic glycolysis.

As muscles relax, the cessation of firing of individual motor units occurs in a groupwise fashion so that a patient exerting an inadequate effort owing to functional weakness (e.g., malingering), lack of motivation, or pain will frequently have a ratchet-like or "give-way" quality on muscle testing. This may permit the distinction between true and feigned weakness.

ELECTROMYOGRAPHY The normal electromyogram The measurement of electric activity arising from muscle fibers is usually performed by inserting a needle electrode percutaneously into a muscle. The electric activity from this electrode is then displayed on a cathode-ray oscilloscope and can be made audible through a loudspeaker. Such studies provide only an average picture of the local electric activity of muscle, and normal electric activity in one area does not exclude the possibility of pathologic phenomena close by.

In a single muscle fiber, as the action potential travels from the neuromuscular junction toward the ends of the muscle fiber, current flows outward through the normally polarized region of the muscle membrane (*sarcolemma*) toward the depolarized zone (Fig. 362-1). The recording electrode initially becomes slightly positive relative to the reference electrode. When the depolarized region moves under the recording electrode, a negative deflection occurs. As the active region moves away from the electrode, the membrane under the electrode become repolarized. The net result is a triphasic action potential (Fig. 362-1). The motor unit comprises many such fibers, and hence firing of many fibers of the motor unit produces a more complex wave form (*the motor unit action potential*) resulting from summation of individual action potentials. Normal muscle is electrically silent when at rest, once *insertional activity*, produced by the trauma of placing the needle, has died down. When a muscle is voluntarily contracted, motor unit action potentials appear. With increasing strength of contraction, the number and size of the motor unit action potentials increase, until with full contraction individual motor unit potentials can no longer be distinguished, and a *complete recruitment (interference) pattern* is produced.

The abnormal electromyogram SPONTANEOUS ACTIVITY DURING COMPLETION RELAXATION　Persistent insertional activity occurs in myotonic disorders, in polymyositis, and in denervated muscles. Spontaneous activity of a single muscle fiber is called *fibrillation*, and of part of or an entire motor unit, *fasciculation*. Triphasic fibrillation potentials and biphasic positive sharp waves can be seen 7 to 25 days after denervation of muscle fibers (depending upon the distance of denervated muscle fibers from the site of the nerve lesion), and may persist for several years unless reinnervation occurs. Fibrillation appears with destruction of the motor neuron or its axon and in muscle diseases where a portion of a muscle fiber is separated from its innervated portions by segmental necrosis.

Fasciculations are seen with slowly progressive disease of the anterior horn cells such as amyotrophic lateral sclerosis and progressive

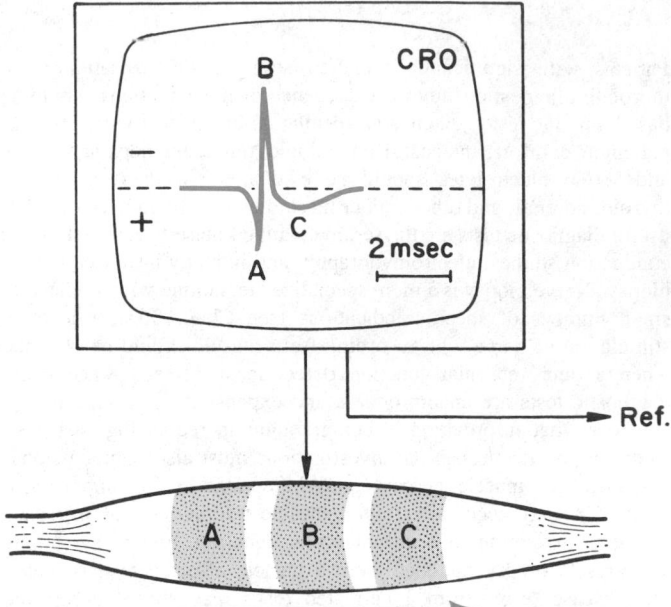

FIGURE 362-1 The triphasic muscle action potential. The shaded area represents the zone of the action potential, which is negative to all other points on the fiber surface. It is shown at three points in its course (from left to right) along the fiber. At each point, the correspondingly lettered portion of the triphasic muscle action potential displayed on the cathode ray oscilloscope (CRO) reflects the potential difference between the active (vertical arrow) and reference (Ref.) electrodes. Polarity in this and subsequent figures is negative upward as depicted. The time calibration is on the CRO screen. (For further details see text.)

spinal muscular atrophy, with compressive nerve root lesions, and in some motor neuropathies. In the syndrome of *benign fasciculations*, the same motor unit tends to fire at a regular rate that is usually faster than that of fasciculations indicative of disease.

In *myotonia*, the sarcolemma is irritable, and repeated muscle depolarization and contraction occur despite voluntary relaxation (see Chap. 365). Such patterns occur in myotonic congenita, myotonic dystrophy, and the periodic paralyses. On electromyography (EMG), myotonia causes high-frequency repetitive discharges that wax and wane in amplitude and frequency, producing a "dive bomber" or "motorcycle" sound on the loudspeaker. Bizarre, *repetitive high-frequency discharges* without waxing and waning are seen in many disorders affecting the motor neurons or muscle. *Coupling of action potentials* into doublets, triplets, or higher multiples of single units occurs in tetany, hemifacial spasm, and myokymia and indicates instability in repolarization of the nerve fiber. Electric silence characterizes *contracture*, as in McArdle's disease and malignant hyperthermia.

ABNORMALITIES IN MOTOR UNIT POTENTIALS　Early in the course of denervation, the remaining motor units are normal, but with the development of reinnervation, the remaining motor units increase in amplitude and become longer in duration and polyphasic (see Fig. 362-2). Conversely, in diseases such as polymyositis, the muscular dystrophies, and other myopathies that destroy scattered fibers within a motor unit (Fig. 362-2), the motor unit action potentials are of lower amplitude and shorter duration and are polyphasic.

In diseases of the central or peripheral nervous system, a *reduced recruitment (interference) pattern* results from maximum voluntary effort because fewer motor units are activated. Conversely, in patients with primary muscle disease, maximum voluntary effort produces a *full recruitment pattern* despite marked weakness. Because fewer muscle fibers are active, however, the amplitude of the pattern is reduced from normal.

A number of advanced electromyographic techniques, such as single-fiber EMG and macro EMG (see Chap. 349), have been

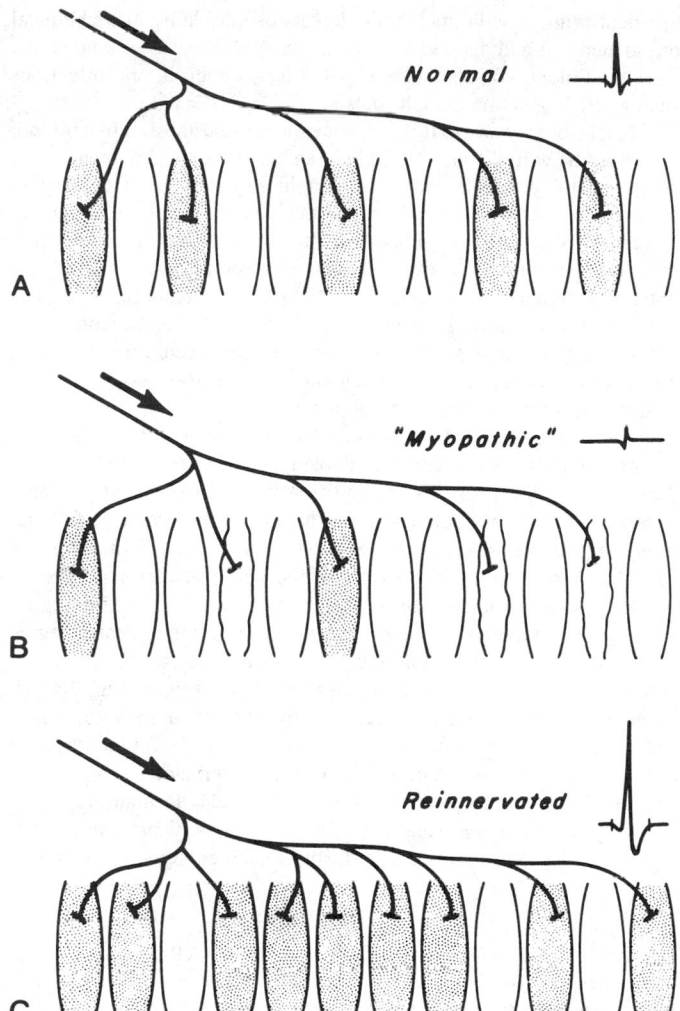

FIGURE 362-2 Motor unit potentials. The shaded muscle fibers are functional members of one motor unit; the axon, which enters from the upper left, branches terminally to innervate the appropriate muscle fibers. The motor unit action potential produced by each motor unit is seen in the upper right; its duration is measured between the two small vertical lines. The normal-appearing but unshaded fibers belong to other motor units. *A.* The normal situation, with five muscle fibers in the active unit. *B.* In this myopathic unit, only two fibers remain active; the other three (shrunken) have been affected by a muscle disease. *C.* Four fibers which belonged to other motor units and had been denervated have now been reinnervated by terminal axon sprouting from the healthy motor unit. Both the motor unit and its action potential are now larger than normal. Note that only under these abnormal circumstances do fibers in the same unit lie next to one another.

developed to investigate the stability of neuromuscular junction and motor unit reinnervation; their description is beyond the scope of this presentation.

Nerve conduction studies Stimulation of the larger peripheral motor and sensory nerves permits the recording of their action potentials and provides objective quantitative data of *latency* and *conduction velocity*. The technique is performed by stimulating the nerve with surface electrodes placed over the nerve. The resulting *compound action potential* is recorded by electrodes placed over the nerve proximally in the case of large sensory nerve fibers, or over the muscle distally in the case of motor nerve fibers in a mixed motor sensory nerve (see Fig. 362-3). The normal maximum motor and sensory nerve conduction velocities vary from 40 to 80 m/s in different peripheral nerves. Values are approximately half in newborn infants, and reach the adult range by 3 to 4 years of age. Normal values have been defined for *distal* or peripheral latencies that represent conduction time from the most distal stimulating electrodes, measured in milli-

seconds from the stimulus artifact to the onset of the response. It is important that the limb be kept warm during nerve conduction studies because subnormal temperatures cause slower conduction velocity. The *compound muscle action potential* obtained by stimulating a mixed motor nerve is of relatively high amplitude (5 to 10 mV) because of the amplification produced by the large number of muscle fibers in each motor unit. Sensory nerve action potentials, lacking this amplification, are of low amplitude (10 to 50 μV), and hence are more difficult to record. In abnormal nerves, sensory nerve action potentials may be small or absent, and sensory conduction measurements may be impossible to record. In contrast, reliable measurement of motor conduction velocities are usually possible even though only a few functional nerve fibers remain intact.

Maximum nerve conduction velocity measurements reflect the status of the best surviving of the largest myelinated nerve fibers and may be normal despite extensive loss of nerve fibers. Hence, nerve conduction velocity is normal or only slightly below normal in many neuropathies, though the amplitude of the evoked action potential is often reduced. In diseases of peripheral nerves causing severe segmental demyelination, such as chronic inflammatory polyneuropathy, diphtheria, metachromatic leukodystrophy, and the hypertrophic neuropathies, the maximum nerve conduction velocities may be reduced to below half of normal. Focal compressions of nerve, as in entrapment syndromes, produce localized slowing of conduction because of demyelination and narrowing of axons at the site of compression. The conduction of proximal segments of the nerves and nerve roots can be studied by F waves and H reflexes (see Chap.

FIGURE 362-3 Measurement of nerve conduction velocity. The median nerve is stimulated through the skin at the wrist (1) or in the antecubital fossa (2), and the resultant compound muscle action potential is recorded as the potential difference between a surface electrode over the thenar eminence (vertical arrow) and a reference electrode (Ref.) more distally. Sweep 1' on the cathode ray oscilloscope (CRO) depicts the stimulus artifact (moment of stimulation at 1) followed by the muscle potential. The distal latency is the time A' on the CRO sweep (3.0 ms, for example) which corresponds to conduction over distance A in the hand. The same is true for sweep 2' where stimulation is at point 2, and the time from artifact to response is A' + B'. The maximal motor conduction velocity from points 2 to 1 is obtained by dividing distance B by time B'.

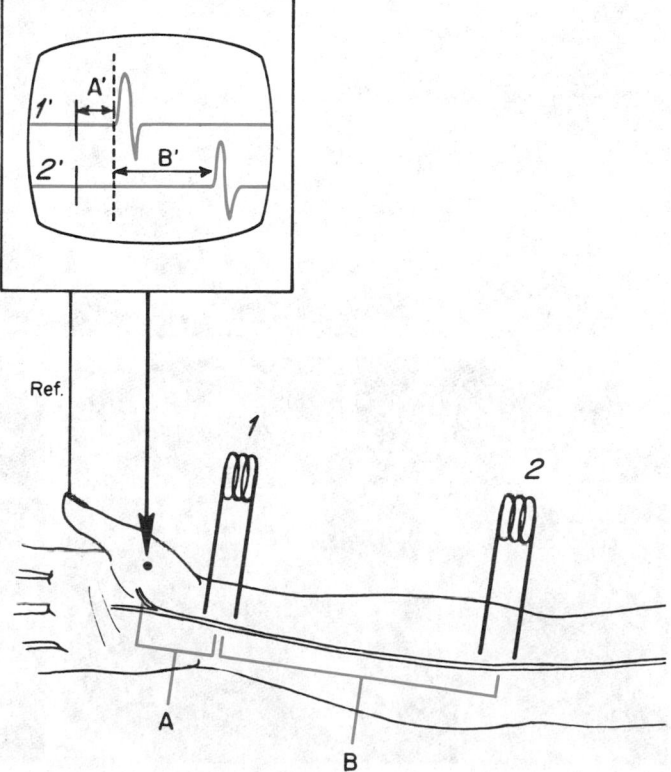

349), or by stimulation of nerve roots by a needle electrode or magnetic stimulator.

Repetitive stimulation tests   In myasthenia gravis, a disorder of the neuromuscular junction, the size of the initial compound muscle action potential produced by a supramaximal electric stimulus to the nerve may be normal. However, after a few stimuli at rates of 2 to 3 Hz the amplitude of compound muscle action potential declines. It then increases again after the fourth or fifth stimulus. This pattern of decrement followed by increment is characteristic of myasthenia gravis. This defect resembles the partial blockade produced by curare and reflects a postjunctional disorder of synaptic function. The defect is reversed by administration of anticholinesterase medications such as intravenous edrophonium hydrochloride (5 to 10 mg). A progressive decline in the compound muscle action potential with repetitive stimulation may also occur in poliomyelitis, amyotrophic lateral sclerosis, myotonia, and other diseases of the motor unit; however, the typical pattern of decrement-increment seen in myasthenia gravis is not present in other disorders.

In the Lambert-Eaton (myasthenic) syndrome, repetitive stimulation causes a facilitation of transmission. Rapid stimulation of nerve (20 to 30 Hz) results in a progressive increase in the amplitude of the muscle action potential, which is small at the first stimulus, to a nearly normal amplitude. This facilitation response is not affected by anticholinesterase drugs.

HISTOPATHOLOGY OF MUSCLE AND NERVE

MUSCLE BIOPSY   Biopsy is useful in (1) distinguishing between neurogenic and myopathic processes; (2) recognizing specific disorders of muscle such as muscular dystrophy or the congenital myopathies;

(3) identifying specific metabolic defects of muscle by histochemical or biochemical techniques; and (4) diagnosing diseases of connective tissue and blood vessels, such as polyarteritis nodosa, and infections such as trichinosis or toxoplasmosis.

Muscle biopsy is performed under local anesthesia. In children and in adults with diffuse conditions, an adequate specimen can often be obtained by needle biopsy. Open biopsy may be necessary to obtain sufficient tissue to diagnose focal, patchy processes such as myositis or vasculitis. In all instances, the muscle chosen for sampling must be appropriate for the condition suspected, and the specimen must be handled by a laboratory skilled in the evaluation of muscle biopsies. If the biopsy is taken from a muscle that has recently been traumatized by an EMG needle or that has been affected by a preexisting disease (e.g., coincidental nerve root compression), misleading information will be obtained.

Muscle fibers are subdivided into two types which have different staining characteristics with the myosin ATPase reaction at pH 9.4. Type 1 fibers (fatigue-resistant and rich in oxidative enzymes) stain lightly with this reaction, and type 2 fibers (fast-contracting, fatigue-prone, and rich in glycolytic enzymes) stain darkly. Normal muscle has a random distribution of fibers of the two histochemical types.

Denervation, reinnervation   A denervated muscle fiber undergoes atrophy, and in the initial stages myofibrils are lost to a greater degree than is sarcoplasm containing the mitochondria, so that muscle fibers appear "super dark" with stains for oxidative enzymes (Fig. 362-4). Such denervated fibers are squeezed by adjacent innervated fibers and therefore become angulated and atrophic. In the initial stages of denervation, because of motor unit overlap, denervated atrophic fibers are distributed randomly throughout the muscle. Remaining motor axons sprout to reinnervate such fibers, eventually producing fiber type grouping. With subsequent death of such enlarged motor units,

FIGURE 362-4   *A.* Normal skeletal muscle biopsy stained for myosin ATPase, pH 9.4. Type 1 fibers are light and type 2 dark. *B.* Chronic denervation-reinnervation showing fiber type grouping. Myosin ATPase, pH 9.4. *C.* Chronic denervation-reinnervation in amyotrophic lateral sclerosis, preparation stained for mitochondrial enzyme, NADH-TR. There are groups of reinnervated type 2 fibers (light), and of denervated angulated atrophic fibers, many of them "superdark" and showing target-fiber changes. *D.* Type 2 fiber atrophy. Myosin ATPase, pH 9.4.

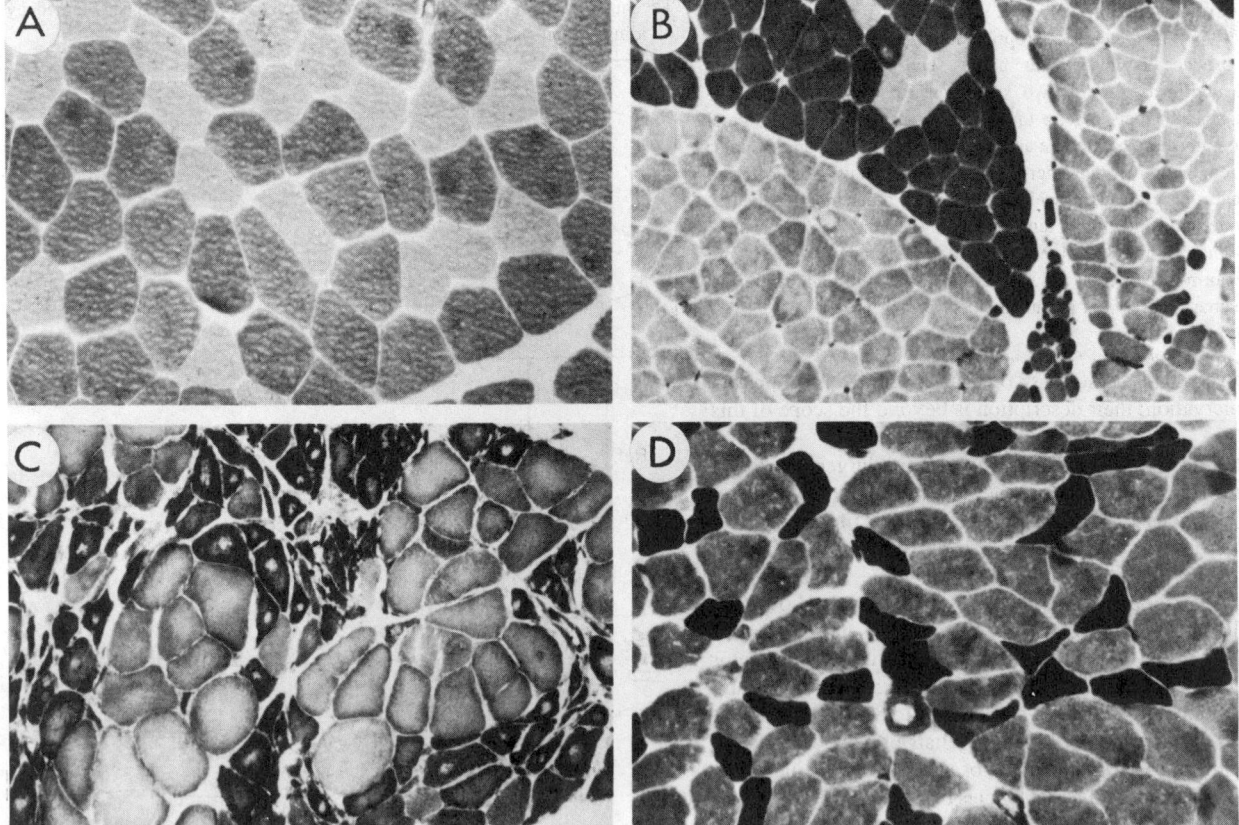

grouped fiber atrophy occurs. The typical appearance of a denervated and reinnervated muscle is shown in Fig. 362-4B and C. The fiber diameter distribution in chronically denervated and reinnervated muscle is bimodal, with the atrophic denervated fibers making up one population and the normal size (or hypertrophied) innervated fibers making up the other population.

Muscle fiber necrosis and regeneration Damage of the sarcolemma of the muscle fiber allows entry of calcium at high extracellular concentration into the low-calcium environment of the sarcoplasm. Calcium entry activates a neutral protease, initiating proteolysis. Calcium also deranges mitochondrial function and can cause cell death. Invading macrophages phagocytize the muscle fibers. Satellite cells, which provide the basis for regeneration of muscle fibers, are spared in most of the processes that damage muscle. They proliferate and fuse to produce multinuclear myotubes leading to regeneration of the muscle fiber. Characteristically, regenerating fibers are small, are basophilic owing to an increased concentration of RNA, and have large vesicular internal nuclei. The distribution of muscle fiber diameters in a typical chronic myopathy is broad and unimodal, very different from the bimodal diameter distribution of denervated and reinnervated muscle.

Muscle fiber necrosis and regeneration are common in trauma, Duchenne muscular dystrophy, polymyositis, and dermatomyositis. Eventually, if the necrosis is sufficiently chronic, regeneration may fail, causing progressive loss of muscle fibers and replacement with fat and fibrous tissue. A chronic myopathy, Duchenne muscular dystrophy, is illustrated in Fig. 362-5. Differences in the extent and tempo of these processes allow histologic distinction among the muscular dystrophies, inflammatory myopathies, and acute rhabdomyolysis.

Structural changes in muscle fibers Degeneration of muscle fibers without frank necrosis produces structural alteration of individual muscle fibers; disorganization of myofibrils and sarcoplasm produces target fibers (Fig. 362-4C), ringbinden (appearance of a portion of the myofibrils wrapped transversely around the remaining longitudinal myofibrils), central cores, cytoid bodies, and nemaline bodies. In one congenital myopathy the fibers resemble myotubes (centronuclear myopathy). In others, abnormal mitochondria suggest an abnormality of mitochondrial biochemistry, while the presence of vacuoles suggests a disturbance of glycogen or lipid metabolism. Rimmed vacuoles (accumulations of degenerating phospholipid material between myofibrils) occur particularly in oculopharyngeal muscular dystrophy and inclusion body myositis.

Inflammatory changes Perivascular and interstitial inflammatory cell infiltration with lymphocytes and macrophages is characteristic of polymyositis and dermatomyositis. Necrosis and regeneration of muscle fibers are also present. In some instances, atrophy of the fibers located on the periphery of muscle fasciculi (*perifascicular atrophy*) is prominent and can be an indicator of inflammatory myopathy, even though a focus of inflammation is not present in the muscle taken at biopsy. Muscle biopsy may show vasculitis in patients with collagen diseases or granulomas in patients with sarcoidosis.

Changes specific to fiber type Pathologic changes may be restricted to one fiber type in the muscle. The most common such condition is type 2 fiber atrophy (Fig. 362-4D), which occurs in a wide range of disorders that limit activity such as disuse, muscle pain, joint pain, and upper motor neuronal dysfunction. Atrophy of type 1 fibers is less frequent and occurs in myotonic dystrophy, rheumatoid arthritis, and some congenital myopathies.

NERVE BIOPSY Nerve biopsy is more difficult and more traumatic than muscle biopsy and is useful in a limited number of specific circumstances (see Chap. 363). The sural nerve in the leg or the superficial radial nerve at the wrist are the usual biopsy sites. Both are sensory nerves and may show no changes in pure motor neuropathies. The biopsy procedure is performed under local anesthesia, and specimens are obtained for light and electron microscopy and for teasing of individual nerve fibers. Nerve biopsy aids in (1) distinguishing between segmental demyelination and axonal degeneration; (2) identifying inflammatory neuropathies; and (3) establishing specific diagnoses such as amyloidosis, sarcoidosis, leprosy, vasculitis, and several metabolic neuropathies. Full evaluation of the nerve biopsy requires the facilities of a laboratory with special interest and experience in peripheral nerve pathology. Light microscopic examination of biopsied nerves is of limited value, showing only gross changes such as vasculitis, inflammation, infiltration by granuloma or amyloid, loss of axons, and axonal degeneration. More information is obtained by electron microscopy and studies of single teased nerve fibers. Some diseases affect specific fiber types. For instance, large myelinated fibers are affected in Friedreich's ataxia and unmyelinated fibers in familial amyloidosis. Quantitative morphometry (measurement of the number of fibers and the distribution of their diameters) can therefore be of additional help. Two basic pathologic processes may be seen in nerve biopsies.

Segmental demyelination Diseases may attack either myelin or the Schwann cell, causing the myelin sheath to undergo degeneration but leaving the axon essentially unchanged. Healing of this segmental demyelination proceeds through a phase of abnormally thin myelin sheaths, which may eventually return to normal thickness. However, even after apparent recovery of segmental demyelination, single teased nerve fiber studies demonstrate short and variable lengths of the internodes (distance between the nodes of Ranvier). If this process is progressive, *onion-bulb formation* occurs with thinly remyelinated fibers lying at the center of concentric lamellae of redundant Schwann cell cytoplasm.

Axonal degeneration Death of the nerve cell body or section of the axon at any level will lead to degeneration of the distal parts of the axon with secondary degeneration of the myelin sheath. If the nerve cell body remains intact proximally there is attempted axonal

FIGURE 362-5 *A.* Normal muscle. Hematoxylin-eosin. *B.* Duchenne muscular dystrophy, showing hyalin fibers, fiber degeneration, loss of fibers and fibrosis. Hematoxylin-eosin.

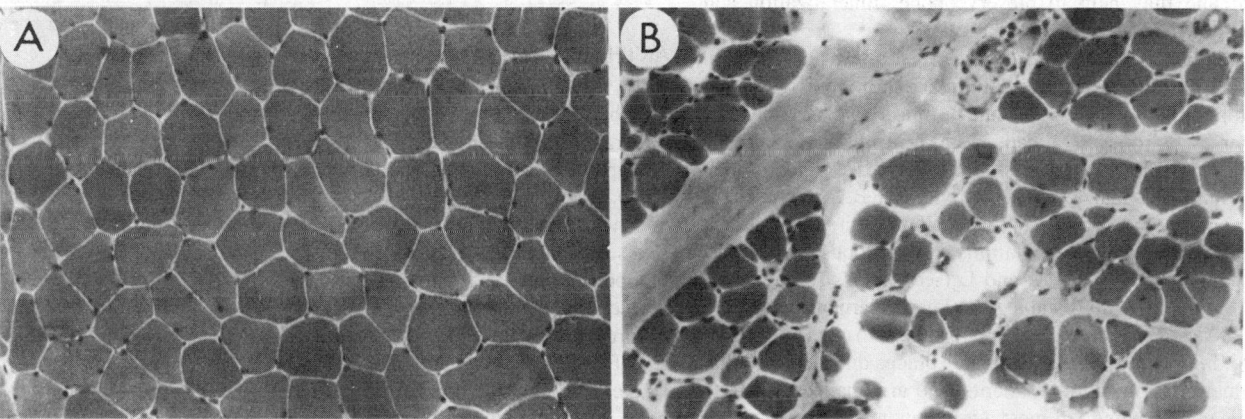

regeneration with sprouting. Such nerve sprouts (*clusters*) are characteristic of degenerating and regenerating axonal neuropathy.

Pathologic changes in neuropathies   Axonal degeneration is most common in toxic, inherited, traumatic, and ischemic diseases. Segmental demyelination may occur in the inherited and autoimmune inflammatory disorders; in the latter condition inflammatory cell infiltration may be seen. A mixed picture of axonal degeneration and segmental demyelination, together with a vasculopathy, is characteristic of diabetes mellitus. Some specific pathologic changes may indicate the probable etiology of a neuropathy. The deposition of IgM on the myelin-associated glycoprotein of the myelin sheaths in IgM gammopathies can be detected by immunofluorescence techniques. The deposition leads to an increase in myelin periodicity. Amyloid fibrils are present in amyloid neuropathy. Specific inclusions may be seen in the Schwann cells in metachromatic leukodystrophy and adrenomyeloleukodystrophy.

GENERAL THERAPEUTIC CONSIDERATIONS

Cardiac   Most disorders of skeletal muscle also involved cardiac muscle. Symptomatic cardiac dysfunction is relatively uncommon, however, perhaps because the limited exercise capacity of the patient with weakness decreases demands on cardiac performance. Relatively specific electrocardiographic abnormalities occur in Duchenne dystrophy and infantile acid maltase deficiency. Cardiac conduction disorders including complete heart block occur in patients with myotonic dystrophy. An electrocardiogram should be obtained in all patients with neuromuscular disease, particularly in patients with myopathies.

Respiratory   Diminished pulmonary function in patients with acute or chronic neuromuscular disease may progress to ventilatory failure. The earliest manifestation of respiratory muscle weakness is a decrease in maximum expiratory and inspiratory pressures. Diaphragmatic weakness, in particular, may be substantial in patients with neuromuscular disease and should be evaluated by examining pulmonary function both while the patient is supine and sitting. Diaphragmatic weakness causes a decrease in pulmonary function when measured in the supine compared with the erect position. Paradoxical abdominal movements may be evident. Patients with chronic respiratory failure may be maintained with home respiratory support. The possible occurrence of cor pulmonale from insidious respiratory failure should be considered in any patient with neuromuscular disease who develops ankle edema or other signs of heart failure.

Physical therapy   Physical therapy is of greatest value in patients with muscle weakness when joint contractures are developing and when enforced immobility, such as an injury, results in decreased activity. Exercises may increase strength in muscles weakened by disease as in normal persons, but there is little evidence that exercise improves functional abilities. However, therapeutic standing in patients with marginal leg and trunk function has considerable psychological benefit and may help to preserve bone mineralization and cardiovascular reflexes.

Dietary modification   Dietary restriction is often necessary in patients with muscle weakness since caloric expenditure is decreased because of immobility and loss of muscle mass. Development of obesity further compromises already reduced mobility, worsens pulmonary function, and may depress ventilatory drive. Unless there is specific evidence for malabsorption of vitamin B_{12} or vitamin E neither these nor any other vitamin has a specific role in the treatment of neuromuscular disease. Certain vitamins are hazardous in excessive dosages, including vitamins B_6, A, and D (see Chaps. 76 and 340).

Bracing   In patients with distal leg weakness, particularly of foot dorsiflexion, ankle-foot orthoses can restore gait to nearly normal. With more proximal weakness, however, leg braces diminish mobility and are of value only in enabling patients who are unable to walk to perform therapeutic standing. In most adults, even this use of braces is impractical because such standing in braces usually requires assistance.

Scoliosis   Spinal deformity complicates many neuromuscular diseases, particularly those that occur before puberty. Duchenne dystrophy, spinal muscular atrophy, and congenital myopathies are particularly liable to this complication. Once full long-bone growth has been achieved, many of these patients should have surgical correction of the scoliosis. Severely impaired pulmonary function is a contraindication to such therapy; therefore, patients with progressive scoliosis need careful sequential follow-up to determine the appropriate timing for surgery.

GENETIC EVALUATION AND COUNSELLING   (See also Chap. 365)   Management of the patient with hereditary muscle disease should include careful family pedigree analysis and genetic counselling. The family history may initially be negative in many patients with autosomal dominant diseases such as Charcot-Marie-Tooth disease, myotonic dystrophy, and facioscapulohumeral dystrophy because of the variable expressivity of the disorders. The availability of chromosomal markers for linkage analysis has made carrier detection, antenatal diagnosis, and early diagnosis of disease feasible in several hereditary neuromuscular diseases (e.g., in Duchenne and myotonic dystrophy). The availability of therapy for disorders such as periodic paralysis, myotonia, and certain metabolic myopathies and of preventive measures in disorders such as malignant hyperthermia provides a strong impetus for early diagnosis. History alone is often inadequate for family evaluation. Physical examination or inspection of photographs of family members will often identify mildly afflicted individuals, providing clues to the characteristic facial or other features of the disorder. Molecular biologic techniques now permit specific diagnosis of certain neuromuscular diseases by identification of an abnormal or missing gene product. Thus, the protein dystrophin is lacking in muscle of patients with Duchenne dystrophy (see Chap. 365).

REFERENCES

BROOKE MH: *A Clinician's View of Neuromuscular Disease*, 2d ed. Baltimore, Williams and Wilkins, 1986

CARPENTER S, KARPATI G: *Pathology of Skeletal Muscle*. New York, Churchill Livingstone, 1984

ENGEL AG, BANKER BQ (eds): *Myology*, New York, McGraw-Hill, 1986

KIMURA J: *Electrodiagnosis in Diseases of Nerve and Muscle*, 2d ed. Philadelphia, Davis, 1989

OH SJ: *Electromyograph; Neuromuscular Transmission Studies*. Baltimore, Williams and Wilkins, 1988

RIGGS JE et al: The periodic paralyses. Neurol Clin 6:485, 1988

SCHAUMBURG HH et al: *Disorders of Peripheral Nerves*. Philadelphia, Davis, 1983

363   DISEASES OF THE PERIPHERAL NERVOUS SYSTEM

ARTHUR K. ASBURY

Peripheral neuropathy is a general term indicating disorder of peripheral nerve of any cause; therefore, knowing that a peripheral neuropathy is present in a particular patient should instigate a search for its basis.

The basic processes affecting nerve and muscle and the approach to diseases of nerve and muscle are fully set forth in Chap. 362. The first purpose here is to build upon that base by providing an overview of the wide array of peripheral neuropathies that afflict humans. Disorders of peripheral nerve exhibit such a bewildering and complex set of manifestations that it is difficult for the physician to know where to begin and how to proceed. Therefore the second purpose here is to develop a logical approach and assessment scheme (summarized in Fig. 363-1) which will guide the examiner to correct diagnoses and management decisions.

GENERAL DESCRIPTION OF NEUROPATHIC SYNDROMES
The prototypical picture of polyneuropathy occurs with acquired toxic or metabolic neuropathic states. From a symptom standpoint, the first noticeable features tend to be sensory and consist of tingling, prickling, burning, or bandlike dysesthesias in the balls of the feet or tips of the toes, or in a general distribution over the soles. Symmetry of symptoms and findings in a distal graded fashion is the rule, but occasionally dysesthesias appear in one foot a brief time before the other or may be more pronounced in one foot. Some care and judgment is needed to avoid confusion with mononeuropathy multiplex. If the polyneuropathy remains mild, no objective motor or sensory signs may be detectable.

With progression, pansensory loss is usually found over both feet, ankle jerks are lost, and weakness of dorsiflexion of the toes, best demonstrated in the great toe, may be present. In some instances, the process begins with weakness in the feet, usually dorsiflexion of the toes and feet without subjective sensory symptoms. As worsening occurs, sensory loss moves centripetally in a graded "stocking" fashion, and the patient may complain that the feet have a numb or "wooden" feeling or may say "I feel as though I'm walking on stumps." Patients experience difficulty walking on their heels during examination and their feet may slap while walking. Later, the knee jerk reflex disappears and foot drop becomes more apparent. By the time sensory disturbance has reached the upper shin, dysesthesias are usually noticed in the tips of the fingers. The degree of spontaneous pain varies, but is often considerable. Light stimuli to hypesthetic areas, once perceived, may be experienced as extremely uncomfortable (hyperpathia). Unsteadiness of gait may be out of proportion to muscle weakness because of proprioceptive loss.

Worsening proceeds in a centripetal, symmetrically graded manner with muscle atrophy, pansensory loss, and areflexia and with motor weakness that is usually greater in the extensor muscles than in corresponding flexor groups. When the sensory disturbance reaches mid thigh, generally a tent-shaped area of hypesthesia on the lower abdomen may be demonstrated. This will grow broader, and the apex will extend rostrally toward the sternum as the neuropathy worsens. By this time, patients generally cannot stand or walk or hold objects in their hands.

In the most extreme cases, ventilatory capacity may be impaired along with sphincteric function. Hypesthesia at the crown of the scalp may be present and spread radially into both the trigeminal and C2 distribution. Considering the entire sequence, nerve fibers are affected according to length of axon without regard to root or nerve trunk distribution—hence, the aptness of the term "stocking-glove" to describe the pattern of sensory deficit. In general, the motor deficit is also graded, distal, and symmetric.

Variations on the general sequence outlined above are manifold and explain the diversity of clinical syndromes encountered. Variations include the rate of evolution; fluctuations in the course; the eventual degree of severity; the presence or absence of positive motor and sensory symptoms; the symmetry of features and their distribution in terms of proximal versus distal, arms versus legs, and motor versus sensory; the relative proportion of dysfunction attributable to large fiber deficit and to small fiber deficit; and the determination, mainly by electrodiagnostic examination, of axonal versus demyelinating processes.

ASSESSMENT AND DIAGNOSIS OF NEUROPATHY Taking the first step Clues to the diagnosis of specific peripheral neuropathies often lie in unnoted or readily forgotten events occurring weeks or months prior to the onset of symptoms. Inquiry should be made about recent viral illnesses; other systemic symptoms; institution of new medications; potentially toxic exposures to solvents, pesticides, or heavy metals; the occurrence of similar symptoms in family members or coworkers; habits concerning alcohol; and the presence of known

FIGURE 363-1 Flowchart approach to the evaluation of peripheral neuropathies. (*After Asbury, 1983.*)

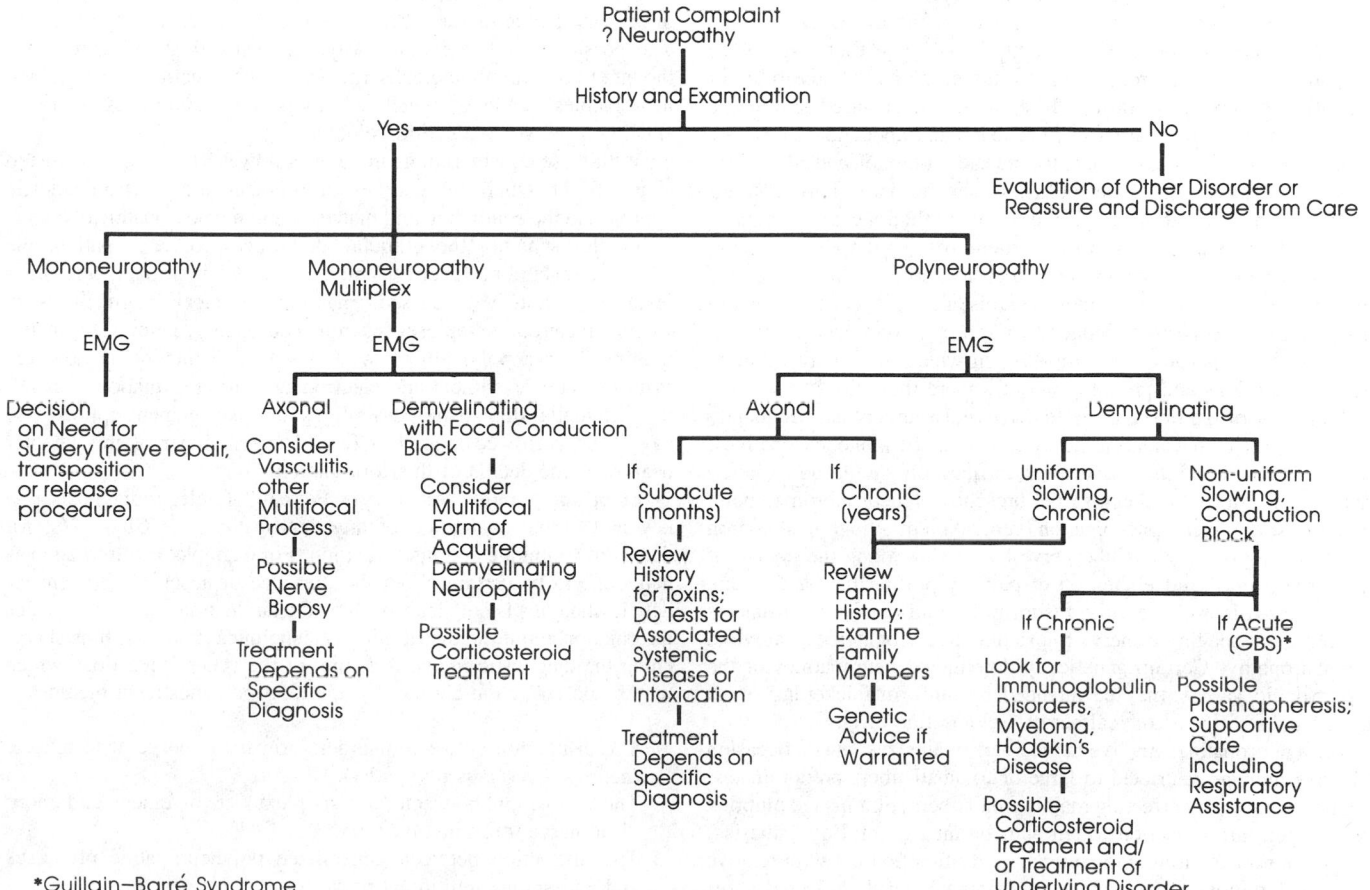

*Guillain–Barré Syndrome

preexisting medical disorders. It is also useful to ask patients if they would otherwise feel well if free of their neuropathic symptoms, to obtain an idea of the presence or absence of an underlying systemic illness.

It is important to learn how symptoms first appeared. Even with distal polyneuropathies, symptoms may appear in the sole of one foot a few days or a week before the other, but usually the patient will describe a distal graded disturbance that moves evenly and symmetrically in centripetal fashion. Tingling dysesthesias will appear in the fingertips only when similar symptoms have reached the level of the knees. It is most important to determine whether symptoms first appeared in the distribution of individual digital nerves involving only one-half of a digit at a time and then gradually spread to become coalescent. This pattern of onset raises strong suspicions of a multifocal process (mononeuropathy multiplex) such as might be encountered with a systemic vasculitis or cryoglobulinemia.

The evolution of neuropathy ranges from rapid worsening over a few days to an indolent process extending many years. Polyneuropathies with a slowly progressive course lasting more than 5 years are most likely to be genetically determined, particularly if the major manifestations are distal atrophy and weakness with few or no positive sensory symptoms. Exceptions are diabetic polyneuropathy and paraproteinemic neuropathies in which the progression may be insidious over 5 to 10 years. Axonal degenerations of toxic or metabolic origin tend to evolve over several weeks to a year or more, and the rate of progression of demyelinating neuropathies is highly variable, ranging from a few days in Guillain-Barré syndrome to many years in others.

Major fluctuations in the course of neuropathy bring to mind two possibilities: (1) relapsing forms of neuropathy, or (2) repeated toxic exposures. A slow fluctuation in symptoms taking place over weeks or months (reflecting changes in the activity of neuropathy) should not be confused with day-to-day variation or diurnal undulation of symptoms. The latter are common to all neuropathic disorders. An example is carpal tunnel syndrome in which dysesthesias may be prominent at night but absent during the day.

In polyneuropathies, the findings can be expected to be quite symmetric on both sides of the body. If only one foot slaps when the patient walks, the process is not symmetric and the possibility of a multifocal process is raised. In addition, in acquired symmetric polyneuropathies, the muscles of extension and abduction tend to be weakened to a greater extent than the muscles of flexion and adduction. Hence, weakness in lower legs often affects the peronei and anterior tibial muscles, with attendant foot drop, more than the gastrocnemius group or foot inverters. In most polyneuropathies the legs are more severely affected than the arms and the distal muscles more than the proximal ones. There are exceptions to this rule, as in lead neuropathy, in which manifestations of bilateral wrist drop may predominate, and occasionally in porphyric neuropathy, in which arms may be more affected than legs and proximal muscles more than distal.

Palpation of the nerve trunk to detect enlargement is a frequently forgotten part of the neurologic examination. In mononeuropathies, the entire course of the nerve trunk in question should be explored manually for focal thickening; the presence of neurofibroma, point tenderness, or Tinel's phenomenon (generation of a tingling sensation in the sensory territory of the nerve by tapping along the course of the nerve trunk); and elicitation of pain by putting the nerve trunk on stretch. In leprous neuritis, fusiform thickening of nerve trunks is frequent, and beading of nerve trunks may be encountered in amyloid polyneuropathy. Certain genetically determined neuropathies of the hypertrophic variety may be attended by uniform thickening of all nerve trunks, often to the caliber of a clothesline or larger.

Most neuropathies involve nerve fibers of all sizes, but on occasion selective damage restricted to large or to small fibers predominates. In a polyneuropathy affecting mainly small fibers, diminished pinprick and temperature sensation, often with burning painful dysesthesias, may predominate along with autonomic dysfunction but with relative sparing of motor power, balance, and tendon jerks. Selected cases

of amyloid and distal diabetic polyneuropathies fall into this category. In contrast, large-fiber polyneuropathy is characterized by areflexia, imbalance, relatively minor cutaneous sensory deficit, and variable but often severe motor dysfunction.

In addition to taking a history and doing a physical examination that bears in mind the points made above, certain other measures can be undertaken routinely in the evaluation of a patient with neuropathy. Electrodiagnostic examination is a key procedure in all patients. For patients with polyneuropathy or mononeuropathy multiplex, standard tests should include a complete blood count and erythrocyte sedimentation rate, urinalysis, chest x-ray, postprandial blood glucose, and serum protein electrophoresis. Further tests should be dictated by the formulation arrived at via the combined history and physical and electrodiagnostic examination (see Fig. 363-1).

Taking the next step   The next step is electrodiagnostic examination. It is not generally possible to make the distinction between axonal versus demyelinating disorders on clinical examination alone; here electrodiagnostic analysis is particularly useful. Electrodiagnostic features of demyelination are slowing of nerve conduction velocity (NCV), dispersion of evoked compound action potentials (CAPs), conduction block (major decrease in amplitude of muscle CAP upon proximal stimulation of its nerve as compared to distal stimulation), and marked prolongation of distal latencies. In contrast, axonal neuropathies are characterized by a reduction in amplitude of evoked CAPs with relative preservation of NCV. The distinction between a primarily demyelinating neuropathy from one which is primarily axonal is crucial because of the differing approaches to diagnosis and management. If in a particular instance of progressive polyneuropathy or subacute or chronic evolution the electrodiagnostic findings are those of an axonopathy, a long list of metabolic states and exogenous toxins come into consideration (see Tables 363-1 and 363-2). If the course is protracted over several years, it raises the likelihood of the neuronal (axonal) form of peroneal muscular atrophy (HMSN-II); family members must be examined and additional attention given to the family history.

Alternatively, if the electrodiagnostic findings are more indicative of primary demyelination of nerve, the approach is entirely different. The possibilities then include acquired demyelinating neuropathy, thought to be immunologically mediated, and genetically determined neuropathies, some of which are marked by uniform and drastic slowing of nerve conduction velocities.

With these considerations in hand, a flowchart can be constructed (Fig. 363-1) which summarizes the clinical and electrodiagnostic approach to the evaluation and management of a neuropathic disorder. Using this scheme, the clinician determines for each patient the tempo, distribution, severity, and functional impairment, and other features previously discussed, making a clinical judgment as to whether the problem represents a mononeuropathy, a mononeuropathy multiplex, or a polyneuropathy. Often this distinction is obvious. With the sum of clinical and electrodiagnostic information in hand, the differential diagnostic possibilities and management options will have been narrowed to only a few. The remainder of this chapter deals with the details of this formulation.

Electrodiagnosis   As seen in Fig. 363-1, electrodiagnosis is a key part of the evaluation of any neuropathy. See Chap. 362 for details of technique and interpretation. For example, electrodiagnosis helps one to be certain about the presence or absence of a sensory deficit when this is not clear by clinical examination alone. It provides information about the distribution of subclinical findings, thus sharpening the diagnostic focus. A listing of the general questions which may be posed by the clinician to the electrodiagnostician includes

1 The distinction between disorders primary to nerve or to muscle (neuropathy versus myopathy).
2 The distinction between root or plexus involvement and more distal nerve trunk involvement.
3 The distinction between generalized polyneuropathic processes and widespread multifocal nerve trunk affection.

TABLE 363-1 Polyneuropathy associated with systemic diseases

Systemic disease	Occur-rence*	Axonal† Acute	Sub-acute	Chron-ic	Demyelinating† Acute	Sub-acute	Chron-ic	Sensory vs. motor‡	Auto-nomic†	Comment
Diabetes mellitus	C	—	±	+	—	±	+	S, SM, rarely M	± to +	Mixed axonal demyelination often seen; see Table 363-4
Uremia	S	±	+	+	—	—	—	SM	±	Controllable with proper dialysis; curable with successful renal transplant
Porphyria (3 types)	R	+	±	—	—	—	—	M	± to +	May be proximal > distal and may have atypical proximal sensory deficits
Hypoglycemia	R	±	+	+	—	—	—	M	—	Usually with insulinoma; arms often > legs; ? anterior horn cells affected
Vitamin deficiency, exclude B₁₂	S	—	+	+	—	—	—	SM	±	Involves at least thiamine, pyridoxine, folate, pantothenic acid; probably others
Vitamin B₁₂ deficiency	S	—	±	+	—	—	—	S	—	Peripheral nerve involvement variable; often overshadowed by myelopathy
Chronic liver disease	S	—	—	—	—	—	+	S or SM	—	Usually mild or subclinical
Primary biliary cirrhosis	R	—	±	+	—	—	—	S	—	Epineurial and subperineurial xanthomatous deposits
Primary systemic amyloidosis	R	—	±	+	—	—	—	SM	+	Also seen with amyloidosis associated with myeloma or macroglobulinemia
Hypothyroidism	R	—	—	—	—	±	+	S	—	May respond to thyroid replacement
Chronic obstructive lung disease	R	—	±	+	—	—	—	S or SM	—	Few reports; a questionable entity
Acromegaly	R	—	—	+	—	—	—	S	—	Carpal tunnel syndrome also frequent
Malabsorption (sprue, celiac disease)	S	—	±	+	—	—	—	S or SM	±	Basis for neuropathy unclear; deficiency suspected
Carcinoma (sensory)	R	—	+	+	—	—	—	Pure S	—	Carcinomatous sensory neuropathy; due to gangliitic neuronopathy; mostly breast carcinoma; paraneoplastic; relatively rare
Carcinoma (sensorimotor)	S	—	+	+	—	—	—	SM	±	Sensorimotor axonal neuropathy; mostly with lung carcinoma; more common than pure sensory, but still infrequent
Carcinoma (late)	C	—	+	+	—	—	—	S>M	±	Mild, late axonal neuropathy, probably related to weight loss and wasting
Carcinoma (demyelinating)	S	—	—	—	+	+	±	SM	—	Acute or relapsing demyelinating neuropathy sometimes seen with carcinoma
Lymphoma including Hodgkin's	S	—	+	+	+	+	±	See above	±	Same as carcinomatous types, although pure sensory type is even rarer
Polycythemia vera	R	—	±	+	—	—	—	S	—	Also many CNS manifestations; often shooting pains in limbs
Multiple myeloma lytic type	S	—	±	+	—	—	—	S, M, or SM	±	Symptomatic neuropathy uncommon, subclinical neuropathy frequent
Multiple myeloma§: osteosclerotic or solitary plasmacytoma	S	—	—	±	—	±	+	SM	—	Although may show severe slowing of nerve conduction velocity recent work suggests this is secondary demyelination

TABLE 363-1   Polyneuropathy associated with systemic diseases (*continued*)

Systemic disease	Occur-rence*	Axonal†			Demyelinating†			Sensory vs. motor‡	Auto-nomic†	Comment
		Acute	Sub-acute	Chron-ic	Acute	Sub-acute	Chron-ic			
Benign monoclonal gammopathy:	S									
IgA		—	±	+	—	—	—	SM	—	IgM_κ (or occasionally
IgG		—	±	+	—	—	—	SM	—	IgM_λ) may bind to
IgM		—	—	—	—	±	+	SM	—	myelin-associated gly-coprotein or glycolipids
Macroglobulinemia	R	—	—	±	—	—	+	SM	—	Usually but not always axonal
Cryoglobulinemia	R	—	±	+	—	—	—	SM	—	May be mononeuropathy multiplex in presenta-tion

* R = rare; S = sometimes; C = common.
† ± = sometimes; + = usual.
‡ S = sensory; M = motor; SM = sensorimotor.
§ Some cases associated with POEMS syndrome (see text).

4 The distinction between upper and lower motor neuron weakness.

5 The distinction, in a given generalized polyneuropathic process, between primary demyelinating neuropathy and axonal degener-ation.

6 The assessment, in both primary axonal and demyelinating neuropathies, of many factors bearing on the nature, activity, and likely prognosis of the neuropathy.

7 The assessment, in mononeuropathies, of the site of the lesion and its major effect on nerve fibers, especially the distinction between demyelinating conduction block and wallerian degener-ation.

8 The characterization of disorders of the neuromuscular junction.

9 The identification, often in muscle of normal bulk and strength, of chronic partial denervation, fasciculations, and myotonia.

10 The analysis of cramp, and its distinction from physiologic contracture.

Nerve biopsy   The sural nerve at the ankle is the preferred site for cutaneous nerve biopsy. There are few indications to employ this invasive technique. The main one is in asymmetric and multifocal neuropathic disorders producing a clinical picture of mononeuropathy multiplex, the basis of which is still unclear after other laboratory investigations are complete. Diagnostic considerations include vas-culitis, amyloidosis, leprosy, and occasionally sarcoidosis. Nerve biopsy is also helpful when one or more cutaneous nerves are palpably enlarged. Another clinical application is in establishing the diagnosis in some genetically determined childhood disorders such as meta-chromatic leukodystrophy, Krabbe's disease, giant axonal neuropathy, and infantile neuroaxonal dystrophy. In all of these recessively inherited diseases, both the central nervous system (CNS) and the peripheral nervous system (PNS) are affected.

There is a tendency to carry out sural nerve biopsy in distal symmetric polyneuropathies of subacute or chronic evolution. This practice is discouraged because it is a low-yield measure. Nerve biopsy in this situation is only useful as part of an approved research protocol when the biopsy will provide crucial information not otherwise obtainable.

POLYNEUROPATHY   Although this term connotes a widespread symmetric process, usually distal and graded, polyneuropathies

TABLE 363-2   Polyneuropathy associated with drugs or environmental toxins

	Axonal*			Demyelinating*			Sensory vs. motor†	Auto-nomic*	CNS*	Comment
	Acute	Subacute	Chronic	Acute	Subacute	Chronic				
DRUGS										
Amiodarone (antiar-rhythmic)	—	—	+	—	—	+	SM	—	—	Dose-dependent neu-ropathy, reversible by decreasing dose; lysosomal dense body accumulation
Aurothioglucose (anti-rheumatic)	±	±	—	+	+	—	SM	—	—	Idiosyncratic reaction, ? immune-mediated
cis-Platinum (antineo-plastic)	—	+	+	—	—	—	S	—	—	Severe sensory neuro-pathy, ? neuronopa-thy; also ototoxicity; dose-related
Dapsone (dermato-logic including lep-rosy)	—	±	+	—	—	—	M	—	—	Dose-related pure mo-tor neuropathy
Disulfiram (antialco-hol)	±	+	+	—	—	—	SM	—	±	Usually occurs after months of treatment
Hydralazine (antihy-pertensive)	—	±	+	—	—	—	S>M	—	—	A pyridoxine antago-nist; only rarely neu-rotoxic
Isoniazid	—	±	+	—	—	—	SM	±	—	A pyridoxine antago-nist; neurotoxic in slow acetylators

* ± = sometimes, + = usual.
† S = sensory; M = motor; SM = sensorimotor.

TABLE 363-2   Polyneuropathy associated with drugs or environmental toxins (*continued*)

	Axonal*			Demyelinating*			Sensory vs. motor†	Autonomic*	CNS*	Comment
	Acute	Subacute	Chronic	Acute	Subacute	Chronic				
DRUGS (*continued*)										
Metronidazole (antiprotozoal	—	—	±	—	—	—	S	—	+	Dose-related central-peripheral distal axonopathy
Misonidazole (radiosensitizer)	—	±	+	—	—	—	S	—	+	Neurotoxicity is the limiting factor
Perhexilene (antiarrhythmic)	—	—	±	—	—	+	SM	±	—	Dose-related neuropathy; lysosomal dense body accumulation
Phenytoin (anticonvulsant)	—	—	+	—	—	—	S>M	—	—	Large-fiber neuropathy, mild, after 20–30 years of phenytoin use
Pyridoxine (vitamin)	—	±	+	—	—	—	S	—	—	Occurs with large intake; >500 mg per day
Thalidomide (antileprous)	—	—	+	—	—	—	S>M	±	+	Red skin and brittle nails; also teratogenic; recovery from neuropathy poor
Vincristine (antineoplastic)	—	+	+	—	—	—	S>M	—	—	Mild sensory neuropathy is nearly universal, hands>feet; motor signs should prompt cessation of treatment
Nitrofurantoin (urinary antiseptic)	—	±	+	—	—	—	SM	—	—	Generally total dose-related; presence of renal failure may enhance toxicity
TOXINS										
Acrylamide (flocculant; grouting agent)	—	±	+	—	—	—	S>M	±	+	Large-fiber neuropathy; sensory ataxia
Arsenic (herbicide; insecticide)	±	+	+	—	—	—	SM	±	±	Skin changes and Mees' lines in nails; if acute intoxication, many systemic effects
Buckthorn (toxic berry)	—	—	—	+	+	—	SM	—	—	Only occurs where berries grow; may mimic GBS
Carbon disulfide, CS₂ (industrial)	—	—	+	—	—	+	SM	—	+	Neurofilamentous accumulation in axons; demyelinating features are secondary
Diphtheria	—	—	—	+	+	—	SM	—	—	Clinically very rare now; can be confused with GBS
Dimethylamino propionitrile (industrial)	—	—	+	—	—	—	S>M	+	—	Small-fiber neuropathy with prominent bladder symptoms and impotence in males
γ-Diketone hexacarbons (solvents)	—	±			—	—	+	SM	±	+	Same features as CS₂; these solvents now in restricted use
Inorganic lead	—	—	+	—	—	—	M>S	—	±	Selective motor neuropathy with prominent wrist drop
Organophosphates	—	±	+	—	—	—	SM	—	+	Brain and spinal cord are also affected, the latter irreversibly
Thallium (rat poison)	—	+	+	—	—	—	SM	—	+	Also alopecia, Mees' lines in nails; ? selective damage to neural mitochondria

* ± = sometimes, + = usual.
† S = sensory; M = motor; SM = sensorimotor.

present a high degree of diversity because of the extreme variability of tempo, severity, mix of sensory and motor features, and presence or absence of positive symptoms. The patient with a fulminant, severely dysesthetic sensory neuropathy and alopecia who is in the early phases of thallium intoxication bears little similarity to the patient with a 40-year history of insidiously progressive clumsiness of gait whose findings are foot drop, lower leg atrophy, pes cavus, and minimal asymptomatic distal sensory deficit (i.e., peroneal muscular atrophy, either type I or II; see Table 363-3). These two patients fall near opposite ends of the spectrum of polyneuropathy.

The classification of peripheral neuropathies has become increasingly complex as the capacity to discriminate new subgroups and identify new associations with toxins and systemic disorders improves. Further, our grasp of the pathophysiologic basis for the clinical phenomena observed in neuropathy has increased rapidly (see Chap. 362). But these advances are primarily descriptive; little or no progress has been made in illuminating the fundamental pathogenetic events in nervous tissue which eventuate in any one of the polyneuropathies.

The important features of each major grouping of polyneuropathies are summarized below and key aspects of specific polyneuropathies may be found in Tables 363-1 to 363-4.

TABLE 363-3   Genetically determined neuropathies

Genetic disorder	Inheritance pattern	Age of onset	Basic process	Other features*	Other systems involved	Metabolic defect	Comment
Peroneal muscular atrophy (HMSN-I)†	Dominant	Decades 2–3	Demyelinating	Hypertrophic change with onion bulb formation; marked ↓ NCV	Some families—Duffy locus linkage	Unknown	Pes cavus, congenital hip problems, motor deficit predominates
Peroneal muscular atrophy (HMSN-II)†	Dominant	Decades 3–5	Axonal	Marked ↓ NAP; NCV sl. decreased	—	Unknown	Same as HSMN-I
Hereditary amyloid neuropathies	Dominant	Decades 3–4	Axonal	Small fiber involvement; endoneurial amyloid deposition	Some families—cornea	Amino acid mutation in transthyretin (prealbumin)	Dysautonomia may be prominent. Genetic defect on chromosome 18.
Hereditary sensory neuropathy (HSN-I)	Dominant	Decades 1–3	Neuronopathic	DRG neurons selectively involved	Sensorineural deafness, some families	Unknown	Frequent distal mutilation—hands and feet
Porphyric neuropathy	Dominant	Adult life	Axonal	Neuropathy part of attacks; may be recurrent	Widespread cellular abnormality	Enzyme defects in porphyrin pathway	Acute intermittent porphyria, variegate porphyria, and erythropoietic porphyria
Hereditary liability to pressure palsy	Dominant	Decades 2–3	? Demyelinating	Tomaculous changes in myelin	—	Unknown	Ulnar, peroneal, and brachial plexus involvement particularly
Fabry's disease	X-linked	Young males	Neuronopathic	Sensory neuronopathy, small DRG neurons	Kidney, skin, lung	Accumulation of ceramide-trihexoside	Neuropathy painful; often die of renal failure
Peroneal muscular atrophy (Phillips et al., 1985)	X-linked	Infancy to 2d decade	Axonal or demyelinating	Heterozygote females may have symptoms		Unknown	Localizes to long arm of X chromosome
Adrenomyeloneuropathy	X-linked	Young males	? Axonal	Mild neuropathy, spastic paraparesis, baldness, hypogonadism	Adrenal cortex, cerebral white matter, spinal cord	Accumulation of very long chain fatty acids	Phenotypic variant of adrenoleukodystrophy; dietary therapy possible
Hereditary sensory neuropathy (HSN-II)	Recessive	Decades 1–3	Neuronopathic	DRG neurons selectively involved	—	Unknown	May be less severe than HSN-I
Déjerine-Sottas neuropathy (HMSN-III)	Recessive	1st decade	Demyelinating	Hypertrophic change with onion bulb formation	May be mentally retarded	Unknown	Marked nerve trunk enlargement
Refsum's disease	Recessive	1st or 2d decade	Demyelinating	Hypertrophic change with onion bulb formation	Retinitis pigmentosa, ichthyosis, sensorineural deafness	Defect in α-oxidation of β-methylated fatty acids	Low phytanate diet, plasmapheresis therapy
Ataxia-telangiectasia	Recessive	Decade 1 or 2	Axonal	Neuropathy moderate	Cell nuclear aneuploidy, skin and scleral telangiectasia, cerebellar atrophy, immunopathy	Basic defect unknown	High incidence of early neoplasia

* DRG, dorsal root ganglia; NAP, nerve action potential; sl, slightly; HMSN, hereditary motor-sensory neuropathy; HSN, hereditary sensory neuropathy.
† Both forms are also collectively referred to as Charcot-Marie-Tooth neuropathy.

TABLE 363-3   Genetically determined neuropathies (continued)

Genetic disorder	Inheritance pattern	Age of onset	Basic process	Other features*	Other systems involved	Metabolic defect	Comment
Abetalipopro-teinemia	Recessive	Decade 1 or 2	Neuronopathic	Large DRG neurons	Retinitis pigmentosa, acanthocytosis of red blood cells	Absence of all lipoprotein-containing apo B	Proprioceptive disturbance marked, minimal small fiber deficit
Giant axonal neuropathy	Recessive	1st decade	Axonal	Massive segmented accumulation of neurofilaments in axons	Slowly progressive encephalopathy with Rosenthal fibers	Generalized disorder of 10-nm filaments	Intermediate filament masses in other cell types
Metachromatic leukodystrophy	Recessive	1st decade	Demyelinating	Schwannopathy with cerebroside accumulation	Cerebral white matter disease predominates	Defect of arylsulfatase A	Infantile, juvenile, and adult onset forms
Globoid cell leukodystrophy	Recessive	1st decade	Demyelinating	Schwannopathy with galacto-cerebroside accumulation	Cerebral white matter disease predominates	Defect of β-galactosidase	Characteristic clefts in Schwann cell cytoplasm
Friedreich's ataxia	Recessive	1st decade	Axonal	Spinocerebellar and corticospinal tracts involved; also 1° sensory neuron	Cardiomyopathy; usual cause of death	Controversial	Ataxia is both sensory and cerebellar

* DRG, dorsal root ganglia; NAP, nerve action potential; sl, slightly; HMSN, hereditary motor-sensory neuropathy; HSN, hereditary sensory neuropathy.
† Both forms are also collectively referred to as Charcot-Marie-Tooth neuropathy.

Acute axonal polyneuropathy In this setting the term acute means evolution over days, making these neuropathies relatively uncommon. Included are porphyric neuropathy and massive intoxications, often suicidal or homicidal in intent. For example, an individual receiving a large dose of arsenic (e.g., 100 mg of arsenous oxide) will become violently ill in a few hours with vomiting, diarrhea, and circulatory collapse. In 1 to 3 days serious renal and liver failure will ensue, and between 14 and 21 days polyneuropathy will appear, often as the systemic disorder abates. Progression occurs for 2 or 3 weeks, but following a plateau, recovery requires months.

Subacute axonal polyneuropathy Subacute, meaning to evolve in weeks, characterizes many instances of toxic and metabolic polyneuropathy, but perhaps even more of these are chronic in evolution (months). Scanning the appropriate columns in Tables 363-1 and 363-2 provides many possibilities. Management in almost all instances involves removing from contact the offending agent or treating the associated systemic order.

Chronic axonal polyneuropathy This category includes many more types of polyneuropathy, in part because the term chronic subsumes neuropathies that have progressed over a period as short as 6 months to as long as 60 years. As a rough approximation, slow worsening for more than 5 years, absence of positive symptoms, mainly motor deficit, and absence of systemic disorder all favor a genetically determined neuropathy. Although these are mostly autosomal dominant in inheritance pattern, recessively inherited and X-linked varieties also occur, including a form phenotypically resembling dominantly inherited peroneal muscular atrophy (HMSN-II) and also

TABLE 363-4   Classification of diabetic neuropathies

A Symmetric
  1 Distal, primarily sensory polyneuropathy
    a Mainly large fibers affected
    b Mixed*
    c Mainly small fibers affected*
  2 Autonomic neuropathy
  3 Chronically evolving proximal motor neuropathy*†
B Asymmetric
  1 Acute or subacute proximal motor neuropathy*†
  2 Cranial mononeuropathy†
  3 Truncal neuropathy*†
  4 Entrapment neuropathy in the limbs

* Often painful.
† Recovery, partial or complete, is likely.

adrenomyeloneuropathy (see Table 363-3). To complete the picture, an array of rare autosomal recessive neuropathies occur in childhood.

Acute demyelinating polyneuropathy For all practical purposes, this category is synonymous with Guillain-Barré syndrome (GBS). This acute, frequently severe and fulminant polyneuropathy occurs at a rate of one case per million population per month, or approximately 3500 cases per year in the United States and Canada. Incidence patterns are similar world-wide. In over two-thirds, a viral infection, either clinically overt or evidenced by serum titer rise, precedes the onset of neuropathy by 1 to 3 weeks. Herpes infections [cytomegalovirus, Epstein-Barr virus (EBV)] account for a large proportion of virus-triggered cases. Another 5 to 10 percent of cases occur within 1 to 4 weeks of a surgical procedure. GBS occurs on a background of lymphoma, including Hodgkin's disease, and in lupus erythematosus more frequently than can be attributed to chance alone. Although the weight of evidence suggests that GBS is immune-mediated, the immunopathogenesis remains obscure. In 1976 to 1977, a flurry of some 500 cases followed in the wake of the national swine flu vaccination program in the United States. This exceeded by severalfold the baseline incidence expected in this period among the vaccines. The epidemiologic features of this outbreak resembled a point-source epidemic with an "incubation" period of 1 to 6 weeks. The reason why swine flu vaccine appeared to trigger GBS in 1976 to 1977 has never been discovered. In subsequent annual flu vaccine programs in the United States, no excess cases of GBS have been identified.

The clinical features of GBS typically include areflexic motor paralysis with mild sensory disturbance coupled with an acellular rise of total protein in the cerebrospinal fluid by the end of the first week of symptoms. Most patients with GBS require hospitalization, and about one-fourth will need ventilatory assistance at some point during the illness. The prognosis is good; approximately 85 percent of patients make a complete or nearly complete recovery. The mortality rate is 3 to 4 percent. Management is generally supportive care, but plasmapheresis also has a role. Large, multicenter, controlled trials in North America and Europe have demonstrated a beneficial effect of plasmapheresis, especially when initiated in the first 2 weeks of illness. In contrast, the utility of glucocorticoid treatment is unproved, and it is generally considered not to be effective.

Other acute demyelinating polyneuropathies are rare and include buckthorn berry intoxication and diphtheritic polyneuritis (see Table 363-2).

Subacute demyelinating polyneuropathy Neuropathies in this category are heterogeneous in origin, although all are acquired. Most common is a relapsing and remitting neuropathy which has many clinical features in common with GBS, but differs from GBS in tempo, course, and absence of discernible triggering events. Previously mentioned toxins (buckthorn berry, diphtheria toxin, aurothioglucose) may also induce a picture of widespread subacute demyelination of peripheral nerves (see Table 363-2).

Chronic demyelinating polyneuropathy Although more common than the subacute neuropathies, chronic polyneuropathy with demyelinating features encompasses a wide diversity of disorders, including hereditary neuropathies, inflammatory neuropathies, and other acquired neuropathies associated with diabetes mellitus, dysproteinemias, other metabolic states, and some chronic intoxications. To complicate matters, many of these disorders present an electrodiagnostic picture of mixed axonal-demyelinative findings. Frequently it is difficult to determine which process, axonal degeneration or demyelination, is the primary event. Aspects of many of these neuropathies are included in Tables 363-1 to 363-3 and in the sections below.

SPECIAL CATEGORIES OF NEUROPATHY   Hereditary neuropathies The major characteristics of this highly variegated group of disorders are summarized in Table 363-3. With the exception of the porphyric neuropathies, the onset of neuropathic dysfunction is insidious and progression is indolent over years or decades. Most of these diseases are quite rare with the striking exception of the dominantly inherited peroneal muscular atrophies (HMSN-I and HMSN-II; see Table 363-3). In peroneal muscular atrophy, phenotypic expression is often variable, so that affected family members of a propositus may have no symptoms and minimal neurologic findings but (in HMSN-I) may still show severe reduction of nerve conduction velocity.

Neuropathies with inflammation Acquired inflammatory demyelinating neuropathies fall into two major groups, the acute form called Guillain-Barré syndrome and more chronic forms, usually referred to as chronic inflammatory demyelinating polyradiculoneuropathy (CIDP). The entire group of acquired inflammatory demyelinating neuropathies constitutes a significant proportion of all cases of polyneuropathy and shares a distinctive clinical, electrophysiologic, and pathologic pattern. The diagnosis rests upon recognition of the clinical pattern and of other features, including elevated cerebrospinal fluid protein level, electrophysiologic changes (marked slowing of conduction velocities, delayed late responses, prolonged distal latencies, dispersion of evoked responses, and evidence of conduction block), and pathologic changes of low-grade inflammation and demyelination-remyelination of peripheral nerves. The course of GBS is acute and monophasic, whereas the more chronic forms pursue either a slowly progressive or a relapsing course. Cases with an intermediate course occur frequently enough to blur the diagnostic delimitation of GBS from the more chronic types of acquired inflammatory demyelinating neuropathy.

Pathogenetically, this group of inflammatory neuropathies is generally agreed to be immune-mediated, but the specific antigens involved and the crucial events of the immune response and why it is activated are uncertain.

Management of chronic, acquired CIPD involves a judicious mix of glucocorticoid therapy, other immunosuppressants, and plasmapheresis. These powerful agents are used only if the disorder is severe enough to threaten walking.

Diabetic neuropathies Classifications of the neuropathies of diabetes mellitus are found in Table 363-4. Although this provides a satisfactory frame of reference, the limitations inherent in classifying diabetic neuropathies should be understood. The most serious limitation is that most patients will not fit neatly into any single category, but rather will have overlapping clinical features of several. For instance, many diabetics with distal, primarily sensory polyneuropathy also can be shown to have autonomic dysfunction, usually in the form of vasomotor disturbance in the limbs and abnormalities of

sweating. Similarly, patients who develop a proximal motor syndrome may have dysautonomic features (including sexual impotence in males) and some degree of distal sensory polyneuropathy. To compound matters, such patients appear at risk to develop a cranial mononeuropathy.

Classifying the diabetic neuropathies tells us nothing of the pathogenesis of the neuropathic lesion. Rather, attempts at classification represent an educated guess at identifying the apparent anatomic sites of disorder and the critical clinical features. Pain is a frequent feature of diabetic neuropathies (see Table 363-4) but is variable in incidence and degree and is subjective in nature. The term diabetic amyotrophy should be avoided because of its ambiguity.

Diabetic neuropathies tend to occur in the setting of long-standing hyperglycemia (decades) whether insulin-dependent or not. By far the most common neuropathies related to diabetes mellitus are the diffuse sensory and autonomic types (categories 1 and 2 under "Symmetric" in Table 363-4). Sensory and autonomic polyneuropathy, chronic and indolent in evolution, may first be noticed in the third or fourth decade in patients with juvenile-onset diabetes but tends to occur after age 50 in patients with adult-onset diabetes. Focal and multifocal types of neuropathy are less common but quite dramatic (categories 1, 2, and 3 under "Asymmetric" in Table 363-4). They rarely occur before the age of 45 and are usually subacute or acute in onset. Cranial mononeuropathies refer to isolated sixth or third nerve palsies. The latter spares the pupil in three-fourths of cases, and some local pain or headache occurs in one-half. Truncal, or thoracoabdominal, neuropathy is painful, involves one or more intercostal or lumbar nerves unilaterally, and frequently coexists with the asymmetric proximal motor neuropathy. Femoral and obturator nerve–innervated muscles (quadriceps femoris, iliopsoas, adductor magnus) and loss of knee jerk on that side are the most evident features of asymmetric proximal motor neuropathy. Sensory deficit is minor, but pain in the hip and anterior thigh may predominate. Common to all of these multifocal and focal neuropathies is the strong likelihood for subsidence of pain within weeks to a year and partial or complete recovery of function. The same is true of symmetric proximal motor neuropathy (category 3 under "Symmetric" in Table 363-4).

Focal and multifocal diabetic neuropathies are considered to be ischemic in origin, and the basis for symmetric polyneuropathies, thought by some to involve abnormality of nerve metabolism, includes the possibility of ischemia.

Management of diabetic neuropathies is directed toward optimal control of hyperglycemia and symptomatic pain suppression. The role of aldose reductase inhibitors in preventing or reversing diabetic complications, including neuropathy, remains unclear. Entrapment neuropathies are frequently amenable to surgical decompression procedures.

Neuropathies with dysproteinemia An association between polyneuropathy and both multiple myeloma and macroglobulinemia has been recognized for many years. With commonly encountered multiple myeloma (MM) having either lytic or diffuse osteoporotic bone lesions, clinically overt polyneuropathy is relatively infrequent, occurring in approximately 5 percent of patients. These neuropathies are sensorimotor, may be severe, and generally do not reverse with successful suppression of the myeloma. In most cases, electrodiagnostic and pathologic features are consistent with a process of axonal degeneration.

In contrast, myeloma with osteosclerotic features, although representing only 3 percent of all myelomas, is associated with polyneuropathy in almost one-half of cases. These neuropathies, which may also occur with solitary plasmacytoma, seem to be different from those linked to MM in that they (1) often respond to radiation or removal of the primary lesion, (2) are more frequently demyelinating in character, (3) are associated with different monoclonal proteins and light chains (almost all lambda as opposed to mostly kappa in MM), and (4) frequently occur in association with other systemic findings. These include skin thickening, hyperpigmentation, hypertrichosis, organomegaly, endocrinopathy, anasarca, papilledema, and clubbing of fingers. (POEMS syndrome: *p*olyneuropathy, *o*rgano-megaly, *e*ndocrinopathy, *m* protein, and *s*kin changes.) A great deal of attention has been paid to this curious syndrome in Japan, where it is prevalent, but the underlying mechanism remains unknown.

Benign monoclonal gammopathy with an IgM serum spike, and usually with kappa light chains, is described in association with demyelinating polyneuropathy that often follows a protracted course and indolent progression. In about one-quarter of cases, the monoclonal serum protein binds to normal human peripheral myelin, specifically to myelin-associated glycoprotein. Immunocytochemical studies show binding of IgM to nerve obtained at biopsy or autopsy of these patients, but in a pattern different from that seen following incubation of sections of nerve with the IgM serum. Incubated nerves show uniform staining of the entire expanse of compact myelin sheath, but in vivo deposited IgM can be demonstrated to localize more selectively, probably at sites of myelin splitting, the latter a phenomenon characteristic of most dysglobulinemic neuropathies. Whether the IgM bound to nerve in vivo plays a role in damaging nerve is unresolved.

Autonomic neuropathy The autonomic nervous system regulates the visceral organs and vegetative functions. Many pharmacologic agents modify specific autonomic functions, but autonomic neuropathy (dysautonomia) with structural changes in pre- and postganglionic neurons can also occur. Usually autonomic neuropathy is a manifestation of a more generalized polyneuropathy also affecting somatic peripheral nervous function, as in diabetic neuropathy, GBS, and alcoholic polyneuropathy, but occasionally syndromes of pure pan-dysautonomia are encountered. Symptoms of dysautonomia are mainly negative (i.e., loss of function) and include postural hypotension with faintness or syncope, anhidrosis, hypothermia, bladder atony, obstipation, dry mouth and dry eyes from failure of salivary and lacrimal glands to secrete, blurring of vision from lack of pupillary and ciliary regulation, and sexual impotence in males. Positive phenomena (hyperfunction) may also occur and include episodic hypertension, diarrhea, hyperhidrosis, and either tachycardia or bradycardia.

Plexopathy This term refers to disorders of either the brachial or lumbosacral plexus. Lesions of the brachial plexus are characterized by motor and sensory signs different from those expected either in mononeuropathies of the upper limb or in polyneuropathies. The usual causes are direct trauma to the plexus, idiopathic brachial neuritis (also called neuralgic amyotrophy), cervical rib or band, infiltration by malignant tumor, or prior radiation therapy. When the upper parts of the brachial plexus, arising from cervical roots 5 through 7, are affected, weakness and atrophy of shoulder girdle and upper arm muscles occur. Injuries to the lower brachial plexus, arising from the eighth cervical and first thoracic roots, produce distal arm weakness, atrophy, and sensory deficit in the forearm and hand. In general, idiopathic brachial neuritis, radiation damage [greater than 60 Gy (6,000 rad)] and particular types of trauma (arm jerked downward) result in damage to the upper portions of the brachial plexus. In contrast, infiltration by malignant tumor, cervical rib or band, and certain other types of trauma (arm jerked upward) cause damage to the lower brachial plexus. Lumbosacral plexopathies are less common; they may be due to idiopathic lumbosacral plexitis, retroperitoneal hemorrhage, malignant tumor infiltration, or occur in association with long-standing diabetes mellitus.

Miscellaneous causes of neuropathy Ischemia of nerve severe enough to produce clinical symptoms has as its basis the widespread compromise of blood flow in the vasa nervorum. Typically, this is the result of small-vessel disease involving the vasa nervorum directly, as occurs with vasculitis, rather than large-vessel disease, such as atherosclerosis. Clinically, widespread disease of the vasa nervorum produces mononeuropathy multiplex, which electrodiagnostically has the features of a patchy axonal process.

Cold exerts deleterious effects on peripheral nerve directly without an intermediate step of ischemia being necessary. Cold injury to nerve occurs after prolonged exposure, usually of a limb, to moderately low temperatures, as with immersion of the feet in seawater; actual freezing of tissue is not required. Axonal degeneration of myelinated fibers is the pathologic expression of cold injury. Frequently limbs affected by cold injury to nerve show sensory deficit and dysesthesias, cutaneous vasomotor instability, pain, and marked sensitivity to minimal cold exposure, which persist for many years. The pathophysiology of these phenomena is uncertain.

TROPHIC CHANGES IN SEVERE NEUROPATHY The array of observable changes in completely denervated muscle, bone, and skin, including hair and nails, is well known, if incompletely understood. It is unclear what portion of the changes is due purely to denervation versus that caused by disuse, immobility, lack of weight bearing, and particularly recurrent, unnoticed, painless trauma. Considerable evidence favors the view that ulceration of skin, poor healing, tissue resorption, neurogenic arthropathy, and mutilation are the result of repeated heedless injury to insensitive parts. This sequence of events is avoidable with proper attention to and care of the insensitive parts by both patient and physician.

RECOVERY FROM NEUROPATHY In contrast to axons in the central nervous system, peripheral nerve fibers have an excellent capability to regenerate under proper circumstances. The process of regeneration following axonal degeneration may take from 2 months to more than a year, depending on the severity of the neuropathy and the length of regeneration required. Whether regeneration takes place depends upon the subsidence of the initial basis for neuropathy. This could be removal from contact with a neurotoxic substance or correction of an abnormal metabolic state. A deficit secondary to demyelination may recover rapidly since intact axons may remyelinate in just a few weeks. For example, a patient with GBS, in whom demyelination but no secondary axonal degeneration has occurred, may recover to normal strength from bedfastness and paralysis of arms and legs in as little as 3 to 4 weeks.

MONONEUROPATHY MULTIPLEX (MULTIFOCAL NEUROPATHY) This term means simultaneous or sequential involvement of individual noncontiguous nerve trunks, either partially or completely, evolving over days to years. Since the disease process underlying mononeuropathy multiplex involves peripheral nerves in a multifocal and random fashion, there is a tendency, as worsening occurs, for the neurologic deficit to become less patchy and multifocal and more confluent and symmetric. Some patients present initially with a distal symmetric neuropathy. Attention to the pattern of early symptoms is therefore important in making the judgment that a particular neuropathy is indeed a mononeuropathy multiplex.

Once that issue is settled, the next question is whether the process is primarily axonal or demyelinating. Almost one-third of all adults with the clinical syndrome of mononeuropathy multiplex have a clear-cut picture of a demyelinating disorder usually with multiple foci of persistent conduction block by electrodiagnostic examination. More intensive study of this subgroup suggests that the multifocal demyelinating neuropathy represents part of the spectrum of chronic acquired demyelinating neuropathy, that is, CIDP. Management of this multifocal subgroup is the same as for CIDP. (See "Neuropathies with Inflammation" above.)

The remaining two-thirds of patients with mononeuropathy multiplex have a picture by electrodiagnostic examination of axonal involvement that is heterogeneously distributed. Although ischemia would be suspected as the basis for neuropathy in these patients, only about one-half can be shown to have a process, usually vasculitis, affecting the vasa nervorum. The others remain undiagnosed even on follow-up, and the basis for their mononeuropathy multiplex is uncertain. Management in this group is conservative, but the management of those with proven vasculitis of vasa nervorum is the same as treatment for systemic vasculitis (see Chap. 276).

In individuals in whom vasculitic change in vasa nervorum can be demonstrated, any one of a large number of underlying disorders may be responsible. The primary vasculitides of the polyarteritis nodosa group constitute the most frequent basis, followed closely by the vasculitis syndrome occurring in the course of other connective tissue disorders. In descending order of frequency, the latter are rheumatoid arthritis, systemic lupus erythematosus, and mixed connective tissue disease. Other rarer causes of mononeuropathy multiplex due to nerve ischemia from occlusion of vasa nervorum include mixed cryoglobulinemia, Sjögren's syndrome, Wegener's granulomatosis, progressive systemic sclerosis, Churg-Strauss allergic granulomatosis, and hypersensitivity angiitides. Management of the neuropathy in each instance is predicated upon the appropriate treatment of the responsible disease.

Mononeuropathy multiplex syndrome may also be seen as a manifestation of leprosy, sarcoidosis, certain types of amyloidosis, hypereosinophilia syndrome, cryoglobulinemia, and multifocal types of diabetic neuropathy.

MONONEUROPATHY Mononeuropathy means focal involvement of a single nerve trunk and therefore implies a local causation.

TABLE 363-5 Some common mononeuropathies

Nerve	Origin (spinal segments)	Muscles innervated	Usual site of lesion	Clinical features	Comments
UPPER EXTREMITY					
Suprascapular	C5,C6	Supraspinatus Infraspinatus	Suprascapular notch of scapula	Weakness of lateral rotation of the humerus	No sensory deficit
Long thoracic	C5–C7	Serratus anterior	Variable	Winging of scapula	No sensory deficit
Axillary	C5,C6	Deltoid, teres minor	Near shoulder joint	Weakness of shoulder abduction; atrophy of shoulder	Sensory deficit similar to C5 dorsal root lesion (see Figs. 28-2 and 28-3)
Radial	C5–T1	Triceps, brachioradialis, wrist, finger, and thumb extensors	Spiral groove of humerus	Wrist drop most obvious, also finger and thumb extensors paralyzed	Saturday night palsy (acute compression) is frequent cause
Posterior interosseous branch	C7,C8	Finger and thumb extensors	Edge of supinator muscle below elbow	Finger drop; wrist relatively spared	No sensory deficit
Ulnar	C8,T1	Ulnar flexor of the wrist, long flexors of 4th and 5th digits, and most intrinsic hand muscles	Ulnar groove at the elbow	Weakness of finger adduction and abduction and thumb adduction (see text); interosseous atrophy, claw-hand	May be acute or insidious; sensory symptoms/signs are distinctive (Figs. 28-2 and 28-3); also see text
			Cubital tunnel	Same as above	Often pain over medial proximal forearm (cubital tunnel)
			Medial base of palm	Intrinsic hand muscles only, interosseous atrophy	No sensory deficit
Median	C6–T1	Abductor pollicis brevis; more proximal muscles include forearm pronator, long finger and thumb flexors	Carpal tunnel	Characteristic sensory symptoms and deficit and inability to make a circle with thumb and index finger	Sensory deficit as per Figs. 28-2 and 28-3 (see text); known as carpal tunnel syndrome
Anterior interosseous branch	C7–T1	Long flexors of thumb and index and middle fingers	Anterior interosseus branch below the elbow	Weakness of pinch; pain in volar forearm	No sensory deficit
LOWER EXTREMITY					
Femoral	L2–L4	Iliopsoas (hip flexor) and quadriceps femoris (knee extensor)	Proximal to inguinal ligament	Knee buckling; absent knee jerk; weak anterior thigh muscles with atrophy	Association with diabetes mellitus; sensory disturbance as per Fig. 28-2
Lateral femoral cutaneous branch	L2,L3	None	Inguinal ligament	Dysesthetic hyperpathia of lateral thigh	Known as meralgia paresthetica
Obturator	L3,L4	Thigh adductors	Intrapelvic or at pubis	Weakness of hip adduction	Sensory deficit on medial thigh
Sciatic	L4–S3	Hamstring muscles, hip abductor and all muscles below the knee	Near sciatic notch	Severe lower leg and hamstring weakness; flail foot; severe disability	Uncommon except from war wounds
Posterior tibial	L5–S2	Calf muscles (proximally), toe flexors and other intrinsic foot muscles	Tarsal tunnel, near medial malleolus	Pain and numbness of sole, weak toe flexors	Known as tarsal tunnel syndrome
Peroneal	L4–S1	Dorsiflexors of toes and foot, evertors of foot	At neck of fibula	Foot drop and weakness of foot eversion	Sensory deficit is similar in distribution to L5, S1 sensory roots

Direct trauma, compression, and entrapment are the usual causes. Ulnar neuropathies, due to lesions either at the ulnar groove or in the cubital tunnel, and median neuropathy due to compression in the carpal tunnel constitute the great majority of mononeuropathies encountered in clinical practice. These are described below, and other common mononeuropathies are listed in Table 363-5.

In the absence of a history of trauma to the nerve trunk, factors favoring conservative management include sudden onset, no motor deficit, few or no sensory findings even though pain and sensory symptoms might be present, and no evidence of axonal degeneration by electrodiagnostic criteria. Factors favoring surgical intervention include chronicity and worsening neurologic deficit on examination, particularly if motor, and electrodiagnostic evidence that the lesion has produced a degree of wallerian degeneration.

Ulnar nerve Complete ulnar paralysis results in a characteristic claw-hand deformity owing to wasting of the small hand muscles and hyperextension of the fingers at the metacarpophalangeal joints and flexion at the interphalangeal joints. The flexion deformity is most pronounced in the fourth and fifth fingers. Sensory loss occurs over the fifth finger, the ulnar aspect of the fourth finger, and the ulnar border of the palm. The superficial location of the nerve at the elbow makes it a common site of pressure palsy. The ulnar nerve may also become entrapped just distal to the elbow in the cubital tunnel formed by the aponeurotic arch linking the two heads of the flexor carpi ulnaris. Prolonged pressure on the base of the palm, as occurs with use of hand tools or bicycle riding, may result in damage to the deep palmar branch of the ulnar nerve, causing weakness of the small hand muscles but no sensory loss.

Median nerve The median nerve in the carpal tunnel lies in close quarters with nine tendons. Entrapment of the nerve at the wrist (carpal tunnel syndrome) may be secondary to excessive use of the wrist, tenosynovitis with arthritis, or local infiltration, for example, by a thickening of connective tissue and deposit of amyloid with multiple myeloma or one of the mucopolysaccharides. Other systemic diseases associated with an increased incidence of carpal tunnel syndrome are acromegaly, hypothyroidism, rheumatoid arthritis, and diabetes mellitus, but these account for only a small fraction of all cases. The main symptoms of carpal tunnel syndrome are nocturnal paresthesias of thumb, index, and middle fingers. With worsening, numbness demonstrable by pin examination occurs in that distribution, and eventually weakness and atrophy of the abductor pollicis brevis (thenar eminence) becomes evident. Treatment of carpal tunnel syndrome is surgical section of the carpal ligament. Incomplete lesions of the median nerve between the axilla and wrist may result in causalgia (a particularly severe type of burning pain; see Chap. 15).

OTHER FOCAL NEUROPATHIES Peripheral nerve tumors These are mostly benign and can arise on any nerve trunk or twig. Although peripheral nerve tumors occur anywhere in the body including the spinal roots and cauda equina, many are subcutaneous in location and present as a soft swelling, sometimes with a purplish discoloration of the skin. Two major categories of peripheral nerve tumors are recognized: neurilemmoma (schwannoma) and neurofibroma. Neurilemmomas are usually solitary and grow within the nerve sheath, rendering the tumor relatively easy to dissect free. In contrast, neurofibromas tend to be multiple, grow within the endoneurial substance, rendering them difficult to dissect, may undergo malignant changes, and are the hallmark of von Recklinghausen's neurofibromatosis. This disease is characterized by an autosomal dominant inheritance pattern, any number of neurofibromas from one to thousands, five or more café au lait–pigmented skin lesions greater than 1.5 cm (80 percent of patients), axillary freckles (93 percent of patients), and an increased incidence of seizure disorder and mental retardation (see Chap. 358).

Herpes zoster This is a sensory neuritis of viral cause characterized by acute inflammation of one or more dorsal root ganglia, due to varicella-zoster virus infection. Lancinating pain and hyperalgesia over the skin surface supplied by affected roots occur for 3 to 4 days, followed by the appearance of herpetic eruption in the same segment characterized by painful raised blisters on reddened bases. If the inflammatory process spreads to involve adjacent motor roots of anterior horns of the cord, segmental motor weakness and wasting appear. Paralysis of the oculomotor nerves may occur in conjunction with ophthalmic division involvement of the trigeminal ganglion (ophthalmoplegic zoster). Facial paralysis may occur with involvement of the geniculate ganglion and herpetic eruption on the ipsilateral tympanic membrane or external ear canal (Ramsay Hunt syndrome).

Leprous neuritis This is a major worldwide cause of neuropathy. *Mycobacterium leprae* organisms readily invade Schwann cells in cutaneous nerve twigs, particularly those associated with unmyelinated nerve fibers. Two major forms of leprous neuritis are recognized, tuberculoid and lepromatous, which actually represent the far ends of a spectrum of disease, the middle of which is called dimorphous leprosy (patchy and multifocal involvement of skin and nerve). Treatment depends upon where in the spectrum a given case is classified (see Chap. 126). Tuberculoid (high-resistance) leprosy is restricted to a single patch of hypesthetic or anesthetic skin in any location. The skin patch is frequently thickened, reddened, or hypopigmented. If a superficially placed nerve trunk, typically a cutaneous nerve, courses just beneath the area of affected skin, it may be engulfed in the inflammatory reaction, resulting in an associated mononeuropathy. Such a nerve may be palpably enlarged and beaded. Lepromatous (low-resistance) leprosy is marked by immunologic tolerance and widespread skin thickening, cutaneous anesthesia, and anhidrosis, sparing only the warmest parts of the body, notably the axilla, groin, and beneath the scalp hair. Motor signs (focal weakness and atrophy) result from damage to mixed nerves lying close to the skin, particularly the median, ulnar, peroneal, and facial nerves.

Bell's palsy This is due to inflammation of the facial nerve in the facial canal, the basis for which remains obscure. Edema may play a part leading to compression of nerve fibers, with resulting acute unilateral paralysis of facial muscles (see Chap. 360).

Sarcoidosis This may involve single or multiple peripheral nerves, producing asymmetric mononeuritis or polyneuritis. Unilateral or bilateral facial paralysis is described in association with parotitis and uveitis (Heerfordt's syndrome).

Polyneuritis cranialis This is a relapsing and remitting mononeuropathy multiplex restricted to cranial nerves. It is usually associated with indolent tuberculous cervical adenitis (scrofula) or sarcoidosis. Treatment of the underlying condition will halt the cranial nerve palsies.

Acknowledgment

By arrangement with the publishers, portions of this section also appear in substantially the same form in Asbury AK: Diseases of peripheral nerve, in *Diseases of the Nervous System*, AK Asbury, GM McKhann, WI McDonald (eds). Philadelphia, Saunders, 1986, and London, Heinemann, 1986.

REFERENCES

ASBURY AK: New aspects of disease of the peripheral nervous system, in *Harrison's Textbook of Internal Medicine, Update IV*. McGraw Hill, New York, 1983, 211 229
———, GILLIATT RW: *Peripheral Nerve Disorders: A Practical Approach*. London, Butterworth, 1984
BENSON MD: Familial amyloidotic polyneuropathy. Trends Neurosci 12: 88, 1989
BROWN MJ (eds): Neuropathy. Semin Neurol 7:1, 1987
DAWSON DM et al: *Entrapment Neuropathies*. Boston, Little, Brown, 1983
DYCK PJ et al (eds): *Peripheral Neuropathy*, 2d ed. Philadelphia, Saunders, 1984
———: *Diabetic Neuropathy*. Philadelphia, Saunders, 1987
LAYZER RB: *Neuromuscular Manifestations of Systemic Disease*, vol 25: *Contemporary Neurology Series*. Philadelphia, Davis, 1984
SPENCER PS, SCHAUMBURG HH (eds): *Experimental and Clinical Neurotoxicology*. Baltimore, Williams & Wilkins, 1980
STEWART JD: *Focal Peripheral Neuropathics*. New York, Elsevier, 1987

364   DERMATOMYOSITIS AND POLYMYOSITIS

WALTER G. BRADLEY / RUP TANDAN

Dermatomyositis and polymyositis are conditions of unknown etiology in which the skeletal muscle is damaged by a nonsuppurative inflammatory process dominated by lymphocytic infiltration. The term *polymyositis* is applied when the condition spares the skin and the term *dermatomyositis* when polymyositis is associated with a characteristic skin rash. One-third of cases are associated with various connective tissue disorders, such as rheumatoid arthritis, lupus erythematosus, mixed connective tissue disorder, and scleroderma, and one-tenth with a malignancy.

ETIOLOGY   The cause of these diseases is unknown. The two main theories are that the diseases are due to a viral infection of the skeletal muscle or to an autoimmune disorder (Chap. 276). Experimental viral myositis can be induced in animals by coxsackievirus. A mild inflammatory myopathy can occur with influenza. The numerous electron-microscope observations of virus-like particles in muscle fibers in dermatomyositis or polymyositis have not been confirmed by virus isolation, rising titers of antiviral antibodies have not been demonstrated, and the disease has not been passed into animals by injection of extracts of affected muscles. One-third of cases have elevated serum antibodies to toxoplasma, but the disease does not generally respond to therapy against toxoplasmosis. A lymphocyte-mediated disease resembling polymyositis has been reported in laboratory animals injected with sterile muscle extracts together with Freund's adjuvant (experimental allergic myositis). Immunohistochemical studies of muscle have shown that fiber necrosis probably results from the action of activated T cells and macrophages in polymyositis, and from T-helper-cell-dependent stimulation of B cells with resultant antibody-mediated cytotoxicity in dermatomyositis. A small proportion of patients have deposition of immunoglobulins on intramuscular blood vessels, suggesting that circulating antibodies may play some role in the disease. The close association of polymyositis and diseases of connective tissue favors the notion of a common autoimmune etiology or pathogenesis. In older patients dermatomyositis is frequently associated with a malignancy. Thus, dermatomyositis-polymyositis is a syndrome which probably has a number of different causes.

CLASSIFICATION   The classification of the dermatomyositis-polymyositis group which is most widely used is given in Table 364-1. This classification is based partly on known differences in etiology and has a number of drawbacks, as noted below. Other uncommon associations of polymyositis are sarcoidosis, giant cell myositis with thymoma, and myositis in systemic infections due to viruses, toxoplasma, or parasites. A focal infective myositis due to streptococcal or staphylococcal infection is mostly seen in the tropics. Focal nodular myositis is a variant of polymyositis where focal areas of myositis cause hot, often painful, multifocal muscle masses. Inclusion body myositis is an inflammatory myopathy with characteristic clinical and pathologic features (see below).

INCIDENCE   Current estimates that the annual incidence of the inflammatory myopathies is about five per million of the population are probably too low.

TABLE 364-1   Classification of polymyositis-dermatomyositis

Group I:	Primary idiopathic polymyositis
Group II:	Primary idiopathic dermatomyositis
Group III:	Dermatomyositis (or polymyositis) associated with neoplasia
Group IV:	Childhood dermatomyositis (or polymyositis) associated with vasculitis
Group V:	Polymyositis (or dermatomyositis) with associated collagen vascular disease

SOURCE: Classification suggested by Bohan et al.

CLINICAL MANIFESTATIONS   Group I: Primary idiopathic polymyositis   This group comprises about one-third of all cases of inflammatory myopathy. It is insidiously progressive over weeks, months, or even years. Rarely the disease is acute, producing severe muscle weakness in a matter of days. The disease may develop at any age and in either sex. Females outnumber males 2:1.

The patients first become aware of weakness of the proximal limb muscles, especially the hips and thighs, and find difficulty in arising from the squatting or kneeling position and in climbing or descending stairs. When shoulder girdle muscles are involved, placing an object on a high shelf or combing the hair becomes difficult. Occasionally the disease is more restricted, affecting only the neck, the shoulder, or the quadriceps muscles. Pain of an aching type in the buttocks, thighs, and calves is experienced in about 10 percent of the cases, and tenderness on palpation in another 20 percent. Early symptoms of dysphagia and weakness of flexor muscles of the neck in a patient with a chronic myopathy suggest the diagnosis of polymyositis.

When the patient is first seen, there may be weakness of the muscles of the trunk, the pectoral and pelvic girdles, the upper arms and thighs, the anterior neck, more so than the posterior, and the pharynx. Ocular muscles are almost never affected except in a rare association with myasthenia gravis. The distal muscles are spared in about 75 percent of cases. Muscle atrophy, contractures, and diminished tendon reflexes are rare in early myositis and never as pronounced as in muscular dystrophies and denervating conditions. When the reflexes are disproportionately reduced, carcinoma with polymyositis and polyneuropathy or the Lambert-Eaton syndrome should be considered. Occasionally, the reflexes may be paradoxically brisk in dermatomyositis-polymyositis, perhaps due to irritation of muscle spindle receptors by the inflammation.

At presentation about 25 percent of patients have dysphagia, about 5 percent have significant respiratory impairment, and 5 percent are unable to walk. Dysphagia is due to involvement of striated muscles of the pharynx and upper esophagus. At some time in the course of the disease cardiac abnormalities are observed in about 30 percent of cases; these include ECG changes, arrhythmias, and heart failure secondary to myocarditis. About half of the fatal cases have pathologic evidence of cardiac disease with necrosis of myocardial fibers, usually with only modest inflammatory reaction. The frequency of myocardial infarction may be increased in those treated for long periods with glucocorticoids. In a few cases there is dyspnea due to lymphocytic pneumonitis, pulmonary edema, or pulmonary fibrosis. Arthralgia, Raynaud's phenomenon, and, rarely, low-grade fever may also be present.

Group II: Primary idiopathic dermatomyositis   This group comprises just over one-third of all cases of myositis. The skin changes may precede or follow the muscle syndrome and include a localized or diffuse erythema, maculopapular eruption, scaling eczematoid dermatitis, or, rarely, an exfoliative dermatitis. The classic lilac-colored (heliotrope) rash is on the eyelids, bridge of the nose, cheeks (butterfly distribution), forehead, chest, elbows, knees and knuckles, and around the nail beds. Itching may be troublesome in some cases. The skin lesions may be subtle and easily overlooked. Periorbital edema is frequent, particularly in acute cases. The skin lesions may occasionally ulcerate. Subcutaneous calcification may occur, especially in children.

The typical rash and myositis allow a diagnosis of dermatomyositis, and such cases may be placed in this category (group II, Table 364-1) if idiopathic and into groups III, IV, and V if there are other features, namely malignancy, vasculitis in children, and an established collagen vascular disease. There should be concern about an underlying malignancy in patients with dermatomyositis over the age of 60.

Group III: Polymyositis or dermatomyositis with neoplasia   This syndrome, which comprises about 8 percent of all cases of myositis, is categorized separately, although muscle and skin changes are indistinguishable from those in the other groups. Malignancy, however, is uncommon in myositis seen in children and in association with a connective tissue disorder. The malignancy may antedate or postdate the onset of the myositis by up to 2 years. The incidence of this paraneoplastic syndrome is higher in patients with dermatomyositis over the age of 60; therefore, in such patients a thorough history and clinical examination (including breast and rectal) must be supplemented by hemogram, biochemical profile, urine analysis for blood and cytology, stool samples for occult blood, chest x-ray, and sputum for cytology seeking clues for an underlying malignancy. This relatively inexpensive search often uncovers most malignancies; undirected radiologic screening procedures are costly and unhelpful in improving the yield. The most common malignancies are lung, ovary, breast, gastrointestinal tract, and myeloproliferative disorders. The myositis is a paraneoplastic syndrome, the cause of which may lie in an altered immune status or an occult viral infection of the muscle.

Group IV: Childhood polymyositis and dermatomyositis associated with vasculitis This group comprises about 8 to 20 percent of all cases of myositis in various series. Inflammatory myopathy in childhood is frequently associated with skin involvement and clinical or pathologic evidence of vasculitis in skin, muscles, gastrointestinal tract, and other organs. There are degeneration and loss of capillaries in a perifascicular distribution in the skeletal muscles; often necrotizing lesions of the skin; and ischemic infarction of kidneys, gastrointestinal tract, and rarely brain. Consequently, some authors have reported mortality rates of up to one-third in childhood dermatomyositis, though most have found that the prognosis is better than in adult dermatomyositis-polymyositis. One limitation of the classification of Bohan et al. is that it is not clear whether or not all cases of childhood myositis should be included in group IV. Subcutaneous calcification is frequently present in childhood dermatomyositis.

Group V: Polymyositis or dermatomyositis with an associated connective tissue disorder This "overlap group" comprises about one-fifth of all cases of myositis. Scleroderma, rheumatoid arthritis, mixed connective tissue disease, and lupus erythematosus are the most common associated conditions; polyarteritis nodosa and rheumatic fever are more rarely associated. Criteria for placement in the overlap group combine the demonstration of the appropriate clinical and laboratory abnormalities required for the diagnosis of the connective tissue disorder together with clinical and laboratory evidence of myositis. The diagnosis of myositis is often difficult in patients with connective tissue disorders producing arthritis, since this may often produce muscle weakness with type II fiber atrophy. Moreover, perivascular inflammatory foci are common in muscle in connective tissue disorders. Demonstration of increased serum creatine kinase (CK), electromyography (EMG), and muscle biopsy are often required to make this diagnosis. Though patients in this overlap group usually respond to glucocorticoid therapy, the prognosis for recovery of function is poorer than in pure dermatomyositis-polymyositis. Dysphagia in group V patients with scleroderma is often due to involvement of the smooth muscle of the distal third of the esophagus.

Other disorders associated with myositis SARCOIDOSIS AND POLYMYOSITIS The skeletal muscle contains noncaseating granulomas with Langhans-type multinuclear giant cells in at least one-quarter of patients with sarcoidosis. Symptomatic polymyositis is, however, uncommon. Regenerating multinuclear myoblasts resemble Langhans' giant cells, which has led to misdiagnosis in many of the cases reported in the literature to have "sarcoid myositis." Giant cell or granulomatous polymyositis and myocarditis, sometimes associated with myasthenia gravis, have been recorded in patients with thymomas.

FOCAL NODULAR MYOSITIS A syndrome of acutely developing and painful focal inflammatory nodules, sometimes occurring sequentially in different muscles, has been termed *focal nodular myositis*. The pathologic appearance and response to therapy are similar to those in generalized polymyositis. The differential diagnosis includes, when single, a muscle tumor (sarcoma or rhabdomyosarcoma) and, when multiple, muscle infarcts such as can occur in polyarteritis nodosa.

INFECTIOUS POLYMYOSITIS Rare cases of polymyositis have clear-cut evidence of being due to known pathogens such as toxoplasma (Chap. 162), viruses (Chap. 144), and spirochetes (Lyme disease). Antibody screening will suggest the diagnosis in such cases. Polymyositis occurs in homosexual men infected with the human immunodeficiency virus (HIV), sometimes as the presenting feature and rarely due to therapy with zidovudine (AZT). Raised serum CK, EMG evidence of a myopathy, and muscle fiber necrosis with or without inflammatory infiltrates are seen. Trichinosis may be confused with iodiopathic polymyositis, particularly if the history of raw pork ingestion is not obtained. The symptoms of trichinosis are variable and depend upon the parasitic load. Low-grade fever, muscle pain of variable degree, conjunctival and periorbital edema, and fatigue are frequent. Weakness is generally mild. Heavy infestation is often associated with central nervous system symptoms of delirium, coma, or focal neurologic deficit. The frequent myocardial involvement is manifested by tachycardia and ECG changes. The diagnosis is made by the history of ingestion of undercooked pork, marked eosinophilia, sensitivity to intradermal *Trichina* antigen, and the appearance of serum antibodies to *Trichina* during the course of the disease. Occasionally the diagnosis is not recognized until a muscle is biopsied. Pyomyositis, a suppurative inflammation of muscle due to staphylococcus or streptococcus, is mainly seen in the tropics. The presentation is that of a diffuse abscess of the muscle.

INCLUSION BODY MYOSITIS The clinical features of this condition are similar to those of chronic idiopathic polymyositis, except that focal and distal muscle involvement are more frequent. Muscle biopsy shows interstitial and occasionally perivascular inflammatory infiltration, necrosis, and regeneration of muscle fibers, but in addition there are "rimmed vacuoles" in the fibers. Electron microscopy reveals paramyxovirus-like filaments in the nuclei and sarcoplasm. The nature of these filaments is still in dispute. This disorder responds poorly to immunosuppressive therapy, and the prognosis is for a chronically progressive disorder with loss of ambulation about 5 to 10 years after presentation.

EOSINOPHILIC MYOSITIS This rare disease probably represents one manifestation of the spectrum of hypereosinophilic syndrome. Subacute onset of muscle pain and proximal weakness, elevated serum CK, myopathic features on electromyogram, and histologic appearances of a myositis with an eosinophilic inflammatory infiltrate are characteristic. Some patients may respond to glucocorticoids, methotrexate, or leukapheresis.

EOSINOPHILIC FASCIITIS This disorder is characterized by painful swelling and thickening of the skin in the extremities, limitation of movement due to contractures, and mild muscle weakness. Raised sedimentation rate, peripheral eosinophilia, hypergammaglobulinemia, and mildly elevated CK are seen. The EMG may show myopathic features. Histologically there is marked thickening and infiltration of the deep fascia with mononuclear cells and eosinophils, some involvement of the epimysium and perimysium, and varying but not striking degeneration of muscle. Most patients respond to treatment with glucocorticoids.

RELAPSING EOSINOPHILIC PERIMYOSITIS In this disease there are recurrent painful and tender areas in the neck or lower extremities, but without muscle weakness. Raised sedimentation rate and peripheral eosinophilia are frequent, serum CK is sometimes raised, and pathologically there is eosinophilic infiltration of the perimysium. Response to glucocorticoids is usually good.

LABORATORY FINDINGS In all forms of polymyositis there may be elevated serum levels of the enzymes present in skeletal muscle, such as CK, aldolase, serum glutamic oxaloacetic transaminase (SGOT), lactic acid dehydrogenase (LDH), and serum glutamic pyruvate transaminase (SGPT). The degree of rise decreases from the first to the last in this series of enzymes, and the pattern is the reverse of that seen in liver disease. Tests for circulating rheumatoid factor and antinuclear antibodies are positive in less than one-half of the cases. Myoglobin can be found in the urine when muscle destruction is acute and extensive; rarely, acute polymyositis causes the full syndrome of rhabdomyolysis and myoglobinuria. The erythrocyte sedimentation rate is elevated in about two-thirds of cases. Most other hematologic indexes are normal. In about 40 percent of cases the electromyogram reveals a markedly increased insertional activity (muscle irritability), together with the typical myopathic triad of motor unit action potentials which are of low amplitude, are polyphasic, and have an abnormally early recruitment. In a further 40 percent of the patients only myopathic changes are present. The ECG is abnormal in about 5 to 10 percent of the cases at presentation. Since the pathologic process in myositis is patchy, greater diagnostic yield is obtained by taking the biopsy from two clinically affected muscles and by skip serial sectioning of all specimens. Muscles recently used for EMG or intramuscular injection must be avoided as these procedures can produce inflammatory changes and muscle fiber damage, leading to false-positive results. In about two-thirds of cases, the biopsies will demonstrate the typical pathologic changes of myositis, but despite following the above recommendations, about 10 percent of cases have normal muscle biopsy.

Skeletal muscle pathology   The principal changes in muscle consist of infiltrates of inflammatory cells (lymphocytes, macrophages, plasma cells, and rare eosinophils and neutrophils) and destruction of muscle fibers with a phagocytic reaction. Perivascular (usually perivenular) inflammatory cell infiltration is the hallmark of polymyositis. Interstitial inflammatory cell infiltration is also a prominent feature of the disease, but lesser degrees of it may be seen in other conditions as a secondary reaction (e.g., in facioscapulohumeral and Becker's muscular dystrophy). The inflammatory infiltrates contain activated T cells of the helper-inducer and cytotoxic-suppressor types, with accompanying macrophages in polymyositis, and B cells in dermatomyositis. Evidence of muscle fiber degeneration and regeneration is almost invariably present. Many of the residual muscle fibers are small, with increased numbers of sarcolemmal nuclei. Either the degeneration of muscle fibers or the infiltration of inflammatory cells may predominate in any given biopsy specimen. Blood vessel changes and perifascicular atrophy are prominent in childhood dermatomyositis, but less so in adult dermatomyositis and polymyositis. Capillary loss due to endothelial cell necrosis occurs particularly in the periphery of fascicles and may explain the perifascular atrophy. Other features include reduplication of capillary basement membrane and the presence of tubular inclusions within endothelial cells. Type II muscle fiber atrophy and muscle infarcts may also be found. Vasculitis is also seen in polymyositis or dermatomyositis associated with connective tissue disorders.

DIAGNOSIS   Patients with dermatomyositis with the characteristic skin rash, muscle weakness, and evidence of muscle damage by EMG and elevation of serum CK may not require a muscle biopsy to confirm the diagnosis. In the case of idiopathic polymyositis, however, a firm diagnosis must be based on the presence of a typical clinical picture, a typical EMG, elevation of serum CK, and a diagnostic muscle biopsy. All four criteria are required to be certain of the diagnosis, since inflammatory changes may occasionally occur in other myopathies (e.g., facioscapulohumeral muscular dystrophy) and in other connective tissue disorders without clear muscle weakness. However, in less than one-third of cases of polymyositis are *all* these criteria satisfied. It may be particularly difficult to obtain a diagnostic muscle biopsy because of the patchy nature of the disease. Thus, a therapeutic trial of glucocorticoids should be given when full investigation of a patient with significant disability leaves a diagnosis of "possible polymyositis," usually because of a nondiagnostic muscle biopsy.

DIFFERENTIAL DIAGNOSIS   The clinical picture of skin rash and proximal or diffuse muscle weakness has few causes other than dermatomyositis. However, proximal muscle weakness without skin involvement can be due to many conditions other than polymyositis and necessitates detailed investigation to establish the correct diagnosis.

Subacute or chronic progressive muscle weakness   This may be due to denervating conditions such as the spinal muscular atrophies

or amyotrophic lateral sclerosis. Upper motor neuron signs in the latter in addition to the muscle weakness aid in the diagnosis. The muscular dystrophies, such as those of Duchenne and Becker and the limb-girdle and facioscapulohumeral types, may appear similar to polymyositis (Chap. 365). However, the muscular dystrophies usually develop more slowly, rarely present after the age of 30, usually involve the pharyngeal and posterior neck muscles only in their later course, and have a pattern of muscle involvement which is selective, involving some muscles such as the biceps and brachioradialis early in the course of the disease, and sparing others, such as the deltoid. Nevertheless, in rare patients it may be difficult, even with a muscle biopsy, to distinguish chronic polymyositis from a rapidly advancing muscular dystrophy. This is particularly true of facioscapulohumeral muscular dystrophy, where interstitial inflammatory cell infiltration is commonly found early in the disease. Such doubtful cases should always be given an adequate trial of glucocorticoid therapy. Dystrophia myotonica produces a characteristic facies with ptosis, facial myopathy, temporalis muscle wasting, and grip myotonia (Chap. 365). Some of the metabolic myopathies, including glycogen storage disease due to myophosphorylase deficiency and the lipid storage diseases due to carnitine and carnitine palmityltransferase deficiency, produce exertional cramps, rhabdomyolysis, and muscle weakness; diagnosis rests upon biochemical studies of the muscle biopsy (Chap. 365). Glycogen storage disease due to acid maltase deficiency also requires muscle biopsy for diagnosis. The endocrine myopathies such as those due to hypercorticosteroidism, hyper- and hypothyroidism, and hyper- and hypoparathyroidism require the appropriate laboratory investigations for diagnosis. Muscle wasting in patients with an underlying neoplasm may be true polymyositis, but it can be due to a protein-wasting state (cachexia), a paraneoplastic neuropathy, or type II fiber atrophy.

Muscle weakness with marked exercise-induced fatigue   Fatigue without much muscle wasting may be due to the neuromuscular junction disorders, myasthenia gravis, or the Lambert-Eaton syndrome. Repetitive nerve stimulation studies aid in the diagnosis of these conditions (Chap. 366).

Acute muscle weakness   This may be caused by an acute neuropathy such as that due to the Guillain-Barré syndrome or a neurotoxin. When combined with painful muscle cramps, rhabdomyolysis, and myoglobinuria, it may be due to known metabolic disorders including some of the glycogen storage diseases such as myophosphorylase deficiency (McArdle's disease), carnitine palmityltransferase deficiency, and myoadenylate deaminase deficiency. Acute viral infections may cause a similar syndrome. Chronic alcoholics may develop a painful myopathy with myoglobinuria after a bout of heavy drinking or may present with a painless acute hypokalemic myopathy which is completely reversible, or may show an asymptomatic elevation of serum CK and myoglobin. Acute muscle weakness with myoglobinuria may occur in prolonged severe hypokalemia due to potassium loss, or with hypophosphatemia and hypomagnesemia, often seen in chronic alcoholics and in patients on nasogastric suction receiving parental hyperalimentation. An acute necrotizing myopathy with myoglobinuria can rarely accompany hypernatremia and hyponatremia.

Drug-induced myopathies   Rhabdomyolysis and myoglobinuria have been associated with intake of amphotericin B, ε-aminocaproic acid, fenfluramine, heroin, and phencyclidine. A predominantly hypokalemic myopathy may result from prolonged use of diuretics, carbenoxolone, and azathioprine. Penicillamine has been reported to produce a myositis. The use of clofibrate, cimetidine, chloroquine, emetine, and, recently, AZT has been associated with a myopathy. Toxic myopathies usually have a different pathology from polymyositis and require a careful drug history for diagnosis. In other cases investigation reveals no etiology, and these may be due to a true acute autoimmune polymyositis or to an as yet undiscovered metabolic defect.

Pain on movement and muscle tenderness   Patients with muscle pain and little or no weakness may be thought to be neurotic or hysterical. A number of conditions including *polymyalgia rheumatica* (Chap. 276) and arthritic disorders of adjacent joints enter into the differential diagnosis of polymyositis. The muscle biopsy either is normal or discloses type II fiber atrophy, but in polymyalgia rheumatica the temporal artery biopsy may show giant cell arteritis (Chap. 276). *Fibrositis* and *fibromyalgia* are syndromes which frequently enter into the differential diagnosis of polymyositis. Patients complain of focal or diffuse muscle tenderness, aching, and weakness, which is sometimes poorly separated from joint pain. In other patients there may be minor signs of a collagen vascular disorder, such as an increased erythrocyte sedimentation rate, antinuclear antibody (ANA), or rheumatoid factor, and occasionally there is slight elevation of the serum CK. The muscle biopsy occasionally shows a few interstitial inflammatory cells. Where there is a focal "trigger point," biopsy may show inflammatory infiltration of the connective tissue. Rarely does this syndrome develop into frank polymyositis, and the prognosis is therefore more benign than that of polymyositis (see below). Many such patients show some response to nonsteroidal anti-inflammatory agents, though most continue to have indolent complaints.

TREATMENT Glucocorticoids in high dosage are the accepted treatment for severe dermatomyositis-polymyositis, though there is no controlled trial to prove their effectiveness. The best results are obtained from the use of prednisone, starting at a dose of 1 to 2 mg/kg body weight per day (60 to 100 mg/d for adults). Improvement may begin within 1 to 4 weeks, though in some patients treatment may need to be continued for 3 months before improvement occurs. When there is significant improvement in the weakness, the daily dose may be reduced by 5 mg every 4 weeks. Repeated manual muscle testing and serum CK determinations should be performed to ensure that the myositis does not relapse. At about 40 mg/d, the schedule is changed gradually to 80 mg every other day in order to reduce the incidence of glucocorticoid side effects. There is some evidence that the use of alternate-day glucocorticoids from the outset may be effective, particularly in patients with milder disease. Children and patients with acute to subacute dermatomyositis-polymyositis tend to improve more rapidly than those with chronic polymyositis. If the dose is reduced too rapidly, or to too low a level, relapse will occur, necessitating return to high dosage. Prednisone therapy may have to be continued for several years, but an attempt should be made every year to withdraw the therapy from patients who are clinically stable in order to determine if the disease is still active.

Cytotoxic drugs should be tried when the disease is severe, when the response to glucocorticoids is inadequate after 1 to 3 months, or when relapses are frequent. Azathioprine (2.5 to 3.5 mg/kg body weight per day in divided doses) is the most commonly used cytotoxic drug in this disease, and in combination with glucocorticoids in preliminary studies has shown a better response than glucocorticoids alone. Cyclophosphamide and methotrexate have also been used with benefit. The aim of cytotoxic therapy with azathioprine or cyclophosphamide is to lower the total lymphocyte count to about 750 per microliter, while maintaining the hemoglobin level above 12 g/dL, the total white cell count above 3000 per microliter, and the platelet count above 125,000 per microliter. Weekly blood counts are required to monitor the cytotoxic drug therapy. Methotrexate is effective at doses that do not produce lymphopenia. The combined use of prednisone and a cytotoxic drug usually allows a lower dose of prednisone to be used. In preliminary studies total-body irradiation has been successfully used in some patients with disease refractory to glucocorticoids and immunosuppressants, but long-term follow-up is lacking. Bed rest has been recommended in the acute phase of the disease but is harmful in the long term. Physiotherapy and rehabilitative devices are important in the long-term treatment of patients with dermatomyositis-polymyositis.

Elderly patients, particularly those with dermatomyositis, should be followed closely for the possibility of malignant disease, and any new symptoms or signs must be appropriately investigated by a directed approach. If a malignant lesion is found, it should be treated, since the muscle weakness may disappear if the neoplasm is eradicated.

However, a response to glucocorticoids can usually be obtained even in patients with polymyositis associated with a malignancy.

The serum CK activity is useful for following patients during reduction of immunosuppressant therapy, since a rise in level generally indicates an incipient clinical relapse. However, it cannot be used to indicate initial response in patients being treated with prednisone for dermatomyositis-polymyositis, since this drug lowers the serum CK activity in a way which is not fully understood, but which is not related to the suppression of muscle inflammation.

Side effects of high-dose daily glucocorticoid therapy (see Chap. 317) are relatively common in patients treated for polymyositis, and these may limit therapy. However, these can be minimized by appropriate use of alternate-day therapy. When patients who have been stable on a static dose of prednisone develop increasing muscle weakness, this may be due to either a relapse of the myositis or to glucocorticoid myopathy. An EMG, serum CK measurement, and, rarely, muscle biopsy may help in differentiating these two conditions if the changes of myositis are present. However, often the only way to separate them is to reduce the dose of prednisone slowly; if glucocorticoid myopathy is the cause of the weakness, it will improve; if a relapse of the myositis is responsible, the weakness will increase.

Side effects of cytotoxic drugs include marrow suppression, alopecia, gastrointestinal tract disorders, damage to the testes and ovaries (including potential genetic damage), disorders of chronic immunosuppression, and potential for malignancy.

PROGNOSIS The overall mortality rate of individuals with dermatomyositis-polymyositis is about four times that of the general population; death is due usually to pulmonary, renal, and cardiac complications. Females, blacks, and those severely affected at presentation have a worse prognosis. Evidence from several series suggests that patients seen at tertiary referral centers may have less favorable outcome when compared with patients seen at smaller community hospitals, probably because they represent a population with more severe disease which shows poorer response to therapy. Nevertheless, the 5-year survival rate is about 75 percent overall, and is better than this in children. The majority of patients improve with therapy. Many patients make a full functional recovery, though some weakness of the shoulders and hips, usually not disabling, remains at the conclusion of treatment. Relapse may occur at any time. Glucocorticoids should not be discontinued too soon, for the relapse which may follow is often more difficult to treat than the original presentation. About one-half of the patients with this disease recover and can discontinue therapy within 5 years after the onset of the symptoms; about 20 percent still have active disease requiring continued therapy. The remaining 30 percent have inactive disease but residual muscle weakness.

REFERENCES

ARAHATA K, ENGEL AG: Monoclonal antibody analysis of mononuclear cells in myopathies. V. Identification and quantitation of T8+ cytotoxic and suppressor cells. Ann Neurol 23:493, 1988

BANKER BQ, ENGEL AG: The polymyositis and dermatomyositis syndromes, in *Myology*, AG Engel, BQ Banker (eds). New York, McGraw-Hill, 1986, pp 1385–1422

BOHAN A et al: A computer-assisted analysis of 153 patients with polymyositis and dermatomyositis. Medicine 56:255, 1977

BRADLEY WG, TANDAN R: Inflammatory diseases of muscle, in *Textbook of Rheumatology*, 3d ed, WN Kelley et al (eds). Philadelphia, Saunders, 1988, chap 72

CARPENTER S, KARPATI G: *Pathology of Skeletal Muscle*. New York, Churchill Livingstone, 1984, pp 515–592

CURIE S: Inflammatory myopathies. Part I: Polymyositis and related disorders, in *Disorders of Voluntary Muscle*, 4th ed, JN Walton (ed). London, Churchill Livingstone, 1981, chap 15

DeVERE R, BRADLEY WG: Polymyositis: Its presentation, mortality, and morbidity. Brain 98:637, 1975

MASTAGLIA FL, OJEDA VJ: Inflammatory myopathies. Ann Neurol 17:215, 317, 1985

PLOTZ PH et al: Current concepts in the idiopathic inflammatory myopathies: polymyositis, dermatomyositis, and related disorders. Ann Int Med 111:143, 1989

RICHARDSON JB, CALLEN JP: Dermatomyositis and malignancy. Med Clin North Am 73:1211, 1989

365 MUSCULAR DYSTROPHY

JERRY R. MENDELL / ROBERT C. GRIGGS

Most myopathies including the hereditary, inflammatory, endocrine, metabolic, and toxic disorders can result in chronic weakness. The approach to differential diagnosis of these disorders is summarized in Chap. 362.

HEREDITARY MYOPATHIES

Muscular dystrophy refers to a group of disorders that have little in common except for their name and the fact that they are inherited. Each type of muscular dystrophy has unique phenotypic and genetic features (Table 365-1).

DUCHENNE MUSCULAR DYSTROPHY This disorder was first described by Edward Meryon (1852) but the disease bears the name of the French neurologist Duchenne. Duchenne's dystrophy is an X-linked recessive disorder affecting males almost exclusively. Estimates of incidence range from 13 to 33 per 100,000 live-born males. In one-third or more of cases the family history is negative, suggesting that many are due to new mutations.

Molecular genetics The gene and gene product, called dystrophin, have recently been identified. The gene, an estimated 2000 kilobases in size, is the largest identified human gene. Dystrophin is a protein of about 400 kDa localized to the plasma membrane of the muscle fiber. Recognition of the gene and gene product was an outgrowth of a series of studies beginning with the recognition that rare females with the Duchenne phenotype had translocations on the short arm of the X chromosome at the Xp21 site. Independent studies accomplished through genetic linkage employing restriction fragment length polymorphisms (RFLPs) as genetic markers confirmed the Duchenne locus at Xp21. In 1985, Kunkle and colleagues isolated the DNA from a male patient with Duchenne's dystrophy who had a large deletion on the X chromosome. The patient also had retinitis pigmentosa, chronic granulomatous disease, and the McCleod red blood cell phenotype. The same year Worton and colleagues cloned the DNA spanning a translocation junction in a female with a Duchenne dystrophy phenotype who had an X;21 translocation. DNA from these patients served as the starting points for chromosomal walking which led to the identification of the Duchenne gene and gene product.

Clinical manifestations Clinical manifestations usually begin at 3 to 5 years of age. The boys fall frequently and have difficulty keeping up with their friends when playing. Running, jumping, and hopping are invariably abnormal. Motor milestones may be delayed even before age 2, but if there is no family history the diagnosis is often not suspected. By age 5 muscle weakness is obvious by muscle testing. On getting up from the floor the patient uses his hands to climb up himself (Gowers' maneuver). In younger children, the calf muscles are usually enlarged from true muscle hypertrophy; later, calf enlargement is appropriately called *pseudohypertrophy* since muscle is replaced by fat and connective tissue.

Contractures of heel cords and iliotibial bands become apparent by age 7 to 8, when toe walking is associated with lordotic posture.

TABLE 365-1 Progressive muscular dystrophies

Type	Usual inheritance	Clinical features	Other organ system involvement
Duchenne's (pseudohypertrophic)	X-linked recessive	Onset by age 5 Progressive weakness of girdle muscles Inability to walk after age 12 Kyphoscoliosis Respiratory failure in second to third decade	Cardiomyopathy Mental impairment
Becker's (benign pseudohypertrophic)	X-linked recessive	Onset in early to late childhood Slowly progressive weakness of girdle muscles Ability to walk after age 15 Respiratory failure after fourth decade	Cardiomyopathy
Myotonic	Autosomal dominant	Onset any decade Slowly progressive weakness of eyelids, face, neck, distal limb muscles Myotonia	Cardiac conduction defects Mental impairment Cataracts Frontal baldness Gonadal atrophy
Facioscapulohumeral	Autosomal dominant	Onset second to fourth decade Slowly progressive face, shoulder girdle, foot dorsiflexion weakness	Hypertension
Limb-girdle (may include several disorders)	Autosomal recessive	Onset early childhood to adult Slowly progressive weakness of shoulder and hip girdle muscles	Cardiomyopathy
Oculopharyngeal	Autosomal dominant (French-Canadian or Hispanic background)	Onset fifth to sixth decade Slowly progressive weakness of extraocular, eyelid, face, and pharyngeal muscles Cricopharyngeal achalasia	
Less well-characterized forms of muscular dystrophies: Congenital (may include several disorders)	Autosomal recessive	Onset at birth Hypotonia, contractures and delayed milestones Early respiratory failure in some; others have static course	Cerebral
Distal (may include several disorders)	Autosomal recessive	Onset second to third decade Slowly progressive weakness of legs beginning with foot drop	
Scapuloperoneal (may include several disorders)	Autosomal dominant	Onset third to fifth decade Progressive shoulder girdle and foot dorsiflexor weakness	Cardiomyopathy

Loss of muscle strength is progressive with predilection for proximal limb muscles and the neck flexors; leg involvement is more severe than arm involvement. Between ages 8 and 10 walking usually requires the use of braces; joint contractures and limitations of hip flexion and knee, elbow, and wrist extension are made worse by prolonged sitting. By age 12 most patients are confined to a wheelchair. Contractures become fixed and a progressive scoliosis often develops which may be associated with considerable discomfort. The chest deformity associated with scoliosis further impairs pulmonary function which is already diminished by the muscle weakness. By age 14 to 18 patients develop serious, sometimes fatal, pulmonary infections. Other causes of death include aspiration of food and acute gastric dilatation.

A cardiac cause of death is uncommon despite the existence of a cardiomyopathy in almost all patients. Congestive heart failure seldom occurs except with severe stress such as pneumonia. Cardiac arrhythmias are rare. The typical ECG shows an increased net RS in lead V_1; deep narrow Q waves in the precordial leads; and RSR′ or polyphasic R waves in V_1.

Intellectual impairment in Duchenne's dystrophy is common and in contrast to the muscle disease is nonprogressive. One-third of patients have intelligence quotients below 75 and the mean is estimated at 85. The intellectual impairment is not the result of physical limitations since verbal skills are impaired before weakness is severe. Its basis is not known but recent findings that dystrophin is found in the brain raise questions about the relationship of intellectual impairment to deficits in the gene product.

Laboratory investigation Laboratory confirmation includes assessment of serum CK level, which is invariably elevated between 20 and 100 times normal. The levels are abnormal at birth, making it possible to diagnose an affected boy early in life. Serum CK activity remains high until late in the disease, when levels decline because of inactivity and loss of muscle mass.

Myopathy can be demonstrated by electromyography (EMG). The muscle biopsy shows muscle fibers of varying size as well as small groups of necrotic and regenerating fibers (see Fig. 362-4). Connective tissue and fat replaces lost muscle fibers.

The understanding of the gene defect in Duchenne's dystrophy has greatly expanded the possibilities for carrier detection and prenatal diagnosis. Serum CK testing is nevertheless still an important initial step and will be elevated in about 50 percent of female carriers. In addition, since about 60 percent of Duchenne boys have a deletion or duplication of one or more exons within the gene, complementary DNA probes are now available for testing potential carriers and for use on amniotic fluid cells or chorionic villi in prenatal diagnosis. In families without deletions or duplications, linkage analysis using probes recognizing RFLPs is also available.

Treatment There is no definitive treatment for Duchenne's dystrophy. Some clinicians advocate administration of glucocorticoids.

BECKER'S MUSCULAR DYSTROPHY This less severe form of X-linked recessive muscular dystrophy was described by Becker and Keiner in 1955. It is often called the benign form of pseudohypertrophic muscular dystrophy. The presentation is similar to that of Duchenne's dystrophy except that the time course is slower. The incidence of Becker's dystrophy is approximately one-tenth that of the Duchenne type. The condition is not usually recognized before age 5 and walking continues well beyond age 15, sometimes into the fourth decade. Calf muscle enlargement is prominent. Death from complications similar to those of Duchenne's dystrophy may occur after age 40.

Until the isolation of the gene for dystrophin, it was not known whether Becker's and Duchenne's dystrophies represented genetically distinct disorders. Recent investigations indicate that these two conditions result from defects of the dystrophin gene and that differences in severity can be attributed to the amount and type of dystrophin deficiency in the muscle.

Carrier detection methods are identical for Duchenne's and Becker's dystrophies. Unlike Duchenne's dystrophy, Becker patients reach child-bearing age; while none of their sons will be affected, the daughters of the Becker patient will all be carriers.

Laboratory confirmation of Becker's dystrophy is the same as that for Duchenne's dystrophy in that high serum CK levels are present early in the course and then gradually decline. The EMG and muscle biopsy changes are similar to those of Duchenne's dystrophy.

FACIOSCAPULOHUMERAL MUSCULAR DYSTROPHY This slowly progressive disorder is usually inherited as an autosomal dominant disorder, affecting males and females equally. It is extremely variable in severity and may start at any age, commonly in the third or fourth decade. Cases starting earlier in life tend to have a worse prognosis. Some patients may remain asymptomatic throughout life. As the name implies, there is characteristic weakness of facial, shoulder girdle, and proximal arm muscles. Scapular winging and sloping shoulders reflect weakness of the serratus anterior, trapezius, and rhomboid muscles; later, the biceps and triceps muscles are affected; the deltoid muscles are usually relatively spared. Facial involvement often produces a lifelong inability to whistle, an expressionless face, and a sullen appearance. Foot drop may occur early in the disease from peroneal and anterior tibial muscle weakness. Leg weakness may eventually progress to loss of ambulation.

Other systems are usually unaffected in facioscapulohumeral dystrophy. Cardiac disease and respiratory compromise are rare, and their occurrence usually suggests a coincidental illness. Patients frequently appear to have exophthalmos but thyroid function is normal; a mild but labile hypertension is common. Intellectual function is intact and life span may be normal.

Diagnostic studies may be unnecessary in typical cases, particularly when a family history is present. CK level may be normal or slightly elevated; EMG and muscle biopsy tend to have mixed features of myopathy and neuropathy and may be misleading. No specific treatment is available; ankle-foot orthoses are occasionally helpful for foot drop. Scapular stabilization procedures improve scapular winging but may not improve function.

LIMB-GIRDLE DYSTROPHY This term encompasses more than one disorder. Inheritance is usually by autosomal recessive transmission. Proximal muscle weakness may begin in either the legs or the arms but usually progresses to all extremities. Weakness may begin before age 5 or as late as the third decade and may be associated with hypertrophy of calf and other muscles. Ambulation continues for over 20 years after the disease first appears. In some patients cardiac involvement results in congestive heart failure or arrhythmias; occasional patients may present with a cardiomyopathy. Respiratory failure ensues after 30 or more years of disease. Intellectual function remains normal. Diagnosis requires the exclusion of inflammatory and metabolic myopathies as well as the phenotypically similar spinal muscular atrophies. The serum CK is elevated in limb-girdle dystrophy although the values are usually lower than in Duchenne's and Becker's dystrophies; the EMG pattern is that of a myopathy. The muscle biopsy shows active myopathy but is not specific.

MYOTONIC DYSTROPHY Clinical manifestations This autosomal dominant disorder affects muscle and numerous other tissues. The incidence is estimated to be 1 per 10,000 and may be higher since many cases escape recognition. Associated features include intellectual impairment, hypersomnia, cardiac disease, posterior subcapsular cataracts, gonadal atrophy, respiratory failure, and gastrointestinal disease. Weakness initially involves eyelid, temporalis, facial, and neck flexor muscles, as well as the distal extremity muscles. Myotonia is demonstrable in hand grip or by percussion of the tongue, the wrist extensors, or the thenar eminence. Disease onset is usually in the second and third decade, but affected individuals may remain free of signs or symptoms throughout life. A severe form of the disease, *congenital myotonic dystrophy*, occurs in some infants of affected mothers and is characterized by severe facial and bulbar weakness; neonatal respiratory insufficiency may occur but is usually self-limited. Affected infants are frequently intellectually impaired.

Molecular genetics   The disorder is transmitted by a mutant gene on the long arm of chromosome 19 which is linked to the genes for apolipoprotein C2, secretor substance, the Lutheran blood group, peptidase D, and the third component of complement. Several RFLPs have been identified that are closely linked to the myotonic dystrophy locus. Early disease detection and antenatal diagnosis are now possible in selected families using linkage techniques.

Diagnosis   Diagnosis is often self-evident because of the distinctive facial appearance; the characteristic pattern of weakness and the abnormalities cause the typical narrow, "hatchet" face; premature frontal balding is frequent. The presence of distal weakness and myotonia confirm the diagnosis. Diagnosis can be made before the onset of symptoms in affected family members by clinical and EMG evaluation for myotonia and by slit-lamp examination for the characteristic cataracts. The CK activity is normal or slightly elevated. Muscle biopsy often shows distinctive type I fiber atrophy; severely involved muscles may have a characteristic appearance including ring fibers, sarcoplasmic masses, and numerous central nuclei.

Cardiac involvement most commonly affects the conduction system; first-degree heart block is present in a majority, and complete heart block may require pacemaker implantation. Since sudden death may occur, patients must be monitored carefully for conduction disturbances, though precise criteria for the timing of pacemaker implantation are lacking. Tachyarrhythmias and congestive failure are less frequent. Respiratory muscle weakness may be severe even in patients with minor limb weakness. Impaired ventilatory drive and hypersensitivity to the depressant effects of small doses of opiates and sedatives may result in sudden ventilatory failure, particularly in the pre- or postoperative setting. Sleep apnea may occur on both a central and peripheral basis (Chap. 217). Chronic hypoxia may lead to cor pulmonale and is the usual cause of heart failure for the patient.

Treatment   Myotonia is seldom so disabling as to require treatment; phenytoin is the therapy of choice since the other antimyotonia agents, quinine and procainamide, may worsen cardiac conduction.

MYOTONIA CONGENITA   This disorder occurs in autosomal dominant (Thomsen) and autosomal recessive forms (Chap. 27). Patients with the autosomal recessive form may develop slight weakness; patients with the dominant form do not develop weakness. Myotonia can be markedly alleviated by antimyotonia agents including quinine, procainamide, phenytoin, acetazolamide, or tocainide. These patients have no involvement of heart or other organs.

OCULOPHARYNGEAL DYSTROPHY   The term *progressive external ophthalmoplegia* describes disorders characterized by slowly progressive ptosis and limitation of eye movements with the sparing of pupil and muscles of accommodation. Patients usually do not complain of diplopia, in contrast to conditions with a more acute onset of ocular muscle weakness. *Oculopharyngeal dystrophy* is an autosomal dominant disorder in which ophthalmoplegia appears in the fifth or sixth decade. Many patients are of French-Canadian or Hispanic ancestry. Pharyngeal weakness leads to cricopharyngeal achalasia, progressive difficulty in swallowing, and frequent, often asymptomatic, aspiration. Severe malnutrition may develop but can be alleviated by surgical correction of cricopharyngeal achalasia.

Additional types of *ocular myopathies* are associated with mitochondrial abnormalities in muscle (see discussion of metabolic myopathies below).

CONGENITAL MUSCULAR DYSTROPHY   This rare disorder appears to represent more than one disease. In most cases inheritance is autosomal recessive but instances of autosomal dominant inheritance have been reported. The usual picture of infantile hypotonia and muscle weakness and wasting is associated with joint contractures. Facial and neck weakness is common with sparing of extraocular muscles. Serum CK is usually elevated and the muscle biopsy shows features typical of muscular dystrophy. The condition is relatively nonprogressive, but many patients are never able to walk. A more severe form of the condition may lead to death from respiratory failure.

In some patients with congenital muscular dystrophy there is also cerebral involvement with hypomyelination of the deep white matter of the brain detectable by computed tomography (CT). Many patients show no clinical manifestations of hypomyelination. A more severe form of congenital muscular dystrophy, associated with cerebral involvement, occurs in Japan, and is called the Fukuyama-type. It is often associated with generalized convulsions, global developmental delay, and death by 10 years of age.

DISTAL MUSCULAR DYSTROPHY   This rare disorder has at least three separate variants. The most frequent is an autosomal recessive or sporadic disorder that presents with distal leg weakness in the second or third decade. Slow progression affecting more proximal muscles occurs. The CK level is markedly elevated. Other distinct forms of a distal myopathy include an autosomal dominant Scandinavian form (Welander) which begins in the hands, and a late-onset (fourth to fifth decade) autosomal dominant disorder that begins in the legs and in which cardiomyopathy is frequent.

SCAPULOPERONEAL DYSTROPHY   Several forms of neuromuscular disease cause foot drop and winging of the scapulas. An autosomal dominant form presents in the third to fifth decade and is variable in its progression; respiratory failure is uncommon, but cardiomyopathy may occur. An X-linked recessive form (Emery-Dreifuss) begins in early childhood and is associated with prominent joint contractures and cardiac conduction disorders. Certain cases of facioscapulohumeral dystrophy may lack facial weakness and resemble scapuloperoneal dystrophy.

CONGENITAL MYOPATHIES

These rare disorders are distinguished from muscular dystrophies by the presence of specific histochemical and structural abnormalities in muscle. A nonprogressive course is common but not invariable. The typical infant has hypotonia and delayed motor milestones. Pectus excavatum, kyphoscoliosis, hip dislocation, and pes cavus are common. The diagnosis is important, since the long-term prognosis and management differ from that of the muscular dystrophies.

Four major forms of congenital myopathies have been described: central core disease, nemaline (rod) myopathy, myotubular (centronuclear) myopathy, and congenital fiber-type disproportion.

CENTRAL CORE DISEASE   This disease, the first congenital myopathy described, was identified by Shy and Magee in 1956. The disorder is inherited as an autosomal dominant disorder but sporadic cases also occur. In infancy hypotonia and delayed motor milestones are typical, but the diagnosis may come to attention in an adult with muscle weakness or skeletal abnormalities.

Short, slender stature and skeletal abnormalities including congenital hip dislocation, scoliosis, pes cavus, and pectus excavatum are characteristic. Weakness of the muscles of the face and limbs, particularly the legs, is mild. The muscle biopsy is diagnostic; it shows fibers with single or multiple central or eccentric discrete zones (cores) devoid of oxidative enzymes. Other laboratory studies are less helpful since the serum CK and the EMG may be normal. Patients with this disorder may be predisposed to develop malignant hyperthermia (Chap. 20).

NEMALINE MYOPATHY   This disorder, also called rod myopathy, was described by Shy and colleagues in 1963. Inheritance is usually as an autosomal dominant trait but it may be recessive or sporadic. Infantile hypotonia is frequent, and death may occur from respiratory failure. The skeletal abnormalities are striking; they include a long face, high arched palate, and slender musculature. Kyphoscoliosis, pectus excavatum, and pes cavus may be present. Muscle weakness affects the face, palate, and limb muscles. The prognosis is variable, with some patients progressing to wheelchair confinement or respiratory failure while in others the disease does not progress.

Muscle histology shows clusters of small rod or nemaline (threadlike) bodies for which the condition was named. Rods, derived from Z-band material, are usually found in type I fibers, and the muscle often shows type I predominance. The serum CK level may be normal or mildly elevated, and the EMG usually shows myopathy.

MYOTUBULAR MYOPATHY This disorder was described by Spiro, Shy, and Gonatas in 1966. The histologic abnormality in myotubular myopathy resembles the embryonic or developmental myotube stage of a muscle fiber. Others have preferred to call the disease *centronuclear myopathy,* arguing that the fibers are not embryonic. The condition is usually sporadic, but inheritance may be as an autosomal dominant, recessive, or X-linked recessive trait. Infantile hypotonia and weakness are common and may cause death. Presentations at an older age include features similar to nemaline myopathy with a long narrow face, pes cavus, and scoliosis. Muscle bulk is reduced, and proximal and distal weakness is of varying severity. The feature that separates these patients from those with other congenital myopathies is the presence of external ophthalmoplegia. The course may or may not be progressive.

Serum CK activity is normal or slightly elevated. The EMG is usually abnormal with excessively recruited small motor unit potentials associated with fibrillations and positive sharp potentials. Muscle biopsy shows muscle fibers with rows of central nuclei often surrounded by a perinuclear clear zone. Type I fibers may be preferentially affected and may be atrophic.

CONGENITAL FIBER-TYPE DISPROPORTION Clinical features of this disorder include hypotonia, weakness, delayed milestones, and skeletal deformities similar to those of other congenital myopathies. The diagnosis is established by the muscle biopsy which shows an increased number of small type I fibers and normal or hypertrophied type II fibers. The pathogenesis is poorly understood. The prognosis is generally good, with most patients showing improvement with age although some residual motor impairment commonly persists; occasional patients may have progressive weakness.

DISORDERS OF MUSCLE ENERGY METABOLISM

Skeletal muscle utilizes two principal sources of energy—fatty acids and glucose. Abnormalities in either glucose or lipid utilization can be associated with distinct clinical features. The more dramatic feature is an acute muscle pain syndrome which can evolve into severe rhabdomyolysis and myoglobinuria. The other is progressive muscle weakness simulating muscular dystrophy. The explanation for the different clinical syndromes is often unknown.

GLYCOGEN STORAGE AND GLYCOLYTIC DEFECTS There are four disorders of glycogen metabolism (types II, III, IV, and V) and four disorders of glycolysis (types VII, IX, X and XI) associated with significant skeletal muscle manifestations (see also Chap. 332).

Acid maltase deficiency (type II glycogenosis) Acid maltase is a lysosomal enzyme, an acid hydrolase, having α-1,4- and α-1,6-glucosidase activity which breaks down glycogen to glucose; however, the enzyme has no well-defined role in carbohydrate metabolism. Three clinical forms of acid maltase deficiency are each inherited as autosomal recessive traits. The biochemical basis for the different clinical presentations is not understood.

In infancy, acid maltase deficiency has features of a generalized glycogenosis. No abnormalities are noted at birth, but shortly thereafter severe muscle weakness, cardiomegaly, hepatomegaly, and tongue enlargement develop. Glycogen accumulation in motor neurons of the spinal cord and brainstem contribute to the muscle weakness. Death usually occurs by 1 year of age.

In children and adults, the picture resembles muscular dystrophy. The childhood form is associated with delayed developmental milestones, proximal limb muscle weakness, and calf enlargement and may progress to respiratory failure and death before the end of the second decade. Cardiac involvement may be present, but hepatomegaly and macroglossia are infrequent.

The adult form begins in the third or fourth decade and may be misdiagnosed as limb-girdle dystrophy or polymyositis. Respiratory failure from diaphragmatic weakness may be the initial manifestation of the disease. The heart, liver, and tongue are not involved. The diagnosis is suggested by muscle biopsy which shows vacuoles containing glycogen and the lysosomal enzyme, acid phosphatase. By electron microscopy, membrane-bound and free tissue glycogen are found. Definitive diagnosis is established by muscle biochemistry. Acid maltase activity is also reduced in the urine. Serum CK level may be as high as ten times normal. EMG distinguishes acid maltase deficiency from muscular dystrophy by the occurrence of bizarre high-frequency and myotonic discharges accompanying short-duration motor unit potentials, fibrillations, and positive sharp potentials.

Debrancher enzyme deficiency (type III glycogenosis) Muscle weakness is uncommon in debrancher enzyme deficiency. This mild disease of childhood is dominated by hepatomegaly, growth retardation, and hypoglycemia. These findings usually diminish or disappear after puberty, and muscle weakness and wasting associated with decreased exercise tolerance may develop. Diagnosis is suggested by a failure of lactic acid level to rise following exercise of the forearm. The serum CK level is elevated. EMG shows myopathy which may be accompanied by membrane irritability with myotonic discharges. Muscle biopsy shows a vacuolar myopathy with increased glycogen. Definitive diagnosis requires muscle biochemistry.

Brancher enzyme deficiency (type IV glycogenosis) Brancher enzyme deficiency is a severe fatal disorder of infancy in which skeletal muscle manifestations are relatively minor in the face of the chronic liver failure. The muscle hypotonia and wasting may, however, suggest the possibility of a primary muscle disease or spinal muscular atrophy.

Muscle phosphorylase deficiency (type V glycogenosis) Exercise intolerance is the dominant feature of muscle phosphorylase deficiency, first described in 1951 by McArdle. The disorder, usually inherited as an autosomal recessive trait, has an unexplained predilection for males. Painful muscle cramps and fatigue after intense exercise such as running or lifting heavy objects usually develops after adolescence. Early infantile and late onset variants have been described. Many patients report a "second wind" phenomenon if they rest briefly or slow down during exercise, which allows them to continue an activity for a longer period of time. Overexertion may lead to rhabdomyolysis and myoglobinuria, and renal failure can result. Persistent weakness and wasting of muscle is rare, and examination of the patient between attacks is usually normal. Other organs are not affected.

Serum CK levels fluctuate widely and may be elevated even during symptom-free periods. The forearm exercise test shows no rise in lactic acid. The EMG is often normal except when taken following an episode of rhabdomyolysis. Muscle biopsy often shows subsarcolemmal blebs containing glycogen. Muscle phosphorylase deficiency can be recognized by a histochemical stain and confirmed by biochemistry. Patients can remain moderately active once they establish their limitations. Dietary supplementation with either glucose or fructose has not alleviated symptoms.

Phosphofructokinase deficiency (type VII glycogenosis) This disorder resembles muscle phosphorylase deficiency and is also an autosomal recessive trait with a male predominance. The precipitating events and the laboratory features also resemble phosphorylase deficiency. A histochemical stain for phosphofructokinase (PFK) can demonstrate the deficiency. Definitive diagnosis requires biochemical analysis of muscle enzymes. Some patients with PFK deficiency have mild hemolysis, increased reticulocyte count, and elevated bilirubin because of a deficiency of a PFK subunit shared by muscle and red blood cells.

New glycolytic enzyme deficiency syndromes Since 1981 deficiencies of three additional glycolytic enzymes have been identified: phosphoglycerate kinase (PGK) deficiency (type IX), phosphoglycerate mutase (PGAM) deficiency (type X), and lactate dehydrogenase deficiency (LDH) (XI). The clinical pictures of the three are similar. In each, episodic myoglobinuria and myalgias precipitated by intense exercise begin in childhood or adolescence. Autosomal recessive inheritance is probable in each disorder. Serum CK level may be elevated during and between episodes. In PGAM and LDH deficiencies, the rise in lactic acid following forearm exercise is lower than normal. PGK deficiency shows no rise in lactate and closely resembles muscle phosphorylase and PFK deficiencies. The muscle histology is unremarkable in these disorders with little evidence of glycogen storage. Diagnosis requires muscle biochemistry.

DISORDERS OF LIPID METABOLISM

Lipid is an important muscle energy source during rest and prolonged, moderately intense exercise (Fig. 365-1).

CARNITINE DEFICIENCY   Carnitine deficiency occurs in myopathic and systemic forms.

Myopathic carnitine deficiency is associated with generalized muscle weakness, usually beginning in childhood. The clinical features overlap with muscular dystrophy and polymyositis. Most cases are sporadic, but the inheritance pattern is thought to be autosomal recessive. Cardiomyopathy may be present. Serum CK level is slightly elevated, and the EMG shows myopathy. The muscle biopsy shows striking lipid accumulation. Serum carnitine is normal. The cause for decreased muscle carnitine is not understood. A defect of transport into muscle has been postulated. Some patients respond to oral carnitine supplements; this should be tried in all cases. Other patients have responded to prednisone for unknown reasons. A diet substituting medium-chain for long-chain triglycerides has been helpful in some cases. Rare patients have also responded to riboflavin.

Systemic carnitine deficiency, an autosomal recessive disease of infancy and early childhood, is characterized by progressive weakness and episodes of hepatic encephalopathy with nausea, vomiting, confusion, coma, and early death. The low *serum* carnitine level distinguishes this condition from the myopathic form. No single cause has been identified to explain the low serum carnitine level. Decreased synthesis explains some cases while increased urinary excretion is seen in others. Serum CK level may be slightly elevated. The muscle biopsy shows lipid storage. In some cases the liver, heart, and kidney also show increased lipid. Treatment with oral carnitine supplements or glucocorticoids has helped some but not all patients.

FIGURE 365-1 Free fatty acids for muscle energy are derived from triglycerides stored in muscle and from circulating very low density lipoproteins (VLDL) which are broken down by endothelial lipoprotein lipase (1) in the capillary. Carnitine, an essential substrate for lipid metabolism, is made in the liver and transported to muscle. In muscle, free fatty acids combine with coenzyme A (CoA-SH) through the action of fatty acylsynthetase (2) found in the outer mitochondrial membrane forming fatty acylcoenzyme A (F-acyl-CoA). Transport through inner mitochondrial membrane requires transfer to carnitine by carnitine palmityltransferase 1 (CPT I) bound to the outer surface of the inner mitochondrial membrane (3). Inside the mitochondrion, fatty acylcarnitine (F-acylcarnitine) is regenerated by CPT II (4) bound to the inner surface of the inner mitochondrial membrane. The fatty acylcoenzyme A then proceeds to beta oxidation.

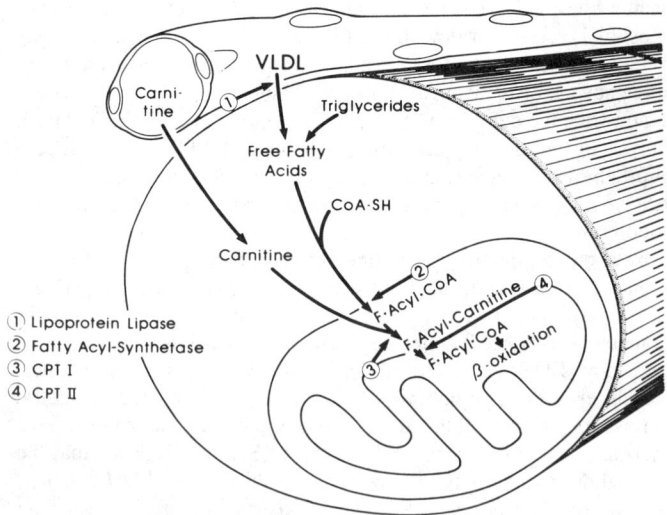

① Lipoprotein Lipase
② Fatty Acyl-Synthetase
③ CPT I
④ CPT II

CARNITINE PALMITYLTRANSFERASE DEFICIENCY   Deficiency of carnitine palmityltransferase (CPT) presents with recurrent myoglobinuria. It is not known if CPT I or CPT II activities are selectively deficient; the deficiency apparently results from disordered regulatory properties of an abnormal enzyme. Rhabdomyolysis may follow prolonged exercise such as soccer, football, or a long hike, but at times no precipitating cause can be found. Initial symptoms often commence in childhood. In contrast to defects in glycolysis where muscle cramps follow short intense bursts of exercise, the muscle pain in CPT deficiency does not occur until the limits of energy utilization have been exceeded and muscle breakdown has begun. Episodes of rhabdomyolysis may produce severe weakness, and some patients require ventilatory assistance. In contrast to carnitine deficiency, strength is normal between attacks and the muscle biopsy does not show lipid accumulation. The diagnosis requires direct measurement of muscle CPT. Treatment consists of increased carbohydrate intake before exercise or of substituting medium-chain triglycerides in the diet. Neither has been entirely satisfactory.

MYOADENYLATE DEAMINASE DEFICIENCY   The enzyme adenylate deaminase converts 5'-adenosine monophosphate (5'AMP) to inosine monophosphate (IMP) with liberation of ammonia and may play a role in regulating adenosine triphosphate (ATP) levels in muscle. In 1978 a group of patients with myalgias and exercise intolerance were found to be deficient in the muscle isoenzyme, adenylate deaminase. The deficiency, however, occurs in as many as 1 percent of the population and can be detected by histochemical staining of muscle tissue as well as by biochemical analysis. Muscle ammonia production is decreased following forearm exercise. Since the original description, a less consistent clinical picture has emerged. Patients with other neuromuscular disorders including anterior horn cell disease, muscular dystrophy, and myasthenia gravis occasionally have the same enzyme deficiency. The full clinical significance of adenylate deaminase deficiency is not established.

MITOCHONDRIAL MYOPATHIES   A heterogeneous group of disorders is characterized by abnormal mitochondria in "ragged-red fibers," named for their appearance in the trichrome stain of biopsied muscle. The most common disorder is characterized by progressive ptosis, external ophthalmoplegia, and proximal weakness and was initially called oculocraniosomatic neuromuscular disease with ragged-red fibers when described by Olson et al. in 1972. Many of these cases show autosomal dominant inheritance. In other cases of sporadic onset, beginning in childhood and referred to as the *Kearns-Sayre syndrome*, there are accompanying cardiac conduction defects which may cause complete heart block, retinal pigmentary degeneration, short stature, and gonadal defects. Another disorder recently assigned the acronym *MERRF syndrome*, because of its myoclonic epilepsy and ragged-red fibers, presents between the first and fifth decades with generalized seizures, myoclonus, dementia, hearing loss, and ataxia. A third disorder, the *MELAS syndrome*, is a slowly progressive disease characterized by mitochondrial myopathy, encephalopathy, lactic acidosis, stroke-like episodes including alternating hemiparesis, hemianopsia or cortical blindness, and focal or generalized seizures.

There is evidence that some of the mitochondrial myopathies are related to abnormalities in mitochondrial, as opposed to nuclear, DNA which appears to be derived solely from the mother through the ovum. In MERRF syndrome which is associated with a defect in cytochrome oxidase, an enzyme of the respiratory chain critical for oxidative phosphorylation, there is unequivocal evidence for maternal inheritance. Affected males do not transmit the condition. In Kearns-Sayre syndrome isolated muscle mitochondria show deletions in mitochondrial DNA, although no examples of transmission of disease to offspring have been reported.

INFLAMMATORY MYOPATHIES

Polymyositis and dermatomyositis (Chap. 364) develop slowly over the course of months. The presence of a characteristic skin rash usually makes the diagnosis of dermatomyositis straightforward. Chronic polymyositis, with slowly progressive proximal weakness, may be impossible to separate on clinical grounds from sporadic cases of limb-girdle dystrophy. Even with detailed EMG and biopsy studies it may prove difficult to establish the diagnosis of polymyositis with confidence. A subgroup of subacute or chronic inflammatory myopathy is termed *inclusion body myositis* because of distinctive cytoplasmic and nuclear inclusions consisting of abnormal filaments. Inclusion body myositis does not respond to glucocorticoid therapy. Chronic myositis may also occur with any of the collagen-vascular diseases and with sarcoidosis.

ENDOCRINE AND METABOLIC MYOPATHIES

Many endocrine disorders cause weakness. Muscle fatigue is more common than true weakness. The cause of weakness in these disorders is not well-defined. It is not even clear that weakness results from disease of muscle as opposed to another part of the motor unit since the CK level is often normal and the muscle histology is characterized by atrophy rather than by destruction of muscle fibers. Nearly all respond to appropriate endocrine management.

THYROID DISORDERS (See Chap. 316) *Hyperthyroidism* may occasionally present as muscle weakness, and the majority of patients are weak. *Hypothyroidism* commonly presents with muscle weakness and pain. The serum CK is often elevated and levels as high as 100 times normal may occur even with minimal clinical evidence of muscle disease. Adult patients may have muscle hypertrophy with cramps (Hoffmann's syndrome) and in children with cretinism a distinctive myopathy with muscle hypertrophy may occur (Kocher-Debré-Sémélaigne syndrome).

PARATHYROID DISORDERS (See Chap. 340) *Hyperparathyroidism* is often associated with muscle weakness and atrophy and may be accompanied by "muscle" pain which is probably from associated bone disease. Hyperreflexia is characteristic. *Hypoparathyroidism* frequently presents with neurologic involvement. The neuromuscular manifestations are usually those of tetany, but since the serum CK level is often elevated such patients are occasionally considered to have polymyositis. Hyporeflexia or areflexia is usually present despite the presence of Chvostek's and Trousseau's signs.

ADRENAL DISORDERS (See Chap. 317) Endogenous elevations of glucocorticoids may produce severe muscle weakness and wasting. Adrenal insufficiency is frequently associated with lassitude and weakness although there is usually little objective reduction in strength.

PITUITARY DISORDERS (See Chap. 313) Acromegaly is occasionally associated with muscle enlargement. Myopathic weakness may occur, but weakness usually results from associated endocrine abnormalities or from neuropathy. The weakness of panhypopituitarism is probably due to coexisting adrenal or thyroid insufficiency.

DIABETES (See Chap. 319) Proximal weakness in the patient with diabetes is usually the result of neuropathy. The finding of evidence on EMG or biopsy for myopathy or of a markedly elevated serum CK level usually suggests coincidental illness.

VITAMIN DEFICIENCY Severe malabsorption, particularly when it occurs in early childhood, may lead to a vitamin E deficiency myopathy. Vitamin E otherwise has no role in the treatment of muscle weakness (Chap. 76). Vitamin D deficiency (Chap. 341), from either decreased intake or decreased absorption, as well as impaired vitamin D metabolism, such as occurs in renal disease, may lead to chronic muscle weakness; pain probably reflects underlying bone disease. Deficiency of other vitamins does not cause myopathy.

OTHER METABOLIC DISORDERS Systemic illnesses such as malignancy and chronic respiratory, cardiac, hepatic, and renal failure are frequently associated with severe muscle wasting and complaints of weakness. Strength testing often demonstrates only mild weakness in such patients, and the problem is often a lack of endurance. Evidence for active muscle degeneration is usually lacking. Electrolyte disturbances such as chronic hypokalemia, hypercalcemia, and hy-

---

TABLE 365-2 Toxic myopathies

I Focal myopathies: Pentazocine, meperidine
II Generalized myopathies
   A Inflammatory: Cimetidine, D-penicillamine, procainamide
   B Muscle weakness and myalgias: Chloroquine, clofibrate, colchicine, glucocorticoids, emetine, ε-aminocaproic acid, labetalol, perhexilene, propranolol, vincristine
   C Rhabdomyolysis and myoglobinuria: Alcohol, azathioprine, heroin, amphetamine, clofibrate, ε-aminocaproic acid, phencyclidine, barbiturates, cocaine
   D Malignant hyperthermia: Halothane, ethylene, diethyl ether, methoxyflurane, ethyl chloride, trichloroethylene, gallamine, succinylcholine, lidocaine, mepivacaine

---

pocalcemia from various causes may produce chronic muscle weakness.

TOXIC MYOPATHIES

A classification of toxic myopathies is shown in Table 365-2. Drugs and chemicals may produce focal or generalized damage of skeletal muscle.

The most common cause of focal damage is the injection of narcotic analgesics. Two agents in particular, pentazocine and meperidine, may cause a severe fibrotic reaction in muscle. Common injection sites include deltoid, triceps, gluteus maximus, and quadriceps muscles. The muscles become indurated and hard and may have local abscess formation. Cutaneous ulcerations and depressions may occur. Severe joint contractures may develop.

Other drugs may induce generalized muscle weakness, particularly affecting the proximal muscles. In most cases the exact mechanism of drug toxicity is poorly understood. D-Penicillamine induces a condition simulating the clinical and pathologic picture of dermatomyositis and polymyositis. A similar condition has been reported with cimetidine. Procainamide may cause myositis as part of a systemic lupus-like reaction. After many months of treatment, chloroquine produces a distinctive vacuolar myopathy that may involve the heart. Clofibrate is associated with muscle pain and weakness either shortly after the start or following several months of treatment. Serum CK elevation may be the only clofibrate-induced abnormality. Emetine hydrochloride (used for treatment of amebiasis), ε-aminocaproic acid (an antifibrolytic agent), and perhexilene (used for angina pectoris) have all been observed to cause weakness and muscle fiber necrosis following several weeks of therapy.

Drug-induced myopathy accompanied by proximal weakness occurs with glucocorticoid therapy. Those fluorinated in the 9α-position, such as triamcinolone, dexamethasone, and betamethasone, are most likely to cause weakness, but chronic administration of all glucocorticoids including prednisone cause weakness. Divided-dose as opposed to single-morning-dose therapy produces more severe weakness. A single-dose, alternate-day regimen has the greatest muscle-sparing effect (Chap. 317). The clinical diagnosis of steroid-induced muscle weakness can be difficult if the medication is being used to treat an underlying inflammatory myopathy. The presence of a normal serum CK level, minimal or no changes of myopathy on EMG, and type II muscle fiber atrophy on biopsy are helpful in suggesting steroid-induced weakness.

In some instances toxic myopathy may be more catastrophic, causing rhabdomyolysis and myoglobinuria. A very serious drug-induced condition, *malignant hyperthermia* (Chap. 20), occurs in susceptible individuals following exposure to certain general anesthetics and depolarizing muscle relaxants (Table 365-2). In local anesthesia, amides including lidocaine and mepivacaine have been implicated as precipitating agents.

REFERENCES

BANKER BQ: The congenital myopathies, in *Myology,* AG Engel, BQ Banker (eds). New York, McGraw-Hill, 1986, vol 2

BROOKE MH: *A Clinician's View of Neuromuscular Disease*, 2d ed. Baltimore, Williams & Wilkins, 1985

DIMAURO S et al: Disorders of lipid metabolism in muscle. Muscle Nerve 3: 369, 1980

ENGEL AG: Acid maltase deficiency, in *Myology*, AG Engel, BQ Banker (eds). New York, McGraw-Hill, 1986, vol 2

GRIGGS RC, MOXLEY RT (eds): Metabolic myopathies. Semin Neurol, 3: 225, 1983

KOENIG M et al: Complete cloning of the Duchenne muscular dystrophy (DMD) cDNA and preliminary genominic organization of the DMD gene in normal and affected individuals. Cell 50: 509, 1987

RIGGS JE (ed): *Neurologic Clinics*, vol 6: *Muscle Disease*. Philadelphia, Saunders, 1988

WALLACE DC et al: Familial mitochondrial encephalomyopathy (MERRF): Genetic, pathophysiological, and biochemical characterization of a mitochondrial DNA disease. Cell 55: 601, 1988

366 MYASTHENIA GRAVIS

DANIEL B. DRACHMAN

Myasthenia gravis (MG) is a neuromuscular disorder characterized by weakness and fatigability of skeletal muscles. The underlying defect is a decrease in the number of available acetylcholine receptors (AChRs) at neuromuscular junctions, due to an antibody-mediated autoimmune attack. Treatment now available for MG is highly effective, although a specific cure has remained elusive.

PATHOPHYSIOLOGY To diagnose and manage patients with MG, it is essential to understand the basic function of the neuromuscular junction and the changes that occur as a result of the disease process (see Fig. 366-1). Acetylcholine (ACh) is synthesized in the motor nerve terminal and stored in vesicles (quanta) containing approximately 10,000 molecules each. Quanta of ACh are released spontaneously, giving rise to miniature end-plate potentials. When an action potential reaches the nerve terminal, ACh from 150 to 200 vesicles is released and combines with AChRs that are densely packed at the peaks of postsynaptic folds. Channels in the AChRs are opened, permitting the rapid entry of cations, chiefly sodium, which produces depolarization at the end-plate region of the muscle fiber. If the depolarization is sufficiently large, it initiates an action potential that is propagated along the muscle fiber, triggering muscle contraction. This process is rapidly terminated by diffusion of ACh away from the receptor, and hydrolysis of ACh by acetylcholinesterase (AChE).

In MG, the fundamental defect is a decrease in the number of available AChRs at the postsynaptic muscle membrane. In addition, the postsynaptic folds are flattened, or "simplified" (Fig. 366-1*B*). These changes result in decreased efficiency of neuromuscular transmission. Therefore, although ACh is released normally, it produces

FIGURE 366-1 Diagrams of (*A*) normal and (*B*) myasthenic neuromuscular junctions. V = vesicles; M = mitochondria. See text for description of normal neuromuscular transmission. The MG junction shows reduced number of AChRs (stippling); flattened, simplified postsynaptic folds; a widened synaptic space; and a normal nerve terminal.

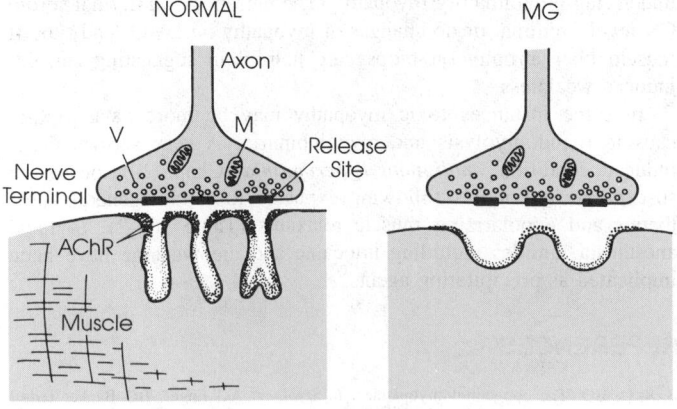

small end-plate potentials which may fail to trigger muscle action potentials. Failure of transmission at many neuromuscular junctions results in weakness of muscle contraction.

The amount of ACh released per impulse *normally* declines on repeated activity (termed *presynaptic rundown*). In the myasthenic patient, decreased efficiency of neuromuscular transmission combined with the normal rundown results in the activation of fewer and fewer muscle fibers by successive nerve impulses and, hence, increasing weakness, or *myasthenic fatigue*. This mechanism also accounts for the decremental response to repetitive nerve stimulation seen on electrodiagnostic testing.

The neuromuscular abnormalities in MG are brought about by an autoimmune response mediated by specific anti-AChR antibodies. The anti-AChR antibodies reduce the number of available AChRs at neuromuscular junctions by three distinct mechanisms: (1) AChRs may be degraded at an accelerated rate by a mechanism involving cross-linking of the receptors; (2) the active site of the AChR, i.e., the site that normally binds ACh, may be blocked by the antibodies; (3) the postsynaptic muscle membrane may be damaged by the antibody in collaboration with complement.

How the autoimmune response is initiated and maintained in MG is not completely understood. However, the thymus appears to play a role in this process. The thymus is abnormal in approximately 75 percent of patients with MG: in about 65 percent of patients the thymus is "hyperplastic," with the presence of active germinal centers, while 10 percent of patients have thymic tumors (thymomas). Musclelike cells within the thymus (myoid cells), which bear AChRs on their surface, may serve as a source of autoantigen and trigger the autoimmune reaction within the thymus gland.

CLINICAL FEATURES Myasthenia gravis is not rare, with a prevalence rate of at least 1 in 10,000. It may affect individuals in any age group, but there are peaks of incidence in women in their twenties and thirties and in men in their fifties and sixties. Overall, women are affected more frequently than men, with a ratio of approximately 3:2. The cardinal features are *weakness* and *fatigability* of muscles. The weakness increases during repeated use (fatigue) and may improve following rest or sleep. The course of MG is often variable. Exacerbations and remissions may occur, particularly during the first few years after the onset of the disease. Remissions are rarely complete or permanent. Unrelated infections or systemic disorders often lead to increased myasthenic weakness, and may precipitate so-called crisis (see below).

The distribution of muscle weakness has a characteristic pattern. The cranial muscles, particularly the lids and extraocular muscles, are often involved early, and diplopia and ptosis are common initial complaints. Facial weakness produces a "snarling" expression when the patient attempts to smile. Weakness in chewing is most noticeable after prolonged effort, as in chewing meat. Speech may have a nasal timbre caused by weakness of the palate or a dysarthric "mushy" quality due to tongue weakness. Difficulty in swallowing may occur as a result of weakness of the palate, tongue, or pharynx, giving rise to nasal regurgitation or aspiration of liquids or food. In approximately 85 percent of patients, the weakness becomes generalized, affecting the limb muscles as well. The limb weakness in MG is often proximal and may be asymmetric. Despite the muscle weakness, deep tendon reflexes are preserved. If weakness of respiration or swallowing becomes so severe as to require respiratory assistance or intubation, the patient is said to be in *crisis*.

DIAGNOSIS AND EVALUATION The diagnosis is suspected on the basis of weakness and fatigability in the typical distribution described above, without loss of reflexes or impairment of sensation or other neurologic function. The suspected diagnosis should always be confirmed definitively before treatment is undertaken; this is essential because (1) other treatable conditions may closely resemble MG, and (2) the treatment of MG may involve surgery and the prolonged use of drugs with adverse side effects.

Anticholinesterase test Drugs that inhibit the enzyme AChE allow ACh to interact repeatedly with the limited number of ACh receptors, producing improvement in the strength of myasthenic muscles. Edrophonium is used most commonly, because of the rapid onset (30 s) and short duration (about 5 min) of its effect. It is essential that an objective endpoint be used to evaluate the effect of edrophonium. The examiner should focus on one or more unequivocally weak muscle groups and evaluate their strength objectively. For example, weakness of extraocular muscles, impairment of speech, or the length of time that the patient can maintain the arms in forward abduction may be useful measures. An initial dose of 2 mg edrophonium is given intravenously. If definite improvement occurs, the test is considered positive and terminated. If there is no change, the patient is given an additional 8 mg intravenously. The dose is administered in two parts because some patients react to edrophonium with unpleasant side effects such as nausea, diarrhea, salivation, fasciculations, and rarely syncope. Atropine (0.6 mg) should be at hand for intravenous administration if these symptoms become troublesome.

False-positive tests occur in occasional patients with other neurologic disorders, such as amyotrophic lateral sclerosis, and in placebo-reactors. False-negative or equivocal tests may also occur. In some cases it is helpful to use a longer-acting drug such as neostigmine, given orally, since this permits more time for detailed evaluation of strength. In virtually all instances, it is desirable to carry out further testing to establish the diagnosis of MG definitively.

Electrodiagnostic testing *Repetitive nerve stimulation* often provides helpful diagnostic evidence of MG. Anticholinesterase medication should be stopped at least 6 h prior to testing. It is best to test weak muscles or proximal muscle groups. Electric shocks are delivered at a rate of 3 or 5 per second to the appropriate nerves, and action potentials are recorded from the muscles. In normal individuals, the amplitude of the evoked muscle action potentials does not change at these rates of stimulation. However, in myasthenic patients there is a rapid reduction in the amplitude of the evoked responses of more than 10 to 15 percent. As a further test, a single dose of edrophonium may be given to prevent or diminish this decremental reaction.

Antiacetylcholine receptor antibody As noted above, anti-AChR antibodies are detectable in the serum of approximately 80 percent of all myasthenic patients, but in only about 50 percent of patients with weakness confined to the ocular muscles. The presence of anti-AChR antibodies is virtually diagnostic of MG, but a negative test does not exclude the disease. The measured level of anti-AChR antibody does not correspond well with the severity of MG in different patients. However, in an individual patient, a treatment-induced fall in the antibody level often correlates with clinical improvement.

Differential diagnosis Several other conditions that cause weakness of the cranial and/or somatic musculature must be considered in the differential diagnosis of MG; these include drug-induced myasthenia, Lambert-Eaton myasthenic syndrome, neurasthenia, hyperthyroidism, botulism, intracranial mass lesions, and progressive external ophthalmoplegia. Treatment with *penicillamine* may result in true MG, but the weakness is mild, and recovery occurs within weeks or months after discontinuing its use. Other drugs such as *aminoglycoside antibiotics* in very large doses and *procainamide* can cause neuromuscular weakness in normal individuals or exacerbation of weakness in myasthenic patients.

The *Lambert-Eaton myasthenic syndrome* is a presynaptic disorder of the neuromuscular junction that can cause weakness similar to that of MG. The proximal muscles of the lower limbs are most commonly affected, but other muscles may be involved as well. Cranial nerve findings, including ptosis of the eyelids and diplopia, occur in up to 70 percent of patients and resemble features of MG. However, the two conditions are readily distinguished as patients with Lambert-Eaton syndrome have depressed or absent reflexes, autonomic changes such as dry mouth and impotence, and show incremental responses on repetitive nerve stimulation. It is now known that Lambert-Eaton syndrome is caused by an autoantibody directed against calcium channels on the motor nerve terminals, resulting in impaired release of ACh. A majority of patients with this syndrome have an associated malignancy, most commonly small cell carcinoma of the lung, which is thought to trigger the autoimmune response. The diagnosis of Lambert-Eaton syndrome may signal the presence of the tumor long before it would otherwise be detected, permitting early removal. Treatment of the neuromuscular disorder involves plasmapheresis and immunosuppression, as for MG.

Neurasthenia may present with weakness and fatigue, but muscle testing usually reveals the ''jerky release'' characteristic of nonorganic disorders, and the complaint of fatigue in these patients means tiredness or apathy rather than decreasing muscle power on repeated effort. *Hyperthyroidism* is readily diagnosed or excluded by tests of thyroid function, which should be routinely carried out in patients with suspected MG. It is worth noting that abnormalities of thyroid function (hyper- or hypothyroidism) may increase myasthenic weakness. *Botulism* can cause myasthenic-like weakness, but the pupils are often affected and repetitive nerve stimulation gives an *incremental*, rather than decremental, response. Diplopia that mimics the symptoms of MG may occasionally be due to *intracranial mass lesions* that compress nerves to the extraocular muscles (e.g., sphenoid ridge meningioma), but computed tomography (CT) or magnetic resonance imaging (MRI) scanning of the head and orbits usually reveals the lesion.

Progressive external ophthalmoplegia is a rare condition resulting in weakness of the extraocular muscles, which may be accompanied by weakness of the proximal muscles of the limbs, and a variety of other systemic features that are beyond the scope of this chapter. Most patients with this condition have mitochondrial disorders that can be detected on muscle biopsy (see Chap. 365).

Search for associated conditions Myasthenic patients have an increased incidence of several associated disorders. *Thymic abnormalities* occur in approximately 75 percent of patients, as noted above. Neoplastic change (thymoma) may produce enlargement of the thymus, which is best detected by CT or MRI scanning of the anterior mediastinum. Enlargement of the thymus in a patient over 40 years of age is highly suspicious of thymoma. *Hyperthyroidism* may occur in 3 to 8 percent of patients and may aggravate the myasthenic weakness. Tests of thyroid function should be obtained. Because of the *association with other autoimmune disorders*, blood tests for rheumatoid factor and antinuclear antibodies should be carried out in all patients. Chronic infection of any kind can exacerbate MG and should be carefully sought. Finally, measurements of *ventilatory function* are valuable because of the frequency and seriousness of respiratory impairment in myasthenic patients.

Because of the side effects of glucocorticoids and other immunosuppressive agents used in the treatment of MG, a thorough medical investigation should be made, searching specifically for evidence of chronic or latent infection (such as tuberculosis or hepatitis), hypertension, diabetes, renal impairment, and glaucoma.

MEDICAL AND SURGICAL THERAPY The prognosis has improved strikingly as a result of advances in treatment; virtually all myasthenic patients can be returned to full productive lives with proper therapy. The most important methods used in the treatment of myasthenia gravis include anticholinesterase medications, immunosuppressive agents, thymectomy, and plasmapheresis.

Anticholinesterase medications Most myasthenic patients can be improved, but few can be brought completely to normal by anticholinesterase medication. There is no substantial difference in efficacy among the various anticholinesterase drugs; oral pyridostigmine is most widely used in the United States. As a rule, the beneficial action of oral pyridostigmine begins within 15 to 30 min and lasts for 3 to 4 h, but the individual response may vary. Treatment is begun with a moderate dose, e.g., 60 mg 3 to 5 times daily. Adjustment of the dosage, i.e., frequency and amount, should be tailored to the patient's individual requirements throughout the day. For example, patients with weakness in chewing and swallowing may benefit by taking the medication before meals so that optimal strength coincides with mealtime. Long-acting pyridostigmine tablets may be helpful to get the patient through the night, but should never be used for daytime medication because of their variable absorption. The maximum useful dose of pyridostigmine rarely exceeds 120 mg every 3 h during daytime. Overdosage with anticholinesterase medication may cause increased weakness and other side effects. In some patients, muscarinic side effects of the anticholinesterase medication (diarrhea, abdominal cramps, salivation, nausea) may limit the dosage tolerated. In these cases, atropine may be used to block the autonomic side effects without altering the beneficial effects on skeletal muscle.

Thymectomy   Two separate issues should be distinguished: surgical removal of thymoma and thymectomy as a treatment for myasthenia gravis. In the case of thymoma, surgical removal is necessary because of the possibility of local tumor spread, although most thymomas are benign. In the absence of a tumor, the available evidence suggests that up to 85 percent of patients improve after thymectomy, and 35 percent may achieve drug-free remission. However, the improvement may begin as long as 1 to 10 years after surgery. The advantage of thymectomy is that it offers the possibility of long-term benefit, in some cases diminishing or eliminating the need for continuing medical treatment. In view of these potential benefits and of the negligible risk in skilled hands, thymectomy has gained widespread acceptance in the treatment of MG. It is the consensus that thymectomy should be carried out in all patients with generalized MG between the ages of puberty and at least 55. Whether thymectomy should be recommended as a rule in children, in adults over 55 years of age, and in patients with weakness limited to the ocular muscles is still a matter of debate. Thymectomy must be carried out in a hospital where this procedure is performed regularly, and where the staff is experienced in the pre- and postoperative management, anesthesia, and surgical techniques of total thymectomy.

Immunosuppression   Immunosuppression using glucocorticoids, azathioprine, and other drugs is effective in nearly all patients with MG. The choice of which drugs to use should be guided by their relative benefits and risks for the individual patient. In general, clinical improvement begins somewhat more rapidly with steroid treatment than with the other immunosuppressive agents. The side effects of each drug may preclude its use in some patients, as indicated below.

STEROID THERAPY   Glucocorticoids, when used properly, produce improvement in myasthenic weakness in the great majority of patients. The initial dose of prednisone should be relatively low (15 to 25 mg/d) to avoid the early weakening that occurs in about one-third of patients treated initially with a high-dose regimen. The dose is increased stepwise, as tolerated by the patient (usually 5 mg/d at 2- to 3-day intervals), until there is marked clinical improvement or the dose of 50 mg/d is reached. This dose is maintained for 1 to 3 months and then is gradually modified to an alternate-day regimen over the course of an additional 1 to 2 months, until the dosage of 100 mg on alternate days is reached. Generally, patients begin to improve within a few months after reaching the maximum dose, and improvement continues to progress for months or years. The prednisone dosage may gradually be reduced, but usually months or years may be needed to determine the minimum effective dose and close monitoring is required by patient and doctor. *Few patients are able to do without prednisone entirely.* Patients on long-term glucocorticoid therapy must be carefully followed to prevent or treat adverse side effects. The commonest errors in the steroid treatment of myasthenic patients include:

1 Insufficient persistence; improvement may be delayed and gradual

2 Too early, too rapid, or excessive tapering of steroid dosage

3 Lack of attention to prevention and treatment of side effects

The management of patients treated with glucocorticoids is discussed in Chap. 317.

OTHER IMMUNOSUPPRESSIVE DRUGS   Azathioprine, cyclosporine (ciclosporin), or occasionally cyclophosphamide is effective in many patients, either alone or in combination with glucocorticoid therapy. Azathioprine is the most widely used because of its relative safety in most patients. Its therapeutic effect may add to that of glucocorticoids and/or allow the steroid dose to be reduced. However, up to 10 percent of patients are unable to tolerate azathioprine because of idiosyncratic reactions consisting of flulike symptoms of fever and malaise, bone marrow depression, or abnormalities of liver function. An initial dose of 50 mg/d should be used to test for adverse side effects. If this is tolerated, the dose is gradually increased until the white blood count falls to approximately 3000 (except in patients concomitantly receiving steroids), or the lymphocyte count falls below 1000 per microliter. The typical dosage range is 2 to 3 mg/kg body weight. The beneficial effect of azathioprine takes at least 3 to 6 months to begin and even longer to reach a maximum level.

Cyclosporine is approximately as effective as azathioprine. It is usually reserved for patients who cannot tolerate azathioprine, as its use is more complicated, requiring measurement of blood levels, and the side effects (particularly nephrotoxicity) are more problematic. Cyclophosphamide is reserved for patients refractory to the other drugs because of the relatively high risk of adverse side effects, including late development of malignancies.

Plasmapheresis   In view of the antibody-mediated pathogenesis of MG, plasmapheresis has been used therapeutically. The plasma, which contains the pathogenic antibodies, is mechanically separated from the blood cells, which are returned to the patient in a suitable fluid medium. Plasmapheresis produces a short-term reduction in anti-AChR antibodies, with clinical improvement in many patients. Thus, it is useful as a temporary expedient in seriously affected patients, or to improve the patient's condition prior to surgery (e.g., thymectomy). The long-term treatment of myasthenic patients requires other methods of therapy outlined in this chapter.

Management of myasthenic crisis   Myasthenic crisis is defined as an exacerbation of weakness sufficient to endanger life. The usual serious threats to life are respiratory failure, caused by diaphragmatic and intercostal weakness, and aspiration, secondary to pharyngeal weakness. Treatment should be carried out in an intensive care unit staffed with physicians experienced in the management of myasthenia gravis, respiratory insufficiency, infectious disease, and fluid and electrolyte therapy. The possibility that the deterioration could be due to excessive anti-ChE medication ("cholinergic crisis") is best excluded by temporarily stopping anti-ChE drugs. The most common cause of crisis is intercurrent infection. This should be treated immediately, because the mechanical and immunologic defenses of the patient can be assumed to be compromised. The myasthenic patient with fever and early infection should be treated like other immunocompromised patients. Early and effective antibiotic therapy, respiratory assistance, and pulmonary physiotherapy are essentials of the treatment program. As discussed above, plasmapheresis is frequently helpful in hastening recovery.

REFERENCES

DRACHMAN DB: Biology of myasthenia gravis. Ann Rev Neurosci 4:195, 1981

——— (ed): Myasthenia gravis: Biology and treatment. Ann NY Acad Sci 505:1, 1987

ENGEL AG et al: The motor endplate in myasthenia gravis and in experimental autoimmune myasthenia gravis: A quantitative ultrastructural study. Ann NY Acad Sci 274:60, 1976

FAMBROUGH DM et al: Neuromuscular junction in myasthenia gravis: Decreased acetylcholine receptors. Science 182:293, 1973

LINDSTROM J et al: Myasthenia gravis. Advances in Immunol 42:233, 1988

TANDAN R et al: Metastasizing thymoma and myasthenia gravis. Favorable response to glucocorticoids after failed chemotherapy and radiation treatment. Cancer 65:1286, 1990

TOYKA KV et al: Myasthenia gravis: Study of humoral immune mechanisms by passive transfer to mice. N Engl J Med 296:125, 1977

367   PERIODIC PARALYSIS

ROBERT C. GRIGGS

Disorders that cause patients of normal strength to become weak intermittently are not common. In contrast, the complaint of intermittent weakness is frequently encountered. The evaluation of such symptoms is challenging because the examination is often normal between attacks and because reliance on history is crucial for diagnosis. This chapter considers the primary periodic paralyses. Other disorders that cause episodic weakness are considered elsewhere (see Chap 27).

All primary periodic paralyses have some features in common. In most patients the disorders are inherited as autosomal dominant traits. Symptoms usually begin early in life and rarely commence after age 25. Attacks typically follow rest or sleep and almost never occur in the midst of vigorous activity, although antecedent exercise frequently provokes weakness. Patients remain alert during the attacks. Early in the course of these disorders interattack strength is normal but after years of attacks progressive weakness may develop. All forms of periodic paralysis are amenable to treatment and progressive weakness can be prevented and even reversed.

Diagnosis is based upon patient history and confirmed by appropriate evaluation of serum electrolytes during attacks and by evaluating the response of strength to provocative testing with glucose, insulin, potassium, and cold.

HYPOKALEMIC PERIODIC PARALYSIS   This disorder occurs as an autosomal dominant condition in two-thirds of cases and as sporadic cases in one-third. Males are more frequently and more severely affected. Attacks of weakness characteristically begin in adolescence but may commence in the first decade. Onset after age 25 is rare; the new onset of episodic paralysis in older individuals is almost never due to periodic paralysis.

Attack frequency varies from daily to yearly. Attacks last from 3 to 4 h to as long as a day or more. Meals high in carbohydrate or high in sodium may provoke attacks. Paralysis involves limb muscles, usually proximal more than distal; rarely ocular, bulbar, or respiratory muscles are weakened, and bulbar and respiratory involvement may prove fatal. Reflexes become hypoactive, and cardiac arrythmias may occur during attacks. Patients may develop persistent proximal weakness after years of attacks. Examination during attack-free intervals is otherwise normal except for the frequent presence of eyelid myotonia.

Diagnosis is established by demonstrating a low serum potassium during a paralytic attack and by excluding secondary causes of hypokalemia (Chap 27). Electrocardiograms during attacks show characteristic features of hypokalemia. Electromyography is not helpful in diagnosis, but muscle biopsy often shows the presence of single or multiple centrally placed vacuoles. Patients whose attacks are so infrequent as to preclude the study of a spontaneous attack require provocative testing with glucose and insulin administration. Such tests are potentially hazardous, and patients must be carefully monitored during their performance. Since these disorders are rare such testing is most appropriately carried out in referral centers.

Pathogenesis   The pathogenesis of paralytic attacks is incompletely understood. There is evidence for an abnormality of muscle membrane, possibly in sodium transport in hypokalemic and other forms of periodic paralysis. The contractile apparatus is normal. Distinctive abnormalities in potassium regulation occur in hypokalemic periodic paralysis. Patients with hypokalemic periodic paralysis often have a decrease in total body potassium but this may reflect muscle wasting. There is no increased excretion of potassium in the urine before or during attacks, but there is excessive flux of potassium from blood into muscle, possibly owing to an abnormality of muscle membrane that causes muscle to become electrically inexcitable.

Muscle from these patients is abnormally sensitive to the effect of insulin on potassium uptake; the significance of this increased sensitivity is not known since weakness is often severe at levels of serum potassium that do not affect normal individuals. Moreover, attacks may occur when insulin levels are low. Therefore, factors other than hypokalemia per se are important in the induction of weakness.

Treatment   ACUTE ATTACKS   The acute paralysis improves following the administration of potassium salts. Oral KCl (0.2 to 0.4 mmol/kg) should be given to patients with severe weakness and repeated at 15 to 30 min intervals depending on the response of the ECG, serum potassium, and muscle strength. Milder attacks usually resolve spontaneously; resolution of weakness is hastened by exercising affected muscles. When patients are unable to swallow or are vomiting, intravenous therapy may be necessary. Small, repeated bolus therapy with KCl (0.1 mmol/kg) may be administered over 5 to 10 min with careful monitoring of the ECG and serum potassium. If potassium is administered as a dilute solution (20 to 40 mmol/L) in 5% glucose or in physiologic saline solution, serum potassium may decline, and weakness may worsen. Mannitol is the preferred vehicle for administering intravenous potassium in such situations since it facilitates rapid return of serum potassium to normal and avoids the hazard of lowering of serum potassium as may occur when glucose or saline solution are given.

PREVENTION OF ATTACKS   The goal of therapy is the elimination of attacks, which also prevents interattack weakness and may improve interattack weakness after it has developed. Prior to availability of effective means of attack prevention, chronic progressive interattack weakness frequently caused serious disability. Prophylactic administration of potassium salts, even in large dosage, does not prevent attacks but acetazolamide (125 to 1000 mg/d in divided dosage) abolishes attacks in the majority of cases. The mechanism of action of acetazolamide is not fully understood, but it may block the flux of potassium from serum into muscle. The metabolic acidosis that it produces may underlie its beneficial effect. Paradoxically, acetazolamide lowers serum potassium; to achieve an adequate response in some patients it may be necessary to give supplementary potassium along with acetazolamide and to avoid high-carbohydrate meals. Chronic acetazolamide treatment may be associated with renal calculi, and patients should be monitored for this complication. In occasional patients attacks may not respond to or may even be worsened by acetazolamide. In such patients triamterene (25 to 100 mg/d or spironolactone 25 to 100 mg/d) may prevent attacks.

THYROTOXIC PERIODIC PARALYSIS   Attacks of hypokalemic periodic paralysis can occur in subjects with thyrotoxicosis, most commonly in young Latin American or oriental men where up to 10 percent of thyrotoxic patients may have periodic paralysis. In many patients thyrotoxicosis has also been overlooked for many months; periodic paralysis has also occurred with T_3-toxicosis and with exogenous thyroid hormone administration. The usual age of onset of the disorder is that of thyrotoxicosis; otherwise the clinical features resemble familial hypokalemic periodic paralysis. Acute attacks respond to potassium administration. Treatment of underlying thyrotoxicosis abolishes attacks and β-adrenergic blocking agents reduce the frequency and severity of attacks while measures to control thyrotoxicosis are being instituted. Acetazolamide is not helpful in preventing attacks. The pathogenesis of thyrotoxic periodic paralysis is uncertain but there is evidence for a decrease in the activity of the calcium pump. The pathogenesis of thyrotoxic periodic paralysis is likely to be different from that of nonthyrotoxic periodic paralysis since thyroid hormone does not worsen the latter.

HYPERKALEMIC PERIODIC PARALYSIS   This disorder differs from hypokalemic periodic paralysis in that attacks are usually brief (1 to 2 h or less) and more frequent; clinical or electromyographic myotonia is often demonstrable. Attacks are usually precipitated by fasting or by rest following exercise. The disease onset is usually at an earlier age than for hypokalemic periodic paralysis, and attacks or myotonia may be evident in the first year of life. The disorder is usually transmitted as an autosomal dominant defect; rare sporadic cases occur.

The name "hyperkalemic" is misleading since patients are often normokalemic during attacks. It is the fact that attacks are *precipitated by potassium administration* that best defines the disorder. "Potassium-sensitive" periodic paralysis is probably preferable terminology. Moreover, the serum potassium is often slightly elevated when patients are not having attacks of weakness. Attacks are characterized by limb weakness predominantly, though cranial and respiratory muscle involvement may occur. Cardiac arrythmias occur occasionally. Paresthesias and muscle pain are present during many attacks, and Chvostek's sign is often present during attacks.

Diagnosis is suggested by a modest elevation of serum potassium during attacks in nearly half of patients; at times, however, the serum potassium is normal or even low. Intravenous glucose-insulin loading does not precipitate weakness but potassium-loading tests (0.05 to 0.15 g/kg) will provoke weakness in such patients. Myotonia may be increased. Potassium-loading tests are potentially hazardous and are contraindicated in patients with renal disease and diabetes. Random serum potassium measurements may suggest the diagnosis since potassium elevations are frequent during attack-free intervals. Electromyographic evidence of myotonia and the finding of vacuoles on muscle biopsy provide supporting data.

Pathogenesis   Hyperkalemia during attacks of hyperkalemic periodic paralysis seldom reaches levels that would be expected to produce paralysis. Furthermore, serum potassium may remain within the normal range. Factors other than hyperkalemia are clearly important in the pathogenesis of attacks. An abnormality of the sarcolemma may cause spontaneous depolarization of the muscle cell and lead both to myotonia and to paralysis. Increased permeability of the muscle membrane to sodium has been noted; a decreased activity of the sodium-potassium pump may be involved in the spontaneous depolarization.

Treatment   Attacks of weakness are seldom severe enough to require emergency treatment and are never fatal. Oral glucose or other carbohydrate hastens recovery. Since interattack weakness may develop after repeated attacks, prophylactic treatment is usually indicated. Remarkably, acetazolamide (125 to 1000 mg/d), the treatment of choice for hypokalemic periodic paralysis, was first found to be beneficial for hyperkalemic periodic paralysis, possibly because of its kaliopenic effect. Thiazide diuretics (e.g., chlorothiazide 250 to 1000 mg/d) are usually more effective and have fewer side effects.

NORMOKALEMIC PERIODIC PARALYSIS   Most subjects with periodic paralysis in whom potassium is normal during attacks, behave like those with typical "hyperkalemic" periodic paralysis, since they are similarly sensitive to potassium administration. In fact, the so-called hyperkalemic and normokalemic forms of this disorder may be a single entity. Treatment is the same as for hyperkalemic periodic paralysis.

Rarely, patients with episodic normokalemic paralysis are not potassium sensitive, but they usually show evidence of muscle destruction or other features suggesting that they should not be classified as having a primary periodic paralysis.

PARAMYOTONIA WITH PERIODIC PARALYSIS   Attacks of paralysis may occur in the paramyotonias, either provoked by cold or spontaneously. Paramyotonia congenita is characterized by paradoxical (i.e., worsening with activity) myotonia, cold provocation, spontaneous attacks, and family history compatible with an autosomal dominant defect. The cold provocation of weakness and muscle stiffness distinguishes this disease from other periodic paralyses. A therapeutically useful subclassification of the paramyotonias has been proposed: (1) paramyotonia congenita, in which spontaneous attacks of weakness are associated with a lowering of serum potassium and in which measures that decrease serum potassium provoke weakness; and (2) paralysis periodica paramyotonia in which spontaneous attacks may be associated with hyperkalemia and may be provoked by oral potassium administration. This potassium sensitivity has led in the past to the classification of this disorder as a variant of hyperkalemic or normokalemic periodic paralysis.

Diagnosis depends upon the provocation of weakness and stiffness with cold. Glucose and insulin loading and potassium challenges aid in the subclassification of the disorder and provide assistance in the choice of medication for treatment.

Pathogenesis   The two types of paramyotonia probably have different etiologies. In paramyotonia congenita cooling of muscle results in an abnormal depolarization, leading first to myotonia and then to inexcitability. Both forms of paramyotonia are characterized by an abnormal uptake of potassium by muscle. Sodium and potassium conductance become abnormal with cooling of muscle. An abnormality of sodium channels with a resulting increase in sodium permeability may account for this alteration.

Treatment   Spontaneous attacks of periodic paralysis in paramyotonia congenita are relatively infrequent. Many patients do not require prophylactic treatment for prevention. In the case of paramyotonia congenita, patients with severe and frequent attacks of weakness may respond to spironolactone, and subjects with paralysis periodica paramyotonica may respond to acetazolamide or thiazides. Acetazolamide may provoke weakness in paramyotonia congenita. Myotonia in both types of paramyotonia improves with 400 to 1200 mg/d of tocainide or with mexiletine hydrochloride (150 to 900 mg/d). These antiarrhythmic agents may work in myotonia by blocking abnormal sodium channels; tocainide also improves weakness and decreases the abnormal uptake of potassium by muscle.

REFERENCES

GRIGGS RC et al: Intravenous treatment of hypokalemic periodic paralysis. Arch Neurol 40:539, 1983

MOXLEY RT et al: Potassium uptake in muscle during paramyotonic weakness. Neurology 39:952, 1989.

RESNICK JS et al: Acetazolamide prophylaxis in hypokalemic periodic paralysis. N Engl J Med 278:582, 1968

RIGGS JE: The periodic paralyses. Neurologic Clinics 6:485, 1988

STREIB EW: Paramyotonia congenita: Successful treatment with tocainide. Clinical and electrophysiological findings in seven patients. Muscle Nerve 10:155, 1987

section 1   Psychiatric disorders

368   PSYCHIATRY AND MEDICINE

This chapter's coverage is divided into major mood disorders (by Lewis L. Judd), schizophrenia (by David L. Braff), anxiety disorders (by Karen Thatcher Britton, S. Craig Risch, and J. Christian Gillin), and personality disorders (by Igor Grant).

MAJOR MOOD (AFFECTIVE) DISORDERS[1]

For centuries it was recognized that some individuals are subject to extremes in mood but, until recently, distinguishing mood alterations that are pathologic from those that are not was elusive. The realization that major mental disorders are psychobiologic phenomena resulting from abnormal brain mechanisms together with the development of an objective, empirically based diagnostic classification system has now made it possible for clinicians to distinguish consistently between abnormal mood states and the normal evanescent changes in emotions that are a part of everyday life.

Recent epidemiologic research has shown that at any instant about 5 percent of the adult population in this country is suffering from clinically significant mood (or affective) disorders. Traditionally, mental disorders in this category were designated as *affective* disorders; however, this has now been replaced by the term *mood* disorder, because the latter refers to a sustained rather than fluctuating emotional state. The mood disorders are a heterogeneous group of mental disorders characterized by extreme exaggerations and disturbances of mood and affect associated with physiologic (vegetative), cognitive, and psychomotor dysfunctions. There is a marked tendency to periodicity and recurrence throughout the patient's lifetime, in which diagnosable affective episodes appear and remit and are followed by symptom-free periods (euthymia) lasting weeks, months, or years. Indeed, recent studies have shown that the disability resulting from mood disorders, even those that are minimally symptomatic, exceeds that of most major chronic medical disorders such as diabetes, arthritis, and angina. The most prevalent and important diagnostic syndromes among the mood disorders are *major depression* (unipolar disorders) and *manic-depressive illness* (bipolar disorders).

The unipolar-bipolar division is a useful distinction in regard to clinical characteristics, life course, and treatment. Evidence continues to accumulate indicating that unipolar and bipolar depressions are, in all likelihood, psychobiologically different but very closely related disorders. For example, bipolar disorders tend to begin, on the average, a decade earlier, pursue a more recurrent course relative to unipolar depression, and respond better to lithium.

An additional distinction that has been helpful in reducing heter-

[1] By Lewis L. Judd. The author gratefully acknowledges the contributions of Robert M. A. Hirschfeld, M.D., Hagop Akiskel, M.D., Robert M. Post, M.D., and Nancy L. Ostrowski, Ph.D.

ogeneity among these disorders is that of primary-secondary. The rationale behind this is that affective disorders occurring in a pure form are likely to be more homogeneous than affective disorders that coexist with other psychiatric or medical conditions. A major affective disorder is *primary* when the affective episode (manic or depressive) is the first-appearing psychiatric illness in a patient's lifetime and is not associated with other psychiatric or medical illnesses. Conversely, a mood disorder is classified as *secondary* when it appears in conjunction with other psychiatric or medical conditions. Depressive episodes can be observed in conjunction with virtually every mental disorder, including schizophrenia, anxiety disorders, alcoholism, substance abuse, dementia, and personality disorders.

Mood disorders can also be associated with such medical diseases as the following: endocrinopathies (Cushing's disease, hyper- or hypothyroidism, hyperparathyroidism), collagen diseases (systemic lupus erythematosus), cardiovascular disease (congestive heart failure, myocardial infarction), neurologic diseases (stroke, Parkinson's disease, Alzheimer's disease, brain tumors, or multiple sclerosis), infections (hepatitis, influenza), malignancies (pancreatic adenocarcinoma, disseminated carcinomatosis), metabolic disorders (porphyria), and vitamin deficiencies (vitamin B_1, nicotinic acid). In addition, the chronic administration of the following medications can also precipitate an affective episode: glucocorticoids, α-methyldopa, propranolol, benzodiazepines, reserpine derivatives, levodopa, neuroleptics, cimetidine, indomethacin, cycloserine, and anti-cancer drugs. Withdrawal from CNS stimulants such as amphetamines or drugs of abuse like cocaine may also be a precipitating factor. It should be noted, however, that even though an affective episode may be classified as being secondary, it can be the most important and compelling aspect of a patient's clinical picture requiring immediate and specific therapeutic intervention (see also Chap. 29).

DIAGNOSTIC CATEGORIES OF MOOD DISORDERS   The diagnosis of a clinically significant affective episode is based upon the criteria contained in the revised third edition of the *Diagnostic and Statistical Manual* (DSM-IIIR). This method of diagnostic classification has been developed and approved by the American Psychiatric Association and is the official standard diagnostic system used in this country today. Two general types of affective episodes can be observed: major depressive episodes (sustained for at least 2 weeks) and manic episodes (sustained for at least 1 week). The diagnostic criteria for major depressive episodes and manic episodes are included in Tables 368-1 and 368-2.

Major depression   The diagnosis of major depression is made when the patient presents with the necessary signs and symptoms of a major depressive episode (see Table 368-1). The diagnostic category of major depression represents the unipolar form of the mood disorders, in which patients manifest only the single pole of affect, that of depression. The diagnosis of recurrent major depression is made when major depressive episodes are repeated throughout a patient's lifetime and is synonymous with the term recurrent unipolar depres-

TABLE 368-1 Diagnostic criteria for major depressive episode*

A At least five of the following symptoms have been present during the same 2-week period and represent a change from previous functioning; at least one of the symptoms is either (1) depressed mood, or (2) loss of interest or pleasure. (Do not include symptoms that are clearly due to a physical condition, mood-incongruent delusions or hallucinations, incoherence, or marked loosening of associations.)
  1 Depressed mood (or can be irritable mood in children and adolescents) most of the day, nearly every day, as indicated either by subjective account or observation by others
  2 Markedly diminished interest or pleasure in all, or almost all, activities most of the day, nearly every day (as indicated either by subjective account or observation by others of apathy most of the time)
  3 Significant weight loss or weight gain when not dieting (e.g., more than 5% of body weight in a month), or decrease or increase in appetite nearly every day (in children, consider failure to make expected weight gains)
  4 Insomnia or hypersomnia nearly every day
  5 Psychomotor agitation or retardation nearly every day (observable by others, not merely subjective feelings of restlessness or being slowed down)
  6 Fatigue or loss of energy nearly every day
  7 Feelings of worthlessness or excessive or inappropriate guilt (not merely self-reproach or guilt about being sick)
  8 Diminished ability to think or concentrate, or indecisiveness, nearly every day (either by subjective account or as observed by others)
  9 Recurrent thoughts of death (not just fear of dying), recurrent suicidal ideation without a specific plan, or a suicide attempt or a specific plan for committing suicide
B 1 It cannot be established that an organic factor initiated and maintained the disturbance
  2 The disturbance is not a normal reaction to the death of a loved one (uncomplicated bereavement)†
C At no time during the disturbance have there been delusions or hallucinations for as long as 2 weeks in the absence of prominent mood symptoms (i.e., before the mood symptoms developed or after they have remitted).
D Not superimposed on schizophrenia or schizophreniform, delusional, or psychotic disorders.

*A major depressive syndrome is defined as criterion A above.
†Morbid preoccupation with worthlessness, suicidal ideation, marked functional impairment or psychomotor retardation, or prolonged duration suggest bereavement complicated by major depression.
SOURCE: Adapted from DSM-IIIR.

TABLE 368-2 Diagnostic criteria for manic episode*

A A distinct period of abnormally and persistently elevated, expansive, or irritable mood.
B During the period of mood disturbance, at least three of the following symptoms have persisted (four if the mood is only irritable) and have been present to a significant degree:
  1 Inflated self-esteem or grandiosity
  2 Decreased need for sleep, e.g., feels rested after only 3 h of sleep
  3 More talkative than usual or pressure to keep talking
  4 Flight of ideas or subjective experience that thoughts are racing
  5 Distractibility, i.e., attention too easily drawn to unimportant or irrelevant external stimuli
  6 Increase in goal-directed activity (either socially, at work or school, or sexually) or psychomotor agitation
  7 Excessive involvement in pleasurable activities that have a high potential for painful consequences, e.g., the person engages in unrestrained buying sprees, sexual indiscretions, or foolish business investments
C Mood disturbance sufficiently severe to cause marked impairment in occupational functioning or in usual social activities or relationships with others, or to necessitate hospitalization to prevent harm to self or others
D At no time during the disturbance have there been delusions or hallucinations for as long as 2 weeks in the absence of prominent mood symptoms (i.e., before the mood symptoms developed or after they have remitted).
E Not superimposed on schizophrenia or schizophreniform, delusional, or psychotic disorders.
F It cannot be established that an organic factor initiated and maintained the disturbance.†

* A manic syndrome is defined as including criteria A, B, and C above. A hypomanic syndrome is defined as including criteria A and B, but not C, i.e., no marked impairment.
† Somatic antidepressant treatment (e.g., drugs, electroconvulsive therapy) that apparently precipitates a mood disturbance should not be considered an etiologic organic factor.
SOURCE: Adapted from DSM-IIIR.

sion. Following the first episode, between 50 and 80 percent of patients will have at least one more major depressive episode. Approximately 20 percent will have a subsequent manic episode, at which point the patient is then reclassified as having a bipolar disorder (manic depressive illness). Major depression is approximately twice as common in women as men. The 1-month prevalence in the adult population (18 years and over) is 2.9 percent for women and 1.6 percent for men. Age at first onset is most often in the late twenties and the thirties, but major depression can occur at any age. Most natural-course studies indicate that unipolar patients average two to three major depressive episodes during their lifetimes, although some patients have only single episodes and others have many more. The average duration of an untreated depressive episode is 8 to 9 months with a range of 1 to 12 months. There is no clear-cut relationship between risk for major depression and socioeconomic class, race, education, or occupation.

There are two other important subtypes of unipolar depression that should be noted: dysthymia and atypical major depression. *Dysthymia* is a chronic, milder form of depression. The diagnosis of dysthymia requires that the range of symptoms has been present for at least 2 years, but often patients describe many years of suffering (see Table 368-3). In the adult population dysthymia is twice as frequent in women as in men, and its 1-month prevalence is 3.3 percent. Clinical studies during the past decade have found that dysthymia occurs in conjunction with a major depression in about 25 percent of patients, a condition labeled *double-depression*. Double-depression is associated with substantially increased risks of recurrence and chronicity for major depression.

The symptoms of *atypical depression* actually match those of "typical" major depression but are distinguished from the latter by the following: reverse vegetative symptoms (e.g., overeating and hypersomnia), interpersonal rejection sensitivity, a sense of "leaden paralysis," or the experience of a significant amount of concurrent anxiety, and/or excessive responsiveness to environmental changes. It is clinically important to identify atypical major depression as distinct from typical major depression, because the former is often very responsive to monoamine oxidase inhibitor (MAOI) antidepressants. Non-psychiatric physicians must be fully aware that the classic manifestations of major depression and the variations described above are primarily based on studies in psychiatric settings. Recent evidence suggests that in medical, especially primary care, setting, many depressed patients initially present with minimal or no psychologic symptoms (e.g., dysphoric mood, low self-esteem, intense guilt, etc.) and instead focus on somatic complaints (e.g., fatigue, bodily

TABLE 368-3 Diagnostic criteria for dysthymia

A Depressed mood (or can be irritable mood in children and adolescents) for most of the day, more days than not, as indicated either by subjective account or observation by others, for at least 2 years (1 year for children and adolescents).
B Presence, while depressed, of at least two of the following:
  1 Poor appetite or overeating
  2 Insomnia or hypersomnia
  3 Low energy or fatigue
  4 Low self-esteem
  5 Poor concentration or difficulty making decisions
  6 Feelings of hopelessness
C During a 2-year period (1-year for children and adolescents) of the disturbance, never without the symptoms in A for more than 2 months at a time.
D No evidence of an unequivocal major depressive episode during the first 2 years (1 year for children and adolescents) of the disturbance.*
E Has never had a manic episode or an unequivocal hypomanic episode (see Table 368-2).
F Not superimposed on a chronic psychotic disorder, such as schizophrenia or delusional disorder.
G It cannot be established that an organic factor initiated and maintained the disturbance, e.g., prolonged administration of an antihypertensive medication.

* There may have been a previous major depressive episode, provided there was a full remission (no significant signs or symptoms for 6 months) before development of the dysthymia. In addition, after these 2 years (1 year in children and adolescents) of dysthymia, there may be superimposed episodes of major depression, in which case both diagnoses are given.
SOURCE: DSM-IIIR.

aches and pains, sleep problems, impotence, etc.). Some uninformed clinicians may refer to these patients somewhat pejoratively as "cracks." Frequently, these patients may initially deny subjective feelings of depression and may even appear superficially cheerful. Diagnosing these individuals is difficult, especially if the clinician is not alert to the possibility of a depressive episode. However, a previous personal history or the presence of a family history of typical mood disorders is an important diagnostic clue that a current mood disorder may be present. The importance of these patients to the primary care physician should not be underestimated as recent studies have indicated that this patient population presents the fourth most common set of complaints in primary care settings. Further, early diagnosis and treatment are vital; these patients and their families experience a great deal of personal suffering with patients often experiencing occupational difficulties, becoming big users of medical services, and tending toward substance abuse (especially alcohol) in misguided attempts at self-medication. Finally, and more ominously, data from "psychological" autopsies of suicide victims indicate that a significant percentage have sought medical advice for the same type of ill-defined somatic complaints previously noted and were unfortunately not diagnosed and hence not treated appropriately.

Bipolar disorders Bipolar disorders are diagnosed using the criteria for both manic and major depressive episodes. In this category of mood disorder, both the affective poles of mania and depression are present. Bipolar disorders are diagnosed as bipolar disorder, manic, if the current episode meets criteria for a manic episode and as bipolar disorder, depressed, if the episode meets criteria for a major depressive episode. Bipolar patients who have depressive and manic features simultaneously (e.g., extreme fatigue with racing thoughts, hypersomnia with increased sexual drive, etc.) are classified as bipolar disorder, mixed. Bipolar depression is slightly more frequent in women than men. Men have significantly more manic than depressive episodes, whereas women have significantly more depressive than manic episodes. The age of risk for bipolar disorder extends from as early as 6 to 7 years to over 65, but the peak age of onset in both men and women for the first attack is in the late twenties and early thirties, with a mean age of onset of 32.5 years. The illness can begin with either a manic or depressive episode. About two-thirds of first episodes are manic and approximately 60 percent of these patients will have a predominantly manic course, while the remaining 25 to 30 percent manifest primarily depressive episodes. Most natural-course studies of untreated bipolar patients generally agree that they will average nine diagnosable affective episodes during their lifetimes (range 1 to more than 20). The pattern is that the cycle length, which is measured from the onset of one episode to the onset of the next, will decrease and the number of episodes will increase over time. For example, in untreated bipolar patients the time between the first and second episode averages from 3.5 to 4 years, between the second and third episodes about 2 years, and between episodes three and four somewhere between 12 and 18 months. Episode duration is from 4 to 13 months, and the average is about 8.5 months but may be shorter during manic phases. Attempts have been made to categorize affective episodes in the bipolar patient based on how often the episodes occur in juxtaposition to those of opposite polarity. The vast majority of episodes are uniphasic, i.e., a manic or depressive episode is preceded by a symptom-free period; however, approximately 10 or 15 percent are biphasic with a depressive episode more often preceding the manic.

There is a small but distinct group of bipolar patients who manifest very rapid cycling patterns (bipolar disorder, mixed). The rapid cycler is a patient who presents with more than four or five episodes in 1 year, but there are patients who have considerably more episodes and there are case reports of patients cycling every 24 h. The rapid-cycling bipolar patient has eight times the number of affective episodes in his or her lifetime in comparison to slow cyclers. Eighty percent of rapid cyclers are women, and the appearance of rapid cycling may be related to impaired thyroid function. Although it is still controversial, there is evidence in a special subgroup of bipolar patients that rapid cycling may be related to previous treatment with tricyclic antidepressants and can only be effectively controlled after the patient is removed from tricyclics and treated with thyroid supplement.

The life-long intensity of illness in bipolar disorder, even among the slow cyclers, is much more extreme than it is in unipolar disorder. Bipolar patients have significantly more episodes of illness, more hospitalizations, spend more total time in the hospital during their lifetimes, are more likely to divorce and, if left untreated, are at significantly higher risk to commit suicide.

ETIOLOGY AND PATHOPHYSIOLOGY OF THE MAJOR MOOD DISORDERS Considerable progress has been made in identifying and characterizing the etiologic factors in major mood disorders, but a comprehensive and detailed understanding of the etiology of these disorders has yet to be achieved. Tremendous advances in knowledge during the past 25 years have provided excellent leads for focused scientific inquiry into the causes of these disorders; these leads, in turn, have led to the development of very specific and effective treatments. Like many other human diseases, the mood disorders are the result of interactions between the patient's genetic makeup and the environment. Evidence continues to mount that significant genetic factors are involved in these disorders, but the genetic components do not appear to be so overwhelming that the disorder is manifested without any environmental challenges. In general, the cause of a major affective episode can be conceptualized by two intersecting continua both with progressive intensities. One involves the patient's inherited constitutional predisposition to develop affective episodes; this interacts with the second continuum of the environmental stresses and life events to which the patient is exposed. Thus, there are those individuals with very high genetic predispositions for mood disorders in whom the disorder will be manifested seemingly without precipitating events. In contrast, there are patients with lower genetic predisposition in whom the disorder is manifested only when the patient is exposed to more serious precipitating life events and cumulative life stresses.

Genetic factors Data derived from virtually every methodologic strategy in human genetics strongly suggest significant genetic influences in the major mood disorders, but as yet the mode of genetic transmission has not been established. The degree of genetic expression varies considerably from patient to patient, and in some patients marked predictable genetic factors are present; in other genetic expression appears to be significantly less influential. *Twin studies* have been used by psychiatric geneticists to attempt to quantify genetic loading in various psychiatric diseases. Studies of mood disorders in twins have reported concordance rates among monozygotic (MZ) twins ranging from 33.3 to 75 percent, with an average of approximately 65 percent. In contrast, the concordance rates for dizygotic (DZ) twins range from 9 to 23 percent, averaging 15 percent. The difference in concordance rates between MZ and DZ twins strongly suggests inherited genetic vulnerability. The concordance rate is highest for recurrent (>3 episodes) mood disorders, which also suggests that the less recurrent mood disorders have less genetic influence. Although no definitive studies are available using the *adoption study* strategy, there is a trend indicating that adoptees with mood disorders have a greater incidence of affective illness in their biologic parents than in their adopted parents.

A large number of *family studies* have been conducted in the mood disorders. The standard paradigm is to make independent and blind diagnoses in the first-degree relatives of mood disorder patients, anticipating that if genetic components are present, the consanguineous relatives will manifest an increased risk for affective illness. First-degree relatives of bipolar patients have a morbidity risk for bipolar disorder ranging from 2.8 to 17.7 percent and a risk of up to 22.4 percent for unipolar depression. The first-degree relatives of unipolar patients have a risk of 6.4 to 17.0 percent for unipolar depression and of 0.3 to 29.0 percent for bipolar disorder. Thus, bipolar patients have both unipolar disorders among their blood relatives, whereas unipolar patients have increased incidence of unipolar, but not bipolar, disorders in their relatives. There is growing evidence that bipolar disorders are an excellent model for molecular genetic investigations. There are a large number of ongoing studies combining careful diagnostic and family pedigree studies with molecular genetics in an attempt to identify the linkage between specific gene markers and the manifestation of major mood disorder in an afflicted or informative family. Several years ago a group reported a genetic linkage on the short arm of chromosome 11 with bipolar disorders in a pedigree of the Old Order Amish. However, a more recent study on an expanded number of subjects in the same pedigree has failed to confirm the original observation. More recently a linkage on the X chromosome has been reported for bipolar disorder in an Israeli pedigree; to date this has not been confirmed by replication studies. In addition, a small subgroup of bipolar patients has been found who have a linkage between protan-deutan (red-green) color blindness, glucose-6-phosphate dehydrogenase deficiency, and the presence of bipolar disorder. Unfortunately this latter pattern has not been present in other families similarly afflicted with bipolar disorders.

In summary, the genetic studies strongly indicate the inheritance of a vulnerability to mood disorders, especially bipolar illness, but the genetic expression is heterogeneous and the degree of vulnerability varies significantly. There is evidence that the genetic factors are stronger in bipolar disorder than in unipolar depression. There is enormous promise for continued molecular genetic studies in the bipolar disorders, but as yet a definitive replicated linkage has not been identified.

Neurotransmitter systems   The earliest investigations of etiologic mechanisms in the mood disorders involved studies of the various neurotransmitter systems in the brain. The original biogenic amine hypothesis focused primarily on the central nervous system (CNS) neurotransmitters norepinephrine, serotonin, and dopamine, attributing depression and mania, respectively, to the deficiency or excess of these neurotransmitters at important synaptic sites in the brain. This hypothesis has stimulated and directed research in the field for many years, and data consistent with the hypothesis continue to emerge. Urinary and cerebrospinal fluid (CSF) studies of norepinephrine, its metabolite 3-methoxy-4-hydroxyphenethyleneglycol (MHPG), and the catalytic enzyme dopamine β-hydroxylase have been reported as being increased or decreased in the predictable direction during depressive and manic episodes. More recently, increases in norepinephrine have been described in both mania and depression. Recent studies identifying alterations in serotonin metabolism have focused attention on 5-hydroxyindole acetic acid (5-HIAA), a serotonin metabolite, that has been found to be reduced in the CSF of depressed patients who make frequent impulsive and aggressive suicide attempts. Deficits in other neurotransmitters such as dopamine and gamma-aminobutyric acid (GABA) have also been identified in some patients with major depression. Finally, another neurotransmitter hypothesis that has directed research in the affective disorders is the cholinergic hypothesis, which postulates increased central cholinergic tone in depression, decreased cholinergic tone in mania, and an imbalance between the cholinergic and adrenergic neurotransmitter systems as being a central pathophysiologic mechanism in affective disorders.

Within the past 10 years, there has been a shift of research focus from the neurotransmitter biosynthetic, storage, and release mechanisms in the presynaptic neuron to the study of receptors on postsynaptic neurons. There is growing evidence that postsynaptic receptor kinetics and activity are predictably and consistently altered during affective episodes and by the psychotropic medications known to ameliorate these disorders. Current research in the pathophysiology of the affective disorders is being concentrated on the role of postsynaptic receptor systems and especially the cascade of intraneuronal molecular and biochemical events that occur in the postsynaptic neuron following the binding of the neurotransmitter to the receptor.

In summary, there is general agreement in the large number of studies that have been conducted to date that the relative functional underactivity of neurotransmitter and/or the down-regulation of postsynaptic receptors have often been correlated with depressive episodes. However, the reciprocal changes that one would predict have not been consistently identified in manic episodes, in part because of the difficulties encountered in the study of these patients, who are extremely hyperactive and noncompliant. Nevertheless, the cumulative data present unequivocal evidence of dysfunctional brain mechanisms in the mood disorders, but a full and precise understanding of the pathophysiology is not yet available.

Environmental factors   There is little systematic data available indicating what role environmental stresses and untoward life events play or what types of stressors might be etiologically significant in the development of major affective episodes. Attempts have been made, for example, to relate early childhood loss and parental separation as predisposing factors for the future development of an affective illness, but the data are inconsistent. In general, studies have shown an overall temporal relationship between stressful and negative life events and the subsequent appearance of affective episodes. Research attempting to characterize qualitative differences in the impact of life stress have been disappointing, although serious life events such as the death of a child or a spouse, job loss, marked changes in social status, and even severe assaults on self-esteem have been linked to affective episodes. While the relationship between environmental stresses and the appearance of affective episodes has not always been demonstrated, generally speaking most experts agree that a single severe or multiple severe adverse events in life can interact with the constitutional predisposition of a patient and result in the triggering of an affective episode.

In further support of the influence of environmental events are the studies that have been conducted in higher primates. In these studies, phenomena that resemble or are analogous to the depressive states in humans are seen in monkeys using both mother/infant and peer separation paradigms. Interestingly, the monkey's "despair" response to the separation can be predictably enhanced by drugs known to specifically alter central concentrations and metabolism of various relevant CNS neurotransmitters (e.g., norepinephrine, dopamine), suggesting that psychosocial and CNS biochemical factors interact in the genesis of affective episodes.

Brain-environmental interactions   One of the brain's most important and central functions is to receive incoming stimuli from the environment for purposes of storage, integration, and interpretation, which in turn provides the basis for an organized and appropriate response. Thus, it should not be surprising to find that environmental events do exert consistent and powerful influences on brain function. However, there is a genuine paucity of testable hypotheses available that offer a plausible explanation of how environmental events could trigger the pathophysiologic brain processes that have been identified with recurrent mood disorders. One of the exceptions is the "kindling" hypothesis of Post and colleagues. From data based on animal models, including stimulant-induced behavioral sensitization (i.e., cocaine-induced seizures) and electrophysiologic kindling (increased sensitivity to electrically induced seizures), the suggestion has been made that a similar sensitization process may be involved in the recurrent episodes characteristic of the cyclic bipolar disorders. This hypothesis is consistent with the observations that spontaneous recurrences of affective episodes late in the progression of the illness seem, at times, to occur without precipitating factors; patients respond differently to pharmacotherapies at different stages of the disorder; there is frequently an increased sensitivity to anticonvulsant medications (i.e., carbamazepine combined with lithium) in some patients at late stages; and there is an increased rate of cycling as the disease progresses. One implication of this line of research is that prophylactic use of pharmacotherapy may be justifiable early in the treatment of unipolar and bipolar mood disorders.

Biologic rhythms   The marked tendency of major mood disorders to periodic manifestation and possibly to seasonal variations has stimulated hypotheses that suggest that the dysregulation of biologic rhythms may be centrally involved in the pathophysiology of affective disorders. There are reports of desynchronization of circadian rhythms in some bipolar patients in which these patients manifested both rapid free-running circadian rhythms (e.g., 23- versus 24-h rhythms) and a phase delay in their rhythms. There is also a special subgroup of patients with major depression in which the depressive episodes are manifested at specific seasons of the year. The most consistently studied groups are those with so-called "winter" depression (also called *seasonal affective disorder*). These patients, while residing in more northern latitudes, experience major depressive episodes during the winter when days are significantly shorter and periods of darkness more prolonged; they do not experience depression of this type when residing in latitudes where the environmental light/dark cycle is not as extreme. Controlled treatment studies, using intense white light (>2000 lux) presented at a specified time during the day and for a precise period of time, have proven to be therapeutically effective in some patients with this syndrome.

BIOLOGIC CORRELATES AND LABORATORY STUDIES   Neu-rohormonal correlates For a number of years probes into the pathophysiologic mechanisms of the affective disorders have used various neurohormones whose secretion is regulated by one or more of the CNS neurotransmitters. One consistent finding from these studies has been that a significant subpopulation of patients with major depression hypersecrete cortisol and have abnormal cortisol circadian secretion patterns. Recent investigations with corticotropin-releasing hormone (CRH) stimulation have yielded blunted adreno-corticotropic hormone (ACTH) responses, suggesting that the corti-costeroid abnormality is of central origin. In addition, even though it is now controversial, the dexamethasone suppression test (DST) has been useful in both diagnosis and monitoring of treatment. The standard DST used in psychiatry involves the administration of 1 mg of dexamethasone at 2300 hours with subsequent cortisol determi-nations at 1600 and 2300 hours the following day. The nonsuppression of cortisol is an abnormal or positive response [>140 nmol/L (>5 μg/dL) cortisol concentration in the 1600 or 2300 sample]. Initial studies reported that up to 50 percent of patients with serious major depression were nonsuppressors on the DST. Further investigations indicate that DST nonsuppression is most likely a state marker, which is positive during the depressive episode but returns to normal after successful resolution of the episode. False-positives on the DST occur in patients with alcoholism, malnutrition, obesity, pregnancy, major physical illnesses, anticonvulsant use, excessive caffeine intake, and in patients over 65 years and this has eroded the usefulness of the test. In addition, more recently a number of studies have appeared in the literature reporting a much smaller percentage of DST non-suppressors associated with major depressive episodes and an in-creased percentage in many other psychiatric illnesses. DST non-suppression among depressed patients has now been reported as low as 10 to 15 percent, especially among depressed outpatients, making this test of no value as a screening test for depression. While the status of this diagnostic marker is still controversial, it is useful in monitoring treatment efficacy in DST-positive depressives, since the DST response reverts to normal when the episode remits. Failure of DST to normalize despite apparent clinical recovery has, in some studies, been associated with suicide.

Other neuroendocrine markers have also been explored, but none as widely as the DST. In major depression, between 25 and 30 percent of patients respond to thyrotropin-releasing hormone (TRH) with blunted thyroid-stimulating hormone (TSH) responses. TSH blunting is not specific to depressive episodes, but an exaggerated TSH response to TRH suggests borderline hypothyroidism and might be useful in identifying those refractory or rapid-cycling bipolar patients who would benefit from thyroid supplementation (e.g., T_3 or T_4). Small subgroups of depressed patients have manifested blunted growth hormone responses to the following challenge agents: cloni-dine, amphetamine, levodopa, 5-hydroxytryptophan, and hypogly-cemia (insulin tolerance test). Even though 15 to 25 percent of depressed patients have blunted growth hormone responses, it has not proved to be diagnostically useful. More recently, blunted prolactin

responses to both TRH and opiate alkaloid challenges have also been reported in subpopulations of depressed patients; while these findings may be of interest in terms of pathophysiologic mechanisms, they are not useful diagnostically.

Sleep studies The disruption of sleep patterns is present in virtually every patient with major affective disorder, and polysom-nographic studies of sleep in these patients have proved to be of interest. In approximately 60 percent of cases of major depression there is a significantly shortened time period between the onset of sleep and the appearance of the first rapid eye movement (REM) (i.e., decreased REM latency). In addition, the density of the REM epoch, measured by the number of eye movements, is increased; there is a tendency for the REM epoch to be increased in duration, and there is a shift of REM activity to an earlier part of the night. These findings from all-night EEG sleep recordings have remained among the most consistent biologic markers for major depression, although they lack specificity, since short REM latency has also been reported in anorexia nervosa, obsessive-compulsive disorders, sleep apnea, and narcolepsy.

Neurotransmitter metabolites and enzymes The neurotrans-mitter hypotheses of mood disorders have stimulated a number of studies correlating biogenic amine metabolites with manic and de-pressive episodes. The data are inconsistent and have not been consistently useful either diagnostically or therapeutically. The one possible exception is MHPG, a metabolite of norepinephrine. Some workers have reported low MHPG excretion as predicting a positive therapeutic response to the antidepressants imipramine, desipramine, etc., and high MHPG excretion as predicting a response to amitrip-tyline, nortriptyline, etc. While these data are of interest and with further study may result in the identification of biochemical subtypes in major depression, these findings have not been regularly replicated in other laboratories.

Investigators who have examined the levels of the enzyme monoamine oxidase (MAO) in platelets, report it to be low in bipolar disorders and high in subjects with anxiety. Further, ^{3}[H]imipramine-binding studies in platelets also have been found to be low in major depressives who were suicidal. Again, these findings, although of interest, lack specificity, since similar results have also been reported to be altered in other psychiatric conditions such as alcoholism, anorexia and bulimia, and impulse control disorders.

TREATMENT OF THE MAJOR MOOD DISORDERS Important advances have been made in the treatment of the major mood disorders, and the majority of these patients can now be treated with a high degree of specificity and success. The most important discoveries have been in the development of potent psychotropic medications for both major depression and the bipolar disorders. The central therapeutic tools in the treatment of the major affective disorders are the antidepressants and lithium. The use of these psychotropic medications is specifically covered in much greater detail in Chap. 369.

Because major affective disorders have strong tendencies for recurrence, an important aspect of the patient's treatment is the comprehensive education of patients and their families about the disorder. It should be emphasized to the patient that these are psychobiologic disorders that involve altered biochemical states in the brain, and that episodes can be triggered by adverse events and stresses in the environment but may occur spontaneously as well. Each patient should be urged to become an expert on his or her own disorder, concentrating on how it manifests and what early signs and symptoms may herald an impending manic or depressive episode. The patient and the family must be urged to take on the responsi-bility for the early recognition of the impending episode, since the earlier a patient presents for treatment, the easier it is to remediate the episode. The absolute necessity of medication compli-ance must be emphasized, and the patient must understand thoroughly the need to take the medications precisely as prescribed and to be aware of side effects and of the potential medical sequelae from the medications.

The counseling and therapeutic techniques the physician uses in dealing with patients who are suffering acute manic or depressive episodes are simple and relatively straightforward. During the acute phase of these episodes, patients respond better to short (10 to 20 min) visits one to three times per week. During these visits the general focus is on monitoring the medication and side effects, but it is also essential that the physician be very reassuring and supportive to the patient. Because patients are functioning essentially in an altered state secondary to the depressive or manic episode, the treatment must be sustained by the physician's optimism and knowledge that, with time, these episodes can be abated or successfully terminated if the right medication and dose are prescribed. Virtually all the mood-stabilizing and -ameliorating psychotropic medications have a significant delay between the time the patient begins the medication and the time of achieving full therapeutic benefits. It is during this time that supportive reassurance and encouragement from the physician is particularly important in sustaining the patient in treatment.

There are approximately 30,000 suicides a year in this country, and clinical surveys have indicated that approximately 70 percent of these patients have major affective disorders. Suicidal ideation is one of the important symptoms that accompany major depression, in both bipolar and unipolar disorders; considerations of suicidal lethality are significant components of the management of these patients. Although it is not possible to distinguish precisely between patients who will attempt suicide and those who will not, there are some factors which should be considered. Generally speaking, many experts agree that patients who have given detailed thought to the method of suicide, who have concomitant alcoholism or drug abuse, and who are socially isolated with few (if any) social supports, in addition to elderly males and patients with terminal medical illnesses, have a greater potential risk for suicide. On the other hand, all of the above characteristics lack true specificity in the assessment of suicidal risk. However, one of the most important risk factors, recently identified, is the presence of an undiagnosed and untreated mental disorder, especially a mood disorder.

Once the acute depressive or manic episode is under control, the switch from supportive to more insight-oriented psychotherapy is a useful adjunct to the pharmacotherapy. Recent studies have established that the combination of psychotherapy with pharmacotherapy is significantly better than either of these two modalities alone. There is also evidence that three types of brief specific psychotherapy, cognitive, behavioral, and interpersonal psychotherapy, specifically designed to treat depression, can be successfully used in the treatment of mild to moderate depressive disorders. However, learning to become a competent psychotherapist in using one of these forms of psychotherapy, requires considerable training and experience to achieve results comparable to those obtained with the relatively simple administration of an antidepressant. Nevertheless, it is recommended that the nonpsychiatric physician rely primarily on the antidepressants or lithium (depending upon the disorder being treated) in combination with educational and supportive psychotherapeutic approaches in the management of patients with major affective disorders (see Chap. 369).

SCHIZOPHRENIC DISORDERS[2]

Schizophrenic disorders are serious mental illnesses that have a duration of 6 months or more and cause significant social, vocational, and personal disability and suffering. The schizophrenic patient often appears to be bizarre, inappropriate, and mentally impaired. Despite its stereotypic presentation, perhaps no other psychiatric disorder has proved as vexing and difficult to define, identify, and treat.

Schizophrenia has a lifetime prevalence rate of about 1 percent across all cultures. In the United States alone there are perhaps 2

[2] By David L. Braff.

million affected individuals who often become ill in their late teenage years and in the third decade of life. Poor outcome frequently leads to extensive and long-term disability, and schizophrenia accounts for a staggering estimated $20 billion per year of lost productivity in 1975 dollars. Most patients with schizophrenic disorders also cause major perturbations for family and social support systems, adding to the economic losses and the toll of human misery. Cumulatively, these factors make schizophrenia one of the most costly and vexing health problems.

DEFINITION AND CLINICAL MANIFESTATIONS In 1919, Emil Kraepelin first made the distinction between dementia praecox, a psychotic illness with progressive deterioration, and manic depressive psychosis. Kraepelin noted, however, that about 13 percent of patients with dementia praecox did not have an inevitably deteriorating outcome, and this favorable outcome has significantly increased largely due to the development and use of antipsychotic medications. Eugen Bleuler concentrated on the putative underlying psychological splitting of personality functions in his classic paper on the "group of schizophrenias." Bleuler's emphasis was on the "four As" of schizophrenia: *a*utism, flattened *a*ffect, loose *a*ssociations, and *a*mbivalence. Other authors have focused on specific symptoms of schizophrenia, such as the sense of being influenced by others and feelings of being controlled by outside forces. To date, research has yet to identify specific and inevitably pathognomonic signs or symptoms of the schizophrenic disorders.

According to DSM-IIIR, after the first and most central criterion of psychotic symptoms is met (see Table 368-4), the schizophrenic individual must show deterioration from a previous level of functioning in such areas as work, social relations, and self-care. The disorder is not attributable to other diagnoses such as mood disorder with psychotic features or organically induced syndromes. Finally, continuous signs of the illness should be present for 6 months at some point during the individual's life with some signs of illness at the time of diagnosis. There may be prodromal, active, and/or residual phases of the illness that are not always clearly demarcated. Prodromal or residual symptoms are somewhat nonspecific and may consist of isolation; marked psychosocial impairment; peculiar behavior; impaired personal hygiene and grooming; blunted, flat, or inappropriate affect; digressive, vague, over-elaborate, circumstantial, or metaphorical speech; odd or bizarre ideation or magical thinking; and unusual perceptual experiences.

TABLE 368-4 Diagnosis of schizophrenic disorders

A Presence of characteristic psychotic symptoms in active phase, either *1*, *2*, or *3* for at least 1 week (unless symptoms are successfully treated):
  1 Two of the following:
    Delusions
    Prominent hallucinations
    Incoherence or marked loosening of associations
    Catatonic behavior
    Flat or grossly inappropriate affect
  2 Bizarre delusions
  3 Prominent hallucinations of a voice with content having no apparent relation to depression or elation, or a voice keeping up a running commentary on the person's behavior or thoughts, or two or more voices conversing with each other
B During the course of disturbance, functioning in areas such as work, social relations, and self-care markedly below highest level achieved before onset of disturbance.
C Schizoaffective disorder and mood disorder with psychotic features have been ruled out.
D Continuous signs of disturbance for at least 6 months. This period must include an active phase (of at least 1 week, or less if symptoms have been successfully treated) during which there were psychotic symptoms characteristic of schizophrenia (see A above), with or without a prodromal or residual phase.
E It cannot be established that an organic factor initiated and maintained the disturbance.
F If a history of autistic disorder exists, the additional diagnosis of schizophrenia can be made only if prominent delusions or hallucinations are also present.

SOURCE: Adapted from DSM-IIIR.

The DSM-IIIR lists four major types of schizophrenic disorders:

1 Catatonic. A relatively rare type with features of stupor, rigidity, excitement, or posturing.

2 Disorganized. A type characterized by incoherence and flat or grossly disorganized affect.

3 Paranoid. A type featuring preoccupation with suspiciousness and one or more systematized delusions.

4 Undifferentiated. A type of disorder with prominent delusions, hallucinations, incoherence, or disorganized behavior, not meeting the criteria for the other three types (see DSM-IIIR for more detailed descriptions).

This emphasis on subtypes carries forward Bleuler's notion of the "group of schizophrenias." There is moderate support for a paranoid/nonparanoid dichotomy as being important in schizophrenia. In an attempt to reduce diagnostic heterogeneity, researchers have identified "type I" schizophrenic patients with a predominance of "positive" symptoms (e.g., hallucinations, paranoid ideation), normal cerebral ventricular size, and symptoms that respond to the hypothesized dopaminergic-blocking effects of antipsychotic drugs. In contrast, "type II" schizophrenic patients seem similar to Kraepelin's dementia praecox patients. Type II patients show a predominance of "negative" symptoms (e.g., anhedonia, social withdrawal, asociality), neuropsychological impairment, and possibly increased cerebral ventricular volume; they do not respond well to antipsychotic medications, but seem to display a "deficit state." The course of the illness is variable, from "in remission" to "chronic."

DIFFERENTIAL DIAGNOSIS Schizophrenic patients have no unique or pathognomonic signs and symptoms; at times, this makes the diagnosis difficult. DSM-IIIR separates psychotic illnesses by a durational criterion into *brief reactive psychoses* lasting 2 weeks or less, *schizophreniform* disorders lasting between 2 weeks and 6 months, and *schizophrenic disorders* lasting more than 6 months. While these distinctions are practical and heuristic, the scientific basis for such a durational criterion is poorly documented. In addition, an acute manic patient may be difficult to distinguish from the schizophrenic patient, especially on a cross-sectional as opposed to longitudinal basis. To complicate matters further, the initial clinical appearance of a patient intoxicated with phencyclidine (PCP) or amphetamines may also be indistinguishable from that of the paranoid schizophrenic patient. It appears then that many functional and organic states may lead to a final common pathway of psychotic symptoms. The diagnosis can only be established reliably by a broad-based multifactorial approach utilizing neurobiologic data (e.g., toxicologic screens, genetic history) and psychosocial data (e.g., premorbid adjustment status) obtained both acutely and over time. Despite these problems, the DSM-IIIR criteria for schizophrenic disorders have undergone extensive and successful field trials for reliability and validity. In general, clinicians using the DSM-IIIR criteria can accurately and consistently diagnose schizophrenia.

PREDISPOSING, PRECIPITATING, AND SUSTAINING FACTORS IN SCHIZOPHRENIA Factors that contribute to the development of schizophrenia can be analyzed in terms of predisposing, precipitating, and sustaining factors. These factors may be analyzed in terms of neuroanatomic and biochemical factors and neurophysiologic, psychophysiologic, intrapsychic, interpersonal, social, and socioeconomic factors. In a complex, multifactorial disorder such as schizophrenia, these neurobiologic and psychosocial factors should be seen as interactive rather than as competing or mutually exclusive. This approach is analogous to comprehensive analyses of diabetes mellitus or hypertension, which also have contributions based on genetics, receptor physiology, and physiologic, familial, psychosocial, and a myriad of other conceptually diverse factors. Within this context, predisposing factors are linked to etiologic variables, precipitating factors are related to the onset of pathophysiology, and sustaining factors are linked to outcome variables.

Etiology GENETIC FACTORS It is clear from twin, family, and adoptive studies that schizophrenia has a significant genetic basis.

Monozygotic twins have roughly a 65 percent or greater concordance rate for schizophrenia, whereas dizygotic twins have a 12 percent concordance rate. Other family studies show that the morbid risk for developing schizophrenia is 5 to 10 percent if one parent is schizophrenic. This figure rises to 46 percent or more if both parents are schizophrenics. Second-degree relatives of schizophrenics run a 2 to 4 percent risk of developing the illness compared to a risk of 1 to 2 percent in the general population.

Adoption studies reveal that these risk factors are largely genetically linked and are not primarily due to the "schizophrenogenic" psychosocial environment of certain families. Still, these figures are fraught with methodologic complexities. For example, reflecting the probable complex mode of inheritance, 89 percent of schizophrenics do not have a parent who is schizophrenic. Eighty-one percent of schizophrenics do not have either a schizophrenic sibling or parent. The appropriate model with which to explain these figures is complex and may include a weighted polygenic model or other sophisticated interpretations of genetic theory. Most recently, there has been an explosion of new knowledge about the genetics of schizophrenia, featuring molecular studies and linkages to chromosome 5 and possibly X (see the entire vol. 15, no. 3, of *Schizophrenia Bulletin,* 1989, and Crow et al.).

The *stress-diathesis model* hypothesizes that there is a vulnerability which is inherited in schizophrenia-prone individuals. These vulnerable individuals are at high risk for developing schizophrenia under certain stressful circumstances. Studies of high-risk children with one or two schizophrenic parents indicate that such children may have a significantly increased incidence of morbidity in utero, at birth, and in the perinatal period. In addition, these infants and children may have psychophysiologic lability, attentional dysfunction, and specific motor disturbances. A number of human and animal studies suggest that such labile attentional mechanisms may result partly or largely from instabilities and increased activity of the mesolimbic and mesocortical dopaminergic systems that have significant connections to the frontal cortex. The literature on neurophysiologically labile and vulnerable children seems to tie the genetic, dopaminergic, and attentional dysfunction hypotheses together. According to the stress-diathesis model, a host of stressful factors may precipitate a psychotic state in a high-risk individual. These factors include intoxication with PCP or amphetamines as well as more nonspecific factors such as medical illnesses and psychosocial life events with concomitant general stress. Further, specific hallucinogens such as lysergic acid diethylamide (LSD) may precipitate a psychotic episode that is ultimately indistinguishable from a schizophrenic disorder. Lastly, there have been a number of hypotheses that a viral vector or early developmental abnormalities may be important as etiologic agents in a least some cases of schizophrenic disorders.

PSYCHOSOCIAL FACTORS There are many psychosocial hypotheses concerning the creation of a predisposition or vulnerability to developing schizophrenia. Empirical support for most of these hypotheses is variable and far from definitive.

In the vulnerable individual, schizophrenia is seen as having its onset in a critical developmental period. The teenager may attempt to leave home and separate from family members for school or work reasons. The onset is often, but not invariably, insidious. In terms of psychosocial approaches to schizophrenia, there is felt to be a developmental or intrapsychic deficit in the vulnerable individual. Once set into motion, the psychosis passes through a series of stages leading to the final common pathway of a psychotic state.

Despite much theorizing, there is no inevitable schizophrenia-prone personality type, although at least a small but significant percentage of schizoid, paranoid, and schizotypal personality-disordered individuals do seem to be vulnerable to developing schizophrenic disorders. In the 1960s, a more family-systems-oriented view emerged. An example of this approach is the "double-bind" hypothesis of Bateson and coworkers who analyzed the formal communications patterns in "schizophrenogenic" families. In this view, communications content is less important than the frequently conflicting and self-contradictory form of communications style of schizophrenic patients' families. It remains unclear whether these familial factors are a cause or a result of having a schizophrenic child in the family. As the importance of biologic factors in schizophrenia have become clearer, family psychosocial factors have been seen more as secondary or epiphenomenal factors.

Psychosocial researchers have also examined the importance of socioeconomic factors in schizophrenia. Lower socioeconomic status correlates with a higher incidence of schizophrenia. There are two possible interpretations of these data. First, there may be a "social drift" of vulnerable individuals to lower socioeconomic status. The second hypothesis is more etiologic—socioeconomic stresses may precipitate schizophrenic episodes, especially in vulnerable individuals.

Pathophysiology NEUROTRANSMITTERS AND NEUROPEPTIDES A number of neurobiologic factors have been correlated with schizophrenic episodes. Which neurobiologic systems underlie the acute psychotic symptoms? Currently, the predominant neurotransmitter hypothesis explaining the pathophysiology of schizophrenic disorders involves dopaminergic overactivity. Evidence supporting the *dopamine hypothesis* comes from several sources. First, the potency of all antipsychotic medications can be roughly predicted by their dopaminergic-blocking capacity. Second, mesolimbic dopamine plays a role in attentional mechanisms and stimulus filtering. When stimulus-filtering mechanisms break down, there is a collapse of the information-processing capacity of the individual, with resulting sensory inundation, cognitive fragmentation, and symptoms of thought disorder.

Despite this support, the dopamine theory of schizophrenia is fraught with complexities when compared with the catecholamine theory of the affective disorders. Affective disorders hypothetically (and oversimplistically) reflect a decrease in norepinephrine tone in hypothalamic nuclei leading to a final common pathway of neurovegetative symptoms. In schizophrenia, there seems to be increased dopamine tone in critical subcortical pathways leading to cognitive fragmentation, thought disorder, and clinical impairment; the impairment and the clinical symptoms are quite complex and highly variable. In this framework, affective disorders may be seen as impinging on the diencephalic "core" of the brain, whereas schizophrenia is conceptualized as a disorder of the mesolimbic-frontal cortical mantle. It is doubtful if any "one neurotransmitter" theory of any psychiatric disorder can reflect the interactive complexity of various neurobiologic and psychosocial systems, although such theories may be useful.

The hypothesis of dopamine overactivity in schizophrenia is generally characterized as a static theory. In reality, dopamine tone is related in a dynamic and variable manner to gamma-aminobutyric acid, serotonin, and other neurotransmitters that are functionally arrayed in a cascade of important brain systems, such as the dorsolateral prefrontal cortex, mesial temporal cortex, nucleus accumbens, ventral pallidum, and the hippocampus. Longer-term correlates of schizophrenia may also involve alterations of neuropeptides with their longer latency and response effects on behavior. At an electrophysiologic level, it has been hypothesized that the initial disturbance in schizophrenia is an aberrant (perhaps excitotoxic-induced) temporal lobe focus that perturbs the homeostasis of the dopamine system. All of these theories are receiving critical experiment scrutiny.

NEUROPATHOLOGIC CHANGES The use of computed tomography (CT) and magnetic resonance imaging (MRI) has been widely employed in studies of schizophrenic patients. Initial reports indicated that a minority of schizophrenic patients had abnormally increased ventricle-brain ratios, reflecting increased ventricular fluid volume associated with brain atrophy. Subsequent studies in identical twins have confirmed increased ventricular size in schizophrenic patients, supporting the contention that schizophrenia is accompanied by brain atrophy. It is quite possible that type II patients have a disorder that is distinct and associated with poor medication response and poor

clinical outcome. Positron emission tomography (PET) data reveal patterns of decreased frontal lobe activity in schizophrenia (hypofrontality) that seem important, especially in view of the close relationship of dopamine activity and frontal lobe function. Future PET studies utilizing new ligands will undoubtedly add to the knowledge of dopamine and other neurotransmitters in the schizophrenic disorders.

PSYCHOPHYSIOLOGY AND INFORMATION PROCESSING Important insights into the pathophysiology of schizophrenia have also been generated by psychophysiologic and information-processing studies. Individuals at high risk for developing schizophrenia and patients with a schizophrenic disorder are frequently psychophysiologically labile and vulnerable to being inundated by stimuli. The proposed mechanism for such vulnerability is an impairment in an individual's ability to screen out irrelevant stimuli and an associated inability to habituate to externally and internally generated cues. Ultimately, this dysfunction, which has been linked to dopamine overactivity in humans and animals, leads to an information-processing overload. The affected person becomes inundated with stimuli and displays cognitive fragmentation and thought disorder. Using attentional tasks, skin conductance habituation, and other measures, investigators have increasingly underscored the importance of these dysfunctions in the schizophrenic disorders. New techniques, such as magnetoencephalography, also offer exciting possibilities for specifying the locus and type of brain disturbance characteristic of the various types of schizophrenic disorders.

Treatment and outcome NEUROBIOLOGIC FACTORS Five-year follow-up studies show that 60 percent of schizophrenic individuals have social recovery and half of those are employed. Thirty percent are handicapped and 10 percent remain hospitalized. This pattern of outcome seems still to be generally accurate. Which factors determine the outcome of the schizophrenic disorders are not clear. It is commonly stated that the outcome of schizophrenia is better when disorientation, affective symptoms, and acute onset are present. The outcome of schizophrenic disorders is thought to be poorer when the patient is well-oriented and has fewer affective symptoms and when the onset is insidious.

The outcome of schizophrenic disorders has been greatly improved by the use of potent and efficacious antipsychotic medications, such as the phenothiazines (see Chap. 369). Studies indicate that antipsychotic medications (often expressed in terms of chlorpromazine equivalents) act selectively against specific target symptoms that are similar to the "positive" symptoms of type I schizophrenia, which include hallucinations and psychotic agitation. In contrast to these responsive target symptoms, antipsychotic medications may not necessarily improve "negative" symptoms such as anhedonia and social withdrawal. The primary treatment modalities for the acute schizophrenic disorders are antipsychotic medication along with psychosocial therapies. The typical schizophrenic patient usually requires at least the equivalent of 600 to 800 mg per day of chlorpromazine administered for 4 to 6 weeks, although higher doses are frequently necessary. Maintenance doses of antipsychotic medications in lower doses and given on a continuous or intermittent basis are often required to prevent relapse.

Antipsychotic medications alter dopaminergic-cholinergic balance in nigrostriatal structures (via dopamine blockade) so that acute extrapyramidal side effects are induced (e.g. dystonia, motor restlessness). These side effects can be treated with anticholinergic medications that restore dopaminergic-cholinergic balance. Aliphatic phenothiazines (such as chlorpromazine) with inherent anticholinergic properties cause fewer extrapyramidal side effects but induce more anticholinergic side effects, such as hypotension or blurred vision. Additionally, blood dyscrasias, liver toxicity, and other idiosyncratic reactions can occur. Also, the long-term use of antipsychotic medications may induce nigrostriatal damage and tardive dyskinesia, a long-lasting and potentially disabling motor syndrome (see Chaps. 25 and 369). Thus the search for new antipsychotic medications with more selective (i.e., nonnigrostriatal) sites of action is critically important for the pharmacologic treatment of schizophrenia. Drugs, such as clozaryl, have been postulated (but not proven) to have such selective properties.

PSYCHOSOCIAL FACTORS   The outcome of schizophrenic patients can be divided into the semi-independent axes of symptoms, rehospitalization, social function, and vocational function. It is possible to treat the specific psychotic symptoms of a schizophrenic individual (affecting the symptomatic axis of outcome), but the patient may be left with major psychosocial deficits (the social axis of outcome). Antipsychotic medications should thus be combined with sensitive psychosocial management including, where appropriate, individual and group psychotherapy, family counseling, and vocational rehabilitation in order to maximize therapeutic outcome and to restore the patient to the premorbid level of adjustment. For example, returning an acutely treated schizophrenic patient to a home filled with hostility, criticisms, and emotional overinvolvement (the so-called high-expressed-emotion family) without the benefit of family therapy is poor psychosocial management and may lead to relapse and poor outcome. Family counseling is often a critical determinant of therapeutic outcome in the schizophrenic disorders.

ANXIETY DISORDERS[3]

Anxiety is a common emotion and as such is often a normal response to the vicissitudes of life. In its mild forms, anxiety may be adaptive. A little anxiety, for example, helps a student prepare for examinations. In its extreme forms, however, anxiety is incapacitating or terrifying. High anxiety may cause the same student to lose concentration, memory, or even his or her voice.

Physicians observe anxiety most commonly in patients experiencing an acute external stress. Although short-term treatment with antianxiety or sedative drugs, such as benzodiazepines, has a place in the management of such patients, physicians often can offer more help by their presence, reassurances, and attitude. Anxiety states often resolve spontaneously with time, although clinicians should be aware that acute stress can lead to chronic anxiety or posttraumatic stress disorder.

The word *anxiety* has more precise diagnostic meaning in psychiatry. It refers to both *paroxysmal* and *persistent* psychological feelings (dread, irritability, ruminations) and physiologic changes (dyspnea, sweating, insomnia, trembling) which endure over time and impair normal functioning. These are often chronic disorders in which symptoms persist in the absence of obvious contemporaneous external stresses or in which the degree of symptoms seems out of proportion to the degree of external stress. Anxiety disorders were formerly lumped together under the term "anxiety neurosis." It is now recognized that a number of relatively distinct syndromes exist under the general rubric of anxiety disorders (Table 368-5).

PANIC DISORDER   Definition   The cardinal feature of panic disorder is the sudden, unexpected, and often overwhelming feeling of terror and apprehension accompanied by somatic symptoms in multiple organ systems such as dyspnea, palpitations, and faintness. The symptoms and signs of panic disorder are similar to those occurring during intense physical exertion or in a life-threatening situation.

Incidence and epidemiology   Panic disorder is estimated to occur in 1 to 2 percent of the population and is equally divided between the sexes. The most frequent age of onset of panic attack is the late teen years and early twenties. Panic disorders tend to be familial, and both panic disorder and affective disorder often coexist in the same family. If an individual has a diagnosed panic disorder, up to 18 percent of first-degree relatives also will have panic disorder. Furthermore, twin studies demonstrate a greater incidence in monozygotic twins, suggesting that panic anxiety may have a genetic basis.

Clinical features   A typical panic attack often begins abruptly and without warning while a patient is involved in a relatively

[3] By Karen Thatcher Britton, S. Craig Risch, and J. Christian Gillin.

TABLE 368-5   Classification of anxiety disorders

Anxiety states:
  Panic disorder
  Generalized anxiety disorder
  Obsessive-compulsive disorder
  Posttraumatic stress disorder
Phobic disorders:
  Agoraphobia (with and without panic attacks)
  Social phobia
  Simple phobia

nonthreatening and nonstressful activity, like entering a store, driving a car, or sitting at a desk working. The patient becomes flushed, lightheaded, and sweaty and is overwhelmed by feelings of terror, apprehension, and impending doom. Dyspnea may occur with a subjective sense of choking or smothering, and palpitations or chest pain are often so severe that patients believe they are having a heart attack or are dying. The symptoms of panic attacks usually peak in less than 10 min and resolve in 20 to 30 min. Most patients experiencing their first panic attack obtain help, sometimes going to a doctor's office or emergency room, but the fear has usually subsided by this time. Fatigue or exhaustion frequently follows a panic attack, and the patient may sleep.

Patients with panic disorder may constitute as many as 15 percent of patients who consult cardiologists and 5 to 25 percent of patients in outpatient psychiatric settings.

The DSM-IIIR criteria for diagnosis of panic disorder are listed in Table 368-6.

Complications   After repeated panic attacks, most patients develop some degree of anticipatory anxiety and try to avoid those situations that have been paired with panic attacks in the past. Many patients, particularly females by a 2:1 ratio to males, develop *agoraphobia*—an irrational fear of being alone or in public places. Without effective treatment, the course of panic attacks and agoraphobia leads to an increasingly restricted life-style marked by preoccupation with avoiding those situations that might trigger an attack. Cases of severe panic disorder with agoraphobia may result

TABLE 368-6   Diagnostic criteria for panic disorder

A At some time during the disturbance, one or more panic attacks (discrete periods of intense fear or discomfort) have occurred that were (1) unexpected, i.e., did not occur immediately before or on exposure to a situation that almost always caused anxiety, and (2) not triggered by situations in which the person was the focus of others' attention.
B Either four attacks, as defined in criterion A, have occurred within a 4-week period, or one or more attacks have been followed by a period of at least a month of persistent fear of having another attack.
C At least four of the following symptoms developed during at least one of the attacks:*
   1 Shortness of breath (dyspnea) or smothering sensations
   2 Dizziness, unsteady feelings, or faintness
   3 Palpitations or accelerated heart rate (tachycardia)
   4 Trembling or shaking
   5 Sweating
   6 Choking
   7 Nausea or abdominal distress
   8 Depersonalization or derealization
   9 Numbness or tingling sensations (paresthesias)
   10 Flushes (hot flashes) or chills
   11 Chest pain or discomfort
   12 Fear of dying
   13 Fear of going crazy or of doing something uncontrolled
D During at least some of the attacks, at least four of the C symptoms developed suddenly and increased in intensity within 10 min of the beginning of the first C symptom noticed in the attack.
E It cannot be established that an organic factor initiated and maintained the disturbance, e.g., amphetamine or caffeine intoxication, hyperthyroidism.

* Attacks involving four or more symptoms are panic attacks; attacks involving fewer than four symptoms are limited symptom attacks.
NOTE: Mitral valve prolapse may be an associated condition, but does not preclude a diagnosis of panic disorder.
SOURCE: Adapted from DSM-IIIR.

in patients remaining house-bound for one or more decades, convinced that leaving the house will induce an attack.

Other complications of panic disorder include major depressive syndrome, higher death rates from both suicide and cardiovascular disease, and drug and alcohol dependency. Losses from unemployment and health care costs are estimated to exceed $100 million a year.

Laboratory findings   Lactate infusions precipitate panic attacks in vulnerable individuals, although at present this is only used as a test in research paradigms. One study employing positron emission tomography demonstrated a decrease rate of blood flow in the left parahippocampus during panic attacks.

Differential diagnosis   Many patients with panic disorder complain of chest pain, cardiac extrasystoles, and palpitations. The diagnostic challenge is to differentiate anxiety with cardiovascular symptoms from the organic diseases it mimics. Because there may be an increased prevalence of mitral valve prolapse in patients with panic disorder this condition should be investigated; however, in the vast majority of patients with panic disorder, no significant cardiac pathology is ever found.

Other diagnostic possibilities include both hyperthyroidism and hypothyroidism, a catecholamine-secreting pheochromocytoma, complex partial seizures, and hypoglycemia. Drug ingestions (amphetamine, cocaine, caffeine, sympathomimetic nasal decongestants) and drug withdrawal (alcohol, barbiturates, opiates, minor tranquilizers) may produce symptoms that simulate panic attacks.

Etiology and pathophysiology   The etiology of panic disorders is uncertain and involves an interplay of multiple psychological and biologic determinants.

PSYCHOLOGICAL FACTORS   In the psychodynamic model, anxiety is considered to be a response to the threatened emergence into consciousness of painful, unacceptable thoughts, impulses, or desires, i.e., psychological conflicts from the past and present. The anxiety response is an attempt to mobilize and ward off danger to the self.

PHYSIOLOGIC FACTORS   Clinical and experimental evidence point to the involvement of noradrenergic neurons, particularly those projecting rostrally from the locus coeruleus in the upper brainstem, in the pathophysiology of panic disorder. Three lines of evidence suggest that hyperactivity of noradrenergic pathways may play a role in the pathogenesis of panic. First, the clinical manifestations of panic attacks are similar to those induced by sudden, massive stimulation of beta-adrenergic receptors. Second, isoproterenol hydrochloride, a beta agonist, and yohimbine, an alpha-adrenergic receptor antagonist that increases noradrenergic function, produce signs and symptoms that mimic panic attacks. Third, clinical studies support a role for noradrenergic beta blockers, such as propranolol, in successful treatment of pathologic anxiety.

Another avenue of investigation is based on the finding that infusions of sodium lactate into patients with a history of panic disorder often provoke a panic attack indistinguishable from a spontaneous one. Normal subjects without a history of panic disorder are unaffected. In addition, patients whose panic attacks are controlled by antidepressants are protected against lactate-induced panic attacks. Inhalation of CO_2 by susceptible persons also precipitates anxiety and panic. Although the mechanism of lactate's effect is unclear, the findings appear to have diagnostic usefulness and provide a good model of anxiety for further clinical investigation.

Overall, the evidence suggests that the main contribution to panic disorder may be a genetic vulnerability to a biologic disease state. Over time, panic attacks may become associated with environmental events that by themselves are able to elicit symptoms. The particular constellation of environmental stimuli that precipitate panic attacks may be influenced by past experience or particular psychological conflicts. A full understanding of the etiology of anxiety probably will require knowledge of a combination of genetic, biologic, and psychological factors.

Treatment   A comprehensive treatment program combines both pharmacologic and psychotherapeutic approaches. The first step is to block the attacks pharmacologically, usually with tricyclic antide-

pressants or monoamine oxidase inhibitors (see Chap. 369). These drugs have 80 to 90 percent effectiveness in the treatment and prevention of spontaneous panic attacks. New antianxiety medications such as alprazolam given in high dose are as effective as antidepressants, have fewer side effects, and work within 1 or 2 days. Other benzodiazepines have not proved uniformly efficacious. Antidepressant medication may take 4 to 6 weeks before being effective. Beta blockers, e.g., propranolol or atenolol, may lock the peripheral manifestations of the panic attacks but have proved ineffective in preventing the psychic fear or panic and may also predispose to or worsen depressive symptomatology. Clonidine may also block panic manifestations, but its efficacy is usually only transient. Relapse is common on discontinuance of pharmacotherapy. More recently, claims have been made for the antipanic capacities of the serotonin-uptake inhibitor fluoxetine.

For some patients with panic disorder, particularly those with debilitating agoraphobia, psychotherapy is indicated. The exact form of psychotherapy needed is controversial, but approaches that seek to understand the anxiety and encourage the patient to confront the feared situations are the most effective.

GENERALIZED ANXIETY DISORDER Definition   Unlike patients with panic disorders whose symptoms come on suddenly, patients with generalized anxiety disorder experience persistent diffuse anxiety, without the specific symptoms that characterize phobic disorders, panic disorders, or obsessive-compulsive disorders. Although the symptoms and signs of anxiety vary from individual to individual, common signs are motor tension, autonomic hyperactivity, apprehensive expectation, and vigilance. Patients with generalized anxiety disorder do not report acute fluctuations in anxiety level and autonomic arousal characteristic of panic disorder.

Incidence and epidemiology   The prevalence of generalized anxiety disorder has been estimated at 2 to 3 percent, but precise epidemiologic data are lacking because of variations in definition and case acquisition. In patients who seek professional help for anxiety, women outnumber men by two to one. There is no evidence to support the popular belief that anxiety is related to the stresses of modern society. In contrast to panic disorder, studies showing a familial or genetic basis for generalized anxiety disorder are inconclusive.

The diagnostic criteria for generalized anxiety disorder are listed in Table 368-7.

Complications   In contrast to panic disorder, generalized anxiety disorder has a more chronic course and favorable outcome. However, the symptoms are persistent and can lead to secondary depression and alcohol and drug abuse, especially of benzodiazepines.

Differential diagnosis   Symptoms and signs resembling anxiety may occur with a number of medical disorders including coronary artery disease, thyroid disease, and drug intoxication or withdrawal. Anxiety may be present in other psychiatric disorders such as depression, schizophrenia, and organic mental states. Diagnosis of these conditions is essential, since the treatment of them is different from that of the anxiety disorders. Because patients with generalized anxiety may abuse alcohol or antianxiety medications to reduce or block anxiety, a careful history of drug use is important. Although the overall degree of psychosocial or occupational impairment is generally less than that noted for the other anxiety disorders, chronic anxiety is an uncomfortable emotion that can restrict a person's ability to enjoy a normal life.

Etiology and pathophysiology   One approach to understanding the etiology of anxiety has been to delineate the mechanisms by which antianxiety drugs exert their therapeutic effects. High affinity, stereospecific receptors for benzodiazepines have been discovered that appear to be coupled to the receptor for the inhibitory neurotransmitter GABA. Considerable evidence supports the hypothesis that the anxiolytic actions of the benzodiazepines are mediated through this receptor.

These findings have several implications. First, the characterization of a benzodiazepine receptor complex implies the existence of a

TABLE 368-7 Diagnostic criteria for generalized anxiety disorder

A Unrealistic or excessive anxiety and worry (apprehensive expectation) about two or more life circumstances, e.g., worry about possible misfortune to one's child (who is in no danger) and worry about finances (for no good reason), for a period of 6 months or longer, during which the person has been bothered more days than not by these concerns. In children and adolescents, this may take the form of anxiety and worry about academic, athletic, and social performance.

B If another anxiety disorder is present, the focus of the anxiety and worry in A is unrelated to it, e.g., the anxiety or worry is not about having a panic attack (as in panic disorder), being embarrassed in public (as in social phobia), being contaminated (as in obsessive-compulsive disorder), or gaining weight (as in anorexia nervosa).

C The disturbance does not occur only during the course of a mood disorder or a psychotic disorder.

D At least 6 of the following 18 symptoms are often present when anxious (do not include symptoms present only during panic attacks):

Motor tension
1 Trembling, twitching, or feeling shaky
2 Muscle tension, aches, or soreness
3 Restlessness
4 Easy fatigability

Autonomic hyperactivity
5 Shortness of breath or smothering sensations
6 Palpitations or accelerated heart rate (tachycardia)
7 Sweating, or cold clammy hands
8 Dry mouth
9 Dizziness or lightheadedness
10 Nausea, diarrhea, or other abdominal distress
11 Flushes (hot flashes) or chills
12 Frequent urination
13 Trouble swallowing or "lump in throat"

Vigilance and scanning
14 Feeling keyed up or on edge
15 Exaggerated startle response
16 Difficulty concentrating or "mind going blank" because of anxiety
17 Trouble falling or staying asleep
18 Irritability

E It cannot be established that an organic factor initiated and maintained the disturbance, e.g., hyperthyroidism, caffeine intoxication.

SOURCE: Adapted from DSM-IIIR.

natural (endogenous) ligand for the receptor. Conceivably, the levels of this substance might correlate with individual differences in anxiety or emotionality or tolerance to stress. Second, pharmacologic antagonists of this receptor block the effects of benzodiazepines and may induce anxiety, a finding that implicates these mechanisms in pathologic anxiety. Third, new *anxiolytic* compounds that influence benzodiazepine receptor binding are being discovered that have fewer and potentially less serious side effects. The possibility exists that *anxiogenic* substances may also be found in the brain. Though major questions remain to be answered, these advances have opened new avenues for understanding the origins and management of anxiety.

Treatment Because feelings of anxiety are normal human emotions with adaptive value, a decision must be made before any treatment or medication is considered concerning whether or not the manifestations of anxiety are within the normal range. There is no justification for the use of anxiolytic drugs in anxiety if it is considered to be within the normal limits of human experience.

Once a decision is made to treat, consideration should be given first to modalities of nonpharmacologic intervention, including supportive or intensive psychotherapy. These approaches may modify maladaptive life-styles, cognition, and avoidance behaviors. Behavior therapy aims at teaching the patient practical means to reduce anxiety and includes techniques like relaxation training, biofeedback, and desensitization. These techniques are of at least temporary benefit for many people.

When generalized anxiety is severe enough to warrant treatment with drugs, benzodiazepines are the agents of choice. In many patients, short courses of anxiolytic drugs (5 to 7 days) are effective, following which the drug should be discontinued. Patients should be warned about the possibility of dependence with long-term use, and the physician should make regular assessments of the need for continuation of medications. Buspirone, a nonbenzodiazepine anx-

iolytic, may become a drug of first choice for these patients. Although it has a delayed onset of action, it lacks many of the problems associated with the benzodiazepines, such as psychomotor impairment, physical dependence, or withdrawal symptoms.

POSTTRAUMATIC STRESS DISORDER Definition Acute and chronic psychological distress following traumatic events have long been recognized. The diagnostic criteria for posttraumatic stress disorders (PTSD), according to DSM-IIIR, are listed in Table 368-8.

PTSD is classified as either acute or chronic (or delayed). In the former, onset of symptoms begin within 6 months of the trauma, or the duration of the symptoms persists less than 6 months. In the latter, symptoms persist more than 6 months (chronic) or start more than 6 months after the trauma (delayed).

Etiology Whether or not PTSD develops appears to depend upon the nature of the trauma, the characteristics of the individual, and the context in which these events take place. The trauma can be anticipated or not, acute or chronic, constant or repetitive, due to natural events (e.g., an earthquake) or malevolence (e.g., rape, child abuse, torture). PTSD can develop in individuals who were apparently healthy, successful, and well-adjusted prior to the traumatic experiences. Among the factors which influence the development of PTSD are (1) the extent to which the individual's life-space is affected, (2) the duration of the impact, (3) the extent to which the individual perceives human malevolence behind the traumatic event (e.g., a fire attributed to arson will probably be more traumatic than one attributed to lightning), and (4) social isolation.

TABLE 368-8 Diagnostic criteria for posttraumatic stress disorder

A The person has experienced an event that is outside the range of usual human experience and that would be markedly distressing to almost anyone, e.g., serious threat to one's life or physical integrity; serious threat or harm to one's children, spouse, or other close relatives and friends; sudden destruction of one's home or community; or seeing another person who has recently been, or is being, seriously injured or killed as the result of an accident or physical violence.

B The traumatic event is persistently reexperienced in at least one of the following ways:
1 Recurrent and intrusive distressing recollections of the event (in young children, repetitive play in which themes or aspects of the trauma are expressed)
2 Recurrent distressing dreams of the event
3 Sudden acting or feeling as if the traumatic event were recurring [includes a sense of reliving the experience, illusions, hallucinations, and dissociative (flashback) episodes, even those that occur upon awakening or when intoxicated]
4 Intense psychological distress at exposure to events that symbolize or resemble an aspect of the traumatic event, including anniversaries of the trauma

C Persistent avoidance of stimuli associated with the trauma or numbing of general responsiveness (not present before the trauma), as indicated by at least three of the following:
1 Efforts to avoid thoughts or feelings associated with the trauma
2 Efforts to avoid activities or situations that arouse recollections of the trauma
3 Inability to recall an important aspect of the trauma (psychogenic amnesia)
4 Markedly diminished interest in significant activities (in young children, loss of recently acquired developmental skills such as toilet training or language skills)
5 Feeling of detachment or estrangement from others
6 Restricted range of affect, e.g., unable to have loving feelings
7 Sense of a foreshortened future, e.g., does not expect to have a career, marriage, or children, or a long life

D Persistent symptoms of increased arousal (not present before the trauma), as indicated by at least two of the following:
1 Difficulty falling or staying asleep
2 Irritability or outbursts of anger
3 Difficulty concentrating
4 Hypervigilance
5 Exaggerated startle response
6 Physiologic reactivity upon exposure to events that symbolize or resemble an aspect of the traumatic event (e.g., a woman who was raped in an elevator breaks out in a sweat when entering any elevator)

E Duration of the disturbance (symptoms in B, C, and D) of at least 1 month.

SOURCE: Adapted from DSM-IIIR.

Epidemiology It is difficult to gauge the extent of PTSD following a traumatic event because the studies that have been done have often followed subjects for only a short period of time, and the nature of the events is often so situation-specific. About 15 percent or more of the civilian population may experience mental distress severe enough to require treatment following a major natural disaster. For example, in a study that followed survivors of a shipboard fire for $3\frac{1}{2}$ to $4\frac{1}{2}$ years, one-third were found to be unable to return to sea because of psychological symptoms. Following extreme prolonged harsh conditions such as combat, prisoner-of-war camps, or Nazi death camps, a higher incidence of both acute and delayed PTSD is likely. Some evidence, based on follow-up of World War II veterans 20 years after the war, indicates an increasing incidence of new patients seeking psychiatric care for war-associated symptoms. The vicissitudes of normal aging may unmask a latent traumatic stress disorder.

Complications Anxiety, depression, alcoholism, drug abuse, impaired marital and occupational activities, and perhaps increased physical morbidity and mortality have been blamed on various forms of PTSD.

Differential diagnosis In adjustment disorder, symptoms such as reexperiencing the trauma are absent. Other considerations include major depressive disorder, generalized anxiety disorder, phobic disorder, organic mental disorders, and other conditions such as "compensation neurosis" and "postconcussion sydrome."

Prophylaxis Military experience suggests that PTSD can be prevented partially if soldiers are taught that a degree of fear and anxiety are normal concomitants of battle rather than signs of cowardice or mental illness. Furthermore, the development of chronic PTSD can often be prevented if the soldier with acute PTSD is seen close to the battle front under the principles of immediate treatment, expectancy of return to normal duties, and brevity of treatment contact.

Treatment The treatment goals of PTSD are reduction of target symptoms, prevention of chronic disability, and occupational and social rehabilitation. An important therapeutic issue is the extent to which the victim of acute PTSD should be allowed to leave the traumatic situation, to regress, and to enjoy the secondary gains of the patient role. The caretakers' unthinking natural sympathy, nurturing instincts, admiration, and, indeed, gratitude (for example, in the case of soldiers who are protecting the homeland) may be as detrimental as an unreasonably cynical, suspicious distrust of someone who is seen as trying to get attention and avoid responsibilities or hoping to collect money from the consequences of the traumatic experience. Successful treatment involves a combination of psychosocial support systems, psychotherapy, behavioral and conditioning techniques, and medications. Group therapy with others who have shared similar experiences may be beneficial.

OBSESSIVE-COMPULSIVE DISORDER **Definition** The major characteristics are recurrent *obsessions* (persistent intrusive thoughts) and *compulsions* (intrusive behaviors) which the patient experiences as involuntary, senseless, or repugnant. The DSM-IIIR diagnostic criteria for obsessive-compulsive disorder are listed in Table 368-9.

Common obsessions include thoughts of violence (e.g., killing a loved one), obsessive slowness, fears of germs or contamination, and doubt (e.g., a priest who worries excessively that he had not said his prayers properly). Examples of compulsions include repeated checking to be assured that something was done properly, hand washing, extreme neatness, and counting rituals, as in numbering steps while walking.

Obsessions and compulsions do not invariably coexist in the same individual. The relationship of the obsessive-compulsive disorder to obsessive or compulsive characterologic traits remains controversial.

Etiology and pathophysiology The etiology of the obsessive-compulsive state is uncertain, but it can be viewed from psychodynamic, psychosocial, and biologic perspectives. Obsessions and compulsions often seem to symbolize unconscious wishes, impulses, and fears and to reflect dynamic adaptations to unwanted aggressive

TABLE 368-9   Diagnostic criteria for obsessive-compulsive disorder

A Either obsessions or compulsions:
  1 Obsessions:
    a Recurrent and persistent ideas, thoughts, impulses, or images that are experienced, at least initially, as intrusive and senseless, e.g., a parent's having repeated impulses to kill a loved child, a religious person's having recurrent blasphemous thoughts
    b The person attempts to ignore or suppress such thoughts or impulses or to neutralize them with some other thought or action
    c The person recognizes that the obsessions are the product of his or her own mind, not imposed from without (as in thought insertion)
    d If another disorder is present, the content of the obsession is unrelated to it, e.g., the ideas, thoughts, impulses, or images are not about food in the presence of an eating disorder, about drugs in the presence of a psychoactive substance use disorder, or guilty thoughts in the presence of a major depression
  2 Compulsions:
    a Repetitive, purposeful, and intentional behaviors that are performed in response to an obsession, or according to certain rules, or in a stereotyped fashion
    b The behavior is designed to neutralize or to prevent discomfort or some dreaded event or situation; however, either the activity is not connected in a realistic way with what it is designed to neutralize or prevent, or it is clearly excessive
    c The person recognizes that his or her behavior is excessive or unreasonable (this may not be true for young children; it may no longer be true for people whose obsessions have evolved into overvalued ideas)
B The obsessions or compulsions cause marked distress, are time-consuming (take more than 1 h/d), or significantly interfere with the person's normal routine, occupational functioning, or usual social activities or relationships with others.

SOURCE: Adapted from DSM-IIIR.

or sexual urges. Biologic factors are suggested by reports of an increased incidence of obsessive-compulsive disorder in monozygotic twins and first-degree relatives of probands, of biologic markers associated with the disorder, and of favorable response to certain tricyclic antidepressants and monoamine oxidase inhibitors.

Epidemiology The lifetime prevalence of obsessive-compulsive disorder, based upon interviews of the general population 18 years and older, varies between 1.9 and 3.0 percent. The prevalence tends to be slightly higher in females than males but does not vary significantly by race, education, or urbanization of area of residence.

Clinical manifestations These disorders usually begin in adolescence or young adulthood, with about 65 percent of cases beginning before age 25. They are rarely seen in children. Clear precipitants are reported in up to 60 percent of cases. Long-term prognosis appears to be variable. Some patients (perhaps 10 percent) show a chronic, unremitting course; some show periods of complete remission; the majority show an episodic course with periods of incomplete remission.

Complications Depression is probably the most common secondary problem but anxiety, avoidant behavior, alcoholism, abuse of sleeping pills and tranquilizers, and impairment of social, marital, and occupational life can be marked.

Laboratory findings No pathognomonic pathologic or laboratory abnormalities have been found.

Differential diagnosis Repetitive self-destructive behaviors, such as gambling, drinking, drug abuse, and overeating, should not be diagnosed as "obsessive-compulsive" disorder since the individual normally derives pleasure from the activity. Stereotyped behavior is also common in schizophrenia, Tourette's syndrome, and depression.

Treatment Clomipramine appears to be the most effective pharmacologic treatment for obsessive-compulsive disorder. The beneficial effects may be delayed 6 to 8 weeks, and it is most effective when specific compulsions are present. Recent reports suggest that fluoxetine, which has effects on the serotoninergic neurotransmitter system, is also successful in the treatment of some patients with obsessive-compulsive disorder.

Obsessive-compulsive patients also may respond to psychotherapeutic intervention. However, in the absence of adequate studies of psychotherapy in this disorder, it is hard to make valid generalizations about its effectiveness. Behavioral therapy can be helpful, and desensitization, flooding, implosion therapy, and aversive conditioning have all been used with variable success.

PHOBIC DISORDERS Phobic disorders comprise a group of disorders having in common persistently recurring, irrational severe anxiety of specific objects, activities, or situations with secondary avoidance behavior of the phobic stimulus. Phobias are relatively commonplace, and the diagnosis of a phobic disorder is made only when fear or avoidance behavior is a significant source of distress to the individual or interferes with social or occupational functioning.

The phobic disorders listed in DSM-IIIR include three separate disorders—agoraphobia, social phobia, and simple phobia.

Agoraphobia DEFINITION Agoraphobia, the fear of being alone or in public places (see Table 368-10), may occur rarely in the absence of panic disorder, but it is almost invariably preceded by that condition.

Social phobias DEFINITION Social phobias are persistent irrational fears and the need to avoid any situation where one might be exposed to scrutiny by others and potentially be embarrassed or humiliated. Even the possibility of such a situation evokes anticipatory anxiety. The individual is aware that this fear is excessive. Common examples are excessive fear of public speaking and anxiety induced by eating in restaurants or by any public performance. The resulting anxiety may actually impair performance and thereby potentiate the phobic disorder.

EPIDEMIOLOGY AND PATHOGENESIS Social phobias are relatively rare, and there is no evidence for a genetic or familial transmission. Social phobias presumably arise from stressful life events occurring during early development. The disorder usually begins in late childhood or early adolescence and tends to be chronic and to wax and wane in severity.

COMPLICATIONS Complications are rare and the disorder is not often incapacitating; it may lead to sedative or hypnotic drug and alcohol abuse and addiction, and to problems in professional advancement.

TREATMENT Treatment of social phobia is primarily behavioral, with use of such techniques as relaxation therapy, systematic desensitization, and related techniques. Pharmacotherapy with beta blockers, i.e., propranolol or atenolol and/or alprazolam, may also be helpful.

Simple phobia DEFINITION Simple phobias are persistent irrational fears and avoidance of specific objects or situations.

CLINICAL FEATURES The individuals experiences significant distress when confronted with the phobic stimulus or even the possibility of confrontation with the phobic stimulus and also recognizes this fear and anxiety as irrational and excessive. When confronted with the phobic stimulus the individual may experience symptoms identical to those of panic attacks. Common examples include fear of heights (acrophobia), fear of closed spaces (claustrophobia), and fear of animals. Fear of the possibility of exposure to the phobic stimulus will often cause the individual to attempt to elicit significant information, e.g., if the party or restaurant is at the top of a high-rise building; if they have a dog.

Age of onset is variable, but the disorder often begins in childhood. Simple phobias that begin in childhood may disappear without treatment, but may persist into adulthood. Although phobias are relatively common in the general population, they rarely result in significant impairment and individuals rarely seek treatment. Simple

---

TABLE 368-10 Diagnosis of agoraphobia

A The individual has marked fear of and thus avoids being alone or being in public places from which escape might be difficult or help not available in case of sudden incapacitation, e.g., crowds, tunnels, bridges, public transportation.

B There is increasing constriction of normal activities until the fear or avoidance behavior dominates the individual's life.

---

phobias are more common in women. Treatment, if required, is behavioral using relaxation therapy and systematic desensitization.

PERSONALITY DISORDERS[4]

Personality denotes characteristic ways of thinking, feeling, behaving, and reacting to the environment. When this "psychological signature" strikes a useful balance between consistency and adaptive flexibility, we speak of personality *traits*. A personality *disorder* is said to exist when a person chronically uses certain mechanisms of coping in an inappropriate, stereotyped, and maladaptive fashion.

DIAGNOSIS OF PERSONALITY DISORDERS DSM-IIIR recognizes 11 distinctive personality disorders. These are grouped into three thematic clusters. *Paranoid, schizoid,* and *schizotypal* personality disorders are characterized by oddness or eccentricity. *Histrionic, narcissistic, antisocial,* and *borderline* personality disorders share a dramatic presentation along with self-centeredness, emotionality, and erratic behavior. Anxiety and fear underlie *avoidant, dependent, compulsive,* and *passive-aggressive* personalities.

The DSM-IIIR diagnostic classification scheme stipulates specific inclusion and exclusion criteria for diagnosis of each disorder. Since the number of specific criteria for individual disorders can be extensive, the descriptions in this chapter are highlights rather than complete expositions. The reader is referred to the DSM-IIIR for the detailed listing of the necessary signs and symptoms required to make the diagnosis of the various personality disorders.

Paranoid personality disorder People with this disorder are suspicious and hypersensitive to perceived slights and injuries. They are hypervigilant to the possibility that someone might trick or harm them and tend to be guarded and secretive and to blame others. They may be jealous and concerned with hidden meanings. They tend to exaggerate difficulties, to take offense and become hostile easily, to hold grudges, and to question the loyalty and fidelity of others.

Schizoid personality disorder Schizoid individuals are loners who seem to have little need for others. They appear emotionally cold and aloof and indifferent to praise and criticism; they lack close friendships, and may be social recluses.

In earlier nomenclatures eccentric thinking was sometimes added to the schizoid picture. DSM-IIIR, however, has split off a second category, schizotypal (see below), to describe persons whose principal difficulties are cognitive rather than interpersonal.

Schizotypal personality disorder Schizotypal persons share with schizophrenics certain eccentricities of thinking, perception, speech, and interpersonal interaction; however, the degree and pervasiveness of such "schizophrenic-like" symptomatology is not sufficient to meet diagnostic criteria for schizophrenia. Odd speech (e.g., vague, circumstantial, metaphorical), ideas of reference (inappropriately inferring that neutral events have some special relevance to the person), magical thinking, and suspiciousness can be prominent. Many schizotypal persons are also socially isolated, and this can lead to confusion with schizoid personality (see above).

Borderline personality disorder Borderline persons have been described as having "stable instability," characterized by chronic difficulty in regulating mood and interpersonal attachments and in maintaining a consistent self-image. Borderline persons can manifest impulsive behavior, some of it self-damaging (e.g., self-mutilation, suicidal behavior). Their mood is unpredictable. Some have brief outbursts of anger, irritability, sadness, and fear. Others suffer from a chronic emptiness. Despite having chaotic interpersonal relationships punctuated by intense love and hate, borderline persons generally are intolerant of being alone. The defense mechanism of "splitting" (regarding persons and events either as "all good" are "all bad") can be prominent.

Histrionic personality disorder People with a histrionic personality have seemingly intense but actually superficial relationships.

[4] By Igor Grant.

They present in a dramatic, engaging, but self-centered fashion. There is an exaggerated expression of emotions, attention seeking, craving for excitement, and a tendency to overreact. While superficially warm and charming, even sexually seductive, histrionic persons are generally perceived as shallow, inconsiderate, self-indulgent, vain, demanding, dependent, and manipulative. Some make frequent suicidal threats or attempts.

Narcissistic personality disorder The narcissistic person has an inflated sense of self-importance, and may be preoccupied with being unique, powerful, and gifted. The patient exaggerates his or her talents and contributions, seeks admiration, feels entitled to preferential treatment, and uses others to achieve a better position, while being indifferent to their feelings and needs. A rejection can produce excessive rage, inferiority, shame, or humiliation.

Antisocial personality disorder Antisocial behavior is characterized by unconcern with the rules and expectations of society and repeated violation of the rights of others. The diagnosis is limited to adults (persons under 18 with antisocial features are classified as having conduct disorder) and requires a history of antisocial behaviors that have their onset before age 15. Such behaviors include truancy, delinquency, running away from home, lying, precocious sexuality, troubles with the law, and alcohol or drug abuse. Beyond such historical considerations, the antisocial diagnosis requires current evidence of certain deviant behaviors which include irresponsibility in work, as a parent, in financial matters, and in personal behavior (e.g., recklessness, driving while intoxicated). Additionally, antisocial persons will usually commit multiple illegal acts, lie and deceive, but lack remorse for such behavior. They manifest an inability to maintain a long-term attachment to a sexual partner, and exhibit irritability and aggressiveness. Alcohol or other substance abuse is common.

Avoidant personality disorder People who are inappropriately concerned with rejection or humiliation, and for this reason avoid close ties with others, are classified as having an avoidant personality disorder. Despite being withdrawn, they give evidence for wishing that they did have intimate relations with others. In contrast with the narcissistic individual, the avoidant person tends to manifest low self-esteem and a tendency to exaggerate his or her shortcomings.

Dependent personality disorder Dependent people allow others to assume responsibility for major aspects of their life and decision making. Because they see themselves as helpless or inept, and fear separation, they are willing to subordinate their needs and wishes to those of others in order to avoid taking personal responsibility.

Passive-aggressive personality disorder Passive-aggressive people resent responsibility, either social or work-related. Rather than expressing their opposition directly, they tend to procastinate, dawdle, behave stubbornly, work inefficiently, and "forget." Additional features may include a tendency to be argumentative or sulky when asked to do something they do not want to do, and to resent authority.

Obsessive-compulsive personality disorder This term describes people who tend to be perfectionistic and inflexible, preoccupied with rules, procedures, and detail. They are often stubbornly insistent on certain things being done a particular way, yet at other times may become indecisive to the point of ineffectiveness. Compulsives tend to value their work and possessions more than interpersonal relationships. They have difficulty expressing warm and tender feelings toward others and are sometimes seen as stiff, cold, and awkward.

Other personality disorders The DSM-IIIR has a category "Personality Disorder Not Otherwise Specified" to accommodate disturbances that do not fit neatly into the foregoing categories. In this residual category are the terms, from the old DSM, *mixed personality disorder* and *atypical personality disorder*. Mixed personality disorder indicates that an individual's behavior fulfills the criteria for more than one personality disorder, e.g., passive-aggressive and dependent. Atypical personality disorder is used when a disorder is suspected but there is insufficient information for a clear classification, and for a disturbance not specifically included in DSM-IIIR, e.g., sadistic, masochistic (self-defeating), impulsive, or immature personality (which are concepts from other diagnostic schemes). One increasingly recognized disorder is *adult attention deficit disorder* (ADD), a residual form of childhood ADD (hyperkinesis). As adults, such individuals continue to have problems in attending and manifest labile mood, explosive temper, impulsivity, stress intolerance, and inability to complete tasks. They may also manifest a paradoxical (calming) reaction to central nervous system (CNS) stimulants.

RELIABILITY OF PERSONALITY DISORDER DIAGNOSES Despite continued research efforts to improve interclinician agreement through specification of diagnostic criteria, reliability is problematic for most personality disorder diagnoses. While trained clinicians tend to agree whether or not some form of personality disorder is present, this reliability breaks down when specific diagnoses are attempted. Best agreement is reported for antisocial and paranoid personality disorders.

DIFFERENTIAL DIAGNOSIS Major mental disorders In its early phases, *schizophrenia* can be mistaken for schizoid, schizotypal, paranoid, and borderline personality disorders. *Affective disorders* can mimic some features of borderline, histrionic, and compulsive personality disorders. *Anxiety disorders* can share features with compulsive, histrionic, and avoidant personalities. *Alcohol and substance abuse disorders* may need to be differentiated from antisocial, borderline, and histrionic personalities. *Paranoid disorders* can sometimes be difficult to differentiate from paranoid, schizotypal, and borderline personalities. Differential diagnostic points are that the major mental disorders tend to have a definite time of onset, that the symptomatology is more severe and causes greater disturbance in everyday functioning, and that specific diagnostic features will be present that transcend the criteria for personality disorders.

Additional personality disorders DSM-IIIR criteria for personality disorders sometimes overlap. "Schizophrenic-like" phenomena, including eccentricity and psychotic experiences, can form part of the picture of paranoid, schizoid, schizotypal, and borderline personalities. Dramatic presentation, emotional outbursts, and erratic behavior can lead to confusion among antisocial, borderline, narcissistic, and histrionic personalities. Impulsivity is found in antisocial, borderline, and histrionic personalities; while anxiety and fearfulness can be part of avoidant, passive-aggressive, dependent, and compulsive behavior. Unfortunately, the DSM-IIIR revision of the criteria for some of the personality disorders has worsened the problem of overlap. In one series it was noted that of patients considered by therapists to have a personality diagnosis almost 52 percent met criteria for two separate disorders.

Medical conditions Medical and neurologic conditions can mimic personality disorders. For example, persons with complex partial seizures with foci in the left temporal lobe can present with excessive orderliness, religiosity, and "viscosity" which might be confused with compulsive personality. Alternatively, they can develop paranoid features or fuzzy thinking suggestive of paranoid or schizotypal personality. Rigid, orderly, and ritualistic behavior mirroring compulsive personality can be part of a dementing process or a sequel of head injury, while irritability, dysregulation of affect, and inappropriate interpersonal behavior in such patients can be confused with borderline personality. Beyond these specific examples, virtually any disease affecting the brain can cause behavioral change suggestive of a personality disorder. The key differential points are that there is a relatively sudden onset and that there are neuropsychological changes indicative of compromised brain function.

ETIOLOGY AND PATHOPHYSIOLOGY It was commonly held that the personality disorders reflected the warping effect of adverse early social environment. Now there is mounting evidence that personality is, in great measure, biologically determined. Both genetic and constitutional (i.e., intrauterine and early physical developmental) factors may be important.

Genetic factors Although not all personality disorders have been examined, for the majority there is a severalfold increase in concordance between monozygotic twins compared with dizygotic twins.

Some of the most careful work has been with antisocial personality. Here it is noted that prevalence among men is three- to fourfold higher than in women, and that first-degree relatives of persons diagnosed as antisocial show increased prevalence of antisocial personality, alcoholism, and somatization disorder (Briquet's syndrome). The latter is characterized by intractable multiorgan system complaints in women who often have a histrionic personality. The association of these two disorders in the same pedigrees has led to suggestions that Briquet's syndrome and antisocial disorder are expressions in women and men of a common biogenetic substrate.

The operation of genetic factors in antisocial personality is further demonstrated by the finding that biologic offspring of antisocial and alcoholic parents have a higher risk of developing antisocial personality disorder even if they are raised by adoptive parents who do not have any antisocial traits. The converse has also been demonstrated; children adopted by antisocial parents tend not to develop antisocial disorder themselves unless they have antisocial personality or alcoholism in their blood relatives.

The XYY chromosomal abnormality was once thought to be related to antisocial personality disorder. More recent studies indicate that although XYY might be overrepresented in certain prison populations, the vast majority of XYY men are not antisocial.

The schizotypal, borderline, and schizoid diagnoses evolved originally from the notion that there ought to be a "preclinical" form of schizophrenia characterized by lesser severity or fewer numbers of the cognitive and interpersonal symptoms of that disorder. Thus, the schizotypal personality might, theoretically, embody earlier forms of the disturbance in thinking, perception, and attention that occur in schizophrenia; whereas the schizoid personality would represent the interpersonal awkwardness inherent in that disorder. Genetic studies have confirmed that there is some increase in schizotypal (but not schizoid) personality in relatives of diagnosed schizophrenics.

The borderline personality is genetically heterogeneous. Up to 50 percent of borderline patients have a family history of affective disorder. Borderline disorder itself, as well as other personality disorders, are also more common in first-degree relatives of borderline patients, but schizophrenia is not consistently related.

There is increased schizophrenia in the families of patients with paranoid personality. For compulsive disorder, twin studies indicate increased concordance for obsessional traits in monozygotic versus dizygotic twins. There is also some evidence that orderliness and rigidity run in families.

The other personality disorders have been studied carefully from a biogenetic standpoint.

Constitutional factors Although there is good evidence that infants are born with certain temperamental characteristics (e.g., high versus low activity level; long versus short attention span), there is little evidence that these temperamental characteristics persist into adolescence. Infant temperament does not appear to predict later personality disorder with the exception that the "difficult child" (irritable, hard to console, irregular rhythms) tends to exhibit more behavioral disturbances. Low intelligence quotient and poor physical health as a child have been noted more frequently in the histories of persons with personality disorders.

Neurophysiologic and neuroendocrine correlates Several neurophysiologic and biochemical changes may be associated with personality disorders. Abnormal slow waves and spikes have been reported in the EEGs of antisocial persons. For borderline patients, patterns suggestive of periodic limbic epileptiform discharges have sometimes been noted.

Some observers suggest that a common neurophysiologic feature of both antisocial and hysterical disorders is reduced cortical arousal to cortical stimulation, secondary to increased inhibition from lower brain regions. This may be coupled with motor disinhibition in antisocial persons and autonomic disinhibition in hysterics.

The schizotypal personality disorder has been associated with disturbance in smooth pursuit eye movement (SPEM). Since many schizophrenics are also poor trackers, it may be that schizotypals share with schizophrenics decreased neural effectiveness in "centering." Some schizophrenics and schizotypals have lowered platelet MAO levels. It has been suggested that lowered MAO activity could be related to inefficient degradation of certain biologically active amines, leading to accumulation of substance with psychotomimetic properties.

Cortisol escape from dexamethasone suppression and shortened REM latency (REM latency is the time between falling asleep and first REM episode) are associated with affective disorder. Both phenomena have also been observed in borderline and obsessive-compulsive personalities, suggesting a link among the affective, borderline, and obsessive-compulsive disorders.

There are no specific data on biologic correlates of the other personality disorders.

Cloninger has postulated that genetically influenced differences in the responsivity and interaction of three chemically coded neural networks—dopaminergic (DA), serotoninergic, and noradrenergic—may explain three broad personality dimensions termed behavioral activation (novelty seeking), behavioral inhibition (harm avoidance), and behavioral maintenance (reward dependence). As an example, someone with DA-dependent high behavioral activation might tend toward the personality characteristics of curiosity, impulsivity, enthusiasm, excitability; those low on activation might tend toward being content, quiet, reserved, slow-tempered, and methodical. Efforts are continuing to validate this "tridimensional neuroadaptive model" of personality.

Environmental factors Early social environment has proved to be an inconsistent predictor of late personality disorder. For example, one study found that 30 percent of men with personality disorders who were investigated reported lack of maternal warmth as children, but so did 24 percent of controls. Multiple problems in the early environment were found in 16 percent of personality-disordered men and 10 percent of those without disorders. Being abused as a child is associated with violence in later life.

The relative weakness of both temperamental and environmental factors as predictors of future personality disorder has led to a "goodness of fit" hypothesis. This theory suggests that later behavioral disorders are more likely when there is a severe mismatch between a child's temperament and childrearing practices and environmental circumstances.

EPIDEMIOLOGY The prevalence of personality disorders ranges from 5 to 23 percent. Antisocial personality is diagnosed more commonly in men than women, whereas borderline and histrionic personalities are diagnosed more commonly in women.

There is increased prevalence of personality disorder in inner cities, prisons, and areas of social disintegration. Personality disorders are three times as common in the lowest social classes as compared to the highest. These sociodemographic patterns are particularly striking for antisocial personality disorder. Among patients attending psychiatric clinics the rates for personality disorder have ranged from 49 to 86 percent, with some studies noting that 50 percent qualified for more than one personality disorder.

NATURAL HISTORY AND PROGNOSIS Compared to controls, a disproportionate number of persons with personality disorders are found to have emotional problems as children. The prevalence of most personality disorders declines with age, the peak being in the age group 20 to 29. This trend is especially prominent for antisocial personality disorder. It is possible that slowly evolving maturational processes during adulthood account for these age effects.

Although only about 20 percent of persons with personality disorders seek psychiatric treatment, the majority evidence long-standing difficulties in maintaining stable employment, marriages, and friendships.

With regard to psychiatric complications, about one-third of persons with personality disorders have significant depression or anxiety. Alcohol abuse is related to personality disorder, with the association being particularly striking for men, whose rate of alcohol problems approaches 50 percent.

TREATMENT Persons with personality disorders generally do not recognize the inner source of their difficulties. They tend to blame others and their environment and make those around them feel badly. Only 20 percent of persons with personality disorders actually present for psychiatric treatment.

Treatment usually consists of psychotherapy in some form. In some specific instances psychopharmacology has been used. Success has been claimed for various types of psychotherapy. Individual, group, couples, and family treatments all have been employed. Despite differences in techniques and orientations, most psychotherapists emphasize the importance (and initial difficulty) of establishing a trusting relationship. The goals tend to be to identify inner sources of maladaptive behavior. From a psychodynamic standpoint this means that the painful feelings which are being avoided need to be identified and their causes traced. Cognitive-behavioral therapists will try to identify the faulty assumptions, lack of foresight regarding consequences of behavior, and ineffectiveness of the existing coping repertoire, with an eye to teaching more useful behavior.

As a broad generalization patients with "dramatic" presentations (borderline, antisocial, histrionic, narcissistic) tend to require a more intrusive, confrontative, limit-setting posture by the therapist. More specifically, antisocial personality probably cannot be treated in an outpatient setting and requires a containing environment (e.g., prison, inpatient unit). In such a setting groups emphasizing mutual interdependence and confrontation appear to produce some success. Regarding the treatment of borderline persons, psychiatrists are divided as to whether a supportive "here and now" versus intensive exploration works best. In either instance, treatment is often punctuated by prolonged periods in which the patient expresses negative feelings toward the therapist, makes suicide attempts, or undergoes psychotic decompensation requiring hospitalization.

In contrast to this more intrusive posture, patients whose personalities fit into the "fearful" and "odd" clusters may benefit from a more gentle, accepting, and clarifying approach.

Psychotherapy tends to be a long-term enterprise, lasting many years. Therapists can expect to feel frustrated, angry, helpless, and inadequate at times. Clinical reports of major improvements are many, but controlled outcome studies are practically nonexistent. This reflects continuing problems in achieving reliable diagnoses and in general methodologic issues in outcome research, especially in prospective studies spanning many years.

There is increasing evidence that psychopharmacologic intervention may be helpful for some of the personality diagnoses. Borderline patients, particularly those with coexisting mood disorder, have benefited from tricyclic antidepressants and MAO inhibitors. Other groups of borderline patients in whom mood dysregulation and impulsiveness are prominent have responded to lithium. Still others with explosive outbursts have benefited from carbamazepine. A few such patients have had EEG abnormalities suggestive of epileptic foci in limbic structures. Both borderline and schizotypal patients undergoing cognitive disorganization can improve with low doses of neuroleptic drugs.

Persons with obsessive-compulsive personality disorder who have obsessional ruminations may benefit from clomipramine, fluoxetine, or fluvoxamine. These agents have specific antiruminative effects that go beyond antidepressive activity. The utility of other antidepressants for this disorder has not been established, although the MAO inhibitors may be useful in compulsives who also experience anxiety or panic attacks.

Methylphenidate may improve inattention and reduce motor overactivity, affective lability, and impulsivity in persons whose personality difficulties are related to adult attention deficit disorder.

REFERENCES

Major affective disorders

BALDESSARINI RJ: Biological hypotheses in psychiatry, in *Chemotherapy in Psychiatry*, Cambridge, Mass, Harvard, 1985, pp 9–12

————: *Biomedical Aspects of Depression*. Washington, DC, APA Press. 1982, pp 1–83

BARON M, RISCH N: X-linkage and genetic heterogeneity in bipolar-related major affective illness: Reanalysis of linkage data. Ann Hum Genet 46 (pt 2):153, 1982

———— et al: Genetic linkage between X-chromosome markers and bipolar affective illness. Nature 326:289, 1987

CLAYTON PJ, BARRETT JE (eds): *Treatment of Depression: Old Controversies and New Approaches*. New York, Raven, 1983

Diagnostic and Statistical Manual of Mental Disorders (3d edition, revised). Washington, DC, American Psychiatric Association, 1987

EGELAND JA et al: Bipolar affective disorders linked to DNA markers on chromosome II. Nature 325:783, 1987

KELSOE JR et al: Re-evaluation of the linkage relationship between chromosome 11p loci and the gene for bipolar affective disorder in the Old Order Amish. Nature 342:238, 1989

KLERMAN GL: History and development of modern concepts of affective illness, in *Neurobiology of Mood Disorders*. RM Post, RC Ballenger (eds). Baltimore, Williams & Wilkins, 1984, pp 1–19

MARTIN JB, REICHLIN S: *Clinical Neuroendocrinology*, 2d ed. Philadelphia, Davis, 1987

POST RM, BALLENGER JC (eds): *Neurobiology of Mood Disorders*. Baltimore, Williams & Wilkins, 1984, vol 1

————, WEISS SRB: Kindling and manic depressive illness, in *The Clinical Relevance of Kindling*. TB Bolwig, MR Trimble (eds). Chichester, England, Wiley, 1989, pp 209–230

ROBINS LN et al: Lifetime prevalence of specific psychiatric disorders in three sites. Arch Gen Psychiatry 41:949, 1984

ROSENTHAL NE et al: Seasonal affective disorder: A description of the syndrome and preliminary findings with light treatment. Arch Gen Psychiatry 41:72, 1984

STEWART AL et al: Functional status and well-being of patients with chronic conditions. Results from the Medical Outcomes Study. JAMA 262(7):907, 1989

WELLS KB et al: The functioning and well-being of depressed patients. Results from the Medical Outcomes Study. JAMA 262(7):914, 1989

Schizophrenic disorders

BRAFF DL: Attention, information processing, and habituation in psychiatric disorders. *Psychiatry III*. Philadelphia, Lippincott, 1985

————, GEYER MA: Sensorimotor gating and schizophrenia. Arch Gen Psychiatry 47:181, 1990

BROWN GW et al: Influence of family life on the course of schizophrenic disorders: A replication. Br J Psychiatry 11:241, 1972

CARLSON G, GOODWIN F: The stages of mania. Arch Gen Psychiatry 28:221, 1973

CHRISTISON GW et al: A quantitative investigation of hippocampal pyramidal cell size, shape, and variability of orientation in schizophrenia. Arch Gen Psychiatry 46:1027, 1989

CROW TJ et al: Schizophrenia as an anomaly of development of cerebral asymmetry: A postmortem study and a proposal concerning the genetic basis of the disease. Arch Gen Psychiatry 46:1145, 1989

DOCHERTY JP et al: Stages of onset of schizophrenic psychosis. Am J Psychiatry 135:420, 1978

JESTE DV, LOHR JB: Hippocampal pathologic findings in schizophrenia. Arch Gen Psychiatry 46:1019, 1989

ROSENBAUM CP: *The Meaning of Madness*. New York, Science House, 1970

ROSENTHAL D, KETY S: *The Transmission of Schizophrenia*. New York, Pergamon, 1968

Special issue: Negative symptoms in schizophrenia. Schizophr Bull 11, 1985

Special issue: Schizophr Bull 15(3), 1989

STRAUSS JS, CARPENTER WT: *Schizophrenia*. New York, Plenum Medical Book Company, 1981

SUDDATH RL et al: Anatomic abnormalities in the brains of monozygotic twins discordant for schizophrenia. N Engl J Med 322:789, 1990

WALKER E et al: Environmental factors related to schizophrenia in psychophysiologically labile high-risk males. J Abnorm Psychol 90:313, 1981

WYSOWSKI DK, BAUM C: Antipsychotic drug use in the United States, 1976–1985. Arch Gen Psychiatry 46:929, 1989

Anxiety disorders

CHARNEY DS et al: Noradrenergic function in panic anxiety. Arch Gen Psychiatry 41:75, 1984

———— et al: Neurobiological mechanisms of panic anxiety: Biochemical and behavioral correlates of yohimbine-induced panic attacks. Am J Psychiatry 144:1030, 1987

DUBOVSKY S: Generalized anxiety disorder: New concepts and psychopharmacologic therapies. J Clin Psychiatry 51(suppl):3, 1990

GOLDBERG J et al: A twin study of the effects of the Vietnam war on posttraumatic stress disorder. JAMA 263:1227, 1990

JENIKE M et al: Obsessive-compulsive disorder: A double-blind, placebo-controlled trial of clomipramine in 27 patients. Am J Psychiatry 146:1328, 1989

LIEBOWITZ MR et al: Lactate provocation of anxiety attacks. Arch Gen Psychiatry 41:764, 1984

MARKOWITZ JS et al: Quality of life in panic disorder. Arch Gen Psychiatry 46:984, 1989

TALLMAN JF et al: Receptors for the age of anxiety: Pharmacology of the benzodiazepines. Science 207:274, 1984

Personality disorders

ALNAES R, TORGERSEN S: DSM-III symptom disorders (Axis I) and personality disorders (Axis II) in an outpatient population. Acta Psychiatr Scand 78:348, 1988

BLUME SB: Dual diagnosis: Psychoactive substance dependence and the personality disorders. *Psychoactive Drugs* 21:139, 1989

CLONINGER CR: A unified biosocial theory of personality and its role in the development of anxiety states: A reply to commentaries. Psychiatr Dev 2:83, 1988

DRAKE RE, VAILLANT GE: A validity study of Axis II of DSM-III. Am J Psychiatry 142:555, 1985

FROSCH JP: The psychosocial treatment of personality disorders, in *Current Perspectives on Personality Disorders*. JP Frosch (ed). Washington, DC, APA Press, 1983, pp 96–112

GRANT I: *Behavioral Disorders: Understanding Clinical Psychopathology*. New York, Spectrum, 1979

GUNDERSON JG: DSM-III diagnoses of personality disorders, in *Current Perspectives on Personality Disorders*. JP Frosch (ed). Washington, DC, APA Press, 1983, pp 68–93

LAHMEYER HW et al: EEG sleep, lithium transport, dexamethasone suppression, and monoamine oxidase activity in borderline personality disorder. *Psychiatry Res* 25:19, 1988

LIEBOWITZ MR: Psychopharmacological intervention in personality disorders. *Current Perspectives on Personality Disorders*. JP Frosch (ed). Washington DC, APA Press, 1983, pp 68–93

LION JR: *Personality Disorders: Diagnosis and Management (Revised for DSM-III)*, 2d ed. Baltimore, Williams & Wilkins, 1981

MILLON T: *Disorders of Personality, DSM-III, Axis II*, New York, Wiley, 1981

MOREY LC: Personality disorders in DSM-III and DSM-III-R: Convergence, coverage, and internal consistency. Am J Psychiatry 145:573, 1988

PERRY JC, VAILLANT GE: Personality disorders, in *Comprehensive Textbook of Psychiatry/V*, HI Kaplan, BJ Sadock (eds). Baltimore, Williams & Wilkins, 1989, pp 1352–1387

PERSE TL et al: Fluvoxamine treatment of obsessive compulsive disorder. Am J Psychiatry 144:1543, 1987

REICH JH: Update on instruments to measure DSM-III and DSM-III-R personality disorders. J Nerv Ment Dis 177:366, 1989

SIEVER LJ et al: Biogenetic factors in personalities, in *Current Perspectives on Personality Disorders*, JP Frosch (ed). Washington, DC, APA Press, 1983, pp 42–65

WENDER PH et al: A controlled study in the treatment of attention deficit disorder, residual type, in adults. Am J Psychiatry 142:547, 1985

WIDIGER TA et al: The DSM-III-R personality disorders: An overview. Am J Psychiatry 145:7, 1988

369 THE THERAPEUTIC USE OF PSYCHOTROPIC MEDICATIONS

LEWIS L. JUDD

Perhaps no other area of pharmacology has experienced the rapid development that has occurred in psychopharmacology during the past several decades. An almost bewildering array of specific and effective psychotropic agents is currently available, with new medications appearing with great frequency. This chapter presents an overview of the major classes of psychopharmacologic drugs to provide the reader with a pragmatic understanding of these potent medications. The most clinically meaningful classification schema is based upon the therapeutic use in patients, as follows: antidepressant medications, lithium and other mood stabilizing medications, anxiolytic or antianxiety medications, and antipsychotic or neuroleptic medications.

ANTIDEPRESSANT MEDICATIONS

The successful search for new and better antidepressant medications has resulted in the two generations of antidepressants that are currently available. The first-generation antidepressants include the tricyclic (TCA) and the monoamine oxidase (MAO) inhibitor antidepressants. To date no newly developed drug has been proven to have greater clinical efficacy than antidepressants in these two major classes. The main benefit of the new generation of antidepressants is that they have provided the physician with an expanded range of pharmacologic options for the treatment of patients who cannot tolerate or who do not respond to the older drugs. The MAO inhibitors are clinically effective and recently have experienced a resurgence in clinical use, but the problems of drug-drug and drug-food interactions have made these the second-line medications in the treatment of depressive disorders. However, the MAO inhibitors appear to be especially effective for depression accompanied by panic attacks or prominent anxiety. The TCAs imipramine and amitriptyline have emerged as the standards for antidepressant efficacy.

No antidepressant is ideal, and currently available drugs have at least one of the following undesirable characteristics: delayed onset of therapeutic action (7 to 28 d), significant anticholinergic side effects, sedation, cardiotoxicity, weight gain, the possible induction of manic or hypomanic episodes in patients with bipolar disorders, or other equally problematic adverse reactions. The search for new medications may yet yield a superior antidepressant, one with a consistently high rate of improvement, rapid onset of action, and fewer side effects.

MECHANISMS OF ACTION TCAs were originally hypothesized to increase synaptic concentrations of central nervous system (CNS) monoaminergic neurotransmitter substances (e.g., norepinephrine, serotonin, and dopamine) by blocking their reuptake by presynaptic monoaminergic neurons. While this assumption is still valid, the focus now is on the regulation of postsynaptic receptor activity of monoaminergic neurons and the down-regulation of neurotransmitter receptors that have been associated with an antidepressant effect. These mechanisms have been hypothesized to account for the activity of most of the established antidepressants, but not of some of the newer antidepressants. At present, therefore, there is a great deal of information available about how antidepressants may ameliorate the pathophysiologic processes associated with depressive disorders, but no precise central mechanism(s) has been identified by which all drugs with antidepressant properties work.

CLINICAL CONDITIONS FOR USE Antidepressants are very effective in treatment of the clinical syndrome of major depression (Chap. 368) but do not affect normal mood changes or make unhappy people into happy ones. Chronic low-grade depression or dysthymic disorders (neurotic depression) generally do not respond well to antidepressants alone, although the combination of antidepressants and psychotherapy has proven effective in some cases. Antidepressants are only rarely prescribed for patients who become temporarily depressed over difficult and stressful life situations (situational depression).

There is growing evidence that antidepressants are effective in the treatment of some anxiety disorders (Chap. 368). TCAs and the MAO inhibitor antidepressants are the drugs of choice for agoraphobia, simple phobias, and panic disorder. Patients with phobic or panic disorders have concomitant anxiety about the recurrence of these attacks; this "anticipatory" anxiety may not respond to antidepressants but may benefit from concomitant treatment with antianxiety medication. There may be a broader role for the antidepressants in the management of pure anxiety disorders, but this possibility requires further study.

CLINICAL USE OF ANTIDEPRESSANTS Table 369-1 lists the more commonly used first-generation antidepressants and the oral doses needed for therapeutic efficacy in the typical patient. Currently imipramine and amitriptyline are the standards for antidepressant potency. Amitriptyline tends to have sedative effects, while imipramine is more energizing. Because of the undesirable side effects observed in these original TCAs, during the past decade growing numbers of experienced clinical psychopharmacologists have gradu-

TABLE 369-1   Commonly used first-generation antidepressants

Antidepressant	Daily oral therapeutic dose range, mg
Tricyclic derivatives:	
Amitriptyline (Elavil, etc.)	150–300
Nortriptyline (Aventyl, etc.)	50–150
Imipramine (Tofranil, etc.)	150–300
Desipramine (Norpramin)	150–250
Doxepin (Sinequan, etc.)	150–300
Monoamine oxidase inhibitors:	
Phenelzine (Nardil)	15–60
Tranylcypromine (Parnate)	20–30
Isocarboxazid (Marplan)	10–30

ally selected the secondary tricyclic amines desipramine and nortriptyline as the antidepressant drugs of choice. Both desipramine and nortriptyline have relatively fewer anticholinergic side effects and are less sedating. Nortriptyline appears to have a clearer relationship between plasma levels and clinical efficacy.

Before antidepressants are prescribed, a patient's physical health must be evaluated by a physical examination. The patient should show normal values on baseline complete blood count (CBC), urinalysis, liver function tests, and (if over 45 years) electrocardiogram (ECG). Patients are started on low doses in a twice daily regimen for a single day (e.g., 25 mg desipramine bid) and checked for side effects (e.g., postural hypotension). The dose is then raised quickly over a few days to that needed for a full therapeutic response. The minimum daily dose for clinical response is the low figure in the ranges listed in Table 369-1, but often higher doses are needed. However, dose schedules in the elderly should be reduced 30 to 50 percent. Physicians inexperienced in psychopharmacology should not exceed the upper dosage limits listed in the table. Treatment from 7 to 28 d is required to achieve a full therapeutic effect. Changes in the depressive symptoms are often noted by friends and family before the patient reports feeling better. A therapeutic trial of an antidepressant requires at least 28 d at the upper end of the dose range. Patients are usually maintained on antidepressants for approximately 9 to 12 months after the depressive symptoms disappear, to reduce the possibility of relapse resulting from premature withdrawal of medication. Highest relapse rates occur during the first 2 months after medication is discontinued, and patients and clinicians should be especially watchful during this time period.

Medications can be given in a single dose an hour before bedtime once an appropriate dose has been established. This procedure improves medication compliance, and sedative side effects are likely to induce sleep in depressed patients, who are often insomniac. Further, if troublesome side effects occur, they do so while the patient is alseep. For patients who cannot tolerate the single bedtime dose, a daytime twice daily or thrice daily schedule is necessary. Tests for plasma levels of the tricyclic antidepressants are routinely available, but unfortunately the relationship of plasma levels to clinical response has been inconsistent. For imipramine, desipramine, and amitriptyline, the relationship is linear, but nortriptyline may have a curvilinear plasma level–response relationship, implying a therapeutic window. Plasma levels may be useful in treatment-resistant patients to evaluate compliance and to see if the dose is sufficient to maintain concentrations above the threshold necessary for response (e.g., imipramine, >180 ng/mL; desipramine, >125 ng/mL; amitriptyline, >95 ng/mL; and nortriptyline, 50 to 150 ng/mL).

After about 10 to 12 months of treatment with an antidepressant, the drug should be withdrawn gradually over a 3- to 4-week period rather than suddenly stopped. Should depressive symptoms reemerge, antidepressant treatment should be restored and maintained for several more months before the withdrawal attempt is repeated.

SIDE EFFECTS AND INTERACTIONS   Listed in Table 369-2 are some of the more common side effects from the tricyclic antidepressants. They include dry mouth, sedation, a fine tremor of the hands,

and mild constipation. More serious are the effects on the cardiovascular system, of which tachycardia and postural hypotension are the most common. The TCAs, especially imipramine, have a quinidine-like action, can induce cardiac arrhythmias, and have been associated with sudden death in a few patients (see section below on overdose). For patients with preexisting cardiac illness, especially those with heart block, TCAs should be used cautiously; drugs with milder cardiac effects should be considered. The most bothersome symptoms are from the anticholinergic effects; while rarely serious, they do cause discomfort and compliance problems.

Some preexisting medical conditions increase the risks associated with using TCAs in certain depressed patients. Tricyclics can produce tachycardia, which may push some patients from asymptomatic congestive failure into symptomatic heart failure. TCAs also lower the seizure threshold and should be used cautiously in patients with seizures. The anticholinergic effects preclude TCA treatment in patients with glaucoma and pose a problem for men with mild to moderate prostatic hypertrophy, who may develop urinary retention. Finally, the use of tricyclic antidepressants in patients with bipolar disorders may shorten the cycle length between affective episodes, may induce an acute manic episode in some patients, and has been related to the phenomenon of rapid cycling.

The tricyclics, especially amitriptyline, imipramine, and doxepin, potentiate the effects of other CNS-depressant medications (e.g., ethanol, benzodiazepines), and patients should be cautioned about ethanol use while on antidepressants. Patients should either not drink or reduce their usual ethanol dose by one-half during tricyclic treatment. Other drug interactions include the potentiation of other anticholinergic agents (e.g., antihistamines, antiparkinsonian agents), which can result in severe constipation, urinary retention, and even paralytic ileus. This combination in the elderly, which can produce a serious anticholinergic blockade (e.g., paralytic ileus, fecal impaction), often has been the cause of frank delirium and confusional states in geriatric patients. Therefore this combination should be avoided in older patients.

Despite the problems, the risk-benefit ratio is overwhelmingly in favor of the antidepressants, and literally hundreds of thousands of patients have been treated with these compounds safely and effectively.

NEWER ANTIDEPRESSANTS   Table 369-3 lists the more prominent second-generation drugs for which some evidence of antidepressant efficacy exists. How these drugs will fare over time under more rigorous scrutiny is unknown. An example of the unforseen problems that arise when promising new drugs are given broader exposure is the experience with zimelidine. This relatively selective serotonin-uptake blocker was originally reported to be an effective antidepressant with milder anticholinergic side effects than others. Increased study has revealed it to be associated with Guillain-Barré syndrome in several patients. Zimelidine has now been withdrawn from the market. Nonetheless, this new generation of psychotropic

TABLE 369-2   Common side effects of tricyclic antidepressants

Anticholinergic (atropine-like) responses:
  Dry mouth
  Nausea and vomiting*
  Constipation
  Urinary retention
  Blurred vision (mydriasis and cycloplegia)
Cardiovascular effects:
  Postural hypotension*
  Tachycardia
  Cardiotoxic side effects—can induce an arrhythmia
Obstructive jaundice—more rare—is reversible when drug is removed
Drowsiness and sleepiness—may want to avoid driving a car until this
  diminishes*
Fine rapid tremor*
Dizziness, ataxia
Hematologic effects:
  Leukopenia

* Side effects seen most commonly

TABLE 369-3 Selected second-generation antidepressants

Antidepressant	Daily oral therapeutic dose range, mg
Tricyclic derivatives:	
Trimipramine (Surmonil)	100–250
Amoxapine (Asendin)	150–300
Tetracyclic derivatives:	
Maprotiline (Ludiomil)	100–225
Derivatives of other chemical classes:	
Fluoxetine (Prozac)	10–40
Bupropion (Wellbutrin)	200–300
Trazodone (Desyrel)	100–600

medications is very promising and has already expanded the physicians' therapeutic choices in the treatment of depressive disorders.

Amoxapine is a tricyclic derivative with clinical efficacy equal to that of the original antidepressants. An unsubstantiated early onset of action has been claimed by the manufacturer (within the first week), although its clinical efficacy at the endpoint of treatment is identical to that of the original TCAs. One of its metabolites (7-hydroxyamoxapine) is a neuroleptic, which accounts for the unwanted extrapyramidal side effects seen with amoxapine including tardive dyskinesia and parkinsonism. Other side effects from amoxapine appear to be similar to those of the original tricyclics, although a disproportionate number of seizures was found in some retrospective studies.

Clomipramine, a tricyclic that inhibits serotonin reuptake, is commonly used worldwide and is now approved for use in the United States. It has been shown in controlled studies to be an effective drug in the treatment of depression and to be effective in obsessive-compulsive disorders, which are frequently disabling and resistant to treatment.

Fluoxetine is a relatively selective serotonin-uptake inhibitor with antidepressant efficacy comparable to imipramine. Improvement in symptoms has been found as early as 1 week. Side effects similar to those observed with other serotonin-uptake blockers include nausea, diarrhea, tremor, headache, agitation, and weight loss, and range from mild to moderate severity. Patients show few signs of cardiotoxicity or dizziness. Fluoxetine is one of the first of a series of highly specific and potent serotonin-uptake inhibitors to be marketed in the United States (e.g., sertraline, fluvoxamine, indalpine) for the treatment of depression. There are also anecdotal reports of successful treatment of obsessive-compulsive disorder by fluoxetine, but no controlled studies have been reported to date.

Maprotiline is a tetracyclic derivative that is equal in antidepressant potency to the original tricyclics and reportedly has fewer anticholinergic side effects. Originally it was offered as a promising drug for use in patients with cardiovascular problems, but this has not been established and it is not recommended for this purpose. It has been reported to cause seizures at two to four times the rate at which the TCAs induce seizures, and a lower dosage schedule is now recommended. Moreover, its use has been associated with more than the expected incidence of blood dyscrasia.

Nomifensine, a potentially interesting antidepressant related to a nonanalgesic opiate derivative, has now been withdrawn from the market worldwide because of serious hypersensitivity reactions.

Trazodone is a triazolopyridine derivative originally introduced for use as an antidepressant. There remains controversy around whether the drug has significant antidepressant properties. The drug produces a high level of sedation and is useful as a hypnotic. It has few, if any, cardiotoxic effects but is associated with increased risk of priapism.

Alprazolam, a benzodiazepine with anxiolytic efficacy, has been reported to be an effective antidepressant, although it may be less potent than the original TCAs in treating major depressive disorders. It is likely to have a place in the treatment of mixed anxiety and depressive syndromes and has the added advantage of relatively rapid

onset. It has no anticholinergic or cardiotoxic effects but causes sedation and lethargy. Since it is a benzodiazepine, withdrawal symptoms, including seizures, may appear after prolonged used so the drug should be withdrawn gradually (i.e., no faster than 0.5 mg every 4 to 5 d; the last milligram should be tapered by 0.25 mg/week) (see Table 369-5 below).

Bupropion was withdrawn from the market because it produced a high rate of seizures in a subpopulation of bulimic patients. It was subsequently re-released when the seizure rate was found to be no greater than that produced by the TCAs (estimated at about 0.4 percent) and is currently used for treating major depression. A role for bupropion in stabilizing patients with rapid-cycling disorders has also been proposed. The mechanism of action may be related to dopamine-reuptake inhibition, although this is not established. Bupropion has energizing properties and consequently is less sedating, with mild side effects including headache, agitation, and some anticholinergic effects.

TRICYCLIC OVERDOSAGE Antidepressants are the fourth most common cause of drug overdose seen in emergency departments in the United States and the third most frequent cause of drug-related death (after alcohol-drug combinations and heroin). Of the antidepressants, tricyclics are the most frequent cause of death. In a California study (Callaham and Kassel) the annual frequency of fatal tricyclic overdose was 1.3 per 100,000 of population; more than two-thirds of the victims were women. Amitriptyline, desipramine, and nortriptyline were the most frequently implicated.

The first 6 h after an overdose of a tricyclic antidepressant are crucial. CNS depression and seizures, respiratory arrest, and cardiovascular arrhythmias are the principal causes of death. ECG changes showing QRS prolongation are early signs of toxicity, and ventricular fibrillation is a common complication. ECG changes are a more sensitive measure for monitoring patients than are blood levels of the drug.

LITHIUM AND OTHER MOOD-NORMALIZING MEDICATIONS

The most important psychotropic medication in this group is lithium. Although lithium possesses some antidepressant properties, it is not, strictly speaking, an antidepressant. Its effectiveness in treating patients with bipolar disorders (see Chap. 368) and other disorders of mood has revolutionized the practice of psychiatry. Lithium's approval by the Food and Drug Administration (FDA) in 1970 for the treatment of acute mania and in 1975 for the maintenance treatment of manic-depressive disorder generated an explosion of basic and clinical research focused on its pharmacologic mechanisms and clinical use.

MECHANISM OF ACTION The central mechanisms by which lithium exerts its clinical effects on extremes of mood are not fully understood. Lithium affects the brain's monoaminergic neurotransmitter concentrations at the synapse, has strong effects on biologic membranes, and intracellularly inhibits the conversion of inositol monophosphate to free inositol. This latter effect may, in turn, reduce neuronal excitability.

CLINICAL CONDITIONS FOR USE Lithium is the drug of choice for treating acute manic/hypomanic episodes and for prevention of recurrent episodes of mania and depression in bipolar illness. Recent studies suggest that the relapse rate among lithium-treated bipolar patients is about one-half that of control patients receiving a placebo. It may also be an effective agent in the prophylaxis of recurrent unipolar depressive disorders. Lithium also has antidepressant properties, especially in depressions seen in bipolar disorders; however, it is not a drug of choice for major depression per se. It has been successfully used in conjunction with neuroleptics in schizoaffective disorders; there may be a subpopulation of schizophrenics responsive to lithium, although most workers feel that such lithium responders are atypical bipolar patients and not schizophrenics. Finally, there are conflicting reports that lithium may be useful in treating alcoholism, a possibility requiring further study.

CLINICAL USE OF LITHIUM   Lithium is a very safe drug with an excellent risk-benefit ratio when it is used knowledgeably. The only genuine contraindication to lithium's use is seriously compromised renal function. The following baseline studies should be obtained before prescribing lithium: CBC, routine urinalysis with a concentration test, thyroxine (T_4), free T_4 index, thyroid-stimulating hormone (TSH), serum creatinine, electrolytes, and (for those over 40) an ECG.

Serum lithium levels peak 1 to 3 h after an oral dose, and the biologic half-life, which averages 24 h, varies with age. Elderly patients frequently have a drug half-life over 30 h, often requiring lower doses. Lithium is monitored by serum levels, which are most informative approximately 10 h after the last dose. Therapeutic efficacy in acute mania is achieved at levels between 0.8 and 1.4 mmol/L. Patients rarely require treatment at serum levels above 1.5 mmol/L. Lithium is always administered orally. Dose ranges are from 600 mg to 3000 mg daily, unless the patient is elderly. A general rule of thumb equates a 0.2 mmol/L rise in serum level with each additional 300-mg tablet of lithium. Unless sustained-release tablets are used, lithium is usually administered twice or three times daily, allowing for smooth, sustained 24-h serum levels. Because there is a 7- to 10-d delay in achieving full therapeutic effects, the addition of antipsychotic medications is often needed during the early phase of treating a manic patient. During acute manic episodes patients often tolerate relatively higher doses of lithium, but once the manic episode remits, it is necessary to reduce the dose.

The current maintenance treatment strategy is to prevent future recurrent episodes of mania and depression in patients with bipolar disorders. Clinicians are advised to seek the lowest possible serum levels in the range from 0.6 to 1.0 mmol/L that will prevent relapse. Lithium's excretion rate is very stable within each patient; as a result patients can be maintained on the same dose day in and day out, with relative certainty that stable levels are present. During maintenance patients are seen every 3 to 6 months, and serum lithium, sodium, potassium, T_4, free T_4 index, TSH, and creatinine are monitored along with urinalysis with a concentration test. The lithium excretion pattern is altered by conditions that change sodium concentrations, and patients on thiazide diuretics or low-salt diets should be warned and monitored more frequently.

SIDE EFFECTS AND INTERACTIONS   Lithium's side effects are listed in a continuum ranging from those seen relatively commonly to those indicating lithium toxicity (see Table 369-4). Many of these are minor side effects, which appear early and disappear as time passes, but some may persist throughout treatment. Because the rapid escalation of serum levels often induces side effects, especially those involving the gastrointestinal tract, smoother, more gradual serum lithium increases are desirable.

Some of the first signs of lithium toxicity are coarsening of tremor, increases in the deep tendon reflexes, and muscle fasciculations. Unusual degrees of sedation and cognitive disruption also may herald lithium toxicity. Lithium toxicity mimics barbiturate intoxication, and when death occurs it is secondary to respiratory depression and its complications. The treatment of lithium toxicity involves good supportive care and excellent hydration. Since lithium's half-life is 24 h, this treatment sustains the patient until the kidneys eliminate the medication. Various methods to improve the treatment of lithium toxicity, such as increasing lithium excretion by aminophylline or alkalinizing the urine, have all been disappointing. For life-threatening cases, the last resort is renal dialysis, but toxicity does not commonly progress to the point where this intervention is needed.

There is some evidence that lithium is a teratogen, particularly when administered during the first trimester of pregnancy. Cardiovascular and valve abnormalities have been detected in 18-week-old fetuses. While there is little evidence for teratogenesis during the second and third trimesters, alternative treatments in pregnant women should be considered.

TABLE 369-4   Common lithium side effects

Severity	Side effect
SIDE EFFECTS COMMONLY SEEN	
Very mild	Thirst
	Nausea (particularly during first few days of treatment)
	Fine tremor of hand
Mild to moderate	Anorexia
	Vomiting
	Diarrhea
	"Upset stomach" or "abdominal pain"
	Polydipsia and/or polyuria
	Muscular weakness and fatigue
SIDE EFFECTS INDICATING TOXICITY	
	Muscle hyperirritability with twitching, muscle fasciculation, or chronic movements
	Sedation, sluggishness, languidness, drowsiness, giddiness
	Coarse tremor
	Ataxia
Moderate to severe	Hypertonic muscles
	Hyperactive deep tendon reflexes
	Hyperextension of arms and legs with grunts and gasping
	Chorea, athetotic movements
	Impairment of consciousness
	Somnolence, confusion, stupor
	Seizures
	Transient focal neurologic signs
	Dysarthria
	Cranial nerve signs
Very severe	Coma
	Complications of coma
	Death

Lithium's interactions with other drugs primarily involve its reciprocal relationship with the sodium ion. Diuretics, which increase sodium excretion, can increase lithium toxicity. There have also been reports that combined neuroleptic and lithium therapy has resulted in a reversible neurotoxicity in a small number of middle-aged and older patients. Clinical observations indicate that this combination is safe and effective provided that both drugs are used in low to moderate doses, carefully monitored, and discontinued as soon as the lithium effect is sufficiently present for the patient to be managed without the neuroleptic.

MEDICAL SEQUELAE OF LITHIUM'S USE   Several medical complications can develop during lithium treatment. Because of its effect on adenylate cyclase activity, lithium inhibits the thyroid gland's secretory function; nontoxic goiters and hypothyroidism can develop, which can be readily corrected during lithium therapy by thyroid supplement. Lithium may induce the following ECG changes especially in older patients: T-wave depression, sinus node dysfunctions, and, very rarely, sinoatrial block and ventricular irritability.

The most important sequelae are the renal complications. About 25 percent of patients develop some degree of vasopressin-resistant nephrogenic diabetes insipidus with polyuria and polydipsia. The lithium inhibition of adenylate cyclase activity is responsible for the disruption of renal tubular transport. These symptoms are usually completely reversible by lithium withdrawal and often can be ameliorated by a reduction in dosage. The most economic and accurate method of monitoring changes in renal function during lithium treatment is by the urine concentration test and serum creatinine level. Consistent urine concentration levels below a specific gravity of 1.025 indicate an early renal effect, and a creatinine clearance test should be obtained. If creatinine clearance is abnormal, the patient's clinical condition should be reevaluated and termination of the lithium treatment considered. There have been reports of renal focal necrosis and interstitial fibrosis in a few long-term lithium patients, and there is evidence, by biopsy, for an increased basal rate of renal pathology among patients with affective disorders. Nonetheless, this nonspecific renal lesion does appear more frequently in patients receiving long-term lithium.

Evidence has emerged linking the more serious renal complications to increased episodes of lithium toxicity and possibly to prolonged combined use of lithium and neuroleptics. While good clinical practice should obviate lithium toxicity, it may be equally important to avoid extremes of high and low serum lithium levels during the day. Despite these concerns, lithium remains one of the most important and effective psychotropic agents and its risk-benefit ratio is excellent.

CARBAMAZEPINE AND OTHER MOOD-STABILIZING MEDICATIONS The anticonvulsant carbamazepine has, in controlled trials, been used successfully in the treatment of manic and, to a lesser extent, depressive episodes in bipolar patients. There is also growing evidence that some bipolar patients (15 to 60 percent) who do not respond to lithium benefit from carbamazepine treatment, and that the combination of lithium and carbamazepine may be therapeutically additive. The drug regimen for bipolar disorders is initiated with 200 mg bid administered orally, increasing to 600 to 1600 mg daily in divided doses and, although not well-correlated with therapeutic response, blood levels may range from 8 to 12 mg/dL.

Carbamazepine is not a completely benign drug; side effects include nausea, blurred vision, and ataxia, and more importantly there have been cases of fatal leukopenia and aplastic anemia reported (incidence $\leq$ 1 in 20,000). Patients treated with carbamazepine must be monitored for renal, liver, and bone marrow functions while they are on the medication. There are also reports of reversible CNS toxicity when this drug is combined with lithium. Therefore patients on this combination should be monitored carefully. Valproic acid, the drug of choice in certain seizure disorders, has also been reported to prevent recurrence of manic episodes in a small number of bipolar patients. The development of this new class of psychotropic compounds is very promising and may herald the future development of a new and useful group of medications.

ANTIANXIETY OR ANXIOLYTIC MEDICATIONS

The development of the benzodiazepines has been a great advance in the pharmacologic management of anxiety. They have also replaced barbiturates as the sedative-hypnotic drugs of choice. The benzodiazepines, unlike the barbiturates, are partial CNS depressants and thus, even at high doses, are rarely associated with lethal respiratory depression or vasomotor collapse. In addition, depending upon the dose, benzodiazepines possess anticonvulsant and muscle relaxant properties.

MECHANISMS OF ACTION There is growing evidence that gamma-aminobutyric acid (GABA), an inhibitory amino acid neurotransmitter, may play a central role in the brain mechanism(s) of anxiety. Benzodiazepines selectively, but indirectly, enhance GABA neurotransmission, possibly by increasing neuronal receptor sensitivity to GABA. Also, a close interaction has been described between GABA and benzodiazepine receptor binding, leading to an increase in neuronal chloride conductance. Despite these observations, the specific mechanism by which benzodiazepines mediate their clinical effects is not completely understood.

CLINICAL CONDITIONS FOR USE The antianxiety medications are most effective in the management of relatively short-lived reactive states of tension and anxiety and are the drugs of choice in the treatment of generalized anxiety disorders (see Chap. 368). Although alprazolam at high doses (4 to 10 mg) can block panic attacks, the TCAs and MAO inhibitors are the drugs of choice for treating panic disorders (see Chap. 368). However, the anxiolytics may have a role in the treatment of anticipatory anxiety, which is almost always present in patients with panic disorders. Sometimes, both a TCA and a benzodiazepine anxiolytic may be necessary in the treatment of panic disorder. The anxiolytics are also useful in treating anxiety symptoms that accompany phobic disorders.

TABLE 369-5 Commonly used benzodiazepines

Benzodiazepine	Daily oral dose range, mg	Half-life, h*
Anxiolytics:		
Chlordiazepoxide (Librium)	20–100†	7–28*
Diazepam (Valium)	5–40†	20–90*
Lorazepam (Ativan)	1–10‡	10–12
Oxazepam (Serax)	30–120‡	3–20
Prazepam (Centrax)	20–60†	40–70*
Alprazolam (Xanax)	0.75–10.0‡	12–15
Sedative-hypnotics:		
Flurazepam (Dalmane)	15–30§	24–100*
Temazepam (Restoril)	30§	8–10
Triazolam (Halcion)	0.125–0.5§	2–5

* Indicates long-acting active metabolites.
† Prescribed in a daily or twice daily regimen.
‡ Prescribed in a three or four times daily regimen.
§ Prescribed in a daily or bedtime regimen.

CLINICAL USE OF ANTIANXIETY MEDICATIONS The benzodiazepines have been most frequently prescribed as anxiolytics. The shorter-acting benzodiazepines, however, are also effective sedative-hypnotics. The more commonly prescribed drugs are listed in Table 369-5 along with the usual oral dose ranges. The pharmacokinetic characteristics of many of the benzodiazepines are complicated by long drug elimination half-lives and the metabolic conversion of parent compounds to active metabolites (see Table 369-5). Diazepam is converted to the active metabolite desmethyldiazepam (nordiazepam) which, in turn, can be hydroxylated to yield oxazepam, also a potent benzodiazepine. This metabolic pathway extends the activity half-life of diazepam threefold. The hypnotic flurazepam is converted to active metabolite N-1-desalkylflurazepam, which has a half-life of more than 48 h; hence, repetitive daily doses given in excess of a week or two can result in the accumulation of the active metabolites of the drug. Prazepam has metabolic breakdown products identical to those of diazepam and has a similar drug elimination half-life. Oxazepam and lorazepam, both of which undergo glucuronide conjugation, have no active metabolites and therefore have the advantage of a shorter half-life. The benzodiazepines temazepam, triazolam, and alprazolam also have the advantage of shorter half-lives and to date, no long-acting active metabolites have been identified.

Diazepam has been the standard against which all anxiolytic drugs are measured, and no other anxiolytics have demonstrated better antianxiety efficacy. The newly developed benzodiazepines appear equally effective and have eliminated certain of the undesirable side effects. Specifically, lorazepam, oxazepam, and alprazolam are without active metabolites and, with proper dosage, cumulative effects of daytime sedation are less noticeable.

Treatment regimens usually last 4 weeks or less, and medications are prescribed continually for 7 to 10 d followed by a 2- to 3-d drug holiday; then this sequence is repeated. This schedule helps avoid the development of tolerance to the anxiolytic effects. The shorter-acting medications (e.g., lorazepam, alprazolam) are prescribed in a three or four times daily regimen, and the longer-acting drugs (e.g., diazepam) are given in a single dose or a twice daily regimen. For example, it is common practice to prescribe one dose of diazepam at bedtime, since it will both promote sleep and reduce anxiety levels the following day.

In prescribing the anxiolytic benzodiazepines clinicians should avoid the possibility of habituating patients to chronic benzodiazepine use. One of the earliest signs is the development of tolerance in which the patient repeatedly requests escalations in drug dose. Since benzodiazepines do produce mild euphoria and a sense of well-being, anxious patients often want to preserve this feeling and request additional medication. However, clinical surveys of prescription practices have shown that clinicians are aware of the problems of benzodiazepine habituation and sometimes respond by being too cautious and by unnecessarily undertreating patients. The use of the drug holiday treatment regimen described above and the physician's resistance to repetitively increasing dosage will help to minimize the problem of drug habituation.

In addition to its role as an anxiolytic, diazepam is also the drug of choice in this class for muscle relaxation and for the treatment of alcohol withdrawal syndromes. It is the benzodiazepine of choice for intractable seizures. Oxazepam, because of the nonaccumulation of active metabolites, is a good choice for anxiolysis in the elderly.

SIDE EFFECTS AND INTERACTIONS The most important adverse effect of the benzodiazepines is the discomfort caused by the withdrawal syndrome, which can occur after chronic treatment. There is little risk of debilitating addiction to these drugs when used appropriately. However, physical dependence does occur since withdrawal symptoms are seen in a high percentage of patients after cessation of chronic benzodiazepine treatment. Motivation to sustain mild feelings of well-being and avoid the discomfort of withdrawal symptoms may contribute to psychological dependence. Withdrawal symptoms include muscle aches, agitation, restlessness, insomnia, and generalized anxious dysphoria. In some patients, more commonly those taking short-acting benzodiazepines, more serious CNS withdrawal symptoms may appear, including confusional and delirium states and, more rarely, grand mal seizures. Rebound anxiety can also be seen in patients with anxiety disorders but is less prevalent when benzodiazepines with long-acting metabolites are used and if medication is gradually discontinued. Risk for withdrawal symptoms increases with the length of treatment; they occur with much greater frequency (e.g., more than 90 percent) among patients who have been treated for 1 year or more. Withdrawal symptoms occur within the first 24 to 48 h after treatment with short-acting benzodiazepines ceases, but for those benzodiazepines with long-acting metabolites (e.g., diazepam, chlordiazepoxide) the withdrawal symptoms can occur 4 to 6 d and even longer after drug cessation. With the usual recommended dosage regimens and the gradual withdrawal technique (e.g., over 3 to 4 weeks), the appearance of a withdrawal syndrome in patients can be minimized significantly. While there is little true addiction potential, patients should be on these medication for only as long as necessary.

The most common minor side effects are daytime sedation, mild cognitive impairment, motor clumsiness, and (e.g., lorazepam, triazolam) specific memory decrements. Another rare but troublesome side effect from some benzodiazepines is paradoxical emotional responses, primarily manifested as aggressive and impulsive behavior.

Unlike barbiturates, the benzodiazepines do not noticeably induce hepatic microsomal enzyme activity and therefore do not affect the metabolism of other medications. The benzodiazepines potentiate the CNS depressant effects of other drugs including barbiturates, general anesthetics, and alcohol. The cross-tolerance with ethanol has made the benzodiazepines ideal medications for the treatment of alcohol withdrawal syndromes. Patients should be cautioned that ethanol's effects are potentiated by benzodiazepines and this combination should be avoided.

NEWER ANXIOLYTIC MEDICATIONS It has been established that certain beta-adrenergic blocking agents, such as *propranolol*, can dampen the peripheral physiologic symptoms of anxiety. Initially, it was felt that these drugs might be better nonsedative anxiolytic compounds, but this promise has not been fulfilled in controlled studies. While propranolol does attenuate somatic manifestations of anxiety (e.g., palpitations, tremor), it appears to have lesser effects on the psychological components (e.g., intense fearfulness). Although propranolol has been used for treating patients extremely fearful of speaking or performing in public (oral dose 40 to 320 mg qd), it is not a comprehensively effective anxiolytic. With additional study, other peripheral blocking agents may prove to be more effective.

A new class of anxiolytic drugs, the azaspirodecanediones, has been developed. One of the first compounds studied clinically is *buspirone*. It has no structural similarity to other anxiolytics or even to other psychotropics. It is not anticonvulsant, does not interact with the benzodiazepine receptor, is not cross-tolerant with other CNS

depressants, and no abstinence syndrome has yet been described. In several controlled trials it has proved to be an effective anxiolytic with significantly less sedation and decrements in psychomotor performance. Because of the near absence of sedation and motor impairment and the relatively long latency for anxiolytic effects to appear (i.e., days to weeks), patients occasionally report that the drug is ineffective. This is most common in individuals who have previously received benzodiazepines such as diazepam. Numerous studies are currently being conducted with buspirone to determine possible side effects.

In addition to the efficacy of *tricyclic antidepressants* in panic and phobic disorders, there are controlled studies reporting that they are anxiolytics as effective as the benzodiazepines in generalized anxiety disorders. It is possible that continued investigations will identify a broader role for TCAs in the treatment of the full spectrum of anxiety disorders.

ANTIPSYCHOTIC OR NEUROLEPTIC MEDICATIONS

The antipsychotics have the capacity to sedate, tranquilize, blunt emotional expression, attenuate aggressive and impulsive behavior, and cause disinterest in the environment and lack of initiative. Unique features of the drugs are that they leave higher intellectual functions relatively intact yet specifically ameliorate the agitation and bizarre behavior and thinking of psychotic patients. Unfortunately no antipsychotic medication currently available even approaches the criteria for an ideal drug in this group. Virtually all have prominent anticholinergic side effects and produce a wide variety of dystonias and extrapyramidal symptoms. Of greater concern is the fact that long-term administration of these agents can cause tardive dyskinesia in some patients (see Chap. 25), a seriously disabling movement disorder that is often irreversible. Nonetheless, the antipsychotics, primarily used in schizophrenia, have helped to reduce enormously the patient populations in mental hospitals and have allowed chronic mentally ill patients who previously would have been lifelong residents of hospitals to live in the community.

MECHANISM OF ACTION With few exceptions, antipsychotic neuroleptics have notable effects on the brain's dopaminergic neurotransmitter system. Specifically, these medications antagonize the effects of the neurotransmitter dopamine in the basal ganglia and in the limbic portions of the forebrain. Since the central characteristic of neuroleptics is their capacity to block dopaminergic neurotransmission, this has led researchers to postulate that an abnormality in the CNS dopaminergic neurotransmitter system is one of the key pathophysiologic mechanisms in the etiology of schizophrenia. Many effects of antipsychotic medications on the brain have been well-described, but the underlying mechanism by which these drugs achieve their antipsychotic efficacy is not yet fully understood.

CLINICAL CONDITIONS FOR USE Because the overall risk of tardive dyskinesia is estimated at 20 to 40 percent with chronic treatment, antipsychotics should only be used when necessary and in those conditions for which they are the drug of choice: in treating schizophrenic disorders (see Chap. 368); in combination with lithium for acute manic episodes (see Chap. 368); and in combination with antidepressants for psychotic and agitated depressions. They are also used in treating Tourette's syndrome and Huntington's disease. Although the antipsychotics should be used with only a relatively narrow spectrum of mental disorders, patients with these disorders make up a significant majority of all patients with serious and chronic mental illness.

CLINICAL USE OF THE ANTIPSYCHOTICS The more commonly used antipsychotics from each pharmacologic class and their average daily oral doses are given in Table 369-6. Chlorpromazine, one of the first drugs of this class to be developed, is the prototypic antipsychotic drug and the potency standard for the others. Dose equivalence for an antipsychotic drug is calculated in comparison with the effect of 100 mg of chlorpromazine. For example, 5 mg of

TABLE 369-6   Some commonly used antipsychotic medications

	Average daily oral dose range, mg	Potency ratio compared to 100 mg of chlorpromazine
Phenothiazines:		
Aliphatics:		
Chlorpromazine (Thorazine)	400–800	1:1
Piperazines:		
Fluphenazine (Prolixin)	4–20	1:50
Fluphenazine enanthate or decanoate	25–100*	
Perphenazine (Trilafon)	8–32	1:10
Trifluoperazine (Stelazine)	6–20	1:20
Piperidines:		
Thioridazine (Mellaril)	200–600	1:1
Butyrophenones:		
Haloperidol (Haldol)	8–32	1:50
Thioxanthenes:		
Chlorprothixene (Taractan)	400–800	1:1 (approx)
Thiothixene (Navane)	15–30	1:25
Oxoindoles:		
Molindone (Moban, Lidone)	40–200	1:10
Dibenzoxazepines:		
Loxapine (Loxitane, Daxolin)	60–100	1:10

* For intramuscular injection only.

trifluoperazine or 2 mg of haloperidol is equivalent in potency to 100 mg of chlorpromazine. Using this ratio as a reference point, acutely psychotic patients usually require an accumulated dose of 500 to 800 mg orally of a chlorpromazine equivalent during the first 24 to 36 h. Following control of the acute agitation, the oral dose is increased over the next week to the chlorpromazine equivalent of between 600 and 1500 mg a day in divided doses. It is uncommon for therapeutic benefits to be measurably increased by exceeding the daily dose equivalent of 1500 mg of chlorpromazine, although it may be necessary to go to two and three times this level in some patients.

Because schizophrenia is a chronic disorder, patients need long-term maintenance on antipsychotics to prevent relapse. In controlled studies as many as 60 percent of schizophrenics relapse within 6 months after discontinuing drug therapy. Patients are maintained on the lowest dose possible that will prevent reemergence of symptoms. This is usually in the range of 20 percent of the peak dose level needed to ameliorate the acute phase of the psychotic symptoms. Compliance is difficult to achieve in this chronically disordered group of patients, and it is often therapeutically advantageous for the clinician to use parenteral long-acting fluphenazine enanthate or decanoate, which can be administered by injection every week or two. Previously it was recommended that drug holidays be used, but this practice has not prevented tardive dyskinesia, and there are few if any advantages to this technique, which is now rarely used.

SIDE EFFECTS AND INTERACTIONS Initially patients are sedated, lethargic, and drowsy, but within days they develop tolerance to these effects. All of the antipsychotics have anticholinergic action, which may produce dry mouth, cycloplegia, postural hypotension, constipation, and urinary retention. Obstructive jaundice, retinal pigmentation (thioridazine), lenticular opacities, skin pigmentation and hypersensitivity to sunlight, and male impotence are also side effects seen with antipsychotics.

The extrapyramidal side effects are the most troublesome, however. During the first five days of treatment, patients may develop acute muscular dystonic reactions but the extrapyramidal Parkinson-like syndrome is the most common. Both the dystonia and the parkinsonism respond well to antiparkinsonian medications (e.g., benztropine mesylate, 1 to 2 mg bid or tid; trihexyphenidyl, 2 to 5 mg bid or tid). Another common side effect is akathisia, a motor restlessness in which patients feel compelled to move their extremities and to move about. It is not uncommon to mistake akathisia for psychotic agitation and increase the antipsychotic dose, exacerbating the prob-

lem. Akathisia may respond to beta blockers (Lipinski et al.) and antiparkinsonian agents but more often requires decreasing the dose of the antipsychotic. It is rarely necessary to continue antiparkinsonian drug treatment beyond the first 3 months of antipsychotic maintenance.

The most serious side effect of the antipsychotics is tardive dyskinesia, which has been seen with virtually every neuroleptic. The specter of tardive dyskinesia has altered the risk-benefit ratio of the antipsychotics; they should only be used for those disorders in which they are clearly the drugs of choice. Usually the symptoms of tardive dyskinesia appear late in treatment and consist of involuntary, repetitive movements of the lips, tongue (e.g., tongue thrusting, lip smacking), and not infrequently of the extremities and trunk. Patients over 60 and those with preexisting CNS pathology are at a higher risk for this disorder (up to 70 percent), but other risk factors have not been confirmed. Although tardive dyskinesia cannot be prevented or reversed once it has developed, newer antipsychotic medications such as clozapine, which can attenuate some of the symptoms, may be substituted for the neuroleptic being used. However, it is too early to determine whether tardive dyskinesia is reduced with some of the newer antipsychotic medications.

The malignant neuroleptic syndrome, a rare complication of neuroleptic drugs, is discussed in Chap. 377.

NEWER ANTIPSYCHOTIC MEDICATIONS Although development of new antipsychotic medications has lagged significantly behind that of the antidepressants and anxiolytic drugs, some promising medications have appeared recently.

Clozapine is a dibenzodiazepine that binds to serotonin and alpha-adrenergic, histaminergic, and dopaminergic receptors. It has been approved by the FDA for use in treatment-refractory psychotic patients and in those who have intolerable side effects with their current medications. Its antipsychotic activity is comparable to the traditional neuroleptics, and it is also effective in attenuating anxiety and tension. Clozapine has proven effective in about 30 percent of treatment-resistant schizophrenics. The drug produces some sedation and muscle relaxation but few extrapyramidal symptoms. It is not known to cause tardive dyskinesia and may, in high doses, attenuate it. Clozapine's side effects include orthostatic hypotension, sinus tachycardia, hypersalivation, temperature elevation, lowered seizure threshold, and constipation. A 1 to 2 percent incidence of potentially fatal agranulocytosis has been reported but this may be considerably higher in eastern European and Jewish subpopulations. Frequent (e.g., weekly) CBCs should be obtained.

Sulpiride, which is available in Europe, is a substituted benzamide that selectively binds to presynaptic, sodium-dependent, D-2 receptors. Its antipsychotic efficacy is comparable to traditional neuroleptics. Moreover, it may cause fewer cases of tardive dyskinesia and extrapyramidal syndrome. This novel structure may herald the development of new classes of safer and better antipsychotics.

REFERENCES

APPLETON WS, DAVIS JM: *Practical Clinical Psychopharmacology*, 2d ed. Baltimore, Williams & Wilkins, 1980

BALDESSARINI RJ: *Chemotherapy in Psychiatry*. Cambridge, Mass, Harvard, 1985

BOEHNERT MT, LOVEJOY FH JR: Value of the QRS duration versus the serum drug level in predicting seizures and ventricular arrhythmias after an acute overdose of tricyclic antidepressants. N Engl J Med 313:474, 1985

CALLAHAM M, KASSEL D: Epidemiology of fatal tricyclic antidepressant ingestion: Implications for management. Ann Emerg Med 14:1, 1985

COOPER TB et al (eds): *Lithium: Controversies and Unresolved Issues*. Amsterdam, Excerpta Medica, 1979

GELENBERG AJ: et al: Comparison of standard and low serum levels of lithium for maintenance treatment of bipolar disorder. N Engl J Med 321:1489, 1989

GILMAN AG et al (eds): *Goodman and Gilman's The Pharmacological Basis of Therapeutics*, 7th ed. New York, MacMillan, 1985

GUZE BH, BAXTER LR JR: Current concepts: Malignant neuroleptic syndrome. N Engl J Med 313:163, 1985

HANESTON PD: *Drug Interactions*, 3d ed. Philadelphia, Lea & Febiger, 1975

HIPPUIS H, WINOKUR G (eds): Part 2, clinical psychopharmacology, in *Psychopharmacology 1*. Amsterdam, Excerpta Medica, 1983

HOLLISTER LE: *Clinical Pharmacology of Psychotherapeutic Drugs*. New York, Churchill Livingston, 1978

IVERSON LL, SNYDER SS (eds): *Handbook of Psychopharmacology*. New York, Plenum, 1977

JARVIK ME: *Psychopharmacology in the Practice of Medicine*. New York, Appleton-Century-Crofts, 1977

KANE J et al (with Clozaril Collaborative Study Group): Clozapine for the treatment-resistant schizophrenic. Arch Gen Psychiatry 45:789, 1988

KLEIN DF et al: *Diagnosis and Drug Treatment of Psychiatric Disorders: Adults and Children*, 2d ed. Baltimore, Williams & Wilkins, 1980

LIEBERMAN JA et al: Clozapine-induced agranulocytosis: Non-cross-reactivity with other psychotropic drugs. J Clin Psychiatry 49(7):271, 1988

LIPINSKI JF JR et al: Propranalol in the treatment of neuroleptic induced akathisia. Am J Psychiatry 141:412, 1984

MELTZER HY (ed): *Psychopharmacology: The Third Generation of Progress*. New York, Raven, 1987

POST RM, BALLENGER JC (eds): Neurobiology of mood disorders, in *Frontiers of Clinical Neuroscience*. Baltimore, Williams & Wilkins, 1984, vol 1

section 2   Alcoholism and drug dependency

370   ALCOHOL AND ALCOHOLISM

MARC A. SCHUCKIT

Ninety percent of people drink alcohol, 40 to 50 percent of men have temporary alcohol-induced problems, and 10 percent of men and 3 to 5 percent of women develop pervasive and persistent alcohol-related problems (alcoholism). The usual alcoholic has a family and a job; only about 5 percent fit the skid row stereotype. Even light drinking may adversely interact with other medications, temporary heavier drinking can exacerbate most medical illnesses, and alcoholism can masquerade as many different medical disorders and psychiatric syndromes. The following sections describe the pharmacology and clinical effects of alcohol and identify circumstances where drinking may cause a major medical or psychiatric problem or exacerbate a preexisting disorder. While these comments apply to the hypothetical "average" person, there is considerable individual variability depending on genetic vulnerability, concomitant drug use, and prior unrelated pathology or disease.

PHARMACOLOGY OF ETHANOL: ABSORPTION AND METABOLISM   Ethanol is a weakly charged molecule that moves easily through cell membranes, rapidly equilibrating between blood and tissues. The effects of drinking depend in part on the amount of ethanol consumed per unit of body weight; the level of alcohol in the blood is expressed as milligrams or grams of ethanol per deciliter (e.g., 100 mg/dL or 0.1000 g/dL). In round figures, 340 mL (12 oz) of beer, 115 mL (4 oz) of nonfortified wine, and 43 mL (1.5 oz) (a shot) of 80-proof beverage each contain approximately 10 g of ethanol; 1 pint of 86-proof beverage contains approximately 160 g and 1 L of wine contains approximately 80 g of ethanol. Congeners found in alcohol beverages may contribute to body damage with heavy drinking; these include low-molecular-weight alcohols (e.g. methanol and butanol), aldehydes, esters, histamine, phenols, tannins, iron, lead, and cobalt.

Ethanol is a central nervous system (CNS) depressant that decreases activity of neurons, although some behavioral stimulation is observed at low blood levels. This drug has cross-tolerance and shares a similar pattern of behavioral problems with other brain depressants, including the benzodiazepines, barbiturates, and other sedatives and hypnotics. Alcohol is absorbed from mucus membranes of the mouth and esophagus (in very small amounts), from the stomach and large bowel (in modest amounts), and from the proximal portion of the small intestine (the major site). The rate of absorption *increases* with rapid gastric emptying; the absence of proteins, fats, or carbohydrates (which interfere with absorption); the absence of congeners; dilution to a modest percentage of ethanol (maximum absorption is seen at about 20 percent by volume); and carbonation (champagne).

Between 2 percent (at low blood alcohol concentrations) and about 10 percent (at high blood alcohol concentrations) of ethanol is excreted directly through the lungs, urine, or sweat, but the greater part is metabolized to acetaldehyde in the liver. At least two metabolic routes, each with different optimal concentrations of ethanol (K_m), result in the metabolism of approximately one drink per hour. The *first* and clinically most important pathway occurs in the cell cytosol via alcohol dehydrogenase (ADH) with a K_m of about 2 mmol. This reaction produces acetaldehyde which is then rapidly destroyed by aldehyde dehydrogenase (ALDH) in the cytosol and mitochondria. Each of these steps requires nicotinamide adenine dinucleotide (NAD) as a cofactor, and it is the increased ratio of the reduced cofactor (NADH) to NAD (NADH:NAD) that is responsible for many of the metabolic derangements observed after drinking. *Second,* microsomes of the smooth endoplasmic reticulum (the microsomal ethanol-oxidizing system or MEOS) with a K_m of about 10 mmol may be responsible for 10 percent or more of ethanol oxidation at high blood alcohol concentrations. Increased activity of this system can be induced after repeated exposure to ethanol.

All pathways result in the production of acetaldehyde, which is oxidized to acetate. The specific clinical significance of acetaldehyde is not fully known, but low levels of this substance may cause stimulation and behavioral reinforcement. Accumulation of higher levels in liver, brain, or other body tissues may cause organ damage.

BEHAVIORAL EFFECTS, TOLERANCE, AND DEPENDENCE   The behavioral and physiologic effects of any drug depend upon the dose, its rate of increase in plasma, the concomitant presence of other drugs or medical problems, and the past experience with the agent. With alcohol, one must also consider whether observation is during rising (where the effects are more intense) or falling blood alcohol levels.

Even though "legal intoxication" requires a blood alcohol concentration of at least 80 to 100 mg/dL (0.1 g/dL), behavioral, psychomotor, and cognitive changes are seen at levels as low as 20 to 30 mg/dL (i.e., after one to two drinks). Narcosis or deep sleep is induced in many people at twice the legal intoxication level, and even in the absence of concomitant medications, death can occur with levels between 300 and 400 mg/dL. Ethanol, either alone or in combination with agents such as benzodiazepines, is probably responsible for more toxic overdose deaths than any other agent.

The mechanisms of action of ethanol on nervous tissues are not fully understood because even modest doses simultaneously change many neurotransmitters and increase the fluidity of neuronal cell membranes. After repeated exposure to the drug, the body compensates in at least three ways to tolerate higher ethanol levels. *First,* after 1 to 2 weeks of daily drinking the liver can increase the metabolic rate of ethanol in humans by as much as 30 percent; i.e., there is *metabolic or pharmacokinetic tolerance,* an adaptation that disappears almost as rapidly as it develops. *Second,* cellular or *pharmacodynamic tolerance* probably occurs through complex neurochemical adaptations or changes in cell membranes with subsequent altered ion flow—

changes that may contribute to physical dependence. *Third*, even at the same blood alcohol concentrations and neuronal adaptation, organisms can learn to adapt behavior and to function better than expected under drug influence (*behavioral tolerance*). For example, practicing driving while intoxicated might result in a psychomotor performance which (*while still impaired*) is better than that observed before practice.

Once the cells have adapted to chronic ethanol exposure, the structural or biochemical changes may not return to normal for several weeks or more. In the face of these adaptations, the neurons require ethanol to function optimally; i.e., the person is physically addicted or drug-dependent. This physical condition is distinct from psychological dependence, a poorly defined concept indicating that the person is psychologically uncomfortable without the drug.

NUTRITIONAL FACTORS   One gram of ethanol has approximately 29.7 kJ (7.1 kcal), and a drink contains between 293.0 and 418.6 kJ (70 and 100 kcal) from ethanol and other carbohydrates. Therefore, 8 to 10 drinks can yield over 4186 kJ (1000 kcal) per day, but these are "empty" of nutrients such as minerals, proteins, and vitamins.

Any vitamin absorbed through the small intestine by active transport or stored in the liver can be deficient in alcoholics. These include folate (folacin or folic acid), pyridoxine (B_6), thiamine (B_1), nicotinic acid or niacin (B_3), and vitamin A. Thiamine deficiency causes Wernicke's and Korsakoff's syndromes (see Chap. 357).

Low blood potassium, magnesium, calcium, zinc, and phosphorus can occur as a consequence of dietary deficiency and acid-base imbalances during excess alcohol ingestion or withdrawal. Hypokalemia can lead to periodic muscle paralysis and areflexia. Deficiencies in magnesium can add to a clouded sensorium and other neurologic symptoms; hypocalcemia can cause tetany and weakness; low levels of zinc are speculated to contribute to gonadal dysfunction, anorexia, problems with wound healing, and immune deficiencies; and low phosphate levels can contribute to myocardial failure, brain dysfunction, weakness of muscles (including those of respiration), and white blood cell and platelet dysfunction.

An ethanol load in a fasting, healthy individual is likely to produce transient hypoglycemia within 6 to 36 h, secondary to the acute actions of ethanol on gluconeogenesis. This impairment is exacerbated by poor diet and by liver and pancreatic disease. As a result, glucose intolerance may be marked until the alcoholic has been abstinent for 2 to 4 weeks. Alcohol ketoacidosis, probably reflecting a decrease in fatty acid oxidation coupled with poor diet or recurrent vomiting, should not be misdiagnosed as diabetic ketosis. With the former, patients show an increase in serum ketones along with a mild increase in glucose but a large anion gap, a mild to moderate increase in serum lactate, and a β-hydroxybutyrate/lactate ratio of between 2:1 and 9:1 (with normal being 1:1).

THE EFFECTS OF ETHANOL ON BODY SYSTEMS

This overview of acute and chronic effects of alcohol on body systems outlines signs and symptoms that can aid in the recognition of the hidden alcoholic. It emphasizes the interactions between drinking and medications and the effects of alcohol on chronic medical conditions, factors that are also important in helping the clinician to understand the effects of alcohol on nonalcoholic patients.

CENTRAL NERVOUS SYSTEM   In addition to acute behavioral effects, an evening of heavy drinking can result in an alcoholic "*blackout*," i.e., an episode of forgetting all or part of what occurred during drinking. This problem is experienced by 30 to 40 percent of men in their late teens and early 20s, most of whom do not go on to develop more serious and pervasive alcohol-related problems. Even after only a few drinks, alcohol acutely decreases *sleep* latency (helping people to fall asleep) and depresses rapid eye movement (REM) sleep early in the night, sometimes followed by later REM rebound associated with bad dreams. The consequence is to "frag-

ment" sleep, causing a more rapid than normal alternation between sleep stages and a deficiency in deep sleep.

Chronic intake of high doses of ethanol can cause *peripheral neuropathy* in 5 to 15 percent of alcoholics (see Chaps. 357 and 363). This syndrome probably results from both thiamine deficiency and direct effects of ethanol and/or acetaldehyde. Patients complain of bilateral limb numbness, tingling, and parasthesias, more pronounced distally than proximally. Although these symptoms can be incapacitating, more often the pain and numbness are mild to moderate in severity. The treatment is abstinence and thiamine supplementation.

Wernicke's and Korsakoff's syndromes are important problems in alcoholics (see Chap. 357). Thiamine deficiency is the major cause in vulnerable individuals (possibly interacting with a genetic transketolase deficiency). Classically, patients with Korsakoff's syndrome present with profound anterograde (unable to learn new material) and retrograde amnesia along with possible impairment in visuospatial, abstract, and conceptual reasoning but with a normal intelligence quotient (IQ). In general, the level of recent memory loss is out of proportion to the global level of cognitive impairment. While most patients demonstrate an acute onset of Korsakoff's syndrome in association with the neurologic stigmata seen with Wernicke's syndrome (e.g., sixth nerve palsy and ataxia), some individuals may have a more gradual development of symptoms probably secondary to repeated bouts of thiamine deficiency. Wernicke's syndrome responds rapidly to oral thiamine replacement of 50 to 100 mg followed by 50 to 100 mg/d. However, only one-quarter of Korsakoff's patients are likely to achieve full recovery, one-half experience partial recovery, and one-quarter show no improvement with thiamine even after many months of supplementation.

About 1 percent of alcoholics with long histories of associated malnutrition develop *cerebellar degeneration*, a syndrome of progressive unsteady stance and gait often accompanied by mild nystagmus (see Chap. 357). Cerebellar atrophy is seen on CT or MRI scan, but the cerebrospinal fluid is usually normal. While ethanol or acetaldehyde might contribute to the problem, the major cause is probably nutritional, and identical symptoms can be seen with some forms of severe malnutrition alone. Treatment consists of abstinence and multiple vitamin supplementation, although improvement is often minimal.

Alcoholics can show severe *cognitive* problems and impairment in recent and remote memory for weeks to months after an alcoholic binge. Cortical functioning (e.g., psychomotor performance and short-term memory) tends to improve with abstinence, but long-term memory problems, perhaps reflecting subcortical damage, may persist. Increased size of the brain ventricles and cerebral sulci are seen in up to 50 percent of chronic alcoholics. These changes are partially reversible, returning toward normal after a year or more of abstinence. Permanent CNS impairment (*alcoholic dementia*) may supervene. Up to 20 percent of chronically demented patients may have had prior alcoholism. There is no single alcoholic dementia syndrome; rather, this label is used to describe patients who have apparently irreversible cognitive changes (possibly from diverse causes) in the midst of chronic alcoholism (see also Chap. 357).

Finally, to borrow a phrase from the past, alcohol could be termed "the great mimicker" because almost every psychiatric syndrome can be seen during heavy drinking or subsequent withdrawal. These include: intense *sadness* lasting for days to weeks in the midst of heavy drinking, a problem that can be viewed as a "normal" effect of alcohol; severe *anxiety* during alcoholic withdrawal, often remaining for many months after cessation of drinking; *psychoses* during the severe form of the alcohol abstinence syndrome; and auditory *hallucinations* and/or *paranoid delusions* in the absence of any obvious signs of withdrawal—a state called alcoholic hallucinosis or alcoholic paranoia. Whatever the cause, the treatment of alcohol-induced psychopathology includes abstinence and supportive care, with the likelihood of full recovery within several days or weeks. Alcohol intake is an important part of the differential diagnosis of *any* patient with one of these psychological symptoms. Another alcohol-related psychiatric syndrome is *pathologic intoxication* or alcohol idiosyncratic intoxication, a state of severe agitation, confusion, and violence lasting minutes to hours which is seen after a very low dose of ethanol (e.g., one to two drinks) and for which the individual is amnestic. This extremely rare phenomenon, seen almost exclusively in individuals with severe preexisting brain damage, is sometimes invoked erroneously for the purposes of legal defense.

THE GASTROINTESTINAL SYSTEM Esophagus and stomach Acute alcoholic intake can result in inflammation of the esophagus (possibly secondary to reflux of gastric contents) and stomach (resulting from damage to the gastric mucosal barrier). Esophagitis can cause epigastric distress, and gastritis, the most frequent cause of gastrointestinal bleeding in heavy drinkers, can present with anorexia and abdominal pain. Chronic heavy drinking, if associated with violent vomiting, can produce a longitudinal tear in the mucosa at the gastroesophageal junction—a Mallory-Weiss lesion. Although many gastrointestinal problems are reversible, two complications of chronic alcoholism, esophageal varices secondary to cirrhosis-induced portal hypertension and atrophy of gastric cells, may be irreversible (see Chaps. 237 and 239).

Small bowel The greater part of the ethanol is absorbed from the proximal small bowel, where it may interfere with absorption of B vitamins and other nutrients. Acutely, ethanol can cause hemorrhagic lesions of the duodenal villi and diarrhea secondary to increased small-bowel motility and decreased water and electrolyte absorption. Chronic alcoholism can contribute to diarrhea through its effects on the pancreas (see Chaps. 240 and 260).

Pancreas Alcoholics commonly develop acute or chronic pancreatitis (see Chap. 260).

Liver Ethanol absorbed from the small bowel is carried directly to the liver, where it becomes the preferred fuel; NADH accumulates and oxygen utilization escalates, gluconeogenesis is impaired (with a resulting fall in the amount of glucose produced from glycogen), lactate production increases, and there is a decreased oxidation of fatty acids in the citric cycle with an increase in fat accumulation within liver cells. In the healthy individual taking no medications these changes are reversible, but with repeated exposure to ethanol more severe changes in liver functioning are likely to occur. These include, in overlapping stages, fatty accumulation, alcohol-induced hepatitis, and cirrhosis (see Chap. 254).

Increased cancer risk Cancer is the second leading cause of death in alcoholics (after cardiovascular disease), who have a rate of carcinoma 10 times higher than that expected in the general population. The sites with the greatest increase over expected rates include the head and neck, esophagus, cardia of the stomach, liver, pancreas, and, according to recent data, breast.

HEMATOPOIETIC SYSTEM Ethanol exerts multiple reversible acute and chronic effects on all blood cells. Alcohol alters acutely the production of red blood cells (RBC), which reaches clinical significance after days to weeks of heavy drinking. The most common finding is an increase in RBC size (mean corpuscular volume, MCV) with a mild anemia. If this is accompanied by folic acid deficiency, there can also be hypersegmented neutrophils, reticulocytopenia, and hyperplastic bone marrow. Other forms of anemia, including sideroblastic changes, can occur concomitantly, especially in the presence of severe malnutrition.

Chronic heavy drinking can also decrease production of most white blood cells (WBC), decrease granulocyte mobility and adherence, and impair the delayed hypersensitivity response to new antigens (with a possible false-negative tuberculin skin test). While the changes in WBCs themselves are usually temporary, they may contribute to the risk of infections, liver damage, and perhaps to the increased risk of cancers in alcoholics. Alcohol can also cause toxic granulocytosis.

Many alcoholics present with mild thrombocytopenia (rarely associated with hemorrhage) due to a decrease in platelet survival and altered function; hypersplenism may occur as a complication of cirrhosis. Alcohol may decrease platelet aggregation and inhibit

release of thromboxane A_2. These problems usually return toward normal within a week of abstinence.

CARDIOVASCULAR SYSTEM Modest doses of alcohol can have both deleterious and beneficial effects in individuals with normal cardiovascular status who take no medications. Ethanol decreases myocardial contractility and causes peripheral vasodilatation resulting in a mild drop in blood pressure and a compensatory increased heart rate and cardiac output. Exercise-induced increases in cardiac oxygen consumption are higher after alcohol. On the other hand, one to two drinks per day over long periods may decrease the risk of cardiovascular death, perhaps through an increase in high density lipoprotein cholesterol (HDL) or changes in clotting mechanisms.

Although ethanol in low doses causes a mild acute drop in blood pressure, the consumption of three or more drinks per day results in a dose-dependent increase in blood pressure which returns to normal within weeks of abstinence. As a result, heavy drinking is an important contributor to reversible causes of mild to moderate hypertension. Chronic heavy drinking can cause cardiomyopathy with symptoms ranging from unexplained arrhythmias in the presence of left ventricular impairment to heart failure with dilatation of all four heart chambers and hypocontractility of heart muscle. Mural thrombi can form in the left atrium or ventricle, while heart enlargement exceeding 25 percent can cause mitral regurgitation. Finally, there is an association between cerebrovascular accidents and alcoholism, especially within 24 h of heavy drinking. Atrial or ventricular arrhythmias, especially paroxysmal tachycardia, can also occur after a binge in individuals showing no other evidence of heart-disease—a syndrome known as the "holiday heart."

GENITOURINARY SYSTEM CHANGES, SEXUAL FUNCTIONING, AND FETAL DEVELOPMENT Acutely, modest ethanol doses (e.g., blood alcohol concentrations of 100 mg/dL or even less) increase sexual drive in men. However, modest ethanol doses may simultaneously decrease erectile capacity. Even in the absence of liver impairment, a significant minority of chronic alcoholic men may show irreversible testicular atrophy with concomitant shrinkage of the seminiferous tubules and loss of sperm cells (see Chap. 321).

The repeated ingestion of high doses of ethanol by women can result in amenorrhea, a decrease in ovarian size, an absence of corpora lutea with associated infertility, and spontaneous abortions. Heavy drinking during pregnancy results in the rapid placental transfer of both ethanol and acetaldehyde, which may have serious consequences for fetal development. The *fetal alcohol syndrome* can include a mixture of any of the following: facial changes with epicanthal eye folds, poorly formed concha, and small teeth with faulty enamel; cardiac atrial or ventricular septal defects; an aberrant palmar crease and limitation in joint movement; and microcephaly with mental retardation (see Chap. 358). The specific amount of ethanol and/or specific time of vulnerability during pregnancy has not been defined, making it advisable for pregnant women to abstain completely.

OTHER EFFECTS OF ETHANOL Heavy drinking can produce an acute *alcoholic myopathy* characterized by painful and swollen muscles, high levels of serum creatine phosphokinase (CK), and rarely myoglobinemia and myoglobinuria. Effects on the *skeletal system* include alterations in calcium metabolism with an increased risk for fractures and osteonecrosis of the femoral head. *Hormonal* changes include an increase in cortisol levels, which can remain elevated during heavy drinking; inhibition of vasopressin secretion at rising blood alcohol concentrations and the opposite at falling blood alcohol concentrations, with the final result that most alcoholics are likely to be slightly overhydrated; a modest and reversible decrease in serum thyroxine (T_4); and a more marked decrease in serum triiodothyronine (T_3).

ALCOHOLISM

Because many drinkers occasionally imbibe to excess, temporary alcohol-related pathology is common in nonalcoholics. The time of heaviest drinking is usually the late teens to the late twenties when between one-third and one-half of male drinkers experience some isolated (although potentially dangerous) alcohol-related social, occupational, or driving difficulty. These include alcohol-related blackouts, a single drunk driving arrest, arguments with friends, and so on. This prevalent alcohol-related morbidity, however, is temporary and a separate problem from alcoholism. The following sections describe diagnostic criteria for alcoholism, offer suggestions for identifying the usual (i.e., middle-class) alcoholic in everyday medical practice, review evidence that alcoholism is a biologic and genetically influenced disorder, and offer advice on confrontation, detoxification, and rehabilitation of alcoholics.

DEFINITIONS AND EPIDEMIOLOGY   The original version of the Third Diagnostic and Statistical Manual of the American Psychiatric Association (DSM-III) and the more recent revision (DSM-IIIR) divide alcoholism into alcohol abuse and alcohol dependence, but this distinction may not be clinically relevant. *Alcohol abuse* indicates psychological dependence, i.e., the need for alcohol for adequate functioning, along with occasional heavy consumption, and continuation of drinking despite social or occupational problems. *Alcohol dependence* encompasses similar impairment *along with* evidence of increased ethanol tolerance or physical signs on withdrawal from alcohol.

A modified approach to a definition of alcoholism is easier to apply in clinical settings. The diagnosis of *alcoholism* is made when an individual ignores the early warning signs that alcohol is causing problems in marriage and goes on to an alcohol-related marital separation or divorce; *or* when alcohol-related problems on the job actually result in the patient being fired or laid off; *or* when there are two or more arrests related to alcohol; *or* when there is physical evidence that alcohol has harmed health (e.g., cardiomyopathy, cirrhosis, alcoholic hepatitis), including signs of alcoholic withdrawal.

It is important to distinguish between *primary and secondary alcoholism*. For example, serious alcohol-related problems occurring during the course of mania or a preexisting antisocial personality disorder (i.e., secondary alcoholism) might be symptomatic of the primary diagnosis, and the course is likely to be that of the primary disorder, not alcoholism. The information on alcoholism offered in this chapter is relevant for *primary alcoholism*. This diagnosis applies to the majority of alcoholics (70 to 80 percent) who develop major life problems from alcohol *before* they fulfill criteria for any other major psychiatric illness.

Using this or similar criteria, the lifetime risk for primary alcoholism in most western countries is about 10 percent for men and 3 to 5 percent for women. When less stringent criteria are used, the rates are substantially higher. Alcoholism is seen in all races, ethnic groups, and socioeconomic strata and, therefore, the average alcoholic (just as the average person) is a blue-collar or white-collar worker or housewife. The homeless or skid row alcoholic represents only 5 percent or less of alcoholics.

GENETICS OF ALCOHOLISM   There is strong evidence that alcoholism is a multifactorial disorder in which biologic and genetic factors interact. The importance of genetic factors in alcoholism is supported by family, twin, and adoption studies. Close relatives of primary alcoholics have an approximately fourfold increased risk for the disorder but are not significantly more vulnerable for other psychiatric illnesses. The probability that the familial nature of the problem is in part a consequence of genetic factors is supported by twin research, where the risk for the identical twin of an alcoholic is much higher than for the fraternal twin of an alcohol abuser. Finally, adoption studies reveal that the fourfold increased risk for children of alcoholics is true even if they were adopted away at birth and raised without knowledge of the problems of their biologic parents.

The evidence supporting genetic influences in alcoholism has stimulated numerous studies of children of alcoholics. The goal is to identify possible trait markers of a vulnerability toward the disorder before alcoholism appears. For example, some studies suggest that these children become significantly less intoxicated at a given blood alcohol concentration than do controls, even before alcoholism develops. After modest alcohol doses, the sons of alcoholics report less intense subjective feelings of intoxication, show less alcohol-related impairment in cognitive and psychomotor tests, and have less intense changes in prolactin and cortisol secretion than do controls. These data may indicate that men at high future risk for alcoholism may be less able than controls to tell when they are beginning to become intoxicated. Taken as a whole these data underscore the probability that alcoholism is biologically influenced and not related to a lack of "moral fiber." It is not surprising that the average alcoholic may continue to work, has a family, and may be difficult to identify if the physician persists with old stereotypes.

NATURAL HISTORY   For the "average" alcoholic, the age of first drink and first minor problems (e.g., an argument with a friend while drunk or an alcoholic blackout) are similar to those in the general population. However, by the mid to late twenties, most men and women moderate their drinking (perhaps learning from minor problems), whereas difficulties for alcoholics are likely to escalate, with the first major life problem from alcohol appearing in the late twenties to early forties. Once established, the course of alcoholism is likely to be one of exacerbations and remissions; the alcoholic becomes frightened when a problem develops and abstains for a period of days to months before experimenting with controlled drinking; this step almost inevitably results in escalation of drinking and problems. The course is not hopeless because a fifth or more achieve permanent abstinence without formal treatment or aid from self-help groups such as Alcoholics Anonymous (AA). However, should the alcoholic continue to drink, the life span is shortened by an average of 15 years with the leading causes of death, in decreasing order, being heart disease, cancer, accidents, and suicide.

IDENTIFICATION AND CONFRONTATION OF THE ALCOHOLIC   The physician should recognize that any patient may have alcoholism and must therefore pay attention to physical findings and laboratory tests that are likely to be abnormal in the alcoholic. These include a high normal or slightly elevated MCV, γ-glutamyl transferase (GGT) (35 to 40 or more units), serum uric acid [greater than 416 μmol/L (7 mg/dL)], and triglycerides [2.0 mmol/L (180 mg/dL) or more]. Mild and fluctuating levels of hypertension (e.g., 140/95), repeated infections such as pneumonia, and otherwise unexplained cardiac arrhythmias all suggest that the patient might be an alcoholic. Certain specific clinical findings also should raise suspicions, including cancer of the head and neck, esophagus, or cardia of the stomach as well as cirrhosis, unexplained hepatitis, pancreatitis, bilateral parotid gland swelling, and peripheral neuropathy.

Once the likelihood of alcoholism is established, only a few moments are needed to gather the history of alcohol-related life problems. The patient *and spouse* should be asked about patterns of accidents, marital difficulties, problems on the job, and driving-related difficulties, after which the role played by alcohol should be identified. All physicians should be able to take the time needed to gather such information. In addition, a simple 25-item form to be answered by the patient, the Michigan Alcohol Screening Test (MAST), is available to aid in identifying the alcoholic.

After an alcoholic is identified, he or she should be confronted with the diagnosis. The presenting complaint can be used as an entrée to the alcohol problem. For instance, the patient complaining of insomnia or hypertension could be told that these are clinically important symptoms and that laboratory tests and physical findings indicate that alcohol appears to have contributed to the complaints and is increasing the risk for further medical and psychological problems. The physician should share information about the course of alcoholism and explore possible avenues of attacking the problem.

The process of confrontation is rarely accomplished in one session. It is helpful to let patients know that they are responsible for their own actions and that the decision to quit drinking rests with them. For the person who refuses to stop drinking at the first confrontation, a logical step is to "keep the door open," establishing future meetings so that help is available as problems escalate. In the meantime the family may benefit from counseling or referral to self-help group such as Alanon (the Alcoholics Anonymous group for family members) and Alateen (for teenage children of alcoholics).

Those patients who refuse to stop but who want to "cut down" should be reminded that the average alcoholic successfully cuts back scores of times but that sooner or later drinking again escalates. The patient who refuses to stop might be offered a guideline of drinking no more than two drinks [115 mL (4 oz) of wine, 340 mL (12 oz) of beer, or 43 mL (1.5 oz) of 80-proof beverage amounts to one drink)] in any 24-h period, but it is very unlikely that this will be effective for an extended period of time. This is another way of keeping the door open in the hope that the patient will return as drinking escalates.

TREATMENT OF THE ALCOHOL-RELATED WITHDRAWAL SYNDROME The clinical syndrome In the presence of ethanol-induced cellular tolerance, any sudden decrease in ethanol may lead to symptoms of withdrawal from the CNS-depressant effects. As with most syndromes, most patients do not develop every symptom and the usual clinical picture is mild. Features include a tremor of the hands (shakes or jitters); autonomic nervous sytem dysfunction such as increases in pulse, respiratory rate, and body temperature; insomnia, possibly accompanied by bad dreams; feelings of generalized anxiety or panic attacks; and gastrointestinal upset. Symptoms begin within 5 to 10 h of decreasing ethanol intake (addicted patients are likely to awaken in the morning with some signs of withdrawal), peak in intensity on day 2 or 3, and improve by day 4 or 5. Anxiety, insomnia, and mild levels of autonomic dysfunction may persist for 6 months or more, as a protracted abstinence syndrome that may contribute to the tendency to return to drinking.

About 5 percent of alcoholics show evidence of severe withdrawal symptoms. These include a state of confusion sometimes accompanied by visual, tactile, or auditory hallucinations. These psychotic symptoms are likely to disappear as the mental state becomes clearer over a period of several days and are distinct from the chronic alcoholic auditory hallucinosis with a clear sensorium described earlier in this chapter. A small percentage of alcoholics also demonstrate one or two generalized seizures ("rum fits"), usually within 48 h of stopping drinking. These are rarely focal in nature (unless there is underlying neuropathology) and electroencephalographic abnormalities are mild and usually return to normal within several days. There is no evidence that withdrawal seizures represent "latent" epilepsy.

The diagnosis of delirium tremens (DTs) is made when the course progresses beyond the usual symptoms of withdrawal to include confusion (with associated delusions and hallucinations), severe agitation, and generalized seizures. The likelihood of developing severe withdrawal symptoms increases with concomitant infections or medical problems, a prior history of withdrawal seizures or DTs, and higher quantity and frequency of drinking. Most periods of severe withdrawal begin and end abruptly, rarely lasting longer than 3 to 5 days. The mortality risk for DTs is quite low but increases with preexisting medical illnesses or organ system failure.

Treatment of withdrawal The *first* and most important step is to perform a *thorough* physical examination in all alcoholics who are considering stopping drinking and in those patients who might be undergoing withdrawal. It is necessary to evaluate organ systems likely to be impaired by heavy drinking, including searching for evidence of liver failure, gastrointestinal bleeding, cardiac arrhythmia, and glucose or electrolyte imbalance.

The *second* step in treating withdrawal is to give patients adequate nutrition and rest. All patients should be administered multiple B vitamins, including 50 to 100 mg of thiamine daily for a week or more. Most patients enter withdrawal with normal levels of body water or mild levels of overhydration, and intravenous fluids should be avoided unless there is evidence of hypotension or a history of recent excessive bleeding, vomiting, or diarrhea. Usually medications can be administered orally.

The *third* step in treatment is to recognize the CNS symptoms caused by removal of the brain-depressant effects of ethanol. Symptoms can be alleviated by administering another CNS depressant and gradually decreasing the levels of the drug over a 3- to 5-day period. While many CNS depressants are effective, the *benzodiazepines* have the highest margin of safety and are, therefore, the preferred class of drugs in the treatment of alcohol withdrawal. Benzodiazepines with short half-lives (see Chap. 369) are especially useful for patients with serious liver impairment or evidence of preexisting encephalopathy or brain damage. On the other hand, short half-life benzodiazepines, e.g., oxazepam or lorazepam, result in rapidly changing drug blood levels; administration every 4 h is required to avoid abrupt fluctuations in blood levels that may increase the risk for seizures. Therefore, most clinicians use drugs with longer half-lives, like diazepam or chlordiazepoxide. The goal is to administer sufficient drug on day 1 to alleviate most of the symptoms of withdrawal and then to decrease the dose by 20 percent on successive days over a period of 3 to 5 days. The dose is increased if signs of withdrawal escalate, and the medication is withheld if the patient is sleeping or shows signs of increasing orthostatic hypotension. The average patient requires 25 to 50 mg of chlordiazepoxide or 10 mg of diazepam given orally every 4 to 6 h on the first day.

The most effective treatment of *severe withdrawal* including delirium tremens remains controversial. Most clinicians use benzodiazepines, but despite as much as 300 mg or more per day of chlordiazepoxide the patient may still remain awake and agitated. Since it is probable that the confused, agitated state will persist for 3 to 5 days regardless of the pharmacologic intervention used, drugs are given to control behavior rather than to change the course of the syndrome. Antipsychotic medications like thioridazine or haloperidol have no place in the treatment of mild withdrawal symptoms.

The generalized seizures or "rum fits" rarely require aggressive pharmacologic intervention beyond that given to the usual patient undergoing withdrawal, i.e., adequate doses of benzodiazepines. There is little evidence that phenytoin is effective in drug withdrawal seizures, and the risk of seizures usually has passed by the time effective drug levels are reached. The rare patient with status epilepticus can be treated initially with intravenous diazepam. If anticonvulsants are used for alcohol withdrawal seizures, they should be stopped within 5 to 7 days unless a cause for a persisting seizure disorder is documented.

While alcohol withdrawal is often treated in a hospital, efforts at reducing costs have resulted in experimentation with outpatient detoxification for alcoholics with mild abstinence syndromes. This outpatient approach is appropriate for patients in good physical condition who demonstrate mild signs of withdrawal despite low blood alcohol concentrations and for those without prior history of DTs or withdrawal seizures. Such individuals still require careful physical examination, evaluation of blood tests, and treatment with vitamin supplementation, and appropriate doses of benzodiazepines might also be used. The latter are given *in a 1- to 2-day supply* to be administered to the patient by a spouse four times a day. Patients are asked to *return daily* for evaluation of vital signs, and the patient's family or friends are told to bring him or her to the emergency room if signs and symptoms of withdrawal escalate.

THE TREATMENT OR REHABILITATION OF ALCOHOLICS After completing alcoholic rehabilitation, 60 percent or more of middle-class alcoholics maintain abstinence for at least a year, many for a lifetime. There is no single best way to rehabilitate the alcoholic, and therapeutic approaches center on general supports which meet commonsense guidelines. Considering the lack of evidence for superiority of any specific treatment type, it is best to keep interventions as simple, safe, and inexpensive as possible.

Maneuvers in rehabilitation fall into two general categories. *First* are attempts to help the alcoholic achieve and maintain a high level of motivation toward abstinence. This includes educating the patient about alcoholism, and teaching the family and/or friends to stop protecting the alcoholic from the problems caused by alcohol. The *second* series of maneuvers help the patient to readjust to life without alcohol and to reestablish a functional life-style through personal counseling, vocational rehabilitation, family support, and sexual counseling.

There is no convincing evidence that inpatient rehabilitation is more effective for the average primary alcoholic than is outpatient care. The decision to hospitalize can be made if (1) the patient has medical problems that are difficult to treat outside a hospital; (2) depression, confusion, or psychosis interfere with outpatient care; (3) the patient has such a severe life crisis that it is difficult to get his or her attention as an outpatient; (4) outpatient treatment has failed; or (5) the patient lives too far from the treatment center. If inpatient care is needed, free-standing treatment programs, units that are divisions of general hospitals, and those in psychiatric hospitals are equally effective. The characteristics of the patient predict outcome more than any specific attribute of the program.

Whether the treatment begins in an inpatient or an outpatient setting, subsequent contact should be maintained for a minimum of 6 months after abstinence is achieved. Counseling with an individual physician or through groups focuses on day-to-day living—emphasizing areas of improved functioning in the absence of alcohol (i.e., why it is a good idea to continue to abstain) and helping the patient to deal with free time without alcohol, develop a nondrinking peer group, and handle stresses on the job without alcohol.

The physician serves an important role in identifying the alcoholic, treating medical or psychiatric syndromes associated with alcoholism, carrying out detoxification, referring to rehabilitation programs, and counseling alcoholics in an inpatient or outpatient setting. The physician must also regulate drug treatment during alcoholism rehabilitation. Once acute detoxification is complete (an average of 3 to 5 days), there is *no place* for hypnotics or antianxiety drugs in the treatment of most alcoholics. The patient has already demonstrated an inability to moderate the use of one brain depressant, alcohol, and is at considerable risk for abusing sleeping pills or tranquilizers. Anxiety and insomnia can be treated with behavior modification such as relaxation training, meditation, and exercise or through increased activity in hobbies or religion.

One medication which has been used in alcohol rehabilitation is disulfiram, usually given as 250 mg/d. This drug inhibits aldehyde dehydrogenase, causing very high levels of acetaldehyde to accumulate after alcohol is consumed. The disulfiram-ethanol reaction includes tremor, hypertension or hypotension, nausea and possibly severe vomiting, and diarrhea. Disulfiram must not be given to persons for whom such a reaction could be dangerous, including patients with portal hypertension, diabetes mellitus, heart disease, or a history of stroke. All drugs have their dangers, and the physician is advised to read carefully about disulfiram and be fully aware of the potential, although rare, serious adverse reactions that can occur. Unfortunately, there is little convincing evidence from carefully controlled studies that the effectiveness of disulfiram is significantly greater than placebo. As result, this drug should not be routinely prescribed.

Finally, an inexpensive, readily available, and dedicated additional support for all alcoholics is available in almost every community. Alcoholics Anonymous is a self-help group of recovering alcoholics (men and women who have stopped drinking, perhaps many years ago) which offers an effective model showing that abstinence can be achieved, provides a sober peer group, and makes crisis intervention available when the drive to drink escalates. No matter what type of rehabilitation program is planned, the alcoholic should be offered the option of joining Alcoholics Anonymous.

REFERENCES

BAUMGARTNER GR et al: Clonidine vs. chlordiazepoxide in the acute alcohol withdrawal syndrome. Arch Intern Med 147:1223, 1987

BLUM K et al: Allelic association of human dopamine D_2 receptor gene in alcoholism. JAMA 263:2055, 1990

CRIQUI MH: Alcohol consumption, blood pressure, lipids, and cardiovascular mortality. Alc: Clin Exp Res 10:564, 1986

DONAHUE RP et al: Alcohol and hemorrhagic stroke. JAMA 255:2311, 1986

FRANK D, RAICHT RF: Alcohol-induced liver disease. Alc: Clin Exp Res 9:66, 1985

FULLER RK et al: Disulfiram treatment of alcoholism. JAMA 256:1449, 1986

GOLDSTEIN DB: *Pharmacology of Alcohol*. New York, Oxford University Press, 1983

GOODWIN DW, GUZE SB: *Psychiatric Diagnosis*, 4th ed. New York, Oxford University Press, 1989

GRANT I: Alcohol and the brain. JCCP 55:310, 1987

GREENSPON AJ, SCHAAL SF: The "holiday heart": Electrophysiologic studies of alcohol effects in alcoholics. Ann Intern Med 98:135, 1983

HARPER C et al: Are we drinking our neurones away? Br Med H 294:534, 1987

IRWIN M et al: Monitoring heavy drinking. Am J Psychiatry 145:595, 1988

LIEBER C: *Metabolic Aspects of Alcoholism*. Lancaster, England, MTP Press, 1977

———: To drink (moderately) or not to drink? N Engl J Med 310:846, 1984

LISHMAN WA: Cerebral disorder in alcoholism: Syndromes of impairment. Brain 104:1, 1981

LISKOW BI, GOODWIN DW: Pharmacological treatment of alcohol intoxication, withdrawal and dependence. J Stud Alc 48:356, 1987

MEAGHER RC et al: Suppression of hematopoietic-progenitor-cell proliferation by ethanol and acetaldehyde. N Engl J Med 307:845, 1982

MELLO NK, BREE MP: Alcohol self-administration disrupts reproductive function in female macaque monkeys. Science 221:677, 1983

MENDELSON JH, MELLO NK: Biologic concomitants of alcoholism. N Engl J Med 301:912, 1979

MUKHERJEE AB et al: Transketolase abnormality in fibroblasts from chronic alcoholics. J Clin Invest 79:1039, 1987

PFEFFERBAUM A et al: Brain CT changes in alcoholics. Alc: Clin Exp Res 12:81, 1988

POTTER JF, BEEVERS DG: Pressor effect of alcohol in hypertension. Lancet: 1:119, 1984

SCHUCKIT MA et al: A simultaneous evaluation of multiple markers of ethanol response in sons of alcoholics. Arch Gen Psychiatr 45:211, 1988

———: Genetic and clinical implications of alcoholism and affective disorder. Am J Psychiatry 143:140, 1986

———: *Drug and Alcohol Abuse: A Clinical Guide to Diagnosis and Treatment*, 3d ed. New York, Plenum, 1989

SCHUCKIT MA: *Alcohol Patterns and Problems*. New Brunswick, Rutgers Press, 1985

———: Genetics and the risk for alcoholism. JAMA 254:2614, 1985

SELLERS EM, KALANT H: Alcohol intoxication and withdrawal. N Engl J Med 294:757, 1976

STREISSGUTH AP, LANDESMAN-DWYER S: Teratogenic effects of alcohol in humans and laboratory animals. Science 209:353, 1980

VAILLANT GE: *The Natural History of Alcoholism*. Cambridge, Mass., Harvard, 1983

VAN THIEL DH: Gastrointestinal and hepatic manifestations of chronic alcoholism. Gastroenterology 81:594, 1981

VICTOR M, ADAMS RD: *The Wernicke-Korsakoff Syndrome*, 2d ed. Philadelphia, Davis, 1989

371 OPIOID DRUG USE

MARC A. SCHUCKIT / DAVID S. SEGAL

The principal effects of the opioids (opiate-like drugs) are a significant damping of pain perception along with modest levels of sedation and euphoria. Tolerance to any one opioid is likely to generalize to the others (i.e., cross-tolerance is likely), and all share a similar pattern of drug-related problems. Each of these substances is capable of producing physical addiction (and thus they all have some legal restrictions), and the abstinence syndrome from any one of the substances can be treated with administration of any of the others.

PHARMACOLOGY The prototypic opiates, morphine and codeine (3-methoxymorphine), are taken directly from the milky juice of the poppy, *Papaver somniferum*. The semisynthetic drugs produced from the morphine or thebane molecules include hydromorphone, codeine, diacetylmorphine (heroin), and oxycodone. The purely synthetic opioids, sharing many of the basic properties of opium and morphine, include meperidine, propoxyphene, diphenoxylate, methadone, and pentazocine. Despite claims to the contrary, all of these substances (including almost all prescription analgesics) are capable of producing euphoria as well as psychological and physical dependence when taken in high enough doses over prolonged periods of time.

The opioids produce their effects by binding to different types of opioid receptors throughout the body including the central nervous system. Endogenous opioid peptides (i.e., enkephalins, endorphins, dynorphin, and others) have been identified that appear to be natural ligands for opioid receptors. These peptides have a distinct distribution in the CNS. Recent evidence suggests that the receptors with which opioid peptides interact may be differentially engaged in production of the various opiate effects such as analgesia, respiratory depression, constipation, and euphoria. Substances capable of antagonizing one or more of these actions include nalorphine, levallophan, cyclazocine, and pentazocine, each of which has mixed agonist and antagonist properties, as well as naloxone and naltrexone, which are pure opiate antagonists. Mixed agonist-antagonist drugs (for example, pentazocine), if administered to a patient addicted to other narcotics, may precipitate opiate withdrawal symptoms. The availability of relatively specific antagonists has helped identify different receptor subtypes including the μ_1 subtype of the classic morphine receptor μ.

Opiate tolerance, dependence, and withdrawal are considered to be related phenomena with common underlying mechanisms. A number of neurochemical systems and psychological processes appear to be implicated in these effects that emerge with chronic administration of morphine or related opiates. Perhaps reflecting the actions of different classes of receptors, tolerance to various opiate actions may develop at different rates, and these same mechanisms might contribute to the diverse signs and symptoms characteristic of withdrawal. Other biochemical systems that might contribute to the development of tolerance and dependence include changes in intracellular modulators such as adenyl nucleotides, calcium and related substances, as well as alterations in neurotransmitters, including acetylcholine, serotonin, and the catecholamines norepinephrine and dopamine. Evidence also implicates environmental and learning factors. For example, clinical observations suggest that classic conditioning plays a role in maintaining dependence in at least some addicts and that conditioning extinction procedures may be useful when integrated into a comprehensive treatment program for opioid addiction. Further research into these phenomena and efforts to elucidate neurochemical mechanisms could significantly facilitate the development of more effective approaches to treatment and prevention.

All of the opioid drugs are easily absorbed from the gastrointestinal system, the lungs, and the muscles. The most rapid and pronounced effects occur following intravenous administration, and the least intense actions are seen after absorption from the digestive tract, at least in part because some of the oral drug is metabolized before it passes into the general circulation. Most of the metabolism of opiates occurs in the liver, primarily through conjugation with glucuronic acid, and only small amounts are excreted directly in the urine or feces. The plasma half-lives of these drugs range from 2.5 to 3 h for morphine to more than 22 h for methadone and even longer for methadyl acetate.

Street heroin typically contains only 5 to 10 percent of the opiate. The remainder consists of materials such as lactose and fruit sugars, quinine, powdered milk, phenacetin, caffeine, antipyrine, and strychnine which are used to "cut" the drug and increase the margin of profit.

THE ACUTE AND CHRONIC EFFECTS OF OPIOID DRUGS ON BODY SYSTEMS   With the exception of overdose conditions and changes associated with physical addiction, most opiate actions are relatively benign and rapidly reversible.

Effects on body systems   Acute changes in the *gastrointestinal system* are the result of decreased GI motility with resulting constipation and anorexia. Chronic GI problems in opiate addicts typically occur as a consequence of impaired liver function resulting from concomitant administration of other drugs and from the development of hepatitis B from shared "dirty" needles.

The direct effects on opiate receptors in the *central nervous system* can result in nausea and vomiting (medulla), decreased pain perception (spinal cord, thalamus, and periaqueductal grey region), euphoria (limbic system), and sedation (reticular activating system and striatum). The adulterants added to street drugs may contribute to some of the more permanent nervous system damage, including peripheral neuropathy, amblyopia, myelopathy, and leukoencephalopathy, while use of contaminated needles can produce abscesses in the CNS and transmit AIDS. Acute opiate administration results in decreases in luteinizing hormone (LH), with a subsequent decrease in testosterone which might contribute to the decreased sex drive reported by most opiate addicts. Other hormonal changes include a decrease in the release of thyrotropin as well as increases in prolactin and possibly in growth hormone (see Chap. 313).

Acute changes in the *respiratory system* include respiratory depression, which results from a decreased response of the brainstem to carbon dioxide tension, a component of the drug overdose syndrome described below. At even low drug doses, this effect can be clinically significant in individuals with compromised lung activity. *Cardiovascular* changes tend to be relatively mild with no direct opiate effect on heart rhythm or myocardial contractility, but there is a potential problem from orthostatic hypotension, probably secondary to dilatation of peripheral vessels. Bacterial infections of both the lungs and heart valves can occur from contaminated needles.

The toxic reaction or overdose syndrome   High doses of opiates taken intentionally (in a suicide attempt) or by the street user who has misjudged the potency of the injected substance can result in a toxic reaction or overdose syndrome with a potentially lethal consequence. The typical syndrome, which occurs immediately with intravenous (IV) overdose, includes shallow respirations of two to four per minute, pupillary miosis (with mydriasis once brain anoxia develops), bradycardia, a decrease in body temperature, and a general absence of responsiveness to external stimulation. If this medical emergency is not treated rapidly, symptoms can progress to cyanosis, and death can ensue from respiratory depression and cardiorespiratory arrest. Postmortem examination reveals few specific changes except for diffuse cerebral edema. An "allergic-like" reaction to adulterants can also occur and is characterized by decreased alertness, a frothy pulmonary edema, and an elevation in the blood eosinophil count.

The preferred treatment for the typical opiate overdose is the narcotic antagonist naloxone, given in an initial dose of 0.4 mg (1 mL) or 0.01 mg/kg intramuscularly (IM) or IV, which can be repeated in 3 to 10 min if no response occurs. Because the effects of this drug diminish within 2 to 3 h, it is important to monitor the individual for at least 24 h after a heroin overdose and 72 h after an overdose of longer-acting drugs such as methadone. Patients who are also physically addicted to an opioid are likely to experience a precipitous onset of an abstinence syndrome within 2 to 8 h after administration of the opioid antagonist, but aggressive treatment of this syndrome is not appropriate until all vital signs are relatively stable.

As with any drug overdose, treatment of either the typical or the "allergic" type of opiate toxic reaction often requires support of vital signs until the body detoxifies the substance. Patients may require a respirator (especially one using oxygen and positive pressure breathing for the "allergic" type of overdose), IV fluids perhaps accompanied by pressor agents to support blood pressure, and gastric lavage to remove any remaining drug, with care taken to use a cuffed endotracheal tube to prevent aspiration if the patient is not alert. Cardiac arrhythmias and/or convulsions, especially likely to be seen with codeine, propoxyphene, or meperidine, also need to be treated.

THE OPIATE ABUSER   The medical abuser   Two groups of individuals are at high risk for abusing analgesics. First, evidence suggests that a majority of people with *chronic pain syndromes* (e.g., back, joint, and muscle disorders) may misuse their prescribed drugs at various times. If physical dependence is established, abstinence syndromes can then intensify the pain, promoting continued drug intake. A few precautions can help the physician to avoid contributing to physical dependence in chronic pain patients, particularly those who have demonstrated a propensity to misuse opioids: (1) the goal is to minimize the debilitating effects of pain with the understanding that discomfort may not be completely eliminated (Chap. 15); (2) all possible efforts must be taken to reinforce the need for the patient to become actively involved in and committed to improvement; (3) analgesic medication should be only one component of treatment and limited to oral administration of the least potent analgesic required to take the "edge off" the pain (e.g., propoxyphene); all such drugs should be coordinated through one physician; (4) behavior modification techniques can include muscle relaxation and meditation, while carefully selected exercises can help increase function and decrease pain; (5) nonmedicinal approaches including electrical transcutaneous neurostimulation for muscle and joint disease can be applied (see also Chap. 15).

The second group at high risk are *physicians, nurses, and pharmacists,* primarily because of their easy access to substances of abuse. Physicians may begin to use opiates to help them sleep or to reduce stress or physical aches and pains. A family history of substance abuse (including alcoholism) probably helps to identify the physician at exceptionally high risk. Because of the growing awareness of these problems, impaired physician programs have been established in many hospitals and by most state medical societies. These groups attempt to identify and aid substance-impaired physicians, giving them peer support and education so as to achieve abstinence before problems escalate to the point of licensure revocation. In general, doctors are advised never to prescribe opiates for themselves or for members of their family—physicians deserve the same level of care and protection from future problems as their patients.

The street abuser   Some opiate addicts satisfy criteria for the antisocial personality disorder as evidenced by serious antisocial problems beginning prior to age 15 and before the first major life problem from drugs (see Chap. 368). However, the majority of opiate addicts have a relatively high level of premorbid functioning. The usual street abuser begins using opiates occasionally, often after experimenting with tobacco, then alcohol, then marijuana, and then brain depressants or stimulants. Occasional opiate use, or "chipping," might continue for some time, and some individuals probably never escalate their intake to the point of developing serious problems. Another pattern of temporary or intermittent abuse is represented by the experiences of Vietnam soldiers, most of whom had little or no prior experience with opiates and who found themselves in a situation of high stress and readily available drugs. Under these circumstances, as many as one-half tried opiates and, although many became physically addicted, those who had not misused drugs before Vietnam tended to return to drug-free status when back in their home communities.

Once persistent opiate use is established, the outcome is often extremely serious. At least 25 percent of such opiate abusers are likely to die within 10 to 20 years of active abuse, with death from suicide, homicide, accidents, and infectious diseases such as tuberculosis or serum hepatitis. The mortality rate has escalated in recent years in response to the epidemic of AIDS among IV drug abusers (see Chap. 264). As many as 50 percent of male and 25 percent of female addicts turn to alcohol when their primary drug is not available, and many of these people meet the criteria for secondary alcohol abuse. The prevalence of alcohol misuse is higher in drug treatment dropouts than in those who stay with therapy, and abuse is more likely in individuals with a history of alcohol problems before they developed opiate-related difficulties.

PHYSICAL ADDICTION AND THE OPIATE ABSTINENCE SYN-DROME   The symptoms of withdrawal   The time to onset as well as the intensity and duration of the acute abstinence syndrome are influenced by a number of factors including the drug's half-life, its dose, and the chronicity of administration. The withdrawal symptoms tend to be opposite to the acute effects of the drug and include nausea and diarrhea, coughing, lacrimation, rhinorrhea, profuse sweating, twitching muscles, and piloerection or "goose bumps"; mild elevations in body temperature, respiratory rate, and blood pressure are also observed. In addition, sensations of diffuse body pain, insomnia, and yawning occur with intense drug craving. Drugs with a short half-life, such as morphine or heroin, cause symptoms typically within 8 to 16 h of the last dose (thus, many addicts awake in mild withdrawal every morning); peak effects are apparent within 36 to 72 h after discontinuation of the drug, and the acute syndrome disappears within 5 to 8 days. However, a protracted abstinence phase of mild symptoms (e.g., slight changes in pupillary size, autonomic dysfunction, changes in sleep pattern) may persist for 6 or more months.

Treatment of the withdrawal syndrome   Patients *must* receive a thorough physical examination which includes an assessment of liver and neurologic function as well as identification of local and systemic infections, especially abscesses. Proper nutrition and rest must be initiated as soon as possible.

Effective treatment of withdrawal, however, also requires readministration of sufficient opiate medication on day one to decrease symptoms, followed by a more gradual withdrawal of the drug, usually over 5 to 10 days. Any opiate will work (they all have some level of cross-tolerance) but for ease of administration many physicians prefer to use a long-acting drug like methadone. In estimating the first day's dose from the patient's history, 1 mg of methadone is approximately equivalent to 3 mg of morphine, 1 mg of heroin, or 20 mg of meperidine. Most patients require between 10 and 25 mg of methadone orally given twice on day one, with higher doses given if prominent symptoms of withdrawal are not damped. After several days of a stabilized drug dose, the opiate is then decreased by 10 to 20 percent of the original day's dose each day.

Most states have restrictions on the prescription of opiates to addicts, and in the absence of special permits, detoxification with opiates is usually limited to 1 month or less. One relatively successful nonopiate approach to the treatment of withdrawal is the use of the alpha$_2$-adrenergic agonist clonidine, used in part to decrease sympathetic nervous system overactivity. Given at doses of approximately 5 µg/kg (up to 0.3 mg given two to four times a day), clonidine causes most patients undergoing opiate withdrawal to experience a decrease in autonomic nervous system dysfunction. Opiates, however, are more effective in relieving discomfort and pain, and clonidine is often not well tolerated because it produces high levels of sedation and orthostatic hypotension. Therefore, under most circumstances opiates are the treatment of choice.

A special case of opiate withdrawal is seen in the newborn, passively addicted by the mother's drug misuse during pregnancy. Some level of addiction develops in 50 to 90 percent of children of heroin-dependent mothers, and the withdrawal syndrome carries a mortality of between 3 and 30 percent if not treated when prominent signs are apparent. In distinction to street addicts, as few as 25 percent of infants of methadone-maintenance-addicted mothers show clinically relevant withdrawal symptoms. The syndrome consists of irritability, crying, a tremor (in 80 percent), increased reflexes, increased respiratory rate, diarrhea, hyperactivity (in 60 percent), vomiting (40 percent), and sneezing/yawning/hiccuping (in 30 percent). The child usually has a low birth weight but may be otherwise unremarkable until the second day, when symptoms are likely to begin.

The treatment follows the same general steps used in the treatment of the physically addicted adult. The child must be carefully evaluated to rule out medical problems such as hypoglycemia, hypocalcemia, infections, and trauma; general supports in a warm, quiet environment and regulation of electrolytes and glucose are also required. The infant with moderate to severe symptoms can be treated with any of the following: paregoric (0.2 mL orally every 3 to 4 h); methadone, (0.1 to 0.5 mg/k per day); phenobarbital (8 mg/kg per day); or diazepam (1 to 2 mg/kg every 8 h). Medication should be given in decreasing levels for 10 to 20 days. It is also possible to treat the addicted infants of mothers on methadone maintenance by having them breast feed while the mothers continue to take methadone.

REHABILITATION OF OPIATE ADDICTS   Despite some differences in demographics, the same general rules for rehabilitation apply to the opiate abuser and to the alcoholic. The basic strategy includes beginning detoxification and general family support. It is also important to establish realistic patient goals and a program of counseling and education to increase motivation toward abstinence. A long-term commitment to rebuilding a life-style without the substance is essential for preventing recidivism.

Identifying and confronting the patient   The first step in treatment requires identification of the opiate abuser—an especially difficult problem with the middle-class street abuser and the medical patient or physician with an iatrogenic addiction. An important step is to gather a clinical history which includes the patterns of opiate usage, information regarding the possible existence of an antisocial personality disorder, or a history of chronic pain. Blood and urine screens can be used to identify opiates in patients in whom misuse is suspected, and clinicians should search for physical stigmata of misuse (e.g., needle marks). One potentially important diagnostic procedure (which should be used carefully because it can precipitate an intense withdrawal) is the opiate antagonist challenge. A 0.4-mg dose of naloxone is given subcutaneously or slowly IV over a 5-min period, and the patient is observed for signs of withdrawal over the next several hours. This challenge test should only be carried out in the presence of a physician and it is important to be prepared to begin treating withdrawal if needed.

After identifying the opiate addict, the next step is confrontation. The need for active treatment of the abstinence syndrome can be presented, and the availability of help in establishing a drug-free life-style can be emphasized. The final decision, of course, rests with the patient.

Rehabilitation Most rehabilitation approaches have common elements. Patients are educated about their responsibility for improving their lives and *motivation for abstinence* is increased by providing information about the medical and psychological problems that can be expected if addiction continues. Patients and families are helped to *establish an opiate-free life-style* by being educated about dealing with chronic pain and developing realistic vocational planning (e.g., this applies to pharmacists, physicians, and nurses). The addict should also be encouraged to establish a drug-free peer group and to participate in self-help groups such as Narcotics Anonymous. Much of this advice and counseling can be given by the physician, but many clinicians refer patients to more formal drug programs, including methadone maintenance clinics, programs using narcotic antagonists, and therapeutic communities. Long-term follow-up of treated patients shows that approximately one-third of addicts are completely drug free in the year before the follow-up interview, and that a total of 60 percent are off opiates, although some may be abusing other substances. Individuals who stay in methadone maintenance or in therapeutic communities show significant decreases in police and social problems and increases in job functioning. In general, the best prognosis for rehabilitation is for those who are employed, who have higher levels of school completion, and who remain in treatment for at least 2 months.

METHADONE MAINTENANCE Methadone and methadyl acetate maintenance should only be used along with education and counseling. It is important to note that drug maintenance is not aimed at "curing" opiate addiction; rather it provides a substitute drug that is legally accessible. The goal is to help the addict who has failed in drug-free programs to improve functioning within the family and job, to decrease legal problems, and to improve health.

Methadone is a long-acting opiate that possesses almost all the physiologic properties of heroin. The addict who has been carefully screened to rule out prior psychiatric disorders may be maintained on a relatively low dose (e.g., 30 to 40 mg/d); a higher dosage schedule (100 to 120 mg/d) can also be used and may be more effective in blocking heroin-induced euphoria. Although the results are not definite, there is some evidence that the higher methadone doses may result in greater retention in treatment and consequently lower levels of arrest and readdiction to street drugs. Methadone is administered in an oral liquid given once a day at the program center, with weekend portions taken by the patient at home. The longer acting analogues, such as methadyl acetate, can be given in lower doses (e.g., 20 to 30 mg) two or three times a week, with levels increased to as high as 80 mg three times a week if needed.

After a period of maintenance (usually 6 months to 1 year or longer), the clinician should work closely with the patient to regulate the rate of drug decrease (by about 5 percent per week). The British have used heroin maintenance with similar goals and following similar guidelines as those used for methadone. There is no evidence that heroin maintenance has any advantages over methadone maintenance, but the heroin approach does add the risk that the drug will be sold on the streets.

OPIATE ANTAGONISTS The opiate antagonists (e.g., naloxone) compete with heroin and other opiates for opioid receptors, reducing the effects of the opiate agonists. Administered over long periods of time in order to block the "high" produced if the patient takes opiates, these drugs can be useful as part of an overall treatment approach that includes counseling and support. Cyclazocine was the first antagonist tested, but its blockade of receptors is incomplete and the level of side effects (including a drunken feeling) are unacceptable. Naloxone is an excellent narcotic antagonist with no agonistic properties, but it has such a short period of action (2 to 3 h) that it is of little use in rehabilitation. The most widely used antagonist in rehabilitation is naltrexone, which is effective for about 24 h with few side effects. A dose of 50 mg of naltrexone per day will block 15 mg of heroin for 24 h, and higher doses (125 to 150 mg) are capable of blocking the effects of 25 mg of IV heroin for up to 3 days. Naltrexone is free of agonist properties, there are no known withdrawal symptoms when the medication is stopped, and side effects tend to be mild. Patients started on this antagonist should be free of opiates for a minimum of 5 days. In addition they must be given a thorough physical examination and should be challenged with 0.4 or 0.8 mg of the shorter-acting naloxone to be certain that they are able to tolerate the long-acting antagonist. Following this procedure, a test dose of 10 mg of naltrexone can be given, with the expectation that any withdrawal symptoms will be seen in $\frac{1}{2}$ to 2 h. Over the next 10 days, the daily dose should be increased to about 100 mg on Mondays and Wednesdays and 150 mg on Fridays. Unfortunately, despite the apparent advantages of this treatment approach, patients demonstrate great resistance to continuing care. In one study, only about 60 percent of the patients completed 6 days of naltrexone induction, and only 10 percent remained in the program at the end of 6 months.

DRUG-FREE PROGRAMS Most existing half-way houses and recovery centers for the opiate abuser utilize the therapeutic community approach. This is an exception to the general preference for short-term inpatient rehabilitation, as care lasts up to a year while the addict is taken out of the street culture and given a new life within the group. In this structure members, including addict leaders, frequently confront participants in an attempt to help them gain insights into more successful life-styles for coping with problems.

REFERENCES

CROWLEY T et al: Naltrexone-induced dysphoria in former opioid addicts. Am J Psychiatry 142:1081, 1985

FINNEGAN L: Neonatal abstinence syndrome, in *Neonatal Therapy*, F Rubatelli (ed). New York, Elsevier, 1986, pp 122–146

FRIEDLAND GH et al: Transmission of the human immunodeficiency virus. N Engl J Med 317:1125, 1987

GREENSTEIN RA et al: Naltrexone: A short-term treatment of opiate dependence. Am J Drug Alcohol Abuse 8:291, 1981

JAFFE JH, MARTIN WR: Opiate analgesics and antagonists, in *Goodman and Gilman's The Pharmacological Basis of Therapeutics*, 7th ed, AG Gilman et al (eds). New York, Macmillan, 1985, pp 491–531

JASINSKI D et al: Clonidine in morphine withdrawal. Arch Gen Psychiat 42:1063, 1985

KLEBER HK, RIORDAN CE: The treatment of narcotic withdrawal: A historical review. J Clin Psychiatry 43:30 1982

McAULIFFE WE et al: Psychoactive drug use among physicians and medical students. N Engl J Med 315:805, 1986

McCUE JD: The effects of stress on physicians and their medical practice. N Engl J Med 306:458, 1982

O'BRIEN CP, WOODY GE: Long-term consequences of opiate dependence. N Engl J Med 304:1098, 1981

—— et al: Classical conditioning is opiate dependence, in *Problems of Drug Dependence*, LS Harris (ed). NIDA Research, Monograph 49, pp 35–46. Washington, DC, US Government Printing Office, 1984

OLIVERIO A et al: Psychobiology of opioids. Int Rev Neurobiol 25:277, 1984

PASTERNAK GW: Multiple morphine and enkephalin receptors and the relief of pain. JAMA 259:1362, 1988

REDMOND DE JR, KRYSTAL JH: Multiple mechanisms of withdrawal from opioid drugs. Annu Rev Neurosci 7:443, 1984

ROUNSAVILLE BJ et al: Identifying alcoholism in treated opiate addicts. Am J Psychiatry 140:764, 1983

SCHUCKIT MA: *Drug and Alcohol Abuse: A Clinical Guide to Diagnosis and Treatment,* 3d ed. New York, Plenum, 1989

SIMON E: Recent studies on opioid receptors: Heterogeneity and isolation, in *Problems of Drug Dependence,* LS Harris (ed). NIDA Research Monograph 49, pp 5–13. Washington, DC, US Government Printing Office, 1984

SIMPSON DD et al: Six-year follow-up of opioid addicts after admission to treatment. Arch Gen Psychiat 39:1318, 1982

VAILLANT GE: A 20-year follow-up of New York narcotic addicts. Arch Gen Psychiat 29:237, 1973

WALLOT H, LAMBERT J: Characteristics of physician addicts. Am J Drug Alcohol Abuse 10:53, 1984

372 COMMONLY ABUSED DRUGS

JACK H. MENDELSON / NANCY K. MELLO

The prevalence of drug abuse in the United States remained at epidemic levels during 1988 and is believed to exceed that of other industrial nations. The extent of drug abuse problems in the United States is illustrated by a December 1988 report from the Division of Epidemiology and Statistical Analysis of the National Institute on Drug Abuse (NIDA): "More than one-half of the American youth try an illicit drug before they finish high school. The number of people admitted to emergency rooms following cocaine use, as reported by the Drug Abuse Warning Network (DAWN), increased more than fivefold over the past five 12-month periods. Further, the number of people who died following cocaine use increased almost fourfold during the same time period. Drug abuse in the United States clearly remains a major public health problem; it is pervasive in extent, diverse in its manifestations, and constantly changing." During the 1980s, drug abuse was the third most frequently reported psychiatric disorder by men (ages 18 to 65) and the second most frequently reported psychiatric disorder by women (ages 18 to 24).

The adverse health consequences of drug abuse are further complicated by AIDS, and drug abuse also increases the risk for HIV exposure. In 1988, NIDA estimated that 31 percent of all AIDS victims are intravenous drug abusers. Drug abuse contributes to the AIDS epidemic by the transmission of HIV infection through needle sharing by intravenous drug users and by direct immunosuppressive and immunomodulatory effects of abused drugs.

The initiation and continuation of drug abuse is determined by a complex interaction of the pharmacologic properties and relative availability of each drug, the personality and expectancy of the user, and the environmental context in which the drug is used. Polydrug abuse, the concurrent use of several drugs with different pharmacologic effects, is increasingly common among individuals from all socioeconomic strata. There has been an alarming increase in a particularly dangerous form of polydrug abuse, the combined use of both heroin and cocaine intravenously, called "speedballing." DAWN reports, based upon emergency room data, indicate that combined heroin and cocaine use increased almost threefold from 1984 to 1988. Deaths due to concurrent use of heroin and cocaine increased fivefold from 1984 through 1988. There is no simple explanation for this change in polydrug use patterns. Sometimes drug abusers attempt to attenuate one drug effect with another, e.g., heroin or alcohol is used to modulate the cocaine high. Sometimes one drug is used to enhance the effects of another, as with benzodiazepines and methadone, or cocaine plus heroin in methadone-maintained patients. Toxic drug interactions associated with polydrug abuse also contribute to the adverse health consequences of drug abuse. This chapter discusses cocaine, marijuana, two hallucinogens (PCP and LSD), and polydrug abuse. Elsewhere there are discussions of alcohol abuse (Chap. 370) and opioid abuse (Chap. 371).

COCAINE Cocaine is a stimulant and a local anesthetic with potent vasoconstrictor properties. The leaves of the coca plant (*Erythroxylon coca*) contain approximately 0.5 to 1 percent cocaine. The drug produces physiologic and behavioral effects when administered orally, intranasally, intravenously, or via inhalation following pyrolysis (smoking). It is now recognized that cocaine has potent pharmacologic effects on dopamine, norepinephrine, and serotonin neurons in the central nervous system. These effects involve alteration and blockade of cellular membrane transport and prevention of the reuptake of biogenic amines. It has been postulated that cocaine-induced euphoria is due to cocaine effects on dopaminergic neurons, but that chronic cocaine use may cause depletion and destruction of crucial dopaminergic pathways in the brain.

Prevalence of cocaine use Cocaine has become more widely available throughout the United States since its cost (relative to disposable income) has decreased considerably. Cocaine is no longer considered a "status" drug since cocaine abuse occurs in virtually all social and economic strata of our society. In 1985 the NIDA National Household Survey on Drug Abuse revealed that 22 million men and women had used cocaine on at least one occasion. Six million persons reported using cocaine at least once during the month prior to the survey, and 12 million individuals had used the drug at least once during the year prior to the survey. Cocaine-related health problems have continued to increase according to DAWN. The number of hospital emergency room cases associated with cocaine abuse increased from 7155 in 1984 to 39,657 in the 12-month period ending June 1988. The number of cocaine-related deaths in major metropolitan areas increased fourfold from 1984 to 1988. The overall increase in cocaine abuse in the general population has been paralleled by an increase in cocaine abuse by heroin-dependent persons, including those in methadone maintenance programs. Intravenous cocaine is often used concurrently with intravenous heroin (the speedball), a combination that purportedly attenuates the postcocaine crash and substitutes the cocaine "high" for the former heroin "high" blocked by methadone. Intravenous use of cocaine plus heroin may further increase risk for HIV infection, both through needle sharing and through the combined immunosuppressive effects of both drugs.

Acute and chronic cocaine intoxication Although cocaine is commonly self-administered by inhalation (snorting), there has been a dramatic increase in both intravenous administration and inhalation of pyrolyzed material via smoking. Following intranasal administration, changes in mood and feeling states are perceived within 3 to 5 min, and peak effects occur at 10 to 20 min. Duration of cocaine effects rarely exceed 1 h following intranasal administration. Inhalation of pyrolyzed materials includes smoking coca paste, a product produced by extracting cocaine preparations with flammable solvents, and cocaine free-base smoking. Coca paste is frequently contaminated with toxic solvents used in its preparation. Cocaine free-base, including the free-base prepared with sodium bicarbonate (crack), is becoming increasingly popular because of the relative high potency of the compounds and their rapid onset of action (8 to 10 s following smoking).

Cocaine produces a brief, dose-related stimulation and enhancement of mood; cardiac rate and blood pressure also increase in a dose-related manner. An increase in body temperature usually occurs following cocaine administration, and high doses of cocaine may induce lethal pyrexia or hypertension. Because cocaine inhibits reuptake of catecholamines at adrenergic nerve endings, the drug potentiates sympathetic nervous system activity. Cocaine has a short plasma half-life of approximately 1 h. In humans, cocaine is primarily metabolized by plasma esterases, and cocaine metabolites are excreted in urine. The very short duration of euphorigenic effects of cocaine observed in chronic abusers is probably due to both acute and chronic tolerance. Frequent self-administration of the drug (two to three times per hour) is often reported by chronic cocaine abusers. Alcohol is used to modulate both the cocaine "high" and the dysphoria associated with the abrupt disappearance of cocaine's effects.

The prevalent assumption that cocaine use is relatively safe is challenged by reports of death from respiratory depression, cardiac arrhythmias, and convulsions after cocaine snorting and intravenous administration. Severe pulmonary disease may develop in individuals who smoke coca paste; this is attributed both to the direct effects of cocaine and to residual solvent contaminants in the smoked material. Hepatic necrosis has also been reported to occur in coca paste smokers. Although men and women who abuse cocaine may report that the drug enhances libidinal drive, chronic cocaine use causes significant decrements in libido and adversely affects reproductive function. Impotence and gynecomastia have been observed in male cocaine abusers, and these abnormalities have persisted for long periods following drug abstinence. Women who abuse cocaine have reported major derangements in menstrual cycle function including galactorrhea, amenorrhea, and infertility. Chronic cocaine abuse may cause persistent hyperprolactinemia as a consequence of cocaine-induced disorders of dopaminergic regulation of prolactin secretion by the pituitary. Cocaine abuse may also adversely affect pregnancy. Infants exposed to cocaine in utero have an increased risk for congenital malformations as well as perinatal cardiovascular and cerebrovascular disease.

Numerous clinical reports, dating from the late nineteenth century, strongly suggest that protracted cocaine abuse may cause paranoid ideation and visual and auditory hallucinations, a state which resembles alcoholic hallucinosis. Psychological dependence upon cocaine, as manifested by inability to abstain from frequent compulsive use, has also been reported. Although occurrence of withdrawal syndromes involving psychomotor agitation and autonomic hyperactivity remains controversial, severe depression ("crashing") following cocaine intoxication may be a concomitant of drug withdrawal.

Treatment of cocaine intoxication and abuse Treatment of cocaine overdose is a medical emergency which involves resuscitation in an intensive care unit. Cocaine toxicity produces hypertension, tachycardia, tonic-clonic seizures, dyspnea, and ventricular arrhythmias. Intravenous diazepam in doses up to 0.5 mg/kg administered over an 8-h period has been shown to be effective for control of seizures. The systemic concomitants of a hypermetabolic state produced by cocaine toxicity with concurrent ventricular arrhythmias have been managed successfully by administration of 0.5 to 1.0 mg propranolol intravenously. Since many instances of cocaine-related mortality have also been associated with concomitant use of other illicit drugs (particularly heroin), the physician must be prepared to institute effective emergency treatment for multiple-drug toxicity.

Treatment of chronic cocaine abuse requires combined efforts by family physicians, psychiatrists, and psychosocial care providers. Early abstinence from cocaine use is often complicated by symptoms of depression and guilt, insomnia, and anorexia, which may be as severe as those observed in major affective disorders. Individual and group psychotherapy, family therapy, and peer group assistance programs are often useful for inducing prolonged remission from drug use. Preliminary reports suggest that tricyclic antidepressant medication (desipramine) may be of value in the treatment of cocaine abuse, even when affective disorder or depression are not present. In fact, depressive illness does not appear to be a frequent antecedent of cocaine abuse.

MARIJUANA AND CANNABIS COMPOUNDS Cannabis sativa contains over 400 compounds in addition to the psychoactive substance, delta-9-tetrahydrocannabinol (THC). Marijuana cigarettes are prepared from the leaves and flowering tops of the plant, and a typical marijuana cigarette contains 0.5 to 1 g of plant material. Although the usual THC concentration varies between 5 and 20 mg, concentrations as high as 100 mg per cigarette have been detected. Hashish is prepared from concentrated resin of Cannabis sativa and contains a THC concentration of between 8 to 12 percent by weight. "Hash oil," a lipid-soluble plant extract, may contain a THC concentration of 25 to 60 percent, and it may be added to marijuana or hashish to enhance their THC concentration. Smoking is the most common mode of marijuana or hashish self-administration. During pyrolysis, over 150 compounds in addition to the THC are released in the smoke. Although most of these compounds do not have psychoactive properties, they do have potential physiologic effects.

THC is quickly absorbed from the lungs into blood and is then rapidly sequestered in tissues. It is metabolized primarily in the liver where it is converted to 11-hydroxy-THC, a psychoactive compound, and more than 20 other metabolites. Most THC metabolites are excreted through the feces at a rate of clearance that is relatively slow in comparison to that of most other psychoactive drugs.

Prevalence of marijuana use The National Institute on Drug Abuse 1985 National Household Survey on Drug Abuse revealed that 62 million persons had used marijuana or hashish at least once in their lifetime and that 18 million individuals reported using the drug at least once during the month prior to the survey. One encouraging datum was a decrease in marijuana use by young persons aged 12 to 17, but 27 percent of persons in this age group reported marijuana use. The DAWN records of marijuana or hashish in emergency room settings increased from 3490 during 1984 to 7934 in 1988. However, the NIDA cautions that "interpreting the trend of marijuana emergencies is problematic since marijuana is often used in conjunction with other substances such as PCP, alcohol, or heroin. In fact, in 1987, 83 percent of all marijuana emergency room mentions were in combination with another substance." Thus, there is a continuing trend for polydrug abuse among young marijuana users, and there are major health hazards associated with this behavior.

Acute and chronic marijuana intoxication Acute intoxication from marijuana and cannabis compounds is related to both THC dose and route of administration. THC is absorbed more rapidly from marijuana smoking than from orally ingesting cannabis compounds. The most frequent form of acute intoxication consists of a subjective perception of relaxation and mild euphoria resembling mild to moderate alcohol intoxication. This condition is usually accompanied by some impairment in thinking, concentration, and perceptual and psychomotor functions. Higher doses of cannabis may produce behavioral effects analogous to severe alcohol intoxication. Although the effects of acute marijuana intoxication are relatively benign in normal users, the drug can precipitate severe emotional disorders in individuals who have antecedent psychotic or neurotic problems. As with other psychoactive compounds, both set (user's expectancy) and setting (environmental context) are important determinants of the type and severity of behavioral intoxication.

As is true of alcoholics, chronic marijuana abusers may lose interest in common socially desirable goals and devote progressively more time to drug acquisition and use. However, it should be emphasized that THC does not cause a specific and unique "amotivational syndrome." The range of symptoms sometimes attributed to marijuana use are difficult to distinguish from mild depression and the maturational dysfunctions often associated with protracted adolescence. Chronic use of marijuana has also been reported to increase the probability of exacerbation of psychotic symptoms in individuals with a past history of schizophrenia.

Physical effects of marijuana Conjunctival injection and tachycardia are the most frequent immediate physical concomitants of smoking marijuana. Tolerance for marijuana-induced tachycardia develops rapidly among regular users; angina may be precipitated by marijuana smoking in persons with a history of coronary insufficiency. Exercise-induced angina may be increased after marijuana use to a greater extent than after tobacco cigarette smoking. Patients with cardiac disease should be strongly advised not to smoke marijuana or use cannabis compounds.

Significant decrements in pulmonary vital capacity have been found in regular daily marijuana smokers. Because marijuana smoking typically involves deep inhalation and prolonged retention of marijuana smoke, marijuana smokers may develop pulmonary disease such as chronic bronchial irritation. Impairment of single-breath carbon monoxide diffusion capacity ($D_{L_{CO}}$) is greater in persons who smoke both marijuana and tobacco than in tobacco smokers. Despite the well-documented association between tobacco smoking and lung cancer, at present there is no direct evidence that marijuana smoking induces lung cancer. However, it should be emphasized that heavy marijuana use among Americans may be of too brief duration for detection of this problem.

Although marijuana has also been associated with adverse effects on a number of other systems, many of these studies await replication and confirmation. For example, the reported correlation between marijuana use and decreased testosterone levels in males has not been confirmed. Decreased sperm count and motility and abnormalities of morphology of spermatozoa following marijuana use have also been reported. Administration of high doses of marijuana to female rhesus monkeys has revealed significant marijuana-induced suppression of pituitary gonadotropins and gonadal steroids. Carefully conducted prospective studies demonstrated a significant correlation between impaired fetal growth and development and heavy marijuana use during pregnancy. Marijuana also has been implicated in derangements of the immune response system, in chromosomal abnormalities, and in inhibition of DNA, RNA, and protein synthesis, but these findings have not been confirmed or related to any specific physiologic effect of marijuana in humans. One report of cannabis-induced brain atrophy in young adults has not been confirmed in computed tomographic studies of young men who had documented histories of heavy marijuana smoking.

Tolerance and physical dependence Habitual marijuana users rapidly develop tolerance to the psychoactive effects of marijuana, often smoking more frequently and trying to secure more potent cannabis compounds. Tolerance for physiologic effects of marijuana develops at different rates; e.g., tolerance for marijuana-induced tachycardia develops rapidly, but tolerance for marijuana-induced conjunctival injection develops more slowly. Tolerance to both behavioral and physiologic effects of marijuana decreases rapidly upon cessation of marijuana use.

Withdrawal signs and symptoms have been reported in chronic cannabis users, with severity of symptoms related to dosage and duration of use. These include tremor, nystagmus, sweating, nausea, vomiting, diarrhea, irritability, anorexia, and sleep disturbances. Withdrawal signs and symptoms observed in chronic marijuana users are usually relatively mild in comparison to those observed in heavy opiate or alcohol users and rarely require medical or pharmacologic intervention. Somewhat more severe and protracted abstinence syndromes may occur after sustained use of high-potency cannabis compounds for long periods.

LYSERGIC ACID DIETHYLAMIDE The serendipitous discovery of psychedelic effects of LSD in 1947 culminated in an epidemic of LSD abuse during the 1960s. Imposition of stringent legal and regulatory constraints on the manufacture and distribution of LSD (classified as a schedule I substance by the FDA), as well as public recognition that psychedelic experiences induced by LSD were a health hazard, has resulted in a significant reduction in LSD abuse. During 1984, relatively few instances of LSD abuse were reported, but the drug still retains some popularity among adolescents and young adults.

LSD is a very potent drug; oral doses as low as 20 μg may induce profound psychological and physiologic effects. Tachycardia, hypertension, pupillary dilation, tremor, and hyperpyrexia occur within minutes following LSD in oral doses of 0.5 to 2 μg/kg. A variety of bizarre and often conflicting perceptual and mood changes, including visual illusions, synesthesias, and extreme lability of mood, usually occur within $\frac{1}{2}$ h after LSD intake. The action of LSD may persist for 12 to 18 h even though the half-life of the drug is only 3 h.

Tolerance develops rapidly for LSD-induced changes in psychological function when the drug is used one or more times per day over a course of 4 days or more. Abrupt abstinence following continued use does not produce withdrawal signs or symptoms. To date there have been no clinical reports of death caused by the direct effects of LSD.

The most frequent acute medical emergency associated with LSD use is panic episodes which may persist up to 24 h ("the bad trip"). Management of this problem is best accomplished by supportive reassurance ("talking down") and, if necessary, administration of small doses of anxiolytic drugs. Adverse consequences of chronic LSD use include enhanced risk for schizophreniform psychosis and derangements in memory function, problem solving, and abstract thinking. Treatment of these disorders is best carried out in specialized psychiatric facilities.

PHENYCYCLIDINE Phencyclidine, a cyclohexylamine derivative, is widely used in veterinary medicine to briefly immobilize large animals and is sometimes described as a dissociative anesthetic. PCP is easily synthesized and is abused, primarily by young people and polydrug users. The true extent of PCP abuse is unknown, but recent national surveys indicate an increase in frequency of use.

Phencyclidine is taken orally, by smoking, or by intravenous injection. It is also used as an adulterant in illicit sales of THC, LSD, amphetamine, or cocaine. The most common street preparation, "angel dust," is a white granular powder which contains 50 to 100 percent of the drug. Low doses (5 mg) produce agitation, excitement, impaired motor coordination, dysarthria, and analgesia. Users may have horizontal or vertical nystagmus, flushing, diaphoresis, and hyperacusis. Behavioral changes include distortions of body image, disorganization of thinking, and feelings of estrangement. Higher doses of PCP (5 to 10 mg) may produce hypersalivation, vomiting, myoclonus, fever, stupor, or coma. PCP doses of 10 mg or more cause convulsions, opisthotonus, and decerebrate posturing which may be followed by prolonged coma.

The diagnosis of PCP overdose is difficult because the patient's initial symptoms may suggest an acute schizophrenic reaction. Confirmation of PCP use is possible by determination of PCP levels in serum or urine. PCP analysis is currently available at most toxicologic centers. Large quantities of PCP remain in urine for 1 to 5 days following high-dosage PCP intake.

PCP overdose requires prompt life support measures including treatment of coma, convulsions, and respiratory depression in a hospital intensive care unit. There is no specific antidote or antagonist for PCP. PCP excretion from the body can be enhanced by acidification of urine and gastric lavage. Death from PCP overdose may occur as a consequence of some combination of pharyngeal hypersecretion, hyperthermia, respiratory depression, severe hypertension, seizures, hypertensive encephalopathy, and intracerebral hemorrhage.

Acute psychosis associated with PCP use should be considered a psychiatric emergency since patients may be at high risk for suicide or extreme violence toward others. Phenothiazines should not be used for treatment of acute PCP psychosis because these drugs potentiate PCP's anticholinergic effects. Haloperidol (5 mg intramuscularly) has been administered on an hourly basis to induce suppression of psychotic behavior. PCP, like LSD and mescaline, produces vasospasm of cerebral arteries at relatively low doses. Chronic PCP use has been shown to induce insomnia, anorexia, severe social and behavioral changes, and, in some cases, chronic schizophrenia.

POLYDRUG ABUSE Although drug abusers often report a preference for a particular drug, such as alcohol or opiates, the concurrent use of other drugs is common. Multiple-drug use often involves substances which may have different pharmacologic effects from the preferred drug. Concurrent use of such dissimilar compounds as stimulants and opiates or stimulants and alcohol is not unusual. The diversity of reported drug use combinations suggests that achieving some perceptible change in state, rather than any particular direction of change (stimulation or sedation), may be the primary reinforcer in polydrug use and abuse. There is also evidence that intoxication with alcohol or opiates is associated with increased tobacco smoking but marijuana smoking does not increase during alcohol intoxication. At present, there is relatively little systematic information available about drug interactions. However, it is known that the combined use of cocaine, heroin, and alcohol increases the risk for toxic effects and adverse medical consequences over risks associated with use of a single drug.

A practical determinant of polydrug use patterns is the relative availability and cost of the drugs. There are many examples of situationally determined drug use patterns, including the fact that soldiers who became dependent on heroin in Vietnam seldom continued heroin use after separation from military service. However, a significant number of men who were heroin addicts in Vietnam abused alcohol and became alcohol-dependent when they returned to the United States. Alcohol abuse, with its attendant medical complications, is one of the most serious problems encountered in former heroin addicts participating in methadone maintenance programs.

The physician must recognize that perpetuation of polydrug abuse and drug dependence is not necessarily a symptom of an underlying emotional disorder. Neither alleviation of anxiety nor reduction of depression accounts for initiation and perpetuation of polydrug abuse. Severe depression and anxiety are as frequently the consequences of polydrug abuse as they are the antecedents. There is also evidence that some of the most adverse consequences of drug use may be reinforcing and contribute to the continuation of polydrug abuse.

Adequate treatment of polydrug abuse, as well as other forms of drug abuse, requires innovative and eclectic programs of intervention. The first step in successful treatment is detoxification, a process which may be difficult because the patient has abused several drugs with different pharmacologic actions (e.g., alcohol, opiates, and cocaine). Since patients may not recall or may deny simultaneous multiple-drug use, diagnostic evaluation should always include urinalysis for qualitative detection of psychoactive substances and their metabolites. Treatment of polydrug abuse requires hospitalization or inpatient residential care during detoxification and the initial phase of drug abstinence. When possible, specialized facilities for the care and treatment of chemically dependent persons should be used. Outpatient detoxification of polydrug abuse patients is likely to be ineffective and may be dangerous.

As in the treatment of alcohol abuse, no single therapeutic modality has been shown to be uniquely effective in inducing remission. Polydrug abuse is a chronic disorder with an unpredictable pattern of remission and recrudescence. Therapeutic management of chronic disorders such as cardiac or neoplastic disease should serve as a model for helping the person with polydrug abuse problems. Even temporary remissions with attendant physical, social, and psychological improvements are preferable to the continuation or progressive acceleration of polydrug abuse and its related adverse medical and interpersonal consequences. In polydrug abuse, as in most chronic disorders, definitive "cures" rarely occur. The concerned physician should continue to assist polydrug abuse patients throughout the cyclic oscillations of this complex behavior disorder, recognizing that resumption of drug use may be the rule rather than the exception.

REFERENCES

BALSTER RL: The behavioral pharmacology of phencyclidine, in *Psychopharmacology: The Third Generation of Progress*, HY Meltzer (ed). New York, Raven, 1987, pp 1573–1579

CREGLER LL, MARK H: Medical complications of cocaine abuse. N Engl J Med 315:1495, 1986

FISCHMAN MW: Cocaine and the amphetamines, in *Psychopharmacology: The Third Generation of Progress*, HY Meltzer (ed). New York, Raven, 1987, pp 1543–1553

GAWIN FH, ELLINWOOD EH JR: Cocaine and other stimulants. Actions, abuse, and treatment. N Engl J Med 318:1173, 1988

————: Cocaine dependence. Ann Rev Med 40:149, 1989

JAFFE JH: Drug addiction and drug abuse, in *The Pharmacological Basis of Therapeutics*, 7th ed, AG Gilman et al (eds). New York, Macmillan, 1985, pp 532–581

KREEK MJ: Multiple drug abuse patterns and medical consequences, in *Psychopharmacology: The Third Generation of Progress*, HY Meltzer (ed). New York, Raven, 1987, pp 1597–1604

MELLO NK: A behavioral analysis of the reinforcing properties of alcohol and other drugs in man, in *The Pathogenesis of Alcoholism, Biological Factors*, B Kissin, H Begleiter (eds). New York, Plenum, 1983, vol 7, pp 133–198

————: Alcohol abuse and alcoholism: 1978–1987, in *Psychopharmacology: The Third Generation of Progress*, HY Meltzer (ed). New York, Raven, 1987, pp 1515–1520

MENDELSON JH: Marijuana, in *Psychopharmacology: The Third Generation of Progress*, HY Meltzer (ed). New York, Raven, 1987, pp 1565–1571

————, MELLO NK (eds): *The Diagnosis and Treatment of Alcoholism*, 2d ed. New York, McGraw-Hill, 1985

PETERSEN RC, STILLMAN RD (eds): *Phencyclidine (PCP) Abuse: An Appraisal*, NIDA Research Monograph Series no 21, US Department of Health, Education and Welfare Publication (ADM) 78-728, 1978

VAN DYKE C, BYCK R: Cocaine use in man, in *Advances in Substance Abuse, Behavioral and Biological Research*, NK Mello (ed). Greenwich, JAI Press, 1983, vol 3, pp 1–24

WEISS RD, MIRIN SM: *Cocaine*. Washington, American Psychiatric Press, 1987

373 TOBACCO

JOHN H. HOLBROOK

Tobacco smoke is a ubiquitous personal and environmental pollutant. Although tobacco has been used in western culture for more than 400 years, human inhalation of cigarette smoke is a twentieth century phenomenon with major medical and economic consequences. In industrialized nations cigarette smoking is the principal cause of preventable disease, disability, and premature death.

Important changes in smoking trends are occurring in the United States. In general, there is less smoking. For example, annual per capita cigarette consumption in adults declined from its 1963 peak of 4345 cigarettes to a 1987 estimate of 3196 cigarettes. In the United States between 1965 and 1987, the prevalence of smoking among aduts declined from 52 to 32 percent of men and 34 to 27 percent of women. There are 48.8 million current adult smokers and 39.9 million former smokers in the United States; the distribution of smokers between the sexes is approximately equal with 25.0 million men and 23.8 million women. Among teenagers, smoking is slightly more prevalent in females than in males. While consumption of cigar and pipe tobacco has decreased, use of smokeless tobacco, especially snuff, has increased among teenage males.

CIGARETTE SMOKE More than 4000 substances have been identified in cigarette smoke, including some that are pharmacologically active, antigenic, cytotoxic, mutagenic, and carcinogenic; these diverse biologic effects provide a framework for understanding the adverse consequences of smoking.

Cigarette smoke is a heterogeneous aerosol produced by incomplete combustion of the tobacco leaf. It is composed of a gas phase in which particulate matter is dispersed. Mainstream smoke emerges from the mouthpiece during puffing. Sidestream smoke is emitted between puffs at the burning cone and from the mouthpiece. The composition of the smoke is influenced by several factors including type of tobacco, temperature of combustion, length of the cigarette, porosity of the paper, additives, and filters. The major tobacco leaf constituents are carbohydrates, nonfatty organic acids, nitrogen-containing compounds, and resins. Cigarette temperatures vary greatly from 30°C at the mouthpiece to 900°C at the burning cone. In the presence of intense heat some tobacco constituents undergo thermic decomposition (pyrolysis). Volatile substances are distilled directly into the smoke. Unstable molecules recombine to generate new compounds (pyrosynthesis). Concentration of smoke constituents occurs as the smoke is filtered by unburnt tobacco and is redistilled by the burning cone. Some substances found in tobacco pass unchanged into cigarette smoke.

Approximately 92 to 95 percent of the total weight of mainstream smoke is present in the gas phase. Nitrogen, oxygen, and carbon dioxide account for 85 percent of the smoke's weight. The remaining gases and particulate matter are the substances of medical importance (Table 373-1). Mainstream smoke contains 0.3 to 3.3 billion particles per milliliter; the mean particle size is 0.2 to 0.5 μm, which is within the respirable range.

A pack-a-day cigarette smoker puffs more than 70,000 times a year, and the membranes of the mouth, nose, pharynx, and trach-

TABLE 373-1 Selected cigarette smoke constituents

Substance	Effect
PARTICULATE PHASE	
"Tar"*	Carcinogen
Polynuclear aromatic hydrocarbons	Carcinogens
Nicotine	Ganglionic stimulator and depressor
Phenol	Cocarcinogen and irritant
Cresol	Cocarcinogen and irritant
β-Naphthylamine	Carcinogen
N-Nitrosonornicotine	Carcinogen
Benzo[a]pyrene	Carcinogen
Trace metals (e.g., nickel, arsenic, polonium 210)	Carcinogens
Indole	Tumor accelerator
Carbazole	Tumor accelerator
Catechol	Cocarcinogen
GAS PHASE	
Carbon monoxide	Impairs oxygen transport and utilization
Hydrocyanic acid	Ciliotoxin and irritant
Acetaldehyde	Ciliotoxin and irritant
Acrolein	Ciliotoxin and irritant
Ammonia	Ciliotoxin and irritant
Formaldehyde	Ciliotoxin and irritant
Oxides of nitrogen	Ciliotoxin and irritant
Nitrosamines	Carcinogen
Hydrazine	Carcinogen
Vinyl chloride	Carcinogen

* The aggregate of particulate matter in cigarette smoke after subtracting nicotine and moisture.

eobronchial tree are exposed repetitively to tobacco smoke. Some constituents act directly on the membranes, while others are absorbed into the blood or are dissolved in saliva and swallowed.

PHARMACOLOGY Tissue and organ system responses to cigarette smoke inhalation are multiple and complex. Most studies in humans have dealt with exposure to whole smoke or to selected constituents thought to pose the greatest risk to health, such as nicotine and carbon monoxide. Relatively little is known about the individual effects and interactions of other potentially toxic smoke constituents that are present in low concentrations.

Nicotine, the component most characteristic of tobacco, is a highly toxic alkaloid that is both a ganglionic stimulant and depressant. Many of its complex effects are mediated by catecholamine release. Acute cardiovascular responses to nicotine observed in normal smokers include increases in systolic and diastolic blood pressure, heart rate, force of myocardial contraction, myocardial oxygen consumption, coronary artery blood flow, myocardial excitability, and peripheral vasoconstriction. Nicotine has also been shown to increase serum concentrations of glucose, cortisol, free fatty acids, vasopressin, and β-endorphin. Nicotine appears to be the major source of addiction to tobacco.

Carbon monoxide is a toxic gas that interferes with oxygen transport and utilization. Because cigarette smoke contains 2 to 6 percent carbon monoxide, smokers inhale concentrations as high as 400 parts per million (ppm) and develop elevated carboxyhemoglobin (COHb) levels. The range of COHb found in smokers is 2 to 15 percent, while levels for nonsmokers are near 1 percent. The average COHb level of moderate cigarette smokers is 5 percent. Carbon monoxide produces its adverse effects by reducing the amount of available oxyhemoglobin and myoglobin, and by displacing the oxygen-hemoglobin dissociation curve to the left. Chronic, mild elevations of COHb due to smoking are a common cause of mild polycythemia and may produce subtle impairment of central nervous system function.

Cigarette smoke and its condensate are carcinogenic in several species of animals. The major identified carcinogens in cigarette smoke are polynuclear aromatic hydrocarbons, aromatic amines, and nitrosamines (Table 373-1). Cocarcinogens present in cigarette smoke,

such as catechol, greatly enhance its carcinogenicity. The sister chromatid exchange rate, a sensitive indicator of mutagenic effects, is higher in the lymphocytes of smokers than in nonsmokers. Cigarette smoke condensate is also mutagenic in a microbial test system.

Potent pulmonary irritants and ciliotoxins are found in cigarette smoke (Table 373-1). These substances increase bronchial mucus secretion and mediate acute and chronic decreases in pulmonary and mucociliary function. Cigarette smoke also increases lung epithelial permeability.

EPIDEMIOLOGY Data from large prospective studies of populations in several countries have shown that cigarette-smoking men have 70 percent higher overall death rates than nonsmokers. The effect on mortality is proportionately greatest in younger age groups. The excess mortality of female smokers has been somewhat less than that of male smokers, but it has increased. Cigarette smoking is the largest single health risk in the United States and is responsible for an estimated 350,000 premature deaths each year; this is equivalent to approximately one-sixth of all deaths. Coronary heart disease (CHD) and lung cancer are the chief contributors to smoking-related excess mortality. In the United States, cigarette smokers also experience more disability due to chronic illness and report significantly more days absent from work than do nonsmokers.

A strong dose-response relationship exists between cigarette smoking and excess mortality, as measured by the age at onset of smoking, the number of cigarettes smoked, the number of years of smoking, and the depth of inhalation. Cessation of smoking is associated with a decrease in the excess mortality. These observations together with clinical, experimental, and pathologic studies indicate that smoking, per se, causes the excess mortality.

CHARACTERISTICS OF SMOKERS Demographic, anthropometric, physiologic, and laboratory features which distinguish cigarette smokers from nonsmokers are due both to baseline differences between these groups and to the effects of smoking. Smokers drink more alcohol, coffee, and tea than do nonsmokers. Their weight and blood pressure are slightly less and their heart rate is slightly faster than those of nonsmokers. In women the menopause comes earlier in smokers than in nonsmokers. Smokers have impaired maximum exercise performance and impaired immune systems compared to nonsmokers. A markedly increased number of pulmonary alveolar macrophages is present in smokers, and the function and metabolism of these cells are abnormal. When compared with nonsmokers, smokers show small increases in the total white blood cell count and serum IgE levels as well as small decreases in leukocyte vitamin C levels, serum uric acid, and albumin. In smokers, the ratio of high-density lipoprotein cholesterol to low-density lipoprotein cholesterol is reduced. Smokers also show reduced levels of prostacyclin (PGI_2).

CLINICAL CORRELATIONS Large population studies have shown a strong association between cigarette smoking and several diseases. Atherosclerotic cardiovascular disease, cancer, and chronic obstructive pulmonary disease account for most of the excess mortality and morbidity due to smoking.

Individual patient risks due to cigarette smoking vary widely. Factors which influence these risks include the duration, intensity, and type of smoke exposure; genetically mediated susceptibility; occupational and environmental exposures; use of medication; and coexisting risk factors and diseases.

Cardiovascular disease Cigarette smoking is a major cause of coronary heart disease (CHD), and premature CHD is one of its most important medical consequences. Approximately 21 percent of the 500,000 CHD deaths occurring each year in the United States is attributable to smoking. Cigarette smoking, hypertension, and hypercholesterolemia are the three major CHD risk factors. Smoking acts both independently of and synergistically with these other CHD risk factors. Two risk factors may produce a fourfold increase in CHD risk and three risk factors may produce an eightfold increase in CHD risk. There is a dose-response relationship between CHD risk and cigarette smoking. These CHD death rates are 60 to 70 percent greater in male smokers than nonsmokers. Sudden death may be the first manifestation of CHD, and it is two to four times more likely to occur in younger male cigarette smokers than in nonsmokers. Women cigarette smokers are also at greater risk of developing CHD than nonsmokers, and the use of both cigarettes and oral contraceptives increases this risk approximately tenfold. Cessation of smoking is associated with decreased CHD mortality, an effect which is measurable within 1 year. Those who continue to smoke after an acute myocardial infarction are more likely to die from CHD than are those who quit smoking. Smokers who undergo coronary artery bypass surgery have increased perioperative mortality compared to nonsmokers. Cigarette smoking may produce an imbalance between myocardial oxygen supply and demand, coronary artery spasm, decrease in the threshold for ventricular fibrillation, a hypercoagulable state, and an increase in platelet aggregation; avoidance of these effects may explain the prompt cardiac benefits of quitting smoking. Cigarette smoking may interfere with the efficacy of medication used to treat CHD, such as propranolol and nifedipine.

Cigarette smoking is an important cause of cerebrovascular disease and accounts for an estimated 18 percent of the 150,000 stroke deaths that occur each year in the United States. Large epidemiologic studies in men and women have shown an increased risk of stroke among smokers compared to nonsmokers, a dose-response relationship between smoking and stroke risk, and a decrease in stroke risk with smoking cessation. Among women, subarachnoid hemorrhage is more likely to occur in smokers than nonsmokers, and the use of both cigarettes and oral contraceptives greatly increases this risk.

Cigarette smoking is the most powerful risk factor for arteriosclerosis obliterans and thromboangiitis obliterans. It also aggravates peripheral ischemia and may adversely affect peripheral bypass grafts. The mortality rate for atherosclerotic aortic aneurysm is greater in male smokers than nonsmokers.

Cigarette smoking is not a risk factor for the development of hypertension; however, hypertensives who smoke are at a greater risk to develop malignant hypertension and to die from hypertension. Cigarette smoking may also interfere with the efficacy of medication used to treat hypertension, such as propranolol. Because of the association with chronic obstructive pulmonary disease, cigarette smoking is an important factor leading to chronic pulmonary heart disease.

Cancer   Cigarette smoking is the single most important cause of cancer mortality in the United States, accounting for 30 percent of all cancer deaths. In spite of the well-documented cause-and-effect relationship between cigarette smoking and lung cancer, more Americans continue to die from this cancer than from any other tumor (see Chap. 215). In 1988 an estimated 139,000 lung cancer deaths occurred in the United States; 87 percent of these deaths were attributable to cigarette smoking. The risk of developing lung cancer is quantitatively related to cigarette smoke exposure. Men who smoke one pack a day increase their risk tenfold compared with nonsmokers; men who smoke two packs a day may increase their risk more than 25 times compared with nonsmokers. Asbestos workers who smoke cigarettes are at especially high risk for developing lung cancer. Cigarette consumption by women increased rapidly in the United States during the past 50 years, and lung cancer mortality among smokers is currently increasing at a faster rate in women than in men. Lung cancer has become the leading cause of cancer death among American women. Because 5-year survival rates for lung cancer are less than 10 percent, emphasis must be placed on prevention. Giving up cigarettes is associated with a gradual decline in the risk of developing lung cancer.

Cigarette smoking is a cause of laryngeal, oral, and esophageal cancer in men and women. Alcohol consumption acts synergistically with cigarette smoking to increase the risk for these neoplasms. Cigarette smoking is an important contributory factor for the development of bladder, kidney, and pancreatic cancer; it is also associated with cancer of the stomach and uterine cervix.

Respiratory disease   Cigarette smoking is the major cause of chronic obstructive pulmonary disease (COPD), that is, chronic

bronchitis and emphysema (see Chap. 210). Of the estimated 70,000 deaths from COPD that occurred in the United States in 1988, 82 percent were attributable to smoking, and many of these deaths were preceded by prolonged respiratory disability. There is a dose-response relationship between COPD death rates and cigarette smoking. Depending upon the extent of smoke exposure, male cigarette smokers experience from 4 to 25 times higher mortality secondary to COPD than do nonsmokers. Although the death rate from COPD among female smokers is somewhat lower than among male smokers, it is increasing much more rapidly in female than in male smokers. Chronic cough, sputum production, and breathlessness are much more common in smokers. Smokers are more likely than nonsmokers to show abnormalities in a number of pulmonary function tests including measurements of elastic recoil, airflow in large and small airways, and diffusing capacity. Mild airflow obstruction in small airways may be present even in teenage smokers. When compared with continuing smokers, ex-smokers experience a decrease in mortality from COPD, a decrease in prevalence of pulmonary symptoms, and a slowing of the rate of decline of lung function to approximately that seen in age-matched nonsmokers. Chronic inhalation of pulmonary irritants and ciliotoxins (Table 373-1) may contribute to the development of COPD. Studies of the pathogenesis of emphysema suggest that smoking results in an excess of pulmonary proteases, which may produce pulmonary damage. The damage is apparently mediated via release of elastase from increased numbers of lung leukocytes and partial inactivation of pulmonary antiproteases by oxidants present in smoke. For most people in the United States cigarette smoking is a more important cause of COPD than are occupational or environmental factors; however, factors such as cotton dust exposure may act independently or conjointly with smoking to produce COPD. In a rare disorder, homozygous α_1-antitrypsin deficiency, smoking greatly accelerates the tendency to panacinar emphysema; furthermore, smoking may play an additive role in individuals heterozygous for this state.

Cigarette smoking has been associated with an increased incidence of respiratory infections and deaths from pneumonia and influenza. Postoperative respiratory complications and spontaneous pneumothorax are also more common in smokers. Because tobacco smoke may increase airway obstruction, asthmatics should be urged not to smoke. Chronic stomatitis and chronic laryngitis occur more frequently in smokers than in nonsmokers.

Pregnancy   Smoking may delay conception, and smoking during pregnancy may affect the fetus adversely. Infants whose mothers smoked during pregnancy weigh, on an average, 170 g less than infants whose mothers did not smoke. This effect probably results from impaired uteroplacental circulation. Maternal smoking during pregnancy increases the risk of spontaneous abortion, fetal death, neonatal death, and the sudden infant death syndrome. This increased risk may be much greater in pregnancies already at high risk due to other factors. Smoking by a woman during pregnancy may also adversely affect the long-term physical growth and intellectual development of the child.

Gastrointestinal disorders   Gastric and duodenal ulcer disease is more prevalent in male than female cigarette smokers and causes more deaths in male smokers than in nonsmokers. Smoking impairs spontaneous and drug-induced healing of peptic ulcers, increases the likelihood of duodenal ulcer recurrence, inhibits pancreatic bicarbonate secretion, and decreases the pressure of esophageal and pyloric sphincters. Histamine-2-receptor antagonist inhibition of nocturnal gastric secretion is also prevented by smoking.

Involuntary smoke inhalation   Indoor atmospheres and other confined spaces are often contaminated by tobacco smoke which is inhaled involuntarily by both smokers and nonsmokers. Most of the atmospheric pollutants arise from sidestream smoke. It contains greater concentrations of many smoke constituents than does mainstream smoke, but since sidestream smoke is diluted in a large volume of air, the smoke exposure from involuntary inhalation is less than that associated with smoking.

Initially, involuntary or passive smoking was thought to cause primarily an irritant effect such as ocular burning. It is now recognized as an important cause of air pollution and a cause of lung cancer in nonsmokers. Parental smoking in the home is associated with an increased risk of acute respiratory illnesses, middle-ear effusions, chronic respiratory symptoms, and slightly impaired lung function in children.

Drug effects   Tobacco smoke constituents induce hepatic microsomal enzyme systems that are important in the metabolism of several drugs. For example, cigarette smoking increases the metabolism of propranolol, propoxyphene, and theophylline. Smoking may also decrease the absorption of subcutaneously administered insulin. Hence, changes in smoking behavior may cause significant alterations of serum drug levels that may result in either drug toxicity or failure of drug treatment.

TYPES OF SMOKING   During the past 20 years the amount of tar and nicotine delivered by cigarettes made in the United States has decreased by more than 50 percent. Filter-tipped cigarettes and lower-tar and -nicotine cigarettes now account for more than 90 and 50 percent of sales, respectively. Lung cancer and laryngeal cancer are the only tobacco-related diseases for which the use of lower-tar and -nicotine cigarettes has been shown to result in risk reduction, compared with the use of higher-tar and -nicotine cigarettes; however, compared with not smoking or quitting, the benefits are minimal. Consumers who choose lower-tar and -nicotine cigarettes and then smoke a larger number of cigarettes or inhale more frequently or deeply may actually increase their exposure to harmful substances. There is also concern because unidentified flavoring agents are added to these cigarettes to enhance consumer acceptance.

Cigar and pipe smokers usually inhale less smoke than cigarette smokers, presumably because the alkaline pH of cigar and pipe tobacco makes it more irritating to the respiratory tract. The smoke exposure and overall mortality rates of pipe and cigar smokers in the United States are substantially less than those of cigarette smokers; however, death rates of cigarette, cigar, and pipe smokers are approximately equal for carcinoma of the oral cavity, larynx, and esophagus, sites where exposures to cigarette, cigar, and pipe smoke are similar. The mortality rates of most cigar and pipe smokers for cancer at other sites, CHD, and COPD are not greatly elevated above the rates of nonsmokers, but cigar and pipe smokers who inhale consistently may experience adverse health effects comparable with those of cigarette smokers. The use of chewing tobacco and snuff may produce plasma nicotine levels comparable to those of cigarette smokers and lead to nicotine dependence or addiction. The use of such smokeless tobacco products also increases the risk for oral cancer.

CESSATION OF SMOKING   Psychosocial forces lead to initiation of smoking, especially among children and teenagers. Later, nicotine addiction and psychological factors help maintain dependence on tobacco. It is estimated that more than 40 million people in the United States have stopped smoking; 95 percent of these succeeded without formal assistance. Smoking cessation reduces the risk of tobacco-related diseases. For example, ten or more years after quitting, the death rate of those who smoked 20 cigarettes a day or less is about the same as that of nonsmokers. For heavier smokers cessation may never reduce the risk to the level of the nonsmoker. Ex-smokers usually experience prompt symptomatic improvement. On the average they also gain approximately 5 lb.

In the United States more than 80 percent of cigarette smokers would like to stop smoking. Many self-care and organized programs are available to assist these individuals. Organized programs employ several techniques including instruction, counseling, withdrawal clinics, behavioral modification, hypnosis, aversive conditioning, self-monitoring, and drug therapy. In these programs 1-year abstinence rates of 20 to 30 percent are common. Relapse usually occurs during the 3-month interval after quitting. Successful programs emphasize maintenance of the nonsmoking state during this critical period. There is a great need for physicians to provide personalized smoking cessation assistance for their patients.

Although less than 10 percent of physicians smoke, a minority of patients report receiving advice from their physician to quit. Controlled trials have shown that physician counseling increases long-term smoking cessation rates. Surveys also show that patients are inadequately informed about the hazards and addictive nature of smoking. All smokers should be encouraged to quit, especially those in high-risk groups. Physicians can help their patients by accepting smoking as a chronic medical problem requiring treatment and by following these guidelines:

1 Obtain a quantitative smoking history.
2 Explain the health risks in a personally relevant fashion.
3 Emphasize the benefits associated with cessation.
4 Assess patient interest in smoking cessation.
5 Assist the patient to quit by setting a target quitting date and by suggesting smoking cessation strategies.
6 Provide self-help reading materials.
7 Support the patient in a maintenance program.

A nicotine-containing chewing gum, which helps alleviate withdrawal symptoms, may be a useful adjunct in medically supervised programs. Preliminary data suggest that clonidine may be of value in a smoking cessation program. Selected patients may benefit from referral to a smoking cessation specialist.

Political, social, and cultural forces play a critical role in the individual decision to start or stop smoking. For this reason, physicians should lead and support efforts to increase tobacco excise taxes, to eliminate all tobacco advertisements and promotional activities, and to ban smoking in public places.

Ultimately, primary smoking prevention in the pediatric and adolescent age groups may be the most effective program. Young people who have been trained to resist social pressures, who understand the consequences of smoking to their health, and who appreciate the difficulty of quitting are less likely to start smoking.

REFERENCES

BENOWITZ NL: Pharmacologic aspects of cigarette smoking and nicotine addiction. N Engl J Med 319:1318, 1988

GRITZ ER: Cigarette smoking: The need for action by health professionals. CA 38:194, 1988

US DEPARTMENT OF HEALTH AND HUMAN SERVICES: *The health consequences of involuntary smoking. A report of the Surgeon General.* DHHS(CDC) Publication no 87-8398, 1987

US DEPARTMENT OF HEALTH AND HUMAN SERVICES: *The health consequences of smoking: Nicotine addiction. A report of the Surgeon General.* DHHS(CDC) Publication no 88-8406, 1988

US DEPARTMENT OF HEALTH AND HUMAN SERVICES: *Reducing the health consequences of smoking: 25 years of progress. A report of the Surgeon General.* DHHS(CDC) Publication no 89-8411, 1989

PART FIFTEEN

374 ACUTE POISON AND DRUG OVERDOSAGE

FREDERICK H. LOVEJOY, JR. / CHRISTOPHER H. LINDEN

A poison (toxin) is a chemical substance capable of producing adverse effects in a living organism. Chemicals may be divided into those intended for human use (foods and their additives, pharmaceuticals, toiletries, cosmetics) and those that are not (household products, industrial chemicals, nonfood nondrug botanicals). An overdose implies exposure to excessive amounts of the former and any amount of the latter; it may or may not result in poisoning.

Poisoning may be local (limited to the eyes, skin, lungs, or gastrointestinal tract), systemic, or both, depending on the dose, extent of absorption and distribution, intrinsic potency of the poison, and host susceptibility. Absorption and distribution are influenced by properties of the chemical itself (molecular size, degree of ionization, lipid and water solubility, protein binding) and of the biologic barriers (membrane composition, pore size, chemical transport systems) through which it penetrates.

Local effects are due to nonspecific chemical reactions such as oxidation, protein denaturation, desiccation, and solvent activity. Their severity and reversibility depend on the dose (concentration), contact time, the potency of the chemical, and the type and condition of the exposed surface. The nature (generalized or limited), severity, and reversibility of systemic effects depend on the dose, potency, and metabolic disposition of the chemical, the functional reserve of the individual or affected tissue, and the presence of secondary complications (shock, hypoxia). Other variables that influence toxicity include coexisting illnesses, previous chemical exposure, and individual differences in biologic response, tissue concentration of a chemical (pharmacodynamics), and/or its pharmacokinetics (absorption, distribution, metabolism, elimination).

EPIDEMIOLOGY

In the United States, poison exposures result in an estimated 5 million requests for medical advice or treatment each year. The common routes of exposure are ingestion (79 percent), dermal (7 percent), ophthalmic (6 percent), inhalation (5 percent), bites and stings (3 percent), and parenteral injections (0.3 percent). Pharmaceutical preparations are involved in 40 percent of exposures. Substances most frequently involved are cleaning agents, analgesics, cosmetics, plants, cough and cold preparations, and hydrocarbons. The majority of exposures are acute, accidental, occur in the home, result in minor or no toxicity, and involve children under 6 years of age.

Accidental exposures also result from the improper use of chemicals at work or at play, product mislabeling, label misreading, mistaken identification of unlabeled chemicals, uninformed self-medication, and dosing errors by nurses, parents, pharmacists, physicians, and

the elderly. Other unintended poisonings are due to the use of drugs for psychotropic effects (abuse) and excessive self-dosing (misuse). Excluding the recreational use of ethanol, attempted suicide is the most common reason for intentional exposure.

Although only 4 percent of victims of exposure require hospitalization, they account for roughly 5 percent of intensive care unit admissions and up to 30 percent of psychiatric admissions. Suicide attempts account for the majority (60 to 90 percent) of serious or fatal poisonings. Most deaths result from carbon monoxide poisoning and occur prior to arrival at a hospital. Antidepresssants, analgesics, stimulants and street drugs, cardiovascular agents, sedative-hypnotics, and asthma medications are responsible for most drug-related fatalities. Nonpharmaceutical agents implicated in fatal poisoning include inorganic chemicals, alcohols and glycols, cleaning agents, and hydrocarbons.

DIAGNOSIS OF POISONING

Although poisoning can mimic other illnesses, the correct diagnosis can usually be established by the history, physical examination, routine and toxicologic laboratory evaluation, and clinical course. The history should include the time, route, duration, and circumstances (location, surrounding events, intent) of exposure; the name and amount of each drug, chemical, or ingredient involved; the time of onset, nature, and severity of symptoms; the time and type of first aid measures provided; and the past medical and psychiatric history. In many cases the victim is confused, comatose, and unaware of an exposure, or unable or unwilling to admit to one. Suspicious circumstances include unexplained illness in a previously healthy person; a history of psychiatric problems (particularly depression); recent changes in health, economic status, or social relationships; and the onset of illness while working with chemicals or after ingesting food, drink (especially ethanol), or medications. Patients who become ill soon after arriving from a foreign country or after arrest for criminal activity should be suspected of having illicit drugs concealed in body cavities (the GI tract). Family, friends, paramedics, police, pharmacists, physicians, and employers may provide valuable information regarding habits, hobbies, behavior changes, available medications, and antecedent events. A search of the victim's clothes and place of discovery may reveal a suicide note or empty container of drugs or chemicals. The imprint code on pills, the label and manufacturer of chemical products, a text or Physicians Desk Reference, or regional poison control center may be used to identify the ingredients and potential toxicity of a suspected poison.

The physical examination should initially focus on the vital signs and cardiopulmonary and neurologic status to assess the need for immediate supportive treatment. These parameters also provide the most important diagnostic clues in poisoning of unknown etiology (Table 374-1). Although vital signs may sometimes be discordant, the clinical picture can usually be characterized by either physiologic stimulation or depression. Examination of the eyes (for nystagmus, pupil size, and reactivity), abdomen (for bowel activity and bladder),

TABLE 374-1 Differential diagnosis of poisoning based on vital signs and CNS activity

Stimulant poisoning	Depressant poisoning
Sympathomimetic syndrome	Sympatholytic syndrome
Amphetamines	Adrenergic blockers
Caffeine	Antiarrhythmics
Cocaine	Antidepressants (tricyclic)
Decongestants	Antihypertensives
Ergot alkaloids	Calcium channel blockers
MAO inhibitors	Digoxin
Theophylline	
Anticholinergic syndrome	Cholinergic syndrome
Antidepressants (tricyclic)	Bethanecol
Antihistamines	Carbamate insecticides
Anti-Parkinsonian agents	Organophosphate insecticides
Antipsychotics	Myasthenia gravis drugs
Antispasmodics (GI, GU)	(e.g., pyridostigmine)
Belladonna alkaloids	Physostigmine
Cyclobenzaprine	
Mydriatics (topical)	
Plants/mushrooms	
Hallucinogenic syndrome	Narcotic syndrome
LSD and synthetic analogues	Analgesics
Marijuana	Antispasmodics (GI)
Mescaline and synthetic	
analogues	
Phencyclidine	
Withdrawal syndrome	Sedative-hypnotic syndrome
Alcohol	Alcohol
Antidepressants	Antiepileptics
Beta-blockers	Barbiturates
Clonidine	Benzodiazepines
Narcotics	Ethchlorvynol
Sedative-hypnotics	Hydrocarbons
	Glutethimide
	Methyprylon

and skin (for burns, bullae, color, warmth, moisture, pressure sores, and puncture marks) often narrow the diagnosis to a particular syndrome. Grading the severity of poisoning (Table 374-2) may be useful for assessing prognosis and for following the clinical course.

The patient should also be examined for evidence of trauma and underlying illnesses. Except with theophylline and drugs that cause hypoglycemia and hypoxia, seizures and neurologic dysfunction due to poisoning are almost never focal. Hence, focal findings should prompt evaluation for a structural CNS lesion. When the history is unclear, all orifices should be examined for the presence of chemical burns and drug packets. The odor of breath or vomitus and the color of nails, skin, or urine may occasionally provide diagnostic clues.

TABLE 374-2 Severity of stimulant and depressant poisoning and drug withdrawal

Severity	Signs and symptoms
STIMULANT POISONING	
Grade 1	Diaphoresis, flushing, hyperreflexia, irritability, mydriasis, tremors
Grade 2	Confusion, fever, hyperactivity, hypertension, tachycardia, tachypnea
Grade 3	Delirium, mania, hyperpyrexia, tachyarrhythmias
Grade 4	Coma, convulsions, cardiovascular collapse
DEPRESSANT POISONING	
Grade 1	Lethargic but arousable; able to answer questions and follow commands
Grade 2	Comatose; withdraws from pain; brainstem and deep tendon reflexes intact
Grade 3	Comatose; no response to pain; most reflexes absent; respiratory depression
Grade 4	Comatose; no response to pain; reflexes absent; respiratory and cardiovascular depression

An increased anion-gap metabolic acidosis is characteristic of methanol, ethylene glycol, and salicylate intoxication, and lactic acidosis may occur in any poisoning that results in hypoxia, hypotension, or seizures. An osmolal gap, the difference between the measured serum osmolality (freezing point depression, not the vapor pressure method) and the calculated osmolality (from the serum sodium, glucose, and BUN), of more than 10 mosmol/kg indicates the presence of a low-molecular-weight solute such as acetone, ethanol, ethylene glycol, isopropyl alcohol, or methanol or an unmeasured electrolyte (magnesium) or sugar (mannitol). An increased anion-gap metabolic acidosis with respiratory alkalosis, ketosis, and tinnitus suggests salicylate poisoning. An increased anion-gap metabolic acidosis and osmolal gap, accompanied by back pain, hypocalcemia, and crystalluria, may be seen with ethylene glycol intoxication, whereas the presence of visual symptoms suggests methanol poisoning. Lists of poisons that cause specific signs, symptoms, and other laboratory abnormalities may be found in the references cited.

Pulmonary edema can occur with carbon monoxide, cyanide, narcotic, paraquat, sedative-hypnotic, and salicylate poisoning; inhalation of irritant gas (chlorine, nitrogen dioxide, metal and polymer fume); or prolonged shock. Aspiration pneumonia is common in patients with coma, seizures, petroleum distillate ingestion, and irritant gas inhalation. Radiopaque densities may be visible on abdominal x-rays following the ingestion of calcium, chloral hydrate, chlorinated hydrocarbons, enteric-coated tablets, heavy metals, phenothiazines, and salicylates.

Bradycardia and AV block may occur in patients poisoned by antiarrhythmic agents, beta blockers, calcium channel blockers, cholinergic agents (carbamate and organophosphate insecticides), digitalis, lithium, phenylpropanolamine, and tricyclic antidepressants. QRS- and QT-interval prolongation may be caused by amantidine, antiarrhythmics, antipsychotics, tricyclic antidepressants, fluorides, heavy metals (arsenic, thallium), lithium, magnesium, or neuroleptics. Ventricular tachyarrhythmias may be seen in poisoning with sympathomimetics and agents that cause QRS and QT prolongation.

Analysis of urine and blood (and occasionally gastric contents and chemical samples) may be useful to confirm or rule out suspected poisoning. Interpretation of laboratory data requires knowledge of the tests used for screening and confirmation (thin layer, gas-liquid, high performance liquid chromatography; colorimetric and fluorometric assays; enzyme-multiplied and radioimmunoassays; gas chromatography; mass spectrometry) and of their sensitivity (limit of detection) and specificity and of the best type and time of sampling of biologic specimens. Personal communication with the laboratory is essential. A negative screen may mean the poison is not detectable at all or its concentration is too low for detection. In such an instance, repeating the test on a sample obtained at a later time will often yield positive results.

Since screening tests require 2 to 6 h for completion, immediate management decisions often must be based on the history, physical examination, and routine ancillary tests. When the patient is asymptomatic or when the clinical picture is consistent with the reported history, qualitative screening is neither clinically useful nor cost-effective. It is of greatest value in patients with severe or unexplained toxicity such as coma, seizures, cardiovascular instability, metabolic or respiratory acidosis, and non-sinus cardiac rhythms. Quantitative analysis is appropriate for acetaminophen, acetone, alcohol (including ethylene glycol), antiarrhythmic, antiepileptic, barbiturate, digoxin, heavy metal, lithium, salicylate, and theophylline poisoning and in carboxyhemoglobinemia and methemoglobinemia. Results are often available within an hour.

Response to antidotes may also be used for diagnostic purposes. Resolution of altered mental status and abnormal vital signs within minutes of intravenous dextrose, naloxone, or flumazenil administration is virtually diagnostic of hypoglycemia, narcotic poisoning, and benzodiazepine intoxication, respectively. The prompt reversal of acute dystonic (extrapyramidal) reactions following an intravenous dose of benztropine or diphenhydramine confirms the diagnosis of benzodiazepine intoxication. *Vin rosé* urine color following a diagnostic dose of deferoxamine can be used to confirm iron poisoning when serum iron and total iron-binding capacity levels are not immediately available. Although reversal of both central and peripheral manifestations of anticholinergic poisoning by physostigmine is diagnostic, physostigmine may cause arousal in patients with central nervous system depression of any etiology.

The absence of signs and symptoms soon after an overdose does not rule out a poisoning. Common poisons whose effects are delayed in onset include acetaminophen, cancer chemotherapeutic agents, carbon tetrachloride, colchicine, digoxin, ethylene glycol, heavy metals, methanol, mushrooms, some plants, narcotics, salicylate, and slow- or sustained-release medications.

TREATMENT

Treatment goals include support of vital signs, prevention of further poison absorption, enhancement of poison elimination, administration of specific antidotes, and prevention of reexposure (Table 374-3). Treatment is based on the identity of the poison, the route and amount of exposure, the time of presentation relative to the time of exposure, and the severity of poisoning. Knowledge of toxin pharmacokinetics and pharmacodynamics is essential.

For patients who present during the preclinical phase, between the time of ingestion and the onset of manifestations, treatment must be based on the history. The maximum potential toxicity based on the greatest possible amount ingested should be assumed. Gastroin-

TABLE 374-3 Fundamentals of poisoning management

I Supportive care
  A Airway protection
  B Oxygenation/ventilation
  C Treatment of arrhythmias
  D Hemodynamic support
  E Treatment of seizures
  F Correction of temperature abnormalities
  G Correction of metabolic derangements
  H Prevention of secondary complications
II Prevention of further poison absorption
  A Gastrointestinal decontamination
    1 Syrup of ipecac–induced emesis
    2 Gastric lavage
    3 Activated charcoal
    4 Whole bowel irrigation
    5 Catharsis
    6 Dilution
    7 Endoscopic/surgical removal
  B Decontamination of other sites
    1 Eye decontamination
    2 Skin decontamination
    3 Body cavity evacuation
III Enhancement of poison elimination
  A Multiple-dose activated charcoal
  B Forced diuresis
  C Alteration of urinary pH
  D Chelation (see heavy metal section)
  E Extracorporal removal
    1 Peritoneal dialysis
    2 Hemodialysis
    3 Hemoperfusion
    4 Hemofiltration
    5 Plasmapheresis
    6 Exchange transfusion
  F Hyperbaric oxygenation
IV Administration of antidotes
  A Neutralization by antibodies
  B Neutralization by chemical binding
  C Metabolic antagonism
  D Physiologic antagonism
V Prevention of reexposure
  A Adult education
  B Child-proofing
  C Notification of regulatory agencies
  D Psychiatric referral

testinal decontamination to minimize absorption and decrease the severity of toxicity is the first priority. Since the decontamination is more effective the sooner it is performed, the history and physical examination should initially be brief. It is also advisable to establish intravenous access and initiate cardiac monitoring, particularly in patients with potentially serious ingestions or unclear histories. The choice of decontamination procedure depends on the predicted toxicity; the availability, efficacy, and contraindications of the procedure; and the nature, severity, and risk of complications. For the home management of patients with accidental ingestions, reliable histories, and mild predicted toxicity, emesis can be induced with ipecac syrup. For patients treated in medical facilities, activated charcoal is administered for most poisons. It has comparable or greater efficacy, fewer contraindications and complications, and is less invasive than ipecac or gastric lavage. Alternative methods should be used if the ingested agent is not well-absorbed by activated charcoal. When the reasons are compelling (e.g., witnessed ingestion of a potentially severe overdose) the use of invasive procedures (gastric lavage) may be justified in an asymptomatic patient. Aspiration or esophageal perforation may result from the forcible use of a lavage tube in an uncooperative patient with a trivial ingestion.

When an accurate history is not obtainable, a poison causing delayed toxicity or irreversible damage is suspected, or the patient develops severe clinical toxicity, toxicologic screening should be accomplished as soon as possible. Obtaining additional blood and urine samples and saving them for future analysis is often helpful. Due to continuing absorption and distribution, blood levels may be greater than those in tissue and not reflect clinical toxicity or the need for additional treatment. However, high blood levels of agents whose metabolites are more toxic than the parent compound (acetaminophen, ethylene glycol, or methanol) may indicate the need for additional interventions (antidotes, dialysis).

After evaluation and GI tract decontamination, some patients may be sent home because the predicted toxicity is minimal or the time of expected maximal toxicity has passed without incident. Observation for at least 4 to 6 h following GI tract decontamination assures that most patients who remain asymptomatic can be discharged safely. Patients ingesting agents that slow gastric emptying and intestinal motility (anticholinergics, narcotics, sedative hypnotics, salicylates), have slow dissolution and absorption characteristics (carbamazepine, phenytoin, enteric-coated tablets, lithium, salicylate, and sustained-release preparations), or tend to form bezoars or concretions (enteric-coated tablets, meprobamate, salicylate) may require longer observation. In such patients, the passage of a charcoal stool prior to discharge should preclude delayed absorption and subsequent toxicity.

During the toxic phase, from the time of onset to the peak clinical or laboratory evidence of poisoning, management is based on clinical and laboratory findings. Resuscitation and stabilization are the first priority. All symptomatic patients should have an intravenous line, supplemental oxygen, cardiac monitoring, continuous observation, and baseline laboratory, ECG, and x-ray evaluation. Patients with altered mental status, particularly those with coma or seizures, should be given an intravenous bolus of glucose, naloxone, and thiamine and additional antidotes as indicated. Further poison absorption should be limited by administering activated charcoal or gastric lavage. Since aspiration is a hazard, ipecac syrup should be used with caution. Patients may be given charcoal by mouth or by a stomach tube. Administering a dose of charcoal both before and after gastric lavage may be more effective than giving charcoal only after lavage. An initial dose of charcoal can be given by small-bore (no. 18 French or less) nasogastric tube while monitoring and supportive measures are being initiated. Once the patient is stable, lavage with a large-bore orogastric tube can be followed with a second dose of charcoal. The rare patient who deteriorates after this regimen should be lavaged and given another dose of charcoal.

Measures that enhance poison elimination may shorten the duration of toxicity and lessen its severity. However, the risks of poison removal must be weighed against the benefits. Diagnostic certainty (usually via laboratory confirmation) is a prerequisite. Intestinal dialysis using activated charcoal is generally safe and effective. The efficacy of diuresis and chelation therapy is limited to a relatively small number of poisons. Extracorporal removal methods are effective for many but not all poisons, but their use should be limited to patients who would otherwise not have a favorable outcome.

Patients with severe poisoning (coma, respiratory depression, hypotension, cardiac conduction abnormalities, cardiac arrhythmias, hypothermia or hyperthermia, seizures), those needing close monitoring or antidotes or enhanced elimination therapy, those showing progressive clinical deterioration, and those with significant underlying medical problems should be admitted to an intensive care unit. Patients with moderate toxicity can be managed on a general medical service, intermediate care unit, or emergency department observation area depending on the anticipated duration and level of monitoring needed (intermittent clinical observation versus continuous clinical, cardiac, and respiratory monitoring). Suicidal patients sometimes require a particularly high level of care.

During the resolution phase, between peak toxicity and full recovery, supportive care should continue until the patient is alert and laboratory and ECG abnormalities are resolved. Repeat charcoal dosing may prevent rebound toxicity when depressed GI function improves and the poison still in the gut is absorbed or additional active metabolites are formed. Since poison is eliminated from the blood before tissues, blood levels are generally lower than tissue levels during this phase and are not necessarily predictive of toxicity. This is particularly true when extracorporal elimination procedures are used. Because of redistribution of poison, relapse and rebound increase in blood level may occur after the termination of such procedures. When a metabolite is responsible for toxic effects, continued treatment of an asymptomatic patient may be necessary because of a previously toxic blood level (acetaminophen and methanol).

Prior to discharge, patients with accidental ingestions (and/or the caregivers) should be instructed about preventive measures, and suicidal patients should receive appropriate psychiatric assessment, disposition, and follow-up.

SUPPORTIVE CARE

The goal of supportive therapy is to maintain physiologic homeostasis until detoxification is accomplished and to prevent and treat secondary complications such as aspiration, bed sores, cerebral and pulmonary edema, pneumonia, rhabdomyolysis, sepsis, and generalized organ dysfunction due to prolonged hypoxia or shock.

In addition to those needing urgent endotracheal intubation, many poisoned patients require semielective endotracheal intubation for protection of the airway against aspiration of gastrointestinal contents and of the poison itself. The gag reflex alone is not a reliable indicator of the need for intubation. Since patients may maintain airway patency while being stimulated but not if left unattended, those who cannot respond to voice or who are unable to sit and drink fluids without assistance are best managed by prophylactic intubation. Patients with severe excitation may also require intubation for airway protection (due to the risk or existence of seizures) and sedation or paralysis for control of agitation and prevention of hyperthermia, acidosis, and rhabdomyolysis. The need for oxygenation and ventilation is best determined by analyses of arterial blood gases.

Drug-induced pulmonary edema is usually secondary to hypoxia, although myocardial depression may contribute. Measurement of pulmonary artery pressure may be necessary to establish the etiology. Arrhythmias can result from direct cardiotoxicity, abnormal cardiovascular reflexes, or metabolic derangements. Supraventricular tachycardia associated with hypertension and CNS excitation is almost always due to sympathetic, anticholinergic, or hallucinogenic stimulation or to drug withdrawal (Table 374-1). Most cases are mild or moderate in severity and require only observation or nonspecific sedation with a benzodiazepine. If severe or associated with hemodynamic instability, chest pain, or ECG evidence of ischemia, specific therapy is indicated. Hypoxia, hypoglycemia, and other metabolic causes of sympathetic stimulation should be ruled out first. For patients with sympathetic hyperactivity, treatment with a combined alpha and beta blocker (labetalol) or a combination of beta blocker and vasodilator (esmolol and nitroprusside) is preferred. For those with anticholinergic hyperactivity, physostigmine is the treatment of choice. Supraventricular tachycardia without hypertension is generally secondary to vasodilation or hypovolemia and responds to fluid administration.

Ventricular tachyarrhythmias may be caused by sympathetic stimulation, myocardial membrane destabilization, or metabolic derangements. Lidocaine and phenytoin are generally safe, but beta blockers can be hazardous unless the arrhythmia is clearly from sympathetic hyperactivity. In tricyclic antidepressant poisoning, quinidine and procainamide are contraindicated (because of similar electrophysiologic effects), but sodium bicarbonate may be therapeutic. Magnesium sulfate and overdrive pacing (by isoproterenol or a pacemaker) may be useful in patients with torsade de pointes and prolonged QT interval. Magnesium and antidigoxin antibodies should be considered for digoxin poisoning. Without invasive (esophageal or intracardiac) ECG recording, it may be impossible to distinguish the origin (ventricular or supraventricular) of wide-complex tachycardias (see Chap. 185). If the patient is hemodynamically stable, it may be prudent to observe rather than to treat with a potentially harmful cardioactive agent. Arrhythmias may be resistant to drug therapy until underlying acid-base and electrolyte derangements, hypoxia, or hypothermia are corrected.

Bradyarrhythmias associated with hypotension should be treated as described in Chap. 184, and the management of hypotension is described in Chap. 39. If hypotension is unresponsive to volume expansion, norepinephrine or high-dose dopamine may be appropriate.

Drug-induced seizures may be due to direct or indirect CNS neuroreceptor stimulation (or inhibition), neuronal membrane destabilization, ischemia, edema, or metabolic abnormalities. Seizures due to excessive stimulation of catecholamine receptors (sympathomimetic or hallucinogen poisoning and drug withdrawal) or decreased activity of inhibitory receptors mediated by gamma-aminobutyric acid (GABA) (isoniazid poisoning) or glycine (strychnine poisoning) are best treated with GABA agonists such as benzodiazepines or barbiturates. Seizures caused by isoniazid, which inhibits the synthesis of GABA, may not respond to agonist therapy until GABA synthesis is restored, because agonists act, at least partially, by promoting the release of GABA from presynaptic vesicles. High doses of pyridoxine, which is necessary for the synthesis of GABA, are often necessary to terminate seizures resulting from isoniazid intoxication. For poisons with central dopaminergic effects (phencyclidine), an agent with opposing activity, such as haloperidol, may be useful. Seizures resulting from membrane destabilization (beta blocker, cyclic antidepressant poisoning) may require a membrane-active agent such as phenytoin as well as a GABA agonist. In rare cases (anticholinergic or cyanide poisoning), specific antidotal therapy may be necessary.

The treatment of seizures secondary to ischemia, edema, or metabolic abnormalities should include correction of the underlying cause. Since prolonged convulsions can lead to rhabdomyolysis and severe acidosis, neuromuscular paralysis is indicated in refractory cases. Aggressive treatment of seizures is necessary to prevent permanent neurologic damage.

Temperature extremes, metabolic, hepatic, and renal abnormalities, and secondary complications should be treated by standard measures. Invasive interventions, such as extracorporal membrane oxygenation, intraaortic balloon pump counterpulsation, and partial (femoral) cardiopulmonary bypass pump circulatory support, should be considered in severe but reversible poisoning.

PREVENTION OF POISON ABSORPTION

GASTROINTESTINAL DECONTAMINATION *Syrup of ipecac* is administered orally in a dose of 30 mL for adults, 15 mL for children, and 10 mL for small infants. Clear liquids should also be given. Ipecac irritates the stomach and stimulates the central chemoreceptor trigger zone. Vomiting usually occurs approximately 22 min following administration. The dose may be repeated if vomiting does not occur. Ipecac decreases drug or poison absorption by an average of 57 percent (range 28 to 73 percent) if given within 5 min of drug ingestion and about 30 percent (range 2 to 45 percent) if given within half an hour. Because there are no suitable control groups, its efficacy in overdose patients is not established. Side effects include lethargy in children (12 percent) and protracted vomiting (8 to 17 percent). Chronic ipecac use (by patients with anorexia nervosa or bulimia) may cause electrolyte and fluid abnormalities, cardiac toxicity, and myopathy. Except for aspiration, serious complications are rare. Isolated cases of gastric and esophageal tears and perforations and stroke have been reported. Ipecac is contraindicated in patients with recent GI surgery, CNS depression, seizures, and ingestions of corrosives and rapidly acting CNS poisons (camphor, cyanide, tricyclic antidepressants, propoxyphene, strychnine).

Gastric lavage is optimally performed using a no. 28 French orogastric tube in children and a no. 40 French tube in adults with about 5 mL fluid per kg body weight. Except for infants, tap water is acceptable. The patient should be placed in Trendelenburg and left lateral decubitus positions to prevent aspiration (even if an endotracheal tube is in place). Lavage decreases poison absorption by an average of 69 percent (range 54 to 84 percent) if performed within 5 min of poison ingestion, 31 percent (range 26 to 38 percent) if performed at 30 min; and 11 percent (range 8 to 13 percent) if performed at 60 min. Its efficacy is similar to that of ipecac. Significant amounts of ingested drug are recovered in a tenth of patients. As with ipecac, its effect on the clinical outcome of poisoned patients is not known. Aspiration is a common complication (up to 10 percent) especially when lavage is improperly performed. Serious complications (tracheal lavage, esophageal and gastric perforation) occur in approximately 1 percent of patients. For this reason, only a physician should insert the lavage tube, and the patient must be restrained (with pharmacologic sedation if necessary) during the procedure. Gastric lavage is contraindicated in patients with ingestion of corrosives and petroleum distillate hydrocarbons because of the risk of aspiration-induced hydrocarbon pneumonia and gastroesophageal perforation.

Activated charcoal, as a suspension in water alone or with a cathartic, is given orally via a nippled bottle (for infants), glass, straw, or small-bore nasogastric tube (for uncooperative patients). The recommended dose is 1 to 2 g/kg body weight, using 8 mL of diluent per gram of charcoal, if a premixed formulation is not available. Palatability may be increased by adding a sweetener (sorbitol) or a flavoring agent (cherry, chocolate, or coke syrup) to the suspension. Charcoal adsorbs ingested poisons within the gut lumen, allowing the charcoal-toxin complex to be evacuated with stool. The complex can also be removed from the stomach by induced emesis or lavage. In vitro, charcoal adsorbs 90 percent or more of most poisons when given in a ratio 10 times that of the toxin. Superactivated charcoal (SuperChar) is two to three times more effective than standard charcoal. Charged (ionized) chemicals such as mineral acids, alkalis, and highly dissociated salts of cyanide, fluoride, iron, lithium, and other inorganic compounds are not well adsorbed by charcoal. Charcoal decreases the absorption of other poisons by an average of 80 percent when given within 5 min of poison administration, 59 percent when given at 30 min, and 33 percent at 60 min. Charcoal is of equal or greater efficacy than ipecac syrup or gastric lavage. Lavage followed by charcoal is more effective than charcoal alone, and charcoal before and after lavage is more effective than charcoal alone or charcoal after lavage. Although the clinical efficacy of charcoal is not known, the outcome of patients treated with charcoal alone is at least as favorable as of those given ipecac followed by charcoal and those treated with lavage followed by charcoal. In those treated sooner than 1 h, the combination of lavage and charcoal is more effective than charcoal alone. Side effects of charcoal include nausea, vomiting, and diarrhea or constipation. Charcoal may also prevent the absorption of orally administered therapeutic agents. Complications include mechanical obstruction of the airway, aspiration, vomiting, and bowel obstruction by inspissated charcoal. Charcoal is contraindicated in patients with corrosive ingestion because it obscures endoscopy.

Whole-bowel irrigation is performed by administering a bowel cleansing solution containing electrolytes and polyethylene glycol (Golytely, Colyte) orally or by gastric tube at a rate of up 0.5 L/h in children and 2.0 L/h in adults until rectal effluent is clear. The patient must be in a sitting position. Although data are limited, whole-bowel irrigation may be more effective than the previously discussed procedures. It may be of particular benefit in patients with foreign body, drug packet, and slow-release medication ingestions.

Cathartic salts (disodium phosphate, magnesium citrate and sulfate, sodium sulfate) or *saccharides* (mannitol, sorbitol) promote the rectal evacuation of gastrointestinal contents. The most effective cathartic is sorbitol in a dose of 1 to 2 g/kg body weight. Alone, cathartics do not prevent poison absorption, except perhaps for the agents used with whole-bowel irrigation. They are of primary use to prevent constipation following charcoal administration. Abdominal cramps, nausea, and vomiting are occasional side effects. Complications include hypermagnesemia and excessive diarrhea. The agents are contraindicated in patients who have ingested corrosives and in those with preexisting diarrhea. Magnesium-containing cathartics should not be used in patients with renal failure.

Dilution is accomplished by having the patient drink 5 mL/kg body weight of water or other clear liquid as soon as possible after the ingestion of a corrosive (acids, alkali). Dilution may also be used as an adjunct to ipecac syrup. Otherwise, it is not indicated because it may increase the dissolution rate (and hence absorption) of capsules, tablets, and other solids.

Endoscopic or surgical removal of poisons may be useful in rare situations such as ingestion of a potentially toxic foreign body that fails to transit the GI tract, a potentially lethal amount of a heavy metal (arsenic, iron, mercury, thallium), or large concretions of pills. Patients who ingest packets of drugs (cocaine) and then become toxic due to packet leakage or rupture require immediate surgical intervention.

DECONTAMINATION OF OTHER SITES Immediate copious flushing with water, saline, or other available clear drinkable liquid is the initial treatment of topical exposures (particularly with corrosives and solvents). Saline is preferred for eye irrigation. A triple wash (water then soap then more water) may be optimal for dermal decontamination. Inhalational exposures should be initially treated with fresh air or oxygen. The removal of liquid poisons from body cavities such as the vagina or rectum is best accomplished by irrigation. Solid poisons (drug packets, pills) should be removed with visual guidance.

ENHANCEMENT OF POISON ELIMINATION

Although the elimination of most poisons can be accelerated by therapeutic interventions, pharmacokinetic efficacy (removal of drug at a rate greater than that accomplished by intrinsic elimination) and the clinical benefits (shortened duration of toxicity, improved outcome) are often more theoretical than proven. Hence, the decision to use a procedure should be based on the actual or predicted toxicity and the potential efficacy and risks.

MULTIPLE-DOSE ACTIVATED CHARCOAL Repeated oral dosing with charcoal (with sorbitol as needed to enhance gastrointestinal motility) enhances the elimination of some poisons. A dose of 1 g/kg body weight every 2 to 4 h, adjusted downward to avoid regurgitation in patients with decreased gastrointestinal motility, is generally recommended. This treatment enhances the elimination of a variety of drugs (carbamazepine, dapsone, diazepam, digoxin, glutethimide, meprobamate, methotrexate, phenobarbital, phenytoin, salicylate, theophylline, valproic acid). Efficacy approaches that of hemodialysis for some agents (theophylline). Multiple-dose therapy is not effective in accelerating elimination of chlorpropamide or imipramine.

FORCED DIURESIS AND ALTERATION OF URINARY pH Diuresis and ion trapping via alteration of urine pH may prevent the renal reabsorption of poisons that undergo excretion by glomerular filtration and active tubular secretion. Since membranes are more permeable to nonionized molecules than to their ionized counterparts, acidic (low pK_a) poisons are ionized and trapped in an alkaline urine, and basic poisons are ionized and trapped in an acid urine. Alkaline diuresis (a urine pH of 7.5 or greater and a urine output of 3 to 6 mL/kg body weight per hour) enhances the elimination of chlorphenoxyacetic acid herbicides, chlorpropamide, phenobarbital (and probably other long-acting barbiturates), and salicylates. Contraindications include congestive heart failure, renal failure, and cerebral edema. Acid-base, fluid, and electrolyte parameters should be carefully monitored. Saline diuresis may enhance the secretion of bromide, lithium, and isoniazid. Acid diuresis enhances the renal elimination of several poisons (amphetamines, cocaine, phencyclidine, quinidine, quinine, sympathomimetics, strychnine), but its use has been largely abandoned because risks are significant and because clinical efficacy has not been established.

EXTRACORPORAL REMOVAL Peritoneal dialysis, hemodialysis, charcoal or resin hemoperfusion, hemofiltration, plasmapheresis, and exchange transfusion are capable of removing any toxin from the bloodstream. Toxins most amenable to enhanced elimination by dialysis have low molecular mass (<500 Da), high water solubility, low protein binding, small volumes of distribution (<1 L/kg body weight), prolonged elimination (long half-life), and high dialysis clearance relative to total body clearance. The efficacy of the other forms of extracorporal removal is not limited by molecular weight, water solubility, or protein binding. Dialysis should be considered in severe poisoning due to bromide, chloral hydrate, ethanol, ethylene glycol, isopropyl alcohol, lithium, heavy metals, methanol, and salicylate. Although hemoperfusion may be effective in removing some of these poisons, it does not correct associated acid-base and electrolyte abnormalities.

Hemoperfusion should be considered in severe poisoning due to chloramphenicol, disopyramide, and hypnotic sedatives (barbiturates, ethchlorvynol, glutethimide, meprobamate, methaqualone, phenytoin, and theophylline). Both techniques require central venous access and systemic anticoagulation and often result in transient hypotension. Hemoperfusion may also cause hemolysis, hypocalcemia, and thrombocytopenia. Peritoneal dialysis and exchange transfusion are less effective but may be used when other procedures are not available, are contraindicated, or are technically difficult (in infants). Exchange transfusion removes poisons affecting red blood cells (e.g., methemoglobinemia or arsine-induced hemolysis). The efficacy of other extracorporeal elimination procedures has not been defined.

Candidates for these invasive treatments include patients with severe toxicity who deteriorate despite aggressive supportive therapy, those with potentially dangerous blood levels of toxins, those who lack the capacity for self-detoxification because of liver or renal failure, and those with serious underlying illnesses or complications that adversely affect recovery.

OTHER TECHNIQUES The enhanced elimination of heavy metals by chelation and urinary excretion of the metal-chelator complex and the accelerated removal of carbon monoxide by hyperbaric oxygenation are discussed with the specific poisons.

ADMINISTRATION OF ANTIDOTES

Antidotes counteract the effects of poisons by neutralizing them (antibody-antigen reactions, chelation, chemical binding) or by an-

tagonizing their physiologic effects (activation of opposing nervous system activity, provision of competitive metabolic or receptor substrate). Antidotes can significantly reduce morbidity and mortality, but most antidotes are potentially toxic. Poisons or conditions with specific antidotes include acetaminophen, anticholinergic agents, anticoagulants, beta blockers, calcium channel blockers, carbon monoxide, cholinergic agents, cyanide, digitalis, drugs that cause dystonic reactions, ethylene glycol, fluoride, heavy metals, hydrogen sulfide, hypoglycemic agents, isoniazid, methemoglobinemia, narcotics, sympathomimetics, and vacor. Since the safe use of antidotes requires correct identification of a specific poisoning or syndrome, antidotal therapy is discussed with the conditions for which they are indicated.

PREVENTION OF REEXPOSURE

Poisoning is a preventable illness. Unfortunately, some adults and children are poison-prone, and recurrences are common. Adults with accidental exposures should be instructed regarding the safe use of medications and chemicals (according to labeling instructions). Confused patients may need assistance with the administration of medications. Errors in dosing by health care providers require special educational efforts. Patients should be advised to avoid circumstances that result in chemical exposure or poisoning. Regulatory agencies and health departments should be notified in cases of environmental or workplace exposure. The best approach with young children and patients with intentional overdose is to limit access to poisons. Indeed, the environment of children must be made poison-proof. Alcoholic beverages, medications, household products (automotive, cleaning, fuel, pet-care, toiletry products), nonedible plants, and vitamins should be kept out of reach or in locked or child-proof cabinets. Depressed or psychotic patients should be given prescriptions for a limited (2 week) supply of drugs and with a limited number of refills. All patients should be monitored for compliance and response to therapy.

SPECIFIC POISONS

The poisons in this section are common, produce life-threatening toxicity, or require unique therapeutic interventions. Poisons not mentioned here are described in the referenced texts. Drug and alcohol abuse are discussed in Chaps. 370 to 372. Heavy metal poisoning is discussed in Chap. 375.

ACETAMINOPHEN At therapeutic doses, acetaminophen is metabolized to sulfate and glucuronide conjugates that are excreted in the urine. Minor amounts are excreted unchanged or as mercapturic acid after conjugation with hepatic glutathione. Following an acute overdose of 140 mg/kg body weight or more, the sulfate and glucuronide pathways become saturated, resulting in an increased fraction of acetaminophen metabolized to mercapturic acid. Once hepatic glutathione is depleted, reactive metabolites are formed that covalently bind to hepatocytes and cause cell lysis. Acetaminophen is rapidly absorbed from the stomach and small bowel and has a volume of distribution of 1 L/kg body weight. Approximately 50 percent is protein bound. The plasma half-life is 1 to 2 h.

Clinical signs Early manifestations of poisoning are nonspecific and not predictive of subsequent hepatotoxicity. Within 2 to 4 h of ingestion, nausea, vomiting, diaphoresis, and pallor develop. Central nervous system depression is absent unless depressant drugs are coingested. Within 24 to 48 h, hepatotoxicity is evidenced by right upper quadrant tenderness and mild hepatomegaly and followed by the appearance of jaundice, clotting abnormalities, and hepatic encephalopathy. Laboratory evidence of hepatic toxicity includes elevation in serum transaminase activity (AST, ALT). With severe ingestion, prolongation of the prothrombin time, elevation of serum bilirubin, and ultimately hyperammonemia may occur. A twofold

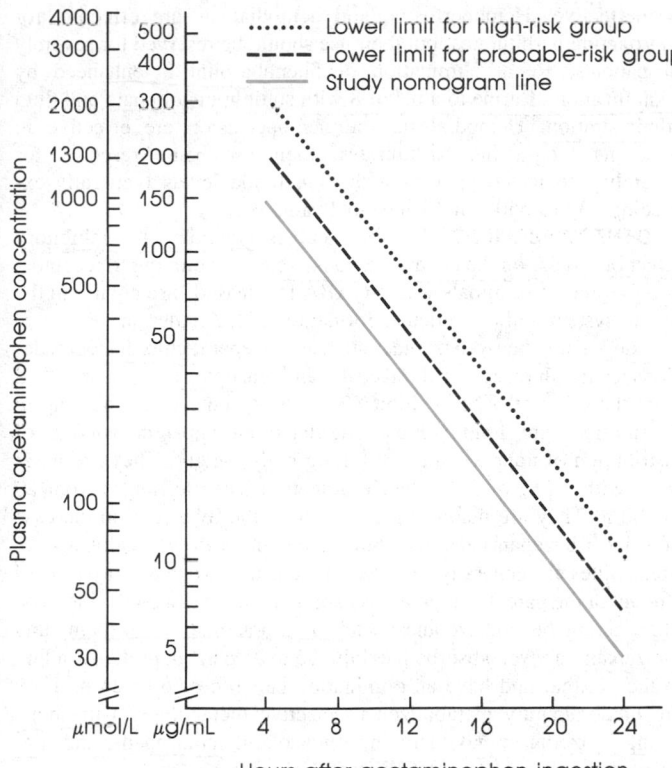

FIGURE 374-1 Nomogram to define risk according to initial plasma acetaminophen concentration. (*After BH Rumack, H Matthew, Pediatrics 55:871, 1975.*)

prolongation of prothombin time and/or serum bilirubin greater than 68 μmol/L (4 mg/dL) on the 3d to 5th day after ingestion indicate severe hepatotoxicity. Histologic evidence of liver damage varies from cytolysis to centrilobular necrosis. Liver histology returns to normal within 3 months. Renal function may also be affected.

Diagnosis A serum acetaminophen level should be determined between 4 and 24 h after ingestion and compared against the Rumack-Matthew nomogram (Fig. 374-1). A level above the two lines on the nomogram is predictive of possible or probable hepatotoxicity. The acetaminophen half-life may be prolonged in patients who develop liver damage.

Treatment Initial treatment involves removal of the ingested product from the gastrointestinal tract. Activated charcoal should be administered. (Charcoal does not significantly interfere with acetylcysteine therapy.) In patients with an acetaminophen level exceeding the lower nomogram line, acetylcysteine therapy is indicated up to 24 h following ingestion. Maximal benefit is achieved if therapy is instituted within 8 to 10 h of the ingestion. Acetylcysteine is given at a loading dose of 140 mg/kg body weight, followed by a maintenance dose of 70 mg/kg body weight every 4 h for 17 doses. Side effects include nausea, vomiting, and epigastric discomfort. If treatment is started prior to availability of the serum level and if the level is subsequently shown to be below the toxic level, therapy may be discontinued. Intravenous acetylcysteine is an investigational drug in this country and requires a protocol for administration. Diuresis has no value.

ACIDS AND ALKALI Burns of the mouth, esophagus, and stomach result from the ingestion of liquid or solid forms of alkali or acids. Common alkaline products include industrial-strength bleach, drain cleaners (sodium hydroxide), surface cleaners (ammonia, phosphates), laundry and dishwasher detergents (phosphates, carbonates), disc batteries, denture cleaners (borates, phosphates, carbonates), and Clinitest tablets (sodium hydroxides). Acids are used in toilet bowl cleaners (hydrofluoric, phosphoric, sulfuric acids), soldering fluxes (hydrochloric acid), antirust compounds (hydrofluoric, oxalic acids),

automobile battery fluid (sulfuric acid), and slate cleaners (hydrofluoric acid).

Alkalies produce liquefactive necrosis with rapidly penetrating tissue burns and higher risk of perforation of the esophagus and stomach than do acids. Acids produce coagulative necrosis. Both burn the mouth, esophagus, and stomach. Liquids tend to produce superficial, often circumferential burns over a larger surface area, while solids and tablets cause localized deeper burns. The severity of the burn relates to the contact time, amount ingested, and the pH (especially <2, >12) of the ingested product.

Clinical signs Burns of the mouth result in excess salivation, pain, dysphonia, and dysphagia. Examination of the mouth shows erythema, edema, ulceration, and necrosis. Deep burns may destroy mucosal nerve endings and produce anesthesia. Esophageal symptoms and signs include drooling, painful swallowing, retrosternal pain, and neck tenderness. Vomiting of blood and mucus may occur. Perforation following alkali ingestion is suggested by increasing severity of chest pain, often with respiratory distress. Epigastric pain, vomiting, and tenderness may occur with burns to the stomach. Aspiration of acids and alkalis results in fulminant tracheitis and bronchial pneumonia. In severe cases hypotension, shock, metabolic acidosis, liver and renal dysfunction, hemolysis, and disseminated intravascular coagulation may be seen. Edema, erythema, and ulceration of the esophagus may be followed by fibrosis with stricture formation and obstruction of the esophagus (in the case of alkalis) or of the gastric outlet (in the case of acids).

Diagnosis A careful history will suggest the ingestion of an acid or an alkali. The lack of oral involvement does not rule out esophageal or gastric injury. Endoscopy is safe within 48 h (optimally 12 to 24 h) of the ingestion and will document the anatomic site and often the severity but not the depth of the injury. The endoscope should be advanced to the site of injury but not past it due to risk of producing perforation. Residual effects of the ingestion can be assessed by barium swallow. Chest x-rays may be necessary to confirm aspiration of the ingested product.

Treatment Treatment consists of immediate dilution to wash the product off the mucosal surface. Weak acid or basic solutions should not be used since the heat of neutralization may cause thermal burns and increase tissue injury. Symptomatic patients should be admitted for endoscopy. If alkali burns of the esophagus exist, glucocorticoids should be started within 48 h and given for 3 weeks followed by tapering. Use of prophylactic broad-spectrum antibiotics is controversial. Antacids should be used for burns of the stomach. For acid burns glucocorticoids are not useful. Esophageal stricture or gastric outlet obstruction may require subsequent dilation and bouginage or surgical reconstruction.

ANTIARRHYTHMIC DRUGS Antiarrhythmic drugs can be divided into three classes: class IA (disopyramide, procainamide, and quinidine), class IB (lidocaine, phenytoin, and tocainide), and class IC (encainide and flecainide). These agents are rapidly absorbed (except for disopyramide and sustained-release formulations), have short half-lives (3 to 11 h, somewhat longer for class IC agents), and are predominantly eliminated by hepatic metabolism.

Clinical signs The acute ingestion of more than twice the usual daily dose is potentially toxic. Onset of toxicity occurs within 1 h, and peak effects are demonstrable within several hours. Manifestations include nausea, vomiting, and diarrhea followed by lethargy, confusion, ataxia, bradycardia, hypotension, and cardiovascular collapse. Anticholinergic effects (blurred vision, dry mucosa) may be seen in disopyramide poisoning. Quinidine and class IB agents may cause agitation, dysphoria, and seizures. Nonspecific ECG findings include bradycardia with AV block and QRS-interval prolongation. Ventricular tachycardia, ventricular fibrillation, (including the polymorphous form, torsade de pointes), and QT-interval prolongation are characteristics of poisoning due to class IA and IC drugs. Depressed myocardial contactility and arrhythmias may lead to decreased cardiac output and pulmonary edema. Laboratory findings are nonspecific (metabolic acidosis), except for hypoglycemia and mild hypokalemia, which may be seen with disopyramide and quinidine intoxication, respectively. Toxicology screening will detect most of these agents. Measurement of serum levels may confirm an overdose and indicate the need for monitoring.

Treatment Treatment consists of gastrointestinal decontamination and supportive therapy. Hypotension, bradyarrhythmias, and seizures are treated with standard measures. Patients with persistent hypotension and bradycardia require monitoring of pulmonary arterial pressure. Cardiac pacing, intraaortic balloon pump counterpulsation, and cardiopulmonary bypass may be necessary. Ventricular tachyarrhythmias should be treated with lidocaine, phenytoin, and bretylium. Sodium bicarbonate or sodium lactate may be effective for tachyarrhythmias due to class IA or IC agents. Mild hypokalemia may be protective, and potassium levels that do not fall below 3.0 mmol/L may be best treated by close monitoring. For torsade de pointes (polymorphous or atypical ventricular tachycardia), magnesium sulfate (4 g or 40 mL of a 10% solution intravenously over 10 to 20 min) and overdrive pacing (with isoproterenol or electricity) may be effective. Hemodialysis and hemoperfusion may enhance the elimination of disopyramide and the active procainamide metabolite, *N*-acetylprocainamide. However, clinical experience is inadequate to support routine use.

BARBITURATES Barbiturates are generally classified into long-acting and short-acting. Long-acting barbiturates include mephobarbital, barbital, phenobarbital, and primidone. Short-acting agents include those with intermediate, short, and ultrashort durations of action such as amobarbital, butabarbital, pentobarbital.

Barbiturates exert their effects through depression of the central nervous system. Long-acting barbiturates are well absorbed from the stomach and the small bowel. Peak plasma concentrations occur within 2 to 4 h. Phenobarbital, as an example of a long-acting barbiturate, is a weak acid with a pK_a of 7.2, a volume of distribution of 0.8 L/kg body weight, and 50 percent protein binding in the plasma. Approximately 75 percent of an ingested dose is metabolized by hydroxylation, and 25 percent is excreted unchanged by the kidneys. Other long-acting barbiturates are converted to active metabolites by the liver prior to excretion (primidone to phenobarbital, mephobarbital to barbital). Phenobarbital is eliminated by first-order kinetics with a half-life of 80 to 120 h in overdose. Intermediate-, short-, and ultrashort-acting barbiturates are rapidly absorbed with an onset of action within 30 min following ingestion and peak concentrations 1 to 2 h following administration. They are lipid soluble and have an apparent volume of distribution ranging from 0.8 to 1.5 L/kg body weight. They have a pK_a of 8, are partly bound to protein in the plasma, and are mainly metabolized in the liver (up to 99 percent). The mean half-life varies from 4 h for ultrashort- to approximately 35 h for intermediate-acting barbiturates.

Clinical signs Barbiturates in low overdose produce confusion and in large overdose cause CNS depression ranging from lethargy to coma, hypotension, pulmonary edema, and cardiac arrest. Hypothermia is common in acute intoxication. Pupils are generally constricted but may dilate in terminal phases. Bullous skin lesions are seen in severe barbiturate overdose. Signs of toxicity usually appear when serum concentrations of long-acting barbiturates exceed 170 µmol/L (4 mg/dL) and short-acting barbiturates exceed 88 µmol/L (2 mg/dL). Maximal toxicity occurs within 4 to 6 h after short-acting barbiturate but may be delayed 10 h or more after overdosage with long-acting barbiturates. The degree of CNS depression relative to ingested dose is dependent upon prior exposure to the drug.

Treatment Initial management involves prompt gastrointestinal decontamination. Barbiturates are well adsorbed by activated charcoal. In the case of long acting barbiturate poisoning, repetitive administration of activated charcoal every 2 to 4 h enhances elimination threefold and decreases half-life by approximately 50 percent. For all barbiturates, attention should be given to hemodynamic and respiratory support, correction of temperature and electrolyte derangement, and monitoring for pulmonary complications. Since short-acting barbiturates are predominantly metabolized by the liver, diuresis

is ineffective. Hemoperfusion and hemodialysis are effective for short-acting barbiturates, but their use should be reserved for severely ill patients. Renal elimination of phenobarbital is enhanced by alkalinization of urine to a pH of 8 with sodium bicarbonate and fluid administration. Hemodialysis and hemoperfusion are effective in removing long-acting barbiturates, their use being reserved for severely intoxicated patients with high blood levels [generally exceeding 430 to 650 µmol/L (10 to 15 mg/dL)].

BENZODIAZEPINES Benzodiazepines potentiate the inhibitory effect of GABA on the central nervous system by binding to receptors at polysynaptic terminals where GABA is released, principally in the limbic system and the reticular formation of the midbrain.

Long-acting benzodiazepines such as diazepam, chlordiazepoxide, clonazepam, flurazepam, clorazepate, and prazepam are well absorbed from the GI tract. They exhibit 85 to 95 percent protein binding in the plasma, are lipid soluble and have an apparent volume of distribution of approximately 1.1 L/kg body weight. They are weak acids with a pK_a of 3.4. Their elimination half-life ranges from 20 to 100 h. They are mainly metabolized by the liver, and in the case of some (diazepam) the metabolites are pharmacologically active. Metabolites are generally excreted in the urine, whereas only a small amount of the parent compound is excreted unchanged by the kidneys. Short-acting benzodiazepines, such as alprazolam, oxazepam, and lorazepam, are well absorbed, exhibit 85 to 95 percent protein binding in the plasma, and have an elimination half-life of 6 to 24 h. They are predominantly metabolized to inactive metabolites. Ultrashort-acting benzodiazepines including midazolam, temazepam, and triazolam have elimination half-lives of 3 to 12 h.

Clinical signs The major effects include weakness, ataxia, drowsiness, and, in severe overdose, coma and respiratory depression. Pupils are generally constricted and unresponsive to naloxone. Respiratory support is rarely needed except in the case of ultrashort-acting agents, massive overdose, or the co-ingestion of other sedative drugs. Ethanol enhances the absorption of benzodiazepine and potentiates the CNS depression. Confirmation of the diagnosis is made by identification of the metabolites in urine.

Treatment Initial management includes prompt gastrointestinal decontamination. Single-dose as well as repeated-dose activated charcoal when metabolites are active (diazepam) is indicated. High protein binding of benzodiazepines limits efficacy of hemodialysis.

BETA-ADRENERGIC BLOCKING AGENTS Beta-adrenergic blocking agents approved for use in the United States include acebutolol, atenolol, esmolol, labetalol, metoprolol, nadolol, pindolol, propranolol, sotalol, and timolol.

Beta blockers act by competitively blocking beta-adrenergic neurohumoral receptors in the bronchial and vascular smooth muscle and myocardium. At therapeutic doses, some beta-blockers act predominantly on beta$_1$ receptors and are "cardioselective" (acebutolol, atenolol, metoprolol), some have partial agonist or sympathomimetic activity (acebutolol, pindolol, timolol), and some have quinidine-like myocardial membrane stabilizing effects (acebutolol, metoprolol, pindolol, propranolol, sotalol). Antiarrhythmic effects are due to a reduction of sodium and calcium influx during membrane depolarization (phase 0) as a consequence of decreased production of cyclic AMP by adenylate cyclase. This activity defines beta blockers as class II antiarrhythmics. Beta blockers decrease cardiac contractility by directly inhibiting the release of calcium from sarcoplasmic reticulum. Following overdose, cardioselectivity is lost, and all beta blockers may cause membrane depressant effects.

Beta blockers are rapidly and well absorbed. They exhibit variable protein binding (5 to 93 percent), low water solubility and variable volumes of distribution (1 to 5.6 L/kg body weight), and are eliminated predominantly by hepatic metabolism (exceptions include nadolol and atenolol).

Clinical signs Manifestations of toxicity usually begin with 1/2 h following an overdose and become maximal within 2 h. Common findings include nausea, vomiting, and diarrhea followed by bradycardia, hypotension, and CNS depression. However, agents with sympathomimetic activity can cause hypertension and tachycardia. Central nervous system effects vary from lethargy and confusion to coma and seizures and tend to be more pronounced with the more lipophilic agents (acebutolol, metoprolol, pindolol, propranol, and timolol). The skin is often pale and cool. Bronchospasm and pulmonary edema may occur in those with a history of asthma, chronic obstructive pulmonary disease, or congestive heart failure. Metabolic abnormalities include hyperkalemia and hypoglycemia (as a direct result of beta-adrenergic receptor blockade) and metabolic acidosis (due to seizures, shock, or respiratory depression). Electrocardiographic manifestations include all degrees of AV block, bundle branch block, prolonged QRS duration, and asystole. Sotalol poisoning may also cause QT-interval prolongation with ventricular tachycardia, ventricular fibrillation, and torsade de pointes. Patients with mild poisoning usually recover within 6 to 12 h whereas those with severe poisoning may be symptomatic for 24 to 48 h. A toxicology screen may identify the presence of beta blockers, but blood levels are not generally available nor helpful in guiding therapy.

Treatment Treatment includes gastrointestinal decontamination, nonspecific supportive measures, and the administration of calcium and glucagon. Because gastric emptying procedures may produce vagal stimulation and exacerbate bradyarrhythmias, monitoring should be instituted first. Treatment of bradycardia and hypotension should begin with atropine, isoproterenol, and dopamine. With severe poisoning these agents may be ineffective, and glucagon, calcium, cardiac pacing (external or internal), and intraaortic balloon pump support may be necessary. Glucagon, which stimulates adenylate cyclase by a nonadrenergic mechanism, should be given at an initial dose of 5 to 10 mg for adults. Patients who respond favorably should then be given an infusion of 1 to 5 mg/L. Calcium, which may reverse nonadrenergic negative inotropic effects, should be given in the same initial dose as described for calcium channel blocker poisoning. Patients with altered mental status or abnormal vital signs should also be given intravenous glucose. Bronchospasm may be treated with inhaled beta agonists, subcutaneous epinephrine, and intravenous aminophylline. Lidocaine or overdrive pacing may be used for sotalol-induced ventricular tachyarrhythmias. Extracorporal elimination procedures are probably not of benefit (exceptions include atenolol, metoprolol, nadolol, and sotalol), but clearcut clinical data are not available.

BLEACH Because of its widespread availability, sodium hypochlorite (bleach, Clorox) is associated with both accidental and purposeful overdose. Bleach solutions for home use generally contain 3 to 6% sodium hypochlorite, and industrial bleaches may have higher concentrations. These solutions have a pH of 10.5 to 11.0, and contain free chlorine, which gives the compound its characteristic odor.

Sodium hypochlorite decomposes rapidly to hypochloric acid on contact with moisture and is irritating but not caustic. Sodium hypochlorite mixed with acid decomposes to chlorine gas and when mixed with ammonia produces chloramine gas. Both chlorine and chloramine gas are highly irritating.

Clinical signs Sodium hypochlorite is irritating to the gastrointestinal mucosa and to mucous membranes of the lips, mouth, and eyes. Household bleach causes superficial injury to the esophagus, but stricture formation does not occur. If the agent is inhaled, chemical pneumonia and pulmonary edema can ensue. Industrial bleaches do cause deep burns of the esophagus with the potential for stricture formation.

Treatment Ingestion of small quantities of sodium hypochlorite should be treated by dilution with milk or water. Neutralization is not necessary, and activated charcoal and cathartics are not indicated. Large ingestions of sodium hypochlorite may require gastric lavage. Care should be taken to prevent vomiting and secondary aspiration. Exposed skin and eyes should be washed.

CALCIUM CHANNEL BLOCKERS Diltiazem, nicardipine, nifedipine, and verapamil are approved for use in the United States. These agents act by decreasing the influx of calcium across slow calcium channels in the membranes of myocardial and vascular smooth muscle cells during phases 2 (plateau) and 4 (spontaneous depolarization) of the action potential (class IV antiarrhythmics). Electrophysiologic effects include decreased cardiac contractility, heart (SA nodal) rate, AV nodal conduction, and vascular tone.

Calcium channel blockers are rapidly absorbed, exhibit high protein binding in the plasma, and have large volumes of distribution (>2 L/kg body weight). They are predominantly eliminated by hepatic metabolism, and their half-lives range from 3 to 8 h.

Clinical signs Toxicity usually develops within $\frac{1}{2}$ to 1 h of ingestion of amounts five to ten times the usual therapeutic dose. Clinical manifestations include bradycardia, hypotension, and cyanosis. Mental status changes range from confusion and drowsiness to coma and seizures and are due both to direct membrane effects and to cerebral hypoperfusion. Depression of cardiac function may lead to pulmonary edema. Electrocardiographic findings include all degrees of AV block, prolonged QRS and QT intervals (mainly with verapamil), evidence of ischemia or infarction, and asystole. Metabolic acidosis (secondary to shock) and hyperglycemia (resulting in the inhibition of insulin release) may be present. Serum calcium levels, however, remain normal.

Treatment Treatment consists of the administration of calcium and glucagon, GI tract decontamination, and supportive measures. Atropine, calcium, isoproterenol, glucagon, and electrical (external or internal) pacing, in order of preference, may be used for symptomatic bradycardia. Calcium, as the 10% chloride or gluconate salt solution, should be given in a dose of 0.2 mL/kg body weight (up to 10 mL) intravenously over 5 min. This dose may be repeated up to four times in patients with a partial, transient, or absent response, provided that serum calcium levels are monitored. A continuous calcium infusion (0.2 mL/kg body weight per hour up to a maximum of 10 mL/h) may be appropriate when relapse occurs after an initial bolus. Although electrical pacing is often required, glucagon, in the same dose as for beta-blocker poisoning, should be tried first. Hypotension that persists despite resolution of bradycardia should be treated with fluids and adrenergic agents. Amrinone, dopamine, dobutamine, glucagon and norepinephrine, alone or in combination, have been used. The benefit of restored perfusion is particularly important in patients with organ ischemia. Intraaortic balloon pump support should be used in patients unresponsive to the above measures. Patients with mild toxicity usually recover within a few hours, whereas those with severe toxicity or overdose with sustained-release preparations may remain symptomatic for 24 h or longer. Extracorporal removal techniques are unlikely to be of benefit.

CARBON MONOXIDE Carbon monoxide is produced in large amounts in industry as well as by gasoline engines, home appliances, and the incomplete combustion of wood, natural gas, and tobacco products. In addition, methylene chloride, a solvent in paint removers, is metabolized to carbon monoxide.

Carbon monoxide is rapidly absorbed through the lungs and binds to hemoglobin (forming carboxyhemoglobin) with an affinity 210 times that of oxygen, resulting in cellular anoxia. This occurs by limiting oxygen-carrying by hemoglobin, by decreasing release of oxygen to tissues (the oxygen dissociation curve shifts to the left), and by binding to various heme proteins (cytochrome oxidase, myoglobin). Once carbon monoxide exposure is discontinued, dissociation of the hemoglobin carbon monoxide complex occurs, and carbon monoxide is excreted through the lungs. At room air this results in a carbon monoxide half-life of 4 to 6 h; the half-life decreases in 100% oxygen to 40 to 80 min and in hyperbaric oxygen to 15 to 30 min. The half-life after methylene chloride exposure is considerably longer.

Clinical signs Manifestations of carbon monoxide poisoning include shortness of breath, dyspnea, tachypnea, headache, emotional lability, confusion, impaired judgment, and clumsiness. Nausea, vomiting, and diarrhea may also occur. Respiratory depression occurs with severe poisoning. Pulmonary edema may result from myocardial failure, and aspiration of vomitus may cause pneumonia. Cardiovascular manifestations include arrhythmias, heart failure, and hypotension. Blisters and bullae may develop over pressure points. The "cherry-red" color of skin and mucous membranes is rare, and cyanosis is usual. Visual field defects, blindness, and venous engorgement with papilledema or optic atrophy may be noted. Neurologic sequelae of acute carbon monoxide poisoning are due to hypoxia.

Sequelae correlate with the level of consciousness on presentation to the hospital. Up to 30 percent of exposed individuals develop multifocal neurologic signs 1 to 3 weeks after initial exposure with varying rates of eventual recovery. While elevated carboxyhemoglobin levels document carbon monoxide exposure, they do not necessarily indicate the severity of the poisoning. Traditionally, levels of 20 to 30 percent are associated with mild symptoms, 30 to 50 percent with moderate symptoms, 50 to 60 percent with severe symptoms, and levels above 60 percent are often fatal. Diffuse slow waves of low voltage on EEG may be noted. Electrocardiographic changes include sinus tachycardia, ST depression, T-wave flattening, premature ventricular contraction, and abnormalities in left ventricular wall function. Serum creatine phosphokinase (CPK) and lactate dehydrogenase (LDH) levels may be elevated. Myoglobinuria, secondary to muscle necrosis, may result in renal failure. Arterial blood gases reveal normal P_{O_2}, decreased oxygen saturation (by direct measurement rather than calculated value), and normal or slightly decreased P_{CO_2}. Metabolic acidosis is generally present.

Treatment   The patients should be removed from the site of exposure. Oxygen (100%) should be administered by a tightly fitting mask at 10 L/min until carbon monoxide levels are less than 10 percent and all symptoms have resolved. Infants and pregnant women may require prolonged treatment because fetal hemoglobin has a high affinity for carbon monoxide. Hyperbaric oxygen at 2 to 3 atm decreases the half-life of carbon monoxide to 15 to 30 min and produces sufficient dissolved oxygen to prevent tissue hypoxia. Hyperbaric oxygen shortens the duration of coma and may diminish the sequelae of carbon monoxide poisoning. While its use is limited by availability, hyperbaric oxygen is recommended for comatose patients with carbon monoxide levels over 40 percent, patients with levels above 25 percent who have seizures or intractable arrhythmias, and patients with delayed onset of sequelae.

COCAINE   (See Chap. 272)

CYANIDE   Hydrogen cyanide is used as a rodenticide and in chemical syntheses. Cyanide salts are used in photography, metallurgy, electroplating, metal cleaning and ore refining. Organic cyanide compounds are used in the synthetic rubber industry as well as in rodenticides. Cyanogenic glycosides are present in the seeds of the chokeberry, cherry, plum, peach, apricot, pear, bean, apple, and crabapple.

Cyanide inhibits mitochondrial ferricytochrome oxidase and other enzyme systems and hence blocks electron transport resulting in decreased oxidative metabolism and oxygen utilization, decreased ATP production, and lactic acidosis. Cyanide is rapidly absorbed from the stomach, lungs, mucosal surfaces, and unbroken skin. In the stomach it reacts with hydrochloric acid, liberating hydrocyanic acid, which is absorbed as cyanide ion. Cyanide is 60 percent protein bound, is concentrated in red cells, and has a volume of distribution of 1.5 L/kg body weight. Cyanide is metabolized by the mitochondrial enzyme rhodanase, which mediates the transfer of sulfur from thiosulfate to the cyanide ion producing thiocyanate, which in turn is excreted in the urine.

Clinical signs   The lethal dose of potassium or sodium cyanide is 200 to 300 mg and of hydrocyanic acid is 50 mg. Early effects of cyanide poisoning include headache, faintness, vertigo, excitement, anxiety, burning sensation in the mouth and throat, and dyspnea. Cardiovascular manifestations include tachycardia and hypertension. Nausea, vomiting, and diaphoresis are common. A bitter almond odor may be detected on the breath. Later effects include coma, convulsions, opisthotonus, trismus, paralysis, respiratory depression, pulmonary edema, arrhythmias, bradycardia, and hypotension. Ther-

apeutic intervention must be initiated on the basis of history and consistent clinical and laboratory findings. Variable correlation exists between blood cyanide levels and symptoms: levels less than 8 μmol/L (0.02 mg/dL) are associated with no symptoms, 20 to 40 μmol/L (0.05 to 0.1 mg/dL) with flushing and tachycardia, 40 to 100 μmol/L (0.1 to 0.25 mg/dL) with obtundation, 100 to 200 μmol/L (0.25 to 0.3 mg/dL) with coma and respiratory depression, and levels greater than 120 μmol/L (0.3 mg/dL) with death. Other laboratory abnormalities include lactic acidosis and narrowing of the arteriovenous oxygen saturation difference. Electrocardiographic abnormalities include both tachyarrhythmias and bradyarrhythmias such as nodal or idioventricular rhythm, atrioventricular dissociation, and progressive slowing of heart rate.

Treatment   Initial management involves general supportive measures and gastrointestinal decontamination. Amyl nitrite, sodium nitrite, and sodium thiosulfate (the Lilly cyanide antidote kit) coupled with oxygen are the cornerstones of therapy. Amyl nitrite is administered by broken ampul and inhaled by the patient for 30 s of each minute. A new ampul should be used every 3 min. The drug produces 5% methemoglobinemia (by converting ferrous iron to its ferric state). Methemoglobin has a higher affinity for cyanide, thereby promoting release of cyanide from mitochondrial cytochrome oxidase sites and forming cyanomethemoglobin. This process is continued while sodium nitrite is being prepared but may be omitted if sodium nitrite is available. Sodium nitrite is then administered intravenously as a 3% solution at a rate of 2.5 to 5.0 mL per minute up to a total dose of 10 to 15 mL (300 to 450 mg) in an effort to produce a 25% methemoglobin concentration. The dose in children is 0.33 mL/kg body weight (10 mg/kg body weight). Finally, sodium thiosulfate is used to remove and bind circulating cyanide from its methemoglobin sites and produce sodium thiocyanate that is excreted by the kidneys. Sodium thiosulfate is administered intravenously as a 25% solution at a dose of 50 mL (12.5 g) given over 1 to 2 min. The dose in children is 1.65 mL/kg body weight (0.5 g/kg body weight). With recurrent symptoms, half of the initial doses of both sodium nitrite and sodium thiosulfate are administered. Sodium thiosulfate is of low toxicity. Oxygen is a safe and important antidote by reversing binding of cyanide to cytochrome oxidase sites and increasing the delivery of oxygen to tissues. It also enhances the efficacy of sodium nitrite and sodium thiosulfate.

DIGOXIN   Cardiac glycoside poisoning occurs most frequently as overdosage during therapeutic use of digitalis preparations and on occasion with plant (oleander) ingestion. Digoxin and other glycosides act by inhibiting the enzyme sodium-potassium ATPase, leading to increased intracellular Na^+ and Ca^{2+} and decreased K^+. Serum levels of digoxin peak 2 to 6 h following ingestion. Digoxin is 25 to 30 percent protein bound in the plasma. Digoxin has a large volume of distribution of 5 to 6 L/kg body weight and is localized in skeletal muscle, liver, and heart. The cardiac-to-plasma ratio for digoxin is approximately 30 to 1; the elimination half-life ranges between 36 and 45 h, is prolonged in renal failure, and may be shortened in overdose. Approximately 60 percent of a dose is excreted unchanged by the kidneys, and the remainder is metabolized by the liver to inactive metabolites. The mean therapeutic serum concentration ranges from 0.6 to 2.5 nmol/L (0.5 to 2.0 ng/mL).

Clinical signs   Symptoms of toxicity include vomiting, confusion, delirium, and occasionally hallucinations, blurred vision, photophobia, scotomata, and disturbed color perception. Cardiac manifestations include sinus arrhythmia, sinus bradycardia and all degrees of atrioventricular block. Premature ventricular contractions, bigeminy, ventricular tachycardia, and fibrillation also occur. The combination of supraventricular tachyarrhythmia and atrioventricular block is highly suggestive of digitalis toxicity. While hypokalemia is commonly associated with chronic intoxication, acute overdose produces hyperkalemia [generally with digoxin serum levels above 13 nmol/L (10 ng/mL)]. Clinical toxicity is seen with digoxin levels in excess of 3.8 to 6.4 nmol/L (3 to 5 ng/mL), and levels as high as

64 to 77 nmol/L (50 to 60 ng/mL) have been seen in the overdose setting. Levels measured sooner than 8 h after ingestion may not reflect complete tissue distributions.

Treatment Gastrointestinal decontamination is carried out with care to avoid vagal stimulation which may worsen existing conduction block. Digitalis is adsorbed effectively by activated charcoal, and repeated doses can be administered to absorb active metabolites as they are excreted by the biliary tract. Diuresis, hemodialysis, and hemoperfusion are ineffective because of the large volume of distribution. Hyerkalemia should be managed with oral sodium polystyrene sulfonate, insulin, and glucose. Atropine is effective for sinus bradycardia and for second and third degree heart block. Electrical pacing may be necessary when heart block is unresponsive to atropine, and magnesium sulfate, phenytoin, and lidocaine may be useful in the treatment of arrhythmias. Cardiac glycoside antibodies are also available for the treatment of severe poisoning. These digoxin-specific Fab fragment antibodies are given intravenously in molar equivalency with the estimated ingested overdose to patients with refractory arrhythmias and significantly elevated serum digoxin concentrations. Following their administration, cardiac arrhythmias and hyperkalemia are corrected within hours; digoxin is bound to Fab fragments and excreted with a half-life of 9 h. The antibodies are given intravenously over 30 min, unless cardiac arrest has occurred, in which case the solution is given as a bolus. The dosage (in 40-mg vials to be given) is estimated by dividing the ingested dose in milligrams by 0.6 mg/vial. (Each milligram of Fab fragments binds 0.015 mg digoxin.) Alternatively, the dose (in vials) can be estimated by multiplying the steady-state serum concentration of digoxin by 0.0093 times the patient's weight (in kilograms). If both dose and serum levels are unknown, an initial dose of 5 to 10 vials may be given to adults. The antibodies cross-react with other cardiac glycosides so that larger doses may be needed for toxicity involving digitoxin.

ETHANOL (See Chap. 370)

ETHYLENE GLYCOL Ethylene glycol is a colorless, odorless, sweet-tasting water soluble liquid that is used as a solvent for paints, plastics, and pharmaceuticals and in the manufacture of explosives, fire extinguishers, foams, hydraulic fluids, windshield cleaners, and de-icer preparations. Most cases of poisoning occur as a result of the ingestion of automobile radiator antifreeze, which contains 95 percent ethylene glycol.

Ethylene glycol is rapidly absorbed. Peak levels occur approximately 2 h following ingestion. Ethylene glycol has a volume of distribution of 0.6 to 0.8 L/kg body weight. Ethylene glycol is oxidized by alcohol dehydrogenase to glycoaldehyde, then metabolized to glycolic acid, glyoxylic acid, and oxalic acid. As much as 20 to 50 percent is excreted unchanged in the urine. The half-life ranges from 3 to 8 h. Since alcohol dehydrogenase has a higher affinity for ethanol than ethylene glycol, ethanol is preferentially metabolized when both alcohols are present. Ethanol inhibits metabolism of ethylene glycol and prolongs its half-life to about 17 h. Ethylene glycol produces CNS depression in overdose. Glycoaldehyde also produces CNS depression, but because of rapid metabolism is unlikely to cause signs and symptoms. Glycolic acid is responsible for decreased serum bicarbonate, metabolic acidosis, and increased anion gap and for interstitial and tubular damage to the kidney. Glyoxylic acid is more toxic than glycolic acid, but because it is oxidized so rapidly to oxalic acid, glycolic acid contributes little to the toxicity of ethylene glycol. Oxalic acid may precipitate as calcium oxalate crystals in the brain, heart, kidney, lung, pancreas, and urine. Precipitation of calcium oxalate may result in hypocalcemia.

Clinical signs As little as 120 mg/kg body weight or 0.1 mL/kg body weight of pure ethylene glycol can result in a serum ethylene glycol concentration of 3 mmol/L (20 mg/dL). Hence, one swallow of ethylene glycol is potentially hazardous. Signs and symptoms appear within 30 min following ingestion and include nausea, vomiting, slurred speech, ataxia, nystagmus, and lethargy. A faint, sweet aromatic odor may be detected on the breath. Coma, seizures,

respiratory depression, cardiovascular collapse, and death may occur. Ethylene glycol metabolites produce signs and symptoms 4 to 12 h following ingestion. At this stage the patient appears more ill than intoxicated. Manifestations include tachypnea, hypotension, agitation, confusion, lethargy, coma, and seizures. Hypocalcemia occurs in a third of patients. Leukocytosis is present in the majority. In severe cases adult respiratory distress syndrome, cyanosis, pulmonary edema, and cardiomegaly may be seen. In this stage the diagnosis is suggested by metabolic acidosis and an abnormal urinalysis (crystalluria). In patients who survive the early stages, acute tubular necrosis manifested by proteinuria, oliguria, and anuria ensues 12 to 24 h following ingestion. Early in intoxication an elevated osmolality is present. Later, an elevated anion gap and decreased serum bicarbonate and chloride are observed. Signs of alcohol-like intoxication suggest a serum ethylene glycol level greater than 8 to 16 mmol/L (50 to 100 mg/dL). Survival has been reported with levels as high as 100 mmol/L (650 mg/dL).

Diagnosis Diagnosis is suggested by a history of exposure to antifreeze in association with CNS depression, an elevated serum osmolality, and a large anion gap. Levels of ethylene glycol (early) and glycolic acid (late) should be determined. Oxalate crystals in the urine suggest the diagnosis.

Treatment Gastrointestinal lavage and then activated charcoal should be administered. Supportive measures include protection of the airway and ventilatory and circulatory support. Seizures should be treated with phenytoin, a short-acting barbiturate, or a benzodiazepine. Hypocalcemia is treated with intravenous calcium salts at a dose of 7 to 14 mL (a 10% solution diluted 10 to 1 with intravenous fluids and given at a rate of 1 mL/min). Metabolic acidosis should be corrected with sodium bicarbonate. Fluids and diuretics may reverse oligura but do not enhance the elimination rate of ethylene glycol. Indications for ethanol therapy include a history or strong suspicion of ethylene glycol ingestion, an ethylene glycol concentration greater than 3 mmol/L (20 mg/dL), and acidosis regardless of the absolute ethylene glycol concentration. A serum ethanol level of at least 20 mmol/L (100 mg/dL) is required to inhibit alcohol dehydrogenase (higher levels may be needed with very high ethylene glycol concentrations). The loading and maintenance doses of ethanol are the same as for methanol poisoning. Serum ethanol and ethylene glycol concentrations should be monitored frequently. Methypyrazole, a competitive inhibitor of alcohol dehydrogenase, is under study as a nontoxic, experimental alternative to ethanol for ethylene glycol poisoning. Hemodialysis reduces ethylene glycol half-life from 17 h on ethanol therapy to 3 h. Indications for hemodialysis include metabolic acidosis not correctable with bicarbonate and ethanol therapy, failure to improve despite treatment, ethylene glycol concentrations greater than 8 mmol/L (50 mg/dL), or renal failure. Supplemental thiamine and pyridoxine may also be beneficial.

HALLUCINOGENS (See also Chap. 372) Hallucinogens occur in three chemical classes, phenylalkylamines, tryptamines, and ergolines, with mescaline, psilocybin, and lysergic acid (LSD) being the prototype for each. Large numbers of synthetic analogues exist in each class. Mescaline is a derivative of the peyote cactus which grows in the southwestern United States. Psilocybin is derived from mushrooms. Lysergic acid is found in the fungus *Claviceps purpurea*, which grows as a contaminant on rye and wheat, and in morning glory seeds. Synthetic LSD is the common source of the street drug.

Mescaline is well absorbed from the gastrointestinal tract and nasal mucosa. It has an apparent volume of distribution of 2 to 3 L/kg body weight and is eliminated by hepatic metabolism. Psilocybin is also rapidly absorbed from the gastrointestinal tract and converted to an active psilocin. Pharmacokinetics of psilocybin are not well worked out. Lysergic acid is generally taken either by ingestion or inhalation ("snorting") and is rapidly absorbed by both the nasal mucosa and gastrointestinal tract. Peak levels of LSD are achieved within 1 to 2 h following ingestion. The drug is protein bound (80 to 90 percent) and has an apparent volume of distribution of 0.8 L/

kg body weight. It is concentrated in kidney, spleen, and liver and in the reticular activating system of the brain. It is metabolized to inactive metabolites that are excreted in the feces and urine. The half-life of LSD is 3 h.

Clinical signs The primary effect of these agents is to produce disordered thought, mood changes, and sensory misperceptions (auditory, gustatory, olfactory, and visual dysesthesias). Mescaline is one four-thousandths as potent as LSD. It is associated with a higher incidence of nausea and vomiting but causes only mild physiologic stimulation (Table 374-2). Psilocybin has one two-hundredths the potency of LSD. Its effects are similar to those of LSD with unique features including fever, hypotonia, and seizures. The effects of LSD may last for 4 to 6 h and include mydriasis, conjunctival injection, piloerection, hypertension, tachycardia, tachypnea, anorexia, tremors, and hyperreflexia. Psychological effects include loss of body image, visual illusions, and alteration of the senses. The psychological effects (''trip'') generally last for 6 to 12 h and can be pleasant or alarming. The EEG may show paroxysmal discharges, and seizures may occur. Flashbacks or recurrences of visual images may appear up to 18 months after ingestion.

Diagnosis Identification of LSD in serum is difficult because of its small quantities. In urine, LSD can be detected for up to 5 days following ingestion, and mescaline can be detected for up to 24 h. Psilocybin is usually not detected in the routine toxic screens.

Treatment Gastrointestinal decontamination is not useful once symptoms are present and may lead to further exacerbation of symptoms. The mainstay of therapy is prevention of physical injury by calming in a quiet room with low lights. Physical restraint may cause hyperthermia, rhabdomyolysis, and acute renal failure. Benzodiazepines are effective for acute panic reaction, and butyrephenones (haloperidol in particular) may be indicated for severe psychotic reactions (see Chap. 372).

HYDROCARBONS Hydrocarbons exist in a number of forms including aromatic hydrocarbons, such as xylene and toluene, halogenated hydrocarbons, such as carbon tetrachloride and trichlorethane, and petroleum distillate hydrocarbons, such as gasoline, lacquer thinner, mineral seal oil, kerosene, and lighter fluid.

All hydrocarbons are CNS depressants. Aromatic and halogenated hydrocarbons are rapidly absorbed and distributed into the central nervous system, myocardium, liver, and kidneys. Petroleum distillate hydrocarbons are toxic to the GI tract, central nervous system, and lungs. The lung involvement is predominantly due to aspiration pneumonitis.

Clinical signs Aromatic hydrocarbons and halogenated hydrocarbons produce excitation in low dose and depression of the central nervous system in high dose. Coma and, rarely, seizures may occur. Other target organs include the GI tract (nausea, vomiting, and abdominal pain), the kidneys (renal tubular acidosis), the hematopoietic system (bone marrow suppression), skeletal muscles (rhabdomyolysis), and brain (permanent psychosis and cerebral atrophy). Sudden death due to myocardial irritability and ventricular fibrillation may occur following hydrocarbon sniffing. Petroleum distillate hydrocarbons cause burning of the mouth and throat with subsequent nausea, vomiting, and diarrhea. Respiratory symptoms include cough, dyspnea, tachypnea, hypoxia, and cyanosis. Lethargy is the most prominent CNS manifestation. Coma and convulsions are rare. Laboratory diagnosis of aromatic, halogenated, or petroleum distillate hydrocarbon poisoning is not available at present.

Treatment Aromatic and halogenated hydrocarbons require prompt gastric lavage. Absorption is rapid and complete within 1 to 2 h following ingestion. Activated charcoal is generally not effective. Supportive therapy includes oxygen, respiratory support, and monitoring of liver, renal, and myocardial function. In the case of petroleum distillate hydrocarbons, unless very large amounts (greater than 18 mL/kg body weight) are ingested, gastric lavage and ipecac-induced emesis are contraindicated. Activated charcoal adsorbs petroleum distillate hydrocarbons, but because administration may result in vomiting and subsequent aspiration their use is contraindicated.

Pulmonary involvement causes consistent symptoms and x-ray changes. If pneumonia is present, supportive therapy and monitoring for superimposed bacterial infection are indicated. Glucocorticoids are ineffective for hydrocarbon pneumonia. CNS effects are relatively short-lived and require careful monitoring and respiratory support.

HYDROGEN SULFIDE Hydrogen sulfide is encountered in the petroleum and mining industry, tanning of leather, vulcanization of rubber, production of synthetic fabrics, metal refining, production of heavy water for atomic reactors, and glue and felt manufacturing. It is encountered in sewers, sulfur springs, the holds of fishing vessels, and as a by-product of manure storage.

The hydrogen sulfide anion inhibits electron transport in the cytochrome oxidase system, thereby inhibiting aerobic metabolism with resultant cellular anoxia and cell death. Hydrogen sulfide is a highly toxic, malodorous, colorless, highly irritating gas that gains access to the blood through the mucous membranes of the tracheobronchial tree. Hydrogen sulfide is detoxified to sulfate products that are principally excreted by the kidneys.

Clinical signs Hydrogen sulfide has a characteristic odor of ''rotten eggs'' at low concentrations. It is highly irritating, resulting in rhinitis, conjunctivitis, and pharyngitis. Systemic effects include headache, vertigo, nausea, confusion, seizures, and coma. As a respiratory depressant, it also produces hypoventilation, hypoxia, cyanosis, and metabolic acidosis. Pneumonia and pulmonary edema are frequent complications of vomiting. The majority of deaths occur at the site of exposure. There is no readily available laboratory test for immediate diagnosis, and the diagnosis is based on history and clinical features.

Treatment Treatment begins with removal of the victim promptly from the site of exposure. The airway should be cleared, assisted ventilation should be used when indicated, and 100% oxygen should be administered. Nitrites may be given (see ''Cyanide'' section above) to bind the sulfide ion by removing it from cytochrome oxidase sites, thereby forming a sulfide-methemoglobin complex (sulfmethemoglobin). Nitrites also enhance detoxification by acting as a catalyst for sulfide oxidation. Absolute indications for nitrite administration do not exist. For optimal effectiveness they must be utilized immediately in symptomatic patients (sulfide oxidation is so rapid that the amount of sulfide bound to cytochrome is minimal by the time the patient presents for treatment). The dosage schedule for nitrites is the same as for cyanide poisoning. The use of thiosulfate is not necessary in sulfide poisoning. Hyperbaric oxygen should be considered in patients who do not respond to the above measures.

IRON Iron preparations may contain one of three ferrous salts (sulfate, fumarate, and gluconate). Toxicity is based on the amount of elemental iron in the salt (20 percent in the sulfate salt, 33 percent in the fumarate, and 12 percent in the gluconate). Ingestion of more than 20 mg/kg body weight of elemental iron produces gastrointestinal toxicity and of more than 60 mg/kg body weight results in systemic toxicity.

Ferrous iron is absorbed into mucosal cells of the duodenum and jejunum and is oxidized to ferric iron where it is bound to ferritin. It is slowly released from ferritin into the plasma where it is bound to transferrin, an iron-specific binding globulin, and transported to tissues for use in hemoglobin, cytochrome, and myoglobin synthesis. Approximately 70 percent of total body iron is present as hemoglobin, 25 percent is stored in liver and spleen as ferritin and hemosiderin, and 5 percent is present in myoglobin and tissue enzymes. Iron bound to transferrin is nontoxic. Free iron that exceeds the iron-binding capacity is toxic to the vasculature and also leads to the release of vasoactive substances such as serotonin and histamine. In addition, excess quantities of ferritin result in vasodilation. All these mechanisms result in increased permeability and fluid loss through the vasculature, with subsequent hypotension and metabolic acidosis. Finally, free iron injures mitochondria, causes lipid peroxidation, and results in renal, tubular, and hepatic necrosis and on occasion in myocardial and pulmonary injury. Iron can also cause irritation and ulceration of the stomach and small bowel. In overdose, iron is deposited in liver, spleen, and kidneys and causes fatty degeneration and necrosis in hepatocytes, renal tubules, and myocardial cells.

Clinical signs   Initial manifestations of iron poisoning include vomiting and diarrhea (often bloody), fever, hyperglycemia, and leukocytosis. Later effects include lethargy, hypotension, and metabolic acidosis and, with severe ingestions, seizures, coma, and vascular collapse. Jaundice, elevated hepatic enzymes, prolongation of prothrombin time, and hyperammonemia are indicative of liver injury. Proteinuria and cells in urine indicate renal injury. Pulmonary edema and hemorrhage are seen with severe overdose. In the recovering patient, gastric outlet scarring may cause obstruction. An overgrowth of *Yersinia enterocolitica* with sepsis is an infrequent complication.

Diagnosis   Iron overdosage may be confirmed by x-ray identification of iron tablets in the stomach or small bowel or by measurement of serum iron. A serum iron concentration above the iron-binding capacity [a serum level generally greater than 50 μmol/L (300 μg/dL)] suggests serious poisoning. A positive urine deferoxamine provocative challenge test (a *vin rosé* color) indicating the presence of ferrioxamine (the complex of free iron bound to deferoxamine) is diagnostic and indicates an iron level greater than the iron-binding capacity. The dose used is 50 mg/kg body weight up to 1 g of deferoxamine given intramuscularly or intravenously. In addition, a white count of greater than 15,000 and a blood sugar greater than 7 mmol/L (120 mg/dL) are associated with serum iron levels greater than 50 μmol/L (300 μg/dL).

Treatment   Removal of ingested iron is best accomplished with either ipecac-induced emesis or a large orogastric tube to remove the iron tablets. An x-ray film following gastric lavage will define the success of the decontamination procedure. Gastrostomy may be necessary for concretion formation or large quantities of iron tablets. Fifty to 100 mL of 1% bicarbonate may be instilled through the gastric tube following lavage in an effort to form an insoluble ferrous carbonate salt. Activated charcoal is ineffective. Oral deferoxamine will complex iron remaining in the stomach in an iron deferoxamine complex (ferrioxamine) which is insoluble. Since the amount of the deferoxamine to be administered is large and since iron is rapidly absorbed, this therapy is rarely used. Intravenous sodium bicarbonate should be used to correct metabolic acidosis. Hypotension may respond to volume expansion. Coagulation abnormalities should be treated with vitamin K or blood products. When serum iron exceeds the iron-binding capacity, deferoxamine should be administered intravenously. A dose of 1 to 2 g is given at an infusion rate not to exceed 10 to 15 mg/kg body weight per hour. The success of therapy is monitored through measurement of serum iron levels and showing a clearing of the *vin rosé* color in the urine. Once the serum iron is less than the iron-binding capacity, deferoxamine therapy can be discontinued. When iron levels exceed 180 μmol/L (1000 μg/dL), larger doses of deferoxamine can be given and followed by exchange transfusion or plasmapheresis to remove the iron-desferal (ferrioxamine) complex.

ISONIAZID   In acute overdose, isoniazid decreases the synthesis of the inhibitory neurotransmitter GABA by inhibiting the pyridoxal phosphate-dependent enzyme glutamic acid decarboxylase. The consequence is CNS stimulation as well as coma. Isoniazid is rapidly absorbed mainly from the small intestine. Peak serum concentrations occur within 1 to 2 h. The volume of distribution is approximately 0.6 L/kg body weight. Serum protein binding is small. Isoniazid is acetylated to acetyl-isoniazid and then hydrolyzed to isonicotinic acid. Approximately 15 percent of an ingested dose of isoniazid is excreted unchanged by the kidneys. The serum half-life of isoniazid in overdose is approximately 1 to 4 h.

Clinical signs   Within 30 min of ingestion symptoms include nausea, vomiting, dizziness, and slurred speech. The major manifestations include coma, generalized seizures, and metabolic acidosis. Seizures are protracted and relatively unresponsive to standard anticonvulsant therapy. Acidosis is transiently responsive to bicarbonate therapy and does not occur when seizures are prevented. CNS

manifestations vary from obtundation to coma and respiratory depression. Diagnosis is made through identification of isoniazid in urine or blood. Toxicity occurs with concentrations as low as 15 μmol/L (2 mg/L). Significant symptoms are seen with serum concentrations greater than 30 to 35 μmol/L (4 to 5 mg/L).

Treatment   Initial therapy consists of prompt gastrointestinal decontamination. Ipecac-induced vomiting should be avoided because of the high incidence of seizures. Isoniazid is well adsorbed by activated charcoal. Pyridoxine (vitamin B6) prevents a decrease in brain GABA concentrations and is efficacious in preventing seizures. Pyridoxine should be given slowly intravenously in weight equivalency with the ingested dose of isoniazid. When the ingested dose is not known, 5 g of pyridoxine should be administered intravenously over 30 min as a 5 to 10% concentration. Cessation of seizures and correction of metabolic acidosis are prompt. Correction of CNS depression occurs more gradually. The dose may be repeated with partial response or when symptoms recur. Diazepam is synergistic with pyridoxine for the control of isoniazid-induced seizures. Due to its low protein binding and small volume of distribution, isoniazid is efficiently removed by hemodialysis, but dialysis is rarely necessary because of the efficacy of pyridoxine.

ISOPROPYL ALCOHOL   Isopropyl alcohol is a component of rubbing alcohol, solvents, after-shave lotions, antifreeze, and window cleaners. Its metabolite, acetone, is found in cleaners, solvents, and nail polish removers.

Isopropyl alcohol, a CNS depressant, is rapidly absorbed from the stomach and the lungs but only minimally through skin. It is distributed in body water and has a volume of distribution of 0.6 L/kg body weight. Its half-life ranges from 3 to 6 h. Isopropyl alcohol is metabolized in the liver by the enzyme alcohol dehydrogenase to acetone, which is excreted by the kidneys and lungs with a half-life of 20 to 30 h. Approximately 20 percent of isopropyl alcohol is excreted unchanged through the kidneys.

Clinical signs   Symptoms occur within 30 min following ingestion. Gastrointestinal effects include vomiting, abdominal discomfort, and hematemesis. A characteristic smell of rubbing alcohol may be noted. Isopropyl alcohol and acetone are two to three times more potent than ethanol as a CNS depressant. Central nervous system manifestations include headache, dizziness, confusion, and excitation. With severe ingestion, obtundation, coma, respiratory depression, hypothermia, and hypotension may occur. Hypoglycemia may be seen. Isopropyl alcohol can cause a falsely elevated serum creatinine. Myopathy and hemolytic anemias are occasionally present. Concentrations of 8 to 17 mmol/L (50 to 100 mg/dL) produce lethargy, concentrations greater than 25 to 33 mmol/L (150 to 200 mg/dL) are associated with coma, and concentrations greater than 66 to 84 mmol/L (400 to 500 mg/dL) are potentially fatal. Serum acetone levels rise during the first 24 h following ingestion and contribute to the observed toxicity. A small anion gap may be seen as well as an increase in the serum osmolality.

Treatment   Gastrointestinal decontamination must be instituted soon following ingestion. Activated charcoal is ineffective in significantly adsorbing isopropyl alcohol. Supportive measures should include intravenous fluids and bicarbonate to correct dehydration, shock, and acidosis. Isopropyl alcohol and acetone are efficiently removed by hemodialysis. The procedure should be considered in patients with levels in the potentially lethal range or in patients inadequately managed by conservative therapy.

LITHIUM   Lithium is most commonly available as the carbonate or the citrate salt. Lithium may substitute for cellular cations (K^+ and Na^+), thereby interfering with adenylate cyclase activation, inhibiting neurotransmitter (norepinephrine) release, and reducing sodium potassium ATPase activity.

The drug is rapidly absorbed from the gastrointestinal tract and reaches peak levels within 2 to 4 h of ingestion (and later with sustained-release preparations). It exhibits low plasma protein binding and has a volume of distribution of approximately 0.6 L/kg body weight. Removal from the body is primarily (95 percent) by glomerular filtration with significant reabsorption (80 percent) by the proximal tubules. Lithium clearance is increased by alkalinization of the urine and decreased by hyponatremia. Serum half-life ranges from 18 to 36 h; the therapeutic levels range from 0.6 to 1.2 mmol/L.

Clinical signs Signs and symptoms occur 1 to 4 h after ingestion. Gastrointestinal effects include nausea, vomiting, and diarrhea; neuromuscular effects include weakness, fasciculations, and twitching; CNS effects include ataxia, tremor, myoclonus, choreoathetosis, seizures, confusion, and coma; and cardiovascular effects include ECG changes and hypotension. Laboratory abnormalities include leukocytosis, hyperglycemia, albuminuria, glycosuria, nephrogenic diabetes insipidus, ECG changes (flattened or inverted T waves, atrioventricular block, prolonged QT interval), and ventricular arrhythmias. Death is due to seizures, coma, cardiovascular collapse, or secondary infection. Chronic intoxication is associated with signs and symptoms at lower serum levels than with acute intoxication. In chronic poisoning, concentrations greater than 1.5 mmol/L are associated with nausea and vomiting; levels between 2 and 2.5 mmol/L cause drowsiness, ataxia, and muscle weakness; levels between 2.5 and 3 mmol/L produce choreoathetosis, myoclonus, and coma; levels between 3 and 4 mmol/L cause seizures and cardiac arrhythmias; and levels greater than 4 mmol/L cause hypotension and coma. In acute poisoning, serum levels may exceed 3 to 4 mmol/L with the patient remaining minimally asymptomatic.

Treatment If seen within 2 to 4 h following ingestion, gastrointestinal decontamination is indicated. Serial lithium levels should be measured until the peak level is achieved because both absorption and tissue distribution occur slowly in the overdose setting. Lithium is poorly adsorbed by activated charcoal. Supportive therapy includes standard treatments for seizures, hypotension, and arrhythmias. Symptomatic patients with serum concentrations greater than 2 to 3 mmol/L require diuretics with saline and osmotic or diuretic agents. Sodium bicarbonate enhances renal excretion of lithium. Hemodialysis is the treatment of choice for acute intoxication and is recommended in symptomatic patients with serum levels above 4.0 mmol/L. Hemodialysis may be indicated in the case of chronic ingestion in patients with serum levels less than 4.0 mmol/L. Hemodialysis may need to be repeated or prolonged due to rebound in serum levels upon cessation of hemodialysis.

MONOAMINE OXIDASE (MAO) INHIBITORS MAO inhibitors used in the treatment of endogenous depression include tranylcypromine, phenelzine, and isocarboxazid. MAO inhibitors block monoamine oxidase, thus inhibiting a major pathway for catabolism of neurotransmitters such as dopamine, norepinephrine, and 5-hydroxytryptamine. Toxicity results from accumulation and hence potentiation of neurotransmitter action.

MAO inhibitors are absorbed efficiently from the GI tract. The volume of distribution is not known but is probably large. The drugs are eliminated predominantly by hepatic metabolism, and less than 5 percent is excreted unchanged in the urine. Plasma half-life of phenelzine and tranylcypromine at therapeutic doses is 24 h.

Clinical signs Signs and symptoms begin 6 to 12 h after ingestion and may not reach peak effect until 24 h following ingestion. Early effects are those of CNS stimulation, hyperpyrexia, tachycardia, hypertension, and tachypnea (Table 374-2). Nausea and vomiting are also early manifestations. Pupils are generally dilated, and nystagmus and papilledema may be present. Agitation, hyperactivity, and confusion may be coupled with fasciculations, twitching, tremor, and rigidity. Cardiovascular and CNS depression occurs in severe overdose. The duration of illness is 3 to 5 days. Toxic concentrations of MAO inhibitors have not been established, and no assay methods are commonly available. The diagnosis is clinical.

Treatment Gastrointestinal decontamination should be vigorous and should be followed by activated charcoal and cathartics. Hyperthermia should be treated with external cooling, sedation, and neuromuscular paralysis. Severe hypertension and tachycardia may require treatment with nitroprusside and propranolol respectively. Dantrolene (2.5 mg/kg body weight by mouth or intravenously every

6 h) may be effective for hyperthermia. Hypotension should be treated with volume expanders, and pressor therapy should be administered with caution and at lower than normal doses because of the possibility of producing an exaggerated pharmacologic response. In fact, before any drug is given potential adverse interactions should be investigated. Convulsions and other severe neuromuscular effects should be treated with anticonvulsant agents. Diuresis, hemodialysis, and hemoperfusion are not effective. No specific antidote exists. Because of persistence of MAO inhibition, both drug therapy and diet should be carefully monitored for 7 to 10 days.

METHANOL Methanol is a component of shellacs, varnishes, paint removers, Sterno, windshield-washer solutions, and copy machine fluid. It is also a denaturant to make ethanol unfit for consumption.

Methanol, a mild CNS depressant, is metabolized to formaldehyde and formic acid, which in turn causes metabolic acidosis and injury to the retina.

Methanol is rapidly and completely absorbed from the GI tract, and peak levels occur within 1 to 2 h of ingestion. It is distributed throughout body water with a volume of distribution of 0.7 L/kg body weight. Its protein binding is negligible. Elimination occurs predominantly by hepatic metabolism, and 3 to 5 percent is excreted unchanged by the kidneys. Elimination follows first-order kinetics at low serum levels and converts to zero-order kinetics [approximately 3 mmol/L per hour (8.5 mg/dL per hour)] at higher levels. The rate of elimination at low overdose is approximately 14 to 20 h and at high overdose 24 to 30 h. Inhibition of alcohol dehydrogenase by ethanol [20 to 30 mmol/L (100 to 150 mg/dL)] increases the elimination time to 30 to 35 h.

Clinical signs Onset of illness is variable and may be delayed. Absence of signs and symptoms should not be equated with absence of subsequent toxicity. Early manifestations are caused by methanol, and late manifestations are due to the methanol metabolite formic acid. Methanol produces nausea, vomiting, and abdominal pain. Central nervous system manifestations include headache, vertigo, and confusion at low overdose [levels of approximately 60 mmol/L (200 mg/dL)]. In large overdose [levels greater than 60 mmol/L (200 mg/dL)] obtundation, convulsions, and coma may be seen. Late manifestations include metabolic acidosis and retinal injury. Metabolic acidosis is secondary to accumulation of formic acid, lactic acid (secondary to poor tissue perfusion), and ketones. A serum HCO_3^- below 12 mmol/L is associated with a large anion gap. Opthalmologic manifestations are present 15 to 19 hours following ingestion and include clouding and diminished vision, dancing and flashing spots, dilated or fixed pupils, hyperemia of the disk, retinal edema, and blindness. These changes are potentially reversible with prompt institution of therapy. Respirations are often rapid due to metabolic acidosis. Cardiac manifestations with severe poisoning include myocardial depression, bradycardia, and shock. Anuria predicts a poor prognosis.

Diagnosis Early diagnosis is suggested by ethanol-like signs of intoxication and an elevated serum osmolality and is confirmed by measurement of serum methanol [usually greater than 6 mmol/L (20 mg/dL)] 12 to 48 h following ingestion. The diagnosis of methanol-derived formic acidosis is suggested by a large anion gap, a low serum bicarbonate, an elevated serum formate level, and an elevated blood methanol.

Treatment Gastrointestinal decontamination is indicated soon after ingestion. Activated charcoal is not routinely used because methanol is poorly adsorbed. Cathartics are not effective. Renal clearance is not increased by diuresis. Systemic acidosis should be corrected with sodium bicarbonate. Seizures should be treated with diazepam and phenytoin. Ethanol therapy is indicated in patients with visual symptoms or a methanol level exceeding 6 to 9 mmol/L (20 to 30 mg/dL). The loading dose and subsequent maintenance dose of ethanol are as follows: loading dose—10 mL/kg body weight of 10% ethanol intravenously or 1 mL/kg body weight of 95% ethanol by mouth; maintenance dose—1.5 mL/kg body weight per hour of

10% ethanol intravenously and 3.0 mL/kg body weight per hour of 10% ethanol intravenously during dialysis. Therapy should be continued until the serum methanol level falls below 6 mmol/L (20 µg/dL) and all clinical signs are resolved. Methanol is efficiently cleared by hemodialysis because of its small volume of distribution and low protein binding. Hemodialysis is indicated for patients with methanol levels exceeding 15 mmol/L (50 mg/dL), for patients with visual signs, and for those patients whose acidosis is unresponsive to bicarbonate. For patients seen late (12 to 24 h or later) after ingestion, ethanol should be used to block further conversion of methanol to formic acid, and sodium bicarbonate should be given to correct metabolic acidosis. Elimination of formic acid is enhanced by alkalization of the urine. A formic acid level at which hemodialysis should be instituted has not been established.

METHEMOGLOBINEMIA Methemoglobinemia results from exposure to a wide variety of chemicals that oxidize ferrous hemoglobin (Fe^{2+}) to its ferric (Fe^{3+}) state. Oxidizing agents include sodium nitrite used as a meat preservative; amyl nitrite and nitroglycerin used as medications; nitrates in contaminated well water; aniline in shoe polish, paints, varnish, and inks; medications such as phenacetin, sulfonamides, pyridium, dapsone, primaquine, lidocaine, and benzocaine; and chemicals such as nitrobenzene, nitrophenol, toluidine, and isobutyl nitrate.

Ferric hemoglobin has a decreased oxygen-carrying capacity, and clinical effects are the result of tissue hypoxia. In addition, the shift of the oxygen dissociation curve to the left limits the release of oxygen to tissues. Oxidant inactivation systems include ascorbic acid and sulfhydryl agents such as glutathione, which combine with oxidizing agents and transform them to less toxic compounds. Mechanisms for the reduction of methemoglobin to oxyhemoglobin include NADH-methemoglobin reductase (responsible for 95% of activity), NADPH-methemoglobin reductase, reduced glutathione, and ascorbic acid. In the presence of NADH-methemoglobin reductase, NADH combines with methemoglobin to form oxyhemoglobin and NAD. The NADPH combines with methemoglobin in the presence of NADPH-methemoglobin reductase to produce oxyhemoglobin and NADP.

Clinical signs Cyanosis occurs with methemoglobin levels greater than 15 percent (15 g/L or 1.5 g/dL absolute methemoglobin). Patients are asymptomatic until methemoglobin levels exceed 30 percent, at which point fatigue, headache, tachycardia, dizziness, and weakness develop. At levels greater than 55 percent, dyspnea, bradycardia, hypoxia, acidosis, seizures, coma, and cardiac arrhythmias may occur. At levels greater than 70 percent, death may ensue secondary to hypoxia. Hemolytic anemia may lead to hyperkalemia and renal failure 1 to 3 days after exposure.

Diagnosis The diagnosis should be suspected in the presence of respiratory distress, brown or gray cyanosis unresponsive to oxygen, and absence of significant CNS depression. Cyanosis in conjunction with a normal P_{O_2} and decreased oxygen saturation (measured by oximeter rather than derived) suggests methemoglobinemia. Blood with high levels of methemoglobin is chocolate colored when placed on filter paper and compared to normal blood. The chocolate color does not revert to pink with oxygen but does return to normal when exposed to 10% potassium cyanide. Methemoglobin is identified by its absorption at a frequency of 630 nm on light spectrometry. Finally, the toxic screen on blood or urine may identify the drug or chemical that serves as the oxidizing agent.

Treatment The toxin, if recently ingested, should be removed by gastrointestinal decontamination followed by administration of activated charcoal and cathartics. Most oxidizing agents are metabolized rapidly, making diuresis ineffective. Dialysis may be effective, depending upon the specific compound. Treatment for methemoglobinemia includes methylene blue, packed red blood cells or exchange transfusion, and oxygen. Indications for methylene blue include a methemoglobin level above 30 g/L (cyanosis alone is not an indication for methylene blue therapy) or methemoglobinemia with hypoxia. In the patient with anemia or cardiovascular disease, methylene blue

may be indicated at lower levels due to a greater risk from tissue hypoxia. Methylene blue is given at a dose of 1 to 2 mg/kg body weight as a 1% solution over 5 min. If a clinical response is not observed within 1 h, the dose may be repeated. A methemoglobin level of 40 g/L can be expected to decrease by half in 1 to 2 h. As long as the oxidizing agent remains in the body methemoglobin will continue to be generated, and additional doses may be necessary. Side effects of methylene blue include precordial pain, dyspnea, restlessness, apprehension, and tremor; a transient blue color to the skin and urine; and the production of methemoglobin at high doses (greater than 7 mg/kg body weight) of methylene blue. Methylene blue is contraindicated in patients with deficiency of glucose-6-phosphate dehydrogenase. Additional approaches to treatment include transfusion with packed red cells optimally to a hemoglobin of 150 g/L to increase oxygen-carrying capacity and administration of 100% oxygen or hyperbaric oxygen to enhance oxygen delivery to tissues. If the methemoglobin level is very high or the patient is deficient in glucose-6-phosphate dehydrogenase exchange transfusion may be indicated.

MUSCLE RELAXANTS Muscle relaxants include orphenadrine, methocarbamol, baclofen, chlorphenesin, cyclobenzaprine, chlorzoxazone, and carisoprodol. Muscle relaxants exert some direct muscle relaxant activity but predominantly act by causing analgesia and sedation (Table 374-2). They depress synaptic reflexes, prolong synaptic recovery time, and reduce repetitive discharges. They are rapidly and completely absorbed, and peak blood levels occur 1 to 2 h following ingestion. The therapeutic half-lives are variable, with most between 1 to 4 h. The majority are metabolized by the liver to derivatives that are generally inactive and are excreted by the kidneys. Baclofen, an exception, is largely excreted unchanged in the urine but is metabolized in the liver to metabolites that undergo enterohepatic circulation.

Clinical signs Manifestations of excess amounts of carisoprodol, chlorphenesin, chlorzoxazone, and methocarbamol include nausea, vomiting, dizziness, headache, nystagmus, hypotonia, and central nervous system depression. Signs and symptoms of excess cyclobenzaprine, baclofen, and orphenadrine are more severe. Cyclobenzaprine produces anticholinergic effects coupled with agitation, hallucination, convulsions, stupor, coma, and hypotension. Baclofen causes CNS depression, hypothermia, excitability, delirium, myoclonus, seizures, conduction abnormalities, tachycardia, bradycardia, and hypotension. Orphenadrine produces anticholinergic effects, tachycardia, arrhythmias, agitation, and depression. The drugs may be identified in blood or urine by toxic screen.

Treatment Initial management includes prompt gastrointestinal decontamination. Muscle relaxants are well adsorbed by single-dose activated charcoal. Repetitive charcoal may be used for baclofen. Cathartics are also indicated. Diuresis is ineffective. The efficacy of hemodialysis or hemoperfusion is not established. Physostigmine is useful for treatment of the anticholinergic effects of orphenadrine and cyclobenzaprine.

NARCOTICS (See Chaps. 371 and 372)

NONSTEROIDAL ANTI-INFLAMMATORY DRUGS Nonsteroidal anti-inflammatory drugs (NSAIDs) fall into two classes: carboxylic acids such as ibuprofen, indomethacin, naproxen, diflunisal, fenoprofen, and tolmetin and enolic acids including phenylbutazone and piroxicam. NSAIDs inhibit prostaglandin synthesis by blocking cyclooxygenase. They are rapidly absorbed with peak blood concentrations achieved within 1 to 2 h following ingestion. They are tightly bound (greater than 95 percent) to plasma protein and have a small volume of distribution of 1.0 L/kg body weight. The pK_a ranges from 3.5 to 6.3. They are predominantly metabolized by conjugation, oxidation, and hydroxylation. Indomethacin and piroxicam undergo enterohepatic recirculation, but the activity of their metabolites is not established. A small portion (1 to 15 percent) is eliminated unchanged by the kidneys. Half-lives vary from 1 h with tolmetin to 50 to 100 h with phenylbutazone.

Clinical signs All NSAIDs may produce gastroenteritis. Other types of toxicity are variable with the carboxylic acid group. Signs and symptoms of ibuprofen toxicity are mild and include nausea, vomiting, abdominal pain, drowsiness, nystagmus, and obtundation. Diflunisal produces, in addition, hyperventilation, tachycardia, and sweating; fenoprofen is toxic to the kidneys. The enolic acid group produces coma, metabolic acidosis, seizures, and renal failure. Hepatic injury has been reported.

Diagnosis   The diagnosis is confirmed by quantification of drug in blood or urine.

Treatment   Therapy for NSAID poisoning includes gastrointestinal decontamination followed by activated charcoal and cathartics. Repeated doses of activated charcoal are of benefit for indomethacin, phenylbutazone, and piroxicam. Renal excretion is not increased by diuresis, and protein binding limits efficacy of hemodialysis. Although experience is limited, hemoperfusion can reduce serum half-life and increase clearance. No antidote is available.

ORGANOPHOSPHATE AND CARBAMATE INSECTICIDES   Organophosphorus compounds such as malathion, parathion, dichlorvos, diazinon, and chlorothion are used as agricultural and household insecticides and in the treatment of animal ectoparasites and human lice infestations. Carbamate insecticides include carbaryl, aldicarb, and propoxur. Organophosphorus insecticides irreversibly inhibit the acetylcholinesterase and cause accumulation of acetylcholine at muscarinic and nicotinic synapses. The exact mechanism by which organophosphorus compounds affect the central nervous system is unclear. Carbamates reversibly inhibit acetylcholinesterase and cause accumulation of acetylcholine at neurosynapses. Organophosphorus compounds are absorbed through the skin, lungs, and gastrointestinal tract and are distributed widely in tissues. They are metabolized in the liver, and the oxidative metabolites are active (paroxon, maloxone). Subsequent hydrolysis of organophosphorus compounds in the liver produces inactive metabolites. The elimination half-life of organophosphorus compounds has not been determined. Absorption, distribution, and elimination of carbamate insecticides are similar to those of organophosphorus insecticides.

Clinical signs   Organophosphorus compounds produce muscarinic, nicotinic, and CNS effects. Carbamates produce a similar picture but have a shorter duration of effect and a lower order of toxicity. Symptoms occur 30 min to 2 h following exposure. Early muscarinic manifestations include nausea, vomiting, abdominal cramps, and urinary and fecal incontinence. Cholinergic stimulation of the respiratory tract produces increased bronchial secretions, cough, and occasionally pulmonary edema. Cholinergic stimulation of sweat, salivary, and lacrimal glands produces sweating, salivation, and lacrimation. Miosis is usual, and blurring of vision may occur. Cholinergic stimulation results in urinary frequency and incontinence. Cholinergic effects on the cardiovascular system include bradycardia, conduction block, and hypotension. In more serious poisoning, nicotinic signs include twitching, fasciculations, weakness, diminished respiratory effort, hypertension, and tachycardia. Central nervous system effects include anxiety, restlessness, tremor, convulsions, confusion, weakness, and coma. Most patients recover within 24 to 48 h, but long-acting agents may cause toxicity for weeks to months. Death is most often due to pulmonary secretions and inadequate ventilation. A reduction of cholinesterase activity in plasma or in red blood cells to less than 50 percent of normal is diagnostic. The activity of red blood cell cholinesterase correlates best with cholinesterase activity in nerve endings and with clinical severity (at least during acute poisoning). Without treatment, return of blood cholinesterase activity to normal may take as long as 4 to 5 weeks.

In the case of carbamate insecticides, depression in plasma or red blood cell cholinesterase levels is rare because of the rapid reversibility of the inhibition. Since cholinesterase assays are not routinely or rapidly available, the initial diagnosis is clinical. Insecticides may be identified in urine on toxic screen.

Treatment   The skin should be rapidly washed with soap and water to remove the toxin, and the patient should be removed from the site of inhalation exposure. In the case of ingestion, gastrointestinal decontamination should be followed by activated charcoal. In the case of symptomatic organophosphorus and carbamate poisoning, large doses of atropine should be administered for muscarinic symptoms. A dose of 0.5 to 2 mg atropine is administered intravenously every 15 to 20 min until complete atropinization is achieved (drying of bronchial and mucous membrane secretions). Pupil size and heart rate cannot be used as end points. Once atropinization is achieved repeated doses or a constant atropine drip is necessary for several days to maintain therapeutic effectiveness. Atropine is useful for muscarinic signs, less so for CNS signs, and ineffective for nicotinic effects. Pralidoxime (2-PAM), an oxime, is effective for most nicotonic symptoms in organophosphate insecticide poisoning. The dose is 1 to 2 g intravenously over several minutes. The dose may be repeated every 8 h until nicotinic signs resolve. Reversal of CNS effects is less pronounced, and pralidoxime is ineffective for muscarinic signs. In carbamate poisoning, controversy exists over the use of pralidoxime. It should not be used in carbaryl poisoning, and in overdosage with other carbamate insecticides it should be used in conjunction with atropine.

PHENOTHIAZINE   The three major classes of phenothiazines are based on side chain substitutions—aliphatic (chlorpromazine, promethazine, promazine), piperidine (mesoridazine, thioridazine), and piperazine (perphenazine, fluphenazine, prochlorperazine, trifluoperazine) derivatives. Phenothiazines block postsynaptic dopamine receptors, exhibit anticholinergic activity, and inhibit reuptake of norepinephrine and 5-hydroxytryptamine. They also exert peripheral alpha-adrenergic blockade, lower the seizure threshold, and exert a quinidine-like effect on the heart. Peripheral anticholinergic effects result from blockade of cholinergic transmission.

Phenothiazines are efficiently absorbed from the GI tract and are metabolized promptly by the liver. Phenothiazines exhibit 95 percent protein binding, and hence the apparent volume of distribution is large (10 to 20 L/kg body weight). Only 1 percent of the administered dose is excreted unchanged in the urine. The majority of metabolites are inactive. The mean half-life for phenothiazines is generally greater than 24 h.

Clinical signs   Phenothiazines are CNS depressants, causing lethargy, obtundation, respiratory depression, and coma. Pupils are often constricted, and hypothermia and hypotension are common. Cardiac effects include hypotension, supraventricular tachycardia, atrioventricular block, and atrial and ventricular arrhythmias. Torsade de pointes, prolonged PR, QRS, and QT intervals, and U- and T-wave abnormalities may be seen especially with thioridazine and its metabolite mesoridazine. The malignant neuroleptic syndrome occurs rarely with the use of phenothiazines. Acute dystonic reactions (extrapyramidal tract signs) are prominent with the piperazine group; signs and symptoms include rigidity, opisthotonus, stiff neck, hyperreflexia, irritability, dystonia, fixed speech, torticollis, tremors, trismus, and oculogyric crisis. The reaction is idiosyncratic rather than dose related.

Diagnosis   The diagnosis is established by toxic screen on blood and urine. In the presence of extrapyramidal tract toxicity, a therapeutic response to diphenhydramine or benztropine confirms the diagnosis.

Treatment   Phenothiazine overdose should be treated with gastrointestinal decontamination followed by activated charcoal and cathartics. Repeated charcoal is not indicated. Diuresis and dialysis are ineffective. Seizures should be treated with anticonvulsants, hypotension should be managed with volume expanders and alpha agonists, and sodium bicarbonate is administered for acidosis. Quinidine and procainamide should be avoided. For treatment of ventricular arrhythmias see Chap. 185. Dantrolene and bromocryptine may be useful in the treatment of neuroleptic malignant syndrome. Extrapyramidal signs respond rapidly and well to intravenous diphenhydramine (1 to 2 mg/kg body weight per dose to a maximum of 50 mg) given over 2 min. Treatment is generally continued for 24 h to prevent recurrence of symptoms.

SALICYLATES   Salicylates increase the sensitivity of respiratory centers in the brain to changes in P_{O_2} and P_{CO_2} resulting in an increased rate and depth of respiration. Salicylates also uncouple oxidative phosphorylation and produce increases in metabolic rate, oxygen consumption, glucose utilization, and heat production. Salicylates inhibit the Krebs tricarboxylic cycle and block carbohydrate and lipid metabolism, resulting in lactic acidosis and ketonemia. Salicylates produce hepatocyte damage, resulting in increased plasma enzyme activity and prolongation of prothrombin time. They also decrease platelet aggregation.

Salicylates are well absorbed both from the stomach and the small bowel. In the plasma, 50 to 80 percent is bound to albumin. Because salicylate is a weak acid with a pK of 3, the unbound portion in the plasma exists in an ionized state. It has a small volume of distribution of 0.2 L/kg body weight which increases with chronic poisoning and with increasing doses. Acidosis increases distribution of salicylate into brain, liver, and other tissues. Salicylates are eliminated by both hepatic metabolism and renal excretion. Saturation of hepatic metabolic pathways partially explains the prolonged half-life (20 to 36 h) in overdose. By alkalinizing the urine to a pH of 8, the drug in the renal tubules is maintained in an ionized state, is not reabsorbed, and is excreted in urine.

Clinical signs Clinical manifestations of mild poisoning include vomiting, tachycardia, hyperpnea, fever, tinnitus, lethargy, and mental confusion. In severe poisoning, convulsions, coma, and respiratory and cardiovascular failure may occur. Vomiting, poor intake, and hyperventilation may cause severe dehydration. Other complications include cerebral and pulmonary edema and myocardial or renal failure. An elevated hematocrit, white blood cell count, and platelet count; hypernatremia; hyperkalemia; and hypoglycemia may be seen. Respiratory alkalosis is commonly coupled with metabolic acidosis (40 to 50 percent), but respiratory alkalosis (20 percent), metabolic acidosis (20 percent), mixed respiratory and metabolic acidosis (5 to 10 percent) may be present. Lactic and other organic acids are responsible for an increased anion gap. Prothrombin time may be prolonged. Salicylates are identified by a positive ferric chloride test on either blood or urine. In the case of an acute single ingestion, a level less than 2.5 mmol/L (35 mg/dL) is associated with no symptoms, 2.5 to 5 mmol/L (35 to 70 mg/dL) with mild to moderate symptoms, 5 to 7 mmol/L (70 to 100 mg/dL) with severe symptoms, and greater than 7 mmol/L (100 mg/dL) with potentially fatal manifestations. In chronic poisoning, symptoms are seen at lower serum levels.

Treatment An ingested dose greater than 150 mg/kg body weight should be removed from the stomach. Concretions may delay absorption, and removal may be helpful up to 12 to 24 h after ingestion. The serum half-life may be shortened and elimination may be increased by repeated administration of activated charcoal. Parenteral fluids should be given to correct fluid losses and to produce a brisk urine flow. Seizures should be controlled with intravenous phenobarbital or diazepam. Myocardial failure should be treated with immediate correction of acidosis, administration of oxygen, and possibly digitalis therapy. Prolongation of prothrombin time should be corrected with intravenous vitamin K. Pulmonary edema should be managed with fluid restriction, osmotic diuresis, and positive end-expiratory ventilation. Cerebral edema requires fluid restriction and often hemodialysis. Sodium bicarbonate should be administered to correct serum pH and thus limit tissue distribution of salicylates. In addition, alkalinization of the urine to a pH of 8 enhances urinary excretion and decreases serum half-life. Potassium losses should be replenished, and sufficient fluids should be given to assure adequate renal perfusion. Salicylates are effectively removed by hemodialysis, which should be considered in severe overdose, cerebral edema, failure of conventional therapy, or compromised renal or hepatic function.

STIMULANTS Amphetamines, phenylpropanolamines, and cocaine are the most commonly used stimulants. Amphetamines have a long record of both abuse and overdose. For cocaine abuse see Chap. 272. Phenylpropanolamine can either be a street drug or a mail-order "legal stimulant." These agents affect both the central and sympathetic nervous systems (Table 374-1).

Amphetamines stimulate alpha- and beta-adrenergic receptors, whereas phenylpropanolamine stimulates only beta-adrenergic receptors. Amphetamines are rapidly absorbed from the GI tract, reaching peak levels 1 to 2 h following ingestion. Amphetamine is a weak base with a pK_a of 8 to 10 and a volume of distribution of 2 to 3 L/kg body weight. The drug is concentrated in brain, lung, and kidneys. Thirty to 40 percent is metabolized by the liver, and the hydroxylated metabolite may be responsible for the psychotic effects. The remainder (60 to 70 percent) is excreted directly by the kidneys. Excretion of amphetamines is enhanced in an acid urine and slowed in an alkaline urine. Plasma half-life is 16 to 31 h at a urine pH greater than 7.5 and falls to 6 to 8 h when the urinary pH is less than 5.0. Phenylpropanolamine is a white crystal powder with a pK_a of 9.4. It is rapidly absorbed from the GI tract. Its apparent volume of distribution is 4.5 L/kg body weight. Only 10 percent of the parent compound is metabolized by the liver, and the bulk is excreted unchanged in the urine. The biologic half-life ranges between 3 h in an acid urine and 6 h in an alkaline.

Clinical signs Effects of amphetamine overdose are seen within 30 to 60 min following ingestion. Gastrointestinal findings include nausea, vomiting, diarrhea, and abdominal cramps. The patient often exhibits excess talkativeness, irritability, confusion, delirium, combativeness, and auditory and visual hallucinations. Tremors and hyperreflexia are common. Hyperpyrexia may precede seizures and rhabdomyolysis. Cardiovascular effects include palpitations, tachycardia, hypertension, and cardiac arrhythmias. Cardiovascular collapse may occur in severe overdose. Sympathomimetic symptoms include dilated pupils, dry mouth, pallor, flushing of the skin, and tachypnea. Fatalities are rare and are usually associated with convulsions, coma, hyperpyrexia, cardiac arrhythmias, cardiovascular collapse, or intracranial hemorrhage. Phenylpropanolamine produces similar clinical findings. Cardiac manifestations include hypertension and reflex bradycardia. Amphetamines and phenylpropanolamine may be identified on toxic screen. Phenylpropanolamine and amphetamine serum levels may be quantitated, but no clear relationship exists between serum level and symptoms.

Treatment Gastric lavage should be followed by administration of activated charcoal and a cathartic. Supportive care includes treatment of seizures with phenytoin or benzodiazepines; hypertension with nitroprusside; hyperpyrexia with cooling blankets, salicylates, and acetaminophen; and agitation with sedatives. Droperidol and haloperidol are particularly effective for acute sedation in the agitated patient. Ventricular tachyarrhythmias should be treated with the appropriate antiarrhythmic drug (see Chap. 185). Seizures may cause myoglobinuria, which in association with an acid urine can lead to acute renal failure. Consequently, acidification of the urine is not recommended. Because of the short duration of effect of phenylpropanolamine, acidification of the urine is not indicated. Extracorporal therapy is of limited value.

THEOPHYLLINE Theophylline causes the release of endogenous catecholamines and prolongs their effects by inhibiting the degradation of cyclic AMP by phosphodiesterase. Theophylline is rapidly and well absorbed from the stomach and upper small bowel. Peak levels are achieved 1 to 2 h after ingestion of liquid preparations and by 2 to 4 h with tablets. Sustained-release preparations reach peak levels 7 to 24 h after ingestion. Theophylline has a pK_a of 9.5. Approximately 60 percent is bound to albumin. Theophylline has a low volume of distribution of 0.6 L/kg body weight, and 95 percent of the parent compound is metabolized by the liver to 1,3-dimethyluric acid, 1-methyluric acid, and 3-methyluric acid. In overdose, the 1-demethylation step of metabolism appears to be saturable. Only 5 percent of the theophylline is excreted unchanged by the kidneys. Theophylline elimination is decreased with impaired liver function, congestive heart failure, viral infections, and concomitantly administered drugs such as cimetidine that interfere with the cytochrome P$_{450}$ system. The serum half-life in overdose is 10 to 12 h.

Clinical signs Vomiting is frequent in overdose, and hematemesis is occasionally seen. Restlessness, irritability, agitation, tachypnea, tachycardia, and muscle tremors are common. Coma and respiratory depression are rare. Generalized tonic-clonic and occasionally focal convulsions occur in severe poisoning. Convulsions are often protracted, repetitive, and resistant to anticonvulsant therapy. Cardiovascular effects include atrial arrhythmias, multifocal premature ventricular contractions, idioventricular rhythms, ventricular tachycardia, and ventricular fibrillation. Rhabdomyolysis with renal failure is occasionally seen. Metabolic abnormalities include ketosis, metabolic acidosis, increased serum amylase, hyperglycemia, and decreased serum potassium, calcium, and phosphorus. Death occurs as a result of cardiovascular collapse or uncontrolled convulsions. Mortality rates are higher after chronic ingestion. Cardiac arrhythmias and seizures may be seen following chronic ingestion with serum levels of 200 to 300 μmol/L (40 to 60 mg/L). With acute ingestions, higher levels are associated with seizures and cardiac arrhythmias. Serial levels should be measured to determine the peak concentration (serving as an important indicator for hemodialysis) and the elimination half-life during recovery.

Treatment Initial therapy involves prompt gastrointestinal decontamination. Theophylline is well adsorbed by activated charcoal. With sustained-release forms of theophylline, removal should be considered up to 6 to 12 h following ingestion, and charcoal may be indicated up to 12 to 24 h following ingestion. When charcoal is administered every 2 to 4 h, serum half-life is shortened by approximately 50 percent. Metaclopramide is useful in controlling theophylline-induced vomiting. Tachycardia should be treated with propranolol or esmolol, and hypotension is treated with volume expansion and propranolol. Benzodiazepines and barbiturates are drugs of choice for convulsions. Phenytoin is ineffective. Arrhythmias should be treated with antiarrhythmic agents, and atropine or epinephrine may be administered for asystole. Diuresis is ineffective for enhancing removal of theophylline. The indication for hemodialysis and hemoperfusion in patients with acute ingestion is a serum level greater than 500 μmol/L (100 mg/L). With chronic ingestion, hemodialysis or hemoperfusion is indicated with serum levels greater than 200 to 300 μmol/L (40 to 60 mg/L). Hemoperfusion should be considered with lower levels in association with refractory seizures or arrythmias, in patients with chronic obstructive lung disease, and in people above age 60.

TRICYCLIC ANTIDEPRESSANTS Commonly available compounds include amitriptyline, imipramine, desipramine, doxepin, and nortriptyline. Tricylic antidepressants block reuptake of synaptic transmitters such as norepinephrine and dopamine in the central nervous system. In addition they have central and peripheral anticholinergic activity, have peripheral alpha-blocking activity, and exert quinidine-like effects on the heart.

Tricyclics are well absorbed from the GI tract, and peak levels are reached within 2 to 4 h of ingestion. In serious overdose, anticholinergic effects may predominate resulting in prolonged absorption and delayed peak levels (6 to 12 h following ingestion). Tricyclics exhibit high protein binding in the plasma. They have large volumes of distribution in the range of 20 to 40 L/kg body weight. Elimination is predominantly by hepatic metabolism with an initial demethylation generating pharmacologically active metabolites. These metabolites generally undergo enterohepatic circulation. Subsequent steps of metabolism result in increasing polarity of metabolites that are then excreted by the kidneys. Less than 5 percent of the parent compound is excreted unchanged in urine. Biliary excretion accounts for up to 15 percent of an ingested dose. The half-life of tricyclics and their demethylated metabolites ranges from 25 to 80 h in the overdose setting.

Clinical signs Symptoms generally develop within 1 to 2 h of ingestion but may be delayed for up to 6 h. In low overdose anticholinergic effects are coupled with agitation and hypertension. In high overdose CNS depression is coupled with depressed myocardial function, seizures, and hypotension. Anticholinergic effects include fever, mydriasis, tachycardia, flushing of the skin, urinary retention,

and decreased bowel activity. Central nervous system manifestations include excitation, restlessness, myoclonus, hyperreflexia, disorientation, confusion, and hallucinations. Lethargy, coma, and seizures occur in large overdose. Both hypertension and hypotension are common. Tachycardia (anticholinergic effect) occurs in low overdose, and ventricular tachyarrhythmias with terminal bradycardia and decreased cardiac output are seen in high overdose. Various degrees of cardiac conduction blocks and atrial arrhythmias also occur. Aspiration pneumonia and pulmonary edema may develop. Death occurs usually within the first 2 to 6 h following ingestion. Prolongation of the QRS complex (greater than 100 ms) in severe overdose is correlated with an increased risk of cardiac arrhythmias and seizures. Serum levels are diagnostic and correlate with severity. Levels less than about 1000 nmol/L (300 ng/mL) are considered therapeutic. Levels over 3300 nmol/L (1000 ng/mL) indicate serious poisoning and are associated with QRS complexes wider than 100 ms. The demethylated metabolite as well as the parent compound should be summed to indicate the total serum concentration.

Treatment Ipecac-induced emesis is contraindicated with tricyclic ingestions. Gastric lavage is indicated for recent ingestions, and activated charcoal every 2 to 4 h may interrupt enterohepatic recycling. Cathartics should be alternated with doses of activated charcoal. Appropriate care includes support of respiration, correction of metabolic acidosis with sodium bicarbonate, and volume expansion and norepinephrine or high-dose dopamine for hypotension. Hypertension is generally limited and does not require specific therapy. Seizures should be treated with phenytoin or diazepam. Treatment of arrhythmias may involve sodium bicarbonate (0.5 to 1 mmol/kg body weight), lidocaine, and phenytoin. Beta-adrenergic blockers and class 1A antiarrhythmics (quinidine, procainamide, and disopyramide) should be avoided. Cardiac pacing may be necessary for the severely depressed myocardium and bradycardia. Correction of acidosis is an important component of the treatment of cardiac arrhythmias. Physostigmine reverses anticholinergic signs, mydriatic pupils, tachycardia, and agitation, thereby helping to establish a clinical diagnosis (diagnostic trial). Physostigmine is contraindicated in the presence of coma, ventricular arrhythmias, or seizures because of unproven efficacy, short duration of effect, and potential for worsening cardiac toxicity.

REFERENCES

General aspects

BRANCATA DJ, NELSON RC: Poisoning mortality in the United States 1980. Vet Hum Toxicol 26:273, 1984

LITOVITZ TL et al: 1987 Annual report of the American Association of Poison Control Centers National Data Collection System. Am J Emerg Med 6:479, 1988

McCARRON MM: Current trends in drug overdose. West J Med 141:98, 1984

Diagnosis

BRETT AS: Implication of discordance between clinical impression and toxicology analysis in drug overdose. Arch Intern Med 148:437, 1988

COUNCIL OF SCIENTIFIC AFFAIRS, AMERICAN MEDICAL ASSOCIATION: Scientific issues in drug testing. JAMA 257:3110, 1987

EMMETT M, NARINS RG: Clinical use of the anion gap. Medicine 56:38, 1977

GLASSER L et al: Serum osmolality and its applicability to drug overdose. Am J Clin Pathol 60:695, 1973

HEPLER BR et al: Role of the toxicology lab in the treatment of acute poisoning. Med Toxicol 1:61, 1986

JAEGER RW et al: Radiopacity of drugs and plants in vivo—limited usefulness. Vet Hum Toxicol 23(Suppl 1):2, 1981

KELLERMANN AL et al: Impact of drug screening in suspected overdose. Ann Emerg Med 16:1206, 1987

MITCHELL AA et al: Drug ingestions associated with miosis in comatose children. J Pediatr 89(2):303, 1977

OLSON KR et al: Physical assessment and differential diagnosis of the poisoned patient. Med Toxicol 2:52, 1987

ROBERTS JR et al: The body stuffer syndrome: A clandestine form of drug overdose. Am J Emerg Med 4:24, 1986

SCHERZ RG: The differential diagnosis of coma due to poisoning and exogenous toxins. Pediatrician 6:190, 1977

SMITHLINE N, GARDNER KD JR: Gaps—anionic and osmolal. JAMA 236:1594, 1976

Treatment

ALBERTSON TE et al: Superiority of activated charcoal alone compared with ipecac and activated charcoal in the treatment of acute toxic ingestions. Ann Emerg Med 18:56, 1989

BRETT AS et al: Predicting the clinical course of intentional drug overdose: Implications for utilization of the intensive care unit. Arch Intern Med 147:133, 1987

BURTON BT et al: Comparison of activated charcoal and gastric lavage in the prevention of aspirin absorption. J Emerg Med 1:411, 1984

CURTIS RA et al: Efficacy of ipecac and activated charcoal/cathartic: Prevention of salicylate absorption in a simulated overdose. Arch Intern Med 144:48, 1984

GOLDBERG MJ et al: An approach to the management of the poisoned patient. Arch Intern Med 146:1381, 1986

GOLDFRANK L et al: Newer antidotes and controversies in antidotal therapy, in Emergency Medicine Annual, DA Rund, BW Wolcott (eds). Norwalk, Conn, Appleton-Century-Crofts, 1984, vol 3, pp 223–266.

KING WD: Syrup of ipecac: A drug review. Clin Toxicol 17:353, 1980

KRENZELOK EP et al: Gastrointestinal transit times of cartharlics combined with charcoal. Ann Emerg Med 14:1152, 1985

KULIG K et al: Management of acutely poisoned patients without gastric emptying. Ann Emerg Med 14:562, 1985

LITOVITZ TL: The anecdotal antidotes. Emerg Med Clin North Am 2:145, 1984

MANNO BR, MANNO JE: Toxicology of ipecac: A review. Clin Toxicol 10:221, 1977

McCARRON MM, WOOD JD: The cocaine "body packer" syndrome: Diagnosis and treatment. JAMA 250:1417, 1983

MINOCHA A, SPYKER DA: Acute overdose with sustained-release drug formulations: Perspectives in treatment. Med Toxicol 1:300, 1986

NEUVONEN PJ: Clinical pharmacokinetics of oral activated charcoal in acute intoxications. Clin Pharmacokinet 7:465, 1982

————, OLKKOLA KT: Oral activated charcoal in the treatment of intoxications: Role of single and repeated doses. Med Toxicol 3:33, 1988

PARK GD et al: Expanded role of charcoal in the poisoned and overdosed patient. Arch Intern Med 146:969, 1986

PETERSON RG, PETERSON LN: Cleansing the blood: Hemodialysis, peritoneal dialysis, exchange transfusion, charcoal hemoperfusion, forced diuresis. Pediatr Clin North Am 33:675, 1986

POND SM: Diuresis, dialysis and hemoperfusion: Indications and benefits. Emerg Med Clin North Am 2:29, 1984

ROSENBERG J et al: Pharmacokinetics of drug overdose. Clin Pharmacokinet 6:161, 1981

SHANNON M et al: Cathartics and laxatives: Do they still have a place in management of the poisoned patient? Med Toxicol 1:247, 1986

SPYKER DA, MINOCHA A: Toxicodynamic approach to the management of the poisoned patient. J Emerg Med 6:117, 1988

STEAD AH, MOFFAT AC: A collection of therapeutic, toxic and fatal blood drug concentrations in man. Hum Toxicol 3:437, 1983

STEWART JJ: Effects of emetic and cathartic agents on the gastrointestinal tract and the treatment of toxic ingestion. Clin Toxicol 20.199, 1983

TENEBEIN M: Whole bowel irrigation as a gastrointestinal decontamination procedure after acute poisoning. Med Toxicol 3:77, 1988

———— et al: Efficacy of ipecac-induced emesis, orogastric lavage, and activated charcoal for acute drug overdose. Ann Emerg Med 16:838, 1987

WHEELER-USHER DH et al: Gastric emptying: Risk versus benefit in the treatment of acute poisoning. Med Toxicol 1:142, 1986

Reference texts

ARENA JM, DREW RH: Poisoning: Toxicology, Symptoms, Treatments, 5th ed. Springfield, Ill., Charles C Thomas, 1986

BASET RC: Disposition of Toxic Drugs and Chemicals in Man, 2d ed. Davis, Calif, Biomedical Publications, 1982

BLOCK JB: The Signs and Symptoms of Chemical Exposure. Springfield, Ill., Charles C Thomas, 1980

BRYSON PD: Comprehensive Review in Toxicology. Rockville, Md, Aspen, 1989

CLAYTON GD, CLAYTON FE (eds): Patty's Industrial Hygiene and Toxicology, 3d ed. New York, Wiley, 1978

DANGAARD J: Symptoms and Signs in Occupational Disease: A Practical Guide, Copenhagen, Year Book Medical Publishers, 1978

ELLENHORN MJ, BARCELOUX DG: Medical Toxicology: Diagnosis and Treatment of Human Poisoning. New York, Elsevier, 1988

FINKEL AJ: Hamilton and Hardy's Industrial Toxicology, 4th ed. Boston, John Wright, 1983

GOLDFRANK LR et al (eds): Goldfrank's Toxicologic Emergencies, 3d ed. Norwalk, Conn, Appleton-Century-Crofts, 1986

GOSSELIN RE: Clinical Toxicology of Commercial Products: Acute Poisoning, 5th ed. Baltimore, Williams & Wilkins, 1984

HADDAD LM, WINCHESTER JF: Clinical Management of Poisoning and Drug Overdose. Philadelphia, Saunders, 1983

HAYES WJ: Pesticides Studies in Man. Baltimore, Williams & Wilkins, 1982

KLASSEN CD et al (eds): Casarett and Doull's Toxicology: The Basic Science of Poisons, 3d ed. New York, Macmillan, 1986

LAMPE KF, McCANN MA (eds): AMA Handbook of Poisonous and Injurious Plants. Chicago, American Medical Association, 1985

RUMACK BH (ed): Poisindex Information System (updated quarterly). Denver, Micromedex

Specific poisons

Acetaminophen

FLANAGAN RJ: The role of acetylcysteine in clinical toxicology. Med Toxicol 2:93, 1987

PRESCOTT LF: Paracetamol overdose. Drugs 25:290, 1983

SMILKSTEIN MJ et al: Efficacy of oral N-acetylcysteine in the treatment of acetaminophen overdose. N Engl J Med 319:1558, 1988

Acids and alkali

FRIEDMAN EM, LOVEJOY FH JR: The emergency management of caustic ingestions. Emerg Med Clin North Am 2:77, 1984

HOWELL JM: Alkaline ingestions. Ann Emerg Med 15:820, 1986

PENNER GE: Acid ingestion: Toxicology and treatment. Ann Emerg Med 9:374, 1980

Antiarrhythmic drugs

BENOWITZ NL: Quinidine, procainamide, and disopyramide, in Clinical Management of Poisoning and Drug Overdose, LM Haddad, JF Winchester (eds). Philadelphia, Saunders, 1983, pp 853–862

FREEDMAN MD et al: Extracorporeal pump assistance—a novel treatment for acute lidocaine poisoning. Eur J Clin Pharmacol 22:129, 1982

HRUBY K, MISSLIVETZ J: Poisoning with oral antiarrhythmic drugs. Int J Clin Pharmacol 23:253, 1985

Barbiturates

HENDERSON LW, MERRILL JP: Treatment of barbiturate intoxication. Ann Intern Med 64:876, 1966

MATTHEW H: Barbiturates. Clin Toxicol 8(5):495, 1975

McCARRON MM et al: Short-acting barbiturate overdosage: Correlation of intoxication score with serum barbiturate concentration. JAMA 248:55, 1982

Benzodiazepines

DIVOLL M et al: Benzodiazepine overdosage: Plasma concentrations and clinical outcome. Psycho Pharmacol 73:381, 1981

GREENBLATT DJ et al: Acute overdosage with benzodiazepine derivatives. Clin Pharmacol Ther 21:497, 1977

PRISCHL F et al: Value of flumazenil in benzodiazepine self-poisoning. Med Toxicol 3:334, 1988

Beta blockers

HEATH A: β-Adrenoceptor blocker toxicity: Clinical features and therapy. Am J Emerg Med 2:518, 1984

HENRY M et al: Cardiogenic shock associated with calcium-channel and β-blockers: Reversal with intravenous calcium chloride. Am J Emerg Med 3:334, 1985

WEINSTEIN RS: Recognition and management of poisoning with beta-adrenergic blocking agents. Ann Emerg Med 13:1123, 1984

Bleach

GAPAY-GAPANAVICUIUS M: Chloramine—induced pneumonitis from mixing household cleaning agents. Br Med J 288:1086, 1982

GAUDREAULT P et al: Predictability of esophageal injury from signs and symptoms. Pediatrics 71:767, 1983

LANDAU GD, SAUNDERS WH: The effect of chlorine bleach on the esophagus. Arch Otolaryngol 80:174, 1964

Calcium channel blockers

HERRINGTON DM et al: Nifedipine overdose. Am J Cardiol 81:344, 1986

SNOVER SW, BOCCHINO V: Massive diltiazem overdose. Ann Emerg Med 15:1221, 1986

ZARITSKY AL et al: Glucagon antagonism of calcium channel blocker induced myocardium dysfunction. Crit Care Med 16:246, 1988

Carbon monoxide

DOLAN MC: Carbon monoxide poisoning. Can Med Assoc J 133:392, 1985

Symposium—carbon monoxide poisoning—mechanism of damage, late sequelae and therapy. Clin Toxicol 23:247, 1985

WINTER PM, MILLER JN: Carbon monoxide poisoning. JAMA 236:1502, 1976

Cocaine

CREGLER LL, MARK H: Medical complications of cocaine abuse. N Engl J Med 315:1495, 1986

JONSSON S et al: Acute cocaine poisoning. Am J Med 75:1061, 1983

Cyanide

GRAHAM DL et al: Acute cyanide poisoning complicated by lactic acidosis and pulmonary edema. Arch Intern Med 137:1051, 1977

HALL AH et al: Clinical toxicology of cyanide: North American clinical experiences, in Clinical and Experimental Toxicology of Cyanides, B Ballantyne, TC Marrs (eds). Bristol, Wright, 1987

Digoxin

EKINS BR, WATANABE AS: Acute digoxin poisonings: Review of therapy. Am J Hosp Pharm 35:268, 1978

SMITH TW: New advances in the assessment and treatment of digitalis toxicity. J Clin Pharmacol 25:522, 1985

———— et al: Treatment of life-threatening digitalis intoxication with digoxin-specific FAB antibody fragments. N Engl J Med 307:1357, 1982

Ethanol

DAVID DJ, SPYKER DA: The acute toxicity of ethanol: Dosage and kinetic nomograms. Vet Hum Toxicol 21:272, 1979

ECKARDT MJ et al: Health hazards associated with alcohol consumption. JAMA 246:648, 1981

HALPERIN ML et al: Metabolic acidosis in the alcoholic: A pathophysiologic approach. Metabolism 32:308, 1983

Ethylene glycol

JACOBSEN D, MCMARTIN KE: Methanol and ethylene glycol poisonings: Mechanism of toxicity, clinical course, diagnosis and treatment. Med Toxicol 1:309, 1986

PARRY MF, WALLACH R: Ethylene glycol poisoning. Am J Med 57:143, 1974

Hallucinogens

BROWN RT, BRADEN NJ: Hallucinogens. Pediatr Clin North Am 34:341, 1987

COHEN S: The hallucinogens and the inhalents. Psych Clin North Am 7:681, 1984

STREICHEN M et al: Syndromes of solvent sniffing in adults. Ann Intern Med 94:758, 1981

Hydrocarbons

ANAS N et al: Criteria for hospitalizing children who have ingested products containing hydrocarbons. JAMA 246:840, 1981

MARKS ME et al: Adrenocorticosteroid treatment of hydrocarbon pneumonia in children—a cooperative study. J Pediatr 81:366, 1972

TRUEMPIER E et al: Clinical characteristics, pathophysiology and management of hydrocarbon ingestion: Case report and review of the literature. Pediatr Emerg Care 3:187, 1987

Hydrogen sulfide

SMITH RP: Management of acute sulfide poisoning. Arch Environ Health 31:166, 1976

STINE RJ et al: Hydrogen sulfide intoxication. Ann Intern Med 85:756, 1976

WHITECRAFT DD et al: Hydrogen sulfide poisoning treated with hyperbaric oxygen. J Emerg Med 3:23, 1985

Iron

PROUDFOOT AT et al: Management of acute iron poisoning. Med Toxicol 1:83, 1986

ROBOTHAM JL, LEITMAN PS: Acute iron poisoning—a review. Am J Dis Child 134:875, 1980

WHITTEN CF et al: Studies in acute iron poisoning: Further observations of desferrioxamine in the treatment of acute experimental iron poisoning. J Pediatr 38:102, 1966

Isoniazid

CHIN L et al: Evaluation of diazepam and pyridoxine as antidotes to isoniazid intoxication in rats and dogs. Toxicol Appl Pharmacol 45:713, 1978

SIEVERS ML, HERRIER RN: Treatment of acute isoniazid toxicity. Am J Hosp Pharm 32:202, 1975

WASON S et al: Single high-dose pyridoxine treatment for isoniazid overdose. JAMA 246:1102, 1981

Isopropyl alcohol

LACOUTURE PG et al: A review of acute isopropyl alcohol intoxication: Diagnosis and management. Am J Med 75:680, 1983

NATOWICZ M et al: Pharmacokinetic analysis of a case of isopropyl intoxication. Clin Chem 31:326, 1985

Lithium

AMDISEN A: Clinical features and management of lithium poisoning. Med Toxicol 3:18, 1988

HANSEN HE, AMDISEN A: Lithium intoxication. Q Med J 47:123, 1978

MAO inhibitors

KAPLAN RF et al: Phenelzine overdose treated with dantrolene sodium. JAMA 255:642, 1986

LINDEN CH: Monoamine oxidase inhibitor overdose. Ann Emerg Med 13:1137, 1984

Methanol

JACOBSEN D, MCMARTIN KE: Methanol and ethylene glycol poisoning: Mechanism of toxicity, clinical course, diagnosis and treatment. Med Toxicol:309, 1986

OSTERLOH JD et al: Serum formate concentrations in methanol intoxication as a criterion for hemodialysis. Ann Intern Med 104:200, 1986

SWARTZ RD et al: Epidemic methanol poisoning: Clinical and biochemical analysis of a recent episode. Medicine 60:373, 1981

Methemoglobinemia

CURRY S: Methemoglobinemia. Ann Emerg Med 11:214, 1982

HALL AH et al: Drug and chemical-induced methaemoglobinaemia. Med Toxicol 1:253, 1986

HARVEY JW, KEITT AS: Studies of the efficacy and potential hazards of methylene blue therapy in aniline-induced methaemoglobinaemia. Br J Haematol 53:29, 1983

Muscle relaxants

DOMINO EF: Muscle relaxants of the mephenesin type. Ann NY Acad Sci 86:238, 1974

VALTONEN EJ: A controlled trial of chlormezanone, orphenadrine, paracetamol and placebo in treatment of painful skeletal muscle spasms. Ann Clin Res 7:85, 1975

Narcotics

CUDDY P: Management of acute opioid intoxication. Crit Care Q 4:65, 1982

FULTZ JM, SENAY EC: Guidelines for the management of hospitalized addicts. Ann Intern Med 82:815, 1975

LAWSON AAH, NORTHRIDGE DB: Dextropropoxyphene overdose. Med Toxicol 2:430, 1987

Nonsteroidal anti-inflammatory drugs

COURT H, VOLANS GN: Poisoning after overdose with nonsteroidal anti-inflammatory drugs. Adverse Drug React Acute Poisoning Rev 3:1, 1984

HALL AH et al: Ibuprofen overdose: 126 cases. Ann Emerg Med 15:1308, 1986

VALE JA, MEREDITH TJ: Acute poisoning due to nonsteroidal anti-inflammatory drugs: Clinical features and management. Med Toxicol 1:11, 1986

Organophosphate and carbamates insecticides

MINTON NA, MURRAY VSG: A review of organophosphate poisoning. Med Toxicol 3:350, 1988

NAMBA T et al: Poisoning due to organophosphate insecticides. Am J Med 50:475, 1971

NATOFF IL, REIFF B: Effect of oximes on the acute toxicity of anticholinesterase carbamates. Toxicol Appl Pharmacol 25:569, 1973

Phenothiazines

BARRY D et al: Phenothiazine poisoning: A review of 48 cases. Calif Med 118:1, 1983

BENOWITZ NL et al: Cardiopulmonary catastrophes in drug-overdosed patients. Med Clin North Am 63:267, 1979

Salicylates

GAUDREAULT P et al: The relative severity of acute vs chronic salicylate poisoning in children: A clinical comparison. Pediatrics 70:566, 1982

MCGUIGAN MA: A two-year review of salicylate deaths in Ontario. Arch Intern Med 147:510, 1987

TEMPLE AR: Acute and chronic effects of aspirin toxicity and their treatment. Arch Intern Med 141:364, 1981

Stimulants

GARY NE, SAIDI P: Methamphetamine intoxication. Am J Med 64:537, 1978

LINDEN CH et al: Amphetamines. Top Emerg Med 7:18, 1985

PENTEL P: Toxicity of over-the-counter stimulants. JAMA 252:1898, 1984

Theophylline

GAUDREAULT P, GUAY J: Theophylline poisoning. Med Toxicol 1:169, 1986

OLSON KR et al: Theophylline overdose: Acute single ingestion versus chronic repeated overmedication. Am J Emerg Med 3:386, 1985

PARK GD et al: Use of hemoperfusion for treatment of theophylline intoxication. Am J Med 74:961, 1983

Tricyclic antidepressants

BOEHNERT MT, LOVEJOY FH JR: Value of QRS duration versus the serum drug level in predicting seizures and ventricular arrhythmias after an acute overdose of tricyclic antidepressants. N Engl J Med 313:474, 1985

CROME P: Poisoning due to tricyclic antidepressant overdose. Med Toxicol 1:261, 1986

FROMMER DA et al: Tricyclic antidepressant overdose; A review. JAMA 257:521, 1987

375   HEAVY METAL POISONING

JOHN W. GRAEF / FREDERICK H. LOVEJOY, JR.

ARSENIC

SOURCE Inorganic arsenic compounds such as arsenic trioxide, arsenic pentoxide, and sodium and potassium arsenite and arsenate are found in insecticides, rodenticides, fungicides, wood preservatives, herbicides, and compounds used in glass manufacturing. Organic arsenic is widely distributed in the environment. Arsine gas is produced in the smelting and refining of metals, in galvanizing and etching, in lead plating, and in making silicon microchips. Historically, organic arsenical compounds have been used in the treatment of syphilis, epilepsy, psoriasis, and amebiasis. Currently, acute toxicity is encountered following accidental ingestion, industrial accidents, or suicidal or homicidal intoxications. Chronic exposures occur most commonly following low-dose exposure in industry or chronic consumption of contaminated food, water, or medications.

METABOLISM   Arsenic is absorbed through the skin, lungs, and gastrointestinal tract. Inorganic compounds are absorbed more readily than organic, with greater than 80 percent of an ingested dose absorbed by the gastrointestinal tract. Arsine gas is absorbed through the lungs. Arsenic is distributed from blood to liver, kidney, lung, and spleen within 24 h of ingestion and to skin, hair, and bone within 2 weeks. Inorganic arsenic compounds are found in high concentrations in leukocytes. Inorganic arsenic does not cross the blood-brain barrier but does cross the placenta. Five to ten percent is excreted in feces, and 90 to 95 percent is excreted in the urine. Small amounts are recovered in bile, feces, and saliva. Arsenic may be detected in urine for 7 to 21 days following an overdose and detected in the serum for a shorter period of time.

CLINICAL TOXICOLOGY   Arsine gas combines with hemoglobin in red blood cells to produce severe hemolysis with anemia, hemoglobinuria, and hematuria within 3 to 4 h of ingestion. Subsequent jaundice may be severe. Signs and symptoms of toxicity include nausea, vomiting and diarrhea, apprehension and malaise, tachycardia, and dyspnea. Acute renal failure is frequent and often fatal.

The reported lethal dose for arsenic ranges from 130 to 300 mg. Manifestations of acute toxicity include for the gastrointestinal tract—burning in the throat, difficulty swallowing, nausea, vomiting, diarrhea, abdominal pain, and a garlic odor on the breath; for the cardiovascular system—cyanosis, difficulty breathing, and hypotension; for the central nervous system—delirium, coma, and seizures; for the kidneys—acute tubular necrosis; for the hematologic system—hemolysis, eosinophilia, and, rarely, bone marrow depression. Manifestations of chronic arsenic poisoning occur 2 to 8 weeks following ingestion and include for the skin and nails—erythroderma, hyperkeratosis, hyperpigmentation, exfoliative dermatitis, and Aldrich-Mees lines (transverse white striae of the fingernails); for the mucous membranes—laryngitis, tracheitis, and bronchitis; for the central nervous system—polyneuritis (sensory and motor). Basal cell carcinomas, squamous cell carcinomas, Bowen's disease of the skin (see Chap. 59), and lung carcinomas have been associated with chronic arsenic exposure.

Arsenic produces its toxicity by binding with tissue sulfhydryl groups. Arsenic also binds to enzymes in the Krebs tricarboxylic acid cycle, thereby interfering with oxidative phosphorylation. Other effects include capillary injury and direct toxic effects on large organs. Pathologic findings include necrosis of the stomach, small bowel, and vasculature and degenerative changes in the liver and kidneys.

LABORATORY FINDINGS   Arsenic is radiopaque and is seen on x-ray of the abdomen. It may also be detected in hair and nails for months following exposure. Specific organ effects include: abnormal liver function tests; anemia, leukocytosis, leukopenia, and hemoglobinemia; proteinuria, hematuria, hemoglobinuria, and cellular casts in the urine. Urine arsenic (As) levels are normally less than 67 nmol $(5 \mu g)/d$.

TREATMENT   Acute ingestion should be treated by inducing vomiting with ipecac syrup if the patient is alert. Gastric lavage is indicated if the patient is obtunded. Activated charcoal is ineffective, and cathartics are contraindicated. Dimercaprol chelates arsenic by producing an insoluble complex that is excreted by the kidneys. For mild symptoms and elevated serum or urinary levels, 2 to 3 mg/kg body weight per dose is given intramuscularly every 6 h for 24 h and then every 12 to 24 h for 10 days. Adequacy of urinary mobilization of arsenic is confirmed and followed during treatment by measurement of serum and urinary levels. Treatment should be continued until 24-h urine As levels are less than 67 nmol $(5 \mu g)/d$. Toxic manifestations of dimercaprol (increased blood pressure, tachycardia, nausea, vomiting, headache, burning sensation in the lips, mucous membrane irritation, coma, and convulsions) occur with increasing doses. For patients with severe symptoms and very high arsenic levels 3 to 5 mg/kg body weight per intramuscular dose of dimercaprol is administered in a similar regime. The water-soluble analogue of dimercaprol,

succimer (DMSA), may be more effective and is less toxic than dimercaprol.

Penicillamine has been successfully used in acute and chronic poisoning, administered orally at a dose of 100 mg/kg body weight per day (the maximum dose not to exceed 1 g/d) in four divided doses for 5 days. Side effects of penicillamine include rash, leukopenia, thrombocytopenia, and nephrotoxicity. Hemodialysis removes arsenic (24 to 100 mg in 24 h) with a clearance of 80 to 90 mL/min and is indicated if renal failure occurs. Hemodialysis early in the clinical course in conjunction with dimercaprol may limit arsenic's distribution phase and enhance clearance of free and complexed arsenic.

Exchange transfusion and, if renal failure develops, hemodialysis are the preferred treatments for arsine gas poisoning. Dimercaprol affords no protection against red cell destruction.

CADMIUM

SOURCE   Exposure to cadmium is usually occupational or via pollution from mining or smelting operations. Cadmium is produced commercially as a by-product of copper and lead or zinc smelting and is used in the manufacture of batteries, in ceramics, in electroplating, and as a pigment in paints and plastics. In contaminated areas, high concentrations may be found in shellfish.

METABOLISM   Absorption occurs via ingestion or inhalation. Normal daily oral intake is up to 200 μg with an estimated mean of 20 to 40 $\mu g/d$. Only 5 to 10 percent of this is absorbed, although like lead, absorption may be increased in the presence of calcium and iron deficiency. About 5 percent of inhaled cadmium is absorbed depending on particle size. Small, highly soluble particles are absorbed at a rate of 25 to 50 percent.

About 50 percent of absorbed cadmium is concentrated in the liver and kidneys. In erythrocytes and soft tissues cadmium is bound to metallothionein, a low-molecular-weight polypeptide containing a large number of available sulfhydryl groups that exert a protective effect. With large single-dose cadmium exposures saturation of the protein may result in loss of protective effect. Cadmium does not pass the placenta and gradually accumulates in the body with age. Biologic half-life has been estimated at more than 20 years except in the presence of kidney damage when urinary excretion is increased. In the kidney, metallothionein-bound cadmium is filtered at the glomerulus and is then reabsorbed by the proximal tubules. The urinary excretion rarely exceeds 5 nmol $(0.5 \mu g)/d$.

CLINICAL TOXICOLOGY   Acute cadmium intoxication may occur after either ingestion or inhalation. Ingestion of water containing concentrations of 15 mg/L or foods containing as little as 30 mg of cadmium can induce vomiting, abdominal pain, and severe diarrhea. Shock may ensue. Acute inhalation of cadmium dust produces dyspnea, weakness, chest pain, shortness of breath, and cough. A chemical pneumonitis produces pulmonary edema and respiratory failure. Clinical symptoms may occur with air exposure as low as 1 mg/m² surface area over 8 h. During the same time period inhalation of 5 mg/m² surface area may be fatal. A latent period of 4 to 24 h from exposure to onset of symptoms may complicate accurate diagnosis. Death usually occurs in 5 to 10 days. Chemical pneumonitis may continue for several months, and pulmonary function can be abnormal for longer than 1 year after exposure.

Chronic intoxication usually occurs by industrial inhalation and produces emphysema and characteristic renal tubular damage with proteinuria and increased urinary excretion of beta₂ microglobulin. Cadmium's inhibitory effect on alpha₁ antitrypsin may be responsible for cadmium-induced emphysema. Relatively minor changes in liver function, a microcytic hypochromic anemia unresponsive to iron therapy, and hypertension are associated findings. Chronic oral intake of contaminated rice and drinking water has produced a syndrome in Japan called *itai-itai* (ouch-ouch) disease with manifestations that include renal tubular damage and osteomalacia.

LABORATORY FINDINGS   Measurement of blood cadmium levels is not useful. Urinary cadmium excretion exceeding 0.1 μmol

(10 µg)/L is associated with renal tubular damage especially when accompanied by elevated urinary beta$_2$ microglobulin and metallothionein levels. Kidney cadmium content obtained by renal biopsy can be assessed by neutron activation analysis. A renal cadmium concentration exceeding 2 µmol/g (200 µg/g) of wet weight is associated with renal disease.

TREATMENT Treatment is controversial. Although chelating agents bind cadmium, they may effectively shift cadmium to the kidney, where further damage can occur. In acute exposure, ethylenediaminetetraacetic acid (edetate) in a dose of 1 g/m^2 surface area daily can be beneficial. Although dimercaprol is not effective, another oral chelating agent, succimer (DMSA), appears promising. Acute inhalation pneumonitis should be treated with glucocorticoids and diuretics. Itai-itai disease appears to respond to large doses of vitamin D. Long-term sequelae of chronic cadmium exposure include emphysema and chronic renal insufficiency.

LEAD

SOURCE Lead is a normal constituent of the earth's crust and is found throughout nature. The increased use of lead during the Industrial Revolution caused extensive disease among lead workers; the addition of lead salts to paints as coloring agents and stabilizers set the stage for the largest epidemic of lead poisoning in history, that of childhood plumbism. This syndrome, caused by ingestion by small children of lead from paint, soil, household dust, and, infrequently, from drinking water, affects an estimated 2,000,000 preschool children annually in the United States alone. Evidence of permanent neurologic sequelae from levels of lead previously thought to be safe has raised fears of possible damage to the fetus and newborn as well. The nature of this epidemic has forced prohibition against the addition of organic lead salts to gasoline as well as extensive prohibitions against the use of lead in consumer products.

METABOLISM Inorganic lead salts are absorbed through ingestion or inhalation. Organic lead salts may also be absorbed through the skin. Generally, gastrointestinal absorption is about 10 percent of an ingested dose, but in children may be as high as 50 percent. It is enhanced by deficiency of iron, calcium, and zinc. Absorption through the lung varies with tidal volume and particle size. Particles smaller than 1 µm may be absorbed if they reach the alveoli. Adults may ingest up to 0.7 µmol (150 µg)/d of lead from normal exposure to food and drinking water. Positive lead balance may occur at these levels since renal excretion normally does not exceed 0.4 µmol (80 µg)/d. In children, no more than 0.02 µmol (5 µg)/kg body weight is tolerated without increasing the body lead burden.

Under steady state conditions, 5 to 10 percent of ingested lead may be found in blood; 95 percent of that fraction is associated with the erythrocyte. Up to 80 to 90 percent is taken up by bone and incorporated into hydroxyapatite crystals, where it is relatively inactive. The remainder is found in soft tissues, principally the kidneys and brain. The principal route of excretion is stool (80 to 90 percent), and the remainder is found in the urine (10 percent). Small amounts are excreted in hair, nails, sweat, and saliva. Lead passes the placenta and blood-brain barrier and may be found in milk. The half-life of lead in blood and soft tissues is 24 to 40 days, and in bone, 104 days.

Lead is a poison of enzymes, binding to the sulfhydryl groups of proteins. In high concentration, lead alters the tertiary structure of intracellular proteins, denaturing them and causing cell death and tissue inflammation.

CLINICAL TOXICOLOGY The toxic effects of lead differ between children and adults. The adult form is generally characterized by abdominal pain, anemia, renal disease, headache, peripheral neuropathy with demyelination of long neurons, ataxia, and memory loss. Symptoms are usually associated with prolonged elevation of lead levels above 4 to 5 µmol/L (80 to 100 µg/dL) of whole blood. A subclinical form in adults affects primarily the peripheral nervous

system and the kidneys. A linear association between hypertension and elevated lead levels [i.e., greater than 1.4 µmol/L (30 µg/dL)] has been reported. Encephalopathy is rare in adults.

Childhood lead poisoning is manifested by abdominal pain and anemia, but the central nervous system effects are most important. As an enzymatic poison, lead affects developing tissues more than tissues with slow turnover. Hence, subclinical lead poisoning is most dangerous to children because its effects emerge without associated symptoms that bring the victim to medical attention. In the acute clinical form, signs and symptoms reflect both the direct effect of high concentrations of lead [(i.e., blood lead greater than 4 µmol/L (80 µg/dL)] and consequent severe alterations in porphyrin synthesis. Signs and symptoms include abdominal pain, irritability followed by lethargy, anorexia, pallor (anemia), ataxia, and slurred speech. In severe cases, convulsions, coma, and death are usually due to severe generalized cerebral edema and renal failure. A history of "high-dose" exposure to lead (usually paint chips), pica (the ingestion of nonfood substances), and malnutrition (iron, calcium, and zinc deficiency) almost always is associated with this syndrome.

The subclinical form of childhood plumbism is associated with elevated blood lead and increased erythrocyte protoporphyrin. However, no symptoms are usually detected. The syndrome is widespread, and its effects on the developing central nervous system are irreversible. These include mental retardation and selective deficits in language, cognitive functions, and behavior, depending on the age and duration of exposure. These latter factors are more important than the height of the lead level.

LABORATORY FINDINGS Laboratory abnormalities include blood lead levels greater than 1.2 µmol/L (25 µg/dL) associated with free erythrocyte protoporphyrin (FEP) greater than 0.6 µmol/L (35 µg/dL). Biochemical and neurodevelopmental abnormalities may occur in association with blood lead levels as low as 0.7 µmol/L (15 µg/dL), particularly in very young children. Although a hemolytic anemia is associated with acute plumbism, chronic plumbism produces a microcytic hypochromic anemia with associated or secondary iron deficiency. Other heme precursors are increased in plasma and urine (e.g., delta aminolevulinic acid).

Renal abnormalities include pyuria, the Fanconi syndrome, and azotemia. In plumbism, urinary excretion of lead exceeds 4 µmol (80 µg)/d. In adults, demyelination of long nerves produces prolonged nerve conduction time and subsequent paralysis of extensor muscles with atrophy (wrist drop or foot drop). While slight prolongation of nerve conduction can be seen in children, it is clinically evident only in those with sickle cell disease. Abnormalities of cardiac, thyroid, and hepatic function occur in adults. In children, a characteristic finding is increased density at the metaphyseal plate of growing long bones, so-called lead lines. These are generally seen in association with levels greater than 2.4 µmol/L (50 µg/dL) of whole blood for a prolonged period. They are not seen in adults.

TREATMENT The *sine qua non* of treatment is removal of the source of exposure. Cases of industrial lead poisoning should be reported to the Occupational Safety Hazards Administration (OSHA). Cases of childhood plumbism should be reported to the local board of health to initiate examination of housing for sources of lead.

Reduction of the body burden of lead is accomplished by use of chelating agents, principally edetate calcium disodium (EDTA), dimercaprol, and penicillamine. The oral chelating agent succimer is undergoing clinical trials and appears to be as effective as parenteral edetate. The lead mobilization test is used to determine the size of the "chelatable" pool of lead. In this test, administration of a calculated dose of chelating agent, usually edetate, induces a lead diuresis that is then compared to the dose of chelating agent. The test is positive when greater than 5 nmol (1 µg) lead is excreted per milligram of chelating agent administered per 24 h. An outpatient modification of this test may be used in which urine is collected for 6 to 8 h. The test is considered positive when greater than 2.5 nmol (0.5 µg) of lead is excreted per milligram of chelating agent. The mobilization test can be useful in determining the utility of chelation therapy in patients with borderline lead levels or in those patients who have been previously treated. The use of x-ray fluorescence of bone to determine the lead burden is under investigation as an alternative to the lead mobilization test.

In acute encephalopathy, double therapy (dimercaprol and edetate) is used until blood lead levels are less than 2 μmol/L (40 μg/dL). Urine flow must be established, and even in the presence of cerebral edema, fluids must be sufficient to produce a lead diuresis. Mannitol and dexamethasone can reduce cerebral edema, but removal of the metal is essential. In symptomatic adults and children, therapy with both dimercaprol and edetate should be used for 5 days at edetate doses of 0.5 to 1 g/m^2 surface area up to 1.5 g/m^2 surface area daily and dimercaprol doses of 12 to 24 mg/kg body weight per day. If further chelation is required, a minimum interval of 48 to 72 h should intervene between courses of therapy. The penicillamine dose is 20 to 40 mg/kg body weight per day, not to exceed 1 g/d. Adverse effects, particularly allergy, may be reduced by beginning therapy with one-quarter of the total dose for 1 week, then doubling and redoubling the dose until full dose is reached. Penicillamine can be administered for 3 to 6 months until the body lead burden is depleted. Only penicillamine and, to a lesser extent, edetate remove lead directly from bone. If edetate is indicated, as many separate 5-day courses as are needed may be given provided that the total safe dose is not exceeded and proper intervals between courses are observed.

MERCURY

SOURCE Humans may encounter mercury in an inorganic (elemental or mercuric salt) or an organic (usually methyl) form. All three are toxic, but organic mercury is most widespread and potentially dangerous. Elemental mercury is used in thermometers, sphygmomanometers, and dental amalgams. It is volatile at room temperature and rapidly oxidizes to mercuric mercury when exposed to oxygen. Toxicity usually occurs from inhalation of mercury vapor during industrial exposure. Mercuric salts are found in topical medicines, in catalytic agents in the manufacture of plastics, in cathartics (e.g., Calomel), and in foodstuffs. Toxicity occurs usually as a result of gastrointestinal exposure. Organic mercury is in paints, fungicides, seeds, foods, medicines, and cosmetic agents. Large amounts of methyl mercury are formed by methylation of mercury salt wastes as occurred in the mercury epidemic in Minamata Bay, Japan.

METABOLISM Elemental mercury is poorly absorbed by the gastrointestinal tract but is absorbed efficiently as vapor through the lungs, with 80 to 100 percent of inhaled mercury entering the bloodstream through the alveoli. Absorbed mercury vapor is lipid-soluble and readily crosses the blood-brain barrier and the placenta. It is rapidly oxidized to its mercuric form and combines with sulfhydryl groups. Excretion is via the urine and feces. Small amounts of mercury vapor may be excreted via the lungs. The half-life of elemental mercury is approximately 60 days.

Inorganic mercury salts are absorbed through the gastrointestinal tract and skin. Large overdoses may produce corrosive effects on the gastrointestinal tract with consequent increased absorption. Normal uptake is less than 10 percent of an ingested dose. Mercuric salts accumulate primarily in the kidney, but are distributed to the liver, erythrocytes, bone marrow, spleen, lung, intestine, and skin. Excretion is via the urine and feces. The half-life of inorganic mercury is approximately 40 days.

Organic (methyl) mercury is readily absorbed through the intestines and the skin. Short-chain alkyl and methyl mercury penetrate the erythrocyte membrane and bind to hemoglobin. The ratio of red blood cell to plasma methyl mercury may be as high as 9:1. Because of its high lipid solubility, methyl mercury freely passes the placenta and blood-brain barrier and enters breast milk. Organic mercury also concentrates in the kidneys and the central nervous system. Metallothionein synthesis is induced by mercury, and the augmented concentration of the protein exerts a protective effect against tissue damage. Excretion is complex. About 1 percent of organic mercury is excreted in urine directly. Methyl mercury is acetylated in the liver or may be conjugated with cysteine or glutathione. The N-acetyl-homocysteine–methyl mercury complex then enters the enterohepatic circulation and is ultimately excreted in the urine. The half-life of organic mercury in humans is about 70 days.

CLINICAL TOXICOLOGY Acute metallic mercury (vapor) poisoning causes inflammation of large and small airways and interstitial pneumonitis. The rapid uptake of mercury vapor into the central nervous system produces tremor and increased excitability. Chronic mercury vapor poisoning primarily affects the central nervous system. Initial symptoms include lassitude, anorexia, weight loss, and gastrointestinal disturbances. Increasing exposure produces the characteristic intention tremor of mercury poisoning and is accompanied by mercurial *erethism* (timidity, memory loss, insomnia, excitability, and, in severe cases, delirium). This neurologic picture in felt-hat workers exposed to mercury vapor and mercuric salts led to the phrase "mad as a hatter."

Chronic inorganic mercury poisoning produces the above neurologic findings as well as excessive salivation, loosening of the teeth, gingivitis, and stomatitis. When applied to the skin, mercuric salts may cause hypersensitivity reactions ranging from mild erythema to exfoliative dermatitis. Acrodynia, or Pink's disease, occurs in young children and may be mistaken for Kawasaki's disease. Symptoms include generalized rash, irritability, photophobia, hypertrichosis, profuse perspiration, and swelling and desquamation of the feet and hands.

Acute inorganic mercury poisoning is characterized by corrosive effects on the gastrointestinal tract, including nausea, vomiting, hematemesis, and abdominal pain followed by tenesmus, bloody diarrhea, and necrosis of intestinal mucosa. Acute fluid redistribution in massive overdose can produce shock and death. Acute inorganic mercury poisoning causes acute tubular necrosis, while chronic inorganic mercury poisoning produces a nephrotic syndrome.

Acute and chronic organic mercury poisoning are indistinguishable. Prenatal poisoning produces cerebral palsy as a result of cortical and cerebellar atrophy. Postnatal poisoning causes paresthesias, headache, pain, visual, hearing, and speech disorders, neurasthenia, loss of memory, incoordination, erethism, spasticity, paralysis, stupor, and coma. These neurologic abnormalities are often permanent.

The daily intake of methyl mercury should not exceed 100 parts per billion. Blood mercury levels above 180 nmol/L (3.5 μg/dL) and urine mercury levels above 0.7 μmol/L (150 μg/L) are abnormal. Symptoms may be seen with blood mercury levels above 1 μmol/L (20 μg/dL) and urine mercury levels above 3 μmol/L (600 μg/L). Clinical findings may be associated with somewhat lower concentrations depending on when exposure occurred.

TREATMENT Treatment is aimed at reducing the absorption of mercury, protecting susceptible tissues, and enhancing elimination. In the case of ingestion of mercuric salts, initial treatment consists of removing mercury from the stomach by inducing emesis or by gastric lavage. Polythiol resins are effective in binding mercury in the gastrointestinal tract. Activated charcoal, however, does not bind metals.

Generally, chelation therapy is indicated when elevated urine or blood mercury levels are present. Chelating agents with active mono- or dithiol groups are most effective. These include dimercaprol and penicillamine. The oral chelating agent succimer shows promise.

In acute inorganic mercury poisoning, dimercaprol should be used at a dose not exceeding 24 mg/kg body weight per 24 h intramuscularly, in divided doses. Generally, therapy should not exceed 5 days at a time but can be reinstituted after a suitable rest period. Penicillamine can be used in the treatment of inorganic mercury poisoning but N-acetyl-DL-penicillamine is equally effective, and less toxic. The dose is 30 mg/kg body weight per day in two to three divided doses. Peritoneal hemodialysis have also been used with some success. Neither is as effective as chelation therapy but may be useful in the presence of renal failure.

In chronic inorganic mercury poisoning, dimercaprol is ineffective. Penicillamine is the drug of choice. The investigational drug N-acetyl-DL-penicillamine is more effective than either dimercaprol or edetate.

THALLIUM

SOURCE Thallium is used as an insecticide and rodenticide, as a catalyst in fireworks, in manufacturing imitation jewelry and optical lenses, in industry as an alloy, and in cardiac perfusion imaging. Accidental as well as purposeful ingestions of thallium occur. Epidemic poisoning has followed the ingestion of grain impregnated with thallium. Thallium is available as iodide, sulfate, acetate, carbonate, and nitrate salts.

METABOLISM Thallium is absorbed percutaneously, by inhalation, and by oral ingestion. It has a large volume of distribution of 4 to 6 L/kg body weight with distribution to body organs including kidney, pancreas, spleen, liver, lung, muscles, and brain. Thallium is bound to sulfhydryl groups on mitochondrial membranes at intracellular sites. The elimination half-life is variable, ranging from 3 to 15 days. The major pathway of elimination is in the urine, conforming to first-order pharmacokinetics; 3 percent of a dose is eliminated per day, or 75 mL/min total-body clearance.

Thallium interferes with oxidative phosphorylation by inhibition of ATPase and substitutes for potassium in many physiologic reactions. Pathologic findings at postmortem include cerebral edema, loss of myelin in peripheral nerves, fatty infiltration of the liver, and degenerative changes in the myocardium.

CLINICAL TOXICOLOGY Severe poisoning occurs following a single ingested dose greater than 1 g or 8 mg/kg body weight. Death has occurred following an ingested dose of 15 mg/kg body weight.

Immediate signs and symptoms (occurring within 3 to 4 h of ingestion) include nausea and vomiting, abdominal pain, diarrhea, and hematochezia. Intermediate manifestations (within 1 week of ingestion) include involvement of the central nervous system with confusion, psychosis, choreoathetosis, organic brain syndrome, convulsions, and coma. Peripheral neurologic involvement is both motor and sensory and includes paresthesias, myalgias, weakness, tremor, and ataxia. Autonomic manifestations are less common and include tachycardia, hypertension, and salivation. Ophthalmologic abnormalities are neuritis, ophthalmoplegia, ptosis, strabismus, and cranial nerve palsies. Late manifestations (occurring 2 to 4 weeks after ingestion) include diffuse hair loss (with sparing of pubic and body hair and the lateral one-third of the eyebrows) with regrowth occurring as body burden decreases over time. Residual effects include memory loss, ataxia, tremor, and foot drop.

LABORATORY FINDINGS Thallium is radiopaque and is evident on an abdomenal x-ray. Thallium levels with severe ingestion range, in blood, from 1.5 to 10 μmol/L (30 to 200 μg/dL) and, in urine, from 0.05 to 0.1 μmol (10 to 20 μg)/d. The electroencephalogram (EEG) is diffusely abnormal, and peripheral nerve conduction may be delayed.

TREATMENT Therapeutic modalities include gastrointestinal decontamination, enhanced renal excretion, and dialysis. Gastric lavage or ipecac syrup is indicated within 4 to 6 h of acute ingestion. Adequacy of removal of thallium can be documented by follow-up abdominal x-ray. Prussian blue absorbs thallium in the gastrointestinal tract by exchanging potassium for thallium on its crystal lattice network thereby preventing absorption. The oral dose is 250 mg/kg body weight, administered once. Activated charcoal is as effective as Prussian blue in increasing fecal elimination by interrupting the enterohepatic circulation of thallium. Mannitol or magnesium citrate is used as a laxative to enhance gastrointestinal removal.

Forced diuresis is the oldest technique in use, and increases urinary excretion by 50 to 100 percent. Potassium chloride promotes renal excretion of thallium through the exchange of potassium for thallium, thereby releasing thallium from tissue sites into blood and augmenting urinary excretion two- to threefold. This therapy shortens thallium half-life in humans but may aggravate neurologic symptoms by redistributing thallium into the brain. The amount of thallium removed as compared to the total ingested dose of potassium is small. Diuretics (furosemide) also increase urinary elimination of thallium. Peritoneal dialysis removes 15 to 20 mg of thallium per day and hemodialysis 8 mg for each 8 h of dialysis. Prolonged hemodialysis can remove up to 25 mg of thallium per day, the total amount removed being relatively small. Charcoal hemoperfusion achieves average blood clearance values of 100 mL/min at a blood flow rate of 300 mL/min. Thus, the combination of forced diuresis, diuretic therapy, and hemoperfusion will most effectively enhance total-body clearance of thallium. This therapy should be combined with oral administration of Prussian blue or activated charcoal plus cathartics.

Ditiocarb has been advocated for early use in overdose because it leads to increased thallium blood levels and a two- to threefold increase in thallium excretion. However, ditiocarb-thallium complexes diffuse into the brain with subsequent clinical and EEG worsening; therefore, ditiocarb is contraindicated in thallium intoxication.

CHELATING AGENTS

Chelating agents are used to bind toxic metals in stable, cyclic compounds with relatively low toxicity and enhanced renal and fecal excretion.

DIMERCAPROL (BRITISH ANTI-LEWISITE, BAL) Dimercaprol was first developed as an antidote for the arsenical war gas lewisite; its chelating property is due to its four sulfhydryl groups which bind in a complex to polyvalent metal ions. Its affinity for metals is strong enough to reverse a significant portion of toxic metal enzyme binding. Dimercaprol diffuses into erythrocytes and enhances fecal as well as urinary metal excretion. It is given intramuscularly in peanut oil every 4 to 8 h in a dose of 12 to 24 mg/kg body weight per 24 h. Toxicity includes mild febrile reactions, nausea, headache, lacrimation, conjunctivitis, salivation, and rhinorrhea. The drug emits a strong sulfide odor, and patients may complain of metallic taste. Contraindications to dimercaprol include glucose-6-phosphate dehydrogenase deficiency, allergy to peanut oil, and concurrent use of medicinal iron, which forms a toxic complex with dimercaprol. Succimer (DMSA), an oral congener of dimercaprol, is under clinical trials in the United States for the treatment of lead and mercury poisoning. It has not been shown to be effective for other metals, although it may work in copper poisoning as well. Its dosage, effectiveness, and safety appear to be comparable to those of parenteral edetate with the advantage of oral administration and more selective excretion of the heavy metal. Mechanism of action appears to be comparable to that of dimercaprol.

EDETATE (EDTA) Because the sodium salt of edetate can produce profound hypocalcemia, only the calcium disodium salt should be used in therapy of metal poisoning. Calcium edetate forms a complex with divalent cations exchanging one atom of calcium for each metal ion. It enhances urinary excretion of lead twenty- to fiftyfold and also increases excretion of zinc and, to a lesser extent, other metals. It does not enter the erythrocyte but removes metals from the extracellular sites. Oral administration is contraindicated because it is variably absorbed and it enhances absorption of metals from the gastrointestinal tract. The drug is given parenterally either by constant intravenous infusion or intramuscular injection in a dose of 500 to 1000 mg/m² surface area per day. The drug can be used safely in conjunction with other chelating agents. Toxicity increases after 4 to 5 days of administration with concomitant reduction in metal excretion; as a consequence, the drug is given for several ''courses'' of from 3 to 5 days each.

Toxicity is principally renal, dose-related, and usually reversible. It can be reduced by maintaining adequate urine flow. During treatment renal function should be carefully monitored.

PENICILLAMINE Penicillamine is the only commercially available oral chelating agent. Not presently approved by the Federal

Drug Administration for treatment of lead poisoning, it is licensed for use in the treatment of rheumatoid arthritis, Wilson's disease, and cystinuria. Nevertheless, there is extensive experience in its use in chelation of other metals. The *N*-acetyl form is particularly helpful in the treatment of inorganic and organic mercury poisoning.

Penicillamine enhances excretion of heavy metals in the urine by an unclear mechanism. The drug is given orally in a dose of 40 mg/kg body weight per day. By initiating therapy at low doses (usually 25 percent of the anticipated maximum dose) and gradually increasing the dose, the frequency of side effects can be reduced substantially.

Side effects may be seen in up to 20 to 30 percent of patients receiving penicillamine and resemble penicillin hypersensitivity, including rash, fever, thrombocytopenia, and leukopenia. Rare side effects include autoimmune hemolytic anemia and Stevens-Johnson syndrome. Anorexia, nausea, sleep disturbances, and urinary frequency may be seen occasionally. Nephrotoxicity is reported in adults receiving large doses and in one case has been reported in a child. Patients receiving penicillamine should, therefore, be carefully monitored for signs of renal, hematologic, or allergic side effects.

REFERENCES

Arsenic

FESMIRE FM et al: Survival following massive arsenic ingestion. Am J Emerg Med 6:602, 1988

FOWLER BA, WEISSBERG JB: Arsine poisoning. N Engl J Med 291:1171, 1974

KLEVAY LM: Pharmacology and toxicology of heavy metals: Arsenic. Pharmacol Ther 1:189, 1976

PETERSON RG, RUMACK BH: D-Penicillamine therapy of acute arsine poisoning. J Pediatr 91:661, 1977

Cadmium

DUNPHY B: Acute occupational cadmium poisoning. J Occup Med 9:22, 1967

FRIBERG L et al: *Cadmium in the Environment*, 2d ed. Cleveland, CRC Press, 1974

——— et al: *Handbook on the Toxicology of Metals*. Amsterdam, Elsevier, 1979

Lead

CARNOW B (ed): *Health Effects of Occupational Lead and Arsenic Exposure, A Symposium*. Chicago, US Department of Health, Education, and Welfare, 1976

NATIONAL ACADEMY OF SCIENCES: *Lead in the Human Environment*, A Report Prepared by the Committee on Lead in the Human Environment, Environmental Studies Board, Commission on Natural Resources, National Research Council, Washington, DC, 1980

KEHOE RA: The metabolism of lead in man in health and disease. The Harben Lectures, 1960. J R Inst Pub Health 24:1, 101; 129; 177, 1961

PIOMELLIS et al: Management of childhood lead poisoning. J Pediatr 105:523, 1984

WALDRON HA, STOFEN D: *Sub-Clinical Lead Poisoning*. New York, Academic, 1974

Mercury

ELHASSANI SB: The many faces of methylmercury poisoning. J Toxicol Clin Toxicol 19:875, 1982–83

FRIBERG L, VOSTAL J (eds): *Mercury in the Environment*. Cleveland, CRC Press, 1972

NATIONAL ACADEMY OF SCIENCES: *An Assessment of Mercury in the Environment*, Washington, DC, 1978

PETERING HG, TEPPER LB: Pharmacology and toxicology of heavy metals: Mercury. Pharmacol Ther 1:131, 1976

WHO Environmental Health Criteria, Mercury. Geneva, World Health Organization, 1976

Thallium

BANK WJ et al: Thallium poisoning. Arch Neurol 26:456, 1972

CHISOLM JJ JR: The use of chelating agents in the treatment of acute and chronic lead intoxication in childhood. J Pediatr 73:1, 1968

DE GROOT G, VAN HEIJST ANP: Toxicokinetic aspects of thallium poisoning. Methods of treatment by toxin elimination. Sci Total Environ 71:411, 1988

——— et al: The evaluation of the efficacy of charcoal hemoperfusion in the treatment of three cases of thallium poisoning. Arch Toxicol 57:61, 1985

Chelating agents

HRUBY R, DONNER A: 2,3-Dimercapto-1-propanesulphonate in heavy metal poisoning. Med Toxicol 2:317, 1987

376 DISORDERS CAUSED BY VENOMS, BITES, AND STINGS

JAMES F. WALLACE

Humans have the propensity to come into contact with a great variety of venomous animals. These contacts occur with many zoologic classes including snakes, lizards, sea animals, spiders, scorpions, and numerous species of insects. In general two types of injuries result: those due to the direct effect of venom on the victim, as exemplified in snakebite, and those due to indirect effects of the poison, of which hypersensitivity reaction to bee stings is an example. Each year in the United States at least 50 persons die as the result of venomous injuries. Three groups of animals—hymenopterous insects, snakes, and spiders—account for over 90 percent of the fatalities. Of even greater public health significance is the loss in economic productivity and human potential resulting from the many serious, nonfatal envenomations that occur annually in otherwise healthy children or working adults.

SNAKE BITE

EPIDEMIOLOGY Fewer than one-tenth of the nearly 3500 known species of snakes are venomous. These poisonous varieties belong to five families or subfamilies: Elapidae (cobras, kraits, mambas, and coral snakes) found in all parts of the world except Europe; Viperidae (true vipers) found in all parts of the world except the Americas; Hydrophidae (sea snakes); Crotalidae (pit vipers) found in Asia and the Americas; and Colubridae (boomslangs, bird snakes) of the African continent. The poisonous varieties of the United States, with the single exception of the coral snake, are pit vipers and include rattlesnakes, the water moccasin, and the copperhead. Although this discussion centers around these species, most of the therapeutic measures outlined are applicable to snakes in all parts of the world.

The number of individuals bitten by poisonous snakes in the United States is estimated to be about 8000 per year, with a relatively large number occurring in the southeastern and Gulf states, particularly Texas. Deaths are not reported separately but are undoubtedly rare, numbering fewer than 20 per year, and most are due to bites of various species of rattlesnake. In many European countries deaths from snakebite have averaged only one every 3 to 5 years for the last half-century. In contrast, the estimate of annual deaths from snakebite throughout the world is between 30,000 and 40,000 with the largest number occurring in the countries of Burma and Brazil, where 2000 deaths are estimated to occur each year.

ETIOLOGY The *coral snake* is found in the southern states from Florida to Arizona. It is usually marked by alternating red and black bands separated by yellow rings; however, black and albino forms exist. Coral snakes are generally nocturnal in their activities, shy and elusive, and rarely bite humans. Their fangs are short and permanently erect; the highly toxic venom is injected into multiple puncture wounds produced by a series of chewing movements.

The *pit vipers* are so named because of a small pit between the eye and the nostril. Large venom glands in the temporal regions give the head a triangular appearance. They are generally aggressive and likely to strike if disturbed. The fangs are long and hinged, folding posteriorly when the mouth is closed. Pit vipers strike suddenly with a forward thrust of the head. The instant that the erect fangs make contact, venom is expressed by sudden muscular contraction.

The *rattlesnakes,* recognized by the horny rattle on the tail, which buzzes when the snake is disturbed, are widely distributed. The diamondbacks (*Crotalus adamanteus* in the southeast and *C. atrox* in the southwest) are the largest and most dangerous snakes in this country. Others include the prairie rattler (*C. confluentus*), the timber rattler (*C. horridus*), and the pigmy rattlers.

The *water moccasin,* or cottonmouth (*Agkistrodon piscivorus*), is found in swampy areas or along the banks of streams. It is a strong swimmer and can bite under water. This snake is notorious for inflicting severe facial bites when disturbed in the branches of small trees. The copperhead, or highland moccasin (*A. mokasen*), is a closely related species. Its bite is painful but rarely fatal.

PATHOGENESIS   Snake venoms   The venoms of most species that have been analyzed have been found to be mixtures of many toxic proteins and enzymes with diversified and complicated pharmacologic effects. As an example, the venom of the Indian cobra (*Naja naja*) contains these distinct and separate substances: a neurotoxin, a hemolysin, a cardiotoxin, a cholinesterase, at least three phosphatases, a nucleotidase, and a potent inhibitor of cytochrome oxidase. Several venoms, including those of the pit vipers, contain hyaluronidase and numerous proteolytic enzymes. Although the exact roles of these components in toxicity are incompletely understood, the venom of a given species is usually predominantly neurotoxic or necrotizing and is frequently associated with hemolysis, abnormalities of blood coagulation, changes in cardiac dynamics, and alterations in vascular resistance. Venoms of elapids, including the coral snake, are neurotoxic, with death resulting from respiratory paralysis probably caused by damage to brain centers and a curariform interference with transmission at the neuromuscular junction. Venoms of crotalid snakes produce local tissue injury, hemorrhage, and hemolysis. Death is often preceded by circulatory collapse associated with a marked fall in circulating blood volume resulting from pooling of blood in the microcirculation, and loss of plasma due to increased capillary permeability. Systemic absorption of venom occurs through the lymphatics, and therapeutic measures designed to reduce lymphatic function are helpful in controlling symptoms.

Factors affecting severity of snake bite   Several factors affect the outcome of snake bite:

1 The age, size, and health of the patient. Envenomation in children is usually serious, and a fatal outcome is more likely, since a relatively large dose of poison is injected into a small victim.
2 Location of bite. Bites on extremities or into adipose tissue are less dangerous than those on the trunk, face, or directly into a blood vessel. A direct strike of the fangs is more dangerous than a scratch, a glancing blow, or one hitting a bone. The discharge orifice of a fang is well above its tip so that the point of the fang can penetrate the skin without envenomation; even a thin layer of clothing may afford great protection. Because of the superficial nature of the wound, as many as one-fifth of patients bitten by venomous snakes will have no evidence of envenomation, even though the fangs have penetrated the skin.
3 The size of the snake (a large pit viper can inject over 1000 mg venom, six times a lethal dose for an adult), the extent of its anger or fear (if hurt it may inject a larger amount of venom), the condition of the fangs (broken or recently renewed), and the condition of the venom glands (recently discharged or full). All these factors are important. Contrary to popular belief, the bite of a snake which has recently killed and fed is not necessarily less venomous for humans; the snake usually does not exhaust its venom in a single bite.
4 The presence of various bacteria, particularly clostridia and other anaerobic organisms, in the mouth of the snake or on the skin of the victim. This may lead to serious infection in the necrotic tissues at the local site.
5 Exercise or exertion, such as running, immediately after the bite. This speeds systemic absorption of toxin.

MANIFESTATIONS   Following the bite of a pit viper, severe burning pain develops within a few minutes at the site of the wound. Local swelling rapidly develops and spreads in all directions, accompanied by the appearance of ecchymoses and bullae over the involved area. As the edema spreads, serosanguinous fluid oozes from the puncture wounds. Later gangrene of the skin and subcutaneous tissues may develop. Systemic effects resulting from the absorption of venom

and local tissue destruction may include fever, nausea and vomiting, circulatory collapse, bleeding into the skin and from all body orifices, low-grade jaundice, neuropathic muscle cramping, pupillary constriction, disorientation, delirium, and convulsions. Death may occur after 6 to 48 h. Survival may be attended by massive local tissue loss from gangrene or secondary infection, or may be complicated by acute renal failure, secondary to disseminated intravascular clotting and cortical necrosis, or by tubular necrosis following circulatory collapse.

The bite of the coral snake causes little pain and local swelling. There are usually multiple fang marks. Within 10 to 15 min numbness and weakness begin in the region of the bite, followed by ataxia, ptosis, pupillary dilatation, palatal and pharyngeal paralysis, slurring of speech, salivation, and occasionally nausea and vomiting. The patient becomes comatose, develops respiratory paralysis and seizures, and dies within 8 to 72 h.

Cobra bites are painful and are often accompanied by severe hemolysis, local necrosis, and sloughing in addition to their neurotoxic effects. There is little pain and no edema at the site of a sea snake bite. Symptoms of systemic envenomation follow a latent period which may vary from 15 min to 8 h. Although the venom is both myotoxic and neurotoxic, the injury to skeletal muscle is most prominent and is characterized by generalized muscle pain, weakness, and myoglobinuria. Hemorrhagic manifestations predominate following envenomation by colubrids (boomslangs and bird snakes) and many pit vipers including certain species of rattlesnake.

LABORATORY ABNORMALITIES   In severe cases, laboratory abnormalities may include progressive anemia, polymorphonuclear leukocytosis of 20,000 to 30,000 cells per microliter, thrombocytopenia, hypofibrinogenemia, disordered tests of coagulation, proteinuria, and azotemia.

TREATMENT   An attempt should be made to determine with certainty that the patient has been bitten by a poisonous snake. Absence of distinct fang punctures and failure of local pain, edema, numbness, or weakness to appear within 20 min are strong evidence against snake venom poisoning. The approximate size of the snake should be noted since larger snakes usually cause more severe envenomation. If the species of snake is not known, the offending reptile should be killed for the purpose of identification.

First aid   This consists of reassuring and calming the victim, instituting measures to retard the absorption of venom and to remove it from the tissues as quickly as possible after the bite, and arranging for transportation to the nearest hospital. The patient should be promptly placed at rest and the bitten extremity immobilized to reduce the rate of spread of the venom. This is best achieved by splinting. If anatomically feasible, a wide constriction band should be placed a few centimeters above the bite and made tight enough to allow one finger to pass beneath with difficulty. The purpose is to impede lymph flow; it is not necessary to obstruct venous return. The band should be loosened and moved proximally when local swelling causes it to tighten. There is no evidence in humans that incision and suction of the wound remove significant amounts of venom or improve outcome. Therefore this procedure is no longer recommended.

In order to help assess the severity of envenomation, the level of swelling should be marked on the skin every 15 min while the patient is being transported to a hospital. Although ice packs relieve pain and slow lymphatic drainage, they do not neutralize venom, and even a small amount of cooling may result in irreparable damage to already injured tissues by causing ischemia. For this reason, it is recommended that no form of cryotherapy be used.

Immediate hospital care   This should include appropriate treatment for shock and respiratory difficulty, antivenin, measures to combat infection, and general supportive care. Initial laboratory studies in a patient with obvious crotalid envenomation should include blood typing and cross-matching, a complete blood count, urinalysis, coagulation screening tests, blood urea nitrogen (BUN), blood glucose, and serum electrolytes. In severe envenomations it is also advisable to obtain an electrocardiogram. None of these tests are particularly helpful in the initial evaluation of a patient with a coral snake bite.

Antivenin is the only specific treatment of snake venom poisoning, and its use in severe bites is vital. In the United States polyvalent crotaline antivenin effective against all American pit vipers and antivenin for North American coral snake poisoning are commercially available. Both products are a lyophilized powder of refined horse serum. Kits are available containing antivenin powder (reconstituted by diluting with water to 10 mL per vial), syringe, normal horse serum for prior sensitivity testing of the patient, and detailed instructions. Intravenously administered antivenin leads to the most rapid and effective response. It is not advisable to infiltrate antivenin at the local site. The initial dose should depend upon an estimate of the amount of envenomation. For pit viper bites accompanied by progressive local swelling but no systemic symptoms (minimal envenomation), 5 vials (50 mL) are usually sufficient. When swelling has progressed beyond the site of the bite, and mild systemic symptoms and/or hematologic and coagulation abnormalities are present, moderate envenomation has occurred, and initial treatment should be 5 to 15 vials (50 to 150 mL). For severe poisonings, associated with rapidly progressive and extensive local effects as well as systemic symptoms and evidence of hemolysis or coagulopathy, 15 to 20 vials (150 to 200 mL) or more should be administered. Up to 50 percent greater doses of antivenin should be given to children or small adults to neutralize the relatively higher venom concentrations. Reconstituted antivenin is diluted in 500 mL of intravenous fluid and administered as rapidly as tolerated over 1 to 2 h. Additional infusions containing 5 to 10 vials (50 to 100 mL) should be repeated every 2 h until progressive swelling in the bitten part ceases and systemic signs and symptoms have disappeared. When an adequate dose has been achieved, improvement in the victim's clinical signs is often extremely rapid.

If *any* evidence of envenomation appears during the first several hours following a coral snake bite, antivenin should be given without waiting for systemic manifestations to develop. Four vials of antivenin should be given intravenously for bites associated only with minimal swelling and/or local paresthesias. If evidence of a bite is more definitive, particularly if there was initial pain, 6 to 10 vials of antivenin should be given as soon as possible. Larger doses should be used in severe bites from large snakes, if the snake bite was prolonged for more than a few seconds, or if the victim is a child.

In the patient with severe envenomation who is allergic to horse serum, the relative risk of death from anaphylaxis rather than from venom poisoning should be carefully weighed before undertaking desensitization with small doses of diluted horse serum.

No antivenin for other snakes is manufactured in the United States, but antiserum for various types is usually kept on hand at large zoos all over the world. A national antivenin index is maintained by the Oklahoma Poison Information Center in cooperation with the Oklahoma City Zoo [(405) 271–5454], and provides 24-h telephone consultation service for physicians needing advice in handling snakebite accidents.

Maintaining *respiration* by mechanical or other means is important. In patients bitten by elapid snakes, respiratory failure is usually reversible. *Tetanus toxoid* or *tetanus immune globulin* of human origin should be given (see Chap. 105). If wound infections appear, antibiotics should be used with the knowledge that the predominant microorganisms in the mouths of snakes are gram-negative pathogens. Treatment should be preceded by appropriate aerobic and anaerobic cultures. *Fasciotomy* occasionally may be necessary to prevent further ischemic injury to a massively swollen limb. Whenever possible, intracompartmental tissue pressures should be monitored, with surgical decompression undertaken only if pressure exceeds 30 to 40 mmHg. *Surgical debridement* of vesicles and superficial necrotic tissue should be instituted near the end of the first week following the bite. *Relief of pain* with salicylates or meperidine, moderate sedation, maintenance of fluid balance, measures to combat shock and hemorrhagic diathesis, and appropriate management of coma or convulsions are all important.

The usefulness of glucocorticoids to prevent tissue damage or systemic intoxication has not been convincingly demonstrated. However, these drugs may be of value in the management of severe shock associated with envenomation and for allergic reactions, particularly serum sickness, following the administration of antivenin.

PREVENTION In snake-infested regions long trousers, high shoes, boots, or leggings, and gloves should be worn. Most important of all is to look where one steps or reaches. A constriction band and antiseptic suffice for an emergency kit, and in inaccessible areas, antivenin should also be carried.

POISONOUS LIZARD BITE

Of the nearly 3000 species of lizard in the world, only two are venomous: the Gila monster (*Heloderma suspectum*) of the arid southwestern United States and the closely related Mexican beaded lizard (*H. horridum*) which inhabits the lowland forests of western Mexico. These reptiles are not aggressive, and virtually every instance of their attacking a human has involved teasing or handling the animals in captivity. The venom is elaborated in eight glands in the floor of the mouth and secreted directly into the oral cavity, where it bathes the teeth, which are grooved posteriorly. The lizard clings tenaciously and is often dislodged only after considerable effort; envenomation occurs by contamination of the wound. The venom contains a potent neurotoxin which is undoubtedly responsible for its lethal effect on experimental animals. Death in humans following a bite is extremely rare. Most often, human envenomation results in tissue injury, excruciating pain, massive edema, and patchy erythema. Acute systemic symptoms may last for 3 to 4 days and include nausea, vomiting, hematemesis, blurred vision, dyspnea, dysphonia, and profound weakness. Intense hyperesthesia of the bitten extremity may persist for several weeks. There is no antivenin available. Treatment should consist of constriction band, cooling of the bitten area, measures to prevent or combat infection, including tetanus, and supportive measures. Parenteral meperidine (Demerol) or infiltration of local anesthetic around the bite may be necessary to relieve pain.

SPIDER BITES

The bite of many spiders is locally irritating, and several species can cause severe, even fatal systemic poisoning in humans. In North America, only two types of spiders are of medical importance: the widow spiders (*Latrodectus* species) and the recluse spiders (*Loxosceles* species).

WIDOW SPIDER BITE The most numerous and important of the venomous spiders are members of the genus *Latrodectus*, widely distributed throughout the world. In the United States and Canada, *L. mactans*, the black widow or shoe-button spider, causes a majority of clinically significant arachnidism. In Florida, *L. bishopi*, the red-legged widow spider, has been reported to produce human poisoning resembling mild black widow bite.

It is the female *L. mactans*, the black widow, that bites humans. She is glossy black with a body 1 cm in diameter, a leg span of 5 cm, and a characteristic red hourglass mark on her abdomen. She spins her web in woodpiles, sheds, basements, or outdoor privies, is very aggressive, and will bite on slight provocation. The venom produces diffuse central and peripheral nervous excitement, autonomic activity, muscle spasm, hypertension, and vasoconstriction.

In the United States, most black widow bites occur between April and October, and many patients are males bitten on the genitalia or buttocks while using a privy. After a momentary sharp pain at the site, there is cramping pain that begins locally within 15 to 60 min and gradually spreads. It may involve all extremities and the trunk. The abdomen is boardlike, and the waves of pain become excruciating, causing the patient to turn, toss, and cry out. Respirations are often labored and grunting. There are also nausea, vomiting, headache, sweating, salivation, hyperactive reflexes, twitching, tremor, paresthesias of the hands and feet, and occasionally, systolic hypertension. A mild polymorphonuclear leukocytosis is usual, and many patients have slight fever. After several hours, the pains subside, although mild recurrences for 2 or 3 days are common. It may be a week before well-being is restored. Deaths due to cardiac or respiratory failure have occurred, mostly in children and the aged.

Because the bite itself is not prominent, patients are often thought to have some abdominal catastrophe such as perforated ulcer, pancreatitis, or appendicitis. Renal colic, myocardial infarction, tetanus, strychnine poisoning, tabetic crisis, lead colic, and porphyria are other conditions to be ruled out. The abdomen is not tender to palpation in arachnidism, and pains in the extremities are not typical of most of these other disorders.

TREATMENT   For *Latrodectus* poisoning, treatment consists of measures to relieve pain and administration of antivenin. Initial treatment should include a hot tub bath which affords prompt, although temporary, relief. A vial (10 mL) of 10% calcium gluconate slowly injected intravenously over 10 to 20 min usually produces dramatic, but transient, cessation of cramps. A solution of 10% methocarbamol administered intravenously also may be effective in treatment of muscle spasms. Opiates are sometimes necessary. When symptoms are severe or when the patient is a small child or is at special risk due to other associated medical problems, treatment with *Latrodectus* antivenin is indicated. An intravenous injection of 1 vial (2.5 mL) diluted in 50 mL of saline and administered over a 15-min period is usually quite effective within a few hours and can be repeated if symptoms recur. Since the antivenin is prepared from horse serum, appropriate testing for hypersensitivity should be undertaken prior to its administration.

LOXOSCELES SPIDER BITE   During the past 30 years in the United States, there have been increasing numbers of reports of severe necrotizing bites due to *Loxosceles* spiders. Originally thought to be a problem only in the midwestern states and associated only with the brown recluse spider, necrotic arachnidism has now been seen in many of the southern and southwestern states as well as in California and has been attributed to at least six species of *Loxosceles* spider. The bite of these spiders may initially produce only a mild stinging discomfort. In severe bites, intense local pain appears within 2 to 8 h, accompanied by bullae formation and erythema at the site of the wound. Subsequently, ischemic necrosis occurs leaving a deep ulcer with a necrotic base. The pathogenetic mechanism for the local reaction is not completely understood but is thought to involve complement-activated tissue damage. Some patients also experience a systemic reaction characterized by fever, myalgias, and a morbilliform rash 24 to 48 h after the bite. Intravascular hemolysis is seen occasionally, and in severe cases hemoglobinuria and acute renal failure may occur. Fatalities have been reported, mostly in children.

Treatment depends upon the severity of the bite. If bullae formation, intense pain, and signs of rapidly progressing ischemic necrosis do not appear within the first 6 to 8 h, the bite is probably not severe and treatment is unnecessary. When symptoms of more serious local reaction are present, the parenteral use of glucocorticoids within the first 24 h following a bite has been advocated to prevent progression of the lesion, but convincing evidence that this is effective is lacking. Dapsone and/or brown recluse antivenin have been reported to prevent extensive ulceration in rapidly progressing *Loxosceles* spider bites. However, use of these forms of therapy should be considered experimental. Other therapeutic measures consist mainly of local wound care including cool compresses, elevation of the bitten extremity, timely surgical debridement, and treatment of secondary infection, if it occurs. The ulcer usually heals spontaneously, although skin grafting may be required on occasion. Patients with systemic loxoscelism should be hospitalized and monitored closely for signs of hemolysis, disseminated intravascular coagulation, and acute renal failure. Although of unproven efficacy, systemic glucocorticoids are usually given only for the duration of the acute phase of the illness,

which lasts 2 to 4 days. Renal failure should be treated as advised in Chap. 223.

SCORPION STING

Scorpions are eight-legged arthropods. Glands in the terminal segment produce venom, which is injected into the victim by a stinger located on the tip of the tail. Scorpions often enter dwellings. During the day they retreat into crevices; emerging at night, they often get into shoes and clothing and even into bedding. They do not deliberately attack humans, but accidental contact results in a sting.

Of about 650 species, roughly 40 occur in the United States, distributed over three-fourths of the nation. They are most numerous in the south from Florida to California, but the only dangerous species, *Centruroides exilicauda,* is limited to Arizona, New Mexico, southern California, parts of Texas, and northern Mexico. This species reaches a maximal length of about 7 cm. Their sting may be fatal to young children or old people, but seldom to a healthy adult.

Most of the nonlethal species of scorpions in the United States cause only minor reactions, like a bee sting. Some in the southwest, however, produce local edema and ecchymosis, with burning pain. In contrast, many species whose venom has potentially lethal systemic effects, including the Arizona *Centruroides*, evoke little or no visible reaction at the site of the sting. There is an immediate burning sensation followed by local paresthesia (''pins and needles''), hyperesthesia, or numbness. These sensations spread to involve the whole extremity, and within an hour or two, malaise, restlessness, neurologic hyperexcitability, lacrimation, rhinorrhea, salivation, perspiration, nausea, and vomiting may appear.

The patient may pass from an agitated state with hyperactive reflexes into coma; convulsions follow. Release of catecholamines may result in tachycardia, various arrhythmias, and hypertension. Myocarditis and pancreatitis have also been reported. Death usually occurs within 12 h, but sometimes as late as 2 days after the sting.

TREATMENT   Despite the reputation for lethality associated with envenomation by *C. exilicauda,* most often the symptoms consist only of pain and paresthesias lasting less than 4 h. These patients can be treated at home with cold compresses and mild analgesics. There is no clear consensus on the management of more severe envenomations. Although the use of constriction bands as in the treatment of snake bite has been recommended, the amount of venom is minute; it produces no local necrotizing effect and is absorbed very rapidly.

Specific antivenin, reconstituted from lyophilized goat serum, is available in some areas and should be considered if the victim develops signs of cranial nerve dysfunction and increased involuntary activity in skeletal muscles other than those innervated by cranial nerves. An intravenous injection of 1 or 2 vials (5.0 or 10.0 mL) administered over 15 to 30 min usually reverses the severe neurologic symptoms within minutes following the infusion. Supportive therapy is directed at combating shock and dehydration. Diazepam or phenobarbital are useful in reducing restlessness, and adrenergic blockers in managing symptoms secondary to catecholamine release.

PREVENTION   This depends upon alertness in avoiding contact with scorpions in infested areas. Clothing and shoes should be well shaken before being put on in the morning. Towels and bedclothes should be inspected. A house infested with scorpions can in time be rid of them by closing all obvious ways of ingress; picking up debris in the environment, such as piles of brush, logs, stones; introducing a mixture of fuel oil or kerosene, containing a small amount of creosote, between the earth and the house foundation; and spraying with a mixture of 2% chlordane, and 0.2% pyrethrins in an oil base.

HYMENOPTERA STINGS

Each year in the United States, nearly twice as many people die as a result of bites by hymenopterous insects (including bees, wasps, hornets, yellow jackets, and fire ants) as from poisonous snake bites. Occasionally, multiple stings in enormous numbers (500 to 1000) are the cause of death. However, the majority of systemic reactions and deaths are due to allergic reactions to the venoms of these insects.

Hymenoptera venoms contain many nonallergenic amines and peptides such as histamine and various kinins which contribute to the local sting reaction through their inflammatory and vasoactive properties. The allergenic venom proteins, which elicit an IgE antibody response in those who are stung, include phospholipases, hyaluronidases, acid phosphatases, and melittin. Venoms are distinctly different for each of the three genera of hymenoptera capable of causing allergic sting reactions: Apidae (various species of bees), Vespidae (hornets, yellowjackets, and wasps), and *Solenopsis* (fire ants).

The usual reaction to a single bee or wasp sting is sharp pain, which lasts for several minutes, local wheal and erythema, followed by intense itching. All signs of the sting normally subside within a few hours. Only in the rare case when a bee is swallowed or inhaled and edema of the laryngopharynx or glottis develops is there danger. A sting directly into a peripheral nerve can destroy its function for a time, much as does an injection of alcohol. Bell's palsy has followed a sting into the trunk of the facial nerve. Unusual reactions such as optic neuritis, generalized polyneuropathy, and myasthenia gravis may follow a sting. The etiology of these reactions is unknown. Acute renal failure has been reported following multiple bee stings. Nephrotoxicity, due to venom-induced rhabdomyolysis, and renal ischemia are thought to be the probable mechanisms.

In hypersensitive individuals, the response to a single sting may vary from an exaggerated local reaction, unassociated with systemic symptoms, to serious anaphylaxis with urticaria, nausea, abdominal or uterine cramps, bronchospasm, massive edema of the face and glottis, dyspnea, cyanosis, hypotension, coma, and death. These symptoms usually appear within a few minutes of the sting. Other patients may experience delayed reactions of the serum-sickness type occurring 10 to 14 days after envenomation. Sensitization is usually the result of previous stings although many fatalities have occurred in individuals who experienced no apparent allergic reaction to earlier envenomation. It has been estimated that 10 to 15 percent of the general population in this country has hymenoptera venom allergy. Those who have experienced a previous systemic allergic reaction to a sting, such as respiratory difficulty, hypotension, or generalized urticaria, are at greatest risk for serious reactions if stung again by the same type of insect.

Since being accidentally introduced into southern Brazil in 1957, African bees have gradually spread through South and Central America. Within the next decade, their northernmost advance will be achieved and is expected to encompass the southern portion of the United States from North Carolina to southern California. Although widely touted as a human health problem, the actual risk is difficult to estimate because of a lack of reliable medical statistics. African bee venom appears to be qualitatively similar to that of European bees, although the median lethal dose may be smaller. Further research is needed to determine its toxocologic and pathologic characteristics.

Many species of ant can produce stinging bites with local redness and swelling. The most notorious of these are the fire ants (*Solenopsis*), particularly two "imported" South American species (*S. invicta* and *S. richteri*). The *invicta* species is now found in thirteen southern states and has largely supplanted all others, including several domestic species. In addition to being a major agricultural pest, fire ants, whose bites may result in extensive vesiculation and skin necrosis or cause serious hypersensitivity reactions, have become a significant health hazard to humans. Unlike other hymenoptera venoms, fire ant venom is mostly a simple insoluble alkaloid rather than a complex mixture of proteins. Although associated with life-threatening allergic reactions of the type seen with IgE-mediated immediate hypersensitivity, there is limited cross-sensitivity between fire ant venom and the venoms of bees, wasps, hornets, and yellowjackets.

TREATMENT The wound site should be examined for a stinger which, if present, should be carefully removed in order to prevent further envenomation from the attached gland. The local reaction to the usual sting is treated by local cool application and antipruritic lotions or oral antihistamines. Fire ant stings, which are frequently multiple, should be thoroughly cleaned with soap and water. Secondary bacterial infection is common and should be anticipated and treated promptly. Epinephrine, 0.3 to 0.5 mL of a 1:1000 aqueous solution subcutaneously repeated every 20 to 30 min, may be lifesaving in patients with an anaphylactic reaction to a sting. A tourniquet to slow the absorption of venom and ice packs to relieve pain may be used. Oxygen, endotracheal intubation, vasopressors, and other supportive measures should be used as needed. In addition, glucocorticoids should be employed in severe cases, although their maximum effect is not achieved until several hours after administration.

PREVENTION Allergic persons should make every effort to avoid contact with these insects, including wearing shoes when outside and not wearing perfumes or bright colors which may attract them. In addition, they should keep epinephrine readily available for immediate use in case of a sting, without waiting for symptoms to develop. Sting kits containing premeasured doses of 1:1000 epinephrine in disposable syringes, tourniquets, and antihistamine tablets are commercially available. Careful instruction in their use should be provided by the person's physician.

IMMUNOTHERAPY Desensitization by injection of preparations containing venom of the specific insect has long been recommended for any patient who has had a systemic or generalized reaction to hymenopterous insect stings. For many years, the only products available for this purpose were extracts of the crushed whole bodies of the stinging insect. However, skin testing with whole-body extracts was frequently unreliable in identifying persons at risk for systemic reactions, and immunization with these materials did not increase IgG-blocking antibodies to venom proteins, a response felt to be essential for protection against insect allergy. In contrast, purified hymenopterous venoms, which were approved for clinical use in the United States in 1979, have proved to be highly accurate in the diagnosis of sting allergy by skin testing. In addition, venom immunotherapy has been shown consistently to stimulate production of circulating venom-specific IgG antibodies, and to provide much better protection than whole-body extracts. The purified venoms have not been associated with a greater number of adverse reactions than treatment with whole-body extracts or with desensitization for pollinosis. These venom antigens are the materials of choice for diagnosis and immunotherapy of high-risk patients, those who have had previous systemic sting reactions and who have positive venom skin tests. The optimal duration of immunotherapy remains to be defined.

TICK BITE

Although ticks may be vectors for such serious diseases as Rocky Mountain spotted fever, Q fever, tularemia, borreliosis, human babesiosis, and Lyme disease, the local reaction to the bite of a tick may be nothing more than an itching papule that subsides within a few days unless there is secondary bacterial infection. However, incomplete removal of a tick, with retention of the mouthparts, may result in the local formation of a nodule that continues to grow and is sometimes annoyingly pruritic. The definitive treatment is surgical excision of the nodule. Histologically, the nodule is a granuloma, but the inflammatory response is sometimes so bizarre and changes in the overlying epithelium are so striking that, in the absence of a history of tick bite, a mistaken diagnosis of malignant tumor may be made.

Ticks should always be removed intact, using gentle, steady traction. Fine tweezers or blunt forceps should be employed if possible. When fingers are used instead, they should be protected with facial tissue and washed afterwards. Application of a drop of oil, petrolatum, nail polish, or other organic solvent may facilitate removal without leaving embedded remnants. However, touching with a hot object such as a glowing cigarette should be discouraged because of the likelihood of injuring the patient.

TICK PARALYSIS   A progressive, ascending, flaccid paralysis, acute ataxia, or a combination of both sometimes develops in humans and certain other mammals while a tick is engorging upon them. Human cases have most frequently been reported from the northwestern United States and western Canada, where the wood tick, *Dermacentor andersoni* Stiles, is responsible. The dog tick, *D. variabilis* Say, has been identified in a number of cases occurring in the southeastern states. *Amblyomma americanum*, the Lone Star tick, *A. maculatum*, the Gulf Coast tick, and *Ixodes scapularis*, the black-legged deer tick, have also been incriminated.

This disorder is caused by a neurotoxin secreted in the saliva of the engorging tick which acts upon spinal and bulbar nuclei, slowing motor nerve conduction without affecting neuromuscular transmission. The tick must feed for several days before symptoms develop.

Most human cases occur in children, generally in young girls. The tick is usually attached to the scalp and hidden by the hair, but may be found on any part of the body, especially the ear, axilla, groin, vulva, or popliteal region.

The patient may be irritable or restless for up to 24 h before frank motor involvement appears. Weakness usually is noted first in the distal muscles of the lower extremities, progressing over the next 24 to 48 h to flaccid paralysis, which may extend to involve the trunk, arms, neck, tongue, pharynx, and bulbar centers. Sensory changes are typically absent, and there is little or no fever unless a secondary infection is present. Results of routine laboratory tests including cerebrospinal fluid examination are normal. Nerve conduction studies may reveal decreased velocities and compound action potentials of nerves and their corresponding muscles.

Tick paralysis is apt to be confused with poliomyelitis, the more so because ticks are active in warm weather when poliomyelitis is most prevalent. Among other diseases which might be considered in differential diagnosis are diphtheritic polyneuropathy, transverse myelitis, the Guillain-Barré syndrome, myasthenia gravis, the Eaton-Lambert syndrome, and botulism.

Definitive treatment is removal of the tick, including any mouth-parts retained in the skin. After this is done, there is striking improvement of motor function within a few hours and complete recovery within 48 h.

The patient should be observed until the recovery trend is established, because if other ticks or retained mouthparts have been overlooked, the paralysis may progress. When bulbar or respiratory paralysis is present, death may occur if the tick is not removed in time. The mortality rate is 10 percent; nearly all who die are children.

OTHER ARTHROPOD BITES AND ENVENOMATIONS

FLEA BITE   There are many fleas that attack humans, including *Pulex irritans* and chicken fleas. In sensitive individuals, the salivary secretion of these bloodsuckers produces large, itching papules. It is thought that much of the papular urticaria of children is probably due to flea bites. Treatment is symptomatic only. Elimination of fleas from the environment may be very difficult, but persistent treatment of animals and of premises with appropriate insecticides is usually successful.

CENTIPEDE BITE   The giant desert centipede, which reaches 15 cm in length, is responsible for most centipede bites in the United States. It is capable of inflicting an intensely painful bite, associated with erythema, edema, and sometimes with regional lymphangitis. Rhabdomyolysis and acute renal failure have occurred following the bite of this arthropod. Pain usually disappears within a few hours, but may require oral or parenteral analgesics. The wound should be washed well with soap and water to help prevent secondary infection.

CATERPILLAR RASH   Contact with the early larval or caterpillar stage of several species of moth produces irritation of skin and mucous membranes resulting in a pruritic, erythematous rash, occasionally accompanied by urticaria and bullae. Symptoms come on rapidly after direct contact with caterpillars, after handling cocoons, or on being exposed to windblown fuzz. The pathogenesis is thought to be due to the direct irritant effects of insect hairs or appendages, although other mechanisms, including intracutaneous injection of toxins or hypersensitivity to insect antigens, have been suggested. The symptoms usually subside within a few days. Local soaks and oral antihistamines are often indicated.

BEDBUG BITE   Members of the genus *Cimex* inflict bites that leave reactions varying from a simple puncture to large urticarial lesions, apparently depending on the sensitivity of the bitten individual. There is no specific treatment.

KISSING BUG BITE   Of the many species of true bugs, those in the family Reduviidae are relatively commonly associated with severe bite reactions. The most important reduviid bug in this country is the kissing bug (genus *Triatoma*), which is found throughout the southern crescent of the United States. The bites of this bug, which is a nocturnal feeder, are characteristically inflicted in multiple groups. Reactions which follow are thought to be allergic in nature and may include intensely pruritic and painful papules with a central punctum, grouped vesicles with moderate swelling and redness but no central lesions, giant urticaria, generalized allergic reactions, including systemic anaphylaxis, and hemorrhagic nodular-to-bullous lesions on a hand or foot, appearing several days after the bite. These may be confused with necrotizing spider bites or with erythema multiforme. However, the former are usually single lesions and the latter rarely has a unilateral distribution. The possibility of kissing bug bites should be considered in patients who awaken in the middle of the night with intense itching, hives, and other signs of a systemic allergic reaction.

Treatment of the local reaction is symptomatic. More severe reactions should be managed similarly to other allergic sting reactions. Patients who have had accelerated reactions to reduviid bites should be provided with sting kits and instructions in their use. Immuno-therapy with whole body extracts of kissing bugs has been attempted but its value is unproven.

CHIGGERS OR REDBUGS   These are tiny mites that are commonly found in foliage or grass in many parts of the world. In the United States, the larval form of *Eutrobicula alfreddugesi* attacks the skin by secreting a substance which digests tissue, creating a red papule that itches intensely. The tiny reddish larva can be seen in the center of the lesion. Treatment is palliative and consists of antipruritic applications. The use of insect repellents, appropriate protective clothing, and prompt bathing after exposure reduce the risk of infestation considerably.

BLOODSUCKING-FLY BITE   Many species of flies, particularly the horsefly and the deerfly, viciously attack and feed upon warm-blooded animals, including humans. Occasionally, transmission of diseases such as anthrax, tularemia, loiasis, and trypanosomiasis has been attributed to horseflies and deerflies. More commonly in North America, however, their bites are responsible for painful, intensely pruritic cutaneous lesions which may be followed by delayed localized allergic reactions characterized by erythema, edema, and urticaria. Treatment should include thorough cleaning of the bite sites, topical glucocorticoids, and oral antihistaminics for severe itching. Antibiotics may be necessary if the wounds become secondarily infected.

MARINE ANIMAL VENOM DISEASES

The venoms of certain marine animals are known to cause illness in humans after injection or inoculation under naturally occurring conditions. Information concerning these toxins is limited; most appear to be composed of proteins and peptides as well as other substances that are pharmacologically active. Although probably less complex than the venoms of reptiles, many marine animal venoms are capable of causing several pathologic effects including neurotoxicity as well as local necrosis.

PORTUGUESE MAN-OF-WAR AND JELLYFISH STINGS The burning discomfort induced by contact with sea nettles or jellyfish is familiar to most surf bathers. Contact with the tentacles of the colorful Portuguese man-of-war (*Physalia* species), which is found mainly in or near the Gulf of Mexico, or the more toxic jellyfish (*Chiropsalmus* of the Indian Ocean and *Rhizostoma* of the Atlantic) is followed by burning pain, swelling, and erythema. Severe, generalized muscular cramps, nausea, vomiting, and pulmonary edema may occur. Victims have died as a result of jellyfish stings, sometimes within minutes after contact. In nonfatal cases, systemic symptoms usually subside within several hours. Treatment consists of bathing the wound in salt water, taking care not to rub the area of the sting. Next, any tentacles still clinging to the skin should be scraped off after first inactivating any remaining nematocysts to prevent discharge of additional venom into the victim. This can be done by sprinkling baking soda over the wound to form a slurry for sea nettle stings or by bathing with vinegar for man-of-war stings. Rinsing with fresh water, isopropyl alcohol, or household ammonia, or rubbing with sand are not recommended since these measures may actually cause nematocysts to discharge. Analgesics should be used for pain control, and antihistaminics if there is an accompanying pruritic rash. Severe envenomations may require advanced life-support measures. Glucocorticoids may be helpful in these cases. An antivenin is now available for treatment of stings by the highly lethal Australian sea wasp, *Chironex fleckeri*.

CORAL WOUNDS AND STINGS The colorful structures known as coral are composed of thousands of small marine animals of the coelenterate phylum, surrounded by a stony exoskeleton of calcium carbonate. Several species, including the fire coral, found in many parts of the world, contain microscopic nematocysts capable of producing painful stings similar to those caused by jellyfish. Often more serious are wounds resulting from abrasions and cuts by the sharp edges of the outer skeleton. These frequently contain small pieces of animal protein and skeletal material that act as foreign bodies and may lead to chronic, suppurative wound infections if not promptly and adequately debrided.

SEA ANEMONE STING ("SPONGE DIVER'S DISEASE") Contact with certain sea anemones (especially *Sargatia elegans*) in Mediterranean and African waters produces extensive dermatitis with chronic ulceration. Occasionally, especially during August and September, systemic symptoms of headache, sneezing, nausea, chills, fever, and collapse are noted. Rare fatalities have occurred. Application of vinegar may inactivate nematocyst discharge. No other specific therapy is known; symptomatic treatment with topical steroids or oral antihistaminics may provide temporary relief.

CONE SHELL POISONING The colorful cone shells are highly prized by collectors. However, many species in the Pacific are venomous, a great danger to unwary hobbyists who pick them up. The poison, a neurotoxin, is delivered into a wound inflicted by pointed hollow teeth resembling darts in the long proboscis of the animal. Local manifestations include sudden intense pain, followed by swelling and numbness, which may persist for several days. Symptoms of serious poisoning include muscular incoordination and weakness progressing to respiratory paralysis. Death may occur within 3 to 6 h, but recovery within 24 h is the rule. There is no specific therapy; recommended treatment is the use of tourniquet, incision, and suction and supportive measures which may include artificial respiration and administration of oxygen.

SPONGE DERMATITIS Direct contact with several species of sponge results in a painful dermatitis, which may persist for several weeks. The lesions appear to be caused by mechanical irritation from the exoskeleton of the sponge as well as by toxins within its tissues. Delayed hypersensitivity reactions may also occur. Topical glucocorticoids or oral antihistamines may provide relief from the pruritus; dilute acetic acid ameliorates local pain, while alkali will intensify it. The lesions are self-limited.

SEA URCHIN WOUNDS AND STINGS Contact with the spines of some species of sea urchin results in painful erythema and ulceration, occasionally accompanied by neurotoxic symptoms of weakness and frank paralysis of lips, tongue, and face lasting for several hours. Treatment is purely symptomatic and supportive. The toxins isolated from sea urchins have produced paralysis in animals and are notably resistant to heat. Deaths from paralysis and drowning have been reported. Occasionally, fragments of sea urchin spines may remain in the skin, leading to granulomatous reactions, or they may migrate into a joint or lodge against a nerve, causing intractable pain. Treatment of these complications is surgical.

PARALYTIC AND NEUROTOXIC SHELLFISH POISONING Certain dinoflagellates, which make up part of the marine phytoplankton, elaborate a potent neurotoxin. Occasionally, conditions in coastal waters become favorable for the growth of excessive numbers of these organisms, causing the water to develop an amber appearance termed the "red tide" and killing massive numbers of fish by exhausting their oxygen supply. When humans ingest shellfish which have themselves ingested toxic dinoflagellates, an illness occurs that is characterized by paresthesias of the face and extremities, dysphonia, and generalized muscular weakness, often accompanied by nausea, vomiting, and diarrhea and occasionally by paralysis and respiratory arrest. The more severe syndrome, known as paralytic shellfish poisoning, is encountered along the Pacific northwest and New England coasts. A milder form, not associated with paralysis in humans, is seen along the Gulf and Atlantic coasts of Florida. Treatment should include induced emesis and purgation to remove unabsorbed toxin from the gastrointestinal tract and whatever additional supportive measures are necessary. Spontaneous recovery usually takes place within 24 h. There is a standardized mouse bioassay procedure for demonstrating and quantitating toxin in shellfish but no diagnostic test for detecting toxin in clinical specimens.

VENOMOUS FISH INJURIES The dorsal fins or spines of bullhead sharks, dogfish, and ratfish and the dorsal and other fins of the lionfish, weeverfish, toadfish, and catfish are grooved, and at their bases are found venom glands. Little is known of the venoms involved except that they contain highly unstable proteins of variable molecular weights and are capable of causing toxic as well as allergic reactions.

Envenomation results in immediate, severe local pain and edema which, if untreated, reaches greatest intensity in 60 to 90 min and resolves within 8 to 12 h. Local necrosis with extensive tissue loss may occur, particularly following lionfish and catfish stings. Systemic reactions, including cardiac arrhythmias, hypotension, muscular weakness, seizures, and paralysis, have been reported and attributed to the effects of the venom.

Treatment should be immediate immersion of the wound in water as hot as the patient can stand for at least 1 h or until symptoms subside. The venoms are extremely heat labile, accounting for the usefulness of this procedure. Although rarely needed, an antivenin is available for patients with severe systemic reactions from stonefish envenomation. It can be obtained from the Health Services Department, Sea World of San Diego [(619) 222–0411]. Tetanus prophylaxis should be given as needed. Narcotics may be required to control pain. Secondary pyogenic infection is a frequent complication.

Probably the most frequent type of fish envenomation in the United States is that produced by the lashing tail of the stingray of the California coast (*Urobatis halleri*). The bony spine is encased in a sheath of epithelial cells containing venom which is expressed into the puncture wound. The wound may be several centimeters deep; portions of the bony spine may break off in it, or, more often, the integumentary sheath remains in the wound. The venom is a circulatory depressant in animals, but local injury predominates in humans. Severe pain and blanching followed by erythema and edema occur immediately. Symptoms due to systemic absorption of venom are infrequent but may include salivation, muscle cramps and weakness, cardiac arrhythmias, seizures, and death. Treatment consists of application of a constriction band (the vast majority of these injuries occur on the legs) and copious syringing of the wound with salt water to remove fragments of sheath. Additional therapeutic measures are the same as for other fish envenomations, including immersion of the injured area in hot water for up to 1 h.

REFERENCES

Hymenoptera stings

GOLDEN DBK et al: Discontinuing venom immunotherapy (VIT): Immunologic and clinical criteria. J Allergy Clin Immunol 79:126, 1987

——— et al: Epidemiology of insect venom sensitivity. JAMA 262:240, 1989

LIGHT WC et al: Unusual reactions following insect stings. J Allergy Clin Immun 59:391, 1977

PATTERSON R, VALENTINE M: Anaphylactic and related allergic emergencies including reactions to insect stings. JAMA 248:2632, 1982

PAULL BR: Imported fire ant allergy: Perspectives on diagnosis and treatment. Postgrad Med 76:155, 1984

TAYLOR OR JR: Health problems associated with African bees, editorial. Ann Intern Med 104:267, 1986

Marine animal venoms

AUERBACH PS, HALSTEAD BW: Hazardous marine life, in *Management of Wilderness and Environmental Emergencies*, PS Auerbach, HR Gee (eds). New York, MacMillan, 1983

BURNETT JW, CARLTON GJ: Jellyfish envenomation syndromes updated. Ann Emerg Med 26:1000, 1987

HUGHES JM, MERSON MH: Fish and shellfish poisoning. N Engl J Med 295:1117, 1976

KIZER KW: Marine envenomations. J Toxicol-Clin Toxicol 21:527, 1983–1984

——— et al: Scorpaenidae envenomation: A 5-year poison center experience. JAMA 253:807, 1985

ROSSON CL, TOLLE SW: Management of marine stings and scrapes. West J Med 150:97, 1989

ZERMAN MG: Catfish stings: A report of 3 cases. Ann Emerg Med 18:211, 1989

Other arthropod bites and stings

FRAZIER CA: *Insect Allergy: Allergic and Toxic Reactions to Insects and Other Arthropods*. St Louis, Grace, 1969

HILLIER FF, WARM RP: Caterpillar dermatitis. Br Med J 1:346, 1967

HUNT GR: Bites and stings of uncommon arthropods: 2. Reduviids, fire ants, puss caterpillars, and scorpions. Postgrad Med 70:107, 1981

LOGAN JL, OGDEN DA: Rhabdomyolysis and acute renal failure following the bite of the giant desert centipede *Scolopendra heros*. West J Med 142:549, 1985

SHELLEY ED et al: The diagnostic challenge of non-burrowing mite bites. JAMA 251:2690, 1984

WIRTZ RA: Allergic and toxic reactions to non-stinging arthropods. Ann Rev Entomol 29:47, 1984

Scorpion stings

CURRY SC et al: Envenomation by the scorpian *Centuroides sculpteratus*. J Toxicol-Clin Toxicol 21:417, 1983–84

LIKES K et al: *Centuroides exilicauda* envenomation in Arizona. West J Med 141:634, 1984

Snake and lizard bites

JURKOVICH GL et al: Complications of Crotalidae antivenin therapy. J Trauma 28:1032, 1988

KITCHENS CS, VAN MIEROP LHS: Envenomation by the eastern coral snake (*Micrurus fulvius fulvius*): A study of 39 victims. JAMA 258, 1615, 1987

LOPRINZI CL et al: Snake antivenin administration in a patient allergic to horse serum. South Med J 76:501, 1983

MITRAKUL C, DHAMKRONG A: Clinical features of neurotoxic snake bite and response to antivenom in 47 children. Am J Trop Med Hyg 33:1258, 1984

RUSSELL FE: *Snake Venom Poisoning*. New York, Scholium International, 1983

———, BOGERT CM: Gila monster: Its biology, venom and bite: A review. Toxicon 19:341, 1981

WINGERT WA, CHAN L: Rattlesnake bites in southern California and rationale for recommended treatment. West J Med 148:37, 1988

Spider bites

HUNT GR: Bites and stings of uncommon arthropods: 1 Spiders. Postgrad Med 70:91, 1981

RAUBER A: Black widow spider bites. J Toxicol-Clin Toxicol 21:473, 1983–84

REES R et al: The diagnosis and treatment of brown recluse spider bites. Ann Emerg Med 16:945, 1987

Tick bite and tick paralysis

GOTHE R et al: The mechanism of pathogenicity in the tick paralysis. J Med Entomol 16:357, 1979

NEEDHAM GR: Evaluation of 5 popular methods for tick removal. Pediatrics 75:997, 1985

SPIELMAN A: How to diagnose and treat tick and mite infestations. Drug Therapy 11:77, 1981

377 HYPOTHERMIA AND HYPERTHERMIA

ROBERT G. PETERSDORF

CONTROL OF BODY TEMPERATURE

In health, the body temperature of humans is maintained within a narrow range despite extremes in environmental conditions and physical activity. This is also true for most birds and mammals, and such animals are termed *homeothermic*, or warm-blooded. An almost invariable accompaniment of systemic illness is a disturbance in temperature regulation, usually an abnormal elevation, or *fever*. Even in the absence of a frank febrile response, interference with heat regulation by disease is evident. This may take the form of flushing, pallor, sweating, shivering, and abnormal sensations of cold or warmth, or it may consist of erratic fluctuations of body temperature within normal limits when a patient is at bed rest. The pathogenesis, diagnosis, and treatment of fever are discussed in Chap. 20.

HEAT PRODUCTION The major sources of basal heat production are through thyroid thermogenesis and the action of adenosine triphosphatase (ATPase) on the sodium pump of all membranes. The muscles are most important in promoting increased heat production through increased shivering. Heat production by muscle is of particular importance because the quantity can be varied according to the need. In most circumstances this variation consists of small increases and decreases in the number of nerve impulses to the muscles, causing inapparent tensing or relaxing. When, however, there is a strong stimulus for heat production, muscle activity may increase to the point of shivering, or even to a generalized rigor. During digestion of food, gastrointestinal production of heat is significant.

HEAT LOSS Heat is lost from the body in several ways. Small amounts are used in warming food or drink and in the evaporation of moisture from the respiratory tract. Most heat is lost from the surface of the body by *convection*. Heat loss by convection depends on the existence of a temperature gradient between the body surface and the ambient air. A second mechanism for heat loss is *radiation*, which may be defined as an exchange of electromagnetic energy between the body and the radiant environment. *Evaporation* is the third major mechanism for dissipating heat and is particularly important when the ambient temperature exceeds that of the body, or when core temperatures are increased by vigorous exercise.

The principal method of regulating heat loss is by varying the volume of blood flowing to the surface of the body. A rich circulation in the skin and subcutaneous tissues carries heat to the surface, where it can escape. In addition, sweating increases heat loss by providing water to be vaporized. The sweat, or eccrine, glands are under the control of the sympathetic nerves which, in this instance, mediate cholinergic stimuli. Heat loss by sweating may be tremendous, and as much as 1 L/h of sweat may be evaporated. The amount of heat loss through sweating is also dependent upon the humidity in the air. The greater the humidity, the less the ability to lose heat through sweat.

When there is need for conservation of heat, adrenergic autonomic stimuli cause a sharp reduction in the blood flow to the surface. This causes vasoconstriction and transforms the skin and subcutaneous tissue into layers of insulation.

HEAT TRANSFER WITHIN THE BODY This depends upon *conduction*, i.e., the transfer of heat between adjacent organs, and upon *circulatory convection*, which is governed by bulk movement of body fluids and which is responsible for the transfer of heat between the cells and the bloodstream. It is useful, although oversimplified, to visualize the body as a central core at uniform temperatures surrounded by an insulating shell. The role of the shell as a mediator for heat conservation and heat loss is determined in part by its blood supply and by vasoconstriction or vasodilatation. Although insulation is relatively uniform throughout the body, some parts, such as the digits, are particularly susceptible to cold because of the increased surface-to-volume ratio. Moreover, blood that reaches the digits has already been cooled on the way. Insulation may be enhanced by the addition of clothing.

NEURAL CONTROL OF TEMPERATURE The control of body temperature, integrating the various physical and chemical processes for heat production or heat loss, is a function of cerebral centers located in the hypothalamus. The temperature-regulating system is a negative feedback control system and possesses three elements essential to such a system: (1) receptors that sense the existing central temperatures; (2) effector mechanisms, consisting of the vasomotor, sudomotor, and metabolic effectors; and (3) integrative structures that determine whether the existing temperature is too high or too low and that activate the appropriate motor response. It is a negative feedback system because a rise in central temperature initiates mechanisms for losing heat while a fall in central temperature activates mechanisms for heat production and heat conservation. The activation of these effector responses is governed by a central integrative mechanism that may be compared with a thermostat and that responds to a variety of stimuli, such as the sensory impulses engendered in flushing or sweating, behavioral impulses, exercise, endocrine influences, and probably the temperature of the blood circulating through the hypothalamic centers. In a sense all these stimuli reset the thermostat, thereby activating compensatory heat loss or heat conservation mechanisms.

A classic example of the neuroendocrine influence on temperature is the effect of menstruation. The mean body temperature of women is higher during the second half of the menstrual cycle than it is between the onset of menstruation and the time of ovulation. The sensations of intense heat followed by diaphoresis that characterize the vasomotor instability experienced by some women at the menopause are most likely the result of neuroendocrine imbalance.

NORMAL BODY TEMPERATURE It is not practical to designate an exact upper level of normal body temperature because there are small differences among normal persons. There are rare individuals whose temperatures are always elevated slightly above accepted "normal" levels, and there is considerable variation in temperature in a given individual. In general, however, it is safe to regard an oral temperature above 37.2°C (99°F) in a person at bed rest as probable indication of disease. The temperature may be as low as 35.8°C (96.5°F) in healthy persons. Rectal temperature is usually 0.3 to 0.6°C (0.5 to 1.0°F) above oral temperature. In very hot weather the body temperature may be elevated by the same amounts.

There is a distinct diurnal variation in body temperature in healthy human beings. Oral readings of 36.1°C (97°F) are relatively common on arising in the morning. Body temperature rises steadily through the day, reaches a peak of 37.2°C (99°F) or greater between 6 P.M. and 10 P.M., and then drops slowly to reach a minimum at 2 A.M. to 4 A.M. Although it has been postulated that this diurnal variation is dependent upon increasing activity during the day and rest at night, the pattern is not reversed in individuals who work at night and sleep during the day. The febrile patterns of most human diseases also tend to follow this normal diurnal variation. Fevers tend to be higher, that is, to "spike," in the evening, and many patients with febrile disease have relatively normal temperatures in the early morning hours.

Body temperature is more labile in young children, and transient elevations after relatively slight exertion in warm weather are frequently observed in them.

Severe or prolonged exercise can produce considerable elevation in body temperature. For example, marathon runners may develop temperatures between 39 and 41°C (103.2 and 105.8°F). Although heat loss may be increased by cutaneous vasodilatation and by hyperventilation, these compensatory mechanisms may fail, leading to hyperpyrexia and, if uncontrolled, to heat stroke. Many of the adverse effects of long-distance running can be prevented by holding races only if the ambient temperature is below 27.8°C (82°F), preferably in the early morning or early evening, and by ensuring ample fluid intake both before and during a race.

DISORDERED THERMOREGULATION In exercise, there is a temporary imbalance between heat production and heat loss with prompt reestablishment of normal temperatures at rest due to continuing activation of heat loss mechanisms. In prolonged exercise, cutaneous vasodilatation in response to an increase in central body temperature ceases in order to preserve central temperature. Less adaptation occurs in fever because once a stable body temperature is reached, heat production equals heat loss, but both are greater than in the basal state. Cutaneous blood flow plays a greater role in controlling heat production and heat loss in fever than does sweating. At the beginning of fever, the body temperature as sensed by the thermoreceptors is low, and the individual responds physiologically as if he or she were cold. *Heat production* is increased by shivering, and *heat loss* is decreased by vasoconstriction. These events explain the sensation of cold or chills that characterizes the beginning of fever. Conversely, when the cause of fever is removed, the temperature returns to normal, and the individual responds as if warm. Cutaneous vasodilatation, sweating, and inhibition of shivering are the compensatory responses.

Deviations of 3°C (approximately 5°F) from the normal body temperature do not interfere appreciably with most bodily functions. Convulsions are common at temperatures higher than 41.1°C (106°F) in children, and irreversible brain damage is common when temperatures of 42.2°C (108°F) are reached. Fortunately, when hyperthermia reaches dangerous levels, the mechanisms for heat loss are suddenly activated; consequently, oral temperatures above 41.1°C (106°F) are relatively rare in humans. Conversely, when temperatures are lowered to 32.8°C (91°F) or below, confusion and loss of consciousness occur; at 30°C (86°F) and below slow atrial fibrillation supervenes. Ventricular fibrillation occurs at extremely hypothermic temperatures and is often a terminal event.

Disease of the regulatory centers in the hypothalamus may affect body temperature. Cases have been observed in which there was destruction of the centers controlling heat-conserving mechanisms, with resulting hypothermia. More commonly, cerebral lesions are manifested by hyperthermia; they include tumors, degenerative diseases, vascular accidents, particularly cerebral hemorrhage, or infections involving the hypothalamus, such as encephalitis. Central fever is accompanied by lack of a diurnal variation, absence of sweating, resistance to antipyretic drugs, excessive response to external cooling, and loss of consciousness.

DISORDERS ASSOCIATED WITH HIGH TEMPERATURES

HEAT SYNDROMES Four clinical syndromes are associated with high environmental temperature: *heat cramps, heat exhaustion, exertional heat injury,* and *heat stroke.* Although each of these entities may be separated from the others on clinical grounds, there is considerable overlap between them, and they may be considered as a series of syndromes along a single spectrum. The incidence of heat syndromes is unknown, but during an ordinary summer about 200 cases of heat stroke are reported. During the heat wave of June 1984, there was a 35 percent increase in mortality in New York City almost exclusively due to a rise in deaths in elderly persons living at home. Heat syndromes occur primarily at elevated ambient temperatures [>32°C (>90°F)] and at high relative humidities (>60%) in elderly individuals, particularly those with mental illness or alcoholism or who receive antipsychotic drugs, diuretics, and anticholinergics, or those who reside in poorly ventilated places without air conditioning. Heat syndromes are especially prevalent during the first days of a heat wave before effective acclimatization can occur. Prophylaxis by augmenting fluid intake prior to exposure and by ensuring that susceptible individuals, particularly the elderly or the very young, wear light clothing, take frequent cool baths, remain in a cool environment, and avoid strenuous physical activity can help prevent the full-blown syndrome, especially heat stroke.

Acclimatization The basic mechanism by which humans accommodate to excessive temperatures is unknown. Acclimatization does not increase the threshold for sweating. However, sweating is the most effective natural means of combating heat stress and can occur with little or no change in the core temperature of the body. As long as sweating continues, humans can withstand remarkably high temperatures, provided water and sodium chloride, the most important physiologic constituents of sweat, are replaced. The concentration of sodium chloride varies between very low concentrations up to that of interstitial fluid. The ability to secrete sweat with a low sodium chloride content, or to increase the quantity of sweat, is a major mechanism for salt conservation in hot weather. Dilatation of the peripheral blood vessels in an attempt to dissipate heat is another major way for the body to acclimatize to hot temperatures. Other alterations include a decrease in total circulating blood volume, a decrease in renal blood flow, an increase of antidiuretic hormone (ADH) as well as aldosterone, a decrease in urine sodium, and an increase in respiratory and pulse rates. Ordinarily, acclimatization takes from 4 to 7 days. The hyperaldosteronism may result in potassium loss, which may be aggravated by replacement of sodium without concomitant repletion of potassium. Initially there is an increase in cardiac output, but as heat stress persists, venous return diminishes and cardiac output may fall. If environmental temperatures in excess of the body's temperature persist, heat is retained and hyperpyrexia develops.

Heat cramps Heat cramps are the most benign heat syndrome. They are characterized by brief, intermittent, and often excruciating cramping pain, and usually follow strenuous exercise in the muscles that have been subjected to extensive work. Individuals who develop this syndrome are usually athletes in excellent physical condition who are well acclimatized. External temperatures do not usually exceed the body temperature, and direct exposure to the sun is not necessary. The body temperature is usually normal, and the victim sweats normally or excessively. Heat cramps may even be precipitated by strenuous exercise in cold environments in untrained persons heavily clothed. Muscles of the extremities bear the brunt of physical activity and hence show the highest incidence of cramps. Treatment consists of rest in a cool environment and replacement of sodium, potassium, and fluid. This syndrome may be prevented by liberal salting of food and ample intake of water. Salt tablets and electrolyte solutions are of no particular value.

Heat exhaustion This is also called heat prostration, or heat collapse, and is probably the most common heat syndrome. It represents a failure of the cardiovascular responses to high external temperatures and is common in elderly individuals who are receiving diuretics. Weakness, anxiety, fatigue, thirst, vertigo, headache, anorexia, nausea, vomiting, the urge to defecate, and faintness may precede collapse. There may be hyperventilation, muscular incoordination, agitation, impaired judgment, and confusion. Heat collapse occurs in both physically active and sedentary individuals. The onset is usually sudden and the duration of collapse brief. During the acute stage, the patient looks ashen-gray. The skin is cold and clammy. The pupils are dilated. The blood pressure may be low and the pulse rate elevated. Since prostration develops before exposure to heat is prolonged, body temperature is subnormal or normal. The duration of exposure and the extent to which sweat is lost determine the treatment, which consists of removing the patient to a cool area and placing him or her in the recumbent position. Spontaneous recovery then usually takes place. Intravenous administration of saline solution is rarely necessary, and, for the most part, water and electrolytes, including sodium and potassium, can be replaced orally.

Exertional heat injury This syndrome occurs in individuals who are exerting themselves in hot ambient temperatures [≥27°C (≥ 80°F)] when the relative humidity is high. It is particularly common in runners who enter races with insufficient acclimatization, inadequate conditioning, or improper hydration (before and during the race).

Obesity, age, and previous heat stroke; hypertension; ingestion of drugs, including diuretics, anticholinergics, vasodilators, antihistamines, tranquilizers, sedatives, beta-blockers and amphetamines; and alcohol consumption are contributing predisposing factors. In contrast to classic heat stroke, individuals with exertional heat injury usually sweat freely, and their temperatures are lower [38.9 to 40°C (102 to 104°F) as opposed to 41.1°C (106°F) and higher in heat stroke]. Symptoms consist of headache, piloerection (gooseflesh) on the chest and upper arms, chills, hyperventilation, nausea, vomiting, muscle cramps, ataxia, unsteady gait, and incoherent speech. In some individuals, loss of consciousness occurs. Physical examination shows tachycardia, hypotension, and evidence of low peripheral resistance. Laboratory data show hemoconcentration, hypernatremia, abnormal liver and muscle enzymes, hypocalcemia, hypophosphatemia, and, in some instances, hypoglycemia. An occasional patient has thrombocytopenia, hemolysis, disseminated intravascular coagulation, rhabdomyolysis, myoglobinuria, and acute tubular necrosis. Injury to the vascular endothelium may be widespread and contribute to these manifestations as well as to organ failure. These severe complications can be avoided by prompt treatment, which consists of placing the victim under wet cold sheets to lower core temperature to 38°C (100.4°F) as quickly as possible, massaging the extremities to improve blood flow from the core to the periphery, and infusing fluids consisting primarily of hypotonic glucose-saline. Patients should be hospitalized for observation.

Exertional heat injury can be prevented by (1) running races early in the morning (before 8 A.M.) when the temperature and humidity are likely to be low, (2) educating runners to enter a race well hydrated by drinking 300 mL of water 10 min before a race and 250 mL every 3 to 4 km (salt and glucose solutions should be avoided), (3) placing aid stations at 5-km intervals, (4) instructing runners not to increase their pace after most of the race has been run, and (5) avoiding alcohol before a race.

Heat stroke Heat stroke can be divided into "exertional" and "classic." Exertional heat stroke occurs in healthy, young individuals and is generally sporadic. The patient usually sweats. Disseminated intravascular coagulation (DIC), acute renal failure, rhabdomyolysis, and lactic acidosis are common complications. Classic heat stroke occurs in older individuals in epidemic form during heat waves. Patients do not sweat. Acute renal failure, rhabdomyolysis, and lactic acidosis are rare. Most persons with classic heat stroke have preexisting chronic disease, including arteriosclerosis and congestive heart failure (particularly when such patients receive diuretics), diabetes mellitus, alcoholism, or have received one or several of the drugs described above. Skin disorders in which it may be difficult to lose heat such as ectodermal dysplasia, congenital absence of the sweat glands, or severe scleroderma predispose to heat stroke. The vasoconstriction that accompanies heat stroke prevents dissipation of heat from the core, but whether this vasoconstriction is cause or effect is not clear. Direct exposure to the sun is not a necessary prerequisite for the development of heat stroke.

There may be few premonitory symptoms, and loss of consciousness may be the first sign. Other patients may complain of headache, vertigo, faintness, abdominal distress, confusion, or hyperpnea. Delirium may develop in more severe cases. Pyrexia and prostration are the significant findings on physical examination. A rectal temperature greater than 41.1°C (106°F) is common, and internal body temperatures as high as 44.4°C (112 to 113°F) have been recorded. The skin is hot and dry, the pulse rate is rapid, and respirations are rapid and weak. The blood pressure is usually low. The muscles are flaccid, and tendon reflexes may be diminished. Lethargy, stupor, or coma, depending on the severity, is present. Shock is common in fatal cases. Coma, hypotension, disseminated intravascular coagulation, and the necessity of intubation are bad prognostic indicators.

Examination of the blood and urine may show few abnormalities. Hemoconcentration is common. Leukocytosis is characteristic, as are proteinuria, cylindruria, and an elevation in BUN. There is usually a respiratory alkalosis which is followed by a metabolic acidosis.

Lactic acidosis is common in classic heat stroke. Serum potassium is normal or low, and there are usually hypocalcemia and hypophosphatemia. The electrocardiogram may show, in addition to tachycardia and sinus arrhythmia, flattening and subsequent inversion of the T waves and depression of the ST segments. Diffuse myocardial necrosis with ECG evidence of myocardial infarction has been reported. Other major laboratory abnormalities include thrombocytopenia; prolonged bleeding, clotting, and prothrombin times; afibrinogenemia and fibrinolysis; and disseminated intravascular coagulation. All these may be responsible for diffuse bleeding. Liver damage is common; it appears 24 to 36 h after admission and is characterized by clinically apparent jaundice and, often, by abnormalities of hepatocellular enzymes. Renal failure is a common complication of exertional heat stroke.

Patients with heat stroke may die within a few hours after being discovered, or may die of complications such as acute renal failure. However, a number of patients will die several weeks after the acute episode, usually of myocardial infarction, heart failure, renal failure, bronchopneumonia, or complicating bacteremia. In such patients autopsy may show extensive parenchymal damage to various organs, either from hyperpyrexia per se or from petechial hemorrhages in the brain, heart, kidneys, or liver.

TREATMENT Heat stroke is a medical emergency, and immediate heroic emergency measures are required. In hot climates, ambulances should be air-conditioned. Once the patient is in the emergency room, time is of the essence. All clothing should be removed. The patient should be wheeled into a shower on a gurney. A successful protocol consists of vigorous massage of the patient, particularly the torso and neck, to decrease peripheral vasoconstriction. At the same time, ice should be applied to the lateral aspects of the trunk while the patient is sprayed with tepid water from the shower. A fan should be directed on the patient to accelerate heat dissipation by convection. Intravenous solutions should be chilled before administration.

After immediate evaluation and measurement of vital signs, the temperature should be measured with an equilibrated thermocouple. Using these measures, the rectal temperature should fall to 37.8 to 38.9°C (100 to 102°F) within 1 h. While immersion of the patient in an ice-water bath is a time-honored treatment, it appears to be no more effective than the less cumbersome measures described above. Massage of the skin should be employed along with cooling because it stimulates return of the cool peripheral blood to the overheated brain and viscera and aids acceleration of heat loss. A Swan-Ganz catheter may be necessary, and urinary output needs to be monitored. Prompt cooling, massage of the limbs, and vigorous hydration along with establishment of a proper airway, avoidance of aspiration, treating coma and convulsions, and watching for arrhythmias will lead to survival of most patients, particularly if they are young and were previously well. Unfortunately, the poor, ill, and elderly, who are often not discovered until heat hyperpyrexia has been present for some hours, have a much less favorable outcome.

MALIGNANT HYPERTHERMIA Etiology and epidemiology Malignant hyperthermia (MH) consists of a group of inherited disorders that are characterized by a rapid increase in temperature to 39 to 42°C (102.2 to 107.6°F) in response to inhalational anesthetics such as halothane, methoxyflurane, cyclopropane, and ethyl ether or muscle relaxants, notably succinylcholine. In one form of the disease in which the mechanism of inheritance is autosomal dominant, the individuals are normal between attacks although some have an elevation in creatine phosphokinase (CPK), and in 90 percent of such cases, biopsied muscle from susceptible individuals contracts on exposure to caffeine or halothane at concentrations that do not alter normal muscle contraction. The incidence of the autosomal dominant form is 1:50,000 to 1:100,000. MH occurs in one per 40,000 adult and one per 15,000 pediatric surgical cases. Interval CPK screening is not effective in detecting susceptible patients. Muscle biopsy followed by the halothane-caffeine contraction reaction is accurate but tedious. A careful history from the patient, including questioning about abnormal reactions during surgery suggestive of MH in relatives,

is the most accurate way to detect and prevent MH. Some anesthesiologists feel that an increase in end-tidal CO_2, unexplained tachycardia, and an increase in core temperature provide early clues.

A second, recessive, form occurs in young boys and, less commonly, girls, with a number of congenital abnormalities including short stature, undescended testes, lumbar lordosis, thoracic kyphosis, pectus carinatum, webbed neck, winged scapulae, small chin, low-set ears, and an antimongoloid obliquity of the palpebral fissures. This form is called the *King syndrome*. MH has also been described in several other myopathies including myotonia congenita, central core disease, and Duchenne's muscular dystrophy.

Pathogenesis The triggering anesthetic releases calcium from the membrane of the muscle cell's sarcoplasmic reticulum, which is defective in storing this ion. The result is a sudden increase in myoplasmic calcium. The calcium activates myosin ATPase, which converts adenosine triphosphate to adenosine diphosphate, phosphate, and heat. There are also inhibition of troponin, uncoupling of oxidative phosphorylation, activation of phosphorylase kinase, and increased glycolysis. Muscular contraction occurs, and it, as well as the chemical events, leads to production of heat.

Manifestations Existence of malignant hyperthermia can be suspected if diminished relaxation is noted during induction of anesthesia and muscle fasciculations become evident when succinylcholine is given. In some patients trismus during intubation is the first sign of a muscle disorder. Although the elevation in temperature is the result of muscular contraction, it may rise very rapidly, and if the temperature is not monitored, the first signs may be a hot skin and tachycardia or a cardiac arrhythmia. In addition to the high fever, muscle rigidity, hypotension, and mottled cyanosis are present.

Early laboratory abnormalities include respiratory and metabolic acidosis, hyperkalemia and hypermagnesemia, and elevation in blood lactate and pyruvate. Late complications include massive skeletal muscle swelling, pulmonary edema, disseminated intravascular coagulation, and acute renal failure.

Treatment Malignant hyperthermia is a medical emergency. The treatment protocol prescribed by the American Society of Anesthesiologists should be followed. It includes prompt interruption of surgery, cessation of the inhalational anesthetic, changing rubber tubing on the anesthesia machine, and external cooling. One hundred percent oxygen should be given, along with sodium bicarbonate (1 to 2 mg/kg), to combat the severe metabolic acidosis. A diuresis should be induced with fluids and diuretics to reduce myoglobinemia and hyperkalemia. Specific treatment consists of dantrolene sodium, 1 mg/kg, by rapid intravenous infusion. The drug should be continued until symptoms have begun to subside or up to a maximum single dose of 10 mg/kg. The regimen can be repeated if symptoms recur. Drugs to combat arrhythmias should be administered under ECG monitoring (see Chap. 185).

Prevention Because of the tendency of this syndrome to run in families, its detection is essential. This can be achieved by monitoring the temperature of all patients under anesthesia; the best way to avert it altogether is to take a thorough family history. Examining patients preoperatively is often not helpful because between attacks persons susceptible to MH are usually entirely normal. In susceptible patients dantrolene should be given prophylactically. The dose is 4 to 8 mg/kg by mouth for 1 to 2 days prior to surgery; the last dose should be administered 3 to 4 h prior to anesthesia. Some favor an additional dose of 2 to 5 mg/kg intravenously immediately prior to induction of anesthesia.

NEUROLEPTIC MALIGNANT SYNDROME (NMS) This syndrome is characterized by autonomic dysfunction, extrapyramidal dysfunction, and hyperthermia. Autonomic dysfunction is characterized by tachycardia, labile blood pressure (range 180 to 40 mmHg systolic), profuse diaphoresis, dyspnea, and urinary incontinence. Extrapyramidal dysfunction is manifested by catatonic behavior, dystonia, generalized muscular rigidity, pseudo-parkinsonism (ptyalism, masked facies, tremors, and brady- or akinesia). The temperature may be as high as 41°C (106°F). Consciousness fluctuates from alertness to coma. Laboratory abnormalities consist of leukocytosis (15,000 to 30,000 per microliter) and elevation in CK. The syndrome occurs after use of potent neuroleptics in therapeutic doses. Most cases have been reported after use of haloperidol, thiothixene, or piperazine phenothiazines. Young adult males with affective disorders predominate. The NMS lasts 5 to 10 days after administration of oral neuroleptics is discontinued, and longer after depot injection. These drugs are not dialyzable, hence the long period necessary for their excretion. The overall mortality is 20 percent and fatalities have occurred as late as 30 days after onset and have been due to renal failure, arrhythmias, pulmonary emboli, or aspiration pneumonia.

The mechanism of action is presumed to be due to blockade of the dopaminic pathways in the basal ganglia and the hypothalamus. Because neuroleptic drugs block dopamine receptors, NMS is attributed to dopamine depletion and this is the rationale for treatment with bromocriptine (a dopamine agonist) in dosage of 7.5 to 60 mg/d divided into 3 daily doses. Dantrolene sodium (as described above for oral prophylaxis of MH) has been successful occasionally, as has amantadine. Supportive measures, including cooling and drug withdrawal, are the *sine qua non* of treatment.

DISORDERS ASSOCIATED WITH LOW TEMPERATURES

HYPOTHERMIA Hypothermia is defined as a central or core temperature of 35°C (95°F) or lower. The central (core) temperature is maintained at the expense of the periphery. During cold weather blood is shunted away from the skin and the extremities to preserve, protect, and maintain core temperatures. Although far less common than is elevation in temperature, hypothermia is of considerable importance because it can represent a medical emergency.

Accidental hypothermia This is a well-known complication of exposure to cold and has been reported frequently during the winter months. It usually occurs after prolonged exposure, not necessarily to excessively low external temperatures. The diagnosis of hypothermia may prove elusive because clinical thermometers do not record temperatures below 35°C (95°F). Whenever a patient presents with a temperature below this level, the true temperature should be determined with an incubator thermometer or a thermocouple. Accidental hypothermia has been found in association with sepsis, hypothyroidism, pituitary insufficiency, adrenal insufficiency, hypoglycemia, cerebrovascular disease, Wernicke's encephalopathy, myocardial infarction, cirrhosis, pancreatitis, and ingestion of drugs—most particularly alcohol. For example, it is not uncommon to find a derelict in a railroad yard or under a bridge following an alcoholic debauch with a core temperature between 28.5 and 32.3°C (85 and 90°F) or lower. From 1976 to 1985, 7450 deaths in the United States were caused by exposure to cold. Most had core temperatures <35°C (<95°F), and individuals older than 60 were at greatest risk. In 428 cases reported from 13 emergency departments, there was a direct correlation between lower body temperatures and outcome.

These patients usually appear cold and pale and, when their temperatures are very low, give the appearance of having rigor mortis, so stiff is their musculature. Patients with temperatures less than 26.7°C (80°F) are usually unconscious. The pupils are usually miotic, respiration tends to be shallow and slow, there is bradycardia, and most patients are hypotensive. Generalized edema is often present. When the temperature falls below 25°C (77°F), coma, areflexia, and lack of pupillary response supervene.

Laboratory data tend to show hemoconcentration, mild azotemia, and metabolic acidosis. The acidosis is due to lactic acidemia, which in turn is a consequence of decreased perfusion and hypoxemia in peripheral tissues. At cold temperatures, the hemoglobin dissociation curve is shifted to the left, and there is decreased unloading of oxygen in the peripheral tissues. Some patients have hypoglycemia while others have hyperglycemia. Thyroid function tests may give results typical of myxedema. Some patients have elevations in serum amylase,

and a few show pancreatitis at autopsy. The electrocardiogram is distorted by muscular tremors and may show bradycardia or slow atrial fibrillation and a characteristic J wave (occurring at the junction of the QRS complex and ST segment). Other arrhythmias are common; ventricular fibrillation is usually a terminal event. The mortality rate is five times higher in people over 75.

TREATMENT Hypothermia is a medical emergency, and therapy should be instituted at once. The following steps are indicated:

1 An airway must be established and maintained, and the patient should be well oxygenated. Warmed oxygen may be helpful. Tracheal intubation of these patients poses no undue risk.
2 Blood gases should be monitored and corrected for temperature.
3 Blood volume should be expanded with warmed glucose and saline, low-molecular-weight dextran, or albumin. Maintenance of blood volume is necessary to prevent the infarctions which have been a hallmark in fatal cases and to avert "rewarming shock." If the patient has persistent hypotension, respiratory failure, or unexplained oliguria, hemodynamic monitoring with Swan-Ganz catheterization may be necessary.
4 Because of the tendency to arrhythmias, serum potassium should be monitored carefully; a transvenous pacemaker may be indicated.
5 Sodium bicarbonate should be given if pH is less than 7.25.
6 Although external rewarming with heating blankets or placing the patient in a warm room is appropriate in patients with mild hypothermia, patients who are moderately hypothermic require reestablishment of core temperature. This can be done effectively by placing the patient in a warm bath or a Hubbard tank at 40 to 42°C (104 to 108°F). This maneuver must be carried out cautiously; physiologic monitoring may be difficult, and if an arrhythmia occurs, resuscitation is hampered. Nevertheless, external warming tends to dilate the constricted peripheral blood vessels and to divert blood from the visceral organs. In severely hypothermic patients, this may result in rewarming shock and restoration of the core temperature may be insufficient to warm the myocardium to make it responsive to antiarrhythmic agents. In this situation extracorporeal circulation with externally warmed blood is the method of choice. Peritoneal dialysis, during which the dialysate is warmed to 37°C (98.6°F), and colonic and gastric lavage with warmed fluids are also helpful. It is particularly important to rewarm the myocardium because in cases of ventricular fibrillation defibrillation will not be successful until myocardial temperature is raised to near normal levels.
7 Many of these patients have systemic infections including sepsis (see Chap. 89); cultures of the blood, urine, and other suspected sites should be obtained and broad-spectrum antibiotic therapy initiated and continued until infection has been excluded. Sepsis should be considered strongly in patients on hemodynamic monitoring who are found to have a lowered systemic vascular resistance and elevated cardiac index.
8 Resuscitative efforts should be vigorous and prolonged despite the poor prognosis which is related primarily to advanced age and associated debilitating disease. In younger individuals, some remarkable rescues have been recorded. Authorities agree that hypothermia victims without vital signs (prolonged asystole) should not be pronounced dead until they have been rewarmed to 36°C (96.8°F) and remain unresponsive to CPR at that temperature. "No one is dead until warm and dead." Mild hypothermia [above 32.2°C (90°F)] has a 25 percent mortality; in moderate hypothermia [26.6 to 32.2°C (80 to 90°F)] the mortality is 50 percent; and below 26.6°C (80°C) it is 60 percent.

Hypothermia secondary to acute illness There is a group of patients who develop moderate hypothermia in association with acute diseases including congestive heart failure, uremia, diabetes mellitus, drug overdose, acute respiratory failure, and hypoglycemia. These patients are generally elderly and upon admission to the hospital are found to have temperatures of 33.3 to 34.4°C (92 to 93.9°F). They also have a severe metabolic acidosis, due to increased production of lactic acid, and cardiac arrhythmias. Most of these patients are comatose. This entity differs from accidental hypothermia only in the absence of exposure; these cases have all occurred at normal ambient temperatures. The mechanism appears to be an acute failure of thermoregulation; shivering did not occur in any of these patients. Usually these patients have been rewarmed within a few hours. Upon return to normal temperature, cardiac arrhythmias, which were present in most of these patients, responded to treatment, and the sensorium returned to normal. With the exception that core rewarming is established by external means, other facets of therapy should follow the steps outlined above. In addition, treatment of the underlying disease such as diabetes with insulin, uremia with dialysis, or congestive heart failure with appropriate cardiac drugs and diuretics, is essential. The prognosis is good provided the syndrome is recognized early and treatment is instituted at once. In general, patients under 60 have the most favorable outcome.

Immersion hypothermia Responses to cold-water immersion may be classified as (1) stimulatory, with deep body temperature normal to 35°C (95°F); (2) depressant, with deep body temperature 35 to 30°C (95 to 86°F); and (3) critical, with deep body temperature 30 to 25°C (86 to 77°F).

The long-distance swimmer is able to maintain a normal body temperature for periods of 15 to 25 h or more in water that may plunge skin temperature to 15°C (59°F) or lower, which is some 15.7°C (28°F) below deep body temperature, lending support to the concept of a body core insulated by a body shell. The vasoconstriction operative in cold water greatly reduces heat loss. However, there is great individual variability in heat loss in cold water. The relatively obese swimmer may maintain a normal rectal temperature for 2 h without shivering in 16°C (61°F) water. A lean person under the same conditions, despite violent shivering, may experience a fall in rectal temperature of several degrees and become incapacitated from the rigor. In hypersensitive persons, immersion in cold water may be followed by vascular spasm, vomiting, and syncope. Other compensatory responses include bradycardia, a slight rise in blood pressure, and an early rise in rectal temperature followed by a fall. At 30°C (86°F), atrial fibrillation is common.

Rewarming in warm water has been recommended as the treatment of immersion hypothermia. In severe cases, extracorporeal circulation or peritoneal dialysis should be instituted.

LOCAL COLD INJURIES Mechanisms of freezing injury These can be divided into phenomena that affect cells and extracellular fluids (direct effects) and those that disrupt the function of organized tissues and the integrity of the circulation (indirect effects).

When tissue freezes, ice crystals form and, concomitantly, solutes in the residual liquid become concentrated. The physical dislocation during slow freezing is extreme. Ice crystals many times the size of individual cells form but are confined to the extracellular spaces. Large ice crystals can develop between cells in soft tissue without producing irreversible injury as long as the percentage of water frozen does not exceed a critical amount. A major source of damage to living cells during freezing and thawing appears to be the strong salt solutions which develop during formation and dissolution of ice; changes in the proportions of lipids and phospholipids in the cell membrane are also of great importance.

The fulminating vascular reaction and stasis that supervene are associated with production of histamine-like substances which increase the permeability of the capillary bed. Within blood vessels, cellular elements aggregate. Irreversible occlusion of small blood vessels by cell masses has been demonstrated in thawed tissue following freezing injury. The damaged frozen tissue simulates tissue damage produced by burns.

Manifestations The mildest form of cold injury is called *frostnip* and tends to occur in organs farthest removed from the core of the body such as the earlobes, nose, cheeks, fingers and toes, and hands and feet. Frostnip represents reversible damage that is characterized by blanching of the skin and numbness. It can be prevented by warm clothing and treated with simple rewarming. More consequential local

cold injuries may be divided into freezing (frostbite) and nonfreezing (immersion foot) injuries. The two types may be observed in the same extremity or in different extremities in the same individual. The diagnosis of freezing versus nonfreezing injury generally can be made on the basis of the history and clinical manifestations.

Immersion foot is an entity observed in shipwreck survivors or in soldiers (trench foot) whose feet have been wet but not freezing cold for prolonged periods. There is primarily injury to nerve and muscle tissue, but no gross or irreparable pathologic changes occur in the blood vessels and skin. The clinical picture reflects primary hypoxic trauma giving rise to three clearly recognizable states: (1) *ischemia*, denoted by a pale, pulseless extremity; (2) *hyperemia*, characterized by a bounding pulsatile circulation in red, swollen, painful feet; and (3) the *posthyperemic* or recovery period. The initial cold-induced vasoconstriction, increased blood viscosity, and impaired oxygen transport in the ischemic state are aggravated by such factors as malnutrition, general hypothermia, dehydration, and trauma from relatively fixed, pendant extremities. The problem of rewarming is critical in these patients during the stage of ischemia, when overheating of tissue may lead to gangrene. In the state of hyperemia, the red, swollen feet require judicious cooling. Severe cases may show muscular weakness, atrophy, ulceration, and gangrene of superficial areas. Sensitivity to cold and pain on weight bearing, which may cause discomfort for many years, are sequelae even of milder injuries.

Frostbite, in contrast to immersion foot, is primarily a vascular problem because the blood vessels may be severely and irreparably injured. The circulation of blood ceases, and the vascular bed of the frozen tissue is occluded by agglutinated cell aggregates and thrombi. The cutaneous injury consists in part of separation of the epidermal-dermal interface. Early the intravascular clumping is reversible. However, with the passage of time, clumped red blood cells within vessels in injured tissue lose their morphologic identity and take on the appearance of a homogeneous, hyalinaceous plug. It has been shown in some, but not all, experimental studies that much of the intravascular aggregation following freezing injury can be reversed and microcirculatory perfusion improved if low-molecular-weight dextran is given intravenously shortly after injury, but the data in humans are less convincing. Tissue damage can be aggravated by trauma to insensitive and friable limbs and by refreezing. Moreover, frostbitten tissues are often neglected and with thawing become macerated. It is important, therefore, not to walk, bear weight or put excessive pressure on a thawed frostbitten area. Thawing followed by refreezing is particularly harmful.

The method of rewarming has been a matter of controversy. It seems most rational to warm the core of the body before treating the local area of frostbite. Following restoration of the core temperature to normal, warming of a frostbitten limb should begin in water at 10 to 15°C (50 to 59°F), which is then increased 5°C (9°F) every 5 min to a maximum of 40°C (104°F). Once the frostbitten limb has been rewarmed, treatment of the areas of tissue damage should be conservative and consist of bed rest, elevation of the injured part, tetanus toxoid administration, and use of antibiotics if infection is present; aseptic early drainage of blebs and bullae; daily washes with chlorhexidine or an iodophor; and early institution of physiotherapy. Alcohol and cigarettes are strongly contraindicated. Except for compartment syndromes that may occur as a result of massive swelling in the early post-thaw period, and that may require surgical release, surgical amputation and reconstruction is usually not necessary. In fact, 3 to 6 months may be required to determine the true level of tissue loss, contraindicating aggressive surgery.

Some patients with frostbite have residua consisting of excessive sweating, pain, cold insensitivity, numbness, abnormal color, dry and cracking skin, arthralgias, and degenerative arthritis. The symptoms are generally worse in the winter and following exposure to cold. These patients also often show abnormal nails, discoloration and pigmentation, hyperhidrosis, and, by x-ray, osteoporosis and cystic defects near the joints. These abnormalities tend to be milder in patients who have had sympathetic blockade. Most cold injuries are preventable by graded exposure to cold, as well as appropriate clothing in freezing temperatures.

REFERENCES

General

MITCHELL D, LABURN HP: Pathophysiology of temperature regulation. Physiologist 28:507, 1985

Heat syndromes

KENNEDY LW: Physiological correlates of heat intolerance. Sports Med 2:279, 1985

TUCKER LE et al: Classical heat stroke. Clinical and laboratory assessment. South Med J 78:20, 1985

Malignant hyperthermia

GRONERT GA et al: Aetiology of malignant hyperthermia. Br J Anaesth 60:253, 1988

PAASUKE RT, BROWNWELL AKW: Serum creatine kinase level as a screening test for malignant hyperthermia. JAMA 255:769, 1986

STEENSON AJ, TORKELSON RD: King syndrome with malignant hyperthermia. Am J Dis Child 141:271, 1987

WARD A et al: Dantrolene. A review of its pharmacodynamic and pharmacokinetic properties and therapeutic use in malignant hyperthermia, the neuroleptic malignant syndrome and an update of its use in muscle spasticity. Drugs 32:130, 1986

Neuroleptic malignant syndrome

ADDONIZIO G et al: Neuroleptic malignant syndrome: Review and analysis of 115 cases. Biol Psychol 22:1004, 1987

GIBB WRG, LEES AJ: The neuroleptic malignant syndrome—a review. Q J Med (ns 56) 220:421, 1985

HARSCH HH: Neuroleptic malignant syndrome. Physiological and laboratory findings in a series of 9 cases. J Clin Psychol 48:328, 1987

LEVENSON JL: Neuroleptic malignant syndrome. Am J Psychiatry 142:1137, 1985

Cold injury

CENTERS FOR DISEASE CONTROL: Hypothermia prevention. Morb Mort Week Rep 37:780, 1988

DANZEL DT, PAZOS RF: Multicenter hypothermia survey. Ann Emerg Med 16:1042, 1987

GRACE TG: Cold exposure injuries in the winter athlete. Orthop Related Res 216:55, 1987

MORRIS DL et al: Hemodynamic characteristics of patients with hypothermia due to occult infection and other causes. Ann Intern Med 102:153, 1985

WHITTLE JL, BATES JH: Thermoregulatory failure secondary to acute illness: Complications and treatment. Arch Intern Med 139:418, 1979

378   DROWNING AND NEAR-DROWNING

JAMES F. WALLACE

EPIDEMIOLOGY In the United States, drowning is the third leading cause of accidental death among all age groups and the second among individuals ages 5 to 44 years. In 1984 there were approximately 5400 drowning deaths or 2.3 per 100,000 persons. This represents a substantial decline from 1978 when there were nearly 7000 deaths. Although no national statistics are available, it has been estimated that as many as 48,000 persons annually are near-drowning victims: those who live at least temporarily following an immersion incident. Children and young adults are most often the victims, and nearly 80 percent are males. Other risk factors are epilepsy, mental retardation, alcohol consumption while swimming or boating, lack of proper swimming training, failure to use personal floating devices, increased use of hot tubs and spas, and use of small, open, or high-speed boats. With the increasing popularity of boating and water sports in this country nearly half the population is at risk of drowning each year, especially during the summer months.

PATHOPHYSIOLOGY Ten to twenty percent of drowning victims have no evidence of water aspiration in their lungs at autopsy ("dry drowning"). Death is due to asphyxia secondary to reflex laryngo-spasm and glottic closure. It is probable that a similar number of near-drowning victims also do not aspirate. If ventilation is reestablished before they sustain irreversible anoxic brain damage, prompt and complete recovery can be anticipated.

When aspiration accompanies drowning ("wet drowning"), the clinical situation is further complicated by the amount of surrounding water that is introduced into the respiratory tract as well as by the solutes and solids contained in it. A severe pulmonary injury often occurs, resulting in persistent arterial hypoxia and metabolic acidosis even after ventilation has been restored.

In the past, an important distinction was made between the pathophysiology of saltwater and freshwater drowning with respect to changes in blood volume, serum electrolyte concentrations, and cardiovascular function. However, it has been established that the most important problem in human near-drowning is hypoxia and that the other disturbances are of considerably less significance in determining survival.

The mechanisms by which hypoxia develops in near-drowning with aspiration are often multiple: laryngospasm, bronchospasm, airway obstruction secondary to aspirated particulate matter, and pulmonary edema following prolonged hypoxia can take place regardless of the composition of the water aspirated, while other types of lung injury causing hypoxia depend upon the osmolar and chemical characteristics of the immersion fluid. Aspiration of seawater, which is hypertonic compared with blood and chemically irritating to the pulmonary alveolocapillary membrane, causes a rapid shift of plasma proteins and water from the circulation into the alveolar lumen. Continued perfusion of these nonventilated, edema-filled alveoli results in an intrapulmonary right-to-left shunt and arterial hypoxia. When hypotonic fresh water is aspirated, fluid is rapidly absorbed from the lung into the circulation. Injury to alveolar lining cells takes place, altering or destroying the property of pulmonary surfactant that maintains surface tension and leading to alveolar collapse. Ventilation-perfusion ratios change in these atelectatic areas of lung, and hypoxia is the result. Metabolic acidosis, which is present in as many as 70 percent of near-drowning victims, is a consequence of tissue hypoxia and may be severe.

Although changes in electrolyte concentrations occur, depending upon the type and volume of fluid aspirated, these disturbances are rarely life-threatening. Most persons who aspirate sufficient quantities to produce marked electrolyte abnormalities do not survive the immersion incident. Similarly, profound changes in circulating blood volume are unusual. However, hypovolemia requiring treatment may be seen in massive saltwater aspiration accompanied by shifts of fluid from the vascular space into the lung.

Although rarely of clinical significance, some hemolysis of red blood cells often takes place, especially with freshwater aspiration. Free hemoglobin may be found in the urine and blood, but the abnormality requires no specific therapy. Disseminated intravascular coagulation has been reported as a complication of freshwater near-drowning. It is thought that with extensive pulmonary injury, "tissue factor" in lung parenchyma and plasminogen activator from pulmonary endothelium are released, triggering the extrinsic clotting and fibrinolytic systems. Other pathophysiologic events in near-drowning include the development of renal failure secondary to acute tubular necrosis, probably due to the combined effects of hypoxia and hypotension, and neurologic deficits secondary to cerebral anoxia. Although the extent of the central nervous system injury tends to correlate with the duration of hypoxia, hypothermia accompanying the incident may be a moderating factor by reducing cerebral oxygen requirements. Complete neurologic recovery has been reported in victims submerged as long as 66 min in water temperatures less than 10°C. However, the mean age of survivors with good neurologic outcomes following ice water submersion accidents is only 10 years.

CLINICAL MANIFESTATIONS The clinical features in near-drowning are variable and depend upon many factors including the amount and type of water aspirated and the promptness and effectiveness of treatment. Pulmonary and neurologic abnormalities usually predominate. Patients may present with mild cough and tachypnea, or with fulminant pulmonary edema. At least a third will require endotracheal intubation and some type of ventilatory therapy for the management of pulmonary injury. Instead of gradual recovery during the first 48 to 72 h of treatment, some patients will develop the adult respiratory distress syndrome, associated with progressive respiratory failure and reduction in lung compliance (see Chap. 218). Other pulmonary complications often include regional atelectasis due to aspirated particulate matter; secondary bacterial pneumonia; lung abscess; empyema; and injuries such as pneumothorax or pneumomediastinum sustained during resuscitation or related to ventilator therapy.

Early neurologic manifestations include seizures, especially during resuscitative efforts, and altered mental status, including agitation, combativeness, or coma. Patients may present with speech, motor, or visual abnormalities or with more diffuse organic brain syndromes. Some of these neurologic deficits will improve gradually and resolve over several months. However, 5 to 20 percent of patients will have permanent sequelae, many of which prove ultimately fatal. Neurologic status usually does not continue to worsen after a near-drowning victim is admitted to the hospital unless there has been a preceding deterioration in pulmonary status. The possibility of unrecognized head trauma coincident with the drowning episode or a subdural hematoma should be considered as well.

Near-drowning victims often require treatment for cardiac as well as respiratory arrest during resuscitation. If this is successfully accomplished, most patients experience few additional cardiovascular problems. Supraventricular arrhythmias are common but usually resolve promptly when acidosis and hypoxia are treated. Heart failure secondary to myocardial ischemia or acutely expanded blood volume is unusual. Instead, pulmonary edema and low cardiac output states are usually due to the pulmonary injury from water aspiration with extravasation of fluid into the lung, resulting in hypovolemia.

Fever, frequently greater than 38°C, is seen in most patients within the first 24 h following significant aspiration. Its appearance later in the hospital course usually indicates a complicating infection. Vomiting is common during and after resuscitation. This often is associated with gastric distention by large quantities of fluid and air swallowed during the near-drowning episode and may result in additional aspiration. Other rare, but clinically important, features which may be encountered include acute renal failure and a severe hemorrhagic diathesis.

LABORATORY FINDINGS Arterial blood gas and pH determinations on admission reveal varying degrees of hypoxia and acidosis; follow-up values are the most reliable indicators of the effectiveness of ventilatory therapy. In 25 percent of near-drowning victims the initial chest x-ray film may be normal; however, this finding does not exclude the possibility that the patient has significant hypoxia. In the remainder of cases, radiologic findings range from fine, symmetric, perihilar infiltrates with relative sparing of apexes, bases, and lateral lung fields to massive bilateral pulmonary edema with little or no areas of sparing. Marked clearing of these abnormalities usually takes place within 72 to 96 h.

Alterations in serum sodium and potassium are generally mild and require no corrective treatment. Leukocytosis up to 40,000 white blood cells per microliter is common during the first 24 to 48 h following near-drowning; significant changes in hematocrit and hemoglobin are rare, irrespective of the type of fluid aspirated. A *falling* hematocrit should raise the possibility of bleeding, not hemolysis, which, if it has occurred, should be apparent at the time of initial evaluation. Thrombocytopenia, prolonged prothrombin and partial thromboplastin times, hypofibrinogenemia, and elevated fibrin degradation products may be seen if disseminated intravascular coagulation takes place (see Chap. 288).

THERAPY The primary objective of therapy is to correct hypoxia and acidosis as rapidly as possible. On-the-scene efforts should include immediate institution of mouth-to-mouth breathing and, if necessary, closed-chest cardiac massage. Time should not be wasted with attempts to drain water from the victim's lungs. However, it is important to establish and maintain a clear airway at the onset of resuscitation in order to avoid accidental overdistention of the stomach, which might result in regurgitation and aspiration. The application of a subdiaphragmatic abdominal thrust (Heimlich maneuver) should be used only if foreign-body obstruction to the airway is suspected and cannot be removed manually or by suction. It is ineffective in removing water from the lower airways and may cause forceful reflux of gastric contents, resulting in aspiration. Victims who are hypothermic may appear dead with no apparent heartbeat or brain function. However, experience from ice-water submersion survivors suggests that full resuscitative efforts can be continued until core body temperature is near normal. One hundred percent oxygen should be administered by inhalation as soon as possible, and other necessary resuscitative efforts continued during evacuation to the hospital. Even if spontaneous ventilation returns and the patient seems coherent, high concentrations of oxygen should be continued, since severe hypoxia and acidosis may be present even in persons who are alert and without cyanosis.

All near-drowning victims should be taken to a hospital for further evaluation. Initial diagnostic studies should include measurement of rectal temperature, arterial blood gas and pH determinations, hemogram, serum electrolytes, and chest x-ray. Patients who are alert, have normal chest x-rays, and show no evidence of hypothermia, hypoxia, or acidosis usually require no further therapy. Nevertheless they should be observed for several hours for evidence of deterioration in blood gas and acid-base status prior to discharge. Hypothermia should be treated as outlined in Chap. 377. Metabolic acidosis should be treated by intravenous administration of sodium bicarbonate ($NaHCO_3$), and hypoxia with supplemental oxygen. If bronchospasm is present, aerosol inhalation of a bronchodilator may be given. Patients with pulmonary edema or hypoxia that fails to respond to increasing inspired oxygen tensions up to 40 percent should be intubated endotracheally and have positive end-expiratory pressure (PEEP) applied to the airways. When respiratory failure is present, lung compliance is markedly reduced, or the patient is unable to breathe spontaneously, mechanical ventilatory support should be used in addition to PEEP. Arterial blood gas tensions and pH should be determined frequently to assess the adequacy of respiratory therapy. Treatment with PEEP should be continued long enough for the lung injury to stabilize before it is withdrawn. This may take 48 to 72 h or even longer. Monitoring the magnitude of the intrapulmonary shunt, the pulmonary wedge pressure, and cardiac output by means of a Swan-Ganz intraarterial catheter is often very helpful in weaning patients from PEEP as well as in managing cases complicated by low cardiac output and hypotension.

Comatose near-drowning victims frequently are found to have elevated intracranial pressure, which is caused by cerebral edema and loss of cerebrovascular autoregulation. Prolonged elevations over 2.0 to 2.7 kPa (15 to 20 mmHg) lead to reductions of cerebral blood flow, adding ischemic injury to already damaged brain tissue. In order to preserve cerebral function in such patients, aggressive therapy termed *cerebral resuscitation*, and including controlled hyperventilation, deliberate hypothermia, and the use of barbiturates, glucocorticoids, and osmotic and loop diuretics, has been advocated while the intracranial pressure is closely monitored via subarachnoid bolts and intraventricular catheters. Although several investigators have reported that there are fewer major neurologic sequelae, particularly in children treated in this manner, these therapeutic interventions are unproven and controversial. Recent studies suggest that neither induced hypothermia, high-dose glucocorticoids, nor barbiturate coma improves survival or neurologic outcome. The need for such aggressive and potentially hazardous therapy requires further study before it can be recommended for all patients in deep coma following near-drowning.

Other therapeutic measures are largely supportive. Patients should be observed closely for evidence of pulmonary infection and treated with appropriate antibiotics on the basis of results of cultures of respiratory secretions. Prophylactic use of antibiotics and glucocorticoids has been of no benefit in near-drowning victims. Fluid and electrolyte balance should be carefully maintained. If hypovolemia is associated with low urinary output or hypotension, plasma expanders may be required. Transfusion with packed red blood cells or whole blood, depending upon circulating blood volume status, may be used for significant anemia. Acute renal failure should be managed as described in Chap. 223.

PROGNOSIS The prognosis depends largely upon the extent and duration of the hypoxic episode. In addition, such factors as the temperature of the submersion medium, the availability and appropriate application of specific treatment, and coexisting medical illness or trauma are often important in determining the outcome. In general, patients who are alert and have normal chest x-rays upon arrival at the hospital can be expected to recover fully. Those who are obtunded but arousable and have normal respirations have nearly as good a prognosis, while approximately two-thirds of those requiring cardiopulmonary resuscitation and who present in coma die or are left with significant neurologic deficits. Prediction of outcome on the basis of other presenting neurologic features or laboratory abnormalities is unreliable. The fact that nearly 90 percent of victims who live long enough to receive definitive hospital care will survive should serve to emphasize that extensive resuscitative efforts are advisable in all cases of near-drowning.

REFERENCES

BOLTE RG et al: The use of extracorporeal rewarming in a child submerged for 66 minutes. JAMA 260:377, 1988

FRATES RC JR: Analysis of predictive factors in assessment of warm-water near-drowning in children. Am J Dis Child 135:1006, 1981

GULAID JA, SATTIN RW: Drownings in the United States, 1978–1984. Morb Mort Week Rep 37(SS-1):27, 1988

MODELL JH: Biology of drowning. Ann Rev Med 29:1, 1978

OAKES DD et al: Prognosis and management of victims of near-drowning. J Trauma 22:544, 1982

ORLOWSKI JP: Drowning, near-drowning, and ice-water drowning (editorial). JAMA 260, 390, 1988

ORNATO JP: The resuscitation of near-drowning victims. JAMA 256:75, 1986

YATSU FM: Cardiopulmonary-cerebral resuscitation (editorial). N Engl J Med 314:440, 1986

379 ELECTRICAL INJURIES

JAMES F. WALLACE

EPIDEMIOLOGY Since the first human fatality from accidental electrocution was reported in 1879, electrical injury has become progressively more common. In recent years, nearly 4000 electricity-related injuries have occurred annually in the United States, and major electrical burns have constituted nearly 5 percent of all admissions to burn centers. There are approximately 1000 deaths each year from electric current accidents, while another 100 persons die as a result of being struck by lightning. Electrical injuries occur most commonly among agricultural workers, utility pole linemen, crane and heavy equipment operators, and construction workers who come into contact with high-tension current, but nearly a third result from accidents in the home or other settings including the hospital with its many electrically powered instruments and appliances.

PATHOGENESIS For an electric current to flow, there must be a closed pathway or circuit, and a difference in potential or voltage must exist between two points in this completed circuit. The flow of current is directly related to the voltage difference and inversely proportional to the electrical resistance between two points in the circuit (Ohm's law). High-resistance paths allow relatively small currents to flow, while low resistances permit large currents to flow. When the voltage is very high, the flow of current will likewise be relatively great, unless the resistance is increased proportionally to the voltage; however, if the potential difference between the two points can be minimized, the current flow can also be minimized regardless of resistance.

Although the end result of passage of an electric current through the human body is unpredictable in the individual case, many factors are known to influence the nature and severity of electrical injuries. Body tissues vary considerably in their resistance to the flow of current, with conductivity being roughly proportional to water content. Bone and skin offer relatively high resistance, while blood, muscle, and nerve are good conductors. The resistance of normal skin can be lowered by moisture, and this factor alone can convert what might ordinarily be a mild injury to a fatal shock. Of importance at the time of contact is grounding which, if effective, can minimize the voltage difference between two points in the electric circuit and lower the intensity of current passing through the body. The pathway of the current through the body is also crucial. An accident involving passage of a current between a point of contact on the leg and the ground is less likely to be injurious than one between the head and the foot, in which the heart lies between the two poles of the circuit. Similarly, a small current leak which would be innocuous when applied to the surface of the intact body may result in a fatal arrhythmia when conducted directly to the heart via a low-resistance intracardiac catheter. Duration of contact also influences the outcome of electrical injury. Alternating current is much more dangerous than direct current, partly because of its ability to produce tetanic muscular contractions, which prevent the victim from being able to release contact with the circuit. The contractions are usually accompanied by sweating, which lowers skin resistance, allowing current of still greater intensity to pass into the body until fatal cardiac arrhythmia results.

In general, when sudden death occurs following low-voltage shock, it is due to the direct effect of relatively small amounts of current upon the myocardium resulting in ventricular fibrillation. With high-tension injury (greater than 1000 V), cardiac asystole and respiratory arrest occur probably as a result of injury to the medullary centers of the brain.

In addition, contact with high-intensity current may cause three types of thermal injuries. Current coursing externally to the body from the contact point to the ground may generate temperatures as high as 10,000°C and cause extensive carbonification of skin and immediately underlying tissues termed *arc* or *flash burns*. Such burns often ignite surrounding clothing or nearby objects which result in *flame burns*. Finally, there is injury due to the *direct heating* of tissues by electric current. As it traverses the skin, energy from current is converted into heat, which produces coagulation necrosis at the points where it enters and exits from the skin as well as in striated muscle and blood vessels through which it passes. The associated vascular injury results in thromboses, often at sites distant from the body surface, and accounts for the observation that a greater amount of tissue destruction characteristically occurs in an electrical injury than is apparent on first inspection.

PATHOLOGY In patients who die immediately, autopsy findings are limited to burns and generalized petechial hemorrhages. If patients survive for a period of days or longer, postmortem examination reveals focal necrosis of bone, large blood vessels, muscle, peripheral nerves, spinal cord, or brain. Renal tubular necrosis may also be seen when acute renal failure follows extensive tissue destruction.

CLINICAL MANIFESTATIONS Immediately after a severe electrical shock, patients are usually comatose, apneic, and in circulatory collapse from ventricular fibrillation or cardiac standstill. If they survive this stage, they often are disoriented, combative, and frequently have seizures. Often they will be found to have fractures of bone caused either by convulsive muscular contractions accompanying the shock or from falls at the time of the accident. Hypovolemic shock often appears soon after high-tension electrical injury and is due to the rapid loss of fluid into areas of tissue damage and from body surface burns. Hypotension, direct injury to the kidneys by the electric current, and renal tubular damage from myoglobin and hemoglobin pigments liberated during massive muscle necrosis and hemolysis may lead to acute renal failure.

Besides the extensive destruction of tissue occurring instantly in electrical burns, additional injury from ischemia produced by swelling of damaged tissues may appear later and is often accompanied by severe metabolic acidosis. Other serious complications are severe ventricular arrhythmias, which typically begin several hours following the burn injury, neurogenic pulmonary edema, gastrointestinal hemorrhage from preexisting or acute Curling-type ulcers, disseminated intravascular coagulation, and both anaerobic and aerobic infections originating in inadequately debrided necrotic muscle masses. Lightning injury may result in cerebral edema with coma lasting from several minutes to several days. Rupture of one or both tympanic membranes is seen in over half of lightning victims.

Late effects include various neurologic disabilities, visual disturbances, and the residual damage left by burns. Nervous system injuries are frequent and include peripheral neuropathies, nerve entrapment syndromes, incomplete transection of the spinal cord, and reflex sympathetic dystrophies, as well as late convulsive disorders and intractable headache. Psychological effects, particularly disturbances in memory and mood, are common in survivors of lightning strikes and may last for several months. The development of cataracts of one or both eyes has been reported to occur up to 3 years following electrical injury.

LABORATORY FINDINGS Immediately following major electrical injury the hematocrit is elevated and the plasma volume reduced, reflecting sequestration of fluid in the wound. Unless extensive flame burns are also present, serial determinations of either of these parameters provide a good means of monitoring the adequacy of fluid replacement therapy. Myoglobinuria is seen frequently in association with severe shocks, and when it persists following establishment of urine flow, usually indicates massive muscle injury. In many patients arterial blood pH determinations will indicate the presence of metabolic acidosis. Lumbar puncture may show elevated pressure associated with cerebral edema or bloody spinal fluid as a result of intracerebral hemorrhage. The electrocardiogram not infrequently shows tachycardia and minor ST-segment alterations, which can persist for several weeks following injury. Unexplained acute hypokalemia leading to respiratory arrest and cardiac arrhythmias has developed in some patients between the second and fourth weeks following injury.

TREATMENT Removal of victims from contact with the current should be accomplished immediately without touching them directly. Rescuers should use a rubber sheet, a leather belt applied as a sling, a wooden pole, or other nonconductive material to detach them, and this should be preceded by cutting off the source of current when possible. If the victim is not breathing, mouth-to-mouth ventilation should be instituted at once. Although most cases who survive develop spontaneous respiration within half an hour, complete recovery after longer periods occurs often enough that respiratory support should be continued for at least 4 h. If there is no evidence of heartbeat, external cardiac massage should accompany ventilatory resuscitation. Persons struck by lightning frequently have cardiac asystole which responds to a manual blow to the chest, or which spontaneously resolves after several minutes of closed-chest cardiac massage and mouth-to-mouth resuscitation, while victims of low-voltage shocks will usually require defibrillation to restore heart action. During cardiopulmonary resuscitation and evacuation to the hospital, attention should be paid to possible broken bones and spinal cord injuries incurred at the time of the accident.

Subsequent hospital management of patients with electrothermal injuries requires considerable specialized care; whenever feasible, they should be referred to an appropriate burn or trauma unit.

Rapid institution of fluid and electrolyte therapy for hypovolemic shock and acidosis is essential, with guidelines being the patient's urine output, hematocrit, osmolality, central venous pressure, and arterial blood gases. Standard burn formulas should not be used to estimate fluid therapy since these are based only upon extent of body surface area injury and do not take into account the extensive damage to muscle which is usually present. Instead, fluid replacement principles used in the treatment of crush injury, which electrical injury closely resembles, should be followed. Large volumes of fluid, preferably lactated Ringer's solution, should be administered in order to maintain urine output greater than 50 mL/h. If myoglobinuria persists after adequate urine flow has been established, the use of furosemide or an osmotic diuretic such as mannitol along with alkalinization of the urine is indicated. Since focal myocardial injury is not uncommon when electrical current has passed through the thorax and since coronary blood flow is decreased in response to burn shock, careful cardiac evaluation should be included in initial hospital care. Even in the absence of diagnostic ECG or enzymatic changes, patients should be monitored electrocardiographically for at least 24 h for significant arrhythmias, which often have a delayed onset. Management of the electrical burn wound should include adequate debridement of necrotic tissue and often will require fasciotomy to prevent further ischemic injury. Tetanus toxoid should be administered to all previously immunized patients. Unimmunized patients who have major burns should be given tetanus antitoxin (3000 units) as well as an initial immunizing dose of toxoid. Topical antimicrobial chemotherapy may be useful in preventing or delaying infections in extensive surface burns. Silver sulfadiazine cream currently is the preferred agent. Systemic antibiotics are poorly delivered to the ischemic areas of the burn wound, therefore their routine use to prevent streptococcal and staphylococcal infections is not recommended. Instead, the patient should be closely monitored, and antimicrobial therapy selected as indicated by the results of routine cultures. Survivors of the acute episode often require extensive treatment for infection, visceral injury, and delayed hemorrhage as devitalized tissues slough. If acute renal failure occurs, it should be managed as described in Chap. 223. Patients who remain comatose after being struck by lightning should undergo monitoring of intracranial pressure and cerebral perfusion and be treated for cerebral edema if it should develop.

PREVENTION Proper installation of appliances, grounding of telephone lines and radio and television aerials, and the use of rubber gloves and dry shoes when working with electric circuits should be routine. Unused wall sockets should be kept plugged and live extension cords not left unattended, particularly in households where there are young children. Electrical appliances used in bathrooms should be disconnected when not in use and never used in wet bathtubs. During a severe thunderstorm, refuge near hilltops, riverbanks, hedges, telephone poles, and trees should be avoided. The safest shelter is the closed house, while a closed automobile, cave, ditch, or even lying on the ground curled up with hands close together is relatively secure. In hospitalized patients, the hazard of ventricular fibrillation precipitated by minute current leaks conducted directly to the myocardium from monitoring equipment via pacemakers or intravascular manometric catheters should be more widely appreciated. Hospital personnel should be aware that, in addition to medical instruments, patient contact with two or more other power line–operated devices such as television sets, radios, electric razors, lamps, and especially electric beds can also result in electrocution if the heart lies within the current path through the patient. These hazards can be minimized by proper grounding of equipment *before* a patient is connected to the instrument, periodic measurement for leakage of current supplied by each device, and by instruction in the principles of electrical safety for hospital personnel who use the complex and dangerous equipment that is so much a part of modern medical practice.

REFERENCES

AMY BW et al: Lightning injury with survival in 5 patients. JAMA 253:243, 1985

APFELBERG DB et al: Pathophysiology and treatment of lightning injuries. J Trauma 14:453, 1974

BAXTER CR: Emergency treatment of burn injury. Ann Emerg Med 17:1305, 1988

HUNT J et al: Acute electrical burns: Current diagnostic and therapeutic approaches to management. Arch Surg 115:434, 1980

JENSEN PJ et al: Electrical injury causing ventricular arrhythmias. Br Heart J 57:279, 1987

ROSENBERG DB, NELSON M: Rehabilitation concerns in electrical burn patients. A review of the literature. J Trauma 28:808, 1988

380 RADIATION INJURY

STUART C. FINCH

Throughout life human beings are continuously exposed to many types of radiation, some harmless and some harmful. The most harmful is *ionizing radiation,* which damages tissue through the action of charged particles. More is known about the acute and late somatic, teratogenic, and genetic effects of ionizing radiation than any other environmental, physical, or chemical agent or force, yet many gaps remain in our knowledge concerning its effects. Most important and least well understood are the late effects of chronic low-dose exposure on humans. There is little reliable direct information, so that it is only possible to estimate such effects by extrapolation from information pertaining to high-dose exposure.

There are two types of ionizing radiation: The first consists of high-frequency electromagnetic waves of relatively short wavelength with particle characteristics, such as naturally occurring gamma rays or machine-made x-rays. These waves are capable of deep tissue penetration and moderate ionization of the tissues along their pathways by indirect mechanisms. Their interactions with the atoms and molecules of tissue structures result in the release of orbital electrons and the formation of ions and reactive radicals that damage cell components and disrupt biologic processes. The second type of ionizing radiation consists of a variety of subatomic particles, the most important of which are electrically charged alpha particles, protons, and electrons and electrically uncharged neutrons. The charged particles densely ionize structures along their pathways in tissues. The depth of penetration is quite limited and varies as a function of particle size, charge, and velocity. Tissue damage is due to the direct ionization of water, oxygen, and other molecules with the formation of free hydroxyl radicals and highly reactive oxygen species. Neutrons penetrate tissues much more deeply than charged particles of equivalent size (such as protons). They indirectly ionize through their interactions with the nuclei of atoms, resulting in the release of protons, alpha particles, and other nuclear fragments that ionize and damage other tissues.

The longer-wavelength waves of the electromagnetic spectrum do not ionize, but some may damage tissues by other mechanisms. For example, ultraviolet light penetrates very little, but it photochemically induces cell damage, some of which may be permanent. Ultrasonic, infrared, radio, and microwave electromagnetic waves are capable of deep tissue penetration with the generation of heat, the effects of which are largely reversible. Weak, low-frequency electromagnetic waves have been shown to modulate ion flow and to interfere with both RNA transcription and DNA synthesis at the cellular level, but the overall effects in humans remain uncertain. This chapter will consider only the acute and late effects of exposure to ionizing radiation.

TERMINOLOGY AND DEFINITIONS Some familiarity with radiation terminology and units is essential for the understanding of radiation effects. An early term for the quantitation of exposure was the *roentgen,* or R, which represents the amount of radiation-induced ionization in a standard volume of air. Much more important is the *rad* (radiation absorbed dose), which represents a unit of absorbed dose in tissue. One rad corresponds to the absorption of one hundred ergs of energy (or about 1 R) in one gram of tissue. Since the same

dose in rads of different kinds of ionizing radiation can produce different biologic effects, the term *rem* (roentgen equivalent man) was introduced. It represents the rad multiplied by its RBE (relative biologic effectiveness), which is a quality factor for the biologic effects of the particular type of radiation used in comparison to a radiation standard. The biologic effect of gamma radiation is the usual standard for comparison. Gamma radiation, therefore, has an RBE of 1, and 1 rad of gamma exposure is roughly equal to 1 rem. Most x-rays have an RBE of 1 or slightly higher, whereas neutrons and some charged particles may have an RBE of 5 to 20 or greater. The terms *gray* (Gy), one unit of which is the equivalent of one hundred rads, and *sievert* (Sv), one unit of which is equal to one hundred rems, have been adopted to replace the rad and rem terminologies, respectively. One-thousandth of a gray is written as mGy (0.1 rad), and one-thousandth of an Sv as mSv (0.1 rem).

The density of tissue ionization produced per unit length along the pathway of ionizing radiation is expressed as its *linear energy transfer* (LET). In general, electrically charged particles or particles of relatively high mass (alpha particles, protons, and neutrons) have high energy transfer (high LET), resulting in relatively large amounts of tissue damage. In contrast, electromagnetic forms of ionizing radiation (gamma rays or x-rays) or charged particles of small mass (electrons) transfer less energy per unit length of travel (have low LET) and produce less tissue damage. There is quite a good correlation between LET and RBE.

The *threshold dose* is the minimum radiation dose that will produce a biologic effect. Radiation effects that vary with dose and frequency but not in severity are called *stochastic* effects. Examples of these are radiation-induced carcinogenic, mutagenic, and teratogenic effects. *Nonstochastic* effects vary in severity above a threshold dose depending on the number of cells injured. Examples of such effects are radiation-induced cataracts of the eye or fibrosis of the bone marrow. The interval of time between exposure and the occurrence of a radiation effect is identified as its *latent period.* The *maximum permissible dose* is that dose of ionizing radiation that, in the light of present knowledge, is not expected to cause any appreciable bodily injury to any person at any time during a lifetime.

TYPES AND SOURCES OF IONIZING RADIATION Most of a person's lifetime radiation exposure is from low-dose background radiation. The average annual effective dose for persons in the United States is estimated to be about 3.6 mSv. About two-thirds of this radiation is from natural sources, of which radon, cosmic rays, radionuclides in the earth, and radioactive elements in the body are the major contributors.

Radon now is believed to contribute about 55 percent of a person's total background radiation exposure. This represents about 2 mSv of exposure per year. Radon is a colorless, odorless, and tasteless alpha particle emitting radioactive gas which is derived from naturally occurring uranium deposits in the earth. It seeps up through soil into the air, where it and its decay products attach to dust, aerosols, or droplets which are inhaled and retained in bronchial epithelium and adjacent structures. The greatest exposures occur in certain indoor areas and mines where there are high adjacent rock concentrations of phosphates, granite, and black shale. Radon itself is not particularly harmful, but some of its alpha-emitting polonium radioactive decay products may heavily irradiate bronchial epithelium cells for many months or years.

Cosmic radiation accounts for about 0.3 mSv of background radiation per year at sea level. It is composed of protons, neutrons, and heavy nuclei from galactic sources and low-energy charged particles from the sun which interact with atmospheric nuclei to produce small secondary particles and electrons that enter the body and ionize tissue. The earth's atmosphere acts as a shield, so that the dose is about doubled with every 1500-m increase in altitude. Radioactive potassium and carbon and other radionuclides within the body contribute about another 0.4 mSv to the average person's annual background radiation exposure. Radioactive decay of thorium and uranium radionuclides in the earth's crust constitute the major sources of terrestrial radiation, which, in most areas, is about 0.3 mSv per year. Amounts of terrestrial radiation may vary by a factor of four to six or more in different geographic locations.

The remaining 18 percent of a person's total background radiation exposure is from man-made sources. Diagnostic x-ray and nuclear medicine account for over 0.5 mSv of the estimated annual total of about 0.65 mSv. Exposure from these sources has doubled in the United States and many other countries during the past 20 years.

Most acute or intermittent excessive exposures to ionizing radiation occur in association with radiation therapy, preparation for organ transplantation, nuclear weapon detonations, nuclear reactor accidents, or accidental ingestion of radionuclides. Most of such exposures are to x- or gamma rays, but direct radiation exposure or fallout from nuclear weapon detonations or reactor accidents or radionuclide ingestion, inhalation, or injection may result in significant exposures to high-LET radiation.

PATHOGENESIS OF RADIATION INJURY There are many types of cellular injury following exposure to ionizing radiation. Most important is damage to the genetic apparatus of the nucleus due to structural alterations of DNA and chromosomes.

Many types of DNA damage may occur, but most common with low-LET radiation are single-strand breaks and base alterations. High-LET radiation produces more double-strand breaks and more complex types of DNA base damage. In both instances, free radicals generated by ionizing radiation are largely responsible for the DNA and chromosome alterations. The extent to which damaged DNA will be responsible for cell death or will become a permanent mutation depends upon the ability of the cells to repair the damage. Repair of DNA damage from low-LET radiation is much more efficient than it is from high-LET radiation. This is extremely important because most of the somatic mutational and late neoplastic effects in replicating cells probably are due to the persistence of radiation-induced unrepaired or misrepaired DNA bases.

Chromosome damage of many types as a function of unrepaired DNA constitutes the other major type of radiation-induced injury to the genetic apparatus of the cell. Chromosomal breaks with rearrangements associated with loss of considerable amounts of chromosomal mass usually are responsible for cell death at the first or one of the first few postirradiation mitotic divisions. Consequently the number of chromosome aberrations present at any one time during the postirradiation period will depend on both the number induced and the rate of cell turnover. Balanced chromosomal rearrangements involving little loss of chromosomal material may persist as stable intracellular markers of radiation injury for many years. There is strong evidence that chromosome rearrangements involving breaks near proto-oncogenes play an important role in the process of radiation-induced malignant transformation (see Chap. 10).

Repair of radiation-induced DNA and chromosomal damage is inversely related to the rate at which the radiation is absorbed. This is particularly true for low-LET radiation, where a high rate of radiation absorption may increase residual tissue damage by factors of 2 to 10 times that experienced with a low rate of radiation absorption.

High doses of radiation may produce direct cell death due to membrane or cytoplasmic structural damage. This type of interphase cell death of autonomic nerve cells, lymphocytes, and capillaries is responsible for most of the early clinical manifestations of high-dose acute radiation exposure. Relatively little direct membrane and cytoplasmic damage occurs following exposure to low doses of ionizing radiation.

HISTORY Most of our knowledge concerning the *late* effects of ionizing radiation exposure for humans has been derived from a series of unfortunate accidents and errors during the past 75 years. In the early 1920s and 1930s about 2000 luminous dial workers, mostly young women in the United States, inadvertently ingested large amounts of radium 226 by means of absorption from their tongues and lips. Many later developed carcinomas of the paranasal sinuses and osteosarcomas. In Germany in the mid-1940s a number of children with bone tuberculosis and many adults with rheumatoid arthritis were injected with radium 224. Five to ten years later many of them also developed osteosarcomas. Increased mortality from leukemia and multiple myeloma was reported for radiologists during the early years of use of medical x-ray equipment. In the 1930s and through the early 1950s thorium dioxide (Thorotrast) was employed as a contrast medium in a number of medical clinics throughout the world. Many injected persons developed hepatic tumors, leukemia, or aplastic anemia in later years. Increased rates of thyroid cancer and leukemia have been reported for children treated with x-rays in the 1940s and 1950s for tinea capitis and presumed thymus enlargement. A sizable number of individuals with ankylosing spondylitis in England who received radiation therapy later developed aplastic anemia and leukemia. Increased incidence of lung cancer has been recognized in uranium miners. Fallout from weapons testing in the Marshall Islands has produced an increased occurrence of hypothyroidism and benign thyroid nodules. Studies of the atomic bomb survivors of Hiroshima and Nagasaki, however, have provided the most extensive and reliable information concerning the late effects of exposure to ionizing radiation.

Most information concerning *acute* radiation exposure derives from two sources: the atomic bomb explosions and radiation accidents. There were approximately 110,000 to 120,000 civilian deaths from the atomic bomb explosions of Hiroshima and Nagasaki, about one-third of which are believed to have been caused by radiation exposure. The Radiation Accident Registry at Oak Ridge has identified 305 major worldwide radiation accidents between 1944 and 1989, involving 122,614 people. There were 1871 significant exposures and 101 deaths. Forty-four of the deaths were attributed to the acute radiation syndrome.

CLINICAL EFFECTS OF RADIATION EXPOSURE *Acute, or early, effects* occur within the first few minutes up to 2 to 3 months following exposure to large amounts of radiation over a short period of time and are due to cell killing, impairment of cell function, inflammation, and infection. *Intermediate effects* occur after the first few months up to a few years following exposure. *Late effects* are the diseases and disorders that develop after the first few months or years for which previous ionizing radiation exposure is responsible.

Acute radiation effects The early clinical manifestations of excessive acute whole-body exposure to ionizing radiation constitute the *acute radiation syndrome*. Its time of onset, severity, and duration will depend on the quality, quantity, and distribution of the radiation absorbed.

There are four classic clinical stages of the complete acute radiation syndrome. The earliest phase is the prodrome, which invariably consists of anorexia, nausea, and vomiting but also may include diarrhea, salivation, abdominal cramps, and dehydration. It commences within minutes to hours of exposure and lasts from a few hours to 1 or 2 days. This usually is followed by a relatively asymptomatic second stage of a few days to a few weeks in duration. The third stage usually begins during the second to fifth weeks following exposure with the abrupt onset of moderate to severe gastrointestinal tract disturbances and manifestations of bone marrow depression. The fourth stage involves recovery, which may take weeks to months, or death.

Persons who receive whole-body radiation in the range of 50 Gy or more invariably will die within 24 to 48 h from complications associated with the *neurovascular syndrome*. This is characterized by the rapid onset of apathy, lethargy, and prostration, frequently followed by seizures ranging from muscle contractions to grand mal convulsions, ataxia, and death. The early occurrence of severe central nervous system problems frequently yields to intractable hypotension, arrhythmias, and shock before death occurs. This sometimes is identified as the *cardiovascular syndrome*.

A significant prodrome also will develop rapidly in persons exposed to whole-body radiation in the range of 10 to 50 Gy. Following a latent period of a few days, the *gastrointestinal syndrome* develops as the result of intestinal tract ulceration, infection, and hemorrhage secondary to mucosal cell atrophy and bone marrow depression. Its clinical manifestations are associated with massive fluid, protein, and electrolyte loss, invariably leading to death within a few more days.

Whole-body exposures in the range of 2 to 10 Gy are characterized by manifestations of the *bone marrow syndrome* due to a loss of marrow stem cells. Following a prodrome of 1 to 3 days and a relatively asymptomatic period of 1 to 3 weeks, buccal and pharyngeal ulcerations, localized and systemic forms of infection, cutaneous petechiae, and possibly generalized bleeding may develop secondary to thrombocytopenia and agranulocytosis. Concomitant loss of gastrointestinal epithelium often results in persistent diarrhea, abdominal distention, dehydration, circulatory collapse, and death. Survivors will experience rapid clinical improvement following partial return of peripheral blood granulocytes and platelets in 6 to 8 weeks, but full recovery may take several months. Epilation usually commences 1 to 2 weeks following exposure and is greatest at 5 to 7 weeks. Regrowth of new hair may take 4 to 6 months or more.

Mild gastrointestinal symptoms are experienced by 25 to 75 percent of persons exposed to less than 2 Gy of whole-body radiation. Hematologic complications rarely develop, because there is only moderate depression of the formed blood elements. Complete recovery of almost everyone in this exposure category is expected within 2 to 5 weeks.

Peripheral blood lymphopenia invariably develops during the first 12 to 48 h following any significant exposure. The rate and magnitude of the drop are reasonably related to radiation exposures up to about 5 to 6 Gy. At higher levels of exposure, lymphopenia is extreme, so that correlations with exposure dose are poor. Reduced lymphocyte levels usually persist for 6 to 8 weeks. There often is a modest increase in numbers of peripheral blood granulocytes during the first 1 to 2 days in response to exposure of more than 2 Gy followed by a continual decline to maximum granulocytopenia in 2 to 5 weeks. The rate of granulocyte decline and the severity of granulocytopenia are functions of the bone marrow exposure dose. The peripheral blood platelet count responses are similar to those of the granulocytes except that early thrombocytosis is rare and rates of both decline and recovery usually are slower. Reversible dose-dependent reticulocytopenia and mild anemia may develop up to radiation doses of about 5 to 6 Gy. Higher exposures usually result in irreversible bone marrow damage.

Early radiation-induced chromosome aberrations observed in peripheral blood lymphocytes include dicentrics, rings, deletions, translocations, inversions, and other types of rearrangements. Other dose-related somatic mutations observed following acute whole-body exposure include loss of hypoxanthine-guanine phosphoribosyl transferase (HPRT) from some circulating lymphocytes and alterations in the structure of erythrocyte membrane glycophorin A.

Reproductive system disturbances are other important early clinical sequelae of acute whole-body radiation exposure. Male oligospermia or aspermia usually is temporary for weeks or months following exposures of 1.5 to 4 Gy, but permanent sterility usually develops at exposures of 5 to 9 Gy or greater. Sterility may be temporary in females exposed to 1.5 to 6.5 Gy and permanent at higher levels.

Intermediate and late radiation effects   The most important late effect of exposure to ionizing radiation is increased incidence of cancer. An increased incidence of leukemia appeared in the Japanese atomic bomb survivors within 2 to 3 years following exposure. Peak rates occurred about 7 to 8 years after the bombings, followed by a steady decline to near-baseline levels during the next 30 to 35 years. Childhood leukemia rates peaked early and returned to normal 15 years after exposure. The latent period for acute leukemia in adults increased with age at the time of exposure. Most of the radiation-induced childhood leukemias were acute lymphocytic in type, but a high incidence of chronic myeloid leukemia also occurred. Acute and chronic myeloid leukemias predominated in adults, but acute lymphocytic leukemia also appeared to be radiation-related. There is no evidence from any studies of human radiation effects that chronic lymphocytic leukemia is radiation-related. Based on atomic bomb survivor information, the expected excess number of deaths from leukemia from low-LET radiation over a period of 40 years is about 10 cases for every 1000 adults exposed to 1 Sv of radiation.

A significant relationship between radiation exposure and the frequency of death from multiple myeloma and cancers of the female breast, esophagus, stomach, colon, lung, ovary, and urinary bladder has been observed in atomic bomb survivors (Table 380-1). Significant increases in mortality have not been observed for lymphomas, bone tumors, and cancers of the rectum, gallbladder, pancreas, uterus, and prostate in this population. Most of the radiation-induced solid tumors have appeared at their usual ages of occurrence, with minimum latent periods ranging from 15 to 35 years. Since the incidence of most cancers increases with aging, it is likely that the increased risk for cancer from radiation exposure lasts for life. There is a dose-dependent shortening of the latent period and a significant increase in cancer risk for children exposed under the age of 10. Excess deaths for specific radiation-induced cancers are about equal in males and females, except for a significant increase in deaths from leukemia in males. The radiation dose-response relationship for solid tumors is linear, but for leukemia it appears to be more linear-quadratic. The radiation response for the induction of tumors is believed to be stochastic, but organ-absorbed doses in the range of 0.2 to 0.49 Gy for leukemia, lung cancer, and several other cancers are the lowest levels for which a significant increase in cancer mortality has been observed (Table 380-1). Excess lifetime mortality from low-LET radiation in adults for cancers other than leukemia is estimated on the basis of atomic bomb survivor information to be about 47 new cases for every 1000 persons exposed to 1 Sv.

Increased incidence of thyroid cancer, benign thyroid adenomas, and hypothyroidism may occur following either external or internal exposure of the thyroid gland to ionizing radiation. The risk of developing thyroid cancer from external irradiation during childhood is about twice that for exposure during adulthood. The female-to-male ratio for radiation-induced thyroid cancer is about 2:1, with latent periods ranging from 4 to 30 years or longer. Persons of Jewish descent appear to be at higher risk than are those of other ethnic backgrounds who have been studied. Thyroid gland exposures to low-LET radiation in the range of 0.2 to 15 Gy have resulted in the increased late occurrence of thyroid cancer. The absolute risk for low-LET radiation–induced thyroid cancer is quite uncertain and depends on many factors, but probably is in the range of 6 to 12 excess cases per 10^4 persons year Gy. The induction rate for benign adenomas is about 30 to 50 percent greater than that for cancer. Radioiodine therapy with thyroid gland doses greater than 15 to 20 Gy kills parenchymal cells and almost invariably results in hypothy-

TABLE 380-1   Significant radiation-induced cancer information for atomic bomb survivors, 1950–1985 (radiation exposure expressed as organ-absorbed dose)

Type of cancer	Excess relative risk at 1 Gy*	Excess deaths per 10^4 persons/ year, Gy*	Minimum dose for increased mortality, Gy	Minimum latent period to death, years
Leukemia	5.2	2.9	0.2–0.5	3–5
Multiple myeloma	2.3	0.3	—	30–34
Ovary	1.3	0.7	0.2–0.3	25–29
Urinary tract	1.3	0.7	—	30–34
Female breast	1.2	1.2	0.5–1.0	20–24
Colon	0.9	0.8	1.0–1.9	30–34
Lung	0.6	1.7	0.2–0.5	20–24
Esophagus	0.6	0.5	—	—
All (except leukemia)	0.4	10.1	0.2–0.5	—
Stomach	0.3	2.4	0.5–1.0	15–19

* Rates from UNSCEAR and Radiation Effects Research Foundation reports have been rounded to the nearest tenth.

roidism rather than cancer. Radioiodine used for diagnostic thyroid studies increases the incidence of benign adenomas but does not increase the incidence of thyroid cancer.

Many types of cancer and other late effects have been related to exposure to ionizing radiation from internally deposited radioisotopes (Table 380-2). The only recognized late effect from excessive radon exposure is lung cancer. The risk of death in the United States from indoor radon exposure is estimated to be 0.4 percent. This would result in the development of 6000 to 25,000 lung cancers per year. The risks of radon exposure and smoking for lung cancer are at least additive.

Bilateral posterior-central dotlike opacities with surrounding granules and vacuoles may develop in the *lens* of the eye within weeks or months following low-LET radiation exposure. The more heavily irradiated persons may have lateral extension of these tiny opacities with central clearing and anterior extension to the anterior surface of the lens. The lesions are defined as cataracts, but they rarely impair vision or progress over the years. Children are more prone to develop radiation-induced lenticular damage than are adults. The lenticular changes induced by radiation are nonstochastic, with a threshold dose of about 0.3 Gy for low-LET radiation.

The early radiation-induced dicentric and ring-form chromosomal aberrations in blood lymphocytes disappear with the first mitosis, so that few remain in later years, but many of the radiation-induced balanced structural rearrangements persist as biologic radiation markers throughout life. Reciprocal translocations and inversions predominate. The radiation dose-response is linear and is not influenced by age at time of exposure. The early radiation-induced structural alterations in erythrocyte membrane glycophorin A persist in later years, but the changes in lymphocyte HPRT disappear with time.

A radiation dose-response relationship for the occurrence of small head size has been observed in newborn infants following in utero exposure of the fetus to atomic bomb radiation during the first 15 weeks of pregnancy. Small head size has been observed in 40 to 50 percent of these infants following exposures of 1 Gy or more. A dose-related risk of mental retardation also has been observed in children following in utero exposure between the eighth and fifteenth weeks of gestation to greater than 0.4 Gy of low-LET radiation. A lower risk for mental retardation exists for exposure between the sixteenth and twenty-fifth weeks of gestation with an apparent threshold at about 0.7 Gy. Prenatal exposure during the eighth to fifteenth weeks of gestation and, to a lesser extent, between the sixteenth and twenty-eighth weeks also is dose-related to an increased incidence of reduced school achievement, lower intelligence test scores, and unprovoked seizures later in life. The crude incidence of

cancer 40 years following intrauterine exposure to radiation above 0.3 Gy is three- to nine-fold greater than for unexposed controls.

Excessive prenatal or childhood radiation exposure in the range of 1 Gy or more has been shown eventually to result in slight reduction in maximum height. Other late effects of whole-body exposure in atomic bomb survivors include accelerated decline in cell-mediated immunity with aging and an increased occurrence of hyperparathyroidism.

There are few direct data for humans concerning the genetic effects of exposure to ionizing radiation. It is believed, however, that the dose-response relationship is linear without a threshold and that the overwhelming majority of induced mutations are damaging. Atomic bomb survivor studies have failed to demonstrate a statistically significant increase in the genetic effects evaluated in the children of exposed persons, but the data suggest that the amount of acute parental radiation required to double the spontaneous mutation rate (*doubling dose*) is about 2 Sv. The Japanese data also suggest a doubling dose for chronic parental radiation exposure of about 4 Sv, in comparison to other estimates from mouse data ranging from 0.5 to 2.5 Sv. All of these estimates have considerable error.

Local or regional radiotherapy   Radiation administered in small intermittent (fractionated) doses is better tolerated by tissue structures than an equivalent amount of radiation given as a single dose. However, since the cumulative total local and regional radiotherapy tissue doses usually are very high, the acute, intermediate, and late effects may be severe and quite different from those due to whole-body exposure. For example, intensive local x-ray therapy to the lung may cause radiation pneumonitis and fibrosis, yet little lung damage will occur following exposure to near lethal amounts of whole-body radiation. Internists should be familiar with the major acute, intermediate, and late effects of radiotherapy, which have been well-documented elsewhere.

TREATMENT   There is no specific therapy for tissue radiation injury, but much can be done to reduce the morbidity and mortality for persons who have been acutely exposed to excessive amounts of whole-body ionizing radiation.

Persons with possible surface contamination from radioactive substances must be evacuated promptly, monitored for external contamination, and decontaminated if necessary. It is extremely important to estimate the dose of radiation exposure as early as possible in order to determine the need for various types of therapy. This may be extremely difficult even under the best of circumstances. The most reliable early indicators of dose in the absence of an actual dosimeter measurement are the exposure history, the severity of clinical symptoms, and the frequency of certain radiation-induced biologic markers in blood cells. The severity and rapidity of the development of lymphopenia may give some early index of exposure dose, but much more reliable is the radiation-induced frequency of dicentric chromosome aberrations in mitogen-stimulated and spontaneously dividing peripheral blood lymphocytes. (An emergency service for lymphocyte chromosome aberrations is available from the Radiation Emergency Assistance Center/Training Site in Oak Ridge, Tennessee.) The rate of granulocyte decline also is a very reliable and practical early biologic radiation dosimeter, but it may take 3 to 5 days or more before the rate is determined accurately. Bone marrow aspirations have limited quantitative relationships to exposure, but if performed in various sites, they may indicate the extent of marrow damage. Measurements of radiation-induced loss of HPRT in lymphocytes and glycophorin A mutations in the red cell membrane also show great promise as biologic dosimeters for the early estimation of radiation dose.

Persons with few symptoms probably are exposed to less than 2 Gy and will require little or no therapy, but should be kept under observation for a few days. Persons with estimated exposures in the range of 2 to 5 or 6 Gy require hospitalization for vigorous supportive therapy. Intravenous fluids and broad-spectrum antibiotic coverage should be instituted if either bacterial infection or severe agranulocytosis develops. Other supportive measures may include the admin-

TABLE 380-2   Late effects of radionuclide exposure

Radionuclide	Route of administration	Late effects
Thorium²³² dioxide (Thorotrast)	Intravenous	Liver angiosarcoma, hemangioendothelioma, hepatic cell carcinoma, and cirrhosis. Bile duct carcinoma, kidney cancer, leukemia, splenic atrophy and fibrosis, and aplastic anemia.
Radium²²⁴	Intravenous	Osteosarcoma, chondroblastic sarcoma, cataracts, leukemia, and renal insufficiency.
Radium²²⁶,²²⁸	Oral	Osteosarcoma, chondroblastic sarcoma, paranasal and mastoid carcinoma, and colon cancer.
Radon²²²	Inhalation	Lung cancer.
Iodine¹²⁵,¹³¹	Oral and intravenous	Hypothyroidism, thyroid adenomas, and thyroid cancer.
Strontium⁹⁰	Topical	Anterior lenticular cataracts from eye applicators; fallout-induced acute beta skin burns may lead to eventual skin necrosis and atrophy.
Phosphorus³²	Topical	Fallout-induced acute beta skin burns may lead to eventual skin necrosis and atrophy.

istration of immunoglobulins, antifungal and antiviral agents, and antibiotics for the reduction of intestinal tract bacterial flora. Platelet transfusions should be administered for either clinical bleeding due to thrombocytopenia or with platelet counts below 20×10^9/L. Blood transfusions are necessary if anemia develops. Bone marrow transfusions are not indicated for persons in this group, but the early and continuous administration of granulocyte colony stimulating factors may be important adjuncts to the other forms of supportive therapy.

If the level of granulocytes falls during the first week to 0.25×10^9/L or less and the level of platelets to less than 30×10^9/L in 10 days, the total-body exposure probably is in the range of 5 to 15 Gy. Exposure doses in this range usually will irreversibly destroy the bone marrow stem cells. Survival with supportive therapy alone usually is not possible, so that the addition of allogeneic bone marrow transplantation and the concomitant administration of granulocyte colony stimulating factors may offer the best hopes for survival (see Chap. 299). Bone marrow transplantations probably are most effective if performed within the first 3 to 5 days of exposure, so early radiation dose estimates are very important. Peripheral blood lymphocytes should be collected as early as is possible for histocompatibility testing, because they disappear rapidly from circulation. Platelets and blood should be irradiated with about 20 Gy prior to transfusion in order to reduce recipient alloantigen sensitization. Preparatory immunosuppression with chemotherapeutic agents and whole-body irradiation probably are not advisable prior to bone marrow transfusion, as permanent engraftment may not be necessary. Furthermore, they will contribute considerably to the severity of the overall illness. Persons with acute exposure to more than 15 to 20 Gy should be admitted to the hospital for supportive therapy only.

It is recommended that persons exposed to fallout in contaminated areas be treated as early as possible with 130 mg/d of potassium iodide for 10 days in order to prevent the accumulation of radioactive iodine in the thyroid gland.

PROGNOSIS Prognosis for survival from the acute manifestations of whole-body exposure to ionizing radiation depends almost entirely upon tissue dose. Mortality without any therapy is negligible at 1 Gy or less and is virtually 100 percent above 15 Gy despite optimal therapy. About 50 percent of persons exposed to between 2 and 4 Gy will succumb without therapy, but most will survive with vigorous support. There is a very high probability of death, even with vigorous general support therapy, at exposures between 5 and 15 Gy, but it seems likely that some people will survive with allogeneic bone marrow transplantation and other forms of supportive therapy.

There are no known forms of therapy for prevention of the late effects of ionizing radiation exposure. They are influenced by tissue dose, rate of exposure, age at time of exposure, concomitant exposure to other carcinogens or radioprotective agents, inherent repair mechanisms, and many other unknown factors. The clinical course and response to therapy of radiation-induced leukemias and solid tumors are not significantly different from those which are not radiation-related.

REFERENCES

COMMITTEE ON THE BIOLOGICAL EFFECTS OF IONIZING RADIATION, NATIONAL RESEARCH COUNCIL: *Health Risks of Radon and Other Internally Deposited Alpha-emitters (BEIR IV)*. Washington, D.C., National Academy Press, 1988

————: *Health Effects of Exposure to Low Levels of Ionizing Radiation (BEIR V)*. Washington, D.C., National Academy Press, 1990

METTLER JR FA, MOSELY JR RD: *Medical Effects of Radiation*. Orlando, Florida, Grune and Stratton, 1985, pp 1–288

NEEL JV et al: The children of parents exposed to atomic bombs: Estimates of the genetic doubling dose of radiation for humans. Am J Human Gen 46:1053, 1990

SHIMUZU Y et al: Studies of the mortality of A-bomb survivors. 9. Mortality, 1950–85, Part 2. Cancer mortality based on the recently revised doses (DS 86). Radiat Res 121:120, 1990.

UNITED NATIONS SCIENTIFIC COMMITTEES ON THE EFFECTS OF ATOMIC RADIATION: *Sources, Effects and Risks of Ionizing Radiation*. Report No. 88. IX. 7. New York, United Nations, 1988

**APPENDIX
AND INDEX**

APPENDIX   LABORATORY VALUES OF CLINICAL IMPORTANCE

INTRODUCTORY COMMENTS

In preparing the Appendix, the editors have taken into account the fact that the system of international units (SI, système international d'unités) is now used in most countries and in virtually all medical and scientific journals including those in the United States.[1] However, many or most clinical laboratories in the United States continue to report values in traditional units. Therefore, in this book we utilize both systems for the Appendix and for the text itself. Values in SI units appear first, and *traditional units appear in parentheses* after the SI units. This dual approach is also used for the large part in the text. In those instances in which the numbers remain the same but only the terminology is changed (mmol/L for meq/L or IU/L for mIU/mL) only the SI units are given. In all other instances the SI unit is followed by the traditional unit in parentheses. The SI base units, SI derived units, other units of measure referred to in the Appendix, and SI prefixes are listed in Tables A-1 to A-3 at the end of the Appendix. Conversions from one system to another can be made as follows:

$$mmol/L = \frac{mg/dL \times 10}{atomic\ weight}$$

$$mg/dL = \frac{mmol/L \times atomic\ weight}{10}$$

ASCITIC FLUID

See Table 48-1, p. 270.

BODY FLUIDS AND OTHER MASS DATA

Body fluid, total volume: 50 percent (in obese) to 70 percent (lean) of body weight
  Intracellular: 0.3–0.4 of body weight
  Extracellular: 0.2–0.3 of body weight
Blood:
  Total volume:
    Males: 69 mL per kg body weight
    Females: 65 mL per kg body weight
  Plasma volume:
    Males: 39 mL per kg body weight
    Females: 40 mL per kg body weight
  Red blood cell volume:
    Males: 30 mL per kg body weight (1.15–1.21 L/m² body surface area)
    Females: 25 mL per kg body weight (0.95–1.00 L/m² body surface area)

[1] Young DS: Implementation of SI Units for Clinical Laboratory Data. Ann Intern Med 106:114, 1987

[2] Since cerebrospinal fluid concentrations are equilibrium values, measurements of the same parameters in blood plasma obtained at the same time is recommended. However, there is a time lag in attainment of equilibrium, and cerebrospinal levels of plasma constituents that can fluctuate rapidly (such as plasma glucose) may not achieve stable values until after a significant lag phase.

CEREBROSPINAL FLUID[2]

		Conversion factor (CF) (C × CF = SI)
Osmolality	292–297 mosmol/kg (292–297 mosmol/L)	—
Electrolytes:		
Sodium	137–145 mmol/L (137–145 meq/L)	—
Potassium	2.7–3.9 mmol/L (2.7–3.9 meq/L)	—
Calcium	1–1.5 mmol/L (2.1–3.0 meq/L)	0.5
Magnesium	1–1.2 mmol/L (2.0–2.5 meq/L)	0.5
Chloride	116–122 mmol/L (116–122 meq/L)	—
CO_2 content	20–24 mmol/L (20–24 meq/L)	—
P_{CO_2}	6–7 kPa (45–49 mmHg)	0.1333
pH	7.31–7.34	—
Glucose	2.2–3.9 mmol/L (40–70 mg/dL)	0.05551
Lactate	1–2 mmol/L (10–20 mg/dL)	0.1110
Total protein:	0.2–0.4 g/L (20–40 mg/dL)	0.01
Prealbumin	2–6 percent	—
Albumin	56–75 percent	—
Alpha₁ globulin	2–7 percent	—
Alpha₂ globulin	4–12 percent	—
Beta globulin	8–16 percent	—
Gamma globulin	3–12 percent	—
IgG	0.01–0.014 g/L (1–1.4 mg/dL)	0.01
IgA	0.001–0.003 g/L (0.1–0.3 mg/dL)	0.01
IgM	0.0001–0.00012 g/L (0.01–0.012 mg/dL)	0.01
Ammonia	15–47 μmol/L (25–80 μg/dL)	0.5872
Creatinine	44–168 μmol/L (0.5–1.9 mg/dL)	88.40
Myelin basic protein	<4 μg/L	—
CSF pressure	50–180 mmH₂O	—
CSF volume (adult)	100–160 mL	—
Leukocytes:		
Total	<4 per mL	—
Differential:		
Lymphocytes	60–70 percent	—
Monocytes	30–50 percent	—
Neutrophils	1–3 percent	—

CHEMICAL CONSTITUENTS OF BLOOD

See also "Function Tests," especially "Metabolic and Endocrine."

	Conversion factor (CF) ($C \times CF = SI$)
Acetoacetate, plasma: <100 μmol/L (<1 mg/dL)	97.95
Albumin, serum: 35–55 g/L (3.5–5.5 g/dL)	10
Aldolase: 0–100 nkat/L (0–6 U/L)	16.67
Alpha$_1$ antitrypsin, serum: 0.8–2.1 g/L (85–213 mg/dL)	0.01
Alpha fetoprotein (adult), serum: <30 μg/L (<30 ng/mL)	—
Aminotransferases, serum:	
Aspartate (AST, SGOT): 0–0.58 μkat/L (0–35 U/L)	0.01667
Alanine (ALT, SGPT): 0–0.58 μkat/L (0–35 U/L)	0.01667
Ammonia, whole blood, venous: 47–65 μmol/L (80–110 μg/dL)	0.5872
Amylase, serum: 0.8–3.2 μkat/L (60–180 U/L)	0.01667
Arterial blood gases:	
[$HCO_3{}^-$]: 21–28 mmol/L (21–28 meq/L)	—
P_{CO_2}: 4.7–5.9 kPa (35–45 mmHg)	0.1333
pH: 7.38–7.44	—
P_{O_2}: 11–13 kPa (80–100 mmHg)	0.1333
Ascorbic acid (vitamin C), serum: 23–57 μmol/L (0.4–1.0 mg/dL)	56.78
Barbiturates, serum: normal, nondetectable	
Phenobarbital, "potentially fatal" level: approximately 390 μmol/L (9 mg/dL)	43.06
Most short-acting barbiturates, "potentially fatal" levels: approximately 150 μmol/L (35 mg/L)	4.419
Base, total, serum: 145–155 mmol/L (145–155 meq/L)	—
β-Hydroxybutyrate, plasma: <300 μmol/L (<3 mg/dL)	96.05
Bilirubin, total, serum (Malloy-Evelyn): 5.1–17 μmol/L (0.3–1.0 mg/dL)	17.10
Direct, serum: 1.7–5.1 μmol/L (0.1–0.3 mg/dL)	17.10
Indirect, serum: 3.4–12 μmol/L (0.2–0.7 mg/dL)	17.10
Bromides, serum: nondetectable	
Toxic levels: >17 mmol/L (>17 meq/L)	—
Bromsulphalein, BSP (5 mg per kg body weight, intravenously): 5 percent or less retention after 45 min	—
Calciferols (vitamin D), plasma:	
1,25-dihydroxyvitamin D [1,25(OH)$_2$D]: 5–14 nmol/L (20–60 pg/mL)	0.2400
25-hydroxyvitamin D [25(OH)D]: 20–100 nmol/L (8–42 ng/mL)	2.496
Calcium, ionized: 1.1–1.4 mmol/L (2.3–2.8 meq/L; 4.5–5.6 mg/dL)	0.2495
Calcium, plasma: 2.2–2.6 mmol/L (9–10.5 mg/dL)	0.2495
Carbon dioxide content, plasma (sea level): 21–30 mmol/L (21–30 meq/L)	—
Carbon dioxide tension (P_{CO_2}), arterial blood (sea level): 4.7–6.0 kPa (35–45 mmHg)	0.1333
Carbon monoxide content, blood: symptoms with over 20 percent saturation of hemoglobin	
Carotenoids, serum: 0.9–5.6 μmol/L (50–300 μg/dL)	0.01863
Ceruloplasmin, serum: 270–370 mg/L (27–37 mg/dL)	10
Chlorides, serum (as Cl^-): 98–106 mmol/L (98–106 meq/L)	—
Cholesterol: see Table A-4	
Complement, serum:	
C3: 0.55–1.20 g/L (55–120 mg/dL)	0.01
C4: 0.20–0.50 g/L (20–50 mg/dL)	0.01

	Conversion factor (CF) ($C \times CF = SI$)
Copper, serum: 11–22 μmol/L (70–140 μg/dL)	0.1574
Creatine phosphokinase, serum (total):	
Females: 0.17–1.17 μkat/L (10–70 U/L)	0.01667
Males: 0.42–1.50 μkat/L (25–90 U/L)	0.01667
Creatinine, serum: <133 μmol/L (<1.5 mg/dL)	88.40
Digoxin serum:	
Therapeutic level: 0.6–2.8 nmol/L (0.5–2.2 ng/mL)	1.281
Toxic level: >3.1 nmol/L (>2.4 ng/mL)	1.281
Ethanol, blood:	
Mild to moderate intoxication: 17–43 mmol/L (80–200 mg/dL)	0.2171
Marked intoxication: 54–87 mmol/L (250–400 mg/dL)	0.2171
Severe intoxication: >87 mmol/L (>400 mg/dL)	0.2171
Fatty acids, free (nonesterified), plasma: <180 mg/L (<18 mg/dL)	10
Ferritin, serum: 15–200 μg/L (15–200 ng/mL)	—
Fibrinogen, plasma: see "Platelets and Coagulation"	—
Fibrinogen split products: see "Platelets and Coagulation"	—
Folic acid, red cell: 340–1020 nmol/L cells (150–450 ng/mL cells)	2.266
Gastrin, serum: 40–200 ng/L (40–200 pg/mL)	—
Globulins, serum: 20–30 g/L (2.0–3.0 g/dL)	10
Glucose (fasting), plasma:	
Normal: 4.2–6.4 mmol/L (75–115 mg/dL)	0.05551
Diabetes mellitus: >7.8 mmol/L [>140 mg/dL (on more than one occasion)]	0.05551
Glucose, 2 h postprandial, plasma:	
Normal: <7.8 mmol/L (<140 mg/dL)	0.05551
Impaired glucose tolerance: 7.8–11.1 mmol/L (140–200 mg/dL)	0.05551
Diabetes mellitus: >11.1 mmol/L on more than one occasion (>200 mg/dL)	0.05551
Hemoglobin, blood (sea level):	
Male: 140–180 g/L (14–18 g/dL)	10
Female: 120–160 g/L (12–16 g/dL)	10
Hemoglobin A$_{1c}$: up to 6 percent of total hemoglobin	—
Immunoglobulins, serum:	
IgA: 0.9–3.2 g/L (90–325 mg/dL)	0.01
IgD: 0–0.08 g/L (0–8 mg/dL)	0.01
IgE: <0.00025 g/L (<0.025 mg/dL)	0.01
IgG: 8.0–15.0 g/L (800–1500 mg/dL)	0.01
IgM: 0.45–1.5 g/L (45–150 mg/dL)	0.01
Iron, serum: 14–32 μmol/L (80–180 μg/dL)	0.1791
Iron-binding capacity, serum: 45–82 μmol/L (250–460 μg/dL)	0.1791
Saturation: 0.2–0.45 (20–45 percent)	
Lactate dehydrogenase, serum:	
200–450 units/mL (Wrobleski)	—
60–100 units/mL (Wacker)	—
0.4–1.7 μkat/L (25–100 units/L)	0.01667
Lactic dehydrogenase isoenzymes, serum (agarose):	
Fraction 1 (of total): 0.14–0.25 (14–26 percent)	0.01
Fraction 2: 0.29–0.39 (29–39 percent)	0.01
Fraction 3: 0.20–0.25 (20–26 percent)	0.01
Fraction 4: 0.08–0.16 (8–16 percent)	0.01
Fraction 5: 0.06–0.16 (6–16 percent)	0.01
Lactate, venous plasma: 0.6–1.7 mmol/L (5–15 mg/dL)	0.1110
Lead, serum: <1.0 μmol/L (<20 μg/dL)	0.04826
Lipids: see Table A-4	—
Lipids, triglyceride, serum: see "Triglycerides"	

	Conversion factor (CF) (C × CF = SI)
Lipoprotein: see Table A-4	—
Lithium, serum:	
Therapeutic level: 0.6–1.2 mmol/L (0.6–1.2 meq/L)	—
Toxic level: >2 mmol/L (>2 meq/L)	—
Magnesium, serum: 0.8–1.2 mmol/L (2–3 mg/dL)	0.4114
Osmolality, plasma: 285–295 mosmol per kg serum water	—
Oxygen content:	
Arterial blood (sea level): 17–21 volume percent	—
Venous blood, arm (sea level): 10 to 16 volume percent	—
Oxygen percent saturation (sea level):	
Arterial blood: 0.97 mol/mol (97 percent)	0.01
Venous blood, arm: 0.60–0.85 mol/mol (60–85 percent)	0.01
Oxygen tension (P_{O_2}) blood: 11–13 kPa (80–100 mmHg)	0.1333
pH, blood: 7.38–7.44	—
Phenytoin, plasma:	
Therapeutic level: 40–80 μmol/L (10–20 mg/L)	3.964
Toxic level: >120 μmol/L (>30 mg/L)	3.964
Phosphorus, inorganic, serum: 1.0–1.4 mmol/L (3–4.5 mg/dL)	0.3229
Potassium, serum: 3.5–5.0 mmol/L (3.5–5.0 meq/L)	—
Proteins, total, serum: 55–80 g/L (5.5–8.0 g/dL)	10
Protein fractions, serum:	
Albumin: 35–55 g/L [3.5–5.5 g/dL (50–60 percent)]	10
Globulin: 20–35 g/L [2.0–3.5 g/dL (40–50 percent)]	10
Alpha$_1$: 2–4 g/L [0.2–0.4 g/dL (4.2–7.2 percent)]	10
Alpha$_2$: 5–9 g/L [0.5–0.9 g/dL (6.8–12 percent)]	10
Beta: 6–11 g/L [0.6–1.1 g/dL (9.3–15 percent)]	10
Gamma: 7–17 g/L [0.7–1.7 g/dL (13–23 percent)]	10
Pyruvate, venous, plasma: 60–170 μmol/L (0.5–1.5 mg/dL)	113.6
Quinidine, serum:	
Therapeutic range: 4.6–9.2 μmol/L (1.5–3 mg/L)	3.082
Toxic range: 15.4–18.5 μmol/L (5–6 mg/L)	3.082
Salicylate, plasma: 0 mmol/L	—
Therapeutic range: 1.4–1.8 mmol/L (20–25 mg/dL)	0.07240
Toxic range: >2.2 mmol/L (>30 mg/dL)	0.07240
Sodium, serum: 136–145 mmol/L (136–145 meq/L)	—
Steroids: see "Metabolic and Endocrine" under "Function Tests"	—
Triglycerides: <1.8 mmol/L (<160 mg/dL)	0.01129
Urea nitrogen, serum: 3.6–7.1 mmol/L (10–20 mg/dL)	0.3570
Uric acid, serum:	
Men: 150–480 μmol/L (2.5–8.0 mg/dL)	59.48
Women: 90–360 μmol/L (1.5–6.0 mg/dL)	59.48
Vitamin A, serum: 0.7–3.5 μmol/L (20–100 μg/dL)	0.03491
Vitamin B$_{12}$, serum: 148–443 pmol/L (200–600 pg/mL)	0.7378
Zinc, serum: 11.5–18.5 μmol/L (75–120 μg/dL)	0.1530

FUNCTION TESTS

Circulation

Arteriovenous oxygen difference: 30–50 mL/L
Cardiac output (Fick): 2.5–3.6 L/m² body surface area per min

	Conversion factor (CF) (C × CF = SI)
Contractility indexes:	
Maximum left ventricular *dp/dt*: 1650 ± 300 mmHg/s	
Maximum (*dp/dt*)/*p*: 44 ± 8.4 s⁻¹	
(*dp/dt*)/DP at DP = 40 mmHg: 37.6 ± 12.2 s⁻¹ (DP = diastolic press.)	
Mean normalized systolic ejection rate (angiography): 3.32 ± 0.84 end-diastolic volumes per second	
Mean velocity of circumferential fiber shortening (angiography) 1.66 ± 0.42 circumferences per second	
Ejection fraction, stroke volume/end-diastolic volume (SV/EDV):	
Normal range: 0.55–0.78; average: 0.67	
End-diastolic volume: 75 ± 15 mL/m²	
End-systolic volume: 25 ± 8 mL/m²	
Left ventricular work:	
Stroke work index: 30–110 (g·m)/m²	
Left ventricular minute work index: 1.8–6.6 [(kg · m)/m²]/min	
Oxygen consumption index: 110–150 mL	
Pressures, intracardiac and intraarterial: see Table A-5	
Pulmonary vascular resistance: 2–12 (kPa·s)/L [20–120 (dyn·s)/cm⁵]	
Systemic vascular resistance: 77–150 (kPa·s)/L [770–1500 (dyn·s)/cm⁵]	
Systolic time intervals: see Table A-6	

Gastrointestinal See also "Stool."

	Conversion factor (CF) (C × CF = SI)
Absorption tests:	
D-Xylose absorption test: After an overnight fast, 25 g xylose is given in aqueous solution by mouth. Urine collected for the following 5 h should contain 33–53 mmol (5–8 g) (or >20 percent of ingested dose). Serum xylose should be 1.7–2.7 mmol/L 1 h after the oral dose (25–40 mg per 100 mL).	
Vitamin A absorption test: A fasting blood specimen is obtained and 200,000 units of vitamin A in oil is given by mouth. Serum vitamin A levels should rise to twice fasting level in 3–5 h.	
Bentiromide test (pancreatic function): 500 mg bentiromide (chymex) orally; *p*-aminobenzoic acid (PABA) measured in plasma and/or urine	
Plasma: >3.6(±1.1) mg/L at 90 min	
Urine: >50 percent recovered as PABA in 6 h	
Gastric juice:	
Volume:	
24 h: 2–3 L	
Nocturnal: 600–700 mL	
Basal, fasting: 30–70 mL/h	
Reaction:	
pH: 1.6–1.8	
Titratable acidity of fasting juice: 4–9 μmol/s (15–35 meq/h)	0.261
Acid output:	
Basal:	
Females (mean ± 1 SD): 0.6 ± 0.5 μmol/s (2.0 ± 1.8 meq/h)	0.2778
Males (mean ± 1 SD): 0.8 ± 0.6 μmol/s (3.0 ± 2.0 meq/h)	0.2778
Maximal (after subcutaneous histamine acid phosphate 0.004 mg/kg body weight and preceded by 50 mg promethazine or after betazole 1.7 mg/kg body weight or pentagastrin 6 μg/kg body weight):	
Females (mean ± 1 SD): 4.4 ± 1.4 μmol/s (16 ± 5 meq/h)	0.2778
Males (mean ± 1 SD): 6.4 ± 1.4 μmol/s (23 ± 5 meq/h)	0.2778
Basal acid output/maximal acid output ratio: 0.6 or less	

	Conversion factor (CF) (C × CF = SI)
Gastrin, serum: 40–200 ng/L (40–200 pg/mL)	—
Secretin test (pancreatic exocrine function): 1 unit per kg body weight, intravenously	
Volume (pancreatic juice): >2.0 mL/kg in 80 min	—
Bicarbonate concentration: >80 mmol/L (>80 meq/L)	—
Bicarbonate output: >10 mmol in 30 min (>10 meq in 30 min)	—

Metabolic and endocrine

	Conversion factor (CF) (C × CF = SI)
Adrenocorticotropin (ACTH) plasma, 8 A.M.: <18 pmol/L (<80 pg/mL)	0.2202
Adrenal cortex function tests: see Chap. 317	—
Adrenal medulla function tests: see Chap. 318	—
Adrenal steroids, plasma:	
Aldosterone, 8 A.M.: <220 pmol/L (patient supine, 100 meq Na and 60–100 meq K intake) (<8 ng/dL)	27.74
Cortisol:	
8 A.M.: 140–690 nmol/L (5–25 µg/dL)	27.59
4 P.M.: 80–330 nmol/L (3–12 µg/dL)	27.59
Dehydroepiandrosterone (DHEA): 7–31 nmol/L (2–9 µg/L)	3.467
Dehydroepiandrosterone sulfate (DHEA sulfate): 1.3–6.7 µmol/L (500–2500 µg/L)	0.002714
11-Deoxycortisol (compound S): <30 nmol/L (<1 µg/dL)	28.86
17-Hydroxyprogesterone:	
Women: follicular phase, 0.6–3 nmol/L (0.20–1 µg/L); luteal phase, 1.5–10.6 nmol/L (0.5–3.5 µg/L)	3.026
Men: 0.2–9 nmol/L (0.06–3 µg/L)	3.026
Adrenal steroids, urinary excretion:	
Aldosterone: 14–53 nmol/d (5–19 µg/d)	2.774
Cortisol, free: 55–275 nmol/d (20–100 µg/d)	2.759
17-Hydroxycorticosteroids: 5.5–28 µmol/d (2–10 mg/d)	2.759
17-Ketosteroids:	
Men: 24–88 µmol/d (7–25 mg/d)	3.467
Women: 14–52 µmol/d (4–15 mg/d)	3.467
Angiotensin II, plasma, 8 A.M.: 10–30 nmol/L (10–30 pg/mL)	—
Arginine vasopressin (AVP), plasma:	
Random fluid intake: 2.3–7.4 pmol/L (2.5–8 ng/L)	0.92
Calcitonin, plasma: <50 ng/L (<50 pg/mL)	
Catecholamines, urinary excretion:	
Free catecholamines: <590 nmol/d (<100 µg/d)	5.911
Epinephrine: <275 nmol/d (<50 µg/d)	5.458
Metanephrines: <7 µmol/d (<1.3 mg/d)	5.458
Vanillylmandelic acid (VMA): <40 µmol/d (<8 mg/d)	5.046
Glucagon, plasma: 50–100 ng/L (50–100 pg/mL)	
Gonadal function tests: see Chaps. 321 and 322	—
Gonadal steroids, plasma:	
Androstenedione:	
Women: 3.5–7.0 nmol/L (1–2 ng/ml)	3.492
Men: 3.0–5.0 mmol/L (0.8–1.3 ng/ml)	3.492
Estradiol:	
Women: 70–220 pmol/L (20–60 pg/mL), higher at ovulation	3.671
Men: <180 pmol/L (<50 pg/mL)	3.671
Progesterone:	
Men, prepubertal girls, preovulatory women, and postmenopausal women: <6 nmol/L (2 ng/mL)	3.180
Women, luteal, peak: >16 nmol/L (>5 ng/mL)	3.180

	Conversion factor (CF) (C × CF = SI)
Testosterone:	
Women: <3.5 nmol/L (<1 ng/mL)	3.467
Men: 10–35 nmol/L (3–10 ng/mL)	3.467
Prepubertal boys and girls: 0.17–0.7 nmol/L (0.05–0.2 ng/mL)	3.467
Gonadotropins, plasma:	
Women, mature, premenopausal, except at ovulation:	
FSH: 5–20 IU/L (5–20 mIU/mL)	—
LH: 5–25 IU/L (5–25 mIU/mL)	—
Ovulatory surge:	
FSH: 12–30 IU/L (12–30 mIU/mL)	—
LH: 25–100 IU/L (25–100 mIU/mL)	—
Postmenopausal women:	
FSH: >12–30 IU/L (>12–30 mIU/mL)	—
LH: >50 IU/L (>50 mIU/mL)	—
Men, mature:	
FSH: 5–20 IU/L (5–20 mIU/mL)	—
LH: 5–20 IU/L (5–20 mIU/mL)	—
Children of both sexes, prepubertal:	
FSH: <5 IU/L (<5 mIU/mL)	—
Growth hormone, after 100 g glucose by mouth: <5 µg/L (<5 ng/mL)	—
Human chorionic gonadotropin, β subunit (β-hCG), plasma:	
Men and nonpregnant women: <3 IU/L (<3 mIU/mL)	
Insulin, serum or plasma, fasting: 43–186 pmol/L (6–26 µU/mL)	7.175
Insulin-like growth factor 1 (somatomedin C, IGF-1/SM-C): see Chap. 314	—
Oxytocin:	
Random: 1–4 pmol/L (1.25–5 ng/L)	0.80
Ovulatory peak in women: 4–8 pmol/L (5–10 ng/L)	0.80
Pancreatic islet function tests: see Chap. 319	—
Parathyroid function tests: see Chap. 340	—
Pituitary function tests: see Chaps. 313 to 315	—
Pregnancy tests: see Chap. 322	—
Prolactin, serum: 2–15 µg/L (2–15 ng/mL)	—
Renin-angiotensin function tests: see Chap. 317	—
Semen analysis: see Chap. 321	—
Thyroid function tests:	
Dynamic tests of thyroid function: see Chap. 316	—
Radioactive iodine uptake, 24 h: 5–30 percent (range varies in different areas due to variations in iodine intake)	
Resin T_3 uptake: 0.25–0.35 (25–35 percent) (varies among laboratories; for calculation of indexes of resin T_3 uptake, see Chap. 316)	0.01
Reverse triiodothyronine (rT_3), plasma: 0.15–0.61 nmol/L (10–40 ng/dL)	0.01536
Thyroid-stimulating hormone (TSH): 0.4–5 mU/L (0.4–5 µU/mL)	—
Thyroxine (T_4), serum radioimmunoassay: 64–154 nmol/L (5–12 µg/dL)	12.86
Triiodothyronine (T_3), plasma: 1.1–2.9 nmol/L (70–190) ng/dL)	0.01536

Pulmonary   See Tables A-9 and A-10.

Renal

	Conversion factor (CF) (C × CF = SI)
Clearances (corrected to 1.72 m² body surface area):	
Measures of glomerular filtration rate:	
Inulin clearance (C1):	
Males (mean ± 1 SD): 2.1 ± 0.4 mL/s (124 ± 25.8 mL/min)	0.01667

	Conversion factor (CF) (C × CF = SI)
Females (mean ± 1 SD): 2.0 ± 0.2 mL/s (119 ± 12.8 mL/min)	0.01667
Endogenous creatinine clearance: 1.5–2.2 mL/s (91–130 mL/min)	0.01667
Urea: 1.0–1.7 mL/s (60–100 mL/min)	0.01667
Measures of effective renal plasma flow and tubular function:	
p-Aminohippuric acid clearance (Cl_{PAH}):	
Males (mean ± 1 SD): 10.9 ± 2.7 mL/s (654 ± 163 mL/min)	0.01667
Females (mean ± 1 SD): 9.9 ± 1.7 mL/s (594 ± 102 mL/min)	0.01667
Concentration and dilution test:	
Specific gravity of urine:	
After 12-h fluid restriction: 1.025 or more	—
After 12-h deliberate water intake: 1.003 or less	—
Protein excretion, urine: <0.15 g/d (<150 mg/d)	0.001
Males: 0–0.06 g/d (0–60 mg/d)	0.001
Females: 0–0.09 g/d (0–90 mg/d)	0.001
Specific gravity, maximal range: 1.002–1.028	—
Tubular reabsorption, phosphorus: 79–94 percent of filtered load	—

HEMATOLOGIC EXAMINATIONS

See also "Chemical Constituents of Blood."

Bone marrow See Table A-12.

Erythrocytes and hemoglobin See also Table A-12.

Carboxyhemoblogin:	
Nonsmoker: 0–0.023 (0–2.3 percent)	0.01
Smoker: 0.021–0.042 (2.1–4.2 percent)	0.01
Erythrocyte "life span":	
Normal survival: 120 days	—
Chromium-labeled, half-life ($t_{\frac{1}{2}}$): 28 days	—
Glucose-6-phosphate dehydrogenase: 12.1 ± 2 IU/gHb (WHO)	—
Ham's test (acid serum): negative	—
Haptoglobin, serum 0.5–2.2 g/L (50–220 mg/dL)	0.01
Hemoglobin, plasma: 0.01–0.05 g/L (1–5 mg/dL)	0.01
Hemoglobin A_2 (HbA_2): 0.015–0.035 (1.5–3.5 percent)	0.01
Hemoglobin, fetal (HbF): <0.02 (<2 percent)	0.01
Hemoglobin H prep: negative	—
Methemoglobin: <0.017 (<1.7 percent)	0.01
Osmotic fragility:	
Slight hemolysis: 0.45–0.39 percent	—
Complete hemolysis: 0.33–0.30 percent	—
Plasma iron turnover: 20–42 mg/d or 0.45 mg/kg body weight per day	—
Protoporphyrin, free erythrocyte (FEP): 0.28–0.64 μmol/L of red blood cells (16–36 μg/dL of red blood cells)	0.0177
Red cell distribution width (Coulter): 13 ± 1.5 percent	
Sedimentation rate:	
Westergren, <50 years of age:	
Males: 0–15 mm/h	
Females: 0–20 mm/h	
Westergren, >50 years of age:	
Males: 0–20 mm/h	
Females: 0–30 mm/h	
Sucrose hemolysis: negative	

Leukocytes See Table A-13.

Platelets and coagulation

Alpha$_2$ antiplasmin: 70–130 percent	
Antithrombin III: 80–120 percent	
Bleeding time:	
Duke method: <4 min	
Simplate: <7 min	
Clot retraction, qualitative: apparent in 60 min, complete <24 h, usually <6 h	
Euglobulin lysis time: >2 h	
Factor II: 60–100 percent	
Factor V: 60–100 percent	
Factor VII: 60–100 percent	
Factor IX: 60–100 percent	
Factor X: 60–100 percent	
Factor XI: 60–100 percent	
Factor XII: 60–100 percent	
Factor XIII: clot stable in urea	
Fibrinogen: 2.0–4.0 g/L (200–400 mg/dL)	0.01
Fibrin split products: <10 mg/L (<10 μg/mL)	—
Plasminogen: 2.4–4.4 CTA U/mL	
Protein C (antigenic assay): 58–148 percent	
Protein S (antigenic assay): 58–148 percent	
Partial thromboplastin time (activated PTT): comparable to control	
Prothrombin time (quick one-stage): control ± 1 s	
Protamine paracoagulation (3P) test: negative	
Platelets: 130,000–400,000 per microliter	
Thrombin time: control ± 3 s	
von Willebrand's antigen: 60–150 percent	

Miscellaneous

Leukocyte alkaline phosphatase (LAP): 0.2–1.6 μkat/L (13–100 U/L)	0.01667
Lysozyme (muramidase), serum: 5–25 mg/L (5–25 μg/mL)	—
Lysozyme, urine: <2 mg/L (<2 μg/mL)	—
Schilling test: excretion in urine of orally administered radioactive vitamin B_{12}: 7–40 percent	—
Viscosity, plasma: 1.7–2.1	—
Viscosity, serum: 1.4–1.8	—

STOOL

Bulk:	
Wet weight: <197.5 (115 ± 41) g/d	—
Dry weight: <66.4 (34 ± 15) g/d	—
Alpha$_1$ antitrypsin: 0.98 (±0.17) mg/g dry weight stool	—
Coproporphyrin: 600–1500 nmol/d (400–1000 μg/d)	1.527
Fat (on diet containing at least 50 g fat): <6.0 (4.0 ± 1.5) g/d when measured on a 3-day (or longer) collection	
Percent of dry weight: <0.30 (<30.4 percent)	0.01
Coefficient of fat absorption: >0.95 (>95 percent)	0.01
Fatty acid:	
Free: 0.01–0.10 (1–10 percent of dry matter)	0.01
Combined as soap: 0.005–0.12 (0.5–12 percent of dry matter)	0.01
Nitrogen: <1.7 (1.4 ± 0.2) g/d	—
Protein content: minimal	—
Urobilinogen: 68–470 μmol/d (40–280 mg/d)	1.693
Water: 0.65 (approximately 65 percent)	0.01

URINE

	Conversion factor (CF) (C × CF = SI)

See also "Metabolic and Endocrine" under "Function Tests."

Acidity, titratable: 20–40 mmol/d (20–40 meq/d)	—
Ammonia: 30–50 mmol/d (30–50 meq/d)	—
Amylase: 35–260 Somogyi units/h	—
Amylase/creatinine clearance ratio [(Cl$_{am}$/Cl$_{cr}$) × 100]: 1–5	—
Bentiromide (pancreatic function): 50 percent excreted in 6 h as *p*-amino benzoic acid (PABA) after 500 mg oral bentiromide	
Calcium (10 meq/d or 200-mg/d calcium diet): <3.8 mmol/d (<7.5 meq/d)	0.5
Catecholamines: <600 nmol/d (<100 μg/d)	5.911
Copper: 0–0.4 μmol/d (0–25 μg/d)	0.01574
Coproporphyrins (types I and III): 150–460 nmol/d (100–300 μg/d)	1.527
Creatine, as creatinine:	
Adult males: <380 pmol/d (<50 mg/d)	7.625
Adult females: <760 pmol/d (<100 mg/d)	7.625
Creatinine: 8.8–14 mmol/d (1.0–1.6 g/d)	8.840
Glucose, true (oxidase method): 0.3–1.7 mmol/d (50–300 mg/d)	0.5551
5-Hydroxyindoleacetic acid (5-HIAA): 10–47 μmol/d (2–9 mg/d)	5.230
Lead: <0.4 μmol/d (<80 μg/d)	0.004826
Protein: <0.15 g/d (<150 mg/d)	0.1
Porphobilinogen: none	—
Potassium: 25–100 mmol/d [25–100 meq/d (varies with intake)]	—
Sodium: 100–260 mmol/d [100–260 meq/d (varies with intake)]	—
Urobilinogen: 1.7–5.9 μmol/d (1–3.5 mg/d)	1.693
Vanillylmandelic acid (VMA): <40 μmol/d (<8 mg/d)	5.046
D-Xylose excretion: 5 to 8 g within 5 h after oral dose of 25 g	—

TABLE A-1 SI and other units

Quantity	Name of unit	Symbol for unit	Derivation of units
SI BASE UNITS			
Length	meter	m	
Mass	kilogram	kg	
Time	second	s	
Thermodynamic temperature	Kelvin	K	
Amount of substance	mole	mol	
SI DERIVED UNITS			
Area	square meter	m²	
Force	newton	N	(m·kg)/g²
Pressure	pascal	Pa	N·m²
Work, energy	joule	J	N·m
Celsius temperature	degree Celsius	°C	K
OTHER UNITS RETAINED FOR USE			
Time	minute	min	
	hour	h	
	day	d	
Volume	liter	L	

TABLE A-2 Radiation derived units

Quantity	Old unit	SI unit	Name for SI unit (and abbreviation)	Conversion
Activity	curie (Ci)	Disintegrations per second (dps)	becquerel (Bq)	1 Ci = 3.7 × 10¹⁰ Bq 1 mCi = 37 mBq 1 μCi = 0.037 MBq or 37 GBq 1 Bq = 2.703 × 10⁻¹¹ Ci
Absorbed dose	rad	joule per kilogram (J/kg)	gray (Gy)	1 Gy = 100 rad 1 rad = 0.01 Gy 1 mrad = 10⁻³ cGy
Exposure	roentgen (R)	coulomb per kilogram (C/kg)	—	1 C/kg = 3876 R 1 R = 2.58 × 10⁻⁴ C/kg 1 mR = 258 pC/kg
Dose equivalent	rem	joule per kilogram (J/kg)	sievert (Sv)	1 Sv = 100 rem 1 rem = 0.01 Sv 1 mrem = 10 μSv

TABLE A-3 SI prefixes and their symbols

Factor	Prefix	Symbol for prefix
10⁹	giga	G
10⁶	mega	M
10³	kilo	k
10²	hecto	h
10¹	deka	da
10⁻¹	deci	d
10⁻²	centi	c
10⁻³	milli	m
10⁻⁶	micro	μ
10⁻⁹	nano	n
10⁻¹²	pico	p
10⁻¹⁵	femto	f
10⁻¹⁸	alto	a

TABLE A-4 Classification of total cholesterol and LDL-cholesterol values

	Total plasma cholesterol	LDL-cholesterol	Conversion factor (C to SI)
Desirable	<5.20 mmol/L (<200 mg/dL)	<3.36 mmol/L (<130 mg/dL)	0.02586
Borderline high	5.20–6.18 mmol/L (200–239 mg/dL)	3.36–4.11 mmol/L (130–159 mg/dL)	0.02586
High	≥6.21 mmol/L (≥240 mg/dL)	≥4.14 mmol/L (≥160 mg/dL)	0.02586

SOURCE: The Expert Panel. Report of the National Cholesterol Education Program Expert Panel on Detection, Evaluation, and Treatment of High Blood Cholesterol in Adults. Arch Intern Med 148:36, 1988

TABLE A-5 Hemodynamic values

Pressures (mmHg):
  Systemic arterial:
    Peak systolic/end-diastolic   100–140/60–90
    Mean   70–105
  Left ventricle:
    Peak systolic/end-diastolic   100–140/3–12
  Left atrium (or pulmonary capillary wedge):
    Mean   2–12
    a wave   3–10
    v wave   3–15
  Pulmonary artery:
    Peak systolic/end-diastolic   15–30/4–14
    Mean   9–17
  Right ventricle:
    Peak systolic/end-diastolic   15–30/2–7
  Right atrium:
    Mean   2–6
    a wave   2–8
    v wave   2–7
Resistances [(dyn·s)/cm^5]:
  Systemic vascular resistance   700–1600
  Total pulmonary resistance   100–300
  Pulmonary vascular resistance   30–130
Flows:
  Cardiac index (liters per minute per square meter)   2.4–3.8
  Stroke index (milliliters per beat per square meter)   30–65
Oxygen consumption (liters per minute per square meter)   110–150
Arteriovenous oxygen difference (milliliters per liter)   30–50

TABLE A-6 Systolic time intervals in normal individuals (in milliseconds)

Regression equation		SD of index
QS$_2$ (M)	= −2.1 HR + 546	14
QS$_2$ (F)	= −2.0 HR + 549	14
PEP (M)	= −0.4 HR + 131	13
PEP (F)	= −0.4 HR + 133	11
LVET (M)	= −1.7 HR + 413	10
LVET (F)	= −1.6 HR + 418	10

NOTE: QS$_2$ = total electromechanical systole, PEP = preejection phase, LVET = left ventricular ejection time, HR = heart rate, M = male, F = female, SD = standard deviation of the systolic time interval index. Systolic ejection period = 220–320 ms per beat; diastolic filling period = 380–500 ms per beat.
SOURCE: AM Weissler, CL Garrard, Mod Concepts Cardiovasc Dis 40:1, 1971.

TABLE A-7 Normal values of echocardiographic measurements in adults*

	Range, cm	Mean, cm	Number of subjects
Age (years)	13 to 54	26	134
Body surface area (m²)	1.45 to 2.22	1.8	130
RVD—flat	0.7 to 2.3	1.5	84
RVD—left lateral	0.9 to 2.6	1.7	83
LVID—flat	3.7 to 5.6	4.7	82
LVID—left lateral	3.5 to 5.7	4.7	81
Posterior LV wall thickness	0.6 to 1.1	0.9	137
Posterior LV wall amplitude	0.9 to 1.4	1.2	48
IVS wall thickness	0.6 to 1.1	0.9	137
Mid IVS amplitude	0.3 to 0.8	0.5	10
Apical IVS amplitude	0.5 to 1.2	0.7	38
Left atrial dimension	1.9 to 4.0	2.9	133
Aortic root dimension	2.0 to 3.7	2.7	121
Aortic cusps' separation	1.5 to 2.6	1.9	93
Percentage of fractional shortening†	34 to 44%	36%	20
Mean rate of circumferential shortening (Vcf)‡, or mean normalized shortening velocity	1.02 to 1.94 circ/s	1.3 circ/s	38

* RVD = right ventricular dimension; LVID = left ventricular internal dimension; d = end diastole; s = end systole; LV = left ventricle; IVS = interventricular septum.

† $\dfrac{\text{LVIDd} - \text{LVIDs}}{\text{LVIDd}}$

‡ $\dfrac{\text{LVIDd} - \text{LVIDs}}{\text{LVIDd} \times \text{ejection time}}$

SOURCE: From H Feigenbaum, Echocardiography, in *Heart Disease—A Textbook of Cardiovascular Medicine,* E Braunwald (ed), Philadelphia, Saunders, 1980.

TABLE A-8 Amplitude of Q, R, S, and T waves in scalar electorcardiogram of 100 normal adults*

	I	II	III	aV$_R$	aV$_l$	aV$_F$	V$_1$	V$_5$	V$_6$
Patients with Q wave	38%	41%	50%	—	38%	40%	0%	60%	75%
Q amplitude:									
Mean	0.4	0.6	0.9	—	0.4	0.7	0	0.3	0.3
Range	0 to 0.10	0 to 1.6	0 to 2.3	—	0 to 1.1	0 to 1.7	0	0 to 1.8	0 to 1.8
R amplitude:									
Mean	5.6	8.9	4.5	1.3	3.4	6.0	1.9	12.6	10.2
Range	1.0 to 10.0	2.0 to 16.9	1.0 to 12.1	0 to 2.9	0 to 8.2	0 to 13.8	1.0 to 6.0	7.0 to 21.0	5.0 to 18.0
S amplitude:									
Mean	2.0	2.1	2.4	7.0	2.6	—	8.0	2.5	1.3
Range	0 to 5.0	0 to 3.7	0 to 6.4	2.2 to 11.8	0 to 5.8	—	3.0 to 13.0	0 to 5.0	0 to 2.0
T amplitude:									
Mean	1.9	2.3	1.0	—	0.3	1.7	1.0	3.3	1.0
Range	1.0 to 3.0	1.0 to 4.0	−2.0 to 2.0	—	−1.0 to 2.0	0 to 4.0	−2.0 to 2.0	2.0 to 7.0	1.0 to 4.0

* Values of Q, R, S, and T amplitudes are in millimeters (1 mm = 0.1 mv).
SOURCE: From J D Cooksey et al, *Clinical Vectorcardiography and Electrocardiography,* 2d ed, Chicago, Year Book Medical Publishers, 1977. Used by permission.

TABLE A-9 Summary of values useful in pulmonary physiology

	Symbol	Typical values Men	Women
PULMONARY MECHANICS			
Spirometry—volume-time curves:			
Forced vital capacity	FVC	≥4.0 liters	≥3.0 liters
Forced expiratory volume in 1 s	FEV_1	>3.0 liters	>2.0 liters
FEV_1/FVC	$FEV_1\%$	>60%	>70%
Maximal midexpiratory flow	MMF (FEF 25–27)	>2.0 liters per second	>1.6 liters per second
Maximal expiratory flow rate	MEFR (FEF 200–1200)	>3.5 liters per second	>3.0 liters per second
Spirometry—flow-volume curves:			
Maximal expiratory flow at 50% of expired vital capacity	$\dot{V}_{max}$ 50 (FEF 50%)	>2.5 liters per second	>2.0 liters per second
Maximal expiratory flow at 75% of expired vital capacity	$\dot{V}_{max}$ 75 (FEF 75%)	>1.5 liters per second	>1.0 liters per second
Resistance to airflow:			
Pulmonary resistance	RL (R_L)	<3.0 cmH_2O/s per liter	
Airway resistance	Raw	<2.5 cmH_2O/s per liter	
Specific conductance	SGaw	>0.13 cmH_2O/s	
Pulmonary compliance:			
Static recoil pressure at total lung capacity	Pst TLC	25 ± 5 cmH_2O	
Compliance of lungs (static)	CL	0.2 L/cmH_2O	
Compliance of lungs and thorax	C(L + T)	0.1 L/cmH_2O	
Dynamic compliance of 20 breaths per minute	C dyn 20	0.25 ± 0.05 liters per cmH_2O	
Maximal static respiratory pressures:			
Maximal inspiratory pressure	MIP	>90 cmH_2O	>50 cmH_2O
Maximal expiratory pressure	MEP	>150 cmH_2O	>120 cmH_2O
LUNG VOLUMES			
Total lung capacity	TLC	6–7 liters	5–6 liters
Functional residual capacity	FRC	2–3 liters	2–3 liters
Residual volume	RV	1–2 liters	1–2 liters
Inspiratory capacity	IC	2–4 liters	2–4 liters
Expiratory reserve volume	ERV	1–2 liters	1–2 liters
Vital capacity	VC	4–5 liters	3–4 liters
GAS EXCHANGE (SEA LEVEL)			
Arterial O_2 tension	Pa_{O_2}	95 ± 5 mmHg	
Arterial CO_2 tension	Pa_{CO_2}	40 ± 2 mmHg	
Arterial O_2 saturation	Sa_{O_2}	97 ± 2%	
Arterial blood pH	pH	7.40 ± 0.02	
Arterial bicarbonate	HCO_3^-	24 ± 2 mmol/L	
Base excess	BE	0 ± 2 mmol/L	
Diffusing capacity for carbon monoxide (single breath)	DL_{CO}	25 mL CO/min/mmHg	
Dead space volume	V_D	50 ± 25 mL	
Physiologic dead space: dead space-tidal volume ratio (rest)	V_D/V_T	≤35% V_T	
(exercise)		≤20% V_T	
Alveolar-arterial difference for O_2	A-a D_{O_2}	≤20 mmHg	

TABLE A-10 Prediction equations for spirometric tests, lung volumes, and gas exchange in adults

Variable	Sex	Age (A)	Height (H)	Weight (W)	Constant (C)	Standard deviation (SD)
PULMONARY MECHANICS						
Spirometry—volume-time curves* (H in inches):						
FVC	M	−0.025	+0.148	—	−4.241	0.74
	F	−0.024	+0.115	—	−2.852	0.52
FEV$_1$	M	−0.032	+0.092	—	−1.260	0.55
	F	−0.025	+0.089	—	−1.932	0.47
MEFR	M	−0.047	+0.109	—	+2.010	1.66
(FEF 200–1200)	F	−0.036	+0.145	—	−2.532	1.19
MMF	M	−0.045	+0.047	—	+2.513	1.12
(FEF 25–75)	F	−0.030	+0.060	—	+0.551	0.80
Spirometry—flow-volume curves† (H in centimeters):						
V̇$_{max}$ 50	M	−0.015	+0.069	—	−5.400	1.422
(FEF 50%)	F	−0.013	+0.035	—	−0.444	1.22
V̇$_{max}$ 75	M	−0.012	+0.044	—	−4.143	1.026
(FEF 75%)	F	−0.014	—	—	+3.042	0.936
Lung volumes‡ (H in meters; W in kilograms):						
TLC	M	—	+6.92	−0.017	−4.30	0.67
	F	−0.015	+6.71	—	−5.77	0.48
FRC	M	+0.015	+5.30	−0.037	−3.89	0.56
	F	—	+5.13	−0.028	−4.50	0.41
RV	M	+0.022	+1.98	−0.015	−1.54	0.38
	F	+0.007	+2.68	—	−3.42	0.32
VC	M	−0.020	+4.81	—	−2.81	0.50
	F	−0.022	+4.04	—	−2.35	0.40
Gas exchange§ (H in meters; W in kilograms):						
DL$_{CO}$	M	−0.20	+32.5	—	−17.6	5.1
	F	−0.16	+21.2	—	−2.66	3.6

NOTE: Answer = (A × age) + (H × height) + (W × weight) + C ± 2 SD. Example: The normal value and lower limit for the FEV$_1$ are sought in a man, age 40 years, height 183 cm, and weight 91 kg. The following equation gives the normal value:
FEV$_1$ = (−0.032 × 40) + (0.092 × 72) + (−1.260) = 4.08 liters
The lower limit of normal:
4.08 − (2 × SD) = 4.08 − (2 × 0.55) = 2.98 liters
Only 2.5% of a normal population will fall below this value (2 SD below the mean).
For other abbreviations, see Table A-9.
* Morris et al, Am Rev Respir Dis 103:57, 1971.
† Knudson et al, Am Rev Respir Dis 113:587, 1976.
‡ Grimby G, Söderholm B, Acta Med Scand 173:199, 1963.
§ Coates JE, *Lung Function and Application in Medicine*, Philadelphia, Davis, 1965.

TABLE A-11 Differential nucleated cell counts of bone marrow

	Normal, mean%*	Range, %†
Myeloid:	56.7	
Neutrophilic series:	53.6	
Myeloblast	0.9	0.2–1.5
Promyelocyte	3.3	2.1–4.1
Myelocyte	12.7	8.2–15.7
Metamyelocyte	15.9	9.6–24.6
Band	12.4	9.5–15.3
Segmented		
Eosinophilic series	3.1	1.2–5.3
Basophilic series	<0.1	0–0.2
Erythroid:	25.6	
Pronormoblasts	0.6	0.2–1.3
Basophilic normoblasts	1.4	0.5–2.4
Polychromatophilic normoblasts	21.6	17.9–29.2
Orthochromatic normoblasts	2.0	0.4–4.6
Megakaryocytes	<0.1	
Lymphoreticular	17.8	
Lymphocytes	16.2	11.1–23.2
Plasma cells	2.3	0.4–3.9
Reticulum cells	0.3	0–0.9

* From MM Wintrobe et al, *Clinical Hematology*, 8th ed, Philadelphia, Lea & Febiger, 1981.
† Range observed in 12 healthy men.

TABLE A-12 Erythrocytes and hemoglobin: Normal values at various ages

| Age | Red blood cell count,* 10^{12}/L | Hemoglobin,* g/L (g/dL) | Vol. packed RBCs,* mL/dL | Corpuscular values | | | |
				MCV, fL	MCH, pg	MCHC, g/L (g/dL)	MCD, μm
Days 1–13	5.1 ± 1.0	195 ± 50 (19.5 ± 5)	54.0 ± 10.0	106–98	38–33	340–360 (36–34)	8.6
Days 14–60	4.7 ± 0.9	140 ± 33 (14 ± 3.3)	42.0 ± 7.0	90	30	330 (33)	8.1
3 months to 10 years	4.5 ± 0.7	122 ± 23 (12.2 ± 2.3)	36.0 ± 5.0	80	27	340 (34)	7.7
11–15 years	4.8	131 (13.14)	39.0	82	28	340 (34)	
Adults:							
Females	4.8 ± 0.6	140 ± 20 (14 ± 2)	42.0 ± 5.0	90 ± 7	29 ± 2	340 ± 20 (34 ± 2)	7.5 ± 0.3
Males	5.4 ± 0.9	160 ± 20 (16 ± 2)	47.0 ± 5.0	90 ± 7	29 ± 2	340 ± 20 (34 ± 2)	7.5 ± 0.3

* The range of values represents almost the extremes of observed variations (93 percent or more) at sea level. The blood values of healthy persons should fall well within these mean ± SD figures.
NOTE: MCV = mean corpuscular volume, MCH = mean corpuscular hemoglobin, MCHC = mean corpuscular hemoglobin concentration, MCD = mean corpuscular diameter.
SOURCE: MM Wintrobe et al, *Clinical Hematology*, 8th ed, Philadelphia, Lea & Febiger, 1981.

TABLE A-13 Normal leukocyte count, differential count, and hemoglobin concentration at various ages

| Age | Leukocytes, total | Neutrophils | | | Eosinophils | Basophils | Lymphocytes | Monocytes |
		Total	Band	Segmented				
12 mo	11.4(6.0–17.5)	3.5(1.5–8.5)	0.35	3.2	0.3(0.05–0.7)	0.05(0–0.20)	7.0(4.0–10.5)	0.55(0.05–1.1)
		31	3.1	28	0.4	0.4	61	4.8
4 yr	9.1(5.5–15.5)	3.8(1.5–8.5)	0.27(0–1.0)	3.5(1.5–7.5)	0.25(0.02–0.65)	0.05(0–0.20)	4.5(2.0–8.0)	0.45(0–0.8)
		42	3.0	39	2.8	0.6	50	5.0
6 yr	4.3(1.5–8.0)	0.25(0–1.0)	4.0(1.5–7.0)	4.0(1.5–7.0)	0.23(0–0.65)	0.05(0–0.20)	3.5(1.5–7.0)	0.40(0–0.8)
		51	3.0	48	2.7	0.6	42	4.7
10 yr	8.1(4.5–13.5)	4.4(1.8–8.0)	0.24(0–1.0)	4.2(1.8–7.0)	0.20(0–0.60)	0.04(0–0.20)	3.1(1.5–6.5)	0.35(0–0.8)
		54	3.0	51	2.4	0.5	38	4.3
21 yr	7.4(4.5–11.0)	4.4(1.8–7.7)	0.22(0–0.7)	4.2(1.8–7.0)	0.20(0–0.45)	0.04(0–0.20)	2.5(1.0–4.8)	0.30(0–0.8)
		59	3.0	56	2.7	0.5	34	4.0

NOTE: Values are expressed as "cells × 10^9/L." The numbers underlined are percentages.
SOURCE: WJ Williams et al (eds), *Hematology*, 3d ed, New York, McGraw-Hill, 1983. By permission.

INDEX

(Page numbers in **boldface** indicate major discussions; numbers preceded by *A* indicate Atlas plates.)

Hemolysis:
  and hyperbilirubinemia, 1317–1318, 1321
  immune
    cold-reactive antibodies and, 1535
    drugs and, 1534–1535
  intravascular, 1499
  laboratory evaluation, 1532–1533
  membrane abnormalities, 1537–1540
    congenital, 1539–1540
  splenomegaly and, 1533–1535
  thrombotic thrombocytopenic purpura, 1536–1537
    (*See also* Thrombocytopenic purpura, thrombotic)
  toxins and, 1537
  transfusion reaction, 1538
  traumatic, A5–7, 1533, 1535–1537, 1538
  and uremia (*see* Hemolytic uremic syndrome)
Hemolytic uremic syndrome, **1193**, 1504, 1537
  differential diagnosis, 1171, 1537
  Escherichia coli and, 523
  rotavirus and, 716
  Shigella and, 615, 616
Hemoperfusion for poisoning, 2168
Hemoperitoneum, 1351
Hemopexin, hemolysis and, 1532
Hemophilia:
  A, **1505–1507**
    therapy, 45, 1493, 1506
    X-linkage, 26, 28, 29, 30
  AIDS and, 1403, 1506, 1507
  B, **1507**
    gene replacement therapy for, 45
  chromosomal mapping, 25, 49
  clinical manifestations, 1505–1506
  complications, 1506–1507
  gene replacement therapy, 45, 1493
  genetic heterogeneity and, 23
  hepatitis and, 1327, 1328, 1333, 1506–1507
  lymphadenopathy and, 354
  molecular diagnosis, 39
  treatment, 45, 56, 1493
Hemoptysis, **219–220**
  endemic (paragonimiasis), 828–829
  vs. hematemesis, 220
  and mitral stenosis, 939
  potentially lethal, 220
  and pulmonary embolism, 1092
  and respiratory disease diagnosis, 1032
Hemorrhage, 348
  adenoviral cystitis, 704
  in agnogenic myeloid metaplasia, 1565
  amebic, 779
  anemia due to, 346
  arboviruses and, 734–738
  brain, 2003–2004
  brainstem, 2004
  clinical evaluation, 351–353
  coagulation and (*see* Coagulation)
  from diverticula, 1284
  Duret, 2004
  esophageal varices, 261, 262, 263
  fever and (*see* Hemorrhagic fever)
  gastrointestinal, **261–264**
    alcohol and, 2148
    amyloidosis and, 1419
    of anorectal lesions, 262
    approach to patient, 262–264
    of arteriosclerotic aortic aneurysms, 262

Hemorrhage:
  clinical manifestation, 261
  of colonic lesions, 262
  colonoscopy and, 1221
  concomitant symptoms, 261
  definitions, 261
  diagnostic and therapeutic approach, 262–264, 1214, 1215
  of diverticula, 262
  drug-induced, 378
  and electrical injuries, 2203
  endoscopy for, 1217–1218
  etiology, 261–262
  of gastric carcinoma, 262
  of gastritis, 261, 1245
  and head trauma, 2008
  and hepatic encephalopathy, 1349
  history taking, 262
  hypersensitivity vasculitis, 1459
  intestinal disorders and, 1282
  intramural, 1288
  and iron loss, 1520–1521
  laboratory studies, 262
  lower, 262
  Mallory-Weiss tear, 261–262
  occult, 261, 264
  of peptic ulcer, 261, 1233, 1237, 1238
  physical examination, 262
  postcholecystectomy, 1364
  and renal failure, 1148, 1149
  and respiratory failure, 1081
  stress ulcers, 1243
  upper, 261–262
  of uremia, 262
  variceal, 261, 262, 263
head trauma and, 2003–2004
hemophilic (*see* Hemophilia)
history taking, 351
hyperkalemia from, 288
infarctions, and cerebral embolism, 1995
intracranial, **1996–2001**
  angiomas/hemangiomas, 2000–2001
  AVM and, 2000–2001
  cerebral, 1006, 1997
  hematology and, 2001
  and hypertension, 1006, 1997–1998
  lobar, 1998
  subarachnoid, 1998–2000
  trauma and, 2001
  tumors and, 2001
keratoconjunctivitis, enterovirus 70 and, 715
laboratory tests, 352–353
leukemia and, 1555
and multiple myeloma, 1413, 1414
necrotizing encephalomyelitis, 2043–2044
occult, differential diagnosis, 505
physical examination, 351–352
platelet defects (*see* Platelets; Thrombocytopenia)
polycythemia vera and, 1564
pontine, 1997
primary and secondary hemostatic disorders, 352
pulmonary
  fibrosis and, 1085–1086
  and glomerular disease, 1182
  and glomerulonephritis, 1173
  Goodpasture's syndrome, 1173, 1182–1183
  (*See also* Hemoptysis)
purpuric (*see* Purpura)

Hemorrhage:
  putamenal, 1997
  relapsing fever and, 667
  retinal
    SLE, 147
    trichinosis and, 808
  and Rift Valley fever, 728
  Rocky Mountain spotted fever lesions, 757
  and shock, 233
  skin necrosis, 1512
  spinal, 2083
  splinter, and endocarditis, 509
  subarachnoid, 1998–2000
    alcoholism and, 2047
    headache of, 108, 110–111, 113
    and smoking, 2160
  and syncope, 137
  thalamic, 1997
  and thrombocytosis, 1567
  transfusions for (*see* Transfusions)
  uterine, abnormal, 299–300
  and Waterhouse-Friderichsen syndrome, 1731
  yellow fever, 734
Hemorrhagic fever, 726
  Argentinian, 723, 726, 739, **740**
  Bolivian, 723, 726, 739, **740**
  Crimean-Congo, 726, **736**
  Ebola, **724**, 741
  Ebola virus, 724
  epidemic, 737–738
  epidemiology, 675
  far eastern, 736–738
  Korean, 736–738
  Kyasanur Forest disease, 726, **736**
  Manchurian endemic, 736–738
  Marburg virus, 724
  Omsk, 726, **736**
  with renal syndrome (HFRS), 726, **736–738**
    of leptospirosis, 664–665
  tick-borne, 726, **736**
Hemorrhoids, **1288–1289**
  bleeding from, 262
  and cancer, 1295
  and constipation, 258, 1287
  differential diagnosis, 1274–1275
  and iron loss, 1520
  and portal hypertension, 1346
Hemosiderin, 1519, 1825–1826
Hemosiderinuria, 1538
  and hemolysis, 1532
Hemosiderosis, 1826
  idiopathic pulmonary, 1086
  and thalassemia, 1551
Hemostasis, **348–353**
  clinical evaluation, 351–353, 1506
  laboratory tests, 352–353
  normal, 348–351
  primary, 348, 352
  and renal failure, 1156
  secondary, 348, 352
Hemostatic plug, 348–351
  vs. thrombus, 351
Hemothorax, 1112–1113
HEMPAS disorder, 1538
Henderson-Hasselbalch equation, 290
Henle's loop, 1141
  Bartter's syndrome and, 1198
  sodium transport and, 1141
Henoch-Schönlein purpura, 337, **1183**, 1459, 1460, 1504
  differential diagnosis, 1171

Myoglobinemia, 175
Myoglobinuria, 273
  and acute tubular necrosis, 1145–1146
  and dermatomyositis-polymyositis,
    2109–2110
  drug-induced, 2110
  and influenza virus, 699
Myokymia, 174
  facial, 174, 2078
Myopathies, **2089–2090, 2114–2117**
  alcoholic, 2148
  central core disease, 2114
  clinical features, 2089–2090
  congenital, 2114–2115
    and scoliosis, 2096
  drug-induced, 379, 2110
  endocrine, 2117
  hereditary, 2112–2114
  inflammatory, 2116–2117
  malignant hyperthermia and, 2197
  metabolic, 2117
  mitochondrial, 1952, 2116
  muscle weakness and, 2090
  myotubular, 2115
  necrotizing, 1643, 1645
  nemaline, 2114
  ocular, 1704, 2114
  toxic, 2117
  (*See also* Muscle; Muscular dystrophy)
Myophosphorylase deficiency, 1857, 1859,
    2092, 2110, 2115
Myopia, 143
  aging and, 75
Myosin:
  cardiac contractility and, 880–881, 882
  heavy chain, 49
  light chain kinase, and platelet activa-
    tion/secretion, 349
Myositis:
  allergic experimental, 2108
  anaerobic streptococcal, 569
  antibodies and, 2108
  clostridial, 582
  drug-induced, 379
  enteroviruses and, 713
  eosinophilic, 2109
  focal nodular, 2108, 2109
  in heroin addicts, 582
  inclusion body, 2109, 2117
    muscle biopsy for, 2095
  and influenza virus, 699
  orbital, 149
  streptococcal, 567
  viral infections and, 2108
  (*See also* Dermatomyositis; Polymyosi-
    tis)
Myotonia, 175, 2089, 2092
  congenita, 174, 2114
    malignant hyperthermia and, 2197
  dystrophy, 174, 2089, 2090, 2110, 2112,
    2113
    cardiomyopathy and, 977
    chromosomal mapping, 24, 1952,
      2096
    clinical manifestations, 2113–2114
    diagnosis, 39, 2114
    ECG, 2096
    genetics, 24, 25, 1952, 2096, 2114
    and hyperglycemia, 1740
    molecular diagnosis, 39
    polyglandular manifestations, 1813
  paradoxica, 1751
  repetitive stimulation tests, 2094
Myringitis, bullous, 763

Myxedema, 1692, 1694, 1701
  anemia of, 1531
  coma, 1701
  differential diagnosis, 1701
  and encephalopathy, 2053
  and intestinal pseudoobstruction, 1285
  and megacolon, 1285
  mumps and, 718
  pericarditis and, 985
  pretibial (localized), 1704
  (*See also* Hypothyroidism)
Myxoma, **988–989**
  catheterization and, 874
  differential diagnosis, 510, 941
  echocardiography and, 862, 863
  fever of, 130
  lentigines and, 329
  murmurs of, 849, 988

N antigen, 1495–1496
Nadolol, 389, 390
  for hypertension, 1011
  overdosage/poisoning, 2170–2171
Naegleria, 458, 781–782
Nafcillin, 479, 484
  adverse reactions, 485
  for bacterial meningitis, 2026
  combination therapy, 482
  for endocarditis, 511
  hepatic clearance, 1315
  for staphylococcal infections, 561
Naftifine, 498
Nail-patella syndrome, 25, 1132, 1186
Nails:
  green, *Pseudomonas* and, 604
  iron deficiency and, 1521
  onychodystrophy, 317
  psoriasis, 309
  reactive arthritis and, 1454
  tinea, 310
  yellow, lymphedema and, 1025
Nairovirus, 725, 728, 734
Nalidixic acid, 492
  adverse reactions to, 376, 378
  bullous eruptions from, 315
  for *E. coli*, 601
  hemolytic reaction, 1542
  photosensitivity and, 314, 342, 376
  for shigellosis, 615
Nalorphine, 2152
Naloxone, 2152, 2154
  and emesis, 1598
  for sepsis, 507
Naltrexone, 2152, 2154
NAME syndrome, 329, 988
Nandrolone for aplastic anemia, 1569
Naproxen:
  and asthma, 1049
  for fever, 127
  for gout, 1840
  overdosage/poisoning, 2177–2178
  for pain, 95, 96
  for rheumatoid arthritis, 1442
Narcissistic personality disorder, 2136
Narcolepsy, 211, **213–214**
  cataplexy and, 176, 214, 1969
  diagnosis, 214
  HLA and, 90, 91
  treatment, 214
Narcotics, 96
  adverse reactions to, 96, 379
  inadequate dosage, 96
  overdosage, and pulmonary edema, 223

Narcotics:
  for pain, 95, 96
  (*See also* Opioids and opiates)
Narcotics Anonymous, 2154
Nasal disorders (*see* Nose)
Nasogastric tubes:
  diagnostic, 1215
  for enteral feeding, 433
Nasopharyngoscope for epiglottitis, 1100
Nasopharynx:
  aspirates, viral diagnosis, 675
  cultures, 456
  flora, and pneumonia, 1064
  neoplasia, **1100**
    and cranial nerve palsies, 2081
    EBV and, 66, 1582
    and ocular motor nerve palsies, 150
    skull pain and, 2021
Natriuresis, polyuria and, 275–276
Natriuretic hormones:
  and renal failure, 1155, 1156
  and sodium excretion, 278
Natriuretic peptide, atrial (ANP), 837,
    838–839
Natural killer cells (NK cells), 450, 1395
  large cellular granulocytes and, 79
  and parasitic infections, 774
  tests, 1398
Nausea, **251–253**
  appendicitis and, 1298
  from chemotherapy, 1596–1598
  differential diagnosis, 252–253
  drug-induced, 378
  treatment, 253
  and uremia, 1156
  (*See also* Vomiting)
Necator americanus (*see* Hookworm disease)
Neck:
  actinomycosis, A2–22, 245, 752
  cancer chemotherapy, 1596
  immobilization, and spinal cord trauma,
    2009
  infections of, 515–516
    anaerobic, 586
  muscle testing, 22089
  pain in, **122–123**
    management, 123–124
  stiff
    and brain abscess, 2029
    and meningitis, 2024
    spondylosis and, 2085
    in viral encephalitis, 2033
  trauma, 2005
Necrobiosis lipoidica, A1–28
  diabetic, 334, 1756, 1758
  ulceration, 338
Needle aspiration:
  body fluids, 458
  lung, 457
Needle biopsy:
  liver, 1311
  lung, 1047
  pleura, 1046
  in pneumonia, 1067
  in pulmonary disease, 1043
nef gene, 679
Negative, 7
Negative predictive value, 7
Negishi, 725
Negri bodies, 721
Neisseria gonorrhoea (*see* Gonorrhea)
Neisseria lactamica, 591

Pericardium:
  tumors, 987
  visceral, 981
Pericholangitis, inflammatory bowel disease and, 1278
Perichondritis, 1099, 1101
  relapsing, 1099
Perihepatitis:
  chlamydial infections and, 766
  gonococcal, 596
  pelvic inflammatory disease and, 535–536
Perimyositis, relapsing eosinophilic, 2109
Periodic disease (see Mediterranean fever, familial)
Periodic paralysis (see Paralysis, periodic syndromes)
Periodontal abscess, 243
  anaerobic, 585, 586
Periodontitis, **243**
  halitosis, 248
  and HIV, 243, 248
  localized juvenile (LJP), 243
  and lung abscess, 587
Periostitis:
  gummatous, 656
  reactive arthritis and, 1455
Peripheral nervous system (see Nervous system, peripheral)
Peristalsis, 249
Peritoneal dialysis, **1159–1160**
  complications, 1160
  continuous ambulatory (CAPD), 1158, 1159–1160
  continuous cyclic (CCPD), 1158, 1159–1160
  intermittent (IPD), 1159
  malaria and, 788
  for poisoning, 2168
  for renal failure
    acute, 1150
    chronic, 1151, 1158, 1159–1160
  (See also Dialysis)
Peritoneal lavage:
  in abdominal pain diagnosis, 108
  pancreatitis and, 1376
Peritoneum:
  abscesses of, **516–517**
  fluid cultures, 458
  inflammation (see Peritonitis)
  macrophages, 80, 462
Peritonitis:
  amebic, 779, 780
  anaerobic, 585, 587–588
  ascites and, 270, 271, 1348
  bacterial, 1348
  benign paroxysmal (see Mediterranean fever, familial)
  chlamydial, 770
  cirrhosis and, 1348
  and cystic fibrosis, 1073
  diverticulitis and, 1284
  E. coli, 600
  gonococcal, 596
  Haemophilus influenzae, 618
  pain from, **105–106**
  periodic (see Mediterranean fever, familial)
  pneumococcal, 555, 556
  Proteus, 603
  pyogenic, 270
  streptococcal, 568
  tuberculous, 270, 271, 640

Peritonitis:
  and volume depletion, 280
  vomiting and, 253
Peritonsillar abscesses, 564
Peritonsillar cellulitis, 564
Peritovenous shunts for ascites, 1348
Perlèche, A1–12
Permethrin for malaria, 786
Pernicious anemia (see Anemia, pernicious)
Pernio (chilblains), 1023
Peroneal artery atherosclerosis, 994, 1019
Peroneal muscular dystrophy, 2102, 2104
  genetics and, 2102
Peroneal neuropathies, 2106
Perphenazine, 2145
  overdosage/poisoning, 2178
Perseveration, 185
Personality, 185
  brain tumor effects on, 2011
  disorders, **2135–2138**
    diagnosis, 2135–2136
    differential diagnosis, 2136
    etiology and pathophysiology, 2136–2137
    treatment, 2138
  examination of, 186
  and ischemic heart disease, 999
  peptic ulcers and, 1233
Personnel (see Health worker precautions)
Pertechnetate radionuclide, 1693, 1698
Pertussis, **620–622**
  and bronchiectasis, 1070
  catarrhal stage, 620
  clinical manifestations, 620–621
  complications, 621
  contact management, 622
  convalescent stage, 621
  diagnosis, 455, 621
  epidemiology, 620
  and G proteins, 397
  immune microscopy, 455
  microbiology, 620
  otitis media, 621
  paroxysmal stage, 620–621
  pathogenesis, 620
  pneumonia and, 621
  prevention, 622
  seizures and, 621
  toxin, 397
  treatment, 621–622
  vaccine, 474, 477, 572, 620, **622**
  virulence, 620
Pes cavus, 2071, 2086
  and myopathies, 2114
PET (see Positron emission tomography)
Petechiae, 336, 352, 1504
  ascariasis, 818
  and brain hemorrhage, 2003
  dengue hemorrhagic fever, 735
  and endocarditis, 509
  and myeloid metaplasia, 1565
  plague, 630
  Rocky Mountain spotted fever, A2–3, A2–4, 757, 758, 1504
  and thrombotic thrombocytopenic purpura, 1536
  (See also Purpura)
Petit mal seizures, 139, 1969, 1974
Petriellidium boydii, 750
Petrous bone fractures, 2002
Peutz-Jeghers syndrome, 1580
  bleeding in, 262

Peutz-Jeghers syndrome:
  intestinal tumors, 1294
  lentigines, 328
  oral lesions, 246
  and ovarian carcinoma, 1622
  and precocious pseudopuberty, 1783
Peyer's patches, viruses and, 673
Peyronie's disease, 298
pH:
  and ammonia metabolism, 1313
  normal concentration, 289
  regulation of, 289
  urinary, and poisoning, 2168
  (See also Acid-base balance)
Phacomatoses, pulmonary fibrosis and, 1086
Phagocytosis, 449–450, 465
  disorders of, **460–464**, 466
    eosinophils, 463–464
    laboratory diagnosis, 464
    monocytes, 463
    neutrophils, 461–462
  skin infections and, 85, 86
  tests, 86, 1398
  (See also Macrophages)
Phagophobia, 249
Phalangeal joint osteoarthritis, 1477, 1478
Pharmaceuticals (see Drugs)
Pharyngitis, **1099–1100**
  adenoviral, 704, 1099
  complications, 1100
  differential diagnosis, 683, 1099
  Ebola virus, 724
  gonococcal, 596, 1099
  herpes simplex, A2–17, 565, 684, 723
  infectious mononucleosis, 689, 690, 692, 1099
  pneumococcal, 553
  streptococcal, 515, **563–566**, 568, 1099
    complications, 564
    course, 564
    cultures, 456
    diagnosis, 564–565
    epidemiology, 563–564
    and glomerulonephritis, 1170–1172
    vs. pyoderma, 566
    and rheumatic fever, 564, 565, 933, 934, 938
    scarlet fever, 564
    symptoms and signs, 564
    treatment, 565–566
  tularemia, 627
Pharyngoconjunctival fever, adenoviral, 704
Pharyngoscopy, laryngeal tumors and, 1102
Pharyngostomy tubes for enteral feeding, 433
Pharynx:
  anaerobic necrotizing infection, 586
  and dysphagia, 249–250
  examination of, 1222–1223
  inflammation (see Pharyngitis)
  motility studies, 1223, 1224
  paralysis, 1223, 1224
  tumors of, **1100**
Phemphigus, syphilitic, 655
Phenacetin:
  adverse reactions to, 376
  hemolytic reaction, 1542
  methemoglobinemia from, 2177
Phenanthrene phototoxicity, 342
Phencyclidine (PCP), 182–183, 2157
  myopathy from, 2110, 2117

TOPICAL TABLE OF CONTENTS